Textbook of
Gastroenterology

SECOND EDITION

Textbook of
Gastroenterology

VOLUME TWO

EDITOR

Tadataka Yamada, MD

John G. Searle Professor and Chairman
Department of Internal Medicine
Professor of Physiology
Physician-in-Chief
University of Michigan Medical Center
Ann Arbor, Michigan

ASSOCIATE EDITORS

David H. Alpers, MD

Professor of Medicine
Chief, Gastroenterology Division
Washington University School of Medicine
St. Louis, Missouri

Chung Owyang, MD

Professor of Internal Medicine
Chief, Division of Gastroenterology
University of Michigan Medical Center
Ann Arbor, Michigan

Don W. Powell, MD

The Edward Randall and Edward Randall, Jr.,
    Chair in Internal Medicine
Professor and Chairman of Internal Medicine
Professor of Physiology and Biophysics
The University of Texas Medical Branch Hospital
    at Galveston
Galveston, Texas

Fred E. Silverstein, MD

Professor of Medicine
Division of Gastroenterology
University of Washington School of Medicine
Director, Endoscopy Training Program
University of Washington Medical Center
Seattle, Washington

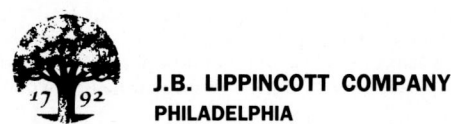

J.B. LIPPINCOTT COMPANY
PHILADELPHIA

Acquisitions Editor: Richard Lampert
Associate Medical Editor: Wendy Greenberger-Czarnecki
Project Editor: Molly E. Dickmeyer
Indexer: Maria Coughlin
Senior Design Coordinator: Kathy Kelley-Luedtke
Interior Designer: Holly Reid McLaughlin
Production Manager: Caren Erlichman
Senior Production Coordinator: Kevin P. Johnson
Compositor: Tapsco, Incorporated
Printer/Binder: Courier Westford
Color Insert Printer: Walsworth

2nd Edition

6 5 4 3

Library of Congress Cataloging-in-Publication Data

Textbook of gastroenterology/editor, Tadataka Yamada; associate
    editors, David H. Alpers . . . [et al.].—2nd ed.
        p.   cm.
    Includes bibliographical references and index.
    ISBN 0-397-51314-3 (set).—ISBN 0-397-51491-3 (v. 1).—ISBN
    0-397-51492-1 (v. 2)
    1. Gastroenterology.   2. Gastrointestinal system—Diseases.
    I. Yamada, Tadataka.
    [DNLM: 1. Gastrointestinal Diseases.   WI 100 T3551   1995]
RC801.T48   1995
616.3'3—dc20
DNLM/DLC
for Library of Congress   94-23213
                                                                    CIP

♾ This paper meets the requirements of ANSI/NISO Z39.48-1992 (permanence of paper).

The authors and publisher have exerted every effort to ensure that drug selection and dosage set forth in this text are in accord with current recommendations and practice at the time of publication. However, in view of ongoing research, changes in government regulations, and the constant flow of information relating to drug therapy and drug reactions, the reader is urged to check the package insert for each drug for any change in indications and dosage and for added warnings and precautions. This is particularly important when the recommended agent is a new or infrequently employed drug.

Preface

In 1988, when we initiated our project to develop a textbook that would be appropriate for students and practitioners of gastroenterology in the 1990s and beyond, we anticipated that we could edit an excellent manuscript, but we were uncertain as to the acceptance it would receive by our colleagues. We have been overwhelmed by the response to our *Textbook of Gastroenterology,* both from its critics who have hailed it as a truly important educational work and from the unexpectedly large number of our readers who have seen fit to obtain the *Textbook.* Personal communications to the Editor of the *Textbook* from our readers have attested to the success of our original concept for the *Textbook* as an encyclopedic reference that combines the important details of clinical problems in gastroenterology with the basic science of our discipline and the exciting diagnostic and therapeutic tools at our disposal.

The success of the first edition has served as an incremental challenge to us as we developed this second edition of the *Textbook of Gastroenterology.* Much has changed in our discipline in the few short years since the First Edition was published in 1991. From the genetics of colon cancer, to the role of *H. pylori* infection in peptic ulcer disease, to the evolution of endoscopic ultrasonography as a widespread diagnostic modality, knowledge of the discipline of gastroenterology continues to grow at an almost unbelievable pace. To keep up with these changes in the second edition of the *Textbook,* several chapters have been added or deleted, every chapter has been updated, and nearly 30% of the chapters have new authors to provide their subjects with a fresh outlook. These changes have helped retain the major assets of the *Textbook,* namely its modernity, its freshness, and its up-to-date accuracy. Throughout the second edition, we have taken great care to maintain the fundamental aims of the *Textbook* in its first edition, to present the scientific basis of gastroenterology in such a fashion that it will provide insight into common clinical problems, to detail the basics of a clinician's approach to common clinical problems, to provide at its core an encyclopedic discussion of virtually all of the disease states encountered in practice, and to describe all of the major diagnostic and therapeutic technologies of gastroenterology, both the long-standing and the very recent, available to clinicians today.

Above all, as in the first edition, the second edition of the *Textbook of Gastroenterology* is planned to integrate the various demands of science, technology, expanding information, good judgment, and common sense in the diagnosis and management of gastrointestinal patients. Because gastrointestinal complaints are among the most commonly encountered in clinical practice, the *Textbook* is not meant solely for the education of practicing or training gastroenterologists and surgeons but also, and most importantly, in the changing health care environment, primary care physicians and physician extenders. We hope that the collective efforts of the authors of the 141 chapters and the five of us who have edited this second edition have succeeded in achieving our goal to provide an outstanding educational work for students and practitioners of the medical science of gastroenterology.

Our efforts were especially facilitated by the expert assistance of Lori Ennis and Marianne Winfield who collaborated as a team to complement editorial talents with interpersonal skills to maintain the high quality of the text and deliver the manuscript in a timely fashion. The editors are indebted to their administrative and secretarial assistants Donna Hall, Pam Borton, Elsa Forero, Katherine Campbell, Norma Urani, Mary Hill, Melanie Meiselbach, and Anita Zinna. In addition, the faculty and fellows of the Gastroenterology Division at the University of Michigan, Washington University at St. Louis, the University of Texas Medical Branch at Galveston, and the University of Washington provided invaluable assistance in reviewing and utilizing all of the chapters in the second edition of the *Textbook.*

The editors wish to express their gratitude to their colleagues at J. B. Lippincott Company who have continued to demonstrate their commitment to quality, integrity, and excellence. Of the many people at Lippincott who have contributed their best efforts to the success of the second edition of the *Textbook,* two deserve special recognition: Rich Lampert and Wendy Greenberger-Czarnecki. This edition would not have been possible without their dedication and extraordinary talent.

Tadataka Yamada, M.D.

Preface to the First Edition

The practice of gastroenterology has changed dramatically during the past 20 years. We have witnessed a logarithmic growth in the volume of information concerning the basic biology and biochemistry of the gut. This wealth of new knowledge not only has provided fresh insight into the pathogenesis of gastrointestinal diseases but also has identified the critical role of the gut in the physiology and pathology of other organ systems. There is every reason to expect that the pace of our scientific growth will continue in the years ahead.

In many instances, advances in the science of gastroenterology have been incorporated directly into clinical practice. This has led to the evolution of a large and ever-expanding armamentarium of diagnostic and therapeutic modalities for management of patients with gastrointestinal diseases. The ability to see the organ of pathology and to treat lesions directly without invasive surgical procedures is an advantage almost unique to gastroenterology. As a result, today's clinicians must think in ways not even imagined by their predecessors. Although the textbooks of the past have served us well, modern gastroenterology dictates a more integrated approach to science, technology, and clinical practice. In the *Textbook of Gastroenterology* the Editors address this need.

The *Textbook* begins with a section of chapters describing the basic mechanisms of normal and abnormal gastrointestinal function. This section of the *Textbook* is written so that fundamental scientific concepts can be understood by a reader who is not scientifically oriented. We hope to present the scientific basis of gastroenterology in such a fashion that it will provide insight into common clinical problems. The section is intended to serve both as a guide for clinicians who need to understand the pathophysiology of their patients' disorders and as a resource for serious students of gastroenterology.

A major shortcoming of textbooks that consist solely of descriptions of diseases is the lack of guidance for the reader in applying the information to the management of patients who present with symptoms or signs rather than diagnoses. Therefore, a major section of the *Textbook* consists of detailed chapters on the clinician's approach to patients presenting with common gastrointestinal problems.

As a fully comprehensive textbook, the *Textbook of Gastroenterology* has at its core an encyclopedic discussion of virtually all of the disease states encountered in practice. These chapters, comprising the bulk of the *Textbook,* have a classical structure that ensures the uniform coverage of all important points.

After the initial evaluation, physicians must choose from a battery of diagnostic and therapeutic modalities as they proceed with patient management. A full section describing all of the major technologies, both the longstanding and the very recent, available to clinicians today comprises the last section of the *Textbook.* This section discusses not only the theory and practical uses of these procedures but also the contraindictions and potential complications, the evaluation and assessment of the data obtained, and the future directions of the modality.

The purposes of the *Textbook of Gastroenterology,* then, are multiple: to teach the scientific basis of gastroenterology, to provide practical approaches to common gastrointestinal problems, to serve as an encyclopedic reference for gastrointestinal diseases, and to indicate the current applications and future directions of the technology of gastroenterology. Above all, the *Textbook* is planned to integrate the various demands of science, technology, expanding information, good judgment, and common sense in the diagnosis and management of gastrointestinal patients. The Editors intend the book to be as useful at the bedside as on an office shelf or a student desk. Because gastrointestinal complaints are among the most commonly encountered in clinical practice, we want our readers to include surgeons, primary care physicians, and nurses as well as gastroenterologists and other internists.

To achieve these goals, the finest experts in the field of gastroenterology have written this *Textbook.* Each chapter is prepared by an authority who is actively engaged in advancing our knowledge of the subject matter of the chapter. We believe that the expertise of this group of physicians and scientists has ensured that the *Textbook* will achieve its aims.

Contents

VOLUME TWO

CHAPTER 80

Miscellaneous Inflammatory and Structural Disorders of the Colon   1806

R. Balfour Sartor, Mark E. Murphy, Edward Rydzak

CHAPTER 81

Irritable Bowel Syndrome   1832

William L. Hasler, Chung Owyang

CHAPTER 82

Motility Disorders of the Colon   1856

Sidney F. Phillips

CHAPTER 83

Diverticulitis   1876

John H. Pemberton, David N. Armstrong, Charles D. Dietzen

CHAPTER 84

Bacterial Infections of the Colon   1891

J. Thomas LaMont

CHAPTER 85

Colonic Polyps: Benign and Premalignant Neoplasms of the Colon   1911

Gordon D. Luk

CHAPTER 86

Polyposis Syndromes   1944

Randall W. Burt

CHAPTER 87

Malignant Tumors of the Colon   1967

C. Richard Boland

Textbook of
Gastroenterology

Textbook of Gastroenterology, second edition, edited by Tadataka Yamada. JB Lippincott Company, Philadelphia © 1995.

C. Small Intestine

CHAPTER 68

Small Intestine: Anatomy and Structural Anomalies

Deborah C. Rubin

Gross Anatomy
Extrinsic Arterial, Venous, and Lymphatic Supply
Neural Supply
Enhancement of Small Intestine Surface Area: Gross and Microscopic Features
Microscopic Anatomy
Serosa and Muscularis Propria
Submucosa
Mucosa
Embryology

Congenital Anomalies
Meckel's Diverticulum
Duplications
Intestinal Atresia and Stenosis
Malrotation
Gastroschisis and Omphalocele
Structural Anomalies
Volvulus
Intussusception
Lymphangiectasia
Celiac Artery Compression

GROSS ANATOMY

The small intestine begins just distal to the stomach's pyloric sphincter and extends to the cecum. Approximately 600 cm long, the small bowel is composed of three major segments: the duodenum, the jejunum, and the ileum. The junction between duodenum and jejunum is anatomically demarcated by the ligament of Treitz. No similar landmark distinguishes jejunum from ileum, but the jejunum is usually defined as the proximal two-fifths of the small bowel, and the ileum, the distal three-fifths.

After the appropriate rotation of the gut and its return to the abdominal cavity in fetal life (see discussion later in this chapter), the normal position of the small bowel loops is attained; the jejunum is generally located in the mid-upper and left upper quadrants, proximal ileum in the middle abdominal region, and the distal ileal loops in the right lower quadrant.[1,2]

The first part of the duodenum, the bulb, is invested with mesentery. The descending, transverse, and ascending retroperitoneal and partially encircles parts of the duodenum are the pancreatic head (Fig. 68-1). The jejunum begins at the ligament of Treitz as the small intestine reenters the peritoneal cavity. Jejunum and ileum are invested with mesentery. The very distal ileum may occasionally be retroperitoneally located.[3]

The gross appearance of the small intestine changes from jejunum to ileum. The jejunum is generally thicker-walled than the ileum. Also, the plicae circulares, or circular folds of mucosa and submucosa that invaginate into the lumen and increase the gut's surface area, are prominent in the duodenum and jejunum and disappear in the middle ileum.[2] Another

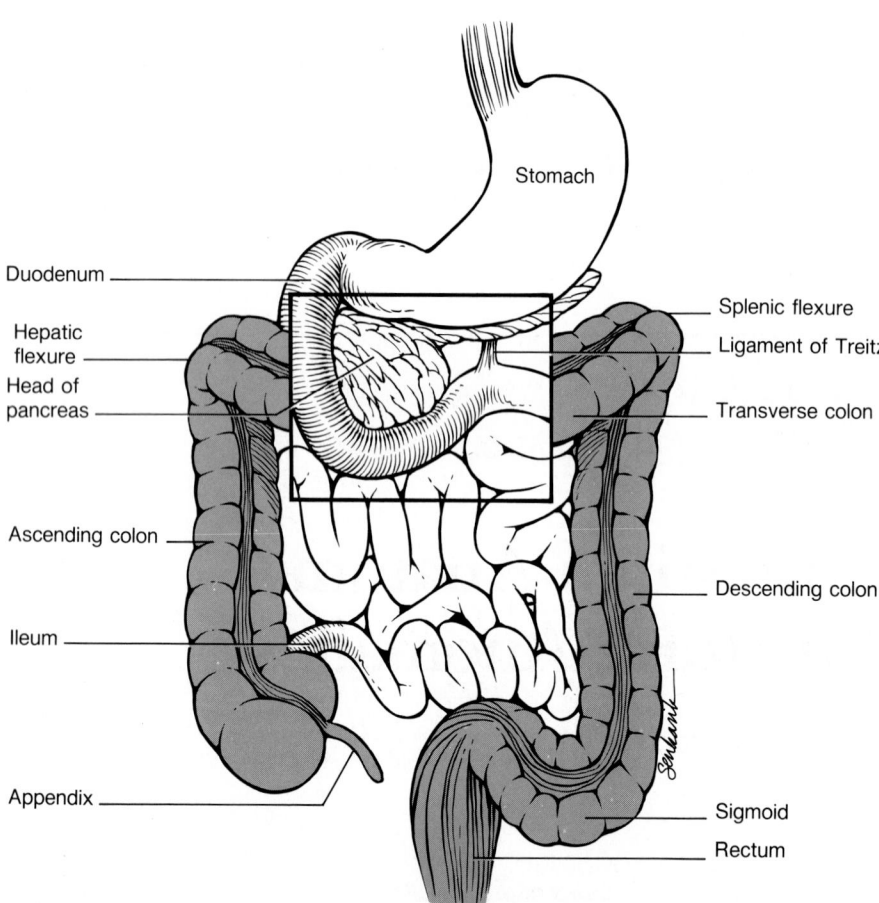

Stomach

Duodenum

Hepatic flexure

Head of pancreas

Ascending colon

Ileum

Appendix

Splenic flexure

Ligament of Treitz

Transverse colon

Descending colon

Sigmoid

Rectum

FIGURE 68-1. Anatomic relations among the stomach, small intestine, and large intestine. The duodenum encircles the head of the pancreas and is retroperitoneal. As the intestine reenters the peritoneal cavity at the ligament of Treitz, it becomes the jejunum. Generally, the jejunal bowel loops are located in the left and middle upper abdomen, the proximal ileum in the middle abdominal region and the distal ileal loops in the right lower quadrant. Inset "window" depicts the retroperitoneal duodenal loop and the ligament of Treitz, located behind the transverse colon.

easily identifiable gross feature are the Peyer's patches, usually found on the antimesenteric border of the small intestine. They are particularly prominent in childhood and atrophy with aging.[2]

Extrinsic Arterial, Venous, and Lymphatic Supply

The arteries, veins, and lymphatics that supply the small bowel travel through the mesentery. The arterial supply of the duodenum derives from several vessels. The hepatic artery gives rise to the gastroduodenal artery, which branches into the anterior and posterior superior pancreaticoduodenal arteries. These anastomose around the duodenum and communicate with the inferior pancreaticoduodenal artery, which arises from the superior mesenteric artery. The superior mesenteric artery also supplies the jejunum and ileum through a series of branches which form numerous arcades in the mesentery and then penetrate the intestine.

The veins that drain the small bowel usually follow the arterial supply. The superior mesenteric vein serves as the major venous conduit and joins the splenic vein to empty into the portal vein. Small lymph channels or villus lacteals drain into mesenteric lymph nodes located near the intestine and along the superior mesenteric and celiac arteries. These drain into the cisterna chyli and the thoracic duct.

Neural Supply

The intestine contains an abundant, complex *intrinsic* neural supply that coordinates motor activities and consists of myenteric (Auerbach's) and submucosal (Meissner's) plexuses (see Chap. 1). The *extrinsic* autonomic innervation of the small intestine consists of components from the parasympathetic and sympathetic systems.[4] The sympathetic motor innervation of the small bowel consists of postganglionic fibers arising from the superior mesenteric ganglion. These synapse with preganglionic fibers from the spinal cord in the region of the tenth and eleventh thoracic roots and travel in the lesser splanchnic nerve. Adrenergic neurons innervate both Auerbach's and Meissner's plexuses. Sensory nerves arise from the dorsal root ganglia. Parasympathetic motor innervation consists of preganglionic nerve fibers that arise from the vagus nerve. Vagal fibers originate from the dorsal motor nucleus and then divide into esophageal, anterior, and posterior vagal trunks. Both the anterior and posterior trunks give rise to celiac branches which directly innervate the small bowel by communicating with the intrinsic nervous system.

The small intestine contains a rich sensory innervation. The extrinsic sensory afferent nerves of the gut arise from either the dorsal root ganglion (sympathetic) or the nodose ganglion (parasympathetic). There is also an abundant intrinsic sensory network; the vast majority of these nerves remain within the gut wall. A small number project their axons out of the intestine to travel with extrinsic nerves and synapse with sympathetic postganglionic neurons at the sympathetic prevertebral ganglia.

Enhancement of Small Intestine Surface Area: Gross and Microscopic Features

The surface area of the small intestine is enhanced by three morphologic features that are peculiar to the gut: the plicae circulares, the villi, and the microvilli[3] (Fig. 68-2). The plicae circulares, or circular folds, consist of mucosal/submucosal invaginations that are predominantly located in the duodenum and jejunum. These infoldings are visible on gross inspection. The intestinal villi, finger-like projections that protrude into the intestinal lumen, are approximately 0.5 to 1.5 mm long and cover the mucosal surface. They can be viewed by close inspection of the mucosa under low-power microscopy and can be appreciated as tiny mucosal protrusions at endoscopy. They consist of a layer of epithelial cells overlying the lamina propria. Their microscopic appearance varies: duodenal villi are characteristically broad and leaf-shaped, jejunal villi are tall and thin, and ileal villi are short and broad. The length and shape of the villi also vary with geographic region; in some underdeveloped regions of the world, villi tend to be shorter than in the United States.[5,6] At the base of the villi, the epithelium enters the lamina propria and forms the crypts of Lieberkühn (Figs. 68-3 and 68-4), which extend almost to the muscularis mucosae. Finally, the microvilli are sub–light microscopic tubular projections that are extensions of the apical cell membrane and compose the brush border. This complex membranous network contains the enzymes, receptors, and carriers required for terminal digestion and absorption.

MICROSCOPIC ANATOMY

The small intestine is composed of four concentric layers, including the serosa, muscularis propria, submucosa, and mucosa. The cellular composition and characteristics of each layer are discussed here, with emphasis on the intestinal mucosa, which is responsible for the terminal absorptive and digestive functions of the gut.

Serosa and Muscularis Propria

The thin serosal lining of the small bowel consists of mesothelial cells overlying loose connective tissue. This outer layer becomes continuous with the mesentery as it joins the small bowel; many large blood vessels course through it. Those portions of the gut that are invested with mesentery are completely covered by serosa, whereas the retroperitoneal segments are invested only on the anterior surface. The muscularis propria consists of two muscle layers, the outer longitudinally oriented layer and the inner circumferential one. Between the two layers lies the myenteric or Auerbach's nerve plexus, composed of intrinsic ganglion cells and nerve fibers. The muscular layers of the gut are responsible for generating coordinated peristaltic movements.

Submucosa

The submucosa is a dense connective tissue layer containing numerous arteries as well as venous and lymphatic plexuses. Typical connective tissue cells are also present, but vascular structures predominate, consistent with the role of this portion of the gut as a conduit for absorptive and digestive products. In the duodenal bulb and descending duodenum are specialized Brunner's glands that secrete mucus and bicarbonate. These are branched epithelial glandular structures that fill the submucosa and are thought to be important in neutralization of stomach acid. The submucosa also contains ganglion cells and nerve fibers termed Meissner's plexus, a collection of autonomic nerves that communicate with Auerbach's plexus. A variety of neuroendocrine substances are produced in Meissner's plexus (see Chap. 1). These plexuses interact to produce regulated, coordinated gut peristalsis.

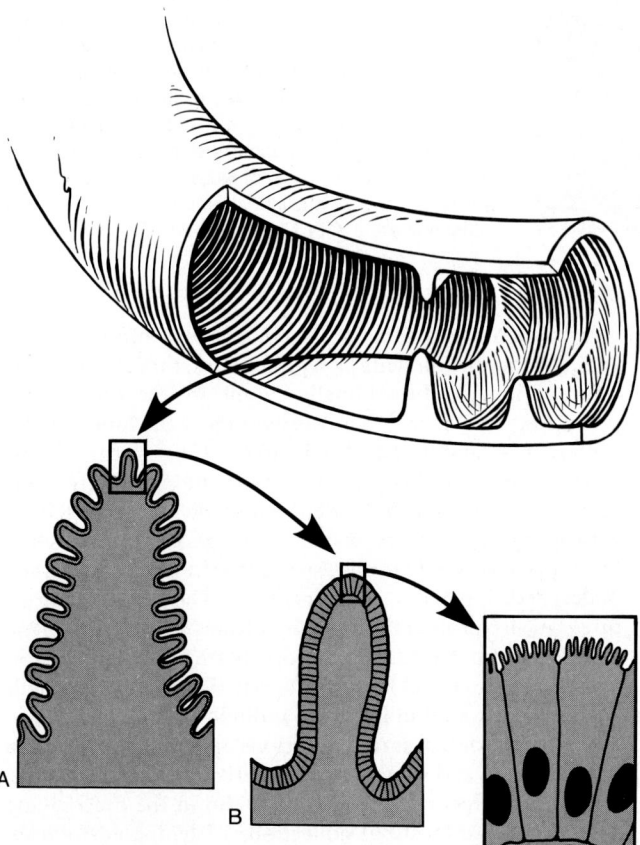

FIGURE 68-2. The surface area of the small intestine is enhanced by three mechanisms: (**A**) the valvulae conniventes; (**B**) the villi; and (**C**) the microvilli. (Adapted from Weaver LT. Anatomy and embryology. In: Walker WA, ed. Pediatric gastrointestinal disease: pathophysiology, diagnosis and management. Philadelphia: BC Decker, 1991:195.)

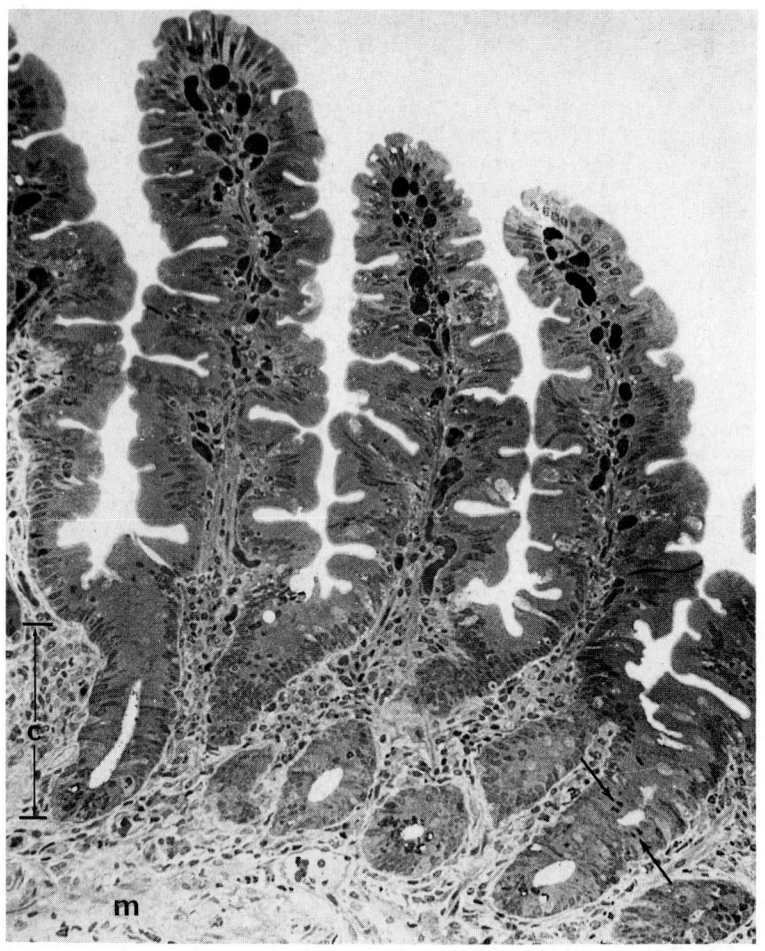

FIGURE 68-3. This semi-thin 1-μm epon section of human jejunum, stained with toluidine blue and viewed by light microscopy, depicts the mucosa. The villi are formed by a continuous sheet of columnar epithelial cells and the underlying connective tissue, the lamina propria. The epithelial sheets are composed primarily of enterocytes; mucus-secreting goblet cells are also present but are much less abundant, as are rare enteroendocrine cells. At the base of the villi, the epithelial cells dip down into the lamina propria to form the crypts, one of which is denoted at left (c). The crypts are lined mainly by undifferentiated crypt cells, which may be observed in mitosis (*arrows*). Differentiation proceeds as these cells migrate up the villus. Paneth's cells at the bases of the crypts are recognized by their dark granules. The muscularis mucosae (m), a thin layer of smooth muscle, separates the mucosa from the submucosa below. (Original magnification ×150; from Rubin W. The epithelial "membrane" of the small intestine. Am J Clin Nutr 1971;24:45.)

Mucosa

The mucosal layer of the gut consists of epithelial cells overlying the lamina propria or connective tissue core and resting on a narrow layer of smooth muscle, the muscularis mucosae (see Fig. 68-3).

Lamina Propria

The connective tissue core of the villus, known as the *lamina propria*, contains a variety of cells and vascular structures (Fig. 68-5). The immune cellular component includes lymphocytes, macrophages, granulocytes, plasma cells, and mast cells. The majority of lamina propria T lymphocytes are T-helper/inducer cells that are surface antigen CD4-positive, although smaller numbers of T-cytotoxic/suppressor cells (CD8+) are also present.[7] In contrast, the *intraepithelial* lymphocytes that reside between villus epithelial cells are primarily CD8-positive and γ/σ T-cell receptor–positive.[8] The lamina propria plasma cells produce immunoglobulin; most importantly, these cells synthesize dimeric immunoglobulin A (IgA), which is taken up into the intestinal epithelium and secreted intralumenally after joining with secretory component.[9] A much smaller number of plasma cells produce IgM or IgG. The maturation of the B cell to an IgA-secreting plasma cell occurs during the course of a migratory journey throughout the body's vascular system. Cells exit the Peyer's patches through lymph vessels, enter the mesenteric lymph nodes, thoracic duct, peripheral blood, and then finally "home" to the gut's lamina propria (as well as to other organs such as the lung, genitourinary tract, and breast).[10] T lymphocytes similarly migrate from one lymphoid organ to another and eventually home to mucosal sites which are determined by their interactions with specific proteins expressed on lymphoid cells as well as the high endothelial venules, specialized vessels of the lymph nodes, Peyer's patches, and appendix.[11] These vascular structures can also proliferate in organs affected by chronic inflammation. Macrophages and eosinophils are present in the normal human intestinal lamina propria. However, neutrophils are primarily found in inflamed and not normal gut.

Lymph follicles are small collections of lymphocytes present in the mucosa and submucosa, scattered throughout the gastrointestinal tract. *Peyer's patches*, found in the mucosa and submucosa, are localized collections of lymphoid follicles, may be as large as 30 cm in diameter,[12] and are most prominent in the ileum. The number of Peyer's patches in the gut increases after birth.[12] The Peyer's patch contains specialized epithelial cells known as M cells that overlie the lymphoid cells and allow entry of lumenal antigens into the mucosa.[13] The dome area of the Peyer's patch lies above the lymph follicles and just below the M cells; it contains lymphocytes and macrophages. The follicular or central region contains large

FIGURE 68-4. High-power views of the crypt. (**A**) A crypt is observed extending to the base of a villus. Note the prominent brush border on the differentiated cells above the villus base and the unapparent brush border on the crypt cells below. The arrow shows a short and irregular brush border on an upper crypt cell. Large, dense Paneth's cell granules are evident at the crypt base; the smaller apical granules higher in the crypt are in undifferentiated crypt cells. (Original magnification ×300.) (**B**) The large granules in Paneth's cells at the base of another crypt are located mainly in the apical cytoplasm. The scantier, lighter apical granules in cells above (*arrows*) are in undifferentiated crypt cells. (Original magnification ×700.) (**C**) The large, dense apical granules in Paneth's cells at another crypt base should be contrasted with the smaller, barely resolvable basal infranuclear granules observed in two endocrine cells (*arrows*). (Original magnification ×700.) (**D**) Differentiated villus epithelial cells and a goblet cell are depicted. Note the tall, prominent brush border. The narrow, light zone below the brush border represents the terminal web. The numerous light structures within the cells are mitochondria. The occasional dense apical structures are lysosome derivatives (*arrowheads*). The apical densities between adjoining cells at the level of the terminal web (*arrows*) are the terminal bars. They represent the junctional complexes of electron microscopy—the tight junctions, intermediate junctions, and desmosomes—specialized structures that serve to bind adjoining epithelial cells at their apices. The accumulation of mucus granules within the apical cytoplasm of the goblet cell distends it into the shape of a "brandy goblet." (Original magnification ×1500; from Rubin W. The epithelial "membrane" of the small intestine. Am J Clin Nutr 1971;24:45.)

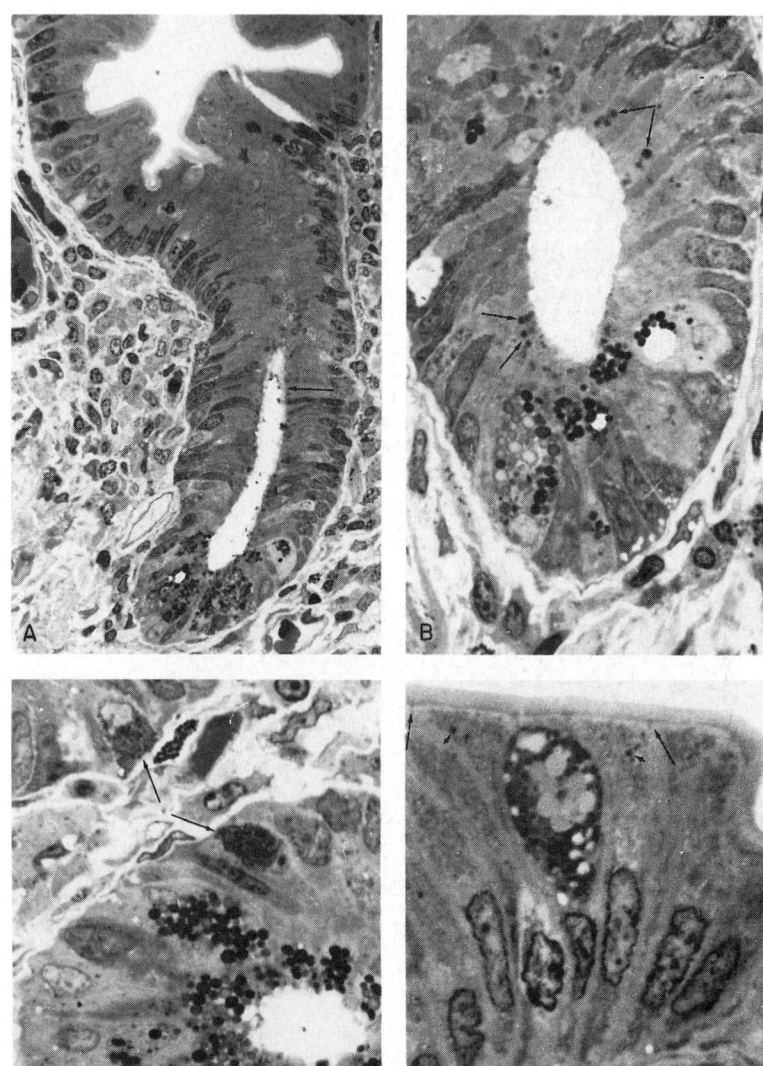

numbers of precursor B cells which undergo active cell division. The interfollicular zone is populated predominantly by T cells.

Other cellular components of the lamina propria include fibroblasts and smooth muscle cells. Arterioles, venules, and a central lacteal are present for delivery of nutrients into the vascular system (see Fig. 68-5).

Epithelium

The intestine contains a complex, rapidly proliferating, and perpetually differentiating epithelium. The epithelium is a continuous sheet of simple columnar cells which rests on a filamentous basal lamina or basement membrane, overlying the villi and forming the crypts (see Figs. 68-3 and 68-4). It constitutes the major barrier between the intestinal lumen and the lamina propria and regulates fluxes between these two compartments. The epithelial cells on the villi vectorially transport the products of digestion into the lamina propria, where they enter the venous capillaries or lymphatic system and are transported to other areas of the body. Tight junctions

(zonula occludens) bind adjacent epithelial cells tightly together near their apices; this restricts fluxes between adjoining cells (the paracellular route) to small ions, small molecules, and water.[14,15]

The crypt and villus form the basic structural and functional unit of the small bowel (Fig. 68-6; see Figs. 68-3 and 68-4). Anchored stem cells located in the crypts of Lieberkühn are the source of the four major terminally differentiated cell types—absorptive enterocyte, mucus-secreting goblet cell, enteroendocrine cell, and Paneth's cell. Cellular differentiation proceeds during a complex, bidirectional process. The presumptive gut epithelial stem cell, postulated to be in the lower crypt region,[16,17] gives rise to proliferating progenitor cells, which differentiate as they migrate up the crypt onto the villus to become enterocytes, goblet cells, and a subset of enteroendocrine cells. In contrast, the Paneth's cells and the other enteroendocrine cells arise as their progenitors journey to the crypt base.[18] Goblet cells are found both in the crypts and on the villi. Several crypts contribute cells to a single villus; the number of crypts supplying each villus varies from duodenum to ileum. Epithelial cell migration and differentiation occurs

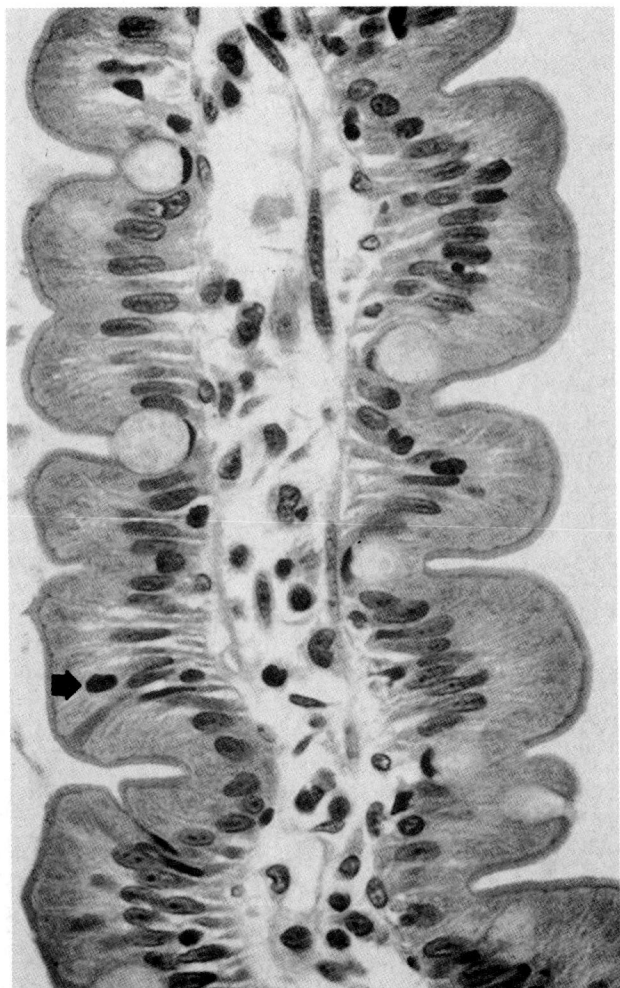

FIGURE 68-5. Upper villus region, featuring the lamina propria, goblet cells, enterocytes, and intraepithelial lymphocytes (*arrow*). (H & E stain; original magnification ×495; from Phillips AD. The small intestinal mucosa. In: Whitehead R, ed. Gastrointestinal and oesophageal pathology. New York: Churchill Livingstone, 1989:29.)

continuously, and the process of cellular renewal takes approximately 3 to 5 days.

Other epithelial cell types include the tuft or caveolated cell, a rare constituent of the villus, and the M cell, a specialized epithelial cell that overlies the Peyer's patch (see following text).

Cellular and topographic organization of the crypt. The present model of the organization of the crypt and its cellular kinetics is derived primarily from studies in the mouse. Although the exact number of stem cells per crypt is unclear, it is postulated that there are between 4 and 16.[16,17,19] However, the number of active stem cells in any one particular crypt is unknown.[20] In the adult gut, these cells are monoclonal.[21,22] The small intestine epithelial stem cell has proven difficult to study because there are no known cell-specific markers, and methods for their isolation and culture have not yet been developed. These cells presumably undergo a process of *asymmetric* division to give rise to actively proliferating progenitor

cells while maintaining the stem cell.[17] Proliferating progenitor cells or transit cells are located in the midcrypt region, above the presumptive stem cell region. In mouse gut, these cells enter the cell cycle every 12 hours.[20] In a process that remains uncharacterized, these progenitor cells subsequently differentiate into the four major cell types. Crypt cells move approximately one to two cell positions per hour at the apex of the crypt.

Undifferentiated crypt cells. Undifferentiated crypt cells have many ribosomes and polysomes but have scant endoplasmic reticulum, mitochondria, and microvilli and undeveloped terminal webs. They are basophilic because they contain large amounts of cytoplasmic RNA. Secretory granules of various sizes are found near the apical surface (see Fig. 68-4*B*), the nature of which are unknown, but which stain with the periodic acid-Schiff (PAS) reaction and are not lysosomes.[23] Undifferentiated crypt cells also synthesize secretory component, the receptor for IgA; this molecule is inserted into the basolateral plasma membrane, binds IgA secreted by plasma cells, internalizes it, and secretes the receptor-IgA complex into the intestinal lumen.[24] These cells contain chloride channels and are capable of secreting chloride in response to cholera toxin or other enterotoxins.[25,26]

Absorptive enterocytes. Upon migration to the upper crypt and villus base, cellular differentiation commences. The cells that are fated to become the absorptive enterocytes, the most abundant and functionally the most important of the epithelial cells, begin to express a variety of specific genes which enable these cells to digest and absorb many different nutrients. These include numerous brush border enzymes such as the disaccharidases, peptidases, and alkaline phosphatase; many genes involved in lipid absorption such as the apolipoproteins and fatty acid-binding proteins; and a host of receptors, carriers, and transporters.[27,28] Immunohistochemical and in situ hybridization analyses indicate that most enterocytic genes, such as those resulting in production of disaccharidases, apolipoproteins, fatty acid-binding proteins, and the sodium-dependent glucose transporter, are initially expressed just as cells emerge above the crypt-villus junction[29–33] and are not found in the crypts. This precise vertical differentiation continues as cells migrate up the villus; microvilli become more prominent and the cells' capacity to absorb lipids, sugars, and amino acids increases.[34]

Despite rapid cellular renewal, complex spatial differentiation in the gut is also maintained from duodenum to colon. Many enterocytic genes are abundantly expressed in the proximal small bowel, but their messenger RNA (mRNA) levels decrease markedly in the distal gut[31,35–38]; other genes are specifically expressed in the ileum.[39,40] The cloning, sequencing, and promotor analysis of these genes have provided some insight into the molecular mechanisms underlying the regulation of regional differentiation in the gut. Specific *cis*-acting DNA elements, as well as the *trans*-acting proteins that regulate cell- and region-specific differentiation along the horizontal and vertical axes of the gut, have begun to be characterized, using transgenic mice or cell culture transfection techniques to map out regulatory promoter elements.[19,32,41–43]

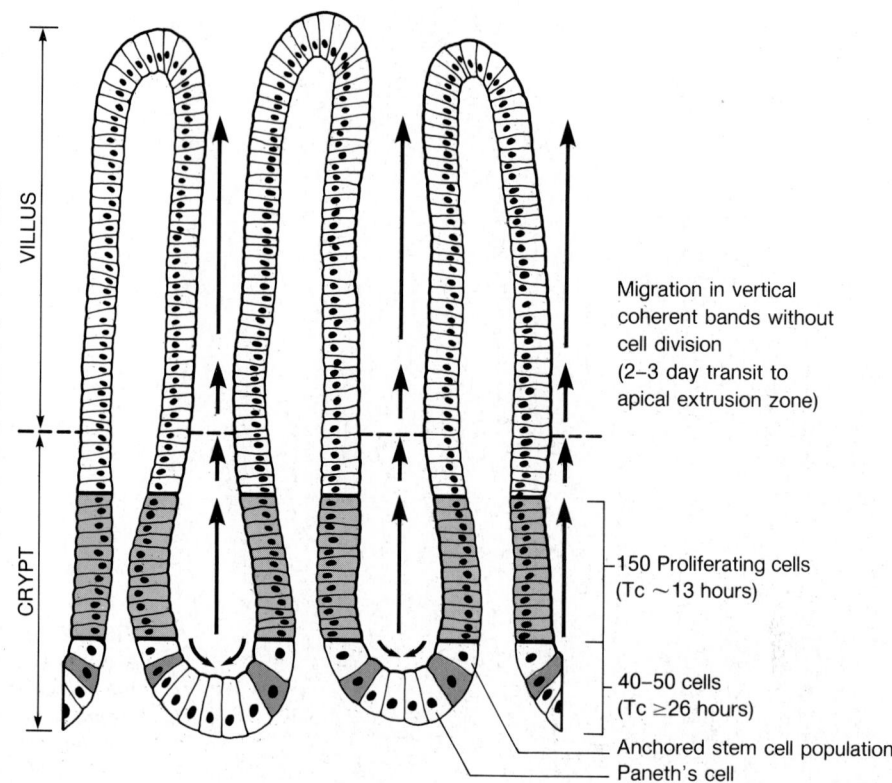

FIGURE 68-6. Model of organization of the crypt-villus axis in the adult mouse small intestine. The small intestinal crypt contains approximately 250 cells. The lower five cell positions contain 40–50 cells which have an average cycle time (Tc) ≥26 hours. This region includes Paneth's cells and is postulated to include undifferentiated, anchored stem cells at the fifth cell position above the base. The undifferentiated cells divide asymmetrically to give rise to proliferating daughter cells (Tc ~ 13 hours) that migrate upward toward the villus and differentiate into enterocytes, goblet cells, and enteroendocrine cells. Paneth's cells also arise from this stem cell during downward translocation to the crypt base. Senescent cells are extruded near the villus tips. (Adapted from Gordon JI. Intestinal epithelial differentiation: new insights from chimeric and transgenic mice. J Cell Biol 1989;108:1187.)

Labels in figure: VILLUS / CRYPT

Migration in vertical coherent bands without cell division (2–3 day transit to apical extrusion zone)

150 Proliferating cells (Tc ~13 hours)

40–50 cells (Tc ≥26 hours)

Anchored stem cell population

Paneth's cell

Ultrastructural features. As undifferentiated crypt cells travel up the villus, they acquire longer, more numerous microvilli, measuring 0.1 μm in width and about 1 μm in height, which produce a prominent striated (brush) border by light microscopy. The development of these long microvilli, finger-like extensions of the apical cell membrane, markedly increases the absorbing surface of the small intestine (Figs. 68-7 and 68-8). The basolateral membrane is relatively smooth in comparison and contains the Na$^+$/K$^+$ exchanger, Na$^+$,K$^+$-ATPase, which pumps sodium from the cell. These cells also develop a terminal web, an organelle-free apical zone below the microvilli, which contains many filaments and some vesicles. They acquire more mitochondria and rough endoplasmic reticulum, they lose their secretory granules, and they acquire large apical dense bodies, which represent lysosomal derivatives[23,44-48] (see Figs. 68-4D and 68-7). The polarity of the enterocyte, with its specific apical and basolateral membrane domains, is strictly maintained, with no mixing of proteins between the two, thereby assuring the vectorial transport of a variety of nutrients and ions from the apical to the basolateral surfaces of these cells. The establishment and maintenance of epithelial cell polarity is a highly regulated process that is not yet well understood.

Filaments composed of actin extend from a dense plaque just beneath the cell membrane at the tip of the microvilli down the core of the microvilli into the terminal web.[44,48,49-52] The terminal web is a dense meshwork of filaments, which contain myosin and other cytoskeletal proteins as well as actin; the meshwork is oriented parallel with the surface and perpendicular to the microvillus filaments, and it is attached to the lateral cell membrane at the intermediate junction (zonula adherens).[49-52] The numerous filaments in the microvilli and terminal web—

known as the cytoskeleton of the brush border—probably confer a structural rigidity to the apices of the differentiated villus cells and may provide for the movement of the microvilli, as far as can be observed in vitro.[49,53] This cytoskeleton probably also affects the uptake of certain nutrients and paracellular permeability.[49,54]

Short, thin, filamentous material extends from the outer leaflet of the cell membrane covering the microvilli into the intestinal lumen, thus producing a surface coat, glycocalyx or "fuzz." The glycocalyx is an integral part of the cell membrane, representing external extensions of proteins and glycoproteins whose hydrophobic portions are rooted in the interior of the microvillus membrane.[49,55] The microvillus membrane of the differentiated villus cells contains many of the enzymes, receptors, and carriers necessary for terminal digestion and absorption, such as the disaccharidases, alkaline phosphatase, peptidases, the ileal cobalamin–intrinsic factor receptor, the bile acid receptor, and the Na$^+$-dependent glucose and amino acid transporters.[40,49,55-57] The active portions of many of these are associated with the glycocalyx. These protein and glycoprotein components of the microvillus membrane and glycocalyx turn over and are replenished by their continual synthesis, primarily in the rough endoplasmic reticulum, and their apparent transport as small carrier vesicles from the Golgi apparatus to the microvillus membrane.[49,55,58-62]

The selective vesicular transport of microvillus constituents from the Golgi's apparatus to the cell apex is dependent on microtubules. Disruption of microtubules in rats and mice with colchicine or vinblastine results in more random routing of these components, with the incorporation of microvillus enzymes into the basolateral surface and even the formation of basolateral microvilli.[58,61] Some of the microvillus enzymes

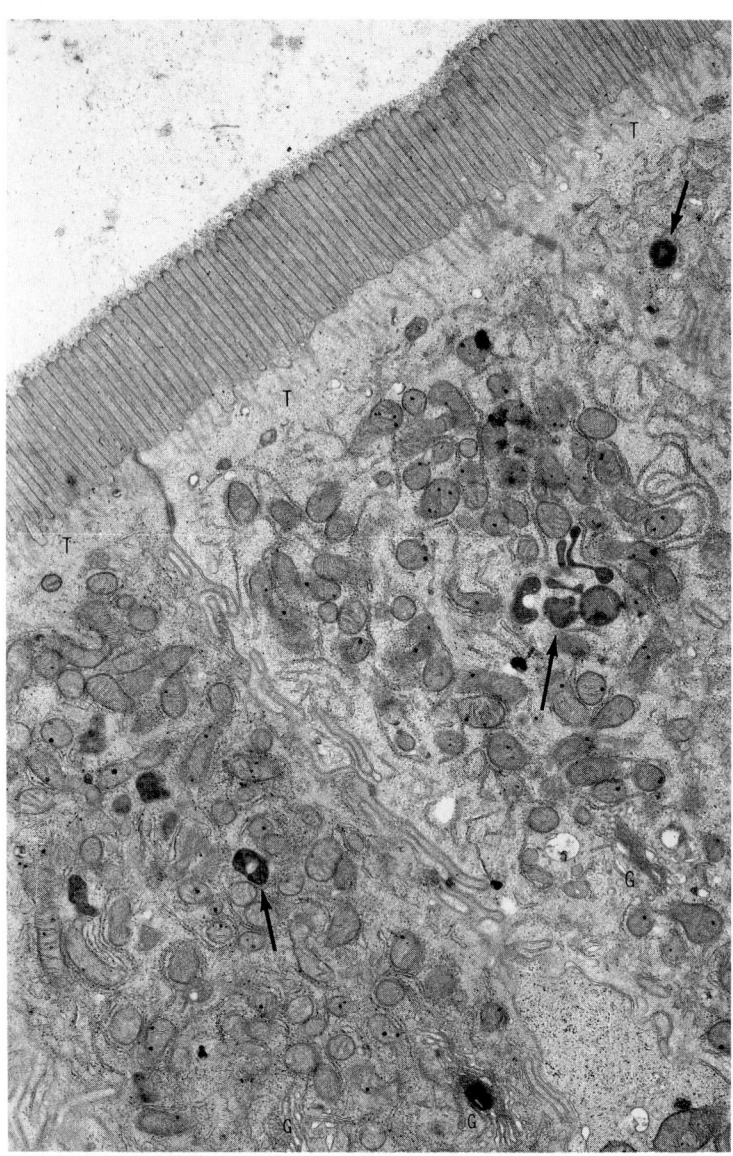

FIGURE 68-7. An electron microscopic picture of the apical halves of differentiated villus epithelial cells. Note the numerous tall microvilli covered with "fuzz" or glycocalyx and an organelle-free apical zone—the terminal web (T)—just below the microvilli. There are abundant mitochondria and profiles of rough endoplasmic reticulum. The irregularly shaped dense bodies (*arrows*) are lysosome derivatives. Supranuclear Golgi profiles are denoted by G. The intercellular space is obliterated between the apices of adjoining cells just below the level of the microvilli by the tight junction (zonula occludens), an apparent fusion of adjoining cell membranes (best seen between the two cells on the *left*). Transport of substances from the lumen between cells (paracellular route) is restricted to water and small molecules and ions. Most products of digestion enter the cell by crossing the microvillar membrane. (Original magnification ×15,000; from Rubin W. The epithelial "membrane" of the small intestine. Am J Clin Nutr 1971;24:45.)

are finally processed in the glycocalyx by the proteolytic activity of pancreatic enzymes, especially elastase, which are adherent to the glycocalyx.[49,55]

Paneth's cells. Paneth's cells are pyramid-shaped cells that reside in the crypt base and contain large eosinophilic secretory granules located in the apical cytoplasm. They have long been recognized in the intestine and have been the focus of intensive investigation, although their function is unclear. Their role in host defense had been suggested by their abundant expression of lysozyme[63] and their ability to degranulate in response to live and heat-killed bacteria.[64] Numerous studies have shown that Paneth's cells produce many proteins related to this putative function. Several of the defensins, a family of small peptides that are abundant in human neutrophils, are also highly expressed in Paneth's cells.[65-67] In particular, defensin-5 and defensin-6 are specific to the small intestine.[66] These peptides are 30 to 35 amino acids in length and show microbicidal activity toward many different microorganisms in vitro. In addition, mRNAs encoding tumor necrosis factor[68]

and α_1-antitrypsin[69,70] have been shown by in situ hybridization to be located in Paneth's cells. Guanylin, an endogenous intestinal protein that activates guanylate cyclase, is a peptide homologue to heat-stable enterotoxins and is also produced by Paneth's cells.[71,72] These studies have opened new vistas of investigation into the function of Paneth's cells and the defensive role of the gut.

Enteroendocrine cells. The intestine contains a remarkably complex enteroendocrine cell population composed of a variety of paracrine-endocrine cell types. These cells were classically characterized as argentaffin or argyrophil cells, depending on their reaction to silver staining in the presence or absence of a reducing agent. Electron microscopic characterization has led to the classification of these cells by the appearance of their granules. Modern immunohistochemical techniques have facilitated the identification of these cells based on their primary neuroendocrine product. The D cell has been shown to produce somatostatin, the L cell produces glucagon-like immunoreactivity, and the EC cell makes se-

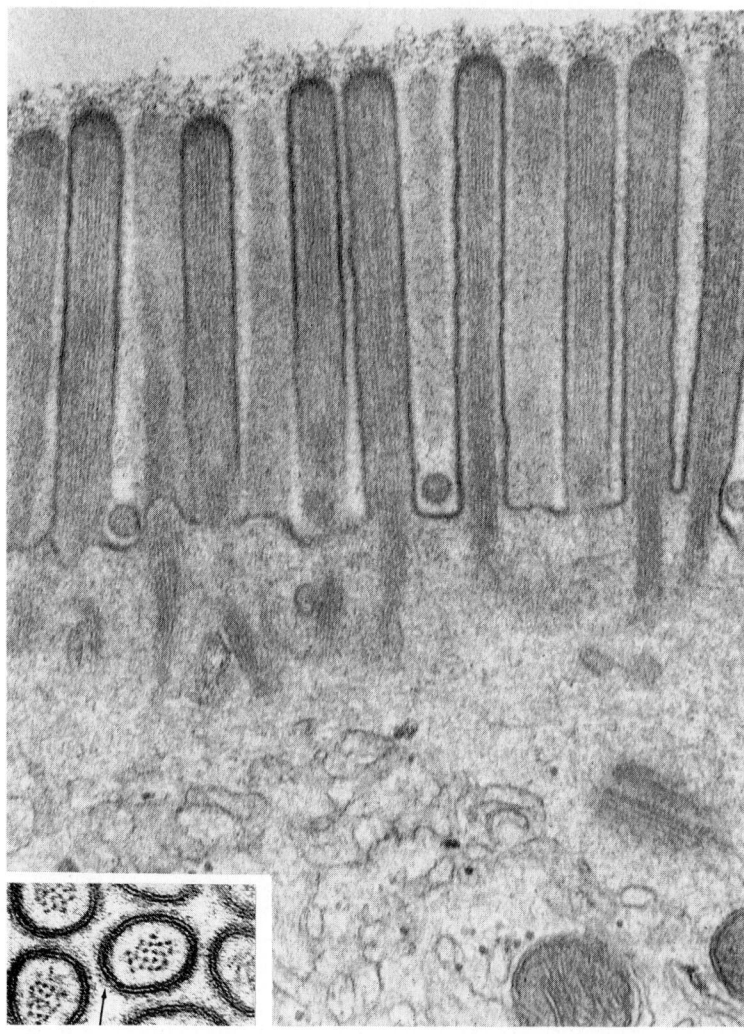

FIGURE 68-8. This electron micrograph illustrates the microvilli in longitudinal section and in cross section (inset). The microvilli are finger-shaped projections of the apical cell membrane that markedly increase the absorbing surface of the enterocytes. The glycocalyx or "fuzz" is indicated by the arrow in the inset. This represents external extensions of proteins and glycoproteins that are anchored in the interior of the microvillus membrane. Terminal digestion of peptides and disaccharides probably occurs at the glycocalyx. In the interior of the microvilli are bundles of actin filaments, seen on end in the inset. The terminal web below the microvilli contains a meshwork of filaments: myosin and other cytoskeletal proteins as well as actin. The terminal web and microvillus filaments constitute the cytoskeleton of the apex of the enterocytes and probably account for their apical rigidity. (Original magnifications ×70,000; *inset* ×130,000; from Rubin W. The epithelial cell "membrane" of the small intestine. Am J Clin Nutr 1971;24:45.)

rotonin. Immunohistochemical analyses have also demonstrated that this cellular population exhibits a very specific spatial distribution along the crypt-to-villus and duodenal-to-colonic axes of the gut. For example, serotonin cells are abundant and are distributed throughout the gastrointestinal tract, whereas secretin and cholecystokinin (CCK) cells are much more frequently found in the duodenum and proximal jejunum.[73-75] In the mouse, secretin cells are predominantly located on the villi, whereas substance P–containing cells are primarily found in the crypts. Each cell type demonstrates its own specific regional localization. Enteroendocrine cells may also coexpress more than one neuroendocrine product[73-76]; this coexpression is developmentally regulated in the rodent.[77]

Although previous data had suggested that enteroendocrine cells were derived from the neural crest,[78] more recent studies have indicated these cells arise from the undifferentiated crypt stem cell.[16,17,19,79,80] The differentiation of endocrine cells seems to be hard-wired, or controlled by an intrinsic genetic program that functions in the absence of lumenal contents, including pancreaticobiliary secretions and dietary factors.[76,81] Although the enteroendocrine cells all arise from a common stem cell, there may be a branch point at which proliferating progenitor cells differentiate into the various en-

docrine cell lineages.[82] The patterns of coexpression of substance P, serotonin, and secretin along the crypt-to-villus axis of the small bowel suggests that these cells are representative of a specific differentiation pathway that arises independently of the other endocrine cell types.[74]

The secretions of these cells may have a multitude of effects on the small bowel. Many act in a paracrine manner and function locally, whereas others are true endocrine products. These peptides and amines may affect bowel motility and intestinal cellular secretion (see Chap. 2).

Ultrastructural features. In contrast to exocrine cells, which secrete apically into the lumen of an organ or the duct of a gland, the morphologic orientation of the endocrine cells is toward the basement membrane. They exhibit an appreciable basal surface, and their widths narrow superiorly so that only narrow bands of apical cytoplasm reach the lumen. Their secretory granules are located predominantly in the basal cytoplasm below the nucleus, ready to be secreted by exocytosis through the basal membrane into the lamina propria (Fig. 68-9; see Fig. 68-4C).

Goblet cells. The mucus-secreting goblet cells are present throughout the entire gastrointestinal tract, but they are more

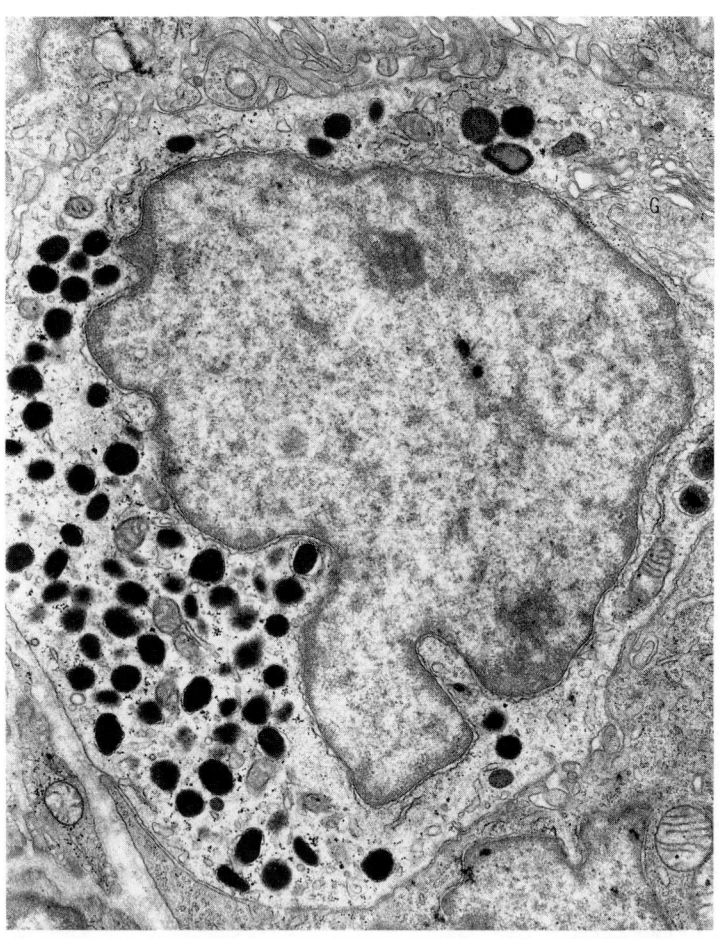

FIGURE 68-9. The endocrine cells, examined by electron microscopy, generally exhibit light cytoplasm, membrane-enclosed granules primarily in the basal cytoplasm between the nucleus and basal cell membrane, and only modest amounts of endoplasmic reticulum and Golgi membranes (G). These cells are the epithelial source of the gut hormones. This endocrine cell, characterized by the presence of dense pleomorphic granules, is an EC cell and is thought to correspond to the enterochromaffin or argentaffin cell that produces serotonin. (Original magnification approximately ×17,000; from Rubin W. The epithelial "membrane" of the small intestine. Am J Clin Nutr 1971;24:45.)

numerous in the ileum than the jejunum. These cells exhibit a brandy-goblet shape and are characterized by apically-located granules filled with mucin. Mucin is their primary secretory product and presumably serves a cytoprotective and lubricant function in the gastrointestinal tract.[83] There are biochemical differences among mucins expressed in the stomach, small intestine, and colon, suggesting heterogeneity among goblet cell populations.[24] A novel goblet cell secretory product has been identified. Intestinal trefoil factor, one of a family of small peptides that includes pS2 and human spasmolysin, was shown to be abundantly expressed in goblet cells of the small intestine and colon, using in situ hybridization techniques.[84] The protein was also present on the intestinal lumenal surface, suggesting its secretion into the lumen by the goblet cell. Detection of its mRNA also revealed that it is expressed in the crypt and may therefore be a marker of early goblet cell differentiation. Although the function of this peptide is unknown, its presence on the epithelial cell surface and the resistance of one of its homologues, porcine spasmolysin, to protease digestion suggest a possible cytoprotective role in the gut.

Goblet cells arise from the same committed stem cell as do the other principal cell types. However, actively proliferating goblet cells have been noted in the crypt; these cells may also contribute to the villus-associated goblet cell population.

M cells. The specialized epithelial membranous or M cells are confined to the epithelium overlying the Peyer's patch. Unlike typical absorptive cells, they have fewer, shorter microvilli and demonstrate numerous apical endocytic vesicles. They serve as antigen sampling cells and endocytose a variety of macromolecules, viruses, and bacteria from the lumen. These molecules are then rapidly transported across the epithelium and come into contact with immune cells.[13,85,86] Although M cells are thought to simply serve a transport function without processing the antigens that they engulf, recent evidence indicates that these cells express class II major histocompatibility complex determinants and have endosomal and lysosomal compartments.[87] The presumptive origin of this cell type is also the multipotent crypt stem cell, as demonstrated by ^{3}H thymidine labeling studies.[85]

EMBRYOLOGY

A complete discussion of the embryology of the gastrointestinal tract is found in Chapter 23. In this section, a brief synopsis of the major events in midgut morphogenesis is presented as a basis for understanding the congenital anomalies discussed below.

The primitive human gut forms when the dorsal part of the yolk sac is incorporated into the embryo at 4 weeks of development, giving rise to the foregut, midgut, and hindgut.[88,89] The foregut is the progenitor of the esophagus, stomach, duodenum up to the biliary duct ampulla, pharynx, respiratory tract, liver, pancreas, and biliary tract. The midgut gives rise to the duodenum distal to the common bile duct, jejunum, ileum, cecum, appendix, ascending colon, and half to two thirds of the transverse colon. The rest of the colon and superior anal canal are derived from hindgut.

The gut endoderm is the precursor of the gastrointestinal tract epithelium. Its endothelium arises from the ectoderm of the stomodeum and proctodeum as well as the endoderm. The splanchnic mesenchyme supplies the muscular and connective tissue components of the gastrointestinal tract. The midgut first freely communicates with the yolk sac and then narrows to be connected by the omphalomesenteric or vitelline duct. The primitive gut forms a U-shaped loop which grows so rapidly compared to the embryo that it herniates into the umbilical cord at the sixth week of gestation. The proximal limb of the loop elongates into multiple intestinal loops, whereas the distal limb simply develops into the cecal diverticulum. The first stage of rotation is 90 degrees counterclockwise around the superior mesenteric artery axis. At 10 weeks, the intestines return into the abdominal cavity and rotate a further 180 degrees counterclockwise in the second stage. Finally, the cecum and appendix descend from the right upper quadrant to the right lower quadrant, and the proximal part of the colon elongates to form the hepatic flexure and ascending colon (third stage of rotation). Fixation occurs as the ascending colonic mesentery fuses with the parietal peritoneum and becomes fixed retroperitoneally. The small bowel mesentery attains a broad-based attachment to the posterior abdominal wall, extending from the duodenal-jejunal junction to the ileocecal region. The end result of this process is the normal location of the small and large intestine as diagrammed in Figure 68-1.

CONGENITAL ANOMALIES

Meckel's Diverticulum

Description and Pathophysiology

During early gestation, the omphalomesenteric or vitelline duct connects the fetal yolk sac to the primitive gut. By 7 to 8 weeks of gestation, this duct is normally completely obliterated. A *Meckel's diverticulum*, the most common congenital anomaly of the gastrointestinal tract, results if this structure fails to resorb completely. The duct remnant most commonly persists as a diverticular sac; alternatively, the diverticulum may be connected to the umbilicus by a fibrous band (Fig. 68-10). Occasionally, only a thick connective tissue band remains attaching the gut to the umbilicus; these bands are clinically relevant because they may lead to volvulus or strangulation of bowel loops. Rarely, a fistula remains patent from ileum to umbilicus, leading to persistent external drainage of ileal contents. Other, more unusual duct remnants are umbilical polyps or vitelline cysts.

Large autopsy series indicate a 2% to 3% prevalence of Meckel's diverticulum in the general population.[90] This

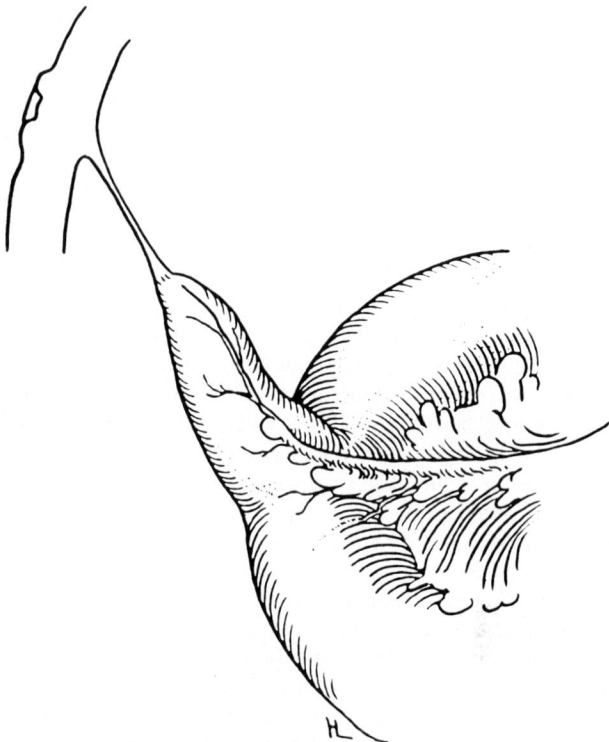

FIGURE 68-10. A Meckel's diverticulum is pictured attached to the umbilicus by the obliterated omphalomesenteric duct. A Meckel diverticulum may be unattached to the umbilicus or abdominal wall; alternatively, the vitelline duct may remain attached and patent, creating a fistula. Fibrous bands may predispose to volvulus and strangulation. (From Johns TNP, Wheeler JR, Johns FS. Meckel's diverticulum and Meckel's diverticular disease: a study of 154 cases. Ann Surg 1959;150:241.)

anomaly is two to three times more common in males.[91] Meckel's diverticula are true diverticula, containing all layers of the bowel from serosa to mucosa. Located on the antimesenteric border of the gut, they are most commonly found within 100 cm of the ileocecal valve but may also exist in other regions of the small bowel. Most diverticula are between 1 and 10 cm in size; giant lesions may be as large as 100 cm in diameter.[92] The two types of giant diverticula are Type I, which is long but of equal caliber to the ileum, and the less common Type II, or ovoid-shaped lesion.[93] Heterotopic tissue is present in approximately 50% of all diverticula.[94] Most common is gastric mucosa, pancreatic tissue, or a combination of the two. Diverticula containing colonic mucosa, Brunner's glands, and hepatobiliary tissue have also been described.[95] The presence of heterotopic mucosa correlates with an increased risk of symptomatic, complicated Meckel's diverticulum. Heterotopic gastric mucosa may lead to diverticular gastrointestinal bleeding in adults and children because of ileal ulceration from acid secretion[96-98]; almost all bleeding diverticula contain gastric mucosa.[99,100] Although there are some conflicting data, recent reports have indicated that *Helicobacter pylori* may rarely colonize the diverticular gastric mucosa and is associated with gastritis in this site.[101,102] Heterotopic tissue is also associated with a modestly increased risk of other complications, including small bowel obstruction and diverticular inflammation.[96,103]

Although early literature suggested a high incidence of complications of Meckel's diverticulum in adults, later studies revealed that the risk of complications dramatically decreases with age and that the majority of adults with Meckel's diverticulum remain asymptomatic.[104] Approximately 2% of all adults with Meckel's diverticulum develop complications.[96,97,104]

The complications of Meckel's diverticulum include bleeding, intestinal obstruction, diverticulitis, perforation, and carcinoma. Obstruction is caused by intussusception of the diverticulum into adjacent bowel; volvulus around or herniation into a fibrous band; entrapment in inguinal, femoral, or umbilical hernia sacs (Littre's hernia); or inflammation and scarring leading to blockage around the diverticular neck and adjacent ileum. The frequency of specific complications differs between adult and pediatric patients. The most common complications in children are gastrointestinal bleeding, most often occurring in infancy and early childhood (<5 years of age),[99,105] and intestinal obstruction. In adults, intestinal obstruction is by far the most frequent presentation, and gastrointestinal bleeding is relatively uncommon.[96,97] Whereas adults most often describe melenic stools, children classically present with red "currant jelly" bowel movements. More unusual complications in the adult include the development of carcinomas such as carcinoids, sarcomas, and, rarely, adenocarcinomas.[106] Carcinoid tumors are typically small and resemble jejunoileal rather than appendiceal carcinoids in their biologic characteristics (e.g., immunohistochemical staining and metastatic potential).[107–109] Patients presenting with carcinoid of a Meckel's diverticulum are older (in the sixth decade) and are frequently asymptomatic. Tumors greater than 5 mm in diameter have a high metastatic potential.[107] Other complications include the development of enteroliths which may become lodged in the diverticulum, causing abdominal pain, vomiting, bleeding, and obstruction.[110]

Diagnosis

The diagnosis of Meckel's diverticulum remains a challenge.[111] Sodium pertechnetate technetium 99m radionuclide scanning is particularly useful in children. The ^{99m}Tc isotope is taken up by the normal stomach and by ectopic gastric mucosa in Meckel's diverticulum. Surface mucus cells accumulate and secrete this anion.[112] To enhance the sensitivity of this test, cimetidine may be administered to decrease anion secretion from the gastric mucosa.[113] Pentagastrin may also be useful, enhancing anion uptake by a poorly understood mechanism.[114] The major drawback of this detection method is that heterotopic gastric mucosa must be present in the diverticulum. In children with lower gastrointestinal bleeding from a Meckel's diverticulum, this test is sensitive and specific because almost all bleeding diverticula contain gastric mucosa, yet in adults this method has high false-positive and -negative rates, even in bleeding patients.[115] Crohn's disease or other inflammatory disorders lead to false-positive scans. In children, Meckel's scan is often followed by a technetium or stannous pyrophosphate red blood cell scan to definitively localize the bleeding site.

Other imaging modalities include small bowel follow-through, which is usually not useful because the diverticulum may not fill with barium and is also rapidly emptied. Enteroclysis examinations improve the sensitivity of barium studies because the administration of contrast material under increased pressure leads to better filling of the diverticulum. Angiography helps to localize the source of hemorrhage and may also demonstrate the vitelline artery and its embryonic branches. This vessel arises from a distal branch of the superior mesenteric artery and ends in a characteristic blush of tortuous small vessels. Frequently, this artery involutes and the diverticulum is directly supplied by branches from the superior mesenteric artery.

Management

The treatment of Meckel's diverticulum complicated by bleeding, obstruction, or perforation is surgical. Diverticulectomy is performed, possibly with concurrent ileal resection if adjacent small bowel is ulcerated, inflamed, or obstructed. These operations can be complicated, and postoperative morbidity occurs in approximately 6% of all cases.[96] The management of asymptomatic diverticula is less clear-cut. Because of the low risk of complications of Meckel's diverticulum in adults and the significant risk of surgery, some have recommended leaving incidentally discovered lesions intact.[96,104] Others prefer to resect asymptomatic diverticula that may have a high probability of complications: large (>2 cm) diverticula, lesions associated with an omphalomesenteric band, which are at risk for volvulus and obstruction, or lesions with a palpable mass within them which may represent tumor or ectopic mucosa.[100,105,116]

Duplications

Duplications of the gastrointestinal tract are rare, congenital cystic anomalies attached to the intestinal mesenteric border (Fig. 68-11). They may be spherical or tubular shaped. They are usually lined by gut mucosa but, as in Meckel's diverticulum, may contain heterotopic gastric mucosa or, less commonly, pancreatic, squamous, thyroid, or bronchial epithelium as well as lymphoid aggregates.[117] They share a common blood supply with the associated native intestine and may also communicate lumenally. Duplications may occur anywhere along the gastrointestinal tract from mouth to anus; those of small bowel origin are most commonly found in the ileum.[117] The embryonic origin of gut duplications is unknown. Postulated mechanisms include aberrant recanalization of the gut lumen during morphogenesis, creating two attached yet distinct gut structures; abnormal notochord-midgut interactions; intrauterine ischemic events; or abortive twinning.[118] Intestinal atresias may be associated with duplications, supporting a possible vascular etiology.[119]

Signs, Symptoms, and Complications

Most patients are diagnosed in infancy and early childhood, but duplications are occasionally newly discovered in the adult. The frequency of symptoms varies inversely with age. Pediatric patients most commonly present with abdominal pain, obstructive symptoms (e.g., nausea, vomiting, pain),

FIGURE 68-11. Tubular duplication of the terminal ileum from a 7-month-old boy. The duplication, lying on the mesenteric border of the bowel, is 29 cm long and communicated with the adjoining bowel near its distal end. The duplication, which is the smaller of the two cross sections, was lined largely by gastric mucosa; an ulcer was present within it, near its point of communication with the bowel. An island of aberrant pancreas was also present in its wall. (From Arey JB, Valdes-Dapena M. Embryology and developmental disorders. In: Ming S, Goldman H, eds. Pathology of the gastrointestinal tract. Philadelphia: WB Saunders, 1992:113.)

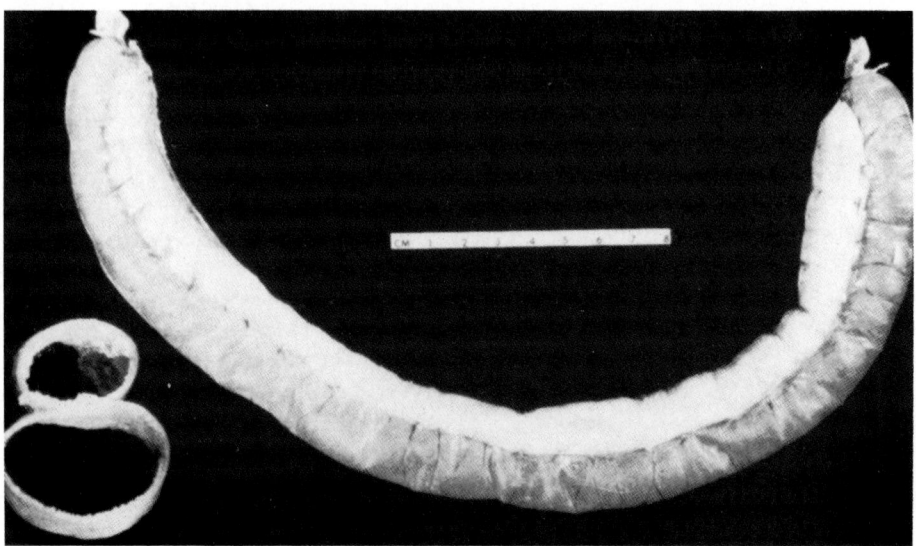

and hemorrhage[118]; much less frequently, these lesions are asymptomatic and are discovered incidentally. Obstruction may result from inflammation of the duplication or from a mass effect produced by a large lesion. Intussusception may be precipitated if duplicated gut acts as a lead point and invaginates into normal intestine. Gastrointestinal hemorrhage may occur from ulceration of the duplicated or surrounding mucosa; very frequently, these lesions contain ectopic gastric mucosa that secretes acid and produces ulceration. A rare complication in adults is the development of carcinoma in the duplication.[120] Carcinoid tumors, adenocarcinoma arising in ectopic gastric mucosa, and squamous cell carcinoma have been reported.[121]

Diagnosis

Small-bowel duplications may be difficult to detect and are seldom diagnosed preoperatively. Plain films may reveal a partially calcified wall of the duplication. Small bowel follow-through or enteroclysis barium examinations may reveal the duplication if it communicates with the gut lumen. Cysts that contain gastric mucosa may be detected by ^{99m}Tc abdominal scintigraphy,[122] which specifically delineates gastric surface mucus cells (see section on Meckel's diverticulum). Ultrasonography or computed tomography (CT) evaluation can provide clues to the diagnosis by revealing the presence of a cystic mass and is also valuable in detecting rare carcinomas which appear as solid tissue within the cyst.[120]

Management

Duplications are treated surgically. If small, these lesions are easily resected with the adjacent small bowel. If duplicated bowel is quite extensive and resection would require the removal of too much normal bowel, the duplication is opened and the mucosa removed, leaving serosa and muscular layers intact. It is important to remove all mucosa, because residual ectopic gastric mucosa could lead to recurrent hemorrhage in the future.

Intestinal Atresia and Stenosis

Intestinal *atresias* are segments of gut in which there is total occlusion of the intestinal lumen. *Stenosis* indicates a narrowing of the gut lumen leading to partial obstruction. Atresia is one of the common causes of bowel obstruction in neonates.[123] Atresias are most often single but may be multiple and are found from esophagus to rectum. The reported incidence of small bowel atresias varies but is approximately 1 in 3000 to 1 in 5000 live births.[124] Several types of small intestine atresias have been described[125] (Fig. 68-12). In type I atresia, a membranous septum or diaphragm of mucosa and submucosa obstructs the lumen, but the bowel wall and mesentery are intact. Type II is characterized by two blind bowel ends connected by a fibrous cord, with intact mesentery in between. In type IIIa lesions, two blind bowel ends are separated by a mesenteric gap, and type IIIb is the "apple peel" atresia, in which there is proximal small bowel atresia and absence of the distal superior mesenteric artery (<5% of all atresias).[126] In this case, the bowel distal to the atresia is foreshortened and coiled and receives retrograde blood supply from the ileocolic, right colic, or inferior mesenteric artery. Finally, type IV denotes multiple atresias, present throughout the small bowel, having the appearance of a "string of sausages"; they may be of types I, II, or IIIa.

Duodenal atresia and stenosis is commonly associated with Down's syndrome, midgut malrotation, esophageal atresia, annular pancreas, imperforate anus, and intrauterine growth retardation.[127] Jejunoileal atresias are much less frequently associated with other congenital anomalies.

Pathophysiology

The pathogenesis of atresia and stenosis is unknown, but ischemic intrauterine events such as midgut volvulus, arterial occlusion, and intussusception have been implicated, especially in single atresia and stenosis. Although vascular events may similarly play a role in multiple intestinal atresias, pathologic examination of neonatal intestine from infants after re-

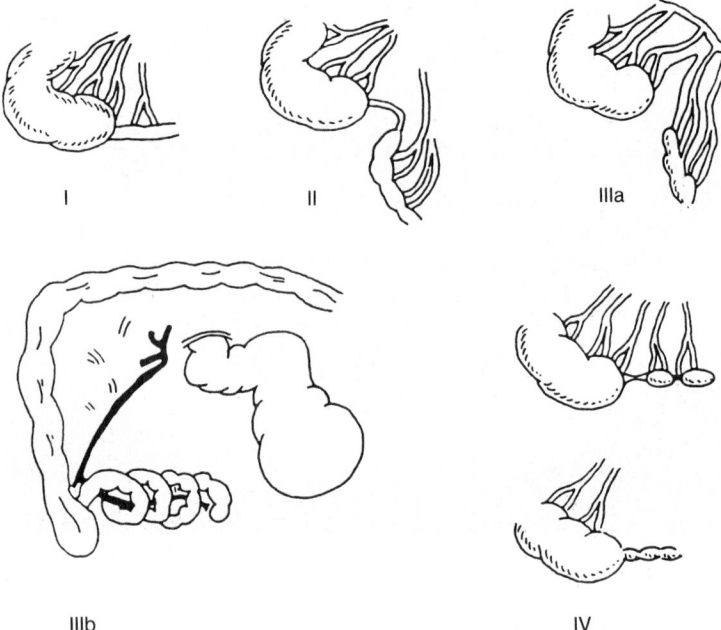

FIGURE 68-12. Classification of intestinal atresias. In type I or membranous atresia, a membranous septum or diaphragm of mucosa and submucosa obstructs the lumen, but the bowel wall and mesentery are intact. In type II, two blind bowel ends are connected by a fibrous cord, with intact mesentery in between. In type IIIa, bowel lesions are separated by a mesenteric gap. Type IIIb is an "apple peel" atresia with proximal small bowel atresia, absence of distal superior mesenteric artery, and coiled and foreshortened bowel. In type IV, there are multiple atresias of any type (I–IIIa). (From Smith GH, Glasson M. Intestinal atresia: factors affecting survival. Aust N Z J Surg 1989;59:151.)

section of atretic segments suggests a different mechanism, one in which there is a defect in recanalization of the gut lumen that is normally obliterated owing to massive epithelial proliferation in the second fetal month.[128] Also, rare familial cases of multiple intestinal atresias and apple peel (type IIIb) atresias have been reported.[123,128,129] An autosomal recessive inheritance pattern has been suggested,[129] but variability in the types of atresia found within families and discordance in a set of monozygotic twins suggest a more complex genetic transmission.[126] Other factors implicated in the pathogenesis of atresia and stenosis are maternal ergotamine use[130] and fetal exposure to methylene blue, which was formerly injected into the amniotic sac during amniocentesis of twin pregnancies to ensure that both sacs have been sampled.[131,132] Multiple intestinal atresias have also been reported to be associated with neonatal immunodeficiency states.[133,134]

Clinical Presentation

Polyhydramnios is frequently detected in fetuses with gastrointestinal obstruction. Neonates with intestinal atresias most commonly present with signs and symptoms of obstruction within hours to 3 days after birth. Bilious vomiting, abdominal distention occasionally associated with visible bowel loops, and failure to pass meconium are frequent presenting complaints. High atresias of the jejunum and duodenum are also associated with jaundice. Infants with intestinal stenoses without atresia may have a much more indolent course because obstruction is usually partial. The diagnosis may therefore be delayed.

Diagnosis

Patients with polyhydramnios are routinely inspected with ultrasonography, which may identify the obstructing defect. Dilated loops of bowel are frequently detected; the presence of fetal ascites and extralumenal calcifications may indicate

aseptic perforation of the bowel. Intralumenal calcifications found in type IV atresias may also be seen. After birth, routine abdominal radiographs may demonstrate multiple air-fluid levels throughout the small bowel or dilated bowel proximal to the obstruction with absence of distal gas. The anatomic defect should always be definitively identified by plain films and cautious contrast radiography before surgical intervention is attempted. It is also important to identify all atretic sites, keeping in mind the risk of multiple atresias.

Important in the differential diagnosis of neonatal bowel obstruction is Hirschsprung's disease, malrotation, meconium ileus associated with cystic fibrosis, duplications, intussusception, Meckel's diverticulum, and mesenteric bands.[135] Barium enema is recommended to rule out Hirschsprung's disease and malrotation with volvulus and to identify other atresias in the bowel distal to the primary obstruction.

Treatment and Prognosis

Initial therapy consists of intravenous hydration, correction of electrolytes, and nasogastric suction to remove accumulated fluid and decompress the bowel. Surgical resection of atretic small intestine is the primary treatment, which may be challenging because bowel preservation is critical and dilation of small bowel proximal to the obstruction makes anastomosis difficult. Several different surgical procedures have been developed to cope with this problem, including tapering enteroplasty and the creation of an ileostomy.[135] Patients with type IIIb and type IV atresias often require extensive resective surgery, resulting in short bowel syndrome and a poorer prognosis. All patients after surgery are placed on total parenteral nutrition and observed for return of normal bowel function as the diet is slowly advanced. Patients with short bowel syndrome frequently require prolonged parenteral nutrition.

The morbidity and mortality rate in infants has dramatically decreased since the 1950s, from 90% to between 11% and 17%.[136] Enhanced survival is a result of improved management of nutritional and pulmonary status. Other factors affecting prognosis include the presence of other congenital anomalies, malrotation, and short bowel syndrome associated with prolonged total parenteral nutrition which may be complicated by sepsis, thrombosis, or liver failure.[136]

Malrotation

Description and Pathophysiology

Alterations in the normal rotation and fixation of the gut during embryogenesis result in a series of anomalies with various clinical manifestations. *Nonrotation* occurs if the embryonic midgut loop does not rotate and the caudal limb of the loop reenters the abdominal cavity first. Subsequently, the small intestine (jejunum and ileum) lies on the right side of the abdomen and the colon is entirely on the left. The cecum is usually located in the left iliac fossa. Frequently, the small bowel mesentery does not attain its broad attachment and remains suspended by a narrow pedicle, leading to the risk of volvulus.[127,137] *Malrotation* or *incomplete rotation* is the most common disorder of rotation and fixation, resulting if the normal 270-degree bowel rotation is not completed. As a result, the cecum may lie in the subpyloric region or may be subhepatic. In addition, the small bowel is not attached by a broad mesentery but instead remains suspended from a narrow vascular pedicle. *Ladd's bands* may form; these are peritoneal bands that may pass from the cecum across the duodenum to the right upper quadrant or may attach to the duodenum. The two major complications of malrotation include volvulus, caused by free rotation of the midgut around the vascular pedicle, and duodenal obstruction secondary to Ladd's bands. *Reversed* rotation results from clockwise instead of counterclockwise rotation of the gut, leading to reentry of the colon into the abdomen first, the colon then taking a position posterior to the superior mesenteric artery and the duodenum. The duodenum becomes placed anterior to the superior mesenteric artery. The small bowel mesentery passes in front of the transverse colon, leading to a mesenteric tunnel that produces colonic compression and obstruction. Finally, failure of the cecum to descend into its normal position in the right lower quadrant may lead to *mobile cecum*; the cecum remains in the right upper quadrant and is unfixed posteriorly, predisposing to cecal volvulus. The ileum may similarly be unfixed and susceptible to volvulus.

Clinical Manifestations

Approximately 50% to 80% of patients with midgut malrotation present in infancy. Related anomalies include atresia and stenosis, omphalocele, congenital heart disease, and diaphragmatic hernia. The most severe complications of malrotation are small bowel obstruction and volvulus. Signs and symptoms that result from these two complications include recurrent bilious vomiting, passage of bloody stools or acute onset of constipation, and bowel loop distention. Those with Ladd's bands may develop symptoms of duodenal obstruction. In patients from 1 month of age through adolescence, symptoms may be more varied and indolent, including intermittent vomiting, failure to thrive, and recurrent abdominal

pain.[138] Adults may be asymptomatic for many years[139] and then present with midgut volvulus with abdominal pain, bloody stools, and distention.[140] Alternatively, adult patients with a long history of recurrent abdominal pain with nausea and vomiting since childhood may never have been diagnosed because the obstruction or volvulus was transient and resolved before presentation.[141]

Diagnosis

Plain films may reveal evidence of duodenal or small bowel obstruction. A classic double bubble sign may be seen, indicating duodenal obstruction. Contrast radiographic studies may demonstrate anomalous small bowel, ligament of Treitz, and cecal locations. In adults with midgut volvulus, upper gastrointestinal contrast series may reveal a dilated stomach and duodenum with a typical corkscrew appearance of the barium in the twisted duodenum and proximal jejunum.[142] CT scan may show reversal of the position of the superior mesenteric artery and vein.[143]

Treatment

Surgical correction of malrotation (incomplete rotation) in symptomatic patients includes relieving obstruction caused by Ladd's peritoneal bands and freeing the duodenum, reducing midgut volvulus, and broadening the mesentery to prevent recurrent rotation of the bowel around a narrow mesentery. In *Ladd's procedure*, the bowel is placed in the position of nonrotation (small bowel on the right side of the abdomen and colon on the left). Variations on this operation are followed for correction of nonrotation and the very rare reversed rotation.

In most patients, bowel function returns to normal. However, there are children with recurrent and prolonged symptoms of nausea, vomiting, and pain before operation who do not fare as well postoperatively, possibly because of persistent dysmotility syndromes associated with malrotation or resulting from damage to the small bowel from long-standing, indolent obstruction.[144,145]

Gastroschisis and Omphalocele

Description and Embryologic Origin

Although gastroschisis and omphalocele both result from abdominal wall defects, these rare disorders are distinct entities (see also Chap. 100). Omphalocele occurs when the abdominal viscera herniates through the umbilical ring and persists outside the body, covered by a membranous sac but not by skin. In gastroschisis, there is a small defect in the abdominal wall, usually to the right of the closed umbilical ring, through which there is massive evisceration of the intestines. The bowel has no membranous covering, has been exposed to amniotic fluid in utero, and is often matted, thickened, foreshortened, and covered with adhesions. The embryologic origins of both gastroschisis and omphalocele are unclear.[146] It has been hypothesized that omphalocele is caused by a failure of embryonic folding at the level of the lateral folds or persistence of the body stalk.[146-148] Gastroschisis may be caused by vascular disruption in utero, leading to failure of differentiation of the somatopleural mesenchyme.[149] An alternative theory proposes that gastroschisis occurs sometime between herniation into the umbilical cord and fixation. A tear develops at the base of the cord, leading to intestinal herniation. The herniation persists as the defect is filled in by skin.[150] The embryologic defect is thought to occur between the fifth and tenth weeks of gestation, but perinatal insults have also been suggested in patients in whom gastroschisis was undetected sonographically.[146,151,152]

Both gastroschisis and omphalocele are associated with other congenital anomalies, although the incidence is higher in omphalocele. Both may present with other intestinal anomalies, including atresia and malrotation. About one third of cases of omphalocele with multiple anomalies have trisomy 13, trisomy 18, or the Beckwith-Wiedemann syndrome, which is characterized by macroglossia, large infant size, and visceromegaly. Other defects associated with gastroschisis include vascular disruptions and renal and gall bladder agenesis.[146]

Prenatal Diagnosis

Improvements in the accuracy of prenatal ultrasonography have led to increased frequency of detection. Presently, the major utility of prenatal diagnosis is to alert the obstetrician so that, at the time of delivery, the mother may proceed to a tertiary care center at which appropriate surgical and neonatal intensive care support are available.[148] Cesarean section is usually not recommended.

Treatment

Surgical closure of omphalocele and gastroschisis is attempted shortly after birth. Primary closure may be possible, using retention sutures and stretching the abdominal wall. If this cannot be achieved, a silo or Silastic sac can be used with successive compression to further reduce the herniation. The material is placed over the herniated bowel or sac and is reduced manually and serially sutured to reintroduce the bowel into the abdominal cavity. Gastroschisis may also be corrected using skin flaps. Advances in surgical correction have greatly improved the prognosis of gastroschisis, despite the fact that the bowel is usually damaged and slow to return to normal function. Survival rates now range from 70% to 90%.[153] The outcome of patients with omphalocele remains poor primarily because of the associated congenital defects. Approximately 25% of infants with omphalocele are stillborn,[146] and 45% of the live-born infants die shortly after birth because of other anomalies.

STRUCTURAL ANOMALIES

Volvulus

A volvulus is an abnormal twisting of the intestine around the axis of its own mesentery, resulting in obstruction of the more proximal bowel. The twisting of the mesentery may involve the mesenteric vessels and thereby make the involved loop particularly susceptible to strangulation and gangrene.

Perforation, peritonitis, and sepsis may result, making this condition potentially catastrophic. In contrast to colonic volvulus, particularly of the cecum and sigmoid colon, small bowel volvulus is relatively rare in the United States and most of Europe.[154] It occurs more frequently in parts of Africa, the Middle East, and the Indian subcontinent.[154–156] Volvulus in these countries occurs in the absence of anatomic abnormalities and is probably related to dietary factors. It has been postulated that eating large amounts of bulky foods after fasting may predispose to torsion of the small bowel loops. In the United States, small bowel volvulus is usually caused by a preexisting defect such as an anomaly of rotation and fixation, postoperative adhesion, or congenital bands.[157]

Clinical Presentation and Diagnosis

Patients present with symptoms of small bowel obstruction and an acute abdomen. In the majority of patients, symptoms are acute in onset. Abdominal pain, nausea, and vomiting are almost always present[154,158]; the severity of pain maybe out of proportion to the physical findings. Signs include abdominal distention, rebound, guarding and rigidity, and occasionally a palpable abdominal mass.

Plain abdominal radiographs taken in supine and upright positions may demonstrate distended bowel with air-fluid levels consistent with obstruction. Perforation may be indicated by the presence of free air. Barium studies can be useful in depicting disorders of rotation. Also, a typical corkscrew-like appearance of barium in the distorted duodenum and jejunum is diagnostic. Angiography may reveal twisting of the branches of the superior mesenteric artery, suggesting the diagnosis of volvulus.

Therapy and Outcome

The treatment of small bowel volvulus is surgical. Resection of ischemic or gangrenous loops of bowel should be performed, although derotation of the bowel may be sufficient therapy in itself. Vascular compromise of the small bowel with subsequent gangrene is common and leads to increased morbidity and mortality postoperatively. Rapid recognition of volvulus and prompt surgical intervention are the keys to decreasing the fatality rate associated with this condition.

Intussusception

Description and Pathophysiology

Intussusception occurs when a segment of bowel invaginates, or telescopes, into adjacent distal bowel, leading to obstruction and possible ischemic injury. The incidence, causes, clinical presentation, and therapy of intestinal intussusception are strikingly different in adult and pediatric patients. Intestinal intussusception is one of the most common causes of small bowel obstruction in children younger than 2 years of age,[159] but it is an unusual cause of bowel obstruction in adults. Most cases in the pediatric age group occur before 5 years of age.[160] Pediatric intussusception is most often idiopathic in origin but may be associated with a pathologic lead point in 8% to 12% of cases.[159,161,162] These include Meckel's diverticulum; a variety of benign and malignant tumors such as polyps, leiomyomas, and lymphomas; duplications; and Henoch-Schönlein purpura, in which vasculitis-affected bowel with an intramural hematoma acts as a lead point. In idiopathic intussusception, an association with prominent Peyer's patches and enlarged mesenteric lymph nodes has been observed but not proven to be causative. In children, ileocolic intussusceptions are most common, followed by ileoileocolic, cecocolic, and, much less frequently, ileoileal involvement.[159]

In adults in the Western world, small bowel intussusception occurs rarely, accounting for approximately 5% of all cases of intestinal obstruction[163] and only 5% to 16% of all intussusceptions.[163,164] Intussusception may occur anywhere along the gastrointestinal tract, but it is most common in the small bowel in adults. Unlike in children, a causative factor can be identified in more than 90% of adult patients.[164] Small intestine intussusception may be precipitated by benign lesions, including leiomyomas, neurofibromas, and lipomas, or by malignant lesions such as lymphomas, small bowel adenomatous polyps, and metastatic tumors with or without peritoneal carcinomatosis. Other causes include Meckel's diverticulum or other diverticular celiac disease, in which the chronically dilated flaccid bowel intussuscepts. Postoperative complications such as adhesions may lead to intussusception. Jejunogastric intussusception may occur after Billroth II surgery, and bypassed bowel may intussuscept after jejunoileal bypass.[164] Patients with acquired immunodeficiency syndrome and Kaposi's sarcoma or diffuse enteritis are also at risk for intussusception.[165,166] Pregnancy and the use of long intestinal or cantor tubes are other predisposing factors.

Signs and Symptoms

The typical pediatric patient is a well-nourished, previously healthy 5-month-old to 5-year-old child. The peak presenting age is 3 to 11 months.[167] Classic signs and symptoms include the acute onset of abdominal pain, vomiting, and hematochezia. A palpable abdominal mass, diarrhea, and somnolence are other frequently associated symptoms.[161,162] In older children, these diagnostic signs and symptoms are often not present.[160,168] In adults, the clinical picture may be confusing. Abdominal pain is almost always present[169] but is often low-grade and chronic; patients may present after several episodes have spontaneously resolved.[163,170] A partial or complete small bowel obstruction may be present, and an abdominal mass is often palpable. Nausea and vomiting are particularly associated with small bowel compared with large bowel intussusception. Weight loss may also occur in patients with chronic, indolent symptoms.

Diagnosis and Therapy

Pediatric patients.   In children, a barium enema is usually considered the diagnostic and therapeutic intervention of choice because the ileocecal region is so frequently involved. It demonstrates the location of the intussusception and is often successful in reducing it. The enema is usually administered with a surgeon in attendance in case of perforation or failure to reduce, which would necessitate immediate surgery. In extremely ill patients in whom peritonitis, perforation, or shock is present, a barium enema is contraindicated.

Plain films may reveal a crescent of gas capping the intussusceptum, outlining its leading edge. A gasless area may also be identified, corresponding with the soft tissue mass of the intussusception. A plain film target sign, consisting of two concentric radiolucent curvilinear lines outlining the intussusception, can occasionally be appreciated.[171] Ultrasonography may also be useful in diagnosing pediatric patients, particularly those with a confusing history or those who are extremely ill. The ultrasonogram may show a classic target or doughnut sign, characterized by multiple concentric rings of sonolucency alternating with 1 or 2 echogenic foci. The edematous outer and inner walls of the intussusception create two hypoechoic areas, ringing the hyperechoic lumenal mucosa.[172,173] CT scan may similarly be useful, but it is usually avoided in children (see discussion following). Upper gastrointestinal contrast series may show proximal intestinal dilatation and a "bird's beak" at the site of obstruction but is contraindicated if perforation or peritonitis is suspected.

As previously mentioned, a barium enema is often sufficient therapy for reducing the intussusception in children.[162] Some centers prefer to use air enemas. If reduction by enema is unsuccessful, the patient is taken to laparotomy for manual reduction if possible. If there is ischemia or gangrene of the bowel, resection must be performed. A careful search is made for a possible pathologic lead point.

Adult patients.   The diagnosis and treatment is quite different in adults than in pediatric patients because the location and causes of intussusception are quite different. The majority of adult intussusception takes place in the small bowel, yet colonic sites also occur frequently. Therefore, a combination of plain film, upper gastrointestinal series, barium enema, and CT scan or ultrasonography are used in the adult. Because of the often puzzling presentation of intussusception in this age group, CT scan is frequently employed. A mass of alternating high and low attenuation may be seen as a target, sausage-shaped, or bilobed lesion.[174,175] Mesenteric fat produces areas of low attenuation, whereas the bowel wall itself produces high attenuation. Thickened bowel loops and an intralumenal soft tissue mass may be seen. However, this technique is not sensitive enough to determine the nature of the pathologic lead point.

Because a pathologic lesion is found so frequently, treatment in the adult consists of surgical intervention with bowel resection. Manual reduction alone may be pursued only if it is certain that no other lesions are present.[169] However, with present diagnostic techniques, it is unlikely that the presence of a tumor or other anatomic cause can be ruled out preoperatively. Therefore, manual reduction of adult intussusception is usually not recommended, because manipulation may lead to tumor seeding intralumenally or intravenously.[168,176] Colonic intussusception is never treated with manual reduction because of the extremely high likelihood of malignancy.[170]

Lymphangiectasia

Description and Pathophysiology

Intestinal lymphangiectasia is characterized by obstruction of lymph drainage from the small intestine and the presence of dilated lacteals and other intestinal lymphatics such as those in the serosa and mesentery, depending on the level of obstruction. As a result of obstruction and increased pressure in the intestinal lymphatics, absorption of chylomicrons and fat-soluble vitamins such as vitamin D is impaired; the recirculation of intestinal lymphocytes into the peripheral circulation is impeded, and excessive intestinal lymph "leaks" into the intestinal lumen. Actual lymphenteric fistulas may form, and intestinal lymph and its chylomicrons, protein, and lymphocytes drain directly into the intestinal lumen. Chylomicrons are sequestered in the lamina propria as well as in the distended lymphatics. Blockage of serosal and mesenteric lymphatics may lead to chylous ascites, and blockage of the thoracic duct to chylous pleural effusions.

Intestinal lymphangiectasia may occur as a primary congenital disorder or secondary to a disease that blocks the intestinal lymph drainage at some level. Causes of secondary lymphangiectasia include extensive abdominal or retroperitoneal carcinoma or lymphoma, retroperitoneal fibrosis, chronic pancreatitis, mesenteric tuberculosis or sarcoidosis,[177] Crohn's disease, Whipple's disease, scleroderma,[178] celiac disease,[179] and even constrictive pericarditis[180] and chronic congestive heart failure.[181] Congenital intestinal lymphangiectasia (Milroy's disease) results from a malformation of the lymphatics, often affecting many areas of the body.

Clinical Presentation

Patients present with varying degrees of steatorrhea and malabsorption; with lymphocytopenia, especially of T lymphocytes; with marked hypogammaglobulinemia with impaired cell-mediated immunity; and most commonly and usually most prominently, with manifestations of protein-losing enteropathy. Patients often have edema and low serum proteins, the reduction in serum albumin usually being most pronounced and usually the only one of clinical significance. Patients with congenital disease present at any time from birth to adulthood, often with asymmetric edema of an extremity caused by peripheral lymphatic obstruction. They may also present, as do the secondary cases, with more diffuse, symmetric edema, usually the result of marked hypoproteinemia. Despite lymphocytopenia and impaired delayed hypersensitivity reactions, opportunistic infections are not common. However, infections with atypical mycobacteria, warts, and cellulitis have been reported.[182,183] Gastrointestinal symptoms are usually not prominent, but some patients may experience diarrhea, abdominal pain, distention, nausea and vomiting, and, occasionally, gastrointestinal bleeding.

Diagnosis

Protein-losing enteropathy should be suspected in any patient with unexplained hypoalbuminemia, and intestinal lymphangiectasia should be especially suspected if the patient also has lymphocytopenia and steatorrhea. The presence of asymmetric lymphedema, especially dating from infancy or childhood, should suggest the congenital (Milroy's) disease. A diagnosis of lymphangiectasia rests on peroral jejunal biopsy demonstrating dilated lymphatic lacteals; several biopsies may be required to demonstrate the diagnostic findings, because the lesions are often patchy and localized.[184] Dilated lacteals may appear as white opaque spots in the duodenum as viewed by endoscopy; these findings aid the endoscopist in selecting appropriate regions to biopsy. Other pathologic findings include moderate villus blunting and mild to moderate inflammatory infiltrate.[184] Other tests that can be performed include those which demonstrate a protein-losing enteropathy by detecting an excessive enteric loss of plasma proteins. Use of radiolabeled plasma proteins, such as those labeled with ^{131}I-albumin, ^{51}Cr-albumin or ^{51}Cr-chloride, has been largely replaced by the measurement of gastrointestinal clearance of α_1-antitrypsin. Small-bowel radiographs usually reveal only some thickening of the folds as a result of intestinal edema. If secondary lymphangiectasia is suspected, appropriate tests such as a CT scan of the abdomen should be performed to diagnose the underlying disease. The degree of malabsorption and nutritional deficiency may be assessed by stool fat quantitation and other nonspecific blood tests such as prothrombin time, serum calcium, and carotene levels. In congenital cases, if necessary, the malformed, hypoplastic lymphatics may be demonstrated by lymphangiography. Pleural effusions and ascites may be tapped for conventional diagnostic studies and examination for chylomicrons.

Therapy

The therapy for lymphangiectasia should be directed toward the underlying diseases as well as the pathophysiologic consequences. In patients with secondary lymphangiectasia, the primary diseases (e.g., lymphoma, tuberculosis, sarcoidosis, constrictive pericarditis) must be diagnosed and treated appropriately. Substitution of short- and medium-chain triglycerides for the usual long-chain triglycerides may reduce the amount of enteric protein loss as well as the degree of malabsorption and diarrhea and may lead to an improvement in serum albumin.[185,186] Short-chain fatty acids are more water-soluble and may be more readily absorbed through portal venous channels rather than through the lymphatics. The concomitant reduction in dietary long-chain fat presumably reduces chylomicrons in obstructed lymphatics and thereby decreases the lymphatic pressure and rate of lymph loss. One case report demonstrated the efficacy of antiplasmin therapy in a patient with increased plasma fibrinolytic activity,[187] yet it is probable that the majority of patients do not respond to this treatment.[188] Peripheral edema can be minimized by postural drainage and elastic stockings to reduce the risk of cellulitis and lymphangitis.

Celiac Artery Compression

The topic of celiac artery compression is covered in the chapter on vascular insufficiency (see Chap. 112).

The reader is directed to Chapter 23, Growth and Development of the Gastrointestinal Tract; Chapter 78, Colon: Anatomy and Structural Anomalies; and Chapter 100, Abdominal Cavity: Anatomy, Structural Anomalies, and Hernias.

REFERENCES

1. Fawcett DW. The intestines. In: Fawcett DW, Bloom W eds. A textbook of histology. 11th ed. Philadelphia: WB Saunders, 1986.

2. Clemente CD. The digestive system. In: Clemente CD, ed. Gray's anatomy of the human body. Philadelphia: Lea and Febiger, 1985:1402.

3. Antonson DL. Anatomy and physiology of the small and large intestine. In: R Wyllie, JS Hyams, eds. Pediatric gastrointestinal disease: pathophysiology, diagnosis, management. Philadelphia: WB Saunders, 1993.

4. Furness J, Costa M. Anatomy of the enteric nervous system. In: Johnson LR, ed. Physiology of the gastrointestinal tract. Vol. 1. 2nd ed. New York: Raven Press, 1987.

5. Sprinz H, Sribhibhadh R, Gangrowa EJ, et al. Biopsy of the small bowel of Thai people. Am J Clin Pathol 1962;38:43.

6. Brunser O, Eidelman S, Klipstein FA. Intestinal morphology of rural Haitians. A comparison between overt tropical sprue and asymptomatic subjects. Gastroenterology 1970;58:655.

7. Cerf-Bensussan N, Guy-Grand D, Griscelli C. TI: intraepithelial lymphocytes of human gut: isolation, characterisation and study of natural killer activity. Gut 1985;26:81.

8. Itohara SA, Farr G, Lafaille JJ, et al. Homing of a gamma delta thymocyte subset with homogeneous T-cell receptors to mucosal epithelia. Nature 1990;343:754.

9. Braendtzaeg P. Overview of the immune system. Curr Top Microbiol Immunol 1989;146:13.

10. Gallatin M, St. John TP, Siegelman M, et al. Lymphocyte homing receptors. Cell 1986;44:673.

11. Holzmann BB, McIntyre W, Weissman IL. Identification of a murine Peyer's patch–specific lymphocyte homing receptor as an integrin molecule with an alpha chain homologous to VLA-4α. Cell 1989;56:37.

12. Cornes JS. Number, size and distribution of Peyer's patches in the human small intestine. Part I. The development of Peyer's patches. Gut 1965;6:225.

13. Owen RI, Jones AL. Epithelial cell specialization within human Peyer's patches: an ultrastructural study of intestinal lymphoid follicles. Gastroenterology 1974;66:189.

14. Farquhar MG, Palade GE. Junctional complexes in various epithelia. J Cell Biol 1963;17:375.

15. Marcial MA, Carlson SL, Madara JL. Partitioning of paracellular conductance along the crypt-villus axis: a hypothesis based on structural analysis with detailed consideration of tight junction structure-function relationships. J Membr Biol 1984;80:59.

16. Cheng H, Leblond CP. Origin, differentiation and renewal of the four main epithelial cell types in the mouse small intestine. Parts I–V. Am J Anat 1974;141:461.

17. Potten CS, Loeffler M. Stem cells: attributes, cycles, spirals, pitfalls, and uncertainties. Lessons for and from the crypt. Development 1990;110:1001.

18. Bjerknes M, Cheng H. The stem-cell zone of the small intestinal epithelium. I. Evidence from Paneth cells in the adult mouse. Am J Anat 1981;160:51.

19. Gordon JI. Intestinal epithelial differentiation: new insights from chimeric and transgenic mice. J Cell Biol 1989;108:1187.

20. Gordon JI. Understanding gastrointestinal epithelial cell biology: lessons from mice with help from worms and flies. Gastroenterology 1993;104:315.

21. Ponder BAJ, Schmidt GH, Wilkinson MM, et al. Derivation of mouse intestinal crypts from single progenitor cells. Nature 1985;313:689.

22. Schmidt GH, Winton DJ, Ponder BAJ. Development of the pattern of cell renewal in the crypt-villus unit of chimeric mouse small intestine. Development 1988;103:785.

23. Rubin W. Maturation of heterotopic intestinal epithelium. Clin Res 1969;17:310.

24. Antonioli DA, Madara JL. Functional anatomy of the gastrointestinal tract. In: Ming, SC, Goldman, H, eds. Pathology of the gastrointestinal tract. Philadelphia: WB Saunders, 1992:14.

25. Welsh MJ, Smith PL, Fromm M, Frizzell RD. Crypts are the site of intestinal fluid and electrolyte secretion. Science 1982;218:1219.

26. Hallback DA, Jodal M, Sjoquist A, Lundgren O. Evidence for cholera secretion emanating from the crypts. Gastroenterology 1982;83:1051.

27. Nordstrom C, Dahlqvist A, Joseffson L. Quantitative determination of enzymes in different parts of the villi and crypts of rat small intestine. Comparison of alkaline phosphatase, disaccharidases and dipeptidases. J Histochem Cytochem 1968;15:713.

28. Norën O, Sjöström H, Danielsen EM, Cowell GM, Skovbjerg H. The enzymes of the enterocyte plasma membrane. In: Desnuelle P, ed. Molecular and cellular basis of digestion. New York: Elsevier, 1986.

29. Traber PG. Regulation of sucrase-isomaltase gene expression along the crypt-villus axis of rat small intestine. Biochem Biophys Res Commun 1990;173:765.

30. Iseki S, Kondo H, Hitomi M, Ono T. Localization of liver fatty acid-binding protein and its mRNA in the liver and jejunum of rats: an immunohistochemical and in situ hybridization study. Mol Cell Biochem 1990;98:27.

31. Rubin DC. Spatial analysis of transcriptional activation in fetal rat jejunal and ileal gut epithelium. Am J Physiol 1992;263(Gastrointest Liver Physiol 26):G853.

32. Sweetser DA, Birkenmeier EH, Hoppe PC, et al. Mechanisms underlying generation of gradients in gene expression within the intestine: an analysis using transgenic mice containing fatty acid-binding protein–human growth hormone fusion genes. Genes Dev 1988;2:1318.

33. Hwang ES, Hirayama BA, Wright EM. Distribution of the SGLT1 Na$^+$/glucose cotransporter and mRNA along the crypt-villus axis of the rabbit small intestine. Biochem Biophys Res Commun 1991;181:1208–1217.

34. Neutra MR. The gastrointestinal tract. In: Weiss L, ed. Cell and tissue biology. Baltimore: Urban and Schwarzenberg, 1988:335.

35. Sweetser DA, Hauft SM, Hoppe PC, et al. Transgenic mice containing intestinal fatty acid-binding protein/human growth hormone fusion genes exhibit correct regional and cell specific expression of the reporter in their small intestine. Proc Natl Acad Sci U S A 1988;85:9611.

36. Elshourbagy NA, Boguski MS, Liao WSL, et al. Expression of rat apolipoprotein A-IV and A-I genes: mRNA induction during development and in response to glucocorticoids and insulin. Proc Natl Acad Sci U S A 1985;82:8242.

37. Asp NG, Gudmand-Hoyer E, Andersen B, et al. Distribution of disaccharidases, alkaline phosphatase, and some intracellular enzymes along the human small intestine. Scand J Gastroenterol 1975;10:647.

38. Freund JN, Duluc I, Raul F. Lactase expression is controlled differently in the jejunum and ileum during development in rats. Gastroenterology 1991;100:388.

39. Sacchettini JC, Hauft SM, Van Camp SL, et al. Developmental and structural studies of an intracellular lipid binding protein expressed in the ileal epithelium. J Biol Chem 1990;265:19199.

40. Levine JS, Allen RH, Alpers DH, Seetharam B. Immunocytochemical localization of the intrinsic factor–cobalamin receptor in dog ileum: distribution of intracellular receptor during cell maturation. J Cell Biol 1984;98:111.

41. Cohn SM, Simon TC, Roth KA, et al. Use of transgenic mice to map cis-acting elements in the intestinal fatty acid-binding protein gene (FABPI) that control its cell lineage-specific and regional patterns of expression along the duodenal-colonic and crypt-villus axes of the gut epithelium. J Cell Biol 1992;119:27.

42. Wu GD, Wang W, Traber PG. Isolation and characterization of the human sucrase-isomaltase gene and demonstration of intestine-specific transcriptional elements. J Biol Chem 1992;267:7863.

43. Gordon JI, Schmidt GH, Roth KA. Studies of intestinal stem cells using normal, chimeric and transgenic mice. FASEB J 1992;6:3039.

44. Rubin W, Ross LL, Jeffries GH, Sleisenger MH. Intestinal heterotopia. A fine structural study. Lab Invest 1966;15:1024.

45. Rubin W, Ross LL, Sleisenger MH, Weser E. An electron microscopic study of adult celiac disease. Lab Invest 1966;15:1720.

46. Palay SL, Karlin LJ. An electron microscopic study of the intestinal villus. I. The fasting animal. J Biophys Biochem Cytol 1959;5:363.

47. Trier JS, Phelps PC, Rubin CE. Electron microscopy of mucosa of small intestine. JAMA 1963;183:768.

48. Weser E, Rubin W, Ross L, Sleisenger MH. Lactase deficiency in patients with the "irritable colon syndrome." N Engl J Med 1965;273:1070.
49. Holmes R, Lobley RW. Intestinal brush border revisited. Gut 1989;30:1667.
50. Mooseker MS. Organization, chemistry and assembly of the cytoskeletal apparatus of the intestinal brush border. Annu Rev Cell Biol 1985;1:209.
51. Bretscher A. The molecular structure of the microvillar cytoskeleton. In: Alvarado F, van Os CH, eds. Ion gradient-coupled transport. INSERM Symp 26. Amsterdam: Elsevier, 1986:13.
52. Maroux S, Coudrier E, Feracci H, et al. Molecular organization of the intestinal brush border. Biochimie 1988;70:1297.
53. Hirokawa N, Keller TCS, Chasan R, Mooseker MS. Mechanism of brush border contractility studied in the quick-freeze, deep-etch method. J Cell Biol 1983;96:1325.
54. Madara JL, Barenberg D, Carlson S. Effects of cytochalasin D on occluding junctions of intestinal absorptive cells: further evidence that the cytoskeleton may influence paracellular permeability and junctional charge selectivity. J Cell Biol 1986;102:2125.
55. Semenza G. Anchoring and biosynthesis of stalked brush border membrane proteins: glycosidases and peptidases of enterocytes and renal tubuli. Annu Rev Cell Biol 1986;2:255.
56. Shirazi-Beechey SP, Davies AG, Tebbutt K, et al. Preparation and properties of brush-border membrane vesicles from human small intestine. Gastroenterology 1990;98:676.
57. Booth IW, Patel PB, Sule D, et al. Glucose-galactose malabsorption: demonstration of specific jejunal brush border membrane defect. Gut 1988;29:1661.
58. Achler C, Filmer D, Merte C, Drenckhahn D. Role of microtubules in polarized delivery of apical membrane proteins to the brush border of the intestinal epithelium. J Cell Biol 1989;109:179.
59. Alpers DH, Tedesco FJ. The possible role of pancreatic proteases in the turnover of intestinal brush border proteins. Biochim Biophys Acta 1975;401:28.
60. Hauri HP, Sterchi EE, Bienz D, et al. Expression and intracellular transport of microvillus membrane hydrolases in human intestinal epithelial cells. J Cell Biol 1985;101:838.
61. Rodriguez-Boulan E, Nelson WJ. Morphogenesis of the polarized epithelial cell phenotype. Science 1989;245:718.
62. Michaels JE, Leblond CP. Transport of glycoprotein from Golgi apparatus to cell surface by means of "carrier vesicles," as shown by radioautography of mouse colonic epithelium after injection of ³H fucose. J Microsc Biol Cell 1976;25:243.
63. Peeters TL, Vantrappen GR. The Paneth cell: a source of intestinal lysozyme. Gut 1975;16:553.
64. Satoh Y, Ishikawa K, Ono K, Vollrath L. Quantitative light microscopic observations on Paneth cells of germfree and ex-germfree Wistar rats. Digestion 1986;34:115.
65. Ouellette AJ, Miller SI, Henschen A, Selsted ME. Purification and primary structure of murine cryptdin-1, a Paneth cell defensin. FEBS Lett 1992;304:146.
66. Jones DE, Bevins CL. Defensin-6 mRNA in human Paneth cells: implications for antimicrobial peptides in host defense of the human bowel. FEBS Lett 1993;315:187.
67. Jones DE, Bevins CL. Paneth cells of the human small intestine express an antimicrobial peptide gene. J Biol Chem 1992;267:23216.
68. Keshav S, Lawson L, Ping Chung L, et al. Tumor necrosis factor mRNA localized to Paneth cells of normal murine intestinal epithelium by in situ hybridization. J Exp Med 1990;171:327.
69. Koopman P, Povey S, Lovell-Badge RH. Widespread expression of human α-1 antitrypsin in transgenic mice revealed by in situ hybridization. Genes Dev 1989;3:316.
70. Molmenti EP, Perlmutter DH, Rubin DC. Cell-specific expression of α-1 antitrypsin in human intestinal epithelium. J Clin Invest 1993;92:2022.
71. Schulz S, Chrisman TD, Garbers DL. Cloning and expression of guanylin. Its existence in various mammalian tissues. J Biol Chem 1992;267:16019.
72. Wiegand RC, Kato J Currie MG. Rat guanylin cDNA: characterization of the precursor of an endogenous activator of intestinal guanylate cyclase. Biochem Biophys Res Commun 1992;185:812.
73. Roth KA, Hertz JM, Gordon JI. Mapping enteroendocrine cell populations in transgenic mice reveals an unexpected degree of complexity in cellular differentiation within the gastrointestinal tract. J Cell Biol 1990;110:1791.
74. Roth KA, Gordon JI. Spatial differentiation of the intestinal epithelium: analysis of enteroendocrine cells containing immunoreactive serotonin, secretin and substance P in normal and transgenic mice. Proc Natl Acad Sci U S A 1990;87:6408.
75. Solcia E, Creutzfeldt W, Falkmer S, et al. Human gastroenteropancreatic endocrine-paracrine cells: Santa Monica 1980 classification. In: Cellular basis of chemical messengers in the digestive system. UCLA Forum in Medical Sciences Series 1981;23:159.
76. Rubin DC, Roth KA, Birkenmeier EH, Gordon JI. Epithelial cell differentiation in normal and transgenic mouse intestinal isografts. J Cell Biol 1991;113:1183.
77. Roth KA, Rubin DC, Birkenmeier EH, Gordon JI. Expression of liver fatty acid-binding protein/human growth hormone fusion genes within the enterocyte and enteroendocrine cell populations of fetal transgenic mice. J Biol Chem 1991;266:5949.
78. Pearse AGE. The cytochemistry and ultrastructure of polypeptide hormone producing cells of the APUD series and the embryologic, physiologic and pathologic implications of the concept. J Histochem Cytochem 1969;17:303.
79. Inokuchi H, Fujimoto S, Kawai K. Cellular kinetics of gastrointestinal mucosa with special reference to gut endocrine cells. Arch Histol Japon 1983;46:137.
80. Inokuchi H, Fujimoto S, Hattori T, Kawai K. Tritiated thymidine radioautographic study on the origin and renewal of secretin cells in the rat duodenum. Gastroenterology 1985;89:1014.
81. Rubin DC, Swietlicki E, Roth KA, Gordon JI. Use of fetal intestinal isografts from normal and transgenic mice to study the programming of positional information along the duodenal-to-colonic axis. J Biol Chem 1992;267:15122.
82. Roth KA, Kim S, Gordon JI. Immunocytochemical studies suggest two pathways for enteroendocrine cell differentiation in the colon. Am J Physiol 1992;263:PG174.
83. Neutra MR, Forstner JF. Gastrointestinal mucus: synthesis, secretion and function. In: Johnson LR, ed. Physiology of the gastrointestinal tract. 2nd ed. New York: Raven Press, 1987:975.
84. Podolsky DK, Lynch M, Devaney K, et al. Identification of human intestinal trefoil factor—goblet-cell specific expression of a peptide targeted for apical secretion. J Biol Chem 1993;268:6694.
85. Bye WA, Allan CH, Trier JS. Structure, distribution, and origin of M cells in Peyer's patches of mouse ileum. Gastroenterology 1984;86:789.
86. Neutra MR, Phillips TL, Mayer EL, Fishkind DJ. Transport of membrane-bound macromolecules by M cells in follicle-associated epithelium of rabbit Peyer's patch. Cell Tissue Res 1987;247:537.
87. Allan CH, Mendrick DL, Trier JS. Rat intestinal M cells contain acidic endosomal-lysosomal compartments and express class II major histocompatibility complex determinants. Gastroenterology 1993;104:698.
88. Moore KL. The digestive system: In: Moore KL, ed. The developing human: clinically oriented embryology. Philadelphia: WB Saunders, 1977:197.
89. Weaver LT. Anatomy and embryology. In: Walker WA, ed. Pediatric gastrointestinal disease: pathophysiology, diagnosis, management. Philadelphia: BC Decker, 1991:195.
90. Soderlund S. Meckel's diverticulum, a clinical and histologic study. Acta Chir Scand Suppl 1959;248:13.
91. Rutherford RB, Akers DR. Meckel's diverticulum: a review of 148 pediatric patients, with special reference to the pattern of bleeding and to mesodiverticular vascular bands. Surgery 1966;59:618.
92. Tisdall FF. Unusual Meckel's diverticulum as a cause of intestinal hemorrhage. Am J Dis Child 1928;36:1218.

93. Miller DL, Becker MH, Eng K. Giant Meckel's diverticulum. A cause of intestinal obstruction. Radiology 1981;140:93.

94. Yamaguchi M, Takeuchi S, Awazu S. Meckel's diverticulum: investigation of 600 patients in the Japanese literature. Am J Surg 1978;136:247.

95. Moses WR. Meckel's diverticulum: a report of 2 unusual cases. N Engl J Med 1947;237:118.

96. Leijonmarck CE, Bonman-Sandelin K, Frisell J, Raf L. Meckel's diverticulum in the adult. Br J Surg 1986;73:146.

97. Diamond T, Russell CFJ. Meckel's diverticulum in the adult. Br J Surg 1985;72:480.

98. Berman EJ, Schneider A, Potts WJ. Importance of gastric mucosa in Meckel's diverticulum. JAMA 1954;156:6.

99. St-Vil D, Brandt ML, Panic S, et al. Meckel's diverticulum in children: a 20-year review. J Pediatr Surg 1991;26:1289.

100. Turgeon DK, Barnett, JL. Meckel's diverticulum. Am J Gastroenterol 1990;85:777.

101. De Cothi GA, Newbold KM, O'Connor HJ. Campylobacter-like organisms and heterotopic gastric mucosa in Meckel's diverticula. J Clin Pathol 1989;42:132.

102. Fich A. Talley NJ, Shorter RG, Phillips SF. Does *Helicobacter pylori* colonize the gastric mucosa of Meckel's diverticulum? Mayo Clin Proc 1990;65:187.

103. Artigas V, Calabuig R, Badia F, et al. Meckel's diverticulum: value of ectopic tissue. Am J Surg 1986;151:631.

104. Soltero MJ, Bill AH. The natural history of Meckel's diverticulum and its relation to incidental removal. Am J Surg 1976;132:168.

105. Mackey WC, Dineen P. A fifty-year experience with Meckel's diverticulum. Surg Gynecol Obstet 1983;156:56

106. Kusumoto H, Yoshitake H, Mochida K, et al. Adenocarcinoma in Meckel's diverticulum: report of a case and review of 30 cases in the English and Japanese literature. Am J Gastroenterol 1992;87:910.

107. Nies C, Zielke A, Hasse C. Carcinoid tumors of Meckel's diverticula. Report of two cases and review of the literature. Dis Colon Rectum 1992;35:589.

108. Weber JD, McFadden DW. Carcinoid tumors in Meckel's diverticula. J Clin Gastroenterol 1989;11:682.

109. Moyana TN. Carcinoid tumors arising from Meckel's diverticulum. A clinical, morphologic and immunohistochemical study. Am J Clin Pathol 1989;91:52.

110. Justus PG, Bergman JJ, Reagan TR. Enteroliths in a Meckel's diverticulum mimicking gallstone ileus. J Fam Pract 1987;24:299.

111. Ghahremani GG. Radiology of Meckel's diverticulum. Crit Rev Diagn Imaging 1986;26:1.

112. Sfanianakis GN, Conway JJ. Detection of ectopic gastric mucosa in Meckel's diverticulum and in other aberrations by scintigraphy: 1. Pathophysiology and 10-year clinical experience. J Nucl Med 1981;22:647.

113. Petrokubi RJ, Baum S, Rohrer GV. Cimetidine administration resulting in improved pertechnetate imaging of Meckel's diverticulum. Clin Nucl Med 1978;3:385.

114. Treves S, Grand RJ, Eraklis AJ. Pentagastrin stimulation of technetium-99m uptake by ectopic gastric mucosa in a Meckel's diverticulum. Radiology 1978;128:711.

115. Schwartz MJ, Lewis JH. Meckel's diverticulum: pitfalls in scintigraphic detection in the adult. Am J Gastroenterol 1984;79:611.

116. Michas CA, Cohen SE, Wolfman EF. Meckel's diverticulum: should it be excised incidentally at operation? Am J Surg 1975;129:682.

117. Ildstad ST, Tollerud DJ, Weiss RG, et al. Duplications of the alimentary tract. Clinical characteristics, preferred treatment and associated malformations. Ann Surg 1988;208:184.

118. Bissler JJ, Klein RL. Alimentary tract duplications in children: case and literature review. Clin Pediatr (Phila) 1988;27:152.

119. Holcomb III GW, Gheissari A, O'Neill Jr JA, et al. Surgical management of alimentary tract duplications. Ann Surg 1989;209:167.

120. Rice CA, Anderson TM, Sepahdari S. Computed tomography and ultrasonography of carcinoma in duplication cysts. J Comput Assist Tomogr 1986;10:233.

121. Smith JHF, Hope PG. Carcinoid tumor arising in a cystic duplication of the small bowel. Arch Pathol Lab Med 1985;109:95.

122. Lecouffe P, Spyckerelle C, Venel H, et al. Use of pertechnetate ^{99m}Tc for abdominal scanning in localising an ileal duplication cyst: case report and review of the literature. Eur J Nucl Med 1992;19:65–67.

123. Teja K, Schnatterly P, Shaw A. Multiple intestinal atresias: pathology and pathogenesis. J Pediatr Surg 1981;16:194.

124. Santulli TV, Chen CC, Schullinger JN. Management of congenital atresia of the intestine. Am J Surg 1970;119:542.

125. Grosfeld JL, Ballantine TVN, Shoemaker R. Operative management of intestinal atresia and stenosis based on pathological findings. J Pediatr Surg 1979;14:368.

126. Seashore JH, Collins FS, Markowitz RI, Seashore MR. Familial apple peel jejunal atresia: surgical, genetic, and radiographic aspects. Pediatrics 1987;80:540.

127. Wesson D. Congenital anomalies. In: Walker WA, ed. Pediatric gastrointestinal disease: pathophysiology, diagnosis, management Philadelphia: BC Decker, 1991:477.

128. Puri P, Fujimoto T. New observations on the pathogenesis of multiple intestinal atresias. J Pediatr Surg 1988;23:221.

129. Guttman FM, Braun P, Garance PH, et al. Multiple atresias and a new syndrome of hereditary multiple atresias involving the gastrointestinal tract from stomach to rectum. J Pediatr Surg 1973;8:633.

130. Graham JM, Marin-Padilla M, Hoefnagel D. Jejunal atresia associated with Cafergot ingestion during pregnancy. Clin Pediatr (Phila) 1983;22:226.

131. Nicolini U, Monni G. Intestinal obstruction in babies exposed in utero to methylene blue (letter). Lancet 1990;336:1258.

132. Van der Pol JG, Wolf H, Boer K. Jejunal atresia related to the use of methylene blue in genetic amniocentesis in twins. Br J Obstet Gynaecol 1992;99:141.

133. Moreno LA, Gottrand F, Turck D. Severe combined immunodeficiency syndrome associated with autosomal recessive familial multiple gastrointestinal atresias: study of a family. Am J Med Genet 1990;37:143.

134. Walker MW, Lovell MA, Kelly TE, et al. Multiple areas of intestinal atresia associated with immunodeficiency and post-transfusion graft-versus-host disease. J Pediatr 1993;123:93.

135. Davenport M, Bianchi A. Congenital intestinal atresia. Br J Hosp Med 1990;44:174.

136. Smith GH, Glasson M. Intestinal atresia: factors affecting survival. Aust N Z J Surg 1989;59:151.

137. Gebara S, Firor HV. Congenital anomalies of the midgut. In: R Wyllie, JS Hyams, eds. Pediatric gastrointestinal disease: pathophysiology, diagnosis, management. Philadelphia: WB Saunders, 1993:493.

138. Yanez R, Spitz L. Intestinal malrotation presenting outside the neonatal period. Arch Dis Child 1986;61:682.

139. Sheridan R. Nonrotation of the midgut presenting in the adolescent and adult. Am J Gastroenterol 1989;84:670.

140. Rowsom JT, Sullivan SN, Girvan DP. Midgut volvulus in the adult. A complication of intestinal malrotation. J Clin Gastroenterol 1987;9:212.

141. Devlin HB. Presentation of midgut malrotation in adults. Br Med J 1968;1:803.

142. Fukuya T, Brown BP, Lu CC. Midgut volvulus as a complication of intestinal malrotation in adults. Dig Dis Sci 1993;38:438.

143. Yang CJC, Lu CC, Murakami J, Franken EA Jr. General case of the day. Radiographics 1987;7:605.

144. Coombs RC, Buick RG, Gornall PG, et al. Intestinal malrotation: the role of small intestinal dysmotility in the cause of persistent symptoms. J Pediatr Surg 1991;26:553.

145. Jolley SG, Tunell WP, Thomas S, et al. The significance of gastric emptying in children with intestinal malrotation. J Pediatr Surg 1985;20:627.

146. Torfs C, Curry C, Roeper P. Gastroschisis. J Pediatr 1990;116:1.

147. Duhamel B. Embryology of exomphalos and allied malformations. Arch Dis Child 1963;38:142.

148. Meller JL, Reyes HM, Loeff DS. Gastroschisis and omphalocele. Clin Perinatol 1989;16:113.

149. DeVries PA. The pathogenesis of gastroschisis and omphalocele. J Pediatr Surg 1980;15:245.

150. Shaw A. The myth of gastroschisis. J Pediatr Surg 1975;10:235.

151. Mercer S, Mercer B, D'Alton MEG, Soucy P. Gastroschisis: ultrasonographic diagnosis, perinatal embryology, surgical and obstetric treatment and outcome. Can J Surg 1988;31:25.

152. Knott PP, Colley NY. Can fetal gastroschisis always be diagnosed prenatally? Prenat Diagn 1987;7:607.

153. Muraji T, Tsugawa C, Nishijima E, et al. Gastroschisis: a 17 year experience. J Pediatr Surg 1989;24:343.

154. Roggo A, Ottinger LW. Acute small bowel volvulus in adults. A sporadic form of strangulating intestinal obstruction. Ann Surg 1992;216:135.

155. Duke JH Jr, Yar MS. Primary small bowel volvulus: cause and management. Arch Surg 1977;112:685.

156. Saidi F. The high incidence of intestinal volvulus in Iran. Gut 1969;10:838.

157. Frazee RC, Mucha P, Farnell MB, van Heerden JA. Volvulus of the small intestine. Ann Surg 1988;208:565.

158. Nicholson O, El Khairi SM, Schreiber H. Primary midgut volvulus in the adult: two case reports. Am J Gastroenterol 1992;87:395.

159. Pang LC. Intussusception revisited. South Med J 1989;82:215.

160. Pollack CV, Pender ES. Unusual cases of intussusception. J Emerg Med 1991;9:347.

161. Luks FI, Yazbeck S, Perreault G, Desjardins JG. Changes in the presentation of intussusception. Am J Emerg Med 1992;10:574.

162. Skipper RP, Boeckman CR, Klein RL. Childhood intussusception. Surg Gynecol Obstet 1990;171:151.

163. Stubenbord WT, Thorjuarnarson B. Intussusception in adults. Ann Surg 1970;172:306.

164. Agha FP. Review: intussusception in adults. AJR Am J Roentgenol 1986;146:527.

165. Balthazar EJ, Reich CB, Pachter HL. The significance of small bowel intussusception in acquired immune deficiency syndrome. Am J Gastroenterol 1986;81:1073.

166. Hofstetter SR, Stollman N. Adult intussusception in association with the acquired immune deficiency syndrome and intestinal Kaposi's sarcoma. Am J Gastroenterol 1988;83:1304.

167. Raudkivi PJ, Smith HLM. Intussusception: analysis of 98 cases. Br J Surg 1981;68:645.

168. Prater JM. Adult intussusception. Am Fam Physician 1993;47:447.

169. Carter CR, Morton AL. Adult intussusception in Glasgow, UK. Br J Surg 1989;76:727.

170. Gordon RS, O'Dell KB, Namon AJ, Becker LB. Intussusception in the adult—a rare disease. J Emerg Med 1991;9:337.

171. Ratcliffe JR, Fong S, Cheong I, O'Connell P. Plain film diagnosis of intussusception: prevalence of the target sign. AJR Am J Roentgenol 1992;158:619.

172. Holt S, Samuel E. Multiple concentric ring sign in the ultrasonographic diagnosis of intussusception. Gastrointest Radiol 1978;3:307.

173. Skaane P, Skjennald A. Ultrasonic features of ileocecal intussusception. J Clin Ultrasound 1989;17:590.

174. Merine D, Fishman EK, Jones B, Siegelman SS. Enteroenteric intussusception: CT findings in nine patients. AJR Am J Roentgenol 1987;148:1129.

175. Lorigan JG, Dubrow RA. The computed tomographic appearances and clinical significance of intussusception in adults with malignant neoplasms. Br J Radiol 1990;63:257.

176. Felix EL, Cohen MH, Bernstein AD, Schwartz JH. Adult intussusception. Case report of recurrent intussusception and review of the literature. Am J Surg 1976;131:758.

177. Popovic OS, Brkic S, Bojic P, et al. Sarcoidosis and protein losing enteropathy. Gastroenterology 1980;78:119.

178. Van Tilburg AJP, van Blankenstein M, Verschoor L. Intestinal lymphangiectasia in systemic sclerosis. Am J Gastroenterol 1988;83:1418.

179. Perisic VN, Kokai G. Coeliac disease and lymphangiectasia. Arch Dis Child 1992;67:134.

180. Wilkinson P, Pinto B, Senior JR. Reversible protein-losing enteropathy with intestinal lymphangiectasia secondary to chronic constrictive pericarditis. N Engl J Med 1965;273:1178.

181. Davidson JD, Waldmann TA, Goodman DS, Gordon RS Jr. Protein-losing enteropathy in congestive heart failure. Lancet 1961;1:899.

182. Ward M, LeRoux A, Small WP, Sirus W. Malignant lymphoma and extensive viral wart formation in a patient with intestinal lymphangiectasia and lymphocyte depletion. Postgrad Med J 1977;53:953.

183. Ross JD, Reid KDG, Ambujatshan VP, et al. Recurrent pleural effusion, protein losing enteropathy, malabsorption, and mosaic warts associated with generalized lymphatic hypoplasia. Thorax 1971;26:119.

184. Abramowsky C, Hupertz V, Kilbridge P, Czinn S. Intestinal lymphangiectasia in children: a study of upper gastrointestinal endoscopic biopsies. Pediatr Pathol 1989;9:289.

185. Jeffries GH, Chapman A, Sleisenger MH. Low-fat diet in intestinal lymphangiectasia: its effect on albumin metabolism. N Engl J Med 1964;270:761.

186. Tift WL, Lloyd JK. Intestinal lymphangiectasia. Long term results with MCT diet. Arch Dis Child 1975;50:269.

187. Mine K, Matsubayashi S, Nakai Y, Nakagawa T. Intestinal lymphangiectasia markedly improved with antiplasmin therapy. Gastroenterology 1989;96:1596.

188. Heresbach D, Raoul JL, Bretagne JF, Gosselin M. Intestinal lymphangiectasia: lack of efficacy of antiplasmin therapy? Gastroenterology 1991;100:1152.

Textbook of Gastroenterology, second edition, edited by Tadataka Yamada. JB Lippincott Company, Philadelphia © 1995.

CHAPTER 69

Dysmotility of the Small Intestine

Sinn Anuras   David Hodges

<table>
<tr><td>

Epidemiology
Etiology
   Primary Causes
   Secondary Causes
Clinical Manifestations
Complications
   Malnutrition
   Bacterial Overgrowth in the Small Intestine
   Pneumatosis Cystoides Intestinalis
Diagnostic Studies

</td><td>

   Blood Tests
   Radiologic Studies
   Other Studies
   Small Intestine Manometric Study
Differential Diagnosis Between Chronic Intestinal
   Pseudoobstruction and Mechanical Obstruction
Treatment
   Medical Treatments
   Surgical Treatment

</td></tr>
</table>

Intestinal motility, the function of intestinal smooth muscle, is controlled mainly by the intrinsic and extrinsic nerves of the gastrointestinal tract and, to a lesser degree, the gastrointestinal hormones (see Chap. 9). Therefore, any abnormality of these factors (i.e., smooth muscle, intrinsic or extrinsic nerves, and gastrointestinal hormones), theoretically, can cause small intestine dysmotility. In clinical situations, we commonly see small intestine dysmotility caused by either smooth muscle or intrinsic and extrinsic nerve dysfunction, but small intestine dysmotility caused by abnormal levels of gastrointestinal hormones has not been reported. Diarrhea in patients with VIPoma or gastrinoma is often attributed to excessive secretion, but there have been no comprehensive motility studies in these patients.

Patients with small intestine dysmotility have a wide range of clinical manifestations, regardless of the underlying cause of the disorder. At one end of the spectrum, the patients may be asymptomatic, and at the other end of the spectrum, they may have chronic intestinal pseudoobstruction. Between the two extremes, patients may have dyspeptic symptoms, including intermittent postprandial epigastric or periumbilical abdominal pain, bloating, nausea, vomiting, and diarrhea (Fig. 69-1).

Patients with small intestine dysmotility usually have dysmotility of other parts of the gastrointestinal tract as well. In this chapter, we focus our discussion on the small intestine, because dysmotility of other parts of the gastrointestinal tract are discussed in other chapters (see Chaps. 54, 60, 81, and 82).

EPIDEMIOLOGY

Incidence of small intestine dysmotility varies according to the underlying disease, and it seems to be less frequent in comparison to esophageal, gastric, or colonic dysmotility. In the past, the lack of a sensitive method to evaluate small intestine motility made it difficult to estimate the incidence of small intestine dysmotility. Today, small intestine manometric studies can be used to evaluate dysmotility. It is a very sensitive method of detecting abnormal motility of the small intestine, and they demonstrate that small intestine dysmotility is not uncommon. Small intestine electromyography has been evaluated in humans, but technical difficulties preclude its usefulness.

During the past 20 years, several hereditary diseases with small intestine dysmotility have been reported, including groups of diseases with smooth muscle degeneration, termed *familial visceral myopathies* (FVM)[1-27] and *childhood visceral myopathies* (CVM),[28-54] and a group of diseases with myenteric plexus degeneration, termed *familial visceral neuropathies* (FVN).[55-66] Although only a small number of families are reported, we believe that FVM, CVM, and FVN are not uncommon. These diseases are reported mostly in Caucasians,

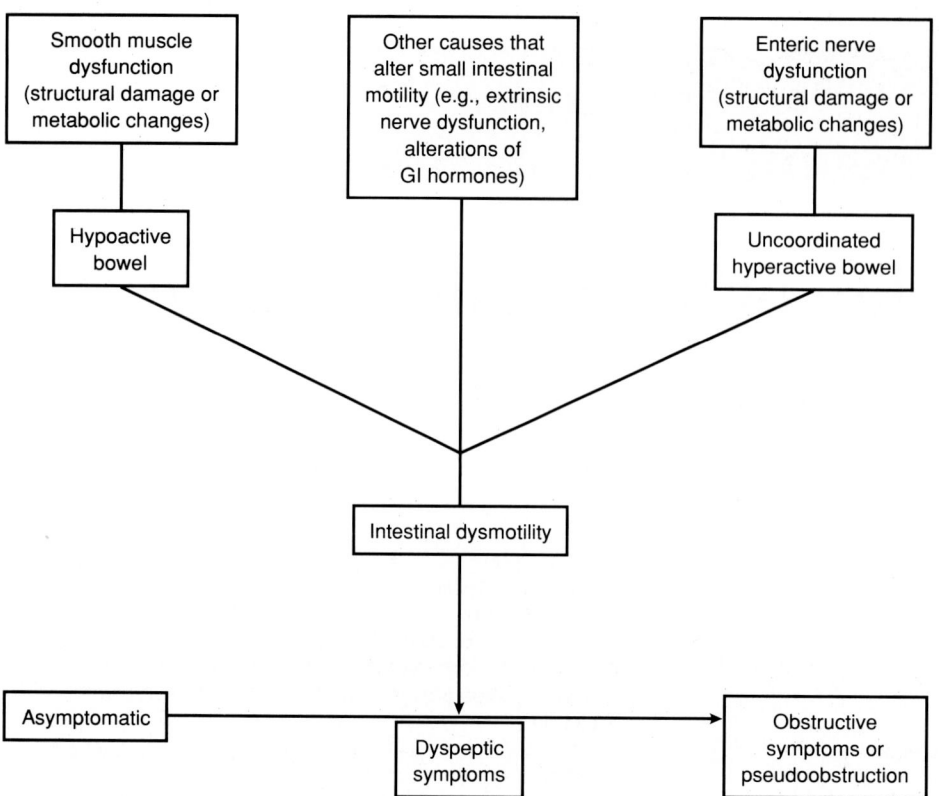

FIGURE 69-1. Mechanisms and manifestations of small intestine dysmotility.

but they are also reported in African Americans[7] and Latinos.[67] We believe that these diseases will be detected worldwide.

ETIOLOGY

Table 69-1 lists the causes of small intestine dysmotility, based mainly on histologic findings. As a result of more careful study of the full thickness of the gastrointestinal wall, many new diseases have been discovered. Smooth muscle is best studied by sectioning across the muscle fibers and using trichrome stain.[68] Myenteric plexus is best evaluated by using silver stains in parallel sections of the gastrointestinal wall, as described by Smith[69] and by Schuffler and Jonak.[70] Certain diseases often will involve only specific parts of the digestive tract with typical gross lesions; therefore, these conditions can be easily missed without thorough study.

Primary Causes

Familial Visceral Myopathies

Familial visceral myopathies (FVM) are a group of genetic diseases characterized by degeneration and fibrosis of gastrointestinal smooth muscle and, in a certain type, the urinary smooth muscle. There are at least three reported types of FVM based on gross lesions of the gastrointestinal tract and the pattern of inheritance (Table 69-2). Pathologically, there is no difference in histologic findings among these three types of FVM.[68] The involved areas show a characteristic change,

consisting of degenerating muscle cells and fibrosis which may involve the full thickness of the muscularis propria but often is more prominent in or limited to the external layer (Fig. 69-2). Degenerating muscle cells appear pale, poorly defined, and fragmented. As residual thread-like remnants become surrounded by collagen, the longitudinal and circular muscles take on a vacuolated appearance that is easily recognized microscopically (Fig. 69-3). Recognition of this change is greatly facilitated by the use of a trichrome stain, and mild lesions may be recognized only with this stain.

Type I.   Type I FVM was first reported by Weiss in 1938 in a German family, but there was no pathologic study in that family.[5] In 1977, Schuffler and Pope identified degeneration of smooth muscle as the cause of this disease[1]; since then, a total of 14 families have been reported.[1-14] The incidence of type I FVM is unknown, but we believe that it is not uncommon. Type I FVM is transmitted by an autosomal dominant gene. Chromosome study of three patients showed no abnormality.

The typical lesions seen in these patients include esophageal dilatation, megaduodenum (Fig. 69-4), redundant colon, and megacystis. In some patients, proximal jejunum may also be slightly dilated. Mydriasis or dilated pupils occurs in more than 50% of patients.

We have followed the largest reported family with type I FVM[3] for 15 years. There were 150 family members in five generations, and we identified 50 affected persons in this family. Approximately one third of the patients were asymptomatic, and two thirds were symptomatic. The asymptomatic

TABLE 69-1
Causes of Small Intestine Dysmotility

Primary Causes
Familial types
    Familial visceral myopathies
        Type I
        Type II
        Type III
    Familial visceral neuropathies
        Type I
        Type II
    Childhood visceral myopathies
        Type I
        Type II (megacystis-microcolon-intestinal hypoperistalsis
            syndrome)
Nonfamilial or sporadic types
    Visceral myopathies
    Visceral neuropathies
    Normal histology
    Irritable bowel syndrome

Secondary Causes
Disease involving the intestinal smooth muscle
    Collagen diseases (e.g., scleroderma, dermatomyositis,
        systemic lupus erythematosus, mixed connective tissue
        disease)
    Muscular dystrophies (e.g., myotonic dystrophy, Duchenne's
        muscular dystrophy)
    Amyloidosis
Neurological diseases
    Chagas' disease
    Ganglioneuromatosis of the intestine
    Visceral neuropathy of carcinomatosis
    Parkinson's disease
    Spinal cord injury
Endocrine disorders
    Diabetes mellitus
    Thyroid disease (i.e., hyperthyroidism, hypothyroidism)
    Hypoparathyroidism
Pharmacologic agents
    Phenothiazines
    Tricyclic antidepressants
    Antiparkinsonian medications
    Ganglionic blockers
    Clonidine
    Narcotics (morphine and meperidine)
Miscellaneous
    Celiac disease
    Small intestine diverticulosis
    Radiation enteritis
    Diffuse lymphoid infiltration of the small intestine
    Jejunoileal bypass
    Postgastrointestinal viral infection
    Anorexia nervosa and bulimia

cases were identified by upper gastrointestinal x-ray films showing megaduodenum. Megaduodenum was usually detected during the early teens; it does not manifest before the age of 10 years. More than 75% of symptomatic cases were girls who became symptomatic following menarche, and their symptoms were also more severe than in those of male patients. Ten percent of patients had chronic intestinal pseudoobstruction syndrome.

Of the symptomatic cases, dysphagia occurred in only 20% of patients, and a few patients had reflux esophagitis and benign esophageal stricture. Esophageal manometric study was abnormal in up to 75% of patients,[1] and it showed low or normal LES pressure and low amplitude of contractions in the lower two thirds of the esophagus, which is the smooth muscle portion. Gastroparesis has not been reported, and we have not seen any cases of gastroparesis in 65 patients in three families. Postprandial abdominal pain, bloating, fullness, and nausea occurred in 15% of cases as a result of retention of contents in the dilated duodenum, and 10% of patients had recurrent obstructive symptoms of the duodenum with vomiting, or chronic intestinal pseudoobstruction syndrome. Chronic constipation occurred in nearly one half of the patient group, and sigmoid volvulus occurred in a few instances. Intermittent diarrhea may occur rarely.

Megacystis occurred in approximately one half of the patients,[71] and nearly all were asymptomatic. Only a few instances of urinary retention and urinary infection required surgical treatment. The uterus in female patients show no increased fibrosis. Some female patients required induction of labor, because they did not experience spontaneous labor after full-term pregnancy.

Treatment depends on the organs involved. Reflux esophagitis requires H_2-receptor antagonists and antacids, and benign esophageal stricture requires dilatation. In patients who have chronic intestinal pseudoobstruction or recurrent postprandial abdominal pain, fullness, and bloating, an operation of the megaduodenum (see Surgical Treatment) may give symptomatic relief. We use milk of magnesia to treat chronic constipation, because fiber laxatives tend to cause more abdominal pain and distention. In patients with severe obstipation or recurrent sigmoid volvulus, sigmoid resection or subtotal colectomy with ileoproctostomy may be required. The prognosis of this group of patients is good, because the patients do well with appropriate operations. We have not had any patients with this disease that require long-term total parenteral nutrition.

Type II. There are five reported families[15,17-20] and three isolated cases with type II FVM.[21-23] The disease is transmitted by an autosomal recessive gene. The patients have severe ptosis and mild external ophthalmoplegia. Gastrointestinal lesions include gastric atony, slight dilatation of the small bowel, and numerous diverticula scattered throughout the entire small bowel (Fig. 69-5). The esophagus, colon, and urinary bladder are normal. A patient in one family[16] had ptosis with normal upper gastrointestinal and small bowel radiographs. This patient refused esophageal and small intestine manometric studies; therefore, we were unable to study gastrointestinal motility in this patient.

All patients with gastrointestinal lesions are malnourished and have chronic intestinal pseudoobstruction. They become symptomatic during their late teens or middle age. Partial gastrectomy and Roux-en-Y gastrojejunostomy in one of our patients[15] did not help to relieve the symptoms. The prognosis is poor, because there is no effective treatment, and patients require long-term parenteral nutrition. Other extragastroin-

TABLE 69-2
Classification of Familial Visceral Myopathies

CHARACTERISTICS	TYPE 1[1–14]	TYPE 2[15–23]	TYPE 3[24–27]
Mode of transmission	Autosomal dominant	Autosomal recessive; isolated cases	Autosomal recessive
Gross lesions	Esophageal dilatation, megaduodenum, redundant colon, and megacystis	Gastric dilatation, slight dilatation of the entire small intestine with numerous diverticula	Marked dilatation of the entire digestive tract from the esophagus to the rectum
Microscopic changes	Degeneration and fibrosis of both muscle layers of the digestive tract	Indistinguishable from type 1	Indistinguishable from type 1
Clinical manifestations			
Age at onset	After the first decade of life	Teens	Middle age
Percentage of symptomatic cases	<50%	>75%	>75%
Symptoms	Variable, from dysphagia and constipation to intestinal pseudoobstruction	Severe abdominal pain and intestinal pseudoobstruction	Intestinal pseudoobstruction
Treatment and prognosis	Symptomatic relief with appropriate operation (side-to-side duodenojejunostomy or partial resection of the duodenum); prognosis good	Does not respond to medical treatment; no effective surgical procedure; prognosis poor	Same as type 2
Extragastrointestinal manifestations	Megacystis, uterine inertia, and mydriasis	Ptosis and external ophthalmoplegia, mild degeneration of striated muscle, peripheral neuropathy, and deafness	None observed

testinal involvements in this disease include various degrees of atrophy and degeneration of both type I and type II striated muscle,[21–22] peripheral neuropathies,[19,21] and deafness.[18,19,22]

Type III.   There are four reported families.[24–27] The disease is probably transmitted by an autosomal recessive gene. In most cases, the patients have dilatation of the entire gastrointestinal tract from the esophagus down to the rectum. However, a patient in the family reported by Jacob and colleagues[24] has nondilated, tubular-appearing small intestine resulting from severe fibrosis of the intestinal wall. The patients do not have urinary bladder or any extragastrointestinal manifestations.

All reported cases have chronic intestinal pseudoobstruction. They become symptomatic during their late teens or middle age, and most of these patients die from malnutrition. The prognosis is poor, because there is no effective medical or surgical treatment. Total parenteral nutrition is required to provide adequate nutritional support.

Familial Visceral Neuropathies

Familial visceral neuropathies (FVN) are a group of genetic diseases characterized by degeneration of the myenteric plexus. There are at least two distinctive types (Table 69-3).

Type I.   There are three reported families with type I FVN.[55–57] This disease is transmitted by an autosomal dominant gene. The patients have dilatations of various lengths of the distal

small intestine (Fig. 69-6) and megacolon. One fourth of the patients have gastroparesis. Histologic study using Smith's method shows a markedly reduced number of argyrophilic neurons and nerve fibers of the myenteric plexus in the distal small intestine (Fig. 69-7). No instances of extragastrointestinal involvement have been reported. Symptoms can become apparent at any age. Type I FVN patients have recurrent postprandial abdominal pain and distention, early satiety, and either diarrhea or constipation. Approximately one half of the patients have chronic intestinal pseudoobstruction syndrome. Colonic pseudoobstruction may precede small intestine dysmotility, and subtotal colectomy is contraindicated, because it will unmask and accelerate small intestine dysmotility.[57] Most patients are mildly to moderately malnourished, and only a small number require parenteral nutrition.

Type II.   There are six reported families[59–64] and one isolated case with type II FVN.[58] This disease is transmitted by an autosomal recessive gene. The patients have hypertrophic pyloric stenosis, dilated short small intestine, and malrotation of the small intestine. Extragastrointestinal involvement includes malformation of the central nervous system and patent ductus arteriosus. Symptoms begin during infancy. All cases present with chronic intestinal pseudoobstruction. Most patients die during infancy.

Other familial visceral neuropathies.   There are a few reported families that do not fit into the two types of FVN discussed previously.[65,66,72]

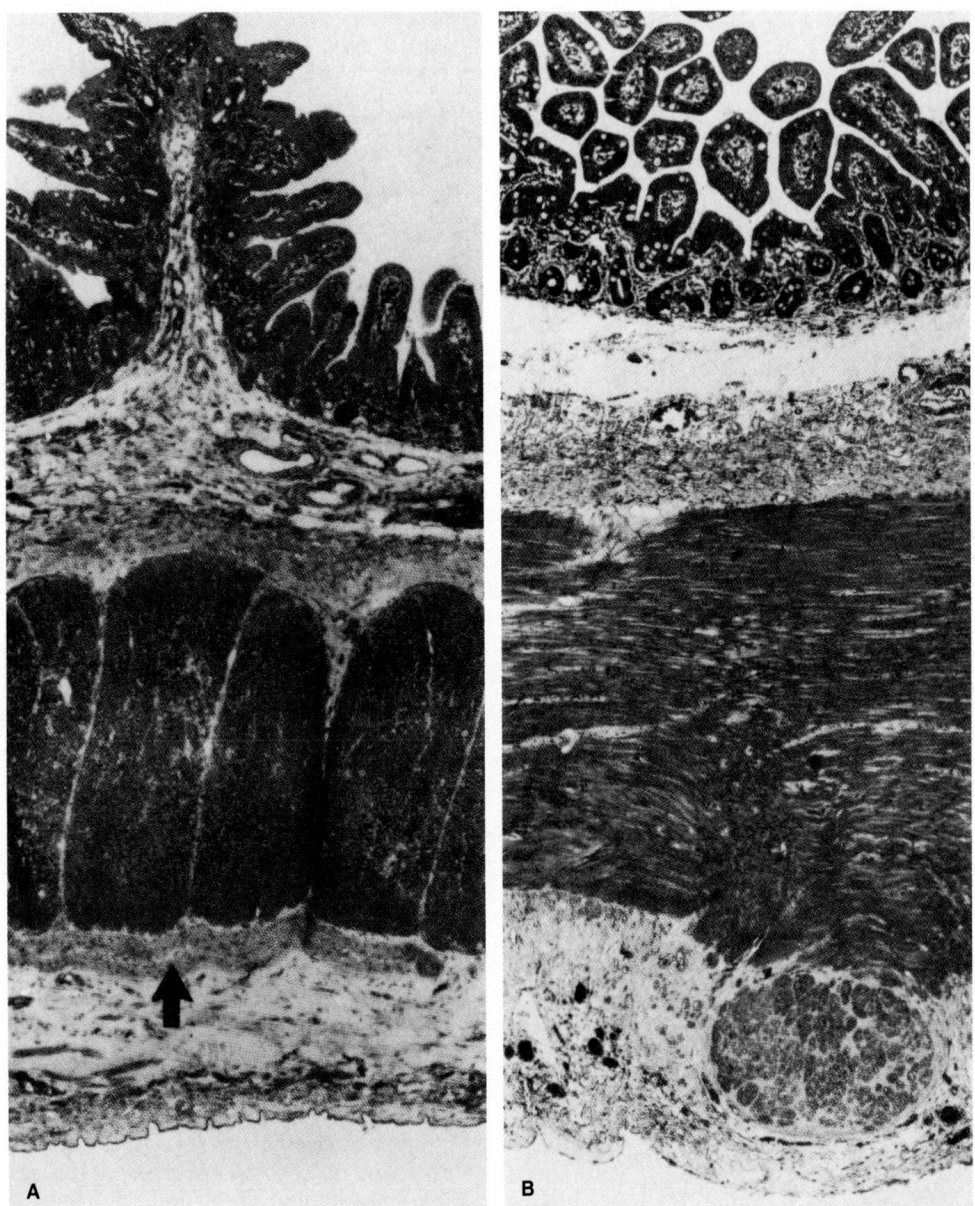

FIGURE 69-2. (**A**) Longitudinal section of jejunum from a patient with familial visceral myopathy shows normal circular muscle layer and a prominent neural bundle (*arrow*). Scattered muscle fibers and collagen are observed in the longitudinal layer. (Trichrome stain; original magnification ×40). (**B**) Cross-section of jejunum from same area depicted in **A**. The outer muscle layer contains one large bundle of preserved smooth muscle fibers and scattered individual fibers throughout the collagen elsewhere. (Trichrome stain; original magnification ×40; from Mitros FA, Schuffler MD, Teja K, et al. Pathologic feature of familial visceral myopathy. Hum Pathol 1982;13:825.)

Schuffler and colleagues[65] reported two siblings who had generalized neurologic disease and intestinal pseudoobstruction. One sibling became symptomatic during adolescence and had a 40-year history of abdominal pain, distention, and vomiting, as well as the systemic symptoms of ataxic gait; small, irregular, poorly reactive pupils; dysarthria; absent deep tendon reflexes; and impaired vibratory and positional senses. Radiographs revealed hyperactive, nonpropulsive contractions in a dilated esophagus and small intestine, and extensive colonic diverticulosis. Postmortem examination showed degeneration of the myenteric plexuses of the esophagus, small intestine, and colon. Myenteric neurons were significantly reduced in number, and about one third of the neurons contained round, eosinophilic, intranuclear inclusions. Neurons and glial cells of the brain and spinal cord, and dorsal root and celiac plexus ganglia also contained identical intranuclear inclusions. Intestinal smooth muscle was normal histologically.

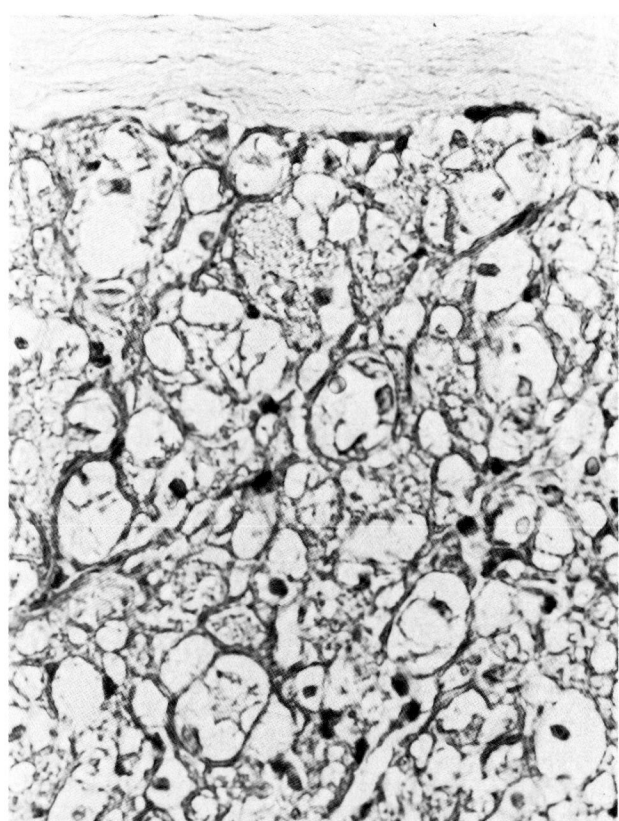

FIGURE 69-3. The characteristic vacuolar change, with collagen fibers encircling spaces filled by fragmented muscle cells, from a patient with familial visceral myopathy. (Trichrome stain; original magnification ×470; from Mitros FA, Schuffler MD, Teja K, et al. Pathologic feature of familial visceral myopathy. Hum Pathol 1982;13:825.)

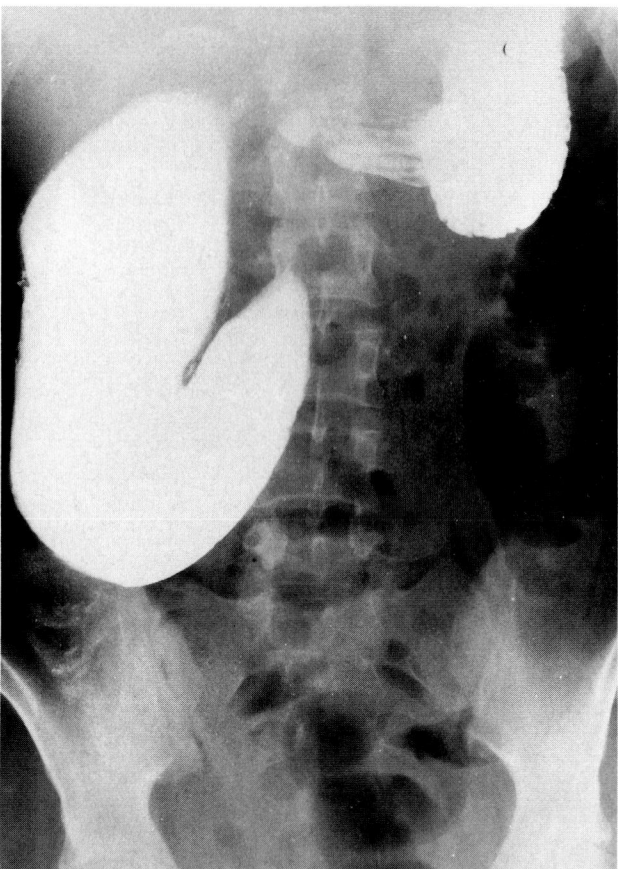

FIGURE 69-4. Upper gastrointestinal radiograph from a patient with type I familial visceral myopathy demonstrates severe megaduodenum.

In the family reported by Cockel and colleagues,[66] affected members had megaduodenum, generalized dilatation of small intestine, malabsorption, redundant colon, mental retardation, and calcification of basal ganglia. Histologic studies showed degeneration of the argyrophobe cells, which produce acetylcholine. The patients became symptomatic for intestinal pseudoobstruction during late childhood, and one patient died during their teenage years.

Faber and colleagues[72] reported five patients with chronic intestinal pseudoobstruction in two families. Conventional histologic examination of the stomach revealed hypertrophy of nerve fibers and an absence of ganglion cells. The disease is transmitted by an autosomal recessive gene. All patients had megaduodenum. One patient had jejunal diverticulosis, and another had dilatation of the entire small intestine. Three patients had gastric dilatation. Most patients had external ophthalmoplegia, ptosis, distal weakness of all extremities, gait disturbances, and acroparesthesia. Symptoms started during the teenage years, and the prognosis was poor.

Childhood Visceral Myopathies

Childhood visceral myopathies (CVM) have been recognized as distinctive diseases; there are two forms of CVM (Table 69-4). These two diseases differ from FVM in their clinical manifestations and modes of inheritance. Degeneration and fibrosis of gastrointestinal and urinary (Fig. 69-8) smooth muscle can be detected in both types of CVM.[26,32,43,71]

Type I. Although there are only a limited number of reported cases of type I CVM,[28-36] we believe that this disease is not uncommon. There are a few instances of cousins reported,[28,30,33] which raises the possibility that this disease is hereditary. Type I CVM affects both genders with equal frequency. The patients usually become symptomatic between infancy and 5 years of age. Nearly all patients have dilatation from the stomach to the rectum, including megacolon. Approximately one third of the patients have esophageal aperistalsis. The patients' first symptoms are usually constipation and abdominal distention, and they progress to chronic intestinal pseudoobstruction. In severe cases, patients have postprandial abdominal pain, nausea, vomiting, obstipation, and signs of intestinal obstruction. A small number of patients may have only constipation and occasional distention of the abdomen. Colonic volvulus causing mechanical obstruction of the colon may occur in some cases. Gastric volvulus and small bowel volvulus occur less frequently. Small bowel perforation occurs in a few cases. Nearly all patients are malnourished and die from complications of malnutrition.

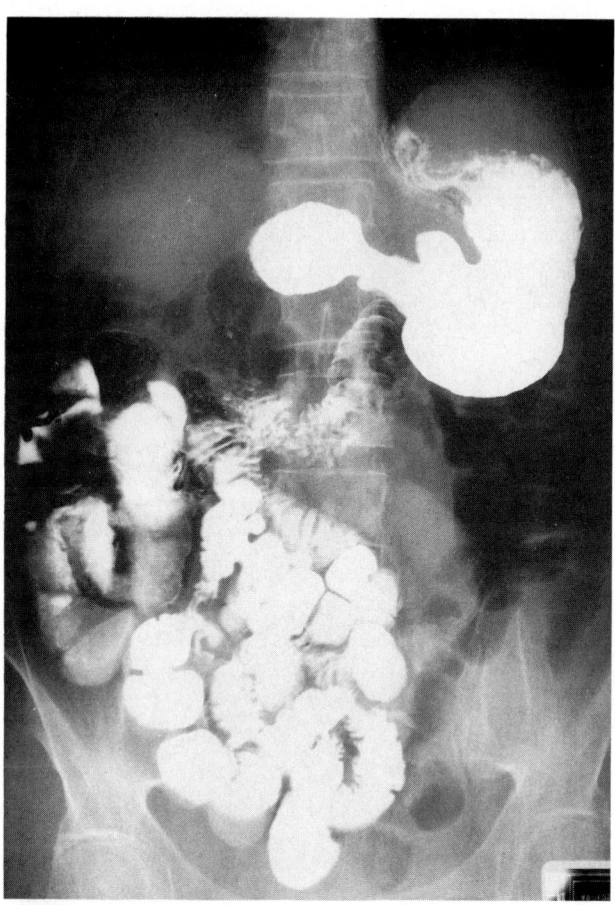

FIGURE 69-5. An enteroclysis from a patient with type II familial visceral myopathy demonstrates numerous diverticula in the small intestine.

Long-term parenteral nutrition will prolong the life of these children. Nearly all patients have megacystis and megaureters (Fig. 69-9). Symptoms include dysuria, recurrent urinary tract infections, and hematuria.

Type II, or megacystis–microcolon–intestinal hypoperistalsis syndrome. Type II CVM is not an uncommon disease.[37–54] It was first recognized by Berdon and colleagues.[37] The disease occurs predominantly in female infants. This form of visceral myopathy may be transmitted by an autosomal recessive gene.[47–49] It has been suggested that prune-belly syndrome, which involves primarily male infants, may have a common pathogenesis with type II CVM,[44] which would make prune-belly syndrome a male counterpart of megacystis–microcolon–intestinal hypoperistalsis syndrome. Type II CVM invariably manifests itself during the first week of infancy. These patients have intestinal hypoperistalsis and pseudoobstruction, microcolon located entirely on the left side of the abdomen, shortening of the small intestine and colon, and malrotation and malfixation of the microcolon. The patients have severe abdominal distention and bilious vomiting. Electron- and light-microscopic examinations of the ileum and urinary bladder show vacuolar degenerative changes in the smooth muscle cells.[43,51] The stomach may be dilated in some patients. There is no effective treatment for this disease, and most patients die during infancy. Some patients may survive past infancy with the use of parenteral nutrition.

All patients have megacystis, and some may have tortuous megaureters. Ultrasonography may allow detection of megacystis and megaureters in the fetus. The patients may have recurrent urinary infections. There are some similarities between type I and type II CVM. Whether they are the variants of the same disease remains to be elucidated.

TABLE 69-3
Classification of Familial Visceral Neuropathies

CHARACTERISTICS	TYPE 1[55–57]	TYPE 2[58–64]
Mode of transmission	Autosomal dominant	Autosomal recessive
Gross lesions	Dilatation of various lengths of small intestine, usually beginning from distal small bowel; megacolon; gastroparesis in one-fourth of patients	Hypertrophic pyloric stenosis, dilated short small intestine, malrotation of small intestine
Microscopic changes	Degeneration of argyrophilic neurons and decrease in numbers of nerve fibers	Deficiency of argyrophilic neurons and increase in neuroblasts
Clinical manifestations		
Age of onset	Any age	Infancy
Percentage of symptomatic cases	>75%	100%
Symptoms	Early satiety; recurrent abdominal pain and distention; diarrhea or constipation; two-thirds of patients have intestinal or colonic pseudoobstruction	All patients have intestinal pseudoobstruction
Treatment and prognosis	No effective medical or surgical treatments, but severely symptomatic patients are uncommon; prognosis fair	No effective medical or surgical treatments; prognosis poor because patients are severely ill
Extragastrointestinal manifestations	None	Malformation of central nervous system in some cases; patent ductus arteriosus

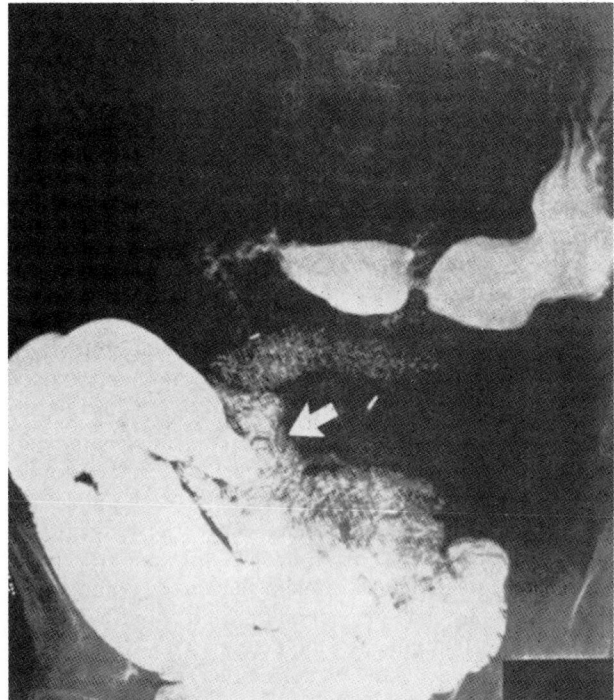

FIGURE 69-6. Small bowel radiograph from a patient with type I familial visceral neuropathy shows a normal stomach, duodenum, and proximal jejunum, but dilated distal small bowel (*arrow*). (From Mayer EA, Schuffler MD, Rotter JI, et al. Familial visceral neuropathy with autosomal dominant transmission. Gastroenterology 1986;91:1528.)

Nonfamilial Visceral Myopathies

There are a handful of reports of nonfamilial visceral myopathies in adults,[73–79] and we have personally seen a few cases. It appears that the disease is heterogeneous. A few cases that we saw have gross lesions and clinical manifestations identical to type III FVM. The case reported by Bannister and Hoyes[76] had gross lesions and clinical manifestations identical to type I FVM. We believe that many cases of apparent nonfamilial visceral myopathy are actually the FVM, because the recessive inheritance may make it appear to be nonfamilial. Histologically, there is no difference between the familial and nonfamilial types. Diffuse mixed inflammatory cell infiltration, including a good number of eosinophils, was observed in one patient.[73] In one reported case,[79] acetylcholinesterase stain of small intestine showed a considerable increase in the amount of positive fibers, but there was no degeneration of neurons in the myenteric plexus. Our view is that the nonfamilial type of visceral myopathy is uncommon; most of cases are actually of an unrecognized familial type. Family history must be carefully obtained in these patients to make a diagnosis of FVM.

Nonfamilial Visceral Neuropathies

Nonfamilial visceral neuropathies are probably much more common than the nonfamilial visceral myopathies, because myenteric plexus damage from chemicals, drugs, or viral infections may occur more frequently. Prolonged delayed gastric

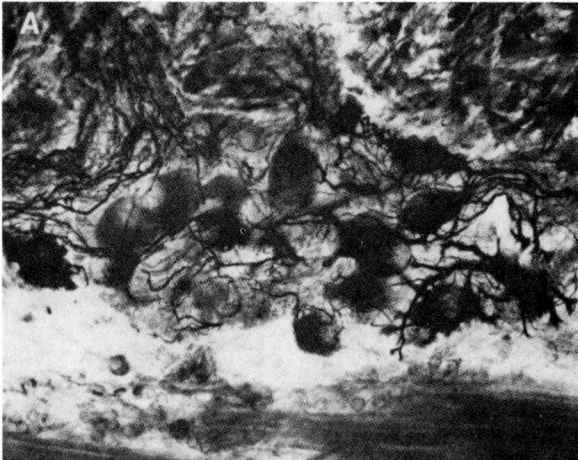
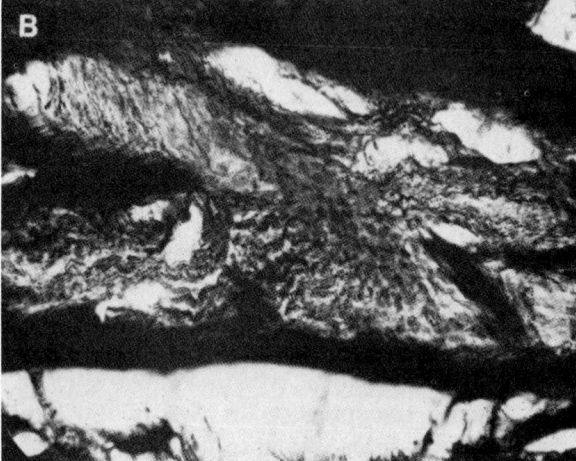
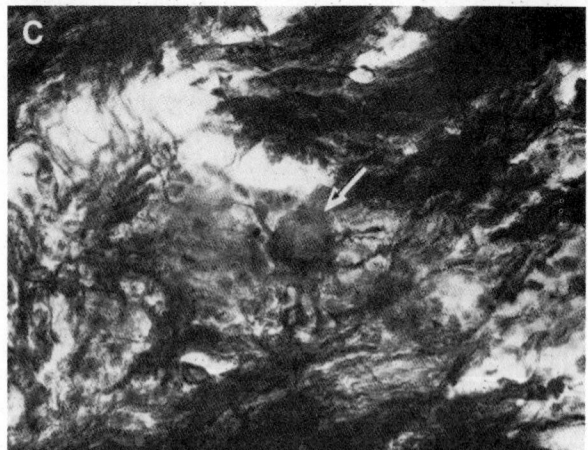

FIGURE 69-7. (**A**) Ganglionic area from normal control ileum demonstrates numerous argyrophilic neurons and nerve fibers. (Silver stain; original magnification ×230.) (**B**) Ganglionic area from a patient with type II familial visceral neuropathy demonstrates absence of argyrophilic neurons and few nerve fibers. There is a faint cluster of small nuclei of unknown cell type. (Silver stain; original magnification ×230.) (**C**) Another ganglionic area from the same patient shows only one, poorly staining, argyrophilic neuron (*arrow*). (Silver stain; original magnification ×362; from Mayer EA, Schuffler MD, Rotter JI, et al. Familial visceral neuropathy with autosomal dominant transmission. Gastroenterology 1986;91:1528.)

TABLE 69-4
Classification of Childhood Visceral Myopathies

CHARACTERISTICS	TYPE 1	TYPE 2
Mode of transmission	Autosomal recessive (?)	Autosomal recessive (?)
Gross lesions	Dilatation of the entire gastrointestinal tract	Short and malrotated small intestine; malrotation and malfixation of the microcolon
Microscopic changes	Degeneration and fibrosis of gastrointestinal and urinary smooth muscle cells	Vacuolar degenerative changes of gastrointestinal and urinary smooth muscle cells
Clinical manifestations		
Age at onset	Infancy and young childhood	Infancy
Gender	Both genders	Predominantly female
Symptoms	Constipation and abdominal distention, which may progress to intestinal pseudoobstruction	Obstipation, intestinal pseudoobstruction
Treatment and prognosis	No effective treatment; prognosis poor	Same
Extragastrointestinal manifestations	Megacystis and megaureters	Megacystis and megaureters

emptying has been observed in patients after viral gastroenteritis.[80,81] Therefore, it is conceivable that some viruses may cause permanent damage to the myenteric plexus in some patients. More cases of visceral neuropathies will be recognized with the use of the Smith's method to examine the myenteric plexus[69] of these patients.

There have been only a handful of reports of nonfamilial visceral neuropathies.[82–89] These patients usually have disturbed motility of the entire gastrointestinal tract, but none have urinary tract involvement. The intestine is dilated but shows active, nonperistaltic contractions.[88] In contrast, patients with visceral myopathies have inactive dilated intestine.[88] Histologic examinations of the myenteric plexus in these patients reveal a reduction in the number of neurons, and those that remain are very abnormal. The neurons are enlarged, with thick, irregular, clubbed processes. There is an

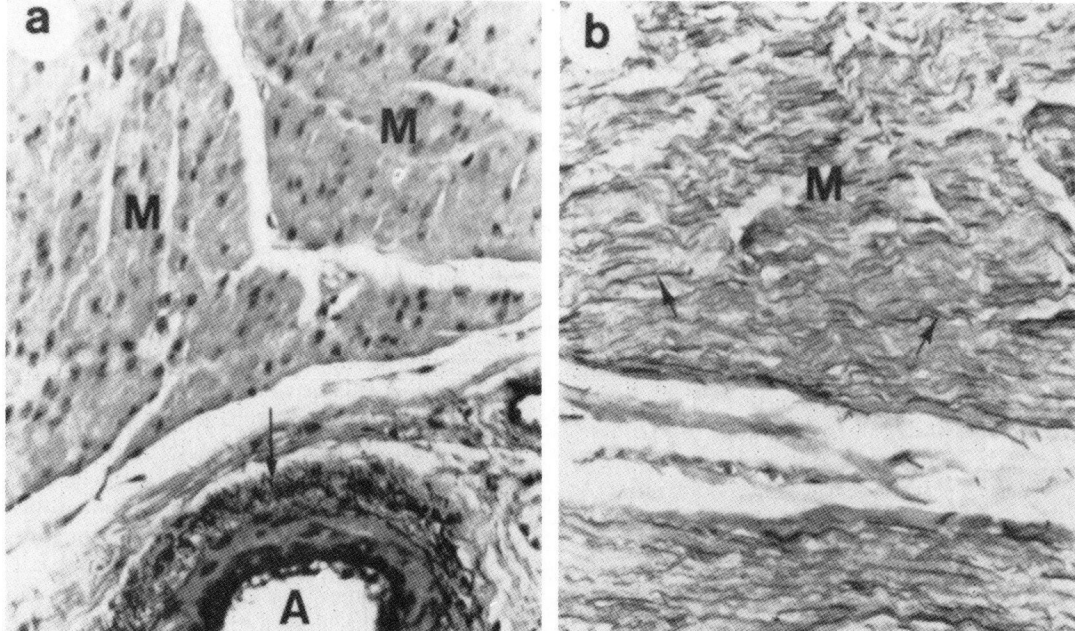

FIGURE 69-8. (**A**) Bladder muscularis from a control specimen demonstrates elastic fibers (*arrow*) in the adventitia of a small artery (A). No elastic fibers are present within muscle bundles (M). (**B**) Bladder muscularis from a type 1 childhood visceral myopathy patient demonstrates numerous, parallel, coarse, wavy, elastic fibers (*arrows*) within muscle bundles (M). (Verhoeff-van Gieson stain; original magnification ×325; from Bonsib SM, Fallon B, Mitros FA, et al. Urologic manifestations of patients with visceral myopathy. J Urol 1984;132:1112.)

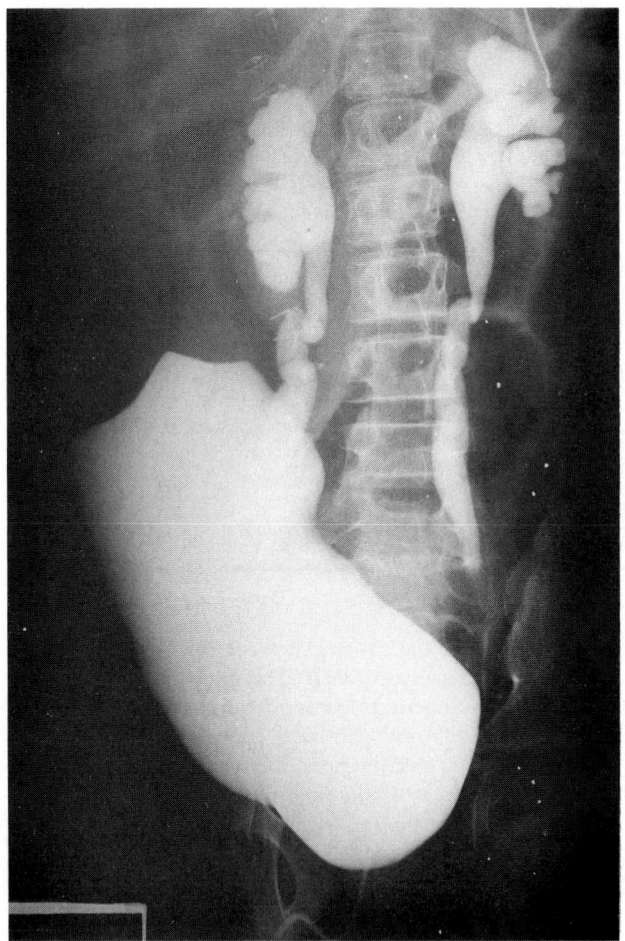

FIGURE 69-9. An intravenous pyelogram of a child with type I childhood visceral myopathy shows megacystis and bilateral ureteral pyelocaliectasis. (From Bonsib SM, Fallon B, Mitros FA, et al. Urologic manifestations of patients with visceral myopathy. J Urol 1984;132:1112.)

increase in the number of Schwann's cells in the nerve trunks and a reduction in the number of axons. Some of the remaining axons are beaded and fragmented. Hypertrophy of the muscularis propria may also be observed. This hypertrophy may involve only one or both muscle layers. All reported cases have chronic intestinal pseudoobstruction. Infants and young children are also affected.[89] We believe that some patients with symptoms of dyspepsia may have a milder form of non-familial visceral neuropathies, because small intestine manometric studies in these patients show changes similar to those with myenteric plexus damages.[90–91] To identify the cause of visceral neuropathies, it is important to take a detailed history of exposure to chemicals and drugs, as well as a history of gastrointestinal viral infections.

Abnormal Intestinal Manometric Studies With Normal Histology of the Gastrointestinal Tract

Some patients may have have abnormal intestinal manometric studies but normal histology of the gastrointestinal tract. How common this entity is is not known. Early reports[92–94] must

be interpreted with caution, because trichrome stain to detect fibrosis of the smooth muscle was not performed, and the Smith's method was not used to examine myenteric plexus. It is likely that abnormal gastrointestinal motility can occur in histologically normal neuromuscular apparatus, presumably as a result of functional disorders of the smooth muscle or neurons in the myenteric plexus. Studies of receptors of smooth muscle cells and histochemical staining of myenteric neurons may uncover the underlying defect in this group of patients.

Irritable Bowel Syndrome

There has been no histologic study of the intestinal wall of patients with irritable bowel syndrome; therefore, it is unknown if there is a pathologic basis for this condition. Small intestine motility studies in patients with irritable bowel syndrome showed abnormalities that suggest small bowel involvement.[95,96] These abnormalities include shorter-than-normal duration of migrating motor complexes (MMCs), prolonged propagated contractions in the ileum, and discrete clustered contractions in the jejunum in some patients.[95] Another study of one patient showed a longer-than-normal duration of MMCs,[96] but irregular clustered contractions were also detected in the jejunum. Manometric findings in irritable bowel patients suggest myenteric plexus dysfunction, but these abnormalities are likely to be functional in origin.

Secondary Causes

Secondary causes of small intestine dysmotility are described in Table 69-5.

Scleroderma, or Progressive Systemic Sclerosis

The small bowel is the second most frequently involved gastrointestinal organ in scleroderma, after the esophagus. Radiographic evidence of gastric sclerosis, intestinal sclerosis, or both occurs in 40% of scleroderma patients.[97–100] Contrast studies reveal dilatation of the duodenum and jejunum, delayed barium transit, and narrow valvulae conniventes, which remain tightly packed together despite bowel dilatation, producing an accordion appearance (Fig. 69-10).[8,100,101] Wide-necked diverticula may be seen but are more frequent in the colon.[102] An uncommon but serious finding is pneumatosis cystoides intestinalis, which signifies a poor prognosis.[103]

Degeneration of smooth muscle with replacement by collagen is responsible for small bowel dysmotility in scleroderma. The circular muscle is involved more often than the longitudinal muscle layer.[8,104,105] The submucosal and myenteric plexuses appear normal by conventional staining. Small bowel dysmotility leads to bacterial overgrowth, resulting in steatorrhea, malabsorption, and weight loss. Intestinal pseudoobstruction is a well-described gastrointestinal complication of scleroderma.[8,106–109]

In scleroderma patients with intestinal involvement, disturbances of small bowel motility have been documented in several studies.[109a,109b] Many patients have a complete absence of the interdigestive MMC; clusters of propagated and non-

TABLE 69-5
Gastrointestinal Lesions in Some Systemic Diseases

DISEASE	CRICOPHARYNX	ESOPHAGUS	STOMACH	SMALL INTESTINE	COLON	ANORECTUM
Scleroderma	Not involved	Dilatation, aperistalsis of lower two-thirds, incompetent LES	Gastroparesis occurs less frequently	Dilatation with narrowed valvulae conniventes	Dilatation with loss of haustral markings, wide-necked diverticula, pneumatosis intestinalis	Incompetent internal anal sphincter
Dermatomyositis and polymyositis	Decreased UES resting tone with nasopharyngeal reflux, tracheal aspiration	Dilatation, dysmotility of proximal portion	Gastroparesis occurs seldomly	Megaduodenum, dilatation distally less frequent	Dilatation of the colon	
Systemic lupus erythematosus	Not involved	Aperistalsis		Dilatation, thumbprinting with ischemia		
Mixed connective tissue disease		Dilatation of lower two-thirds, aperistalsis	Not involved	Megaduodenum	Diverticula	
Myotonic dystrophy	Decreased peristalsis, incompetent UES	Decreased peristalsis, dilatation	Delayed emptying, dilatation	Dilatation	Dilatation	External anal sphincter dysfunction
Duchenne's muscular dystrophy	Decreased pharyngeal muscles	Dilatation	Dilatation	Dilatation	Dilatation	
Amyloidosis	Not involved	Aperistalsis, incomplete LES relaxation	Delayed emptying	Dilatation	Dilatation	
Chagas' disease	Not involved	Dilatation, aperistalsis, incomplete LES relaxation	Dilatation	Proximal dilatation	Dilatation	Incompetent internal anal sphincter
Neurofibromatosis	Not involved		Gastroparesis occurs less frequently	Dilatation	Dilatation	Not involved
Visceral neuropathy in carcinomatosis		Aperistalsis	Gastroparesis	Dilatation	Dilatation	
Parkinson's disease	Impaired peristalsis	Diffuse spasm, dilatation, aperistalsis	Gastroparesis occurs less frequently	Dilatation	Dilatation, sigmoid volvulus	
Diabetes mellitus	Decreased pharyngeal peristalsis	Decreased peristalsis, normal LES	Dilatation, delayed emptying	Delayed, normal, or rapid transit	Dilatation	Decreased sensation, incompetent external sphincter, low resting tone
Spinal cord injury	Not involved	Not involved	Gastroparesis infrequent	Increased gas occasionally seen	Delayed transit mainly in left colon	Sensation absent or decreased, low resting tone, impaired external sphincter

LES, lower esophageal sphincter; NR, not reported; UES, upper esophageal sphincter.

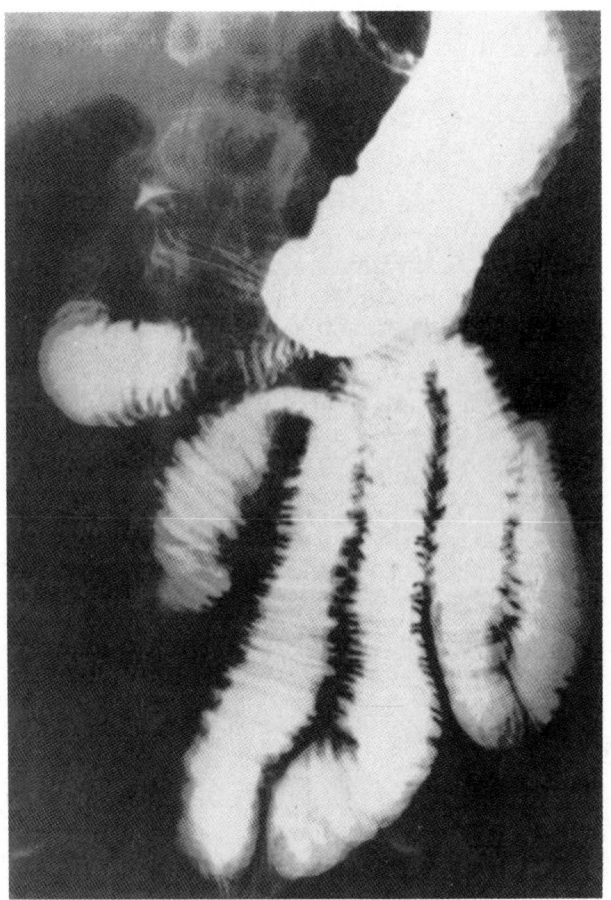

FIGURE 69-10. Upper gastrointestinal series in a patient with scleroderma shows dilatation of the small bowel with normal appearance of the stomach. In some cases, the valvulae conniventes are not thickened, as is usually seen in disorders that produce dilatation. In contrast, they remain narrow and crowded, producing the accordion appearance shown here. (From Cohen S, Laufer I, Snape WJ Jr. The gastrointestinal manifestation of scleroderma; pathogenesis and management. Gastroenterology 1980;79:155.)

propagated contractions may be the only finding in others. Abnormally long MMC cycle, diminished activity of phase III, and hypomotility of the fed pattern are other abnormal findings.[110-112] Scleroderma patients without gastrointestinal involvement demonstrate normal small bowel manometry[110] and normal small bowel transit time.[113]

Treatment with cisapride, a prokinetic agent, has improved gastric emptying and upper abdominal symptoms in scleroderma patients.[114] Octreotide, a long-acting somatostatin analogue, induces phase III activity in patients with previous complete absence of MMCs and also reduces bacterial overgrowth and symptoms (Fig. 69-11).[115] More studies are needed to confirm these observations.

Dermatomyositis and Polymyositis

The inflammatory disorders dermatomyositis and polymyositis are characterized by weakness and atrophy of skeletal muscles; an associated skin rash distinguishes the former from the latter. The gastrointestinal tract is involved in one half of the cases. Esophageal involvement causes dysphagia, which often is a presenting symptom in these diseases.

Studies of the small bowel in these patients are mainly limited to radiographic and histologic examinations. Megaduodenum and delayed intestinal transit of barium are prominent features.[116-118] Autopsy findings have shown atrophy and fibrosis of intestinal smooth muscle, suggesting a visceral myopathy.[117,118] Acute pseudoobstruction has been reported in one patient with dermatomyositis but was limited to the colon.[119]

Systemic Lupus Erythematosus

Abdominal pain is the most common gastrointestinal symptom in systemic lupus erythematosus, occurring in 10% to 20% of patients. Autopsy studies disclose a 60% to 70% incidence of previous peritoneal inflammation, but documented cases of serositis as the sole cause of abdominal pain are rare.[120] *Lupus enteritis* is a term used to describe bowel changes from

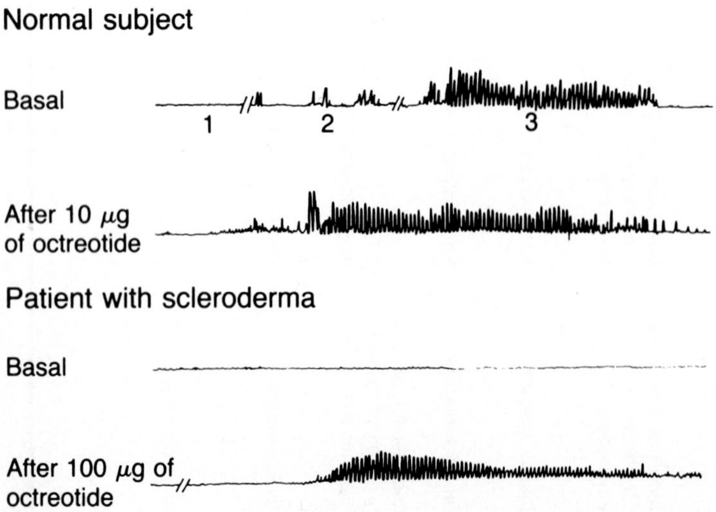

Normal subject

Basal

      1   2   3

After 10 μg
of octreotide

Patient with scleroderma

Basal

After 100 μg of
octreotide

FIGURE 69-11. Effect of octreotide on healthy persons and scleroderma patients. In the normal person, octreotide stimulates phase 3 activity. In patients with scleroderma and pseudoobstruction, octreotide induces phase 3 activity when no migrating motor complex activity was present in basal state. (From Soudah HC, Hasler WL, Owyang C. Effect of octreotide on intestinal mobility and bacterial overgrowth in scleroderma. N Engl J Med 1991;325:1461.)

lupus-induced vasculitis of small and, to a lesser extent, large blood vessels. Ischemia leads to intestinal angina, mucosal ulceration, edema, and hemorrhage. Smooth muscle dysfunction results in dilatation of the small bowel and ileus. In severe cases, there is necrosis of the bowel wall with perforation or infarction.

Diagnosis of lupus enteritis is made radiographically. Small bowel changes include dilatation, coarsened folds, and thumbprinting secondary to submucosal edema and hemorrhage.[121,122] Diarrhea occurs in 5% to 10% of lupus patients. Unusual intestinal manifestations can cause diagnostic difficulties. Small bowel involvement in lupus may simulate Crohn's ileitis in some cases.[123,124] A severe protein-losing enteropathy was described in one lupus patient who demonstrated vasculitis and basement membrane thickening on full-thickness jejunal biopsy.[125] Transit or manometric studies of the small bowel in lupus patients have not been performed.

Mixed Connective Tissue Disease

Mixed connective tissue disease is a clinical entity characterized by overlapping features of scleroderma, polymyositis, and rheumatoid arthritis. It has a distinct serologic finding of high titers of antinuclear antibody against ribonucleoprotein. The extent of gastrointestinal involvement is unknown but appears to resemble that of scleroderma. Duodenal and jejunal dilatation are seen radiographically, and pneumatosis cystoides intestinalis may complicate severe disease.[126]

Myotonic Dystrophy

Myotonic muscular dystrophy is a slowly progressive disease characterized by myotonia, or difficulty in muscle relaxation. Besides muscle wasting, the patient often has a nasal voice as a result of pharyngeal and palatal weakness, early onset of cataracts, and cardiac conduction defects. Dysphagia is the most common gastrointestinal symptom resulting from esophageal involvement. Diarrhea and abdominal cramping are common and occur in up to one third of those affected. Malabsorption and steatorrhea have been reported in a few cases.[127-129] Constipation also is a frequent occurrence and can alternate with diarrhea. Intestinal pseudoobstruction is rare and has been reported in two patients.[130,131] The small bowel may demonstrate abnormal but nonspecific radiographic changes, including dilatation, diminished motility, and delayed transit of barium.[132]

Dysmotility of the small intestine may play a significant role in the production of intestinal symptoms. In a group of 10 patients with symptoms of intestinal dysmotility but normal small bowel contrast examinations, abnormal small bowel motility was found in all subjects. Manometric findings included low-amplitude contractions in fasting and fed states, retrograde propagation of phase III, interruption of phase III, and increased incidence of tonic contractions.[133] In one patient with chronic pseudoobstruction and dilated small bowel, manometry revealed low-amplitude duodenal contractions and an increased maximal rate of contraction in the duodenum.[131]

Histologically, small intestine smooth muscle discloses changes similar to those found in dystrophic skeletal muscle.

The smooth muscle cells have been described as swollen, partially destroyed, decreased in size, and replaced by fat.[134,135] These studies did not examine the histology of the myenteric plexuses, however. Using silver stain, degenerative changes of the myenteric plexus of the colon were found in a patient with megacolon,[136] indicating that intestinal dysmotility may be caused by smooth muscle as well as enteric nerve dysfunction. We believe that in most patients, the predominant cause of dysmotility is smooth muscle damage.

Duchenne's Muscular Dystrophy

Duchenne's muscular dystrophy is a severe, pseudohypertrophic muscular dystrophy that follows an X-linked recessive pattern, affecting young boys early in childhood. Skeletal and cardiac fibers are infiltrated and eventually replaced by connective and fatty tissue. Similarly, smooth muscle of the gastrointestinal tract also is involved. Histologic changes comprise degeneration and atrophy of smooth muscle fibers, and separation of fibers by connective tissue.[137-139] The myenteric plexus is not involved.

Despite typical dystrophic changes in the small bowel in most postmortem specimens, gastrointestinal symptoms are usually related to dysmotility of the esophagus and stomach, which are more severely affected than the small bowel. Dysphagia is the predominant symptom (36% in one series), followed less often by vomiting, diarrhea, and constipation.[139] Orocecal transit time is normal in asymptomatic subjects[140]; however, severe bowel dysmotility can occur. Episodes of acute intestinal pseudoobstruction, manifested by abdominal distention, persistent vomiting, and gastric or small bowel dilatation, can be life-threatening.[141-143] Chronic intestinal pseudoobstruction has also been reported in this disease.[144]

Amyloidosis

Amyloid protein is deposited in the small bowel in all forms of amyloidosis: primary, secondary, myeloma-associated, and hereditary (i.e., familial Mediterranean fever). The severity of dysmotility is related to the amount and distribution of amyloid deposited. In all forms, amyloid is deposited in blood vessel walls, leading to ischemic ulcers, infarction, and occasionally perforation.

In primary and myeloma-associated forms of amyloidosis, the muscle layers of the small bowel are more severely affected than the mucosa, resulting in dysmotility. In the secondary and hereditary forms, the mucosa is predominantly involved, resulting in malabsorption. Amyloid deposits are infrequently found in the myenteric plexus, although in hereditary forms, neuropathy may result from deposition in major nerve trunks supplying the bowel.[145,146]

Gastrointestinal symptoms include diarrhea; constipation, which is often present for years then followed by diarrhea; malabsorption; and pseudoobstruction. Diarrhea can exist without malabsorption and appears to be secondary to small bowel bacterial overgrowth, as evidenced by improvement after antibiotic therapy.[147] Radiographically, there is coarsening of the small bowel mucosal pattern, dilatation, and diminished motility with prolonged transit of barium.[148] These changes are nonspecific and can be mistaken for scleroderma.

In a mixed group of amyloid patients, orocecal transit time

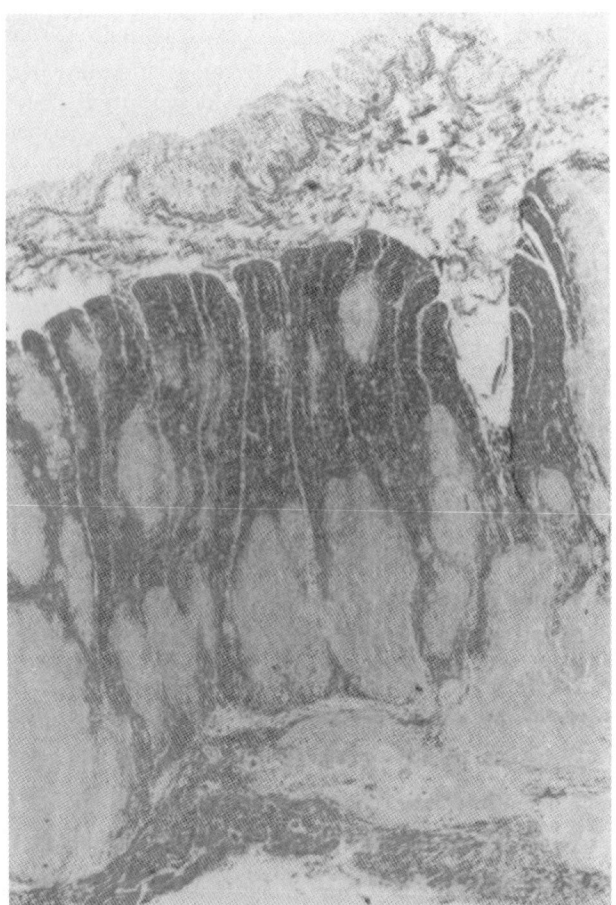

FIGURE 69-12. Small bowel myopathy in a patient with amyloidosis and pseudoobstruction. The large, pale areas in the muscle layer represent heavy amyloid deposition. The myenteric plexus is less frequently involved than the mucosa and muscle layers. (From Mitros FA. Motor and mechanical disorders. In: Ming S, Goldman H, eds. Pathology of the gastrointestinal tract. Philadelphia: WB Saunders, 1992:208).

was prolonged to more than twice that of controls.[149] This suggests delayed small bowel transit, because the hydrogen breath test using liquid lactulose is not dependent on gastric emptying. However, wide variability between and within normal subjects has been observed with this technique.[150] With heavy infiltration of the small bowel muscle layers, acute intestinal pseudoobstruction is a serious and often fatal complication (Fig. 69-12).[109,151–153]

Chagas' Disease

Chronic infection with *Trypanosoma cruzi* leads to destruction of the submucosal and myenteric plexuses along the entire length of the gastrointestinal tract. Megacolon and megaesophagus are the most common presentations, although the small bowel may be similarly affected with megaduodenum and megajejunum. Small intestine manometric studies in these patients demonstrate normal frequency of the MMC, but the velocity of propagation of the activity front is significantly slowed, to about one half that of normal.[154] Patients with

small bowel involvement may be entirely asymptomatic despite significant neuronal destruction.[155] Diarrhea or constipation can occur, as can intestinal pseudoobstruction in severe cases.

Neurofibromatosis, or von Recklinghausen's Disease

Gastrointestinal neurofibromas are most commonly found in the small intestine. They are reported to occur in up to 10% of patients with neurofibromatosis; the true incidence is probably underestimated, however, because of their generally asymptomatic nature. Small bowel neurofibromas may be single or multiple and are most frequently found in the ileum. These tumors are submucosal, and they may become quite large and extend to the serosa. Their presence is usually established by a small bowel series.[156,157] Ulceration through the mucosa can cause acute or chronic bleeding. Mechanical small bowel obstruction or intussusception requires exploratory surgery.

Chronic intestinal pseudoobstruction has been described in one patient with neurofibromatosis. Small bowel manometry was abnormal, and small bowel transit was markedly delayed.[158] Pathologic studies on the nerves and muscles in the small bowel are lacking in this disease. In the colon, neurogenic changes consisting of nerve fiber proliferation in the myenteric and submucosal plexuses were found in a patient with megacolon.[159] Similar changes have not been described in the small bowel in neurofibromatosis patients.[160]

Visceral Neuropathy of Carcinomatosis

Chronic intestinal pseudoobstruction has been reported in small cell carcinoma of the lung[161–163] and epidermoid carcinoma of the lip.[164] This phenomenon represents a paraneoplastic syndrome caused by visceral neuropathy. The small bowel, like the colon, shows widespread neuronal and axonal degeneration of the myenteric and submucosal plexuses. There is also mononuclear cell infiltration and Schwann's cell proliferation. Tumor metastasis to the bowel is not present.

Pseudoobstruction symptoms are the presenting features in patients with visceral neuropathy and small cell carcinoma. The lung cancer is usually occult and is often found at autopsy. The small bowel is usually not dilated on x-ray films, but there is delay of barium passage through the small bowel. In one patient with small cell carcinoma who underwent small bowel manometry, no interdigestive MMCs were found; only short periods of activity similar to phase II MMCs were present.[163] In older patients with intestinal pseudoobstruction of unknown cause, a search for malignancy, especially small cell carcinoma of lung, must be sought.

Parkinson's Disease

Symptoms of gastrointestinal dysmotility are common in patients with Parkinson's disease. Dysphagia, nausea, bloating, constipation, and difficulty with evacuation occur frequently.[165] Dilatation of the small bowel may be seen radiographically.[166] Small bowel dysmotility does occur; however, its frequency is not known. Manometric studies in Parkinson's disease patients reveal infrequent MMCs, which may even be absent in some cases; hypomotility in the fed state; and an increased incidence of retrograde and tonic contractions compared to controls.[167] The contribution of these abnormalities to symptoms is not clear.

The pathogenesis of small bowel dysmotility is unknown. In patients with dysphagia and megacolon, Lewy's bodies, which are neurons containing cytoplasmic hyaline inclusions, have been found in the myenteric plexus of the esophagus and colon.[168,169] Lewy's bodies were originally identified in the brain and are highly characteristic of Parkinson's disease. To our knowledge, Lewy's bodies have not been reported in the small bowel.

Therapy for Parkinson's disease patients includes drugs that adversely affect gut motility, leading some gastroenterologists to conclude that drug therapy is responsible for gastrointestinal symptoms. However, these symptoms are as common in untreated as in treated patients, suggesting that the disease itself is the primary factor producing dysmotility and resultant symptoms.[165]

Diabetes Mellitus

The small bowel is not as frequently or severely affected in diabetes as the stomach or colon. Many diabetics experience diarrhea, which has a variety of causes (e.g., bacterial overgrowth, pancreatic exocrine insufficiency, bile salt malabsorption, impaired absorption, alterations in gut hormones). Early radiographic studies of the small bowel demonstrated variable findings, including normal, delayed, or rapid transit. Similarly discrepant results are found using the hydrogen breath test, and there is a poor correlation of rapid transit with diarrhea.[170–172] This probably reflects the multiple causes of diarrhea outlined previously.

Pathologically, demyelination of the proximal vagus nerve and sympathetic nerves supplying the bowel occurs in diabetes. The intrinsic nervous system of the gut appears to be unaffected, because no morphologic abnormalities of the myenteric or submucosal plexuses have been observed.[173,174] Although thickening of the small bowel muscle layers and eosinophilic hyaline bodies in smooth muscle cells have been observed,[175–177] most authorities believe that myopathy is not a cause of gastrointestinal dysmotility in diabetes patients.

Motility studies of the small bowel in diabetes patients have shown mixed results. Normal MMCs are found in many patients with documented gastroparesis.[178] Absence of intestinal phase III has been demonstrated in some patients.[170,179,180] Other abnormalities include diminished amplitude of contractions, decreased duration of phase III, MMCs originating in the distal duodenum or jejunum, and occasional bursts of up to 2 minutes of nonpropagated, powerful contractions (Fig. 69-13).[170,179,181] The clinical relevance of these abnormal findings is uncertain. In one study, both manometry and small bowel transit were measured in the same patients, and there was no correlation between abnormal transit time and manometric abnormalities.[170] Hyperglycemia, which can delay gastric emptying, does not affect MMC of the small bowel.[182]

Thyroid Disease

Thyroid dysfunction may present primarily as gastrointestinal disease. Hyperthyroid patients may have diarrhea and steatorrhea, whereas hypothyroid patients frequently complain of constipation.[183–185] Intestinal dysmotility from the altered thyroid state has been historically recognized as the cause of symptoms. This is supported by abnormalities found in the

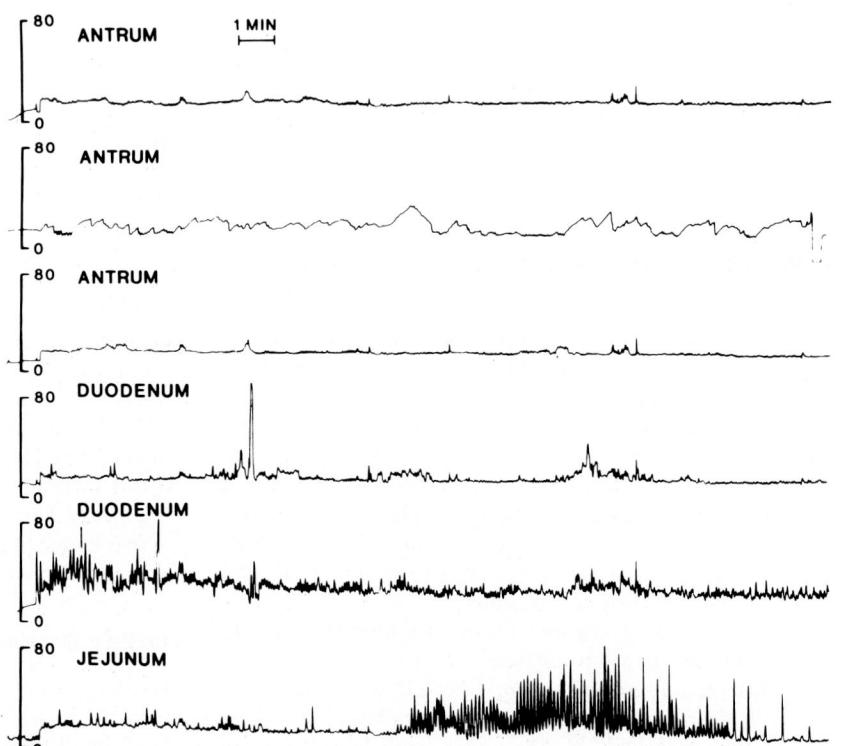

FIGURE 69-13. Small bowel dysmotility in diabetes. In this patient, phase 3 of the migrating motor complex begins in the jejunum with no antecedent activity in the antrum or duodenum. Other patients may have a complete absence of phase 3 activity. (From Dooley CP, El Newihi HM, Zeidler A, et al. Abnormalities of the migrating motor complex in diabetics with autonomic neuropathy and diarrhea. Scand J Gastroenterol 1986;81:217).

intrinsic electrical control of gut motor activity. In the duodenum, slow wave frequencies are increased in hyperthyroid patients and decreased in hypothyroid patients.[186,187] These abnormalities return to normal after correction of the thyroid dysfunction.

Hyperthyroidism. Early radiographic studies using the crude barium meal test reported rapid gastric emptying and small bowel transit.[188,189] Later studies using the hydrogen breath test confirm a rapid orocecal transit time; this is a consequence of accelerated small bowel transit, because the rate of gastric emptying is actually unchanged.[183,190–192] Hyperthyroid patients may present with a malabsorption syndrome; in fact, more than 25% of hyperthyroid patients excrete more than 7 g of fat in their stool daily.[193,194] This is apparently caused by decreased contact time of lumenal contents with small bowel mucosa as a result of rapid transit; this abnormality improves after correction of the hyperthyroid state.

Hypothyroidism. In contrast to hyperthyroidism, small bowel transit is significantly slowed in patients with hypothyroidism.[183] With adequate hormone replacement, transit may be normalized. Many, but not all hypothyroid patients develop constipation; this is probably more a result of colonic rather than small bowel dysmotility. Manometric studies reveal decreased amplitude of small bowel contractions and an overall decreased motility index.[195] With severe hypothyroidism (i.e. myxedema), paralytic ileus and intestinal pseudoobstruction can occur.[196–200]

Hypoparathyroidism

The mechanism by which parathyroid hormone affects gastrointestinal motility is not known. However, calcium is essential for smooth muscle contraction, and the hypocalcemia of hypoparathyroidism may impair gut contractile activity. Intestinal pseudoobstruction and malabsorption have been reported with small bowel dysmotility in hypoparathyroid subjects.[201] Barium studies reveal dilated loops of small bowel and prolonged transit time. Symptoms improve with calcium administration; glucocorticoids may benefit some patients with severe ileus and steatorrhea.

Drug-Induced Small Intestine Dysmotility

Many drugs profoundly affect gastrointestinal motility. Although the colon is usually recognized as the main target organ for drug-induced dysmotility, the small bowel is frequently affected as well. Phenothiazines and some antiparkinsonian drugs decrease colonic and small bowel motility and can cause constipation, colonic pseudoobstruction, and adynamic ileus.[202–205] Tricyclic antidepressants in particular are noted for causing iatrogenic ileus. The anticholinergic agents atropine and scopolamine and related belladonna alkaloids decrease intestinal tone as well as the amplitude and frequency of peristaltic contractions.[206]

Opiate analgesics are well known to suppress motility throughout the gastrointestinal tract. Morphine enhances the amplitude of nonpropulsive small bowel contractions and markedly decreases propulsive contractions by way of receptors in the gut wall.[207,208] The upper small bowel is more prone to these effects than the ileum. The net effect is a decrease in motility and delayed small bowel transit. Using nuclear imaging techniques, morphine and nalbuphine significantly delay small bowel transit compared to placebo.[209]

Ketorolac, a nonsteroidal antiinflammatory agent used for postoperative pain, has significantly less effect on small bowel transit compared with morphine.[210] Whether ketorolac slows motility compared to controls is not known; however, it is generally agreed the nonsteroidal antiinflammatory agents have no effect on gut motility. Loperamide, a synthetic opiate used to treat diarrhea, also reduces small bowel motility and delays transit time. This effect is antagonized by the concomitant administration of naloxone, which by itself has no effect on transit time.[211,212]

Calcium channel antagonists cause constipation in 6% to 10% of patients. In a recent study, small bowel transit time in subjects taking verapamil was unchanged from pretreatment values. Transit through the colon was slowed, however, and this effect likely accounts for the constipation seen with this drug.[213] Clonidine, an α_2-adrenergic agent used as an antihypertensive, prolongs small bowel transit by up to 70% as measured by the lactulose hydrogen breath test.[214,215] Clonidine has been used successfully to treat diabetic diarrhea; however, its therapeutic benefit may also result from its known action of increasing fluid and electrolyte absorption from the gut.[216]

Drugs that stimulate small bowel motility include cisapride, octreotide, erythromycin, and cholinergic agonists. Erythromycin binds to motilin receptors on the smooth muscle of the gastric antrum and duodenum. Motilin, in physiologic doses, induces interdigestive motor complexes in the upper gut. Erythromycin has been used to treat diabetic gastroparesis; the long-term beneficial effects are not as pronounced as the short-term effects.[217] Cholinergic agonists, such as bethanechol, augment the amplitude of small bowel contractions and overall motility.[218]

Octreotide is a long-acting synthetic analog of somatostatin. In normal individuals, it increases the frequency of MMCs by significantly shortening the duration of phase II.[219,220] It was shown to be useful in a small group of scleroderma patients by inducing previously absent phase III contractions and reducing small bowel bacterial overgrowth.[115] When given after a meal, intravenous somatostatin interrupts the fed pattern of motility and induces bursts of propagated activity similar to phase III.[221]

Cisapride is a nondopaminergic prokinetic agent that works by increasing acetylcholine release in the myenteric plexus. It accelerates transit of both liquids and solids through the small intestine[222] and has been found useful in treating patients with chronic intestinal pseudoobstruction.[159] Cisapride induces phase II–type activity in the fasted state and also augments small bowel motility after a meal.[223,224] The latter effect is generated after a small (1000 kcal) meal but is not present with a larger (4200 kcal) meal. Cisapride's prokinetic effects are more pronounced than those of metoclopramide.[225]

Celiac Disease

Four cases of intestinal pseudoobstruction have been reported to occur in association with nontropical sprue.[109,226–228] Dilated small bowel loops with delayed passage of barium are observed radiographically. In one patient who underwent exploratory laparotomy with full-thickness jejunal biopsy, the nerves and muscle coats appeared normal on both light and electron microscopy.[228] Parenteral nutrition may be required during prolonged attacks of pseudoobstruction. To our knowledge, no small bowel motility studies have been performed in patients with celiac disease.

Jejunal Diverticulosis

Diverticula can occur anywhere in the small intestine, but they are most common in the jejunum. Like their counterparts in the colon, they represent herniations through the mesenteric side of the bowel and are usually acquired.[153] Jejunal diverticulosis is associated with many diseases, including scleroderma, celiac disease, Fabry's disease, type II FVM, and Cronkhite-Canada syndrome.[229] Patients present with diarrhea, steatorrhea, weight loss, and megaloblastic anemia. Chronic intestinal pseudoobstruction occurs in jejunal diverticulosis and can mimic mechanical obstruction.[109,230]

Altered small bowel motility underlies the formation of diverticula and bacterial overgrowth, with subsequent malabsorption and steatorrhea. The concept that dysmotility causes diverticula formation and not vice versa is supported by one case report in which resection of the small bowel segment containing diverticula failed to resolve the patient's pseudoobstruction symptoms.[8]

Small bowel manometry shows that all phases of the MMC are present; however, phase I is dominated by spastic contractions all along the bowel. These contractions may be antegrade, simultaneous, or retrograde.[229] Histology of the bowel reflects the heterogenous causes of dysmotility (e.g., visceral neuropathy, visceral myopathy).[231]

Irradiation

Ionizing radiation damages all structures of the small intestine, including mucosa, blood vessels, connective tissue, enteric nerves, and smooth muscle. Radiation damage to the bowel can be separated into acute and chronic injury.

Acute injury. Above a certain threshold dose of radiation to the abdomen, symptoms of nausea, vomiting, abdominal pain, and diarrhea are common. These symptoms abate soon after exposure is discontinued. Reversible changes in small bowel absorptive function have been considered as the main cause of diarrhea. However, newer studies disclose that small bowel dysmotility occurs and may play a significant role in acute radiation enteropathy. In dogs, a large, single dose of radiation abolishes the interdigestive MMC.[232] Smaller, fractionated doses, the method employed for radiation treatment in humans, also result in dysmotility in the dog model. In the fasting state, manometric changes during exposure include an increased frequency of giant migrating contractions and retrograde contractions, with only a mild decrease in MMC cycle length.[233] These changes revert to normal within a few days after exposure. Other studies, however, show decreased intestinal motility, particularly in the distal small bowel, in the fasting and fed state which persists up to 1 month after the last exposure.[234,235]

Motility studies in humans in the acute phase of radiation sickness have not been performed. One study demonstrated accelerated small bowel transit in a group of patients undergoing abdominopelvic irradiation compared with pretreatment values.[236] More than 75% of the patients exhibited diarrhea during treatment.

Chronic injury. Delayed gastrointestinal complications may occur months, years, or even decades after radiation exposure. Both neuronal and muscular structures of the small bowel are affected. The resulting dysmotility leads to bacterial overgrowth, diarrhea, and malabsorption. Edema, atrophy, and fibrosis of smooth muscle fibers is a characteristic histologic finding.[237–240] The myenteric plexus can appear normal on routine staining; however, proliferation of submucosal neurons with extension into the circular muscle coat has been observed.[239,240]

Latent gastrointestinal symptoms from previous radiation damage have been attributed to altered gut motility. Recurrent episodes of intestinal pseudoobstruction have been described in two patients many years after they received abdominal radiation.[240,241] Small bowel contrast studies show dilated loops of bowel with air-fluid levels and thickened bowel wall. Manometric evaluation in one patient revealed normal MMCs in the proximal duodenum, decreased amplitude and frequency of contractions in the distal duodenum, and absence of peristaltic contractions in the jejunum. Subsequent histologic examination of the bowel suggested visceral myopathy as the cause of dysmotility.[240]

Diffuse Lymphoid Infiltration

Four cases of chronic intestinal pseudoobstruction in association with diffuse lymphoid infiltration of the small bowel have been described.[242] All four patients were women who presented with diarrhea at an early age. Histology revealed lymphocytic infiltration of the lamina propria, muscularis propria, and myenteric plexus. The infiltrates were seen to be polyclonal by immunochemical stains, reflecting a pseudolymphoma rather than a true neoplasm. The myenteric plexus appeared normal with routine and silver stains. An absence of smooth muscle cells was found in areas of lymphoid infiltration; therefore, the dysmotility is attributed to a myopathic process.

Jejunoileal Bypass

Recurrent episodes of intestinal pseudoobstruction can occur in patients after jejunoileal bypass for morbid obesity.[109,243] Symptoms begin as early as 1 week postoperatively and consist of abdominal distention and pain, diarrhea, vomiting, and fever. X-ray films reveal massively dilated small bowel loops and occasional pneumatosis cystoides intestinalis. Bacterial overgrowth of the bypassed small intestine causes this enteropathy; small bowel cultures typically grow fecal flora and anaerobes similar to those described in blind loop syndrome. Over time, most patients become either symptom-free or have a significant decrease in the frequency or severity of pseudoobstruction. Intermittent antibiotic therapy may benefit patients with chronic symptoms.

In contrast to intestinal pseudoobstruction, mechanical obstruction secondary to ileal volvulus at the anastomotic site can occur and presents a difficult diagnostic challenge.[244] Contrast radiography may aid in establishing the correct diagnosis. Recurrent acute colonic pseudoobstruction also has been reported after jejunoileal bypass.[245,246]

The effect of bypassing a long segment of small bowel on intestinal motility is unknown. In patients reoperated on for various metabolic or hepatic complications (not the enteropathy described previously), the bypassed segment appears normal, and normal small bowel function is restored after reversal of the bypass.[247]

Spinal Cord Injury

Extrinsic denervation of the small bowel by spinal cord injury usually produces only mild and probably insignificant dysmotility in the small intestine. The only changes revealed in manometric studies performed in a group of patients with spinal cord injury were a greater number of phase III contractions beginning in the duodenum rather than the antrum in patients with high spinal cord lesions.[248] Patients with injury to the lower spinal cord demonstrated no abnormal findings. Another report describes a woman with cervical spinal stenosis and paraplegia who displayed normal MMCs but a twofold to threefold prolonged interval between MMCs.[249] One case of intestinal pseudoobstruction in a spinal cord injury patient has been observed.[109]

Immediately after spinal cord injury, a state of spinal shock develops. This is characterized by complete loss of all sensory, motor, and reflex function below the level of injury. Paralytic ileus with abdominal distention follows and usually resolves in a few days. Chronically, postprandial abdominal distention and discomfort are common, occurring in more than 40% of spinal cord injury patients in one series.[250] The exact cause of these symptoms is unknown. Many stable spinal cord injury patients exhibit increased amounts of gas in the small and large intestine on routine abdominal x-ray films (Fig. 69-14).[251] Colonic dysmotility is well recognized, and is responsible for the high incidence of constipation and difficulty of evacuation in these patients.[252]

Anorexia Nervosa and Bulimia

Both anorexic and bulemic patients frequently complain of bloating and constipation. Delayed gastric emptying of solids is a well-established abnormality in these patients. Recent studies using the lactulose hydrogen breath test in anorexia nervosa patients also reveal a modest delay in orocecal transit.[253,254] This method of measuring small bowel transit is not dependent on gastric emptying of solids, because lactulose is given as a liquid meal. However, wide variability between and within normal subjects has been observed with this technique.[150]

Bulemic patients also have an increased orocecal transit time. Whole-gut transit time, measured by radiopaque markers, is also significantly delayed compared with controls.[254] Additional transit and manometric studies are needed in these patients.

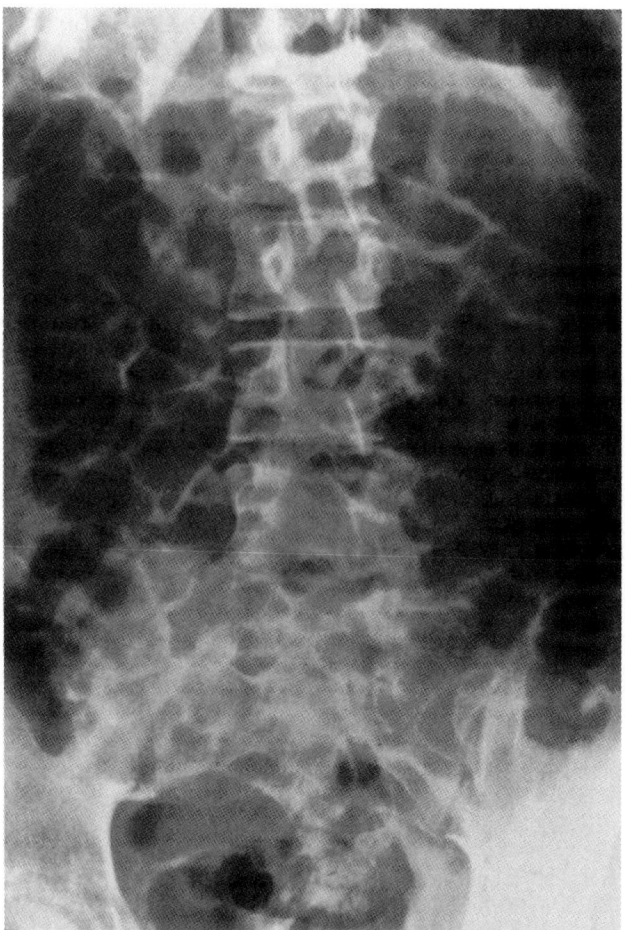

FIGURE 69-14.   Abdominal radiograph from a stable, healthy, spinal cord injury patient. A nonobstructive gassy abdomen is frequently observed, even in the absence of abdominal complaints. (From Gore RM, Mintzer RA. Gastrointestinal complications. In: Calenoff L, ed. Radiology of the spinal cord. St. Louis: CV Mosby, 1981:287.)

CLINICAL MANIFESTATIONS

The small intestine is a vital organ for the absorption of nutrients; therefore, individuals will not survive if a long segment of small intestine does not function or functions poorly. Fortunately, the small intestine is usually the last organ in the gastrointestinal tract to be affected by severe dysmotility. Severe dysmotility of the esophagus, colon, and even the stomach occur much more frequently than dysmotility of the small intestine. It is very unusual to see isolated severe small intestine dysmotility, because most patients with small intestine dysmotility will have dysmotility of other parts of the digestive tract as well. In this chapter, the discussion is limited to the small intestine. Dysmotility of other organs of the digestive tract are discussed in Chapters 54, 60, 81, and 82.

With a few exceptions, most patients with small intestine dysmotility have similar clinical manifestations regardless of the underlying causes. The spectrum of clinical manifestations varies widely (see Fig. 69-1). At one end of the spectrum, the patients may be asymptomatic, and at the other end, the patients may have recurrent symptoms and signs of small intestine obstruction, termed *chronic intestinal pseudoobstruction*. In between these two ends of the spectrum, patients may have recurrent symptoms of postprandial, crampy, periumbilical and epigastric abdominal pains; abdominal bloating; nausea; and vomiting. The symptoms, as a rule, are usually related to eating. Diarrhea can occur in patients with bacterial overgrowth and malabsorption. In severe cases, the patients have episodes of small intestine obstruction or chronic intestinal pseudoobstruction syndrome. These patients have severe postprandial abdominal pain, abdominal distention, nausea, and vomiting. Plain abdominal x-ray films of patients with intestinal pseudoobstruction during attack show multiple air-fluid levels and dilatation of the small intestine. The incidence and severity of recurrent obstructive episodes vary from patient to patient and from episode to episode in the same patient. In some patients, the obstructive episodes may only occur once or twice per year, but in very severe cases, the obstructive symptoms may be persistent.

Physical examinations vary according to the severity of the symptoms. The patients may be cachectic and malnourished as a result of malnutrition because they are unable to take in adequate nutrients, or malabsorption because of bacterial overgrowth in small intestine. The abdomen may be distended and mildly tender. Bowel sounds are inactive and infrequent in patients with smooth muscle dysfunction, but are hyperactive and high pitched in patients with myenteric plexus dysfunction. Borborygmi may be detected in some patients. In less symptomatic patients, abdominal examination may be normal. In patients with chronic intestinal pseudoobstruction, during an obstructive episode, abdominal examination may be indistinguishable from true mechanical obstruction.

As mentioned previously, patients with small intestine dysmotility usually have symptoms of dysmotility of other parts of gastrointestinal tract as well. Therefore, the patients with chronic intestinal pseudoobstruction may have symptoms and signs of multiorgan dysmotility.

Extragastrointestinal manifestations may be detected in some patients, depending on their underlying diseases. Megacystis and megaureters are commonly seen in type I FVM and CVM; these patients may have urinary retention and infection. Mydriasis, ptosis and external ophthalmoplegia may be seen in patients with certain forms of FVM. Ataxia, dysautonomia, and neurologic symptoms may be seen in patients with certain forms of visceral neuropathies. In the secondary forms of small intestine dysmotility, patients may also have systemic manifestations of the underlying disease (e.g., scleroderma, muscular dystrophies).

COMPLICATIONS

Malnutrition

Malnutrition occurs in patients with severe dysmotility of the small intestine as a result of inadequate intake of food and vomiting. Postprandial abdominal pain and bloating limit the patient's oral intake. The patients may be anemic due to iron, folate, and vitamin B_{12} deficiency. Serum cholesterol, calcium, and albumin levels may be low. Supplemental formulas such as Ensure or Vivonex are useful to improve nu-

trition. In severe cases, long-term parenteral nutrition may be the only method to provide adequate nutrients to these patients.

Bacterial Overgrowth in the Small Intestine

Bacterial overgrowth in the small intestine may complicate patients with severe intestinal dysmotility.[28,75,93,255] The small intestine is usually dilated and atonic in these patients. These patients have malabsorption and steatorrhea, which causes additional weight loss. The diagnosis can be made by culturing intestinal aspirate for both aerobic and anaerobic bacteria. A number of different species can be found, and the total concentration of bacteria generally exceeds 10^5 organisms/mL. Another approach to diagnosing bacterial overgrowth is the timed analysis of breath excretion of volatile metabolites produced by intralumenal bacteria. Both measurement of expired labeled CO_2 after oral administration of ^{14}C- or ^{13}C-labeled substrates and breath hydrogen after administration of nonlabeled substrates have been employed. The patients may have macrocytic anemia caused by vitamin B_{12} deficiency. Tetracycline, metronidazole, or ampicillin can be used to treat patients with intestinal bacterial overgrowth. We usually prescribe an antibiotic for 7 to 10 days intermittently, depending on the recurrence of diarrhea. In some cases, an antibiotic may be given for 1 week of every 3 to 4 weeks. Abdominal bloating may improve with antibiotics in some patients.

Pneumatosis Cystoides Intestinalis

Pneumatosis cystoides intestinalis is a rare condition characterized by multiple, gas-filled cysts in the wall of the small and large intestine. Pneumoperitoneum may occur. Pneumatosis cystoides intestinalis can occur in some patients with small intestine dysmotility and dilatation. In most cases, this condition is an incidental finding on radiographs. The pathogenesis is not known, and there is no specific treatment for this condition. Surgery should be avoided in these patients, because it usually causes deterioration of the patient's condition.[108]

DIAGNOSTIC STUDIES

Diagnostic studies for patients with small intestine dysmotility are outlined in Table 69-6.

Blood Tests

A complete blood count may reveal anemia as a result of malnutrition and bacterial overgrowth. Blood chemistries also reflect malnutrition and malabsorption. Diabetic patients have hyperglycemia, and hypoparathyroid patients may have hypocalcemia. Patients with connective tissue disease have a positive antinuclear antibody. Patients with thyroid disease have changes in serum T_3, T_4 and TSH levels. Muscular dystrophy patients may have elevated creatine phosphokinase

(CPK) and isoenzymes. Hemagglutination and compliment fixation for Chagas' disease may be positive in patients with a history of living in Central or South America.

Radiologic Studies

Plain abdominal x-ray films are very useful in patients who complain of abdominal distention and bloating, because they may show gaseous distention of of the gastrointestinal tract. Upper gastrointestinal and small bowel x-ray films may show typical lesions seen in certain types of diseases. Areas affected by severe dysmotility usually are dilated.

Enteroclysis, or small bowel enema,[256] is very useful to detect lesions in the small intestine and rule out mechanical obstruction. Experienced radiologists can identify structural lesions in the small intestine in up to 98% of patients with mechanical obstruction. Barium enema and intravenous pyelogram may be useful in detecting abnormalities of the colon and urinary tract, respectively.

Other Studies

Striated muscle biopsy should be obtained in patients suspected of having muscular dystrophy. Cultures of small bowel aspirates must be obtained in patients with suspected bacterial overgrowth in the small bowel. Small intestine manometric study should be obtained to detect the patterns of the abnormalities.

If a full-thickness biopsy of the dysfunctional part of the intestine is available, careful pathologic examination for abnormalities in the smooth muscle or myenteric plexus with special trichrome and silver stain must be carried out.

Since Szurszewski discovered migrating myoelectric complex in canine small intestine in 1969,[257] a similar phenomenon has been described in various species, including humans. Most of the studies in human small intestine use intralumenal pressure sensors to detect the contractile activities; therefore, the term *migrating motor complex* has been used in place of *migrating myoelectric complex* in these situations. A low-compliance water infusion technique is the most common method used, but miniature transducers[258,259] and radiotelemetry[260] have also been employed.

The small intestine has a unique pattern of motility. During fasting, there is a cyclical pattern of motility called the migrating motor complex (MMC). The MMC is divided into three phases. Phase I is a quiescent period that lasts for about 15 to 30 minutes. Phase II, which lasts for about 60 minutes, is a period of intermittent contractions that increase in frequency with time until phase III is initiated. During phase III, there are intense contractions that propagate aborally from the duodenum to the ileum. Phase III lasts for 4 to 7 minutes. After phase III, the small intestine become quiescent again (i.e., enters phase I) to start a new cycle of the MMC. This cyclical pattern continues until the subject eats. After eating, the MMC is replaced by frequent intermittent contractions, or the fed pattern. The fed pattern usually lasts for 4 to 6 hours, and after it is complete, the fasting pattern or MMC returns.

Small intestine manometric study is a very sensitive method to detect dysmotility of the small intestine, and it has been used to study patients with various types of small intestine dysmotility.[90–91,110–111,133,255,259–277] However, there are no specific motility patterns that are diagnostic for any diseases. Many studies were done in patients with various clinical syndromes instead of specific diseases, which make the results difficult to interpret. Small intestine motility studies have been performed in patients with small bowel bacterial overgrowth,[255] chronic intestinal pseudoobstruction,[261–263] nonulcer dyspepsia,[90–91] orthostatic hypotension,[264] and irritable bowel syndrome.[95–96] Several patterns of small intestine motility were detected in each clinical syndrome, because each of these clinical syndromes is caused by heterogeneous groups of diseases. More meaningful data have been obtained in studies of specific diseases such as FVM,[3,15,25,269–271] nonfamilial visceral myopathy,[28,271] familial visceral neuropathy (FVN),[56,57] nonfamilial visceral neuropathy,[163] scleroderma,[110,111] myotonic dystrophy,[133,277] and diabetes mellitus with gastroparesis.[259,273–276] Several patterns have been recognized in these diseases.

Visceral Myopathic Pattern

In patients with smooth muscle dysfunction, manometry demonstrates a decrease in frequency and amplitude of contractions in the affected segment. This is generally found during both the fast and fed periods. During fasting, the MMC is usually present but is diminished in amplitude. Myoelectric recordings may reveal abnormalities of the slow wave, such as variability in rate or rhythm, and abnormalities in propagation, such as loss of coupling or shortening in the length or even changes in the direction of propagation. These recordings are characteristic of diseases involving the smooth muscle, such as FVM, advanced scleroderma, dermatomyositis, muscular dystrophies, and amyloidosis.[145,148,149,278]

Visceral Neuropathic Pattern

Neurologic disorders tend to produce disorganization and incoordination of motor activity. The MMC is often absent or abnormal in these patients. The MMC is clearly abnormal if no phase III activity occurs within 5 hours of recording after an overnight fast. An abnormal rate of migration, as well as retrograde propagation of the activity front (phase III), also may be noted. Activity fronts may appear to be normal proximally and then arrest or disappear in the more distal segments of the small intestine. In neurologic disorders, the normal fed pattern may not replace the fasted pattern as it should. These abnormalities occur because these motility patterns are regulated by the enteric nervous system. Amplitude and frequency of contractions actually may be increased when the inhibitory innervation and the coordinating function of the enteric nervous system are perturbed. Many of these abnormalities can be seen best during sleep, when motor activity is quite stereotyped. The list of neurologic disorders that have been described as producing manometric abnormalities include diabetes mellitus, Chagas' disease, early scleroderma and amyloidosis, neurofibromatosis, paraneoplastic neuropathy, primary autonomic neuropathy, Parkinson's disease, brain tumors, and multiple sclerosis.[56,154,167,170,181,279–280]

Mechanical Obstruction Pattern

Recurring episodes of intense contractions followed by periods of rest have been observed radiographically in part of the intestine proximal to an obstruction. This phenomenon can be detected manometrically as clustered contractions in conjunction with periods of intervening quiescence lasting longer than 1 minute (Fig. 69-15).[281] The clustered contractions disappear after the obstruction is relieved surgically. In addition to the clustered contractions, occasional simultaneous, prolonged, high-amplitude or giant contractions have been reported in patients with obstruction.[282] It should be empha-

sized that manometry is not the usual way to establish the diagnosis of mechanical obstruction.

Overall, we believe that small intestine manometry is a very sensitive technique in detecting small bowel dysmotility, but it lacks the specificity to diagnose the underlying disease. However, a few patterns described previously may provide some clues as to the underlying causes of the small intestine dysmotility. More studies directed to specific diseases will enable researchers to gather more data on small intestine manometry so it can be used in clinical practice in the future.

DIFFERENTIAL DIAGNOSIS BETWEEN CHRONIC INTESTINAL PSEUDOOBSTRUCTION AND MECHANICAL OBSTRUCTION

Patients with severe dysmotility of the small intestine may develop chronic intestinal pseudoobstruction. Partial small bowel obstruction from adhesions, tumors, intussusception, or stricture can mimic chronic intestinal pseudoobstruction. Features listed in Table 69-7 will help differentiate between these two problems. Enteroclysis is probably the most helpful study to differentiate chronic intestinal pseudoobstruction from mechanical obstruction. In our experience, however, enteroclysis may not be conclusive in differentiating chronic intestinal pseudoobstruction from mechanical obstruction in some patients. In those cases, exploratory laparotomy is necessary to rule out a obstructing lesion.

TREATMENT

Medical Treatments

Drug Therapy to Improve Small Intestine Motility

Theoretically, it is difficult to envision a drug that can either stimulate damaged muscle to contract effectively or normalize the coordinating functions of a damaged myenteric plexus.

Fed - Mechanical Obstruction

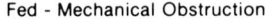
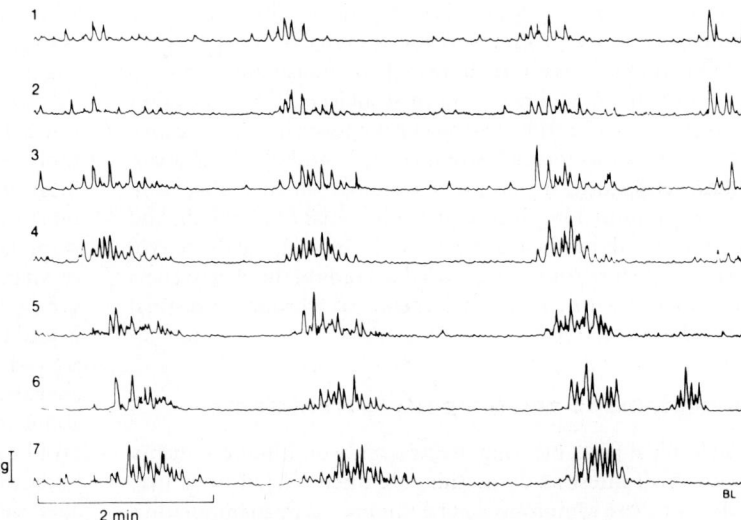

FIGURE 69-15. An example of intestinal contractile activity after a meal in a patient with mechanical obstruction. Multiple clustered contractions separated by long quiescent periods migrate aborally. (From Summers RW, Anuras S, Green J. Jejunal manometry patterns in health. Gastroenterology 1983;85:1297.)

TABLE 69-7
Features That Differentiate Chronic Intestinal Pseudoobstruction From True Mechanical Obstruction

CHRONIC INTESTINAL PSEUDOOBSTRUCTION	MECHANICAL INTESTINAL OBSTRUCTION
Diarrhea or constipation	Constipation and obstipation
May have other gastrointestinal symptoms (e.g., dysphagia or symptoms of gastric atony)	No esophageal or gastric problems
Symptoms of abdominal pain, nausea, vomiting or dysphagia between the attacks	Usually symptom-free between attacks
Cachectic appearance	Seldomly cachectic
May have urinary retention and infection	No urinary symptoms
Symptoms and signs of systemic disease (e.g., scleroderma or muscular dystrophies) if secondary	No underlying systemic disease
May have family history of similar problems	No family history
Plain abdominal radiographs may show air throughout the small bowel and colon	Plain abdominal radiographs show no air beyond the point of obstruction
Esophagram may show esophageal aperistalsis and dilatation	Esophagram is normal
Upper gastrointestinal roentgenograms may show gastric atony and megaduodenum	Upper gastrointestinal may show dilatation of proximal small bowel if the obstruction is in proximal bowel
Small bowel roentgenograms may show gastric atony and megaduodenum	Small bowel roentgenograms show dilatation of bowel proximal to the obstructing lesion
Enteroclysis shows no obstructing lesion	Enteroclysis may show obstructing lesion
Barium enema may show redundant colon or wide-mouthed diverticula	Barium enema may show obstructing lesion
Intravenous pyelogram may show megacystis or megaureter	Intravenous pyelogram is normal
Esophageal manometric studies may show diminished lower esophageal sphincter tone and low amplitude of contractions of lower two-thirds of esophagus	Esophageal manometric studies are normal
Jejunal manometric studies: fasting—absence of one or more phases of migrating motor complexes, low amplitude of contractions, or retrograde and simultaneous contraction; fed—inactive contractions after feeding	Jejunal manometric studies show clusters of contractions during both fasting and fed periods, but migrating motor complexes are present during fasting
No obstructing lesion found during exploratory laparotomy	Obstructing lesion can be identified during exploratory laparotomy

Drugs that stimulate intestinal motility in normal subjects (e.g., bethanechol, prostigmine, metoclopramide, erythromycin) have no beneficial effects in patients with small intestine dysmotility. No information is available on the use of domperidone. Cisapride decreased the transit time of meal through the small bowel in normal subjects,[283] but the effect of short-term cisapride therapy in patients with small intestine dysmotility was inconclusive in a small study.[284] In a small, short-term study, octreotide, a somatostatin analogue, stimulated intestinal motility, reduced bacterial overgrowth, and improved abdominal symptoms in patients with scleroderma.[115] More studies are needed to confirm the effectiveness of these agents in the treatment of chronic intestinal pseudoobstruction.

Symptomatic and Supportive Treatments

Abdominal pain, bloating, nausea, and vomiting in patients with small intestine dysmotility are often related to eating. Most of these symptoms can be minimized by manipulating the amount, nature, and frequency of meals. The important point to keep in mind is to give the patients sufficient calories without overloading the inefficient bowel. A rule of thumb is to give approximately 25 cal/kg of the patient's ideal body weight per day. Adult patients should consume 1500 to 1800 cal/day divided into three or four equal feedings. At least one half of the calories should come from supplemental formulas such as Ensure, Isocal, or Vivonex, because a liquid meal empties faster from the stomach and probably progresses more easily through the small bowel than a solid meal. These formulas are lactose-free and contain the daily requirements of vitamins and minerals. We prefer Vivonex, because it is very low in fat content, does not require any digestion, and is readily absorbable in the small bowel. The patients should try various types of supplemental formulas to find a few that are palatable to them. A dietitian should instruct the patients about the caloric content in each type of food. They must avoid carbonated beverages to prevent adding excessive gas to the digestive tract. When patients still feel full several hours after the first meal, it is important that they do not force themselves to eat subsequent meals to avoid aggravating their symptoms. Some fluid may suffice for that day.

In patients who have chronic intestinal pseudoobstruction, recurrent symptoms and signs of intestinal obstruction may occur despite the previously described regimens. In these situations, nasogastric suction and intravenous fluids are needed when the patients have obstructive symptoms. When the obstructive symptoms and pain persist or occur several times per week despite dietary manipulation, long-term parenteral nutrition is the only treatment that will improve the patients' symptoms and nutrition.

Abdominal pain unrelated to eating is uncommon in patients with small intestine dysmotility. During episodes of obstruction, patients may require parenteral administration of narcotics such as morphine or meperidine. Long-term narcotic use should be discouraged, because the patients will become addicted to them, and narcotics may further disturb gastrointestinal motility.

Constipation is common in patients who also have colon involvement. It is important to make certain that the patients have a good bowel movement at least once every few days, because constipation tends to increase symptoms of intestinal dysmotility. We prescribe 30 to 60 mL of milk of magnesia per day. Tap water enemas may be used if the patients have no bowel movement for 3 days. Bulk-forming laxatives should be avoided in patients with severe small intestine dysmotility, because they only add more load to an inefficient intestine and cause more symptoms.

Treatment of Secondary Causes

A few types of secondary small intestine dysmotility, such as myxedema, celiac sprue, and drug-induced dysmotility, can be treated with thyroid replacement, gluten-free diet, and discontinuation of the offending drugs, respectively. There are no specific treatments for most of the secondary causes of small intestine dysmotility.

Surgical Treatment

Patients who have dysmotility limited to short segments of the small intestine, such as those with megaduodenum, have a better prognosis than those with dysmotility throughout the length of the bowel, because the dysfunctional segment can be resected or bypassed.[285] Megaduodenum, which is commonly seen in type I FVM, scleroderma, and systemic lupus erythematosus patients, can be drained using a side-to-side duodenojejunostomy, which usually gives symptomatic relief to most patients. In some patients with a massively dilated duodenum, a side-to-side duodenojejunostomy may be inadequate to drain the duodenum. In these cases, resection of as much of the duodenum as possible with preservation of the papilla of Vater and anastomosing the opened jejunum to the cut edge of duodenum to create a small conduit may be required to treat these patients.[11,286]

For patients with long segments of small intestine dysmotility (i.e., >1.2 m), there is no effective surgical treatment. Any unnecessary surgery should be avoided in such patients, because it may create adhesions and additional difficulties.

The reader is directed to Chapter 9, Motility of the Small Intestine; Chapter 37, Approach to the Patient With Ileus and Obstruction; Chapter 68, Small Intestine: Anatomy and Structural Anomalies; Chapter 81, Irritable Bowel Syndrome; and Chapter 132, Evaluation of Gastrointestinal Motility: Methodologic Considerations.

REFERENCES

1. Schuffler MD, Pope CE II. Studies of idiopathic intestinal pseudoobstruction. II. Hereditary hollow visceral myopathy: family studies. Gastroenterology 1977;73:339.
2. Lewis TD, Daniel EE, Sarna SK, et al. Idiopathic intestinal pseudoobstruction. Report of a case, with intraluminal studies of mechanical and electrical activity, and response to drugs. Gastroenterology 1978;74:109.
3. Faulk DL, Anuras S, Gardner GD, et al. A familial visceral myopathy. Ann Intern Med 1978;89:600.
4. Shaw A, Shaffer H, Teja K, et al. A perspective for pediatric surgeons: chronic idiopathic intestinal pseudoobstruction. J Pediatr Surg 1979;14:719.
5. Weiss W. Zur Atiologie des Megaduodenums. Deutsch Ztschr Chir 1938;251:317.
6. Law DH, Ten Eyck EA. Familial megaduodenum and megacystis. Am J Med 1961;33:911.
7. Newton WT. Radical enterectomy for hereditary megaduodenum. Arch Surg 1968;96:549.
8. Schuffler MD, Rohrmann CA, Chaffer RG, et al. Chronic intestinal pseudoobstruction. A report of 27 cases and review of the literature. Medicine 1981;60:173.
9. Ducastelle T, Tranvouez JL, Lerebours E, et al. Myopathie viscerale hereditaire: une entité au sein des pseudo-qobstructions intestinales idiopathiques. Gastroenterol Clin Biol 1986;10:355.
10. Rodrigues CA, Shepherd NA, Lennard-Jones JE, et al. Familial visceral myopathy: a family with at least six involved members. Gut 1989;30:1285.
11. Anuras S, Baker CRF Jr, Carter J, et al. Subtotal duodenectomy for massive dilatation of duodenum in patients with type I familial visceral myopathy. Gastroenterology 1990;98:A323.
12. Eaves ER, Schmidt GT. Chronic idiopathic megaduodenum in a family. Aust N Z J Med 1985;15:1.
13. Jones SC, Dixon MF, Lintott DJ, et al. Familial visceral myopathy: a family with involvement of four generations. Dig Dis Sci 1992;37:464.
14. Bannister R, Hoyes AD. Generalised smooth-muscle disease with defective muscarinic-receptor function. Br Med J 1981;282:1015.
15. Anuras S, Mitros FA, Nowak TV, et al. A familial visceral myopathy with external ophthalmoplegia and autosomal recessive transmission. Gastroenterology 1983;84:346.
16. Ionasescu VV, Thompson HS, Aschenbrener C, et al. Late-onset oculogastrointestinal muscular dystrophy. Am J Med Genet 1984;18:781.
17. Anuras S. A new family of small intestinal diverticulosis and external ophthalmoplegia. Gastroenterology 1986;90:1328.
18. Faber J, Fich A, Steinberg A, et al. Familial intestinal pseudoobstruction dominated by a progressive neurologic disease at a young age. Gastroenterology 1987;92:786.
19. Igarashi M, MacRae D, O-Uchi T, et al. Cochleo-Saccular degeneration in one of three sisters with hereditary deafness, absent gastric motility, small bowel diverticulosis and progressive sensory neuropathy. J Otorhinolaryngol Relat Spec 1981;43:4.
20. Mulder NH, Que GS, Bartelink A, et al. Triad of duodenal megabulbus, diverticula and gastric atony in four siblings. Neth J Med 1983;26:120.
21. Bardosi A, Creutfeldt W, DiMauro S, et al. Myo-, neuro-, gastrointestinal encephalopathy (MNGIE syndrome) due to par-

tial deficiency of cytochrome-c-oxidase. A new mitochondrial multisystem disorder. Acta Neuropathol (Berl) 1987;74:248.

22. Cervera R, Bruix J, Bayes A, et al. Chronic intestinal pseudoobstruction and ophthalmoplegia in a patient with mitochondrial myopathy. Gut 1988;29:544.

23. Cave DR, Compton CC. Case records of the Massachusetts General Hospital, Case 12-1990. N Engl J Med 1990;322:829.

24. Jacob E, Ardichvili D, Perissino A, et al. A case of familial visceral myopathy with atrophy and fibrosis of the longitudinal muscle layer of the entire small bowel. Gastroenterology 1979;77:745.

25. Anuras S, Mitros FA, Milano M, et al. A familial visceral myopathy with dilatation of the entire gastrointestinal tract. Gastroenterology 1986;90:385.

26. Alstead EM, Murphy MN, Flanagan AM, et al. Familial autonomic visceral myopathy with degeneration of muscularis mucosae. J Clin Pathol 1988;41:424.

27. Strosberg JM, Peck B, Harris ED Jr. Scleroderma with intestinal involvement: fatal in two of a kindred. J Rheumatol 1977;4:46.

28. Anuras S, Mitros FA, Soper RT, et al. Chronic intestinal pseudoobstruction in young children. Gastroenterology 1986;91:62.

29. Kapila L, Haberkorn S, Nixon HH. Chronic adynamic bowel simulating Hirschsprung's disease. J Pediatr Surg 1975;10:885.

30. Bagwell CE, Filler RM, Cutz E, et al. Neonatal intestinal pseudoobstruction. J Pediatr Surg 1984;19:732.

31. Stafford SJ, Ulshen MH, Mandell J. Familial visceral myopathy. J Urol 1983;131:978.

32. Schuffler MD, Pagon RA, Schwartz R, et al. Visceral myopathy of the gastrointestinal and genitourinary tracts in infants. Gastroenterology 1988;94:892.

33. Glassman M, Spivak W, Mininberg D, et al. Chronic idiopathic intestinal pseudoobstruction: a commonly misdiagnosed disease in infants and children. Pediatrics 1989;83:603.

34. Kaschula RDC, Cywes S, Katz A, et al. Degenerative leiomyopathy with massive megacolon. Myopathic form of chronic idiopathic intestinal pseudoobstruction occurring in indigenous Africans. Perspect Pediatr Pathol 1987;11:193.

35. Jayachandra J, Frank JL, Jonas MM. Isolated intestinal myopathy resembling progressive systemic sclerosis in a child. Gastroenterology 1988;95:1114.

36. Nonaka M, Goulet O, Arahan P, et al. Primary intestinal myopathy, a cause of chronic idiopathic intestinal pseudoobstruction syndrome (CIPS): clinico-pathological studies of seven cases in children. Pediatr Pathol 1989;9:409.

37. Berdon WE, Baker DH, Blanc WA, et al. Megacystis-microcolon-intestinal hypoperistalsis syndrome: a new cause of intestinal obstruction in the newborn. Report of radiologic findings in five newborn girls. AJR Am J Roentgenol 1976;126:957.

38. Wiswell TE, Rawlings JS, Wilson JL, et al. Megacystis-microcolon-intestinal hypoperistalsis syndrome. Pediatrics 1979;63:805.

39. Jona JA, Werlin SL. The megacystis microcolon intestinal hypoperistalsis syndrome: Report of a case. J Pediatr Surg 1981;16:749.

40. Amoury RA, Fellows RA, Goodwin CD, et al. Megacystis-microcolon-intestinal hypoperistalsis syndrome: a cause of intestinal obstruction in the newborn period. J Pediatr Surg 1977;12:1063.

41. Vezina WC, Morin FR, Winsberg F. Megacystis-microcolon-intestinal hypoperistalsis syndrome: antenatal ultrasound appearance. AJR Am J Roentgenol 1979;133:749.

42. Young LW, Yunis EJ, Girdamy BR, et al. Megacystis-microcolon-intestinal hypoperistalsis syndrome: additional clinical, radiologic, surgical and histopathologic aspects. AJR Am J Roentgenol 1981;137:749.

43. Puri P, Lake BD, Gorman F, et al. Megacystis-microcolon-intestinal hypoperistalsis syndrome: a visceral myopathy. J Pediatr Surg 1983;18:64.

44. Oliveira G, Boechat MI, Ferreira MA. Megacystis-microcolon-intestinal hypoperistalsis syndrome in the newborn girl whose brother had prune belly syndrome: common pathogenesis? Pediatr Radiol 1983;13:294.

45. Gillis DA, Grantmyre EB. Megacystis-microcolon-intestinal hypoperistalsis syndrome: survival of a male infant. J Pediatr Surg 1985;20:279.

46. Tomomasa T, Itoh Z, Koizumi T, et al. Manometric study on the intestinal motility in a case of megacystis-microcolon-intestinal hypoperistalsis syndrome. J Pediatr Gastroenterol Nutr 1985;4:307.

47. Winter RM, Knowles SAS. Megacystis-microcolon-intestinal hypoperistalsis syndrome: confirmation of autosomal recessive inheritance. J Med Genet 1986;23:360.

48. Penman DG, Lilford RJ. The megacystis-microcolon-intestinal hypoperistalsis syndrome: a fatal autosomal recessive condition. J Med Genet 1989;26:66.

49. Farrell SA. Intrauterine death in megacystis-microcolon-intestinal hypoperistalsis syndrome. J Med Genet 1988;25:350.

50. Taguchi T, Ikeda K, Shono T, et al. Autonomic innervation of the intestine from a baby with megacystis microcolon intestinal hypoperistalsis syndrome. I. Immunohistochemical study. J Pediatr Surg 1989;24:1264.

51. Kubota M, Ikeda K, Ito Y. Autonomic innervation of the intestine from a baby with megacystis microcolon intestinal hypoperistalsis syndrome. II. Electrophysiological study. J Pediatr Surg 1989;24:1267.

52. Young ID, McKeever PA, Brown LA, et al. Prenatal diagnosis of the megacystis-microcolon-intestinal hypoperistalsis syndrome. J Med Genet 1989;26:403.

53. Dogruyol H, Gunay U, Esmer A, et al. Megacystis-microcolon-intestinal hypoperistalsis syndrome in a newborn after clomiphene ingestion during pregnancy. Z Kinderchir 1987;42:321.

54. Vinograd I, Mogle P, Lernau OZ, et al. Megacystis-microcolon-intestinal hypoperistalsis syndrome. Arch Dis Child 1984;59:169.

55. Roy AD, Bharucha H, Nevin NC, et al. Idiopathic intestinal pseudoobstruction: a familial visceral neuropathy. Clin Genet 1980;18:291.

56. Mayer EA, Schuffler MD, Rotter JI, et al. Familial visceral neuropathy with autosomal dominant transmission. Gastroenterology 1986;91:1528.

57. Anuras S, Mukherjee SK, Dunn D, et al. A new family with autosomal dominant transmitted visceral neuropathy. Gastroenterology 1988;94:A10.

58. Kern IB, Harris MJ. Congenital short bowel. Aust N Z J Surg 1973;42:283.

59. Royer P, Ricour C, Nihoul-Fekete C, et al. Le syndrome familial de grele court avec malrotation intestinale et stonose hypertrophique du pylore dhez le nourrison. Arch Franc Pediatr 1974;31:223.

60. Tanner MS, Smith B, Lloyd JK. Functional intestinal obstruction due to deficiency of argyrophil neurones in the myenteric plexus. Familial syndrome presenting with short small bowel. Gastroenterology 1976;84:346.

61. Laugier MMJ, Mercier C, Robert M, et al. Syndrome de grele court avec malrotation intestinale et stenose hypertrophique der pylore. Bordeaux Med 1975;8:419.

62. Nezelof C, Jaubert F, Lyon G. Syndrome familial associant grele court, malrotation intestinale, hypertrophie du pylore et malformation cerebrale: etude anatomo-clinique de trois observations. Ann Anat Pathol 1976;21:401.

63. Sansaricq C, Chen WJ, Manka M, et al. Familial congenital short small bowel with associated defects. Clin Pediatr 1983;23:453.

64. Harris DJ, Ashcraft KW, Beatty EC, et al. Natal teeth, patent ductus arteriosus and intestinal pseudoobstruction: a lethal syndrome in the newborn. Clin Genet 1976;9:479.

65. Schuffler MD, Bird TD, Sumi M, et al. A familial neuronal disease presenting as intestinal pseudoobstruction. Gastroenterology 1978;75:889.

66. Cockel R, Hill EE, Rushton DI, et al. Familial steatorrhea with calcification of the basal ganglia and mental retardation. Q J Med 1973;42:771.

67. Byrne WJ, Cipel L, Euler AR, et al. Chronic idiopathic intestinal pseudoobstruction syndrome in children—clinical characteristics and prognosis. J Pediatr 1977;90:585.
68. Mitros FA, Schuffler MD, Teja K, et al. Pathologic feature of familial visceral myopathy. Hum Path 1982;13:825.
69. Smith BF. The neuropathology of the alimentary tract. London: Edward Arnold, 1972.
70. Schuffler MD, Jonak Z: Chronic idiopathic intestinal pseudoobstruction caused by a degenerative disorder of the myenteric plexus: the use of Smith's method to define the neuropathology. Gastroenterology 1982;82:476.
71. Bonsib SM, Fallon B, Mitros FA, et al. Urologic manifestations of patients with visceral myopathy. J Urol 1984;132:1112.
72. Faber J, Fich A, Steinberg A, et al. Familial intestinal pseudoobstruction dominated by a progressive neurologic disease at a young age. Gastroenterology 1987;92:786.
73. Murley RS. Painful enteromegaly of unknown aetiology. Proc Roy Soc Med 1959;52:479.
74. Paul CA, Tomiyasu U, Mellinkoff SM. Nearly fatal pseudoobstruction of the small intestine. A case report of its relief by subtotal resection of the small bowel. Gastroenterology 1961;40:498.
75. Naish JM, Capper WM, Brown NJ. Intestinal pseudoobstruction with steatorrhea. Gut 1960;1:62.
76. Bannister R, Hoyes AD. Generalized smooth muscle disease with defective muscarinic-receptor function. Br Med J 1981;282:1015.
77. Smith JA, Hauser SC, Madara JL. Hollow visceral myopathy. Am J Surg Path 1982;6:269.
78. Jayachandar J, Frank JL, Jonas MM. Isolated intestinal myopathy resembling progressive systemic sclerosis in a child. Gastroenterology 1988;95:1114.
79. Smout AJPM, De Wilde K, Kooyman CD, et al. Chronic idiopathic intestinal pseudoobstruction: Coexistence of smooth muscle and neuronal abnormalities. Dig Dis Sci 1985;30:282.
80. Rhodes JB, Robinson RG, McBride N. Sudden onset of slow gastric emptying of food. Gastroenterology 1979;77:569.
81. Meiroff JC, Schreiber DS, Trier JS, et al. Abnormal gastric motor function in gastroenteritis. Ann Intern Med 1980;92:370.
82. Dyer NH, Dawson AM, Smith BF, et al. Obstruction of bowel due to lesion in the myenteric plexus. Br Med J 1969;1:686.
83. Shilkin KB, Gracey M, Joske RA. Idiopathic intestinal pseudoobstruction. Report of a case with neuropathological studies. Aust Paediatr J 1978;14:102.
84. Bogomoletz WV, Birembaut P, Gaillard D, et al. Chronic idiopathic intestinal pseudoobstruction with myenteric plexus damage. Lancet 1979;1:679.
85. Hanks JB, Meyers WC, Andersen DK, et al. Chronic primary intestinal pseudoobstruction. Surgery 1981;89:175.
86. Achem SR, Owyang C, Schuffler MD, et al. Neuronal dysplasia and chronic intestinal pseudoobstruction: rectal biopsy as a possible aid to diagnosis. Gastroenterology 1987;92:805.
87. Nahai F. Pseudoobstruction of the small bowel. Bristol Medico-Chirurgical Journal 1969;84:209.
88. Schuffler MD, Rohrmann CA Jr, Templeton FE. The radiologic manifestations of idiopathic intestinal pseudoobstruction. Am J Roentgenol Radium Ther Nucl Med 1976;127:729.
89. Krishnamurthy S, Heng Y, Schuffler MD. Chronic intestinal pseudoobstruction in twenty-six infants and young children caused by a spectrum of abnormalities of the myenteric plexus. Gastroenterology 1992;102:A471.
90. Malagelada JR, Stanghellini. Manometric evaluation of functional upper gut symptoms. Gastroenterology 1985;88:1223.
91. Abell TL, Kim CH, Malagelada JR. Idiopathic cyclic nausea and vomiting—a disorder of gastrointestinal motility. Mayo Clin Proc 1988;63:1169.
92. Moss AA, Goldberg HI, Brotman M. Idiopathic intestinal pseudoobstruction. Am J Roentgenol Radium Ther Nucl Med 1972;115:312.
93. Lukie BE, Sanders MG. Chronic idiopathic intestinal pseudoobstruction with malabsorption, a scleroderma-like disorder. Can Med Assoc J 1973;109:1222.
94. Kesavarzian A, Isaacs P, McColl I, Sladen GE. Idiopathic intestinal pseudoobstruction and contaminated small bowel syndrome—treatment with metronidazole, ileostomy and indomethacin. Am J Gastroenterol 1983;78:562.
95. Kellow JE, Phillips SF. Altered small bowel motility in irritable bowel syndrome is correlated with symptoms. Gastroenterology 1987;92:1885.
96. Thompson DG, Laidlow JM, Wingate DL. Abnormal small bowel motility demonstrated by radiotelemetry in a patient with irritable colon. Lancet 1979;2:1321.
97. Hoskins LC, Norris HT, Gottlieb LS, et al. Functional and morphological alterations of the gastrointestinal tract in progressive systemic sclerosis (scleroderma). Am J Med 1962;33:459.
98. Bluestone R, MacMahon M, Dawson JM. Systemic sclerosis and small bowel involvement. Gut 1969;10:185.
99. Poirier TJ, Rankin GB. Gastrointestinal manifestations of progressive systemic scleroderma based on a review of 364 cases. Am J Gastroenterol 1972;58:30.
100. Cohen S, Laufer I, Snape WJ Jr. The gastrointestinal manifestation of scleroderma: pathogenesis and management. Gastroenterology 1980;79:155.
101. Horowitz AL, Meyers MA. The "hide-bound" small bowel of scleroderma: characteristic mucosal fold pattern. Am J Roentgenol 1973;119:332.
102. Queloz JM, Woloshin HJ. Sacculation of the small intestine in scleroderma. Radiology 1972;105:513.
103. Meihoff WE, Hirschfield JS, Kern F Jr. Small intestinal scleroderma with malabsorption and pneumatosis cystoides intestinalis. J Am Med Assoc 1968;204:102.
104. Schuffler MD, Beagle RG. Progressive systemic sclerosis of the gastrointestinal tract and hereditary hollow visceral myopathy: two distinguishable disorders of intestinal smooth muscle. Gastroenterology 1979;77:664.
105. D'Angelo WA, Fries JF, Masi AST, et al. Pathologic observations in systemic sclerosis (scleroderma): a study of fifty-eight matched controls. Am J Med 1969;46:428.
106. Arcilla R, Bandler M, Morton F, et al. Gastrointestinal scleroderma simulating chronic and acute intestinal obstruction. Gastroenterology 1956;31:764.
107. Treacy WL, Bunting WL, Gambill EE, et al. Scleroderma presenting as obstruction of the small bowel. Proc Staff Meet Mayo Clin 1962;37:607.
108. Miercort CD, Merrill FG. Pneumatosis and pseudoobstruction in scleroderma. Radiology 1969;92:359.
109. Hirsh EH, Bradenburg D, Hersh T, et al. Chronic intestinal pseudoobstruction. J Clin Gastroenterol 1981;3:247.
109a. Rees WDW, Leigh RJ, Christofides ND, Bloom SR, Turnberg LA. Interdigestive motor activity in patients with systemic sclerosis. Gastroenterology 1982;83:575.
109b. Soudah HC, Hasler WL, Owyang C. Effect of octreotide on intestinal motility and bacterial overgrowth in scleroderma. N Engl J Med 1991;325:1461.
110. Rees WDW, Leigh RJ, Christofides ND, et al. Interdigestive motor activity in patients with systemic sclerosis. Gastroenterology 1982;83:575.
111. Greydanus MP, Camilleri M. Abnormal postcibal antral and small bowel motility due to neuropathy or myopathy in systemic sclerosis. Gastroenterology 1989;96:110.
112. Bortolotti M, Turba E, Tosti A, et al. Gastric emptying and interdigestive antroduodenal motility in patients with esophageal scleroderma. Am J Gastroenterol 1991;86:743.
113. Madsen JL, Hendel L. Gastrointestinal transit times of radiolabeled meal in progressive systemic sclerosis. Dig Dis Sci 1992;37:1404.
114. Horowitz M, Maddern GJ, Maddox A, et al. Effect of cisapride on gastric and esophageal emptying in progressive systemic sclerosis. Gastroenterology 1987;93:311.
115. Soudah HC, Hasler WL, Owyang C. Effect of octreotide on intestinal motility and bacterial overgrowth in scleroderma. N Engl J Med 1991;325:1461.
116. Kleckner FS. Dermatomyositis and its manifestations in the gastrointestinal tract. Am J Gastroenterol 1970;53:141.
117. Feldman F, Marshak RH. Dermatomyositis with significant

involvement of the gastrointestinal tract. Am J Roentgenol 1963;90:746.

118. Malkinson FD, Rothman S. Changes in the gastrointestinal tract in scleroderma and other diffuse connective tissue diseases. Am J Gastroenterol 1956;26:414.

119. Swenson WM, Witkowski LJ, Roskelley RC. Total colectomy for dermatomyositis. Am J Surg 1968;115:405.

120. Hoffman BI, Katz WA. The gastrointestinal manifestations of systemic lupus erythematosus: a review of the literature. Semin Arthritis Rheum 1980;9:237.

121. Brown CH, Shirey EK, Haserick JR. Gastrointestinal manifestations of systemic lupus erythematosus. Gastroenterology 1956;31:364.

122. Shapeero LG, Myers A, Oberkircher PE, et al. Acute reversible lupus vasculitis of the gastrointestinal tract. Radiology 1974;112:569.

123. Dubrow MH, McPherson JR, Bowie JW. Lupus erythematosus presenting as an acute abdomen. Minn Med 1966;49:577.

124. Shafer RB, Gregory DH. Systemic lupus erythematosus presenting as regional enteritis. Minn Med 1970;53:789.

125. Weiser MM, Andres GA, Brentjens JR, et al. Systemic lupus erythematosus and intestinal venulitis. Gastroenterology 1981;81:570.

126. Norman DA, Fleischmann RM. Gastrointestinal systemic sclerosis in serologic mixed connective tissue disease. Arthritis Rheum 1978;21:811.

127. Chiu VSW, Englert E. Gastrointestinal disturbances in myotonia dystrophica. Gastroenterology 1962;42:745.

128. Lups S. Dystrophia myotonica with steatorrhea. Acta Med Scand 1941;106:557.

129. Kemp A. Some metabolic aspects of myotonia dystrophica. Folia Psychiatr Neurol Neurochir Neerlandica 1957;60:88.

130. Harvey JC, Sherbourne DH, Siegel CI. Smooth muscle involvement in myotonic dystrophy. Am J Med 1965;39:81.

131. Lewis TD, Daniel EE. Gastroduodenal motility in a case of dystrophia myotonica. Gastroenterology 1981;81:145.

132. Simpson AF, Khilnani MT. Gastrointestinal manifestations of the muscular dystrophies. Am J Roentgenol 1975;125:948.

133. Nowak TV, Anuras S, Brown BP. Small intestinal motility in myotonic dystrophy patients. Gastroenterology 1984;86:808.

134. Pruzanski W, Huvos AG. Smooth muscle involvement in primary muscle disease. Arch Pathol 1967;83:229.

135. Keschner M, Davison D. Dystrophica myotonica: a clinicopathologic study. Arch Neurol Psychiatr 1933;30:1259.

136. Yoshida MM, Krishnamurthy S, Wattchow DA. Megacolon in myotonic dystrophy caused by a degenerative neuropathy of the myenteric plexus. Gastroenterology 1988;95:820.

137. Bevans M. Changes in the musculature of the gastrointestinal tract and in the myocardium in progressive muscular dystrophy. Arch Pathol 1945;40:225.

138. Huvos AG, Pruzanski W. Smooth muscle involvement in primary muscle disease. II. Progressive muscular dystrophy. Arch Pathol 1967;83:234.

139. Jaffe KM, McDonald CM, Ingman E, et al. Symptoms of upper gastrointestinal dysfunction in Duchenne muscular dystrophy: case-control study. Arch Phys Med Rehab 1990;71:742–44.

140. Korman SH, Bar-Oz B, Granot E, et al. Orocaecal transit time in Duchenne muscular dystrophy. Arch Dis Child 1991;66:143.

141. Crowe GG. Acute dilatation of stomach as a complication of muscular dystrophy. Br Med J 1961;1:1371.

142. Robin GC, de La Falewski G. Acute gastric dilatation in progressive muscular dystrophy. Lancet 1963;2:171.

143. Barohn RJ, Levine EJ, Olson JO, et al. Gastric hypomotility in Duchenne's muscular dystrophy. N Engl J Med 1988;319:15.

144. Leon SH, Schuffler MD, Kettler M, et al. Chronic intestinal pseudoobstruction as a complication of Duchenne's muscular dystrophy. Gastroenterology 1986;90:455.

145. Gilat T, Revach M, Sohar E. Deposition of amyloid in the gastrointestinal tract. Gut 1969;10:98.

146. Gilat T, Spiro HM. Amyloidosis and the gut. Am J Dig Dis 1968;13:619.

147. Feurle GE. Pathophysiology of diarrhea in patients with familial amyloid neuropathy. Digestion 1987;36:13.

148. Legge DA, Carlson HC, Wollaeger EE. Roentgenologic appearance of systemic amyloidosis involving gastrointestinal tract. AJR Am J Roentgenol 1970;110:406.

149. Matsumoto T, Iida M, Hirakawa M, et al. Breath hydrogen test using water-dilated lactulose in patients with gastrointestinal amyloidosis. Dig Dis Sci 1991;36:1756.

150. Amin A, Bilder CR, DiLorenzo C, et al. Inability to standardize the lactulose-hydrogen breath test by feeding (abstract). Gastroenterology 1990;98:322.

151. Legge DA, Wollaeger EE, Carlson HC. Intestinal pseudoobstruction in systemic amyloidosis. Gut 1970;11:764.

152. Wald A, Kichler J, Mendelow H. Amyloidosis and chronic intestinal pseudoobstruction. Dig Dis Sci 1981;26:462.

153. Mitros FA. Motor and mechanical disorders. In: Ming S, Goldman H, eds. Pathology of the gastrointestinal tract. Philadelphia: WB Saunders, 1992:208.

154. Oliveira RB, Meneghelli UG, de Godoy RA, et al. Abnormalities of interdigestive motility of the small intestine in patients with Chagas' disease. Dig Dis Sci 1983;28:294.

155. Köberle F. Enteromegaly and cardiomegaly in Chagas' disease. Gut 1963;4:399.

156. Marshak RH, Freund S, Maklansky D. Neurofibromatosis of the small bowel. Am J Dig Dis 1963;8:478.

157. Davis GB, Berk RN. Intestinal neurofibromas in von Recklinghausen's disease. Am J Gastroenterol 1973;60:410.

158. Camilleri M, Brown ML, Malagelada JR. Impaired transit of chyme in chronic intestinal pseudoobstruction. Correction by cisapride. Gastroenterology 1986;91:619.

159. Feinstat T, Tesluk H, Schuffler MD, et al. Megacolon and neurofibromatosis. A neuronal intestinal dysplasia. Gastroenterology 1984;86:1573.

160. Carney JD, Go VLW, Sizemore GW, et al. Alimentary-tract ganglioneuromatosis, a major component of the syndrome of multiple endocrine neoplasia, type 2b. N Engl J Med 1976;295:1287.

161. Chiappa KH, Young RR. A case of paracarcinomatous pandysautonomia (abstract). Neurology 1973;23:423.

162. Ahmed MN, Carpenter S. Autonomic neuropathy and carcinoma of the lung. Can Med Assoc J 1975;113:410.

163. Schuffler MD, Baird HW, Fleming CR, et al. Intestinal pseudoobstruction as the presenting manifestation of small-cell carcinoma of the lung. Ann Intern Med 1983;98:129.

164. Lhermitte F, Gray F, Lyon-Caen O, et al. Paralysis of digestive tract with lesions of myenteric plexus: a new paraneoplastic syndrome. Rev Neurol (Paris) 1980;136:825.

165. Edwards LL, Pfeiffer RF, Quigley EMM et al. Gastrointestinal symptoms in Parkinson's disease. Mov Disord 1991;6:151.

166. Lewitan A, Nathanson L, Slade WR. Megacolon and dilatation of the small bowel in Parkinsonism. Gastroenterology 1952;17:367.

167. Bozeman T, Anuras S, Hutton T, et al. Small intestinal manometry in Parkinson's disease (abstract). Gastroenterology 1990;99:1202.

168. Qualman SJ, Haupt HM, Yang P, et al. Esophageal Lewy bodies associated with ganglion cell loss in achalasia. Similarity to Parkinson's disease. Gastroenterology 1984;87:848.

169. Kupsky WJ, Grimes MM, Sweeting J, et al. Parkinson's disease and megacolon: concentric hyaline inclusions (Lewy bodies) in enteric ganglion cells. Neurology 1987;37:1253.

170. Dooley CP, El Newihi HM, Zeidler A, et al. Abnormalities of the migrating motor complex in diabetics with autonomic neuropathy and diarrhea. Scand J Gastroenterol 1988;23:217.

171. Keshavarzian A, Iber FL. Intestinal transit in insulin-dependent diabetes mellitus. Am J Gastroenterol 1986;81:257.

172. Scarpello HJB, Greaves M, Sladen GE. Small intestinal transit in diabetes. Br Med J 1976;2:1225.

173. Yoshida MM, Schuffler MD, Sumi SM. There are no morphologic abnormalities of the gastric wall or abdominal vagus in patients with diabetic gastroparesis. Gastroenterology 1988;94:907.

174. Hensley GT, Soergel KH. Neuropathologic findings in diabetic diarrhea. Arch Pathol 1968;85:587.

175. Smith HB. Neuropathology of the esophagus in diabetes mellitus. J Neurol Neurosurg Psychiatr 1974;37:1155.
176. Whalen GE, Soergel KH, Geenen JE. Diabetic diarrhea. A clinical and pathophysiological study. Gastroenterology 1969;56:1021.
177. Duchen LW, Anjorin A, Watkins PJ, et al. Pathology of autonomic neuropathy in diabetes mellitus. Ann Intern Med 1980;92:301.
178. Malagelada JR, Rees WDW, Mazzotta LJ, et al. Gastric motor abnormalities in diabetic and post-vagotomy gastroparesis: effect of metoclopramide and bethanechol. Gastroenterology 1980;78:286.
179. Horowtiz M, Harding PE, Chatterton BE, et al. Acute and chronic effects of domperidone on gastric emptying in diabetic autonomic neuropathy. Dig Dis Sci 1985;30:1.
180. Achem-Karam SR, Funkcoshi A, Vinik AI, et al. Plasma motilin concentration and interdigestive migrating motor complex in diabetic gastroparesis: effect of metoclopramide. Gastroenterology 1985;88:492.
181. Camilleri M, Malagelada JR. Abnormal intestinal motility in diabetics with gastroparesis syndrome. Eur J Clin Invest 1984;14:420.
182. Hsu JJ, Kim CH. The effect of diabetes and hyperglycemia on the interdigestive migrating motor complex (MMC) in man (abstract). Gastroenterology 1990;99:1218.
183. Shafer R, Prentiss R, Bond J. Gastrointestinal transit in thyroid disease. Gastroenterology 1984;86:852.
184. Miller L, Gorman C, Go V. Gut-thyroid interrelationships. Gastroenterology 1978;75:901.
185. Middleton W. Thyroid hormones and the gut. Gut 1971;12:172.
186. Christensen JH, Schedl H, Clifton J. The basic electrical rhythm of the duodenum in normal human subjects and in patients with thyroid disease. J Clin Invest 1964;43:1659.
187. Christensen JH, Clifton J, Schedl H. Variations in the frequency of the human duodenal basic electrical rhythm in health and disease. Gastroenterology 1966;51:200.
188. Shirer JW. Hypermotility of the gastrointestinal tract in hyperthyroidism. Am J Med Sci 1933;186:73.
189. Brown RB, Pendergrass EP, Burdick ED. Hypermotility of the gastrointestinal tract in hyperthyroidism. Surg Gynecol Obstet 1941;73:766.
190. Wegener M, Wedmann B, Langhoff T, et al. Effect of hyperthyroidism on the transit of a caloric solid-liquid meal through the stomach, the small intestine, and the colon in man. J Clin Endocrinol Metab 1992;75:745.
191. Wiley ZD, Larigne ME, Liu KM, et al. The effect of hyperthyroidism on gastric emptying rates and pancreatic exocrine and biliary secretion in man. Dig Dis Sci 1978;23:1008.
192. Miller LJ, Owang C, Malagelada JR, et al. Gastric, pancreatic and biliary responses to meals in hyperthyroidism. Gut 1980;21:695.
193. Middleton WRJ, Thompson GR. Steatorrhea in hyperthyroidism. Gut 1968;9:725.
194. Thomas FB, Caldwell JH, Greenberger NJ. Steatorrhea in thyrotoxicosis. Relation to hypermotility and excessive dietary fat. Ann Intern Med 1973;78:669.
195. Duret RL, Bastenie MD. Intestinal disorders in hypothyroidism. Clinical and manometric study. Am J Dig Dis 1971;16:723.
196. Bastenie PA. Paralytic ileus in severe hypothyroidism. Lancet 1946;1:413.
197. Hohl RD, Nixon RK. Myxedema ileus. Arch Intern Med 1965;115:145.
198. Abbasi AA, Douglass RC, Bissell GW, et al. Myxedema ileus. A form of intestinal pseudoobstruction. J Am Med Assoc 1975;234:181.
199. Boruchow IB, Miller LD, Fitts WT. Paralytic ileus in myxedema. Arch Surg 1966;92:960.
200. Salerno N, Grey N. Myxedema pseudoobstruction. AJR Am J Roentgenol 1978;130:175.
201. Taybi H, Keele D. Hypoparathyroidism: a review of the literature and report of two cases in sisters, one with steatorrhea and intestinal pseudoobstruction. AJR Am J Roentgenol 1962;88:432.
202. Davis JT, Nusbaum M. Chlorpromazine therapy and functional large bowel obstruction. Am J Gastroenterol 1973;60:635.
203. Spiro RK, Kysilewskyj RM. Iatrogenic ileus secondary to medication. J Med Soc N J 1973;70:565.
204. Warnes H, Lehmann HE, Ban TA. Adynamic ileus during psychoactive medication: a report of three fatal and five severe cases. Can Med Assoc J 1967;96:1112.
205. Milner G. Gastrointestinal side effects and psychotropic drugs. Med J Aust 1969;2:153.
206. Taylor P. Atropine, scopolamine, and related antimuscarinic drugs. In: Gilman AG, Goodman LS, Rall TW, Murad F, eds. Goodman and Gilman's the pharmacological basis of therapeutics. 6th ed. New York: MacMillan, 1985:136.
207. Jaffe JH, Martin WR. Opioid analgesics and antagonists. In: Gilman AG, Goodman LS, Rall TW, Murad F, eds. Goodman and Gilman's the pharmacological basis of therapeutics. 6th ed. New York: MacMillan, 1985:503.
208. Burks TF, Galligan JJ, Porreca F. Gastrointestinal drug receptors. J Clin Gastroenterol 1983;5(Suppl 1):29.
209. Yukioka H, Rosen M, Evans KT, et al. Gastric emptying and small bowel transit times in volunteers after intravenous morphine and nalbuphine. Anaesthesia 1987;42:704.
210. Yee MK, Evans WD, Facey PE, et al. Gastric emptying and small bowel transit in male volunteers after i.m. ketorolac and morphine. Br J Anaesth 1991;67:426.
211. Kachel G, Ruppin H, Hagel J, et al. Human intestinal motor activity and transport: effects of a synthetic opiate. Gastroenterology 1986;90:85.
212. Basilisco G, Bozzani A, Camboni G, et al. Effect of loperamide and naloxone on mouth-to-caecum transit time evaluated by lactulose hydrogen breath test. Gut 1985;26:200.
213. Krevsky B, Maurer AH, Niewiarowski T, et al. Effect of verapamil on human intestinal transit. Dig Dis Sci 1992;37:919.
214. Rubinoff MJ, Piccione PR, Holt PR. Clonidine prolongs human small intestine transit time: use of lactulose-breath hydrogen test. Am J Gastroenterol 1989;84:36.
215. Morali GA, Braverman DZ, Lissi J, et al. Effect of clonidine on gallbladder contraction and small bowel transit time in insulin-treated diabetics. Am J Gastroenterol 1991;86:995.
216. Fedorak RN, Field M, Chang EB. Treatment of diabetic diarrhea with clonidine. Ann Intern Med 1985;102:197.
217. Janssens J, Peeters TL, Van Trappen G, et al. Improvement of gastric emptying in diabetic gastroparesis by erythromycin. N Engl J Med 1990;322:1028.
218. Taylor P. Cholinergic agonists. In: Gilman AG, Goodman LS, Rall TW, Murad F, eds. Goodman and Gilman's the pharmacological basis of therapeutics. 6th ed. New York: MacMillan, 1985:103.
219. Peeters TL, Janssens J, Van Trappen GR. Somatostatin and the interdigestive migrating motor complex in man. Regul Pept 1983;5:209.
220. Peeters TL, Romanski KW, Janssens J, et al. Effect of the long-acting somatostatin analogue SMS 201-995 on small intestinal interdigestive motility in the dog. Scand J Gastroenterol 1988;23:769.
221. Neri M, Cuccurullo F, Marzio L. Effect of somatostatin on gallbladder volume and small intestinal motor activity in humans. Gastroenterology 1990;98:316.
222. Edwards CA, Holden S, Brown C, et al. Effect of cisapride on the gastrointestinal transit of a solid meal in normal human subjects. Gut 1987;28:13.
223. Stacher G, Steinringer H, Schneider G, et al. Effects of cisapride on jejunal motor activity in fasting healthy humans. Gastroenterology 1986;90:1210.
224. Stacher G, Gaupmann G, Steinringer H, et al. Effect of cisapride on postcibal jejunal motor activity. Dig Dis Sci 1989;24:1405.
225. Lux G, Katschinski P, Lederer P, et al. Digestive and interdigestive antroduodenal motility—influence of cisapride (c) and metoclopramide (m) in man (abstract). Gastroenterology 1986;90:1527.

226. Ingelfinger FJ. The diagnosis of sprue in non-tropical areas. N Engl J Med 1963;228:180.

227. Naish JM, Capper WM, Brown NJ. Intestinal pseudoobstruction with steatorrhea. Gut 1960;1:62.

228. Dawson DJ, Sciberras CM, Whitwell H. Coeliac disease presenting with intestinal pseudoobstruction. Gut 1984;25:1003.

229. Case Records Massachusetts General. Abdominal pain and vomiting in a 64 year-old man with chronic malabsorption and diarrhea. N Engl J Med 1990;322:1796.

230. Nelson PA, Schmitz RL, Narsete EM. Jejunal diverticulosis complicated by chronic "non-mechanical" obstruction. Ill Med J 1954;106:371.

231. Krishnamurthy S, Kelly MM, Rohrmann CA, et al. Jejunal diverticulosis. Gastroenterology 1983;85:538.

232. Summers RW, Flatt AJ, Prihoda M, et al. Small intestinal motility in dogs after irradiation injury. Dig Dis Sci 1987;32:1402.

233. Otterson MF, Sarna SK, Moulder JE. Effects of fractionated doses of ionizing radiation on small intestinal motor activity. Gastroenterology 1988;95:1249.

234. Otterson MF, Sarna SK, Lee MB. Fractionated doses of ionizing radiation after postprandial small intestinal motor activity. Dig Dis Sci 1992;37:709.

235. Summers RW, Glenn CE, Flatt AJ, et al. Does irradiation produce irreversible changes in canine jejunal myoelectric activity? Dig Dis Sci 1992;37:716.

236. Fernández-Bañares F, Villá S, Esteve M, et al. Acute effects of abdominopelvic irradiation on the orocecal transit time: its relation to clinical symptoms, and bile salt and lactose malabsorption. Am J Gastroenterol 1991;86:1771.

237. Novak JM, Collins JT, Donowitz M, et al. Effects of radiation on human intestinal tract. J Clin Gastroenterol 1979;1:9.

238. Warren S, Friedman NB. Pathology and pathologic diagnosis of radiation lesions in the gastrointestinal tract. Am J Pathol 1942;18:499.

239. Schier J, Symmonds RF, Dahlin DC. Clinicopathologic aspects of actinic enteritis. Surg Gynecol Obstet 1964;199:1019.

240. Perino LE, Schuffler MD, Mehta SJ, et al. Radiation-induced recurrent intestinal pseudoobstruction. Gastroenterology 1986;91:994.

241. Conklin JL, Anuras S. Radiation-induced recurrent intestinal pseudoobstruction. Am J Gastroenterol 1981;75:440.

242. McDonald GB, Schuffler MD, Kadin ME, et al. Intestinal pseudoobstruction caused by diffuse lymphoid infiltration of the small intestine. Gastroenterology 1985;89:882.

243. Drenick EJ, Ament ME, Finegold SM, et al. Bypass enteropathy: an inflammatory process in the excluded segment with systemic complications. Am J Clin Nutr 1977;30:76.

244. Ackerman NB, Abou-Mourad NN. Obstructive, pseudoobstructive and enteropathic syndromes after jejunoileal bypass. Surg Gynecol Obstet 1979;148:168.

245. Barry RE, Benfield JR, Nicell P, et al. Colonic pseudoobstruction: a new complication of jejunoileal bypass. Gut 1975;16:903.

246. Fikri E, Cassella RR. Jejunoileal bypass for morbid obesity; results and complications in fifty-two patients. Ann Surg 1974;179:460.

247. Sherman CD Jr, Faloon WW, Flood MS. Revision operations after bowel bypass for obesity. Am J Clin Nutr 1977;30:98.

248. Fealy RD, Szurszewski JH, Meritt JL, et al. Effect of spinal cord transection on human upper gastrointestinal motility and gastric emptying. Gastroenterology 1984;87:69.

249. Hellstrom PM, Aly A, Johansson CJ. Cisapride stimulates small intestinal motility and relieves constipation in myelopathy due to cervical stenosis: case report. Paraplegia 1990;28:261.

250. Stone JM, Nino-Murcia M, Wolfe VA, et al. Chronic gastrointestinal problems in spinal cord injury patients: a prospective analysis. Am J Gastroenterol 1990;85:1114.

251. Gore RM, Mintzer RA. Gastrointestinal complications. In: Calenoff L, ed. Radiology of the spinal cord. St. Louis: Mosby, 1981;278.

252. Hodges DS. Extrinsic nerve dysfunction causing gastrointestinal dysmotility. In: Anuras S, ed. Motility disorders of the gastrointestinal tract. New York: Raven Press, 1992;262.

253. Hirakawa M, Okada T, Iida M, et al. Small bowel transit time measured by hydrogen breath test in patients with anorexia nervosa. Dig Dis Sci 1990;35:733.

254. Kamal N, Chami T, Andersen A, et al. Delayed gastrointestinal transit times in anorexia nervosa and bulimia nervosa. Gastroenterology 1991;101:1320.

255. Vantrappen G, Janssens J, Hellemans J, et al. The interdigestive motor complex of normal subjects and patients with bacteria overgrowth of the small intestine. J Clin Invest 1977;59:1158.

256. Miller RE, Sellink JL. Enteroclysis: the small bowel enema. Radiology 1979;4:269.

257. Szurszewski JH. A migrating electric complex of the canine small intestine. Am J Physiol 1969;217:1757.

258. Mathias JR, Sninsky CA, Millar HD, et al. Development of an improved multipressure-sensor probe for recording muscle contractions in human intestine. Dig Dis Sci 1985;30:119.

259. Malagelada JR, Rees WDW, Mazzotta LJ, et al. Gastric motor abnormalities in diabetic and postvagotomy gastroparesis: effect of metoclopramide and bethanechol. Gastroenterology 1980;78:286.

260. Thompson DG, Wingate DL, Archer L, et al. Normal patterns of human upper small bowel motor activity recorded by prolonged radiotelemetry. Gut 1980;21:500.

261. Summers RW, Anuras S, Green J. Jejunal manometry patterns in health, partial intestinal obstruction, and pseudoobstruction. Gastroenterology 1983;85:1290.

262. Kumpuris DD, Brannan PG, Goyal RK. Characterization of motor activity in the jejunum of normal subjects and two patients with idiopathic intestinal pseudo-obstruction syndrome (IPPS) (abstract). Gastroenterology 1979;76:1177.

263. Stanghellini V, Camilleri M, Malagelada JR. Chronic idiopathic intestinal pseudo-obstruction: clinical and intestinal manometric findings. Gut 1987;28:5.

264. Camilleri M, Malagelada JR, Stanghellini V, et al. Gastrointestinal motility disturbance in patients with orthostatic hypotension. Gastroenterology 1983;88:1852.

265. Stanghellini V, Malagelada JR, Zinsmeister AR, et al. Stress-induced gastroduodenal motor disturbances in humans: possible humoral mechanisms. Gastroenterology 1983;85:83.

266. Thompson DG, Richelson E, Malagelada JR. Perturbation of gastric emptying and duodenum motility through the central nervous system. Gastroenterology 1982;83:1200.

267. Anuras S, Sutherland J. Small intestinal manometry in health elderly subjects. J Am Geriatr Soc 1984;32:581.

268. Huston WR, Rockrkasse RL, Wald A. Influence of gender and menopause on gastric emptying and motility. Gastroenterology 1989;96:11.

269. Sugerbaker DJ, May RJ, Goyal RK. The spectrum of small bowel motility abnormalities in patients with familial hollow visceral myopathy (HVM) (abstract). Gastroenterology 1984;86:1269.

270. Anuras S. Small intestinal manometric studies in patients with familial visceral myopathies (FVM's). Gastroenterology 1986;90:1269.

271. Tomomasa T, Itoh Z, Koizumi T, et al. Manometric study on the intestinal motility in a case of megacystis-microcolon-intestinal hypoperistalsis syndrome. J Pediatr Gastroenterol Nutr 1985;4:308.

272. Soffer EE, Strottmann MP, Anuras S. Elevated ANA titers in patients with severely abnormal gastrointestinal motility. Dig Dis Sci 1984;29(8):735.

273. Camilleri M, Malagelada JR. Abnormal intestinal motilin in diabetics with the gastroparesis syndrome. Eur J Clin Invest 1984;14:420.

274. Achem-Karam SR, Funakoshi A, Vinik AI, et al. Plasma motilin concentration and interdigestive migrating motor complex in diabetic gastroparesis: effect of metoclopramide. Gastroenterology 1985;88:492.

275. Mearin F, Camilleri M, Malagelada JR. Pyloric dysfunction in diabetics with recurrent nausea and vomiting. Gastroenterology 1986;90:1919.

276. Dooley CP, El Newihi HM, Zeidler A, et al. Abnormalities of migrating motor complex in diabetics with autonomic neuropathy and diarrhea. Scand J Gastroenterol 1988;23:217.

277. Lewis TD, Daniel EE. Gastroduodenal motility in a case of dystrophy myotonica. Gastroenterology 1981;81:145.

278. Battle WM, Rubin MR, Cohen S, et al. Gastrointestinal motility dysfunction in amyloidosis. N Engl J Med 1979;301:24.

279. Malagelada JR, Camilleri M, Stanghellini V. Manometric diagnosis of gastrointestinal motility disorders. New York: Thieme, 1986.

280. Summers RW, Karacis JJ, Anuras S. Pseudo-obstruction syndrome in multiple sclerosis. J Gastrointest Motil 1991;3(3):144.

281. Summers RW, Anuras S, Green J. Jejunal manometry patterns in health, partial intestinal obstruction and pseudoobstruction. Gastroenterology 1983;85:1290.

282. Camilleri M. Jejunal manometry in distal subacute mechanical obstruction: significance of prolonged simultaneous contractions. Gut 1989;30:468.

283. Edwards CA, Holden S, Brown C, et al. Effect of cisapride on gastrointestinal transit of a solid meal in normal subjects. Gut 1987;28:13.

284. Camilleri M, Malagelada JR, Abell TL, et al. Effects of six week treatment with cisapride in gastroparesis and intestinal pseudoobstruction. Gastroenterology 1989;96:704.

285. Anuras S, Shirazi S, Gardner GD, et al. Surgical treatments familial visceral myopathy. Ann Surg 1979;189:306.

286. Anuras S, Shirzai SS. Severe gastrointestinal motility disturbance mimicking bowel obstruction. Clin Surg Int 1987;13:1253.

Textbook of Gastroenterology, second edition, edited by Tadataka Yamada. JB Lippincott Company, Philadelphia © 1995.

CHAPTER 70

Small Intestine: Infections With Common Bacterial and Viral Pathogens

Herbert L. DuPont
Abraham G. Miranda

Methods of Diarrhea Production in the Gastrointestinal Tract
Travelers' Diarrhea
  Source and Etiology
  Prevention and Treatment

Food Poisoning and Common-Source Outbreaks
  Epidemiology
  Etiology

Infections of the gastrointestinal tract can be manifested by a number of different symptoms and signs that include generalized complaints (malaise, backache, headache, lassitude), fever, abdominal pain or cramps, nausea, vomiting, and diarrhea. Of these, diarrhea is by far the most widely recognized and constant marker of intestinal infection. Hence, the study of diarrhea and its etiologies make up the bulk of the data accumulated thus far on the subject of gastrointestinal infections.

Although there are many definitions of diarrhea that take into consideration stool volume, weight, and frequency of effluent, the simplest and most amenable to interpretation is one proposed by Alonso Palmer in 1887: "when a person has abnormally profuse, frequent, and liquid intestinal evacuations, not the immediate effect of a cathartic medicine, he is said to have diarrhea."[1] The true scope of diarrheal illness is difficult to assess; however, estimates of enteric infections in the United States reveal an annual incidence of 25 million illness cases.[2] In the world as a whole, diarrheal disease is calculated to cause more than 1 billion illness episodes and 5 million deaths per year.[3] Table 70-1 lists the average frequencies of specific pathogens in the United States, developing nations, and those commonly found in the diarrhea of travelers. The epidemiology of these enteropathogens, however, can vary significantly with the particular season, geographic location, and the age group being surveyed (e.g., rotavirus is probably the most common cause of diarrhea in infants during the winter months in the United States). No comprehensive surveys exist that accurately reflect the prevalence of specific pathogens in multiple areas of the world, taking into account season- and age-related differences. Such an undertaking would be impossible, or at least superficial given the major differences in geographic, climatic, and host factors that exist.

METHODS OF DIARRHEA PRODUCTION IN THE GASTROINTESTINAL TRACT

Our understanding of the small bowel pathophysiologic mechanisms that lead to diarrhea has expanded tremendously in just two decades. A full discussion of these mechanisms under normal and pathologic states is beyond the scope of this chapter, and they are dealt with elsewhere in this book (see Chap. 38). A brief discussion follows.

Significant diarrheal disease of small bowel origin is usually associated with active secretion or malabsorption of cations and water.[4] Under normal circumstances, the small intestine absorbs between 5 to 9 L of fluid in a day, and the colon is able to retain approximately 2 L of this fluid before emptying. These two factors (presence of intralumenal fluid and electrolytes plus reservoir capacity of the colon) explain why diarrhea of small bowel origin is characterized by the passage of a small number of voluminous stools. In contrast, small-volume stools, often containing blood, pus, and mucus, are characteristic of colonic involvement. Intestinal secretion characteristically occurs as a result of elaborated bacterial exotoxins that work through cyclic nucleotides and intracellular calcium-dependent pathways (see Chap. 14). The agents that produce such exotoxins include *Vibrio cholerae*, enterotoxigenic *Escherichia coli* (ETEC), *Clostridium perfringens*, *Shigella* species, *Yersinia enterocolitica* and *Aeromonas* species. The prototypic small bowel pathogen producing secretory diarrhea is *V cholerae*. In Figure 70-1, the action of cholera toxin is schematically depicted.

Malabsorption results when the intestine is unable to digest its contents secondary to destruction of brush border enzymes (disaccharidase deficiency characteristically produced by viral agents, *Giardia* species, or ETEC) or to destruction of the digestive cells themselves by invasive microorganisms (*Salmonella* species, enteroinvasive *E coli*, protozoa, or viral agents). Finally, abnormal motility patterns may influence gastrointestinal symptoms in enteric infection. The contribution of motility alteration to acute diarrhea is largely an unstudied area.

TRAVELERS' DIARRHEA

International travelers are estimated in the range of 300 million, with an annual expenditure of over $100 billion.[5] A varying frequency of occurrence of diarrhea in travelers has led to the formulation of maps that essentially divide the world into high-, intermediate-, and low-risk areas for the development of travelers' diarrhea.[6] It is not by chance that high-risk areas correspond to developing areas of the world where rates of endemic diarrhea are highest, and include Latin America, Africa, the Middle East, and Asia.[7,8] Conversely, highly developed nations such as the United States, Canada, Northern Europe, New Zealand, Australia, South Africa, and some Caribbean islands pose the lowest risk for development of travelers' diarrhea.[9,10] Intermediate-risk areas include Southern Europe, China, the Soviet Union, and a few Caribbean is-

---

TABLE 70-1
Epidemiology of Infectious Diarrhea: Approximate Frequency of Etiologic Agent by Geographic Location

	GEOGRAPHIC LOCATION AND SPECIFIC POPULATION (%)		
ETIOLOGIC AGENT	U.S. Children	Developing Tropical Countries	U.S. Travelers to Developing Countries
Shigella sp	3–15	3–15	10
Salmonella sp	4	4	7
Campylobacter jejuni	3–15	3–15	3–15
Aeromonas sp	1	1–8	1–8
Plesiomonas shigelloides	<1	1–3	1–4
ETEC	<2	10–20	5–40†
EPEC	4	4	<1
Rotavirus	20–30‡	15–30	<10
Giardia lamblia	4	4	<2
Unknown	60	30–40	20

ETEC, enterotoxigenic *Escherichia coli*; EPEC, enteropathogenic *E. coli* (classic serotypes).

* Lower frequency in rainy summer, higher in drier winter.

† Lower frequency in drier winter, higher in rainy summer.

‡ Higher frequency in winter.

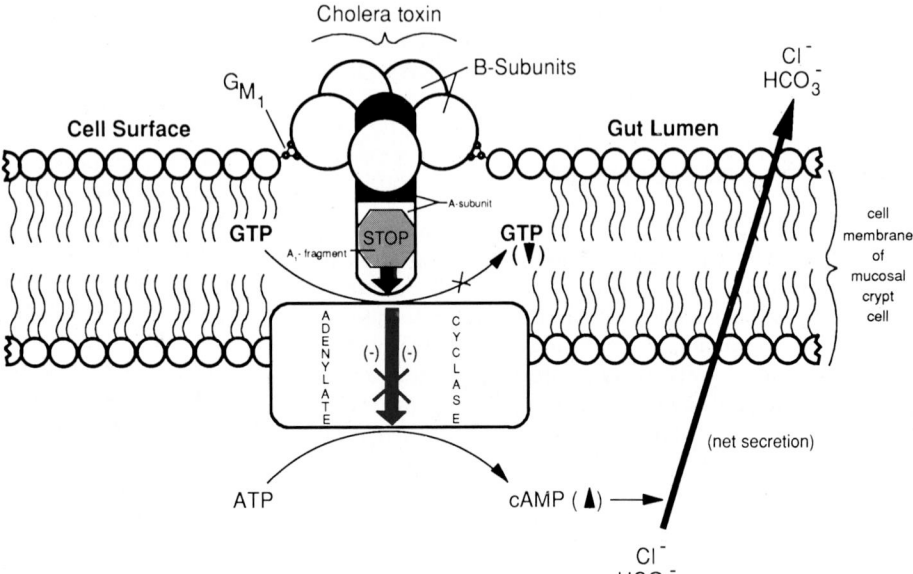

FIGURE 70-1. Mechanism of action of cholera toxin. The five B-subunits of cholera toxin bind to G_{M_1} on the cell surface. The A-subunit is internalized, where the A_1-fragment inhibits the GTPase activity, which regulates production of cAMP by adenylate cyclase. By turning off GTPase activity, adenylate cyclase is no longer inhibited, and cAMP is perpetually produced. This process is irreversible. (ATP, adenosine triphosphate; cAMP, cyclic adenosine monophosphate; GTP, guanosine triphosphate.)

lands.[9,11] Travelers at risk for development of diarrhea mostly comprise those people from industrialized countries traveling to high-risk areas of the world for periods of up to 1 month, and number at least 16 million per year from the United States alone.[5] Attack rates, which can range from 20% to 50% depending on the region visited, become lower as travelers remain in these countries for longer periods of time. Mortality is low to nonexistent, but morbidity can be considerable, confining the traveler to bed in up to 30% of cases, or altering 40% of itineraries.[12] It also is true that travelers from high-risk areas of the world have diarrhea in destinations within the developed world. This illness, however, tends to be mild, clinically unimportant, and may relate to more frequent reliance on public rather than private eating establishments, alterations in diet, alcohol consumption, and emotional disturbances.[10,13]

The features of travelers' diarrhea are quite variable. In general, men and women are equally affected, but travelers' diarrhea is more common in younger than in older people, which may well be the result of adventurous dietary and living habits. Most travelers' diarrhea occurs within the first week of travel and can occur once or more than once at any time during the visit or on returning home. The typical duration of diarrhea is 3 to 4 days, and the patient passes an average of four to five unformed stools per day. Abdominal cramping is common and 15% may experience fever, bloody stools, or both.[5]

Source and Etiology

Travelers' diarrhea usually is acquired by way of the fecal–oral route through ingestion of contaminated food or drink. Studies have suggested that, contrary to popular belief, it is the food, and not the water, that contributes most frequently to the development of travelers' diarrhea.[14,15] This is not to say that water can be discounted as a potential source of enteric pathogens. In studies conducted in Guadalajara, and elsewhere

in Mexico, tap water samples were shown to contain large numbers of coliforms, enteric viruses, and rotavirus.[16]

The fact that most diarrhea of travelers is caused by pathogenic bacteria, including culture-negative cases, is supported by antibiotic prophylactic studies that demonstrate greater than 90% protection rate against development of illness.[17] Also, antimicrobials have been shown to be effective in treating the illness regardless of whether an etiologic bacterial pathogen is identified.

The single most important etiologic agent in travelers' diarrhea in most countries where studies have been carried out remains ETEC, accounting for approximately 28% to 72% of travelers' diarrhea, as shown in Table 70-1. The organism was shown to have a striking seasonal pattern in two semitropical areas (Mexico and Morocco), being common in the more rainy summertime and unusual in the dryer wintertime.[18,19] In contrast, *Campylobacter jejuni* occurs in up to 15% of cases in the dryer wintertime in these areas and is less commonly found in the summer. *Shigella* sp account for 3% to 25% of cases of travelers' diarrhea. Nontyphoid *Salmonella* species are found with a slightly lower frequency.

Rotavirus has been implicated in travelers' diarrhea in adults in Mexico, and was the most commonly identified cause of diarrhea during winter among U.S. troops in South Korea. Rates of viral diarrhea in travelers are not known with certainty, but estimates range between 0% and 36%.[5] Norwalk virus seroconversion has been reported in 10% to 15% of travelers. Rotavirus, Norwalk virus, and other enteric viruses including astrovirus, calicivirus, adenovirus, and coronavirus may play a role in travelers' diarrhea, and may comprise a percentage of diarrhea for which an organism cannot ordinarily be identified.

Parasitic infections are not major causes of travelers' diarrhea, but parasites occasionally can be important pathogens in prolonged or recurrent infections. Together, parasites may comprise between 0% and 9% of travelers' diarrhea. *Giardia lamblia* should be suspected in people traveling to Russia or mountainous areas of the United States or Canada (especially if exposed to surface water), or when diarrhea is prolonged or recurrent. *Cryptosporidium* species also has been shown to be an important cause of diarrhea among travelers to St. Petersburg, Russia.[20]

Prevention and Treatment

With food being the major culprit, it is reasonable to pay close attention to what is consumed where, to prevent this illness. In general, foods should be selected that are served piping hot. Raw vegetables, raw meat or seafood, and other moist foods maintained at room temperature are high-risk items. In addition, milk, dairy products, tap water, and ice usually can be considered unsafe. Safe food items include boiled or iodine- or chlorine-treated water, carbonated beverages and beer, wine, hot coffee or tea, fruits that can be peeled, dry breads (not pastries), and canned products. Likewise, food prepared by oneself is safe, but risk for development of travelers' diarrhea increases when eating at restaurants, and particularly when eating food purchased from street vendors.[15]

Prophylaxis studies show that doxycycline, trimethoprim-sulfamethoxazole (TMP-SMX), trimethoprim alone, or norfloxacin are effective in significantly reducing the incidence of travelers' diarrhea.[21-25] The use of prophylactic antibiotics, however, carries the risk of adverse effects such as photosensitivity (primarily with doxycycline), hematologic and skin disorders, and antibiotic-associated colitis, particularly if use is prolonged. One nonantibiotic drug, bismuth subsalicylate (Pepto-Bismol), whether in liquid form (2 ounces four times a day) or tablet form (two tablets four times a day), has been shown to impart protection rates against travelers' diarrhea of 62% to 65%.[26,27] Apart from blackened stools and occasional minimal tinnitus, this product is well tolerated by most travelers. Prophylaxis can be used for people with important underlying diseases (achlorhydria associated with previous gastric surgery or drugs like omeprazole, active inflammatory bowel disease, immunodeficiency states, or serious medical disorders). For others who have inflexible travel itineraries and cannot tolerate even minor inconvenience, and in others who wish prophylaxis after accepting the associated problems, bismuth subsalicylate may be used. For most travelers, self-therapy is preferred to prophylaxis as an approach to illness.

In the treatment of travelers' diarrhea, as in other forms of the illness, drugs that work symptomatically and antimicrobial agents play a role in selected cases. Antimotility agents, such as diphenoxylate (Lomotil) and loperamide (Imodium) are synthetic opiates effective in relieving abdominal cramping and frequency of diarrhea; however, they should not be used if fever or dysentery is present or for periods in excess of 48 hours.

The following are general recommendations to follow in the treatment of diarrhea:

1. Oral fluids and prevention of dehydration should always be the mainstay of therapy in all forms of diarrhea.
2. With mild to moderately severe symptoms, bismuth subsalicylate (1 ounce every 30 minutes for a total of 8 ounces) or an antimotility agent such as loperamide (4 mg initially, followed by 2 mg after each unformed stool, not to exceed 8 mg/day [over-the-counter doses] or 16 mg/day [prescription dose]) may be given.

3. For severe illness (more than six unformed stools in 24 hours together with disabling symptoms) or that associated with fever or passage of bloody, mucoid stools, an antimicrobial agent probably should be used: TMP-SMX (160 mg TMP/800 mg SMX) for travel to the interior of Mexico in summer and a quinolone for other places and other times of the year; norfloxacin 400 mg, or ciprofloxacin 500 mg, or ofloxacin 300 mg, with each drug given twice daily for 3 days. For milder cases without fever or dysentery, single-dose therapy is effective. For the patient without fever or dysentery, the combination of the antimicrobial agent with loperamide may be optimal therapy. For pregnant women, oral fluid therapy is the preferred treatment of travelers' diarrhea. For more severe cases occurring during travel to central Mexico during the summer, TMP-SMX is appropriate. The quinolones are not used in pregnancy because of possible damage to articular cartilage in the fetus.

FOOD POISONING AND COMMON-SOURCE OUTBREAKS

Epidemiology

Food can easily serve as a culture medium and vehicle of transmission for microbial agents, particularly if it is improperly cooked or left unrefrigerated before consumption. Water also frequently serves as a vehicle for common-source outbreaks of gastroenteritis (and other illnesses).

The Centers for Disease Control (CDC), which publishes annual summaries of food-borne illness in the United States, in 1987 reported 136 outbreaks in the United States.[28] During that time, the total number of illness cases from the various reported outbreaks amounted to 9652. In 61% of the outbreaks, a bacterial agent was identified, with chemicals causing 8%, parasitic agents (*Trichinella spiralis*) 3%, and viral agents 7% (Table 70-2). Mortality from this type of illness is rare, with 5 deaths reported in 1987.

Water-borne disease outbreaks (also reported by the CDC) in 1985 revealed *G lamblia* to be the most commonly involved organism, followed by *Campylobacter jejuni*.[29] Large community outbreaks of water-borne enteric infection may occur as a result of water contamination by *Cryptosporidium* species, as occurred in Milwaukee in 1993. Viruses, particularly Norwalk and others (i.e., rotavirus), are frequently transmitted through water and likely accounted for part of the 57% of cases in which no agent was isolated that year. Although water-borne disease seems to be experiencing a decline in the United States, this trend has not been observed for food-borne illness, and, in fact, the figures presented herein may underestimate the scope of the problem by a factor of 10 to 100. The epidemiology of food- and water-borne disease also varies with geographic location and dietary and sanitation standards. For example, in the United States, *Salmonella* species is the primary cause of food-borne illness, whereas *Vibrio parahaemolyticus* causes 70% of the outbreaks of gastroenteritis in Japan, presumably because of the higher consumption of raw seafood in that country.[30]

Although the sufferer of food-borne illness may or may not recognize the symptoms as being related to the ingestion

TABLE 70-2
Partial List of Etiologies of Confirmed Food-Borne Outbreaks of Gastroenteritis Reported to the Centers for Disease Control—1987

ETIOLOGY	PERCENTAGE OF OUTBREAKS	PERCENTAGE OF CASES
Bacterial		
Salmonella sp	38	19.1
Staphylococcus aureus	0.7	1
Clostridium perfringens	1.5	3
Clostridium botulinum	8.1	0.2
Bacillus cereus	1.5	0.1
Shigella sp	6.6	67.3
V. parahaemolyticus	1.5	0.1
Campylobacter sp	2.2	0.4
Total for all bacterial pathogens	61	92.5
Viral		
Norwalk	0.7	3.8
Hepatitis A	6.6	1.9
Chemical		
Ciguatoxin	8.1	0.4
Scombrotoxin	16.2	1
Mushrooms	1.5	0
Heavy metals	1.5	0.2
Other	1.5	0.1

Etiology of Confirmed Water-Related (Intended for Drinking) Outbreaks of Gastroenteritis Reported to the Centers for Disease Control—1985

Giardia sp	20	48.3
Campylobacter sp	13.3	11.2
Salmonella typhi	6.7	1.8
Shigella sp	6.7	3.9
Virus	0	0
Unknown	53.3	34.8

Adapted from Centers for Disease Control. Food-borne disease outbreaks, 5-year summary, 1983–1987. MMWR, 1990;39:15; and adapted from St. Louis ME. Water-related disease outbreaks, 1985. MMWR CDC Surveill Summ 1988; 37(SS-2):15.

of a particular contaminated food item, certain established guidelines aid in the diagnosis of this syndrome. For the purposes of standardization, food-borne disease can, in most cases, be established if two or more people have a similar illness after consuming a common meal; an epidemiologic survey implicates a particular food item(s) as the probable cause of an outbreak; or microbiologic studies identify the same organism (in some cases threshold quantities are required) or epidemic strain from a common food, food source sample (i.e., handler, preparation area), or clinical specimens obtained in a suspected outbreak. In spite of careful studies designed to establish the source of contamination, the causative agent remains undetected in a large percentage of cases—a fact that probably will change for the better as technological advances continue to provide newer and better methods of diagnosing this illness (e.g., DNA hybridization, toxin assays, commercial diagnostic kits, and serologic markers). Table 70-

3 summarizes the clinical features of agent-specific food-borne disease.

Etiology

Toxins Associated With Bacterial Food Poisoning

Bacterial pathogens frequently elaborate toxins that can cause symptoms in the gastrointestinal tract. Two prominent examples are S aureus[31,32] and Bacillus cereus,[31,33] both of which can produce similar illnesses marked by profuse vomiting with a short time of onset (i.e., less than 12 hours).

S aureus is a gram-positive coccus that frequently colonizes the mucous membranes and skin of humans and animals. Thirty to 50% of healthy people are carriers of the organism, and they serve as the most frequent sources of food contamination. S aureus is known to produce at least seven antigenic types of "classic" enterotoxin and a delta-toxin previously known as a hemolysin, all of which are capable of causing net fluid secretion in the intestine.[32] S aureus is the second most commonly implicated agent in bacterial food poisoning in the United States. Outbreaks of S aureus food-borne disease can occur during all seasons, but are most frequent during warm weather, a fact perhaps explained by the association between S aureus outbreaks and large gatherings (i.e., school and club activities, and picnics), which tend to take place during the warmer months. Foods with high salt or sugar content select for the growth of S aureus and include those foods listed in Table 70-3. The primary mode of transmission usually entails foods that have been prepared or mixed by people who are carriers of enterotoxin-producing strains, and in which adequate time and temperature are provided for the multiplication of the organism (advance preparation and lack of refrigeration). Once produced in food, the toxin is not inactivated by heating. Attack rates among people consuming contaminated foods are usually high, reaching 80% to 100%. The emetic response so characteristic of S aureus food poisoning seems to be related to toxin stimulation of neural receptors in the intestine as part of an immunologic response. The clinical features of S aureus food poisoning are profuse vomiting, nausea, and abdominal cramping within 6 to 8 hours after ingestion of preformed enterotoxin, often followed by diarrhea. In the extreme, blood can be observed in the vomitus or stool. Full recovery from the usual syndrome usually occurs within 24 to 48 hours. Fever is not part of the syndrome. The diagnosis is made on clinical grounds and can be confirmed by culturing the epidemiologically incriminated food or the skin or nasopharynx of the food handler. Phage-typing allows comparison of the strains isolated from food and food handler.

In 1987, B cereus ranked as the fifth most common bacterial pathogen implicated in food-borne disease. The incidence of this disease, however, may be underestimated, because many laboratories do not routinely test for B cereus. The organism is an aerobic, motile, spore-forming gram-positive rod that produces clinical symptoms through the elaboration of several enterotoxins. The syndromes produced by this organism can be divided into a vomiting-type illness almost exclusively associated with the consumption of fried rice, and a diarrhea-

(text continues on p. 1614)

TABLE 70-3
Clinical and Epidemiologic Features of Agent-Specific Food-Borne Disease

ORGANISM OR AGENT	INCUBATION PERIOD	DURATION OF ILLNESS (RANGE)	DIARRHEA	FEVER	VOMITING	ENTEROTOXIN	INVASION	FOODS MOST COMMONLY IMPLICATED	COMMENTS
Staphylococcus aureus	1–8 h	24 h (8–48 h)	+	–	+++	++	–	Salads, cream-filled pastries, meats (pork, beef, poultry)	High attack rates (80–100%) Outbreaks most frequent during summer months Vomiting is a more prominent finding than diarrhea
Bacillus cereus Emetic illness	1–6 h	9 h (2–10 h)	+	–	+++	++	–	Fried rice	Abdominal cramps often experienced Vomiting occurs more often than diarrhea
Diarrheal illness	6–14 h	20 h (16–48 h)	+++	–	+	+	–	Meats, vanilla sauce, cream baked goods, salads, chicken soup	Diarrhea occurs more often than vomiting Organism may be found in stool of healthy people
Clostridium botulinum	12–36 h (may be as long as 8 d)	Weeks to months	±	–	±	++ (Neurotoxin)		Raw honey (infants), improperly canned products	Neurologic symptoms are results of parasympathetic and neuromuscular blockade 15% Mortality rate Treatment is early administration of antitoxin Infants < 1 y of age should not be fed raw honey
Clostridium perfringens	8–24 h	24 h (8–72 h)	+++	–	±	++	–	Improperly stored beef, fish, or poultry dishes (after preparation), pasta salads, dairy products, Mexican foods	"Pig-bel" or necrotizing enterocolitis is a rare variant Stool contains no WBCs or blood Commercial kit available for detection of toxin in stool
Puffer fish	<2 h	Variable	+	–	+	+ Tetrodotoxin (neurotoxin)		Fugu (especially prepared Japanese puffer fish), other puffer fish, vividly colored frogs of South America, blue-ringed octopus	Symptoms include paresthesias, ataxia, hypotension, seizures, cardiac arrhythmias, respiratory and skeletal muscle paralysis 30%–60% Mortality rate Treatment: gastric lavage and cardiac/respiratory support Prognosis greatly improves if patient survives first 6 h

Illness	Onset	Duration				Toxin		Food sources	Comments
Paralytic shellfish	1–3 h	3 d (0.5–7 d)	–	–	+	+ Saxitoxin (Neurotoxin)	–	Most bivalved mollusks (shellfish), especially from endemic waters experiencing red tide blooms	Symptoms and treatment similar to puffer fish poisoning; 5%–18% Mortality rate; Etiology is concentration of toxic dinoflagellates in mollusks during "red tide" season (i.e., spring and fall)
Ciguatera	1–6 h	Variable (can persist for months)	+	–	+	+ Ciguatoxin (Neurotoxin)	–	Barracuda, grouper, snapper, jacks, reef sharks	Most common form of fish intoxication in United States; Commonly seen in Florida, Hawaii, and the Caribbean; Symptoms similar to puffer fish poisoning; ELISA assay available for detection of toxin; Treatment suggested with Amitrityline
Scombroid	<2 h	Variable (2–10 h)	±	–	+	– (Preformed saurine) histamine-like substance causes symptoms. Not an allergic reaction	–	"Blood fish" (tuna, albacore, mackerel, skip jacks) under spoiling conditions	Symptoms: flushing, generalized or localized erythema, vertigo, generalized burning sensation; Histamine levels can be assayed in implicated fish; Treatment with antihistamines effective; Fish with unpleasant odor or clouded eyes should be avoided
Salmonella sp	8–48 h	3 d (1–14 d)	+++	++	+++	+	+ (little mucosal damage)	Eggs, poultry, beef, dairy products	Infection with some serotypes can lead to severe complications in certain patients (i.e., patients with malignancy, atherosclerosis, and AIDS); Treatment not recommended except in severe or disseminated disease because it prolongs carriage of organism; Stool contains WBCs and may contain blood
Shigella sp	24–72 h (up to 7 d)	3 d (1–14 d)	+++	+++	±	+	+	Salads (egg, tuna, poultry), milk	Low infective dose (10^2 organisms); Person-to-person transmission common; Stools often contain blood, mucus, and pus; Systemic symptoms (i.e., headache, malaise, lethargy) common

(continued)

TABLE 70-3. *(Continued)*

ORGANISM OR AGENT	INCUBATION PERIOD	DURATION OF ILLNESS (RANGE)	DIARRHEA	FEVER	VOMITING	ENTEROTOXIN	INVASION	FOODS MOST COMMONLY IMPLICATED	COMMENTS
Yersinia sp	24–72 h (up to 6 d)	7 d (2–30 d)	+++	++	±	+	+	Milk (raw or chocolate), tofu	Abdomen pain is a very prominent feature of illness and may be confused with appendicitis. Presence of pharyngitis common in children. Rheumatologic postinfectious complications have been reported (see text)
Vibrio parahaemolyticus	4–96 h	3 d (2–10 d)	++	±	+	+	± (Not documented in humans)	Oysters, crabs, shellfish, sea-water-contaminated food	Antimicrobials do not shorten illness. Fecal WBC and blood uncommon
Non-0:1 *Vibrio cholerae*	6–72 h	2 d (2–12 d)	++	±	±	+ (A few produce cholera toxin)	±	Seafood, grated eggs, potatoes	25% can have bloody diarrhea. Illness similar to cholera but much less dehydration
Vibrio cholerae	12–72 h	3 d (2–14 d)	+++	–	+	+++	–	Seafood, fecally contaminated water	Disease usually of abrupt onset. Severe dehydration can lead to death within hours. Hypoglycemia can be seen in children. Treatment primarily focused on replacing fluid and electrolyte losses. Effective vaccine undergoing field trials

Organism								Vehicle	Comments
Campylobacter sp	2–11 d	3 d (2–30 d)	+++	++	±	+	+	Raw milk, poultry, beef, clams, pet animals	Stool contains RBCs and WBCs; Mostly resistant to TMP-SMX; Complications include meningitis and Guillain-Barré syndrome
Escherichia coli (enterotoxigenic)	24–72 h	3 d (1–14 d)	+++	+	−	+	−	Salads, peeled fruits, meat dishes, pastries	At least two toxins elaborated: heat-labile (similar to choleratoxin) and heat-stable; Most common bacterial agent of travelers' diarrhea
Escherichia coli (enteroinvasive)	24–72 h	3 d (1–14 d)	+++	+++	±	−	++	Salads, cheese	Stools often contain blood, mucus, and pus; Systemic symptoms (i.e., headache, malaise, lethargy) common
Rotavirus	48–72 h	5 d (3–14 d)	+++	+ (Low grade)	++	−	− (Superficial damage to mucosa)	Fresh water, seafood	Primarily an illness of infants and children; Endemic in nature; Respiratory symptoms common; Can cause severe dehydration in children; Vaccine under development
Norwalk virus	24–48 h	1 d (1–3 d)	++	+ (Low grade)	++	−	− (Superficial damage to mucosa)	Shellfish, drinking water	Affects primarily older children and adults; Industrialized regions; occurs earlier in life in developing regions

AIDS, acquired immunodeficiency syndrome; ELISA, enzyme-linked immunosorbent assay; RBCs, red blood cells; TMP-SMX, trimethoprin–sulfamethoxazole; WBCs, white blood cells.

Adapted from Syndman DR. Bacterial food poisoning. In: Gorbach SL, ed. Infectious diarrhea. Boston: Blackwell, 1986:201; Sanders WE Jr. Intoxications from the seas: ciguatera, scombroid, and paralytic shellfish poisoning. Infect Dis Clin North Am 1987;1:665; and Dupont HL, Pickering LK. Infections of the gastrointestinal tract. Microbiology, pathophysiology, and clinical features. New York: Plenum, 1980.

type illness associated with a number of foods (see Table 70-3). Separate toxins appear to be involved in each.[34,35] It is not known whether these syndromes are a result of ingestion of preformed toxins or if the organisms elaborate the toxin after multiplication in the gut.

The emetic illness caused by *B cereus* usually has an incubation period of 1 to 6 hours and in almost all cases produces vomiting and abdominal cramping. Diarrhea can be seen in up to one third of patients. The diarrheal illness caused by *B cereus*, on the other hand, usually has a longer incubation period (range, 6–14 hours) and is characterized by watery diarrhea, abdominal cramping, and, to a lesser extent, vomiting. Fever is rarely seen in this or the vomiting type of illness. The duration of illness is usually 2 to 10 hours for the emetic syndrome and 16 to 48 hours for the diarrheal syndrome.

Many foods are found to contain *B cereus* (25%–50% of foods tested in different studies), and the organism may be found in the stools of healthy people. Therefore, a diagnosis is based primarily on clinical information and food ingestion history. Heavy contamination of food (i.e., greater than 10^5 organisms per gram) or negative stool cultures in a well selected control group during an outbreak can be confirmatory. Given the self-limited nature of this illness, treatment is not required. Prevention lies in the adherence to standard food handling techniques, with particular attention paid to avoiding multiplication of the organism within food (i.e., proper heating and the prompt refrigeration after cooking of food items).

Clostridium botulinum[36] is a ubiquitous, gram-positive, anaerobic, spore-forming bacteria that produces a heat-labile neurotoxin capable of blocking acetylcholine at the neuromuscular junction. *C botulinum* spores are heat resistant and are produced only under anaerobic conditions and pH above 4. Such conditions exist particularly in improperly prepared canned products, but can occur in any food that is contaminated and meets the criteria for spore germination. Symptomatic disease caused by ingestion of preformed toxin develops within 12 to 36 hours after ingestion, but may take as long as 8 days. The clinical features consist of nausea, vomiting, abdominal pain, and diarrhea, all of which tend to be mild. The neurologic symptoms include diplopia and ophthalmoplegia, dysarthria, dysphagia and dysphonia, descending bilateral weakness or paralysis, postural hypotension, and respiratory muscle paralysis that can be fatal if the patient is not supported with mechanical ventilation. Botulism has a 15% case fatality rate. Mental status usually remains clear, and there is no fever. Full recovery may take months, but muscle involvement usually recovers first. Assaying of stool, vomitus, or suspected food for botulinum toxin may be helpful. Electromyography is useful in distinguishing this syndrome from Guillain-Barré syndrome, an ascending paralysis. Treatment includes supportive measures and early administration of antitoxin. The antitoxin, however, is made from horse serum and produces an allergic reaction in up to 10% of patients. Antibiotics are of no benefit, and aminoglycosides may worsen the paralysis.

One form of this disease, described in infants younger than 6 months of age, is associated with the ingestion of raw honey containing *C botulinum* spores. Because of this syndrome, raw honey should not be fed to infants younger than 1 year of age, and home canning should be done by properly trained people.

Given the seriousness of this illness, and potential for widespread involvement, a single case of botulism (or any type of chemical poisoning) is considered an outbreak by public health authorities, and protection for other people therefore dictates prompt reporting of the disease to local public health officials. Asymptomatic, exposed people should not be treated with antitoxin to minimize the risk of anaphylaxis.

Toxins Associated With Seafood Consumption

Three clinical entities have been described associated with neurologic abnormalities after ingestion of toxin-containing fish. These are puffer fish poisoning (tetrodotoxin); paralytic shellfish poisoning (saxitoxin); and ciguatera (ciguatoxin).[37,38] The unifying clinical features of these syndromes has led to their being described as causing "pelagic paralysis," from the ancient Greek word *pelagos*, meaning "open sea." Mills and Passmore,[38] who suggested this term, point out that these three entities cannot be distinguished clinically, and all three toxins involved cause alterations of sodium conductance in myelinated and nonmyelinated nerves—hence the categorical denomination. In two instances (saxitoxin and ciguatoxin), the toxins can be traced through the food chain to unicellular, plant-like organisms called dinoflagellates. A fourth syndrome (scombroid fish poisoning) is caused by *Proteus* and *Klebsiella* sp decarboxylation of histidine-producing saurine (histamine-like substance), which occurs in spoiling fish.[37] Table 70-3 summarizes the clinical features of these intoxications.

Bacterial Infection

The conventional invasive bacterial pathogens *Shigella, Salmonella,* and *Campylobacter* species may be spread through contaminated foods. This is particularly true for *Salmonella* and *Campylobacter*, which are commonly found to contaminate poultry. *Shigella* and *Campylobacter* usually are colonic pathogens, and are considered in Chapter 84.

Clostridium perfringens.   *C perfringens* is one of the most common causes of bacterial food poisoning in the world, and consistently numbers among the first four major etiologic agents for this disease in the United States.[31,39,40] This organism is an obligate anaerobe, but it can tolerate exposure to oxygen for up to 72 hours, and is the only nonmotile species of *Clostridium*.

The pathogenesis of *C perfringens* food poisoning resides in the organism's ability to elaborate exotoxins. *C perfringens* enterotoxin (CPE) is a heat-labile protein toxin capable of producing fluid accumulation in animal ileal loop models, and is elaborated by *C perfringens* types A, C, and D. The mechanism by which CPE produces clinical symptoms seems to be related to cytotoxic action in the intestinal epithelial cells.[41] Intralumenal CPE binds to mucosal cell surfaces, where it causes structural damage to these cells with subsequent loss of intracellular substances, primarily sodium, chloride, protein, and fluid. This effect probably leads to impaired macromolecular synthesis, further structural damage, and eventual cell death. Sporulation of viable cells (at least 10 organisms) within the small intestine is commonly believed to be the cause of the resulting diarrhea.

Most *C perfringens* outbreaks occur during the fall and winter months (unlike *Salmonella* species and *S aureus* outbreaks), and typically involve those foods listed in Table 70-3. When involved, these foods usually have been prepared in advance and allowed to cool without prompt refrigeration. In this fashion, heat-resistant spores that survive the cooking process germinate within the food during the cooling period (reduced redox potential within the food favors this process). On reheating before consumption, not all viable cells are killed, and heat-induced sporulation of the cells and enterotoxin production within the intestine causes diarrhea.

C perfringens causes a watery diarrhea (two to four stools) that frequently is accompanied by pronounced abdominal cramping and pain characteristically 8 to 24 hours (mean, 12 hours) after ingestion of the contaminated food. Attack rates during epidemics usually are high, and in the United States the median number of people affected in an outbreak ranges between 23% and 35%. Constitutional symptoms such as vomiting, fever, chills, and malaise are not commonly seen. The disease is self-limited and full recovery is expected within 24 hours. A fatal outcome is rare and usually associated with older age groups and secondary dehydration. Although serum antibody to CPE has been demonstrated in asymptomatic adults and in some but not all volunteers challenged with CPE, the development of protective immunity has not been shown. Local production of anti-CPE antibody in the gut, however, may confer immunity in previously exposed people.[42]

C perfringens food poisoning cannot be distinguished easily from other noninfectious, enterotoxigenic intoxications such as those caused by *B cereus* and *S aureus*. Because *C perfringens* organisms are regularly found in small numbers in raw food and in the gastrointestinal tract of humans, confirmation of an outbreak relies on quantitation of organisms in food (i.e., greater than 10^5 organisms per gram) or excreta of ill people (greater than 10^6 spores per gram). Simple-to-perform assays of great sensitivity and specificity for CPE (reverse passive latex agglutination and slide-latex agglutination) have proven very useful in accurately diagnosing illness caused by *C perfringens*.

Several reports have implicated *C perfringens* as the cause of antibiotic-associated diarrhea[43–45] and prolonged and recurrent infectious diarrhea in the elderly and patients under chronic care conditions.[46] It has been demonstrated that many otherwise healthy hosts (particularly the elderly) can harbor high numbers of *C perfringens* organisms in the large intestine without experiencing a pathologic condition; however, when symptoms develop, they always are associated with the presence of enterotoxin-producing strains. In addition, a significant association with prior antibiotic exposure has been reported in patients in whom symptoms of enterocolitis develop, and whose stools contain *C perfringens* and its enterotoxin but no other identifiable common pathogen.[43,44] The illness thus resembles that associated with *Clostridium difficile*, and although pseudomembranous enterocolitis per se has not been demonstrated in any of the patients in whom endoscopic ex-

amination has been performed, the presence of fecal blood and biopsy-proven mucosal hemorrhage and edema in some patients speaks in favor of a "colitis." A favorable clinical and microbiologic response to oral metronidazole (400 mg three times a day for 7 to 10 days) has been demonstrated.[44,47] Nevertheless, the experience with oral antibiotic therapy for *C perfringens* antibiotic-associated diarrhea is small and not all patients so treated display resolution of symptoms or eradication of the organism from their excreta. It seems reasonable, however, to treat those cases of prolonged diarrhea in which *C perfringens* and its enterotoxin are identified or presumed given the history of prior antibiotic use.

A different clinical syndrome related to the production of various other toxins (i.e., beta-toxin and alpha-toxin) and characterized by a necrotizing enterocolitis, ileus, and pneumatosis intestinalis has been described with *C perfringens* type C and, more recently, with type A (also see Chap. 77).[48,49] Although *Darmbrand*, as it was called, was initially reported in war-torn northern Germany in the mid-1940s and ascribed to *C perfringens* type F (now included under type C), the illness may date back to descriptions of enteric disease documented by Hippocrates. This disease, which appeared in epidemic numbers, is no longer observed in Germany and is seen only rarely in Western countries. By contrast, a similar condition—"pig-bel," as it is commonly referred to in Papua, New Guinea—still causes significant morbidity and mortality (estimated at 40%) in that country's highlands, in frequent association with native feasts in which large amounts of ceremonial pork are ingested. Malnutrition and sudden changes in dietary intake of protein may place people at risk, with those affected primarily children and the elderly. Bowel resection frequently was required to treat this disease, but accumulated data indicate that passive immunization with *C perfringens* type C antiserum (i.e., beta-antitoxin)[49] and active immunization before the fact with Wellcome pig-bel toxoid vaccine[50] significantly reduces both morbidity and mortality from this illness.

Listeria monocytogenes.   *L monocytogenes* is an uncommon cause of food-borne infection, but several outbreaks have been reported.[51,52] In 1985, poorly pasteurized Mexican-style soft cheese was implicated in 142 cases of *Listeria* food poisoning, 66% of which involved pregnant women and their infants, and nearly all of the remaining cases had a predisposing health problem.[53] As shown by this outbreak, unpasteurized milk is a common vehicle of transmission and populations at risk predominantly include pregnant women and their infants, the latter acquiring *Listeria* through vertical transmission. Both cellular and humoral immunity play important roles in defense against *L monocytogenes*. The organism preferentially causes illness in immunocompromised people (i.e., patients with hematologic malignancies, cirrhosis, diabetes, corticosteroid therapy, acquired immunodeficiency syndrome, and renal failure), although the elderly, veterinarians, and laboratory workers also are at risk. The organism is ubiquitous in animals and the environment, and it appears that many people can carry the organism asymptomatically. The primary portal of entry in all cases except fetal and neonatal infections appears to be the gastrointestinal tract. The clinical syndromes caused by *L monocytogenes* can range between a mild febrile illness to frank bacteremia and sepsis. Meningoencephalitis, granulomatosis infatiseptica (granulomas and abscess in multiple internal organs), cervical adenitis, subacute endocarditis, arthritis, osteomyelitis, brain abscesses, peritonitis, and cholecystitis also have been described. Diarrhea and other gastrointestinal symptoms can precede the onset of systemic listeriosis. Given the seriousness of this illness (meningitis, for example, has a mortality rate of 13%–43%) and the particular population at risk, it is no wonder that successful therapy has been associated with early diagnosis and initiation of treatment. Ampicillin is currently the first choice of therapy followed by trimethoprim/sulfamethoxazole.

Diarrheagenic *Escherichia coli*. *E coli* is a common inhabitant of the gastrointestinal tracts of both humans and animals. Although most *E coli* strains do not possess known virulence characteristics, a subset exists that can be pathogenic to humans, specifically through the induction of gastroenteritis. Since the 1940s, knowledge about these enteropathogens has led to the use of many descriptive terms to denote the particular pathogens associated with acute diarrhea. In the interest of simplicity, these pathogens are herein collectively referred to as diarrheagenic *E coli*, and the particular syndromes produced by each are discussed in the following sections.

The members of the species *E coli* belong to the family *Enterobacteriaceae*, and are characteristically facultative, anaerobic, non–spore-forming, mostly motile, gram-negative bacteria that grow well at 37°C in nonenriched media. The distinction of *E coli* from other members of the *Enterobacteriaceae* family is made by demonstration of characteristic biochemical reactions; however, the identification of different strains within the same species of *E coli* is done serologically and by virulence testing. Serologically distinct antigens have been identified on different structures of the bacterium. The H antigen (H-Ag) or flagellar protein is located on the peritrichous flagellum common to this organism. Similarly, the O-antigen or lipopolysaccharide antigen (O-Ag) and the K-antigen are located on the cell wall and capsule or envelope (when present), respectively. In addition, fimbria or pili and other attachment factors of these organisms can be determinants of pathogenicity. There are four well defined diarrheagenic *E coli* that show specific clinical and epidemiologic features: ETEC, enteropathogenic *E coli* (EPEC), enteroinvasive *E coli* (EIEC), and enterohemorrhagic *E coli*.

Enterotoxigenic **E coli.** ETEC produces disease by adherence to the gut mucosa and elaboration of one (or more) of at least three enterotoxins differing in susceptibility to heat: LT (heat-labile toxin), ST_a, and ST_b (heat-stable toxin).[54,55] The characteristics of LT are remarkably similar to those of cholera toxin (see section on *Vibrio*), including a molecular weight of 84,000 daltons, five identical binding B subunits, and an enzymatically active A subunit, which activates the cyclic adenosine monophosphate (cAMP) system (see Fig. 70-1). LT and cholera toxin also share antigenic properties, and cholera antitoxin neutralizes the fluid-evoking capacity of *E coli* enterotoxin. ST_a stimulates the guanylate cyclase system, and ST_b may not be important in human disease. The ability of ETEC to adhere to the human intestinal epithelium seems to relate to specific attachment fimbriae known as colonization factor antigens (CFA I and II and E8775), many of which probably have not yet been identified.

ETEC, as mentioned, has a worldwide distribution and is a major etiologic agent of diarrhea affecting children in the developing world (20%–50%). Although ETEC is a rare cause of diarrhea in the United States, it accounts for most cases of illness in the traveler to developing countries. Acquisition of ETEC is primarily through ingestion of contaminated food or water. Person-to-person transmission probably occurs only rarely, because a large inoculum is required to produce illness in healthy people (10^6–10^8 organisms).

The illness produced by ETEC is characterized mainly by watery diarrhea. Other symptoms may include cramping, abdominal pain, and, rarely, low-grade fever. Headache, arthralgias, myalgias, vomiting, and chills also occur. The illness usually is self-limiting, and when untreated usually lasts 3 to 5 days; those affected pass an average of 8 to 12 unformed stools per day. Dehydration tends to be severe only in the very young and very old. Fatalities are rare and treatment with antimicrobials (see section on "Prevention and Treatment" of travelers' diarrhea) shortens the duration of disease. Fluid and electrolyte replacement is emphasized, especially in the populations at risk. It is known that natural immunity to ETEC occurs, and many patients with ETEC diarrhea demonstrate antibodies against the somatic antigen as well as LT.[56] Given these findings and the fact that older people and residents from endemic areas display a decreased susceptibility to ETEC infection,[57] and the additional fact that asymptomatic Latin American students rarely excrete this organism in their stool (unlike asymptomatic students from the United States),[58] it seems likely that ETEC infection could be prevented by a number of immunologic mechanisms. Trials conducted to evaluate vaccines that target specific virulence properties have met with variable success.

Enteropathogenic **E coli.** EPEC organisms lack *Shigella*-like invasive properties and fail to produce classic ETEC-type enterotoxins.[54,55] The organism's mechanism of pathogenesis appears to reside primarily in its enteroadherence properties.[59] The in vitro model for EPEC's ability to adhere to intestinal epithelial cells is mannose-resistant adherence to HEp-2 cells in tissue culture. Classically, the EPEC strains show focal attachment to HEp-2 cells. Other forms of attachment (diffuse or aggregative) have been described and may be associated with pathogenicity of *E coli* strains. ETEC and normal-flora *E coli* strains rarely display this ability, in contrast to most EPEC strains.. The relation between particular serotypes and pathogenicity remains undefined.

EPEC was discovered to be a distinct pathogenic strain of *E coli* in the 1950s, based on several diarrhea outbreaks in hospital nurseries. Based on these outbreaks, a clinically distinct syndrome was observed. EPEC diarrhea seems to affect primarily the very young (<2 years of age), and most studies point to increased frequency of outbreaks among hospitalized infants. Epidemic EPEC strains have been isolated from the oropharynx and the excreta of asymptomatic contacts of ill cases during several outbreaks. Older children and adults, particularly mothers of hospitalized infants, may serve as reservoirs for this organism. It is estimated that 10% of infantile diarrhea in developing countries and in the United States may be caused by EPEC strains. Further studies are needed to better identify and correlate EPEC diarrhea in specific populations. *E coli* showing EPEC-like attachment to HEp-2 cells have been implicated as causes of persistent diarrhea in infants in developing tropical regions, and these enteroadherent *E coli* also have been identified as common causes of travelers' diarrhea.

Primarily in infants, illness with EPEC is marked by watery diarrhea, which may become profuse and protracted. EPEC enteritis is one of the few identifiable causes of prolonged diarrhea in infancy. A variable percentage of patients display vomiting, fever, failure to thrive, and metabolic acidosis. Dehydration can be severe and life threatening if the disease is allowed to progress without fluid and electrolyte replacement. Bloody stools have been reported with EPEC infection. Stool culture and serotyping (O-Ag and H-Ag), documenting characteristic tissue culture adherence, or detection of adherence factor by DNA probe if *E coli* is identified, are the only ways of incriminating EPEC strains in the particular diarrhea episode.

Treatment of EPEC usually is not required given the self-limiting nature of the illness; however, careful attention always should be paid to the replacement of fluids and electrolytes through oral or intravenous routes. This has proven to be the most important nonspecific therapy. The use of antimicrobial agents is advocated in severe illness, but which ones and for how long remain to be firmly established.[60,61] In vitro antimicrobial susceptibilities should be routinely used with isolated strains, particularly because these organisms tend to show a surprisingly high rate of antimicrobial resistance.[62]

***Enteroinvasive* E coli.**   Disease from strains of *E coli* that display the ability to invade the intestinal mucosa has been described primarily in large outbreaks of food-borne enteric infection. Imported Camembert and Brie cheeses were the cause in a widespread outbreak in 1971,[63] and a second outbreak of EIEC was documented in 1981 aboard a cruise ship.[64] Although EIEC is thought to be a rare cause of diarrhea (except in Brazil and Eastern Europe), and is not commonly spread through person-to-person contact, the epidemiology of this illness is unclear, although food appears to be the major vehicle of transmission. EIEC organisms have been associated with specific somatic antigens (O-Ag) and by definition are Sereny test positive. EIEC possess the same 140-megadalton plasmid that is associated with invasiveness in *Shigella* strains. The Sereny test (production of keratoconjunctivitis in guinea pigs) and tissue culture invasion were previously the only methods available to detect EIEC. DNA probes and an enzyme-linked immunosorbent assay (ELISA) developed for EIEC may prove useful in detecting these strains in the near future. EIEC shares extensive DNA homology and antigenic and biochemical characteristics with *Shigella* organisms. Furthermore, the illness produced is indistinguishable from the dysentery-like disease caused by *Shigella*. Unlike most *E coli* strains, EIEC ferments lactose slowly, and most organisms are nonmotile. Because EIEC are primarily colonic pathogens, they will not be considered here further.

***Enterohemorrhagic* E coli.**   It has become evident that yet another clinical syndrome, this one characterized by hemorrhagic colitis and bloody diarrhea, can be attributed to a different strain of *E coli*.[55,65,66] Investigations of food-borne outbreaks of diarrhea in 1982 in Oregon and Michigan have incriminated *E coli* serotype 0157:H7 as the etiologic agent in this syndrome.[65] Since then, studies have shown that this particular organism is responsible for both sporadic and epidemic illness cases in Canada and the United States. Epidemiologic studies point to the consumption of ground beef and raw milk as risk factors for the acquisition of this disease, and person-to-person transmission among household members has been documented.[65,67] Bloody diarrhea caused by *E coli* 0157:H7 can be complicated by the hemolytic uremic syndrome and thrombotic thrombocytopenic purpura, and can result in a high mortality rate.[65,68] Because *E coli* 0157:H7 does not invade the epithelium (Sereny test negative), does not produce ST or LT enterotoxins, and does not display CFA I or II (adherence factors), its primary virulence factor appears to be the production of at least two toxins with similar properties to the one elaborated by *Shigella dysenteriae* type 1 (Shiga toxin), called Shiga-like toxin I and II or verotoxins I and II. Although Shiga-like toxin II remains poorly characterized, it is known that Shiga-like toxin I has the same biologic properties of, and is immunologically and genetically indistinguishable from Shiga toxin.[69] As has been well established, Shiga toxin is lethal to certain cells in culture, can cause fluid secretion in the small intestine, and causes limb paralysis when injected parenterally into animals.[70] The toxin also has been shown to be cytotoxic to vascular endothelial cells in vitro. It is perhaps through vascular endothelial damage that infection with *E coli* 0157:H7 is capable of producing hematologic abnormalities (i.e., hemolysis and thrombosis). Shiga-like toxin production is not limited to the 0157:H7 strain of *E coli*. Other serotypes that normally are thought to belong to enteropathogenic and enterotoxigenic groups of *E coli* have been shown to produce Shiga-like toxins.[66,71] Conversely, culture-confirmed infections with *E coli* 0157:H7 can produce a nonbloody diarrhea, and can also cause asymptomatic infection. Nonbloody diarrhea infections tend to be milder and less likely to be complicated by hemolytic uremic syndrome. It is likely, then, that the amount, the site of production, and the chemical structure of the toxin, and perhaps the organism's ability to adhere to the intestinal mucosa, all play a role in the development of the particular clinical syndromes. Further study of Shiga-like toxin-producing *E coli* strains is needed to elucidate their clinicopathologic features. The clinical illness produced by Shiga-like toxin-producing *E coli* is described in Chapter 84.

***Salmonella* species.**   Few bacteria are more genetically diverse than *Salmonella* organisms, or more tenacious in finding new ways of entering the food chain. The classification scheme for the different species and particular bioserotypes within each species is complicated and is similar to that described for *E coli*. Some *Salmonella* serotypes (i.e., *Salmonella typhi* and *Salmonella paratyphi*) display an envelope antigen, Vi ("virulence") antigen, which serves as a virulence marker (see following discussion). By identifying the O-Ag and the H-Ag, 2200 serotypes of *Salmonella* (this number will undoubtedly grow in the future) have been identified that display varying degrees of host-specific adaptation and the ability to cause different clinical syndromes. The 10 most frequently isolated *Salmonella* serotypes are listed in Table 70-4, and account for about 70% of total isolates. The genus *Salmonella* is divided into three species: *S typhi*, (2) *Salmonella cholerasuis*, and (3)

TABLE 70-4
Ten Most Frequently Isolated *Salmonella* Serotypes

1. *S. typhimurium*
2. *S. heidelberg*
3. *S. enteriditis*
4. *S. newport*
5. *S. agona*
6. *S. infantis*
7. *S. saint-paul*
8. *S. montevideo*
9. *S. oranienburg*
10. *S. thompson*

Adapted from Rubin RH, Weinstein L. Salmonellosis: microbiologic, pathologic, and clinical features. New York: Stratton, 1977.

Salmonella enteriditis. Serotypes within the species *S enteriditis* are named.

Nontyphoid salmonellosis. Nontyphoidal *Salmonella* sp have been, and continue to be, one of the most frequent causes of food-borne enteric infection in the industrialized world, and account for 25% to 40% of outbreaks in the United States. Paradoxically, the organisms do not cause a comparatively great percentage of pediatric diarrhea in developing countries, of endemic diarrhea in the United States, or of travelers' diarrhea (see Table 70-1). There is a curious increase, however, in occurrence of nontyphoid salmonellosis in infants younger than 1 year of age. Also, these infants characteristically have intraintestinal infections (e.g., meningitis or sepsis) that represent important management problems. The incidence of nontyphoidal salmonellosis has been rising in the United States; this may in part be the result of better awareness and reporting of disease caused by *Salmonella* species, and the progressive trend toward mass processing and distribution of food products. This is especially true of those foods derived from animals in which these organisms are widely distributed. *Salmonella* serotypes, particularly those belonging to *S enteriditis*, have been isolated from a wide variety of animals, including poultry and all types of farm animals. Apart from food (and milk), other notable outbreaks have occurred in which the *Salmonella* organism was traced to pet turtles and carmine red dye (made from insect pigment) in food coloring. Aerosols, various fomites, marijuana, thermometers, fiberoptic endoscopes, and platelet transfusions also have been found to transmit the disease. The major reservoir for *Salmonella* organisms that cause human illness, however, is poultry and domestic livestock. Commercially prepared meats, particularly chickens and their eggs, have been notorious culprits. One study found poultry in retail stores to be contaminated with viable *Salmonella* sp in 50% of cases.[72] Eggs and egg products often have been identified as sources of epidemic salmonellosis. Small cracks offer passage of the organism into the egg's interior while it is being laid (contact with feces) or being cleaned, or through vertical contamination in utero before the shell calcifies. Person-to-person transmission of salmonellosis is thought to be minor, but may be important in institutional settings (including day care centers) where fecal contamination of the environment and inadequate hygiene

are common. About 85% of all outbreaks, however, occur through consumption of contaminated food or drink, and only 10% through cross-infection. Both *S typhi* and nontyphoidal *Salmonella* species show a seasonal variation and reach peak frequencies of illness in summer and fall. There is no sex preponderance, and attack rates are greatest in infants younger than 1 year of age, followed by age groups younger than 20 and older than 70 years. Patients with malignancies, immunosuppression, alcoholism, postsurgical state, sickle cell disease, abnormal cardiovascular system, hemolytic anemias, schistosomiasis, and the presence of a major underlying disease are predisposed to progressive salmonellosis with bacteremia. A case fatality rate of 0.2% has been reported in epidemics, but the overall mortality rate averages 2% to 3% if any of the predisposing factors exist. Nursing home patients and infants in nurseries have the highest case fatality rates (7%–9%).

The development of salmonellosis hinges on the number of organisms ingested (10^3–10^8) and on predisposing host factors. Lack of gastric acidity seems to play a particularly important role in the development of this illness. The production of diarrhea requires that viable organisms reach the small intestine and there invade the intestinal mucosa. Unlike the case with *Shigella* species, invasion of *Salmonella* organisms usually does not cause epithelial damage and is accomplished through an invagination of the mucosal cell membrane and formation of a phagosome around the organism. Pathologic studies reveal organisms intracellularly and in the lamina propria early in the course of the illness, with subsequent development of patchy inflammation in the deeper submucosa. Rarely, nontyphoidal *Salmonella* species can produce more extensive lesions consisting of an intense colitis, with small hemorrhages and ulcerations of the surface epithelium and multifocal microabscesses. Some nontyphoidal *Salmonella* serotypes, especially *S cholerasuis*, show a much greater ability to invade, and this may explain their propensity to cause enteric fever and bacteremia. Invasion by most nontyphoidal *Salmonella* species is restricted to lymphoid follicles and draining mesenteric lymph nodes. Isolation of nontyphoidal *Salmonella* species from blood during illness occurs in just under 10% of cases. The continuous presence of *Salmonella* organisms in the bloodstream, indicated by more than 50% of blood cultures being positive during the course of the illness, suggests the presence of intravascular focal infection. Men older than 50 years of age, and patients with sickle cell disease, atherosclerotic aortic aneurysms, or neoplastic, hemolytic, and valvular heart disease are particularly at risk for development of *Salmonella* bacteremia. The fatality rate of infections with *S cholerasuis*, the most systemically invasive *Salmonella* species, is 23 times that of *S typhi*, and 5 to 6 times that of nontyphoidal *Salmonella* infections.[73] Strict control of pork products in the United States has dramatically reduced the incidence of infection with *S cholerasuis*.

The pathogenic mechanism of *Salmonella* gastroenteritis is poorly understood, but both inflammatory and toxigenic properties have been described.[74] The clinical features of salmonellosis reflect the pathogenesis of the organism and site of infection. *Salmonella* infection in humans is divided into four clinical syndromes: gastroenteritis, enteric fever, bacteremia, and asymptomatic carriage.

The features of *Salmonella* gastroenteritis, usually the result of food-borne infection primarily with *S enteriditis* serotypes, constitutes a spectrum. At one end is a very mild, self-limiting disease consisting of one to a few loose stools and only minimal symptoms. At the opposite end is a cholera-like illness with profuse diarrhea and significant dehydration. A dysentery-like syndrome also can be seen, consisting of paste-like stools that may contain blood, mucus, and pus and be associated with significant tenesmus. This latter entity reflects distal colonic involvement. In up to 50% of cases, fever, usually lower than 39°C (102°F), is observed along with abdominal pain and cramping, general malaise, headache, nausea, and vomiting. Physical signs include lower abdominal tenderness and peristaltic rushes. Symptoms usually develop within 8 to 48 hours, frequently on awakening, and coincide with active bacterial invasion after ingestion of contaminated food. The diarrhea usually lasts 2 to 3 days and is preceded by the previously mentioned symptoms by a few hours. Improvement is expected after the initial 36 hours. Bacteremia is not common with this type of illness (6%–8%), but is seen more frequently in children and in people with underlying health defects (15%). Also, the disease tends to be more severe and associated with a higher mortality rate in children and the elderly (i.e., >50 years of age). Serious complications can occur in association with underlying disorders, as seen in the case of osteomyelitis in patients with sickle cell disease and other hemolytic disease processes. Bacteremia and focal abscesses, which can result in septic shock, are complications seen in patients with acquired immunodeficiency syndrome and patients with malignancies or receiving therapy for malignancies. Finally, infected aortic or iliac aneurysms in patients with preexisting atherosclerotic vascular disease can result in mortality rates of over 60%. These complications notwithstanding, salmonellosis is most commonly a benign disease in otherwise healthy human hosts.

Antimicrobials should not be used routinely in mild to moderately ill patients with gastroenteritis because their use may prolong the intestinal carriage of nontyphoidal *Salmonella* species.[75] Untreated and asymptomatic people also can excrete the organism for short periods of time (up to 2 months) and thereby further contribute to the reservoir of infection. The chronic carrier state (excretion for 1 year or longer) is seen most often with *S typhi* and *S paratyphi* infections (3%) in patients recovering from typhoid infection, and is commonly associated with children younger than 1 year of age, adults older than 60 years of age, concomitant biliary tract disease, and presence of schistosomiasis (important in urinary tract carriage of *Salmonella* species). The biliary tract commonly serves as a focus of *Salmonella* organism multiplication in typhoid carriers, especially if concomitant derangements are present (i.e., stones, obstruction). Chronic carriage of *Salmonella* species in the urinary tract also occurs, and should prompt an investigation into possible obstructive uropathy.

Drug resistance among *Salmonella* species (including *S typhi*, *S typhimurium*, and certain serotypes of *S enteriditis*) is well recognized and can have significant impact in the general population, especially where treatment of severe disease is concerned. Multiply resistant strains of *S typhi* and *Salmonella typhimurium* have been documented in the United States, Britain, Mexico, Thailand, Southeast Asia, Peru, and elsewhere.[76-78] *Salmonella* resistance to such antimicrobials as chloramphenicol, tetracycline, ampicillin, TMP-SMX, and the aminoglycosides seems to be mediated by plasmids that can be interchanged among the same organisms, or through interspecies and intergenus spread.[78,79]

In *Salmonella* infections, indications for antimicrobial therapy are presence of predisposing factors that can complicate salmonellosis, including extremes of age and in the face of an immunodeficiency condition; signs and symptoms of sepsis; infection with organisms likely to produce bacteremia (i.e., *S typhi*, *S paratyphi*, *S cholerasuis*; focal infections (e.g., osteomyelitis, abscess diseases); and chronic typhoid carrier states.

Appropriate drugs for enteric fever, septicemia, and focal infections include ampicillin, amoxicillin, chloramphenicol, and TMP-SMX for 10 to 14 days orally or parenterally, or the new fluoroquinolones (e.g., ciprofloxacin or ofloxacin) for 7 to 10 days. For typhoid carriers, norfloxacin or ciprofloxacin are given orally for 3 weeks. For adult patients with severe *Salmonella* gastroenteritis which may be complicated by sepsis, a quinolone (e.g., ciprofloxacin or ofloxacin) given orally for five days is suggested. As with all diarrheal illness, fluid and electrolyte replacement should be routinely undertaken, particularly in the small child and elderly individual.

Typhoid (enteric) fever.   Apart from the common gastrointestinal manifestation of salmonellosis, a clinical syndrome denoted as enteric fever can also occur with any *Salmonella* serotype, but most commonly with *S typhi* and *S paratyphi*. The hallmarks of enteric fever are prolonged fever, sustained bacteremia in the absence of endothelial and endocardial involvement, marked stimulation of the reticuloendothelial system, and metastatic spread leading to multiple organ dysfunction.

The pathogenesis of *S typhi* (and other enteric fever-causing *Salmonella* serotypes) infection may reside, in part, with the Vi antigen. This antigen appears to protect the somatic antigens (O-Ag) from being identified and targeted by the immune cells by forming an envelope around the cell wall. In this fashion, it may prevent antibody binding and subsequent phagocytosis. Alternatively, *S typhi* may inhibit normal leukocyte metabolism, because the organism is able to grow unrestrictedly within nonactivated macrophages.

S typhi usually is transmitted through ingestion of material contaminated by human feces, either from ill people or asymptomatic carriers. Because humans are the only reservoir of *S typhi*, the factors that directly relate to the prevalence of this organism in the environment are lack of water sanitation and number of carriers. In the United States, the rate of typhoid has dramatically decreased (in contrast to nontyphoidal salmonellosis) in the latter part of this century, whereas it continues to be a prevalent endemic problem in developing nations.

Bacteremia after gastrointestinal invasion is the hallmark of typhoid or enteric fever. The route taken by the organism after penetration of the intestinal mucosa is most likely through the lymphatic drainage after their release from dying macrophages in Peyer patches. After reaching the bloodstream, the organisms are quickly cleared by circulating macrophages and other cells of the reticuloendothelial system, and therefore this initial bacteremia is transient. Persistence of *S typhi* in the macrophages usually leads to the transfer of viable organisms to distant body sites, from where they reenter the bloodstream. This second phase of bacteremia usually coincides with the clinical manifestations of the illness, and accounts for the characteristic stepwise rise in temperature.

The clinical features of typhoid are those of an acute febrile illness lasting an average of 3 to 5 weeks and accompanied by specific and nonspecific signs and symptoms. The nonspecific symptoms appear early, are usually insidious, and can include frontal headache, general malaise, prostration, mental confusion (and at times delirium), anorexia, and abdominal discomfort and bloating. Upper respiratory tract symptoms, particularly dry cough, coryza, and sore throat, can be prominent presenting complaints and may lead the physician to misdiagnose the illness. Constipation is common initially but may give way to diarrhea in the late phase of the illness. The typical time course of typhoid begins with an incubation period of approximately 1 week (range, 3–60 days), followed by an active phase characterized by a stepwise increment in temperature, which plateaus at 39°C to 40°C and persists for 2 to 3 weeks in untreated illness. During this active phase, blood cultures are positive in more than 90% of patients, and characteristic clinical signs develop. The liver and spleen frequently are enlarged, and abdominal tenderness can be observed, particularly over the lower quadrants (at times mimicking appendicitis) and over the liver. Typical "rose spots" usually appear within the first 1 to 2 weeks, last only 3 to 4 days, and characteristically are distributed in general clusters of small numbers over the upper anterior trunk. This rash is probably the result of embolized bacteria causing a vasculitis, and consists of 2- to 4-mm, slightly raised macules that blanch on pressure. Rose spots can be present in 30% to 90% of patients, but are difficult to identify in highly pigmented people and are not specific for typhoid (i.e., they have been reported with psittacosis, shigellosis, brucellosis, and other illnesses). Symptoms usually begin to abate after the third week of untreated illness, but in 3% to 13% of untreated patients (and about 20% of treated patients), relapse can occur, usually after a variable period of time has elapsed (average, 2 weeks) from subsidence of symptoms. Relapse tends to be a milder and shorter illness compared to the full-blown syndrome. Development of antibodies against specific antigens (i.e., O-Ag, H-Ag, Vi) does not correlate with risk of relapse.

Complications of typhoid, although rare, can result in high mortality rates, and usually occur late in the illness, after the second or third week. These complications are caused by infectious lesions associated with mononuclear inflammation primarily in the biliary tract and intestines, but also in bone marrow, lung, bone, kidney, and meninges. Intestinal perforation and hemorrhage are the most common complications of typhoid, and both show an incidence of approximately 2% to 3%. Hemorrhage is caused by erosion of blood vessels in the inflamed and necrotic Peyer patches of the small and large intestines. When deep ulcerations develop from this process, intestinal perforation can occur with resulting peritonitis. Perforation accounts for 75% of all deaths due to typhoid. Jaundice and acute (and chronic) cholecystitis and hepatic cell necrosis also are complications. The almost invariable presence of *S typhi* in the biliary tree causes enormous shedding of organisms in the feces and may lead to the chronic carrier state, particularly in patients with cholelithiasis.

Immunization against typhoid has proven successful with a number of vaccines. The strategies used have entailed both parenteral and oral vaccines. The immunizing agents include attenuated and genetically modified strains of *S typhi* and *S typhimurium*. A Ty21a attenuated *S typhi* oral vaccine was 95% effective in one study after 3 years.[80] The oral vaccine, given every other day for four doses, or a single parenteral injection of Vi antigen vaccine, both appear to be effective and are preferable to the older, more reactogenic acetone-inactivated preparation.

Yersinia species.   *Yersinia* species, members of the *Enterobacteriaceae* family, are gram-negative, non–lactose-fermenting coccobacilli that are motile at 25°C and grow best in cooler environments.[81–84] The classification scheme of *Yersinia* species relies on surface antigens (somatic [O-Ag] and flagellar [H-Ag]). On this basis, more than 50 serotypes of *Y enterocolitica* and 6 serotypes of *Yersinia pseudotuberculosis* are recognized, with specific geographic distributions.

Gastrointestinal illness due to *Yersinia* species is primarily a problem of children, with most reported cases originating from Europe, and specifically the Scandinavian countries. Disease caused by this organism, however, can affect people of all ages and is distributed widely throughout the world. In the United States, the incidence of *Y enterocolitica* infection is not known, but isolation rates have increased dramatically during the 1980s, and serologic data also suggest that the actual frequency of this disease is on the rise. Typical isolation rates of *Y enterocolitica* from patients with diarrheal illness in Europe, Canada, and Japan range between 2% and 4%.[85] *Y pseudotuberculosis* is not commonly isolated in the United States, but is more frequently reported in Europe, and disease in humans presumably occurs through direct or indirect contact with animals, particularly swine.

It is widely believed that *Yersinia* infection is an epizootic phenomenon, with both wild and domestic animals serving as the major reservoir; however, organisms isolated from animals commonly differ biochemically and serologically from human pathogenic strains. *Y enterocolitica* disease is mainly transmitted by the fecal–oral route, and numerous food-borne outbreaks due to this pathogen have been reported. Apart from animals (dogs have been implicated) and outbreak-associated foods (prominent outbreaks have involved chocolate milk, ice cream, and tofu), *Y enterocolitica* has been linked to disease produced by contaminated surface water, and person-to-person transmission has been documented.

The two most common features of *Y enterocolitica* infection are diarrhea and abdominal pain. The latter can localize sharply to the right lower quadrant, mimicking acute appendicitis to the extent that many unnecessary appendectomies are performed in patients suffering from this illness. Localized right lower quadrant pain rarely is seen in children younger than 5 years of age. Other common symptoms, in order of decreasing frequency, include fever, vomiting, dysentery, arthritis, and no symptoms. Pharyngitis can occur in half of children and 10% of adults.

The course of the illness tends to be self-limiting, although chronic diarrhea persisting for months is observed in a small number of patients, usually children. Most patients experience a *Shigella*-like illness with a few watery stools per day, often blood streaked, accompanied by abdominal pain, low-grade fever, and constitutional symptoms, which tend to improve by the second or third day of illness. Examination of the stool reveals many fecal white blood cells, and frequently red blood cells, and the peripheral blood smear characteristically shows a leukocytosis with early forms. These findings may not be present in infants. Complete recovery usually is achieved by the second week of illness in uncomplicated cases. The diagnosis can be made by using both bacteriologic and serologic techniques. The laboratory personnel should be alerted if *Yersinia* infection is suspected because standard processing of stool specimens may overlook this organism.

Rarely, *Y enterocolitica* infection assumes a more malignant course, with fulminant ulcerative enterocolitis, mesenteric adenitis, peritonitis, and, very rarely, small bowel gangrene and massive intestinal hemorrhage. These features are seen almost exclusively in children and young adults. The mesenteric lymph nodes can be enlarged, forming a large conglomerate mass that can progress to a suppurative lesion. In a small percentage of patients, culture-positive acute or subacute appendicitis has been reported.

Septicemia due to *Y enterocolitica* is uncommon and usually is seen in patients with a predisposing illness, particularly iron overload states such as hemochromatosis, cirrhosis, and hemolytic processes (the ability of *Yersinia* species to use iron denotes a particular virulence factor). Similarly, *Y enterocolitica* infections can lead to extraintestinal focal suppurative lesions that may involve any region of the body, including meninges, joints, bone, sinuses, and pleural spaces. Infants younger than 6 months of age are particularly prone to development of extraintestinal disease.

Postinfectious complications can lead to thyroiditis, glomerulopathy, Reiter's syndrome, carditis, reactive arthritis, erythema nodosum, skin rashes, ankylosing spondylitis, and inflammatory bowel disease (IBD). These complications are not commonly seen in the United States, but are reported more frequently in Scandinavian countries. Except for cases of thyroiditis and glomerulopathy, these patients tend to be HLA-B27-positive, and may have their disease precipitated by an acute *Yersinia* infection. Indeed, antibodies to *Y enterocolitica* cross-react with many native mammalian tissues, and this may be one mechanism by which an autoimmune disorder is initiated in genetically susceptible people.

There is no evidence that antimicrobial therapy for *Yersinia* enteritis alters the course of this usually self-limiting illness, and therefore treatment is not commonly advocated. This is in sharp contrast to septicemic illness, in which antibiotics should be administered, but where mortality rates of 50% for *Y enterocolitica* and 75% for *Y pseudotuberculosis* infections are the rule despite antibiotic therapy. Antibiotics have no effect on the postinfectious complications.

Aminoglycosides, tetracycline, chloramphenicol, and TMP-SMX usually are effective, although resistance is seen in rare strains. A 3-week (or longer) course of antibiotic therapy is recommended for the treatment of extraintestinal disease. *Y pseudotuberculosis* usually is susceptible to ampicillin in addition to the antimicrobials already listed.

Vibrio species. Cholera is the commonly accepted prototype of enterotoxigenic diarrhea. The illness is caused by *V cholerae* O-group 1, a member of the *Vibrionaceae* family, which also includes *Aeromonas* species and other *Vibrio* species, some of which are pathogenic to humans. Cholera is endemic in southern Asia, Africa, and Latin America, where the disease

still takes a high toll in mortality. Cholera epidemics and pandemics are well documented since the early 1800s. The discovery in 1959 that cell-free stool filtrates from *V cholerae* could cause fluid secretion in rabbit intestinal loops led to an intense research effort into the mechanisms of enterotoxigenic diarrhea.

Vibrio, Aeromonas, and *Plesiomonas* are three genera within the same family of bacteria that cause illness in humans. Gastroenteritis can be caused by 7 of the 10 known pathogenic *Vibrio* species (*V cholerae, Vibrio parahaemolyticus, Vibrio fluvialis, Vibrio mimicus, Vibrio hollisae, Vibrio furnisii,* and probably *Vibrio vulnificus*), of which *V cholerae* and *V parahaemolyticus* are the most important. *V cholerae* is a motile, monoflagellated, short, gram-negative curved rod that grows best in thiosulfate–citrate–bile salts (TCBS) agar; and although it can grow on nonselective agar, it is inhibited by the selective media commonly used in routine stool cultures.[86,87] According to the classification used by the CDC, *V cholerae* is subdivided into 70 or more serogroups distinguished by the O-Ag (somatic) antigen. Those strains associated with endemic or epidemic cholera are designated as O:1 and the rest are commonly described in general as non-O:1 *V cholerae*.

Three subtypes of O:1 *V cholerae* exist, of which Ogawa and Inaba are the most important. Each subtype can be further differentiated into one of two biovars: Classical and El Tor, which react differently in standard biochemical and immunochemical reactions. Although the pathogenesis of the classic cholera syndrome has long been attributed to the effects of an elaborated enterotoxin, it is now known that *Vibrio* can produce illness even if the bacteria do not possess the cholera toxin gene. Also, some strains of *V cholerae* appear to produce other enterotoxins, such as zonula occludens toxin and accessory cholera toxin, that may play a role in disease pathogenesis. Water, and specifically fecally contaminated water, is the major vehicle of transmission for O:1 *V cholerae*; although food, especially seafood, is increasingly implicated in disease transmission. Where endemic, cholera affects primarily children between the ages of 2 to 9 years, with a second peak occurring in women of childbearing age. In endemic areas, which tend to be overcrowded and have poor water and waste sanitation, a distinct seasonal pattern is observed that varies with geographic location. Peaks of disease correlate better with the living conditions than with any weather pattern. Also in these endemic areas, women have higher attack rates than men, perhaps owing to cultural norms whereby women may have greater exposure to the organism through domestic chores such as washing or the rearing of small children. All age groups and both sexes are affected equally when cholera is introduced into a previously uninfected area.

Person-to-person transmission is not thought to play a major role in the propagation of cholera. Chronic human carriage has been demonstrated but is rare, more often seen with El Tor than with Classical biovars. There is evidence, however, that suggests that the organism may persist in the aquatic environment in a free-living state in close association with particulate matter and other organisms such as plankton, marine crustaceans, and copepods.[88] This perhaps explains the frequency with which seafood is associated with cholera transmission,[89] and also why epidemic strains reemerge after their apparent disappearance between epidemics. Several reports have documented *V cholerae* in the waters and seafood (i.e., crabs) of the Gulf of Mexico since 1973, establishing endemity of this organism (El Tor biovar) in those areas, and human cases of cholera have occurred. Since early 1991, when an outbreak of El Tor cholera occurred in Peru, hundreds of thousands of cases have been diagnosed throughout Latin America.

Apart from children in endemic areas, people with decreased stomach acid content and nonimmune adults are at high risk for acquiring cholera. For as yet undiscovered reasons, people with blood type O tend to experience clinically more severe cholera. The disease process itself is in a continuing state of evolution. The elaboration of an enterotoxin by O:1 *V cholerae* and its effect on the surface epithelial cells of the gut has been well studied and has contributed much to the understanding of the pathophysiology of diarrhea. The fluid losses seen in cholera can be staggering, and can result in the purge of 10% to 15% of body weight over several hours (i.e., more than 7 L of isotonic saline). In extreme cases, 100% of body weight can be lost within 4 to 7 days.

Choleratoxin is a protein with a molecular weight of 84,000 daltons and six structural subunits: five binding "B" subunits and one active "A" subunit composed of two peptides (A-1 and A-2).[90] All B subunits bind to specific receptors on the cell surface (GM-1 ganglioside is the best studied) in a circular manner and, through a conformational change of the toxin, enable the A subunit to be internalized into the cell membrane or cytosol. Once internalized, the A-1 peptide irreversibly locks the adenylate cyclase enzyme into a perpetual active state that constantly converts adenosine triphosphate into cAMP molecules, thereby raising intracellular cAMP levels. Choleratoxin inhibits the guanosine triphosphatase "turnoff" mechanism that helps regulate the internal concentration of cAMP at the level of adenylate cyclase. It is well established that choleratoxin elevates cellular levels of cAMP and alters the net absorptive tendency of the small intestine to one of net secretion. At the cellular level, a rise in cAMP concentrations stimulates secretion of Cl^- and HCO_3^- from mucosal crypt cells and inhibits the absorption of Cl^- through NaCl cotransport by villus cells. This situation inevitably leads to fluid loss as water passively follows the electrolyte solute into the lumen of the bowel and then to the exterior. Altered cAMP levels elsewhere in the body also may serve to amplify this local effect by disrupting the closely integrated hormonal system that regulates normal intestinal function. The colon also may participate in the illness by decreasing its absorptive capacity and increasing the secretion of potassium and bicarbonate ions. For choleratoxin to produce its effects, the organism must be ingested and be able to survive the "acid trap" present in the stomach.

V cholerae is very sensitive to a low pH. The inoculum size required to produce illness in volunteers is comparatively large (10^6 organisms), but fewer organisms can produce disease in people with hypochlorhydria from various causes, such as stomach resection and chronic antacid use. Once in the small intestine, the organisms multiply and colonize the gut. They do so by adhering to the mucosal surface through poorly understood mechanisms. The organism also produces different toxins, various enzymes (e.g., mucinases), and extracellular proteins (e.g., hemagglutinin and neuraminidase), which may contribute to its virulence.[87] The clinical symptoms of the illness present as a spectrum comprising subclinical gastroenteritis at one end, to severe cholera at the other end. In adults, these symptoms can vary somewhat from those experienced by children. The mild to moderate illness caused by cholera cannot be distinguished from other forms of enterotoxigenic diarrhea, and many sufferers do not seek medical attention. By contrast, severe, complicated cholera, now relatively rare if oral fluid therapy is made available, can lead to hypovolemic shock within 1 hour and death within 2 to 3 hours if left untreated. The key feature is that fluid and electrolyte loss leads to serious complications in children, including severe metabolic acidosis, hyponatremia, hypokalemia, lethargy, altered sensorium, and seizures. Clinical signs of such profound dehydration include wrinkled skin with minimal turgor, eyes sunken within their sockets, cold extremities, restlessness, thirst, dry mucous membranes, depressed fontanelles in infants, weakened voice, thready pulse, and systolic hypotension. Usually, severe cholera starts abruptly with diarrhea, which for the first few motions will contain fecal material but which later evolves into the well known "rice water" of cholera. The incubation period is between a few hours to 7 days, during which the patient may feel premonitory symptoms of abdominal cramping or anorexia, although most severe cholera is of sudden onset. The rate of diarrhea production, which can exceed 1 L/hour, usually peaks within the first 24 hours and slowly declines thereafter. Vomiting may complicate and exacerbate dehydration but usually abates when the patient is properly hydrated. Fever is rare. The explanation for the hypoglycemia occasionally seen (particularly in children) is unclear because no glucose is found in the stool of patients. Cultural practices that withhold nourishment from children during their illness may contribute to this problem. As a corollary, malnutrition in children places them at higher risk for development of severe dehydration and prolonged diarrhea despite antibiotics. Full recovery without the use of antibiotics can be expected in 1 to 6 days if rehydration is administered. If rehydration strategies are delayed, prolonged hypotension can lead to acute renal tubular necrosis. Hypoglycemia in children can result in grand mal seizures. Hypoglycemia and altered consciousness are risk factors for death. Paralytic ileus, muscle cramping, weakness, and cardiac arrhythmias may herald hypokalemia, the most common electrolyte abnormality of children in the tropics. Pulmonary edema has been reported in severely acidotic children rehydrated with normal saline not containing base, unless augmented with standard oral rehydration salts.

The simple rule of thumb in the treatment of cholera is to replace those elements lost and reduce the amount of purging. The first goal is easily accomplished in 92% to 95% of cases with early institution of oral rehydration solutions endorsed by the World Health Organization.[91] Patients with severe dehydration or incessant vomiting, however, necessitate intravenous rehydration therapy, and the World Health Organization suggests that lactated Ringer's is the best commercial solution available if it is supplemented with potassium. The rate of replacement should match the clinical presentation, with severely dehydrated patients receiving a rapid infusion of 2 L of fluid within the first 30 minutes. A slower rate of hydration, or even a switch to oral rehydration solutions can be initiated if clinical improvement is achieved. Oral rehydration solutions owe their success to in vivo experiments that demonstrated enhanced intestinal absorption of sodium and fluid in patients with cholera who were administered oral solutions containing glucose and electrolytes. This well recognized glucose–amino acid–sodium cotransport, leading to fluid and electrolyte absorption, is not affected by the secretory intestine in cholera. Absorption of sodium (and water) occurs during the process of absorption of glucose and other organic molecules such as amino acids, dipeptides, or tripeptides. Cereal-based oral rehydration solutions are being evaluated because they offer advantages: The large polymers provide slowly digested glucose and additional calories, whereas the proteins in the cereals are digested into smaller peptides and amino acids. Cereal-based solutions are cheap and easy to prepare in the home. Their biggest problem is their potential to become contaminated if not properly processed and stored.

The diagnosis can be made presumptively based on clinical manifestations and by examining the stool under dark-field or phase microscopy. *V cholerae* display a typical shooting-star motility, but unless specific antisera (Ogawa or Inaba) are added to the stool preparation, a diagnosis of cholera cannot be made with certainty. The diagnosis is established by isolating the causative organism from stool; however, when cholera is suspected, the laboratory should be alerted to use the proper media.

Antibiotic therapy shortens the period of excretion of *V cholerae* and reduces the volume and duration of diarrhea, thereby also diminishing the cumulative amount of fluid loss. The drug of choice for adults is tetracycline, 250 to 500 mg every 6 hours for 3 days, although streptomycin, chloramphenicol, TMP-SMX, nalidixic acid, and ampicillin all have proven effective. Furazolidone also is effective, and is particularly useful in pregnant women who already are at higher risk for abortion because of cholera.

It is clear that primary infection with O:1 *V cholerae* confers long-term immunity to development of recurrent illness. Illness in adults and recurrent illness in children is rare in endemic areas. Immunity in adult volunteers has been shown to last for at least 3 years. This makes the study of the immunobiology of cholera crucial to the development of effective vaccines. Natural infection with one biovar (i.e., Classical or El Tor) often leads to protection against illness from both. Moreover, serologic responses in humans occur to both the organisms and its toxin. It is likely that both antitoxin antibodies and antibodies directed primarily against somatic O-Ag function synergistically to confer immunity. Parenteral and oral vaccines are under investigation that use various components of *V cholerae*, including the B subunit of the choleratoxin, lipopolysaccharide antigens on the bacterial cell wall, and whole-cell killed and live attenuated organisms. Oral B-subunit and whole-cell preparations show promise, especially if used in combination. Immune prophylaxis has shown efficacy, and the future looks bright for the development of successful cholera vaccines.

Apart from O:1 *V cholerae*, a number of other *Vibrio* sp can produce illness in humans. These pathogenic noncholera vibrios are encountered frequently in the marine environment or associated with seafood, and are known to cause or are suspected of causing gastroenteritis. They can be conveniently divided into three groups: *V parahaemolyticus*; non-O:1 cholera vibrios; and other pathogenic vibrios.

V parahaemolyticus is a halophilic (i.e., salt-loving) vibrio, meaning it will grow only in media containing salt.[86,92] It is commonly isolated from marine waters, their sediment, their inhabitants (fish, crustaceans, and shellfish), and less commonly from soft tissue infections of people who have come in contact with seawater. Isolation of the organism from asymptomatic people is rare.

V parahaemolyticus is a major etiologic agent of bacterial diarrhea in Japan. Furthermore, it has been implicated frequently as a causative agent of food poisoning outbreaks in the United States, where nearly all confirmed cases have been associated with either consumption of raw or improperly stored (after cooking) seafood, or with contamination of food with seawater. Nearly all isolates associated with human illness (97%), but virtually none of the environmental isolates (1%), produce hemolysin (i.e., production of β-hemolysis on modified blood agar, also known as the Kanagawa phenomenon). But, although hemolysin can produce fluid secretion in suckling mice and has mouse-lethal activity, it most likely does not account for the organism's entire ability to produce illness. *V parahaemolyticus* has the ability to elaborate an uncharacterized enterotoxin and also can produce an inflammatory response in the small intestine. The organism has been recovered from blood in laboratory animals after oral challenge. It is likely that these other mechanisms play a role in the organism's pathogenetic capabilities, and may help explain the variable clinical presentations, which can range between a mild, watery diarrhea to a dysentery-like syndrome. Typically, most cases present with an acute onset of diarrhea after an incubation period of less than 24 hours (range, 4–96 hours) that resembles nontyphoidal salmonellosis. Nausea, vomiting, headache, and low-grade fever are common, but severe dehydration as seen with cholera is rare. Mortality rates are low, and the elderly and very young are at greatest risk, particularly if concomitant underlying illness exists. The diarrheal effluent is most commonly watery, but may contain a few leukocytes and, less often, frank blood (<15%). The diagnosis is confirmed by culturing the organism from stool, a procedure that usually requires the use of selective media (i.e., TCBS agar).

Treatment should be directed at prompt replacement of lost fluid and electrolytes, usually orally but intravenously if the clinical situation requires it. The correct antimicrobial therapy has not been well established; usually, none is required given the self-limiting nature of the illness. In addition, the use of antibiotics has not been shown to shorten the natural course of the illness or the duration of pathogen excretion. Some experts suggest that tetracycline may be used in those rare occasions when illness is severe. As with any organism involved in food poisoning, prevention lies in proper food preparation technique (i.e., appropriate cooking and storage temperatures and avoidance of raw or poorly cooked seafood, including oysters and clams).

Non-O:1, also known as nonagglutinable, cholera vibrios are known as such because, despite their biochemical resemblance to *V cholerae*, they do not agglutinate in antiserum against the O-group 1 (somatic) antigen.[86,93] Non-O:1 *V cholerae* have been found to cause gastroenteritis in many parts of the world such as Asia, Africa, and the Americas, including the United States. They also have been isolated from wound and ear infections, biliary tract and blood cultures, and pneumonias. They grow well in waters with increased salinity, commonly being found in the estuarine environment during the warm months, and in marine animals, particularly filter feeders such as oysters, but also other shellfish, in which they may be concentrated. Although illness is strongly associated with consumption of seafood (especially raw oysters), a number of other foods have been implicated in disease outbreaks, including grated eggs and potatoes. Non-O:1 cholera vibrios are associated with cases of travelers' diarrhea, and have been isolated from animals, including dogs. Transmission appears to be primarily by way of the fecal–oral route through contaminated food and water; furthermore, the general environment, including both fresh and sea water, as well as animals, may provide reservoirs for the organism.

The clinical manifestations of the illness range between a cholera-like syndromes to frank dysentery. Non-O:1 *V cholerae* has the capacity to produce cholera toxin or another heat-labile toxin that is active in biologic assays. Most organisms in the United States, however, are not enterotoxigenic, and illness tends to be less severe than typical cholera. Epidemiologic studies show that up to 25% of patients in the United States infected by nonagglutinable vibrios manifest bloody diarrhea, and in some cases more than 20 stools per day can be passed.[93] The illness usually begins with diarrhea, followed by abdominal cramping, fever, and nausea and vomiting after a 12-hour incubation period (range, 6 hours to 3 days), and lasts 1 to 6 days. Diagnosis is made by culturing the stool for the organism, preferably in TCBS agar, because colonies of non-O:1 cholera vibrios will not be identified when stools are submitted for routine culture. Antimicrobial treatment has not been shown to reduce the course or severity of the disease, but, as with *V parahaemolyticus*, tetracycline seems a logical choice in cases of severe diarrhea.

The other pathogenic vibrios include *V fluvialis* and *V furnisii* (also *V hollisae* and *V mimicus*), which are associated with diarrheal illness more frequently than their counterparts *Vibrio damsella* and *V vulnificus*, which are more commonly seen as pathogens in wound infections and sepsis. The epidemiology and features of the diarrheal illness caused by these organisms resembles those seen with *V parahaemolyticus* and the non-O:1 *V cholerae*, being found commonly in the marine environment and associated with seafood consumption. No direct evidence exists that *V vulnificus*, a potentially lethal cause of wound infections and sepsis in the patient with immune disorders, diabetes, or liver disease, causes gastroenteritis. The organism has been recovered and identified as the sole pathogen in stool cultures of patients with gastroenteritis, however, some of whom had predisposing conditions such as unrecognized colon cancer and heavy alcohol consumption.[94]

Aeromonas species and Plesiomonas shigelloides. *Aeromonas* sp[86,95] and *Plesiomonas shigelloides*[96,97] (both members of the *Vibrionaceae* family) appear to be important causes of diarrheal illness in certain settings. The strongest evidence is provided by epidemiologic and microbiologic data that implicate both *Aeromonas* species and *P shigelloides* as human pathogens on the basis of recovery of these organisms as predominant pathogens in patients with gastroenteritis and other infections (i.e., wounds, meningitis). In addition, both organisms have been implicated in travelers' diarrhea and are commonly isolated from fresh- and salt-water environments. *P shigelloides* also has been associated with food-borne outbreaks, particularly those involving oysters and other seafoods.

Aeromonas species are non–lactose-fermenting, facultatively anaerobic, gram-negative rods that grow well on nonselective media. No consensus exists as to the classification of *Aeromonas* species, but a generally agreed-on speciation of this organism recognizes *Aeromonas hydrophila*, *Aeromonas sobria*, and *Aeromonas caviae* as three distinct species within the heterogenous mesophilic group. Of these, *A caviae* appears to show reduced pathogenic potential. New species undoubtedly will be identified as better biochemical assays become available. *A hydrophila* and *A sobria* are the most frequently isolated enteropathogenic species, although *A caviae* also has been implicated in diarrheal disease, particularly with a cholera-like illness. *Aeromonas* species also can be isolated from asymptomatic patients, and in some populations rates of recovery in infected people with and without diarrhea parallel each other. A study of 1000 children with diarrhea in Australia, however, demonstrated *Aeromonas* strains in 10% of children with diarrhea, as opposed to an incidence of only 1% in age- and sex-matched controls.[98] Furthermore, treatment of gastrointestinal symptoms with antibiotics directed against *Aeromonas* species has resulted in clinical improvement, and serologic conversions have been demonstrated after clinical infection. Infection with *A hydrophila* is commonly associated with exposure to water, and the organism often is demonstrated as a pathogen in immunocompromised and otherwise healthy adults, and in wound infections, endocarditis, and meningitis. The pathogenesis of *A hydrophila* infection is incompletely understood, but virulence probably relates to production of enterotoxin and natural cytotoxic activity. The organism produces both heat-stable and heat-labile enterotoxins (the actions of the latter resemble those of choleratoxin) and other extracellular products such as α- and β-hemolysins, proteases, and peptidases, which may account for cytotoxicity. The features of enteric illness with *A hydrophila* usually are self-limiting, with a tendency to occur during the warmer months, and frequently include watery diarrhea that may contain blood and mucus in up to 22% of cases, mild fever, and vomiting. Symptoms usually last less than 1 week, but may persist as long as 2 or more weeks in the case of short-term illness, and more than 1 year in the case of chronic illness. A study of symptomatic patients in whom *Aeromonas* species were the only identifiable pathogens in stool specimens found that persons aged 12 through 73 years were more likely to experience prolonged illness (mean duration, 42 days) than children younger than 12 years of age, in whom the illness tended to be shorter (mean duration, 19 days) but more severe.[99] Four of the adults experienced chronic symptoms for longer than 1 year. Five patients in whom gastrointestinal symptoms had lasted a mean of 47 days experienced resolution of their illness after taking antimicrobials to which the organism was susceptible. The role of antimicrobial therapy in this illness, however, remains undefined. In vitro studies have demonstrated these organisms to be sensitive to the fluoroquinolones, aminoglycosides (except streptomycin), TMP-SMX, tetracycline, third-generation cephalosporins, and chloramphenicol.

The classification of *P shigelloides* also is unresolved, with some studies suggesting this organism be classified with the *Enterobacteriaceae* family rather than *Vibrionaceae*.[100] *P shigelloides* is a non–lactose-fermenting, facultatively anaerobic, gram-negative rod that grows on commonly used enteric media. Based on O-Ag and H-Ag antigens, 107 serovars exist, some of which cross-react with antigens common to *Shigella* and *Aeromonas* sp. *P shigelloides* gastroenteritis affects both children and adults, and 70% of identifiable cases are associated with an underlying illness or risk factor such as consumption of contaminated food (i.e., seafood) or foreign travel. The features of this illness can vary, taking on an invasive character similar to that caused by *Shigella* species in some reports, or manifesting itself as a cholera-like illness or less severe enterotoxigenic diarrhea. The most common symptom is abdominal cramps, followed by vomiting, dehydration, and fever, and many patients experience bloody diarrhea. The untreated illness can last from 1 to 14 days (mean, 11 days), but antimicrobial therapy has been associated with elimination of the organism from stool with concomitant improvement in clinical symptoms. A number of extraintestinal manifestations are associated with *P shigelloides* infection, including septicemia, meningitis, endophthalmitis, arthritis, cellulitis, and cholecystitis. The pathogenic properties responsible for illness production remain obscure. Although some strains of *P shigelloides* demonstrate the ability to invade the intestinal mucosa, the Sereny test has always demonstrated negative results. Some strains have been shown to produce heat-labile or heat-stable enterotoxins. Although large clinical trials with antimicrobial agents are lacking, in vitro experience shows the organism to be susceptible to chloramphenicol, the aminoglycosides, TMP-SMX, tetracycline, imipenem, some third-generation cephalosporins, and the fluoroquinolones.

Viral Gastroenteritis

Viruses were first confirmed as etiologic agents in acute diarrhea in 1972, with the report of virus particles identified by immune electron microscopy in the stool of a volunteer made ill when fed bacteria-free stool filtrates originally obtained during an outbreak of gastroenteritis in an elementary school in Norwalk, Ohio.[101] Since then, a number of other viral agents have been implicated in diarrheal illness of both children and adults. The literature on this subject recognizes at least five classes of virus that produce illness in humans (i.e., rotavirus, Norwalk virus, enteric adenoviruses, calicivirus, and other small round viruses) and a number of other viruses suspected of causing illness (astrovirus and breda-like viruses, and enteric coronavirus-like viruses).[102,103] Rotavirus and Norwalk viruses are discussed in the following section.

Although exact figures do not exist, probably owing to difficulty in diagnosis, viral gastroenteritis is estimated to be responsible for approximately 25% to 40% of the mortality due to gastrointestinal infection worldwide. Certainly, rotavirus is the single most important cause of infant death in non–cholera-endemic areas. New and improving diagnostic techniques, including immune electron microscopy, various assays (radioimmunoassay and ELISA), and analysis of genetic material (polyacrylamide gel electrophoresis and dot hybridization) will no doubt aid in placing these agents into proper perspective.

Rotavirus. Rotavirus, first recognized as pathogenic in 1973, is a nonenveloped, spherical, 70-nm virus that possesses a protein core enclosing a double-stranded RNA genome, RNA-dependent RNA polymerase, and other enzymes.[104,105] This

core is surrounded by an inner capsid connected by spoke-like capsomeres to an outer capsid, giving the appearance of a spoked wheel under electron microscopy (*rota* in Latin means "wheel"). Numerous rotaviruses, all sharing a common appearance and representing a separate genus of the family *Reovirideae*, can be found in different mammalian and avian species. Most human and animal disease is caused by group A rotavirus; furthermore, by using RNA polyacrylamide gel electrophoresis techniques, it has been possible to identify different rotaviral strains such as pararotavirus (or rotavirus group B) and other non-group A rotaviruses. Group B rotavirus is rare in the United States, but has been responsible for large outbreaks of diarrhea in adults and children in China, one of which involved over 7000 cases.[106]

Rotavirus principally produces sporadic episodes of gastroenteritis in children between the ages of 6 and 24 months, has a worldwide distribution, and occurs more frequently during the winter months in temperate climates, but year-round in tropical areas. It also has been documented occasionally as an etiologic agent in adult gastroenteritis and travelers' diarrhea.[18,107] Symptomatic rotavirus infection occurs rarely in newborns, although asymptomatic infection has been documented. Rotavirus accounts for 15% to 50% of hospital admissions for diarrheal disease in tropical areas, and 35% to 60% of the gastroenteritis cases in industrialized countries. These figures can be substantially higher (i.e., 80%–100%) if determined by season (i.e., winter months), by age specificity (i.e., 6–24 months), and economic status. Rotaviral infection rates are lower in the outpatient and the general community, 25% and 13%, respectively. The predominant mode of transmission of rotavirus seems to be through the fecal–oral route, most likely person to person, with children and probably asymptomatic adults serving as major reservoirs in the community. The virus can survive for weeks on environmental surfaces and hence has been an important factor in the development of nosocomial infections, particularly in pediatric and geriatric wards. Intrafamilial spread has likewise been shown to be important; furthermore, rotavirus has been identified in seafood, drinking and environmental water, and in asymptomatic adults and children.

Epidemiologic studies show that 80% to 100% of people older than the age of 2 years living in endemic areas have acquired serum antibody to rotavirus, likely reflecting past symptomatic or asymptomatic infection. In addition, over 80% of human colostral and milk samples tested in several studies contained anti-rotavirus secretory α-immunoglobulin (IgA), and it is recognized that breast feeding decreases both the incidence and severity of gastrointestinal illness in children. Local secretory IgA production correlates well with protection, unlike humoral antibody levels; however, secretory IgA is serotype specific, and protection against one specific rotavirus serotype does not provide protection against other serotypes. Sequential infections with rotavirus of same and differing serotypes is known to occur, particularly in children younger than 5 years of age; however, it is likely that a booster response of mucosal immunity occurs, which may account for the self-limiting nature of most rotaviral infections in older age groups.

Rotavirus causes damage to the mucosal cells of the proximal small intestine, thereby promoting morphologic changes in the structure of the epithelial lining. The result is shortened villi, hypertrophied crypts, mitochondrial swelling, decreased numbers of and irregularly shaped microvilli, and mononuclear infiltration of the lamina propria. The immature cells, which quickly replace and lack the absorptive capacity of the lost mature enterocytes, are greatly impaired in the ability to absorb sodium and water through glucose-coupled sodium transport and sodium–potassium adenosine triphosphatase activity. Disaccharidase function also is impaired. This process leads to sodium, water, and carbohydrate malabsorption. The osmotic diarrhea resulting from disaccharidase deficiency can be prolonged. Other features include fat malabsorption and delayed emptying, the latter likely accounting for the nausea and vomiting frequently seen in this illness.

Most symptomatic illness occurs in infants and children and can be marked by profound dehydration, frequently with a compensated metabolic acidosis and electrolyte imbalance, all important factors in the mortality of this disease. The high rates of rotaviral diarrhea among children presenting to the hospital reflects the tendency of this pathogen to cause significant dehydration in the very young. The typical rotavirus gastroenteritis syndrome begins with large-volume, watery diarrhea accompanied by vomiting, after a 48- to 72-hour incubation period. Low-grade fever is common, and abdominal cramping also may be seen; however, systemic symptoms and bloody diarrhea are rare. Respiratory tract symptoms, such as pharyngitis and otitis media, have been reported in up to 60% of pediatric patients. The disease is usually self-limiting when attention is paid to fluid and electrolyte replacements. Diarrhea (i.e., 3–12 stools per day) can persist for 4 to 5 days, and complete recovery is expected within 10 to 14 days. Examination of the stool usually fails to reveal either fecal white or red blood cells, but fatty, pasty, mucoid, brown, or yellow-green stools may be seen. Outside cholera-endemic areas, rotavirus is the most important cause of dehydration, and it is estimated that 1 million of the 5 million diarrhea-related deaths occurring annually in the developing world are a result of rotavirus infection.

Symptomatic infection in children is associated with viral shedding in large numbers, making the diagnosis with conventional fecal assay techniques feasible. Adults excrete lower concentrations of virus, making commercial kits less useful. Antibody-dependent assays cannot detect non-group A rotavirus, but are nevertheless the most widely used assays available for diagnostic purposes. A number of these assays are available as commercial kits for routine diagnostic requirements and to screen large numbers of stool specimens. These kits (e.g., Rotazyme; Enzygnost; Bio-Enzabead; Rotalex) are more sensitive and specific than electron microscopy (Rotazyme has 95% sensitivity and specificity), although some false-positive reactions may occur.

The ability to propagate rotavirus in tissue culture (unlike Norwalk and other viruses) has been instrumental in establishing inroads into vaccine development. Through the use of attenuated oral vaccines that use rotavirus strains that infect animals (bovine and simian), protection rates of 88% have been reported against homologous strain-induced illness, although these rates may be lower in developing countries.[108] Further study and genetic manipulation of the virus may produce a safe and effective vaccine.

There is no available antiviral agent against rotaviral gastroenteritis. Treatment is predicated on prevention and management of clinical dehydration and electrolyte abnormalities through the use of oral rehydration formula and intravenous replacement. Because mucosal recovery depends on adequate nutrition, refeeding should not be withheld for more than 24 hours. Avoidance of milk products in adults and older children and the use of dilute milk preparations in infants is recommended to avoid aggravating the osmotic diarrhea resulting from disaccharidase deficiency.

Norwalk virus. Despite being the best recognized and one of the most extensively studied viral agents of acute gastroenteritis, many features of the Norwalk virus[109,110] remain obscure, primarily because it cannot be cultivated in in vitro systems, and no animal model exists. Nevertheless, a great deal of information has been gathered regarding the gastroenteritis syndrome caused by this 27-nm, nonenveloped, round particle. Furthermore, studies have shown that a number of morphologically similar but antigenically distinct agents also can cause acute gastroenteritis. They are categorized as "Norwalk-like" or "other small round viruses," of which Norwalk is the prototype. Some of those are named according to where the naturally occurring outbreak first took place, such as Snow Mountain (Colorado), Paramatta (Australia), and others.

Norwalk virus is a significant cause of epidemic diarrhea in developed countries, and seroepidemiologic studies have shown it to be a common infection worldwide. From studies at the National Institutes of Health and the CDC, it appears that one third to one half (or more) of outbreaks of epidemic nonbacterial gastroenteritis can be attributed to Norwalk or serologically related viruses.[109] In one outbreak caused by contaminated water in an elementary school in Washington state in 1978, 72% of students and teachers who consumed water from the implicated source became ill.[110] A secondary attack rate of 32% was noted in family contacts. This outbreak serves to illustrate several important points about Norwalk-induced diarrheal illness: high attack rates; a great propensity for secondary (and even tertiary) transmission, most likely through person-to-person contact; and the fact that water is the most frequently implicated common-source origin for development of illness. The primary form of viral transmission is through the fecal–oral route, although airborne transmission of aerosolized vomitus has been suggested to explain the rapidity of secondary spread. Respiratory tract symptoms are less common in Norwalk virus illness compared to rotavirus gastroenteritis. Apart from disease outbreaks implicating water from swimming pools, lakes, and municipal supplies, large food-borne outbreaks of Norwalk virus (particularly involving shellfish) have been documented in the United States and Australia. The virus also has been demonstrated as an agent of gastroenteritis in institutional outbreaks (i.e., schools, nursing homes), cruise ships, travelers' diarrhea, and intrafamilial disease.

Norwalk virus, in contrast to rotavirus in the United States, primarily affects older children and adults, and does not display a seasonal pattern. In developed countries, antibody to Norwalk virus is unusual during childhood, and generally appears after the child is 5 years of age, reaching a prevalence of 50% to 80% by late adolescence and adulthood. In developing countries, however, the antibody is acquired at an earlier age, suggesting that, unlike in developed nations, Norwalk may be an important etiologic agent in the severe diarrheal illness of infants and children.

The clinical manifestations of Norwalk gastroenteritis are those of a mild illness, characteristically epidemic in nature, with an incubation period of 24 to 48 hours and symptoms that last approximately the same time span. In fact, many outbreaks of "intestinal influenza" or "stomach virus" are actually Norwalk viral infections. The illness may last anywhere from 2 hours to several days, with vomiting and diarrhea being the two most notable symptoms of this disease. Other features include nausea, abdominal cramping or discomfort, low-grade fever, myalgias, anorexia, and headache. Dysentery, or bloody stools, are not features of this illness. Although morbidity can be high, the illness rarely requires hospitalization, and deaths occur infrequently.

Development of illness correlates with particular lesions detected on small bowel biopsy specimens of ill, but not well, volunteers. Although Norwalk virus cannot be visualized in the cells of the intestinal epithelium (unlike rotavirus), during illness these cells appear abnormal, with decreased cell height and increased vacuolation. There also is increased leukocyte infiltration of the lamina propria and villous tips. Adenylate cyclase levels remain normal, but intestinal brush border enzyme levels are decreased. These features implicate decreased absorptive capacity as the pathogenic mechanism of diarrhea production by this organism. The delayed gastric emptying observed during Norwalk illness may help explain, in part, why vomiting is such a prominent feature of this syndrome.

The diagnosis of Norwalk (and Norwalk-like) viral gastroenteritis is difficult primarily because there are no commercially available diagnostic tests, and the diagnostic techniques in use (i.e., immune electron microscopy, radioimmunoassay, and ELISA) are labor and reagent intensive, and largely relegated to investigative use. Norwalk virus has been cloned independently in two laboratories, and reagents for detection of the virus are being developed. The particular clinical and epidemiologic features of the illness are helpful in arriving at the diagnosis but are not specific enough to differentiate this entity from other short-lived diarrheal illnesses. Confirmation can be achieved by detection of the viral particles in feces or vomitus or by demonstrating a fourfold or greater antibody titer rise in convalescent sera of ill people; however, this usually requires that the specimen be sent to a specialized reference laboratory.

No antiviral agent exists against Norwalk or Norwalk-like viruses, and therefore fluids, electrolytes, and symptomatic treatment represent the major forms of therapy.

Diarrhea of Uncertain Etiology

Regardless of completeness of study, the etiology of most cases of nonepidemic diarrheal disease remains unestablished. Much of the illness is undoubtedly caused by as yet inadequately defined enteropathogens. A variety of poorly characterized bacterial enteropathogens may on occasion be identified by the research laboratory, including enterotoxigenic or cytotoxigenic *Bacteroides fragilis*, *Klebsiella pneumoniae*, and other miscellaneous gram-negative bacilli. Additional small, round viruses resembling Norwalk or astroviruses will be identified in these patients. Finally, newly described parasitic agents such as *Cyclospora* (previously called cyanobacter-like

organisms) will be found.[111-117] These represent examples of some of the agents identified. Numerous other agents have been implicated as causes of small bowel infection and diarrhea in a limited number of patients. Future study will determine the importance of these new agents.

The reader is directed to Chapter 38, Approach to the Patient With Diarrhea; Chapter 51, Advice to Travelers; Chapter 84, Bacterial Infections of the Colon; and Chapter 131, Microbiologic Studies.

REFERENCES

1. Palmer AB. Diarrhea and dysentery: modern views of their pathology and treatment. Detroit: George S. Davis, 1887.
2. Bennett JV, Holmberg SD, Rogers MF, Solomon SL. Infectious and parasitic diseases. In: Amler RW, Dull HB, eds. Closing the gap: the burden of unnecessary illness. New York: Oxford University Press, 1987:102.
3. Snyder JD, Merson MH. The magnitude of the global problem of acute diarrhoeal disease: a review of active surveillance data. Bull WHO 1982;60:605.
4. Davenport HW, ed. Physiology of the digestive tract. 4th ed. Chicago: Year Book Medical Publishers, 1977:161:198.
5. National Institutes of Health. Travelers' diarrhea: consensus conference. JAMA 1985;253:2700.
6. DuPont HL, Pickering LK. Infections of the gastrointestinal tract: microbiology, pathophysiology, and clinical features. New York: Plenum Medical Book Company, 1980:218.
7. Kendrick MA. A study of illness among Americans returning from international travel, July 11–August 24, 1971 (preliminary data). J Infect Dis 1972;126:684.
8. Lowenstein MS, Balows A, Gangarosa EJ. Turista at an International Congress in Mexico. Lancet 1973;1:529.
9. Kendrick MA. Summary of study on illness among Americans visiting Europe, March 31, 1969–March 30, 1970. J Infect Dis 1972;126:685.
10. Ryder RW, Wells JG, Gangarosa EJ. A study of travelers' diarrhea in foreign visitors to the United States. J Infect Dis 1977;136:605.
11. Steffen R. Epidemiologic studies of travelers' diarrhea, severe gastrointestinal infections, and cholera. Rev Infect Dis 1986;8(Suppl 2):S122.
12. Gorbach SL. Travelers' diarrhea. In: Gorbach SL, ed. Infectious diarrhea. Boston: Blackwell, 1986:179.
13. Dandoy S. The diarrhea of travelers: incidence in foreign students in the United States. California Medicine 1966;104:458.
14. Tjoa WS, DuPont HL, Sullivan P, et al. Location of food consumption and travelers' diarrhea. Am J Epidemiol 1979;106:61.
15. Ericsson CD, Pickering LK, Sullivan P, DuPont HL. The role of location of food consumption in the prevention of travelers' diarrhea in Mexico. Gastroenterology 1980;79:812.
16. Keswick BH, Gerba CP, DuPont HL, et al. Detection of enteric viruses in treated drinking water. Appl Environ Microbiol 1984;47:1290.
17. DuPont HL, Ericsson CD, Johnson PC, et al. Antimicrobial agents in the prevention of travelers' diarrhea. Rev Infect Dis 1986;8(Suppl 2):S167.
18. Ericsson CD, DuPont HL. Travelers' diarrhea: approaches to prevention and treatment. Clin Infect Dis 1993;16:616.
19. Mattila L, Siitonen A, Kyrönseppa H, et al. Seasonal variation in etiology of travelers' diarrhea. J Infect Dis 1992;165:385.
20. Jokipii L, Pohjola S, Jokipii AMM. Cryptosporidium: a frequent finding in patients with gastrointestinal symptoms. Lancet 1983;2:358.
21. DuPont HL, Ericsson CD. Prevention and treatment of traveler's diarrhea. N Engl J Med 1993;328:1821.

22. DuPont HL, Galindo E, Evans DG, et al. Prevention of travelers' diarrhea with trimethoprim–sulfamethoxazole and trimethoprim alone. Gastroenterology 1983;84:75.

23. Ericsson CD, DuPont HL, Galindo E, et al. Efficacy of bicozamycin in preventing travelers' diarrhea. Gastroenterology 1985;88:473.

24. Johnson PC, Ericsson CD, Morgan DR, et al. Lack of emergence of resistant fecal flora during successful prophylaxis of travelers' diarrhea with norfloxacin. Antimicrob Agents Chemother 1986;30:671.

25. Sack DA, Froehlich JL, Zulich AW, et al. Prophylactic doxycycline for travelers' diarrhea: results of a prospective double-blind study of Peace Corps volunteers in Morocco. Gastroenterology 1979;76:1368.

26. DuPont HL, Sullivan P, Evans DG, et al. Prevention of travelers' diarrhea (emporiatric enteritis): prophylactic administration of subsalicylate bismuth. JAMA 1980;243:247.

27. DuPont HL, Ericsson CD, Johnson PC, et al. Prevention of travelers' diarrhea by the tablet formulation of bismuth subsalicylate. JAMA 1987;247:1347.

28. Centers for Disease Control. Food-borne disease outbreaks: 5-year summary, 1983–1987. MMWR Surveill Summ 1990;39:15.

29. St. Louis ME. Water-related disease outbreaks, 1985. MMWR CDC Surveill Summ 37(SS-2):15, 1988.

30. Sakazaki R. *Vibrio parahaemolyticus*: a non-choleragenic enteropathogenic *Vibrio*. In: Bushnell OA, Brookhyser CS, eds. Proceedings of the Cholera Research Symposium. Washington, DC: U.S. Department of Health, Education, and Welfare, 1965:30.

31. Syndman DR. Bacterial food poisoning. In: Gorbach SL, ed. Infectious diarrhea. Boston: Blackwell, 1986:201.

32. Holmberg SD, Blake PA. Staphylococcal food poisoning in the United States: new facts and old misconceptions. JAMA 1984;251:487.

33. Terranova W, Blake PA. *Bacillus cereus* food poisoning. N Engl J Med 1978;298:143.

34. Melling J, Capel BJ, Turnbull PCB, Gilbert RJ. Identification of a novel enterotoxigenic activity associated with *Bacillus cereus*. J Clin Pathol 1976;29:938.

35. Turnbull PCB. Studies on the production of enterotoxins by *Bacillus cereus*. J Clin Pathol 1976;29:941.

36. Hughes JM, Blumenthal JR, Merson MH, et al. Clinical features of types A and B food-borne botulism. Ann Intern Med 1981;95:442.

37. Sanders WE Jr. Intoxications from the seas: ciguatera, scombroid, and paralytic shellfish poisoning. Infect Dis Clin North Am 1987;1:665.

38. Mills AR, Passmore R. Pelagic paralysis. Lancet 1988;1:161.

39. Birkhead G, Vogt RL, Heun EM. Characterization of an outbreak of *Clostridium perfringens* food poisoning by quantitative fecal culture and fecal enterotoxin measurement. J Clin Microbiol 1988;26:471.

40. Larson HE, Borriello SE. Infectious diarrhea due to *Clostridium perfringens* (letter). J Infect Dis 1988;157:390.

41. McDonel JL. Mechanism of action of *Clostridium perfringens* enterotoxin. Food Technol 1980;34:91.

42. Skjelkvale R, Uemura T. Experimental diarrhoea in human volunteers following oral administration of *Clostridium perfringens* enterotoxin. J Appl Bacteriol 1977;43:281.

43. Borriello SP, Larson HE, Welch AR, et al. Enterotoxigenic *Clostridium perfringens*: a possible cause of antibiotic-associated diarrhea. Lancet 1984;1:305.

44. Williams R, Piper M, Borriello P, et al. Diarrhoea due to enterotoxigenic *Clostridium perfringens*: clinical features and management of a cluster of ten cases. Age Ageing 1985;14:296.

45. Borriello SP, Barclay FE, Welch AR, et al. Epidemiology of diarrhoea caused by enterotoxigenic *Clostridium perfringens*. J Med Microbiol 1985;20:363.

46. Jackson SG, Vip-Chuck DA, Clark JB, Brodsky MH. Diagnostic importance of *Clostridium perfringens* enterotoxin analysis in recurring enteritis among elderly, chronic care psychiatric patients. J Clin Microbiol 1986;23:748.

47. Borriello SP, Williams RKT. Treatment of *Clostridium perfrin-*

gens enterotoxin-associated diarrhoea with metronidazole. J Infect 1985;10:65.

48. Van Kessel LJP, Verbrugh HA, Stringer MF, Hoekstra JBL. Necrotizing enteritis associated with toxigenic type A *Clostridium perfringens* (letter). J Infect Dis 1985;151:947.

49. Murrell TGC, Roth L, Egerton J, et al. Pig-bel: enteritis necroticans. A study in diagnosis and management. Lancet 1966;1:217.

50. Lawrence G, Shann F, Freestone DS, Walker PD. Prevention of necrotising enteritis in Papua, New Guinea by active immunisation. Lancet 1979;1:227.

51. Schlech WF III, Lavigne PM, Bortolussi RA, et al. Epidemic listeriosis evidence for transmission by food. N Engl J Med 1983;308:203.

52. Bojsen-Moller J. Human listeriosis: diagnostic, epidemiological, and clinical studies. Acta Pathol Microbiol Scand [Suppl] 1972;229:1.

53. Linnan MJ, Mascola L, Xiao Dong L, et al. Epidemic listeriosis associated with Mexican-style cheese. N Engl J Med 1988;319:823.

54. DuPont HL, Pickering LK, eds. Infections of the gastrointestinal tract: microbiology, pathophysiology, and clinical features. New York: Plenum Medical Book Company, 1980;239.

55. Levine MM. *Escherichia coli* that cause diarrhea: enterotoxigenic, enteroinvasive, enterohemorrhagic, and enteroadherent. J Infect Dis 1987;155:377.

56. Satterwhite TK, Evans DG, DuPont HL, et al. Role of *Escherichia coli* colonization factor in acute diarrhea. Lancet 1978;2:181.

57. DuPont HL, Olarte J, Evans DG, et al. Comparative susceptibility of Latin American and United States students to enteric pathogens. N Engl J Med 1976;295:1520.

58. Pickering LK, DuPont HL, Evans DG, et al. Isolation of enteric pathogens from asymptomatic students from the United States and Latin America. J Infect Dis 1977;135:1003.

59. Donnenberg MS, Kaper JB. Enteropathogenic *Escherichia coli*. Infect Immun 1992;60:3953.

60. Rothbaum R, McAdams J, Giannella R, Partin JC. A clinicopathologic study of enterocyte-adherent *Escherichia coli*: a cause of protracted diarrhea in infants. Gastroenterology 1982;83:441.

61. Thoren A. The role of enteropathogenic *E. coli* in infant diarrhea: aspects on bacteriology, epidemiology, and therapy. Scand J Infect Dis [Suppl] 1983;37:1

62. Yamamoto T, Echeverria P, Yokota T. Drug resistance and adherence to human intestines of enteroaggregative *Escherichia coli*. J Infect Dis 1992;165:744.

63. Tulloch EF Jr, Ryan KJ, Formal SB, Franklin FA. Invasive enteropathic *Escherichia coli* dysentery: an outbreak in 28 adults. Ann Intern Med 1973;79:13.

64. Snyder JD, et al. Outbreak of invasive *Escherichia coli* gastroenteritis on a cruise ship. Am J Trop Med Hyg 1984;33:281.

65. Griffin PM, Ostroff SM, Tauxe RV, et al. Illness associated With *Escherichia coli* 0157:H7 infections: a broad clinical spectrum. Ann Intern Med 1988;109:705.

66. 26th Interscience Conference on Antimicrobial Agents and Chemotherapy. Epidemiology of sporadic diarrhea due to verocytotoxin-producing *Escherichia coli*: a two-year prospective study. J Infect Dis 1988;157:1054.

67. Ratnam S, March SB, Sprague WD, et al. Are humans a source of *Escherichia coli* 0157:H7, the agent of hemorrhagic colitis? N Engl J Med 1986;315:1612.

68. Karmali MA, Petric M, Lim C, et al. The association between idiopathic hemolytic uremic syndrome and infection by verotoxin-producing *Escherichia coli*. J Infect Dis 1985;151:775.

69. Strockbine NA, Jackson MP, Jung LM, et al. Cloning and sequencing of the genes for shiga toxin from *Shigella dysenteriae* type 1. J Bacteriol 1988;170:1116.

70. Keusch GT. Shigella in infectious diarrhea. In: Gorbach SL, ed. Infectious diarrhea. Boston: Blackwell, 1986:32.

71. Levine MM, Xu J-G, Kaper JB, et al. A DNA probe to identify enterohemorrhagic *Escherichia coli* of 0157:H7 and other serotypes that cause hemorrhagic colitis and hemolytic uremic syndrome. J Infect Dis 1987;156:175.

72. Wilder AN, MacCready RA. Isolation of *Salmonella* from poul-

try, poultry products, and poultry processing plants in Massachusetts. N Engl J Med 1966;274:1453.

73. Rubin RH, Weinstein L. Salmonellosis: microbiologic, pathologic, and clinical features. New York: Stratton, 1977.

74. Baloda SB, Faris A, Krovacek K, Wadstrom T. Cytotonic enterotoxins and cytotoxic factors produced by *Salmonella enteriditis* and *Salmonella typhimurium*. Toxicon 1988;21:785.

75. Aserkoff B, Bennett JV. Effect of antibiotic therapy in acute salmonellosis on the fecal excretion of *Salmonella*. N Engl J Med 1969;281:636.

76. Murray BE. Resistance of *Shigella*, *Salmonella*, and other selected enteric pathogens to antimicrobial agents. Rev Infect Dis 1986;8(Suppl 2):S172.

77. Rowe B, Threlfall EJ. Drug resistance in gram-negative aerobic bacilli. Br Med Bull 1984;40:68.

78. Goldstein FW, Chumpitaz JC, Guevara JM. Plasmid-mediated resistance to multiple antibiotics in *Salmonella typhi*. J Infect Dis 1986;153:261.

79. Murray BE. Problems and mechanism of antimicrobial resistance. Infect Dis Clin North Am 1989;3:423.

80. Wahdan MH, Serie C, Cerisier Y, et al. A controlled field trial of live *Salmonella typhi* strain Ty21a oral vaccine against typhoid: three year results. J Infect Dis 1982;145:292.

81. Gutman LT. *Yersinia enterocolitica* and *Yersinia pseudotuberculosis*. In: Gorbach SL, ed. Infectious diarrhea. Boston: Blackwell, 1986:65.

82. Feeney GF, Kerlin P, Sampson JA. Clinical aspects of infection with *Yersinia enterocolitica* in adults. Aust N Z J Med 1987;17:216.

83. Bottone EJ, ed. *Yersinia enterocolitica*. Boca Raton, FL: CRC Press, 1981.

84. Cover TL, Aber RC. *Yersinia enterocolitica*. N Engl J Med 1989;321:16.

85. Van Noyen RV, Selderslaghs R, Wauters G, Vandepitte J. Comparative epidemiology of *Yersinia enterocolitica* and related speciesq in patients and healthy controls. Contrib Microbiol Immunol 1987;9:61.

86. Morris JG Jr. *Vibrio* and *Aeromonas*. In: Gorbach SL, ed. Infectious diarrhea. Boston: Blackwell, 1986:101.

87. Rabbani GH. Cholera. Clin Gastroenterol 1986;15:507.

88. Colwell RR, Seidler RJ, Kaper J, et al. Occurrence of *Vibrio cholerae* serotype 01 in Maryland and Louisiana estuaries. Appl Environ Microbiol 1981;41:555.

89. Centers for Disease Control. Cholera associated with international travel. MMWR 1992;141:664.

90. Gemmell CG. Comparative study of the nature and biological activities of bacterial enterotoxins. J Med Microbiol 1984;17:217.

91. The management of acute diarrhea in children: oral rehydration, maintenance and nutritional therapy. MMWR 1992;41:1.

92. Joseph SW, Collwell RR, Kaper JB. *Vibrio parahaemolyticus* and related halophilic vibrios. CRC Crit Rev Microbiol 1983;10:77.

93. Morris JG, et al. Non-O group 1 *Vibrio cholerae* gastroenteritis in the United States. Ann Intern Med 1981;94:656.

94. Johnston JM, Becker SF, McFarland LM. Gastroenteritis in patients with stool isolates of *Vibrio vulnificus*. Am J Med 1986;80:336.

95. delaMorena ML, Van R, Singh K, et al. Diarrhea associated with *Aeromonas* species in children in day care centers. J Infect Dis 1993;168:215.

96. Brenden RA, Miller MA, Janda JM. Clinical disease spectrum and pathogenic factors associated with *Plesiomonas shigelloides* infections in humans. Rev Infect Dis 1988;10:303.

97. Holmberg SD, Wachsmuth JK, Hickman-Brenner FW, et al. *Plesiomonas* enteric infections in the United States. Ann Intern Med 1986;105:690.

98. Burke V, Gracey M, Robinson J, et al. The microbiology of childhood gastroenteritis: *Aeromonas* species and other infective agents. J Infect Dis 1983;148:68.

99. Holmberg SD, Schell WL, Fanning GR, et al. *Aeromonas* intestinal infections in the United States. Ann Intern Med 1986;105:683.

100. Basu S, Tharanathan RN, Kantrohr T, et al. Chemical structure of the lipid A component of *Plesiomonas shigelloides* and its taxonomical significance. FEMS Microbiol Lett 1985;28:7.

101. Kapikian AZ, Wyatt RG, Dolin R, et al. Visualization by immune electron microscopy of a 27-nm particle associated with acute infectious nonbacterial gastroenteritis. J Virol 1972;10:1075.

102. Blacklow NR, Greenberg HB. Viral gastroenteritis. N Engl J Med 1991;325:252.

103. Green KY, Lew JF, Jiang X, et al. Comparison of reactivities of baculovirus-expressed recombinant Norwalk virus capsid antigen with those of the native Norwalk virus antigen in serologic assays and some epidemiologic observations. J Clin Microbiol 1993;31:2185.

104. Christensen ML. Human viral gastroenteritis. Clin Microbiol Rev 1989;2:51.

105. Bartlett AV, Bednarz-Prashad AJ, DuPont HL, Pickering LK. Rotavirus gastroenteritis. Annu Rev Med 1987;38:399.

106. Tao H, Changan W, Zhaoying F. Waterborne outbreak of rotavirus diarrhoea in China caused by a novel rotavirus. Lancet 1984;1:1139.

107. Hardy DB. Epidemiology of rotavirus in adults. Rev Infect Dis 1987;9:461.

108. Vesikari T, Kapikian AZ, Delem A, Zissis G. Protection of infants against rotavirus diarrhoea by RIT 4327 attenuated bovine rotavirus strain vaccine. Lancet 1984;1:977.

109. Kaplan JE, Gary GW, Baron RC, et al. Epidemiology of Norwalk gastroenteritis and the role of Norwalk virus in outbreaks of acute nonbacterial gastroenteritis. Ann Intern Med 1982;96:756.

110. Taylor JW, Gary GW, Greenberg HB. Norwalk-related viral gastroenteritis due to contaminated water. Am J Epidemiol 1981;114:584.

111. Rennie RP, Anderson CM, Wensley BG, et al. *Klebsiella pneumoniae* gastroenteritis masked by *Clostridium perfringens*. J Clin Microbiol 1990;28:216.

112. Albert MJ, Alam K, Ansaruzzaman M, et al. Pathogenesis of *Providencia alcalifaciens*-induced diarrhea. Infect Immun 1992;60:5017.

113. Schmidt H, Montag M, Biochemuhl J, et al. Shiga-like toxin II-related cytoxins in *Citrobacter freundii* strains from humans and beef samples. Infect Immun 1993;61:534.

114. Grohmann G, Glass RI, Gold J, et al. Outbreak of human calicivirus gastroenteritis in day-care center in Sydney, Australia. J Clin Microb 1991;29:544.

115. Esahli H, Brebäck K, Bennet R, et al. Astroviruses as a cause of nosocomial outbreaks of infant diarrhea. Pediatr Infect Dis J 1991;10:511.

116. Udkow MP, Markell EK. *Blastocystis hominis*: prevalence in asymptomatic versus symptomatic hosts. J Infect Dis 1993;168:242.

117. Ortega YR, Sterling CR, Gilman RH, et al. *Cyclospora* species: a new protozoan pathogen of humans. N Engl J Med 1993;328:1308.

Textbook of Gastroenterology, second edition, edited
by Tadataka Yamada. JB Lippincott Company,
Philadelphia © 1995.

CHAPTER 71

Chronic Infections of the Small Intestine

William O. Dobbins III

Tropical Sprue	*Epidemiology*
Epidemiology	*Etiology*
Etiology	*Clinical and Pathologic Manifestations*
Clinical Manifestations	*Differential Diagnosis and Diagnostic Studies*
Laboratory Findings	*Clinical Course and Treatment*
Differential Diagnosis	**Tuberculosis**
Treatment	**Histoplasmosis**
Whipple's Disease	

Most viral and bacterial infections of the gastrointestinal tract cause brief, self-limited episodes of acute diarrhea. Although the distinction between acute and chronic diarrhea is an arbitrary one, the persistence of diarrhea for longer than 2 or 3 weeks should lead the clinician to consider other pathogenic factors. Among these are infections with specific organisms that can cause symptoms that last for months; these include *Yersinia enterocolitica* (see Chap. 70), *Clostridium difficile* (see Chap. 84), the parasites *Giardia lamblia, Isospora belli* (see Chap. 106), *Strongyloides stercoralis,* and *Capillaria philippinensis,* and helminths (see Chap. 107). Among immunocompetent persons, consideration should also be given to the possible presence of a noninfectious disorder such as a chronic inflammatory or motility disturbance. Among immunocompromised patients, such as those who test positive for the human immunodeficiency virus (HIV) or have acquired immunodeficiency syndrome (AIDS), infections with organisms such as *Campylobacter jejuni,* which are usually brief in immunocompetent persons, can become chronic, and infection with cryptosporidia, *Mycobacterium avium* complex, and cytomegalovirus must be considered (see Chap 105).

There are two other mechanisms that can be responsible for chronic diarrhea associated with an intestinal infection: the postenteritis syndrome and chronic infection of the small bowel with microorganisms. Diarrhea persists for more than 2 weeks in about 10% of children who have experienced an acute enteric infection. This ill-defined syndrome, sometimes referred to as the postenteritis syndrome, occurs most often among the very young and the malnourished.[1] Lactose intolerance is its most common manifestation, but malabsorption of monosaccharides and other substances can occur, sometimes having an adverse effect on nutritional status. A

similar syndrome, in which diarrhea and diffuse abnormalities of the small bowel function can persist for up to several months, has also been described in a few adults.[2]

The causes of these various postinfectious syndromes are unclear and probably multifactorial. Antigen sensitization can occur during gastroenteritis, with the resultant development of transient cow's milk protein intolerance in some children. Infection with a variety of enteric pathogens can be associated with the development of transient small bowel abnormalities in some infected persons. Certain pathogens, such as rotavirus, can directly injure the intestinal mucosa, causing reduction in brush border disaccharidase activities. In addition, most children and adults with acute infectious diarrhea, irrespective of the identity of the initial pathogenic agent, have contamination of their proximal small bowel with coliform bacteria during the acute episode, and this persists in those with the postenteritis syndrome.[1] The role of these bacteria and their metabolites in perpetuating symptoms and intestinal abnormalities remains to be clarified.

In the various postinfectious syndromes, symptoms and small bowel abnormalities eventually return to normal in the absence of specific treatment. In other cases of chronic diarrhea, chronic bacterial or fungal infections of the small bowel are present that cause intestinal abnormalities that persist until the bacteria are eradicated by antimicrobial therapy. In this chapter, four such disorders are described. The first disease discussed, tropical sprue, is confined to the gastrointestinal tract, occurs only in certain tropical localities, and appears to be caused in most instances by chronic small bowel contamination with coliform bacteria that elaborate toxins that are injurious to the intestinal mucosa. The second disease discussed, Whipple's disease, is caused by a bacillus which was identified in 1992 and named *Tropheryma whippelii*.[3] The other two infections, enteric histoplasmosis and tuberculosis, are usually the result of disseminated spread from pulmonary foci and involve principally the ileocecal region.

TROPICAL SPRUE

Tropical sprue is a disease involving the entire small intestine that causes malabsorption of progressive severity which eventually results in the development of severe nutritional deficiencies. This disorder occurs only among persons who visit or become residents of certain tropical areas. First recognized as a clinical entity among Europeans colonizing India and Southeast Asia during the 18th century, tropical sprue was next observed in the early 1900s among Americans living in Puerto Rico and the Philippines. Since then, it has been described, although infrequently, among persons in some African countries, in the Middle East, and in Central America. It has a particularly scattered distribution in the West Indies: it is common in Puerto Rico, Cuba, Haiti, and the Dominican Republic but has not been recognized elsewhere.

Epidemiology

For unexplained reasons, tropical sprue is primarily a disease of adults, occurring only rarely in children. It usually appears in isolated cases, but epidemics have occurred among British forces serving in Burma during World War II, American military personnel serving in the Philippines, and villagers living in South India.[4] In these epidemics, tropical sprue developed among some persons as a sequel to large outbreaks of acute undifferentiated diarrhea. Several reports have indicated that there is a peak seasonal occurrence of tropical sprue, both among sporadic cases and in epidemics, the timing of which is unrelated to the rainy season.[5]

Although tropical sprue can afflict visitors within weeks or months after their arrival in an endemic region, it usually occurs among those who have lived there for more than a year.[6] The prevalence of tropical sprue among residents of developed countries visiting endemic areas for long periods of time appears to be decreasing; this may be related in part to the frequent use of self-medication with antibiotics for episodes of acute diarrheal disease among such persons. Tropical sprue also appears to occur more often among native and non-native residents and who live under poor sanitary conditions (e.g., among people traveling overland to Nepal).[7] In rare instances, tropical sprue does not become clinically apparent among native or non-native residents until months or even years after they have moved to a temperate climate.[8]

Etiology

The available evidence suggests that tropical sprue is an infectious disease resulting from persistent contamination of the small bowel by toxigenic strains of coliform bacteria. Supporting this theory are several additional observations. Although extensive studies have failed to identify a single specific viral, bacterial, fungal, or algal agent as the causative factor, most persons with tropical sprue, including both native and non-native residents, have bacterial overgrowth in the jejunum with strains of *Klebsiella pneumoniae* or, less often, *Enterobacter cloacae* or *Escherichia coli*[9-11]; eradication of these bacteria by antimicrobial therapy results in cure of the intestinal abnormalities.[9,11] These coliform bacteria are clearly not just a manifestation of living in a contaminated environment, because they are not present in the small bowels of healthy residents of the tropics; furthermore, among foreigners who have acquired tropical sprue, the bacterial contamination persists after their return to a temperate climate until they receive antibiotic treatment.[11]

The contaminating bacterial population in the small bowel of patients with tropical sprue is not heterogeneous; there are no anaerobic bacteria, as there are in the blind loop syndrome, and the coliforms present consist of only one or a few species, serotypes, and biotypes in each individual patient.[10] These coliform bacteria have pathogenic properties that are not shared by similar isolates obtained from the small bowel of persons with the blind loop syndrome.[12] The coliforms isolated from patients with tropical sprue are not invasive, but cell-free supernatants of their cultures contain toxins that cause structural abnormalities, net water secretion, and reduced absorption of solutes such as xylose in rats and rabbits.[12,13] The studies that demonstrated these pathogenic properties were performed before specific techniques and assays to precisely identify the characteristics of these toxins became available; therefore, it remains unknown whether they are structure-damaging cytotoxins or enterotoxins, although the former seems likely.

Most non-native residents develop tropical sprue after an attack of acute watery diarrhea. Episodes of acute infectious diarrhea caused by a variety of enteric pathogens are often associated with transient jejunal contamination by coliform bacteria.[1] This event may be the precipitating factor in tropical sprue, and the basic defect may be that, rather than being expelled within a matter of days or weeks as usually occurs, the coliform bacteria are able to permanently colonize the small intestine, with the result that prolonged exposure of the small bowel intestinal mucosa to their toxins causes progressively more severe abnormalities of intestinal structure and function.

The factors responsible for the persistent bacterial colonization in tropical sprue are unknown. There is evidence to suggest that these coliforms may be unusually adherent to the intestinal mucosa,[14] but light and electron microscopy of jejunal biopsy specimens obtained from patients with untreated tropical sprue have failed to show bacteria adherent on the intestinal lumenal surface, in contrast to the case with children infected with enteroadherent strains of *E coli*.[15] Studies regarding the integrity of the immunologic protective systems responsible for clearing the gut of pathogenic microbes have been uniformly normal in persons with tropical sprue.[16] Certain epidemiologic and in vitro studies raise the question of whether variation in dietary ingredients, specifically long-chain unsaturated fatty acids such as linoleic acid, can alter the intestinal bacterial ecosystem in a manner that is permissive to coliform colonization,[5] but it remains to be determined whether this is actually clinically relevant.

Although the information available suggests that tropical sprue is an example of postinfectious malabsorption caused by chronic persistence of toxigenic coliform bacteria, this is an oversimplification because it fails to answer a number of aspects of the disorder, such as its rarity among children and its scattered geographic distribution. Furthermore, whereas bacterial contamination has been found to be common among patients with tropical sprue in North India, elsewhere in Asia, and in the West Indies, such has not been the case among those investigated in South India or South Africa, raising the question as to whether another cause, such as an unidentified virus, may be the pathogenic factor in these cases.[17] The unique role of folate deficiency in the etiology of tropical sprue also remains to be clarified. Intestinal structure and function remain normal in persons who develop a megaloblastic anemia from folate deficiency caused by inadequate dietary intake alone. On the other hand, treatment with pharmacologic doses of folic acid (or of vitamin B_{12}) results in structural and functional improvement of the small bowel in patients with tropical sprue.[6] The structural response in tropical sprue may perhaps be explained by the concurrence of folate deficiency with the intralumenal elaboration of ethanol by the contaminating coliform bacteria in tropical sprue.[10] The combination of folate deficiency with excessive ethanol intake is known to cause intestinal injuries.

Clinical Manifestations

Many visitors to endemic regions can identify the onset of their disease as an episode of acute watery diarrhea, often associated with abdominal cramps and excessive gas. After about a week, these symptoms become milder and chronic. Jejunal structure remains normal or is only slightly deranged during the first few weeks of the illness; thereafter, morphologic abnormalities become progressively more prominent and are accompanied by the development of functional changes. The onset of brush border abnormalities reduces disaccharidase enzyme activities, and the development of lactase deficiency results in milk intolerance. Some patients also become intolerant to alcohol. Within 2 to 4 months, jejunal malabsorption results in depletion of body folate stores; this causes anorexia, resulting in decreased food intake, which together with malabsorption is responsible for the onset of weight loss. After a variable period of time, usually about 6 months but sometimes earlier in poorly nourished native residents who develop this disorder, severe depletion of folate coupled with the development of vitamin B_{12} deficiency causes symptoms associated with megaloblastic anemia, such as weakness, as well as glossitis in some. These deficiencies and their manifestations can develop in about 10% of patients with tropical sprue who have never experienced any gastrointestinal symptoms.

Most changes on physical examination are manifestations of nutritional deficiencies and therefore are present only late in the course of the disease. They include pallor, glossitis, and edema. Stomatitis, hyperpigmentation, and neurologic manifestations of vitamin B_{12} deficiency can occur but are rare.

The clinical and pathologic picture of tropical sprue must be differentiated from the usually milder abnormalities of intestinal structure and function that are present among a variable proportion of native residents and others who have lived in tropical areas longer than 6 to 12 months, a condition that is usually referred to as tropical enteropathy. The key difference is that, without specific treatment, the course of tropical sprue is not ameliorated by removal to a temperate climate, and the intestinal abnormalities become inexorably more severe, eventually resulting in severe nutritional deficiencies.[8] In contrast, the intestinal abnormalities in tropical enteropathy vary, getting better or worse over time; they usually do not cause nutritional deficiencies unless the person is living on a suboptimal dietary intake, and they revert to normal within a year after moving to a temperate climate, even without specific therapy.[18] It is thought that the varying intestinal abnormalities of tropical enteropathy are a manifestation of repeated, transient episodes of intestinal infection caused by varied enteric pathogens.

Laboratory Findings

Nutritional Deficiencies

The megaloblastic anemia of advanced tropical sprue is usually caused by combined deficiencies of folate and vitamin B_{12}. Serum concentrations of carotene, vitamin A, albumin, cholesterol, and calcium are also usually subnormal. Marked elevation of the prothrombin time is unusual.

Intestinal Function

Most persons with tropical sprue have net secretion of water, sodium, and chloride into the small bowel and defective absorption of water and electrolytes from the colon. Xylose, fat, and vitamin B_{12} are the substances most commonly used to test absorptive capacity. Xylose absorption is uniformly reduced. Steatorrhea is present in 50% to 90% of patients; this is caused by defective transport through the enterocyte and not by intralumenal events because, in contrast to the blind loop syndrome, anaerobic bacteria are not present in the proximal small bowel to deconjugate bile salts, and the bile salt pool is only moderately reduced by ileal malabsorption.[19] Cobalamin (vitamin B_{12}) malabsorption is present in nearly all cases. It is not corrected by the addition of intrinsic factor, because impaired ileal transport is the usual cause. In a few cases, however, prompt improvement of vitamin B_{12} absorption occurs after the institution of antibiotic therapy, incriminating uptake of this vitamin by the coliform bacteria within the lumen of the small bowel.

Carbohydrate absorption is reduced secondary to impaired brush border enzyme activity in all patients and impaired transport through the enterocyte in some; results of the glucose tolerance test are subnormal in about 50% of cases. Folate malabsorption is consistently present as a result of both impaired hydrolysis of the dietary polyglutamate form within the brush border and malabsorption of the monoglutamate form through the enterocyte. The absorption of both amino acids and dipeptides through the enterocyte is reduced; in some cases, excessive albumin loss into the gut (protein-losing enteropathy) also contributes to the development of protein deficiency. Calcium absorption is usually reduced owing both to impaired absorption and to deficiency (malabsorption) of vitamin D.

Radiologic Examination

Thickening and coarsening of the mucosal folds of the small bowel can be seen in about one half of patients with tropical sprue. This finding is nonspecific and contributes to the diagnosis largely by excluding the presence of other, specific chronic disorders of the small bowel.

Intestinal Morphology

Structural abnormalities are more prominent in the jejunum during the early phase of tropical sprue, but the entire small bowel is equally affected thereafter. The histologic changes consist of lengthening of the crypt area, broadening and shortening of the villi with infiltration of the lamina propria by chronic inflammatory cells, and variable degrees of abnormality of the surface epithelium[15,20] (Fig. 71-1). A completely flat mucosa, such as is seen in untreated celiac disease, is found in fewer than 10% of biopsy specimens from patients with tropical sprue. The basement membrane usually appears thickened, staining as collagen on light microscopy[20]; electron microscopy shows that this represents an accumulation of dense material, of unknown composition, subjacent to a normal basal lamella.[15]

Differential Diagnosis

Clinically, tropical sprue can be divided into two phases: during the first several months, only intestinal symptoms and abnormalities are present, and thereafter, manifestations of nutritional deficiencies become prominent. Most non-resident visitors seek medical attention while in the first phase, and this disorder should be considered in any person returning from the tropics who has experienced diarrhea for more than 1 month, particularly if anorexia or weight loss is present.

The finding of reduced xylose absorption and, if tested, fat or vitamin B_{12} malabsorption should lead to a jejunal biopsy. The diagnosis is made firmer by the demonstration of the characteristic changes in villus architecture. Also included in the differential diagnosis should be chronic infection with either *Y enterocolitica*, which can be excluded by culture on cold-enrichment medium, or *G lamblia*. Because *Giardia* are notoriously difficult to detect in stool samples, if these are negative a jejunal biopsy and imprint should be examined for the presence of these organisms. As a final recourse, the effect of treatment, with metronidazole (Flagyl) or quinicrine (Atabrine) for giardiasis or with folic acid and tetracycline for tropical sprue, can be evaluated. Lastly, the clinician must remember that diarrhea can persist for several weeks in some persons who were afflicted with an enteric infection while visiting the tropics, and that symptoms caused by any form of gastrointestinal disorder, such as irritable bowel disease or inflammatory bowel disease, can commence while that person is visiting or living in the tropics; these disorders must be excluded by tests such as radiologic examination or colonoscopy.

Among native residents, diarrhea is common, and these persons usually defer seeking medical attention until after the onset of symptoms of nutritional deficiencies, most commonly those related to anemia. The finding of megaloblastic anemia should lead to tests of absorption and a jejunal biopsy. The diagnosis of tropical sprue is confirmed by the prompt clinical and laboratory response to the institution of treatment with folic acid, tetracycline, or both. On the other hand, it is sometimes difficult to be certain of the diagnosis of tropical sprue among populations who have an inadequate nutritional intake, often with hypoalbuminemia, and live in areas such as Haiti where there is also a high prevalence of tropical enteropathy.[21] We have found the presence of megaloblastic anemia and response to specific therapy for tropical sprue to be helpful in this circumstance.

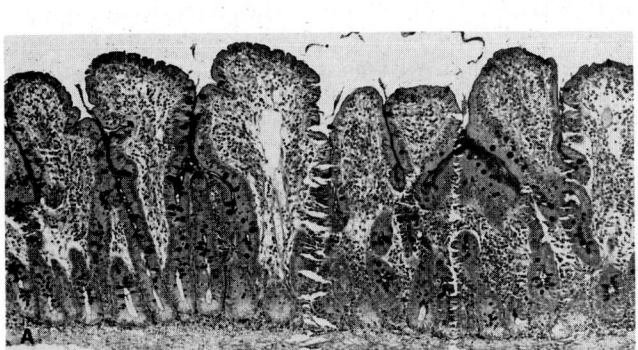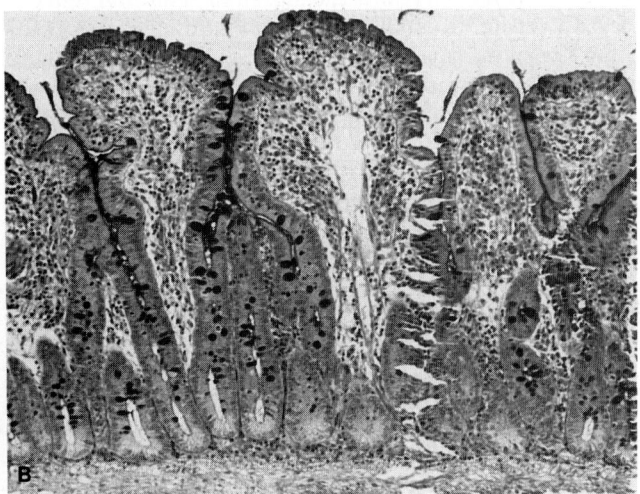

FIGURE 71-1. (A) Light microscopic appearance of the moderate villous abnormality of tropical sprue acquired by a North American on a 2-week visit to the Philippines. Note the broadened villi, the infiltrate of the lamina propria by plasma cells and lymphocytes, and the lymphocytic infiltrate of the epithelium. (PAS and hematoxylin stain; original magnification ×80). (B) Enlargement of a portion of A reveals the epithelial changes. (Original magnification ×132.)

Treatment

Until relatively recent times, tropical sprue was usually a fatal disease. The mortality rate was high among those living in the tropics, although spontaneous remissions did occur rarely, and return to a temperate climate was usually associated with chronic invalidism. This changed after treatment with liver extract was introduced in 1931, followed a decade later by folic acid treatment and then, in the 1960s, by antimicrobial therapy.

Treatment with pharmacologic doses of folic acid (or of vitamin B_{12}) alone produces a prompt hematologic remission of the megaloblastic anemia and return of appetite, followed by the onset of weight gain in those with advanced disease. Intestinal morphologic abnormalities improve after a surge of mitotic activity in the crypts. Subsequently, gastrointestinal symptoms become less severe, brush border enzyme activity improves, and the absorption of xylose increases. This therapy alone may be curative for those in the early stage of the disease, although treatment for up to 2 years may be required for intestinal structure and function to return to normal completely.[6] In contrast, although folic acid improves gastrointestinal symptoms and abnormalities in those with advanced, chronic disease, it usually fails to completely reverse the intestinal abnormalities, and chronic symptoms often persist.[22]

Treatment with antimicrobials eradicates the contaminating coliform bacteria.[9,11] Tetracycline and nonabsorbable sulfonamides are equally effective[23,24]; other antimicrobials have not been evaluated. If given alone, antimicrobial therapy causes improvement in gastrointestinal symptoms within 1 to 2 weeks and slow, progressive improvement of the intestinal abnormalities; improved absorption of folate results in a hematologic response and return of appetite within several weeks.

The logical approach to the treatment of tropical sprue is combined therapy. This usually consists of 5 mg of folic acid given orally per day, together with 1000 µg vitamin B_{12} given parenterally once a week for several weeks in order to replete tissue stores and tetracycline, 250 mg, given orally four times a day. This results in complete healing of the intestinal lesion within several months in those with early disease, including most visitors, but treatment for up to 6 months is often needed for those with chronic disease.[23,24] Among some native residents who have been so treated, intestinal abnormalities and gastrointestinal symptoms may recur within 5 years after cessation of therapy[25]; such is not the case for treated visitors who have returned to a temperate climate.[8]

WHIPPLE'S DISEASE

This disease, so well described in Whipple's original report,[26] is a systemic bacterial illness of middle-aged white men. The manifestations are protean, although the organs showing predominant pathologic changes are the gut and its lymphatic drainage, the heart, and the central nervous system (CNS). Involved tissues are infiltrated by macrophages, which stain intensely with the periodic acid-Schiff (PAS) reaction. Persons with the disease may suffer from arthralgias, which are sometimes disabling, for years before the development of diarrhea and malabsorption, pericarditis or endocarditis, or dementia.

They may present with fever of undetermined cause, with a sarcoid-like illness, or with wasting syndrome. Because the illness is usually insidious in onset and has a varied presentation, and because of its low incidence, the disease is often diagnosed late in its course. The etiologic agent, Whipple's bacillus, has been observed free and within macrophages in the intestinal mucosa, liver, mesenteric and peripheral lymph nodes, heart, CNS, eye, kidney, synovium, and lung. A poorly defined immune deficiency may predispose some persons to the infectious agent. Antibiotics are the treatment of choice.

Epidemiology

Six hundred ninety-six patients with this disease have been reported in the literature or in a survey that ended on May 31, 1986.[27] Since then, data have been obtained on 65 additional patients. Of the 696 patients surveyed, the age and sex were available in 664. There were 574 men (86.4%) and 90 women (13.6%). The average age of male patients at diagnosis was 49.1 years and that of the women was 51 years. The youngest patient was 7 years old and the oldest 80 years old. Of the 65 patients reported more recently, 25% were women, with an average age of 55.9 years, and 75% were men, with an average age of 49.5 years. The range in age was 23 to 80 years. More striking than the curious male predominance is the almost exclusive development of the illness in Caucasians. The illness has been reported in only 12 people of African descent, 1 Native American, 3 patients from India, and 1 Japanese; the remainder are Caucasian. There are no reports of the disease from China, Taiwan, or the Far East. The distribution of the disease in the United States is shown in Figure 71-2, and the worldwide distribution shown in Figure 71-3.

Etiology

The disease is clearly a bacterial one even though the causative agent has not been cultured in vitro, nor has the disease been reproduced in animals. Whipple described the presence of great numbers of a rod-shaped organism in silver-stained sections of a small mesenteric lymph node. This observation was not confirmed until 1960–1961, when three electron microscopic reports clearly showed the presence of bacilli in involved tissues of patients with the disease.[28–30] The organism described was stained by the PAS, Gram, and Giemsa methods and had the fine structural features of bacteria (Fig. 71-4). It provoked a predominantly macrophage inflammatory response. It reacted with tissue stains specific for bacteria (Brown's and Brenn's) and was stained by the silver method but was not acid-fast. Its size was 0.25 µm by 1.0 to 2.0 µm.

Using a polymerase chain reaction (PCR) technique, the bacillus has been shown to have a consistent and unique ribosomal sequence which identifies the bacillus.[3] This PCR technique may become, in the future, a specific test for the disease.[3] There are two remarkable histologic features of this disease in the intestinal mucosa: one is that the lamina propria is packed with macrophages that contain bacilli in varying stages of digestion (see Fig. 71-4), and the second is the profuse presence of free (extracellular) bacilli just below the ep-

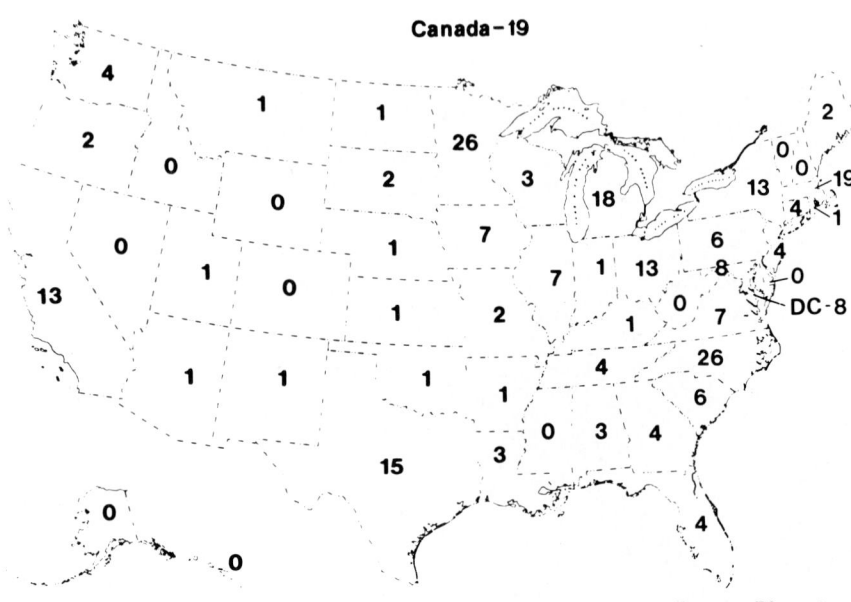

FIGURE 71-2. Distribution of patients with Whipple's disease in North America. (From Dobbins WO. Whipple's disease. Springfield, IL: Charles C Thomas, 1987.)

ithelial cell basal lamina, with a progressive decrease in numbers of bacilli toward the submucosa.

Electron microscopy shows that the core of the bacillus is enclosed within a plasma membrane. External to the plasma membrane is a 20-nm thick cell wall consisting of three distinct areas.[31,32] The dense inner layer contains polysaccharides (? teichoic acid), which accounts for the PAS staining reaction, and is the final remnant of bacilli within macrophages.[32] The dense outer layer has a trilaminar appearance similar to that of plasma membranes,[31] is conceivably of host origin,[32] and may account for the apparent antigenic tolerance to the bacillus, that is, the failure to mount a humoral antibody response to the bacillus, and for its indolent growth pattern.

The bacillus has been found in the intestine, colon, lymph nodes, CNS, eye, heart, liver, lung, synovium, kidney, bone marrow, and skin. The organism has low virulence in humans. Large numbers of organisms may be present even though evidence of tissue injury is minimal. The inflammatory response to the organism appears to be muted and consists largely of macrophages.

There is one notable, although unconfirmed, report of successful culture of Whipple's bacillus. Clancy's report of culture of a "cell wall–deficient," α-hemolytic *Streptococcus dysgalactiae* in hypertonic sucrose media bears merit because electron microscopy of the isolated organism revealed, for the first time in a report of culture of the putative Whipple's

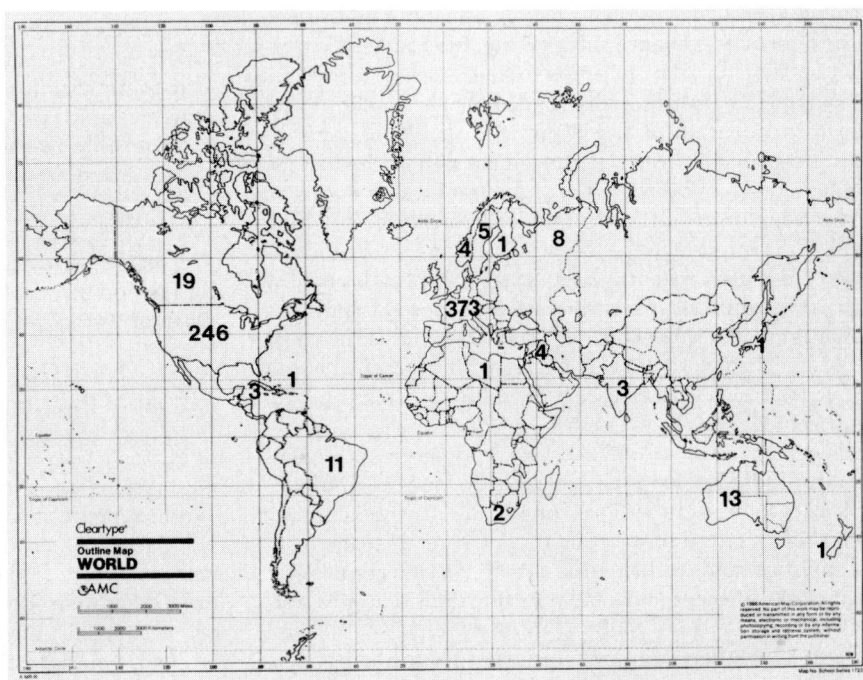

FIGURE 71-3. Worldwide distribution of patients with Whipple's disease. (From Dobbins WO. Whipple's disease. Springfield, IL: Charles C Thomas, 1987.)

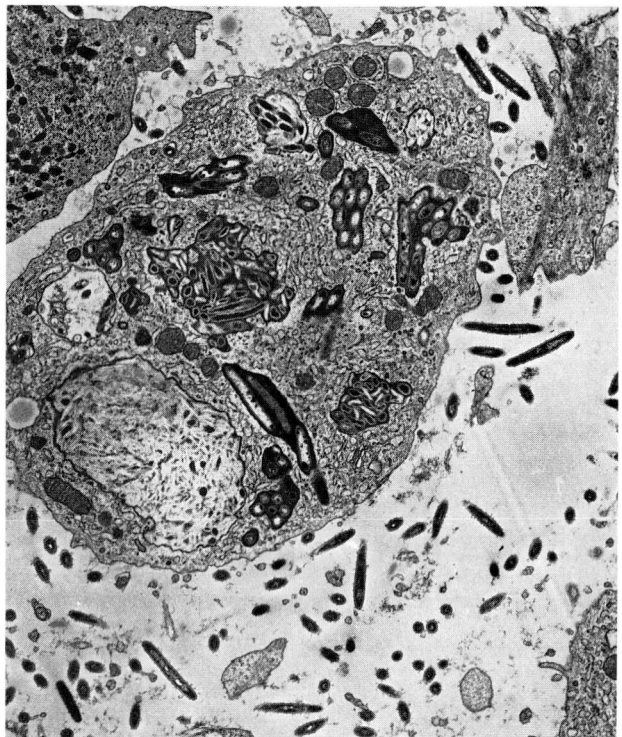

FIGURE 71-4. Electron micrograph showing numerous bacilli (B) in the extracellular spaces and ingested bacilli in varying stages of breakdown within a macrophage (M). (Original magnification ×11,000; from Dobbins WO. Whipple's disease. Springfield, IL: Charles C Thomas, 1987.)

bacillus, a strong resemblance to Whipple's bacillus as seen in tissues.[33] The electron microscopic appearance of the bacillus is the gold standard for its identification. Numerous attempts to culture the bacillus in animals have been unsuccessful.[27] All of the many reports of successful culture of the bacillus, identifying it as a known organism, must be assumed to be reports of contaminants.[27] Whipple's bacillus is a separate species and, like the leprosy bacillus, still uncultured.

Whipple's bacillus shares strong antigenic similarity with streptococcal groups B and G and with *Shigella flexneri*.[27,34] This is explained by the fact that similar polysaccharides are found in different bacteria. These immunologic reactions do not give a clue as to the identity of the organism involved. Rather, the importance of these observations is that there is a distinctive bacterial antigen profile, as defined with a battery of bacterial antisera, that further supports the concept that a unique, antigenically definable bacterial species is the cause of Whipple's disease.[27] This "fingerprint" of reactivity with bacterial antisera may be used to establish or confirm the diagnosis of Whipple's disease.[34]

There may be an unusual host susceptibility to Whipple's bacillus. Indeed, there is considerable evidence of immunodeficiency in the untreated patient, but this may be secondary to malnutrition, to obstruction of lymphatic drainage from the intestine, and to the transient anergy of infection. After successful treatment, most immune functions return to normal, but there is no or minimal antibody response to Whipple's bacillus, suggesting immune tolerance to the bacillus,

and there may be defective ability of monocytes to degrade ingested antigen.[27,35] There is clear evidence that the clinically well patient has a subtle defect in cellular immunity. There is a persistent lymphocytopenia (with normal ratios of helper to suppressor T cells), there is diminished responsiveness of T cells to nonspecific mitogens, and the cutaneous response to antigens (delayed hypersensitivity) is depressed. Immune complexes may play a role in the pathogenesis of arthralgias.[27] There is a clear association of Whipple's disease with HLA-B27. Sixteen (26%) of 62 patients tested were HLA-B27 positive, whereas the gene frequency in the ethnic groups most likely to develop Whipple's disease ranges from 0.3% to 6.9%.

The immunopathology of Whipple's disease is that of a striking infiltrate of involved tissues with macrophages that contain a myriad of ingested bacilli in varying states of degradation (see Fig. 71-4). Occasionally, there is a prominent infiltrate by granulocytes. The response may be granulomatous; 9% of patients have granulomatous changes, largely present in the liver and in mesenteric and peripheral lymph nodes but sometimes in the intestine, brain, and lung. The similarity of the disease to sarcoidosis is often emphasized, and a number of patients have been thought at first to have sarcoidosis. The differentiation of the two diseases is sometimes difficult because in Whipple's disease the noncaseating granulomas may be PAS-negative.[27,36]

Clinical and Pathologic Manifestations

General Features

The most prominent presenting manifestations are those of weight loss, diarrhea, arthralgia, and abdominal pain.[27,37–39] Variations on this theme have been reported by Duke University, the Mayo Clinic, and the University of Heidelberg in 19, 29, and 22 patients, respectively.[37–39] Less frequent presenting manifestations are chills and fever, cardiovascular symptoms, and neurologic abnormalities. Weight loss and diarrhea are observed less commonly in patients who present before 40 years of age. The weight loss usually occurs in the year before diagnosis and is about 20 to 30 pounds, but it may be as much as 100 pounds. Diarrhea has the usual features of steatorrhea but may be watery and sometimes nocturnal. Occult gastrointestinal bleeding is common, and gross bleeding is occasionally seen.[27] Arthralgias are migratory, involve large joints, and may be intermittently present for years. Weight loss, diarrhea, and fever usually precede the diagnosis by a period of 1 to 4 years, whereas arthralgias are present a mean of 9 years before diagnosis.[38]

Physical Findings

Evidence of weight loss and hypotension (<100/60 mm Hg) is consistent. Peripheral lymphadenopathy is present in 50%, and mesenteric adenopathy, sometimes presenting as a palpable abdominal mass, is found in 25% of patients. Abdominal tenderness to palpation and distended loops of bowel may be apparent. Low-grade fever is present in 40% to 50%, and occasionally the fever may be spiking. Cardiac murmurs are found in 25%, but pericardial friction rubs are rare. Increased skin pigmentation is present in one third and may be associated with hyperkeratosis and purpura. Glossitis, peripheral edema, and ascites are sometimes present if there is severe malabsorption. Hepatomegaly and splenomegaly are rare. Neurologic features may be prominent.

Radiologic Features

Marked but nonspecific coarsening of duodenal and jejunal folds is the most common feature seen on barium study. Results of the upper gastrointestinal tract series may be entirely normal. Enlarged retroperitoneal lymph nodes may widen the duodenal loop or displace the stomach. These nodes are more often detected with ultrasound, computed tomography (CT), or magnetic resonance imaging (MRI). CT and MRI are essential to detection of CNS lesions. Chest films may, rarely, detect evidence of fibrosis, focal lesions, and pleural effusions. Radiographs of joints are usually normal but may show bone erosions and narrowing of joint spaces. Ankylosis is very rare. Radiologic sacroiliitis is sometimes seen, but spondylitis is most unusual.

Laboratory Findings

Anemia is present in 90% of patients; it is usually related to chronic disease but may occasionally be caused by iron deficiency and, rarely, by folate or cobalamin (vitamin B_{12}) deficiency. Leukocyte counts tend to be high-normal, and neutrophilia is found in one third of patients. Mild lymphocytopenia is to be expected. Eosinophilia and thrombocytosis are sometimes present. Hypoalbuminemia is common, with a mean value of 2.7 g/dL (range 1.0–4.4 g/dL) in one series.[27,37] Serum globulin levels, including those of immunoglobulins, are usually normal. Mild prolongation of the prothrombin time is common. Steatorrhea is present in the majority—43 (93%) of 46 patients in one series.[37] Absorption of D-xylose was diminished in 25 (78%) of 32, whereas only 2 (13%) of 11 had malabsorption of vitamin B_{12}.

System Review

Gastrointestinal tract.   The gut and its mesentery are almost always involved in this systemic disease. Indeed, duodenojejunal biopsy is the diagnostic procedure of choice. The duodenum, jejunum, and ileum are almost always infiltrated by characteristic PAS-positive macrophages. The infiltrate is usually mucosal and rarely submucosal. The stomach and colon are rarely involved.[40,41] More importantly, mucosal biopsy specimens of both stomach and colon frequently contain PAS-positive macrophages in conditions other than Whipple's disease (i.e., muciphages in the colon and lipophages in the stomach).[27]

Histologically, intestinal villi are usually clubbed (Fig. 71-5) but may be normal in shape. Occasionally, a severe intestinal mucosal lesion comparable to that seen in untreated celiac sprue may be present.[37] The lamina propria is packed with macrophages, numerous bacilli (demonstrated with bacterial stains), and many large free lipid inclusions. The macrophages and bacilli are most frequently found at the apex of villi but are occasionally present in the submucosa. Lacteals are dilated and rarely contain lipid inclusions. The macrophages contain numerous sickle-shaped inclusions that are unique to Whipple's disease (Fig. 71-6). These membrane-bound inclusions contain a myriad of bacilli in various stages of digestion. It is the polysaccharide content of these inclusions that permits the intense PAS staining reaction.[32] After treatment, bacilli clear rapidly but the macrophages clear slowly. The macrophage infiltrate may still be prominent at the end of a year's course of antibiotic treatment and is still present in small numbers as much as 11 years after completion of treatment.[42]

The mesentery tends to be markedly thickened and contains numerous enlarged lymph nodes that have a characteristic histologic appearance.[27] Retroperitoneal and mesenteric adenopathy may be such that the patient presents with an abdominal mass. Liver biopsy specimens, frequently obtained in those patients who present with chronic fever or obscure systemic illness, are usually not helpful. Granulomas,

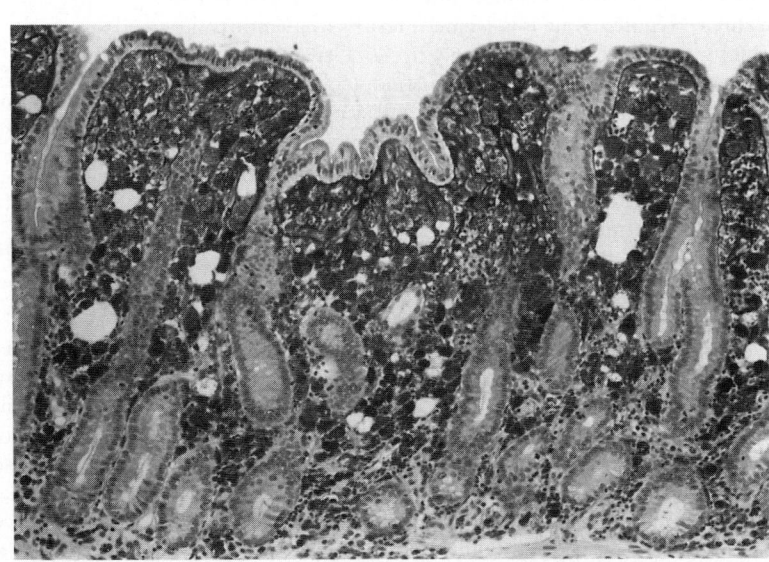

FIGURE 71-5. Light microscopic appearance of the intestinal mucosa in a patient with Whipple's disease. The villi are clubbed, and the lamina propria is packed with PAS-positive macrophages (PAS and hematoxylin stain; original magnification ×250; from Dobbins WO. Whipple's disease. Springfield, IL: Charles C Thomas, 1987.)

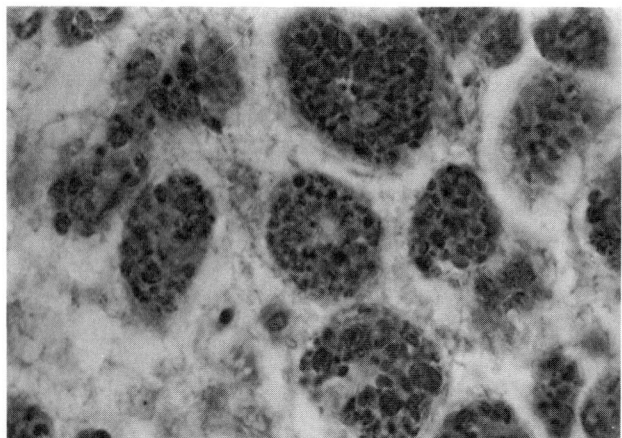

FIGURE 71-6. Light microscopic appearance of macrophages in the intestinal lamina propria in Whipple's disease. Note that most of the PAS-stained inclusions are rounded or sickle-shaped. This appearance is virtually diagnostic, especially if seen in the intestinal mucosa (PAS and hematoxylin stain; original magnification ×1000; from Dobbins WO. Whipple's disease. Springfield, IL: Charles C Thomas, 1987.)

which in Whipple's disease are often PAS-negative, delay diagnosis.[27,36]

Cardiovascular system. Pericarditis and endocarditis are prominent findings at autopsy in untreated patients, whereas clinically important cardiac manifestations are infrequent.[27] The clinical findings include apical systolic murmur in about 25%, pericardial friction rubs in 10%, and, rarely, congestive heart failure. Pathologically, adhesive pericarditis is present in 75%, fibrosis or deformity of cardiac valves with presence of marantic lesions in about 50%, and myocardial fibrosis in 10%. Replacement of aortic and mitral valves has sometimes been required.[43] Vasculitis is uncommon.

Central nervous system and eye. The clinical manifestations of CNS involvement are protean and reflect the widespread distribution of lesions. Hemispheric involvement results in dementia, personality change, and, rarely, hemiparesis and seizures. Hypothalamic involvement results in insomnia, hypersomnia, hyperphagia, or polydipsia. Cerebellar ataxia, mesencephalic lesions causing ophthalmoplegia or nystagmus, and Wernicke's encephalopathy are all reported complications.[27] Dementia, ophthalmoplegia, and myoclonus are the most common manifestations and, if present simultaneously, constitute a virtually diagnostic triad. Hypothalamic changes are the fourth most frequent CNS manifestation. Rhythmic convergence of the eyes associated with synchronous contractions of masticatory muscles—oculomasticatory myorhythmia—although rare, is unique to Whipple's disease.[44]

A number of patients with CNS disease have had minimal gastrointestinal tract signs and symptoms even though characteristic histologic changes were found in intestinal biopsy specimens.[27] More importantly, a small number of persons have had CNS disease without gut involvement.[27] Finally, many patients have developed, years after initially successful treatment, disease relapse manifested by irreversible and progressive dementia leading to death.[27,45]

CT and MRI have been used to detect CNS lesions and even to make a biopsy diagnosis.[27,46] Cerebrospinal fluid analysis is rarely helpful but occasionally shows presence of PAS-positive macrophages. The eye manifestations include uveitis, vitreitis, retinitis, retrobulbar neuritis, and papilledema.

Musculoskeletal system. The disease often presents as a seronegative enteropathic arthritis, with 65% of patients having arthralgias or arthritis affecting the large joints during the course of their disease. In 50%, the joint manifestations precede the intestinal ones, sometimes by as much as 10 to 30 years. The articular attacks are usually acute in onset and last for hours to a few days. Rarely, the pain is chronic. The characteristic pattern is that of a migratory polyarthritis or oligoarthritis involving usually the ankles, knees, shoulders, elbows, and fingers. There is usually no change on examination. Sometimes there may be swelling, effusion, and increased warmth. The clinical combination of polyarthralgias and fever occurring before intestinal symptoms may lead to early diagnosis. Destructive joint changes are unusual, and synovial fluid analysis reveals only nonspecific changes of inflammatory arthropathy.

Axial arthritis is also associated with the disease. Clinical and radiologic sacroiliitis are common (20%–30%), but ankylosing spondylitis is rare, even though 16 (26%) of 62 patients examined were HLA-B27 positive.

Pulmonary system. Chronic nonproductive cough, dyspnea on exertion, and pleuritic chest pain are common. The disease can mimic sarcoidosis, both clinically and radiologically. Pleural effusions and the presence of diffuse and focal infiltrates may be seen on the chest film.[47]

Skin and peripheral lymph nodes. Increased skin pigmentation, not involving the buccal mucosa and of undefined mechanism, is present in one third of patients and is one of the hallmarks of the disease. Several patients have had scurvy.[27] Peripheral lymphadenopathy, localized in 25% and generalized in 15%, may be a prominent feature. Node biopsy in the workup of obscure illnesses has occasionally led to the diagnosis.[27]

Endocrine system. Endocrine involvement almost never occurs. The patient with Whipple's disease often presents clinically with features similar to those of Addison's disease, but the latter diagnosis has not been established in such patients.

Differential Diagnosis and Diagnostic Studies

The disease should be suspected in patients with weight loss, diarrhea, arthralgias, and abdominal pain. If the arthralgias precede the other symptoms or the patient has increased skin pigmentation, then the likelihood of Whipple's disease deserves very serious consideration. The disease is a great mimic and may be confused with abdominal lymphoma, sarcoidosis, or collagen vascular disease. The astute clinician should have a high index of suspicion in the following situations[27]:

TABLE 71-1
Differential Diagnosis of PAS-Positive Macrophages

DISORDER	ORGAN	MACROPHAGE MORPHOLOGY	
		Light Microscopy (PAS-positive Inclusions)	Electron Microscopy (Organisms Present)
None	Intestine	Nonsickled; occasional	None
Whipple's disease	Intestine	Sickle-shaped; round; frequent	Bacilli 0.25 × 1–2 μm
Mycobacterium avium complex infection	Intestine	Round; frequent; acid-fast bacilli	Mycobacteria
Histoplasmosis	Intestine	Large, round, encapsulated organisms; frequent	Encapsulated fungi
Macroglobulinemia	Intestine	Faint, homogeneous stain; no inclusions	None
Miscellaneous disease states	Stomach	Faintly stained; lipid-containing	None: bacilli needed to make diagnosis of Whipple disease
	Rectum	Strongly stained; mucin-containing	

PAS, periodic acid–Schiff.

Presentation with a fever of undetermined origin, often with arthralgias and peripheral lymphadenopathy, even with a paucity of gastrointestinal symptoms

Chronic pericarditis or pleuropericarditis of obscure origin

Dementia, especially if associated with paralysis of gaze, convergent nystagmus, myoclonus, or hypothalamic symptoms

Visual change or loss from chronic idiopathic bilateral retinitis or vitritis, especially if associated with the CNS manifestations discussed previously

Chronic obscure arthropathy, particularly if migratory and involving the ankles, knees, shoulders, elbows, or fingers

Recurrent chest pain and chronic cough of unknown cause, especially if associated with pleural effusions or lung parenchymal infiltrates simulating sarcoidosis

Generalized peripheral lymphadenopathy in a patient with an obscure illness

In a patient with atypical sarcoidosis.

The diagnostic procedure of choice is *peroral intestinal biopsy*. The disease process is usually diffuse, but because it may be focal, four to six biopsy specimens should be obtained endoscopically. The duodenoscopic appearance is characteristic—there are thickened mucosal folds that are coated with a yellow granular material, or with 1- to 2-mm yellow-white plaques, in a diffuse or patchy distribution.

The appearance alone of the PAS-stained section is sufficient to establish the diagnosis in the majority of cases, and electron microscopic demonstration of bacilli is not essential (see Fig. 71-4). Macrophages are occasionally found in the normal intestinal lamina propria; they may stain with the PAS reaction, usually faintly or even strongly, but the inclusions are not sickle-shaped (see Fig. 71-6). There are three infrequent situations in which the presence of numerous PAS-positive macrophages in the intestinal lamina propria may be misleading: in AIDS with *M avium* complex infection, in systemic histoplasmosis, and in macroglobulinemia (summarized in Table 71-1). The pathologist should be able to easily distinguish between the faintly staining, homogeneously PAS-positive macrophages of macroglobulinemia, or the large, PAS-positive, rounded, encapsulated *Histoplasma* organisms

in macrophages, and the histologic appearance found in Whipple's disease. More care must be taken to differentiate the appearance of Whipple's disease from that of the intestinal mucosa in patients with AIDS with a lamina propria filled with macrophages containing *M avium* complex (Fig. 71-7). In the latter case, the lamina propria is packed with macrophages that, with the hematoxylin and eosin stain and with the PAS stain, clearly resemble those seen in Whipple's disease. However, *M avium* complex bacilli are acid-fast (see Fig. 71-7), are easily cultured, and have an electron microscopic appearance quite different from that of Whipple's bacilli.[27,39]

Very rarely (10/760 patients) the diagnosis has been established in the absence of intestinal involvement. In these

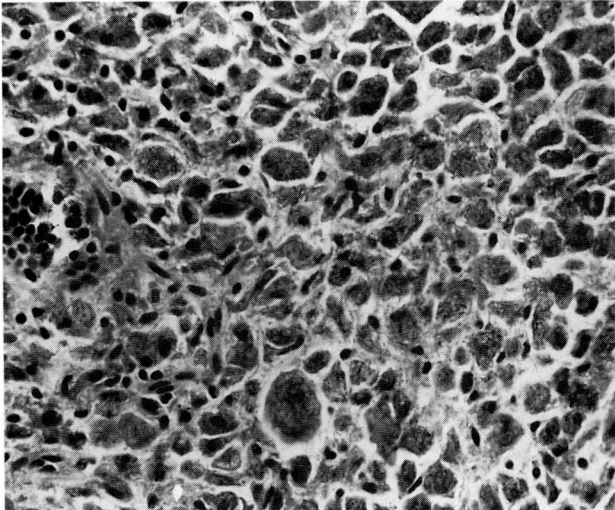

FIGURE 71-7. Light microscopic appearance of macrophages in the intestinal lamina propria of a patient with acquired immunodeficiency syndrome and *Mycobacterium avium-intracellulare* involvement of the gut. Note the easily identified bacilli within the macrophages (Acid-fast stain: original magnification ×500; from Dobbins WO. Whipple's disease. Springfield, IL: Charles C Thomas, 1987.)

cases, the diagnosis was established by the electron microscopic demonstration of bacilli in cerebrospinal fluid, in CT-guided or surgical brain biopsy specimens, or in peripheral lymph nodes.

Considerable caution is required in the interpretation of gastric and rectal biopsy specimens. PAS-positive macrophages are often present in the normal gastric and rectal mucosa and in many disease states of the stomach and rectum. The stomach often contains faintly PAS-positive, lipid-containing macrophages (lipophages), and the rectal mucosa usually contains strongly PAS-positive muciphages and pigment-containing macrophages. Usually, electron microscopic demonstration of Whipple's bacilli in these tissues is necessary in order to establish the diagnosis.

Clinical Course and Treatment

Antibiotics are the treatment of choice. The typical early response is frequently described as "spectacular." Because there seems to be a higher rate of relapse after short courses of treatment, it is appropriate to continue treatment for 1 year. The long-term outlook is more guarded.[45] Follow-up of 88 patients for 1 or more years after completion of treatment showed that 57 patients remained well but 31 had a relapse. Histologic documentation of relapse (demonstration of presence of Whipple's bacilli on electron microscopy) was not obtained, and many of these relapses are questionable. Of more serious nature are the 13 patients who had a CNS relapse, always 2 or more years after completion of original treatment, manifested by irreversible dementia and death in 10 of the patients. The pathogenesis of the late CNS relapse is not defined, because autopsy was performed in only 1 of the 13 patients and no viable bacilli were found. Only 2 of the 13 patients responded to additional antibiotic treatment. It is likely that the CNS damage was the result of original injury leading to neuronal loss and to gliosis. Finally, a large number of persons who died before treatment (10/11 in one series) were found at autopsy to have CNS involvement in the absence of CNS signs and symptoms. The physician should therefore assume that all persons with the disease have CNS involvement.

Careful long-term follow-up of all treated patients is necessary. There is no need for routine invasive diagnostic studies such as annual intestinal biopsy. The patient's progress should be monitored with routine clinical evaluation and laboratory studies. If the patient is clinically well and laboratory tests are normal, repeat intestinal biopsy is not indicated. Repeat biopsy should only be done if the patient fails to respond or relapses. Documentation of the presence of extracellular bacilli confirms either failure to respond or relapse. PAS-positive macrophages persist in the intestinal lamina propria for years after successful treatment, and monitoring their presence or absence as a guide to therapy is not helpful.

Initial recommended treatment is oral administration of double-strength trimethoprim-sulfamethoxazole (TMP/SMX) twice daily for 1 year. TMP/SMX penetrates the blood-brain barrier well and should effectively eradicate CNS involvement.[45] Neither penicillin nor streptomycin crosses the blood-brain barrier in the presence of uninflamed meninges, as is the case in Whipple's disease. Parenteral penicillin is especially helpful in patients initially too ill to tolerate oral medications. In the patient who is unable to tolerate TMP/SMX or who is allergic to sulfonamides, treatment with parenteral penicillin for 10 to 14 days followed by oral penicillin (penicillin VK 250 mg four times per day) for 1 year is recommended. These patients may be severely malnourished and may require supplements of folic acid, vitamin B_{12}, fat-soluble vitamins, and iron.

Treatment of relapse is more complex. If relapse is suspected, an intestinal biopsy specimen should be examined for presence of free bacilli. Biopsy of other tissues, such as lymph nodes, should be done if there is evidence of their involvement. This may include biopsy of focal CNS lesions guided by CT or MRI. If CNS relapse is suspected, a lumbar puncture with examination of the cerebrospinal fluid for PAS-positive macrophages is indicated. Presence of free bacilli in tissue samples clearly establishes relapse. If clinical evidence of relapse is strong, and especially if there is evidence of CNS disease, then empiric treatment should be given in the absence of histologic proof of relapse. Treatment of CNS relapse should also be a repetition of initial therapy. Failure to respond requires a course with chloramphenicol (250 mg four times a day) for up to 1 year. Chloramphenicol, like TMP/SMX, results in relatively high CNS concentrations of the drug.

Treatment of non-CNS relapse should be that recommended for initial therapy. If there is no response, then a trial with oral penicillin (penicillin VK, 250 mg four times daily) or with tetracycline (250 mg four times daily) is indicated. If the patient responds, the treatment should continue for 6 to 12 months.

TUBERCULOSIS

Gastrointestinal tuberculosis is commonly recognized in developing countries and is seen increasingly in the United Kingdom and North America. Abdominal tuberculosis is relatively unusual in nonimmunocompromised hosts in the Western hemisphere (see Chap. 105 for a discussion of AIDS-related tuberculosis) but is still encountered in certain subgroups, especially Asians and elderly alcoholics.[48] Tuberculous enteritis may develop as a primary focus of infection or secondary to pulmonary involvement. The likelihood of intestinal involvement in pulmonary tuberculosis increases with the severity of the pulmonary lesion and can be present in as many as 10% of cases.[49] Intestinal involvement occurs from swallowing infected sputum, from miliary spread, or from direct extension from adjacent organs. The human strain commonly is the cause, and direct infection from bovine milk is very unusual in Western countries.

Gastrointestinal tuberculosis can be confused with either ileocecal Crohn's disease[48] or colonic carcinoma,[50] because the ileocecal area and the colon are most commonly involved. Duodenum, stomach, and esophagus are rarely infected. Symptoms are nonspecific and include fever, night sweats, weight loss, anorexia, nausea, abdominal pain, and diarrhea. An abdominal mass, usually in the right lower quadrant can be present in more than half of patients. If intestinal symptoms occur in a patient with active pulmonary tuberculosis, intestinal involvement must be suspected.

Definitive diagnosis of tuberculosis may be more difficult

to achieve than the clinical suspicion of the disease. A strongly positive intradermal test and active pulmonary disease on a chest film are helpful clues, but these are often entirely negative.[51] Contrast radiographs of the intestine may resemble those in Crohn's disease, lymphoma, or ameboma. Features that suggest tuberculosis include an empty, contracted ileocecal area with ulceration and nodularity (Fig. 71-8). The ileocecal area is usually involved as a unit, and ileal disease alone should suggest another diagnosis. Strictures are usually shorter than in Crohn's disease and are often multiple. The mucosa is thickened with ulceration that is often circumferential, rather than longitudinal as it is in Crohn's disease. The cecum is contracted, and distortion of folds, stenosis, and pseudopolyps may be seen on both sides of the ileocecal valve. Colonoscopy[52] and CT evaluation[53] may aid in the diagnosis. Laparoscopy with peritoneal biopsy may be useful in some cases. If surgery is performed, the bowel wall is found to be thickened and inflamed, and the serosa may be studded with tubercles. Regional nodes may be enlarged and show caseating necrosis after sectioning. The external bowel appearance can be similar to that in Crohn's disease or in infection with *Y*

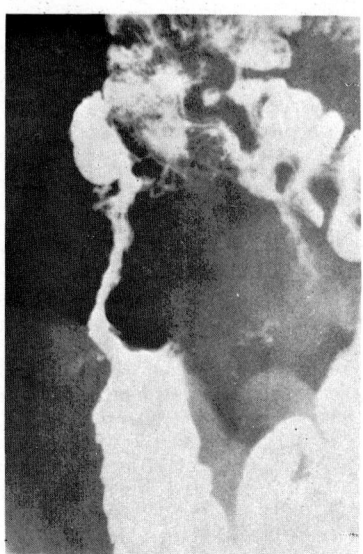

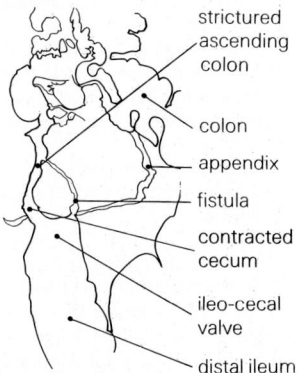

strictured ascending colon
colon
appendix
fistula
contracted cecum
ileo-cecal valve
distal ileum

FIGURE 71-8. Barium study in a patient with hypertrophic tuberculosis shows a dilated distal ileum leading into a contracted cecum and strictured ascending colon. (From Misiewicz JJ, et al. Atlas of clinical gastroenterology. London: Gower, 1985;6:9.)

enterocolitica, although the latter disease has a much shorter course.

Complications include obstruction, hemorrhage, and malabsorption, with the latter symptoms caused by bacterial overgrowth in the presence of obstruction.[54] The segments of small bowel involved by tuberculosis are never sufficiently extensive to be the primary cause of malabsorption. Free perforation occurs rarely.

Treatment is that required for miliary or extrapulmonary disease and includes three antibacterial agents initially, usually isoniazid (300 mg/day), ethambutol (15 mg/kg/day), and Rifampicin (600 mg/day). Although sclerosing lesions are common, intestinal obstruction is now rarely a cause for surgical intervention. Hypertrophic forms of the disease can produce a mass that can mimic carcinoma and may need to be excised for diagnosis as well as for obstructing symptoms.

Intestinal atypical mycobacteriosis is seen in immunocompromised states (e.g., AIDS) in which *M avium* complex is common (see Chap. 105). Atypical mycobacteria have been suggested to be related to Crohn's disease but may also occur in normal persons.[55] Three cases of primary intestinal typical mycobacterial infection have been reported to have affected the colon; these involved *Mycobacterium nonchromegenicium* in two cases and *Mycobacterium chelonae* in one case.[56] The patients presented with the appearance of colonic Crohn's disease, tuberculosis, and rectal ulcers. Biopsy revealed noncaseating granulomas. Atypical mycobacteriosis must be considered in the differential diagnosis of chronic colonic inflammatory conditions.

HISTOPLASMOSIS

Progressive disseminated histoplasmosis has been recognized since the 1930s, but it is not realized how often it may, like Whipple's disease, present with multiple system involvement, including liver, gastrointestinal tract, or CNS rather than pulmonary disease.[57] Liver involvement is a prominent feature in most cases; anemia, thrombocytopenia, and pulmonary abnormalities are present in about half the patients. Age at presentation can vary from infancy to old age. Initial symptoms usually include fever, chills, malaise, anorexia, and weight loss. Histoplasmosis can cause an ulcerative enteritis, most commonly in the terminal ileum or colon.[58] In most reported cases, the patients have simultaneous involvement of the various levels of the gastrointestinal tract.[59] The ulcerations can present with bleeding, obstruction, perforation, or malabsorption.[60] Rarely, the disease can present as a protein-losing enteropathy with enlarged intestinal villi, simulating Whipple's disease.[61] Disseminated histoplasmosis occurs in normal hosts[62] but can also complicate AIDS, in which it presents with caseating hepatic lesions or with rectal or ileocecal involvement.[57]

Diagnosis can be difficult, because histoplasmosis is as protean in its manifestations as tuberculosis. Ileocecal involvement can mimic Crohn's disease.[63] Biopsy of the rectum or involved portion of the gastrointestinal tract is best, demonstrating *Histoplasma capsulatum* in the tissue. Histoplasmin skin tests are not helpful, because they are often positive in endemic regions. Positive complement fixation tests may be useful if obtained serially. Treatment regimens have been directed at eradicating pulmonary involvement and have included amphotericin B (2 g over 10 weeks for adults) or ketoconazole (200–400 mg daily for 6 months). Presumably these doses would be useful for enteric involvement, but good documentation of this is not available.

The reader is directed to Chapter 38, Approach to the Patient With Diarrhea; Chapter 74, Bacterial Overgrowth; and Chapter 105, Gastrointestinal Complications of the Acquired Immunodeficiency Syndrome.

REFERENCES

1. Klipstein FA. Jejunal bacterial overgrowth in acute and persistent infectious diarrhea. J Pediatr Gastroenterol Nutr 1986;5:683.
2. Montgomery RD, Beale DJ, Sammons HG, Schneider R. Postinfective malabsorption: a sprue syndrome. Br Med J 1973;2:265.
3. Relman DA, Schmidt TM, MacDermott RA, Falkow S. Identification of the uncultured bacillus of Whipple's disease. New Engl J Med 1992;327:293.
4. Jones TC, Dean AG, Parker GW. Seasonal gastroenteritis and malabsorption at an American military base in the Philippines: II. Malabsorption following the acute illness. Am J Epidemiol 1972;95:128.
5. Klipstein FA, Corcino JJ. Seasonal occurrence of overt and subclinical tropical malabsorption in Puerto Rico. Am J Trop Med Hyg 1974;23:1189.
6. Klipstein FA. Tropical sprue in travelers and expatriates living abroad. Gastroenterology 1981;80:590.
7. Tomkins AM, James WPT, Walters JH, Cole ACE. Malabsorption in overland travellers to India. Br Med J 1974;3:380.
8. Klipstein FA, Falaiye JM. Tropical sprue in expatriates from the tropics living in the continental United States. Medicine (Baltimore) 1969;48:475.
9. Gorbach SL, Mitra R, Jacobs B, et al. Bacterial contamination of the upper small bowel in tropical sprue. Lancet 1969;1:74.
10. Klipstein FA, Holdeman LV, Corcino JJ, Moore WEC. Enterotoxigenic intestinal bacteria in tropical sprue. Ann Intern Med 1973;79:632.
11. Tomkins AM, Drasar BS, James WPT. Bacterial colonisation of jejunal mucosa in acute tropical sprue. Lancet 1975;1:59.
12. Klipstein FA, Engert RF, Short HB. Enterotoxigenicity of colonising coliform bacteria in tropical sprue and blind-loop syndrome. Lancet 1978;2:342.
13. Klipstein FA, Horowitz IR, Engert RF, Schenk EA. Effect of *Klebsiella pneumoniae* enterotoxin on intestinal transport in the rat. J Clin Invest 1975;56:799.
14. Montgomery F, Tomkins AM. Adhesion of enteropathogenic bacteria to cells in tissue culture. Dev Biol Stand 1980;46:83.
15. Brunser O, Eidelman S, Klipstein FA. Intestinal morphology of rural Haitians: a comparison between overt tropical sprue and asymptomatic subjects. Gastroenterology 1970;58:655.
16. Ross IN, Mathan VI. Immunological changes in tropical sprue. Q J Med 1981;200:435.
17. Bhat P, Shantakumari S, Rajan D, et al. Bacterial flora of the gastrointestinal tract in southern Indian control subjects and patients with tropical sprue. Gastroenterology 1972;62:11.
18. Gerson CD, Kent TH, Saha JR, et al. Recovery of small-intestinal structure and function after residence in the tropics: II. Studies in Indians and Pakistanis living in New York City. Ann Intern Med 1971;75:41.
19. Bevan G, Engert R, Klipstein FA, et al. Bile salt metabolism in tropical sprue. Gut 1974;15:254.
20. Schenk EA, Samloff IM, Klipstein FA. Morphologic characteristics of jejunal biopsies in celiac disease and in tropical sprue. Am J Pathol 1965;47:765.
21. Klipstein FA, Samloff IM, Schenk EA. Tropical sprue in Haiti. Ann Intern Med 1966;64:575.
22. Sheehy TW, Baggs B, Perez-Santiago E, Floch MH. Prognosis of tropical sprue: a study of the effect of folic acid on the intestinal aspects of acute and chronic sprue. Ann Intern Med 1962;57:892.
23. Guerra R, Whelby MS, Bayless TM. Long-term antibiotic therapy in tropical sprue. Ann Intern Med 1965;63:619.
24. Maldonado N, Horta E, Guerra R, Perez-Santiago E. Poorly absorbed sulfonamides in the treatment of tropical sprue. Gastroenterology 1969;57:559.
25. Rickles FR, Klipstein FA, Tomasini J, et al. Long-term follow-up of antibiotic-treated tropical sprue. Ann Intern Med 1972;76:203.
26. Whipple GH. A hitherto undescribed disease characterized anatomically by deposits of fat and fatty acids in the intestinal and mesenteric lymphatic tissues. Bull Johns Hopkins Hosp 1907;18:382.
27. Dobbins WO III. Whipple's disease. Springfield, IL: Charles C Thomas, 1987.
28. Cohen AS, Schimmel EM, Holt PR, Isselbacher KJ. Ultrastructural abnormalities in Whipple's disease. Proc Soc Exp Biol Med 1960;105:411.
29. Chears WC Jr, Ashworth CT. Electron microscopic study of the intestinal mucosa in Whipple's disease—demonstration of encapsulated bacilliform bodies in the lesion. Gastroenterology 1961;41:129.
30. Yardley JH, Hendrix TR. Combined electron and light microscopy in Whipple's disease. Bull Johns Hopkins Hosp 1961;109:80.
31. Dobbins WO III, Kawanishi H. Bacillary characteristics in Whipple's disease: an electron microscopic study. Gastroenterology 1981;80:1468.
32. Silva MT, Macedo PM, Moura Nunes JF. Ultrastructure of bacilli and the bacillary origin of the macrophagic inclusions in Whipple's disease. J Gen Microbiol 1985;131:1001.
33. Clancy RL, Tomkins WAF, Muckle TJ, et al. Isolation and characterization of an aetiological agent in Whipple's disease. Br Med J 1975;3:568.
34. Keren DF, Weisburger WR, Yardley JH, et al. Whipple's disease: demonstration by immunofluorescence of similar bacterial antigens in macrophages from three cases. Bull Johns Hopkins Hosp 1976;139:51.
35. Bjerknes R, Laerum OD, Odegaard S. Impaired bacterial degradation by monocytes and macrophages from a patient with Whipple's disease. Gastroenterology 1985;89:1139.
36. Cho C, Linscheer WG, Hirschkorn MA, Ashutosh K. Sarcoid-like granulomas as an early manifestation of Whipple's disease. Gastroenterology 1984;87:941.
37. Maizel H, Ruffin JM, Dobbins WO III. Whipple's disease: a review of 19 patients from one hospital and a review of the literature since 1950. Medicine (Baltimore) 1970;49:175.
38. Fleming JL, Wiesner RH, Shorter RG. Whipple's disease. Clinical biochemical, and histopathologic features and assessment of treatment in 29 patients. Mayo Clin Proc 1988;63:539.
39. Herbay A von, Otto HF. Whipple's disease: a report of 22 patients. Klin Wochenschr 1988;66:533.
40. Cruz Martinez A, Gonzalez P, Garza E, et al. Electrophysiologic follow-up in Whipple's disease. Muscle Nerve 1987;10:616.
41. Gonzalez-Licea A, Yardley JH. Whipple's disease in the rectum: light and electron microscopic findings. Am J Pathol 1968;52:1191.
42. Martin FF, Vilseck J, Dobbins WO III, et al. Immunological alterations in patients with treated Whipple's disease. Gastroenterology 1972;63:6.
43. Ratliff NB, McMahon JT, Nabb TJ, Cosgrove DM. Whipple's disease in the porcine leaflets of a Carpentier-Edwards prosthetic mitral valve. N Engl J Med 1984;311:902.
44. Grotta JC, Pettigrew LC, Schmidt WA, et al. Oculomasticatory myorhythmia. Ann Neurol 1987;22:395.
45. Keinath RD, Merrel DE, Vlietstra R, Dobbins WO III. Antibiotic treatment and relapse in Whipple's disease: long-term follow-up of 88 patients. Gastroenterology 1985;88:1867.
46. Adams M, Rhyner PA, Day J, et al. Whipple's disease confined to the central nervous system. Ann Neurol 1987;21:104.
47. Symmons DPM, Shepherd AN, Boardman PL, Bacon PA. Pulmonary manifestations of Whipple's disease. Q J Med 1985;56:497.

48. Palmer KR, Patil DH, Basren GS, et al. Abdominal tuberculosis in urban Britain: a common disease. Gut 1988;26:1296.
49. Yasawy MI, Karawi MA, Mohamed AE. Alimentary tract tuberculosis: a continuing challenge to gastroenterologists—report of 55 cases. J Gastroenterol Hepatol 1987;2:137.
50. Panton ONM, Sharp R, English RA, Atkinson KG. Gastrointestinal tuberculosis—the great mimic still at large. Dis Colon Rectum 1985;28:446.
51. Schulze K, Warner HA, Murray D. Intestinal tuberculosis: experience at a Canadian teaching institution. Am J Med 1977;63:735.
52. Kalvaria I, Kottler RE, Marks IN. The role of colonoscopy in the diagnosis of tuberculosis. J Clin Gastroenterology 1988;10:516.
53. Balthazar EJ, Gordon R, Hulnick D. Ileocecal tuberculosis: CT and radiologic evaluation. AJR Am J Roentgenol 1990;154:499.
54. Sherman S, Rohwedder JJ, Ravikrishnan KP, Weg JG. Tuberculous enteritis and peritonitis: report of 36 general hospital cases. Arch Intern Med 1980;140:506.
55. Graham DY, Markesic DC, Yoshimura HH. Mycobacteria and inflammatory bowel disease: result of culture. Gastroenterology 1987;92:4.
56. Fujisawa K, Watanabe H, Wamamoto K, et al. Primary atypical mycobacteriosis of the intestine: a report of three cases. Gut 1989;30:541.
57. Cappell MS, Mandell W, Grimes MM, Neu HC. Gastrointestinal histoplasmosis. A review. Dig Dis Sci 1988;33:353.
58. Parsons RJ, Jarafonatis CD. Histoplasmosis in man—report of seven cases and a review of seventy-one cases. Arch Intern Med 1945;75:1.
59. Shull HJ. Human histoplasmosis: disease with protean manifestations often with digestive system involvement. Gastroenterology 1953;25:582.
60. Goodwin RA Jr, Shapiro JL, Thurman GH, et al. Disseminated histoplasmosis: clinical and pathological correlations. Medicine (Baltimore) 1980;59:1.
61. Banks S, Trey C, Gans I, et al. Histoplasmosis of the small bowel with "giant" intestinal villi and secondary protein losing enteropathy. Am J Med 1965;39:492.
62. Goodwin RA Jr, Loyd JE, Des Prez RM. Histoplasmosis in normal hosts. Medicine (Baltimore) 1981;60:231.
63. Alberti-Flor JJ, Granada A. Ileocecal histoplasmosis mimicking Crohn's disease in a patient with Job's syndrome. Digestion 1986;33:176.

Textbook of Gastroenterology, second edition, edited by Tadataka Yamada. JB Lippincott Company, Philadelphia © 1995.

CHAPTER 72

Celiac Disease

Martin F. Kagnoff

Epidemiology
Etiology and Pathogenesis
Models of Pathogenesis
Environmental Factors
Genetics
Humoral and Cell-Mediated Immunity
Pathology
Clinical Manifestations
Gastrointestinal Symptoms
Extraintestinal Manifestations
Physical Findings
Diagnostic Studies
Screening Tests
Radiologic Studies
Small Intestine Mucosal Biopsy
Noninvasive Screening Tests
Differential Diagnosis
Diseases and Disorders Associated With Celiac Disease
Dermatitis Herpetiformis
Other Disease Associations
Complications
Malignancy
Ulcerative Jejunoileitis
Refractory Sprue and Collagenous Sprue
Neuropathy
Therapy
Prognosis

Celiac disease, also known as celiac sprue, adult celiac disease, nontropical sprue, and gluten-sensitive enteropathy, is characterized by damage to the mucosa of the small intestine and malabsorption of most nutrients. Disease is activated by the dietary ingestion of wheat gluten and similar proteins in rye, barley, and oats. Symptoms reflect the consequences of malabsorption and often appear during the first three years of life after the introduction of cereals into the diet. A second peak in incidence occurs in adults during the third decade.[1-4]

Celiac disease was recognized in the second century A.D.

by Aretaeus the Cappadocian who described a chronic malabsorptive disorder in adults. In 1888, Samuel Gee, in the classic paper entitled "On the Coeliac Affection," described childhood celiac disease.[5] During World War II, wheat and rye flour were in very short supply in Holland. As those products became more available after the war, Dicke noted an increase in celiac disease among children. Shortly thereafter, gluten, a water-insoluble protein in wheat flour, was described as the major component of wheat flour that activates disease.[6,7] Paulley described the characteristic intestinal lesion of celiac disease in 1954.[8] With the introduction of peroral intestinal suction biopsy in the late 1950s, and its common use, it was soon realized that celiac disease in children and nontropical sprue in adults shared the same clinical and pathologic features.[9] The recognition in the 1970s that genes encoded in the HLA region are strongly associated with disease susceptibility, coupled with the histopathologic picture of celiac disease, indicated that immune mechanisms play an important role in the pathogenesis of this disease.[2-4,10] The clinical presentation of celiac disease can be highly variable in adults. Small intestine mucosal biopsy is the current gold standard for diagnosis, and a gluten-free diet is the mainstay of therapy.

EPIDEMIOLOGY

The reported incidence and prevalence of celiac disease increased markedly after 1960 in the United States, Europe, and Australia, paralleling the increased clinical application of mucosal biopsy of the small intestine. However, the true incidence and prevalence of celiac disease are unknown because mildly symptomatic disease and asymptomatic disease (i.e., subclinical or latent disease) make ascertainment difficult. The estimated prevalence of celiac disease in Great Britain and Northern Europe ranges from 1 in 400 to 1 in 2000 adults. In the United States, clinically diagnosed celiac disease affects 1 in 3000 to 1 in 10,000 of the adult population. In Western Ireland, the prevalence of celiac disease was as high as 1 in 300,[11] but it has decreased by approximately 60% since 1975.[12] Although the incidence of celiac disease in children appears to be falling in parts of Scandinavia such as Finland, this has not been the case in Sweden.[13,14] Celiac disease is also found outside North America, Europe, and Australia, in geographic areas as diverse as India and West Pakistan, Cuba, Mexico, and the Middle East.[1] However, disease is rare in Japan and Southeast Asia and in those of African descent.

Celiac disease in children usually is diagnosed after weaning and the introduction of cereals into the diet. Breast feeding has been reported to delay the age of onset of clinically symptomatic disease and has been suggested to decrease the risk of developing celiac disease.[15] However, the delayed introduction of gluten into the diet of children, such as occurred in Holland during World War II, did not prevent the later development of clinically active celiac disease.[16] The declining incidence of celiac disease in Western Ireland has been paralleled by changes in the pattern of breast feeding and in the composition of cow's milk formulas in that region, although a definite cause and effect relation has not been established. Celiac disease that develops in childhood frequently remits, in terms of clinical symptoms, during adolescence. However,

a second peak of recurrent disease often occurs in later decades in those whose childhood disease remitted. The onset of disease in adults with no past history of childhood celiac disease most often occurs in the third or fourth decades, although disease may be discovered as late as the seventh or eighth decade.

ETIOLOGY AND PATHOGENESIS

Models of Pathogenesis

There are several competing hypotheses regarding the pathogenesis of celiac disease. The most favored one envisions an interplay of genetic factors, environmental factors, and the immune system.[2,3,17,18] A less favored hypothesis proposes that gliadins and other grain prolamins have a direct toxic effect on the mucosa of the small intestine in celiac disease patients as a result of a deficiency of a small intestine peptidase.[19] However, biochemical abnormalities and small intestine peptidase activities usually return to normal after patients are treated with a gluten-free diet, indicating that such abnormalities do not have a primary role in disease pathogenesis.[20] Further, the small intestine mucosa contains multiple peptide hydrolases with overlapping substrate specificities. In addition, abnormal host responses to gliadin are not restricted to the small intestine mucosa, because exposure of the colonic mucosa of celiac disease patients to gliadin also can initiate an inflammatory response in that site.[21-23]

Another hypothesis envisions that the carbohydrate side chains on gliadins are important in disease pathogenesis. However, this is unlikely, because some α-gliadins that are known to activate celiac disease lack carbohydrate side chains.[24] In addition, experimental evidence does not support the suggestion that gluten, when purified, has lectin-like properties or that possible lectin-like properties of gluten are important in disease pathogenesis.[25,26] A further hypothesis proposes that celiac disease results from a primary defect in intestinal mucosal permeability. However, this seems unlikely because, in some patients, abnormalities in mucosal permeability that are documented during active disease can normalize during treatment with a gluten-free diet.

Environmental Factors

Celiac disease is activated in susceptible individuals by the ingestion of food products that contain wheat, rye, barley, or oats. The alcohol-soluble gliadin fraction of wheat gluten and similar alcohol-soluble proteins called prolamins in rye, barley, and oats are the disease-activating moieties in these grains.[27]

Cereal grains belong to the grass family, Gramineae. As shown in Figure 72-1, grains other than wheat that activate celiac disease (e.g., rye, barley) bear a close taxonomic relation to wheat. Oats, which in large quantities can activate disease, are further removed from wheat, rye, and barley. Grains that do not activate disease (e.g., rice, maize, millet, sorghum) are still further separated from wheat in terms of their derivation from the primitive grasses.[24,28,29]

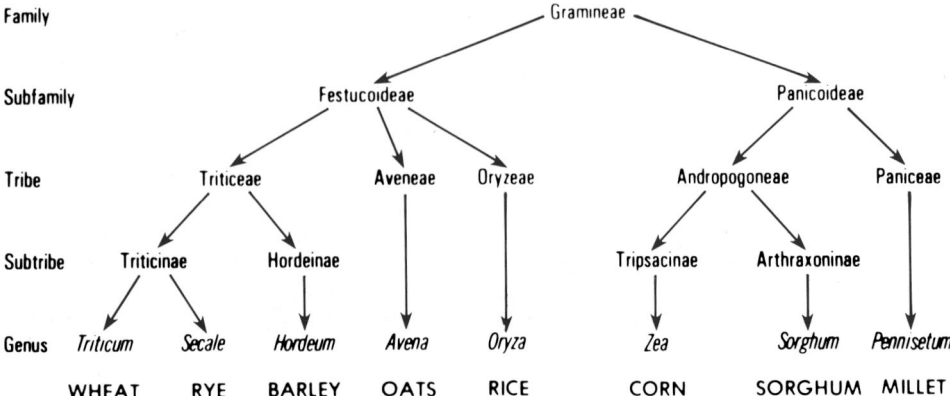

FIGURE 72-1. Taxonomic relationships among major cereal grains. (Adapted from Bietz JA. Cereal prolamin evolution and homology revealed by sequence analysis. Biomed Genet 1982; 20:1039.)

Gluten is a major component of the wheat endosperm and serves as a source of nitrogen for the germinating wheat embryo.[24,28] Its elastic properties are important in the production of bread. Gliadins and glutenins are the major protein components of gluten, but only the gliadins have clearly been demonstrated to activate celiac disease. Minor constituents that contaminate gluten extracts (e.g., wheat albumins, globulins, membrane proteins, lipids, carbohydrates) do not appear important in disease activation. In rye, barley, and oats, the alcohol-soluble proteins associated with the activation of disease are termed secalins, hordeins, and avenins, respectively.

Gliadins range in molecular weight from 30,000 to 70,000 d and exist as single polypeptide chains. They have a low charge[28] and a high glutamine and proline content (32–56 glutamine and 15–30 proline residues per 100 amino acid residues). A single variety of wheat may contain 40 or more different, but closely related, gliadins,[28] which can be categorized into four major electrophoretic fractions based on gel electrophoresis: α-gliadins, β-gliadins, γ-gliadins, and ω-gliadins.[28,30] Each fraction in turn contains several subcomponents.[31] The complete amino acid sequence of several of the gliadins and related prolamins in other grains is known.[32-36] This information should allow investigators to determine the specific amino acid sequences in these proteins that are responsible for disease activation.

In addition to dietary grains, other environmental factors have been postulated to be important in the pathogenesis of celiac disease. In this regard, A-gliadin, a major α-gliadin component that can activate celiac disease, and the E1b protein of human adenovirus serotype 12 (Ad12), an adenovirus usually isolated from the human intestinal tract, have a region of predicted amino acid sequence similarity.[37] The region of A-gliadin that shares amino acid sequence homology with the Ad12 E1b protein can be recognized as an antigenic determinant by populations of celiac disease patients.[38-41] Further, populations of celiac disease patients have been reported to have a significantly higher prevalence of past Ad12 infection than controls,[39,42] and peptides that encompass the region of shared sequence between A-gliadin and the Ad12 E1b protein have been reported to activate disease pathology in the small intestine of celiac disease patients.[43,44] This suggests that molecular mimicry may be involved in the immunopathogenesis of celiac disease.[43]

Genetics

Family and Twin Studies

Celiac disease, often asymptomatic, can occur in as many as 5% to 15% of first-degree relatives of celiac patients.[45-48] Although abnormalities in intestinal permeability have been noted in some first-degree relatives of celiac disease patients,[49] addition of gluten to the diet of healthy siblings of probands with celiac disease did not precipitate histologic abnormalities in the small intestine.[50]

Among 24 pairs of twins thought to be identical, 18 (75%) were concordant for celiac disease.[51] However, not all of these twin pairs were proven to be monozygotic and, in some, the diagnosis of celiac disease was not unequivocally documented. Nonetheless, it appears there are monozygotic twins who are discordant for celiac disease.

HLA and Non-HLA Markers

Celiac disease is strongly associated with HLA class II D region genes in the major histocompatibility complex (MHC) on chromosome 6.[17,18,52] Within the HLA-D region, the DQ subregion alleles, *DQA1*0501* and *DQB1*0201*, code for a specific DQ2 molecule that is present in 95% or more of celiac disease patients from geographically different areas.[53-55] Most individuals with celiac disease inherit these alleles in *cis* pattern on HLA-DR17 haplotypes (old nomenclature, DR3; Fig. 72-2) or in *trans* pattern on heterozygous DR11/DR7 or DR12/DR7 haplotypes (old nomenclature DR5/DR7).[52-54] In a small number of individuals, these alleles are inherited in *trans* or *cis* pattern on other HLA haplotypes. Although the DQ2 molecule encoded by these alleles is necessary for disease susceptibility in most persons, it is not sufficient for disease expression, because fewer than 0.1% of individuals carrying this molecule develop clinically symptomatic celiac disease.[17,18,52] Based on the increased prevalence of DR17/DR7 heterozygotes in the celiac disease population, and the fact that both DR17 and DR7 haplotypes carry the celiac disease-associated *DQB1*0201* allele, it has been postulated that the gene dosage of *DQB1*0201* also may increase susceptibility to celiac disease.[56] The HLA-DQ alleles associated with celiac disease are markedly overrepresented in the celiac disease

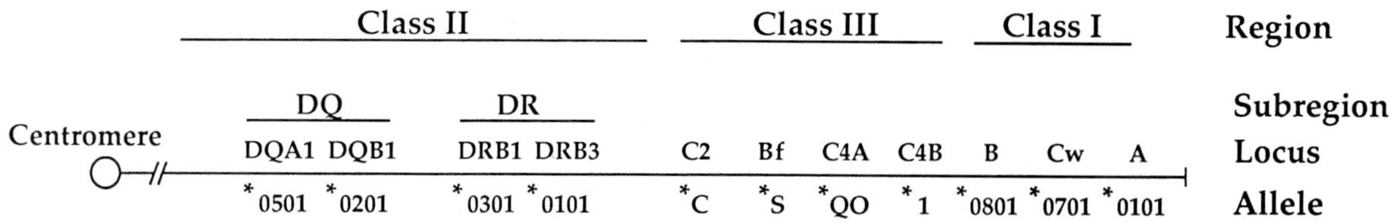

	Class II		Class III			Class I		Region
	DQ	DR						Subregion
Centromere	DQA1 DQB1	DRB1 DRB3	C2	Bf	C4A C4B	B	Cw A	Locus
	*0501 *0201	*0301 *0101	*C	*S	*QO *1	*0801	*0701 *0101	Allele

FIGURE 72-2. Schematic representation of the loci and alleles on an extended HLA DR17 haplotype that is frequently present in northern European Caucasians with celiac disease. The alleles *DQA1*0501* and *DQB1*0201* encode the α and β chains, respectively, of the celiac disease-associated DQ2 molecule. The allele *DRB1*0301* encodes the β chain of the DR17 molecule. Other DR haplotypes also carry *DQA1*0501* and *DQB1*0201* but have different alleles at the DRB3 locus and at loci within the class III and class I regions.

population but appear to be structurally normal.[54] Most celiac disease patients who lack the DQ2 molecule encoded by *DQA1*0501* and *DQB1*0201* have an HLA-DR4 haplotype that carries the alleles *DQA1*0301* and *DQB1*0302* that encode a DQ8 molecule.[57-59] Other genes that map within the HLA region may also increase susceptibility to celiac disease.[3,17,18,54] This raises the possibility that the susceptibility to celiac disease associated with genes in the HLA region may be multigenic, with more than one MHC-encoded gene contributing to disease pathogenesis.

Among sibling pairs in which both siblings have celiac disease, more than 95% share one or both of their HLA haplotypes.[60] Among siblings who share one or two HLA haplotypes with a proband, approximately 28% and 40%, respectively, develop celiac disease.[51,61] The difference in concordance rates for celiac disease among monozygotic twins (i.e., 75% concordant) compared with HLA-identical siblings (approximately 40% concordant) suggests that genes outside the HLA locus also determine susceptibility to celiac disease. The observation that celiac disease occurs more often in family members who share a celiac disease-associated HLA haplotype than in nonfamily members who appear to have the same HLA haplotype[62] further supports this notion. Furthermore, approximately 25% of identical twins and approximately 60% of siblings who are thought to be HLA-identical to the patient on both chromosomes do not develop celiac disease.[51,61] Thus, genes in the HLA region are important markers for celiac disease susceptibility, but other host background genes or environmental factors also clearly influence the phenotypic expression of clinical disease.

Genes that code for immunoglobulin heavy chain allotype markers on human IgG heavy chain (Gm markers) may mark a second genetic region associated with susceptibility to celiac disease.[63-65] The G2m(n) allotype marker on *IgG2* has been associated with the persistence of anti-gliadin antibody in celiac disease patients maintained on a gluten-free diet,[64] and the Gm(f;n;b) phenotype may be a predisposing factor to celiac disease among selected subgroups of individuals.[65] However, these associations are weak compared with the association between HLA genes and celiac disease. Other candidate genes concerned with the regulation of the immune response also can be postulated to be associated with celiac disease susceptibility. These include T-cell receptor genes and a broad array of host genes that are important in modulating the immune response.

Humoral and Cell-Mediated Immunity

Humoral Immunity

IgA and IgG serum antibody to purified gliadin and to all the major electrophoretic fractions of gliadin (i.e., α, β, γ, and ω) can be detected in the sera of most patients with clinically active celiac disease,[66,67] in some patients with treated celiac disease, and in some patients with asymptomatic celiac disease.[64,66-70] Significant elevations in IgA antigliadin antibody titers are more common in untreated than in treated celiac disease patients, and they are unusual in healthy controls.[67,71] Antigliadin antibodies are not specific for celiac disease, because IgG and, to a lesser extent, IgA antigliadin antibody also can be found in individuals with other intestinal diseases and disorders[64,72] and in IgA mesangial glomerulonephritis.[73,74] In children with celiac disease, more than one half of the serum IgA antigliadin antibody is polymeric, suggesting its mucosal origin.[75] Serum IgG antigliadin antibody directed against any one or more of the four major electrophoretic fractions of gliadin can persist for long periods (up to 20 years) in clinically asymptomatic celiac disease patients maintained on a gluten-free diet.[64,67]

Most patients with active celiac disease, but also as many as 15% to 20% of individuals with other gastrointestinal diseases and disorders, have detectable IgM and IgA antigliadin antibodies in small intestine secretions.[76] In celiac disease patients, this is paralleled by increased numbers of IgM-, IgA-, and IgG-producing cells in the lamina propria of the small intestine, as assessed by immunohistochemistry.[77] IgG- and IgM-producing cells are disproportionately increased in the mucosa relative to IgA-producing cells,[77-79] and by virtue of their ability to participate in inflammatory responses, these cells are thought to play an important role in the ongoing inflammatory response in the celiac mucosa. Specific increases in mucosal production of IgM, IgA and IgG antigliadin antibody also can be demonstrated after gliadin challenge of small intestine mucosal biopsies from celiac disease patients in vitro.[79-81] Approximately 2% of celiac disease patients are IgA deficient,[82,83] and they usually have a compensatory increase in IgM-producing cells in the lamina propria.

Antigliadin antibody may play a role in the pathogenesis of celiac disease by forming immune complexes that, in turn, activate tissue-damaging effector mechanisms,[84,85] including the complement cascade. In addition, antigliadin antibody could cause mucosal injury by a cell-mediated cytotoxic re-action in which antigliadin antibodies recognize gliadin pep-tides bound to mucosal structures and direct an antibody-dependent, cell-mediated cytotoxic reaction.[67] Many celiac disease patients have serum antibodies against food proteins in addition to gliadins. These include antibodies to milk (e.g., β-lactoglobulin, casein), egg, and soy proteins.[86,87] Such an-tibodies may reflect increased permeability of the celiac mucosa[71] or, alternatively, an abnormality in immunoregu-lation of the host response to dietary antigens.

Cell-Mediated Immunity

Cell-mediated immune mechanisms appear to play an im-portant role in the pathogenesis of celiac disease. Soluble me-diators (i.e., putative cytokines) which are active in leukocyte migration inhibition assays are produced when small intestine mucosal biopsies from patients with clinically active disease are cultured with α-gliadin or other gluten fractions.[88–91] Proinflammatory cytokines (e.g., tumor necrosis factor-α [TNFα], interferon-γ [IFNγ]) secreted by T cells or mono-nuclear phagocytes in the mucosa of celiac disease patients after the exposure to gliadin are thought to contribute to the pathogenesis of the mucosal tissue injury seen in this disease.

The density of intraepithelial lymphocytes (IELs) in the small intestine mucosa is increased in celiac disease patients with clinically symptomatic disease and abnormalities in mu-cosal architecture. Consistent with this, IEL numbers increase within hours of gluten exposure in celiac disease patients.[92,93] The proportion of IELs bearing the γ/δ T-cell receptor, rel-ative to those bearing the α/β T-cell receptor, is increased during clinically active disease and remains increased during remission. The finding of an increased proportion of γ/δ to α/β IELs also may suggest the presence of latent celiac disease in asymptomatic individuals, although that finding is not spe-cific for celiac disease.[76,94,95] The role of γ/δ IELs in the pathogenesis of celiac disease currently is not known. In the lamina propria, the ratio of CD4 T cells (i.e., helper/inducer phenotype) to CD8 T cells (i.e., suppressor/cytotoxic phe-notype) is similar in celiac disease patients and controls,[96,97] although there may be impaired suppressor function of the CD8 T cells in celiac disease.[98,99] CD4 T cells bearing the α/β T-cell receptor are the major population of T cells that are activated in the lamina propria of celiac disease patients after gluten challenge. These cells are thought to contribute to disease pathogenesis through the release of cytokines which result in epithelial cell damage or alterations in the growth characteristics of crypt epithelial cells.

HLA class II DR molecules and, to a lesser extent, DP molecules are constitutively expressed on the villous epithelial cells in normal small intestine. In celiac disease patients with subtotal or total villous atrophy and crypt elongation, these molecules are newly expressed on epithelial cells in the crypt region.[100-104] The expression of HLA class II molecules on epithelial cells appears to be regulated by cytokines (e.g., IFNγ, TNFα) that are produced by activated mucosal mononuclear cells. HLA-DQ molecules which are associated with increased susceptibility to celiac disease are poorly expressed on normal villous small intestine epithelial cells and on villous and crypt epithelial cells in celiac disease patients.[103,104] In contrast, after gliadin challenge and during clinically active disease, HLA-

DQ molecules are expressed at increased levels on mucosal mononuclear cells, including activated T cells, in the lamina propria.[105,106] The distribution of HLA molecules on epithelial cells and on cells in the lamina propria reverts to normal in celiac disease patients in remission. The specific role played by HLA class II molecules on mucosal epithelial and lamina propria mononuclear cells in the pathogenesis of celiac disease is not known, but it is thought these molecules present gliadin peptides to mucosal T lymphocytes.

PATHOLOGY

The pathologic lesion of celiac disease involves the mucosal layer of the small intestine and has characteristic features, but it is not disease-specific. The submucosa, muscular layers, and serosa are spared. The length of small intestine involved and the severity of the lesion vary markedly among patients, and, within each patient, they vary depending on the activity of the disease. The lesion usually involves only the duodenum and proximal jejunum and, although it can involve the entire length of small intestine, disease characteristically is most se-vere proximally in the duodenum and jejunum. Nonetheless, the distal and proximal small bowel of celiac disease patients react similarly to the direct instillation of gluten or gliadin, and rectal instillation of gluten or gliadin in celiac disease patients results in mucosal inflammation in that site.[21-23,107] The distal intestine is usually spared because the proteins that activate disease largely are digested or absorbed before they reach that region.

During clinically active disease, histologic examination can reveal a complete loss of normal villous structure, a flat ab-sorptive surface, and marked elongation of the intestinal crypts.[108] (Fig. 72-3). Crypt elongation is associated with in-creased numbers of crypt mitoses, reflecting the proliferative activity in that region. Increased lymphocyte mitotic activity can also be seen. In addition to the striking decrease in the epithelial surface area available for absorption, there are marked abnormalities in surface epithelial cells. The columnar epithelial cells that line the surface of the normal mucosa are replaced by cuboidal or squamoid cells which have lost the normal basal polarity of the nucleus and have a more baso-philic cytoplasm. In addition, there is a loss of brush border which, in normal mucosa, contains enzymes required for digestion and absorption. The total thickness of the mucosa remains relatively unchanged, despite the loss of intestinal villi, because of the marked crypt hyperplasia.

The surface epithelium in celiac disease appears heavily infiltrated with IELs by histologic examination. Although the density of IELs in the mucosa may be increased on a quan-titative basis, the total number of IELs may not be increased because of the concurrent decrease in mucosal surface area.[109,110] The lamina propria is infiltrated with increased numbers of plasma cells, lymphocytes, eosinophils, and mast cells.[111-114] Increased numbers of enterochromaffin cells can also be seen.[115,116]

The mucosal lesion in the proximal small intestine is less severe in some patients with celiac disease or with partially treated disease, and in these individuals mucosal abnormalities are also less severe in the more distal compared with the prox-imal small intestine. In some, mucosal biopsies show subtotal

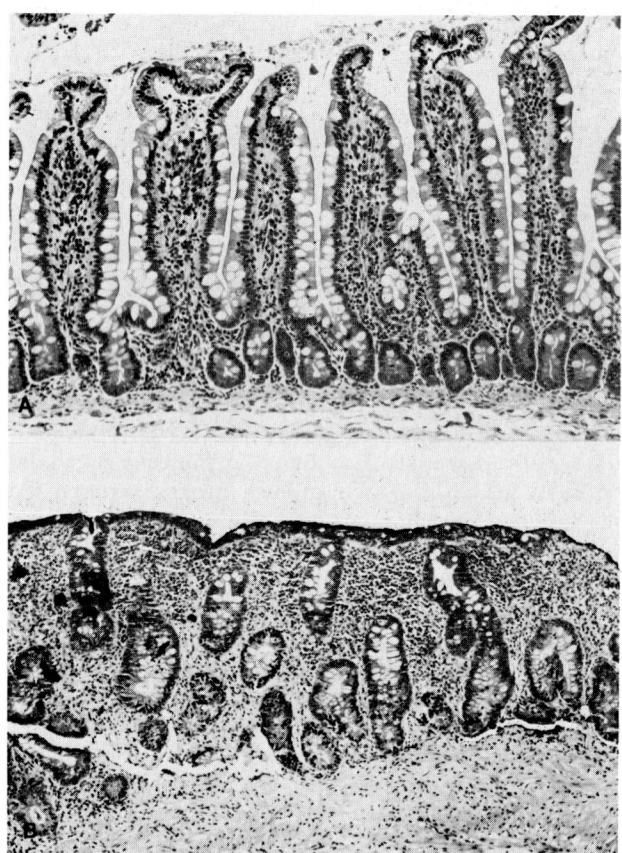

FIGURE 72-3. **(A)** Normal jejunal mucosa. Note the tall villi, columnar epithelial cells with basally oriented nuclei, and the crypt:villous ratio of approximately 4:1 or 5:1. **(B)** Jejunal mucosa in celiac disease. Note the flat surface, absent villi, hyperplastic crypts, and increased cellularity of the lamina propria. (Original magnification 150×; courtesy of K. Miyai, M.D., University of California at San Diego, San Diego, CA.)

villous atrophy with villus blunting. Characteristically, villi are fused and club-shaped, the crypts are hyperplastic, surface cells are abnormal, and there is increased cellularity of the lamina propria. Caution is required in interpreting biopsies from children because as many as 30% of normal children have shorter villi and longer crypts than normal adults.[117] In other adults with clinically mild or asymptomatic celiac disease, all that may be seen is an abnormally high density of IELs in the villous epithelium, with an increased proportion of these cells having the γ/δ T-cell receptor.[118,119] After oral gluten challenge of celiac disease patients in remission, changes in the initial few hours include increases in crypt lymphocytes, surface IELs, and crypt volume.[20] The more classic celiac-like lesion with villous atrophy is seen later. By electron microscopy, there are decreased numbers of microvilli and microvilli that are irregular and shorter than normal (Fig. 72-4). In addition, there are fewer microvillus intramembrane particles and abnormal tight junctions between epithelial cells.[120] The latter contribute to the abnormalities in intestinal permeability seen in celiac disease.

After initiation of a gluten-free diet, abnormalities in the surface absorptive cells usually are the first to improve. There

is a return toward normal in columnar epithelial cells, which have basally oriented nuclei within the first few days. This is accompanied by a decrease in the infiltrate of IELs. Over the ensuing weeks to months, there is improvement in the villous architecture with lengthening of villi, shortening of the crypts, and a concomitant return toward normal in the cellularity of the lamina propria. The distal small intestine mucosa improves more rapidly than proximal mucosa. This is consistent with the less severe lesions being distal and the more severe lesions being proximal. A complete return to normal mucosal architecture does not always take place, and residual abnormalities in histology may persist in up to 50% of celiac disease patients for months or years after gluten withdrawal. Moreover, even patients whose small intestine biopsies appear normal may have a persistent increase in IEL density and persistent abnormalities in jejunal permeability.[118,119,121]

CLINICAL MANIFESTATIONS

The clinical presentation of celiac disease can vary markedly, particularly in adults. At one end of the spectrum, patients may present with diarrhea characterized by large, bulky, pale, foul-smelling stools that have a loose consistency and float because of an increased content of air and fat.[122] These symptoms may be accompanied by abdominal distention, borborygmi, flatus, abdominal cramps, and marked weight loss. Abdominal pain is unusual and, in patients with long-standing celiac disease, should invoke the consideration of a complicating lymphoma. At the other end of the spectrum, adults may be relatively asymptomatic and present with only nonspecific complaints such as malaise, lassitude, and weakness. Children often present with failure to gain weight, diarrhea, and abdominal distention.

Many of the symptoms in celiac disease patients reflect the consequences of malabsorption. These symptoms reflect abnormalities in systems outside the gastrointestinal tract. The more extensive the small intestine lesion, the greater the severity of the malabsorption and the ensuing clinical manifes-

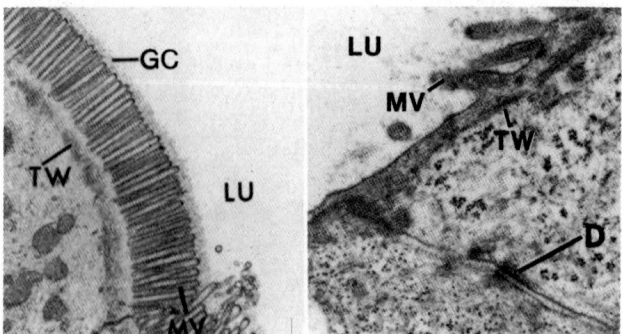

FIGURE 72-4. Transmission electron microscopic view of **(A)** normal epithelial cell brush border compared with **(B)** destroyed brush border on epithelial cells of an untreated celiac patient. (TW, terminal web; GC, glycocalyx; LU, lumen; MV, microvilli; D, desmosomes; from Biempica L, Toccalino H, O'Donnell JC. Cytochemical and ultrastructural studies of the intestinal mucosa of children with celiac disease. Am J Pathol 1968;52:4.)

tations. Persons with minimal disease, involving the duodenum and proximal jejunum, may present simply with anemia secondary to iron or folic acid deficiency or with osteogenic bone disease secondary to malabsorption of calcium and vitamin D.[123,124] Such patients may have no gastrointestinal complaints. Alternatively, individuals with extensive small intestine involvement, including the ileum, may have symptoms that reflect multiple nutrient deficiencies, including megaloblastic anemia and neurologic disease secondary to vitamin B_{12} deficiency.

Celiac disease in children most commonly has its onset between the first and third year of life. Clinical symptoms often diminish or disappear during adolescence, although biochemical or morphologic abnormalities may persist, and symptoms may reoccur in early adult life. Alternatively, celiac disease may have its first clinical onset in adulthood, often during the third or fourth decade or later. These individuals lack a clear past history of celiac disease or a history suggestive of celiac disease during childhood. Nonetheless, some of these patients may have had asymptomatic disease earlier in life. The observations that the intestinal lesion of celiac disease can be found on biopsy in some asymptomatic relatives of celiac disease patients and that celiac disease can be unmasked in otherwise asymptomatic patients after gastric surgery, intercurrent infections, or other major metabolic stress suggest that disease can be present for many years without clinically apparent symptoms. Because of the many ways in which celiac disease can present, the diagnosis frequently is not considered and the disease is missed. This is particularly the case in those who present primarily with constitutional symptoms, anemia or osteomalacia, neurologic complaints, psychologic disturbances, infertility, or growth disturbances.

Gastrointestinal Symptoms

Progressive weight loss, diarrhea, flatulence, and abdominal distention are classic findings in the gastrointestinal presentation of celiac disease. Stools can be bulky, pale, foul-smelling, and floating, or there may be a watery diarrhea. Often, patients simply complain of soft stools and do not have diarrhea, whereas a small number of patients may actually be constipated. Some patients complain of anorexia, whereas others maintain a voracious appetite.

Multiple factors contribute to the diarrhea associated with celiac disease. These include an increased osmotic load secondary to malabsorption of carbohydrates, fats,[125] and proteins accompanied by a decrease in the absorption of water and electrolytes in the upper small intestine. In addition, abnormalities in motility may result from the altered production or release of gastrointestinal hormones.[126–128] In the colon, hydroxy fatty acids produced by the action of bacteria on nonabsorbed dietary fat have cathartic properties. Further, patients with ileal involvement may experience the cathartic effects of bile acid malabsorption on the colon.[125]

The extent of weight loss varies depending on the severity of the intestinal lesion and the degree to which the patient compensates for malabsorption by increasing dietary intake. Some patients have rapid weight loss, whereas others lose little or no weight.

Extraintestinal Manifestations

Many of the symptoms and clinical findings in celiac disease reflect abnormalities outside the gastrointestinal tract. Patients may develop anemia, osteogenic bone disease, neurologic symptoms, menstrual abnormalities, mood or mental changes, or, in the case of children, an abnormal growth pattern.

Anemia usually is secondary to impaired iron or folate absorption. In patients with long-standing ileal disease, vitamin B_{12} malabsorption can also be an important factor.

Osteogenic bone disease develops secondary to abnormal absorption of calcium and vitamin D, a fat-soluble vitamin. Calcium malabsorption may be further exacerbated by the binding of intralumenal calcium to unabsorbed dietary fatty acids and the formation of calcium soaps. Patients may present with bone pain or, less commonly, pathologic fractures. Hypocalcemia and hypomagnesemia may be associated with paresthesias, muscle cramps, and tetany. Further, with prolonged calcium malabsorption, patients may develop secondary hyperparathyroidism.

Hemorrhagic manifestations, if present, are secondary to the malabsorption of the fat-soluble vitamin, vitamin K. This is accompanied by a prolonged prothrombin time. Patients may bleed into the skin or mucous membranes or may develop hematuria, epistaxis, and gastrointestinal bleeding. Thrombocytosis and hyposplenism have also been observed in some celiac disease patients.[129,130]

Peripheral neuropathy with paresthesias and sensory abnormalities are the most common neurologic manifestations of celiac disease. Muscle weakness with a proximal myopathy and resultant ataxia also can be seen. It is important to exclude hypokalemia owing to stool potassium loss as a factor contributing to the muscle weakness. Rarely, a patchy demyelinization of the spinal cord and cerebellar atrophy have been observed. Deficiency of vitamin A, if prolonged and severe, may be associated with night blindness. However, the role of specific vitamin deficiencies in the neurologic abnormalities that accompany celiac disease often is not clear and, unless long-standing ileal disease is present, these individuals usually have normal serum vitamin B_{12} levels. Before removal of gluten from the diet, celiac disease patients may also experience neuropsychiatric symptoms, including mood changes, irritability, and depression. The underlying basis for these abnormalities is not known. However, it is important to note that the diagnosis of celiac disease is easily missed in patients whose primary symptoms are neurologic or neuropsychiatric, especially if gastrointestinal symptoms are not prominent.

In women with celiac disease, abnormalities in menstruation, particularly amenorrhea and delayed menarche, and disturbances in fertility have been observed. These are largely improved by exclusion of gluten from the diet.[131] In men, impotence and infertility can be seen.[132] Malnutrition may contribute to these changes, possibly through abnormalities in centrally mediated hormonal regulation.

Physical Findings

Physical findings in celiac disease are not specific and depend on the severity of the disease. In mild disease, there are no striking physical findings. In severe cases, patients become emaciated. The nails may be clubbed, and there may be edema of the lower extremities or ascites secondary to hypoproteinemia. The skin may develop ecchymoses secondary to vitamin K malabsorption and hypoprothrombinemia. Anemia secondary to iron or folic acid deficiency can be associated with pallor, and there may be cheilosis and glossitis with decreased papillation of the tongue, reflecting vitamin deficiencies. Hyperkeratosis follicularis can be seen in patients with vitamin A deficiency. The abdomen may be protuberant, tympanitic, and of a doughy consistency with dilated intestinal loops filled with fluid and gas. Patients may have decreased sensation to touch, vibration, and position and a decrease in deep tendon reflexes secondary to peripheral neuropathy. A positive Chvostek or Trousseau sign may be present in patients with severe hypocalcemia or magnesium depletion. Lymphadenopathy is unusual in the absence of complicating lymphoma.

DIAGNOSTIC STUDIES

A diagnosis of celiac disease in adults with clinical symptoms or laboratory abnormalities requires the demonstration by histology of an intestinal mucosal lesion on jejunal biopsy that is compatible with celiac disease as well as clinical and morphologic improvement on a gluten-free diet. Similar diagnostic criteria apply in children.[133] Small intestine mucosal biopsy is the gold standard for diagnosis but requires an invasive procedure. Therefore, small intestine biopsy usually is done after patients have undergone simpler screening and noninvasive diagnostic tests.

Screening Tests

Screening tests for celiac disease are the same as those used to assess the presence of other malabsorption disorders. Assuming the individual is eating carotene-containing foods, fat malabsorption is suggested by a low serum carotene or by an increased qualitative fecal fat excretion as indicated by Sudan III stain. More definitive documentation of fat malabsorption can be obtained during balance studies by documenting quantitative fecal fat loss. The hemogram may reveal microcytosis associated with iron deficiency, macrocytosis associated with folic acid (i.e., vitamin B_{12}) deficiency, or a mixed picture. The serum calcium may be low and, if osteopenic bone disease is present, accompanied by a low serum phosphorus and an elevated serum alkaline phosphatase. The serum prothrombin time may be prolonged because of malabsorption of vitamin K and is corrected by parenteral vitamin K therapy. There may be a metabolic acidosis secondary to stool bicarbonate loss if diarrhea is severe, and serum electrolytes, including magnesium, can be depleted. Serum albumin and globulin levels may be low, reflecting the enteric loss of protein. It is not unusual to see mild abnormalities in liver function tests, which may reflect a nonspecific reactive hepatitis or fatty infiltration of the liver.[134] D-xylose or other monosaccharide absorption tests have been used to help distinguish mucosal disease from abnormalities in intralumenal digestion. However, these tests are not specific for celiac disease and have a relatively low positive and negative predictive value for disease. If celiac disease is suspected based on the patient's history and other screening tests, it is best to proceed directly to small intestine mucosal biopsy.[135,136]

Radiologic Studies

Characteristic changes on radiologic examination of the small intestine usually parallel the extent of the disease and include dilatation of the small intestine, which is most marked proximally. In addition, barium often is segmented and there is a prolonged transit time. The normal feathery jejunal mucosal pattern may be replaced by a coarsened pattern, and there may be obliteration of mucosal folds. These changes are not specific for celiac disease. Patients with minimally symptomatic or clinically asymptomatic disease may have totally normal small bowel barium contrast studies.

Small Intestine Mucosal Biopsy

Small intestine mucosal biopsy is the gold standard for the diagnosis of celiac disease. Its importance is underscored by a high false-positive rate of diagnosis, with the concomitant unnecessary institution of a gluten-free diet, when it is not performed.

Small intestine mucosal biopsy specimens are easily obtained using endoscopic forceps at the time of flexible gastroduodenoscopy. If properly handled and oriented, villus side up on a supportive matrix, and serially sectioned, this approach provides adequate tissue for diagnosis. In patients with active disease, visual inspection of the duodenum at the time of endoscopy often reveals a loss of the normal duodenal folds, suggesting the presence of villous atrophy.[137–139] Further, inspection of the biopsy with a hand lens or dissecting microscope may reveal a flat mucosal surface (Fig. 72-5). Alternatively, manual multipurpose suction biopsy instruments and hydraulic instruments can be used to obtain larger peroral suction biopsies of small intestine mucosa. Biopsies are best performed at a defined site (e.g., near the ligament of Treitz) in order to ensure a consistent biopsy site. This is important, particularly when assessing changes in mucosal morphology on rebiopsy after therapy.

Each patient should undergo a small intestine mucosal biopsy before initiating a gluten-free diet, to demonstrate the characteristic mucosal morphology of celiac disease, and a biopsy while on a gluten-free diet to demonstrate improvement. There is no justification for deliberately administering a gluten challenge and obtaining a third set of biopsies to demonstrate subsequent relapse, and that approach involves unwarranted risk. In practice, however, many patients conduct their own rechallenge experiment through dietary indiscretion with a return of symptoms or laboratory abnormalities.

Controlled gluten challenge and biopsy can be justified in some adults who have been placed on a gluten-free diet for presumptive celiac disease without a prior mucosal biopsy[140] and in the very few patients for whom the diagnosis based on biopsy and noninvasive screening tests is in doubt. There is marked individual variability in the clinical and laboratory response to reintroduction of gluten into the diet. Moreover, there are no absolute criteria for what constitutes an appropriate gluten challenge, either with respect to the amount of

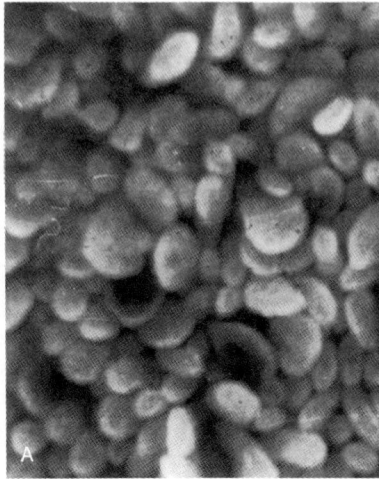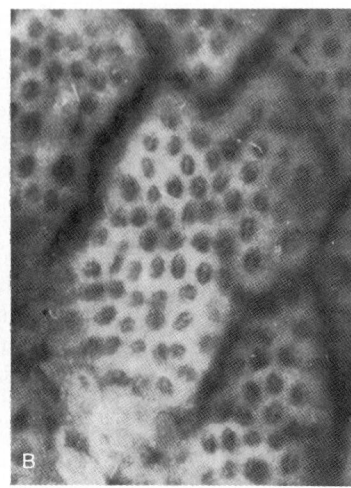

FIGURE 72-5. Dissecting microscopic view of (**A**) normal leaf-like villi in a healthy individual, compared with (**B**) a flat mucosal surface in a patient with celiac disease. (From Thompson H. Pathology of coeliac disease. Curr Top Pathol 1976;63:49.)

gluten administered or its duration[140,141] or with respect to the morphologic and laboratory criteria required to define a relapse.[142] Rectal mucosal biopsy after a rectal gluten challenge demonstrates a time-dependent inflammatory response in many celiac disease patients but not in controls, and this ultimately may provide a useful substitute for oral gluten re-challenge.[21,22,107] However, colonic biopsy sometimes reveals lymphocytic infiltration of the colon surface epithelium in the absence of overt rectal gluten challenge (i.e., lymphocytic colitis).[143] Similarly, biopsy of the gastric mucosa may reveal lymphocytic gastritis characterized by increased numbers of lymphocytes between epithelial cells.[144]

Noninvasive Screening Tests

Noninvasive screening tests provide information that can assist decision making in difficult cases in which the diagnosis is in doubt and that, when serially determined, can help in the assessment as to whether patients are adhering to a gluten-free diet. None of the noninvasive tests currently available should be substituted for small intestine mucosal biopsy in establishing the diagnosis.

Antibody Tests

Several antibody tests are useful as adjuncts to small intestine mucosal biopsy for establishing the diagnosis of celiac disease. These tests are also useful in screening selected target populations, (e.g., family members) suspected of having celiac disease and in the follow-up of patient compliance with the gluten-free diet. Serum antigliadin antibodies can be detected in as many as 90% of patients with untreated clinically symptomatic celiac disease and in many patients with treated or asymptomatic celiac disease.[67–70] However, antigliadin antibodies can also be found in persons with other disorders that affect the small intestine mucosa (e.g., small bowel Crohn's disease). In general, IgA antigliadin antibody has greater specificity for the detection of celiac disease than IgG antigliadin antibody.[69] Serial measurements of serum antigliadin antibodies can be useful to monitor the effectiveness of, and

compliance with, dietary therapy in individual patients because titers decrease as disease improves on a gluten-free diet and increase on gluten rechallenge.[69,145–147] After institution of a gluten-free diet, IgA antigliadin antibodies return to normal more rapidly than those of the IgG class.[145,146] In children, detection of increased levels of polymeric IgA antigliadin antibody in serum appear to be more specific for celiac disease than increased titers of monomeric IgA or IgG antigliadin antibody.[148] Since children with celiac disease who are negative for HLA-DR17 or HLA-DR7 haplotypes have lower serum antigliadin antibody titers than those who have those haplotypes, antigliadin antibody screening is not as useful an indicator of disease activity in that subpopulation.[149] Direct assay of small intestine secretions rather than of serum for antigliadin antibody does not appear to add to the diagnostic usefulness of the antigliadin antibody test.

A second antibody test for the diagnosis of celiac disease is the antiendomysial antibody, an antibody that is directed to extracellular matrix components.[150–156] Elevated titers of IgA antiendomysial antibodies are present in 95% of patients with clinically active celiac disease who have subtotal or total villous atrophy.

Antiendomysial antibodies are more specific for celiac disease than antigliadin antibodies, and they are as sensitive as antigliadin antibodies in those patients who have moderate to marked abnormalities in mucosal architecture. They commonly are not elevated in individuals whose mucosal architecture has returned to normal on a gluten-free diet. Consistent with this, antiendomysial antibody titers decrease as patients with the classic mucosal lesion improve on a gluten-free diet. Because antiendomysial antibodies currently are assayed by immunofluorescence using tissue sections of monkey esophagus, absolute titers are subject to greater interobserver variation than enzyme-linked immunosorbent assay (ELISA)-based methods, such as those used to assay for antigliadin antibody.

Antireticulin antibodies have also received much attention in the diagnosis of celiac disease. The R1 pattern of antireticulin antibody, as assayed by immunofluorescence, has a low level of sensitivity in detecting disease (<40%–50%) but a higher degree of specificity than does the antigliadin antibody.[157,158]

Combined determination of IgG and IgA antigliadin and IgA antiendomysial antibody titers, together with IgA anti-reticulin antibody titers, if available, provides a greater level of sensitivity and specificity for the detection of celiac disease than the measurement of each antibody by itself. Individuals with elevated antigliadin antibody titers but normal or near normal histology of the small intestine mucosa may have latent celiac disease, and on later rebiopsy they may, in some cases, exhibit characteristic mucosal changes of celiac disease.[159] IgA antigliadin, antiendomysial, and antireticulin antibodies are not elevated in the approximately 2% of celiac disease patients with accompanying IgA deficiency. In those persons, assays for elevated titers of IgG antigliadin antibody can be useful.

Absorption Tests

The intestinal mucosa in celiac disease is relatively impermeable to small polar molecules such as mannitol and rhamnose (i.e., monosaccharides) but not to intermediate-size polar molecules (e.g., disaccharides). This forms the basis for differential monosaccharide-disaccharide absorption tests, in which celiac disease patients, relative to healthy controls, can be demonstrated to underabsorb small polar molecules and paradoxically absorb the larger polar molecules.[160] In such tests, a small polar molecule and a disaccharide are administered simultaneously by the oral route, and the absorption of each is compared and expressed as a ratio. For example, the absorption of cellobiose, a disaccharide, compared with that of mannitol;[161] lactulose, a disaccharide, compared with L-rhamnose, a monosaccharide;[162] or lactulose, a disaccharide, compared with mannitol[49,163] can be determined. These tests have an advantage over those that only assess monosaccharide absorption. Extraneous factors that can influence the results of oral absorption tests that rely on urine collections (e.g., variations in gastric and bladder emptying or the presence of renal disease) are less important, because both molecules are administered concurrently and the results of absorption are expressed as a ratio. Moreover, these tests, particularly the lactulose-mannitol test, are relatively easy to perform and are more sensitive and specific for celiac disease than monosaccharide absorption tests such as D-xylose.[136,164] If used in combination with antibody tests, their utility is increased. Absorption tests based on intestinal uptake of chromium-labeled ethylenediaminetetraacetic acid (EDTA) also can be used to assess mucosal malabsorption in celiac disease, but such tests involve the administration of radioactivity and do not offer any significant advantage over the differential absorption tests just described.[165,166] Altered intestinal permeability, like an increased ratio of γ/δ to α/β IEL T cells, increased production of IgA and IgM antigliadin antibody in intestinal secretions,[76] and increased antigliadin or antireticulin antibody in serum,[167-170] may be a marker for latent celiac disease[49]

HLA Genes

More than 95% of celiac disease patients have an HLA-DQ2 molecule encoded by the HLA class II alleles, *DQA1*0501* and *DQB1*0201*.[53-55] Most celiac disease patients who lack that DQ2 molecule have a DQ8 molecule coded by the HLA class II DQ alleles, *DQA1*0301* and *DQB1*0302,* present on DR4 haplotypes.[57-59] HLA class II typing by PCR for the DQ2 molecule encoded by those alleles and for DR4 can therefore be a useful adjunct to help exclude celiac disease in individuals in whom the diagnosis based on biopsy, antibody tests, or absorption tests is in doubt. Thus, celiac disease is unusual in persons who lack *DQA1*501* in combination with *DQB1*0201*, or *DQA1*0301* in combination with *DQB1*0302.* HLA typing also can be useful for identifying which family members are at risk for the development of celiac disease. Because celiac disease can be asymptomatic, family members who carry the relevant susceptibility genes are candidates for further screening tests and, if positive, for small intestine mucosal biopsy.

DIFFERENTIAL DIAGNOSIS

The differential diagnosis of celiac disease includes other causes of malabsorption and other gastrointestinal disorders that are associated with changes in jejunal morphology. Pancreatic insufficiency, most often secondary to chronic pancreatitis, is a common cause of malabsorption but, unlike celiac disease, frequently is accompanied by abdominal pain; also, the pancreas may be calcified on radiographic examination, and the small bowel biopsy is normal. In some celiac disease patients, pancreatic insufficiency may be present concurrently with celiac disease. It is relevant to evaluate this possibility in patients who do not respond to treatment with a gluten-free diet. On clinical grounds, celiac disease in adults is easily distinguished from Whipple disease, which is a multisystem disease, and from malabsorption secondary to infiltration of the mucosa with *Mycobacterium avium-intracellulare,*[72] and the histologic findings on small intestine biopsy are distinctly different in these diseases.

Several diseases are associated with mucosal biopsy abnormalities that can resemble celiac disease. The common variable immunodeficiency syndromes can be associated with subtotal villous atrophy. However, in those disorders, plasma cells are markedly diminished or absent in the lamina propria, rather than increased as in celiac disease. In tropical sprue, the history usually reveals travel to, or residence in, an endemic area. Finally, at times, the small intestine mucosal lesion associated with diffuse lymphoma of the small intestine, gastric acid hypersecretion secondary to gastrinoma, eosinophilic gastroenteritis, or small intestine bacterial overgrowth may resemble celiac disease. In children, a small intestine lesion similar to celiac disease may follow an acute episode of viral gastroenteritis. In addition, jejunal mucosal abnormalities similar to those in celiac disease, but usually less severe, can be seen in cow's milk or soy protein intolerance.[171,172] In the former, the diagnosis may be problematic because children with untreated celiac disease also may be milk intolerant and may not remit until after milk is removed from the diet. In contrast, mucosal abnormalities associated with cow's milk protein intolerance revert on withdrawal of milk, despite the continued ingestion of gluten. Soy protein can be used as a substitute for milk protein in cow's milk protein intolerance. However, some children develop mucosal abnormalities resembling those of celiac disease on ingestion of soy protein.[172]

Parasitic infection can be associated with malabsorption and changes in jejunal morphology. Abnormal villous architecture resembling that of celiac disease can be seen during infestation of the small intestine with the protozoan parasite, *Giardia lamblia*, and mucosal architecture usually improves following eradication of the parasite. *G lamblia* infection is more frequent also in patients with common variable immunodeficiency syndrome. Although changes in mucosal morphology also can be seen in strongyloidiasis, coccidiosis, and hookworm disease, these changes rarely include a flat mucosal biopsy.

Some patients develop diarrhea on gluten ingestion, but their mucosa, when biopsied, is normal or only mildly edematous, with a minimal infiltrate of inflammatory cells. Such gluten-sensitive diarrhea responds to a gluten-free diet but differs from celiac disease.[173] Still other persons have characteristic findings of celiac disease but fail to respond to a gluten-free diet. These patients are said to have refractory sprue.[174] In most, the problem is the inadvertent presence of gluten in the diet or failure to adhere to the diet. However, a small number of patients thought to have refractory sprue may have a complicating lymphoma or collagenous sprue, characterized by deposits of collagen-like material in the subepithelial layer of the intestinal mucosa and progressive malabsorption.[175,176]

DISEASES AND DISORDERS ASSOCIATED WITH CELIAC DISEASE

Many of the diseases that occur more frequently among the celiac disease population are also associated with HLA-DR17 haplotypes. These haplotypes not only carry the celiac disease-associated DQ alleles but appear to carry, in addition, susceptibility genes for several different diseases.

Dermatitis Herpetiformis

Dermatitis herpetiformis (DH) is a skin disease characterized by papulovesicular lesions which are usually located symmetrically on the elbows, knees, buttocks, sacrum, face, scalp, neck, and trunk. The lesions are accompanied by profound itching and burning. Most patients with DH, when biopsied, have a celiac disease-like small intestine lesion[177-179] which often is patchy and varies in severity from area to area. Because the mucosal lesions can be patchy, multiple biopsies may be required to detect the lesion and, in a small number of DH patients, gluten ingestion may be required to provoke the small intestine histologic abnormalities. Usually the small bowel mucosal abnormality in DH is morphologically and functionally not as severe as in celiac disease. Consistent with this, many DH patients have no intestinal symptoms and the majority do not have severe nutrient malabsorption, although isolated nutrient deficiencies (e.g., iron, folic acid) can be seen. As in celiac disease, an increased incidence of lymphoma is seen in DH.[180,181]

Two different patterns of IgA deposits are seen at the dermal-epidermal junction of the uninvolved skin in DH patients. A granular or speckled pattern occurs in most patients, with a linear pattern occurring less often.[178,179] Partial or total villous atrophy of the small intestine mucosa is found exclusively in patients with the granular or speckled pattern of skin IgA deposits.[178,179] Characteristically, complement components (C3, C5) are found in association with these IgA deposits.[179] It is not clear whether the IgA in the skin of DH patients is directed against specific skin and connective tissue proteins or against dietary proteins that have been deposited in the skin or cross-react with skin proteins. Since IgA deposits occur in both involved and uninvolved skin, additional factors are required to produce the localized rash.

DH in patients having granular or speckled type IgA deposits is associated with HLA-DQ2, which, in most patients, is encoded in *cis* pattern on an HLA-DR17 haplotype.[179,182] As in celiac disease, there is an increased density of IELs and an increased proportion of γ/δ relative to α/β IEL within the small intestine epithelium.[183] Antigliadin antibodies can be found in the circulation,[184,185] and most DH patients have elevated titers of antiendomysial antibody.[186,187] Further, like patients with clinically active celiac disease, a large proportion of DH patients have evidence of past exposure to Ad12 as assessed by neutralizing antibody titers.[41] Nonetheless, the precise relation between celiac disease and DH is not known. It also is not known why only 5% of celiac disease patients have clinically evident DH.

Treatment with dapsone usually results in prompt clinical improvement of the skin lesions but does not affect the intestinal mucosal lesions. The skin lesions also respond, albeit slowly, to treatment with a gluten-free diet, which permits a reduction or discontinuation of dapsone over a period of months.[188-190] However, improvement of the skin lesions on a gluten-free diet does not appear to be related to the ability to absorb dapsone more effectively. In persons whose skin rash responds to a gluten-free diet, jejunal morphology also improves, and subepidermal deposits of IgA in the skin decrease, although they often do not disappear. DH skin lesions may improve on a gluten-free diet even in patients whose small intestine mucosa is thought to be normal, although it is possible that jejunal lesions were present in these patients but missed by biopsy because of their patchy nature. DH patients whose rash is controlled on a gluten-free diet usually experience recurrence of the rash after rechallenge with gluten.[191] A minority of patients with DH obtain no relief of their skin lesions from a gluten-free diet despite morphologic improvement in the small intestine mucosa.

Other Disease Associations

There is an established association between celiac disease and insulin-dependent diabetes mellitus (IDDM)[192-195] and between celiac disease and thyroid disease.[196] The incidence of celiac disease in IDDM patients is increased as much as 50-fold, and control of diabetes in these individuals can be difficult because of variable nutrient absorption. IDDM is strongly associated with heterozygous DR4/DR17 haplotypes, with the celiac disease-associated DQ alleles being encoded in *cis* pattern on the DR17 haplotype.[197]

Selective IgA deficiency is the most common immunodeficiency known and has a prevalence of 1 in 500 to 1 in 700 among Northern European Caucasians. This disorder occurs 10 times as often in celiac disease patients, with as many as 2% of these patients being IgA deficient.[82,198] Selective IgA deficiency has been associated with several different HLA haplotypes, one of the common ones being the celiac disease-associated DR17 haplotype.[199-201]

Hyposplenism and splenic atrophy have been noted in some celiac disease patients.[202] The mechanism responsible is not known, but such individuals have an increased risk of developing bacterial infections[203] and should be treated prophylactically with antibiotics before invasive manipulations, including dental procedures. In addition, several cases of mesenteric lymph node cavitation have been associated with celiac disease.[204,205]

Celiac disease has been reported in some patients with Sjögrens syndrome and, rarely, in patients with systemic lupus erythematosus, the former also being associated with a DR17 haplotype.[206,207] Although a small number of adult celiac disease patients have been reported to develop a nonspecific arthritis, the relation between the arthritis and the bowel disease is unknown. Mixed cryoglobulinemia and vasculitis also have been reported in some celiac disease patients,[208-210] and it is tempting to speculate that the absorption of exogenous antigens across an abnormal small intestine mucosa may play a role in the pathogenesis of these disorders. Although associations have been reported between a variety of pulmonary diseases and celiac disease,[211-214] between idiopathic recurrent pericarditis and celiac disease,[215] and between celiac disease and inflammatory bowel disease,[216-219] the underlying mechanisms that are responsible for these associations are not known.

Neurologic disorders including encephalopathy, polymyositis, distal axonopathy, and a progressive cerebellar syndrome have been associated with celiac disease.[220-223] Further, ocular abnormalities and renal abnormalities have been reported in this disease.[224,225] With regard to the latter, some cases of primary IgA mesangial nephropathy have been associated with the deposition of IgA antigliadin antibodies in the kidney.[225] Celiac disease does not have strong associations with other gastrointestinal disorders. However, cases of primary sclerosing cholangitis and primary biliary cirrhosis have been reported to accompany celiac disease.[226-228] Such associations also appear to reflect the increased frequency of a shared HLA haplotype among these diseases.

COMPLICATIONS

Malignancy, ulcerative jejunoileitis, refractory sprue, collagenous sprue, and neuropathy are among the major complications that occur in celiac disease.

Malignancy

The incidence of malignancy, in general, is approximately twofold greater in celiac disease than in the general population, but the risk of specific gastrointestinal malignancies is markedly increased (see Chap. 76).[229,230] Ten percent to 15% of celiac disease patients, mostly older patients, develop neoplastic disease. These patients often have carried diagnoses of celiac disease for 20 to 40 years.[231]

Lymphoma of the small intestine, often multifocal and diffuse, comprises approximately 50% of the malignancies that complicate celiac disease, and most are of T-cell origin.[232-235] The onset of symptoms in these patients may be insidious. For example, a patient with celiac disease may be doing well and then develop symptoms of weight loss, malabsorption, abdominal pain, or intestinal bleeding, despite adhering to a gluten-free diet. In others, the onset may be acute and related to a complication of the lymphoma such as intestinal perforation, obstruction, or hemorrhage. In some, lymphoma is diagnosed concurrently or shortly after the onset of celiac disease symptoms, and it appears that, in some, lymphoma can be a complication of latent celiac disease.[236] It may be difficult to determine whether the small intestine disease is caused by lymphoma superimposed on celiac disease or, alteratively, is directly related to the lymphoma. Lymphoma is frequently difficult to diagnose by small bowel biopsy because superficial biopsies may not reveal the presence of the malignant cells.

One half of the nonlymphoma solid tumors complicating celiac disease arise from the gastrointestinal tract. Carcinoma of the esophagus, mouth, pharynx, and small bowel are the most common. The average age of patients affected is greater than 50 years. Presenting symptoms are related to the primary location and complications of the tumor. For example, adenocarcinoma of the duodenum or upper jejunum may present with abdominal pain, anemia, bleeding, an abdominal mass, or symptoms of obstruction.

The mechanisms responsible for the increased prevalence of malignancy in celiac disease are not known. However, it has been suggested that, alone or in combination, increased crypt mitotic activity, abnormalities of the surface epithelium, increased turnover of lymphoid cells within the mucosa, underlying abnormalities in the mucosal immune system, penetration of the damaged jejunal mucosa by carcinogens, or infections with oncogenic viruses play a role. Evidence strongly suggests that adherence to a gluten-free diet reduces the subsequent incidence of malignancy associated with celiac disease[230] and, in the absence of data to the contrary, it seems prudent to advise celiac disease patients to adhere to a strict gluten-free diet.

Ulcerative Jejunoileitis

Ulcerative jejunoileitis, also known as chronic nongranulomatous ulcerative enterocolitis, and nongranulomatous jejunitis, is a serious complication characterized by ulceration and strictures of the small intestine (see Chap. 77).[237-239] Chronic multiple ulcers appear in the jejunum or, less commonly, in the ileum or colon. These ulcers may perforate and cause peritonitis, may bleed, or may be associated with the formation of small intestine strictures and resultant obstructive complications. Patients with ulcerative jejunoileitis often are refractory to treatment with a gluten-free diet and may not respond to corticosteroids. Further, lymphoma may develop in some of these individuals. Ultimate treatment frequently involves intestinal resection of the ulcerated area. Ulcerative jejunoileitis is associated with a high mortality rate. The mechanisms responsible for this complication are not known, although it has been suggested that an autoimmune reaction directed to intestinal epithelial cells develops, superimposed on the background of celiac disease.[240]

Refractory Sprue and Collagenous Sprue

Patients who initially respond to a gluten-free diet may subsequently relapse despite maintaining their diet. Such patients are then refractory to further dietary therapy. In contrast, others are refractory to dietary therapy from its inception and, assuming they are truly on a gluten-free diet, may not have celiac disease; these patients are said to have unclassified sprue. Some refractory patients with celiac disease, typical or atypical, respond to treatment with corticosteroids or other immunosuppressive drugs such azathioprine, cyclophosphamide, or cyclosporine.[241–243,243a] In others, there is no response and malabsorption may be progressive.

Collagenous sprue is characterized by the development of a thick band of collagen-like material directly under the intestinal epithelial cells and has been regarded by some as a separate entity from celiac disease.[176] However, subepithelial collagen deposition has been noted in up to 36% of patients with classic celiac disease and in tropical sprue.[244] Although individuals with large amounts of subepithelial collagen may be refractory to therapy, the presence of subepithelial collagen does not, a priori, preclude a successful response to a gluten-free diet.[244] Collagenous colitis accompanying celiac disease also has been observed.[245–247] and should be considered in the differential diagnosis of diarrhea occurring in celiac disease patients on a gluten-free diet.[248,249]

Neuropathy

Neuropathic complications of celiac disease occur in approximately 5% of patients. Their cause is unknown, and there is not a clear link with vitamin B_{12} or other vitamin deficiencies. Clinically, such individuals may present with a rapidly developing sensory ataxia, often associated with numbness, tingling, pain, and weakness of the legs. Distal deep tendon reflexes are often diminished, and sensory impairment with a glove and stocking distribution can be seen. This disorder may not respond to gluten withdrawal from the diet and has also been seen to develop in patients who were on a gluten-free diet.[250]

THERAPY

The mainstay of treatment for celiac disease is a gluten-free diet. Because celiac disease is a permanent condition, commitment to a gluten-free diet in adults is lifelong. The diet excludes not only gluten-containing wheat products but also rye, oats, and barley, which also contain disease-activating prolamins. Maintenance of a strict gluten-free diet requires considerable diligence on the part of the patient and support and knowledge of what constitutes a gluten-free diet on the part of the physician. Patients must be educated to exercise considerable caution in their food purchases in stores and restaurants and to carefully read food labels, because gliadins and other disease-activating prolamins are ubiquitous, particularly in processed foods. In those whose antigliadin or antiendomysial antibody titers were elevated and fell toward normal on a gluten-free diet, a recurrent increase in titers suggests a problem in dietary compliance. Commercial laboratory tests and home test kits are becoming available to assay questionable foods as to whether they contain prolamins associated with activation of disease.

Wheat is often used as an extender and is present in many commercially available products (e.g., some salad dressings, canned vegetables and soups, ice cream, candy bars). Even wheat starch flour, which forms a basis for the preparation of gliadin-free breads, depending on its source, is frequently contaminated with gluten. Durum wheat, a tetraploid variety, is used in the preparation of pasta and has been suggested to be less injurious to the small intestine mucosa than common bread wheats. Nonetheless, durum wheat also causes mucosal damage in celiac disease patients and should be avoided. Corn, rice, buckwheat, millet, and sorghum do not activate celiac disease. Triticale is a hybrid of wheat and rye, and spelt and semolina are varieties of wheat. These products often are sold in health food stores and should be avoided.[251]

Gluten is not present in distilled spirits. Therefore, rye whiskey, scotch whiskey, and other cereal-derived spirits can be consumed. Similarly, brandy and wine are made from fruit and should cause no problem. Beer and ale, on the other hand, are produced from barley and contain hordeins (i.e., barley prolamin),[252,253] but there is a lack of clinical evidence that they activate disease. Malt made from barley should be avoided. Barley malt often is a component of foods thought otherwise to be predominantly corn- or rice-based. In contrast, the proteins that activate celiac disease are removed in the production of malt extracts and malt flavoring. Hydrolysed vegetable proteins (HVP) are flavor enhancers in processed foods but may be made from wheat, soy, corn, or other cereal proteins. Their source usually is not provided on food labels, and therefore foods containing HVP are best avoided.

Persons with untreated celiac disease may have accompanying brush border lactase deficiency secondary to damage to the surface intestinal epithelial cells. Therefore, milk and milk products should be avoided at the initiation of treatment. However, after response to the diet, these products can be added, if they are tolerated. Celiac disease societies and support groups are an excellent source for lists of gluten-free products and their manufacturers and for useful books of recipes for cooking with gluten-free ingredients. After starting a gluten-free diet, most patients improve within a few weeks. In many, improvement in the state of well-being is noticed within 48 hours, although it may take weeks or months to achieve full remission. Clinical symptoms usually improve before the return toward normal of mucosal architecture as assessed by histology. In approximately 50% of adults on a gluten-free diet, biopsies show a partial, but not complete, return toward normal.[254–256]

A strict gluten-free diet should be maintained throughout life. This clearly is the case in children, in whom growth and stature may be seriously affected in the absence of complete treatment. In adults, many physicians titrate the strictness of the diet with the patient's clinical symptoms. Nonetheless, individuals on a partial gluten-free diet may have ongoing inflammation and damage with minimal clinical symptoms. Studies on the relation between diet and malignancy in celiac disease[230] suggest that a strict gluten-free diet is a more prudent approach.

Supplemental therapy with iron or folate is needed in individuals with malabsorption of those nutrients. Rarely, vitamin B_{12} may be required. Patients with prolongation of the prothrombin time require supplemental vitamin K. Others require appropriate replacement of fluids and electrolytes, including calcium and magnesium. Individuals with osteopenic bone disease require vitamin D replacement. In some patients, improvement has been seen with correction of zinc deficiency.

Steroids are rarely needed in the therapy of celiac disease, although the response to the institution of steroids can be striking.[241] Steroids should be reserved for patients who have not responded to a gluten-free diet or, occasionally, those with complicating disorders such as ulcerative jejunoileitis. Cyclosporine also may be useful in selected cases of atypical sprue.[243,243a]

PROGNOSIS

Celiac disease has a favorable prognosis if diagnosed early. Conversely, if not recognized and treated, it can be a progressive disorder characterized by malnutrition and debilitation. In adults, there usually is a return of absorptive functions to normal and a disappearance of many of the manifestations of disease after initiation of a gluten-free diet. However, complications of the disease, such as peripheral neuropathy or pathologic fractures secondary to osteopenic bone disease, may not be completely reversible.

Although celiac disease usually remits during the teenage years, the extent of true remission is not certain; many patients can be shown to have persistent hematologic and morphologic abnormalities.[257–259] It may be the clinical symptoms rather than the disease that remits.

The reader is directed to Chapter 5, The Immune System; Chapter 14, Electrolyte Secretion and Absorption: Small Intestine and Colon; Chapter 38, Approach to the Patient With Diarrhea; Chapter 76, Tumors and Other Neoplastic Diseases of the Small Bowel; Chapter 77, Miscellaneous Diseases of the Small Intestine; and Chapter 130, Endoscopic Mucosal Biopsy.

REFERENCES

1. Cole SG, Kagnoff MF. Celiac disease. Annu Rev Nutr 1985;5:241.
2. Kagnoff MF. A model of an immunologically mediated intestinal disease. In: Kagnoff MF, ed. Immunology and allergy clinics of North America. Philadelphia: WB Saunders, 1988:505.
3. Kagnoff MF. Celiac disease: a gastrointestinal disease with environmental, genetic and immunologic components. In: MacDermott RP, Elson CO, eds. Gastroenterology clinics of North America. Philadelphia: WB Saunders, 1992:405.
4. Kagnoff MF. Celiac disease. In: Targan SR, Shanahan F, eds. Immunology and immunopathology of the liver and gastrointestinal tract. New York: Igaku-Shoin, 1990:487.
5. Gee S. On the coeliac affection. St Barth Hosp Rep 1888;24:17.
6. Dicke WK, Weijers HA, van de Kamer JH. Coeliac disease. II. The presence in wheat of a factor having a deleterious effect in cases of coeliac disease. Acta Paediatr 1953;42:34.
7. Van de Kamer JH, Weijers HA, Dicke WK. Coeliac disease. IV. An investigation into the injurious constituents of wheat in connection with the action on patients with coeliac disease. Acta Paediatr 1953;42:223.
8. Paulley LW. Observations on the aetiology of idiopathic steatorrhea. Br Med J 1954;2:1318.
9. Rubin CE, Brandborg LL, Phelps PC, Taylor HC Jr. Studies of celiac disease. I. The apparent identical and specific nature of the duodenal and proximal jejunal lesion in celiac disease and idiopathic sprue. Gastroenterology 1960;38:28.
10. Kagnoff MF. Celiac disease. Pathogenesis and clinical features. In: Shaffer E, Thomson ABR, eds. Modern concepts in gastroenterology. New York: Plenum Publishing, 1989:227.
11. Mylotte M, Egan-Mitchell B, McCarthy CF, McNicholl B. Incidence of coeliac disease in the west of Ireland. Br Med J 1973;1:703.
12. Stevens FM, Egan-Mitchell B, Cryan E, et al. Decreasing incidence of coeliac disease (abstract). In: Kumar PJ, Walker-Smith JA, eds. Coeliac disease: 100 years. London: Proceedings for the International Coeliac Symposium, 1991:306.
13. Cavell B, Stenhammar L, Ascher H, et al. Increasing incidence of childhood coeliac disease in Sweden. Results of a national study. Acta Paediatr Scand 1992;81:589.
14. Ascher H, Krantz I, Kristiansson B. Increasing incidence of coeliac disease in Sweden. Arch Dis Child 1991;66:608.
15. Auricchio S. Gluten-sensitive enteropathy and infant nutrition. J Pediatr Gastroenterol Nutr 1983;2:S304.
16. Stevens FM, Pena AS. A further lesson from war time Holland. In: Kumar PJ, Walker-Smith JA, eds. Coeliac disease: 100 years. London: Proceedings for the International Coeliac Symposium, 1991:306.
17. Kagnoff MF. Genetic basis of celiac disease. Role of HLA genes. In: Marsh M, ed. Coeliac Disease. London: Blackwell Scientific, 1992:215.
18. Kagnoff MF. Role of environmental and genetic factors in celiac disease. In: Branski D, Kagnoff M, Rozen P, eds. Frontiers of gastrointestinal research: gluten sensitive enteropathy. Basel: S Karger, 1992:15.
19. Cornell HJ, Maxwell RJ. Amino acid composition of gliadin fractions which may be toxic to individuals with celiac disease. Clin Chim Acta 1982;123:311.
20. Bailey DS, Freedman AR, Price SC, et al. Early biochemical responses of the small intestine of coeliac patients to wheat gluten. Gut 1989;30:78.
21. Loft DE, Marsh MN, Sandle GI, et al. Studies of intestinal lymphoid tissue. XII. Epithelial lymphocyte and mucosal responses to rectal gluten challenge in celiac sprue. Gastroenterology 1989;97:29.
22. Loft DE, Marsh MN, Crowe PT. Rectal gluten challenge and diagnosis of coeliac disease. Lancet 1990;335:1293.
23. Dobbins WO, Rubin CE. Studies of the rectal mucosa in celiacsprue. Gastroenterology 1964;47:471.
24. Kasarda DD. Toxic proteins and peptides in celiac disease: relations to cereal genetics. In: Walker DN, Kretchmer N, eds. Food, nutrition and evolution. New York: Masson, 1981:201.
25. Colyer J, Farthing MJ, Kumar PJ, et al. Reappraisal of the "lectin hypothesis" in the aetiopathogenesis of coeliac disease. Clin Sci 1986;71:105.
26. Colyer J, Kumar PJ, Waldron NM, et al. Gliadin binding to rat and human enterocytes. Clin Sci 1987;72:593.
27. Shewry PR, Tatham AS, Kasarda DD. Cereal proteins and coeliac disease. In: Marsh M, ed. Coeliac disease. London: Blackwell Scientific, 1992:305.
28. Kasarda DD, Bernardin JE, Nimmo CC. Wheat proteins. In: Pomerancz Y, ed. Advances in cereal science and technology. St. Paul: American Association of Cereal Chemists, 1976:158.
29. Kasarda DD, Nimmo CC, Bernardin JE. Structural aspects and genetic relationships of gliadins. In: Hekkems WTJM, Pena AS, eds. Proceedings of the Second International Celiac Symposium. Leiden: HE Stenfert Korese, 1974:25.
30. Woychik JH, Boudy JA, Dimler RJ. Starch gel electrophoresis of wheat gluten proteins with concentration urea. Arch Biochem Biophys 1961;94:477.

31. Kagnoff MF, Austin RK, Johnson HC, et al. Celiac sprue: correlation with murine T-cell responses to wheat gliadin components. J Immunol 1982;129:2693.

32. Kasarda DD, Okita TW, Bernardin JE, et al. Nucleic acid (cDNA) and amino acid sequences of α-type gliadins from wheat (*Triticum aestivum L.*). Proc Natl Acad Sci U S A 1984;81:4712.

33. Bartels D, Thompson RD. The characterization of cDNA clones coding for wheat storage proteins. Nucleic Acids Res 1983;11:2961.

34. Rafalski JA, Scheets K, Metzler M, et al. Developmentally regulated plant genes: the nucleotide sequence of a wheat gliadin genomic clone. EMBO J 1984;3:1409.

35. Kim WT, Okita TW. Nucleotide and primary sequence of a major rice prolamin. FEBS Lett 1988;231:308.

36. Chesnut RS, Shotwell MA, Boyer SK, Larkins BA. Analysis of avenin proteins and the expression of their mRNAs in developing oat seeds. The Plant Cell 1989;1:913.

37. Kagnoff MF, Austin RK, Hubert JJ, et al. Possible role for a human adenovirus in the pathogenesis of celiac disease. J Exp Med 1984;160:1544.

38. Karagiannis JA, Priddle JD, Jewell DP. Cell-mediated immunity to a synthetic gliadin peptide resembling a sequence from adenovirus 12. Lancet 1987;1:884.

39. Kagnoff MF, Paterson YJ, Kumar PJ, et al. Evidence for the role of a human intestinal adenovirus in the pathogenesis of coeliac disease. Gut 1987;28:995.

40. Mantzaris GJ, Karagiannis JA, Priddle JD, Jewell DP. Cellular hypersensitivity to a synthetic dodecapeptide derived from human adenovirus 12 which resembles a sequence of A-gliadin in patients with coeliac disease. Gut 1990;31:668.

41. Lahdeaho ML, Lehtinen M, Rissa HR, et al. Antipeptide antibodies to adenovirus E1b protein indicate enhanced risk of celiac disease and dermatitis herpetiformis. Int Arch Allergy Appl Immunol 1993;101:272.

42. Arato A, Kosnai I, Szonyi L, Toth M. Frequent past exposure to adenovirus 12 in coeliac disease. Acta Paediatr Scand 1991;80:1101.

43. Kagnoff MF. Celiac disease: adenovirus and alpha gliadin. Curr Top Microbiol Immunol 1989;145:67.

44. Mantzaris G, Jewell DP. In vivo toxicity of a synthetic dodecapeptide from A gliadin in patients with coeliac disease. Scand J Gastroenterol 1991;26:392.

45. MacDonald WC, Dobbins WO, Rubin CE. Studies on the familial nature of celiac sprue using biopsy of the small intestine. N Engl J Med 1968;272:448.

46. Mylotte M, Egan-Mitchell B, Fottrell PF, et al. Family studies in coeliac disease. Q J Med 1974;171:359.

47. Stokes PL, Ferguson R, Holmes GKT, Cooke WT. Familial aspects of coeliac disease. Q J Med 1976;180:567.

48. Auricchio S, Mazzacca G, Tosi R, et al. Coeliac disease as a familial condition: identification of asymptomatic coeliac patients within family groups. Gastroenterol Int 1988;1:25.

49. Van Elburg RM, Uil JJ, Mulder CJ, Heymans HS. Intestinal permeability in patients with coeliac disease and relatives of patients with coeliac disease. Gut 1993;34:354.

50. Polanco I, Mearin ML, Larrauri J, et al. Effect of gluten supplementation in healthy siblings of children with celiac disease. Gastroenterology 1987;92:678.

51. Polanco I, Biemond I, van Leeuwen A, et al. Gluten-sensitive enteropathy in Spain: genetic and environmental factors. In: McConnell RB, ed. The genetics of coeliac disease. Lancaster: MTP Press, 1981:211.

52. Kagnoff MF. Understanding the molecular basis of coeliac disease. Gut 1990;31:497.

53. Sollid LM, Markussen G, Ek J, et al. Evidence for a primary association of celiac disease to a particular HLA-DQ alpha/beta heterodimer. J Exp Med 1989;169:345.

54. Kagnoff MF, Harwood JI, Bugawan TL, Erlich HA. Structural analysis of the HLA-DR, -DQ, and -DP alleles on the celiac disease-associated -DR3 (DRw17) haplotype. Proc Natl Acad Sci U S A 1989;86:6274.

55. Mazzilli MC, Ferrante P, Mariani P, et al. A study of Italian pediatric celiac disease patients confirms that the primary HLA association is to the DQ(α1*0501,β1*0201) heterodimer. Hum Immunol 1992;33:133.

56. Rioski R, Ek J, Thorsby E, Sollid LM. On the HLA-DQ(α1*0501, β1*0201) associated susceptibility in celiac disease: A possible gene dosage effect of DQB1*0201. Tissue Antigens 1993;41:173.

57. DeMarchi M, Carbonara AO, Ansaldi N, et al. HLA-DR3 and DR7-negative celiac disease. In: Albert ED, ed. Histocompatibility testing. Berlin: Springer-Verlag, 1984:359.

58. Tosi R, Tanigaki N, Polanco I, et al. A radioimmunoassay typing study of non-DQw2-associated celiac disease. Clin Immunol Immunopathol 1986;39:168.

59. Spurkland A, Sollid LM, Polanco I, et al. HLA-DR and -DQ genotypes of celiac disease patients serologically typed to be non-DR3 or non-DR5/7. Hum Immunol 1992;35:188.

60. Scholz S, Albert E. HLA and diseases: involvement of more than one HLA-linked determinant of disease susceptibility. Immunol Rev 1983;70:77.

61. Mearin ML, Biemond I, Pena AS, et al. HLA-DR phenotypes in Spanish coeliac children: their contribution to the understanding of the genetics of the disease. Gut 1983;24:532.

62. Alper CA, Fleischnick E, Awdeh Z, et al. Extended major histocompatibility complex haplotypes in patients with gluten-sensitive enteropathy. J Clin Invest 1987;79:251.

63. Kagnoff MF, Weiss JB, Brown RJ, et al. Immunoglobulin allotype markers in gluten-sensitive enteropathy. Lancet 1983;1:952.

64. Weiss JB, Austin RK, Schanfield MS, Kagnoff MF. Gluten-sensitive enteropathy. Immunoglobulin G heavy-chain (Gm) allotypes and the immune response to wheat gliadin. J Clin Invest 1983;72:96.

65. Carbonara AO, DeMarchi M, van Loghem E, Ansaldi N. Gm markers in celiac disease. Hum Immunol 1983;6:91.

66. Ciclitira PJ, Ellis HJ, Evans DJ. A solid-phase radioimmunoassay for measurement of circulating antibody titres to wheat gliadin and its subfractions in patients with adult coeliac disease. J Immunol Methods 1983;62:231.

67. Levenson SD, Austin RK, Dietler MD, et al. Specificity of antigliadin antibody in celiac disease. Gastroenterology 1985;89:1.

68. Friis SU, Gudmand-Hoyer E. Screening for coeliac disease in adults by simultaneous determination of IgA and IgG gliadin antibodies. Scand J Gastroenterol 1986;21:1058.

69. Kelly CP, Feighery C, Gallagher RB, et al. Mucosal and systemic IgA anti-gliadin antibody in celiac disease. Contrasting patterns of response in serum, saliva, and intestinal secretions. Dig Dis Sci 1991;36:743.

70. Ciclitira PJ, Ellis HJ, Richards D, Kemeny DM. Gliadin IgG subclass antibodies in patients with coeliac disease. Int Arch Allergy Appl Immunol 1986;80:258.

71. Scott H, Brandtzaeg P. Gluten IgA antibodies and coeliac disease. Lancet 1989;1:382.

72. Gillin JS, Urmacher C, West R. Disseminated mycobacterium avium-intracellulare in acquired immunodeficiency syndrome mimicking Whipple's disease. Gastroenterology 1983;85:1187.

73. Laurent J, Branellec A, Heslan JM, et al. An increase in circulating IgA antibodies to gliadin in IgA mesangial glomerulonephritis. Am J Nephrol 1987;7:178.

74. Rostoker G, Laurent J, Andre C, et al. High levels of IgA antigliadin antibodies in patients who have IgA mesangial glomerulonephritis but not coeliac disease. Lancet 1988;1:356.

75. Mascart-Lemone F, Cadranel S, Van den Broeck J, et al. IgA immune response patterns to gliadin in serum. Int Arch Allergy Appl Immunol 1988;86:412.

76. Arranz E, Ferguson A. Intestinal antibody pattern of celiac disease: occurrence in patients with normal jejunal biopsy histology. Gastroenterology 1993;104:1263.

77. Baklien K, Brandtzaeg P, Fausa O. Immunoglobulins in jejunal mucosa and serum from patients with adult coeliac disease. Scand J Gastroenterol 1977;12:149.

78. Scott BB, Goodall A, Stephenson P, Jenkins D. Small intestinal plasma cells in coeliac disease. Gut 1984;25:41.

79. Scott H, Ek J, Baklien K, Brandtzaeg P. Immunoglobulin-producing cells in jejunal mucosa of children with coeliac dis-

ease on a gluten-free diet and after gluten challenge. Scand J Gastroenterol 1980;15:81.

80. Falchuk ZM, Strober W. Gluten-sensitive enteropathy: synthesis of antigliadin antibody in vitro. Gut 1974;15:947.

81. Ciclitira PJ, Ellis HJ, Wood GM, et al. Secretion of gliadin antibody by coeliac jejunal mucosal biopsies cultured in vitro. Clin Exp Immunol 1986;64:119.

82. Crabbe PA, Heremans JF. Selective IgA deficiency with steatorrhoea. A new syndrome. Am J Med 1967;42:319.

83. Fassett RT, Kagnoff MF. Clinical significance of selective IgA deficiency. Internal Medicine for the Specialist 1987;8:90.

84. Shiner M. Ultrastructural changes suggestive of immune reactions in the jejunal mucosa of coeliac children following gluten challenge. Gut 1973;14:1.

85. Halstensen TS, Hvagtum M, Scott H, et al. Association of subepithelial deposition of activated complement and immunoglobulin G and M response to gluten in celiac disease. Gastroenterology 1992;102:751.

86. Haeney MR, Goodwin BJ, Barratt ME, et al. Soya protein antibodies in man: their occurrence and possible relevance in coeliac disease. J Clin Pathol 1982;35:319.

87. Volta U, Lazzari R, Bianchi FB, et al. Antibodies to dietary antigens in coeliac disease. Scand J Gastroenterol 1986;21: 935.

88. Howdle PD, Bullen AW, Losowsky MS. Cell-mediated immunity to gluten within the small intestinal mucosa in coeliac disease. Gut 1982;23:115.

89. Corazza GR, Rawcliffe PM, Frisoni M, et al. Specificity of leucocyte migration inhibition test in coeliac disease. A reassessment using different gluten subfractions. Clin Exp Immunol 1985;60:117.

90. O'Farrelly C, Hekkens WT, Feighery C, Weir DG. The specificity of wheat protein reactivity in coeliac disease. Scand J Gastroenterol 1983;18:603.

91. Horvath K, Graf L, Walcz E, et al. Naloxone antagonizes effect of alpha-gliadin on leucocyte migration in patients with coeliac disease. Lancet 1985;2:184.

92. Flores AR, Winter HS, Bhan AK. In vitro model to assess immunoregulatory T lymphocyte subpopulations in gluten sensitive enteropathy (GSE) (abstract). Gastroenterology 1982;82:1058.

93. Freedman AR, Macartney JC, Nelufer JM, Ciclitira PJ. Timing of infiltration of T lymphocytes induced by gluten into the small intestine in coeliac disease. J Clin Pathol 1987;40:741.

94. Maki M, Holm K, Collin P, Savilahti E. Increase in gamma/delta T cell receptor bearing lymphocytes in normal small bowel mucosa in latent coeliac disease. Gut 1991;32:1412.

95. Spencer J, Isaacson PG, MacDonald TT, et al. Gamma/delta T cells and the diagnosis of coeliac disease. Clin Exp Immunol 1991;85:109.

96. Jenkins D, Goodall A, Scott BB. T-lymphocyte populations in normal and coeliac small intestinal mucosa defined by monoclonal antibodies. Gut 1986;27:1330.

97. Malizia G, Trejdosiewicz LK, Wood GM, et al. The microenvironment of coeliac disease: T cell phenotypes and expression of the T2 "T blast" antigen by small bowel lymphocytes. Clin Exp Immunol 1985;60:437.

98. Pignata C, Troncone R, Monaco G, et al. Impaired suppressor activity in children affected by coeliac disease. Gut 1985;26: 285.

99. Corazza GR, Sarchielli P, Londei M, et al. Gluten specific suppressor T cell dysfunction in coeliac disease. Gut 1986;27: 392.

100. Sarles J, Gorvel JP, Olive D, et al. Subcellular localization of class I (A,B,C) and class II (DR and DQ) MHC antigens in jejunal epithelium of children with coeliac disease. J Pediatr Gastroenterol Nutr 1987;6:51.

101. Kelly J, Weir DG, Feighery C. Differential expression of HLA-D gene products in the normal and coeliac small bowel. Tissue Antigens 1988;31:151.

102. Ciclitira PJ, Nelufer JM, Ellis HJ, Evans DJ. The effect of gluten on HLA-DR in the small intestinal epithelium of patients with coeliac disease. Clin Exp Immunol 1986;63:101.

103. Scott H, Sollid LM, Fausa O, et al. Expression of major histocompatibility complex class II subregion products by jejunal epithelium in patients with celiac disease. Scand J Gastroenterol 1987;26:563.

104. Marley NJ, Macartney JC, Ciclitira PJ. HLA-DR, DP and DQ expression in the small intestine of patients with coeliac disease. Clin Exp Immunol 1987;70:386.

105. Schweizer JJ, Mearin ML, Pena AS, et al. Expression of HLA-DQ antigens in the small-intestinal mucosa of patients with coeliac disease. Scand J Gastroenterol 1991;26:605.

106. Lundin KE, Scott H, Hansen T, et al. Gliadin-specific, HLA-DQ (alpha1*0501, beta1*0201) restricted T cells isolated from the small intestinal mucosa of celiac disease patients. J Exp Med 1993;178:187.

107. Ensari A, Ager A, Marsh MN, et al. Time-course of adhesion molecule expression in rectal mucosa of gluten-sensitive subjects after gliadin challenge. Clin Exp Immunol 1993;92:303.

108. Rosekrans PC, Meijer CJ, Polanco I, et al. Long-term morphological and immunohistochemical observations on biopsy specimens of small intestine from children with gluten-sensitive enteropathy. J Clin Pathol 1981;34:138.

109. Niazi NM, Leigh R, Crowe PT, Marsh MN. Morphometric analysis of small intestinal mucosa. I. Methodology, epithelial volume compartments and enumeration of inter-epithelial space lymphocytes. Virchows Arch 1984;404:49.

110. Marsh MN. Studies of intestinal lymphoid tissue. III. Quantitative analyses of epithelial lymphocytes in the small intestine of human control subjects and of patients with celiac sprue. Gastroenterology 1980;79:481.

111. Marsh MN, Hinde J. Inflammatory component of celiac sprue mucosa. I. Mast cells, basophils and eosinophils. Gastroenterology 1985;89:92.

112. Strobel S, Busuttil A, Ferguson A. Human intestinal mucosal mast cells: expanded population in untreated coeliac disease. Gut 1983;24:222.

113. Wingren U, Hallert C, Norrby K, Enerback L. Histamine and mucosal mast cells in gluten enteropathy. Agents Actions 1986;18:266.

114. Colombel JF, Torpier G, Janin A, et al. Activated eosinophils in adult coeliac disease: evidence for a local release of major basic protein. Gut 1992;33:1190.

115. Sjolund K, Alumets J, Berg NO, et al. Enteropathy of coeliac disease in adults: increased number of enterochromaffin cells in the duodenal mucosa. Gut 1982;23:42.

116. Pietroletti R, Bishop AE, Carlei F, et al. Gut endocrine cell population in coeliac disease estimated by immunocytochemistry using a monoclonal antibody to chromogranin. Gut 1986;27:838.

117. Penna FJ, Hill ID, Kingston D, et al. Jejunal mucosal morphometry in children with and without gut symptoms and in normal adults. J Clin Pathol 1981;34:386.

118. Ferguson A, Arranz E, O'Mahony S. Clinical and pathological spectrum of coeliac disease—active, silent, latent, potential. Gut 1993;34:150.

119. Savilahti E, Arato A, Verkasalo M. Intestinal gamma/delta receptor-bearing T lymphocytes in celiac disease and inflammatory diseases in children. Pediatr Res 1990;28:579.

120. Madara JL, Trier JS. Structural abnormalities of jejunal epithelial cell membranes in celiac sprue. Lab Invest 1980;43: 254.

121. Bjarnason I, Peters TJ, Veall N. A persistent defect in intestinal permeability in coeliac disease demonstrated by a ^{51}Cr-labelled EDTA absorption test. Lancet 1983;1:323.

122. Levitt MD, Duane WC. Floating stools—flatus versus fat. N Engl J Med 1972;286:973.

123. Stahlberg MR, Savilahti E, Siimes MA. Iron deficiency in coeliac disease is mild and it is detected and corrected by gluten-free diet. Acta Paediatr Scand 1991;80:190.

124. Depla AC, Bartelsman JF, Mulder CJ, Tytgat GN. Anemia: monosymptomatic celiac disease. A report of 3 cases. Hepatogastroenterology 1990;37:90.

125. Vuoristo M, Miettinen TA. The role of fat and bile acid malabsorption in diarrhea of coeliac disease. Scand J Gastroenterol 1987;22:289.

126. Rhodes RA, Tai HH, Chey WY. Impairment of secretin release in celiac sprue. Am J Dig Dis 1978;23:833.

127. Maton PN, Selden AC, Fitzpatrick ML, Chadwick VS. Defec-

tive gallbladder emptying and cholecystokinin release in celiac disease. Reversal by gluten-free diet. Gastroenterology 1985;88:391.

128. Kilander AF, Dotevall G, Lindstedt G, Lundberg PA. Plasma enteroglucagon related to malabsorption to coeliac disease. Gut 1984;25:629.

129. Nelson EW, Ertran A, Brooks FP, Cerda JJ. Thrombocytosis in patients with celiac sprue. Gastroenterology 1976;70:1042.

130. O'Grady JG, Stevens FM, Harding B, et al. Hyposplenism and gluten-sensitive enteropathy. Natural history, incidence, and relationship to diet and small bowel morphology. Gastroenterology 1984;87:1326.

131. Ferguson R, Holmes GK, Cooke WT. Coeliac disease, fertility, and pregnancy. Scand J Gastroenterol 1982;17:65.

132. Farthing MJ, Rees LH, Dawson AM. Male gonadal function in coeliac disease. III. Pituitary regulation. Clin Endocrinol (Oxf) 1983;19:661.

133. Walker-Smith JA, Guandalini S, Schmitz J, et al. Revised criteria for diagnosis of coeliac disease. Arch Dis Child 1990;65:909.

134. Hagander B, Berg NO, Brandt L. Hepatic injury in adult coeliac disease. Lancet 1988;109:713.

135. Sladen GE, Kumar PJ. Is the xylose test still a worth-while investigation? Br Med J 1973;3:223.

136. Lamabadusuriya SP, Packer S, Harries JT. Limitations of xylose tolerance test as a screening procedure in childhood coeliac disease. Arch Dis Child 1975;50:34.

137. Jabbari M, Wild G, Goresky CA, et al. Scalloped valvulae conniventes: an endoscopic marker of celiac sprue. Gastroenterology 1988;95:1518.

138. McIntyre AS, Ng DP, Smith JA, et al. The endoscopic appearance of duodenal folds is predictive of untreated adult celiac disease. Gastrointest Endosc 1992;38:148.

139. Brocchi E, Corazza GR, Caletti G, et al. Endoscopic demonstration of loss of duodenal folds in the diagnosis of celiac disease. N Engl J Med 1988;319:741.

140. Kumar PJ, O'Donoghue DP, Stenson K, Dawson AM. Reintroduction of gluten in adults and children with treated coeliac disease. Gut 1979;20:743.

141. Bramble MG, Zucoloto S, Wright NA, Record CO. Acute gluten challenge in treated adult coeliac disease: a morphometric and enzymatic study. Gut 1985;26:169.

142. Marsh MN. Coeliac disease. In: Marsh MN, ed. Immunopathology of the small intestine. Chichester: John Wiley & Sons, 1987:371.

143. Wolber R, Owen D, Freeman H. Colonic lymphocytosis in patients with celiac sprue. Hum Pathol 1990;21:1092.

144. Wolber R, Owen D, DelBuono L, et al. Lymphocytic gastritis in patients with celiac sprue or spruelike intestinal disease. Gastroenterology 1990;98:310.

145. Scott H, Ek J, Brandtzaeg P. Changes of serum antibody activities to various dietary antigens related to gluten withdrawal or challenge in children with coeliac disease. Int Arch Allergy Appl Immunol 1985;76:138.

146. Kilander AF, Nilsson LA, Gillberg R. Serum antibodies to gliadin in coeliac disease after gluten withdrawal. Scand J Gastroenterol 1987;22:29.

147. Carswell F, Ferguson A. Plasma food antibodies during withdrawal and reintroduction of dietary gluten in coeliac disease. Arch Dis Child 1973;48:583.

148. Mascart-Lemone F, Delacroix DL, Cadranel S, et al. Size distribution of serum IgA antibodies to food proteins: bovine beta-lactoglobulin (BGL), bovine serum albumin (BSA) and gliadin (GL). Adv Exp Med Biol 1987;216A:841.

149. Bonamico M, Morellini M, Mariani P, et al. HLA antigens and antigliadin antibodies in coeliac disease. Dis Markers 1991;9:313.

150. Chorzelski TP, Beutner EH, Sulej T, et al. IgA anti-endomysium antibody. A new immunological marker of dermatitis herpetiformis and coeliac disease. Br J Dermatol 1984;111:395.

151. Kapuscinska A, Zalewski T, Chorzelski TP, et al. Disease specificity and dynamics of changes in IgA class anti-endomysial antibodies in celiac disease. J Pediatr Gastroenterol Nutr 1987;6:529.

152. Rossi T, Kumar V, Lerner A, et al. Relationship of endomysial antibodies to jejunal mucosal pathology: specificity towards both symptomatic and asymptomatic celiacs. J Pediatr Gastroenterol Nutr 1988;7:858.

153. Burgin-Wolff A, Gaze H, Hadziselimovic F, et al. Antigliadin and antiendomysium antibody determination for coeliac disease. Arch Dis Child 1991;66:941.

154. Ferreira M, Davies SL, Butler M, et al. Endomysial antibody: is it the best screening test for coeliac disease? Gut 1992;33:1633.

155. Volta U, Molinaro N, Fusconi M, et al. IgA antiendomysial antibody test. A step forward in celiac disease screening. Dig Dis Sci 1991;36:752.

156. Karpati S, Meurer M, Stolz W, et al. Ultrastructural binding sites of endomysium antibodies from sera of patients with dermatitis herpetiformis and coeliac disease. Gut 1992;33:191.

157. Eade OE, Lloyd RS, Lang C, Wright R. IgA and IgG reticulin antibodies in coeliac and non-coeliac patients. Gut 1977;18:991.

158. Dias J, Unsworth DJ, Walker-Smith JA. Antigliadin and antireticulin antibodies in screening for coeliac disease. Lancet 1987;2:157.

159. Collin P, Helin H, Maki M, et al. Follow-up of patients positive in reticulin and gliadin antibody tests with normal small-bowel biopsy findings. Scand J Gastroenterol 1993;28:595.

160. Cobden I, Rothwell J, Axon AT. Intestinal permeability and screening tests for coeliac disease. Gut 1980;21:512.

161. Juby LD, Rothwell J, Axon AT. Cellobiose/mannitol sugar test—a sensitive tubeless test for coeliac disease: results on 1010 unselected patients. Gut 1989;30:476.

162. Santana IA, Talbot MB, Sharma BK, Pounder RE. Screening for small intestine mucosal damage using the lactulose/L rhamnose sugar permeability test. Gut 1984;25:A546.

163. Juby LD, Rothwell J, Axon ATR. Lactulose/mannitol test: an ideal screen for coeliac disease. Gastroenterology 1989;96:79.

164. Bode S, Gudmand-Hoyer E. The diagnostic value of the D-xylose absorption test in adult coeliac disease. Scand J Gastroenterol 1987;22:1217.

165. Martines D, Morris AI, Gilmore IT, et al. Comparison between the cellobiose/mannitol and ^{51}CR-labeled ethylenediaminetetra-acetate absorption tests in the detection of coeliac disease. Clin Sci 1988;75:375.

166. Fotherby KJ, Wraight EP, Neale G. ^{51}Cr-EDTA/^{14}C-mannitol intestinal permeability test. Clinical use in screening for coeliac disease. Scand J Gastroenterol 1988;23:171.

167. Corazza GR, Valentini RA, Frisoni M, et al. Gliadin immune reactivity is associated with overt and latent enteropathy in relatives of celiac patients. Gastroenterology 1992;103:1517.

168. Grodzinsky E, Franzen L, Hed J, Strom M. High prevalence of celiac disease in healthy adults revealed by antigliadin antibodies. Ann Allergy 1992;69:66.

169. Maki M, Holm K, Lipsanen V, et al. Serological markers and HLA genes among healthy first-degree relatives of patients with coeliac disease. Lancet 1991;338:1350.

170. Ferguson A, Arranz E, O'Mahony S. Spectrum of expression of intestinal cellular immunity: proposal for a change in diagnostic criteria of celiac disease. Ann Allergy 1993;71:29.

171. Walker-Smith JA, Harrison M, Kilby A, Phillips A, France N. Cows' milk-sensitive enteropathy. Arch Dis Child 1978;53:375.

172. Ament ME, Rubin CE. Soy protein—another cause of the flat intestinal lesion. Gastroenterology 1972;62:227.

173. Cooper BT, Holmes GK, Ferguson R, et al. Gluten-sensitive diarrhea without evidence of celiac disease. Gastroenterology 1980;79:801.

174. Rubin CE, Eidelman S, Weinstein WM. Sprue by any other name. Gastroenterology 1970;58:409.

175. Trier JS, Falchuk ZM, Carey MC, Schreiber DS. Celiac sprue and refractory sprue. Gastroenterology 1978;75:307.

176. Weinstein WM, Saunders DR, Tytgat GN, Rubin CE. Collagenous sprue—an unrecognized type of malabsorption. N Engl J Med 1970;283:1297.

177. Gillberg R, Kastrup W, Mobacken H, et al. Endoscopic duodenal biopsy compared with biopsy with the Watson capsule

from the upper jejunum in patients with dermatitis herpetiformis. Scand J Immunol 1982;17:305.

178. Katz SI, Hall RP, Lawley TJ, Strober W. Dermatitis herpetiformis: the skin and the gut. Ann Intern Med 1980;93:857.

179. Lawley TJ, Strober W, Yaoita H, Katz SI. Small intestinal biopsies and HLA types in dermatitis herpetiformis patients with granular and linear IgA skin deposits. J Invest Dermatol 1980;74:9.

180. Reunala T, Helin H, Kuokkanen K, Hakala T. Lymphoma in dermatitis herpetiformis: report on four cases. Acta Derm Venereol (Stockh) 1982;62:343.

181. Tucker WF, Leonard JN, Fry L. Increased risk of lymphoma in dermatitis herpetiformis. J R Soc Med 1983;76:95.

182. Fronek Z, Cheung MM, Kagnoff MF. Molecular analysis of HLA DP and DQ genes associated with dermatitis herpetiformis. J Invest Dermatol 1991;97:799.

183. Savilahti E, Reunala T, Maki M. Increase of lymphocytes bearing the gamma/delta T cell receptor in the jejunum of patients with dermatitis herpetiformis. Gut 1992;33:206.

184. Unsworth DJ, Leonard JN, McMinn RM, et al. Anti-gliadin antibodies and small intestinal mucosal damage in dermatitis herpetiformis. Br J Dermatol 1981;105:653.

185. Vainio E, Collin P, Lehtonen OP. Avidity of antigliadin IgA and IgG antibodies in gluten-sensitive enteropathy and dermatitis herpetiformis. Clin Immunol Immunopathol 1986;41:295.

186. Reunala T, Chorzelski TP, Viander M. IgA anti-endomysial antibodies in dermatitis herpetiformis: correlation with jejunal morphology, gluten-free diet and anti-gliadin antibodies. Br J Dermatol 1987;117:185.

187. Beutner EH, Chorzelski TP, Kumar V, et al. Sensitivity and specificity of IgA-class antiendomysial antibodies for dermatitis herpetiformis and findings relevant to their pathogenic significance. J Am Acad Dermatol 1986;15:464.

188. Frodin T, Gotthard R, Hed J, et al. Gluten-free diet for dermatitis herpetiformis: the long-term effect on cutaneous, immunological and jejunal manifestations. Acta Derm Venereol (Stockh) 1981;61:405.

189. Fry L, Leonard JN, Swain AF, et al. Long-term follow-up of dermatitis herpetiformis with and without dietary gluten withdrawal. Br J Dermatol 1982;107:631.

190. Reunala T, Blomqvist K, Tarpila S, et al. Gluten-free diet in dermatitis herpetiformis. I. Clinical response of skin lesions in 81 patients. Br J Dermatol 1977;97:473.

191. Leonard JN, Haffenden G, Tucker W, et al. Gluten challenge in dermatitis herpetiformis. N Engl J Med 1983;308:816.

192. Maki M, Hallstrom O, Huupoonen T, et al. Increased prevalence of coeliac disease in diabetes. Arch Dis Child 1984;59:739.

193. Cacciari E, Salardi S, Volta U, et al. Prevalence and characteristics of coeliac disease in type 1 diabetes mellitus. Acta Paediatr Scand 1987;76:671.

194. Savilahti E, Simell O, Koskimies S, et al. Coeliac disease in insulin-dependent diabetes mellitus. J Pediatr 1986;108:690.

195. Collin P, Salmi J, Hallstrom O, et al. High frequency of coeliac disease in adult patients with type-I diabetes. Scand J Gastroenterol 1989;24:81.

196. Mulder CJJ, Tytgat GN, Groenland F, Pena AS. Combined coeliac disease and thyroid disease, a study of 17 cases. J Clin Nutr Gastroenterol 1988;3:89.

197. Svejgaard A, Ryder LP. HLA genotype distribution and genetic models of insulin-dependent diabetes mellitus. Ann Hum Genet 1981;45:293.

198. Mawhinney H, Tomkin GH. Gluten enteropathy associated with selective IgA deficiency. Lancet 1971;2:121.

199. Hammarstrom L, Smith CI. HLA-A, B, C and DR antigens in immunoglobulin A deficiency. Tissue Antigens 1983;21:75.

200. Wilton AN, Cobain TJ, Dawkins RL. Family studies of IgA deficiency. Immunogenetics 1985;21:333.

201. Volanakis JE, Zhu ZB, Schaffer FM, et al. Major histocompatibility complex class III genes and susceptibility to immunoglobulin A deficiency and common variable immunodeficiency. J Clin Invest 1992;89:1914.

202. Robinson PJ, Bullen AW, Hall R, et al. Splenic size and function in adult coeliac disease. Br J Radiol 1980;53:532.

203. O'Donoghue DJ. Fatal pneumococcal septicaemia in coeliac disease. Postgrad Med J 1986;62:229.

204. Matuchansky C, Colin R, Hemet J, et al. Cavitation of mesenteric lymph nodes, splenic atrophy, and a flat small intestinal mucosa. Gastroenterology 1984;87:606.

205. Freeman HJ, Chiu BK. Small bowel malignant lymphoma complicating celiac sprue and the mesenteric lymph node cavitation syndrome. Gastroenterology 1986;90:2008.

206. Rustgi AK, Peppercorn MA. Gluten-sensitive enteropathy and systemic lupus erythematosus. Arch Intern Med 1988;148:1583.

207. Pittman FE, Holub DA. Sjogren's syndrome and adult celiac disease. Gastroenterology 1965;48:869.

208. Doe WF, Evans D, Hobbs JR, Booth CC. Coeliac disease, vasculitis and cryoglobulinaemia. Gut 1972;13:112.

209. Meyers S, Dikman S, Spiera H, et al. Cutaneous vasculitis complicating coeliac disease. Gut 1981;22:61.

210. Simila S, Kokkonen J, Kallioinen M. Cutaneous vasculitis as a manifestation of coeliac disease. Acta Paediatr Scand 1982;71:1051.

211. Turton CW, Turner-Warwick M, Owens R, et al. Red cell folate levels, food antibodies and reticulin antibodies in Farmers lung—is there an association with coeliac disease? Br J Dis Chest 1983;77:397.

212. Edwards C, Williams A, Asquith P. Bronchopulmonary disease in coeliac patients. J Clin Pathol 1985;38:361.

213. Reading R, Watson JG, Platt JW, Bird AG. Pulmonary haemosiderosis and gluten. Arch Dis Child 1987;62:513.

214. Pacheco A, Casanova C, Fogue L, Sueiro A. Long-term clinical follow-up of adult idiopathic pulmonary hemosiderosis and celiac disease. Chest 1991;99:1525.

215. Laine LA, Holt KM. Recurrent pericarditis and celiac disease. JAMA 1984;252:3168.

216. Curtis WD, Schuman BM, Griffin JW Jr. Association of gluten-sensitive enteropathy and Crohn's colitis. Am J Gastroenterol 1992;87:1634.

217. Kitis G, Holmes GKT, Cooper BT, et al. Association of coeliac disease and inflammatory bowel disease. Gut 1980;21:636.

218. Breen EG, Coghlan G, Connoly EC, Increased association of ulcerative colitis and coeliac disease. Ir J Med Sci 1987;156:120.

219. Shah A, Mayberry JF, Williams G, et al. Epidemiological survey of coeliac disease and inflammatory bowel disease in first-degree relatives of coeliac patients. Q J Med 1990;74:283.

220. Henriksson KG, Hallert C, Norrby K, Walan A. Polymyositis and adult coeliac disease. Acta Neurol Scand 1982;65:301.

221. Kinney HC, Burger PC, Hurwitz BJ, et al. Degeneration of the central nervous system associated with celiac disease. J Neurol Sci 1982;53:9.

222. Kristoferitsch W, Pointner H. Progressive cerebellar syndrome in adult coeliac disease. J Neurol 1987;234:116.

223. Kaplan JG, Pack D, Horoupian D, et al. Distal axonopathy associated with chronic gluten enteropathy: a treatable disorder. Neurology 1988;38:642.

224. Saari KM, Keyrilinen O. Immunological disorders of the eye complicating coeliac disease. Lancet 1984;1:968.

225. Fornasieri A, Sinico RA, Maldifassi P, et al. IgA-antigliadin antibodies in IgA mesangial nephropathy (Berger's disease). Br Med J 1987;295:78.

226. Hay JE, Wiesner RH, Shorter RG, et al. Primary sclerosing cholangitis and celiac disease. A novel association. Ann Intern Med 1988;109:713.

227. Behr W, Barnert J. Adult celiac disease and primary biliary cirrhosis. Am J Gastroenterol 1986;81:796.

228. Ginn P, Workman RD. Primary biliary cirrhosis and adult celiac disease. West J Med 1992;156:547.

229. Selby WS, Gallagher ND. Malignancy in a 19-year experience of adult celiac disease. Dig Dis Sci 1979;24:684.

230. Holmes GK, Prior P, Lane MR, et al. Malignancy in coeliac disease—effect of a gluten free diet. Gut 1989;30:333.

231. Cooper BT, Holmes GK, Cooke WT. Lymphoma risk in coeliac disease of later life. Digestion 1982;23:89.

232. Isaacson PG, O'Connor NT, Spencer J, et al. Malignant his-

tiocytosis of the intestine: a T-cell lymphoma. Lancet 1985;1:688.

233. Salter DM, Krajewski AS, Dewar AE. Immunophenotype analysis of malignant histiocytosis of the intestine. J Clin Pathol 1986;39:8.

234. Loughran TP Jr, Kadin ME, Deeg HJ. T-cell intestinal lymphoma associated with celiac sprue. Ann Intern Med 1986;104:44.

235. Swinson CM, Slavin G, Coles EC, Booth CC. Coeliac disease and malignancy. Lancet 1983;1:111.

236. Freeman HJ, Chiu BK. Multifocal small bowel lymphoma and latent celiac sprue. Gastroenterology 1986;90:1992.

237. Seliger G, Goodman AB, Firoozhia H, Lawrence LR. Ulceration of the small intestine complicating celiac disease. Am J Dig Dis 1973;18:820.

238. Baer AN, Bayless TM, Yardley JH. Intestinal ulceration and malabsorption syndromes. Gastroenterology 1980;79:754.

239. Mills PR, Brown IL, Watkinson G. Idiopathic chronic ulcerative enteritis. Report of five cases and review of the literature. Q J Med 1980;49:133.

240. Strober W, Falchuk ZM, Rogentine GN, et al. The pathogenesis of gluten-sensitive enteropathy. Ann Intern Med 1975;83:242.

241. Wall AJ, Douglas AP, Booth CC, Pearse AG. Response of the jejunal mucosa in adult coeliac disease to oral prednisolone. Gut 1970;11:7.

242. Sinclair TS, Kumar PJ, Dawson AM. Azathioprine responsive villous atrophy. Gut 1983;24:A494.

243. Bernstein EF, Whitington PF. Successful treatment of atypical sprue in an infant with cyclosporine. Gastroenterology 1988;95:199.

243a. Longstreth GF. Successful treatment of refractory sprue with cyclosporine. Ann Intern Med 1993;119:1014.

244. Bossart R, Henry K, Booth CC, Doe WF. Subepithelial collagen in intestinal malabsorption. Gut 1975;16:18.

245. Hamilton I, Sanders S, Hopwood D, Bouchier IA. Collagenous colitis associated with small intestinal villous atrophy. Gut 1986;27:1394.

246. Breen EG, Farren C, Connolly CE, McCarthy CF. Collagenous colitis and celiac disease. Gut 1987;28:364.

247. Eckstein RP, Dowsett JF, Riley JW. Collagenous enterocolitis: a case of collagenous colitis with involvement of the small intestine. Am J Gastroenterol 1988;83:767.

248. O'Mahony S, Nawroz IM, Ferguson A. Coeliac disease and collagenous colitis. Postgrad Med J 1990;66:238.

249. Perisic VN, Kokai G, Pavlovic M. Coeliac disease and collagenous colitis. Ital J Gastroenterol 1992;24:418.

250. Cooke WT, Smith WT. Neurological disorders associated with adult coeliac disease. Brain 1966;89:683.

251. Campbell JA. Foods for patients with celiac disease. Can Med Assn J 1982;127:963.

252. Ellis HJ, Freedman AR, Ciclitira PJ. Detection and estimation of the barley prolamin content of beer and malt to assess their suitability for patients with coeliac disease. Clin Chim Acta 1990;189:123.

253. Bell L, Hoffer M, Hamilton JR. Recommendations for foods of questionable acceptance for patients with celiac disease. J Can Diet Assoc 1981;42:143.

254. MacDonald WC, Brandborg LL, Flick AL, et al. Studies of celiac sprue. IV. The response of the whole length of the small bowel to a gluten-free diet. Gastroenterology 1964;47:573.

255. Benson GD, Kowlessar OD, Sleisenger MH. Adult celiac disease with emphasis upon response to the gluten-free diet. Medicine (Baltimore) 1964;43:1.

256. Montgomery AM, Goka AK, Kumar PJ, et al. Low gluten diet in the treatment of adult coeliac disease: effect on jejunal morphology and serum anti-gluten antibodies. Gut 1988;29:1564.

257. Mortimer PE, Stewart JS, Norman AP, Booth CC. Follow-up study of coeliac disease. Br Med J 1968;3:7.

258. McCrae WM, Eastwood MA, Martin MR, Sircus W. Neglected coeliac disease. Lancet 1975;1:187.

259. Sheldon W. Prognosis in early adult life of coeliac children treated with a gluten-free diet. Br Med J 1969;2:401.

Textbook of Gastroenterology, second edition, edited by Tadataka Yamada. JB Lippincott Company, Philadelphia © 1995.

CHAPTER 73

Disorders of Epithelial Transport in the Small Intestine

Mark L. Lloyd   Ward A. Olsen

Disorders of Carbohydrate Absorption
  Pathophysiology of Carbohydrate Malabsorption
  Lactase Deficiency
  Sucrase–Isomaltase Deficiency
  Trehalase Deficiency
  Glucose–Galactose Malabsorption
  Intolerance to Other Dietary Carbohydrates
Disorders of Protein and Amino Acid Absorption
  Enterokinase Deficiency

  Disorders of Amino Acid Transport
Disorders of Fat Absorption
  General Remarks
  Abetalipoproteinemia
Miscellaneous Defects
  Genetic Disorders of Electrolyte and Mineral Transport
  Microvillous Inclusion Disease
  Disorders of Vitamin B$_{12}$ Absorption
  Primary Bile Salt Malabsorption

The intestinal mucosa is an active tissue with respect to protein synthesis. A considerable portion of that synthetic activity is directed toward the production of proteins that provide for the digestion and uptake of dietary nutrients. Disorders in the synthesis and processing of these mucosal proteins often are associated with maldigestion or malabsorption of specific components of the diet. The clinical sequelae of such disorders include conditions ranging from life threatening to insignificant. This chapter focuses on specific mucosal protein deficiency states that result in impaired epithelial transport.

DISORDERS OF CARBOHYDRATE ABSORPTION

Pathophysiology of Carbohydrate Malabsorption

Starch, sucrose, and lactose are the major forms of dietary carbohydrate. Their assimilation requires the hydrolysis of each to its component monosaccharides and subsequent uptake of the individual hexoses at the mucosal surface of the small intestine. When there is a defect in this mechanism, independent of the cause, the resulting presence of unabsorbed sugars within the intestinal lumen has predictable consequences. Intralumenal unabsorbed carbohydrate draws fluid into the small intestine by virtue of its osmotic effect, and the amount of fluid entering the gut is substantially greater than that expected on the basis of osmolarity of the sugar alone. Equilibrium is reached only after an influx of additional fluid and electrolytes, with the sugar accounting for only one third of the total solute load.[1] The extra intralumenal fluid is the result of the inability of the intestine to maintain a high electrochemical gradient for sodium between intralumenal contents and blood. This excess fluid contributes to the symptoms of distention and borborygmi experienced on consumption of unabsorbable carbohydrate. On delivery to the colon, the unabsorbed sugar becomes a substrate for bacterial fermentation and, in the case of disaccharides or oligosaccharides, cleavage to individual monosaccharides. Because the colon, unlike the small bowel, cannot absorb monosaccharides, the osmotic load is further increased. Fortunately, however, further fermentation is possible with the conversion of carbohydrate to short-chain fatty acids (acetate, propionate, and butyrate) that are readily absorbed by the colon.[2] Additional byproducts of fermentation include carbon dioxide and

hydrogen and, in some subjects, methane (Fig. 73-1). Because the fatty acids are rapidly absorbed in the colon, a substantial portion of the caloric value of the carbohydrate is salvaged and the osmotic effect of carbohydrate malabsorption may be reduced or eliminated.[3,4] There is considerable individual variability in the efficiency of this process, and with the delivery of a sufficient amount of unabsorbed carbohydrate to the colon, the salvage mechanism is overwhelmed. The result is an osmotic diarrhea often accompanied by distention, bloating, and flatulence related to the gaseous fermentation products.

Lactase Deficiency

Deficiency of intestinal lactase is the most common mucosal enzyme deficiency state; in fact, adult-type hypolactasia represents the most frequent genetic deficiency syndrome in humans, affecting over half of the world's population. The causes of lactase deficiency fall into three categories: congenital, primary with delayed onset, and secondary (Table 73-1). The association of low levels of intestinal lactase with malabsorption of dietary lactose was first reported by Holzel and colleagues in two patients with intolerance to the disaccharide since birth (congenital lactase deficiency).[5] This rare autosomal recessive condition typically presents as severe, watery diarrhea in the newborn period and absence of measurable specific enzyme activity in the intestinal mucosa. The condition is distinguished from congenital glucose–galactose malabsorption in that it responds to the introduction of a glucose-based formula diet and lactose restriction.

The much more common disorder with the delayed loss of lactase activity to levels 5% to 10% of those at birth in otherwise normal intestine was subsequently described independently by Auricchio and associates and Dahlqvist and colleagues.[6,7] This condition appears to parallel the situation in all other land mammals in which there is a physiologic decline in lactase activity coincident with weaning. Indeed, an examination of population groups worldwide supports the contention that delayed lactase deficiency represents the norm—affecting more than 90% of the members of many population groups (Table 73-2).[8] It has been suggested that retained lactase activity and the capacity therefore to use milk in the diet developed as a genetically selected mutation that provided a survival advantage in populations that domesticated dairy animals.[8] Thus, although adult lactase deficiency might be viewed as an autosomal recessive trait, it may be

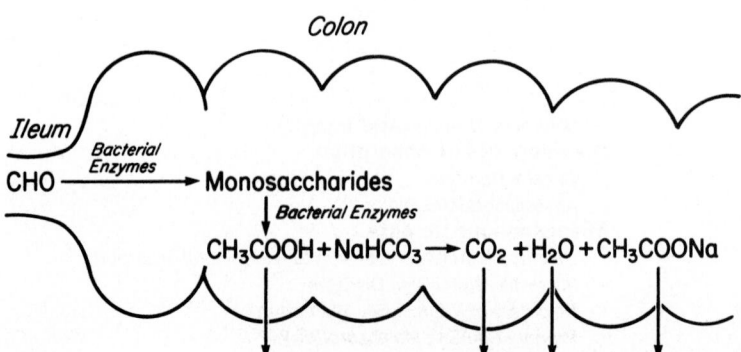

FIGURE 73-1. Colonic salvage of unabsorbed carbohydrate. Colonic bacteria hydrolyze unabsorbed carbohydrates to monosaccharides, which then undergo further fermentation with the generation of hydrogen, carbon dioxide, and short-chain fatty acids. Acetate production is depicted, although propionate and butyrate also are formed. The organic acids are rapidly absorbed, and the osmotic load to the colon is reduced. Colonic salvage thereby lessens the diarrhea associated with carbohydrate malabsorption.

TABLE 73-1
Lactase Deficiency

TYPE	PATHOGENESIS
Congenital	Enzyme activity absent from birth
Primary—delayed onset	Genetically predetermined reduction of enzyme activity during childhood or adolescence
Secondary	Reduced enzyme activity in response to diffuse intestinal insult— giardiasis, rotavirus, tropical sprue, celiac disease, bacterial overgrowth, Crohn's disease, intestinal resection

TABLE 73-2
Ethnic Distribution of Lactase Deficiency

POPULATION	PREVALENCE OF LACTASE DEFICIENCY (%)
Northern European	5–15
Mediterranean	60–85
African Black	85–100
American Black	45–80
American Caucasian	10–25
Native American	50–95
Mexican American	40–75
Asian	90–100

Data from Simoons FJ. The geographical hypothesis and lactose malabsorption: a weighing of the evidence. Am J Dig Dis 1978;23:963.

more appropriate to consider the converse—that the persistence of high levels of lactase activity in adulthood represents a mutation with an autosomal dominant pattern of inheritance.[9]

Enzyme activity in delayed-onset lactase deficiency (adult lactase deficiency) generally declines in early childhood but may persist into adolescence. Most human studies have demonstrated that lactase activity cannot be maintained or induced by continued feeding of lactose.[10,11] The mechanism by which this genetically predetermined loss occurs is not well understood. Although lactase-deficient and lactase-persistent subjects appear to have an identical lactase gene and identical upstream regulatory sequences,[12,13] lactase expression in most deficient subjects appears to be reduced coordinate with the level of mRNA abundance (at least in the proximal intestine).[13,14] This is accompanied by diminished biosynthesis of the protein,[13,15,16] and results in characteristic diminished and patchy immunostaining for lactase over the brush border surface of the intestine.[17,18] Several adult deficient subjects have been described, however, in whom altered processing of the precursor protein appears to be partially or solely responsible for reduced lactase activity.[15,16] The relative ethnic distribution of these mechanistic variations is unknown. Furthermore, it is not clear that the regulatory mechanism dictating lactase expression is invariable over the longitudinal axis of the gut. In adult lactase-deficient subjects from whom jejunal tissue was sampled at surgery rather than by endoscopic biopsy, there was a poor correlation between transcript abundance and lactase activity.[19]

Lactose intolerance also may occur in the setting of insults to the intestine that result in insufficient absorptive surface area, insufficient contact time between the mucosa and disaccharide, or reduced mucosal levels of the enzyme. The latter often are associated with histologic changes on biopsy and diminished levels of other mucosal hydrolases. Although the digestion of other oligosaccharides also may be reduced in the setting of diffuse intestinal diseases, the hydrolysis of lactose is particularly affected, and recovery of normal lactase activity often is prolonged after adequate treatment of the underlying condition. In regions of the world where intestinal infections are common, lactase deficiency may be the result of both primary and secondary causes.

The development of milk intolerance after a gastrointes-

tinal infection, however, does not necessarily imply lactase deficiency. In particular, the intolerance to cow's milk that follows rotavirus infections in infants may be linked to sensitization to a protein component of cow's milk rather than lactase deficiency.[20] Breast milk and lactose-containing formulas that are less antigenic than cow's milk are frequently well tolerated in this setting (see Chap. 110 for discussion of food allergy).

Lactose intolerance is the symptomatic response to lactose malabsorption and includes distention, bloating, abdominal pain, flatulence, and diarrhea. There is great individual variability in the perception of symptoms. Lactase-deficient subjects generally show symptoms with the ingestion of 12 to 18 g of lactose (the equivalent of 1 to 1½ glasses of milk), although the threshold may be less in patients with underlying functional bowel disease.[21,22] The awareness of the association between milk ingestion and symptoms also is highly variable.[23] The diagnosis of lactose intolerance should be considered in all patients with chronic gastrointestinal complaints compatible with lactose intolerance in the setting of some degree of lactose ingestion. Although the diagnostic yield is greatest in population groups with a high prevalence of lactase deficiency, even low-prevalence populations selected for these symptoms may have a substantial number of malabsorbers.[24]

In infants with diarrhea and in whom milk is the primary dietary staple, the diagnosis of lactase deficiency is suggested by the finding of an acidic pH and the presence of reducing substances on stool testing. These findings are not reliable in the first 2 months of life or with the mixed diet of older children and adults. Intestinal mucosal biopsy with disaccharidase assay represents the standard by which other methods of detection are judged, but it is seldom necessary to subject the patient to biopsy unless tissue is required to exclude other disorders. Indeed, in practice it is frequently unnecessary to perform any formal testing to make the diagnosis of lactase deficiency. In a patient from a high-prevalence population with a history of compatible symptoms and significant consumption of milk products, an empiric trial of dietary withdrawal is reasonable.

The lactose tolerance test is a method that has been commonly used to secure the diagnosis of lactase deficiency. After a 50-g oral dose of lactose, blood glucose levels are determined at serial time points over 2 hours. Adequate hydrolysis of the disaccharide and subsequent absorption of the component sugars are reflected by a greater than 20 mg/dL rise in blood glucose and the lack of symptoms (Table 73-3). A response of this magnitude, however, may occur in the person with diabetes despite lactase deficiency, as a result of impaired regulation of glucose metabolism. Altered gastric emptying also may influence the results and lead to spurious interpretations of oral tolerance testing, because the normal blood glucose response may be relatively higher with rapid emptying and lower in the patient with delayed emptying. A variation of the oral tolerance test can be performed with the quantitative determination of galactose measured in blood or urine. This may give more reliable results, but requires the administration of a small amount of ethanol with the lactose to inhibit the rapid hepatic metabolism of absorbed galactose. Because symptoms may accompany oral tolerance testing despite an apparently normal blood glucose response, it may be best simply to withhold dietary lactose as the diagnostic study in all but confusing cases. If symptoms are not improved, the demonstration of a low blood glucose response to an oral challenge will be of no help.

Breath hydrogen testing is an alternative, noninvasive method for diagnosing lactose malabsorption, one that uses a gas chromatograph to detect hydrogen liberated during the colonic fermentation of the unabsorbed carbohydrate.[25] Detection of a rise in breath hydrogen of greater than 20 ppm after the administration of oral lactose is considered diagnostic, and the magnitude of the rise correlates with the degree of malabsorption in a semiquantitative fashion.[1] False-negative examination results may occur in a minority of subjects who have colonic flora that do not produce appreciable amounts of hydrogen during fermentation.

Dietary manipulation represents the cornerstone of management of the lactose-intolerant patient. Because most lactase-deficient subjects are tolerant of the sugar up to some threshold level, it is sometimes possible simply to reduce the amount of exposure at a given time, such as consuming two glasses of milk over the course of a day rather than all at breakfast. Milk products are a valuable source of calcium, and absolute restriction is not recommended unless necessary. The prescribed diet is thus a low-lactose not a "no-lactose" diet. Milk in which 70% of the lactose has been prehydrolyzed is readily available in many food stores, and active enzyme preparations have been marketed that can be added to refrigerated milk at home to convert most of the lactose to glucose and galactose. Such milk tastes rather sweet and is not tolerated in large amounts. Substitute milks also are available (made from corn syrup) that contain no lactose, but are more difficult for patients with diabetes to tolerate. Lactase enzyme is also available in capsule and tablet form. Two to four tablets or capsules consumed with lactose-containing products provide sufficient amounts of enzyme to avoid symptoms of lactose intolerance. Yogurt is a unique source of lactose in that concentrations of the disaccharide are similar to those found in whole milk, yet yogurt is well tolerated by lactase-deficient subjects. This has been attributed to the intraintestinal digestion of lactose by lactase released from bacteria that participate in the yogurt fermentation process.[26]

Sucrase–Isomaltase Deficiency

Congenital sucrase–isomaltase deficiency is considered to be an autosomal recessive disorder characterized by undetectable levels of intestinal sucrase activity and reduced isomaltase activity in otherwise normal intestine. Although relatively rare in the United States and Western Europe, the incidence of this condition is 5% to 10% among native Greenlanders.[27] Typically, patients present with chronic diarrhea and failure to thrive during infancy, although frequently the diagnosis is not made until early childhood.

Of all the congenital disorders of carbohydrate absorption, the biochemical defects of sucrase–isomaltase deficiency have been best characterized. Sucrase–isomaltase is encoded by a gene on chromosome 3,[28] and under normal conditions its intestinal expression is regulated at the level of mRNA abundance.[29] As an integral brush border membrane glycoprotein, however, the precursor from which mature sucrase–isomaltase arises must undergo extensive posttranslational processing (see Chap. 17).[30] In studying one deficient person, Lloyd and Olsen demonstrated translation and early glycosylation of an immature precursor protein that failed to undergo completion of glycosylation.[31] Eight additional cases were studied by Naim and colleagues using a combination of metabolic labeling studies and immunoelectron microscopy.[32] The molecular nature of the deficiency states was characterized by three phenotypes: one in which the sucrase–isomaltase precursor accumulated in the endoplasmic reticulum after failing to undergo initial trimming reactions, another in which the precursor accumulated in the Golgi apparatus, and a third in which a catalytically altered sucrase–isomaltase was transported to the brush border membrane. Fransen and colleagues subsequently described two more affected subjects phenotypically unique with respect to their molecular disorder.[33] In one person, precursor sucrase–isomaltase accumulated in the endoplasmic reticulum but also was missorted to the basolateral membrane, and in the other, intracellular precursor was prematurely cleaved and only the isomaltase subunit was directed to the brush border membrane. The variable nature of the defects in these cases suggests that in each case studied,

---

TABLE 73-3
Interpretation of Lactose Tolerance Test Results

Plasma Glucose Response > 20 mg/dL and No Symptoms
Normal response with normal lactase levels

Plasma Glucose Response < 20 mg/dL and Symptoms
Lactase deficient and lactose intolerant

Plasma Glucose Response > 20 mg/dL and Symptoms
Consider lactase deficiency with diabetes mellitus
Consider rapid intestinal transit with lactose malabsorption despite normal lactase levels (e.g., postgastrectomy, irritable bowel syndrome)

Plasma Glucose Response < 20 mg/dL and No Symptoms
Consider delayed gastric emptying
Consider lactase deficiency without lactose intolerance (colonic compensation)

the deficiency state arose from different allelic mutations of the sucrase–isomaltase gene.

In congenital sucrase–isomaltase deficiency, symptoms develop with the introduction of sucrose into the diet. Therefore, infants fed sucrose-containing formulas will present earlier than breast-fed infants. This condition must be distinguished from congenital lactase deficiency and from glucose–galactose malabsorption. The diagnosis can be made by an oral sucrose tolerance test, by breath hydrogen examination after sucrose challenge, or by intestinal biopsy and measurement of disaccharidase activities. Institution of a sucrose-free diet is associated with cessation of diarrhea and prompt weight gain. Lifelong maintenance of a diet free of sucrose usually is necessary, although one report suggests that symptoms of sucrose intolerance may be attenuated by the ingestion of lyophilized baker's yeast as an exogenous source of the enzyme.[34] Results from a Food and Drug Administration trial using an oral sucrase supplement from this source have been reported.*[34a] Although intestinal isomaltase activity usually is markedly reduced in this disease, dietary starch usually is well tolerated. Although isomaltase plays a pivotal role in the digestion of alpha-limit dextrins, products of intralumenal starch digestion, the limited contribution of these dextrins to the total starch load and the preserved hydrolytic capacity of mucosal maltase–glucoamylase probably account for the lack of starch intolerance in this setting.

Trehalase Deficiency

Selective intolerance to the disaccharide trehalose has been described in only a few cases.[35,36] This probably reflects the fact that this sugar represents an insignificant contribution to the normal diet, because young mushrooms are the only source. Features typical of carbohydrate intolerance (abdominal pain, bloating, and diarrhea) have been provoked by trehalose loading in identified affected people. No detectable trehalase activity was detected in jejunal biopsy material from those subjects. Relative trehalase deficiency may be rather common in Greenland.[37] In this population, more than 8% of adult patients undergoing upper gastrointestinal surgery had mucosal trehalase activities less than the lowest values found in Danish and American control groups.

Glucose–Galactose Malabsorption

Congenital glucose–galactose malabsorption is characterized by a selective defect in the intestinal transport of these two monosaccharides. More than 30 cases have been reported in the literature since this autosomal recessive condition was described. In vivo perfusion studies have demonstrated impaired absorption of glucose and galactose but normal fructose uptake. Results of in vitro mucosal uptake of these sugars and Ussing chamber studies are consistent with defective sodium-coupled glucose–galactose transport.[38] Vesicle studies have confirmed a brush border membrane defect.[39] The molecular basis of this disease was demonstrated with the identification of a single missense mutation in the gene that encodes the sodium–glucose cotransporter.[40,41]

Typically, affected infants present with profuse, watery diarrhea and dehydration in the first week of life. Stool analysis reveals a low pH and the presence of fecal reducing substances. Patients usually show immediate improvement with the institution of a fructose-based formula and withdrawal of glucose and galactose from their diet. Despite the persistence of the defect, the development of tolerance to some dietary glucose has been noted in older children.

Transient glucose malabsorption also has been described in neonates after gastrointestinal surgery and in infants as a sequela to acute gastroenteritis.[42] Rotavirus infection has been identified as the most frequent etiology. Usually, the monosaccharide intolerance resolves rapidly, although protracted illness occasionally may occur.

Intolerance to Other Dietary Carbohydrates

The following conditions are not related to mucosal deficiencies, but similar clinical presentations warrant their discussion here. Fructose is an important dietary carbohydrate found in its free form in fruit and as one of the component monosaccharides of sucrose (Table 73-4). High-fructose corn syrup has become increasingly common as a sweetener in the manufacture of soft drinks. Although early perfusion studies suggested that the intestinal absorption of fructose was quite efficient, it now appears that in some people the absorptive capacity of the intestine may be overwhelmed by doses of this

---

TABLE 73-4
Content of Potentially Malabsorbed Carbohydrate in Food

CARBOHYDRATE	AMOUNT
Lactose	
Milk	12 (g/8 oz)
Yogurt	4.6 (g/100 g)
Cottage cheese	1.4 (g/100 g)
Ice cream	3.6 (g/100 g)
Chocolate	8.1 (g/100 g)
Fructose	
Figs	30 (g/100 g dry weight)
Prunes	15 (g/100 g dry weight)
Grapes	8 (g/100 g dry weight)
Soft drinks	25 (g/12 oz)
Sorbitol	
Pears	4.6 (g/100 g dry weight)
Prunes	2.4 (g/100 g dry weight)
"Sugarless" gum	1.3–2.2 g/piece
"Sugarless" mints	1.7–2.0 g/piece
Stachyose/Raffinose	
Navy beans	4 (g/100 g)

Data from Ravich WJ, Bayless TM, Thomas M. Fructose: incomplete intestinal absorption in humans. Gastroenterology 1983;84:26; Hyams JS. Sorbitol intolerance: an unappreciated cause of functional gastrointestinal complaints. Gastroenterology 1983;84:30; Levitt MD, Hirsh P, Fetzer CA, et al. H₂ excretion after ingestion of complex carbohydrates. Gastroenterology 1987;92:383; and Levitt MD, Savaiano DA. Lactose intolerance and yogurt: diagnosis and treatment. Practical Gastroenterology 1985;9:41.

---

* Treem W, personal communication, May 1993.

suga ountered in normal dietary practices. Andersson and Nygr identified four patients with chronic diarrhea and abdominal pain related to eating fruit and documented reproduction of their symptoms with the oral administration of 100 g of fructose.[43] Using breath hydrogen analysis, Ravich and associates demonstrated incomplete absorption of 50 g of a 10% fructose solution (approximately equivalent to two 12-ounce cans of soda) in 37% of otherwise healthy subjects.[44] Abdominal symptoms of gas, cramping, and diarrhea were recorded in several of these subjects. The threshold for symptoms in the setting of incomplete fructose absorption may be further reduced for those patients with underlying functional bowel disease.[45]

Sorbitol is a polyalcohol sugar found naturally in fruits. Its slow fermentation by oral flora and incomplete absorption by the intestine have led to its widespread use as a sweetener in dietetic foods and "sugar-free" products (approximately 1.5 g per piece of sugarless gum or mint). Osmotic diarrhea has been associated with the consumption of large doses of sorbitol (20–50 g), but symptomatic malabsorption may occur at much smaller doses.[46,47] In one study, ingestion of 5 to 10 g of sorbitol was associated with elevated breath hydrogen and symptoms of gas and bloating in most of the study population.[47]

Although dietary starch traditionally has been thought to be completely absorbed, work by Levitt and colleagues questions this position.[48,49] After ingestion of complex carbohydrate from a variety of foods, breath testing revealed hydrogen production consistent with malabsorption of up to 19% of the ingested carbohydrate in otherwise healthy subjects. Significant malabsorption was documented with wheat, corn, oats, potatoes, and beans, but not rice (Fig. 73-2). The magnitude of hydrogen production exceeded that attributable to fiber or indigestible oligosaccharides such as stachyose and raffinose. Starch from refined and gluten-free flours was more completely absorbed, suggesting that fiber or the protein complexed with starch may interfere with absorption. The reported symptomatic improvement in patients with apparent functional bowel disease after gluten restriction suggests that incomplete starch absorption may have clinical relevance in some populations.

Measures that have been advocated to lessen the symptoms of distention and flatulence associated with unabsorbed carbohydrate, whether from starchy foods or from high-fiber foods, include the use of simethecone and activated charcoal. Although the efficacy of simethicone is doubtful, evidence supporting the utility of charcoal is mixed.[50,51] A preparation of a mold-derived α-galactosidase (Beano) has been marketed as a food additive to be used to hydrolyze oligosaccharides otherwise indigestible within the small intestine, but evidence for its effectiveness is limited.[52]

Finally, carbohydrate malabsorption may represent the desired response in certain clinical settings. Inhibitors of α-amylase (starch blockers) and α-glucosidase have been studied to determine their potential as therapeutic agents in the treatment of diabetes and obesity. The nonabsorbable carbohydrates, lactulose and mannitol, are used for their cathartic effect, but their use is limited by the production of gas and bloating, presumably related to colonic fermentation.

Paradoxically, patients with celiac disease may have enhanced uptake of certain poorly absorbed carbohydrates compared to healthy controls. This observation led to the development of the differential sugar test as a noninvasive screening tool for celiac disease.[53] Affected patients are thought to have enhanced uptake of larger molecules through "leaky" paracellular routes. This probably reflects an increased number of sites for paracellular transport (tight junctions), which are at highest density in the crypt compartment—which in turn is expanded in this condition—as well as functional changes that enhance permeability at those sites as a response to inflammatory cells and cytokines.[54] Uptake of small molecules is reduced because of diminished intestinal surface area. Thus, ratios of absorbed lactulose or cellobiose to absorbed mannitol are elevated compared with ratios in the normal population. Similar findings have been noted in patients with Crohn's disease.[55] Because there is evidence that increased intestinal permeability also may be present in unaffected relatives of patients with Crohn's disease, it has been suggested that this

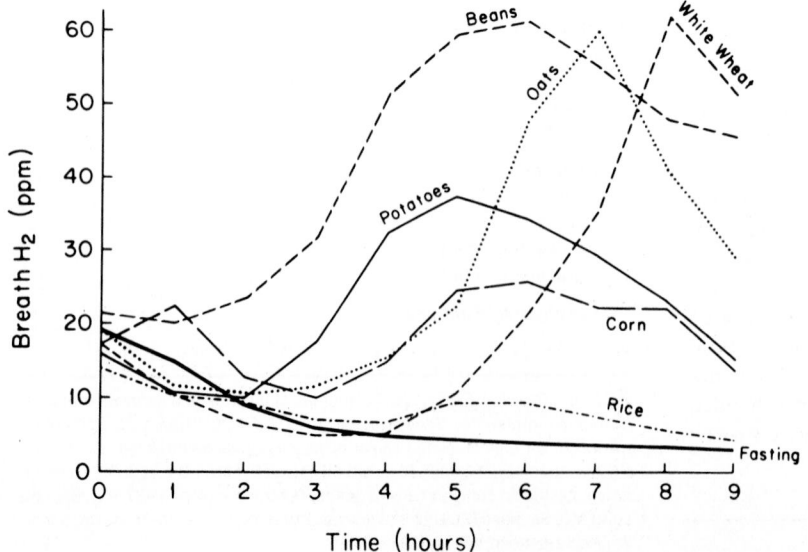

FIGURE 73-2. Breath H_2 concentrations after ingestion of 100 g of carbohydrate in the form of various complex carbohydrates. With the exception of rice, starch was malabsorbed from all sources, with the amount of fermentation ranging from 7% to 20% of the total ingested carbohydrate. (From Levitt MD, Hirsh P, Fetzer CA, et al. H_2 excretion after ingestion of complex carbohydrates. Gastroenterology 1987;92:383.)

defect may be a primary contributor to the etiology of the enteritis rather than a consequence of inflammation.[56] The basis of differential permeability testing and its application to human intestinal disease are discussed in a comprehensive review.[57]

DISORDERS OF PROTEIN AND AMINO ACID ABSORPTION

Enterokinase Deficiency

Congenital enterokinase deficiency is a rare disorder of protein malabsorption. In 1969, Hadorn and colleagues first described the disorder in a child whose duodenal juice showed very low levels of enterokinase and proteolytic activity despite normal levels of lipase and amylase.[58] The addition of exogenous enterokinase resulted in the appearance of normal levels of trypsin, chymotrypsin, and carboxypeptidase. This disorder is attributed to the absence of mucosal enterokinase activity. Enterokinase is a brush border membrane protein that is released from the membrane by the action of bile salts to initiate the conversion of the proenzyme trypsinogen to trypsin. Because trypsin further autoactivates trypsinogen as well as the other pancreatic protease proenzymes, the consequences are analogous to severe pancreatic insufficiency with respect to protein digestion. Those affected present in infancy with diarrhea, growth retardation, and hypoproteinemia with edema. Steatorrhea may be present, because secondary mucosal changes and pancreatic insufficiency may accompany the hypoproteinemia.[59] Diagnostic considerations include cystic fibrosis and Shwachman's syndrome. Diagnosis is confirmed by failure to detect enterokinase activity on assaying a mucosal biopsy or by the demonstration of in vitro activation of proteolytic activity in duodenal fluid by added enterokinase. Symptomatic improvement and satisfactory growth can be maintained with oral pancreatic enzyme supplementation.

Disorders of Amino Acid Transport

Clinically significant protein deficiencies usually do not occur as a consequence of primary defects of enterocyte amino acid transport (Table 73-5). The capacity of the intestine to absorb amino acids in the form of dipeptides and tripeptides provides insurance against the development of nutritional insufficiency, even though the intestinal transport of several essential amino acids may be defective. Although the greatest clinical impact of these diseases may be on organ systems other than the gut (e.g., the genitourinary tract and nervous system), the study of affected people has resulted in important observations concerning the mechanisms of intestinal amino acid and peptide uptake.

Hartnup's disease and cystinuria are both autosomal recessive disorders characterized by transport defects for free amino acids in the mucosa of the small intestine and proximal renal tubule.[60,61] In Hartnup's disease, neutral amino acids are affected, whereas in the latter the transport of cystine and the dibasic amino acids are impaired. In these diseases the absorption of affected amino acids has been shown to be normal, when they are presented in the form of dipeptides; therefore, malnutrition is not observed.

TABLE 73-5
Disorders of Intestinal Amino Acid Transport

DISORDER	SUBSTRATES	CLINICAL ASSOCIATIONS
Hartnup's disease	Neutral amino acids	Pellagra-like rash Neuropsychiatric symptoms
Cystinuria	Dibasic amino acids Cystine	Renal calculi Chronic pancreatitis
Lysinuric protein intolerance	Dibasic amino acids	Failure to thrive Growth retardation Hepatosplenomegaly Hyperammonemia
Blue diaper syndrome	Tryptophan	Bluish-discolored diapers Hypercalcemia Nephrocalcinosis
Oasthouse urine disease	Methionine	Mental retardation Seizures
Lowe's syndrome	Lysine Arginine	Mental retardation Cataracts Renal failure
Joseph's syndrome (iminoglycinuria)	Glycine Proline Hydroxyproline	Aminoaciduria

Data from Freeman HJ, Sleisinger MH, Kim YS. Human protein digestion and absorption: normal mechanisms and protein-energy malnutrition. Clin Gastroenterol 1983;12:357; and Silk DBA. Disorders of nitrogen absorption. Clin Gastroenterol 1982;11:47.

The neuropsychiatric symptoms of Hartnup's disease may be related to the gut's absorption of indoles and toxic amines derived from the decarboxylation of free tryptophan by intestinal bacteria. These same metabolites also may be potent inhibitors of the conversion of tryptophan to nicotinamide in the body. This could explain the pellagra-like rash that occurs in this condition, despite adequate uptake of tryptophan from dipeptides.

In cystinuria, nephrolithiasis is the most common presenting complaint, owing to the relative insolubility of cystine in urine. Lysinuric protein intolerance also is characterized by impaired intestinal transport of dibasic amino acids, but unlike the case in cystinuria, patients are affected with failure to thrive and severe growth retardation. The reason for this difference is that the transport defect in this disorder is located at the basolateral membrane of the enterocyte. Therefore, affected amino acids are not absorbed across the enterocyte, despite intact dipeptide transport at the brush border membrane.[62,63]

DISORDERS OF FAT ABSORPTION
General Remarks

The efficient digestion and assimilation of dietary fat depend on the integrated participation of several organ systems (see Chap. 18). In this schema, the enterocyte has a pivotal function in that it provides for the uptake and intracellular transport of solubilized fatty acids and monoglycerides, the resynthesis of the absorbed lipids into triglycerides, and finally the packaging of lipid into chylomicron particles, which are discharged into the extracellular space for lymphatic uptake and subsequent tissue distribution. Important steps in this process are the synthesis and processing of the specific apolipoproteins that will become components of the chylomicrons. In particular, apolipoprotein B appears to play a critical role, because defective synthesis of this apoprotein results in the inability to construct chylomicrons and the failure to transport dietary triglyceride from the intestinal mucosa to the plasma. Organ-specific forms of apolipoprotein B have been identified in intestine (B48) and liver (B100).[64]

Abetalipoproteinemia

Abetalipoproteinemia is a rare autosomal recessive disease presenting with fat malabsorption and abnormal red blood cell morphology (acanthocytosis) at birth. In affected people, plasma apolipoprotein B-containing lipoproteins (both B100 and B48) are absent, and concentrations of plasma cholesterol and triglycerides are very low. Fasting intestinal biopsy shows the mucosa to be engorged with lipid droplets. These findings reflect the intestine's ability to absorb monoglycerides and free fatty acids but failure to synthesize and secrete triglyceride-rich chylomicrons. Originally, it was believed that either defective synthesis or aberrant posttranslational processing of apolipoprotein B represented the molecular defect in this disorder.[65,66] Using restriction length polymorphisms, however, Talmud and colleagues demonstrated the absence of linkage between abetalipoproteinemia and the apolipoprotein B gene.[67] They suggested that this condition arose from a defect in another gene responsible for the assembly or secretion of apolipoprotein B-containing lipoproteins from intestine and liver, a contention supported by the observation that apolipoprotein B mRNA undergoes normal editing and may be present in increased abundance in this condition.[68–70] Wetterau and colleagues identified that abnormal microsomal triglyceride transfer protein, a carrier responsible for the transport of triglycerides, cholesteryl ester, and phosphotidyl choline in intestine and liver, is the likely molecular defect in abetalipoproteinemia.[71]

Clinical variants of abetalipoproteinemia include chylomicron retention disease, or Anderson's disease, and normotriglyceridemic abetalipoproteinemia, conditions in which only apolipoprotein B48 or B100, respectively, are absent from the plasma.[72,73] Unlike classic abetalipoproteinemia, acanthocytosis is absent and fasting triglyceride concentrations are normal. Also included in the differential diagnosis of abetalipoproteinemia is the autosomal codominant disorder, familial hypobetalipoproteinemia. Although the homozygous form of hypobetalipoproteinemia is biochemically indistinguishable from abetalipoproteinemia, the molecular defects accounting for this condition are distinctly different.[74] Mutations of the apolipoprotein B gene have been identified in several kindreds.[75,76] The clinical manifestations of the disease are sometimes milder than those of abetalipoproteinemia and may occur at a later age. The diagnosis is facilitated by the identification of first-degree relatives who are heterozygotes. They usually are asymptomatic, and have plasma apo-

lipoprotein B and low-density lipoprotein cholesterol levels that are approximately half of normal.

Long-term sequelae of abetalipoproteinemia are a result of malabsorption of fat-soluble vitamins (particularly vitamin E), and include the eventual development of retinopathy and spinocerebellar degeneration. These complications can be avoided by supplementation with large oral doses of vitamin E (100 mg/kg/day). Management also includes fat restriction and supplementation with vitamins A and K.

MISCELLANEOUS DEFECTS

Genetic Disorders of Electrolyte and Mineral Transport

Infants with congenital diarrhea characterized by high fecal chloride concentrations were first reported independently by Darrow[77] and Gamble and associates[78] in 1945. Over 100 cases of congenital chloridorrhea have now been recognized. This autosomal recessive disease is the result of defective active Cl^-/HCO_3^- exchange in the distal ileum and colon. Although the primary defect leads to the loss of chloride and acidification of intestinal contents, secondary impairment of sodium absorption also occurs. The clinical consequence of these effects is lifelong watery diarrhea that is present from birth. If untreated, the disease rapidly results in hyponatremia, hypochloremia, and dehydration. Metabolic alkalosis and hypokalemia may develop later in response to protracted loss of acid in the stool and volume contraction. The diagnosis of congenital chloridorrhea is confirmed by the documentation of high fecal chloride concentrations. In affected newborns, fecal chloride concentrations are above 100 mmol/L (more than twice the typical chloride concentration in diarrheal stool from neonates), and by 3 months of age, fecal chloride concentrations characteristically exceed the sum of fecal sodium and potassium concentrations (NH_4^+ accounts for the missing cations).[79] Treatments directed at correction of the diarrhea accompanying this disorder have been uniformly unsuccessful, and therefore replacement of fluid and electrolyte losses is the therapeutic goal. Normal growth and development is expected with the adequate oral administration of a combination of NaCl and KCl solutions despite persistent diarrhea.

Isolated cases of congenital diarrhea characterized by defective sodium absorption have been reported.[80,81] Unlike the case in congenital chloridorrhea, these patients have mild metabolic acidosis and persistent watery diarrhea characterized by sodium losses in excess of chloride and elevated fecal bicarbonate. Results of jejunal perfusion and vesicle studies in one affected person suggested defective brush border membrane Na^+/H^+ exchange. Fluid and electrolyte replacement with sodium citrate provide for normal growth and development.

Familial hypomagnesemia is a condition characterized by the onset of tetany and seizures in the first month of life in association with low serum levels of magnesium and calcium. The primary defect appears to be impaired intestinal absorption of magnesium.[82] Normal growth and development can be expected with the initiation of oral magnesium therapy, which corrects both the primary deficiency as well as secondary hypocalcemia.

Acrodermatitis enteropathica is a rare autosomal recessive disease presenting in infancy with the onset of a characteristic rash involving the skin of the perioral region, the perianum, and the distal extremities, with associated diarrhea, alopecia, and failure to thrive.[83] Reflecting altered intestinal uptake, serum zinc levels are low, as is the activity of the zinc-dependent enzyme, alkaline phosphatase. The condition rapidly responds to the oral administration of supplemental zinc.

Originally thought to be a defect in intestinal copper uptake, Menkes' (steely hair) syndrome is now recognized to represent a generalized disorder of cellular copper transport, thereby mimicking copper deficiency.[84] This rare, x-linked recessive disease is characterized by growth retardation, abnormal hair, hypopigmentation, bone changes, and progressive cerebral degeneration. Death usually occurs by the age of 3 years.

Microvillous Inclusion Disease

Microvillous inclusion disease or congenital microvillous atrophy also presents with intractable, watery diarrhea within a few days of birth. Unlike the congenital defects of electrolyte transport, this condition is associated with a generalized enteropathy characterized by intestinal villous atrophy and specific ultrastructural abnormalities (Fig. 73-3).[85,86] The pathologic features suggest that this disease is the result of defective brush border assembly and differentiation. Electron microscopy of intestinal mucosal biopsy specimens reveals well preserved crypt epithelium containing increased amounts of secretory granules, which are thought to contain brush border-related glycoproteins. The enterocytes of the surface epithelium, however, lack microvilli or have irregularly arranged, shortened microvilli in diminished number, and contain numerous vesicular bodies. Intracytoplasmic vacuoles lined by inwardly facing brush border microvilli may be detected within some enterocytes, and are considered diagnostic of this disorder. There is evidence that the basic defect in microvillous inclusion disease involves an abnormality of the cytoskeletal elements that are necessary for orderly intracellular trafficking.[85]

Affected infants have severe diarrhea despite restriction of oral intake, and lifelong total parenteral nutrition is required to support nutrient and fluid requirements. In an isolated case, the chronic administration of the long-acting somatostatin analog, octreotide, resulted in a marked reduction of stool volumes.[86] Subtotal enterectomy has been advocated as a further option to address the problem of refractory, life-threatening fluid and electrolyte losses.[87] Intestinal transplantation has been successfully used in this setting, and may ultimately represent accepted therapy for this disease.[88] The requirement for jejunal biopsy in affected infants may be circumvented by performing electron microscopy on a rectal mucosal biopsy specimen, because diagnostic microvillous inclusions have been detected within the rectal epithelium.

Disorders of Vitamin B₁₂ Absorption

Deranged B_{12} absorption and transport due to specific defects of the ileal enterocytes represent a rare set of disorders. Selective congenital B_{12} malabsorption associated with protein-

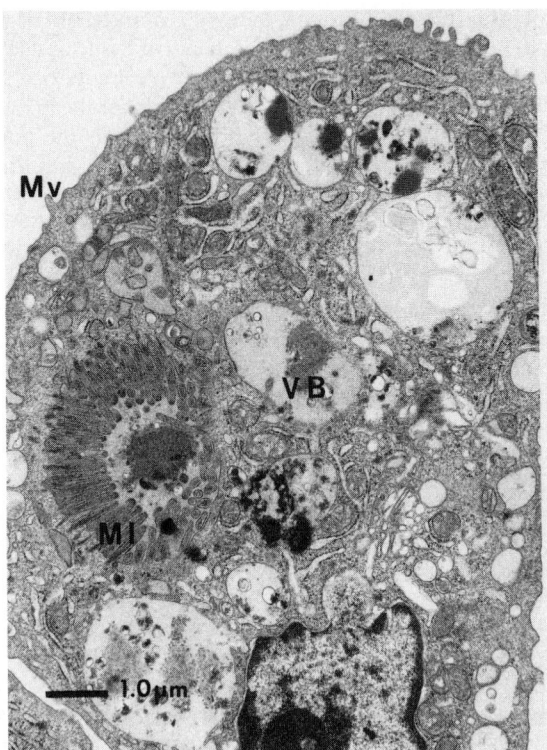

FIGURE 73-3. Ultrastructural abnormalities of the enterocyte in microvillus inclusion disease. The apical plasma membrane lacks an organized brush border surface; instead, a few rudimentary microvilli (Mv) are present. The supranuclear cytoplasm contains a characteristic microvillus inclusion (MI) with well developed, inwardly facing brush border microvilli. Numerous vesicular bodies (VB) are present, and although their role is unknown, they may represent either precursors of the microvillus inclusions or part of a degradative pathway for the missorted brush border proteins. (From Cutz E, Rhoads JM, Drumm B, et al. Microvillous inclusion disease: an inherited defect of brush-border assembly and differentiation. N Engl J Med 1989;320:646.)

uria was described independently in 1960 by Imerslund[89] and by Grasbeck and colleagues.[90] This is an autosomal recessive disorder characterized by the onset of hematologic and neurologic sequelae of vitamin B_{12} deficiency during childhood. Serum B_{12} levels are low in the presence of normal values for folate. The Schilling test shows impaired absorption of the vitamin despite administration of intrinsic factor, pancreatic extract, or antibiotics. The nature of the defect remains obscure. Mackenzie and colleagues demonstrated uptake of intrinsic factor-bound B_{12} by ileal homogenates from an affected person, and therefore postulated a postreceptor defect.[91] Burman and associates were unable to demonstrate the in vivo uptake of radiolabeled B_{12} into ileal biopsy specimens, and concluded that the defect was at the level of the intrinsic factor–B_{12} receptor.[92] Affected patients respond to monthly injections of cyanocobalamin with complete reversal of neurologic and hematologic symptoms if treated promptly.

Transcobalamin II deficiency is a disorder characterized by absence of the transport protein for B_{12}. Although fetal development is normal as a consequence of maternally derived transcobalamin II, profound megaloblastic anemia develops in infancy. Serum B_{12} levels usually are normal, however, reflecting vitamin sequestered in the circulation by binding to haptocorrin (plasma R-protein, transcobalamin I and III) and unavailable for transcobalamin II-dependent tissue uptake. It has been suggested that the failure of the ileal enterocyte to synthesize the transport protein is responsible for the inability to transport dietary B_{12} across the mucosa into the portal circulation.[93] Treatment requires the parenteral administration of huge doses of B_{12} so that the vitamin may enter tissues by passive diffusion.

These disorders should be distinguished from congenital intrinsic factor deficiency. This condition also presents with the manifestations of B_{12} deficiency in early childhood. Serum B_{12} levels are low, and on testing, absorption is impaired unless exogenous intrinsic factor is included. Although these laboratory findings are identical to those with classic pernicious anemia, this condition occurs in the absence of achlorhydria, atrophic gastritis, or parietal cell antibodies. Functional intrinsic factor is absent from gastric secretions or present in greatly reduced amounts. Variants of this disease with no intrinsic factor synthesis, synthesis of structurally altered proteins that result in low ileal receptor affinity, and synthesis of intrinsic factor susceptible to alteration by acid and proteolysis, have been described.[94,95]

Primary Bile Salt Malabsorption

The conservation of bile salts through ileal absorption is an integral feature in the enterohepatic circulation of these compounds. This process depends on the efficient uptake of bile salts by a sodium-dependent transporter in the ileal brush border membrane.[96] Impaired absorption with the presentation of increased amounts of bile salts to the large intestine may result in the stimulation of colonic water and electrolyte secretion. This mechanism can be a major cause of the diarrhea accompanying limited ileal resection or bypass and a contributing factor in the setting of ileal inflammatory disease.

Thaysen and Pedersen first suggested that a selective defect in the uptake of bile acids accounted for a chronic diarrheal illness in certain patients with no other evidence of ileal disease.[97] These patients demonstrated bile acid malabsorption when assessed by ^{14}C-cholylglycine breath tests, despite normal ileal structure by radiologic examinations and preserved B_{12} absorption by Shilling tests. All improved markedly on treatment with cholestyramine, relapsing on discontinuation of sequestration therapy. Further support for this distinct clinical syndrome came from the in vitro demonstration of impaired taurocholic acid uptake in ileal biopsy specimens that were ultrastructurally normal from two boys with suspected primary bile salt malabsorption and congenital diarrhea.[98] It is possible, however, that primary bile salt malabsorption in the pediatric population represents a disorder distinct from that of adults. Three adult patients have been described who exhibit the clinical features of this syndrome associated with subtotal villous atrophy of the ileal mucosa and mononuclear infiltration of the lamina propria.[99] The presence of markers for altered immune function raises the possibility that the condition is immunologically mediated in some patients.

Primary bile salt malabsorption, if it occurs, is a rare disorder. Most patients with idiopathic chronic diarrhea are reported to have bile salt malabsorption when evaluated by the measurement of fecal excretion of labeled taurocholate, but

this probably is an epiphenomenon, and these patients do not usually respond to cholestyramine.[100] A number of diagnostic tests have been used to demonstrate exaggerated fecal losses of bile salts. These include the measurement of radioactivity in expired air and stool after ingestion of ^{14}C-labeled cholylglycine, the quantitation of fecal radioactivity after the administration of radiolabeled taurocholate, and the measurement of the total excretion and aqueous concentration of fecal bile acids. The usefulness of these tests is limited by their lack of general availability and the complexity of their interpretation. Alternatively, whole-body counting after ingestion of the taurine conjugate of a synthetic bile acid containing a γ-emitting isotope of selenium (the SeHCAT test) has been advocated as a superior method for identifying bile salt malabsorption. Regardless, the failure to respond to cholestyramine with a significant reduction in stool volume suggests that the diagnosis is unlikely.

> The reader is directed to Chapter 17, Carbohydrate Assimilation; Chapter 49, Genetic Counseling for Gastrointestinal Patients; and Chapter 108, Gastrointestinal Manifestations of Specific Genetic Disorders.

REFERENCES

1. Bond JH, Levitt MD. Quantitative measurement of lactose absorption. Gastroenterology 1976;70:1058.
2. Miller TL, Wolin MJ. Fermentations by saccharolytic intestinal bacteria. Am J Clin Nutr 1979;32:164.
3. Saunders DR, Wiggins HS. Conservation of mannitol, lactulose, and raffinose by the human colon. Am J Physiol 1981;241:G397.
4. Hammer HF, Fine KD, Santa Ana CA, et al. Carbohydrate malabsorption, its measurement and its contribution to diarrhea. J Clin Invest 1990;86:1936.
5. Holzel A, Schwarz V, Sutcliffe KW. Defective lactose absorption causing malnutrition in infancy. Lancet 1959;1:1126.
6. Auricchio S, Rubino A, Landolt M, et al. Isolated intestinal lactase deficiency in the adult. Lancet 1963;2:324.
7. Dahlqvist A, Hammond JB, Crane RK, et al. Intestinal lactase deficiency and lactose intolerance in adults. Gastroenterology 1963;45:488.
8. Simoons FJ. The geographic hypothesis and lactose malabsorption: a weighing of the evidence. Am J Dig Dis 1978;23:963.
9. Johnson JD, Simoons FJ, Hurwitz R, et al. Lactose malabsorption among the Pima Indians of Arizona. Gastroenterology 1977;1:1299.
10. Cuatrecasas P, Lockwood DH, Caldwell JR. Lactase deficiency in the adult: a common occurrence. Lancet 1965;1:14.
11. Gilat T, Russo S, Gelman-Malachi E, Aldor TAM. Lactase in man: a nonadaptable enzyme. Gastroenterology 1972;62:1125.
12. Boll W, Wagner P, Mantei N. Structure of the chromosomal gene and cDNAs coding for lactase-phlorizin hydrolase in humans with adult-type hypolactasia or persistence of lactase. Am J Hum Genet 1991;48:889.
13. Lloyd M, Mevissen G, Fischer M, et al. Regulation of intestinal lactase in adult hypolactasia. J Clin Invest 1992;89:524.
14. Escher JC, deKoning ND, van Engen CGJ, et al. Molecular basis of lactase levels in adult humans. J Clin Invest 1992;89:480.
15. Witte J, Lloyd M, Lorenzsonn V, et al. The biosynthetic basis of adult lactase deficiency. J Clin Invest 1990;86:1338.
16. Sterchi EE, Mills PR, Fransen JAM, et al. Biogenesis of intestinal lactase–phlorizin hydrolase in adults with lactose intolerance. J Clin Invest 1990;86:1329.
17. Maiuri L, Raia V, Potter J, et al. Mosaic pattern of lactase

expression by villous enterocytes in human adult-type hypolactasia. Gastroenterology 1991;100;359.

18. Lorenzsonn V, Lloyd M, Olsen W. Imunocytochemical heterogeneity of lactase–phlorizin hydrolase in adult lactase deficiency. Gastroenterology 1993;105:51.

19. Sebastio G, Villa M, Sartorio R, et al. Control of lactase in human adult-type hypolactasia and in weaning rabbits and rats. Am J Hum Genet 1989;45:489-497.

20. What has happened to carbohydrate intolerance following gastroenteritis (editorial)? Lancet 1987;1:23.

21. Newcomer AD, McGill DB, Thomas PJ, Hofmann AF. Tolerance to lactose among lactase-deficient American Indians. Gastroenterology 1978;74:44.

22. Bedine MS, Bayless TM. Intolerance of small amounts of lactose by individuals with low lactase levels. Gastroenterology 1973;65:735.

23. Bayless TM. Lactose malabsorption, milk intolerance, and symptom awareness in adults. In: Paige DM, Bayless TM, eds. Lactose digestion, clinical and nutritional implications. Baltimore: The Johns Hopkins University Press, 1981;117.

24. DiPalma JA, Naravaez RM. Prediction of lactose malabsorption in referral patients. Dig Dis Sci 1988;33:303.

25. Levitt MD, Donaldson RM. Use of respiratory hydrogen (H_2) excretion to detect carbohydrate malabsorption. J Lab Clin Med 1970;75:937.

26. Kolars JC, Levitt MD, Mostafa A, Savaiano DA. Yogurt: an autodigesting source of lactose. N Engl J Med 1984;310:1.

27. Gudmand-Hoyer E, Fenger HJ, Kern-Hansen P, Madsen PR. Sucrase deficiency in Greenland: incidence and genetic aspects. Scand J Gastroenterol 1987;22:24.

28. Green F, Edwards Y, Hauri H-P, et al. Isolation of a cDNA probe for a human jejunal brush-border hydrolase, sucrase–isomaltase and assignment of the gene locus to chromosome 3. Gene 1987;57:101.

29. Traeber PG, Yu L, Wu GD, Judge TA. Sucrase–isomaltase gene expression along crypt–villus axis of human small intestine is regulated at the level of mRNA abundance. Am J Physiol 1992;262:G123.

30. Naim HY, Sterchi EE, Lentze MJ. Biosynthesis of the human sucrase–isomaltase complex differential O-glycosylation of the sucrase subunit correlates with its position within the enzyme complex. J Biol Chem 1988;263:7242.

31. Lloyd ML, Olsen WA. A study of the molecular pathology of sucrase–isomaltase deficiency a defect in the intracellular processing of the enzyme. N Engl J Med 1987;316:438.

32. Naim HY, Roth J, Sterchi EE, et al. Sucrase–isomaltase deficiency in humans different mutations disrupt intracellular transport, processing, and function of an intestinal brush border enzyme. J Clin Invest 1988;82:667.

33. Fransen JAM, Hauri HP, Ginsel LA, Naim HY. Naturally occurring mutations in sucrase–isomaltase provide evidence for the existence of an intracellular sorting signal in the isomaltase subunit. J Cell Biol 1991;115:45.

34. Harms H-K, Bertele-Harms R-M, Bruer-Kleis D. Enzyme-substitution therapy with the yeast *Saccharomyces cerevisiae* in congenital sucrase–isomaltase deficiency. N Engl J Med 1987;316:1306.

34a. Treem WR, Ahsan N, Sullivan B, et al. Evaluation of liquid yeast-derived sucrase enzyme replacement in patients with sucrase–isomaltase deficiency. Gastroenterology 1993;105:1061.

35. Bergoz R. Trehalose malabsorption causing intolerance to mushrooms: report of a probable case. Gastroenterology 1971;60:909.

36. Madzarovova-Nohejlova J. Trehalase deficiency in a family. Gastroenterology 1973;65:130.

37. Gudmand-Hoyer E, Fenger HJ, Skovbjerg H, et al. Trehalase deficiency in Greenland. Scand J Gastroenterol 1988;23:775.

38. Evans L, Grasset E, Heyman M, et al. Congenital selective malabsorption of glucose and galactose. J Pediatr Gastroenterol Nutr 1985;4:878.

39. Booth IW, Patel PB, Sule D, et al. Glucose–galactose malabsorption: demonstration of specific jejunal brush border membrane defect. Gut 1988;29:1661.

40. Hediger MA, Turk E, Wright EM. Homology of the human Na^+/glucose and *Escherichia coli* Na^+/proline cotransporters. Proc Natl Acad Sci USA 1989;86:5748.

41. Turk E, Zabel B, Mundlos S, et al. Glucose/galactose malabsorption caused by a defect in the Na^+/glucose cotransporter. Nature 1991;350:354.

42. Manuel PD, Mukhtar DJL, Walker-Smith JA. Transient monosaccharide intolerance in infants with acute and protracted diarrhea. J Pediatr Gastroenterol Nutr 1984;3:41.

43. Andersson DEH, Nygren A. Four cases of long-standing diarrhea and colic pains cured by fructose-free diet: a pathogenic discussion. Acta Med Scand 1978;203:87.

44. Ravich WJ, Bayless TM, Thomas M. Fructose: incomplete intestinal absorption in humans. Gastroenterology 1983;84:26.

45. Rasmussen JJ, Gudman-Hoyer. Absorption capacity of fructose in healthy adults: comparison with sucrose and its constituent monosaccharides. Gut 1986;27:1161.

46. Ravry MJR. Dietetic food diarrhea. JAMA 1980;244:270.

47. Hyams JS. Sorbitol intolerance: an unappreciated cause of functional gastrointestinal complaints. Gastroenterology 1983;84:30.

48. Anderson IH, Levine AS, Levitt MD. Incomplete absorption of the carbohydrate in all-purpose wheat flour. N Engl J Med 1981;304:891.

49. Levitt MD, Hirsh P, Fetzer CA, Sheahan M, Levine AS. H^2 excretion after ingestion of complex carbohydrates. Gastroenterology 1987;92:383.

50. Jain NK, Patel VP, Pitchumoni CS. Activated charcoal, simethecone, and intestinal gas. Ann Intern Med 1986;105:61.

51. Potter T, Ellis C, Levitt MD. Activated charcoal: in vivo and in vitro studies of the effect on gas formation. Gastroenterology 1985;88:620.

52. Alpha-galactosidase to prevent gas. Med Lett Drugs Ther 1993;35:29.

53. Juby LD, Rothwell J, Axon ATR. Lactulose/mannitol test: an ideal screen for celiac disease. Gastroenterology 1989;96:79.

54. Madara J. Loosening tight junctions, lessons from the intestine. J Clin Invest 1989;83:1089.

55. Ukabam SO, Clamp JR, Cooper BT. Abnormal small intestinal permeability to sugars in patients with Crohn's disease of the terminal ileum and colon. Digestion 1983;27:70.

56. Hollander D, Vadheim CM, Brettholz E, et al. Increased Intestinal permeability in patients with Crohn's disease and their relatives: a possible etiologic factor. Ann Intern Med 1986;105:883.

57. Travis S, Menzies I. Intestinal permeability: functional assessment and significance. Clin Science 1992;82:471.

58. Hadorn B, Tarlow MJ, Lloyd JK, Wolff OH. Intestinal enterokinase deficiency. Lancet 1969;1:812.

59. Hadorn B. Disease of the pancreas in children. Clin Gastroenterol 1972;1:125.

60. Freeman HJ, Sleisenger MH, Kim YS. Human protein digestion and absorption: normal mechanisms and protein-energy malnutrition. Clin Gastroenterol 1983;12:357.

61. Silk DBA. Disorders of nitrogen absorption. Clin Gastroenterol 1982;11:47.

62. Ragantie J, Simell O, Perheentupa J. Basolateral membrane transport defect for lysine in lysinuric protein intolerance. Lancet 1980;1:1219.

63. Desjeux JF, Ragantie J, Simell O, et al. Lysine fluxes across the jejunal epithelium in lysinuric protein intolerance. J Clin Invest 1980;65:1382.

64. Kane JP, Hardman DA, Paulus HE. Heterogeneity of apolipoprotein B: isolation of a new species from human chylomicrons. Proc Natl Acad Sci USA 1980;77:2465.

65. Glickman RM, Green PHR, Lees RS, et al. Immunofluorescence studies of apolipoprotein B in intestinal mucosa: absence in abetalipoproteinemia. Gastroenterology 1979;76:288.

66. Dullaart RPF, Speelberg B, Schuurman H-J, et al. Epitopes of apolipoprotein B-100 and B-48 in both liver and intestine: expression and evidence for local synthesis in recessive abetalipoproteinemia. J Clin Invest 1986;78:1397.

67. Talmud PJ, Lloyd JK, Muller DPR, et al. Genetic evidence from

two families that the apolipoprotein B gene is not involved in abetalipoproteinemia. J Clin Invest 1988;82:1803.

68. Lackner KJ, Monge JC, Gregg RE, et al. Analysis of the apolipoprotein B gene and messenger ribonucleic acid in abetalipoproteinemia. J Clin Invest 1986;78:1707.

69. Black DD, Hay RV, Rohwer-Nutter PL, et al. Intestinal and hepatic apolipoprotein B gene expression in abetalipoproteinemia. Gastroenterology 1991;101:520.

70. Glickman RM, Glickman JN, Magun A, Brin M. Apolipoprotein synthesis in normal and abetalipoproteinemic intestinal mucosa. Gastroenterology 1991;101:749.

71. Wetterau JR, Aggerbeck LP, Bouma M-E, et al. Absence of microsomal triglyceride transfer protein in individuals with abetalipoproteinemia. Science 1992;258:999.

72. Roy CC, Levy E, Green PHR, et al. Malabsorption, hypocholesterolemia, and fat-filled enterocytes with increased intestinal apoprotein B: chylomicron retention disease. Gastroenterology 1987;92:390.

73. Hardman DA, Pullinger CR, Hamilton RL, et al. Molecular and metabolic basis for the metabolic disorder normotriglyceridemic abetalipoproteinemia. J Clin Invest 1991;88:1722.

74. Ross RS, Gregg RE, Law SW, et al. Homozygous hypobetalipoproteinemia: a disease distinct from abetalipoproteinemia at the molecular level. J Clin Invest 1988;81:590.

75. Young SG, Hubl ST, Chappell DA, et al. Familial hypobetalipoproteinemia associated with a mutant species of apolipoprotein B (B-46). N Engl J Med 1989;320:1604.

76. Collins DR, Knott TJ, Pease RJ, et al. Truncated variants of apolipoprotein B cause hypobetalipoproteinemia. Nucleic Acids Res 1988;16:8361.

77. Darrow DC. Congenital alkalosis with diarrhea. J Pediatr 1945;26:519.

78. Gamble JL, Fahey KR, Appleton J, MacLachlan E. Congenital alkalosis with diarrhea. J Pediatr 1945;26:509.

79. Holmberg C. Congenital chloride diarrhoea. Clin Gastroenterol 1986;15:583.

80. Holmberg C, Perheentupa J. Congenital Na$^+$ diarrhea: a new type of secretory diarrhea. J Pediatr 1985;106:56.

81. Booth IW, Murer H, Strange G, et al. Defective jejunal brush-border Na$^+$/H$^+$ exchange: a cause of congenital secretory diarrhoea. Lancet 1985;1:1066.

82. Stromme JH, Steen-Johnsen J, Harnaes K, et al. Familial hypomagnesemia: a follow-up examination of three patients after 9 to 12 years of treatment. Pediatr Res 1981;15:1134.

83. Bohane TD, Cutz E, Hamilton JR, Gall DG. Acrodermatitis enteropathica, zinc, and the Paneth cell: a case report with family studies. Gastroenterology 1977;73:587.

84. Danks DM. Of mice and men, metals and mutations. J Med Genet 1986;23:99.

85. Carruthers L, Dourmashkin R, Phillips A. Disorders of the cytoskeleton of the enterocyte. Clin Gastroenterol 1986;15:105.

86. Cutz E, Rhoads JM, Drumm B, et al. Microvillous inclusion disease: an inherited defect of brush-border assembly and differentiation. N Engl J Med 1989;320:646.

87. Rhoads JM, Vogler RC, Lacey SR, et al. Microvillus inclusion disease: in vitro jejunal electrolyte transport. Gastroenterology 1991;100:811.

88. Todo S, Tzakis AG, Abu-Elmagd, et al. Intestinal transplantation in composite visceral grafts or alone. Ann Surg 1992;216:223.

89. Imerslund O. Idiopathic chronic megaloblastic anemia in children. Acta Paediatr 1960;49(Suppl 119):1.

90. Grasbeck R, Gordin R, Kantero I, Kuhlback B. Selective vitamin B$_{12}$ malabsorption and proteinuria in young people: a syndrome. Acta Med Scand 1960;167:289.

91. MacKenzie IL, Donaldson RM Jr, Trier JS, Mathan VI. Ileal mucosa in familial selective B$_{12}$ malabsorption. N Engl J Med 1972;286:1021.

92. Burman JF, Jenkins WJ, Walker-Smith JA, et al. Absent ileal uptake of IF-bound vitamin B$_{12}$ in vivo in the Imerslund-Grasbeck syndrome (familial vitamin B$_{12}$ malabsorption with proteinuria). Gut 1985;26:311.

93. Chanarin I. Disorders of vitamin absorption. Clin Gastroenterol 1982;11:73.

94. Katz M, Mehlman CS, Allen RH. Isolation and characterization of an abnormal human intrinsic factor. J Clin Invest 1974;53:1274.

95. Yang Y, Ducos R, Rosenberg AJ, et al. Cobalamin malabsorption in three siblings due to an abnormal intrinsic factor that is markedly susceptible to acid and proteolysis. J Clin Invest 1985;76:2057.

96. Wilson FA. Intestinal transport of bile acids. Am J Physiol 1981;241:G83.

97. Thaysen EH, Pedersen L. Idiopathic bile acid catharsis. Gut 1976;17:965.

98. Heubi JE, Balistreri WF, Fondacaro JD, et al. Primary bile salt malabsorption: defective in vitro active bile acid transport. Gastroenterology 1982;83:804.

99. Popovic OS, Kostic KM, Milovic VB, et al. Primary bile acid malabsorption histologic and immunologic study in three patients. Gastroenterology 1987;92:1851.

100. Schiller LR, Hogan RB, Morawski SG, et al. Studies of the prevalence and significance of radiolabeled bile acid malabsorption in a group of patients with idiopathic chronic diarrhea. Gastroenterology 1987;92:151.

Textbook of Gastroenterology, second edition, edited by Tadataka Yamada. JB Lippincott Company, Philadelphia © 1995.

CHAPTER 74

Bacterial Overgrowth

Ellen Li

Conditions Favoring Bacterial Overgrowth
  Small Intestinal Stasis
  Abnormal Connection Between Proximal and Distal Bowel
  Immunodeficiency
  Age
Pathogenesis
  Malabsorption of Fats and Fat-Soluble Vitamins

  Carbohydrate Intolerance
  Hypoproteinemia
  Malabsorption of Water-Soluble Vitamins
  Extraintestinal Manifestations
Pathology
Clinical Manifestations
Diagnosis
Treatment

Small bowel bacterial overgrowth is a syndrome characterized by nutrient malabsorption associated with excessive numbers of bacteria in the small intestine.[1,2] Other terms that have been used to describe this syndrome are blind loop syndrome, contaminated small bowel, small bowel stasis, and stagnant loop syndrome. Recognition of this syndrome dates back to 1897, when Faber reported an association between pernicious anemia and small intestinal strictures.[3] In 1939, Barker and Hummel first postulated that the association of macrocytic anemia with intestinal strictures or anastomoses was the result of bacterial overgrowth or "putrefaction."[4] Patients with a variety of structural or functional disorders of the gastrointestinal tract are predisposed to the development of bacterial overgrowth.[1,2] There is evidence that bacterial overgrowth may develop in the absence of an anatomic lesion or a severe motility disorder in the elderly and pediatric populations.[5,6] Bacterial overgrowth should be considered as a possible cause of diarrhea, malabsorption, or abdominal pain in these clinical settings. Because the diagnosis of bacterial overgrowth presents several difficulties and limitations, empiric treatment of bacterial overgrowth often is used in clinical practice.

CONDITIONS FAVORING BACTERIAL OVERGROWTH

The conditions favoring bacterial overgrowth can be classified in terms of the mechanisms involved in the normal control of the enteric flora (Table 74-1). Furthermore, the presence of a single condition may not result in clinically significant small intestinal overgrowth until the development of another condition favoring bacterial overgrowth.

Small Intestinal Stasis

Small intestinal peristalsis plays a major role in preventing bacterial overgrowth. A number of anatomic or structural disorders that interfere with intestinal peristalsis frequently lead to small bowel bacterial overgrowth. These include chronic small intestinal obstruction secondary to intestinal strictures, such as those arising from Crohn's disease, lymphoma, and radiation injury.[7-9] Surgical alterations of the intestinal anatomy with creations of blind pouches or long segments of diverted small bowel, such as end-to-side enteroenteric anastomosis, the Billroth II anastomosis, jejunoileal bypass, and the Koch distal ileal pouch (for continent ileostomies), have been associated with clinically significant bacterial overgrowth.[10-12] These procedures produce stagnant pouches and loops resulting in marked proliferation of bacteria. Small intestinal diverticula also serve as pockets of stagnation, and become clinically significant particularly in the setting of hypochlorhydria or achlorhydria.[10]

Generalized impairment in small intestinal motor function (see Chap. 9) also may lead to small bowel bacterial overgrowth. Malabsorption resulting from small intestine bacterial overgrowth has been documented in patients with intestinal hypomotility associated with scleroderma, idiopathic intestinal pseudoobstruction, and diabetic autonomic neuropathy.[13-15] The absent or disordered migrating motor complex has been associated with bacterial overgrowth[16]; in one patient,

> **TABLE 74-1**
> **Conditions Favoring Bacterial Overgrowth**

Intestinal Stasis
Anatomic
    Strictures (e.g., Crohn's disease, radiation enteritis)
    Small intestinal diverticulosis
    Surgical operations
        End-to-side enteroenteric anastomoses
        Billroth II anastomoses
        Jejunoileal bypass
        Koch's distal ileal pouches
Small intestinal motility disorders
    Scleroderma
    Idiopathic intestinal pseudoobstruction
    Diabetic autonomic neuropathy

Abnormal Connection Between Proximal and Distal Bowel
Fistulas (secondary to peptic ulcer disease, carcinoma)
    Gastrocolic
    Gastrojejunocolic
Resection of the ilealcecal valve

Hypochlorhydria
Chronic atrophic gastritis
Hypochlorhydric medications
Surgical therapy of peptic ulcer disease

Immunodeficiency
Primary immunodeficiency states
Acquired immunodeficiency syndrome
Malnutrition

Age

the return of phase 3 of the migrating motor complex preceded resolution of bacterial overgrowth.[17]

Abnormal Connection Between Proximal and Distal Bowel

Small intestinal bacterial overgrowth may arise from abnormal connections between the proximal bowel and the colon that lead to seeding of the proximal bowel with colonic flora. Resection of the ileocecal valve may lead to retrograde seeding of the small intestine with colonic flora and contribute to the development of small intestinal bacterial overgrowth.[18,19] There also is evidence that resection of the ileocecal valve (as well as a portion of the terminal ileum and cecum) results in alterations in motility that may play an important role in the development of bacterial overgrowth.[20] Gastrocolic or gastrojejunocolic fistulas may arise in patients with gastric ulcers and ulcerating carcinomas of the stomach or colon. In this situation, malabsorption results from reflux of colonic contents into the proximal bowel.[21]

Gastric acid is responsible for decreasing the bacterial inoculum reaching the proximal small intestine. A significant increase in the proximal gastrointestinal bacterial concentration is observed in patients with achlorhydria due to chronic gastritis, compared with control subjects.[22] Gastric acid secretion also is impaired as a result of medical and surgical therapy of peptic ulcer disease. Increased bacterial counts and

overgrowth have been reported in association with cimetidine therapy[23]; these may be even more significant clinically with the use of more potent hypochlorhydric medications, such as omeprazole. Gastric surgery affects bacterial proliferation by impairing gastric acid secretion and by altering intestinal motility. The results from animal models and from humans tested postsurgery suggest that impaired gastric acid secretion alone is not sufficient to produce clinically significant bacterial overgrowth.[11,24] Hypochlorhydria, however, may promote intestinal overgrowth in patients who also have intestinal disorders that promote stasis (e.g., diverticula, delayed intestinal transit).

Immunodeficiency

Chronic diarrhea, malabsorption, and weight loss have been observed in a number of immunodeficiency states (see Chap. 46). For example, 60% of patients with common variable immunodeficiency have chronic diarrhea. Frequently, malabsorption is associated with *Giardia lamblia* infestation and responds to treatment of giardiasis. Overgrowth of bacteria is a common finding in these patients; however, the bacterial counts (particularly those of anaerobic organisms) are lower than those observed in cases associated with intestinal stasis.[25] Bacterial overgrowth also may be related to decreased acid secretion in these patients.[25] Chronic diarrhea is a prominent symptom in patients suffering from acquired immunodeficiency syndrome. These patients may have multiple opportunistic infections (see Chap. 105); however, the etiology of their diarrhea and malabsorption frequently cannot be identified. Bacterial colonization of the proximal bowel has been observed in these patients, but the role this colonization plays in the pathogenesis of acquired immunodeficiency syndrome-related diarrhea remains speculative, because the concentration of anaerobic organisms is far lower than is usually observed in bacterial overgrowth associated with stasis.[26]

Age

Bacterial overgrowth of the small intestine is an important cause of malabsorption in the elderly.[5,27,28] Overall, both asymptomatic and symptomatic elderly subjects have increased duodenal bacterial counts. Possible explanations for this finding are reduced gastric acidity, impaired intestinal motility, or both. In addition, many of these patients are malnourished, and malnutrition itself has been associated with bacterial overgrowth.[19]

PATHOGENESIS

The pathogenesis of small bowel bacterial overgrowth can be discussed in terms of the consequences of misplacing the colonic flora into the small intestine. The enteric flora, which normally is located principally within the colon, plays an important role in the metabolism of intralumenal substances (Table 74-2). The amount of intralumenal substances the bacteria normally would encounter, however, is limited by small intestinal absorption. With small bowel bacterial over-

TABLE 74-2
Pathogenesis of Bacterial Overgrowth

Bacterial Metabolism of Intraluminal Substances

Impaired deconjugation of bile acids
Impaired vitamin B_{12} metabolism
Impaired metabolism of carbohydrates
Malabsorption of fats, vitamins A, D, E, generation of
    secretagogues
Malabsorption of vitamin B_{12}
Intestinal gas (H_2, CO_2), osmotic diarrhea

Mucosal Injury

Decreased brush border enzyme activity
    Lactase
    Enterokinase, peptidase
Impaired uptake of monosaccharides
Impaired uptake of peptides
Impaired uptake of lipids
Lactose intolerance
Hypoproteinemia
Carbohydrate intolerance
Hypoproteinemia
Fat malabsorption

CONSTRUCTION OF BLIND LOOP

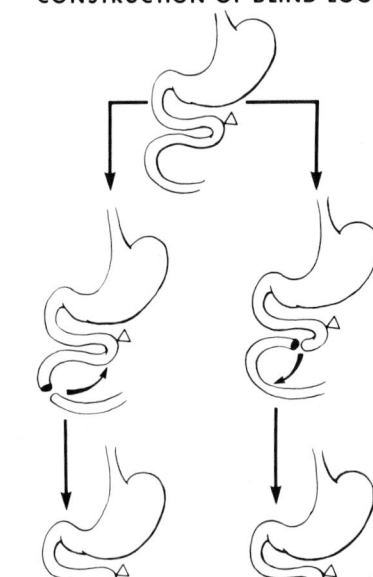

SFBL   SEBL

FIGURE 74-1. Animal model of small bowel overgrowth. Diversion of an isoperistaltic segment of jejunum results in the formation of a self-filling blind loop (SFBL). The SFBL is often used to characterize the pathophysiology of bacterial overgrowth in the small bowel because it results in proliferation of colonic-type bacterial flora and sequelae that mimic those observed in human disease. A short, patent, antiperistaltic segment of jejunum, referred to as a self-emptying blind loop (SEBL), serves as an operated control, because bacterial overgrowth and its sequelae do not develop postoperatively. (From Sherman P, Lichtman S. Small bowel bacterial overgrowth syndrome. Surv Dig Dis 1987;5:157.)

growth, the bacteria have much greater access to nutrients and other intralumenal substances. In addition to intralumenal bacterial metabolism, there is evidence that mucosal injury also results in the malabsorption of fats, carbohydrates, and proteins[29,30]; however, there is no evidence that bacterial invasion is involved.[31]

The surgical formation of a self-filling blind loop (Fig. 74-1) in a variety of animal models has resulted in marked proliferation of both aerobic and anaerobic bacteria and reproduces many of the manifestations of overgrowth observed in humans.[32,33] Much of the experimental work defining the pathogenesis of small bowel bacterial overgrowth is based on these models.

Malabsorption of Fats and Fat-Soluble Vitamins

Bacterial deconjugation of bile acids is the primary mechanism for malabsorption of fats and fat-soluble vitamins.[34,35] Normal fat absorption requires a critical concentration of conjugated bile acids for the assembly of mixed micelles. Bacterial deconjugation of bile acids by lumenal bacteria, particularly anaerobic organisms,[36] reduces the level of conjugated bile acids below the critical micellar concentration. Steatorrhea has been improved in patients[34] and experimental animals[35] with bacterial overgrowth after conjugated bile acids were administered; however, the observation that complete biliary diversion in animals does not produce the steatorrhea seen in bacterial overgrowth suggests that other factors may play a role.[19] Vitamin D, A, and E deficiencies have been reported as complications.[37,38] The synthesis of vitamin K by lumenal bacteria, however, accounts for the absence of coagulopathy in patients with bacterial overgrowth. It has been suggested that bacterial metabolites (e.g., hydroxylated fatty acids and unconjugated

bile acids) may have a toxic effect on the intestinal mucosa, resulting in malabsorption of fats, carbohydrates, and proteins. Many of these metabolites serve as secretagogues that contribute to the development of diarrhea.

Carbohydrate Intolerance

Bacterial overgrowth results in carbohydrate intolerance secondary to reduction of brush border disaccharidases and decreased uptake of monosaccharide.[39–42] Lactase activity is the first to be reduced and is the last disaccharidase activity to recover after antibiotic therapy has been administered.[40,42] There is evidence that anaerobic organisms produce proteases and glycosidases that release or destroy hydrolases on the brush border.[39,40,43] Carbohydrate intolerance results in an increased delivery to the small intestine of osmotically active carbohydrate fragments, contributing to the pathogenesis of diarrhea associated with bacterial overgrowth. Bacterial metabolism of carbohydrates to hydrogen and carbon dioxide may play a role in the pathogenesis of abdominal pain, and is the basis of various breath tests used to diagnose bacterial overgrowth.

Hypoproteinemia

Hypoproteinemia is common in bacterial overgrowth, although severe protein nutrition is rarely seen.[44] Disruption of normal protein assimilation is caused by multiple factors. Bacteria compete with the host for protein substrates[41]; decreased amino acid and peptide uptake has been demonstrated in experimental models, perhaps reflecting mucosal injury[43]; decreased levels of enterokinase have been measured in patients with bacterial overgrowth, and may impair the activation of pancreatic proteases[45]; and, finally, a protein-losing enteropathy has been described in patients and experimental animals with bacterial overgrowth.[46]

Malabsorption of Water-Soluble Vitamins

The association of macrocytic anemia with bacterial overgrowth is the result of direct competition between the intestinal flora and the host for vitamin B_{12}. The anaerobic organisms are primarily responsible because only anaerobicidal therapy reversed vitamin B_{12} deficiency in an experimental stasis model.[19] Anaerobic organisms, in contrast to aerobic organisms, can use vitamin B_{12} in either the free form or when complexed with intrinsic factor.[47,48] When bacteria take up the vitamin, not only does it become unavailable to the host, but inactive metabolites are produced that compete with normal vitamin B_{12} binding and absorption.[49] In contrast, folate levels are normal or elevated in bacterial overgrowth, because bacteria synthesize folate that subsequently is absorbed by the host. Thiamine[50] and nicotinamide[51] are two other water-soluble vitamins that have been reported to be low in patients with bacterial overgrowth.

Although iron deficiency anemia has not been clearly associated with bacterial overgrowth in humans, increased intestinal losses of iron and blood were documented in animal models.[52] Mineral and trace element deficiencies have not been reported in patients with bacterial overgrowth.

Extraintestinal Manifestations

The pathogenesis of extraintestinal manifestations of bacterial overgrowth is not well understood. Hepatobiliary injury has been observed in experimental models of bacterial overgrowth in susceptible rat strains.[53,54] The injury can be prevented by antibiotic treatment.[55] It has been suggested that bacterial cell wall polymers or other bacterial toxins from the blind loop cause hepatic lesions in genetically susceptible hosts.[53]

PATHOLOGY

Lumenal bacteria clearly influence intestinal morphology. Many of the normal morphologic characteristics of the intestinal epithelium are seen only in association with a resident bacterial flora (see Chap. 26). In the germ-free state, the villi are thinner and longer, and crypts are shallower. The mucosal cells are cuboidal rather than columnar. The lamina propria consists of a sparse stroma infiltrated with a few lymphocytes and macrophages, plasma cells are absent, and Peyer patches are smaller, with fewer germinal centers. On light microscopy, the histologic appearance of the small intestine with bacterial overgrowth usually is not significantly different from that observed in the intestine with a normal enteric flora. The main purpose of obtaining a mucosal biopsy in the evaluation of these patients is therefore to rule out mucosal diseases such as celiac sprue. Histologic evidence of mucosal damage, however, has been observed in some cases of bacterial overgrowth, including subtotal villus atrophy and increased inflammatory cells within the lamina propria.[30] Focal areas of ulceration and erosion have been observed in some instances, and may be important in understanding the symptoms of "pouchitis" associated with bacterial overgrowth after surgical formation of a continent ileostomy (Koch pouch) or ileoanal anastomosis.[56,57] Ultrastructural studies of experimental models of bacterial overgrowth revealed vacuolization of microvillus membranes and swelling of the mitochondria (Fig. 74-2), suggesting that bacterial overgrowth does result in damage to the enterocyte.[29]

CLINICAL MANIFESTATIONS

Many of the clinical features of bacterial overgrowth can be predicted based on the pathogenesis of the disorder (Table 74-3). Diarrhea and weight loss are prominent symptoms due

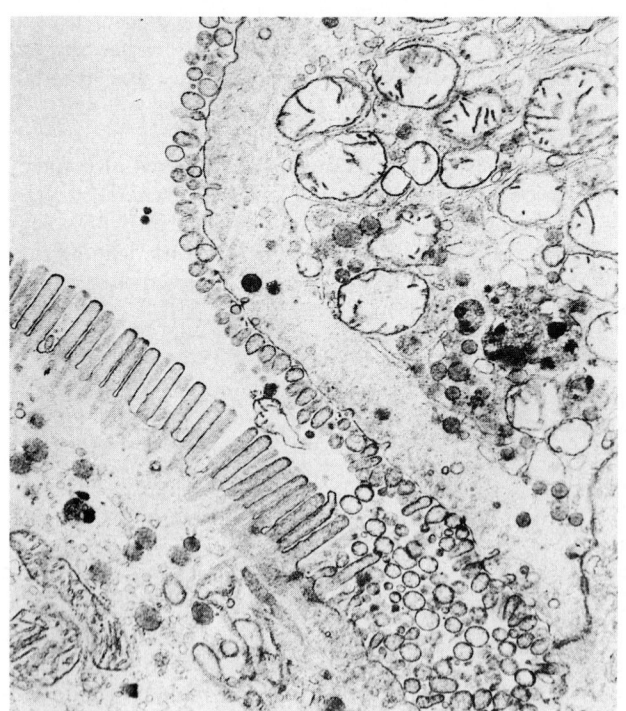

FIGURE 74-2. Electron micrograph of columnar cells in the midvillus area of a self-filling blind loop. The cell at *lower left* shows regular microvilli, unaltered mitochondria, and endoplasmic reticulum. The cell at *upper right* shows altered microvilli, swollen mitochondria, and endoplasmic reticulum. Alterations of microvilli include blunting, swelling, budding, and ballooning. (Original magnification ×22,000; from Toskes PP, Giannella RA, Jeruis HR, et al. Small intestinal mucosal injury in the experimental blind loop syndrome. Gastroenterology 1975;68:1193.)

TABLE 74-3
Clinical Manifestations of Bacterial Overgrowth

Diarrhea
Steatorrhea
Malnutrition
Macrocytic anemia
Abdominal pain
Peripheral neuropathy
Tetany
Osteomalacia
Night blindness
Dermatitis, hepatic injury, nephrotoxicity, and arthritis
  (observed in jejunoileal bypass)

largely to the malabsorption and maldigestion of fats, carbohydrates, and proteins. In addition, many patients with bacterial overgrowth curtail their intake to reduce symptoms.[2] The association of macrocytic anemia with intestinal strictures is a manifestation of vitamin B_{12} deficiency. Patients also may present with the neurologic changes associated with vitamin B_{12} deficiency. Recurrent abdominal pain may be reported, particularly among young children, as a presenting symptom.[6] Other presentations include night blindness, osteomalacia, tetany, peripheral neuropathy, and edema,[58,59] reflecting malabsorption of micronutrients such as vitamins A, D, and E, as well as the water-soluble vitamins thiamine and nicotinamide.

Extraintestinal manifestations of bacterial overgrowth have been observed especially in patients who have undergone jejunoileal bypass. These include dermatitis, hepatic injury, nephrotoxicity, and arthritis.[60–62]

DIAGNOSIS

The diagnosis of bacterial overgrowth should be considered in patients with chronic diarrhea who have the predisposing conditions discussed previously in this chapter. The differential diagnostic considerations include other causes of malabsorption and maldigestion: intestinal mucosal diseases (e.g., celiac sprue), infections (particularly parasitic diseases such as giardiasis), and pancreatic insufficiency. In patients with underlying diseases that favor bacterial proliferation, such as Crohn's disease or scleroderma, it may be difficult to distinguish whether clinical deterioration in these patients is caused by the development of bacterial overgrowth or worsening of the primary intestinal disease.

Microbiologic cultures of small bowel aspirates are considered the most direct method for diagnosing bacterial overgrowth (Table 74-4).[1,2] In general, the diagnosis of bacterial overgrowth is considered to be confirmed if the count exceeds 10^5 colonies/mL after duodenal intubation.[2] A variety of techniques have been reported, using sterile and nonsterile tubes,[63] the capsule method,[64] direct needle aspiration of gut contents,[65] and the string test.[66] The feasibility of collecting aspirates from the proximal small bowel under direct visualization at the time of endoscopy has been demonstrated, which could facilitate the collection of samples during routine en-

doscopy.[67] Small intestinal aspirates were obtained using a sterile suction catheter placed inside a sterile overtube, which was passed through the suction channel of the endoscope after the desired collection site was reached. The aspirates should be transferred immediately to an anaerobic transport vial, and the contents plated for both aerobic and anaerobic organisms.[67] Significant bacterial overgrowth usually is associated with detection of anaerobic organisms. Because of the technical difficulties in culturing fastidious anaerobic organisms, the presence of more than 10^5 colony-forming units/mL in the duodenum is considered diagnostic of bacterial overgrowth.[2] Analyses of unconjugated bile acids[68] and short-chain fatty acids[69] in the fluid also have been performed, but are largely investigational tools. In addition to the technical difficulties of collecting the specimen properly, without contamination by mouth flora, as well as transporting and culturing the fluid, an aspirate of the proximal bowel may not reflect distal bacterial overgrowth.[70] Furthermore, bacterial colonization of the duodenum in the elderly appears to be relatively common, and was not associated with clinical improvement after administration of antibiotics.[28] This observation raises the question of how to interpret elevated bacterial counts in the elderly population.[28]

Breath tests were devised as a less invasive alternative to intubation of the proximal bowel. These tests measure the breath excretion of CO_2 or H_2 produced by intralumenal bacterial metabolism of an administered substrate (see Chap. 35). Breath tests that measure $^{14}CO_2$ in the expired air require the administration of radiolabeled substrates, whereas the H_2 breath tests do not involve radiation. The initial bile acid or ^{14}C-cholylglycine breath test was one of the first breath tests developed, but cannot distinguish bacterial overgrowth from ileal malabsorption.[71] Because of its poor sensitivity and specificity, this test largely has been abandoned. The radiolabeled pentose, ^{14}C-D-xylose, is a more ideal substrate for a breath test because it is minimally metabolized by the host after absorption. Because xylose is absorbed in the proximal bowel, as opposed to bile acids, which are absorbed in the ileum, there is less chance of a false-positive measurement from colonic metabolism.[19] The sensitivity of this test compared to that of microbiologic culturing ranges from 30% to 100%.[28,72] The specificity of the test appears to be high (89%–100%), and it is well tolerated.[28,72]

TABLE 74-4
Diagnostic Tests for Bacterial Overgrowth

TESTS	LIMITATIONS
Culture of small intestinal aspirate	Invasive, possible contamination with oral flora, difficulty in transport of anaerobic cultures, can miss distal intestinal overgrowth
^{14}C-Xylose breath test	Radioactivity, decreased sensitivity
H_2 Breath tests	
Glucose-H_2	20% Of the population unable to produce H_2, decreased sensitivity
Lactulose-H_2	Can miss distal intestinal overgrowth because of overlap between early and late peak

The hydrogen breath tests have the advantage of not involving radioactive substrates. A major problem with these tests is that 15% to 20% of the human population harbor flora that does not produce hydrogen.[71] Lactulose and glucose are two substrates often used for the purpose of diagnosing bacterial overgrowth. Patients with bacterial overgrowth who are administered lactulose exhibit an early breath hydrogen peak from small intestinal bacterial fermentation, followed by a prolonged peak from colonic bacterial metabolism.[73] With distal intestinal overgrowth, it may be difficult to resolve the two peaks. In a study comparing the 10-g lactulose-H_2 breath test to the Enterotest string test in Burma, only 2 of 15 children with more than 10^5 organisms/mL exhibited a positive breath test.[74] A comparison of the glucose-H_2 and lactulose-H_2 tests showed sensitivities of 62% and 68%, respectively, and specificities of 83% and 44%, respectively, compared with jejunal culture.[75] Elevated levels of fasting breath hydrogen have been observed in some patients with bacterial overgrowth, but this is a relatively insensitive indicator of bacterial overgrowth.[76] The ^{14}C-xylose breath test is the only breath test recommended by the Clinical Efficacy Committee of the American College of Physicians for diagnosing bacterial overgrowth.[1]

Analysis of unconjugated bile acids in the serum has been performed in patients with bacterial overgrowth, and may provide a noninvasive test for bacterial overgrowth.[77]

In summary, the available diagnostic tests all have their limitations. Many of the tests are used primarily as investigational tools, and are not available in many institutions. Barium studies may be useful for documenting an anatomic defect or suggesting the presence of a severe motility disorder. In certain clinical settings, such as documentation of fat malabsorption, or vitamin B_{12} malabsorption in the setting of an anatomic defect or severe motility disorder, it may be reasonable to consider a course of empiric antibiotic therapy without further confirmation of the diagnosis. In the absence of a documented predisposing abnormality of the gastrointestinal tract, however, it is recommended that further diagnostic tests be performed. Routine upper endoscopy with small bowel biopsy and culture of the aspirate obtained using a sterile overtube[67] may be the most efficient means of confirming the diagnosis and excluding other causes of malabsorption such as celiac sprue and giardiasis.

TREATMENT

Initial management consists of fluid and nutritional support, including the replacement of vitamin deficiencies. After the diagnosis of bacterial overgrowth is made, an attempt to identify an underlying cause should be made. Surgical correction of anatomic causes of intestinal stasis should be considered. Severe motility disorders are more difficult to manage. Octreotide administered to patients with scleroderma for 3 weeks has been shown to clear bacterial overgrowth, as demonstrated by reversal of abnormal breath hydrogen excretion.[78] Octreotide stimulated intestinal motor activity in these patients. This is a very significant observation, because other clinical trials using higher doses of octreotide have suggested that this drug may cause steatorrhea secondary to hypomotility and bacterial overgrowth.[79] Prokinetic agents such as cisapride

TABLE 74-5
Treatment for Bacterial Overgrowth

Nutritional Supplementation
Increase calorie intake
Correction of micronutrient deficiencies (e.g., vitamin B_{12})

Correction of Intestinal Stasis
Surgery (e.g., resection of strictures)
Prokinetic agents (e.g., octreotide in scleroderma)

Antibiotic Treatment

have been shown to normalize intestinal motility in patients with motor disorders,[80] but their role in treating bacterial overgrowth remains to be explored (Table 74-5).

Often, the underlying lesion is not correctable, and the primary treatment is directed at suppressing the bacterial overgrowth with antibiotics. Numerous antibiotics have been reported to be effective, including tetracycline, chloramphenicol, ampicillin, erythromycin, clindomycin, metronidazole, and oral aminoglycosides. Most patients experience a sustained remission after a single 7- to 10-day course of therapy.[2] Some patients experience recurrence of symptoms after completion of a course of antibiotics. For these patients, rotating antibiotic regimens are recommended as treatment, such as 2 weeks of metronidazole followed by 2 weeks of oral gentamycin.[2] The dramatic response that some patients with chronic underlying gastrointestinal disease have to a brief course of antibiotic treatment makes bacterial overgrowth an important entity to consider in their management.

The reader is directed to Chapter 9, Motility of the Small Intestine; Chapter 26, The Gastrointestinal Microflora; Chapter 45, Approach to Gastrointestinal Problems in the Elderly; Chapter 48, Approach to the Patient Requiring Nutritional Supplementation; and Chapter 131, Microbiologic Studies.

REFERENCES

1. Kirsch M. Bacterial overgrowth. Am J Gastroenterol 1990;85: 231.
2. Sherman PM. Bacterial overgrowth. In: Yamada T, Alpers DH, Owyang C, et al., eds. Textbook of gastroenterology. 1st ed. Philadelphia: JB Lippincott, 1991:1530.
3. Faber K. Perniciöse Anämie bei Dunndarmstricturen. Berl Klin Wochenschr 1897;34:643.
4. Barker WH, Hummel LE. Macrocytic anemia in association with intestinal strictures and anastomoses. Bull Johns Hopkins Hosp 1939;46:215.
5. Roberts SH, Janes O, Jarvis EH. Bacterial contamination of the small intestine is an important cause of occult malabsorption in the elderly. Lancet 1977;2:1194.
6. Davidson GP, Robb TA, Kirubakaran CP. Bacterial contamination of the small intestine as an important cause of chronic diarrhea and abdominal pain: diagnosis by breath hydrogen test. Pediatrics 1984;74:229.
7. Bishop RF, Anderson CM. Bacterial flora of stomach and small intestine in children with intestinal obstruction. Arch Dis Child 1960;35:487.
8. Swan RW. Stagnant loop syndrome resulting from small bowel

irradiation injury and intestinal bypass. Gynecol Oncol 1974;8:441.

9. Russell RM, Abadi P, Ismail-Beigi F. Role of bacterial overgrowth on the malabsorption syndrome of primary small intestinal lymphoma. Cancer 1977;89:8579.

10. Toskes PP, Donaldson RM. The blind loop syndrome. In: Sleisinger MH, Fordtran JS, eds. Gastrointestinal disease: pathophysiology, diagnosis, management. Philadelphia: WB Saunders, 1989;1289.

11. Browning GG, Buchan KA, Mackay C. The effect of vagotomy and drainage on the small bowel flora. Gut 1974;15:139.

12. Schonsby H., Halvorsen JF, Hofstad T, Hovdenak N. Stagnant loop syndrome in patients with continent ileostomy (intraabdominal ileal reservoir). Gut 1983;18:795.

13. Goldstein F, Wirts CW, Kowlessar OD. Diabetic diarrhea and steatorrhea: microbiologic and clinical observations. Ann Intern Med 1970;72:215.

14. Kahn IJ, Jeffries GH, Sleisenger MH. Malabsorption in intestinal scleroderma: correction by antibiotics. N Engl J Med 1966;274:1339.

15. Pearson AJ, Brezechwa-Ajdukiewicz, McCarthy CF. Intestinal pseudo-obstruction with bacterial overgrowth in the small intestine. Am J Dig Dis 1969;14:200.

16. Vantrappen G, Hanssens J, Hellemans J, et al. The interdigestive motor complex of normal subjects and patients with bacterial overgrowth of the small intestine. J Clin Invest 1977;59:1158.

17. Vantrappen G, Janssens J, Coremans G, et al. Gastrointestinal motility disorders. Dig Dis Sci 1986;31(Suppl):5S.

18. Griffin WO Jr, Richardson JD, Medley ES. Prevention of small bowel contamination by ileocecal valve. South Med J 1971;64:1056.

19. King CE, Toskes PP. Small intestinal bacterial overgrowth. Gastroenterology 1979;76:1035.

20. Dowling RH. The short bowel syndrome. Gastroenterology 1979;77:572.

21. Atwater JS, Butt HR, Priestly JT. Gastrojejunocolic fistulae with special reference to associated nutritional deficiencies and certain surgical aspects. Ann Surg 1943;117:414.

22. Drasar BS, Shiner M, McCleod GM. Studies on the intestinal flora. I. The bacterial flora of the gastrointestinal tract in healthy and achlorhydric persons. Gastroenterology 1969;56:71.

23. Ruddell WSJ, Losowsky MS. Severe diarrhoea due to small intestinal colonization during cimetidine treatment. Br Med J 1980;281:273.

24. Greenlee HB, Gelbart SM, DeOrio AJ, et al. The influence of gastric surgery on the intestinal flora. Am J Clin Nutr 1977;30:1826.

25. Brown WR, Savage DC, Dubois RS, et al. Intestinal microflora of immunoglobulin-deficient and normal human subjects. Gastroenterology 1972;62:1143.

26. Budhraja M, Levendoglu MD, Kocka F, et al. Duodenal mucosal T cell subpopulation and bacterial cultures in acquired immune deficiency syndrome. Am J Gastroenterol 1987;82:427.

27. McEvoy A, Dutton J, James OFW. Bacterial contamination of the small intestine is an important cause of occult malabsorption in the elderly. Br Med J 1983;287:789.

28. Donald JP, Kitchingham G, Donald F, Kupfer RM. The diagnosis of small bowel bacterial overgrowth in elderly patients. J Am Geriatr Soc 1992;40:692.

29. Toskes PP, Giannella RA, Jervis HR, et al. Small intestinal mucosal injury in the experimental blind loop syndrome. Gastroenterology 1975;68:1193.

30. Ament ME, Shimoda SS, Saunders DR, et al. Pathogenesis of steatorrhea in three cases of small intestinal stasis syndrome. Gastroenterology 1972;63:728.

31. Sherman P, Fleming N, Forstner J, et al. Bacteria and the mucus blanket in experimental small bowel bacterial overgrowth. Am J Pathol 1987;126:527.

32. Cameron DG, Watson GM, Witts LJ. The experimental production of macrocytic anemia by operations of the intestinal tract. Blood 1949;4:803.

33. King CE, Toskes PP. The experimental rat blind loop preparation: a model for small-intestine bacterial overgrowth in man.

In: Pfeiffer CJ, ed. Animal models for intestinal disease. Boca Raton, FL: CRC Press, 1985:217.

34. Tabaqchi S., Hatzioanuou J, Booth CC. Bile-salt deconjugation and steatorrhea in patients with the stagnant loop syndrome. Lancet 1968;2:12.

35. Kim YS, Spritz N, Blum M, et al. The role of altered bile acid metabolism in the steatorrhea of experimental blind-loop syndrome. J Clin Invest 1966;45:956.

36. Simon GL, Gorbach SL. The human intestinal microflora. Dig Dis Sci 1986;31(Suppl):147S.

37. Schonsby H. Osteomalacia in the stagnant loop syndrome. Acta Med Scand [Suppl] 1977;603:39.

38. Brin MF, Fetell MR, Green PHA, et al. Blind loop syndrome, vitamin E malabsorption and spinocerebellar degeneration. Neurology 1985;35:338.

39. Riepe SP, Goldstein J, Alpers DH. Effect of secreted *Bacteroides* proteases on human intestinal brush border hydrolases. J Clin Invest 1980;66:314.

40. Sherman P, Wesley A, Forstner G. Sequential disaccharidase loss in rat intestinal blind loops: impact of malnutrition. Am J Physiol 1985;248:G626.

41. Giannella RA, Rout WR, Toskes PP. Jejunal brush border injury and impaired sugar and amino acid uptake in the blind loop syndrome. Gastroenterology 1974;67:95.

42. Sherman P, Lichtman S. Small bowel bacterial overgrowth syndrome. Dig Dis 1987;5:157.

43. Jonas A, Krishnan C, Forstner G. Pathogenesis of mucosal injury in the blind loop syndrome: release of disaccharidases from brush border membrane extracts of bacteria obtained from intestinal blind loops in rats. Gastroenterology 1978;75:791.

44. Jones EA, Craigie A, Tavill AS, et al. Protein metabolism in the intestinal stagnant loop syndrome. Gut 1968;9:466.

45. Rutgeerts L, Mainguet P, Tytgat G, et al. Enterokinase in contaminated small-bowel syndrome. Digestion 1974;10:249.

46. King CE, Toskes PP. Protein-losing enteropathy in the human and experimental rat blind-loop syndrome. Gastroenterology 1981;80:834.

47. Giannella RA, Broitman SA, Zamchek N. Competition between bacteria and intrinsic factor for vitamin B_{12}: implications for vitamin B_{12} malabsorption in intestinal bacterial overgrowth. Gastroenterology 1972;62:255.

48. Welkos SL, Toskes PP, Baer H. Importance of anaerobic bacteria in the cobalamin malabsorption of the experimental rat blind loop syndrome. Gastroenterology 1981;80:313.

49. Brandt LJ, Bernstein LH, Wagle A. Production of vitamin B_{12} analogues in patients with small bowel bacterial overgrowth. Ann Intern Med 1977;87:546.

50. Lervol L, Eugene C, Anciaux ML, et al. Polynevrite compliquant une colonisation bacterienne chronique du grele an cours d'une diverticulose jejunale. Gastroenterol Clin Biol 1988;12:585.

51. Tabaqchali S, Pallis C. Reversible nicotinamide deficiency encephalopathy in a patient with jejunal diverticulosis. Gut 1970;11:1024.

52. Giannella RA, Toskes PP. Gastrointestinal bleeding and iron absorption in the experimental loop syndrome. Am J Clin Nutr 1976;29:754.

53. Lichtman SN, Sartor RB, Keku J, Schwab JH. Hepatic inflammation in rats with experimental small intestinal bacterial overgrowth. Gastroenterology 1990;98:414.

54. Lichtman SN, Keku J, Clark RL, et al. Biliary tract disease in rats with experimental small bowel bacterial overgrowth. Hepatology 1991;13:766.

55. Lichtman SN, Keku J, Schwab JH, Sartor RB. Hepatic injury associated with small bowel bacterial overgrowth in rats is prevented by metronidazole and tetracycline. Gastroenterology 1991;100:513.

56. Luukkonen P, Valtonen V, Sivonen A, et al. Fecal bacteriology and reservoir ileitis in patients operated on for ulcerative colitis. Dis Colon Rectum 1988;31:864.

57. O'Connell PR, Rankin DR, Weiland LH, Kelly KA. Enteric bacteriology, absorption, morphology and emptying after ileal pouch–anal anastomosis. Br J Surg 1986;73:909.

58. Bjornekett A, Hoverstad T, Hovig T. Bacterial overgrowth. Scand J Gastroenterol 1985;109:123.

59. Banwell JG, Kister LA, Giannella RA, et al. Small intestinal bacterial overgrowth syndrome. Gastroenterology 1981;80:834.
60. Ely PH. The bowel bypass syndrome: a response to bacterial peptidoglycans. J Am Acad Dermatol 1980;2:473.
61. Jorizzo RL, Apisarnthanarax P, Subrt P, et al. Bowel by-pass syndrome without bowel by-pass. Arch Intern Med 1983;143:457.
62. Hocking MP, Duerson MC, O'Leary JP, Woodward ER. Jejuno-ileal bypass for morbid obesity. N Engl J Med 1983;308:995.
63. Gracey M. The contaminated small bowel syndrome: pathogenesis, diagnosis and treatment. Am J Clin Nutr 1979;32:234.
64. Drasar BS Shiner M. Studies on the intestinal flora. II. Bacterial flora of the small intestine in patients with gastrointestinal disorders. Gut 1969;10:812.
65. Thadepallie H, Lou SMA, Bach VT, et al. Microflora of the small intestine. Am J Surg 1979;138:845.
66. Liebman WM, Rosenthal P. Evaluation of the string test in intestinal bacterial overgrowth. Am J Dis Child 1983;13-7:1177.
67. Bardhan FK, Gyr K, Begliner C, et al. Diagnosis of bacterial overgrowth after culturing proximal small-bowel aspirate obtained during routine upper gastrointestinal endoscopy. Scand J Gastroenterol 1992;27:253
68. Northfield TC, Drasar BS, Wright JT. Value of small intestinal bile acid analysis in the diagnosis of the stagnant loop syndrome. Gut 1973;14:341.
69. Hoverstad T, Bjorneklett A, Fausa O, Midtvedt T. Short-chain fatty acids in the small-bowel bacterial overgrowth syndrome. Scand J Gastroenterol 1985;20:492.
70. Orenstein SR, Whitington PF. Intestinal bacterial overgrowth in the pediatric patient. J Tenn Med Assoc 1984;77:198.
71. King CE, Toskes PP. Breath tests in the diagnosis of small intestinal bacterial overgrowth. CRC Crit Rev Clin Lab Sci 1984;21:269.
72. Pruthi HS, Mehta SK, Pathak CM, et al. Evaluation of ^{14}C-D-xylose breath test to diagnosis of small intestinal bacterial overgrowth. Indian J Med Res 1984;80:598.
73. Rhodes JM, Middleton P, Jewell DP. The lactulose hydrogen breath test as a diagnostic test for small-bowel bacterial overgrowth. Scand J Gastroenterol 1979;14:333.
74. Khin-Maung-U, Tin-Aye, Du-Tin-Myint, et al. In vitro hydrogen production by enteric bacteria cultured from children with small bowel bacterial overgrowth. J Pediatr Gastroenterol Nutr 1992;14:192.
75. Corazza GR, Menozzi MG, Strocchi A, et al. The diagnosis of small bowel bacterial overgrowth: reliability of jejunal culture and inadequacy of breath hydrogen testing. Gastroenterology 1990;98:302.
76. Kerlin P, Wong L. Breath hydrogen testing in bacterial overgrowth of the small intestine. Gastroenterology 1988;95:982.
77. Setchell KDR, Harrison DL, Gilbert JM, Mupthy GM. Serum unconjugated bile acids: qualitative and quantitative profiles in ileal resection and bacterial overgrowth. Clin Chim Acta 1985;152:297.
78. Soudah HC, Hasler WL, Owyang C. Effect of octreotide on intestinal motility and bacterial overgrowth in scleroderma. N Engl J Med 1991;325:1461.
79. Witt K, Pedersen NT. The long-acting somatostatin analogue SMS 202-995 causes malabsorption. Scand J Gastroenterol 1989;24:1248
80. Camilleri M, Malagelada JR, Abell TL, et al. Effect of six weeks of treatment with cisapride in gastroparesis and intestinal pseudoobstruction. Gastroenterology 1989;96:704.

Textbook of Gastroenterology, second edition, edited by Tadataka Yamada. JB Lippincott Company, Philadelphia © 1995.

CHAPTER 75

Short Bowel Syndrome

Thomas A. Brasitus   Michael D. Sitrin

With improvements in surgical, anesthetic, and postoperative techniques, an increasing number of patients undergo and survive resection of an extensive amount of the small intestine. A large patient population now exists with the short bowel syndrome, a term used to refer to the clinical consequences of small bowel resection, with or without some additional loss of colon. Even this definition is somewhat misleading, however, because it implies that there is a well recognized clinical pattern in patients with intestinal resections. The clinical consequences of removing a portion of the small intestine are, in fact, extremely variable and depend on a number of well known factors (see Factors Influencing the Metabolic Consequences of Intestinal Resection).

DISEASE COMMONLY LEADING TO SHORT BOWEL SYNDROME

Adults

As shown in Table 75-1, there are a number of different causes of the short bowel syndrome in adults. In these patients, the most common disorders leading to this syndrome are intestinal resection after a vascular insult to the small bowel, and regional enteritis with multiple bowel resections.[1,2] Risk factors for intestinal vascular insults include age, long-standing congestive heart failure, atherosclerotic and valvular heart disease, chronic diuretic use, hypercoagulable states, and use of oral contraceptives. Although no longer routinely recommended or performed, jejunoileal bypass operations for morbid obesity still account for a number of cases of this syndrome. Less common causes of short bowel syndrome include abdominal trauma, primary and secondary neoplasms of the gut, and radiation enteropathy. Rarely, inadvertent gastroileal anastomosis for peptic ulcer disease may produce a clinical picture indistinguishable from that seen after massive intestinal resection.[1]

Children

The etiology of the short bowel syndrome in children can be divided into prenatal and postnatal causes (Table 75-2), with most underlying conditions originating in intrauterine life.[3,4]

TABLE 75-1
Causes of Short Bowel Syndrome in Adults

Vascular Insults to Small Intestine
Thrombosis or embolus of superior mesenteric artery
Thrombosis of superior mesenteric vein
Volvulus of small intestine
Strangulated hernia

Postsurgical
Jejunoileal bypass for morbid obesity
Abdominal trauma with resultant bowel resection
Inadvertent gastroileal anastomosis for peptic ulcer
    disease

Miscellaneous Conditions
Regional enteritis
Radiation enteropathy
Primary and secondary neoplasms involving the gut

TABLE 75-2
Causes of Short Bowel Syndrome in Infants and Children

Prenatal
Vascular accidents
Intestinal atresia
Midgut or segmental volvulus
Abdominal wall defect

Postnatal
Necrotizing enterocolitis
Trauma
Inflammatory bowel disease
Midgut segmental volvulus
Hirschsprung's disease
Radiation enteritis
Venous thrombosis
Arterial thrombosis
    or embolus

Antenatal vascular accidents presenting as intestinal atresia are a particularly common etiology for this syndrome. Midgut or segmental volvulus secondary to malfixation and malrotation also quite frequently lead to this syndrome, and may arise in utero or at any time postnatally. Necrotizing enterocolitis increasingly has been recognized as a cause of the short bowel syndrome in neonatal units.[3,4] Other, less common etiologic postnatal factors include Hirschsprung's disease involving the small bowel, mesenteric vascular embolism or thrombosis secondary to hypercoagulable states, cardiac valvular lesions with vegetations, and abdominal trauma. Radiation enteritis or Crohn's disease also can cause this syndrome, but generally affect an older age group.

FACTORS INFLUENCING THE METABOLIC CONSEQUENCES OF INTESTINAL RESECTION

Several important factors have been shown to influence nutrient absorption after small bowel resection.[2,5-7] These include the extent and site of resected bowel; the presence of the ileocecal valve; the condition of the remaining bowel and other digestive organs such as the pancreas and liver; and the degree of adaptation in the residual small and large intestine.

Extent and Site of Resected Bowel

A priori, the more extensive the resection of bowel, the greater the loss of absorbing surface for nutrients, water, and electrolytes transported by active and diffusional mechanisms, and, therefore, the greater the mortality and morbidity of the operation. Although this rule is generally true, because the length of intestine varies among individuals, it is clear that the length of the *residual* intestine and its function are more important than the amount of small bowel removed per se.[7] The amount of small bowel remaining after resection determines the degree of absorbing surface for lumenal nutrients as well as the transit time of the lumenal intestinal contents. In this regard, another confounding variable is that in vivo measurements of the bowel at surgery may be very difficult secondary to the variable extent of relaxation or spasm.[7] Thus, although survival without parenteral nutrition is unusual if less than 1 foot of jejunum or ileum is present in addition to the patient's duodenum, a number of cases have been reported with long-term survivals in patients with 6 to 18 inches of remaining jejunum plus the duodenum.[2] It appears that approximately half of the small intestine may be resected in patients without significant problems in sustaining normal nutritional requirements.[2] Patients with 75% or greater small intestinal resections, however, almost invariably have severe malabsorption problems and are the most difficult to manage.[2]

The site of intestinal resection also is of prime importance in determining its metabolic consequences in these patients.[2,5–7] Proteins, carbohydrates, fats, and most water-soluble vitamins as well as minerals usually are absorbed along the length of the small intestine, but particularly in the duodenum and jejunum. After loss of the proximal intestine, a normal ileum usually will take over most of these absorptive functions; however, because the proximal small intestine is also the site of cholecystokinin and secretin synthesis and release, loss of this segment may result in decreased release of biliary and exocrine pancreatic secretions, further compounding the decreased transit time and loss of absorptive surfaces in these patients.[6] In humans, ileal nutrients have been shown to be important regulators of gastric emptying and small bowel transit.[5] The loss of this segment of the small intestine may therefore lead to decreased intestinal transit time in such patients.

The loss of ileum also is metabolically more important than loss of jejunum because it is the selective site for absorption of both conjugated bile salts and intrinsic factor-bound vitamin B_{12}.[2,6,7] The jejunum may compensate, at least partially, for bile salt losses after ileal resection by increased diffusion across its mucosa.[6] Loss of less than 100 cm of ileum leads to a reduction in the enterohepatic circulation of bile salts and excess entry of bile salts into the colon, with production of "cholerrheic" diarrhea (Table 75-3). In these patients, the liver is able partially to compensate for the loss of these bile salts by increasing its synthesis rate.[6] Thus, steatorrhea usually is mild (<20 g/day of fat). More extensive loss of ileum (>100 cm), however, may result in severe bile salt malabsorption.[6] Under these circumstances, because the hepatic synthesis of bile salts is limited (fourfold to eightfold increases are possible), a marked reduction in the circulating pool of bile salts is seen, thereby markedly decreasing micelle formation, leading to severe steatorrhea (>20 g/day of fat) and steatorrheic diarrhea (see Table 75-3). In addition, hepatic synthesis of glycine-conjugated bile salts is decreased in these patients, resulting in increased passive–nonionic uptake of bile salts, further compounding this problem.

Patients usually tolerate removal of short lengths of ileum (<50 cm) without significant malabsorption of intrinsic factor-bound vitamin B_{12}.[7] Loss of larger amounts of ileum (>60–100 cm), however, leads to inadequate absorption of this water-soluble vitamin.[7] A deficiency of this vitamin, if uncorrected, can result in the development of megaloblastic anemia and peripheral neuropathy, and ultimately lead to subacute combined degeneration of the spinal cord.[6]

Clinical experience also has shown that patients with combined small and large intestinal resections fare much worse than those with small intestinal resections alone.[7] The large intestine is an important organ with respect to the absorption of water, electrolytes, and even certain nutrients such as short-chain fatty acids. Normally, an adult ingests approximately 2 L of fluids per day and produces about 7 L of endogenous fluids through gastric, pancreatic, biliary, and small bowel secretions. Only 100 to 200 mL of this fluid volume is not reabsorbed. In patients who have a partial or total colectomy as well as extensive small bowel resections, critical dehydration and sodium and potassium depletion are more likely to develop.[6,7]

Presence of an Ileocecal Valve

After partial or total colectomy, the surgical removal of the ileocecal valve also appears to have important metabolic consequences. Removal of this valve results in decreased transit time of the lumenal contents within the small intestine.[6,7] Loss of this valve also may result in increased bacterial colonization of the remaining small intestine, deconjugation of bile salts, reduced absorption of fat and fat-soluble vitamins, and an increased entry of bile acids into the colon.[7] Vitamin B_{12} also may be metabolized by the increased bacteria in the small intestine, thereby reducing its absorption. Hence, shorter lengths of remaining intestine are therefore better tol-

---

TABLE 75-3
Features of Cholerrheic and Steatorrheic Diarrhea After Ileal Resection

VARIABLE	CHOLERRHEIC	STEATORRHEIC
Length of resection	<100 cm	>100 cm
Fecal bile acid output	Increased	Increased
Fecal bile acid loss compensated by hepatic synthesis	Partially compensated	Uncompensated
Decreased bile acid pool size	No	Yes
Steatorrhea	Variable, usually minimal	Yes
Response to low-fat diet	None	Yes
Response to cholestyramine	Yes, but variable	None, may even be exacerbated

erated with fewer metabolic problems in patients with intact ileocecal valves.

Condition of Remaining Bowel and Other Digestive Organs

After loss of small intestine, the function of residual bowel is critical to the patient's survival and long-term health.[6,7] For example, in patients whose intestine has been resected because of Crohn's disease, lymphoma, or radiation enteritis, diseased or functionally impaired remaining intestine will have reduced absorptive capacity, and management difficulties will be increased. Pancreatic exocrine function also may be significantly impaired in severely malnourished patients.[6] Gastric hypersecretion may occur after extensive small bowel resection (see Gastric Hypersecretion and Peptic Ulcer Disease). In such cases, the reduced small bowel lumenal pH also interferes with exocrine pancreatic digestion.[2,6,7]

Degree of Adaptation in the Residual Small and Large Intestine

Changes in Structure and Function After Resection

Morphologic and functional adaptive changes in the residual small intestine have been extensively studied in animals, whereas similar studies in humans have been relatively sparse.[6,8-10] In the rat, resection of the proximal and middle intestine has been shown to lead to an increase in the circumference, thickness, and height of villi in the residual ileum.[8] Moreover, hyperplasia of residual ileal mucosa after jejunal resection appears to occur from accelerated cellular proliferation and migration with a concomitant reduction in the life span of individual cells.[8] Similar but less impressive and more variable morphologic alterations have been noted in the jejunum of animals after ileal resection.[8] In humans, proximal

mucosal cell hyperplasia also has been found in intestinal biopsy specimens after resection.[8] There is no evidence, however, suggesting that intestinal villi became taller in humans, unlike in animal studies.[8]

Experiments in animals have suggested that enhanced segmental absorption, as a consequence of adaptive ileal mucosal hyperplasia (Fig. 75-1), may permit normal growth and development by compensating for the loss of intestinal transport functions. After proximal intestinal resection, increased absorption of glucose, maltose, sucrose, bile acids, vitamin B$_{12}$, and calcium all have been documented.[8] These phenomena, with the possible exception of calcium absorption, appear to be proportional to the number of epithelial cells per unit length or to the mucosal weight, suggesting that these functional transport adaptive changes are secondary to an increase in the number of absorption cells, rather than to an increased capacity of individual cells. It has even been suggested that individual cells may be functionally immature,[8] although this concept has been questioned.[11] Calcium transport, however, may indeed be increased in individual cells.[8]

Enzymatic and metabolic alterations have been noted in the hyperplastic mucosa seen after proximal intestinal resection in animals.[8] The specific activities of sodium–potassium-dependent adenosine triphosphatase, peptide hydrolases, enterokinase, and enzymes involved in DNA and pyrimidine synthesis all have been shown to be increased, whereas the activities of disaccharidase- and lipid-reesterifying enzymes of individual cells are reduced.[8] The metabolism of glucose by means of the pentose phosphate pathway also has been found to be significantly increased in this hyperplastic mucosa.[8] After extensive bowel resection in humans, studies have shown that there is a gradual improvement in absorption of fat, nitrogen, and carbohydrates, particularly glucose.[8] Although the mechanisms involved in these functional adaptive changes are likely to represent an increased number of absorptive cells, at least in part, they remain to be elucidated.[8] In contrast to these findings, however, lactose absorption clearly is impaired in patients after extensive resection, probably secondary to reduced total lactase activity and rapid transit.[8]

Even less is known about the adaptive response of the colon

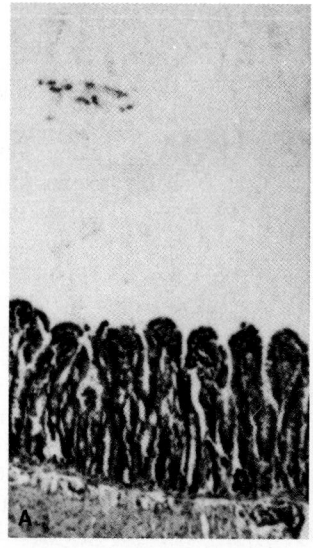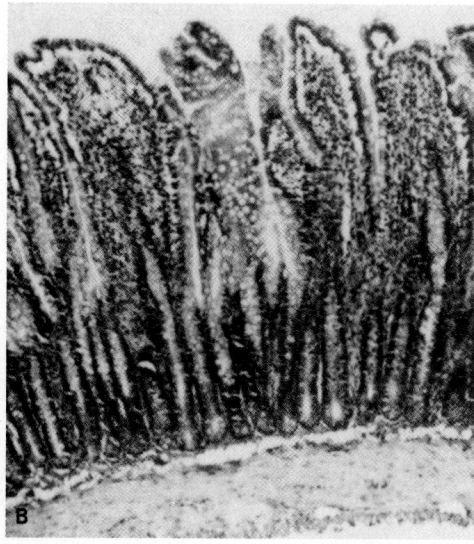

FIGURE 75-1. Ileal hyperplasia after jejunal resection in rats fed chow diet. **(A)** Normal ileum. **(B)** Ileum 1 month after jejunal resection. (Hematoxylin and eosin stain, formalin-fixed sections, original magnification ×1000.)

than about enteric adaptation after intestinal resection in animals and humans (for reviews, see references 9 and 10). Thus, in humans, functional adaptation by the colon has been relatively poorly documented.[9,10] Preliminary studies suggest that after intestinal resection or jejunoileal bypass for obesity, the colon may increase its absorption of glucose and amino acids.[9,10]

Potential Stimuli for Adaptation

Several possible mechanisms have been proposed for stimulating small bowel mucosal hyperplasia after intestinal resection (for reviews, see references 6, 9, and 10). These include increased exposure of the residual bowel to dietary nutrients; stimulation by biliary and pancreatic secretions; trophic effects of hormones and other factors; stimulation by polyamines; neural factors; and increased blood flow to the residual bowel. As with the morphologic and functional data discussed in previous sections, most of the experiments in this area of investigation have involved animals rather than humans.

Considerable experimental evidence has accumulated indicating that an increased concentration of nutrients in the intestinal lumen of residual bowel plays an important role in intestinal adaptation.[6,7] It has been shown repeatedly that without intestinal nutrients in the lumen, adaptation does not occur, and, in fact, hypoplasia may develop.[6,7] Intestinal hypoplasia also has been shown to occur even in patients with short bowel syndrome receiving total parenteral nutrition. The mechanisms responsible for this phenomenon remain unclear. Bulk or nonnutritive agents, however, usually do not appear to stimulate mucosal growth; therefore, absorption and metabolism of lumenal nutrients appear necessary for intestinal adaptation.[6]

Nutrients in the intestinal lumen also stimulate biliary and exocrine pancreatic secretions, which may produce mucosal hyperplasia directly, especially when present in higher-than-usual concentrations in the residual ileum.[6,7] Ileal mucosal growth is markedly enhanced when the bile and pancreatic ducts are transplanted into this segment in normal rats.[8] Pancreatic secretions appear to have the most impressive effects with respect to stimulation of mucosal hyperplasia. Pancreatic secretions also alter the activities of certain brush border membrane enzymes in the intestine.[8] Again, however, it is unclear how these intralumenal factors induce intestinal hyperplasia after resection.

Lumenal nutrients also may cause the release of hormones or other factors with trophic effects on the small bowel.[6,8] Alternatively, intestinal resection might remove inhibitory enteric factors, causing the response of trophic factors to be exaggerated.[6] Parabiotic studies in rats,[12] moreover, have strongly suggested that hormonal agents stimulate mucosal growth after intestinal resection. Although several different hormones have been suggested as candidate trophic hormones, gastrin has received the most attention.[6,8] Based on investigations from a number of different laboratories,[6] however, it is unlikely that this hormone plays an important role in the adaptive hyperplasia of the residual intestine, with the possible exception of the duodenum. Parenteral administration of secretin and cholecystokinin has been shown to stimulate mucosal growth in total parenteral nutrition-treated animals,[6] but it appears that this effect of these hormones is

most likely mediated through their action on biliary and pancreatic secretions, rather than by direct trophism.[6] Other hormones, including corticosteroids and, in particular, enteroglucagon, appear to be important in the induction of intestinal hyperplasia.[8] Similarly, prostaglandins, epidermal growth factor, and growth hormone-releasing factor (somatocrinin) all appear to stimulate epithelial cell proliferation in the small intestine.[8] Whether enteroglucagon or any of these other factors, given as pharmacons, will prove clinically useful for the stimulation of intestinal hyperplasia in patients with the short bowel syndrome, remains to be determined.

The growth-associated polyamines, putrescine, spermidine, and spermine, have received increasing attention with respect to their possible role in adaptation after intestinal resection.[7,13,14] Initial studies suggested that ornithine decarboxylase, the rate-limiting enzyme in polyamine biosynthesis, might be critical for adaptive hyperplasia in this organ.[13] This concept has been questioned,[14] however, and it appears that the levels of the polyamines or the activities of other biosynthetic enzymes such as S-adenosylmethionine decarboxylase may be more important in this phenomenon. Studies of the possible role of polyamines in adaptive mucosal growth are at an early stage, and much needs to be learned before they conclusively can be assigned a role in the adaptive process seen after intestinal resection.

Still other possible mechanisms, such as altered innervation or blood flow to the residual intestine, may play a part in intestinal adaptation,[6] but need to be studied further.

Regardless of the exact mechanisms involved, which are likely to be multiple, it appears that adaptation of the remaining bowel occurs after intestinal resection over the course of several months to a year after surgery.[6,7] This factor is clearly important to the overall health, nutrition, and survival of patients with the short bowel syndrome.

CLINICAL FEATURES

Overview of Clinical Course

The clinical course of patients with short bowel syndrome involves three phases—early, intermediate, and late—that tend to merge with one another[7]:

In patients with extensive (75% or greater) small bowel resections, diarrhea is the predominant early clinical feature. In the immediate postoperative period, therefore, dehydration and electrolyte deficiencies, particularly hyponatremia, hypokalemia, hypocalcemia, and even hypomagnesemia, may be troublesome.

An intermediate phase then follows, during which malabsorption predominates, at times with major weight loss and the development of nutritional deficiencies. During the late phase, despite continuing diarrhea and steatorrhea, body weight frequently stabilizes, although at a lower level than before resection. In certain patients, however, even with optimal dietary and drug regimens as well as fully developed adaptive changes, the length of their intestine is inadequate to maintain overall nutrition without supplementary support (see Nutritional Therapy of the Patient With Short Bowel Syndrome). Even in these patients, adequate replacement therapy usually is compatible with a normal life expectancy.

Specific Clinical Features

Diarrhea

Diarrhea is almost invariably seen in patients after extensive bowel resection. The pathogenesis of the diarrhea is multifactorial,[6,7] and may involve: decreased transit time secondary to removed bowel and to motility disturbances (Fig. 75-2); an increase in the osmolarity of the lumenal contents secondary to malabsorption of lactose and other carbohydrates, which may be accentuated in patients with bacterial overgrowth due to decreased enterocyte brush border membrane disaccharidase activities caused by the bacteria; increased secretion of water and electrolytes, particularly in patients with ileal resections, secondary to increased colonic dihydroxy bile acids that, in turn, stimulate adenylate cyclase activity—in this regard, studies have emphasized that the fecal pH was the most important determinant of diarrhea in bile acid malabsorption due to ileal resection, because pH determines the amount of bile salts with secretory effects in solution[15]; loss of ileal and right colonic absorptive capacity for sodium chloride,[16] which may account for the subset of patients in which postresection stool weight and diarrhea do not respond to cholestyramine or a low-fat diet (see Dietary Management); and steatorrhea, leading to an increase in lumenal distal small intestinal and colonic fatty acids that in turn stimulates adenylate cyclase activity in these organs, resulting in secretion of water and electrolytes.

Given the complex nature of the diarrhea in patients with the short bowel syndrome, it is critical to evaluate thoroughly the possible cause of this clinical feature in each patient to

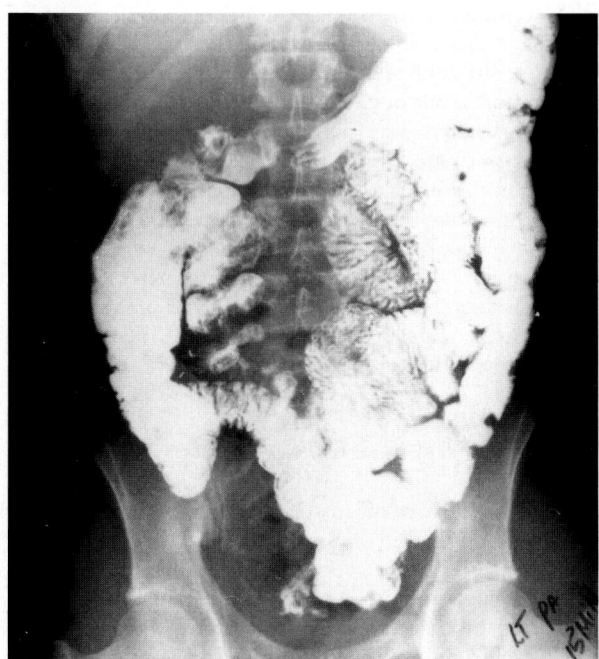

FIGURE 75-2. Small bowel radiograph of a patient after resection of all but 100 cm of small intestine after a midgut volvulus with infarction. There is a paucity of small bowel and a rapid intestinal transit, with barium reaching the colon within 15 minutes after ingestion.

use appropriate dietary and drug therapy (see Medical Management of Short Bowel Syndrome, and Nutritional Therapy of the Patient With Short Bowel Syndrome).

Gastric Hypersecretion and Peptic Ulcer Disease

Gastric hypersecretion is a well recognized feature of extensive small bowel resection in both humans and animals.[6,7,17-19] This phenomenon may at times not only lead to serious peptic ulcer disease, but contribute to the already compromised small intestinal absorption in patients with short bowel syndrome by inducing diffuse mucosal damage, impairing micelle formation, and reducing intralumenal lipid digestion by means of pH-induced inhibition of pancreatic enzymes.[6] These latter effects of hypersecretion as well as the large volumes of gastric juice may increase postresection diarrhea. In addition, breakdown of surgical anastomoses occasionally has been reported in these patients.[6] Gastric hypersecretion has been documented to occur within 24 hours after resection, almost always gradually lessens with time, and can be managed medically.[6,7] Therefore, surgery is rarely if ever necessary to treat patients with gastric hypersecretion and should be avoided, because it may lead to additional nutritional management problems. Although it appears that the length of small bowel removed correlates roughly with the degree of hypersecretion, it is not clear whether jejunal or ileal resection is the more potent stimulus to gastric hypersecretion.[7]

Serum gastrin concentrations have been reported to be elevated in humans and dogs with resected bowels,[17] suggesting that acid hypersecretion may be secondary to increased stimulation by this hormone or to its trophic effects on the gastric mucosa.[17] Others have proposed that removal of the small bowel might affect gastrin catabolism or that another hormone that normally inhibits gastrin effects on the stomach might be removed with the resected bowel.[6] In other cases of hypersecretion after resection, however, serum gastrin levels have not been found to be elevated.[20] Normal acid secretion also has been noted in patients with hypergastremia[6]; moreover, certain patients even manifest hypochlorhydria after intestinal resection.[7] Hence, the exact mechanisms involved in gastric hypersecretion after intestinal resection are unclear.

Nutritional Deficiencies

As noted, after extensive resection of the small bowel there is reduced absorption of virtually all nutrients, including protein and, particularly, fat and carbohydrates.[6,21,22] The caloric deprivation caused by impaired absorption of these nutrients results in severe weight loss, lassitude, weakness, and fatigue. In children, growth retardation also can be expected. Fluid loss is especially common during the first few weeks after surgery, with fecal effluents often greater than 5 L/day, particularly with concomitant partial or total colectomy. Unless replacement therapy is promptly instituted, severe hypovolemia, hyponatremia, and hypokalemia, with attendant weakness, may develop. The consequences of impaired absorption of other electrolytes and nutrients become manifest with time. Calcium and magnesium deficiencies also may occur in these patients secondary to the malabsorption of fatty acids that form soap complexes with these divalent cations.[21] Calcium depletion can be further exacerbated by malabsorption of vitamin D. Although calcium deficiency normally results in an increased secretion of parathyroid hormone, in patients with concomitant calcium and magnesium depletion, release of this hormone is decreased secondary to magnesium deficiency.[21] Reduced absorption of these divalent cations in patients not only compounds their weakness, but may lead to tetany. Osteomalacia and osteoporosis also can occur as the duration of calcium, vitamin D, and protein malabsorption increases.

Steatorrhea is associated with decreased absorption of the fat-soluble vitamins, particularly vitamin D, but also vitamins A, K, and, rarely, E. Because serum levels of vitamin A are not always a dependable measure of deficiency of this vitamin, functional tests such as dark adaptation for vitamin A should be considered.[21] Although relatively uncommon, perhaps secondary to lumenal bacterial synthesis, vitamin K deficiency in these patients may cause purpura and even generalized bleeding.[21]

Although vitamin B[12] deficiency is likely after all but the smallest ileal resection, the other water-soluble vitamins are generally well absorbed.[21,22] Occasionally, however, folate deficiency with the development of megaloblastic anemia has been reported, but is fairly uncommon.[22] Deficiencies of these fat-soluble vitamins as well as of iron, which is seen particularly after proximal intestinal resections, therefore all can be involved in anemia seen after intestinal resection.[22]

As with the water-soluble vitamins, trace metal absorption usually is sufficient in most patients after intestinal resection.[21,22] Zinc deficiency, with its attendant hypogeusia and dermatitis, may be seen occasionally, especially in those patients with extensive ileal resections.

Enteric Hyperoxaluria and Renal Calculi

An increase in the incidence of nephrolithiasis has been well documented in patients with ileal resections or ileal disease.[23–26] Hyperoxaluria frequently is present in these patients, and the calculi are predominantly calcium oxalate.[26] Moreover, the hyperoxaluria appears to be secondary to an increased absorption of dietary oxalate, particularly in the colon, involving at least two distinct mechanisms.[26] First, it would appear that the steatorrhea seen in certain of these patients may contribute to the increased absorption of oxalate through an increase in lumenal fatty acid, which by complexing to calcium prevents the formation of insoluble calcium oxalate.[26] The presence of hyperoxaluria in patients with steatorrhea of diverse etiologies lends further support to this contention. Second, bile salts and fatty acids in these patients also appear to cause nonspecific alterations in the colonic mucosal permeability, thereby again increasing oxalate absorption in this organ.[25,26] In this regard, oxalate always had been thought to be absorbed in the small intestine and colon through a passive, non–carrier-mediated pathway.[25] Studies by Knickelbein and colleagues,[27] however, have shown that both oxalate : OH and oxalate : Cl exchange occur on the brush border membranes of rabbit ileal epithelial cells. The importance of these transmembrane carrier-mediated pathways of oxalate transport in the pathogenesis of calcium oxalate nephrolithiasis, however, remains to be determined.

The mechanisms involved in the pathogenesis of calcium oxalate stones in these patients also need to be better defined. It is quite likely that other urinary factors, in addition to hyperoxaluria, are responsible for the increased renal calcium oxalate calculi.[28] These factors include a decreased urinary concentration of calcium-binding anions such as phosphate and citrate, and diminished urinary volume in these patients.

Risk of Bacterial Overgrowth

Patients with jejunoileal bypass procedures and ileocolonic resections appear to be at increased risk for the development of bacterial overgrowth. In patients with bypass, this appears to be the result of increased stasis in the excluded loop.[6] In patients with ileocolonic resections, bacterial overgrowth has been attributed to the loss of the ileocecal valve.[6] The latter explanation, however, has been questioned, because this valve almost certainly is not bacteriologically competent.[7] Some studies[7] have suggested that alterations in motility after resection of the terminal ileum/ileocecal valve–cecal complex are far more important in the pathogenesis of bacterial overgrowth in these patients.

Gallstones

It has been well documented that the incidence of gallstones is increased twofold to threefold in patients after ileal resection.[29,30] It generally has been assumed that interruption of the enterohepatic circulation of bile with attendant bile acid malabsorption leads to an increase in hepatic synthesis of cholesterol, thereby producing bile supersaturated with cholesterol and gallstones.[7] Although appealing, this explanation appears to be simplistic. For example, up to 40% of patients with ileectomies have had calcium-containing, radiopaque gallstones rather than radiolucent (cholesterol-rich) stones.[29] Moreover, although studies have shown that cholesterol supersaturation in bile or cholesterol gallstones occurs after this operation,[31] others have suggested that the bile actually becomes hyposaturated with cholesterol, with increasing loss of bile acids in the feces.[32] In addition, it appears that interruption of the enterohepatic circulation predisposes to an increased incidence of pigment stones.[32–34] Taken together, patients with ileal resections clearly have an increased number of gallstones, probably both cholesterol and pigment stones, but that further elucidation is needed of the mechanisms involved in these formations.

Jejunoileal Bypass Complications

Although an effective means of long-term weight reduction in patients with morbid obesity, jejunoileal bypass operations are being replaced as the procedure of choice in these patients by gastric bypass and gastroplasty in most hospitals, because of the problems that developed from exclusion of 90% of the small bowel from intestinal continuity and function.[35,36]

Many of the problems noted in patients after jejunoileal bypass operations are seen in patients with short bowel syndrome per se.[35,36] These include diarrhea leading to electrolyte disturbances, particularly hypokalemia and hypomagnesemia; fat malabsorption resulting in fat-soluble vitamin deficiencies, metabolic bone disease, renal calculi, and retinopathy; folate and vitamin B_{12} deficiencies; protein and carbohydrate malabsorption and maldigestion; and gallstones.

Another group of problems is unique or more commonly seen in patients with bypass operations. Although the exact etiology for these latter complications remains unclear, they appear to develop secondary to bacterial overgrowth in the bypassed bowel. This may in turn lead to bypass enteritis syndrome[37]; D-lactic acidosis and encephalopathy secondary to increased production of D-lactate by certain bacteria[38]; and possible immune-complex–mediated diseases, including papulopustular or nodular skin lesions,[39] liver disease including cirrhosis,[40] myalgia and nondeforming arthritis,[41] focal interstitial nephritis[42] and renal tubular acidosis[43], and hemolytic anemia.[44] Although many of these complications occur within the first year after the bypass procedure, Hocking and associates[36] have shown that side effects and complications continue for at least 5 years, mandating careful follow-up of these patients indefinitely.

MEDICAL MANAGEMENT

The primary goal of medical therapy of the patient with the short bowel syndrome must be control of diarrhea. This is necessary to permit adequate contact time between the mucosal surface and the intestinal contents for nutrient absorption, and to diminish nutrient losses in diarrheal fluid. Of equal importance is the need to control diarrhea to encourage adequate food intake. Many patients with a short bowel experience immediate, severe postprandial diarrhea, cramps, and even incontinence, and will limit their eating to avoid these troublesome symptoms.

Narcotic agents or their derivates are the most effective antidiarrheal medications for patients with short bowel syndrome. These drugs act mainly on intestinal smooth muscle to decrease transit time and increase intestinal capacity, and have been demonstrated to diminish ileostomy output.[45,46] Enterocytes contain opiate and other receptors on their membrane surfaces, and it is possible that these drugs also exert some effect on ion transport.[47] It is advisable to begin treatment with medications such as loperamide that have little addiction potential, but some patients require potent constipating narcotics such as codeine or tincture of opium to achieve adequate control of diarrhea. Liquid forms of medications sometimes are more effective because the rapid transit through the short bowel may not permit adequate dissolution and absorption of drugs in tablet or capsule form. In extreme cases, parenteral narcotics have been required.[2] Other antidiarrheal preparations, such as kaolin–pectin mixtures or psyllium fiber preparations, may be useful in patients with mild diarrhea or as adjunctive therapy in those receiving antimotility agents. Bile acid-binding resins such as cholestyramine may be useful in controlling the watery diarrhea of patients with small ileal resections.

Somatostatin and its synthetic analog, octreotide, have been used in the management of diarrhea in patients with the short bowel syndrome. In several studies, an octreotide dose of 50 μg twice or three times daily by subcutaneous injection significantly decreased stool fluid and electrolyte losses.[48–50]

In some, but not all patients, long-term octreotide treatment permitted discontinuation or reduction of intravenous fluids. Increasing the octreotide dose beyond 50 μg twice or three times daily has not been shown to be beneficial. Octreotide also has been administered in parenteral nutrition fluids.

The mechanism of action of octreotide in patients with short bowel syndrome is uncertain; various investigators have invoked antimotility effects, decreased secretion of digestive juices, and influences on mucosal fluid and electrolyte transport to explain the antidiarrheal effect.[48] In addition to pain associated with the subcutaneous injection, abdominal discomfort and even obstruction have been associated with octreotide use in patients with short bowel syndrome.[48] Cooper and associates found increased fecal fat excretion with octreotide treatment.[49] Chronic octreotide use has been associated with cholelithiasis,[48] and it is of potential concern that use of this agent in patients with short bowel, who already are at increased risk for gallstones, may further increase the risk for this complication. In addition, octreotide could potentially decrease the production of gastrointestinal peptide hormones that are important for intestinal adaptation.

As discussed, gastric acid hypersecretion often occurs transiently after intestinal resection, and in a few patients the hypersecretory state persists. After resection, patients usually receive H_2 blockers, first intravenously and then orally, to prevent peptic ulceration, diminish nasogastric tube and ostomy fluid and electrolyte losses, and control metabolic alkalosis. This practice has reduced the need for emergency peptic ulcer surgery in patients recovering from intestinal resection, which when combined with the short bowel syndrome often greatly worsened diarrhea and absorptive deficits. Several studies have indicated that H_2 blockers or omeprazol may be useful in decreasing diarrhea in stable, ambulatory patients with a short bowel.[51,52] Significant decreases in fecal or ostomy fluid and electrolytes and, in some cases, fat losses have been noted even in patients who did not manifest hypersecretion with formal gastric acid analysis. H_2 blockers can be administered in total parenteral nutrition solutions.[53]

Small bowel bacterial overgrowth in conjunction with a short bowel could magnify diarrhea, malabsorption, and nutritional deficits. Patients with the short bowel syndrome from inflammatory bowel diseases such as Crohn's disease or radiation enteritis may have enteroenteric fistulas, intestinal strictures, or bypassed segments that produce stasis leading to bacterial proliferation. In addition, resection of the ileocecal valve and terminal ileum also may permit greater reflux of colonic bacteria into the small intestine. Detection of bacterial overgrowth in patients with short bowel syndrome, however, is difficult. Quantitative culture of small intestinal fluid remains the gold standard for diagnosis, but is somewhat invasive and requires special care to avoid contamination and to ensure accurate culture of anaerobes and fastidious aerobic intestinal organisms. Other noninvasive tests commonly used to diagnose bacterial overgrowth, such as the bile acid breath test or the Schilling test with intrinsic factor, will produce abnormal results in patients with ileal resections. New breath tests such as the ^{14}C-xylose breath test[54] and the glucose–hydrogen breath test[55] may be able to distinguish between bacterial overgrowth and mucosal disease. If bacterial overgrowth is suspected, a therapeutic trial of a broad-spectrum antibiotic is warranted.

Secretion of pancreatic enzymes may be impaired in patients with severe protein-calorie malnutrition. In addition, those with extensive proximal small intestinal resections may have a blunted release of secretin and cholecystokinin–pancreozymin, leading to diminished pancreatic stimulation and functional pancreatic insufficiency. For selected patients, therefore, pancreatic enzyme replacement may improve nutrient absorption. In most patients with short bowel syndrome, however, intralumenal nutrient digestion proceeds normally, and pancreatic enzyme replacement is unnecessary.

NUTRITIONAL THERAPY

As discussed, the clinical course of the patient with the short bowel syndrome can be divided into three phases that require different types of nutritional management.[56] The first phase is characterized by severe diarrhea that becomes apparent when the patient is given oral intake. Total parenteral nutrition is required to prevent dehydration and electrolyte and acid–base disturbances. The second phase corresponds to the period during which small bowel adaptation occurs. Diarrhea stabilizes and the patient usually can maintain fluid and electrolyte balance with oral intake. The major clinical problem during the second phase is malabsorption of nutrients that can result in nutritional deficiency if proper replacement therapy is not initiated. Enteral formulas often are used to supplement a restricted diet. With time, the third phase of full intestinal adaptation is achieved, and the patient is able to maintain adequate nutritional status by oral intake. Some patients with large resections of small bowel will not be able to maintain adequate nutritional status and avoid dehydration, electrolyte, and acid–base disturbances on oral intake alone, and require prolonged parenteral nutrition.[57]

Total Parenteral Nutrition

During the first phase of the short bowel syndrome, the patient requires total parenteral nutrition. Premature attempts at oral feeding only result in massive diarrhea, dehydration, and electrolyte and acid–base disturbances. These problems are particularly severe in the patient with a marked secretory response to food intake, whose shortened intestine is not capable of absorbing even endogenous secretions. Food intake must be limited to small amounts with the goal of beginning to stimulate intestinal adaptation.

The techniques of total parenteral nutrition have been reviewed in detail elsewhere,[58] and are beyond the scope of this chapter, but several points deserve special attention. Total parenteral nutrition is most safely and effectively conducted by multidisciplinary groups, including physicians, pharmacists, nurses, and dietitians, who are experienced in the required procedures and the potential complications. Meticulous care must be given to inserting and maintaining a central venous catheter for total parenteral nutrition, particularly because many patients with the short bowel syndrome, such as those with chronic inflammatory bowel disease, have had repeated previous venous catheterizations that limit vascular access. Complications such as pneumothorax, hemothorax, vascular thrombosis, and catheter-related sepsis can be min-

imized by proper surgical technique and by the use of strict aseptic procedures for cleaning the catheter insertion site and administering the nutrient solutions. A careful nutritional assessment must be performed to determine the calorie, protein, electrolyte, and micronutrient requirements of the patient. Inadequate parenteral nutrition support results in further nutritional depletion and may contribute to postoperative problems including wound infections, poor wound healing, and sepsis. Administration of parenteral nutrition beyond the patient's requirements also results in serious complications, such as hyperglycemia, respiratory compromise, and fatty infiltration of the liver from excessive glucose administration.[59–61] In the initial phase, particular attention must be paid to careful monitoring of fecal, ostomy, and urinary fluid and electrolyte losses and serum electrolyte, creatinine, and blood urea nitrogen levels to permit accurate assessment of the adequacy of intravenous fluid and electrolyte replacement, and adjustment of the parenteral nutrition formula as needed. Periodic nutritional assessments, including anthropometric measurements and laboratory evaluation of the serum levels of proteins such as albumin, minerals, and vitamins, are necessary to evaluate the adequacy of the parenteral nutrition formula.

The length of time a patient with the short bowel syndrome requires parenteral nutrition support is quite variable, and depends on the factors that determine the severity of the metabolic consequences of intestinal resection. Gouttebel and colleagues reported that patients with as little as 30 to 50 cm of healthy small bowel and most of their colon remaining usually could be weaned off total parenteral nutrition within 1 year.[62] In their experience, patients with a short bowel and no colon required more than 60 cm of small bowel to avoid permanent total parenteral nutrition.[62] Caniano and associates reported the clinical course of 14 neonates with severe short bowel syndrome, less than 25% of the expected length for gestational age.[63] The survival rate was 86%, and 67% of survivors had sufficient intestinal adaptation to permit discontinuation of total parenteral nutrition within 6 to 45 months. Once stabilized on a total parenteral nutrition program, many patients can successfully continue this therapy at home while oral feeding is gradually resumed and intestinal adaptation is occurring (see Home Total Parenteral Nutrition).

Enteral Formulas

Limited oral intake should be resumed as soon as the patient is stable after surgery and stool output is less than about 2 L/day. Feeding is begun soon after surgery, primarily to induce intestinal adaptation. Routine postoperative liquid diets are of limited value because they are grossly nutritionally inadequate and are severely hyperosmolar and commonly provoke an osmotic diarrhea. Full liquid diets often contain much lactose and are poorly tolerated by most patients with the short bowel syndrome who are lactose intolerant.

Many clinicians recommend the use of elemental or semielemental formulas as the initial oral intake after intestinal resection.[2,64] These diets contain mainly carbohydrate in the form of sucrose and glucose polymers, easily digestible protein sources, or, in some cases, free amino acids or small peptides, and vitamins and minerals. These formulas are very low in fat, often providing minimal amounts to meet essential fatty acid requirements. They are quite efficiently absorbed within the proximal 100 cm of jejunum,[64] and have been demonstrated to be effective in stimulating adaptation of the proximal small intestine.[65] In addition, some elemental diets contain the amino acid glutamine, which is a major fuel for the small intestine and has been suggested to be particularly important in inducing intestinal adaptation.[66] The poor taste of the elemental or semielemental formulas often limits oral intake, and they are quite hyperosmolar and may provoke considerable worsening of diarrhea. Therefore, these formulas may be used more effectively for nasogastric or nasointestinal tube feedings, where they can be administered as slow, constant infusions permitting more complete absorption and better tolerance.[64,67]

Some have reported that the problems of poor taste and diarrhea with elemental and semielemental diets outweigh their potential advantages, and have been more successful using polymeric formula diets.[68] Polymeric supplements generally provide approximately 30% of calories as fat, and contain intact protein sources. They are more palatable than elemental diets, less hyperosmolar, and are considerably less expensive. Polymeric formulas are suitable for both oral use and as tube feedings.

Dietary Management

After nutritional repletion and stabilization of the fluid and electrolyte status is achieved with parenteral nutrition and formula diets, the patient with the short bowel syndrome is ready to resume some food intake. During the second phase of the short bowel syndrome, malabsorption is the predominant feature, and the goal of dietary management is to control symptoms such as diarrhea, bloating, and cramps while increasing food intake and diminishing reliance on specialized nutritional support. There is considerable controversy, however, over dietary recommendations for patients with the short bowel syndrome.

It has been common clinical practice to use a low-fat, high-carbohydrate diet for patients with a short bowel, with some experts suggesting limiting dietary fat intake to as little as 25 g per day.[2] This recommendation is based on the many adverse effects of steatorrhea, especially diarrhea caused by stimulation of fluid and electrolyte secretion. Hydroxy fatty acids produced by bacterial metabolism of unabsorbed dietary fat are particularly potent secretagogues.[69] The proximal colon is the bowel segment that demonstrates the most significant secretory response to fatty acids.[70] Patients with a short bowel ending in a jejunostomy or ileostomy, therefore, have been shown to have the same ostomy output of water, sodium, and potassium on high-fat and high-carbohydrate diets.[71] Presumably, a patient with a jejunostomy or ileostomy will have an osmotic diarrhea from a high-carbohydrate diet that is similar in magnitude to the secretion induced by high dietary fat. It also has been suggested that dietary fat induces secretion of gastrointestinal hormones that slow intestinal motility and thereby improve absorption.[72] Divalent cations, including calcium, magnesium, zinc, and copper, may bind to fatty acids in stool, and some, but not all studies have demonstrated excessive fecal losses of these minerals when patients with

short bowel syndrome are on high-fat diets.[71,73] Steatorrhea also would be expected to accentuate malabsorption of fat-soluble vitamins, although the magnitude of this effect has not been quantitated in patients with short bowel syndrome. As discussed, increased fecal fat losses also enhance dietary oxalate absorption, oxaluria, and the tendency for renal stone formation. The primary site for intestinal oxalate absorption is the colon, and patients with malabsorption and small bowel ostomies rarely demonstrate hyperoxaluria.[74] It therefore seems appropriate to individualize recommendations for dietary fat intake based on the patient's symptoms. The patient with a short bowel and a small intestinal ostomy probably tolerates dietary fat quite well, and should be restricted only to the extent necessary to avoid mineral and fat-soluble vitamin depletion. This should be monitored with periodic measurement of serum and urinary mineral levels, serum levels of retinol, tocopherol, and 25-hydroxyvitamin D, prothrombin time, and perhaps assessment of bone density. In contrast, the patient with the short bowel syndrome and preservation of much of the colon likely requires a more severe fat restriction. Limitation of dietary fat intake to 60 g/day or less may be required to control diarrhea and to reduce enteric hyperoxaluria. It always is important, however, to balance the beneficial effects of fat restriction in these patients against the limitations of food palatability and caloric intake imposed by low-fat diets.

Preparations containing medium-chain triglycerides often are used as caloric supplements for patients with the short bowel syndrome. Medium-chain triglycerides are rapidly hydrolyzed in the intestinal lumen, and the medium-chain fatty acids produced are water soluble and are easily absorbed even in the absence of bile salts.[75] Medium-chain fatty acids are not resynthesized into triglyceride in the enterocytes and incorporated into chylomicrons, but instead are released directly into the portal circulation, where they are rapidly extracted by the liver and other tissues for use as a fuel source.[75] Medium-chain triglyceride preparations may therefore be well absorbed and tolerated by patients with a short bowel and significant malabsorption of dietary long-chain triglyceride. Medium-chain triglycerides have an unpleasant taste, produce diarrhea in some patients when given at doses more than about 35 g/day, and do not provide a source of essential fatty acids.

Most patients with the short bowel syndrome have significant lactose malabsorption and poor tolerance of lactose-containing dairy products. Lactose malabsorption is caused by the reduced mucosal surface area, and perhaps by functional immaturity of the enterocytes in the remaining intestine undergoing adaptation. Restriction of lactose-containing dairy products is necessary to avoid worsening of diarrhea, bloating, and abdominal cramps. These food restrictions, however, limit available sources of calcium, vitamin D, riboflavin, and protein, and necessitate inclusion of other sources of these nutrients in the diet or supplementation. Bacterial and yeast lactases have been developed for production of low-lactose dairy products that are well tolerated by patients with short bowel syndrome. The degree of lactose malabsorption in a patient with a short bowel and a preserved colon can be readily quantitated by hydrogen breath tests after graded doses of lactose.[76]

Clinicians have commonly prescribed a low-fiber diet for patients with the short bowel syndrome.[2] This recommendation was based on the observation that some types of dietary fiber, such as wheat bran, decrease intestinal transit time and increase fecal weight.[77] It is now appreciated that dietary fiber is quite heterogeneous, with different types of fiber demonstrating variable effects on the intestine.[78] Soluble fibers, such as pectin, can delay gastric emptying and increase intestinal transit time, which often is desirable in patients with short bowel syndrome.[79,80] Some fibers bind bile salts and have significant water-retaining capacity, which could be beneficial in the management of diarrhea. In addition, bacterial fermentation of some fiber sources generates short-chain fatty acids, which are a major fuel source for the colon and can stimulate mucosal cell proliferation of colon and small intestine.[81] It therefore seems appropriate to allow patients with the short bowel syndrome to experiment with different sources of dietary fiber, and to individualize fiber intake to maximize symptom control.

Patients with enteric hyperoxaluria and calcium oxalate renal calculi often require additional dietary modifications. High-oxalate foods such as chocolate, cola drinks, tea, carrots, celery, spinach, pepper, nuts, plums, figs, and strawberries need to be limited. Oxalate is widely distributed in foods, however, and avoidance of high-oxalate foods alone usually does not reduce the urinary oxalate to an acceptable level. As discussed, dietary fat needs to be restricted in an effort to minimize oxalate absorption.[24] An increase in dietary calcium achieved through calcium-containing foods or supplements often is recommended to promote intralumenal formation of insoluble calcium oxalate.[82] Cholestyramine has been used in the management of hyperoxaluria because this resin binds oxalate as well as the bile salts that increase colonic permeability for oxalate.[83] These beneficial effects of cholestyramine need to be weighed against its negative effects on absorption of dietary fat and fat-soluble vitamins.

Rarely, a metabolic encephalopathy associated with increased serum levels of D-lactate develops in patients with the short bowel syndrome.[38] Immediate treatment consists of intravenous fluids and stopping oral intake. Long-term management centers on carbohydrate-restricted diets and nonabsorbable antibiotics to diminish production by colonic bacteria of D-lactate and other substances that may produce encephalopathy.

Vitamin and Mineral Supplementation

In phase three of the short bowel syndrome, the patient's residual small intestine has adapted to the extent that adequate energy and protein nutritional status is maintained on a modified diet, and gastrointestinal symptoms are controlled. Long-term follow-up of patients with short bowel syndrome has demonstrated that they usually can attain ideal body weight and maintain a normal serum albumin.[22] Significant malabsorption of specific micronutrients frequently persists, however, necessitating mineral or vitamin replacement therapy.[22] Inadequate dietary intake, loss of micronutrients in diarrheal fluid, and drug-induced malabsorption also contribute to development of vitamin and mineral deficiencies.

Clinical deficiency of water-soluble vitamins, with the exception of vitamin B_{12} and folate, are observed only rarely in patients with a short bowel. Water-soluble vitamins except B_{12} are well absorbed throughout the small intestine, and deficiency syndromes such a pellagra from niacin malabsorption have been observed only with massive resection.[84] Folate deficiency may occur more frequently in patients with short bowel due to Crohn's disease because the drug sulfasalazine used in the treatment of inflammatory bowel disease acts as a competitive inhibitor of folate absorption.[85] Vitamin B_{12} absorption occurs in the ileum, which contains a membrane receptor that recognizes that intrinsic factor–B_{12} complex. With an ileal resection of more than 90 cm, Schilling test results are always abnormal.[86] There is a significant enterohepatic circulation of vitamin B_{12} that is interrupted with ileal resection and accelerates development of deficiency.[87]

Deficits of fat-soluble vitamins are more frequently noted in patients with short bowel syndrome. Bile salts are required for micellar solubilization of fat-soluble vitamins, and absorption is impaired in patients with large ileal resections resulting in depletion of the bile salt pool.[88] In addition, steatorrhea depresses fat-soluble vitamin absorption, and cholestyramine may worsen absorption by further reducing the intralumenal bile salt concentration and by binding the vitamins. Vitamin D deficiency and osteomalacia have been reported as common complications of ileal resection for Crohn's disease,[89,90] and in patients who have undergone jejunoileal bypass for morbid obesity.[91,92] Vitamin A deficiency causing night blindness, vitamin K deficiency with bleeding, and vitamin E deficiency resulting in neurologic deficits, all have been reported in patients with short bowel syndrome.[22,93]

Patients with the short bowel syndrome usually are advised to take a daily multiple-vitamin preparation typically providing two to five times the Recommended Dietary Allowances. Those with ileal resection of more than 90 cm require intramuscular vitamin B_{12} supplementation because the remaining jejunum does not adequately increase its absorptive capacity for B_{12}. Doses of 100 μg per month or 1000 μg every 3 to 4 months are adequate. Patients with severe malabsorption may require larger doses of fat-soluble vitamins than are provided in multiple-vitamin preparations. Because substantial toxicity can occur with excess vitamins A and D, therapy should be guided by monitoring serum levels of retinol and 25-hydroxyvitamin D, and serum and urinary calcium concentrations.

Deficiencies of minerals and trace elements present difficult diagnostic and therapeutic challenges in the patient with short bowel syndrome. Severe calcium malabsorption has been demonstrated, and appears to correlate with the extent of resection.[94] Vitamin D deficiency and steatorrhea both contribute to calcium malabsorption. Calcium absorption in the small bowel and colon may improve somewhat with time after intestinal resection, but remains significantly impaired.[94] Patients with short bowel frequently have severe reductions in bone mineral content that predispose them to debilitating fractures.[95] It seems prudent to encourage a generous calcium intake of 1000 to 1500 mg/day through the use of calcium-rich foods and calcium supplements, but the efficacy of this approach in maintaining bone mass has not been demonstrated. For those patients who are noted to have significantly reduced bone mass, more aggressive therapeutic measures may be indicated. Women with the short bowel syndrome probably should receive estrogen replacement after menopause if permitted by their underlying medical condition. Other therapies used in the treatment of osteoporosis such as fluoride supplements need to be evaluated further in patients with short bowel syndrome. Hypomagnesemia is noted frequently in patients with short bowel syndrome, and may present with muscle cramps, tetany, cardiac rhythm disturbances, and other symptoms.[96,97] A greater number of patients with short bowel syndrome have depletion of cellular magnesium stores, assessed by measuring the magnesium content of muscle biopsies.[96] Cellular magnesium depletion significantly contributes to a variety of common symptoms, including muscle weakness, fatigue, renal stones, and depression. Oral replacement therapy with salts such as magnesium oxide, magnesium gluconate, or magnesium chloride can be attempted, but is often limited by the well known cathartic effect of magnesium-containing preparations, necessitating parenteral magnesium supplementation.

Iron deficiency occurs in 25% to 50% of patients with short bowel syndrome, and is particularly prevalent in those with disorders such as Crohn's disease that are likely to have continuing blood loss.[22] Oral iron supplementation often produces distressing gastrointestinal symptoms, and therapy with intramuscular or intravenous iron dextran often is needed to maintain an adequate hemoglobin level. Fecal zinc losses in patients with the short bowel syndrome parallel the volume of diarrheal fluid.[98] Although florid clinical zinc deficiency with acral skin lesions and other findings is rare,[99] many patients with short bowel have zinc malabsorption, are in negative balance, and appear to have a marginal zinc status.[100] Assessment of zinc nutritional status is difficult because the serum zinc concentration is affected by many factors in addition to zinc nutriture, including the serum albumin level and inflammatory mediators.[101] Newer measures, such as white blood cell zinc and measurement of zinc-dependent enzymes, offer promise as improved assessment techniques.[102] Deficiencies of other essential trace elements such as copper, selenium, chromium, and molybdenum also have been reported in a few patients with short bowel syndrome.[103–106] Therapy with combined multiple-vitamin and mineral preparations usually is adequate to prevent trace element deficiency.

Home Total Parenteral Nutrition

A small number of patients with severe short bowel are unable to maintain adequate nutritional status and avoid dehydration and electrolyte disturbances on oral intake, and require permanent parenteral nutrition support. Since the early 1970s, increasing numbers of patients have been trained to administer parenteral nutrition at home. The development of the technology and services necessary for home total parenteral nutrition has permitted the nutritional and social rehabilitation of many patients with severe short bowel who previously would have required prolonged hospital confinement or died of nutritional complications. Home total parenteral nutrition, however, is associated with all of the difficulties of short-term hospital parenteral nutrition and additional metabolic complications of prolonged intravenous feeding.

The details of home total parenteral nutrition are described in depth in other publications, and are considered only briefly here.[57,58,107] Home total parenteral nutrition is most commonly administered through a Silastic central venous catheter that has been tunneled subcutaneously to provide easy access for cleaning the insertion site and connecting the administration tubing. The long subcutaneous tunnel also serves as a barrier against infection. Arteriovenous fistulas similar to those used for chronic hemodialysis also have been used successfully by some. Patients most commonly infuse their nutrient solutions overnight, permitting resumption of normal work or school activities during the day. Adequate education of the patient and his or her family is essential for successful home total parenteral nutrition, and is best performed by a nutrition support team experienced in home therapy. The patient and family must be trained in aseptic technique for catheter care and solution compounding, proper use of sophisticated pumps that control the infusion rate, and appropriate procedures for handling emergencies such as catheter rupture to prevent air embolus and other devastating complications. In addition, the patient must be trained to monitor urinary glucose and ketones. With proper patient education and management, the outcome of home parenteral nutrition is extremely gratifying. Nutritional status can be well maintained, even permitting normal growth and development in children with the short bowel syndrome.[108] Social rehabilitation is often excellent, and many patients are able to resume a high level of functioning in their employment, home, and school settings. Some children on home total parenteral nutrition have demonstrated deficits in perceptual–motor functions that may be related to frequent, lengthy hospitalizations.[109] Some on prolonged home total parenteral nutrition also experience significant psychiatric disturbances such as depression and sexual dysfunction.[57] Drug abuse through the indwelling catheter and suicide attempts can be major management problems. Important financial and insurance implications of this expensive therapy may significantly limit a patient's ability to resume previous employment.

Catheter-related infection remains the most common serious complication of home total parenteral nutrition. Organisms that typically reside on the skin, including *Staphylococcus* species and fungi, are the most frequent organisms cultured from catheters,[110] and presumably infect the lines during catheter manipulation and by migration along the catheter tract. Gram-negative bacterial catheter infections are more commonly observed in patients with ostomies whose skin is colonized by these organisms. With maintenance of good aseptic technique, episodes of catheter-related infection can be minimized. Infection rates of one episode per 3 years of catheter use or better can be achieved.[111] Bacterial catheter-related infections usually can be treated with antibiotic administration without removal of the line, whereas fungal infections almost always require catheter removal.[112]

Vascular thrombosis is a troublesome complication of home total parenteral nutrition, and patients may present with arm swelling from subclavian vein occlusion or with the superior vena cava syndrome. Thrombolytic therapy with urokinase sometimes restores venous patency,[113] but in many cases catheter replacement is required. With repeated episodes of venous occlusion, vascular access may become severely limited, and drastic measures such as direct implantation of the catheter in the right atrium might be required.

Patients on home total parenteral nutrition manifest the metabolic complications of intravenous feeding such as hyperglycemia, electrolyte disorders, and hypertriglyceridemia that are well recognized with short-term parenteral nutrition. In addition, however, several complications have been recognized in patients maintained on prolonged intravenous feeding. Table 75-4 presents some of the vitamin and trace element deficiencies that have been observed in patients on home total parenteral nutrition.[93,103,105,106,114]

Abnormalities of hepatic function and structure that may ultimately progress to cirrhosis have been described in patients on prolonged total parenteral nutrition. Children on home parenteral nutrition are prone to severe cholestasis that may evolve into biliary cirrhosis.[115] Adult patients on home total parenteral nutrition have developed steatonecrosis that can progress to a micronodular cirrhosis, changes that are indistinguishable from alcoholic liver disease.[116] The relative importance of adverse metabolic effects of total parenteral nutrition versus the patient's underlying medical problems in the pathogenesis of these liver diseases remains uncertain. There is a high prevalence of biliary tract disease in patients on long-term total parenteral nutrition. With 4 to 6 weeks of parenteral nutrition, most patients will have ultrasonographic evidence of gallbladder sludge.[117] In one study, gallstones, which usually were symptomatic, developed in 35% of patients on home total parenteral nutrition.[118] Thirty-nine percent of those with ileal disorders receiving prolonged parenteral nutrition had gallstones, a higher prevalence than has been observed in those with similar ileal disease who were not on parenteral nutrition.[118] In addition, patients on total parenteral nutrition for Crohn's disease had gallstones sooner after diagnosis than other patients with Crohn's disease. Acalculous cholecystis also has been noted in patients on home total parenteral nutrition. Gallbladder stasis has been implicated as an important pathogenic factor in biliary tract disease associated with parenteral nutrition.[118] Food-stimulated gastrointestinal hormone secretion is lacking in these patients, and may result in decreased bile flow and diminished gallbladder contraction. Patients on total parenteral nutrition in whom gallstones develop are more likely to use medications such as narcotics and anticholinergic drugs that interfere with gallbladder contractility.[118] Effects of total parenteral nutrition on bile composition affecting lithogenicity have been reported by some, but remain controversial.[119]

Severe metabolic bone disease has been noted in patients on home total parenteral nutrition. Some patients had incapacitating bone pain, hypercalcemia, hypercalciuria, and osteomalacia documented by iliac crest bone biopsy.[120] This clinical syndrome was apparently caused by aluminum contamination of protein hydrolysates used in some total parenteral nutrition formulations, and has not been observed with use of free amino acid preparations that contain little aluminum.[121] Some have suggested that a toxic effect of intravenously administered vitamin D also contributed to osteomalacia seen with total parenteral nutrition.[122] The major metabolic bone disease observed in home total parenteral nutrition patients has been osteoporosis, which in some cases is associated with a low bone turnover rate.[123,124] Hypercalciuria and negative calcium balance has been described in patients on total parenteral nutrition, and may be influenced by the amino acid, phosphate, and acetate content of the nutritional solution.[125,126] Because patients requiring home total parenteral nutrition often have had chronic malnutrition and have required medications such as corticosteroids, many have a significantly diminished bone mass before the initiation of intravenous feedings.[127]

SURGICAL THERAPY

A number of surgical procedures have been devised to slow intestinal transit in patients with severe short bowel syndromes.[128] A small intestinal reversal procedure has been used most commonly, in which a segment of bowel is turned in the antiperistaltic direction. Although success with this operation has been reported, particularly in young children, the outcome is very unpredictable.[128,129] If too short an intestinal segment is reversed, there is little effect on transit time, whereas if too long a segment is used, functional obstruction occurs. Colon interposition in either the isoperistaltic or antiperistaltic direction also has slowed intestinal transit in some cases. Construction of intestinal valves, by intussuscepting or submucosally tunneling intestinal segments, and creation of recirculating loops have been used to increase transit time in experimental short bowel syndromes, but have not achieved much success in clinical trials. Retrograde electrical pacing of the distal small intestine produces reverse peristalsis and improved absorption in dogs, but experience in humans is limited. Patients with the short bowel syndrome may have a markedly dilated maximal bowel, which interferes with effective peristalsis and promotes bacterial overgrowth. Tapering enteroplasty has been reported to improve intestinal function.[128] An attractive variation of this procedure uses the intestine that is tapered to provide additional length, but may be limited by the quality of the vascular supply. Growing neointestinal mucosa on patched bowel defects holds promise, but has not been adequately tested clinically. Surgical procedures should be considered only in patients who continue to have severe short bowel symptoms in spite of maximal dietary and pharmacologic therapy, and who have waited sufficient time for intestinal adaptation to occur.

Small bowel transplantation is an exciting new treatment modality for selected patients with severe short bowel syndrome. Early attempts at small intestinal transplantation were uniformly unsuccessful because of severe graft rejection or graft-versus-host disease.[130] With the availability of newer immunosuppressive agents such as cyclosporine and FK506, however, long-term graft survival has been achieved in experimental animal models and in humans.[130,131] Research in animal models has made substantial progress in defining the

---

TABLE 75-4
Vitamin and Trace Element Deficiency Syndromes in Patients on Home Total Parenteral Nutrition

NUTRIENT	SYMPTOMS AND SIGNS
Vitamin E	Neurologic deficits; muscle weakness[93]
Biotin	Alopecia, skin rash, lethargy, organic aciduria[115]
Chromium	Glucose intolerance[105]
Selenium	Muscle weakness, liver dysfunction, hematologic abnormalities[103]
Molybdenum	Encephalopathy, hypouricemia[106]

optimal surgical methods, in devising immunosuppressive strategies to prevent rejection and graft-versus-host disease, and in developing approaches for organ preservation.[130]

Most of the long-term successes in human small intestinal transplantation have occurred in those who received combined small bowel and liver transplants for short bowel and total parenteral nutrition-associated liver disease or for antithrombin III deficiency causing bowel infarction.[130-134] Some patients have been able to discontinue total parenteral nutrition and to maintain an excellent nutritional status after successful transplantation. Much experimental and clinical evidence suggests that liver transplantation significantly affects rejection of other organs, perhaps by altering antigen processing, releasing major histocompatibility antigens in a soluble form that block cytotoxic antibodies, or other immunologic mechanisms.[130] Rejection of the intestinal graft is characterized by cryptitis, loss of mucosal goblet cells, and blunting of the villi, which progresses to vasculitis and mononuclear cell infiltration of the lamina propria, followed by mucosal sloughing. There is loss of the intestinal barrier function, and bacterial translocation and sepsis is a common complication.[131] With chronic rejection, there is villous atrophy, subintimal vascular thickening, and muscular fibrosis. Diagnosis of rejection by mucosal biopsy can be difficult because of the patchy nature of the process and because nonspecific inflammatory changes at stomas and mucosal atrophy in defunctionalized bowel can cause diagnostic difficulties. Various functional tests to diagnose rejection are being investigated, including the maltose absorption test, tests of intestinal permeability, and others.[130,131] Graft-versus-host disease is of potential concern because of the large number of lymphoid cells in the donor intestine, but this complication generally has been mild and easily controlled in human small bowel transplantation using modern immunosuppressants.[130,131] Within a few months after transplantation, the lymphoreticular cells of the graft lamina propria are replaced by the recipient's lymphoreticular cells.[132] Lymphomas associated with Epstein-Barr virus infection have been observed quite frequently after small intestinal transplantation, particularly in those with multivisceral grafts.[131]

In the initial period after small intestinal transplantation, various abnormalities in motor and absorptive function are observed, which may be related to lymphatic disruption and denervation as well as damage during organ preservation, rejection, and toxic effects of immunosuppressive agents.[130,131] Usually, however, motility and barrier function improve so that enteral alimentation is possible within a few weeks posttransplantation.[130-132] Episodes of rejection are associated with a marked decline in small intestinal function. Detailed studies of successful small bowel transplants in experimental animals have found mild abnormalities of absorption and secretion, but the limited experience in humans has indicated that absorption and motility in successful grafts are excellent.[130]

The most important aspect of surgery in the short bowel syndrome clearly lies in the use of operative techniques to minimize the extent of resection. Whenever possible, bowel-preserving procedures such as stricturoplasty or serosal patches for perforation should be used instead of extensive resection. In diseases such Crohn's disease and radiation enteropathy, resection should be limited to the minimum amount necessary for treatment of complications such as obstruction, bleeding, or fistulas. The detection of mesenteric vascular disease often is difficult clinically, and prompt use of angiography must be encouraged in high-risk patients to allow early diagnosis and vascularization before extensive bowel infarction has occurred.

The reader is directed to Chapter 20, Vitamins and Minerals; Chapter 21, General Nutritional Principles; Chapter 38, Approach to the Patient With Diarrhea; Chapter 79, Inflammatory Bowel Disease; Chapter 112, Mesenteric Vascular Insufficiency; and Chapter 113, Radiation Injury.

REFERENCES

1. Greenberger NJ. The management of patients with short bowel syndrome. Am J Gastroenterol 1978;70:528.
2. Weser E. The management of patients after small bowel resection. Gastroenterology 1976;71:146.
3. Zeigler MM. Short bowel syndrome in infancy: etiology and management. Clin Perinatol 1986;13:163.
4. Schwartz MZ, Maeda K. Short bowel syndrome in infants and children. Pediatr Clin North Am 1985;32:1265.
5. Welch McL, Cunningham KM, Read NW. Regulation of gastric emptying by ileal nutrients in humans. Gastroenterology 1988;94:401.
6. Weser E, Fletcher JT, Urban E. Short bowel syndrome. Gastroenterology 1979;77:572.
7. Dowling RH. The short bowel syndrome. Endoscopy Review 1988;1:47.
8. Weser E. Intestinal adaptation after small bowel resection. Viewpoints Dig Dis 1978;10:1.
9. Williamson RCN, Chir M. Intestinal adaptation: structure, functional and cytokinetic changes. N Engl J Med 1978;298:1393.
10. Williamson RCN, Chir M. Intestinal adaptation: mechanisms of control. N Engl J Med 1978;198:1444.
11. Urban E. Further insights into mucosal adaptation. Gastroenterology 1988;95:248.
12. Williamson RCN, Buchholtz TW, Malt RA. Hormonal stimulation of cell proliferation in small bowel after transection and resection in rats. Gastroenterology 1978;75:249.
13. Luk GD, Yang P. Polyamines in intestinal and pancreatic adaptation. Gut 1987;28:95.
14. Luk GD, Yang P. Distribution of polyamines and their biosynthetic enzymes in intestinal adaptation. Am J Physiol 1988;254:G194.
15. McJunkin B, Fromm H, Sarva RP, et al. Factors in the mechanism of diarrhea in bile acid malabsorption: fecal pH—a key determinant. Gastroenterology 1981;80:1454.
16. Arrambide KA, Santa Ana CA, Schiller LR, et al. Loss of absorptive capacity for sodium chloride as a cause of diarrhea following partial ileal and right colon resection. Dig Dis Sci 1989;34:193.
17. Buxton B. Small bowel resection and gastric acid hypersecretion. Gut 1974;15:229.
18. Winawer SJ, Zamcheck N. Pathophysiology of small intestinal resection. In: Progress in gastroenterology. New York: Grune and Stratton, 1968:395.
19. Windsor CWO, Fejfar J, Woodward DAK. Gastric secretion after massive small bowel resection. Gut 1969;10:779.
20. Murphy JP, King DR, Dubois A. Treatment of gastric hypersecretion with cimetidine in the short-bowel syndrome. N Engl J Med 1979;300:80.
21. Andersson H, Bosaeus I, Brummer R-J, et al. Nutritional and metabolic consequences of extensive bowel resection. Dig Dis 1986;4:193.
22. Compston JE, Creamer B. The consequences of small intestinal resection. Q J Med 1977;46:485.
23. Smith LH, Fromm H, Hofmann AF. Acquired hyperoxaluria,

nephrolithiasis, and intestinal disease. N Engl J Med 1972;286: 1371.

24. Earnest DL, Johnson G, Williams HE, et al. Hyperoxaluria in patients with ileal resection: an abnormality in dietary oxalate absorption. Gastroenterology 1974;66:1114.
25. Binder HJ. Intestinal oxalate absorption. Gastroenterology 1974;67:441.
26. Dobbins JW, Binder HJ. Effect of bile salts and fatty acids on the colonic absorption of oxalate. Gastroenterology 1976;70: 1096.
27. Knickelbein RG, Aronson PS, Dobbins JW. Oxalate transport by anion exchange across rabbit ileal brush-border. J Clin Invest 1986;77:170.
28. Elliot JS, Soles WP. Excretion of calcium and citric acid in patients with small bowel disease. J Urol 1974;111:810.
29. Heaton KW, Read AE. Gallstones in patients with disorders of the terminal ileum and disturbed bile salt metabolism. Br Med J 1969;3:494.
30. Hill GL, Mair WSH, Goligher JC. Gallstones after ileostomy and ileal resection. Gut 1975;16:932.
31. Dowling RH, Bell GD, White J. Lithogenic bile in patients with ileal dysfunction. Gut 1972;13:415.
32. Farkkila MA. Biliary cholesterol and lithogenicity of bile in patients after ileal resection. Surgery 1988;104:18.
33. Bickerstoff K, Moossa AR. Effects of resection or by-pass of the distal ileum on the lithogenicity of bile. Am J Surg 1983;145: 34.
34. Pitt HA, Lewinski MA, Muller EL, et al. Ileal resection-induced gallstones: altered bilirubin or cholesterol metabolism? Surgery 1984;96:154.
35. Griffen WO, Bivins BA, Bell RM. The decline and fall of jejunoileal bypass. Surg Gynecol Obstet 1983;157:301.
36. Hocking MP, Duerson MC, O'Leary P, et al. Jejunoileal bypass for morbid obesity. N Engl J Med 1983;308:995.
37. Passaro E, Dresnick E, Wilson SE. Bypass enteritis. Am J Surg 1976;131:169.
38. Thurn JL, Pierpont GL, Ludvigsen CW, et al. D-lactate encephalopathy. Am J Med 1985;79:717.
39. Dresnick EJ, Ahmed AR, Greenway F, et al. Cutaneous lesions after intestinal bypass. Ann Intern Med 1980;93:557.
40. Baker AL, Monroe P, Glagov S, et al. Management of liver failure in a patient following jejunoileal bypass. Gastroenterology 1980;78:1593.
41. Dicken CH. Bowel-associated dermatosis-arthritis syndrome: bowel bypass syndrome without bowel bypass. Mayo Clin Proc 1984;59:43.
42. Dresnick ET, Stanley TM, Border WA, et al. Renal damage with intestinal bypass. Ann Intern Med 1978;89:594.
43. Schaffalitzky de Muckadell DE, Ladefoged J, et al. Renal tubular acidosis secondary to jejunoileal bypass for morbid obesity. Scand J Gastroenterol 1985;20:823.
44. Moake JL, Kageler WV, Cimo PL, et al. Intravascular hemolysis, thrombocytopenia, leukopenia, and circulating immune complexes after jejunoileal bypass surgery. Ann Intern Med 1977;86: 576.
45. Schiller LR, Davis GR, Santa Ana CA, et al. Studies of the mechanism of the antidiarrheal effect of codeine. J Clin Invest 1982;70:999.
46. Sandhu BK, Tripp JH, Candy CA, et al. Loperamide: studies on its mechanism of action. Gut 1981;22:658.
47. Dobbins J, Racusen L, Binder HJ. Effect of D-alanine methionine enkephalin amide on ion transport in the rabbit ileum. J Clin Invest 1980;66:19.
48. Rosen GH. Somatostatin and its analogs in the short bowel syndrome. Nutrition in Clinical Practice 1992;7:81.
49. Cooper JC, Williams NS, King RFGJ, et al. Effects of a long-acting somatostatin analogue in patients with severe ileostomy diarrhoea. Br J Surg 1986;73:128.
50. Ladefoged K, Christensen KC, Hegnhoj J, et al. Effect of a long acting somatostatin analogue SMS 201-995 on jejunostomy effluents in patients with severe short bowel syndrome. Gut 1989;30:943.
51. Aly A, Barany F, Kollberg B, et al. Effect of an H2-receptor blocking agent on diarrhoeas after extensive small bowel resection in Crohn's disease. Acta Med Scand 1980;207:119.
52. Jacobsen O, Ladefoged K, Stage JG, et al. Effects of cimetidine on jejunostomy effluents in patients with severe short-bowel syndrome. Scand J Gastroenterol 1986;21:824.
53. Baptista RJ. Role of histamine H2 receptor antagonists in total parenteral nutrition patients. Am J Med 1987;83(Suppl 6A): 53.
54. King CE, Toskes PP, Guilarte TR, et al. Comparison of the one-gram D-[14C]xylose breath test to the [14C] bile acid breath test in patients with small-intestine bacterial overgrowth. Dig Dis Sci 1980;25:53.
55. King CE, Toskes PP. Comparison of the 1-gram [14C]xylose, 10-gram lactulose-H2, and 80-gram glucose-H2 breath tests in patients with small intestinal bacterial overgrowth. Gastroenterology 1986;91:1447.
56. Rombeau JL, Rolandelli RH. Enteral and parenteral nutrition in patients with enteric fistulas and short bowel syndrome. Surg Clin North Am 1987;67:551.
57. Fleming CR, Beart RW, Berkner S, et al. Home parenteral nutrition for management of the severely malnourished adult patient. Gastroenterology 1980;79:11.
58. Rombeau JL, Caldwell MD. Parenteral nutrition. Philadelphia: WB Saunders, 1986:1.
59. Askanazi J, Rosenbaum SH, Hyman AI, et al. Respiratory changes induced by the large glucose loads of parenteral nutrition. JAMA 1980;243:1444.
60. Wolfe RR, O'Donnell TF, Stone MD, et al. Investigation of factors determining the optimal glucose infusion rate in total parenteral nutrition. Metabolism 1980;29:892.
61. Lowry SF, Brennan MF. Abnormal liver function during parenteral nutrition: relation to infusion excess. Surg Res 1979;26: 300.
62. Gouttebel MC, Saint-Aubert B, Astre C, et al. Total parenteral nutrition needs in different types of short bowel syndrome. Dig Dis Sci 1986;31:718.
63. Caniano DA, Starr J, Ginn-Pease ME. Extensive short-bowel syndrome in neonates: outcome in the 1980s. Surgery 1989;105:119.
64. Heymsfield SB, Bethel RA, Ansley JD, et al. Enteral alimentation: an alternative to central venous hyperalimentation. Ann Intern Med 1979;90:63.
65. Morin CL, Linq V, Bourassa D. Small intestinal and colonic changes induced by a chemically defined diet. Dig Dis Sci 1980;25:123.
66. Souba WW, Smith RJ, Wilmore DW. Glutamine metabolism by the intestinal tract. JPEN J Parenter Enteral Nutr 1985;9: 608.
67. Dobbie RP, Hoffmeister JA. Continuous pump-tube enteric hyperalimentation. Surg Gynecol Obstet 1976;143:273.
68. Fairfull-Smith R, Abunassar R, Freeman JB, et al. Rational use of elemental and nonelemental diets in hospitalized patients. Ann Surg 1980;192:600.
69. Bright-Asare P, Binder HJ. Hydroxy fatty acids (OHFA) stimulate colonic secretion of water and electrolytes. Gastroenterology 1972;62:727.
70. Ammon HV, Phillips SF. Inhibition of colonic water and electrolyte absorption by fatty acids in man. Gastroenterology 1973;65:744.
71. Ovesen L. Chu R, Howard L. The influence of dietary fat on jejunostomy output in patients with severe short bowel syndrome. Am J Clin Nutr 1983;38:270.
72. Simko V, McCarroll AM, Goodman S, et al. High fat diet in a short bowel syndrome. Dig Dis Sci 1980;25:333.
73. Woolf GM, Miller C, Kurian R, et al. Diet for patients with a short bowel: high fat or high carbohydrate. Gastroenterology 1983;84:823.
74. Dobbins JW. Binder HJ. Importance of the colon in enteric hyperoxaluria. N Engl J Med 1977;296:298.
75. Zurier RB, Campbell RG, Hashim SA, et al. Use of medium-chain triglyceride in management of patients with massive resection of the small intestine. N Engl J Med 1966;274:490.
76. Newcomer AD, McGill DB, Thomas PJ, et al. Prospective com-

parison of indirect methods for detecting lactase deficiency. N Engl J Med 1975;293:1232.

77. McCance RA, Prior KM, Widdowson EM. A radiologic study of the rate of passage of brown and white bread through the digestive tract of man. Br J Nutr 1953;7:98.

78. Eastwood MA, Kay RM. A hypothesis for the action of dietary fiber along the gastrointestinal tract. Am J Clin Nutr 1979;32:364.

79. Lawetz O, Blackburn AM, Bloom SR. Effect of pectin on gastric emptying and gut hormone release in the dumping syndrome. Scand J Gastroenterol 1983;18:327.

80. Hillman L, Peters S, Fisher A, et al. Differing effects of pectin, cellulose, and liquid on stool pH, transit time, and weight. Br J Nutr 1983;50:189.

81. Sakata T, Yajima T. Influence of short chain fatty acids on the epithelial cell division of digestive tract. Q J Exp Physiol 1984;69:639.

82. Barilla DE, Notz C, Kennedy D, et al. Renal oxalate excretion following oral oxalate loads in patients with ileal disease and with renal and absorptive hypercalciurias: effect of calcium and magnesium. Am J Med 1978;64:579.

83. Sitrin MD, Rosenberg IH, Chawla K, et al. Nutritional and metabolic complications in a patient with Crohn's disease and ileal resection. Gastroenterology 1980;78:1069.

84. Pollack S, Enat R, Harim S, et al. Pellagra as the presenting manifestation of Crohn's disease. Gastroenterology 1982;82:948.

85. Franklin JL, IH Rosenberg. Impaired folic acid absorption in inflammatory bowel disease: effects of salicylazosulfapyridine (Azulfidine). Gastroenterology 1973;64:517.

86. Gerson CD, Coben N, Janowitz HD. Small intestinal absorptive function in regional enteritis. Gastroenterology 1973;64:907.

87. Green R, Jacobsen DW, Van Tonder SV, et al. Enterohepatic circulation of cobalamin in the non-human primate. Gastroenterology 1981;81:773.

88. Hollander D. Intestinal absorption of vitamins A, E, D and K. J Lab Clin Med 1981;97:449.

89. Compston JE, Ayers AB, Horton LWL, et al. Osteomalacia after small intestinal resection. Lancet 1978;1:9.

90. Driscoll RH, Meredith SC, Sitrin M, et al. Vitamin D deficiency and bone disease in patients with Crohn's disease. Gastroenterology 1982;83:1252.

91. Teitelbaum SL, Halverson JD, Butts M, et al. Abnormalities of circulating 25-OH vitamin D after jejunal-ileal bypass for obesity. Ann Intern Med 1977;86:289.

92. Hey H, Stokholm KH, Lund B, et al. Vitamin D deficiency in obese patients and changes in circulating vitamin D metabolites following jejunoileal bypass. Int J Obes 1982;6:473.

93. Howard L, Ovesen L, Satya-Murti S, et al. Reversible neurological systems caused by vitamin E deficiency in a patient with short bowel syndrome. Am J Clin Nutr 1982;36:1243.

94. Colette C, Gouttebel MC, Monnier LH, et al. Calcium absorption following small bowel resection in man: evidence for an adaptive response. Eur J Clin Invest 1986;16:271.

95. Hylander E, Ladefoged K, Madsen S. Calcium balance and bone mineral content following small-intestinal resection. Scand J Gastroenterol 1981;16:167.

96. Hessov I, Hasselblad C, Fasth S, et al. Magnesium deficiency after ileal resection for Crohn's disease. Scand J Gastroenterol 1983;18:643.

97. Gelland L. Magnesium and inflammatory bowel disease. Magnesium 1988;7:78.

98. Wolman SL, Anderson GH, Marliss EB, et al. Zinc in total parenteral nutrition: requirements and metabolic effects. Gastroenterology 1979;76:458.

99. McClain C, Soutor C, Zieve L. Zinc-deficiency: a complication of Crohn's disease. Gastroenterology 1980;78:272.

100. Sturniolo G, Molukhia MM, Shields R, et al. Zinc absorption in Crohn's disease. Gut 1980;21:387.

101. Ainby CC, Cason J, Carlsson LK, et al. Zinc status in inflammatory bowel disease. Clin Sci 1988;75:277.

102. Jones RB, Keeling PWN, Hilton PJ, et al. The relationship between leukocyte and muscle zinc in health and disease. Clin Sci 1981;60:237.

103. Fleming CR, McCall JT, O'Brien JF, et al. Selenium status in patients receiving home parenteral nutrition. JPEN J Parenter Enteral Nutr 1984;8:258.

104. Dunlap WM, James JC, Hume DM. Anemia and neutropenia caused by copper deficiency. Ann Intern Med 1974;80:470.

105. Brown RO, Forloines-Lynn S, Cross RE, et al. Chromium deficiency after long-term total parenteral nutrition. Dig Dis Sci 1986;31:661.

106. Abumrad NN, Schneider AJ, Steel D, et al. Amino acid intolerance during prolonged total parenteral nutrition reversed by molybdate therapy. Am J Clin Nutr 1981;34:2551.

107. Stokes MA, Almond DJ, Pettil SH, et al. Home parenteral nutrition: a review of 100 patient years of treatment in 76 consecutive cases. Br J Surg 1988;75:481.

108. Lin CH, Rossi TM, Heitlinger LA, et al. Nutritional assessment of children with short-bowel syndrome receiving home parenteral nutrition. Am J Dis Child 1987;141:1093.

109. O'Connor MJ, Ralston CW, Ament ME. Intellectual and perceptual–motor performance of children receiving prolonged home–total parenteral nutrition. Pediatrics 1988;81:231.

110. Steiger E, Srp F. Morbidity and mortality related to home parenteral nutrition in patients with gut failure. Am J Surg 1983;145:102.

111. Fuchs PC, Gustafson ME, King JT, et al. Assessment of catheter-associated infection risk with the Hickman right atrial catheter. Infect Control 1984;5:226.

112. Schuman ES, Winters VN, Gross GF, et al. Management of Hickman catheter sepsis. Am J Surg 1985;149:627.

113. Smith NL, Ravo B, Soroff HS, et al. Successful fibrinolytic therapy for superior vena cava thrombosis secondary to long-term total parenteral nutrition. JPEN J Parenter Enteral Nutr 1985;9:55.

114. Mock DM, De Lorimer AA, Liebman WM, et al. Biotin deficiency: an unusual complication of parenteral alimentation. N Engl J Med 1981;304:870.

115. Whitington PF. Cholestasis associated with total parenteral nutrition in infants. Hepatology 1985;5:693.

116. Bowyer BA, Fleming CR, Ludwig J, et al. Does long-term home parenteral nutrition in adult patients cause chronic liver disease? JPEN J Parenter Enteral Nutr 1985;9:11.

117. Messing B, Bories C, Kunstlinger F, et al. Does total parenteral nutrition induce gallbladder sludge formation and lithiasis? Gastroenterology 1983;84:1012.

118. Roslyn JJ, Pitt HA, Mann LL, et al. Gall bladder disease in patients on long-term parenteral nutrition. Gastroenterology 1983;84:148.

119. Gimmon Z, Kelley RE, Simko V, et al. Total parenteral nutrition solution increases bile lithogenicity in rat. J Surg Res 1982;32:256.

120. Klein GL, Ament ME, Bluestone R, et al. Bone disease associated with total parenteral nutrition. Lancet 1980;2:1041.

121. Ott SM, Maloney NA, Klein GL, et al. Aluminum is associated with low bone formation in patients receiving chronic parenteral nutrition. Ann Intern Med 1983;98:910.

122. Shike M, Harrison JE, Sturtridge WC, et al. Metabolic bone disease in patients receiving long-term total parenteral nutrition. Ann Intern Med 1980;92:343.

123. De Vernejoul MC, Messing B, Modrowski D, et al. Multi-factorial low bone remodeling bone disease during cyclic total parenteral nutrition. J Clin Endocrinol Metab 1985;60:109.

124. Shike M, Shils ME, Heller A, et al. Bone disease in prolonged parenteral nutrition: osteopenia without mineralization defect. Am J Clin Nutr 1986;44:89.

125. Bengoa JM, Sitrin MD, Wood RJ, et al. Amino acid induced hypercalciuria in patients on total parenteral nutrition. Am J Clin Nutr 1983;38:264.

126. Berkelhammer CH, Wood RJ, Sitrin MD. Acetate and hypercalciuria during total parenteral nutrition. Am J Clin Nutr 1988;48:1482.

127. Epstein S, Traberg H, Levine G, et al. Bone and mineral status of patients beginning total parenteral nutrition. JPEN J Parenter Enteral Nutr 1986;10:263.

128. Thompson JS. Surgical considerations in the short bowel syndrome. Surg Gynecol Obstet 1993;176:89.

129. Warden MJ, Wesley JR. Small bowel reversal procedure for treatment of the "short gut" baby. J Pediatr Surg 1978;13:321
130. Sigalet D, Kneteman NM, Thomson ABR. Small bowel transplantation: past, present and future. Dig Dis 1992;10:258.
131. Grant DR. Small bowel transplantation. Gastrointestinal Journal Club 1992;1:3.
132. Todo S, Tzakis AG, Abu-Elmagd K, et al. Cadaveric small bowel and small bowel–liver transplantation in humans. Transplantation 1992;53:369.
133. Grant DR, Wall W, Mimeault R, et al. Successful small-bowel/liver transplantation. Lancet 1 1990;335:181.
134. Busuttil RW, Farmer DG, Shaked A, et al. Successful combined liver and small intestine transplantation for short-gut syndrome and liver failure. West J Med 1993;158:184.

Textbook of Gastroenterology, second edition, edited by Tadataka Yamada. JB Lippincott Company, Philadelphia © 1995.

CHAPTER 76

Tumors and Other Neoplastic Diseases of the Small Bowel

Peter Lance

Epidemiology
Etiology—Possible Pathophysiologic Mechanisms
Clinical Manifestations of Small Bowel Tumors
   Relative Numbers of Symptomatic and Asymptomatic Tumors
   Relative Numbers of Benign and Malignant Symptomatic Tumors
   Histologic Varieties of Small Bowel Tumor and Their Distribution
   Symptoms and Signs of Small Bowel Tumor and Their Distribution

Differential Diagnosis
Diagnostic Modalities
   Barium Contrast Studies
   Arteriography
   Noninvasive Studies
   Endoscopy
Varieties of Small Bowel Tumor
   Adenoma and Adenocarcinoma
   Carcinoid Tumors and Syndrome
   Lymphoma
   Leiomyoma and Leiomyosarcoma

Tumors of the duodenum, jejunum, and ileum are the subject of this chapter. Although benign and malignant tumors of the small bowel are uncommon by comparison with those in other parts of the gastrointestinal tract, they exhibit a diversity that reflects all the histologic components, epithelial and mesenchymal, of the organ (Table 76-1). In addition to tumors that grow as discrete masses in the wall of the small bowel, some diffuse lesions of small intestinal lymphoid tissue are discussed; examples of the latter are lymphoid hyperplasia and the lymphomas.

Investigators have been intrigued by the relative rarity of small bowel tumors partly because of the insights that a better understanding of this phenomenon might bring to determining the cause of the more common gastrointestinal tumors, especially those of the colon. The small and the large bowel are often involved in patients with familial adenomatous polyposis (FAP), which are described in detail in Chapter 86 along with other polypoid tumors, especially hamartomas; FAP is discussed here only to emphasize that adenocarcinoma of the small bowel, typically in the periampullary region, is an important feature of these syndromes.

Small bowel tumors are often asymptomatic and without clinical significance; almost all Brunner's gland hamartomas, many lipomas, and some carcinoids are in this category. Certain nonneoplastic intestinal diseases, such as celiac sprue and Crohn's disease, may predispose the individual to malignant neoplasms of the small bowel. Small bowel tumors give rise to systemic as well as local symptoms; flushing may be the first symptom of a carcinoid tumor, and a primary lymphoma of the small bowel may present as a malabsorption syndrome.

TABLE 76-1
Classification of Small Bowel Tumors

Benign Epithelial Tumors
Adenoma

Malignant Epithelial Tumors
Primary adenocarcinoma
Secondary carcinoma
Carcinoid tumors (enterochromaffin cells)

Lymphoproliferative Disorders
Lymphoid hyperplasia
Immunoproliferative small intestinal disease
Malignant lymphoid tumors
    Hodgkin's and non-Hodgkin's lymphoma
    Plasma cell tumors of gastrointestinal tract
    Leukemias
    Primary macroglobulinemia

Benign and Malignant Mesenchymal Tumors
Myogenous (smooth muscle)
Lipomatous
Fibromatous
Neurogenic

Hamartomas
Peutz-Jeghers syndrome
Brunner's gland
Cronkhite-Canada syndrome
Neurofibromatosis

Adapted from Morson BC, Dawson IMP. Gastrointestinal pathology. 2nd ed. Oxford: Blackwell Scientific, 1979:400.

Local symptoms are stereotyped and usually not indicative of the histologic nature of the offending tumor.

Barium radiology, refined by enteroclysis, remains the primary diagnostic modality for small bowel tumors, but endoscopy and noninvasive imaging procedures have assumed important roles. The clinical outcome in many cases of small bowel malignancy is poor. If surgical resection fails, alternative therapy is usually unsuccessful.

EPIDEMIOLOGY

Most malignant tumors of the small bowel become symptomatic and are eventually fatal, in contrast to the asymptomatic majority of benign small bowel tumors. Consequently, reliable epidemiologic data are available for the former but not the latter. In 1993, approximately 3600 new cases and 925 deaths from malignant small bowel tumors were expected in the United States.[1] A total of 1832 primary small bowel malignancies were reported by nine cancer registries participating in the Surveillance, Epidemiology, and End Results Program for the period 1973 to 1982, to give an overall annual incidence rate for these tumors of 9.6 per million, or less than 1 per 100,000.[2] In descending order, the most common histologic varieties of malignant small bowel tumor were adenocarcinoma, carcinoid, lymphoma, and sarcoma; respective average annual incidence rates for these tumors were 3.9, 2.9, 1.6, and 1.2 per million. Carcinoma, carcinoid, and sarcoma were slightly more common in men than in women, but the

incidence of small bowel lymphoma among men was nearly double the rate among women. Carcinoma was 1.4 times more common in those of African descent than in Caucasians, and the incidence of carcinoid was 1.7-fold higher, but the incidence of lymphoma among Caucasians exceeded the rate among those of African descent by almost twofold. The incidences of carcinoma, carcinoid, and lymphoma increased progressively with age; the incidence of sarcoma reached a plateau after the sixth decade. To emphasize the relative rarity of small bowel malignancies, incidences for men and women combined have been reported to be 79 per 100,000 for all malignancies of the digestive tract, 34 per 100,000 for colon cancer, and 15 per 100,000 for cancers of the rectum and rectosigmoid. Small bowel tumors account for little more than 1% of all gastrointestinal malignancies.

With the exception of one form of lymphoma (immunoproliferative small intestine disease, or IPSID), malignant small bowel tumors are more common in Western developed countries than in other parts of the world.[3] There is a strong correlation between the incidences of small and large bowel cancer in a given country,[4] although a similar correlation does not exist between the incidences of small bowel cancer and cancer of the stomach or esophagus. As is the case with large bowel cancer, Japanese persons living in Hawaii have a higher incidence of small bowel cancer than do Japanese living in Japan, and the incidence is similar to that for the Caucasian population of Hawaii.[3]

ETIOLOGY—POSSIBLE PATHOPHYSIOLOGIC MECHANISMS

Relatively little is known of the mechanisms that are responsible for the development of small bowel tumors. Although the cause almost certainly varies with the type of tumor, certain factors may predispose an individual to more than one kind of neoplasm; the increased frequency of both adenocarcinoma and lymphoma of the small bowel in patients with preexisting celiac sprue is an example. Various aspects of the anatomy and physiology of the organ have been plausibly invoked, for the most part without supporting evidence, to explain the rarity of all varieties of small bowel tumor.[4]

It has been argued that the neutral or alkaline pH in the lumen of the small bowel prevents formation of the nitrosamines that may be carcinogenic in the acid environment of the stomach.[5] However, the lumenal pH is essentially the same in the small and large bowel, so this mechanism cannot explain the different incidences for malignant neoplasms in the two organs. Rapid transit, the liquid nature of the contents, and the presence of detoxifying enzymes such as benzopyrene hydroxylase that nullify putative carcinogens may minimize the risk of neoplastic change in small intestine epithelium.[6]

The metabolites of anaerobic bacteria are thought by some to play an important role in the causation of colorectal cancer,[7] and bacteria constitute about one third by weight of the contents of the colon.[8] Bacterial counts in the small bowel, typically less than 10^4 per gram of contents in the jejunum and less than 10^8 in the ileum, are much lower than in the colon, and anaerobes are usually completely absent.[9,10] It is therefore

TABLE 76-2

TABLE 76-2
Most Frequently Encountered Varieties of Small Bowel Tumor

BENIGN	MALIGNANT
Adenoma	Primary adenocarcinoma
	Carcinoid
	Primary lymphoma
Leiomyoma	Leiomyosarcoma
Brunner's gland hamartoma	
Lipoma	

17,070 autopsies performed from 1913 to 1957 at a single institution, 93 patients (0.6%) who had died from unrelated causes were found to have small bowel tumors, of which 26% were malignant.[14] In comparison, approximately 1 of 10,000 inpatients (0.0001%) is admitted because of a symptomatic small bowel tumor.[15] Although a statistically rigorous comparison between these figures is not permissible, they indicate the preponderance of asymptomatic over symptomatic small bowel tumors.

Several further generalizations can be made: the majority of asymptomatic tumors are benign; almost all of the malignant asymptomatic tumors are carcinoids that have not metastasized[16]; and the majority (>80%) of malignant small bowel tumors become symptomatic.[16]

argued that the milieu of the small bowel, unlike that of the colon, is not conducive to the formation of carcinogens from bile, thus explaining the relative rarity of malignant neoplasms of the small bowel.[4]

Apoptosis, the physiologic process of programmed cell death or cell suicide, has attracted considerable interest.[11,12] Inhibition of apoptosis causes aberrant cell survival and thereby contributes to oncogenesis. Expression of the *BCL2* gene is thought to prevent apoptosis. The 26-kd protein encoded by the *BCL2* gene is expressed abundantly by murine colonic crypt cells but only poorly by murine small intestine crypt cells.[13] Confirmation of these observations in human intestine would be consistent with the wide disparity between the incidences of small and large bowel cancer.

Certain conditions are associated with particular histologic types of small bowel tumor. They are discussed in the sections devoted to the individual varieties of tumor.

CLINICAL MANIFESTATIONS OF SMALL BOWEL TUMORS

Relative Numbers of Symptomatic and Asymptomatic Tumors

The data from which it would be possible to determine accurately the ratio of symptomatic to asymptomatic small bowel tumors do not exist, but there is little doubt that the majority are clinically silent. In a retrospective survey of

Relative Numbers of Benign and Malignant Symptomatic Tumors

Estimates of the ratio of benign to malignant symptomatic small bowel tumors are based on series of surgically managed cases,[15,16] in which malignant tumors modestly outnumber benign ones; the proportion of malignant tumors is in the range of 50% to 65%.

Histologic Varieties of Small Bowel Tumor and Their Distribution

A histologic classification is given in Table 76-1. Some of the tumors listed are extremely rare and are not discussed in any detail here. The relatively few histologic varieties that account for most small bowel tumors are listed in Table 76-2. The relative frequencies and anatomic distributions of the four most common malignant small bowel tumors are shown in Tables 76-3 and 76-4.

Symptoms and Signs of Small Bowel Tumor and Their Distribution

The clinical features of benign and malignant small bowel tumors are summarized in Table 76-5.

TABLE 76-3
Relative Frequencies of the Four Commonest Malignant Small Bowel Tumors*

	RELATIVE FREQUENCY (%)	5-YEAR SURVIVAL (%)
Primary adenocarcinoma	33–50	Resectable: 10–20
		Unresectable: <1
Malignant carcinoid	17–39	50
Primary lymphoma	12–24	Resectable: 40–50
		Unresectable: <25
Leiomyosarcoma	11–20	20–50

* The ranges for the percentages of each variety of tumor from four US series[14–16,138] and overall 5-year survival rates are given.

TABLE 76-4
Distribution of Malignant Small Bowel Tumors*

	DUODENUM (%)	JEJUNUM (%)	ILEUM (%)
Primary adenocarcinoma (n = 116)	40	38	22
Malignant carcinoid (n = 67)	18	4	78
Primary lymphoma (n = 47)	6	36	58
Leiomyosarcoma (n = 32)	3	53	44

* Combined data from four US series.[14-16,138] The percentages of each tumor located in each segment of small bowel are given.

Benign Tumors

It is uncommon for benign small bowel tumors to become symptomatic in subjects younger than 50 years of age. Fluctuating pain caused by intermittent partial small intestine obstruction is the most common presenting manifestation of the minority of benign tumors that do become symptomatic and is present in up to 70% of cases.[5] However, the pain is often vague. Intussusception is the most common cause of obstruction from benign small bowel tumors, which account for half of all cases of adult intussusception.[14,17] In contrast to children, in whom the intussusceptum is rarely a mass lesion, intussusception in adults typically is not an acute surgical emergency, and a thorough diagnostic evaluation can usually be undertaken before surgical intervention. Few benign small bowel tumors are palpable on abdominal examination. Occult gastrointestinal blood loss is reported in one quarter to one half of patients with symptomatic benign small tumors. Hematemesis and rectal bleeding are rare, as are weight loss and other symptoms.

Malignant Tumors

Most malignant small bowel tumors become symptomatic during the sixth and seventh decades; in one series, 86% of patients were older than 50 years of age on presentation.[15] Abdominal pain, which may be colicky or more constant in nature, is the most common initial symptom. About one third of patients with malignant small bowel tumors develop partial or complete small bowel obstruction, which can arise in several ways. Adenocarcinomas cause obstruction through infiltration and annular constriction of the intestinal wall. In addition to encroachment on the intestinal lumen by the tumor itself, the desmoplastic reaction in the adjacent mesentery that often accompanies the growth of a carcinoid tumor[18,19] may lead to kinking of the bowel and episodes of obstruction.

On the rare occasions that obstruction caused by a malignant small bowel tumor is the result of intussusception, the tumor is likely to be a polypoid lymphoma or leiomyosarcoma. Intramural metastases have also been reported as a very rare cause of intussusception.[20] As with benign tumors, obstruction caused by malignant small bowel tumors is usually intermittent, and the episode that leads to diagnosis of the tumor will most likely have been preceded by earlier similar episodes over a period of months that resolved spontaneously.

Weight loss and hemorrhage have each been reported in as many as one half of cases of small bowel malignancy. Weight loss is most severe and likely to be a major symptom with lymphoma. Hemorrhage is usually apparent only if the stool is tested for occult blood. However, leiomyosarcomas occasionally cause massive hemorrhage with frank rectal bleeding, and duodenal tumors are a rare cause of painless hematemesis.[14,21] An abdominal mass, consisting of tumor or distended bowel or both, is palpable in up to 41% of cases of small bowel malignancy.[14] Intestinal perforation occurs in about 10% of cases, almost all of which are lymphomas or leiomyosarcomas.

The clinical features of periampullary tumors are distinctive. In one retrospective series of 126 patients who were

TABLE 76-5
Clinical Features of Small Bowel Tumors

SYMPTOM	BENIGN	MALIGNANT
Abdominal pain	Most frequent symptom	Most frequent symptom; one third of patients develop partial or complete obstruction
Intussusception	Most common cause of intussusception in adults, lipomas are the leading cause.	Rare
Occult blood loss	25%–50% of cases	Up to 50% of cases
Frank bleeding	Rare	Rare; leiomyosarcoma is most likely tumor
Weight loss	Very rare	Up to 50% of cases; most severe with lymphoma
Palpable abdominal mass	Uncommon	40% of cases
Perforation	Very rare	About 10% of cases, almost all of which are lymphomas or leiomyosarcomas.
Jaundice	Rare occurrence with benign periampullary tumor	Occurs with nearly 80% of malignant periampullary tumors
Flushing	Carcinoid syndrome does not occur	Carcinoid syndrome occurs in minority of cases of metastatic carcinoid tumor
Diarrhea	Very rare	Common in cases of lymphoma; occurs with carcinoid syndrome

treated surgically, the tumors were malignant in all but 6, and 78% of patients were clinically jaundiced on presentation.[22]

The symptoms of carcinoid tumors most often derive from the local effects of tumor growth, which are indistinguishable from those caused by other varieties of tumor. Symptoms from these tumors may arise in two other ways, to be discussed more fully in later sections: first, desmoplasia, local peritoneal and mesenteric fibrosis that is a reaction to the tumor sometimes causes kinking of the bowel and obstructive symptoms, and second, disseminated hormone-secreting tumors give rise to symptoms of the carcinoid syndrome.

DIFFERENTIAL DIAGNOSIS

Depending on the age of the patient, patient history, and other clinical features, small bowel tumors may be considered as one of the less frequent causes in the differential diagnoses of intestinal obstruction, occult gastrointestinal blood loss, weight loss, and unexplained abdominal pain. The diagnosis of a small bowel tumor is often not made before laparotomy, for which the most frequent indication is obstruction.

Some other causes of small bowel obstruction are listed in Table 76-6, and for several of these the term pseudotumor is sometimes applied. Endometriosis involving the bowel is easily overlooked as a cause of acute complete or, more typically, recurrent partial obstruction in women. The distinction between obstruction of a purely inflammatory nature in patients with Crohn's disease and that caused by a supervening malignant small bowel tumor can often not be made preoperatively (see discussion elsewhere in this chapter). Masses or pseudotumors composed of worms are among the rare causes of obstruction that occasionally come into the differential diagnosis of small bowel tumors.

TABLE 76-6
Differential Diagnosis of Small Intestine Obstruction

Extrinsic
Adhesions
Hernias
Intussusception
Volvulus
Intraabdominal abscess and hematoma
Annular pancreas
Endometriosis and pelvic inflammatory disease
Anomalous vessels

Bowel Wall
Crohn's disease
Ischemia
Hematoma (e.g., associated with oral anticoagulant therapy)
Radiation enteritis
Amyloidosis

Intraluminal
Ingested foreign body
Gallstones
Bezoars
Worms

Most cases of intussusception in adults are caused by benign small bowel tumors. This diagnosis should be suspected if rectal bleeding accompanies an episode of obstruction, although the absence of bleeding does not exclude it. Besides benign and malignant tumors, other causes of intussusception in adults include duplication, ectopic pancreas, foreign body, and Meckel's diverticulum.[17,23]

Occasionally, the cause of jaundice is a periampullary tumor of the duodenum. Because the incidence of these tumors is increased in patients with one of the familial polyposis syndromes, a periampullary tumor should be included in the differential diagnosis of jaundice in such patients.

DIAGNOSTIC MODALITIES

In almost all cases, some form of barium study is the first diagnostic investigation to be performed. The indications for further investigation after barium radiology depend on what kind of tumor is suspected; these indications are summarized in Table 76-7.

Barium Contrast Studies

With the exception of tumors in the proximal and descending duodenum, which are accessible to the endoscopist, barium contrast radiology is the method that is most likely to lead to the diagnosis of a small bowel tumor before surgery. The small bowel follow-through (SBFT), an extension of the conventional barium meal in which the contrast is ingested orally, remains the most widely used of the barium techniques that are employed for the investigation of small bowel disease. Abdominal compression as the column of barium approaches the cecum increases the diagnostic sensitivity for tumors and mucosal abnormalities of the terminal ileum, but results in other parts of the small bowel are inferior to those obtained with duodenal intubation.[24]

The terms enteroclysis and small bowel enema are synonymous for techniques in which the duodenum is intubated for the purpose of administering dilute barium directly to the small bowel.[25] They are not double (air) contrast techniques. To perform enteroclysis, approximately 1 L of barium suspension with a specific gravity of 1.25 to 1.3 is infused at a rate of 100 mL per minute. Bowel distention is key to achieving satisfactory results with enteroclysis. To this end, contrast should be infused at a constant rate until the column of barium reaches the terminal ileum.

Except for lesions of the terminal ileum, where unavoidable dilution of barium reduces its sensitivity, enteroclysis is superior to SBFT in the diagnosis of small bowel disease. In one series of 45 patients who had each had a normal SBFT, a surgically confirmed small bowel lesion was diagnosed within 3 months by enteroclysis.[26] The lesions included ten tumors, of which two were jejunal adenocarcinomas and three were metastases. In a consecutive series of 88 patients who underwent the examination, enteroclysis gave the correct diagnosis in 96%, compared with 65% accuracy for SBFT in the same patients.[27] In light of such evidence, the reluctance of many radiologists to perform enteroclysis is surprising.

A rational diagnostic approach to patients with suspected

TABLE 76-7
Indications for Additional Studies After Barium Radiology

Endoscopy
Usually indicated for any duodenal lesions that might be accessible with the gastroduodenoscope
Suspected immunoproliferative small intestinal disease for biopsy
Terminal ileal lesions accessible with the colonoscope

Computed Tomography
To determine spread, including hepatic involvement, by putatively malignant tumors
To detect tumor-specific appearances: vascularity (after intravenous contrast) of smooth muscle tumors, and central necrosis of leiomyosarcomas; low attenuation of lipomas

Arteriography
Investigation of cases of obscure gastrointestinal bleeding
If barium radiology suggests a lesion that has characteristic arteriographic appearances: carcinoids have stellate pattern on arteriography; smooth muscle tumors have characteristic hypervascularity

Serotonin and Metabolities
Measurement of urinary 5-hydroxyindoleacetic acid and serum serotonin if carcinoid syndrome is suspected

Scintigraphy
Scanning with ^{125}I-labeled Tyr^3-octreotide or metaiodobenzylguanidine for visualization of carcinoid tumors

---

structural lesions of the small bowel is first to request SBFT, including compression views of the terminal ileum. If that examination is negative or inconclusive, enteroclysis should be performed. Characteristic examples of barium radiographs of the common benign and malignant small bowel tumors are shown in Figures 76-1 through 76-5.

Two other barium techniques are sometimes advocated, although not widely used, for the diagnosis of small bowel tumors. In the complete reflux examination, a single-contrast study of the colon is performed first, with dilute barium, and after the column reaches the ileocecal valve, a smooth muscle relaxant is administered.[24] The ileum is visualized as barium refluxes through the valve. In most cases, enteroclysis is superior to the complete reflux examination, but the latter is occasionally useful in the investigation of intestinal obstruction. For the peroral pneumocolon examination of the il-eocecal region, after barium has been given by mouth, air is administered rectally when the column reaches the ileocecal region. Lesions of the terminal ileum, such as those found in Crohn's disease, are well demonstrated by this method.[24]

Arteriography

Although arteriography is not routinely performed in patients with suspected small bowel tumors, it is often indicated if the cause of gastrointestinal bleeding is not revealed by barium studies and endoscopy. Lesions of the small bowel, including

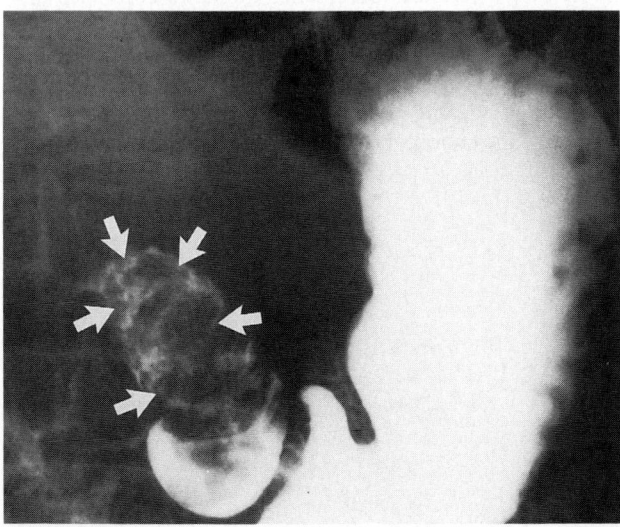

FIGURE 76-1. Villous adenoma of duodenal bulb. Barium radiograph shows a large, lobulated filling defect (*arrows*). (Courtesy of ML Andres, M.D., Buffalo, NY.)

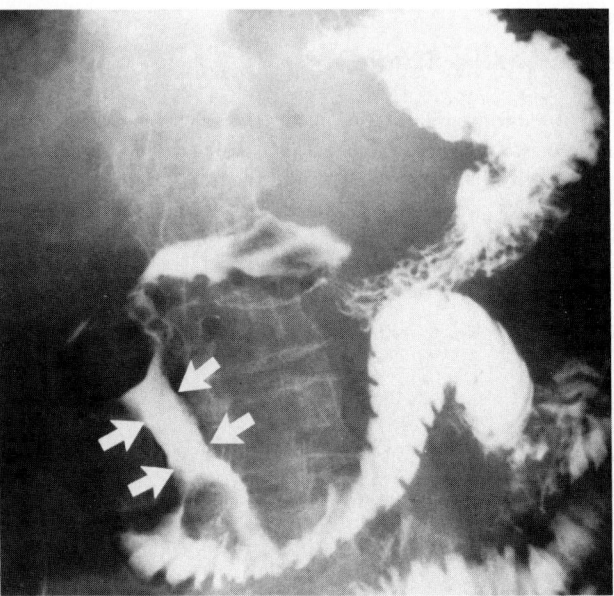

FIGURE 76-2. Periampullary adenocarcinoma of the duodenum. Barium radiograph shows annular constriction (*arrows*), overhanging edges, and complete loss of normal mucosal pattern. (Courtesy of ML Andres, M.D., Buffalo, NY.)

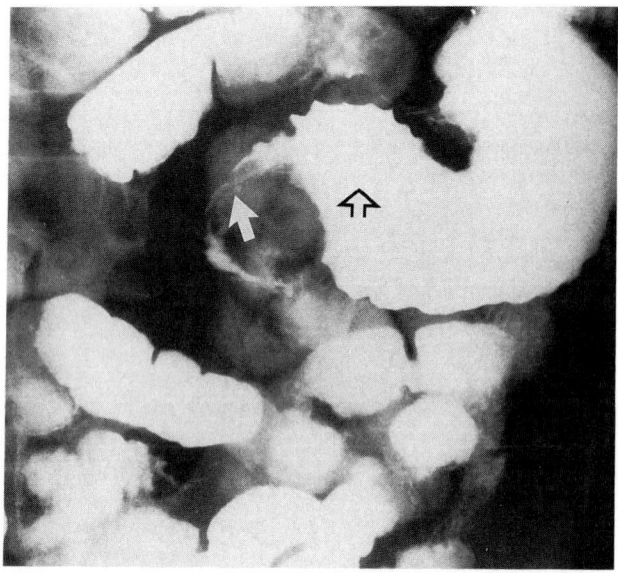

FIGURE 76-3. Carcinoid tumor of distal jejunum demonstrated on barium radiograph. Characteristic desmoplastic reaction has caused kinking (*solid arrow*) with dilated proximal bowel (*open arrow*). (Courtesy of ML Andres, M.D., Buffalo, NY.)

tumors, account for 17% of cases of obscure gastrointestinal bleeding in which a diagnosis is eventually made arteriographically.[28] Superselective catheterization of specific branches of the celiac or superior mesenteric arteries enhances the diagnostic yield. Some small bowel tumors have characteristic arteriographic features.[29] Leiomyomas are hypervascular and have a dense, well-circumscribed blush. Arterial tortuosity and narrowing draws carcinoid tumors into a stellate pattern. Adenocarcinomas are usually seen as hypovascular masses with arteries that are occluded or encased.

Noninvasive Studies

Computed tomography (CT) delineates the local invasiveness and metastatic spread of carcinomas and sarcomas more accurately than barium studies, and it identifies involvement of lymph nodes and other organs in cases of primary small bowel lymphoma (PSBL).[29] The vascularity of leiomyomas and

leiomyosarcomas is well demonstrated after intravenous administration of contrast, and visualization of the central necrosis that occurs in leiomyosarcomas is another way by which CT may contribute to their diagnosis. It has been claimed that the CT finding of a mass with low attenuation, characteristic of fat, is diagnostic of intestinal lipoma.[30] The cause was correctly predicted by CT in 73% of cases in a recent series of 84 patients with small bowel obstruction.[31] CT may become the imaging method of choice in patients with prolonged obstruction and a diffusely dilated small bowel.[32]

Endoscopy

Several endoscopic approaches are useful in the diagnosis of small bowel tumors. The first and second parts of the duodenum, including the ampulla of Vater, are accessible by routine upper endoscopy, and the distal 5 to 25 cm of terminal ileum is accessible by colonoscopy. In the accepted though not widely used technique of push-enteroscopy, a clean pediatric colonoscope is passed through the mouth and advanced as far as two feet beyond the ligament of Treitz. However, even if push-enteroscopy and retrograde ileoscopy are combined, the majority of the small bowel remains inaccessible to endoscopic examination by routine methods.[33] To fill this gap and make total enteroscopy possible, long endoscopes that are passed through the nose and advanced by peristalsis (the sonde method) have been developed. Total enteroscopy must therefore be included in a discussion of the role that endoscopy should play in the diagnosis of small bowel tumors. Finally, the pediatric colonoscope is sometimes used intraoperatively to inspect the small bowel; an assistant maneuvers the endoscope and the surgeon facilitates the procedure by telescoping bowel over the instrument.

It is possible to visualize and biopsy most duodenal mucosal tumors, including nearly all periampullary lesions, with conventional instruments, and endoscopy is routine if a duodenal tumor is suspected on symptomatic grounds. Most authorities now recommend that asymptomatic patients with FAP undergo periodic surveillance duodenoscopy (see discussion elsewhere in this chapter).

Endoscopic pinch biopsies are usually unhelpful for the diagnosis of submucosal lesions such as lipomas and smooth muscle tumors. Depending on the size of the lesion, the experience of the endoscopist, and other circumstances, resort-

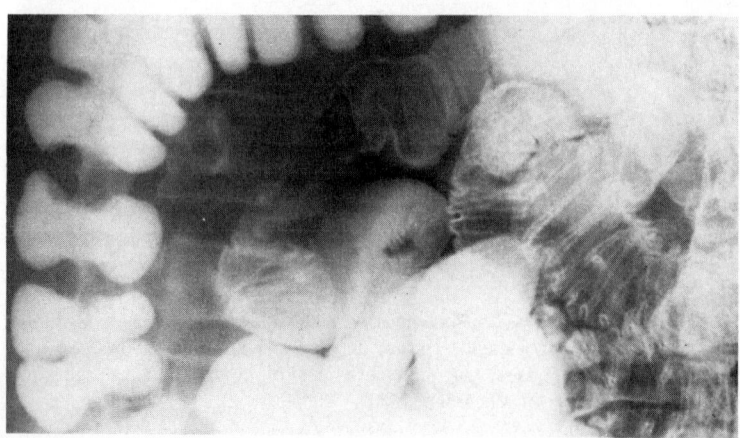

FIGURE 76-4. Primary non-Hodgkin's lymphoma of proximal ileum. Short segment of narrowed bowel seen on enteroclysis. Preceding barium small bowel follow-through with compression views was negative. (Courtesy of ML Andres, M.D., Buffalo, NY.)

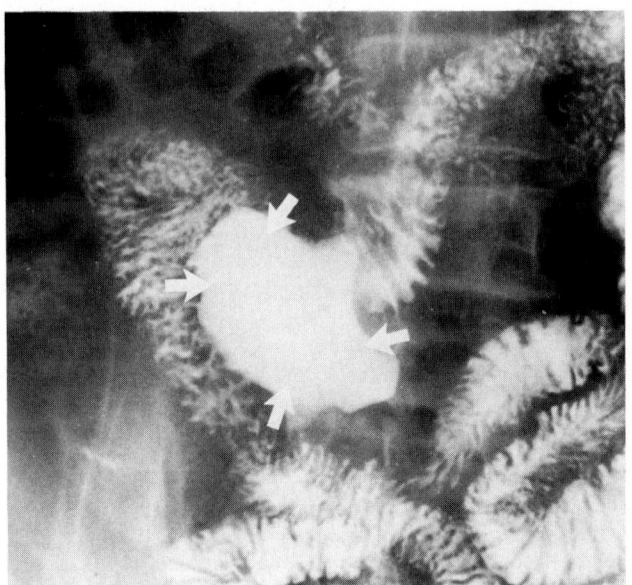

FIGURE 76-5. Leiomyosarcoma of proximal jejunum. Barium radiograph shows a large, extraluminal, ulcerating cavity that indicates the intramural origin of this tumor. (Courtesy of ML Andres, M.D., Buffalo, NY.)

ing to the riskier procedure of loop biopsy of submucosal lesions may occasionally be indicated if conventional mucosal biopsy has not yielded a satisfactory diagnosis.

Endoscopy is indicated in suspected cases of IPSID. Using colonoscopes for push-enteroscopy or forward-viewing gastroduodenoscopes, investigators from Tunisia reached the jejunum in 91% of a prospective series of 80 patients.[34] Endoscopic biopsies were diagnostic of IPSID in 85% of cases. An infiltrated pattern, in which the bowel wall is motionless, is not readily distended on insufflation, and feels firm under biopsy forceps, was noted by the endoscopist in 80% of cases. By contrast, endoscopy does not usually contribute to the diagnosis of intestinal lymphomas of the Western variety, PSBL.

Chronic gastrointestinal bleeding of obscure origin is the principal indication for total enteroscopy. The procedure is diagnostic in up to 50% of cases. Bleeding arises from arte-

riovenous malformations in 40% of the cases in which total enteroscopy is diagnostic. A previously undiagnosed small bowel tumor was diagnosed in 5% of a recent series of 258 patients undergoing total enteroscopy.[35] The tumors that were diagnosed enteroscopically included adenocarcinomas, lymphomas, a carcinoid, and a leiomyosarcoma. Obstruction is a contraindication to enteroscopy.

VARIETIES OF SMALL BOWEL TUMOR

Adenoma and Adenocarcinoma

The histogenesis of small bowel adenocarcinoma is probably analogous to the adenoma-carcinoma or dysplasia-carcinoma sequence through which most colorectal cancers are thought to evolve[36]; the distributions of adenomas and adenocarcinomas within the small bowel coincide, and approximately 30% of small bowel adenomas include malignant foci. More than 40% of patients who have had a total colectomy because of FAP have polyps in the upper gastrointestinal tract; the majority are duodenal adenomas,[37] and they usually develop or are diagnosed 10 to 20 years later than the colonic lesions.[38] About 5% of patients with FAP develop invasive upper gastrointestinal adenocarcinoma, and more than 90% of these tumors are in the duodenum itself or at the ampulla of Vater.[39] The relative risks of duodenal and ampullary adenocarcinoma in patients with FAP have been estimated as approximately 300 and 100, respectively.[40] Whether all adenocarcinomas of the small bowel arise from adenomas is uncertain.

Increased Risk of Adenoma and Adenocarcinoma

Several other conditions, in addition to FAP, are associated with increased risk for adenocarcinoma of the small bowel (Table 76-8).[41] Nineteen cases were reported in a retrospective series of 116 nonlymphomatous malignancies from patients with celiac sprue, compared with 0.23 cases expected.[42]

Adenocarcinoma of the small bowel is more common in patients with Crohn's disease of the small intestine than in normal subjects, with an estimated odds ratio of 8 for this complication.[41] More than 80 examples have been reported,

TABLE 76-8
Clinical Conditions Associated With Increased Risk of Small Bowel Tumor

ASSOCIATED CONDITION	TYPE OF TUMOR	USUAL SITE
Celiac sprue	Adenocarcinoma	Duodenum or jejunum
Crohn's disease	Adenocarcinoma	Ileum
Familial adenomatous polyposis	Adenoma	Duodenum
	Adenocarcinoma	
Ileal conduit or ileocystoplasty	Adenocarcinoma	Adjacent to anastomosis
Ileostomy after colectomy	Adenocarcinoma	Ileocutaneous junction
Neurofibromatosis	Adenocarcinoma; leiomyoma	Ileum
Celiac sprue	Non-Hodgkin's lymphoma (T-cell)	Jejunum
Immunoproliferative small intestine disease	Non-Hodgkin's lymphoma (B-cell)	Jejunum
Nodular lymphoid hyperplasia	Non-Hodgkin's lymphoma	Ileum
Acquired immunodeficiency syndrome	Non-Hodgkin's lymphoma; Kaposi's sarcoma	Ileum

and the majority of adenocarcinomas were ileal.[43,44] The risk is increased further in segments of excluded bowel and in association with fistulas.[45] There is some histologic evidence to support a dysplasia-carcinoma sequence in the development of small bowel adenocarcinomas that complicate Crohn's disease.[44]

Ileal adenocarcinoma is an uncommon late complication after urologic surgery in which the ureters or bladder are anastomosed to the ileum. Adenomas and adenocarcinomas have been reported in an ileal conduit after cystectomy for adenocarcinoma of the urethra[46] and in the ileal components of augmentation ileocystoplasties that were performed in the course of treatment for genitourinary tuberculosis.[47,48] Several cases of ileal adenocarcinoma adjacent to the ileocutaneous junction have been reported in patients with permanent ileostomies.[49,50] A minimum of 25 years lapsed between the original colectomy, performed in all cases for ulcerative colitis or FAP, and development of the ileal tumor.

Dysplasia is recognized in the anorectal mucosal strippings obtained for examination at the time of restorative proctocolectomy with ileal reservoir in patients with FAP or ulcerative colitis.[51] Furthermore, a case of cancer developing in an ileoanal reservoir has been reported.[52] This cancer was diagnosed 4 years after total colectomy and pelvic pouch anastomosis for severely dysplastic colitis. Complete mucosectomy is obligatory for patients with FAP who undergo an ileoanal procedure. The same is true for patients with ulcerative colitis undergoing proctocolectomy because they have already developed, or are thought to be at high risk for developing, colorectal cancer.

Five cases of ileal tumors in patients with neurofibromatosis have been reported.[53] All had an ileal adenocarcinoma and concurrent leiomyomas.

Pathology

Adenomas of the small bowel have similar histologic characteristics to those of the large bowel. Tubular and villous features are recognized. A photomicrograph of a villous adenoma of the duodenum is shown in Figure 76-6. Adenomas

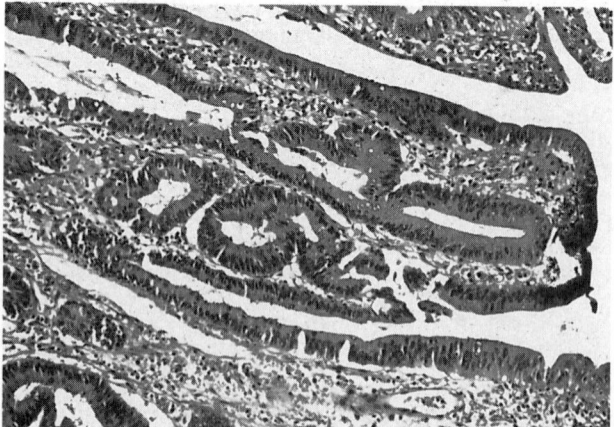

FIGURE 76-6. Villous adenoma of the duodenum. Nuclei are enlarged and hyperchromatic. Goblet cells are scarce. (Hematoxylin and eosin stain; original magnification ×150; courtesy of SK Satchidanand, M.D., Buffalo, NY.)

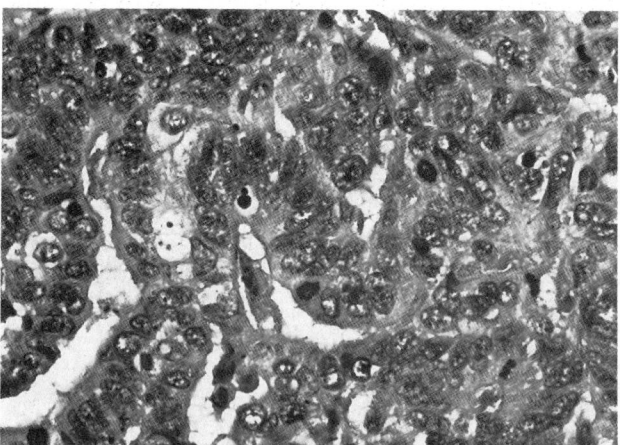

FIGURE 76-7. Adenocarcinoma of the duodenum. The tumor is well differentiated. Nuclear pleomorphism and mitoses are seen in back-to-back glands. (Hematoxylin and eosin stain; original magnification ×600; courtesy of SK Satchidanand, M.D., Buffalo, NY.)

of the ampulla of Vater should be differentiated from those of the duodenum. The former are excluded from most series of small bowel tumors, whereas periampullary tumors are included. The propensity of patients with familial polyposis syndromes to develop periampullary adenomas has been mentioned,[37] and sporadic villous adenomas of the duodenum have a predilection for the same area; in one series, almost 90% of such tumors were in the second portion of the duodenum.[38]

Primary adenocarcinomas grow variously as flat, stenosing, infiltrating, ulcerating, and polypoid tumors. Microscopically, they are similar to other gastrointestinal adenocarcinomas, and they are usually well differentiated, even after metastatic spread has occurred. A photomicrograph of a duodenal adenocarcinoma is shown in Figure 76-7.

Clinical Features and Diagnosis

Adenomas. The location of most small bowel adenomas in the second part of the duodenum (periampullary region) has been emphasized. This applies to sporadic adenomas as well as those in patients with FAP, and to tubular and villous adenomas alike. Reliable data concerning the natural history of duodenal adenomas are limited. In a Japanese series, 20 patients with FAP were followed for an average of 7.1 years with upper gastrointestinal examinations.[54] Eighteen patients had asymptomatic tubular adenomas of less than 8 mm in diameter, and in 17 the adenomas were multiple. One patient, who eluded adequate surveillance, had, in addition to multiple small adenomas, a 17-mm polypoid lesion of the duodenal bulb that progressed to an advanced adenocarcinoma over a 22-month period. In the remaining 17 patients, the number, size, and histologic nature of the adenomas did not change significantly, implying that most small tubular adenomas of the duodenum have a benign clinical course and remain asymptomatic. Invasive adenocarcinoma is found in 25% to 50% of resected villous adenomas.[38]

The limited evidence available indicates that tubular adenomas out number tubulovillous and villous lesions in patients with FAP who have duodenal adenomas; in one prospective series, 79% of such patients had only tubular lesions.[55] It is likely that tubular adenomas predominate in patients with sporadic duodenal adenomas, but this has not been formally studied.

Besides malignancy, other clinical problems that are caused by duodenal villous adenomas include partial gastric outlet obstruction, pancreatitis, bleeding, and obstructive jaundice.[56,57] Most villous adenomas that are resected for these problems are 3 cm or more in diameter. However, little is known of the histologic evolution and rate of growth of the duodenal villous adenoma.

Adenocarcinoma.   The clinical features of small bowel adenocarcinoma include abdominal pain, chronic gastrointestinal bleeding, and progressive weight loss. Most patients with periampullary lesions are jaundiced at the time of presentation.

The diagnosis of a small bowel adenocarcinoma is usually made on SBFT or enteroclysis, supplemented by endoscopic examination and biopsy for duodenal and terminal ileal tumors. A hypovascular mass and encasement of tumor vessels may be seen on arteriography. A periampullary tumor may first be suspected because of characteristic appearances on sonography and percutaneous cholangiography in patients with biliary tract obstruction; endoscopic retrograde cholangiopancreatography (ERCP) should usually be included in the further evaluation of these cases.

Diagnosis of Small Bowel Tumors in Patients with Crohn's Disease

The diagnosis of a small bowel tumor may be especially problematic in patients with preexisting Crohn's disease. Indeed, adenocarcinoma complicating Crohn's disease is usually not suspected before surgery.[43,44,58] The typical patient has longstanding inflammatory bowel disease with recurrent obstructive episodes, and the radiologic appearances of the tumor cannot be distinguished from those of the Crohn's disease. Adenocarcinomas of the small bowel in this setting are almost invariably poorly differentiated and incurable. Diagnostic approaches that might lead to an earlier diagnosis and, conceivably, a better prognosis have yet to be proposed.

Treatment and Prognosis

Adenomas.   The location, size, shape (pedunculated or sessile), and histologic nature (tubular or villous) of the lesion determine what therapy is most appropriate for a small bowel adenoma. Endoscopic biopsy should be performed for adenomas that are accessible, and because most small bowel adenomas are in the duodenum, this is often possible. A useful practical distinction can be made between those adenomas that are diagnosed incidentally (e.g., during endoscopy for unrelated symptoms) and those that cause symptoms; the former are usually tubular and the latter villous adenomas.[57]

Most pedunculated adenomas in the first and second parts of the duodenum with a diameter of up to about 1.5 cm are amenable to resection by endoscopic snare polypectomy. However, the specifications that determine which polyps may safely be removed endoscopically vary with the clinical circumstances and experience of the endoscopist. All resected

adenomas must be submitted for meticulous histologic examination; if there is a villous component, the pathologist should look carefully for foci of adenocarcinoma. In practice, most of the adenomas that are removed endoscopically are tubular, and, for these, polypectomy alone is sufficient treatment.

The rate of development of further small bowel neoplasms in patients from whom sporadic small bowel tubular adenomas have been removed endoscopically has not been definitively studied, but the cancer risk is probably minimal. It is reasonable to repeat the endoscopy if removal was incomplete, for ablation or for snare polypectomy of residual adenomatous tissue, but long-term endoscopic surveillance is not indicated.

Endoscopic surveillance of individuals with FAP is indicated for the purpose of detecting duodenal adenomas before they become adenocarcinomas, but it is not clear how frequently these examinations should be performed. A reasonable schedule includes upper endoscopy in patients about to have a prophylactic colectomy, again at the age of 30 years, and every 5 years thereafter.[37] At these examinations, all polyps should be biopsied, as should the ampulla of Vater if it looks abnormal (i.e., in case of adenomatous change).

Because of the existence of foci of invasive adenocarcinoma in 25% to 50% of small bowel villous adenomas,[38] it is imperative that resection of these tumors should be complete. The size and sessile nature of most villous adenomas, particularly those that are symptomatic, make complete resection by endoscopic methods impossible. A few duodenal villous adenomas that could not be resected in one piece with snare polypectomy have been ablated by laser, electrocautery, or the heater probe over a course of several endoscopies.[38] However, this approach should not be used in routine practice, and surgical resection is usually indicated for the treatment of villous small bowel adenomas.

Local resection is considered adequate for the treatment of villous adenomas that do not include carcinoma, but the surgical literature is made confusing by the fact that in some series of villous adenomas, invasive adenocarcinomas existing within villous adenomas are included. Wide excision is indicated for invasive adenocarcinoma within a villous adenoma, amounting to pancreaticoduodenectomy (the Whipple procedure) for periampullary lesions. The presence of invasive adenocarcinoma in a villous adenoma may not be detected in preoperative endoscopic biopsies and frozen sections of material obtained during surgery. Accordingly, prophylactic duodenectomy has been advocated by some for patients with large duodenal adenomas if high-grade dysplasia is identified.[40,59]

The limited data available suggest that about 30% of patients develop recurrent adenomas within 12 months of endoscopic or surgical resection of a benign duodenal villous adenoma.[38] However, the respective contributions to the apparent recurrence rate by true metachronous adenomas and residual adenomatous tissue that was not resected initially are not known. Adenocarcinomas have been reported among recurrent small bowel tumors in patients whose original tumors were benign villous adenomas; again, some of the recurrences may have developed from neoplastic tissue remaining after an incomplete original resection. A 5-year survival rate of 87% has been reported after resection of duodenal villous adenomas that did not contain invasive adenocarcinoma.

Adenocarcinoma.   Surgical resection is the only treatment for small bowel adenocarcinoma that has curative potential. It is appropriate to attempt curative surgery only if extranodal metastases are not seen at operation. Although many authors recommend radical excision, with the exception of tumors of the terminal ileum the vascular supply and lymphatic drainage of the small bowel are such that true regional cancer resection is not feasible.[15] Resection of the tumor, a 10-cm margin of normal bowel on either side of it, and a wedge of adjacent mesentery is adequate treatment for adenocarcinomas of the jejunum and all but the terminal portion of the ileum.[60] For surgical purposes, malignant tumors of the terminal ileum should be treated as colonic tumors; right hemicolectomy and careful resection of the regional lymph nodes are favored. As discussed in the section on treatment of villous adenomas, pancreaticoduodenectomy (the Whipple procedure) is the appropriate surgical treatment for adenocarcinomas of the duodenum.

In many cases, it is clear at the time of surgery that curative treatment is not possible. Palliative resection and anastomosis to relieve or avoid the development of obstruction are then indicated. In practice, the operative approach is often similar whether the intent is curative or palliative.

Neither chemotherapy nor radiotherapy has a proven role in the management of small bowel adenocarcinoma. Benefit has been claimed on a case-by-case basis for 5-fluorouracil and the nitrosoureas, but objective evidence of an improved survival rate is lacking, and it is hard to justify the use of chemotherapy or radiotherapy outside the setting of a controlled trial.

The 5-year survival rate for adenocarcinoma of the small bowel is no better than 10% to 20% even after curative resection has been attempted. Most patients undergoing palliative resection (i.e., those with extranodal metastases) die within 6 months of surgery. The prognosis after potentially curative resections is strongly influenced by the presence or absence of nodal involvement in the surgical specimens. Eighty-eight percent of patients with positive nodes are reported to die of their disease, compared with 45% of those with negative nodes.[61] Recurrence of malignancy later than 5 years after surgical resection is extraordinarily rare.

Carcinoid Tumors and Syndrome

Pathology

Strictly, all carcinoid ("similar to carcinoma"[62]) tumors, of which about 70% are in the appendix,[63] are malignant. Although distant metastasis from an appendiceal carcinoid of diameter less than 1 cm has been reported,[64] this is such a rare event[65] that for practical purposes appendiceal carcinoids are often regarded as benign. After the appendix, the small bowel is the most common location for carcinoid tumors, and small bowel carcinoids are most often located in the ileum.[62] All small bowel carcinoids have metastatic potential and are, therefore, classified as malignant. Microscopically, the tumor cells are arranged in characteristic clumps, with rims composed of cells that are smaller than the rest and have hyperchromatic nuclei (Fig. 76-8).

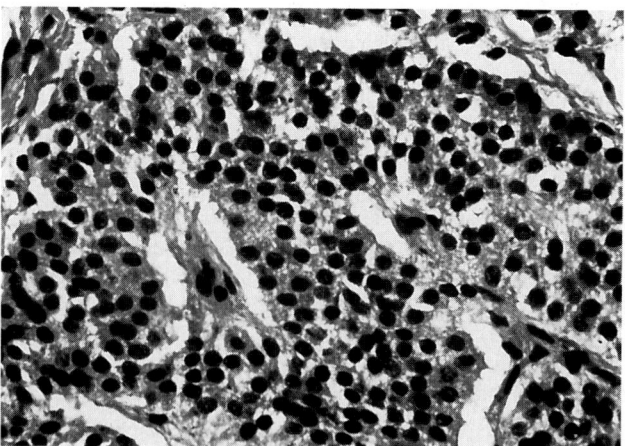

FIGURE 76-8. Carcinoid tumor of duodenum. Uniform cells with hyperchromatic nuclei are arranged in solid clumps. (Hematoxylin and eosin stain; original magnification ×600; courtesy of SK Satchidanand, M.D., Buffalo, NY.)

Clinical Features

Asymptomatic carcinoid tumors of the small bowel may be discovered incidentally at endoscopy, laparotomy, or autopsy, and in some series up to 70% of carcinoids have been in this category.[66] Among patients with clinically significant small intestine carcinoids encountered by the gastroenterologist or general surgeon, local obstructive symptoms predominate; in one series, 13 of 15 patients presented with obstruction.[14] Overt metastases are reported in about one third of symptomatic small bowel cases,[67] and the size of the primary tumor is an important influence on the metastatic spread of carcinoids, which occurs with only 6% of tumors that are less than 1 cm in diameter.[68,69]

The intense fibroplastic or desmoplastic response that often occurs in the vicinity of carcinoid tumors has for long been attributed, without conclusive supporting evidence, to demonstrable local elevations of serotonin level.[18,19,70] The mesenteric shortening and thickening that accompanies desmoplasia is an important contributor to intestinal obstruction in patients with carcinoid tumors of the small bowel. The clinical features of the desmoplastic response adjacent to carcinoid tumors of the small bowel are similar to those of retractile mesenteritis.[71]

Clinical symptoms of the carcinoid syndrome are rare unless metastatic spread, usually to the liver, has taken place. Occasionally, very small foregut carcinoids that secrete active hormones cause symptoms of the carcinoid syndrome in the absence of hepatic metastases. About 10% of patients with symptomatic small bowel carcinoids develop the carcinoid syndrome, the main features of which are flushing, diarrhea, abdominal pain, and valvular cardiac lesions.[62]

The immunohistochemical and hormonal profiles differ among carcinoids located in the foregut (respiratory tract, pancreas, stomach, and duodenum), midgut (jejunum, ileum, and appendix), and hindgut (colon and rectum).[62,72,73] All produce serotonin, which is thought to be responsible for many, but not all, of the features of the carcinoid syndrome.

Foregut carcinoids may secrete various other hormones, causing symptoms, for example, of hypoglycemia, gastric hypersecretion, and Cushing's syndrome in addition to those of the carcinoid syndrome.

A rare association has been recognized, in several case reports, between neurofibromatosis and somatostatin-rich carcinoids in the ampulla of Vater.[74]

Diagnosis of Carcinoid Tumors

Narrowing and kinking of the bowel as a result of mesenteric desmoplasia contribute to the features of carcinoid tumors seen on SBFT and enteroclysis.[29] Desmoplasia is also responsible for characteristic appearances on CT and arteriography.[75,76] Foreshortening of the mesentery causes tortuosity and a stellate pattern of the arteries in the region of the tumor.

Carcinoids, like other neuroendocrine tumors, are notoriously difficult to localize by CT, magnetic resonance imaging, or ultrasonography.[77] Alternative noninvasive imaging techniques take advantage of the large numbers of somatostatin receptors expressed by most carcinoid tumors.[78,79] In one series, primary tumors or metastases, many of them previously undiagnosed, were visualized in 12 of 13 patients with carcinoid tumors by scanning with ^{123}I-labeled Tyr[3]-octreotide (TOCT), a somatostatin analogue.[78] The optimum time for identifying tumor uptake of TOCT is 10 to 30 minutes after injection.[80] In a complementary scintigraphic technique, the radiopharmaceutical used is ^{123}I-labeled metaiodobenzylguanidine, and the optimum time for tumor visualization is 24 to 48 hours after injection.[80]

Diagnosis of the Carcinoid Syndrome

The major contribution of serotonin to the manifestations of the carcinoid syndrome has been discussed. 5-Hydroxyindoleacetic acid (5-HIAA) is a urinary metabolite of serotonin. A diagnosis of the carcinoid syndrome is confirmed if the urinary 5-HIAA level is more than 10 mg in 24 hours.[62] Serotonin-containing foods and drugs, such as phenothiazines, that increase serotonin levels should be withheld immediately before and during the collection of urine for measurement of 5-HIAA. Malabsorption (e.g., from celiac sprue) and chronic intestinal obstruction can cause modest elevations of urinary 5-HIAA levels in the absence of the carcinoid syndrome. Although not routinely measured in most centers, plasma and platelet serotonin levels are increased in the carcinoid syndrome, and serial plasma serotonin levels can be used to monitor for tumor recurrences.[81] In addition to the typical histologic appearance, serotonin-producing cells are demonstrable by immunocytochemical methods in carcinoid tumors after resection from patients with the syndrome.[82]

Treatment and Prognosis

Tumors that are causing bowel symptoms and asymptomatic tumors larger than 1 cm in diameter should be treated as frankly malignant and capable of metastasizing. Patients with the carcinoid syndrome already have widespread metastases. The approach to curative resection in patients without obvious metastases is similar to that for adenocarcinomas.[83] Ileocecectomy and a radical regional lymph node resection are performed for tumors of the terminal ileum. Tumors in the remainder of the ileum and jejunum are treated by wide segmental resection, and a Whipple procedure is usually indicated for duodenal carcinoids. Local excision may be permissible for asymptomatic small bowel carcinoids that are less than 1 cm in diameter.[83]

Most authorities recommend aggressive debulking of unresectable intestinal and hepatic metastatic carcinoids in the hope of alleviating symptoms of the carcinoid syndrome, and there is some retrospective evidence to suggest that this approach may also prolong survival.[84] However, liver involvement is usually diffuse, fewer than 10% of patients with the carcinoid syndrome have resectable hepatic metastases, and evidence to suggest that partial hepatic resection could be curative is lacking. Hepatic artery embolization and ligation and hepatic dearterialization procedures have also been advocated for patients with hepatic metastatic carcinoids.[83]

Somatostatin inhibits the release of various endogenous peptides. A synthetic somatostatin analog, octreotide, injected subcutaneously in doses of 50 to 250 μg two or three times a day, alleviates the clinical features and biochemical abnormalities of the carcinoid syndrome.[85,86] Symptoms are improved or abolished in more than 90% of patients.[87] Although plasma serotonin levels are not altered, octreotide reduces urine 5-HIAA excretion in 66% of patients. Claims that long-term octreotide therapy alone retards or even reverses the growth of carcinoid tumors have not been substantiated. Patients with the carcinoid syndrome are prone to hypotensive crises, particularly during the induction of general anesthesia. Octreotide may reverse such crises or, if given prophylactically before the induction of anesthesia, may prevent them.

Other drugs with antisecretory or antihormonal activity that have been used to treat the gastrointestinal symptoms of the carcinoid syndrome include methysergide, cyproheptadine, and ketanserin.[62] β-Blockers, phenothiazines, histamine H$_1$- and H$_2$-receptor antagonists, and kallikrein inhibitors have been given for the flushing,[62] but with only limited success. The availability of octreotide, now approved by the U. S. Food and Drug Administration for treatment of the carcinoid syndrome, has greatly curtailed the use of other agents for this purpose.

A combination of streptozocin and 5-fluorouracil has been the usual chemotherapeutic approach in patients with metastatic carcinoid tumors. Although response rates as high as 40% have been reported, it is doubtful whether this regimen significantly increases the survival rate.[88] More recently, a combination of interferon-α and octreotide in escalating doses has been advocated for treatment of metastatic carcinoid tumors.[89] Biochemical responses and tumor regression have been claimed by some,[90,91] but others have been less impressed.[92] It remains to be seen whether interferon-α, alone or in combination with other therapies, will significantly prolong survival in patients with metastatic carcinoid tumors. Carcinoids respond poorly if at all to radiotherapy.

The overall 5-year survival rate of patients with small bowel carcinoids in one large series was 54%.[65] With local disease that was completely resected, 5-year survival rate was 75%, compared with 19% in patients with distant metastases. Survival time is shorter in patients with the carcinoid syndrome compared with those without the syndrome who have equivalently disseminated carcinoid tumors.[93]

Lymphoma

It is useful to distinguish two major categories of extranodal lymphoma involving the small bowel. In Western countries, PSBLs are discrete tumors, almost all of the non-Hodgkin's variety. In developing countries, a diffuse primary lymphoma of the small bowel, IPSID, is recognized.

Etiology of Immunoproliferative Small Intestine Disease

The evidence, though circumstantial, is quite compelling that microbial colonization of the small bowel is of major etiologic significance for IPSID.[94] Also known as α-chain disease, Mediterranean lymphoma, or diffuse primary small intestinal lymphoma,[95] IPSID is well recognized in impoverished parts of the world such as the Middle East, Africa, Southeast Asia, and South and Central America. It is virtually unknown in the developed world except among immigrants from these regions, although a single case has been reported in an American who had never left the United States.[96]

IPSID is characterized by an intense lymphoplasmacytic infiltrate of the lamina propria and, sometimes, the regional lymph nodes of the proximal small bowel. The proliferating cells are IgA-secreting B lymphocytes. The α-heavy chain paraprotein that is detectable in the peripheral blood of 20% to 69% of patients, usually during the early stages of the disease,[97] derives from an expanded abnormal clone of these cells. In the early stages of IPSID, the intestinal infiltrate is characterized by mature plasma cells. Subsequently, dystrophic cells appear, and eventually, after a period of years, frank lymphomatous proliferation may develop. The lymphoma is usually of the B-immunoblast sarcoma variety. In at least one study, it has been demonstrated that the malignant cells, the prelymphomatous lymphoplasmacytic infiltrate, and the α-heavy chain paraprotein all arise from the same clone.[98] Several lines of evidence suggest that infection may be important in the development of IPSID-related lymphoma.

Poor standards of hygiene and endemic parasitic and other enteric infections are characteristic of the geographic regions in which IPSID is common.[94,99] The incidence rate for IPSID is much lower among Jews of North African and Asian descent who were born and live in Israel than among their counterparts who were born in North Africa or Asia and subsequently migrated to Israel.[94] Perhaps most compelling, however, is the evidence that IPSID is reversible if treated at the early prelymphomatous stage. Tetracycline induces complete remission if it is given before dystrophic changes in the lymphoplasmacytic infiltrate have occurred.[94] The response is less predictable if it is not given until the late prelymphomatous stage.[100]

It is not known which microbial pathogens may be implicated in IPSID and, if they predispose to or cause malignant transformation, how they do so. Through cellular (T-cell) and humoral (secretory IgA) immune mechanisms of the gut-associated lymphoid tissue and Peyer's patches, the normal small bowel is well protected from bacterial and viral attack.

Impairment of the normal immunologic and mechanical barriers that protect the host from harmful antigens in the gut lumen may be of pathophysiologic significance in IPSID and related conditions.

Increased Risk of Primary Small Bowel Lymphomas

Intestinal lymphoma was first recognized as a complication of celiac sprue in 1962.[101] The causative mechanism for this association is not known, but lymphoma usually presents in the fifth decade or later as a clinical relapse of sprue that was diagnosed many years previously. In one retrospective series of 385 patients with celiac sprue collected over a 30-year period, 17 cases of intestinal lymphoma were diagnosed.[102] Originally classified as a reticulum cell sarcoma, this form of lymphoma was then thought to be a malignant histiocytosis[103] and now has been reclassified as a T-cell lymphoma.[104] Ulcerative enteritis, another complication of longstanding celiac sprue, is probably a variant form of intestinal lymphoma.[105] The profile of T-cell subsets has been analyzed in lymphomatous small bowel and in small bowel from the same patients that shows typical changes of celiac sprue but no histologic evidence of lymphoma.[106] The profiles are identical to each other but are characteristically different from those found in normal jejunum and mucosa that shows villus atrophy of uncertain etiology. This has been interpreted as a further strong indication that celiac sprue is a potentially prelymphomatous condition. Indeed, it has been suggested that some patients with adult-onset celiac disease may have low-grade lymphoma from the outset of their illness.[107]

Nodular lymphoid hyperplasia (NLH) of the terminal ileum occurs as an incidental and apparently innocent finding in some normal children and young adults from developed countries of the Western world. Diffuse NLH involving the entire small bowel is associated with primary immunodeficiency syndromes,[108] and a rare association of NLH in immunodeficient subjects with non-Hodgkin's lymphoma of the small bowel has been suggested.[109] More recently, an association between symptomatic diffuse NLH and non-Hodgkin's lymphoma of the affected bowel has been documented in patients without an immunodeficiency syndrome from the developed world.[110]

Individuals infected with the human immunodeficiency virus (HIV) are at increased risk of developing non-Hodgkin's lymphoma, and the cumulative incidence rate of this complication of HIV infection has been estimated at 8% among Danish AIDS patients.[111] Extranodal presentation is seen in the majority of patients with HIV-related non-Hodgkin's lymphoma. In the United States, the estimated relative risk of non-Hodgkin's lymphoma among patients with HIV infection is 100-fold greater than in the general population, and the gastrointestinal tract accounts for 10% to 20% of extranodal locations.[112]

Pathology

The following criteria should be met before designating a lymphoproliferative malignancy as a primary gastrointestinal lymphoma[113,114]: absence of palpable lymphadenopathy; normal total and differential leukocyte counts; absence of mediastinal lymphadenopathy on chest radiograph; and grossly demonstrable disease confined to the affected segment or segments of the gastrointestinal tract. The stomach is the primary site of involvement in more than 70% of cases of primary gastrointestinal lymphoma in the United States, and the remaining cases are divided equally between the small and large bowel.[115]

As mentioned, PSBLs are localized tumors, in contrast to the diffuse nature of IPSID-related lymphomas. The Ann Arbor system has been used to stage PSBL (Table 76-9)[95,115] and has been modified for IPSID lymphomas.[116] Virtually all PSBLs are non-Hodgkin's lymphomas, although Hodgkin's disease of the duodenum has been reported.[117] PSBLs have usually been classified according to the Rappaport classification.[118] In some more recent reports, the Working Formulation of the National Cancer Institute for classifying non-Hodgkin's lymphomas[119] has been applied to PSBL. However, neither classification takes account of the cell lineage and immunologic markers of these tumors.

Apart from the T-cell lymphomas that arise from the diseased small bowel in patients with celiac sprue, the great majority of PSBLs are of B-cell origin. Isaacson and colleagues have observed common clinical and histologic features among B-cell malignant lymphomas of the gastrointestinal tract, salivary glands, lung, and thyroid and have applied the term mucosa-associated lymphoid tissue (MALT) collectively to the histogenesis of these lymphomas.[120] MALT B-cell lymphomas express a heterogeneous array of leukocyte differentiation antigens.[121] Centrocyte-like (CCL) cells are a characteristic feature of MALT lymphomas, so named for their resemblance to the small cleaved cells (centrocytes) of the follicle center-cell lymphomas of peripheral lymph nodes. CCL cells invade individual glands and form the lymphoepithelial lesions that are characteristic of MALT lymphomas. The lineage of CCL cells is controversial.[122]

The presence in gastric and other primary gastrointestinal lymphomas of well-defined follicles, the long clinical course, and the late dissemination to other parts of the body have led some to argue that gastrointestinal lymphomas of the PSBL variety, like the IPSID-related lymphomas, are reactive lesions.

TABLE 76-9
Staging of Non-Hodgkin's Primary Small Bowel Lymphomas

Stage IE	Involvement of a localized segment of bowel without nodal involvement
Stage IIE	Involvement of a localized segment of bowel with involvement of regional nodes
Stage IIIE	Involvement of bowel and lymph nodes on both sides of the diaphragm; the spleen may be involved (stage IIIES)
Stage IV	Diffuse involvement of more than one extralymphatic organ or tissue, with or without nodal involvement

Data from Gray GM, Rosenberg SA, Cooper AD, et al. Lymphomas involving the gastrointestinal tract. Gastroenterology 1982;82:43, and National Cancer Institute sponsored study of classification of non-Hodgkin lymphomas. Cancer 1982;49:2112.

The prevailing view has been that CCL cells are key to the development of malignancy, that they are analogous to follicle center cells, and that gastrointestinal lymphomas are follicular tumors.

Further evidence from Isaacson's group suggests otherwise.[123] Leukocyte antigen studies indicate that B cells external to the mantle zone of Peyer's patches, in the dome epithelium, and not follicular center cells are probably the normal counterparts of CCL cells. Their phenotype may also be identical with cells from the splenic marginal zone. The latter cells constitute a discrete population of B cells that, although derived from circulating precursors, do not recirculate; this, it has been speculated, might explain the relative indolence of PSBLs. Additional evidence that MALT B-cell lymphomas, including PSBLs, are not of follicle center-cell lineage comes from a molecular hybridization study with cDNAs for the *BCL2* gene.[124] A characteristic rearrangement of the gene that occurs in 75% of nodal follicular lymphomas was absent from all cases of PSBL that were examined.

The pathologic features of PSBL and IPSID-related lymphomas are compared in Table 76-10. A photomicrograph of PSBL is shown in Figure 76-9.

Clinical Features and Diagnosis

Patients with PSBL usually present before 10 or after 50 years of age.[118] The clinical features are similar to those of other small bowel malignancies.[115] Abdominal pain is prominent, and weight loss and intestinal obstruction are common. Some patients present acutely as a result of perforation of an involved viscus, and almost all present within a few months of the onset of symptoms. A palpable abdominal mass is reported in approximately one third to one half of cases.[118] The association between PSBL and preexisting celiac sprue has been discussed.[42,101-104] PSBL should be suspected in middle-aged and older patients who present as new cases of celiac sprue and in those with stable celiac sprue who relapse despite compliance with a gluten-free diet.[102] Abdominal pain, diarrhea, and weight loss are the usual symptoms.

IPSID presents earlier than PSBL, usually in the second or third decade. The interval between the first symptom and time of diagnosis ranges from a few months to more than 12 years.[118] In contrast to PSBL, diarrhea is a prominent early symptom in addition to abdominal pain. The diarrhea is initially watery but later changes to steatorrhea. Clubbing of the fingers is reported in one half to three quarters of cases, but a palpable abdominal mass is rarely detectable.[118] Severe weight loss is almost invariable with IPSID. An α-heavy chain paraprotein is detectable in the peripheral blood of 20% to 69% of patients.[97]

The radiologic appearances of the small bowel are abnormal in almost all cases of small bowel lymphoma. The length of abnormal bowel is restricted in cases of PSBL and extensive in IPSID. Endoscopically obtained biopsies are diagnostic of IPSID in 85% of patients.[34]

Treatment and Prognosis

Primary small bowel lymphoma. Segmental resection of the involved bowel and associated lymphatics is usually advocated for PSBL,[125] and it is advisable to obtain confirmation of the

TABLE 76-10
Pathological Features of PSBL and ISPID-Related Lymphomas

	PSBL	IPSID-RELATED
Cell lineage	Majority, B cell; celiac sprue; T cell	B cell
Macroscopic	Localized tumors	Diffuse, longer segments of bowel
Distribution	Mainly ileum	Mainly duodenum and jejunum
Microscopic	Follicles, centrocyte-like cells (cleaved), and plasma cells; cytologic monotony.	Dense mucosal infiltrate of plasmacytic or lymphoid cells ranging from low- to high-grade malignancy
Spread	Late and indolent; to spleen, liver, and extraabdominal nodes	Local spread to adjacent organs, involvement of spleen, liver, and extraabdominal nodes is rare

IPSID, immunoproliferative small intestine disease; PSBL, Western-type primary small bowel lymphomas.

diagnosis of lymphoma from surgical biopsies. It is recommended by some that biopsies be taken from the liver and periaortic nodes and that the spleen be removed for staging purposes.[125] Surgeons differ as to whether it is prudent to proceed directly, during the same operation, to an extensive staging exercise, on the basis of frozen-section small bowel biopsies, or whether staging should be performed later at a second operation, after thorough examination of fixed and embedded sections. Resection is potentially curative if complete excision of lymphomatous bowel can be achieved and only contiguous nodes are involved (stage IE or IIE disease).

If curative resection is not feasible, palliative resection of as much diseased bowel as possible has usually been recommended before administering combination chemotherapy, although evidence to support this approach is inconclusive. Life-threatening complications such as perforation and hemorrhage that arise from residual lymphomatous bowel are a well-recognized problem early in the course of chemotherapy. Protagonists of palliative resection emphasize avoidance of this risk.[126] Others have found no evidence of measurable benefit from surgical resection before the administration of combination chemotherapy in patients with aggressive primary gastrointestinal lymphomas.[127]

Radiotherapy provides effective palliation for extensive unresectable disease. It is not clear whether adjuvant radiotherapy should be given to patients with localized disease after potentially curative surgical resection of PSBL.[115] Similarly, the role of adjuvant chemotherapy for localized disease has not been fully defined. It is common practice to treat disseminated disease with radiotherapy and combination chemotherapy.

The results of chemotherapy in patients with PSBL are similar to those for comparable lymphomas that do not involve the gastrointestinal tract. In patients who had a complete response to combination chemotherapy, a 4-year disease-free survival rate of 85% was predicted in one report,[127] suggesting a considerably more optimistic prognosis than has usually been associated with PSBL.

The reported 5-year survival rate for patients with PSBL after complete surgical resection (stages IE and IIE1) is in the range of 24% to 47%.[118,128] The 5-year survival rate for those with unresectable disease is less than 25%. Relapses that do not manifest until more than 5 years after resection are well recognized.[128] The prognosis for PSBL is worse in patients with preexisting celiac sprue than in those without previous small bowel disease. Fifty-five percent of all patients with celiac sprue who develop PSBL die within 6 months of diagnosis, and only 10% survive 5 years.[42]

Immunoproliferative small intestine disease. Tetracycline therapy, if given at the early prelymphomatous stage, reverses the histologic and clinical features of IPSID.[94,118] Radiotherapy, often supplemented with combination chemotherapy, is the accepted treatment for established intestinal lymphomas of the IPSID variety. Therapeutic responses are well documented, but the extent to which treatment increases life expectancy is not clear. The 5-year survival rate in patients with established IPSID is little more than 20%.[129]

Leiomyoma and Leiomyosarcoma

Pathology

Leiomyomas are often lobulated. Arising from the muscle coat or blood vessel walls, they may project to the lumenal or serosal surfaces, or in both directions. They consist of bundles of smooth muscle cells.

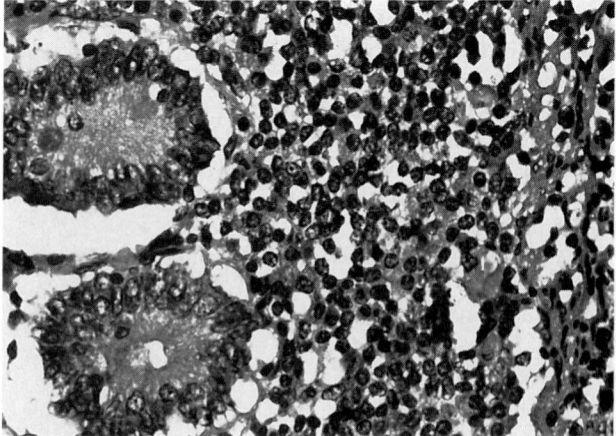

FIGURE 76-9. Primary small bowel non-Hodgkin's lymphoma is characterized by large cells with cleaved nuclei. Glands are spared. (Hematoxylin and eosin stain; original magnification ×300; courtesy of SK Satchidanand, M.D., Buffalo, NY.)

A simple staging scheme is used for leiomyosarcomas. Tumors are graded from Stage I (disease completely confined to the bowel wall) to Stage IV (local spread and distant metastases).[130] The malignant cells in Stage I and II tumors are well differentiated, and these tumors may be difficult to distinguish from benign smooth muscle tumors (leiomyomas). The relative abundance of mitoses in leiomyosarcomas may be the only feature that distinguishes them from leiomyomas. The resemblance to smooth muscle cells is progressively lost in Stage III and IV tumors. A photomicrograph of a leiomyosarcoma is shown in Figure 76-10.

Clinical Features

It is asserted by some that most leiomyomas become symptomatic and by others that most remain small and asymptomatic.[131] They grow as bundles of smooth muscle cells within the intestinal wall, and it can be difficult to differentiate benign (leiomyomatous) from malignant (leiomyosarcomatous) smooth muscle tumors. Central ulceration and erosion of the overlying epithelium are common, causing occult gastrointestinal bleeding or melena.[132] Intestinal obstruction, sometimes acute, is also a common mode of presentation for leiomyomas. Central ulceration may be obvious as umbilication on barium radiograph and at endoscopy. Hypervascularity that can be visualized arteriographically is characteristic of leiomyomas and leiomyosarcomas.

It is unusual for leiomyosarcomas to cause symptoms in patients younger than 50 years of age; in one series, 14 of 16 patients were older than 50 years of age at presentation.[130] The symptoms of abdominal pain, bleeding, and weight loss do not definitively distinguish leiomyosarcomas from other malignant small bowel tumors. However, melena or frank rectal bleeding is quite common, and the history, with symptoms sometimes present for more than 1 year before diagnosis, tends to be longer than with other small bowel malignancies.[130] Most patients have a palpable mass at the time of diagnosis. A case of leiomyosarcoma presenting as a fever of unknown origin has been reported.[133]

An intralumenal mass is almost always obvious on barium study. Leiomyomas and leiomyosarcomas are both vascular tumors and may be difficult to differentiate arteriographically, but the presence of vascular liver metastases, if seen on hepatic arteriography, makes the distinction possible.[134]

Treatment and Prognosis

For therapy to be curative, surgical resection of these tumors must be complete. Leiomyosarcomas have a low potential for lymphatic spread, and an extensive lymph node resection is not required.[125] Useful palliation is claimed for radiation therapy and combination chemotherapy with doxorubicin and other drugs in patients whose disease is not resectable. An aggressive surgical approach is advocated for the treatment of hepatic and pulmonary metastases, which are often solitary or few in number.

The overall 5-year survival rate in patients with a leiomyosarcoma ranges from 20% to 50% in different reports.[125,135] The size and histologic grade of tumor have a major bearing on the long-term prognosis. Five-year survival rates of 71% and 27% have been reported in patients whose resected tumors were, respectively, less than or more than 5 cm in diameter.[136] Five-year survival rates of 75% and 7% have been reported for patients with stage I and stage IV disease, respectively. Sixty percent of recurrences occur within 2 years of surgical resection.[137]

The reader is directed to Chapter 24, Neoplasia of the Gastrointestinal Tract; Chapter 86, Polyposis Syndromes; and Chapter 87, Malignant Tumors of the Colon.

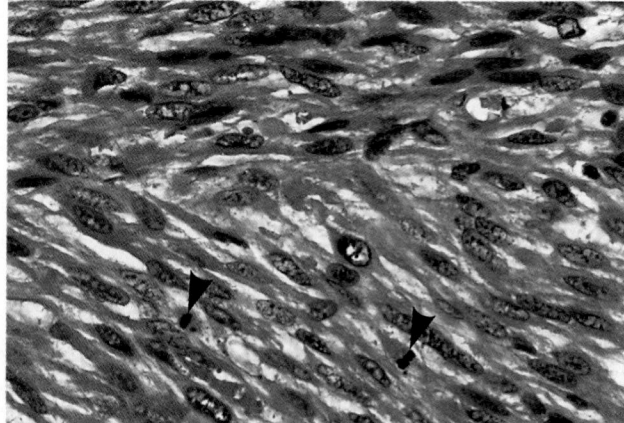

FIGURE 76-10. Leiomyosarcoma of ileum. The tumor consists of bundles of spindle cells. The presence of more than 10 mitoses (*arrowhead*) per 50 high-power fields distinguishes leiomyosarcoma from leiomyoma. (Hematoxylin and eosin stain; original magnification ×600; courtesy of SK Satchidanand, M.D., Buffalo, NY.)

REFERENCES

1. Boring CC, Squires TS, Tong T. Cancer statistics, 1993. CA Cancer J Clin 1993;43:7.
2. Weiss NS, Yang C-P. Incidence of histologic types of the small intestine. J Natl Cancer Inst 1987;78:653.
3. Lightdale CJ, Koepsell TD, Sherlock P, et al., eds. Cancer epidemiology and prevention. Philadelphia: WB Saunders, 1982:692.
4. Lowenfels AB. Why are small-bowel tumors so rare?. Lancet 1973;1:24.
5. Herbsman H, Wetstein L, Rosen Y, et al. Tumors of the small intestine. Curr Probl Surg 1980;17:121.
6. Wattenberg LW. Studies of polycyclic hydrocarbon hydroxylases of the intestine possibly related to cancer. Cancer 1971;28:99.
7. Zaridze DG. Environmental etiology of large-bowel cancer. J Natl Cancer Inst 1983;70:389.
8. Moore WE, Cato EP, Holdeman LV. Some current concepts in intestinal bacteriology. Am J Clin Nutr 1978;31(10 Suppl):S33.
9. Savage DC. Gastrointestinal microflora in mammalian nutrition. Annu Rev Nutr 1986;6:155.
10. Simon GL, Gorbach SL. The human intestinal microflora. Dig Dis Sci 1986;31(9 Suppl):147S.
11. Williams GT. Programmed cell death: apoptosis and oncogenesis. Cell 1991;65:1097.
12. Wyllie AH. Apoptosis and the regulation of cell numbers in normal and neoplastic tissue: an overview. Cancer Metastasis Rev 1992;11:95.

13. Potten CS. The significance of spontaneous and induced apoptosis in the gastrointestinal tract of mice. Cancer Metastasis Rev 1992;11:179.
14. Darling RC, Welch CE. Tumors of the small intestine. N Engl J Med 1959;260:397.
15. Zollinger RM, Sternfeld WC, Schreiber H. Primary neoplasms of the small intestine. Am J Surg 1986;151:654.
16. Wilson JM, Melvin DB, Gray GF, Thorbjarnarson B. Primary malignancies of the small bowel: a report of 96 cases and review of the literature. Ann Surg 1974;180:175.
17. Stubenbord WT, Thorbjarnarson B. Intussusception in adults. Ann Surg 1970;172:306.
18. Hallen A. Fibrosis in the carcinoid syndrome. Lancet 1964;1:746.
19. Horsley BL, Baker RR. Fibroblastic response to intestinal carcinoids. Am Surg 1970;36:676.
20. Haynes IG, Wolverson RL, O'Brien JM. Small bowel intussusception due to metastatic renal carcinoma. Br J Urol 1986;58:460.
21. Lynch-Nyhan A, Fishman EK, Kadir S. Diagnosis and management of massive gastrointestinal bleeding owing to duodenal metastasis from renal cell carcinoma. J Urol 1987;138:611.
22. Tarazi RY, Hermann RE, Vogt DP, et al. Results of surgical treatment of periampullary tumors: a thirty-five year experience. Surgery 1986;100:716.
23. Harkins HN. Intussusception due to invaginated Meckel's diverticulum: report of two cases with a study of 160 cases collected from the literature. Ann Surg 1933;98:1070.
24. Nolan DJ. Barium examination of the small intestine. Gut 1981;22:682.
25. Miller RE, Sellink JL. Enteroclysis: the small bowel enema. How to succeed and how to fail. Gastrointest Radiol 1979;4:269.
26. Maglinte DDT, Hall R, Miller RE, et al. Detection of surgical lesions of the small bowel by enteroclysis. Am J Surg 1984;147:225.
27. Gurian L, Jendrzejewski J, Katon R, et al. Small bowel enema. An underutilized method of small-bowel examination. Dig Dis Sci 1982;27:1101.
28. Allison DJ, Hemingway AP, Cunningham DA. Angiography in gastrointestinal bleeding. Lancet 1982;2:30.
29. Nolan DJ. Radiology of the small intestine. In: Nelson RL, Nyhus LM, eds. Surgery of the small intestine. Norwalk: Appleton & Lange, 1987:59.
30. Farah MC, Jafri SZH, Schwab RE, et al. Duodenal neoplasms: role of CT. Radiology 1987;162:839.
31. Megibow AJ, Balthazar EJ, Cho KC, et al. Bowel obstruction: evaluation with CT. Radiology 1991;180:313.
32. Rubesin SE, Herlinger H. CT evaluation of bowel obstruction: a landmark article—Implications for the future. Radiology 1991;180:307.
33. Lewis BS, Waye JD. Small bowel enteroscopy in 1988: pros and cons. Am J Gastroenterol 1988;83:799.
34. Halphen M, Najjar T, Jaafoura H, Cammoun M. Diagnostic value of upper intestinal fiber endoscopy in primary small intestinal lymphoma. Cancer 1986;58:2140.
35. Lewis BS, Kornbluth A, Waye JD. Small bowel tumours: yield of enteroscopy. Gut 1991;32:763.
36. Sellner F. Investigations on the significance of the adenoma-carcinoma sequence in the small bowel. Cancer 1990;66:702.
37. Kurtz RC, Sternberg SS, Miller HH, DeCosse JJ. Upper gastrointestinal neoplasia in familial polyposis. Dig Dis Sci 1987;32:459.
38. Galandiuk S, Hermann RE, Jagelman DG, et al. Villous tumors of the duodenum. Ann Surg 1988;207:234.
39. Jagelman DG, DeCosse JJ, Bussey HJ. Upper gastrointestinal cancer in familial adenomatous polyposis. Lancet 1988;1:1149.
40. Offerhaus GJA, Giardiello FM, Krush AJ, et al. The risk of upper gastrointestinal cancer in familial adenomatous polyposis. Gastroenterology 1992;102:1980.
41. Lashner BA. Risk factors for small bowel cancer in Crohn's disease. Dig Dis Sci 1992;37:1179.
42. Swinson CM, Slavin G, Coles EC, Booth CC. Coeliac disease and malignancy. Lancet 1983;1:111.
43. Collier PE, Turowski P, Diamond DL. Small intestinal adenocarcinoma complicating regional enteritis. Cancer 1985;55:5116.
44. Petras RE, Mir-Madjlessi SH, Farmer RG. Crohn's disease and intestinal carcinoma. Gastroenterology 1987;93:1307.
45. Ribeiro MB, Greenstein AJ, Heimann TM, et al. Adenocarcinoma of the small intestine in Crohn's disease. Surg Gynecol Obstet 1991;173:343.
46. Meretyk S, Landau EH, Okon E, et al. Adenocarcinoma in an ileal conduit: a late recurrence of urethral adenocarcinoma. J Urol 1987;138:859.
47. Stone AR, Davies N, Stephenson TP. Carcinoma associated with augmentation cystoplasty. Br J Urol 1987;60:236.
48. King PH, Osborn DE, Mackay EH. Tubulovillous adenoma arising 30 years after ileocystoplasty. J Clin Pathol 1992;45:928.
49. Vasilevsky C-A, Gordon PH. Adenocarcinoma arising at the ileocutaneous junction occurring after proctocolectomy for ulcerative colitis. Br J Surg 1986;73:378.
50. Suarez V, Alexander-Williams J, O'Connor HJ, et al. Carcinoma developing in ileostomies after 25 or more years. Gastroenterology 1988;95:205.
51. Tsunoda A, Talbot IC, Nicholls RJ. Incidence of dysplasia in the anorectal mucosa in patients having restorative proctocolectomy. Br J Surg 1990;77:506.
52. Stern H, Walfisch S, Mullen B, et al. Cancer in an ileoanal reservoir: a new late complication? Gut 1990;31:473.
53. Jones TJ, Marshall TL. Neurofibromatosis and small bowel adenocarcinoma: an unrecognized association. Gut 1987;28:1173.
54. Iida M, Yao T, Itoh H, et al. Natural history of duodenal lesions in Japanese patients with familial adenomatosis coli (Gardner's syndrome). Gastroenterology 1989;96:1301.
55. Sarre RG, Frost AG, Jagelman DG, et al. Gastric and duodenal polyps in familial adenomatous polyposis: a prospective study of the nature and prevalence of upper gastrointestinal polyps. Gut 1987;28:306.
56. Burt RW, Rikkers LF, Gardner EJ, et al. Villous adenoma of the duodenal papilla presenting as necrotizing pancreatitis in a patient with Gardner's syndrome. Gastroenterology 1987;92:532.
57. Ryan DP, Shapiro RH, Warshaw AL. Villous tumors of the duodenum. Ann Surg 1986;203:301.
58. Senay E, Sachar DB, Keohane M, Greenstein AJ. Small bowel carcinoma in Crohn's disease. Distinguishing features and risk factors. Cancer 1989;63:360.
59. Chappuis CW, Divincenti FC, Cohn I. Villous tumors of the duodenum. Ann Surg 1989;209:593.
60. Nelson RL. Adenocarcinoma of the small intestine. In: Nelson RL, Nyhus LM, eds. Surgery of the small intestine. Norwalk: Appleton & Lange, 1987:223.
61. Bridge MF, Perzin KH. Primary adenocarcinoma of the jejunum and ileum: a clinicopathologic study. Cancer 1975;36:1876.
62. Creutzfeldt W, Stockmann F. Carcinoids and carcinoid syndrome. Am J Med 1987;82(Suppl 5B):4.
63. Moertel CG, Dockerty MB, Judd ES. Carcinoid tumors of the vermiform appendix. Cancer 1968;21:270.
64. MacGillivray DC, Heaton RB, Rushin JM, Cruess DF. Distant metastasis from a carcinoid tumor of the appendix less than one centimeter in size. Surgery 1992;111:466.
65. Godwin DJ. Carcinoid tumors: an analysis of 2,837 cases. Cancer 1975;36:560.
66. Moertel CG, Sauer WG, Dockerty MB, et al. Life history of the carcinoid tumor of the small intestine. Cancer 1961;14:901.
67. Wilson H, Cheek RC, Sherman R, Storer EH. Carcinoid tumors. Curr Probl Surg 1970;7:1.
68. Zeitels J, Naunheim K, Kaplan EL, Straus F. Carcinoid tumors. A 37-year experience. Arch Surg 1982;117:732.
69. MacGillivray DC, Synder DA, Drucker W, ReMine SG. Carcinoid tumors: the relationship between clinical presentation and the extent of disease. Surgery 1991;110:68.
70. Gupta A, Saibil F, Kassim O, McKee J. Retroperitoneal fibrosis caused by carcinoid tumour. Q J Med 1985;56:367.

71. Case records of the Massachusetts General Hospital (Case 20-1986). N Engl J Med 1986;314:1369.

72. Williams ED, Sandler M. The classification of carcinoid tumors. Lancet 1963;1:238.

73. Sanders RJ. Carcinoids of the gastrointestinal tract. Springfield: Charles C Thomas, 1973.

74. Stephens M, Williams GT, Jasani B, Williams ED. Synchronous duodenal neuroendocrine tumors in von Recklinghausen's disease--a case report of co-existing gangliocytic paraganglioma and somatostatin-rich glandular carcinoid. Histopathology 1987;11:1331.

75. Boitsen E, Kaude J, Tylen U. Radiologic diagnosis of ileal carcinoid tumors. Acta Radiol [Diagn] 1974;65:15.

76. Seigel RS, Kuhns LR, Borlaza GS, et al. Computed tomography and angiography in ileal carcinoid tumor and retractile mesenteritis. Radiology 1980;134:437.

77. Patel YC. Somatostatin-receptor imaging for the detection of tumors. N Engl J Med 1990;323:1274.

78. Lamberts SWJ, Bakker WH, Reubi J, Krenning EP. Somatostatin-receptor imaging in the localization of endocrine tumors. N Engl J Med 1990;323:1246.

79. Lamberts SWJ, Krenning EP, Reubi J-C. The role of somatostatin and its analogs in the diagnosis and treatment of tumors. Endocr Rev 1991;12:450.

80. Bomanji J, Ur E, Mather S, et al. A scintigraphic comparison of iodine-123-metaiodobenzylguanidine and an iodine-labeled somatostatin analog (Tyr-3-octreotide) in metastatic carcinoid tumors. J Nucl Med 1992;33:1121.

81. Feldman JM, Davis JA. Radioenzymatic assay of platelet serotonin, dopamine and norepinephrine in subjects with normal and increased serotonin production. Clin Chim Acta 1981;109:275.

82. Martensson H, Nobin A, Sundler F, Falkmer S. Endocrine tumors of the ileum. Pathol Res Pract 1985;180:356.

83. Udekwu A, Kaplan EL. Carcinoid tumors of the small intestine and their carcinoid syndromes. In: Nelson RL, Nyhus LM, eds. Surgery of the small intestine. Norwalk: Appleton & Lange, 1987:231.

84. Soreide O, Berstad T, Bakka A, et al. Surgical treatment as a principle in patients with advanced abdominal carcinoid tumors. Surgery 1992;111:48.

85. Kvols LK, Moertel CG, O'Connell MJ, et al. Treatment of the malignant carcinoid syndrome. Evaluation of a long-acting somatostatin analogue. N Engl J Med 1986;315:663.

86. Wynick D, Bloom SR. The use of the long-acting somatostatin analog octreotide in the treatment of gut neuroendocrine tumors. J Clin Endocrinol Metab 1991;73:1.

87. Gorden P, Comi RJ, Maton PN, Go VLW. Somatostatin and somatostatin analogue (SMS 201-995) in treatment of hormone-secreting tumors of the pituitary and gastrointestinal tract and non-neoplastic diseases of the gut. Ann Intern Med 1989;110:35.

88. Moertel CG, Hanley JA. Combination chemotherapy trials in metastatic carcinoid tumor. Cancer Clin Trials 1979;2:327.

89. Oberg K, Eriksson B. The role of interferons in the management of carcinoid tumours. Br J Haematol 1991;79(Suppl)1:74.

90. Veenhof CHN, De Wit R, Taal BG, et al. A dose-escalation study of recombinant interferon-alpha in patients with a metastatic carcinoid tumour. Eur J Cancer 1992;28:75.

91. Joensuu H, Kumpulainen E, Gröhn P. Treatment of metastatic carcinoid tumour with recombinant interferon alfa. Eur J Cancer [A] 1992;28A:1650.

92. Välimäki M, Järvinen H, Salmela P, et al. Is the treatment of metastatic carcinoid tumor with interferon not as successful as suggested? Cancer 1991;67:547.

93. Davis Z, Moertel CG, McIlrath DC. The malignant carcinoid syndrome. Surg Gynecol Obstet 1973;137:637.

94. Khojasteh A, Haghshenass M, Haghighi P. Immunoproliferative small intestinal disease. A "third-world" lesion. N Engl J Med 1983;308:1401.

95. Gray GM, Rosenberg SA, Cooper AD, et al. Lymphomas involving the gastrointestinal tract. Gastroenterology 1982;82:143.

96. Blumstein M, Bank S, Greenberg RE, et al. Immunoproliferative small intestinal disease in an American patient with lymphoma and macroamylasemia. Gastroenterology 1992;103:1071.

97. Rambaud J-C, Modigliani R, Nguyen Phuoc BK, et al. Non-secretory alpha-chain disease in intestinal lymphoma. N Engl J Med 1980;303:53.

98. Panagalis GA, Rappaport H. Common clonal origin of lymphoplasmacytic proliferation and immunoblastic lymphoma in intestinal α-chain disease. Lancet 1977;2:880.

99. Al-Saleem TI. Evidence of acquired immune deficiencies in Mediterranean lymphoma: a possible aetiological link. Lancet 1978;2:709.

100. Galian A, Lecestre M-J, Scotto J, et al. Pathological study of alpha-chain disease with special emphasis on evolution. Cancer 1977;39:2081.

101. Gough KR, Read AE, Naish JM. Intestinal reticulosis as a complication of idiopathic steatorrhea. Gut 1962;3:232.

102. Cooper BT, Holmes GKT, Ferguson R, Cooke WT. Celiac disease and malignancy. Medicine (Baltimore) 1980;59:249.

103. Isaacson PG, Wright DH. Malignant histiocytosis of the intestine. Its relationship to malabsorption and ulcerative jejunitis. Hum Pathol 1978;9:661.

104. Loughran TP, Kadin ME, Deeg J. T-cell intestinal lymphoma associated with celiac sprue. Ann Intern Med 1986;104:44.

105. Jewell DP. Ulcerative enteritis. Br Med J 1983;287:1740.

106. Spencer J, MacDonald TT, Diss TC, et al. Changes in intraepithelial lymphocyte subpopulations in coeliac disease and enteropathy associated T cell lymphoma (malignant histiocytosis of the intestine). Gut 1989;30:339.

107. Wright DH, Jones DB, Clark H, et al. Is adult-onset coeliac disease due to a low-grade lymphoma of intraepithelial T lymphocytes?. Lancet 1991;337:1373.

108. Ajdukiewicz AB, Youngs GR, Bouchier IAD. Nodular lymphoid hyperplasia with hypogammglobulinemia. Gut 1972;13:589.

109. Gonzales-Vitale JC, Gomez LG, Golblum RM, et al. Immunoblastic lymphoma of small intestine complicating late-onset immunodeficiency. Cancer 1982;49:445.

110. Matuchansky C, Touchard G, Lemaire M, et al. Malignant lymphoma of the small bowel associated with diffuse nodular lymphoid hyperplasia. N Engl J Med 1985;313:166.

111. Hamilton-Dutoit SJ, Pallesen G, Franzmann MB, et al. AIDS-related lymphoma: histopathology, immunophenotype, and association with Epstein-Barr virus as demonstrated by in situ nucleic acid hybridization. Am J Pathol 1991;138:149.

112. Safai B, Diaz B, Schwartz J. Malignant neoplasms associated with human immunodeficiency virus infection. CA Cancer J Clin 1992;42:74.

113. Dawson IMP, Cornes JS, Morson BC. Primary malignant lymphoid tumors of the intestinal tract: a report of 37 cases with a study of factors influencing prognosis. Br J Surg 1961;49:80.

114. Najem AZ, Porcaro JL, Rush BF. Primary non-Hodgkin's lymphoma of the duodenum. Cancer 1984;54:895.

115. Weingrad DN, DeCosse JJ, Sherlock P, et al. Primary gastrointestinal lymphoma: a 30-year review. Cancer 1982;49:1258.

116. Salem P, El-Hashimi L, Anaissie E, et al. Primary small intestinal lymphoma in adults. A comparative study of IPSID versus non-IPSID in the Middle East. Cancer 1987;59:1670.

117. Devaney K, Jaffe ES. The surgical pathology of gastrointestinal Hodgkin's disease. Am J Clin Pathol 1991;95:794.

118. Al-Mondhiry H. Primary lymphomas of the small intestine: East-West contrast. Am J Hematol 1986;22:89.

119. National Cancer Institute sponsored study of classification of non-Hodgkin's lymphomas. Cancer 1982;49:2112.

120. Isaacson PG, Wright DH. Malignant lymphoma of mucosa-associated lymphoid tissue. Cancer 1983;52:1410.

121. Mielke B, Möller P. Histomorphologic and immunophenotypic spectrum of primary gastro-intestinal B-cell lymphomas. Int J Cancer 1991;47:334.

122. Isaacson PG, Spencer J. Malignant lymphoma of mucosa-associated lymphoid tissue. Histopathology 1987;11:445.

123. Myhre MJ, Isaacson PG. Primary B-cell gastric lymphoma—a reassessment of its histogenesis. J Pathol 1987;152:1.

124. Pan L, Diss TC, Cunningham D, Isaacson PG. The bcl-2 gene in primary B cell lymphoma of mucosa-associated lymphoid tissue (MALT). Am J Pathol 1989;135:7.

125. Walker MJ. Sarcomas of the small intestine. In: Nelson RL, Nyhus LM, eds. Surgery of the small intestine. Norwalk: Appleton & Lange, 1987:243.

126. Pettengell R, Bishop PW, Crowther D. Clinical oncology: case presentations from oncology centres. Intensive treatment of poor prognosis gastrointestinal lymphoma. Eur J Cancer [A] 1992;28A:1742.

127. Salles G, Herbrecht R, Tilly H, et al. Aggressive primary gastrointestinal lymphomas: review of 91 patients treated with the LNH-84 regimen. A study of the Groupe d'Etude des Lymphomes Agressifs. Am J Med 1991;90:77.

128. Radaszkiewicz T, Dragosics B, Bauer P. Gastrointestinal malignant lymphomas of the mucosa-associated lymphoid tissue: factors relevant to prognosis. Gastroenterology 1992;102:1628.

129. Al-Bahranai ZR, Al-Mondhiry H, Bakir F, Al-Saleem T. Clinical and pathologic subtypes of primary intestinal lymphoma. Experience with 132 patients over a 14 year period. Cancer 1983;52:1666.

130. Ricci A, Ciccarelli O, Cartun RW, Newcomb P. A clinicopathologic and immunohistochemical study of 16 patients with small intestinal leiomyosarcoma. Cancer 1987;60:1790.

131. Reddy RR, Schuman BM, Priest RJ. Duodenal polyps: diagnosis and management. J Clin Gastroenterol 1981;3:139.

132. Wilson JM, Melvin DB, Gray G, Thorbjarnarson B. Benign small bowel tumors. Ann Surg 1975;181:247.

133. Dendale P, Devis G, Goossens A. Leiomyosarcoma of the small intestine presenting as fever of unknown origin. Gut 1992;33:411.

134. Cho KJ, Reuter SR. Angiography of duodenal leiomyomas and leiomyosarcomas. AJR Am J Roentgenol 1980;135:31.

135. Ranchod M, Kempson RL. Smooth muscle tumors of the gastrointestinal tract and retroperitoneum: a pathologic analysis of 100 cases. Cancer 1977;39:255.

136. Shiu MH, Farr GH, Egeli RA, et al. Myosarcomas of the small and large intestine: a clinicopathologic study. J Surg Oncol 1983;24:67.

137. Ng E-H, Pollock RE, Romsdahl MM. Prognostic implications of patterns of failure for gastrointestinal leiomyosarcomas. Cancer 1992;69:1334.

138. Ciccarelli O, Welch JP, Kent GG. Primary malignant tumors of the small bowel. The Hartford Hospital experience, 1969–1983. Am J Surg 1987;153:350.

Textbook of Gastroenterology, second edition, edited by Tadataka Yamada. JB Lippincott Company, Philadelphia © 1995.

CHAPTER 77

Miscellaneous Diseases of the Small Intestine

Marc S. Levin

The diseases discussed in this chapter should be considered in patients presenting with gastrointestinal hemorrhage, abdominal pain, diarrhea, intestinal obstruction, or perforation that eludes diagnosis by routine gastroduodenal endoscopy and radiographic studies. Topics include ulceration of the small intestine, small intestine complications of drug therapy, necrotizing enterocolitis (NEC), and protein-losing gastroenteropathy (PLGE). Although most of these are infrequently encountered in clinical practice, differentiating them from more common diseases can produce important therapeutic benefits.

ULCERS OF THE SMALL INTESTINE

Many causes of small intestine ulcerations distal to the duodenum have been identified (Table 77-1). Most of these produce solitary ulcers with sharp borders and normal surrounding mucosa. With surgical resection or removal of offending agents, these ulcers seldom recur and are associated with a benign clinical course. The mortality from multiple ulcers occurring in an abnormal mucosa, as is occasionally seen with gluten-sensitive enteropathy or unclassified sprue, chronic ulcerative (nongranulomatous) jejunoileitis, or lymphoma, can be as high as 75%.[1] It is essential to attempt to define the underlying cause of small intestinal ulcers if possible.

Primary (Idiopathic) Small Bowel Ulcers

Epidemiology and Etiology

The diagnosis of primary small bowel ulcers is made after known causes of small bowel ulcers have been eliminated. It is a diagnosis of exclusion, and it is unlikely to represent a distinct etiologic entity. The cause of this disorder remains a mystery, and no animal model has been described. With increasing recognition of secondary causes of small intestine ulceration, the residuum of patients falling into this diagnostic category is diminishing. The actual incidence of idiopathic small bowel ulceration is unknown, although it is clearly an uncommon disorder. Because asymptomatic and uncomplicated intestinal ulcers are rarely detected, the true incidence of this entity is certainly higher than estimates based on clinical experience. A review of the Mayo Clinic records from 1959 to 1979 (59 patients, including 6 who were taking enteric potassium preparations) found an incidence of 4 small bowel ulcers per 100,000 new patients.[2] In this study and in several others summarized in Table 77-2, males and females were affected equally, and all age groups were affected.

Clinical Features

Symptomatic complications of small bowel ulcers include bleeding, perforation, and obstruction. The incidence of these complications is not known. Intestinal obstruction is apparently more frequent than it is with duodenal ulcers. Intermittent crampy abdominal pain resulting from partial small bowel obstruction is the most frequent presenting complaint (63% to 100% of patients; see Table 77-2). Histories often include symptoms of intermittent partial small bowel obstruction present for a period of 3 days to 20 years.[2] Small intestine obstruction or perforation can also present with an acute abdomen. Although ulcers are more commonly seen in the ileum, perforated ulcers are more common in the jejunum; in the Mayo Clinic series, 78% of perforated ulcers were jejunal and 11% were ileal.[2] Evidence of gastrointestinal bleeding is also common, especially in younger patients. These patients may present with intestinal hemorrhage or with occult blood loss. In the Mayo Clinic series, 50% of patients were anemic, and the incidence was over 90% in those with proven gastrointestinal bleeding.[2] Patients presenting with gastrointestinal bleeding often have symptoms consistent with a history of intermittent intestinal obstruction as well. The diagnosis of small intestine ulceration should be considered if intestinal bleeding and evidence of small intestine obstruction coexist.

Pathology

Most primary small intestinal ulcers (75%) are located in the middle to distal ileum.[1] In the Mayo Clinic series, a solitary ulcer was found in 70%, two or three ulcers in 20%, and more

---

TABLE 77-1
Causes of Small Intestine Ulceration

Infectious	Tuberculosis, typhoid, cytomegalovirus, syphilis, parasites, strongyloidosis hyperinfection, *Campylobacter* infection, yersiniosis
Toxic	Acute jejunitis (β-toxin–producing *Clostridium perfringens*), arsenic
Inflammatory	Crohn's disease, systemic lupus erythematosus with high serum antiphospholipid levels, diverticulitis
Mucosal lesions	Gluten-sensitive enteropathy (jejunoileitis)
Tumors	
Primary	Malignant histiocytosis, lymphoma
Secondary	Adenocarcinoma, melanoma, Kaposi's sarcoma
Vascular	Mesenteric insufficiency, giant cell arteritis, vasculitis, vascular abnormality, amyloidosis (ischemic lesion)
Hyperacidity	Zollinger-Ellison syndrome, Meckel's diverticulum, stomal ulceration
Metabolic	Uremia
Drugs	Potassium chloride, nonsteroidal antiinflammatory drugs, antimetabolites
Radiation	Therapeutic, accidental
Idiopathic	Primary ulcer, Behçet's syndrome

TABLE 77-2
Profile and Presenting Symptoms of Primary Small Bowel Ulcers

STUDY AND YEAR	NUMBER OF PATIENTS	GENDER (M:F RATIO)	AGE (y)	SBO* (%)	BLEEDING (%)	ACUTE ABDOMEN (%)	DURATION OF SYMPTOMS
Davies, Brightmore (1970)[3]	8†	5:3	16–62	63	38	25	No data
Boydstun et al. (1981)[2]	59‡	31:28	17–77	78	25	12	3 d–20 y
Reid et al. (1982)[4]	3	1:2	12–64	0	100	0	6 mo–30 y
Glynn et al. (1984)[5]	2	1:1	57–71	0	100	0	No data
Thomas, Williamson (1985)[6]	6	4:2	4 mo–76 y	66	83	17	No data
Ballantyne et al. (1986)[7]	3§	1:2	6 wk–12 y	100	100	0	6 wk–12 y

* SBO, small bowel obstruction.

† Included 2 subjects taking potassium chloride.

‡ Included 6 subjects taking potassium chloride.

§ Included 1 subject taking nonsteroidal antiinflammatory drugs.

than three in 10% of patients.[1] Ulcers typically have sharply demarcated borders and can vary in diameter from 0.3 to 5 cm.[2] The pathologic features are nonspecific and are identical to those of peptic ulcerations.[8] A marked eosinophilic infiltrate is sometimes present.[9] The surrounding mucosa is usually normal. Granulomas, sinus tracts, and pathologic vascular changes are not seen. Granulation tissue and fibrosis that extend deep into the bowel wall may produce intestinal stenosis. The absence of granulomas and the normal surrounding mucosa are features that help to distinguish idiopathic ulcers from those seen in Crohn's disease and in chronic ulcerative jejunoileitis (discussed further elsewhere in this chapter).

Diagnosis

Both detection of intestinal ulceration and exclusion of known etiologic agents are required to support a diagnosis of primary small bowel ulcers. A careful history is necessary to identify exposure to potentially ulcerogenic substances such as nonsteroidal antiinflammatory drugs (NSAIDs) and enteric-coated potassium preparations (see discussion in following sections). Prior abdominal surgery and other risk factors that predispose to intestinal ischemia should be identified. Assessment of immune status may also be useful. For example, it is important to exclude cytomegalovirus infection in immunocompromised patients because of the propensity for cytomegalovirus ulcers to bleed or perforate.

There are no pathognomonic biochemical abnormalities, and the only laboratory tests that are useful for diagnostic purposes are those that help to establish an alternative diagnosis. Small intestine ulcers can be detected radiographically, endoscopically, or at laparotomy.

Although small intestine ulcers cannot be detected by plain abdominal radiographs, small bowel dilatation suggestive of obstruction and pneumoperitoneum indicative of perforation may be detected. Conventional contrast radiography of the small intestine rarely identifies primary ulcers of the small intestine. In the Mayo Clinic series, the ulcer site was identified by small bowel barium series in only 6 of 38 patients.[2] Enteroclysis is a superior technique for demonstrating small intestine mucosal lesions (see Chap. 119). It should be consid-

ered the radiographic procedure of choice in the evaluation of suspected ulcers of the small intestine. Although intestinal strictures may be readily detected, small intestine ulcers are seldom demonstrated radiographically. Ileal ulcers can, on rare occasions, be detected if contrast is refluxed into the terminal ileum; however, the yield from barium enemas does not justify their use for detecting small bowel ulcers. Other radiographic techniques such as ^{99m}Tc-labeled red cell scanning and mesenteric angiography, if used for the evaluation of gastrointestinal bleeding, may lead indirectly to the detection of small intestine ulcerations. For example, diagnosis of a Meckel's diverticulum with ^{99m}Tc pertechnetate would identify the likely site of intestinal ulcers.

Small intestine enteroscopy is becoming a useful adjunct for the diagnosis of small intestine lesions because of improvements in equipment and technique. In the setting of obscure gastrointestinal bleeding, for example, a diagnosis was made in 50% of 258 patients, all of whom had a negative enteroclysis.[10] These data suggest that enteroscopy is useful in the evaluation of small bowel ulcers, although it has not been specifically evaluated for this purpose. Intraoperative enteroscopy can also be a valuable adjunct in difficult cases.[11]

Despite the refinement of enteroclysis and enteroscopy, most symptomatic idiopathic small intestine ulcers are not detected without surgical intervention. Exploratory laparotomy is valuable for both diagnostic and therapeutic purposes. In the patient with persistent gastrointestinal blood loss or abdominal pain with evidence of small bowel obstruction, surgical exploration of the abdomen should be given serious consideration (see Chap. 140).

Therapy

The therapy for primary small intestine ulcers is dictated by the severity of complications. Emergent surgical intervention is required if an acute abdomen or pneumoperitoneum indicative of intestinal perforation is present. Life-threatening intestinal bleeding is an indication for diagnostic and therapeutic mesenteric angiography or surgical exploration (see Chap. 30). The best therapy for ulcers that present with less serious complications is also surgical resection. Detection of small bowel ulcers is usually readily accomplished at laparotomy. Intraoperative enteroscopy may be required occasionally. Most ulcers can be easily managed by surgical resection with end-to-end anastomosis. Advantages of this approach include the ability to obtain adequate material for pathologic analysis and the low incidence of complications and ulcer recurrences. Because of their idiopathic nature, it is not desirable to simply oversew small bowel ulcers. With such an approach, the amount of material available for pathologic analysis is limited, and the risk of ulcer recurrence is high. Medical management with antiinflammatory or immunosuppressive agents is not effective therapy for intestinal ulcers or strictures. Furthermore, unsuspected perforation is often found at surgery.[2] The incidence of perforation with primary jejunal ulcers is approximately 78%, and with ileal ulcers it is 11%.[2] The overall incidence is only 22%, because most ulcers are found in the ileum and are unlikely to perforate.

Drug-Induced Small Bowel Ulcers

The entrapment of a pill or capsule before dissolution or the release of large concentrations of a drug in a segment of intestine can result in localized ulceration as a result of physical pressure or specific cytotoxic effect. In recent years, NSAIDs have been the most common cause of drug-induced small intestine ulcers. In the 1960s, enteric-coated potassium chloride (KCl) was introduced and was soon recognized to be an intestinal ulcerogen. Ferrous salts, digoxin, corticosteroids, zirconium, and clofazimine have all been implicated as ulcerogens as well.[12]

Nonsteroidal Antiinflammatory Drugs

NSAIDs are a heterogenous group of organic acids that inhibit prostaglandin synthesis and have analgesic antiinflammatory and antipyretic properties.[13] Although they have been used for decades in the treatment of inflammatory arthropathies, their use has been extended in recent years to include many nonrheumatologic problems.[13] As a result, NSAIDs are among the most commonly used drugs worldwide. A number of recent publications have addressed the magnitude and cost of NSAID-associated gastrointestinal complications, which have been described as an emerging epidemic.[14–18]

Perhaps as a consequence of the increased usage of NSAIDs and certainly as a result of improved small intestine diagnostic methods, small bowel enteropathy is a frequently diagnosed complication of NSAID use. Multiple ulcerations, mucosal diaphragms, strictures, and perforations have all been associated with NSAID use.[18–21]

The epidemiology of NSAID-induced enteropathy is not well characterized. Up to 70% of patients on NSAIDs have evidence of increased intestinal permeability or inflammation,[22–24] but the majority are asymptomatic. An autopsy study showed the presence of nonspecific small intestine ulcers in 8.4% of 249 patients who had NSAIDs prescribed during the 6 months before death, compared with an incidence of 0.6% in 464 patients who had not used NSAIDs.[25] Three of the long-term users of NSAIDs were found to have died of perforated nonspecific small intestine ulcers. Small intestine erosions or ulcerations were detected by small bowel enteroscopy

in 7 of 15 iron-deficient patients on long-term NSAID therapy for rheumatoid arthritis.[26] All of the patients had negative upper and lower endoscopies. These studies indicate a high prevalence of unsuspected gastrointestinal lesions in patients taking NSAIDs. A meta-analysis of studies examining the association between NSAIDs and serious adverse gastrointestinal events indicated that NSAID users are at three times greater risk than are nonusers.[25,27] Independent risk factors seem to be age exceeding 60 years, previous NSAID complications, and concomitant steroid use. Gender was not a risk factor. This study did not analyze small bowel effects independently, so it is not certain whether this risk profile is applicable to NSAID-induced small intestine enteropathy. Risk factors specific for the development of NSAID-induced complications of the small intestine have not been identified.

Pathology. The mechanisms by which NSAIDs injure the small intestine mucosa are unknown. It has been proposed that reduction of mucosal prostaglandins through cyclooxygenase inhibition increases intestinal permeability, rendering it susceptible to lumenal macromolecules and toxins.[28] This defect in permeability is evident within hours after NSAID administration[18,29] and in rats may be ameliorated by pretreatment or simultaneous treatment with glucocorticoids, sulfasalazine, or tetracycline.[30] The relative importance of local and systemic effects in the pathogenesis of the NSAID-induced change in permeability was addressed in 12 human volunteers who received either indomethacin or nabumetone for 1 week.[31] Nabumetone requires metabolism for activation and has no significant enterohepatic circulation, so direct effects on the intestinal mucosa are unlikely. Only indomethacin increased intestinal permeability. In another study, the prodrug sulindac was compared to indomethacin with similar results.[32] These studies suggest that NSAIDs alter intestinal permeability through local rather than systemic effects.

Changes in intestinal permeability and local effects are clearly not the only mechanisms by which NSAIDs induce intestinal injury, because the risk profiles of pro-drugs and indomethacin are similar. Another proposed mechanism for NSAID damage is direct toxicity that is independent of changes in cyclooxygenase activity.[33–35] Inhibition of glycolysis and the tricarboxylic acid cycle, reducing cellular ATP production and uncoupling oxidative phosphorylation, have been demonstrated in vitro. Coadministration of glucose and citrate with indomethacin to humans was shown to prevent the increased permeability seen with indomethacin alone.[33] This observation—that provision of the primary substrates for glycolysis and the tricarboxylic acid cycle provided protection against indomethacin-induced changes in intestinal permeability—is compatible with this hypothesized mechanism.

NSAID-associated intestinal injury primarily affects the distal small intestine. Intestinal ulcers induced by NSAIDs are pathologically identical to primary ulcers and to other drug-induced ulcers. Strictures are seen in up to 5% of patients on chronic NSAID therapy for arthritis.[18] In addition to strictures that are indistinguishable from those seen in Crohn's disease and other disorders, apparently unique, diaphragm-like strictures have been described (Fig. 77-1).[19,21,36–38] These strictures encroach on and narrow the lumen to an opening as small as 1 mm in diameter.[36] They usually occur as multiple strictures separated by a length of normal bowel a few cen-

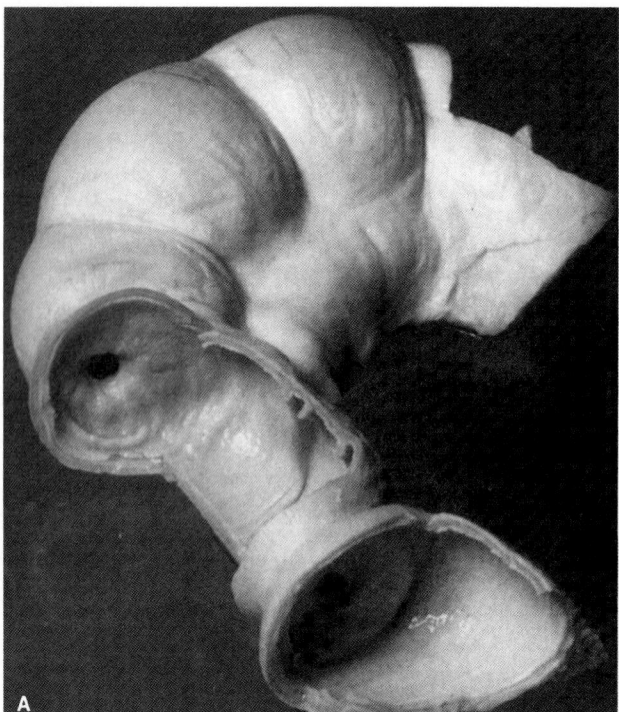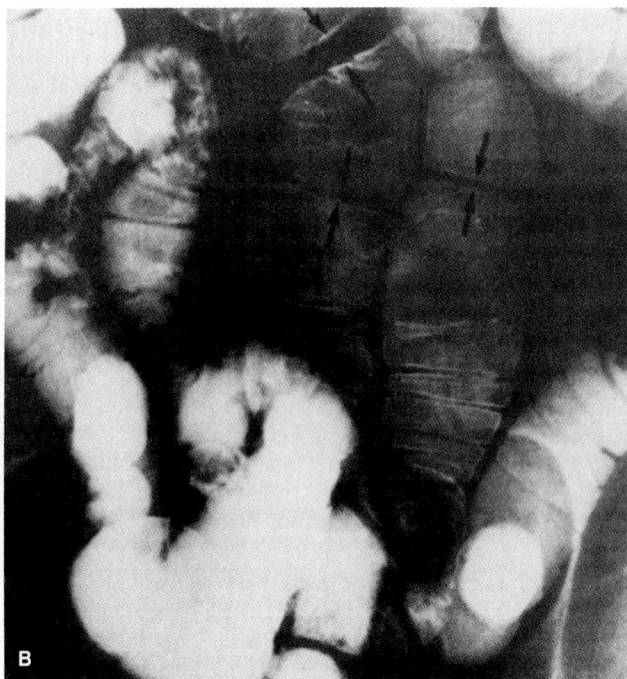

FIGURE 77-1. Nonsteroidal antiinflammatory drug–induced small intestine strictures. **(A)** Diaphragm strictures of the small intestine are apparent in resected intestine. **(B)** Enteroclysis study in a patient on nonsteroidal antiinflammatory drugs. Diaphragm strictures (*arrows*), which were found at surgery, are difficult to appreciate and resemble exaggerated plica circularis. (From Bjarnason I, Hayllar J, Macpherson AJ, Russell AS. Side effects of nonsteroidal antiinflammatory drugs on the small and large intestine in humans. Gastroenterology 1993;104:1832.)

timeters long.[36] Submucosal fibrosis replacing or merging with the muscularis mucosa is characteristic.[19,36] Mild inflammation of the overlying mucosa is invariably present with or without shallow ulceration.[19] The adjacent mucosa is usually completely normal. Patients with this "diaphragm disease" present with weight loss, hypoalbuminemia, anemia, and intermittent vague abdominal pain.[36] The diaphragm-like strictures are difficult to detect radiologically and can be missed at laparotomy unless an enterotomy is performed.[36–38] The role of small bowel enteroscopy, which is useful for detecting intestinal ulcers,[26] has not been defined in NSAID-related intestinal strictures. The success of surgical enterotomy and the demonstration of ileal diaphragms by sigmoidoscopic examination in 7 patients with a subtotal colectomy and an ileorectal anastomosis[38] suggest that enteroscopy is useful.

Morphologically, the presentation of NSAID-related enteropathy is often similar to that of Crohn's disease, because both disorders are associated with transmural injury that can cause stricture formation.[34,35] In addition, although most patients with NSAID-associated small intestine enteropathy are asymptomatic, some patients on long-term treatment present with clinical features of Crohn's disease.[13] In a prospective study, 10% of patients with colitis not secondary to Crohn's disease were thought to have NSAID-induced colitis.[39] It has also been reported that NSAIDs may exacerbate Crohn's disease and ulcerative colitis.[16,40–42] These reports emphasize the importance of obtaining an accurate drug history for all pa-

tients presenting with an illness resembling Crohn's disease. NSAIDs have been reported to be associated with a variety of other intestinal disorders, including collagenous colitis,[43] nonceliac flattening of small intestinal mucosa,[44] celiac sprue, and intestinal malignancies.[45] Reports that NSAIDs can cause perforation and other complications of diverticular disease suggest it may be prudent to avoid NSAIDs in patients with diverticulitis.[34] Nevertheless, the available data are not sufficient to establish a true association between NSAID use and any of these conditions.[35]

Therapeutic considerations. The majority of patients on NSAIDs appear to have intestinal inflammation as indicated by ^{111}In leukocyte scans and fecal excretion,[23] and they have increased intestinal permeability as indicated by ^{51}Cr-EDTA absorption. These abnormalities usually resolve after the medications are discontinued. However, inflammation may persist for up to 16 months.[18] Discontinuation of NSAIDs should also be sufficient for treatment of uncomplicated ulcers. Surgical intervention is required for therapy of intestinal perforation or symptomatic strictures.

The optimal regimen for patients for whom there is no good alternative to continued NSAID use has not been established. Based on the observation that nabumetone and sulindac did not increase intestinal permeation to ^{51}Cr-EDTA, switching to these or other pro-drugs may be beneficial. Observations in rats indicate that switching to NSAIDs that are less potent inhibitors of cyclooxygenase may also be helpful.[46,47] Delivery of NSAIDs encapsulated in liposomes was protective in a rat study.[48] High intestinal concentrations caused by biliary excretion and enterohepatic circulation of some NSAIDs are also thought to contribute to intestinal toxicity. The degree of ulceration in rats was related to the amount of active drug excreted in bile.[46,47,49] Human studies investigating the incidence of small intestine enteropathy using pro-drugs or NSAIDs with decreased biliary excretion of active drug have not been reported. In the case of the pro-drugs, it is clear that the incidence of upper gastrointestinal bleeding is not decreased.

Although the role of the gut flora in NSAID enteropathy is equivocal, germ-free rats are resistant to indomethacin-induced intestinal lesions,[50] and antibiotics reduced the incidence of small intestinal ulcers in rats given indomethacin.[51] In human studies, metronidazole[35] and sulfasalazine[52] have been shown to reduce intestinal inflammation—a response not yet proven to correspond to prevention of or recovery from NSAID-induced complications.

Prophylaxis of small intestine NSAID injury has been the subject of several experimental and clinical studies. In studies using rats, pretreatment or concurrent treatment with glucocorticoids, sulfasalazine, tetracycline, sucralfate,[53] pentagastrin,[54] naloxone (tested because morphine potentiates the ulcerogenic effect of indomethacin),[55] clonidine,[56] or thromboxane synthetase inhibitors[30] reduced indomethacin-induced permeability and inflammatory changes in rats. Drugs that exacerbated the intestinal toxicity of indomethacin in rats include cyclosporin[57] and morphine. Although prostaglandin E analogues such as misoprostol and enprostil are efficacious in NSAID-associated injury of the stomach and duodenum,[58-62] their effects in the small intestine are not known. Protection was demonstrated in animal models.[63-65] In human subjects, misoprostol prevented NSAID-induced permeability changes in one study[66] but not in another.[32]

Potassium Chloride

The introduction of enteric-coated KCl tablets in the 1960s was associated with an unacceptably high incidence of small intestine ulceration. This was attributed to high lumenal concentrations of KCl resulting from the rapid dissolution of the tablets in the small intestine. Slow-release formulations employing a wax-polymer matrix (dissolution in approximately 4 hours) or microencapsulation (dissolution in 8-10 hours) were developed in an attempt to eliminate this adverse effect. As a result, the incidence of gastrointestinal ulceration was reduced but not eliminated. In a retrospective study in Stockholm,[67] 2 cases of small intestine ulceration were identified in the period 1970 through 1983, which was equivalent to 3 cases per 100,000 patient-years of slow-release wax matrix tablet use, but there were 56 cases from the period 1960 through 1965 when enteric preparations were used, or 65 cases per 100,000 patient-years. Regardless of the preparation used, the risk of ulceration is increased if intestinal transit is delayed by concurrent medications, general debility, or advanced age.[68]

The clinical presentation, diagnosis, and treatment of patients with KCl-induced small intestine ulcers or strictures are the same as those for patients with primary or NSAID-induced ulcers. Although the ulcers can occur anywhere along the gastrointestinal tract, they are most common in the distal ileum.[69]

Other drugs for which there are reports of small intestine ulcers or perforation include corticosteroids,[70] cytarabine[71] and other chemotherapeutic agents, digoxin,[72] and ferrous sulfate preparations.[12]

Small Bowel Ulcers Associated With Systemic Disorders

Behçet's Syndrome

Behçet's syndrome is a systemic disease that affects the skin, joints, vascular system, central nervous system, and intestinal tract. Oral and genital ulcers are a common feature of the syndrome; intestinal ulceration has also been described[73] in fewer than 1% of all patients with Behçet's syndrome. The ileocecal region is most frequently involved.[74] Multiple deep ulcers in a background of minimally inflamed mucosa are characteristic. The ulcers bleed easily and are often penetrating. The abnormalities are readily differentiated from those of Crohn's disease or ulcerative colitis.[74,75]

The optimal treatment of Behçet's syndrome has yet to be established, although surgery with wide resection margins should not be delayed in complicated cases.[74,76] No medical treatment significantly alters the natural course, and ulcer recurrence is common after surgery.[76] Additional details of intestinal involvement in Behçet's syndrome can be found in Chapter 109.

Systemic Lupus Erythematosus

A number of case reports have described the pathologic changes in patients with systemic lupus erythematosus who had intestinal ulcerations.[77] Microthrombosis and vasculitis with intestinal ischemia are the likely mechanisms for this uncommon complication of systemic lupus erythematosus.

Diffuse Small Bowel Ulceration and Concurrent Malabsorption

A rare clinical syndrome consisting of malabsorption, abdominal pain, and multiple nonmalignant ulcers of the small intestine has been described. Typically, these patients are in the sixth or seventh decade and have long-standing gluten-sensitive enteropathy (GSE). In such patients, the disorder is characterized by extensive villus atrophy and small bowel ulcerations that fail to improve on gluten withdrawal. There is also a distinct subgroup of patients who do not have GSE. The term *chronic ulcerative (nongranulomatous) jejunoileitis* (CUJ) and synonyms such as idiopathic mucosal enteropathy, idiopathic chronic ulcerative enteritis, unclassified sprue, malignant histiocytosis, and enteropathy-associated T-cell lymphoma have been applied to this latter group of patients. The nomenclature reflects the poor understanding of the etiology and pathophysiology of CUJ. For the purposes of this chapter, the term CUJ is used to describe this disease in patients with and without evidence of GSE.

Etiology

The typical histologic features of CUJ are partial or total villus atrophy, mucosal ulceration, crypt hyperplasia, and an inflammatory cell infiltrate.[78,79] The loss of intestinal villi results in a marked decrease in the absorptive area of the intestine, and the aborted maturation of the enterocytes results in lower levels of digestive enzymes on the intestinal brush border. The effect of these disturbances is malabsorption of all dietary components and a variable degree of protein-losing enteropathy. Although the mechanism is poorly understood, villus atrophy appears to be related to infiltration by activated T cells.[80]

Relation to gluten-sensitive enteropathy.   CUJ that occurs without a prior history of GSE is usually more extensive in distribution and fails to respond to gluten withdrawal. CUJ and GSE are both associated with splenic atrophy of unknown origin, and most cases of CUJ are preceded by a variable period of suspected or proven GSE.[1,81–83] Nevertheless, it seems clear that CUJ can develop without GSE.

Relation to small bowel lymphoma.   Although small bowel lymphoma can resemble GSE clinically,[84] there is strong evidence that lymphomas arise in chronic GSE.[85–89] The incidence of malignant degeneration may be decreased by a strict gluten-free diet.[90] In contrast to primary small intestine lymphomas, the typical lymphoma associated with GSE is derived from T cells.[91–93] These lymphomas, which are referred to as *enteropathy-associated T-cell lymphomas* (EATL), are difficult to differentiate from those of CUJ. Histologically, both EATL and CUJ exhibit villus atrophy, ulceration, and mucosal infiltration by activated T cells. Both disorders usually present with splenic atrophy. The major difficulty results from the observations that EATL may be indolent in its early stages and that patients with CUJ can develop lymphoma several years after diagnosis. In some cases, retrospective examination of biopsies obtained at the time of diagnosis of CUJ have revealed typical malignant cells.[78,81,94] In one series, all of the patients with CUJ had metastatic disease at the time of diagnosis,[78] but in a different retrospective study, no evidence of preexisting lymphoma was detected.[82] These data indicate that CUJ is a significant risk factor for the development of lymphoma and suggest that this development may be invariable.

Non–T-cell lymphomas, such as immunoproliferative small intestinal disease (IPSID) and Mediterranean (B-cell) lymphoma, can also be accompanied by mucosal atrophy and ulceration and may have all of the features of CUJ (see Chap. 76). This group may have a dramatic response to antibiotics or cytotoxic agents.[95–98] These lymphomas cannot be differentiated solely on the basis of morphology; it is important to determine cell surface markers for proper diagnosis.

Clinical Features

The age at diagnosis of CUJ tends to be older than it is for typical GSE. Childhood cases have not been reported. The onset of CUJ is indolent. CUJ patients with and without known GSE were symptomatic for a mean of 13 and 4.5 years, respectively. Most patients present with chronic symptoms that are typical of malabsorption syndromes. Midepigastric

pain and weight loss associated with steatorrhea and diarrhea are common.[82] Shortly after presentation, 20% to 30% of patients have ulcer complications such as small bowel obstruction (30%), melena (25%), and perforation (22%). In addition to symptoms caused by these complications, patients with CUJ may have low-grade fever and signs of malnutrition.

Pathology

Multiple superficial or deep ulcers are invariably present in the jejunum. Involvement of the ileum is also common. Gastric and colonic ulcers are occasionally present as well.[82,99] Splenic atrophy is often present. Lymphomatous infiltration of lymph nodes, liver, spleen, and bone marrow is common with concurrent lymphoma.[78]

According to Isaacson, there are "variable degrees (usually severe) of villus atrophy, crypt hyperplasia, intraepithelial lymphocytic infiltration, irregularity of surface enterocytes, and a dense lamina propria infiltrate consisting almost solely of plasma cells with a variable number of eosinophils and occasional neutrophils" (Fig. 77-2).[79] Invasion of the epithelial layer may cause ulceration (Fig. 77-3). Subepithelial collagen deposition, which is also seen in GSE, and marked fibrosis of the ulcer base may also be present. Crypt hyperplasia and villus atrophy are seen in the surrounding mucosa; the distant mucosa is usually normal. It is imperative that multiple sections be exhaustively examined for malignant cells to avoid missing the diagnosis of lymphoma. Neoplastic cells are derived from T cells.[91–93,100] They are histiocyte-like, with minimal or no atypia, and the presence of intracellular erythrocytes, platelets, and cell debris is a common feature (Fig. 77-4).[78] Confusion with Hodgkin's disease may occur because of similarities with Reed-Sternberg cells.[84,85,101]

Diagnosis

The diagnosis of CUJ should be considered in patients with GSE who present with worsening malabsorption despite continued compliance with gluten-free diets. CUJ is essentially

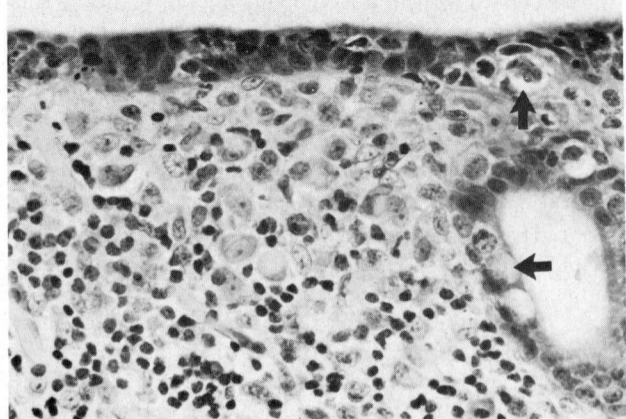

FIGURE 77-2.   Jejunal resection of chronic ulcerative nongranulomatous jejunoileitis: Aggregates of what were supposed to be histiocytes, now known to be malignant T cells, can be seen invading the surface epithelium (*arrows*). (Original magnification ×400; from Isaacson P. Malignant histiocytosis of the intestine: the early histological lesion. Gut 1980;21:381.)

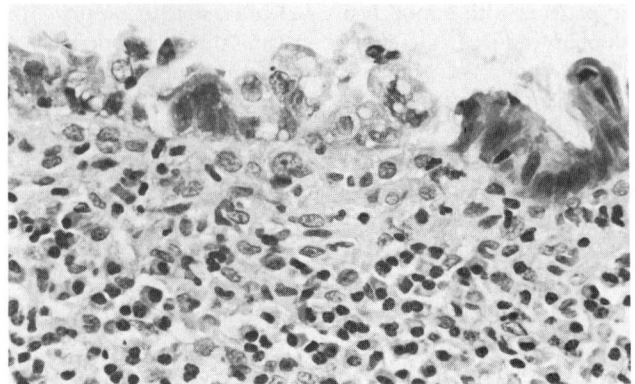

FIGURE 77-3. The malignant chronic ulcerative nongranulomatous jejunoileitis cells have invaded the surface epithelium and produced an ulcer. An exuberant plasma cell infiltrate is seen in the subepithelial tissue. (Original magnification ×400; from Isaacson P. Malignant histiocytosis of the intestine. The early histological lesion. Gut 1980;21:381.)

a diagnosis of exclusion, whether or not a history of celiac disease is present. Disorders presenting with malabsorption and intestinal ulceration that must be excluded include Crohn's disease, ischemic enteritis, radiation enteritis, lymphoma, drug-induced ulceration, vasculitis, Zollinger-Ellison syndrome, and Whipple's disease.

The patient with suspected CUJ should be assessed for malnutrition, and a careful evaluation of the extent of disease should be undertaken. Malabsorption and protein-losing enteropathy account for hypoalbuminemia, and hypoglobulinemia and deficiencies of divalent cations, iron and folate are common. Hyposplenism is often present.[83] Intestinal perforation should be ruled out if leukocytosis with or without fever and peritoneal signs is present.

Roentgenographic studies. The diagnosis of CUJ is rarely made radiographically. Evidence of bowel thickening and of

complications such as small bowel perforation or obstruction may be present on plain films. Demonstration of small bowel strictures by contrast studies (Fig. 77-5) helps to distinguish CUJ from uncomplicated GSE: small bowel dilatation is typical of the latter.[102–104] The presence of bowel thickening, mesenteric lymphadenopathy, and splenic atrophy are consistent with CUJ. However, lymphadenopathy in patients with GSE is not diagnostic of lymphoma.

Small bowel biopsy. Small bowel biopsies are essential for establishing the presence of CUJ. Although the yield from blind biopsies is poor, improvements in the ability to obtain endoscopic biopsies should markedly reduce the need for surgery to establish the diagnosis. In one case report,[104] endoscopy revealed a normal proximal duodenum, but the distal duodenum and the jejunum were markedly edematous and friable, and numerous punched-out ulcers were seen. Biopsies obtained from ulcerated regions are the most desirable.

As has been discussed, it is essential that adequate tissue is obtained, sectioned extensively, and examined by an experienced pathologist before excluding the diagnosis of EATL.[79] A careful search for disseminated lymphoma at the time of presentation is essential.[78] It is also important to assess for the presence of B-cell surface markers, because B-cell lymphomas and IPSID may be associated with villus atrophy.

Therapy

No specific therapy has been shown to modulate the course of CUJ. Most patients have unresponsive malabsorption, and life expectancy at diagnosis is less than 2 years. Surgical resection of severely affected bowel has been of benefit in some cases.[82,94] Although patients with CUJ are at increased risk for intestinal perforation, prednisone therapy should be considered in all symptomatic patients with no evidence of lymphoma. The dose should be reduced to the minimum nec-

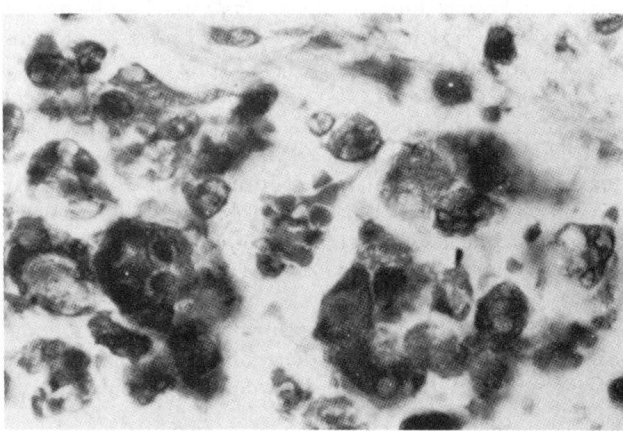

FIGURE 77-4. Chronic ulcerative nongranulomatous jejunoileitis tumor cells show typical erythrophagocytosis. (Original magnification ×1000; from Isaacson P, Wright DH. Malignant histiocytosis of the intestine; its relationship to malabsorption and ulcerative jejunitis. Human Pathol 1978;9:661.)

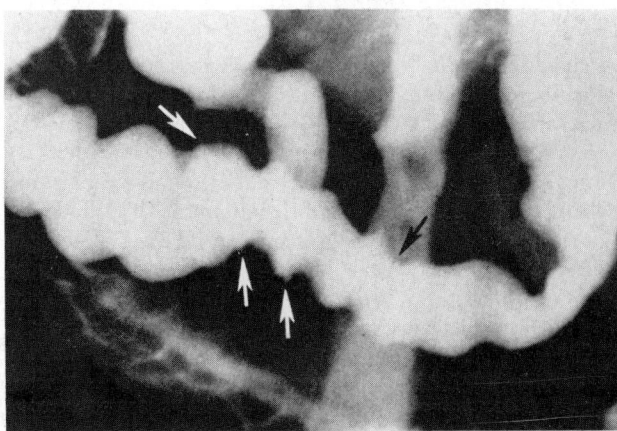

FIGURE 77-5. Chronic ulcerative nongranulomatous jejunoileitis (CUJ). Thirty-minute small bowel follow-through shows prominent intestinal folds, thickening of the bowel wall, diffuse luminal narrowing, and mucosal ulceration (*arrows*). Dilatation, which is typical of gluten-sensitive enteropathy, is not a feature of CUJ. (From Freeman M, Cho S-R. Nongranulomatous ulcerative jejunoileitis. Am J Gastroenterol 1984;79:446.)

essary to maintain a symptomatic response with tolerable side effects.

It has been hypothesized that continued immune stimulation by gliadin, at least in patients with GSE, may promote the progression to lymphoma.[90] Although CUJ does not respond to removal of dietary gluten, it is possible that this measure may impede the development of lymphoma. If a localized lymphomatous infiltrate is found, local excision is mandatory. Although some patients have been cured by resection alone,[105] most remain symptomatic after surgery. Mortality in these cases is very high, presumably because of progression of the lymphoma. The impacts of adjuvant radiation and chemotherapy have not been evaluated. Disseminated T-cell lymphoma should be treated with aggressive chemotherapy. No trials have been done, but the principles are probably similar to those used in the treatment of other lymphomas, employing combinations such as CHOP (cyclophosphamide, hydroxyadriamycin, vincristine, and prednisone).[106]

DRUG-INDUCED SMALL BOWEL DISEASE

Many of the drugs used today have a variety of effects on the small intestine. The mechanisms of injury include erosive damage by NSAIDs and KCl; ischemic damage by cardiac drugs, cocaine, ergotamine alkaloids, and oral contraceptives; hematomas from anticoagulants; motility disorders from opiates; malabsorption; and inhibition of epithelial cell turnover by chemotherapeutic agents. Unfortunately, many of these medications produce side effects or complications without much warning, but these adverse reactions may be reversible if the drug is discontinued. Some medications produce permanent effects. This section focuses on drugs that have a profound or permanent effect on the small intestine, with the exception of those causing erosive damage, which were discussed above.

Drugs Causing Ischemia

Mechanisms by which drugs and toxins can produce intestinal ischemia include induction of arterial vasoconstriction, systemic or splanchnic hypotension, and thrombosis of mesenteric vessels. Some of the more common agents that act through one or more of these mechanisms to induce intestinal ischemia are discussed after a brief summary of the clinical features of intestinal ischemia (see Chap. 112).

Regardless of cause, the mortality rate from small bowel ischemia ranges from 70% to 90%.[107] Delays in presentation and diagnosis and coexistent health problems account for this high mortality. Patients with drug-induced mesenteric ischemia usually present with severe, poorly localized abdominal pain, low-grade fever, and hematochezia. Signs of peritonitis or abdominal distention secondary to ileus may be present. Evidence of intestinal perforation, obstruction, or ileus can be obtained by radiographic studies. The demonstration of bowel wall edema and thumbprinting, pneumatosis intestinalis, or portal venous gas are consistent with mesenteric infarction (Fig. 77-6).[107] In several studies, computed tomography scanning has proven to be a reliable method to make this diagnosis.[108,109] Radiographic studies may be normal

in patients with nonocclusive ischemia, such as occurs with digitalis-induced mesenteric spasm and antihypertensive medications.[110,111] Mesenteric angiography may be needed to document digitalis-induced ischemia.[112]

In addition to measures specific to the offending agent, general supportive measures include administration of fluids and oxygen, correction of electrolyte and acid-base disorders, and antibiotic therapy.[107] Surgical resection of infarcted small bowel is necessary, although most patients are very high-risk surgical candidates.

Cardiac Drugs

Intestinal ischemia or infarction may result from drugs that produce or potentiate arterial either vasoconstriction or hypotension.[113] The incidence of these side effects is greatest if the splanchnic circulation is already compromised, such as occurs with congestive heart failure. Antihypertensive agents and diuretics can induce intestinal ischemia secondary to hypotension and hypovolemia. Drugs with direct vasoconstrictive effects, such as norepinephrine, dopamine, and intraarterial or intravenous vasopressin, reduce intestinal blood flow and can cause mesenteric infarction.[114,115] Digitalis glycosides reduce splanchnic flow in patients with congestive heart failure. Intestinal ischemia resulting from digoxin use may be reversed with nitroprusside and calcium channel blockers.[112,116]

Cocaine

Cocaine is a lipophilic drug that is readily absorbed by mucosal surfaces, including the intestinal mucosa. It has potent stimulatory effects on the central nervous system because of inhibition of presynaptic reuptake of norepinephrine, dopamine, and serotonin as well as increased synthesis of norepinephrine and dopamine.[117,118] Excessive sympathetic stimulation produces peripheral vasoconstriction and tachycardia, which can cause hypertension and nonocclusive intestinal ischemia.[119] Rebound vasodilation after intense vasoconstriction can further compromise intestinal perfusion.

Intestinal ischemia is a serious but rare complication of cocaine and crack abuse.[120,121] Gastrointestinal problems are more likely to be encountered by "body packers." Such individuals transport illicit drugs by ingesting drug-containing packets or condoms or by inserting them in the rectum.[119,122,123] Complications include mechanical intestinal obstruction and rupture of a packet, which can release a lethal quantity of cocaine.[123,124] Signs of drug toxicity, mechanical intestinal obstruction, or marked leukocytosis, which may indicate the presence of gangrenous bowel, are indications for laparotomy.[114] Asymptomatic patients should be treated with activated charcoal to bind any leached drug and with mild cathartics to stimulate gastrointestinal transit.[114,122] Abdominal radiographs may reveal evidence of intestinal obstruction or ileus as well the pathognomonic "double condom sign."[125]

Ergotamines

Ergot alkaloids such as ergotamine, dihydroergotamine, methylergonovine, and methysergide are used in the symptomatic treatment or prevention of migraine headaches.[126] Common intestinal complications of ergots include abdom-

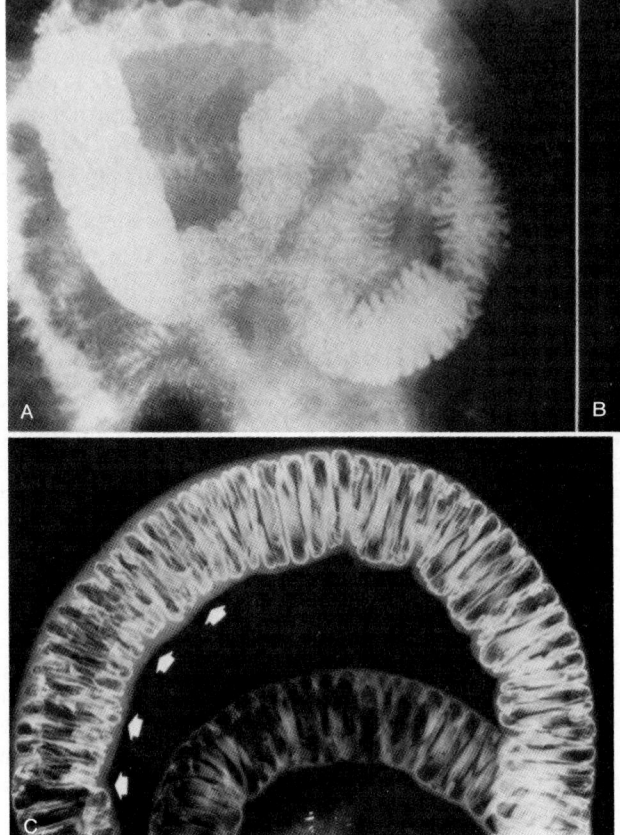
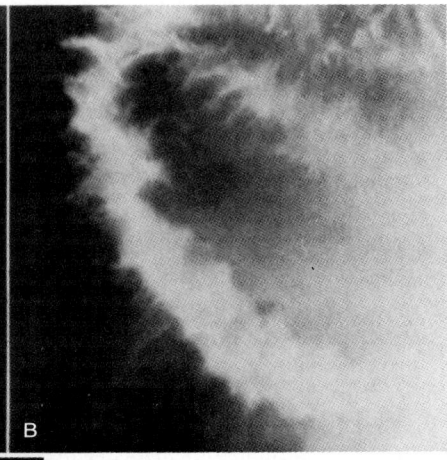

FIGURE 77-6. Acute spontaneous mesenteric venous thrombosis. (**A**) Involved jejunum shows separation of loops and thumbprinting. (**B**) Blurring of mucosal folds is seen in a distal zone of involvement. (**C**) Barium study of a surgical specimen shows thickening of mucosal wall and folds, thumbprinting, and pseudomembrane formation (*arrows*). (From Pringot J, Bodart P. Inflammatory Diseases. In: Margulis AR, Burhenne HJ, eds. Alimentary tract radiology. St Louis: CV Mosby, 1989:804.)

inal pain, nausea, and vomiting. Symptomatic vasospasm affecting the extremities is a common complication of ergot toxicity, whereas severe splanchnic vasoconstriction is rare.[127,128] There are several reports of bowel infarction after administration of large doses of ergots.[127,128] Ergots have high affinity for α-adrenergic and 5-hydroxytryptamine receptor subtypes.[129] Ergot-induced vasospasm is thought to occur as a result of peripheral adrenergic stimulation.[127,129] The diagnosis of ergot-induced intestinal ischemia is based on the presence of abdominal symptoms in a patient on ergotamines. Arteriographic demonstration of mesenteric vascular spasm and collateralization supports the diagnosis.[128] Discontinuation of ergots and supportive care with fluids are usually sufficient therapy. Intravenous sodium nitroprusside may be beneficial in severe cases.[130] Emergency laparotomy is essential if there is evidence of gangrenous bowel.

Oral Contraceptives

Oral contraceptives have been reported to cause small intestine infarction. The pathophysiologic mechanisms are not known, although mesenteric arterial occlusion[131–134] or mesenteric venous thrombosis[135–138] is often present. It appears that progestins cause arterial occlusion, whereas estrogens can produce both arterial and venous occlusion.[139,140] Mechanisms that have been implicated include hypercoagulability, reduced mesenteric venous blood flow, and endothelial proliferation.[133,141] The risk is increased by ancillary factors such as collagen vascular disease, hypercoagulable states, smoking, and hypertension.[142] The duration of contraceptive usage is

not an independent risk factor and does not correlate with the severity of symptoms.[133]

The diagnosis should be considered in contraceptive users presenting with poorly localized colicky abdominal pain, bloody diarrhea, or hematochezia. Fever is often present, and presenting symptoms may also include nausea and vomiting.[134] Although abdominal pain may be present for several weeks or months, pain serious enough to warrant hospitalization is usually of recent onset. Laboratory studies, including platelet count, prothrombin time, and partial thromboplastin time, are usually normal.[134] The diagnosis depends on the demonstration of intestinal ulceration or ischemia in contraceptive users. Abdominal radiographs may demonstrate bowel wall thickening or ileus. Ulceration, which may be detected with contrast studies, is usually continuous in involved segments.[134]

Oral contraceptives should be discontinued and supportive therapy initiated. Although mesenteric ischemia may be reversible, the mortality rate in severe cases is almost 50%.[134] The risk of thromboembolic complications decreases to normal levels within 1 month of discontinuation of oral contraceptives.[141]

Anticoagulants

Gastrointestinal hemorrhage is a common complication of anticoagulant therapy. The incidence of this complication depends on intensity of therapy, adequacy of monitoring and dosage adjustment, route of administration, concurrent drug therapy, and the gender, age, and underlying condition of the patient. The incidence of gastrointestinal bleeding requiring transfusion for medical inpatients without predisposing illness in the Boston Collaborative Drug Surveillance Program was 1.2% and 0.2% for heparin and warfarin, respectively.[143] Minor gastrointestinal bleeding occurred in 8.3% and 3.3%, respectively. Gastrointestinal bleeding should be thoroughly investigated, even if it is a minor symptom, and regardless of the prothrombin time.[144-148] Most episodes of gastrointestinal bleeding in patients on anticoagulants are attributable to a demonstrable gastric or intestinal lesion.[147,148]

The most common hemorrhagic small intestine complication is spontaneous or trauma-induced intramural hematoma.[149] This is most likely to occur in the jejunum in the absence of abdominal trauma. The relative fixation of the descending duodenum is responsible for a higher susceptibility to intramural hematoma in response to blunt abdominal trauma.[149] Hematomas may cause colicky abdominal pain and symptoms secondary to intestinal obstruction. Biliary symptoms or pancreatitis may result from obstruction of the biliary or pancreatic ducts. Minor intestinal bleeding is detected in 25% and major bleeding in 3.5%.[150] Patients may present with an acute abdomen that can be differentiated from that owing to other causes by the more gradual onset of symptoms and the acute decrease in hematocrit.[151]

Abdominal tenderness, low-grade fever, and a palpable abdominal mass are common physical findings. Evidence of proximal small bowel obstruction may be present on plain abdominal radiographs. The most useful diagnostic test is an upper gastrointestinal series demonstrating the classic coiled-spring, picket-fence, or stack-of-coins sign (Fig. 77-7).[144,149] This radiographic appearance is caused by extravasation of blood into the valvulae conniventes, narrowing the lumen with spike-like projections of barium outlining the normal caliber of the lumen.[144] Serial ultrasound examinations can be useful for monitoring the behavior of the hematoma.[152]

Conservative medical management is usually sufficient because most hematomas undergo spontaneous reabsorption,

with resolution of symptoms within 3 weeks (Fig. 77-8). Reversal of anticoagulation with fresh frozen plasma and vitamin K, intravenous hydration, and continuous nasogastric suction are sufficient for management of most patients. Surgical intervention may be required if there is complete intestinal obstruction or if conservative medical management fails to resolve intestinal bleeding, obstructive symptoms, or fever.[146,150]

Drugs Causing Motility Disorders

Drug-induced intestinal pseudoobstruction can occur with the use of anticholinergic drugs, drugs with anticholinergic effects such as phenothiazines and tricyclic antidepressants, opioids, verapamil, and clonidine and also, occasionally, with initiation of cyclosporine therapy. Neurotoxicity induced by such drugs as vincristine can also produce intestinal pseudoobstruction,[153] which frequently appears within 3 days of the initiation of therapy and resolves within 2 weeks after the cessation of therapy. Direct toxicity to the enteric nervous system is probable because evidence of peripheral nerve dysfunction is not always present in patients with this complication.

The persistent use of narcotic analgesics can produce the narcotic bowel syndrome. This clinical syndrome is characterized by abdominal pain, intermittent vomiting, weight loss, and other symptoms suggestive of intermittent pseudoobstruction.[154] Poorly localized chronic abdominal pain that is colicky in nature, with acute exacerbations, is typically the major symptom. The pain is initially responsive to narcotic analgesics, but, with continued narcotic use, progressively larger doses are required for pain relief. Although the differential diagnosis includes biliary colic, pancreatitis, peptic ulcer disease, and renal calculi, the history, physical examination, and laboratory tests are usually not consistent with these entities. Abdominal radiographs typically are consistent with ileus and, on rare occasions, with mechanical small bowel obstruction.[154] The diagnosis of narcotic bowel syndrome is

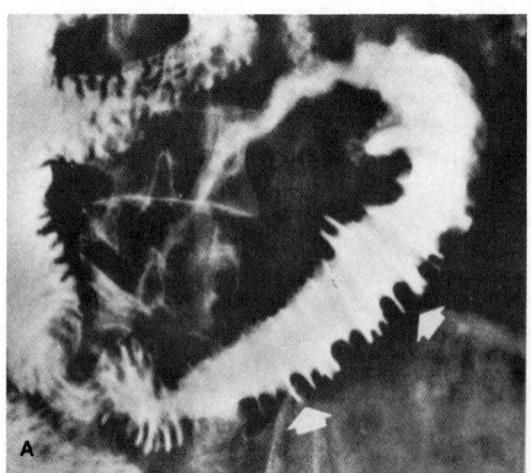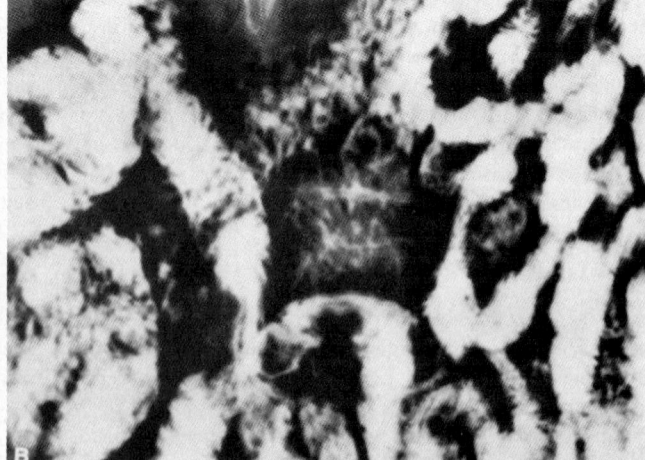

FIGURE 77-7. Small intestine ischemia. **(A)** Segmental ischemia in a picket-fence pattern of regular thickening of small bowel folds (*arrows*). **(B)** Complete resolution of the ischemic process is achieved after conservative therapy. (From Eisenberg R. Regular thickening of small bowel folds. In: Eisenberg R, ed. Gastrointestinal radiology: a pattern approach. Philadelphia: JB Lippincott, 1989:459.)

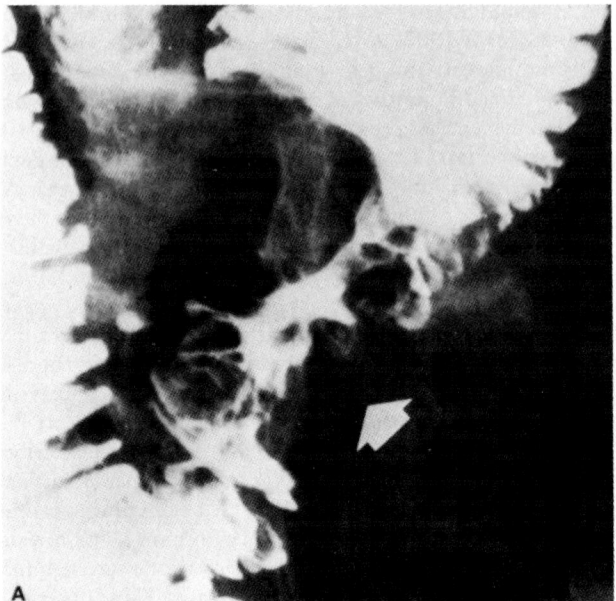 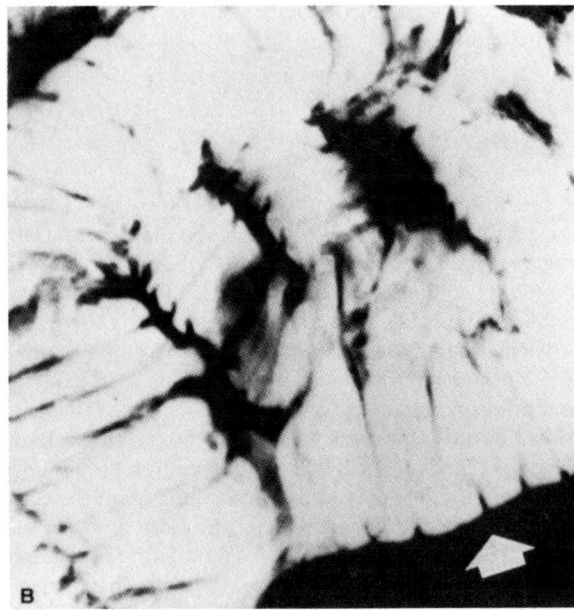

FIGURE 77-8. Intramural hemorrhage in a patient on Coumadin (warfarin). (**A**) Mass effect with shouldering and partial obstruction (*arrow*), suggests a neoplastic process. (**B**) Complete resolution is achieved after discontinuing of the drug and applying conservative therapy. The *arrow* corresponds to the previously involved loop. (From Eisenberg R. Regular thickening of small bowel folds. In: Eisenberg R, ed. Gastrointestinal radiology: a pattern approach. Philadelphia: JB Lippincott, 1989:457.)

readily made with an intake history of more than 2 weeks of moderate to heavy doses of narcotics and a work-up that excludes more serious disorders.[154]

Narcotic withdrawal is essential for treatment of narcotic bowel syndrome. On withdrawal, the patient may experience vomiting, diarrhea, and cramping resulting from increased intestinal motility.[154] These symptoms can be markedly reduced or abolished by the α_2-adrenergic receptor agonist, clonidine.[155] Opiates are discontinued after an initial clonidine dose of 0.1 mg. The dose is gradually increased from 0.1 mg twice daily to 0.1 mg four times daily.[155] After 1 week of therapy, the dose is tapered over 3 days. Narcotic bowel syndrome and withdrawal symptoms can be successfully treated in 90% to 95% of patients with this regimen. Metoclopramide therapy has been of benefit in patients with cancer.[156]

Drugs Causing Malabsorption

Drug-induced malabsorption of nutrients, electrolytes, and concurrently-used medications occurs by several different mechanisms.[110,134,157] These include intralumenal interactions that interfere with the solubilization, digestion, or transport of nutrients; increased rate of intestinal transit; mucosal injury; direct inhibition of absorptive processes; and inhibition of gastric, biliary, or pancreatic secretions. Drugs that impede nutrient assimilation by direct interaction include tetracycline, which chelates calcium ions; cholestyramine, which binds to iron and vitamin B_{12}; mineral oil, which reduces the solubilization of β-carotene and fat-soluble vitamins; and aluminum and magnesium hydroxide, which precipitate calcium and phosphate ions. Prokinetic agents and cathartics can impair fat absorption by increasing intestinal transit.[158] Mucosal in-

jury resulting in diminished nutrient absorption has been reported with drugs such as colchicine, neomycin, and methotrexate. In addition to causing diffuse intestinal injury by inhibiting mitosis, colchicine is thought to directly inhibit brush-border disaccharidases.[159] Colchicine can impair absorption of fat, vitamin B_{12}, β-carotene, D-xylose, lactose, bile salts, and steroids.[159] Neomycin in doses of 6 to 12 g per day is thought to cause brush-border damage by inhibiting enterocyte protein synthesis.[160,161] Neomycin is also thought to impair micellar solubilization of bile salts, cholesterol, fatty acids, and fat-soluble vitamins by directly binding to bile salts. Azotorrhea and decreased D-xylose absorption can also be seen with neomycin. The degree of malabsorption with neomycin is dose-related and can been seen with as little as 3 g/day.[160] Discontinuation of the drug typically reverses the malabsorption and diarrhea. Methotrexate decreases the height of intestinal microvilli and brush-border membrane protein and lipid content. Other drugs that produce histologic changes in the jejunal mucosa associated with fat malabsorption include methyldopa[162] and allopurinol.[163] Sodium aminosalicylate[164] and thiazide diuretics, which impair ileal vitamin B_{12} and sodium transport, respectively, are examples of drugs that directly inhibit nutrient transport.

The clinical significance of drug-induced malabsorption is influenced by such variables as baseline nutritional status and dietary intake, underlying disorders that interfere with intestinal function, and pharmacologic considerations such as drug dosage and schedule and duration of therapy. Awareness of the nutritional consequences of drug therapy facilitates their prevention and early detection. For some drugs, prophylactic nutritional supplementation is reasonable. For example, patients treated chronically with sulfasalazine, phenytoin, or colestipol should receive folic acid, and patients receiving the latter two drugs should also receive vitamin D supplementation.

Chemotherapeutic Agents

Most chemotherapeutic agents produce cytotoxic effects in normal cells because they have low therapeutic indices. Cells that have a high turnover rate, such as those of the small intestine crypt epithelium, are particularly vulnerable to drugs that inhibit cell proliferation. The magnitude of gastrointestinal toxicity is highly variable between patients and is affected by dose, duration of treatment, specific agents used, concurrent radiotherapy, and nutritional status of the patient. Nausea and vomiting are common acute side effects of antineoplastic drugs and are mediated in part by the chemoreceptor trigger zone in the brain. These symptoms predominate in the early stages of therapy, and not those resulting from direct injury to the small intestine mucosa. After a single course of therapy, mucosal damage is usually evident within the first 3 days. Regeneration and repair occur rapidly after cessation of therapy, with grossly normal mucosa present by 14 days, although inflammatory changes may be present for several weeks.[165]

Erosive enteritis, with or without stomatitis, presents with abdominal pain, bleeding, vomiting, ileus, or diarrhea. It is most common with methotrexate therapy but is also seen with 5-fluorouracil, actinomycin D, doxorubicin, cytosine arabinoside, bleomycin, and vincristine. These chemotherapeutic agents are also associated with other complications. Methotrexate is associated with malabsorption (discussed in the previous section). The erosive enteritis associated with Ara-C when it is used in combination regimens occurs within 8 to 11 days from the start of therapy. This syndrome is also associated with hypokalemia, hypocalcemia, and protein-losing enteropathy. Ara-C can also produce a syndrome characterized by telangiectasis and intramural hematomas.[166] Vincristine can induce acute intestinal pseudoobstruction (as already discussed). Preconditioning for bone marrow transplantation with cyclophosphamide and total body irradiation produces diffuse intestinal injury. Symptoms, including crampy abdominal pain, watery diarrhea, and anorexia, are common within the first 3 weeks after transplantation. Symptoms that persist beyond 3 weeks should be investigated to rule out enteric infection or other intestinal disorders. Neutropenic enterocolitis or typhlitis is most frequently encountered after chemotherapy for leukemia or lymphoma. Diffuse patchy mucosal necrosis involving the ileocecal region is associated with nonspecific symptoms and fever, nausea, vomiting, right lower quadrant pain, and hematochezia. The effect of these drugs in the colon complication is discussed in Chapter 80.

NECROTIZING ENTEROCOLITIS

Acute Jejunitis

Acute jejunitis is also referred to as pig-bel, enteritis necroticans, darmbrand, nonspecific jejunitis, epidemic regional jejunitis, Pasini's regional jejunitis, and necrotizing jejunitis.

Although there were a number of European outbreaks during and after World War II,[167] acute jejunitis is largely a problem in nonindustrialized nations.[168–170] Outbreaks are most frequent in communities in which protein deprivation and poor food hygiene are prevalent. For example, the illness was documented in 62 Khmer children along the Thai-Kampuchean border from June 1985 to July 1986.[171] The disease was a major cause of illness and death among children in the highlands of Papua New Guinea until immunization against the β-toxin of the causative organism, *Clostridium perfringens*, was begun in 1980.[172] *C perfringens* type C (initially identified as *Clostridium welchii* type F) is a heat-resistant bacterium that can often be isolated from the tissues, stool, and food of affected patients.[173–176] One sixth of normal persons were shown to harbor a less pathogenic strain. A similar illness attributed to pathogenic strains of this organism has been described in a number of animal species,[177,178] and experimental instillation of *C perfringens* into the small intestine of guinea pigs causes jejunal necrosis. Immunization against the β-toxin resulted in a reduction in hospital admissions for acute jejunitis to less than one fifth of previous figures.[172] These observations have firmly established that this organism is a causative agent of acute jejunitis. The agent has also been isolated from children in Bangladesh with nonnecrotizing diarrheal illnesses.[179]

Acute jejunitis occurs sporadically and in epidemics. Illness is characterized by bloody diarrhea, fever, and abdominal pain. In the outbreak in Kampuchea, the mortality rate was 58%.[171] Small intestine necrosis of varying severity, with areas of full-thickness necrosis, is usually found.

Neonatal Necrotizing Enterocolitis

The pathogenesis of acute jejunitis and other necrotizing enteropathies has not been determined. A discussion of neonatal NEC is included because similar pathophysiologic mechanisms may be operative in necrotizing enteropathies that are encountered in adult gastroenterology. Neonatal NEC is a disease of focal or diffuse small intestine ulceration and necrosis that is seen almost exclusively in premature infants and low-birth-weight neonates. The causes, clinical presentation, differential diagnosis, pathology, and management of NEC have been discussed in several excellent reviews.[180–182]

The cause of NEC is unknown. However, several pathogenic factors appear to be implicated.[180,183] These include prematurity, intestinal ischemia, infectious agents, and the initiation of enteral nutrition. Not all cases of NEC occur in premature or low-birth-weight infants, and institution of enteral nutrition is not an absolute requirement. Intestinal ischemia, hypoxia, and possibly direct injury by hypertonic fluids are important causes of intestinal mucosal injury that appear to predispose individuals to NEC.[184–191] Hypothermia,[187,192,193] exchange transfusion,[194,195] umbilical artery catheterization,[196] and the use of indomethacin[197,198] are additional causes of mucosal injury that have been implicated in the pathogenesis of NEC. It is thought that the neonatal intestine is predisposed to ischemic injury because its collateral blood supply is not well developed.[199,200] The high prevalence of NEC in infants whose mothers used cocaine during pregnancy is also consistent with a pathogenic role for hypoxic and ischemic injury.[117,118,201–204]

Clinical and experimental data support the hypothesis that bacteria have a significant role in the development of NEC. Bacterial precolonization is a requirement in experimental models of NEC.[184,187] For example, Musemeche and colleagues,[205] using germ-free rats, showed that bacteria were the major determinant of necrosis after surgically created ileal loops were made ischemic and injected with different bacteria or infant formulas.[183] Bacterial endotoxin production, with stimulation of inflammatory cytokines such as tumor necrosis factor and platelet aggregating factor, may be one of the mechanisms by which bacteria contribute to the development of NEC.[206] Clinical evidence supporting a pathogenic role for bacteria includes the observation that NEC often occurs in epidemics within a single intensive care unit.[207] Nevertheless, blood cultures, which are positive in 30% to 35% of cases, mirror the colonic flora,[208-209], and no organisms have consistently been identified in NEC.[183,209-211]

The importance of enteral nutrition in the pathogenesis of NEC is well established. In 95% of affected infants, enteral feedings were initiated before the onset of clinically recognizable NEC. Introduction of bacteria into the intestine by enteral feeding is a possible explanation for this association. NEC is rarely seen in infants who are fed with breast milk, although a protective role for breast milk has not been definitively established.[209,212-213] The ability of enteral commercial IgA-IgG preparations to protect infants from NEC suggests that antibodies are active components of human milk.[213]

Several case-control studies support the theory that stressed infants are at greater risk of developing NEC if enteral feedings are advanced rapidly or if excessive volumes are used.[214-217] Intestinal distention resulting from overfeeding may result in local intestinal hypoxemia by interfering with mesenteric blood flow.[209] Intestinal distention and ischemia secondary to fermentation of malabsorbed lactose may also be a consequence of overfeeding.[209] Large quantities of hydrogen gas resulting from lactose metabolism by lumenal bacteria have been detected in the lumen and in pneumatosis intestinalis cysts.[218]

The pathogenesis of NEC is clearly multifactorial, and susceptibility of individuals to NEC is probably also dependent on host factors.[183] Such factors have not, however, been identified. Successful delineation of these factors and other pathogenic mechanisms should improve the ability to prevent and treat NEC and also provide insight into the mechanisms of intestinal disorders seen in adults.

PROTEIN-LOSING GASTROENTEROPATHY

Definition

PLGE is a syndrome characterized by enteric loss of plasma proteins in abnormal amounts. A large number of intestinal and extraintestinal diseases may be associated with PLGE, and treatment is aimed almost exclusively at the underlying disorder. The recognition of PLGE mandates a careful search for an associated illness.

The defining characteristic of PLGE is hypoproteinemia resulting from gastric or intestinal losses. Studies of ^{131}I-albumin secretion into the stomach of a patient with hypertrophic gastritis first identified the gastrointestinal tract as a site of excessive protein loss.[219] Before recognition of the pathogenesis of this disorder, it was thought that catabolic processes were responsible for hypoproteinemia that could not otherwise be ascribed to malnutrition, renal disease, or hepatic disease.

Under physiologic conditions, sloughed enterocytes and pancreatic and biliary secretions account for almost all of the endogenous protein that is found in the intestine. Most of these proteins are digested, and the constituent amino acids are reabsorbed.[220-221] Gastrointestinal loss of serum proteins, as indicated by measuring serum albumin kinetics, accounts for less than 10% of daily protein catabolism.[222-226] This may increase four- to fivefold in patients with PLGE. Hypoproteinemia results if the capacity to increase protein synthesis is not sufficient to compensate for increased intestinal protein losses. For example, albumin synthesis is increased no greater than twofold in patients with PLGE.[227]

Etiology

Most diseases associated with PLGE cause exudative protein losses secondary to ulcerative or nonulcerative enteropathies or secondary to lymphatic obstruction or increased lymphatic hydrostatic pressure (Table 77-3).

TABLE 77-3
Classification of Protein-Losing Enteropathy

Increased Interstitial Pressure (Intestinal Lymphatic Obstruction)
Congenital intestinal lymphangiectasia
Mesenteric lymphatic obstruction
    Tuberculosis
    Sarcoidosis
    Lymphoma
    Retroperitoneal fibrosis
Increased right-sided heart pressure
    Constrictive pericarditis
    Congestive heart failure
Whipple's disease
Crohn's disease

Breakdown of the Enterocyte Barrier
Ulcerative Diseases
    Erosive gastritis or enteritis
    Neoplasia-carcinoma or lymphoma
    Crohn's disease
    Pseudomembranous enterocolitis
    Acute graft-versus-host disease
Nonulcerative Diseases
    Giant hypertrophic gastropathy (Menetrier's disease)
    Hypertrophic hypersecretory gastropathy
    Viral enteritides
    Bacterial overgrowth
    Parasitic diseases (malaria, giardiasis, schistosomiasis)
    Whipple's disease (see also lymphatic obstruction)
    Allergic enteritis
    Eosinophilic gastroenteritis
    Gluten-sensitive enteropathy
    Tropical sprue
    Systemic lupus erythematosus

Intestinal Inflammatory and Ulcerative Disorders

Enteropathies resulting in PLGE include ulcerating gastrointestinal carcinomas and inflammatory disorders such as Crohn's disease and ulcerative colitis. The cause of the hypoalbuminemia and reduced protein pools that are seen in these disorders is multifactorial. In the case of inflammatory bowel disease, the magnitude of enteric protein loss is significant, and it is directly related to the extent and activity of mucosal inflammation.[228-229]

Nonulcerative Intestinal Enteropathies

Nonulcerative diseases such as Ménétrier's disease,[219] atrophic gastritis, hypertrophic hypersecretory gastropathy, tropical sprue, celiac disease, allergic gastroenteritis, eosinophilic gastroenteritis, collagenous colitis, and colonic polyposis syndromes have also been associated with PLGE.[219,230-236]

Infectious Causes

Acute and chronic intestinal infections can result in PLGE. Examples include acute staphylococcal, salmonella,[220] and shigella[237] infections. The incidence of PLGE seems to be species- and strain-dependent. For example, *Shigella dysenteriae* type 1 infections cause greater loss of enteric protein than do other strains.[237] PLGE has also been documented in small bowel bacterial overgrowth.[238] Pseudomembranous colitis and colonization by *Clostridium difficile* without symptoms can result in enteric loss of protein. As an example, colonization with *C difficile* and fecal excretion of α_1-antitrypsin were correlated in asymptomatic infants.[239] In a study of elderly nursing home patients, PLGE was documented in all 12 patients with pseudomembranous colitis, in 6 of 14 with *C difficile* diarrhea but no pseudomembranes, and in 6 of 12 who were colonized with *C difficile* without toxin or diarrhea; none of the 15 normal control patients had evidence of excessive enteric protein loss.[240] Parasitic diseases with documented PLGE include *Strongyloides stercoralis* infection,[241] schistosomiasis,[242-243] and giardiasis.[244-246] Acute viral illnesses have also been linked to PLGE.[247-249]

Collagen Vascular Diseases

PLGE has been well documented in patients with systemic lupus erythematosus.[250-253] It occurs most commonly in young women, and it may be the initial clinical manifestation of lupus. Fifty percent present with steroid-responsive diarrhea without steatorrhea.[254] Mixed connective tissue disease[255-256] and other collagen vascular diseases can also be complicated by PLGE.[257]

Diseases Associated With Lymphatic Dysfunction

Diseases that produce disruption of intestinal lymphatic vessels or obstruction of lymph flow are an additional cause of PLGE. Tortuous, dilated mucosal and submucosal lymphatic vessels are the hallmark of primary intestinal lymphangiectasia (see Chap. 68). Most patients with this disease present by 30 years of age with edema, diarrhea, hypoproteinemia, and lymphocytopenia resulting from epithelial leakage and lymphatic rupture.[258] A similar lesion has been implicated as the mechanism of enteric protein loss in systemic sclerosis and systemic lupus erythematosus.[259-260]

PLGE is seen with many diseases that impair lymphatic egress from the intestine by causing mechanical obstruction or increased hydrodynamic pressure. Examples include Whipple's disease,[261,262] lymphoma,[263] and Crohn's disease.[228,264] By producing retroperitoneal lymph node enlargement or fibrosis, inflammatory granulomatous diseases such as sarcoidosis and mesenteric tuberculosis cause PLGE.[265-266] Additional retroperitoneal processes including pancreatitis, pancreatic cancer, and other retroperitoneal tumors can also present with PLGE. Right-sided congestive heart failure, constrictive pericarditis, superior vena caval obstruction, and other causes of elevated central venous pressure[267,268] commonly produce PLGE.

Clinical Features

The major clinical manifestation of PLGE is dependent edema resulting from decreased plasma oncotic pressure. Although all plasma proteins are lost, those such as albumin, immunoglobulins, fibrinogen, and α_1-antitrypsin that have long circulating half-lives and a limited capacity for increased synthesis are most likely to exhibit depressed levels. Decreased levels of proteins other than albumin are rarely symptomatic, although in the setting of lymphatic obstruction, symptomatic lymphopenia and steatorrhea may be present.

Diagnosis

Although edema and hypoproteinemia resulting from enteric protein loss may be the presenting manifestations of disease, often the magnitude of protein loss is a minor aspect. The diagnosis of PLGE is established by the documentation of excessive intestinal protein losses. The diagnosis should always be considered in hypoalbuminemic patients if other causes such as malnutrition or protein loss from other sites are not apparent. If it is necessary to document intestinal protein losses, the preferred method is to quantitate fecal α_1-antitrypsin concentration or clearance. Alternative methods employing radiolabeled substrates for quantitating enteric protein loss remain useful research tools but they are seldom used for clinical purposes. Sites of albumin loss can occasionally be determined scintigraphically using ^{99m}Tc-labeled albumin.[269-270]

α_1-Antitrypsin is particularly valuable because it constitutes approximately 4% of serum proteins, has a molecular weight similar to that of albumin, is resistant to proteolysis, is not actively absorbed or secreted, is normally present in low quantities in stool, and is easy to assay. The test cannot be used for analyzing gastric protein losses because α_1-antitrypsin is degraded at a pH below 3.[271] The α_1-antitrypsin concentration in stool and the plasma clearance of α_1-antitrypsin were compared in normal subjects and in consecutive patients with chronic diarrhea, malabsorption, or unexplained hypoalbuminemia.[272] The plasma clearance is the product of daily stool volume and stool α_1-antitrypsin concentration divided by the serum α_1-antitrypsin concentration.[273] In contrast to earlier studies,[274-276] fecal α_1-antitrypsin concentration was not a reliable index of abnormal α_1-antitrypsin clearance.[272] However, the more accurate clearance test demonstrated a highly significant correlation between α_1-antitrypsin clearance and serum albumin concentration. If the α_1-antitrypsin clearance was elevated more than threefold, serum albumin levels were below 3.0 g/dL. Induction of diarrhea by ingestion of lactulose, sorbitol, sodium sulfate, or phenolphthalein in otherwise healthy subjects caused α_1-antitrypsin clearance levels to increase.[272] Clearance levels may also be overestimated if hematochezia or meconium are present. These observations need to be considered in establishing normal values.

Therapy

There is no specific therapy for PLGE. Optimal therapy of the primary illness is the only effective remedy. Prophylactic measures to avoid complications resulting from peripheral edema should be instituted. In the setting of lymphangiectasia, reduction of lymphatic transport may reduce enteric protein loss. Low-fat diets supplemented with medium-chain triglycerides may be beneficial in this setting.[277,278] Surgical drainage of dilated lymphatic channels (lymphovenous anastomosis) is occasionally helpful.[264,279]

The reader is directed to Chapter 80, Miscellaneous Inflammatory and Structural Disorders of the Colon; Chapter 109, Gastrointestinal Manifestations of Systemic Diseases; and Chapter 110, Gastrointestinal Manifestations of Immunologic Disorders.

REFERENCES

1. Baer AN, Bayless TM, Yardley JH. Intestinal ulceration and malabsorption syndromes. Gastroenterology 1980;79:754.
2. Boydstun JS, Gaffey TA, Bartholomew LG. Clinicopathologic study of nonspecific ulcers of the small intestine. Dig Dis Sci 1981;26:911.
3. Davies DR, Brightmore T. Idiopathic and drug-induced ulceration of the small intestine. Br J Surg 1970;57:134.
4. Reid J, Gilmour HM, Holt S. Primary non-specific ulcer of the small intestine. J R Coll Surg Edinb 1982;27:228.
5. Glynn MJ, Pendower J, Shousha S, et al. Recurrent bleeding from idiopathic ulceration of small bowel. Br Med J 1984;288:975.
6. Thomas WEG, Williamson RCN. Nonspecific small bowel ulceration. Postgrad Med 1985;61:587.
7. Ballantyne KC, Morris DL, Hawkey CJ, et al. Haemorrhage from idiopathic annular ulcers of the small intestine. Ann R Coll Surg Engl 1986;68:168.
8. Guest JL. Nonspecific ulceration of the intestine. Int Abstr Surg 1963;117:409.
9. Morgenstern L, Frelich M, Panish JF. The circumferential small bowel ulcer: clinical aspects in 17 patients. JAMA 1965;191:637.
10. Lewis BS, Kornbluth A, Waye JD. Small bowel tumors: yield of enteroscopy. Gut 1991;32:763.
11. Lau WY, Fan ST, Chu KW, et al. Intra-operative fibreoptic enteroscopy for bleeding lesions in the small intestine. Br J Surg 1986;73:217.
12. Iatropoulos MJ, Davis TE. Ulcerative and inflammatory lesions. In: Rozman K, Hanninen O, eds. Gastrointestinal toxicology. Amsterdam: Elsevier, 1986:267.
13. Biscarini L. Anti-inflammatory analgesics and drugs used in gout. In: Dukes MNG, ed. Meyler's side effects of drugs: an encyclopedia of adverse reactions and interactions. 12th ed. Amsterdam: Elsevier, 1992:181.
14. Fries JF, Miller SR, Spitz PW, et al. Toward an epidemiology of gastropathy associated with non-steroidal anti-inflammatory drug use. Gastroenterology 1989;96:647.
15. Langman MJS. Epidemiologic evidence on the association between peptic ulceration and antiinflammatory drug use. Gastroenterology 1989;96:640.
16. Aabakken L: Review article: non-steroidal, anti-inflammatory drugs—the extending scope of gastrointestinal side effects. Aliment Pharmacol Ther 1992;6:143.
17. Gabriel SE, Bombardier C. NSAID induced ulcers: an emerging epidemic. J Rheumatol 1990;17:1.
18. Bjarnason I, Zanelli G, Smith T, et al. Non-steroidal anti-inflammatory drug-induced intestinal inflammation in humans. Gastroenterology 1987;93:480.
19. Lang J, Price AB, Levi AJ, et al. Diaphragm disease: pathology of disease of the small intestine induced by non-steroidal anti-inflammatory drugs. J Clin Pathol 1988;41:516.
20. Langman MJS, Morgan L, Worrall A. Use of anti-inflammatory drugs by patients admitted with small or large bowel perforations and hemorrhage. Br Med J 1985;290:347.
21. Bjarnason I, Price AB, Zanelli G, et al. Clinicopathological features of non-steroidal anti-inflammatory drug-induced small intestinal strictures. Gastroenterology 1988;94:1070.
22. Bjarnason I, Williams P, Su A, et al. Intestinal permeability and inflammation in rheumatic arthritis: effects of non-steroidal anti-inflammatory drugs. Lancet 1984;2:1171.
23. Bjarnason I, Williams P, Smethurst P, et al. Effect of non-steroidal anti-inflammatory drugs and prostaglandins on the permeability of the human small intestine. Gut 1986;27:1292.
24. Rooney PJ, Jenkins RJ, Smith KM, et al. [111]Indium-labeled polymorphonuclear leukocyte scans in rheumatoid arthritis—an important clinical cause of false positive results. Br J Rheumatol 1986;25:167.
25. Allison MC, Howatson AG, Torrance CJ, et al. Gastrointestinal damage associated with the use of nonsteroidal antiinflammatory drugs. N Engl J Med 1992;327:749.
26. Morris AJ, Madhok R, Sturrock RD, et al. Enteroscopic diagnosis of small bowel ulceration in patients receiving non-steroidal anti-inflammatory drugs. Lancet 1991;337:520.
27. Gabriel SE, Jaakkimainen L, Bombardier C. Risk for serious gastrointestinal complications related to use of nonsteroidal anti-inflammatory drugs: a meta-analysis. Ann Intern Med 1991;115:787.
28. Jenkins RT, Rooney PJ, Jones DB, et al. Increased intestinal permeability in patients with rheumatoid arthritis: a side-effect of oral non-steroidal anti-inflammatory drug therapy? Br J Rheumatol 1987;26:103.
29. Bjarnason I, Zanelli G, Prouse P, et al. Effect of non-steroidal anti-inflammatory drugs on the human small intestine. Drugs 1986;32(Suppl 1):35.
30. Banerjee AK, Peters TJ. Experimental non-steroidal anti-inflammatory drug-induced enteropathy in the rat: similarities to inflammatory bowel disease and effect of thromboxane synthetase inhibitors. Gut 1990;31:1358.
31. Bjarnason I, Fehilly B, Smethhurst P, et al. Importance of local versus systemic effects of non-steroidal anti-inflammatory drugs in increasing small intestinal permeability in man. Gut 1991;32:275.
32. Davies GR, Rampton DS. The pro-drug sulindac may reduce the risk of intestinal damage associated with the use of conventional non-steroidal anti-inflammatory drugs. Aliment Pharmacol Ther 1991;5:593.
33. Bjarnason I, Smethurst P, Macpherson A, et al. Glucose and citrate reduce the permeability changes caused by indomethacin in humans. Gastroenterology 1992;102:1546.
34. Bjarnason I, Hayllar J, Macpherson AJ, Russell AS. Side effects

of nonsteroidal anti-inflammatory drugs on the small and large intestine in humans. Gastroenterology 1993;104:1832.

35. Erickson RA. NSAIDs and the small intestine: is there any cause for concern? Pract Gastroenterol 1991;105:39.

36. Levi S, de Lacey G, Price AB, et al. "Diaphragm-like" strictures of the small bowel in patients treated with non-steroidal anti-inflammatory drugs. Br J Radiol 1990;63:186.

37. Matsuhashi N, Yamada A, Hiraishi M, et al. Multiple strictures of the small intestine after long-term nonsteroidal anti-inflammatory drug therapy. Am J Gastroenterol 1992;87:1183.

38. Hershfield NB. Endoscopic demonstration of non-steroidal anti-inflammatory drug-induced small intestinal strictures. Gastrointest Endosc 1992;38:388.

39. Tanner AR, Raghunat H. Colonic inflammation and NSAID administration. Digestion 1988;41:116.

40. Del Favero A. Anti-inflammatory drugs used in rheumatoid arthritis and gout. In: Dukes MNG, Aronson JK, eds. Side effects of drugs annual 15: a worldwide yearly survey of new data and trends. Amsterdam: Elsevier, 1991:92.

41. Rampton DS, Sladen GE. Relapse of ulcerative proctocolitis during treatment with NSAID. Postgrad Med J 1981;57:297.

42. Kaufman HJ, Taubin HL. Nonsteroidal anti-inflammatory drugs activate quiescent inflammatory bowel disease. Ann Intern Med 1987;107:513.

43. Giardiello FM, Hansen FC III, Lazenby AJ, et al. Collagenous colitis in setting of nonsteroidal antiinflammatory drugs and antibiotics. Dig Dis Sci 1990;35:257.

44. Batt M. Non-coeliac flat jejunal mucosa. Gut 1989;30:67.

45. Cooper BT, Holmes GKT, Cooke WT. Celiac disease and malignancy. Medicine (Baltimore) 1980;59:249.

46. Brune K, Dietzel K, Nuernberg B, et al. Recent insight into the mechanism of gastrointestinal tract ulceration. Scand J Rheumatol Suppl 1987;65:135.

47. Beck WS, Schneider HT, Dietzel K, et al. Gastrointestinal ulcerations induced by anti-inflammatory drugs in rats. Arch Toxicol 1990;64:210.

48. Soehngen EC, Godin-Ostro E, Fielder FG, et al. Encapsulation of indomethacin in liposomes provides protection against both gastric and intestinal ulceration when orally administered to rats. Arthritis Rheum 1988;31:414.

49. Brune K, Nuernberg B, Szelenyi I, et al. The enterohepatic circulation of some anti-inflammatory drugs may cause intestinal ulcerations. In: Rainsford KD, Velo GP, eds. Side-effects of anti-inflammatory drugs. Part 2: Studies in major organ systems. Lancaster, UK: MTP Press, 1987:29.

50. Robert A, Asano T. Resistance of germ free rats to indomethacin-induced intestinal lesions. Prostaglandins 1977;14:331.

51. Kent TH, Cardeli RM, Stanler FU. Small intestinal ulcers and intestinal flora in rats given indomethacin. Am J Pathol 1969;54:237.

52. Bjarnason I, Hopkinson N, Zanelli G, et al. Treatment of nonsteroidal anti-inflammatory drug induced enteropathy. Gut 1990;31:777.

53. Waisman Y, Zahavi I, Marcus H, et al. Sucralfate is protective against indomethacin-induced intestinal ulceration in the rat. Digestion 1988;41:78.

54. Harel L, Zahavi I, Marcus H, et al. Pentagastrin protects the proximal small intestine against indomethacin-induced ulcers in the rat. Digestion 1987;38:156.

55. Waisman Y, Marcus H, Ligumski M, et al. Modulation by opiates of small intestinal prostaglandin E2 and 3′, 5′ cyclic adenosine monophosphate levels and of indomethacin-induced ulceration in the rat. Life Sci 1991;48:2035.

56. Kiro A, Zahavi I, Marcus H, et al. L-dopa is protective against indomethacin-induced small intestinal ulceration in the rat: possible role of an α-2-adrenergic mechanism. Life Sci 1992;51:1151.

57. Whiting PH, Burke MD, Thomson AW. Drug interactions with cyclosporine: implications from animal studies. Transplant Proc 1986;11(Suppl 5):56.

58. Graham DY, Agarwal N, Roth SH. Prevention of NSAID-induced gastric ulcer with the synthetic prostaglandin, misoprostol—a multicenter, double-blind placebo-controlled trial. Lancet 1988;2:1277.

59. Graham DY. Prevention of gastroduodenal injury induced by chronic nonsteroidal antiinflammatory drug therapy. Gastroenterology 1989;96:675.

60. Graham DY, White RH, Moreland LW, et al. Duodenal and gastric ulcer prevention with misoprostol in arthritis patients taking NSAIDs. Misoprostol Study Group. Ann Intern Med 1993;119:257.

61. Sontag SJ, Schnell JG, Mak E, et al. Enprostil heals NSAID induced gastric ulcers. Gastroenterology 1990;98:A129.

62. Jaszewski R, Graham DY, Stromatt SC. Treatment of nonsteroidal antiinflammatory drug-induced gastric ulcers with misoprostol. A double-blind multicenter study. Dig Dis Sci 1992;37:1820.

63. Tabata K, Okabe S. Effects of 16,16-dimethyl-PEG2-methyl ester on aspirin- and indomethacin-induced gastric and intestinal lesions in mini pigs. Digestion 1983;26:61.

64. Romain N, Dandrifosse G, Forget P, Lepoint A. Effect of prostaglandin E2 on the small intestine of indomethacin-treated rats. Life Sci 1987;41:1199.

65. Robert A. An intestinal disease produced experimentally by prostaglandin deficiency. Gastroenterology 1975;69:1045.

66. Bjarnason I, Zanelli G, Smith T, et al. The pathogenesis and consequence of non-steroidal anti-inflammatory drug induced small intestinal inflammation in man. Scand J Rheumatol (Suppl) 1987;64:55.

67. Leijonmarck CE, Raf L. Ulceration of the small intestine due to slow-release potassium chloride tablets. Acta Chir Scand 1985;151:273.

68. Graham DY. Effectiveness and tolerance of solid vs. liquid potassium replacement therapy. In: Whelton PK, Whelton A, eds. Potassium in cardiovascular and renal medicine. New York: Marcel Dekker, 1987:435.

69. Venho, VMK. Toxicants in the gastrointestinal tract: drugs. In: Rozman K, Hanninen O, eds. Gastrointestinal toxicology. Amsterdam: Elsevier, 1986:363.

70. Remine SG, McIlrath DC. Bowel perforation in steroid-treated patients. Ann Surg 1980;192:581.

71. Stentoft J. The toxicity of cytarabine. Drug Saf 1990;5:7.

72. Ferrer MI, Bradley SE, Wheeler HO, et al. Effect of digoxin in splanchnic circulation in ventricular failure. Circulation 1965;32:524.

73. Baba S, Maruta M, Ando K, et al. Intestinal Behçet's disease: report of 5 cases. Dis Colon Rectum 1976;19:428.

74. Sayek I, Aran O, Uzunaliamoglu B, et al. Intestinal Behçet's disease: surgical experience in seven cases. Hepatogastroenterology 1991;38:81.

75. Whitehead R. The alimentary tract in systemic disease and miscellaneous lesions. In: Whitehead R, ed Gastrointestinal and oesophageal pathology. New York: Churchill Livingstone, 1989:827.

76. Kashara Y, Tanaka S, Nishino M, et al. Intestinal involvement in Behçet's disease. Dis Colon Rectum 1981;24:103.

77. Sasamura H, Nakamoto H, Ryuzaki M, et al. Repeated intestinal ulcerations in a patient with systemic lupus erythematosus and high serum antiphospholipid antibody levels. South Med J 1991;84:515.

78. Isaacson P, Wright DH. Malignant histiocytosis of the intestine: its relationship to malabsorption and ulcerative jejunitis. Hum Pathol 1978;9:661.

79. Isaacson P. Malignant histiocytosis of the intestine: the early histological lesion. Gut 1980;21:381.

80. MacDonald TT, Spencer J. Evidence that activated mucosal T cells play a role in the pathogenesis of enteropathy in human small intestine. J Exp Med 1988;167:1341.

81. Klaeveman HL, Gebhard RL, Sessoms C, et al. In vitro studies of ulcerative ileojejunitis. Gastroenterology 1975;68:572.

82. Mills PR, Brown IL, Watkinson G. Idiopathic chronic ulcerative enteritis. Q J Med 1980;49:133.

83. Robertson DAF, Dixon MF, Scott BB, et al. Small intestinal ulceration: diagnostic difficulties in relation to coeliac disease. Gut 1983;24:565.

84. Fairley NH, Mackie FP. A clinical and biochemical syndrome in lymphadenoma and allied diseases involving the mesenteric lymph glands. Br Med J 1937;1:375.

85. Harris OD, Cooke WT, Thompson H, et al. Malignancy in adult coeliac disease and idiopathic steatorrhoea. Am J Med 1967;42:899.

86. Austad WI, Cornes JS, Gough KR, et al. Steatorrhoea and malignant lymphoma. Am J Dig Dis 1983;12:475.

87. Cooper BT, Holmes GKT, Cooke WT. Lymphoma risk in coeliac disease of later life. Digestion 1982;23:89.

88. Haagen Nielsen O, Jacobsen O, Rask Pedersen E, et al. Non-tropical sprue. Malignant diseases and mortality rate. Scand J Gastroenterol 1985;20:13.

89. Logan RF, Rifkind EA, Turner IA, et al. Mortality in celiac disease. Gastroenterology 1989;97:265.

90. Holmes GKT, Prior R, Lane MR, et al. Malignancy in coeliac disease—effect of a gluten free diet. Gut 1989;30:333.

91. Isaacson PG, Spencer J, Connolly CE, et al. Malignant histiocytosis of the intestine: a T-cell lymphoma. Lancet 1985;2:688.

92. Salter DM, Krajewski AS, Dewar AE. Immunophenotype analysis of malignant histiocytosis of the intestine. J Clin Pathol 1986;39:8.

93. Spencer J, Cerf-Bensussan N, Jarry A, et al. Enteropathy-associated T cell lymphoma (malignant histiocytosis of the intestine) is recognized by a monoclonal antibody (HML-1) that defines a membrane molecule on human mucosal lymphocytes. Am J Pathol 1988;132:1.

94. Jeffries GH, Steinberg H, Sleisenger MH. Chronic ulcerative (nongranulomatous) jejunitis. Am J Med 1968;44:47.

95. Gilinsky NH, Mee AS, Beatty DW, et al. Plasma cell infiltration of the small bowel: lack of evidence for a non-secretory form of alpha heavy chain disease. Gut 1985;26:928.

96. McDonald GB, Schuffler MD, Kadin ME, et al. Intestinal pseudolymphoma caused by diffuse lymphoid infiltration of the small intestine. Gastroenterology 1985;89:882.

97. Smith W, Price SK, Isaacson PG. Immunoglobulin gene rearrangement in immunoproliferative small intestinal disease (IPSID). J Clin Pathol 1987;40:1291.

98. Matuchansky C, Cogne M, Lemaire M, et al. Nonsecretory alpha-chain disease with immunoproliferative small-intestinal disease. N Engl J Med 1989;320:1534.

99. Roehrkasse RL, Roberts IM, Wald A, et al. Celiac sprue complicated by lymphoma presenting with multiple gastric ulcers. Gastroenterology 1986;91:740.

100. Loughran TP, Marshall E, Kadin E, et al. T-cell lymphoma associated with celiac sprue. Ann Intern Med 1986;104:44.

101. Gough KR, Read AE, Naish JM. Intestinal reticulosis as a complication of idiopathic steatorrhoea. Gut 1962;3:232.

102. Lamont CM, Adams FG, Mills PR. Radiology in idiopathic chronic ulcerative enteritis. Clin Radiol 1982;33:283.

103. Brunton F, Guyer PB. Malignant histiocytosis and ulcerative jejunitis of the small intestine. Clin Radiol 1983;34:291.

104. Freeman M, Cho S-R. Nongranulomatous ulcerative jejunoileitis. Am J Gastroenterol 1984;79:446.

105. Swinson CM, Coles EC, Slavin G, et al. Coeliac disease and malignancy. Lancet 1983;1:111.

106. Sussman NL, Sutton FM Jr. Miscellaneous diseases of the small intestine. In: Yamada T, ed. Textbook of gastroenterology. Philadelphia: JB Lippincott, 1991:1555.

107. Young JP. Abdominal catastrophes. Emerg Med Clin North Am 1989;7:699.

108. Federle MP, Chun G, Jeffrey RB, et al. Computed tomography findings in bowel infarction. Am J Radiol 1984;142:91.

109. Clavien PA, Huber O, Mirescy D, et al. Contrast enhances CT scan as a diagnostic procedure in mesenteric ischaemia due to mesenteric venous thrombosis. Br J Surg 1989;76:93.

110. Lewis JH. Gastrointestinal injury due to medicinal agents. Am J Gastroenterol 1986;81:819.

111. Sachs SM, Morton JH, Schwartz SI. Acute mesenteric ischemia. Surgery 1982;92:646.

112. Bowerman RE, Steinmetz EF, Schwarten D, et al. Reversal of digitalis-induced mesenteric vasospasm by sodium nitroprusside. Ann Intern Med 1982;142:403.

113. Goglin WK, Elliott BM, Deppe SA. Nifedipine-induced hypotension and mesenteric ischemia. South Med J 1989;82:274.

114. Mueller PD, Benowitz NL. Toxicologic causes of acute abdominal disorders. Emerg Med Clin North Am 1989;7:667.

115. Kirkeby OJ, Rise C. Intestinal ischemia after a single intravenous injection of deslanoside. Acta Chir Scand 1984;150:91.

116. Young GP. Calcium channel blockers in emergency medicine. Ann Emerg Med 1984;13:712.

117. Hall WC, Talbert RL, Ereshefsky L. Cocaine abuse and its treatment. Pharmacotherapy 1990;10:47.

118. Young SL, Vosper HJ, Phillips SA. Cocaine: its effects on maternal and child health. Pharmacotherapy 1992;12:2.

119. VanDette JM, Cornish LA. Medical complications of illicit cocaine use. Clin Pharm 1989;8:401.

120. Hon DC, Salloum LJ, Hardy III HW, Barone JE. Crack-induced enteric ischemia. N J Med 1990;87:1001.

121. Garfia A, Valverde JL, Borondo JC, et al. Vascular lesions in intestinal ischemia induced by cocaine-alcohol abuse: report of a fatal case due to overdose. J Forensic Sci 1990;35:740.

122. Caruana DS, Weinbach B, Goerg JD, et al. Cocaine-packet ingestion—diagnosis, management and natural history. Ann Intern Med 1984;100:73.

123. Suarez CA, Arango A, Lester JL. Cocaine-condom ingestion. JAMA 1977;238:1391.

124. Introna F Jr, Smialek JF. The "mini-packer" syndrome. Fatal ingestion of drug containers in Baltimore, Maryland. Am J Forensic Med Pathol 1989;10:21.

125. Beerman R, Nunez D, Wetli CV. Radiographic evaluation of the cocaine smuggler. Gastrointest Radiol 1986;11:351.

126. Schulman EA, Silberstein SD. Symptomatic and prophylactic treatment of migraine and tension-type headache. Neurology 1992;42:16.

127. Merhoff GC, Porter JM. Ergot intoxication: historical review and description of unusual clinical manifestations. Ann Surg 1974;180:773.

128. Rogers DA, Mansberger JA. Gastrointestinal vascular ischemia caused by ergotamine. South Med J 1989;82:1058.

129. Goldstein J. Ergot pharmacology and alternative delivery systems for ergotamine derivatives. Neurology 1992;42:45.

130. Rogers AI, Vloedman DA, Bloom EC, et al. Neomycin-induced steatorrhoea. JAMA 1966;197:185.

131. Brennan MF, Clarke AM, Macbeth AAG. Infarction of the midgut associated with oral contraceptives. N Engl J Med 1968;279:1213.

132. Nothmann BJ, Chittinand S, Schuster MM. Reversible mesenteric vascular occlusion associated with oral contraceptives. Am J Dig Dis 1973;18:361.

133. Lamy AL, Roy PH, Morissette JJ, et al. Intimal hyperplasia and thrombosis of the visceral arteries in a young woman: possible relation with oral contraceptives and smoking. Surgery 1988;103:706.

134. Schneiderman D, Cello JP. Intestinal ischemia and infarction associated with oral contraceptives. West J Med 1986;145:350.

135. Greig JD. Oral contraceptives and intestinal ischemia. J R Coll Gen Pract 1989;39:76.

136. Maung R, Kelly JK, Schneider MP, et al. Mesenteric venous thrombosis due to antithrombin III deficiency. Arch Pathol Lab Med 1988;112:37.

137. Naraynsingh V, Raju GC, Busby G. Mesenteric venous thrombosis and oral contraceptive use. Trop Geogr Med 1985;37:192.

138. Graubard ZG, Friedman M. Mesenteric venous thrombosis associated with pregnancy and oral contraception. S Afr Med J 1987;71:453.

139. Haramburu F. Hormonal contraceptives In: Dukes MNG, ed. Meyler's side effects of drugs: an encyclopedia of adverse reactions and interactions, 12th ed. Amsterdam: Elsevier, 1992:995.

140. Kay CR. Progestogens and arterial disease—evidence from the Royal College of General Practitioners' study. Am J Obstet Gynecol 1982;142:762.

141. Porter JB, Hunter JR, Danielson S, et al. Oral contraceptives and nonfatal vascular disease—recent experience. Obstet Gynecol 1982;59:299.

142. Gelfaud MD. Ischemic colitis associated with a depot synthetic progesterone. Am J Dig Dis 1972;17:275.

143. Jick H, Porter J. Unwanted effects of drugs. Drug-induced gastrointestinal bleeding. Lancet 1978;2:87.

144. Wiot JF, Weinstein AS, Felson B. Duodenal hematoma induced by coumarin. AJR Am J Roentgenol 1961;86:70.
145. Eiland M, Han SY, Hicks GM. Intramural hemorrhage of the small intestine. JAMA 1978;239:139.
146. Freeark RJ, Corley RD, Norcross WJ, et al. Intramural hematoma of the duodenum. Arch Surg 1966;92:463.
147. Jaffin BW, Bliss CM, Lamont JT. Significance of occult gastrointestinal bleeding during anticoagulation therapy. Am J Med 1987;83:269.
148. Gurwitz JH, Goldberg RJ, Holden A, et al. Age-related risks of long-term oral anticoagulant therapy. Arch Intern Med 1988;148:1733.
149. Hughes CE, Conn J Jr, Sherman JO. Intramural hematoma of the gastrointestinal tract. Am J Surg 1977;133:276.
150. Birns MT, Katon RM, Keller F. Intramural hematoma of the small intestine presenting with major upper gastrointestinal hemorrhage. Gastroenterology 1979;77:1094.
151. Cocks JR. Anticoagulants and the acute abdomen. Med J Aust 1970;1:1138.
152. Chau WK, Na AT, Loh IW, et al. Real-time ultrasound diagnosis of intramural intestinal hematoma. J Clin Ultrasound 1989;17:392.
153. Mannes, P, Derriks R, Moens R, et al. Multidisciplinary curative treatment for disseminated carcinoma of the breast. Cancer Treat Rep 1976;60:85.
154. Cerda JJ. The narcotic bowel syndrome (editorial). J Clin Gastroenterol 1989;11:132.
155. Sandgren JE, McPhee MS, Greenberger NJ. Narcotic bowel syndrome treated with clonidine—resolution of abdominal pain and intestinal pseudo-obstruction. Ann Intern Med 1984;101:331.
156. Bruera E, Brenneis C, Michaud M, et al. Continuous subcutaneous infusion of metoclopramide for treatment of narcotic bowel syndrome. Cancer Treat Rep 1987;71:1211.
157. Roe DA. Drug effects on nutrient absorption, transport, and metabolism. Drug-Nutrient Interactions 1985;4:117.
158. Read NW. Speculations on the role of motility in the pathogenesis and treatment of diarrhea. Scand J Gastroenterol 1983;18:45.
159. Race TR, Paes IC, Faloon WW. Intestinal malabsorption induced by oral colchicine: comparison with neomycin and cathartic agents. Am J Med Sci 1970;259:32.
160. Dobbins WO, Herrero BA, Mansback CM. Morphologic alterations associated with neomycin-induced malabsorption. Am J Med Sci 1968;255:63.
161. Reiner E, Patterson M. The effect of neomycin on disaccharidase activity of the small bowel. Clin Res 1966;14:49.
162. Schneerson JM, Gazzard BG. Reversible malabsorption syndrome caused by methyldopa. Br Med J 1977;2:1456.
163. Chen B, Shapira J, Ravid M, et al. Steatorrhoea induced by allopurinol. Br Med J 1982;284:1914.
164. Palva IP, Heinivaara O, Mattila M. Drug-induced malabsorption of vitamin B_{12}: 3. Interference of PAS and folic acid in the absorption of vitamin B_{12}. Scand J Haematol 1966;3:149.
165. Riddell RH. The gastrointestinal tract. In: Riddell RH, ed. Pathology of drug induced and toxic disease. New York: Churchill Livingstone, 1982:515.
166. Slavin RE, Dias MA, Saral R. Cytosine, arabanoside-induced gastrointestinal toxic alterations in sequential chemotherapeutic protocols—a clinical, pathological study of 33 patients. Cancer 1978;42:1747.
167. Hertzberg J. Jejunitis acuta. Acta Chir Scand (Suppl) 1954;194:150.
168. Murrell TGC, Roth L, Egerton J. Pig-bel: enteritis necroticans. A study in diagnosis and management. Lancet 1966;1:217.
169. Davis MW. A review of pigbel (necrotising enteritis) in Papua New Guinea, 1961–1984. P N G Med J 1985;28:75.
170. Murrell TG, Walker PD. The pigbel story of Papua New Guinea. Trans R Soc Trop Med Hyg 1991;85:119.
171. Johnson S, Echeverria P, Taylor DN, et al. Enteritis necroticans among Khmer children at an evacuation site in Thailand. Lancet 1987;2:496.
172. Lawrence GW, Lehmann D, Anian G, et al. Impact of active immunisation against enteritis necroticans in Papua New Guinea. Lancet 1990;336:1165.
173. Zeissler J, Rassfeld-Sternberg L. Enteritis necroticans due to Clostridium welchii type F. Br Med J 1949;1:267.
174. Oakley CL. The toxins of Cl. welchii type F. Br Med J 1949;1:269.
175. Hain E. Origin of Cl. welchii type F infection. Br Med J 1949;1:271.
176. Hain E. On the occurrence of Cl. welchii type F in normal stool. Br Med J 1949;1:271.
177. Field HI, Goodwin REW. The experimental reproduction of enterotoxemia in piglets. J Hyg 1959;57:81.
178. Bullen JJ, Scarisbrick R. Enterotoxemia of sheep: experimental reproduction of the disease. J Pathol Bacteriol 1957;73:495.
179. Van Loon FP, Van Schaik S, Banik AK, et al. Clostridium perfringens type C in bloody and watery diarrhea in Bangladesh. Trop Geogr Med 1990;42:123.
180. Kliegman RM, Walsh MC. Neonatal necrotizing enterocolitis: pathogenesis, classification and spectrum of disease. Curr Probl Pediatr 1987;17:213.
181. Kliegman RM. Neonatal necrotizing enterocolitis. In: Wyllie R, Hyams JS, eds. Pediatric gastrointestinal disease: pathophysiology, diagnosis, management. Philadelphia, WB Saunders, 1993:788.
182. Israel EJ. Necrotizing enterocolitis. In: Walker WA, Durie PR, Hamilton JR, et al., eds. Pediatric gastrointestinal disease. Philadelphia: BC Decker, 1991:639.
183. Kosloske AM. A unifying hypothesis for pathogenesis and prevention of necrotizing enterocolitis. J Pediatr 1990;117:S68.
184. De Lemos RA, Rogers JH, McLaughlin GW. Experimental production of necrotizing enterocolitis in newborn goats. Pediatr Res 1974;8:380.
185. Book LS, Herbst J, Atherton SO, et al. Necrotizing enterocolitis in low-birth-weight infants fed an elemental formula. J Pediatr 1975;87:602.
186. Willis DM, Chabot J, Radde I, et al. Unsuspected hyperosmolality of oral solutions contributing to necrotizing enterocolitis. Pediatrics 1977;60:535.
187. Barlow B, Santulli TV. Importance of multiple episodes of hypoxia or cold stress on the development of enterocolitis in an animal model. Surgery 1975;77:687.
188. Szabo JS, Mayfield SR, Oh W, et al. Postprandial gastrointestinal blood flow and oxygen consumption: effects of hypoxemia in neonatal piglets. Pediatr Res 1987;21:93.
189. Nowicki PT, Miller CE. Autoregulation in the developing postnatal intestinal circulation. Am J Physiol 1988;254:G189.
190. Nowicki PT, Miller CE, Haun SE. Effects of arterial hypoxia and isoproterenol on in vitro postnatal intestinal circulation. Am J Physiol 1988;255:H1144.
191. Nowicki P. Intestinal ischemia and necrotizing enterocolitis. J Pediatr 1990;117:S14.
192. Kleinman PK, Winchester P, Brill PW. Necrotizing enterocolitis after open heart surgery employing hypothermia and cardiopulmonary bypass. AJR Am J Roentgenol 1976;127:757.
193. Silane MF, Symchych PS. Necrotizing enterocolitis after cardiac surgery: a local ischemic lesion? Am J Surg 1977;133:373.
194. Orme RLE, Eader SM. Perforation of the bowel in the newborn as a complication of exchange transfusion. Br Med J 1968;4:349.
195. Lucy JF. Colonic perforation after exchange transfusion. N Engl J Med 1969;280:724.
196. Lehmiller DJ, Kanto WP. Relationship of mesenteric thromboembolism, oral feeding, and necrotizing enterocolitis. J Pediatr 1978;92:96.
197. Nagaraj HS, Sandhu AS, Cook LN, et al. Gastrointestinal perforation following indomethacin therapy in very low birthweight infants. J Pediatr Surg 1981;16:1003.
198. Morgard M, Nylander G, Enochsson L. Effect of hyperosmotic feeding and indomethacin upon the gastrointestinal regional blood flow of the rat. Surg Gynecol Obstet 1982;154:841.
199. Crissinger KD, Granger DN. Characterization of intestinal collateral blood flow in the developing piglet. Pediatr Res 1988;24:473.
200. Crissinger KD, Granger DN. Mucosal injury induced by isch-

emia and reperfusion in the piglet intestine: influences of age and feeding. Gastroenterology 1989;97:920.

201. Telsey AM, Merrit TA, Dixon SD. Cocaine exposure in a term neonate, necrotizing enterocolitis as a complication. Clin Pediatr (Phila) 1988;27:547.

202. Hoyme HE, Jones K, Dixon SD, et al. Prenatal cocaine exposure and fetal vascular disruption. Pediatrics 1990;85:743.

203. Czyrko C, Del Pin CA, O'Neill JA Jr, et al. Maternal cocaine abuse and necrotizing enterocolitis: outcome and survival. J Pediatr Surg 1991;26:414.

204. Sehgal S, Ewing C, Waring P, et al. Morbidity of low-birthweight infants with intrauterine cocaine exposure. J Natl Med Assoc 1993;85:20

205. Musemeche CA, Kosloske AM, Bartow SA, et al. Comparative effects of ischemia, bacteria, and substrate on the pathogenesis of intestinal necrosis. J Pediatr Surg 1986;21:536.

206. Caplan MS, Hsueh W. Necrotizing enterocolitis: role of platelet activating factor, endotoxin, and tumor necrosis factor. J Pediatr 1990;117:S47.

207. Kliegman RM, Fanaroff AA. Necrotizing enterocolitis. N Engl J Med 1984;310:1093.

208. Palmer S, Biffen A, Gamsu H. Outcome of neonatal necrotizing enterocolitis: results of the BAPM/CDSC surveillance study 1981–84. Arch Dis Child 1989;64:388.

209. Kliegman RM. Models of the pathogenesis of necrotizing enterocolitis. J Pediatr 1990;117:S2.

210. Gerber AR, Hopkins RS, Lauer BA, et al. Increased risk of illness among nursery staff caring for neonates with necrotizing enterocolitis. Pediatr Infect Dis J 1985;4:246.

211. Kliegman RM. Neonatal necrotizing enterocolitis: bridging the basic science with the clinical disease. J Pediatr 1990;117:833.

212. Hoy C, Millar MR, MacKay P, et al. Quantitative changes in faecal microflora preceding necrotizing enterocolitis in premature neonates. Arch Dis Child 1990;65:1057.

213. Eibl MM, Wolf HM, Furnkranz H, et al. Prevention of necrotizing enterocolitis in low-birth-weight infants by IgA-IgG feeding. N Engl J Med 1988;319:1.

214. Spritzer R, Koolen AMP, Baerts W, et al. A prolonged decline in the incidence of necrotizing enterocolitis after the introduction of a cautious feeding regimen. Acta Paediatr Scand 1988;77:909.

215. Zabielski PB, Groh-Wargp SL, Moore JJ. Necrotizing enterocolitis: feeding in endemic and epidemic periods. J Parenter Enter Nutr 1989;13:520.

216. Anderson DM, Kliegman RM. The relationship of neonatal alimentation practices to the occurrence of endemic necrotizing enterocolitis. Am J Perinatol 1991;8:62

217. McKeown RE, Marsh D, Amarnath U, et al. Role of delayed feeding and of feeding increments in necrotizing enterocolitis. J Pediatr 1992;121:764.

218. Engel RR, Virnig NL, Hunt CE, et al. Origin of mural gas in necrotizing enterocolitis. Pediatr Res 1973;7:292.

219. Citrin Y, Sterling K, Halsted JA. Mechanism of hypoproteinemia associated with giant hypertrophy of gastric mucosa. N Engl J Med 1957;257:906.

220. Jeffries GH, Holman HR, Sleisenger MH. Plasma proteins and the gastrointestinal tract. N Engl J Med 1962;266:652.

221. Waldmann TA, Wochner RD, Strober W. The role of the gastrointestinal tract in plasma protein metabolism. Studies with ^{51}Cr-albumin. Am J Med 1986;46:275.

222. Gitlin D, Klinenberg JR, Hughes WL. Site of catabolism of serum albumin. Nature 1958;181:1064.

223. Jeejeebhoy KN, Jarnum S, Singh B, et al. ^{95}Nb-labelled albumin for the study of gastrointestinal albumin loss. Scand J Gastroenterol 1968;3:449.

224. Katz J, Rosenfeld S, Sellers AL. Sites of plasma albumin catabolism in the rat. Am J Physiol 1961;200:1301.

225. Van Tongeren JHM, Reichert WJ. Demonstration of protein-losing gastro-enteropathy: the quantitative estimation of gastrointestinal protein loss, using ^{51}Cr-labelled plasma proteins. Clin Chim Acta 1966;14:42.

226. Waldmann TA, Wochner RD, Strober W. The role of the gastrointestinal tract in plasma protein metabolism. Studies with ^{51}Cr-albumin. Am J Med 1969;46:275.

227. Wochner, RD, Weissman, SM, Waldman, TA, et al. Direct measurement of the rates of synthesis of plasma proteins in control subjects and patients with gastrointestinal protein loss. J Clin Invest 1968;47:3

228. Steinfeld JL, Davidson JD, Gordon RS, et al. Mechanism of hypoproteinemia in patients with regional enteritis and ulcerative colitis. Am J Med 1960;29:405.

229. Beeken WL, Busch HJ, Sylwester DL. Intestinal protein loss in Crohn's disease. Gastroenterology 1972;62:207.

230. Overholt BF, Jeffries GH. Hypertrophic, hypersecretory protein losing gastropathy. Gastroenterology 1979;58:80.

231. Waldmann TA, Wochner RD, Laster L, et al. Allergic gastroenteropathy. A cause of excessive gastrointestinal protein loss. N Engl J Med 1967;276:761.

232. Klein NC, Hargrove RL, Sleisenger MH, et al. Eosinophilic gastroenteritis. Medicine (Baltimore) 1970;49:299.

233. Gordon RS. Protein-losing enteropathy in the sprue syndrome. Lancet 1961;1:55.

234. Rubini ME, Sheehy TW, Meroney WH, et al. Exudative enteropathy II. Observations in tropical sprue. J Lab Clin Med 1961;58:902.

235. Stark ME, Batts KP, Alexander GL. Protein-losing enteropathy with collagenous colitis. Am J Gastroenterol 1992;87:780.

236. Meuwissen SG, Ridwan BU, Hasper HJ, et al. Hypertrophic protein-losing gastropathy. A retrospective analysis of 40 cases in The Netherlands. The Dutch Menetrier Study Group. Scand J Gastroenterol Suppl 1992;194:1.

237. Bennish ML, Salem MA, Wahed MA. Enteric protein loss during shigellosis. Am J Gastroenterol 1993;88:53.

238. King CE, Toskes PP. Protein-losing enteropathy in the human and experimental rat blind loop syndrome. Gastroenterology 1981;80:504.

239. Cooperstock M, Riegle L, Fabacher D, et al. Relationship between fecal α_1-antitrypsin and colonization with *Clostridium difficile* in asymptomatic infants. J Pediatr 1985;107:257.

240. Rybolt AH, Bennett RG, Laughon BE, et al. Protein-losing enteropathy associated with *Clostridium difficile* infection. Lancet 1989;1:1353.

241. Sullivan PB, Lunn, PG, Northrop-Clewes CA, et al. Parasitic infection of the gut and protein-losing enteropathy. J Pediatr Gastroenterol Nutr 1992;15:404.

242. Kiire CF, Gwavava N. Protein losing enteropathy: an unusual presentation of intestinal schistosomiasis. Gut 1987;28:616.

243. El Aggan HA, Marzouk S. Fecal alpha-1-antitrypsin concentration in patients with schistosomal hepatic fibrosis. J Egypt Soc Parasitol 1992;22:195.

244. Sherman P, Liebman WM. Apparent protein-losing enteropathy associated with giardiasis. Am J Dis Child 1980;134:893.

245. Sutton DL, Kamath KR. Giardiasis with protein-losing enteropathy. J Pediatr Gastroenterol Nutr 1985;4:56.

246. Korman SH, Bar-Oz B, Mandelberg A, et al. Giardiasis with protein-losing enteropathy: diagnosis by fecal alpha-1-antitrypsin determination. J Pediatr Gastroenterol Nutr 1990;10:249.

247. Schreiber DS, Blacklow NR, Trier JS. The mucosal lesion of the proximal small intestine in acute infectious nonbacterial gastroenteritis. N Engl J Med 1973;288:1318.

248. Dossetor JFB, Whittle HC. Protein-losing enteropathy and malabsorption in acute measles enteritis. Br Med J 1975;2:592.

249. Sarker SA, Wahad MA, Rahaman MM, et al. Persistent protein losing enteropathy in post measles diarrhoea. Arch Dis Child 1986;61:739.

250. Wood ML, Foulds IS, French MA. Protein losing enteropathy due to systemic lupus erythematosus. Gut 1984;25:1013.

251. Edmunds SE, Ganju V, Beveridge BR, et al. Protein-losing enteropathy in systemic lupus erythematosus. Aust N Z J Med 1988;18:868.

252. Benner KG, Montanaro A. Protein-losing enteropathy in systemic lupus erythematosus. Diagnosis and monitoring immunosuppressive therapy by alpha-1-antitrypsin clearance in the stool. Dig Dis Sci 1989;34:132.

253. Kobayashi K, Asakura H, Yoshida S, et al. Protein-losing enteropathy in systemic lupus erythematosus. Observations by magnifying endoscopy. Dig Dis Sci 1989;34:1924.

254. Perednia DA, Curosh NA. Lupus-associated protein-losing enteropathy. Arch Intern Med 1990;150:1806.
255. Terren P. Protein-losing enteropathy and mixed connective-tissue disease. Med J Aust 1988;149:558.
256. Furuya T, Suzuki T, Onoda N, et al. Mixed connective tissue disease associated with protein losing enteropathy: successful treatment with intravenous cyclophosphamide therapy. Intern Med 1992;31:1359
257. Tsutsumi A, Sugiyama T, Matsumura R, et al. Protein losing enteropathy associated with collagen vascular diseases. Ann Rheum Dis 1991;50:178.
258. Mistilis SP, Skyring AP, Stephen DD. Intestinal lymphangiectasia. Mechanism of enteric loss of plasma protein and fat. Lancet 1965;1:77.
259. Van Tillburg AJ, van Blankenstein M, Verschoor L. Intestinal lymphangiectasia in systemic sclerosis. Am J Gastroenterol 1988;83:1418.
260. Edworthy SM, Fritzler MJ, Kelly JK, et al. Protein-losing enteropathy in systemic lupus erythematosus associated with intestinal lymphangiectasia. Am J Gastroenterol 1990;85:1398.
261. Laster L, Waldmann TA, Fenster LF, et al. Reversible enteric protein loss in Whipple's disease. Gastroenterology 1962;42:762.
262. Southern JF, Moscicki RI, Magro C, et al. Lymphedema, lymphocytic myocarditis and sarcoid-like granulomatosis. Manifestations of Whipple's disease. JAMA 1989;261:1467.
263. Konar A, Brown CB, Hancock BW, Moss S. Protein losing enteropathy as a sole manifestation of non-Hodgkins lymphoma. Postgrad Med 1986;62:399.
264. Wellman W, Luska G, Stender HS, et al. Reduced intestinal protein loss in Crohn's disease after lymphovenous anastomosis. Digestion 1985;32:149.
265. Popovic OS, Brkic S, Bojic P, et al. Sarcoidosis and protein losing enteropathy. Gastroenterology 1980;78:119.
266. Godeau B, Farcet JP, Delchier JC, et al. Protein-losing enteropathy in gastrointestinal sarcoidosis associated with malignant lymphoma. J Clin Gastroenterol 1992;14:78.
267. Davidson JD, Waldmann RA, Goodman DS, et al. Protein-losing enteropathy in congestive heart failure. Lancet 1961;1:899.
268. Wilkinson P, Pinto B, Senior JR. Reversible protein-losing enteropathy with intestinal lymphangiectasia secondary to chronic constrictive pericarditis. N Engl J Med 1965;273:1178.
269. Divgi CR, Lisann NM, Yeh SDJ, et al. Technetium-99m albumin scintigraphy in the diagnosis of protein-losing enteropathy. J Nucl Med 1986;27:1710.
270. Oommen R, Kurien G, Balakrishnan N, et al. Tc-99m albumin scintigraphy in the localization of protein loss in the gut. Clin Nucl Med 1992;17:787.
271. Florent C, L'Hirondel C, Dexmazures C, et al. Intestinal clearance of α_1-antitrypsin. A sensitive method for the detection of protein-losing enteropathy. Gastroenterology 1981;81:777.
272. Strygler B, Nicor MJ, Santangelo WC, et al. α_1-Antitrypsin excretion in stool in normal subjects and in patients with gastrointestinal disorders. Gastroenterology 1990;99:1380.
273. Perrault J, Markowitz H. Protein-losing gastroenteropathy and the intestinal clearance of serum alpha-1-antitrypsin. Mayo Clin Proc 1984;59:7278.
274. Thomas DW, Sinatra FR, Merrit RJ. Random fecal alpha-1-antitrypsin concentration in children with gastrointestinal disease. Gastroenterology 1981;80:776.
275. Thomas DW, Sinatra FR, Merrit RJ. Fecal alpha-1-antitrypsin excretion in young people with Crohn's disease. J Pediatr Gastroenterol Nutr 1983;2:491.
276. Maguzzu G, Jacono G, Di Pasquale G, et al. Reliability and usefulness of random fecal alpha-1-antitrypsin concentration: further simplification of the method. J Pediatr Gastroenterol Nutr 1985;4:402.
277. Jeffries GH, Chapman A, Sleisenger MH. Low-fat diet in intestinal lymphangiectasia: its effect on albumin metabolism. N Engl J Med 1964;270:761.
278. Tift WL, Lloyd JK. Intestinal lymphangiectasia. Long term results with MCT diet. Arch Dis Child 1975;50:269.
279. Mistilis SP, Skyring AP. Intestinal lymphangiectasia. Therapeutic effect of lymph venous anastomosis. Am J Med 1966;40:634.

Textbook of Gastroenterology, second edition, edited by Tadataka Yamada. JB Lippincott Company, Philadelphia © 1995.

D. Colon

CHAPTER 78

Colon: Anatomy and Structural Anomalies

Steven Mark Cohn   Elisa H. Birnbaum

COLONIC DEVELOPMENT

The primitive foregut, midgut, and hindgut develop during the fourth week in utero. The midgut lengthens, herniates out of the abdominal cavity, and rotates 90 degrees counterclockwise around the superior mesenteric artery during the sixth week in utero. By the tenth week, the midgut rotates an additional 180 degrees as it returns to the abdominal cavity. The cecum descends to the right iliac fossa, where it becomes fixed. The base of the small bowel mesentery then runs from the ligament of Treitz in the left upper quadrant to the ileocecal valve in the right lower quadrant.[1,2]

The small intestine distal to the entrance of the common bile duct, cecum, appendix, ascending colon, and proximal transverse colon arise from the midgut and are supplied by the superior mesenteric artery. The distal transverse colon, descending colon, sigmoid colon, rectum, upper portion of the anal canal, and part of the lower urogenital tract are derivatives of the hindgut and are supplied by the inferior mesenteric artery. The lower third of the anal canal is ectodermal in origin and is supplied by branches of the internal pudendal artery.[3]

The cloaca is located at the distal end of the hindgut and by the end of the sixth week is separated by the anorectal septum into a ventral urogenital sinus and a dorsal rectum.[3] The anal membrane covering the cloaca ruptures at the end of the eighth week, forming the anal canal. The dentate line is the approximate location of the transition from endoderm to ectoderm, at the junction of the upper two thirds of the anal canal with the lower one third.

The enteric nervous system forms during early fetal life. Neural crest cells, precursors of ganglion cells, migrate from cephalad to caudad during the first 12 weeks in utero.[4] The migration from the midtransverse colon to the anus takes 4 weeks to complete. Interruption of this migration results in a congenital absence of the myenteric plexus in a distal segment of bowel and is thought to be the cause of Hirschsprung's disease (see section on Structural and Congenital Abnormalities). In vitro studies have suggested that components of the extracellular matrix, including laminin and type IV collagen, promote neuronal outgrowth, migration, and survival. Qualitative differences in laminin and type IV collagen have been found in some patients with Hirschsprung's disease, suggesting a potential role for abnormalities in fetal extracellular matrix components in the pathogenesis of this disease.[5] Smooth muscle cells begin to appear within the mesenchymal layer around the tenth week of gestation. The developing circular muscle layer spreads cranially. The outer longitudinal bands of smooth muscle (taenia coli) and haustra begin to appear between the tenth and eleventh weeks of gestation.[6] By the twelfth week of gestation, Auerbach's and Meissner's plexuses and the circular and longitudinal muscle layers of the colon are well formed, and colonic motility may be observed in isolated fetal colon as early as this developmental stage.[6,7]

In many respects, the development of the colonic epithelium parallels that of the small intestine (Fig. 78-1; see Chap. 68). At 8 to 9 weeks of gestation, the developing colon consists of a pseudostratified columnar epithelium several cell layers deep, with a slit-like lumen surrounded by mesenchymal tissue forming a simple tubular structure.[8-10] Epithelial ridges form between 10 and 11 weeks of gestation, giving the colonic lumen a stellate appearance. Small secondary lumens form at the base of the pseudostratified epithelium and subsequently extend to the primary lumen, resulting in the formation of broad primary villi. Between the thirteenth and fifteenth weeks of gestation, the formation of cyst-like spaces within these primary villi and the accompanying upward growth of mesenchymal tissue result in the division of primary villi into numerous secondary villi. During this developmental stage, epithelial cells near the bases of the primary villi undergo rapid proliferation and bud into the surrounding mesenchyme to form the developing colonic crypts. Numerous goblet cells, columnar epithelial cells with well-developed microvilli, and enteroendocrine cells can be observed in the epithelium by this time.[11,12] The fetal enteroendocrine cell population has been found to secrete a variety of neuroendocrine mediators,

some of which may have important trophic effects on the developing epithelium. The mesenchymal tissue underlying the developing colonic epithelium appears to play a crucial role in the induction of appropriate regional differentiation in the gut epithelium.[13] Prominent supranuclear inclusion bodies can be observed in the principal epithelial cells lining the fetal colon. These inclusion bodies were originally termed meconium corpuscles because it was thought that they arose from uptake of lumenal contents present in the developing colon. However, more recent studies have found that these membrane-bound inclusion bodies are a result of apoptosis, emphasizing the role of programmed cell death in the morphologic restructuring of the epithelium that occurs during fetal life.[14] Colonic villi are present through at least the twenty-ninth week of gestation but are not found in the colon of term infants.[12,15] During fetal life, the colonic epithelium is also similar to the developing small intestine in its biochemical characteristics. For instance, the initial appearance and the activity of many brush border hydrolases found in the fetal colonic epithelium, including sucrase-isomaltase complex and at least five dipeptidases, are similar to those found in the developing small intestine.[8,15-18] However, by term, the activities of these brush border hydrolases have declined to levels similar to those found in the adult colon.

HISTOLOGY

The colonic wall consists of mucosa, submucosa, inner circular muscle, outer longitudinal muscle, and serosa (Fig. 78-2). The colonic mucosa is similar in organization to the small intestine mucosa except that it lacks villi. The mucosa is lined by a simple columnar epithelium that forms straight tubular crypts that are about 0.5 mm in length (Fig. 78-3). The lamina propria extends from the simple columnar epithelium to the muscularis mucosae and contains many cells involved in immunologic functions of the gut (see Chap. 5). Numerous immunoglobulin-secreting plasma cells, macrophages, and lymphocytes are present, in addition to abundant lymphoid nodules which often extend through the muscularis mucosae into the underlying submucosa (Fig. 78-4). Subepithelial fibroblasts surround each crypt and produce the collagen table, and many of the extracellular matrix components that underlie the basal lamina of the epithelium (Fig. 78-5). These fibroblasts and the extracellular matrix that they secrete appear to have an important role in regulating cell proliferation and differentiation events within the overlying epithelium.[19-23] The submucosa contains numerous small veins, arteries, and lymphatic channels surrounded by loose connective tissue. The inner circular muscle fibers form a continuous layer around the colon. The outer longitudinal smooth muscle fibers are condensed into three bands (taenia coli) equidistant around the circumference of the colon. Haustra are the bulging sacculations that form between adjacent taenia coli. The serosa is a mesothelial-derived cell layer that covers the peritoneal surface of the colonic wall. Therefore, regions of the ascending colon, the descending colon, and the rectum that lie outside the peritoneal cavity have no outer serosal layer (see section on Anatomy).

The colonic epithelium undergoes continuous and rapid renewal; epithelial cells are sloughed from the flat lumenal

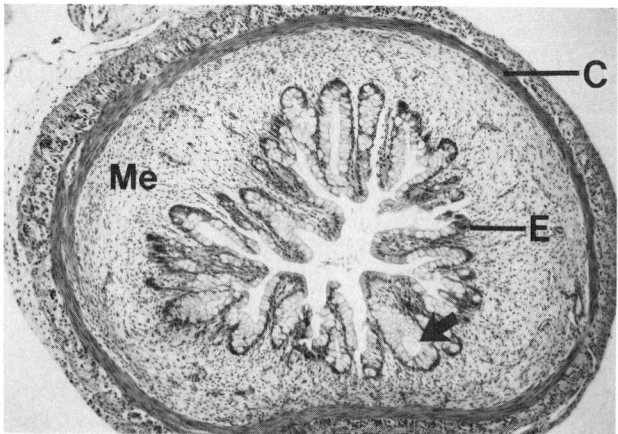

FIGURE 78-1. Human fetal colon at 14 weeks of gestation. Note the villus architecture of the developing epithelium. The circular smooth muscle layer is already well formed. (*Arrowhead,* secondary lumen; E, columnar epithelium; C, circular smooth muscle layer; Me, mesenchymal tissue; paraffin-embedded 4-μm section stained with hematoxylin and eosin; original magnification ×100.)

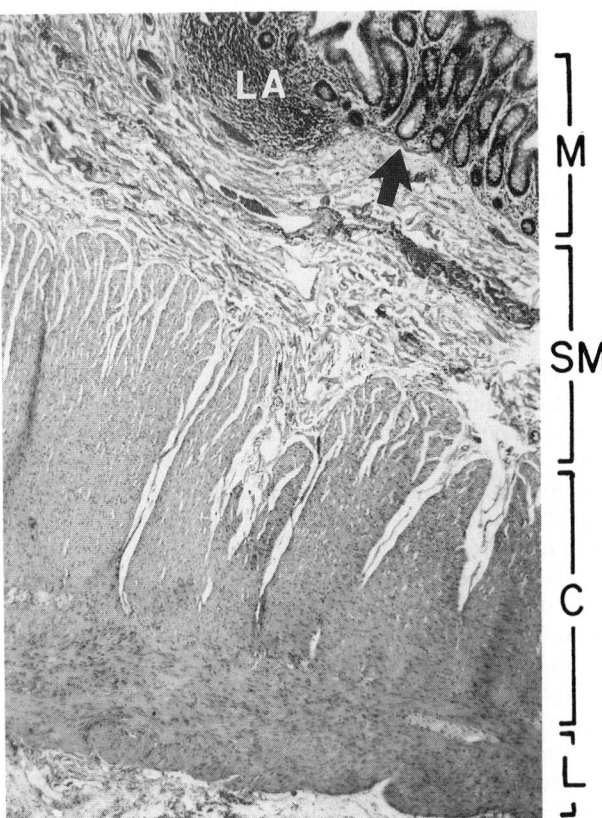

FIGURE 78-2. Anatomy of the colonic wall. The muscularis mucosae is indicated (*arrow*). (C, circular smooth muscle layer; L, longitudinal smooth muscle layer; LA, lymphoid aggregate; M, mucosa; SM, submucosa; paraffin-embedded 4-μm section stained with hematoxylin and eosin; original magnification ×40.)

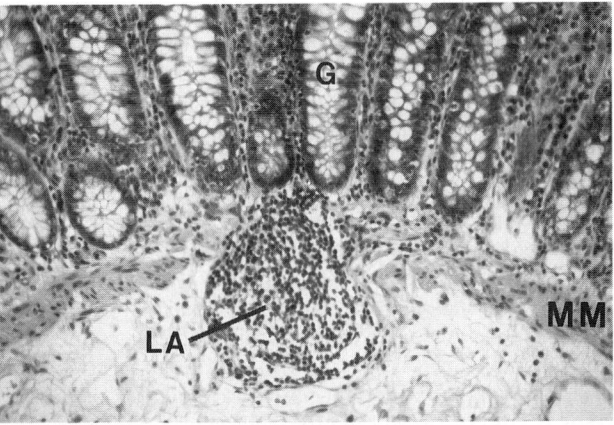

FIGURE 78-4. A lymphoid aggregate arises in the lamina propria and extends through the muscularis into the submucosa. (Paraffin-embedded 4-μm section stained with hematoxylin and eosin; original magnification ×200.)

surface of the colon and are replaced by replication of the descendants of epithelial stem cells located in the bottom one third of each crypt. There are three principal differentiated epithelial cell types present in the adult colonic epithelium: absorptive colonocytes, goblet cells, and enteroendocrine cells. All of these cell lineages appear to be derived from a common epithelial cell stem cell precursor. Undifferentiated cells, replicating cells, and enteroendocrine cells predominate near the base of each colonic gland (crypt).[24] Cells belonging to each of the principal cell lineages differentiate during a highly ordered migration away from the zone of proliferation. The average life span of goblet cells and absorptive cells, from their birth deep in the crypt to the point where they are sloughed into the lumen, is approximately 6 days.[25] Some enteroendocrine cell subtypes appear to have a much longer

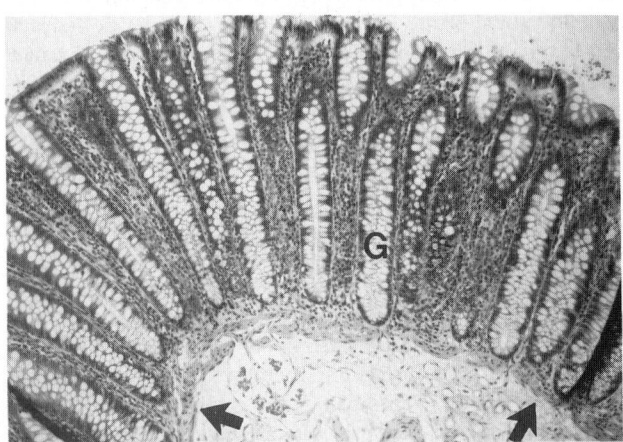

FIGURE 78-3. Histology of the colonic mucosa. Straight, simple colonic glands (G) extend from the muscularis mucosae (*arrows*) to the lumenal surface of the colon. Note the numerous small arteries, veins, and lymphatics coursing through the loose conective tissue stroma in the submucosa. (Paraffin-embedded 4-μm section stained with hematoxylin and eosin; original magnification ×100.)

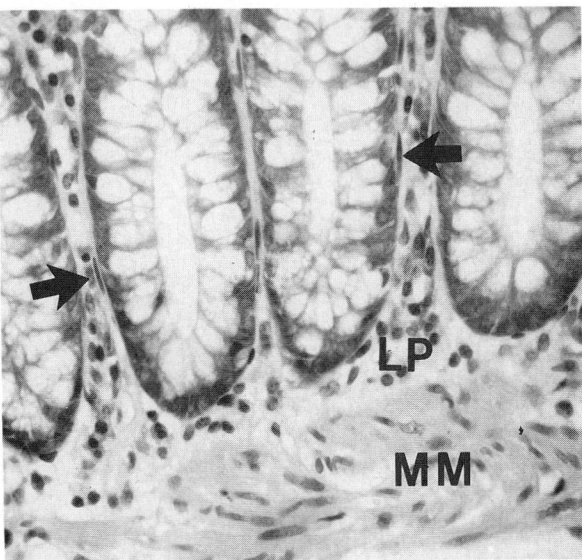

FIGURE 78-5. Colonic crypts. Note the subepithelial fibroblasts (*arrows*). Numerous plasma cells, macrophages, and lymphocytes are seen in the lamina propria (LP). (Paraffin-embedded 4-μm section stained with hematoxylin and eosin; original magnification ×400.)

life span, suggesting that their migration up the crypt to the surface epithelium must be uncoupled from that of adjacent epithelial cells.[25] Recent animal studies using X-linked enzyme markers, chimeric mice, and transgenic mice have suggested that the epithelial cell population of each small intestine or colonic crypt is derived from a single or at most a very small number of stem cells.[26-30] If normal homeostasis of the epithelial cell populations within the colonic mucosa is to be maintained, the rate of epithelial cell production within each crypt must be closely matched to the rate of cell loss from the surface epithelium. Although the mechanisms that regulate epithelial cell renewal have yet to be fully elucidated, peptide growth factors, including transforming growth factors α and β, are emerging as important potential regulators of the dynamic balance between cell proliferation and cell loss in the intestinal and colonic epithelium (see Chap. 23).[31]

One of the principal functions of absorptive columnar cells is the regulation of water and electrolyte content of the feces. The mature adult absorptive columnar cell in the colon absorbs sodium, chloride, and water; potassium and bicarbonate are secreted (see Chap. 14).[32] However, in contrast to the enterocytes of the small intestine, colonocytes are not able to absorb significant amounts of glucose or amino acids. Under normal conditions, lipid absorption is complete in the small intestine, but under pathologic conditions in which small intestine lipid absorption is incomplete, the surface columnar cells of the colon have a limited capacity for uptake of fatty acids and subsequent packaging of them into chylomicrons.[33] As these cells differentiate during their migration up the crypt, they develop short microvilli and clear, apically-oriented vesicles containing a fibrillar, glycoprotein-rich secretory product that may contribute to the glycocalyx.[33] These apical vesicles are lost, and microvilli elongate and increase in number, as the maturing absorptive cells emerge onto the surface epithelium (Fig. 78-6). At this point, alkaline phosphatase activity

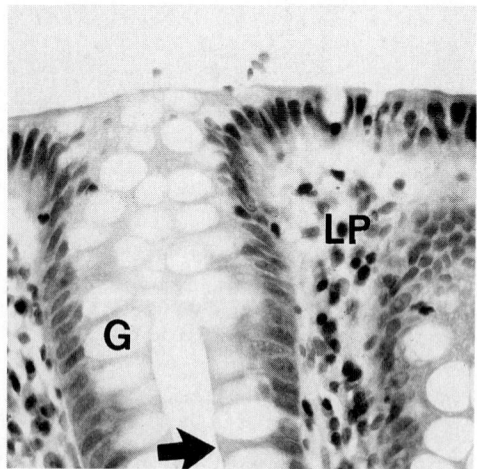

FIGURE 78-6. Surface epithelium of the colon. The mature absorptive columnar epithelial cells (*arrow*) lose their apical vesicles as they migrate into the upper regions of the colonic glands and emerge onto the luminal surface. Goblet cells (G) elongate as they emerge onto the surface epithelium because of accelerated secretion of their mucus granules. (Paraffin-embedded 4-μm section stained with hematoxylin and eosin; original magnification ×400.)

appears on the brush border, and the basolateral membranes have acquired a considerable amount of Na$^+$,K$^+$-ATPase activity, reflecting their function in water and electrolyte transport.

Goblet cells are flask-shaped cells with large apical vesicles that store and secrete mucus.[34] Mucus secreted by the goblet cell forms a viscous gel that functions as a lubricant and also protects the surface epithelium against adherence of invading pathogens. Mucins are a family of large, sulfated glycoproteins that are synthesized in the rough endoplasmic reticulum (see Fig. 78-6). Glycosylation and sulfation of these proteins occur posttranslationally in the Golgi apparatus. The composition of mucus shows regional variability along the cephalocaudal axis of the gut.[34] The membrane-bound vesicles bud off the Golgi apparatus and are slowly transported to the apical cell surface, where they secrete their contents into the lumen by exocytosis. Mucus granules accumulate during the migration of goblet cells toward the lumenal surface of the colon, distending the apical aspect of the cell and giving it its broad, flask-like appearance. As goblet cells emerge onto the surface epithelium, the secretion of mucus occurs more rapidly, depleting the apically-stored granules and causing the goblet cells to elongate (see Fig. 78-6). Increased cholinergic stimulation can cause accelerated secretion of mucus from crypt-associated goblet cells, leading to deep invaginations of the apical surface. Certain components of mucus may become depleted in pathologic conditions such as ulcerative colitis (see Chap. 79).

Originally thought to be of neuroectodermal origin, the enteroendocrine cells found in the intestinal and colonic epithelium are now recognized to arise from the same common stem cell precursor as do the other principal cell lineages found in the gut epithelium. A number of different enteroendocrine cell types are found within the colonic epithelium, including L cells, which contain both enteroglucagon and peptide YY (PYY); cells that secrete only PYY; EC$_1$ cells, which secrete serotonin, substance P, and leu-enkephalin; pancreatic polypeptide–secreting cells; and rare somatostatin-secreting cells.[11,35] These enteroendocrine cells are characterized by their polygonal shape, their broad base, and the numerous membrane-bound secretory granules present in their basilar portions (Fig. 78-7). Enteroendocrine cells are identified in pathologic specimens using argentaffin or agyrophilic silver staining techniques or through immunohistochemical methods using antibodies to the particular neuroendocrine products stored in each enteroendocrine cell subtype. The narrow apical process of the enteroendocrine cell communicates with the lumen of the crypt and may serve to sense changes in the lumenal environment. Each enteroendocrine cell is joined to other adjacent cells in the epithelium through junctional complexes located near the apical pole.[25] Despite these intracellular attachments, each enteroendocrine cell appears to migrate within the glandular colonic epithelium independently its neighbors (see previous discussion of migration). The regulatory peptides or bioamine products stored in the basally-located secretory granules are secreted through the basolateral membrane and act through paracrine or endocrine mechanisms as mediators of gastrointestinal secretion, absorptive function, and motility in response to lumenally- or basolaterally-derived signals (see Chap. 2). Enteroendocrine cells are more numerous in the appendix and the rectum than

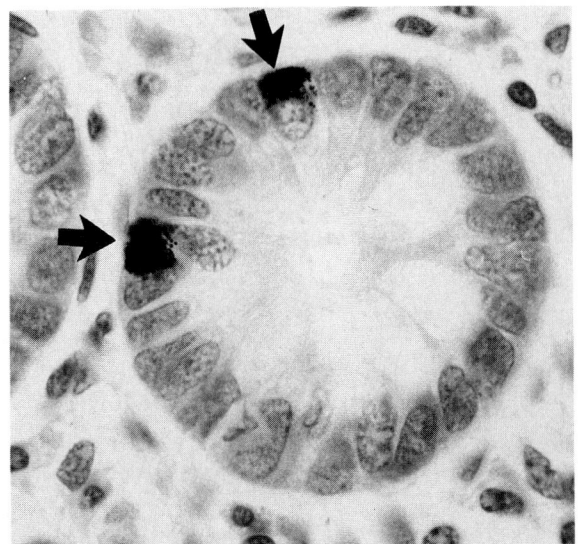

FIGURE 78-7. Enteroendocrine cells (*arrows*) seen in a cross section of a colonic crypt have a narrow apical process and a broad base filled with membrane-bound granules containing the neuroendocrine secretory product. (Paraffin-embedded 4-μm section, argentaffin stain, Fontanna-Mason technique; original magnification ×1000.)

in the rest of the colon. This may, in part, explain the more frequent occurrence of certain subtypes of neuroendocrine tumors at these sites.

The appendix is similar in histologic organization to the rest of the colon. The mucosa of the appendix consists of deep folds lined by a columnar epithelium forming simple tubular or forked glands.[33] This epithelium contains abundant goblet cells and enteroendocrine cells. Numerous lymphoid nodules are found in the lamina propria. The normal histologic architecture of the adult appendix is often replaced by fibrous scar tissue as a result of subclinical bouts of appendicitis.

ANATOMY

The colon extends from the ileocecal valve to the proximal rectum and is approximately 3 to 5 feet in length. The terminal ileum enters the cecum on its posteromedial border at the ileocecal valve. The cecum is a large, blind pouch approximately 7.5 to 8.5 cm in diameter which projects from the antimesenteric side of the ascending colon. The colon progressively diminishes in size toward the sigmoid colon, which is approximately 2.5 cm in diameter and is the narrowest portion of the colon. This size discrepancy accounts for the fact that cecal tumors often grow to be large and bulky before the onset of symptoms but sigmoid tumors are symptomatic at smaller sizes. In addition, tension on the bowel wall is directly proportional to the diameter of the bowel, as explained by the law of Laplace: $T = PR$ (where T is tension in the wall of the bowel, P is internal pressure, and R is the radius of the bowel). Because the cecum has the largest diameter, it is usually the first part of the bowel to rupture as a result of distal obstruction.

The omentum is attached to the transverse colon on its anterior superior edge. The ascending colon, descending colon, rectum, and posterior surface of the hepatic and splenic flexures are fixed retroperitoneal structures. The cecum, transverse colon, and sigmoid colon are intraperitoneal and are prone to volvulus because of their location and relative lack of fixation.

The longitudinal muscle is an incomplete layer and is seen as three bands of muscle, called taenia coli, located 120 degrees apart around the circumference of the colon. The taenia converge proximally at the appendix and disappear as distinct bands at the level of the sacral promontory. Haustra coli are sacculations between the taenia and are separated by crescent-shaped folds called plicae semilunares. Appendices epiploicae are fatty appendages covered by peritoneum and have no anatomic or pathologic significance.

The rectal wall consists of mucosal, submucosal, inner circular, and outer longitudinal muscular layers (Fig. 78-8). There is no serosal layer in the rectum. The rectum is approximately 12 to 15 cm in length and extends from the sigmoid colon to the anal canal, following the curve of the sacrum. The proximal rectum begins at the sacral promontory (third sacral vertebra), at which point the taenia fan out to form a complete layer of longitudinal muscle.

The anal canal is approximately 4 cm long and appears as a collapsed anteroposterior slit in the normal patient (see Fig. 78-8). The anal verge is the junction between anal and perianal skin. Anal epithelium (anoderm) lacks hair follicles, sebaceous glands, and sweat glands. The dentate line is a true mucocutaneous junction located 1 to 1.5 cm above the anal verge. A 6 to 12 mm transitional zone exists above the dentate line, in which the squamous epithelium of the anoderm becomes cuboidal and then columnar epithelium. The columns of Morgagni are eight to fourteen mucosal folds located just above the dentate line which surround by anal crypts. Small, rudimentary glands open into some of the crypts. These glands go through the internal sphincter into the intersphincteric groove but do not penetrate the external sphincter. The anorectal ring is 1 to 1.5 cm above the dentate line and is the palpable upper border of the anal sphincter complex. The anatomic anal canal extends from the anal verge to the dentate line. The surgical anal canal extends from the anal verge to the anorectal ring.

Arterial Supply

The superior mesenteric artery arises from the ventral surface of the aorta below the celiac axis, passes behind the pancreas, and crosses in front of the third portion of the duodenum (Fig. 78-9). The cecum, ascending colon, and transverse colon are supplied through its ileocolic, right colic, and middle colic branches. The inferior mesenteric artery arises from the infrarenal aorta and supplies the descending colon, sigmoid colon, and upper rectum through its left colic, sigmoidal, and superior rectal branches.

Collaterals exist between the superior and inferior mesenteric arteries in the region of the splenic flexure.[36] The arcades of the ileocolic, right, middle, and left colic arteries are peripherally connected by the marginal artery of Drummond, which runs along the mesenteric border of the colon and pro-

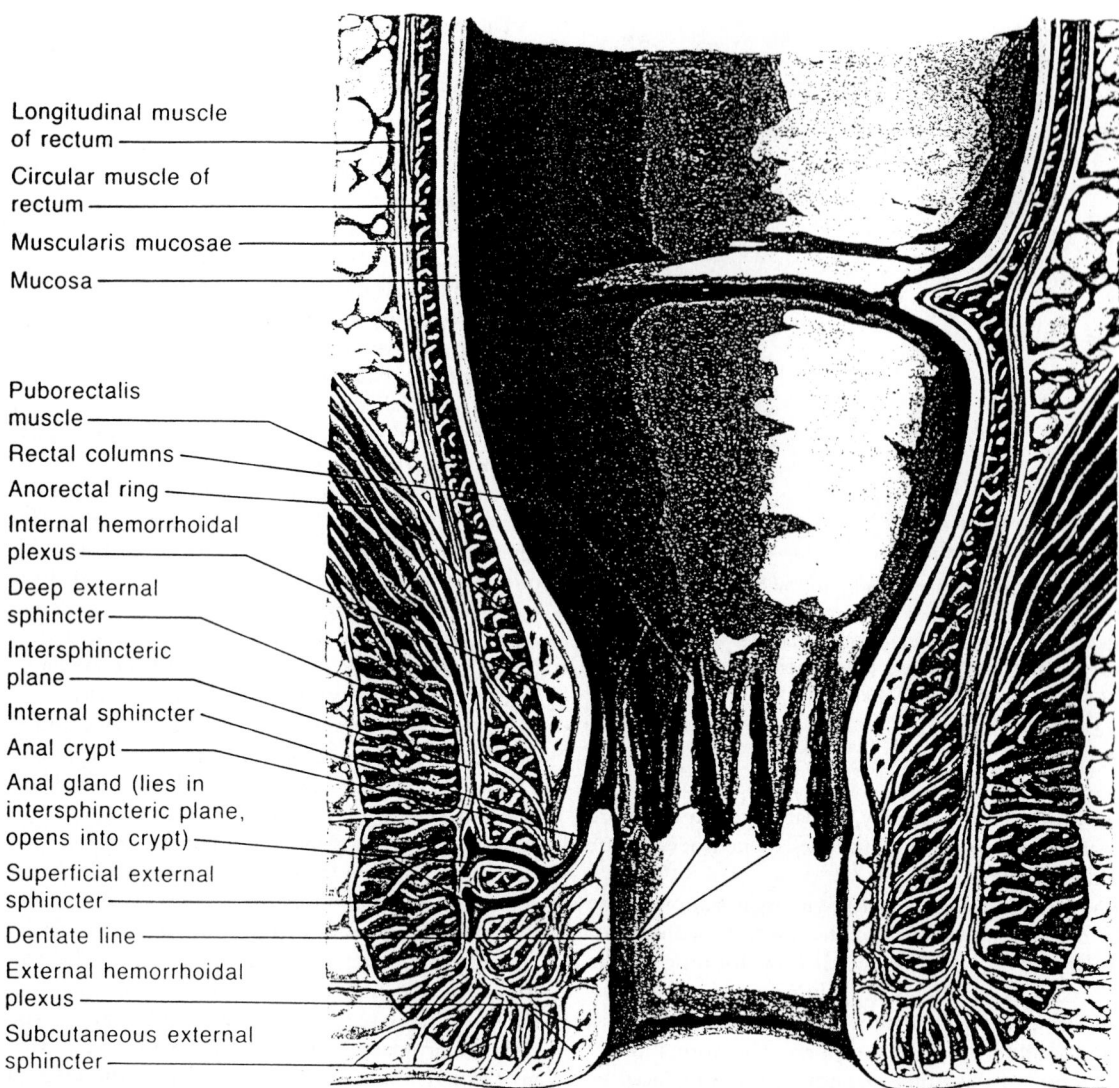

Longitudinal muscle
of rectum

Circular muscle of
rectum

Muscularis mucosae

Mucosa

Puborectalis
muscle

Rectal columns

Anorectal ring

Internal hemorrhoidal
plexus

Deep external
sphincter

Intersphincteric
plane

Internal sphincter

Anal crypt

Anal gland (lies in
intersphincteric plane,
opens into crypt)

Superficial external
sphincter

Dentate line

External hemorrhoidal
plexus

Subcutaneous external
sphincter

FIGURE 78-8. Anorectal anatomy. (From Fry RD, Kodner IJ. Anorectal disorders. CIBA Clinical Symposia 1985;37:6.)

vides the vasa recta to the colon. The arc of Riolan is a tortuous, inconstant vessel that exists between the left colic branch of the inferior mesenteric artery and the middle colic branch of the superior mesenteric artery. It is frequently referred to as the meandering mesenteric artery and is best visualized if there is an occlusion of either the inferior or superior mesenteric artery.

The terminal branch of the inferior mesenteric artery becomes the superior rectal artery, which descends in the sigmoid mesocolon and bifurcates at the level of third sacral vertebra (Fig. 78-10A). Branches of the superior rectal artery supply the upper and middle rectum. The middle rectal arteries arise from the internal iliac arteries, and the inferior rectal arteries are branches of the internal pudendal arteries. These arteries supply the lower two thirds of the rectum.[37] The middle sacral artery arises just before the aortic bifurcation and provides very little blood supply to the rectum. Anastomosis exists between the middle and superior rectal arteries; there are no anastomoses with the inferior rectal arteries. Preservation of the middle rectal arteries is necessary to maintain viability of

the rectal stump after high ligation of the inferior mesenteric artery.[37]

Venous Drainage

The veins draining the colon follow the same course as the corresponding arteries except for the inferior mesenteric vein. The inferior mesenteric vein drains the descending colon, sigmoid colon, and proximal rectum and runs in a retroperitoneal location to the left of the ligament of Treitz, at which point it enters the splenic vein. The superior mesenteric vein drains the cecum, ascending colon, and transverse colon and joins the splenic vein to form the portal vein.

The venous drainage of the rectum enters the portal or systemic (caval) system. The upper and middle rectum are drained by the superior rectal vein, which enters the portal system through the inferior mesenteric vein. The lower rectum and upper anal canal are drained by the middle rectal vein, which empties into the internal iliac veins and then into the

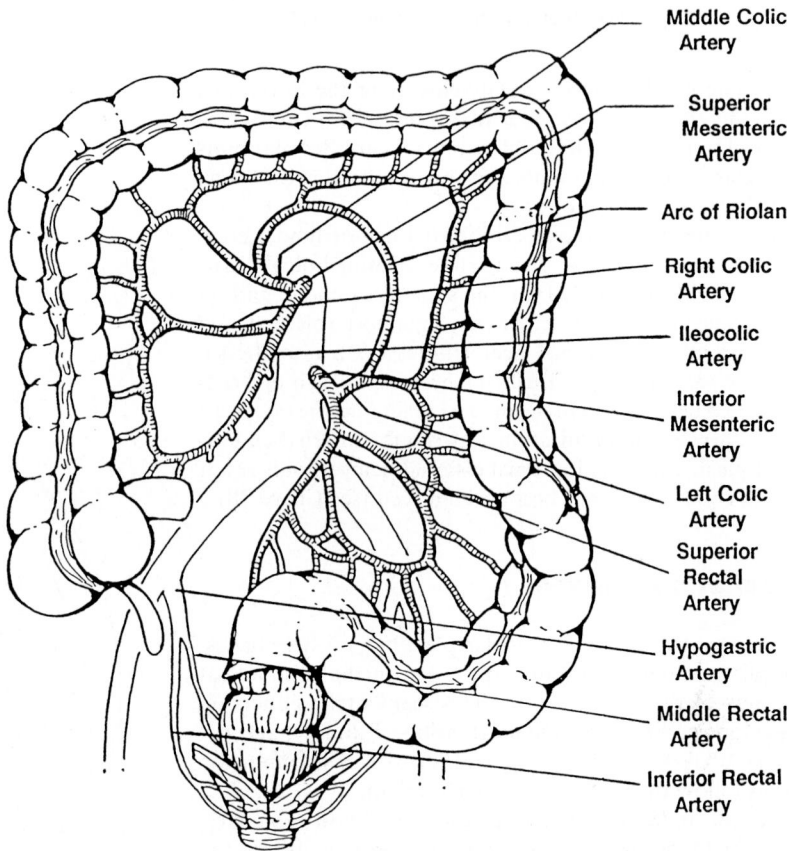

Middle Colic
Artery

Superior
Mesenteric
Artery

Arc of Riolan

Right Colic
Artery

Ileocolic
Artery

Inferior
Mesenteric
Artery

Left Colic
Artery

Superior
Rectal
Artery

Hypogastric
Artery

Middle Rectal
Artery

Inferior Rectal
Artery

FIGURE 78-9. Arterial blood supply of colon and rectum. (From Kodner IJ, Fry RD, Fleshman JW, Birnbaum EH. Colon, rectum and anus. In: Schwartz SI, ed. Principles of surgery. 6th ed. New York: McGraw-Hill, 1993.)

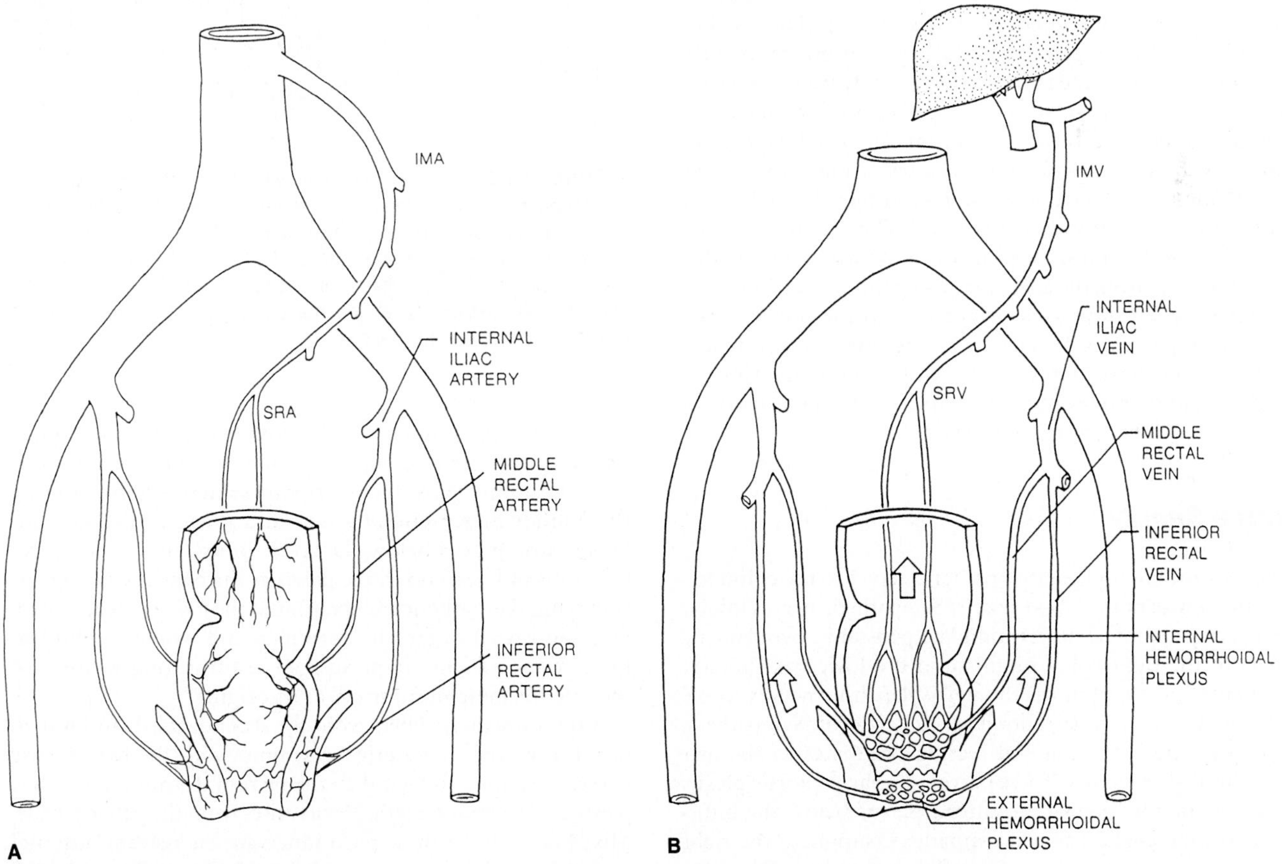

IMA

INTERNAL
ILIAC
ARTERY

SRA

MIDDLE
RECTAL
ARTERY

INFERIOR
RECTAL
ARTERY

A

IMV

INTERNAL
ILIAC
VEIN

SRV

MIDDLE
RECTAL
VEIN

INFERIOR
RECTAL
VEIN

INTERNAL
HEMORRHOIDAL
PLEXUS

EXTERNAL
HEMORRHOIDAL
PLEXUS

B

FIGURE 78-10. Vascular supply of the anus and rectum (**A**) Arterial supply. (**B**) Venous drainage. (IMA, inferior mesenteric artery; IMV, inferior mesenteric vein; SRA, superior rectal artery; SRV, superior rectal vein; from Kodner IJ, Fleshman JW, Fry RD. Anal and rectal cancer principles of management. In: Schwartz SI, Ellis H, eds. Maingot's abdominal operations. 9th ed. Norwalk, CT: Appleton & Lange, 1989.)

caval system. The inferior rectal veins drain the lower anal canal and empty into the pudendal veins, which empty into the caval system through the internal iliac veins. Rectal tumors can metastasize through venous channels into either the portal or systemic venous systems.

There are three submucosal internal hemorrhoidal complexes located above the dentate line. Hemorrhoidal tissue receives its blood supply from the superior, middle, and inferior rectal arteries. The left lateral, right posterolateral, and right anterolateral internal hemorrhoids drain into the superior rectal vein (Fig. 78-10*B*). The external hemorrhoids are located below the dentate line and drain into the pudendal veins. There is communication between the internal and external plexi, and mixed internal-external hemorrhoids result if these communications become engorged (see Chap. 88).

Lymphatic Drainage

Colonic mucosa has rich vascular plexi but no lymphatics. Lymphatic capillaries encircle the colon in the submucosal and muscularis mucosae layers. This segmental architecture limits longitudinal intramural extension of tumors, and circumferential extension results in annular lesions. Lymphatic vessels follow the blood supply of the colon.

Lymph nodes are located on the bowel wall (epicolic), along the inner margin of the bowel (paracolic), around the named mesenteric arteries (intermediate), and along the origin of the superior and inferior arteries (main) (Fig. 78-11). Lymph from the upper and middle rectum drains into the inferior mesenteric nodes. The lower rectal lymphatics follow the superior rectal artery and enter the inferior mesenteric nodes. Lymph from the lower rectum can also flow laterally along the middle and inferior rectal arteries, posteriorly along the middle sacral artery, or anteriorly through channels in the rectovesical or rectovaginal septum.[38] These channels drain to the iliac nodes and subsequently to periaortic lymph nodes.

Lymphatics from the anal canal above the dentate line drain through the superior rectal lymphatics to the inferior mesenteric lymph nodes or laterally to the internal iliac lymph nodes. Below the dentate line, the lymphatics drain primarily to the inguinal nodes but they can drain to the inferior or superior rectal lymph nodes as well.[38]

Nerve Supply

The sympathetic and parasympathetic nerves to the colon follow the course of the blood vessels. Sympathetic nerves inhibit and parasympathetic nerves stimulate peristalsis. Sympathetic fibers to the right colon originate in the lower six thoracic segments and travel in the thoracic splanchnic nerves to the celiac and then to the superior mesenteric plexus. Sympathetic supply to the left colon and rectum originates in the first three lumbar segments. These nerves join the preaortic plexus and become the inferior mesenteric plexus below the bifurcation of the aorta. The parasympathetic supply to the right colon is presumed to come from the right vagus. The parasympathetic nerves to the left colon ascend from the pelvis, pass through the sigmoid mesocolon, and spread out toward the sigmoid and the descending colon.

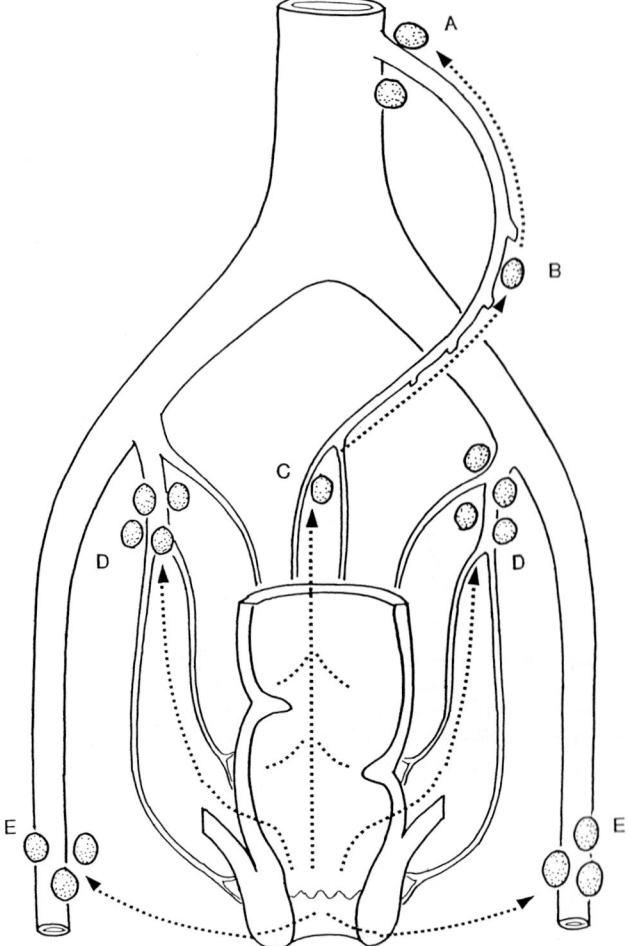

FIGURE 78-11. Lymphatic drainage of the rectum and anus. (A, nodes at origin of inferior mesenteric artery; B, nodes at origin of sigmoid branches; C, sacral nodes; D, internal iliac nodes; E, inguinal nodes; from Kodner IJ, Fleshman JW, Fry RD. Anal and rectal cancer: principles of management. In: Schwartz SI, Ellis H, eds. Maingot's abdominal operations. 9th ed. Norwalk, CT: Appleton & Lange, 1989.)

The rectum is innervated by both sympathetic and parasympathetic nerves.[39] Sympathetic nerves from thoracolumbar segments unite below the inferior mesenteric artery, forming the inferior mesenteric plexus, and descend to the superior hypogastric plexus below the aortic bifurcation. The nerves bifurcate and descend in the pelvis as the hypogastric nerves, supplying sympathetic innervation to the lower rectum, bladder, and sexual organs in both men and women. Injury to the inferior mesenteric plexus can result during ligation of the inferior mesenteric artery at its origin.

Parasympathetic fibers from the second, third, and fourth sacral roots (the nervi erigentes) unite with the hypogastric nerves anterior and lateral to the rectum, forming the pelvic plexus.[39] The periprostatic plexus arises from the pelvic plexus. Mixed fibers from these plexi innervate the rectum, internal anal sphincter, prostate, bladder, and penis. The pudendal nerve (originating from the second, third, and fourth sacral nerves) mediates sensory stimuli from the penis or clitoris through the dorsal nerve. Damage to the periprostatic plexus may occur during dissection of the rectum. Injury to the pelvic autonomic nerves may result in bladder dysfunction, impotence, or both.

Below the dentate line, cutaneous sensations of temperature, pain, and touch are conveyed by afferent fibers of the inferior rectal and perineal branches of the pudendal nerve. Numerous free nerve endings make this area very sensitive to sensations.[40] Above the dentate line, a poorly defined dull sensation, experienced if the mucosa is pinched or if internal hemorrhoids are ligated, is probably mediated by parasympathetic fibers.

STRUCTURAL AND CONGENITAL ABNORMALITIES

Congenital abnormalities of the intestine are common; most arise from errors in rotation or fusion of the mesenteries or from failure of neural crest cells to complete their migration during fetal colonic development. Imperforate anus, duplication, and malrotation are usually identified in the neonatal period. Hirschsprung's disease may present in the neonatal period, in childhood, or, more rarely, in the young adult.

Omphaloceles and Gastroschisis

Abdominal wall defects are present at birth. Omphaloceles are identified by a mass of bowel and viscera in the central abdomen covered by a translucent membrane. The size of the defect varies, and it can be associated with other congenital anomalies. Gastroschisis is usually a small defect that occurs at the junction of the umbilicus and normal skin. The bowel is not covered by a membrane and there are usually no associated anomalies. Both need immediate operation. Reduction of the bowel and primary closure of the defect are usually possible only in gastroschisis. If the bowel is edematous and thickened or the defect is too large to close primarily, a Silastic silo can be constructed to achieve gradual reduction of the bowel.

Hirschsprung's Disease and Congenital Megacolon

Hirschsprung's disease is a result of the failure of neural crest cells (precursors of ganglion cells) to complete their caudal migration during normal colonic development (see the section on Colonic Development). The aganglionic segment does not relax and causes a functional obstruction. The normal proximal bowel hypertrophies and eventually dilates. The rectosigmoid is involved in approximately 75% to 80% of cases.[41] The entire colon and various lengths of small bowel are aganglionic in 5% to 10% of cases.[42] A very short aganglionic segment is the typical finding in adult Hirschsprung's disease.

Delayed passage of meconium and abdominal distention are often the presenting symptoms in the newborn.[43] Chronic constipation, abdominal distention, volvulus, or perforation may be symptoms of the disease in a child. Hirschsprung's disease in the adult is rare but must be considered in the evaluation of patients with chronic constipation dating back

to childhood.[44-47] Patients with total colonic aganglionosis may present with less dramatic intermittent symptoms of constipation.[42]

Digital rectal examination aids in the diagnosis. The rectal vault is empty in patients with Hirschsprung's disease and is full of stool in patients with idiopathic megacolon. Abdominal radiographs usually show colonic dilatation and a paucity of gas in the rectum. Barium enema may suggest the presence of a short, narrow segment or transition zone (Fig. 78-12). Patients with total aganglionosis or very-short-segment Hirschsprung's disease may have a normal-appearing barium enema. Newborns may have a normal-appearing barium enema because the proximal bowel has not had time to dilate.

The rectoanal inhibitory reflex is the relaxation of the internal sphincter in response to rectal distention. This reflex is easily identified using anal manometry. The internal sphincter does not relax in response to rectal distention in patients with Hirschsprung's disease, and an abnormal reflex during manometry aids in the diagnosis.[48,49] The rectoanal inhibitory reflex may be normal in patients with short-segment Hirschsprung's disease.

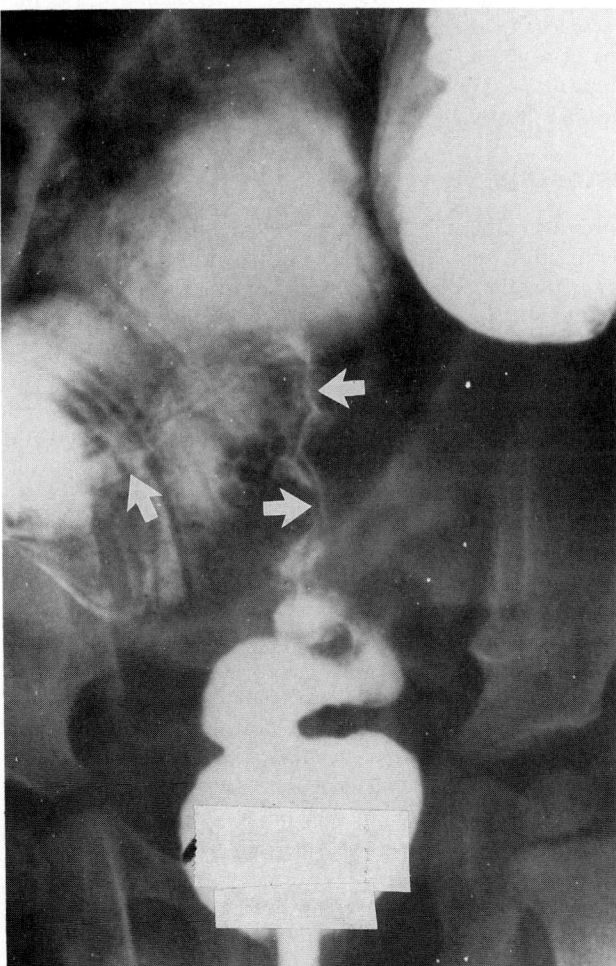

FIGURE 78-12. Radiologic study from a patient with Hirschsprung's disease. The short, collapsed, aganglionic segment (*arrows*) is evident on this radiograph of a barium enema performed on a 28-month-old infant with constipation. The colon proximal to the aganglionic segment is often dilated and filled with stool.

Histologic evaluation is necessary to make the diagnosis of Hirschsprung's disease. Hyperplasia or hypertrophy of nerve fibers can be seen, but ganglion cells are absent in the submucosa and myenteric plexus of these patients. Suction biopsies are simple to perform, but the mucosa and submucosa must be identifiable to have an adequate specimen. Full-thickness rectal biopsies may be necessary for confirmation. Routine hematoxylin and eosin staining misses ganglion cells in almost 40% of normal patients.[66] Acetylcholinesterase staining has been found to be more accurate in identifying patients with Hirschsprung's disease. Acetylcholinesterase-positive nerve fibers are increased in number in the lamina propria and the muscularis propria in these patients. A positive diagnosis may be obtained even by evaluation of superficial suction biopsies.

Colostomies are usually performed after the diagnosis is made in newborns. This allows a period of stabilization and growth before definitive repair. A colostomy may be used in the older child or adult to allow hypertrophied bowel to resume a more normal caliber. Pull-through operations (Swenson's technique, Duhamel's procedure, or Soave's procedure) have been devised to anastomose normally innervated bowel to the anus with or without resection of the abnormal bowel.[43,46] Intraoperative biopsies must demonstrate the presence of ganglion cells at the level of the colostomy and the proximal margin of the colonic resection. Rectal myectomy may be curative in patients with short-segment Hirschsprung's disease.

Intestinal Duplications

Intestinal duplications are rare congenital anomalies that can occur anywhere along the gastrointestinal tract. There are many theories regarding the cause of intestinal duplication, including failure of the bowel to recanalize in utero, caudal twinning, and incomplete separation of the notochord from the entoderm. The resultant structures may either be tubular, communicating with the intestinal lumen, or, more commonly, closed cystic duplications. These cysts are lined with gastrointestinal mucosa and contain a layer of smooth muscle within their walls. Duplications are usually found on the mesenteric side of the intestine. They frequently share a common wall and blood supply with the involved bowel. All regions of the gastrointestinal tract may be involved; the esophagus and ileum are the most commonly involved sites. The colon and rectum account for 5% to 10% of all gastrointestinal duplications.[51]

Duplications are usually symptomatic during childhood. They can produce symptoms of obstruction, volvulus, or hemorrhage. Duplications in adults are often asymptomatic and may be discovered incidentally. They can be complicated by infection, bleeding, or malignant degeneration. Plain abdominal radiographs, barium enemas, and computed tomography scans may reveal soft tissue masses or the point of communication with normal bowel. Evaluation of the genitourinary tract should be performed to rule out associated anomalies.

Resection is indicated for rectal duplications because of the risk of neoplasia, even for asymptomatic duplications. Cystic duplications can often be excised. Tubular duplications can be treated by dividing the common wall. Mucosal excision may be necessary if heterotopic gastric mucosa is present.[51]

Malrotation

Malrotation occurs if the midgut fails to complete the 270-degree counterclockwise rotation as it returns from herniation (10–12 weeks gestation).[2,52] The base of the small bowel mesentery normally stretches from the ligament of Treitz in the left upper quadrant to the ileocecal valve in the right lower quadrant. In malrotation, the entire midgut and its vascular pedicle have a narrow-based mesenteric attachment in the right upper quadrant. The duodenojejunal junction (ligament of Treitz) comes to lie to the right of the spine. The cecum and right colon overlie the duodenum in the right upper quadrant, and Ladd's bands form over the duodenum in an attempt to peritonealize the cecum. Associated anomalies, such as small bowel atresias, intussusception, Hirschsprung's disease, and abdominal wall defects, have been reported in 30% to 60% of patients.[52,53]

Most infants present with evidence of malrotation within 1 month of birth.[52,53] The clinical picture is one of a high small bowel obstruction, volvulus, or ischemia. One should suspect the diagnosis in an infant with bilious vomiting and a flat abdomen. Bloody stools indicate vascular compromise. Less severe forms of malrotation can present in childhood or later in adult life.

Plain abdominal radiographs may show evidence of a complete gastric or duodenal obstruction with a paucity of gas in the distal small bowel. A barium upper gastrointestinal series shows the ligament of Treitz to the right of midline. A barium enema is rarely needed, but it may demonstrate the cecum in the right upper quadrant.

The treatment of malrotation is operative. Most neonates with an obstruction from malrotation have a midgut volvulus.[53] The volvulus is reduced by untwisting it in a counterclockwise rotation.[54] Ladd's bands overlying the right colon and duodenum are lysed. The duodenum is placed in the right upper quadrant and the cecum in the left upper quadrant. An appendectomy is performed because the alteration in anatomy would make future diagnosis of appendicitis difficult.[53]

Imperforate Anus

Imperforate anus occurs in 1 of 20,000 live births and is associated with other congenital anomalies in 50% of cases. Genitourinary anomalies and sacral abnormalities are frequently seen. Cardiac and gastrointestinal anomalies (primarily esophageal atresia) are also associated with imperforate anus.

Imperforate anus is classified according to the relation of the rectum to the levator ani muscles.[55] High lesions are those in which bowel of normal or greater caliber terminates above the levator muscle complex. The rectum often ends in the prostatic urethra in males. In low lesions, the rectum terminates distal to the levators, often ending in a fistula. Low lesions are more common in females. Fistula tracts may connect the distal rectum with the perineum, vagina, or other hollow organs. Intermediate lesions are found within the levator complex and may be associated with a partial anal canal or perineal fistula.

The diagnosis is usually made by physical examination at birth. Most infants with imperforate anus fail to pass meconium at birth unless a fistula is present. Radiographs can be used to determine the type of defect. Air invertograms can be used to identify the location of the rectum in relation to the perineum but are difficult to interpret. Fistulograms may be performed, and computed tomography and magnetic resonance imaging are useful in evaluating high lesions. The urinary tract should be evaluated with an intravenous pyelogram and voiding cystourethrogram because of the associated urogenital anomalies.

Treatment is dependent on the type of lesion.[55] Low lesions can be treated by dilation of fistula tracts with or without anoplasty. Most healthy infants with low lesions do not require colostomies. Intermediate and high lesions are treated with an initial diverting colostomy to allow a period of stabilization and growth. A number of pull-through operations have been advocated. The posterior sagittal approach developed by Peña and deVries identifies and divides the levator muscle complex.[56] The rectal segment is then identified and brought through the center of the divided muscles. A coloanal anastomosis is performed in the location of the anal dimple. Most series have claimed a 70% to 80% success rate with intermediate and high lesions.[50] A greater success rate can be expected with low lesions.

Volvulus

Volvulus occurs whenever an air-filled segment of bowel twists about its mesentery and almost never occurs if the colon is filled with solid stool. A dilated, redundant colon with a nar-row-based mesocolon is a prerequisite for colonic volvulus. In the United States, fewer than 10% of colonic obstructions are caused by colonic volvulus. In countries with high-fiber diets, volvulus has been reported as the most common cause of intestinal obstruction.[57] Volvulus is classified and treated according to its location in the colon.

Sigmoid volvulus accounts for approximately 60% of all volvulus seen in the United States.[58] It usually occurs in elderly or institutionalized patients or in patients with various neuropsychiatric disorders. Chronic constipation, laxative abuse, and colonic atony have been implicated as the cause of the dilated, redundant sigmoid colon.

Patients usually present with abdominal pain, distention, and obstipation. Evidence of peritoneal irritation on physical examination, fever, or an elevated leukocyte count indicates gangrenous bowel. Plain abdominal radiographs showing an inverted, U-shaped, sausage-like loop with a dense line running toward the point of torsion are diagnostic for sigmoid volvulus. In questionable cases, barium or Gastrografin enema may be diagnostic. The "bird's beak" deformity forms where the contrast tapers to a point at the site of obstruction. Reduction of the volvulus can occur during these examinations. If the patient has signs of peritoneal irritation or gangrene is suspected, barium or Gastrografin enema should not be attempted, and the patient should undergo emergency exploration.

If peritonitis is not present, sigmoidoscopy should be performed. The volvulus can often be reduced by inserting a soft rectal tube past the point of obstruction. This results in dramatic decompression, and the rectal tube is left in place to

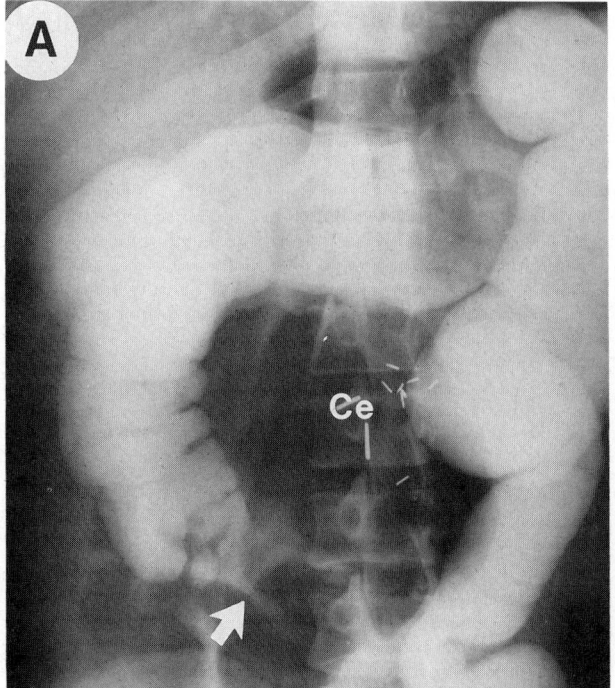 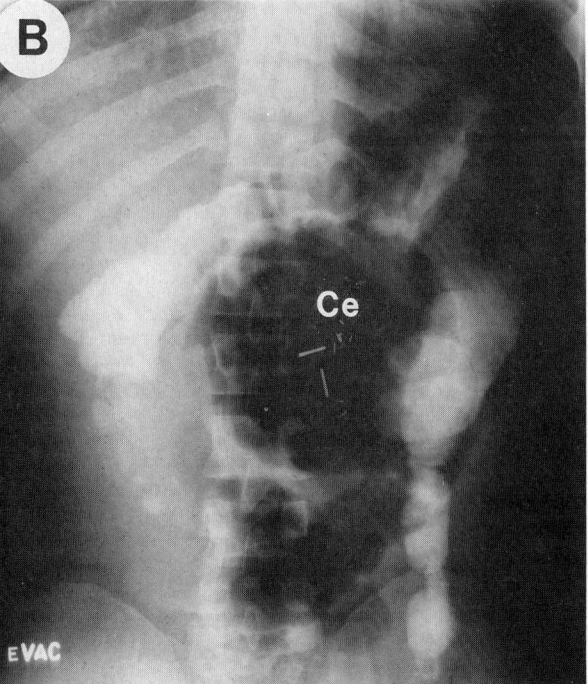

FIGURE 78-13. Cecal volvulus. (**A**) Hypaque enema shows tapering of the column of contrast at the site of torsion (*arrow*) and displacement of the cecum toward the epigastrum. (**B**) The gas-filled, dilated cecum (CE) is evident in the epigastrum in this postevacuation radiograph. Note the paucity of gas in the normal location of the cecum in the right lower quadrant of the abdomen.

assist with further decompression. Volvulus beyond the limits of the rigid sigmoidoscope may be reduced by flexible sigmoidoscopy or colonoscopy.[59] A 43% recurrence rate after nonoperative reduction can be expected.[60] Therefore, after reduction, medically stable patients should undergo mechanical bowel preparation and an elective resection. Evidence of mucosal ischemia, bloody discharge, or unsuccessful detorsion indicates strangulation and possibly gangrene. If this occurs, sigmoidoscopy should be terminated, and the patient should undergo an emergency exploration. Mortality is related to the presence of gangrenous bowel.[60]

Cecal volvulus accounts for fewer than 20% of all cases of colonic volvulus and is generally seen in younger patients.[59] It is thought to be caused by anomalous fixation of the right colon, leading to a freely mobile cecum.[61] Other precipitating factors include adhesions from previous surgeries, pregnancy, and obstructing lesions of the left colon. Ninety percent of patients with cecal volvulus have a full axial volvulus twisting the associated mesentery and blood vessels.[57] In the remaining patients, the cecum folds in an anterior cephalad direction (cecal bascule). The cecal bascule is not a true volvulus around a mesentery, but gangrene can result from tension on the bowel wall.

Abdominal pain, nausea, vomiting, and obstipation are common symptoms of cecal volvulus. Patients with cecal volvulus clinically appear to have a small bowel obstruction. Many patients give a history of similar, chronic, intermittent symptoms.[57] A plain abdominal radiograph may show the cecum as a kidney-shaped, air-filled structure in the left upper quadrant. Multiple air-filled levels may be seen and indicate a distal small bowel obstruction. Barium or Gastrografin enema may show obstruction of the column of contrast at the level of the volvulus (Fig. 78-13). The tapered edge of the contrast points toward the site of torsion. Barium studies should not be routinely performed if the diagnosis is clear. Colonoscopy has been used to treat cecal volvulus with limited success and should rarely be attempted.[59,62]

Operative detorsion alone, cecopexy, and cecostomy are associated with variable rates of recurrence.[57,63] Right hemicolectomy with primary anastomosis or cecopexy and cecostomy is recommended if there is no evidence of gangrenous bowel. Resection, ileostomy, and mucous fistula are indicated if there is evidence of gangrene. Mortality is increased in the presence of gangrenous bowel.

Volvulus of the transverse colon is rare because the mesentery is short and broad-based. Failure of the mesentery to fuse normally or narrowing of the mesenteric attachments may predispose the transverse colon to volvulus. Patients present with a clinical picture of large bowel obstruction. Barium enema is diagnostic and reveals the point of obstruction. Although rare successful attempts at colonoscopic detorsion have been reported, most patients require operative detorsion and resection of the redundant transverse colon.[64,65]

NOTE ADDED IN PROOF

A number of recent studies have identified some of the genes involved in the susceptibility and development of Hirchsprung's disease. A recessive susceptibility locus for Hirchsprung's disease that encodes the endothelin-B receptor has been mapped to human chromosome 13.[67] Targeted and naturally occuring mutations of the mouse endothelin-B re-

ceptor gene or in the mouse endothelin-3 ligand gene also result in aganglianosis and a megacolon phenotype as well as defects in development or migration of other neural crest–derived cell lineages, including epidermal melanocytes.[68,69] Together, these studies suggest that defects in the endothelin-B receptor or its ligand can cause an hereditary form of Hirchsprung's disease. Other studies have identified mutations in the *RET* receptor tyrosine kinase gene located on human chromosome 10 in an autosomal dominant form of Hirchsprung's disease.[70,71] Segregation analysis in a Menonite family indicate the existence of other major loci for susceptability to Hirchsprung's disease.[67] These findings confirm the multigenic nature of this disease.

The reader is directed to Chapter 10, Motility of the Large Intestine; Chapter 14, Electrolyte Secretion and Absorption: Small Intestine and Colon; Chapter 39, Approach to the Patient With Constipation; and Chapter 88, Anorectal Diseases.

REFERENCES

1. Moore K. The developing human: clinically oriented embryology. 4th ed. Philadelphia: WB Saunders, 1988.
2. Snyder W, Chaffin L. Embryology and pathology of the intestinal tract: presentation of 40 cases of malrotation. Ann Surg 1954;140:368.
3. Rowe J, Skandalakis J, Gray S, et al. The surgical anal canal. Contemp Surg 1974;5:107.
4. Okamoto E, Ueda T. Embryogenesis of intramural ganglia of the gut and its relation to Hirschsprung's disease. J Pediatr Surg 1967;2:437.
5. Parikh DH, Tam PKH, Velzen DV, Edgar D. Abnormalities in the distribution of laminin and collagen type IV in Hirschsprung's disease. Gastroenterology 1992;102:1236.
6. Pace JL. The age of appearance of the haustra of the human colon. J Anat 1971;109:75.
7. Ruckebusch Y. Motility of the gut during development. In: Lebenthal E, ed. Human gastrointestinal development. New York: Raven Press, 1989:183.
8. Potter GD. Development of colonic function. In: Lebenthal E, ed. Human gastrointestinal development. New York: Raven Press, 1989:545.
9. Johnson F. The development of the mucous membrane of the large intestine and vermiform process in the human embryo. Am J Anat 1913;14:187.
10. Bell L, Williams L. A scanning and transmission electron microscopical study of the morphogenesis of human colonic villi. Anat Embryol (Berl) 1982;165:437.
11. Bryant MG, Buchan AMJ, Gregor M, et al. Development of intestinal regulatory peptides in the human fetus. Gastroenterology 1982;83:47.
12. Ménard D. Growth-promoting factors and the development of the human gut. In: Lebenthal E, ed. Human gastrointestinal development. New York: Raven Press, 1989:123.
13. Kedinger M, Simon-Assmann PM, Lacroix B, et al. Fetal gut mesenchyme induces differentiation of cultured intestinal endodermal and crypt cells. Dev Biol 1986;113:474.
14. Williams L, Bell L. An ultrastructural study of meconium corpuscles in human foetal colon. Anat Embryol (Berl) 1985;171:373.
15. Raul F, Lacroix B, Apranhamian M. Longitudinal distribution of brush border hydrolases and morphological maturation in the preterm infant. Early Hum Dev 1986;13:225.
16. Triadou N, Zweibaum A. Maturation of sucrase-isomaltase complex in human fetal small and large intestine during gestation. Pediatr Res 1985;19:136.
17. Dahlqvist A, Lindberg T. Development of the intestinal disaccharidase and alkaline phosphatase activities in the human foetus. Clin Sci (Colch) 1966;30:517.

18. Lindberg T. Intestinal dipeptidases: characterization, development and distribution of intestinal dipeptidases of the human foetus. Clin Sci (Colch) 1966;30:505.

19. Haffen K, Lacroix B, Kedinger M, Simon-Assmann PM. Inductive properties of fibroblastic cell cultures derived from rat intestinal mucosa on epithelial differentiation. Differentiation 1983;23:226.

20. Haffen K, Kedinger M, Simon-Assmann P. Mesenchyme-dependent differentiation of epithelial progenitor cells in the gut. J Pediatr Gastroenterol Nutr 1987;6:14.

21. Marsh MN, Trier JS. Morphology and cell proliferation of subepithelial fibroblasts in adult mouse jejunum. I. Structural features. Gastroenterology 1974;67:622.

22. Marsh MN, Trier JS. Morphology and cell proliferation of subepithelial fibroblasts in adult mouse jejunum. II. Radioautographic studies. Gastroenterology 1974;67:636.

23. Maskens AP, Rahier JR, Meersseman FP, Dujardin-Loits RM, Haot JG. Cell proliferation of pericryptal fibroblasts in the rat colon mucosa. Gut 1979;20:775.

24. Lorenzsonn V, Trier JS. The fine structure of the human rectal mucosa. The epithelial lining of the base of the crypt. Gastroenterology 1968;55:88.

25. Tsubouchi S, Leblond CP. Migration and turnover of enteroendocrine and caveolated cells in the epithelium of the descending colon, as shown by radioautography after continuous infusion of ^{3}H-thymidine into mice. Am J Anat 1979;156:431.

26. Cohn SM, Roth KA, Birkenmeier EH, Gordon JI. Temporal and spatial patterns of transgene expression in aging adult mice provide insights about the origins, organization and differentiation of the intestinal epithelium. Proc Natl Acad Sci U S A 1991;88:1034.

27. Griffiths DFR, Davies SJ, Williams D, et al. Demonstration of somatic mutation and crypt clonality by X-linked enzyme histochemistry. Nature 1988;333:461.

28. Ponder BAJ, Schmidt GH, Wilkinson MM, et al. Derivation of mouse intestinal crypts from single progenitor cells. Nature 1985;313:689.

29. Schmidt GH, Garbutt DJ, Wilkinson MM, Ponder BAJ. Clonal analysis of intestinal crypt populations in mouse aggregation chimaeras. J Embryol Exp Morph 1985;85:121.

30. Winton DJ, Ponder BAJ. Stem cell organization in mouse small intestine. Proc R Soc Lond B Biol Sci 1990;241:13.

31. Podolsky DK. Regulation of intestinal epithelial proliferation: a few answers, many questions. Am J Physiol 1993;264:G179-G186.

32. Binder HJ, Sandle GI. Electrolyte absorption and secretion in the mammalian colon. In: Johnson LR, ed. Physiology of the gastrointestinal tract. 2nd ed. New York: Raven Press, 1987:1389.

33. Neutra MR. The gastrointestinal tract. In: Weiss L, ed. Cell and tissue biology: a textbook of histology. Baltimore: Urban & Schwarzenberg, 1988:643.

34. Neutra MR, Forstner JF. Gastrointestinal mucus: synthesis, secretion, and function. In: Johnson LR, ed. Physiology of the gastrointestinal tract. 2nd ed. New York: Raven Press, 1987:975.

35. Dayal Y. Neuroendocrine cells of the gastrointestinal tract: introduction and historical perspective. In: Dayal Y, ed. Endocrine pathology of the gut and pancreas. Boca Raton, FL: CRC Press, 1991.

36. Sonneland J, Anson B, Beaton L. Surgical anatomy of the arterial supply to the colon from the superior mesenteric artery based upon a study of 600 specimens. Surg Gynecol Obstet 1958;106:385.

37. Boxall TA, Smart P, Griffiths JD. The blood-supply of the distal segment of the rectum in anterior resection. Br J Surg 1963;50:399.

38. Block I, Enquist I. Lymphatic studies pertaining to local spread of carcinoma of the rectum in the female. Surg Gynecol Obstet 1961;112:41.

39. Church JM, Raudkivi PJ, Hill GL. The surgical anatomy of the rectum—a review with particular relevance to the hazards of rectal mobilisation. Int J Colorect Dis 1987;2:158.

40. Duthie HL, Gairns FW. Sensory nerve-endings and sensation in the anal region of man. Br J Surg 1960;206:585.

41. Grosfeld J, Ballantine TN, Csicsko J. A critical evaluation of the Duhamel operation for Hirschsprung's disease. Ann Surg 1978;113:454.

42. Careskey J, Weber T, Grosfeld J. Total colonic aganglionosis. Analysis of 16 cases. Am J Surg 1982;143:160.

43. Nixon H. Hirschsprung's disease: progress in management and diagnostics. World J Surg 1985;9:189.

44. Starling J, Croom R, Thomas C. Hirschsprung's disease in young adults. Am J Surg 1986;151:104.

45. Wheatley M, Wesley J, Coran A, Polley T. Hirschsprung's disease in adolescents and adults. Dis Colon Rectum 1990;33:622.

46. Natsikas N, Sbarounis C. Adult Hirschsprung's disease. An experience with the Duhamel-Martin procedure with special reference to obstructed patients. Dis Colon Rectum 1987;30:204.

47. Barnes P, Lennard-Jones JE, Hawlwy PR, Todd IP. Hirschsprung's disease and idiopathic megacolon in adults and adolescents. Gut 1986;27:534.

48. Meunier P, Marechal J, Molfard P. Accuracy of the manometric diagnosis of Hirschsprung's disease. J Pediatr Surg 1978;13:411.

49. Rosenberg A, Vela A. A new simplified technique for pediatric anorectal manometry. Pediatrics 1983;71:240.

50. Iwai N, Yanagihara J, Tokiwa K, et al. Results of surgical correction of anorectal malformations. A 10–30 year follow-up. Ann Surg 1988;207:219.

51. Ildstad S, Tollerud D, Weiss R, et al. Duplications of the alimentary tract. Clinical characteristics, preferred treatment, and associated malformations. Ann Surg 1988;208:184.

52. Filston H, Kirks D. Malrotation—the ubiquitous anomaly. J Pediatr Surg 1981;16:614.

53. Stewart D, Colodny A, Daggett W. Malrotation of the bowel in infants and children: a 15 year review. Surgery 1976;79:716.

54. Ladd W. Congenital obstruction of the duodenum in children. N Engl J Med 1932;206:277.

55. DeVries P, Cox K. Surgery of anorectal anomalies. Surg Clin North Am 1985;65:1139.

56. Peña A, deVries P. Posterior sagittal anorectoplasty: important technical considerations and new applications. J Pediatr Surg 1982;17:796.

57. Ballantyne GH, Brandner MD, Beart RW, Ilstrup DM. Volvulus of the colon. Incidence and mortality. Ann Surg 1985;202:83.

58. Ballantyne GH. Volvulus of the splenic flexure: report of a case and review of the literature. Dis Colon Rectum 1981;24:630.

59. Brothers TE, Strodel WE, Eckhauser FE. Endoscopy in colonic volvulus. Ann Surg 1987;206:1.

60. Ballantyne GH. Review of sigmoid volvulus. History and results of treatment. Dis Colon Rectum 1982;25:494.

61. Wolfer JA, Beaton LE, Anson BJ. Volvulus of the cecum. Anatomical factors in its etiology; report of a case. Surg Gynecol Obstet 1942;74:882.

62. Anderson MJ, Okike N, Spencer RJ. The colonoscope in cecal volvulus: report of three cases. Dis Colon Rectum 1978;21:71.

63. Rabinovici R, Simansky DA, Kaplan O, et al. Cecal volvulus. Dis Colon Rectum 1990;55:765.

64. Fishman EK, Goldman SM, PG Patt, et al. Transverse colon volvulus: diagnosis and treatment. South Med J 1983;76:185.

65. Joergensen K, Kronborg O. The colonoscope in volvulus of the transverse colon. Dis Colon Rectum 1980;23:357.

66. Ikawa H, Kim S, Hendren H, Dunahoe P. Acetylcholinesterase and manometry in the diagnosis of the constipated child. Arch Surg 1986;121:435.

67. Puffenberger EK, Hosda K, Washington SS, et al. A missense mutation of the endothelin-B receptor gene in multigenic Hirschsprung's disease. Cell 1994;79:1257.

68. Hosoda K, Hammer RE, Richardson JA, et al. Targeted and natural (piebald-lethal) mutations of endothelin-B receptor gene produce megacolon associated with spotted coat color in mice. Cell 1994;79:1267.

69. Baynash AG, Hosada K, Giaid A, et al. Interaction of endothelin-3 with endothelin-B receptor is essential for development of epidermal melanocytes and enteric neurons. Cell 1994;79:1277.

70. Edery P, Lyonnet S, Mulligan L, et al. Mutation for the RET proto-oncogene in Hirschsprung's disease. Nature 1994;367:378.

71. Romeo G, Ronchetto P, Luo Y, et al. Point mutations affecting the tyrosine kinase domain of the RET proto-oncogene in Hirchsprung's disease. Nature 1994;367:377.

Textbook of Gastroenterology, second edition, edited by Tadataka Yamada. JB Lippincott Company, Philadelphia © 1995.

CHAPTER 79

Inflammatory Bowel Disease

William F. Stenson

Ulcerative colitis and Crohn's disease are chronic inflammatory diseases of the gastrointestinal tract.[1-3] They are identified and diagnosed by the appearance of a set of clinical, endoscopic, and histologic characteristics. The inflammatory response in ulcerative colitis is largely confined to the mucosa and submucosa, but in Crohn's disease inflammation extends all the way through the intestinal wall from mucosa to serosa. Ulcerative colitis is confined to the colon, and colectomy is a curative procedure. Crohn's disease, in contrast, has the potential to involve the patient's entire gastrointestinal tract,

even though only a small segment is involved initially. Resection of the inflamed segment is not curative in Crohn's disease, and inflammation is likely to recur in the gastrointestinal tract sometime after resection. Despite these differences in distribution, there is no single finding that is absolutely diagnostic of one disease or the other. Moreover, there is a group of patients who have a clinical picture that falls between the two diseases; these patients are said to have indeterminate colitis.

There is an increased incidence of Crohn's disease in the

relatives of Crohn's disease patients and an increased incidence of ulcerative colitis in the relatives of ulcerative colitis patients.[4] However, there is also an increased incidence of ulcerative colitis in the relatives of Crohn's disease patients and an increased incidence of Crohn's disease in the relatives of ulcerative colitis patients. These patterns of family aggregation suggest that there is a genetic basis to both diseases and that the genetic basis is at least partially shared.

In view of the similarities in clinical and histologic presentation and the shared genetic background, these two diseases are presented in a single chapter. In the absence of established etiologic agents or definitive markers, it is possible that what is designated as ulcerative colitis or Crohn's disease may in fact be a mixture of diseases of diverse causes but common clinical presentation. There may actually be more than two diseases under the title of inflammatory bowel disease (IBD). Presentation in a single chapter emphasizes the common characteristics of these diseases and minimizes splitting into groups that may not be valid. This combined presentation allows the areas of similarity to be presented without repetition and allows comparisons in areas of dissimilarity.

EPIDEMIOLOGY

The incidence and prevalence of Crohn's disease and ulcerative colitis vary greatly with geographic location. The rates given in Table 79-1 are for Caucasian populations in northern Europe and North America. Rates in central and southern Europe are somewhat lower, and in South America, Asia, and Africa they are much lower. Within geographic areas, there are ethnic and racial variations in the incidence of IBD.[5-7] Crohn's disease is three to eight times more common in Jews than non-Jews. Similarly, the incidence of ulcerative colitis is two to four times higher in Jews. However, the incidence among Israeli Jews is much lower than among American and European Jews. Furthermore, in Israel, the incidence is lower among Sephardic or Oriental Jews of Asian or African origin than among Ashkenazi Jews of European or American origin.[7] In the United States, the incidence of both ulcerative colitis and Crohn's disease in the black population has been one fifth to one half that in the Caucasian population, but in recent years that gap appears to be narrowing.[8]

TABLE 79-1
Epidemiology of Inflammatory Bowel Disease

FACTOR	ULCERATIVE COLITIS	CROHN'S DISEASE
Incidence (per 100,000)	2–10	1–6
Prevalence (per 100,000)	35–100	10–100
Racial incidence	High in caucasians	High in caucasians
Ethnic indicence	High in Jews	High in Jews
Gender	Slight female preponderance	Slight female preponderance
Age at onset	15–25 ?55–65	15–25 ?55–65
Smoking	Fewer smokers than expected	More smokers than expected

It is hard to make firm statements about changes in the incidence of IBD over time because some of the apparent increase in incidence may come from greater awareness of these diseases, better diagnostic studies, and better reporting. Moreover, some patients now diagnosed as having Crohn's colitis may have been diagnosed as having ulcerative colitis in the past. Despite these ambiguities, certain trends are apparent.[9,10] In geographic areas in which the incidence of these diseases has been slight, it is now increasing. In northern Europe and North America, where the incidence of both diseases has been substantial, the incidence of ulcerative colitis has leveled off but that of Crohn's disease is still increasing.

Some series show an approximately equal incidence of both diseases in men and women, but other studies show an incidence that is greater in women by up to 30%.[8] The peak age of onset for both diseases is between 15 and 25 years of age. In some, but not all, series there is a second, lesser peak of incidence between 55 and 65 years of age.[8] Both diseases occur in childhood, although the incidence is much lower before 15 years of age than after. Ulcerative colitis is more common than Crohn's disease in children younger than 10 years of age. The similarities between ulcerative colitis and Crohn's disease in geographic distribution, racial and ethnic distribution, distribution by sex, and age of onset support the contention that the two diseases are related.

One fascinating but unexplained difference between patients with these two diseases is the incidence of smoking. Among patients with ulcerative colitis, the incidence of smoking is less than in the general population. In several studies, the risk of developing ulcerative colitis was found to be increased among both nonsmokers and former smokers, compared with current smokers.[11,12] In contrast, the incidence of smoking among Crohn's disease patients was found to be as high or higher than in the general population.[12] Whether cessation of smoking improves the clinical picture in Crohn's disease or initiation of smoking improves the clinical picture in ulcerative colitis has not been determined.

ETIOLOGY AND PATHOGENESIS

Genetics

Any theory of the pathogenesis of IBD must deal with the evidence for a genetic basis of the disease. The most firmly established and quantitatively greatest risk factor for developing IBD is a positive family history.[13] Approximately 15% of patients with IBD have first-degree relatives who also have IBD.[14,15] The best estimates of the lifetime risk of developing IBD among first-degree relatives of affected individuals is 8.9% for offspring, 8.8% for siblings, and 3.5% for parents.[16] The incidence of IBD among first-degree relatives of IBD patients is 30 to 100 times that of the general population. Moreover, although the relatives of patients with Crohn's disease are more likely to have Crohn's disease than ulcerative colitis, the incidence of ulcerative colitis in this group is also higher than in the general population.[4] Similarly, relatives of patients with ulcerative colitis have a higher incidence of both ulcerative colitis and Crohn's disease than the general population. These data support the contention that ulcerative colitis and Crohn's disease are related diseases. The increased incidence among first-degree relatives contrasts with the absence of any evidence for an increased incidence of IBD in spouses of patients. The spouse data support the theory that the presence of many affected individuals in a family relates to genetic factors rather than common exposure to some environmental agent.

Twin studies also support the presence of a genetic basis for these diseases. A study of unselected twins from a Swedish twin registry demonstrated that dizygotic twins have the same rate of concordance as would be expected for siblings, whereas monozygotic twins have higher rates of concordance for both diseases.[17] There is no reported case of monozygotic twins in which one twin had Crohn's disease and the other ulcerative colitis, suggesting that these diseases have a similar but not identical genetic background.

There is no clear-cut mendelian pattern of inheritance in IBD. There are, however, HLA class II genes that have been associated with Crohn's disease and ulcerative colitis. The DR1/DQw5 haplotype has been associated with Crohn's disease,[18] and HLA-DR2 has been associated with ulcerative colitis.[19]

Another approach to understanding the genetic basis of IBD is the search for subclinical markers, that is, parameters used to detect the abnormal genotype in the absence of the full clinical phenotype. The two subclinical markers that have received the most attention are increased intestinal epithelial permeability in Crohn's disease and antineutrophil cytoplasmic antibodies (ANCA) in ulcerative colitis. There is a report of increased intestinal permeability to PEG-400 in Crohn's disease patients and their first-degree relatives.[20] A genetic defect of intestinal epithelial cells allowing permeation of lumenal antigens across the epithelial monolayer could result in nonspecific activation of the intestinal immune system. However, subsequent studies using a variety of probes under different conditions have yielded somewhat inconclusive data.[21,22] The other subclinical marker that has received considerable attention is the presence of ANCA in the sera of patients with ulcerative colitis.[23] About 70% of patients with ulcerative colitis are ANCA-positive, with no correlation with disease extent or activity. The antigen with which the antibody reacts and the role, if any, of the antibody in the pathogenesis of the disease are unknown. However, clinically healthy relatives of patients with ulcerative colitis have an increased incidence of positive ANCA compared with the general population, suggesting that ANCA is more than just a marker for colonic inflammation.[24]

Potential Etiologic Agents and Antigenic Triggers

There is clear evidence for the activation of the immune response in IBD. The lamina propria is infiltrated with lymphocytes, macrophages, and other cells of the immune system. In any immune response there is a specific antigen that serves as a trigger for the response and as a target for the effector arm of the response. Over the past 30 years, there has been an intensive search for the antigens that trigger the immune response in IBD. Immune activation in IBD is largely confined to the gastrointestinal tract; therefore, the search for the antigenic trigger has focused on the intestinal lumen. Most of the antigens in the intestinal lumen are of either microbial or dietary origin.

There are three major hypotheses as to the antigenic triggers in IBD. One hypothesis is that the antigenic triggers are microbial pathogens that have not yet been identified because of fastidious culture requirements. According to this hypothesis, the immune response in IBD is an appropriate but ineffective response to these pathogens. Various viruses and bacteria have been proposed as candidate organisms, but there is little evidence to support any of them as having a causative role in IBD. An organism that has created much interest is a species of mycobacterium similar to or identical with *Mycobacterium paratuberculosis*. This organism has been isolated from a number of Crohn's disease surgical specimens.[25,26] *M paratuberculosis* causes Johne's disease, an intestinal disorder in ruminants that clinically and histologically resembles Crohn's disease. Mycobacteria isolated from a Crohn's disease surgical specimen were administered orally to a young goat and caused a disease similar to Johne's disease.[27] This is the closest any infectious agent has come to fulfilling Koch's postulates in IBD. However, although this organism is pathogenic for goats, it is probably nonpathogenic in humans. There are several pieces of evidence that suggest that this mycobacterium is not a causative agent in Crohn's disease. First, despite intensive efforts, this organism has been isolated from relatively few patients with Crohn's disease and has been isolated from patients with other intestinal diseases.[28] Second, there is no evidence for either a humeral or a cellular response directed against this organism in Crohn's disease. Finally, patients with Crohn's disease improve clinically after treatment with immunosuppressives, a response that would not be expected in a disease caused by mycobacteria.

The second hypothesis as to the antigenic trigger in IBD is that it is some common dietary antigen or usually nonpathogenic microbial agent against which the patient mounts an abnormal immune response. In healthy individuals, there is a finely tuned, low-grade chronic inflammation in the intestinal lamina propria. Presumably, this chronic inflammation is a product of chronic exposure of the lamina propria to lumenal antigens. Failure to suppress this inflammatory response could result in the uncontrolled immune activation seen in IBD. As a result of failure of normal suppressor mechanisms, immune activation in IBD may be an inappropriately vigorous and prolonged response to some normal lumenal antigen. The genetic basis of IBD may relate to a genetically determined ability to mount an immune response to a specific lumenal antigen. It may be that patients with IBD are genetically programmed to mount an intense immune response to some common lumenal antigen—either dietary or microbial—to which most people do not respond.

Other than bacteria, the major source of antigens in the intestinal lumen is the diet. Dietary antigens can trigger an immune response, as is seen in the response to wheat gliadin in patients with celiac sprue. One of the foods implicated as playing a role in the pathogenesis of IBD is cow's milk. There is an increased incidence of antibodies to cow's milk protein both in patients with ulcerative colitis and in those with Crohn's disease.[29,30] However, these antibodies may merely reflect a normal immune response to cow's milk proteins. In IBD, cow's milk proteins and other dietary antigens have an abnormal access to the lamina propria because of the defect in the epithelial cell monolayer caused by inflammation. The immune response to cow's milk protein serves as an example of a general problem in sorting out the pathogenesis of IBD. In health, the intestinal epithelium serves as a barrier between the immune cells of the lamina propria and lumenal antigens. The immune cells see only lumenal antigens that have been selected and processed by the M cells. However, in IBD, because of the destruction of the epithelium, the immune cells of the lamina propria are exposed to numerous lumenal antigens. These lumenal antigens, although they may have no specific role as etiologic agents, are capable of triggering immune responses if seen by the immune cells of the lamina propria. Molecular genetic analysis of immunoglobulin and T-cell receptor genes has shown that the lymphocyte population in IBD is polyclonal.[31] As a result, the specific immune response to the etiologic agent may be drowned out by the immune responses to the thousands of lumenal antigens that pass through the damaged epithelium. It would be difficult to separate the secondary immune response from response directed against the primary etiologic agent.

The third hypothesis as to the antigenic trigger in IBD is that it is an antigen expressed on the patient's own cells, particularly on intestinal epithelial cells. This is an autoimmune theory for the pathogenesis of IBD. In this theory, the patient mounts an appropriate immune response against some lumenal antigen—either dietary or microbial. However, because of similarities between proteins on the epithelial cells and the lumenal antigen, the patient's immune system also attacks the epithelial cells. Under the autoimmune theory, the immune response is directed specifically toward the epithelial cell, and the epithelial cell is destroyed by one of two immune effector mechanisms—either antibody-dependent cellular cytotoxicity, which requires an antibody directed against an epithelial cell surface antigen, or direct cell-mediated cytotoxicity. In support of the autoimmune theory, several investigators have reported the presence of anticolon antibodies in the sera of ulcerative colitis patients.[32,33] However, similar antibodies have been found in the sera of normal individuals and in patients with systemic lupus erythematosus in whom there was no intestinal inflammation.[34] Das and colleagues have demonstrated the presence of a tissue-bound antibody that could be eluted from ulcerative colitis surgical resections. This antibody is directed against a 40-kd protein that has been identified as tropomyosin.[35–37] The presence of an anticolon antibody does not necessarily mean that the antibody plays a pathogenetic role. A more convincing case for a pathogenetic role could be made by the demonstration that this antibody participates in antibody-dependent cellular cytotoxicity.

The Immune Response

The first step in the immune response to an antigen is the uptake and processing of the antigen by macrophages or other antigen presenting cells (Fig. 79-1). CD4 (helper/inducer) T cells recognize soluble antigens in conjunction with HLA class II molecules (HLA-DP, -DQ, and -DR) present on macrophages. Class II antigens on intestinal epithelial cells may also play a role in antigen processing within the intestinal immune compartment. In the normal human, class II molecules are present on epithelial cells of the small intestine but not those of the colon, and Class II antigen expression on small intestine epithelial cells is retained in patients with Crohn's disease. HLA-DR–like molecules on human intestine epithelial cells may be involved in antigen-induced triggering of intraepithelial lymphocytes. Marked enhancement of colon epithelial cell HLA-DR staining occurs in active ulcerative colitis and Crohn's colitis, and intestinal epithelial cells from patients with IBD are capable of processing and presenting antigens in vitro.[38]

The activated macrophage, in addition to presenting antigen to the T cell, releases interleukin-1 (IL-1), which activates the T cell. The activated T cell releases IL-2, which promotes the clonal expansion of cytotoxic T cells and increased function of helper T cells and B cells. Cell-mediated immune responses may be involved in the pathogenesis of IBD. Various approaches have been taken to define such a role, including descriptive studies of T-cell number and surface antigen phenotype in the intestine, comparison of the functional activity of intestinal cells isolated from IBD patients with controls, and studies on T cells from other sites such as the peripheral blood. Early studies disagreed on the quantitative changes in peripheral blood lymphocyte subpopulations in Crohn's disease. The conflicting studies were clarified by the studies of Auer,[39,40] who showed that patients with newly diagnosed Crohn's disease had the same distribution of lymphocyte subpopulations as normal individuals and that changes in distribution occurred only with drug therapy or the development of malnutrition.

Antibody Secretion

In view of the increased access of lumenal antigens to the immune cells of the lamina propria, it is not surprising that there is increased antibody secretion by the intestinal mononuclear cells in IBD. Not only is the number of antibody secreting cells increased, but the distribution of immunoglobulin classes is changed. In healthy individuals, the vast majority of the immunoglobulin secreted by intestinal mononuclear cells is IgA. In IBD, there is markedly increased production of IgM and IgG. IgA does not fix complement, whereas IgM and IgG do. A transition from IgA production to IgM and IgG production, combined with antibody binding to a local antigen, could result in increased fixation of complement to antigen-antibody complexes and the development of inflammation. The tissue-bound antibody eluted from ulcerative colitis colon resections by Das and colleagues is an IgG.[36] This raises the question of whether this antibody binds complement participates in antibody-dependent cellular cytotoxicity. There are subclasses of IgG that are defined by the structure of their constant regions. There is some subclass specificity in the increase in IgG production seen in IBD. Ulcerative colitis is associated with increased production of IgG1 and IgG3, whereas Crohn's disease is associated with increased production of IgG2. IgG1 and IgG3 antibodies account for the predominant IgG response to proteins and T cell–dependent antigens. IgG2 provides the predominant IgG response to carbohydrates and many bacterial antigens. Delineation of the stimuli and antigens that induce the increased

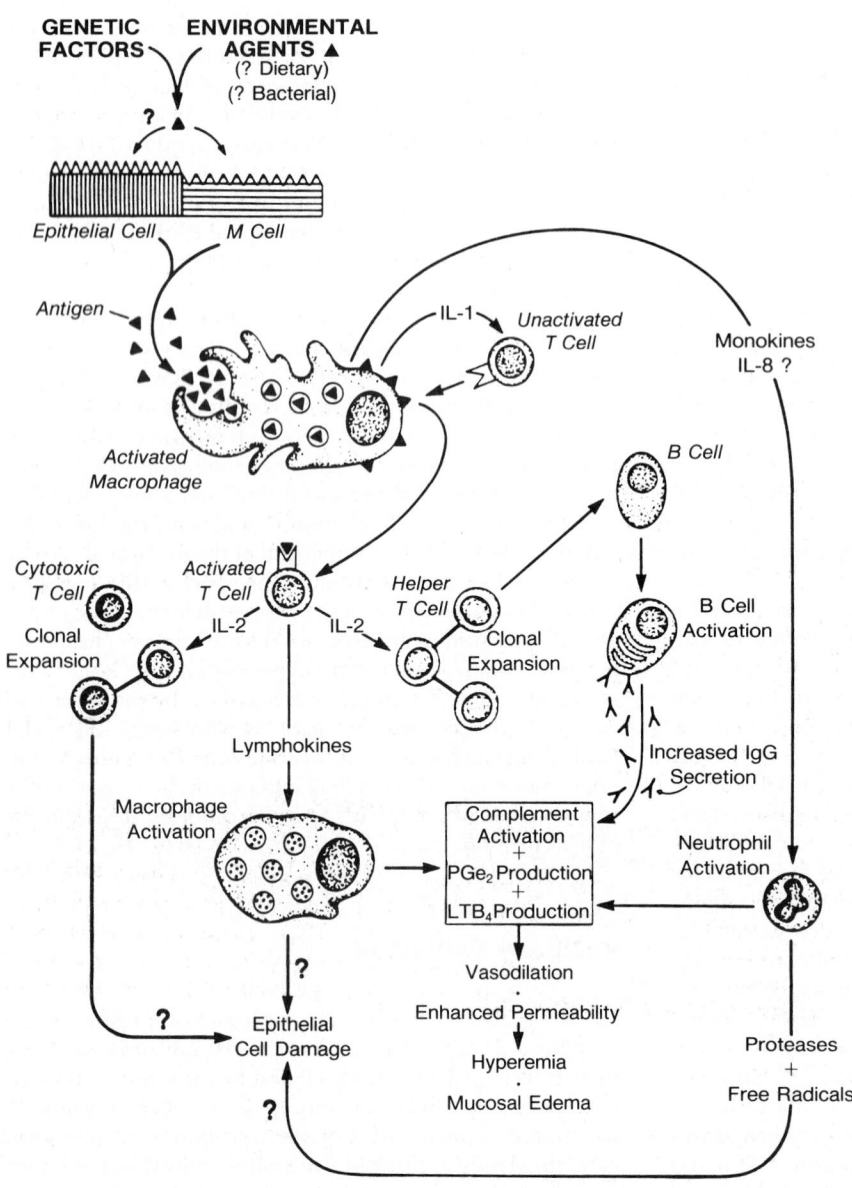

FIGURE 79-1. An immunologic sequence that has been postulated to account for the inflammatory responses observed in inflammatory bowel disease starts with an exogenous sensitization to lumenal antigens, possibly facilitated by undefined genetic influences. The first cell population involved would be the intestinal macrophage, which would phagocytose and process an antigen and present it to a T lymphocyte. In combination with a signal in the form of interleukin-1 (IL-1), this would lead to a population of sensitized and activated T cells capable of interleukin-2 (IL-2) secretion. This, in turn, would stimulate clonal expansion of specific cytolytic T cells and a helper T-cell/B-cell collaboration resulting in increased antibody secretion (particularly IgG subclasses). At the same time, monokines would activate neutrophils, and T-cell lymphokines would induce further macrophage activation. Thus, an attack on the bowel epithelium would be mounted by a broad array of inflammatory cells and soluble mediators. (Adapted from MacDermott RP, Stenson WF. Hosp Pract 21:97, 1986.)

secretion of IgG subclasses may provide insight into the etiology and pathogenesis of IBD.

Cytokines

Cytokines are glycosylated proteins that mediate potent biologic function at low concentrations in a hormone-like fashion. Like hormones, they act through receptors, but unlike hormones, which act on cells at a distance from their cell of origin, cytokines act on neighboring cells. They were originally described as being produced by immune cells and acting on immune cells, but it is now clear that they are also both produced by and act on nonimmune cells. Cytokines almost certainly play important regulatory roles in IBD, just as they do in other chronic inflammatory states.[41,42] The state of knowledge of the role of cytokines in IBD is rapidly advancing but is still at a fairly early stage. The best developed data is that

demonstrating increased production of most of the major proinflammatory cytokines (IL-1, IL-6, IL-8). There are conflicting reports as to the level of production of the other major proinflammatory cytokine, tumor necrosis factor (TNF). The major cell source of the proinflammatory cytokines is almost certainly activated macrophages in the lamina propria, although there may be important contributions from other cell types. Cytokines, particularly IL-1, TNF, and interferon-γ, stimulate epithelial, endothelial, and mesenchymal cells and activate immune cells.[43] They are also involved in the regulation of wound healing and fibrosis.[44] Cytokines may be useful as markers of disease activity, especially tissue IL-1 levels in ulcerative colitis and serum IL-2 receptor levels in Crohn's disease.[45,46] There is also a possibility that drugs specifically designed to affect cytokine production or activity may be useful in the management of IBD. There is already evidence that a naturally occurring IL-1 receptor antagonist is effective in reducing inflammation in a rabbit model of colitis.[47]

IBD is commonly viewed as a disorder of chronic inflammation, a view reinforced by the large numbers of lymphocytes and histiocytes in the diseased mucosa and submucosa. More recently, there has been increased awareness that these diseases also have histologic characteristics of acute inflammation, including an intense infiltration of the mucosa and submucosa with neutrophils. Large numbers of neutrophils leave the bloodstream and enter the inflamed mucosa and submucosa of the bowel.[48,49] Some neutrophils migrate across the epithelium into the lumen and are passed in the stool, and others are destroyed in the inflamed tissue before they have a chance to migrate into the lumen. This constant flux of neutrophils is mediated by the expression of adhesion molecules on circulating neutrophils and vascular endothelial cells which allow the neutrophil to bind to the endothelium before migrating into the tissue. Both the expression of adhesion molecules and the migration of neutrophils are regulated by inflammatory cytokines (IL-8 and TNF) and lipid mediators of inflammation, including platelet activating factor and leukotriene B_4 (LTB$_4$). Neutrophil activation in the inflamed gut results in the release of granule-bound proteases and the production of superoxide and other reactive oxygen species. These products of activated neutrophils probably play a role in the destruction of epithelial cells in IBD.

Some of the functional and macroscopic changes seen in IBD, including mucosal hyperemia and edema, are typical of changes seen in any inflammatory state, no matter which organ system is involved. These changes are the products of soluble mediators released in the process of inflammation. Mediators cause tissue edema by increasing vascular (postcapillary venule) permeability to albumin and other macromolecules; hyperemia results from mediators that induce vasodilation. Progress has been made in characterization of the soluble mediators of inflammation and their role in the amplification of the immune response in IBD. There are two reasons for defining their pathogenic role. First, the soluble mediators appear to be largely responsible for the clinical and histologic changes seen in the disease. Second, the drugs that have proved to be beneficial for ulcerative colitis and Crohn's disease appear to exert their therapeutic effects by blocking the synthesis of those mediators. Corticosteroids and sulfasalazine block the synthesis of prostaglandins and leukotrienes in vivo and in vitro.[50,51] Furthermore, until the etiologic agents of ulcerative colitis and Crohn's disease are identified, it is likely that advances in medical therapy will be in the area of regulation of the synthesis of soluble mediators of inflammation.

Prostaglandins are produced by almost all mammalian cells, including intestinal epithelium and cells associated with inflammatory events (e.g., mast cells, macrophages, platelets). Prostaglandins, particularly those of the E series, have biologic properties that are proinflammatory, including enhanced vascular permeability, vasodilation, and production of pain. Prostaglandin levels are elevated in mucosa and serum in IBD and correlate with disease activity.[52,53] However, there is substantial evidence against a significant role for prostaglandins as mediators of inflammation in IBD. This evidence comes from a few small clinical studies of nonsteroidal antiinflammatory drugs (NSAIDs), particularly indomethacin, which are potent inhibitors of prostaglandin production.[54,55] Small trials of indomethacin administered orally and rectally revealed no improvement in ulcerative colitis; there was even some suggestion that indomethacin caused clinical deterioration despite decreasing prostaglandin production. The failure of NSAIDs to induce clinical improvement suggests that prostaglandins do not play important roles as mediators of inflammation in IBD.

Attention has now turned to the 5-lipoxygenase pathway, a pathway of arachidonic acid metabolism found primarily in cells of bone marrow origin involved in the inflammatory process—mast cells, neutrophils, monocytes, and macrophages. Neutrophils metabolize arachidonic acid to LTB$_4$, a potent chemotactic agent for neutrophils. Lipid extracts of IBD colonic mucosa contain large amounts of LTB$_4$,[56] and the concentrations of LTB$_4$ are markedly higher in rectal dialysates from ulcerative colitis patients than from controls.[57] The presence of large numbers of neutrophils in IBD mucosa suggests that there is a chemotactic factor (or factors) present in IBD mucosa that induces neutrophils to migrate out of the circulation and into the tissue. In vitro studies indicate that LTB$_4$ is the major neutrophil chemotactic agent in IBD mucosa.[58] Extrapolation to the in vivo situation would imply that LTB$_4$ is the mediator primarily responsible for neutrophils leaving the circulation and entering the intestinal tissue in IBD. One approach to improved therapy for IBD may be inhibition of neutrophil migration from the circulation into the mucosa and submucosa, which would diminish the intensity of the inflammatory response and, in turn, the degree of clinical disease activity. Drugs that block LTB$_4$ synthesis or inhibit LTB$_4$ binding to neutrophil receptors might be expected to diminish the inflammatory response and disease activity in IBD. Similarly, dietary supplementation with fish oil, containing eicosapentaenoic acid, which reduces LTB$_4$ production by acting as a competitive substrate for 5-lipoxygenase, results in significant but modest improvements in ulcerative colitis symptoms.[59] Other approaches to blocking neutrophil and monocyte migration may be useful in the management of IBD. Parenterally administered antibodies against adhesion molecules or soluble agents that bind to adhesion molecules may have clinical utility.

ULCERATIVE COLITIS: CLINICAL FINDINGS AND NATURAL HISTORY

Symptoms and Physical Findings

The dominant symptom in ulcerative colitis is diarrhea, which is usually, but not always, associated with blood in the stool.[60] Bowel movements are frequent but small in volume as a result of irritability of the inflamed rectum.[61] If inflammation is confined to the rectum, blood is seen only on the surface of the stool, but if inflammation is more extensive, blood is mixed in with the stool. Other symptoms include fever and pain, which may be in either lower quadrant or in the rectum. Many patients also experience noticeable weight loss. The patient's symptoms are a function, in part, of the extent of the disease. Systemic symptoms—fever, malaise, and weight loss—are more common if all or most of the colon is involved. If disease is confined to the rectum, the patient may complain only of bloody diarrhea with or without urgency, tenesmus, or rectal pain. Although diarrhea is the dominant complaint, some patients, especially elderly persons, complain of constipation. In these individuals, rectal spasm may prevent the passage of stool.

Classification by Severity

Truelove and Witts[62] devised a system for dividing ulcerative colitis patients into those with mild, moderately severe, and severe disease based on their symptoms, physical findings, and laboratory values (Table 79-2). This is a useful classification which helps the clinician predict both the anatomic extent of the patient's disease and the range of likely outcomes based on the presentation. This classification also helps the clinician judge how vigorously the patient needs to be treated.

Edwards and Truelove found that in 54% of their ulcerative colitis patients, the first attack was mild.[63] Mild disease is usually associated with inflammation confined to the rectum and sigmoid but can occur even in the presence of pancolonic involvement. Diarrhea and rectal bleeding are usually the only complaints in mild disease. Those patients with diarrhea but without rectal bleeding may be misdiagnosed as having irritable bowel syndrome, and those with rectal bleeding but without diarrhea may be misdiagnosed as bleeding from hemorrhoids. Mild disease, especially if confined to the rectum, is frequently associated with a normal physical examination.

Most patients with ulcerative proctitis have disease of mild severity. Ulcerative proctitis should not be viewed as a separate entity but rather as part of the spectrum of ulcerative colitis. Although most patients who present with proctitis continue to have disease confined to the rectum, there is extension to involve the more proximal colon in 15% of cases followed for 10 years,[64] with extension to the hepatic flexure in 7%.

In 27% of patients with ulcerative colitis, the first attack is of moderate severity. These patients typically present with five or six bloody bowel movements per day. Abdominal pain, which is uncommon in mild disease, may be present. Patients are fatigued and may have a low-grade fever. In moderate disease, there is often some degree of abdominal tenderness, but bowel sounds are usually normal. Initial attacks of moderate severity may be misdiagnosed as infectious colitis.

Edwards and Truelove found that 19% of their patients with ulcerative colitis presented with severe disease. In addition to having frequent episodes of bloody diarrhea, a patient with severe colitis is likely to be weak and may even be bedridden. If the attack is sustained, the patient develops weight loss, marked anemia, and hypoalbuminemia. Severe disease is marked by fever, tachycardia, and postural hypotension. Some abdominal tenderness is common even in mild disease, but significant abdominal tenderness, particularly with rebound over the colon, suggests severe disease. Markedly hypoactive or absent bowel sounds, indicating that the colon has lost all motility, is also a sign of severe disease. Protuberance of the abdomen, reflecting atony and dilation of the colon, raises the possibility of toxic megacolon.

Initial Attack

The initial attack of ulcerative colitis may be fulminant with bloody diarrhea present from the beginning; more commonly, the disease begins indolently, with nonbloody diarrhea progressing to bloody diarrhea.[65] Symptoms often gradually worsen over the course of a few weeks. Ulcerative colitis can present initially with any extent of anatomic involvement, from disease confined to the rectum to pancolitis, and with any degree of activity, from mild diarrhea to toxic megacolon. At initial presentation, colitis extending all the way to the cecum is seen in only about 20% of patients. Limited colitis is more common, with 75% of patients having no disease proximal to the sigmoid.[66] The greater the anatomic extent of the disease at the time of the first presentation, the more severe the symptoms are likely to be (Table 79-3).[65] Extraintestinal manifestations, most commonly arthralgias and mild arthritis, are present in fewer than 10% of patients at initial presentation.

Endoscopic examination of the colon is important at the time of the initial presentation both to establish the diagnosis and to determine the anatomic extent of the disease. In mild ulcerative colitis, the rectal mucosa is erythematous and edematous. In more severe disease, edema is more marked, the mucosa bleeds spontaneously, and there is an extensive purulent exudate. In the most severe cases, frank ulceration is seen.

The outcome of the first attack of ulcerative colitis can be predicted on the basis of the extent of the disease and the severity of the symptoms (Table 79-4).[66] More than 90% of patients with mild disease go into remission after the first attack. Among patients with more severe disease, a significant number require colectomy, and a few worsen and die; death occurs primarily in patients who present with toxic megacolon.

Clinical Evaluation

Management of ulcerative colitis involves repeated evaluation of the patient's clinical condition over time. These evaluations are required at the initial presentation, at the beginning of

---

TABLE 79-2
Truelove and Witts' Classification of Ulcerative Colitis

Severe

Diarrhea: six or more bowel movements per day, with blood
Fever: mean evening temperature higher than 37.5°C, or higher than 37.7°C on at least 2 of 4 days at any time of day
Tachycardia: mean pulse rate higher than 90 beats/minute
Anemia: hemoglobin of 75 mg/dL or less compared with normal values, allowing for recent transfusions
Sedimentation rate: more than 30 mm/h

Mild

Mild diarrhea: fewer than four bowel movements per day, with only small amounts of blood
No fever
No tachycardia
Mild anemia
Sedimentation rate: below 30 min/hour

Moderately Severe

Intermediate between mild and severe

Adapted from Truelove SS, Witts LJ. Cortisone in ulcerative colitis: final report on a therapeutic trial. Br Med J 1955;2:1041.

TABLE 79-3
Incidence of Severe First Attacks Related to Clinical Extent of Disease

EXTENT OF DISEASE	TOTAL NUMBER OF PATIENTS	NUMBER OF PATIENTS WITH SEVERE ATTACKS	INCIDENCE OF SEVERE ATTACKS (%)
Rectum	72	9	12.5
Sigmoid-splenic flexure	75	28	37.3
Total colon	41	24	58.5

Adapted from Watts JMcK, de Dombal FT, et al. Early course of ulcerative colitis. Gut 1966;7:16.

each subsequent attack to define the severity of the attack, and at multiple points during each attack to determine if the clinical picture is worsening or improving. The extent of the clinical evaluation is guided by the presentation; the milder the presentation, the less extensive the required evaluation. The most important part of the clinical evaluation is the history and physical examination. The frequency and severity of diarrhea is a good first guide to the severity of the disease. More than six bowel movements per day is usually associated with severe disease; however, comparison of the number of bowel movements with the patient's normal bowel habits may be more informative than the absolute number. Moreover, the number of bowel movements is a more useful indication of severity in acute than in chronic disease. Systemic signs and symptoms (fever, hypotension, tachycardia) are markers for the presence of severe disease and demand a more extensive evaluation. Coexistence of irritable bowel syndrome or infectious diarrhea with ulcerative colitis makes evaluation of the patient's symptoms more difficult.

Endoscopic examination is required at the initial presentation to help establish the diagnosis and define the extent of disease.[67] Endoscopic examination may be useful at the presentation of subsequent attacks if there is a question as to whether the attack is a recrudescence of ulcerative colitis. In patients with a past history of ulcerative colitis who develop diarrhea, proctoscopy is a useful method for distinguishing recurrences of ulcerative colitis from infectious diarrhea. Endoscopic examination may also be indicated if a recurrence of ulcerative colitis is more severe than earlier occurrences, suggesting anatomic extension of the disease. For patients with long-standing disease, colonoscopic examination is used for surveillance for dysplasia.[68,69] Some clinicians routinely follow the course of ulcerative colitis exacerbations by repeated proctoscopy, with the thought that the endoscopic picture provides important information about the response to drug therapy; however, there is no definitive evidence that this yields any more useful information than asking the patient about the severity of his or her symptoms. The usefulness of this practice is particularly questionable if the clinical picture is stable or improving. Similarly, with the possible exception of dysplasia surveillance, the usefulness of routine endoscopy as part of the periodic evaluation of patients with inactive ulcerative colitis has not been established.

One of the most important functions of clinical evaluation in exacerbations of ulcerative colitis is the identification of those patients who are progressing to toxic megacolon.[70,71] Fever, leukocytosis, and marked abdominal tenderness all indicate severe disease. Plain films of the abdomen demonstrate whether there is colonic dilatation consistent with toxic megacolon.

Laboratory studies also play a role in the clinical evaluation of ulcerative colitis. If the history and physical examination indicate mild disease activity, laboratory studies are likely to add little to the evaluation. They are most useful in confirming a clinical impression of severe disease and in following the clinical course of a severe exacerbation. The laboratory studies most likely to reflect disease activity are hemoglobin level, leukocyte count, and erythrocyte sedimentation rate. An elevated leukocyte count, however, may be difficult to interpret in patients treated with corticosteroids. Other biochemical abnormalities may be apparent. Hypoalbuminemia is a sign of severe disease, usually of long duration. Electrolyte disorders, particularly hypokalemia, are seen with severe diarrhea.

The role of microbial agents in inducing exacerbations of

TABLE 79-4
Outcome of First Attack of Ulcerative Colitis Versus Severity

	MILD	MODERATE	SEVERE
Total patients	364	138	33
Remission	333 (91.5%)	118 (84.9%)	13 (38.2%)
Surgical treatment	0 (0.0%)	5 (3.6%)	10 (29.0)%
Continuing symptoms	29 (8.0%)	11 (7.9%)	1 (2.9%)
Death (total)	5 (1.4%)	4 (2.9%)	8 (23.0%)
Death caused by colitis	0 (0.0%)	1 (0.7%)	8 (23.0%)

Adapted from Sinclair TS, Brunt PW, Mowat NAG. Nonspecific proctocolitis in northeastern Scotland: a community study. Gastroenterology 1983:85:1.

IBD has been a somewhat controversial area. Intercurrent intestinal infections, either bacterial (*Clostridium difficile, Campylobacter* species, *Yersinia* species) or viral (cytomegalovirus), have been implicated in inducing exacerbations. Although one study reported very high levels of recovery of *C difficile* toxin from patients with symptomatic relapses,[72] other studies have reported low rates.[73] There is no uniformity of opinion as to when patients with exacerbations of IBD should be tested for *C difficile*. A reasonable approach is to test patients if they are currently receiving or have recently received antibiotics. Routine stool culture for all exacerbations of IBD is not indicated.[72] Cytomegalovirus causes gastrointestinal infection and is fairly common in the immunosuppressed host (e.g., patients taking corticosteroids). The typical presentation is abdominal pain and watery diarrhea. Endoscopic biopsies show cytomegalovirus vasculitis within the lamina propria. Typical intranuclear inclusions are seen in endothelial cells. If cytomegalovirus is found, corticosteroids and immunosuppressives should be tapered and stopped if possible.

Natural History

Most commonly, ulcerative colitis follows a chronic intermittent course, marked by long periods of quiescence interspersed with acute attacks lasting weeks to months (Table 79-5).[63] In 18% of patients diagnosed as having ulcerative colitis, there is a single acute attack of colitis with no recurrences. However, one suspects that in some of these patients the diagnosis is not correct. A small but significant percentage of patients suffer a chronic continuous course with persistent symptoms and no complete remission. Patients who require continuous treatment with steroids to maintain them in remission are also part of this group.

Figure 79-2 presents the risk of relapse after the first attack of ulcerative colitis as a function of the patient's age at the time of the first attack.[66] Older patients are more likely than younger ones to go long periods of time without relapse. For those younger than 50 years of age, the median time for relapse after the first attack is 2 to 3 years. Neither the severity of the first attack nor the extent of colonic involvement at the time of diagnosis has any effect on the frequency of recurrence. However, the severity and extent of the disease at the time of

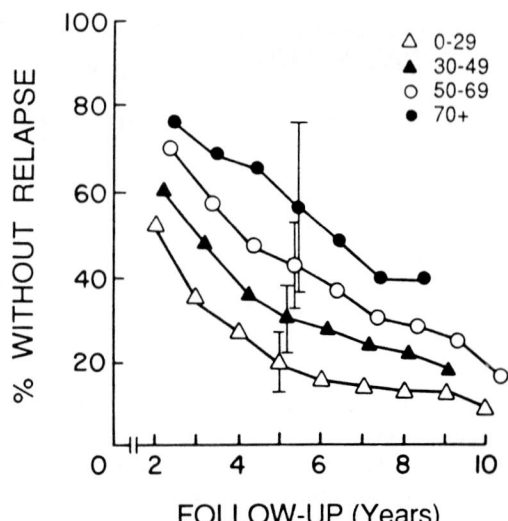

FIGURE 79-2. Risk of relapse following first attack of ulcerative colitis versus age. (From Sinclair TS, Brunt PW, Mowat NAG. Nonspecific proctocolitis in northeastern Scotland: a community study. Gastroenterology 1983;85:1.)

initial presentation has a great effect on the likelihood and timing of subsequent colectomy.[66] For those with severe disease at first presentation, the rate of colectomy reaches 50% by 2 years after the initial attack (Fig. 79-3). For those with pancolitis, the rate of colectomy reaches 50% after 5 years. In contrast, fewer than 10% of patients who present with mild disease or with proctitis alone have undergone colectomy after 10 years. As with the risk of relapse, the cumulative resection rate among patients with ulcerative colitis is inversely proportional to age. Those in the oldest age group are the least likely to suffer relapse and the least likely to undergo resection.

TABLE 79-5
Clinical Course of Ulcerative Colitis

CLINICAL COURSE	NUMBER OF PATIENTS	PERCENTAGE
Acute fulminating	20	8.0
Chronic intermittent	161	64.4
Chronic continuous	18	7.2
One attack only	45	18.0
Total colectomy in first attack	2	0.8
Died in first attack of other causes	1	0.4
Unknown	2	0.8
Total	249	100.0

Adapted from Edwards FC, Truelove SC. The course and prognosis of ulcerative colitis. Gut 1963;4:299.

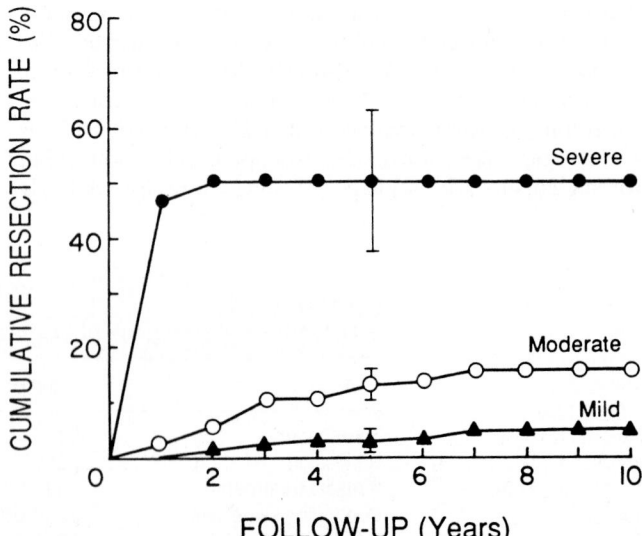

FIGURE 79-3. Cumulative resection rate in ulcerative colitis versus severity of first attack. (From Sinclair TS, Brunt PW, Mowat NAG. Nonspecific proctocolitis in northeastern Scotland: a community study. Gastroenterology 1983;85:1.)

CROHN'S DISEASE: CLINICAL FINDINGS AND NATURAL HISTORY

Disease Location

Crohn's disease is a more complex and difficult clinical entity than ulcerative colitis, partially because of the diversity of anatomic locations in which it is detected and the effects of this diversity on presentation, clinical course, and therapeutic options. There are three major patterns of disease distribution: disease present in the ileum and cecum, a pattern seen in 40% of patients at presentation; disease confined to the small intestine, a pattern seen in 30% of patients at presentation; and disease confined to the colon, a pattern seen in 25% of patients at presentation.[74] Among those with colonic disease, most have pancolitis but about a third have segmental disease. Much less commonly, Crohn's disease involves more proximal parts of the gastrointestinal tract—the mouth, the tongue, the esophagus, the stomach, and the duodenum.

The predominant symptoms in Crohn's disease are diarrhea, abdominal pain, and weight loss.[74,75] Any one of these three symptoms may be most prominent in a given individual. This is in contrast to ulcerative colitis, in which diarrhea is almost universally the most prominent complaint. The initial presentation of Crohn's disease may not be dramatic. Patients may complain for months or years with vague abdominal pain and intermittent diarrhea before the diagnosis of Crohn's disease is considered.

Diarrhea occurs in almost all those with Crohn's disease, but the pattern varies with the anatomic location of the disease (Table 79-6).[74] In patients with colonic disease, especially with rectal involvement, diarrhea may be of small volume and associated with urgency and tenesmus; in disease confined to the small intestine, stools are of larger volume and not associated with urgency or tenesmus. Patients with severe involvement of the terminal ileum and those who have had surgical resections of the terminal ileum may have elements of bile salt diarrhea or, in more severe cases, frank steatorrhea.[76] Strictures in the small intestine may lead to bacterial overgrowth with deconjugation of bile salts and fat malab-

sorption. If diarrhea is a product of fat malabsorption, the timing and severity of the diarrhea are a function of the pattern of fat ingestion. Finally, internal fistulas are common in Crohn's disease and can lead to diarrhea either by colonization of the small bowel with bacteria, as in enterocolonic fistulas, or through bypass of large segments of absorptive epithelium, as in enteroenteric or enterocolonic fistulas.

The location and pattern of pain in Crohn's disease often correlate with disease location. One common pain pattern is cramping right lower quadrant pain in patients with ileocolonic disease.[77] This pain usually occurs after eating and is probably related to partial intermittent obstruction of a narrowed intestinal lumen. Pain is caused by stretching of the wall in the dilated segment proximal to the obstruction and by powerful contractions of the small bowel musculature attempting to push intestinal contents through the obstructed segment. Abdominal distention, nausea, and vomiting may accompany pain in this circumstance. Visceral pain may result from inflammation of the serosa, as is seen in transmural Crohn's disease. The pathophysiologic basis of abdominal pain in other forms of Crohn's disease is less clear. Pain management is a prominent therapeutic problem in many patients with Crohn's disease.

Weight loss of some degree occurs in most patients with Crohn's disease irrespective of anatomic location. Loss of more than 20% of body weight is less common, occurring in 10% to 20% of affected individuals. Some weight loss is a product of malabsorption, but for most individuals, weight loss is a product of diminished intake. Patients, especially those with small bowel disease, may avoid food because eating brings on pain or diarrhea or, more commonly, because they are anorectic. Colonic disease is associated with a high incidence of rectal bleeding and perianal involvement but a low incidence of internal fistulas and obstruction (see Table 79-6). In contrast, disease confined to the small intestine is associated with a lower incidence of bleeding and perianal involvement but a higher incidence of obstruction.

Physical findings in Crohn's disease also vary with the distribution and severity of the disease.[78,79] When the disease is active, the patient looks pale, weak, and chronically ill. Longstanding severe disease with malnutrition results in temporal and interosseous wasting. The abdomen may be tender, typically over the area of disease activity. Thickened bowel loops, thickened mesentery, or an abscess may cause a sense of fullness or a mass, often in the right lower quadrant. The presence of perianal Crohn's disease is suggested by fistulous openings, induration, redness, or tenderness near the anus.

Laboratory findings in Crohn's disease are largely nonspecific.[80] The peripheral blood count may reveal anemia resulting from chronic disease, blood loss, or nutritional deficiencies (iron, folate, or vitamin B_{12}). A modestly elevated leukocyte count is indicative of active Crohn's disease, but a marked elevation suggests the presence of an abscess or other suppurative complication. Thrombocytosis may occur with active disease. Bleeding or thrombotic complications may seen secondary to thrombocytosis. The erythrocyte sedimentation rate has been used to follow disease activity in Crohn's disease, and it tends to be higher in colonic disease than ileal disease. Hypoalbuminemia is a good indication of disease severity and malnutrition. Ileal disease or ileal resection results in a diminished serum vitamin B_{12} level because of malabsorption.

TABLE 79-6
Frequency of Clinical Features in Crohn's Disease

CLINICAL FEATURE	DISEASE LOCATION (%)		
	Ileitis (%)	Ileocolitis (%)	Colitis (%)
Diarrhea	~100	~100	~100
Abdominal pain	65	62	55
Bleeding	22	10	46
Weight loss	12	19	22
Perianal disease	14	38	36
Internal fistulae	17	34	16
Intestinal obstruction	35	44	17
Megacolon	0	2	11
Arthritis	4	4	16
Spondylitis	1	2	5

Adapted from Farmer RG, Hawk WA, Turnbull RB. Clinical patterns in Crohn's disease: a statistical study of 615 cases. Gastroenterology 1975;68:627.

Crohn's disease may rarely involve the stomach and duodenum. In these cases, more distal involvement, particularly of the ileum, is usually also present. Gastroduodenal Crohn's disease may present with epigastric pain like that of duodenal ulcer. Upper gastrointestinal series may show ulceration and narrowing of the antrum and duodenum (Fig. 79-4). Aphthous ulcers and linear ulcers in the gastric antrum may be seen on endoscopy.[81] Therapy is the same as for ileal Crohn's disease, although a trial of H_2-receptor antagonists is useful for those with ulcers. Duodenal Crohn's disease often leads to stenosis, obstruction, and postprandial vomiting.[82] Gastrojejunostomy without resection may be required to bypass the obstruction but should be avoided if possible.

Disease Activity Indices

It is often difficult to assess the course of disease activity in Crohn's disease. There are usually a number of different disease manifestations (increased number of bowel movements, diminished general sense of well-being, fistula formation, weight loss, decreased hematocrit, endoscopic appearance, histology, increased sedimentation rate, increased orosomucoid levels), which do not necessarily improve or worsen in parallel. This problem becomes particularly obvious in comparing medical therapies or in assessing the efficacy of new medical therapies. There are many markers of disease activity that can be followed, and it is difficult to interpret studies in which some markers improve but others do not. Several attempts have been made to establish numerical systems for evaluating disease severity and response to therapy in Crohn's disease.[83-87] The National Cooperative Crohn's Disease Study devised the Crohn's Disease Activity Index (CDAI) for evaluating response to therapy in that study.[83] The CDAI was calculated by assigning numerical scores to the number of diarrheal stools, abdominal pain, general well-being, systemic manifestations, use of antidiarrheal agents, presence of abdominal mass, hematocrit, and body weight. These factors are quantified and weighted, and a final score is generated by adding up the scores for the eight parameters. This scoring system is complicated and has been criticized for placing excessive weight on the number of bowel movements per day, a parameter that is influenced by factors other than disease activity. For example, a patient who had significant diarrhea caused by an ileocolic resection could have a high CDAI even if the disease were inactive. Other groups have proposed and used alternative numerical indices to quantify Crohn's activity, but these indices, although promoted as simplified, are not especially easy to use, nor are they necessarily more valid than the CDAI.[80,85-87]

Natural History

Crohn's disease, like ulcerative colitis, is a relapsing and remitting disease. About 30% of placebo-treated patients with Crohn's disease of mild to moderate activity go into remission within 4 months.[88,89] Conversely, if a group of patients with Crohn's disease in remission and on no therapy is followed, about 70% remain in remission at 1 year and 50% at 2 years. Within 10 years of diagnosis, 60% of Crohn's patients have surgery. Postoperatively, there are endoscopic signs of recurrence in 70% of patients at 1 year, and there is recurrence of symptoms in 40% to 50% within 4 years of operation. Of those patients who have one surgical resection for Crohn's disease, 45% will eventually require reoperation.

Many patients with Crohn's disease suffer significant disability because of their disease. Although employment rates for Crohn's patients are high, half of Crohn's patients make significant changes in their employment as a result of their disease.[90] These changes include decreased hours, leaves of absence, and career changes.

EXTRAINTESTINAL MANIFESTATIONS

Although ulcerative colitis and Crohn's disease primarily involve the bowel, they are both associated with manifestations in other organ systems. For some patients, especially those with sclerosing cholangitis or ankylosing spondylitis, the extraintestinal manifestations may be more problematic than the bowel disease. The extraintestinal manifestations can be divided into two major groups: those in which the clinical activity follows the activity of the bowel disease and those in which the clinical activity is unrelated to the clinical activity of the bowel disease. Most extraintestinal manifestations occur more commonly with ulcerative colitis or Crohn's colitis than with Crohn's disease confined to the small intestine.

The most common extraintestinal manifestation of IBD is arthritis (Table 79-7).[91-94] The two arthritic complications of IBD are colitic arthritis and ankylosing spondylitis. Colitic arthritis is a migratory arthritis that affects knees, hips, ankles, wrists, and elbows; usually, fewer than six joints are involved.[92] Colitic arthritis is more common with Crohn's colitis than ulcerative colitis and is uncommon with Crohn's disease confined to the small intestine. The majority of arthritic flares

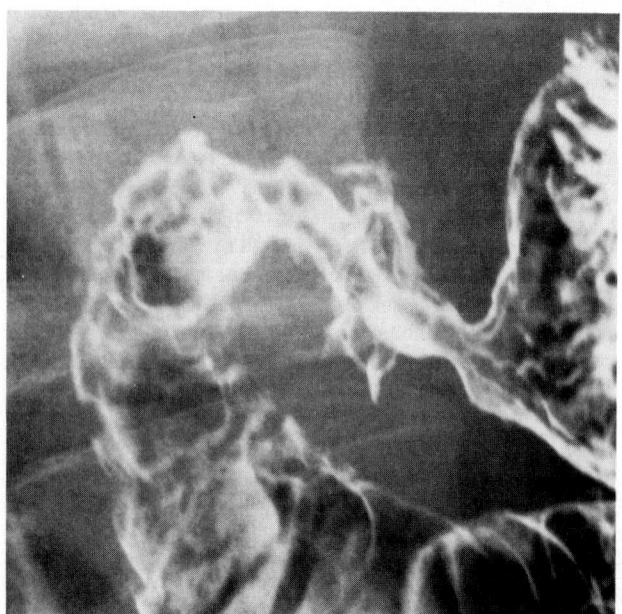

FIGURE 79-4. Crohn's disease involving the antrum and duodenum. (Courtesy of Dennis Balfe, M.D., St. Louis, MO.)

TABLE 79-7
**Extraintestinal Manifestations in 202 Patients
With Ulcerative Colitis**

ORGAN INVOLVED	NUMBER OF PATIENTS	PERCENTAGE OF TOTAL
Joint	53	26
Polyarthralgia	27	13
Spine	8	4
Extremities	18	9
Skin	39	19
Erythema nodosum	9	4
Pyoderma gangrenosum	10	5
Other	20	10
Mouth	8	4
Eye	9	13
Total patients	202	

Adapted from Greenstein AJ, Janowitz HD, Sachar DB. Extra-intestinal complications of Crohn's disease and ulcerative colitis: Study of 700 patients. Medicine (Baltimore) 1979;55:401.

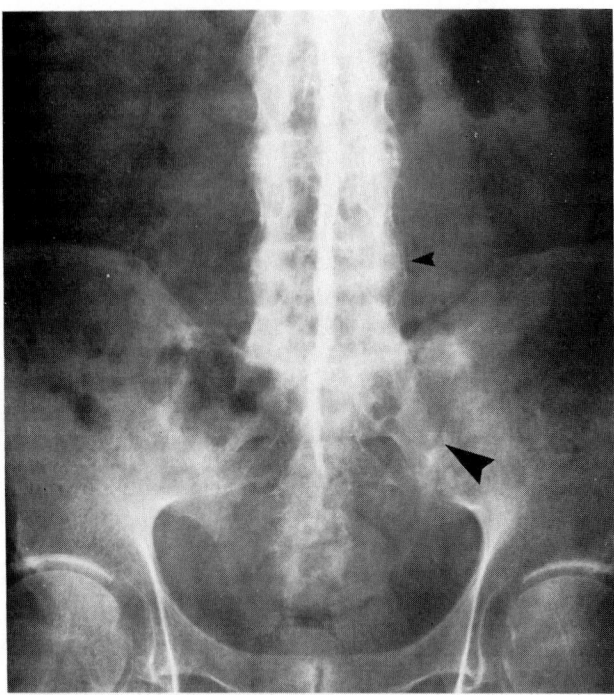

FIGURE 79-5. Sacroiliitis and ankylosing spondylitis demonstrating obliteration of the sacroiliac joints (*large arrow*) and bamboo spine with syndesmophytes (*small arrow*). (Courtesy of Dennis Balfe, M.D., St. Louis, MO.)

last only a few weeks. Deformity with radiologic changes occurs in fewer than 25% of cases. The joint pain, swelling, and stiffness parallel the course of the bowel disease. Successful treatment of the intestinal inflammation results in improvement in the arthritis. Colitic arthritis responds well to corticosteroids. Often, treatment of bowel disease with corticosteroids results in a dramatic improvement in the associated arthritis. Colitic arthritis, uveitis, and erythema nodosum are often seen together.

Sacroiliitis with ankylosing spondylitis is seen in patients with IBD, but its activity does not follow that of the bowel disease, and treatment of the bowel disease does not affect the spondylitis.[93,94] Ankylosing spondylitis presents with morning stiffness, low back pain, and stooped posture. Radiographs of the pelvis in sacroiliitis reveal blurring of the margins of the sacroiliac joints, with patchy sclerosis. Radiography of the spine in ankylosing spondylitis shows squaring of the vertebrae and straightening of the spine. Syndesmophytes appear along the lateral and anterior portions of the intervertebral discs, giving the picture of "bamboo spine" (Fig. 79-5).

Patients with ulcerative colitis have a 30-fold increase in the incidence of ankylosing spondylitis compared with the general population. Even though there is not an increased incidence of HLA-B27 in ulcerative colitis, 80% of those with both ulcerative colitis and ankylosing spondylitis are B27-positive.[95] In contrast to colitic arthritis, which is episodic and usually nondeforming, ankylosing spondylitis can be relentlessly progressive and crippling. The results of medical management of ankylosing spondylitis in IBD are poor. Nonsteroidal antiinflammatory drugs reduce inflammation and pain in spondylitis and in colitic arthritis but do not halt the progression of the disease. There is also considerable anecdotal evidence that nonsteroidal antiinflammatory drugs can exacerbate IBD. Physical therapy plays a major role in maintaining function. Regular range of motion exercises prevent the development of contractures and preserve joint function. A physical or occupational therapist can teach patients to bend

or to carry objects in ways that are least likely to damage inflamed joints. Pain management is a problem, and narcotic addiction is common. Medical treatment of the IBD and colectomy are not helpful in managing the ankylosing spondylitis. Sacroiliitis alone is more common than sacroiliitis with ankylosing spondylitis in patients with ulcerative colitis. Many patients with sacroiliitis alone are asymptomatic, and the diagnosis is frequently made incidentally on radiographs of the pelvis.[96]

The hepatic complications of IBD include fatty liver, pericholangitis, chronic active hepatitis, and cirrhosis. The biliary tract complications are sclerosing cholangitis and gallstones. Cholesterol gallstones occur in patients with ileal disease or ileal resections owing to malabsorption of bile salts and the resultant decrease in the size of the bile salt pool. The combination of gallstones and an ileal stricture in Crohn's disease can give rise to ileal obstruction by a gallstone impacted in the stricture (Fig. 79-6).

Pericholangitis is the most common hepatic complication of IBD, with prevalences as high as 50% to 80% reported.[97,98] Patients with pericholangitis are usually asymptomatic. Elevations of alkaline phosphatase are seen frequently; elevations of bilirubin are less common. Histologically, there is inflammation of the portal tracts, with lymphocyte and eosinophil infiltrates and degenerative changes of the bile ductules.[99] In more advanced cases, there can be progressive fibrosis. The diagnosis of pericholangitis is made by liver biopsy. Some studies have suggested that pericholangitis may be a part of the spectrum of sclerosing cholangitis, and the histologic manifestations of sclerosing cholangitis and pericholangitis on liver biopsy may be indistinguishable.[100] For this reason,

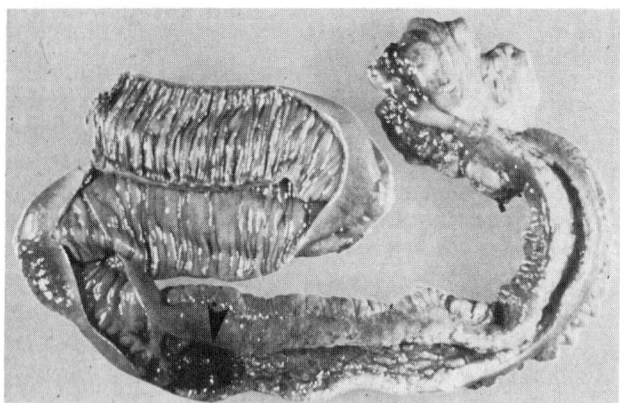

FIGURE 79-6. Crohn's ileitis with gallstone (*arrow*) impacted in stricture. (Courtesy of Ira Kodner, M.D., St. Louis, MO.)

patients diagnosed as having pericholangitis on liver biopsy may need to undergo endoscopic retrograde cholangiopancreatography (ERCP) to rule out sclerosing cholangitis. There is no effective therapy for pericholangitis.

Sclerosing cholangitis is a chronic cholestatic liver disease marked by fibrosing inflammation of the intrahepatic and extrahepatic bile ducts; it occurs in 1 to 4% of patients with ulcerative colitis and with lower frequency in Crohn's disease.[101,102] The majority of patients with sclerosing cholangitis have IBD. The prevalence of IBD is so high in patients with sclerosing cholangitis that colonoscopy should be performed even on those without intestinal symptoms. Endoscopic and histologic evidence of IBD are not uncommonly found in sclerosing cholangitis patients without intestinal symptoms. Sclerosing cholangitis can affect intrahepatic bile ducts, extrahepatic bile ducts, or both. In patients with IBD and sclerosing cholangitis, usually both intrahepatic and extrahepatic ducts are affected. Early in the disease, liver biopsy shows enlargement of the portal tracts, with edema and bile duct proliferation. Later on, biopsies show extension of fibrosis out of the portal space, eventually leading to cirrhosis.

Bile duct strictures are the major clinical problem in sclerosing cholangitis; strictures can occur in both intrahepatic and extrahepatic bile ducts (Fig. 79-7). Patients may be asymptomatic until the disease is far advanced and then present with fever, right upper quadrant pain, and jaundice. More often, sclerosing cholangitis is first recognized in the evaluation of abnormal laboratory studies—elevated alkaline phosphatase, bilirubin, and transaminases. The differential diagnosis of sclerosing cholangitis includes biliary tumors and common duct gallstones; diagnosis is made by ERCP or transhepatic cholangiography. Sclerosing cholangitis progresses to cirrhosis, hepatic failure, and death in 5 to 10 years.[103] Endoscopic balloon dilatation or stenting of extrahepatic strictures may be palliative. Cholestyramine, a bile salt–binding resin, may help relieve pruritus. Colectomy and medical therapy of the bowel disease are without benefit in the management of sclerosing cholangitis. Liver transplantation has been used with success, and sclerosing cholangitis is now one of the most common indications for liver transplantation in adults. Cholangiocarcinoma develops in 10% to 15% of IBD patients with long-standing sclerosing chol-

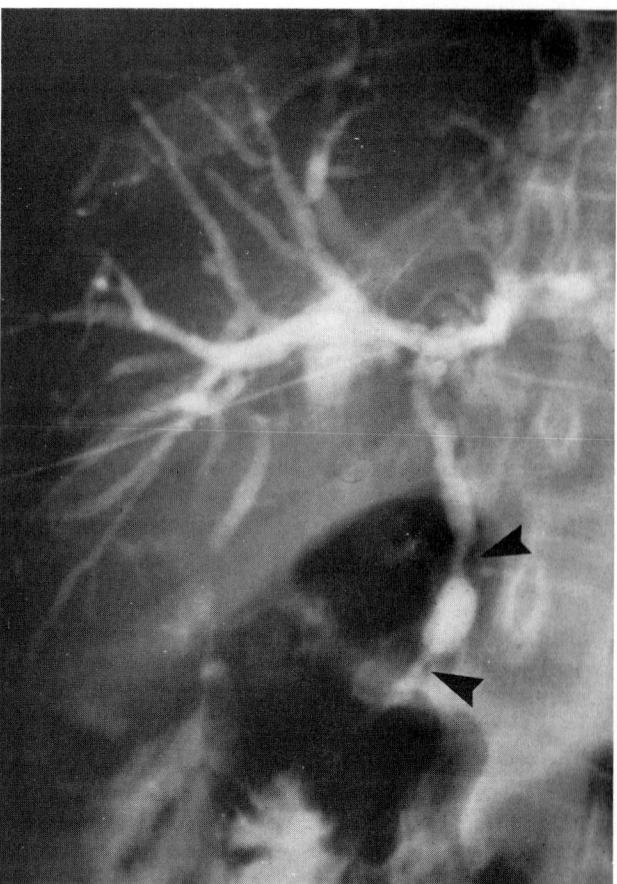

FIGURE 79-7. Sclerosing cholangitis with segmental strictures (*arrows*) in common bile duct. There are also strictures in the intrahepatic bile ducts. (Courtesy of Dennis Balfe, M.D., St. Louis, MO.)

angitis. Differentiating cholangiocarcinoma from the benign strictures of sclerosing cholangitis is difficult. ERCP with brushing or cholangioscopy with biopsy may help to make this distinction.

The incidence of kidney stones in IBD patients is several times that in the general population.[104,105] Calcium oxalate stones are seen in patients with small intestine Crohn's disease. Ileal resections or ileal disease leads to fat malabsorption, and unabsorbed fatty acids bind calcium in the lumen. In normal individuals, oxalate in the lumen is bound to calcium. Calcium oxalate is poorly soluble and poorly absorbed. However, if calcium is bound to malabsorbed fatty acids, oxalate combines with sodium to form sodium oxalate which is soluble and is absorbed in the colon.[106] The development of calcium oxalate stones in Crohn's disease requires an intact colon to absorb oxalate; patients with ileostomies do not develop calcium oxalate stones. However, the presence of an ileostomy predisposes to other kinds of kidney stones, particularly urate stones, because of the diminished urine volumes in patients with significant ileostomy volume losses.[104,107]

There are two urinary tract complications associated specifically with Crohn's disease. Inflammation from the bowel extending into the retroperitoneal space can occlude the ureters, leading to obstruction and hydronephrosis.[354] This process most commonly extends from the area of the cecum and terminal ileum and involves the right ureter. Also in Crohn's disease, fistulas can form between inflamed bowel and the urinary bladder, leading to urinary tract infections.[305,306]

The two dermal complications of IBD are pyoderma gangrenosum and erythema nodosum. Pyoderma gangrenosum is seen with colitis and ileocolitis and is associated with extensive disease of long standing. The incidence of pyoderma in ulcerative colitis is low (1%–5%), and it is even lower in Crohn's disease; however, 36% to 50% of all patients with pyoderma gangrenous have IBD.[108,109] The typical lesion is a discrete ulcer with a necrotic base, usually found on the lower extremities (Fig. 79-8). The ulcers may drain purulent material, but the drainage is sterile on culture. These ulcers can become large and deep, with destruction of surrounding soft tissues. Activity of pyoderma gangrenosum may or may not follow the activity of the bowel disease, but these lesions almost always develop during a bout of acute colitis. They usually resolve with control of the colitis by use of oral corticosteroids. Alternatively, corticosteroids can be injected directly into the skin lesions. Therapy with periactin, dapsone, cyclosporine, and azathioprine have all been reported.[110,111] In rare cases, colectomy is required to control the pyoderma. Erythema nodosum is seen particularly in association with Crohn's disease in children.[112] The lesions are raised, tender nodules which are usually found over the anterior surface of the tibia. Activity of erythema nodosum follows the activity of the bowel disease and responds to treatment of the bowel disease. Most patients have just a single episode of erythema nodosum.

The ocular complications of IBD are uveitis and episcleritis.[113] Uveitis (iritis) is an inflammatory lesion of the anterior chamber, presenting with blurred vision, headache, eye pain, photophobia, and conjunctival injection. Diagnosis is made by slit-lamp examination, which demonstrates perilimbic edema and cells in the anterior chamber. Local therapy with corticosteroids and atropine or other agents that dilate the pupil helps to prevent scarring and blindness. Episcleritis is a less serious problem, presenting with burning eyes and scleral injection. Treatment with topical steroids is effective.

Amyloidosis is seen in patients with Crohn's disease and has caused death from renal insufficiency.[114] Renal amyloidosis does not respond to conventional medical therapy for Crohn's disease and, for the most part, does not improve after the inflamed section of intestine is resected.

Thromboembolic events occur in ulcerative colitis and Crohn's disease. Activation of clotting factors and thrombocytosis are common. In ulcerative colitis, increased levels of factor V, factor VIII, and fibrinogen and decreased levels of antithrombin III have been demonstrated.[115,116] Deep vein thrombosis and pulmonary emboli affect patients with severe disease and may occur after colectomy. Thromboembolic events in the eye and in intracranial vessels have also been described.[115,117]

PATHOLOGY

Ulcerative colitis and Crohn's disease each have a characteristic pathologic appearance, but in any given case the pathologic picture may not be specific enough to distinguish between them, or to differentiate these forms of IBD from other diseases such as infectious colitis or ischemic colitis. In both ulcerative colitis and Crohn's disease, the pathologic picture is influenced by the degree of disease activity; the pathologic assessment of disease activity may or may not correlate with the clinical and endoscopic assessments.

Macroscopic features of pathologic specimens in ulcerative colitis depend on the severity and duration of the disease. In severe disease, the mucosa is edematous and deep purple owing to congestion with blood (Fig. 79-9). The distribution of the involved mucosa is also characteristic of ulcerative colitis. The inflammation begins in the rectum, extends proximally a certain distance, and then abruptly stops, with a clear demarcation between involved and uninvolved mucosa (see Fig. 79-9). In mild disease, there are superficial erosions, whereas

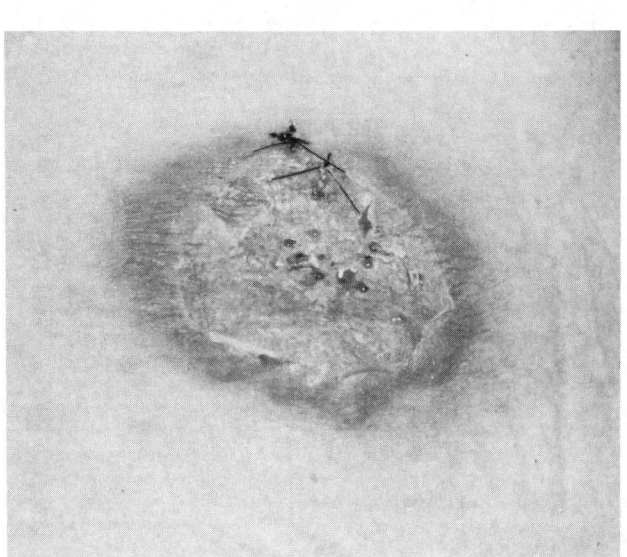

FIGURE 79-8. Pyoderma gangrenosum (with stitches after biopsy). (Courtesy of Ira Kodner, M.D., St. Louis, MO.)

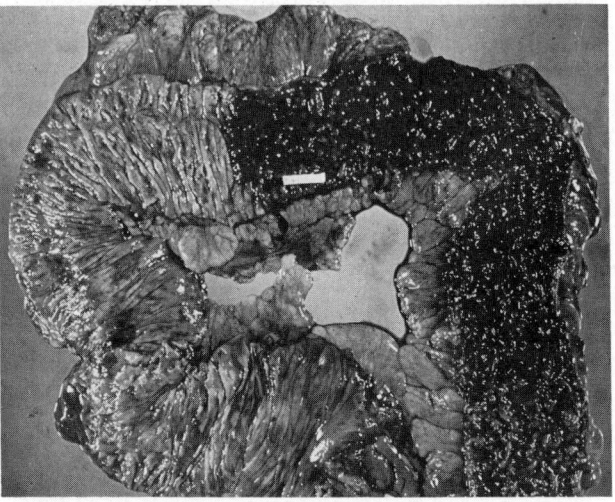

FIGURE 79-9. Colectomy specimen from patient with ulcerative colitis demonstrates sharp demarcation in the midtransverse colon between involved and uninvolved mucosa. (Courtesy of Ira Kodner, M.D., St. Louis, MO.)

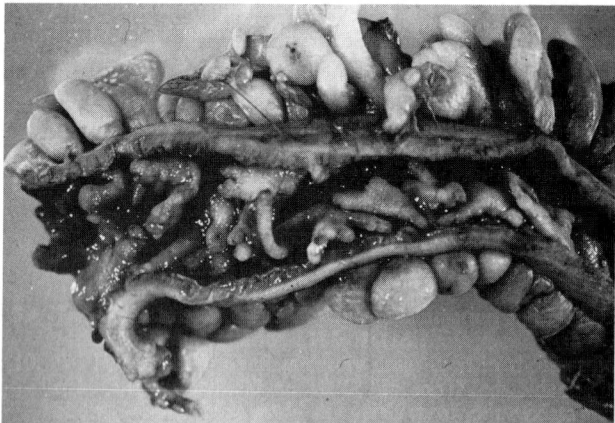

FIGURE 79-10. Filiform pseudopolyps. (Courtesy of Ira Kodner, M.D., St. Louis, MO.)

in severe disease, there may be large ulcers or areas in which the mucosa is completely denuded. In chronic disease, the mucosa loses its normal folds and becomes flat. Inflammatory polyps or pseudopolyps may be present; rarely, these polyps may be long (filiform polyps) and occur in groups (Fig. 79-10).

Most of the pathologic findings in ulcerative colitis are limited to the mucosa and submucosa (Fig. 79-11); the muscularis propria is affected only in fulminant disease. Active ulcerative colitis is marked by an intense infiltrate, with neutrophils in the mucosa and submucosa and clumps of neutrophils in crypt lumens (crypt abscesses) (Fig. 79-12). Although characteristic of active ulcerative colitis, the presence of a neutrophil infiltrate with crypt abscesses may also be seen in Crohn's disease and infectious colitis. In active ulcerative colitis, there is mucus depletion and mucosal edema; vascular congestion with focal hemorrhage is seen in more severe cases. There may be a villous character to the mucosal surface in ulcerative colitis. Ulcers, if present, tend to be superficial, only penetrating the muscularis mucosa in severe disease. In addition to signs of acute activity, there are usually also signs of chronicity, with lymphoid aggregates, plasma cells, mast cells, and eosinophils in the lamina propria. In quiescent ulcerative colitis, the inflammatory infiltrate is less intense than in active disease, but the mucosa is usually architecturally abnormal. The crypts are reduced in number and often branched. Shortening and branching of the crypts is typical of ulcerative colitis, although it may also be seen in Crohn's disease. In quiescent disease, goblet cell mucin content is restored to normal.

Histologic evaluation of rectal biopsy may be helpful in differentiating ulcerative colitis from acute self-limited colitis and from Crohn's disease (Table 79-8).[118] Distorted crypt

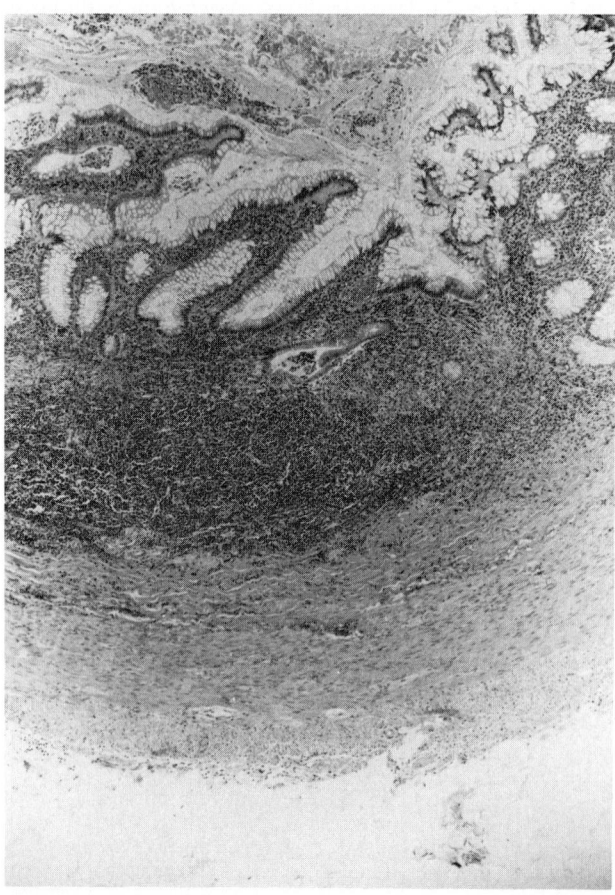

FIGURE 79-11. Ulcerative colitis in the appendix showing mucosal inflammation with crypt abscesses. Note the absence of inflammation in the muscularis propria. (Courtesy of David Lacey, M.D., St. Louis, MO.)

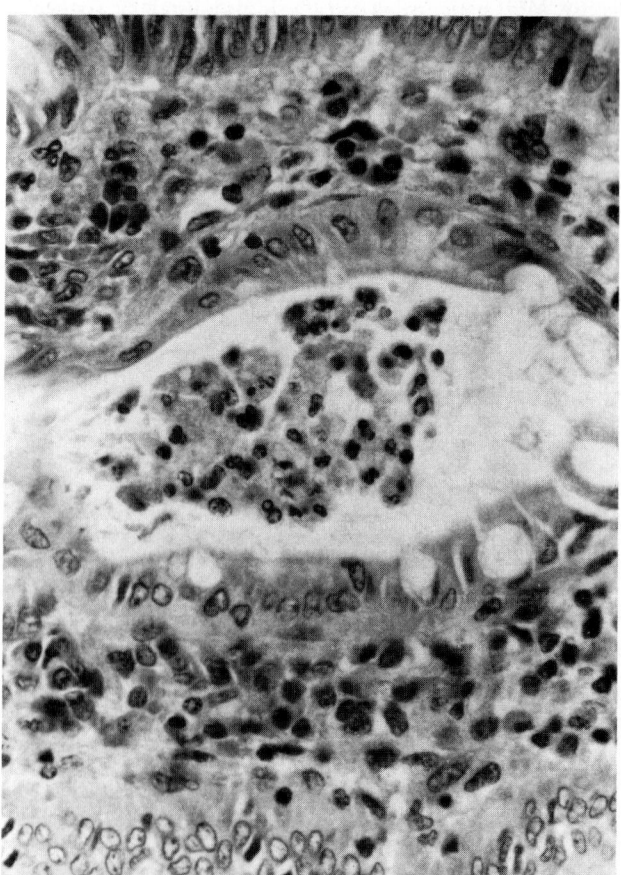

FIGURE 79-12. Crypt abscess from the specimen shown in Figure 79-11. (Courtesy of David Lacey, M.D., St. Louis, MO.)

TABLE 79-8
Histologic Features That Allow the Physician to Distinguish Among Acute Self-Limited Colitis (ASLC), Ulcerative Colitis (UC), and Crohn's Disease (CD)*

FEATURE	ASLC (44)	UC (56)	ASLC vs. UC (P*)	CD (26)	ASLC vs. CD (P*)	UC vs. CD (P*)
Distorted crypt architecture	0	32	<0.00001	7	<0.0005	0.01
Mixed lamina propria inflammation	0	15	<0.001	7	<0.001	NS
Villous surface	0	22	<0.00001	3	<0.047	<0.11
Granuloma	1†	3†	NS	16	<0.0017	<0.00001
Crypt atrophy	0	16	<0.0001	3	<0.048	<0.047
Basal lymphoid aggregates	0	12	<0.0011	3	NS	NS
Surface erosions	4	21	<0.0011	2	NS	<0.007
Superficial isolated giant cell	7	3	NS	0	NS	NS
Basal isolated giant cell	1	6	NS	3	NS	NS
Polymorphonuclear cells in surface epithelium	9	19	NS	3	NS	<0.04

NS, not significant; P, probability

* Statistics compared ASLC with UC and with CD, and UC with CD, using the Pearson χ^2 test.

† The presence of granulomas in three UC cases probably reflects the fact that rectal biopsy information was not used in the clinical categorization of cases.

From Surawicz CM, Belic L, Rectal biopsy helps to distinguish acute self-limited colitis from idiopathic inflammatory bowel disease. Gastroenterology 1984;86:104.

architecture, mixed acute and chronic inflammation in the lamina propria, a villous mucosa, and crypt atrophy are all far more common in ulcerative colitis than in acute self-limited colitis. The best histologic distinction between Crohn's colitis and ulcerative colitis is the presence of granulomas, which, in one series, were seen in 16 of 26 patients with Crohn's colitis but in only 3 of 56 patients with ulcerative colitis. Crypt atrophy, polymorphonuclear leukocytes in the epithelium, and surface erosions are each significantly more common in ulcerative colitis than Crohn's colitis. Despite these distinctions, ulcerative colitis and Crohn's disease cannot be distinguished histologically in 15% to 25% of cases.[119]

Gross examination of the intestine in Crohn's disease shows the bowel wall to be thickened and stiff. The mesentery is thickened and edematous and may be contracted, which fixes the intestine in one position. Adipose tissue extends from the mesentery and "creeps" over the serosal surface of the intestine. Transmural inflammation may cause loops of intestine to be matted together. Opening of a segment of involved intestine shows that all the layers of the intestine are thickened and the lumen is narrowed (Fig. 79-13). Deep linear ulcers with intervening normal mucosa give the mucosal surface the appearance of having been clawed (Fig. 79-14). The distribution of inflammation in the gross specimen may suggest

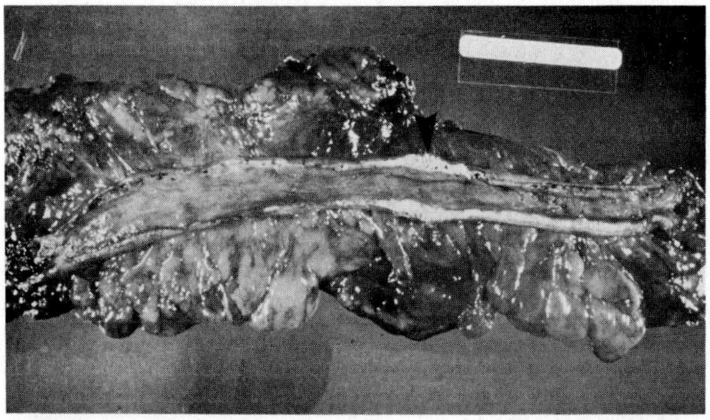

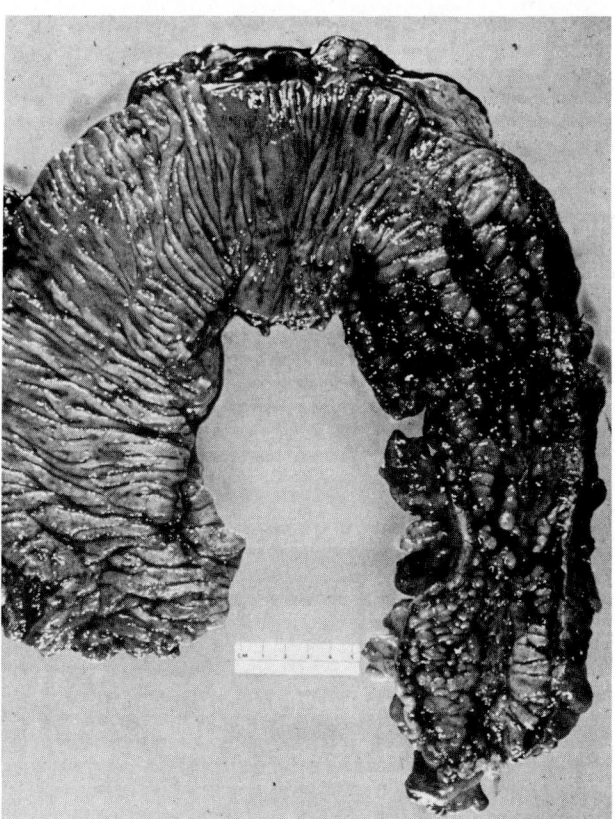

FIGURE 79-14. Crohn's colitis colectomy specimen shows deep, clawed linear ulcers in the transverse and descending colon. (Courtesy of Ira Kodner, M.D., St. Louis, MO.)

FIGURE 79-13. Crohn's disease of the small intestine showing lumenal narrowing and thickening of the intestinal wall (*arrow*). There is also a large amount of fat on the serosa. (Courtesy of Ira Kodner, M.D., St. Louis, MO.)

the diagnosis of Crohn's disease. Colonic inflammation with rectal sparing is more consistent with Crohn's disease than with ulcerative colitis.

The earliest lesion of Crohn's disease is the aphthoid ulcer. In the small intestine, aphthoid ulcers typically occur over Peyer patches, and in the colon over lymphoid aggregates. However, aphthoid ulcers can occur anywhere in the epithelium, even where there is no lymphoid tissue. As the disease progresses, aphthoid ulcers enlarge and become stellate. Eventually, the stellate ulcers coalesce to form longitudinal and transverse linear ulcers. The remaining islands of nonulcerated mucosa give a cobblestone appearance. Fissures develop from the base of aphthoid ulcers, extending down through the muscularis to the serosa. Free perforation is uncommon because serositis induces the adherence of other bowel loops into which the fissure extends.

Transmural inflammation is the histologic hallmark of Crohn's disease (Fig. 79-15).[120] Lymphoid aggregates are found in the submucosa and external to the muscularis propria. Occasional lymphoid aggregates in the muscularis propria complete the transmural pattern. Granulomas are found in most surgical resections for Crohn's disease (Fig. 79-16), but the exact percentage of positive specimens is not clear. The likelihood of finding granulomas in biopsies is a function

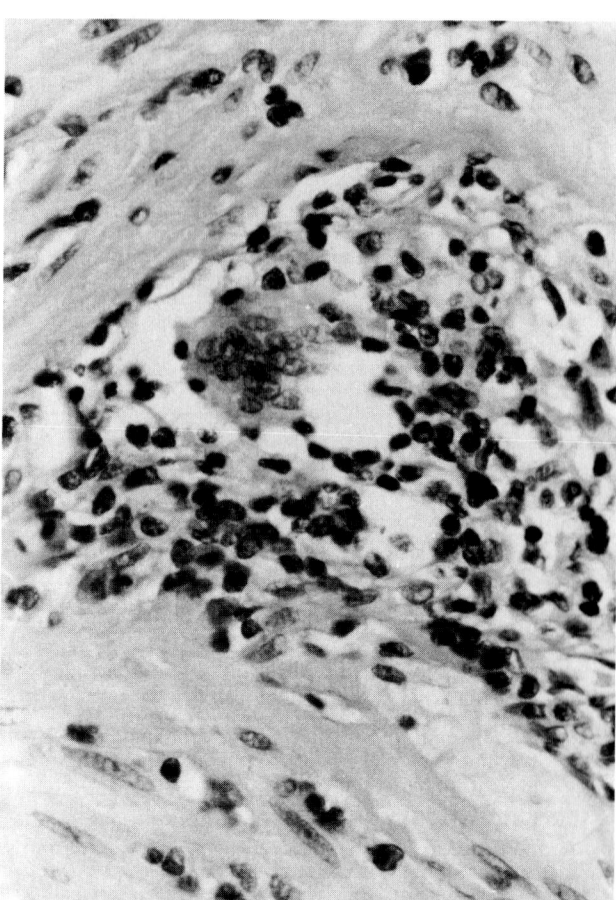

FIGURE 79-16. Granuloma in a surgical resection specimen from a patient with Crohn's disease. (Courtesy of David Lacey, M.D., St. Louis, MO.)

of the number of biopsies taken, the number of sections examined, and the definition of a granuloma.[121] Granulomas occur more commonly in the submucosa than the mucosa and are therefore more easily found on surgical specimens than on mucosal biopsies. Granulomas can also be found in lymph nodes, mesentery, peritoneum, and liver. In most cases, clinical, endoscopic, and pathologic characteristics allow the diagnosis of Crohn's disease even if no granulomas are found. Intestinal granulomas can be found in a number of infectious diseases, including tuberculosis, fungal infections, yersiniosis, and chlamydial infections. They are also seen in sarcoidosis and foreign body reactions. Granulomas in Crohn's disease resemble those in sarcoidosis and lack the caseating necrosis seen in tuberculosis. Granulomas are less commonly part of the pathologic picture in ulcerative colitis. If pathologic findings are used to differentiate ulcerative colitis from Crohn's colitis, the presence of granulomas suggests Crohn's colitis, but the absence of granulomas is not helpful. One pathologic finding thought to be characteristic of Crohn's disease is the presence of axonal necrosis of autonomic nerves.[122]

RADIOGRAPHY

The two major diagnostic techniques used in IBD are endoscopy and contrast radiography. These are complementary techniques with their own strengths and weaknesses.[123,124] The

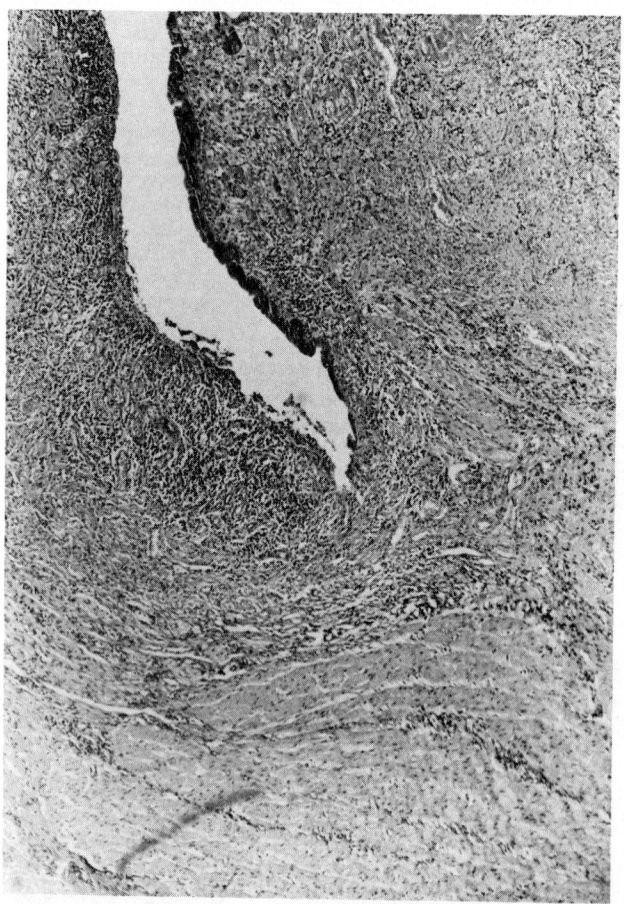

FIGURE 79-15. Fissure in a patient with Crohn's disease. The fissure extends into the muscularis propria. There is a chronic inflammatory infiltrate that extends into the muscularis propria. (Courtesy of David Lacey, M.D., St. Louis, MO.)

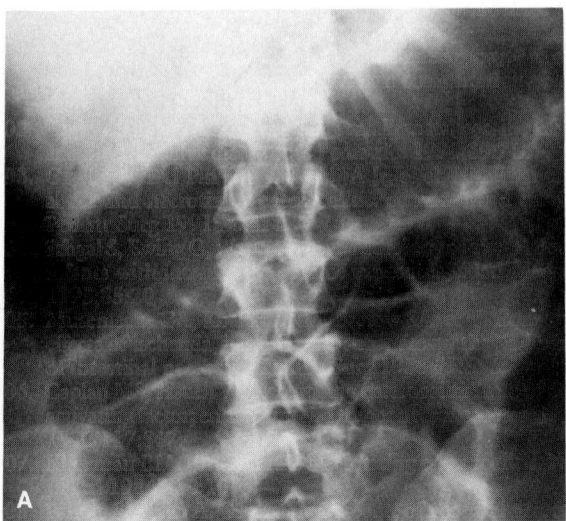 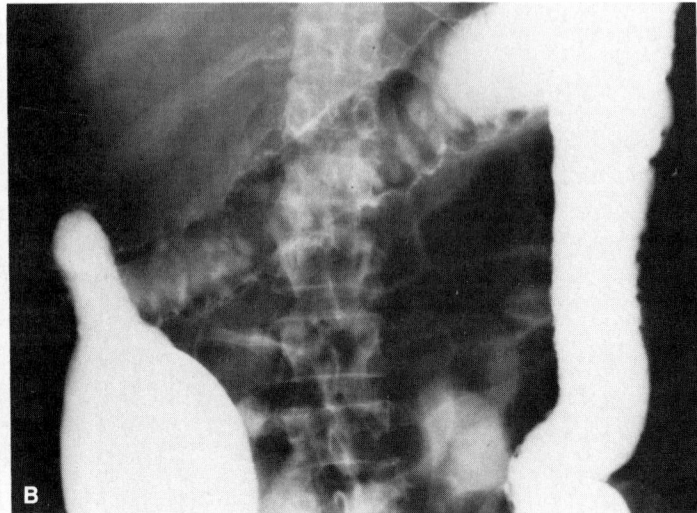

FIGURE 79-17. Toxic megacolon. **(A)** Plain film radiograph shows colonic dilatation; **(B)** contrast radiography reveals large ulcerations. (Courtesy of Dennis Balfe, M.D., St. Louis, MO.)

decision as to which one to use is made on the basis of the question being addressed. Air contrast radiography is better for assessing colonic distensibility, the presence of strictures, and the presence of fistulas. Endoscopy is better for defining the extent of mucosal disease and the presence of superficial mucosal abnormalities. Radiography without contrast serves two functions in IBD: the assessment of colonic dilatation in suspected toxic megacolon (Fig. 79-17) and the definition of the location and completeness of intestinal obstruction.

For the most part, air contrast or double-contrast studies are preferred to single-contrast studies because they give much better definition of fine mucosal detail. Single-contrast studies are more useful, however, for the definition of fistulas, strictures, and tumors.[125] Although contrast studies are usually well tolerated, there are some precautions that should be observed. Barium enema is contraindicated in patients with moderate or severe colitis (either ulcerative colitis or Crohn's colitis), because injection of air and barium into the inflamed colon may precipitate toxic megacolon. Even patients with significant diarrhea usually need laxatives to clean the bowel in preparation for barium enema. Harsh, irritative laxatives should be avoided, but osmotic laxatives such as citrate of magnesia are usually tolerated. Oral contrast agents should be used with caution whenever obstruction may be present.

In both ulcerative colitis and Crohn's disease, radiographic findings may not correlate well with disease activity.[126] In particular, asymptomatic patients may have markedly abnormal radiographic studies because of fibrosis of the bowel wall with resultant loss of distensibility. Contrast radiographic studies are, for the most part, not useful in following the patient's response to medical management over relatively short periods of time. The patient's clinical response or endoscopic findings are more useful for this purpose.

In early ulcerative colitis, the barium enema may be normal. The most sensitive radiologic finding in ulcerative colitis is limited distensibility of the involved segment, resulting in a narrowed, shortened, and tubular form of the lumen. The haustral markings disappear, and the normally tortuous appearance of the colon is straightened. Air contrast examination

reveals a fine granular appearance to the mucosa, with a slightly irregular surface (Fig. 79-18). In more severe disease, the granularity becomes coarser and eventually nodular. These changes may be more obvious on evacuation films. In addition to the granularity, small discrete ulcers surrounded by mounds

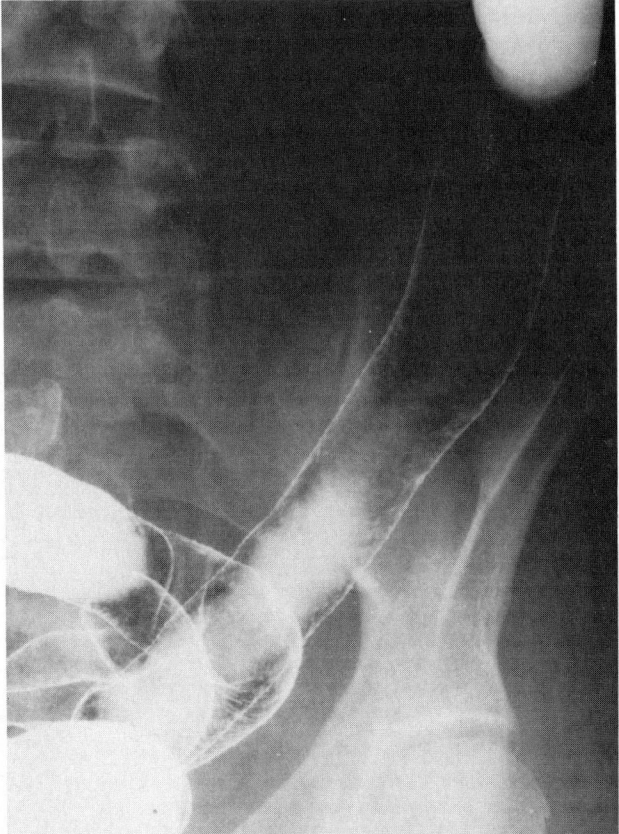

FIGURE 79-18. Mild-to-moderate, left-sided, ulcerative colitis shows granularity of mucosa without ulceration. (Courtesy of Dennis Balfe, M.D., St. Louis, MO.)

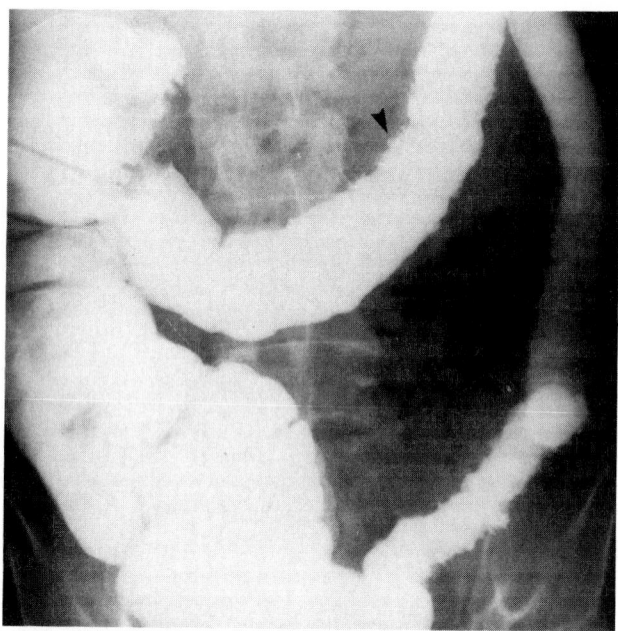

FIGURE 79-19. Ulcerative colitis with collar-button ulcerations seen in profile (*arrow*). (Courtesy of Dennis Balfe, M.D., St. Louis, MO.)

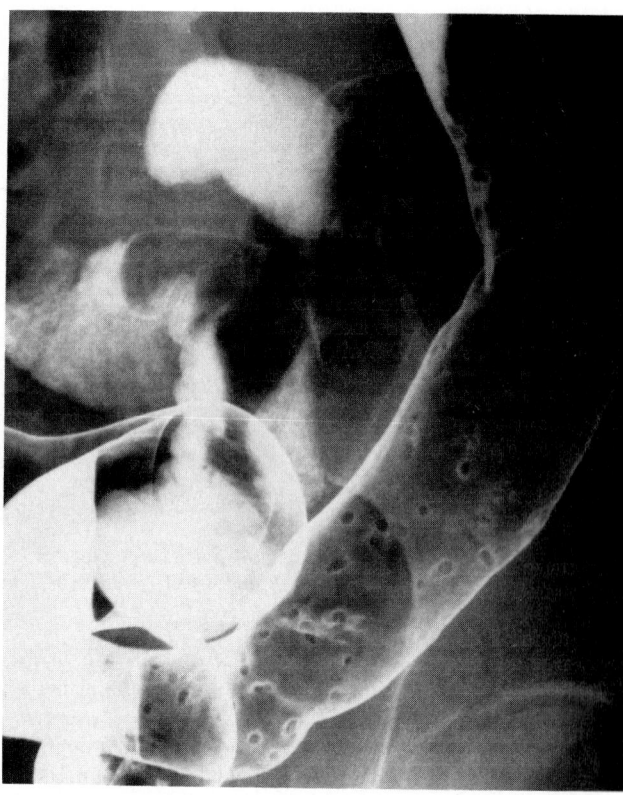

FIGURE 79-20. Inflammatory polyps are present in an otherwise featureless colon. (Courtesy of Dennis Balfe, M.D., St. Louis, MO.)

of inflamed tissue may be seen. In more severe disease, ulcers penetrate through the mucosa and can be seen in profile as small collar-button collections of barium extending beyond the colonic lumen (Fig. 79-19). Inflammatory polyps, either nodular or filiform, may be seen in either active or quiescent disease (Fig. 79-20). Inflammation and fibrosis in the rectum increase the presacral space—the distance from the sacrum to the rectal lumen—on lateral views. An enlarged presacral space (>2 cm) is consistent with severe rectal inflammation. In chronic ulcerative colitis, the colon becomes shortened and loses it haustral markings (Figs. 79-21 and 79-22). In

cases of burnt-out ulcerative colitis, markedly abnormal radiographs may be seen in patients who are asymptomatic.

In 15% to 20% of ulcerative colitis patients with pancolitis, the terminal ileum appears abnormal radiographically. The ileocecal valve is deformed and open, the terminal ileum is

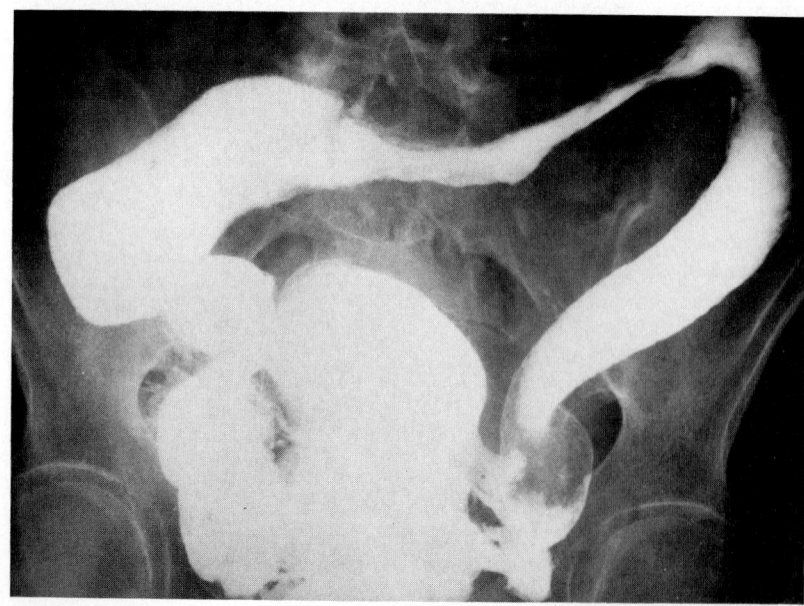

FIGURE 79-21. Full-column barium enema in a patient with ulcerative colitis shows shortening of the colon and loss of haustral markings. (Courtesy of Dennis Balfe, M.D., St. Louis, MO.)

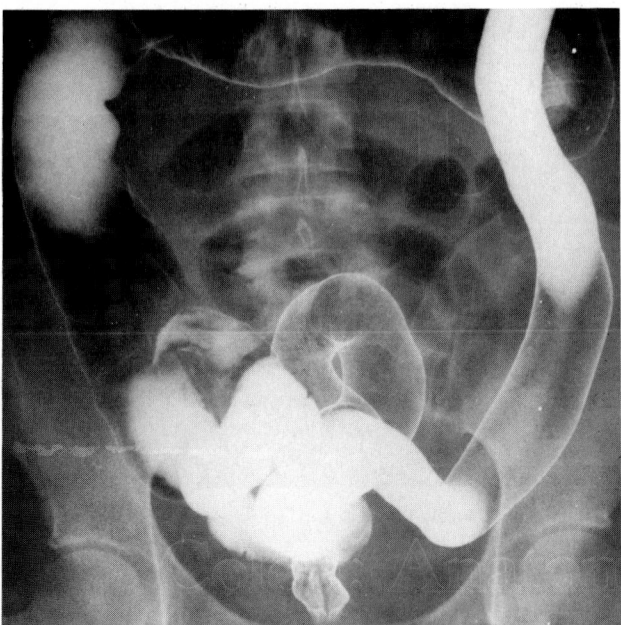

FIGURE 79-22. Air-contrast study of chronic ulcerative colitis with ahaustral colon. (Courtesy of Dennis Balfe, M.D., St. Louis, MO.)

dilated, and the mucosa is irregular, but there are no ulcerations. This process, termed backwash ileitis, should be differentiated from terminal ileal involvement in Crohn's disease, which is marked by lumenal narrowing, wall thickening, ulceration, and fistula formation.[127]

Carcinoma in ulcerative colitis can appear as a mass protruding into the lumen, as it may in those without ulcerative colitis, but in ulcerative colitis carcinoma is more often an infiltrating process that appears on radiography either as a flattened, rigid area of bowel wall or, in more advanced cases, as a stricture. Radiologic methods fail to detect cancer in patients with ulcerative colitis about 15% of the time.[125,128] Benign strictures may be indistinguishable from malignancy radiographically (Fig. 79-23). The presence of a flattened, rigid area or a stricture necessitates colonoscopy with biopsy. Because of the infiltrating nature of carcinoma in ulcerative colitis, colonic biopsies may be negative even if malignancy is present. If the radiograph is suggestive of carcinoma, surgery may be necessary despite a negative endoscopic biopsy.

The earliest form of Crohn's disease detectable by air contrast barium enema is marked by the presence of aphthous ulcers, which appear as small discrete collections of barium surrounded by radiolucent halos of inflammatory infiltrate (Fig. 79-24). These small ulcers are usually multiple, and the intervening mucosa is normal. Aphthous ulcers are not, however, unique to Crohn's disease; they are seen in amebiasis, Behçet's syndrome, shigellosis, and other conditions. As Crohn's disease becomes more severe, the aphthous ulcers enlarge, deepen, and connect with one another to form stellate and linear ulcers; the intervening mucosa develops a nodular appearance on radiograph, a process termed cobblestoning.

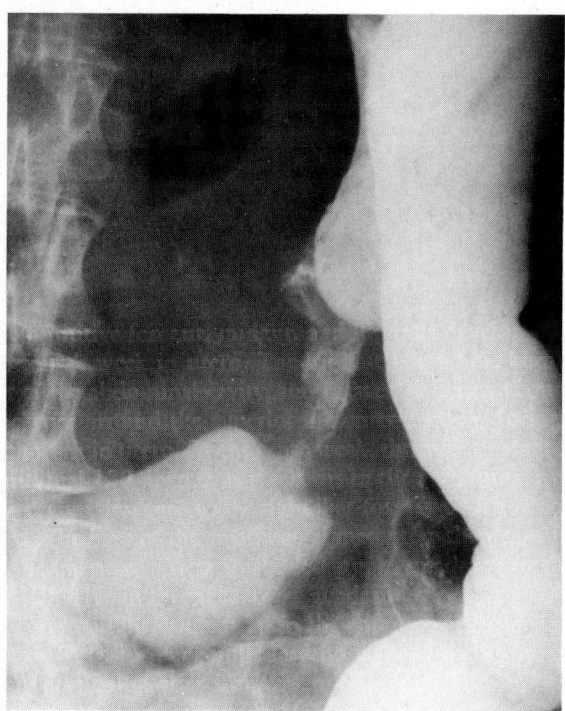

FIGURE 79-23. Benign stricture in transverse colon of patient with chronic ulcerative colitis. This lesion is radiographically indistinguishable from a malignancy. (Courtesy of Dennis Balfe, M.D., St. Louis, MO.)

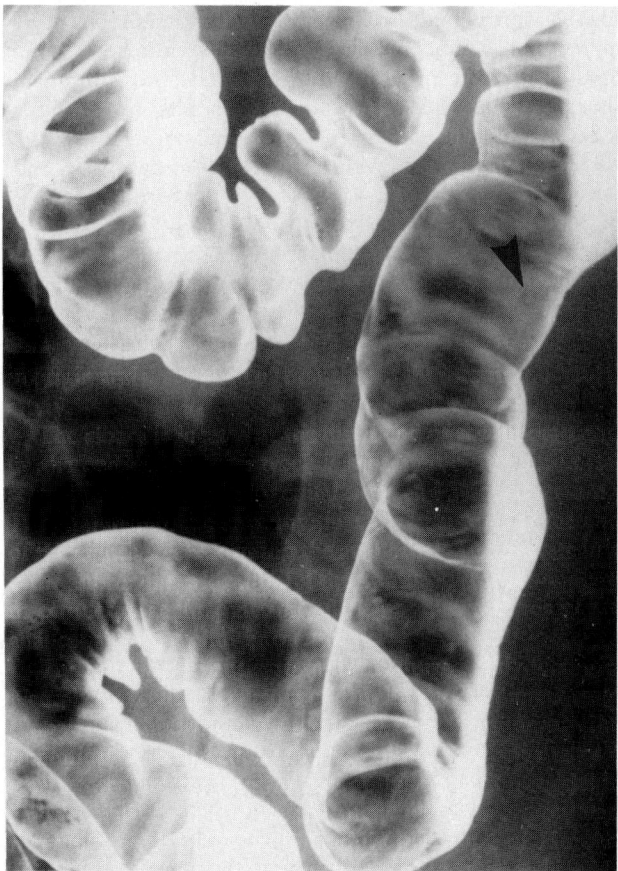

FIGURE 79-24. Crohn's colitis with numerous aphthous ulcers (*arrowhead*). (Courtesy of Dennis Balfe, M.D., St. Louis, MO.)

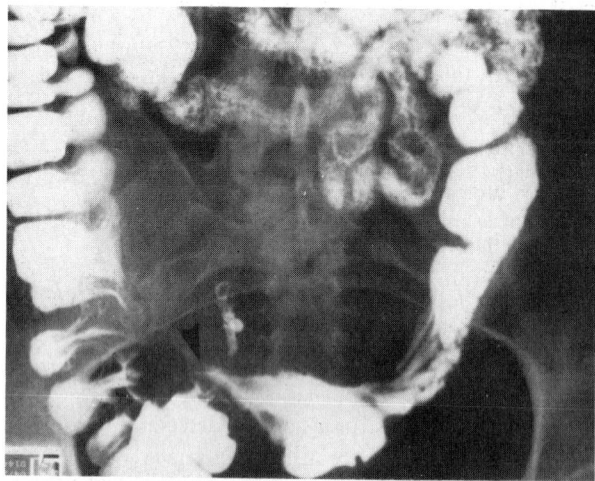
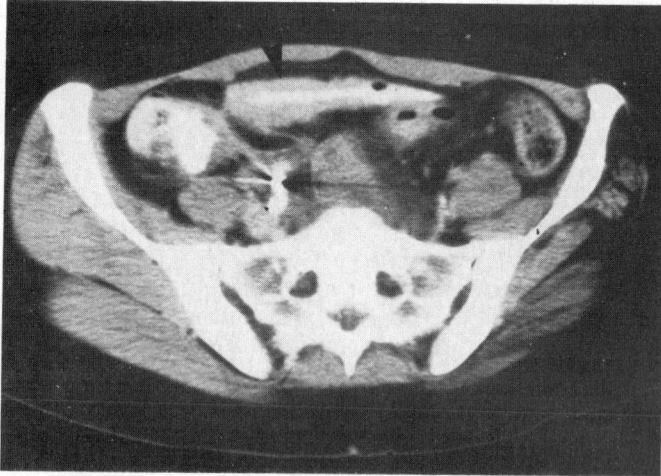

FIGURE 79-25. Crohn's disease of the terminal ileum (*arrows*) on small bowel follow-through and computed tomography (CT) scan in the same patient. Thickening of the intestinal wall is easily appreciated on the CT scan. On small bowel follow-through, wall thickening is indicated by the separation of the columns of barium. (Courtesy of Dennis Balfe, M.D., St. Louis, MO.)

Progressive deepening of ulcers can lead to abscess formation or fistulization. Contrast studies are far more likely than endoscopic studies to identify fistulas. Transmural inflammation and fibrosis lead to limited distensibility, with decreased lumenal diameter. If transmural inflammation and fibrosis is circumferential, the result is stricture formation and possible obstruction. Like fistulas, strictures are more easily appreciated on radiographic studies than by endoscopy. Long areas of circumferential inflammation and fibrosis result in long areas of lumenal narrowing; if this process occurs in the ileum, the result is the "string sign." Transmural inflammation and fibrosis result in thickening of the bowel wall, and as a result there are wide gaps between the barium-filled lumens of loops of inflamed small bowel (Figs. 79-25 and 79-26). The distribution of radiographic abnormalities can support the diagnosis of Crohn's disease. Findings typical of diffuse colitis may be consistent with either Crohn's disease or ulcerative colitis, but distal sparing is more consistent with Crohn's disease. Thickening of the bowel wall and retraction and thickening of the mesentery make the bowel rigid, stiff and immobile on fluoroscopy.

Computed axial tomography (CT) and ultrasonography are useful in identifying abscesses and other fluid collections and in assessing the thickness of the bowel wall. Thickened bowel wall, which is appreciated on barium studies as separation of the columns of barium, is easily seen on CT scan (see Fig. 79-25). CT and ultrasonography can also be used to direct percutaneous drainage of abscesses.

Nuclear medicine also may occasionally have a role in the management of IBD. In IBD, there is a markedly increased migration of neutrophils into the inflamed tissue and then out into the intestinal lumen. This process can be followed by harvesting a patient's peripheral blood neutrophils, labeling them in vitro with ^{111}In or ^{99}Tc, and then injecting them intravenously into the patient.[48,49] The radiolabeled neutrophils are carried by the bloodstream to the bowel, where they migrate into the inflamed tissue. A gamma camera can then be used to identify the sites of inflammation. This method not only allows the definition of the anatomic extent of inflammation but also allows an assessment of the severity of the inflammatory response by defining the number of neutrophils leaving the circulation and entering the bowel wall. This is largely a research technique now but may eventually find more general clinical applicability.

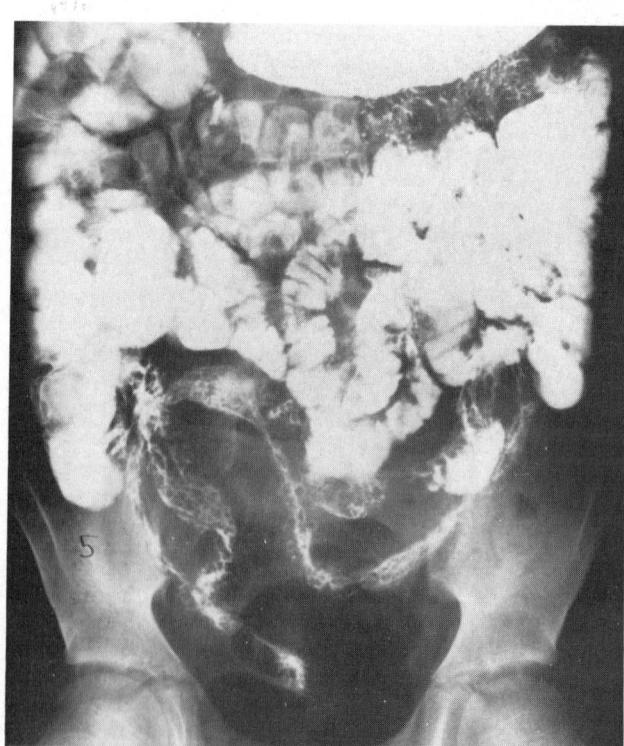

FIGURE 79-26. In Crohn's ileitis with a long segment of involved ileum, the barium columns are widely separated as a result of wall thickening. (Courtesy of Dennis Balfe, M.D., St. Louis, MO.)

ENDOSCOPY

For the most part, the precautions to be taken in performing endoscopy in patients with IBD are similar to those for the general population; however, there are some considerations that are peculiar to IBD. Perforation during colonoscopy is more likely; the bowel wall is inflamed and its integrity may be weakened by penetrating ulcers and fistulas, particularly in Crohn's disease. Severe inflammation with deep ulceration is a relative contraindication to colonoscopy. Similarly, toxic megacolon is an absolute contraindication to colonoscopy because the colonic wall is paper-thin. Scarring and fibrosis, often present in IBD, make the colon less elastic and distensible and more prone to perforation from pressure. Great care should be taken not to use excessive force in advancing the scope. The risk of perforation in severe ulcerative colitis makes it unwise to attempt a complete colonoscopy. Examination of the rectum with a proctoscope or flexible sigmoidoscope should yield enough information to confirm the diagnosis.

If considering the use of endoscopy in IBD, it is important to think about the specific clinical question being addressed, because endoscopy may or may not be able to provide an answer. Strictures and fistulas, for example, are more easily visualized by a radiologic approach (see previous section). If using colonoscopy to help establish the diagnosis of IBD, it is important to realize that none of the endoscopic findings associated with IBD are absolutely specific. The endoscopic findings in several varieties of infectious colitis are indistinguishable from those seen in IBD.[67,129,130] These similarities in endoscopic appearance probably reflect the similar spectra of inflammatory mediators involved in these conditions.

The earliest endoscopic manifestation of ulcerative colitis is loss of the fine vascular pattern seen in the normal rectal mucosa and the development of diffuse erythema (see Color Fig. 31).[67] Erythema is usually accompanied by mucosal edema, which is manifested endoscopically by blunting of the rectal valves, loss of normal vasculature, and development of granular-appearing mucosa. In the normal colon, finely branching vessels are easily seen through the mucosa. In mild colitis, the vessels are still seen but may be tortuous. As colitis becomes more severe, the more prominent edema blunts the haustral pattern, and vessels cannot be seen at all (see Color Fig. 32). Normal rectal mucosa is flat and smooth and reflects light in large patches. If the mucosa becomes edematous, little mounds of swollen tissue surround the crypts, creating an uneven surface (see Color Fig. 33). Light reflects off the uneven surface as numerous small spots rather than large patches. This pattern of reflection is termed granularity (Table 79-9). Inflammation is associated with the presence of collections of yellowish exudate on the mucosa. The exudate is called mucopus, and the more active the disease, the larger the area of mucosa that is covered with it. The inflamed mucosa bleeds easily if touched with the endoscope or a cotton swab. This easy bleeding is termed friability. In more severe disease, the mucosa bleeds spontaneously and small ulcerations appear. In the presence of inflammation and spasm, the rectum does not distend easily when insufflated with air. This is the equivalent of the loss of distensibility seen on radiography. An important aspect of the endoscopic findings in ulcerative colitis is their distribution. Inflammation begins in the rectum, extends proximally a certain distance, and then stops; all the

TABLE 79-9
Colonoscopic Mucosal Features and Their Diagnostic Specificity in Inflammatory Bowel Disease*

LESION	ULCERATIVE COLITIS	CROHN'S DISEASE
Inflammation		
Distribution		
Colon		
Contiguous	+++	+
Symmetric	+++	+
Rectum	+++	+
Friability	+++	+
Topography		
Granularity	+++	+
Cobblestoned	+	+++
Ulceration		
Location		
Overt colitis	+++	+
Ileum	0	++++
Discrete lesion	+	+++
Features		
Size > 1 cm	+	+++
Deep	+	++
Linear	+	+++
Aphthoid	0	++++
Bridging	+	++

* Specificity index range: 0 (not seen) to ++++ (diagnostic).

From Hogan WJ, Henshey GT, Geenen JE, Endoscopic evalution of inflammatory bowel disease. Med Clin North Am 1980;64:1084.

mucosa proximal to that point is normal, and all the mucosa distal to it is abnormal (see Fig. 79-9). As ulcerative colitis heals, there is residual mucosal edema, absent vasculature, and postinflammatory polyps in a tubular ahaustral lumen (see Color Fig. 34).

The earliest endoscopic manifestation of Crohn's disease is the aphthous ulcer (see Color Fig. 35), a small discrete ulcer a few millimeters in diameter surrounded by a thin red halo of edematous tissue (see Table 79-9).[131,132] Aphthous ulcers are usually multiple, and the intervening mucosa is normal. They can grow to form large stellate or linear ulcers. Ulcers may be rounded (see Color Fig. 36) or long and serpiginous. Longitudinal and transverse ulcers may intersect to form a grid with intervening cobblestone-like areas of nonulcerated mucosa. In Crohn's disease, large, deep, penetrating ulcers can be surrounded by areas of normal-appearing mucosa. The diffuse mucosal irregularities of erythema, edema, and granularity, prominent in ulcerative colitis, occur less commonly and later in the course of Crohn's disease. The rectum may or may not be involved in Crohn's disease. Areas of involvement are typically interspersed with normal "skip areas."

Yersinia, Campylobacter, Shigella, and cytomegalovirus infections can all have endoscopic pictures not very different from that of ulcerative colitis: mucosal edema, granularity, erythema, and easy friability.[129,130] Pseudomembranous colitis in its later stages may produce diffuse mucosal changes like those of ulcerative colitis, but the characteristic raised, yellow, plaque-like pseudomembranes should be diagnostic. Amebiasis is the infectious disease most likely to result in discrete, punched-out ulcers with normal intervening mucosa, as seen in Crohn's colitis.[133,134]

Endoscopy also plays a role in the assessment of disease extent and in defining the severity of inflammation. Endoscopy is more sensitive than radiographic contrast studies in defining the margins of inflammation. Comparisons of double-contrast radiography with colonoscopy show that radiography underestimates the extent of colonic involvement in two thirds of cases.[135] However, in the older literature, radiography was the basis for assessment of disease extent and subsequent recommendations for therapy. Colonoscopic assessment of the extent of inflammation is frequently part of preoperative evaluations, especially for Crohn's disease. This examination helps the surgeon decide on the extent of resection so that all the severely involved tissue is removed. Colonoscopic examination can also assure the surgeon that the segments chosen for the creation of an ileostomy or colostomy are not involved.

Endoscopy is also useful in following the course of disease. Arbitrary values of 0 to 4+ can be assigned to erythema, granularity, edema, and friability to yield an endoscopic severity score. These scores correlate reasonably well with the patient's clinical condition as assessed by symptoms in ulcerative colitis. However, there are many cases in which the colonoscopic picture is either much better or much worse than would be predicted by the patient's symptoms. In these cases, the usual approach is to base management decisions primarily on the patient's clinical presentation rather than the endoscopic findings. Some clinicians, however, place greater reliance on the endoscopic appearance in making therapeutic decisions. In patients with exacerbations of ulcerative colitis treated with steroids, some clinicians begin to taper the steroid dose after the patient's symptoms have resolved, but others confirm that there is also endoscopic improvement before tapering steroids. There are no data to support one approach over the other, although greater reliance on endoscopy is more expensive. If symptoms are severe and the endoscopic findings are minimal, it is possible that the symptoms are manifestations of functional disease rather than inflammation. Endoscopic assessments are routinely used in drug trials in ulcerative colitis and may be useful in following the response of patients to medical therapy in clinical practice. Endoscopy can also be used in ulcerative colitis to follow disease activity by assessing the proximal extent of inflammation. As ulcerative colitis improves, not only does the general endoscopic picture improve, but the proximal limit of inflammation moves toward the rectum.

Strictures and mass lesions in the colon in patients with IBD are suspicious for carcinoma, especially if the disease has been present for longer than 10 years. These lesions should be investigated colonoscopically and biopsied.[136–138] Carcinoma causing a stricture usually appears as an eccentric, friable mass. Malignant strictures have these endoscopic features: rigidity, nodules within the stricture or at its margins, an eccentric lumen, and a shelf-like margin. Sometimes in ulcerative colitis, the bulk of the tumor may be submucosal even though the tumor starts in the epithelium. In these cases, epithelial biopsies may be negative. Strictures that appear malignant by endoscopy should probably be resected regardless of the histologic appearance on biopsy. Colonoscopy for dysplasia surveillance is discussed elsewhere in this chapter.

Colonoscopy also has therapeutic potential in IBD. Polypectomy is approached much the same way in patients with IBD as in the general population; however, pseudopolyps are not premalignant and do not need to be resected. Pseudopolyps can be resected colonoscopically if they are bleeding or causing obstruction. Colonoscopic dilatation of strictures is sometimes possible; dilatation is performed with a balloon passed through the colonoscope. The best results have been achieved with short, uninflamed strictures. Longer strictures are less likely to be successfully dilated and more likely to perforate during attempted dilatation.

DIFFERENTIAL DIAGNOSIS

Differentiating Crohn's Disease From Ulcerative Colitis

For many therapeutic decisions, it is not particularly important to know whether the patient has ulcerative colitis or Crohn's disease. However, there are circumstances in which the distinction is important. For example, an ileoanal anastomosis could be recommended with much more enthusiasm if the physician were confident the patient had ulcerative colitis rather than Crohn's colitis. Similarly, colectomy could be more confidently recommended as a curative procedure if it were certain that the patient had ulcerative colitis.

The clinical presentations of ulcerative colitis resemble those of Crohn's disease, especially Crohn's colitis.[139,140] Diarrhea may be the most prominent symptom in both diseases, although it is more likely to be bloody in ulcerative colitis. The presence of pain as a prominent symptom is more suggestive of Crohn's disease, although patients with severe ulcerative colitis may also have significant pain, usually in the rectum. Malaise, fever, and weight loss are more common with Crohn's disease. The presence of a right lower quadrant mass and tenderness are also more suggestive of Crohn's disease. Certain complications are far more common in Crohn's disease than in ulcerative colitis; among these are fistulas (enteroenteric, enterocutaneous, enterovesicular, enterovaginal), intraabdominal abscesses, strictures, and malabsorption. Extensive perianal involvement with fistulas and abscess point to Crohn's disease as the diagnosis.

Usually, ulcerative colitis and Crohn's disease can be differentiated endoscopically (see Table 79-9).[67,141] The anatomic distribution of the inflammatory response is suggestive of the diagnosis. In ulcerative colitis, inflammation is seen in the rectum and extends proximally for some distance; in extensive disease, inflammation extends all the way to the cecum. Although ulcerative colitis does not involve the small intestine, there may be a few centimeters of inflamed mucosa without ulceration in the terminal ileum. If the rectum is spared or if there are areas of uninflamed mucosa (skip areas) between areas of inflamed mucosa, then Crohn's colitis is more likely. Ulcerative colitis is not only continuous along the longitudinal axis of the colon, but the degree of inflammation is also consistent and symmetric circumferentially at any level. In contrast, in Crohn's colitis, deep linear ulcers may be separated by areas of normal mucosa. Involvement of more than a few centimeters of the terminal ileum or ulceration in the terminal ileum is also indicative of Crohn's disease.

In addition to the presence of skip areas and asymmetric involvement, there are other endoscopic findings that suggest Crohn's colitis. Ulcers are more likely to be large, deep, and have discrete margins in Crohn's colitis than in ulcerative colitis. Aphthoid ulcers occur commonly in Crohn's disease but infrequently, if at all, in ulcerative colitis.

The pathologic changes seen in Crohn's disease and ulcerative colitis are discussed elsewhere in this chapter (see Table 79-8). A major distinguishing mark in favor of Crohn's disease is the presence of transmural inflammatory changes; in ulcerative colitis, inflammation is confined to the mucosa and submucosa. The presence of noncaseating granulomas suggests Crohn's disease, but even in Crohn's disease, most patients have no granulomas on biopsy.

Despite all these differences, there is a small but significant number of patients with IBD who cannot be assigned with confidence to one disease category or the other.[142] These patients are considered to have indeterminate colitis. As for the patients who seem to fall definitively into one category or the other, it is important to keep an open mind about the diagnosis. Later developments may require that it be reconsidered.

Differentiating Inflammatory Bowel Disease From Other Diseases

Much has been written about the necessity for differentiating the initial episode of ileocolonic Crohn's disease from acute appendicitis; however, in practice, this distinction is seldom a major problem.[143] Patients with Crohn's disease usually give a history of diarrhea of significant duration before the episode of severe pain. Appendicitis is marked by more severe pain, guarding, and a more rapid course. If the surgeon operates and finds ileocolic Crohn's disease rather than appendicitis, he or she must decide whether to resect the inflamed intestine. If there is no compelling reason for resection, medical management of the condition should be attempted. Another consideration in this differential diagnosis is acute ileitis caused by *Yersinia* infection.[144] *Yersinia* infection may present with a clinical picture resembling appendicitis or the initial onset of Crohn's disease. At laparotomy, the acute *Yersinia* ileitis may be indistinguishable from Crohn's ileitis. The diagnosis of this infection is made by stool culture, and antibiotic therapy is curative. The possibility of *Yersinia* infection is another reason to avoid hasty resections for what is thought to be the acute onset of Crohn's ileitis.

The most common problem in the differential diagnosis of the recent onset of IBD is ruling out infectious colitis (see Chap. 84).[145,146] Infections with shigella, amoeba, *Giardia*, and *Campylobacter* organisms can all cause symptoms very similar to those of ulcerative colitis. Moreover, the endoscopic picture of infections with *Shigella* or *Campylobacter* organisms can be identical to that seen in ulcerative colitis. The endoscopic picture of amebiasis may also resemble that of ulcerative colitis, but in amebiasis there are usually scattered ulcers, 5 to 15 mm in diameter, covered with a yellow exudate that contains organisms. These ulcers may occur anywhere in the colon but are most common in the cecum and ascending colon. An important distinction between these infectious diseases and IBD is that the diarrhea in the infectious diseases tends to be limited to a period of days to a few weeks, whereas the diarrhea of IBD is typically of longer duration. Stool cul-

tures for bacterial pathogens and serologic tests for amebiasis help distinguish infectious diarrhea from IBD. In patients who present with prolonged diarrhea, the diagnosis of giardiasis must be considered. Giardiasis, like Crohn's disease, can present with cramping abdominal pain, weight loss, and lactose intolerance.

Intestinal tuberculosis resembles Crohn's disease both clinically and pathologically (see Chap. 71).[147,148] The areas most commonly involved with intestinal tuberculosis are the cecum and the ileum. If pulmonary tuberculosis is also present, the diagnosis of intestinal tuberculosis is not difficult, but intestinal tuberculosis can occur without pulmonary involvement. It is important not to mistake tuberculosis for IBD because steroid treatment exacerbates tuberculosis.

Sexual transmission of enteric pathogens by anal intercourse in homosexual men can lead to proctitis resembling ulcerative proctitis.[149,150] *Neisseria gonorrhea*, *Chlamydia* organisms, herpes simplex, and *Treponema pallidum* can all cause proctitis. Chlamydial infections of the lymphogranuloma venereum immunotype can result in diffuse rectal ulceration that is difficult to distinguish from Crohn's colitis. The increased prevalence of the human immunodeficiency virus (HIV) has broadened the number of potential enteric pathogens to include *Cryptosporidia* and *Isospora* species, *Mycobacterium avium* complex, and cytomegalovirus. In patients without risk factors for HIV infection, the only diagnostic studies needed to rule out infectious colitis are routine stool cultures, examination of stool for ova and parasites (on three separate days), and sigmoidoscopy. However, patients who are at risk for HIV infection require a more elaborate evaluation. Cytomegalovirus and herpesvirus can be identified by viral culture and histologic examination of biopsy specimens. Chlamydial infections are diagnosed by serology and culture. Intestinal involvement in HIV infection is discussed more fully in Chapter 105.

Intestinal lymphoma can produce symptoms similar to those of Crohn's disease—fever, weight loss, diarrhea, and abdominal pain. Small bowel radiographs in lymphoma may show diffuse involvement with masses in the bowel wall, but in Crohn's disease there is usually more localized involvement of the ileum, with ulceration and narrowing of the lumen.

Collagenous or lymphocytic colitis is a chronic inflammatory disease marked pathologically by the presence of a thick collagen deposition in the subepithelial layer of the colonic mucosa.[151,152] The typical clinical presentation is chronic watery diarrhea in a middle-aged woman. Endoscopically, the mucosa appears mildly inflamed or, more commonly, absolutely normal. The histologic picture provides the diagnosis. Collagenous colitis is discussed more fully in Chapter 80.

Ischemic colitis is part of the differential diagnosis of the initial bout of IBD and should be considered in elderly persons or others at particular risk for ischemic disease.[153,154] Bloody diarrhea and abdominal pain are common with ischemic colitis. Colonoscopy reveals mucosal edema and erythema, and there may be discrete ulcers similar to those seen in Crohn's colitis. Usually, ischemic colitis spares the rectum because of collateral circulation there. Differentiation of ischemic colitis from IBD, especially Crohn's colitis, may be impossible on clinical, histologic, or endoscopic grounds. However, in contrast to IBD, ischemic colitis usually resolves spontaneously over a few weeks.

Another condition that may be difficult to separate from acute Crohn's colitis, especially in the elderly, is diverticulitis.[155-157] Both diseases can present with abdominal pain, fever, diarrhea, and rectal bleeding. Endoscopically, the presence of inflammation over a long segment of colon or in the rectum, where there are no diverticula, suggests Crohn's disease, as does the presence of perianal disease or extracolonic disease. Diverticulitis, like ischemic colitis, tends to be an acute problem and does not lead to a chronic inflammatory state as does IBD. Diverticulosis can be associated with rectal bleeding, but the bouts of bleeding are abrupt in onset and the blood loss is great, whereas in ulcerative colitis or Crohn's colitis, blood loss is usually chronic and small in volume.

Pseudomembranous colitis presents with profuse watery diarrhea and may last from a few days to 2 months (see Chap. 84).[158,159] The presence of small membranous plaques adherent to the mucosa on sigmoidoscopy is pathognomonic. However, not all patients with pseudomembranous colitis have the characteristic sigmoidoscopic picture. As part of the evaluation of the initial acute presentation of IBD, it is appropriate to check the stool for *C difficile* toxin, especially if there has been recent antibiotic exposure.

Mild ulcerative colitis in which rectal bleeding is the primary manifestation can be confused with hemorrhoids or anal fissures. The presence of urgency or diarrhea is more consistent with ulcerative colitis. Sigmoidoscopy should easily differentiate ulcerative colitis from these perianal problems.

If IBD, especially Crohn's disease of the small intestine, has a long, indolent course with relatively mild symptoms, it may be difficult to differentiate from irritable bowel syndrome.[160,161] It should be easy to distinguish between irritable bowel syndrome and ulcerative colitis by proctoscopy, which is normal in irritable bowel syndrome. Chronic, cramping abdominal pain and diarrhea are typical of both irritable bowel syndrome and Crohn's disease. The presence of fever, abdominal tenderness, and weight loss all suggest Crohn's disease. This differential diagnosis may be particularly troublesome in that some patients with Crohn's disease also have irritable bowel syndrome. Making the diagnosis of irritable bowel syndrome in a patient with coexisting IBD is difficult because of the overlapping symptoms and the absence of any definitive histologic or biochemical marker for either IBD or irritable bowel syndrome. For many patients with IBD, there are symptoms, typically pain and diarrhea, that appear not to correlate with disease activity as assessed endoscopically or histologically. Whether these symptoms are products of undetected disease activity, "functional" symptoms of IBD, or signs of irritable bowel syndrome is difficult to establish. A confounding issue is the high incidence of depression in both irritable bowel syndrome and IBD and the influence of depression on the patient's symptoms. The coexistence of these diseases is of importance not only in making the diagnosis but also in following therapy. Patients who have both Crohn's disease and irritable bowel syndrome have been treated aggressively (and unsuccessfully) with corticosteroids for abdominal pain and diarrhea that were, in fact, products of irritable bowel syndrome. Diversion colitis is a nonspecific inflammation of segments of colon excluded from the fecal stream. Diversion colitis sometimes occurs in patients who have had surgery for Crohn's colitis with creation of a Hartman pouch. In these cases, diversion colitis may be difficult to differentiate from recurrence of Crohn's disease in the excluded segment. Many patients with diversion colitis have severe endoscopic findings with minimal symptoms. A clinical response to enemas of short-chain fatty acids should differentiate diversion colitis from active Crohn's disease.[162]

NUTRITIONAL MANAGEMENT

Malnutrition is an important clinical problem in IBD, particularly in Crohn's disease. At the time of diagnosis, most patients with Crohn's disease have lost weight. Hypoalbuminemia, anemia, and vitamin D deficiency can all result from malnutrition in Crohn's disease.

There are five factors that lead to malnutrition in Crohn's disease.

1. Diminished oral intake, primarily due to loss of appetite, is the most important cause of malnutrition in patients with Crohn's disease.[163] Anorexia may result from inflammation, depression, or the side effects of medication. Even in the absence of anorexia, many patients diminish food intake because eating brings on pain, cramps, and diarrhea; this is seen particularly in patients with small bowel obstruction.

2. There are increased caloric requirements in Crohn's disease because of the catabolism associated with fever and inflammation.[164]

3. There is malabsorption of nutrients owing to reduction of the absorptive area by extensive surgical resections or involvement of large areas of small bowel with inflammation. Rarely, fistulas can result in malabsorption as a result of nutrients bypassing absorptive epithelium. The nutrients most likely to be affected are fats and vitamin B_{12}, because bile salts and vitamin B_{12} are selectively absorbed in the distal ileum, the area of the small intestine most commonly involved in Crohn's disease and the area most commonly resected. Malabsorption of bile salts leads to a decrease in the total bile salt pool and thus to fat malabsorption. Bacterial overgrowth in the small intestine proximal to strictures leads to deconjugation of bile salts by bacteria. The deconjugated bile salts are rapidly absorbed and so are not available in the lumen to participate in fat absorption. Fat malabsorption also impairs the absorption of the fat-soluble vitamins.

4. There is loss of proteins and electrolytes into the intestinal lumen in areas of inflammation. Bleeding into the intestinal lumen results in iron deficiency. Potassium, magnesium, and zinc can all be depleted by losses into the intestine.

5. The drug therapy of IBD can lead to nutritional problems. Sulfasalazine impairs folate absorption but uncommonly leads to anemia. Corticosteroids induce negative nitrogen balance and decrease intestinal calcium absorption.

For most patients with IBD, the only nutritional therapy required is the instruction to eat adequate amounts of a well-balanced diet. Patients look for a nutritional basis to their disease and for nutritionally based therapy. These expectations lead many to decide that exacerbations of pain or diarrhea were caused by the foods they ate before the exacerbation. They exclude from their diets a lengthy list of foods that were temporally associated with an exacerbation of disease. As a result, these patients place themselves on a diet that has limited variety and is likely to be nutritionally unbalanced. They need to be instructed that foods should only be eliminated from the diet if they consistently and reproducibly result in symptoms. Some patients have lactose intolerance and should avoid dairy products or use lactase-containing products such as LactAid. Patients with strictures, especially in the small intestine, should avoid fibrous, high-residue foods such as popcorn, bean sprouts, and celery.

More involved nutritional therapy in Crohn's disease can be directed at one of two ends—treating nutritional deficiencies or reducing inflammation. Treatment of nutritional deficiencies is straightforward and noncontroversial. Deficiencies of specific nutrients can usually be managed by supplementation. Oral iron supplementation may be necessary in patients with significant intestinal bleeding. Specific supplementation with calcium, magnesium, zinc, vitamin B_{12}, vitamin D, and vitamin K may be required if there are clinical or biochemical manifestations of deficiency. These are nutrients that may be malabsorbed if there is extensive involvement of the small bowel mucosa. Bone densitometry will reveal evidence of calcium loss from bone caused by calcium malabsorption or steroid therapy. Even in the absence of clinical or biochemical evidence of micronutrient deficiency, it is reasonable to give multivitamin supplements to patients with small bowel Crohn's disease. Extensive (>100 cm) resections of the terminal ileum, or lesser resections combined with active disease or scarring in the remaining ileum, lead to vitamin B_{12} malabsorption. Some clinicians evaluate patients with serum vitamin B_{12} levels, but others empirically treat all patients with significant ileal resections with parenteral vitamin B_{12} (1000 μg once a month). Ileal resection and ileal disease also lead to malabsorption of bile salt and fat. Diarrhea induced by bile salts can be managed with cholestyramine, a resin that binds bile salts and prevents them from inducing water and electrolyte secretion from the colonic mucosa. Cholestyramine therapy, however, further depletes the bile salt pool and can worsen fat malabsorption. Fat malabsorption induces diarrhea because unabsorbed fatty acids entering the colon are hydroxylated by bacteria, and the hydroxylated fatty acids induce colonic water and electrolyte secretion. Fat-induced diarrhea is managed by reducing the fat content of the diet. Caloric deficiencies are made up by increasing the intake of complex carbohydrates. Alternatively, medium-chain triglycerides, which do not require bile salts for absorption, can be substituted for part of the conventional long-chain triglycerides in the diet. The usefulness of medium-chain triglycerides is limited, however; if used in large quantities, they themselves induce diarrhea.

Anorexia leads to inadequate nutritional intake and malnutrition in many patients with IBD even if absorptive function is normal. Supplementation of the patient's oral intake with defined formula diets can prevent or reverse malnutrition. Defined formula diets can be taken orally or administered by nasogastric tube, gastrostomy tube, or jejunostomy tube (see Chap. 48). Most IBD patients who require nutritional supplementation can be managed with enteral therapy. However, there are cases in which parenteral nutrition is required: in the presence of chronic small intestine obstruction that is not amenable to surgical resection; after massive small bowel resection, especially if the amount of remaining small intestine is insufficient for absorption of daily caloric needs; or if enteral nutrition results in severe, uncontrollable diarrhea.

The use of dietary therapy (either enteral or parenteral) to manage malnutrition in IBD is universally accepted. More controversial is the use of total parenteral nutrition (TPN) or the enteral administration of an elemental diet as specific therapy in IBD. Elemental diets consist of amino acids, monosaccharides, vitamins, minerals, and essential fatty acids. A number of studies, most of them uncontrolled,[165–167] suggest that elemental diets reduce disease activity in Crohn's disease. Four controlled trials have compared elemental diets with corticosteroids alone or with corticosteroids plus sulfasalazine in achieving remissions in Crohn's disease. Two of these studies found that the two approaches achieved equal rates of remission.[168,169] In the other two studies, drug therapy was significantly superior to elemental diet.[170,171] In another controlled study, a low-residue diet had no advantage over a normal diet.[172]

Two suggestions have been put forth for mechanisms by which an elemental diet may be useful in Crohn's disease. One postulates that the absence of peptides reduces the antigenic load and thereby removes a stimulus to immune activation; the other states that the components of the elemental diet are absorbed in the proximal small intestine, providing bowel rest for the distal small intestine, where involvement with Crohn's disease is more likely. Nutritional therapy clearly has a role in treating the malnutrition associated with Crohn's disease; whether elemental diets or TPN induce a short-term clinical improvement is less clearly established. There is no evidence that nutritional therapy affects the course of the disease over the long term.

Malnutrition is less commonly problematic in ulcerative colitis than in Crohn's disease, in part because malabsorption of nutrients is not a problem in ulcerative colitis. Diminished food intake, however, is a problem in ulcerative colitis. Patients with ulcerative colitis reduce calorie intake because of loss of appetite and because eating worsens their diarrhea. Nutritional requirements are increased in severe ulcerative colitis because of the catabolism associated with fever and inflammation. TPN has been used to improve the nutritional status and reduce the symptoms of patients with severe ulcerative colitis.[173] This approach has been especially successful in improving the nutritional status of patients before colectomy. Improved nutritional status decreases the likelihood of complications for surgical procedures in general and, presumably, for IBD surgery in particular. There is no evidence that TPN reduces the necessity for colectomy. Two studies compared the rates of colectomy in ulcerative colitis patients receiving TPN with those on regular hospital food. In both studies, the rates for colectomy were the same in the two groups.[174,175]

DRUGS USED IN IBD

General Supportive Therapy

There is a role in the management of IBD for drugs (antidiarrheal agents, antispasmodics, and analgesics) that reduce the patient's symptoms without affecting the level of disease activity. The use of these drugs should not be a matter of routine for all; rather, their use should be individualized for each patient. Moreover, they should supplement antiinflammatory drugs, not substitute for them.

Antidiarrheal agents, usually loperamide or diphenoxylate, are useful in patients with mild disease activity to reduce the number of bowel movements and to relieve rectal urgency. In addition to controlling disease-related diarrhea, these agents can control diarrhea caused by bile salt and fat malabsorption, as is seen in patients with surgical resections of the terminal ileum. For patients who have undergone an ileocolic resection treatment with cholestyramine (up to six scoops per day) may be particularly useful. Cholestyramine is a resin that binds bile salts in the lumen and prevents bile salt–induced colonic secretion. Depending on the clinical presentation, antidiarrheal agents can be given on a regular schedule or on an as-needed basis. Antidiarrheal agents may allow reduction of steroid dosage in patients with chronic steroid requirements. In moderate and especially in severe colitis, antidiarrheal agents are contraindicated because they predispose to the development of toxic megacolon.

Abdominal cramping is often a prominent complaint in IBD. Anticholinergics (tincture of belladonna, clidinium, propantheline bromide, and dicyclomine hydrochloride) may reduce cramps, pain, and rectal urgency. They are best given before meals to depress peristalsis brought on by eating. As with antidiarrheal agents, antispasmodics are contraindicated in severe colitis because of the risk of precipitating toxic megacolon. Antispasmodics should also be avoided if obstruction is present. Analgesia can be a difficult problem in IBD. In general, the best approach to pain management is the control of disease activity. Narcotics can cause dependency and, by reducing bowel motility, induce toxic megacolon.

Sulfasalazine

Mechanism of Action

Attempts to define the mechanism of action of sulfasalazine are intertwined with definition of its pharmacokinetics.[51] Sulfasalazine is composed of sulfapyridine and 5-aminosalicylate (5-ASA) joined by an azo bond. Twenty percent to 30% of orally-administered sulfasalazine is absorbed in the small intestine; much of this is taken up by the liver and excreted unmetabolized in the bile.[176] About 75% of the ingested sulfasalazine enters the colon, where the azo bond is cleaved by colonic bacteria to yield 5-ASA and sulfapyridine. 5-ASA is the therapeutic agent in sulfasalazine[177]; clinical trials with 5-ASA administered as a rectal suppository or as a retention enema have demonstrated improvement in the signs and symptoms of ulcerative colitis and a decline in the activity index in patients with Crohn's colitis. In each of these trials, sulfapyridine had no effect. 5-ASA is poorly absorbed from the colon and remains in the colonic lumen until excreted in the feces. Sulfapyridine appears to have little or no therapeutic effect. Its absorption from the colon is relatively efficient, and when transported to the liver it is acetylated, hydroxylated, and conjugated with glucuronic acid. The rate of acetylation of sulfapyridine, which varies considerably among individual patients, is a major determinant of serum sulfapyridine levels.

The adverse effects of sulfasalazine are largely related to sulfapyridine; many toxic side effects correlate with serum sulfapyridine levels and thus with the rate of acetylation.[178] Hypersensitivity reactions are not directly related to serum levels. Sulfapyridine and its metabolites are excreted in the urine.

Table 79-10 lists the serum and stool concentrations of sulfasalazine, sulfapyridine, and 5-ASA in treated patients with ulcerative colitis. The serum concentration of sulfasalazine is significant but low compared to the stool concentration; the serum concentration of 5-ASA is very low and the stool concentration very high. In treated patients, the lumenal surface of the inflamed colonic mucosa is exposed to high levels of sulfasalazine and 5-ASA, whereas the basolateral surface is exposed to much lower levels from the circulating blood. However, the concentrations of these agents actually achieved in the inflamed mucosa are not known. Definition of the effective concentrations of both sulfasalazine and 5-ASA in this tissue might help in establishing the mechanism of action of sulfasalazine.

The mechanism of action is currently unknown. One earlier theory was that sulfasalazine acts as a vehicle for the delivery of 5-ASA to the colon, where it blocks prostaglandin production (Fig. 79-27).[53,179] 5-ASA is a salicylate and, like aspirin, an inhibitor of cyclooxygenase, the enzyme that catalyzes the conversion of arachidonic acid to prostaglandins. If patients with IBD are treated with sulfasalazine, the levels of prostaglandins in their serum and mucosa decline and their clinical condition improves. If patients with IBD are treated with indomethacin or other nonsteroidal antiinflammatory drugs, the prostaglandin levels in their serum and mucosa decline but their clinical condition does not improve. This suggests that the inhibition of prostaglandin synthesis is not the mechanism of action of sulfasalazine.

A more recent proposal for the mechanism of action of sulfasalazine relates to the other major class of arachidonic acid metabolites—leukotrienes. Sulfasalazine and 5-ASA have been shown to inhibit lipoxygenase and thus the synthesis of LTB_4 in both peripheral blood neutrophils and in IBD mucosa.[180,181] The concentration of sulfasalazine and 5-ASA required for inhibition of LTB_4 synthesis is 1 to 2 mM, well within the range of concentrations found in the stool of treated patients but far higher than the serum concentrations.

TABLE 79-10
Concentrations of Sulfasalazine and Metabolites in Serum and Stool*

	SULFASALAZINE	SULFAPYRIDINE	5-ASA
Serum	18 (45)†	44 (149)†	1 (7)†
Stool	780 (1959)‡	480 (1907)†	1500 (9800)‡

* Concentrations are µg/mL; numbers in parentheses are µmol.

† Data from Das KM, Eastwood MA, McManus JPA. Metabolism of salicylazo-sulphapyridine in ulcerative colitis: relationship between metabolites and response to treatment in patients. Gut 1973;14:631. Serum values are from patients with ulcerative colitis who respond to an oral dose of 3 to 6 g of sulfasalazine per day.

‡ Data from Peppercorn MA, Goldman P. Distribution studies of salicylazosulfapyridine and its metabolites. Gastroenterology 1973;64:240. Stool values are for patients taking 3 to 12 g of sulfasalazine per day.

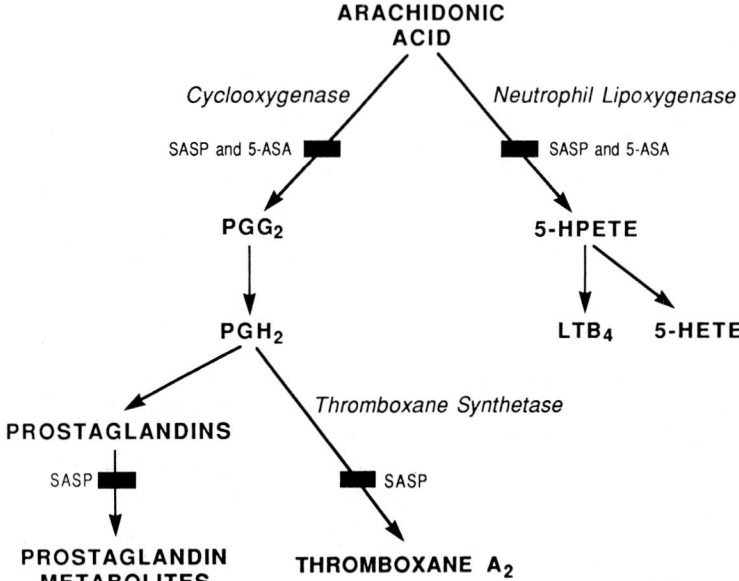

FIGURE 79-27. Effect of sulfasalazine (SASP) and 5-aminosalicylate (5-ASA) on arachidonic acid metabolism. Thick bars (▬) indicate inhibition.

Whether this concentration is achieved in the colonic mucosa is unknown. Sulfasalazine and 5-ASA inhibit both the lipoxygenase and cyclooxygenase pathways, whereas indomethacin and other nonsteroidal antiinflammatory drugs inhibit only the cyclooxygenase pathway. The efficacy of sulfasalazine in the treatment of IBD and the inefficacy of nonsteroidal antiinflammatory drugs suggest that lipoxygenase products are important mediators of inflammation in IBD and cyclooxygenase products are not. A clinically useful selective inhibitor of the lipoxygenase pathway would provide a suitable test for this hypothesis.

Ulcerative colitis and Crohn's disease are marked by a massive flux of neutrophils out of the circulation into the inflamed mucosa and then on into the intestinal lumen. An important component of neutrophil activation is the respiratory burst, a process that results in the production of superoxide, hydroxyl radicals, and peroxides. These products of the respiratory burst are important in the microbicidal properties of neutrophils and may be important in neutrophil-induced epithelial cell damage. 5-ASA has been shown to act as a free radical scavenger and to inactivate the products of the respiratory burst.[182] This pharmacologic property of 5-ASA has been proposed as a potential mechanism for its therapeutic efficacy.

There are markedly increased levels of immunoglobulin and increased numbers of immunoglobulin-secreting cells in the lamina propria in IBD. These immunoglobulins are thought to play an important role in immune-mediated injury. 5-ASA, but not sulfasalazine, was found to inhibit immunoglobulin secretion by peripheral blood and intestinal mononuclear cells.[183]

Sulfasalazine in Ulcerative Colitis

Sulfasalazine has been used successfully as a single agent in mild to moderate acute attacks of ulcerative colitis. Most clinicians view sulfasalazine as the drug of choice in mild cases if the patient tolerates it. Three different series reported fa-

vorable responses in 64% to 80% in patients treated with sulfasalazine, compared with 35% to 40% favorable responses in controls.[184–186] In these series, the patients were treated with 4 to 6 g per day in four divided doses. Success rates with sulfasalazine in acute ulcerative colitis are dose-related. Most clinicians do not use doses above 4 g/day, yet several studies have demonstrated better success rates with doses of 6 g/day or more. The incidence of side effects also increases with dose, but if a patient tolerates 4 g/day and has not fully responded clinically, there is no reason not to push the dose higher.

To lessen the side effects, sulfasalazine is given in gradually increasing doses, beginning at 500 mg twice a day and increasing to 1 g four times a day over the course of a week or so. Taking sulfasalazine with food in four divided doses lessens gastric symptoms in most individuals; but, if the patient tolerates the drug, the schedule can be changed to 2 g twice a day. Patients who respond to sulfasalazine usually do so in 2 to 3 weeks, although some take 4 weeks or longer. After remission has been achieved, the dose of sulfasalazine can be tapered to 2 to 3 g/day and the patient maintained on that dose indefinitely. If the disease flares as the drug is tapered, the dose can be raised again to 4 to 6 g/day.

There are no studies to support the use of sulfasalazine as a sole agent in more severe ulcerative colitis. In comparisons of sulfasalazine and corticosteroids in acute severe attacks of colitis, steroids induced remissions in a higher percentage of patients and induced them more quickly than did sulfasalazine.[187,188] For this reason, most clinicians use corticosteroids, either alone or with sulfasalazine, as the treatment of choice for moderate to severe attacks. There is no evidence to suggest that the combination is better than corticosteroids alone. The dosage schedule for sulfasalazine combined with steroids is the same as for sulfasalazine alone. One advantage of combined therapy is that when the time comes to taper steroids, the patient is already on sulfasalazine. If patients on combined therapy go into remission, the usual approach is to taper and stop steroids and then to taper sulfasalazine until the patient is on a maintenance dose of 2 to 3 g/day.

Sulfasalazine in Crohn's Disease

Sulfasalazine is also useful in acute attacks of Crohn's disease. In the National Cooperative Crohn's Disease Study, sulfasalazine at a dose of 1 g per 15 kg of body weight per day for 17 weeks was superior to placebo, inducing symptomatic improvement for patients with colonic involvement whether or not the small bowel was involved.[189] However, sulfasalazine was not effective against disease confined to the small bowel. Patients were less likely to respond to sulfasalazine if they had been on prednisone before being randomized to sulfasalazine. The European Cooperative Crohn's Disease Study also found sulfasalazine therapy beneficial in patients with active colonic disease.[190] In that study, treatment with sulfasalazine (3 g/day) resulted in a modest but statistically significant improvement in the Crohn's Disease Activity Index. The National Cooperative Crohn's Disease Study did not find any advantage with the combination of corticosteroids and sulfasalazine over corticosteroids alone. However, many clinicians treat acute Crohn's disease, especially Crohn's colitis, with a combination of corticosteroids and sulfasalazine. The usual procedure is to treat with the combination until the disease becomes inactive and then to taper the corticosteroids.

The efficacy of sulfasalazine in preventing relapse in ulcerative colitis is well established. In one study,[191] patients with ulcerative colitis in remission were randomized to placebo or 2 g of sulfasalazine per day. Recurrence was defined as a flare of symptoms. Over the course of 1 year, 24 of 33 placebo-treated patients relapsed, but only 7 of 34 who received sulfasalazine relapsed. In a second study, maintenance doses of 1, 2, and 4 g per day were compared (Fig. 79-28).[192] These patients had recurrence rates of 33%, 14%, and 9%, respectively. This indicates a dose-response effect in the prevention of relapse by sulfasalazine. However, the recommended dose for maintenance therapy is 2 g, because more patients tolerate 2 g than 4 g. Some patients have flares of their disease while on a maintenance program of 2 g/day and yet their flares are controlled by raising the dose to 3 or 4 g/day. If these patients tolerate the higher dose, it is worth a trial of the higher dose as maintenance therapy. The risks of

long-term maintenance therapy with sulfasalazine are modest. There are no definitive guidelines for the duration of maintenance therapy. The usual approach has been to continue therapy for several years in those who have had a single attack of mild to moderate severity and to continue maintenance therapy indefinitely in those with multiple relapses.

Several studies have investigated the usefulness of sulfasalazine in preventing relapse in patients with Crohn's disease. The National Cooperative Crohn's Disease Study examined the effects of sulfasalazine in patients who achieved remission during the initial study.[189] The majority of patients in both the sulfasalazine- and placebo-treated groups remained in remission, with no significant differences between the groups. Similarly, the European Cooperative Crohn's Disease Study showed no benefit of sulfasalazine treatment for patients with quiescent disease at entry into the study.[190] Despite the lack of support in the literature, many physicians use sulfasalazine as maintenance therapy in Crohn's disease, especially in patients with Crohn's colitis in whom acute disease responded to sulfasalazine.

Adverse Effects

The side effects most commonly reported with sulfasalazine are nausea, vomiting, anorexia, headache, fever, rash, and abdominal discomfort. There are two groups of side effects caused by sulfasalazine: dose-related toxic effects, thought to be related to serum sulfapyridine levels, and hypersensitivity reactions, which are not related to serum sulfapyridine levels. The dose-related toxic effects (headache, nausea, vomiting, and abdominal discomfort) are far more common and are associated with serum sulfapyridine levels of greater than 50 μg/mL. Sulfapyridine is metabolized by acetylation, so slow-acetylators have high serum levels of free sulfapyridine and low levels of acetylated sulfapyridine, whereas fast-acetylators have low levels of free sulfapyridine and high levels of acetylated sulfapyridine. The dose-related side effects are more common in slow-acetylators, and the incidence of side effects increases with dosages of 4 g or more per day. Another common dose-related adverse reaction to sulfasalazine is low-grade hemolysis. In one series, 19 of 36 patients taking 4 to 5 g of sulfasalazine per day had biochemical evidence of hemolysis, although only four had overt hemolytic anemia, which was associated with high serum sulfapyridine levels and slow-acetylator status. Most of the toxic dose-related side effects of sulfasalazine develop in the first few weeks of therapy and resolve with discontinuation of therapy. Because these side effects are dose-related, most patients can avoid them if given a low enough dose. A patient who develops headaches or nausea taking 4 g of sulfasalazine per day for an acute attack may well tolerate a 2-g maintenance dose without problems. For those whose only side effect is dyspepsia, relief may be obtained by taking the drug with meals or by using the enteric-coated preparation.[193,194]

The second group of side effects, hypersensitivity reactions, includes rash, fever, aplastic anemia, agranulocytosis, and autoimmune hemolysis. In contrast to toxic reactions, these are not related to the dose of sulfasalazine, acetylator status, or serum sulfapyridine concentrations. Hypersensitivity reactions occur less commonly than toxic reactions, but they tend to occur with greater severity. Myeloblastic anemia, presumably

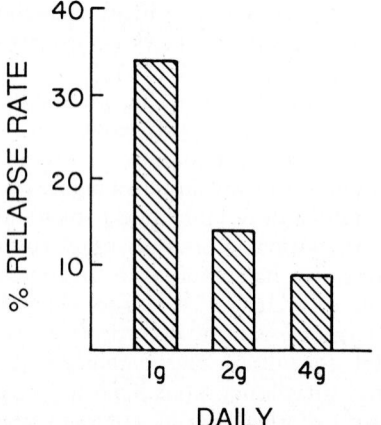

FIGURE 79-28. Relapse rate with maintenance sulfasalazine. (From Azad Khan AK, Howes DT, Piris J, Truelove SC. Optimum dose of sulphasalazine for maintenance treatment of ulcerative colitis. Gut 1980;21:232.)

a result of folate deficiency, has been reported with sulfasalazine but is much less common than a reduction in the serum folate concentration.[195,196] Although uncommon, agranulocytosis, with a mortality rate of 35% reported in one series, is probably the most common fatal side effect. In addition to numerous cases of dose-related toxic hemolysis, there are also reports of a few cases of non–dose-related autoimmune hemolysis.

Sulfasalazine commonly causes changes in sperm morphology and decreased sperm counts, leading to infertility.[197,198] The incidence of abnormalities in sperm morphology and number appear to be high in slow-acetylators. The effects are reversible within 3 months of sulfasalazine withdrawal. It has been speculated that the effects of sulfasalazine on sperm relate to its antifolate activity.

Bloody diarrhea has been described as a rare toxic complication of sulfasalazine. This hypersensitivity reaction has endoscopic and histologic features similar to those of ulcerative colitis.[199] All patients reported to have this complication have improved with withdrawal of sulfasalazine and treatment with corticosteroids. In contrast to the other side effects described, bloody diarrhea appears to be a product of 5-ASA rather than sulfapyridine.

Drug Interactions

Broad-spectrum antibiotics that markedly reduce the bacterial flora of the colon would be expected to diminish the cleavage of sulfasalazine to 5-ASA and sulfapyridine.[200] Whether this is a significant problem in clinical practice has not been established. Sulfasalazine inhibits folic acid absorption and is a competitive inhibitor of folate conjugase in the jejunal brush border.[201] Malabsorption of folate with reduced serum folate levels has been described in patients on sulfasalazine therapy, and some clinicians routinely recommend folic acid supplementation of 1 to 2 mg/day for patients treated with sulfasalazine. Concomitant administration of sulfasalazine and digoxin has been demonstrated to interfere with the bioavailability of digoxin, with mean reduction of serum digoxin levels of 25%.

Pregnant Women and Children

There have been a number of studies of the effects of sulfasalazine on infants in utero and nursing children. No evidence of harmful effects has been found, and the usual recommendation is that the drug can be used safely either in acute or maintenance therapy in pregnant and lactating women.[202–207] Children can be treated safely with sulfasalazine. For acute disease in children older than 2 years of age, the initial dose is 25 to 40 mg/kg/day in three to six doses; this can be increased gradually to 75 mg/kg/day.[208] For maintenance therapy in children older than 2 years of age, the dose is 20 mg/kg/per day in divided doses. An oral suspension is available.

5-ASA Preparations

5-ASA is the active therapeutic moiety in sulfasalazine. A number of pharmaceutical preparations of 5-ASA for oral and rectal use have been developed. All these formulations allow the patient to take 5-ASA without also taking sulfapyridine, the component of sulfasalazine that causes most of the adverse reactions; however, some patients have adverse reactions to 5-ASA. The rectal formulations of 5-ASA achieve a higher concentration of 5-ASA in the rectum than can be attained with oral sulfasalazine. The clinical response to sulfasalazine increases with increasing dose, so it is likely that 5-ASA enemas are more effective than sulfasalazine in proctitis owing to the higher concentration achieved. Some of the oral 5-ASA preparations allow slow release in the small intestine, raising the possibility of treating small intestine Crohn's disease. The newer 5-ASA formulations offer potential benefits over sulfasalazine in the form of decreased toxicity, increased concentration at the site of action, and extended distribution.

5-ASA is currently available in the United States as a 4-g enema (Rowasa), as a suppository, and in several oral formulations (Dipentum, Asacol, Pentasa). In one large double-blind study of proctitis,[209] 4-g 5-ASA enemas were compared with 100-mg hydrocortisone enemas in 86 patients for a period of 2 weeks. The 5-ASA enemas induced remission by clinical standards in 93% of patients, by sigmoidoscopic standards in 93%, and by histologic standards in 77%. For the hydrocortisone group, the comparable numbers were 57%, 54%, and 53%, respectively. Prolonged treatment with daily 5-ASA enemas does not result in significant blood levels of 5-ASA. Although 5-ASA enemas induce clinical improvement in patients with proctitis, withdrawal of the enemas results in prompt recrudescence of disease activity. There are anecdotal reports of severe recurrences after 5-ASA enemas were abruptly stopped. In some of these cases, the colitis extended to involve the entire colon and colectomy was required. To prevent recrudescence, the frequency of enema administration is diminished gradually. After a clinical remission has been firmly established with daily enemas, the frequency is reduced to every other day and then every third day; however, many patients flare as the enemas are withdrawn. Administration of sulfasalazine along with the enemas tends to even out the amount of 5-ASA in the colon and may reduce the risk of recurrence as the enemas are withdrawn. 5-ASA enemas have also been used to maintain remission in patients with quiescent disease[210]; patients were treated with enemas for 1 week out of each month for a year with good results. If maintenance therapy is required, most patients prefer an oral agent such as sulfasalazine rather than an enema. Maintenance therapy with enemas should be considered in patients with distal disease who have adverse reactions to sulfasalazine or who cannot be maintained in remission with sulfasalazine.

If 5-ASA alone is administered orally, it is rapidly absorbed and significant lumenal concentrations are not achieved. Several approaches have been taken to formulate oral 5-ASA to yield high lumenal concentrations with little systemic absorption. One approach has been to covalently bond 5-ASA through an azo linkage to another 5-ASA (Dipentum, Olsalazine) or to 4-aminobenzoyl-β-alanine (Balsalazide). Like sulfasalazine, these compounds release their 5-ASA in the colon when bacteria cleave the azo bond. Olsalazine causes secretion from the small intestine, resulting in watery diarrhea in 5% to 10% of treated patients.[211] An alternate approach is to formulate 5-ASA in coated granules that release 5-ASA slowly and in a pH-dependent fashion (Pentasa, Asacol, Salofalk, Claversal). Asacol is 5-ASA coated with Eudragit-S; it dissolves at pH 7 or above and releases 5-ASA primarily in the colon and terminal ileum. Pentasa is 5-ASA in a semipermeable membrane which releases the 5-ASA at pH 6 and above. Pentasa releases 35% of its 5-ASA in the small intestine and may be useful for small intestine Crohn's disease. However, release in the small intestine results in increased absorption and therefore increased risk of toxicity. High doses of oral 5-ASA are nephrotoxic in rats, but this has not been a major problem in human clinical studies. Thus far, oral 5-ASA preparations have been found to be as effective as sulfasalazine in the management of acute exacerbation of ulcerative colitis.[212,213] Asacol at a dose of 2.4 g/day was superior to placebo in patients with mildly to moderately active ulcerative colitis.[214] These newer formulations of 5-ASA have also been found to be effective in the maintenance of remissions in both ulcerative colitis and Crohn's disease. Both Olsalazine[215] and Pentasa (1500 mg/day) were as effective as sulfasalazine (3 g/day) in the maintenance of remission in ulcerative colitis.[216] Asacol at a dose of 2.4 g/day was found to be superior to placebo in the maintenance of remission in patients with Crohn's disease, particularly those with ileitis.[217]

The exact role of 5-ASA preparations, both rectal and oral, in the management of IBD remains to be seen. The incidence of side effects is clearly less with these compounds than with sulfasalazine. The increased level of tolerability allows patients to achieve higher colonic lumenal concentrations of 5-ASA with these preparations than with sulfasalazine and thus increases the likelihood of a clinical response. At the least, these compounds should be useful as substitutes for sulfasalazine for patients with adverse reactions to sulfapyridine. They may, in addition, have a broader therapeutic role in circumstances in which increased local concentrations of 5-ASA or an increased area of distribution are important.

Corticosteroids

Mechanism of Action

Corticosteroids prevent or suppress inflammation induced by chemical, mechanical, infectious, and immunologic agents. The wide range of inflammatory events in which corticosteroids are effective suggests that the final pathway in the production of inflammation is similar regardless of the initiating event and that corticosteroids act on that final pathway. Moreover, because corticosteroids are useful in the treatment of inflammatory diseases of widely ranging causes, the fact that IBD responds to corticosteroids is not at all helpful in establishing a cause. In IBD, as in other inflammatory diseases, the administration of steroids appears to be palliative therapy: the inflammatory response is suppressed but the etiologic agent remains.

Corticosteroids block the early manifestations of inflammation—enhanced vascular permeability, vasodilation, and neutrophil infiltration (Table 79-11). However, they also block the later stages of the inflammatory process—vascular proliferation, fibroblast activation, and collagen deposition. Corticosteroids have in vitro effects on events that are considered to be immunologic, such as T-cell response to antigens, as well as on events considered inflammatory, such as

TABLE 79-11
Effects of Corticosteroids on Inflammation

Lymphocytes
Redistribution of lymphocytes from vascular space to lymphoid organs
Decreased peripheral blood lymphocyte count
Inhibition of T-cell proliferation in response to mitogens and specific antigen
Decreased interleukin-2 production

Monocytes and Macrophages
Redistribution of monocytes from vascular space to lymphoid organs
Decreased peripheral blood monocyte count
Decreased margination of monocytes and thus decreased migration into inflamed tissue
Diminished response to chemotactic factors and lymphokines including migration inhibiting factor
Decreased phagocytosis and microbial killing
Decreased expression of IgG and C3b receptors
Decreased production of interleukin-1
Inhibition of secretion of proteins including collagenase, elastase, and plasminogen activator

Neutrophils
Increased release from bone marrow
Increased peripheral blood neutrophil count
Decreased margination and thus decreased migration into inflamed tissue.

Soluble Mediators
Increased production of lipomodulin with a resultant decrease in arachidonic acid release from phospholipids
Decreased produciton of leukotrienes and prostaglandins as a result of increased lipomodulin production

neutrophil migration and mediator production.[218–221] Because it is unknown whether the therapeutic effects of corticosteroids in IBD relate to their effects on inflammation or to their effects on immunologic events, the response to corticosteroids does not help to determine whether the primary event in IBD is a defect in immunoregulation.

Corticosteroids are physiologic products of the adrenal gland. Therapeutically administered exogenous steroids interact with the same receptors as naturally produced corticosteroids do. Steroids diffuse freely through the plasma membrane to bind to receptors in the cytosol. After the binding of a steroid molecule to the steroid receptor in the cytosol, the ligand-receptor complex travels to the nucleus, where it attaches to DNA, derepresses certain genes, and results in the production of messenger RNA specific for particular proteins. The proteins synthesized in response to corticosteroids are specific for each cell type. Steroid receptors are widely distributed, and pharmacologic doses of corticosteroids affect the function of almost all mammalian cells, including those involved in immunologic and inflammatory responses. Because the wide distribution of steroid receptors in the immune system and the variety of proteins whose synthesis is affected result in a complex response of the immune system to steroids, it is difficult to sort out which effects are most relevant to the therapeutic response. Similarly, the wide distribution of steroid receptors in other organ systems results in a host of undesirable side effects in response to pharmacologic doses of steroids.

Administration of a single dose of steroids results in a prompt decline in the number of circulating lymphocytes (see Table 79-11). In humans, the fall in circulating lymphocytes is caused by redistribution of lymphocytes from the circulation to lymphoid organs. Part of the human lymphocyte population, mostly T cells, normally shuttles back and forth between the vascular space and lymphoid organs, including lymph nodes and bone marrow. Steroids cause a larger than normal proportion of this recirculating lymphocyte population to enter the lymphoid organs. In addition to affecting lymphocyte distribution, corticosteroids also impair the proliferative response of T cells to specific antigens. Steroid-treated lymphocytes have diminished synthesis of IL-2, a lymphokine that amplifies T-cell proliferation. The impaired proliferative capacity of steroid-treated lymphocytes may relate in part to decreased IL-2 production. Administration of corticosteroids causes a redistribution of monocytes similar to that seen with lymphocytes. Monocytes leave the intravascular space and enter lymphoid organs. Circulating monocyte levels fall from 300 to 400/cm^3 to 50/cm^3; the circulating monocyte count reaches its lowest level 4 to 6 hours after steroid administration and is back to normal at 24 hours. A decrease in the population of circulating monocytes results in a decrease in the number of macrophages found in the inflamed tissue. Macrophages are thought to play an important role in the formation of granulomas in diseases such as Crohn's disease. Therefore, a steroid-induced decrease in the number of circulating monocytes may affect granuloma formation. Steroids are known to reduce the febrile response in inflammatory diseases. The endogenous pyrogen responsible for the febrile response is IL-1, a product of activated macrophages. Steroids reduce IL-1 production by macrophages and thus reduce the febrile response.

Macrophages and monocytes kill microorganisms most efficiently if the microorganisms are opsonized, complexed with IgG and C3b, a product of the complement cascade. Macrophages and monocytes attach to opsonized microorganisms through cell surface receptors for the Fc portion of IgG and for C3b. Treatment with corticosteroids reduces the number of receptors for IgG and C3b expressed on the plasma membranes of macrophages and monocytes and reduces their ability to bind opsonized microorganisms. In response to stimulation, monocytes and macrophages release a number of proteins thought to be important in the inflammatory response. These proteins include collagenase and elastase, which degrade portions of the extracellular matrix. Macrophages also release tissue plasminogen activator, which converts plasminogen to plasmin, a process that is thought to facilitate the migration of leukocytes into areas of inflammation by breaking down fibrin and other proteins. Secretion of all these proteins is impaired by steroid administration.

In contrast to the decrease in the number of circulating lymphocytes and monocytes induced by steroids, the number of circulating neutrophils increases markedly. The increase in circulating neutrophils is caused by enhanced release of neutrophils from the bone marrow and decreased migration out of the circulation. The first step in the process of neutrophil migration out of the circulation and into an inflamed tissue is the adherence of neutrophils to the postcapillary venule

endothelium. This process, called margination or pavementing, is inhibited by corticosteroids. This effect is of particular interest in IBD, in which there is known to be a massive flux of neutrophils out of the circulation into the inflamed mucosa and then out into the colonic lumen. The neutrophils that migrate into the inflamed mucosa are thought to be important mediators of epithelial destruction. The inhibition of neutrophil and monocyte migration out of the circulation and into the intestinal tissue may be the most important component of the therapeutic efficacy of corticosteroids in IBD.

Products of arachidonic acid metabolism through both the cyclooxygenase and lipoxygenase pathways are important soluble mediators of inflammation. There is little free arachidonic acid in mammalian cells. The rate-limiting step in the production of both cyclooxygenase and lipoxygenase products is the release of arachidonic acid from phospholipids by phospholipase A_2. In immune cells, phospholipase A_2 is activated by the binding of lymphokines and other soluble mediators to cell surface receptors. Corticosteroids promote the synthesis of a protein called lipomodulin which inhibits phospholipase A_2 and thus blocks the release of arachidonic acid.[50]

It is not clear which of the specific effects of corticosteroids on the inflammatory process contribute most to therapeutic efficacy in IBD. The decreased margination of monocytes and neutrophils, with the resultant decrease in the number of monocytes and neutrophils entering the inflamed colon, is clearly of potential relevance to the therapeutic efficacy of steroids in IBD. Similarly, diminished production of IL-1 and IL-2 could contribute to a loss of amplification of the inflammatory response and a clinical improvement in IBD. In particular, decreased IL-2 production could block T-cell proliferation and result in fewer helper T cells to promote antibody production and fewer cytotoxic lymphocytes to participate in epithelial cell cytotoxicity. Finally, lipomodulin production would result in decreased LTB_4 production. LTB_4 has been shown to be an important neutrophil chemotactic factor in IBD. In this manner, corticosteroid administration would also reduce neutrophil migration into IBD mucosa by decreasing the synthesis of an important chemotactic factor.

Corticosteroids in Ulcerative Colitis

Studies dating back almost 40 years document the efficacy of corticosteroids in ulcerative colitis. In 1955, Truelove compared patients treated with cortisone (100 mg/day) with subjects treated with placebo for 6 weeks.[62] Cortisone was found to be superior to placebo in patients with disease ranging in severity from mild to severe; the difference was less striking in the more severely ill patients. Corticosteroids have been demonstrated to be effective in ulcerative colitis if given either orally or parenterally; oral steroid therapy is effective in the majority of patients with mild to moderate disease.[187] Few studies have assessed the relative value of various dosage regimens of oral corticosteroids. In one study (Fig. 79-29), two thirds of outpatients treated with 40 to 60 mg of prednisolone per day improved over a period of 3 weeks, compared with just one third of those receiving 20 mg/day.[222] Most responders improved within 2 weeks. As a result of this study, 40 mg/day has been widely recommended as an initial dose of prednisone for patients with moderately severe ulcerative colitis (prednisone and prednisolone are effectively equal in

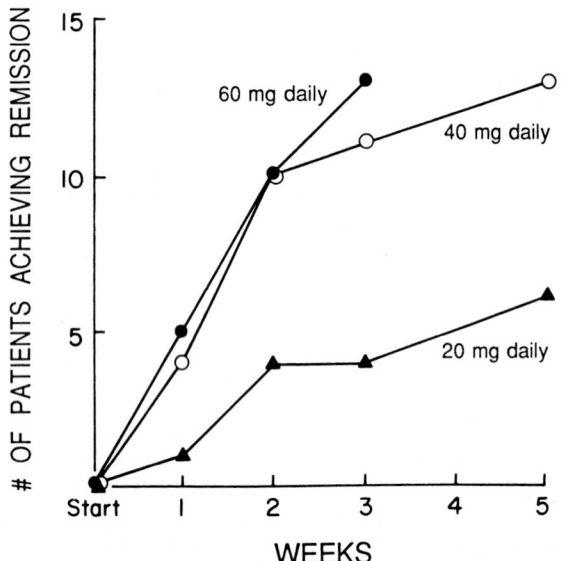

FIGURE 79-29. The number of patients with active ulcerative colitis achieving remission over a 5-week period with increasing doses of prednisolone. (From Baron JH, Connell AM, Kamaghinis TG, et al. Outpatient treatment of ulcerative colitis. Br Med J 1962;2:441.)

antiinflammatory potency). For most patients, administration of oral prednisone in a single morning dose is as effective as divided doses[223]; however, use of divided doses may be appropriate in selected patients. Several studies have compared parenteral corticosteroids with parenteral adrenocorticotropic hormone (ACTH) for severe ulcerative colitis. For the most part, they have been found to be equally effective. However, in the largest controlled trial, intravenous ACTH (120 U/day) was found to be somewhat more effective than intravenous hydrocortisone (300 mg/day) in patients with severe ulcerative colitis who had never previously received oral corticosteroids, whereas hydrocortisone was more effective in those who had previously received steroid therapy.[224] Despite the results of this one study, most clinicians seldom or never use ACTH for IBD. The expense, the requirement for parenteral administration, and the failure of earlier studies to find a significant benefit compared with steroid treatment all contribute to the limited use of ACTH in practice. Corticosteroid enemas have been demonstrated to be useful in left-sided colitis.[225,226] In most individuals, a 100-mL corticosteroid enema reaches the mid-descending colon, although in some the enema reaches the mid-transverse colon. About 80% of patients with proctitis obtain a remission or significant improvement with one enema per night for 2 to 3 weeks. The extent of systemic absorption varies with the corticosteroid preparation and with the severity of inflammation. In general, systemic absorption is much less than with orally administered steroids; however, in some cases as much as 75% of the dose administered rectally is absorbed.[227,228] Several corticosteroid enema preparations have been designed to minimize systemic side effects. Beclomethasone enemas have been used with clinical effectiveness but without suppressing the adrenal-pituitary axis.[229] A second topical steroid under study is tixocortol pivalate, which is absorbed if given as an enema and is

so rapidly metabolized that no systemic effects are seen.[230,231] A third corticosteroid under study for topical application in ulcerative colitis is budesonide, which, if given as an enema, has a high degree of topical potency with modest side effects.[232,233] Neither beclomethasone nor tixocortol pivalate is available in enema formulation in the United States at this time. In addition to enema preparations, corticosteroids are also available in foam suspension. Proximal penetration with foam is not as great as with enemas, so foam can only be used for disease confined to the rectum; however, foam preparations are less bothersome for the patient than enema preparations.

Corticosteroids in Crohn's Disease

The National Cooperative Crohn's Disease Study found that a 17-week course of prednisone (.25–.75 mg/kg/day) was more effective than placebo in Crohn's disease of the small bowel.[189] Sixty percent of prednisone-treated patients achieved remission, compared with 30% of those receiving placebo. The European Cooperative Crohn's Disease Study found similar benefits with oral corticosteroids in Crohn's disease.[190] In that study, 6-methylprednisolone, beginning with a dose of 48 mg daily, was more effective than placebo in Crohn's disease of the small bowel or colon. In a large series of 142 patients with active Crohn's disease, treatment with prednisolone (1 mg/kg/day) resulted in clinical remission in 92% of patients within 7 weeks, although the rate of endoscopic remission was much lower.[234] Considering the prominent role that corticosteroids have played in the management of Crohn's disease, there have been few studies addressing the issues of optimal doses, duration of therapy, and parameters for adjusting dosages. The physician must be sure that there is no abscess present if considering the use of corticosteroids. An abscess requires surgical drainage and antibiotics, and the use of corticosteroids in a patient with an undrained abscess may lead to uncontrolled sepsis. In addition, the physician must also be certain that the patient's symptoms relate to inflammation and not to a stricture or other fibrotic process that will not respond to steroids. The usual starting dose is 20 to 40 mg of prednisone per day, depending on the severity of disease. Prednisone is given orally if the patient can tolerate and absorb oral medication, or steroids are given parenterally if the patient cannot tolerate oral medication. The patient is left on high doses of corticosteroids until symptoms begin to diminish, after which the dose of corticosteroids is very gradually reduced.

Maintenance therapy with corticosteroids for the prevention of recurrences in patients in clinical remission has been demonstrated to be ineffective in both ulcerative colitis and Crohn's disease.[189] In both diseases, however, there are patients with continuously active disease that responds to corticosteroids but flares up if the dose of steroids is reduced.

Adverse Effects

The many side effects of corticosteroids are the major factor limiting their use in IBD.[190,235] Although the side effects of corticosteroids are dose-dependent, there is a wide range of patient susceptibility to these side effects. Some patients tolerate prolonged courses of high-dose corticosteroid therapy without ill effects, but others develop devastating side effects with short courses of low-dose therapy. The range of patient susceptibility to developing corticosteroid side effects is a function of differences in plasma protein binding (with hypoalbuminemic patients being at risk) and of variations in rates of metabolism and clearance of synthetic steroids. The major differences between the manifestations of iatrogenic steroid administration and the manifestations of spontaneous Cushing's syndrome are related to the increased levels of androgens and mineralocorticoids in spontaneous Cushing's syndrome.[236] Features more common in spontaneous Cushing's syndrome include hypertension, virilism, hirsutism, striae, and purpura. Features more common in iatrogenic steroid administration include posterior subcapsular cataracts, avascular necrosis of bone, and glaucoma. Patients taking 10 mg or more of prednisone daily for longer than 3 weeks should be viewed as having a suppressed hypothalamic-pituitary-adrenal axis for 1 year after cessation of therapy and should receive supplemental glucocorticoids for surgery or severe illness. Patients should be instructed about adrenal suppression and the need for glucocorticoid supplementation for surgery and severe illness even after cessation of therapy.

Patients also need to be educated about the benefits and toxicities of glucocorticoids. They should understand the trade-offs between efficacy and toxicity. In particular, they should understand the more predictable side effects of osteoporosis and cataract formation and the necessity of observing for their occurrence. Common predictable side effects include increased appetite, centripetal obesity, moon facies, acne, insomnia, increased risk of infection, and, in children, growth arrest. Less common problems for which the patient should be monitored include hypertension and glucose intolerance. Psychiatric problems occur, including depression and psychosis. Avascular bone necrosis, particularly of the femoral heads, occurs and can result in permanent disability.

Osteoporosis is a common and potentially devastating side effect of corticosteroid therapy. Every patient treated with glucocorticoids develops negative calcium balance. The effects of corticosteroids on bone include both enhanced bone resorption and diminished bone formation.[236] Steroid-induced bone loss is a particular problem in small intestine Crohn's disease, in which malabsorption of vitamin D and calcium can also accelerate calcium loss from bone. Bone loss characteristically involves trabecular bone in ribs, vertebrae, and distal radius. Rib fractures and vertebral compression fractures are common. The incidence of symptomatic bone loss is higher in children and postmenopausal women. There are conflicting data on the effects of low-dose corticosteroids on bone loss. Dykman and colleagues reported significant bone loss with doses as low as 8 to 10 mg of prednisone per day,[237] but Sambrook and associates reported no increase in bone loss over a period of 7 years using an equivalent dose of prednisolone.[238] Alternate-day glucocorticoid therapy appears not to increase bone loss and thus has an advantage over daily therapy. Unfortunately, many patients with IBD cannot be successfully switched to alternate-day therapy. Patients on significant doses of prednisone over a long period of time should have their calcium stores monitored by bone densitometry. Diet supplementation with calcium and vitamin D

may diminish the rate of bone calcium loss. The adequacy of therapy with calcium and vitamin D is assessed by measuring urinary calcium. For amenorrheic or postmenopausal women with IBD and osteoporosis, estrogen therapy may reduce bone loss. The lowest effective dose is the equivalent of 0.625 mg/day of conjugated equine estrogens. Posterior subcapsular cataracts occur frequently with corticosteroid therapy, and their incidence correlates with dose and duration of therapy.[239] Of patients receiving 15 mg of prednisone for 1 year, 25% developed lenticular changes. Glucocorticoids also increase intraocular pressure in up to 40% of patients. Irreversible glaucoma and blindness can occur in susceptible individuals. Referral to an ophthalmologist for baseline measurement of intraocular pressure and slit-lamp examination should be considered if long-term corticosteroid management is expected. Periodic examinations should be performed if therapy is continued.

Immunosuppressive Drugs

Immunosuppressives are a loosely defined group of drugs that act by blocking lymphocyte proliferation, activation, or effector mechanisms. There is fairly extensive experience in the use of two immunosuppressives, azathioprine and its metabolite 6-mercaptopurine (6-MP), in the treatment of IBD and lesser experience with other immunosuppressives, including cyclosporine and methotrexate. The mechanisms of action for the therapeutic efficacy of these compounds in IBD are not precisely defined. The role of immunosuppressive drugs has been a major source of controversy in Crohn's disease therapy. The National Cooperative Crohn's Disease Study found that azathioprine was no more effective than placebo in a 17-week trial.[189] However, the therapeutic effects of immunosuppressives are not seen until after 3, 4, or more months of therapy, and the 17-week treatment period in this study was too short to demonstrate the maximal effect. There have been a number of studies in which azathioprine or 6-MP has been shown to be efficacious in the treatment of Crohn's disease.[240-243] In these trials, the usual dose was 2 to 2.5 mg/kg/day. More recently, there has been a tendency to use immunosuppressives in somewhat lower doses to minimize toxicity. An initial dose of 50 mg/day is given, and blood counts are monitored for 3 weeks. If the patient tolerates the drug, the dose is gradually increased to 1.5 mg/kg/day. Although most investigators and clinicians agree that immunosuppressives have a role to play in the management of Crohn's disease, there is a divergence of opinion as to what that role should be. Patients in whom the use of immunosuppressives is widely accepted include those who have active disease poorly controlled by steroids but who are not surgical candidates, and those with active disease that is controlled by steroids but in whom steroids have caused significant side effects. In these patients, an immunosuppressive is added to steroid therapy. After 3 or 4 months, when the immunosuppressives are likely to have taken effect, the dose of steroids is gradually tapered. With immunosuppressives, as with other medical therapies for IBD, disease activity is likely to worsen after the drug is withdrawn. A few clinicians use immunosuppressives, rather than corticosteroids, as first-line therapy in Crohn's disease. Immunosuppressives have also been promoted as primary therapy for fistulas in Crohn's disease. Although immunosuppressives heal some fistulas, the fistulas tend to recur after the drugs are stopped.

The major limiting factor in the use of immunosuppressives is their toxicity.[244] Immunosuppressives commonly cause leukopenia, and the leukocyte count of patients receiving them must be carefully monitored. These drugs should be tried only in patients who are likely to be compliant with the required laboratory monitoring. The largest review of the toxicity of 6-MP in IBD cataloged experience with 396 patients followed for an average of 60 months.[245] Significant but reversible morbidity included pancreatitis (3.3%), bone marrow depression (2%), and allergic reactions (2%). Infectious complications were seen in 7%, including one case of herpes zoster encephalitis. There were 12 neoplasms, but probably only one, a diffuse histiocytic lymphoma of the brain, was associated with the drug. Certainly the risk of neoplasm is a worrisome problem; lymphomas have been described in patients taking these drugs for other diseases, but the magnitude of the risk is not yet clear.[244,246]

Cyclosporine is a powerful immunosuppressive that is widely used to prevent rejection in transplant patients. There is increasing experience with the use of cyclosporine (parenteral, oral, and enema formulations) in IBD. Renal toxicity is a major problem with cyclosporine; both serum cyclosporine levels and renal function must be carefully monitored. One clear advantage of cyclosporine over azathioprine and 6-MP is that the onset of action is seen in a few days rather than several months. Cyclosporine has been tested in a double-blind study in chronic Crohn's disease.[247] Patients were treated for 3 months with a fairly low dose (5–7.5 mg/kg/day) of oral cyclosporine. Cyclosporine was superior to placebo in achieving treatment goals designated for each patient but was not superior to placebo in reducing the Crohn's Disease Activity Index. Further studies are needed to determine whether cyclosporine has a role in the management of IBD.

Immunosuppressives play a smaller role in the management of ulcerative colitis than in Crohn's disease. Azathioprine and 6-MP can be used in ulcerative colitis to achieve the same steroid-sparing effects described for Crohn's disease. The long delay in the onset of a therapeutic response with these drugs is a problem in ulcerative colitis as in Crohn's disease. There is some experience with the use of intravenous cyclosporine in ulcerative colitis. Here, the major indication is an attempt to avoid colectomy in severe disease that is unresponsive to intravenous corticosteroids. In one series, patients who failed to respond to 7 to 10 days of intravenous corticosteroids were given placebo or cyclosporine at a dose of 4 mg/kg/day by continuous infusion. Nine of eleven patients who received cyclosporine responded, but none of the nine placebo-treated patients responded.[248] How many of these cyclosporine-treated patients can remain under control after being switched to oral cyclosporine is unknown. The approach to the use of cyclosporine in ulcerative colitis is to control disease activity with 1 to 2 weeks of parenteral cyclosporine and then switch to oral cyclosporine for 3 months. During that time, the patient is begun on 6-MP with the hope that after 3 months the cyclosporine can be stopped and the 6-MP continued. The decision to use long-term immunosuppressives in ulcerative colitis is somewhat more difficult because of the availability of a curative therapy—colectomy.

Antibiotics

Except in cases of overt sepsis, there appears to be little role for antibiotics in the management of ulcerative colitis. Antibiotics do not affect the remission rate,[249] and a trial of metronidazole in ulcerative proctitis showed it to be ineffective.[250] Moreover, the risk of inducing antibiotic-associated pseudomembranous colitis must be considered.

The role of antibiotic therapy in Crohn's disease is more confused. Clearly, broad-spectrum antibiotics play a role in the management of the suppurative complications of Crohn's disease, especially abscess formation and perianal disease. In addition, antibiotics play a role in the management of diarrhea caused by overgrowth of bacteria in the small bowel. This problem usually occurs because of stasis behind a stricture. If the stricture is not amenable to surgical or endoscopic management, the symptoms of pain, gaseousness, and diarrhea can be managed with courses of broad-spectrum antibiotics such as tetracycline. Even though broad-spectrum antibiotics have commonly been used in the management of uncomplicated Crohn's disease, there have been no controlled trials to justify this approach.

Metronidazole is one antibiotic with a somewhat better defined role in the management of Crohn's disease. The efficacy of metronidazole has been demonstrated in perianal Crohn's disease (discussed in a previous section) and in colonic Crohn's disease. A Swedish trial compared metronidazole (800 mg/day) and sulfasalazine (3 g/day) in patients with Crohn's disease.[251] The two drugs were equally effective, and both were more effective in disease confined to the colon. Patients who failed on sulfasalazine often improved after being switched to metronidazole, whereas those who failed on metronidazole did not respond to sulfasalazine. Side effects of metronidazole in this study were less common and less severe than those reported in other studies. In particular, peripheral neuropathy was not a major problem in this study. The low dose of metronidazole and the short duration of the study may account for the low incidence of side effects. A second study compared metronidazole at 10 mg/kg and 20 mg/kg with placebo in Crohn's disease and found dose-related improvements in disease activity, but the incidence of side effects was high and only half the patients completed the study.[252]

The mechanism of action of metronidazole in Crohn's colitis is not known. Other antimicrobials with similar patterns of bacterial killing are not effective in Crohn's disease, suggesting that the efficacy of metronidazole is not a product of its antimicrobial properties. If metronidazole has immunsuppressive or antiinflammatory properties, they are yet to be described.

MEDICAL MANAGEMENT OF ULCERATIVE COLITIS

Active Proctitis

There are several reasonable approaches to the initial treatment of active ulcerative proctitis; however, there are no data to support one approach over another. One relatively effective and rapidly acting approach is the use of local corticosteroids in the form of retention enemas (Cortenema) or, for more limited disease, rectal foam (Cortifoam or Proctofoam-HC) administered once a day at bedtime for 2 to 3 weeks. If there is a good clinical response, this therapy is continued for another few weeks on an every-other-night basis. An equally acceptable alternative is the nightly administration of 5-ASA (Rowasa) retention enemas or suppositories. If the patient responds, the frequency of the enemas or suppositories can be reduced from nightly to every other night after 2 to 3 weeks. Rowasa enemas are often supplemented with oral sulfasalazine or an oral 5-ASA preparation. Either 5-ASA suppositories or corticosteroid foam is appropriate for disease in up to 20 cm of distal colon; 5-ASA or corticosteroid retention enemas can be used for active disease in up to 60 cm of distal colon. A third acceptable initial therapeutic approach to proctitis or distal colitis is oral sulfasalazine or an oral 5-ASA preparation. Sulfasalazine is begun at a dose of 500 mg twice daily and gradually increased every few days until a dose of 3 to 4 g/day is reached. Oral 5-ASA preparations that can be used instead of sulfasalazine include mesalamine (Asacol or Pentasa) and olsalazine (Dipentum), although Dipentum is not approved by the United States Food and Drug Administration for acute disease. The initial dose of Asacol is 800 mg three times a day; this can be increased up to 4.8 g/day if necessary. The response to oral sulfasalazine or 5-ASA compounds may not be seen for 3 to 4 weeks, which is slower than the response to corticosteroid or 5-ASA enemas.

The patient with proctitis who does not respond to corticosteroid enemas can be tried on Rowasa's enemas, oral sulfasalazine, or 5-ASA. Conversely, those not responsive to Rowasa enemas, sulfasalazine, or oral 5-ASA can be tried on corticosteroid enemas. Patients not responding to any of these modalities should be tried on oral corticosteroids; treatment with prednisone can be started with a dose of 30 to 40 mg/day. Those who do not respond to any of the initial therapies or to oral corticosteroids can be tried on 6-MP, although there is usually a delay of several months before a clinical response is seen with 6-MP. There are also some favorable preliminary reports on the use of cyclosporine enemas for the management of refractory proctitis.[253]

For patients with mild disease activity, whether with proctitis or more extensive disease, there is likely to be a role for symptomatic antidiarrheal therapy, usually with loperamide or diphenoxylate. They can be used to reduce the number of bowel movements or to reduce rectal urgency. Most patients use them on an as-needed basis after diarrheal stools, but some find it useful to take them on a prophylactic basis, for example, with meals in patients in whom eating induces diarrhea.

After the proctitis is in remission, maintenance therapy should be considered. There is no compelling evidence that patients with a single, easily managed bout of proctitis need maintenance therapy; however, those with difficult to manage disease or with frequent or early relapses should have chronic maintenance therapy. The largest experience with maintenance therapy is with sulfasalazine. The usual maintenance dose of sulfasalazine is 2 g/day; however, there is convincing evidence that maintenance with 4 g/day is more effective.[252] For patients who have undesirable side effects with sulfasalazine, maintenance therapy with olsalazine (1 g/day) or other oral 5-ASA formulations should be considered. If active disease is controlled with 5-ASA enemas, maintenance therapy with the same enemas may be appropriate. Typically, mainte-nance therapy with 5-ASA enemas is given every other day or every third day. Because of the expense and inconvenience, maintenance therapy with 5-ASA enemas is reasonable only in patients who have failed maintenance therapy with sulfasalazine and oral 5-ASA compounds.

Active Extensive Colitis

For patients with colitis of mild to moderate activity and extension proximal to the sigmoid colon, the initial drug of choice is either sulfasalazine or an oral 5-ASA compound. The dosages and the scheduling of dose changes are similar to those discussed under proctitis. However, not every patient responds to sulfasalazine or 5-ASA, and the response, if it occurs, may take 3 or 4 weeks. For patients with more active disease (>5–6 bowel movements per day) or in whom a therapeutic response is desired in less than 3 to 4 weeks, the initial treatment of choice is oral prednisone. This is also the drug of choice for those who have not responded to 3 to 4 weeks of therapy with oral sulfasalazine or 5-ASA preparations. The initial dose of prednisone is determined by the severity of the symptoms. Patients with severe diarrhea, systemic symptoms, or significant amounts of blood in the stool may be started on 40 mg/day; those with lesser symptoms may be started on slightly lower doses. Most patients respond to oral corticosteroids within a few days to 3 weeks. After the symptoms are controlled, the dose of prednisone can be gradually reduced. One standard approach is to cut the daily dose by 5 mg every 1 to 2 weeks. It is usually relatively easy to reduce the corticosteroid dose to 20 mg/day, but the disease is more likely to flare as the dose is reduced further. It may be necessary to taper the dose more slowly below 20 mg/day or to use alternate-day dosing as part of the tapering protocol. Those who respond to oral prednisone and who can be fully withdrawn from prednisone should be maintained on sulfasalazine or an oral 5-ASA preparation.

Severely Active Colitis

Some patients develop incapacitating disease that requires hospitalization. The most common reason for hospitalization is intractable diarrhea, although blood loss is also a common problem. Incapacitating symptoms may develop acutely over a period of a few days or insidiously over weeks to months. Management with oral corticosteroids has usually been tried before admission. Patients with severe active ulcerative colitis should be evaluated for toxic megacolon, the management of which is discussed in a following section. Anticholinergics and antidiarrheal agents are contraindicated in moderate to severe ulcerative colitis because of the risk of precipitating toxic megacolon. The mainstays of therapy for severe ulcerative colitis are bed rest, rehydration with intravenous fluids, and intravenous steroids (hydrocortisone 300 mg/day, prednisolone 60–80 mg/day, or methylprednisolone 48–60 mg/day). Patients with significant anemia should be transfused, and those with peritoneal signs or signs of systemic infection should be treated with parenteral antibiotics. Because active ulcerative colitis is often associated with a moderate leukocytosis and a low-grade fever, it may be difficult to identify those who have bacterial infection in addition to ulcerative colitis. If there is any doubt, cultures should be obtained, and the patient should be given broad-spectrum antibiotics such as ampicillin, metronidazole, or an aminoglycoside. Dehydration with or without hypokalemia occurs in those with severe diarrhea. Fluids should be administered aggressively to replenish water and electrolytes. The patient is given nothing by mouth, and nasogastric suction is used if there is an ileus or colonic dilatation. Nutrition is often a major problem in severe active ulcerative colitis. Those whose disease has been active for a considerable time may enter the hospital malnourished; these patients and those who are likely to be unable to take adequate oral nutrition for an extended period should be placed on TPN. If the bout of acute colitis has been of short duration, the patient's current nutritional status is good, and the history of his previous exacerbations suggests that this one will be of short duration, then TPN is probably unnecessary. However, if the patient is already malnourished or will probably be unable to take oral nutrition for a prolonged period, TPN should be initiated. Patients with severe active ulcerative colitis should be given a trial of bed rest, TPN, and intravenous steroids for 7 to 10 days. Those who do not improve during this period should be considered for either colectomy or a trial of intravenous cyclosporine, which is given at a dose of 4 mg/kg/day by continuous infusion, aiming for serum levels of 100 to 400 ng/mL.[248] For patients who do respond to cyclosporine, the average time to response is 7 days. If therapeutic success is achieved with intravenous cyclosporine, the patient is switched to oral cyclosporine (8 mg/kg/day).

Refractory Disease

A small but problematic group of ulcerative colitis patients includes those who do not respond to corticosteroids and those who do respond but whose disease flares whenever the corticosteroids are withdrawn. In these cases, the clinician is faced with three potential courses of action: a trial of immunosuppressive agents; colectomy; and, if the patient has responded but can't be withdrawn from corticosteroids, indefinite continuation of corticosteroids. The option of continued chronic corticosteroid therapy is frequently the least appealing of the three because of the long-term side effects, including osteoporosis and cataract formation. Continuation of high-dose corticosteroid therapy for too long a time is the most common serious error in the management of ulcerative colitis. If the patient is on a substantial dose (>15 mg of prednisone per day) for more than 6 months, a trial of immunosuppressives or surgery should be given serious consideration. The use of immunosuppressive agents, usually 6-MP or azathioprine, is worthy of consideration in many cases. For patients who have been on high-dose steroid therapy, the steroids are continued, and 6-MP or azathioprine is added at a dose ranging from 50 mg/day up to 1.5 or 2.0 mg/kg/day. The combination of immunosuppressive agent plus steroids is continued for 3 to 4 months, and then the steroids are gradually tapered. If the steroids cannot be tapered after 6 months on immunosuppressive therapy, then the immunosuppressive drug should be stopped. For patients who respond to immunosuppressives in this circumstance, the next question is how long they should be maintained on the drug and what happens if it is withdrawn. Most clinicians attempt to withdraw the patient from immunosuppressives after 1 to 3 years of therapy. However, in many cases, disease activity flares after the drug is withdrawn. The clinician and patient are then faced with the difficult choice of restarting immunosuppressive therapy with the plan of lifetime administration or choosing colectomy. Given the risks of malignancy associated with long-standing ulcerative colitis and the risks associated with long-term immunosuppressive therapy, the prospect of colectomy, especially if the creation of an ileoanal anastomosis is possible, is more appealing than it might appear initially.

Maintenance Therapy

There is compelling evidence that sulfasalazine and oral 5-ASA preparations can reduce the incidence of recurrences in patients with ulcerative colitis. Most patients with ulcerative colitis should be viewed as candidates for chronic maintenance therapy. For the patient with a single episode of easily managed ulcerative colitis, it may be difficult to justify long-term maintenance therapy. In this case, the usual course is to maintain the patient on maintenance therapy for 1 year and then discontinue it. However, for patients who have difficulty controlling the disease, or who have multiple recurrences, it is reasonable to recommend lifetime maintenance therapy. Sulfasalazine and oral 5-ASA agents are probably equally effective. However, the efficacy of sulfasalazine as maintenance therapy in ulcerative colitis is a function of the dose. The efficacy of sulfasalazine at 3 to 4 g/day is greater than the efficacy of 2 g/day even though 2 g/day is the usual recommended maintenance dose. The dose of sulfasalazine should be pushed to the higher levels in patients who tolerate higher doses. Oral 5-ASA agents can achieve higher lumenal concentrations of 5-ASA than are usually achieved with sulfasalazine and, on that basis, may be more effective as maintenance therapy. Corticosteroids are not effective as maintenance therapy and should not be used. Most of the experience with 6-MP as maintenance therapy in ulcerative colitis is in patients whose acute disease has been brought under control with 6-MP; withdrawal of 6-MP from these patients has resulted in a high incidence of exacerbation. The efficacy of sulfasalazine and 5-ASA in preserving remissions induced by 6-MP has never been directly addressed.

MEDICAL MANAGEMENT OF CROHN'S DISEASE

General Approach

It is more difficult to develop generally applicable guidelines for management of Crohn's disease, compared with ulcerative colitis, because of the greater variety of anatomic locations, more varied clinical presentations, and greater importance of gastrointestinal complications such as fistulas, abscesses, strictures, and perforations. The guidelines given here are for active disease without complications; management of specific complications is discussed separately.

Symptomatic therapy plays an important role in the management of mild Crohn's disease. Antidiarrheal agents can reduce the number of bowel movements in patients with mild disease activity or in those with diarrhea secondary to surgical resections, bile salt malabsorption, or fat malabsorption. Loperamide and diphenoxylate are the antidiarrheal agents most commonly prescribed. Appropriate symptomatic therapy can reduce steroid requirements; however, antispasmodics and antidiarrheal agents should be used with caution in patients with severe disease because of the risk of precipitating toxic megacolon. Psychotropic drugs, particularly tricyclic antidepressants, can be useful adjunctive therapy in Crohn's disease. The incidence of depression is high among patients with Crohn's disease, and the manifestations of depression can make management of Crohn's disease more difficult. A trial of low-dose tricyclic antidepressants is indicated in patients who have clinical manifestations of significant depression.

A common problem in the management of Crohn's disease is a marked discrepancy between the severity of the patient's symptoms and the objective signs of disease. Patients with severe pain and diarrhea may have minimal findings on endoscopy or radiographic studies. In these cases, several possible explanations may need to be considered. Patients who have undergone ileal resections may have significant diarrhea on the basis of their surgery alone. Removal of the ileocecal valve increases transit and can increase the number of bowel movements. Surgical removal of the distal ileum can result in failure to reabsorb bile acids. Bile acids induce colonic chloride secretion, leading to diarrhea. More extensive ileal resections may result in enough bile salt malabsorption to decrease the size of the bile salt pool, resulting in fat malabsorption. Malabsorbed fatty acids can be hydroxylated by colonic bacteria; hydroxyfatty acids also induce colonic chloride secretion and contribute to diarrhea. Crohn's disease patients with a history of ileal resection who present with diarrhea may deserve a trial of cholestyramine plus a low-fat diet to determine how much of their diarrhea is a product of their surgery rather than active Crohn's disease.

For therapy with sulfasalazine, corticosteroids, or immunosuppressives, response is monitored by empiric clinical assessment directed at the problem that is most troublesome for the patient. If the major complaint is pain, then the success of therapy is assessed by the severity of pain; if diarrhea is the major problem, then the success is measured by the frequency of diarrhea. In assessing the patient's response to drug therapy, it is important to understand the basis of the chief complaint. If abdominal pain is a result of obstruction behind a fibrotic stricture, it is not reasonable to expect sulfasalazine or corticosteroids to relieve the pain. Similarly, if diarrhea is caused by small bowel overgrowth behind a stricture, it is unlikely that sulfasalazine or corticosteroids will improve the diarrhea.

Mildly to Moderately Active Ileitis, Ileocolitis, or Colitis

For colonic or ileocolic disease with mild to moderate activity, sulfasalazine or an oral 5-ASA formulation is a reasonable first approach to therapy. The dosage and treatment schedules are the same as those described for ulcerative proctitis or ulcerative colitis of mild to moderate activity. Pentasa, an oral 5-ASA preparation with greater availability of 5-ASA in the ileum than sulfasalazine or Asacol, may be a better choice for patients with ileitis or ileocolitis.[254] An alternative to sulfasalazine or the 5-ASA preparations is metronidazole, given by mouth at a dose of 10 to 20 mg/kg/day. A disadvantage of sulfasalazine, the 5-ASA preparations, and metronidazole is that a clinical response may not be seen for 3 to 4 weeks.

Oral prednisone may be used as first-line therapy for patients with ileal disease or for patients with colonic or ileocolic disease with higher levels of disease activity. Prednisone is also the drug of choice for patients who have failed to respond to sulfasalazine, 5-ASA preparations, or metronidazole. The response to prednisone is usually more rapid than that to sulfasalazine or 5-ASA formulations. In a Crohn's disease patient with abdominal pain, fever, and a high leukocyte count, an abdominal CT scan should be obtained to rule out the presence of an abscess before corticosteroids are given. Corticosteroid therapy in a Crohn's patient with an abscess, especially in the absence of antibiotic therapy, can lead to serious septic complications. The most common clinical indication for the use of prednisone in Crohn's disease is the presence of a ileal narrowing caused by mucosal inflammation. If the patient's ileum is only partially obstructed, he or she is managed as an outpatient with bed rest, a low-residue diet, and oral prednisone at dose of 40 mg/day. If the symptoms come under control, the dose of prednisone is tapered as has been described in previous sections. If disease activity flares after the dose of prednisone is tapered, then the possibility of surgery or a trial of immunosuppressives should be considered.

Severely Active Ileitis, Ileocolitis, or Colitis

The approach to severe Crohn's disease is similar to the approach to severe ulcerative colitis. The patient is hospitalized, given nothing by mouth, rehydrated with intravenous fluids, and given parenteral steroids in the dosages listed in the previous section. For patients who do not respond to corticosteroids or for patients who require large doses of corticosteroids for a long time to control disease activity, a trial of immunosuppressives may be indicated. Addition of immunosuppressives allows many patients to reduce the dose of steroids required to maintain a clinical remission. The long period of treatment before the onset of a clinical response must be considered when contemplating the use of immunosuppressives. The decision between continuing corticosteroid therapy and the trial of immunosuppressives is influenced by the dose of corticosteroids, the duration of corticosteroid therapy, and the presence of side effects from corticosteroids. The starting dose of 6-MP or azathioprine is 50 mg/day, which can be gradually increased to a maximum dose of 2 mg/kg/day if the patient tolerates the medication. The development of mild leukopenia indicates that the patient is at or approaching the maximal tolerable dose. Corticosteroids are continued with the immunosuppressive until a clear clinical response is seen or until the patient has been on an immunosuppressive for 4 to 6 months. Lack of a clinical response and inability to taper steroids indicate that the immunosuppressives have not been effective and should be withdrawn. Patients who do respond to immunosuppressives should be maintained on the medication for 1 to 3 years. Many patients have flares of their disease after the drug is withdrawn.[240,243]

If prolonged courses of steroids or immunosuppressives are required to maintain a clinical remission, the possibility of surgical intervention should be considered. Would a surgical procedure allow the corticosteroids or immunosuppressives to be withdrawn? What is the likely morbidity of the surgery, and how does it compare with the likely morbidity of prolonged medical therapy? Will the continuation of medical therapy actually save the patient from a surgical procedure, or is it merely delaying the inevitable?

Maintenance Therapy

There are little useful data available on maintenance therapy in Crohn's disease. Although there are no definitive studies to support its use, many clinicians use sulfasalazine as maintenance therapy in Crohn's colitis, especially in patients whose active disease was brought under control with sulfasalazine. In one study,[255] Pentasa (2 g/day) was found to be more effective then placebo in maintaining remission in Crohn's disease patients. This study included patients with ileal, ileocolic, and colonic disease. In a similar study, Asacol (800 mg three times daily) was found to be superior to placebo in maintaining remission in Crohn's disease. 5-ASA preparations may also be useful in maintaining remission in Crohn's disease after surgical resections.[256,257] The role of 5-ASA preparations in maintenance therapy in Crohn's disease should become better defined over the next few years. There is no role for corticosteroids as maintenance therapy in Crohn's disease. Many Crohn's disease patients who are brought under control with immunosuppressives, particularly azathioprine and 6-MP, are maintained on these drugs for years. There are now trials under way to assess the role of immunosuppressives in maintenance therapy in Crohn's disease.

SURGICAL MANAGEMENT

Ulcerative Colitis

About 20% to 25% of patients with extensive ulcerative colitis eventually undergo colectomy, usually because their disease has not responded adequately to medical therapy.[258,259] For some, the indications for colectomy are urgent and compelling, but more commonly the decision for or against colectomy is made at a time when the disease is active but stable. The decision between surgery and continued medical therapy is often not clear-cut, and in many cases defensible arguments can be made for either course. It is important in these cases to attempt to balance the risks and benefits of the two approaches. Excessive enthusiasm for or avoidance of operative therapy are both inconsistent with the patient's best interests. At the time of first diagnosis, the patient may absolutely reject even the consideration of eventual colectomy. However, a single prolonged episode of severe colitis or multiple recurrent episodes of more moderate severity increase the patient's desire to get rid of this debilitating disease with its restrictions on activity, and the prospect of colectomy becomes less intolerable.

In ulcerative colitis, colectomy is a curative procedure, in contrast to the situation in Crohn's disease, in which there is a significant likelihood of recurrence sometime after colectomy.[260,261] The assurance of a permanent cure increases the appeal of colectomy in ulcerative colitis. The development of the ileoanal anastomosis, eliminating the need for an ostomy, has made the thought of colectomy more tolerable for many. The decision for or against colectomy is influenced by the patient's age, social circumstances, and duration of disease. The morbidity of severe ulcerative colitis in childhood and the morbidity of corticosteroids in childhood combine to lead to the early consideration of colectomy as definitive therapy. For young adults with moderately severe disease, colectomy may be more acceptable for those in stable marriages than for those who are single. The risk of developing malignancy enters into the equation when considering colectomy in those with long-standing ulcerative colitis; if the other indications are equivocal, the risk of malignancy may push the balance in favor of colectomy.

Indications for Surgery in Ulcerative Colitis

Urgent Indications. Emergency colectomy may be required in toxic megacolon or in a severe fulminating attack without toxic megacolon.[262] Although colectomy for acute attacks of ulcerative colitis is more commonly associated with toxic megacolon, it is clear that acute fulminating ulcerative colitis in the absence of colonic dilatation can also proceed to perforation. The goal is to recognize the necessity for surgical intervention before perforation occurs. If perforation does occur, it is an absolute indication for surgery. Perforation in this circumstance is a medical disaster with a 40% mortality rate.[263] The indications for surgery in toxic megacolon are discussed under that heading. For fulminant colitis, in the absence of toxic megacolon, the general indications for operation are similar. Before the patient undergoes colectomy for intractable ulcerative colitis, it is important to rule out complicating conditions that can be treated. The possibilities of infection with *Giardia* organisms, amoeba, *C difficile*, and cytomegalovirus should be considered and, if indicated, tested for. The presence of worsening colitis and especially worsening systemic signs (e.g., fever, prostration, tachycardia, hypotension) in the face of aggressive medical therapy is a sign that surgical intervention may be indicated. Severe hemorrhage is another indication for emergency colectomy. Hemorrhage in ulcerative colitis can usually be managed by conservative measures but may occasionally necessitate colectomy.

Nonurgent indications. The failure of medical therapy to control the activity of ulcerative colitis, resulting in an unacceptable lifestyle, is the most common indication for colectomy in ulcerative colitis. There are several varieties of intractability. In one variety, the disease enters a chronic continuous phase in which the patient no longer achieves remission even with maximal medical therapy, and chronic diarrhea is severe enough that the quality of life is severely compromised. Frequent bowel movements prevent the patient from moving far from a bathroom and do not allow normal travel or employment. In some cases, the patient's or the physician's aversion to colectomy results in months or years of functional disability far worse than would have existed if a colectomy had been performed. Another type of intractability occurs when adequate control of the patient's symptoms requires high doses of corticosteroids over a long period of time. Attempts should be made, if possible, to reduce corticosteroid requirements by use of sulfasalazine or 5-ASA preparations. In some cases, it may be appropriate to attempt to reduce steroid requirements by administering azathioprine or 6-mercaptopurine, but the morbidity of those drugs must also be considered. The side effects of corticosteroids are dose- and time-dependent and vary considerably from patient to patient. Unacceptable side effects (e.g., psychosis, accelerated hypertension) occur in some individuals even with modest doses given over a short period of time. In these cases, the decision for surgery is clear-cut. A more difficult and more common problem is the patient who requires moderate to high doses of corticosteroids to control disease activity but who has had no specific problem with the corticosteroid treatment. Although this is a decision in which factors specific to the individual patient play a large role, some general guidelines may be useful. In patients who have taken large doses of prednisone (>15 mg/day) for more than 6 months, even if no specific corticosteroid side effects are present, the morbidity of continued steroid therapy must be weighed against the morbidity of surgery. Ophthalmologic examination for cataract and bone densitometry may help identify those with clinically silent corticosteroid side effects. The identification of asymptomatic but clinically important corticosteroid side effects may make the decision for colectomy easier. Growth failure in children is another form of intractability. Adequate nutritional support aids in most young patients, but some require colectomy. Surgical intervention should be strongly considered if growth retardation persists despite maximal nutritional and medical therapy.[264] In such a case, it is important to initiate therapy before puberty and the closing of epiphyses.

Extraintestinal manifestations.   Uveitis, pyoderma gangrenosum, and arthritis usually resolve with colectomy. Some other extraintestinal manifestations including ankylosing spondylitis and sclerosing cholangitis, do not. The extraintestinal manifestations that respond to colectomy usually respond to medical management as well. Extraintestinal manifestations are an infrequent indication for colectomy.

Dysplasia and carcinoma.   The role of colectomy in the management of dysplasia and carcinoma is discussed in the section on cancer.

Choice of Operation in Ulcerative Colitis

The standard operation for ulcerative colitis is a proctocolectomy and Brooke's ileostomy. The utility of newer procedures is measured against this standard. Proctocolectomy and ileostomy can be performed in one or two stages. In a two-stage procedure, the first stage is colectomy and ileostomy, and the second is proctectomy. The two-stage procedure is favored if the patient is severely ill, as in toxic megacolon, or if the degree of perirectal inflammation is such that careful dissection is difficult and the risk of impaired sexual function in the male is increased. The two-stage procedure may also be useful if the patient has not fully accepted the idea of a permanent ileostomy. However, the one-stage procedure is preferred if it is possible. Proctocolectomy and ileostomy has a number of advantages: it is a definitive, curative procedure, and additional surgery is seldom required; the patient's functional status with the operation can be predicted with confidence; most patients make a remarkably good adjustment to the ileostomy and lead full, useful lives; it is a procedure that many surgeons can perform successfully.

The major disadvantage of the proctocolectomy and ileostomy is that the patient has an ostomy and is totally incontinent of gas and stool; an appliance must be worn at all times. Some patients develop mechanical problems with their stomas—prolapse, retraction, hernia, stenosis—which may require surgical revision. The incidence of these problems is low if the procedure is properly done. One recently popularized alternative operation is the ileoanal anastomosis. In this procedure, the colon is removed completely but the mucosa and submucosa of the rectum are dissected from the muscularis; the mucosa and submucosa are removed and the muscularis, including the internal and external sphincters, are left in place. A pouch is constructed from the terminal 30 cm of ileum. The distal end of the pouch is pulled through the anal canal, and the ileal mucosa is sewed to the dentate line. The advantage of this procedure is that the patient has no ostomy and no appliance. However, a proximal temporary diverting loop ileostomy is commonly used to protect the ileoanal anastomosis until it heals.

For several months after the creation of an ileoanal anastomosis, the patient has numerous bowel movements. The number gradually declines so that, at 12 months, most patients are having five or six bowel movements per day. Twelve months after operation, complete daytime continence is achieved by 75%, 23% have seepage (minor staining of underclothes), and 2% are incontinent.[265] The corresponding numbers for nighttime continence are 48%, 47%, and 5%, respectively. Results are better for patients younger than 50 years of age than for older patients. Six percent of patients need to have their ileal reservoirs excised and a permanent ileostomy created because of pelvic sepsis, intractable diarrhea, or the appearance of Crohn's disease in the neorectum. One complication is the formation of an abscess in the ileal pouch (Fig. 79-30). In creating an ileoanal anastomosis, some surgeons leave a few centimeters of rectal mucosa in place; this residual rectal mucosa may cause acute symptoms if the ulcerative colitis flares up or may develop malignancy over time. An in-depth discussion of these surgical alternatives is presented in Chapter 40.

Crohn's Disease

Within 10 years of diagnosis, approximately 60% of patients with Crohn's disease undergo surgery for their disease.[266] The surgical approach to Crohn's disease is markedly different from the approach to ulcerative colitis. Surgical resection is not curative in Crohn's disease as colectomy is in ulcerative colitis. As a consequence, there has been a more conservative approach to the amount of tissue removed, in the knowledge that recurrences are likely and that additional surgical resections in the future may be necessary. Intractability, or failure of medical management, is a common cause for resection in Crohn's disease, as it is in ulcerative colitis, but complications

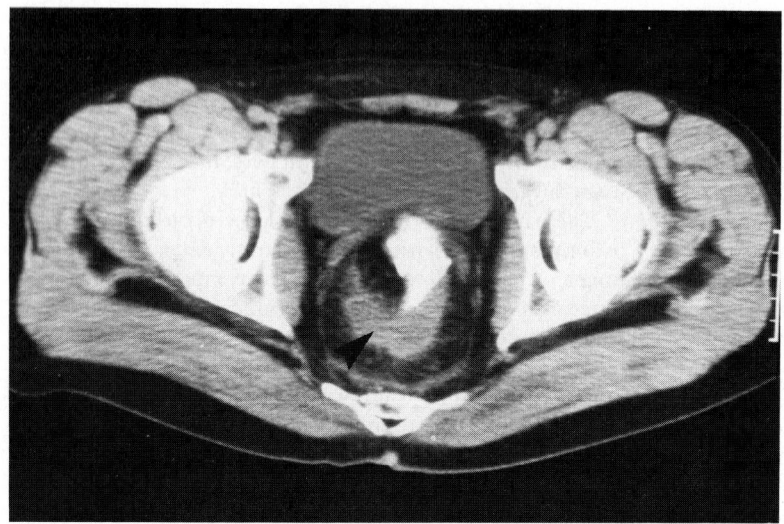

FIGURE 79-30. Computed tomographic scan through ileal pouch in a patient with ileoanal anastomosis. There is an abscess (*arrow*) in the ileal pouch. (Courtesy of Dennis Balfe, M.D., St. Louis, MO.)

(e.g., obstruction, fistula, abscess) are often indications for resection in Crohn's disease. The line between failure of medical management and a more defined complication such as obstruction is often not distinct. If a patient with a radiographically identifiable stricture has symptoms consistent with intermittent partial obstruction (i.e., diarrhea and pain brought on by eating) and does not respond to medical management, it is hard to say whether the indication for surgery is obstruction or failure of medical management.

Defining the point at which medical management has failed in Crohn's disease is somewhat more involved than in ulcerative colitis, because in Crohn's disease symptoms may not be caused by disease activity. Diarrhea and weight loss may be a result of fatty acid malabsorption, bile salt–induced colonic secretion, or small bowel bacterial overgrowth. Optimal medical management requires recognition and treatment of these disorders. If these problems are not identified, patients may be subjected to unnecessary surgery.

As in ulcerative colitis, surgery for failure of medical management in Crohn's disease falls into two groups. In the first group, surgery is required because the progression of the disease has led the patient to a condition of unacceptable disability and invalidism despite optimal medical management. Whereas in ulcerative colitis the major source of disability is diarrhea, in Crohn's disease there is more commonly a combination of diarrhea, pain, weight loss, and malnutrition. In evaluating the possibility of surgical intervention in ulcerative colitis, the patient's current morbidity from disease activity is balanced against the relatively predictable morbidity of a colectomy. In Crohn's disease, however, the current morbidity must be balanced against the less well defined morbidity of more limited surgery and also against the projected long-term morbidity as the disease progresses. Another distinction between surgical therapy in ulcerative colitis and Crohn's disease is that in ulcerative colitis, surgery is almost always performed to remove actively inflamed tissue, but in Crohn's disease, surgery may be required either for active disease or for sequelae of earlier inflammation. For example, strictures requiring surgical intervention may occur in Crohn's disease at the site of earlier activity or earlier surgical anastomosis even though there is not much active inflammation. This is an important

distinction, because there is no point in treating a stricture with a therapeutic trial of steroids if the stricture is caused by scarring and fibrosis. In addition, if the problem is known to be caused by scarring and fibrosis, a stricturoplasty can be done or the extent of the surgical resection can be limited to the area of narrowing without worry about maintaining adequate uninflamed margins.

The second group of patients operated on for failure of medical management in Crohn's disease are those suffering side effects from drugs, usually corticosteroids. The guidelines for surgical intervention in patients with complications of medical therapy are exactly the same as for patients with ulcerative colitis. A problem frequently faced by physicians treating Crohn's disease is the patient whose disease is controlled with corticosteroids but flares if the dose of corticosteroids is reduced below a certain level. The level varies from patient to patient, but one study put the average at 0.15 mg of prednisone per kilogram per day.[267] If this happens, it is usually reasonable to treat the patient again with steroids but to taper the steroids more slowly. Patients typically go through several cycles consisting of disease flare, prednisone therapy, tapering to the critical level, and then another flare. There are several options available in this circumstance. One approach is to maintain the patient at a steroid dose above the critical level and to follow the patient carefully for manifestations of steroid toxicity. This follow-up includes bone densitometry and ophthalmologic examinations. A second approach, not exclusive of the first, is the use of immunosuppressives to achieve a steroid-sparing effect. This approach trades potential complications of corticosteroids for those of immunosuppressives. A third approach is to resect the involved segment knowing, that the chance of eventual recurrence is high. In the future, there may be some role for orally administered 5-ASA, methotrexate, or cyclosporine in this circumstance. Each of these approaches has its own advantages and disadvantages, all of which should be explained to the patient before a decision is made.

For small bowel Crohn's disease, the most common surgical procedure is segmental resection for obstruction or fistula. The length of small bowel to be resected is a subject of considerable controversy. Soon after the first surgical resections for Crohn's disease, it was noted that disease activity recurred at the site of the anastomosis. One response to this observation was to resect wide margins of apparently normal tissue on each side of the involved segment, with the hope of achieving a cure by removing not only the tissue that was macroscopically involved but also the tissue that was microscopically involved. However, Crohn's disease recurred at the anastomosis even after wide margins of normal tissue were resected.[268,269] Increasing the length of microscopically normal intestine resected did not reduce the incidence of recurrence (Fig. 79-31).[270]

The incidence of recurrence after ileal resection for ileitis or ileocolic resection for ileocolic disease is about 50% after 10 years and 75% after 15 years, as assessed by rates of reoperation.[270] If the presence of recurrence is assessed endoscopically, it is clear that recurrence after resection occurs more rapidly than previously appreciated. Routine colonoscopic surveillance 1 year after ileocolic resections revealed a 72% incidence of recurrence, as manifested by the presence of aphthous ulcers on the ileal side of the ileocolic anastomosis.[271]

A surgical alternative to resection for small intestine strictures, termed stricturoplasty, involves longitudinal incision of the strictured segment, followed by transverse closure.[272,273] This method preserves bowel and has a low rate of complications.

Surgical approaches to Crohn's colitis include segmental resection, subtotal colectomy with ileoproctostomy, and total colectomy with ileostomy. Segmental resection of Crohn's colitis is appropriate if a relatively short segment of colon is involved. Recurrence rates are high, approximating those described for ileal and ileocolic disease. Subtotal colectomy with ileoproctostomy should be considered only in patients with an absolutely normal rectum.[274,275] Even in selected patients, the recurrence rate after this procedure is high, approximately 75% at 10 years.[276,277] For patients with extensive disease including the rectum, the procedure of choice is total proctocolectomy with a Brooke's ileostomy. Total colectomy with ileoanal anastomosis is not appropriate in Crohn's colitis because recurrence of Crohn's disease in the ileal segment forming the new pouch would require a repeat operation and loss of a long segment of ileum.

COMPLICATIONS OF ULCERATIVE COLITIS

Perforation

Free perforation of the colon commonly complicates toxic megacolon but can occur in severe ulcerative colitis even without toxic megacolon. Perforation occurs more often during first episodes of colitis, perhaps because of lack of fibrosis and scarring from previous attacks. Most perforations occur in the left colon, particularly the sigmoid. Steroid therapy has been suggested to be a risk factor for colonic perforation, but some investigators have not found this to be the case.

Stricture

Clinically important strictures are relatively uncommon in ulcerative colitis, but some degree of narrowing may be seen in as many as 12% of surgical specimens.[278] Careful histologic examination of strictures demonstrates hypertrophy and thickening of the muscularis mucosa without fibrosis. Strictures most often occur in patients with extensive disease and continuous symptoms without remission. They tend to appear later in the course of the disease, typically between 5 and 25 years after onset, most commonly in the sigmoid and rectum. Most strictures are short, typically 2 to 3 cm in length, but they may be much longer. Symptoms associated with strictures include an increase in diarrhea and fecal incontinence. Strictures have been associated with malignancy in ulcerative colitis and should be viewed as potentially malignant lesions. Unfortunately, biopsy of strictures containing malignancy does not always yield malignant tissue. Development of a stricture in a patient with long-standing ulcerative colitis should be a source of concern and may necessitate resection because of the risk of malignancy.

Toxic Megacolon

If the inflammatory process extends beyond the submucosa into the muscularis, the colon loses its ability to contract and as a result becomes dilated. Dilatation of the colon is associated with a worsening of the patient's clinical condition and the development of fever and prostration. Jalan and associates defined criteria for the clinical diagnosis of toxic megacolon.[70] These include radiographic evidence of colonic distention (see Fig. 79-17) in addition to at least three of the four following conditions: fever higher than 38.6° C; heart rate greater than 120 beats per minute; neutrophil leukocytosis greater than 10,500 cells/mm^3; anemia. At least one sign of toxicity—dehydration, mental changes, electrolyte disturbance, or hypotension—must also be present. Physical examination of

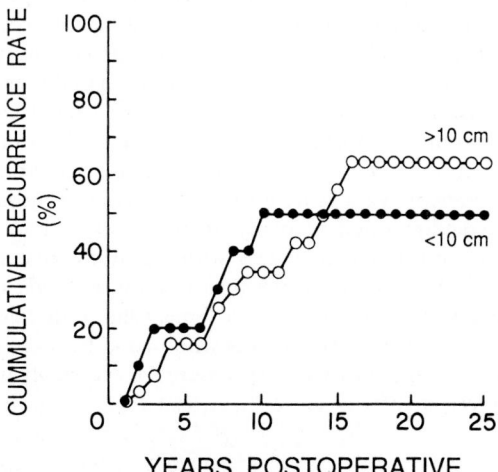

FIGURE 79-31. Calculated cumulative recurrence rates for resections in patients with ileitis having proximal resection margins greater or less than 10 cm. The curves are not significantly different. (From Trnka YM, Glotzer DJ, Kasdon EJ, et al. The long-term outcome of restorative operation on Crohn's disease: influence of location, prognostic factors and surgical guidelines. Ann Surg 1982;196:345.)

the patient with toxic megacolon reveals fever and postural hypotension. The abdomen is tender over the distribution of the colon, and there may be rebound tenderness. Colonic dilatation causes abdominal distention. Bowel sounds are markedly hypoactive or absent because of loss of colonic motility.

Toxic megacolon usually occurs in patients with pancolitis, but has been reported in those with more limited disease. Patients are at greatest risk for developing toxic megacolon early in the course of their disease, and it can even occur as the initial presentation. In one series of 55 patients who developed toxic megacolon, 23 developed it within 3 months of the initial presentation of ulcerative colitis.[70]

Pharmacologic agents that impair colonic motility are likely to initiate or exacerbate toxic megacolon.[279] Anticholinergic drugs diminish muscular tone in the colon and inhibit motility. Narcotic analgesics and antidiarrheals also inhibit the propulsive activity of the colonic musculature. Many cases of toxic megacolon are temporally associated with the initiation of therapy with anticholinergics or opiates or with increases in the doses of those drugs.[279,280] For this reason, anticholinergic agents and antidiarrheals are contraindicated in patients with severe ulcerative colitis. Even in disease of moderate activity, these drugs should be used with caution and the patient should be instructed to discontinue them if symptoms worsen. Toxic megacolon has also been temporally associated with barium enema examination and with colonoscopy.[281] The distention of the colon with barium or with air during colonoscopy is thought to further impair the already limited blood supply to the colonic wall. The rapid distention of the colon with barium or air may force bacteria and other intestinal contents into the ulcerated bowel wall, resulting in further exacerbation of colonic inflammation. Barium enema and colonoscopic examination are contraindicated in patients with severe ulcerative colitis. However, the patient can be safely examined by rigid proctoscopy or by limited flexible sigmoidoscopy so long as the physician takes care not to insufflate air into the already dilated colon.

Radiographic examinations are useful both for establishing the diagnosis and for following the course of toxic megacolon. X-ray films of the abdomen reveal colonic dilation, usually maximal in the transverse colon, which exceeds 6 cm in diameter.[80,81] Segments of the right and left colon may also be dilated. Although the transverse colon may not be the site of the most severe disease, it is usually the most dilated segment, because colonic gas tends to accumulate in the highest portion of the colon, and the transverse colon is the highest portion when the patient is supine. Repositioning the patient moves the site of maximal dilatation to some other segment. Serial flat plate films of the abdomen taken at 12- to 24-hour intervals are useful in following the clinical course.

Although laboratory findings are not diagnostic in toxic megacolon, there is a pattern of laboratory abnormalities that is commonly seen. Patients with toxic megacolon may be anemic because of blood loss, and there is usually a leukocytosis with predominance of neutrophils. Hypokalemia and hypoalbuminemia as a result of losses in diarrhea are also seen.

Medical therapy is designed to reduce the likelihood of perforation and to return the colon to normal motor activity as rapidly as possible. The patient is given nothing by mouth, and a nasogastric tube is placed in the stomach. Nasogastric

suction decompresses the patient's upper gastrointestinal tract, and the amount of gas or liquid intestinal contents entering the dilated colon is diminished. Some clinicians use a longer tube, such as a Miller-Abbott or Cantor's tube, but there is no evidence to suggest that these are more efficacious than a nasogastric tube.

Intravenous fluids should be administered to replete water and electrolytes.[282] Fluid and electrolyte disorders impair the normal motility of the colon and increase the risk of perforation from toxic megacolon. There are frequently large deficits of water, sodium, chloride, and, especially, potassium. Patients with toxic megacolon often receive broad-spectrum antibiotics in anticipation of peritonitis resulting from perforation. The value of corticosteroids in the treatment of toxic megacolon has not been established in controlled studies. However, most clinicians treat patients who have the condition with parenteral corticosteroids at a dose equivalent to more than 40 mg of prednisone per day.[283,284] Medical therapy for toxic megacolon is most likely to be successful if the condition is recognized early and appropriate steps are taken. The patient should be monitored carefully. Signs of improvement include a decrease in abdominal girth and the return of bowel sounds. Deterioration is marked by the development of rebound tenderness, increasing abdominal girth, and cardiovascular collapse. Loss of hepatic dullness on percussion suggests the presence of air over the liver and is a sign of perforation.

If medical therapy is successful during the first 24 to 48 hours, both an improvement in the signs of clinical toxicity and a decrease in the diameter of the dilated colon on radiographic examination should be seen. Persistence of fever after 48 hours on high-dose steroids suggests perforation or abscess. If the patient does not begin to show signs of clinical improvement during the first 24 to 48 hours of medical therapy, the risk of perforation increases markedly, and surgical intervention is indicated.[285] The most usual procedure is colonic resection with creation of an ileostomy. The rectum may be left in place and removed at a later date; however, single-stage proctocolectomy is now more commonly done. The key steps in management are early recognition of the condition and identification of those patients who do not respond to medical therapy. Surgical therapy after perforation is likely to have a poor outcome.[262] Mortality in that group is 44%, compared with 2% in those who were operated on before perforation. Among patients with toxic megacolon, many of those who are successfully treated medically are likely to undergo colonic resection for intractable disease within a year. Toxic megacolon is a sign of severe disease that may not respond to medical therapy over a long period of time. One study followed the clinical course of 38 patients who had been successfully treated medically for toxic megacolon; 18 eventually underwent colectomy.[286]

COMPLICATIONS OF CROHN'S DISEASE

Abscesses and Fistulas

Abscesses and fistulas are both products of the extension of a mucosal fissure or ulcer through the intestinal wall and into extraintestinal tissue. Leakage of intestinal contents through a tract into the peritoneal cavity results in an abscess. Extension of the tract through the wall of adjacent viscera or through the abdominal wall to the exterior results in a fistula.

Abscesses occur in 15% to 20% of patients with Crohn's disease.[287] They can arise from any affected area, but the terminal ileum is an especially likely point of origin. If confined to the abdominal cavity, abscesses form between loops of intestine, within the mesentery, or between the intestine and the parietal peritoneum. Abscesses also extend into the iliopsoas and retroperitoneal regions. One pattern is extension of an abscess from the terminal ileum to the right iliopsoas; such a lesion presents as pain on flexion of the right hip, which can be mistaken for sciatica.[288] Hepatic and splenic abscesses also occur. Abscesses may develop postoperatively at the site of an anastomosis after resection. Development of an abscess soon after resection usually results from an anastomotic leak, whereas development of an abscess several months after surgical resection is a result of disease recurrence.[289] The typical clinical presentation of intraabdominal abscess associated with Crohn's disease is fever and abdominal pain. The location and quality of the pain is determined by the location of the abscess. Tenderness and abdominal mass may accompany the pain and fever. Leukocytosis is the most common laboratory abnormality. Spontaneous rupture of an abscess through the abdominal wall can occur and results in an enterocutaneous fistula.

Abdominal abscess is most often diagnosed by CT scan, but barium enema, ultrasonography, and radionucleotide scanning with ^{67}Ga are also useful.[290-292] The frequently encountered organisms in Crohn's abdominal abscesses are *Escherichia coli*, *Bacteroides fragilis*, enterococcus, and α-hemolytic *Streptococcus* species.[289] Many different organisms may be found in a single abscess. Broad-spectrum antibiotic therapy, including anaerobic coverage, is indicated. Antibiotic coverage should be adjusted on the basis of results of culture of blood and abscess contents. Corticosteroids are not effective in the treatment of these abscesses and may impair the host response to infection. If the patient has not been on steroids, they should not be started until the infection has been brought under control with drainage and antibiotics. If the patient has been on steroids and the dose is being tapered, he or she may require higher doses to deal with the stress of infection.

Simple drainage of abscesses in patients with Crohn's disease may not provide adequate therapy because of persistent communication between the abscess cavity and the intestinal lumen. In fact, drainage in such circumstances commonly results in the formation of an enterocutaneous fistula. Resection of the portion of involved intestine containing the communication is usually required for definitive therapy. The abscess is first drained percutaneously under guidance by ultrasound or CT scan. After the abscess is adequately drained and inflammation is reduced, the involved segment of bowel is resected. The site of communication is not always obvious, and radiographic examination after oral administration of contrast material or injection of contrast into the abscess cavity may help in its identification.

The prevalence of fistulas is 20% to 40% in Crohn's disease.[287] Most fistulas are enteroenteric or enterocutaneous, with smaller numbers that are enterovesical or enterovaginal. Irrespective of the location, the mechanism of fistula formation appears to be the same. A deep abscess penetrates through the intestinal wall and into an adjacent organ or the skin. Enteroenteric fistulas develop either between a loop of involved bowel and a loop of uninvolved bowel or between two loops of involved bowel. The terminal ileum is the segment most commonly involved; fistulas from the terminal ileum may extend to other loops of small intestine or to the sigmoid. Fistulas develop when the disease is active but frequently persist even after the disease is no longer active. Enteroenteric fistulas by themselves seldom cause significant symptoms and are often found incidentally by barium contrast studies (Fig. 79-32).[293] Most enteroenteric fistulas are of small diameter and do not have significant flow rates; however, those of larger diameter may allow a flow great enough to cause malabsorption, diarrhea, and weight loss.

Pain and diarrhea in patients with enteroenteric fistulas are usually caused by active Crohn's inflammation and not by the mere presence of the fistula. Patients should be treated as they would be in the absence of a fistula; asymptomatic fistulas require no treatment. If an enteroenteric fistula is thought to be responsible for significant symptoms, administration of TPN or immunosuppressive therapy may induce fistula closure.[294-296] However, the fistulas often recur after the TPN or immunosuppressives is stopped. Korelitz and Present performed a double-blind, placebo-controlled study using 6-mercaptopurine at a dose of 1.5 mg/kg/day to close fistulas.[294] Of the 29 patients who received 6-mercaptopurine, 9 completely healed their fistulas, compared with 1 of 17 in the placebo group. The mean time required for healing with 6-mercaptopurine was 3 months. However, the fistulas reopened after 6-mercaptopurine was stopped. Although nutritional and medical therapy may play a role in the management of some fistulas in Crohn's disease, the problem of recurrence with the discontinuation of these treatments leaves surgery as the major therapeutic modality.[297-299] Surgical therapy includes resection of the segment involved with active disease. If both loops are involved, then both need to be resected; if only one is involved, that one should be resected and the other oversewn. Fistulas commonly develop in the high-pressure zone proximal to a stricture. Successful management of the fistula and prevention of recurrence are more likely if the stricture is resected with elimination of the high-pressure zone.

Enterocutaneous fistulas are more often problematic than enteroenteric fistulas. They commonly occur as a result of anastomotic leaks after resections for active disease.[300] In these cases, the cutaneous end of the fistula is in the scar (Fig. 79-33), and the enteric end is at the anastomosis. Enterocutaneous fistulas also occur spontaneously in the absence of previous surgery. Although the presence of an enterocutaneous fistula does not constitute an absolute indication for surgery, most patients find significant persistent drainage through the abdominal wall to be intolerable. The decision in favor of surgical therapy depends on the amount of drainage, the extent of disease activity, and the patient's nutritional status. More than one cutaneous opening may be present, but usually the enteric ends of the fistulas are close together, and the amount of bowel requiring resection may be no more than if only one cutaneous opening were present.

Rectovaginal fistulas are most commonly seen in active rectal Crohn's disease.[301] Smaller fistulas cause only a foul vaginal discharge, but larger fistulas result in the passage of

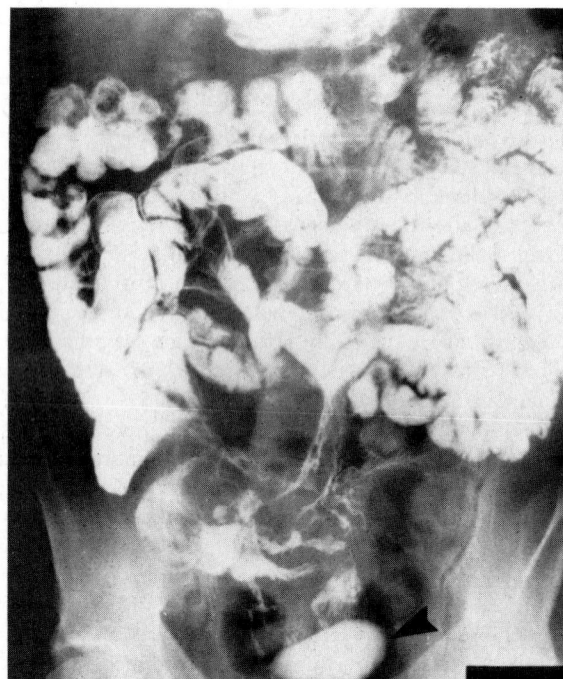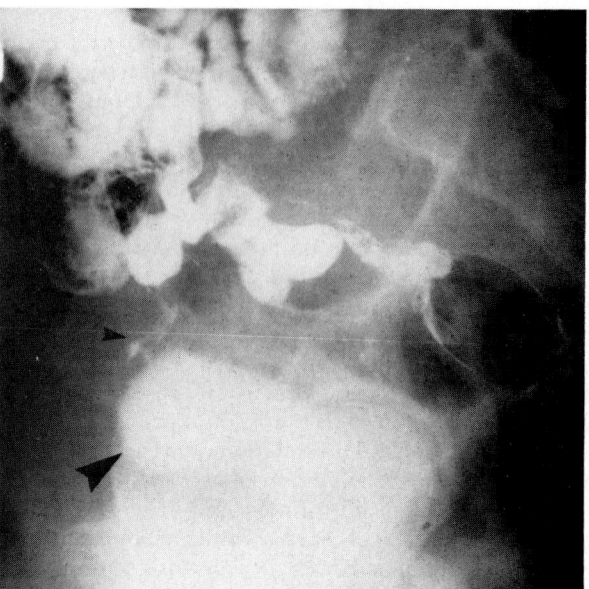

FIGURE 79-32. Crohn's disease with a complex of enteroenteric fistulae arising from an involved area in the distal ileum. There is also an enterovesicular fistula (*small arrow*) arising from the ileum. The contrast-filled urinary bladder (*large arrow*) is seen on both views. (Courtesy of Dennis Balfe, M.D., St. Louis, MO.)

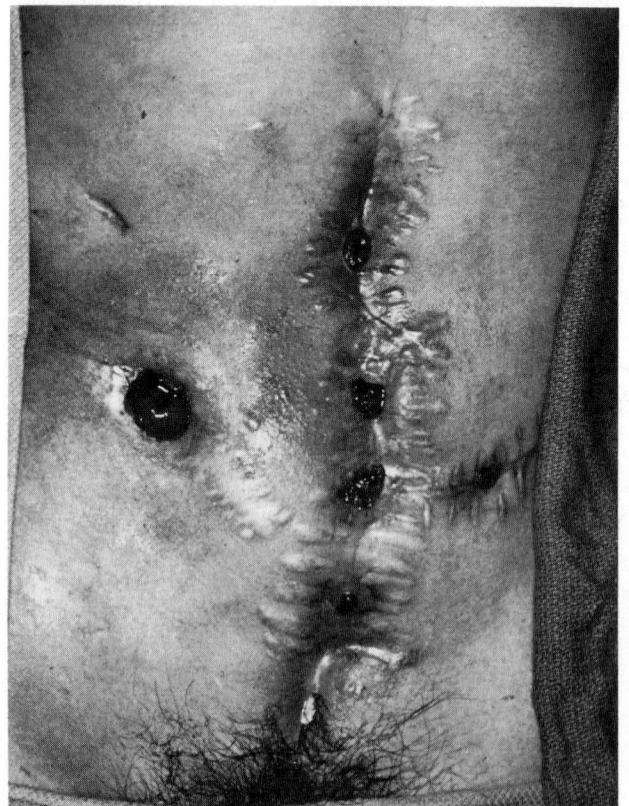

FIGURE 79-33. Enterocutaneous fistulae in abdominal scars in a patient with Crohn's disease. (Courtesy of Ira Kodner, M.D., St. Louis, MO.)

gas and stool through the vagina. Rectovaginal fistulas can usually be identified by proctoscopy or by speculum examination of the vagina; however, some are apparent only on barium enema (Fig. 79-34). If the symptoms are minimal, no therapy is necessary. Metronidazole leads to healing in some[302,303]; however definitive therapy usually requires surgical intervention.[304] Primary closure has been successful in some patients, diverting colostomy or abdominal perineal resection have been necessary in others. Enterovesicular fistulas usually involve diseased segments of ileum or sigmoid.[305,306] Signs include gas in the urine (pneumaturia) and recurrent urinary tract infections. Diagnosis may be made by barium enema, upper gastrointestinal series with small bowel follow-through (see Fig. 79-32), cystoscopy, or intravenous pyelogram. Definitive surgical management is usually recommended, especially if there are recurrent urinary tract infections, because of the risk of irreversible kidney damage. Surgical therapy includes resection of the involved segment of bowel. The bladder defect may be closed primarily or, more rarely, resected.

Obstruction

Obstruction is a common complication of Crohn's disease, particularly in the small intestine, and is a leading indication for surgery.[74,307] Small bowel obstruction in Crohn's disease may be caused by mucosal thickening from acute inflammation, by muscular hyperplasia and scarring as a result of previous inflammation, or by adhesions. Obstruction may also occur because of impaction of a bolus of particularly fibrous

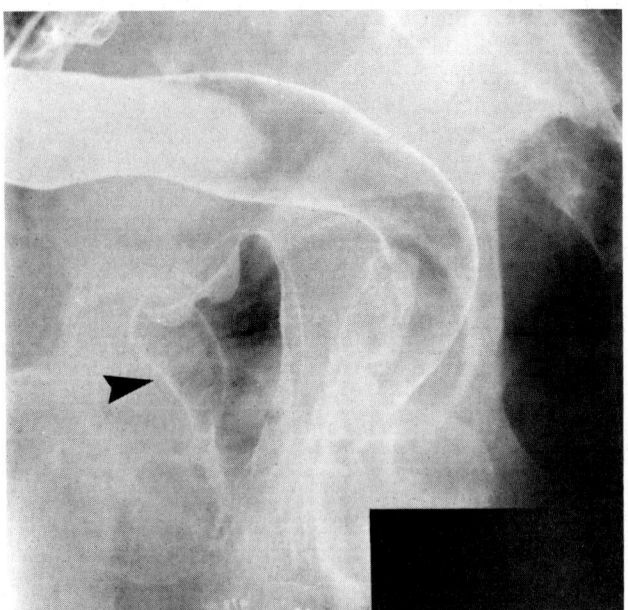

FIGURE 79-34. Rectovaginal fistula in a patient with Crohn's disease. The vagina (*arrow*) is coated with barium after barium enema. (Courtesy of Dennis Balfe, M.D., St. Louis, MO.)

the severity of the patient's complaints. Some patients have minimal complaints with near-obstructing strictures, but others have severe complaints with only modest narrowing. Lesions that block the passage of food particles may allow liquid contrast agents to pass freely; as a result, functionally significant strictures and adhesions may be totally missed by radiographic studies. Initial therapy is to give nothing by mouth, to apply nasogastric suction, and to give intravenous fluids. Anticholinergics should not be used in patients with obstruction. If acute inflammation is an important component of the obstructive process, parenteral corticosteroids may help; however, corticosteroids are not useful in the management of fibrotic strictures. A common error in the management of Crohn's disease is treatment of patients with obstructive symptoms from fixed anatomic lesions with long courses of corticosteroids. If the obstruction does not resolve with nasogastric suction and corticosteroids, dilation or surgery is necessary. If the fibrotic stricture is short and accessible, endoscopic balloon dilatation can be attempted; more likely, surgical intervention, either resection or stricturoplasty, will be required.[308]

Perianal Disease

material in a stable, long-standing stricture. Obstruction presents with cramping abdominal pain and diarrhea that worsen after meals and resolve with fasting. Symptoms worsen as the obstruction tightens. A common history is that of intermittent episodes of mild cramps and diarrhea, followed by prolonged episodes of severe pain and diarrhea accompanied by nausea and vomiting. The prolonged episodes of symptoms may be brought on by fibrous meals. Strictures may be evaluated by oral contrast studies, barium enema, or colonoscopy, depending on the anatomic location. Evaluation of strictures includes assessment of location, length, and lumenal diameter. Dilation of the intestine proximal to the stricture suggests chronicity. There is often an apparent discrepancy between the tightness of the stricture as assessed radiographically and

Perianal disease is an especially difficult complication of Crohn's disease.[309,310] Patients with IBD are subject to the same perianal problems as the general population, primarily hemorrhoids and anal fissures. However, patients with Crohn's disease also develop a complex of problems marked by ulcers in the anal canal which result in perirectal abscesses or fistulas that extend from the ulcers. The fistulous openings are most commonly in the perianal skin but can be in the groin, the vulva, or the scrotum (Fig. 79-35). A single rectal ulcer can give rise to a fistulous tract with multiple openings. The mucosal ends of fistulas often arise from anorectal glands. There are 10 to 12 anorectal glands at the level of the dentate line (see Chap. 88). These glands extend through the internal sphincter to the intermuscular plane. Two of these glands,

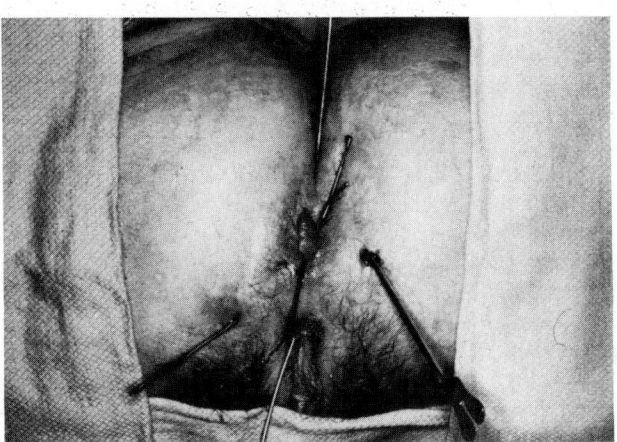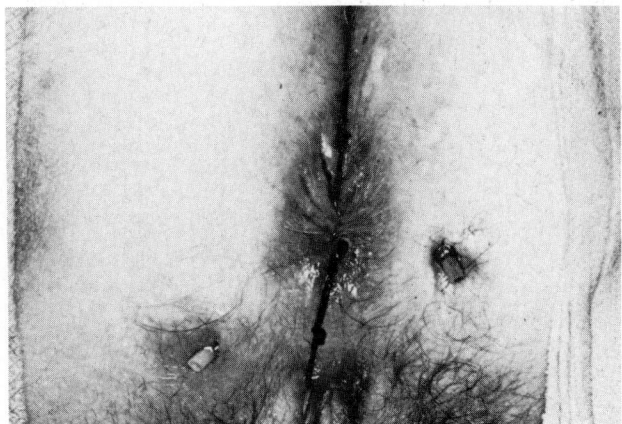

FIGURE 79-35. Perianal Crohn's disease with fistulae. Probes are placed intraoperatively to define fistulae (*left*). Mushroom catheters and setons allow adequate drainage (*right*). (Courtesy of Ira Kodner, M.D., St. Louis, MO.)

one in the anterior midline and one in the posterior midline, are the source of most fistulas and rectal abscesses.

Fistulas present with drainage of serous or mucous material. If the fistula does not drain freely, there is local accumulation of pus with redness, pain, and induration. Perianal abscesses present with pain that is exacerbated by defecation, sitting, or walking. The typical presentation of abscess is redness and pain in the perianal region with tenderness on digital examination; however, supralevator and pelvirectal abscesses may have no local manifestations and may present with fever alone. Usually, perirectal fistulas and abscesses are seen in conjunction with disease activity, but they may occur in the absence of other symptoms and may be the initial presentation of the disease.

Adequate assessment of perianal disease usually requires proctoscopic examination under anesthesia. Barium enema may reveal the course of fistulas (Fig. 79-36). CT scans are useful in defining the presence and extent of perianal abscesses. Persistent severe perianal Crohn's disease can result in destruction of the anal sphincter and fecal incontinence. The goals of therapy in perianal disease are relief of local symptoms and preservation of the sphincter. The mere presence of a fistula does not require therapy; if it is not causing problems, it does not need to be treated. The aggressiveness of therapy is determined by the severity of the perianal disease. Careful local cleansing with sitz baths is an important first step in management. Limited disease can be approached with sitz baths and antibiotics, but in most cases, adequate external drainage is also required. Setons or drains in the fistulous tracts allow for continuing drainage (see Fig. 79-35). Optimum management of perianal complications includes control of disease activity. Good control of disease activity reduces

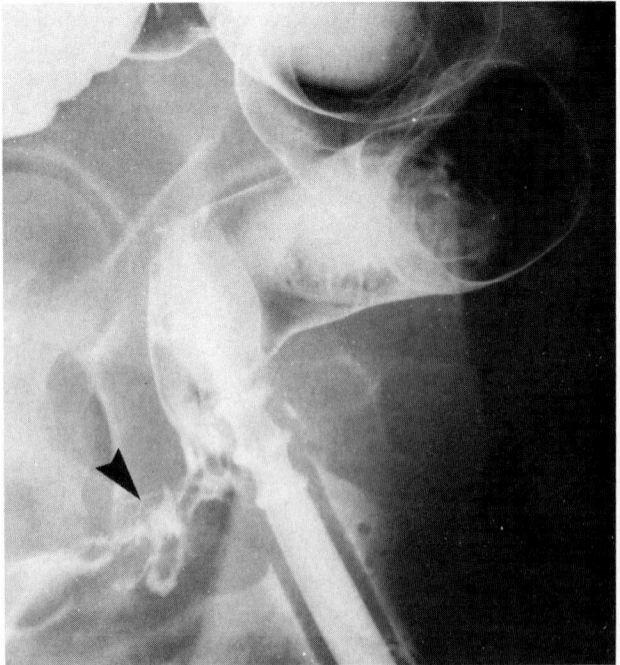

FIGURE 79-36. Perianal Crohn's disease. A fistula (*arrow*) to perianal skin is demonstrated by barium enema. (Courtesy of Dennis Balfe, M.D., St. Louis, MO.)

the amount of diarrhea passing through the perianal area. Every effort should be made to minimize disease activity with medical management before any consideration is given to further surgical intervention for perianal disease.

Metronidazole plays a role in the management of perianal disease. Bernstein and colleagues treated perianal Crohn's disease with metronidazole at a dose of 20 mg/kg/day in divided doses and found complete healing in 45% of patients and improvement without complete healing in another 23%.[302,303] Other investigators have also had success with metronidazole, but with a lower response rate then that found by Bernstein.[311] Prolonged therapy at this dosage is associated with a high rate of side effects, of which peripheral neuropathy is the most troublesome. Numbness and tingling are seen in as many as 75% of patients after 3 months of therapy.[311,312] Patients complain that their feet are cold and numb in the winter and they are unable to warm them. Paresthesias usually resolve if the dose is reduced or the drug discontinued. In an attempt to minimize side effects, particularly paresthesias, clinicians initiate therapy at a somewhat lower dose (250 mg four times daily). Discontinuation of metronidazole therapy results in recurrence of perianal disease in the majority of patients, even if complete healing has been achieved. Despite these problems, a trial of metronidazole is recommended if the patient still has significant symptoms after adequate surgical drainage of perianal disease.

If simple drainage and medical management are unsuccessful, there are a number of possible surgical approaches to perianal disease. Many patients respond well to careful surgical drainage and placement of setons and mushroom catheters, which can be left in place for months as the perianal disease slowly heals. Partial internal anal sphincterotomy can be used to remove the cryptoglandular epithelium from which the fistulas arise.[313] An alternative approach is to marsupialize all the fistulous tracts and lay open the crypt of origin. Fecal diversion by colostomy has also been used; however, the general experience is that fecal diversion does not lead to healing of perianal disease.[314,315]

COLON CANCER, DYSPLASIA, AND COLONOSCOPIC SURVEILLANCE

Patients with extensive ulcerative colitis have a markedly increased risk for colon cancer compared with the general population. The magnitude of this risk is uncertain. Early reports of extremely high incidences of colon cancer among ulcerative colitis patients (50% cumulative risk at 30 years) were biased by the use of referral-based populations that were not representative of the general population.[138] A report of the experience of a private gastroenterology practice in New York probably comes closer to the experience in the general population. In this practice, the probability that colon cancer would develop in patients with extensive colitis was 11.7% at 26 years.[316] Retrospective studies have revealed cumulative risks as high as 34% at 25 years in Sweden and as low as 1.4% at 18 years in Denmark. Several series have put the lifetime risk of cancer in ulcerative colitis patients in the 3% to 5% range.[317–319] The risk of developing cancer becomes appreciable 8 to 10 years after diagnosis and increases with time. Age of onset of ulcerative colitis seems to have little impact on the annual incidence of colon cancer. However, the risk of malignancy is a larger issue for those who develop ulcerative colitis earlier in life because they have a longer period in which they are at risk and thus a higher cumulative incidence of cancer. Colon cancer in the general population is a disease of late middle age and old age, but in ulcerative colitis, colon cancer occurs earlier and is commonly seen in the fourth decade of life. The risk of malignancy is also a function of the anatomic extent of the disease; the risk is much greater with pancolitis than with left-sided disease. Patients with long-standing ulcerative colitis are at risk for developing cancer even if their symptoms have been relatively mild.[138,260,320] Patients are seen with colon cancer whose ulcerative colitis has been quiescent for 10 to 15 years.

The response of the medical community to the risk of colon cancer in ulcerative colitis has been that the increased risk is too high to ignore but not high enough to recommend prophylactic colectomy at some arbitrary time after diagnosis. These circumstances have led to a desire to be able to identify those patients at special risk for colon cancer so that they can be offered a colectomy before the development of malignancy—or after malignancy has developed but curative resection is still possible. Examination of stool for occult blood is a widely used screening test for colon cancer in the general population, but it is useless in ulcerative colitis because of colitis-induced bleeding. Even overt symptoms are of less use in identifying colon cancer in ulcerative colitis than in the general population. Rectal bleeding, a symptom associated with left-sided colon cancers in the general population, is a common feature of ulcerative colitis and thus is not a reliable marker for the presence of malignancy.

The situation in ulcerative colitis is somewhat similar to that seen in patients who have colonic polyps. Both groups are at high risk for the development of colon cancer, and surveillance is used in both groups with the expectation that, if asymptomatic individuals can be identified before they develop malignancy or when the malignancy is in its early stages, the likelihood of cure is much higher than if the malignancy is identified only after symptoms have developed. However, there are important differences between patients with polyps and those with ulcerative colitis. In patients with colonic polyps, surveillance involves the search for adenomatous polyps, premalignant lesions that are relatively easily identified and removed. Even if that fails and a cancer develops, colon cancers in this population are easily identified at colonoscopy. In ulcerative colitis, surveillance colonoscopy is used to search for malignancies and to obtain random mucosal biopsies to be examined for dysplasia. In patients with ulcerative colitis, colon cancers are often submucosal and may easily be missed at colonoscopy. Dysplasia, if present, does not occur universally throughout the colon but only in certain areas, and it cannot be identified by visual inspection but only by microscopic examination of biopsies. The utility of surveillance in patients with ulcerative colitis is therefore more problematic than in patients with adenomatous polyps.

The pathology of colon cancers in ulcerative colitis is also different from that in the general population. In the general population, multicentric tumors account for only 2% to 3% of all colon cancers, but in ulcerative colitis, multicentric tumors are reported in up to 26% of all malignancies.[317,321,322] As mentioned, cancers in ulcerative colitis are more likely to

be largely submucosal. The tumor may be indistinguishable from the surrounding mucosa; it may appear as a flat, plaque-like lesion, or it may present as a stricture. The large exophytic masses with sharp margins seen in colon cancer in the general population are less common in ulcerative colitis.

Dysplasia is a pathologic condition marked by nuclear stratification, loss of nuclear polarity, and nuclear and cellular pleomorphism (Fig. 79-37). Dysplasia appears to be a premalignant lesion, but the chronology of its development and the extent to which it is reversible are unclear. In 1967, Morson and Pang reported a group of nine ulcerative colitis patients who were found to have dysplasia on rectal biopsy and underwent colectomy.[323] Of these nine patients, five were found to have malignancies elsewhere in the colon. The investigators then reviewed 23 colon specimens removed for cancer in ulcerative colitis patients and found that all of them had areas of dysplasia. Other groups have confirmed these observations, and it is now clear that about 88% of colons resected for malignancy in ulcerative colitis have dysplasia somewhere in the specimen.[324] These findings suggest that dysplasia may precede the development of carcinoma and that dysplasia may be a marker to identify patients with ulcerative colitis who have developed or are at risk of developing carcinoma. This, in turn, has led to the suggestion that patients with long-standing ulcerative colitis undergo periodic colonoscopy with biopsies and, if the biopsies show high-grade dysplasia, prophylactic colectomy.

There are, however, several problems with this plan of action. The first is that dysplasia is not easy to read on colonic biopsy, and interobserver variation is considerable. A group of pathologists has now developed a classification for dysplasia which should help to resolve this problem.[325] This classification divides biopsies into negative, indefinite, and positive groups; the positive group is further divided into those of high-grade and low-grade dysplasia. A second problem is that the presence of inflammation often makes it effectively impossible to decide whether dysplasia is present. A third problem is that, although dysplasia may be extensive, it is more

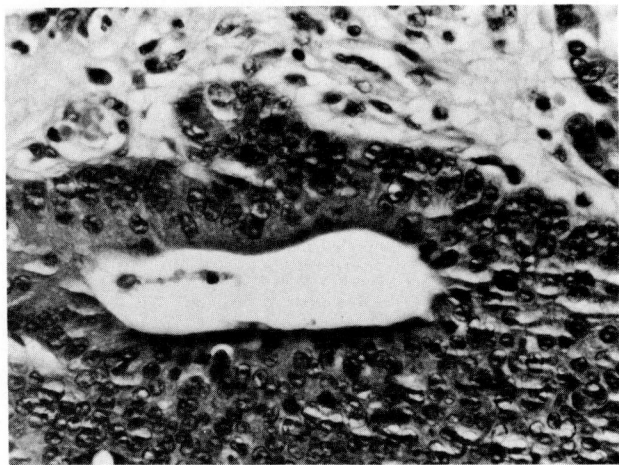

FIGURE 79-37. High-grade dysplasia with nuclear stratification, nuclear and cellular pleomorphism, and loss of nuclear polarity. Compare with Figure 79-12, in which nuclear polarity is clearly preserved despite the presence of inflammation. (Courtesy of David Lacey, M.D., St. Louis, MO.)

often patchy and can be missed entirely if blind biopsies are taken at 10-cm intervals through the colon. In some cases, dysplasia exists only in small patches in the immediate vicinity of the tumor. Although 88% of carcinomas are associated with dysplasia elsewhere in the specimen, that does not mean that colonoscopy with biopsies will always find the dysplastic area.

There is a group of patients in whom the finding of dysplasia appears to have special meaning—those in whom dysplasia is found in the vicinity of a suspicious lesion or mass.[326,327] This condition is called DALM (dysplasia-associated lesion or mass). Preliminary figures suggest that if an endoscopically visible lesion and low-grade dysplasia are present together on a first colonoscopy, there is a 40% chance the lesion will be carcinoma; if high-grade dysplasia and an endoscopically visible lesion are present, the incidence of colon cancer increases to 60%. In this selected group, the finding of dysplasia, even low-grade dysplasia, is highly significant.

The association of dysplasia and colon cancer in ulcerative colitis is firmly established, but the benefits of surveillance for dysplasia are less clear. The usual approach to surveillance has been to perform colonoscopy with biopsy at intervals of 1 to 2 years in patients with ulcerative colitis of at least 8 to 10 years' duration. If the biopsies show high-grade dysplasia, the procedure is repeated, and if high-grade dysplasia is confirmed, the patient undergoes colectomy. If the biopsy shows low-grade dysplasia, colonoscopy and biopsy are repeated after a short interval (3 months). If high-grade dysplasia is found on the second colonoscopy the patient undergoes colectomy. There are, however, some who recommend colectomy even for those with low-grade dysplasia.

Table 79-12 shows the results of four large studies of surveillance in ulcerative colitis.[326,329–334] These results are difficult to interpret. The most obvious success is the identification of seven patients with Dukes' stage A carcinoma. However, how

does one interpret the 46 patients who, as a result of surveillance studies, had colectomies that contained dysplasia but no carcinoma? Some would declare these all to be surveillance successes, but we do not know how many of them would have developed carcinoma if untreated. We know that there is a high incidence of dysplasia in ulcerative colitis colons resected for carcinoma. However, both the sensitivity (how many ulcerative colitis patients with early cancer will have biopsies positive for dysplasia) and the specificity (how many people who test positive for dysplasia will go on to develop cancer) for dysplasia surveillance are unknown. Thus, despite huge amounts of effort over a long period of time, we do not have the information to make clear recommendations about the usefulness or the timing of surveillance. Developing guidelines for surveillance would be much easier if we had a clearer idea of the magnitude of the risk of developing carcinoma in ulcerative colitis. It would be easier to be enthusiastic about a program that called for prophylactic colectomy in ulcerative colitis patients with dysplasia if the cumulative lifetime risk of ulcerative colitis patients developing colon cancer were 25% than if it were 2%.

The present system of surveillance is not ideal, but no more definitive or more useful alternative markers of malignancy in ulcerative colitis have been identified. There is also no clear evidence that surveillance improves survival. How should the practitioner deal with the issue of surveillance in the face of inadequate data? The first step is to inform the patient of the risks of malignancy. Patients with long-standing quiescent disease need this information as much as those with active disease because they too are at increased risk. Similarly, patients with subtotal colectomies and retained rectums need to know that they are at risk. The second step is to explain the purpose of surveillance. If the patient would refuse colectomy even if high-grade dysplasia were found, there is no purpose in initiating surveillance. Conversely, knowledge of

---

TABLE 79-12
Summary of Four Surveillance Studies in Patients With Ulcerative Colitis

STUDY	NUMBER OF PATIENTS	DYSPLASIA OR DALM BEFORE COLECTOMY*	NO CANCER AT COLECTOMY	CANCER AT COLECTOMY†	DUKES' STAGE OF CANCER		
					A	B	C or D
Lennard-Jones[330–331]	303	16	9	7	6	1	0
Nugent[332–334]	151	20	14	6	0	2	4
Rosenstock[329]	248	22	15	7	1	3	3
Blackstone[326]	112‡	15	8	7§	0	4	2
Total	814	73	46	27	7	10	9‖

DALM, dysplasia-associated lesion or mass

* In some patients, dysplasia or DALM was the principal indication for colectomy; in other patients, other factors predominated.

† Patients in whom cancer developed but who had not known dysplasia before colectomy are not included.

‡ Only 66 of these patients were actually in a surveillance program.

§ The Dukes' stage was not provided for one patient.

‖ The number of Dukes' stage C or D lesions would increase to 12 if the most recent progress from the Lennard-Jones group were included.

From Collins RH Jr, Feldman M, Fordtran JS. Colon cancer, dysplasia, and surveillance in patients with ulcerative colitis. N Engl J Med 1987;316:1654.

the increased risk of malignancy may drive the patient to seek a prophylactic colectomy, especially if he or she has already suffered severe problems from disease activity. Another consideration is the availability of a pathologist competent to evaluate dysplasia. Many pathologists have little or no experience in identifying and grading dysplasia in ulcerative colitis.

If the patient is willing to undergo surveillance and competent pathology support is available, the next question is the design of the surveillance protocol. Most protocols involve taking one or two biopsies every 10 cm throughout the colon. It is important that the entire colon be examined. Biopsies should be taken from uninflamed areas if possible.[325] The colon should also be examined for masses, strictures, and plaque-like lesions, which should all be biopsied, and for polyps, which should be removed. However, pseudopolyps are not premalignant lesions and need not be removed. Surveillance should begin about 8 to 10 years after the start of pancolitis and can be delayed longer than that for left-sided disease. Some protocols call for colonoscopy every year, but that is probably excessive. One group calculated the optimal screening interval on a cost-benefit basis and suggested surveillance every 3 years initially and then more frequently as the duration of the disease and the risk of malignancy increase.[335] The algorithms for most surveillance programs are similar, and the specifics of one are given in Figure 79-38.[331] High-grade dysplasia associated with a mass or lesion is a strong indication for colectomy. High-grade dysplasia even without an associated lesion is also reason for colectomy. Low-grade dysplasia, if persistent, would be viewed by some as an adequate indication for colectomy. Despite the absence of evidence for increased survival, most clinicians use a surveillance program for patients with long-standing extensive dis-ease. Although most gastroenterologists use some surveillance protocol, it would be difficult to fault one who, because of the absence of a well-documented benefit to surveillance, did not engage in any surveillance program.

There is much less information available on cancer in Crohn's disease than in ulcerative colitis.[336] For those with Crohn's colitis, the incidence of colon cancer appears to be higher than in the general population but lower than in patients with ulcerative colitis. As with ulcerative colitis, the incidence of colon cancer in Crohn's colitis increases with the duration of the disease. Also, as in ulcerative colitis, colon cancers occur in patients with Crohn's disease at a younger age than in the general population. Although malignancy may develop in areas remote from active disease, usually it appears in areas of active inflammation. As in ulcerative colitis, the development of colon cancer in Crohn's disease is associated with dysplasia. Nonetheless, there are currently no data to support a role for surveillance, and the lower incidence of colon cancer in Crohn's disease than in ulcerative colitis would make it even more difficult to establish a favorable cost-benefit ratio.

There is an association between small intestine Crohn's disease and adenocarcinoma of the small intestine.[337] Most adenocarcinomas occur in areas of the small intestine actively involved with Crohn's disease. Adenocarcinoma of the small intestine occurs at an earlier age in patients with Crohn's disease than in the general population. There is also an association of small intestine adenocarcinoma with surgically bypassed loops of small bowel. It is not clear whether the high incidence of cancer in bypassed bowel is a product of the bypass procedure or merely reflects the long duration of the disease.

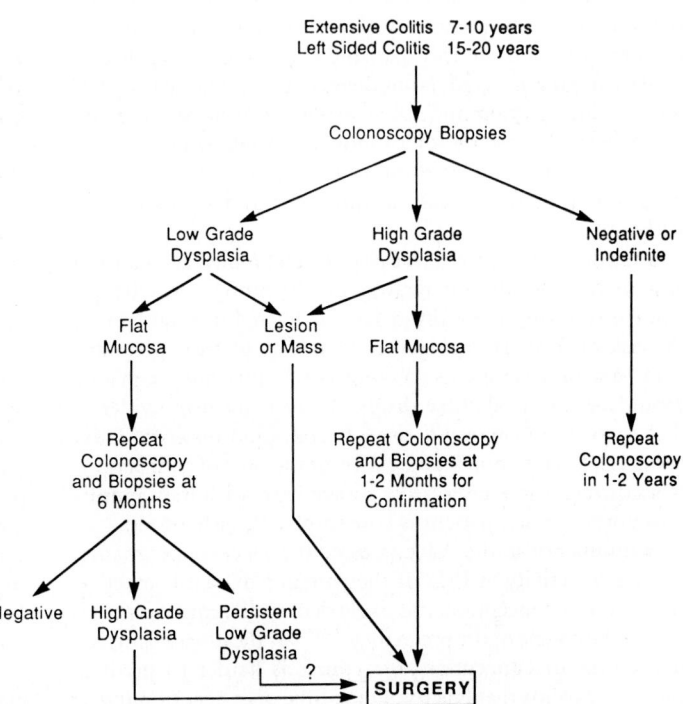

FIGURE 79-38. A proposed system of surveillance for cancer in patients with ulcerative colitis using colonoscopy and biopsy. (Adapted from Lennard-Jones J, Ritchie J, Morson B, Williams C. Cancer surveillance in ulcerative colitis. Lancet 1983;2:149).

PREGNANCY AND INFLAMMATORY BOWEL DISEASE

Because IBD affects many women in early adulthood, the effect of IBD on pregnancy is an important clinical issue. Fertility in women with IBD is normal or only minimally impaired.[338,339] Fertility in men taking sulfasalazine is diminished but returns to normal a few months after cessation of the drug.[198,340]

Most pregnancies in women with IBD produce healthy babies. The incidences of prematurity, stillbirth, and developmental defects are similar to those of the general population.[205] However, the incidence of spontaneous abortion is slightly higher in women with IBD (12.2%) than in the general population (9.9%). There is some suggestion that the incidence of fetal complications is somewhat higher in cases in which the mother's disease is clinically active, irrespective of drug therapy.[205] The incidences of prematurity and spontaneous abortion are both higher in patients with more active disease. Previous proctocolectomy or the presence of an ileostomy is not an impediment to the successful completion of a pregnancy.[341]

Many women with IBD take medication on a chronic basis, and the possibility of the fetus' suffering undesirable effects from the drugs is a matter of concern. Many women have taken sulfasalazine throughout the course of pregnancy, and there is no evidence for its causing harm to the fetus or newborn. In one series of 174 patients, sulfasalazine was found to have no effect on spontaneous abortion, prematurity, or fetal weight.[203] Pregnant women have an increased requirement for folic acid, and sulfasalazine interferes with folate absorption. Women taking sulfasalazine who are pregnant or considering pregnancy should receive folate supplementation (1 mg twice daily) to ensure that the fetus receives amounts adequate for normal development. The use of corticosteroids by pregnant women with IBD is not associated with an increased rate of fetal complications.[203] In general, it appears that the risks to the pregnancy of treatment with sulfasalazine or corticosteroids are less than the risks of allowing disease activity to go untreated. Nonetheless, it is advisable for pregnant women to minimize their exposure to drugs, and sulfasalazine and corticosteroids should be withdrawn if possible. Even better, the patient should, if she can, delay becoming pregnant until her disease is quiescent and drugs can be withdrawn.

Immunosuppressives (azathioprine and 6-mercaptopurine) and metronidazole are teratogenic in animals. Although women receiving these drugs have delivered normal babies, the risk of fetal damage makes it unwise to treat pregnant women with these agents. Women contemplating pregnancy should be taken off these drugs. There is no firm evidence that there is an increased risk of fetal abnormalities if the father is taking immunosuppressives at the time of conception. Nonetheless, the conservative stance is to withdraw immunosuppressives if a patient is contemplating fatherhood.

A number of studies have assessed the effects of pregnancy on disease activity in IBD. If the patient's disease is inactive at the time of conception, it is likely that it will remain inactive during the course of the pregnancy.[342,343] If the disease is active at the time of conception, the course is harder to predict. Ulcerative colitis that is active at the time of conception tends to get worse. In two thirds of Crohn's disease cases that are active at conception, the degree of activity remains the same; among the other third, some improve clinically and others deteriorate.

INFLAMMATORY BOWEL DISEASE IN CHILDHOOD AND ADOLESCENCE

Although the peak incidence of IBD is in young adulthood, 15% of patients with ulcerative colitis and 25% to 33% of patients with Crohn's disease present before 20 years of age.[344,345] For the most part, IBD presenting in childhood is similar to the disease in adults. The clinical presentation of ulcerative colitis in childhood, as in adulthood, is marked by diarrhea and rectal bleeding. The clinical presentation of Crohn's disease, however, is somewhat different in childhood.[346] Abdominal pain, weight loss, and diarrhea are common in both adults and children, but extraintestinal manifestations (e.g., arthritis, iridocyclitis, clubbing, erythema nodosum) are more likely to be major components of the initial clinical presentation in children than in adults. Abdominal pain in Crohn's disease tends to be periumbilical and colicky in character and may easily be confused with the pain of functional disease.

Growth failure is a major presenting complaint in 30% of children with Crohn's disease.[346-348] In mild disease of short duration, growth failure manifests itself as reduced weight for height; but, in disease of long standing, linear growth may be markedly retarded. Retarded bone development and delayed sexual maturation can also be manifestations of growth failure. In one third of children with impaired growth and Crohn's disease, the failure of linear growth antedates the onset of intestinal symptoms. Malnutrition appears to be the major cause of growth retardation. Poor oral intake and malabsorption both contribute to malnutrition. Poor oral intake results from anorexia and food avoidance as a result of pain and diarrhea associated with eating. Hypoalbuminemia is common, as is anemia, which may result from blood loss or from diminished intake of iron and folate. In addition to malnutrition, the presence of inflammation may contribute to growth failure. Extensive inflammation increases caloric requirements. Whether cytokines and other factors produced during inflammation contribute to growth retardation is unknown. Corticosteroid therapy can also contribute to growth failure. Growth retardation is less common in children with ulcerative colitis than in those with Crohn's disease.

Diagnosis of Crohn's disease in children is commonly delayed. The prominence of extraintestinal manifestations and growth retardation and the lesser role of intestinal symptoms contributes to the delay in the consideration of Crohn's disease as a diagnosis. Recurrent abdominal pain with or without diarrhea is a common complaint in childhood and usually reflects no significant pathology. However, in Crohn's disease, pain and diarrhea are seldom the only presenting symptoms.[346] Urgency, rectal bleeding, fever, and weight loss are signs that the child's abdominal pain is not on a functional basis and suggest that evaluation for IBD is indicated. Findings of perianal disease, uveitis, clubbing, or arthritis should suggest the possibility of Crohn's disease.

Nutritional supplementation plays a major role in the management of IBD, particularly Crohn's disease, in childhood. Children have smaller nutritional reserves and higher nutritional requirements per kilogram than adults. Moreover, nutritional deficiencies are a major source of growth retardation in childhood IBD. Oral supplementation with liquid formulas,[349] continuous supplementation by nasogastric tube,[166,350] and TPN have all been successful in reducing symptoms and reversing growth retardation. Irrespective of the method of delivering nutrition, all programs attempt to administer a number of calories in excess of the number recommended for healthy children, because the children with Crohn's disease have lost weight. Calorie intake on the various regimens ranges from 50 to 93 kcal/kg/day and protein intake ranges from 1.6 to 3.5 grams/kg/day.

Medical management of IBD in childhood is largely the same as in adulthood. All of the major controlled studies of therapy in IBD purposefully excluded children. Treatment in children is extrapolated from those studies. The indications for sulfasalazine therapy in children are the same as in adults. In children, sulfasalazine is begun at 25 to 40 mg/kg/day and increased to 75 mg/kg/day. The indications for corticosteroid therapy are also the same as for adults with IBD. Typical starting doses for moderate to severe disease would be 1.0 to 2.0 mg of prednisone per kilogram per day. Continuous therapy with prednisone in doses as low as 10 mg/day can inhibit normal growth. After acute symptoms are under control, an attempt should be made to convert the patient to an every-other-day prednisone regimen.[351,352] If prednisone is given as a single dose every other day, the side effects are markedly reduced. In particular, prednisone at doses as high as 40 to 50 mg every other morning allows normal growth.[351] However, not all patients can be converted to an alternate-day regimen. In some patients, the disease flares on the day off prednisone.

Immunosuppressives have been used in childhood Crohn's disease much as they have been used in the adult disease. Reservations about side effects are, if anything, greater if these drugs are used in children. The possibility of malignancy is particularly worrisome in children, who have the potential for longer exposure.

Indications for colectomy in ulcerative colitis in childhood are the same as for adults, with the addition of growth failure as an indication. Growth failure may be the result of either disease activity or corticosteroid administration. Surgical resection of localized areas of disease activity may be useful in children with Crohn's disease. However, the success of surgical resections in reversing growth retardation has been disappointing.[353]

The reader is directed to Chapter 38, Approach to the Patient With Diarrhea; Chapter 40, Approach to the Patient With Ileostomy and Ileal Pouch; Chapter 49, Genetic Counseling for Gastrointestinal Patients; Chapter 80, Miscellaneous Inflammatory and Structural Disorders of the Colon; Chapter 116, Colonoscopy and Flexible Sigmoidoscopy; and Chapter 119, Contrast Radiology.

REFERENCES

1. Kirsner JB, Shorter RG. Inflammatory bowel disease. 3rd ed. Philadelphia: Lea & Febiger, 1988.
2. Bayless TM. Current management of inflammatory bowel disease. Philadelphia: BC Decker, 1989.
3. Kirsner JB, Shorter RG. Recent developments in "nonspecific" inflammatory bowel disease. N Engl J Med 1982;306:775.
4. Monsen U, Brostrom O, Nordenvall B, et al. Prevalence of inflammatory bowel disease among relatives of patients with ulcerative colitis. Scand J Gastroenterol 1987;22:214
5. Shohat T, Vadheim CM, Rotter JI. The genetics of inflammatory bowel disease. In: Gitnick G, ed. Inflammatory bowel diseases: a physician's guide. New York: Igaku-Shoin, 1989.
6. Mendeloff AI. Newer concepts of IBD epidemiology. In: Rachmilewitz D, ed. Inflammatory bowel diseases. The Hague: Martinus Nijhoff, The Hague 1982.
7. Gilat T, Grossman A, Fireman Z, Rozen P. Inflammatory bowel disease in Jews. In: McConnell R, Rozen R, Langman M, Gilat T, eds. The genetics and epidemiology of inflammatory bowel disease. New York: Karger, 1986.
8. Calkins BM, Lilienfeld AM, Garland CF, Mendeloff AI. Trends in the incidence rates of ulcerative colitis and Crohn's disease. Dig Dis Sci 1984;29:913.
9. Sedlack RE, Nobrega FR, Kurland LT, Sauer WG. Inflammatory colon disease in Rochester, Minnesota, 1935–1964. Gastroenterology 1972;62:935.
10. Miller DS, Keighley AC, Langman MJS. Changing patterns in epidemiology of Crohn's disease. Lancet 1974;2:691.
11. Harries AD, Baird A, Rhodes J. Non-smoking. A feature of ulcerative colitis. Br Med J 1982;284:706.
12. Calkins B. Smoking factors in ulcerative colitis and Crohn's disease in Baltimore. Am J Epidemiol 1984;120:498.
13. Yang H, Shohat T, Rotter JI. The genetics of inflammatory bowel disease. In: MacDermott RP, Stenson WF, eds. Inflammatory bowel disease. New York: Elsevier, 1992:17.
14. Farmer RG, Michener WM, Mortimer EA. Studies of family history among patients with inflammatory bowel disease. Clin Gastroenterol 1980;9:271.
15. Weterman IT, Pena AS. Familial incidence of Crohn's disease in the Netherlands and a review of the literature. Gastroenterology 1984;86:449.
16. Roth, MP, Petersen GM, McElree C, et al. Familial recurrence risk estimates of inflammatory bowel disease in Ashkenazi Jews. Gastroenterology 1989;96:1016.
17. Tysk C, Lindberg E, Jarnerot G, Floderus-Myrhed B. Ulcerative colitis and Crohn's disease in an unselected population of monozygotic and dizygotic twins. A study of heritability and the influence of smoking. Gut 1988;29:990.
18. Neigut D, Proujansky R, Trucco M, et al. Association of an HLA-DQB-1 genotype with Crohn's disease in children. Gastroenterology 1992:102:A671.
19. Toyoda H, Wang S-J, Yang H, et al. Distinct association of HLA class II genes with inflammatory bowel disease. Gastroenterology 1992;104:741.
20. Hollander D, Vadheim CM, Brettholtz E, et al. Increased intestinal permeability in Crohn's patients and their relatives: an etiological factor? Ann Intern Med 1986;105:883.
21. Teahon K, Smethurst P, Levi AJ, et al. Intestinal permeability in patients with Crohn's disease and their first-degree relatives. Gut 1992;33:320.
22. Ruttenberg D, Young GO, Wright JP, Isaacs S. PEG-400 excretion in patients with Crohn's disease, their first-degree relatives, and healthy volunteers. Dig Dis Sci 1992;37:705.
23. Duerr RH, Targan SR, Landers CJ, et al. Antineutrophil cytoplasmic antibodies in ulcerative colitis. Comparison with other colitides/diarrheal illnesses. Gastroenterology 1991;100:1590.
24. Shanahan F, Duerr RH, Rotter JI, et al. Neutrophil autoantibodies in ulcerative colitis: familial aggregation and genetic heterogeneity. Gastroenterology 1992;103:456.
25. Chiodini RJ, Van Kruiningen HJ, Thayer WR, et al. Possible role of mycobacteria in inflammatory bowel disease. I. Unclassified mycobacterium species isolated from patients with Crohn's disease. Dig Dis Sci 1984;29:1073.
26. Chiodini RJ, Van Kruiningen HJ, Thayer WR, Coutu JA. Spheroplastic phase of mycobacteria isolated from a patient with Crohn's disease. J Clin Microbiol 1986;24:357.

27. Van Kruiningen HJ, Chiodini RJ, Thayer WR, et al. Experimental disease in infant goats induced by a mycobacterium isolated from a patient with Crohn's disease. A preliminary report. Dig Dis Sci 1986;31:1351.
28. Graham DY, Markesich DC, Yoshimura HH. Mycobacteria and inflammatory bowel disease. Results of culture. Gastroenterology 1987;92:436.
29. Taylor KB, Truelove SC. Circulating antibodies to milk proteins in ulcerative colitis. Br Med J 1961;2:924.
30. Knoflach P, Park BH, Cunningham R, et al. Serum antibodies to cow's milk proteins in ulcerative colitis and Crohn's disease. Gastroenterology 1987;92:479.
31. Kaulfersch W, Fiocchi C, Waldmann TA. Polyclonal nature of the intestinal mucosal lymphocyte populations in inflammatory bowel disease: a molecular genetic evaluation of the immunoglobulin and T-cell antigen receptors. Gastroenterology 1988;95:364.
32. Harrison WJ. Autoantibodies against intestinal and gastric mucous cells in ulcerative colitis. Lancet 1965;1:1346.
33. Hibi T, Aiso S, Ishikawa M, et al. Circulating antibodies to the surface antigens on colon epithelial cells in ulcerative colitis. Clin Exp Immunol 1983;54:163.
34. Deodhar SD, Michener WM, Farmer RG. A study of the immunologic aspects of chronic ulcerative colitis and transmural colitis. Am J Clin Pathol 1969;51:591.
35. Das KM, Dubin R, Nagai T. Isolation and characterization of colonic tissue-bound antibodies from patients with idiopathic ulcerative colitis. Proc Natl Acad Sci U S A 1978;75:4528.
36. Takahashi F, Das KM. Isolation and characterization of a colonic autoantigen specifically recognized by colon tissue-bound immunoglobulin G from idiopathic ulcerative colitis. J Clin Invest 1985;76:311.
37. Vecchi M, Sakamaki S, Diamond B, Das KM. A human colon specific antigen reactive with ulcerative colitis colon tissue-bound IgG: Immunohistochemical localization by the use of monoclonal antibody. Gastroenterology 1986;90:1679.
38. Mayer L, Shlien R. Evidence for function of Ia molecules on gut epithelial cells in man. J Exp Med 1987;166:1471.
39. Auer IO, Gotz S, Ziemer E, et al. Immune status in Crohn's disease. III. Peripheral blood B lymphocytes, enumerated by means of F(ab)2-antibody fragments, Null and T lymphocytes. Gut 1979;20:261.
40. Auer IO, Wechsler W, Ziemer E, et al. Immune status in Crohn's disease. I. Leukocyte and lymphocyte subpopulations in peripheral blood. Scand J Gastroenterol 1978;13:561.
41. Isaacs KL, Sartor RB, Haskill S. Cytokine mRNA profiles in inflammatory bowel disease mucosa detected by PCR amplification. Gastroenterology 1992;103:1587.
42. Lowes JR, Radwan P, Priddle JD, Jewell DP. Characterisation and quantification of mucosal cytokine that induces epithelial histocompatibility locus antigen-DR expression in inflammatory bowel disease. Gut 1992;33:315.
43. Fiocchi C. Cytokines. In: MacDermott RP, Stenson WF, eds. Inflammatory bowel disease. New York: Elsevier, 1992:137.
44. Stallmach A, Schuppan D, Riese HH, et al. Increased collagen type III synthesis by fibroblasts isolated from strictures of patients with Crohn's disease. Gastroenterology 1992;102:1920.
45. Brynskov J, Tvede N, Andersen CB, Villen M. Increased concentrations of interleukin 1, interleukin 2, and soluble interleukin 2 receptors in endoscopical mucosal biopsy specimens with active inflammatory bowel disease. Gut 1992;33:55.
46. Matsuura T, West GA, Klein JS, et al. Soluble interleukin 2 and CD8 and CD4 receptors in inflammatory bowel disease. Gastroenterology 1992;102:2006.
47. Cominelli F, Nast CC, Duchini A, Lee M. Recombinant interleukin 1 receptor antagonist blocks the proinflammatory activity of endogenous interleukin 1 in rabbit immune colitis. Gastroenterology 1992;103:365.
48. Saverymuttu SH, Chadwick VS, Hodgson HJ. Granulocyte migration in ulcerative colitis. Eur J Clin Invest 1985;15:60.
49. Saverymuttu SH, Peters AM, Lavender JP, et al. In vivo assessment of granulocyte migration to diseased bowel in Crohn's disease. Gut 1985;26:378.
50. Flower RJ, Blackwell CJ. Anti-inflammatory steroids induce biosynthesis of a phospholipase A2 inhibitor which prevents prostaglandin generation. Nature 1979;278:456.
51. Stenson WF. Pharmacology of sulfasalazine. Viewpoints Dig Dis 1984;16:13.
52. Gould SR. Assay of prostaglandin-like substances in faeces and their measurement in ulcerative colitis. Prostaglandins 1981;11:489.
53. Sharon P, Ligumsky M, Rachmilewitz D, et al. Role of prostaglandins in ulcerative colitis. Enhanced production during active disease and inhibition by sulfasalazine. Gastroenterology 1978;75:638.
54. Campieri M, Lanfranchi GA, Bazzochi G, et al. Prostaglandins, indomethacin, and ulcerative colitis. Gastroenterology 1980;78:193.
55. Gilat T, Ratan J, Rosen P, et al. Prostaglandins and ulcerative colitis. Gastroenterology 1979;77:1083.
56. Sharon P, Stenson WF. Enhanced synthesis of leukotriene B4 by colonic mucosa in inflammatory bowel disease. Gastroenterology 1984;86:453.
57. Lauritsen K, Laursen LS, Bukhave K, et al. In vivo effects of orally administered prednisolone on prostaglandin and leukotriene production in ulcerative colitis. Gut 1987;28:1095.
58. Lobos EA, Sharon P, Stenson WF. Chemotactic activity in inflammatory bowel disease. Dig Dis Sci 1987;32:1380.
59. Stenson WF, Cort D, Rodgers J, et al. Dietary supplementation with fish oil in ulcerative colitis. Ann Intern Med 1992;33:323.
60. Both H, Torp-Pedersen K, Kreiner S, et al. Clinical appearance at diagnosis of ulcerative colitis and Crohn's disease in a regional patient group. Scand J Gastroenterol 1983;18:987.
61. Sparberg M, Fennessy J, Kirsner JB. Ulcerative proctitis and mild ulcerative colitis: a study of 220 patients. Medicine (Baltimore) 1966;45:391.
62. Truelove SC, Witts, LJ. Cortisone in ulcerative colitis. Final report on a therapeutic trial. Br Med J 1955;2:1041.
63. Edwards EC, Truelove SC. The course and prognosis of ulcerative colitis. Gut 1963;4:299.
64. Powell-Tuck J, Ritchie JK, Lennard-Jones JE. The prognosis of idiopathic proctitis. Scand J Gastroenterol 1977;12:727.
65. Watts JMcK, de Dombal FT, Watkinson G, Goligher JC. Early course of ulcerative colitis. Gut 1966;7:16.
66. Sinclair TS, Brunt PW, Mowat NAG. Nonspecific proctocolitis in northeastern Scotland: a community study. Gastroenterology 1983;85:1.
67. Waye J. The role of colonoscopy in the differential diagnosis of inflammatory bowel disease. Gastrointest Endosc 1977;23:150.
68. Riddell R, Morson B. Value of sigmoidoscopy and biopsy in detection of carcinoma and premalignant change in ulcerative colitis. Gut 1979;20:575.
69. Nugent FW, Haggett RC, Gilpin PA. Cancer surveillance in ulcerative colitis. Gastroenterology 1991;100:1241.
70. Jalan KN, Sircus W, Card WI, et al. An experience of ulcerative colitis. I. Toxic dilation in 55 cases. Gastroenterology 1969;57:68.
71. Truelove SC, Marks CG. Toxic megacolon. Part I: Pathogenesis, diagnosis and treatment. Clin Gastroenterol 1981;10:107.
72. Trnka YM, La Mont JT. Association of Clostridium difficile toxin with symptomatic relapse of chronic inflammatory bowel disease. Gastroenterology 1981;80:693.
73. Greenfield C, Aguilar-Ramirez JR, Pounder RE, et al. Clostridium difficile and inflammatory bowel disease. Gut 1983;24:713.
74. Farmer RG, Hawk WA, Turnbull RB. Clinical patterns in Crohn's disease: a statistical study of 615 cases. Gastroenterology 1975;68:627.
75. Hellers G. Crohn's disease in Stockholm County, 1955–1974. A study of epidemiology, results of surgical treatment and longterm prognosis. Acta Chir Scand (Suppl) 1979;490:1.
76. Hofmann AF. Bile acid malabsorption caused by ileal resection. Arch Intern Med 1972;130:597.
77. Summers RW, Anuras S, Green J. Jejunal manometry patterns in health, partial intestinal obstruction and pseudo-obstruction. Gastroenterology 1983;85:1290.
78. Mekhijian HS, Switz DM, Melnyk CS, et al. Clinical features

and natural history of Crohn's disease. Gastroenterology 1979;77:898.

79. Farmer RG. Clinical features and natural history of inflammatory bowel disease. Med Clin North Am 1980;64:1103.

80. Myren J, Bouchier IA, Watkinson G, et al. The O.M.G.E. Multinational inflammatory bowel disease survey, 1976–1982. A further report of 2657 cases. Scand J Gasroenterol (Suppl) 1984;95:1.

81. Danzi JT, Farmer RG, Sullivan BH, Rankin GB. Endoscopic features of gastroduodenal Crohn's disease. Gastroenterology 1976;70:9.

82. Farmer RG, Hawk WA, Turnbull RB. Crohn's disease of the duodenum (transmural duodenitis). Clinical manifestations. Report of 11 cases. Am J Dig Dis 1972;17:191.

83. Best WR, Becktel JM, Singleton JW. Development of a Crohn's disease activity index: National Cooperative Crohn's Disease Study. Gastroenterology 1976;70:439.

84. Best WR, Becktel JM, Singleton JW. Rederived values of the eight coefficients of Crohn's Disease Activity Index (CDAI). Gastroenterology 1979;77:843.

85. Van Hees PAM, Van Elteren PH, Van Lier JJ, Van Tongeren JHM. An index of inflammatory activity in patients with Crohn's disease. Gut 1980;21:279.

86. Harvey RG, Bradshaw JM. A simple index of Crohn's disease activity. Lancet 1980;1:514.

87. Cooke WT, Prior P. Determining disease activity in inflammatory bowel disease. J Clin Gastroenterol 1984;6:17.

88. Salomon R, Kornbluth A, Aisenberg J, Janowitz HD. How effective are our current drugs for Crohn's disease? A metaanalysis. J Clin Gastroenterol 1992;14:211.

89. Meyers S, Janowitz HD. "Natural history" of Crohn's disease. An analytic review of the placebo lesson. Gastroenterology 1984;87:1189.

90. Wyke RJ, Edwards FC, Allan RN. Employment problems and prospects for patients with inflammatory bowel disease. Gut 1988;29:1229.

91. Haslock I, Wright V. Musculoskeletal complications of Crohn's disease. Medicine (Baltimore) 1973;52:217.

92. McEwen JC, Ling C, Kirsner JB. Arthritis accompanying ulcerative colitis. Am J Med 1962;33:923.

93. Fernandez-Herlihy L. The articular manifestations of chronic ulcerative colitis. An analysis of 555 cases. N Engl J Med 1959;261:259.

94. Miller MM. Ankylosing spondylitis, Reiter's syndrome, psoriatic arthritis and arthritis of inflammatory bowel disease. Prim Care 1984;11:271.

95. Brewerton DA, Nicholls A, Caffrey M, et al. HLA-B27 and arthropathies associated with ulcerative colitis and psoriasis. Lancet 1974;1:956.

96. Wright R, Lumsden K, Luntz, MH, et al. Abnormalities of the sacro-iliac joints and uveitis in ulcerative colitis. Q J Med 1965;34:229.

97. Christophi C, Hughes ER. Hepatobiliary disorders in inflammatory bowel disease. Surg Gynecol Obstet 1985;160:187.

98. Mistilis SP. Pericholangitis and ulcerative colitis. 1. Pathology, aetiology and pathogenesis. Ann Intern Med,1965;63:1.

99. Dew MJ, Thompson H, Allan RN. The spectrum of hepatic dysfunction in inflammatory bowel disease. Q J Med 1979;48:113.

100. Weisner RH, LaRusso NF. Clinicopathologic features of the syndrome of primary sclerosing cholangitis. Gastroenterology 1980;79:200.

101. Mihas AA, Murad TM, Hirshowitz BI. Sclerosing cholangitis associated with ulcerative colitis. Am J Gastroenterol 1978;70:614.

102. Cooperman AM, Judd ES. The role of colectomy in hepatic disease accompanying ulcerative and granulomatous colitis. Mayo Clin Proc 1972;47:36.

103. Cutler B, Donaldson GA. Primary sclerosing cholangitis and obliterative cholangitis. Am J Surg 1969;117:502.

104. Deren JJ, Porush JG, Levitt MF, Khilnani MT. Nephrolithiasis as a complication of ulcerative colitis and regional enteritis. Ann Intern Med 1962;56:843.

105. Gelzayd EA, Breuer RI, Kirsner JB. Nephrolithiasis in inflammatory bowel disease. Am J Dig Dis 1968;13:1027.

106. Dobbins JW, Binder HJ. Importance of the colon in enteric hyperoxaluria. N Engl J Med 1977;296:298.

107. Grossman MS, Nugent FW. Urolithiasis as a complication of chronic diarrheal disease. Am J Dig Dis 1967;12:491.

108. Thorton JR, Teague RH, Low-Beer TS, Read AE. Pyoderma gangrenosum in ulcerative colitis. Gut 1980;21:247.

109. Perry HO. Pyoderma gangrenosum. South Med J 1969;62:899.

110. Soto LD. Diaminodiphenylsulfone and steroids in the treatment of pyoderma gangrenosum. Int J Dermatol 1970;9:293.

111. Gelernt IM, Kreel I. Pyoderma gangrenosum in ulcerative colitis: prevention of the gangrenous component. Mt Sinai J Med 1976;43:467.

112. Samitz MH. Skin complications of ulcerative colitis and Crohn's disease. Cutis 1973;16:533.

113. Baioco PJ, Gorman BD, Korelitz BJ. Uveitis occurring after colectomy and ileal rectal sleeve anastomosis for ulcerative colitis. Dig Dis Sci 1984;29:570.

114. Verbanck J, Lameire N, Praet M, et al. Renal amyloidosis as complication of Crohn's disease. Acta Clin Belg 1979;34:6.

115. Talbot RW, Heppell J. Dozois RR, Beart RW. Vascular complications of inflammatory bowel disease. Mayo Clin Proc 1986;61:140.

116. Lam A, Borda I, Inwood M. Coagulation studies in ulcerative colitis and Crohn's disease. Gastroenterology 1975;68:245.

117. Yassinger S, Adelman R, Cantor D, et al. Association of inflammatory bowel disease and large vascular lesions. Gastroenterology 1976;71:844.

118. Surawicz CM, Belic L. Rectal biopsy helps to distinguish acute self-limited colitis from idiopathic inflammatory bowel disease. Gastroenterology 1984;86:104.

119. Magulis AB, Goldberg HI, Lawson TL, Montgomery CK. The overlapping spectrum of ulcerative and granulomatous colitis: A roentgenographic-pathologic study. AJR Am J Roentgenol 1971;113:325.

120. Chong SK, Blackshaw AJ, Boyle S, et al. Histological diagnosis of chronic inflammatory bowel disease in childhood. Gut 1985;26:55.

121. Surawicz CM, Meisel JL, Ylvisaker T, et al. Rectal biopsy in the diagnosis of Crohn's disease: value of multiple biopsies and serial sectioning. Gastroenterology 1981;81:66.

122. Dvorak AM, Silen W. Differentiation between Crohn's disease and other inflammatory conditions by electron microscopy. Ann Surg 1985;201:53.

123. Gabrielsson N, Granqvist S, Sundelin P, Thorgeirsson T. Extent of inflammatory lesions in ulcerative colitis assessed by radiology, colonoscopy, and endoscopic biopsies. Gastrointest Radiol 1979;4:395.

124. Williams HJ Jr, Stephens DH, Carlson HC. Double-contrast radiography: colonic inflammatory disease. Am J Radiol 1981;137:315.

125. Johnson CD, Carlson HC, Taylor WF, Weiland LP. Barium enemas of carcinoma of the colon: sensitivity of double- and single-contrast studies. Am J Radiol 1983;140:1143.

126. Ekberg O, Fort FT, Hildell J. Predictive value of small bowel radiography for recurrent Crohn's disease. Am J Radiol 1980;135:1051.

127. Saltzstein SL, Rosenberg BF. Ulcerative colitis of the ileum and regional enteritis of the colon, a comparative histopathologic study. Am J Clin Pathol 1963;40:610.

128. James EM, Carlson HC. Chronic ulcerative colitis and colon cancer: can radiographic appearance predict survival patterns? Am J Radiol 1978;130:825.

129. Tedesco J, Moore S. Infectious diseases mimicking inflammatory bowel disease. Am Surg 1982;48:242.

130. Tedesco F, Hardin R, Harper R, Edwards B. Infectious colitis endoscopically simulating inflammatory bowel disease: a prospective evaluation. Gastrointest Endosc 1983;29:195.

131. McGovern V, Goulston S. Crohn's disease of the colon. Gut 1968;9:164.

132. Morson B. The early histological lesion of Crohn's disease. Proc R Soc Med 1972;65:71.

133. Crowson T, Hines C. Amebiasis diagnosed by colonoscopy. Gastrointest Endosc 1978;24:254.

134. Tucker P, Webster P, Zachary M, Kilpatrick A. Amebic colitis mistaken for inflammatory bowel disease. Arch Intern Med 1975;135:681.

135. Gabrielsson N, Granqvist S, Sundeline P, Thorgeirsson T. Extent of inflammatory lesions in ulcerative colitis assessed by radiology, colonoscopy, and endoscopic biopsy. Gastrointest Radiol 1979;4:395.

136. Waye J. Endoscopy in inflammatory bowel disease. Clin Gastroenterol 1980;9:279.

137. Hunt R, Teague R, Swarbrick E, Williams G. Colonoscopy in the management of colonic strictures. Br Med J 1975;2:360.

138. Greenstein A, Sachar DB, Smith H, et al. Cancer in universal and left-sided ulcerative colitis: factors determining risk. Gastroenterology 1979;77:290.

139. Kirsner JB. Problems in the differentiation of ulcerative colitis and Crohn's disease of the colon: the need for repeated diagnostic evaluation (editorial). Gastroenterology 1975;68:187.

140. Clamp SE, Myren J, Bouchier IA, et al. Diagnosis of inflammatory bowel disease: an international multicentre scoring system. Br Med J 1982;284:91.

141. Hogan WJ, Hensley GT, Geenen JE. Endoscopic evaluation of inflammatory bowel disease. Med Clin North Am 1980;64:1083.

142. Schacter H, Kirsner J. Definitions of inflammatory bowel disease of unknown etiology. Gastroenterology 1975;68:591.

143. Kovalcik P, Simstein L, Weiss M. The dilemma of Crohn's disease: Crohn's disease and appendectomy. Dis Colon Rectum, 1977;20:377.

144. Vantrappen G, Agg HO, Geboes K, et al. *Yersinia* enteritis. Med Clin North Am 1982;66:639.

145. Lindeman RJ, Weinstein L, Lavitan R, Patterson JF. Ulcerative colitis and intestinal salmonellosis. Am J Med Sci 1967;254:855.

146. Shorter RG, Huizenga KA, Spencer RJ. A working hypothesis for the etiology and pathogenesis of nonspecific inflammatory bowel disease (editorial). Am J Dig Dis 1972;17:1024.

147. Schulze K, Warner HA, Murray D. Intestinal tuberculosis: experience at a Canadian teaching institution. Am J Med 1977;63:735.

148. Hoon JR, Dockerty MB, Pemberton J de J. Collective review: ileocecal tuberculosis including comparison of this disease with nonspecific regional enterocolitis and noncaseous tuberculated enterocolitis. Int Abstr Surg 1950;91:417.

149. Quinn TC, Corey L, Chaffee RG, et al. The etiology of anorectal infections in homosexual men. Am J Med 1981;71:395.

150. Quinn TC, Stamm WE, Goodell SE, et al. The polymicrobial origin of intestinal infections in homosexual men. N Engl J Med 1983;309:576.

151. Lindstrom CG. "Collagenous colitis" with watery diarrhoea—a new entity? Pathol Eur 1976;11:87.

152. Pieterse AS, Hecker R, Rowland R. Collagenous colitis: a distinctive and potentially reversible disorder. J Clin Pathol 1982;35:338.

153. Fagin RR, Kirsner JB. Ischemic diseases of the colon. Adv Intern Med 1971;17:343.

154. Reinus JF, Brandt LJ, Boley SJ. Ischemic diseases of the bowel. Gastroenterol Clin North Am 1990;19:319.

155. Carr N, Schofield PF. Inflammatory bowel disease in the older patient. Br J Surg 1982;69:223.

156. Berman IR, Corman ML, Coller JA, Veidenheimer MC. Late onset Crohn's disease in patients with colonic diverticulitis. Dis Colon Rectum 1979;22:524.

157. Schmidt GT, Lennard-Jones JE, Morson BC, Young AC. Crohn's disease of the colon and its distinction from diverticulitis. Gut 1968;9:7.

158. Bartlett JG, Gorbach SL. Pseudomembranous enterocolitis (antibiotic-related colitis). Adv Intern Med 1977;22:455.

159. Kappas A, Shinagawa N, Arabi Y, et al. Diagnosis of pseudomembranous colitis. Br Med J 1978;1:675.

160. Isgar B, Harman M, Kaye MD, et al. Symptoms of irritable bowel syndrome in ulcerative colitis in remission. Gut 1983;24:190.

161. Bayless TM. Coexistent irritable bowel syndrome and inflammatory bowel disease. In: Bayless TM, ed. Current management of inflammatory bowel disease. Toronto: BC Decker, 1989:59.

162. Harig JM, Woergel KH, Komorowski RA, Wood CM. Treatment of diversion colitis with short-chain fatty acid irrigation. N Engl J Med 1989;320:23.

163. Sitrin MD, Rosenberg IH, Chawla K, et al. Clinical conference: nutritional and metabolic complications in a patient with Crohn's disease and ileal resection. Gastroenterology 1980;78:1069.

164. Chan ATJ, Fleming CR, O'Fallon WM, Huizenga KA. Estimated versus measured basal energy requirements in patients with Crohn's disease. Gastroenterology 1986;91:75.

165. O'Morain C. Elemental diets in the treatment of Crohn's disease. Proc Nutr Soc 1979;38:403.

166. Navarro J, Vargas J, Cezard JP, et al. Prolonged constant rate elemental enteral nutrition in Crohn's disease. J Pediatr Gastroenterol Nutr 1982;1:541.

167. Lochs H, Egger-Schodl M, Schuh R, et al. Is tube feeding with elemental diets a primary therapy of Crohn's disease? Klin Wochenschr 1984;62:821.

168. O'Morain C, Segal AW, Levi AJ. Elemental diet as primary treatment of acute Crohn's disease: a controlled trial. Br Med J 1984;288:1859.

169. Saverymuttu S, Hodgson HJF, Chadwick VS. Controlled trial comparing prednisolone with an elemental diet plus non-absorbable antibiotics in active Crohn's disease. Gut 1985;26:994.

170. Lochs H, Steinhardt HJ, Klaus-Wentz B, et al. Comparison of enteral nutrition and drug treatment in active Crohn's disease. Gastroenterology 1991;101:881.

171. Lindor KD, Fleming R, Burnes JU, et al. A randomized prospective trial comparing a defined formula diet, corticosteroids, and a defined formula diet plus corticosteroids in active Crohn's disease. Mayo Clin Proc 1992;67:328.

172. Levenstein S, Prantera C, Luzi C, D'Ubaldi A. Low residue or normal diet in Crohn's disease: a prospective controlled study in Italian patients. Gut 1985;26:989.

173. Rombeau JL, Afonso JJ. Clinical and scientific basis for nutritional support of patients with inflammatory bowel disease. In: MacDermott RP, Stenson WF, eds. Inflammatory bowel disease. New York: Elsevier, 1992:525.

174. Dickinson RJ, Ashton MG, Axon ATR, et al. Controlled trial of intravenous hyperalimentation and total bowel rest as an adjunct to the routine therapy of acute colitis. Gastroenterology 1980;79:1199.

175. Jarnerot G, Rolny P, Sandberg-Gertzen H. Intensive intravenous treatment of ulcerative colitis. Gastroenterology 1985;89:1005.

176. Das KM, Dubin R. Clinical pharmacokinetics of sulfasalazine. Clin Pharmacokinet 1976;1:406.

177. Van Hees PAM, Bakker JH, Van Tongeren JHM. Effect of sulphapyridine, 5-aminosalicylic acid, and placebo in patients with idiopathic proctitis. A study to determine the active therapeutic moiety of sulphasalazine. Gut 1980;21:632.

178. Das KM, Eastwood MA, McManus JPA, Sircus W. Adverse reactions during salicylazosulfapyridine therapy and the relation with drug metabolism and acetylator phenotype. N Engl J Med 1973;289:491.

179. Gould SR, Brash AR, Conolly ME, Lennard-Jones JE. Studies of prostaglandins and sulphasalazine in ulcerative colitis. Prostaglandins and Medicine 1981;6:165.

180. Stenson WF, Lobos E. Sulfasalazine inhibits the synthesis of chemotactic lipids by neutrophils. J Clin Invest 1982;69:494.

181. Allgayer H, Stenson WF. A comparison of effects of sulfasalazine and its metabolites on the metabolism of endogenous vs. exogenous arachidonic acid. Immunopharmacology 1988;15:39.

182. Lauterburg BH. 5-aminosalicylic acid (5-ASA) scavenges superoxide anion radicals: an additional mode of action in ulcerative colitis. Gastroenterology 1986, 90:1514

183. MacDermott RP, Schloemann SR, Bertovich MJ, et al. Inhibition of antibody secretion by 5-aminosalicylic acid. Gastroenterology 1989;96:442.

184. Moertel CG, Bargen JA. A critical analysis of the use of sali-

cylazosulfapyridine in chronic ulcerative colitis. Ann Intern Med 1959;51:879.

185. Baron JH, Connell AM, Lennard-Jones JE. Sulphasalazine and salicylazo-sulphadimidine in ulcerative colitis. Lancet 1962;1: 1094.

186. Dick AP, Grayson MJ, Carpenter RG, Petrie A. Controlled trial of sulphasalazine in the treatment of ulcerative colitis. Gut 1964;5:437.

187. Lennard-Jones JE, Longmore AJ, Newell AC, et al. An assessment of prednisone, salazopyrine, and topical hydrocortisone used as outpatient treatment for ulcerative colitis. Gut 1960;1: 217.

188. Truelove SC, Watkinson G, Draper G. Comparison of corticosteroid and sulphasalazine therapy in ulcerative colitis. Br Med J 1962;2:1708.

189. Summers RW, Switz DM, Sessions JT Jr, et al. National Co-operative Crohn's Disease CD Study: results of drug treatment. Gastroenterology 1979;77:847.

190. Malchow H, Ewe K, Brandes JW, et al. European Cooperative Crohn's Disease Study (ECCDS): results of drug treatment. Gastroenterology 1984;86:249.

191. Misiewicz JJ, Lond MB. Controlled trial of sulphasalazine in maintenance therapy for ulcerative colitis. Lancet 1965;2:185.

192. Azad Khan AK, Howes DT, Piris J, Truelove SC. Optimum dose of sulphasalazine for maintenance treatment of ulcerative colitis. Gut 1980;21:232.

193. Pieniaszek HJ, Resetarits DE, Wilferth WW, et al. Relative systemic availability of sulfapyridine from commercial enteric-coated and uncoated sulfasalazine tablets. J Clin Pharmacol 1979;19:39.

194. Nielsen OH. Sulfasalazine intolerance: a retrospective survey of the reasons for discontinuing treatment with sulfasalazine in patients with chronic inflammatory bowel disease. Scand J Gastroenterol 1982;17:389.

195. Halsted CH, Gandhi G, Tamura T. Sulfasalazine inhibits the absorption of folates in ulcerative colitis. N Engl J Med 1981;305:1513.

196. Longstreth GF, Green R. Folate status in patients receiving maintenance doses of sulfasalazine. Arch Intern Med 1983;143: 902.

197. Birnie GG, McLeod TIF, Watkinson G. Incidence of sulphasalazine-induced male infertility. Gut 1981;22:452.

198. Toovey S, Hudson E, Hendry WF, Levi AJ. Sulphasalazine and male infertility: reversibility and possible mechanism. Gut 1981;22:445.

199. Werlin SL, Grand RJ. Bloody diarrhea—a new complication of sulfasalazine. J Pediatr 1978;92:450.

200. Peppercorn MA, Goldman P. Distribution studies of salicylazosulfapyridine and its metabolites. Gastroenterology 1973;64: 240.

201. Franklin JL, Rosenberg JH. Impaired folic acid absorption in inflammatory bowel disease: effects of salicylazopyridine (Azulfidine). Gastroenterology 1973;64:517.

202. Willoughby CP, Truelove SC. Ulcerative colitis and pregnancy. Gut 1980;21:469.

203. Mogadam M, et al. Pregnancy in inflammatory bowel disease: effect of sulfasalazine and corticosteroids on fetal outcome. Gastroenterology 1981;80:72.

204. Nielsen OH, Andreasson B, Bondesen S, Jarnum S. Pregnancy in ulcerative colitis. Scand J Gastroenterol 1983;18:735.

205. Baiocco PJ, Korelitz BI. The influence of inflammatory bowel disease and its treatment on pregnancy and fetal outcome. J Clin Gastroenterol 1984;6:221.

206. Jarnerot G, Into-Malmberg MB. Sulphasalazine treatment during breast feeding. Scand J Gastroenterol 1979;14: 869.

207. Lewis JH, Weingold AB. The use of gastrointestinal drugs during pregnancy and lactation. Am J Gastroenterol 1985;80:912.

208. Goldstein PD, Alpers DH, Keating JP. Sulfapyridine metabolites in children with inflammatory bowel disease receiving sulfasalazine. J Pediatr 1979;95:638.

209. Campieria M, Lanfranchi GA, Bazzocchi G, et al. Treatment of ulcerative colitis with high-dose 5-aminosalicylic acid enemas. Lancet 1981;2:270.

210. D'Albaso G, et al. Long-term maintenance therapy in ulcerative

colitis. A controlled trial with intermittent 5-aminosalicylic acid (5-ASA) enemas. Second International Symposium on Inflammatory Bowel Diseases, Jerusalem, 1985.

211. Meyers S, Sachar DB, Present DH, Janowitz HD. Olsalazine sodium in the treatment of ulcerative colitis among patients intolerant of sulfasalazine: a prospective randomized, placebo-controlled double-blind, dose-ranging clinical trial. Gastroenterology 1987;93:1255.

212. Meyers S, Sachar DB, Present DH, Janowitz HD. Olsalazine sodium in the treatment of ulcerative colitis among patients intolerant of sulfasalazine. Gastroenterology 1987;93:1255.

213. Dew MJ, Highes P, Haris AD, et al. Maintenance of remission with oral preparation of 5-aminosalicylic acid doses by mouth. Gastroenterology 1988;95:1679.

214. Sninsky CA, Cort DH, Shanahan F, et al. Oral mesalamine (Asacol) for mildly to moderately active ulcerative colitis. Ann Intern Med 1991;115:350.

215. Kiilerich S, Ladefoged K, Rannem T, Ranlov PJ. Prophylactic effects of olsalazine v sulphasalazine during 12 months maintenance treatment of ulcerative colitis. Gut 1992;33:252.

216. Hanauer S, Schwartz J, Robinson M, et al. Mesalamine capsules for treatment of active ulcerative colitis: results of a controlled trial, Pentasa study group. Am J Gastroenterol 1993;88:1188.

217. Prantera C, Pallone F, Brunetti G, et al. Oral 5-aminosalicylic acid (Asacol) in the maintenance treatment of Crohn's disease. Gastroenterology 1992;103:363.

218. Claman HN. Glucocorticosteroids I. Anti-inflammatory mechanisms. Hosp Pract 1983;18:123.

219. Cupps TR, Fauci AS. Corticosteroid-mediated immunoregulation in man. Immunol Rev 1982;65:133.

220. Parrillo JE, Fauci AS. Mechanisms of glucocorticoid action on immune processes. Annu Rev Pharmacol Toxicol 1979;19:179.

221. Schleimer RP. The mechanisms of anti-inflammatory steroid actions in allergic diseases. Annu Rev Pharmacol Toxicol 1985;25:381.

222. Baron JH, Connell AM, Kanaghinis TG, et al. Out-patient treatment of ulcerative colitis. Br Med J 1962;2:441.

223. Powell-Tuck J, Brown RL, Lennard-Jones JE. A comparison of oral prednisolone given as single or multiple daily doses for active proctocolitis. Scand J Gastroenterol 1978;13:833.

224. Meyers S, Sachar DB, Goldberg JD, Janowitz HD. Corticotropin versus hydrocortisone in the intravenous treatment of ulcerative colitis. A prospective, randomized, double-blind clinical trial. Gastroenterology 1983;85:351.

225. Truelove SC. Treatment of ulcerative colitis with local hydrocortisone hemisuccinate sodium: a report on a controlled therapeutic trial. Br Med J 1958;2:1072.

226. Watkinson G. Treatment of ulcerative colitis with topical hydrocortisone hemisuccinate sodium. Br Med J 1958;2:1077.

227. Halvorsen S, Myren J, Aakvaag A. On the absorption of prednisone and prednisolone disodium phosphate after rectal administration. Scand J Gastroenterol 1969;4:581.

228. Lee AH, Taylor GM, James VHT, Walker G. Plasma prednisolone levels and adrenocortical responsiveness after administration of prednisolone-21 phosphate as a retention enema. Gut 1979;20:349.

229. Levine DS, Rubin CE. Topical beclomethasone dipropionate enemas improve distal ulcerative colitis and idiopathic proctitis without systemic toxicity. Gastroenterology 1985;88:1473.

230. Larochelle P, Du Souich P, Bolte E, et al. Tixocortol pivalate, a corticosteroid with no systemic glucocorticoid effect after oral, intrarectal, and intranasal application. Clin Pharmacol Ther 1983;33:343.

231. Hanauer SB, Kirsner JB, Barrett WE. The treatment of left sided ulcerative colitis with tixocortol pivalate. Gastroenterology 1986;90:1449.

232. Danielsson A, Lofberg R, Persson T, et al. A steroid enema, budesonide, lacking systemic effects for the treatment of distal ulcerative colitis or proctitis. Scand J Gastroenterol 1992;27:9.

233. Matzen P. Budesonide enema in distal ulcerative colitis: a randomized dose-response trial with prednisolone enema as positive control. Scand J Gastroenterol 1991;26:1225.

234. Modigliani R, Mary JY, Simon JF, et al. Clinical, biological,

and endoscopic picture of attacks of Crohn's disease: evolution on prednisolone. Gastroenterology 1990;98:811.

235. Singleton JW, Law DH, Kelley ML Jr, et al. National Cooperative Crohn's Disease Study: adverse reactions to study drugs. Gastroenterology 1979;77:870.

236. Axelrod L. Glucocorticoid therapy. Medicine (Baltimore) 1976;55:39.

237. Dykman TR, Gluck OS, Murphy WA, et al. Evaluation of factors associated with glucocorticoid-induced osteopenia in patients with rheumatic diseases. Arthritis Rheum 1985;28:361.

238. Sambrook PN, Eisman JA, Champion GD, et al. Determinants of axial bone loss in rheumatoid arthritis. Arthritis Rheum 1987;30:721.

239. Levine SB, Leopold IH. Advances in ocular corticosteroid therapy. In: Azarnoff DL, ed. Steroid therapy. Philadelphia: WB Saunders, 1975.

240. Present DH, Korelitz BI, Wisch N, et al. Treatment of Crohn's disease with 6-mercaptopurine. A long-term, randomized, double-blind study. N Engl J Med 1980;302:981.

241. Klein M, Binder HJ, Mitchell M, et al. Treatment of Crohn's disease with azathioprine: a controlled evaluation. Gastroenterology 1974;66:916.

242. Rosenberg JL, Wall AJ, Levin B. A controlled trial of azathioprine in Crohn's disease. Am J Dig Dis 1975;20:721.

243. O'Brien JJ, Bayless TM, Bayless JA. Use of Azathioprine or 6-MP in the treatment of Crohn's disease. Gastroenterology 1991;101:39.

244. Kinlen LJ, Sheil AGR, Peto J, Doll R. Collaborative United Kingdom-Australian study of cancer in patients treated with immunosuppressives drugs. Br Med J 1979;2:1461.

245. Present DH, Meltzer SJ, Krumholz MP, et al. 6-Mercaptopurine in the management of inflammatory bowel disease: short- and Long-term toxicity. Ann Intern Med 1989;111:641.

246. Kinlen LJ. Incidence of cancer in rheumatoid arthritis and other disorders after immunosuppressive treatment. Am J Med 1985;78:44.

247. Brynskov J, Freund L, Rasmussen SN, et al. A placebo-controlled, double-blind, randomized trial of cyclosporine therapy in active chronic Crohn's disease. N Engl J Med 1989;321:845.

248. Lichtiger S, Present DH, Kornbluth A, Hanauer S. Cyclosporine A in the treatment of severe refractory ulcerative colitis: a double-blinded placebo controlled trial. Gastroenterology 1983;104:A732.

249. Rice-Oxley JM, Truelove SC. Ulcerative colitis. Course and prognosis. Lancet 1950;1:663.

250. Davis PS, Rhodes J, Heatley RV, Owen E. Metronidazole in the treatment of chronic proctitis: a controlled trial. Gut 1977;18:680.

251. Ursing B, Alm T, Barany F, et al. A comparative study of metronidazole and sulfasalazine for active Crohn's disease: the cooperative Crohn's disease study in Sweden. II. Result. Gastroenterology 1982;83:550.

252. Sutherland L, Singleton J, Sessions J, et al. Double-blind, placebo controlled trial of metronidazole in Crohn's disease. Gut 1991;32:1071.

253. Sandborn WJ, Tremaine WJ, Schroeder KW, et al. A randomized, double-blind, placebo-controlled trial of cyclosporine enemas for mildly to moderately active left-sided ulcerative colitis. Gastroenterology 1993;104:A775.

254. Singleton J, Gitnick G, Hanauer S, et al. Response of Crohn's disease to oral Pentasa (controlled release mesalamine) as a function of disease location and prior therapy. Results of a randomized trial (abstract). Gastroenterology 1991;100:A251.

255. Gendre JP, Mary JY, Florent C, et al. Oral mesalamine (Pentasa) as maintenance treatment in Crohn's disease: a multicenter placebo-controlled study. Gastroenterology 1993;104:435.

256. Caprilli R, Andreloi A, Capurso L, et al. 5-ASA in the prevention of Crohn's disease post-operative recurrence: an interim report of the Italian Study Group of the Colon (GISC) (abstract). Gastroenterology 1992;102:A601.

257. Thomson ABR. International mesalamine study group coated oral 5-aminosalicylic acid vs. placebo in maintaining remission in inactive Crohn's disease. Aliment Pharmacol Ther 1990;4:55.

258. Bonnevie O, Binder V, Anthonisen P, Riis P. The prognosis of ulcerative colitis. Scand J Gastroenterol 1974;9:81.

259. Ritchie JK, Powell-Tuck J, Lennard-Jones JE. Clinical outcome of the first ten years of ulcerative colitis and proctitis. Lancet 1978;1:1140.

260. Devroede GJ, Taylor WF, Sauer WG, et al. Cancer risk and life expectancy of children with ulcerative colitis. N Engl J Med 1971;285:17.

261. Daly DW. Outcome of surgery for ulcerative colitis. Ann R Coll Surg Engl 1968;42:38.

262. Greenstein, AJ, Sachar DB, Gibas A, et al. Outcome of toxic dilatation in ulcerative and Crohn's colitis. J Clin Gastroenterol 1985;7:137.

263. Greenberger NJ. Indications for surgery in inflammatory bowel disease: A gastroenterologist's opinion. In: Kirsner JB, ed. Inflammatory bowel disease. 3rd ed. Philadelphia: Lea & Febiger, 1988:565.

264. Berger M, Gribetz D, Korelitz BI. Growth retardation in children with ulcerative colitis: the effects of medical and surgical therapy. Pediatrics 1975;55:459.

265. Dozois RR, Kelly KA. Newer operations for ulcer colitis and Crohn's disease. In: Kirsner JB, ed. Inflammatory bowel disease. 3rd ed. Philadelphia: Lea & Febiger, 1988:660.

266. Sales DJ, Kirsner JB. Prognosis of inflammatory bowel disease. Arch Intern Med 1983;143:294.

267. Whittington PF, Barnes HV, Bayless TM. Medical management of Crohn's disease in adolescence. Gastroenterology 1977;72:1338.

268. Garlock JH, Crohn, BB, Klein SH, Yarnia H. An appraisal of the long-term results of surgical treatment of regional enteritis. Gastroenterology 1951;19:414.

269. Van Patter WN, Bargen AJ, Dockerty MB, et al. Regional enteritis. Gastroenterology 1954;26:347.

270. Trnka YM, Glotzer DJ, Kasdon EJ, et al. The long-term outcome of restorative operation on Crohn's disease. Influence of location, prognostic factors and surgical guidelines. Ann Surg 1982;196:345.

271. Rutgeerts P. Natural history of recurrent Crohn's disease at the ileocolonic anastomosis after curative surgery. Gut 1984;25:665.

272. Alexander-Williams J. New directions for future research: surgical/clinical. In: Rachmilewitz D, ed. Inflammatory bowel diseases. Vol. 3. London: Martinus Nijhoff, 1982.

273. Lee ECG, Papaionnou N. Minimal surgery for chronic obstruction in patients with extensive or universal Crohn's disease. Ann R Coll Surg Engl 1982;64:229.

274. Jones PF, Munro A, Ewen SWB. Colectomy and ileorectal anastomosis for colitis: report on a personal series with a critical review. Br J Surg 1977;64:615.

275. Khubchandani IT. Ileorectal anastomosis for ulcerative and Crohn's colitis. Am J Surg 1978;135:751.

276. Glotzer DJ, Gardner RC, Goldman H, et al. Comparative features and course of ulcerative and granulomatous colitis. N Engl J Med 1960;282:582.

277. Fawaz KA, Glotzer DJ, Goldman H. Ulcerative colitis and Crohn's disease of the colon: a comparison of the long-term postoperative courses. Gastroenterology 1976;71:372.

278. De Dombal FT, Watts JMcK, Watkinson G, Goligher JC. Local complications of ulcerative colitis: strictures, pseudopolyposis and carcinoma of colon and rectum. Br Med J 1966;1:1442.

279. Garret JM, Sauer WG, Moertel CG. Colonic motility in ulcerative colitis after opiate administration. Gastroenterology 1967;53:93.

280. Brown JW. Toxic megacolon associated with Loperamide therapy. J Am Med Assoc 1979;241:501.

281. Odyniec NA, Judd ES, Sauer WG. Toxic megacolon. Significant improvement in surgical management. Arch Surg 1967;94:638.

282. Caprilli R, Colaneri VO, Frieri G. Risk factors in toxic megacolon. Dig Dis Sci 1980;25:817.

283. Binder HJ. Steroids and toxic megacolon. Gastroenterology 1979;76:888.

284. Meyers S, Janowitz HD. The place of steroids in the therapy of toxic megacolon. Gastroenterology 1978;75:729.

285. Hartong WA, Arvanitakis C, Skibba RM, Klotz AP. Treatment

of toxic megacolon. A comparative review of 29 patients. Dig Dis Sci 1977;22:195.

286. Grant CS, Dozois RR. Toxic megacolon: ultimate fate of patients after successful medical management. Am J Surg 1984;147:106.

287. Steinberg DM, Cooke WT, Alexander-Williams J. Abscess and fistulae in Crohn's disease. Gut 1973;14:865.

288. Van Dongen LM, Lubbers EJC. Psoas abscess in Crohn's disease. Br J Surg 1982;69:589.

289. Keighley MRB. Incidence and microbiology of abdominal and pelvic abscess in Crohn's disease. Gastroenterology 1982;83:1271.

290. Chennells PM, Simpkins KC. The barium enema diagnosis of paracolic abscess. Clin Radiol 1981;32:73.

291. Holdstock G, Ligorria JE, Krawitt EL. Gallium-67 scanning in patients with Crohn's disease: an aid to the diagnosis of abdominal abscess. Br J Surg 1982;69:277.

292. Chintapalli K, Thorsen MK, Foley WD, Unger GF. Abdominal abscesses with enteric communications: CT findings. AJR Am J Roentgenol 1983;141:27.

293. Broe PJ, Bayless TM, Cameron JL. Crohn's disease: are enteroenteral fistulas an indication for surgery? Surgery 1982;91:249.

294. Korelitz BI, Present DH. Favorable effect of 6-mercaptopurine on fistulae of Crohn's disease. Dig Dis Sci 1985;30:58.

295. Bos LP, Nabe M, Weterman IT. Total parenteral nutrition in Crohn's disease; a clinical evaluation. In: Pena AS, Weterman IT, Booth CC, Strober W, eds. Recent advances in Crohn's disease. Boston: Martinus Nijhoff, 1981.

296. Elson CO, Layden TJ, Nemchausky BA, Rosenberg IH. An evaluation of total parenteral nutrition in the management of inflammatory bowel disease. Dig Dis Sci 1980;25:42.

297. Broe PJ, Cameron JL. Surgical management of ileosigmoid fistulas in Crohn's disease. Am J Surg 1982;143:611.

298. Block GE, Schraut WH. The operative treatment of Crohn's enteritis complicated by ileosigmoid fistula. Ann Surg 1982;196:356.

299. Heimann T, Greenstein AJ, Aufses AH. Surgical management of ileosigmoid fistula in Crohn's disease. Am J Gastroenterol 1979;72:21.

300. McIntyre JK, Ritchie JK, Hawley PR, et al. Management of enterocutaneous fistulas: a review of 132 cases. Br J Surg 1984;71:293.

301. Rothenberger DA, Goldberg SM. The management of rectovaginal fistula. Surg Clin North Am 1983;63:61.

302. Bernstein LH, Frank MS, Brandt LJ, Boley SJ. Healing of perineal Crohn's disease with metronidazole. Gastroenterology 1980;79:357.

303. Brandt LJ, Bernstein LH, Boley SJ, Frank MS. Metronidazole therapy for perineal Crohn's disease: a follow-up study. Gastroenterology 1982;83:383.

304. Tuxen PA, Castro AF. Rectovaginal fistula in Crohn's disease. Dis Colon Rect 1979;22:58.

305. Greenstein AJ, Sachar DB, Tzakis A, et al. Course of enterovesical fistulas in Crohn's disease. Am J Surg 1984;147:788.

306. Talamini MA, Broe PJ, Cameron JL. Urinary fistulas in Crohn's disease. Surg Gynecol Obstet 1982;154:553.

307. Farmer RG, Hawk WA, Turnbull RB Jr. Indications for surgery in Crohn's disease: analysis of 500 cases. Gastroenterology 1976;71:245.

308. Alexander-Williams J. Conservative nonresection operations for Crohn's disease. In: Najarian JS, Delaney JP, eds. Advances in gastrointestinal surgery. Chicago: Year Book Medical Publishers, 1984.

309. Williams DR, Coller JA, Corman ML, et al. Anal complications in Crohn's disease. Dis Colon Rectum 1981;24:22.

310. De Dombal FT, Watts JMcK, Watkinson G, Goligher JC. Incidence and management of anorectal abscess, fistula and fissure, in patients with ulcerative colitis. Dis Colon Rectum 1966;9:201.

311. Jakobovits J, Schuster MM. Metronidazole therapy for Crohn's disease and associated fistulae. Am J Gastroenterol 1984;79:533.

312. Duffy LF, Daum F, Fisher SE, et al. Peripheral neuropathy in Crohn's disease patients treated with metronidazole. Gastroenterology 1985;88:861.

313. Parks AG. Pathogenesis and treatment of fistula in ano. Br Med J 1961;1:463.

314. Williams NS, MacFie J, Celesin LR. Anorectal Crohn's disease. Br J Surg 1979;66:743.

315. Jones JH, Lennard-Jones JE, Lockhart-Mummery HE. Experience in the treatment of Crohn's disease of the large intestine. Gut 1966;7:448.

316. Katzka I, Brody RS, Morris E, Katz S. Assessment of colorectal cancer risk in patients with ulcerative colitis: experience from a private practice. Gastroenterology 1983;85:22.

317. Edwards FC, Truelove SC. The course and prognosis of ulcerative colitis. Part 4. Carcinoma of the colon. Gut 1964;5:15.

318. Johnson WR, McDermott FT, Hughes ES, et al. Carcinoma of the colon and rectum in inflammatory bowel disease of the intestine. Surg Gynecol Obstet 1983;156:193.

319. Thompson H, Waterhouse JAH, Allan RN. Cancer morbidity in ulcerative colitis. Gut 1982;23:490.

320. Devroede GJ, Taylor WF. On calculating cancer risk and survival of ulcerative colitis patients with the life table method. Gastroenterology 1976;71:505.

321. Goldgraber MB, Kirsner JB. Carcinoma of the colon in ulcerative colitis. Cancer 1964;17:657.

322. Greenstein AJ, Sachar DB, Pucillo A, et al. Cancer in universal and left sided ulcerative colitis: clinical and pathological features. Mt Sinai J Med 1979;46:25.

323. Morson BC, Pang LSC. Rectal biopsy as an aid to cancer control. Gut 1967;8:423.

324. Dobbins WO III. Current status of the precancer lesion in ulcerative colitis. Gastroenterology 1977;73:1431.

325. Riddle R, Goldman H, Ransohoff DF, et al. Dysplasia in inflammatory bowel disease: standardized classification with provisional clinical applications. Hum Pathol 1983;14:931.

326. Blackstone M, Riddell R, Rogers B, Levin B. Dysplasia-associated lesion or mass (DALM) detected by colonoscopy in longstanding ulcerative colitis: an indication for colectomy. Gastroenterology 1981;80:366.

327. Butt J, Konishi F, Morson BC, et al. Macroscopic lesions in dysplasia and carcinoma complicating ulcerative colitis. Dig Dis Sci 1983;28:18.

328. Collins RH Jr, Feldman M, Fordtran JS. Colon cancer, dysplasia, and surveillance in patients with ulcerative colitis: a critical review. N Engl J Med 1987;316:1654.

329. Rosenstock E, Farmer RG, Petras R, et al. Surveillance for colonic carcinoma in ulcerative colitis. Gastroenterology 1985;89:1342.

330. Lennard-Jones JE, Morson BC, Path FRC, et al. Cancer in colitis: assessment of the individual risk by clinical and histological criteria. Gastroenterology 1977;73:1280.

331. Lennard-Jones J, Ritchie J, Morson BC, Williams C. Cancer surveillance in ulcerative colitis. Lancet 1983;2:149.

332. Nugent FW, Haggitt RC, Colcher H, Kutteruf GC. Malignant potential of chronic ulcerative colitis: preliminary report. Gastroenterology 1979;76:1.

333. Nugent FW. Surveillance of patients with ulcerative colitis. Lahey Clinic results. In: Winawer SJ, Schottenfeld D, Sherlock P, eds. Colorectal cancer prevention, epidemiology, and screening. New York: Raven Press, 1980:375.

334. Nugent FW, Haggin RC. Results of a longterm prospective surveillance program for dysplasia in ulcerative colitis. Gastroenterology 1984;86:1197.

335. Lashner BA, Hanauer SB, Silverstein MD. Optimal timing of colonoscopy to screen for cancer in ulcerative colitis. Ann Intern Med 1988;108:274.

336. Greenstein AJ, Sachar DB, Smith H, et al. A comparison of cancer risk in Crohn's disease and ulcerative colitis. Cancer 1981;48:2742.

337. Darke SG, Parks AG, Grogano SL, Pollock DN. Adenocarcinoma and Crohn's disease. A report of two cases and analysis of the literature. Br J Surg 1973;60:169.

338. Webb MJ, Sedlack RF. Ulcerative colitis in pregnancy. Med Clin North Am 1974;55:823

339. Khosla R, Willoughby CP, Jewell DP. Crohn's disease and pregnancy. Gut 1984;25:52.
340. Toth A. Reversible toxic effect of salicylazosulfapyridine on semen quality. Fertil Steril 1979;31:538.
341. Priest FO, Gilchrist RK, Long JS. Pregnancy in the patient with ileostomy and colectomy. J Am Med Assoc 1959;169:213.
342. De Dombal FT, Cantab MB, Watts JM, et al. Ulcerative colitis and pregnancy. Lancet 1965;2:599.
343. Mogadam M, Korelitz BI, Ahmed SW, et al. The course of inflammatory bowel disease during pregnancy and postpartum. Am J Gastroenterol 1981;75:265.
344. Goligher JC, et al. Ulcerative colitis. Baltimore: Williams & Wilkins, 1968.
345. Kyle J. Crohn's disease. New York: Appleton-Century-Crofts, 1972.
346. Burbidge EJ, Huang S, Bayless TM. Clinical manifestations of Crohn's disease in children and adolescents. Pediatrics 1975;55:866.
347. Gryboski JD, Spiro HD. Prognosis in children with Crohn's disease. Gastroenterology 1978;74:807.
348. Motil KJ, Grand RJ, Davis-Kraft E. The epidemiology of growth failure in children and adolescents with inflammatory bowel disease. Gastroenterology 1983;84:1254.
349. Kirschner BS, Klich JR, Kalman SS, et al. Reversal of growth retardation in Crohn's disease with therapy emphasizing oral nutritional restitution. Gastroenterology 1981;80:10.
350. O'Morain C, Segal AW, Levi AJ. Elemental diets in the treatment of acute Crohn's disease. Br Med J 1980;281:1173.
351. Sadeghi-Nejad A, Senior B. The treatment of ulcerative colitis in children with alternate-day corticosteroids. Pediatrics 1968;43:840.
352. Whittington PF, Barns HV, Bayless TM. Medical management of Crohn's disease in adolescence. Gastroenterology 1977;72:1338.
353. Wesson DE, Shandling B. Results of bowel resection for Crohn's disease in the young. J Pediatr Surg 1981;16:449.
354. Present D, Rabinowitz J, Banks P, Janowitz H. Obstructive hydronephrosis—A frequent but seldom recognized complication of granulomatous disease of the bowel. N Engl J Med 1969;280:573.

Textbook of Gastroenterology, second edition, edited by Tadataka Yamada. JB Lippincott Company, Philadelphia © 1995.

CHAPTER 80

Miscellaneous Inflammatory and Structural Disorders of the Colon

R. Balfour Sartor   Mark E. Murphy   Edward Rydzak

A variety of stimuli and idiopathic syndromes produce inflammation and structural abnormalities of the colon which can be differentiated from ulcerative colitis and Crohn's disease by clinical, endoscopic, and histologic characteristics. This chapter discusses conditions distinct from idiopathic inflammatory bowel disease, radiation, ischemic, and infectious enterocolitis. Because the colon has a limited repertoire of pathologic and physiologic responses to injury, many of these syndromes have overlapping clinical, endoscopic, and histologic features (Table 80-1). However, we have attempted to provide distinguishing characteristics to aid in the differential diagnosis and therapeutic approach to these miscellaneous

TABLE 80-1
Clinical and Pathologic Characterization of Inflammatory Disorders of the Colon*

CONDITIONS	PRIMARY LOCATION	SYMPTOMS	ENDOSCOPIC FINDINGS	HISTOLOGIC FINDINGS
Lymphocytic colitis	Diffuse	Diarrhea	Normal	Mucosal inflammation with mononuclear cells, increased intraepithelial lymphocytes, few neutrophils
Collagenous colitis	Diffuse	Diarrhea	Normal	Similar to lymphocytic colitis, plus subepithelial collagen band >10 μm
Diversion colitis	Bypassed segment	Mucoid discharge, bleeding	Erythema, granularity, friability	Follicular lymphoid hyperplasia, neutrophilic and mononuclear infiltration
Endometriosis	Rectosigmoid	Dysmenorrhea, dyspareunia, partial obstruction, rare hematochezia	Usually normal, rare extrinsic compression	Serosal implants of endometrial cells, muscular hypertrophy, fibrosis
Caustic enema-induced colitis	Rectosigmoid	Hematochezia, pain, diarrhea	Diffuse distal mucosal injury	Necrosis, ranging from epithelial to transmural, acute injury
Drug-induced ischemic colitis	Splenic flexure, descending	Pain, diarrhea, hematochezia	Friability, granularity, necrosis	Necrosis, acute inflammation
NSAID-induced ulcers	Diffuse, especially rectosigmoid	Diarrhea, bleeding	Erythema, discrete ulcers, exudate	Acute and chronic inflammation, discrete ulcers
Nonspecific ulcers	Cecum, ascending colon	Pain, bleeding	Solitary, round ulcer	Acute and chronic inflammation
Stercoral ulcer	Rectosigmoid	Pain, bleeding, fever	Discrete ulcer, sharp margins	Transmural necrosis
Solitary rectal ulcer	Anterior rectum	Constipation, bleeding, pain	Demarcated ulcer	Fibromuscular obliteration of lamina propria
Typhlitis	Cecum	Pain, fever	Mucosal ulceration, necrosis	Mucosal necrosis, hemorrhage, submucosal edema, no inflammatory cells
Colitis cystica profunda	Anterior rectum	Bleeding, mucoid discharge	Polypoid submucosal mass, erythema, friability	Epithelial-lined cysts, fibrosis
Pneumatosis cystoides intestinalis	Idiopathic—left colon; secondary—right colon	None, rare pain	Multiple, soft, round submucosal masses	No epithelial lining, foreign-body giant cells, acute and chronic inflammation
Malakoplakia	Descending, rectosigmoid	None, diarrhea, pain, bleeding	Yellow, soft plaque or nodule	PAS-positive macrophages containing basophilic calculospherules (Michaelis-Gutmann bodies)

* Excluding inflammatory bowel disease and radiation, infections, and ischemic colitis.

NSAID, nonsteroidal antiinflammatory drug; PAS, periodic acid–Schiff.

conditions. Pathophysiology and etiologic theories are emphasized, although current knowledge is limited for most of these disorders.

COLLAGENOUS AND LYMPHOCYTIC COLITIS

Clinical Features

Collagenous and lymphocytic colitis are syndromes characterized by chronic watery diarrhea with histologic evidence of chronic mucosal inflammation but normal endoscopic and radiographic evaluations. These histologically distinguishable disorders may represent two extremes of the spectrum of "microscopic colitis." Collagenous colitis, originally described by Lindstrom in 1976,[1] is diagnosed by increased subepithelial collagen deposition and chronic mucosal inflammation. Microscopic colitis was originally reported by Read and colleagues[2] in 1980 as a subset of patients with idiopathic chronic diarrhea whose only histologic abnormality was increased numbers of mucosal mononuclear cells. The term lymphocytic colitis was later proposed by Lazenby et al. to distinguish this syndrome from mild inflammatory bowel disease and infectious colitis.[3] In both of these disorders, the mean age of patients is 60 to 65 years, with a female predominance and a frequent association of arthritis, autoimmune disorders, and celiac disease.[4] Collagenous colitis and lymphocytic colitis have been described in children, who have similar clinical presentations.[5,6] The predominant symptom is chronic nonbloody diarrhea, 300 to 1700 g/24 hours,[4,7] associated with nocturnal stools, occasional fecal incontinence, and decreased stool volume with fasting. Variable symptoms include crampy abdominal pain, nausea, weight loss, and abdominal distention. Fever and gross rectal bleeding are atypical features. Routine laboratory tests are usually normal, although patients may occasionally exhibit mild anemia, hypoalbuminemia, increased sedimentation rate, and, rarely, steatorrhea. The onset of diarrhea is usually insidious, although some patients have abrupt onset of diarrhea after a presumed infection. Diarrhea is persistent, between 2 months and 20 years in duration, with a fluctuating clinical course marked by spontaneous relapses and remissions. The exact prevalence is unknown. Although increased use of colonoscopic biopsies in the evaluation of patients with chronic diarrhea has increased the rate of diagnosis, these disorders remain relatively unusual. At Johns Hopkins Hospital, 12 patients were diagnosed with lymphocytic colitis in a group of 1314 patients undergoing colorectal biopsy for nonneoplastic conditions in 1987.[3]

Pathology

Both disorders are characterized by moderate numbers of mononuclear cells infiltrating the mucosa, with epithelial cell damage and preservation of the crypt architecture (Fig. 80-1). Intraepithelial lymphocytes are increased five- to tenfold (20–25 lymphocytes/100 epithelial cells).[3] Flattened surface epithelial cells, occasionally with a syncytial appearance, a mild decrease in number of goblet cells, Paneth cell hyperplasia, and increased numbers of epithelial mitoses are common histologic features. Lamina propria cells are typically lymphocytes, plasma cells, and macrophages; in some studies, eosinophils and mast cells[8] are increased. Neutrophils are rarely present, and there is a notable absence of crypt distortion and cryptitis.

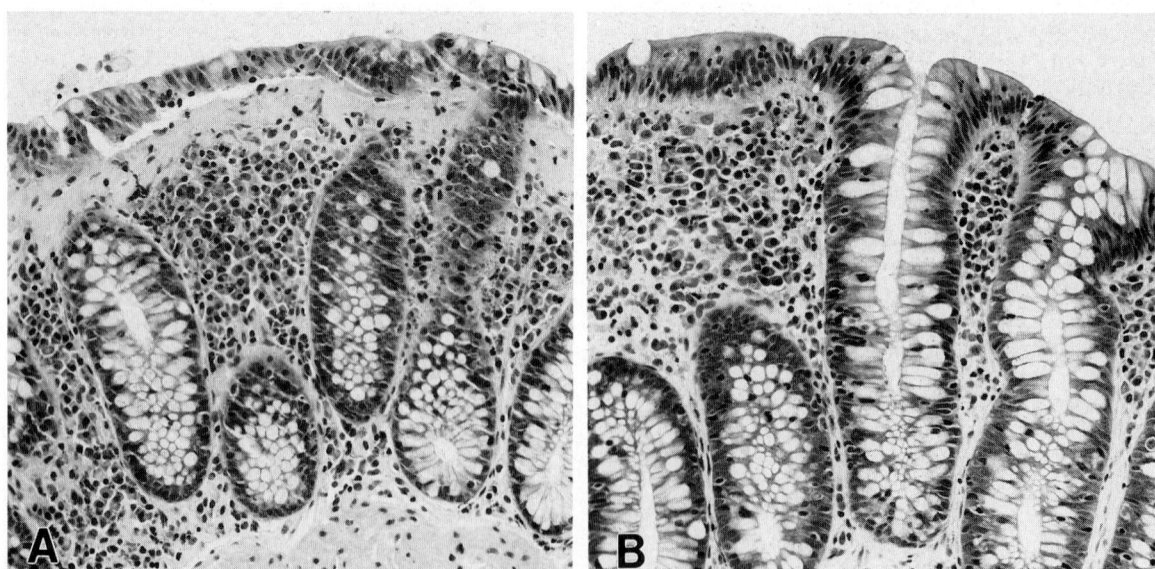

FIGURE 80-1. Histologic comparison of lymphocytic and collagenous colitis. **(A)** Collagenous colitis is characterized by a thickened subepithelial collagen layer as well as the inflammatory features of increased plasma cells in the lamina propria and a damaged surface epithelium with increased epithelial lymphocytes. **(B)** Lymphocytic colitis shows all the inflammatory features of collagenous colitis but lacks the subepithelial collagen layer. (Hematoxylin and eosin stains; original magnification ×225; courtesy of Audrey Lazenby, M.D., Baltimore, MD.)

Collagenous colitis is histologically differentiated from lymphocytic colitis by a linear subepithelial collagen layer (Fig. 80-1A). The normal basement membrane is less than 4 μm thick, whereas in collagenous colitis the subepithelial collagen band is greater than 10 μm thick and can extend to 100 μm.[9] Linearly arranged type IV collagen constitutes the basement membrane in normal subjects; however, the band in collagenous colitis is composed of types I and III collagen and fibronectin.[10] The thickened collagen layer is most prominent beneath the surface epithelium between crypts and is frequently penetrated by capillaries. Although cellular infiltration in both disorders is pancolonic, distribution of the thickened collagen table is spotty, being most prevalent in the cecum (82% of cases) and transverse colon (83% of cases) and least likely to be detected in the rectum (27% of cases).[9] Marked variability in simultaneous samples from the same patient and regional distribution of lesions raise serious questions in interpreting reports of resolution and development of collagenous colitis over time with serial biopsies.[11,12] Clearly, these reports of changes in thickness of subepithelial collagen bands could reflect sampling error.

Etiology and Pathogenesis

These disorders, though idiopathic, appear to be caused by immunologic events. The chronic, diffuse, and superficial nature of mucosal inflammation suggest an immune response to lumenal constituents or epithelial antigens, although the nature of the stimulant remains obscure. Increased intraepithelial lymphocytes, epithelial damage, and cellular infiltration in these disorders closely resemble certain histologic features of celiac disease, and both lymphocytic colitis and collagenous colitis can be associated with typical or refractory celiac disease. Approximately 20% to 30% of patients with typical celiac disease had evidence of lymphocytic colitis on investigation by colonic biopsies.[13,14] Conversely, 4 of 10 patients with collagenous colitis had small intestine biopsies compatible with celiac disease.[15] However, colonic inflammation does not typically respond to a gluten-free diet, and the majority of lymphocytic colitis and collagenous colitis patients do not exhibit clinical evidence of malabsorption. Moreover, these disorders are not associated with HLA-B8 and -DR3, as is celiac disease. Arthritis, thyroid abnormalities, and other possibly autoimmune disorders frequently accompany microscopic colitis, but no consistent evidence of autoimmune HLA haplotypes or serum markers has been found. In small studies, lymphocytic colitis has been associated with HLA-A1 and collagenous colitis with HLA-A2.[16,17]

The strong association of arthritis with these disorders raises the possibility that nonsteroidal antiinflammatory drugs (NSAIDs) may play an etiologic role. In a well-controlled study, significantly more collagenous colitis patients (61%) had used NSAIDs for more than 6 months than age- and gender-matched controls (13%; p<.02).[18] In an uncontrolled study, 21% of patients in a collagenous colitis registry had used NSAIDs.[19] NSAIDs can cause gastric, small bowel, and colonic inflammation in patients and experimental animals.[20] Given the high frequency of NSAID use in a 60-year-old population and the relative rarity of collagenous colitis and lymphocytic colitis, other factors must be important. The possibility of genetically determined host susceptibility factors was raised by reports of collagenous colitis in multiple members of two families[21] and of differential susceptibility of inbred rat strains to indomethacin.[22] No pathogen has yet been incriminated, but it is possible that nonspecific infection could initiate mucosal injury that evolves into chronic inflammation in the genetically susceptible individual. The possibility that bile acid malabsorption injures colonic epithelia in these disorders is raised by the occasional response to cholestyramine and the demonstration of bile salt malabsorption in some patients.[23,24] Finally, the ability of ingested substances to injure the colon is illustrated by clinical and experimental inflammation induced by L-tryptophan.[25] Future studies must concentrate on the role of environmental agents, especially NSAIDs, and host genetic factors in the etiology of these disorders.

Diarrhea in the small number of patients investigated with microscopic colitis is caused by defective active and passive absorption of sodium and chloride and reduced chloride-bicarbonate exchange.[7] Two of six patients displayed coexisting abnormal small intestine fluid and electrolyte absorption. Active colonic chloride secretion associated with increased lumenal prostaglandin E_2 concentrations[26] and prevention of diarrhea by an H_1 antagonist in a patient with increased numbers of mast cells[8] suggest that soluble mediators produced by activated immune and mesenchymal cells mediate epithelial cell absorptive dysfunction. This hypothesis is supported by correlation of diarrhea with increased numbers of mucosal inflammatory cells rather than thickness of the collagen table.[27] The latter observation argues against the theory that subepithelial collagen blocks electrolyte and water absorption.

Diagnosis and Differential Diagnosis

Lymphocytic colitis and collagenous colitis are diagnosed by compatible histologic features in a patient with chronic watery diarrhea whose endoscopic, radiographic, microbial, and endocrine evaluations are normal. Multiple biopsies must be taken from different colonic segments to reliably diagnose collagenous colitis.[9,28] Colonoscopy with biopsy of multiple segments demonstrated only one site positive in 5 of 17 patients and a greater than 50% variability of collagen thickness in multiple samples taken simultaneously from the cecum of one patient.[9] Rectal biopsy is a poor predictor of this disease because only 27% of patients with documented collagenous colitis had diagnostic biopsies from the rectum, although 82% of pooled biopsies from the descending colon, sigmoid colon, and rectum showed a thickened collagen plate.[9] Ninety-four percent of these patients had evidence of chronic inflammation on biopsies from these sites, demonstrating that a flexible sigmoidoscopy is an adequate screening examination. However, a full colonoscopy with multiple segmental biopsies is necessary to exclude these diagnoses. Proper orientation of the specimen is essential to prevent artifactual thickening of the subepithelial basement membrane caused by tangential sectioning; the presence of associated lamina propria inflammation is an important codiagnostic feature of collagenous colitis.[29]

Ulcerative colitis and Crohn's disease can be differentiated by diagnostic colonoscopy and radiography as well as by different histologic features. Infectious agents must be excluded by stool ova and parasite examinations, standard fecal bacterial cultures, and *Clostridium difficile* toxin assays. Chronic diarrhea secondary to *Giardia* infestation can be most definitively evaluated by jejunal aspirates, which can also determine bacterial overgrowth; these may be taken at the time of small bowel biopsies performed to rule out celiac disease and Whipple's disease. Malabsorption and secretory diarrhea are not characteristic features of lymphocytic colitis and collagenous colitis but may be present. Hormone producing tumors, laxative abuse, ischemic colitis, amyloidosis, and hyperthyroidism must be considered in the differential diagnosis. Irritable bowel syndrome can be differentiated by normal stool volume and colonic biopsies.

Several disorders resembling lymphocytic colitis and collagenous colitis can be differentiated by careful histologic analysis.[4,29] Acute infectious colitis is associated with mucosal edema, neutrophilic infiltration, and a paucity of intraepithelial lymphocytes. Ulcerative colitis and Crohn's disease biopsies have crypt abscesses, neutrophils, and possible granulomas with few intraepithelial lymphocytes. Pericrypt eosinophilic enterocolitis is characterized by chronic watery diarrhea and normal endoscopy but can be differentiated from lymphocytic colitis by the absence of increased numbers of intraepithelial and superficial lamina propria lymphocytes and the presence of eosinophilic infiltration, crypt foreshortening, and inflammation in the deep lamina propria and muscularis mucosa.[30] Fibrosis in ischemic colitis, radiation colitis, and solitary rectal ulcer syndrome (SRUS) is diffuse in the lamina propria, and colonic collagen deposition in progressive systemic sclerosis occurs along all basement membranes and may be transmural. Similarly, amyloid deposits occur along the basement membrane of the crypts and blood vessels as well as the surface epithelium; amyloidosis can be diagnosed by histochemical staining.

Treatment

Treatment of these disorders remains empiric because of the lack of controlled trials and insight into the pathogenesis of colonic inflammation. Clinical symptoms of lymphocytic colitis and collagenous colitis can spontaneously relapse and remit, which makes interpretation of the small, mostly retrospective, treatment courses reported to date quite difficult. The majority of patients have decreased diarrhea and improved histologic scores after therapy with 5-aminosalicylate (5-ASA), sulfasalazine, and prednisone, but at least one third of patients respond to symptomatic therapy. In the only controlled trial,[31] six patients with collagenous colitis (43%) had significantly decreased number of stools (p = 0.03) and a decrease in the degree of mucosal inflammation (not quantitated) with 3 months of prednisolone therapy. However, stool frequency returned to pretherapy levels within 2 to 4 weeks after cessation of therapy, and thickness of the collagen band was unchanged by treatment in 5 of 6 patients. In a recent retrospective study, 8 (57%) of 18 collagenous colitis patients treated for 14 months with 5-ASA, sulfasalazine, prednisolone, or a combination of therapy had histologic remission of inflammation; 7 of these patients had an associated clinical remission.[28]

Based on current data, the following progressive approach is suggested for therapy of these disorders. Initial treatment should be symptomatic, including administration of antidiarrheal agents and withdrawal of all drugs potentially contributing to mucosal injury, such as NSAIDs. If symptoms continue, sulfasalazine (or 5-ASA in the sulfasalazine-intolerant patient) can be added. Corticosteroid therapy should be reserved for patients who are not responding to these measures and who have debilitating symptoms. Celiac disease should be excluded in patients refractory to antiinflammatory drugs, and antihistamine therapy should be considered in patients with large numbers of mast cells on biopsy.[8]

Overlap or Distinct Diseases

Whether lymphocytic and collagenous colitis are two separate but similar disorders or different presentations of a single disorder is the subject of an unresolved debate.[16,27,32] These diseases share similar clinical, demographic, and histologic characteristics and differ primarily by the presence or absence of a thickened subepithelial collagen plate. Serial biopsies have shown resolution or development of this collagen band with time[11,12]; however, the spotty nature and segmental distribution of the collagen plate[9,27] raise serious questions regarding the conclusion that lymphocytic colitis can develop into collagenous colitis. Type III collagen in the subepithelial band suggests that collagen is deposited as a result of inflammation in the lamina propria or as a primary defect in the permeability of subepithelial capillaries.[10] Advocates of the separatist theory argue that thickness of the collagen table follows a multimodel distribution and does not increase with age or with duration of symptoms,[27] suggesting that collagen deposition is not merely a consequence of active inflammation and a natural progression of long-standing lymphocytic colitis. Moreover, in small studies, the HLA associations of lymphocytic colitis (HLA-A1) and collagenous colitis (HLA-A2) are distinct,[16,17] and a higher female/male gender ratio is present in collagenous colitis.[16] This controversy can only be resolved by more complete understanding of the origin, pathogenesis, and natural history of these disorders.

DIVERSION COLITIS

Clinical Features and Natural History

Inflammation insidiously develops in the distal bypassed colon within Hartmann's pouches or mucus fistulas after exclusion of the fecal stream. Most patients with proximal colostomies or ileostomies created for treatment of cancer, diverticulitis, Crohn's disease, ulcerative colitis, or trauma have no symptoms referable to the bypassed colonic segment. However, approximately one third of patients develop frequent mucoid discharges which may progress to rectal bleeding and pain 1 to 9 months after fecal diversion.[33] Symptoms have been reported to be more prevalent in patients operated on for inflammatory bowel disease (89%) than for carcinoma (23%) or other indications (50%).[34] Endoscopic evidence of inflammation is found in 60% to 80% of patients in most series[33–37] and in most, if not all, patients with inflammatory bowel disease.[38] Endoscopic features include diffuse erythema, granularity, friability, aphthous ulcers, and exudate. Nodularity and diffuse ulceration are features of more advanced lesions. Histologic abnormalities are apparent in 90% to 100% of bypassed segments.[33–39] Lymphoid follicular hyperplasia is a nearly universal finding, and neutrophils and crypt inflammation are present in at least 60% of patients by 3 months. Clinical, endoscopic, and histologic abnormalities appear to be progressive, with mild changes at 3 months[35] and more severe findings by 6 to 9 months after proximal fecal diversion.[33,36–38] Most patients, however, particularly those without preoperative Crohn's disease, do not develop debilitating symptoms. Anal sphincter function remains normal, although rectal volume diminishes by 3 months postoperatively.[35] In almost all cases, the inflammatory process completely resolves soon after restoration of the fecal stream. This syndrome was first noted by Morson in 1972[40] and was named and publicized by Glotzer and colleagues[41] in 1981.

Pathology

A histologic spectrum of inflammation is present, ranging from mild follicular hyperplasia and lymphoplasmacytic infiltrates to severe inflammation. Diffuse follicular lymphoid hyperplasia with frequent germinal centers is a characteristic feature of all stages of diversion colitis (Fig. 80-2).[39,42,43] Early inflammatory changes consist of mucosal infiltration by lymphocytes, plasma cells, and neutrophils, aphthous ulcers overlying lymphoid aggregates, and reactive epithelial cells. More advanced lesions consist of crypt abscesses, relatively mild crypt architectural changes, and Paneth cell metaplasia.

Mucin granulomas are present in a minority of cases. In severely involved resected tissues, gross abnormalities include diffuse nodularity and minute ulcerations with exudate.[43] Large ulcers and transmural changes are not typically present.

Pathogenesis

Considerable clinical and experimental evidence incriminates lumenal nutrient deficiency as the cause of diversion colitis. Roediger and colleagues[44,45] have demonstrated that lumenal short-chain fatty acids (SCFAs), metabolic products of carbohydrate, and peptide fermentation by anaerobic bacteria, are the principal fuels for the distal colonocyte. Butyrate provides 70% of oxidative energy for the rectal epithelial cell; acetate, ketone bodies, and glutamine are alternative sources. Elegant studies by Harig and colleagues[46] demonstrated that excluded colonic segments contained negligible concentrations of SCFAs and that infused carbohydrates were not metabolized to SCFAs. Moreover, institution of SCFA enemas twice daily induced clinical, endoscopic, and histologic remissions in four patients with diversion colitis. Although this theory has achieved widespread acceptance, in part supported by the observations that colonic epithelia in ulcerative colitis also exhibit aberrant SCFA metabolism and respond to SCFA enemas,[47,48] it should be noted that SCFA therapy of diversion colitis is not always successful.[49] Additional evidence exists that factors other than SCFAs are involved in the pathogenesis of diversion colitis. Atrophy, rather than rectal inflammation, occurs in germ-free rodents and patients receiving long-term parenteral nutrition or elemental diets,[50] conditions in which lumenal SCFAs would be predicted to be quite low. Moreover,

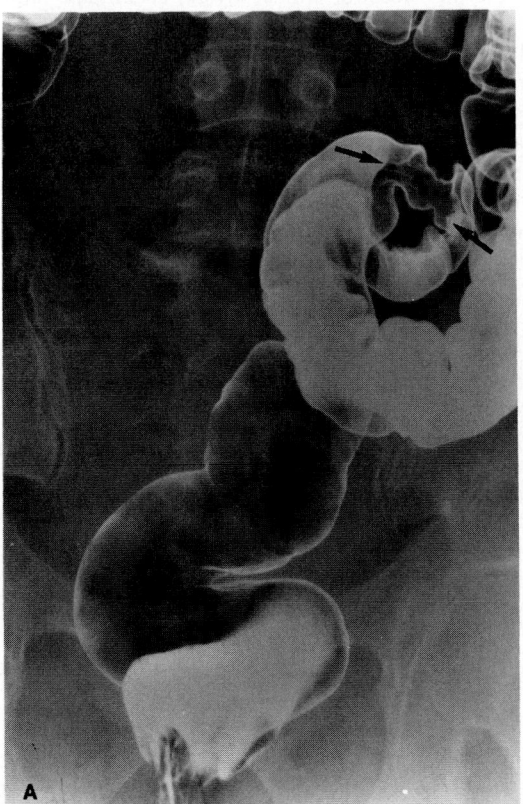

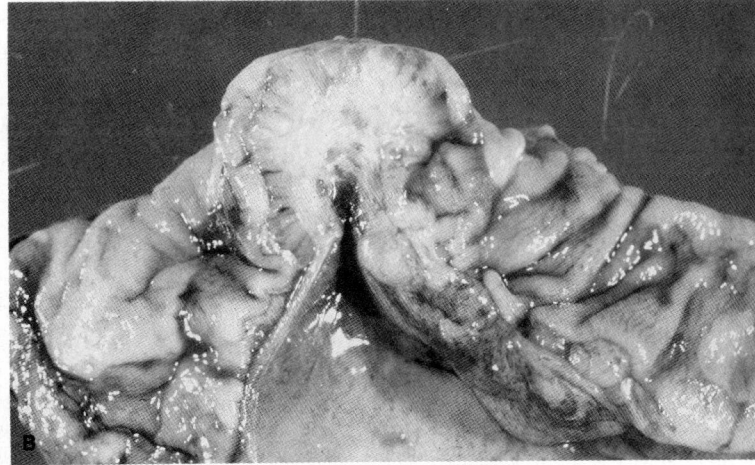

FIGURE 80-2. (**A**) Air contrast barium enema shows an intramural filling defect in the sigmoid colon (*arrows*) which produced stenosis of the lumen. (**B**) Operative specimen of the sigmoid colon demonstrates an intramural endometrium. The mucosa is intact but thinned, and the muscle layer is dramatically thickened. (From Croom RD, Donovan ML, Schweisinger WH. Intestinal endometriosis. Am J Surg 1984;148:660.)

inflammation does not develop in urinary colon conduits (ureterosigmoidostomies) that are not in continuity with the fecal stream.[51] Urine does not contain detectable SCFAs. The fact that diversion colitis rapidly resolves after reanastomosis to restore bowel continuity suggests that lumenal factors provide protection from inflammation. Entirely speculative alternatives to the SCFA hypothesis are that lumenal growth factors, dietary constituents, or other bacterial metabolic products are necessary to maintain optimal colonocyte function, or that alterations in bacterial profiles after exclusion induce damage. There is no evidence for pathogenic microbial agents, although normal anaerobic bacterial concentrations are significantly diminished and certain enterobacterial strains proliferate in the excluded colon.[52]

Diagnosis and Differential Diagnosis

Evaluation of inflammation in the diverted colon is relatively straightforward in the patient who had no preoperative intestinal inflammation. Flexible sigmoidoscopy with biopsies and examination of lumenal aspirates for ova and parasites, bacterial culture, and C *difficile* toxin is usually adequate to establish the diagnosis and evaluate activity of inflammation. Radiographic contrast studies can be performed but add little additional information unless a fistula or abscess is suspected, in which case a computed tomography (CT) scan may be helpful. Visualization of the bypassed colonic segment must be included as part of periodic screening after resection of colonic adenocarcinomas, because recurrent cancers and polyps can cause bleeding in the excluded bowel.[34] Radiation or ischemic colitis must be considered in appropriate clinical situations.

The major diagnostic challenge is to differentiate recurrent Crohn's disease from severe diversion colitis, which is an important distinction if reanastomosis is being considered. Advanced diversion colitis has a nodular appearance because of lymphoid follicular hyperplasia, which can mimic Crohn's disease.[42] Endoscopic features favoring recurrent Crohn's disease are longitudinal ulcers and possibly strictures,[38] because mucosal ulcers are usually quite small, even in advanced diversion colitis.[43] The utility of CT scanning and endoscopic ultrasonography to measure rectal wall thickness has not yet been investigated in this setting. Histologic features suggesting Crohn's disease are transmural inflammation, marked crypt architectural changes, and epithelioid granulomas. Granulomas can occur in diversion colitis but are usually mucinous. Lymphoid hyperplasia can occur in both disorders but is particularly prominent in diversion colitis. The absence of preoperative rectal involvement in the patient with Crohn's disease can also be useful information; all four patients in Korelitz's study[38] regained their normal rectal appearance after reanastomosis. The operative morbidity of performing an anastomosis with mild to moderately active diversion colitis is quite low.[38]

Treatment

Because most patients are asymptomatic or have only mild mucus discharge, therapy is rarely indicated. As has been discussed, SCFA enemas (60 mmol/L acetate, 30 mmol/L pro-

prionate, and 40 mmol/L butyrate) induce a remission in some patients.[46] However, SCFA enemas have not been beneficial in other studies[48,49] and are not yet commercially available. Hydrocortisone enemas are usually not successful.[38,49] 5-ASA enemas are reported to have induced an endoscopic and histologic remission in one patient[53] and have been successful in the authors' practice.*

ENDOMETRIOSIS

Endometriosis, defined as the presence of endometrial glands and stroma outside the uterine cavity and musculature (myometrium), is a common disorder, occurring in approximately 15% of menstruating women.[54] Intestinal implants have been described in up to 37% of patients who undergo surgical exploration for endometriosis.[55] In these patients, the majority (95%) have rectosigmoid involvement, with appendiceal (10%), ileal (5%), and proximal colon locations uncommon.[55] Meyer described the first case of rectal endometriosis in 1909.[56]

Clinical Features

Most patients with serosal endometrial implants in the rectosigmoid have no specific intestinal symptoms apart from those symptoms typically experienced with pelvic endometriosis. The majority of patients with intestinal endometriosis have associated implants on their ovaries, anterior and posterior cul-de-sacs, uterus and uterine ligaments.[54] Pelvic symptoms of dysmenorrhea, dyspareunia, infertility, and dysfunctional uterine bleeding almost always accompany and frequently overshadow intestinal symptoms. Patients with serosal implants may have localized tenderness and palpable nodules on rectovaginal exam. Penetration of endometriomas into the bowel wall and adhesions can lead to symptoms of partial obstruction, including intermittent abdominal pain and constipation. Obstruction is rarely complete and is caused by extensive compression of the lumen by submucosal endometriomas, fibrosis, and contraction of the mesentery. Partial obstruction usually occurs in the rectosigmoid area but may involve the ileum. Diarrhea and rectal bleeding have variable incidences, with grossly evident hematochezia present in 3% to 33% of patients who undergo surgical bowel resection.[57–60] Bleeding is a rare event in nonoperative series. Cyclic episodes of intestinal symptoms corresponding with menses occur in less than half of patients carefully evaluated, although the vast majority (80%) of patients with intestinal endometriosis have associated gynecologic symptoms.[61] There have been reports of acute appendicitis, caused by intussusception or obstruction by an endometrioma.[62,63]

The average age of women undergoing surgical resection for intestinal endometriosis is 32 to 41 years, but ages range from 16 to 60 years.[59–61] Endometriosis is found almost exclusively in women of reproductive age, with mean age of diagnosis at 25 to 29 years.[1] The somewhat older age of patients undergoing bowel resection probably is related to the

---

*Sartor JB, personal communication.

chronic nature of the inflammation, which progresses to obstructive complications. Although it is unusual, postmenopausal women can develop symptomatic colonic obstruction, especially if they are treated with estrogen replacement. Intestinal symptoms can persist after hysterectomy and oophorectomy if partially obstructing lesions are not resected at the time of initial surgical treatment.[61,64]

Pathology

Serosal implants are common but usually do not produce specific symptoms unless they invade the intestinal wall. Peritoneal or serosal implants are classically described as bluish-gray nodules ranging from 2 mm to 2 cm in diameter.[54] Secretory glands lined by cuboidal endometrial epithelial cells are surrounded by endometrial stroma embedded in fibrotic tissue. These glands can become cystic or be filled with blood. Endometrial deposits invading the bowel wall usually do not involve the mucosa but are associated with localized muscular hypertrophy and fibrosis (Fig. 80-2B),[65] which may lead to strictures or asymmetric kinking of the bowel. Histologic mucosal abnormalities are confined to the region of invading endometrial nodules and range from mild crypt distortion to active inflammation with crypt abscesses.[65] Mucosal ulceration is an unusual feature.

Pathophysiology

Three theories of the genesis of endometriosis have clinical and experimental support.[54,66]

Transplantation

Dissemination of viable uterine epithelial and stromal cells by retrograde menstruation, vascular, lymphatic, or iatrogenic spread could lead to implantation of cells in ectopic locations. Epithelial and stromal cells then proliferate under hormonal stimulation to form invasive nodules. Retrograde menstruation is an almost universal occurrence, and dissemination by this route is supported by the frequency of endometrial implants in the ovaries and dependent areas of the pelvis.[67] Hematogenous and lymphatic spread account for remote implants such as those in pleural, pericardial, and lymph node tissues, and operative dissemination leads to lesions within surgical scars.

Coelomic Metaplasia

Endometrial and peritoneal cells are derived from the coelomic-wall epithelium, raising the possibility that peritoneal cells can undergo metaplastic transformation to related endometrial epithelial cells. This metaplasia would have to be driven by estrogen to be consistent with epidemiologic observations. The rarity of endometriosis in anovulatory women with persistently elevated estrogen levels and the low frequency of endometrial nodules within the thoracic cavity, which is also derived from the coelomic wall, make this theory unlikely.

Induction Theory

This theory, a combination of the first two, states that unknown factors within the shed endometrium induce endometrial metaplasia. Evidence of endometrial-like glands adjacent to millipore chambers containing endometrial cells in rodents support this theory.

Regardless of which theory is correct, proliferation of endometrial glands and stroma appears to be under hormonal influence. Estrogen stimulates growth, and progesterone inhibits it. A large variety of growth factors modulate hormonal influences, providing a mechanism by which local inflammatory and stromal cells can regulate growth of implanted tissues. Progressive invasion of intestinal muscle and submucosal layers leads to muscular hypertrophy and fibrosis. These changes result in segmental narrowing of the intestinal lumen adjacent to the proliferating endometrial nodule, leading to obstructive symptoms. Smooth muscle hyperplasia, hypertrophy, and collagen deposition are almost certainly the result of stimulation by the same growth factors that regulate endometrial proliferation.

Diagnosis

Clinical diagnosis of intestinal endometriosis can be difficult because of nonspecific symptoms. The classic presentation is partial obstruction of the colon in an infertile woman of reproductive age with progressive dysmenorrhea and dyspareunia. A cyclic occurrence of symptoms is suggestive but not required, because fewer than 50% of patients exhibit this feature. Some 70% to 80% of patients have symptoms of pelvic endometriosis. Tender nodules palpable in the rectovaginal septum (posterior cul-de-sac) on rectovaginal examination are highly suggestive of endometriosis, but fixation of the rectum is nonspecific. Barium enema and endoscopic examination are normal in the presence of noninvasive serosal implants. The vast majority of patients with obstructing endometriosis have extrinsic compression or smooth strictures with normal mucosa (see Fig. 80-2A) and normal biopsy specimens. If rectal bleeding is present, endoscopic evaluation with biopsies has been reported to be diagnostic in 4 of 6 patients.[68] Histologic examination confirmed mucosal endometrial involvement in 5 of these patients. CT and magnetic resonance imaging scans are usually nonspecific because of the small size of implants. Endorectal ultrasonography can detect intestinal wall invasion by endometrial implants,[69] but experience with this technique is quite limited to date.

Definitive diagnosis is made by surgical exploration, either by laparoscopy or by celiotomy, and by tissue diagnosis.[61] The vast majority of patients with intestinal endometriosis have multiple associated implants on the surface of pelvic organs and multiple serosal nodules on the intestine.

Differential Diagnosis

Intestinal endometriosis with altered bowel habits is difficult to differentiate from irritable bowel syndrome. The distinction can be suggested by a cyclic nature of pain and bowel symptoms, associated infertility, dysmenorrhea and dyspareunia, presence of tender nodules on rectovaginal examination, and evidence of extrinsic rectosigmoid compression on flexible sigmoidoscopy or barium enema examinations. Laparoscopy may be necessary to establish the diagnosis. Strictures secondary to Crohn's colitis usually have associated mucosal ulceration and histologic evidence of inflammation; these findings are rare in endometriosis. Primary colonic carcinoma must be considered in all cases of bowel stricture regardless of age. Endoscopic and radiologic features favoring adenocarcinoma include mucosal ulceration and sharp margins; endometriosis is usually submucosal.[58] Additional clinical features suggesting carcinoma are advanced age (postmenopausal), hematochezia, multiparity, and lack of dysmenorrhea and tenderness. However, none of these features is absolute, and resection with transmural histologic examination is the only way to definitively rule out carcinoma. Malignant degeneration of extraovarian endometriosis, including the colon, is well documented, although the incidence is unknown and probably quite unusual.[70] Rarely, mucosal involvement by endometriosis can simulate adenomatous polyps.[68] Ischemic strictures are usually in the descending colon, whereas endometrial strictures are more distal. Diverticular masses and radiation induced strictures occur in older age groups and can usually be differentiated on clinical grounds.

Treatment

Superficial serosal implants without compromise of the intestinal lumen can be treated by hormonal therapy or nonresective surgery. Current medical therapeutic options diminish estrogen stimulation by inducing pseudopregnancy, pseudomenopause, or chronic anovulation. Danazol, a 17α-ethinyltestosterone derivative, medroxyprogesterone, and gonadotropin-releasing hormone analogs are clinically comparable and superior to placebo in diminishing pain and size of pelvic endometrial nodules,[54,71] but results in patients with intestinal endometriosis remain anecdotal. Ablation of infiltrating endometrial implants on the anterior rectum and rectovaginal septum can be safely accomplished with a laparoscopic carbon dioxide laser,[72] but results have not been subjected to controlled trials. Most authors advocate segmental resection of partially obstructed colons because of poor results with medical therapy or superficial ablation and the inability to exclude carcinomas associated with endometriosis by clinical assessment.[55,60,61,64] In postmenopausal women and those women who do not desire pregnancy, hysterectomy and bilateral oophorectomy should be performed at the time of intestinal resection to treat associated pelvic endometriosis and to minimize the risk of recurrent disease. Low-dose estrogen replacement can be considered if all macroscopic nodules are removed. Patients who desire to preserve fertility should have excision or laser ablation of associated endometriosis in the pelvic organs in conjunction with bowel resection. Reports of successful pregnancies after surgical treatment vary, but results seem to be superior to those achieved with medical therapy.[54] However, recurrence of symptoms of endometriosis after preservation of ovarian function is substantial, and patients may subsequently develop obstructive intestinal symptoms that require definitive surgical therapy.

DRUG- AND CHEMICAL-INDUCED COLONIC INJURY

Drug- and chemical-induced toxic colitis has been associated with numerous orally and rectally administered agents; in addition, certain drugs have been implicated as causative factors in ischemic colitis, melanosis coli, and cathartic colon (Table 80-2). This section reviews the various types of chemical-induced colonic injury, with an emphasis on clinical findings and pathogenesis.

Syndromes Associated With Enema Use

Colitis with a broad spectrum of clinical and endoscopic findings may result from various chemicals administered in enema form. High-risk groups for toxic colitis include patients with a history of self-mutilation or of self-medication for constipation, members of certain African tribes who ritualistically use herbal enemas, and those who have been treated with soap enemas or water-soluble contrast media. Generally, individuals with chemical colitis may present with abdominal pain, bloody or nonbloody diarrhea, tenesmus, and fever; rectal and abdominal tenderness, with or without peritoneal signs, may be seen on physical examination. Leukocytosis is often present.[73–75] Endoscopic findings are nonspecific and range from friable, granular mucosa to frank ulceration, with or without pseudomembrane formation. One endoscopic clue to toxin-induced colitis is the association of perianal excoriation with a predominantly distal colitis.[73] Treatment is primarily supportive, with intravenous fluids, bowel rest, and, if clinically indicated, broad-spectrum antibiotics. However, surgery may be necessary in some cases.[73,75,76]

Soap Colitis

Syndromes of soap-associated colitis range from mild inflammation with increased stool frequency to severe acute colitis with bloody diarrhea resembling idiopathic ulcerative colitis.[74] Acute colitis may heal with scarring and colonic cicatrization[76,77] or may progress to transmural necrosis and perforation.[78,79] Endoscopic findings range from mucosal edema (with loss of normal vascular pattern) to mucosal

---

TABLE 80-2
Colonic Injury Induced by Therapeutic Agents

Enemas
Soap, water-soluble contrast media (Gastrografin), hydrogen peroxide

Laxatives
Melanosis coli, cathartic colon

Agents Inducing Ischemia
Oral contraceptives, vasopressin, ergotamine, cocaine, dextroamphetamine, neuroleptics, digitalis

Miscellaneous
Nonsteroidal antiinflammatory drugs, gold, isotretinoin, antibiotics, chemotherapy, methyldopa, flucytosine

sloughing and ulceration.[74] Damage may extend into the muscular layers of the colon.[76] The pathophysiology of soap-induced colonic injury centers on its detergent effects on the colonic mucosa. Kirchner and colleagues[76] described a case of caustic colitis caused by a detergent enema in a pediatric patient and subsequently reproduced the observed acute injury by using the same detergent enemas in animals. Liquefaction necrosis, as seen in alkaline-induced mucosal injury, was the predominant acute histologic picture. Histologically and radiographically, the injury resembled corrosive esophagitis, with an acute necrotic phase (days 1–4), an ulceration/granulation phase (days 3–5), and a cicatrization phase (beginning in weeks 3–4). The severity of damage in soap-induced colitis is related to both the soap concentration and the duration of mucosal contact.[74]

Water-Soluble Contrast Media

Colitis, ranging from minimal focal inflammation to severe colitis with necrosis and perforation, is associated with several hyperosmolar water-soluble contrast media, including Gastrografin, Hypaque, and Renografin-76.[75] These agents are used to opacify partially obstructed colons and avoid the potential complications of barium. Gastrografin is also used to treat meconium ileus in neonates with cystic fibrosis and severe fecal impactions in adults; its hypertonicity and the presence of the detergent Tween 80 are thought to facilitate stool passage by drawing fluid into the gut lumen. Gastrografin had a greater propensity for inducing colitis in animals than Hypaque, Renografin-76, or barium.[80] Tween 80 may damage the gut mucosa in a manner similar to soap enemas. Enemas containing Tween 80 in addition to Hypaque sodium 25%—which by itself did not cause substantial inflammation—increased the incidence and severity of colonic inflammation in rats.[80] These results were not borne out in later animal studies, however. Lumenal distention may be the major predisposing factor to the development of experimental colitis. Animals without lumenal distention suffered no ill effects regardless of the medium used to fill the colon, causing Wood to postulate the pathogenetic importance of compromised mucosal blood flow in the distended gut.[81] In virtually all reports of contrast medium–induced colitis in humans, damage occurred proximal to obstructing lesions, mainly in the cecum and ascending colon.[75,82] Prolonged mucosal exposure and preexisting mucosal injury may also predispose patients to damage induced by water-soluble contrast media.[75]

Hydrogen Peroxide

Hydrogen peroxide enemas are not currently in widespread use; however, they have been used in the disintegration of impacted feces, treatment of meconium ileus, and removal of intestinal gas in preparation for radiologic study.[83] Hydrogen peroxide enemas have been associated with bloody diarrhea, pneumatosis coli, colonic perforation, sepsis, and death.[83] The colitis may be caused by ischemic destruction of the mucosa, submucosa, and muscularis as a result of the entrance of gas into the loose connective tissues of the mucosa and submucosa and, eventually, into the vasculature, resulting in abolition of mucosal blood flow. Sheehan[84] and Shaw and

colleagues[85] investigated the ischemic hypothesis in animal models: hydrogen peroxide enemas resulted in the rapid formation of gas cysts in the mucosa, submucosa, and serosa, with subsequent absorption of the gas into the local circulation and eventual mucosal ischemia. Oxygen free radicals released by hydrogen peroxide may also contribute to mucosal damage.

Other Miscellaneous Substances

Inadvertent ethanol enema administration has been reported to cause an acute hemorrhagic colitis with associated lower abdominal pain.[86] Self-administration of a hydrofluoric acid enema resulted in rectal pain and bloody diarrhea; after unsuccessful treatment with calcium carbonate enemas, a segment of necrotic, ulcerated sigmoid colon was resected.[73] Segal and associates[87] reported an unusual series of cases in which the ritual use of enemas by South African tribesmen—traditionally involving roots, herbs, tree bark, and other natural constituents—had been adapted to more modern agents, including vinegar, potassium dichromate, potassium permanganate, copper sulfate, unknown herbal medicines, and chloroxylenol (Dettol). The vinegar enema induced extensive bowel infarction with destruction of the rectovaginal septum. Effects of other substances ranged from mild rectal inflammation to transmural coagulative necrosis.

Syndromes Associated With Laxatives

Melanosis Coli

Melanosis coli is a dark pigmentation of the colonic mucosa frequently seen in patients who use anthraquinone laxatives (cascara sagrada, aloe, rhubarb, senna, and frangula). Its gross appearance is a reticulated pattern of striations and spots that resembles alligator skin (Fig. 80-3; see Color Figs. 37 and 38).[88,89] Dark pigmentation of the colonic mucosa was first described in 1825 by Billiard and was named melanosis coli by Rudolph Virchow in 1857. The association between melanosis coli and anthraquinone laxatives was first advanced by Bartle in 1928. This association is now well-established; 73% of patients using anthracene laxatives develop melanosis.[90] Melanosis can appear as rapidly as 4 months after the initiation of anthraquinone laxatives, with an average time to appearance of 9 months. Withdrawal of anthraquinones results in resolution of pigment changes in an average of 9 months.[88] The overall reported incidence of melanosis coli in endoscopy and autopsy series ranges from 0.25% to 23.6%, with an increased frequency among those older than 40 years of age. Most studies demonstrate a female predominance.[89] Melanosis coli is found mainly in the cecum and the rectum, although it may involve the entire colon. Melanosis can often be detected in biopsy specimens stained with hematoxylin and eosin even if it is not grossly visible.[88]

Histologically, melanosis coli is associated with the deposition of a brown, granular pigment within macrophages in the lamina propria (Fig. 80-4). The number and size of macrophages within the lamina propria are increased, and they are situated between the colonic crypts. Two distinct groups of macrophages are evident; those nearest the lumen have the least pigment, and those furthest from the lumen

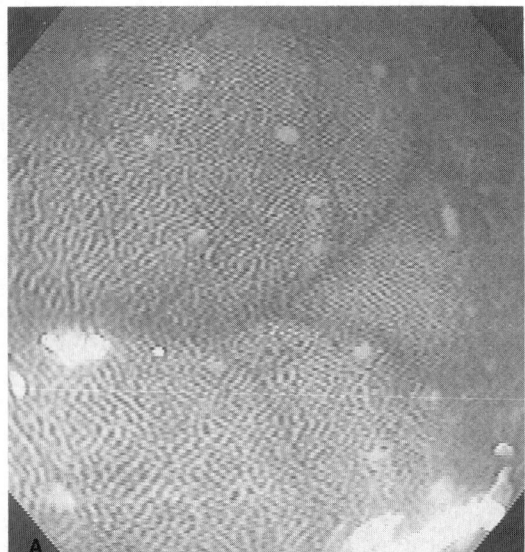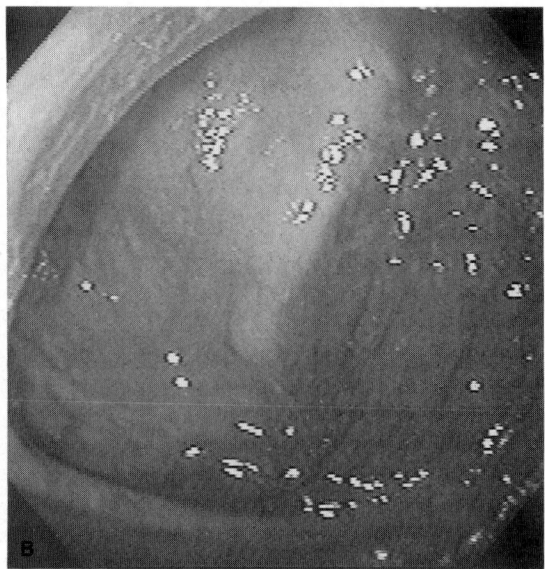

FIGURE 80-3. (See Color Figs. 37 and 38.) Endoscopic photographs of melanosis coli. (**A**) The reticulated, alligator-skin appearance is characteristic of this condition. (**B**) Melanosis coli with a sharp line of demarcation at the small bowel–colonic anastomosis.

have the most pigment.[91] The colonic epithelial cells are normal by light microscopic examination. However, electron microscopy has revealed decreased numbers of microvilli, vacuolization of the apical cellular surface, lipid droplets near the basal membrane, and small vesicles near the lateral cell membrane.[92] The source of the pigment in melanosis coli is unclear. It has biochemical features of both lipofuscin and melanin,[89] and there is some evidence that it is similar to the pigment of Dubin-Johnson syndrome.[93] Some have suggested that it is an absorbed pigment derived from anthraquinone laxatives[88]; others have suggested an origin from degenerating mitochondria or lysosomes.[91] Walker and colleagues[94] reported the induction of a condition resembling human melanosis coli in guinea pigs who were fed danthron, an anthraquinone laxative. Each treatment resulted in transient large-

scale apoptosis of colonic surface epithelial cells. Cellular debris was phagocytosed by macrophages and carried into the lamina propria, where it was transformed into the typical lipofuscin-like pigment seen in melanosis coli. This may well provide an explanation of the mechanism of pigment formation in melanosis coli.[94]

The clinical significance of melanosis coli, apart from its association with anthracene laxative abuse, is uncertain; however, there is universal agreement that it is a benign condition. Colonic adenomas in patients with melanosis coli are not pigmented, and neoplastic tissues lack pigment-laden macrophages.[89,95] Biopsy of islands of unpigmented tissue in patients with background melanosis is therefore advised. Melanosis coli has also been reported in patients with carcinoma of the colon; in these patients, the pigment is deposited prox-

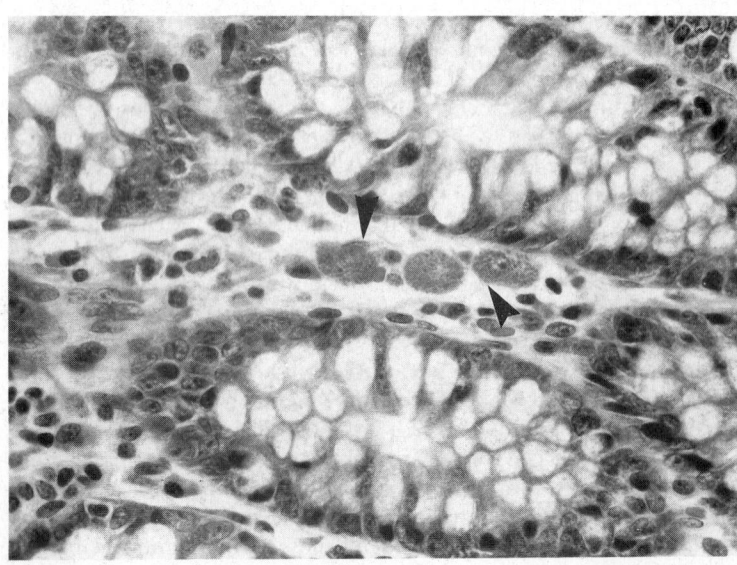

FIGURE 80-4. High-power photomicrograph demonstrates lipofuscin-like pigment within macrophages (*arrows*) in the lamina propria of a rectal biopsy specimen from a patient with melanosis coli.

imal to the tumor, leading to speculation that colonic stasis may contribute to pigment deposition.[89] However, Badiali and associates[90] found no correlation between the presence of melanosis and colorectal transit. There does not appear to be a greater risk of colon cancer in patients with melanosis.

Cathartic Colon

In 1943, Heilbrun described the index case of what is now known as cathartic colon, a young woman who had chronically used laxatives for two decades with distinctly abnormal contrast radiographic studies.[96] Cathartic colon is now a well-recognized entity. Most patients are women who have abused laxatives, either overtly or surreptitiously, for 15 or more years.[97] Habitual laxative users may complain of bloating, abdominal fullness, vague lower abdominal pain, and symptoms of incomplete evacuation without laxative use. They frequently use laxatives to achieve the regular bowel movement pattern that they consider ideal. Laxative dosing gradually escalates until these patients cannot defecate normally without cathartic use.[98] Ninety percent of surreptitious laxative abusers are women; many are emotionally disturbed.[98] These patients may present with chronic idiopathic diarrhea and undergo multiple diagnostic evaluations without success.

Additional complaints include vague abdominal discomfort, thirst, and weakness.[99] Electrolyte and fluid abnormalities, particularly hypokalemia and hypovolemia, may be evident; steatorrhea has been reported. Heizer and colleagues[100] detailed two cases of protein-losing enteropathy with hypoalbuminemia which resolved after cessation of cathartic abuse.

The most striking abnormalities in cathartic colon are seen on contrast radiographs (Fig. 80-5). Mild cases have findings limited to a foreshortened, conical cecum and loss of the typical beak-like appearance of the ileocecal valve. More severe cases are characterized by a dilated, tubular colon distal to the cecum, with loss of haustral markings; segments of bowel may appear narrowed, but these pseudostrictures are transient in nature.[97] The radiographic appearance of cathartic colon is similar to that of long-standing ulcerative colitis. The critical features used to differentiate these disorders are the distensibility of the bowel in cathartic colon and the lack of evidence of mucosal inflammation.[96,97] The radiographic abnormalities in cathartic colon may extend to the descending colon; however, the rectosigmoid region is usually spared. Complete resolution of these abnormalities within 4 months of cessation of laxative use has been reported.[101]

Cathartic colon is related to chronic use of irritant laxatives (primarily anthraquinones); however, the precise mechanism

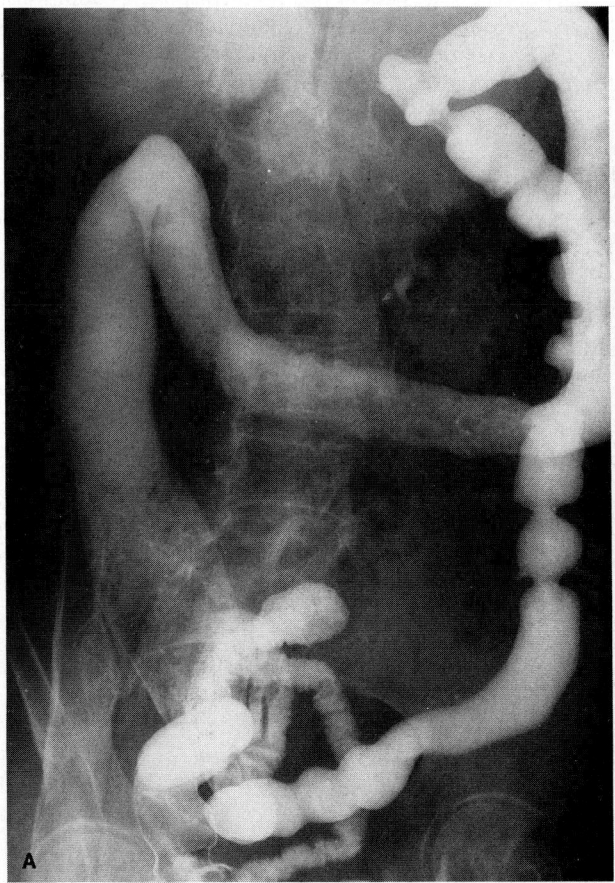 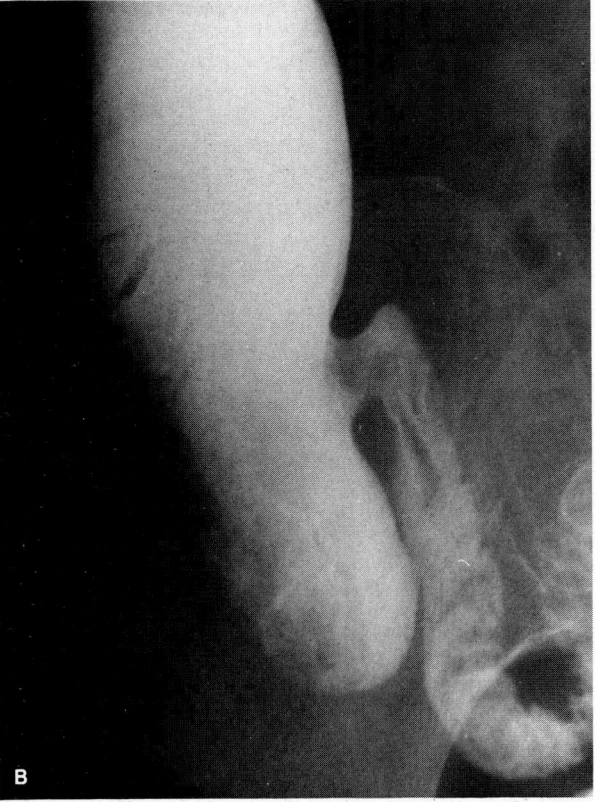

FIGURE 80-5. Cathartic colon. **(A)** Barium enema study reveals that the right and transverse colon are devoid of haustrations. No ulcerations are seen. **(B)** Detail of the cecum and proximal ascending colon reveals a gaping ileocecal valve. The lack of haustration in the right colon is striking. (From Campbell WL. Cathartic colon: reversibility of roentgen changes. Dis Colon Rectum 1983;26:445–448.)

is unknown. Anthraquinones are potent cellular toxins. Intravenous or oral administration of syrup of senna to mice causes damage to the myenteric plexus.[102] Resected human specimens show hypertrophy of the muscularis mucosae, thinning of the muscularis propria, excessive submucosal fat deposition, loss of myenteric plexus neurons, and replacement of ganglia by Schwann cells.[102] Reversible abnormalities in colonic nerve plexuses exist in chronic laxative abusers who have not yet developed typical radiographic changes.[103] Toxic effects of anthraquinones on the colonic myenteric plexus nerves are the likely cause of the cathartic colon syndrome, although it is possible that a subgroup of patients with chronic idiopathic constipation have a developmental anomaly of the myenteric plexus.[104]

Treatment of cathartic colon centers on withdrawal of irritant laxatives, particularly anthraquinones. Bulking agents, a high-fiber diet, and bowel retraining are the most effective measures. In the early phases of bowel retraining, use of an osmotic laxative or Fleet's enemas may be helpful. Patient cooperation is critical; lack of compliance is a common problem.[98] In refractory cases, surgical approaches have been used, the most effective being total or subtotal colectomy.[105] However, in light of the apparent reversibility of some cases,[101] surgical treatment should be considered only after failure of maximal medical therapy.

Drugs Resulting in Ischemic Colonic Injury

Several substances have been described which cause ischemic colonic injury by compromising mucosal blood flow. This may occur through vasospasm, thrombosis, or both. Although ischemic colitis is not uncommon in elderly patients with mesenteric atherosclerotic disease, its presence in a younger patient should prompt a search for a predisposing cause, such as medications.[106] The symptom complex manifested by these patients is fairly uniform, consisting of severe abdominal pain, bloody or nonbloody diarrhea, tenesmus, nausea, vomiting, and fever. Rebound tenderness and guarding, with hypoactive or absent bowel sounds, may be noted, although less striking physical findings may be found. Leukocytosis is variably present, and plain or contrasted abdominal radiographs may reveal "thumbprinting." Endoscopy may show mucosal friability, edema, erythema, granularity, ulceration with or without pseudomembranes, or necrosis.[107-109] As in atherosclerotic mesenteric vascular disease, the junction of the distributions of the superior and inferior mesenteric vessels (from the distal end of the transverse colon to the proximal descending colon) is a common site of injury in drug-induced ischemic colitis.

Oral Contraceptives

Transient ischemic colitis in otherwise healthy young women taking oral contraceptives was first described in 1968.[107] Mesenteric thrombosis, both arterial and venous, has been extensively described in association with oral contraceptives; arterial thrombosis carries twice the mortality of venous thrombosis but is half as common.[108] Although the typical presentation is that of classic ischemic colitis, Tedesco and associates[109] described one group of five patients with symptoms indistin-

guishable from those of Crohn's disease. Estrogens can cause a hypercoagulable state, vasospasm in the mesenteric vessels, and endothelial proliferation with subendothelial fibrosis, all of which may play a role in estrogen-induced ischemic colitis.[108] High-dose estrogen preparations, high-dose progesterone combinations, depot progesterone dosages, and sequential estrogen/progesterone therapy have all been implicated in mesenteric thrombosis.[108,109] The duration of oral contraceptive use in these patients ranges from 10 days to 11 years. The dose of the estrogenic fraction correlates with thrombogenicity.[75,107,108]

Vasopressin

Vasopressin, a vasoconstrictor used to treat bleeding esophageal varices, decreases colonic blood flow in a dose-dependent fashion. A case of reversible ischemic colitis associated with intravenous vasopressin infusion has been reported.[110]

Ergotamine

The association between ergot preparations and ischemic colitis is presumably related to vasospasm. Stillman described a 50-year-old woman who developed acute bloody diarrhea and acute colitis in the splenic flexure area while taking ergotamine tartarate; her symptoms resolved after discontinuation of ergotamine.[111] The patient had no predisposing conditions for the development of mesenteric ischemia. Rectal ulceration, with obliteration of small blood vessels, endothelial proliferation, and vascular wall thickening, can develop in patients using ergotamine suppositories.[112]

Cocaine

Several reports of severe, right-sided ischemic colitis in patients using high doses of cocaine have been published.[113,114] The putative mechanism of cocaine-related ischemic colitis is catecholamine-induced mesenteric vasospasm by this powerful sympathomimetic agent.[113]

Dextroamphetamine

A case of reversible ischemic colitis attributed to intense mesenteric vasoconstriction has been described in a 47-year-old man taking dextroamphetamine as his only medication.[106] This patient presented with the acute onset of abdominal pain and bloody diarrhea, which resolved after cessation of dextroamphetamine therapy. Mesenteric angiography was normal.

Neuroleptics

Ischemic colitis has been linked to the use of neuroleptics, especially tricyclic antidepressants, in some case reports.[115]

Digitalis Preparations

Digitalis preparations have been associated with intestinal ischemia in several published reports. Most of these detail ischemia in the small or small and large intestine; isolated colonic ischemia has not been reported. It is likely that these reports represent a manifestation of the clinical setting of digitalis use (i.e., systemic hypoperfusion). Digitalis preparations have been shown to cause mesenteric vasoconstriction in laboratory animals, however, and may directly contribute to mesenteric ischemia.[116]

Miscellaneous Drug-Induced Colitides

Nonsteroidal Antiinflammatory Drugs

Several inflammatory syndromes have been associated with the use of NSAIDs. Colitis in previously asymptomatic individuals has been associated with numerous NSAIDs, including mefenamic and flufenamic acid, diclofenac, indomethacin, enteric-coated aspirin, ibuprofen, phenylbutazone, naproxen, and piroxicam.[20,117,118] It has been estimated that 10% of newly diagnosed colitis cases may be related to NSAID use.[119] Forty cases of NSAID-associated colitis were reviewed by Gibson and associates.[118] Typically, these patients were elderly (average age, 63 years); no gender predilection was noted. Most presented with diarrhea and either occult or gross lower gastrointestinal bleeding. Some had weight loss or fever. The majority were anemic; many had an elevated erythrocyte sedimentation rate and leukocytosis. Endoscopic findings were variable and ranged from mild proctitis to ulcerative pancolitis. Ulcerations or other inflammatory changes could occur at any point in the colon, and could be focal or diffuse. Treatment was primarily withdrawal of the offending NSAID, although surgery for complications such as bleeding and perforation was required in 25% of cases. Medical treatment with steroids and sulfasalazine was used on several occasions. All 12 patients who were rechallenged with NSAIDs had relapses. Relapse of quiescent inflammatory bowel disease was described in 19 patients; these patients were significantly younger than those with de novo NSAID-induced colitis (average age, 42 years), and the median latency period between NSAID exposure and colitis symptoms was less than 1 week. Eighty percent of those relapsing were ulcerative colitis patients. Relapse occurred in all eight patients rechallenged with NSAIDs after reinduction of remission.[118] A mild segmental ischemic colitis has been described in two middle-aged patients taking NSAIDs. Histologic findings were consistent with a nongangrenous ischemic colitis.[117] An increased rate of spontaneous colonic perforation or hemorrhage is associated with NSAID use.[20,118] NSAIDs have been associated with an increased risk of perforation of colonic diverticula in numerous case reports and in controlled studies.[20,120] Other reported colonic complications include proctitis[20,120] related to NSAID suppository use, eosinophilic colitis,[20] and diaphragm disease of the colon. This last entity appears to be similar to the small intestine diaphragm disease previously associated with nonsteroidal usage.[121]

The pathogenesis of NSAID-induced colonic injury is uncertain but probably is mediated by the effects of cyclooxygenase inhibition. Loss of the mucosal cytoprotection and immunosuppression afforded by prostaglandins, coupled with the shifting of arachadonic acid metabolites into the proinflammatory lipoxygenase pathway, could induce colonic injury and inflammation.[118,120] Loss of vasodilating prostaglandins and production of vasoconstricting leukotrienes and cytotoxic oxyradicals associated with lipoxygenase activation could impair mesenteric blood flow. Epithelial injury and enhancement of colonic mucosal permeability by NSAIDs, with resultant increased susceptibility to lumenal toxins, may also play a role.[20,117]

Gold

Gold salt-induced colitis in rheumatoid arthritis patients is probably caused by local toxicity of the drug. Up to 95% of orally-administered gold is excreted in the feces, and stainable gold is present in mucosal biopsy specimens.[122] Most patients are women; clinical manifestations may include bloody diarrhea, abdominal pain, tenesmus, fever, and leukocytosis. Diagnosis is usually made endoscopically. Endoscopy may reveal ulceration and friability, often with hemorrhage; lesions are most often found in the rectosigmoid, although colitis may be diffuse.[122] Biopsies may reveal nonspecific acute and chronic inflammation; some have histologic findings that might cause confusion with Crohn's disease.[122,123] Treatment is primarily withdrawal of gold therapy and supportive care, although surgery, steroids, British anti-Lewisite (BAL), and sulfasalazine have been used with success.[122] One case of eosinophilic gold-induced colitis responded to oral cromolyn therapy.[124] The older literature reports a 40% mortality with this complication; however, a more recent review reveals no deaths in 14 cases reported between 1980 and 1986.[122] The average time to recovery is 2 weeks after suspension of gold therapy.[122,125]

Isotretinoin

Isotretinoin, a synthetic analogue of vitamin A used in treatment of severe cystic acne, has been linked to acute colitis and to the reactivation of quiescent inflammatory bowel disease. Martin and colleagues[126] reported that cessation of therapy resulted in prompt colitis resolution, whereas rechallenge caused an almost identical recurrence. The pathogenesis of this inflammatory response is unknown.

Antibiotics

Hemorrhagic colitis has been associated with ampicillin, amoxicillin, and erythromycin. This colitis differs from typical *C difficile* colitis in that patients present with bloody diarrhea, generally do not have pseudomembranes, have predominantly right-sided colitis, rapidly improve with discontinuation of antibiotics, and test negative for *C difficile* toxin.[75,127,128] The pathogenesis is unknown, although this may represent a variant of *C difficile* disease or an overgrowth of unrecognized pathogens.[127]

Chemotherapeutic Agents

The rapidly dividing cells of the gastrointestinal epithelium are particularly susceptible to the toxic effects of cancer chemotherapeutic agents. DNA synthesis is almost completely blocked in both human and animal gastrointestinal epithelia by cytotoxic doses of antimetabolites.[129] Multiple chemotherapeutic agents cause colonic damage, including cytosine arabinoside, methotrexate, cyclophosphamide, and 5-fluorouracil. Clinical manifestations range from mild segmental colitis to fulminant ulcerative colitis with toxic megacolon.[129-132] The pathogenesis is probably multifactorial and includes direct epithelial injury by chemotherapeutic agents, invasion of the mucosa by intestinal pathogens, and ischemic injury.[129-131] Cytosine arabinoside induces a three-stage pattern of damage consisting of initial injury—replacement of normal mucosal cells with atypical undifferentiated cells, with conspicuous absence of mitotic figures; progressive injury—cellular necrosis and glandular dilatation, with persistent lack of mitosis; and regeneration—resumption of normal mitotic activity, with mature goblet cells in the bases of crypts.[130] Similar histologic findings, persisting for up to 18 days, follow administration of 5-fluorouracil.[131] These changes can probably be extrapolated to most chemotherapeutic agents.

Methyldopa

Colitis, presenting as bloody or nonbloody diarrhea, has been associated with methyldopa therapy. All reported cases were notable for prompt resolution of symptoms with drug withdrawal; moreover, three patients who were rechallenged with methyldopa demonstrated symptom recurrence.[133]

Flucytosine

Flucytosine, an antifungal agent, been associated with the development of colonic inflammation resembling idiopathic ulcerative colitis.[134]

COLONIC ULCERS

In addition to medication use, a number of other conditions can be associated with colonic ulceration (Table 80-3). Common presenting symptoms include hematochezia, abdominal pain, and a mucopurulent rectal discharge. Diarrhea is variable depending on the surface area affected and is uncommon with isolated ulceration. A careful endoscopic and histologic examination can provide useful information to distinguish these conditions using the criteria established in Table 80-3.

Isolated Nonspecific Colonic Ulcer

Isolated nonspecific ulceration in the colon was first described by Cruveilhier in 1832, although the first histologically proven case was not described until 1895.[135] The group of 127 pa-

tients reviewed by Ona had an average age of 45 years, with a range of 8 to 84 years and a 55% female predominance.[136] Sixty-seven percent were cecal ulcers, another 18% were ascending or transverse colonic lesions, and 15% were descending or sigmoid ulcers. Virtually all were solitary ulcers located on the antimesenteric side of the lumen, ranging from 0.5 to 6.5 cm in diameter.[135-138] Cecal ulcerations are most often found near the ileocecal valve. Most of these lesions are round or oval in configuration, with sharply-demarcated margins and relatively normal surrounding mucosa.[136,139,140] Histologically, biopsies are nonspecific, with the predominant findings being those of acute and chronic inflammation.[136,140]

Pathogenesis

The cause of nonspecific colonic ulceration remains unknown. Therefore, nonspecific colonic ulceration may be diagnosed only after other causes of colonic ulceration have been ruled out. Some of the more interesting hypotheses for the origin of nonspecific colonic ulceration include the following.

The ischemic hypothesis.   Vascular abnormalities, including thickening of vascular walls, thrombosis, thrombus organization, and recanalization within local vessels, as well as microvascular thrombosis, have been described in areas underlying and adjacent to nonspecific colon ulcers.[138-141] These findings may implicate a localized form of ischemic colitis,[138] perhaps promoted by fecal stasis.[137-139] However, this explanation is less plausible if one considers that ischemic injury usually occurs in the watershed area of the colons (descending colon and splenic flexure), not the cecum. Moreover, right-sided fecal impaction is relatively rare.[142,143] Finally, thrombosis may be secondary to the adjacent inflammation, making determination of cause and effect difficult.

Cecal diverticulosis.   Based on the observation that 5 out of 10 cases of cecal ulceration had histologic evidence of cecal diverticula, Williams proposed that cecal diverticulitis could result in ulcer formation.[144] However, one would expect to see a greater percentage of colonic ulcers in the sigmoid colon, given the higher incidence of diverticulosis there. Furthermore, cecal nonspecific ulcers are almost invariably located on the antimesenteric border of the lumen, whereas cecal diverticula are usually found on the mesenteric side of the cecum.[138,142]

The acid-peptic hypothesis.   Some statistical correlations between peptic ulcer disease and colonic ulceration have been

TABLE 80-3
Clinical Characteristics of Colonic Ulcers

TYPE OF ULCER	PRIMARY LOCATION	SIZE	DISTINGUISHING FEATURES
Solitary rectal ulcer	Anterior rectum	≤1 cm	Associated with rectal prolapse, pelvic floor motor disturbances
Nonspecific ulcers	Cecal	0.5–6.5 cm	Antimesenteric location, oval, round
Dieulafoy's ulcer	Variable	<2 mm	Erosion into large submucosal artery
Stercoral ulcer	Sigmoid, rectosigmoid	1–4 cm	Associated with fecal impaction, antimesenteric location
Crohn's disease	Right colon	0.2–2 cm	Multiple, nodularity, strictures
Ischemic ulcer	Splenic flexure, descending colon	1–10 cm	Circumferential, shallow, diffuse, dusky mucosa
Malignant ulcer	Variable	Variable	Associated with mass, stricture

made.[135,137] It has been postulated that, because nonspecific ulcers frequently occur in the cecum just distal to the ileocecal valve (where colonic contents are usually neutral to slightly acidic in pH), a disturbance in the acid-base status of this region could lead to cecal ulceration. One author posited that digestive enzymes in the cecal area could also contribute to ulcer formation.[138]

Other associations. Correlations have been noted between the use of corticosteroids, NSAIDs, oxyphenbutazone, and oral contraceptives and the occurrence of colonic ulcers.[136,139,142] However, causation has not been established for any of these substances, and they cannot be implicated in a substantial majority of colonic ulcers. Other potential causative explanations include foreign body trauma,[135] neurologic stress,[143] lipomas,[145] bacterial or viral infections,[138,143] and unknown toxins.[138] The cause of nonspecific colon ulceration at this point remains unclear. It seems unlikely that a single explanation can be made to fit all cases.

Clinical Features

Most of the historical and physical examination findings are nonspecific. In Ona's 1982 review,[136] the signs or symptoms most frequently cited were acute or chronic right lower quadrant abdominal pain (50% of cases) with symptoms similar to those of appendicitis; lower gastrointestinal bleeding (33% of cases) most commonly presenting as hematochezia; perforation, with acute surgical abdomen (19%); and abdominal mass (16%), which is most common in left-sided or transverse colonic ulcers. Other reported findings include obstruction, fever, and leukocytosis. Hemoccult positive stool was seen in one case of nonspecific cecal ulceration in the absence of any other demonstrable source of gastrointestinal blood loss.[†]

Diagnosis

Because of the lack of specific historical and physical examination findings, appropriate selection of tests is important to obtain the proper diagnosis. Colonoscopy is the diagnostic test of choice, with 100% sensitivity in one recent review.[136] The use of colonoscopy has shifted management of this condition from the surgical to the medical realm. The findings on air contrast barium enema are abnormal in 69% to 75% of cases but are nonspecific. They may include lumenal narrowing, filling defects, mucosal irregularities, localized colonic spasm, or mass effects.[135,136,145] Sigmoidoscopy misses most colonic ulcers by virtue of their predilection for cecal location.[136] In the setting of brisk bleeding from a colonic ulcer, mesenteric angiography is sensitive (89%) but nonspecific.[136] A CT scan is useful primarily in cases with associated perforation or abscess.

Differential Diagnosis

Because colonic ulcers are histologically nonspecific, diagnosis is based on exclusion of other potential entities. Solitary rectal ulcers occur in the rectum and have a characteristic histologic

---

[†]Murphy ME, personal observation.

appearance (see discussion in a following section). Ulcers associated with Crohn's disease are usually multiple, may be longitudinal, and are often associated with evidence of Crohn's disease elsewhere in the gastrointestinal tract.[139] Infectious causes of colonic ulceration include tuberculosis, *Entamoeba histolytica*, cytomegalovirus (especially in immunocompromised patients), and *Salmonella typhi* and are usually multiple in number. Diagnosis can often be made by biopsy.[136] Tuberculosis of the colon usually results in multiple transverse cecal ulcers. Nodularity and deformity of the ileocecal valve were seen in 100% of cases in one study.[146] This same study demonstrated that 7 of 11 patients had colonoscopic biopsies diagnostic of tuberculosis, either by culture or histology. Ischemic ulcers occur in older patients; frequently, these are multiple lesions with a serpiginous or linear configuration, with irregular margins and abnormal surrounding mucosa. The most common areas of involvement are the splenic flexure and the rectosigmoid junction.[139] Biopsy is nonspecific. Stercoral ulcers usually occur in the sigmoid area in association with fecal impactions (see discussion in a following section). Malignancy (including carcinoma and lymphoma) must be ruled out histologically, because gross appearance is not diagnostic.[139] Other miscellaneous causes of colonic ulceration which have been reported include systemic lupus erythematosus, Behcet's disease, Wegener's granulomatosis, essential mixed cryoglobulinemia, and Churg-Strauss syndrome.[136,147–149] These can usually be differentiated by the setting of their underlying disease.

Prognosis and Therapy

The earliest reports of nonspecific colonic ulceration were of ulcers discovered during surgery for complications (perforation, abscess, or bleeding) or during postmortem examination. Barron's 1928 review described an 82% incidence of perforation, with 100% mortality without surgical therapy.[137] As recently as 1974, surgery was the recommended treatment for all nonspecific colon ulcers. However, in 1990, Blundell described four patients who had nonspecific ulcers discovered at colonoscopy.[142] Three of these patients were managed conservatively, with satisfactory clinical outcomes. Currently, it is recommended that uncomplicated colonic ulcers be followed endoscopically, with multiple biopsies taken during each endoscopy to document healing and to rule out malignancy and infection. The optimal interval between colonoscopies is uncertain; 4 to 6 weeks seems a reasonable period based on healing rates.[136,138,142] Surgery is recommended for ulcers complicated by perforation, substantial bleeding, or associated intraabdominal abscess, or which fail to heal with observation. Surgical procedures that have been used include oversewing of the ulcer, local ulcer excision, and right hemicolectomy.[136,140,150]

Dieulafoy's-Type Colonic Ulceration

In 1898, Georges Dieulafoy described three cases of asymptomatic patients exsanguinating from minute gastric ulcerations which he termed exulceratio simplex. The initial description was of an ulcer less than 2 mm in diameter in the gastric mucosa, with rupture of a relatively large submucosal artery into the gut lumen. Several reports have been published detailing bleeding from colonic lesions similar to those described by Dieulafoy.[151-154] All of the patients described thus far with Dieulafoy-type colonic ulcers have been men, with ages ranging from 20 to 74 years. The colonic lesions are histologically identical to Dieulafoy-type gastric ulcers—a solitary mucosal defect, extending no deeper than the upper submucosal layer, with erosion of an underlying submucosal large-caliber artery (Fig. 80-6). This artery is tortuous and curved toward the mucosa, with erosion at the apex of its curve. There is no associated arterial aneurysm, vasculitis or other vascular anomaly. Inflammation in the ulcerated area is minimal to nonexistent.[151,152] The cause is unknown, although some have postulated that the pulsations of a large submucosal artery may cause mechanical damage to the overlying mucosa, allowing an inflammatory reaction to the lumenal contents to further erode the exposed arterial wall.[151] Clinically, patients present with the acute onset of massive

bleeding; they are otherwise asymptomatic. The mucosal lesions are notoriously difficult to visualize on endoscopy; selective mesenteric angiography has been useful in localization. Systemic vasopressin infusion has not been successful in managing bleeding from these lesions. The definitive therapy is segmental surgical resection, although successful endoscopic sclerotherapy of a rectal lesion has been reported.[151-154]

Stercoral Ulcer (Huntley's Syndrome)

Colonic ulceration caused by ischemic pressure necrosis from a stercoraceous mass may result in colonic perforation, with resultant peritonitis.[155] In Serpell and Nicholls' review of stercoral perforation,[156] the median age of patients was 60 years, with a range of 16 to 89 years. There was a slight female predominance. Risk factors included chronic constipation (61%) and conditions associated with constipation, such as confinement to a nursing home or other chronic care facility (23%), renal failure, or transplantation (13%); use of constipating medications (aluminum hydroxide-containing antacids, narcotics, phenothiazines); hypothyroidism; and colonic strictures. Foreign bodies have also been implicated.[155-157] The actual incidence is unknown. In an early review of 175 unselected autopsies, 4.6% were found to have stercoral ulcerations; half of these had perforations.[158] However, later autopsy studies revealed one case among 2500 psychiatric patients[159] and a 0.3% incidence in a second series of unselected 375 patients.[160] A later review found only 64 reported cases of colonic perforation as a consequence of stercoral ulcer.[156]

Patients who have perforated usually present with complaints of abdominal pain and signs of peritoneal irritation (80%–100%).[156,161] An abdominal mass (23%) or a fecal mass on rectal examination (6%) may be palpable. Plain radiographic findings include pneumoperitoneum (53%), marked fecal loading (30%), and calcified fecaliths within the colon (21%). Contrast radiography is rarely helpful.[156] The correct preoperative diagnosis is rarely made,[156] although survival is improved if the diagnosis is established.[161] Nonperforating stercoral ulcers are rarely diagnosed but must be considered in a constipated patient presenting with abdominal pain, rectal bleeding, and leukocytosis.

Perforating stercoral ulcers are usually located on the antimesenteric border of the sigmoid or rectosigmoid colon (77%), with 47% of these within the sigmoid alone.[156] Other reported sites include the cecum (9%), the descending colon (5%), and the splenic flexure (2%). Resected specimens reveal sharply demarcated, irregular ulcers that conform to the contours of the fecal masses present. Histologically, the colonic mucosa is necrotic and denuded, with acute and chronic inflammatory changes.[158]

The pathophysiology of stercoral ulceration is related directly to the presence of a hard mass of feces (scybalum), which may be present for months to years.[156] The pressure of the scybalum on the colonic wall exceeds the capillary perfusion pressure, which causes ischemic necrosis, with resultant ulceration and eventual perforation.[156,162] The sigmoid predominance is probably caused by progressive desiccation of the fecal mass in the distal colon, the narrower lumenal di-

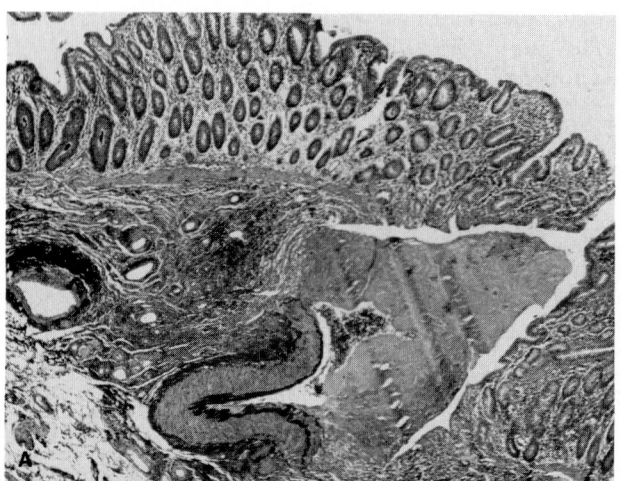
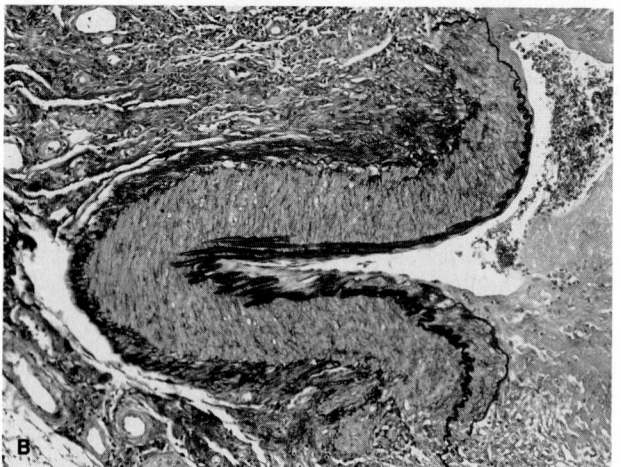

FIGURE 80-6. Dieulafoy ulcer of the colon. (**A**) Low magnification shows a thick-walled, tortuous muscular artery just below the muscularis mucosa, with fresh ulceration overlying the artery at the site of bleeding. (**B**) Higher magnification reveals details of the site of bleeding, at the apex of the artery's curve toward the mucosa. (From Barbier P, Luder P, Triller J, et al. Colonic hemorrhage from a solitary minute ulcer. Gastroenterology 1985;88: 1065.)

ameter of the sigmoid, and the relatively poor colonic blood supply in this area.[156]

The differential diagnosis of stercoral ulceration is limited and includes idiopathic (spontaneous) colonic perforation and perforation from trauma, malignancy, infection, or other cause. Spontaneous colonic perforation, in particular, may be confused with stercoral perforation. It often occurs during a difficult bowel movement and appears grossly as a tear in the mucosa (as opposed to the round or ovoid perforations seen in the bases of stercoral ulcerations). Histologically, there is no evidence of inflammation.[161]

Surgery is required for definitive therapy of both perforated and nonperforated stercoral ulcers. Intravenous antibiotics are indicated as adjunctive therapy; the majority of deaths occur as the result of uncontrolled sepsis.[156] Resection with primary anastomosis; resection with end colostomy, mucous fistula, or Hartmann's pouch; loop colostomy with exteriorization of the perforation; and plication of the perforation with proximal loop colostomy have all been employed. Resection of the perforation with end colostomy and Hartmann's pouch or mucous fistula has been associated with a lower mortality (23%) than other procedures (53%) and has been recommended as the surgical procedure of choice.[162] The overall mortality for patients undergoing resection was 35% in two reviews of surgical treatment.[156,162] Lavage of the peritoneal cavity to reduce fecal contamination is mandatory.[157] Intraoperative colonic lavage is useful in removing scybala proximal to the site of the perforation and may prevent recurrence of ulceration.[163]

Solitary Rectal Ulcer Syndrome

Although first described by Cruveilheir in 1829, the classic 1969 review by Madigan and Morson[164] established the diagnostic criteria for what is now known as the SRUS. This syndrome, with more than 400 cases reported in the literature, primarily affects young adults; the average age is in the third and fourth decades, with a range from 10 to more than 80 years. There is a slight female predominance.[165]

Patients with SRUS typically present with symptoms related to bowel disturbance; 70% to 90% present with constipation, tenesmus, incomplete evacuation, straining at stool, or lower abdominal pain.[165-167] Rectal bleeding is observed in 56% to 89% of patients in published series.[165,166] Passage of mucus per rectum, overt rectal prolapse, and fecal incontinence are less frequent.[165] One large review found that 26% of patients with endoscopic discovery of a solitary rectal ulcer were asymptomatic.[163] Systemic symptoms are uncommon, and bleeding is rarely significant enough to warrant transfusion.

Gross endoscopic appearance of SRUS is variable; the lesion may appear as a single, well-demarcated ulcer up to 5 cm in size, as multiple ulcers, as a polypoid lesion, or as a flat region of erythematous mucosa. Typically, the lesion appears on the anterior rectal wall (68%–95% of cases) approximately 6 to 10 centimeters from the anal verge.[165,167,168] Specific histologic criteria are used to establish the diagnosis, as defined by Madigan and Morson.[164] The lamina propria is replaced by fibroblasts, smooth muscle, and collagen, with associated hypertrophy and disorganization of the muscularis mucosa,

termed fibromuscular obliteration of the lamina propria (Fig. 80-7). Displacement of the mucosal glands into the submucosa and erosion of the mucosal surface may also be seen; the occasional presence of submucosal cystic glands has led to speculation that SRUS and colitis cystica profunda are identical or closely related syndromes with a common cause.[168] Levine and colleagues[169] noted that diffuse collagen infiltration of the lamina propria is seen almost exclusively in SRUS and can be used to differentiate this syndrome from Crohn's disease, ulcerative colitis, and chronic ischemic colitis. Malignancy, amebiasis, lymphogranuloma venereum, and secondary syphilis must also be considered in the differential diagnosis.

The pathophysiology of solitary rectal ulcer syndrome is uncertain. Self-digitation (seen in up to 50% of SRUS patients) has been suggested as a cause,[166] as have a congenital anomaly of the anterior rectal wall, a localized form of inflammatory bowel disease, and infectious agents, although convincing support of these hypotheses is lacking. Prolapse-induced rectal mucosal trauma or ischemia has been strongly implicated as a possible cause of SRUS.[168] The incidence of mucosal or full-thickness rectal prolapse ranges from 13% to 100% in pub-

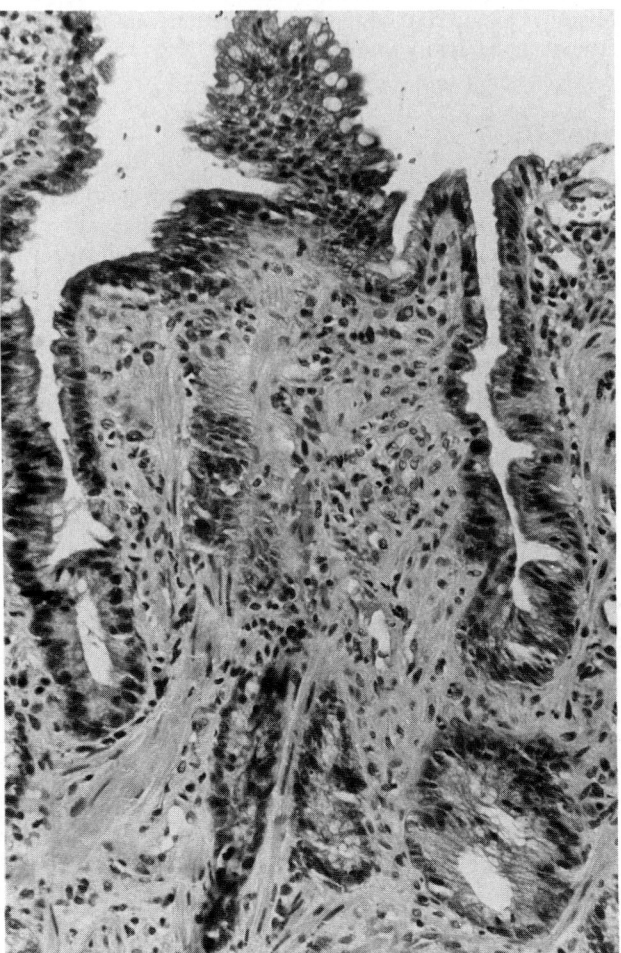

FIGURE 80-7. Solitary rectal ulcer syndrome is characterized by fibromuscular obliteration of the lamina propria with crypt distortion. (Hematoxylin and eosin stain; original magnification ×200); (Courtesy of John Woosley, M.D., Chapel Hill, NC.)

lished series of SRUS patients.[165] A combination of rectal prolapse and a high fecal voiding pressure (caused by overactivity of the external anal sphincter or failure of puborectalis relaxation during defecation) has been theorized to cause local ischemic injury and trauma to the rectal mucosa, resulting in ulceration.[170,171] However, other studies have failed to find electromyographic evidence of a hyperactive anal sphincter in a majority of patients.[165]

Treatment of SRUS depends on the gross morphology of the lesion and on the presence or absence of rectal prolapse. Patients with polypoid lesions usually are younger and are more likely to be asymptomatic, to have a better prognosis, and to respond to conservative medical therapy.[165] Such therapy includes bowel retraining, the use of bulk laxatives, and reassurance. Antiinflammatory drugs (i.e., corticosteroids, salicylates, sucralfate enemas) have been used with varying degrees of success, but none can be routinely recommended. Surgery is advised for patients with rectal prolapse because of their poor response to medical therapy. A 65% overall response rate to surgical intervention was noted in Tjandra's review, with best results in patients with polypoid lesions. The procedure of choice in patients with rectal prolapse is abdominal rectopexy. Anteroposterior rectopexy, local excision, colonic resection, and, rarely, diverting colostomies have been successfully employed in nonprolapsing patients with intractable symptoms refractory to medical therapy.[165,172]

Typhlitis

Typhlitis (from the Greek "typhlos," meaning blind sac), an acute necrotizing colitis principally involving the cecum, was originally described in 1970 by Wagner and colleagues in terminally ill leukemic children with severe neutropenia.[173,174] Synonymous terms include neutropenic enterocolitis, necrotizing enterocolitis, and ileocecal syndrome because inflammation may involve the terminal ileum, ascending colon, and appendix.[175] Although typhlitis occurs primarily in severely immunosuppressed children and adults with leukemia, it has been described in patients with immunosuppression caused by combination chemotherapy for other malignancies, renal transplant, autologous bone marrow transplant, drug-induced granulocytopenia, aplastic anemia, cyclic neutropenia, and possibly the acquired immunodeficiency syndrome (AIDS).[175–177] The incidence rate in autopsy series of children with acute leukemia ranges from 10% to 24%.[174,175] There is a suggestion of increasing frequency, attributed to more aggressive chemotherapeutic regimens. No race or gender predilection or specific regimen of chemotherapy is apparent.[178]

The clinical spectrum of disease varies from mild, self-limited cecal inflammation to fulminant necrosis and perforation. Symptoms may be nonspecific, and typhlitis is commonly diagnosed at laparotomy or autopsy. Symptoms and signs usually develop at the nadir of neutropenia 1 to 2 weeks after completion of chemotherapy. Typhlitis is more common during induction of chemotherapy than during consolidation. Virtually all patients are neutropenic and febrile. Most patients have abdominal pain (localized to the right lower quadrant in approximately 40% to 60% of cases) and many have nausea, vomiting, abdominal distention, diarrhea (20%–45% bloody), and associated stomatitis and necrotizing pharyngitis, indic-

ative of diffuse mucositis. Peritoneal signs or shock suggest the possibility of perforation or sepsis. Positive blood cultures usually grow enteric bacteria, especially *Pseudomonas* or *Candida* organisms.

Typhlitis is difficult to diagnose because of nonspecific symptoms, signs, and radiographic findings.[174] In the appropriate clinical setting, certain radiographic patterns may be helpful. Plain films of the abdomen may show a fluid-filled, distended cecum with dilated small bowel loops, diminished or absent gas in the right lower quadrant (and often the entire colon), "thumbprinting" of the ascending colon, evidence of a right lower quadrant soft tissue mass with small bowel displacement, or cecal pneumatosis. CT scan may reveal symmetrical cecal wall thickening (average about 10 mm) with pericecal fluid or a soft tissue mass if an abscess is present (Fig. 80-8). Ultrasound examination of the right lower quadrant may show the target or halo sign of a solid mass with echogenic center (collapsed mucosa and intestinal contents) and hypoechoic periphery (thickened bowel wall). This finding is nonspecific and has been seen with intestinal hemorrhage, ischemic colitis, intussusception, and lymphoma.[179] Barium enema and arteriography have been reported to be useful in diagnosing typhlitis but are hazardous in the presence of potentially necrotic bowel with a risk of cecal perforation.[180] Instillation of air by endoscopy may be similarly hazardous; however, a gentle, flexible sigmoidoscopy may be useful to detect inflammatory bowel disease or pseudomembranous or ischemic colitis.

In general, typhlitis must be considered in any neutropenic patient with fever, abdominal pain, and diarrhea. The differential diagnosis includes pseudomembranous colitis secondary to *C difficile*, drug-induced or infectious colitis, appendicitis, diverticulitis, ischemic colitis, intussusception, inflammatory bowel disease, intramural hemorrhage, leukemic infiltrate, or Ogilvie's syndrome.

Inflammation almost always involves the cecum but may

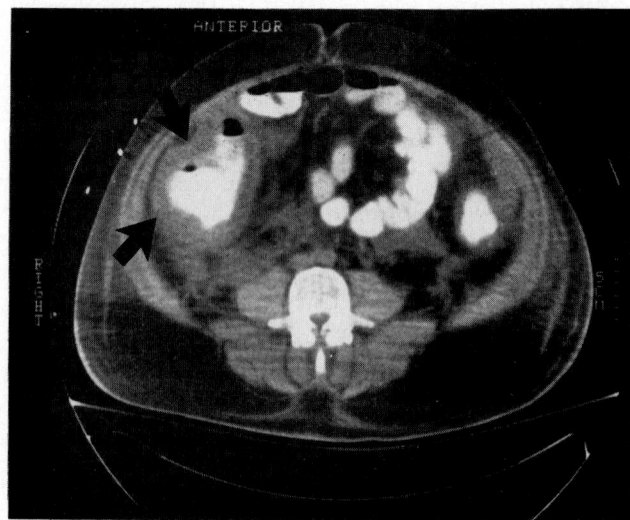

FIGURE 80-8. Computed tomographic scan reveals a massively dilated cecum with thickened walls, spiculation of pericolic fat, and inflammatory changes in the soft tissues of the right flank of a patient with typhlitis. (Courtesy of David Warshauer, M.D., Chapel Hill, NC.)

additionally affect the terminal ileum or ascending colon, or the patient may have sporadic ulcers throughout the large and small intestine. The involved segments are dilated, edematous, and often hemorrhagic on external appearance. The cecal wall is thickened and hemorrhagic; necrotic material covers the ulcerated mucosa. Superficial ulcers can coalesce to form larger lesions. The serosal surface usually remains intact despite severe mucosal damage. Microscopically, there is marked edema of the submucosa, with hemorrhagic necrosis of the mucosa but without a significant inflammatory reaction or leukemic infiltrate. Fungal organisms may be seen, and bacteria (usually gram-negative rods) may surround and infiltrate small blood vessels.[174,175,180]

The pathogenesis is unknown, but many causes have been proposed, including leukemic infiltration of the bowel, intramural hemorrhage and necrosis, local ischemia, toxic effects of chemotherapy, gastrointestinal stasis with bowel erosion, or a combination of these factors. The following sequence of events may occur: failure to maintain an intact epithelial barrier of the right colon (from the listed factors); bacterial invasion of bowel wall; intramural proliferation of bacteria secondary to decreased phagocytosis (neutropenia); production of bacterial endotoxins with subsequent necrosis, hemorrhage and perforation; sepsis. It is unclear why the cecum is always affected.[174,175,181]

Survival in this illness depends on prompt recognition of the condition, appropriate management, and rapid return of normal levels of neutrophils. Management is primarily medical, with selective surgical intervention. Medical therapy includes nasogastric suction for bowel rest, intravenous hydration, broad-spectrum antimicrobial therapy with *Pseudomonas* coverage, and avoidance of antimotility agents. If fever persists for more than 72 hours after antibiotics are begun, antifungal therapy with amphotericin B should be considered and a CT scan performed to identify an abscess. Granulocyte transfusions have been used with some success, but their benefit has not been proven. Surgery has been effective in patients failing medical therapy, and its use should depend on prognosis of underlying primary disease. Indications for surgery include evidence of free intraperitoneal perforation, persistent or life-threatening gastrointestinal hemorrhage, clinical deterioration despite intensive support suggesting uncontrolled sepsis, and evidence of an intraabdominal process that would normally require surgery. The preferred procedure is a right hemicolectomy with ileostomy and mucous fistula formation. Total excision of the necrotic focus is imperative because incomplete removal uniformly results in death in these immunocompromised patients.[182,183] Typhlitis has a high mortality rate (averaging 40%–50%) whether treated medically or surgically. Patients who develop typhlitis during induction and are medically treated are likely to relapse during subsequent chemotherapy (up to 67%).[184] Allowance of complete healing is advocated before resumption of chemotherapy to minimize risk of relapse.

COLITIS CYSTICA PROFUNDA

Colitis cystica profunda is a rare, benign disease most often involving the rectum, characterized by the presence of submucosal, mucus-filled cysts. This lesion was first reported by Stark in 1766 and was termed colitis cystica polyposa by Virchow in 1863. In 1957, the term colitis cystica profunda was used to differentiate this condition from colitis cystica superficialis, in which multiple mucus-filled cysts are limited to the mucosa in association with pellagra and celiac sprue.[185,186] The cysts of colitis cystica profunda are typically large and located below the muscularis mucosae, and they may mimic a malignant process.

Colitis cystica profunda can be solitary or multiple in a localized, segmental, or diffuse distribution. In a review of 144 cases, 85% were localized lesions, typically involving the rectum; there was a slight female preponderance and a median age of 30 years.[187] Symptoms most often include blood or mucus discharge per rectum. At times, diarrhea; abdominal, rectal, or sacral pain; and tenesmus may be present. Bulky or fibrotic lesions may rarely produce either partial or complete obstruction.[188] Physical examination findings vary according to distribution of disease; the localized form is often found on digital rectal examination, which reveals one or more smooth firm masses not adherent to the underlying muscle layer, a thickened rectal wall, or stenosis.

Lesions are usually found within 12 cm of the anal verge and are commonly located on the anterior rectal wall. Endoscopic findings range from normal overlying mucosa to mucosal edema, erythema, friability, or even ulceration overlying a polypoid submucosal mass with or without umbilication. Obvious cysts may be present. If lesions are multiple, they can form a mass up to 3 cm in size. Rectal stricture or prolapse may be seen. Barium enema may demonstrate no abnormalities or may show thickened valves of Houston, increased presacral space, various mucosal abnormalities, filling defects, circumferential stricture, or visible prolapse.[189] Transrectal ultrasound may be useful, although further evaluation is needed.[190] The differential diagnosis of these symptoms and findings is extensive and includes broad categories of inflammatory, infectious, and neoplastic diseases.[185] Definitive diagnosis of colitis cystica profunda is based on typical histologic findings and absence of malignant features. Microscopically, the submucosal layer is enlarged by cysts which occasionally involve the muscularis propria and serosa (Fig. 80-9). Submucosal cysts are found in a variety of conditions[189] and must be differentiated from a well-differentiated mucinous adenocarcinoma. The cysts may be bordered by normal colonic mucosa with a well-differentiated epithelial lining ranging from tall columnar to squamous cells, or they may have no lining at all. The lamina propria stroma may be replaced with collagen and misoriented smooth muscle cells. Adjacent mucosal edema, superficial ulceration, acute and chronic inflammation, pseudomembranes, and distorted crypt architecture may be present.

The pathogenesis is not known; however, three mechanisms have been proposed.[184,189] A congenital origin and herniation of epithelium owing to a weakened muscularis mucosa are two unsubstantiated theories. An acquired origin is supported by the absence of colitis cystica profunda in large pediatric autopsy series, an association with conditions causing trauma of the bowel wall, regression after diverting colostomy, and experimental studies implicating an inflammatory cause. Colitis cystica profunda may be one manifestation of a spectrum of disease states that includes SRUS and internal rectal prolapse. Rectal prolapse has been reported in up to 54% of

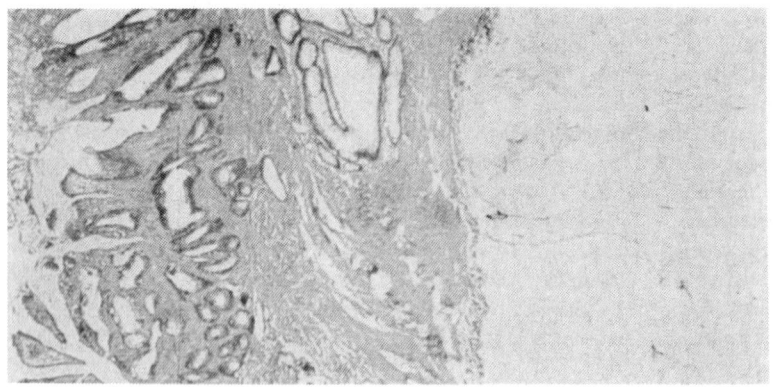

FIGURE 80-9. Submucosal mucin-filled cysts are characteristic of colitis cystica profunda.

patients with colitis cystica profunda, and the anterior location and lamina propria fibrosis resemble SRUS.[164,165,189] Localized colitis cystica profunda is probably caused by ischemia, most often secondary to trauma induced by rectal prolapse. Defecography showing prolapse and abnormal pelvic electromyography are frequently seen,[187,191] but these findings are not always present, suggesting that inflammation and mucosal trauma also contribute to the pathogenesis of this lesion.

The diagnosis of colitis cystica profunda must be considered to avoid inappropriate or radical surgery for suspected cancer. Because shallow mucosal biopsies are usually inadequate, definitive diagnosis may require a surgical excision. The usual course of this disease is a chronic, stable appearance of the rectal mucosa; however, cysts, ulcers and symptoms may come and go. The lesions are not always progressive and are not premalignant. However, for unclear reasons, adenocarcinoma may be located adjacent to colitis cystica profunda.[192] The severity and duration of symptoms should guide choice of treatment options. Most patients can tolerate symptoms with treatment consisting of reassurance, dietary fiber to soften bowel movements, and education to stop straining during defecation and to avoid digital manipulation of the rectum. Only a small preliminary experience has reported the benefits of rectal prolapse repair. Local surgical procedures to excise cysts and ulcers, such as transanal excision, posterior proctectomy, electrocautery, or injection sclerosis, are usually adequate, although lesions may reoccur.[185,188–194] Resectional surgery is usually unnecessary and overly aggressive. Diverting colostomy, performed in the most disabled patients, alleviates the symptoms. Complications such as hemorrhage, obstruction, severe pain, or rectal stenosis need surgical intervention.

PNEUMATOSIS CYSTOIDES INTESTINALIS

This is an uncommon condition characterized by multiple, thin-walled, noncommunicating, gas-filled cysts with no epithelial lining in the wall of the small or large intestine, or both. Less frequently, other areas can be involved, including the stomach, duodenum, and extraintestinal structures (e.g., mesentery, lymph nodes, omentum, gastrohepatic/falciform ligaments, peritoneum).[195] One of the earliest descriptions was by Du Vernoi in 1730, and the term was coined by Mayer in 1925. Usually pneumatosis cystoides is discovered unex-

pectedly in an asymptomatic or minimally symptomatic patient and follows a benign course. Occasionally, it is associated with more fulminant illness such as bowel infarction, pseudomembranous enterocolitis, or necrotizing enterocolitis. After serious illness is excluded, pneumatosis intestinalis can be classified as either primary (idiopathic) or secondary, the latter being associated with a variety of conditions. Pneumatosis is most commonly associated with chronic obstructive pulmonary disease, intestinal obstruction, collagen vascular diseases (scleroderma), and iatrogenic conditions (after surgery or endoscopy). In Koss's review in 1952, only 15% of cases were classified as idiopathic. He also reported an increased male prevalence of 3.5:1, but more recent reports suggest an equal male to female ratio. Pneumatosis intestinalis may be seen at any age, but in adults it usually occurs between 30 and 50 years of age.[196]

If symptoms are present, the most common complaints are diarrhea, vague abdominal discomfort, and abdominal distention. At times, hematochezia, mucus per rectum, and weight loss can occur. Typically, the condition is discovered incidentally during radiographic or endoscopic evaluation or at laparotomy. The abdomen may be tender, and occasionally an abdominal mass is palpable; however, fever and peritoneal signs are unusual.[197] Secondary cases of pneumatosis intestinalis typically involve the small bowel and ascending colon, whereas idiopathic cases tend to involve the left colon. The rectum is infrequently involved, but colonic pneumatosis is becoming more commonly reported.[196,198] The cysts range in size from a few millimeters to several centimeters and are typically found in clusters. A segmental distribution with skip areas is common, and from a few centimeters to a meter of bowel can be involved. An association with sigmoid colon redundancy has been suggested.[198] Complications can occur in about 3% of cases and include volvulus, pneumoperitoneum, intestinal obstruction, intussusception, tension pneumoperitoneum, hemorrhage, and intestinal perforation.[196] Pneumatosis intestinalis is one cause of prolonged recurrent asymptomatic pneumoperitoneum.[196]

Diagnosis is most commonly made on plain radiograph of the abdomen, on which linear, curvilinear, or cystic lucencies are seen in the bowel wall (Fig. 80-10). Additionally, pneumoperitoneum or retroperitoneal air may be found. Barium studies may help confirm location within bowel wall. However, CT scan of the abdomen is more sensitive than conventional radiography in detecting intramural gas, which

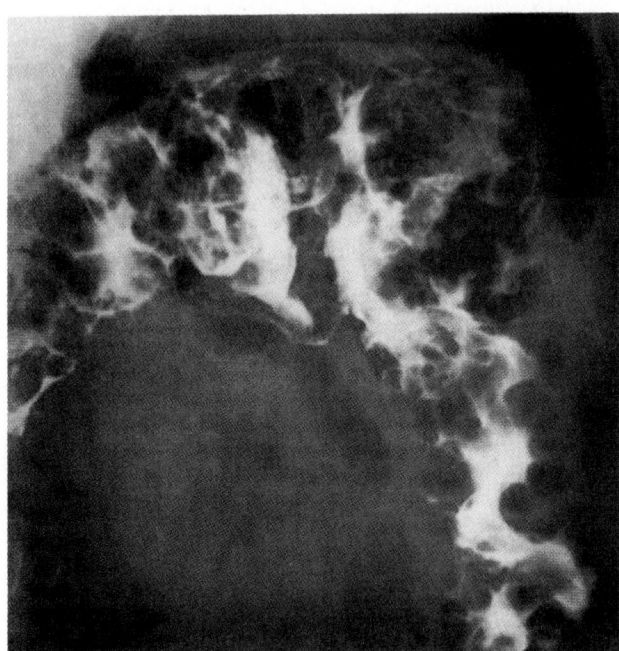

FIGURE 80-10. Pneumatosis cystoides intestinalis in an asymptomatic person. The intramural collections of gas simulate multiple colonic filling defects. Note that the filling defects in this condition appear to be more radiolucent than the soft-tissue masses in the intestinal polyposis syndromes.

parallels the bowel wall.[198] CT scan can also detect portal or mesenteric venous gas, which, when associated with pneumatosis, is highly suggestive of bowel infarction. Endoscopically, pneumatosis appears as multiple, pale to bluish, rounded, soft polyploid masses protruding into the lumen. Because the cysts contain air under pressure, they deflate with a pop or hiss sound if punctured.[196] Submucosal pneumatosis of the colon can mimic polyposis, pseudopolyposis, or intramural hematomas on barium study; endoscopy can help differentiate causes. Enterogenous intestinal cysts are rare and occur in children and young adults. They are usually single, intramural, and most often involve the terminal ileum; their normal intestinal mucosal lining helps to differentiate them from pneumatosis. Lymphangiomas of the peritoneum differ in that lymph and not gas is present within cysts and no giant cells line these areas. Diffuse emphysema caused by infection with gas-producing organisms is distributed in all tissue spaces. In fat necrosis and sclerosing lipogranulomatosis, a fat stain is positive.

The cysts in pneumatosis cystoides intestinalis have a submucosal or subserosal location and contain a high concentration of hydrogen (up to 50%).[196,197] The serosal cysts usually occur near the mesenteric border.[196] They may be partially lined by endothelial cells and are surrounded by foreign body multinucleated giant cells. Inflammation with neutrophils, eosinophils, plasma cells, lymphocytes, and epithelioid granulomas can be observed. Koss postulated that fibrosis progresses until cysts disappear. The cause of pneumatosis is unknown, but several theories exist. The mechanical theory suggests that gas is forced into the bowel by one of several routes: pulmonary, trauma, mucosal breaks, anastomoses,

obstruction, increased pressure, or increased peristalsis. The bacterial theory proposes that gas-producing bacteria invade the bowel wall. Finally, the biochemical theory postulates that excessive gas produced by bacterial fermentation of carbohydrate in the intestinal lumen is absorbed and trapped within the intestinal wall.

In asymptomatic patients, treatment is indicated only for associated illnesses present, because the cysts usually resolve spontaneously. Medical therapy may be tried for symptomatic lesions, but recurrences may ensue.[199] High-flow oxygen breathing using 55% to 75% oxygen to achieve partial pressure of oxygen (PO2) values between 200 and 350 millimeters of mercury for 4 to 10 days may result in cyst resolution.[196,197] To avoid pulmonary and central nervous system toxicity, hyperbaric oxygen at 2.5 atmospheres for 2.5 hours on 2 or 3 consecutive days has also been successful.[200] Antibiotic treatment with metronidazole or ampicillin and elemental diet therapy have been used to resolve cysts.[196,197,200–203] Surgical resection should be reserved for severe symptoms not responding to medical therapy or to manage complications. Unfortunately, surgery is not always successful, and pneumatosis may become more extensive after resection.[204] Surgery is indicated in fulminant cases of pneumatosis in which delay may lead to extensive necrosis of bowel, sepsis, and death. History, physical examination, CT scan of the abdomen, and evaluation for the presence of metabolic acidosis (especially lactic acidosis) and marked hyperamylasemia may help differentiate the patient with intestinal infarction. Mortality is high in these cases, even with surgery.[196,197,204,205] Finally, pneumatosis occurs in organ transplant patients; if present without an underlying systemic illness, it is probably a self-limited and benign illness. However, in the setting of a systemic complication it is a poor prognostic sign.[206]

MALAKOPLAKIA

This is a rare chronic, granulomatous, inflammatory disorder first described in 1902 by Michaelis and Gutmann and named by von Hansemann in 1903 (from the Greek: malakos, "soft"; plakos, "plaque"). It most commonly affects the urinary tract, but it can involve many other organs, including the male or female genital tract, skin, lung, bone, brain, and gastrointestinal tract.[207]

McClure[208] reviewed 34 cases of gastrointestinal malakoplakia; the most common site was the descending/sigmoid colon and rectum, although virtually every area of the gastrointestinal tract may be involved. In this review, there was a bimodal distribution of age incidence, with a small cluster of children younger than 13 years of age and a later peak among middle-aged adults. The average age of the adults was 57 years (range, 18–88 years), with a slight male preponderance[208]; most were Caucasian. The patient may be asymptomatic or may have diarrhea, abdominal pain, rectal bleeding, or symptoms of intestinal obstruction. Physical findings may include abdominal tenderness, rectal tumor, abdominal mass, or weight loss.

The lesions are yellowish, soft plaques or nodules 1 to 20 mm in size or larger, usually elevated and sometimes with a central depression.[208–210] They can be single or multiple and have been noted to involve adjacent structures (i.e., lymph nodes, mesentery, or retroperitoneum). Malakoplakia can present as an intestinal mass, stricture, or fistula, thereby mimicking other inflammatory or neoplastic processes.

Diagnosis is usually made on histologic examination of biopsy material. Diagnosis by fine-needle aspiration has been reported.[211] Histologically, there is a diffuse histiocytic infiltrate with a strongly periodic acid-Schiff (PAS)–positive eosinophilic granular cytoplasm (von Hansemann's cells) containing the characteristic basophilic, laminated cytoplasmic calculospherules called Michaelis-Gutmann's bodies.

Predisposing conditions include chronic infections by coliform bacteria (especially *Escherichia coli*)[212,213] and granulomatous processes such as sarcoidosis and tuberculosis.[207] In addition, malakoplakia has been identified in patients who are immunosuppressed by steroids, immunosuppressant agents (transplant patients), hypogammaglobulinemia, or AIDS.[214–216] McClure's review found that about a third of patients with gastrointestinal malakoplakia had associated colorectal carcinoma, and up to one half had a coexistent malignancy.[207,208]

Although the pathogenesis is unclear, some theories exist. Many authors believe that there is a defect in the phagocytic or digestive activity of the macrophages.[217,218] One patient had low levels of intracellular cyclic GMP with poor release of β-glucuronidase during phagocytosis. More recently, two kidney transplant patients with malakoplakia improved significantly after immunosuppressive therapy was tapered or discontinued, lending support to an immune origin.[214]

Because this condition is rare, no systematic evaluation of treatment has been undertaken. The possibility of associated malignancy or infection mandates a thorough history and physical examination. Localized intestinal malakoplakia can be treated by excisional biopsy or fulguration. If involvement is more diffuse or extensive, empiric trials of antituberculosis medications, antibiotics (e.g., trimethoprim-sulfamethoxazole, ciprofloxacin), or cholinergic agonists (bethanechol, especially in patients with hypogammaglobulinemia) have been used with varying degrees of success.[209,215,218–220]

The reader is directed to Chapter 77, Miscellaneous Diseases of the Small Intestine; Chapter 109, Gastrointestinal Manifestations of Systemic Diseases; and Chapter 110, Gastrointestinal Manifestations of Immunologic Disorders.

REFERENCES

1. Lindstrom CG. "Collagenous colitis" with watery diarrhea. A new entity. Pathol Eur 1976;11:87.
2. Read NW, Krejs GJ, Read MG, et al. Chronic diarrhea of unknown origin. Gastroenterology 1980;68:264.
3. Lazenby AJ, Yardley JH, Giardiello FM, et al. Lymphocytic ("microscopic") colitis: a comparative histopathologic study with particular reference to collagenous colitis. Hum Pathol 1989;20:18.
4. Stampfl DA, Friedman LS. Collagenous colitis pathophysiologic consideration. Dig Dis Sci 1991;36:705.
5. Mashako MNL, Sonsino E, Navarro J, et al. Microscopic colitis: a new cause of chronic diarrhea in children? J Pediatr Gastroenterol Nutr 1990;10:21.
6. Gremse DA, Boudreaux CW, Manci EA. Collagenous colitis in children. Gastroenterology 1993;104:906.
7. Bo-Linn GW, Vendrell DD, Lee E, Fordtran JS. An evaluation of the significance of microscopic colitis in patients with chronic diarrhea. J Clin Invest 1985;75:1559.
8. Baum CA, Bhatia P, Miner PB. Increased colonic mucosal mast cells associated with severe watery diarrhea and microscopic colitis. Dig Dis Sci 1989;34:1462.
9. Tanaka M, Mazzoleni G, Riddell RH. Distribution of collagenous colitis: utility of flexible sigmoidoscopy. Gut 1992;33:65.
10. Flejou JF, Grimaud JA, Molas G, et al. Collagenous colitis: ultrastructural study and collagen immunotyping of four cases. Arch Pathol Lab Med 1984;108:977.
11. Teglbjaerg PS, Thaysen EH, Jensen HH. Development of collagenous colitis in sequential biopsy specimens. Gastroenterology 1984;87:703.
12. Giardiello FM, Lazenby AJ, Bayless TM, et al. Lymphocytic (microscopic) colitis. Clinicopathologic study of 18 patients and comparison to collagenous colitis. Dig Dis Sci 1989;34:1730.
13. DuBois RN, Lazenby AJ, Yardley JH, et al. Lymphocytic enterocolitis in patients with "refractory sprue." JAMA 1989;262:935.
14. Wolber R, Owen D, Freeman H. Colonic lymphocytosis in patients with celiac sprue. Hum Pathol 1990;21:1092.
15. Armes J, Gee DC, Macrae FA, et al. Collagenous colitis: jejunal and colorectal pathology. J Clin Pathol 1992;45:784.
16. Giardiello FM, Lazenby AJ, Yardley JH, et al. Increased HLA A1 and diminished HLA A3 in lymphocytic colitis compared to controls and patients with collagenous colitis. Dig Dis Sci 1992:37:496.
17. Sylwestrowicz T, Kelly JK, Hwang WS, et al. Collagenous colitis and microscopic colitis: the watery diarrhea-colitis syndrome. Am J Gastroenterol 1989;84:763.
18. Riddell RH, Tanaka M, Mazzoleni G. Non-steroidal anti-inflammatory drugs as a possible cause of collagenous colitis: a case-control study. Gut 1992;33:683.
19. Giardielo FM, Hansen FC, Lazenby AJ, et al. Collagenous colitis in setting of nonsteroidal antiinflammatory drugs and antibiotics. Dig Dis Sci 1990;35:257.
20. Bjarnason I, Hayllar J, MacPherson AJ, Russel AS. Side effects of nonsteroidal anti-inflammatory drugs on the small and large intestine in humans. Gastroenterology 1993;104:1832.
21. Van Tilburg AJP, Lam HGT, Seldenrijk CA, et al. Familial occurrence of collagenous colitis. J Clin Gastroenterol 1990;12:279.
22. Sartor RB, Bender DE, Holt LC. Susceptibility of inbred rat strains to intestinal and extraintestinal inflammation induced by indomethacin. Gastroenterology 1992;102:A690.
23. Rampton DS, Baithun SI. Is microscopic colitis due to bile-salt malabsorption? Dis Colon Rectum 1987;30:950.
24. Giardiello FM, Bayless TM, Jessurun J, et al. Collagenous colitis: physiologic and histopathologic studies in seven patients. Ann Intern Med 1987;106:46.
25. De Schryver-Kecskemeti K, Bennert KW, Cooper GS, Yang P. Gastrointestinal involvement in L-Tryptophan (L-Trp) associated eosinophilia-myalgia syndrome (EMS). Dig Dis Sci 1992;37:697.
26. Rask-Madsen J, Grove O, Hansen MGJ, et al. Colonic transport of water and electrolytes in a patient with secretory diarrhea due to collagenous colitis. Dig Dis Sci 1983;28:1141.
27. Lee E, Schiller LR, Vendrell D, et al. Subepithelial collagen table thickness in colon specimens from patients with microscopic colitis and collagenous colitis. Gastroenterology 1992;103:1790.
28. Carpenter HA, Tremaine WJ, Batts KP, et al. Sequential histologic evaluation in collagenous colitis. Dig Dis Sci 1992:1903.
29. Lazenby AJ, Yardley JH, Giardiello FM, Bayless TM. Pitfalls in the diagnosis of collagenous colitis: experience with 75 cases from a registry of collagenous colitis at The Johns Hopkins Hospital. Hum Pathol 1990;21:905.
30. Clouse RE, Alpers DH, Hockenbery DM, et al. Pericrypt eosinophilic enterocolitis and chronic diarrhea. Gastroenterology 1992;103:168.

31. Sloth H, Bisgaard C, Grove A. Collagenous colitis: a prospective trial of prednisolone in six patients. J Intern Med 1991;302:443.

32. Jessurum J, Yardley JH, Lee EL, et al. Microscopic and collagenous colitis. Different names for the same condition? (letter). Gastroenterology 1986;91:1583.

33. Ma CK, Gottlieb C, Haas PA. Diversion colitis: a clinicopathologic study of 21 cases. Hum Pathol 1990;21:429.

34. Haas PA, Fox TA, Szilag EJ. Endoscopic examination of the colon and rectum distal to a colostomy. Am J Gastroenterol 1990;85:850.

35. Roe AM, Warren BF, Brodribb AJM, Brown C. Diversion colitis and involution of the defunctioned anorectum. Gut 1991;34:382.

36. Geraghty JM, Talbot IC. Diversion colitis: histological features in the colon and rectum after defunctioning colostomy. Gut 1991;32:1020.

37. Orsay CP, Kim DO, Pearl RK, Abcarian H. Diversion colitis in patients scheduled for colostomy closure. Dis Colon Rectum 1993;36:366.

38. Korelitz BI, Cheskin LJ, Sohn N, Sommers SC. The fate of the rectal segment after diversion of the fecal stream in Crohn's disease: its implications for surgical management. J Clin Gastroenterol 1985;7:37.

39. Haque S, Eisen RN, West AB. The morphologic features of diversion colitis: studies of a pediatric population with no other disease of the intestinal mucosa. Hum Pathol 1993;24:211.

40. Morson BC, Dawson IMP. Gastrointestinal pathology. 1st ed. London: Blackwell Scientific, 1972:485.

41. Glotzer DJ, Glick ME, Goldman H. Proctitis and colitis following diversion of the fecal stream. Gastroenterology 1981;80:438.

42. Yeong ML, Bethwaite PB, Prasad J, Isbister WH. Lymphoid follicular hyperplasia—a distinctive feature of diversion colitis. Histopathology 1991;19:55.

43. Murray FE, O'Brien MJ, Birkett DH, et al. Diversion colitis. Pathologic findings in a resected sigmoid colon and rectum. Gastroenterology 1987;93:1404.

44. Roediger WEW. Role of anaerobic bacteria in the metabolic welfare of the colonic mucosa in man. Gut 1980;21:793.

45. Roediger WEW. Utilization of nutrients by isolated epithelial cells of the rat colon. Gastroenterology 1982;83:424.

46. Harig JM, Soergel KH, Komorowski RA, Wood CM. Treatment of diversion colitis with short-chain-fatty acid irrigation. N Engl J Med 1989;320:23.

47. Roediger WEW. The starved colon—diminished mucosal nutrition, diminished absorption, and colitis. Dis Colon Rectum 1990;33:858.

48. Guillemot F, Colombel JF, Neut C, et al. Treatment of diversion colitis by short-chain fatty acids. Dis Colon Rectum 1991;34:861.

49. Ordein JJ, Lorenzo CD, Flores A, Hyman PE. Diversion colitis in children with severe gastrointestinal motility disorders. Am J Gastroenterol 1992;87:88.

50. Morin CL, Ling V, Bourassa D. Small intestinal and colonic changes induced by a chemically defined diet. Dig Dis Sci 1980;25:123.

51. Tomasino RM, Latteri MV, et al. Histological and histochemical changes in the colon mucosa after ureterosigmoidostomy or colon conduit. Eur Urol 1988;15:248.

52. Neut C, Colombel JF, Guillemot F, et al. Impaired bacterial flora in human excluded colon. Gut 1989;30:1094.

53. Tripodi J, Gorcey S, Burakoff R. A case of diversion colitis treated with 5-aminosalicylic acid enemas. Am J Gastroenterol 1992;87:645.

54. Olive DL, Schwartz LB. Endometriosis. Medical progress. N Engl J Med 1993;328:1759.

55. Williams TJ, Pratt JH. Endometriosis in 1,000 consecutive celiotomies: incidence and management. Am J Obstet Gynecol 1977;129:245.

56. Meyer R. Uber entzundliche heterotope Epithelwucherungen im weiblichen Genitalgebiete and uber eine bir in die Wurzel des Mesocolon ausgedehnte benigne Wucherung des Darme-

57. Panganiban W, Cornog J. Endometriosis of the intestines and vermiform appendix. Dis Colon Rectum 1972;15:253.

58. Macafee CHG, Greer HLH. Intestinal endometriosis. J Obstet Gynecol 1960;67:539.

59. Weed JC, Ray JE. Endometriosis of the bowel. Obstet Gynecol 1987;69:727.

60. Coronado C, Franklin RR, Lotze RC, et al. Surgical treatment of symptomatic colorectal endometriosis. Fertil Steril 1990;53:411.

61. Collin GR, Russell JC. Endometriosis of the colon. Its diagnosis and management. Am Surg 1990;56:275.

62. Jevon GP, Dayo D, Qizilbash AH. Intussusception of the appendix. A report of four cases and review of the literature. Arch Pathol Lab Med 1992;116:960.

63. Heupel HW, Reece RL, Pincus M. Stromal endometrioma mimicking acute appendicitis. Minn Med 1970;53:153.

64. Gray LA. Endometriosis of the bowel: role of bowel resection, superficial excision and oophorectomy in treatment. Ann Surg 1973;177:580.

65. Rowland R, Langman JM. Endometriosis of the large bowel: a report of 11 cases. Pathology 1989;21:259.

66. Rock JA, Markham SM. Pathogenesis of endometriosis. Lancet 1992;340:1264.

67. Jenkins S, Olive DL, Haney AF. Endometriosis: pathogenetic implications of the anatomic distribution. Obstet Gynecol 1986;67:335.

68. Bozdech JM. Endoscopic diagnosis of colonic endometriosis. Gastrointest Endosc 1992;38:568.

69. St Ville EW, Jafri SZH, Madrazo BL, et al. Endorectal sonography in the evaluation of rectal and perirectal disease. AJR Am J Roentgenol 1991;157:503.

70. Hitti IF, Glasberg SS, Lubicz S. Clear cell carcinoma arising in extraovarian endometriosis: report of three cases and review of the literature. Gynecol Oncol 1990;39:314.

71. Shaw RW. Treatment of endometriosis. Lancet 1992;340:1267.

72. Nezhat C, Nezhat F, Pennington E. Laparoscopic treatment of infiltrative rectosigmoid colon and rectovaginal septum endometriosis by the technique of videolaparoscopy and the CO_2 laser. Br J Obstet Gynaecol 1992;99:664.

73. Cappell MS, Simon T. Fulminant colitis following a self-administered hydrofluoric acid enema. Am J Gastroenterol 1993;88:122.

74. Hardin RD, Tedesco FJ. Colitis after Hibiclens enema. J Clin Gastroenterol 1986;8:572.

75. Fortson WC, Tedesco FJ. Drug-induced colitis: a review. Am J Gastroenterol 1984;79:878.

76. Kirchner SG, Buckspan GS, O'Neill JA, et al. Detergent enema: a cause of caustic colitis. Pediatr Radiol 1977;6:141.

77. Kim SK, Cho C, Levinsohn EM. Caustic colitis due to detergent enema. AJR Am J Roentgenol 1980;134:397.

78. Pike BF, Phillippi PJ, Lawson EH Jr. Soap colitis. N Engl J Med 1971;285:217.

79. Bendit M. Gangrene of the rectum as a complication of an enema. Br Med J 1945;1:664.

80. Lutzger LG, Factor SM. Effects of some water-soluble contrast media on the colonic mucosa. Radiology 1976;118:545.

81. Wood BP, Katzberg RW, Ryan DH, Karch FE. Diatrizoate enemas: facts and fallacies of colonic toxicity. Radiology 1978;126:441.

82. Seltzer SE, Jones B. Cecal perforation associated with Gastrografin enema. AJR Am J Roentgenol 1978;130:997.

83. Meyer CT, Brand M, Deluca VA, Spiro HN. Hydrogen peroxide colitis: a report of three patients. J Clin Gastroenterol 1981;3:31.

84. Sheehan JF, Brynjolfsson G. Ulcerative colitis following hydrogen peroxide enema. Lab Invest 1960;9:150.

85. Shaw A, Cooperman A, Fusco J. Gas embolism produced by hydrogen peroxide. N Engl J Med 1967;277:238.

86. Herrerias JM, Muniain MA, Sanchez S, Garrido M. Alcohol-induced colitis. Endoscopy 1983;15:121.

87. Segal I, Tim LO, Hamilton DG, Lawson HH, et al. Ritual-enema-induced colitis. Dis Colon Rectum 1979;22:195.

pithels. Virchows Arch Path Anat Band 195, Folge IXI. Berlin: Band Verlag 1909:487.

88. Speare GS. Melanosis coli: experimental observations of its production and elimination in twenty-three cases. Am J Surg 1951;82:631.

89. Wittoesch JH, Jackman RJ, McDonald JR. Melanosis coli: general review and a study of 887 cases. Dis Colon Rectum 1958;1:172.

90. Badiali D, Marcheggiano A, Pallone F, et al. Melanosis of the rectum in patients with chronic constipation. Dis Colon Rectum 1985;28:241.

91. Steer HW, Colin-Jones DG. Melanosis coli: studies of the toxic effects of irritant purgatives. J Pathol 1975;115:199.

92. Balazs M. Melanosis coli: ultrastructural study of 45 patients. Dis Colon Rectum 1986;29:839.

93. Park C, Cho NH, Jeong HJ. Melanosis coli: histochemical and immunohistochemical comparison of the pigments of melanosis coli and Dubin-Johnson Syndrome. Yonsei Med J 1990;31:27.

94. Walker NI, Bennett RE, Axelsen RA. Melanosis coli: a consequence of anthraquinone-induced apoptosis of colonic epithelial cells. Am J Path 1988;131:465.

95. Morganstern L, Shemen L, Allen W, et al. Melanosis coli: changes in appearance when associated with colonic neoplasia. Arch Surg 1983;118:62.

96. Heilbrun N. Roentgen evidence suggesting enterocolitis associated with prolonged cathartic abuse. Radiology 1943;41:486.

97. Heilbrun N, Bernstein C. Roentgen abnormalities of the large and small intestine associated with prolonged cathartic ingestion. Radiology 1955;65:549.

98. Moriarty KJ, Silk DBA. Laxative abuse. Dig Dis Sci 1988;6:15.

99. Smith B. Pathology of cathartic colon. Proc R Soc Med 1972;65:288.

100. Heizer WD, Warshaw AL, Waldmann TA, Laster L. Protein-losing gastroenteropathy and malabsorption associated with factitious diarrhea. Ann Intern Med 1968;68:839.

101. Campbell WL. Cathartic colon: reversibility of roentgen changes. Dis Colon Rectum 1983;26:445.

102. Smith B. Pathologic changes in the colon produced by anthraquinone purgatives. Dis Colon Rectum 1973;16:455.

103. Rieman JF, Zimmerman W. Ultrastructural studies of colonic nerve plexuses in chronic laxative abuse. Gastroenterology 1978;74:1085.

104. Krishnamurthy S, Schuffler MD, Rohrmann CA, Pope CE II. Severe idiopathic constipation is associated with a distinctive abnormality of the colonic myenteric plexus. Gastroenterology 1985;88:26.

105. Todd IP. Cathartic colon: surgical aspects. Proc R Soc Med 1973;66:244.

106. Beyer XL, Bickel JT, Butt JH. Ischemic colitis associated with dextroamphetamine use. J Clin Gastroenterol 1991;13:198.

107. Cotton PB, Thomas ML. Ischaemic colitis and the contraceptive pill. Br Med J 1971;3:27.

108. Parker WA, Morris ME, Shearer CA. Oral contraceptive-induced ischemic bowel disease. Am J Hosp Pharm 1979;36:1103.

109. Tedesco FJ, Volpicelli NA, Moore FS. Estrogen-and progesterone-associated colitis: a disorder with clinical and endoscopic features mimicking Crohn's colitis. Gastrointest Endosc 1982;28:247.

110. Lambert M, de Peyer R, Muller AF. Reversible ischemic colitis after intravenous vasopressin therapy. JAMA 1982;247:666.

111. Stillman AE, Weinberg M, Mast WC, Palpant S. Ischemic bowel disease attributable to ergot. Gastroenterology 1977;72:1336.

112. Wormann B, Bochter W, Seib HJ, Ottenjann R. Ergotamine-induced colitis. Endoscopy 1985;17:165.

113. Fishel R, Hamamoto G, Barbul A, et al. Cocaine colitis: is this a new syndrome? Dis Colon Rectum 1985;28:264.

114. Nalbandian H, Sheth N, Dietrich R, Georgiou J. Intestinal ischemia caused by cocaine ingestion: report of two cases. Surgery 1985;97:374.

115. Basse P, Rordam P. Ischemic colitis complicating imipramine overdose and alcohol ingestion. Eur J Surg 1992;158:187.

116. Capell MS, Simon T. Colonic toxicity of administered medications and chemicals. Am J Gastroenterol 1993;88:1684.

117. Carratu R, Parisi P, Agozzino A. Segmental ischemic colitis associated with nonsteroidal antiinflammatory drugs. J Clin Gastroenterol 1993;16:31.

118. Gibson GR, Whitacre EB, Ricotti CA. Colitis induced by nonsteroidal anti-inflammatory drugs: report of four cases and review of the literature. Arch Intern Med 1992;152:625.

119. Tanner AR, Raghunath AS. Colonic inflammation and non-steroidal anti-inflammatory drug administration. Digestion 1988;41:116.

120. Aabakken L, Osnes M. Non-steroidal anti-inflammatory drug induced disease in the distal ileum and large bowel. Scand J Gastroenterol 1989;24(suppl 163):48.

121. Halter F, Weber B, Huber T, et al. Diaphragm disease of the ascending colon: association with sustained-release diclofenac. J Clin Gastroenterol 1993;16:7480.

122. Langer HE, Hartmann G, Heinemann G, Richter X. Gold colitis induced by auranofin treatment of rheumatoid arthritis: case report and review of the literature. Ann Rheum Dis 1987;46:787.

123. Lavy A, Militianu D, Eidelman S. Diseases of the intestine mimicking Crohn's disease. J Clin Gastroenterol 1992;15:17.

124. Martin DM, Goldman JA, Gilliam J, Nasrallah SM. Gold-induced eosinophilic enterocolitis: response to oral cromolyn sodium. Gastroenterology 1981;80:1567.

125. Marcuard SP, Ehrinpreis MN, Fitter WF. Gold induced ulcerative proctitis: report and review of the literature. J Rheumatol 1987;14:142.

126. Martin P, Manley PN, Depew WT, Blakeman JM. Isotretinoin associated proctosigmoiditis. Gastroenterology 1987;93:606.

127. McKinley M, Toffler RB. Antibiotic-associated hemorrhagic colitis. Dig Dis Sci 1980;25:812.

128. Sakurai Y, Tsuchiya H, Ikegami F, et al. Acute right-sided hemorrhagic colitis associated with oral administration of ampicillin. Dig Dis Sci 1979;24:910.

129. Mitchell EP, Schein PS. Gastrointestinal toxicity of chemotherapeutic agents. Semin Oncol 1982;9:52.

130. Slavin RE, Dias MA, Saral R. Cytosine arabinoside induced gastrointestinal toxic alterations in sequential hemotherapeutic protocols: a clinical-pathologic study of 33 patients. Cancer 1978;42:1747.

131. Milles SS, Muggia AL, Spiro HM. Colonic histologic changes induced by 5-fluorouracil. Gastroenterology 1962;43:391.

132. Atherton LD, Leib ES, Kaye MD. Toxic megacolon associated with methotrexate therapy. Gastroenterology 1984;86:1583.

133. Graham CF, Gallagher K, Jones JK. Acute colitis with methyldopa. N Engl J Med 1981;304:1044.

134. Bennett JE. Flucytosine. Ann Intern Med 1977;86:319.

135. Mark HI, Ballinger WF. Nonspecific ulcer of the colon, report of a case and review of 51 cases from the literature. Am J Gastroenterol 1964;41:266.

136. Ona FV, Allende HD, Vivenio R, et al. Diagnosis and management of nonspecific colon ulcer. Arch Surg 1982;117:888.

137. Barron ME. Simple, nonspecific ulcer of the colon. Arch Surg 1928;17:375.

138. Butsch JL, Dockerty MB, McGill DB, Judd ES. "Solitary" nonspecific ulcers of the colon. Arch Surg 1969;98:171.

139. Khawaja FI, Vakil N. Colonoscopy as an aid in the diagnosis of nonspecific ulcers of the colon. Gastrointest Endosc 1987;33:43.

140. Shallman RW, Kuehner M, Williams GH, et al. Benign cecal ulcers. Dis Colon Rectum 1985;28:732.

141. Hardie JR, Nicoll P. Localized ulceration of the caecum due to microcirculatory thrombosis. Aust N Z J Surg 1973;42:149.

142. Blundell CR, Earnest DL. Idiopathic cecal ulcer: diagnosis by colonoscopy followed by nonoperative management. Dig Dis Sci 1980;25:494.

143. Mahoney TJ, Bubrick MP, Bitchcock CR. Nonspecific ulcers of the colon. Dis Colon Rectum 1978;21:623.

144. Williams KL. Acute solitary ulcers and acute diverticulitis of caecum and ascending colon. Br J Surg 1960;47:351.

145. Gardiner GA, Bird CR. Nonspecific ulcers of the colon resembling annular carcinoma. Radiology 1980;137:331.

146. Bhargava DK, Tandon HD, Chawla TC, et al. Diagnosis of ileocecal and colonic tuberculosis by colonoscopy. Gastrointest Endosc 1985;31:68.

147. Shimamoto C, Hirata I, Ohshiba S, et al. Churg-Strauss syn-

drome (allergic granulomatous angiitis) with peculiar multiple colonic ulcers. Am J Gastroenterol 1990;85:316.

148. Wilson RT, Dean PJ, Upshaw JD, Wruble LD. Endoscopic appearance of Wegener's granulomatosis involving the colon. Gastrointest Endosc 1987:33:388.

149. Baxter R, Nino-Murcia M, Bloom RJ, Kosek J. Gastrointestinal manifestations of essential mixed cryoglobulinemia. Gastrointest Radiol 1988;13:160.

150. Lazarovich I, Michowitz M, Lowenthal M, Solowiejczyk M. Nonspecific ulcers of the cecum. Dis Colon Rectum 1974;17: 381.

151. Barbier P, Luder P, Triller J, et al. Colonic hemorrhage from a solitary minute ulcer. Gastroenterology 1985;88:1065.

152. Richards WO, Grove-Mahoney D, Williams LF. Hemorrhage from a Dieulafoy-type ulcer of the colon: a new cause of lower gastrointestinal bleeding. Am Surg 1988;54:121.

153. Franko E, Chardavoyne R, Wise L. Massive rectal bleeding from a Dieulafoy's type ulcer of the rectum: a review of this unusual disease. Am J Gastroenterol 1991;86:1545.

154. Abdulin JD, Santoro MJ, Chen YK, Collen MJ. Dieulafoy-like lesion of the rectum presenting with exsanguinating hemorrhage: successful endoscopic therapy. Am J Gastroenterol 1993;88:1939.

155. Lalla R, Enquist I, Oloumi M, Velez FJ. Stercoraceous perforation of the right colon. South Med J 1989;82:80.

156. Serpell JW, Nicholls RJ. Stercoral perforation of the colon. Br J Surg 1990;77:1325.

157. Grundill WL, Klompje J. Spontaneous rupture and stercoral perforation of the colon. S Afr Med J 1986;69:203.

158. Grinvalsky HT, Bowerman CI. Stercoraceous ulcers of the colon: relatively neglected medical and surgical problem. JAMA 1959;171:1941.

159. Wang S, Sutherland JC. Colonic perforation due to fecal impaction. Dis Colon Rectum 1977;20:355.

160. Lal S, Brown GN. Some unusual complications of fecal impaction. Am J Proctol 1967;18:226.

161. Gekas P, Schuster MM. Stercoral perforation of the colon: case report and review of the literature. Gastroenterology 1981;80: 1054.

162. Guyton DP, Evans D, Schreiber H. Stercoral perforation of the colon: concepts of operative management. Am Surg 1985;51: 520.

163. Serpell JW, Giddins SG, Nicholls RJ, Bradfield WJD. Stercoral perforation of the colon proximal to an end colostomy. Postgrad Med J 1991;67:299.

164. Madigan MR, Morson BC. Solitary ulcer of the rectum. Gut 1969;10:871.

165. Tjandra JT, Fazio VW, Church JM, et al. Clinical conundrum of solitary rectal ulcer. Dis Colon Rectum 1992;35:227.

166. Niv Y, Bat L. Solitary rectal ulcer syndrome-clinical, endoscopic, and histological spectrum. Am J Gastroenterol 1986;81:486.

167. Pescatori M, Maria G, Mattana C, et al. Clinical picture and pelvic floor physiology in the solitary rectal ulcer syndrome. Dis Colon Rectum 1985;28:862.

168. Levine DS. "Solitary" rectal ulcer syndrome. Gastroenterology 1987;92:243.

169. Levine DS, Surawicz CM, Ajer TN, et al. Diffuse excess mucosal collagen in rectal biopsies facilitates differential diagnosis of solitary rectal ulcer syndrome from other inflammatory bowel disease. Dig Dis Sci 1988;33:1345.

170. Snooks SJ, Nicholls RJ, Henry MM, Swash M. Electrophysiological and manometric assessment of the pelvic floor in the solitary rectal ulcer syndrome. Br J Surg 1985;72:131.

171. Womack NB, Williams NS, Holmfield JHM, Morrison JFB. Pressure and prolapse—the cause of solitary rectal ulceration. Gut 1987;28:1228.

172. Nicholls RJ, Simson JNL. Anteroposterior rectopexy in the treatment of solitary rectal ulcer syndrome without overt rectal prolapse. Br J Surg 1986;73:222.

173. Wagner ML, Rosenberg HS, Fernbach OJ, Singleton ED. Typhlitis: complication of leukemia in childhood. AJR Am J Roentgenol 1970;109:341.

174. Jones B, Wall SD. Gastrointestinal disease in the immunocompromised host. Radiol Clin North Am 1992;30:555.

175. Katz JA, Wagner ML, Gresik MV, et al. Typhlitis: an 18-year experience and post mortem review. Cancer 1990;65:1041.

176. Nagler A, Pavel L, Naparstek E, et al. Typhlitis occurring in autologous bone marrow transplantation. Bone Marrow Transplant 1992;9:63.

177. Cutrona AF, Blinkhorn RJ, Crass J, Spagnudo PJ. Probable neutropenic enterocolitis in patients with AIDS. Rev Infect Dis 1991;13:828.

178. Kunkel JM, Rosenthal D. Management of the ileocecal syndrome. Dis Colon Rectum 1986;29:196.

179. Merine D, Nussbaum AR, Fishman EK, Sanders RC. Sonographic observation in a patient with typhlitis. Clin Pediatr 1989;28:377.

180. Taylor AJ, Dodds WJ, Gonyo JE, Komorowski RA. Typhlitis in adults. Gastrointest Radiol 1985;10:363.

181. Prolla JC, Kirsner JB. The gastrointestinal lesions and complications of the leukemias. Ann Intern Med 1964;61:1084.

182. Moir CR, Scudamore CH, Benny WB. Typhlitis: selective surgical management. Am J Surg 1986;151:563.

183. Shamberger RC, Weinstein HJ, Delorey MJ, Levey RH. The medical and surgical management of typhlitis in children with acute nonlymphocytic leukemia. Cancer 1986;57:603.

184. Keidan RD, Fanning J, Gatenby RA, Weese JL. Recurrent typhlitis. Dis Colon Rectum 1989;32:206.

185. Guest CB, Reznick RK. Colitis cystica profunda: review of the literature. Dis Colon Rectum 1989;32:983.

186. Epstein SE, Ascari WA, Ablow RC, et al. Colitis cystica profunda. Am J Clin Pathol 1966;45:186.

187. Lowry AC, Goldberg SM. Internal and overt rectal procidentia. Gastroenterol Clin North Am 1987;16:47.

188. Bentley E, Chandrasoma P, Cohen H, et al. Colitis cystica profunda: presenting with complete intestinal obstruction and recurrence. Gastroenterology 1985;89:1157.

189. Levine DS. "Solitary" rectal ulcer syndrome: are "solitary" rectal ulcer syndrome and "localized" colitis cystica profunda analogous syndromes caused by rectal prolapse? Gastroenterology 1987;92:243.

190. Hulsmans FJH, Tio TL, Reeders JWA, Tytgat GNJ. Transrectal US in the diagnosis of localized colitis cystica profunda. Radiology 1991;181:201.

191. Kuijpers HC, Schreve RH, Hoedemakers HTC. Diagnosis of functional disorders of defecation causing the solitary rectal ulcer syndrome. Dis Colon Rectum 1986;29:126.

192. Silver H, Stolar J. Distinguishing features of well differentiated mucinous adenocarcinoma of the rectum and colitis cystica profunda. Am J Clin Pathol 1969;51:493.

193. Walker JP, Wiener I, Rowe EB. Colitis cystica profunda: diagnosis and management. South Med J 1986;79:1167.

194. Guy PJ, Hall M. Colitis cystica profunda of the rectum treated by mucosal sleeve resection and colo-anal pull through. Br J Surg 1988;75:289.

195. Koss LG. Abdominal gas cysts (pneumatosis cystoides intestinalis hominis). Arch Pathol 1952;53:523.

196. Galandink S, Fazio VW. Pneumatosis cystoides intestinalis: a review of the literature. Dis Colon Rectum 1985;29:358.

197. Sequeira W. Pneumatosis cystoides intestinalis in systemic sclerosis and other diseases. Semin Arthritis Rheum 1990;19:269.

198. Moote DJ, Fried LA, LeBrum GP, Fraser DB. Pneumatosis coli: Is there a relationship with sigmoid colon redundancy. Gastrointest Radiol 1989;14:79.

199. Caudill JL, Rose BS. The role of computed tomography in the evaluation of pneumatosis intestinalis. J Clin Gastroenterol 1987;9:223.

200. Van der Linden W. Reappearance of intestinal gas cysts after oxygen treatment. Lancet 1974;2:1388.

201. Masterson JST, Fratlin LB, Osler TR, Trapp WG. Treatment of pneumatosis cystoides intestinalis with hyperbaric oxygen. Am Surg 1975;187:245.

202. Ellis BW. Symptomatic treatment of primary pneumatosis coli with metronidazole. Br Med J 1980;250:763.

203. Van der Linden W, Marsell R. Pneumatosis cystoides coli associated with high H_2 excretion: treatment with an elemental diet. Scand J Gastroenterol 1979;14:173.

204. Witowshi LJ, Pontius GV, Anderson RE. Gas cysts of the intestine. Surgery 1955;37:959.
205. Knechtle SJ, Davidoff AM, Rice RP. Pneumatosis intestinalis. Surgical management and clinical outcome. Ann Surg Aug 1990;212:160.
206. Andorsby RI. Pneumatosis cystoides intestinalis after organ transplantation. Am J Gastroenterol 1990;85:189.
207. McClure J. Malakoplakia. J Pathol 1983;140:275.
208. McClure J. Malakoplakia of the gastrointestinal tract. Postgrad Med J 1981;57:95.
209. Sanusi ID, Tio FO. Gastrointestinal malakoplakia. Am J Gastroenterol 1974;62:356.
210. Gozalez-Angulo A, Corral E, Garcia-Torres R, Quijano M. Malakoplakia of the colon. Gastroenterology 1965;48:383.
211. Kumar PV, Hambarsoomina B, Banani SA, Vaezzadeh K. Diagnosis of intestinal malakoplakia by fine needle aspiration cytology. Acta Cytol 1987;31:53.
212. Lou TY, Teplitz C. Malakoplakia: pathogenesis and ultrastructural morphogenesis. Hum Pathol 1974;5:191.
213. Lewin KJ, Harell GS, Lee AS, Crowley L. Malakoplakia. An electron microscopic study. Gastroenterology 1974;66:28.
214. Biggar WD, Crawford L, Cardella C, et al. Malakoplakia and immunosuppressive therapy. Am J Pathol 1985;119:5.
215. Webb M, Pincott JR, Marshall WC, et al. Hypogammaglobulinaemia and malakoplakia: response to bethanechol. Eur J Pediatr 1986;145:297.
216. Schwartz DA, Ogden PO, Blumberg HM, Honig E. Pulmonary malakoplakia in a patient with acquired immunodeficiency syndrome. Arch Pathol Lab Med 1990;114:1267.
217. Lewin KJ, Fair WR, Steigbegel RT, et al. Clinical and laboratory studies into pathogenesis of malakoplakia. J Clin Pathol 1976;29:354.
218. Abdou NI, NaPombejara C, Sagawa A, et al. Malakoplakia: evidence for monocyte lysosomal abnormality correctable by cholinergic agonist in vitro and in vivo. N Engl J Med 1977;297:1413.
219. Fraser I, Smart JG, Watkin EM, MacKay EH. Successful treatment of upper urinary tract malakoplakia. Br J Urol 1987;59:485.
220. Van Furth R, van't Wout JW, Wertheimer PA, Zwartendijk J. Ciprofloxacin for treatment of malakoplakia. Lancet 1992;339:148.

Textbook of Gastroenterology, second edition, edited by Tadataka Yamada. JB Lippincott Company, Philadelphia © 1995.

CHAPTER 81

Irritable Bowel Syndrome

William L. Hasler   Chung Owyang

The irritable bowel syndrome (IBS) is a gastrointestinal disorder characterized by alterations in bowel habits with or without abdominal pain in the absence of detectable organic disease. Studies of the pathogenesis of IBS have been unrevealing to date, and no clear diagnostic markers exist, so all definitions of IBS are based on characteristic clinical presentations. International working teams have developed standardized definitions of IBS, based on abdominal symptomatology, which can be employed by clinicians to more accurately diagnose their patients and by researchers to better investigate well-defined study populations. The symptom criteria for the diagnosis of IBS from a 1992 working team include, first, at least 3 months of continuous or recurrent abdominal pain or discomfort relieved by defecation or associated with a change in the frequency or consistency of the stool, and second, two or more of the following at least 25% of the time: altered stool frequency, altered stool form, altered stool passage, passage of mucus, and bloating or abdominal distention (Table 81-1).[1] However, other criteria have been used by both clinicians and investigators, some of which are more inclusive than the current definition. Therefore, in reviewing a publication on IBS, the characteristics of the particular patient population must be carefully ascertained by the reader.

EPIDEMIOLOGY

IBS is the most common digestive disease encountered by gastroenterologists, representing up to 50% of outpatient referrals. If all office-based practices are included, IBS is the seventh most common diagnosis, with a rate of 10.6 patient visits per thousand population per year.[2] IBS is the second leading cause of absenteeism after the common cold.[3] Although usually considered to be an outpatient disorder, IBS was the major discharge diagnosis in 96,000 hospitalized patients as recently as 1976.[4] However, as awareness of the disease has increased and hospital admission criteria have become stricter, hospital admissions for IBS have markedly decreased over the past decade.[5] Classically, IBS is considered a disorder of young people, especially in whites, with the majority of new cases presenting in patients younger than 45 years of age

---

TABLE 81-1
Criteria for Diagnosing Irritable Bowel Syndrome

At least 3 months of the following continuous recurrent symptoms:
   Abdominal pain or discomfort that is relieved by defecation or is associated with change in frequency or consistency of stool
                         and
Disturbed defecation involving two or more of the following characteristics at least 25% of the time:
   Altered stool frequency
   Altered stool form (e.g., lumpy or hard, or loose or watery)
   Altered stool passage (e.g., straining, urgency, or feeling of incomplete evacuation)
   Passage of mucus
   Bloating or feeling of abdominal distention

(Fig. 81-1).[2] However, recent epidemiologic studies suggest that the elderly are troubled by IBS symptoms up to 92% as often as middle-aged persons.[6] Indeed, patients older than 65 years of age make approximately 500,000 physician visits per year for care of IBS.[7] It has been postulated that many of the diagnoses of "painful diverticular disease" given to elderly patients in fact represent IBS.[8] Women are diagnosed with IBS at 2.4 times the rate of men, although this may be related to a greater tendency of women to seek medical care for abdominal symptom complexes.[2,9,10]

The number of IBS patients seeking medical care is dwarfed by the actual number of individuals who experience symptoms of IBS. Using mailed questionnaires, investigators have found that approximately 25% of healthy persons have more than six episodes of abdominal pain per year and that 14% to 24% of the population complain of chronic constipation or diarrhea.[11,12] Using strict clinical criteria, 9% to 22% of the population note symptoms which would be considered diagnostic for IBS, yet most studies find that only a small fraction (9%–33%) of these individuals seek medical attention, suggesting that other factors are important in the decision to obtain the advice of a physician.[11-14]

CLINICAL FEATURES

Gastrointestinal Symptoms

IBS is a heterogeneous disorder with numerous different symptom presentations. Different subsets of IBS can be devised, based on the dominant symptom or symptoms, to aid in the evaluation and treatment of the IBS patient, but the hallmark of IBS remains the presence of chronic symptoms of abdominal pain or disturbances in bowel function.

Abdominal Pain

The intensity and location of abdominal pain in IBS are highly variable, even at different times within a single patient. In one report, the pain of IBS was localized to the hypogastric area in 25%, to the right side in 20%, to the left side in 20%, and to the epigastrium in 10% of patients.[15] Although it may be so mild as to be ignored, the abdominal pain of IBS is often severe enough to interfere with daily activities. Despite this, malnutrition caused by inadequate caloric intake is exceedingly rare with painful IBS. Similarly, sleep deprivation solely as a result of IBS is unusual because abdominal pain is almost always present only during waking hours. Abdominal pain is usually characterized as crampy or as a generalized ache with superimposed periods of abdominal cramps, although sharp, dull, gas-like, or nondescript pains are also common.[16]

Several factors exacerbate or reduce the pain of IBS. Many IBS patients report increased symptoms during periods of stress or emotional upset such as job or marital difficulties. Defecation may provide temporary relief from the abdominal pain of IBS, whereas ingestion of food may exacerbate the discomfort, usually 60 to 90 minutes after the meal. Pain that is progressive, that prevents sleep, that leads to anorexia or inability to eat, or that is associated with weight loss is not

Females

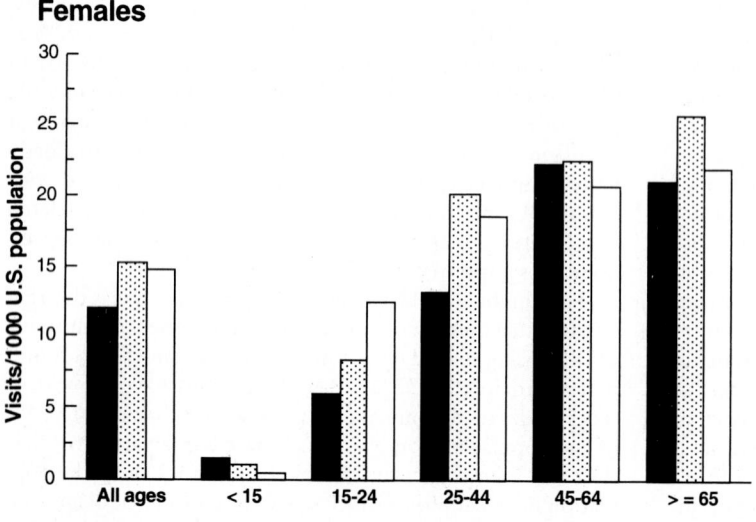

Males

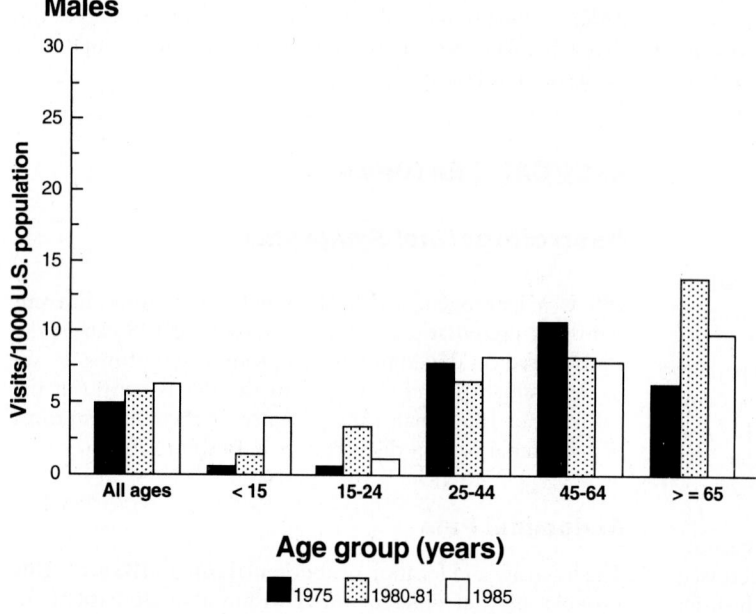

Age group (years)

■ 1975   ▨ 1980-81   □ 1985

FIGURE 81-1. Estimated rates of visits to office-based physicians of patients with the diagnosis of irritable bowel syndrome per 1000 US population per year. (From Everhart JE, Renault PF. Irritable bowel syndrome in office-based practice in the United States. Gastroenterology 1991;100:998–1005.)

consistent with IBS and warrants evaluation for other organic disease.

Alteration in Bowel Habits

The range of normal defecatory patterns is broad. In a combined series of 1455 subjects from a British industrial community and general medical practice, 99% reported a defecation frequency of between three per week and three per day, documenting a wide range of normal in an unselected population.[17] Nonetheless, complaints of altered bowel habits are almost uniformly volunteered by IBS patients. Chaudhary and Truelove first distinguished between patients with spastic abdominal pain and alterations in defecation, which represented 83% of their group, and patients with painless diarrhea, which was noted by 17% of their population.[16] Because this report was released in 1962, it is possible that many patients with painless and pain-associated diarrhea in their population exhibited manifestations of other diseases, such as lactase de-

ficiency or microscopic or collagenous colitis, which were poorly understood at the time but are now known to cause "functional" diarrhea. Nonetheless, it is well recognized that IBS patients present with either constipation, diarrhea, or constipation alternating with diarrhea. With constipation, stools usually are hard and may be scybalous or pellet-like. Long periods of straining on the toilet may be required to note a satisfactory stool passage, especially in constipation-predominant cases but also with some diarrhea-prone patients.[18] Constipation can persist for weeks to months, interrupted by brief periods of diarrhea. A sensation of incomplete fecal evacuation may lead the IBS patient to make multiple attempts at stool passage over a short span of time. In diarrhea-prone patients, the stools characteristically are loose and frequent but of normal total daily volume, and they may or may not be associated with pain. Usually, diarrheal stools occur only during waking hours, often early in the day, and an urgent desire to defecate after a meal is often noted, being reported in 36% of IBS patients in one study.[19] Mucus discharge has been reported in up to 50% of IBS patients.[19] As with complaints of abdominal pain, patients may experience fecal urgency and loose stools during periods of stress. Complaints that are noted more frequently in IBS than in organic gastrointestinal disease include relief of abdominal pain with defecation, looser stools at the onset of pain, and more frequent stools at the onset of pain.[20] Symptoms that are not associated with IBS include nocturnal diarrhea, rectal bleeding, malabsorption, and weight loss. The presence of any of these symptoms should prompt a thorough evaluation for organic disease.

Other Gastrointestinal Symptoms

Symptoms of upper gastrointestinal dysfunction are common in IBS, with 25% to 50% of patients reporting heartburn, early satiety, nausea, and vomiting and up to 87% noting intermittent dyspepsia. Many IBS patients note a sensation of increased gas production and abdominal distention, although the majority do not, in fact, produce excessive amounts of gas.[21] A study comparing abdominal dimensions of IBS patients to those of healthy volunteers using computerized tomography did indeed show increased lateral profiles in the IBS group, although no increases in visceral gas retention were seen.[22] The authors postulated that the demonstrable finding of abdominal distention in their patient group resulted from changes in gastrointestinal motility or tone.

Extraintestinal Symptoms

Although symptoms referable to the gastrointestinal tract predominate, extraintestinal complaints are commonly reported by IBS patients. Compared with healthy individuals, patients with functional gastrointestinal disorders visit primary care physicians three times as often for nongastrointestinal problems.[23,24] Additionally, patients with functional gastrointestinal complaints are more likely to have undergone hysterectomy or appendectomy.[25,9] A high incidence of genitourinary dysfunction, including dysmenorrhea, dyspareunia, impotence, urinary frequency, nocturia, and a sensation of incomplete bladder emptying, has been noted, including one study in which 83% of IBS patients experienced impaired sexual function, compared with 30% of inflammatory bowel disease patients and 16% of peptic ulcer patients.[16,26] Two groups have noted an association between IBS and primary fibromyalgia, with approximately two thirds of IBS patients reporting rheumatologic symptoms. In a telephone survey, patients with functional bowel disorders reported a higher incidence of peptic ulcer disease, hypertension, low back pain, headaches, and rashes than the general population.[27] Finally, IBS patients often report nonspecific fatigue, loss of concentration, insomnia, palpitations, and an unpleasant taste in the mouth.[15,28]

PATHOPHYSIOLOGY

The pathogenesis of IBS is poorly understood, although investigators have postulated roles for abnormal gut motor and sensory activity as well as for stress and psychologic disturbances. The following sections detail the current state of knowledge about what causes or contributes to symptoms in IBS. Unfortunately, despite intensive investigation, there remains no one abnormality that clearly separates IBS from organic gastrointestinal disease or even from normal bowel function.

Gastrointestinal Motor Abnormalities

Role of Abnormal Colonic Motor Activity

Before discussing the role of colon motor abnormalities in the pathogenesis of IBS, the normal myoelectric and motor physiology of the colon should be reviewed. Two types of myoelectrical activity are documented in the colon, slow waves and spike potentials. Slow waves, also referred to as electrical control activity, serve to regulate the frequencies of some colonic contractions, whereas spike potentials increase the membrane potential above the threshold needed for initiation of contraction.[29] In contrast to slow wave activity in the small intestine and stomach, colonic slow wave frequencies in normal volunteers are extremely variable, ranging from 2 to 13 cycles per minute (cpm) in different anatomic regions and at different times.[29,30] Spike potentials may occur in the form of short spike bursts (SSB), alternately known as electrical response activity, which are patterns of 5 to 15 seconds' duration temporally in phase with the slow wave (Fig. 81-2). Additionally, long spike bursts (LSB), alternately referred to as the contractile electrical complex, are spike potential patterns which last 15 to 60 seconds and are unrelated to the slow wave (see Fig. 81-2).[10,31,32] SSBs are the electrical patterns responsible for short-duration contractions in the colon, whereas LSBs lead to generation of long-duration contractions. Short-duration contractions and most long-duration contractions are nonpropagating and are believed to represent the segmenting activity that mixes and increases resistance to fecal flow.[29] Some long-duration contractions, however, are propagative and may result in propulsion of feces in both oral and aboral directions. Long-duration contractile activity is generally maximal after meals and disappears during sleep, but short-duration contractions persist throughout the day and night.[32] A third motor pattern, the giant migrating contraction, is a high-amplitude, intensely propagative contraction that usually begins in the right colon and results in mass movements of feces and defecation.[29] Giant migrating contractions occur only once or twice a day in healthy volunteers; their role in IBS is unknown. Most measurements of colonic motor function in IBS patients or healthy controls have employed lumenally placed rectosigmoid manometry catheters. Manometry tracings at adjacent 5-cm recording sites in the sigmoid rarely document progressive or simultaneous motor activity, and therefore most studies of colonic motor activity in IBS measure segmenting activity, which would serve to delay the passage of the fecal bolus, and not propagative movements.[33]

Studies of colonic myoelectrical and motor activity under unstimulated conditions have not yielded consistent abnormalities in IBS. Snape described a predominant 3-cpm slow wave cycling pattern in IBS patients, in both diarrhea- and constipation-predominant patients, associated with increased

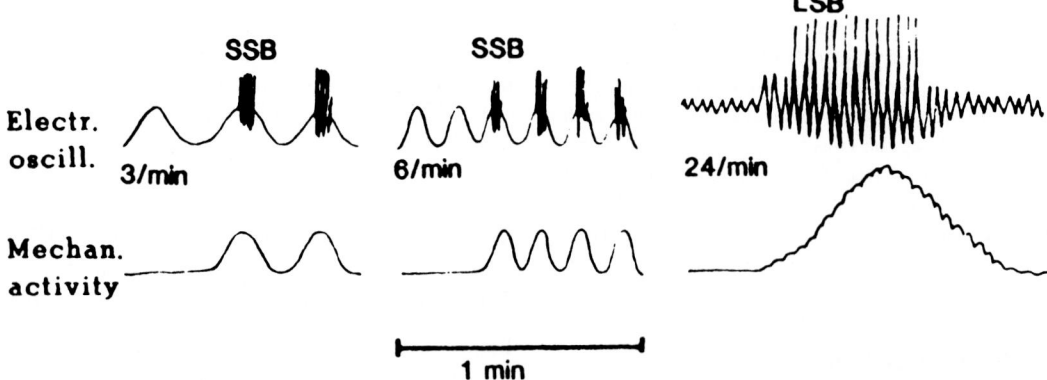

FIGURE 81-2. Colonic myoelectric (*top*) and motor (*bottom*) activity in normal individuals. Short spike bursts (SSB) occur in phase with the colonic slow wave and induce contractions with a maximal frequency equal to the colonic slow wave. Long spike bursts (LSB) are prolonged bursts of electrical activity that induce intense, prolonged contractile activity that is not in phase with the slow wave. (From Abrahamsson H. Gastrointestinal motility in patients with the irritable bowel syndrome. Scand J Gastroenterol (Suppl) 1987;130:21–26.)

3-cpm motor activity, in contrast to a 6-cpm pattern noted in his normal controls.[34,35] Other investigators were not able to reproduce these findings, because the normal colonic slow-wave pattern is so variable. Furthermore, Latimer found that the slow-wave abnormalities noted by Snape could also be demonstrated in psychoneurotic patients without bowel symptoms, suggesting that the myoelectrical disturbance was neither diagnostic for IBS nor particularly meaningful from symptom standpoint.[36] Some investigators have proposed that IBS can be categorized based on the spike potential pattern, although this is not universally accepted. Bueno reported that patients with constipation-predominant disease exhibit an increased number of SSBs but diarrhea-prone patients have reduced SSB activity.[31] Most investigators have shown no reproducible motor abnormalities in the colon under basal conditions, although Welgen and Latimer reported increases in basal motility.[34–38] More recently, colonic scintigraphy has provided means for the noninvasive assessment of regional colon transit using physiologic radiolabeled compounds. Using this technique, investigators demonstrated selective acceleration in right colon transit in some IBS patients with diarrhea.[39] It is unknown whether this represents a marker for a pathogenic motor abnormality in IBS or if all diarrhea patients exhibit this finding. No similar studies have been reported in constipation-predominant IBS, although patients with idiopathic constipation exhibit delayed right colon transit.[40]

In contrast to studies of the unstimulated colon, colonic motor abnormalities are more easily demonstrated under stimulated conditions in IBS. Rectosigmoid myoelectrical and manometric studies show a characteristic pattern in response to a meal. In normal volunteers, ingestion of a meal induces a rapid increase in spike potential and contractile activity. The frequency of spike potential activity begins to increase 10 minutes after ingestion of the meal and returns to basal at 50 minutes.[31] The amplitude and frequency of motor activity increase 20 to 30 minutes after a solid meal, decrease to a basal level at 1 hour, and may exhibit a second increase at 80 minutes (Fig. 81-3). Manometric recordings in IBS show

increased rectosigmoid motor activity, which may persist up to 3 hours after ingestion of a meal (see Fig. 81-3).[32,41] The onset of this increased activity may be delayed or blunted in some IBS patients. Although these patterns are characteristic of diarrhea-prone patients, constipated IBS patients also exhibit an exaggerated gastrocolonic response, albeit to a lesser degree.[42] In contrast to healthy volunteers, sham feeding induces increased rectosigmoid motility in IBS, suggesting the presence of a cephalic phase for the gastrocolonic response.[43–45] Provocative stimuli induce exaggerated colonic motor responses in IBS patients compared with healthy volunteers. Inflation of rectal balloons in IBS patients leads to marked distention-evoked contractile activity, especially in diarrhea-predominant patients but also in some constipated patients.[32,46] In addition to the immediate contractile response, IBS patients may experience ten or more delayed contractions after rectal distention. Patients with painful IBS exhibit greater increases in rectosigmoid motility after cholinergic stimulation than do patients with painless diarrhea.[47] Intravenous cholecystokinin induces painful rectosigmoid contractions which reproduce the presenting symptoms in a subset of IBS patients complaining of postprandial pain.[48] An exaggerated colonic motor response can be demonstrated in IBS patients after perfusion of deoxycholic acid within the colon.[49] These studies suggest that characteristic disturbances in colonic myoelectrical and motor activity can be demonstrated in different subsets of IBS, especially under conditions in which the colon is stimulated.

Role of Abnormal Small Bowel Motor Activity

As with the colon, investigators have examined motor activity in the small intestine to search for pathognomonic abnormalities in IBS. In contrast to the colon, motility patterns in the small intestine under unstimulated conditions are organized and well characterized. The major small intestine motor pattern in the interdigestive period is the migrating motor complex (MMC), which consists of three phases cycling every

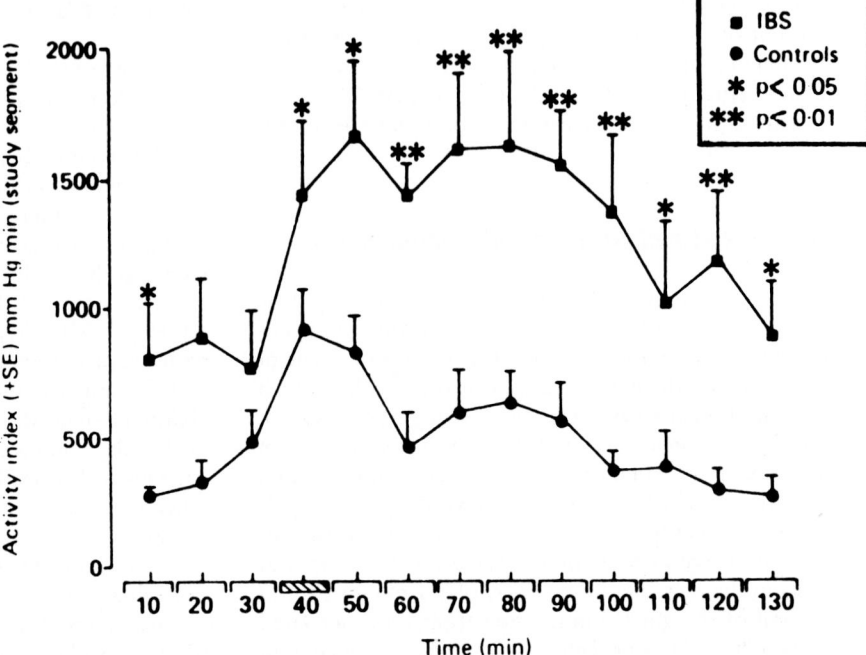

FIGURE 81-3. Colonic motor activity after ingestion of a 1040 kcal meal is plotted as a function of time in normal controls and irritable bowel syndrome (IBS) patients. IBS patients exhibited both an increased amplitude and a prolonged duration of the gastrocolonic response, in some cases persisting for up to 3 hours. (From Rogers J, Henry MM, Misiewicz JJ. Increased segmental activity and intraluminal pressures in the sigmoid colon of patients with the irritable bowel syndrome. Gut 1989;30:634–641.)

90 to 120 minutes that serve to cleanse the proximal gut of undigested debris.[50] Studies employing continuous manometry have suggested subtle abnormalities in fasting small intestine motility. Kellow and colleagues demonstrated decreases in the amplitudes of the phases of the MMC in constipation-predominant IBS patients and reductions in MMC cycle length in diarrhea-predominant individuals; however, these abnormalities have not been universally described.[51,52] Interdigestive intestinal motility was normal during sleep. Other physiologic motor patterns include discrete clustered contractions (DCC), also known as the minute rhythm, which are clusters of phasic contractions occurring roughly every minute in the duodenum or jejunum, and prolonged propagated contractions (PPC), which are intense complexes originating in the ileum that serve to clear the ileum and prevent coloileal reflux.[50] DCCs and PPCs occur infrequently, often less than once a day, and at irregular intervals in healthy volunteers. In IBS patients, DCCs and PPCs occur more often and make up a larger fraction of fasting recording time.[18,53] Although these studies show quantitative but not qualitative differences in intestinal motor patterns between IBS patients and normal individuals, it is unlikely that these complexes have pathogenic significance because they are similar in patients with constipation and with diarrhea.

As in the colon, motor abnormalities of the small intestine under stimulated conditions have been described in IBS. The fed motor pattern, a period of intense irregular phasic contractions that occurs for 2 to 3 hours after a meal, is the most important of these stimulated conditions. In both constipation- and diarrhea-predominant IBS, the duration of the fed pattern has been shown to be shorter than in healthy volunteers.[18] Other stimuli have been used to study small intestine motor abnormalities in IBS. Intravenous cholecystokinin produces exaggerated high-amplitude ileal contractions in diarrhea-predominant IBS patients, whereas the anticholin-

esterase neostigmine induces frequent DCCs in both diarrhea-predominant and constipated patients.[54] In addition to manometry, transit of a meal through the small intestine has been studied using radioactive technetium tracers. Using this technique, intestinal transit of a meal is delayed in patients with constipation or distention plus abdominal pain. In contrast, transit is characteristically accelerated in diarrhea-predominant IBS patients.[8] Similarly, using radiolabeled bran, investigators have demonstrated delayed emptying of the ileum and decreased ileocecal clearance in IBS patients compared with healthy individuals.[55] Therefore, IBS is associated with abnormal motor patterns, especially under stimulated conditions, throughout the gut.

Other Motor Abnormalities

In addition to disturbances seen in the large and small intestine, IBS is associated with motor abnormalities in other smooth muscle sites in the body. Esophageal manometry reveals decreased lower esophageal sphincter pressures as well as abnormalities in esophageal peristalsis, including increased spontaneous motor activity, repetitive contractions, and simultaneous waves in the esophageal body.[32,56] In contrast, the upper esophageal sphincter, which is striated muscle, exhibits no manometric abnormalities in IBS. In the stomach, gastric slow-wave dysrhythmias (tachygastria, bradygastria) have been reported in dyspeptic patients with symptoms of IBS.[32] Fasting gallbladder volumes and residual volumes after contraction are greater in IBS patients, although there is no increase in gallbladder disease with IBS.[57] One study has reported that constipation-predominant patients exhibit enhanced gallbladder contraction and patients with diarrhea exhibit impaired contraction compared with controls.[58] Outside of the gut, urodynamic studies have been employed to demonstrate abnormal bladder function with IBS. Detrusor instability was noted in 10 of 30 IBS patients, compared with 1 of 10 controls.[59] Similarly, IBS patients exhibit hyperreactive airway function after administration of the smooth muscle stimulant methacholine.[60] These findings suggest IBS is a disorder with diffuse disturbances in smooth muscle motor activity.

Gastrointestinal Sensory Abnormalities

The studies mentioned in the previous sections would be meaningless if they could not be related to the symptoms being experienced by the IBS patient, and a major focus of investigators is on the perceptual abnormalities in IBS which lead to sensations of pain, gas, or bloating. Perception of abdominal symptoms is accomplished through activation of a complex afferent neural pathway by visceral stimuli acting on chemoreceptors (which sense osmolarity, temperature, pH, and so on), mechanoreceptors (which are located in the gut wall and discharge in response to changes in tension), and receptors in the mesentery which may play a role in painful stimulation of the gut.[61] Information from these activated receptors is carried in spinal afferent nerves which synapse in the dorsal horn of the spinal cord. From there, the impulses are transmitted to the brain, where perception occurs.[61] It has been postulated that IBS results from sensitization of afferent pathways such that normal physiologic gut stimuli, which are not perceived by healthy individuals, induce pain in the IBS patient. An experimental model for such an afferent sensitization comes from studies from Japan of the compound clioquinol, which causes subacute myelooptic neuropathy as well as abdominal pain, constipation, and bloating. Studies of testicular nerves show that clioquinol can sensitize afferent pathways to subsequent stimulation such that other insults such as mechanical or thermal irritation are perceived much more severely.[62] Although it is unknown what might sensitize visceral afferents in IBS, this hypothesis remains intriguing and worthy of further investigation.

Disturbed Sensation Under Basal Conditions

A number of studies have looked at the temporal association of myoelectrical and motor disturbances with abdominal pain and other symptoms. Myoelectrical recordings have shown good correlation between the appearance of intense fused colonic SSB and abdominal pain in constipation-predominant IBS patients, inferring a colonic source of pain.[32] Studies of jejunal motility have noted irregular contractile activity coincident with the development of abdominal pain, although some investigators have detected no abnormal motor patterns.[62–64] Kellow reported that 61% of PPCs were associated with symptoms in IBS patients, compared with 17% in controls.[53] Similarly, the presence of DCCs in association with abdominal pain was reported in 4 of 12 IBS patients but in no healthy volunteers (Fig. 81-4).[53] More recently, Kellow has shown that nearly half of patients with IBS can perceive different phases of the MMC as discomfort, a tugging sensation, or frank pain.[18] These studies suggest that, in contrast to healthy individuals, IBS patients possess the ability to sense physiologic motor events in the gastrointestinal tract.

These findings may provide a partial explanation for older studies postulating a role for intestinal gas in the generation of unpleasant abdominal symptoms. It was once believed that patients with abdominal symptoms but no structural lesions had abnormal amounts or distributions of intestinal gas as a source of their pain. Early investigators described an entity called the splenic flexure syndrome which consisted of severe abdominal pain, usually in the left upper quadrant, that was associated with apparent collections of gas in the splenic flexure on abdominal radiographs.[65] Relief could be obtained by defecation, passage of flatus, or administration of an enema, and symptoms were reproducible by inflation of a balloon in the splenic flexure. Subsequent studies have shown that the absolute volume of gas in patients who complain of gas and bloating is normal. In a study by Levitt using a washout technique, the total volume of intestinal gas was similar in asymptomatic individuals and in subjects with complaints of excess

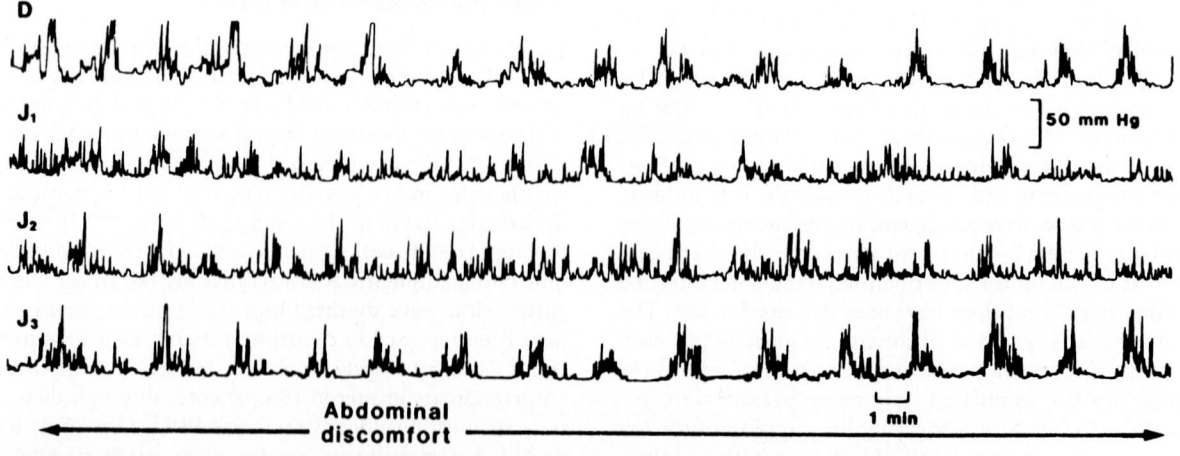

FIGURE 81-4. Manometric recordings of intraluminal pressure from the jejunum of a patient with irritable bowel syndrome shows 30 minutes of discrete clustered contractions in the duodenum and jejunum which were associated with discomfort. (D, duodenal pressure recording; J$_1$, J$_2$, J$_3$, jejunal pressure recordings; from Kellow JE, Phillips SF. Altered small bowel motility in irritable bowel syndrome is correlated with symptoms. Gastroenterology 1987;92:1885–1893.)

gas.[21] Furthermore, the transit time for infused gas to reach the rectum was the same in both groups. The only significant differences between the two groups were that patients with complaints of excess gas refluxed more gas from the intestine to the stomach and complained of distention and pain at low volumes of gas infusion that did not affect the controls (Fig. 81-5). In addition to showing possible abnormal propulsion of intestinal gas, this report demonstrates an abnormal sensitivity to the presence of physiologic amounts of gas in the intestine in patients with functional symptoms.

Disturbed Sensation Under Stimulated Conditions

As with studies of motor activity, IBS patients frequently exhibit exaggerated sensory responses on visceral stimulation. Postprandial symptoms in IBS are associated with characteristic motor patterns. Cann reported that postprandial pain was temporally related to entry of the food bolus into the cecum in 74% of patients.[8] A subgroup of patients with non-ulcer dyspepsia and IBS experienced postprandial abdominal pain in association with increased pressure activity in the rectosigmoid.[33] Using radiotelemetry capsules in the jejunum, food has been shown to induce bursts of intestinal pressure activity that correlate temporally with periods of abdominal pain.[66]

Exaggerated symptoms in IBS can be induced by visceral distention. Inflation of a rectal balloon produces nonpainful and painful sensations at significantly lower volumes in IBS

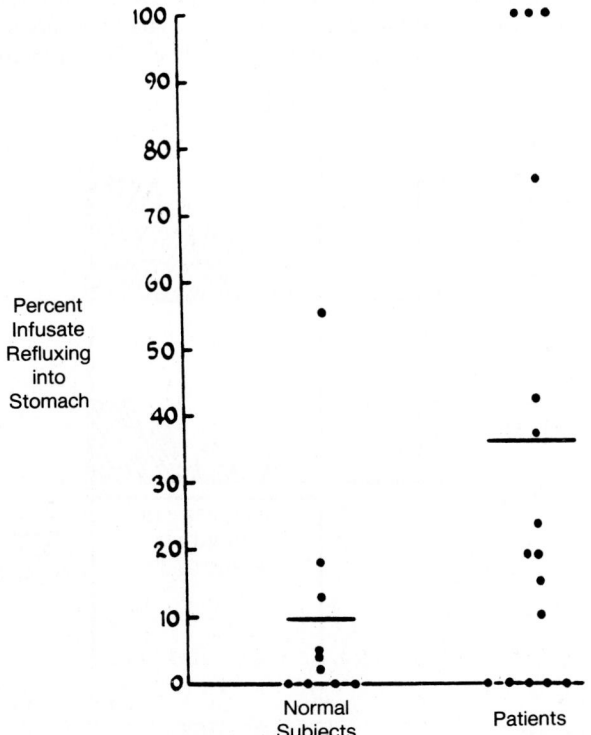

FIGURE 81-5. Percentage of gas infused into the intestine that refluxed back into the stomach was greater in patients with complaints of abdominal pain than in normal subjects. (From Lasser RB, Bond JH, Levitt MD. The role of intestinal gas in functional abdominal pain. N Engl J Med 1975;293:524–526.)

patients than in healthy controls, but with no associated changes in rectal wall tension, suggesting that afferent pathways which mediate perception of uncomfortable sensations are disturbed in IBS.[67] This visceral hypersensitivity was initially seen in both constipation- and diarrhea-predominant patients and correlated well with studies showing gastric and esophageal perceptual hypersensitivity in patients with non-ulcer dyspepsia and noncardiac chest pain, respectively.[67,68] More recently, investigators have reported that IBS patients can be categorized into three groups based on the response to rectal distention.[69] These include patients with a sensitive rectum, a low sensory threshold to distention, and normal to low intrarectal pressures; patients with a stiff rectum, normal to low sensory thresholds, and high pressures; and patients with an insensitive rectum, a high sensory threshold, and normal or high pressures (Fig. 81-6). The sensitive rectum subtype was found in 57% of diarrhea-predominant patients but only 7% of patients with constipation.[69] Diarrhea-predominant patients exhibited abnormal balloon distention responses in 75% of cases, compared with 30% in patients with constipation, suggesting that, although quite common, visceral sensory abnormalities are not universal in IBS. Intralumenal balloon inflation of the stomach, small intestine, or colon can reproduce presenting complaints of abdominal pain, bloating, and fecal urgency.[29,70,71] However, in contrast to healthy controls who experience discomfort localized to only one quadrant after colonic balloon inflation, patients with IBS experience symptoms diffusely with pain in the right upper and lower quadrants, right flank, hypochondrium, and epigastrium as well as in the back, shoulders, thighs, and chest.[70] These studies indicate that, in addition to exhibiting greater levels of discomfort for a given level of distention, IBS patients experience abnormal anatomic distributions of pain, suggesting diffuse disturbances of afferent function.

Other provocative stimuli have been employed to provide insight into the mechanisms responsible for symptoms in IBS. Stimulation of rectosigmoid or small bowel activity by cholinergic agonists or cholecystokinin induces pain in some patients.[10,66] In contrast to enhanced sensitivity of the gastrointestinal tract to hormonal and physical stimulation, IBS patients may experience reduced sensitivity elsewhere in the body. Using electrocutaneous stimulation, investigators demonstrated that individuals with IBS or Crohn's disease had higher touch and pain thresholds than a matched group of normal volunteers.[72] The afferent pathway disturbances found in IBS span a wide variety of intralumenal and neurohormonal stimuli, but the defects appear to be selective for visceral sensory innervation with sparing of somatic pathways.

Effects of Stress on Visceral Motor and Sensory Function

The role of the central nervous system in the mediation of physiologic function has intrigued researchers for decades. Because stress is an important promoter or enhancer of symptoms in IBS, the work of these investigators may be pivotal in the understanding of the pathophysiology of IBS. The early studies by Almy reinforce the importance of the brain-gut axis in the regulation of colonic activities. While observing the colonic response through a proctoscope, he studied the

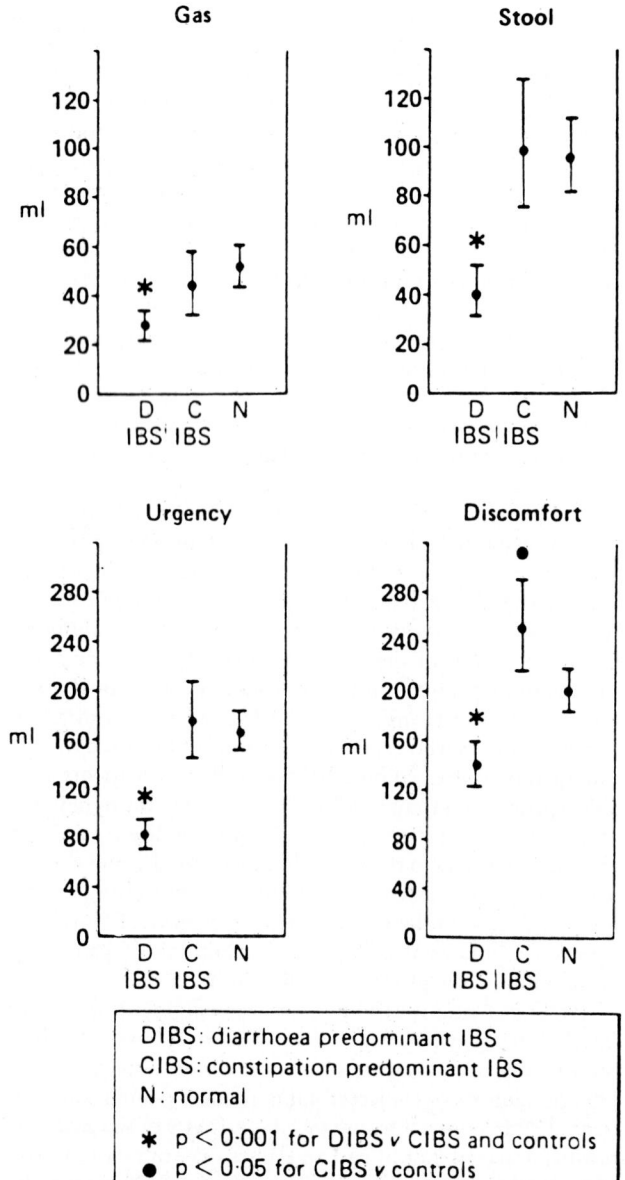

FIGURE 81-6. Comparison of rectal sensory thresholds for perception of gas, stool, fecal urgency, and rectal discomfort in diarrhea-predominant irritable bowel syndrome (IBS) patients, constipation-predominant IBS patients, and normal controls. Diarrhea-predominant patients noted all levels of perception at lower volumes than controls, suggesting sensory hypersensitivity. Constipated patients, in contrast, were more similar to healthy controls, although volumes required to elicit discomfort were greater. (From Prior A, Maxton DG, Whorwell PJ. Anorectal manometry in irritable bowel syndrome: differences between diarrhea and constipation predominant patients. Gut 1990;31:458–462.)

a medical student during a proctoscopic examination that a rectal cancer had been found.[74] The medical student was then shown a piece of potato which he was told was a biopsy of the alleged malignancy. As with the painful stimuli, the rectal wall exhibited intense contractions and reddening of the mucosa, which disappeared when the hoax was revealed (Fig. 81-7). Almy also studied patients with symptoms consistent with IBS. In seven constipated subjects and eight with diarrhea, changes in rectosigmoid motility were inducible with stressful interviews.[75] Increased motor activity was observed with hostile or aggressive reactions, whereas passive reactions or dejection led to relative motor quiescence. More recently, stressors such as anger, ball sorting, and stimulus differentiation testing have been shown to cause increases in colonic motility or spike potential activity in IBS patients and controls.[37,38,76]

In addition to its effects on the colon, stressful stimuli induce physiologic responses elsewhere in the gastrointestinal tract. In the stomach, vertigo induced by vestibular stimulation with cold water infusion into the external ear leads to delayed gastric emptying and conversion of a fed motor pattern to a fasting pattern.[77] In the small bowel, barium studies performed on subjects during stressful interviews show segmentation, widening of the mucosal folds, and areas of distention.[78] Goin performed serial barium studies on a Jewish woman who insisted she followed no religious restrictions in her diet but complained of a pork allergy which caused nausea, pain, and diarrhea.[79] When the patient was fed pork followed by barium, spasm and segmentation of the small bowel barium column was noted. In contrast, when ground pork was mixed in with the barium solution without the patient's knowledge, a normal radiographic pattern was seen, suggesting that her perception of what she had ingested modified the contractile

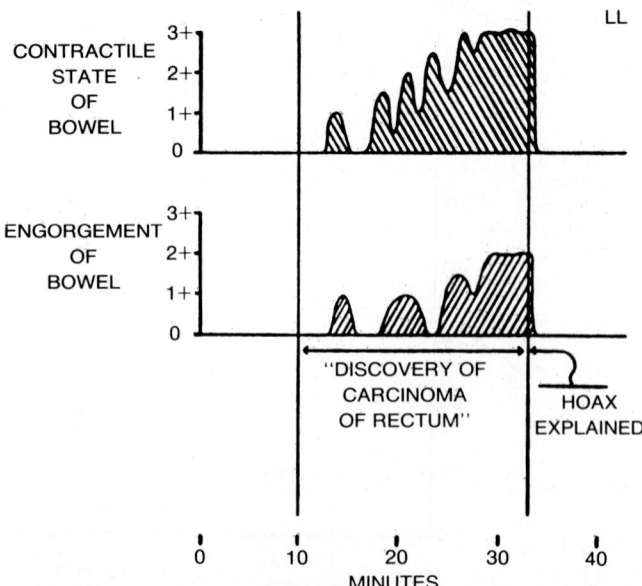

FIGURE 81-7. Changes in rectosigmoid motility and engorgement in a medical student during a hoax in which he was falsely led to believe carcinoma had been discovered. (From Almy TP. Experimental studies on the irritable colon. Am J Med 1951;10: 60–67.)

effects of painful stimuli such as forearm immersion in ice water or use of a device called a headscrew in which screws in a circumferential metal band around the forehead were successively tightened until they induced severe headaches.[73] Induction of pain led to engorgement of the rectal mucosa and intense muscular spasm. Psychologic stressors were employed to induce the same effect. One hoax involved telling

pattern of her small bowel. In a recent report, psychologic stress with intense participation in a video game or driving in rush hour traffic decreased cycling of the intestinal MMC in healthy volunteers.[80] In contrast, nocturnal stress induced by repetitively waking the subjects from a sound sleep did not alter small bowel motility despite being perceived by the subjects as more stressful than the daytime stressors. This suggests that small bowel motility is regulated in a different manner depending on whether a person is awake or asleep. The relative effects of stress on small intestine motility in IBS patients compared with healthy individuals have been a matter of controversy. In a comparison of IBS patients with controls using radiotelemetry capsules in the small bowel, long periods of mental stress induced motor abnormalities in 19 of 22 IBS patients compared with 1 of 10 controls.[64] In 7 patients, MMC cycling was eliminated, and in 18 patients, there were episodes of irregular motor activity lasting from 1 to 6 hours that altered the normal cycling frequency. In contrast, Kellow showed equivalent suppression of MMC activity in IBS patients and controls.[81] Furthermore, he demonstrated inhibition, rather than induction, of DCCs in both subject groups, suggesting that IBS patients may not be more susceptible to stress than asymptomatic controls.

These studies demonstrate convincingly that motor activity in the gastrointestinal tract is closely dependent on central nervous system events. It is now apparent that the central nervous system also modifies visceral perception through unknown mechanisms that suppress or enhance afferent impulses from the gastrointestinal tract.[61] In a study of 15 IBS patients, hypnosis reduced perception of rectal distention in diarrhea-predominant patients, with a lesser effect on constipated patients.[82] The lack of effect of hypnotherapy on rectal compliance or motor activity suggested that afferent pathways were being actively suppressed by central nervous system activity.

The role of the brain-gut axis in the initiation or enhancement of motor and sensory abnormalities in IBS requires further study. Based on the absence of motility disturbances in sleep in IBS, Wingate has postulated that central nervous system arousal is required for symptoms to develop in IBS.[83] It is unknown whether IBS represents a primary gut disturbance with inappropriate input from the central nervous system or a central nervous system disorder with centrally directed changes in gut motor and sensory activity.[83] New technologies are being developed to study this issue. Using the technique of cerebral evoked potential recording, investigators have recently reported findings suggesting that peripheral afferent pathways stimulated by esophageal distention are not abnormal in noncardiac chest pain and that perceptual disturbances result from abnormalities in the central nervous system.[84] Similar studies in IBS are likely to be forthcoming.

Abnormal Psychiatric Features

Of the 25% of the population who experience bowel symptoms consistent with IBS, only a small fraction present to a physician for evaluation of their complaints. Investigators have attempted to characterize differences between symptomatic individuals who seek medical attention and those who do not, known as nonreporters. In one study, IBS patients exhibited more frequent abnormal personality patterns and greater illness behavior than symptomatic individuals who did not seek medical attention.[23] Nonreporters were intermediate in illness behavior and personality patterns and coped better with stress, experiencing their symptoms as less disruptive than individuals who sought medical care. A second study using psychometric inventories noted that IBS patients exhibited characteristics of psychiatric disturbances far in excess of the general population but that nonreporters were not different from asymptomatic individuals.[85] Patients with lactose intolerance were shown to have a prevalence of psychiatric diagnoses similar to that of IBS patients and greater than that of normal controls. The presence of abnormal psychiatric features is a major determinant of which symptomatic individuals present to a physician for medical care, and most symptomatic individuals without psychologic disturbances do not become IBS patients.

Abnormal psychiatric features have been recorded in up to 80% of patients with IBS, although formal diagnoses of mental illness are given in only a small fraction of cases.[2,67,86,87] IBS is reported by patients twice as often as other digestive diseases during visits for treatment of mental disorders.[2] Despite the high prevalence of psychologic disease in IBS, there is no single psychiatric diagnosis that predominates. The total lifetime incidences for major depression, somatization disorder, generalized anxiety disorder, panic disorder, and phobias are higher in IBS patients than in healthy controls.[88,89] However, recent studies note that major depression represents one third of all psychiatric diagnoses in IBS patients. Eighty percent of the original population described by Chaudhary and Truelove had underlying depression or anxiety, and another study reported hysteria or depression in 72% of IBS patients compared with 18% of normal volunteers.[16,87,90] An evaluation of 41 IBS patients showed an increase in scores for neuroticism and a decrease in extroversion compared with controls.[90] Additional psychiatric disorders associated with IBS include hostility, hypochondriasis, and increased interpersonal sensitivity.[67] Esler and Goulston found that only diarrhea-prone IBS patients are neurotic, whereas Whitehead found no differences in psychological profiles in diarrhea versus constipation-predominant patients.[67] Many of these psychiatric findings are similar to those noted with other chronic pain syndromes. Furthermore, investigators have found that psychiatric features predate or occur simultaneously with the onset of bowel symptoms in 67% to 85% of patients, suggesting that it is not the bowel symptoms of IBS which induce psychiatric disease.[67,85,91,92] Unfortunately, IBS patients with psychiatric disorders tend to respond less well to medical therapy than do patients without psychiatric features.

Current or recent stressful events have been observed to exacerbate symptoms in more than half of IBS patients, although the role of stress as a precipitant of IBS is not universally accepted.[16,93] Mendeloff found that stressful life events were more common in IBS patients compared with normal subjects or with ulcerative colitis patients. Chaudhary and Truelove noted a pattern of marital difficulties, interactive problems with children or parents, and career stresses to be more prevalent and severe in IBS patients; however, Hislop found no increase in life stresses in his study of IBS patients.[90] A history of severe emotional stress in the distant past or early in life often is elicited on careful questioning. Two studies have shown that loss of a parent, either through death or marital dissolution, was an important stressor in one third of patients.[94,95] A more recent survey of 206 women patients with functional bowel disorders reported a 44% incidence of physical or sexual abuse in childhood, which was 3 to 11 times the rate in a control population.[96] Recent or past life stressors may be more common in IBS patients than in the population as a whole, but they do not cause IBS in most patients, a finding which is supported by a recent prospective study.[97]

How a person responds to his or her symptoms determines whether he or she presents to a physician. Pain-predominant IBS patients view minor respiratory infections as more severe and seek medical care for less serious ailments than patients with peptic ulcer disease or asymptomatic volunteers.[27] IBS patients may have histories of more frequent and more serious illnesses as children resulting in school absences and pediatrician visits.[98] Furthermore, patients with IBS often report that gifts or treats were provided during periods of illness as children, suggesting that their expectations for illness behavior involve a form of reward.[27] These studies provide evidence that IBS patients view the "sick" role differently than do symptomatic individuals in the community who do not pursue medical evaluation.

Other Studies on Pathogenesis

Role of Malabsorption or Intolerance to Specific Foods

Several investigators have evaluated the role of carbohydrate malabsorption as a cause of bloating, pain, and diarrhea in IBS. Lactase deficiency is a well-described syndrome in which ingestion of milk products causes symptoms similar to those in IBS. A report of Mexican patients found that 8 of 12 patients diagnosed with IBS malabsorbed 12.5 g of lactose; however, symptoms were independent of lactase supplementation in a placebo-controlled trial, suggesting that lactase deficiency was not the cause of IBS in these patients.[99] The role of malabsorption of other sugars was studied in 25 patients with either IBS or complaints of excess gas.[100] Ingestion of fructose and sorbitol, two sugars found in fruits as well as soft drinks and candy, led to prominent symptoms in most subjects; however, dietary exclusion of these sugars to assess their causal role was not performed. More recently, studies of basal breath hydrogen levels in IBS patients revealed no excess gas production compared with controls, suggesting that carbohydrate malabsorption was not responsible for symptoms in these patients.[101] There is no firm evidence to implicate carbohydrate malabsorption as the cause of symptoms in the majority of IBS patients.

Intolerance to other foods has also been studied as a possible cause of IBS. Alun Jones reported on patients with diarrhea-predominant IBS who noticed symptom exacerbation after ingestion of wheat, dairy products, coffee, tea, or citrus fruits.[102] In 6 of 14 patients, a blinded challenge with the offending food led to worsening of the symptoms; this was associated with elevations in rectal prostaglandin E_2. The investigators concluded that food hypersensitivity was responsible for symptoms in a large subset of IBS patients. Subse-

quent studies, however, have reported that only a small fraction of diarrhea-prone IBS patients can expect improvement on an exclusion diet, which may not be greater than a placebo effect.[103,104] Even those individuals with positive skin test responses to particular foods have not shown diminution of their symptoms on dietary exclusion of those foods.[105] Although a small subset of diarrhea-predominant patients may indeed exhibit true food hypersensitivity and benefit from an exclusion diet, symptoms in the vast majority of IBS patients do not result from food intolerance.

Disturbed Neurohumoral Activity

The possibility of systemic disturbances in neural and hormonal activity in IBS has been addressed in several studies. Defects in efferent vagal nerve function have been suggested by reports showing reductions in vagally-mediated increases in lower esophageal sphincter pressure after abdominal compression, impaired pulse variability with inspiration, and reduced ratios of insulin-induced peak gastric acid output to pentagastrin-stimulated maximal acid output in subsets of IBS patients.[106] Studies revealing decreased digital temperatures and enhanced peripheral electromyographic activity have led investigators to postulate a diffuse autonomic neural disturbance in IBS.[107] A recent report of prolongation of rapid eye movement (REM) sleep with episodes of sleep apnea in IBS suggests that the central nervous system in IBS exhibits abnormalities outside of the brain-gut axis.[108] Blunting of α-adrenergic pathways in the central nervous system has been suggested by a report showing impaired growth hormone release in IBS patients, but not in ulcer patients or in healthy controls, in response to the α_2 receptor stimulant desipramine.[109] Hormonal disturbances have been postulated, but not proven, as a cause of symptoms in the subset of IBS patients who experience symptom exacerbations at the time of the menses.[25,110] Abnormal levels of circulating pancreatic polypeptide, neurotensin, insulin, motilin, and gastrin have been reported in some IBS patients.[111,112] The roles of subtle neurohumoral disturbances in the pathogenesis of IBS are unclear.

Abnormal Characteristics of the Stool

Abnormal characteristics of the fecal material have been postulated as inducers of symptoms in IBS. Because bile acids increase colonic motor activity in IBS, investigators have proposed that diarrhea-predominant IBS patients may have underlying bile acid malabsorption.[31] Bile acid–binding agents such as cholestyramine have been used in IBS with anecdotal reports of success; however, this may be a result of the general constipating effects of the resin. Others have proposed that elevated levels of short-chain fatty acids in the stools may mediate the diarrhea of IBS; however, symptoms have not correlated with fecal levels of these compounds.[113] Recently, disturbances in gut flora have been suggested as the cause of symptoms in IBS, and trials to modify the dominant colonic organisms have met with some success in reducing symptoms.[114,115] Nonetheless, these unsubstantiated reports do not offer convincing evidence that stool characteristics are abnormal in IBS.

DIAGNOSTIC APPROACH TO THE PATIENT WITH PRESUMED IBS

The diagnosis of IBS is based on the recognition of characteristic symptom patterns combined with the exclusion of organic gastrointestinal diseases which might have a more serious long-term prognosis. Symptoms reported by IBS patients are also common complaints in a number of other conditions. Organic disorders that result in abdominal pain and changes in bowel habits include malignancies, inflammatory diseases, infections, and ischemic diseases of the gastrointestinal tract as well as some nongastrointestinal conditions. Peptic ulcer disease, intestinal ischemia, and gastric or pancreatic carcinoma produce pain in the upper abdomen, whereas lower abdominal pain is more common with inflammatory bowel disease, colonic ischemia, diverticular disease, and colon carcinoma. Postprandial pain with bloating or nausea suggests possible gastroparesis or lumenal obstruction. Genitourinary diseases should be considered if there is pain in relation to the menstrual cycle or if there are abnormalities on urinalysis. Lactase deficiency, laxative abuse, malabsorption, hyperthyroidism, inflammatory bowel disease, parasitosis such as giardiasis, and infectious colitis should be considered in the patient with diarrhea. If constipation is an important symptom, hypothyroidism, hypercalcemia, colonic malignancies, and medication side effects from anticholinergics, antihypertensives, or antidepressants should be considered. Rare disorders such as lead poisoning or acute intermittent porphyria may present in a similar fashion to IBS; therefore, one must consider these possibilities in selected patients.

Historical Features

Although the differential diagnosis of the patient with presumed IBS is broad, there are historical features that can help differentiate IBS from organic disease. This issue was comprehensively addressed by Manning and colleagues, who distributed a questionnaire to 109 outpatients to determine which symptoms were selective for IBS and which for organic disease.[20] A prospective review of case records after 17 to 26 months revealed that four symptoms were significantly more common in IBS than in organic disease. These were relief of abdominal pain on defecation, looser stools with onset of pain, more frequent stools with the onset of pain, and abdominal distention. Ninety-one percent of IBS patients had two or more of these symptoms, compared with 30% of patients with organic disease. Other symptoms that were common in IBS patients included passage of mucus, a sensation of incomplete evacuation, fecal urgency, defecation before breakfast or at night or between meals, harder or less frequent stools at pain onset, and pain eased by passage of flatus; however, these symptoms did not differentiate IBS from organic disease. A similar study by Kruis and colleagues investigated patients with abdominal pain, flatulence, and altered bowel habits.[116] Symptoms that were found to correlate with the absence of organic disease included the combination of pain, flatulence, and irregular defecation; symptoms persisting for more than 2 years; pain described as burning, cutting, very strong, or terrible; a defecation pattern of alternating defecation and constipation; pencil-like or pellet-like stools; and

the passage of mucus in the stools. Although these historical criteria suggest symptom profiles for IBS that are distinct from those for organic disease, the history alone is often inadequate for a confident diagnosis. A report studying the diagnostic value of the Manning criteria found that IBS could be differentiated from organic disease with a sensitivity of only 58% and a specificity of 74%.[117] Additionally, IBS was differentiable from all non-IBS gastrointestinal diseases with a sensitivity of 42%. Further investigations suggest that the Manning criteria are considerably more reliable for the diagnosis of IBS in women than in men.[118] In the evaluation of the patient with presumed IBS, a careful history should be complemented with a thorough physical examination and judicious use of laboratory and structural tests.

Physical Findings

In general, the physical examination of the patient with IBS is unimpressive. The patient may appear anxious and may have cold, clammy hands. Abdominal compression often elicits tenderness which may be vague and poorly localized. In one report, a tender bowel loop was palpable in 45 of 50 patients with IBS.[9] Mass lesions, lymphadenopathy, hepatosplenomegaly, jaundice, ascites, a succession splash, blood in the stool, and evidence of autonomic or peripheral neuropathy are suggestive of organic disease and are not compatible with the diagnosis of IBS.

Laboratory Studies and Structural Findings

In most instances, a minimal laboratory and structural evaluation should be performed to rule out organic gastrointestinal disease in the patient with presumed IBS. A complete blood count can assess for anemia, leukocytosis, or leukocytopenia, which are consistent with systemic disease but not IBS. Similarly, infectious processes, malignancy, or other inflammatory conditions may be indicated by an elevation in the sedimentation rate. It has been reported that the presence of symptoms consistent with IBS, the absence of historical features or physical findings of organic disease, and the presence of a normal complete blood count and sedimentation rate are 83% sensitive and 97% specific for the diagnosis of IBS.[15]

Sigmoidoscopy should be performed in most individuals with presumed IBS, regardless of whether the patient has diarrhea or constipation. In constipated patients, sigmoidoscopy serves to rule out distal obstructive lesions, and in diarrhea-prone patients, sigmoidoscopy can assess for inflammatory conditions of the colon that might mimic the symptoms of IBS. In these instances, random rectosigmoid biopsies should be performed to rule out microscopic or collagenous colitis, which usually presents with normal-appearing mucosa. In fact, sigmoidoscopy routinely shows normal anatomy in IBS, although increased mucus secretion or engorged mucosa may be apparent. Spasm on sigmoidoscopic examination is frequently reported and, in one study, sigmoidoscopy induced pain similar to the presenting symptoms in 40 of 41 IBS patients.[9] In addition to its diagnostic utility, performance of sigmoidoscopy may promote good patient-physician rapport by providing evidence that the physician is aggressively evaluating the patient's complaints.[15]

In most instances, the evaluation described is sufficient to rule out organic gastrointestinal diseases. Patients who might require additional evaluation are described in more detail in the sections on the approach to different subsets of IBS. Additionally, many clinicians recommend a complete colonic evaluation, either with air contrast barium enema or with colonoscopy, in any patient with the new onset of symptoms after the age of 40 to 45 years because of the increased likelihood of colonic neoplasm in this age group. Although usually normal in IBS, barium studies may show nonspecific findings such as areas of hypertonicity and spasm, regions of narrowing and segmentation, and increased and irregular haustra.[19]

TREATMENT

Because the treatment of the IBS patient can be frustrating to the clinician and patient as well, the physician should strive to gain the patient's confidence with a concise, appropriate work-up and by offering reassurance and education that IBS is a functional disorder without significant long-term health risks. A fraction of IBS patients, especially those presenting with new onset of symptoms, express relief that their symptoms are not caused by a serious condition such as malignancy. Whenever possible, the physician should resist the temptation to try a broad range of medications which might have limited efficacy and erode the patient's confidence. Nonetheless, a recent survey revealed that medications were prescribed at 75% of outpatient visits of IBS patients.[2]

A number of medications have been proposed for the treatment of IBS, but none has been shown convincingly to have positive therapeutic effects in the IBS population as a whole. Because IBS is a symptom complex without clear pathophysiologic markers, the efficacy of drug therapy is difficult to measure. Furthermore, the placebo response ranges up to 70% in various studies, thereby making the detection of positive treatment effects very difficult.[119] Drug therapy is best used in patients with severe symptoms refractory to physician counseling and dietary manipulations. A review and critique of published drug trials for IBS has been reported by Klein, who evaluated all studies from 1966 to 1988 on the basis of entry criteria, study design and length, placebo responsiveness, and validity of statistical analysis.[119] He concluded that there was no convincing evidence to indicate significant efficacy for any drug regimen for the IBS population as a whole and that most of the studies of the medical therapy of IBS were too short in duration to detect efficacy, had poorly designed crossover protocols in which adequate washout periods between active drug and placebo administration were not provided, employed inappropriate statistical methods, or exhibited such large placebo effects that only studies enrolling hundreds of patients would be able to detect a statistically significant drug effect. Nonetheless, most physicians who care for patients with IBS believe there is a role for certain medical treatments in patients with distinct symptom profiles. The sections to follow detail the different classes of medications that have been proposed for the treatment of IBS and offer

suggestions as to which subsets of IBS patients might benefit from different medical interventions.

Dietary Measures

Occasionally, a meticulous dietary history reveals foods that exacerbate symptoms in an individual patient; however, most studies of dietary exclusion as a treatment of IBS have yielded negative results. Nonetheless, a subset of patients with excess gas with or without diarrhea, after lactase deficiency is ruled out, should be considered for dietary modification. It is every normal person's experience that certain foods induce intestinal gas production. In healthy volunteers, one report quantitated that ingestion of a diet rich in pork and beans increased colonic gas passage from 15 to 176 mL/hour.[120] Analysis of the ingested foodstuff revealed that a low-molecular-weight fraction containing mono-, di-, and oligosaccharides such as stachyose and raffinose was responsible for the excess gas production. Levels of dietary fiber may also induce intestinal gas production. In one study, patients on a high-fiber diet with beans produced 49.4 mL of gas per hour, compared with 26.7 mL/hour for patients on a crude fiber diet and 10.9 mL/hour for those on a liquid diet low in fiber.[121] Although most IBS patients with complaints of excess flatus produce normal amounts of gas, one study reported the case of a man who averaged 34 flatus events per day.[122] He was not lactase deficient, and his symptoms were not caused by aerophagia, because his expelled gas was predominantly hydrogen and carbon dioxide with relatively little nitrogen. After certain foods were excluded from his diet, his flatus frequency decreased to 16 per day, which is close to the normal mean value of 14.[122] Subsequent studies led to lists of foodstuffs associated with increased flatulence, including beans, onions, celery, carrots, raisins, bananas, apricots, prunes, Brussels sprouts, wheat germ, pretzels, and bagels (Table 81-2).[122] Although it is unlikely to afford significant relief to most IBS patients, exclusion of these foods should be considered in some patients with excess gas.

Bulking Agents

The most widely recommended agents for treatment for IBS are fiber preparations which serve to enhance the water-holding properties of the stool, form gels to provide stool lubrication, provide bulk for the stool, and bind agents such as bile acids that may be responsible for some of the symptoms in IBS.[123] There is some physiologic basis for use of these agents. Studies in pigs have shown that colonic motor and electrical activity are critically dependent on the dietary fiber content. Pigs exhibit similar colonic myoelectrical characteristics to humans, with a slow wave at 10.3 cpm, nonpropagative SSB of 0.5 to 2 seconds' duration, and propagative LSB of 7 seconds' duration.[124] On a high-fiber diet, propagative LSB were frequent and SSB were present 15% of the time; on a low-fiber diet, some pigs became constipated and exhibited an LSB frequency that was one fifth as great and segmenting SSB activity that occupied 44% of the recording time. This study suggests that dietary fiber reduces segmenting myoelectrical activity, which leads to fecal retention and de-

TABLE 81-2
Foods and Flatus Production

Normoflatulogenic Foods

Meat, fowl, and fish

Vegetables (e.g., lettuce, cucumber, broccoli, pepper, avocado, cauliflower, tomato, asparagus, zucchini, okra, olives)

Fruits (e.g., cantaloupe, grapes, berries)

Carbohydrates (e.g., rice, corn chips, potato chips, popcorn, graham crackers)

Nuts

Miscellaneous (e.g., eggs, nonmilk chocolate, flavored gelatin, fruit ice)

Moderately Flatulogenic Foods

Pastries

Potatoes

Eggplant

Citrus fruit

Apple bread

Extremely Flatulogenic Foods

Milk and milk products

Vegetables (e.g., onions, beans, celery, carrots, Brussels sprouts)

Fruit (e.g., raisins, bananas, apricots, prune juice)

Miscellaneous (e.g., pretzels, bagels, wheat germ)

Adapted from VanNess MM and Cattau EL. Flatulence: pathophysiology and treatment. Am Fam Physician 1985;31:198.

hydration, and increases propulsive activity, which effects fecal elimination. Human studies of the effects of bran supplements on colonic motor function correlate well with these findings. In a comprehensive literature review, Muller-Lissner found that bran ingestion led to increased fecal weight in 18 of the 20 studies evaluated and accelerated fecal transit in 16.[125] A study of healthy humans noted that volunteers with an initial transit time of 3 or more days exhibited accelerated colonic transit on bran, whereas those with an initial transit time of only 1 day showed a delay in colonic transit with ingestion of bran, suggesting that dietary fiber leads to a more uniform pattern of fecal transit in normal individuals.[126] Normal volunteers and patients with constipation, diverticulosis, and IBS exhibited qualitatively similar responses in Muller-Lissner's literature review.[125] Unfortunately, constipated patients showed a lesser increase in stool weight and less acceleration of transit than normal subjects. It is unknown why IBS patients would need increased levels of dietary fiber, because there are no detectable differences in fiber intake in controls and patients with IBS.[127]

Several fiber preparations are available for the treatment of IBS. Soluble fiber, such as pectin, psyllium, or oat bran, offers the theoretical advantage of enhancing water-retentive properties of the stool, whereas insoluble fiber, such as cellulose or lignin, are likely to be more effective bulking agents.[123] Clinical trials using these different fiber preparations in IBS populations have reported placebo responses of 63% to 71%.[119] Additionally, most studies of fiber supplementation have enrolled fewer than 100 patients, and the large placebo response may have obscured any therapeutic effect. Reports by Taylor and Manning provided evidence of symptomatic improvement using bran preparations, showing increased

stool weights, decreased transit times, improvement in bowel habits, and slight reductions in pain.[128,129] In contrast, studies by Soltoft, Arffmann, and Lucey showed symptomatic improvement with bran that was not greater than with placebo.[130–132] The Lucey and Arffmann groups demonstrated increased stool weight, and Arffmann documented accelerated transit, but pain, bowel habits, distention, and borborygmi were not improved. However, the Lucey study enrolled relatively few constipation-predominant IBS patients, possibly obscuring a real therapeutic effect. Commercially prepared fiber supplements that have been studied in placebo-controlled fashion include psyllium and processed flea seed husk (ispaghula). Longstreth, using psyllium, showed no difference in symptomatic response compared with placebo.[133] In contrast, Kumar demonstrated dose-dependent reductions in pain and constipation using ispaghula in an uncontrolled trial, and controlled studies by Prior using ispaghula alone and by Ritchie using ispaghula with an anticholinergic or tranquilizer showed improvement predominantly in constipated patients.[134–136] Prior noted that two patients with diarrhea experienced symptom exacerbation with ispaghula. The best conclusion that can be drawn from these studies is that fiber supplementation is no better than placebo for treatment of IBS as a whole but that patients with constipation may show some response to intensive fiber treatment. In contrast, patients with predominant pain, diarrhea, or bloating are no more likely to respond to fiber than to placebo.

Antispasmodic Agents

After fiber preparations, antispasmodic agents are the next most commonly prescribed group of medications for the treatment of IBS. Included in the antispasmodic class are medications that block the cholinergic nerve function responsible for much of the contractile activity of the gut, agents that prevent calcium movements that are needed for intestinal contraction, direct gut smooth muscle relaxants, and agents that act by unknown pathways. The rationale for their use is that, because IBS patients exhibit exaggerated patterns of gut motor activity, inhibition of this activity might provide an effective treatment for symptoms caused by these motility abnormalities. Indeed, both anticholinergics and calcium channel blockers are effective inhibitors of the gastrocolonic response.[137–141] Despite these potent motor effects, the utility of antispasmodic agents in the treatment of IBS as a whole is poorly substantiated by the literature.[119]

Anticholinergics

Anticholinergic agents represent the major class of antispasmodic medications used in the United States. Several controlled trials of anticholinergics have been performed in IBS. Dicyclomine, prifinium, and cimetropium have been reported to reduce symptoms in IBS compared with placebo, with dicyclomine showing improvement in both fecal urgency and pain.[142–144] However, both dicyclomine and cimetropium induced greater side effects than placebo, thus raising the issue of whether the blinding of the studies was truly effective. Furthermore, the prifinium trial lasted only 3 weeks and used inappropriate statistical methods, thereby throwing into question its conclusions.[119,143] A more recent 3-month trial of cimetropium showed reduction of abdominal pain and improvement in the global sense of well-being compared with placebo.[145] In contrast, the anticholinergic tricyclamol did not lead to a global reduction of symptoms compared with placebo in one report.[146] These reports do not provide firm evidence that anticholinergic agents are efficacious in the IBS population as a whole; however, because of their physiologic effects on the gastrocolonic response, it is possible that IBS patients with abdominal pain or fecal urgency, especially after a meal, may benefit from their use.

Calcium Channel Blockers

Calcium channel blockers have been proposed for the treatment of IBS by virtue of their smooth muscle relaxant properties and their inhibitory effects on the gastrocolonic response. However, there is little data on their use in IBS. A report of three cases of IBS with crampy abdominal pain and diarrhea exacerbated by stress suggested that verapamil was effective in symptom reduction.[147] However, in a trial of nifedipine in 13 patients with IBS, 6 expressed a preference for placebo and only 2 preferred nifedipine.[148] Similarly, a double blind trial of diltiazem in 18 IBS patients did not show global improvement, although there was a trend toward resolution of diarrhea and abdominal pain.[149] Octylonium bromide, a direct smooth muscle relaxant that inhibits gut calcium mobilization, led to improvement in two of five symptom parameters; however, 83% of the patients had neither constipation nor diarrhea and therefore did not meet the diagnostic criteria for IBS.[119] Peppermint oil is a naturally occurring carminative that relaxes gastrointestinal smooth muscle by reduction of calcium influx.[150] Two small trials by Rees and Dew showed preference for peppermint oil over placebo; however, each performed global assessments rather than looking at specific symptoms, and each study noted an atypically low placebo response.[119,151,152] In contrast, there was no reduction in abdominal pain with peppermint oil in the largest trial to date.[153] The newest agent, pinaverium, a purported gut selective slow calcium channel blocker with minimal systemic effects, inhibits colonic contractile activity and affects colonic transit.[154–156] However, no studies to date have demonstrated clinical efficacy for pinaverium in IBS. As with anticholinergics, there are no controlled studies to support the use of calcium channel blockers in the treatment of IBS as a whole. However, as with anticholinergics, calcium channel blockers inhibit postprandial motility and could conceivably be useful in persons with postprandial symptoms.

Other Antispasmodics

A number of antispasmodic agents, available outside the United States, that do not act by inhibition of cholinergic activity or calcium flux have been prescribed for IBS. Mebeverine is a smooth muscle relaxant similar to papaverine that is nearly devoid of anticholinergic side effects. Three times as potent as papaverine, it can inhibit ileal peristalsis and colon motility in IBS patients.[157] In two small studies by Connell and Tasman-Jones, IBS patients expressed a preference for mebeverine over placebo, with improvement of pain noted in one study.[157,158] In contrast, a 16-week study by Kruis

showed no benefit of mebeverine over placebo.[159] Trimebutine is an antispasmodic that stimulates small intestine motility by acting on peripheral opioid receptors as morphine does but inhibits colonic motility by a naloxone-insensitive pathway.[160] In both constipation- and diarrhea-predominant IBS patients, trimebutine reduces LSB activity in the transverse and descending colon.[160] A 3-day study of trimebutine in IBS patients resulted in improvements in abdominal pain, flatulence, and sensations of fullness.[161] Moshal reported reductions in pain, constipation, and transit time at 8 weeks in 20 IBS patients, but there was no overall preference for trimebutine over placebo.[162] In the largest placebo-controlled trial, involving 60 IBS patients, there were no differences in pain relief with trimebutine compared with placebo.[163] Therefore, neither of these antispasmodic medications has convincingly been shown to provide therapeutic benefit in IBS.

Antidiarrheal Agents

In many IBS patients, a major goal of treatment is to reduce diarrhea. The use of medications that act through peripheral opioid pathways is based on the finding that morphine and the enkephalins cause segmenting colonic contractions. Three studies have compared the opioid medication loperamide with placebo in IBS. Cann reported that loperamide slowed small bowel and whole gut transit, decreased stool frequency and the passage of unformed stools, and reduced diarrhea, fecal urgency, and borborygmi in 28 patients.[164] For symptoms other than constipation, loperamide was as good or better than placebo. In a study of 21 patients, Lavo demonstrated improvement in stool consistency, abdominal pain, fecal urgency, and overall well-being.[165] Hovandek reported improved stool frequency and consistency in patients with painless diarrhea and reduced diarrhea and abdominal pain in pain-predominant patients with alternating constipation and diarrhea.[166] Patients with alternating bowel habits but no pain showed no improvement, and patients with constipation experienced exacerbation on loperamide. These studies provide a forceful argument for the use of peripheral opiate-related medications such as loperamide in diarrhea-predominant IBS.

Agents other than the opioids have been proposed for use in diarrhea-predominant IBS. Cholestyramine, a resin that binds endogenous bile acids, produced marked symptom improvement in an uncontrolled trial of five patients with unexplained painless diarrhea.[167] A more recent evaluation of the serotonin receptor (5-HT$_3$) antagonist ondansetron, an agent that delays colonic transit in healthy volunteers, showed relief of loose stools and a delay in colonic transit in diarrhea-predominant IBS patients.[168,169] Unfortunately, some individuals noted increased abdominal pain with ondansetron, suggesting that some IBS patients may not be appropriate candidates for the drug. No prolonged placebo-controlled trials with either of these medications have been reported.

Prokinetic Agents

Medications that stimulate gastrointestinal motor function, known as prokinetic agents, have been proposed for use in IBS patients with predominant constipation. Additionally, because many IBS patients experience dyspepsia (and one unconfirmed study reports delayed gastric emptying in IBS),[170] prokinetic agents have been proposed for patients with upper gut symptoms. Agents studied in IBS include domperidone, a selective dopamine receptor antagonist, and cisapride, which acts through cholinergic, serotonergic, and direct smooth muscle effects. Domperidone is most effective as a prokinetic agent in the upper gastrointestinal tract, having been demonstrated to enhance gastric emptying and small bowel transit.[171] Domperidone has no prokinetic effects in the colon; on the contrary, it blocks dopamine-induced rectosigmoid contractions and reduces the gastrocolonic response to a meal.[172] Three placebo-controlled trials of domperidone have been performed in IBS. Milo, in a 4-week trial, demonstrated that 80% of IBS patients noted decreases in flatulence, abdominal pain, and disorders of defecation on domperidone.[173] However, all patients had preexisting dyspepsia or delayed gastric emptying. In contrast, domperidone trials by Fielding and Cann showed no improvement in transit time, stool weight, symptom frequency, or symptom intensity in patients with IBS.[174,175] The usefulness of domperidone in IBS remains to be established, although the Milo trial suggests that patients with dyspepsia may benefit. In contrast to domperidone, cisapride exhibits motor stimulatory effects in the colon. In constipation-predominant IBS patients, Passaretti noted an increase in stool frequency and acceleration of whole gut transit with cisapride.[176] A second placebo-controlled 12-week trial in constipated IBS patients showed that 71% of patients on cisapride reported good to excellent results with reduced abdominal pain, increased stool frequency, and improved stool consistency, compared with 39% of those receiving placebo.[177] Although these results require confirmation, there are encouraging signs that cisapride and newer prokinetic agents may have therapeutic utility in IBS patients with predominant constipation.

Agents to Selectively Reduce Visceral Perception

Because drugs designed to modify gut motor activity have limited efficacy and because many IBS patients exhibit sensory hypersensitivity to visceral stimulation, some investigators have redirected their attention to medications that reduce gut perception. Such antiafferent agents may act through one or more mechanisms to reduce visceral sensation, including modification of release of pain-inducing mediators in the gut wall, blockade or activation of peripheral afferent nerve receptors, inhibition of afferent nerve transmission, and modification of afferent activity in the central nervous system.[61] It is possible that such medications to reduce visceral perception may also have effects on gut motor activity. This has been demonstrated for the calcium channel blocker nicardipine, which has the dual effect of increasing the threshold for painful sensation of rectal balloon inflation and reducing the gastrocolonic response.[178] Opiate medications may be considered the classic agent to inhibit gut perception through sensory pathways in the central nervous system. Codeine, for example, reduces perception of rectal distention.[179] However, newer opiate drugs, which act only on peripheral opiate pathways, have been shown to reduce perception of gastric distention, suggesting that such antiafferent properties may be unrelated to central analgesia.[180] Serotonin (5-HT) has been proposed as a mediator of visceral wall pain. In rats, the cardiovascular response to gut distention is inhibited by blockade at the 5-HT$_3$ receptor subtype.[181] More recently, the 5-HT$_3$ receptor antagonist ondansetron was shown to reduce perception of esophageal distention in patients with noncardiac chest pain.[182] The most thorough work to date on medications designed to inhibit visceral afferent pathways has been with the somatostatin analog octreotide. Hasler and colleagues demonstrated that octreotide reduces perception of rectal distention by inhibition of visceral afferent pathways in healthy volunteers.[183] In a follow-up study, IBS patients with fecal urgency were shown to exhibit a similar response to octreotide.[184] Additionally, octreotide reduced the increased pressures that resulted from rectal distention in these patients. The only report of its therapeutic use was in a 52-year-old woman with bromocriptine-treated acromegaly who noted complete resolution of associated symptoms of abdominal pain and distention on octreotide.[185] Subsequent work by Roberts, using the technique of cortical and spinal evoked potential measurement, showed that octreotide specifically inhibits spinal afferent pathways from the rectum, documenting a peripheral site of action for the somatostatin analog.[186] Although these investigations are conceptually intriguing, no placebo-controlled trials have been performed, and the use of medications designed to reduce visceral perception remains an option that requires further study.

Antidepressants and Anxiolytics

Because many IBS patients exhibit abnormal psychiatric features which predate the onset of their bowel symptoms, many investigators have evaluated the use of antidepressant and anxiolytic medications in IBS. In addition to their central nervous system effects, these drugs may alter intestinal motility. For example, tricyclic antidepressants exhibit anticholinergic activity, and benzodiazepines can relax peripheral smooth muscle.

Among the classes of antidepressant medications, the tricyclics have been most extensively evaluated in IBS. In an uncontrolled study by Hislop of 56 patients with IBS, 29 became symptom-free and 16 others showed improvement on amitriptyline.[96] Furthermore, improvement of bowel symptoms on amitriptyline occurred more rapidly than improvement in depression and at doses subtherapeutic for the treatment of depression. A 4-week study of trimipramine reported significant improvement in vomiting, depression, sleeplessness, and mucus in stools compared with placebo; however, abdominal pain and other bowel complaints were not improved.[187] Heefner demonstrated improvement in abdominal pain in 86% of patients given 2 months of desipramine, compared with 59% of the placebo group, but stool characteristics showed the same improvement in both groups.[188] A similar study of 28 IBS patients showed improvement in stool frequency, diarrhea, pain, and depression.[189] If stratified according to the predominant symptoms, improvements were confined to diarrhea-predominant patients, with no improvement being noted in constipated patients.[189] Statistical methods used in each of these studies have been questioned. The utility of tricyclic antidepressant therapy in IBS is unknown, but it is possible that patients with predominant diarrhea with or without pain may experience some benefit with this class of medications.[119] Additionally, it is likely that IBS patients with well-defined depression will experience clinical improvement on tricyclic therapy.

Tranquilizers have been used for decades in the treatment of IBS. Older studies using phenaglycodol and meprobamate in IBS demonstrated global improvement compared with placebo, although specific symptoms were not evaluated.[190] In one study of 21 IBS patients, the combinations of heteronium plus amobarbital or propantheline plus phenobarbital led to improvement in overall well-being compared with placebo.[191] In contrast, another report of five sedative-anticholinergic combinations showed no benefit compared with placebo.[192] The utility of benzodiazepines in the treatment of IBS has been evaluated by several groups. Narducci demonstrated prevention of stress-induced increases in rectosigmoid motility with chlordiazepoxide.[76] In an investigation of 52 patients, diazepam led to greater relief of anxiety and related symptoms than placebo.[193] A placebo-controlled study of medazepam reported symptom improvement in 15 of 19 patients with aerophagia and in 14 of 22 patients with abdominal pain.[194] Aprazolam, in an uncontrolled study of IBS patients with concomitant anxiety disorder, resulted in an 89% reduction in gastrointestinal symptoms which was maintained after drug withdrawal.[195] Unfortunately, in most of these studies, the usefulness of benzodiazepines in treating IBS has been incompletely characterized because of poorly defined symptoms and patient populations. Coupled with the clear abuse potential of these medications and the rapid development of tolerance to their anxiolytic effects, the use of sedatives in IBS is not indicated in most patients. Perhaps newer agents such as the purportedly nonaddicting compound buspirone will be important therapies for IBS, but this requires confirmation with well-designed placebo-controlled trials.

Miscellaneous Medical Treatments

Because the pathogenesis of IBS is so poorly understood, it is not surprising that numerous other medications have been proposed for IBS, including antigas preparations, various neurotransmitter receptor antagonists and agonists, hormonal analogs, medications designed to prevent presumed gut allergic responses, anticonvulsants, and medications designed to alter the gut flora.

Because complaints of gas and abdominal distention are major symptoms in some IBS patients, an effective antigas preparation would be an extremely useful compound. Several agents have been promoted to reduce gaseous symptoms. Anticholinergics reduce the gastrocolonic response to a meal and reduce the increase in flatus production after ingestion of beans.[122] Silicone preparations change properties of gas bubbles such that 1 ounce of simethicone can defoam 250,000 pounds of molasses.[196] Uncontrolled studies using silicone agents show reduction of excess bloating and flatus production in patients with complaints of excess gas.[196] Activated charcoal has an enormous surface area to mass ratio (450–1800 m^2/g) which allows it to be an excellent adsorbent of gas.[197] Small

doses of activated charcoal can decrease the number of flatus passages after ingestion of a bean meal in healthy volunteers.[197] Recently a compound released under the trade name of Beano was proposed for treatment of patients with gaseous complaints. Beano, which consists of microbial α-galactosidases not present in the human gut, has been shown to reduce hydrogen gas production after ingestion of black beans in healthy volunteers.[198] No randomized controlled trials have been performed with these agents in the specific study of IBS patients with complaints of excess gas.

Dysfunctional neurotransmission has been postulated as a cause of IBS, and many investigators have searched for agents that act on known gut neurotransmitter receptors. β-Adrenergic pathways may be physiologic mediators of colonic motility. Based on the finding that the β-antagonist propranolol increases rectosigmoid pressure, it has been postulated that β-adrenoceptor antagonists may have therapeutic roles in patients with reduced rectosigmoid motility.[199,200] Marzuk described a 26-year-old patient with diarrhea-predominant IBS who experienced dramatic symptomatic improvement with atenolol.[201] In placebo-controlled trials, neither atenolol nor timolol provided symptom relief in IBS compared with placebo.[202,203] Recently, the β-adrenoceptor agonist ritodrine was shown to delay orocecal transit, suggesting possible utility in diarrhea-prone patients with accelerated upper gut transit. Nonetheless, at this time, there is no evidence to suggest that agents which act on β-adrenoceptors have utility in IBS.

Because symptoms may worsen during the postovulatory phase of the menstrual cycle, investigators have searched for hormonal means of treating IBS. Continuous administration of gonadotropin releasing hormone (Gn-RH) leads to reduced synthesis of the gonadotropins, follicle-stimulating hormone and luteinizing hormone, with subsequent inhibition of cyclic variations in the gonadal hormones. Recently the Gn-RH analog, leuprolide, was studied in four women with abdominal pain, nausea, vomiting, and altered stool habits.[204] Subcutaneous administration for 3 months led to complete symptom resolution in three women and improvement in the fourth. Progesterone was given every 3 months to induce menses, and estrogen supplements with calcium were given to reduce osteoporosis. Obviously, this regimen for IBS has several potential complications, and until a well-controlled trial is performed, this aggressive treatment plan cannot be routinely recommended.

Despite the controversy over the role played by food hypersensitivity in the genesis of symptoms in IBS, a number of groups have evaluated the utility of medications designed to reduce allergic phenomena in the gut in IBS patients with predominant diarrhea. In one uncontrolled study, five of seven patients noted improvement with oral disodium chromoglycate treatment.[104] A larger study evaluated 101 patients with diarrhea-predominant IBS who showed evidence of dietary hypersensitivity on the basis of exclusion diets.[205] Of those patients who exhibited evidence of food allergy based on skin prick test results, 67% noted symptomatic improvement with disodium chromoglycate. In contrast, only 41% of patients with negative skin tests experienced symptomatic relief. These results, however, require confirmation in placebo-controlled fashion.

Diphenylhydantoin was considered at one time as therapy for IBS because it had been shown to relax colonic smooth muscle. Unfortunately, a 20-week double-blind crossover trial in 12 IBS patients showed no differences in symptomatic response compared with placebo.[206]

A few investigators have hypothesized that IBS is caused by subtle alterations in colonic microbial flora. One group administered a colonic lavage solution to IBS patients to remove their bowel flora and subsequently replaced the flora with samples from healthy donors, with reported symptom improvement.[114] More recently, freeze-dried cultures of the bacterium *Streptococcus faecium* (trade name Paraghurt) were administered in placebo-controlled fashion in IBS.[115] Eighty-one percent of patients noted an improved sense of well-being with Paraghurt, compared with 41% with placebo. Obviously, treatments such as this are very much unproven and require confirmation.

Psychotherapy, Biofeedback, and Hypnosis

The involvement of psychiatrists in the management of IBS has been reserved for patients with clear psychologic features who do not respond to standard therapeutic maneuvers; however, some investigators recommend a wider role for psychiatric intervention. Psychotherapy has shown promise of reduced symptoms in patients who do not show improvement on medications. In a population of 101 IBS patients, 3 months of dynamically-oriented psychotherapy in addition to medications provided greater improvement in somatic symptoms than medical treatment alone.[207] A second psychotherapy study on 102 patients who had failed medications showed improvement in depression and reduced abdominal pain and diarrhea, but not constipation.[208] Group psychotherapy, including techniques such as psychodrama, has not been shown to reduce abdominal pain or improve bowel habits, although anxiety levels may decrease.[209]

Biofeedback and stress reduction techniques have been employed by some clinicians. Muscle relaxation training and education into means of decreasing stress was used successfully by Blanchard to reduce bowel symptoms in an uncontrolled study, especially in those individuals who exhibited improvement in depression and anxiety.[210,211] At follow-up after 4 years, 50% of the population reported sustained improvements in pain, diarrhea, nausea, and flatulence.[212] Similarly, Shaw demonstrated reduced frequency and severity of painful attacks of IBS with these techniques, compared with an antispasmodic regimen.[213] In contrast, a study by Bennett comparing relaxation and stress reduction to medications showed no improvement in bowel symptoms.[214] In a novel study, patients were trained to reduce bowel symptoms by listening to their bowel sound pattern through a stethoscope and attempting to modify their borborygmus.[215] This bowel sound biofeedback led to improved symptomatology in three of five patients enrolled, with long-term success in two of the five.

Hypnosis has been proposed for refractory cases of IBS. In an initial study of 30 patients with refractory IBS randomized to hypnosis or psychotherapy, the hypnosis group showed a small improvement in abdominal pain, distention, and well-being but not bowel pattern after 3 months of treatment.[216] Eighteen months after instruction in autohypnosis was given,

sustained remission was demonstrated in most individuals, although patients older than 50 years of age or with underlying psychopathology were less likely to respond.[217] Subsequently, the authors reported a success rate of 85% in more than 200 IBS patients treated with hypnosis.[218] A study using anorectal manometric monitoring of 15 IBS patients demonstrated reduced perception of rectal distention with hypnosis, suggesting that hypnosis may inhibit afferent pathways that mediate perception of visceral discomfort.[82]

Despite these encouraging findings, many of the studies using psychotherapy, biofeedback, stress reduction, or hypnosis provide poor definitions of symptomatic responses and have inadequate control populations. Their roles in IBS require further characterization. It is likely, however, that IBS patients with depression or anxiety can benefit from aggressive psychiatric intervention.

APPROACH TO DIFFERENT SUBSETS OF IBS PATIENTS

The Constipation-Predominant Patient

The principles of management of the IBS patient with predominant constipation are to increase stool water and bulk and to reduce the effort needed for defecation. The previous sections indicate that the most widely used and most efficacious compounds for this purpose are the bulking agents in concert with a high-fiber diet. Additionally, any medications that inhibit colonic motor function should be discontinued. Patients should be cautioned that fiber supplementation may take several weeks to produce a satisfactory result and that fiber should be introduced gradually to prevent excess distention and gas. Those patients with an inadequate response should be given an osmotic agent such as milk of magnesia or lactulose in addition to the fiber program. Stimulant laxatives should be avoided because of the potential for long-term damage to colonic motor function. The role of prokinetic agents is undefined at this time, although agents such as cisapride may have utility in a subgroup of patients.

In the patient with refractory symptoms of constipation, further diagnostic evaluation may be needed to rule out organic disease not detected by the work-up detailed in previous sections (see Chap. 39). Endocrinologic causes of constipation can be assessed with determination of thyroid-stimulating hormone levels to rule out hypothyroidism and serum calcium to rule out hyperparathyroidism. Other studies can screen for porphyria or lead toxicity. Using radioopaque markers or the recently developed technique of colonic scintigraphy, diffuse delays in colonic transit suggest colonic inertia, whereas localized delays suggest functional outlet obstruction, usually in the distal colon. Defecography, or cinefluoroscopy of the defecation process, can identify individuals with puborectalis muscle dysfunction, rectocele, or rectal prolapse. Anorectal manometry, in addition to demonstrating sensory abnormalities, can screen for Hirschsprung's disease. These techniques are useful for detecting patient populations who might be better treated surgically or with a biofeedback program of bowel retraining.

The Diarrhea-Predominant Patient

The management of the diarrhea-prone IBS patient centers on reduction of defecation frequency or urgency and improvement in stool consistency. The agents most commonly employed and the drugs shown to be most effective are the opiate derivatives such as loperamide or diphenoxylate. Many clinicians prescribe agents such as fiber to add bulk to the stool, but controlled trials do not show a greater response to this therapy in diarrhea-predominant IBS than to placebo. Those individuals with a prominent gastrocolonic response may achieve additional benefit from antispasmodic agents such as anticholinergics or calcium channel blockers which inhibit this physiologic response. Other drugs with some efficacy in diarrhea-prone patients include cholestyramine and antidepressant medications. The role of newer antidiarrheal agents such as ondansetron is undefined at this time. A careful dietary history should screen for foods containing compounds such as lactose, sorbitol, or fructose that cause diarrhea. Other dietary manipulations usually are without benefit and are not encouraged in most individuals. The use of disodium chromoglycate, directed at treatment of food hypersensitivity, is unsubstantiated in most diarrhea-prone patients.

Subsequent evaluation of the diarrhea-predominant IBS patients is dictated by the history (see Chap. 38). In patients with a travel history, recent antibiotic use, or ingestion of well water, evaluation for an infectious cause should be pursued, including collection of stool samples for leukocytes, culture for enteric pathogens including *Clostridium difficile*, and examination for ova and parasites. Subsequent examination of duodenal aspirates for *Giardia* may be needed in some individuals. Small bowel biopsy and barium studies are useful in some patients to rule out inflammatory conditions such as Crohn's disease or celiac sprue, although most of these individuals also exhibit anemia, hypoalbuminemia, or an elevated sedimentation rate on laboratory screening. If malabsorption is suspected, stool samples should be obtained for fecal fat determination. Patients with palpitations or tachycardia should undergo laboratory testing to rule out hyperthyroidism. In patients with bloating, diarrhea, and gas, lactase deficiency should be ruled out with a hydrogen breath test or a trial on a lactose-free diet. The total stool volume over a 24-hour period in diarrhea-prone IBS patients should fall within the normal range, with very few individuals exceeding 300 g/day.[8,219] The diarrhea of IBS often is postprandial. If diarrhea persists after a 24-hour fast, this suggests a secretory process and not IBS. Finally, screening for laxatives should not be overlooked, because a surprisingly large subset of diarrhea-prone patients intentionally abuse these compounds.

The Patient With Painful IBS

Severe abdominal pain represents one of the most difficult symptoms to treat in IBS and is compounded by the lack of convincingly effective medications for this complaint. Perhaps the most useful treatment that can be offered by the physician is reassurance and counseling about the nonthreatening nature of IBS. Use of addictive pain killers should be avoided because their use is counterproductive. Many clinicians recommend bulking agents for painful IBS, although the data supporting efficacy for this symptom is weak. Antispasmodic drugs, especially the anticholinergics, are most commonly employed in pain-predominant IBS, and some patients, especially those with postprandial pain, may benefit from such therapy. Antidepressant medications may benefit an additional subset of patients. Antigas agents or low-gas diets are used for bloating, with variable results. Prokinetic agents such as metoclopramide or cisapride may be of use in the patient with upper gut pain with nausea.

Most pain-predominant IBS patients require only the screening work-up detailed previously, but some individuals may need further evaluation (see Chap. 34). If dyspepsia or heartburn is severe, upper gastrointestinal barium studies or esophagogastroduodenoscopy may be indicated to exclude structural disease such as ulcers or inflammation. If biliary tract disease is suspected, liver chemistries and right upper quadrant abdominal ultrasonography should be performed. Computerized tomography or small bowel radiography is occasionally obtained. If nausea, vomiting, or early satiety suggest the possibility of gastroparesis or intestinal pseudoobstruction, a nuclear medicine gastric emptying scan or a gastroduodenal motility study may be indicated. Rare individuals may need screening to rule out lead toxicity or porphyria.

PATIENT OUTCOME

IBS, although not a cause of patient mortality, usually persists in a waxing and waning fashion for long periods. Although few studies have provided long-term follow-up of well-defined patient populations, most investigators have shown that symptoms in IBS may not resolve completely, even after many years. This is corroborated by studies demonstrating a high incidence of functional gastrointestinal complaints in the elderly.[2] Of the group of patients studied by Chaudhary and Truelove, only 34 of 103 patients were symptom-free on long-term follow-up.[220] Similarly, Waller and Misiewicz followed 50 IBS patients at 2-month intervals for 12 to 31 months.[221] In 44 of these patients, the qualitative nature of the symptoms did not change with long-term follow-up, although the severity of the symptoms was quite variable.

Despite these pessimistic reports, the quality of life for many IBS patients can be enhanced by appropriate physician intervention. Of the 44 patients with persistent symptoms in the study reported by Waller and Misiewicz, 18 patients showed some reduction in symptom intensity with continued medical follow-up.[221] Of 34 fully employed patients, 20 lost no work in the first year after diagnosis and only 7 patients lost more than 2 weeks as a result of their symptoms. The authors commented that, although there often was little or no change in symptom severity, most patients were better able to cope with their symptoms. A more recent study of 43 IBS patients reported that, of all the abdominal symptoms reported, only abdominal pain was significantly reduced after 5 years of follow-up.[222] However, 65% of their population noted an improved sense of well-being. Those individuals who improved exhibited markedly reduced levels of anxiety compared with those who did not. Perhaps the best outcome was seen in a group of 97 patients with IBS who were studied for a period of 5 to 7 years on a treatment regimen of an antispasmodic, bulking agents, and a high-fiber diet.[220] Of these patients, 26% remained symptom-free and an additional 42% experienced only occasional minor symptoms. Patients who were male, had a short history of symptoms, had a history of recent acute onset of symptoms, exhibited predominant constipation, and showed a good initial response to treatment were most likely to achieve good long-term improvement. Taken as a whole, these studies suggest that a significant fraction of the patient population with IBS can expect to achieve symptomatic reduction over the course of weeks to years. It is likely that the ongoing counseling, reassurance, and education provided by the physicians, the judicious use of medications, and the continued interest in the patients' well-being all contributed to the successful outcomes in these long-term investigations.

In conclusion, the pathophysiology of IBS is complex and is unlikely to result from a single etiologic factor. Until the pathogenesis is understood, it is advisable to customize the treatment plan according to each patient's individual symptom complex. In addition, the importance of physician education and reassurance to the patient cannot be overemphasized.

The reader is directed to Chapter 9, Motility of the Small Intestine; Chapter 10, Motility of the Large Intestine; Chapter 34, Approach to the Patient With Abdominal Pain; Chapter 35, Approach to the Patient With Gas and Bloating; Chapter 38, Approach to the Patient With Diarrhea; Chapter 39, Approach to the Patient With Constipation; Chapter 60, Disorders of Gastric Emptying; Chapter 61, Acid-Peptic Disorders: Chapter 69, Dysmotility of the Small Intestine; Chapter 79, Inflammatory Bowel Disease; Chapter 82, Motility Disorders of the Colon; and Chapter 83, Diverticulitis.

REFERENCES

1. Thompson WG, Creed F, Drossman DA, et al. Functional bowel disorders and functional abdominal pain. Gastroenterol Int 1992;5:99.
2. Everhart JE, Renault PF. Irritable bowel syndrome in office-based practice in the United States. Gastroenterology 1991;100:998.
3. Schuster MM. Diagnostic evaluation of the irritable bowel syndrome. Gastroenterol Clin North Am 1991;20:269.
4. Mendeloff AI. Epidemiology of the irritable bowel syndrome. Practical Gastroenterology 1979;3:12.
5. O'Keefe E, Talley NJ. The irritable bowel syndrome in the elderly. Gastroenterol Clin North Am 1991;20:369.
6. Thompson WG, Heaton KW. Functional bowel disorders in apparently healthy people. Gastroenterology 1980;79:283.
7. Sandler RS. Epidemiology of irritable bowel syndrome in the United States. Gastroenterology 1990;99:409.
8. Cann PA, Read NW, Brown C, et al. Irritable bowel syndrome: relationship of disorders in the transit of a single meal to symptom patterns. Gut 1983;21:405.
9. Keeling PWN, Fielding JF. The irritable bowel syndrome: a review of 50 consecutive cases. J Irish Coll Phys and Surg 1975;4:91.
10. Thompson WG. The irritable bowel. Gut 1984;25:305.
11. Talley NJ, Zinsmeister AR, Van Dyke C, Melton LJ. Epidemiology of colonic symptoms and the irritable bowel syndrome. Gastroenterology 1991;101:927.
12. Talley NJ, O'Keefe EA, Zinsmeister AR, Melton LJ. Prevalence of gastrointestinal symptoms in the elderly: a population-based study. Gastroenterology 1992;102:895.
13. Heaton KW, O'Donnell LJ, Braddon FE, et al. Symptoms of irritable bowel syndrome in a British urban community: consulters and nonconsulters. Gastroenterology 1992;102:1962.
14. Jones R, Lydeard S. Irritable bowel syndrome in the general population. BMJ 1992;304:87.
15. Crouch MA. Irritable bowel syndrome: toward a biopsychosocial systems understanding. Prim Care 1988;15:99.
16. Chaudhary NA, Truelove SC. The irritable colon syndrome: a study of the clinical features, predisposing causes, and prognosis in 130 cases. Q J Med 1962;31:307.
17. Connell AM, Hilton C, Irvine G, et al. Variation of bowel habit in two population samples. Br Med J 1965;2:1095.
18. Kellow JE, Gill RC, Wingate DL. Prolonged ambulant recordings of small bowel motility demonstrate abnormalities in the irritable bowel syndrome. Gastroenterology 1990;98:1208.
19. Kalser MH, Zion DE, Bockus HL. Functional diarrhea: an analysis of the clinical and roentgen manifestations. Gastroenterology 1956;31:629.
20. Manning AP, Thompson WG, Heaton KW, Morris AF. Towards positive diagnosis of the irritable bowel. Br Med J 1978;2:653.
21. Lasser RB, Bond JH, Levitt MD. The role of intestinal gas in functional abdominal pain. N Engl J Med 1975;293:524.
22. Maxton DG, Martin DF, Whorwell PJ, Godfrey M. Abdominal distention in female patients with irritable bowel syndrome: exploration of possible mechanisms. Gut 1991;32:662.
23. Drossman DA, McKee DC, Sandler RS, et al. Psychosocial factors in the irritable bowel syndrome. A multivariate study of patients and nonpatients with irritable bowel syndrome. Gastroenterology 1988;95:701.
24. Sandler RS, Drossman DA, Nathan HP, McKee DC. Symptom complaints and health care seeking behavior in subjects with irritable bowel syndrome. Gastroenterology 1984;87:314.
25. Whitehead WE, Cheskin LJ, Heller BR, et al. Evidence for exacerbation of irritable bowel syndrome during menses. Gastroenterology 1990;98:1485.
26. Guthrie E, Creed FH, Whorwell PJ. Severe sexual dysfunction in women with the irritable bowel syndrome: comparison with inflammatory bowel disease and duodenal ulceration. Br Med J 1987;295:577.
27. Whitehead WE, Winget C, Fedoravicius AS, et al. Learned illness behavior in patients with irritable bowel syndrome and peptic ulcer. Dig Dis Sci 1982;27:202.
28. Whorwell PJ, McCallum M, Creed FH, Roberts CT. Non-colonic features of irritable bowel syndrome. Gut 1986;27:37.
29. Sarna SK. Physiology and pathophysiology of colonic motor activity. Dig Dis Sci 1991;36:827.
30. Snape WJ. Irritable bowel syndrome: progress in understanding and management. Postgrad Med 1987;81:291.
31. Weber J, Ducrotte P. Colonic motility in health and disease. Dig Dis 1987;5:1.
32. Abrahamsson H. Gastrointestinal motility in patients with the irritable bowel syndrome. Scand J Gastroenterol Suppl 1987;130:21.
33. Connell AM, Avery Jones F, Rowlands EN. Motility of the pelvic colon. Part IV. Abdominal pain associated with colonic hypermotility after meals. Gut 1965;6:105.
34. Snape WJ, Carlson GM. Colonic myoelectric activity in the irritable bowel syndrome. Gastroenterology 1976;70:326.
35. Snape WJ, Carlson GM, Matarazzo SA, Cohen S. Evidence that abnormal myoelectric activity produces colonic motor dysfunction in the irritable bowel syndrome. Gastroenterology 1977;72:383.
36. Latimer P, Sarna S, Campbell D, et al. Colonic motor and myoelectrical activity: a comparative study of normal subjects, psychoneurotic patients, and patients with irritable bowel syndrome. Gastroenterology 1981;80:893.
37. Welgan P, Meshkinpour H, Beeler M. Effect of anger on colon motor and myoelectric activity in irritable bowel syndrome. Gastroenterology 1988;94:1150.
38. Welgan P, Meshkinpour H, Hoehler F. The effect of stress on

colon motor and electrical activity in irritable bowel syndrome. Psychosom Med 1985;47:139.

39. Vassallo M, Camilleri M, Phillips SF, et al. Transit through the proximal colon influences stool weight in the irritable bowel syndrome. Gastroenterology 1992;102:102.

40. Stivland T, Camilleri M, Vassallo M, et al. Scintigraphic measurement of regional gut transit in idiopathic constipation. Gastroenterology 1991;101:107.

41. Rogers J, Henry MM, Misiewicz JJ. Increased segmental activity and intraluminal pressures in the sigmoid colon of patients with the irritable bowel syndrome. Gut 1989;30:634.

42. Waller SL, Misiewicz JJ, Kiley N. Effect of eating on motility of the pelvic colon in constipation or diarrhoea. Gut 1972;13:805.

43. Jepsen JM, Skoubo-Kristensen E, Elsborg L. Rectosigmoid motility response to sham feeding in irritable bowel syndrome: evidence of a cephalic phase. Scand J Gastroenterol 1989;24:53.

44. Sun EA, Snape WJ, Cohen S, Renny A. The role of opiate receptors and cholinergic neurons in the gastrocolonic response. Gastroenterology 1982;82:689.

45. Keinath R, Wiley J, Tatum D, et al. Mechanism for the gastrocolonic response: participation of gastric and intestinal mechano- and chemoreceptors. Gastroenterology 1987;90:1488.

46. Mitra R, Chura C, Rajendra GR, Schuster MM. Abnormal responses to rectal distension in irritable bowel syndrome. Gastroenterology 1974;66:770.

47. Wangel AG, Deller DJ. Intestinal motility in man: III. mechanisms of constipation and diarrhea with particular reference to the irritable colon syndrome. Gastroenterology 1965;48:69.

48. Harvey RF, Read AE. Effect of cholecystokinin on colonic motility and symptoms in patients with the irritable-bowel syndrome. Lancet 1973;1:1.

49. Taylor I, Basu P, Hammond P, et al. Effect of bile acid perfusion on colonic motor function in patients with the irritable colon syndrome. Gut 1980;21:843.

50. Hasler WL. Motility of the small intestine. In: Yamada T, ed. Textbook of gastroenterology. Philadelphia: JB Lippincott, 1991:158.

51. Kellow JE, Eckersley GM, Jones M. Enteric and central contributions to intestinal dysmotility in irritable bowel syndrome. Dig Dis Sci 1992;37:168.

52. Kingham JGC, Bown R, Colson R, Clark ML. Jejunal motility in patients with functional abdominal pain. Gut 1984;25:375.

53. Kellow JE, Phillips SF. Altered small bowel motility in irritable bowel syndrome is correlated with symptoms. Gastroenterology 1987;92:1885.

54. Kellow JE, Phillips SF, Miller LJ, Zinsmeister AR. Dysmotility of the small intestine in irritable bowel syndrome. Gut 1988;29:1236.

55. Trotman IF, Price CC. Bloated irritable bowel syndrome defined by dynamic ^{99m}Tc bran scan. Lancet 1986;2:364.

56. Whorwell PJ, Clouter C, Smith CL. Oesophageal motility in the irritable bowel syndrome. Br Med J 1981;282:1101.

57. Braverman DZ. Gallbladder contraction in patients with irritable bowel syndrome. Isr J Med Sci 1987;23:181.

58. Kellow JE, Miller LJ, Phillips SF, et al. Altered sensitivity of the gallbladder to cholecystokinin octapeptide in irritable bowel syndrome. Am J Physiol 1987;253:G650.

59. Whorwell PJ, Lupton EW, Erduran D, Wilson K. Bladder smooth muscle dysfunction in patients with irritable bowel syndrome. Gut 1986;27:1014.

60. White AM, Stevens WH, Upton AR, et al. Airway responsiveness to inhaled methacholine in patients with irritable bowel syndrome. Gastroenterology 1991;100:68.

61. Andrews PLR. Modulation of visceral afferent activity as a therapeutic possibility for gastrointestinal disorders. In: Read NW, Ed. Irritable bowel syndrome. London, Blackwell Scientific Publications, 1991:91.

62. Kumazawa T, Mizumura K. Abnormal activity of polymodal receptors induced by clioquinol. Brain Res 1984;310:185.

63. Thompson DG, Laidlow JM, Wingate DL. Abnormal small-bowel motility demonstrated by radiotelemetry in a patient with irritable colon. Lancet 1979;2:1321.

64. Kumar D, Wingate DL. The irritable bowel syndrome: a paroxysmal motor disorder. Lancet 1985;2:973.

65. Machella TE, Dworken HJ, Biel FJ. Observations on the splenic flexure syndrome. Ann Intern Med 1952;37:543.

66. Holdstock DJ, Misiewicz JJ, Waller SL. Observations on the mechanism of abdominal pain. Gut 1969;10:19.

67. Whitehead WE, Engel BT, Schuster MM. Irritable bowel syndrome: physiological and psychological differences between diarrhea-predominant and constipation-predominant patients. Dig Dis Sci 1980;25:404.

68. Mayer EA, Raybould HE. Role of visceral afferent mechanisms in functional bowel disorders. Gastroenterology 1990;99:1688.

69. Prior A, Maxton DG, Whorwell PJ. Anorectal manometry in irritable bowel syndrome: differences between diarrhoea and constipation predominant patients. Gut 1990;31:458.

70. Swarbrick ET, Hegarty JE, Bat L, et al. Site of pain from the irritable bowel. Lancet 1980;2:443.

71. Moriarty KJ, Dawson AM. Functional abdominal pain: further evidence that whole gut is affected. Br Med J 1982;284:1670.

72. Cook IJ, van Eeden A, Collins SM. Patients with irritable bowel syndrome have greater pain tolerance than normal subjects. Gastroenterology 1987;93:727.

73. Almy TP, Tulin M. Alterations in colonic function in man under stress: experimental production of changes simulating the "irritable colon". Gastroenterology 1947;8:616.

74. Almy TP. Experimental studies on the irritable colon. Am J Med 1951;10:60.

75. Almy TP, Abbot FK, Hinkle LE. Alternations in colonic function in man under stress: IV. hypomotility of the sigmoid colon, and its relationship to the mechanism of functional diarrhea. Gastroenterology 1950;15:95.

76. Narducci F, Snape WJ, Battle WM, London RL, Cohen S. Increased colonic motility during exposure to a stressful situation. Dig Dis Sci 1985;30:40.

77. Thompson DG, Richelson E, Malagelada J-R. Perturbation of gastric emptying and duodenal motility through the central nervous system. Gastroenterology 1982;83:1200.

78. Friedman J. Roentgen studies of the effects on the small intestine from emotional disturbances. AJR Am J Roentgenol 1954;72:367.

79. Goin LS. Some obscure factors in the production of unusual small bowel patterns. Radiology 1952;59:177.

80. Valori RM, Kumar D, Wingate DL. Effects of different types of stress and of "prokinetic" drugs on the control of the fasting motor complex in humans. Gastroenterology 1986;90:1890.

81. Kellow JE, Langeluddecke PM, Eckersley GM, et al. Effects of acute psychologic stress on small-intestinal motility in health and irritable bowel syndrome. Scand J Gastroenterol 1992;27:53.

82. Prior A, Colgan SM, Whorwell PJ. Changes in rectal sensitivity after hypnotherapy in patients with irritable bowel syndrome. Gut 1990;31:896.

83. Wingate DL. The irritable bowel syndrome. Gastroenterol Clin North Am 1991;20:351.

84. Smout AJPM, DeVore MS, Dalton CB, Castell DO. Cerebral potentials evoked by oesophageal distention in patients with non-cardiac chest pain. Gut 1992;33:298.

85. Whitehead WE, Bosmajian L, Zonderman AB, et al. Symptoms of psychologic distress associated with irritable bowel syndrome. Comparison of community and medical clinic samples. Gastroenterology 1988;95:709.

86. Liss JL, Alpers D, Woodruff RA. The irritable colon syndrome and psychiatric illness. Dis Nerv Syst 1973;34:151.

87. Young SJ, Alpers DH, Norland CC, Woodruff RA. Psychiatric illness and the irritable bowel syndrome: practical implications for the primary physician. Gastroenterology 1976;70:162.

88. Walker EA, Katon WJ, Jemelka RP, Roy-Byrne PP. Comorbidity of gastrointestinal complaints, depression, and anxiety disorders in the Epidemiologic Catchment Area (ECA) study. Am J Med 1992;92:26S.

89. Walker EA, Roy-Byrne PP, Katon WJ, et al. Psychiatric illness and irritable bowel syndrome: a comparison with inflammatory bowel disease. Am J Psychiatry 1990;147:1656.

90. Creed F, Guthrie E. Psychological factors in the irritable bowel syndrome. Gut 1987;28:1307.
91. Wise TM, Cooper JN, Ahmed S. The efficacy of group therapy for patients with irritable bowel syndrome. Psychosomatics 1982;23:465.
92. West KL. MMPI correlates of ulcerative colitis. J Clin Psychol 1970;26:214.
93. Hislop IG. Psychological significance of the irritable colon syndrome. Gut 1971;12:452.
94. Hill OW, Blendis L. Physical and psychological evaluation of "nonorganic" abdominal pain. Gut 1971;12:452.
95. Hislop IG. Childhood deprivation: an antecedent of the irritable bowel syndrome. Med J Aust 1979;1:372.
96. Drossman DA, Leserman J, Nachman G, et al. Sexual and physical abuse in women with functional or organic gastrointestinal disorders. Ann Intern Med 1990;113:828.
97. Paykel ES, Prusoff BA, Uhlenhuth EH. Scaling of life events. Arch Gen Psychiatry 1971;25:340.
98. Lowman BC, Drossman DA, Cramer EM, McKee DC. Recollection of childhood events in adults with irritable bowel syndrome. J Clin Gastroenterol 1987;9:324.
99. Lisker R, Solomons NW, Perez Briceno R, Ramirez Mata M. Lactase and placebo in the management of the irritable bowel syndrome: a double-blind, cross-over study. Am J Gastroenterol 1989;84:756.
100. Rumessen JJ, Gudmand-Hoyer E. Functional bowel disease: malabsorption and abdominal distress after ingestion of fructose, sorbitol, and fructose-sorbitol mixtures. Gastroenterology 1988;95:694.
101. Haderstorfer B, Psycholgin D, Whitehead WE, Schuster MM. Intestinal gas production from bacterial fermentation of undigested carbohydrate in irritable bowel syndrome. Am J Gastroenterol 1989;84:375.
102. Alun Jones V, McLaughlan P, Shorthouse M, et al. Food intolerance: a major factor in the pathogenesis of irritable bowel syndrome. Lancet 1982;2:1115.
103. McKee AM, Prior A, Whorwell PJ. Exclusion diets in irritable bowel syndrome: are they worthwhile? J Clin Gastroenterol 1987;9:526.
104. Paganelli R, Fagiolo V, Cancian M, et al. Intestinal permeability in irritable bowel syndrome. Effect of diet and sodium cromoglycate administration. Ann Allergy 1990;64:377.
105. Zwetchkenbaum J, Burakoff R. The irritable bowel syndrome and food hypersensitivity. Ann Allergy 1988;61:47.
106. Smart HL, Atkinson M. Abnormal vagal function in irritable bowel syndrome. Lancet 1987;2:475.
107. McAllister C, McGrath F, Fielding JF. Altered skin temperature and electromyographic activity in the irritable bowel syndrome. Biomed Pharmacother 1990;44:399.
108. Kumar D, Thompson PD, Wingate DL, et al. Abnormal REM sleep in the irritable bowel syndrome. Gastroenterology 1992;103:12.
109. Dinan TG, Barry S, Ahkion S, et al. Assessment of central noradrenergic functioning in irritable bowel syndrome using a neuroendocrine challenge test. J Psychosom Res 1990;34:575.
110. Heitkemper MM, Jarrett M. Pattern of gastrointestinal and somatic symptoms across the menstrual cycle. Gastroenterology 1992;102:505.
111. Besterman HS, Sarson DL, Rambaud JC, et al. Gut hormone responses in the irritable bowel syndrome. Digestion 1981;21:219.
112. Sjolund K, Ekman R. Are gut peptides responsible for the irritable bowel syndrome (IBS)? Scand J Gastroenterol Suppl 1987;130:15.
113. Mortensen PB, Andersen JR, Arffmann S, Krag E. Short-chain fatty acids and the irritable bowel syndrome: the effect of wheat bran. Scand J Gastroenterol 1987;22:185.
114. Borody TJ, George L, Andrews P, et al. Bowel-flora alteration: a potential cure for inflammatory bowel disease and irritable bowel syndrome? (letter). Med J Aust 1989;150:604.
115. Gade J, Thorn P. Paraghurt for patients with irritable bowel syndrome. A controlled clinical investigation from general practice. Scand J Prim Health Care 1989;7:23–26.
116. Kruis W, Thieme C, Weinzierl M, et al. A diagnostic score for the irritable bowel syndrome: its value in the exclusion of organic disease. Gastroenterology 1984;87:1.
117. Talley NJ, Phillips SF, Melton LJ, et al. Diagnostic value of the Manning criteria in irritable bowel syndrome. Gut 1990;31:77.
118. Smith RC, Greenbaum DS, Vancouver JB, et al. Gender differences in Manning criteria in the irritable bowel syndrome. Gastroenterology 1991;100:591.
119. Klein KB. Controlled clinical trials in the irritable bowel syndrome: a critique. Gastroenterology 1988;95:232.
120. Steggerda FR. Gastrointestinal gas following food consumption. Ann N Y Acad Sci 1968;150:57.
121. Davies PJ. Influence of diet on flatus volume in human subjects. Gut 1971;12:713.
122. Van Ness MM, Cattau EL. Flatulence: pathophysiology and treatment. Am Fam Physician 1985;31:198.
123. Friedman G. Diet and the irritable bowel syndrome. Gastroenterol Clin North Am 1991;20:313.
124. Fioramonti J, Bueno L. Motor activity in the large intestine of the pig related to dietary fibre and retention time. Br J Nutr 1980;43:155.
125. Muller-Lissner SA. Effect of wheat bran on weight of stool and gastrointestinal transit time: a meta analysis. Br Med J 1988;296:615.
126. Payler DK, Pomare EW, Heaton KW, Harvey RF. The effect of wheat bran on intestinal transit. Gut 1975;16:209.
127. The bran wagon (editorial). Lancet 1987;1:782.
128. Taylor I, Darby C, Hammond P. Comparison of rectosigmoid myoelectrical activity in the irritable colon syndrome during relapses and remissions. Gut 1978;19:923.
129. Manning AP, Heaton KW, Harvey RF, Uglow P. Wheat fibre and irritable bowel syndrome: a controlled trial. Lancet 1977;2:417.
130. Soltoft J, Gudmand-Hoyer E, Krag B, et al. A double-blind trial of the effect of wheat bran on symptoms of irritable bowel syndrome. Lancet 1976;1:270.
131. Arffmann S, Andersen JR, Hegnhoj J, et al. The effect of coarse wheat bran in the irritable bowel syndrome: a double-blind crossover study. Scand J Gastroenterol 1985;20:295.
132. Lucey MR, Clark ML, Lowndes JO, Dawson AM. Is bran efficacious in irritable bowel syndrome? a double blind placebo controlled crossover study. Gut 1987;28:221.
133. Longstreth GF, Fox DD, Youkeles L, et al. Psyllium therapy in the irritable bowel syndrome: a double blind trial. Ann Intern Med 1981;95:53.
134. Kumar A, Kumar N, Vij JC, et al. Optimum dosage of ispaghula husk in patients with irritable bowel syndrome: correlation of symptom relief with whole gut transit time and stool weight. Gut 1987;28:150.
135. Ritchie JA, Truelove SC. Treatment of irritable bowel syndrome with lorazepam, hyoscine butylbromide, and ispaghula husk. Br Med J 1979;1:376.
136. Prior A, Whorwell PJ. Double blind study of ispaghula in irritable bowel syndrome. Gut 1987;28:1510.
137. Snape WJ, Wright SH, Battle WM, Cohen S. The gastrocolic response: Evidence for a neural mechanism. Gastroenterology 1979;77:1235.
138. Lanfranchi GA, Bazzocchi G, Campieri M, et al. Reduction by cimetropium bromide of the colonic motor response to eating in patients with the irritable bowel syndrome. Eur J Clin Pharmacol 1988;33:571.
139. Prior A, Harris SR, Whorwell PJ. Reduction of colonic motility by intravenous nicardipine in irritable bowel syndrome. Gut 1987;28:1609.
140. Narducci F, Bassotti G, Gaburri M, et al. Nifedipine reduces the colonic motor response to eating in patients with the irritable colon syndrome. Am J Gastroenterol 1985;80:317.
141. Narducci F, Bassotti G, Granata MT, et al. Colonic motility and gastric emptying in patients with irritable bowel syndrome. Dig Dis Sci 1986;31:241.
142. Page JG, Dirnberger GM. Treatment of the irritable bowel syndrome with Bentyl (dicyclomine hydrochloride). J Clin Gastroenterol 1981;3:153.

143. Piai G, Mazzacca G. Prifinium bromide in the treatment of the irritable colon syndrome. Gastroenterology 1979;77:500.

144. Centonze V, Imbimbo BP, Campanozzi F, et al. Oral cimetropium bromide, a new antimuscarinic drug, for long-term treatment of irritable bowel syndrome. Am J Gastroenterol 1988;83:1262.

145. Dobrilla G, Imbimbo BP, Piazzi L, Bensi G. Long-term treatment of irritable bowel syndrome with cimetropium bromide: a double blind placebo controlled trial. Gut 1990;31:355.

146. Kasich AM, Rafsky JC. Clinical evaluation of an anticholinergic in the irritable colon syndrome: a double blind study of tricyclamol. Am J Gastroenterol 1959;31:47.

147. Byrne S. Verapamil in the treatment of irritable bowel syndrome (letter). J Clin Psych 1987;48:388.

148. Powell-Tuck J, MacRae KD, Healy MJR, et al. A defence of the small clinical trial: evaluation of three gastroenterological studies. Br Med J 1986;292:599.

149. Perez-Mateo M, Sillero C, Cuesta A, et al. Diltiazem in the treatment of the irritable bowel syndrome. Int J Clin Pharmacol Res 1986;6:425.

150. Hills JM, Aaronson PI. The mechanism of action of peppermint oil on gastrointestinal smooth muscle. Gastroenterology 1991;101:55.

151. Rees WDW, Evans BK, Rhodes J. Treating irritable bowel syndrome with peppermint oil. Br Med J 1979;2:835.

152. Dew MJ, Evans BK, Rhodes J. Peppermint oil for the irritable bowel syndrome: a multicentre trial. Br J Clin Pract 1984;38:394.

153. Walsh P, Gould SR, Barnardo DE. Peppermint oil does not relieve the pain of irritable bowel syndrome. Br J Clin Pract 1986;40:292.

154. Froguel E, Chaussade S, Roche H, et al. Effects of an intestinal smooth muscle calcium channel blocker (pinaverium bromide) on colonic transit time in humans. J Gastrointest Motil 1990;2:176.

155. Cristen MO. Action of pinaverium bromide, a calcium-antagonist, on gastrointestinal motility disorders. Gen Pharmacol 1990;21:821.

156. Passaretti S, Sorghi M, Colombo E, et al. Motor effects of locally administered pinaverium bromide in the sigmoid tract of patients with irritable bowel syndrome. Int J Clin Pharmacol Ther Toxicol 1989;27:47.

157. Connell AM. Physiological and clinical assessment of the effect of the musculotropic agent mebeverine on the human colon. Br Med J 1965;2:848.

158. Tasman-Jones C. Mebeverine in patients with the irritable colon syndrome: double blind study. N Z Med J 1973;77:232.

159. Kruis W, Weinzierl M, Schussler P, Holl J. Comparison of the therapeutic effect of wheat bran, mebeverine and placebo in patients with the irritable bowel syndrome. Digestion 1986;34:196.

160. Frexinos J, Fioramonti J, Bueno L. Effect of trimebutine on colonic myoelectrical activity in IBS patients. Eur J Clin Pharmacol 1985;28:181.

161. Luttecke K. A trial of trimebutine in spastic colon. J Int Med Res 1978;6:86.

162. Moshal MG, Herron M. A clinical trial of trimebutine (Mebutin) in spastic colon. J Int Med Res 1979;7:231.

163. Fielding JF. Double blind trial of trimebutine in the irritable bowel syndrome. Ir Med J 1980;73:377.

164. Cann PA, Read NW, Holdsworth CD, Barends D. Role of loperamide and placebo in management of irritable bowel syndrome. Dig Dis Sci 1984;29:239.

165. Lavo B, Stenstam M, Nielsen A-L. Loperamide in treatment of irritable bowel syndrome—a double blind placebo controlled study. Scand J Gastroenterol Suppl 1987;130:77.

166. Hovdenak N. Loperamide treatment of the irritable bowel syndrome. Scand J Gastroenterol Suppl 1987;130:81.

167. Schapiro RH, Heizer WD, Goldfinger SE, Aserkoff BR. Cholestyramine responsive idiopathic diarrhea. Gastroenterology 1970;58:993.

168. Talley NJ, Phillips SF, Miller LJ, Haddad A. A specific 5-HT$_3$ antagonist delays colonic transit and inhibits postprandial neurotensin release. Gastroenterology 1988;95:891.

169. Steadman CJ, Talley NJ, Phillips SF, Mulvahill C. Trial of a selective serotonin type 3 (5-HT$_3$) receptor antagonist ondansetron (GR38032F) in diarrhea predominant irritable bowel syndrome (IBS). Gastroenterology 1990;98:A394.

170. Van Wijk HJ, Smout AJ, Akkermans LM, et al. Gastric emptying and dyspeptic symptoms in the irritable bowel syndrome. Scand J Gastroenterol 1992;27:99.

171. Baeyens R, Van de Velde E, De Schepper A, et al. Effects of intravenous and oral domperidone on the motor function of the stomach and small intestine. Postgrad Med J 1979;55(Suppl 1):19.

172. Wiley J, Owyang C. Dopaminergic modulation of rectosigmoid motility: action of domperidone. J Pharmacol Exp Ther 1987;242:548.

173. Milo R. Use of the peripheral dopamine antagonist, domperidone, in the management of gastrointestinal symptoms in patients with irritable bowel syndrome. Curr Med Res Opin 1980;6:577.

174. Fielding JF. Domperidone treatment in the irritable bowel syndrome. Digestion 1982;23:125.

175. Cann PA, Read NW, Holdsworth CD. Oral domperidone: double blind comparison with placebo in irritable bowel syndrome. Gut 1983;24:1135.

176. Passaretti S, Tittobello A, Capozzi C, Verlinden M. Cisapride accelerates total intestinal transit in patients with irritable bowel syndrome-associated constipation. Progr Med 1987;43(Suppl 1):121.

177. Van Outryve M, Milo R, Toussaint J, Van Eeghem P. "Prokinetic" treatment of constipation-predominant irritable bowel syndrome: a placebo-controlled study of cisapride. J Clin Gastroenterol 1991;13:49.

178. Sun WM, Edwards CA, Prior A, et al. Effect of oral nicardipine on anorectal function in normal human volunteers and patients with irritable bowel syndrome. Dig Dis Sci 1990;35:885.

179. Coremans G, Vergauwe P, Vantrappen G. How do analgesic mixtures contribute to constipation? J Gastrointest Motil 1991;3:178.

180. Coffin B, Jian R, Lemann M, et al. Fedotozine increases threshold of discomfort to gastric distention in healthy subjects. Gastroenterology 1992;102:A437.

181. Moss H, Sanger GJ. Antagonism by BR-43694 of pseudoaffective reflexes evoked by duodenal distention. Br J Pharmacol 1987;92:531P.

182. Stark M, Maher K, Gupta P, et al. Visceral afferent blockade with ondansetron (Zofran) increases nociceptive thresholds in patients with chest pain of undetermined etiology. Am J Gastroenterol 1991;82:1305.

183. Hasler WL, Soudah HC, Owyang C. A somatostatin analogue inhibits afferent pathways mediating perception of rectal distention. Gastroenterology 1993;104:1390.

184. Hasler WL, Soudah HC, Owyang C. Somatostatin analog inhibits afferent response to rectal distention in diarrhea-predominant irritable bowel patients. J Pharmacol Exp Ther 1994;268:1206.

185. Talley NJ, Turner I, Middleton WRJ. Somatostatin and symptomatic relief of irritable bowel syndrome (letter). Lancet 1987;2:1144.

186. Roberts D, Chey WD, Hasler W, et al. Somatostatin analog reduces perception of rectal distention by specific inhibition of spinal afferent pathways (abstract). Gastroenterology 1993;104:A571.

187. Myren J, Groth H, Larssen S-E, Larsen S. The effect of trimipramine in patients with the irritable bowel syndrome: a double-blind study. Scand J Gastroenterol 1982;17:871.

188. Heefner JD, Wilder RM, Wilson ID. Irritable colon and depression. Psychosomatics 1978;19:540.

189. Greenbaum DS, Mayle JE, Vanegeren LE, et al. Effects of desipramine on irritable bowel syndrome compared with atropine and placebo. Dig Dis Sci 1987;32:257.

190. Kasich AM, Fein HD, Miller JW. Comparative effect of phenaglycodol, meprobamate, and a placebo on the irritable colon. Am J Dig Dis 1959;4:229.

191. Kasich AM. A double-blind study of heteronium bromide and

amobarbital in the management of gastrointestinal conditions associated with anxiety. Curr Ther Res 1968;10:508.

192. Rhodes JB, Abrams JH, Manning RT. Controlled trial of sedative-anticholinergic drugs in patients with the irritable bowel syndrome. J Clin Pharm 1978;18:340.

193. Deutsch E. Relief of anxiety and related emotions in patients with gastrointestinal disorders: a double-blind controlled study. Dig Dis 1971;16:1091.

194. Baume P, Cuthbert J. The effect of medazepam in relieving symptoms of functional gastrointestinal distress. Aust N Z J Med 1973;3:457.

195. Tollefson GD, Luxenberg M, Valentine R, et al. An open label trial of aprazolam in comorbid irritable bowel syndrome and generalized anxiety disorder. J Clin Psychiatry 1991;52:502.

196. Rider JA, Moeller HC. Use of silicone in the treatment of intestinal gas and bloating. JAMA 1960;174:2052.

197. Hall RG, Thompson H, Strother A. Effects of orally administered activated charcoal on intestinal gas. Am J Gastroenterol 1981;75:192.

198. Friedman G. Treatment of the irritable bowel syndrome. Gastroenterol Clin North Am 1991;20:325.

199. Abrahamsson H, Lyrenas E, Dotevall G. Effects of beta-adrenoceptor blocking drugs on human sigmoid colonic motility. Dig Dis Sci 1983;28:590.

200. Abrahamsson H, Dotevall G. Effects of propranolol on colonic pressure in patients with irritable bowel syndrome. Scand J Gastroenterol 1981;16:1021.

201. Marzuk PM. Atenolol in irritable bowel syndrome (letter). Lancet 1987;2:1143.

202. McIntyre AS, Burnham WR, Thompson DG. Atenolol in irritable bowel syndrome (letter). Lancet 1988;1:67.

203. Fielding JF. Timolol treatment in the irritable bowel syndrome. Digestion 1981;22:155.

204. Mathias JR, Ferguson KL, Clench MH. Debilitating "functional" bowel disease controlled by leuprolide acetate, gonadotropin-releasing hormone (GnRH) analog. Dig Dis Sci 1989;34:761.

205. Stefanini GF, Prati E, Albini MC, et al. Oral disodium cromoglycate treatment of irritable bowel syndrome: an open study on 101 subjects with diarrheic type. Am J Gastroenterol 1992;87:55.

206. Greenbaum DS, Ferguson RK, Kater LA, et al. A controlled therapeutic study of the irritable bowel syndrome: effect of diphenylhydantoin. N Engl J Med 1973;288:13.

207. Svedlund J, Sjodin I, Ottosson J-O, Dotevall G. Controlled study of psychotherapy in irritable bowel syndrome. Lancet 1983;2:589.

208. Guthrie E, Creed F, Dawson D, Tomenson B. A controlled trial of psychological treatment for the irritable bowel syndrome. Gastroenterology 1991;100:450.

209. Arn I, Theorell T, Uvnas-Moberg K, Jonsson CO. Psychodrama group therapy for patients with functional gastrointestinal disorders—a controlled long-term follow-up study. Psychother Psychosom 1989;51:113.

210. Blanchard EB, Schwarz SP. Adaptation of a multicomponent treatment for irritable bowel syndrome to a small-group format. Biofeedback Self Regul 1987;12:63.

211. Blanchard EB, Radnitz C, Schwarz SP, et al. Psychological changes associated with self-regulatory treatments of irritable bowel syndrome. Biofeedback Self Regul 1987;12:31.

212. Schwarz SP, Taylor AE, Scharff L, Blanchard EB. Behaviorally treated irritable bowel syndrome patients: a four-year follow-up. Behav Res Ther 1990;28:331.

213. Shaw G, Srivastava ED, Sadlier M, et al. Stress management for irritable bowel syndrome: a controlled trial. Digestion 1991;50:36.

214. Bennett P, Wilkinson S. A comparison of psychological and medical treatment of the irritable bowel syndrome. Br J Clin Psychol 1985;24:215.

215. Radnitz CL, Blanchard EB. Bowel sound biofeedback as a treatment for irritable bowel syndrome. Biofeedback Self Regul 1988;13:169.

216. Whorwell PJ, Prior A, Faragher EB. Controlled trial of hypnotherapy in the treatment of severe refractory irritable-bowel syndrome. Lancet 1984;2:1232.

217. Whorwell PJ, Prior A, Colgan SM. Hypnotherapy in severe irritable bowel syndrome: further experience. Gut 1987;28:423.

218. Whorwell PJ. Hypnotherapy in irritable bowel syndrome (letter). Lancet 1989;1:622.

219. Vernia P, Latella G, Magliocca FM, et al. Seeking clues for a positive diagnosis of the irritable bowel syndrome. Eur J Clin Invest 1987;17:189.

220. Harvey RF, Mauad EC, Brown AM. Prognosis in the irritable bowel syndrome: a 5-year prospective study. Lancet 1987;1:963.

221. Waller SL, Misiewicz JJ. Prognosis in the irritable-bowel syndrome: a prospective study. Lancet 1969;2:753.

222. Fowlie S, Eastwood MA, Ford MJ. Irritable bowel syndrome: the influence of psychological factors on the symptom complex. J Psychosom Res 1992;36:169.

Textbook of Gastroenterology, second edition, edited by Tadataka Yamada. JB Lippincott Company, Philadelphia © 1995.

CHAPTER 82

Motility Disorders of the Colon

Sidney F. Phillips

The human colon displays widely divergent patterns of motility and transit. In severely constipated persons, mean transit times can be measured in days, even up to a week or more[1], yet propulsive, peristaltic motility can move contents over long distances very rapidly, with an efficiency approaching that of the esophagus.[2] It has been proposed that the colon is programmed to move its contents efficiently and rapidly, like the rest of the gut. Only by being under strong inhibitory influences for much of the time can colonic transit be slowed and fecal contents solidified. The well-developed muscular wall of the colon exhibits basal tone but, at the same time, has a pronounced propensity to relax.[3] Afferent nervous signals arising from the colon readily reach consciousness, where they are perceived as visceral pain.[4] This wide range of functions establishes the large intestine as a potential site from which many symptoms could originate. In particular, as the organ responsible for the final stages of absorption and elimination, the colon is highly relevant to diarrhea and constipation. Moreover, colonic fermentation of dietary residues, mainly the unavailable carbohydrates, generates hydrogen, carbon dioxide, short-chain fatty acids, and methane by the anaerobic action of bacterial enzymes[5]; distention of the abdomen and flatulence can follow. Finally, for imagined, cultural, and psychosocial reasons, many populations focus on their habits of elimination. Constipation is a major concern of many persons, and fecal incontinence is an understandable social fear of others. For all of these reasons, disturbances of colonic motility figure prominently in the minds of patients and physicians.

Although the precise pathogenic mechanisms responsible for disorders of colonic motility are still obscure, a few clues are available. The material presented here cannot address all issues in equal depth; related chapters on the brain and the gut (see Chap. 3), the motor physiology of the colon (see Chap. 10), abdominal pain (see Chap. 34), gas and bloating (see Chap. 35), constipation (see Chap. 39), irritable bowel syndrome (see Chap. 81), and the clinical evaluation of gastrointestinal motility (see Chap. 132) should also be consulted. The only clinical conditions to be addressed specifically here are those of acute colonic pseudoobstruction (Ogilvie's syndrome) and chronic intestinal pseudoobstruction.

REVIEW OF COLONIC MOTOR FUNCTION

The mammalian large intestine is a highly versatile organ that maintains fluid and electrolyte balance, salvages the products of intracolonic fermentation, and stores feces until elimination is convenient. These functions all depend ultimately on the colon's capacity to control the distal progression of contents. As chyme enters the colon from the ileum, it is retained in the proximal colon while colonic microorganisms degrade indigestible food residues such as cellulose; water and electrolytes are absorbed actively. The colonic contents are desiccated during further transit, and solid feces can be formed because colonic transit normally requires hours, even days, for completion.

Much of the early information on colonic motility and transit came from direct observations. At laparotomy, animals were studied after high obliterations of the spinal cord[6] that were necessary so that activity of the normally quiet colon was increased. Distention of the colon in herbivores caused the circular muscle to contract and the cecum to empty; aborad transit was often observed. In carnivores, with their smaller proximal colons, distention of the proximal third of the colon caused antiperistalsis, and distention in the intermediate and distal colons provoked aborad propulsive contractions. Fluoroscopy of the cat colon had previously shown antiperistalsis in vivo in response to water enemas.[7]

Colonic Function in Humans

The human colon, though unessential for normal health, serves many functions. Its anatomy is adapted to an omnivorous diet; as in herbivores, the human proximal colon is voluminous and has prominent haustrations. The proximal colon contains fermentative bacteria which degrade organic material, principally complex carbohydrates, to short-chain fatty acids. The predominant products are acetate, propionate, and butyrate. Short-chain fatty acids are rapidly absorbed from the colon; they also augment sodium, chloride, and water absorption[8], and they are a source of energy for human colonic epithelial cells.[9] These fermentative and absorptive processes appear to be facilitated by motor activity that stirs and mixes the contents.

In healthy persons, the colon absorbs approximately 1.5 L of ileal effluent each day,[10] probably mainly in the proximal colon. Further desiccation of colonic contents occurs as they are propelled distally, and the end result is the convenient elimination of approximately 100 to 200 g of formed stool in one or two bowel movements per day. If stressed by increased volumes of ileal effluent, the healthy colon can absorb up to 4 to 6 L/day before diarrhea develops.[11] The contribution of changes in motility to the colonic absorptive reserve is uncertain.

Colonic Manometry

Pressure waves recorded manometrically are generally equated with contractile forces. Colonic contractions are often irregular, of varying frequency and amplitude, and subject to many perturbing influences. Individual emotional states, the types of meals that are eaten, and the composition of chyme entering the colon from the ileum are all known to modulate colonic contractile activity, but they vary significantly in their importance in any person from hour to hour and day to day.[12] Colonic manometry has developed considerably from early attempts that used compressible balloons and open-ended, air-filled tubes[13,14]; today, high-fidelity techniques, internal

strain gauges, electronic transducers, and pneumohydraulic capillary infusion systems linked to external transducers are available. Records can be retained for analysis by a variety of direct writing and computerized data storage systems. The refinement of ambulatory systems for prolonged recording allows motor patterns to be sampled day and night for several days outside of the laboratory environment.[15]

Despite better recording and analytic technology, colonic manometry provides only general insights into the control of contractile events. There are few clearly recognizable patterns, access to the colonic lumen is sometimes difficult, and the colon must be cleansed for reliable records to be obtained. For many years, difficulties with access restricted most studies of colonic motility to the rectum and distal sigmoid region, the extent to which a rigid sigmoidoscope could be inserted. However, colonoscopy is now used to place motility sensors throughout the cleansed colon.[3]

Cyclic contractile activity with a periodicity of 20 to 30 minutes (Fig. 82-1) and perhaps analogous to the migrating motor complex of the small intestine is found in the colon of dogs.[16,17] Bursts of contractile activity occur in the fasting and fed states. Most migrate in the caudad direction, a few are retrograde, and stationary bursts also occur. In humans, however, colonic cyclic contractile activity has not been demonstrated. Recordings of resting colonic motility made for short periods suggest that the colon is often quiescent or that contractions are often isolated (perhaps reflecting a dominant inhibitory control); sometimes, pressure waves are recorded in continuous bursts ranging in duration from 10 to 30 minutes.[18] These bursts have a dominant frequency of approximately 6 contractions per minute in the right colon, but higher and lower frequencies have also been observed. In the distal colon, contractions are present at two frequencies, about 3 and about 7 per minute (Fig. 82-2), but marked intra- and interindividual variations are seen.[18]

Phasic pressure waves are the most common manometric phenomenon, but their role in enhancing colonic absorption or facilitating propulsion is not well defined. Phasic colonic contractions are stimulated by meals, the response being characterized by increased numbers of pressure waves. These are usually expressed as a colonic motility index (a representation of the cumulative number and amplitude of pressure waves occurring in a predetermined period of time). Motility indices increase 20 to 30 minutes after a meal, and they remain elevated for up to 3 hours, sometimes showing a biphasic pattern with a second peak of activity at approximately 70 and 90 minutes postprandially.[19,20] This response to eating, termed the gastrocolic reflex, remains after gastrectomy and after vagotomy.[21] Even in the absence of the stomach, food arriving in the small intestine elicits increased activity in the colon. If the stomach is intact, gastric distention and the

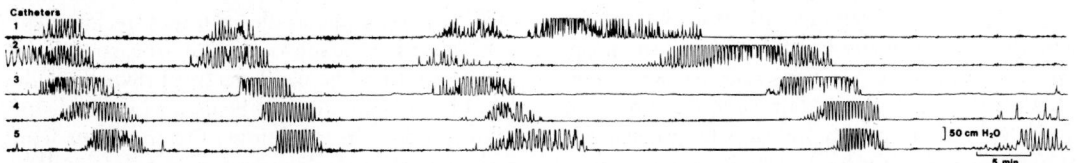

FIGURE 82-1. Manometric recordings from five sites in canine colon (1 through 5, proximal to distal). Cycles of motility occur each 20 to 30 minutes.

Terminal Ileum

Ascending Colon

Recto-sigmoid
Colon & Rectum

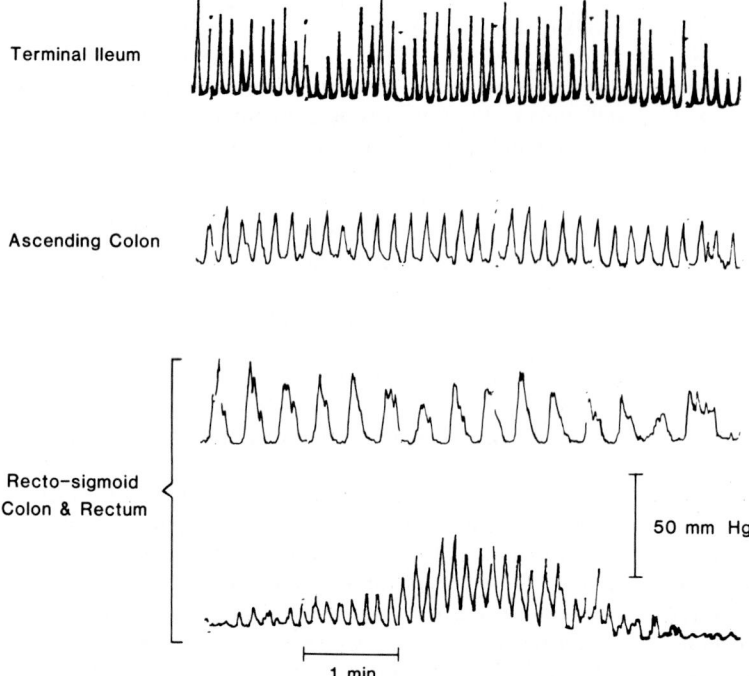

50 mm Hg

1 min

FIGURE 82-2. Regular phasic waves recorded from the human terminal ileum and three colonic segments illustrate different patterns within the large intestine.

chemical stimulation by nutrients elicits a comparable response; lipids are the most potent stimulus.[22] The colonic response to eating occurs in all parts of the colon, but contractile events differ quantitatively from segment to segment.[18]

Control of the colonic response to eating involves neural and, possibly, hormonal mechanisms. That part of the response mediated by gastric mechanoreceptors is very sensitive to blockade by atropine, but that which originates in the small intestine is only partially under muscarinic control. Cholecystokinin (CCK), which is normally secreted after meals, has been thought to play a role in the response, because high blood concentrations of CCK stimulate contractile activity in both the small and large intestine. However, the CCK_A receptor antagonist, Loxiglumide, did not block the gastrocolonic response to food.[23] Increased phasic contractile activity also occurs in response to drugs, particularly morphine and prostigmine, but it is reduced by meperidine and largely abolished by muscarinic blockers (anticholinergics).[24,25]

Longer periods of observation may help elucidate colonic motility, but there are still relatively few data of this type. Like pieces of a puzzle, data gained from shorter studies must be viewed as part of the overall diurnal cycle. Low-amplitude contractions, appearing in bursts (at frequencies of 3 or 7 per minute) or singly, constitute most of each day's contractile activity. The early concept of categorizing intestinal contractile activity into segmentation and peristalsis is still useful in understanding colonic motility. Irregular phasic activity does not appear to propagate, and this activity probably equates with segmentation; on the other hand, high-pressure, propagating waves are the equivalent of peristalsis. Isolated, high-amplitude (up to 200 mg Hg) peristaltic contractions (Fig. 82-3), propagating at 1 cm per second over long distances, are thought to be important for transit; these are uncommon and are most often seen after waking and after meals.[26] However, peristaltic waves occur reliably after instillation of irri-

tants such as bisacodyl into the colonic lumen.[27] Oleic acid, infused into the colon to simulate steatorrhea, stimulated high-pressure (>60 mm Hg) propagating waves of long duration (>10 seconds).[2]

An important variant of manometry is the electromechanical *barostat*. Originally developed for the detection of volume changes in the gastric fundus, the methodology is well suited to identify relaxation in any hollow viscus. The barostat bag is of large volume and infinite compliance up to a volume of 500 to 600 mL. Air is introduced or withdrawn from the bag by a servomechanism to maintain a preset, low pressure in the bag. Changes in volume are reflections of changes in wall tone. Basal tone in the proximal and distal colon exhibits rhythmic fluctuations (Fig. 82-4), and food induces an immediate and prolonged increase in tone.[3,28] The rectum also exhibits tonic changes which feature prominent relaxation.[29] Isobaric methodology is also being applied to the sensitivity of the rectum to distention.[30] It is now known that some patients with irritable bowel syndrome (IBS) have reduced compliance ("stiff rectum") and excessive sensitivity to rectal distention.[31]

Colonic Electromyography

The recording of electrical signals generated by the longitudinal and circular muscle layers of the colon is an important facet of physiologic studies, but these techniques have not yet achieved a significant role in clinical gastroenterology. In the small intestine, the basal electrical rhythm ("slow wave") is highly consistent and can be used as a reliable index of physiology and pathophysiology. On the other hand, electrical activity in the colon is complex and variable.[32]

The slow wave frequency of the colon ranges widely (4–48 per minute) and is present only inconsistently. Moreover,

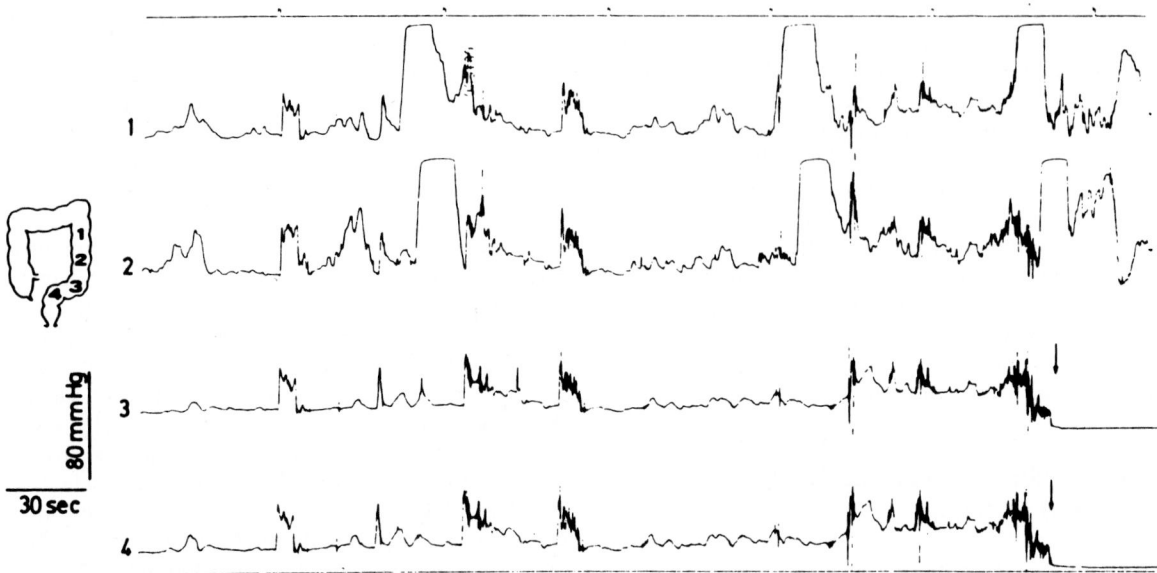

FIGURE 82-3. High pressure waves recorded sequentially from four sites in the human colon. These giant migrating contractions are thought to correspond to mass movements of colonic content. They occur less frequently in patients with constipation. (From Narducci F, Bassotti G, Gaburri M, Morelli A. Twenty-four hour manometric recording of colonic motor activity in healthy man. Gut 1987;28:17.)

a study of isolated rings of human colonic circular muscle found their mechanical activity to be only occasionally synchronized with the frequency of slow waves or with the electrical spiking.[32] Cholinergic stimulation of these preparations by carbachol evoked synchronized, periodic slow waves with superimposed spikes. Regular phasic contractions, at the frequency of the bursts of electrical activity (about 1 per minute), were blocked by atropine but not by tetrodotoxin, a nonspecific neurotoxin. This was thought to be consistent with a stimulus-induced pattern of myogenic activity resembling long spike bursts, recorded in vivo.[32] In longitudinal muscle, spontaneous electrical activity at a mean frequency of 26 cycles

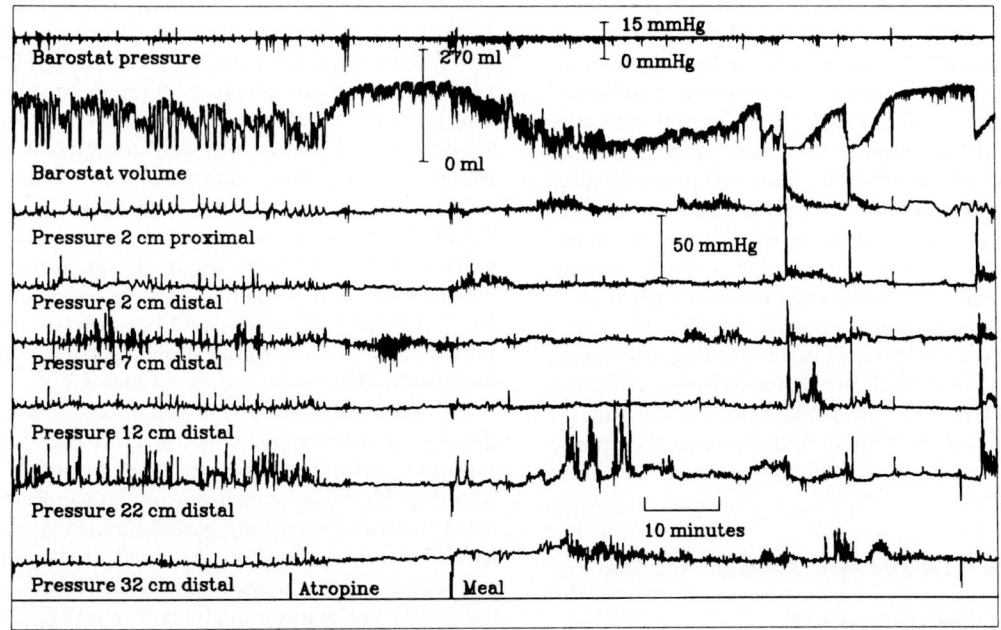

FIGURE 82-4. Barostat recording from the descending colon of a healthy person. The volume in the barostat increased after an injection of atropine, indicating relaxation of the wall of the colon. After a meal, the volume decreased as a result of increased tone in the wall of the colon. This increase in tone was not accompanied by manometric evidence of colonic motor activity. (From Steadman CJ, Phillips SF, Camilleri M, Talley NJ, Haddad A, Hanson R. Control of muscle tone in the human colon. Gut 1992;33:541.)

per minute and an amplitude of 8 mV has been recorded, with spiking superimposed on the oscillations. Contractions in the longitudinal muscle corresponded to the frequency of these bursts but not to the frequency of individual oscillations. Coupling appears to exist between the circular and longitudinal muscle layers in humans, possibly by the electrotonic spread of slow wave potentials through the smooth muscle cells; however the anatomic basis for this interaction (e.g., intermingled smooth muscle fibres or intercellular connections such as gap junctions) is uncertain. Slow waves in the colon may spread toward the serosal surface from a specialized layer, the interstitial cells of Cajal, located on the inner (mucosal) surface of the circular muscle layer. These structures have been identified in human tissues.[33]

In Vivo Recording of Human Colonic Myoelectrical Activity

In vivo recordings of human colonic myoelectrical activity are characterized by variability over time, among subjects, and among laboratories. Electrical control activity (slow waves) at the rectosigmoid has been reported to be either continuous[34,35] or intermittent[36,37] and to consist of two prominent frequency bands, 2 to 4 cycles per minute and 6 to 12 cycles per minute. Spiking has been reported to be both unrelated and related to the slow wave, and contractions may or may not accompany spiking. There are a number of reasons why such variability could exist. Electrical activities arising from other parts of the gut may be recorded in the colon.[38] Moreover, the intrinsic frequency of slow waves in vitro appears to vary more widely in humans than in animals.[32]

Technical factors are also germane to this variability. Recording methods have included bipolar electrodes on the serosal surface under the taenia coli[34,37] and monopolar or bipolar electrodes attached to the colonic mucosa by suction. Electrodes have also been mounted on intralumenal tubes[39] or clipped to the mucosal surface.[40] Poor mucosal contact by intralumenal electrodes impairs the recording of spiking activity. Most intralumenal recordings have been from the distal colon, although more proximal segments have been sampled by colonoscopic placement of electrodes.[41] The time of day, the timing of meals, and the nature of the colonic contents all may affect colonic contractile and myoelectrical activity.[25] Colonic myoelectrical activity is diurnal; there is little activity during sleep, but activity increases in the morning, after meals, and during periods of stress. Postprandial activity is influenced by the composition of meals: a high-calorie meal causes a greater increase in colonic activity, and ingestion of an amino acid mixture has been found to inhibit myoelectrical activity.[40]

POTENTIAL PATHOGENIC MECHANISMS

Disorders of Colon Transit

Historical Methods

As early as Cannon's (1902) observations on the movement of bismuth subnitrate in the feline colon,[7] it has been clear that colonic contents do not leave the colon in the same order

in which they enter. In healthy humans, glass beads of different colors given on successive days appear in the stool about 24 to 72 hours from the time of ingestion, but they are mixed together.[42] Cinefluorography of barium-impregnated colonic contents[43] has demonstrated mixing, storage, and propulsion. Interhaustral shuttling, propulsion, retropulsion, and to-and-fro movements mix the colonic contents. Propulsion and retropulsion appear to occur in similar ways: contents move from one haustrum to the next, through multihaustral segments, or within a single segment. During multihaustral propulsion, three or more haustral segments become contiguous, and the mass of contents moves onto the next segment while the original haustration is reformed. Peristaltic contractions usually start as interhaustral constrictions, travel further along the colon, and are able to propel feces distally. Defecation usually empties only the distal colon, and colonic contents orad to those that are expelled may be relatively unaffected at the end of defecation. The rectum is usually the only region that empties completely although, at times, material from the distal transverse colon can also be eliminated.[44]

Marker substances used to track the movement of colonic contents are usually taken orally and can be given as a single bolus, repeated boluses, or continuously. Observing the appearance and disappearance of markers in stools (mouth-to-anus transit) quantifies total colonic transit, but does not assess segmental transit, or the changes in transit through colonic segments.

Radiopaque Marker Techniques

Whole-gut transit. Discrete, barium-impregnated polythene markers that move with the colonic contents have become simple but robust measures of transit. Hinton and colleagues[45] measured gastrointestinal transit times using solid, 2- to 5-mm polythene pellets containing barium sulphate and small (2.7–4.5 mm diameter) pieces of radiopaque polythene tubing. These inert, nonabsorbable markers had a specific gravity similar to gut contents and were completely recoverable in the stool. Followed by either abdominal radiographs or stool radiography, the movement of such markers was taken to represent the transit of meal residues through the gut. No significant differences were found in the transit of markers whether they were given immediately before or with a meal. In 25 normal male subjects, all but one had passed 80% of the markers by the fifth day after ingestion, although none had passed 80% by the end of the first day.[45]

All subsequent work with radiopaque markers has been directed at refining this range of normality, reducing x-ray exposure, and minimizing inconvenience (such as stool collections). Methods involving many radiopaque markers (15 per day) taken over a long period (6 weeks) were compared with Hinton's single-dose method.[46] This continuous technique used a simple mathematical transformation to convert the number of markers in stools to a transit time in hours, by taking into account the period between marker ingestion and appearance of markers in the stools. Calculation of the colonic transit time utilized the turnover of markers accumulated in the colonic pool at equilibrium—that is, after daily elimination equalled the number ingested. Comparison of continuous and single-dose marker methods showed a good correlation. A test for whole gut transit requiring collection of only a single stool was subsequently developed.[47]

Segmental colonic transit. The rate of disappearance of radiopaque markers from colonic segments can be monitored with daily abdominal radiographs after a single dose of radiopaque markers.[48,49] Right and left colonic, sigmoid, and rectal segments can be defined by simply drawing lines between bony landmarks of the vertebral column and pelvis and confirming the validity of the segments using gas shadows. Methods were then developed to calculate actual segmental transit times rather than the rate of disappearance of markers from colonic segments.[50] A mathematical expression based on the time interval between serial abdominal radiographs described the continuous change in numbers of markers at any location in the colon.

Metcalf and associates[51] simplified the method so that only one radiograph with a fast film, high-kilovoltage technique is necessary, and radiation exposure is therefore minimal. By this method, radiopaque markers are taken in fixed numbers, at the same time (arbitrarily, 9:00 A.M.) each day for 3 days. On the fourth day, again at the same time, a radiograph is taken. The results obtained from this technique correlate well with the daily radiograph approach. The method works on the assumption that a 24-hour sampling interval approximates continuous observation. Rapid transit can cause all the markers to be lost in the feces before radiography on the fourth day; conversely, in slow transit, all 60 markers may be present on the single radiograph. A film on day 7 can then give more information. At present, this technique[51] is the most practical way of measuring segmental and total colonic transit. Capsules of marker rings are available as Sitz-Mark (Konsyl Pharmacological, Fort Worth, TX).

Radioisotope Methods

The transit of gamma-emitting radioisotopes through the colon can be quantified using a gamma camera linked to a computerized recording and processing system. In contrast to radiographic methods, the isotope can be monitored continuously for long periods without increasing radiation exposure. The transit of solids and liquids can be measured simultaneously[52] if different isotopes are used to label liquid and solid bowel contents, and segmental regions of interest in the colon can be easily defined.

Krevsky[53] and Spiller[54] and their associates instilled liquid isotope directly into the colon and Camilleri's group[55] followed labeled solids from the stomach, through the small bowel, and across the ileocolonic junction. Colonic filling usually featured bolus movements of isotope separated by plateaus, during which little isotope moved from the small to large bowel. This finding raised the possibility that if a bolus of isotope could be delivered to the distal ileum it might be possible to define a zero-time, the time at which the majority of isotope entered the cecum. Such a starting time could then serve as a suitable base from which emptying curves could be constructed. A pH-sensitive polymer that dissolves at the pH of the ileum can be used to coat capsules containing isotopically labeled beads.[56] By this approach, it has been possible to image the unprepared colon without the use of intubation; it is likely that such methods allow more physiologic mea-surements of colonic transit. Some have placed isotopes into capsules or tablets that were designed to pass intact through the small intestine and colon.[57,58] Gastric retention of larger capsules and possible differences in how the colon handles large capsules compared with food residues probably limit the usefulness of such approaches.

A few studies have attempted to correlate colonic motility and transit. If myoelectrical activity, intralumenal pressure, and flow of an infused fluid are recorded together in the distal colon, rhythmic, short (3-second) bursts of spiking electrical activity are observed in association with small rises in intralumenal pressure but no increase in flow.[39] Sporadic, long spike bursts (12 seconds and longer) are associated with higher intralumenal pressures and rapid flow to the rectum.[39] The most clear relation between colonic motility and transit is seen in colonic peristalsis, when distally propagating high-pressure waves propel boluses of colonic contents toward the rectum in mass movements. Instillation of oleic acid into the ascending colon induced high-pressure waves (>60 mm Hg) that moved colonic contents distally over long distances in several minutes (Fig. 82-5) and resulted in defecation.[2,26] However, propagating waves do not always move colonic contents distally. Radioisotope instilled at the splenic flexure moved away from the flexure in both directions during the recording of propagating pressure waves.[59]

Consequences of Rapid Transit

The net effects of fast or slow colonic transit are most clearly seen in the consistency of the stools. O'Donnell and colleagues[60] developed a seven-point scale for describing stool form and consistency, ranging from liquids to hard solids. These authors also were able to relate stool consistency to the overall mouth-to-anus transit time. A refinement of this approach enabled stool form to be related to colonic transit times.[52] If colonic transit times were altered experimentally by rapid cecal infusions of fluid, a good correlation was found between stool consistency and colonic transit time (Fig. 82-6).

Pain of Colonic Origin

Conditions usually thought to be associated with disorders of motility and transit, such as IBS, diarrhea, and constipation, are often accompanied by abdominal pain. Indeed, pain is a prerequisite for most definitions of IBS.[61] These patients are almost universally sensitive to distention of the small or large bowel by balloons or gas.[62] Visceral hypersensitivity has been proposed as an important component of IBS, and these patients experience widespread abdominal discomfort when the colon is distended at colonoscopy.[63] Moreover, IBS patients, especially those who complain of diarrhea, have lower thresholds for anorectal sensation; they experience gas, the call to stool, and rectal discomfort at lower volumes of distention than do patients with constipation or healthy controls.[64] Increased rectal sensitivity to distention is accompanied by an excessive motor response of the rectum,[31] confirming the important interaction between excessive sensation and quantitative motor responsiveness. Much attention has been given to an altered peripheral function of visceral afferents or central

RELATIONSHIP BETWEEN MOTILITY TRACING AND TRANSIT

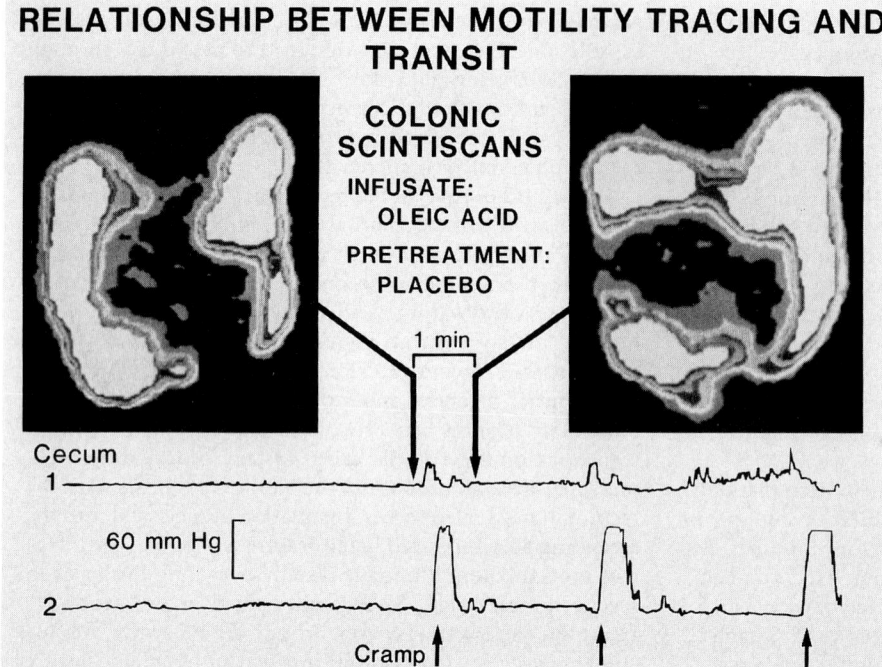

FIGURE 82-5. Two colonic scintiscans taken 1 minute apart from infusing oleic acid into the cecum. Comparison of the scans show almost complete emptying of the cecum and ascending colon, with distal movement of contents. A mass movement occurred during the 1-minute time lag between these scans. A high-pressure wave was recorded from the ascending colon at the same time, and the subject complained of abdominal cramps. (From Kamath PS, Phillips SF, O'Connor MK, Brown ML, Zinsmeister AR. Colonic capacitance and transit in man: modulation by luminal contents and drugs. Gut 1990;31:443.)

processing of afferent information in the altered somatovisceral sensation of patients with functional bowel disorders such as IBS.[4] Understanding what it is that alters visceral afferent function in IBS may uncover new therapeutic strategies aimed at blunting the excessive visceral perception or motor reflex responses evoked by visceral stimuli.[65-68]

Pathways of Visceral Pain

Like other segments of the gastrointestinal tract, the colon has dual innervation by the sympathetic and parasympathetic systems. On the afferent or sensory side, the vagus nerve is a major pathway for parasympathetic afferents, and the vagus overall is now thought to contain 90% afferent fibers. Vagal afferents have cell bodies in the nodose ganglion, and signals are relayed to the nucleus of the solitary tract. Spinal afferents have cell bodies in the dorsal root ganglion, which is reached by the main sympathetic or pelvic parasympathetic trunks. From the dorsal root ganglion, central transmission is through the dorsal horn. An additional afferent system arises from cell bodies in the submucous or myenteric plexus, with axons traveling with the sympathetic nerves to the prevertebral ganglia.

Although several pathways exist, specialized sensory endings have not been described. Nevertheless, the information carried by these systems includes tension in the gut wall, as recognized by mechanoreceptors, which are thought to be in series with circular muscle fibers; mesenteric tension or distention; and certain physical and chemical features of the contents such as temperature, osmolality, and nutrient composition.[4]

Modulation of Afferent Signals

Although patients with IBS are hypersensitive to colonic distention, their heightened pain response is not caused by generalized hyperalgesia, because somatic pain thresholds are normal.[64] Moreover, heightened sensitivity to colonic or rectal distention in IBS patients induces sensations similar to the common symptoms experienced by patients with functional bowel disorders. The pharmacology of afferents arising from the gut has been reviewed in detail.[69] Two approaches to modifying afferent input have been tested recently, using 5-HT$_3$ receptor antagonists and somatostatin analogues. The 5-HT$_3$ antagonist, granisetron, was able to reduce rectal hypersensitivity in a subgroup of IBS patients,[66] although a related compound, Ondansetron, was not.[30] The somatostatin analogue, octreotide, reduced rectal sensitivity to distention in healthy subjects[65] and those with IBS.[67]

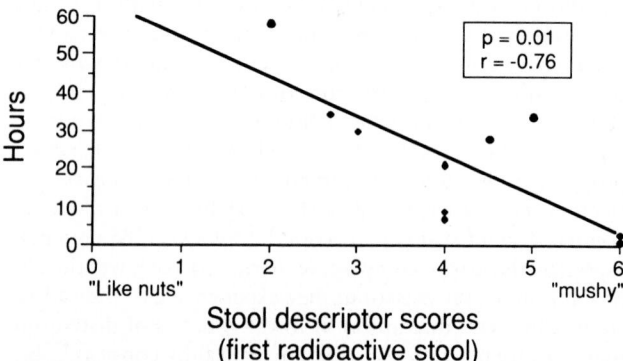

FIGURE 82-6. Relation between colonic transit time and physical appearance of stools; slow transit was associated with hard stools. (From Hammer J, Phillips SF. Fluid loading of the human colon: Effects of segmental transit and stool composition. Gastroenterology 1993;105:988.)

Pathogenic Mechanisms of Bloating and Distention

Abdominal distention is a frequent complaint of patients diagnosed with IBS. Typically, the complaint is episodic, often developing during the course of the day, and being variably aggravated by eating and relieved by defecation.[70] Visible distention and the need to loosen clothing are often described. Explanations proposed in the past included the presence of excessive volumes of intralumenal gas, unusual depression of the diaphragm, lumbar lordosis, and hysteria. None of these mechanisms adequately explains abdominal distention. Whorwell's group proposed that changes in motility or tone of gastrointestinal smooth muscle offer a more likely explanation,[71] although a physiologic basis for any such mechanism was not identified.

Viscerosomatic motor reflexes are known to exist; stimulation of abdominal viscera evokes reflex contractions of the abdominal wall and limb muscles.[72] Relaxation of the abdominal wall viscera was noted in response to visceral stimulation, using gastric distention in anesthetized dogs.[73] Bloating was also associated with delayed emptying from the terminal ileum of a radiolabeled bran meal.[74] This common constellation of symptoms in IBS, although usually assumed to be related to dysmotility, has no validated mechanism but is worthy of further study.

DISORDERS OF COLONIC MOTILITY

Constipation

Patients complain of constipation if stools are passed infrequently or if more effort (straining) is needed than they think appropriate. Difficult evacuation of feces, especially if noted for stools of softer than the normal consistency, is more likely to result from disorders of the pelvic floor or the anorectum than from slow colonic transit. Disorders of the pelvic floor (e.g., dyschezia, obstructed defecation) are disturbances of evacuation and are more appropriately dealt with in Chapters 39 and 88.

Slow transit through some or all segments of the colon leads to hard fecal masses that are also passed infrequently and often with great difficulty. This condition, called colonic inertia or slow transit constipation (STC), can probably be considered as being separate from IBS and should be diagnosed only if abdominal pain is not a prominent feature. On the other hand, STC certainly merges with IBS if pain, abdominal distention, excessive rectal mucus, and intermittent episodes of frequent, looser stools also occur (see Chap. 81). This section deals with STC; the motility features of IBS are discussed in a later section.

Slow Transit

Figure 82-7 shows radioopaque markers retained predominantly in the distal colon (rectosigmoid segment) 96 hours after their ingestion.[51] The marker technique is simple, inexpensive, and of proven value in the documentation of STC.[75] Gamma scintigraphy is another approach that can be made shorter (24 or 48 hours) and is practical and comple-

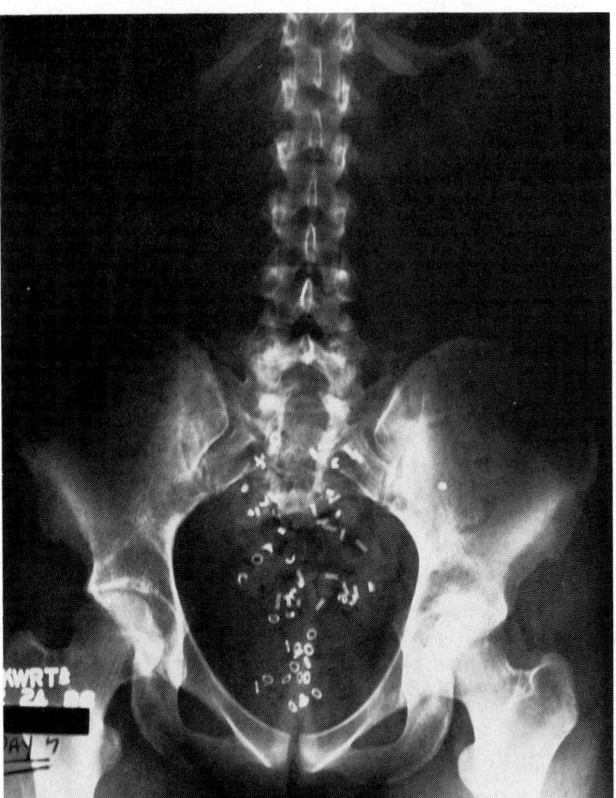

FIGURE 82-7. Radiograph of radioopaque markers as a measure of colonic transit. Most markers are in the rectosigmoid colon in this patient.

mentary to the marker method.[56,76] Whichever method is used, the implications for therapy are potentially important. Surgical resection of portions of the colon is occasionally necessary for severe STC, and, if patients are screened extensively and selected carefully, the results are very good.[75] Currently, subtotal colectomy and ileorectal anastomosis is the preferred surgical approach for this highly selected subgroup that represents 10% or less of those patients referred for tertiary opinion.[75] If tests of pelvic floor function identify a clinically relevant abnormality, colectomy is not indicated even in the presence of slow transit. Retraining programs for the pelvic floor should first be used to correct the defect in expulsion, after which transit could be retested.[75] Only then should resective surgery be considered.

Manometry

Attention has also focused on the pathogenic role in STC of the lack of normal high-amplitude pressure waves in the colon.[77] These propagating waves are thought to cause the mass movement of contents. Attention was first drawn to them by Narducci and his colleagues during their overnight studies.[26] Though not completely absent in STC, reduced numbers of high-amplitude pressure waves have been reported in these patients.[77]

Hirschsprung's disease, or congenital megacolon, is a special case. In this condition, a segment of anorectum, of variable length, fails to relax and thus offers a functional obstruction to the distal passage of fecal boluses. The pathophysiologic diagnosis is made by demonstrating absence of the rectoanal inhibitory reflex. If the rectum is distended to a volume of 10 to 100 mL, the internal anal sphincter normally relaxes; this is often accompanied by contraction of the external anal sphincter. In Hirschsprung's disease, the physiologic abnormality is accompanied by the histopathologic absence of ganglion cells from the myenteric plexus. Demonstration of the rectoanal inhibitory reflex is a major step in the evaluation of any young patient with severe constipation. Although usually a disease of infants and children, less severe variants of the disease can present in later life (see Chap. 88 for additional details).

Myoelectrical Patterns

The concept of paradoxical colonic motility was first proposed by Alistair Connell,[78] who observed that patients with diarrheal disease often had colons that demonstrated relatively little overall motility, whereas those with constipation often had very active motor patterns. He explained this by suggesting that not all pressure waves or myoelectrical activity resulted in aboral propulsion. Rather, many of the motor

phenomena created pressure gradients that favored a delay in transit of contents, and these contractions should be considered as mixing or retarding rather than propulsive forces. Myoelectrical recordings have confirmed this general principle. Bueno and his colleagues[79-81] reported the most elegant observations in this regard (Fig. 82-8).

Many patients with STC severe enough to warrant subtotal colectomy display histologic changes in the enteric nervous system of the resected colon.[82] Neurons in the myenteric plexus may be absent or abnormal morphologically on silver staining. It is assumed that these patients have a morphologic abnormality of the neural control of colonic motility. These clinical and histopathologic features appear to merge with the syndromes of intestinal pseudoobstruction (discussed elsewhere in this chapter).

Chronic Diarrhea

Diarrhea represents the other end of the clinical spectrum of altered colonic transit. Diarrhea is more frequent defecation or the passage of stools that are less well formed than is thought to be normal by the individual. In patients with IBS

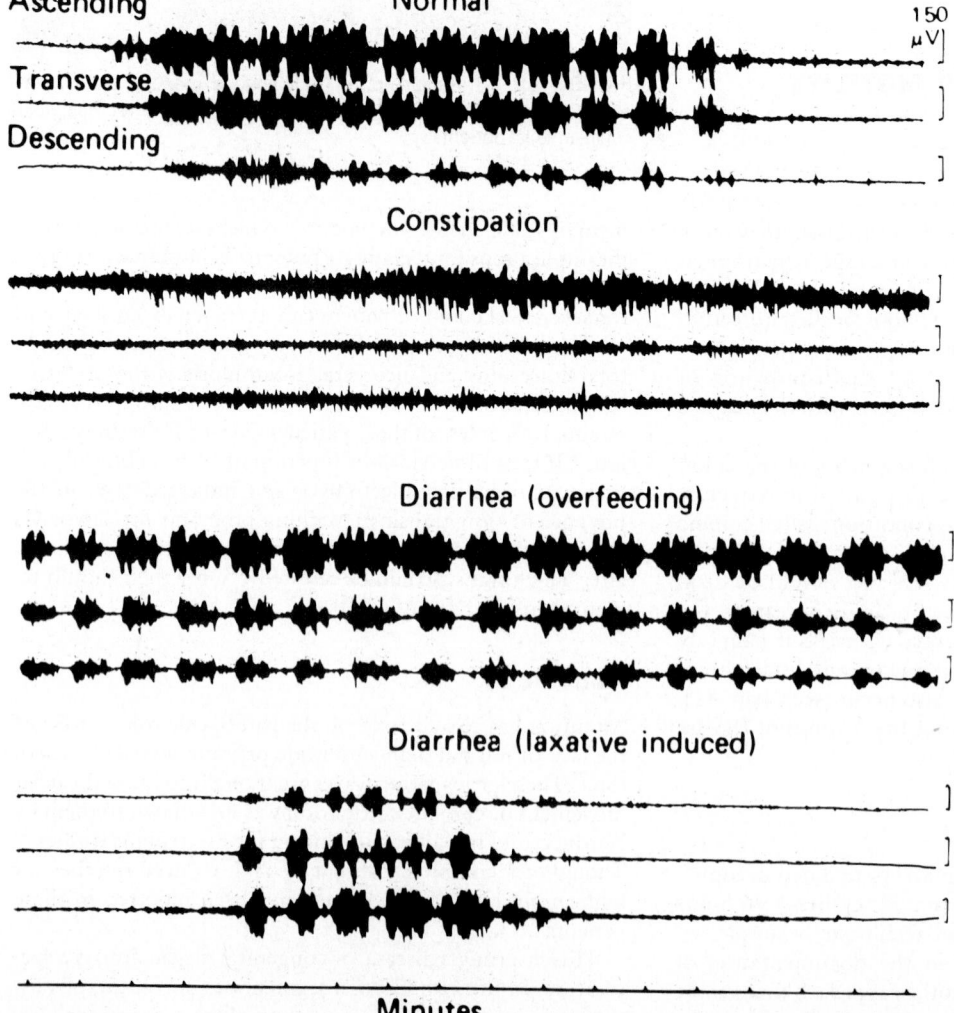

FIGURE 82-8. Electromyogram of the canine colon. After constipation was induced, short spike bursts predominated. After diarrhea was induced, long spike bursts were prominent. (Courtesy of Lionel Bueno, M.D., Toulouse, France.)

and diarrhea, transit through the proximal colon is accelerated, and the rate at which the ascending and transverse colons empty is related to fecal weight.[76] Stools that are less solid (fragmented, semisolid, or liquid) are associated with more rapid transit through the colon.[52] The most characteristic bowel pattern in IBS is one of wide fluctuations of stool frequency and consistency. Presumably, the speed of colonic transit changes dramatically to produce these stooling patterns.[52,60]

Our laboratory has also used the scintigraphic method to quantify small bowel and colonic transit in diarrhea associated with carcinoid syndrome.[83] Small bowel transit was found to be accelerated, so any increase in secretions from the small bowel (a putative effect of serotonin) should increase the fluid load entering the proximal colon. There was a fivefold increase in the emptying rate of the ascending and transverse colons; this was associated with storage of a reduced volume in the ascending colon, as measured by the scintigraphic method. The rapid transit and reduced capacitance of the proximal colon were associated with increased postprandial tone as measured by the barostat (Fig. 82-9).

Irritable Bowel Syndrome

IBS is usually defined by the Manning criteria,[61] as modified by an international panel that reevaluated the symptomatic features of this extremely common condition.[84] The major features are altered bowel habits and abdominal pain that is directly related to a change in the pattern of bowel movements. The colon has been incriminated as the origin of these symptoms.

Transit

Colonic transit was evaluated in patients with IBS and diarrhea,[76] and rapid transit of solids through the proximal colon was documented. It had earlier been reported that small bowel transit was also rapid in IBS with diarrhea.[85] The variable consistency of the stools, so characteristic of IBS, presumably is the result of slow transit of some of the fecal residue and rapid transit of other portions.

The constipation that is experienced by some patients with IBS appears to blend imperceptibly into the syndrome of idiopathic constipation. Transit of radioopaque markers in constipated IBS patients is prolonged. In a group of nearly 300 persons referred to a tertiary center with a major complaint of constipation,[75] the majority had normal or only modest slowing of colonic transit and were considered to be examples of IBS.

Colonic Sensation

Attention has focused on the afferent, or sensory, side of intestinal innervation in IBS. One of the few consistent findings in clinical studies of IBS has been the finding that the bowel, at all levels, is intolerant of distention.[62–64,86] Visceral hyperalgesia is not caused merely by a low overall tolerance for pain, for patients with IBS are no more sensitive to somatic pain than are controls.[64]

Balloon distention of the colon was revealing with regard to the pain experienced by IBS patients. If their colons were distended at different loci, the pain experienced by them was more diffuse than it was in asymptomatic controls.[63] Sensitivity of the rectum in IBS is also important because many persons suffer from urgency and unsatisfied defecation.[30,31]

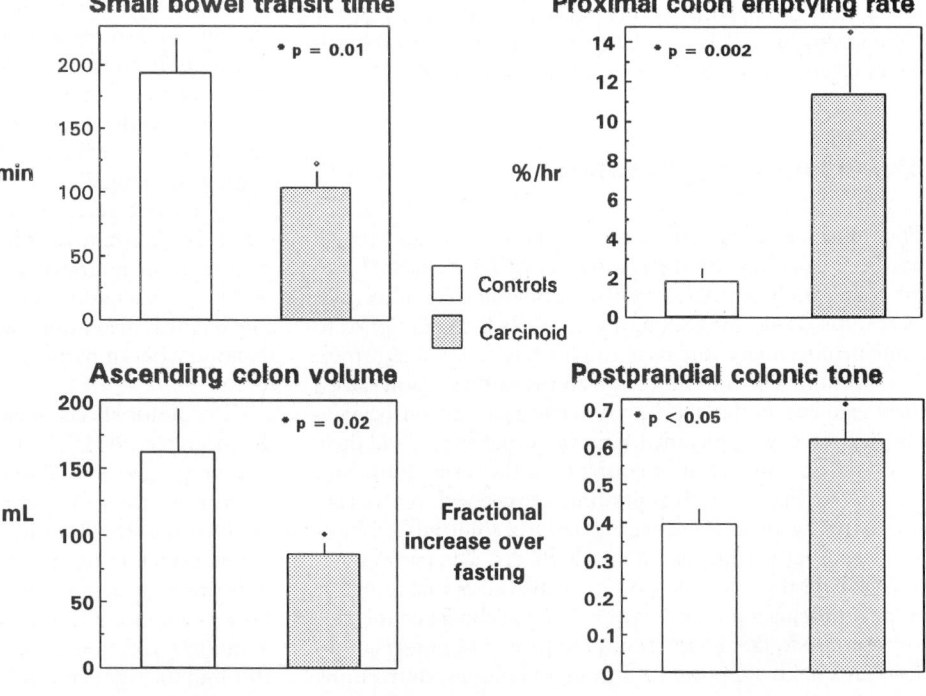

FIGURE 82-9. Summary of pathophysiologic findings in patients with carcinoid syndrome with diarrhea. The proximal colon showed increased tone, impaired accommodation, and rapid emptying. (Adapted from von der Ohe M, Camilleri M, Kvols LK, Thomforde GM. Motor dysfunction of the small bowel and colon in patients with the carcinoid syndrome and diarrhea. N Engl J Med 1993;329:1073.)

The rectal wall also demonstrates decreased compliance in IBS.[30,31] Some have proposed that IBS patients can be subdivided, on the basis of rectal sensitivity, into those with and those without a heightened awareness of rectal distention.[66] Rectal sensitivity in asymptomatic subjects and patients with IBS can be reduced by 5-HT$_3$ antagonists[66] and by analogues of somatostatin.[65,67]

Manometry and Myoelectrical Studies

Several laboratories recorded colonic manometry in IBS in the 1950s and 1960s. Initially, these experiments were performed with manometric probes placed through the rigid sigmoidoscope, and most observations were restricted to the upper rectum and sigmoid colon. The advent of fiberoptic endoscopy facilitated the positioning of recording probes into the descending colon and even more proximal segments. This extensive literature was fully summarized, up to 1988, by Whitehead and Schuster.[62]

The essential findings are that differences between IBS patients and controls have not always been demonstrable under basal conditions. The quiescent colon in IBS does not have a predictable motor abnormality, although stimulation with drugs, food, and emotional or other stresses has often brought out differences from health. Early studies concentrated on the effects of stimulant drugs (usually parasympathomimetic agents), but later the more physiologic stimulus of a meal has been employed. Two patterns of response have been noted in IBS, one being a more pronounced stimulation of motility within minutes of the meal, the second being loss of the immediate response but an exaggerated motility later in the postprandial period (30–90 minutes after a meal).

Myoelectrical recordings from the rectosigmoid region in patients with IBS showed a greater predominance of slow waves at a reduced frequency (3–4 cycles per minute), compared with healthy controls. Though the phenomenon was reported from several groups, divergent results were also noted, and the hypothesis of a primary abnormality of the colonic slow wave has now fallen from favor. The subject is reviewed completely by Whitehead and Schuster.[62]

Malabsorption Syndromes

The influence of steatorrhea on colonic motility and transit has been examined by the instillation of fatty acids[2,54] into the colon. In these studies, emulsions of long-chain fatty acids were infused into the cecum, the mixtures being designed to simulate intestinal contents in moderately severe steatorrhea. The infusion of fat into the cecum and ascending colon caused these segments of the large bowel to contract vigorously; high-pressure waves were recorded, pain was experienced, and there was rapid aboral transit of contents to the distal colon and rectum (see Fig. 82-5). It is presumed that chemosensors are stimulated by lumenal fat, because control solutions, without long-chain fatty acids, had no such effects. The pathway responsible for the colon's response involves an opioid receptor, because pharmacologic doses of morphine abolished the motor response to fat and the cramping pain.[2,54] Long-chain dietary fatty acids are powerful stimuli of colonic contractions

and transit, possibly explaining the pain and urgency experienced by many patients with malabsorption syndromes.

Inflammatory Disease of the Colon

The diarrhea of inflammatory colitis is primarily caused by exudation of fluid and mucus, bleeding, and impaired absorption; however, disordered motility and transit should be considered also.[14] Connell first proposed that the colon in advanced ulcerative colitis may behave as a semi-rigid tube, showing fewer phasic pressure waves than is normal.[78] Moreover, it is well recognized clinically that haustral contractions are absent in the late stage of colitis. These radiologic phenomena (haustra) are thought to be produced by repetitive, nonpropagated, phasic contractions. Snape's group[87] used combined manometric and scintigraphic techniques to study transit in ulcerative colitis. They confirmed the paucity of phasic pressure activity in the fasting state. However, postprandially, low-amplitude pressure waves were more frequent in colitis and, if these were propagated, they always moved contents in an antegrade direction. Movement of isotope from the splenic flexure to the sigmoid colon was usually rapid, perhaps reflecting the absence of retarding pressure waves.

Another important disorder of motility is seen in ulcerative proctitis, in which a heightened sensitivity of the rectum to distention has been reported.[88] Clinically, such patients are often sensitive to very small amounts of feces or mucus in the rectum. Pressure waves of high amplitude in the rectum have been recorded in proctitis and implicated in the symptom of tenesmus.[88]

Response of the Colon to Drugs

This last section is arranged according to the major clinical actions of two groups of pharmacologic agents, those that are thought to hasten colonic transit (laxatives and prokinetics) and those that slow transit (antidiarrheals). The most complete study of laxative agents and drugs that have diarrhea as a major side effect was that of Karaus and Sarna.[89] In dogs with strain gauges sewn onto the colon, they studied the effects of hypertonic glucose, castor oil, neostigmine, and guanethidine. In all instances, if the agents induced diarrhea, powerful contractions migrated around most or all of the colon and led to an evacuation. On the other hand, a local stimulus to the rectum (distention) was able to provoke expulsion of the balloon without participation of the whole colon in the motor event.

The motor effects of local instillation of stimulant laxatives has been recorded from the human colon,[27] and the myoelectrical responses to oral senna have been reported.[90] The effects of laxative doses of castor oil on the colon should be similar to those reported for oleic acid,[2,54] because oleic acid and the active principle of castor oil (ricinoleic acid) are both C-18 aliphatic fatty acids. Lactulose has also been used experimentally as a stimulant to colonic transit; in doses that induced a modest increase in stool frequency, it hastened transit through the right colon.[91] The prokinetic drug, cisapride, has been reported to have contrasting effects on colonic transit,[92,93] and its clinical efficacy has not been well established.

The most effective antidiarrheals currently available are agents that are related to opioids. Opiates are said to augment the mixing contractions that inhibit transit and to increase colonic tone, both of which might be expected to favor absorption. These actions should retard transit and help alleviate diarrhea. Morphine's effects on colonic tone have also been explored in dogs and humans with the electromechanical barostat. Under baseline conditions in the dog, the drug increased tone sharply,[28] in association with an increase in phasic contractions. In the human colon,[94] the effects of morphine were more complex; it relaxed a segment showing high postprandial tone and caused a late decrease in spontaneous tone (40 minutes after injection). The effects of opiates on the colon are therefore complex and perhaps species dependent. Although morphine increased tone in the dog, the human colon can be relaxed by morphine, especially if it has previously been stimulated to increase its tone.[2,94]

PSEUDOOBSTRUCTION SYNDROMES

Acute Megacolon

Acute toxic megacolon occurs in patients with severe, fulminant inflammatory bowel disease or during infectious colitis (see Chaps. 79 and 84); the colon also dilates in response to acute distal obstruction (e.g., volvulus). However, acute megacolon also occurs in patients without evidence of intrinsic colonic disease or mechanical obstruction. In this latter instance, the patient has a form of acute colonic pseudoobstruction named after Ogilvie.[95] In fact, the condition Ogilvie described in two patients was of long standing and was caused by malignant infiltration of mesenteric nerves. Regardless of the misnomer, the syndrome now given Ogilvie's name should be considered as a form of pseudoobstruction localized to the colon; the characteristic time course is an acute or subacute one. Most examples are clearly associated with an underlying disease. The most common predisposing conditions described in a meta-analysis of 400 cases were trauma, orthopedic surgery, obstetric procedures, pelvic and abdominal surgery, metabolic imbalance, and neurologic conditions.[96]

Pathophysiology

The precise cause of acute colonic pseudoobstruction is unknown. However, Ogilvie's syndrome is the clearest example of the human colon dilating in response to nonmechanical factors, and the original author proposed that an imbalance of intrinsic autonomic neural control was the basis for the syndrome.[95] This propensity of the colon to relax and dilate has been explored experimentally using the barostat.[3] In these experiments, wall tone decreased markedly during sleep and in response to glucagon but increased after neostigmine and morphine. The concept that the wall of the colon is able to relax or constrict readily in response to physiologic and pharmacologic stimuli is perhaps important as a basis for megacolon.

Clinical Presentation

The typical patient is middle-aged or older, is recovering quite uneventfully from surgery a few days previously, and is already eating a general diet. In one report,[97] more than half the patients had recent surgery or manipulation of the spine or retroperitoneum. The abdomen becomes grossly distended and breathing becomes labored but, early in the course, no peritoneal signs are present, and the leukocyte count is normal. An abdominal film shows massive gaseous distention of the colon with air distributed throughout, including the rectum. Usually the small bowel is not seen. The diameter of the cecum at this point is often 9 to 10 cm.

Initial Management

Oral feedings should be stopped, parenteral fluids started, and a nasogastric tube passed; all nonessential drugs should be discontinued.[97] A Hypaque (water-soluble contrast) enema is administered; in this way, mechanical obstruction can be excluded and pseudoobstruction confirmed. As a side benefit, hyperosmolar Hypaque usually evacuates the colon during the diagnostic maneuvers. After confirmation, acute colonic pseudoobstruction should be treated aggressively, with a rectal decompression tube and enemas. Any associated metabolic abnormalities or electrolyte disorders (e.g., hypokalemia) must be corrected, because these are prominent in 20% to 30% of cases.[97] Pharmacologic blockade of ganglia with guanethidine followed by cholinergic stimulation with neostigmine has been reported to help[98]; however, in many patients, the condition resolves with simple measures.[99] Treatment with cisapride[100] and erythromycin[101] has been reported also to help.

Subsequent Management

Most patients who do not respond to enemas, nasogastric decompression, and drug therapy continue to have a normal leukocyte count and to develop no fever or peritoneal signs. If the cecum measures greater than 11 cm, the next step is colonoscopic decompression. The previous enema often has emptied the colon, facilitating endoscopy. Gas and liquid stool are aspirated while small amounts of additional air (or carbon dioxide) are insufflated. Mucosal detail is often obscured by the contents, but an obstructing lesion can usually be seen. It is not necessary to reach the cecum to accomplish adequate decompression; positioning the colonoscope at the hepatic flexure with aspiration of distal contents usually collapses the right colon. An abdominal film should then be obtained; the collapsed cecum can be documented, and the patient can then be kept on enemas until stool and flatus pass spontaneously. Although it may need to be repeated, more than 80% of patients respond ultimately to colonoscopic decompression and require no further management.[97,98]

An operation is advisable for patients with a very large cecum (>11 cm) and those who remain intractable to medical and endoscopic management; the most useful and efficacious approach is tube cecostomy. In addition, if at any time a patient manifests fever, leukocytosis, or peritoneal signs, abdominal exploration is mandatory. In these situations, the right colon is often nonviable or has already perforated. For perforation, right hemicolectomy, ileostomy, and a mucous fistula is the operation of choice. In patients with nonviable bowel but without perforation, right hemicolectomy and primary anastomosis can be performed with little risk of serious complications.

Chronic Intestinal Pseudoobstruction

Definition and Clinical Variants

Chronic intestinal pseudoobstruction (CIP) is a rare and heterogenous clinical syndrome manifested by recurrent episodes of symptoms and signs of intestinal obstruction. As implied in the definition, these symptoms occur in the absence of mechanical bowel obstruction, and CIP is thought to result from impaired gut motility. The characteristic symptoms are nausea, vomiting, abdominal pain and distention, and an alteration in bowel habit (most typically, constipation). Total gut failure with weight loss and malnutrition may occur in the more advanced stages. CIP may be associated with symptoms caused by the involvement of smooth muscle in organs other than the small and large intestines; these include the esophagus, stomach, ureter, and urinary bladder.

The evolution of the disease and the regions of the gut affected determine the clinical presentation. Esophageal involvement can produce dysphagia, esophagitis, regurgitation, and heartburn; gastric and small bowel involvement results in nausea, vomiting, bloating, distention, and abdominal discomfort; and colonic involvement leads to distention and constipation. The heterogenous nature of CIP is well illus-

trated by the fact that 4 of 42 patients in one series had previously undergone colectomy for constipation.[102] On the other hand, many young, usually female, patients who present primarily with severe idiopathic constipation have evidence of esophageal, gastric, or small bowel dysmotility[103,104] at the time of colectomy or subsequently. The condition may be focal; localized variants of CIP include megaduodenum, the superior mesenteric artery syndrome, and selective left colonic pseudoobstruction.

Pathophysiology

Chronic intestinal pseudoobstruction may be caused by a number of underlying diseases.[105,106] In practice, identification of an underlying process (e.g., progressive systemic sclerosis) may be all that is necessary to diagnose the associated gut dysmotility. For those patients in whom the cause is not immediately apparent, classification tables can be consulted (Table 82-1). Although an array of possible differential diagnoses may be helpful, more rational is an approach that addresses the pathophysiology of the motility disturbance.[107] The pathophysiologic features of CIP can be broadly subdivided into a *myopathic variety* (e.g., progressive systemic sclerosis, amyloidosis, hollow visceral myopathy) and a *neuropathic variety* (e.g., diabetes mellitus). The idiopathic variant, which is thought to result from disorder of the myenteric plexus, usually has the features of a neuropathy.

The normal patterns of gastric and small bowel motility in health are generally well recognized[107,108] and provide a basis for defining the pathophysiologic type of CIP. The myopathic variant is characterized by low-amplitude pressure wave

---

TABLE 82-1
Classification of Chronic Intestinal Pseudoobstruction

TYPE	MYOPATHIC	NEUROPATHIC	COMMENTS
Familial	Familial visceral myopathies (autosomal dominant or recessive)	Familial visceral neuropathies; von Recklinghausen's disease	Rare disorders, usually present in neonatal period or childhood; neurofibromas may also cause mechanical obstruction
Sporadic			
Infiltrative	Progressive systemic sclerosis Amyloidosis	Progressive systemic sclerosis (early); amyloidosis	Manometry essential to differentiate pathophysiology
General neurologic disease	Myotonic and other dystrophies	Diabetes mellitus, porphyria, brainstem tumor, multiple sclerosis, spinal cord transection, dysautonomias	
Infectious		Chagas' disease, cytomegalovirus	Nonspecific "postviral" causes appear to be common
Drug-induced		Tricyclic antidepressants, narcotics, anticholinergics, antihypertensives, vincristine, laxative abuse	Exclusion of drug side effects is essential in all patients
Neoplastic		Paraneoplastic (bronchial small cell carcinoma)	May require chest computed tomography scan to exclude bronchial cancer if chest roentgenogram is negative
Idiopathic	Nonfamilial hollow visceral myopathy	Hirschsprung disease	Variable manifestations and severity in CIP

CIP, chronic idiopathic intestinal pseudoobstruction.

activity in the duodenojejunum, whereas the neuropathic type tends to produce excessive or uncoordinated manometric profiles throughout the small bowel (Figs. 82-10 and 82-11). Similar features have also been observed in dysmotilities of the esophagus: low-amplitude pressure waves characterize myopathic processes, and motor incoordination is seen in neuropathic disorders. Comparable data are not available for the colon. Some conditions, such as amyloidosis and progressive systemic sclerosis, can produce a neuropathic pattern initially, followed by a myopathic one.[109]

Knowledge of the pathophysiology confirms and extends clinical suspicions and leads to a more logical approach to the diagnosis. For example, postural dizziness, visual disturbances, and sweating abnormalities suggest an autonomic neuropathy; the associated manometric findings of marked incoordination necessitate a search for the underlying process. A positive family history suggests a congenital disorder, and urinary symptoms suggest genitourinary involvement, most commonly seen in a generalized visceral myopathy. Patients should also be questioned about the use of anticholinergic drugs, phenothiazines, antihypertensive agents, narcotics, and tricyclic antidepressants. The role of drugs cannot be overemphasized, and the motor effects of opiates must always be kept in mind because these patients often have chronic abdominal pain requiring long-term analgesia. Important physical signs should be sought by a complete neurologic examination, measurement of the blood pressure with the patient in both supine and standing positions, and a search for abdominal distention or a succussion splash.

Identification of the neuropathic variant of CIP necessitates a more detailed search for the underlying cause. The cause may be a disturbance in the extrinsic neural supply, as with a brain tumor or an autonomic neuropathy, or a disorder of the intrinsic or enteric nervous system (e.g., idiopathic or postviral syndromes, paraneoplasia). The extrinsic neural supply may need to be assessed by computed tomographic or magnetic resonance imaging or by noninvasive tests of autonomic function. These include pupillary pharmacology, thermoregulation and sweating, screening of autonomic reflexes, the pancreatic polypeptide response to hypoglycemia or sham feeding (for vagal integrity), and plasma norepinephrine levels.[110] Such studies should help identify the level at which the neural supply is deranged, and this information in turn may uncover a treatable lesion.

Disorders of the enteric nervous system should be suspected if a neuropathic form of CIP is recorded manometrically but a disorder of the extrinsic neural supply cannot be documented. The clearest example of an intrinsic disorder is Hirschsprung's disease, in which localized aganglionosis results in impairment of colonic transit proximal to the obstructed segment, dilatation of the bowel, and megacolon. This is also the best example of a condition with a clear-cut morphologic lesion. To date, histologic studies of the myenteric plexus in other patients with gastrointestinal motility disturbances, usually based on silver staining techniques, are incomplete.[82,111,112] These have demonstrated either neuronal intranuclear inclusions, reductions in the number of ganglion cells and replacement by glial cells, abnormalities in the neuronal processes (dendritic or axonal), or inflammatory cell infiltration of the enteric plexuses. At least two forms of fa-

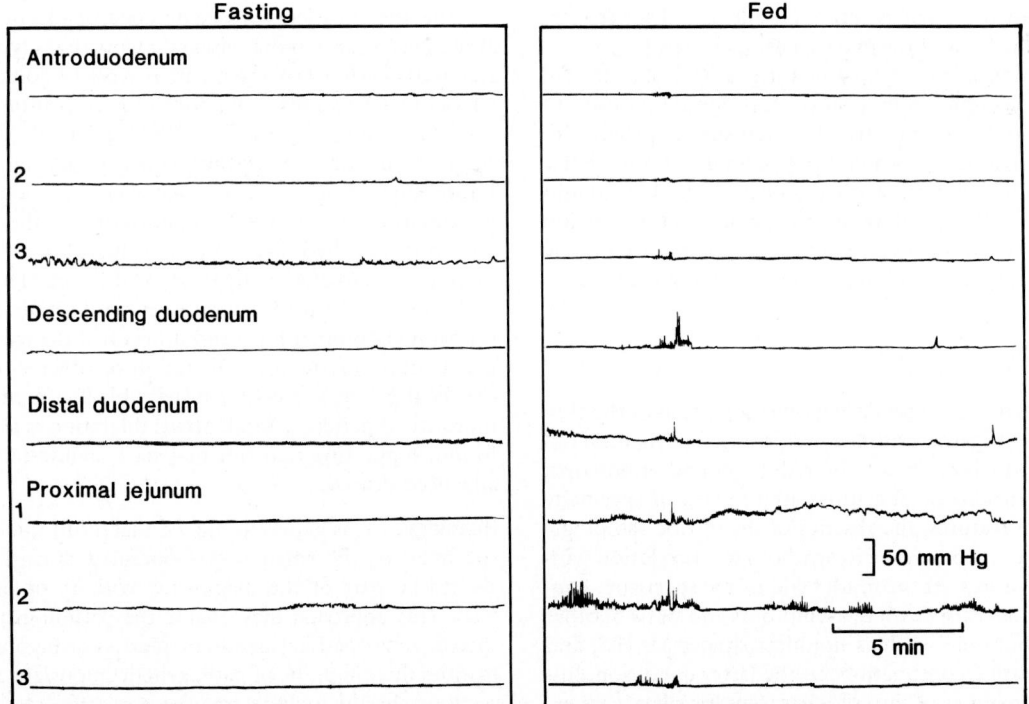

FIGURE 82-10. Tasting and postprandial manometric profiles, show pronounced hypomotility in a 30-year-old man with hollow visceral myopathy. Eating causes no change in the featureless record. (From Colemont J, Camilleri M. Chronic intestinal pseudo-obstruction: diagnosis and treatment. Mayo Clinic Proc 1989;64(1):60.)

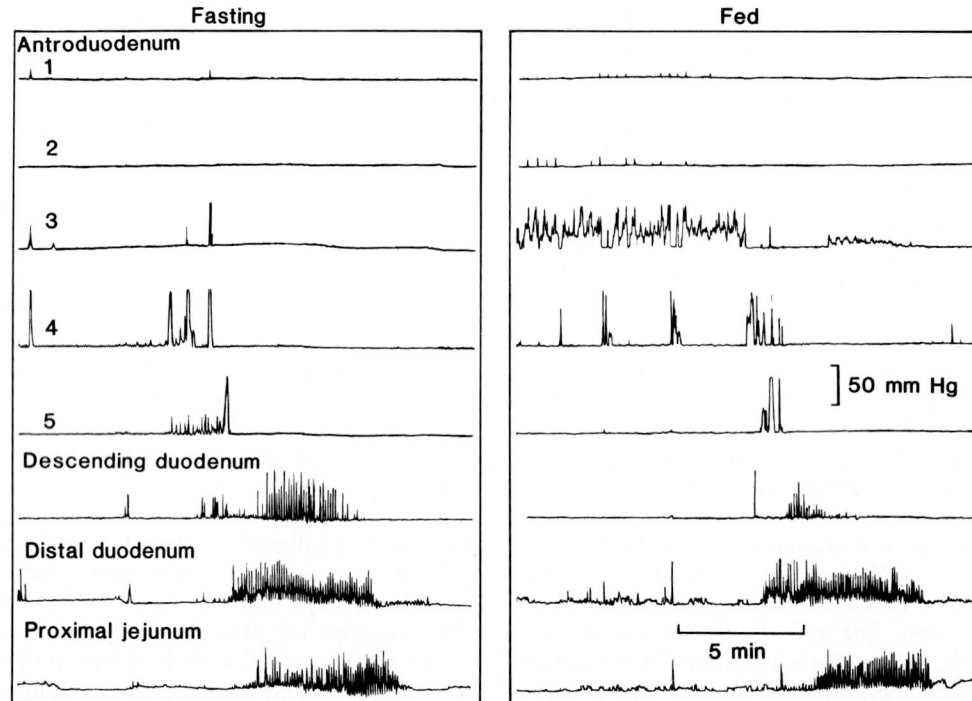

FIGURE 82-11. Manometric profile in 26-year-old woman with diabetes and autonomic neuropathy shows abnormal propagation of phase III of the interdigestive motor complex and lack of a well-developed antral component in the fasting tracing. Postprandially, there is antral hypomotility, pylorospasm (*lead 3*), and failure of the meal to induce a fed pattern. (From Colemont J, Camilleri M. Chronic intestinal pseudo-obstruction: diagnosis and treatment. Mayo Clinic Proc 1989;64(1):60.)

milial visceral neuropathy have been described[113]; the number of families is still small, one form appears to be autosomal dominant and the other is recessive, and the disorders are probably at the level of the enteric nevous system.

Identification of the myopathic form of CIP should lead to a more thorough family history, appropriate biopsies to look for amyloid and infiltrative disorders such as progressive systemic sclerosis, and a search for a generalized muscle disease. The familial visceral myopathies have been divided into several types[114,115] depending on the age of onset, the region of the gut affected, the involvement of other smooth muscle (usually megacystitis), and numerous associated features.

Diagnosis

The diagnosis of CIP depends first on recognition of the clinical syndrome, together with the exclusion of mechanical obstruction or mucosal disease, by radiology and endoscopy. The greatest diagnostic difficulties are the lack of specificity of the clinical features, the absence of diagnostic radiologic criteria, and an incomplete histopathologic correlation with the clinical features. At the milder end of the spectrum, considerable overlap exists with the symptoms and signs of other functional syndromes such as nonulcer dyspepsia, IBS, and chronic idiopathic constipation. In the latter condition, histologic abnormalities of the colonic myenteric plexus are extremely common.[104]

Radiologic studies. The most important contribution of radiology to the diagnosis of CIP is the exclusion of mechanical

obstruction. The radiologic findings are related to the anatomic regions affected, although they may also suggest whether the disorder is caused by a neuropathy or a myopathy. It has been reported that visceral myopathy is typified by pronounced duodenal enlargement, increased colonic caliber with a lack of haustrations, and poor to absent contractions.[116] On the other hand, visceral neuropathy is mainly characterized by disorganized contractility, which is best appreciated on fluoroscopy. Progressive systemic sclerosis produces close approximation of the valvulae conniventes in the small bowel and wide-mouthed sacculations in the colon.

In the group of 42 patients with CIP studied by Rohrmann and associates,[116] some patients had findings of paralytic ileus on plain abdominal film, and others had the features of true mechanical obstruction. Dilatation of other viscera such as the renal pelvis, ureters, or urinary bladder is identified in a minority of patients. Small bowel dilatation is not invariably found, suggesting that this may be a manifestation of more advanced disease.

Histology. It is generally agreed that a full-thickness biopsy specimen of the small bowel obtained during laparotomy should be part of the diagnostic work-up of patients with CIP. This approach may enable the pathologist to identify specific neuropathic (myenteric plexus) or myopathic abnormalities that might be of pathogenetic importance. Histologic sections should include transverse paraffin sections stained with hematoxylin and eosin, as well as thicker and larger sections cut in the plane of the myenteric plexus. To date, most published studies have used Smith's silver staining technique for neural tissues.[111,112,113]

Unfortunately, histology, even of full-thickness biopsy specimens, does not always provide a clear-cut diagnosis. For example, cases are described in which the histologic features cannot differentiate systemic sclerosis from visceral myopathy,[117,118] and the histologic changes in familial visceral myopathy can be quite variable.[119] In some adults[120] and children,[121] tissue specimens may show no specific neural or muscular morphologic abnormality. It has been proposed that rectal biopsy may be of value in selected patients in whom the diagnosis of intestinal neuronal dysplasia is considered.[122] Such an approach would clearly be advantageous. Further development awaits larger numbers of clinicopathologic correlations on the regular use of immunohistochemical techniques for the study of peptidergic innervation.

Motility studies. Qualitative analysis of manometric recordings provides complementary evidence of a motility disorder. The stomach and small bowel are most frequently involved with CIP and, because patterns of gastric and small bowel motility in normal subjects have been well established,[107,108] gastrointestinal manometry provides the usual basis for identification of dysmotility states. Availability of this information represents a substantial advance over the less specific abnormalities observed by esophageal and anorectal motility studies. The relevant abnormalities include aberrant configuration or propagation of phase III of the interdigestive migrating motor complex, sustained uncoordinated pressure activity, intense bursts of phasic pressure activity, and the failure of a meal to induce a "fed pattern" or to interrupt cyclic interdigestive motor activity.[102,107]

Gastrointestinal transit. The availability of noninvasive tests of gastric emptying and small bowel and colonic transit can also facilitate the diagnosis of CIP. Techniques have been developed in which radiolabeled liquids and solids (separate isotopes) can be monitored scintigraphically from their entry into the stomach to their elimination in feces. The most useful techniques measure gastric emptying, small bowel transit, and regional colonic transit simultaneously.[56] Slow colonic transit by the radioopaque marker technique[51] in constipated patients is the most frequent indication for further studies. The concurrence of abnormal gastric emptying or small bowel transit in such patients should raise the possibility of a more generalized disorder, such as CIP. One technique uses a labeled test meal and an encapsulated, second isotope directed toward colonic contents.[56] The methodology has been simplified and made sufficiently cost-effective to justify its use in the routine setting.[123]

Localized Forms of Pseudoobstruction

Localized forms of CIP may affect isolated colonic segments[124] or the duodenal loop.[125] The superior mesenteric artery syndrome is usually diagnosed in young women with recurrent vomiting and abdominal pain. It has been suggested that duodenal dilatation in these patients results from a localized disorder of motility, and that the radiologically observed obstruction of the duodenum is caused by dilatation secondary to hypomotility. This must be differentiated from true obstruction of the duodenum by the superior mesenteric artery, which occurs in immobilized patients with prominent

weight loss (e.g., after spinal injury). Surgical treatment is sometimes justifiable and efficacious in localized forms of pseudoobstruction.

Pseudoobstruction in the Pediatric Age Group

In a survey conducted by members of the North American Society of Pediatric Gastroenterology and Nutrition, 87 pediatric patients were identified; 22% had symptoms at birth, 43% within their first month, and 64% in the first year of life.[126] This survey excluded Hirschsprung's disease, which must always be considered in the differential diagnosis of abnormal colonic motility or distention in the pediatric age group. The predominant clinical features were distention, vomiting, constipation, diarrhea, failure to thrive, and urinary tract abnormalities. Esophageal manometry was abnormal in all of 14 patients in whom it was studied. Anorectal manometry was generally unhelpful, being abnormal in only 1 of 16. Full-thickness biopsy specimens of the intestine were abnormal in all 12 reported in this series (8 plexus disorders, 4 muscle degeneration). Twenty-two other miscellaneous gut biopsies were noncontributory. Among the group in whom follow-up was adequate, more than 30% died, with almost half of these deaths being attributed to complications of central parenteral nutrition within the first 6 months.

Although this retrospective experience is the most comprehensive, specific reports highlight other features of pediatric pseudoobstruction. Hyman and colleagues found qualitative abnormalities in the patterns of antroduodenal pressure profiles in all of 13 patients, features that were similar to those reported in adults.[121] Pathologic abnormalities were detected in only 4 of 7 patients who underwent full-thickness biopsy. The histologic features of visceral neuropathy and myopathy were essentially similar to those reported in adults. In the pediatric age group, the underlying disease processes that result in pseudoobstruction also include Kawasaki's disease[127] and Duchenne's muscular dystrophy.[128] The familial forms of pseudoobstruction[115] are frequently manifest in the pediatric age group; of 87 cases in the North American pediatric group series, 15 were familial. Neonatal pseudoobstruction rarely occurs in isolation and is more often in association with other anomalies requiring surgical correction; these include gastroschisis, duodenal atresia, and megacystitis.

Treatment

The goals of treatment for CIP are to maintain adequate nutrition and to restore normal intestinal propulsion. However, it must be appreciated that the clinical spectrum varies enormously, from nuisance value to a life-threatening condition.

Nutritional support. In those with mild to moderate symptoms, simple measures should be used, oral feeding should be prolonged as much as possible, and deficiencies of trace elements and vitamins should be identified and corrected.

Food that is soft, blenderized, or liquid is tolerated better in patients with impaired gastric emptying. More advanced measures include the use of low-lactose, low-fiber, polypeptide or hydrolyzed protein diets with multivitamins. Specific supplementation with iron, folate, calcium, and vitamins D, K, and B_{12} may be required. Despite these measures, only a minority of well-advanced patients can be controlled adequately.

The next stage relies on tube feedings, often requiring bypass of the stomach by a jejunostomy feeding tube (see Chaps. 48 and 136). Eventually, many patients with advanced CIP require home central parenteral nutrition (CPN) owing to ineffective dietary and medical treatments and because surgical intervention is indicated in only a few selected cases. In particular, CPN is the mainstay of treatment for patients with myopathic pseudoobstruction, in whom prokinetic agents are seldom beneficial. CPN can maintain weight and reverse deficiencies in trace elements and vitamins. However, treatment is costly and is associated with significant morbidity and mortality. During a 10-year period, 4 of 10 infants with neonatal intestinal pseudoobstruction in one series died, 2 of sepsis and 2 of hepatic failure related to CPN.[129] Nevertheless, these and other potentially disastrous complications have to be accepted, because the prognosis of patients with severe forms of CIP, particularly the myopathic variants, is extremely poor.

Bacterial overgrowth. Treatment of bacterial overgrowth with broad-spectrum antibiotics is often helpful, although benefit has been well documented only in a small number of patients.[130] In some instances, the clinical benefit can be immediate and dramatic. Antibiotics are usually given for 10 to 14 days and, because the flora is diverse, antibiotic sensitivities are of little use. A broad-spectrum agent is needed, and tetracycline or doxycycline are used commonly.

Pharmacologic agents. Cholinergic agents have usually been ineffective in the treatment of CIP; their brief duration of action and side effects preclude long-term treatment. Metoclopramide has been used to treat familial visceral myopathy,[105] idiopathic CIP, and scleroderma,[131,132] but its overall efficacy has been disappointing. Anecdotal reports have suggested that other drugs may be beneficial in restoring the disturbed gastrointestinal motility in patients with CIP.[133] Subcutaneous administration of the opiate antagonist naloxone resulted in an increase in gastric emptying of solids and a decrease of small intestinal transit time. In two brothers with CIP, intravenous neostigmine and cholecystokinin normalized intestinal activity, as judged by cinematography.[134] Intravenous administration of trimebutine, a peripheral opiate agonist, induced phase 3-like activity in four children with intestinal pseudoobstruction.[135] However, more substantive controlled trials of those agents are necessary before their clinical efficacy can be assessed. Cisapride is a nondopaminergic, noncholinergic, prokinetic drug that has been shown to enhance the release of acetylcholine from the myenteric nerve endings in the digestive tract.[136] Because of its selective action on the gut, cisapride is devoid of the systemic side effects that frequently occur with other cholinergic agonists (such as bethanechol) and inhibitors of acetylcholinesterase (such as neostigmine). In patients with CIP, cisapride was effective in reducing the delayed intestinal transit time to within the normal range.[137] It also increased considerably the rate of gastric emptying of solids when administered for 6 weeks.[138] Unfortunately, its beneficial effects on symptoms are less clear; further long-term studies of clinical efficacy still must be undertaken.

The somatostatin analog, octreotide, stimulates phase 3-like bursts of phasic contractions in healthy persons and in patients with scleroderma.[139] In short-term studies, octreotide reduced symptoms and evidence of bacterial overgrowth in patients with CIP. Erythromycin and its various analogs (including those with no antibacterial activity) interact with motilin receptors and stimulate phase 3-like antroduodenal motility.[140] Although initial results in gastroparesis can sometimes be dramatic,[141] tachyphylaxis is common, and efficacy of the agents declines sharply. The analog of gonadotrophin-releasing hormone, leuprolide, has been suggested as therapy for CIP, based on possible effects in functional bowel disorders.[142]

Surgical treatment. Surgical bypass of affected segments might be beneficial in selected patients. Schuffler and Deitch[143] reviewed 73 operations performed on 12 patients with CIP and found that although some procedures were not helpful (e.g., gastrojejunostomy and resection of the small bowel), others were beneficial if a short segment of the bowel was involved (e.g., side-to-side duodenojejunostomy for megaduodenum or colectomy for colonic pseudoobstruction). In patients with familial visceral myopathy, Anuras and colleagues[144] reported variable results from duodenojejunostomy for megaduodenum. Sometimes, intractable and incapacitating symptoms arising from a dilated, immobile segment may necessitate radical resection of the small bowel[145]; enterectomy has even been advocated.[146]

Venting. A venting enterostomy creates an effective means of relieving gaseous distention and bloating and thereby providing symptomatic relief for patients being managed on CPN.[147] Venting can reduce the need for nasogastric intubation and hospitalization for precipitous obstructive episodes commonly suffered by these patients.

> The reader is directed to Chapter 10, Motility of the Large Intestine; Chapter 39, Approach to the Patient With Constipation; Chapter 69, Dysmotility of the Small Intestine; Chapter 81, Irritable Bowel Syndrome; Chapter 88, Anorectal Diseases; and Chapter 132, Evaluation of Gastrointestinal Motility: Methodologic Considerations.

REFERENCES

1. Steadman CJ, Phillips SF. Measurement of colonic motor function. In: Kumar D, Waldron DJ, Williams NS, eds. Clinical measurement of coloproctology. New York: Springer-Verlag, 1991:19.
2. Kamath PS, Phillips SF, O'Connor MK, et al. Colonic capacitance and transit in man: modulation by luminal contents and drugs. Gut 1990;31:443.
3. Steadman C, Phillips SF, Camilleri M, et al. Variation of muscle tone in the human colon. Gastroenterology 1991;101:373.
4. Mayer EA, Tache Y. Role of visceral afferent mechanisms in functional bowel disorders. Gastroenterology 1990;99:1688.
5. McFarlane GT, Cummings JH. The colonic flora, fermentation and large bowel digestive function. In: Phillips SJ, Pemberton JH, Shorter RG, eds. The large intestine. New York: Raven Press, 1991:51.
6. Elliott TR, Barclay-Smith E. Antiperistalsis and other muscular activities of the colon. J Physiol 1904;31:272.
7. Cannon WB. The movements of the intestines studied by means of the roentgen rays. Am J Physiol 1902;6:251.

8. Ruppin H, Bar-Meir S, Soergel KH, Wood CM, Schmitt MG. Absorption of short chain fatty acids by the colon. Gastroenterology 1980;78:1500.

9. Roediger WE. Utilization of nutrients by isolated epithelial cells of the rat colon. Gastroenterology 1982;83:424.

10. Phillips SF, Giller J. The contribution of the colon to electrolyte and water conservation in man. J Lab Clin Med 1973;81:733.

11. Debongnie JC, Phillips SF. Capacity of the human colon to absorb fluid. Gastroenterology 1978;74:698.

12. Misiewicz JJ. Human colonic motility. Scand J Gastroenterol 1984;19(Suppl 93):43.

13. Connell AM. The motility of the pelvic colon. 1. Motility in normals and in patients with asymptomatic duodenal ulcer. Gut 1961;2:175.

14. Spriggs EA, Code CF, Bargen JA, et al. Motility of the pelvic colon and rectum of normal persons and patients with ulcerative colitis. Gastroenterology 1951;19:480.

15. Soffer EE, Scalabrini P, Wingate DK. Prolonged ambulatory monitoring of human colonic motility. Am J Physiol 1989;257: G601.

16. Sarna SK. Cyclic motor activity; migrating motor complex: 1985. Gastroenterology 1985;89:894.

17. Flourie B, Phillips SF, Richter H, Azpiroz F. Cyclic motility in canine colon: responses to feeding and perfusion. Dig Dis Sci 1989;34:1185.

18. Kerlin P, Zinsmeister A, Phillips S. Motor responses to food of the ileum, proximal colon, and distal colon of healthy humans. Gastroenterology 1983;84:762.

19. Holdstock DJ, Misiewicz JJ. Factors controlling colonic motility: colonic pressures and transit after meals in patients with total gastrectomy, pernicious anemia or duodenal ulcer. Gut 1970;11:100.

20. Holdstock DJ, Misiewicz JJ, Smith T, Rowlands EN. Propulsion (mass movements) in the human colon and its relationship to meals and somatic activity. Gut 1970;11:91.

21. Duthie HL. Colonic response to eating. Gastroenterology 1978;75:527.

22. Wiley J, Tatum D, Keinath R, Owyang C. Participation of gastric mechanoreceptors and intestinal chemoreceptors in the gastrocolonic response. Gastroenterology 1988;94:1144.

23. Niederan C, Faber S, Karaus M. Cholecystokinin's role in regulation of colonic motility in health and in irritable bowel syndrome. Gastroenterology 1992;102:1889.

24. Painter NS, Truelove SC. The intraluminal pressure patterns in diverticulosis of the colon. Part I: Resting patterns of pressure. Part II: The effect of morphine. Gut 1964;5:201.

25. Painter NS, Truelove SC. The intraluminal pressure patterns in diverticulosis of the colon. Part III: The effect of prostigmine. Gut 1964;5:365.

26. Narducci F, Bassotti G, Gaburri M, Morelli A. Twenty-four hour manometric recording of colonic motor activity in healthy man. Gut 1987;28:17.

27. Preston DM, Lennard-Jones JE. Pelvic motility and response to intraluminal bisacodyl in slow transit constipation. Dig Dis Sci 1985;30:289.

28. Neri M, Phillips SF, Fich AF. Measurement of tone in the canine colon. Am J Physiol 1991;260:G505.

29. Bell AM, Pemberton JH, Hanson RB, Zinsmeister AR. Variation of muscle tone of the human rectum: recordings with an electromechanical barostat. Am J Physiol 1991;23:G17.

30. Hammer J, Phillips SF, Talley NJ, Camilleri M. Effect of a 5-HT$_3$ antagonist (Ondansetron) on rectal sensitivity and compliance in health and the irritable bowel syndrome. Aliment Pharmacol Ther 1993;7:543.

31. Prior A, Maxton DG, Whorwell PJ. Anorectal manometry in irritable bowel syndrome: differences between diarrhea- and constipation-predominant subjects. Gut 1990;31:458.

32. Huizinga JD, Daniel EE. Motor functions of the colon. In: Phillips SF, Pemberton JH, Shorter RG, eds. The large intestine: physiology, pathophysiology and disease. New York: Raven Press, 1991:93.

33. Rumessen JJ, Thuneberg L. Interstitial cells of Cajal in human small intestine. Gastroenterology 1991;100:1417.

34. Sarna SK, Waterfall WE, Bardakjian BL, Lind JF. Types of human colonic electrical activities recorded postoperatively. Gastroenterology 1981;81:61.

35. Sarna S, Latimer P, Campbell D, Waterfall WE. Electrical and contractile activities of the human rectosigmoid. Gut 1982;23: 698.

36. Snape WJ, Carlson GM, Cohen S. Colonic myoelectric activity in the irritable bowel syndrome. Gastroenterology 1976;70: 326.

37. Taylor I, Duthie HL, Smallwood R, Linkens D. Large bowel myoelectrical activity in man. Gut 1975;16:808.

38. Fioramonti J, Bueno L, Sarna SK, Ruckebusch Y. Origin of high slow wave frequency in the dog colon. Reprod Nutr Dev 1982;20:983.

39. Schang JC, Devroede G. Fasting and postprandial myoelectric spiking activity in the human sigmoid colon. Gastroenterology 1983;85:1048.

40. Battle WM, Cohen S, Snape WJ. Inhibition of postprandial colonic motility after ingestion of an amino acid mixture. Dig Dis Sci 1980;25:647.

41. Dapoigny M, Trolese JF, Bommelaer G, Tournut R. Myoelectric spiking activity of right colon, left colon and rectosigmoid of healthy humans. Dig Dis Sci 1988;33:1007.

42. Alvarez WC, Freedlander BL. The rate of progress of food residues through the bowel. J Am Med Assoc 1924;83:576.

43. Ritchie JA, Truelove SC, Ardran GM, Tuckey MS. Propulsion and retropulsion of normal colonic contents. Dig Dis 1971;16: 697.

44. Edwards DAW, Beck LR. Movement of radiopacified feces during defecation. Dig Dis 1971;16:709.

45. Hinton JM, Lennard-Jones JE, Young AC. A new method for studying gut transit times using radiopaque markers. Gut 1969;10:842.

46. Cummings JH, Jenkins DJ, Wiggins HS. Measurement of the mean transit time of dietary residue through the human gut. Gut 1976;17:210.

47. Cummings JH, Wiggins HS. Transit through the gut measured by analysis of a single stool. Gut 1976;17:219.

48. Martelli H, Devroede G, Arhan P, et al. Some parameters of large bowel motility in normal man. Gastroenterology 1978;75: 612.

49. Martelli H, Devroede G, Arhan P, Duguay C. Mechanisms of idiopathic constipation: outlet obstruction. Gastroenterology 1978;75:623.

50. Arhan P, Devroede G, Jehannin B, et al. Segmental colonic transit time. Dis Colon Rectum 1981;24:625.

51. Metcalf AM, Phillips SF, Zinsmeister AR, et al. Simplified assessment of segmental colonic transit. Gastroenterology 1987;92:40.

52. Hammer J, Phillips SF. Fluid loading of the human colon: effects of segmental transit and stool composition. Gastroenterology 1993;105:988.

53. Krevsky B, Malmud LS, D'Ercole F, et al. Colonic transit scintigraphy. A physiologic approach to the quantitative measurement of colonic transit in humans. Gastroenterology 1986;91: 1102.

54. Spiller RC, Brown ML, Phillips SF. Decreased fluid tolerance, accelerated transit, and abnormal motility of the human colon induced by oleic acid. Gastroenterology 1986;91:100.

55. Camilleri M, Colemont LJ, Phillips SF, et al. Human gastric emptying and colonic filling of solids characterized by a new method. Am J Physiol 1989;257:G284.

56. Proano M, Camilleri M, Phillips SF, et al. Transit of solids through the human colon: regional quantification in the unprepared bowel. Am J Physiol 1990;258:G856.

57. Kirwan WO, Smith AN. Gastrointestinal transit estimated by an isotope capsule. Scand J Gastroenterol 1974;9:763.

58. Hardy JG, Healey JNC, Lee SW, Reynolds JR. Gastrointestinal transit of an enteric-coated delayed-release 5-aminosalicylic acid tablet. Aliment Pharmacol Ther 1987;1:209.

59. Moreno-Osset E, Bazzocchi G, Lo S, et al. Association between postprandial changes in colonic intraluminal pressure and transit. Gastroenterology 1989;96:1265.

60. O'Donnell LJD, Virjee J, Heaton KW. Detection of pseudo-

diarrhea by simple clinical assessment of intestinal transit rates. Br Med J 1990;300:439.

61. Manning AP, Thompson GW, Heaton KW, et al. Towards a positive diagnosis of the irritable bowel syndrome. Br Med J 1978;2:653.

62. Whitehead WE, Schuster MM. Irritable bowel syndrome: physiological and psychological mechanisms. In: Whitehead WE, Schuster MM, eds. Gastrointestinal disorders. New York: Academic Press, 1985:179.

63. Swarbrech ET, Hegarty JE, Bat L, et al. Sited pain from the irritable bowel. Lancet 1980;2:443.

64. Whitehead WE, Holtkotter B, Enck P, et al. Tolerance for rectosigmoid distension in irritable bowel syndrome. Gastroenterology 1990;98:1187.

65. Hasler WL, Soudah HC, Owyang C. A somatostatin analogue inhibits afferent pathways mediating perception of rectal distension. Gastroenterology 1993;104:1390.

66. Prior A, Read NW. Reduction of rectal sensitivity and post-prandial motility by granisetron, a $5-HT_3$-receptor antagonist, in patients with irritable bowel syndrome. Aliment Pharmacol Ther 1993;7:175.

67. Hasler WL, Soudah HC, Owyang C. Somatostatin analogue inhibits afferent response to rectal distension in diarrhea predominant irritable bowel patients. J Pharmacol Exp Ther (in press).

68. Plourde V, Lembo T, Shui Z, et al. Effects of the somatostatin analogue Octreotide on rectal afferent nerves in humans. Am J Physiol 1993;265:G742.

69. Andrews PLR. Modulation of visceral afferent activity as a therapeutic possibility for gastrointestinal disorders. In: Read NW, ed. Irritable bowel syndrome. Boston: Blackwell Scientific, 1991:91.

70. Maxton DG, Whorwell PJ. Abdominal distension in irritable bowel syndrome: the patient's perception. Eur J Gastroenterol Hepatol 1992;4:241.

71. Maxton DG, Martin DF, Whorwell PJ, Godfrey M. Abdominal distension in female patients with irritable bowel syndrome: exploration of possible mechanisms. Gut 1991;32:662.

72. Miller FR. Viscero-motor reflexes. Am J Physiol 1924;71:84.

73. Tong EY, Tjioe DT. Effects of gastric distention on activity of abdominal muscles in dogs. Am J Physiol 1971;221:1652.

74. Trotman IF, Price CC. Bloated irritable bowel syndrome defined by dynamic ^{99m}Tc bran scan. Lancet 1986;2:364.

75. Pemberton JH, Rath DM, Ilstrup DM. Evaluation and surgical treatment of severe chronic constipation. Ann Surg 1991;214:403.

76. Vassallo M, Camilleri M, Phillips SF, et al. Transit through the proximal colon influences stool weight in irritable bowel syndrome. Gastroenterology 1992;102:102.

77. Bassotti G, Gaburri M, Imbimbo BP, et al. Colonic mass movements in idiopathic chronic constipation. Gut 1988;29:1173.

78. Connell AM. The motility of the pelvic colon. II. Paradoxical motility in diarrhea and constipation. Gut 1962;3:342.

79. Bueno L, Fioramonti J, Ruckebusch Y, et al. Evaluation of colonic myoelectrical activity in health and functional disorders. Gut 1980;21:480.

80. Frexinos J, Bueno L, Fioramonti J. Diurnal changes in myoelectrical spiking activity of the human colon. Gastroenterology 1985;88:1104.

81. Frexinos J, Fioramonti J, Bueno L. Colonic myoelectrical activity in IBS painless diarrhea. Gut 1987;28:1613.

82. Krishnamurthy S, Schuffler M, Rohrmann C, Pope CI. Severe idiopathic constipation is associated with a distinctive abnormality of the myenteric plexus. Gastroenterology 1985;85:26.

83. Von der Ohe M, Camilleri M, Kvols LK, et al. Motor dysfunction of the small bowel and colon in patients with the carcinoid syndrome and diarrhea. N Engl J Med 1993;329:1073.

84. Thompson WG, Dotevall G, Drossman DA. Irritable bowel syndrome: guidelines for the diagnosis. Gastroenterology International 1989;2:92.

85. Cann PA, Read NW, Brown C, et al. Irritable bowel syndrome: relationship of disorders in the transit of a single solid meal to symptom patterns. Gut 1983;24:405.

86. Kellow JE, Phillips SF. Altered small bowel motility in irritable

bowel syndrome is correlated with symptoms. Gastroenterology 1987;98:1885-1893.

87. Reddy SN, Bazzocchi G, Chan S, et al. Colonic motility and transit in health and ulcerative colitis. Gastroenterology 1991;101:1289.

88. Rao SSC, Read NW, Stobhart JAH, et al. Anorectal contractility under basal conditions and during rectal infusion of saline in ulcerative colitis. Gut 1988;29:769.

89. Karaus M, Sarna SK. Giant migrating contractions during defecation in the dog colon. Gastroenterology 1987;92:925.

90. Frexinos J, Staumont G, Fioramonti J, Bueno L. Effects of sennosides on colonic myoelectrical activity in man. Dig Dis Sci 1989;34:214.

91. Barrow L, Steed KP, Spiller RC, et al. Scintigraphic demonstration of lactulose-induced accelerated proximal colon transit. Gastroenterology 1992;103:1167.

92. Madson JL. Effects of Cisapride on gastrointestinal transit in healthy humans. Dig Dis Sci 1990;35:1500.

93. Krevsky B, Maurer AH, Malmud LS, Fisher RS. Cisapride accelerates colonic transit in constipated patients with colonic inertia. Am J Gastroenterol 1989;84:882.

94. Steadman CJ, Phillips SF, Camilleri M, et al. Control of muscle tone in the human colon. Gut 1992;33:541.

95. Ogilvie H. Large intestinal colic due to sympathetic deprivation: a new clinical syndrome. Br Med J 1948;2:671.

96. Vanek VW, Al-Salti M. Acute pseudo-obstruction of the colon (Ogilvie's syndrome): an analysis of 400 cases. Dis Colon Rectum 1986;29:203.

97. Jetmore AB, Timmcke AE, Gathright JB, et al. Ogilvie's syndrome: colonoscopic decompression and analysis of predisposing factors. Dis Colon Rectum 1992;35:1135.

98. Hutchinson R, Griffiths C. Acute colonic pseudo-obstruction: a pharmacological approach. Ann R Coll Surg Engl 1992;74:364.

99. Sloyer AF, Panella VS, Demas BE, et al. Ogilvie's syndrome. Successful management without colonoscopy. Dig Dis Sci 1988;33:1391.

100. MacColl C, MacConnell KL, Baylis B, Lee SS. Treatment of acute colonic pseudo-obstruction (Ogilvie's syndrome) with cisapride. Gastroenterology 1990; 98:773.

101. Bonacini M, Smith OI, Pritchard T. Erythromycin as therapy in acute colonic pseudo-obstruction (Ogilvie's Syndrome). J Clin Gastroenterol 1991;13:475.

102. Stanghellini V, Camilleri M, Malagelada JR. Chronic idiopathic intestinal pseudo-obstruction: clinical and intestinal manometric findings. Gut 1987;28:5.

103. Preston DM, Hawley PR, Lennard-Jones JE, et al. Results of colectomy for severe idiopathic constipation in women (Arbuthnot Lane's disease). Br J Surg 1984;71:547.

104. Leon SH, Krishnamurthy S, Schuffler MD. Subtotal colectomy for severe idiopathic constipation: a follow-up study of 13 patients. Dig Dis Sci 1987;32:1249.

105. Faulk DL, Anuras S, Christensen J. Chronic intestinal pseudo-obstruction. Gastroenterology 1978;74:922.

106. Camilleri M, Phillips SF. Acute and chronic intestinal pseudo-obstruction. Adv Intern Med 1991;36:287.

107. Malagelada JR, Camilleri M, Stanghellini V. Manometric diagnosis of gastrointestinal motility disorders. New York: Thieme-Stratton, 1986.

108. Kellow JE, Borody TJ, Phillips SF, et al.Human interdigestive motility: variations in patterns from esophagus to colon. Gastroenterology 1986;91:386.

109. Greydanus MP, Camilleri M. Abnormal postcibal antral and small bowel motility due to neuropathy or myopathy in systemic sclerosis. Gastroenterology 1989;96:110.

110. Camilleri M. Disorders of gastrointestinal motility in neurologic diseases. Mayo Clin Proc 1990;65:825.

111. Krishnamurthy S, Schuffler MD. Pathology of neuromuscular disorders of the small intestine and colon. Gastroenterology 1987;93:610.

112. Krishnamurthy S, Heng Y, Schuffler MD. Chronic intestinal pseudo-obstruction in infants and children caused by diverse abnormalities of the myenteric plexus. Gastroenterology 1993;104:1398.

113. Anuras S. Familial visceral neuropathies. In: Anuras S, ed. Motility disorders of the gastrointestinal tract. New York: Raven Press, 1992:189.
114. Anuras S. Familial visceral myopathies. In: Anuras S, ed. Motility disorders of the gastrointestinal tract. New York: Raven Press, 1992:165.
115. Anuras S. Childhood visceral myopathies. In: Anuras S, ed. Motility disorders of the gastrointestinal tract. New York: Raven Press, 1992:197.
116. Rohrmann CA Jr, Ricci MT, Krishnamurthy S, et al. Radiologic and histologic differentiation of neuromuscular disorders of the gastrointestinal tract. Visceral myopathies, visceral neuropathies, and progressive systemic sclerosis. AJR Am J Roentgenol 1984;143:933.
117. Jayachandar J, Frank JL, Jonas MM. Isolated intestinal myopathy resembling progressive systemic sclerosis in a child. Gastroenterology 1988;95:1114.
118. Venizelos IO, Shousha S, Bull TB, et al. Chronic intestinal pseudo-obstruction in two patients. Overlap of features of systemic sclerosis and visceral myopathy. Histopathology 1988;12: 533.
119. Fitzgibbons PL, Chandrasoma PT. Familial visceral myopathy. Evidence of diffuse involvement of intestinal smooth muscle. Am J Surg Pathol 1987;11:846.
120. Loening-Baucke VA, Anuras S, Mitros FA. Changes in colorectal function in patients with chronic colonic pseudo-obstruction. Dig Dis Sci 1987;32:1104.
121. Hyman PE, McDiarmid SV, Napolitano J, et al. Antroduodenal motility in children with chronic intestinal pseudo-obstruction. J Pediatr 1988;112:899.
122. Achem Sr, Owyang C, Schuffler MD, et al. Neuronal dysplasia and chronic intestinal pseudo-obstruction: rectal biopsy as a possible aid to diagnosis. Gastroenterology 1987;92:805.
123. Camilleri M, Zinsmeister AR. Towards a relatively inexpensive, non-invasive, accurate test for colonic motility disorders. Gastroenterology 1992;103:36.
124. Suzuki H, Amano S, Matsumoto K, et al. Chronic idiopathic intestinal pseudo-obstruction caused by acquired visceral neuropathy localized in the left colon: report on two cases. Jpn J Surg 1987;17:302.
125. Cohen LB, Field SP, Sachar DB. The superior mesenteric artery syndrome. The disease that isn't, or is it? J Clin Gastroenterology 1985;7:113.
126. Vargas JH, Sachs P, Ament ME. Chronic intestinal pseudo-obstruction syndrome in pediatrics. Results of a national survey by members of the North American Society of Pediatric Gastroenterology and Nutrition. J Pediatr Gastroenterol Nutr 1988;7:323.
127. Miyake T, Kawamori J, Yoshida T, et al. Small bowel pseudo-obstruction in Kawasaki disease. Pediatr Radiol 1987;17:383.
128. Leon SH, Schuffler MD, Kettler M, et al. Chronic intestinal pseudo-obstruction as a complication of Duchenne's muscular dystrophy. Gastroenterology 1986;90:455.
129. Bagwell CE, Filler RM, Cutz E, et al. Neonatal intestinal pseudo-obstruction. J Pediatr Surg 1984;19:732.
130. Keshavarzian A, Isaacs P, McColl I, et al. Idiopathic intestinal pseudo-obstruction and contaminated small bowel syndrome—treatment with metronidazole, ileostomy, and indomethacin. Am J Gastroenterol 1983;78:562.
131. Lipton AB, Knauer CM. Pseudo-obstruction of the bowel: therapeutic trial of metoclopramide. Am J Dig Dis 1977;22: 263.
132. Lewis TD, Daniel EE, Sarna SK, et al. Idiopathic intestinal pseudo-obstruction: report of a case, with intraluminal studies of mechanical and electrical activity, and response to drugs. Gastroenterology 1978;74:107.
133. Schang JC, Devroede G. Beneficial effects of naloxone in a patient with intestinal pseudo-obstruction. Am J Gastroenterol 1985;80:407.
134. Laustsen J, Haling H, Fallingborg J. Treatment of chronic idiopathic intestinal pseudo-obstruction, letter to the editor. Dig Dis Sci 1987;32:222.
135. Boige N, Cargill G, Mashako L, et al. Trimebutine-induced phase III-like activity in infants with intestinal motility disorders. J Pediatr Gastroenterol Nutr 1987;6:548.
136. Schuurkes JAJ, Van Nueten JM, Van Daele PGH, et al. Motor-stimulating properties of cisapride on isolated gastrointestinal preparations of the guinea pig. J Pharmacol Exp Ther 1985;234: 775.
137. Camilleri M, Brown ML, Malagelada JR. Impaired transit of chyme in chronic intestinal pseudo-obstruction: correction by cisapride. Gastroenterology 1986;91:619.
138. Camilleri M, Malagelada JR, Abell TL, et al. Effect of six weeks of treatment with cisapride in gastroparesis and intestinal pseudo-obstruction. Gastroenterology 1989;96:704.
139. Soudah HC, Hasler WL, Owyang C. Effect of octreotide on intestinal motility and bacterial overgrowth in scleroderma. N Engl J Med 1991;325:1461.
140. Peeters T, Matthiss G, Depoortere I, et al. Erythromycin is a motilin receptor agonist. Am J Physiol 1989;257:G470.
141. Janssen SJ, Peeters TL, Van Trappen G, et al. Improvement of gastric emptying in diabetic gastroparesis by erythromycin. N Engl J Med 1990;322:1028.
142. Mathias JR, Ferguson KL, Clench MH. Debilitating functional bowel disease controlled by leuprolide acetate, gonadotrophin releasing hormone analog. Dig Dis Sci 1989;34:761.
143. Schuffler MD, Deitch EA. Chronic idiopathic intestinal pseudo-obstruction: a surgical approach. Ann Surg 1980;192:752.
144. Anuras S, Shirazi S, Faulk DL, et al. Surgical treatment in familial visceral myopathy. Ann Surg 1979;189:306.
145. Schuffler MD, Leon SH, Krishnamurthy S. Intestinal pseudo-obstruction caused by a new form of visceral neuropathy: palliation by radical small bowel resection. Gastroenterology 1985;89:1152.
146. Mughal MM, Irving MH. Treatment of endstage chronic intestinal pseudo-obstruction by subtotal entrectomy and home parenteral nutrition. Gut 1988;29:1613.
147. Pitt HA, Mann LL, Berquist WE, et al. Chronic intestinal pseudo-obstruction: management with total parenteral nutrition and a venting enterostomy. Arch Surg 1985;120:614.

Textbook of Gastroenterology, second edition, edited by Tadataka Yamada. JB Lippincott Company, Philadelphia © 1995.

CHAPTER 83

Diverticulitis

John H. Pemberton   David N. Armstrong
Charles D. Dietzen

The term diverticular disease is derived from the Latin word *diverticulum*, which means "a small diversion from the normal path." With diverticular disease, balloon-like sacs or pouches called diverticula develop in the walls of the colon. These tiny pouches are formed when pressure causes the inside wall of the colon to bulge out through weak spots in the outer wall.

Originally the term *diverticular disease* was used to indicate the presence of diverticula, symptomatic or not, in the large bowel. However, the term *diverticulosis* indicates only the presence of diverticula. Symptomatic diverticular disease may present as bleeding, inflammation (diverticulitis), or other abdominal symptoms in the absence of inflammation.

This chapter describes diverticular disease of the colon, including its epidemiology, etiology, pathologic and clinical manifestations; provides a differential diagnosis; and enumerates the important diagnostic tests used for evaluation. Finally, the management of diverticular disease is detailed together witn the complications that may arise.

EPIDEMIOLOGY

The infrequency of reports of clinically important diverticular disease before 1900 suggests that it was an uncommon problem until the 20th century.[1] However, the methods of diagnosis, by radiologic contrast study, operative discovery, or autopsy, are flawed by measurement and source selection biases, making the accuracy of prevalence estimates unreliable.

Reports on the prevalence of diverticulosis in this century have noted the disease to be common in highly industrialized countries and infrequent in economically underdeveloped nations.[1-3] A male preponderance was documented by early studies, but this difference has not been seen since the mid-1950s, and a slight female preponderance is suggested by more recent reports. In areas where the disease is common, age is an important variable, with diverticulosis unusual in the first four decades and common in later years.[4-6]

Radiographic and autopsy studies from the United States,[7-12] United Kingdom,[13-16] Australia,[3,17] Greece,[18] and other developed countries[19] report prevalence rates that vary between 5% and 45%. This wide range is explained by differing methods of measurement and by selection biases related to both age and symptoms. Most of the later studies indicate that in industrialized nations, 33% to 50% of the population older than 50 years of age and more than 50% of those older than 80 years of age have colonic diverticula.[5] In addition, the incidence of diverticulitis also increases with the age of the patient. In one longitudinal study, the incidence of diverticulitis increased from 10% to 35% after 20 years of observation.

The high prevalence rates in the technologically advanced countries is in sharp contrast to the rates in more primitive societies in parts of Africa and Asia.[20,21] Carefully performed studies from both Africa and Asia document prevalence rates

DIVERTICULAR DISEASE
A Disease of 20th Century Western Civilization

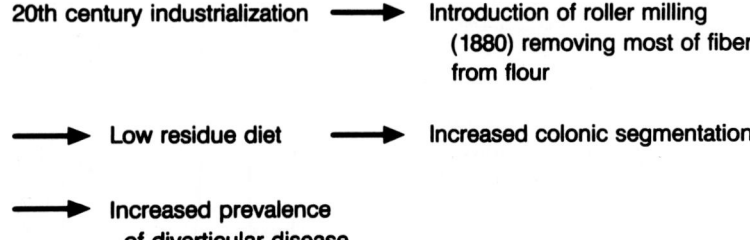

FIGURE 83-1. Painter and Burkitt's concept of the source of diverticular disease.

of less than 0.2%.[1,21,22] These statistics are supported by the rare occurrence of diverticulitis, a clinical indicator for the presence of colonic diverticula.[1] Japan represents an interesting exception to these observations. In keeping with recent adoption of a more Western lifestyle, the prevalence of diverticulosis in Japan is on the rise, especially among the elderly.[23] However, in contrast to patients in most other developed countries, Japanese patients with right-sided diverticulosis outnumber those with left-sided disease 5 to 1.[3]

Painter and Burkitt[1] noted that persons from highly industrialized societies tended to consume diets low in fiber, an observation also made by other investigators.[24,25] Moreover, dietary fiber consumption has been associated with the absence of diverticulosis.[1] Painter and Burkitt postulated that a low-fiber diet was the major factor responsible for the emergence of diverticular disease in the 20th century (Fig. 83-1). This concept has, however, been criticized by Mendeloff for its simplicity and lack of scientific basis.[26]

PATHOLOGIC FEATURES

Histologic studies have established that colonic diverticula are of the false or pseudodiverticula type, consisting of mucosa and serosa with no intervening muscular coat (Fig. 83-2). These pulsion diverticula are acquired, and the occurrence of a congenital, true diverticulum or of a duplication of the large bowel is rare.

Although usually present in clusters, diverticula may be solitary. The distribution of diverticula over the different segments of the colon is unequal (Fig. 83-3). Ninety-five percent of all patients harbor diverticula in the sigmoid colon.[27] A classification according to location places most patients in one of four categories: diverticula limited to the sigmoid colon (65%); diverticula involving the sigmoid and other segments of colon (24%); diverticula dispersed over the entire colon (7%); and diverticula limited to a segment proximal to the sigmoid colon (4%).[27] A number of Asian countries, including

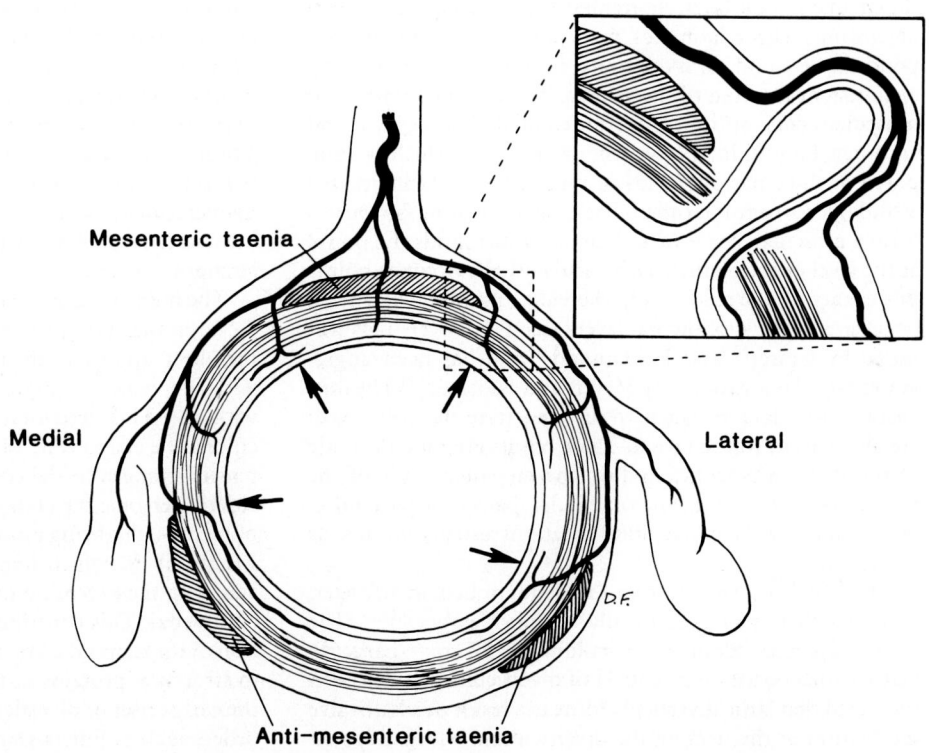

FIGURE 83-2. Diverticula occur where the vasa recti penetrate the submucosa of the colon.

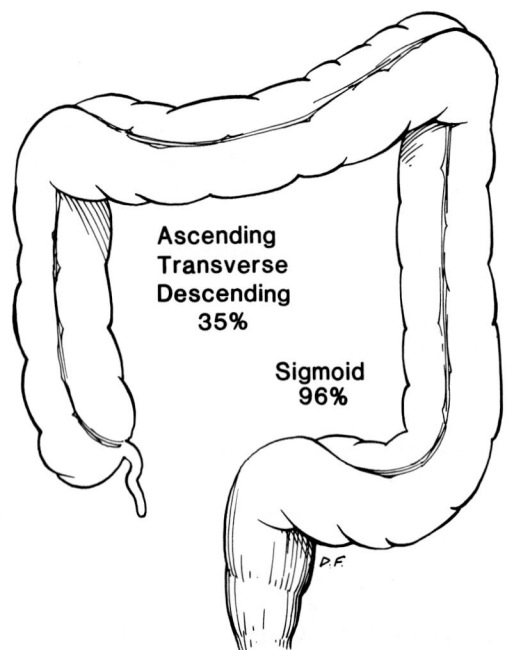

**Ascending
Transverse
Descending
35%**

**Sigmoid
96%**

D.F.

FIGURE 83-3. Frequency distribution of diverticulosis: 96% of patients with diverticulosis have sigmoid involvement; 35% also have more proximal disease.

Japan, Korea, and Thailand, represent an interesting exception to these findings. In these countries, patients with right-sided diverticula outnumber those with left-sided diverticula by a large ratio. Right-sided diverticula tend to occur earlier in life than left-sided diverticula.[28,29] The underlying cause for these findings is unknown.

Most patients with sigmoid diverticula have thickening of the circular muscle layer, shortening of the taenia, and lumenal narrowing. The relation of myochosis to diverticulosis is poorly understood. Cross-sectional examination demonstrates a consistent location of diverticula. The colon contains two muscular coats, an inner, circumferential circular layer and an outer, longitudinal layer (the taenia coli), which is composed of three narrow bands of muscle fibers, each situated 120 degrees from the other. The taenia, in turn, fan out to form a muscular sleeve that completely surrounds the bowel at the level of the rectum. Diverticula usually occur at points of weakness in the colon wall, where the intramural vasa recta penetrate to the submucosal layers (see Fig. 83-2). This was noted by Graser[30] and Drummond[31] and has been angiographically demonstrated by Meyers and associates.[32] The four characteristic loci at which vessels penetrate the colon wall are all adjacent to the taenia. These points are on either side of the taenia mesocolica and on the mesenteric side of the taenia libera and the taenia omentalis. Exceptions are infrequent, and diverticula at other locations usually are not as prominent.

Diverticula vary in size from 1 or 2 mm to 1 cm in diameter, although they may occasionally be much larger.[3,13,27] The largest reported colonic diverticulum was 27 cm.[33] Large diverticula may occur as a sequela of diverticulitis. It has been theorized that large diverticula form as a result of a ball-valve mechanism at the neck of the diverticulum, which traps air

with resultant enlargement of the diverticulum. Because of surrounding inflammation, the mucosal lining of giant diverticula is invariably absent.[33] The external appearance of the diverticular colon is distinctive. Diverticula adjacent to the antimesenteric taenia (taenia libera and taenia omentalis) are often seen. Epiploic appendices sometimes cover the diverticula, which, in some patients, make the colon appear to be free of diverticula. The orifices that mark the neck or base of diverticula are easily identified endoscopically, often with fecaliths projecting from the opening.

Diverticula of the rectum are rare. The presence of a circumferential longitudinal muscle layer probably offers added resistance to mucosal herniation. Walstad and Sahibzada estimated that rectal diverticula occur 50 times less frequently than colonic diverticula,[34] although this may be an overestimate. As with colonic diverticulosis, bleeding or diverticulitis (with abscess, obstruction, or a clinical picture similar to a carcinoma) can complicate rectal diverticula.[34–36] Acquired diverticulosis of the appendix also occurs. In a large autopsy/surgery study, approximately 1.4% of all appendices had diverticula.[37] Diverticulitis, likewise, can occur in an appendiceal diverticulum. Although the clinical presentation is similar to that of acute appendicitis, appendiceal diverticulitis and acute appendicitis are two distinctly different pathologic entities.[38,39]

ETIOLOGY

Herniation of the colonic mucosa through the muscular layer of the colon is a function of two factors: the strength of the bowel wall and the pressure differential between the lumen of the colon and the peritoneal cavity.[6]

The nature of the bowel wall in diverticulosis cannot be fully understood without considering myochosis, the thickening found in many patients with diverticulosis. If found without diverticula, myochosis probably represents a prediverticular state.[40] Myochosis is most often seen in sigmoid diverticulosis, also referred to as spastic colon diverticulosis.[27] Neither hypertrophy nor hyperplasia of the colonic wall has been found in myochosis; however, increased elastin deposition in the taenia has been documented.[41] The cause of myochosis is unknown; however, the characteristic decrease in diameter of the colon creates conditions that produce high intralumenal pressures with no compensatory increase in wall strength.

The mechanical properties of the colonic wall are a possible factor in the etiology of diverticular disease. Consistent with the observation that the frequency of diverticulosis increases with age, tensile strength and elasticity of the colon decrease with age. This deterioration is most marked in the sigmoid colon, the narrowest, thickest segment. Collagen provides tensile strength to the colonic wall: in the sigmoid colon of elderly persons, the collagen fibers become smaller and more numerous, this being more pronounced in diverticular disease. Elastin fibers, which impart elasticity, also deteriorate with age, with the exception of those in the taenia, which become contracted. This contributes to the sacculation and contraction of the sigmoid colon in diverticular disease. Deterioration in structural proteins in the colonic wall are consistent with the early onset of diverticular disease in connective tissue disorders such as Ehlers-Danlos and Marfan's syndromes.

Anatomic variations in regions of the colon determine pressure gradients between the peritoneal cavity and the colonic lumen. Intralumenal colonic pressure in any given segment is determined by the law of Laplace, which states that pressure is directly proportional to wall tension and inversely proportional to bowel radius. In mathematical form, $P = kT/R$ (where P is the colonic pressure, T is the wall tension, R is the colon radius, and k is a conversion factor). The sigmoid has the smallest diameter of any part of the human colon and, consequently, the highest pressure. It is not surprising that diverticula are most common in this part of the colon.

A motility disorder has been suggested as the cause of diverticulosis.[42,43,44] A number of motility studies performed on the diverticular colon, both at rest and stimulated, have been reported.[45-49] These support motor dysfunction as one factor in the development of diverticulosis. The role of disturbed motility in diverticular disease was demonstrated by Eastwood and colleagues,[42] who identified exaggerated colonic pressure responses to selected drugs and feeding in patients with symptomatic diverticulosis, compared with patients without symptoms.

Other investigators have reported that patients with symptomatic diverticular disease have patterns of intralumenal pressure activity and responses to balloon distention that resemble those of irritable bowel syndrome (IBS).[45] On the other hand, the colonic myoelectrical patterns seen in diverticular disease differ from those in IBS.[50,51] The relation between IBS and diverticulosis remains controversial. It is possible that diverticulosis is an entirely asymptomatic condition and that those diverticulosis patients with pain have coexisting IBS.

Painter and Burkitt have suggested that segmentation, a form of nonpropulsive colonic contraction, plays a major role in the pathogenesis of diverticula (Fig. 83-4).[1,52] They argued that during periods of segmentation, contraction rings partition the colon into obstructed sectors; localized, abnormally

high pressures could then cause mucosal herniation characteristic of pulsion diverticula.

Studies of the effect of fiber also lend credence to motility disturbance as an etiologic factor in diverticulosis. Animal experiments demonstrate that diverticula are produced with a diet low in fiber and are prevented with high fiber intake.[53,54] It is uncertain how these findings translate to the development of diverticulosis in man. Combined with the apparent protective effect of fiber in human populations and the observed high prevalence of diverticula in populations with low bulk diets, the evidence indicates that dietary fiber, perhaps through an effect on colonic pressure and motility, may play a role in diverticulosis.

In summary, the cause of colonic diverticulosis seems to be multifactorial. The roles of colonic muscle changes, abnormal intralumenal pressure, motor dysfunction, and dietary fiber in the pathogenesis of diverticulosis are probably interrelated but remain to be elucidated.

UNCOMPLICATED DIVERTICULOSIS

Clinical Manifestations

At least 80% to 85% of individuals with diverticulosis never present with a clinical problem. This majority of affected people either have no symptoms whatsoever or have such low-grade or intermittent problems they never seek medical attention[55] (Table 83-1). A small fraction of these patients have symptoms such as intermittent abdominal pain, bloating, excessive flatulence, and irregular defecation. The cause of these symptoms is unknown and could well be secondary to coexistent irritable bowel.[56] Of the remaining 15% to 20% of diverticular patients, roughly three quarters develop diverticulitis and one quarter have some degree of hemorrhage.[55]

Differential Diagnosis

Virtually any disease causing abnormal intestinal motility may be confused with diverticular disease (Table 83-2). The following describes the most important of these.

Irritable Bowel Syndrome

Symptoms of abdominal pain and altered bowel habits may be indistinguishable from those of irritable bowel disease (see Chap. 81). Whether the pain is intrinsic to diverticulosis or

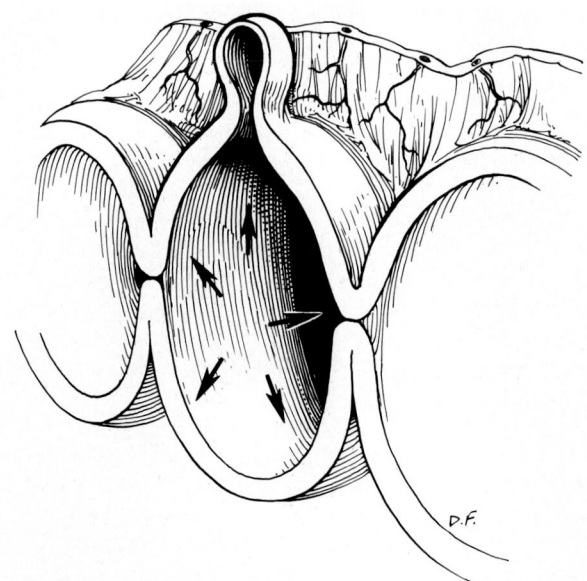

FIGURE 83-4. Painter and Burkitt's concept of segmentation causing pulsion diverticula to form.

TABLE 83-1	
Diverticular Disease	
TYPE OF DISEASE	**RELATIVE FREQUENCY (%)**
Uncomplicated	
Asymptomatic	70
Symptomatic	
Complicated	
Diverticulitis	10–25
Diverticular hemorrhage	5

TABLE 83-2
Differential Diagnosis of Diverticular Disease

Irritable bowel syndrome
Cancer
Appendicitis
Inflammatory bowel disease (e.g., Crohn's colitis, chronic ulcerative
  colitis)
Other colitides (e.g., ischemic colitis)
Gynecologic inflammatory or neoplastic diseases
Vascular ectasia
Anorectal disease

caused by coexisting IBS remains unanswered. This issue is more academic than practical, however, because the management of symptomatic diverticulosis and IBS are similar.

Colonic Carcinoma

Colorectal carcinoma and diverticular disease may present in remarkably similar manners. Both are common and are most frequently seen in the elderly in technologically advanced countries. Both can exist in any segment of the colon but are often found in the sigmoid. Both tend to constrict the lumen of the colon with advancement of disease and result in abdominal colic which can progress to obstruction or perforation. Finally, both can be clinically silent except for rectal bleeding (although carcinoma rarely causes massive hemorrhage, and diverticulosis is not known to cause occult rectal bleeding). To further confound the problem, the external appearance of a colon mass at operation often cannot differentiate colon cancer from smoldering diverticulitis. Radiologic and endoscopic evaluation of the colon are central to making a correct diagnosis.

Diagnostic Studies

Plain Films

In patients with uncomplicated diverticular disease or diverticular bleeding, plain abdominal radiographs are usually normal and, therefore, of little value. However, patients with diverticulitis often have localized ileus in adjacent small bowel and evidence of some degree of colon obstruction. Occasionally, if perforation has occurred, pneumoperitoneum on upright chest or lateral decubitus films is seen. Although these findings are not specific to diverticulitis, their presence lends credence to the clinical diagnosis.

Contrast Enema

The use of barium or one of the water-soluble contrast agents to visualize the colon is probably more reliable than colonoscopy in simply documenting presence or absence of diverticula in patients with asymptomatic diverticulosis.

Diverticula appear as barium-filled globular protrusions from the external surface of the colon outlined by the barium column (Fig. 83-5). On postevacuation films, retention of the contrast in the diverticula is common and is not a sign

of active diverticulitis. Every diverticulum is not always visualized on barium enema. Colonic spasm occluding the diverticular orifice, obscuring of diverticula by the barium-filled colon, and other factors make identification of every diverticulum on every examination unlikely. Sacculation seen on one study and not on subsequent studies is common.

Frequently, barium studies are performed not so much to confirm the diagnosis but to rule out colonic neoplasm. The accuracy of barium enema in the diagnosis of concomitant lesions in a diverticular colon is as low as 50% in some series.[57,58] One reason for this problem is illustrated in Figure 83-6; whether or not a carcinoma lies in the narrowed diverticular segment is difficult to determine. Moreover, diverticula may masquerade as polyps on barium enema, either by inversion of the diverticulum into the colonic lumen, or the en face appearance of contrast forming a ring in the stool-filled diverticulum (Fig. 83-7).[59-62] Careful study of multiple views, compression spot films, and postevacuation films helps to improve the diagnostic accuracy of barium studies.

Endoscopy

Lower gastrointestinal endoscopy is probably more valuable in assessing the large bowel for coexisting pathology than for the actual diagnosis of diverticular disease. Often, the orifices of diverticula are not seen; however, patient discomfort and difficulty with advancement of the endoscope because of sigmoid tortuosity and thickened rugae suggest previous episodes of diverticulitis.

Clinical Course and Complications

The majority of patients with colonic diverticula have an uncomplicated course. However, a significant number of patients, 10% to 25%, are afflicted with diverticulitis and its

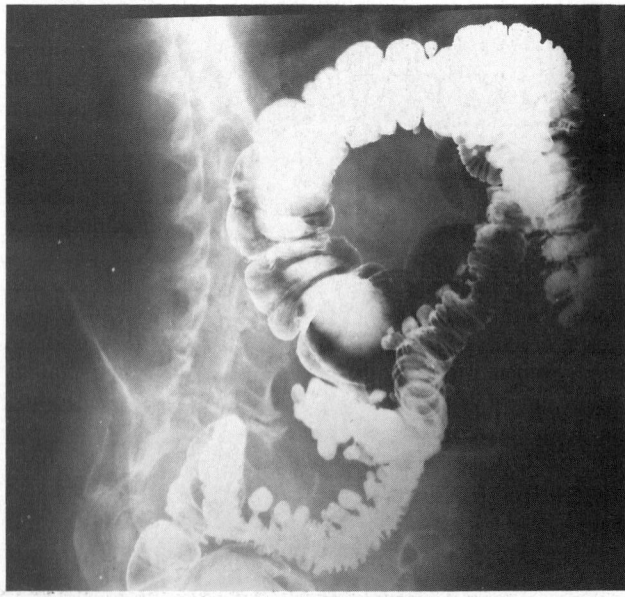

FIGURE 83-5. Radiologic appearance of pancolonic diverticulosis (oblique view; barium enema study).

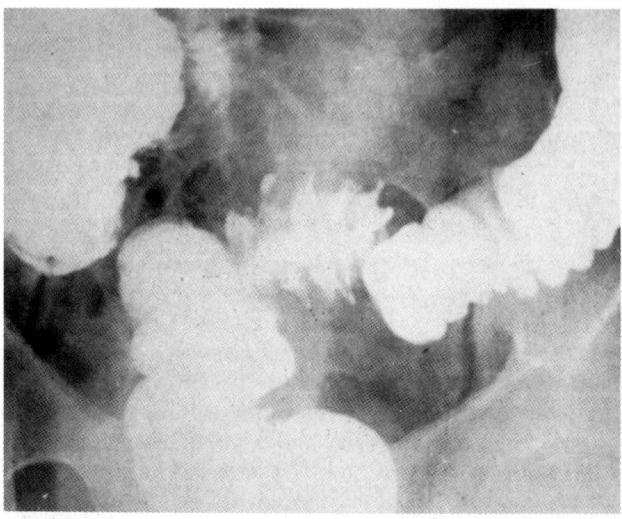

FIGURE 83-6. Barium enema study shows narrowed diverticular segment of sigmoid colon. Presence or absence of a neoplasm in this segment of bowel is difficult to determine by contrast exam.

sequelae; additionally, about 5% of patients with diverticulosis eventually have massive bleeding from a diverticulum.[5,6,63] Either diverticulitis or massive bleeding can develop in a patient with known, long-standing diverticulosis or in a previously undiagnosed and completely asymptomatic patient. Coexistent diverticulitis and diverticular bleeding is rare.

Treatment

There is support in the literature for treatment of uncomplicated but symptomatic diverticular disease with fiber.[49] In this subset of patients, bulk-forming agents may prevent the development of diverticula.[25,50,53,54,64]

The treatment of uncomplicated, asymptomatic diverticular disease is more controversial. Some retrospective studies provide circumstantial evidence to suggest that a high-fiber diet may prevent complications such as diverticular hemorrhage or diverticulitis.[65,66] Surgical treatment for uncomplicated diverticular disease, symptomatic or asymptomatic, is not indicated.

COMPLICATED DIVERTICULAR DISEASE: DIVERTICULITIS

Clinical Manifestations

The term complicated diverticular disease implies inflammation or bleeding has occurred. It is highly unusual for both to be present in the same patient. Inflammation (diverticulitis) occurs in 10% to 25% of patients with diverticulosis and begins as peridiverticulitis caused by a microperforation of the bowel.[5,6] Some patients with early diverticulitis, who have no physical or laboratory findings to suggest inflammation, may be mistakenly diagnosed as having uncomplicated but symptomatic diverticulosis. Early symptoms and signs of divertic-

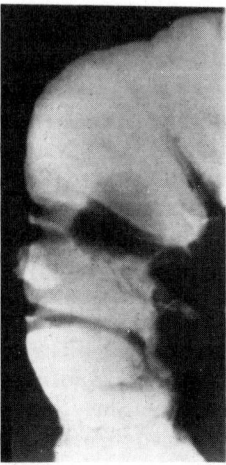

FIGURE 83-7. Barium enema study depicts an inverted diverticulum masquerading as a polyp.

ulitis include abdominal pain over the area of inflammation, nausea and vomiting, ileus, fever, localized abdominal tenderness with or without a mass, and, on rectal examination, tenderness with possible mass effect. As the clinical course evolves, manifestations may change (Fig. 83-8). If inflammation resolves, the early symptoms and signs subside. However, the inflammation often progresses, and abscess (either mesenteric or abdominopelvic), free perforation (with suppurative or fecal peritonitis), fistulization or obstruction (with distention, obstipation, colic, and, if unattended, perforation) may occur.

Differential Diagnosis

Acute Appendicitis

Appendicitis can be confused with diverticulitis involving any part of the colon. The inflamed sigmoid may lie in the right lower quadrant, mimicking appendicitis. Appendicitis is more common than diverticulitis and affects younger people. If appendicitis cannot be excluded, urgent surgery is mandatory. If diverticulitis is found, appropriate surgical management, usually resection, is undertaken. For this reason computed tomography (CT) scanning has assumed an increasing important role in diagnosing right-sided abdominal pain of un-

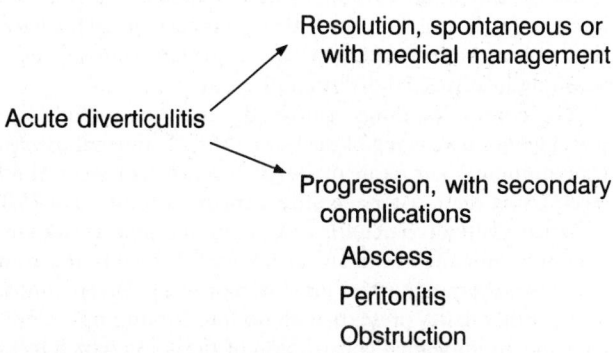

FIGURE 83-8. Clinical course of diverticulitis.

certain origin. It is emerging as the investigation of choice in diagnosing suspected diverticulitis.[67]

Inflammatory Bowel Disease

Symptoms and signs common to inflammatory bowel disease and diverticular disease include abdominal colic, altered bowel habits, rectal bleeding, fever, and abdominal tenderness. Chronic ulcerative colitis (CUC) is easier to differentiate from diverticular disease than is Crohn's colitis. Rectal sparing is rare in CUC, making proctoscopy an easy and reliable method for ruling out ulcerative colitis. Granulomatous (Crohn's) colitis, like diverticulitis, is associated with fistulization, obstruction, and, occasionally, formation of an abscess. Diverticulitis in combination with arthritis and pyoderma gangrenosum has been reported, and the presence of extraintestinal manifestations should not be used as the sole basis for differentiating granulomatous colitis from diverticulitis.[68] Radiologic and endoscopic evaluation render the correct diagnosis in most cases.[69,70]

Other Diseases

Ischemic colitis, radiation-induced colitis, and the infectious colitides can present with symptoms and signs similar to those of diverticulitis. As the clinical course evolves and the radiographic, endoscopic, and laboratory evaluation proceeds, the correct diagnosis usually becomes readily apparent. Other abdominal conditions are also sometimes confused with diverticulitis. What appears to be a simple small bowel obstruction from postoperative adhesions may, in fact, be diverticulitis with a loop of small intestine adherent to the inflamed segment of the colon.[71] The proximity of the pelvic organs to the sigmoid colon makes inflammatory and neoplastic diseases of the uterus, tubes, and ovaries part of the differential diagnosis of diverticulitis in women.[72]

Diagnostic Studies

Contrast Barium Enema

Barium enema is not recommended in patients with acute diverticulitis.[73] The risk of exacerbating an acute attack or precipitating a barium peritonitis from an unsuspected perforation is real. If there is doubt about the diagnosis, limited studies of the sigmoid colon, using water-soluble agents, can be done safely and with some degree of accuracy. However, this has been largely superseded by the greater accuracy of CT scanning in suspected diverticulitis.

The contrast findings seen in diverticulitis include displacement or narrowing of the bowel; altered mucosal pattern (sawtoothing); soft tissue mass; gas lucencies; or an air-fluid level. Using these criteria, contrast enema is accurate in 75% of patients with diverticulitis.[74] A carcinoma appears as a mucosa-breaching mass with an abrupt, well-defined border and a relatively short segment of lumenal narrowing. Diverticulitis, on the other hand, presents with no interruption in the mucosa and an ill-defined constriction of the colon which lacks the "shoulder effect" produced by a carcinoma. Moreover,

after diverticulitis subsides, the radiologic appearance improves, a finding that never occurs with carcinoma. Despite these differences, carcinoma of the colon can be missed on contrast enema if it is located in a myochotic segment with multiple diverticula and concomitant spasm. Schnyder and associates found that contrast enema correctly diagnosed patients with diverticulosis or diverticulitis with an associated carcinoma, only 50% of the time.[57]

Computed Tomography

CT of the abdomen and pelvis has been used increasingly to evaluate patients with diverticulitis. As with contrast enemas, the inflammatory changes seen with CT during an episode of diverticulitis are nonspecific and are not pathognomonic of the condition. Hulnick and colleagues[75] described the characteristic CT findings, which include thickening of the colon wall, pericolic inflammation, fistula, sinus, abscess, and obstruction. CT evidence of pericolic inflammation was seen in 98% of patients with diverticulitis, which demonstrates the high sensitivity of the scan.[75] Contrast studies delineate lumenal changes but frequently underestimate pericolic inflammation; CT is the method of choice for demonstrating pericolic and extracolonic extension, such as abscess and fistula[67,76] (Fig. 83-9). Another advantage of CT is that it gives a more accurate estimate of the degree of inflammation than other imaging studies.

In spite of its increasing popularity, all patients with acute diverticulitis do not require CT for successful management. However, CT should be performed in the following conditions: there is significant uncertainty about the diagnosis of diverticulitis; there is clinical suspicion that an abscess or fistula is present; medical treatment of the acute phase has not resulted in clinical improvement; the patient is immunocompromised (e.g., steroid-dependent) and clinical evaluation, therefore, is not a reliable indicator of the patient's condition; or an unusual clinical situation exists, such as right-sided diverticulitis[77] or giant diverticulum of the colon.[78]

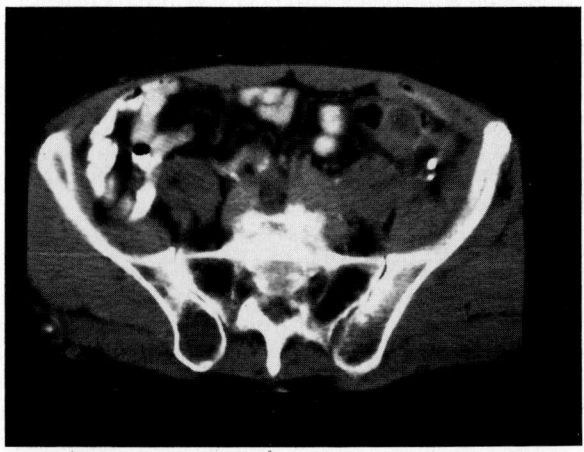

FIGURE 83-9. Computed tomographic scan of the pelvis in a patient with a diverticular abscess. The scan localized the abscess as a contrast-enhanced, walled structure juxtaposed to the sigmoid colon just beneath the left abdominal wall.

Ultrasonography

There are few descriptions of the use of ultrasound for diagnosing diverticulitis.[79,80] However, ultrasonography provides a useful, noninvasive means of imaging extracolonic fluid collections and may be used to direct percutaneous drainage of pelvic and paracolic abscesses. The advantages of ultrasonography include ease of operation and its relative cost compared with CT scan. One disadvantage is that the technique and interpretation of the images are more operator-dependant than are CT scans.

Endoscopic Studies

Flexible sigmoidoscopy is often used during an episode of suspected diverticulitis.[73] Its main usefulness arises in the event of colonic obstruction, to differentiate an obstructing carcinoma from an obstructing diverticular mass. Minimal insufflation of air is used, to prevent rupturing the already fragile colon. Colonoscopy is not indicated in active, acute diverticulitis. However, it is useful after the inflammatory process subsides.

Clinical Course and Complications

Morson[81] reported that the earliest microscopic evidence of diverticular inflammation caused by inspissated fecal matter is lymphoid hyperplasia at the apex of the diverticulum. Peridiverticulitis from microperforation with pericolic abscess (microscopic or macroscopic) follows. At this point, either spontaneous or medically-induced resolution is possible, as is progression to localized or generalized sepsis.

Hinchey and colleagues,[82] modifying the classification of Hughes' group,[83] described four stages of perforated diverticular disease (Table 83-3). Each successive stage represents more advanced disease and a poorer prognosis:

1. Pericolic abscess, frequently intramesenteric
2. Pelvic abscess, or extension of a pericolic abscess
3. Generalized (suppurative) peritonitis, or rupture of a pelvic abscess
4. Fecal peritonitis, or free perforation of an inflamed diverticulum.

The second stage, pelvic abscess, almost always requires either percutaneous or operative drainage. The last two stages, generalized peritonitis and fecal peritonitis, mandate urgent surgical treatment.

**TABLE 83-3
Stages of Diverticulitis**

Pericolic abscess
Pelvic abscess
Generalized suppurative peritonitis*
Fecal peritonitis*

---

* Associated with high morbidity and mortality rates.

Adapted from Hinchey EJ, Schaal PGH, Richards GK. Treatment of perforated diverticular disease of the colon. Adv Surg 1978;12:85.

Two clinical situations deserve detailed discussion, diverticulitis in the immunocompromised patient and diverticulitis with fistula formation. Spontaneous colon perforation and perforated diverticulitis occur more frequently in a variety of compromised patients: patients on prolonged steroid therapy[84-86]; chronic renal failure patients[87]; renal transplant patients[88,89]; and patients taking nonsteroidal antiinflammatory drugs.[90,91] Although the incidence of diverticulitis is no greater in this population,[92] the disease runs a more sinister course in immunocompromised patients. Early in the illness, symptoms are masked, often delaying diagnosis. The peritoneal organs and tissues fail to contain and wall off the infectious process, resulting in a high rate of generalized suppurative or fecal peritonitis. In these instances, medical management is rarely successful. The majority of these patients require aggressive surgical management early, with resection of the affected colon and exteriorization of the proximal colon.[89,92]

Fistula formation is common in patients with diverticulitis. The bladder is the most commonly involved organ, being affected in 10% to 15% of patients.[93,94] However, the skin (buttock, flank, perineum, scrotum, lower extremity, hip),[95] vagina,[93] bowel (small intestine, colon, appendix),[93,96,97] uterus,[93] ureter,[98] and portal venous system[99,100] may all be sites of fistulas. If fistulas connect with the bladder, pneumaturia is a classic symptom. The clinical status of these patients depends on the size of any associated abscess and how well this is drained by the fistula. It is unusual for these fistulas to close spontaneously, and resection of the tract and involved segment of colon is indicated. However, there is some evidence to suggest that conservative treatment of colovesical fistulas may be well tolerated in the short to medium term,[94] and it may be appropriate treatment for patients with prohibitive operative risks.

Treatment

Management of diverticulitis includes the standard measures for assessing fluid status and its replacement, nasogastric suction for ileus or obstruction, and broad-spectrum antibiotics. The antibiotic regimen should be one that covers the major colonic pathogens, anaerobes (*Bacteroides fragilis*), gram-negative bacilli (*Escherichia coli*), and gram-positive coliforms (*Streptococcus fecalis*). In spite of the development of new broad-spectrum antibiotics, the gold standard of treatment in the unstable septic patient remains "triple therapy" (e.g., ampicillin, gentamicin, and metronidazole). In more stable patients with local peritoneal signs, the newer single-agent antibiotic regimes include ampicillin/sulbactam, a carbapenum such as Imipenum/cilastatin, or ticarcillin clavulanate. Clindamycin remains an alternative to metronidazole for coverage of anaerobic organisms, vancomycin substitutes for penicillin in allergic patients, and the monobactam aztreonam may substitute for gentamycin in renal impairment. In the absence of peritoneal signs, oral administration of a flouroquinolone, amoxicillin clavulanate, or a cephalosporin may be appropriate. Further evaluation and management depend on the clinician's assessment of the patient and the response to initial treatment.

A favorable clinical response to medical treatment is usually seen within 2 to 4 days. If fever, abdominal signs, and leukocytosis have resolved or substantially abated and if bowel function (flatus) has returned, liquids can be started, cautiously graduating to solid food. The antibiotic course should be maintained for 7 to 10 days. Elective evaluation of the colon may be performed after the inflammatory process resolves. Recurrence of diverticulitis has been reported to occur in 27% to 45% of patients.[73,101] If a favorable response to medical management is not forthcoming, if clinical signs point to secondary complications (e.g., pelvic or abdominal abscess, fistula, obstruction), or if there is doubt about the diagnosis, a CT scan should be performed.

Surgical management is usually necessary in 15% to 30% of patients with diverticulitis.[5] The classic surgical indications are free perforation with fecal peritonitis, suppurative peritonitis secondary to ruptured abscess, abdominal or pelvic abscess, fistula, obstruction, recurrent diverticulitis, and inability to rule out carcinoma.[82]

Peritonitis, whether fecal (from colonic perforation) or suppurative (from abscess rupture), always requires urgent surgery. Both conditions run a fulminant course. After hemodynamic stabilization, operation should proceed without further delay. In the urgent case, resection of the involved segment is all that is required; there is no place for extensive and unnecessary dissections that open up tissue planes to infection and increase blood loss.

It is an important surgical principle to avoid a primary anastomosis in the urgent situation, because anastomotic breakdown can almost be assured. Adverse factors in this situation include an elderly patient, sepsis or hemodynamic instability, an unprepped colon, local contamination, friable tissues, malnutrition, steroids, and poor anastomotic blood supply, to cite only a few. In the absence of these, and if all other factors are favorable, a one-stage resection (primary anastomosis without colostomy) may be considered (Fig. 83-10).[101,102] A two-stage resection is a more conservative

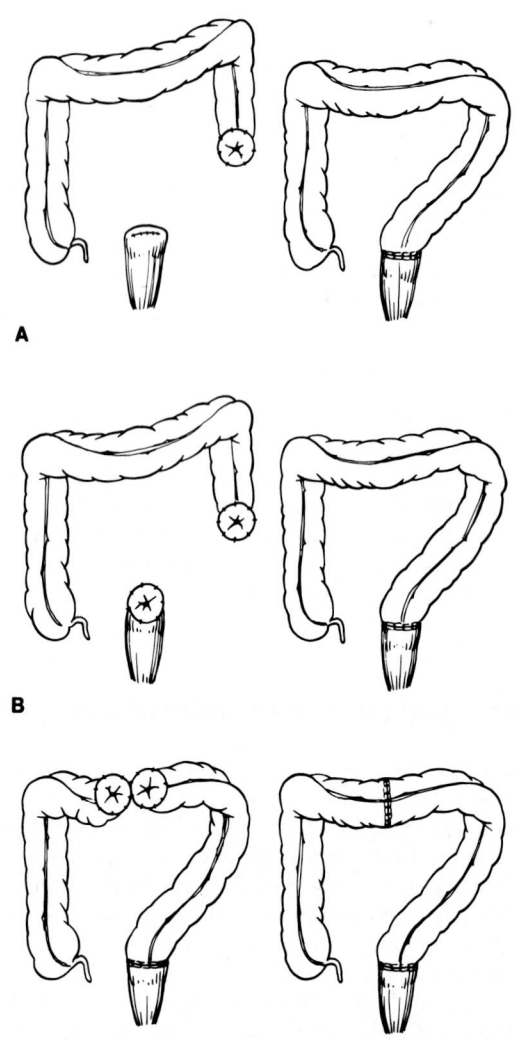

FIGURE 83-11. Two-stage approaches to resection of diverticular disease. Common among the approaches is that the offending segment of diverticular disease is resected at the first operation. (**A**) Stage one: the Hartman operation: diseased sigmoid colon is removed, the fecal stream is diverted, and the rectum is oversewn. Stage two: Intestinal continuity is reestablished by a descending colorectostomy. (**B**) Stage one: diseased sigmoid is removed, and both ends of bowel are brought to the surface as stomas. In stage two, intestinal continuity is reestablished as in **A**. (**C**) Stage one: diseased sigmoid colon is resected, and a colorectostomy is constructed and protected by a diverting transverse colostomy. Stage two is closure of the transverse colostomy.

option. This involves exteriorizing of the proximal colon (colostomy) and resection of the involved segment.[26,82,103–105] (Fig. 83-11). The colostomy is closed electively in 3 months after the patient is fully recovered.

Formerly, a three-stage approach, consisting of proximal colostomy and drainage, resection, and colostomy closure, was recommended for free perforation and suppurative or feculent peritonitis (Fig. 83-12). However, two-stage resections carry lower morbidity and mortality rates.[106,107] Nagorney and colleagues reported a mortality of 26% with the three-stage procedure and 7% percent with two-stage resection.[107]

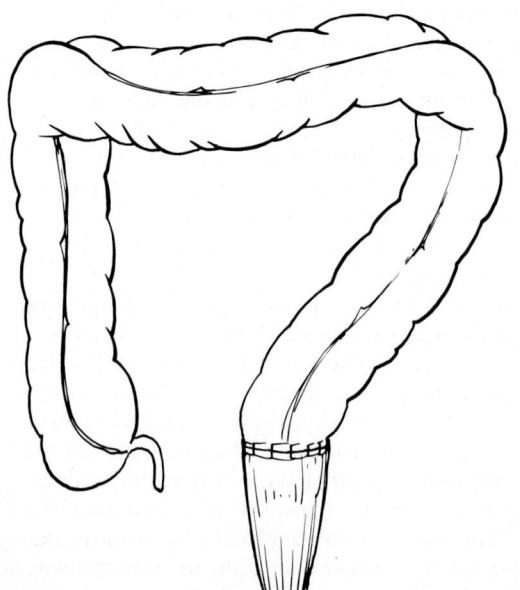

FIGURE 83-10. One-stage resection and anastomosis for uncomplicated diverticular disease.

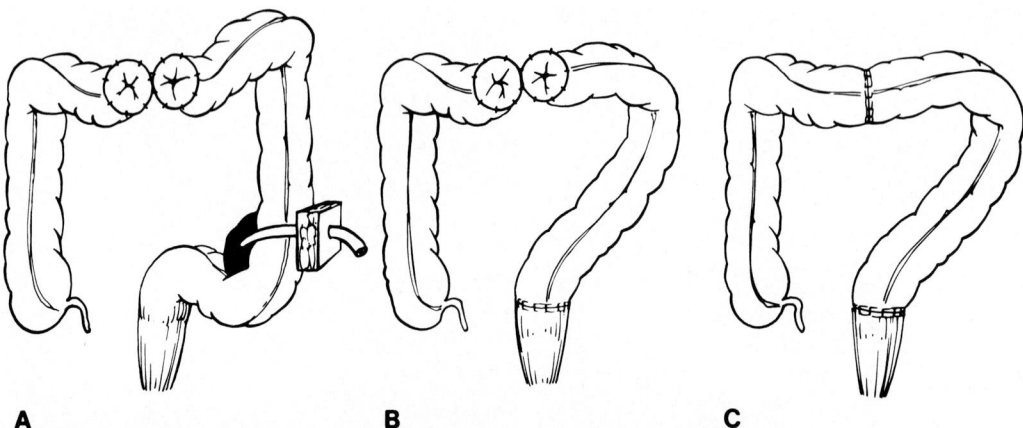

FIGURE 83-12. Three-stage resection of diverticular disease. (**A**) Diverticular abscess is drained, and the fecal stream is diverted by a double-barreled colostomy (stage one). (**B**) Sigmoid diverticular disease and abscess are resected, and a colorectostomy is constructed (stage two). (**C**) The colostomy is closed, and intestinal continuity is restored (stage three).

The authors hypothesized that removal of the septic process and elimination of the need for a second procedure may be two reasons for the lower mortality.

Diverticulitis with abscess formation but without perforation has traditionally been resected using a two-stage approach. These abscesses have been treated successfully with initial percutaneous abscess drainage under CT guidance (Fig. 83-13).[108] After the sepsis subsides, mechanical colon preparation and a one-stage resection are possible. Usually, the definitive operation is performed during the same hospitalization. A recent study by Stabile and colleagues[76] reported successful percutaneous drainage of diverticular abscess in 84% of patients, with subsequent elective resection and primary anastomosis. The following criteria must be met, before consideration is given to percutaneous drainage and single-stage resection: the patient must be stable and without signs of persistent sepsis; the abscess must be approachable by a direct route, avoiding vascular structures and other noninvolved organs; the abscess should be nonloculated and filled with fluid material. If percutaneous drainage fails to control sepsis, definitive surgery should not be postponed unnecessarily.

Fistula secondary to diverticulitis almost always mandates operative resection. A one-stage elective resection and anastomosis is feasible in most patients if the colon can be mechanically prepared and local sepsis controlled. Otherwise, in more urgent cases, multiple-staged treatment may be warranted. In medically unfit patients with stable colovesical fistulas from diverticulitis, observation without operation may be a reasonable course.[94]

Obstruction from acute diverticulitis necessitates urgent two-stage surgical treatment. However, if medical management relieves the obstruction, mechanical preparation of the bowel may be possible and one-stage resection performed. Mechanical cleansing of the colon intraoperatively, followed by primary resection and anastomosis, has been reported,[109] but its popularity is limited. Infrequently, endoscopic and imaging techniques cannot distinguish carcinoma from a diverticular mass. If a mass persists after medical management and carcinoma cannot be excluded, resection is indicated.

Because morbidity and mortality increase with each subsequent episode of diverticulitis, these patients are candidates for elective resection. A more aggressive approach is warranted after the first attack in younger people; because of the greater likelihood of recurrence,[110,111] these patients should undergo resection after the first episode.

Elective and urgent surgical management carry mortality rates of 1% to 4% and 5% to 15%, respectively. Recurrent diverticulitis occurs in 30% of patients after successful medical management. Recurrent diverticulitis after surgical resection is infrequent, in the range of 5% to 10%. Investigations indicate that in order to prevent recurrence, resection of all diverticula-bearing colon is not important.[112] However, if distal sigmoid colon remains, the chance of recurrence is significantly increased.[111,113,114] Benn and associates[113] found a recurrence rate of 12.5% if any distal sigmoid colon remained, but 6.7% if none did. Therefore, resection of the entire distal sigmoid colon and anastomosis to the rectum is the procedure of choice.

COMPLICATED DIVERTICULAR DISEASE: DIVERTICULAR HEMORRHAGE

Clinical Manifestations

Painless rectal bleeding associated with diverticulosis is reported in up to 47% of patients.[80] Many of these patients have minor bleeding, but massive bleeding from diverticula occurs in about 5%[115] Passage of large amounts of bright blood per rectum with signs of hypovolemic shock (hypotension, tachycardia, and syncope) are the usual clinical manifestations. Spontaneous cessation of hemorrhage, however, is common.

Differential Diagnosis

Any gastrointestinal lesion that has the potential for massive hemorrhage, such as duodenal ulcer or Meckel's diverticulum, can present in a manner similar to diverticular bleeding. Because bright red bleeding per rectum indicates rapid loss of blood, the signs of hemorrhagic shock are usually present.

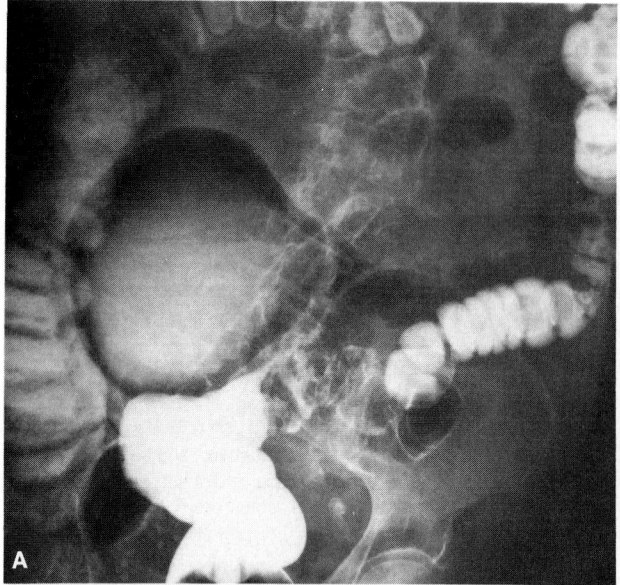

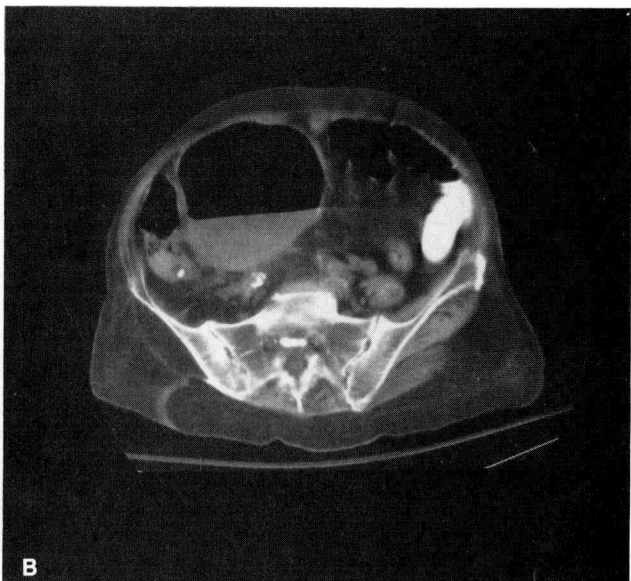

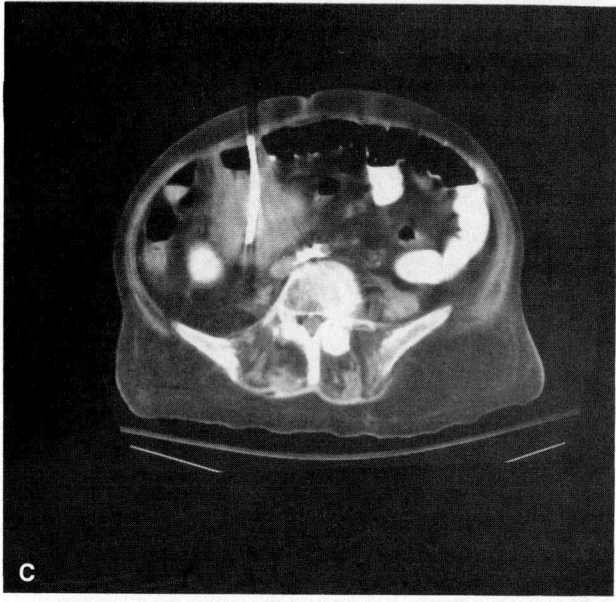

FIGURE 83-13. Nonoperative management of a diverticular abscess. **(A)** Appearance of a large diverticular abscess on barium enema study. The abscess is full of air, and barium is seen escaping into it from the sigmoid colon. **(B)** Computed tomographic scan appearance of the abscess. **(C)** A large-bore drainage catheter has been percutaneously placed into the abscess by computed tomographic guidance. The patient defervesced, and an elective resection was performed subsequently.

These physical findings, the patient's history, and the character of the nasogastric aspirate, along with the judicious use of esophagogastroduodenoscopy, small bowel contrast studies, arteriography, and nuclear scans can confirm or rule out an upper gastrointestinal source of bleeding.

Angiodysplasias and Other Causes of Lower Gastrointestinal Hemorrhage

Vascular ectasias (angiodysplasia, arteriovenous malformation, vascular malformation, telangiectasia, and angioma) are acquired lesions that most often occur in the cecum and ascending colon in elderly persons. As with colonic diverticula, the true prevalence of vascular ectasias and the frequency with which they bleed are not well documented. It is only in the past 30 years that vascular ectasia has been identified as a common cause of lower gastrointestinal bleeding.[116] In series reviewing experience with lower gastrointestinal bleeding, vascular ectasia and diverticulosis have been the most frequent

sources, causing hemorrhage in approximately equal numbers of patients.[116,117] In contrast to the bleeding in diverticulosis (which is almost always massive), the bleeding from vascular ectasia can range from occult to torrential. Although colonoscopy and nuclear scans are helpful, selective mesenteric angiography during active bleeding best differentiates ectasia from diverticular disease.[117]

Rarely, anorectal lesions, usually hemorrhoids, bleed heavily. The diagnosis would seem to be obvious; however, an invasive, time-consuming, and expensive radiographic and endoscopic work-up can be avoided if anoscopy is performed early in the patient's evaluation.

Diagnostic Studies

Colonoscopy

The means of localizing the site of colonic hemorrhage depend primarily on the extent of the bleed. Slow, intermittent bleeds are best approached endoscopically, whereas torrential bleeds

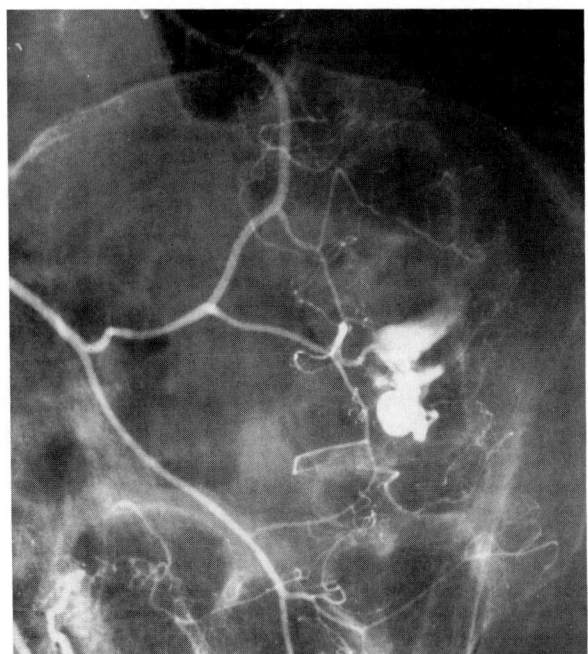

FIGURE 83-14. Arteriogram in a patient with diverticular bleeding illustrates extravasation of contrast medium from a diverticular bleeding source into the lumen of the descending colon.

often obscure the view through the colonoscope, necessitating scintigraphic or angiographic localization. Emphasis has recently been placed on accurate endoscopic localization of the site of the colonic bleed, even in the face of substantial bleeding. These methods include colonoscopy and high-flux irri-

gation, or intraoperative colonoscopy and antegrade colonic lavage through a surgical cecostomy. These modalities enable a limited resection of the appropriate segment, with little chance of rebleed. This compares with a 60% rebleed rate associated with blind subtotal colectomy.[118]

Angiography

The principal use of selective mesenteric angiography is in patients with massive hemorrhage from diverticulosis. The procedure is highly sensitive if performed during major bleeds (i.e., >0.5 mL of blood per minute). Extravasation of angiographic contrast media in a diverticulum is the diagnostic radiographic finding (Fig. 83-14) and is distinctly different from the features seen with colonic bleeding caused by vascular ectasia—dilated, slowly emptying, submucosal veins, vascular tufts, and early filling submucosal veins.[116]

The principal value of arteriography is its ability to locate the site of hemorrhage and to serve as a conduit for infusion of vasopressin to halt the bleeding (Fig. 83-15). The angio-catheter may also be used to embolize isolated bleeding sites in patients considered unfit for surgery, although this risks infarction of the bowel. Elective resection of the segment of colon from which the bleeding has occurred has a much lower rate of morbidity than emergency total abdominal colectomy.[24]

Nuclear Scans

Scintigraphic studies with technetium 99m sulfur colloid and ^{99m}Tc-tagged red blood cells are used in conjunction with angiography in the evaluation of lower gastrointestinal bleed-

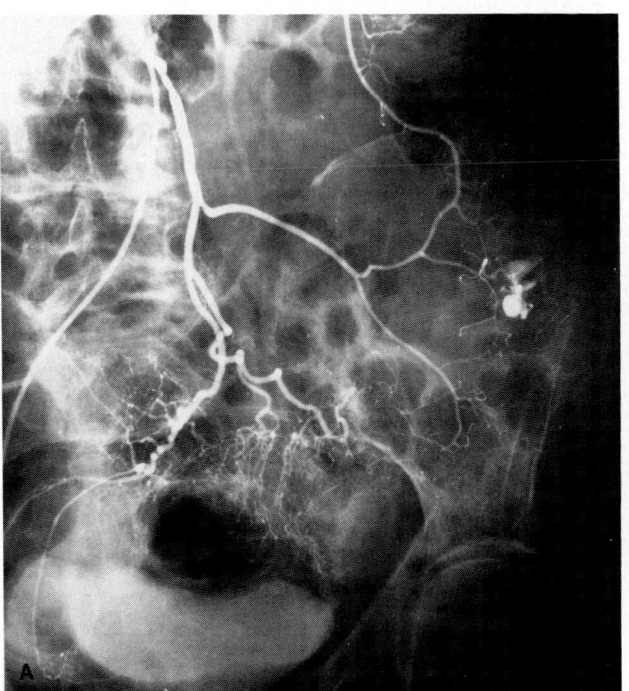
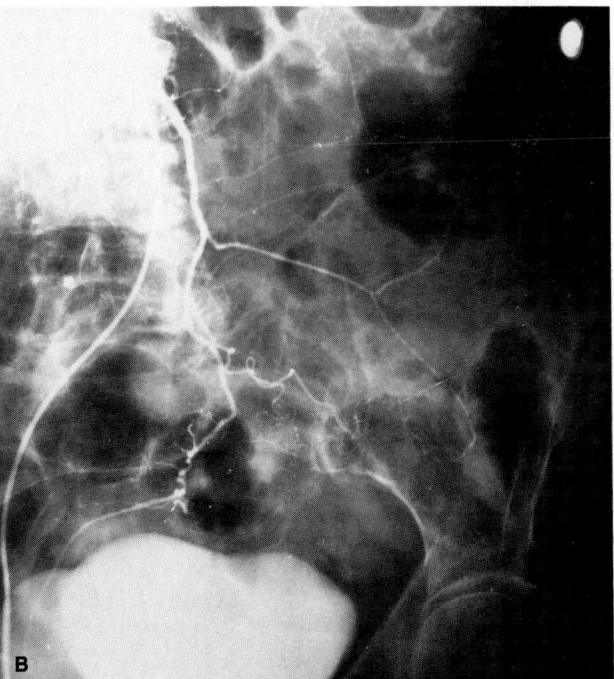

FIGURE 83-15. (**A**) Arteriogram of the same patient as in Figure 82-14, before infusion of vaso-pressin. (**B**) Arteriogram of the same patient after vasopressin was infused. Note the markedly reduced flow in the left colonic and sigmoidal branches of the inferior mesenteric artery.

ing. No scintigraphic findings are specific for diverticular bleeding. However, the ^{99m}Tc sulfur colloid scan is capable of detecting bleeding that is as slow as 0.1 mL/minute. One drawback is that uptake of the colloid by the liver may obscure a bleeding site. The technetium-tagged red cell study is particularly helpful in patients with intermittent bleeding because the red cells are not cleared from the circulation as rapidly as is the sulfur colloid. A profound disadvantage of the red cell study is that background counts often obscure the precise location of the site of hemorrhage.[115,119] Such studies, therefore, cannot be relied on to plan operative strategy. Their usefulness is controversial, but they are frequently used to confirm the presence of active bleeding before a more definitive, but invasive, mesenteric arteriography.

Clinical Course and Complications

Hemorrhage from diverticular disease originates from an arterial source (vasa recta) at an asymmetric part of the diverticulum. Bleeding, as in diverticulitis, usually arises from one diverticulum. The pathophysiology of the bleeding is uncertain, but it has been suggested that traumatic factors within the diverticulum or the colon lumen induce intimal proliferation, scarring, and rupture of the vasa recta. In histologic studies, most cases of bleeding show no associated inflammation in the bleeding diverticulum.[120]

Massive bleeding occurs in about 5% of all patients with diverticulosis.[63] The hemorrhage is usually massive and often necessitates transfusion. Spontaneous cessation of bleeding occurs in about 80% of patients. Recurrence of the bleeding after one episode occurs in about 20% of patients. Of those with recurrent diverticular bleeding, the chance of a second recurrence is at least 50%.[121]

The complications of diverticular hemorrhage are related to hypovolemia and circulatory collapse. Early on, diverticular bleeding is often insidious and thus dangerous. The colon may fill with large amounts of blood before being passed per rectum. In the elderly patient with massive bleeding, the tolerance for even transient hypovolemia may be limited. The major organs sensitive to ischemia (i.e., heart, brain, kidneys, and lungs) are at risk for temporary or permanent injury with each bleeding episode.

Treatment

The evaluation and treatment of diverticular bleeding are interrelated. Circulating volume should be restored and hemoglobin and coagulation studies checked. Proctoscopy to rule out anal or rectal bleeding should also be part of the initial management.

Minor bleeds (<2 units transfused) with spontaneous cessation of hemorrhage occur commonly and are best followed by abbreviated colon purgation to remove clot, followed by colonoscopy.[26] If the colonoscopy is negative and bleeding does not recur, a repeat colonoscopy or a barium enema is the next test.

Persistent bleeds (2–4 units transfused) merit angiographic or scintigraphic studies.[84] The order in which these tests should be performed is controversial. However, three-vessel angiog-

raphy is the study most likely to determine the exact site and source of the bleeding. Should a source of active bleeding be identified, angiography facilitates selective infusion of vasopressin to the site (see Fig. 82-15). This may buy time during which the patient may be resuscitated and the responsible segment resected on a semielective basis.[115,122]

The source of major colonic bleeds (>4 units transfused) should be evaluated first using angiography or nuclear scan. If these studies are inconclusive, colonoscopy with high flux irrigation or antegrade colonic irrigation may localize the bleed. Failure to visualize the bleeding site forces the surgeon to perform blind (total abdominal) colectomy.[115,118]

In summary, in the management of bleeding diverticular disease, several points should be emphasized. First, colonoscopy should be performed initially if bleeding has ceased, but, conversely, angiography should be performed initially if bleeding persists. Second, a barium enema should never be the initial test in patients with diverticular bleeding because it precludes angiography or colonoscopy until the contrast medium is purged. Third, newer techniques such as intraoperative panendoscopy and intraoperative angiography for localization of the indeterminate bleeding site are still under evaluation.[118,123] Finally, angiographic embolization frequently controls colonic bleeding but a major complication, ischemic colitis, can occur.[122] The prognosis of diverticular bleeding is generally good. Most bleeding stops spontaneously and does not recur. If surgery is necessary, segmental colectomy carries a 9% mortality rate.[115]

The reader is directed to Chapter 10, Motility of the Large Intestine; Chapter 30, Approach to the Patient With Gross Gastrointestinal Bleeding; Chapter 31, Approach to the Patient With Occult Gastrointestinal Bleeding; Chapter 34, Approach to the Patient With Abdominal Pain; Chapter 36, Approach to the Patient With Acute Abdomen; Chapter 37, Approach to the Patient With Ileus and Obstruction; Chapter 39, Approach to the Patient With Constipation; Chapter 78, Colon: Anatomy and Structural Anomalies; Chapter 79, Inflammatory Bowel Disease; Chapter 80, Miscellaneous Inflammatory and Structural Disorders of the Colon; Chapter 81, Irritable Bowel Syndrome; Chapter 82, Motility Disorders of the Colon; Chapter 87, Malignant Tumors of the Colon; Chapter 112, Mesenteric Vascular Insufficiency; Chapter 116, Colonoscopy and Flexible Sigmoidoscopy; Chapter 119, Contrast Radiology; and Chapter 127, Angiography.

REFERENCES

1. Painter NS, Burkitt DP. Diverticular disease of the colon: a deficiency disease of western civilization. Br Med J 1971;2:450.
2. Horner JL. Natural history of diverticulosis of the colon. Am J Dig Dis 1958;3:343.
3. Hughes LE. Postmortem survey of diverticular disease of the colon. Gut 1969;10:336.
4. Connell AM. Pathogenesis of diverticular disease of the colon. Adv Intern Med 1977;22:377.
5. Parks TG. Natural history of diverticular disease of the colon. Clin Gastroenterol 1975;4:53.
6. Almy TP, Howell DA. Diverticular disease of the colon. N Engl J Med 1980;302:324.
7. Mayo WJ. Diverticula of the sigmoid. Ann Surg 1930;92:739.
8. Ochsner HC, Bargen JA. Diverticulosis of the large intestine;

an evaluation of historical and personal observations. Ann Intern Med 1935;9:282.

9. Rankin FW, Brown PW. Diverticulitis of the colon. Surg Gynecol Obstet 1930;50:836.

10. Kocour EJ. Diverticulosis of the colon: its incidence in 7000 consecutive autopsies with reference to its complications. Am J Surg 1937;37:433.

11. Smith CC, Christensen WR. The incidence of colonic diverticulosis. AJR Am J Roentgenol 1959;82:996.

12. Eggers C. Acute diverticulitis and sigmoiditis. Ann Surg 1941;113:15.

13. Spriggs EI, Marxer OA. Intestinal diverticula. Q J Med 1925;19:1.

14. Manousos ON, Truelove SC, Lumsden K. Prevalence of colonic diverticulosis in general population of Oxford area. Br Med J 1967;3:762.

15. Parks TG. Post-mortem studies on the colon with special reference to diverticular disease. Proc R Soc Med 1968;61:932.

16. Edwards HC. Diverticulosis and diverticulitis of the intestine. Postgrad Med J 1953;29:20.

17. Cleland JB. Incidence of diverticulosis. Br Med J 1968;1:579.

18. Manousos ON, Vrachliotis G, Papaevangelon G, et al. Relation of diverticulosis of the colon to environmental factors in Greece. Am J Dig Dis 1973;18:174.

19. Sim GPG, Scobie BA. Large bowel diseases in New Zealand based on 1118 air contrast enemas. N Z Med J 1982;95:611.

20. Bremner CG, Ackerman LV. Polyps and carcinoma of the large bowel in the South African Bantu. Cancer 1970;26:991.

21. Kyle J, Adesola AO, Tinckler LF, de Beaux J. Incidence of diverticulitis. Scand J Gastroenterol 1967;2:77.

22. Kim EH. Hiatus hernia and diverticulum of the colon: their low incidence in Korea. N Engl J Med 1964;271:764.

23. Sugihara K, Muto T, Morioka Y, Asano A, Yamamoto T. Diverticular disease of the colon in Japan: a review of 615 cases. Dis Colon Rectum 1984;27:531.

24. Brodribb AJM, Humphreys DM. Diverticular disease: three studies. Part 1—Relation to other disorders and fibre intake. Br Med J 1976;1:424.

25. Gear JSS, Fursdon P, Nolan DJ, et al. Symptomless diverticular disease and intake of dietary fibre. Lancet 1979;1:511.

26. Mendeloff AI. A critique of "fiber deficiency." Am J Dig Dis 1976;21:109.

27. Parks TG. Natural history of diverticular disease of the colon. A review of 521 cases. Br Med J 1969;4:639.

28. Kubo A, Ishiwata J, Maeda Y, et al. Clinical studies on diverticular disease of the colon. Jpn J Med 1983;22:185.

29. Vajrabukka T, Saksornchai K, Jimakorn P. Diverticular disease of the colon in a far-eastern community. Dis Colon Rectum 1980;23:151.

30. Graser E. Das Falsche darm Divertikel. Arch Klin Chir 1899;59:638.

31. Drummond H. Sacculi of the large intestine, with special reference to their relations to the blood-vessels of the bowel wall. Br J Surg 1916;4:407.

32. Meyers MA, Volberg F, Katzen B, et al. The angioarchitecture of colonic diverticula: significance in bleeding diverticulosis. Radiology 1973;108:249.

33. Gallagher JJ, Welch JP. Giant diverticula of the sigmoid colon: a review of differential diagnosis and operative management. Arch Surg 1979;114:1079.

34. Walstad PM, Sahibzada AR. Diverticula of the rectum. Am J Surg 1968;116:937.

35. Chiu TCT, Bailey HR, Hernandez AJ Jr. Diverticulitis of the midrectum. Dis Colon Rectum 1983;26:59.

36. Giffin HZ. Diverticulitis of the rectum: a report of two cases operated upon, one of them with carcinomatous degeneration. Ann Surg 1911;53:533.

37. Collins DC. A study of 50,000 specimens of the human vermiform appendix. Surg Gynecol Obstet 1955;101:437.

38. Delikaris P, Teglbjaerg PS, Fisker-Sorensen P, Balslev I. Diverticula of the vermiform appendix: alternatives of clinical presentation and significance. Dis Colon Rectum 1983;26:374.

39. Buffo GC, Clair MR, Bonheim P. Diverticulosis of the vermiform appendix. Gastrointest Radiol 1986;11:108.

40. Fleischner FG. Diverticular disease of the colon: new observations and revised concepts. Gastroenterology 1971;60:316.

41. Watters DAK, Smith AN. Strength of the colon wall in diverticular disease. Br J Surg 1990;77:257.

42. Eastwood MA, Watters DAK, Smith AN. Diverticular disease—is it a motility disorder? Clin Gastroenterol 1982;11:545.

43. Keith A. Diverticula of the alimentary tract of congenital or of obscure origin. Br Med J 1910;1:376.

44. Edwards HC. Diverticula of the colon and vermiform appendix. Lancet 1934;1:221.

45. Weinreich J, Andersen D. Intraluminal pressure in the sigmoid colon. II. Patients with sigmoid diverticula and related conditions. Scand J Gastroenterol 1976;11:581.

46. Arfwidsson S. Pathogenesis of multiple diverticula of the sigmoid colon in diverticular disease. Acta Chir Scand 1964[ppl 342:1.

47. Painter NS, Truelove SC. The intraluminal pressure patterns in diverticulosis of the colon. Gut 1964;5:201.

48. Painter NS, Truelove SC, Ardran GM, Tuckey M. Effect of morphine, prostigmine, pethidine, and probanthine on the human colon in diverticulosis studied by intraluminal pressure recording and cineradiography. Gut 1965;65:57.

49. Srivastava GS, Smith AN, Painter NS. Sterculia bulk-forming agent with smooth-muscle relaxant versus bran in diverticular disease. Br Med J 1976;1:315.

50. Taylor I, Duthie HL. Bran tablets and diverticular disease. Br Med J 1976;1:988.

51. Snape WJ Jr, Carlson GM, Cohen S. Colonic myoelectric activity in the irritable bowel syndrome. Gastroenterology 1976;70:326.

52. Painter NS. The aetiology of diverticulosis of the colon with special reference to the action of certain drugs on the behaviour of the colon. Ann R Coll Surg Engl 1964;34:98.

53. Carlson AJ, Hoelzel F. Relation of diet to diverticulosis of the colon in rats. Gastroenterology 1949;12:108.

54. Hodgson WJB. An interim report on the production of colonic diverticula in the rabbit. Gut 1972;13:802.

55. Thompson WG. Do colonic diverticula cause symptoms? (editorial) Am J Gastroenterol 1986;81:613.

56. Otte JJ, Larsen L, Andersen JR. Irritable bowel syndrome and Cheskin LJ, Bohlman M, Schuster MM. Diverticular disease in the elderly. Gastroenterol Clin North Am 1990;19(2):391.

57. Schnyder P, Moss AA, Thoeni RF, Margulis AR. A double-blind study of radiologic accuracy in diverticulitis, diverticulosis, and carcinoma of the sigmoid colon. J Clin Gastroenterol 1979;1:55.

58. Boulos PB, Cowin AP, Karamanolis DG, Clark CG. Diverticula, neoplasia, or both? Early detection of carcinoma in sigmoid diverticular disease. Ann Surg 1985;202:607.

59. Freeny PC, Walker JH. Inverted diverticula of the gastrointestinal tract. Gastrointest Radiol 1979;4:57.

60. Schuman BM. Endoscopic diverticulectomy in the sigmoid colon. Gastrointest Endosc 1982;28:189.

61. Lappas JC, Maglinte DD, Kopecky KK, et al. Diverticular disease: imaging with post-double-contrast sigmoid flush. Radiology 1988;168:35.

62. Ribchester JM, Ward A. Solitary diverticulum of transverse colon masquerading as polyp. Br Med J 1978;2:665.

63. Knight CD. Massive hemorrhage from diverticular disease of the colon. Surgery 1957;42:853.

64. Brodribb AJM. Treatment of symptomatic diverticular disease with a high-fibre diet. Lancet 1977;1:664.

65. Leahy AL, Ellis RM, Quill DS, Peel ALG. High fibre diet in symptomatic diverticular disease of the colon. Ann R Coll Surg Engl 1985;67:173.

66. Hyland JMP, Taylor I. Does a high fibre diet prevent the complications of diverticular disease? Br J Surg 1980;67:77.

67. Doringer E. Computerized tomography of colonic diverticulitis. Crit Rev Diagn Imaging 1992;33:421.

68. Klein S, Mayer L, Present DH, et al. Extraintestinal manifestations in patients with diverticulitis. Ann Intern Med 1988;108:700.

69. Schmidt GT, Lennard-Jones JE, Morson BC, Young AC.

Crohn's disease of the colon and its distinction from diverticulitis. Gut 1968;9:7.

70. Marshak RH, Eliasoph J. Inflammatory lesions of the small bowel secondary to colonic diverticulitis. Am J Dig Dis 1961;6: 423.

71. Frager D, Wolf EL, Frager JD, Beneventano TC. Small intestinal complications of diverticulitis of the sigmoid colon. JAMA 1986;256:3258.

72. Balz FF. Diverticulitis as a diagnostic problem in gynecology. Am J Obstet Gynecol 1968;101:372.

73. Ertan A. Colonic diverticulitis. Recognizing and managing its presentations and complications. Postgrad Med 1990;88:67.

74. Johnson CD, Baker ME, Rice RP, et al. Diagnosis of acute colonic diverticulitis: comparison of barium enema and CT. AJR Am J Roentgenol 1987;148:541.

75. Hulnick DH, Megibow AJ, Balthazar EJ, et al. Computed tomography in the evaluation of diverticulitis. Radiology 1984;152: 491.

76. Stabile BA, Puccio E, vanSonnenberg E. Preoperative percutaneous drainage of diverticular abscess. Am J Surg 1990;159: 99.

77. Crist DW, Fishman EK, Scatarige JC, Cameron JL. Acute diverticulitis of the cecum and ascending colon diagnosed by computed tomography. Surg Gynecol Obstet 1988;166:99.

78. Fields SI, Haskell L, Libson E. CT appearance of giant colonic diverticulum. Gastrointest Radiol 1987;12:71.

79. Parulekar SG. Sonography of colonic diverticulitis. J Ultrasound Med 1985;4:659.

80. Machan L, Pon MS, Wood BJ, Wong AD. The "coffee bean" sign in periappendiceal and peridiverticular abscess. J Ultrasound Med 1987;6:373.

81. Morson BC. The muscle abnormality in diverticular disease of the sigmoid colon. Br J Radiol 1963;36:385.

82. Hinchey EJ, Schaal PGH, Richards GK. Treatment of perforated diverticular disease of the colon. Adv Surg 1978;12:85.

83. Hughes ESR, Cuthbertson AM, Carden ABG. The surgical management of acute diverticulitis. Med J Aust 1963;1:780.

84. Canter JW, Shorb PE Jr. Acute perforation of colonic diverticula associated with prolonged adrenocorticosteroid therapy. Am J Surg 1971;121:46.

85. Steriofff S, Orringer MB, Cameron JL. Colon perforations associated with steroid therapy. Surgery 1974;75:56.

86. ReMine SG, McIlrath DC. Bowel perforation in steroid-treated patients. Ann Surg 1980;192:581.

87. Starnes HF Jr, Lazarus JM, Vineyard G. Surgery for diverticulitis in renal failure. Dis Colon Rectum 1985;28:827.

88. Lao A, Bach D. Colonic complications in renal transplant recipients. Dis Colon Rectum 1988;31:130.

89. Church JM, Fazio VW, Braun WE, et al. Perforation of the colon in renal homograft recipients: a report of 11 cases and a review of the literature. Ann Surg 1986;203:69.

90. Corder A. Steroids, non-steroidal anti-inflammatory drugs, and serious septic complications of diverticular disease. Br Med J 1987;295:1238.

91. Langman MJS, Morgan L, Worrall A. Use of anti-inflammatory drugs by patients admitted with small or large bowel perforations and haemorrhage. Br Med J 1985;290:347.

92. Perkins JD, Shield CF III, Chang FC, Farha GJ. Acute diverticulitis: comparison of treatment in immunocompromised and nonimmunocompromised patients. Am J Surg 1984;148:745.

93. Woods RJ, Lavery IC, Fazio VW, Jagelman DG, Weakley FL. Internal fistulas in diverticular disease. Dis Colon Rectum 1988;31:591.

94. Amin M, Nallinger R, Polk HC Jr. Conservative treatment of selected patients with colovesical fistula due to diverticulitis. Surg Gynecol Obstet 1984;159:442.

95. Ravo B, Khan SA, Ger R, et al. Unusual extraperitoneal presentations of diverticulitis. Am J Gastroenterol 1985;80:346.

96. Van Hillo M, Fazio VW, Lavery IC. Sigmoidoappendiceal fistula—an unusual complication of diverticulitis: report of a case. Dis Colon Rectum 1984;27:618.

97. Libson E, Bloom RA, Verstandig A, et al. Sigmoid-appendiceal fistula in diverticular disease. Diagn Imag Clin Med 1984;53: 262.

98. Ney C, Cruz FS Jr, Carvajal S, et al. Ureteral involvement secondary to diverticulitis of the colon. Surg Gynecol Obstet 1986;163:215.

99. Jensen JA, Tsang D, Minnis JF, et al. Pneumo-pylephlebitis and intramesocolic diverticular perforation. Am J Surg 1985;150: 284.

100. Sonnenshein MA, Cone LA, Alexander RM. Diverticulitis with colovenous fistula and portal venous gas: report of two cases. J Clin Gastroenterol 1986;8:195.

101. Madden JL. Primary resection in the treatment of acute perforations of the colon with abscess or diffuse peritonitis. In: Delaney JP, Varco RL, eds. Controversies in Surgery II. Philadelphia: WB Saunders, 1983:349.

102. Ravo B, Mishrick A, Addei K, et al. The treatment of perforated diverticulitis by one-stage intracolonic bypass procedure. Surgery 1987;102:771.

103. Chappuis CW, Cohn I Jr. Acute colonic diverticulitis. Surg Clin North Am 1988;68:301.

104. Rodkey GV, Welch CE. Changing patterns in the surgical treatment of diverticular disease. Ann Surg 1984;200:466.

105. Hackford AW, Veidenheimer MC. Diverticular disease of the colon: current concepts and management. Surg Clin North Am 1985;65:347.

106. Greif JM, Fried G, McSherry CK. Surgical treatment of perforated diverticulitis of the sigmoid colon. Dis Colon Rectum 1980;23:483.

107. Nagorney DM, Adson MA, Pemberton JH. Sigmoid diverticulitis with perforation and generalized peritonitis. Dis Colon Rectum 1985;28:71.

108. Mueller PR, Saini S, Wittenburg J, et al. Sigmoid diverticular abscesses: percutaneous drainage as an adjunct to surgical resection in 24 cases. Radiology 1987;164:321.

109. Saadia R, Schein M. The place of intraoperative antegrade colonic irrigation in emergency left-sided colonic surgery. Dis Colon Rectum 1989;32:78.

110. Freischlag J, Bennion RS, Thompson JE Jr. Complications of diverticular disease of the colon in young people. Dis Colon Rectum 1986;29:639.

111. Church JM. Surgical treatment of sigmoid diverticulitis. Schweiz Med Wochenschr 1991;121:744.

112. Wolff BG, Ready RL, MacCarty RL, et al. Influence of sigmoid resection on progression of diverticular disease of the colon. Dis Colon Rectum 1984;27:645.

113. Benn PL, Wolff BG, Ilstrup DM. Level of anastomosis and recurrent colonic diverticulitis. Am J Surg 1986;151:269.

114. Fowler C, Aaland M, Johnson L, Sternquist J. Perforated diverticulitis in a Hartmann rectal pouch. Dis Colon Rectum 1986;29:662.

115. Browder W, Cerise EJ, Litwin MS. Impact of emergency angiography in massive lower gastrointestinal bleeding. Ann Surg 1986;204:530.

116. Boley SJ, Brandt LJ. Vascular ectasias of the colon—1986. Dig Dis Sci 1986(Suppl)31:26.

117. Welch CE, Athanasoulis CA, Galdabini JJ. Hemorrhage from the large bowel with special reference to angiodysplasia and diverticular disease. World J Surg 1978;2:73.

118. Berry AR, Campbell WB, Kettlewell RG. Management of major colonic hemorrhage. Br J Surg 1988;75:637.

119. Simpson AJ, Previti FW. Technetium sulfur colloid scintigraphy in the detection of lower gastrointestinal tract bleeding. Surg Gynecol Obstet 1982;155:33.

120. Meyers MA, Alonso DR, Baer JW. Pathogenesis of massively bleeding colonic diverticulosis: new observations. AJR Am J Roentgenol 1976;127:901.

121. McGuire HH Jr, Haynes BW Jr. Massive hemorrhage from diverticulosis of the colon: guidelines for therapy based on bleeding patterns observed in fifty cases. Ann Surg 1972;175: 847.

122. Kadir S, Ernst CB. Current concepts in angiographic management of gastrointestinal bleeding. Curr Probl Surg 1983;20: 281.

123. Robertson HD, Gathright JB Jr. The technique of intraoperative segmental artery arteriography to localize vascular ectasias. Dis Colon Rectum 1985;28:274.

Textbook of Gastroenterology, second edition, edited by Tadataka Yamada. JB Lippincott Company, Philadelphia © 1995.

CHAPTER 84

Bacterial Infections of the Colon

J. Thomas LaMont

The large intestine is the primary target of five important bacterial pathogens: *Shigella* species, *Campylobacter* species, enterohemorrhagic and enteroinvasive *Escherichia coli*, and *Clostridium difficile*. The first three produce an acute diarrheal syndrome, "bacillary dysentery," characterized by abdominal cramps and bloody, mucoid diarrhea. *C difficile* is the causative agent of an increasingly common condition, antibiotic-associated colitis. In addition to these three major pathogens, the rectum and anus may be infected by *Chlamydia trachomatis, Neisseria gonorrhoeae, Treponema pallidum, Entamoeba histolytica*, and herpes simplex virus (HSV). Infection with one or more of these organisms by sexual transmission in homosexual men causes an acute proctitis with pain, rectal discharge, and bleeding, the gay bowel syndrome. This chapter focuses on the pathophysiology, diagnosis, and treatment of acute infectious colitis and the gay bowel syndrome. Infections of the small intestine with bacteria and enteric viruses are discussed in Chapter 70.

Acute infectious colitis produces a different clinical picture than infection of the small intestine. The signs and symptoms listed in Table 84-1 may help the physician determine the location of the infection. These features are not absolute, and considerable overlap occurs. Small-volume diarrhea (<1 L/day) usually indicates colonic infection; large-volume diarrhea (>1 L/day) is more likely to result from small intestinal infection. Pain in the lower abdomen and tenesmus are indicative of bacterial colitis, in contrast to the crampy, central abdominal pain of small intestinal infection. Colonic infections produce acute inflammatory changes that can be visualized by sigmoidoscopy or colonoscopy.

The gross and microscopic appearance of the stool also may provide clues to the presence of infectious colitis. Grossly bloody stools or bloody mucus in patients with acute dysentery indicate the likely presence of bacterial or amebic colitis, because these symptoms are rare in viral or bacterial infections of the small intestine. In one multicenter study in the United States, a history of grossly bloody stool was highly correlated with the finding of *Campylobacter jejuni* by culture. In field studies, the presence of fecal leukocytes and blood in patients with acute diarrhea is highly correlated with a positive stool culture for either *Campylobacter, Salmonella,* or *Shigella* species.[1,2] Fecal leukocytes are also found in ulcerative colitis, Crohn's colitis, and amebic colitis, but these conditions usually are subacute or chronic in nature compared to acute ba-

TABLE 84-1
Comparative Features of Small Intestine Versus Colonic Infection

FEATURES	SMALL INTESTINE	COLON
Location of pain	Diffuse or periumbilical	Lower abdomen
Tenesmus	Absent	Present
Stool volume	>1 L/day	<1 L/day
Type of stool	Watery	Mucoid or bloody
Fecal leukocytes	Uncommon	Common
Proctosigmoidoscopy	Normal	Erythema, ulceration, hemorrhage
Typical pathogens	*Salmonella* species, pathogenic *Escherichia coli*, *Vibrio* sp	*Shigella* species, *Campylobacter* species, *Clostridium difficile*

cillary dysentery. Leukocytes may be identified by adding a drop of methylene blue to the liquid stool sample before examination. The fecal leukocyte test is considered positive when three or more leukocytes are present per high-power field in four or more fields. The presence of occult fecal blood can be conveniently tested by using guaiac-impregnated test cards (Hemoccult) or by microscopy of fresh liquid stool specimen.

Many patients with bacterial enteritis present to their physicians with acute bloody diarrhea, crampy abdominal pain, and fever. The usual bacterial pathogens are *Shigella*, *Campylobacter*, and *Salmonella* species, and toxigenic *E coli* 0157: H7. Amebic dysentery and certain forms of the gay bowel syndrome also may present with acute bloody diarrhea. Also to be considered are idiopathic ulcerative colitis and, in older patients, acute ischemic colitis. Accurate diagnosis may be quite difficult, especially early in the course of disease before the results of stool cultures are available. Careful examination of the stool for parasites, and flexible sigmoidoscopy or colonoscopy with biopsy may help differentiate idiopathic ulcerative colitis and ischemic colitis from the acute bacillary dysenteries.

Shigella INFECTION

Etiology

Shigella species are aerobic, nonmotile, gram-negative rods that ferment glucose but usually not lactose. The original isolation and description of the "Shiga bacillus" (later called *Shigella dysenteriae*) was made by Shiga in 1898.[3] The genus *Shigella* is subdivided into four major groups, A, B, C, and D, on the basis of biochemical and antigenic traits.[4] Group A contains *S dysenteriae*, of which 10 types are described. *S dysenteriae* type 1 has caused major epidemics and pandemics of dysentery in Japan, Africa, and Central America. Type 1 strain is considered particularly virulent, and outbreaks have been associated with considerable morbidity and mortality compared to other serotypes. Group B contains *Shigella flex-*

neri (six types), a common isolate in tropical countries. Group C contains 15 serotypes of *Shigella boydii*. Group D comprises the *Shigella sonnei* serotype, which accounts for most of the reported cases of shigellosis in the United States and Western Europe.

Epidemiology

Approximately 15,000 cases of shigellosis are reported annually in the United States.[5] If, as has been suggested, only 1 in 20 cases of bacterial dysentery is reported, the actual incidence may approach 300,000 cases annually. *S sonnei* (60%–70%) and *S flexneri* (20%–30%) together account for more than 90% of isolates reported to the Centers for Disease Control. Shigellosis is primarily a disease of children between the ages of 6 months and 5 years, with a peak incidence at the age of 2 years. The type of *Shigella* isolated is related in part to the age of the patient. *S sonnei* is more common before the age of 15 years; *S flexneri* is more common in patients older than 15 years.

Shigellosis is transmitted primarily by way of the fecal-oral route through close personal contact, or in developing countries by way of infected food or water. The persistence of this pathogen in humans is attributed to its ability to survive for long periods in the environment (soil, water, wooden surfaces) and to a small number of chronic human carriers. Outbreaks of shigellosis have been traced to contaminated food,[6] although point-source outbreaks of this type are quite unusual. Shigellosis is often endemic in custodial institutions, nursing homes, and day-care centers.[7] In adults, *Shigella* infection is occasionally associated with foreign travel.

Shigella species are highly contagious; ingestion of only 180 *S flexneri* organisms resulted in diarrhea and fever in 22% of healthy volunteers.[8] Ingestion of 5000 organisms resulted in an attack rate of 57%, but higher doses (10^4 or 10^5 organisms) did not increase the attack rate above 60%. By comparison, ingestion of 10^7 cells of certain *Salmonella* species is required to achieve a 50% attack rate.[9] The typical stool of a patient with acute shigellosis contains 10^9 pathogens per gram of stool, enough to infect thousands of other individuals.[4] Host resistance factors include gastric acidity and normal colonic microflora, although neither has been carefully studied. The protective role of *Shigella* antibodies is discussed in a following section.

Several pandemics of shigellosis have been described during the 20th century. The most dramatic occurred in Japan in the early 1900s when waves of *S dysenteriae* type 1 swept the islands, causing thousands of deaths each year.[10] Between 1968 and 1970, a pandemic of *S dysenteriae* involved a large percentage of the population in Guatemala and San Salvador.[11] This pandemic strain was characterized by rapid spread, increased virulence, and resistance to antibiotics. The Central American pandemic was probably accounted for, at least in part, by primitive sanitary facilities, extensive pollution of water supplies, and crowded living conditions in rural villages. Shigellosis is endemic in Mexico, Central America, the Indian subcontinent, and Southeast Asia. *S flexneri* and *S dysenteriae* infections occur frequently in these areas, and isolates are almost always highly resistant to antibiotics.[12]

Pathophysiology

Shigella species produce intestinal damage by two mechanisms: invasion of the colonic epithelium, and production of enterotoxin. Of these two mechanisms, the property of invasiveness is essential for virulence.[13] All *Shigella* species (except laboratory mutants) contain a plasmid-mediated virulence factor, which enables the organism to invade and multiply within intestinal epithelial cells. *Shigella* species also elaborate a potent enterotoxin, but this does not appear to be essential for colitis. Lipopolysaccharide (endotoxin) production is also a feature of virulent *Shigella* strains, but is not required for virulence.

The histopathologic findings in *Shigella* infection are nonspecific and resemble the changes observed in other acute infections of the colon. Biopsies of the rectum during acute shigellosis reveal an intense inflammatory infiltrate with polymorphonuclear leukocytes, hemorrhage, mucus depletion, and occasional abscesses. Small ulcers occur where necrotic epithelial cells have split open. The lamina propria is edematous, congested, and heavily infiltrated with neutrophils and mononuclear cells. Bacterial cells can be demonstrated within colonocytes, but not all damaged colonocytes contain bacteria, suggesting that some tissue damage may be secondary to enterotoxin or to inflammatory mediators released by neutrophils and monocytes. The distribution of colonic damage in acute shigellosis as determined by colonoscopy[14] reveals severe inflammation in the rectosigmoid, with diminished severity in the proximal colon. The entire colon is involved in 15% of patients and, in these patients, the terminal ileum may be mildly inflamed as well.

The relative importance of epithelial invasiveness versus toxin production has been documented in human volunteers inoculated with either fully virulent or attenuated strains of *S dysenteriae* type 1.[13] The fully virulent strains were both invasive and toxigenic, whereas the attenuated strains lacked either the invasiveness factor or the ability to make toxin. The fully virulent strains produced acute diarrhea after oral inoculation of 10^1 to 10^4 organisms (attack rate 10%–83%). Similar rates of infection and disease severity were observed with the invasive, nontoxigenic strain. In contrast, the noninvasive, toxigenic strain produced no disease in 85 to 86 volunteers ingesting up to 10^{11} organisms.

Genetic engineering studies indicate that invasiveness, but not toxin production, may be essential for virulence. Several virulence-associated plasmids of 180 to 220 kilobases are required for *Shigella* species to invade and multiply within intestinal epithelial cells.[15] These plasmids encode a series of polypeptides that mediate enterocyte invasion, intracellular multiplication, and killing of host cells.[16] Fontaine and colleagues[17] prepared isogenic mutant strains of *S dysenteriae* that lacked either the invasiveness plasmid or the toxin gene, but were otherwise genetically identical. The invasive, nontoxigenic mutants caused dysentery in macaque monkeys that was equal in severity to that caused by the invasive, toxigenic strain. Those animals infected with the toxigenic strains had somewhat bloodier diarrhea compared to those infected with the nontoxigenic strains. Bloody diarrhea is also more frequent in humans infected with high toxin-producing strains than those infected with low toxin-producing strains.[18] These observations suggest that the severity of diarrhea and degree of bleeding are related to the amount of toxin produced by different *Shigella* strains.

All strains of *Shigella* elaborate protein exotoxins with enterotoxic, cytotoxic, and neurotoxic properties.[19,20] *S dysenteriae* type 1 has been the subject of nearly all studies on *Shigella* toxin, and it is assumed that other *Shigella* strains produce identical or closely related toxins.

Shigella toxin has an A-B subunit structure, a feature common to many other bacterial toxins. Each molecule of *Shigella* holotoxin (molecular weight 70,000 d) contains a single A (catalytic) subunit of molecular weight 32,000 d and five B (binding) subunits of molecular weights 7700 d each. The receptor for shigatoxin on rabbit jejunal brush border has been identified as globotriaosylceramide.[21] This receptor is lacking on enterocytes from rabbits younger than 20 days old, and the number of receptors per cell in older animals is closely related to the rate of fluid secretion after exposure to *Shigella* toxin.[22] The absence of the toxin receptor in newborn rabbits suggests that the infrequency of shigellosis in human newborns may likewise be related to absence of the toxin receptor.

After binding to its glycolipid receptor of HeLa cells, *Shigella* toxin is internalized by receptor-mediated endocytosis.[23] The catalytic A subunit is released inside the cell and causes a profound inhibition of total protein synthesis.[24] The mechanism by which *Shigella* toxin elicits intestinal fluid secretion may not be related to protein synthesis inhibition, however, because other inhibitors of protein synthesis do not elicit intestinal secretion. *Shigella* toxin does not activate adenyl or guanyl cyclases as do other enterotoxins. Rather, inhibition of protein synthesis in surface absorptive cells appears to cause a secondary failure of fluid absorption.

Immunity

Serum and secretory (intestinal) antibodies to *Shigella* have been demonstrated in patients after experimental inoculation with *Shigella* and also in populations with a high incidence of naturally occurring shigellosis.[25] It has been assumed, but not convincingly proven, that immunity to *Shigella* infection primarily involves secretory IgA antibody released into the intestinal lumen at the site of infection. Because serum and secretory antibody production are regulated independently, the clinician must be cautious in interpreting the significance of serum antibody levels to *Shigella* or other enteric pathogens.

Epidemiologic data suggest that prior infection with *Shigella* appears to protect against subsequent infection. In institutions for the mentally retarded, where shigellosis is common, the rate of infection is considerably higher in the first year of residence than in subsequent years.[7] A similar trend toward high infectivity among new recruits has been observed in military populations.[26] This resistance to infection among long-term residents has been attributed to acquired immunity. Prior infection with *S flexneri* conferred protection in human volunteers subjected to a second oral challenge with the same strain.[8] The incidence of acute bloody diarrhea and fever after oral challenge was only 20% in volunteers with previous infection, versus 56% in volunteers without previous exposure. The rate of positive stool cultures, however, was virtually identical in the two groups (67% vs. 69%, respectively), suggesting that some immune people may become colonized without manifesting symptoms of infection.

Development of an effective oral vaccine against *Shigella* would profoundly influence worldwide morbidity and mortality, particularly among children in developing countries. Although several vaccines have been tested, none is considered effective enough for clinical use. One vaccine was prepared from a bivalent strain of *Salmonella typhi—S sonnei* that expressed antigens from both pathogens but was attenuated and did not itself cause diarrhea.[27] After three oral doses of this vaccine, 25% of volunteers demonstrated increased levels of serum IgA and 35% had increased secretory IgA in intestinal secretions. Compared with nonvaccinated control subjects, the vaccinated group experienced a significant reduction of diarrhea and fever after challenge with a virulent strain. In another study, higher levels of serum IgG and non-IgM antibody to *Shigella* lipopolysaccharide appeared to protect military personnel against naturally acquired *S sonnei* and *S flexneri* infections.[26]

The virulence-associated peptides required for tissue invasion by *Shigella* species also may be important in acquired immunity. IgG and IgA antibodies to these peptides are present in acute and convalescent sera from patients with *Shigella* dysentery.[28] In one survey from an endemic area, serum antibody to virulence peptides was often present in children older than 5 years of age, but absent or in low titer in younger children except after infection.[29] These observations suggest that vaccination with *Shigella* virulence peptides may provide better protection than vaccination with other *Shigella* antigens.

Clinical Features

Most patients with *Shigella* dysentery have acute diarrhea with blood or bloody mucus, and fever.[30] Much of the information on shigellosis has been derived from human volunteer studies in healthy young men.[8,27] Fever developed in human volunteers from 22 hours to 3 days after ingestion of *S flexneri*. Abdominal cramps and diarrhea followed fever within 24 hours, and, in half the volunteers, the diarrhea was bloody. Without antibiotic treatment, diarrhea abated by the seventh day on average, although some untreated volunteers remained symptomatic for up to 30 days.

Stool cultures usually were positive for *S flexneri* within 3 days of oral challenge, and, in untreated patients, stool cultures remained positive for an average of 27 days. A curious finding in several volunteer studies and in community outbreaks of shigellosis was the observation that not all volunteers with positive stool cultures had symptoms. Conversely, not all those with typical fever and bloody diarrhea had positive stool cultures for *Shigella*. Thus, a negative stool culture does not necessarily exclude the diagnosis of shigellosis.

Naturally occurring shigellosis presents with a much wider spectrum of symptoms than is reported in volunteers.[30] *Shigella* dysentery may be very severe, especially in malnourished children or debilitated adults without access to medical treatment. On the other end of the spectrum are patients who complain only of a few loose stools and seldom seek medical attention. Adults with severe rectal inflammation from shigellosis may complain of tenesmus, a sensation of not having evacuated the rectum completely after a bowel movement.

Shigella dysentery may present as a two-phase illness, especially during epidemics or large outbreaks. The initial or small intestinal phase is characterized by the abrupt onset of watery diarrhea every 20 or 30 minutes. The second or dysenteric phase commences 12 to 72 hours later with passage of smaller volumes of blood-tinged mucus or a few small blood clots. In many patients with *Shigella* dysentery, rectal bleeding is occult or microscopic.

Physical examination during acute shigellosis reveals lower abdominal tenderness, with normal or increased bowel sounds. Rebound tenderness or prolonged ileus are unusual and should suggest an alternate diagnosis. Some patients, especially young children, may become dehydrated, especially if diarrhea and vomiting have been present for more than 48 hours. Evidence of volume depletion, including elevation of the hematocrit or serum sodium, and mild azotemia, may be present. Leukocytosis is unusual, and bacteremia is rarely seen except in infants with fulminant infection (see section on Complications).

The laboratory diagnosis of *Shigella* infection is made by stool culture of a fresh sample. The recommended approach is to collect a liquid stool specimen in a sterile container and to inoculate this as soon as possible on selective media for *Shigella* and *Salmonella* species. The percentage of positive stool cultures for bacterial pathogens is greatly increased by selectively culturing only those stool specimens that contain fecal leukocytes and erythrocytes, but this would miss some infections. Nonselective stool cultures from all adults presenting with acute diarrhea are positive for bacterial pathogens (*Salmonella, Shigella, Campylobacter,* and *Yersinia* sp) in less than 20% of samples. In contrast, selective culturing of only those stool specimens containing leukocytes increases the yield to 75% or higher and greatly reduces the total cost of obtaining a single positive stool culture for *Salmonella* or *Shigella*.[31] All patients with bloody diarrhea, particularly those with a history of foreign travel, should have a careful examination of fresh stool to exclude *E histolytica* infection.

Clinical Course

Shigellosis usually runs a shorter course in children (2–3 days) than in adults (5–7 days). Some adult patients may have a 2- to 3-week illness with waxing and waning diarrhea. This subacute presentation may be confused with new-onset ulcerative colitis, especially because the proctosigmoidoscopic findings may be identical. Isolation of *Shigella* and prompt response to antibiotic therapy should allow differentiation of these two entities.

Fecal shedding of *S sonnei* and *S flexneri* has been reported in adults after clinical recovery from typical acute dysentery.[32] Investigation of the *Shigella* carrier state has been limited because of the rarity of this condition.

Complications

Shigella bacteremia is a severe complication usually observed in malnourished children. In a large study from Bangladesh, the incidence of *Shigella* bacteremia was 7.2% in infants younger than 1 year of age, 3.9% in children between the ages of 1 and 14 years, and 1.4% in patients aged 15 years or older.[33] *Shigella* bacteremia carries an approximately 20%

mortality from renal failure, hemolytic anemia, thrombocytopenia, gastrointestinal bleeding, and shock.[34]

Reiter's syndrome is a triad of arthritis, urethritis, and conjunctivitis after bacillary dysentery or venereal disease. The syndrome is most common between the ages of 20 and 40 years, and has a strong predilection for men with the human leukocyte antigen (HLA)-B27 phenotype. Careful follow-up investigations of localized outbreaks of shigellosis indicate that 1% or 2% of infected people subsequently have Reiter's syndrome.[35,36] *S flexneri* is frequently implicated in Reiter's syndrome, as are certain strains of *Salmonella, Yersinia,* and *Campylobacter.* Approximately 80% of patients with Reiter's syndrome are positive for the HLA-B27 antigen.[37] Conversely, approximately 20% of HLA-B27-positive patients have Reiter's syndrome after a bout of bacillary dysentery. Several other "enteric arthropathies" are associated with the HLA-B27 phenotype, including ankylosing spondylitis with ulcerative colitis, sacroiliitis complicating Whipple's disease, and Behçet's syndrome.

Reiter's syndrome is quite variable in its clinical expression, and limited forms are common. Urethritis or balanitis may be minimal or absent. In addition to arthritis, in many patients periostitis, tendonitis, heel spurs, and plantar fasciitis develop. The typical presentation is asymmetric arthritis or periarthritis of a lower extremity occurring 2 to 4 weeks after a bout of shigellosis or other bacterial dysentery. By the time the patient complains of articular or other manifestations, the enteric infection has almost always resolved and antibiotic therapy is not indicated. The arthritic manifestations tend to be chronic and relapsing, even in the absence of recurrent dysentery. Treatment of Reiter's syndrome is aimed at symptomatic relief of arthritis with nonsteroidal antiinflammatory compounds.

The occurrence of hemolytic-uremic syndrome (HUS) in children with severe *S dysenteriae* infection was first described in the Central American pandemic in 1974[38] and in Bangladesh in 1975.[39] HUS also has been observed in children with hemorrhagic colitis due to infection with verotoxin-producing strains of *E coli.*[40] The syndrome is characterized by acute hemolytic anemia, renal failure, and uremia associated with disseminated intravascular coagulation. Pathologic examination of the kidneys reveals microangiopathic damage and cortical necrosis secondary to thrombosed interlobular arteries. HUS is a serious complication of shigellosis and hemorrhagic *E coli* colitis, with a mortality rate in excess of 50%. Severe dehydration, bacteremia, and leukemoid reaction may occur in association with HUS.

The pathogenic mechanism underlying postdysenteric HUS is unknown. The development of HUS in Bangladeshi children with shigellosis was correlated with serum levels of endotoxin, which presumably gained access into the systemic circulation across the damaged colonic epithelium.[41] Endotoxin is thought to cause renal microvascular damage by way of a Shwartzman-like reaction. An animal model of HUS has been reported[42] in rabbits injected with lipopolysaccharides (endotoxin) of *S dysenteriae* and *S flexneri.*

Therapy

One of the more confusing topics in bacterial diarrheas is that of therapy. Part of the confusion arises from the fact that some, but not all, enteric infections respond to antibiotic therapy (Table 84-2). In addition, many enteric infections are self limited, and the patient already may have recovered by the time the results of stool culture are available. Antibiotic therapy has been clearly shown to reduce the duration and severity of symptoms in shigellosis and to shorten the period of fecal excretion of the organism. Thus, antibiotic therapy is recommended for all patients with *Shigella* diarrhea except those with mild, self-limited disease.

The main problem in treatment of shigellosis is antibiotic resistance.[43] *Shigella* species rapidly develop resistance to antibiotics, and in India and Southeast Asia, most strains are resistant to nearly all antibiotics. Even in Great Britain and the United States, many *Shigella* strains demonstrate multiple drug resistance. As illustrated in Figure 84-1, *Shigella* organisms gradually develop resistance to antibiotics after their introduction to clinical practice. Sulfonamides and streptomycin were first introduced in the 1940s, but by the 1970s and 1980s more than 75% of *Shigella* in Britain were resistant to these antibiotics. The experience with tetracyclines, ampicillin, and trimethoprim-sulfamethoxazole (TMP-SMZ) is similar. When first introduced in 1975, TMP-SMZ was effective against all *Shigella* strains, but by the early 1990s approximately 25% to 40% of strains were resistant. In general, *S flexneri, S boydii,* and *S dysenteriae* are more likely to be multiply drug resistant than *S sonnei,* the strain that accounts for approximately 75% of all infections in the United States. For this reason, travelers to Mexico, the Indian subcontinent, or Southeast Asia are more likely to be infected with a resistant strain than patients who are infected with local *S sonnei* strains.[44]

Several antibiotics have been convincingly demonstrated in placebo-controlled trials to reduce the duration of diarrhea and eliminate *Shigella* from the stool. The following therapeutic recommendations are based on the assumption that the *Shigella* isolate is sensitive in vitro to the antibiotic under discussion. Tetracycline, 500 mg four times daily for 5 days, is effective in adults, and a single oral dose of 2.5 g of tetracycline is as effective as 5-day therapy.[45] Tetracycline is contraindicated in pregnancy, and in young children because it may discolor the teeth. Ampicillin, 500 mg four times daily, and TMP 160 mg/SMZ 800 mg every 12 hours for 5 days also are effective against acute *Shigella* dysentery.[46]

TABLE 84-2
Effectiveness of Antibiotic Therapy in Enteric Infections

DEGREE OF EFFECTIVENESS	INFECTION
Very effective	Typhoid fever
Effective	Shigellosis
	Cholera
	Clostridium difficile
	Travelers' diarrhea
	Giardiasis
	Amebiasis
Ineffective or minimally effective	*Campylobacter* diarrhea
	Intestinal salmonellosis
	Cryptosporidiosis
	Enterohemorrhagic *Escherichia coli*

Adapted from DuPont HL, Ericsson CD, Robins A, et al. Current problems in antimicrobial therapy for bacterial enteric infection. Am J Med 1987;(Suppl 4A) 82:324.

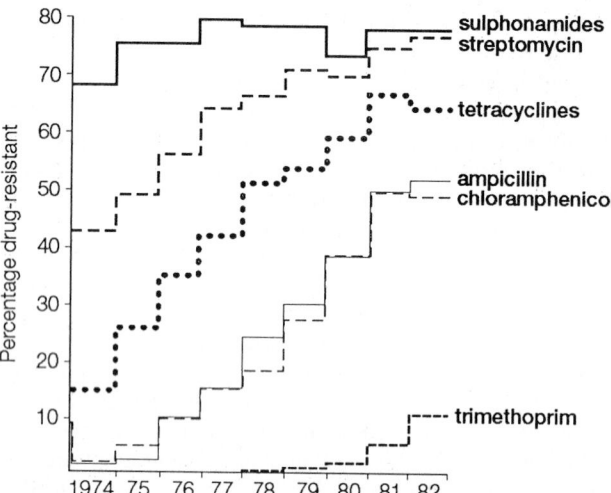

FIGURE 84-1. Resistance of *Shigella* species to various antibiotics in Great Britain from 1974 to 1982. (From Rowe B, Threllfall EJ. Drug resistance in gram negative aerobic bacilli. Br Med Bull 1984;40:68.)

The most recent addition to the therapeutic armamentarium against *Shigella* species is the quinolone group of antibiotics, which includes norfloxacin and ciprofloxacin. These antibiotics are highly effective against many enteric pathogens, including *Shigella, Salmonella*, enterotoxigenic *E coli*, and *C jejuni*. In clinical trials, ciprofloxacin, 500 mg twice daily for 5 days, was as effective as TMP-SMZ in treating acute *Shigella* dysentery acquired in Mexico.[47] In Bangladesh, a single 1-g dose of ciprofloxacin was as effective as 500 mg twice daily for 5 days in the treatment of acute shigellosis due to all strains except *S dysenteriae*. Effective treatment of the latter species required a full 5 days of therapy.[48]

The choice of antibiotic for *Shigella* infections ideally should be based on in vitro sensitivity testing, although in severely ill patients, the physician may feel pressured to begin antibiotic therapy before these results are available. In this situation, the physician must choose an antibiotic that is likely to be effective based on the predicted pathogen and its previous pattern of antibiotic resistance in the local community. The initial antibiotic may be altered when in vitro sensitivity results are available.

In addition to antibiotic therapy, treatment of dehydration is an important aspect of therapy. Oral rehydration may be effective in mild disease, whereas more severely ill patients at the extremes of age may require intravenous rehydration. Antidiarrheal medications are not recommended because they may prolong the duration of symptoms and delay clearance of the pathogen.[49] Patients with mild shigellosis often are well by the time stool culture results are available and do not require antibiotic therapy.

Campylobacter INFECTION

In the last two decades, *C jejuni* has emerged as a major cause of acute dysentery, in some surveys accounting for up to 20% of positive stool cultures in patients with acute bacillary diarrhea.[50] Like *Shigella, C jejuni* primarily affects the colon, and

produces a clinical syndrome of acute febrile illness in children and adults that resembles shigellosis.

Etiology

Campylobacter species have many subgroups, but two of these, *C jejuni* and *Campylobacter coli*, account for the majority of human infections.[51] *Helicobacter pylori*, formerly *Campylobacter pylori*, is a cause of type B gastritis and may be involved in the pathogenesis of peptic ulcer disease (see Chap. 61).

Nearly all clinical laboratories are capable of routinely identifying *Campylobacter* in stool cultures, using selective media and microaerophilic conditions. *Campylobacter* species are motile, gram-negative rods or spirals that possess oxidase and catalase activity. They grow optimally at 42°C in 5% oxygen, 10% carbon dioxide. Isolation is improved if the stool sample is placed quickly into special transport media and promptly inoculated onto the plating media, or held at 4°C for not more than 24 hours.

Epidemiology

Campylobacter resembles *Salmonella* in its modes of transmission. Although person-to-person spread by way of fecal-oral transmission is most common, the major source of human infection is ingestion of poultry and eggs.[52] In addition, ingestion of raw or contaminated milk and exposure to sick pets, especially puppies,[53] has been associated with disease outbreaks. *Campylobacter* species including *C jejuni*, have been isolated from many species of domestic and wild animals, and, under certain circumstances, animal hosts appear to serve as important reservoirs of human infection. Point-source epidemics of *Campylobacter* have also been traced to contaminated water supplies.

Pathogenesis

The pathophysiologic mechanisms by which *C jejuni* causes intestinal disease still are not known, but two potential virulence factors have been suggested: invasiveness and toxin production.[50,51] The classic test for invasiveness, the Sereny test, measures the ability of a pathogen to cause keratoconjunctivitis in rabbits. Although this test is negative for *C jejuni*, the histopathologic course of experimental enteritis in animals suggests that *C jejuni* invades and destroys epithelial cells, much like *Shigella* species.[54] Some strains of *C jejuni* produce a heat-labile enterotoxin that stimulates adenylate cyclase and is neutralized by antibodies to cholera toxin and *E coli* heat-labile toxin.[55] Certain strains of *C jejuni* also produce a cytotoxin active against tissue culture cells.[56]

Strain differences among *C jejuni* isolates may account for some of the variability of disease expression in humans.[57] *C jejuni* strains isolated from asymptomatic carriers do not release enterotoxins and are negative in rabbit ileal loop assays. In contrast, strains recovered from patients with watery diarrhea produce variable amounts of enterotoxin, and strains from patients with bloody diarrhea produce a cytotoxin.

Ingestion of *C jejuni* by human volunteers produces acute

diarrhea and fever, although the severity of the diarrhea is clearly strain dependent.[58] As in *Shigella* infection, the occurrence of diarrhea is not closely related to the number of *Campylobacter* organisms ingested. All volunteers who became ill had fecal leukocytes in their stool, suggesting that the absence of leukocytes makes *C jejuni* infection most unlikely. Rechallenge of volunteers with the same strain 1 month after recovery failed to elicit disease, indicating that acute infection confers short-term, homologous immunity. Serum titers of IgA and IgM antibodies peaked at 11 days postinoculation, but IgG antibody levels did not reach statistical significance. Secretory antibody to several *C jejuni* antigens appears in stools after naturally acquired infection.[59] Whether serum or secretory antibodies protect against *Campylobacter* reinfection is uncertain.

Clinical Features

Children younger than 5 years of age appear to be most susceptible to *Campylobacter* infection, with young adults the next most susceptible group. Acute colitis of *Campylobacter* infection resembles *Shigella* dysentery. The spectrum of disease produced by *C jejuni* ranges from asymptomatic carriage to severe, life-threatening colitis with toxic megacolon.[52,53] After an incubation period of 1 to 6 days, a syndrome of fatigue and myalgia develops, lasting for 24 hours. This is followed by nausea, anorexia, lower abdominal cramping, and diarrhea. The diarrhea may be watery or bloody, and passage of 10 or more stools per day is not uncommon. Abdominal pain and tenderness are typical and may be so localized as to mimic acute appendicitis or other causes of a "surgical abdomen." Tenesmus occurs in approximately 25% of patients, and up to 80% exhibit evidence of proctocolitis by sigmoidoscopy. Some patients with *Campylobacter* infection have a relapsing course with hematochezia, resembling idiopathic ulcerative colitis or Crohn's disease.[52] In addition, some patients with recent onset of ulcerative colitis or Crohn's disease may be infected with *C jejuni* or other bacterial pathogens.[60]

Fecal leukocytes and erythrocytes are present in most patients with *C jejuni* infection. Peripheral blood leukocytosis and laboratory evidence of dehydration are observed in some moderately to severely ill patients. Positive stool cultures for *C jejuni* seldom persist for more than 2 weeks, and more than 90% of patients are culture-negative after 5 weeks.

Complications

Although most patients with *Campylobacter* enteritis have a self-limited illness of less than a week's duration, some patients have a more protracted illness resembling acute ulcerative colitis. Extraintestinal infection resulting from bacteremia has been described and appears to be more frequent in patients with lowered host resistance.[61] Toxic megacolon has been reported secondary to *Campylobacter* infection, as has severe pseudomembranous colitis (PMC). Reiter's syndrome[62] and HUS[63] may follow *Campylobacter* enteritis, with clinical features resembling those described for *Shigella* enteritis. Recurrent infection with *Campylobacter* infection in patients with acquired immunodeficiency syndrome (AIDS) has been at-

tributed to impaired antibody response or to persistence of the organism in gallbladder bile.[64]

Therapy

The mainstay of therapy in *Campylobacter* infection is replacement of fluid and electrolytes. In most patients with mild or moderate disease, the symptoms are already waning or gone entirely by the time the results of stool culture are available. Some patients have severe dysentery or a relapsing course, however, which may require hospitalization or extended absence from work, and in these patients the question of antibiotic therapy is often raised. Although *C jejuni* is susceptible to several antibiotics in vitro, erythromycin has emerged as the most frequently recommended antibiotic for *Campylobacter* diarrhea. There is no compelling evidence from the medical literature that antibiotic therapy with erythromycin or other antibiotics reduces the duration or severity of symptoms. In four controlled trials of erythromycin therapy for *C jejuni* enteritis, duration of diarrhea after starting therapy was comparable in the placebo versus antibiotic-treated groups[65]; however, the duration of *Campylobacter* shedding was definitely reduced in the erythromycin-treated group. Some authorities have suggested that prompt treatment with erythromycin within 3 days of onset of diarrhea reduces the duration of symptoms. Adult patients, especially debilitated or immunocompromised people with severe *Campylobacter* enteritis or relapsing disease, appear to benefit from long-term antibiotic therapy, although the evidence to support this is primarily anecdotal.[52,66] If antibiotic therapy is initiated, erythromycin, 250 mg four times daily for 5 days, is effective in eradicating the organism from feces. Ciprofloxacin, 500 mg twice daily, is an alternate choice and has the additional advantage of being very effective against enterotoxic *E coli*, *Shigella* species, and *Salmonella*.[67] Quinolone-resistant strains of *C jejuni* have been described after treatment with ciprofloxacin.[68]

Clostridium difficile ENTEROCOLITIS

C difficile (originally called *Bacillus difficilis*) was discovered in 1935 in the stools of healthy newborns.[69] The organism was considered "difficult" by its discoverers because of its slow growth on conventional media and tendency to die during attempts at isolation. Although it was pathogenic for guinea pigs and rabbits, the organism was considered part of the normal gut flora that disappeared after weaning. *C difficile* remained a laboratory curiosity until 1978, when Bartlett and colleagues[70] identified it as the source of cytotoxin in the stools of patients with antibiotic-associated PMC. *C difficile* is now recognized as a common nosocomial infection and the major cause of antibiotic-associated colitis and diarrhea.

Etiology

C difficile is a gram-positive, obligate anaerobic rod that grows best in selective media containing cycloserine and cefoxitin and enriched with fructose and egg yolk.[71] This selective medium can detect as few as 2000 organisms in stool samples. As noted, *C difficile* is frequently cultured from the stools of healthy newborns, but in older children and adults, it is considered a pathogen. Individual strains of *C difficile*, identified by agglutinating antisera[72] or DNA fingerprinting,[73] appear to differ with regard to pathogenicity. Hospital outbreaks have been attributed to epidemic strains that are high toxin producers, although nontoxigenic or weakly toxigenic strains are becoming increasingly recognized. The organism is a spore former, allowing it to survive in harsh environments and even in patients during antibiotic therapy.

C difficile does not readily colonize the gastrointestinal tract of older adults and children unless the endogenous microflora has been altered by antibiotics, cancer chemotherapy, or the presence of another pathogen, such as *Salmonella* or *Shigella*. Similarly, *C difficile* cannot be introduced into normal adult hamsters unless the animals have been pretreated with antibiotics. Presumably, the normal colonic microflora competes with *C difficile* for nutrients, and, unless this microflora has been altered by antibiotics, *C difficile* cannot colonize the bowel. Cats, dogs, horses, and donkeys are colonized by *C difficile*, but there is no evidence that animals serve as reservoirs of human disease.[74]

Pathogenesis

C difficile produces intestinal damage by release of two potent exotoxins called toxins A and B. Toxin B, a cytotoxin, was first detected in the stools of several patients with antibiotic-associated PMC. Initially, the toxin was incorrectly attributed to *Clostridium sordellii*, but subsequently it was shown to be produced in culture by *C difficile*.[75]

Toxin B is heat-labile, trypsin-sensitive protein whose molecular weight is approximately 250,000 d, as deduced from the cloned gene.[76] Toxin B possesses cytopathic activity against fibroblasts and other cells in culture and is lethal when injected parenterally into mice or rabbits. Highly purified toxin B, however, does not produce secretion or tissue damage when placed into rabbit ileal loops.

Toxin A, the enterotoxin of *C difficile*, is also a heat-labile,

protease-sensitive protein of molecular weight 308,000 d.[77] Like toxin B, it possesses lethal properties for laboratory animals and is cytotoxic for cultured fibroblasts, but at much higher concentrations than observed for toxin B. Analysis of the cDNA sequence of the toxin genes reveals considerable homology, suggesting a shared mechanism of action.[76,77] The effects of toxin A on rabbit, rat, or mouse intestine differ considerably from those of other enterotoxins. In common with cholera toxin and *E coli* enterotoxin, toxin A elicits secretion of fluid from rabbit ileal loops; however, in contrast to the watery fluid obtained with cholera toxin, the fluid released after toxin A exposure is a typical inflammatory exudate containing neutrophils, lymphocytes, and erythrocytes, as well as serum proteins and mucus.[78] In addition, highly purified toxin A elicits a profound inflammatory response in the lamina propria and severe epithelial necrosis in rabbit ileal loops, findings not observed with the classic enterotoxins.

The cellular mechanisms of toxin A action appear to be quite complex. Highly purified toxin A stimulates a prompt increase in intracellular calcium in human neutrophils and also exerts a strong chemotactic response in these cells,[79] a property that may underlie its ability to elicit an intestinal inflammatory response. Toxin A also has a direct effect on enterocytes in vitro. Human colon cancer cell lines exposed to toxin A demonstrate decreased electrical resistance, increased permeability, and profound disorganization of the cytoskeleton in the area of the intercellular tight junctions.[80] Neither toxin alters adenylate or guanylate cyclase in target cells. In summary, available experimental evidence from animal studies suggests that toxin A rather than toxin B is primarily responsible for intestinal damage.

Immunity

Serum IgG antibodies to toxins A and B are found in 60% to 70% of children and adults in the United States[81] (Fig. 84-2). The titers of serum IgG and IgA and secretory IgA-specific antitoxins are elevated in patients convalescing from recent infection, but antibody levels are not well correlated with recovery as opposed to relapse,[82] and it is not clear if

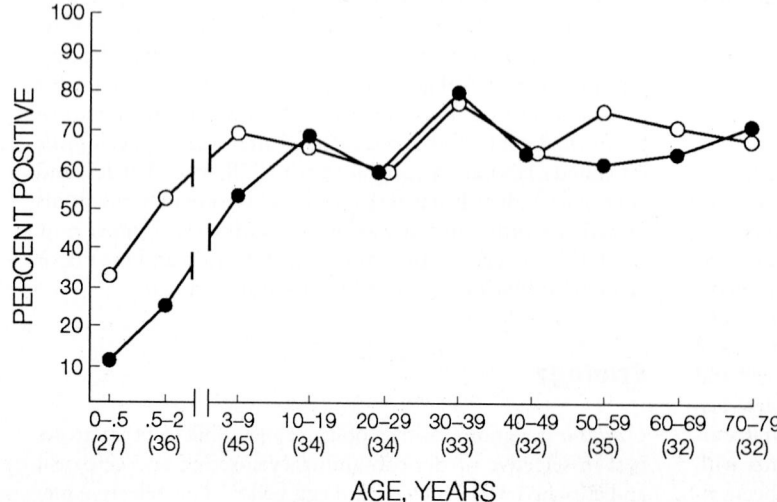

FIGURE 84-2. Age-related prevalence of antibodies to toxin A (*closed circles*) and toxin B (*open circles*) in 340 hospital patients. (From Viscidi R, Laughon BE, Yoken R, et al. Serum antibody response to toxins A and B of *Clostridium difficile*. J Infect Dis 1983;148:93.)

patients with serum or secretory antibody to toxins A or B are protected from disease.

Immunization of experimental animals with *C difficile* toxins protects against subsequent infection. Female hamsters immunized with toxoid A alone or a combination of toxoid A and B are protected against subsequent *C difficile* colitis, but toxoid B alone is not protective. The serum and breast milk of immunized hamsters contains neutralizing antitoxins, and infant hamsters can be protected by passive transfer of antitoxin in breast milk.[83]

Epidemiology

C difficile diarrhea and colitis result primarily from nosocomial (hospital-acquired) infection. Outbreaks of symptomatic infection have been reported in many hospitals in North America and Europe, but infection is rather uncommon in ambulatory patients treated at home with antibiotics. Although asymptomatic carriage of *C difficile* is rare in healthy adults, the incidence of *C difficile* carriage appears to be surprisingly high among hospital inpatients. In one survey, 7% of patients had positive stool cultures for *C difficile* on admission, and another 21% became culture positive during their hospital stay[84] (Fig. 84-3). Diarrhea developed in only one third of those patients with *C difficile* in their stools.

Environmental surveys based on wipe tests indicate that *C difficile* is a common contaminant in hospitals, especially in rooms or units where infected patients have been recently treated.[85,86] The organism can be cultured from bathrooms, toilets, scales, dust mops, and shoes of hospital personnel. *C difficile* can be cultured 40 days after an infected patient was moved from a hospital room.[87] Clustering of *C difficile* infection has been described in hospital rooms or special care units occupied by a succession of infected patients. Transmission of identical strains of *C difficile* between hospital roommates[84] and children at day care centers[88] suggests that direct person-to-person spread is also possible.

Hand carriage of *C difficile* by hospital personnel often follows contact with infected patients. The organism can be cultured from fingernails, fingertips, and the underside of rings.[84] Healthy hospital personnel rarely become fecal carriers of *C difficile*, and infection with this organism does not appear to be more common in hospital or laboratory workers who take antibiotics.

C difficile is a frequent cause of antibiotic-associated diarrhea and colitis in chronic care hospitals and nursing homes.[89]

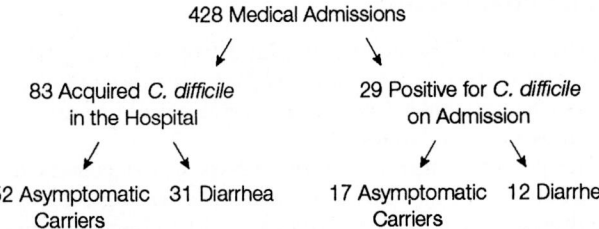

FIGURE 84-3. Hospital-acquired *Clostridium difficile* infection. (From McFarland LV, Mulligan ME, Kwok RY, et al. Nosocomial acquisition of *Clostridium difficile* infection. N Engl J Med 1989;320:240.)

At the time of hospital discharge or transfer to a chronic care facility, 82% of asymptomatic carriers of *C difficile* have positive stool cultures for *C difficile*.[84]

Newborns also acquire *C difficile* from the hospital environment. *C difficile* is commonly cultured from environmental surfaces in newborn nurseries and neonatal intensive care units.[85] The asymptomatic carriage rate of *C difficile* among infants appears to be very high.[90] A prospective study of three postnatal hospital wards in London indicated that the colonization rate of infants with *C difficile* as determined by daily stool culture ranged from 2% to 52%.[91] The rate of colonization in infants was correlated with length of hospital stay. Most of the isolates produced toxin B in culture, but toxin A production was not tested. It has been suggested that breastfeeding protects infants from *C difficile* colonization,[92] but this has not been confirmed.[93]

Many infant carriers of toxigenic *C difficile* have high titers of toxin B in their stools yet are completely asymptomatic. This could be explained if the infant intestine lacks specific receptors for toxin A, which develop later in the first year of life. Specific toxin A receptors have been identified on hamster intestinal brush border membranes.[94] The binding receptor in human intestine has not yet been identified, but specific binding sites for toxin A are absent in newborn rabbit brush border membranes and gradually reach adult levels by day 30.[95]

Another possible explanation for the asymptomatic carrier state is that infant carriers may be colonized by nontoxigenic or weakly toxigenic strains, whereas patients with colitis are colonized by highly toxigenic strains. Fecal toxin titers in healthy infants, however, are similar to those found in adult patients with *C difficile* infection.[96]

Clinical Features

PMC was originally associated with bowel obstruction, uremia, and sepsis. In the 1960s, *Staphylococcus aureus* was implicated as an etiologic agent in PMC.[97] After the introduction of lincomycin and clindamycin into clinical practice in the early 1970s, the incidence of PMC increased dramatically. Of 200 consecutive hospital inpatients treated with clindamycin and evaluated by proctosigmoidoscopy, PMC was observed in 10%.[98] In retrospect, this high incidence of PMC probably represented a hospital outbreak of *C difficile* colitis. After the discovery of *C difficile* as the cause of antibiotic-associated colitis, it became apparent that *C difficile* infection resulted in a disease spectrum ranging, in order of decreasing severity, from PMC, antibiotic-associated colitis without pseudomembranes, antibiotic-associated diarrhea, to the asymptomatic carrier state. As shown in Table 84-3, the cytotoxin assay is positive in almost all patients with PMC, but in a smaller percentage of patients with less florid manifestations of *C difficile* infection.

Pseudomembranous Colitis

Diarrhea and crampy abdominal pain typically begin during the first week of antibiotic therapy, although the range of onset is 2 days to 3 weeks.[70,75,99] Some patients complain of a sensation of incomplete evacuation (tenesmus), diffuse lower

TABLE 84-3
Clostridium difficile and Its Cytotoxin in Patients With Various Manifestations of *C difficile* Infection

CONDITION	*C difficile* CULTURE (% POSITIVE)	*C difficile* CYTOTOXIN (% POSITIVE)
Pseudomembranous colitis	95–100	95–100
Colitis without pseudomembranes	75–90	60–75
Antibiotic-associated diarrhea	20–40	15–30
Hospitalized adults, asymptomatic	10–15	2
Healthy adults	0–3	0
Healthy neonates and infants	30–80	25–50

Adapted from references 70, 75, 84, 90, and 96.

abdominal cramps, nausea, and occasional vomiting. Fever, chills, and dehydration may accompany severe colitis. Physical examination in PMC reveals abdominal distention and diffuse abdominal tenderness. The rectal examination may reveal occult gastrointestinal bleeding, but hematochezia is rarely observed. Fecal leukocytes are present in approximately 50% of patients. The diagnosis of PMC can be confirmed in some patients by sigmoidoscopy, which reveals the characteristic yellow-white, raised plaques, approximately 2 to 5 mm in diameter, scattered over the mucosal surface (Fig. 84-4; see Color Fig. 39). Pseudomembranes may at times become confluent, giving the appearance of a white or yellowish membrane covering the entire mucosa.[100] Biopsy of a pseudomembranes reveals the typical "summit lesion," an outpouring of fibrin, mucus, and inflammatory cells from a microulceration of the surface epithelium (Fig. 84-5; see Color Fig. 40). The diagnosis of PMC is not excluded by the absence of rectal pseudomembranes, because they may spare the rectum and occur higher up in the colon in 30% of patients.[101] Colonoscopy, however, is seldom required to make the diagnosis of PMC, and is not recommended except when ordinary diagnostic measures have failed.

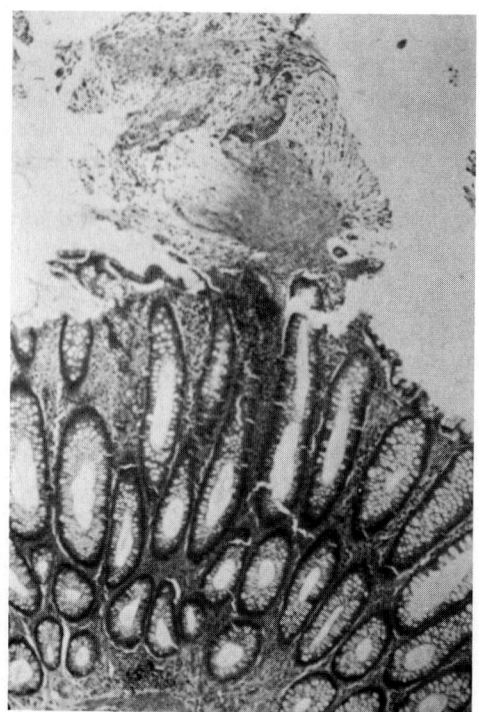

FIGURE 84-5. (See Color Fig. 40.) Biopsy specimen of a pseudomembrane shows the typical summit lesion.

Fulminant Colitis

Fulminant *C difficile* colitis involves transmural extension of the inflammatory process, resulting in perforation of the bowel and localized peritonitis.[102] In fulminant colitis, the colon may lose its muscular tone, resulting in toxic megacolon. Fulminant *C difficile* colitis may begin suddenly in a patient previously well or may develop during the course of milder infection. The patient appears toxic and may complain of steady, localized pain in contrast to the crampy pain of milder disease. Fever, tachycardia, localized tenderness, guarding, ascites, decreased bowel sounds, and signs of toxemia are present. As acute toxic dilation and paralytic ileus develop, diarrhea may lessen without any corresponding improvement in the general condition. Plain abdominal films may show accumulation of gas in a dilated colon (Fig. 84-6), and computed tomography scan often reveals a massively thickened colonic wall.[103]

Antibiotic-Associated Colitis Without Pseudomembranes

Approximately 50% of patients with diarrhea who are cytotoxin and culture positive for *C difficile* have pseudomembranes; the remainder have lesser degrees of colitis without typical pseudomembranes.[104]

The clinical features of antibiotic-associated colitis are similar to those seen with PMC, but of lesser degree.[104,105] The disease usually begins insidiously, with an increased urgency to defecate, lower abdominal cramps, and watery diarrhea. Malaise, fever, abdominal tenderness, leukocytosis, and dehydration may be present. Sigmoidoscopy may reveal diffuse or patchy erythema, friability, or purulent exudate without

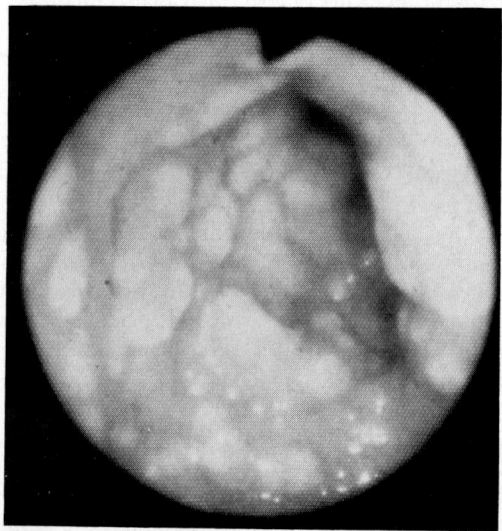

FIGURE 84-4. (See Color Fig. 39.) Colonoscopic appearance of pseudomembranous colitis.

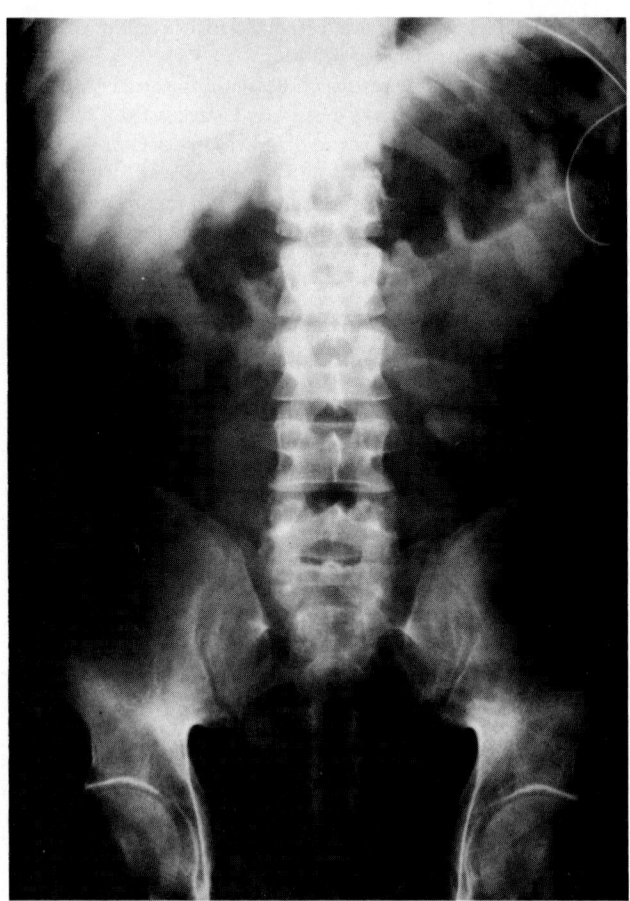

FIGURE 84-6. Acute toxic dilatation of the transverse colon in a patient with fulminant pseudomembranous colitis.

typical pseudomembranes. Sparing of the rectum with involvement of the proximal colon also may occur.

Antibiotic Diarrhea Without Colitis

In this common condition, diarrhea and crampy abdominal pain begin within a week of starting antibiotics, but usually the symptoms are milder and less frequent than in patients with colitis.[106] Systemic findings are absent, and the diarrhea usually subsides when antibiotics are stopped. Approximately 15% to 25% of patients with antibiotic diarrhea without colitis have cytotoxin in their stools, and up to 40% are culture positive for *C difficile*.

C difficile Colitis Complicating Inflammatory Bowel Disease

C difficile infection can occasionally occur in patients with ulcerative colitis or Crohn's disease, sometimes without prior use of antibiotics.[107,108] A 5% to 25% incidence of cytotoxin positivity or positive stool culture has been reported in relapsed patients with inflammatory bowel disease, mostly after antibiotic exposure. The symptoms of severe diarrhea, bleeding, abdominal pain, and fever may be confused with the symptoms of chronic inflammatory bowel disease. The endoscopic features of *C difficile* infection are difficult to distinguish from the underlying inflammatory bowel disease, and pseudomembranes usually are not present. It is recommended

that stool toxin assay for *C difficile* be obtained on all patients with inflammatory bowel disease during acute relapses, especially after recent exposure to antibiotics.

Diagnosis

The current diagnostic test of choice for *C difficile* is the stool cytotoxin assay. A sterile, cell-free filtrate of diarrheal stool is added to a culture plate of human fibroblasts, which are examined for cellular rounding or detachment after 24 and 48 hours' incubation at 37°C.[70,75] As little as several picograms of *C difficile* toxin B produces a very characteristic rounding of the cell body (cytotoxin effect), which is easily recognized under light microscopy by an experienced observer. The test is made specific by preincubating the stool sample with neutralizing antitoxin. The disadvantages of the assay are the 1- or 2-day incubation period and the requirement for a tissue culture facility, often unavailable in smaller community hospitals. As noted, both toxins A and B possess cytotoxic activity against cultured fibroblasts. Because toxin B is at least 100 times more potent than toxin A on a molar basis, it is likely that stool cytotoxic activity is attributable to toxin B.

Many clinical laboratories report a cytotoxin titer expressed as a dilution factor in stool samples. Cytotoxin titer was correlated in one study with the presence or absence of pseudomembranes,[109] but other investigators have not confirmed a clear-cut relationship between fecal cytotoxin titer and disease severity.[110]

Some hospital laboratories use a commercially available latex bead agglutination assay to detect *C difficile* in stool samples.[111] Originally designed to detect toxin A, the latex assay was subsequently shown to cross-react with antigenic determinants from nontoxigenic strains of *C difficile*, and for this reason the test is not recommended.[112] A new clinical assay, rapid enzyme immunoassay, has been introduced to replace the tissue culture assay in clinical laboratories.[113–115] These assays are based on specific and sensitive antibodies and provide same-day results. Although not quite as sensitive as the tissue culture assay, enzyme immunoassays will probably soon become the test of choice in most hospital laboratories.

Stool culture is a very sensitive test for *C difficile*, but does not differentiate carriers from patients with colitis. A significant portion of hospitalized patients with diarrhea are found to be culture positive but toxin negative for *C difficile*.[84,116] These patients do not have endoscopic evidence of colitis and usually recover without specific therapy. Although sigmoidoscopy and colonoscopy are not required to make the diagnosis of *C difficile* infection, these endoscopic procedures may allow a presumptive diagnosis in patients with diarrhea after antibiotic therapy. This is occasionally important in very ill hospitalized patients in whom it may not be prudent to wait for stool toxin assay. A limited bedside sigmoidoscopy is well tolerated by almost all patients and may provide useful diagnostic information in very ill patients.

Therapy

The natural history of untreated *C difficile* enterocolitis suggests that discontinuation of antibiotic therapy usually results in complete recovery. In one study,[98] diarrhea remitted in less than 10 days when the initiating antibiotics were discontinued promptly, but lasted for 3 to 4 weeks if antibiotics were continued after onset of diarrhea. This suggests that patients with mild antibiotic-associated diarrhea and colitis recover when the precipitating antibiotics are stopped and the colonic microflora is reconstituted.

Because of significant morbidity and mortality from *C difficile*-associated colitis, most patients are treated with antibiotics capable of eradicating *C difficile* from stools. The original mainstay of therapy was vancomycin, a poorly absorbed antibiotic that is highly effective against *C difficile* in vitro. Nearly all strains of *C difficile* are sensitive in vitro to vancomycin in concentrations of 10 μg/mL or less.[117] Concentrations 100- to 500-fold higher than this are present in stools when vancomycin is given orally at doses of 250 mg four times daily. Because vancomycin-resistant strains of *C difficile* have not been reported, this antibiotic is very effective in treating *C difficile* infection. The typical response to vancomycin therapy in patients with documented infection is disappearance of toxin from stools and improvement in diarrhea within 2 to 3 days, and complete disappearance after 1 week of therapy.[118,119] Initial treatment failure is rare with vancomycin. The lower dose of vancomycin, 125 mg four times daily, is as effective as 500 mg four times daily.[120] Despite the fact that *C difficile* is universally sensitive to vancomycin in vitro, the organism may still be cultured from stools during vancomycin therapy, even though symptoms have improved.

The major drawback to vancomycin therapy is expense. Mainly for this reason, metronidazole has emerged as the drug of choice for *C difficile*, in a dosage of 250 mg orally four times daily for 10 days. Metronidazole was known to be effective in vitro against *C difficile*. An initial uncontrolled trial of metronidazole of 1.5 to 2.0 g/day for 7 to 14 days resulted in complete disappearance of diarrhea in 13 patients with cytotoxin-positive PMC.[121] A subsequent prospective, randomized trial of metronidazole versus vancomycin showed excellent clinical response with both agents and a relapse rate of approximately 16% for both.[122] The incidence of side effects was low with both drugs, but metronidazole costs only a tenth as much as vancomycin.

Metronidazole, unlike vancomycin, is significantly absorbed in the upper intestine after oral therapy, and only very low levels are measured in the feces in otherwise healthy subjects.[123] In patients with colitis, metronidazole reaches the colonic lumen primarily by way of the bloodstream because of the increased permeability of the inflamed colonic mucosa. Therapeutic concentrations of metronidazole in feces are also obtained after intravenous administration of 125 mg every 6 hours,[124] and intravenous treatment has been effective in a small number of patients. This is a distinct advantage over vancomycin in seriously ill patients with adynamic ileus or megacolon, because intravenous vancomycin therapy does not achieve therapeutic concentrations in the colon.

Bacitracin is also effective against *C difficile* in vitro and is poorly absorbed from the intestinal tract, thus producing high stool concentrations of the drug. At a dosage of 20,000 units orally every 6 hours, bacitracin produced symptomatic relapse as effectively as vancomycin 125 mg every 6 hours, but vancomycin was more likely than bacitracin to eradicate *C difficile* and its toxin from the stool.[125] Oral teicoplanin 100 mg twice

daily for 10 days also was as effective as vancomycin in treating a small series of patients with PMC.[126]

The anion exchange resins, cholestyramine and colestipol, bind the toxins, and have been used successfully to treat antibiotic-associated colitis and diarrhea. In doses of 4 g three times daily, colestipol and cholestyramine are effective in patients with mild colitis.[127,128] Resins are not recommended as first-line treatment for patients with documented *C difficile* colitis, but they may be useful in treatment of relapse after metronidazole or vancomycin therapy (see section on Relapse). Because resins also bind vancomycin and metronidazole, they should be given several hours apart if used in the same patient.

Diphenoxylate and other antidiarrheal agents are not recommended in the treatment of severe *C difficile* colitis,[129] but may be useful in mild cases. As in other bacterial dysenteries, diphenoxylate may reduce the frequency but not the duration of diarrhea, and theoretically might predispose to ileus and megacolon by inhibiting colonic motility.

A novel approach to therapy of antibiotic-associated diarrhea is administration of nonpathogenic microorganisms, which inhibit the growth of *C difficile*. For example, *Saccharomyces boulardii*, a nonpathogenic yeast used widely in Europe to prevent antibiotic-associated diarrhea, protects hamsters from clindamycin-associated colitis.[130] The same organism, when administered concurrently to hospitalized patients receiving antibiotics, reduced the incidence of antibiotic-associated diarrhea from 22% to 10%.[131]

An unusual remedy for antibiotic-associated colitis or diarrhea in surgical practice has been the administration of fecal enemas to restore the normal flora. Although not esthetically attractive, this form of therapy has a strong rational appeal. Stools from a healthy person (usually a house officer or medical student) are suspended in water and given by enema to patients with antibiotic-associated diarrhea or colitis. This novel approach has been reported to cure relapsing *C difficile* enterocolitis.[132]

Relapse

Approximately 15% to 20% of patients treated successfully with vancomycin relapse after the initial course of therapy. Multiple recurrences in the same patient are not uncommon and may necessitate repeated courses of antibiotic therapy and hospitalizations for severe symptoms. Relapse of *C difficile* colitis typically occurs within 1 to 5 weeks after completion of therapy. Persistence or recurrence of diarrhea during vancomycin or metronidazole therapy is unlikely to be caused by *C difficile*, and should alert the physician to exclude other causes of diarrhea. The signs and symptoms of relapse resemble those of the original infection, and sigmoidoscopic evidence of colitis with or without pseudomembranes may be present. Cytotoxin is present in stools, and *C difficile* cultures are positive.

The mechanisms of symptomatic relapse after metronidazole or vancomycin therapy are unclear. Antibiotic resistance is not a factor because *C difficile* is highly sensitive in vitro to both of these antibiotics. Vancomycin therapy results in elimination of *C difficile* and its cytotoxin from stools of 80% or more of patients, usually within 5 days.[125] In some patients, *C difficile* can still be cultured from stool during and after vancomycin therapy.[133] Persistence of the pathogen during vancomycin therapy may reflect persistence of spores that are insensitive to antibiotics and that can revert to vegetative forms after cessation of antibiotic therapy. Another possibility is that very small numbers of vegetative forms persist during vancomycin therapy and increase in number after the course of treatment.

Reinfection from environmental sources also has been postulated to explain relapse after effective antibiotic therapy. *C difficile* spores survive in the hospital environment for long periods of time and might recolonize hospitalized patients after treatment for *C difficile* infection. Biotyping of *C difficile* isolates from patients with recurrent diarrhea after treatment indicates true relapse with the same strain, rather than reinfection with a different strain.[134]

Many treatment regimens for relapsing *C difficile* colitis have been tried, but none has been completely effective in randomized, clinical trials. One approach favored by the author is to withhold a second course of antibiotics (metronidazole or vancomycin) for mild relapse. The rationale for therapeutic nihilism in this situation is that *C difficile* cannot colonize the bowel in the presence of the normal flora, which reconstitutes itself more quickly if antibiotics are withheld. In one report, withdrawal of antibiotics alone resulted in complete recovery without relapse in patients with mild colitis secondary to *C difficile*.[133] This management plan is obviously not appropriate for hospitalized, acutely ill patients.

When relapse is accompanied by moderately severe symptoms such as high fever, severe abdominal pain, ileus, or significant dehydration, a second course of antibiotic therapy is indicated (Table 84-4). In a study[135] of 22 patients who had experienced a total of 74 relapses, a decreasing dosage schedule of vancomycin followed by pulse therapy every third day for 21 days was successful in all patients, and no further relapses occurred during follow-up of 2 to 12 months. Intermittent or pulse therapy may allow antibiotic-resistant spores to convert to antibiotic-sensitive vegetative forms on the off days. Another treatment regimen for relapse is to repeat a 2-week course of vancomycin or metronidazole in the usual dosages followed by a 2- to 4-week course of an anion-binding resin. Resin and vancomycin should not be taken at the same time, but separated by several hours, because the resins are able to bind the antibiotic and neutralize its effects. The combination

of vancomycin, 125 mg four times daily, and rifampin, 600 mg twice daily, for 7 days was reported to cause disappearance of symptoms within 2 to 3 days and eradication of *C difficile* and its toxins from the stools of patients with symptomatic relapse.[134]

Hospital Control Measures

C difficile is recognized as one of the most common nosocomial infections, colonizing or infecting up to 20% of hospitalized patients. Measures to control the spread of this pathogen have not yet been carefully tested, but standard enteric isolation measures are recommended to limit hospital spread.[84] Patients with *C difficile* diarrhea who are incontinent of feces should be isolated because of the likelihood of spread to roommates. Because *C difficile* can be carried transiently on the hands of hospital personnel, the use of disposable gloves when handling stools or linen and careful handwashing after patient contact are strongly recommended. Environmental contamination can be reduced with disinfectants effective against *C difficile*, such as phosphate-buffered hypochlorite.[84]

COLITIS SECONDARY TO *Escherichia coli* INFECTION

Diarrhea can result from intestinal infection with five distinct strains of *E coli*: *enterotoxigenic, enteropathogenic, enteroadherent, enteroinvasive,* and *enterohemorrhagic*.[136] The latter two strains affect mainly the colon and produce signs and symptoms of disease similar to shigellosis or other dysenteric organisms. These *E coli* strains share certain common features, including plasmid-associated virulence factors, specific interaction with the intestinal mucosa, toxigenicity, and a narrow range of 0:H serotypes within each category.

Colitis Secondary to Enteroinvasive Strains of *Escherichia coli*

Etiology

The enteroinvasive strains of *E coli* (EIEC) were first described by DuPont and colleagues[137] in 1971 and subsequently have been reported as an occasional cause of traveler's diarrhea, and of outbreaks of food-borne gastroenteritis.[138] EIEC account for approximately 5% of children in developing countries who present with bloody diarrhea.[139] These EIEC were reported to cause dysentery in human volunteers that was similar to *Shigella*-associated dysentery.[137] The major pathogenic feature of EIEC is their ability to proliferate within colonocytes, eventually resulting in cell death. This invasive property of *Shigella* species and EIEC is carried on large virulence plasmids that code for production of outer membrane proteins involved in cell invasion.[140] Loss of the virulence plasmid results in loss of invasive phenotype and loss of pathogenicity. Antisera against these factors recognize two virulence antigens, IpaB and IpaC, which are expressed by *Shigella* and EIEC.[141] Most EIEC strains also produce low levels of cytotoxins and enterotoxins, but the relation of these toxins, which are not related to the shiga-like toxins elaborated

TABLE 84-4
Treatment Regimens for Relapse of Antibiotic-Associated Colitis

STUDY	REGIMEN
Tedesco et al, 1978[119]	Vancomycin 125 mg q 6 h for 1 wk 125 mg q 12 h for 1 wk 125 mg q 24 h for 1 wk 125 mg q 48 h for 1 wk 125 mg every third day for 2 wk
Tedesco, 1979[110]	Vancomycin in tapering dosage (as above) plus colestipol 4 g bid
Buggy et al, 1987[134]	Vancomycin 125 mg qid for 1 wk Rifampin 600 mg bid for 1 wk

by enterohemorrhagic strains of *E coli*, to pathogenesis is unknown.[142]

Clinical and Laboratory Features

Typical signs and symptoms of dysentery accompany EIEC infection.[136,137,139] Patients complain of fever, malaise, anorexia, crampy lower abdominal pain, and watery diarrhea followed by passage of small amounts of blood-tinged stool or mucus. Fecal leukocytes are present, as in other bacterial dysenteries. In one study, fecal occult blood and fecal leukocytes were documented in a third of children with EIEC, compared to two thirds of those infected with *Shigella* species.[143] Severe complications of chronicity are not observed with EIEC-associated disease.

Laboratory identification of EIEC requires serotyping of *E coli* 0 and H antigens. Most strains belong to eight different serotypes; strain 0143:H− has been associated with outbreaks in Texas and Mexico.[138] Additional bacteriologic studies for EIEC include the Sereny test, which tests for invasion of the organism in rabbit conjunctivae, Congo red dye binding, and an enzyme-linked immunosorbent assay for membrane proteins associated with invasiveness.[141] DNA probes for identification of the invasion plasmid are diagnostic for EIEC and *Shigella* species, and have been used to identify invasive strains in food-related outbreaks.[138] These more sophisticated molecular probes are not yet available for routine clinical use, however.

Controlled trials of antibiotic therapy in EIEC have not been carried out, and thus specific recommendations regarding treatment are not available. Because EIEC resemble invasive *Shigella* species, antibiotics recommended for the latter also may be effective in EIEC infection.[65] A reasonable approach for the treatment of patients with suspected bacterial dysentery, characterized by bloody stools or mucus containing leukocytes, is to obtain a stool culture and begin empiric treatment with TMP 160 mg/SMZ 800 mg, twice daily, ampicillin 500 mg four times a day, or ciprofloxacin 500 mg twice daily.

Colitis Secondary to Enterohemorrhagic Escherichia coli

Colitis caused by infection with a specific strain of *E coli*, identified as 0157:H7, was first recognized in 1982 in an outbreak of bloody diarrhea traced to contaminated fast-food hamburgers.[144] Since then, numerous outbreaks and sporadic cases of this serious infection have been reported.[145]

Etiology

The strain responsible for hemorrhagic colitis, enterohemorrhagic *E coli* (EHEC), does not invade the gut epithelium, does not produce typical *E coli* heat-labile or heat-stable toxins, and does not display the typical adherence factors found in other pathogenic strains. The primary virulence factor appears to be the production of at least two potent toxins. Shiga-like toxins I and II (also called verotoxins I and II) bear a striking resemblance to the toxins of *S dysenteriae*.[146] Toxin I is nearly identical to shigatoxin, both biochemically and immunologically. Toxin II is antigenically distinct, although its mecha-

nism of action and protein structure are similar to toxin I. These shiga-like or verotoxins share a common mechanism of action with shigatoxin: inactivation of 60 S ribosomes in receptor-bearing cells resulting in inhibition of protein synthesis. Like shigatoxin, EHEC toxins also cause enterotoxicity in ligated ileal loops, cytotoxicity in HeLa and Vero cells, and mouse lethality after parenteral injection.[147] It is thought that intestinal uptake of these toxins may lead to the severe systemic complications of *E coli* 0157:07 infection, including thrombotic thrombocytopenic purpura and HUS.

The genes encoding shiga-like toxins I and II are carried on specific phages. The toxin genes have approximately 50% to 60% overall homology with each other, and encode proteins with typical toxin subunits consisting of five binding subunits of 7.7 kDa and a single catalytic subunit of 33.1 kDa. All strains of *E coli* 0157:H7 associated with hemorrhagic colitis produce large amounts of these toxins. Curiously, all wild strains of *E coli*, including nonpathogenic strains, can be classified as high-, moderate-, or low-toxin-producing based on release of toxins in vitro. Clearly, low toxin production, as occurs in most *E coli* strains, has no apparent pathologic significance.

Clinical and Laboratory Features

A broad clinical spectrum of disease has been described in patients infected with *E coli* 0157:H7.[148] In the typical case, the infection first causes watery diarrhea and abdominal cramps, followed by bloody diarrhea 12 to 24 hours later. Approximately 50% of patients describe blood in the stools. Stools may be streaked with blood or bloody mucus, but in severe cases passage of gross blood and clots may occur. Fever and vomiting occur in less than a fourth of all cases, although in a higher percentage of hospitalized patients. The illness may be confused with intussusception in children, or with inflammatory bowel disease and ischemic colitis in adults.

HUS and thrombotic thrombocytopenic purpura occur in a small percentage of patients during outbreaks of EHEC infection. Children younger than 5 years of age and older adults appear to be particularly susceptible to this dreaded complication, which carries a high mortality rate.[149,150] Most patients in whom these complications develop have bloody diarrhea and white blood counts above 20,000/mm[3].

Examination of stools in this infection generally reveals the presence of fecal leukocytes and red cells. *E coli* 0157:H7 can be cultured on sorbitol-MacConkey culture medium, where it grows as sorbitol-negative colonies. Specific identification requires antibody testing for production of shiga-like toxins. Stool specimens tested 6 days or more after the onset of illness are less likely to be positive for the organism than those tested within 6 days. Hence, a single negative stool culture does not necessarily exclude infection, and two or three samples should be obtained from patients who have had diarrhea longer than 6 days.[151]

Epidemiology

Outbreaks of bloody colitis secondary to 0157:H7 infection have been linked to ground beef served at fast-food restaurants, unpasteurized dairy products, and fecal contamination of a municipal water system.[145] Clusters of cases in elementary schools, day care centers, and nursing homes have been reported. Because dose-response studies have not been performed in human volunteers, it is not known if the infecting dose is related to the severity of diarrhea or complications. Short-term fecal carriers (1 month or less) have been described after outbreaks of disease, but long-term carriage as in *Salmonella* species infection has not been described. Cattle appear to be a reservoir of infection and ingestion of beef or dairy products is often implicated as a risk factor in epidemics. Sporadic cases of EHEC infection occur.[152] In one prospective study of sporadic diarrhea in a health maintenance organization in Washington State, *E coli* 0157:H7 was isolated from stools more frequently than was *Shigella*.[153] In patients with acute bloody diarrhea of infectious origin not associated with outbreaks, EHEC is a frequently isolated pathogen.

Treatment

Recovery without sequelae is the usual outcome in this infection, except for patients with HUS or thrombotic thrombocytopenic purpura, in whom chronic renal failure or neurologic deficit may persist after subsidence of colitis. The effectiveness of antibiotic therapy has not been documented.[145] Some strains of *E coli* 0157:H7 may increase toxin production when exposed to antibiotics, raising the theoretical risk that antibiotics may worsen the condition.[154] Antibiotics are not recommended for this infection, although the organism is usually sensitive to TMP-SMZ, ampicillin, tetracycline, and norfloxacin.[155,156]

SEXUALLY TRANSMITTED ENTERIC INFECTIONS

Homosexual or bisexual men with multiple sexual partners appear to be at high risk for the development of enteric infections, sometimes referred to collectively as the gay bowel syndrome.[157,158] This term is a misnomer inasmuch as women may acquire similar infections (e.g., gonorrheal proctitis) after heterosexual anal intercourse. Gay bowel syndrome should not be confused with the opportunistic enteric infections that occur commonly in patients with AIDS (see Chap. 105). The gay bowel syndrome occurs in immunocompetent homosex-ual men and was first described in 1976,[159] before the discovery of AIDS.

The gay bowel syndrome produces two clinical patterns based on sexual practice and type of pathogen isolated (Table 84-5). The most common form, acute proctitis, is associated with recent anal-receptive intercourse with an infected partner and produces symptoms of anal discharge and bleeding, pain, tenesmus, and diarrhea. The pathogens most frequently associated with proctitis are *N gonorrhoeae*, *C trachomatis*, HSV, and *T pallidum*. Not uncommonly, several pathogens are isolated from a single patient. A diarrheal syndrome in gay men is closely associated with anilinction or fellatio with a partner with a fecally contaminated penis. Multiple enteric pathogens are often isolated from such patients, including *Giardia lamblia*, *E histolytica*, *Shigella* species, and *Campylobacter* species. Both of these conditions are more prevalent in urban gay men with multiple sexual partners. Gay bowel syndrome should be suspected in homosexual men with symptoms of proctitis or dysentery. Failure to take a careful history of sexual preference and practice is often related to the physician's discomfort in asking such questions. Physical examination in some homosexual men may reveal an unusually lax anal sphincter. Routine studies in patients suspected of gay bowel syndrome should include a fecal leukocyte test, a Venereal Disease Research Laboratory antigen test, smears and culture for *N gonorrhoeae*, stool culture for enteric pathogens, stool culture for ova and parasites, and flexible sigmoidoscopy. Additional studies for suspected pathogens should be based on signs or symptoms for specific anorectal infections, as described in the following sections.

Gonorrheal Proctitis

Asymptomatic rectal carriage of *N gonorrhoeae* is common in promiscuous urban gay men. In one study, 53% of patients with positive cultures for this organism were asymptomatic.[160] Rectal carriers may have no symptoms or only mild complaints, such as hemorrhoidal bleeding or constipation, not attributable to this pathogen. Acute rectal gonorrhea in gay men produces symptoms of creamy rectal discharge, rectal bleeding, hematochezia, and anal dyspareunia. Constipation or obstipation is more common than diarrhea. Sigmoidoscopy reveals evidence of mild proctitis with erythema and friability,

TABLE 84-5
Clinical Patterns of the Gay Bowel Syndrome

CONDITION	RISK FACTORS	SYMPTOMS	PATHOGENS
Acute proctitis	Promiscuity Anal-receptive intercourse	Anal discharge or bleeding Anorectal pain Tenesmus Diarrhea	*Neisseria gonorrhoeae* *Chlamydia trachomatis* Herpes simplex virus *Treponema pallidum*
Diarrheal syndrome	Promiscuity Anilinction	Diarrhea Abdominal pain Weight loss	*Giardia lamblia* *Entamoeba histolytica* *Shigella* species *Campylobacter* species

especially around the anal crypts and the anorectal junction. Anorectal gonorrhea is rarely complicated by perirectal abscess or fistula formation, rectal stricture, and septicemia.

Diagnosis of gonococcal proctitis is based on positive culture obtained from rectal swabs.[161] A sterile cotton swab is passed through the anal canal and rotated a few times. Swabs that show visible pus are more likely to be culture positive than swabs coated with feces. Some authorities recommend that rectal swabs be taken through the sigmoidoscope, but it is not clear that this improves recovery of *N gonorrhoeae*. Swabs should be plated directly on Thayer-Martin media or into special transport media. Prompt handling of rectal swabs greatly increases the yield of positive cultures. A second rectal swab should be smeared on a microscope slide and stained with Gram's stain; however, this misses approximately half of gonococcal infections documented by culture and is of diagnostic value only when positive.[158]

Therapy for anorectal gonorrhea is either single intramuscular injection of 4.8 million units of aqueous procaine penicillin G with 1.0 g of probenecid orally, or spectinomycin 2.0 g intramuscularly. Both regimens are associated with cure rates above 95%.[162] Follow-up rectal swab culture in 10 days is highly recommended. Antibiotic-resistant strains of gonococcus are isolated with increasing frequency from patients with acute infection. These strains produce penicillinase, and may also be resistant to tetracycline. Therapy with a third-generation cephalosporin usually is effective for penicillin-resistant strains. Persistence of symptoms after eradication of the gonococcus usually is related to the presence of other pathogens such as herpes virus or *Chlamydia* species.

Chlamydial Proctitis

Infection with *C trachomatis*, the causative agent of lymphogranuloma venereum (LGV), accounts for up to 20% of proctitis in gay men.[157-160] *C trachomatis* is an obligate intracellular organism that is divided into several serotypes; LGV strains L1, L2, and L3 are responsible for proctitis. As with other infections of the anorectum in gay men, asymptomatic carriage of *C trachomatis* infection occurs in 2% to 5%. Acute chlamydial proctitis is accompanied by bloody diarrhea, passage of a mucopurulent discharge, and, less commonly, rectal pain, tenesmus, and constipation. Chronic diarrhea and fistula formation mimicking Crohn's disease may occur.

The pathologic presentation of *C trachomatis* proctitis is distinctive in that granulomatous inflammation with giant cells is found as well as inflammatory changes with neutrophils, eosinophils, and crypt abscesses.[163] Chronic infection leading to fistula formation and stricture is not uncommon. Tender, enlarged lymph nodes or "buboes" can be palpated in the inguinal area. These occur much more commonly in women infected by way of vaginal intercourse but may also be found in men with proctitis. The causative organism can sometimes be demonstrated by Giemsa stain in rectal biopsies or excised lymph nodes. *C trachomatis* infection is determined by culture of the organism from rectal swabs. Rectal swabs should be placed in 0.2 M sucrose-phosphate medium for transport and storage and plated onto McCoy's cells. Immunofluorescent staining of rectal biopsies with specific LGV antisera is also highly sensitive[164] but not widely available.

The treatment of choice of *C trachomatis* proctitis and other forms of LGV is tetracycline 500 mg four times a day for 2 to 3 weeks.

Herpes Simplex Proctitis

HSV is associated with acute proctitis but can also be cultured from asymptomatic people. In one study of nongonococcal proctitis, HSV was isolated from the rectum in 15 of 52 patients, but only 4 had visible mucocutaneous lesions.[157] The clinical features of HSV proctitis are anal pain and tenderness, tenesmus, discharge, and constipation. Herpetic proctitis may be associated with urinary symptoms (retention, poor stream), lower abdominal buttock and thigh pain, impotence, and sacral paresthesias.[165] HSV proctitis produces such exquisite rectal pain and tenderness that many patients cannot tolerate a digital rectal examination or sigmoidoscopy without local or general anesthesia. Sigmoidoscopy during acute infection may reveal the typical small focal ulcers and vesicles of HSV infection. Biopsy reveals acute and chronic inflammatory changes with focal microabscesses and superficial ulcerations.[163]

Diagnosis of HSV infection is based on viral isolation from rectal swabs or biopsies. Approximately 80% to 90% of patients with HSV proctitis are infected with HSV-2; the remainder are infected with HSV-1.[150] Therapy of this condition with acyclovir in standard doses appears to hasten clinical recovery.[166]

Anorectal Syphilis

Proctitis caused by *T pallidum* produces symptoms similar to those seen in other forms of infectious proctitis: rectal pain, discharge, and tenesmus.[157,158] In a screening study of gay men in Sweden,[167] 18 of 133 men showed serologic evidence of syphilis, and all but 2 had been previously treated for syphilis. Primary syphilis of the anorectum produces a chancre of the squamous epithelium in the anal canal. Chancres are indurated lesions approximately 1 to 2 cm in diameter with a raised border. Exudate from chancres should be examined by dark-field microscopy to reveal the presence of the spirochete. Chancres may be multiple, and symmetric lesions on opposite walls of the anal canal are sometimes seen. Inguinal adenopathy is present during the acute stage. Secondary syphilis produces flat, wart-like perianal and penile lesions called condylomata lata. The diagnosis of syphilis is confirmed by serologic testing, although a negative test does *not* exclude early disease. Repeat serologic testing 4 weeks after the primary lesion should be positive if syphilis is present.

Spirochetal organisms similar to *T pallidum* are often found in rectal biopsy specimens of symptomatic and asymptomatic gay men.[168] The organisms can be detected by careful microscopic examination of biopsy specimens and appear as a thick band of filamentous material adherent to surface epithelial cells. The relationship of these spirochetes to intestinal disease is not clear because they are usually found in conjunction with other known pathogens. The taxonomy of these organisms is still unsettled, and many are believed to be related to *T pallidum*.

The treatment of anorectal syphilis is a single intramuscular dose of benzathine penicillin, 2.4 million units, or tetracycline, 500 mg four times daily for 15 days.[169]

Diarrheal Pathogens

Homosexual men are much more likely to harbor certain intestinal parasites, especially *E histolytica* and *G lamblia*, and bacterial pathogens, particularly *Shigella* and *Campylobacter* species.[170] These pathogens may produce a typical diarrheal syndrome in gay men that resembles the signs and symptoms encountered in heterosexual adults. In addition, gay patients may harbor one or more of these pathogens without any symptoms. For example, in one survey of asymptomatic homosexual men attending a venereal disease clinic, 30% harbored *E histolytica*, *G lamblia*, or both.[167] Several other studies[171,172] have documented that symptomatic amebic colitis is rarely observed in gay men. Two unusual features were noted in asymptomatic homosexual men who were positive for *E histolytica*: serum antibodies to amebae were absent, and the stools contained cysts, but not trophozoites. Long-term follow-up of homosexual men who are asymptomatic cyst passers suggests that symptomatic episodes are rare and that antibiotic therapy is not required. Gay male patients with *E histolytica* trophozoites in their stools and evidence of acute colitis, however, should receive standard therapy for acute amoebic dysentery (see Chap. 106). Nonpathogenic amebae are commonly found in gay men with or without *E histolytica*. These include *Entamoeba hartmanni*, *Entamoeba coli*, *Endolimax nana*, *Iodamoeba buetschlii*, and *Dientamoeba fragilis*. None of these commensal organisms requires antibiotic therapy.

G lamblia is often identified in the stools of both symptomatic and asymptomatic gay men. This parasite colonizes the duodenum and produces a syndrome of subacute or acute diarrhea and crampy abdominal pain. In one survey,[167] *G lamblia* was identified in 7.5% of asymptomatic gay men attending a venereal disease clinic. This parasite is often discovered in combination with other pathogens in the stools of patients with proctitis, but it probably has no pathogenic role, unless diarrhea or other symptoms of giardiasis are present (see Chap. 106).

Anal Warts

Anal warts or condyloma accuminata are skin lesions of the anal canal resulting from the human papilloma virus (HPV) infection. Warts in different locations on the body are caused by separate strains of HPV. Common warts or plantar warts are associated with HPV types 1, 2, and 4, whereas genital and anal warts usually are related to HPV type 6.[173] In men, warts are most commonly found on the glans penis; in women, they are most common on the labia, vulva, and cervix. In some patients, genital warts are spread by autoinoculation to the perineal area and anus. Anal warts in men are frequently, but not always, associated with anal-receptive intercourse. The virus is transmitted through intercourse and has a latency period of 1 to 6 months.

Anal warts appear as verrucous, skin-colored or pink papilliform lesions. Often, the lesions are multiple and extend up the anal canal, causing stricture, discharge, and bleeding. Condyloma accuminata must be differentiated from condyloma lata, the warty lesions of secondary syphilis. In comparison to the typical venereal wart, condyloma lata are flatter and have a velvet-like texture. Dark-field examination for spirochetes and serologic tests for syphilis are required for definitive diagnosis. Squamous carcinoma of the anal canal may sometimes be confused with warts but can be easily differentiated by biopsy.

Treatment of anal warts is complicated by a high rate of reinfection and recurrence, especially in patients with numerous sexual partners.[173,174] Podophyllin is a caustic agent that causes regression of warts when applied directly to the lesions, but should not be applied to healthy tissues because it may cause burns. Cryotherapy and surgical fulguration also have been used successfully to treat venereal warts. All forms of treatment are occasionally complicated by formation of anal stricture, which may require dilatation.

The reader is directed to Chapter 26, The Gastrointestinal Microflora; Chapter 38, Approach to the Patient With Diarrhea; Chapter 51, Advice to Travelers; Chapter 70, Small Intestine: Infections With Common Bacterial and Viral Pathogens; and Chapter 131, Microbiologic Studies.

REFERENCES

1. Blaser M, Wells JG, Feldman RA, et al. *Campylobacter* enteritis in the United States: a multicenter study. Ann Int Med 1983;98: 360.
2. Siegel D, Cohen PT, Neighbor M, et al. Predictive value of stool examination in acute diarrhea. Arch Pathol Lab Med 1987;111:715.
3. Shiga K. Ueber den Dysenteriebacillus (*Bacillus dysenteriae*). Zentralblat für Bakteriologie 1898;24:817.
4. DuPont HL. *Shigella* species (bacillary dysentery). In: Mandell GL, Douglas RG, Bennett JE, eds. Principles and practice of infectious diseases. New York: John Wiley & Sons, 1979:1751.
5. Centers for Disease Control. Shigellosis, United States, 1984. MMWR 1985;34:600.
6. Hedberg CN, Levine WC, White KE, et al. An international foodborne outbreak of shigellosis associated with a commercial airline. JAMA 1992;268:3208.
7. Centers for Disease Control. Shigellosis in child day care centers. MMWR 1992;42:440.
8. DuPont HL, Hornick RB, Snyder MJ, et al. Immunity in shigellosis. II. Protection induced by oral live vaccine or primary infection. J Infect Dis 1972;125:12.
9. Hornick RB, Greisman SE, Woodward TE, et al. Typhoid fever: pathogenesis and immunologic control. N Engl J Med 1970;283:686.
10. Shiga K. The trend of prevention, therapy and epidemiology of dysentery since the discovery of its causative organism. N Engl J Med 1936;215:1205.
11. Mata LJ, Gangarosa EJ, Caceres A, et al. Epidemic shiga bacillus dysentery in Central America. I. Etiologic investigations in Guatemala. J Infect Dis 1970;122:170.
12. Lolekha S, Vibulbandhitkit S, Poonyarit P. Response to antimicrobial therapy for shigellosis in Thailand. Rev Infect Dis 1991;13(Suppl 4):S342.
13. Hale TL, Keren DF. Pathogenesis and immunology in shigellosis: applications for vaccine development. Curr Top Microbiol Immunol 1992;180:117.
14. Speelman P, Kabir I, Islam M. Distribution and spread of colonic

lesions in shigellosis: a colonoscopic study. J Infect Dis 1984;150:899.

15. Maurelli AT, Samsonetti PJ. Genetic determinants of *Shigella* pathogenicity. Annu Rev Microbiol 1988;42:127.

16. Hale TL, Oaks EV, Formal SB. Identification and antigenic characterization of virulence-associated, plasmid-coated proteins of *Shigella* spp. and enteroinvasive *Escherichia coli*. Infect Immun 1983;39:505.

17. Fontaine A, Arondel J, Samsonetti PJ. Role of shiga toxin in the pathogenesis of bacillary dysentery, studied by using a tox-mutant of *Shigella dysenteriae*. Infect Immun 1988;56:3099.

18. Prado D, Clary TG, Pickering LK. The relation between productions of cytotoxins and clinical features in shigellosis. J Infect Dis 1986;154:149.

19. O'Brien AD, Holmes RK. Shiga and shiga-like toxins. Microbiol Rev 1987;51:206.

20. Keusch GT, Donohue-Rolfe A, Jacewicz M. *Shigella* toxin and the pathogenesis of shigellosis. Ciba Found Symp 1985;112:193.

21. Keusch GT, Jacewicz M, Mobassaleh M, et al. Shiga toxin: intestinal cell receptors and pathophysiology of enterotoxic effects. Rev Infect Dis 1991;13(Suppl 4):5304.

22. Mobassaleh M, Donohue-Rolfe A, Jacwicz M, et al. Pathogenesis of *Shigella* diarrhea: evidence for a developmentally-regulated glycolipid receptor for *Shigella* toxin involved in the fluid secretory response of rabbit small intestine. J Infect Dis 1988;157:1023.

23. Eiklid K, Olsnes S. Entry of *Shigella dysenteriae* toxin into Hela cells. Infect Immun 1983;42:771.

24. Reisbig R, Olsnes S, Eiklid K. The cytotoxic activity of *Shigella* toxin: evidence of catalytic inactivation of the 60s ribosomal subunit. J Biol Chem 1981;256:8739.

25. Holmgren J, Svennerholm AM. Bacterial enteric infections and vaccine development. Gastroenterol Clin North Am 1992;21:283.

26. Cohen D, Green MS, Block, et al. Serum antibodies to lipopolysaccharide and natural immunity to shigellosis in an Israeli military population. J Infect Dis 1988;157:1068.

27. Black RE, Levin MM, Clements ML, et al. Prevention of shigellosis by a *Salmonella typhi-Shigella sonnei* bivalent vaccine. J Infect Dis 1987;155:1260.

28. Winsor DK, Matthewson JJ, DuPont JL. Comparison of serum and fecal antibody responses of patients with naturally acquired *Shigella sonnei* infection. J Infect Dis 1988;158:1108.

29. Oaks EV, Hale TL, Formal SB. Serum immune response to *Shigella* protein antigens in rhesus monkeys and humans injected with *Shigella* spp. Infect Immun 1986;53:57.

30. Halpern Z, Dan M, Giladi M, et al. Shigellosis in adults: epidemiologic clinical and laboratory features. Medicine 1989;68:210.

31. Guerrant RL, Shields DS, Thorson SM, et al. Evaluation and diagnosis of acute infectious diarrhea. Am J Med 1985;78(Suppl 6B):91.

32. Levine MM, DuPont HL, Khodabandelou M, et al. Long-term *Shigella*-carrier state. N Engl J Med 1973;288:1169.

33. Strulens MJ, Patte D, Kabir I, et al. *Shigella* septicemia: prevalence, presentation risk factors and outcome. J Infect Dis 1985;152:784.

34. Bennish ML. Potentially lethal complications of shigellosis. Rev Infect Dis 1991;13(Suppl 4):5319.

35. Simon DG, Kaslow RA, Rosenbaum J, et al. Reiter's syndrome following epidemic shigellosis. J Rheumatol 1981;8:969.

36. Finch M, Rodey G, Lawrence D, et al. Epidemic Reiter's syndrome following an outbreak of shigellosis. Eur J Epidemiol 1986;2:26.

37. Arnett FC. HLA and the spondyloarthropathies. In: Calin A, ed. Spondyloarthropathies. New York: Grune & Stratton, 1984:297.

38. Gulline-Alvarez G, Bolanos EV. Sindrome hemolitcco uremico: reporte de 60 casos asociados a una epidemica de enterocolitis hemorrhagia. Rev Colombiana Pediatr 1974;28:414.

39. Rahman MM, Alan A, Islam MR, et al. Shiga bacillus dysentery associated with marked leukocytosis and erythrocyte fragmentation. Johns Hopkins Med J 1975;136:65.

40. Karmali MA, Petric M, Lin C, et al. The association between idiopathic hemolytic-uremic syndrome and infection by verotoxin-producing *Escherichia coli*. J Infect Dis 1985;151:775.

41. Koster F, Levin J, Walker L, et al. Hemolytic uremic syndrome after shigellosis. N Engl J Med 1978;298:927.

42. Butler T, Rahman H, Al-Mahmud KA, et al. An animal model of haemolytic-uraemic syndrome in shigellosis: lipopolysaccharides of *Shigella dysenteriae* type 1 and *S. flexneri* produce leukocyte-mediated renal cortical necrosis in rabbits. J Exp Pathol 1985;66:7.

43. Rowe B, Threllfall EJ. Drug resistance in gram negative aerobic bacilli. Br Med Bull 1984;40:68.

44. Lin SR, Chang SF. Drug resistance and plasmid profile of shigellae in Taiwan. Epidemiol Infect 1992;108:87.

45. Pickering L, DuPont HL, Olarte J. Single dose tetracycline therapy for shigellosis in adults. JAMA 1978;239:853.

46. Nelson JD, Kusmiesz H, Jackson LH, et al. Trimethoprim/sulfamethoxazole therapy for shigellosis. JAMA 1976;235:1239.

47. Ericsson CD, Johnson PC, DuPont HL, et al. Ciprofloxacin or trimethoprin-sulfamethoxazole as initial therapy for traveler's diarrhea. Ann Intern Med 1987;106:216.

48. Bennish ML, Salam MA, Khan MA, Khan AM. Treatment of shigellosis. III. Comparison of one- or two-dose ciprofloxacin with standard 5-day therapy: a randomized, blinded, trial. Ann Intern Med 1992;117:727.

49. DuPont HL, Hornick RB. Adverse effect of Lomotil therapy in shigellosis. JAMA 1973;226:1525.

50. Blaser MJ. *Campylobacter* enteritis. In: Ellner PD, ed. Infectious diarrheal diseases. New York: Marcel Dekker, 1984:1.

51. Perez-Perez GI, Blaser MJ. *Campylobacter* and *Helicobacter*. In: Baron S, ed. Medical microbiology. 3rd ed. New York: Churchill-Livingstone, 1991:337.

52. Blaser MJ, Berkowitz ID, LaForce FM, et al. *Campylobacter* enteritis: clinical and epidemiologic features. Ann Intern Med 1979;91:179.

53. Blaser MJ, Reller LB. *Campylobacter* enteritis. N Engl J Med 1981;305:1444.

54. Duffy MC, Benson JB, Dubin SJ. Mucosal invasion in *Campylobacter* enteritis. Am J Clin Pathol 1980;73:706.

55. Ruiz-Palcios GM, Torres J, Torres NI, et al. Cholera-like enterotoxin produced by *Campylobacter jejuni*. Lancet 1983;2:250.

56. Yeen WD, Puthucheary SD, Pang T. Demonstration of a cytotoxin form *Campylobacter jejuni*. J Clin Pathol 1983;36:1237.

57. Klipstein FA, Evgert RF, Short H, et al. Pathogenic properties of *Campylobacter jejuni*: assay and correlation with clinical manifestations. Infect Immun 1985;50:43.

58. Black RE, Levin MM, Clements ML, et al. Experimental *Campylobacter jejuni* infection in humans. J Infect Dis 1988;157:472.

59. Winsor DK, Mathewson JJ, DuPont HL. Western blot analysis on intestinal secretory immunoglobin A response to *Campylobacter jejuni* antigens in patients with naturally acquired *Campylobacter* enteritis. Gastroenterology 1986;90:1217.

60. Newman A, Lambert JR. *Campylobacter jejuni* causing flare-up in inflammatory bowel disease. Lancet 1980;2:919.

61. Blaser MJ, Perez GP, Smith PF, et al. Extraintestinal *Campylobacter jejuni* and *Campylobacter coli* infections: host factors and strain characteristics. J Infect Dis 1986;153:552.

62. Urman JD, Zuerier RB, Rothfield NF. Reiter's syndrome associated with *Campylobacter fetus* infection. Ann Intern Med 1977;86:444.

63. Delans RJ, Biuso JD, Saba SR, et al. Hemolytic-uremic syndrome after *Campylobacter*-induced diarrhea in an adult. Arch Intern Med 1984;144:1074.

64. Perlman DM, Ampel NM, Schifman RB, et al. Persistent *Campylobacter jejuni* infections in patients infected with human immunodeficiency virus (HIV). Ann Intern Med 1988;108:540.

65. Levine MM. Antimicrobial therapy for infectious diarrhea. Rev Infect Dis 1986;8(Suppl 2):5207.

66. Pitkanen T, Ponka A, Petersson T, et al. *Campylobacter* enteritis in 188 hospitalized patients. Arch Intern Med 1983;143:215.

67. DuPont HL, Ericsson CD, Robins A, et al. Current problems

in antimicrobial therapy for bacterial enteric infection. Am J Med 1987;82(Suppl 4A):324.

68. Segreti J, Gootz TD, Goodman LT, et al. High level quinolone resistance in clinical isolates of *Campylobacter jejuni*. J Infect Dis 1992;165:667.

69. Hall IC, O'Toole E. Intestinal flora in newborn infants. Am J Dis Child 1935;49:390.

70. Bartlett JG, Moon N, Chang TW, et al. Role of *Clostridium difficile* in antibiotic-associated pseudomembranous colitis. Gastroenterology 1978;75:778.

71. George WL, Sutter VL, Citron D, et al. Selective and differential medium for isolation of *Clostridium difficile*. J Clin Microbiol 1979;9:214.

72. Delmee M, Homel M, Wauters G. Serogrouping of *Clostridium difficile* strains of slide agglutination. J Clin Microbiol 1985;21:323.

73. Kupier EJ, Oudbier JH, Stuifbergen WN, et al. Application of whole-cell DNA restriction endonuclease profiles to the epidemiology of *Clostridium difficile*-induced diarrhea. J Clin Microbiol 1987;25:751.

74. Hafiz S, Oakley CL. *Clostridium difficile*: isolation and characteristics. J Med Microbiol 1976;9:136.

75. Bartlett JG, Chang TW, Gurwith M, et al. Antibiotic-associated pseudomembranous colitis due to toxin-producing clostridia. N Engl J Med 1978;298:531.

76. Eichel-Streiber C, Laufeinberg-Feldman R, Sartingen S, et al. Cloning of *Clostridium difficile* toxin B gene and demonstration of high N-terminal homology between toxin A and B. Med Microbiol Immunol 1990;179:271.

77. Dove CH, Wang S, Price SB, et al. Molecular characterization of the *Clostridium difficile* toxin A gene. Infect Immun 1990;58:480.

78. Triadafilopoulos G, Pothoulakis C, O'Brien MJ, et al. Differential effects of *Clostridium difficile* toxins A and B in rabbit ileum. Gastroenterology 1987;93:273.

79. Pothoulakis C, Sullivan R, Melnick DA, et al. *Clostridium difficile* toxin A stimulates intracellular calcium release and chemotactic response in human granulocytes. J Clin Invest 1988;81:1741.

80. Hecht G, Pothoulakis C, LaMont, JT, et al. *Clostridium difficile* toxin A perturbs cytoskeletal and tight junction permeability of cultured human intestinal epithelial monolayers. J Clin Invest 1988;82:1516.

81. Viscidi R, Laughon BE, Yoken R, et al. Serum antibody response to toxins A and B of *Clostridium difficile*. J Infect Dis 1983;148:93.

82. Johnson S, Gerding DN, Janoff EN. Systemic and mucosal antibody responses to toxin A in patients infected with *Clostridium difficile*. J Infect Dis 1992;166:1287.

83. Kim P-H, Iaconis JP, Rolfe RD. Immunization of adult hamsters against *Clostridium difficile*-associated ileocecitis and transfer of protection of infant hamsters. Infect Immun 1987;55:2984.

84. McFarland LV, Mulligan ME, Kwok RY, et al. Nosocomial acquisition of *Clostridium difficile* infection. N Engl J Med 1989;320:240.

85. Kim R-H, Fekety R, Batts DH, et al. Isolation of *Clostridium difficile* from the environment and contacts of patients with antibiotic-associated colitis. J Infect Dis 1981;143:42.

86. Fekety R, Kim K-H, Brown D, et al. Epidemiology of antibiotic-associated colitis: isolation of *Clostridium difficile* from the hospital environment. Am J Med 1981;70:906.

87. Mulligan ME, Rolfe RD, Finegold SM, et al. Contamination of the hospital environment by *Clostridium difficile*. Current Microbiology 1979;3:173.

88. Kim K, DuPont HL, Pickering LK. Outbreaks of diarrhea associated with *Clostridium difficile* and its toxin in day-care centers: evidence of person-to-person spread. J Pediatr 1983;102:376.

89. Bender BS, Laughon BE, Grydos C, et al. Is *Clostridium difficile* endemic in chronic care facilities? Lancet 1986;2:11.

90. Al-Jumaili IJ, Shibley M, Lishman AH, et al. Incidence and origin of *Clostridium difficile* in neonates. J Clin Microbiol 1984;19:77.

91. Larson HE, Barclay FE, Honour P, et al. Epidemiology of *Clostridium difficile* in infants. J Infect Dis 1982;146:727.

92. Cooperstock M, Steffan E, Yolken R, et al. *Clostridium difficile* in normal infants and sudden death syndrome: an association with infant formula feeding. Pediatrics 1982;70:91.

93. Donta ST, Nyers MG. *Clostridium difficile* toxin in asymptomatic neonates: fetal and neonatal medicine. J Pediatr 1982;100:431.

94. Krivan HC, Clark GF, SMith DF, et al. Cell surface binding site for *Clostridium difficile* enterotoxin: evidence for a glycoconjugate containing the sequence Galα 1-3 Galβ 1-4 GlcNac. Infect Immun 1986;53:573.

95. Eglow R, Pothoulakis C, Itzkowitz S, et al. Diminished *Clostridium difficile* toxin A sensitivity in newborn rabbit ileum is associated with decreased toxin A receptor. J Clin Invest 1992;90:822.

96. Viscidi R, Willey S, Bartlett JG. Isolation rates and toxigenic potential of *Clostridium difficile* isolates from various patient populations. Gastroenterology 1981;81:5.

97. Altemeier WA, Hammel RP, Hill EO. Staphylococcal enterocolitis following antibiotic therapy. Ann Surg 1963;157:847.

98. Tedesco FJ, Barton RW, Alpers DH. Clindamycin-associated colitis: a prospective study. Ann Intern Med 1974;81:429.

99. Fekety R, Shah AB. Diagnosis and treatment of *Clostridium difficile* colitis. JAMA 1993;269-71.

100. Price AB, Davies DR. Pseudomembranous colitis. J Clin Pathol 1977;30:1.

101. Tedesco FJ, Corless JK, Brownstein RE. Rectal sparing in antibiotic-associated pseudomembranous colitis: a prospective study. Gastroenterology 1982;83:1259.

102. Waddell TK, Macleod RS, Rotstein OD, et al. Surgical management of fulminant pseudomembranous colitis. Can J Surg 1992;35:555.

103. Medich DS, Lee KK, Simmons RL et al. Laparotomy for fulminant pseudomembranous colitis. Arch Surg 1992;127:847.

104. Gerding DN, Olson MM, Peterson LR, et al. *Clostridium difficile* associated diarrhea and colitis in adults. Arch Intern Med 1986;146:95-100.

105. Totter MA, Gregg JA, Fremont-Smith P, et al. Clinical and pathologic spectrum of antibiotic-associated colitis. Am J Gastroenterol 1978;69:311.

106. Lishman AH, Al-Jumaili IJ, Record CO. Spectrum of antibiotic-associated diarrhea. Gut 1981;22:34.

107. LaMont JT, Trnka Y. Therapeutic implications of *Clostridium difficile* toxin during relapse of inflammatory bowel disease. Lancet 1980;1:381.

108. Bolton RP, Sherriff RJ, Read AE. *Clostridium difficile*-associated diarrhea: a role in inflammatory bowel disease? Lancet 1980;1:383.

109. Burdon DW, George RH, Mogg GA, et al. Faecal toxin and severity of pseudomembranous colitis. J Clin Pathol 1981;34:548.

110. Tedesco FJ. Antibiotic-associated pseudomembranous colitis with negative proctosigmoidoscopy examination. Gastroenterology 1979;77:295.

111. Peterson LR, Holter JJ, Shanholtzer CW, et al. Detection of *Clostridium difficile* toxins A (enterotoxin) and B (cytotoxin) in clinical specimens. Am J Clin Pathol 1986;86:208.

112. Lyerly DM, Wilkins TD. Commercial latex test for *Clostridium difficile* toxin A does not detect toxin A. Am J Clin Microbiol 1986;23:622.

113. DePersio JR, Varga FJ, Conwell DL, et al. Development of a rapid enzyme immunoassay for *Clostridium difficile* toxin A and its use in the diagnosis of *C. difficile*-associated disease. J Clin Microbiol 1991;29:2724.

114. Delmee M, Mackey T, Hamitou A. Evaluation of a new commercial *Clostridium difficile* toxin A enzyme immunoassay using diarrheal stools. Eur J Clin Microbiol Infect Dis 1992;11:246.

115. DeGirolami PC, Hanff PA, Eichelberger K, et al. Multicenter evaluation of a new enzyme immunoassay for detection of *Clostridium difficile* enterotoxin A. J Clin Microbiol 1992;30:1085.

116. Lashner BA, Todorczuk J, Sahm DF, et al. *Clostridium difficile* culture-positive toxin-negative diarrhea. Am J Clin Gastroenterol 1986;81:940.

117. Burdon DW, Brown JD, Youngs DJ, et al. Antibiotic suscep-

tibility of *Clostridium difficile*. J Antimicrob Chemother 1979;5:307.

118. Keighley MR, Burdon DW, Arabi Y, et al. Randomized controlled trial of vancomycin for pseudomembranous colitis and post-operative diarrhea. Br Med J 1978;2:1667.

119. Tedesco FJ, Markham R, Gurwith M, et al. Oral vancomycin for antibiotic-associated pseudomembranous colitis. Lancet 1978;2:226.

120. Fekety R, Silva J, Kauffman C, et al. Treatment of antibiotic-associated *Clostridium difficile* colitis with oral vancomycin: comparison of two dosage regimens. Am J Med 1989;86:15.

121. Cherry RD, Porthroy D, Jabbari M, et al. Metronidazole: an alternate therapy for antibiotic-associated colitis. Gastroenterology 1982;82:849.

122. Teasley DG, Olson MM, Gebbhard RL, et al. Prospective randomized trial of metronidazole versus vancomycin for *Clostridium difficile*-associated diarrhea and colitis. Lancet 1983;2:1043.

123. Arabi Y, Dimock F, Burdon DW, et al. Influence of neomycin and metronidazole on colonic microflora of volunteers. J Antimicrob Chemother 1979;5:531.

124. Bolton RP, Culshaw MA. Faecal metronidazole concentrations during oral and intravenous therapy for antibiotic-associated colitis due to *Clostridium difficile*. Gut 1986;27:1169.

125. Young GP, Ward PB, Bagley N, et al. Antibiotic colitis due to *Clostridium difficile*: double-blind comparison of vancomycin with bacitracin. Gastroenterology 1985;89:1038.

126. de Lalla F, Nicolin R, Rinaldi E, et al. Prospective study of oral teicoplanin vs oral vancomycin for therapy of pseudomembranous colitis and *Clostridium difficile*-associated diarrhea. Antimicrob Agents Chemother 1992;36:2192.

127. Chang TW, Onderdonk AB, Bartlett JG. Anion-exchange resins in antibiotic-associated colitis. Lancet 1978;2:258.

128. Kreutzer EW, Miligan FD. Treatment of antibiotic-associated pseudomembranous colitis with cholestyramine resin. Johns Hopkins Med J 1978;143:67.

129. George WL, Rolfe RO, Finegold SM. Treatment and prevention of antimicrobial agent-induced colitis and diarrhea. Gastroenterology 1980;79:366.

130. Toothaker RD, Elmer GW. Prevention of clindamycin-induced mortality in hamsters by *Saccharomyces boulardii*. Antimicrob Agents Chemother 1984;26:552.

131. Surawicz CM, Elmer GW, Speelman P, et al. Prevention of antibiotic-associated diarrhea by *Saccharomyces boulardii*: a prospective study. Gastroenterology 1989;96:981.

132. Schwan A, Sjolin S, Trottestarn U, et al. Relapsing *Clostridium difficile* enterocolitis cured by rectal infusion of normal faeces. Scand J Infect Dis 1984;16:211.

133. Walters BA, Roberts R, Stafford R, et al. Relapse of antibiotic-associated colitis: endogenous persistence of *Clostridium difficile* during vancomycin therapy. Gut 1983;24:206.

134. Buggy BP, Fekety R, Silva J. Therapy of relapsing *Clostridium difficile*-associated diarrhea and colitis with the combination of vancomycin and rifampin. J Clin Gastroenterol 1987;2:155.

135. Tedesco FJ, Gordon D, Fortson WC. Approach to patients with multiple relapses of antibiotic-associated pseudomembranous colitis. Am J Gastroenterol 1985;80;867.

136. Levine MM. *Escherichia coli* that cause diarrhea: enterotoxigenic, enteropathogenic, enteroinvasive, enterohemorrhagic and enteroadherent. J Infect Dis 1987;155:377.

137. DuPont HL, Formal SB, Hornick RB, et al. Pathogenesis of *Escherichia coli* diarrhea. N Engl J Med 1971;285:1.

138. Gordillo ME, Reeve GR, Pappas J, et al. Molecular characterization of strains of enteroinvasive *Escherichia coli* 0143, including isolates from a large outbreak in Houston, Texas. J Clin Microbiol 1992;30:889.

139. Escheverria P, Sethabutr O, Serichantalergs O, et al. *Shigella* and enteroinvasive *Escherichia coli* infections in households of children with dysentery in Bangkok. J Infect Dis 1992;165:144.

140. Small PL, Falkow S. Identification of regions on a 230-kilobase plasmid from enteroinvasive *Escherichia coli* that are required for entry into Hep-2 cells. Infect Immun 1988;56:225.

141. Pal T, Formal SB, Hale TL. Characterization of virulence marker antigen of *Shigella* spp. and enteroinvasive *Escherichia coli*. J Clin Microbiol 1989;27:561.

142. Fasano A, Kay BA, Russell RG, et al. Enterotoxin and cytotoxin production by enteroinvasive *Escherichia coli*. Infect Immun 1990; 58:3717.

143. Echeverria P, Sethabutr O, Pitarangsi C. Microbiology and diagnosis of infections with *Shigella* and enteroinvasive *Escherichia coli*. Rev Infect Dis 1991;13(Suppl 4):5220.

144. Riley LW, Remis RS, Helgerson SD, et al. Hemorrhagic colitis associated with a rare *Escherichia coli* serotype. N Engl J Med 1983;308:681.

145. Griffin PM, Tauxe RV. The epidemiology of infections caused by *Escherichia coli* 0157:H7, other enterohemorrhagic *E. coli*, and the associated hemolytic uremic syndrome. Epidemiol Rev 1991;13:60.

146. Karmali MA. Infection by verocytotoxin-producing *Escherichia coli*. Clin Microbiol Rev 1989;2:15.

147. O'Brien AD, Holmes RK. Shiga and shiga-like toxins. Microbiol Rev 1987;51:206.

148. Griffin PM. Illness associated with *Escherichia coli* 0157:H7 infections: a broad clinical spectrum. Ann Intern Med 1988;109:705.

149. Cordovez A, Prado V, Maggi L, et al. Enterohemorrhagic *Escherichia coli* associated with hemolytic uremic syndrome in Chilean children. J Clin Microbiol 1992;30:2153.

150. Martin DL, MacDonald KL, White KE, et al. The epidemiology and clinical aspects of the hemolytic uremic syndrome in Minnesota. New Engl J Med 1990;323:1161.

151. Wells JG, Pavis BR, Wachsmuth IK, et al. Laboratory investigation of hemorrhagic colitis outbreaks associated with a rare *Escherichia coli* serotype. J Clin Microbiol 1983;18:512.

152. Remis RS, MacDonald KL, Riley LW, et al. Sporadic cases of hemorrhagic colitis associated with *Escherichia coli* 0157:07. Ann Intern Med 1984;101:624.

153. MacDonald KL, O'Leary MJ, Cohen ML, et al. *Escherichia coli* 0157:H7, an emerging gastrointestinal pathogen: results of a one year, prospective, population-based study. JAMA 1988;259:3567.

154. Carter AO, Borczyk AA, Carlson JA, et al. A severe outbreak of *Escherichia coli* 01567:07-associated hemorrhagic colitis in nursing home. N Engl J Med 1987;317:1496.

155. Ratnam S, March SB, Ahmed R, et al. Characterization of *Escherichia coli* serotype 0157:H07. J Clin Microbiol 1988;26:2006.

156. Pai CH, Gordon R, Sims HV, et al. Sporadic cases of hemorrhagic colitis associated with *Escherichia coli* 0157:07. Ann Intern Med 1984;101:738.

157. Quinn TC, Corey L, Chaffee RG, et al: The etiology of anorectal infections in homosexual men. Am J Med 1981;71:395.

158. Baker RW, Peppercorn MA. Gastrointestinal ailments of homosexual men. Medicine 1982;61:390.

159. Kazal HL, Sohn N, Corrasco JI, et al. The gay bowel syndrome: clinicopathologic correlation in 260 cases. Ann Clin Lab Sci 1976;6:184.

160. Rompalo AM, Price CB, Roberts PL, et al. Potential value of rectal-screening cultures for *Chlamydia trachomatis* in homosexual men. J Infect Dis 1986;153:888.

161. Klein EJ, Fisher LS, Chou AW, et al. Anorectal gonococcal infection. Ann Intern Med 1977;86:340.

162. Lebedoff DA, Hochman EB. Rectal gonorrhea in men: diagnosis and treatment. Ann Intern Med 1980;92:463.

163. Surawicz CM, Goodell SE, Quinn TC, et al. Spectrum of rectal biopsy abnormalities in homosexual men with intestinal symptoms. Gastroenterology 1986;91:651.

164. Klotz SA, Drutz DJ, Tam MR, et al. Hemorrhagic proctitis due to lymphogranuloma venereum serogroup L2. N Engl J Med 1983;308:1563.

165. Goldmeier D. Proctitis and herpes simplex virus in homosexual men. Br J Vener Dis 1980;56:111.

166. Rompalo AM, Mertz GJ, Davis LG, et al. Oral acyclovir for treatment of first-episode herpes simplex virus proctitis. JAMA 1988;259:2879-2881.

167. Hakansson C, Kjell T, Norkrans G, et al. Intestinal parasitic

infection and other sexually transmitted diseases in asymptomatic homosexual men. Scand J Infect Dis 1984;16:199.

168. Surawicz CM, Roberts PL, Rompalo A, et al. Intestinal spirochetosis in homosexual men. Am J Med 1987;82:587.

169. Centers for Disease Control. Syphilis: recommended treatment schedules. MMWR 1976;25:101.

170. Quinn TC, Goodell SE, Fennell C, et al. Infections with *Campylobacter jejuni* and *Campylobacter*-like organisms in homosexual men. Ann Intern Med 1984;101:187.

171. Allason-Jones E, Mindel A, Sargeaunt P, et al. *Entamoeba histolytica* as a commensal intestinal parasite in homosexual men. N Engl J Med 1986;315:353.

172. Allason-Jones E, Mindel A, Sargeaunt P, et al. Outcome of untreated infection with *Entamoeba histolytica* in homosexual men with and without HIV antibody. Br Med J 1988;297:654.

173. Koutsky LA, Wolner-Hanssen P. Genital human papillomavirus infections: current knowledge and future prospects. Obstet Gynecol Clin North Am 1989;16:541.

174. MacLeod JH. A method of proctology. Hagerstown, MD: Harper & Row, 1979:64.

Textbook of Gastroenterology, second edition, edited by Tadataka Yamada. JB Lippincott Company, Philadelphia © 1995.

CHAPTER 85

Colonic Polyps: Benign and Premalignant Neoplasms of the Colon

Gordon D. Luk

Epidemiology
  Prevalence
  Hereditary Factors
  Anatomic Distribution
  Association With Other Diseases
  Nonneoplastic Polyps
Etiology
  Polyp Formation Theories
  Contributory Factors
  Adenoma (Dysplasia)—Carcinoma Sequence
  Genetic Factors
Clinical Manifestations
  Signs and Symptoms
  Neoplastic Polyps
  Nonneoplastic Polyps
  Submucosal Lesions
Differential Diagnosis
Screening Studies
  Sigmoidoscopy

  Radiography
  Colonoscopy
Diagnostic Studies
  Radiography
  Colonoscopy
  Biopsy and Histopathologic Examination
Biochemical and Molecular Markers
Clinical Course and Complications
  Natural History
  Metachronous Adenomas
  Malignant Polyps
Therapy
  Polypectomy
  Laser Ablation
  Surgical Resection
  Noninvasive Carcinoma
  Malignant Polyp
  Follow-Up

The term *polyp* refers to any tissue protrusion above the mucosal surface. In the colon, polyps are protrusions into the lumen. Polyps may assume varying sizes and shapes. A polyp can be described by the texture of its mucosal surface, color, or presence of a stalk, ulcerations, or bleeding. The most important characteristic is the histologic type. Colonic polyps (or polypoid lesions) may be classified into three main subgroups (Table 85-1). These are the neoplastic polyps, which consist of the adenomatous polyps (adenomas) and the carcinomas; the nonneoplastic polyps; and submucosal lesions (which produce a polypoid lesion). Interest in colonic polyps has increased for several clinically relevant reasons.

TABLE 85-1
Classification of Colonic Polyps

NEOPLASTIC	NONNEOPLASTIC	SUBMUCOSAL TUMORS
Premalignant	Mucosal	Lymphoid
(adenomas)	Hyperplastic	Pneumatosis cystoides intestinalis
Tubular	Inflammatory	Colitis cystica profunda
Tubulovillous	Pseudopolyp	Lipoma
Villous	Hamartoma	Carcinoid
Malignant	Juvenile	Metastatic lesions
(carcinomas)	Peutz-Jeghers	Leiomyoma
Noninvasive carcinoma	Other	Hemangioma
Malignant polyp		Fibroma
		Other

The availability of flexible fiberoptic endoscopic instruments has facilitated the detection and removal of colonic polyps (see Chap. 116). Interest in the adenomas has also increased with the understanding of their role as premalignant precursors of colonic carcinomas (see Chap. 87). The nonneoplastic polyps do not share this high premalignant potential. Recent work in adenomas and in the inherited polyposis syndromes has identified the *APC* gene, which is mutated or lost in patients with adenomatous polyposis coli and with sporadic colorectal neoplasms, and other genes involved in colorectal cancer (see Chaps. 86 and 87). Owing to this increasing significance of the colonic adenoma, trials in large-scale screening and detection for occult gastrointestinal bleeding (see Chap. 31) and in early detection of colorectal neoplasms are ongoing (see Chap. 87).

Colonic polyps may be divided into three separate groups, neoplastic, nonneoplastic, and submucosal lesions. The neoplastic polyps are of greatest clinical significance because of their premalignant nature, and their potential to progress to carcinoma. Submucosal lesions are uncommon, and their clinical significance depends on the underlying etiology.

Colonic polyps usually are asymptomatic. They are frequently found during screening or early detection testing for colorectal cancers. When the presence of colonic polyps is highly suspected, the definitive diagnostic, and often therapeutic, test is complete colonoscopy and polypectomy. Endoscopic polypectomy will adequately treat most adenomatous polyps, including those with severe focal atypia or intramucosal carcinoma. Malignant polyps with poor prognostic features, however, may require surgical resection.

Adenomas and their malignant counterparts—the carcinomas—constitute the colonic polyps with malignant potential. Nonneoplastic polyps have little or no malignant potential. As discussed later in this chapter and in Chapters 86 and 87, nonneoplastic polyps, especially when they occur in a setting of inherited polyposis syndromes, are associated with cancers of the gastrointestinal tract and other organs. The malignant potential of submucosal lesions depends on their underlying etiology.

The malignant potential of the adenomatous polyp depends on size, number, architectural type, and degree of atypia. Those polyps larger than 1 cm, multiple, with a large villous architectural component or with severe atypia are those with a high frequency of malignancy. The natural history of the progression of the adenomatous polyp is unclear, but it appears that most adenomas take at least 3 to 7 years to progress to frank malignancy.

To properly manage the patient with a colonic polyp, the physician should have an understanding of the different histologic types of polyps, their epidemiology, etiology, clinical manifestations and course, as well as the appropriate diagnostic studies and therapeutic options.[1,2] This chapter provides an approach to the understanding and management of colonic polyps.

EPIDEMIOLOGY

Prevalence

The true prevalence of colonic polyps, or, more important, colonic adenomas, in the general population is not known. Large population studies with complete colonoscopy have not been done. The data available are from autopsy studies or from small-scale colonoscopy surveys. In general, autopsy studies show a much higher prevalence rate of polyps and adenomas than endoscopic studies. In the United States, autopsy studies suggest an overall polyp prevalence of 50%,[3–6] but colonoscopic surveys suggest no more than 40%.[7–12] The difference is probably the result of methodology. In autopsy studies, fixation of the colon and use of a magnifying glass allows detection of small polyps that are not easily detected during colonoscopy. Furthermore, autopsy subjects generally are older. As described later, usually only the larger polyps, or more specifically, adenomas, are clinically important, and colonoscopic surveys provide reasonable data for the practicing physician.

More than 80% to 90% of colonic polyps detected on colonoscopy are adenomas or hyperplastic polyps.[7–12] Of this number, approximately 75% are adenomas. When diminutive polyps (<5 mm) are considered, about half are hyperplastic polyps. Anatomic location is also an important factor because most diminutive and hyperplastic polyps are found in the rectosigmoid.[13,14]

Autopsy studies show that the prevalence of adenomas varies widely among countries. In general, the prevalence of colonic adenomas in a given country parallels the frequency of colon cancer in that country.[3-6,15-21] Some results in men, in the age group of 40 to 59 years, are shown in Table 85-2. Because of different study designs and techniques used in the various studies, there are some discrepancies, especially when the results for the countries with moderate colon cancer frequency are examined carefully. This occasional discrepancy, however, actually highlights the highly correlative nature between colonic adenoma prevalence and colon cancer frequency. In two prefectures in Japan, Akita and Miyagi, for example, the results demonstrate this striking difference. In Akita, where the colon cancer frequency is moderate, the adenoma prevalence is 31%; in Miyagi, where the colon cancer frequency is low, the adenoma prevalence is 9%. This difference in adenoma prevalence occurs in the same country, where the ethnic and cultural background of the population is highly preserved,[18] whereas for Japanese men in Hawaii, the frequencies of colon cancer and adenoma are both high.[5,22] These results suggest an environmental contribution to adenoma prevalence, and perhaps also to colon cancer frequency.

Age is the major determinant of colon adenoma frequency. The rates in men and women are very similar. The prevalence of adenomas increases with age,[3,6,22] with the peak prevalence usually after the age of 60 years, and their size at detection also increases with age.[21] Colonic adenomas are uncommon in people younger than 30 years of age, with the exception of the adenomatous polyposis syndromes (see Chap. 86).

As described in the next section, virtually all colon carcinomas arise from adenomas. In addition, adenomas are closely associated with colon carcinomas. As described, the prevalence of adenomas increases in parallel with the frequency of colon cancer (see Table 85-2). Among patients who have one colonic adenoma, 30% to 50% have at least one other synchronous adenoma.[23-27] For those patients with at least two synchronous adenomas, the likelihood of finding metachronous adenomas and cancers is further increased.[26,28,29] In patients with colon cancer, up to 30% have at least one synchronous adenoma.

In those with two or more synchronous cancers, 50% to 85% have a synchronous adenoma. These adenomas found in association with colon carcinoma are more likely to show greater degrees of atypia.[24,28-30] The colon cancer far outweighs the adenoma in terms of clinical significance, but the coexistence of synchronous carcinomas and adenomas is correlated with an increased frequency of subsequent metachronous adenomas and carcinomas.

Hereditary Factors

Hereditary factors clearly play an important role in adenomatous polyposis coli syndromes (see Chap. 86) as well as in hereditary nonpolyposis colorectal carcinoma (see Chap. 87). Adenomatous polyposis coli syndromes account for less than 1% of all colonic neoplasms. But there is increasing evidence that hereditary factors may also play a role in the more common sporadic adenomas. Perhaps as many as 30% of adenomas, and presumably the subsequent carcinomas, are hereditary in nature.[31-33]

Studies have shown that patients with colonic adenomas are two to five times more likely than unaffected controls to have a first-degree relative with colorectal neoplasms. Conversely, first-degree relatives of those with colonic neoplasms (adenomas or carcinomas) are two to five times more likely to have colorectal cancer than the general population, especially if more than one first-degree relative is affected.[34-36]

Analysis of family pedigrees in the state of Utah have identified an autosomal dominant hereditary pattern of adenomas. About 200 members of a large pedigree with familial clustering of colon cancer, without evidence of the known inherited syndromes of colorectal cancer, were systematically examined by flexible fiberoptic sigmoidoscopy. Twenty-one percent of family members, but only 9% of spouses, were found to have one or more adenomas. In comparison, hyperplastic polyps were found in 24% of family members and 29% of spouses.[31]

Subsequent analyses of additional pedigrees continue to

TABLE 85-2
Prevalence of Colonic Adenomas in Men

POPULATION	COLON CANCER INCIDENCE (PER 100,000/y)	ADENOMA PREVALENCE (%, ~AGE 50y)
Hawaiian-Japanese	34	65
New Orleans-Caucasian	28	40
New Orleans-African American	26	30
Sweden (Trellaborg)	17	30
Japan (Akita)	16	30
Spain (Barcelona)	13	20
Brazil	12	15
Sweden (Bollnas)	10	10
Japan (Miyagi)	8	10
Colombia (Cali)	5	5
Costa Rica	3	5
Iran	<2	<5
Bolivia	<2	<5

TABLE 85-3
Anatomic Distribution of Colonic Adenomas

	ASCENDING (%)	TRANSVERSE (%)	DESCENDING (%)	SIGMOID (%)	RECTUM (%)
Colonoscopy	10	10	30	45	5
Autopsy (all adenomas)	30	20	15	15	20
Autopsy (adenomas >1 cm)	15	15	25	35	10

demonstrate a twofold to threefold increase in adenomas in family members compared with spouse controls.[32] Pedigree analysis using likelihood methods was used to estimate which of the possible mechanisms of familial clustering (autosomal dominant, autosomal recessive, decreased penetrance of mendelian factors, polygenic inheritance, or shared environmental factors) may account for the familial clustering of adenomas seen. It was found that an autosomal dominant inheritance of susceptibility to adenoma (and colon carcinoma) best explained the pattern of adenoma and carcinoma occurrence in the pedigrees. In addition, the population gene frequency was estimated to be 19% in that population. These results suggest strongly that familial and hereditary factors play a role in 20% or more of adenomas.

Anatomic Distribution

Colonoscopic studies and some autopsy studies show that colonic adenomas are more common in the left colon, similar to the distribution of colon cancer (Table 85-3). In autopsy studies, adenomas appear more uniformly distributed throughout the entire colon. When only large adenomas (>1 cm) are considered, the left-sided predominance is again observed.[6-8,37-39]

Clinical studies suggest that left-sided adenomas are more likely to be detected by fiberoptic endoscopy, and more likely to come to clinical attention. Autopsy studies suggest that many more of the presumably asymptomatic or smaller adenomas are in the right colon and that this right-sided accentuation increases with age, especially after the age of 60 years.[6,7,38,39] An overall proximal shift of colonic adenomas has not been shown conclusively.[40]

Association With Other Diseases

Table 85-4 summarizes the associations between colonic polyps and other diseases, which are discussed in detail in the following sections.

Strong to Moderate Association

Ureterosigmoidostomy. Ureterosigmoidostomy sites, and any other colonic or rectosigmoid segments used for urinary diversion or reservoirs, are prone to development of neoplasms, including adenomatous polyps and adenocarcinomas.[41-43] Juvenile polyps[44,45] and inflammatory polyps[45] have also been observed, often with adenomatous foci.[44] Some studies have shown that these lesions may develop in as many as 30% of these patients.[41] The adenomatous polyps and adenocarcinomas have been found an average of 20 and 26 years, respectively, after the surgical operation,[41] but latency periods as short as 2 years[41] and even 4 months[42] have been described. In addition, a duration of exposure of the sigmoid mucosa to urine for less than 1 year has resulted in subsequent adenoma and cancer.[46] It has been suggested that these neoplasms are induced by nitrosamines produced by the action of fecal flora on urinary amines.[42,43,47] Because of the high frequency of neoplasms, lifelong risk, and the small number of at-risk patients, surveillance has been advocated, and appears justified.[43,48]

Acromegaly. Acromegaly has been associated with a twofold to sixfold increase in colorectal cancer and adenomatous polyps.[49,50] The association appears to be especially strong in those patients with skin tags (acrochordons)[49] or with a family history of colorectal cancer.[50] The risk appears to persist even in patients who have been treated or cured. Studies suggest that the colon mucosa exhibits increased proliferative indices in acromegaly.[51,52] Because the number of patients with acromegaly is small, and they are already under chronic medical care, surveillance by periodic colonoscopy might be considered.

Breast cancer. Although an association between breast cancer and colorectal cancer has been described, the association

TABLE 85-4
Association of Colonic Polyps With Other Diseases

DISEASE	ASSOCIATION	SCREENING
Ureterosigmoidostomy	Very strong	Yes
Acromegaly	Moderate	Probably
Breast cancer	Moderate	Unclear
Streptococcal infections	Moderate	No
Skin tags	No	No
Atherosclerosis	Uncear	No
Cholecystectomy	Unclear	No
Lymphoid follicles	Unclear	No
Diverticular disease	Unclear	No
Inguinal hernias	Unclear	Unclear

of breast cancer and adenomatous polyps has not been established.[53] In a study of 95 women hospitalized for breast cancer and 95 control subjects, all of whom underwent colonoscopy, 10.5% of the patients with breast cancer and 8.5% of the controls were found to have adenomas, and 5.3% and 3.9%, respectively, were found to have colon cancer.[54] In another case-control study, 14.2% of 161 women with breast cancer were found to have adenomas, compared to 4.7% of controls.[55] A more recent case-control study of 128 patients with adenomas and 284 controls. however, found no association with a history of breast cancer.[53]

Streptococcal infection. Adenomas, adenomatous polyposis coli, and even colonic cancer have been associated with *Streptococcus bovis* bacteremia and endocarditis.[56–58] *S bovis* has been found in the feces of people with adenomas or carcinomas at a higher rate than in otherwise healthy control subjects.[59] There are also case reports of *Streptococcus agalactiae* endocarditis in two patients with rectal villous adenomas.[60]

Unclear Association

Skin tags. In patients with acromegaly, the presence of skin tags (acrochordons) is associated with the presence of colonic adenomas.[49] These studies have been extended to the general population. In an early study of 94 men undergoing colonoscopy, skin tags were associated with the presence of polyps. Of the 48 men with skin tags, 77% had polyps, and only 20% of the 46 men without skin tags had polyps.[61] These studies, however, were done in patients who presumably had some signs or symptoms because they were undergoing colonoscopy. Other studies were performed in older patients, in whom skin tags occur frequently.[62,63] In a subsequent study of 492 unselected men in a primary clinic, 10% of patients with skin tags were found to have rectosigmoid polyps, but 8% of those without skin tags also had polyps.[64] In screening asymptomatic family members in adenomatous polyposis coli, no such correlation was found.[65] This lack of correlation has now been confirmed in an autopsy study,[66] a meta-analysis of published studies,[67] and a prospective study of 218 patients older than 40 years of age.[68]

Atherosclerosis. In autopsy studies, one of which was in Japanese men in Hawaii (in whom the frequency of colonic adenoma and cancer is very high), an association was found between colonic adenomas and atherosclerosis.[69,70] These results suggest that these two diseases of developed industrial nations may share certain risk factors, such as an increase in serum cholesterol; however, studies attempting to correlate serum cholesterol levels and the presence of adenomas have not been conclusive. Serum cholesterol levels in patients with adenomas were high in some studies[71,72] but normal in others.[73,74] The possible association of cholesterol levels with the presence of adenomas awaits further studies.

Cholecystectomy. Cholecystectomy has been associated with an increased prevalence of colonic adenomas[75] and cancers.[76] It has been theorized that cholecystectomy results in greater delivery of bile acids to the intestine and colon. In mice, the mucosa after cholecystectomy shows an increased mitotic index.[77,78] Although the hypothesis appears plausible, most studies have not confirmed the association between cholecystectomy and colon adenomas[79–81] or cancers.[82,83] More recent studies suggest that the risk factor might be cholelithiasis and not cholecystectomy.[84]

Other diseases. Cirrhosis appears to be an independent but small risk factor for colonic adenomas, with a twofold to threefold increase in associated polyps.[85] Diverticular disease has been associated with colonic polyps.[19] A case-control study of 150 patients with colonic diverticular disease found 36% with colonic adenomas and carcinomas, compared to 17% in matched controls, a significant but small twofold to threefold increase in associated colonic neoplasms.[86]

An association between colonic lymphoid follicles and colonic neoplasms has been suggested. A radiographic study found colonic lymphoid follicles in 2.6% of patients aged 40 years or older. Of these, 69% were found to have synchronous or previous colonic neoplasms, compared to 8.5% of those without lymphoid follicles.[87] An association between inguinal hernias and colonic neoplasms has been suggested, but controlled studies are not available. An uncontrolled study of 110 patients undergoing hernia repair found polyps in 25% and cancers in 4%, with less than half of affected patients testing positive for fecal occult blood.[88] Another uncontrolled study found colonic neoplasms in 6.5% of 202 patients with inguinal hernias, and lumenal obstruction did not appear to be the cause of the inguinal hernias.[89]

Nonneoplastic Polyps

The epidemiology of non-neoplastic polyps is not well studied because they account for a much smaller percentage of colonic polyps. One nonneoplastic polyp that has been studied to some extent is the hyperplastic polyp, the second most common colon polyp.[13,90] Hyperplastic polyps usually are diminutive, that is, smaller than 5 mm in diameter, and usually found in the rectosigmoid area. They are rarely, if ever, villous in structure, show high-grade atypia, or contain invasive carcinoma. Some studies have found an association between distal hyperplastic polyps and more proximal adenomas and colon cancer,[91–97] but others have not.[9,98–102] The evidence is not conclusive. It is possible that hyperplastic polyps, especially with the extensive screening examinations being done, are being found in older people who also harbor proximal adenomas by reason of age alone. The predominant evidence from the larger and better controlled studies would suggest that hyperplastic polyps are not premalignant and are not of great clinical concern.[40] Unless other risk factors are present, asymptomatic patients found to have diminutive distal hyperplastic polyps on sigmoidoscopy probably do not need complete colonoscopy.

ETIOLOGY

Polyp Formation Theories

The etiology of colonic polyps depends on their histologic type. For instance, inflammatory polyps result from the inflammatory and regenerative response to injury. Because of their clinical significance and prevalence, the remainder of this section focuses on the potential etiology of adenomas.

Adenomas are benign neoplasms. Although they have differing architectural appearances and histologic features, adenomas have in common a characteristic neoplastic epithelial appearance. This neoplastic epithelial appearance has been called dysplasia, characterized by cells with enlarged, hyperchromatic, elongated, and stratified nuclei arranged in a picket-fence pattern, with variably decreased amounts of cellular mucin and increased numbers of mitotic cells. These changes result in a more basophilic appearance to the adenomatous epithelium in hematoxylin and eosin-stained sections.[103,104]

The healthy colon epithelium is characterized by constant cell proliferation and differentiation, resulting in total renewal of the surface epithelial cells approximately every 6 days. The process of cell proliferation and differentiation is normally highly regulated, resulting in a homeostasis between cell production and cell maturation and death, thus maintaining the normal colonic epithelium at the same thickness and level of maturity, with a proper mix of different cell types.[105]

Cell proliferation, as marked by cell mitosis, and DNA and RNA synthesis, predominates in the basal third of crypts in the healthy colon epithelium. The new cells that are generated then migrate upward toward the top of the crypt. As the cells migrate, cellular proliferation ceases and maturation begins. The middle third of the crypt is a transition zone in which cell proliferation slows and DNA and RNA synthesis decreases until the process of proliferation is virtually halted. Cell maturation then begins gradually, with the cells taking on a more mature phenotype as they continue to migrate toward the top of the crypt. The cells complete the maturation process in the top third of the crypt. Here the cells gradually become senescent, die, and are then extruded into the lumen.[105-107] The mesenchymal tissue that surrounds the epithelial cells in the crypt, and which has been termed the pericryptal fibroblast sheath, also undergoes a similar process of proliferation and maturation, although its kinetics are not well understood.[106,108]

The normal process of cell proliferation and differentiation is altered and disordered in adenomatous epithelium. There is continued cell proliferation as the cells migrate up the crypt, so that there is an extension of the proliferative compartments into the middle and even the upper third of the crypt. The epithelial cells therefore retain their proliferative status and immaturity, with cell mitosis seen all the way to the crypt surface. There is also a delayed maturation, with decreased senescence and extrusion of the cells into the lumen.[103,107] Results suggest that the entire colonic mucosa in patients with colon adenomas and cancers may show increased epithelial cell proliferation compared to the colonic mucosa of control patients.[108] A disorganization in cell proliferation also has been described for the pericryptal fibroblast sheath.[109,110]

This disorderly and persistent cell replication near the crypt surface coupled with retarded cell maturation and extrusion into the lumen results in an increase in the number of surface epithelial cells, which then continue to replicate. This continued replication of epithelial cells is then thought to result in a downward infolding of the epithelial cells, which interpose and branch between the normal crypt elements. The process of infolding and branching results in the typical branching

glandular pattern seen in tubular adenomas.[103,106] This epithelial infolding process has been described for adenomatous epithelium, adenomas, and for adenomatous polyposis coli.[111]

Mesenchymal proliferation is also thought to play a role in the formation of adenomas. Where mesenchymal proliferation is less than epithelial proliferation, there is mesenchymal resistance to epithelial growth, resulting in continued branching and infolding. This results in a network of branching and infolding glands, characteristic of the appearance of a tubular adenoma. This mesenchymal resistance to continued outward epithelial expansion may also help to limit the size of the tubular adenoma. Where mesenchymal proliferation is increased to a degree commensurate with epithelial proliferation, resistance to continued epithelial expansion is reduced, and there may be unimpeded cell proliferation, resulting in long, finger-like projections of glandular elements all the way from the center of the adenoma to its outer surface. These long, finger-like epithelial projections are characteristic of villous adenomas. This relative lack of impedance to continued epithelial expansion may then result in a villous adenoma of large size. More commonly, adenomas demonstrate a combination of tubular and villous architecture, possibly reflecting regional differences between epithelial and mesenchymal proliferation.[106,109,110]

The disordered cellular proliferation and differentiation seen in adenomas usually is not observed in hyperplastic or inflammatory polyps. In hyperplastic and inflammatory polyps, cell proliferation is increased, with increased cell mitosis and cell production, but the process of cell proliferation generally remains confined to the basal third of the crypt, the normal proliferative compartment. With increased cell production, there are increased epithelial cell elements and some infolding, leading to the characteristic polypoid appearance. Cell proliferation, however, stops appropriately by the time cells migrate to the middle third of the crypt, and cell maturation proceeds normally, producing a normal distribution of glandular and absorptive cell elements. Furthermore, dysplasia is not seen in pure hyperplastic or inflammatory polyps.[104,106]

Contributory Factors

The potential roles of geography, age, diet, and inherited factors have been discussed in the section on epidemiology. Primary genetic factors appear to be important in at least 20% to 30% of adenomas.[31,32] The results from epidemiologic studies suggest that environmental factors play an important role in the other apparently nonhereditary adenomas. Based again on epidemiologic studies, it appears that diet is probably the most important environmental factor. The dietary factors that predispose to adenoma formation are similar to those that have been associated with colon cancer (see Chap. 87), but the evidence is less extensive for adenomas.

Diet

There is marked variation in the prevalence of colonic adenomas in different countries (see Table 85-2). Additional epidemiologic analyses have suggested that these geographic variations usually are caused not by racial, ethnic, or climatic factors, but probably by dietary factors. Many dietary factors have been proposed as potential causative agents, but the strongest evidence points to dietary fat, bile acids, and fecal bacteria.[112,113] There also is evidence of roles for dietary fiber and carcinogens.

The prevalence of colon adenomas, as well as cancers, has been correlated with high dietary fat intake (greater than 40% of total caloric intake). Conversely, dietary fat intake of less than 15% of total caloric intake has been correlated with a low frequency of colon adenomas and cancers.[114–117] In Japanese men in Hawaii a significant correlation has been found between the presence of colon adenomas and atherosclerosis.[70] As discussed, it has been suggested that these two common conditions in developed countries may share similar causative factors, increased dietary fat consumption and elevated serum cholesterol levels. In fact, increased dietary fat has been shown in experimental animals to lead to increased hepatic synthesis of cholesterol and bile acids, and their increased presence in the colon contents and feces. Bacteria flora in the colon may then convert these sterols into cholesterol metabolites and oxidized bile acids, which have tumor-promoting activity.[113]

Higher fecal concentrations of bile acids and oxidized bile acids have been found in populations at higher risk for development of colon adenomas and cancers, compared to those at lower risk. Subjects living in areas with high prevalence of colonic adenomas have higher concentrations of fecal bile acids. Similarly, subjects in these geographic areas have been found to have higher numbers of fecal anaerobic bacteria. Studies have also demonstrated an association between high numbers of fecal anaerobic bacteria, increased amounts of metabolized cholesterol and oxidized bile acids in the feces, and the high prevalence of colon neoplasms in different populations.[112,113] These results suggest, but do not prove, that increased dietary fat intake, increased intralumenal bile acid and cholesterol synthesis, and increased fecal anaerobic bacteria may be important causative factors in the development of colon adenomas and cancers. It is also possible that increased dietary fat leads to increased anaerobic bacteria, or that the anaerobic flora and the high bile acid and cholesterol synthesis are hereditary or environmentally related.

Fiber

Lack of dietary fiber is receiving increased attention as an etiologic factor in colon adenomas and cancers. Fiber is a heterogeneous group of plant carbohydrates and noncarbohydrates that is resistant to digestion in the upper digestive tract. Thus, epidemiologic data and experimental animal studies have been complicated by the different types and mix of actual fiber components. Nevertheless, studies show that subjects consuming diets high in fiber and who also have large, bulky stools tend to have a lower frequency of colon adenomas and cancers.[114–116,118] The types and amount of dietary fiber that may confer a protective effect is unknown, however.[119]

Carcinogens

Studies also have demonstrated increased fecal mutagenic activity in the stools of patients at higher risk for development of colon adenomas and cancers.[113,120] Whether the increased fecal mutagenic activity is related to dietary fat intake, fecal

bile acids, or bacteria is still unclear. Studies have attempted to use potential antioxidants, such as vitamins A, C, and E in an attempt to decrease the production of mutagens in the stool as a way of decreasing colon adenomas and cancers. Final results from these studies are not yet available.[121] There is also preliminary evidence to show that calcium, perhaps by binding fecal fat, bile acids, and cholesterol, may confer a protective effect.[122]

Genetics

Multiple DNA alterations have been noted in adenomas. Aneuploidy, tetraploidy, and DNA hypomethylation have been defined in adenomas and in adenomatous polyposis coli.[123,124] Other studies have found decreased DNA repair synthesis in the circulating leukocytes of patients at higher risk for development of colonic neoplasms.[125] Studies of colon adenomas have suggested an altered pattern of expression of oncogenes, such as *fos*, *myc*, and *ras*. Studies have implicated increasing genetic alterations, including DNA methylation changes and chromosomal allelic deletions and mutations, such as *K-ras* gene mutations, and deletions of *DCC*, *p53*, and other genes, in concert with the progression of normal colon epithelium to adenoma and to carcinoma[126,127](Fig. 85-1). This is described in greater detail in Chapter 87.

Adenoma (Dysplasia)— Carcinoma Sequence

It is generally accepted that, with rare exceptions, virtually all colon carcinomas arise from colonic adenomas (or at the very least, dysplasia). It is also clear that most colonic adenomas do not develop into colon carcinomas. The exact frequency and time course of this neoplastic progression is not yet clearly defined. The evidence for the adenoma-carcinoma sequence is derived from epidemiologic, morphologic, biologic, clinical, and therapeutic data. Studies in adenomatous polyposis syndromes also tend to confirm this sequence.

Epidemiology

The strong correlation between the frequency of colon adenomas and colon carcinomas in terms of geography, age, and anatomic distribution has been described in detail in the section on epidemiology (see Table 85-2). In general, the frequency of adenomas parallels the frequency of colon cancer in various countries. The increasing frequency of colon adenomas with increasing age parallels, and precedes, the increasing frequency of colon cancer. There appears to be approximately a 7-year difference in time between the onset of adenomas and the development of cancer.[3,24,28,128]

The anatomic distribution for large colon adenomas and colon cancers is similar, showing a moderate left-sided predominance. There is also an association of colon adenomas and colon carcinomas within the same colon.[3,7,129] As described in the epidemiology section, patients in whom more than two adenomas are found have an increased risk of metachronous adenomas and colon cancers.[26,28,29] Thirty percent of patients with colon cancers have a synchronous adenoma.

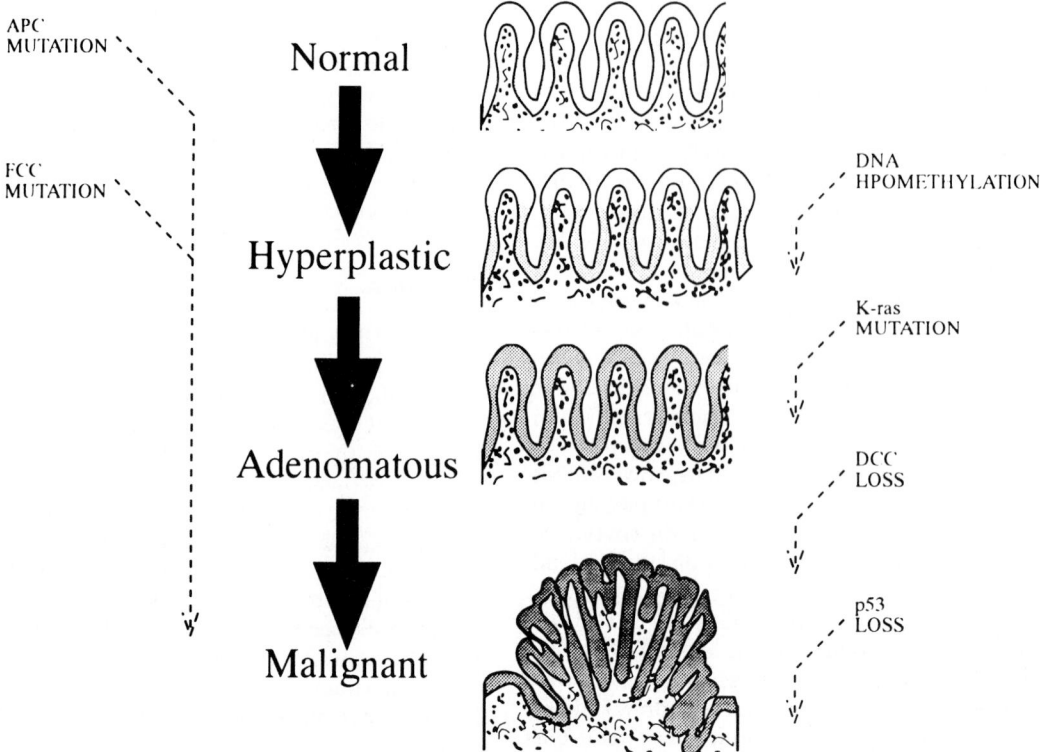

APC
MUTATION

FCC
MUTATION

Normal

Hyperplastic

Adenomatous

Malignant

DNA
HPOMETHYLATION

K-ras
MUTATION

DCC
LOSS

p53
LOSS

FIGURE 85-1. A genetic model for the colorectal adenoma–carcinoma sequence. Colorectal carcinomas arise through a sequence (or an accumulation) of genetic alterations, in concert with histopathologic progression through adenomas with increasing severity of atypia. Inherited or somatic mutations in *APC*, *FCC*, or other as yet undiscovered genes may be responsible for a predisposition to colorectal carcinoma development. Mutations or losses of other genes, such as *K-RAS*, *DCC*, and *P53* are increasingly seen in later stages of the adenoma–carcinoma sequence. Some genetic alterations, such as *P53* loss, have been shown to be critical for the carcinoma phenotype, and restitution of the lost genetic elements may normalize colon carcinoma cells in vitro. (Data from refs 126, 146, and 147.)

Up to 85% of patients with two or more synchronous colon cancers have a synchronous adenoma.[24,28,30]

Morphology

If the adenoma-carcinoma sequence is correct, one would expect to find minute adenocarcinomas arising in adenomas. If the adenoma-carcinoma sequence does not occur, then one would expect to find minute adenocarcinomas arising de novo. In fact, systematic morphologic studies of colon carcinomas and of resection specimens from patients with adenomatous polyposis coli show that minute adenocarcinomas are frequently found within adenomas, whereas the de novo minute carcinoma is extremely rare.[130]

If the adenoma-carcinoma sequence is correct, then carcinomas arising within adenomas should gradually increase in size and ultimately replace all the adenomatous elements with carcinoma. Indeed, this has been found to be the case. The frequency of finding adenomatous tissue in a carcinoma varies inversely with the size and extent of invasion of the carcinoma. Associated adenomatous tissue is found in more than 50% of carcinomas with some mucosal invasion, less than 20% of carcinomas with invasion of the muscularis propria, and less than 10% of carcinomas with serosal invasion.[131,132]

Biology

Colon adenomas and carcinomas also share similar biologic features. Both adenomas and carcinomas have been shown to be monoclonal.[133] Approximately half of colon adenomas larger than 1 cm and half of colon cancers have been found to have *K-ras* gene mutations, primarily in the codon 12 position.[126] Large adenomas frequently have allelic loss of chromosomes. Approximately one third of large adenomas and carcinomas have allelic loss of chromosome 5, and half have allelic loss of chromosome 18.[126] In all instances, the rate of *ras* gene mutations and chromosomal lesions shows a progressive increase from apparently healthy mucosa to adenomas to carcinomas, suggesting a neoplastic progression.

Clinical History

The adenoma-carcinoma sequence is also supported by the natural history of adenoma progression. Although it is unethical and impossible to follow an untreated adenoma for its progression to carcinoma, the available evidence suggests that this progression occurs. Adenomas have occasionally been left untreated because of patient noncompliance or technical difficulties. Invasive carcinomas have been found to develop at the site of these adenomas.[132,134,135] These sporadic and anecdotal cases have strongly implicated the progression from adenoma to carcinoma.

The peak age at which adenomas develop, 50 years, precedes the peak age of development of colon carcinomas, 57 years, by 7 years.[136] In untreated and unscreened patients with adenomatous polyposis coli, the age of diagnosis of symptomatic adenomas, 36 years, also precedes the age of onset of carcinoma, 39 years.[132] The more rapid time course in adenomatous polyposis coli may be the result of the younger age of the patients, earlier age of detection of cancers, or nature of the disease itself.

The frequency of finding carcinoma within an adenoma also increases proportionally with increasing size, more severe atypia, and greater villous component of the adenoma (Table 85-5). This again supports a natural progression from adenoma to carcinoma. In addition, an increasing number of adenomas also is associated with increasing risk for development of carcinomas.

Therapy

In a large, uncontrolled study, patients underwent periodic sigmoidoscopies and all polyps that were found were removed. Most polyps removed were found to be adenomatous. The frequency of carcinomas occurring in a subsequent 7- to 14-year period was found to be about a third of the expected rate in an untreated population.[137] This has been confirmed in a recent retrospective study[138] and the National Polyp Study.[139] In the National Polyp Study, in which patients undergo colonoscopy and polypectomy on enrollment, and then at 3 and 6 years (and also at 1 year for half the patients), no symptomatic cancers and five asymptomatic malignant polyps have been found after almost 6000 patient-years of follow-up over more than 4 years.[139] In a study in patients with adenomatous polyposis coli who had colectomies and ileorectal anastomoses, it was found that periodic removal of adenomas from the rectal stump prevented the subsequent development of

TABLE 85-5
Malignant Potential of Colonic Adenomas

	PERCENT WITH CARCINOMA
Size	
<0.5 cm	<0.5
0.5–1 cm	2
1–2 cm	10
>2 cm	40
Histology	
Tubular	5
Tubulovillous	20
Villous	40
Dysplasia*	
Mild	5
Moderate	20
Severe	40

* This is an artificial distinction. An adenoma with carcinoma present usually is classified as a malignant polyp. This table enumerates the frequency of finding carcinoma in an adenoma with different degrees of overall dysplasia (the predominant epithelial component).

rectal carcinoma.[24] This evidence suggests that the removal of adenomas before they have a chance to become carcinomas results in decreased carcinoma formation, again validating the adenoma-carcinoma sequence.

Adenomatous Polyposis Coli

The increasing risk of colon carcinoma with increasing numbers of adenomas is well proven in the polyposis syndromes. Adenomatous polyposis coli is characterized by the development of more than 100 adenomas. The risk for development of colon carcinomas is virtually 100% if the colon is not removed. In addition, adenomas precede the appearance of carcinoma by about 5 years. In this condition, minute carcinomas have been found within adenomas, and apparently benign adenomas have been found to enlarge and progress to carcinomas.[132]

Exceptions

A few exceptions to this adenoma-carcinoma sequence may occur. Rare minute carcinoma have been described as developing de novo in apparently nonadenomatous epithelium.[140,141] It is possible, however, that the carcinoma may have arisen in a focus of adenomatous epithelium that had not yet assumed a polypoid appearance (which has been found in adenomatous polyposis coli), and the subsequent carcinomatous development had replaced and obliterated the adenomatous epithelium.

It also has been suggested that in the hereditary nonpolyposis colorectal carcinoma (Lynch's) syndromes, carcinomas may arise without passing through a polyp phase. Other studies, however, have observed small precursor adenomas and "flat adenomas" in these syndromes.[142,143]

Although there is no precursor polyp, colon carcinoma in the setting of long-standing ulcerative colitis is believed to develop from a dysplastic focus. The progression from inflammation-injury-regeneration to dysplasia to carcinoma is believed to be analogous to the adenoma (dysplasia)-carcinoma sequence. In addition, the dysplastic lesion in long-standing ulcerative colitis often assumes a raised plaque-like appearance.[144]

It would appear from these lines of evidence that most carcinomas arise from adenomas or an analogous dysplastic change in the colonic epithelium.

Genetic Factors

Our understanding of the genetic mechanisms underlying the development of colon adenomas and, hence, colon carcinomas is advancing rapidly (see section on Epidemiology, and Chap. 87). Studies have identified the adenomatous polyposis coli (*APC*) gene on chromosome 5 (5q 21–22).[145-149] This *APC* gene also appears to be involved in apparently nonhereditary sporadic colon carcinomas, as noted by somatic mutations. Most mutations appear to result in the expression of truncated *APC* gene products, and preliminary studies suggest that genetic analyses may be helpful in the preclinical diagnosis of familial adenomatous polyposis. In addition, the accumulation of genetic alterations appear to accompany the sequential progression of adenomas to cancer.[127] This is discussed in Chapters 24 and 87.

CLINICAL MANIFESTATIONS

Signs and Symptoms

Most patients with colonic polyps are asymptomatic. Most often, the polyps are discovered only as an incidental finding during examination for nonspecific abdominal complaints or for other unrelated disorders. This is in keeping with the fact that most polyps are small or are hyperplastic polyps and do not cause symptoms. Even in the case of the adenomatous polyposis coli syndromes, where adenomas number in the hundreds to thousands, symptoms occur late or are the result of coexisting colon carcinomas.

A true picture of the clinical findings associated with colonic adenomas could be determined only in large population studies by screening all members with complete colonoscopy. Such studies are not available. In available studies, subjects are often screened for specific reasons, are symptomatic, or are seeking treatment. These studies may thus give an overestimate of the clinical findings. Even in such groups, most patients are still asymptomatic.[150,151] In a report of more than 800 hospitalized patients with colon polyps, 32% were found to be asymptomatic.[150] When symptoms occur, they tend to be in patients who have colonic polyps of 1 cm in size or larger.[152] The most common symptoms are rectal bleeding, both overt and occult, change in bowel habits, abdominal pain, and rectal prolapse. Symptoms, however, have little correlation with histologic status, pathologic condition, or location.[150,151]

Bleeding is the symptom most commonly attributed to colon adenomas. Histologic studies have shown that, as opposed to colon carcinomas, which often ulcerate on the surface and result in persistent rectal bleeding, adenomas tend to have minimal ulceration and have an intact lumenal surface. Any bleeding that occurs is often into the stroma. Thus, any rectal bleeding tends to be intermittent and small in amount, only rarely resulting in anemia.[153] Studies have demonstrated that only patients with polyps of 1.5 cm in size or larger consistently have higher amounts of fecal blood loss than healthy control subjects.[154] In patients with no adenomas, about 20% are found to have positive fecal occult blood on screening. The number of patients with a positive fecal occult blood test (FOBT) result increases with the presence of polyps and also with larger and more distal adenomas. But even in the group of the more than 800 hospitalized patients, only 44% were found to have either overt or occult rectal bleeding.[150] Conversely, overt rectal bleeding is often not caused by colon adenomas. Less than 20% of patients presenting with hematochezia, frank rectal bleeding, were subsequently found to have colon adenomas.[155]

Colonic polyps, especially juvenile polyps, may occasionally undergo autoamputation, resulting in rectal bleeding. One of the most common presenting complaints in children with juvenile polyps is rectal bleeding with defecation.[156] The presence of polyp tissue in the feces is extremely rare.[156,157]

Changes in bowel habits have been associated with the presence of colonic polyps. Constipation has been attributed

to colonic polyps, especially when they are bulky lesions and occur in the distal colon. Colocolic intussusception due to large polyps has been found in children.[158] Diarrhea has also been described, particularly for large villous adenomas. A rare syndrome of profuse, watery diarrhea, resulting in massive fluid and electrolyte depletion, has been described for large villous adenomas, especially those located in the distal colon and rectum.[150,159] Diffuse, nonspecific abdominal pain has been at times attributed to intussusception, particularly of larger polyps. Rectal prolapse of larger polyps has also been reported.[150] Other nonspecific abdominal symptoms such as discomfort and flatulence also have been associated with polyps.[150] It is important to note that these symptoms often remain even after polypectomy, suggesting that the symptoms were probably not caused by the colonic polyps.

Physical examination rarely uncover signs of colon polyps. Digital rectal examination often fails to discern rectal polyps because they may be small, pliable, and movable.[150,151] The signs and symptoms of rectal bleeding usually are late findings and are more often associated with colorectal cancers.[160,161] Rectal bleeding, especially in patients older than 40 years of age or those with other risk factors, should never be ascribed solely to coexisting hemorrhoids without a thorough evaluation of the colorectum.[161]

Table 85-6 lists the appearances and clinical features of the nonhereditary colonic polyps.

Neoplastic Polyps

The initial diagnosis of a colon polyp is often made by direct endoscopic visualization of the polyp tissue mass protruding into the bowel lumen. The polyp is then sampled for biopsy or removed by polypectomy, and its histologic type determined by pathologic examination. Even at the time of endoscopic examination, certain morphologic features may help classify the polyp, although these features can be misleading.[162]

Adenomas

Adenomas account for about two thirds of all resected colorectal polyps. Adenomas may show a spectrum of atypical changes ranging from mild atypia to severe atypia or carcinoma. Because adenomas are by definition dysplastic, it may be less confusing to use the term *atypia* to describe them. Adenomas may thus be classified accordingly to the most atypical focus within the lesion. Mild atypia includes the histologic changes of slightly enlarged and elongated nuclei that still retain relatively uniform size and basal polarity. Adenomas with severe atypia have markedly enlarged pleomorphic and hyperchromatic nuclei, an increased nuclear : cytoplasmic ratio, loss of basal polarity, and loss of nuclear stratification and stroma. Moderate atypia signifies those changes intermediate between mild and severe degrees of atypia. The term *severe focal atypia* has been used synonymously with, and is preferred over, *carcinoma in situ* when the atypical cells (carcinoma) are confined within the basement membrane. Once the basement membrane has been breached, but the atypical cells remain within the lamina propria, without extension through the muscularis mucosae, the lesions may be termed *intramucosal carcinoma*. Both severe focal atypia and intra-

TABLE 85-6
Features of Colonic Polyps (Nonhereditary)

TYPE	AGE (y)	LOCATION	SIZE (cm)	APPEARANCE	HISTOLOGY	CANCER RISK (%)
Tubular adenoma	>40	Distal	0.5–2	Dark red, stalk smooth or lobulated	Epithelial tubules	5
Tubulovillous adenoma	>40	Throughout	0.5–5	Intermediate between tubular and villous	Tubules and villi	20
Villous adenoma	>40	Rectum	>2	Dark red, sessile, shaggy, friable	Villi	>40
		Cecum			Dysplasia	
Mucosal	Any	Distal	<0.5	Mucosal pearls	Normal	0
Hyperplastic	Any	Distal	<0.5	Mucosal pearls	Elongated crypts, serrated surface	0
Inflammatory	Any	Distal	<1	Inflamed, friable	Inflammation, regeneration	0*
Juvenile	Any	Rectum	<2	Cherry red, stalk smooth, friable	Mucus-filled glands, edematous lamina propria	0
	Usually <10					
Peutz-Jeghers†	10–30	Throughout	<2	Smooth or lobulated	Hamartoma, normal	0‡
Lymphoid	<30	Rectum	<0.5	Mucosal pearls	Lymphocytes, follicles	0
Pneumatosis	Any§	Throughout	<1	Air blebs	Cysts with giant cells	0
Colitis cystica	Any	Throughout	<1	Mucosal elevation	Mucous cysts	0
Lipoma	>40	Proximal	<3	Round, soft, glossy	Adipose tissue	0
Hemangioma	Any	Throughout	<2	Cherry red, vascular	Hemangioma	0

* Inflammatory polyps may occur in the setting of inflammatory bowel disease with dysplasia, when cancer risk is substantial.

† Peutz-Jeghers polyps are hereditary and are included for comparison with juvenile polyps only.

‡ The Peutz-Jeghers polyps themselves may not be premalignant, but the syndrome is associated with increased frequency of malignancies.

§ Pneumatosis in the setting of colonic ischemia or necrosis occurs in the pediatric setting.

mucosal carcinoma are noninvasive, and patients are cured by excision of the lesions without additional therapy (see Therapy).[163,164]

The atypical carcinomatous cells remain above the muscularis mucosae. The lymphatics in the colon usually do not extend above the muscularis mucosae; hence, atypical carcinomatous cells that have not invaded the muscularis mucosae do not result in invasive metastatic disease. Such evaluation of invasiveness must include complete polypectomy and serial sectioning of the adenoma. Studies have demonstrated that partial removal of the polyp and partial biopsies have missed invasive malignancies, when subsequent complete removal and histologic analysis of the adenoma demonstrated carcinomatous invasion through the muscularis mucosae.[165,166]

Occasionally, pseudoinvasion, also termed epithelial displacement or misplaced epithelium, has been described. In this instance, islands of adenomatous tissue are found in the submucosa, but the condition is considered benign, and hence the term *epithelial displacement* may be preferred. The displaced epithelium is frequently cystic and occasionally shows extravasation of pools of mucin and evidence of bleeding into the submucosa. Epithelial displacement may be distinguishable from invasive carcinoma by several histologic features. In general, the displaced epithelial cells are surrounded by lamina propria and not by desmoplastic reaction, the displaced epithelium is histologically similar to that of the overlying adenomatous epithelium, and there may be presence of extravasated blood and mucin in the submucosa.[130,167–169]

Adenomas also are classified by their architecture. The architectural types all show dysplasia (with varying degrees of atypia) but with a different morphologic glandular arrangement within the polyp. Tubular adenomas are those that contain branching and infolding of the glandular epithelium, so they form a tubule-like picture. Villous adenomas tend to have long, finger-like projections extending from the surface of the adenoma all the way to the center. As described in a previous section, it has been hypothesized that the adenoma architecture depends on the associated mesenchymal proliferation. When mesenchymal proliferation matches epithelial proliferation, the result may be a villous adenoma. When mesenchymal proliferation is restricted, it may result in impedance of glandular elongation and produce marked infolding of the epithelium, leading to a tubular architecture. The frequency of distribution of adenoma architectural types depends on how they are classified. A pure architectural type is extremely rare.[170,171] In general, if one were to classify an adenoma by its predominant architecture (>80%[168] or >75%[172]), tubular adenomas would be the most common, comprising approximately 80% to 85% of all adenomas. The mixed type of tubulovillous adenomas would then comprise approximately 10%, with villous adenomas comprising the remaining 5%.[172] The association with carcinoma and the risk of carcinoma development appear to increase proportionately with the size of the villous component. Villous adenomas have the highest risk, and tubular adenomas the lowest risk.[132,173]

The distribution of adenoma size depends on the method of size estimation. As described, autopsy studies include smaller adenomas that are visible only with fixation of the colon and examination with a magnifying glass. When adenomas removed by polypectomy only are considered, more

than a third are diminutive (5 mm or smaller), more than another third are between 5 and 10 mm in size, and the remaining (about 25%) are larger than 1 cm.[172] Studies suggest that adenoma size is an independent risk factor for subsequent colorectal cancer. In 1618 patients followed for a mean period of 14 years after initial sigmoidoscopy and polypectomy, the risk of subsequent rectal cancer depended on size, histologic type, and multiplicity, with a size greater than 1 cm and villous architecture being the strongest risk factors. Conversely, patients with small tubular adenomas without severe atypia had no increased risk for colon cancer.[173] Small polypoid cancers and small polyps containing invasive carcinomas, however, even though extremely rare, have been described.[174]

Tubular adenomas. These tend to be smaller adenomas. They appear to be darker red in color than the surrounding mucosa and tend to have a smooth surface, although a granular to lobulated surface has also been described. There is also occasional surface erosion and ulceration, although much less frequently than in carcinomas (Figs. 85-2 and 85-3; see Color Figs. 41 and 42).

The histologic architecture shows the presence of infolding tubules. These adenomas may display the entire spectrum of atypia, ranging from mild to severe[24,103,164,172] (Figs. 85-4 and 85-5; see Color Figs. 43 and 44). The term *severe focal atypia* is often used to describe an atypical or carcinomatous focus confined within the basement membrane. The term *intramucosal carcinoma* is used when the carcinomatous cells have invaded into the lamina propria, but not through the muscularis mucosae. Because severe focal atypia and intramucosal carcinoma do not invade the muscularis mucosae, lymphatic metastasis should be extremely rare. In one study of more than 1600 adenomas with focal noninvasive carcinoma, not a single case of regional lymph node metastasis was found.

Villous adenomas. As described, the malignant potential of an adenoma is proportional to its villous component as well as to its size.[170] Villous adenomas comprise approximately 5% of all adenomas, and tend to occur more in patients older

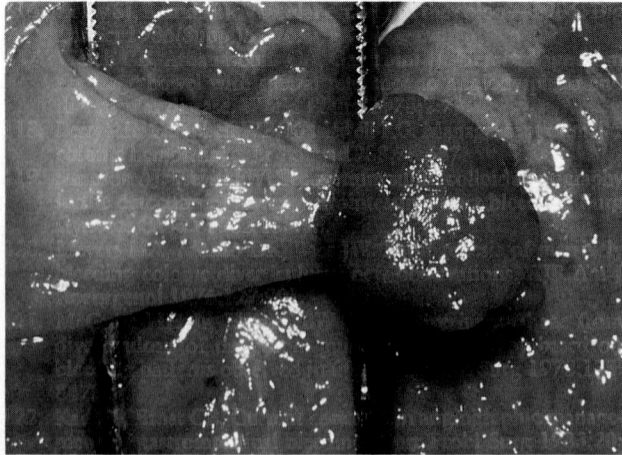

FIGURE 85-2. (See Color Fig. 41.) Macroscopic appearance of a pedunculated tubular adenoma. The forceps marks the base and the neck of the stalk.

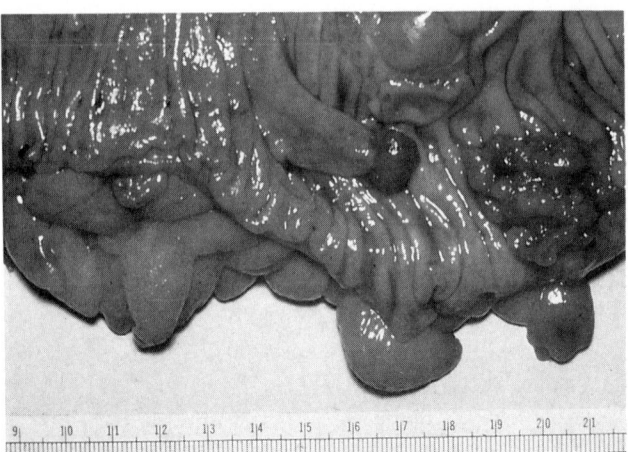

FIGURE 85-3. (See Color Fig. 42.) A synchronous, pedunculated, tubular adenoma adjacent to a sessile, tubulovillous adenoma. Synchronous adenomas not infrequently are found adjacent to each other. In this instance, a 1-cm, pedunculated, tubular adenoma is found about 5 cm away from a 3-cm, sessile, tubulovillous adenoma. Note the smooth surface of the tubular adenoma and the smooth, lobulated surface of the tubulovillous, primarily tubular adenoma.

than 60 years of age[171,172,175,176] (Figs. 85-6 and 85-7; see Color Fig. 45).

When seen during endoscopy, they usually are larger and typically sessile. The surface has a shaggy, cauliflower-like or frond-like appearance, may be soft and velvety, and often is friable. For adenomas with a large villous component, a finely granular surface pattern and a reddish color with white spots may be seen, and dye spraying may show a characteristic pattern.[177] Villous adenomas tend to be distal in location, large, and bulky, and have resulted in constipation and rectal prolapse.[175]

Foci of noninvasive carcinoma are found in up to 30% to 50% of villous adenomas. In addition, synchronous and

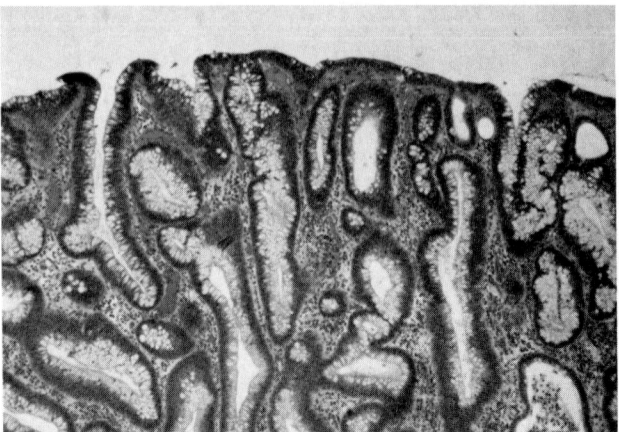

FIGURE 85-5. (See Color Fig. 44.) Histologic appearance of a tubular adenoma with moderate dysplasia. There is increased cellular crowding, pleomorphic, hyperchromatic nuclei with some loss of basal polarity, and an increased nuclear : cytoplasmic ratio.

metachronous colon carcinomas are frequently found in association with villous adenomas. Villous adenomas, especially large rectal lesions, have been associated with profuse, watery diarrhea, resulting in marked electrolyte and fluid depletion, with resultant hypokalemia and hyponatremia.[175,178,179]

Tubulovillous adenomas. Tubulovillous adenomas have been defined as containing at least a 25% villous component and at least a 25% tubular component, without either architectural type predominating.[172] Their clinical behavior tends to be intermediate between that of tubular and villous adenomas[168] (Figs. 85-8 and 85-9; see Color Figs. 46 and 47). Because the malignant potential of any adenoma is usually proportional to its size, its villous component, and degree of atypia, an adenoma might be described pathologically by its size, the percentage of its villous component, as well as the

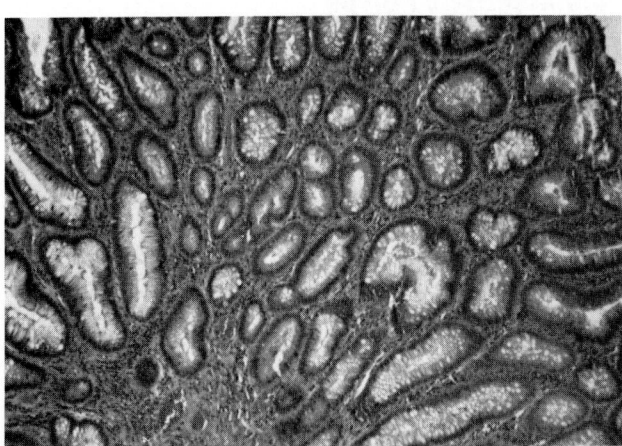

FIGURE 85-4. (See Color Fig. 43.) Histologic appearance of a tubular adenoma with minimal dysplasia. Architectural features include closely packed epithelial tubules with hyperchromatic, elongated nuclei but still with a predominant basal orientation and a normal nuclear : cytoplasmic ratio.

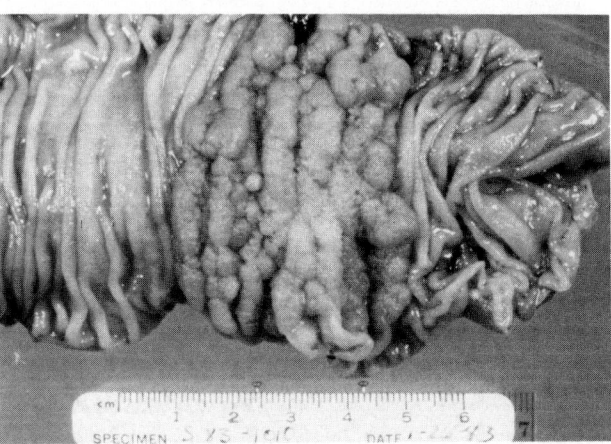

FIGURE 85-6. (See Color Fig. 45.) This cecal villous adenoma is virtually circumferential with submucosal carcinomatous invasion. The lesion is sessile in nature, and has a cauliflower appearance with a shaggy, frond-like, friable surface that contrasts with the smoother, lobulated surface seen in Figure 85-2.

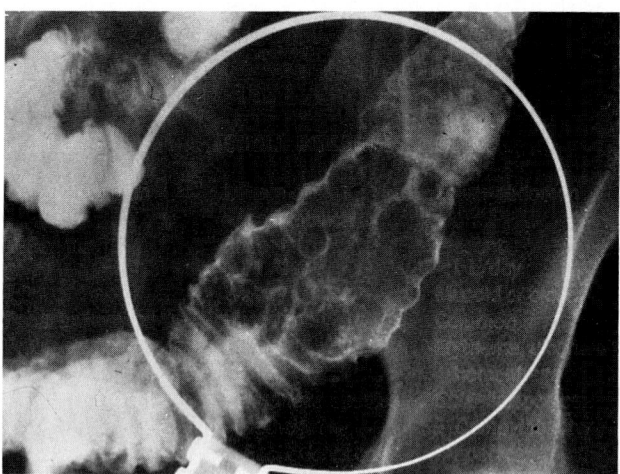

FIGURE 85-7. A very large, multilobulated, polypoid mass is demonstrated in the colon by radiography. Note the shaggy-appearing mucosal surface. The mass was subsequently found to be a large, sessile, villous adenoma that was virtually circumferential, similar to the lesion in Figure 85-6. It is easy to see how these lesions may produce colonic obstruction.

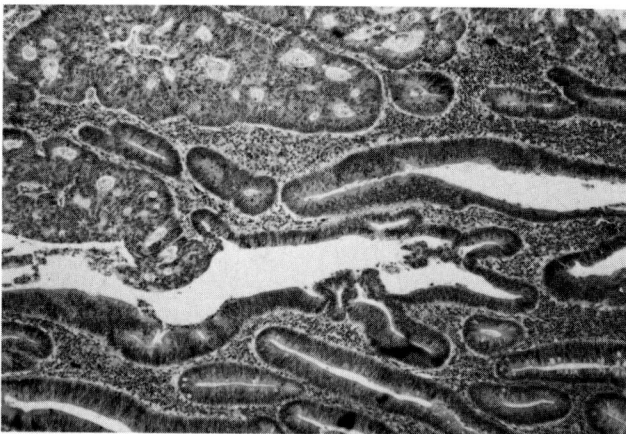

FIGURE 85-9. (See Color Fig. 47.) Histologic appearance of a tubulovillous adenoma with severe dysplasia and contiguous carcinoma. Note the hyperchromatic elongated nuclei with loss of basal polarity and the increased nuclear : cytoplasmic ratio. There is a sharp and drastic transition between these adenomatous features and carcinoma.

percentage of epithelium containing severe atypia, to provide improved clinical utility.[170,171]

Flat adenomas. The nonpolypoid adenoma, or flat adenoma, has been described, particularly in some cancer-prone families. These flat adenomas tend to be minimally raised if at all, small (usually <1 cm), discoid plaques, and are often erythematous. Because they are not polypoid they are often missed during colonoscopy.[142,180,181] A familial syndrome with flat adenomas has been described by Lynch and colleagues.[143,182] Despite their small size, more than a third of these flat adenomas have associated foci of high-grade atypia. In addition, flat adenomas are often multiple and associated with small adenocarcinomas.[180–184]

Mixed hyperplastic (serrated) adenomas. Mixed hyperplastic-adenomatous polyps with the architectural features of hyperplastic polyps and the cytologic features (dysplasia) of adenomas have been recognized.[185] They account for less than 1% of colorectal polyps,[186] and show the typical serrated surface and glandular epithelial appearance, but also dysplasia characterized by nucleolar prominence, increased mitoses, hyperchromasia, and nuclear pleomorphism.[187] The borders between hyperplastic and dysplastic cells are sharply demarcated.[188] These mixed (serrated) adenomas are associated with a high frequency of high-grade atypia (up to 40%) and intramucosal carcinoma (10%). They should probably be considered a variant of adenoma; hence, the terms *mixed adenoma* or *serrated adenoma* may be useful.

Nonneoplastic Polyps

The neoplastic polyps, or adenomas, all share a common histologic feature of dysplasia, and all carry the potential for progression to carcinoma. The nonneoplastic polyps, on the other hand, consist of distinct and often unrelated histologic groups. These are mucosal, hyperplastic, and inflammatory polyps (including pseudopolyps); a variety of hamartomas, including juvenile polyps; and other submucosal polypoid lesions.

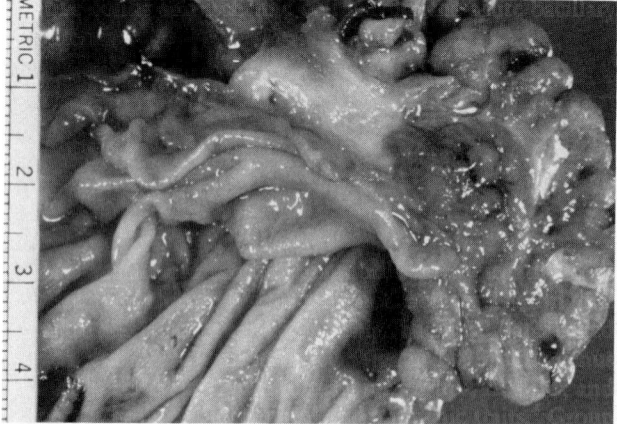

FIGURE 85-8. (See Color Fig. 46.) Sectioned surface of a tubulovillous adenoma with early carcinoma extending into the neck of the stalk. Note the large size (4 cm) of the adenoma and the extent of carcinomatous tissue extending from the head of the adenoma into the stalk, obliterating the muscularis propria layers.

Mucosal Polyps

These are small, pearl-like excrescences with coloration and appearance similar to adjacent normal mucosa. They are usually smaller than 5 mm. Histologically, they represent normal colonic mucosa that has been elevated by the submucosa, without any change in histologic status or architecture. They pose no known clinical significance.[168]

Hyperplastic Polyps

Hyperplastic polyps are among the most common of small colonic polyps, accounting for 15% or more of all colonic polyps.[168,172] They usually are small (<5 mm), sessile polyps, found predominantly in the distal colon,[189] with the same or paler coloration and appearance as the adjacent normal mucosa. Depending on the method of study, these hyperplastic polyps can be found in more than 80% of subjects. Studies that use a magnifying glass to examine a resected colon specimen, as well as studies that use sigmoidoscopy, tend to provide a higher estimate of the frequency of hyperplastic polyps. The frequency of hyperplastic polyps appears to increase with age.[16]

Histologically, hyperplastic polyps consist of well differentiated epithelium without any evidence of dysplasia. They are characterized by elongated glands with papillary infolding and increased mucus, which often gives a serrated appearance to the surface of the polyp. The crypt bases are hyperplastic with increased mitosis (Figs. 85-10 and 85-11; see Color Figs. 48 and 49).[110,190]

Studies demonstrate normal cell proliferation and maturation but do suggest delayed cell migration toward the top of the crypt that, together with delayed senescence and decreased extrusion of cells into the lumen, results in papillary infolding at the upper portion of the crypt, giving the typical serrated surface appearance.[191,192] Although they are not believed to be neoplastic, hyperplastic polyps share several histochemical and biochemical characteristics with adenomas. Like adenomas, they are associated with an increased expression of carcinoembryonic antigen (CEA) and a reduction in and low IgA secretory activity.[193]

Hyperplastic polyps have been associated with the presence of adenomas and even carcinomas in the same colon.[91–93,163] In one study, adenomas were found in more than 90% of patients with hyperplastic polyps.[194] These results, however,

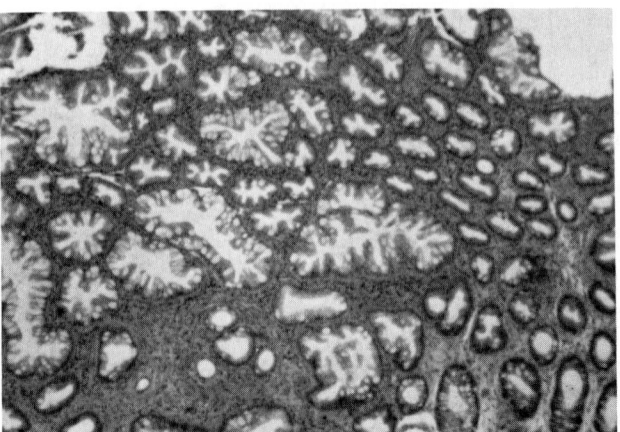

FIGURE 85-11. (See Color Fig. 49.) Histologic appearance of adenomatous epithelium in a predominantly hyperplastic polyp. This polyp should be managed as if it were an adenoma, because the adenomatous areas are presumed to be premalignant.

need to be interpreted in the context that distal hyperplastic polyps are extremely common, occurring in 80% or more of the population, with even higher frequencies in the elderly. All these features of hyperplastic polyps suggest that they may indeed be found in the population that is also at risk for adenomas and carcinomas, and the association may be purely coincidental. A number of studies have shown that the association may indeed be serendipitous[9,98–102] (see section on Epidemiology).

Despite their lack of malignant potential, hyperplastic polyps often are removed because they are endoscopically impossible to distinguish from premalignant adenomas. It is probably not necessary, except in those with other strong risk factors, to have patients with rectosigmoid hyperplastic polyps undergo complete colonoscopy.

Inflammatory Polyps

Inflammatory polyps are found in the setting of inflammatory diseases of the colon mucosa. The polypoid lesions may be one of two types. First, they may represent residual islands of intact colonic mucosa arising from the sea of colonic lumenal surface denuded of mucosa. In this instance, the term *pseudopolyp* is often applied. Inflammatory polyps can also represent exuberant masses of granulation tissue and regenerating mucosa. These inflammatory polyps may be large and solitary, with marked inflammation and ulceration, and can thus appear malignant endoscopically.[195]

Histologically, pseudopolyps often represent normal-appearing mucosa with inflammatory and regenerative changes. Large, solitary inflammatory polyps often show marked inflammation and granulation tissue with distortion of architecture. Inflammatory polyps are most commonly seen with any form of severe inflammatory colitis,[196–198] including ulcerative colitis,[195,199] Crohn's disease,[199,200] amebiasis,[201] strongyloidiasis,[202] tuberculosis,[203] severe diverticular disease,[204] or schistosomiasis.[205,206] In schistosomiasis, the inflammatory polyp may contain, in addition to the inflammation and granulation tissue, schistosome eggs or adult worms.[205] Some schistosome egg-induced polyps show in-

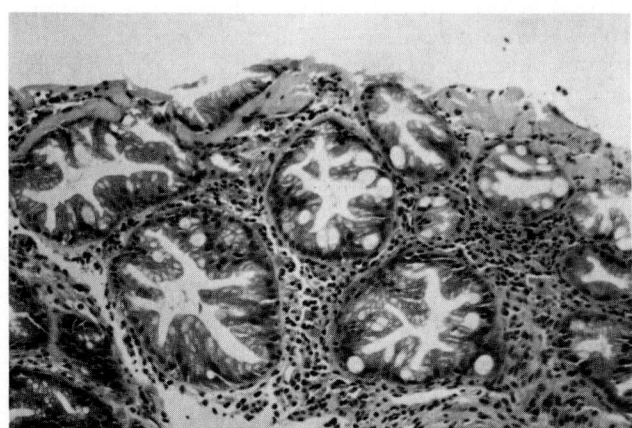

FIGURE 85-10. (See Color Fig. 48.) Histologic appearance of a hyperplastic polyp is characterized by the typical elongated glands with papillary infolding and increased mucus, which produce a serrated surface appearance. The epithelial cells are well differentiated with abundant cytoplasm, a normal nuclear : cytoplasmic ratio, and abundant secreted mucus. The nuclei are not hyperchromatic, retain their basal polarity, and show no dysplasia. The starfish appearance of the hyperplastic crypts seen in cross section is characteristic.

creased epithelial proliferation, with features of dysplasia, including crypt elongation, nuclear pleomorphism, disordered cell crowding, and nuclear stratification. Although there are inadequate data, these dysplastic schistosomiasis-associated polyps may be premalignant.[206]

Inflammatory polyps may be large,[198,199] produce symptoms of pain and obstruction,[207] and may even become pedunculated[208] or filiform.[197,209] They may also occur in settings with only minimal or healed inflammation, such as ulcerative colitis in remission,[207] solitary rectal ulcer syndrome,[210,211] ischemic colitis,[212] or even without any clinically apparent inflammatory bowel disease.[213]

Inflammatory polyps and pseudopolyps have no intrinsic malignant potential; however, they often occur in settings at high risk for development of colon cancer (ulcerative colitis), and must be carefully distinguished from dysplastic or neoplastic mass lesions (Fig. 85-12). An infiltrating adenocarcinoma in a large pseudopolyp without surface dysplasia has been described.[214]

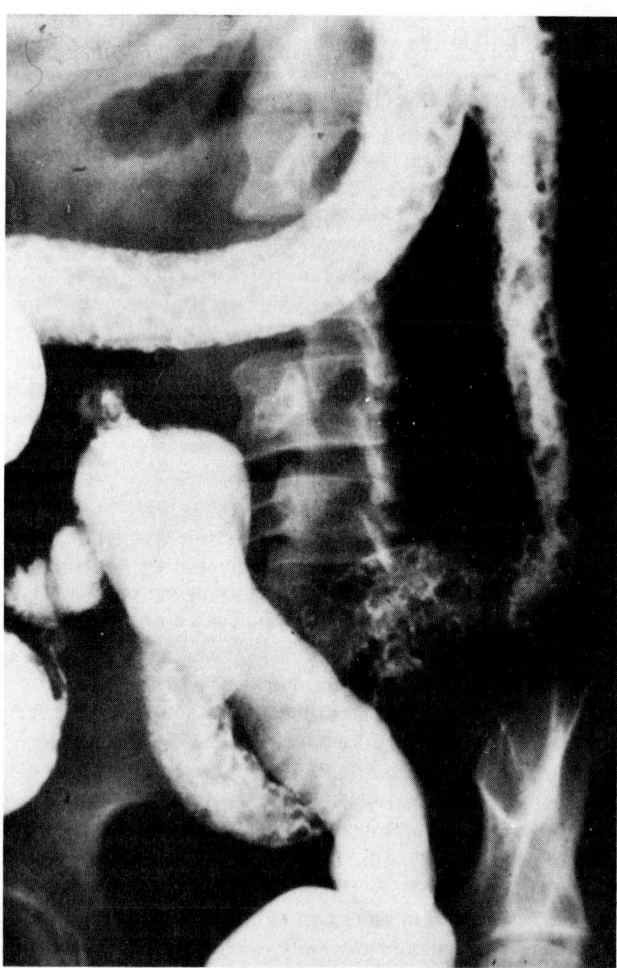

FIGURE 85-12. Multiple inflammatory polyps are present throughout the colon in a patient with ulcerative colitis. Colonoscopy and biopsy are necessary for proper identification of the lesions. During colonoscopy, the endoscopist must take biopsy specimens not just from the polyps but also from suspect plaque-like areas, because dysplastic lesions are the premalignant sites in this instance (see Chap. 87).

Rare cases of recurrent multiple inflammatory polyps producing pain, intussusception, and obstruction have been reported.[207] A family has been described in which three women, one from each of three successive generations, were found to have multiple inflammatory polyps of the ileum and gastric antrum without any malignancy reported.[215]

An unusual inflammatory polyp arising in the anorectal mucosa, the inflammatory cloacogenic polyp, has been described.[210,211] Inflammatory cloacogenic polyps have been found in all age groups and both sexes, and often present with rectal bleeding. Histologically, the polyps consist of a tubulovillous pattern of crypt hyperplasia with no dysplasia, with the superficial mucosa often showing ulceration. An association with the solitary rectal ulcer syndrome and mucosal prolapse, thought to be an etiologic factor, has been postulated.

The inflammatory cap polyp, found in the rectal area, is also thought to be a result of mucosal prolapse. The cap polyp is covered by a cap of inflammatory and granulation tissue, with intramucosal elastin at the edge of the cap. Macroscopically there often is associated hemorrhage into cap polyps, with hemorrhagic polyps separated by normal intervening mucosa. Some associated symptoms that have been described include mucous diarrhea, tenesmus, and rectal bleeding. Symptoms resolve after polypectomy.[216,217]

Another inflammatory polyp has been termed the *inflammatory myoglandular polyp* because of the presence of inflammatory and granulation tissue in the lamina propria with abundant smooth muscle proliferation, and hyperplastic glands with occasional cystic dilation. Unlike the cap polyp, it has no fibrin cap and is found more proximally, usually in the left colon or sigmoid. More than half of the patients were asymptomatic. When symptoms were present, they consisted of overt or occult rectal bleeding.[218]

Hamartomatous Polyps

Juvenile polyps. Juvenile polyps, also known as retention polyps because of their histologic characteristics, are so termed because three quarters of them are found in children younger than 10 years of age.[219,220] They tend to be single, pedunculated, cherry-red, round polyps with a smooth surface and contour. They are often friable and ulcerated, bleed frequently, and tend to prolapse because of their predominant location in the rectum and their pedunculated nature.[156,221–223] They are subject to volvulus with resultant ulceration and hemorrhage, autoinfarction, and autoamputation. Polyp tissue may be found in the stool.[157] Histologically, juvenile polyps are hamartomas with distended, mucus-filled glands that often show cystic dilation and edematous lamina propria containing abundant vasculature. This apparent mucin retention has also led to the term *retention polyps.* Juvenile polyps also frequently show foci of severe inflammation with ulceration.[219,220,224]

Juvenile polyps are rare in the first year of life and are most frequently seen from ages 1 to 10 years. They are thus presumed to be acquired and not congenital. Beyond the first decade, they are found only rarely in the second decade of life, but are again commonly found in adulthood.[225] The true prevalence is difficult to determine because there are no large population studies of asymptomatic children or large autopsy series of children. In one study, a frequency of approximately

2% was found in asymptomatic children.[226] In a series of children seen for rectal bleeding, solitary juvenile polyps were found in 20% and multiple juvenile polyps in 10%.[227] In other studies, however, only about 25% of children with juvenile polyps were found to have multiple polyps.[222] The presenting symptom is most commonly rectal bleeding. In fact, rectal bleeding is the symptom that leads to the diagnosis of juvenile polyps in more than 90% of cases. In other studies, up to 70% of children with rectal bleeding were found to have juvenile polyps by colonoscopy, and about a fourth had multiple polyps.[223] Of all polyps found in children younger than 15 years of age, up to 97% can be juvenile polyps.[156] Rectal prolapse of the polyp or autoamputation of the polyp[157] is the presenting complaint in about one third to one fourth of patients, and diarrhea and constipation are found in about 10%.[221]

Isolated juvenile polyps usually are not dysplastic and have no intrinsic malignant potential. Juvenile polyps may also occur in a familial setting,[228,229] however, and familial juvenile polyposis of the colon is characterized by autosomal dominant inheritance (see Chap. 86). In multiple juvenile polyposis, adenomatous and carcinomatous changes have been reported.[226,229–235] The association may be coincidental, because colorectal cancer occurring in families with juvenile polyposis is not always associated with the polyposis trait.[232] Studies suggest, however, that even solitary juvenile polyps may have associated adenomatous changes, sometimes seen in children as young as 3 years.[236] Thus all juvenile polyps, just like all other polypoid lesions, should be excised in toto if they can be removed safely. After removal, juvenile polyps recur only infrequently, with a rate of about 3% in 3 years.[226] If extensive adenomatous changes or severe atypia is seen, the patient may be considered for surveillance.[234]

Peutz-Jeghers polyps. Peutz-Jeghers polyps are the multiple hamartomatous polyps found throughout the gastrointestinal tract in Peutz-Jeghers syndrome.[237] The polyps are hamartomas, usually with prominent branching of smooth muscle. The syndrome is a rare autosomal dominant syndrome of gastrointestinal hamartomatous polyposis associated with melanin spots of the lips, buccal mucosa, and extremities[237,238] (see Chap. 86). Peutz-Jeghers polyps are not considered premalignant, although the syndrome has been associated with an increase in carcinomas,[239,240] mostly extracolonic.[241,242] A patient with multiple colon cancers, however, was found to have foci of carcinoma arising in hamartomatous Peutz-Jeghers polyps.[243] In this case, the other noninvolved hamartomatous polyps showed no dysplasia. Thus, the association of dysplasia and cancer with the Peutz-Jeghers polyps may be coincidental.

Unusual hamartomas with abundant adipose tissue have been described. These include angiomyolipomas, which are usually found in patients with tuberous sclerosis, and are hamartomas originating from the kidney that have invaded the colon. These angiomyolipomas are filled with adipose tissue as well as increased vasculature, and also have been found in patients without tuberous sclerosis. They appear to be benign, and complete removal may not be necessary.[244] Another variant hamartoma with mature stromal adipose tissue and simple benign glands, considered benign, also has been described.[245]

Submucosal Lesions

Submucosal lesions represent polypoid lesions that result from elevation of the mucosal surface by submucosal tumors. They are a group of diverse and generally unrelated entities.

Lymphoid Hyperplasia

There is lymphoid tissue throughout the entire gastrointestinal tract, including the colon. In the colon, lymphoid tissue exists as lamina propria lymphocytes and as lymphoid follicles. Lymphoid hyperplasia can involve either the diffuse lamina propria lymphocytes or the lymphoid follicles. When a focus of diffuse lamina propria lymphocytes is involved in the hyperplastic process, the result is focal lymphoid hyperplasia, also termed lymphoid polyp or benign lymphoid polyp.[246,247] When the lymphoid follicles are involved, usually an entire region of lymphoid tissue is involved, resulting in (diffuse) nodular lymphoid hyperplasia.[248,249]

Lymphoid polyps. Lymphoid polyps present commonly as distal, sessile, smooth polyps. Although they often appear pale yellow or white they may have the same color as normal adjacent mucosa. They usually are single, but can be multiple and occasionally present as mucosal cobblestoning. The extent of involvement is usually limited to the rectosigmoid area. Microscopically, lymphoid polyps are formed by elevation and occasional distention and stretching of the overlying epithelium by dilation of the underlying lamina propria from marked lymphocyte infiltration. Occasionally, lymphoid follicles are also present in the lamina propria, straddling the mucosa and the submucosa.[247,250,251]

Lymphoid polyps occur in all age groups but appear to be most common between the second and fifth decades, when adenomas are uncommon.[252,253] Lymphoid polyps are usually asymptomatic, but large lymphoid polyps in the rectum may occasionally prolapse. Although symptoms such as bleeding, abdominal distress, anal discomfort, constipation, and diarrhea have been reported, they are likely unrelated to the underlying lymphoid polyps.[247,254,255]

Diffuse nodular lymphoid hyperplasia. When the lymphoid follicles throughout a long segment of the colon or the small intestine become hyperplastic, a picture of diffuse polypoid lesions appears.[248,249,256] The colonic (or small intestinal) mucosa is covered with polypoid nodules, generally 5 mm in size or smaller. These polyps usually are sessile, appear pale yellow or white, or have coloration similar to that of adjacent normal mucosa. Although occasional umbilication may be observed, there usually is no ulceration, erosion, friability, or bleeding.[248,249,256,257]

Histologically, the nodules are composed of one or a cluster of hyperplastic lymphoid follicles with prominent germinal centers, often confined to the lamina propria and the superficial submucosa. There usually is elevation as well as distention of the overlying epithelium. When nodular lymphoid hyperplasia is associated with hypogammaglobulinemia, a decrease in the number of lamina propria lymphocytes and plasma cells is also observed. In nodular lymphoid hyperplasia, the histologic picture appears to represent hyperplasia of the preexisting solitary lymphoid follicles that are normally present in the colonic mucosa.

Diffuse nodular lymphoid hyperplasia is a common finding in children and usually is thought of as an incidental finding, without any clinical significance.[248,256] In a series of 1000 consecutive autopsies, nodular lymphoid hyperplasia was found in 3%. When nodular lymphoid hyperplasia was found, about half was found in the colon only, about half found in both the colon and small intestine, and 10% or so was found in the small intestine only.[258] In none of the patients in this autopsy series was the cause of death attributed to the nodular lymphoid hyperplasia. Furthermore, none of the patients studied had gastrointestinal symptoms or symptoms attributable to hypogammaglobulinemia.

Although diffuse nodular lymphoid hyperplasia is not considered premalignant, it must be distinguished from multiple adenomas and the adenomatous polyposis coli syndromes. Because the finding of multiple polypoid lesions on radiographic or endoscopic studies may prompt the incorrect diagnosis of adenomatous polyposis coli, care must be taken to make a definitive diagnosis. Unnecessary colectomies have been performed for this type of lymphoid polyposis.[259,260] The distinction between malignant lymphoma and multiple polyps is difficult,[261,262] and lymphoma has developed in a few patients with apparent nodular lymphoid hyperplasia.[249,263] A number of cases have also shown some response to chemotherapy.[264] It is unclear whether the malignant lymphoma represents a progression from the lymphoid hyperplasia or a de novo development of lymphoma. The diagnosis occasionally requires confirmation with immunocytochemical and gene rearrangement analysis.[262]

Pneumatosis Cystoides Intestinalis

Pneumatosis cystoides intestinalis refers to multiple air-filled cysts found within the submucosa. The cysts may be found in the colon or small intestine. The air-filled cysts are easily recognizable by radiographic examination as well as endoscopy (Fig. 85-13). At endoscopy, they are seen as multiple polypoid lesions in the colonic mucosa, which on closer examination appear to be translucent polyps that may look like air blebs just underneath the mucosa. Occasionally hemorrhage into the cysts may be observed. On biopsy, there is often a release of the submucosal air and deflation of the polypoid lesion.[265,266]

Pneumatosis intestinalis is generally asymptomatic,[265,267] but can also be associated with pneumoperitoneum.[267,268] Occasional cases associated with scleroderma or chronic obstructive pulmonary disease have been seen.[266] In these cases, the air-filled cysts may resolve after treatment with oxygen.[268]

Pneumatosis intestinalis also may be seen as part of the clinical picture associated with fulminant intestinal ischemia, especially in children. In that setting, the pneumatosis represents gas produced from gas-forming organisms during the course of ischemia, necrosis, or necrotizing enterocolitis, and is often fatal.[265]

Colitis Cystica Profunda

The radiographic appearance of colitis cystica profunda is virtually indistinguishable from that of solitary or multiple colonic polyps. The polyps are sessile and consist of dilated,

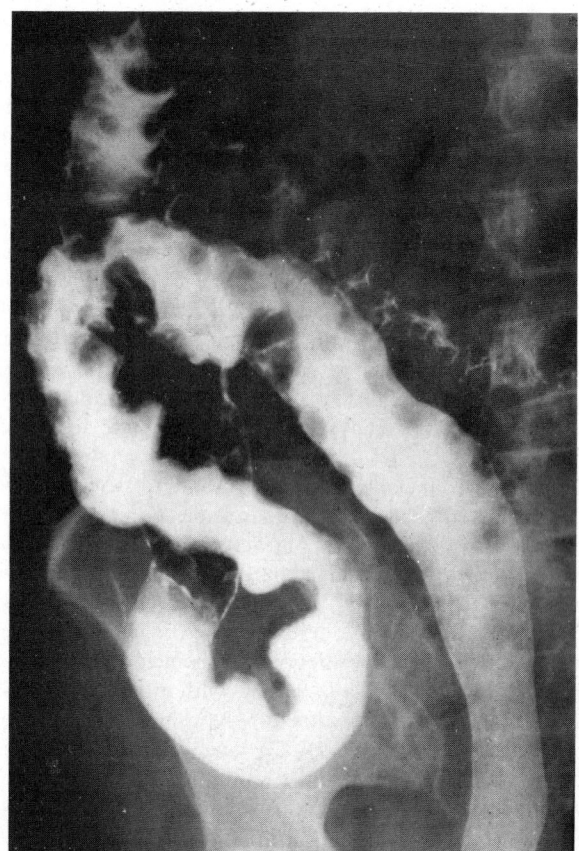

FIGURE 85-13. Pneumatosis cystoides intestinalis seen on barium-enhanced radiography. The intramural gas-filled cysts could have been identifiable on a plain abdominal radiograph.

epithelium-lined mucous cysts within the muscularis mucosae. They are found most often in the rectum in association with inflammatory colitis, or after surgery,[269,270] but also have been found more proximally in the descending colon.[271] It has been postulated that colitis cystica profunda is a result of the displacement of normal colonic glands into the muscularis mucosae during healing after surgical manipulation or after inflammatory colitis.[269] Some investigators also postulate that colitis cystica profunda is analogous to the solitary rectal ulcer and may also be a result of rectal prolapse.[272] Rarely, the lesions are large and produce obstruction.[273]

Their greatest clinical significance is their endoscopic and radiographic similarity to adenomas, and their histologic similarity to colloid carcinoma (because of the presence of mucus in the submucosa). When colitis cystica profunda is seen within an adenoma, it has been referred to as "pseudoinvasion" or "misplaced epithelium."[130,167,274] Most pathologists prefer the term *misplaced epithelium* because the process is benign. Careful histologic examination should reveal no adenomatous changes in the epithelium.

Lipomas

Lipomas within the gastrointestinal tract are found most commonly within the colon, usually in the right colon on or near the ileocecal valve. These lesions tend to be solitary but may be multiple in 20% or more of cases. Radiographically, because of the lower density of lipomas, they often show up as slightly radiolucent submucosal lesions. Lipomas, especially if they lie close to the mucosal surface, may appear light yellow or whitish endoscopically; this appearance is known as the naked-fat sign. These submucosal lesions occasionally may be found to be soft, pliable, and deformable by biopsy forceps; this appearance is known as the pillow sign. Biopsies may be needed when visual identification and distinction from adenomas cannot be ascertained. Once the diagnosis of lipoma is confirmed, removal of the lesion is not necessary because it has no clinical significance.[275,276]

Other Submucosal Lesions

A number of other rare submucosal lesions may also present radiographically or endoscopically as polypoid lesions. Virtually any disease process that can result in a mucosal or submucosal mass could present as a polypoid lesion in the colon. In general, biopsies of the surface would reveal normal colonic epithelium. Deeper biopsies, or sequentially deeper biopsies at the same biopsy site, biopsy with hot biopsy forceps, or biopsy after submucosal saline injection to elevate the mass may be required to reach the submucosal mass.

Malignant submucosal lesions include carcinoids,[277,278] metastatic carcinomas, most commonly malignant melanoma[279] and lymphoma,[262] gastric cancer,[280] Kaposi's sarcoma,[276] and plasma cell leukemia.[281] Benign lesions include lymphangiomas, fibromas, neurofibromas,[282] leiomyomas, myoblastomas, hemangiomas, and endometriosis.[283] Clinical signs and symptoms, when they are present, are often those of the underlying lesion; however, small lesions are commonly asymptomatic.

Other colorectal lesions may occasionally masquerade as polyps. Such lesions include hemorrhoids, condylomata,[284] enlarged anal papillae, inverted diverticula,[285] enteroenteric and ureteroenteric anastomoses,[286] and the residual stalk of a pedunculated polyp after polypectomy.[287] This residual stalk polyp shows recanalized vasculature, hemosiderin, and scarring on histologic examination, but is difficult to distinguish from an adenoma endoscopically.[287]

All polypoid lesions need to be distinguished from adenomas or carcinomas, and biopsies are mandatory. Biopsies often reveal normal mucosa, and deeper biopsies may be needed with hot biopsy forceps, larger forceps, or snare biopsy with or without submucosal saline injection to elevate the lesion. Care should be taken, however, not to sample vascular or vascular-like lesions aggressively.

DIFFERENTIAL DIAGNOSIS

The differential diagnosis of polypoid lesions found in the colon and rectum includes neoplastic polyps, nonneoplastic polyps, and submucosal lesions. Some of the distinctive clinical, morphologic, and histologic features have been described. The most important modality in arriving at a correct diagnosis is microscopic histologic analysis. Thus, colonoscopy and biopsy of all polypoid lesions is virtually mandatory.

SCREENING STUDIES

Screening for colonic adenomatous polyps is done in the setting of screening, surveillance, and early detection of colorectal cancer,[84,288–291] and is discussed in Chapter 87.

Sigmoidoscopy

Data suggest that 10% or more of colonic neoplasms are located in the rectum and an additional 35% to 45% arise in the sigmoid colon (see Table 85-3). The standard rigid sigmoidoscope has a potential depth of insertion of 25 cm, although on the average a 17- to 20-cm depth of insertion is achieved. A 60-cm flexible sigmoidoscope could achieve an average length of insertion of 48 to 55 cm and thus potentially detect up to 60% of all colonic neoplasms.[292] In general, flexible sigmoidoscopy provides a two to three times higher yield than rigid sigmoidoscopy. Flexible sigmoidoscopy, however, is more expensive, requires more skill, and takes longer to perform than rigid sigmoidoscopy. Nevertheless, it is preferred over rigid sigmoidoscopy because of its higher yield and greater patient acceptance.[292,293] A 30-cm flexible sigmoidoscope has been introduced for the screening of rectosigmoid neoplasms. This instrument is easier for generalists to use and is less time consuming. It appears that up to 40% of all colonic neoplasms could be detected with the 30-cm sigmoidoscope.[294,295] Because patient discomfort and preparation are identical for both types of flexible sigmoidoscopic examinations, and the necessary skill is easily acquired, the longer instrument is preferred. Complications of flexible sigmoidoscopy are extremely rare. Patient preparation is simple. A single, self-administered tap water or phosphate enema 2 hours before the procedure usually suffices. A complete examination of the lower rectal area and anal region may require anoscopy in some cases.

A large number of studies on the use of sigmoidoscopy have accumulated over the past two decades.[296] Although most studies before 1979 used a rigid sigmoidoscope, more recent series have reported experience with flexible sigmoidoscopy. These studies vary in number, age, and type of patients included (i.e., symptomatic or asymptomatic). Most of these studies describe only the findings at sigmoidoscopy, and do not provide follow-up information. Most important, none of the published studies is a randomized, controlled trial. As expected, studies that include symptomatic patients have higher yield for neoplastic lesions. Among screened asymptomatic patients, cancer was detected in less than 1% of subjects, and adenoma in 5%.[297,298] In symptomatic patients, cancer was detected in 3% and adenomas in up to 35%. Studies that used the flexible sigmoidoscope gave higher yield for both carcinomas and adenomas.

Radiography

Single-contrast barium enema is relatively insensitive for the detection of early colorectal neoplasms.[299] Air-contrast studies have better sensitivity but still are less sensitive than fiberoptic colonoscopy in most hands.[300] Most series have indicated that colonoscopy is 10% to 12% more accurate than air-contrast barium enema and gives fewer false-positive results.[301,302] Patient discomfort with barium enema is about the same as with colonoscopy. Barium enema is not recommended for the screening of asymptomatic, average-risk people.

Colonoscopy

Fiberoptic colonoscopy is not recommended as a screening tool for average-risk, asymptomatic people. Although it is highly sensitive and specific for colorectal neoplasia, its expense, discomfort, and potential complications can be prohibitive. Colonoscopy may be an appropriate means of screening for selected high-risk groups: family members in adenomatous polyposis coli syndromes and hereditary colorectal cancer syndromes, patients with long-standing, extensive ulcerative colitis, and those with previous history of adenomas and cancers.

DIAGNOSTIC STUDIES

Digital rectal examination, FOBT, and sigmoidoscopy are properly considered as screening studies and not diagnostic studies. They are discussed in Chapter 87.

Radiography

Single-contrast barium enema has been shown to have approximately 75% sensitivity and specificity for detection of colonic polypoid lesions. With the improved definition of the air-contrast barium enema, sensitivity and specificity are increased to more than 90% and 85%, respectively.[303,304] But artifacts still occur, especially in those patients whose bowel preparation is less than totally satisfactory.[305] Although most studies have found that even double-contrast barium enemas miss polypoid lesions subsequently detected on colonoscopy,[225,302,306] the converse has also been observed. Some studies found that double-contrast barium enema can detect polyps missed during colonoscopy.[307,308] Most studies show that colonoscopy has a higher detection rate, albeit at a higher cost.[306,309–311] The accuracy of both procedures, however, depends on the expertise of the examiner. Also, there are patients in whom colonoscopy cannot be completed to the cecum because of anatomic or clinical reasons. In these patients, the air-contrast barium enema remains the only diagnostic method to detect colonic polyps proximal to the rectosigmoid (Fig. 85-14).

Although radiography has been advocated as a primary diagnostic test for colonic polyps, colonoscopy may still be the preferred method of follow-up after a positive FOBT or sigmoidoscopy.[9,312–314] Colonoscopy allows the therapeutic removal of any polypoid lesions found, whereas a positive radiologic examination still necessitates subsequent follow-up colonoscopy for biopsy or endoscopic removal of the lesion.[314,315]

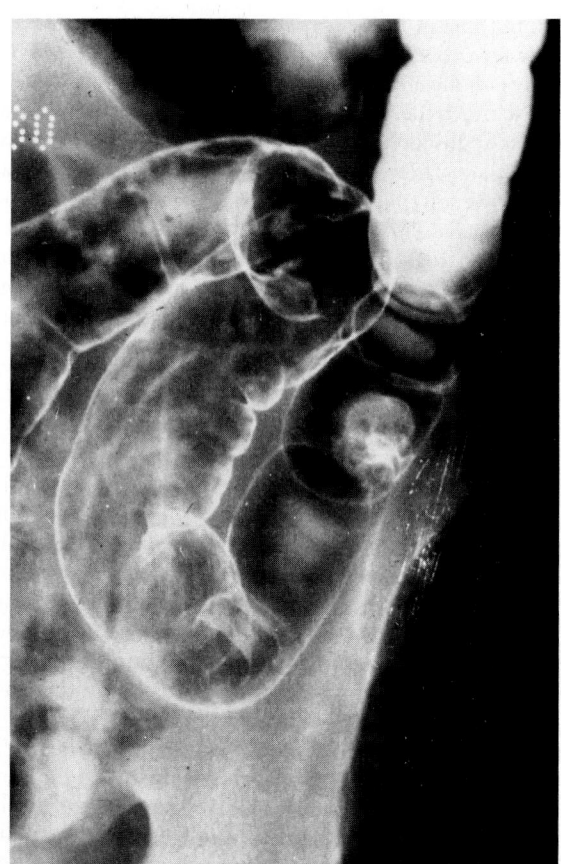

FIGURE 85-14. A pedunculated polyp demonstrated by double-contrast radiography. A carefully done single-contrast examination, especially with postevacuation films, can also demonstrate polypoid lesions. Note the lobulated appearance of the polyp surface. The mass was subsequently found to be a tubulovillous adenoma. Colonoscopy and biopsy or polypectomy must be done, because the histologic status and appropriate management and follow-up cannot be established otherwise.

Colonoscopy

When a patient is suspected of having colonic neoplasms by signs, symptoms, or physical examination, colonoscopy is the procedure of choice to evaluate the colon (see Chap. 116). Even if a neoplasm has been documented by sigmoidoscopy, total colonoscopy of the entire colon is recommended because synchronous adenomas and cancers may be present at other sites in the colon and may affect the extent of surgical resection performed. Many studies have documented that colonoscopy is superior to barium enema (both single and double contrast) in detecting both polyps and cancers.[306,309–311] Colonoscopy also allows for polypectomy or biopsy of all suspect lesions at the time of the procedure. The fiberoptic colonoscope has been improved greatly in design and ease of maneuverability in the last two decades, and most practitioners agree that barium enema is less sensitive and less specific than colonoscopy.[306,309] Colonoscopy in experienced hands has a sensitivity and specificity exceeding 95%, and is extremely safe even in young children, with a major complication rate of less than 3%, with less than 0.5% of patients requiring surgical intervention, and virtually no mortality.[316,317]

Before colonoscopic evaluation, a careful history with close attention to family history (for the identification of other family members at high risk) and symptoms should be obtained. A thorough physical examination should be performed, specifically looking for dermatomyositis or cutaneous and subcutaneous metastases, and for lymph node involvement, particularly in the inguinal and supraclavicular area. Enlarged lymph nodes may be difficult to interpret because these nodes drain large areas. For inguinal nodes, enlargement is most often without obvious etiology or associated with anorectal inflammatory diseases. Close attention to the abdomen may reveal an abdominal mass or evidence of liver involvement. In women, a pelvic examination may be necessary to exclude contiguous involvement of pelvic organs. The breast and prostate should be carefully examined to exclude these sites as potential primary sources of a metastatic lesion.

Biopsy and Histopathologic Examination

Biopsy or polypectomy of all polypoid lesions should be done because histopathologic analysis is the definitive diagnostic test. Histopathologic examination is required to establish the nature of the polyp and the presence of adenomatous epithelium or malignancy, and is critical in determining management.

The histologic features of the spectrum of colonic polyps are described in the section on Clinical Manifestations of the various polypoid lesions, and are not discussed here. It should be clear from the preceding discussions, and the subsequent discussions of clinical course and therapy, that the pathologist should be enlisted as a partner in the management team for colonic polyps.[318]

Discussions with the pathologist are necessary to determine the optimal methods for biopsy and polypectomy, the handling of the specimens, the use of the proper fixative, and the provision of requisite clinical information, especially previous biopsies and the anatomic location of the current specimen. It is important to use separate specimen containers when specimens are obtained from different anatomic sites; otherwise, lesions may be interchanged and it may be difficult to determine which of several anatomically distinct lesions is the one showing adenomatous changes or malignancy on histologic examination.

Discussions with the pathologist should also include the use of special stains and examinations, such as determinations of biochemical and genetic markers. Some of these techniques require special handling, such as frozen sections and special fixatives. In some cases, the pathology staff may want to come to the endoscopy suite to prepare the specimen. Attempts also should be made to take part in the histopathologic examination together with the pathologist. With this cooperative effort, gastroenterologists and pathologists (and radiologists where radiography was performed) can work together to discuss clinicopathologic interpretations and management, and help each other to complement and build skills.

BIOCHEMICAL AND MOLECULAR MARKERS

These biochemical markers usually are studied in the context of colorectal cancers and not adenomas, and are discussed in Chapter 87.

CEA, initially described in 1965,[319] belongs to a class of proteins referred to as *oncofetal proteins* that are normally expressed in the fetus but only in very small amounts in healthy adults. CEA is actually a group of related glycoproteins whose immunoreactivity resides on the protein moieties. The sensitivity of serum CEA for diagnosing colonic adenomas is low.[320] Specificity is also low because serum CEA is elevated in patients with nongastrointestinal epithelial tumors, as well as in smokers and patients with nonmalignant conditions, including liver disease, renal failure, and fibrocystic disease.[320,321] CEA is thus not useful in screening or detection of colonic neoplasms.

CA-19-9 is a commercially available monoclonal antibody to a tissue glycoprotein that also recognizes a mucin-type glycoprotein in serum.[322] This antibody, originally developed against colon cancer to aid in its serologic diagnosis, is more sensitive for gastric, pancreatic, and hepatobiliary tumors and has a very high specificity for these tumors in some studies.[323,324] CA-19-9, however, has not proven useful in screening or detection of colonic neoplasms.

Other new biochemical markers such as blood group antigens and carbohydrate antigens are under active investigation.[325,326]

CLINICAL COURSE AND COMPLICATIONS

Natural History

Nonneoplastic polyps may enlarge, decrease in size, or even regress, but they are not premalignant. Nevertheless, most nonneoplastic polyps are removed by endoscopic polypectomy, because it is difficult to distinguish them from neoplastic polyps during endoscopy.

The natural history of submucosal lesions depends on the type of lesion. Metastatic lesions, such as malignant melanomas and lymphomas, are aggressive tumors. Other lesions, such as lipomas and fibromas, usually are truly asymptomatic and pose no clinical concern.

Because of their premalignant nature and the adenoma-carcinoma sequence, the natural history of the adenomatous polyp is of major clinical importance, and the remainder of this section refers specifically to the adenoma. Although the evidence is clear (see previous sections) that virtually all colon carcinomas arise from adenomas, the natural history and the growth rate of adenomas are still not completely defined. Because of the inherent risks of colonoscopy, there has not been a large-scale, randomized, population-based, prospective colonoscopy study to determine the natural clinical history of adenomas. In addition, it is unethical and impossible to follow the unimpeded growth of an adenoma or its progression to a malignant carcinoma. Even if one were to undertake such a study, the complete removal and histologic study of the polyp would be required to ascertain that a polyp is indeed an adenoma and does not contain any carcinoma. Thus an attempt at a natural history follow-up is difficult on clinical grounds as well. Because of patient noncompliance and occasional technical and surgical difficulties, however, a small number of patients with adenomas have been followed over a number of years.

Studies examining the ages at which adenomas of differing degrees of atypia are found, as well as the ages of patients in whom colon carcinomas develop, have been performed in Japan (where the colon adenoma and carcinoma frequency is lower than in the United States). It was estimated that it takes approximately 11 years for an adenoma with mild atypia, and approximately 4 years for an adenoma with severe atypia, to progress to carcinoma.[327] This is consistent with the estimated period of 7 years between the peak age of onset of adenomas and the peak age of onset of carcinomas.[132,136] These results are also consistent with those estimated from patients with unresected adenomas, where the period for progression to carcinoma appears to be 5 to 10 years.[24]

Some limited studies, however, have suggested that there is great variation among the growth rates of colon adenomas. A study using serial sigmoidoscopy to follow asymptomatic rectal polyps smaller than 1 cm found that most did not increase in size. Over the course of 3 to 5 years, only 4% of the polyps increased in size. Seventy percent remained unchanged in size, 8% were smaller, and 18% were found to have disappeared spontaneously.[328] Studies using serial barium enemas also suggest that most of polyps grow very slowly, if at all.[329,330] The histologic status of these polyps, however, and whether they were even adenomas, is of course unknown.

Using the available data on the growth rate of colon adenomas and carcinomas, a mathematical model has suggested that it takes 2 to 3 years for a small adenoma (<0.5 cm) to grow to 1 cm in size, and another 2 to 5 years for the 1-cm adenoma to progress to carcinoma.[331,332]

A retrospective study examined the risk for development of colon carcinoma at the site of an adenoma 1 cm or larger left in situ. A total of 226 patients was followed for an average of more than 5 years with an average of five barium enemas. During the course of follow-up, 37% of the polyps increased in size, colon carcinomas developed at the site of the index polyp in 10% of the patients, and carcinoma developed at sites removed from the index polyp in another 5%. The cumulative risk for development of carcinoma at the site of a polyp 1 cm or larger was estimated to be 3% at 5 years, 8% at 10 years, and 24% at 20 years. The data for the 5- and 10-year follow-ups are of course more accurate than those for the 20-year follow-up.[134]

A prospective follow-up of 215 polyps less than 5 mm in diameter has been done. At polypectomy 2 years later, approximately 50% were found to be hyperplastic polyps, 25% were mucosal polyps, and only 25% were adenomatous polyps. There was both regression and enlargement of polyps from the time of initial observation. Usually, mucosal polyps regressed and the adenomas and hyperplastic polyps enlarged, with a doubling in size in the 2-year period; however, no polyp was significantly larger than 5 mm, and no high-grade atypia or cancer was found.[333]

In the National Polyp Study, the polyp recurrence rate in patients followed by periodic colonoscopy and polypectomies was about 3% at 1 year and 35% at 3 years, and the absolute 2-year recurrence rate (between year 1 and year 3) was 20%. These results suggest an adenoma recurrence rate of about 10% per year on the average. The data also suggest that patients with multiple adenomas with villous histology and marked atypia were more likely to have recurrence, as were older men with a family history of colorectal neoplasms.[334]

These results, when taken together, suggest that most polyps enlarge slowly if at all. Because the histologic type of the polyp cannot be determined without polypectomy, however, all polyps probably should be removed (see section on Therapy). In addition, a small but consistent number of adenomas do pose significant cancer risk over periods as short as 3 years.

Metachronous Adenomas

Synchronous and metachronous adenomas occur commonly. New adenomas also develop when most or all existing adenomas are removed. Most studies document a new polyp occurrence rate of 10% to 50% in 2 to 3 years, with higher rates in patients whose adenomas were larger or present in greater numbers.[335–337] More recent studies suggest that follow-up colonoscopy at 3 years postpolypectomy is as effective for detecting and removing new adenomas as at 1 year.[338]

Malignant Polyps

As discussed in previous sections, larger adenomas (>1 cm) and those with a predominant villous architecture demonstrate a higher frequency of severe focal atypia. The atypical or carcinomatous cells also can be locally invasive within the mucosa (intramucosal carcinoma). Such noninvasive carcinomas are the pathologist's cancers (i.e., those with no clinical significance) because neither severe focal atypia nor intramucosal carcinoma breach the muscularis mucosae. The lymphatics in the colon usually do not extend beyond the muscularis mucosae, and thus these noninvasive carcinomas within adenomatous polyps are unlikely to result in invasive metastatic disease and require no additional therapy after they are removed by polypectomy. There have not been any confirmed reports of lymphatic invasion resulting from severe focal atypia or intramucosal carcinoma.[165,336,339] Hence, most pathologists prefer the terms *adenoma with severe focal atypia* or *noninvasive carcinoma* because the terms carcinoma in situ and intramucosal carcinoma have all too often resulted in unnecessary additional therapy.

The carcinomatous focus can further invade through the muscularis mucosae and then the remainder of the submucosa. The adenoma is then termed a malignant polyp. Malignant polyps have the potential to develop into a malignancy with metastasis.[340] As discussed, distinction from pseudoinvasion (i.e., misplaced epithelium) may need to be made.[130,167–169]

THERAPY

Polypectomy

Since the advent of fiberoptic endoscopy and the introduction of colonoscopic snare polypectomy, a simple and cost-effective procedure has been available to manage colonic polyps.[7,315,341,342] As described in previous sections, adenomatous polyps have a potential for malignant degeneration, and virtually all colorectal cancers arise form adenomatous polyps.[132] Thus, all adenomas encountered during colonoscopy should be removed if possible (see Chap. 116).

In practice, all polyps are considered abnormal and should be removed. Polyps that are smaller than 5 mm, also referred to as diminutive polyps, usually are benign, rarely produce bleeding, and may be left in place if they are multiple. But at least three to five of the polyps should be removed for histologic examination[343,344]; they should all be removed if found to be adenomas. Although hot biopsy[345] and bipolar electrocoagulation[346] have been advocated for eradication of diminutive polyps, it appears that they all can leave behind residual polyp (adenomatous) tissue more than 20% of the time,[345–348] even if tissue necrosis was visualized.[347] Cold snare polypectomy or garroting of small polyps may be effective.[349]

It may not be possible to determine the histologic type by gross visual appearance, but polyps larger than 2 cm in size usually are adenomatous and, thus, premalignant. These large polyps should be removed in toto if pedunculated. If sessile, they may need to be removed piecemeal,[350] although the histologic evaluation of the presence or degree of invasion of any carcinomatous foci would then be difficult or impossible. If there is any concern that residual polyp tissue may be left, the polypectomy site should be tattooed with sterilized India ink to facilitate follow-up evaluation.[351] The number of polyps that can be removed safely depends on their location and size. In the patient with a diagnosis of adenomatous polyposis coli or related hereditary polyposis syndromes, colectomy, not polypectomy, is indicated. For multiple adenomatous polyps, where there is the possibility of removing them endoscopically, the colon should be cleared of polyps a section at a time to reduce the chance of complications. The wall thickness of the cecal area and right colon is thinner than that of the left, which also must be considered when removing polyps through cautery. Although the optimal type of cautery current has been debated, it appears they are equally safe.[352] If polyps are inflammatory, hyperplastic, or otherwise nonadenomatous by histologic examination, complete removal is unnecessary, but a sampling of several polyps from each cluster is required.

Polypectomy is safe in adults[316] and children[317] when done by experienced physicians. The major complication rate is less than 3%, the requirement for hospitalization or surgical intervention less than 0.3%, and death is virtually nonexistent.[316] Colonoscopic polypectomy may be associated with higher complication rates in patients in whom a safe colonoscopy is difficult to perform, such as those with long redundant colons, intraabdominal adhesions, or multiple large diverticula. Polypectomy should be deferred in patients with severe bleeding diatheses, unstable cardiac arrhythmias, recent myocardial infarctions, acute colitis, pregnancy (second or third trimester), recent colonic surgery, or abdominal abscess or perforation.[353]

When an adenoma is found without evidence of severe atypia, a repeat colonoscopy every 3 years suffices. One study shows that repeat colonoscopy at 3 years is as effective as two colonoscopies done at 1 and 3 years postpolypectomy.[338] For patients at higher risk for colorectal cancers, more frequent examinations may be in order. If colon cancer is found, a definitive colonoscopic or surgical procedure is indicated. If the colon was adequately examined before surgery, follow-up colonoscopy can be performed at intervals as long as every 3 years in the asymptomatic patient if repeated examinations are negative.

The procedural aspects of colonoscopy and polypectomy, including patient preparation, premedication, antibiotic prophylaxis, polypectomy, and polyp retrieval techniques, are discussed in Chapter 116.

Laser Ablation

Laser ablation with the neodymium–yttrium-aluminum garnet laser is an alternative method for the rapid removal of large numbers of small polyps from segments of the colon.[43,354–358] In experienced hands it is efficacious, rapid, and safe. The complications of hemorrhage and stenosis occur in about 5% of cases.[358] Perforation is extremely rare, even in the thin-walled cecal area.[357] Its particular applications are for the removal of multiple polyps after the histologic diagnosis has been confirmed by previous biopsies or polypectomies. It is extremely useful for the ablation of the multiple tiny polyps in the rectal stump of patients with adenomatous polyposis coli who have undergone total colectomy with ileorectal anastomosis.[358] It also may be used for large-scale removal of hyperplastic polyps when at least one of the hyperplastic polyps has been found to have mixed adenomatous elements. Laser ablation is also useful in patients who are not surgical candidates, and often results in rapid symptomatic relief.[358] The disadvantages, of course, are that laser ablation is destructive and does not yield specimens for pathologic evaluation, and may rarely result in colonic perforation.[357] It is also possible that a focus of invasive malignancy in the polyp may be missed, and appropriate management may not be provided.

Surgical Resection

In cases in which a polyp is large and sessile, or otherwise cannot be removed by endoscopic polypectomy, surgical resection may be necessary. Surgical resection is also indicated for large villous adenomas in the rectum, as well as for some adenomas with invasive carcinoma (malignant polyps).[359–361] Large rectal adenomas may be extirpated by transanal excision. Other large polypoid lesions and malignant polyps need to be removed by laparotomy. Advances in laparoscopic surgery have led to a report of laparoscopic resection of a large villous adenoma of the colon, which was delivered laparoscopically to outside the abdominal wall through a small skin incision.[362] Once laparotomy is indicated, many surgeons advocate the use of a formal segmental colectomy including lymph node dissection. The rationale is that when a laparotomy is required for lesions above the peritoneal reflection, a formal hemicolectomy adds little or no additional anesthesia time or perioperative mortality and morbidity.[361] The patient's willingness, however, to assume some risk for potential undertreatment for disease and the patient's ability to maintain surveillance also are factors that should be considered in any therapeutic decision.

Noninvasive Carcinoma

The presence of severe focal atypia (carcinomatous cells contained by the basement membrane) or intramucosal carcinoma (carcinomatous cells beyond the basement membrane and into the lamina propria, but still contained within the muscularis mucosae) does not make an adenoma malignant because the cancerous cells have not penetrated the muscularis mucosae (see Chap. 87). It is commonly assumed that adenomas with severe focal atypia or intramucosal carcinoma do not metastasize owing to the lack of lymphatic channels within the mucosa of such lesions, thus eliminating the route by which many colonic malignancies seem to spread. Adenomas with severe focal atypia and intramucosal carcinoma are uniformly thought to be cured by polypectomy. Hence, most pathologists prefer *severe focal atypia* or equivalent terms rather than carcinoma in situ, and the term *noninvasive carcinoma* for both types of lesions, because the word carcinoma has all too often resulted in unnecessary additional therapy.

The occurrence of severe focal atypia, intramucosal carcinoma, and malignancy makes evaluation of a polyp by fragmental biopsy or brush cytology a practice fraught with inaccuracy and one to be avoided.[165,363] Although biopsy of a polyp may reveal its nonneoplastic nature, the presence of cancerous cells on a biopsy or cytology specimen does not reveal the malignant nature of a polyp. Furthermore, biopsy may miss an area of invasive carcinoma or be too superficial to make this diagnosis. Only careful examination of serial sections of the entire polyp after removal is adequate for proper evaluation.

Malignant Polyp

When a polyp contains malignant cells that have penetrated the muscularis mucosae, it is termed a malignant polyp. Malignant invasion usually is not diffuse, and removal of the entire polyp with careful examination of multiple sections must be done, especially when malignant cells or severe atypia are noted and have been found on the mucosal surface. Care must be taken to distinguish invasive carcinoma from misplaced epithelium (pseudoinvasion).[274,364]

The proper management of malignant polyps remains controversial.[342] Many features of malignant polyps have been studied for their predictive potential. Poor prognostic features include incomplete resection, venous or lymphatic invasion, invasion of the submucosa of the colonic wall, the absence of or the short length of a stalk, poorly differentiated carcinoma, involvement of or within 2 mm of polypectomy margins, replacement of the bulk of the adenoma by carcinoma, and large polyp size. The presence of poor prognostic features should lead the physician to favor colectomy (Table 85-7).[165,166,365-368]

There have been no prospective trials evaluating the natural history of malignant polyps or their optimal management strategy. Studies usually are retrospective and patients have not been randomized to either endoscopic resection or surgical excision. It may well be unethical to implement such a trial, because clinical evidence suggests that the risk of cancer recurrence or metastasis may be as high as 10% within 5 years for polyps with poor prognostic features, and operative mortality in otherwise healthy patients can be much lower.

TABLE 85-7
Poor Prognostic Features of Malignant Polyps in Decreasing Order of Importance

Incomplete endoscopic resection
Venous or lymphatic invasion
Invasion of submucosa of colonic wall
Sessile or very short stalk
Poorly differentiated carcinoma
Involvement of or within 2 mm of polypectomy margins
Cancer larger than half of polyp volume
Polyp size >2 cm

Most studies suggest that the presence of venous or lymphatic invasion is a grave prognostic factor, and that these patients should undergo colon resection.[365,368] Some studies suggest that lymphatic invasion may be subject to observer variability.[369] Malignant polyps with venous (or lymphatic) invasion are associated with higher-grade cancers, recurrences, and metastases, but the studies have been mostly retrospective reviews.[368] Sessile polyps are also considered to have a worse prognosis. In one study, 7 of 34 patients with sessile polyps had local recurrence or distant metastases within 6 years, compared to none of 47 patients with pedunculated polyps.[370] Of those with pedunculated polyps, most had invasion limited to the head (level 1), neck (level 2), or stalk (level 3), although 1 patient had invasion to the base of the stalk (level 4). In another study, even patients with pedunculated polyps with venous invasion in the stalk fared poorly. Of 62 evaluatable patients who also had endoscopic polypectomy, 4 had recurrence (or cancer of unknown origin) within 5 years, giving a recurrence rate of less than 7% over 5 years.[369] In other studies, patients who underwent endoscopic polypectomy for pedunculated malignant polyps did better. In one study, 19 patients with pedunculated malignant polyps (average size 3 cm), with one polyp showing venous invasion, were all asymptomatic after 1 to 6 years.[371] In another retrospective review of 43 patients with pedunculated malignant polyps who were followed for almost 5 years, 19 patients initially underwent colon resection because of physicians' "clinical judgment." Of these 19 patients, as well as the 24 who had polypectomy alone, none had cancer recurrence. Of the 13 evaluatable patients with sessile polyps, all underwent colon resection, when Dukes' B or C cancer was found in 11. None has had cancer recurrence after almost 5 years.[372]

These results are based on flawed studies and it is difficult to formulate rigid guidelines based on them. The studies do suggest that most patients with pedunculated malignant polyps, without venous invasion or other poor prognostic features, are cured by endoscopic polypectomy alone.[370-372] They also suggest that patients with sessile malignant polyps do well after colon resection,[372] but quite poorly after endoscopic polypectomy alone.[165,370] We are left to speculate on whether these patients, or a subgroup with less grave prognostic features, might have done almost as well without surgery. It would appear prudent to weigh the known risks of surgery against the potentially poor but uncertain risks of an endoscopically resected malignant polyp. A patient whose perioperative mortality risk is less than 2% to 5% might benefit from a colon resection, whereas another patient whose perioperative mortality risk is higher than 7% to 10% or whose life expectancy is less than 5 years might benefit from polypectomy alone.

Recommendations concerning the management of malignant polyps must take into account the successes and risks of resectional surgery compared to the risks of residual cancer in the colon or lymph nodes after polypectomy. When both the endoscopist and the pathologist agree that the resection margin is endoscopically and microscopically free of cancer, no additional surgery may be needed. Surgery is probably indicated for treating residual cancer remaining after polypectomy, or when cancer involves the polypectomy resection margin. In 90% or more of cases, however, there is no residual tumor in a surgical specimen at the polypectomy site, even in cases in which polypectomy was considered incomplete clinically or where cancer extends to the resection margin histologically. The cautery used during the polypectomy may extirpate small amounts of residual carcinoma in the bowel wall.[373] Nonetheless, the risk of residual tumor is significant and colectomy offers the best chance of cure, even though some authors have suggested further endoscopic polypectomy in this situation.[166,364,366,374–376]

Colectomy is of course not without risks. Operative mortality ranges from 2% to 10%, increasing with the age of the patient.[361,377] Because most patients with malignant polyps are in their seventh and eighth decades, the risk of colectomy is significant. Nonetheless, the apparent benefit of surgery generally outweighs the surgical risk in otherwise healthy patients when the risk of residual cancer is great. Surgery may also provide palliative benefits (i.e., the prevention of bowel obstruction or local cancer spread) even if not curative. Colectomy would be of little or no benefit for distant metastases that are already present at the time of surgery.

Decision making about surgery or other therapeutic interventions must involve careful evaluation of the patient and his or her polyp. This requires maximum cooperation between the gastroenterologist, endoscopist, pathologist, and surgeon. The endoscopist must provide a careful description of the polyp in the colon (including an accurate description of the polyp's anatomic location), expert polypectomy technique, and careful determination of the completeness of excision. Marking the polypectomy site with sterilized India ink is helpful to the surgeon.[351] The pathologist must make sure that the polyp is appropriately processed and thoroughly evaluated. Good methodology for polyp processing has been described.[166,364] Most important, the pathologist must be careful and precise in his or her terminology, and be certain that the pathologic diagnosis and its implications are carefully communicated to the responsible physicians.[165] Despite great care, some polyps, particularly sessile ones and those removed in piecemeal fashion, cannot be adequately assessed for resection margin and degree of invasion. The surgeon must be certain of the location of the resected polyp in the colon, and again, endoscopic tattooing with India ink can be helpful in this respect.[351]

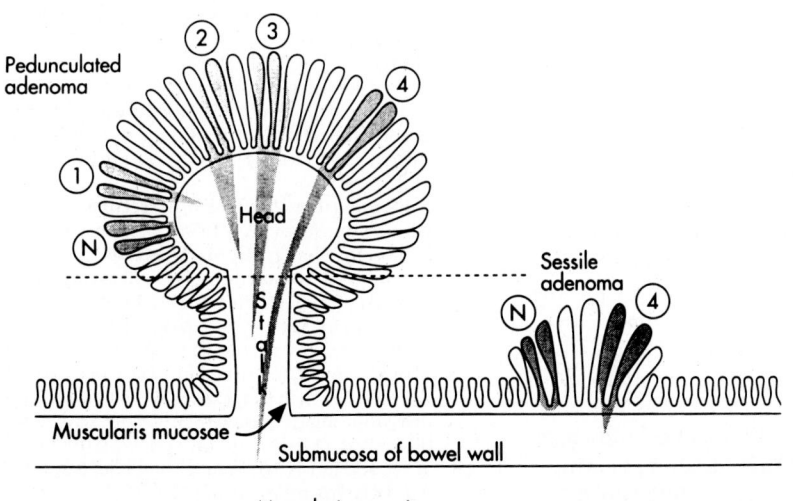

FIGURE 85-15. Level of carcinoma involvement in malignant polyps—pedunculated versus sessile adenomas. When carcinomatous cells are contained within the mucosa, without breaching the muscularis mucosae, the lesions are known as noninvasive carcinomas—severe focal atypia and intramucosal carcinoma (N). Once cancer has invaded through the muscularis mucosae into the submucosa of the bowel wall, the polyp is then termed a malignant polyp. Because lymphatics are present in the submucosa, metastatic spread is then possible. Increasing levels of invasion of the carcinoma, to the head (level 1), neck (level 2), stalk (level 3), and base of the stalk–submucosa (level 4) may carry worsening prognostic implications. A malignant sessile adenoma has, by definition, invaded the submucosa of the bowel wall (level 4). Noninvasive carcinomas (N) require no additional therapy after polypectomy. Usually, malignant polyps with invasions only of the head, neck, and stalk (1, 2, 3) and with clear resection margins and no poor prognostic features (see Table 7) are adequately treated by polypectomy alone. In malignant polyps with invasion of the submucosa of the bowel wall (4) or with poor prognostic features, colectomy should be seriously considered for potential cure. (Data from references 165, 166, and 369.)

Based on current evidence, the following recommendations can be made (Fig. 85-15; see Table 85-7):

A pedunculated malignant polyp with invasion of the head, neck, or stalk (levels 1, 2, and 3) is adequately treated by polypectomy alone if the polypectomy did not require piecemeal resection; there is no apparent blood vessel or lymphatic vessel involvement by cancer, and no invasion of the submucosa of the colonic wall; the cancer is not poorly differentiated; and the resection margin is free of cancer.

Malignant polyps with invasion of the stalk (level 3) with involvement of the margin of resection or with non-assessable margins; those with invasion of the submucosa of the bowel wall (level 4); and those containing evidence of blood vessel or lymphatic involvement or poorly differentiated invasive carcinoma should be treated by colectomy, unless the surgical risk is prohibitive. For sessile malignant polyps, invasion of the submucosa of the colonic wall (level 4) is present by definition, and surgery should be entertained.

Malignant polyps treated by polypectomy alone should be followed in 1 to 3 months and at 1 year with endoscopy and biopsy to assess for recurrence at the polypectomy site.

In all cases, patients must be informed of the rationale behind the physician's therapeutic decision, and the patient should participate in that decision. Patients must be aware that strict guidelines have not yet been established for the treatment of malignant polyps.[342]

Follow-Up

Current recommendations for following patients with adenomatous polyps are not clear.[342] Several prospective studies are addressing this issue. The St. Mark's Neoplastic Follow-up study reexamined 305 patients with previous polypectomies for adenomatous polyps at three different time intervals (1, 3, and 5 years).[378] Patients were followed with either colonoscopy or flexible sigmoidoscopy plus double-contrast barium enema. Thirty-seven percent of patients had a neoplastic lesion detected at a mean follow-up of 3.6 years after polypectomy. Recommendations from this study are to document that the colon is free of polyps by colonoscopy and then follow the patient with annual FOBT, and colonoscopy every 3 years or sooner if positive FOBT, bleeding, or symptoms are present. This interval of 3 years after initial polypectomy for adenomas has been confirmed to be as effective as follow-up colonoscopy after both 1 and 3 years.[338] Even longer intervals might be equally effective, but definitive data are not available.[379–381] The role of FOBT for adenoma surveillance remains unclear.[84]

Patients who have undergone surgical resection of a primary colorectal cancer are at risk not only for recurrence of their first cancer, but they are at about a threefold to fourfold risk for development of metachronous adenomas and cancer.[26,27,382] Therefore, follow-up should assess not only for evidence of metastatic disease and recurrent disease at the surgical margins of resection, but also for development of a second primary cancer. If the entire length of the colon was not completely visualized before surgery (owing to tumor obstruction or poor preparation), a complete colonoscopy to look for synchronous lesions is indicated after 3 to 6 months. Once the colon has been documented to be free from neoplasms, follow-up may be continued every 3 years, as in the follow-up after polypectomy for adenomatous polyps.

The reader is directed to Chapter 24, Neoplasia of the Gastrointestinal Tract; Chapter 31, Approach to the Patient With Occult Gastrointestinal Bleeding; Chapter 86, Polyposis Syndromes; Chapter 87, Malignant Tumors of the Colon; and Chapter 116, Colonoscopy and Flexible Sigmoidoscopy.

REFERENCES

1. Itzkowitz SH. The adenomatous polyp. Semin Gastrointest Dis 1992;3:3.
2. Itzkowitz SH, Kim YS. Polyps and benign neoplasms of the colon. In: Sleisenger MH, Fordtran JS, eds. Gastrointestinal disease: pathophysiology, diagnosis, management. Philadelphia: WB Saunders, 1993:1401.
3. Correa P. Epidemiology of polyps and cancer. In: Morson BC, ed. The pathogenesis of colorectal cancer. Philadelphia: WB Saunders, 1978:126.
4. Correa P, Strong JP, Reif A, et al. The epidemiology of colorectal polyps: prevalence in New Orleans and international comparisons. Cancer 1977;38:2258.
5. Stemmermann GN, Yatani R. Diverticulosis and polyps of the large intestine: a necropsy study of Hawaii Japanese. Cancer 1973;31:1260.
6. Clark JC, Collan Y, Eide TJ, et al. Prevalence of polyps in an autopsy series from areas with varying incidence of large-bowel cancer. Int J Cancer 1985;36:179.
7. Shinya H, Wolff WI. Morphology, anatomic distribution, and cancer potential of colonic polyps: an analysis of 7000 polyps endoscopically removed. Ann Surg 1979;190:679.
8. Granqvist S. Distribution of polyps in the large bowel in relation to age: a colonoscopic study. Scand J Gastroenterol 1981;16:1025.
9. Lieberman DA, Smith FW. Screening for colon malignancy with colonoscopy. Am J Gastroenterol 1991;86:946.
10. Disario JA, Foutch PG, Mai HD, et al. Prevalence and malignant potential of colorectal polyps in asymptomatic, average-risk men. Am J Gastroenterol 1991;86:941.
11. Johnson DA, Gurney MS, Volpe RJ, et al. A prospective study of the prevalence of colonic neoplasms in asymptomatic patients with an age-related risk. Am J Gastroenterol 1990;85:969.
12. Rex DK, Lehman GA, Hawes RH, et al. Screening colonoscopy in asymptomatic average-risk persons with negative fecal occult blood tests. Gastroenterology 1991;100:64.
13. Waye JD, Lewis BS, Frankel A, Geller SA. Small colon polyps. Am J Gastroenterol 1988;83:120.
14. Church JM, Fazio VW, Jones IT. Small colorectal polyps: are they worth treating? Dis Colon Rectum 1988;31:50.
15. Eide TJ, Stalsberg H. Polyps of the large intestine in northern Norway. Cancer 1978;42:2839.
16. Vatn MH, Stalsberg H. The prevalence of polyps of the large intestine in Oslo: an autopsy study. Cancer 1982;49:819.
17. Williams AR, Balasooriya BAW, Day DW. Polyps and cancer of the large bowel: a necropsy study in Liverpool. Gut 1982;23:835.
18. Sato E, Ouchi A, Satano N, Ishidate T. Polyps and diverticulosis of large bowel in autopsy population of Akita prefecture, compared with Miyagi. Cancer 1976;37:1316.
19. Coode PE, Chan YT. Polyps and diverticula of the large intestine: a necropsy survey in Hong Kong. Gut 1985;26:1045.
20. Isbister WH. Colorectal polyps: an endoscopic experience. Aust N Z J Surg 1986;56:717.

21. Johannsen LGK, Momsen O, Jacobsen NO. Polyps of the large intestine in Aarhus, Denmark: an autopsy study. Scand J Gastroenterol 1989;24:799.
22. Correa P, Haenszel W. The epidemiology of large-bowel cancer. Adv Cancer Res 1978;27:1.
23. Chapman I. Adenomatous polyps of large intestine: incidence and distribution. Ann Surg 1963;157:223.
24. Muto T, Bussey HJR, Morson BC. The evolution of cancer of the colon and rectum. Cancer 1975;36:2251.
25. Warden MJ, Petrelli NJ, Herrera L, Mittelman A. The role of colonoscopy and flexible sigmoidoscopy in screening for colorectal carcinoma. Dis Colon Rectum 1987;30:52.
26. Carlsson G, Petrelli NJ, Nava H, et al. The value of colonoscopic surveillance after curative resection for colorectal cancer or synchronous adenomatous polyps. Arch Surg 1987;122:1261.
27. Sollenberger LL, Eisenstat TE, Rubin RJ, Salvati EP. Is preoperative colonoscopy necessary in carcinoma of the colon and rectum? Am Surg 1988;54:113.
28. Morson BC, Bissey HJR. Magnitude of risk for cancer in patients with colorectal adenomas. Br J Surg 1985;72:S23.
29. Schuman BM, Simsek H, Lyons RC. The association of multiple colonic adenomatous polyps with cancer of the colon. Am J Gastroenterol 1990;85:846.
30. Isler JT, Brown PC, Lewis FG, Billingham RP. The role of preoperative colonoscopy in colorectal cancer. Dis Colon Rectum 1987;30:435.
31. Burt RW, Bishop DT, Cannon LA, et al. Dominant inheritance of adenomatous colonic polyps and colorectal cancer. N Engl J Med 1985;312:1540.
32. Cannon-Albright LA, Skolnick MH, Bishop DT, et al. Common inheritance of susceptibility to colonic adenomatous polyps and associated colorectal cancers. N Engl J Med 1988;319:533.
33. Burt RW. Hereditary polyposis syndrome and inheritance of adenomatous polyps. Semin Gastrointest Dis 1992;3:13.
34. Bonelli L, Martines H, Conio M, et al. Family history of colorectal cancer as a risk factor for benign and malignant tumors of the large bowel: a case-control study. Int J Cancer 1988;41:513.
35. Guillem JG, Neugut AI, Forde KA, et al. Colonic neoplasms in asymptomatic first-degree relatives of colon cancer patients. Am J Gastroenterol 1988;83:271.
36. Guillem JG, Forde KA, Treat MR, et al. Colonoscopic screening for neoplasms in asymptomatic first-degree relatives of colon cancer patients: a controlled, prospective study. Dis Colon Rectum 1992;35:523.
37. Cronstedt J, Carling L, Will'en R, et al. Geographic differences in the prevalence and distribution of large-bowel polyps: colonoscopic findings. Endoscopy 1987;19:110.
38. Jass JR. Subsite distribution and incidence of colorectal cancer in New Zealand. Dis Colon Rectum 1991;34:56.
39. Vukasin AP, Ballantyne GH, Flannery JH, et al. Increasing incidence of cecal and sigmoid carcinoma: data from the Connecticut Tumor Registry. Cancer 1990;66:2442.
40. Luk GD. Epidemiology and etiology of colorectal neoplasia. Current Opinion in Gastroenterology 1992;8:19.
41. Stewart M, Macrae FA, Williams CB. Neoplasia and ureterosigmoidoscopy: a colonoscopic survey. Br J Surg 1982;69:414.
42. Stillwell TJ, Myers RP. Adenomatous polyp in defunctional colonic segment used as a urinary bladder. Urology 1988;32:538.
43. Husmann DA, Spence HM. Current status of tumor of the bowel following ureterosigmoidostomy: a review. J Urol 1990;144:607.
44. Ali MH, Satti MB, Al-Nafussi A. Multiple benign colonic polyps at the site of ureterosigmoidostomy. Cancer 1984;53:1006.
45. van Driel MF, Zwiers W, Grond J, et al. Juvenile polyps at the site of a ureterosigmoidostomy: report of five cases. Dis Colon Rectum 1988;31:553.
46. Sohn M, Fuzesi L, Deutz F, et al. Signet ring cell carcinoma in adenomatous polyp at site of ureterosigmoidostomy 16 years after conversion to ileal conduit. J Urol 1990;143:805.
47. Stewart M, Hill MJ, Pugh RCB, Williams JP. The role of N-nitrosamine in carcinogenesis at the ureterocolic anastomosis. Br J Surg 1981;53:115.
48. Qvist N, Kronborg O, Hage E, Fenger C. Benign colonic neoplasm at the site of ureterosigmoidostomy. Eur Urol 1986;12:360.
49. Klein I, Parveen G, Gavaler JS, VanThiel DH. Colonic polyps in patients with acromegaly. Ann Intern Med 1982;97:27.
50. Brunner JE, Johnson CC, Zafar S, et al. Colon cancer and polyps in acromegaly: increased risk associated with family history of colon cancer. Clin Endocrinol 1990;32:65.
51. Murphy J, Schaaf M, Luk G, et al. Mucosal proliferation is increased in patients with active acromegaly. Gastroenterology 1993;104:A433.
52. Tobi M, Hassan N, Memon N, et al. Zollinger Ellison syndrome (ZES), acromegaly and colorectal neoplasia: increased expression of a premalignant marker. Proc Am Assoc Cancer Res 1993;34:241.
53. Murray TI, Neugut AI, Garbowski GC, et al. Relationship between breast cancer and colorectal adenomatous polyps: a case-control study. Cancer 1992;69:2232.
54. Toma S, Giacchero A, Bonelli L, et al. Association between breast and colorectal cancer in a sample of surgical patients. Eur J Surg Oncol 1987;13:429.
55. Jouin H, Baumann R, Derlon A, et al. Is there an increased incidence of adenomatous polyps in breast cancer patients? Cancer 1989;63:599.
56. Klein RS, Catalano MT, Edberg SC, et al. *Streptococcus bovis* septicemia and carcinoma of the colon. Ann Intern Med 1979;91:560.
57. Busby WJ, Campbell AJ, Ilsley CD. *Streptococcus bovis* infection of the pulmonary valve in an elderly woman with a colonic polyp. J Am Geriatr Soc 1987;35:166.
58. Tabibian N, Clarridge JE. *Streptococcus bovis* septicemia and large bowel neoplasia. Am Family Physician 1989;39:227.
59. Burns CA, McCaughey R, Lauter CB. The association of *Streptococcus bovis* fecal carriage and colon neoplasia: possible relationship with polyps and their premalignant potential. Am J Gastroenterol 1985;80:42.
60. Wiseman A, Rene P, Crelinsten GL. *Streptococcus agalactiae* endocarditis: an association with villous adenomas of the large intestine. Ann Intern Med 1985;103:893.
61. Leavitt J, Lein I, Kendricks F, et al. Skin tags: a cutaneous marker for colonic polyps. Ann Intern Med 1983;93:928.
62. Kune GA, Gooey J, Penfold C, Sali A. Association between colorectal polyps and skin tags. Lancet 1985;2:1062.
63. Chobanian SJ, Van Ness MM, Winters C Jr, Cattau EL Jr. Skin tags as a marker for adenomatous polyps of the colon. Ann Intern Med 1985;103:892.
64. Gould BE, Ellison RC, Greene HL, et al. Lack of association between skin tags and colon polyps in a primary care setting. Arch Intern Med 1988;148:1799.
65. Luk GD and the Colon Neoplasia Work Group. Colonic polyps and acrochordons (skin tags) do not correlate in familial colonic polyposis kindreds. Ann Intern Med 1986;104:209.
66. Dalton ADA, Coghill SB. No association between skin tags and colorectal adenomas. Lancet 1985;1:1332.
67. Piette AM, Meduri B, Fritsch J, et al. Do skin tags constitute a marker for colonic polyps? Gastroenterology 1988;95:1127.
68. Brendler SJ, Watson RD, Katon RM, et al. Skin tags are not a risk factor for colorectal polyps. J Clin Gastroenterol 1989;11:299.
69. Correa P, Strong JP, Johnson WD, et al. Atherosclerosis and polyps of the colon: quantification of precursors of coronary heart disease and colon cancer. J Chron Dis 1982;35:513.
70. Stemmerman GN, Heilbrun LK, Nomura A, et al. Adenomatous polyps and atherosclerosis in autopsy study of Japanese men in Hawaii. Int J Cancer 1986;38:789.
71. Mannes GA, Maier A, Thieme C, et al. Relation between the frequency of colorectal adenoma and the serum cholesterol level. N Engl J Med 1986;315:1634.
72. O'Sullivan KR, Mathias PM, Tobin A, O'Morain C. Risk of adenomatous polyps and colon cancer in relation to serum antioxidants and cholesterol status. Eur J Gastroenterol Hepatol 1991;3:775.
73. Neugut AI, Johnsen CM, Fink DJ. Serum cholesterol levels in

adenomatous polyps and cancer of the colon. JAMA 1986;255: 365.

74. Demers RY, Neale AV, Demers P, et al. Serum cholesterol and colorectal polyps. J Clin Epidemiol 1988;41:9.
75. Mannes AG, Weinzierl M, Stellaard F, et al. Adenomas of the large intestine after cholecystectomy. Gut 1984;25:863.
76. Mamianetti A, Cinto RO, Altolaguirre D, et al. Relative risk of colorectal cancer after cholecystectomy: a multicentre case-control study. Int J Colon Dis 1988;3:215.
77. Hickman MS, Salinas HC, Schwesinger WH. Does cholecystectomy affect colonic tumorigenesis? Arch Surg 1987;122:334.
78. Bandettini L, Filipponi F, Romagnoli P. Increase of the mitotic index of colonic mucosa after cholecystectomy. Cancer 1986;58:685.
79. Sandler RS, Martin ZZ, Carlton NM, et al. Adenomas of the large bowel after cholecystectomy: a case-control study. Dig Dis Sci 1988;33:1178.
80. Llamas KJ, Torlach LG, Ward M, Bain C. Cholecystectomy and adenomatous polyps of the large bowel. Gut 1986;27:1181.
81. Neugut AI, Murray TI, Garbowski GC, et al. Cholecystectomy as a risk factor for colorectal adenomatous polyps and carcinoma. Cancer 1991;68:1644.
82. Ekbom A, Yuen J, Adami H-O, et al. Cholecystectomy and colorectal cancer. Gastroenterology 1993;105:142.
83. Giovannucci E, Colditz GA, Stampfer MJ. A meta-analysis of cholecystectomy and risk of colorectal cancer. Gastroenterology 1993;105:130.
84. Luk GD. Epidemiology, etiology, and diagnosis of colorectal neoplasia. Current Opinion in Gastroenterology 1993;9:19.
85. Naveau S, Chaput JC, Bedossa P, et al. Cirrhosis as an independent risk factor for colonic adenomas. Gut 1992;33:535.
86. Morini S, de Angelis P, Manurita L, Colavolpe V. Association of colonic diverticula with adenomas and carcinomas: a colonoscopic experience. Dis Colon Rectum 1988;31:793.
87. Glick SN, Teplick SK, Ross WM. Colonic lymphoid follicles associated with colonic neoplasms. Radiology 1988;168:603.
88. Rubin BG, Ballantyne GH, Zdon MJ, et al. The role of flexible sigmoidoscopy in the preoperative screening of patients with inguinal hernia: a high yield of neoplasms. Arch Surg 1987;122:296.
89. Pratt SM, Weaver FA, Potts JR III. Preoperative evaluation of patients with inguinal hernia for colorectal disease. Surg Gynecol Obstet 1987;165:53.
90. Farinon AM, De Masi E, Percudani M, Stroppa I, Nardi F. Dysplasia-carcinoma sequence in diminutive polyps of the large bowel. Ital J Surg Sci 1988;18:35.
91. Achkar E, Carey W. Small polyps found during fiberoptic sigmoidoscopy in asymptomatic patients. Ann Intern Med 1988;109:880.
92. Ansher AF, Lewis JH, Fleischer DE, et al. Hyperplastic colonic polyps as a marker for adenomatous colonic polyps. Am J Gastroenterol 1989;84:113.
93. Stoltenberg PH, Kirtley DW, Culp KS, et al. Are diminutive colorectal polyps (DCP) clinically significant? Gastrointest Endosc 1988;34:172.
94. Foutch PG, Disario JA, Pardy K, et al. The sentinel hyperplastic polyp: a marker for synchronous neoplasia in the proximal colon. Am J Gastroenterol 1991;86:1482.
95. Opelka FG, Timmcke AE, Gathright JB Jr, et al. Diminutive colonic polyps: an indication for colonoscopy. Dis Colon Rectum 1992;35:178.
96. Matter SE, Campbell DR. Significance of distal polyps detected with flexible sigmoidoscopy in asymptomatic patients. Arch Intern Med 1992;152:1776.
97. Ellis CN, Boggs HW, Slagle GW, et al. Clinical significance of diminutive polyps of the rectum and sigmoid colon. Dis Colon Rectum 1993;36:8.
98. Zauber AG, Winawer SJ, Diaz B, et al. The National Polyp Study: the association of colonic hyperplastic polyps and adenomas. Am J Gastroenterol 1988;83:1060.
99. Ryan ME, Norfleet RG, Kirchner JP, et al. The significance of diminutive colonic polyps found at flexible sigmoidoscopy. Gastrointest Endosc 1989;35:85.
100. Provenzale D, Garrett JW, Condon SE, Sandler RS. Risk of colon adenomas in patients with rectosigmoid hyperplastic polyps. Ann Intern Med 1990;113:760.
101. Rex K, Smith JJ, Ulbright TM, Lehman GA. Distal colonic hyperplastic polyps do not predict proximal adenomas in asymptomatic average-risk subjects. Gastroenterology 1992;102:317.
102. Pines A, Bat L, Rosenbaum J, et al. Are tiny polyps important when found on sigmoidoscopy in asymptomatic people? J Clin Gastroenterol 1992;15:113.
103. Maskens AP. Histogenesis of adenomatous polyps in the human large intestine. Gastroenterology 1979;77:1245.
104. Kaye GI, Fenoglio CM, Pascal RR, et al. Comparative electron microscopic features of normal, hyperplastic and adenomatous human colonic epithelium. Gastroenterology 1973;64:926.
105. Lipkin M. Proliferation and differentiation of normal and neoplastic cells in the colon of man. Cancer 1971;28:38.
106. Fenoglio CM, Lane N. The anatomical precursor of colorectal carcinoma. Cancer 1974;34:819.
107. Lipkin M. Phase 1 and phase 2 proliferative lesions of colonic epithelial cells in diseases leading to colonic cancer. Cancer 1974;34:878.
108. Terpstra OT, van Blankenstein M, Dees J, Eilers GAM. Abnormal pattern of cell proliferation in the entire colon mucosa of patients with colon adenoma or cancer. Gastroenterology 1987;92:704.
109. Kaye GI, Pascal RR, Lane N. The colonic pericryptal fibroblast sheath: replication, migration and cytodifferentiation of a mesenchymal cell system in adult tissue. III. Replication and differentiation in human hyperplastic and adenomatous polyps. Gastroenterology 1971;60:515.
110. Lane N, Kaplan H, Pascal RR. Minute adenomatous and hyperplastic polyps of the colon: divergent patterns of epithelial growth with specific associated mesenchymal changes. Gastroenterology 1971;60:537.
111. Bleibrg H, Mainguet P, Galand P. Cell renewal in familial polyposis: comparison between polyp and adjacent healthy mucosa. Gastroenterology 1972;63:240.
112. Wynder LE, Reddy BS. Metabolic epidemiology of colorectal cancer. Cancer 1974;34:801.
113. Hill MJ. Bacteria and the etiology of colonic cancer. Cancer 1974;34:815.
114. Kune GA, Kune S, Read A, et al. Colorectal polyps, diet, alcohol, and family history of colorectal cancer: a case-control study. Nutr Cancer 1991;16:25.
115. Giovannucci E, Stampfer MJ, Colditz G, et al. Relationship of diet to risk of colorectal adenoma in men. J Natl Cancer Inst 1992;84:91.
116. Neugut AI, Garbowski GC, Lee WC, et al. Dietary risk factors for the incidence and recurrence of colorectal adenomatous polyps: a case-control study. Ann Intern Med 1993;118:91.
117. Kono S, Imanishi K, Shinchi K, Yanai F. Relationship of diet to small and large adenomas of the sigmoid colon. Jpn J Cancer Res 1993;84:13.
118. Macquart-Moulin G, Riboli E, Corn'ee J, et al. Colorectal polyps and diet: a case-control study in Marseilles. Int J Cancer 1987;40:179.
119. Slattery ML, Sorensoin AW, Mahoney AW, et al. Diet and colon cancer: assessment of risk by fiber type and food source. J Natl Cancer Inst 1988;80:1474.
120. Peuchant E, Salles C, Jensen R. Relationship between fecal neutral steroid concentrations and malignancy in colon cells. Cancer 1987;60:994.
121. McKeown-Eyssen G, Holloway C, Jazmaji V, et al. A randomized trial of vitamins C and E in the prevention of recurrence of colorectal polyps. Cancer Res 1988;48:4701.
122. Lipkin M, Newmark H. Effect of added dietary calcium on colonic epithelial-cell proliferation in subjects at high risk for familial colonic cancer. N Engl J Med 1985;313:1381.
123. Sciallero S, Bruno S, DiVinci A, et al. Flow cytometric DNA ploidy in colorectal adenomas and family history of colorectal cancer. Cancer 1988;61:114.
124. Silverman AL, Park JH, Hamilton SR, et al. Abnormal methylation of the calcitonin gene in human colonic neoplasms. Cancer Res 1989;49:3468.

125. Pero RW, Ritchie M, Winawer SJ, et al. Unscheduled DNA synthesis in mononuclear leukocytes from patients with colorectal polyps. Cancer Res 1985;45:3388.
126. Vogelstein B, Fearon ER, Hamilton SR, et al. Genetic alterations during colorectal-tumor development. N Engl J Med 1988;319:525.
127. Hamilton SR. The molecular genetics of colorectal neoplasia. Gastroenterology 1993;105:3.
128. Wegener M, Borsch G, Schmidt G. Colorectal adenomas: distribution, incidence of malignant transformation, and rate of recurrence. Dis Colon Rectum 1986;29:383.
129. Eide TJ. The age-, sex-, and site-specific occurrence of adenomas and carcinoma of the large intestine within a defined population. Scand J Gastroenterol 1986;21:1083.
130. Lev R, Grover R. Precursors of human colon carcinoma: a serial sections study of colectomy specimens. Cancer 1981;47:2007.
131. Morson BC. Factors influencing the prognosis of early cancer of the rectum. Proc R Soc Med 1966;59:607.
132. Morson BC. The polyp-cancer sequence in the large bowel. Proc R Soc Med 1974;67:451.
133. Fearon ER, Hamilton SR, Vogelstein B. Clonal analysis of human colorectal tumors. Science 1987;238:193.
134. Stryker SJ, Wolff BG, Culp CE, et al. Natural history of untreated colonic polyps. Gastroenterology 1987;93:1009.
135. Rawlinson J, Tate JJ, Brunton FJ, Royle GT. Radiological evidence for the polyp/cancer sequence in the colon. Clin Radiol 1989;40:386.
136. Enterline HT. Polyps and cancer of the large bowel. Curr Top Pathol 1976;63:75.
137. Gilbertsen VA. Proctosigmoidoscopy and polypectomy in reducing the incidence of rectal cancer. Cancer 1974;34:936.
138. Murakami R, Tsukuma H, Kanamori S, et al. Natural history of colorectal polyps and the effect of polypectomy on occurrence of subsequent cancer. Int J Cancer 1990;46:159.
139. Winawer SJ, Zauber AG, Gerdes H, et al. Reduction in colorectal cancer incidence following colonoscopic polypectomy: report from the National Polyp Study. Gastroenterology 1991;100:A410.
140. Shamsuddin AM. Microscopic intraepithelial neoplasia in large bowel mucosa. Hum Pathol 1982;13:510.
141. Spjut HJ, Frankel NB, Appel MF. The small carcinoma of the large bowel. Am J Surg Pathol 1979;3:39.
142. Muto T, Kamiya J, Sawada T, et al. Small "flat adenoma" of the large bowel with special reference to its clinicopathologic features. Dis Colon Rectum 1985;28:847.
143. Lynch HT, Smyrk T, Lanspa SJ, et al. Flat adenomas in a colon cancer-prone kindred. J Natl Cancer Inst 1988;80:278.
144. Dobbins WO III. Dysplasia and malignancy in inflammatory bowel disease. Annu Rev Med 1984;35:33.
145. Kinzler KW, Nilbert MC, Su L-K, et al. Identification of FAP locus genes from chromosome 5q21. Science 1991;253:661.
146. Nishisho I, Nakamura Y, Miyoshi Y, et al. Mutations of chromosome 5q21 genes in FAP in colorectal cancer patients. Science 1991;253:665.
147. Joslyn G, Carlson M, Thliveris A, et al. Identification of deletion mutations and three new genes at the familial polyposis locus. Cell 1991;66:601.
148. Miyoshi Y, Ando H, Nagase H, et al. Germ-line mutations of the APC gene in 53 familial adenomatous polyposis patients. Proc Natl Acad Sci USA 1992;89:4452.
149. Stella A, Lonoce A, Resta N, et al. Familial adenomatous polyposis: identification of a new frameshift mutation of the APC gene in an Italian family. Biochem Biophys Res Commun 1992;184:1357.
150. Welch CE, Hedberg SE. Polypoid lesions of the gastrointestinal tract. 2nd ed. Philadelphia: WB Saunders, 1975.
151. Olsen HW, Lawrence WA, Shook CW, Mutch WM. Risk factors and screening techniques in 500 patients with benign and malignant colon polyps. Dis Colon Rectum 1988;31:216.
152. Welch CE. Polyps and cancer of the colon. Am J Surg 1979;138:625.
153. Sobin LH. The histopathology of bleeding from polyps and carcinomas of the large intestine. Cancer 1985;55:577.
154. Ahlquist DA, McGill DB, Schwartz S, et al. Fecal blood levels in health and disease: a study using HemoQuant. N Engl J Med 1985;312:1422.
155. Macrae F, St John DJB. Relationship between patterns of bleeding and Hemoccult sensitivity in patients with colorectal cancers or adenomas. Gastroenterology 1982;82:891.
156. Mougenot JF, Baldassarre ME, Mashako LM, et al. Recto-colic polyps in the child: analysis of 183 cases. Arch Fr Pediatr 1989;46:245.
157. Paul RE Jr, Gherardi GJ, Miller HH. Autoamputation of benign and malignant polyps: report of two cases. Dis Colon Rectum 1974;17:331.
158. Arthur AL, Garvey R, Vaness DG. Colocolic intussusception in a three-year-old child caused by a colonic polyp. Conn Med 1990;54:492.
159. Steven K, Lange P, Bukhave K, Rask-Madsen J. Prostaglandin E_2-mediated secretory diarrhea in villous adenoma of rectum: effect of treatment with indomethacin. Gastroenterology 1981;80:1562.
160. Goulston KJ, Cook I, Dent OF. How important is rectal bleeding in the diagnosis of bowel cancer and polyps? Lancet 1986;2:261.
161. Pines A, Shemesh E, Bat L. Prolonged rectal bleeding associated with hemorrhoids: the diagnostic contribution of colonoscopy. South Med J 1987;80:313.
162. Neale AV, Demers RY, Budev H, Scott RO. Physician accuracy in diagnosing colorectal polyps. Dis Colon Rectum 1987;30:247.
163. Ekelund G, Lindstrom C. Histopathological analysis of benign polyps in patients with carcinoma of the colon and rectum. Gut 1974;15:654.
164. Konishi F, Morson BC. Pathology of colorectal adenomas: a colonoscopic survey. J Clin Pathol 1982;35:830.
165. Haggitt RC, Glotzbach RE, Soffer EE, et al. Prognostic factors in colorectal carcinomas arising in adenomas: implications for lesions removed by endoscopic polypectomy. Gastroenterology 1985;89:328.
166. Morson BC, Whiteway JE, Jones EA, et al. Histopathology and prognosis of malignant colorectal polyps treated by endoscopic polypectomy. Gut 1984;25:437.
167. Morson BC. Some peculiarities in the histology of intestinal polyps. Dis Colon Rectum 1962;5:337.
168. Jass JR, Sobin LH. World Health Organization: histological typing of intestinal tumours. 2nd ed. New York: Springer-Verlag, 1989.
169. Pascal RR, Hertzler G, Hunter S, Goldschmid S. Pseudoinvasion with high-grade dysplasia in a colonic adenoma: distinction from adenocarcinoma. Am J Surg Pathol 1990;14:694.
170. Appel MF, Spjut HJ, Estrada RG. The significance of villous component in colonic polyps. Am J Surg 1977;134:770.
171. Shinya H, Wolff WI. Morphology, anatomic distribution and cancer potential of colonic polyps. Ann Surg 1979;190:679.
172. O'Brien MJ, Winawer J, Zauber AG, et al. The national polyp study. Patient and polyp characteristics associated with high-grade dysplasia in colorectal adenomas. Gastroenterology 1990;98:371.
173. Atkin WS, Morson BC, Cuzick J. Long-term risk of colorectal cancer after excision of rectosigmoid adenomas. N Engl J Med 1992;326:658.
174. Cosgrove JM, Wolff WI, Tanenbaum N, Margolis IB. An appraisal of small and diminutive colonic polyps. Surg Endosc 1991;5:143.
175. Quan SHQ, Castro EB. Papillary adenomas (villous tumors): a review of 215 cases. Dis Colon Rectum 1971;14:267.
176. Horn RC Jr. Malignant potential of polypoid lesions of the colon and rectum. Cancer 1971;28:146.
177. Iida M, Iwashita A, Yao T, et al. Endoscopic features of villous tumors of the colon: correlation with histological findings. Hepatogastroenterology 1990;37:342.
178. Welch JP, Welch CE. Villous adenomas of the colo-rectum. Am J Surg 1976;131:185.
179. Hanley PH, Hines MO, Ray JE. Villous tumors: experience with 217 patients. Am Surg 1971;37:190.
180. Wolber RA, Owen DA. Flat adenomas of the colon. Hum Pathol 1991;22:70.

181. Shimoda T, Ikegami M, Fujisaki J, et al. Early colorectal carcinoma with special reference to its development de novo. Cancer 1989;64:1138.

182. Lynch HT, Smyrk TC, Lanspa SJ, et al. Phenotypic variation in colorectal adenoma/cancer expression in two families: hereditary flat adenoma syndrome. Cancer 1990;66:909.

183. Chuong JJH, DuBovik S, McCallum RW. Achalasia as a risk factor for esophageal carcinoma: a reappraisal. Dig Dis Sci 1984;29:1105.

184. Kuramoto S, Oohara T. Flat early cancers of the large intestine. Cancer 1989;64:950.

185. Urbanski SJ, Kossakoiwska AE, Marcon N, et al. Mixed hyperplastic adenomatous polyps: an underdiagnosed entity. Am J Surg Pathol 1984;8:551.

186. Deschner EE, Lytle JS, Wong G, et al. The effect of dietary omega-3 fatty acids (fish oil) on azoxymethanol-induced focal areas of dysplasia and colon tumor incidence. Cancer 1990;66:2350.

187. Longacre TA, Fenoglio-Preiser CM. Mixed hyperplastic adenomatous polyps serrated adenomas: a distinct form of colorectal neoplasia. Am J Surg Pathol 1990;14:524.

188. Veress B, Gabrielsson N, Granqvist S, Billing H. Mixed colorectal polyps: an immunohistologic and mucin-histochemical study. Scand J Gastroenterol 1991;26:1049.

189. Levine MS, Barnes MJ, Bronner MP, et al. Atypical hyperplastic polyps at double-contrast barium enema examination. Radiology 1990;175:691.

190. Fenoglio CM, Richart RM, Kaye GI. Comparative electron-microscopic features of normal, hyperplastic and adenomatous human colonic epithelium. Gastroenterology 1975;69:100.

191. Hayashi T, Yatani R, Apostol J, Stemmermann GN. Pathogenesis of hyperplastic polyps of the colon: a hypothesis based upon ultrastructural and in vitro cell kinetics. Gastroenterology 1974;66:347.

192. Kaye GI, Fenoglio CM, Pascal RP, Lane N. Comparative electron microscopic features of normal, hyperplastic and adenomatous human colon epithelium: variations in cellular structure relative to the process of epithelial cell differentiation. Gastroenterology 1973;64:926.

193. Jass JR. Relation between metaplastic polyp and carcinoma of the colorectum. Lancet 1983;1:28.

194. Provenzale D, Martin ZZ, Holland KL, et al. Colon adenomas in patients with hyperplastic polyps. J Clin Gastroenterol 1988;10:46.

195. Teague RH, Read AE. Polyposis in ulcerative colitis. Gut 1975;16:792.

196. Szolgay-Daniel E, Carlsson J, Zierlold K, et al. Effects of amiloride treatment on U-118 and U-251 MG human glioma and HT-29 human colon carcinoma cells. Cancer Res 1991;51:1039.

197. Buck JL, Dachman AH, Sobin LH. Polypoid and pseudopolypoid manifestations of inflammatory bowel disease. Radiographics 1991;11:293.

198. Balazs M. Giant inflammatory polyps associated with idiopathic inflammatory bowel disease: an ultrastructural study of five cases. Dis Colon Rectum 1990;33:773.

199. Archibald GR, Scholz FJ, Larsen CR. Computed tomographic findings of giant intestinal pseudopolyposis. Gastrointest Radiol 1988;13:155.

200. Foderaro AE, Barloon TJ, Murray JA. Giant pseudopolyposis in Crohn's disease with computed tomography correlation. J Comput Tomogr 1987;11:288.

201. Berkowitz D, Bernstein LH. Colonic pseudopolyps in association with amebic colitis. Gastroenterology 1975;68:786.

202. Carp NZ, Nejman JH, Kelly JJ. Strongyloidiasis: an unusual cause of colonic pseudopolyposis and gastrointestinal bleeding. Surg Endosc 1987;1:175.

203. Peh WC. Filiform polyposis in tuberculosis of the colon. Clin Radiol 1988;39:534.

204. Kelly JK. Polypoid prolapsing mucosal folds in diverticular disease. Am J Surg Pathol 1991;15:871.

205. Nebel OT, El Masry NA, Castell DO, Farid Z, Fornes MF, Sparks HA. Schistosomal disease of the colon: a reversible form of polyposis. Gastroenterology 1974;67:939.

206. Yu XR, Chen PH, Xu JY, et al. Histological classification of schistosomal egg induced polyps of colon and their clinical significance. Chin Med J 1991;104:64.

207. Adelson JW, deChadar'evian JP, Azouz EM, Guttman FM. Giant inflammatory polyposis causing partial obstruction and pain in "healed" ulcerative colitis in an adolescent. J Pediatr Gastroenterol Nutr 1988;7:135.

208. Nakano H, Miyachi I, Kitagawa Y, et al. Crohn's disease associated with giant inflammatory polyposis. Endoscopy 1987;19:246.

209. Rozenbajgier C, Ruck P, Jenss H, Kaiserling E. Filiform polyposis: a case report describing clinical, morphological, and immunohistochemical findings. Clin Invest 1992;70:520.

210. Lobert PF, Appelman HD. Inflammatory cloacogenic polyp: a unique inflammatory lesion of the anal transition zone. Am J Surg Pathol 1981;5:761.

211. Saul SH. Inflammatory cloacogenic polyp: relationship to solitary rectal ulcer syndrome/mucosal prolapse and other bowel disorders. Hum Pathol 1987;18:1120.

212. Levine DS, Surawicz CM, Spencer GD, et al. Inflammatory polyposis two years after ischemic colon injury. Dig Dis Sci 1986;31:1159.

213. Tan KH, Meijer S, Donner R. Giant localized pseudopolyp of the colon without colonic inflammatory disease: case report. Neth J Surg 1989;39:95.

214. Kasunoki M, Nishigami T, Yanagi H, et al. Occult cancer in localized giant pseudopolyposis. Am J Gastroenterol 1992;87:379.

215. Anthony PO, Morris DS, Vowles KDJ. Multiple and recurrent inflammatory fibroid polyps in three generations of a Devon family: a new syndrome. Gut 1984;25:854.

216. Williams GT, Bussey HJR, Morson BC. Inflammatory "cap" polyps of the large intestine. Br J Surg 1985;72 (Suppl):322A.

217. Campbell AP, Cobb CA, Chapman RWG, et al. Cap polyposis: an unusual cause of diarrhoea. Gut 1993;34:562.

218. Nakamura S, Kino I, Akagi T. Inflammatory myoglandular polyps of the colon and rectum: a clinicopathological study of 32 pedunculated polyps, distinct from other types of polyps. Am J Surg Pathol 1992;16:772.

219. Roth SI, Helwig EG. Juvenile polyps of the colon and rectum. Cancer 1973;16:468.

220. Silberberg SG. "Juvenile" retention polyps of the colon and rectum. Am J Dig Dis 1970;15:617.

221. Horrilleno EG, Edkert C, Ackerman LV. Polyps of rectum and colon in children. Cancer 1957;10:1210.

222. Holgersen LO, Miller RE, Zintel HA. Juvenile polyps of the colon. Surgery 1971;69:288.

223. Kirberg A, Morales X. Diagnosis and treatment of juvenile polyp of the colon. Rev Chil Pediatr 1991;62:34.

224. Goodman ZD, Yardley JH, Milligan FD. Pathogenesis of colonic polyps in multiple juvenile polyposis. Cancer 1979;43:1906.

225. Morosi C, Ballardini G, Pisani P, et al. Diagnostic accuracy of the double-contrast enema for colonic polyps in patients with or without diverticular disease. Gastrointest Radiol 1991;16:345.

226. Turrell R, Maynard A de L. Adenomas of rectum and colon in juvenile patients. JAMA 1956;161:57.

227. Kerr JG. Polyposis of colon in children. Am J Surg 1948;76:667.

228. Haggitt RC, Reid BJ. Hereditary gastrointestinal polyposis syndromes. Am J Surg Pathol 1986;10:871.

229. Grotsky HW, Rickert RR, Smith WD, Newsome JF. Familial juvenile polyposis coli. A clinical and pathologic study of a large kindred. Gastroenterology 1982;82:494.

230. Stemper JT, Kent TH, Summers RW. Juvenile polyposis and gastrointestinal carcinoma: a study of a kindred. Ann Intern Med 1975;83:639.

231. Beacham CH, Shields HM, Raffensperger ED, Enterline HT. Juvenile and adenomatous gastrointestinal polyposis. Am J Dig Dis 1978;23:1137.

232. Jarvinen H, Franssila KO. Familial juvenile polyposis coli: increased risk of colorectal cancer. Gut 1984;25:792.

233. Bentley E, Chandrasoma P, Radin R, Cohen H. Generalized

juvenile polyposis with carcinoma. Am J Gastroenterol 1989;84: 1456.

234. Longo WE, Touloukian RJ, West AB, Ballantyne GH. Malignant potential of juvenile polyposis coli: report of a case and review of the literature. Dis Colon Rectum 1990;33:980.

235. Atsumi M, Kawamoto K, Ebisui S, et al. A case report of juvenile polyposis with adenomatous change and a review of 34 cases reported in Japan. Gastroenterol Jpn 1991;26:523.

236. Giardiello FM, Hamilton SR, Kern SE, et al. Colorectal neoplasia in juvenile polyposis or juvenile polyps. Arch Dis Child 1991;66:971.

237. Jeghers H, McKusick VA, Katz KH. Generalized intestinal polyposis and melanin spots of the oral mucosa, lips and digits. N Engl J Med 1949;241:993.

238. Burdick D, Prior JT. Peutz-Jeghers syndrome: a clinicopathologic study of a large family with a 27-year follow-up. Cancer 1982;50:2139.

239. Perzin KH, Bridge MF. Adenomatous and carcinomatous changes in hamartomatous polyps of the small intestine (Peutz-Jeghers syndrome). Cancer 1982;49:971.

240. Gardner EJ, Burt RW, Freston JW. Gastrointestinal polyposis: syndromes and genetic mechanisms. West J Med 1980;132: 488.

241. Scully RE. Sex cord tumor with annular tubules: a distinctive ovarian tumor of the Peutz-Jeghers syndrome. Cancer 1970;25: 1107.

242. Giardiello FM, Welsh SB, Hamilton SR, et al. Increased risk of cancer in the Peutz-Jeghers syndrome. N Engl J Med 1987;316:1511.

243. Niimi K, Tomoda H, Furusawa M, et al. Peutz-Jeghers syndrome associated with adenocarcinoma of the cecum and focal carcinomas in hamartomatous polyps of the colon: a case report. Jpn J Surg 1991;21:220.

244. Hikasa Y, Narabayashi T, Yamamura M, et al. Angiomyolipoma of the colon: a new entity in colonic polypoid lesions. Gastroenterol Jpn 1989;24:407.

245. Davis E, Chow C, Miyai K. A hamartoma of the colon with unusual features. Endoscopy 1991;23:349.

246. Holtz F, Schmidt LA. Lymphoid polyps (benign lymphoma) of the rectum and anus. Surg Gynecol Obstet 1958;106:639.

247. Ranchod M, Lewin KJ, Dorfman RF. Lymphoid hyperplasia of the gastrointestinal tract: a study of 26 cases and review of the literature. Am J Surg Pathol 1978;2:383.

248. Capitano MA, Kirkpatrick JA. Lymphoid hyperplasia of the colon in children. Radiology 1970;94:323.

249. Fernandes BJ, Amato D, Goldfinger M. Diffuse lymphomatous polyposis of the gastrointestinal tract. Gastroenterology 1985;88:1267.

250. Keeling WM, Beatty GL. Lymphoid polyps of the rectum. Arch Surg 1956;73:753.

251. Louw JW. Polypoid lesions of the large bowels in children with particular reference to benign lymphoid polyposis. J Pediatr Surg 1968;3:195.

252. Reid BJ, Weinstein WM, Lewin KJ, et al. Endoscopic biopsy can detect high-grade dysplasia or early adenocarcinoma in Barrett's esophagus without grossly recognizable neoplastic lesions. Gastroenterology 1988;94:81.

253. Gilbert DA, Hallstrom AP, Shaneyfelt SL, et al. The national ASGE colonoscopy study: complications of colonoscopy (abstract). Gastrointest Endosc 1984;30:156.

254. Cornes JS, Wallace H, Morson BC. Benign lymphomas of the rectum and anal canal: a study of 100 cases. J Pathol Bacteriol 1961;83:371.

255. Sheehan DB, Martin F, Baginsky S, et al. Multiple lymphomatous polyposis of the gastrointestinal tract. Cancer 1971;28: 408.

256. Franken EA. Lymphoid hyperplasia of the colon. Radiology 1970;94:329.

257. Benchimol D, Frileux P, Herve de Sigalony JP, Parc R. Benign lymphoid polyposis of the colon: report of a case in an adult. Int J Color Dis 1991;6:165.

258. Robinson MJ, Padron S, Rywlin AM. Enterocolitis lymphofollicularis. Arch Pathol 1973;96:311.

259. Collins JO, Falk M, Guibone R. Benign lymphoid polyposis of the colon: a case report. Pediatrics 1966;38:897.

260. Gruenberg J, Mackman S. Multiple lymphoid polyps in familial polyposis. Ann Surg 1972;175:552.

261. Norum J, Wist E. Intestinal lymphoma presented as multiple intestinal polyposis. Tidsskr Nor Laegeforen 1992;112:1956.

262. Ohri SK, Keane PF, Sackier JM, et al. Primary rectal lymphoma and malignant lymphomatous polyposis: two cases illustrating current methods in diagnosis and management. Dis Colon Rectum 1989;32:1071.

263. Matuchansky C, Morchau-Beauchant M, Touchard G, et al. Nodular lymphoid hyperplasia of the small bowel associated with primary jejunal malignant lymphoma. Gastroenterology 1982;78:1587.

264. Sagar SM, Karp SJ, Falzon M. Malignant lymphomatous polyposis: diagnosis and response to chemotherapy. Clin Oncol 1990;2:230.

265. Smith BH, Welter LH. Pneumatosis intestinalis. Am J Clin Pathol 1967;48:455.

266. Shailal JA, van Heerden JA, Bartholomew LG, Cain JC. Pneumatosis cystoides intestinalis. Mayo Clin Proc 1974;49:180.

267. Born A, Inouye T, Diamant N. Pneumatosis coli: case report documenting time from x-ray appearance to onset of symptoms. Dig Dis Sci 1981;26:855.

268. Mirables M, Hinojosa J, Alonso J, Berenguer J. Oxygen therapy in pneumatosis coli: what is the minimum oxygen requirement? Dis Colon Rectum 1983;26:458.

269. Wayte DM, Helwig EB. Colitis cystica profunda. Am J Clin Pathol 1967;48:159.

270. Magidson JG, Lewin KJ. Diffuse colitis cystica profunda. Am J Surg Pathol 1983;5:393.

271. Kim WH, Choe GY, Kim YI, Kim JP. Localized form of colitis cystica profunda: a case of occurrence in the descending colon. Journal of Korean Medical Science 1992;7:76.

272. Levine DS. "Solitary" rectal ulcer syndrome: are "solitary" rectal ulcer syndrome and "localized" colitis cystica profunda analogous syndromes caused by rectal prolapse? Gastroenterology 1987;92:243.

273. Bentley E, Chandrasoma P, Cohen H, et al. Colitis cystica profunda presenting with complete intestinal obstruction and recurrence. Gastroenterology 1984;89:157.

274. Qizilbash AH, Meghji M, Castelli M. Pseudocarcinomatous invasion in adenomas of the colon and rectum. Dis Colon Rectum 1980;23:529.

275. DeBeer RA, Shinya H. Colonic lipoma. Gastrointest Endosc 1975;22:90.

276. Manfrini R, Bonini CA. Submucosal polyps of the large intestine: observations on 2 cases and review of the literature. Minerva Dietol Gastroenterol 1990;36:43.

277. Maruyama M, Fukayama M, Koike M. A case of multiple carcinoid tumors of the rectum with extraglandular endocrine cell proliferation. Cancer 1988;61:131.

278. Beaton HL. Carcinoid tumors of the alimentary tract. CA 1982;32:92.

279. Jubelirer SJ. Multiple colonic polyps as the initial presentation of malignant melanoma. West Virginia Medical Journal 1992;88:279.

280. Metayer P, Antonietti M, Oumrani M, et al. Metastases of a gastric adenocarcinoma presenting as colonic polyposis: report of a case. Dis Colon Rectum 1991;34:622.

281. Sakai H, Sawamura M, Tamura J, et al. A patient with primary plasma cell leukemia accompanied by an extensive polypoid infiltration of the gastrointestinal tract. J Med Clin Exp Theor 1991;11:195.

282. Haff RC, San Diego AG. Ganglioneuroma of the ileocecal valve: review of the literature. Arch Pathol 1972;93:549.

283. McSwain B, Kinn RJ, Haley RL, et al. Endometriosis of the colon: report of 14 patients requiring partial colectomy. Medicine 1974;67:651.

284. Patel PH, Lakshman S, Farnum JB, Thomas E. Condyloma acuminata presenting as rectal polyp in a heterosexual man: importance of CT scan of the pelvis. Am J Gastroenterol 1987;82:479.

285. Hollander E, David G. Inverted sigmoid diverticulum simulating polyps. Orv Hetil 1993;134:639.

286. Williams JG, Williams LA, Colhoun EN. Changes of uteroenteric anastomoses masquerading as a neoplastic polyp: report of two cases. Dis Colon Rectum 1988;31:313.

287. Kelly JK, MacCannell KL, Price LM, Hershfield NB. Residual stalks of pedunculated adenomas: an underrecognized type of colonic polyp. J Clin Gastroenterol 1987;9:227.

288. Mettlin C, Dodd GD. The American Cancer Society Guidelines for the cancer-related checkup: an update. CA 1991;41:279.

289. American Cancer Society. Update January 1992. The American Cancer Society guidelines for the cancer-related checkup. CA 1992;42:44.

290. Levin B, Murphy GP. Revision in American Cancer Society Recommendations for the early detection of colorectal cancer. CA 1992;42:296.

291. Ransohoff DF, Lang CA. Screening for colorectal cancer. N Engl J Med 1991;325:37.

292. Magliate DT, Keller KJ, Miller RE, et al. Colon and rectal carcinoma: spatial distribution and detection. Radiology 1983;147:669.

293. Wanebo HJ, Fang WL, Mills AS, Sfass AM. Colorectal cancer: a blueprint for disease control through screening by primary care physicians. Arch Surg 1986;121:1347.

294. Dubow RA, Katon RM, Benner KG, et al. Short (35-cm) versus long (60-cm) flexible sigmoidoscopy: a comparison of findings and tolerance in asymptomatic patients screened for colorectal neoplasia. Gastrointest Endosc 1985;31:305.

295. Weissman GS, Winawer SJ, Baldwin MP, et al. Multicenter evaluation of training of non-endoscopists in 30 cm flexible sigmoidoscope. CA 1987;37:26.

296. Cole P, Morrison AS. Basic issues in population screening for cancer. J Natl Cancer Inst 1980;64:1263.

297. Neugut AL, Pita S. Role of sigmoidoscopy in screening for colorectal cancer: a critical review. Gastroenterology 1988;95:492.

298. Gupta T, Jaszewski R, Luk GD. Efficacy of screening flexible sigmoidoscopy for colorectal neoplasia in asymptomatic subjects. Am J Med 1989;86:547.

299. Bader J. Screening of colon cancer. Dig Dis Sci 1986;31:43S.

300. Tedesco FJ, Gottfried EB, Corless JK, et al. Prospective evaluation of hospitalized patients with nonactive lower intestinal bleeding: timing and role of barium enema and colonoscopy. Gastrointest Endosc 1984;30:281.

301. de Roos A, Hermans J, Shaw PC, et al. Colon polyps and carcinomas: prospective comparison of the single and double-contrast examination in the same patients. Radiology 1985;154:11.

302. Bolin S, Franz'en L, Nilsson E, Sjödahl R. Carcinoma of the colon and rectum: tumors missed by radiologic examination in 61 patients. Cancer 1988;61:1999.

303. Ott DJ, Scharling ES, Chen YM, et al. Positive predictive value and posttest probability of diagnosis of colonic polyp on single- and double-contrast barium enema. AJR 1989;153:735.

304. Spencer NJ, Richards DG, Bartlett P, et al. Colorectal polyps: a correlation of radiological and pathological findings. Clin Radiol 1988;39:407.

305. Tawil S, Brandt LJ. Chili bean colonic pseudopolyp. Gastrointest Endosc 1992;37:106.

306. Norfleet RG, Ryan ME, Wyman JB, et al. Barium enema versus colonoscopy for patients with polyps found during flexible sigmoidoscopy. Gastrointest Endosc 1991;37:531.

307. Glick SN, Teplick SK, Balfe DM, et al. Large colonic neoplasms missed by endoscopy. AJR 1989;152:513.

308. Gelfand DW, Chen MY, Ott DJ. Benign colorectal neoplasms undetected by colonoscopy. Gastrointest Radiol 1992;17:344.

309. Warnecke J, Petrelli N, Herrera L, Nava H. Accuracy of colonoscopy for the detection of colorectal polyps. Dis Colon Rectum 1992;35:981.

310. Pesce CM, Colacino R. Relative growth of adenomatous polyps of the colon: sterology and allometry of multiple polyposis. Virchows Arch [A] 1987;412:151.

311. Mecklin JP, Sipponen P, Jarvinen H. Histopathology of colorectal carcinomas and adenomas in cancer family syndrome. Dis Colon Rectum 1986;29:849.

312. Lindsay DC, Freeman JG, Cobden I, Record CO. Should colonoscopy be the first investigation for colonic disease? Br Med J 1988;296:167.

313. Barry MJ, Mulley AG, Richter JM. Effect of workup strategy on the cost-effectiveness of fecal occult blood screening for colorectal cancer. Gastroenterology 1987;93:301.

314. Mosvold J, Osnes M, Serck-Hanssen A. Colonoscopy in the diagnosis of colorectal cancer. Scand J Gastroenterol [Suppl] 1988;149:43.

315. Williams CB, Whiteway JE, Jass JR. Practical aspects of endoscopic management of malignant polyps. Endoscopy 1987;1:31.

316. Waye JD, Lewis BS, Yessayan S. Colonoscopy: a prospective report of complications. J Clin Gastroenterol 1992;15:347.

317. Jalihal A, Misra SP, Arvind AS, Kamath PS. Colonoscopic polypectomy in children. J Pediatr Surg 1992;27:1220.

318. Demers RY, Neale AV, Budev H, Schade WJ. Pathologist agreement in the interpretation of colorectal polyps. Am J Gastroenterol 1990;85:417.

319. Gold P, Freeman SO. Demonstration of tumor specific antigens in human colonic carcinomata by immunological tolerance and absorption techniques. J Exp Med 1965;121:439.

320. Fletcher RH. Carcinoembryonic antigen. Ann Intern Med 1986;104:66.

321. Fishbach W, Mössner J. Do size, histology, or cytology of colorectal adenomas and their removal influence serum CEA? Dis Colon Rectum 1987;30:595.

322. Magnani JL, Steplewski Z, Koprowski H, et al. Identification of the gastrointestinal and pancreatic cancer associated antigen detected by monoclonal antibody CA-19-9 in the sera of patients as a mucin. Cancer Res 1983;43:5489.

323. Afdhal NH, Long A, Tobbia I, et al. Immunohistochemical CA19-9 in primary colonic polyps and polyps synchronous with colorectal cancer. Gut 1987;28:594.

324. Steinberg WM, Gelfand R, Anderson KK, et al. Comparison of the sensitivity and specificity of CA19-9 and carcinoembryonic antigen assays in detecting cancer of the pancreas. Gastroenterology 1986;90:343.

325. Itzkowitz SH, Kim YS. New carbohydrate tumor markers. Gastroenterology 1986;90:491.

326. Boland CR, Chen Y-F, Rinderle SJ, et al. Use of the lectin from *Amaranthus caudatus* as a histochemical probe of proliferating colonic epithelial cells. Cancer Res 1991;51:657.

327. Kozuka S, Nogaki M, Ozeki T, Masumori S. Premalignancy of the mucosal polyp in the large intestine. II. Estimation of the periods required for malignant transformation of mucosal polyps. Dis Colon Rectum 1975;18:894.

328. Knoernschild HE. Growth rate and malignant potential of colonic polyps: early results. Surg Forum 1963;14:137.

329. Welin S, Youker J, Spratt JS Jr. The rates and patterns of growth of 375 tumors of the large intestine and rectum observed serially by double contrast enema study (Malmo technique). AJR 1963;90:673.

330. Tada M, Misaki F, Kawai K. Growth rates of colorectal carcinoma and adenoma by roentgenologic follow-up observations. Gastroenterol Jpn 1984;19:550.

331. Carroll RLA, Klein M. How often should patients be sigmoidoscoped? A mathematical perspective. Prev Med 1980;9:741.

332. Figiel LS, Figiel SJ, Wieterson FK. Roentgenologic observation of growth rates of colonic polyps and carcinoma. Acta Radiol Diagn 1965;3:417.

333. Hoff G, Foerster A, Vatn MH, et al Epidemiology of polyps in the rectum and colon: recovery and evaluation of unresected polyps 2 years after detection. Scand J Gastroenterol 1986;21:853.

334. Winawer SJ, Diaz B, Zauber A, et al. The National Polyp study: colorectal adenomas and hyperplastic polyps. Gastroenterology 1988;94:A499.

335. Holtzman R, Poulard JB, Bank S, et al. Repeat colonoscopy after endoscopic polypectomy. Dis Colon Rectum 1987;30:185.

336. DeCosse JJ. Malignant colorectal polyps. Gut 1984;25:433.

337. Woolfson IK, Eckholdt GJ, Wetzel CR, et al. Usefulness of performing colonoscopy one year after endoscopic polypectomy. Dis Colon Rectum 1990;33:389.

338. Winawer SJ, Zauber AG, O'Brien MJ, et al. Randomized comparison of surveillance intervals after colonoscopic removal of newly diagnosed adenomatous polyps. N Engl J Med 1993;328:901.

339. Enterline HT, Evans GW, Mercado-Lugo R, et al. Malignant potential of adenomas of colon and rectum. JAMA 1962;179:322.

340. Wilcox GM, Anderson PB, Colacchio TA. Early invasive carcinoma in colonic polyps: a review of the literature with emphasis on the assessment of the risk of metastasis. Cancer 1986;57:160.

341. Waye JD. Endoscopic treatment of adenomas. World J Surg 1991;15:14.

342. Bond JH. Polyp guideline: diagnosis, treatment, and surveillance for patients with nonfamilial colorectal polyps. Ann Intern Med 1993;119:836.

343. Granquist S, Gabrielsson W, Sundelin P. Diminutive colonic polyps: clinical significance and management. Endoscopy 1979;11:36.

344. Waye JD, Frankel A, Braunfeld SF. The histopathology of small colon polyps. Gastrointest Endosc 1980;75:80A.

345. Gilbert DA, DiMarino AJ, Jensen DM, et al. Status evaluation: hot biopsy forceps. American Society for Gastrointestinal Endoscopy, Technology Assessment Committee. Gastrointest Endosc 1992;38:753.

346. Woods A, Sanowski RA, Wadas DD, et al. Eradication of diminutive polyps: a prospective evaluation of bipolar coagulation versus conventional biopsy removal. Gastrointest Endosc 1989;35:536.

347. Vanagunas A, Jacob P, Vakil N. Adequacy of "hot biopsy" for the treatment of diminutive polyps: a prospective randomized trial. Am J Gastroenterol 1989;84:383.

348. Peluso F, Goldner F. Follow-up of hot biopsy forceps treatment of diminutive colonic polyps. Gastrointest Endosc 1991;37:604.

349. Tappero G, Gaia E, De Giuli P, et al. Cold snare excision of small colorectal polyps. Gastrointest Endosc 1992;38:310.

350. Walsh RM, Ackroyd FW, Shellito PC. Endoscopic resection of large sessile colorectal polyps. Gastrointest Endosc 1992;38:303.

351. Fennerty MB, Sampliner RE, Hixson LJ, Garewal HS. Effectiveness of India ink as a long-term colonic mucosal marker. Am J Gastroenterol 1992;87:79.

352. Van Gossum A, Cozzoli A, Adler M, et al. Colonic snare polypectomy: analysis of 1485 resections comparing two types of current. Gastrointest Endosc 1982;38:472.

353. Chung RS. Therapeutic endoscopy gastrointestinal surgery. New York: Churchill-Livingstone, 1987.

354. Mathus-Vliegen EMH, Tytgat GNJ. Nd:YAG laser photocoagulation in colorectal adenoma: evaluation of its safety, usefulness and efficacy. Gastroenterology 1986;90:1865.

355. Kiefhaber P. Indications for endoscopic neodymium-YAG laser treatment in the gastrointestinal tract: twelve years' experience. Scand J Gastroenterol 1987;139:53.

356. Low DE, Kozarek RA, Ball TJ, Ryan JA Jr. Nd-YAG laser photoablation of sessile villous and tubular adenomas of the colorectum. Ann Surg 1988;208:725.

357. Low DE, Kozarek RA, Ball TJ, et al. Colorectal neodymium-YAG photoablative therapy: comparing applications and complications on both sides of the peritoneal reflection. Arch Surg 1989;124:684.

358. Mathus-Vliegen EM, Tytgat GN. The potential and limitations of laser photoablation of colorectal adenomas. Gastrointest Endosc 1991;37:9.

359. Wilcox GM, Beck JR. Early invasive cancer in adenomatous colonic polyps ("malignant polyps"): evaluation of the therapeutic options by decision analysis. Gastroenterology 1987;92:1159.

360. Sackier JM, Wood CB. Ulcerative colitis and polyposis coli: surgical options. Surg Clin North Am 1988;68:1319.

361. Nicholls RJ. Surgical treatment of adenomas. World J Surg 1991;15:20.

362. Cooperman AM, Katz V, Simmon D, Botero G. Laparoscopic colon resection: a case report. J Laparoendosc Surg 1991;1:221.

363. Wolff WI, Shinya A. Definitive treatment of "malignant" polyps of the colon. Ann Surg 1975;182:516.

364. Cranley JP, Petras RE, Carey WD, et al. When is endoscopic polypectomy adequate therapy for colonic polyps containing invasive carcinoma? Gastroenterology 1986;91:419.

365. Russell JM, Chu DZ, Russell MP, et al. When is polypectomy sufficient treatment for colorectal cancer in a polyp? Am J Surg 1990;160:665.

366. Eckardt VF, Fuchs M, Kanzler G, et al. Follow-up of patients with colonic polyps containing severe atypia and invasive carcinoma: compliance, recurrence, and survival. Cancer 1988;61:2552.

367. Coverlizza S, Risio M, Ferrari A, et al. Colorectal adenomas containing invasive carcinoma: pathologic assessment of lymph node metastatic potential. Cancer 1989;64:1937.

368. Muller S, Chesner IM, Egan MJ, et al. Significance of venous and lymphatic invasion in malignant polyps of the colon and rectum. Gut 1989;30:1385.

369. Geraghty JM, Williams CB, Talbot IC. Malignant colorectal polyps: venous invasion and successful treatment by endoscopic polypectomy. Gut 1991;32:774.

370. Pollard CW, Nivatvongs S, Rojanasakul A, et al. The fate of patients following polypectomy alone for polyps containing invasive carcinoma. Dis Colon Rectum 1992;35:933.

371. Alonso AP, Vasquez-Iglesias JL, Arnal MF, et al. The endoscopic polypectomy of colonic polyps with invasive adenocarcinoma: a series of 19 cases. Rev Esp Enferm Dig 1991;80:376.

372. Pines A, Bat L, Shemesh E, et al. Invasive colorectal adenomas: surgery versus colonoscopic polypectomy. J Surg Oncol 1990;43:53.

373. Morson BC, Bussey HJR, Samoorian S. Policy of local excision for early cancer of the colorectum. Gut 1977;18:1045.

374. Richards WO, Webb WA, Morris SJ, et al. Patient management after endoscopic removal of the cancerous colon adenoma. Ann Surg 1987;205:665.

375. Conte CC, Welch JP, Tennant R, et al. Management of endoscopically removed malignant colon polyps. J Surg Oncol 1987;36:116.

376. Chantereau MJ, Faivre J, Boutron MC, et al. Epidemiology, management, and prognosis of malignant large bowel polyps within a defined population. Gut 1992;33:259.

377. Greenburg AG, Saik RP, Coyle JJ, et al. Mortality and gastrointestinal surgery in the aged. Arch Surg 1981;116:788.

378. Williams CB, Macrae FA. The St. Mark's neoplastic polyp follow-up study. Frontiers of Gastrointestinal Research 1986;19:226.

379. Christie JP. Polypectomy or colonectomy? Management of 106 consecutively encountered colorectal polyps. Am Surg 1988;54:93.

380. Rossini FP, Ferrari A, Coverlizza S, et al. Large bowel adenomas containing carcinoma: a diagnostic and therapeutic approach. Int J Colorectal Dis 1988;3:47.

381. Nava H, Carlsson G, Petrelli NJ, Mittelman A. Follow-up colonoscopy in patients with colorectal adenomatous polyps. Prog Clin Biol Res 1988;279:79.

382. Chu DZJ, Giacco G, Martin RG, Guinee VF. The significance of synchronous carcinoma and polyps in the colon and rectum. Cancer 1986;57:445.

Textbook of Gastroenterology, second edition, edited
by Tadataka Yamada. JB Lippincott Company,
Philadelphia © 1995.

CHAPTER 86

Polyposis Syndromes

Randall W. Burt

Adenomatous Polyposis Syndromes
  Familial Adenomatous Polyposis
  Gardner's Syndrome
  Turcot's Syndrome
  Attenuated Adenomatous Polyposis Coli
Hamartomatous Polyposis Syndromes
  Peutz-Jeghers Syndrome

Familial Juvenile Polyposis Coli
Extremely Rare Hamartomatous Polyposis Syndromes
Noninherited Polyposis Syndromes
  Cronkhite-Canada Syndrome
  Nodular Lymphoid Hyperplasia
  Inflammatory Polyposis
  Miscellaneous Polyposis Conditions

The first reports of intestinal polyposis appeared in the medical literature in 1861 and 1873.[1] These reports described what is now known as familial adenomatous polyposis coli. The hereditary nature of this disease was recognized by 1882, and cases of associated malignancy were published in 1887 and 1890.[1] The autosomal dominant inheritance of colonic adenomatous polyposis was clearly established by 1934.[2]

A large body of literature subsequently has addressed gastrointestinal polyposis conditions, which are now considered important diagnostic entities in clinical medicine. Clinical and pathologic observations have shown that there are a number of distinct syndromes. Most of them are inherited. Most also exhibit a significant risk of colon cancer. Present knowledge has led to detailed screening and management guidelines for both patients with polyposis and their relatives. Application of these guidelines can lead to prevention of cancer and other complications of the polyposis conditions.

The polyposis syndromes also have provided a unique opportunity to study the biologic mechanisms of colonic polyps and malignancy. A number of cellular and biochemical abnormalities have been demonstrated in patients with inherited polyposis. Most importantly, the gene that gives rise to familial adenomatous polyposis and Gardner's syndrome when mutated has been identified and characterized. Continued work should soon reveal the molecular basis of polyp formation and cancer predisposition in these syndromes and in turn provide clues to the mechanisms of polyp and cancer occurrence in the general population.

The polyposis syndromes are differentiated on the basis of histologic and clinical criteria. There are inherited and noninherited types (Table 86-1). The inherited syndromes can be further divided histologically into those that express adeno-

matous polyposis and those that exhibit multiple hamartomatous polyps. In this chapter, the adenomatous polyposis syndromes are addressed first, followed by a discussion of the hamartomatous syndromes and finally the noninherited polyposis conditions.

ADENOMATOUS POLYPOSIS SYNDROMES

The adenomatous polyposis syndromes include familial adenomatous polyposis (FAP), Gardner's syndrome (GS), and Turcot's syndrome. FAP is a disease that is inherited in an autosomal dominant pattern and is characterized by the presence of hundreds to thousands of colorectal adenomatous polyps and the inevitable development of colon cancer if left untreated. Synonymous terms for FAP include adenomatous polyposis coli (APC) and familial polyposis coli. FAP is the term most commonly used to refer to the clinical disease, preferred because adenomas often occur in the upper gastrointestinal tract as well as in the colon. Geneticists, on the other hand, have elected to call the gene for FAP and GS the *APC* gene. If FAP occurs with clinically manifest extraintestinal lesions, classically osteomas or benign soft tissue tumors and cysts, the disorder is called GS. In common usage, FAP often is used to refer to all patients with inherited adenomatous polyposis, both FAP and GS.

The majority of available information on FAP has been derived from studies that have examined all patients with colonic adenomatous polyposis, without regard to the presence or absence of extraintestinal lesions. Investigations of GS, by definition, have examined patients and families in whom le-

TABLE 86-1
Gastrointestinal Polyposis Syndromes

Inherited Polyposis Syndromes
Adenomatous polyposis syndromes
    Familial adenomatous polyposis
    Gardner's syndrome
    Turcot's syndrome
    Attenuated adenomatous polyposis coli
Hamartomatous polyposis syndromes
    Peutz-Jeghers syndrome
    Familial juvenile polyposis
    Extremely rare syndromes
        Cowden's disease
        Intestinal ganglioneuromatosis
        Ruvalcaba-Myhre-Smith syndrome
        Devon family syndrome

Noninherited Polyposis Syndromes
Cronkhite-Canada syndrome
Nodular lymphoid hyperplasia
Lymphomatous polyposis
Hyperplastic polyposis
Inflammatory polyposis
Miscellaneous conditions

sions specific to that disease were observed. The recent demonstration that subtle extraintestinal lesions are often present in persons otherwise thought to have FAP has clouded the separation between these conditions. The section on FAP therefore reviews intestinal polyposis, and the section on GS presents data on the extraintestinal lesions found in these syndromes. Debate continues on whether separation of patients with extraintestinal lesions is clinically or investigationally useful.

Turcot's syndrome is defined as the occurrence of central nervous system (CNS) tumors associated with colonic adenomatosis polyposis. This syndrome is considered separately because of recent evidence that it does not arise from *APC* gene mutations.

Attenuated adenomatous polyposis coli (AAPC) represents a variant of FAP that arises from mutations in the *APC* gene. It is expressed as a variable number of colonic adenomas, usually less than 100.

Familial Adenomatous Polyposis

Epidemiology

Estimates of the frequency of FAP vary from 1 in 6850 to 1 in 30,000 people.[3,4] The frequency is fairly constant throughout the world, although most descriptions come from Western countries and Japan. Men and women are affected equally by this disease. It is estimated that one third of newly diagnosed cases (i.e., those not belonging to previously identified families) appear to represent new mutations.[3] In such cases, parents and siblings are not affected, but children have the same risk of developing adenomatous polyposis as children of any other affected parent. Approximately 0.5% of colon cancer cases arise from FAP.[4]

Etiology

FAP is an autosomal dominantly inherited disorder with an 80% to 100% penetrance.[5] The disease results from inactivating germ line mutations of the *APC* gene. The normal function of the *APC* gene and protein are not yet known, but certain cellular and physiologic abnormalities that result from *APC* mutations are observed in patients with this disease.

Molecular genetics. The *APC* gene is located on the long arm of chromosome 5.[6–10] The coding portion of the gene contains 8538 base pairs and gives rise to an approximately 300 kd protein with 2843 amino acids.[11] Immunohistochemical analysis of the protein in normal colonic mucosa demonstrates cytoplasmic staining most intensely in the basolateral margins of the epithelial cell. Staining also is more pronounced in the upper portions of the crypt, suggesting increased expression with maturation. Expression of the APC protein is found in many other tissues,[11] and mutations of the *APC* gene have been described in malignancies other than colon cancer.[12]

The majority of FAP families tested have been found to have unique and different mutations of the *APC* gene.[13] Although these different mutations are found scattered throughout the gene, a unifying feature is that they almost all result in truncation of the APC protein. The mutations described are mostly single base pair substitutions or short deletions or insertions; almost all result in novel stop codons. Stop codons are DNA base pair triplets that signal for the translation of mRNA to protein to cease, thereby truncating the protein in the case of an accidental stop signal. These truncated APC proteins have been found to oligomerize to the normal or wild type protein.[14] A current hypothesis based on these observations is that the truncated protein inactivates the protein from the normal allele by dominant negative inhibition.

The *APC* gene is thus believed to be a tumor suppressor gene. This implies that the gene normally acts to suppress cell growth. Inactivation of the gene results in deregulation of cell growth control. Inactivation may occur either by mutation of both copies of the gene[15] or by dominant negative inhibition. A mouse model of FAP has been developed in which intestinal polyposis arises from a mutation in the murine homolog of the *APC* gene.[16] As in the human situation, the mutation is a base pair change that gives rise to an unexpected stop codon.

Missense mutations, those that cause simple amino acid substitutions, are believed to occur much more frequently in nature than mutations that give rise to protein truncation. Such mutations appear insufficient to cause FAP, however, and truncating mutations are almost always identified in FAP families. Tissues from sporadic adenomas and cancers of the colon also often exhibit *APC* gene mutations (see Chaps. 85 and 87). In this setting, the mutations are acquired rather than inherited, because they are not found in normal tissues. The tumor mutations are nonetheless almost all mutations that cause truncation of the protein, similar to the inherited mutations of FAP.[17]

These severe mutations of the *APC* gene are of central importance to the pathogenesis of all types of colorectal cancer. Inherited *APC* mutations result in FAP, whereas acquired

APC mutations are an early and integral step in sporadic adenomas and colon cancer. Subsequent mutations frequently found in colon cancer tissues, including those of *K-ras*, the *p53* transformation-associated gene, and the chromosome 18 deleted-in-colon-cancer gene, appear to be the same in FAP and sporadic malignancies.[18,19] The mutations that give rise to GS do not differ in location or character from those that cause FAP. In one case, an identical mutation was observed to cause GS in one family and FAP in another.[20] It is hypothesized that modifying genes probably play a role in the expression of the extraintestinal manifestations of these conditions. One study does suggest that families that exhibit a colonic adenoma density greater than 5000 polyps per person are found to have mutations in the middle portion of the *APC* gene, whereas those with 2000 or fewer polyps have mutations proximal or distal to that area.[21]

Environmental factors. Environmental factors do not appear to be of primary importance in the pathogenesis of FAP. Nonetheless, there is evidence that the genetic defects of FAP are modulated by certain environmental factors. Polyps, for example, have been seen to resolve after subtotal colectomy,[22] pregnancy,[23] oral calcium,[24] oral fiber,[25] and oral sulindac.[26]

Cellular and metabolic abnormalities. The proliferative compartment of the colonic crypt in persons with FAP is expanded to include the entire crypt, as with the growth patterns observed in adenomatous polyps.[27] It is postulated that this proliferative pattern is the earliest discernible change in the progression from benign to malignant and that adenomas arise in this setting. An alternative hypothesis is that adenomas arise from a clone of mutant cells that begin in the lower crypt but are not preceded by the expanded proliferative compartment phenotype.[28]

A number of cellular abnormalities found in colonic adenomas and cancers also are observed in normal-appearing colonic epithelial cells from patients with FAP. These include elevated levels of ornithine decarboxylase, an enzyme essential for intestinal mucosal proliferation[29]; the appearance of certain cytokeratins, which are normally found only in the upper crypt levels, at all levels of the colonic crypt[30]; abnormalities of mucin structure, expressed as abnormal lectin binding[31]; and increased in vitro sensitivity to tumor promoters[32].

Cultured cutaneous fibroblasts from FAP patients likewise exhibit features of neoplasm and susceptibility to neoplastic change.[33,34] Fibroblasts exhibit an increased neoplastic transformation from tumor promoters, transforming viruses,[34] carcinogens, and irradiation. They also demonstrate increased production of plasminogen activator and disordered actin fibers. Loss of contact inhibition and decreased serum requirements for fibroblast growth also have been observed, although not consistently. Spontaneous or mutagen-induced chromosomal instability in FAP fibroblast cultures has been observed directly and has been implicated through an increased sensitivity of fibroblasts to x-radiation, ultraviolet (UV) radiation, mitomycin C, and alkylating agents. Chromosomal tetraploidy[35] and other numerical chromosomal aberrations also have been seen in FAP adenoma cells.[5,36] Because bile appears to be a promoter in colon carcinogenesis and because adenomas often cluster around the duodenal papilla in FAP patients, bile acids have been examined for their possible role in FAP adenoma formation. Low fecal bile and neutral sterol concentrations have been demonstrated.[37] Additionally, there appears to be no degradation of fecal cholesterol in FAP patients.[38] Biliary bile acid profiles are also abnormal, including a higher bile acid concentration, a greater proportion of chenodeoxycholic acid, and a lower proportion of deoxycholic acid.[39]

Clinical Manifestations

Extensive data concerning the details of the FAP phenotype first came from the St. Mark's registry in London.[3] This registry includes a very large number of patients with FAP (617 persons from almost 300 families) and a long period of follow-up. Observations from a number of other registries also are available and together comprise the current knowledge of FAP.[4,40–46]

Colonic adenomatous polyposis. The hallmark of the FAP phenotype is the presence of 100 or more colonic adenomatous polyps, although the average number of adenomatous polyps in a person with fully expressed FAP is 1000, with some persons exhibiting more than 5000 polyps (Fig. 86-1).

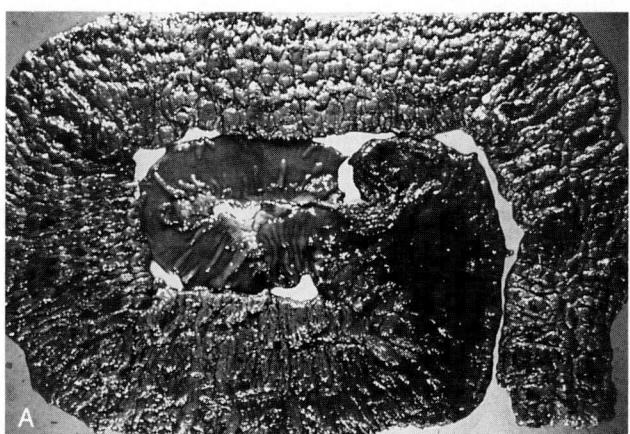

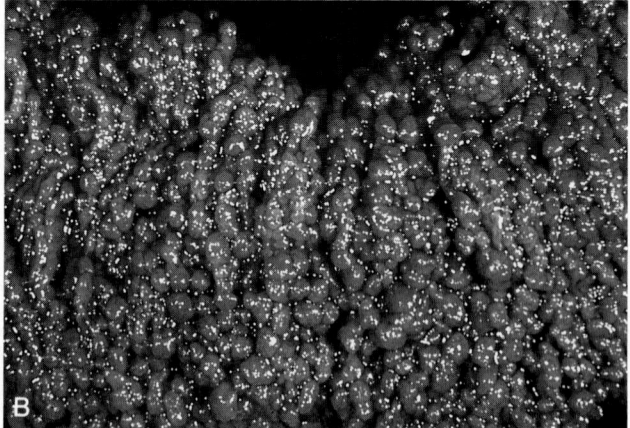

FIGURE 86-1. **(A)** Colon removed from a patient with fully developed familial adenomatous polyposis coli. This colon exhibits the carpeting pattern of polyp growth. (From Gardner EJ, Burt RW, Freston JW. Gastrointestinal polyposis: syndromes and genetic mechanisms. West J Med 1980;132:488.) **(B)** Section of a second colon exhibiting the carpeting pattern with even smaller polyps. (Courtesy of Robert Flinner, M.D., Salt Lake City, UT.)

The number 100 was originally established as a diagnostic reference because no one with fully developed FAP in the St. Mark's registry had fewer than this number and no one with sporadic adenomas had more than 100 polyps.[3] Recent colonoscopic surveys have confirmed that it is unusual to find more than 6 polyps and rare to find more than 50 polyps in persons with sporadic adenomas. However, the diagnosis of FAP is often established in young persons from FAP families when only a few polyps are present.

Polyposis usually develops in the second or third decade of life. The mean age of polyp occurrence assessed by rigid sigmoidoscopy in a study that combined the St. Mark's and Perth FAP registries was 15.9 ± 5.4 years[47] (Fig. 86-2). The youngest at-risk person developing polyps in that study was 8, and the oldest was 34 years of age. All subjects were required to have had a previous negative examination, thus giving a reasonably accurate estimate of the age of adenoma expression. It is likely, however, that studies employing fiberoptic or video endoscopy will find a still younger age of adenoma development. Other studies have reported adenomas to occur as early as 4 and 7 years,[3,48] and microscopic adenomatous change of the epithelium has been seen at an even younger age.[49] There are reports of polyposis developing after 40 years of age,[50] but this is extremely unusual. The average age of diagnosis of polyposis in patients presenting because of symptoms in the St. Mark's registry was 35.8 years, with a range of 4 to 72 years.[3] The average age of polyposis diagnosis among relatives subsequently contacted for screening was 24.5 years (range, 9–57 years). Polyps are distributed evenly throughout the colon, with a slight distal colonic excess.[3] The size of the polyps depends on the stage at which the patient is examined. Even in fully developed cases, however, 90% of adenomas are less than 0.5 cm in diameter. Less than 1% of polyps are larger than 1 cm in diameter at that stage. There is usually some variation in polyp size in individual patients. Two patterns of polyp formation are recognized. The carpeting pattern is characterized as myriads of tiny polyps which uniformly cover the entire surface of the colon (see Fig. 86-1). Also seen is a pattern of more discrete, but fewer, polyps which are slightly larger (Fig. 86-3). Striking heterogeneity of polyp number and growth rate has been observed in some kindreds,[51,52] although this appears to be unusual. The genetic basis of these differences in phenotype is not defined. As has already been described, however, a clustering of APC mutations in the middle portion of the APC gene corresponds in one study to a phenotype producing more than 5000 polyps in a colon.

The colonic polyps in FAP are usually tubular adenomas, indistinguishable from common or sporadic adenomas. Villous and tubulovillous histologies are also seen, but much less frequently and usually in larger polyps. A histologic feature of FAP not observed in the general population is dysplastic or adenomatous epithelial cells in single crypts or even portions of single crypts. Such structures are called microadenomas.[3] They are often seen in biopsy specimens of normal-appearing flat mucosa in individuals with FAP. Budding of dysplastic epithelium from normal crypts is also observed. Aberrant crypt foci also have been reported to occur with increased frequency in FAP.[53] These lesions are similar to microadenomas but are identified with methylene blue staining of the colonic mucosal surface. This method remains investigational but may potentially offer a noninvasive way to identify phenotypic expression of the APC gene and other types of colon cancer predisposition before adenomas are visible.

Colon cancer. Adenocarcinoma is the inevitable consequence of FAP unless the colon is removed (Fig. 86-4). In the St. Mark's series, the average age at cancer diagnosis was 39 years. By 45 years of age, 87% had developed cancer, and by 50 years, 93%. Multiple colonic malignancies were present in about 48% of those with cancer (41% synchronous, 7% metachronous). Eighty-four percent of malignancies were at or distal to the splenic flexure, a fraction almost identical to that found in their series of random colorectal malignancies. Average life expectancy after diagnosis of cancer was 2.6 years. Colon cancer has been reported as early as 9 years of age, although the occurrence of malignancy before adolescence is very unusual.[49]

Upper gastrointestinal polyps. Upper gastrointestinal polyps are a common pleiotropic manifestation of FAP.[54-56] Some studies indicate a slight correlation with extraintestinal lesions, but this is generally not significant. Upper gastrointestinal cancer has been reported to occur in 4.5% of FAP patients, with an average age at diagnosis of 52 years.[44]

Gastric polyps occur in 30% to 100% of FAP patients.[54] In the gastric fundus and body, the polyps are nonneoplastic fundic gland polyps (Fig. 86-5). These polyps are histologically seen to consist of simple hyperplasia of the fundic glands with microcysts. Endoscopically, the polyps are multiple sessile lesions, 1 to 5 mm in diameter, that are the same color as surrounding mucosa. Considerable variation in size and number is observed. The polyps are sometimes so numerous that they coalesce, forming areas of irregular, matted surface mucosa. Fundic gland polyps rarely cause symptoms. They have been observed to occur as early as 8 years of age. Size and number may gradually increase, remain static, or even decrease.[57]

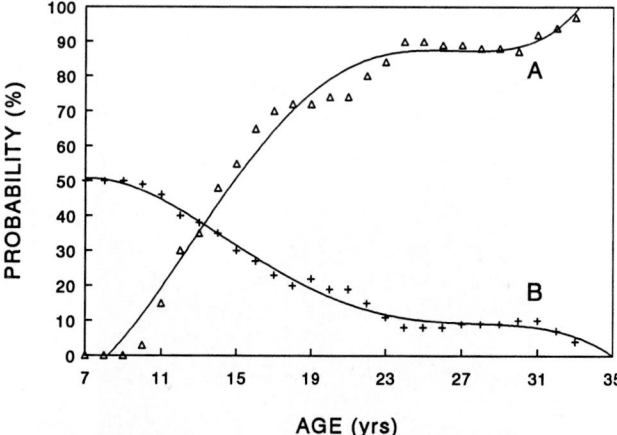

FIGURE 86-2. **(A)** Probability of finding adenomas with rigid sigmoidoscopy in a relative at a given age if he or she has inherited the gene for adenomatous polyposis coli. **(B)** Probability that an at-risk relative will be affected if a prior sigmoidoscopic result at a given age was negative. (From Petersen GM, Slack J, Nakamura Y. Screening guidelines and premorbid diagnosis of familial adenomatous polyposis using linkage. Gastroenterology 1991;100:1658.)

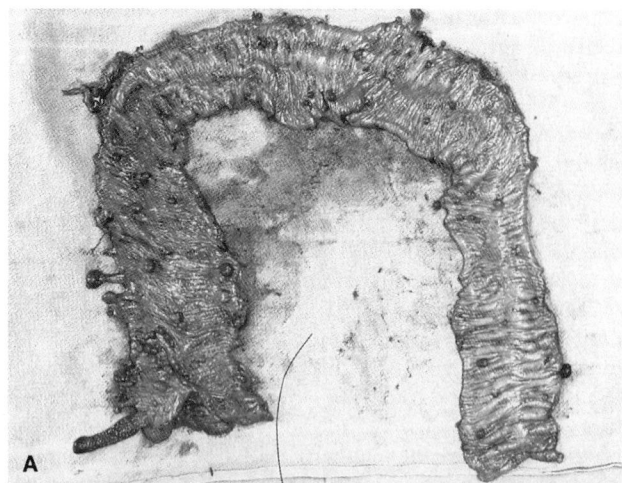

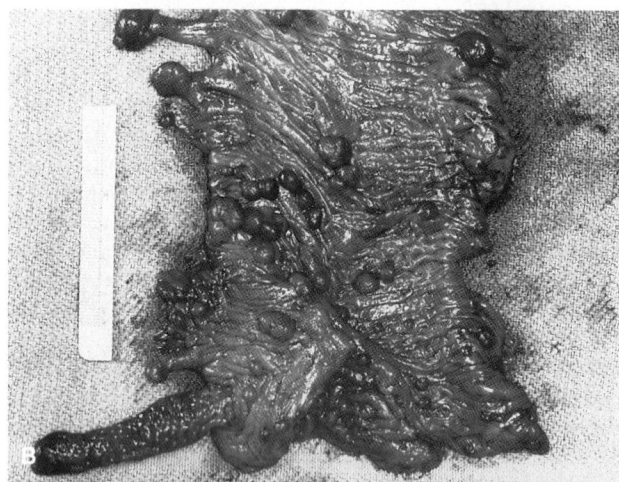

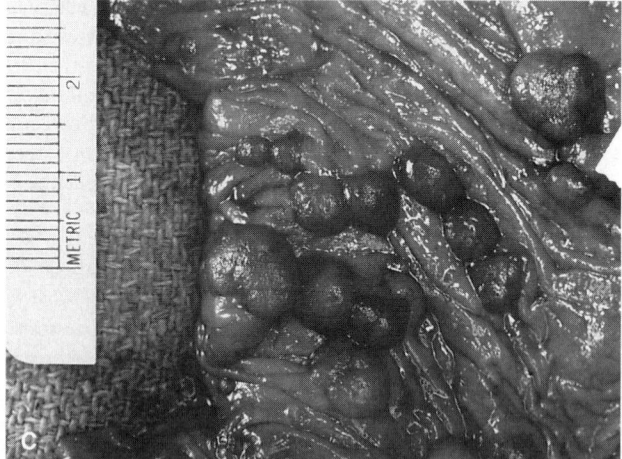

FIGURE 86-3. (**A**) Colon removed from a patient with Gardner's syndrome. This colon demonstrates the pattern of discrete polyp formation. Both the carpeting pattern and the discrete polyp formation pattern are known to occur in familial adenomatous polyposis and Gardner's syndrome. (**B**) and (**C**) close-up views of the polyposis in the discrete polyp pattern. (From Gardner EJ, Burt RW, Freston JW. Gastrointestinal polyposis: syndromes and genetic mechanisms. West J Med 1980;132:488.)

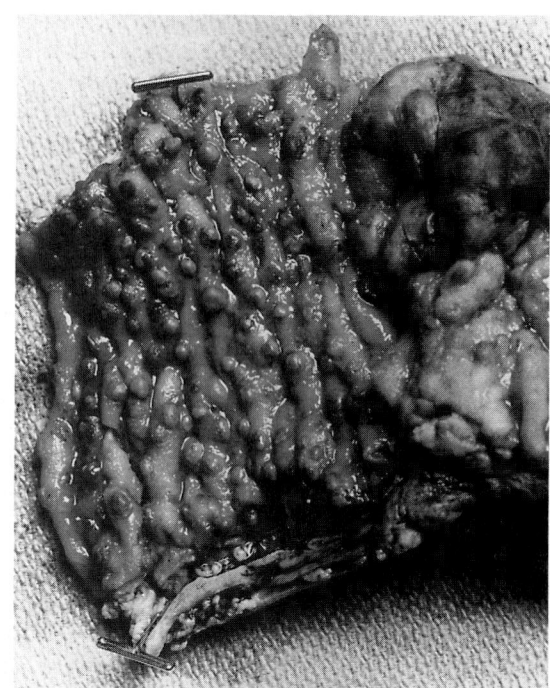

FIGURE 86-4. Section of colon exhibiting adenomatous polyposis and an adjacent carcinoma.

Fundic gland polyps do not appear to have malignant risk. Similar polyps, although fewer in number, also are sometimes observed in the general population.[58]

Adenomatous polyps may also occur in the stomach of persons with FAP, but are almost always confined to the gastric antrum.[55,56,59] They are commonly observed in FAP patients in Japan but are very unusual in other countries. There is little, if any, increased risk of gastric cancer in FAP patients outside Japan.[60]

Duodenal polyps are found in 46% to 93% of polyposis patients.[54–56] The polyps are multiple adenomas, 1 to 5 mm

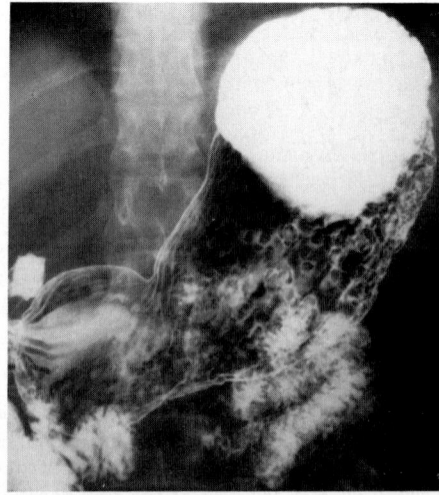

FIGURE 86-5. Upper gastrointestinal radiograph of a patient with familial adenomatous polyposis coli. Fundic gland polyps are seen in the proximal stomach, the fundus, and the body.

in diameter, and are almost always asymptomatic. They may sometimes grow large and exhibit villous histology but often change little over time.[61] There is a significant risk of malignancy in the duodenum, with a 4% to 12% lifetime incidence of duodenal cancer.[44] This frequency is estimated to be more than 300-fold greater than that of the general population.[3,44,60,62] Some studies find the risk of duodenal cancer to be greater than that of rectal cancer in patients who have had a subtotal colectomy with ileorectal anastomosis.[42,55] The average age at diagnosis of periampullary cancer in patients with polyposis is 46 years, compared with 39 years for the age at colon cancer diagnosis.[3]

The duodenal papilla has a particular propensity for adenomatous change in polyposis patients.[60-64] Fifty percent or more of FAP patients exhibit adenomatous histology of the papilla, although the polyps are often small and difficult to appreciate without a side-viewing endoscope. More than one third of the duodenal cancers reported occur at the papilla,[44] and the risk of malignancy is more than 100-fold greater than in the general population.[60] Obstruction of the pancreatic duct has been observed from benign and malignant tumors of the papilla.[65] These papillary neoplasms may account for the excess incidence of pancreatitis reported in some series of FAP.[66]

Reports from Japan have revealed jejunal adenomatous polyps in up to 40% and ileal polyps in 20% of those with FAP.[67,68] The polyps occur throughout the small bowel but are concentrated for the most part in the proximal jejunum and distal ileum. Transformation to malignancy is very unusual, but a few cases of small bowel cancer distal to the duodenum have been reported.[5,44,54,69]

Adenomatous polyps are also known to occur, possibly with increased frequency postoperatively, in the distal ileum after subtotal colectomy, colectomy with ileostomy, and colectomy with ileoanal pull-through.[70-72] Distal ileal cancer also has been reported in these settings, but it is rare.[71] Prominent lymphoid polyps may occur frequently in the terminal ileum of younger patients with FAP and should be differentiated from adenomas by biopsy.[73,74] Gallbladder and bile duct adenomas and cancer have also been reported, as has pancreatic cancer, but these appear to be very rare.[44,54]

Differential Diagnosis

All of the polyposis syndromes are included in the differential diagnosis of a patient found to have gastrointestinal polyposis. Histology is the key to differentiating these syndromes (see Table 86-1). Lymphoid hyperplasia and hyperplastic polyposis, in particular, may mimic FAP endoscopically and require biopsy diagnosis. Additional parameters to be considered in differentiating the various polyposis conditions include the distribution of polyps in the gastrointestinal tract, the number of polyps present, the presence of extraintestinal growths or lesions, the presence of malignancy, and the family history. Each of the polyposis syndromes in this chapter is characterized in terms of these parameters. The features that differentiate the major polyposis syndromes are summarized in Tables 86-2 and 86-3.

FAP and GS also must be differentiated from the other causes of adenomatous polyps. These include AAPC, hereditary nonpolyposis colorectal cancer, and common or sporadic adenomatous polyps. Persons with AAPC exhibit many, albeit usually fewer than 100, colonic adenomas (see Attenuated Adenomatous Polyposis Coli). Persons with hereditary nonpolyposis colorectal cancer (HNPCC) usually exhibit only a few colonic adenomas and yet show an autosomal dominant pattern of colon cancer inheritance.[75] The polyps in HNPCC occur at a relatively young age and on average are larger and histologically more advanced than sporadic polyps. Extensive kindred study is often needed to verify this syndrome, although evidence suggests that it arises from mutations on chromosome 2. Common or sporadic colonic adenomas and cancer also often cluster in families. Inherited syndromes are unlikely if polyps are few, inheritance patterns are not readily apparent, the colon cancer occurrence in the family is not extreme, and the age of cancer diagnosis is close to that observed in the general population.[76]

Screening and Diagnostic Studies

The justification for screening as a method of cancer prevention in FAP is well established.[43] The cancer risk in FAP patients presenting with symptoms varies from 32% to 57%,

TABLE 86-2
Polyp Features That Distinguish the Major Polyposis Syndromes

SYNDROME	INHERITANCE	POLYP HISTOLOGY	POLYP DISTRIBUTION (%)	AGE OF APPEARANCE OF COLONIC POLYPS
Familial adenomatous polyposis (FAP)	Autosomal dominant	Adenomatous	Colon (100) Stomach (30–100) Duodenum (46–93) Jejunum (40) Ileum (20)	16 y (range, 8–34 y)
Gardner's syndrome	Autosomal dominant	Adenomatous	Same as FAP	Same as FAP
Peutz-Jeghers syndrome	Autosomal dominant	Peutz-Jeghers	Small bowel (64–96) Stomach (24–49) Colon (60)	First decade
Familial juvenile polyposis	Autosomal dominant	Juvenile	Colon, usually Stomach, may occur Small bowel, may occur	First decade

TABLE 86-3
General Features That Distinguish the Major Polyposis Syndromes

SYNDROME	AVERAGE ONSET OF GASTROINTESTINAL SYMPTOMS	RISK OF COLON CANCER	OTHER CANCERS	ASSOCIATED LESIONS
Familial adenomatous polyposis coli	33 y	100%	Same as in GS	Desmoids, CHRPE
Gardner's syndrome (GS)	33 y	100%	Periampullary and duodenal—10% CNS—rare Thyroid—rare Hepatoblastoma—rare Adrenal—rare	Desmoids, CHRPE, osteoma, benign soft tissue tumors, dental abnormalities
Peutz-Jeghers syndrome	23–26 y	Slightly increased	Stomach and duodenum—2%–13% Breast, cervical, ovarian, testicular, pancreatic	Orocutaneous melanin pigment spots
Familial juvenile polyposis	10 y (5 y in nonfamilial form)	At least 9%	Gastric? Duodenal? Pancreatic?	Congenital abnormalities in 20% of nonfamilial type

CHRPE, congenital hypertrophy of the retinal pigment epithelium; CNS, central nervous system.

whereas the cancer risk in call-up groups ranges from 0% to 33%. Cancer is almost never present at the time of polyposis diagnosis in patients who undergo interval prospective screening. Appropriate screening could conceivably prevent all colon cancer in persons known to be at risk of FAP. This outcome depends mostly on family notification and regular follow-up. Screening of FAP should be done by video or fiberoptic endoscopy because of the usual small polyp size and the requirement of histology for diagnosis.

Children of affected parents should be screened regularly to detect the emergence of colonic polyposis. Flexible proctosigmoidoscopy is sufficient for screening in view of the colonic polyp distribution. Examinations should begin by 10 to 12 years of age and should continue every 1 or 2 years until 35 years of age; thereafter, examinations should be performed every 3 years. An extensive family history should always be obtained, and pedigree charts should be constructed so that members of the extended family who are at risk can be identified and offered appropriate screening. Full colonoscopy should be performed on the person who is first diagnosed with polyposis that is already well developed, because larger polyps and malignancy may be present in the proximal colon in this situation.

Genetic testing for FAP using the DNA obtained from peripheral blood samples is available at regional DNA diagnostic laboratories. Testing employs DNA linkage markers to the *APC* gene. The use of linkage markers requires that two family members already have a firm diagnosis of FAP. Such markers can diagnose more than 95% of persons at risk of FAP, with greater than 98% accuracy.[13] Direct detection of mutations may eventually allow diagnosis of FAP in individuals without regard to the family setting. This approach is not yet practical because most FAP families have unique *APC* mutations. A few mutations, however, have been found to be common to a number of families.[77] Although testing for these specific mutations is possible, it is predicted that only

about 10% to 20% of FAP patients could be diagnosed in this way at present.[13] A method for detection of abnormal APC protein is available and can detect up to 87% of gene carriers.[77a]

Genetic testing should first be performed at 10 to 12 years of age. Those who test positive should undergo sigmoidoscopy, as has been outlined, to examine for the development of adenomas. Persons testing negative should nonetheless have sigmoidoscopy every 3 to 5 years until 40 years of age. As genetic testing approaches 100% accuracy, follow-up of this group becomes unnecessary. Testing of children younger than 10 years of age should be avoided because it is not clinically important and may lead to problems with parental bonding, peer rejection, and poor self-image.

Upper gastrointestinal screening should begin when the diagnosis of colonic polyposis is made.[54-56,65] Benign or malignant complications of duodenal adenomas are rare before the onset of colonic adenomatosis. Screening consists of upper gastrointestinal endoscopy every 1 to 3 years. The longer interval is adequate if polyps are not present. The presence of antral or duodenal adenomas, and especially adenomatous change on the duodenal papilla, justifies endoscopic inspection every 1 or 2 years, depending on the number and size of polyps.[61] Side-viewing endoscopy should be used during the examination to accurately assess the duodenal papilla. Although definitive guidelines for screening the small bowel distal to the duodenum have not been developed, small bowel radiography should be obtained in those found to have prominent duodenal polyps or if the patient is to have surgery.[69]

Clinical Course and Complications

The majority of individuals with FAP remain asymptomatic until colon cancer occurs. Adenomatous polyp development is slow and insidious. There are usually only a few, minute polyps when adenomas are first detected in at-risk persons.

Polyp number and size increase gradually over ensuing years. Symptoms from the disease are seldom experienced if a timely colectomy is performed. If the disease is left untreated, however, nonspecific symptoms eventually develop from the polyposis or the inevitable colon cancer. The majority of patients in the St. Mark's registry (196 of 293) presented with symptoms that included rectal bleeding (79%), diarrhea (70%), and abdominal pain (40%). The average age of onset of symptoms was 32.8 years. Sixty-six percent of individuals who presented with symptoms had already developed cancer. For this reason, the central focus of disease management in FAP is prevention of colon cancer through appropriate screening of asymptomatic family members. Upper gastrointestinal polyps likewise usually are asymptomatic until cancer occurs, with the exception of polyps at the duodenal papilla. These may cause obstructive jaundice or pancreatitis.[65] Of 1255 patients followed by the registries enrolled in the Leeds Castle Polyposis Group, invasive upper gastrointestinal cancer occurred in 57 (4.5%).[44] Cancer cases included 7 gastric, 10 ampullary, 26 second duodenum, 3 third and fourth duodenum, 5 jejunum, 1 ileum, 2 bile duct, and 3 pancreas. The median age of cancer diagnosis was 52 years (range, 17–81 years). Symptoms were nonspecific and included abdominal pain, weight loss, gastrointestinal blood loss, palpable mass, and lumenal obstruction.

The average life expectancy for persons with untreated FAP has been estimated to be 42 years. Life expectancy is thought to be much longer with colectomy, but accurate figures are not available. The major causes of death after colectomy are upper gastrointestinal cancer and desmoid tumors.[42,55] Thirty-six FAP patients were identified from the Cleveland Clinic records who had undergone total or subtotal colectomy and died at some time thereafter. The major causes of death in that group were desmoid tumors, in 11 (31%) of 36 patients; periampullary cancer in 8 (22%); rectal cancer in 3 (8%); adrenal cancer in 1 (3%); and carcinomatosis in 1 (3%). The remainder died of causes not directly related to FAP. Those with desmoid tumors died an average of 6.6 years after colectomy, whereas those with periampullary cancer died an average of 23.1 years after surgery. The average age at death for the entire group was 41.6 years. This must not be equated with overall life expectancy, because only patients who had died were studied.

Therapy

Colectomy should be anticipated to minimize cancer risk after a diagnosis of colonic adenomatosis is made. Colectomy can usually be delayed a short time to accommodate school and work schedules, especially if polyps are small and few in number. Interval colonoscopy should be performed if a delay longer than a few months is anticipated. The procedure should be repeated every 6 to 12 months, depending on the size and number of polyps present. Persons first screened at an older age may have more fully developed polyposis, and expeditious surgical intervention is important in such persons.

Surgical options include subtotal colectomy with ileorectal anastomosis, total proctocolectomy with ileostomy, and colectomy with mucosal proctectomy and ileoanal pouch.[43,78–80] Proctocolectomy with ileostomy is rarely required unless cancer is already present in the distal rectum. Subtotal colectomy

with ileorectal anastomosis is a relatively simple procedure, with mortality of less than 1% and morbidity less than 10%.[43] The primary concern with this procedure is continued adenoma formation in the rectum and attendant cancer risk. Rectal adenomas often regress after colectomy,[22] possibly because of changes in bile acids,[81] but they almost always recur. Sigmoidoscopy with ablation of recurrent adenomas is therefore needed every 3 to 6 months.[80] Despite planned follow-up, the incidence of rectal cancer is reported between 6% at 20 years and 55% at 30 years postsurgery.[43] The mean age of rectal cancer development is 48 years.[80] Up to 30% of these postsurgical patients also need eventual rectal resection because of inability to control polyps medically.

Colectomy with mucosal proctectomy and ileoanal pouch has been introduced as a method of complete colonic mucosal removal that retains rectal function.[82] This procedure now is considered the procedure of choice in many centers.[83] Several problems, however, are more common than with ileorectal anastomosis, including more nighttime incontinence and more sexual dysfunction.[80] An intermediate approach has been suggested that includes selecting patients with fewer rectal polyps for ileorectal anastomosis and then later revision to ileoanal pouch if warranted. This approach may become particularly attractive if sulindac and other nonsteroidal antiinflammatory drugs (NSAIDs) prove successful in maintaining polyp suppression in patients with a remaining rectum.

The management of upper gastrointestinal polyps is more problematic, since long-term studies of polyp treatment only recently have begun.[55,60] It is agreed, however, that radical surgical treatment is not indicated for numerous small gastric or duodenal polyps alone. Villous adenomas, large tubular adenomas (>5 mm), and symptomatic adenomas, regardless of histology, warrant removal because of the potential for malignant change and nonmalignant complications.[65] Endoscopic removal of polyps should be considered if the polyp is pedunculated and separate from the papilla.[84] Villous polyps and symptomatic tubular adenomas of the duodenal papilla require surgical excision.[85] Endoscopic removal of such lesions has been attempted in one study with some success, but the investigators suggest that such therapy be attempted only in the setting of a controlled trial.[86] One group recommended that pancreaticoduodenectomy be considered in the otherwise fit patient with extensive benign ampullary villous adenomas and localized cancers. This recommendation was made because of the high incidence of malignancy in villous adenomas of the papilla and duodenum and because of the recurrence of villous polyp tissue if only local resection was performed.[85]

Sulindac, an NSAID with prostaglandin inhibitory properties, has been shown in a number of studies to cause adenoma regression.[26,86–88] This has been observed both in the rectums of FAP patients who have undergone subtotal colectomy with ileorectal anastomosis and in the colons of unoperated FAP patients. Most, but not all, colonic adenomas regress; it is uncertain whether colon cancer risk is decreased. Although it is premature to recommend sulindac as a primary therapy for unoperated FAP, there seems little reason not to use the medication for those who have had colectomy with ileorectal anastomosis. Close follow-up is required in those patients in any case, and pharmacologic treatment would simply reduce the number of polyps that must otherwise be ablated. Effective polyp control might also delay the need for eventual proctectomy and possibly reduce cancer risk. If second-generation drugs can be developed that have less long-term toxicity than present NSAIDs, such drugs could possibly also be used for prevention of adenomas after polypectomy of sporadic polyps. It is not yet known whether upper gastrointestinal polyps are affected by NSAIDs. In one study, sulindac reduced duodenal cell proliferation but failed to cause adenoma regression.[89]

Gardner's Syndrome

In the early 1950s, Gardner and his colleagues described a large kindred that exhibited autosomal dominant inheritance of colonic adenomatous polyposis and colon cancer, together with a high occurrence of certain benign extracolonic lesions.[90–92] These included multiple osteomas, multiple epidermoid cysts, and soft fibromas of the skin. Dental abnormalities, desmoid tumors, and mesenteric fibromatosis were later added as additional pleiotropic manifestations of the underlying genetic defect.[93] Other accompanying lesions subsequently have been described, and the constellation of inherited colonic adenomatosis together with these extracolonic lesions has become known as Gardner's syndrome (GS).

General Features

GS is inherited as an autosomal dominant disorder with 100% penetrance.[94] Like FAP, it arises from mutations of the *APC* gene. It is considered to be less common than FAP, with an occurrence estimated at 1 in every 14,025 births.[95] The difficulty in distinguishing between FAP and GS, however, has made prevalence figures more a result of arbitrary definitions than of true prevalence differences between the two disorders. Furthermore, the epidemiology and presently defined genetics of the two syndromes are similar. The clinical characteristics, differential diagnosis, course, and treatment of the colonic polyposis and upper gastrointestinal polyps are essentially the same. The separation of GS from FAP on the basis of extraintestinal lesions thus appears somewhat arbitrary.

The expression of extraintestinal lesions may differ markedly between families and yet is usually quite homogeneous within families. In some kindreds, such as the one originally described by Gardner, affected persons exhibit numerous and obvious lesions, whereas in others extraintestinal growths are subtle and found only occasionally. Kindreds with intermediate expression of findings are common. These observations argue for distinct genetic differences between families, even though these differences do not particularly coincide with the traditional categories of FAP and GS. The genetic basis for the variable expression of extraintestinal lesions remains to be defined. Because there appears to be no obvious correlation between extraintestinal lesions and the type or location of mutations in the *APC* gene, some have postulated the involvement of modifier genes. Until genetic research defines the basis for the observed differences, extraintestinal lesions must be considered a disease risk in all persons with FAP. And although the clinical separation of GS from FAP appears imprecise, the term GS undoubtedly will continue to be used to describe families in which extraintestinal lesions are prom-

inently expressed. This section describes the extraintestinal lesions that occur in FAP and traditionally define GS.

Extraintestinal Lesions

Osteomas.   Multiple osteomas were the first extracolonic lesion associated with GS.[3,91,93] They are found most commonly on the skull and mandible but may occur on any bone of the body (Fig. 86-6). The size ranges from imperceptible to several centimeters in diameter, and the number from one to dozens. Osteomas may occur in children who are at risk of FAP before the onset of colonic polyposis. Osteomas have no malignant potential and are not a clinical problem except in a few cases in which removal is undertaken for cosmetic reasons. Subtle radiopaque jaw lesions are often evident by panoramic dental radiographs in patients with FAP and no other apparent extraintestinal lesions of GS.[96–98] There is disagreement as to whether these lesions are useful predictors of polyposis, because they are often found in control subjects.[98–101]

Dental abnormalities.   Various dental abnormalities also have been described in GS, including unerupted teeth, supernumerary teeth, dentigerous cysts, and odontomas.[93,102] These all may precede the development of colonic polyposis. Early caries and early complete loss also have been described but are probably features that occur secondary to osteomas and the other dental abnormalities.[1]

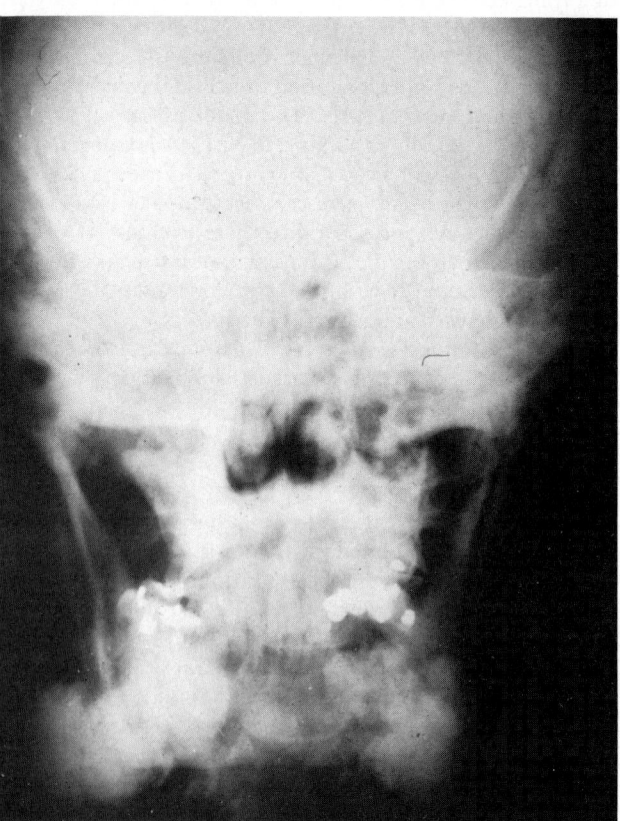

FIGURE 86-6. Skull x-ray film of a patient with Gardner's syndrome. Prominent large osteomas are seen at the angle of the mandible bilaterally. Osteomas are frequently found in this location, although they are often more subtle.

Benign cutaneous lesions. Benign soft tissue tumors were the second extracolonic manifestation described as a part of GS.[92] These included epidermoid cysts and fibromas. Epidermoid cysts occur most commonly on the legs, face, scalp, and arms, in that order, but may appear anywhere on the body surface.[103] They range in size from millimeters to several centimeters. The largest in Gardner's original description was 8 cm in diameter. Epidermoid cysts are common in the general population but are very unusual before puberty. In GS, they often occur before puberty and may also precede the onset of polyposis. Numerous fibromas, ranging in size from millimeters to centimeters, were also found on the cutaneous surface of the scalp, shoulders, arms, and back of all affected persons in Gardner's original kindred.[92] Fibromas have been found, albeit less commonly, in other GS kindreds.[103,104] Epidermoid cysts and fibromas are of little clinical significance except as occasional cosmetic problems and as a marker for colonic polyposis.

Desmoid tumors. Connective tissue abnormalities associated with GS include desmoid tumors and mesenteric fibromatosis. Desmoid tumors are defined as locally invasive, benign fibrous tissue tumors that arise in musculoaponeurotic structures throughout the body.[3,105–107] Multiple desmoids or fibrous tissue tumors in the mesentery are termed mesenteric fibromatosis. Desmoids are histologically benign and do not metastasize. They nonetheless infiltrate adjacent structures, extend along facial planes, attach to and erode bones, and may engulf and compress blood vessels, nerves, ureters, and other hollow organs of the abdomen. Severe and even fatal clinical problems are sometimes caused by these tumors, especially if mesenteric vessels or other abdominal organs are obstructed.[104,108] In GS, desmoids often occur after colectomy as discrete masses in surgical scars of the abdominal wall or as infiltrating fibroblast sheets within the abdominal mesentery or retroperitoneum.[107] Trauma, estrogens and genetic factors have been implicated in desmoid formation.[106,107] There is a very strong predisposition for desmoids in some GS kindreds, with many or most persons in the kindreds exhibiting these lesions.[105,108] There appears to be no relation between desmoids and the presence or absence of other extraintestinal lesions.

The prevalence of desmoid tumors in patients with GS or FAP is 4% to 13%.[107] A mortality rate of 18% to 38% has been reported from intraabdominal desmoids. The mean age of diagnosis is approximately 30 years, with an average duration from diagnosis to mortality of 4 to 6 years. Desmoid tumors have become a significant cause of death in FAP patients, in one series accounting for 11% of overall mortality. Desmoid tumors usually enlarge very gradually, and they sometimes stop growing altogether. The most common symptom is abdominal pain. Intraabdominal desmoids sometimes become massive, occupying much of the abdominal cavity and encasing many segments of viscera. Diagnosis is usually on the basis of physical examination or abdominal computed tomography scan when unexplained abdominal symptoms are present.

Treatment is conservative. A number of medical therapies have been attempted with variable success, including the antiestrogen tamoxifen, progesterone, prednisone, ascorbate, the NSAIDs sulindac and indomethacin, combination chemo-

therapy, and radiation therapy.[109–111] Definitive recommendations for treatment await further investigation, but most authors recommend that tamoxifen or sulindac be used initially, followed by chemotherapy, radiation therapy, or surgery only as necessary. Simple but adequate local resection is recommended if removal becomes necessary.[112,113] If the small bowel mesentery is involved, surgery is difficult or impossible; surgery is therefore reserved for intestinal or ureteral obstruction.[108] Postsurgical recurrence of desmoids is common because of the local invasive character of the tumor.

Congenital hypertrophy of the retinal pigment epithelium. Multiple and bilateral patches of congenital hypertrophy of the retinal pigment epithelium (CHRPE) have been described as manifestation of FAP or GS.[114] The lesions are discrete, darkly pigmented, and round, oval, or kidney-shaped, and they range in size from 0.1 to 1.0 disc diameters.[115] Some of the lesions appear to represent hamartomas of the retinal epithelium.[116] The presence of bilateral or multiple (>4) lesions is highly specific (94%–100%) but only moderately sensitive (58%–84%) for FAP.[41,117] These findings reflect the observation that CHRPE is closely associated with the polyposis phenotype in kindreds in which it occurs but may be present in as few as 65% of FAP kindreds.[118,119] The lesion appears to be congenital and has been detected in a 3-month-old at-risk infant. CHRPE may be the earliest clinically detectable lesion of GS, although careful slit-lamp examination is often required for detection. It is seen independently of other manifestations of GS.[120]

Extracolonic malignancies. There are several extracolonic malignancies associated with FAP. Most prominent are periampullary and duodenal carcinoma, discussed in a previous section. Other less common associated cancers include papillary carcinoma of the thyroid[121]; hepatoblastoma[122]; CNS cancer, or Turcot syndrome; biliary neoplasia, both benign and malignant[123]; and adrenal neoplasia, both benign and malignant.[124,125] Except for duodenal cancers, these malignancies are so unusual in FAP that their relation, if any, to other extraintestinal growths has not been established.

Turcot's Syndrome

Turcot's syndrome is a rare hereditary disease in which brain tumors are associated with colonic adenomatous polyposis.[126] Approximately 55 cases of this syndrome have been reported.[127] The brain tumors of Turcot's syndrome are gliomas pathologically and have included, for the most part, glioblastomas, medulloblastomas, and astrocytomas. These usually occur in the first or second decade of life.

Turcot's syndrome can be divided into three groups based on differences in the number and character of colonic polyps.[128] Group 1 comprises patients with 20 to 100 polyps that tend to be large, often more than 3 cm in diameter. Malignant transformation usually occurs in the second or third decade of life. In several such cases, the parents have been consanguineous. In other cases, polyposis has not been seen in previous or subsequent generations, although occasionally a same generation sibling also has been affected, strongly suggesting an autosomal recessive mode of inheritance.[128,129] Individuals in the group 2 are characterized by the presence of small colonic polyps numbering fewer than 10. The mode of inheritance is unclear. Persons in group 3 exhibit numerous small colonic adenomas, often more than 100. The syndrome in group 3 strongly resembles classical FAP. Furthermore, all patients in the third group have a family history of FAP, implying an autosomal dominant mode of inheritance.[128,129] Extraintestinal manifestations of GS have been observed in groups 1 and 3 but are more common in group 3 individuals.

A recent genetic study found no linkage between Turcot's syndrome patients with the characteristics of group 1 and the *APC* gene.[130] A genetic etiology separate from FAP therefore appears likely. No linkage studies to date have been performed in families with characteristics of groups 2 or 3. Molecular genetic analysis also has shown the *p53* tumor suppressor gene on chromosome 17 to be intact in germ line cells of two individuals with group 1 characteristics. This gene was, however, mutated in colonic tumor cells from the same individuals.[127] Mutated *p53* therefore appears to play a role in Turcot's syndrome with regard to tumor progression but not to inheritance.

The evaluation and treatment of all categories of Turcot's syndrome is identical to that of FAP, with the addition of neurologic evaluation as part of the regular surveillance and with the recognition that fewer, larger adenomas may be evidence of affected status. It also has been suggested that survivors of childhood CNS tumors undergo colonic screening at least once before they reach 20 years of age.[131]

Attenuated Adenomatous Polyposis Coli

AAPC is an attenuated form of FAP in which affected persons develop a variable number of adenomas.[132] Seven large kindreds with this condition have been described.[133] More than half of those with AAPC exhibit fewer than 100 adenomas, even at older ages. Adenomas are usually smaller than 5 mm in diameter and are sometimes found more prominently in the proximal colon. The age of onset appears to be about 10 years later than for classical FAP, but further definition of the phenotype is required. Gastric hamartomas and duodenal adenomas also are observed in some patients, as is the case with FAP. The risk of colon cancer is extremely high in affected individuals, with a mean age at diagnosis of 54 years.

AAPC arises from mutations of the *APC* gene.[133] As in FAP, the mutations give rise to stop codons, but all mutations found to date have occurred at the extreme 5' end of the *APC* gene, which is not the case with FAP. Screening of AAPC should include complete colonoscopy of family members at risk, starting at an age 10 years younger than the earliest case of colon cancer in the family. Colonoscopy is needed because of the paucity of polyps and their possible proximal location. Repeat examination every 2 to 3 years is recommended. Genetic testing with linkage markers or mutation detection based on polymerase chain reaction (PCR) is also now possible. Colectomy with ileorectal anastomosis may be a more viable treatment in this disease than in FAP because of the colonic distribution of adenomas. Nonetheless, total colectomy with mucosal proctectomy and ileoanal pouch is the surest prevention for colorectal cancer. This condition appears to be the same as the flat adenoma syndrome.[134]

HAMARTOMATOUS POLYPOSIS SYNDROMES

Hamartomatous polyposis syndromes are a collection of separate and distinct conditions in which multiple hamartomatous polyps are present in the gastrointestinal tract. As a group, these syndromes are substantially less common than FAP. The hamartomatous syndromes traditionally have been considered to have little if any malignant potential because hamartomatous polyps are nonneoplastic. Data, however, indicate that most of the hamartomatous syndromes exhibit significant cancer risk, with cancers sometimes arising in the hamartomatous polyps.

Peutz-Jeghers Syndrome

Epidemiology and Etiology

Peutz-Jeghers syndrome is an inherited disorder expressed as intestinal hamartomatous polyposis in association with characteristic mucocutaneous pigmentation.[103,135–138] It is a rare syndrome, encountered in polyposis registries in the United States about one tenth as often as FAP. The inheritance is autosomal dominant, with a high penetrance of both polyposis and skin pigmentation. The occurrence in males and females is essentially equivalent.[136] Gene mapping studies are underway to identify the chromosomal location of the responsible DNA defect.

Clinical Manifestations

Pigment spots. The mucocutaneous pigmentation, or melanin spots, of Peutz-Jeghers syndrome is a distinctive feature that is observed in more than 95% of affected persons (Fig. 86-7).[136] The melanin spots are described as multiple, brownish to black macules, 1 to 5 mm in diameter, that look like dark freckles but are unusual because of their location. They are most common on the lips where, unlike common freckles, they cross the vermilion border, and on the perioral region (94%). They also occur on the buccal mucosa (66%), face, forearms, palms, soles, digits, perianal area, and, rarely, the intestinal mucosa.[135] The spots often appear during the first 1 or 2 years of life and then increase in number and cover a wider area of the skin over ensuing years. Lesions on the lips may fade after puberty, requiring the clinician to examine the buccal mucosa and other parts of the cutaneous surface.[136]

Polyps. Gastrointestinal hamartomatous polyps occur in 88% to 100% of individuals with Peutz-Jeghers syndrome.[136] They most commonly are present in the small intestine (64%–96%) but also frequently occur in the stomach (24%–49%) and colon (60%). The number of polyps varies from 1 to 20 per gastrointestinal segment.[136] Polyps range in size from 0.1 cm to 3 cm in diameter and have a coarsely lobulated surface. Larger polyps are pedunculated, but smaller polyps are sessile, except in the stomach, where polyps are most often sessile

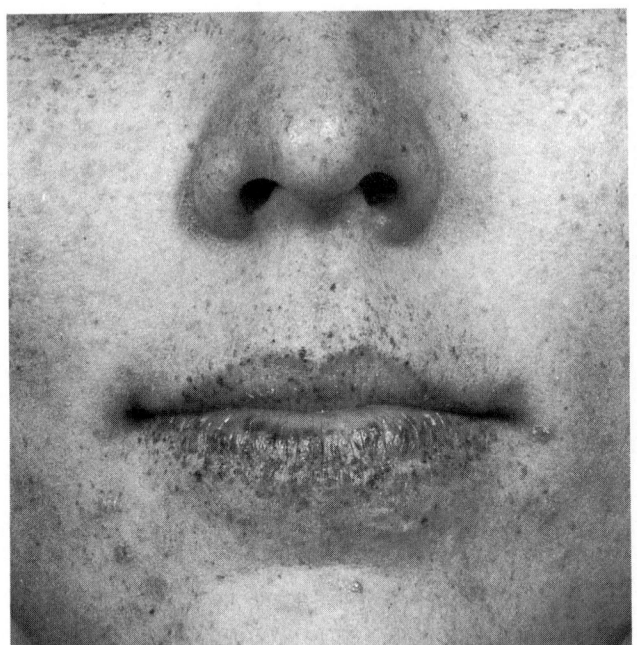

FIGURE 86-7. Mucocutaneous pigmentation of a patient with Peutz-Jeghers disease. The melanin spots are most prominent in the perioral area and on the lips. In this patient, they are also seen across the bridge of the nose and under the eyes.

regardless of size. Polyp growth begins in the first decade of life, but patients typically do not become symptomatic until the second or third decade. Symptoms arise from larger polyps, which may infarct, ulcerate, bleed, and cause intestinal obstruction and intussusception. Microscopically, Peutz-Jeghers polyps are distinct[5] (Fig. 86-8). They are nondysplastic and have normal overlying epithelium specific to the gastrointestinal site in which they are found. The architecture, however, is very abnormal and consists of an arborizing pattern of growth with muscularis mucosa extending into branching fronds of the polyp. A unique feature of these polyps is that benign glands may be surrounded by smooth muscle and may extend into the submucosa or muscularis propria. This growth pattern sometimes has led to the mistaken diagnosis of malignant invasion. There is usually no cellular atypia or malignant behavior, although adenomatous changes have been reported.[138] This characteristic has been classified as pseudoinvasion.

Gastrointestinal malignancy. There have been numerous reports of gastrointestinal cancers in patients with Peutz-Jeghers syndrome despite the fact that the polyps are not generally considered neoplastic.[138,139-141] Although some of the earlier reports may have misinterpreted pseudoinvasion or reported fortuitous cancer associations, present evidence suggests an incidence of gastrointestinal malignancy that is several times that of the general population. Two observations have led to this conclusion. First, adenomatous change and cancer have been documented to occur in Peutz-Jeghers polyps from all areas of the gastrointestinal tract.[138] The incidence of neoplastic change in these polyps is between 3% and 6%.[139] Second, many of the reported gastrointestinal malignancies have occurred at an age much younger than expected in the general

population.[5] There is also the suggestion that Peutz-Jeghers patients may fare worse from their cancers than the general population.[141] Considering these factors, the incidence of attributable gastrointestinal malignancy has been estimated at between 2% and 13%.[138,141] The most common sites of cancer are the stomach and duodenum.

Extraintestinal malignancy. Several extraintestinal tumors, both benign and malignant, also have been reported to have an association with Peutz-Jeghers syndrome.[5,138,140,142] In women, these lesions include breast carcinoma which is often bilateral; cervical adenocarcinoma; and benign and malignant ovarian tumors.[138,142] The benign ovarian tumors observed have been described as sex cord tumors with annular tubules. In patients with Peutz-Jeghers syndrome, these are usually asymptomatic, small, multifocal, bilateral, and characterized by tubules surrounding central hyaline cores.[5] These lesions are almost always present in the ovaries of affected females and therefore are considered one of the phenotypic characteristics of the syndrome. In males, there is an association with testicular tumor. An excess occurrence of pancreatic adenocarcinoma has been described in both genders. Malignancies in addition to those mentioned have been reported, but the validity of their relation to the syndrome remains in question. The overall malignancy risk in Peutz-Jeghers syndrome is substantial, with almost 50% of affected individuals in one registry report developing some type of cancer.[140]

Clinical Course

The average age of diagnosis in Peutz-Jeghers syndrome is 23 years in males and 26 years in females. Presenting complaints in one large series included obstruction (43%), abdominal pain (23%), blood in the stool (14%), and anal extrusion of a polyp (7%).[136] Twenty-three percent of patients were diagnosed because of the presence of typical cutaneous pigmentation. The clinical course is characterized by recurrent bouts of small bowel intussusception, obstruction, and bleeding. These complications begin in the second or third decade of life and usually require repeated abdominal surgeries.[136] Multiple surgeries may lead to further problems, especially adhesions with bowel obstruction and short bowel syndrome. Despite these potential problems, one study reported the actuarial survival of patients with Peutz-Jeghers syndrome to be identical to that of the general population.[143] Another report from Japan, however, found survival substantially decreased compared with a control population.[136] The same study also found that 43% of the deaths that occurred before 30 years of age resulted from complications of the polyposis, whereas 60% of the deaths after that age were caused by malignancy. A recent study from London of 72 Peutz-Jeghers patients reported that 48% had died from a malignancy, most of which were gastrointestinal, by 57 years of age.[141]

Management

The diagnosis of Peutz-Jeghers syndrome is based on examination of the cutaneous surface for typical melanin spots and evaluation of the gastrointestinal tract for polyps. Upper and lower gastrointestinal endoscopy and small bowel radiography

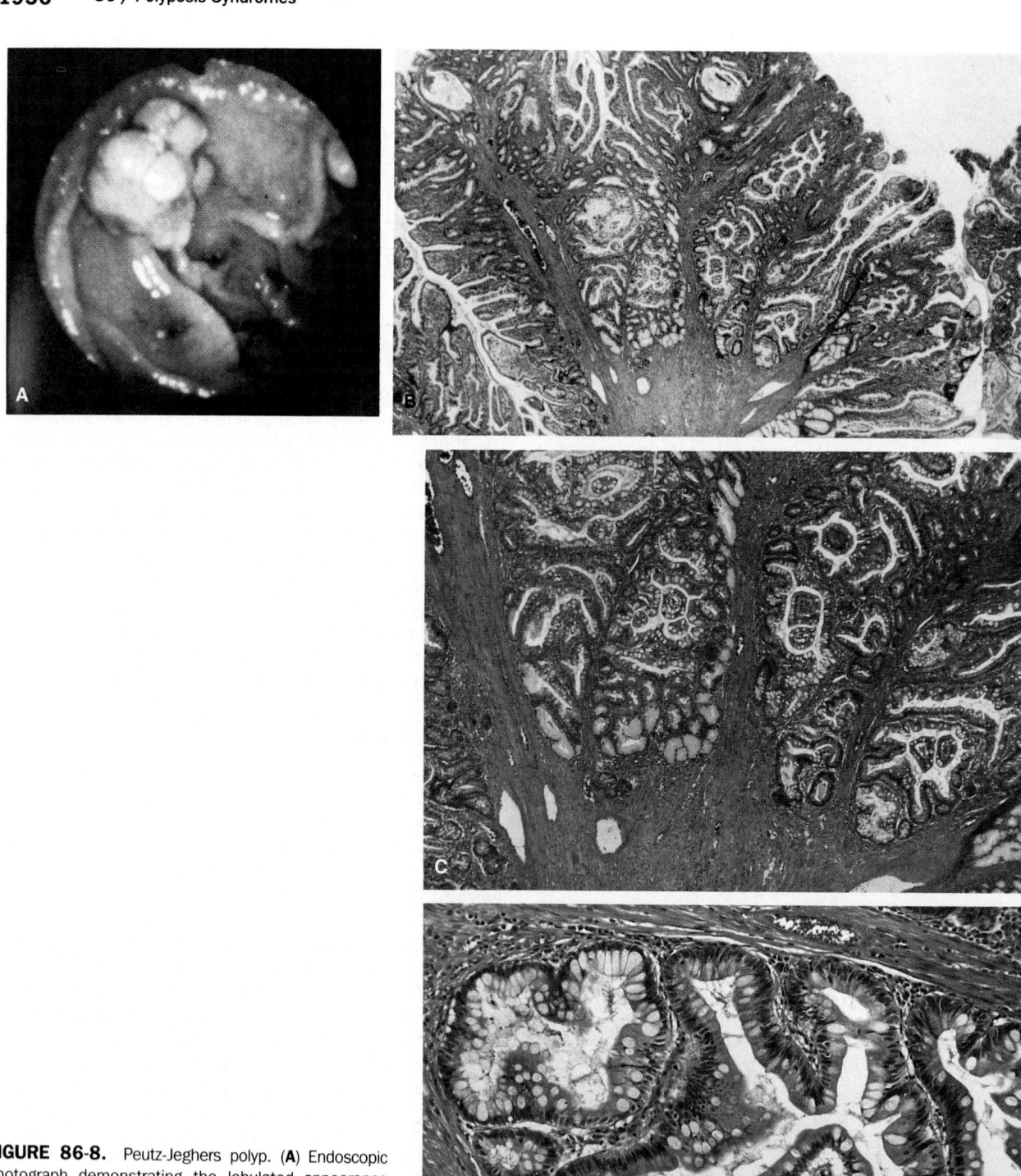

FIGURE 86-8. Peutz-Jeghers polyp. (**A**) Endoscopic
photograph demonstrating the lobulated appearance
of the Peutz-Jeghers polyp. (**B**) Low-power microscopic
view in which the arborizing, or branching, pattern of
muscularis is observed. (**C**) In a higher-power view,
the glands are seen within the branching strands of
muscularis. (**D**) Higher-power view demonstrates the
normal epithelium of the Peutz-Jeghers polyp. (Courtesy of Wade S. Samowitz, M.D.)

are the recommended studies. All three studies are indicated if a person at risk or with characteristic pigmentation develops gastrointestinal symptoms. These studies should be repeated every 2 years after a diagnosis is made.[144] Endoscopic polypectomies are performed for any hemorrhagic or large polyps (>1 cm). Smaller polyps that are grossly suspicious should be biopsied or removed in view of the associated cancer risk. Surgery is indicated for removal of any small bowel polyps that are symptomatic or larger than 1.5 cm. It has been suggested that the time between surgeries could be extended by performing small bowel endoscopy and polypectomy during laparotomy.[145] In this way, all polyps could be removed from the small bowel, achieving a clean intestine and allowing longer asymptomatic periods. Routine breast and gynecologic examinations have been recommended as a part of the surveillance.[138,140] Annual fecal occult blood testing and flexible proctosigmoidoscopy every 3 years beginning in the second decade would also seem prudent in the asymptomatic person at risk of developing Peutz-Jeghers syndrome. Endoscopic and radiographic evaluations could then begin after bleeding or small polyps were detected, thus avoiding serious complications as the initial presentation.

Familial Juvenile Polyposis Coli

Description

Familial juvenile polyposis coli is a rare syndrome defined as the familial occurrence of 10 or more juvenile polyps.[5] Juvenile polyps are nonneoplastic hamartomatous polyps that usually occur in the colons of children between 4 and 14 years of age.[146] One percent to 2% of children express such polyps. A solitary polyp is found in 70% of these cases, but in 30%, two or three are observed. Rarely, 10 or more polyps are present, in which case the condition is labeled juvenile polyposis coli. Juvenile polyposis coli appears to represent a separate entity rather than just part of the spectrum of juvenile polyp occurrence. In about one third of juvenile polyposis cases, the condition is familial.[147] The distribution of affected persons in family groupings is consistent with an autosomal dominant pattern of inheritance with high penetrance. The cause of polyposis in the nonfamilial cases in not known but could relate to new genetic mutations or environmental factors. Juvenile polyposis appears to be even less common than Peutz-Jeghers syndrome.

Polyps

The polyps in juvenile polyposis are typical juvenile polyps that vary in size from small sessile nodules to pedunculated lesions 3.0 cm in diameter.[146] The surface is smooth and rounded without fissures or lobulations. On cut section, the polyps have multiple cystic spaces filled with mucin. Microscopically, there is abundant lamina propria with benign but often elongated and cystically dilated glands (Fig 86-9). Inflammation is sometimes present. The epithelial lining of the surface and the cysts is nondysplastic and reflects the area of the gastrointestinal tract where the polyp is located.[5,148,149] The polyps in both the familial and nonfamilial forms of juvenile polyposis usually are found in the colon but also may

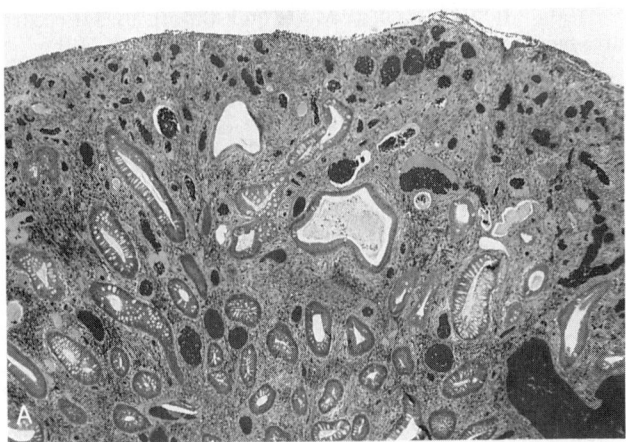

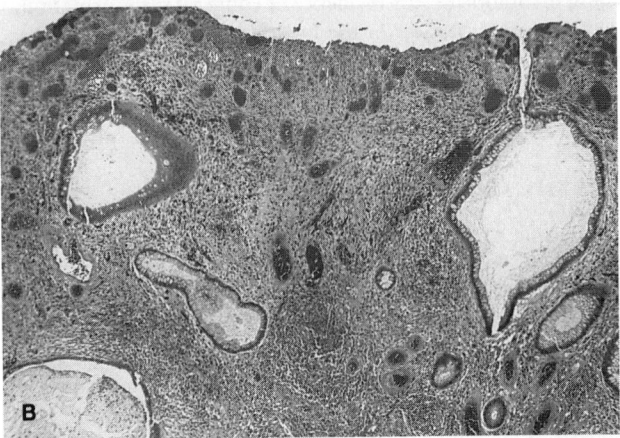

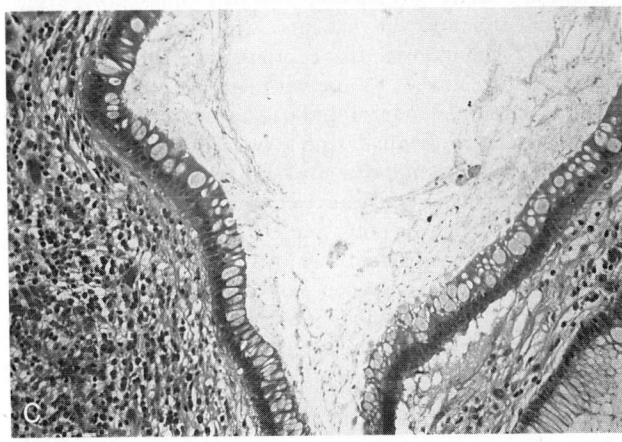

FIGURE 86-9. Juvenile polyp. (**A**) Low-power photomicrograph demonstrates the smooth surface and multiple mucous-filled cystic spaces of the juvenile polyp. (**B**) In a higher-power view, the abundant stroma is seen. (**C**) Higher-power magnification demonstrates the normal epithelial lining of a cyst. (Courtesy of Wade S. Samowitz, M.D., Salt Lake City, UT.)

occur throughout the gastrointestinal tract.[150] A condition termed "generalized juvenile polyposis" previously was thought to represent a separate entity but is now believed to be the same disease as colonic juvenile polyposis.[150] Polyp growth begins in the first decade of life. Dozens to many hundreds of polyps are present in the fully developed syndrome. Unlike solitary juvenile polyps, the polyps in juvenile polyposis often are seen in adults and almost always recur after removal.[146]

Clinical Features

Signs and symptoms in affected persons may occur in infancy and almost always are present by 30 years of age. In the non-familial form of polyposis, the average age at presentation of symptoms is 4.5 years, and in the familial cases, it is 9.5 years.[149] The most common manifestation is rectal bleeding and anemia, which may occur in as many as 75% of patients.[146,150,151] Other common symptoms include rectal prolapse of a polyp, abdominal pain, diarrhea, and failure to thrive. Protein loss, malnutrition, cachexia, and intussusception are additional symptoms that are particularly life-threatening in infants. A 20% incidence of congenital abnormalities, including malrotation of the bowel, hydrocephalus, cardiac lesions, Meckel's diverticulum, and mesenteric lymphangioma, has been noted in the nonfamilial cases of juvenile polyposis but not in the familial ones.[5]

Cancer

Carcinoma of the colon has been reported with increasing frequency in individuals with familial juvenile polyposis.[5,146,147,150,152-156] The exact risk of colon cancer is not known, but it is at least 9% and may be as high as 23%.[153,155] The median age of colon cancer diagnosis in one large series was 34 years. It appears that the malignancy arises from the juvenile polyps, because carcinomatous and especially adenomatous changes have been documented in the polyps of a substantial fraction of patients with juvenile polyposis.[147,149,155] An increased risk of colon cancer also is observed among adult relatives of those with familial juvenile polyposis.[148,150] Gastric, duodenal, and pancreatic cancers also have been reported in individuals with juvenile polyposis,[150,157-159] although the association with these other malignancies is less certain. Colon malignancies, as well as adenomatous and carcinomatous change in polyps, also have been observed in nonfamilial cases of juvenile polyposis[5] and, rarely, in solitary juvenile polyps.[155] The frequency of neoplastic occurrence in this setting, however, is thought to be much lower than that found in the familial form of the disease.

Evaluation and Therapy

Juvenile polyps should be suspected in a person who has rectal bleeding and familial risk of this disease, or who has rectal bleeding and is younger than 20 years of age. The diagnosis is made with colonoscopy and biopsy. Upper gastrointestinal endoscopy and small bowel radiography should be done if colonic juvenile polyposis is diagnosed. Colonoscopic polypectomy is often adequate therapy for a small number of polyps.[149,155] Colectomy with ileorectal anastomosis may be more appropriate if a large number of polyps are present, particularly if blood or protein loss is not easily controlled.[154,156] Appreciation of the substantial risk of colon cancer as well as the significant medical problems has led to a recommendation for colectomy as the therapy of choice in this syndrome.[152] Continued surveillance of the remaining rectum to remove recurrent polyps is then necessary. Removal of the rectal mu-

cosa with ileoanal pouch anastomosis additionally has been necessary in some patients because of continued symptoms after colectomy.[146,160] One group recommends that prophylactic colectomy to prevent cancer be strongly considered at 20 years of age if it has not already been necessary for medical problems.[152] These investigators document a substantial cancer risk in patients with juvenile polyposis and also observe that younger patients exhibit more colonic polyps, whereas older patients have fewer polyps but more polyps with adenomatous change. Interval upper endoscopic examination is also recommended after a diagnosis of juvenile polyposis has been made.

Surveillance

It would seem prudent to periodically screen children of a parent affected with the familial form of juvenile polyposis. Screening should begin after 12 years of age if symptoms have not already led to a diagnosis. Asymptomatic adult relatives should likewise be screened because of their increased risk of cancer.[152] Screening in both these groups should include at least annual fecal occult blood tests and flexible proctosigmoidoscopy every 3 to 5 years. These screening recommendations are interim guidelines based on the risk of malignant and nonmalignant complications of juvenile polyposis.

Extremely Rare Hamartomatous Polyposis Syndromes

Cowden's Disease

Cowden's disease, also called multiple hamartoma syndrome, is a condition inherited in an autosomal dominant pattern and characterized by multiple hamartomatous polyps of the skin and mucous membranes.[161] Approximately 130 cases have been reported, although many cases may go undiagnosed because the most common manifestation is asymptomatic skin papules.[162] A high penetrance and a substantial incidence of new mutations are features of this genetic disease. Growth factors are suspected of being involved in the pathogenesis of Cowden's disease because multiple hamartomatous neoplasms of ectodermal, mesodermal, and endodermal origin are observed. Measurements of epidermal growth factor, however, have been normal.[163] In addition, genetic linkage studies, DNA amplification studies and karyotype analyses have failed to elucidate the chromosomal location of the responsible gene.[162,164]

Several reviews have detailed both the gastrointestinal and other characteristics of this syndrome.[162,165,166] Approximately 35% of affected patients exhibit gastrointestinal polyps, although the gastrointestinal tract has been examined in only a fourth of reported cases.[165] If the gastrointestinal tract is involved, numerous hamartomatous polypoid lesions are found throughout, including the esophagus. The polyps range in size from 1 mm to several centimeters in diameter.[167] A number of different types of hamartomas occur, including lipomas, juvenile polyps, inflammatory polyps, ganglioneuromas, and lymphoid hyperplasia. The most common polyp observed consists of a protuberance of normal epithelium, which reflects the intestinal location of the lesion, cystic dilatation of glands, fibrosis of the lamina propria, and extension of the muscularis mucosa into the lamina propria.[5] Glycogenic acanthosis has been reported in the esophageal lesions. There does not appear to be an increased risk of gastrointestinal cancer, and gastrointestinal symptoms are uncommon.[165,166]

The hallmark of the syndrome is the presence of multiple facial trichilemmomas. They are described as smooth or keratotic papules from pinpoint to pea-sized[162] that develop insidiously late in the second decade. They most commonly occur around the mouth, nose, and eyes but also are frequently observed on the distal extremities, including the palms and soles. A number of less common skin lesions have been described, including café-au-lait spots, vitiligo, cysts, and squamous cell and basal cell carcinomas. Oral mucosal lesions develop a few years after the skin growths and are present in approximately 85% of patients. They include pinpoint, red, flat-topped papules on the outer lips and small, flat, papillomatous or verrucous papules of the oral mucosa, gingiva, and tongue. Two thirds of patients have a goiter, histologically arising from nodular hyperplasia or follicular adenomas. A 10% incidence of thyroid carcinoma has been observed.[168] Three fourths of affected females have breast lesions, including fibrocystic disease and fibroadenomas. There is a 50% incidence of breast carcinoma reported, with frequent bilateral occurrence and a median age at diagnosis of 41 years.[168] The occurrence of multiple cancers in the same individual is not uncommon.[169] A variety of additional benign soft tissue and visceral tumors have been observed, including hemangiomas, lipomas, lymphangiomas, neurofibromas, uterine leiomyomas, and meningiomas. Developmental or congenital abnormalities also occur and most commonly include hypoplastic mandible, a prominent forehead, and a high-arched palate.[162]

It is important to recognize Cowden's disease so that periodic screening for breast, thyroid, cutaneous, and other malignancies can be performed on all affected persons in the family. Gastrointestinal investigations do not appear necessary unless referable symptoms are present.

Intestinal Ganglioneuromatosis

Intestinal ganglioneuromatosis is defined as an overgrowth of nerve tissue in the mucosa, submucosa, or muscle layers of the gastrointestinal tract. The overgrowth may be polypoid or cause diffuse thickening of the bowel wall. Ulcerations may occur in the overlying mucosa. Intestinal ganglioneuromatosis has been observed in von Recklinghausen's neurofibromatosis, in multiple endocrine neoplasia type 2b (i.e., mucosal neuroma syndrome), in Cowden's disease, in association with adenocarcinoma of the colon, in juvenile polyposis and multiple adenomatous polyps, and also as an isolated abnormality. In each instance, the disease is inherited as an autosomal dominant. Transmural ganglioneuromatosis with involvement of the myenteric plexus predominates in individuals with multiple endocrine neoplasia type 2b, whereas involvement limited to the mucosa characterizes the disease in von Recklinghausen's disease, although overlap does occur.[170]

About 25% of individuals affected with von Recklinghausen disease exhibit multiple intestinal polypoid neurofibromas or ganglioneuromas. The small bowel is affected most often, followed by the stomach and finally the colon.[171] Neurofibrosarcoma rarely has been reported in von Recklinghausen disease.

Ganglioneuromatosis was reported to occur commonly with multiple endocrine neoplasia type 2b in one series.[170] Histologically, lesions were found throughout the gastrointestinal system, from the lips to the rectum, in all patients from whom tissue was obtained. Many of these patients had clinical evidence of gastrointestinal dysfunction as well, but polypoid lesions of the gastrointestinal tract were not observed. The tissue examined microscopically was acquired surgically or at autopsy. Barium studies did not show polypoid lesions, and polyps were not mentioned in the descriptions of surgical or autopsy tissues. Endoscopic studies are awaited to determine whether visible polyps are actually a part of this syndrome of microscopic ganglioneuromas.

Multiple colonic ganglioneuromas also were observed in a family and in isolated cases unrelated to von Recklinghausen's disease or to multiple endocrine neoplasia type 2b.[170] The observed ganglioneuromas were both microscopic and polypoid. There were dozens of visible colonic polyps ranging up to 0.5 cm in diameter. A single 1.5-cm polyp was seen. Other parts of the gastrointestinal tract were not examined. The distribution of affected persons in the one family described was typical of autosomal dominant inheritance.

Ruvalcaba-Myhre-Smith Syndrome

Ruvalcaba-Myhre-Smith syndrome is characterized by hamartomatous intestinal polyps, together with unusual craniofacial appearance, developmental delay, macrocephaly, and pigmented macules on the shaft and glans of the penis.[172] Intussusception is an observed complication. In one pedigree, 7 of 12 affected individuals also displayed Hashimoto's thyroiditis.[173] The occurrence of this syndrome in each of six generations in this pedigree, along with the occurrence in a mother and son in another family, suggests autosomal dominant inheritance. Review of pathologic material from polyps led to the suggestion that this syndrome is probably a variant of juvenile polyposis.[5]

Devon Family Syndrome

A single female member in two successive generations and three females in the third generation of a family developed multiple inflammatory fibroid polyps of the ileum.[174] The polyps varied in size from 0.5 cm to 8.0 cm. Each affected person experienced intussusception or small bowel obstruction from the polyps. Similar polyps were found in the gastric antrum of one of the patients. No associated findings or malignancies were present, and chromosome studies were not revealing. Histologically, the polypoid lesions were found to be self-limiting proliferations of histiocytes.

NONINHERITED POLYPOSIS SYNDROMES

All of the noninherited polyposis syndromes are exceptionally rare. They are important, however, because several of the conditions require specific therapy and several exhibit significant cancer associations. Additionally, they need to be differentiated from the inherited polyposis conditions, especially FAP.

Cronkhite-Canada Syndrome

Cronkhite-Canada syndrome is a noninherited condition characterized by generalized gastrointestinal polyposis, cutaneous hyperpigmentation, hair loss, and nail atrophy.[175,176] The syndrome has a worldwide distribution, and more than 60 cases have been described.[177] Sixty percent of reported cases occur in males. The average age at symptom onset is 59 years, with a range of 31 to 86 years. No familial occurrences have been observed. Nutritional, infectious, and immunologic associations have been discussed, but the cause of this illness remains unknown.[178,179]

The polyposis of Cronkhite-Canada syndrome is present throughout the gastrointestinal tract except for the esophagus.[176] Hundreds of polyps are observed, with polyp size ranging from a few millimeters to 3 cm in diameter. Colonic polyps are almost always sessile, even when large, which can often differentiate them from juvenile polyps. This is not, however, a reliable feature of the gastric polyps, because these often become pedunculated and cannot be reliably differentiated from hyperplastic polyps.[178] Ulceration and friability are surface features of some of the polyps. Microscopically, the polyps are almost identical to juvenile polyps, with normal surface epithelium, proliferated tortuous glands with frequent cystic dilation, and edematous chronically inflamed lamina propria. In contrast to juvenile polyposis, however, the mucosa between polyps is also histologically abnormal, with edema, congestion, and inflammation of the lamina propria and focal glandular ectasia. Polyps may appear over several years or several months. They usually resolve after remission of symptoms, but they may persist for years. Adenomatous change and colon cancer have been reported in the hamartomatous polyps of this syndrome.[177,180,181] The overall incidence of colon cancer appears to be about 15%.[176] A number of ectodermal manifestations are observed in almost all patients with Cronkhite-Canada syndrome.[176] Nails of the fingers and toes exhibit various degrees of dystrophy, described as thinning, splitting, and partial separation from the nail bed (i.e., onycholysis). Hair loss occurs over a few weeks on the scalp, eyebrows, face, axillae, pubic area, and extremities. Hyperpigmentation is described as dark, brownish macules, ranging from a few millimeters to 10 cm in diameter. The pigmentation results from an increase of melanin in the basal layer of the skin. It occurs most commonly over the upper extremities, followed by the lower extremities, face, palms, soles, neck, back, chest, and scalp, in that order. The nail, hair, and pigmentation abnormalities are all reversible on remission of the disease.

Prominent diarrhea and weight loss are the presenting symptoms in almost all patients. The diarrhea results from protein loss caused by excess mucous secretion by crypt cells.[178] Variable degrees of fat and disaccharide malabsorption also occur because of a somewhat decreased absorptive surface, but not from damage to the absorptive epithelium. Other common symptoms include abdominal pain, anorexia, fatigue, weakness, edema, nausea, and vomiting.

Cronkhite-Canada syndrome is a disease with a fairly acute onset and a rapidly progressive course.[176] The illness begins with diarrhea, abdominal discomfort, and anorexia. Weight loss and edema ensue, and ectodermal changes occur in a few weeks to a few months. Gastrointestinal bleeding also may occur and may be severe in some cases. Intussusception from small bowel polyps has been reported but is unusual. The diarrhea and protein-losing enteropathy may be extremely severe, resulting in profound malnutrition. Complications resulting from malnutrition are a major cause of morbidity and mortality in this syndrome. They include severe cachexia, anemia, congestive heart failure, and impaired immunity, resulting variously in pneumonia, sepsis, and septic shock. The disease may be fatal within a few months, although a more protracted course is also possible, especially if the patient responds to therapy or remits spontaneously. In a review of Cronkhite-Canada patients, 20 of 55 reported patients had expired of causes directly attributable to the disease, and 10 had died of other causes.[176] Of the 25 patients reported as still living, 16 had been followed 6 months or less, 3 had been followed for 7 to 24 months, and 6 had been followed for more than 24 months. Survival of many years was observed in 2 patients.

A number of spontaneous remissions have been reported in this disease, and partial or complete remissions have resulted from several different interventions.[176,182-184] Therapies have included corticosteroids, antibiotics, surgery, hyperalimentation, and combinations of these. Each therapy has been successful in some cases but unsuccessful in others. Present recommendations are for aggressive supportive therapy, including enteral or intravenous alimentation. Corticosteroid therapy is undertaken if deterioration continues, and antibiotic therapy may be attempted, although its usefulness is questionable. Surgery is most often used to treat complications, including bleeding, malignancy, and intussusception. Colonoscopy should be performed, if feasible, to consider the possibility of malignancy. Periodic examination of the colon seems to be indicated in long-term survivors with persistent polyps to screen for adenomatous change and colon cancer.

Nodular Lymphoid Hyperplasia

Nodular lymphoid hyperplasia is a rare lymphoproliferative disorder of unknown cause that, in most cases, is not related to any distinct disease.[185] It is found in the terminal ileum of some patients with GS,[74] in about 20% of patients with common variable immunodeficiency syndrome,[185-190] as a rare association with intestinal lymphoma,[191-193] and in some otherwise healthy children.[194,195] It has been reported in a patient with human immunodeficiency virus (HIV) infection who had not yet progressed to AIDS.[196] Nodular lymphoid hyperplasia also has been described in the duodenums and small bowels of adults without immunodeficiency.[197,198] It has been suggested that hyperplasia of the lymphoid nodules occurs as a local immune response to antigens in the gut lumen.

The relation of nodular lymphoid hyperplasia to immunodeficiency is of particular interest. Common variable immunodeficiency, also known as adult-onset immunoglobulin deficiency or common variable hypogammaglobulinemia, is characterized by hypogammaglobulinemia, defective terminal differentiation of B lymphocytes, recurrent sinopulmonary infections, gastrointestinal symptoms, and an increased incidence of malignancies. Recurrent pneumonia and bronchiectasis are the most common pulmonary problems. Lymphoma and gastric carcinoma are the most frequently associated malignancies, with 30-fold and 50-fold increased risk, respectively. Gastrointestinal abnormalities include watery diarrhea with or without malabsorption, frequent *Giardia lamblia* infestations, chronic-atrophic gastritis, and nodular lymphoid hyperplasia. Nodular lymphoid hyperplasia appears to be more pronounced in individuals with steatorrhea but is probably independent of *Giardia* infections.[185] In this disease, lymphoid follicles may become hyperplastic secondary to chronic stimulation of defective or inhibited B lymphocytes.[190]

The hyperplastic lymphoid nodules of nodular lymphoid hyperplasia are most often found in the small bowel but may also occur in the stomach and colon. They are described as numerous, 3 to 6 mm in diameter, and exhibiting the same color as surrounding mucosa. Occasionally, polyps may reach 10 mm in diameter and even larger. The enlarged lymphoid follicles are morphologically indistinguishable from lymphoid follicles that occur normally in the gastrointestinal tract. The polyps themselves do not usually cause symptoms, although large pedunculated polyps may in rare cases lead to intussusception or bleeding. Symptoms usually are related to the underlying conditions, such as malabsorption and *Giardia* infections in the immune deficiency syndromes and other gastrointestinal infections in children. Nodular lymphoid hyperplasia also must be considered in the setting of normal lymphoid tissue of the gastrointestinal tract. Normal lymphoid follicles range in size from 0.6 to 3 mm in diameter and are found throughout the gastrointestinal tract. They are sometimes observed by air contrast radiography or endoscopic examination. In one study, the results of sequential air contrast barium enema examinations were reviewed for the presence of lymphoid tissue.[199] Multiple lymphoid follicles were detected in 52% of patients younger than 30 years of age and in 17% of patients older than 30 years of age. The follicles were 1 to 3 mm in diameter and were distributed throughout the colon, with a proximal colonic predilection. It is sometimes difficult to know when to label lymphoid polyps as hyperplastic. In the study just cited, a group of patients with inflammatory bowel disease or diarrhea was selected on the basis of the presence of lymphoid hyperplasia of the colon. The lymphoid follicles in this group were larger than 4 mm and exhibited a distal colonic distribution. Normal lymphoid tissue in the colon is less frequently detected by colonoscopy but becomes very apparent in melanosis coli.[197,200]

Lymphoid hyperplasia often is found in the terminal ileum. Almost half of patients examined in a colonoscopic study exhibited multiple hyperplastic lymphoid follicles of the terminal ileum.[201] Follicles ranged from 1 to 10 mm or more in diameter. They were larger, more numerous, and more frequent in younger individuals. It appears that the prominent gastrointestinal lymphoid tissue of childhood often regresses with age. On the other hand, nodular lymphoid hyperplasia associated with common variable immunodeficiency and lymphoma is usually detected in older age groups.

Nodular lymphoid hyperplasia, lymphoid hyperplasia of the terminal ileum, and normal lymphoid tissue must be differentiated from other polyposis conditions, especially FAP.

Confusion of lymphoid polyps with FAP has led to unnecessary colectomy in several patients. The terminal ileum of FAP patients likewise has been sometimes inappropriately resected during colectomy because of hyperplastic lymphoid tissue. Endoscopic or surgical biopsy should always precede surgical resection. Nodular lymphoid hyperplasia as an entity does not require therapy. It is most important to define associated diseases so that they may be treated and to differentiate hyperplastic lymphoid tissue from other conditions.

The concern that primary follicular lymphomas of the gastrointestinal tract could be mistaken for follicular lymphoid hyperplasia led to the investigation of immunohistochemical markers to differentiate the two. An initial study reported 75% expression of the *BCL2* oncogene in follicular lymphomas[202] but was contradicted by a subsequent demonstration that this marker appeared in only 22% of primary intestinal lymphomas,[203] making this marker of limited usefulness for lymphoma.

Lymphomatous Polyposis

About 30% of primary extranodal lymphomas occur in the gastrointestinal tract. Most of these present as a single lesion. Lymphomatous polyposis and Mediterranean-type lymphoma are the two types of lymphoma in which diffuse involvement of the gastrointestinal tract is observed together with multiple nodular lesions.[204,205] Lymphomatous polyposis is a rare intestinal malignancy characterized by the presence of numerous polypoid lesions of malignant lymphoma. The polyps are usually 5 to 7 mm in diameter and often involve the entire gastrointestinal tract. The lymphoma arises from uncommitted B lymphocytes,[204,206] although a lymphoma of T-cell origin has been reported.[207] This condition occurs in elderly persons, is not associated with intestinal malabsorption, and usually exhibits extraabdominal dissemination, especially to peripheral lymph nodes.

Multiple nodular lesions of the gut also may be seen in Mediterranean-type lymphoma. This disease begins as an intense proliferation of plasma cells in the lamina propria. It eventually proceeds to an overt malignant lymphoma with extension beyond the lamina propria and occurrence of nodular lesions. The lymphoma is a plasma cell tumor or an immunoblastic sarcoma. An abnormal paraprotein is frequently present, which represents the α-chain fragment of IgA. Unlike lymphomatous polyposis, it is confined to the gut and is most often present in the small bowel. The disease is further characterized by occurrence in younger persons, a predominance in the Mediterranean region, and an association with malabsorption.

Hyperplastic Polyposis

Hyperplastic polyps are nonneoplastic mucosal excrescences that are commonly found in the colon. They rarely are larger than 4 or 5 mm and account for 50% or more of the diminutive polyps of the large bowel. Hyperplastic polyps are not believed to have cancer potential, although rare instances of adenomatous and carcinomatous change in these polyps have been described. In 10% of cases, hyperplastic polyps are multiple, and it is not uncommon to find up to five or ten polyps, particularly in the distal colorectum. Rarely, hundreds of hyperplastic polyps are present in the colon, simulating FAP. The St. Mark's registry in London encountered seven patients with such a condition.[208] Six of them were males whose ages ranged from 27 to 59 years, with a mean of 37.4 years. They exhibited between 50 and 150 polyps each. Most polyps were sessile and ranged from 1 to 7 mm in diameter, although a few polyps were larger than 1 cm and pedunculated. In two patients, polyps were distributed equally throughout the colon; a left colonic predominance was noted in the other five. Patients were managed conservatively, with periodic colonic examination and biopsy and removal of larger lesions. There were no symptoms attributable to the polyposis.

Solitary adenomas may sometimes occur in the background of hyperplastic polyposis and complicate its management. The author has observed one such case in which a subtotal colectomy was eventually required because of recurrence of adenomas and even a villous adenoma in the setting of hundreds of hyperplastic polyps. It is important to differentiate hyperplastic polyposis from FAP by biopsy, because the radiologic and endoscopic appearance of the two entities may be indistinguishable.

Inflammatory Polyposis

Numerous inflammatory polyps, or pseudopolyps, may occur in long-standing inflammatory bowel disease, particularly ulcerative colitis (see Chap. 79). The polyps are not neoplastic and do not exhibit any intrinsic cancer risk, although there is a cancer risk associated with inflammatory bowel disease. The radiographic and endoscopic appearance of inflammatory polyps may simulate adenomatous polyposis, but confusion is seldom encountered because of the setting and the characteristic histology.

Miscellaneous Polyposis Conditions

A case of leiomyomatosis of the colon was reported in which a single benign leiomyoma extended over 40 cm of bowel.[209] Multiple 3- to 15-mm nodules were present on the lumenal surface of the involved bowel. Multiple lipomas of the bowel have also been reported.[210,211] Pneumatosis cystoides intestinalis is characterized by multiple air-filled cysts of the wall of the gastrointestinal tract.[212] The diagnosis is made by abdominal radiography.

The reader is directed to Chapter 49, Genetic Counseling for Gastrointestinal Patients; Chapter 85, Colonic Polyps: Benign and Premalignant Neoplasms of the Colon; and Chapter 87, Malignant Tumors of the Colon.

REFERENCES

1. Gardner EJ, Burt RW, Freston JW. Gastrointestinal polyposis: syndromes and genetic mechanisms. West J Med 1980;132: 488.
2. Lockhart-Mummery JP, Dukes CE. Familial adenomatosis of colon and rectum. Lancet 1939;237:586.
3. Bussey HJR. Familial polyposis coli. Family studies, histopathology, differential diagnosis and results of treatment. Baltimore: The Johns Hopkins University Press, 1975.
4. Järvinen HJ. Epidemiology of familial adenomatous polyposis in Finland: impact of family screening on the colorectal cancer rate and survival. Gut 1992;33:357.
5. Haggitt RC, Reid BJ. Hereditary gastrointestinal polyposis syndromes. Am J Surg Pathol 1986;10:871.
6. Bodmer WF, Bailey CJ, Bodmer J, et al. Localization of the gene for familial adenomatous polyposis on chromosome 5. Nature 1987;328:614.
7. Leppert M, Dobbs M, Scambler P, et al. The gene for familial polyposis coli maps to the long arm of chromosome 5. Science 1987;238:1411.
8. Joslyn G, Carlson M, Thliveris A, et al. Identification of deletion mutations and three new genes at the familial polyposis locus. Cell 1991;66:600.
9. Groden J, Thliveris A, Samowitz W, et al. Identification and characterization of the familial adenomatous polyposis coli gene. Cell 1991;66:589.
10. Kinzler KW, Nilbert MC, Su L-K, et al. Identification of FAP locus genes from chromosome 5q21. Science 1991;253:661.
11. Smith KJ, Johnson KA, Bryan TM, et al. The APC gene product in normal and tumor cells. Proc Natl Acad Sci U S A 1993;90: 2846.
12. Neuman WL, Wasylyshyn ML, Jacoby R, et al. Evidence for a common molecular pathogenesis in colorectal, gastric, and pancreatic cancer. Genes Chromosom Cancer 1991;2:468.
13. Burt RW, Groden J. The genetic and molecular diagnosis of adenomatous polyposis coli. Gastroenterology 1993;104: 1211.
14. Su L-K, Johnson KA, Smith K, et al. Association between wild type and mutant APC gene products. Cancer Res 1993;53: 2728.
15. Ichii S, Horii A, Nakatsuru S, et al. Inactivation of both APC alleles in an early stage of colon adenomas in a patient with familial adenomatous polyposis (FAP). Hum Mol Genet 1992;1:387.
16. Su L-K, Kinzler KW, Vogelstein B, et al. Multiple intestinal neoplasia caused by a mutation in the murine homolog of the APC gene. Science 1992;256:668.
17. Powell SM, Zilz N, Beazer-Barclay Y, et al. APC mutations occur early during colorectal tumorigenesis. Nature 1992;359: 235.
18. Miyaki M, Seki M, Okamoto M, et al. Allele loss and KRAS mutation involved in the development of colorectal tumors in patients with familial adenomatous polyposis. In: Utsunomiya J, Lynch HT, eds. Hereditary colorectal cancer. New York: Springer-Verlag 1990:445.
19. Shirasawa S, Urabe K, Yanagawa Y, et al. P53 gene mutations in colorectal tumours from patients with familial polyposis coli. Cancer Res 1991;51:2874.
20. Nishisho I, Nakamura Y, Miyoshi Y, et al. Mutations of chromosome 5q21 genes in FAP and colorectal cancer patients. Science 1991;253:665.
21. Nagase H, Miyoshi Y, Horii A, et al. Correlation between the location of germ-line mutations in the APC gene and the number of colorectal polyps in familial adenomatous polyposis patients. Cancer Res 1992;52:4055.
22. Feinberg SM, Jagelman DG, Sarre RG, et al. Spontaneous resolution of rectal polyps in patients with familial polyposis following abdominal colectomy and ileorectal anastomosis. Dis Colon Rectum 1988;31:169.
23. Stevenson JK, Reid BJ. Unfamiliar aspects of familial polyposis coli. Am J Surg 1986;152:81.
24. Lipkin M, Newmark H. Effect of added dietary calcium on colonic epithelial-cell proliferation in subjects at high risk for familial colonic cancer. N Engl J Med 1985;313:1381.
25. DeCosse JJ, Miller HH, Lesser ML. The effect of wheat fiber and vitamins C and E on rectal polyps in patients with familial adenomatous polyposis. J Natl Cancer Inst 1989;81:1290.
26. Giardiello FM, Hamilton SR, Krush AJ, et al. Treatment of colonic and rectal adenomas with sulindac in familial adenomatous polyposis. N Engl J Med 1993;328:1313.

27. Lipkin M, Blattner WA, Gardner EJ, et al. Classification and risk assessment of individuals with familial polyposis, Gardner's syndrome, and familial non-polyposis colon cancer from [^{3}H] thymidine labeling patterns in colonic epithelial cells. Cancer Res 1984;44:4201.

28. Nakamura S, Kino I, Baba S. Cell kinetics analysis of background colonic mucosa of patients with intestinal neoplasms by ex vivo autoradiography. Gut 1988;29:997.

29. Luk GD, Baylin SB. Ornithine decarboxylase as a biological marker in familial colonic polyposis. N Engl J Med 1984;311:80.

30. Chesa PG, Rettig WJ, Melamed MR. Expression of cytokeratins in normal and neoplastic colonic epithelial cells. Implications for cellular differentiation and carcinogenesis. Am J Surg Pathol 1986;10:829.

31. Sams JS, Lynch HT, Burt RW, Boland CR. Abnormalities in lectin binding profiles in familial colon cancer and familial polyposis coli. Gastroenterology 1985;88:1568.

32. Friedman E, Gillin S, Lipkin M. 12-0-tetradecanoyl-phorbol-13-acetate stimulation of DNA synthesis in cultured preneoplastic familial polyposis colonic epithelial cells but not in normal colonic epithelial cells. Cancer Res 1984;44:4078.

33. Kopelovich L. Tissue culture studies in familial adenomatous polyposis: biomarkers, genetics, and cancer. In: Herrera L, ed. Familial adenomatous polyposis. New York: Alan R Liss, 1990:267.

34. Friedman EA. Familial polyposis colonic epithelial cells respond inappropriately to endogenous modulators of colonic cell growth. In: Herrera L, ed. Familial adenomatous polyposis. New York: Alan R Liss, 1990:275.

35. Danes BS. Increased in vitro tetraploidy: tissue specific within the heritable colorectal cancer syndromes with polyposis coli. Cancer 1978;41:2330.

36. Quirke P, Dixon MF, Day DW, et al. DNA aneuploidy and cell proliferation in familial adenomatous polyposis. Gut 1988;29:603.

37. Bone E, Drasar BS, Hill MJ. Gut bacteria and their metabolic activity in familial polyposis. Lancet 1975;1:117.

38. Lipkin M, Reddy BS, Weisburger J, Schecter L. Nondegradation of fecal cholesterol in subjects at high risk for cancer of the large intestine. J Clin Invest 1981;67:304.

39. Spigelman AD, Owen RW, Hill MJ, Phillips RK. Biliary bile acid profiles in familial adenomatous polyposis. Br J Surg 1991;78:321.

40. Utsunomiya J, Iwama T, Taimura M, Hirayama R. Clinical and population genetics of the hereditary gastrointestinal polyposes. In: Rotter JI, Samloff IM, Rimoin DL, eds. The genetics and heterogeneity of common gastrointestinal disorders. New York: Academic Press, 1980:391.

41. Giardiello FM, Offerhaus GJA, Traboulsi EI, et al. Value of combined phenotypic markers in identifying inheritance of familial adenomatous polyposis. Gut 1991;32:1170.

42. Arvantis ML, Jagelman DG, Fazio VW, et al. Mortality in patients with familial adenomatous polyposis. Dis Colon Rectum 1990;33:639.

43. Rhodes M, Bradburn DM. Overview of screening and management of familial adenomatous polyposis. Gut 1992;33:125.

44. Jagelman DG, DeCosse JJ, Bussey HJR. Upper gastrointestinal cancer in familial adenomatous polyposis. Lancet 1988;1:1149.

45. Herrera L, ed. Familial adenomatous polyposis. New York: Alan R Liss, 1990.

46. Blow S. The Danish polyposis register. Description of the methods of detection and evaluation of completeness. Dis Colon Rectum 1984;27:351.

47. Petersen G, Slack J, Nakamura Y. Screening guidelines and premorbid diagnosis of familial adenomatous polyposis using linkage. Gastroenterology 1991;100:1658.

48. Pierce ER. Pleiotropism and heterogeneity in hereditary intestinal polyposis. Birth Defects 1972;8:52.

49. Naylor EW, Lebenthal E. Gardner's syndrome. Recent developments in research and management. Dig Dis Sci 1980;25:945.

50. Knapp GM. Diffuse polyposis of the colon. Rocky Mountain Med J 1965;62:36.

51. Lynch HT, Lynch PM, Follett KL, Harris RE. Familial polyposis coli: heterogeneous polyp expression in 2 kindreds. J Med Genet 1979;16:1.

52. Nelson RL, Orsay CP, Pearl RK, Abcarian H. The protean manifestations of familial polyposis coli. Dis Colon Rectum 1988;31:699.

53. Roncucci L, Stamp D, Medline A, et al. Identification and quantification of aberrant crypt foci and microadenomas in the human colon. Hum Pathol 1991;22:287.

54. Kurtz RC, Sternberg SS, Miller HH, Decosse JJ. Upper gastrointestinal neoplasia in familial polyposis. Dig Dis Sci 1987;32:459.

55. Spigelman AD, Williams CB, Talbot IC, et al. Upper gastrointestinal cancer in patients with familial adenomatous polyposis. Lancet 1989;2:783.

56. Sarre RG, Frost AG, Jagelman DG, et al. Gastric and duodenal polyps in familial adenomatous polyposis: a prospective study of the nature and prevalence of upper gastrointestinal polyps. Gut 1987;28:306.

57. Iida M, Yao T, Itoh H, et al. Natural history of fundic gland polyposis in patients with familial adenomatosis coli/Gardner's syndrome. Gastroenterology 1985;89:1021.

58. Iida M, Yao T, Watanabe H, Itoh H, Iwashita A. Fundic gland polyposis in patients without a familial adenomatosis coli: its incidence and clinical features. Gastroenterology 1984;86:1437.

59. Iida M, Yao T, Itoh H, et al. Natural history of gastric adenomas in patients with familial adenomatosis coli/Gardner's syndrome. Cancer 1988;61:605.

60. Offerhaus GJC, Giardiello FM, Krush AJ, et al. The risk of upper gastrointestinal cancer in familial adenomatous polyposis. Gastroenterology 1992;102:1980.

61. Iida M, Yao T, Itoh H, et al. Natural history of duodenal lesions in Japanese patients with familial adenomatosis coli (Gardner's syndrome). Gastroenterology 1989;96:1301.

62. Pauli RM, Pauli ME, Hall JG. Gardner's syndrome and periampullary malignancy. Am J Med Genet 1980;6:205.

63. Alexander JR, Andrews JM, Buchi KN, et al. High prevalence of adenomatous polyps of the duodenal papilla in familial adenomatous polyposis. Dig Dis Sci 1989;34:167.

64. Iada M, Yao T, Itoh H, et al. Endoscopic features of adenoma of the duodenal papilla in familial polyposis of the colon. Gastrointest Endosc 1981;27:6.

65. Burt RW, Rikkers LF, Gardner EJ, et al. Villous adenoma of the duodenal papilla presenting as necrotizing pancreatitis in a patient with Gardner's syndrome. Gastroenterology 1987;92:532.

66. Sever SF, Miller HH, De Cosse JJ. The spectrum of polyposis. Surg Gynecol Obstet 1984;159:525.

67. Iida M, Yao T, Ohsato K, et al. Diagnostic value of intraoperative fiberscopy for small-intestinal polyps in familial adenomatosis coli. Endoscopy 1980;12:161.

68. Watanabe H, Enjoji M, Yao T, et al. Accompanying gastroenteric lesions in familial adenomatosis coli. Acta Pathol Jpn 1977;27:823.

69. Buchi KN, Becker JM, Burt RW. Duodenal polyposis and malignancy in a case of familial polyposis coli. Am J Gastroenterol 1988;83:985.

70. Hamilton SR, Bussey HJR, Mendelsohn G, et al. Ileal adenomas after colectomy in nine patients with adenomatous polyposis coli/Gardner's syndrome. Gastroenterology 1979;77:1252.

71. Primrose JN, Quirke P, Johnston D. Carcinoma of the ileostomy in a patient with familial adenomatous polyposis. Br J Surg 1988;75:384.

72. Iida M, Itoh H, Matsui T, et al. Ileal adenomas in postcolectomy patients with familial adenomatosis coli/Gardner's syndrome. Incidence and endoscopic appearance. Dis Colon Rectum 1989;32:1034.

73. Thomford NR, Greenberger NJ. Lymphoid polyps of the ileum associated with Gardner's syndrome. Arch Surg 1968;96:289.

74. Shull LN Jr, Fitts CT. Lymphoid polyposis associated with

familial polyposis and Gardner's syndrome. Ann Surg 1974;180:319.

75. Lynch HT, Smyrk TC, Watson P, et al. Genetics, natural history, tumor spectrum, and pathology of hereditary nonpolyposis colorectal cancer: an updated review. Gastroenterology 1993;104:1535.

76. Cannon-Albright LA, Thomas TC, Bishop DT, et al. Characteristics of familial colon cancer in a large population data base. Cancer 1989;64:1971.

77. Ando H, Miyoshi Y, Nagase H, et al. Detection of 12 germline mutations in the adenomatous polyposis coli gene by polymerase chain reaction. Gastroenterology 1993;104:989.

77a. Powell SM, Petersen GM, Krush AJ. Molecular diagnosis of familial adenomatous polypsis. N Engl J Med 1993;329:1982.

78. Jagelman DG. Ileorectal anastomosis—familial adenomatous polyposis. Hepatogastroenterol 1991;38:535.

79. Skinner MA, Tyler D, Granum GD, et al. Subtotal colectomy for familial polyposis. Arch Surg 1990;125:621.

80. Nugent KP, Phillips RKS. Rectal cancer risk in older patients with familial adenomatous polyposis and an ileorectal anastomosis: a cause for concern. Br J Surg 1992;79:1204.

81. Cats A, Kleibeuker JH, Kuipers F, et al. Changes in rectal epithelial cell proliferation and intestinal bile acids after subtotal colectomy in familial adenomatous polyposis. Cancer Res 1992;52:3552.

82. Hrabovsky EE, Watne AL, Carrier JM. Changing management in familial polyposis. Role of ileoanal endorectal pull-through. Am J Surg 1984;147:130.

83. Dayton MT, Faught WE, Becker JM, Burt R. Superior results of ileoanal pullthrough (IAPT) in polyposis coli vs ulcerative colitis patients. J Surg Res 1992;52:131.

84. Reddy RR, Schuman BM, Priest RJ. Duodenal polyps: diagnosis and management. J Clin Gastroenterol 1981;3:139.

85. Ryan DP, Shapiro RH, Warshaw AL. Villous tumors of the duodenum. Ann Surg 1986;203:301.

86. Van Stolk R, Sivak MV Jr, Petrini JL, et al. Endoscopic management of upper gastrointestinal polyps and periampullary lesions in familial adenomatous polyposis and Gardner's syndrome. Endoscopy 1987;19:19.

87. Labayle D, Fischer D, Vielh P, et al. Sulindac causes regression of rectal polyps in familial adenomatous polyposis. Gastroenterology 1991;101:635.

88. Rigau J, Pique JM, Rubio E, et al. Effects of long-term sulindac therapy on colonic polyposis. Ann Intern Med 1991;115:952.

89. Nugent KP, Farmer KCR, Spigelman AD, et al. Randomised double blind placebo controlled clinical trial of the effect of sulindac on duodenal and rectal polyposis and cell proliferation in familial adenomatous polyposis. Br J Surg 1993;80:1618.

90. Gardner EJ. A genetic and clinical study of intestinal polyposis—a predisposing factor for carcinoma of the colon and rectum. Am J Hum Genet 1951;3:167.

91. Gardner EJ, Plenk HP. Hereditary pattern for multiple osteomas in a family group. Am J Hum Genet 1952;4:31.

92. Gardner EJ, Richards RC. Multiple cutaneous and subcutaneous lesions occurring simultaneously with hereditary polyposis and osteomatosis. Am J Hum Genet 1953;5:139.

93. Gardner EJ. Follow-up study of a family group exhibiting dominant inheritance for a syndrome including intestinal polyps, osteomas, fibromas and epidermoid cysts. Am J Hum Genet 1962;14:376.

94. Naylor EW, Gardner EJ. Penetrance and expressivity of the gene responsible for the Gardner syndrome. Clin Genet 1977;11:381.

95. Wennstrom J, Pierce ER, McKusick VA. Hereditary benign and malignant lesions of the large bowel. Cancer 1974;34:850.

96. Ushio K, Sasagawa M, Doi H, et al. Lesions associated with familial polyposis coli: studies of lesions of the stomach, duodenum, bones, and teeth. Gastrointest Radiol 1976;1:67.

97. Bülow S, Sndergaard JO, Witt I, et al. Mandibular osteomas in familial polyposis coli. Dis Colon Rectum 1984;27:105.

98. Johan G, Offerhaus A, Levin LS, et al. Occult radiopaque jaw lesions in familial adenomatous polyposis coli and hereditary nonpolyposis colorectal cancer. Gastroenterology 1987;93:490.

99. Woods RJ, Sarre RG, Ctercteko GC, et al. Occult radiologic changes in the skull and jaw in familial adenomatous polyposis coli. Dis Colon Rectum 1989;32:304.

100. Katou F, Motegi K, Baba S. Mandibular lesions in patients with adenomatous coli. J Craniomaxillofac Surg 1989;17:354.

101. Kaffe I, Rozen P, Horowitz I. The significance of idiopathic osteosclerosis found in panoramic radiographs of sporadic colorectal neoplasia patients and their relatives. Oral Surg Oral Med Oral Pathol 1992;74:366.

102. Kubo K, Miyatani H, Takenoshita Y, et al. Widespread radiopacity of jaw bones in familial adenomatosis coli. J Craniomaxillofac Surg 1989;17:350.

103. Bussey HJR, Veale AMO, Morson BC. Genetics of gastrointestinal polyposis. Gastroenterology 1978;74:1325.

104. Sener SF, Miller HH, DeCosse JJ. The spectrum of polyposis. Surg Gynecol Obstet 1984;159:525.

105. Naylor EW, Gardner EJ, Richards RC. Desmoid tumors and mesenteric fibromatosis in Gardner's syndrome. Arch Surg 1979;114:1181.

106. Klemmer S, Pascoe L, DeCosse J. Occurrence of desmoids in patients with familial adenomatous polyposis of the colon. Am J Med Genet 1987;28:385.

107. Berk T, Cohen Z, McLeod RS, Stern HS. Management of mesenteric desmoid tumours in familial adenomatous polyposis. Can J Surg 1992;35:393.

108. Jones IT, Jagelman DG, Fazio VW, et al. Desmoid tumors in familial polyposis coli. Ann Surg 1986;204:94.

109. Tsukada K, Church JM, Jagelman DG, et al. Systemic cytotoxic chemotherapy and radiation therapy for desmoid in familial adenomatous polyposis. Dis Colon Rectum 1991;34:1090.

110. Tsukada K, Church JM, Jagelman DG, et al. Noncytotoxic drug therapy for intra-abdominal desmoid tumor in patients with familial adenomatous polyposis. Dis Colon Rectum 1992;35:29.

111. Waddell WR, Kirsch WM. Testolactone, sulindac, warfarin, and vitamin K_1 for unresectable desmoid tumors. Am J Surg 1991;161:416.

112. Reitamo JJ, Scheinin TM, Häyry P. The desmoid syndrome. New aspects in the cause, pathogenesis and treatment of the desmoid tumor. Am J Surg 1986;151:230.

113. Hunt RTN, Morgan HC, Ackerman LV. Principles in the management of extra-abdominal desmoids. Cancer 1960;13:825.

114. Blair NP, Trempe CL. Hypertrophy of the retinal pigment epithelium associated with Gardner's syndrome. Am J Ophthalmol 1980;90:661.

115. Traboulsi EI, Krush AJ, Gardner EJ, et al. Prevalence and importance of pigmented ocular fundus lesions in Gardner's syndrome. N Engl J Med 1987;316:661.

116. Traboulsi EI, Murphy SF, de al Cruz ZC. A clinicopathologic study of the eyes in familial adenomatous polyposis with extracolonic manifestations (Gardner's syndrome). Am J Ophthalmol 1990;110:550.

117. Morton DG, Gibson J, Macdonald F, et al. Role of congenital hypertrophy of the retinal pigment epithelium in the predictive diagnosis of familial adenomatous polyposis. Br J Surg 1992;79:689.

118. Moore AT, Maher ER, Koch DJ, Charles SJ. Incidence and significance of congenital hypertrophy of the retinal pigment epithelium (CHRPE) in familial adenomatous polyposis coli (FAPC). Ophthalmic Paediatr Genet 1992;13:67.

119. Heyen F, Jagelman DG, Romania A, et al. Predictive value of congenital hypertrophy of the retinal pigment epithelium as a clinical marker for familial adenomatous polyposis. Dis Colon Rectum 1990;33:1003.

120. Berk T, Cohen Z, McLeod RS, Parker JA. Congenital hypertrophy of the retinal pigment epithelium as a marker for familial adenomatous polyposis. Dis Colon Rectum 1988;31:253.

121. Thompson JS, Harned RK, Anderson JC, et al. Papillary carcinoma of the thyroid and familial polyposis coli. Dis Colon Rectum 1983;26:583.

122. Giardiello FM, Offerhaus JA, Krush AJ, et al. Risk of hepa-

toblastoma in familial adenomatous polyposis. J Pediatr 1991;119:766.

123. Walsh N, Qizilbash A, Banergee R, Waugh GA. Biliary neoplasia in Gardner's syndrome. Arch Pathol Lab Med 1987;111:76.

124. Painter TA, Jagelman DG. Adrenal adenomas and adrenal carcinomas in association with hereditary adenomatosis of the colon and rectum. Cancer 1985;55:2001.

125. Naylor EW, Gardner EJ. Adrenal adenomas in a patient with Gardner's syndrome. Clin Genet 1981;20:1.

126. Turcot J, Despres J-P, St. Pierre F. Malignant tumors of the central nervous system associated with familial polyposis of the colon. Dis Colon Rectum 1959;2:465.

127. Kikuchi T, Rempel SA, Rutz H-P, et al. Turcot's syndrome of glioma and polyposis occurs in the absence of germ line mutations of exons 5 to 9 of the P53 gene. Cancer Res 1993;53:957.

128. Jarvis L, Bathurst N, Mohan D, Beckly D. Turcot's syndrome. A review. Dis Colon Rectum 1988;31:907.

129. Mastronardi L, Ferrante L, Lunardi P, et al. Association between neuroepithelial tumor and multiple intestinal polyposis (Turcot's syndrome): report of a case and critical analysis of the literature. Neurosurgery 1991;28:449.

130. Tops CMJ, Vasen HFA, Henegouwen GvB, et al. Genetic evidence that Turcot syndrome is not allelic to familial adenomatous polyposis. Am J Med Genet 1992;43:888.

131. Anseline PF. Turcot's syndrome. Aust N Z J Surg 1992;62:587.

132. Leppert M, Burt R, Hughes JP, et al. Genetic analysis of an inherited predisposition to colon cancer in a family with a variable number of adenomatous polyps. N Engl J Med 1990;322:904.

133. Spirio L, Olschwang S, Groden J, et al. Alleles of the APC gene: an attenuated form of familial polyposis. Cell 1993;75:951.

134. Lynch HT, Smyrk TC, Watson P, et al. Hereditary flat adenoma syndrome: a variant of familial adenomatous polyposis? Dis Colon Rectum 1992;35:411.

135. Jeghers H, McKusick VA, Katz KH. Generalized intestinal polyposis and melanin spots of the oral mucosa, lips and digits. A syndrome of diagnostic significance. N Engl J Med 1949;241:993.

136. Utsonomiya J, Gocho H, Miyanaga T, et al. Peutz-Jeghers syndrome: its natural course and management. The Johns Hopkins Med J 1975;136:74.

137. Burdick D, Prior JT. Peutz-Jeghers syndrome. A clinicopathologic study of a large family with a 27-year follow-up. Cancer 1982;50:2139.

138. Foley TR, McGarrity TJ, Abt AB. Peutz-Jeghers syndrome: a clinicopathologic survey of the "Harrisburg Family" with a 49-year follow-up. Gastroenterology 1988;95:1535.

139. Narita T, Eto T, Ito T. Peutz-Jeghers syndrome with adenomas and adenocarcinomas in colonic polyps. Am J Surg Pathol 1987;11:76.

140. Giardiello FM, Welsh SB, Hamilton SR, et al. Increased risk of cancer in the Peutz-Jeghers syndrome. N Engl J Med 1987;316:1511.

141. Spigelman AD, Murday V, Phillips RKS. Cancer and the Peutz-Jeghers syndrome. Gut 1989;30:1588.

142. Chen KTK. Female genital tract tumors in Peutz-Jeghers syndrome. Hum Pathol 1986;17:858.

143. Linos DA, Dozois RR, Dahlin DC, Bartholomew LG. Does Peutz-Jeghers syndrome predispose to gastrointestinal malignancy? A later look. Arch Surg 1981;116:1182.

144. Williams CB, Goldblatt M, Delaney PV. "Top and tail endoscopy" and follow-up in Peutz-Jeghers syndrome. Endoscopy 1982;14:82.

145. Van Coevorden F, Mathus-Vliegen EMH, Brummelkamp WH. Combined endoscopic and surgical treatment in Peutz-Jeghers syndrome. Surg Gynecol Obstet 1986;162:426.

146. Grosfeld JL, West KW. Generalized juvenile polyposis coli. Clinical management based on long-term observations. Arch Surg 1986;121:530.

147. Ramaswamy G, Elhosseiny AA, Tchertkoff V. Juvenile polyposis of the colon with atypical adenomatous changes and carcinoma in situ. Report of a case and review of the literature. Dis Colon Rectum 1984;27:393.

148. Veale AMO, McColl I, Bussey HJR, Morson BC. Juvenile polyposis coli. J Med Genet 1966;3:1.

149. Grotski HW, Rickert RR, Smith WD, Newsome JF. Familial juvenile polyposis coli. A clinical and pathologic study of a large kindred. Gastroenterology 1982;82:494.

150. Stemper TJ, Kent TH, Summers RW. Juvenile polyposis and gastrointestinal carcinoma. A study of a kindred. Ann Intern Med 1975;83:639.

151. Gilinsky NH, Elliot MS, Price SK, Wright JP. The nutritional consequences and neoplastic potential of juvenile polyposis coli. Dis Colon Rectum 1986;29:417.

152. Jarvinen H, Franssila KO. Familial juvenile polyposis coli: increased risk of colorectal cancer. Gut 1984;25:792.

153. Jass JR, Williams CB, Bussey HJR, Morson BC. Juvenile polyposis—a precancerous condition. Histopathology 1988;13:619.

154. O'Riordain DS, O'Dwyer PJ, Cullen AF, et al. Familial juvenile polyposis coli and colorectal cancer. Cancer 1991;68:889.

155. Giardiello FM, Hamilton SR, Kern SE, et al. Colorectal neoplasia in juvenile polyposis or juvenile polyps. Arch Dis Child 1991;66:971.

156. Longo WE, Touloukian RJ, West AB, Ballantyne G. Malignant potential of juvenile polyposis coli. Dis Colon Rectum 1990;33:980.

157. Sassatelli R, Bertoni G, Serra L, et al. Generalized juvenile polyposis with mixed pattern and gastric cancer. Gastroenterology 1993;104:910.

158. Platell C, Levitt S. Juvenile polyposis: a premalignant condition? Aust N Z J Surg 1990;60:481.

159. Bentley E, Chandrasoma P, Radin R, Cohen H. Generalized juvenile polyposis with carcinoma. Am J Gastroenterol 1989;84:1456.

160. Golladay ES. Diffuse juvenile polyposis: management by ileoendorectal pull-through. South Med J 1988;81:1571.

161. Lloyd KM II, Dennis M. Cowden's disease: a possible new symptom complex with multiple system involvement. Ann Intern Med 1963;58:136.

162. Scully RE, Mark EJ, McNeely WF, McNeely BU. Case records of the Massachusetts General Hospital. Case 24-1987. N Engl J Med 1987;316:1531.

163. Carlson HE, Burns TW, Davenport SL, et al. Cowden's disease: gene marker studies and measurements of epidermal growth factor. Am J Hum Genet 1986;38:908.

164. Williard W, Borgen P, Bol R, et al. Cowden's disease. A case report with analyses at the molecular level. Cancer 1992;69:2969.

165. Salem OS, Steck WD. Cowden's disease (multiple hamartoma and neoplasia syndrome): a case report and review of the English literature. J Am Acad Dermatol 1983;8:686.

166. Starink TM. Cowden's disease: analysis of fourteen new cases. J Am Acad Dermatol 1984;11:1127.

167. Weinstock JV, Kawanishi H. Gastrointestinal polyposis with orocutaneous hamartomas (Cowden's disease). Gastroenterology 1978;74:890.

168. Elston DM, James WD, Rodman OG, Graham GF. Multiple hamartoma syndrome (Cowden's disease) associated with non-Hodgkin's lymphoma. Arch Dermatol 1986;122:572.

169. Haibach H, Burns TW, Carlson HE, et al. Multiple hamartoma syndrome (Cowden's disease) associated with renal cell carcinoma and primary neuroendocrine carcinoma of the skin (Merkel cell carcinoma). Am J Clin Pathol 1992;97:705.

170. D'Amore ESG, Manivel JC, Pettinato G, et al. Intestinal ganglioneuromatosis: mucosal and transmural types. Hum Pathol 1991;22:276.

171. Hochberg FH, Dasilva AB, Galdobini J, Richardson JP. Gastrointestinal involvement in van Recklinghausen's neurofibromatosis. Neurology 1974;24:1144.

172. DiLiberti JH, Weleber RG, Budden S. Ruvalcaba-Myhre-Smith syndrome: a case with probable autosomal-dominant inheritance and additional manifestations. Am J Med Genet 1983;15:491.

173. Gorlin RJ, Cohen MM, Condon LM, et al. Bannayan-Riley-Ruvalcaba syndrome. Am J Med Genet 1992;44:307.
174. Allibone RO, Nanson JK, Anthony PP. Multiple and recurrent inflammatory fibroid polyps in a Devon family ("Devon polyposis syndrome"): an update. Gut 1992;33:1004.
175. Cronkhite LW Jr, Canada WJ. Generalized gastrointestinal polyposis: an unusual syndrome. Postgrad Med J 1973;252:1011.
176. Daniel ES, Ludwig SL, Lewin KJ, et al. The Cronkhite-Canada syndrome: an analysis of clinical and pathologic features and therapy in 55 patients. Medicine (Baltimore) 1982;61:293.
177. Malhotra R, Sheffield A. Cronkhite-Canada syndrome associated with colon carcinoma and adenomatous changes in C-C polyps. Am J Gastroenterol 1988;83:772.
178. Burke AP, Sobin LH. The pathology of Cronkhite-Canada polyps. A comparison to juvenile polyposis. Am J Surg Pathol 1989;131:940.
179. Lin H-J, Tsai Y-T, Lee S-D, et al. The Cronkhite-Canada syndrome with focus on immunity and infection. J Clin Gastroenterol 1987;9:568.
180. Katayama Y. Cronkhite-Canada syndrome associated with rectal cancer and adenomatous changes in colonic polyps. Am J Surg Pathol 1985;9:65.
181. Rappaport LB, Sperling HV, Stavrides A. Colon cancer in the Cronkhite-Canada syndrome. J Clin Gastroenterol 1986;8:199.
182. Peart AG Jr, Sivak MV, Rankin GB, et al. Spontaneous improvement of Cronkhite-Canada syndrome in a postpartum female. Dig Dis Sci 1984;29:470.
183. Russell DM, Bhathal PS, St. John DJB. Complete remission in Crohkite-Canada syndrome. Gastroenterology 1983;85:180.
184. Russell DM, Bhathal PS, St. John DJB Sr. Sustained remission in Cronkite-Canada syndrome. Gastroenterology 1986;91:1580.
185. Bästlein C, Burlefinger R, Holzberg E, et al. Common variable immunodeficiency syndrome and nodular lymphoid hyperplasia in the small intestine. Endoscopy 1988;20:272.
186. Webster ADB, Kenwright S, Ballard J, et al. Nodular lymphoid hyperplasia of the bowel in primary hypogammaglobulinemia: study of in vivo and in vitro lymphocyte function. Gut 1977;18:364.
187. Bennett WG, Watson RA, Heard JK, Vesely DL. Home hyperalimentation for common variable hypogammaglobulinemia with malabsorption secondary to intestinal nodular lymphoid hyperplasia. Am J Gastroenterol 1987;82:1091.
188. Laszewski MJ, Kemp JD, Goeken JA, et al. Clonal immunoglobulin gene rearrangement in nodular lymphoid hyperplasia of the gastrointestinal tract associated with common variable immunodeficiency. Am J Clin Pathol 1990;94:338.
189. Tytgat GN, Huibregtse K, Schellekens PTA, Feltkamp-Vroom TH. Clinical and immunologic observations in a patient with late onset immunologic observations in a patient with late onset immunodeficiency. Gastroenterology 1979;76:1458.
190. Van den Brande P, Geboes K, Vantrappen G, et al. Intestinal nodular lymphoid hyperplasia in patients with common variable immunodeficiency: local accumulation of B and CD8(+) lymphocytes. J Clin Immunol 1988;8:296.
191. Matuchansky C, Touchard G, Lemaire M, et al. Malignant lymphoma of the small bowel associated with diffuse nodular lymphoid hyperplasia. N Engl J Med 1985;313:166.
192. Aguilar FP, Alfonso V, Rivas S, et al. Jejunal malignant lymphoma in a patient with adult-onset hypo-γ-globulinemia and nodular lymphoid hyperplasia of the small bowel. Am J Gastroenterol 1987;82:472.
193. Cammoun M, Jaafoura H, Tabbane F, et al. Immunoproliferative small intestinal disease without α-chain disease: a pathological study. Gastroenterology 1989;96:750.
194. Atwell JD, Burge D, Wright D. Nodular lymphoid hyperplasia of the intestinal tract in infancy and childhood. J Pediatr Surg 1985;20:25.
195. Capitanio MA, Kirkpatrick JA. Lymphoid hyperplasia of the colon in children. Roentgen observations. Radiology 1970;94:323.
196. Levendoglu H, Rosen Y. Nodular lymphoid hyperplasia of gut in HIV infection. Am J Gastroenterol 1992;87:1200.
197. Blackstone MO. Endoscopic Interpretation. Normal and pathologic appearances of the gastrointestinal tract. New York: Raven Press, 1984.
198. Rambaud JC, de Saint-Louvent P, Marti R, et al. Diffuse follicular lymphoid hyperplasia of the small intestine without primary immunoglobulin deficiency. Am J Med 1982;73:125.
199. Kenney PJ, Koehler RE, Shackelford GD. The clinical significance of large lymphoid follicles of the colon. Radiology 1982;142:41.
200. Burbige EJ, Sobky RZF. Endoscopic appearance of colonic lymphoid nodules: A normal variant. Gastroenterology 1977;72:524.
201. Nagasako K, Takemoto T. Endoscopy of the ileocecal area. Gastroenterology 1973;65:403.
202. LeBrun DP, Kamel OW, Cleary ML, et al. Follicular lymphomas of the gastrointestinal tract. Pathologic features in 31 cases and BCL-2 oncogenic protein expression. Am J Pathol 1992;140:1327.
203. Shepherd NA, McCarthy KP, Hall PA. 14;18 translocation in primary intestinal lymphoma: detection by polymerase chain reaction in routinely processed tissue. Histopathology 1991;18:415.
204. Fernandes BJ, Amato D, Goldfinger M. Diffuse lymphomatous polyposis of the gastrointestinal tract. A case report with immunohistochemical studies. Gastroenterology 1985;88:1267.
205. Triozzi PL, Borowitz MJ, Gockerman JP. Gastrointestinal involvement and multiple lymphomatous polyposis in mantle-zone lymphoma. J Clin Oncol 1986;4:866.
206. Stessens L, van den Oord JJ, Geboes K, de Wolf-Peeters C, Desmet VJ. GI lymphomatous polyposis. Gastroenterology 1986;90:2041.
207. Hirokazu N, Sakamoto H, Tanaka T, et al. UCHL1-positive extranodal lymphoma resembling multiple lymphomatous polyposis of the gastrointestinal tract. Cancer 1989;64:1500.
208. Williams GT, Arthut JF, Bussey HJR, Morson BC. Metaplastic polyps and polyposis of the colorectum. Histopathology 1980;4:155.
209. Freni SC, Keeman JN. Leiomyomatosis of the colon. Cancer 1977;39:263.
210. Ling CS, Leagus C, St. Ahlgren LH. Intestinal lipomatosis. Surgery 1959;46:1054.
211. Swain VAJ, Young WF, Pringle EM. Hypertrophy of the appendices epiploicae and lipomatous polyposis of the colon. Gut 1969;10:587.
212. Finelli DS, McClary R, Cerda JJ. Pneumatosis cystoides intestinalis: report of two cases and review of the literature. Mil Med 1987;152:574.

Textbook of Gastroenterology, second edition, edited by Tadataka Yamada. JB Lippincott Company, Philadelphia © 1995.

CHAPTER 87

Malignant Tumors of the Colon

C. Richard Boland

An explosion of new information in both basic and clinical research in colorectal cancer began in the 1980s and has continued to the present. Epidemiologic studies have clarified the roles of certain dietary constituents in cancer causation and unexpectedly suggested a possible role for aspirin in cancer prevention.[1,2] A genetic scheme for the pathogenesis of colorectal cancer has been proposed, and a large body of evidence has accumulated that validates the concept of multistep carcinogenesis in the colon and rectum.[3,4] The gene for familial adenomatous polyposis (FAP) has been cloned,[5-8] and its role in sporadic colorectal cancer is becoming clear.[9] The gene for hereditary nonpolyposis colorectal cancer (HNPCC) has been located by linkage analysis,[10] and its cloning and characterization are anticipated. Genetic characteristics of HNPCC tumors suggest that they may develop through a different pathogenetic pathway than do most other colorectal cancers.[11] It is clear that tumor suppressor genes, which normally serve to regulate cell proliferation, are inactivated by a complex process that requires two separate types of genetic damage. Variable occurrences and timing of these multiple genetic

lesions may account for the diversity in pathologic and clinical outcomes seen in patients with cancer. As these processes become better understood, new therapeutic approaches will be forthcoming, including chemopreventive therapy for patients with recurrent adenomas or those at especially high risk for cancer. Important clinical advances have been made in the management of colorectal neoplasia, including a better understanding of the roles of screening for cancer, surveillance for recurrent neoplasia, and adjuvant therapy for surgically excised cancers of the colon and rectum. All this progress has made it a challenge to keep current in the field.

Colorectal cancer is one of the most common potentially lethal gastrointestinal diseases encountered in clinical practice and is readily cured with proper management. Most of the neoplastic lesions in this organ are adenomas and adenocarcinomas, and the comments made in this chapter are directed toward these tumors, unless specifically stated otherwise. Colorectal neoplasia is a multifaceted problem. The basic biology of gastrointestinal neoplasia has been discussed in Chapter 24, including discussion of concepts such as tumor genetics, multistage carcinogenesis, protooncogene activation, inactivation of tumor suppressor genes, clonal expansion of neoplastic cells, and the generation of cellular diversity in tumor progression as a background for understanding colonic neoplasia. Additional details regarding the performance and interpretation of tests for occult fecal bleeding are found in Chapter 31. Small intestine tumors share some of the characteristics of colonic tumors but are addressed specifically in Chapter 76. Benign colonic polyps and gastrointestinal polyposis syndromes are discussed here in the context of cancer but are described in more detail in Chapters 85 and 86, respectively. Management of malignant polyps is discussed in the context of adenomatous polyps in Chapter 85 of this edition. Carcinoma of the anus has not been described in this chapter, but it is covered in Chapter 88. The use of colonoscopy in the diagnosis of colonic neoplasia is discussed here, but additional details regarding the mechanics of this procedure may be obtained from Chapters 116 and 139. Colonic lymphoma and carcinoid tumors of the colon are quite distinct from adenocarcinomas and are discussed separately at the end of this chapter, together with rarer pathologic forms of colon cancer.

EPIDEMIOLOGY

Cancer is considered to be an acquired genetic disease produced by exposure to environmental carcinogens which cause damage that accrues over many years. Exposure to environmental carcinogens is a constant and cumulative process. Because colonic carcinogenesis appears to be a multistep process, the passage of time is required for these chance events to accumulate. Gut epithelia are dynamic tissues, constantly undergoing proliferation and renewal. Each mutation or genetic alteration involved in carcinogenesis produces a new cell which has a slight survival advantage over the previous ones. This growth advantage permits clonal expansion of the cells. Additional genetic events occur to cells within the clone, which then give rise to new clones that, in turn, overgrow their progenitors. A critical but currently undefined nuclear event eventually occurs that results in genomic instability, giving rise to a tremendous degree of genetic diversity within expanded clones of cells. After this critical event, additional chromosomal changes continue spontaneously without the apparent necessity for additional exogenous carcinogens. Eventually, clones emerge which are capable of forming metastatic colonies.

The likelihood of producing a neoplastic clone, i.e., one that can free itself from homeostatic growth controls, increases with time and total carcinogen exposure (which is constant, and perhaps inevitable), and the clinical result is that cancer incidence rises as an exponential function of age.[12] Deaths from colorectal cancers typically begin to increase slowly in the fifth decade of life, rising steeply with advancing age, as depicted in Figure 87-1.[13] In the Western world, incidence of cancers of the colon and rectum increases between 50 and 80 years of age as a function of the sixth power of age.[14] Any consideration of cancer epidemiology must therefore be corrected for differences of age in the study populations.

In the United States in 1993, there were an estimated 152,000 new cases of colorectal cancer and 57,000 deaths

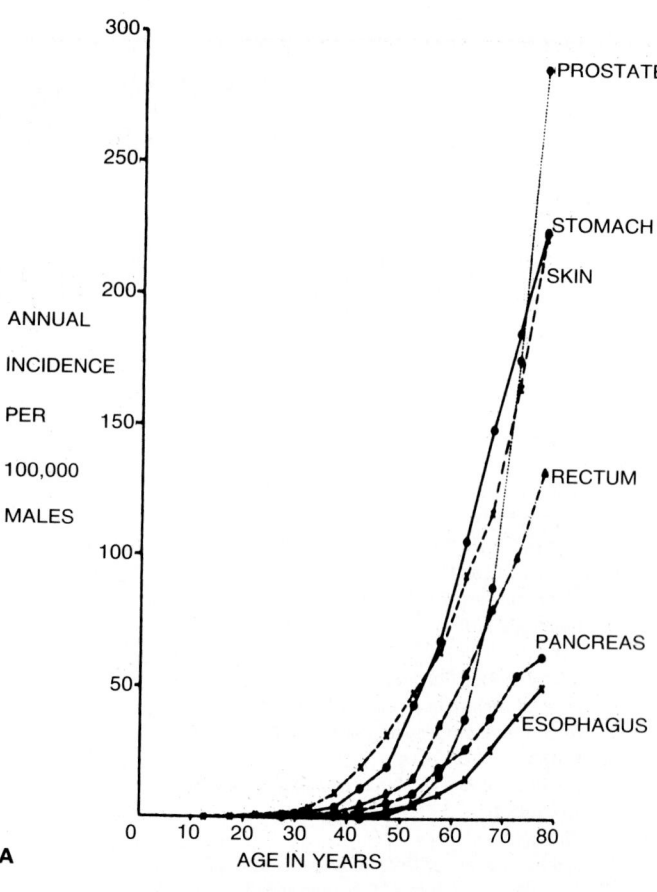

TOTAL	<15	15–24	25–34	35–44	45–54	55–64	65–74
306.7	12.4	36.3	118.9	200.9	407.9	789.6	1,344.0

FIGURE 87-1. The relation between cancer incidence and age. **(A)** Site-specific increases in cancer incidence with advancing age. **(B)** Crude age-specific total cancer incidence per 100,000 population for all sites. (From Miller AB. Trends in cancer mortality and epidemiology. Cancer 1983;51:2413.)

from this disease (38% of the incidence rate).[15] In 1989, there were approximately half a million cancer deaths per year in the United States, and almost 12% (>57,000) were caused by colorectal cancer.[15] Several countries in Europe have incidence and mortality rates higher than this. Attack rates for colon cancer are considerably lower in Japan and in most developing nations.

Rectal cancer is a distinct disease from colon cancer in its epidemiology, in its pathogenesis, and in the way we treat it. The incidence of rectal cancer in Japan is similar to that in the United States. Mortality from rectal cancer in the United States appears to be declining, even though incidence is slowly increasing.[16,17] The divergence between incidence and mortality is associated with a shift to cancers with a more favorable stage, suggesting the impact of early detection of tumors and removal of premalignant lesions from the distal colon and rectum.

GEOGRAPHIC PATTERNS

An essential feature of colorectal cancer is its wide geographic variation in incidence at the international level. As illustrated in Table 87-1, the age-adjusted incidence of colorectal cancer varies by as much as a factor of 15 between different population groups.[14] With the notable exception of Japan, industrialized nations are at greatest risk. These differences appear not to be caused by genetic factors, because populations migrating from low- to high-incidence regions experience an increase in their rate of colorectal cancer.[18] Also, there is a marked difference in risk between African-Americans and black African populations.[19,20] This is strong evidence for the impact of environmental factors on colon cancer incidence, which is a source of optimism that the high rates seen in the Western world might be reduced by identifying and removing critical causative factors from the diet or environment.

The estimated incidence rates of cancer vary widely, depending on the means of ascertainment used by the epidemiologist. It is often not possible to compare incidence rates estimated by different studies. In addition to considerations of accuracy in diagnosis and completeness of data retrieval, some studies do not correct the raw incidence figures for differences in age between populations. One can only reliably interpret differences in disease incidence that have been determined using the same methodologies. Accepting the inherent difficulties in collecting accurate data, it has been estimated that gastrointestinal cancers (i.e., colonic, gastric, esophageal, and oral) account for four of the seven most frequent cancer deaths observed worldwide and that lethal tumors of the colorectum rank just below cancers of the lung and stomach.[21] The rates are skewed in the United States, where colorectal cancer plays a more important role in cancer incidence and mortality (Table 87-2).

Figure 87-2 helps to illustrate an important point regarding the epidemiology of colorectal cancer in the United States. Whereas the incidence of these cancers has slowly drifted upwards, there has been a slight downward drift in mortality, suggesting that some recently introduced factor (perhaps the use of screening and colonoscopic polypectomy) has resulted in better patient outcome from this disease.[16] The simultaneous trends toward increased incidence and falling mortality has been confirmed by other studies which examined either rectal cancer individually or the entire colorectum.[15–17,22] Any study that uses historical controls must take into consideration the problem of changing trends for incidence and mortality over time.

In certain parts of the world, foci of increased colon cancer risk may be identified amid a background of relatively low incidence. In China, for example, colon cancer occurs in association with the polypoid lesions in the colon caused by *Schistosoma japonicum*; however, similar lesions are not seen with *Schistosoma mansoni* or *Schistosoma hematobium* in Africa.[23] Unlike the very wide ranges found in the international incidence of colorectal cancer, the rates are relatively uniform throughout North America. Although urban populations and people of higher socioeconomic status show slightly more colorectal cancers, the impact of this on public health is minor. There have been no consistent observations of high-risk industries or occupations, and smoking, for example, does not

(text continues on p. 1972)

TABLE 87-1
Age-Adjusted International Colorectal Cancer Death Rates per 10^5 Population*

COUNTRY	MALE	FEMALE
United States	17.2 (22)	12.0 (21)
Argentina†	13.3 (33)	9.7 (32)
Australia	21.6 (9)	15.4 (10)
Austria	22.0 (8)	14.5 (14)
Belgium†	19.5 (14)	14.1 (17)
Bulgaria	14.4 (28)	10.0 (30)
Canada	18.1 (19)	12.9 (19)
Chile‡	6.9 (41)	6.9 (41)
China‖	7.6 (40)	6.8 (43)
Costa Rica	6.8 (42)	7.5 (39)
Cuba	9.7 (38)	10.8 (25)
Czechoslovakia	29.4 (1)	16.4 (6)
Denmark	23.6 (5)	17.5 (3)
Ecuador	3.1 (47)	3.4 (47)
England and Wales	20.2 (12)	14.2 (16)
Finland‖	11.9 (36)	8.7 (36)
France	18.1 (20)	10.6 (26)
German Dem.	18.7 (16)	14.5 (13)
Germany, Fed.	21.4 (10)	15.9 (8)
Greece	6.1 (43)	5.3 (45)
Hong Kong‡	15.3 (24)	10.6 (28)
Hungary	26.9 (2)	17.9 (2)
Iceland	12.4 (35)	11.1 (24)
Ireland	23.3 (6)	16.6 (4)
Israel‡	14.2 (30)	12.2 (20)
Italy	15.5 (23)	10.3 (29)
Japan	14.2 (29)	9.3 (34)
Korea Republic‡	4.2 (46)	2.5 (49)
Kuwait‡	2.4 (49)	6.9 (42)
Luxembourg	25.5 (3)	14.4 (15)
Malta	14.5 (27)	8.3 (38)
Mexico†	3.1 (48)	3.2 (48)
Netherlands	19.0 (15)	13.7 (18)
New Zealand‡	24.3 (4)	21.5 (1)
Northern Ireland	23.0 (7)	16.5 (5)
Norway	20.1 (13)	14.6 (12)
Panama‡	5.6 (44)	5.4 (44)
Poland	13.9 (31)	10.0 (31)
Portugal	13.6 (32)	9.4 (33)
Puerto Rico‡	9.0 (39)	7.2 (40)
Scotland	21.2 (11)	15.9 (7)
Singapore‡	18.6 (17)	15.1 (11)
Spain†	11.8 (37)	8.6 (37)
Sweden§	14.7 (25)	11.2 (23)
Switzerland	18.6 (18)	11.3 (22)
Thailand‡	1.6 (50)	1.0 (50)
Uruguay‡	18.1 (21)	15.5 (9)
USSR	14.6 (26)	10.6 (27)
Venezuela‡	5.0 (45)	5.3 (46)
Yugoslavia	13.0 (34)	8.9 (35)

* Age-adjusted to the WHO world standard population. Figures in parentheses are order of rank within site and sex group.

†, 1986 only; ‡, 1986–1987 only; §, 1987 only; ‖, 1987–1988 only.

From Boring CC, Squires TS, Tong T. Cancer Statistics, 1993. CA Cancer J Clin 1993;43:7.

TABLE 87-2
Estimated Crude Rates of Cancer Incidence Per 10^5 Population, 1985

	MOUTH/PHARYNX		ESOPHAGUS		STOMACH		COLON/RECTUM		LIVER		PANCREAS		LARYNX		LUNG		MELANOMA	
	M	F	M	F	M	F	M	F	M	F	M	F	M	F	M	F	M	F
1. Eastern Afica	6.1	4.4	5.8	1.9	4.3	4.9	2.2	1.9	7.9	3.7	0.8	0.6	1.1	0.2	1.5	0.5	1.7	3.2
2. Middle Africa	2.0	1.7	0.6	0.1	2.5	2.2	0.8	1.0	3.1	2.1	0.2	0.4	0.4	0.2	1.1	0.3	1.0	1.5
3. Northern Africa	5.6	3.4	2.3	1.5	2.1	1.5	3.2	2.9	2.5	1.3	0.9	0.6	4.5	0.7	5.8	1.7	0.8	0.4
4. Southern Africa	1.5	0.4	4.4	1.6	1.3	0.8	1.3	1.2	1.7	0.6	0.5	0.4	0.8	0.1	3.7	1.0	0.2	0.3
5. Western Africa	1.5	1.4	0.4	0.6	3.1	1.9	1.1	1.2	10.8	3.9	0.4	0.5	0.5	0.1	1.0	0.5	0.5	0.6
6. Caribbean	1.7	0.5	0.8	0.3	1.9	1.0	1.9	2.0	0.5	0.4	0.7	0.5	1.0	0.2	4.4	1.5	0.2	0.1
7. Central America	1.3	0.8	0.7	0.4	4.4	3.5	2.3	2.5	0.5	0.4	1.2	0.8	1.2	0.3	4.6	2.0	0.4	0.5
8. South America (Temperate)	1.7	0.6	2.3	1.1	5.5	3.1	3.7	3.8	0.9	0.8	0.4	0.2	1.6	0.2	8.6	1.7	0.4	0.5
9. South America (Tropical)	12.9	3.7	7.4	2.2	26.7	14.1	10.6	10.9	2.5	2.1	3.7	2.8	7.3	0.9	19.4	5.5	2.1	2.2
10. North America	21.4	9.4	7.7	2.8	14.1	9.2	78.5	79.4	4.5	2.6	14.1	13.6	11.5	2.4	116.7	55.9	14.0	13.5
11. Eastern Asia: China	37.9	26.7	89.3	52.4	176.3	84.8	45.0	46.2	96.9	40.6	25.7	25.8	11.6	4.8	115.4	53.1	1.7	1.9
12. Eastern Asia: Japan	3.2	1.6	6.4	1.5	53.8	31.2	19.5	16.4	16.5	6.0	6.6	4.9	2.3	0.2	25.9	9.7	0.3	0.2
13. Eastern Asia: other	2.2	0.9	2.0	0.5	11.8	7.2	2.9	2.7	8.0	2.7	0.8	0.6	1.2	0.3	6.9	2.9	0.1	0.1
14. Southeastern Asia	17.9	13.7	3.6	1.9	8.7	6.1	11.2	13.1	20.7	8.6	2.0	1.5	4.3	1.4	27.1	11.0	0.8	1.4
15. Southern Asia	90.5	52.4	32.0	24.4	27.2	14.1	16.1	12.6	10.3	5.7	4.0	2.6	26.7	4.5	46.3	7.5	0.9	0.8
16. Western Asia	3.3	2.7	1.1	1.1	3.7	3.1	3.3	4.0	1.6	1.0	1.1	1.1	5.2	0.8	15.5	3.1	0.6	0.7
17. Eastern Europe	6.8	2.0	2.4	0.6	17.0	11.1	15.8	16.4	4.7	3.9	5.8	5.4	5.9	0.5	41.0	8.1	1.8	2.4
18. Northern Europe	3.8	2.0	3.5	2.6	10.7	7.2	20.2	21.3	1.5	1.1	5.1	5.1	2.4	0.5	38.0	14.6	2.5	3.8
19. Southern Europe	10.0	2.7	4.1	1.1	22.5	15.2	23.7	24.0	7.5	4.9	5.9	4.8	10.3	0.8	47.8	8.2	2.3	2.8
20. Western Europe	16.1	4.3	7.3	1.7	18.9	15.2	40.5	47.8	4.5	2.5	7.4	7.3	8.5	0.8	60.2	11.1	5.1	6.8
21. Australia/New Zealand	1.6	0.6	0.5	0.3	1.4	0.8	4.9	4.7	0.2	0.1	0.8	0.7	0.6	0.1	5.8	1.9	2.2	2.4
22. Melanesia	0.6	0.3	0.0	0.0	0.1	09.0	0.1	0.0	0.3	0.1	0.0	0.0	0.0	0.0	0.1	0.0	0.1	0.0
23. Micronesia/Polynesia	0.0	0.0	0.0	0.0	0.0	0.0	0.0	0.0	0.0	0.0	0.0	0.0	0.0	0.0	0.1	0.0	0.0	0.0
24. USSR	20.0	6.7	11.2	7.1	54.2	44.2	22.2	30.5	6.4	5.7	8.4	8.3	11.7	0.8	79.6	17.5	2.1	3.7
All areas	269.6	142.8	195.9	107.6	472.5	282.3	331.0	346.5	214.2	100.7	96.6	88.5	120.5	20.7	676.5	219.3	41.8	49.9

	BREAST F	CERVIX F	CORPUS UTERI F	OVARY F	PROSTATE M	BLADDER M	BLADDER F	KIDNEY M	KIDNEY F	LYMPHOMA M	LYMPHOMA F	LEUKEMIA M	LEUKEMIA F	ALL SITES EXCLUDING SKIN M	ALL SITES EXCLUDING SKIN F
1. Eastern Africa	9.2	21.8	2.0	3.4	7.0	2.5	1.6	0.7	0.9	6.2	3.7	0.9	0.7	64.1	81.9
2. Middle Africa	4.5	6.6	1.5	1.4	2.8	1.1	0.4	0.3	0.2	2.2	1.8	0.3	0.2	26.3	34.0
3. Northern Africa	21.7	6.2	1.0	1.8	2.1	7.5	2.2	0.8	0.6	6.9	3.7	2.0	1.1	59.1	63.6
4. Southern Africa	3.8	6.6	0.5	0.8	1.9	0.8	0.3	0.2	0.2	0.8	0.5	0.7	0.5	23.8	22.2
5. Western Africa	5.5	10.3	0.9	2.8	3.8	1.8	0.5	0.8	1.0	5.2	3.2	0.8	1.5	38.4	45.4
6. Caribbean	4.9	3.0	0.8	0.7	4.2	1.2	0.4	0.3	0.2	1.2	1.2	0.8	0.8	24.5	22.6
7. Central America	8.6	13.7	2.0	1.9	5.2	1.5	0.5	0.8	0.7	3.1	2.3	2.5	2.0	41.6	56.0
8. South America (Temperate)	10.7	5.8	1.8	0.8	5.5	2.3	0.7	1.1	0.4	2.4	2.0	1.4	1.2	51.7	54.5
9. South America (Tropical)	36.8	29.5	6.6	6.4	17.5	6.9	1.8	2.7	1.7	9.1	6.5	5.5	3.9	168.8	174.9
10. North America	153.6	16.0	33.5	21.4	105.0	37.4	13.1	16.0	9.8	29.7	26.1	15.5	12.7	547.7	527.7
11. Eastern Asia: China	67.2	78.2	17.9	27.8	4.7	25.5	11.6	9.4	7.6	28.5	19.3	30.7	21.6	815.5	707.8
12. Eastern Asia: Japan	17.9	9.4	2.2	4.1	5.6	4.9	1.9	3.1	1.4	5.2	3.7	3.6	2.7	170.3	132.4
13. Eastern Asia: other	4.6	6.6	0.6	0.9	0.4	1.4	0.4	0.4	0.3	1.6	1.2	1.7	1.3	52.0	46.2
14. Southeastern Asia	33.5	42.5	4.3	11.0	5.0	4.4	2.0	1.5	1.3	7.8	7.2	6.8	7.3	150.1	201.4
15. Southern Asia	71.4	109.5	4.5	18.0	11.1	10.0	2.1	4.9	2.4	21.4	10.0	13.5	8.3	396.0	410.9
16. Western Asia	14.6	2.8	3.4	3.3	2.3	4.7	1.3	1.1	0.8	4.1	3.2	2.4	1.8	62.7	63.1
17. Eastern Europe	28.0	12.4	8.7	8.3	11.5	7.9	2.2	5.9	4.2	5.0	4.1	4.1	3.6	150.7	147.9
18. Northern Europe	38.1	6.3	6.4	8.0	20.8	11.6	4.4	4.2	2.8	7.5	6.6	4.2	3.5	155.2	154.8
19. Southern Europe	47.6	8.7	10.8	7.8	17.2	19.4	4.7	5.1	3.1	10.1	8.2	6.0	4.8	228.1	202.6
20. Western Europe	79.2	11.9	14.7	14.0	43.0	17.3	5.6	9.2	6.7	13.5	12.4	7.7	6.9	311.1	318.3
21. Australia/New Zealand	7.0	1.3	1.2	1.1	4.5	1.8	0.6	0.8	0.6	1.7	1.5	1.0	0.7	32.0	29.0
22. Melanesia	0.2	0.5	0.1	0.1	0.0	0.0	0.0	0.0	0.0	0.2	0.1	0.1	0.0	2.2	2.1
23. Micronesia/Polynesia	0.1	0.0	0.0	0.0	0.0	0.0	0.0	0.0	0.0	0.0	0.0	0.0	0.0	0.4	0.3
24. USSR	50.2	27.7	14.8	15.8	10.0	9.9	2.8	5.4	4.6	7.6	6.8	8.2	8.4	277.4	274.5
All areas	719.1	437.3	140.0	161.5	291.2	181.7	61.4	74.8	51.7	180.8	135.2	120.5	95.5	3859.4	3774.2

From Parkin DM, Disani P, Ferlay J. Estimates of The Worldwide incidence of eighteen major cancers in 1985. Int. J Cancer 1993;54:594.

seem to play a role, despite the fact that tobacco use is associated with two- to threefold increases in adenoma prevalence generally.[24] Alcohol use, and specifically beer drinking, is associated with a two- to threefold increase in risk for colorectal adenomas[24–26] and a significant increase in risk of colorectal cancer.[27,28] There is a 2.0- to 3.6-fold elevated risk for colorectal cancers among women who have been irradiated for gynecologic cancer.[29] Asbestos exposure (either inhaled or ingested in the water supply) does not appear to increase the risk for colorectal cancer.[30,31]

DIETARY PATTERNS

Macronutrient Considerations

Investigators are most suspicious of the role of diet in the causation of colorectal cancer.[32] Dietary composition has been compared among populations with divergent incidences of colorectal cancer. Studying diet to identify colonic carcinogens is a complicated undertaking. The human diet contains a great variety of naturally occurring mutagens and carcinogens, as well as blockers and antagonists of each. Because proximate carcinogens are by their very nature highly reactive and short-lived molecules, the procarcinogens in the diet are probably a more appropriate target to study, but these are difficult to identify out of the context of the fecal contents and activating enzymes present in the mucosa.[33]

It is difficult to dissect the components of the diet that are most important in conferring cancer risk. To begin with, the estimated risk of colon cancer increases by 2.3% for each 100

calories per day, and the total energy intake may be powerful enough to overwhelm other individual components of the diet.[34] Compelling epidemiologic leads have come from studies of the dietary intakes of fat, meat, and fiber,[35] and there is a very strong, dose-related association between per capita intake of total dietary fat or meat and incidence of colorectal cancer (Fig. 87-3).[36,37]

Meat and Fat

Large epidemiologic studies have examined the role of diet in cancer. In a study of more than 88,000 women, the intake of animal fat was positively associated with colon cancer incidence, with a relative risk of 1.89 for the highest quintile compared with the lowest (p=0.01). The relative risk among daily eaters of beef, pork, or lamb compared with those reporting consumption less often than once a month was 2.49. Animal fat from dairy sources was not a risk factor, because the relative risk for consumption of more than 18 g/day, compared with less than 7 g/day, was 0.91. There was no apparent risk for ingestion of vegetable fat or linoleic acid. Fat intake was not independent of total energy intake as a risk factor in this study. Eating fish or skinned chicken was associated with lower risk as well. Lower intake of fiber appeared to be a contributing dietary factor but was not independent of meat consumption.[38] A note of caution is in order: nutritional assessments outside of the metabolic ward are notoriously difficult, frequently inaccurate, and there is considerable variation in results among the studies. The role of diet

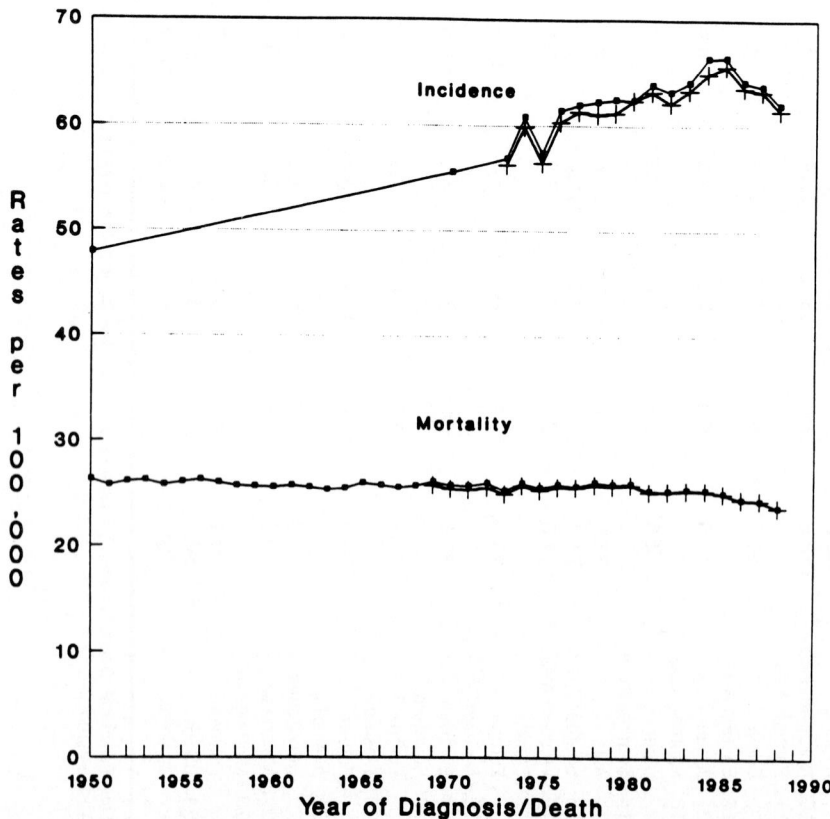

FIGURE 87-2. Incidence of colorectal cancer from five geographic regions of the United States from 1950 to 1988 (*top*), and the mortality rates for the entire United States during that time (*bottom*). Both curves are age-adjusted to a 1970 standard population (Adapted from Greenwald P. Colon cancer overview. Cancer 1992;70:1206.)

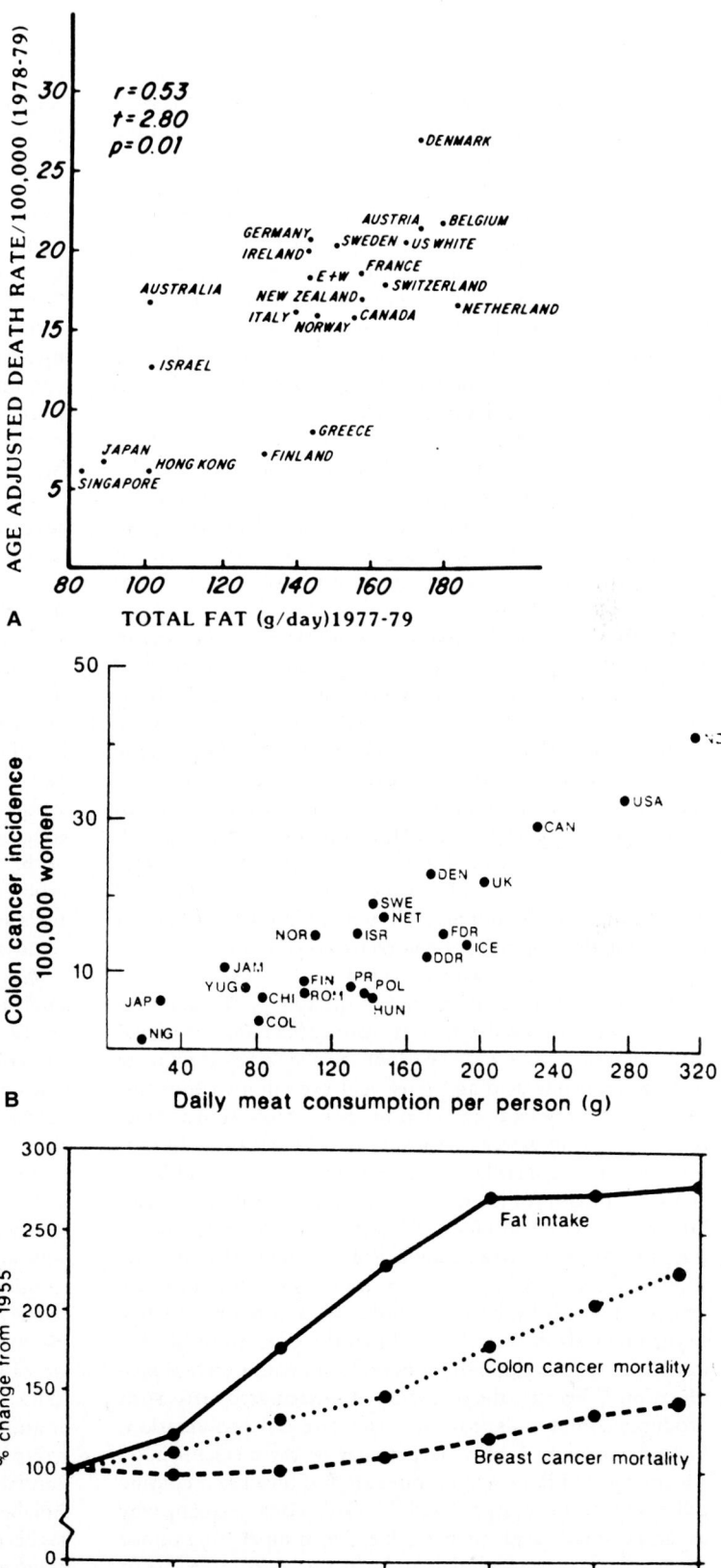

FIGURE 87-3. Influence of meat and fat intake on colorectal cancer incidence. (**A**) Correlation between incidence of colon cancer and per capita fat consumption. (From Armstrong B, Doll R. Environmental factors and cancer incidences and mortality in different countries with special reference to dietary practices. Int J Cancer 1975;15:617.) (**B**) Correlation between per capita meat consumption and colon cancer. (**C**) Correlation between changing fat intake and age-adjusted mortality from cancer of the colon and breast from 1955 to 1985 in Japan, during which time an increase in fat intake of 180% occurred. From Willett W. The search for the causes of breast and colon cancer. Nature 1989;338:389.)

in cancer causation is complex, but the trends noted above are recurring themes in epidemiologic and laboratory research.

Serum cholesterol is, in part, a reflection of total dietary intake of fat, and two large studies have shown a direct relation between cholesterol levels and colon cancer. After excluding patients with colon cancer at the time of blood collection, a prospective study of 8000 Hawaiian-Japanese men indicated that higher cholesterol values were significantly associated with later tumor development, particularly in the proximal colon.[39] A prospective study of more than 92,000 Swedish subjects revealed a positive association between serum cholesterol level and the risk of rectal cancer in men, with a relative risk of 1.65 for levels greater than 276 mg/dL. Similar trends were observed in women, although they were not statistically significant.[40] Decreased levels of high-density lipoprotein cholesterol and increased levels of low-density cholesterol have been reported in patients with colorectal adenomas.[41] Obesity in middle age is associated with increased colon cancer risk in men (relative risk for heaviest compared with lightest quintiles = 2.40); however, increased physical activity appears to eliminate the risk associated with obesity.[42] Women were not examined in this study.

Curiously, studies from several countries have reported an inverse relation between serum cholesterol and colorectal cancer risk,[43-45] and the Framingham Study reported a fourfold increase in risk for colon cancer among men who were both obese and had low serum cholesterol.[46] This may be explained, at least in part, by a case-control study that demonstrated an average decline of 13% in the serum cholesterol of colon cancer patients over a 10-year period, compared with controls, who experienced a 2% rise during the same time frame.[47] Serum cholesterol may therefore reflect the increased risk of a high-fat diet but may fall by an unknown mechanism during the development of colorectal neoplasia.

The mechanism by which a high-fat diet enhances tumor production appears to be related to the role of bile acids on colonic epithelial proliferation. Increasing the intake of animal fat from 62 to 152 g per day produced a significant increase in total fecal bile acid and fatty acid excretion in humans, without affecting fecal weight, number of stools, transit time, fecal β-glucuronidase, or fecal steroid degradation.[48] In rats, the intracolonic instillation of deoxycholic acid (DOC) increased cellular proliferation as measured by ornithine decarboxylase activity and new DNA synthesis. The proliferative response to DOC may be abolished by agents that destroy superoxide (such as superoxide dismutase) or inhibit lipoxygenase activity. It has been shown that DOC produces reactive oxygen radicals in the colon and that the generation of such molecular species can independently stimulate mucosal proliferation.[49] Because the oxidation of unsaturated fatty acids produces compounds that may stimulate cell proliferation, the generation of reactive oxygen may be the mechanism by which oxidized fatty acid residues are produced and colonic cell proliferation is stimulated.[50,51] This could explain why unsaturated fatty acids are more effective in supporting tumor production in animal models and why the coordinate role of bile acids and fat in the pathogenesis of colorectal cancer.

Certain fats can induce mitogenesis in neoplastic colonic epithelial cells but not in the normal colon. Diglycerides containing stearic, oleic, palmitic, and myristic acid side chains have been found in human fecal extracts in concentrations that stimulate mitogenesis in cultured explants of human adenomas and carcinomas. The potency of mitogenesis was correlated with the chain length of the saturated aliphatic chains up to 16 carbons long. Oleic acid (C18:1) was the most active mitogen, but its saturated counterpart, stearic acid (C18:0), had greatly reduced activity. This is of particular interest because of the structural similarity of these diglycerides to the phorbol ester class of tumor promoters.[52] Phorbol esters activate protein kinase C and stimulate enhanced proliferative activity and reactive oxygen production in the rodent colon.[53] A high-fat diet, even administered as a bolus, can lead to an increase in the proliferation of human colonic epithelium, confirming the above observations.[54] Therefore, fats may play a critical role in regulating proliferation of both normal and transformed epithelium; however, the specific lipids involved may depend on the maturational status of the epithelial cell.

It has been suggested that fish oil contains fats that protect against colorectal neoplasia. Marine fish oils are rich in unsaturated fatty acids, including n-3 or ω-3 fatty acids (which refers to the location of the double bonds being 3 positions from the end of the chain), in contrast to the n-6 or ω-6 fatty acids that predominate in unsaturated plant lipids. Geographic regions in which people have large amounts of marine fish in the diet tend to have lower incidences of colorectal cancer. Furthermore, supplemental marine oils do not promote cancer in animal models. After treatment for 12 weeks with 4.1 g/day of eicosapentaenoic acid and 3.6 g/day of docosahexaenoic acid, subjects with adenomatous polyps showed a rapid contraction of the zone of proliferation into the lower portion of the colonic crypt, although no change in the total rate of proliferation was seen.[55] The mechanism by which ω-3 fatty acids suppress proliferation in the superficial portion of the crypt is not known.

As mentioned above, increased ingestion of dietary fat results in an elevation of fecal bile acids.[48] Fecal steroid excretion has been examined for relations between specific bile acids and colonic cancer. A significant elevation in fecal bile acid concentration has been reported in 82% of patients with large bowel cancer, compared with 17% of patients with other diseases.[56] This observation has been confirmed in a wide range of population groups.[57] Patients with colorectal cancer have relatively high levels of unconjugated primary bile acids and neutral animal sterols and relatively low levels of esterified neutral sterols and saponifiable bile acids in their feces when compared with a group of nonvegetarian patients without cancer. These differences are even more profound if cancer patients are compared with vegetarians, who have a lower risk of colorectal cancer than omnivores.[58] A population from Akita, Japan, at low risk for colon cancer also had lower levels of animal sterols and cholesterol in their stools than did a group of ethnic Japanese living in Hawaii who were at a substantially higher risk for this cancer.[59] By administering radiolabeled bile acids and measuring their excretion in bile, it has been found that patients with adenomatous polyps absorb significantly more primary and secondary bile acids than do controls.[60] It also has been suggested that the presence of clostridial species capable of metabolizing the steroid nucleus plays a role in the abnormal fecal bile acid profiles seen in colorectal cancer patients.[56]

Fiber

The Western diet is relatively deficient in fiber compared with the diet of non-Western populations, and this may be important in the pathogenesis of colon cancer.[36,61] However, countries with high fiber intake also tend to have lower intakes of fat, and often lower life expectancy, which introduces confounding variables. Although data obtained in laboratory animals have been somewhat confusing, the epidemiologic observations are more consistent.[62] Some case-control studies have demonstrated protective effectives of dietary fiber,[63] but other studies have failed to confirm this.[37,64] If one considers the entire body of data accumulated on the subject, the majority of papers show a consistent protective effect of fiber, a small number of studies show no effect, and no study shows a deleterious effect of fiber on colon cancer.[65] In a prospective questionnaire study of more than 760,000 people, the ingestion of a diet rich in vegetables and high-fiber grains was found to be significantly protective against fatal colorectal cancer, and the highest quintile of intake had relative risks of 0.62 (for women) and 0.76 (for men) compared with the lowest quintile.[1] A meta-analysis of 13 case-control studies that examined the impact of dietary fiber intake on colorectal cancer incidence revealed relative risks of 0.53, 0.63, 0.69, and 0.79 after comparing the four highest quintiles of fiber intake with the lowest ($P = 0.0001$). After adjustment for fiber intake, relatively weak independent protective effects were also seen for vitamin C and β-carotene, which underscores the complexity of the role of diet in cancer causation.[66]

The intake of nonstarch polysaccharides (i.e., fiber) correlates directly with fecal weight in studies from diverse international populations, and the incidence of colorectal cancer shows a significant inverse correlation with fecal weight (Fig. 87-4). Fecal weights in Great Britain were found to be approximately 106 g/day (corresponding to a fiber intake of 12.8 g/day). Based on the observation that high-risk Western nations have fecal weights in the range of 80 to 120 g/day, these investigators suggested that an increase in fiber intake to >18 g/day would increase fecal weights to >150 g/day and might reduce cancer incidence.[67] One trial has demonstrated that the addition of 13.5 g of bran fiber to the diet (equal to a 1.5-oz bowl of a commercially available bran cereal) resulted in a significant reduction in rectal epithelial proliferation in a group of high-risk patients with a past history of resected colorectal cancers.[68]

A number of mechanisms have been proposed for the protective effect of fiber against colorectal cancer. Fiber decreases fecal transit time and, by virtue of its sheer presence in stool, tends to dilute the concentration of other colonic constituents. Both of these would tend to minimize contact between carcinogens and colonic epithelium. Secondly, fiber polymers may bind toxic substances and remove them from contact with epithelium. Thirdly, fiber is neither digested nor absorbed in the small intestine but undergoes fermentation in the presence of the colonic flora, which reduces fecal pH and generates short-chain (volatile) fatty acids.[69] Certain short-chain organic acids derived from the fermentation of fiber can protect isolated colonic epithelial cells from DOC-induced injury in culture.[70] One of these, butyric acid, present in high concentrations in the colonic lumen, is thought to be an important energy source for colonic epithelium and has the ability to induce cellular differentiation in certain cultured cell lines.

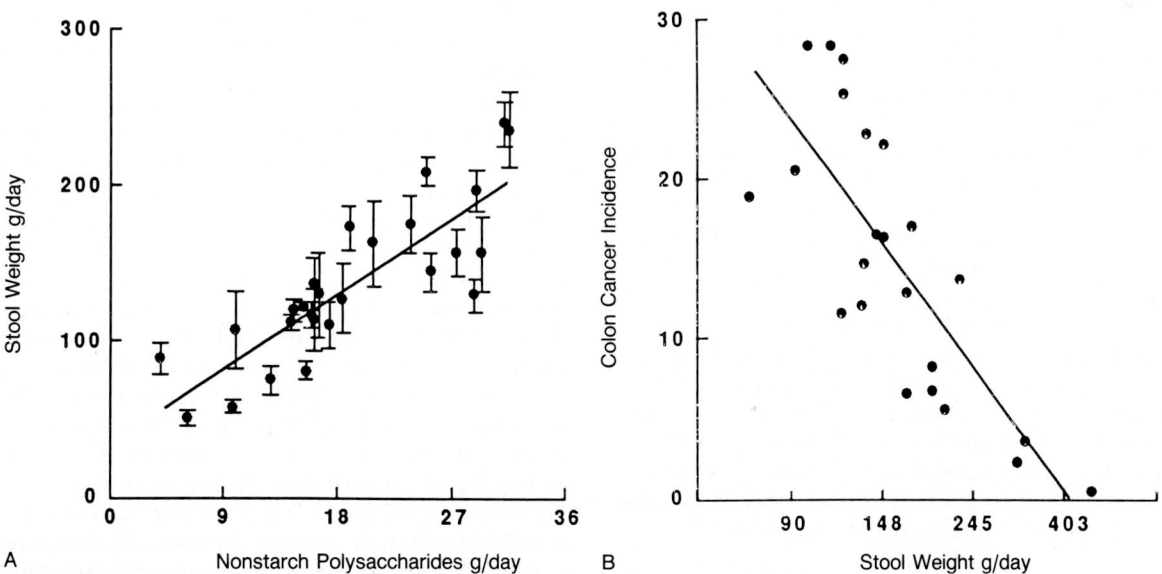

FIGURE 87-4. (**A**) The mean stool weights ± SEM in 11 groups of healthy subjects (n = 206) on controlled diets containing different amounts of dietary fiber. (**B**) The relation between colon cancer incidence (age-adjusted cases per 100,000 population) from 23 population groups in 12 countries, plotted against stool weight in grams per day (r = 0.78). (From Cummings JH, Bingham SA, Heaton KW, et al. Fecal weight, colon cancer risk, and dietary intake of nonstarch polysaccharides (dietary fiber). Gastroenterology 1992;103:1983.)

Micronutrient Considerations

Calcium

Cell proliferation normally takes place in the lower half of the colonic crypt. Early colorectal neoplasia has been associated with a shift of the proliferative zone from the lower to the upper portion of the crypt.[71] A generalized disturbance in the normal regulation of cell proliferation has been reported throughout the colons of patients with adenomatous polyps or cancers.[72] Groups at low risk for colorectal cancer, such as Seventh-Day Adventist vegetarians,[73] have low levels of colonic epithelial cell proliferation, and this has been used as an intermediate endpoint biomarker for interventions in high-risk groups. Dietary calcium appears to participate in the regulation of colonic epithelial cell proliferation, although the mechanism of this control, and its interaction with bile acids, is not entirely clear. For example, colonic cell damage and epithelial proliferation may be stimulated by the addition of a bile acid, and both of these may be minimized by the supplementation of the diet with calcium.[74,75] It has been hypothesized that the damaging and mitogenic effects of free fatty acids and bile acids could be reduced in the presence of supplemental calcium by precipitating free fatty acids as calcium soaps.[76] However, correction of the hyperproliferative indices by supplemental calcium can also be achieved using epithelial explants in vitro.[77] This indicates that calcium may play an additional role that is not explained by modification of the lumenal concentrations of fatty acids.

Proliferative indices in the colons of a small group of patients at high risk for familial colonic cancer have been studied on a conventional diet (assumed to contain approximately 700 mg calcium per day) and then restudied after adding 1.25 grams of calcium carbonate to the daily diet. Repeat study after 2 to 3 months indicated a reduction of the abnormal colonic proliferative indices to almost normal levels.[78] Although this result has been confirmed in another high-risk population,[79] contradictory results have been reported by other controlled trials.[80]

The dose of calcium administered and the underlying proliferative activity of the epithelium may be important issues. Supplements of 1200 mg/day of elemental calcium did not reduce colonic epithelial cell labeling index in patients with adenomatous polyps,[81] but a daily dose of 2000 mg of calcium (i.e., 5 g of calcium carbonate) significantly suppressed rectal proliferation.[82] As previously mentioned, the mechanism by which supplemental calcium corrects the hyperproliferative states seen in patients at high risk for colon cancer has been questioned because of the ability to inhibit DNA synthesis with supplemental calcium in vitro.[77,83] However, although proliferation may be inhibited by supplemental calcium in normal tissues in vitro, growth inhibition is not observed in neoplastic tissues (i.e., adenomas and carcinomas).[83]

Other Minerals

Low levels of selenium have been associated with an increased risk for colorectal neoplasia.[84] Selenium is a constituent of glutathione peroxidase, which prevents free radical damage to tissue and, by an independent mechanism, antagonizes toxicity caused by certain heavy metals. Attempts to assess interventions with supplemental selenium in geographic locations in which the selenium content of soil and foods is poor are in progress. Excessive doses of selenium can be toxic to humans.

Blood samples were obtained from a group of healthy subjects who were followed prospectively for the development of cancer. This approach demonstrated significantly lower levels of serum selenium among patients who later developed gastrointestinal cancers, but no excess risk was found among patients with lower levels of serum retinoids, carotenoids, or vitamin E, all of which are potent antioxidants and were hypothesized to play a protective role against cancer.[85] Threshold limits for lower levels of these micronutrients are not known, and their roles in cancer prevention remain open questions. Selenium intake has been estimated in 27 countries and has been correlated with cancer incidence at various body sites. Significant inverse correlations were found between selenium intake and cancer of the colon and rectum.[84,86]

Vitamins

A number of vitamins may have anticancer effects. Vitamin A, β-carotene, and vitamin E are known to have powerful antioxidant activities, and retinoids function in certain laboratory models as differentiating agents. Also, a meta-analysis of five cohort studies suggested that those in the highest quartile for serum α-tocopherol (vitamin E) had a matched odds ratio of 0.6 for colorectal cancer compared with the lowest quartile (confidence interval 0.4–1.0).[87]

Although it has long been suggested that individuals with low serum levels of antioxidants may be at greater risk of developing certain cancers, prospective studies have been unable to confirm significant negative relationships between serum levels and subsequent risk of gastrointestinal cancer.[85] A 6-month chemopreventive interventional program using daily doses of 30,000 IU vitamin A, 1 g vitamin C, and 70 mg vitamin E (D,L-α-tocopherol acetate) in patients with colorectal adenomas demonstrated a reduction in certain proliferation indices, but prevention of recurrent neoplasia has not yet been proven.[88] A small study of the effects of 400 mg of ascorbic acid and 400 mg of α-tocopherol per day has suggested a small reduction in the rate of colonic polyp recurrence over a period of 2 years. The minor benefit suggests that large numbers of people must be examined over a long period to detect significant benefits from this type of intervention.[89] In another study, a group of patients with FAP was treated with 4 g of vitamin C plus 400 mg of α-tocopherol per day with or without 22.5 g/day of supplemental fiber from bran cereal. There appeared to be a modest regression of rectal polyps among patients treated with vitamin C, vitamin E, and the high-fiber diet compared with patients given vitamins and a low-fiber diet or only placebo. However, this benefit did not quite reach statistical significance using rigorous analysis.[90]

Hypomethylation of DNA has been proposed to play a role in carcinogenesis, and dietary folate and methionine are required for this process. Higher levels of dietary folic acid have been associated with lower risks of colorectal adenomas.[91] A high level of alcohol intake may reduce levels of S-adenosylmethionine, which is required for methylation, and, as already mentioned, alcohol intake has been correlated with risk for colorectal neoplasia.[91]

Other Micronutrient Anticarcinogens

A growing list of dietary micronutrients and synthetic compounds have anticancer activity in animal models of cancer.[92] Many of these are blocking agents that prevent carcinogenesis by a variety of mechanisms. For example, benzyl isothiocyanate, a naturally-occurring constituent of cruciferous vegetables, prevents the activation of certain procarcinogens. Organosulfur compounds from *Allium* species (i.e., garlic and onion families) also prevent procarcinogen activation, as do monoterpenes found in citrus fruits. A second class of blocking agents enhances the detoxification of carcinogens through phase 1 or 2 enzymatic pathways, and are referred to as type A and B inhibitors, respectively.[92] A third class of blocking agents is effective by inhibiting the increased cell proliferation that plays a role in promoting tumor formation, and they are effective inhibitors after carcinogen exposure. Many compounds share this activity, including phenols, flavones, tannins, curcumin, glycyrrhetinic acid, and glucarates. Other agents, referred to as suppressing agents, and also act to suppress tumor development after carcinogen exposure, but through poorly understood mechanisms distinct from those of the third class of blocking agents. This group includes protease inhibitors, terpenes, and other compounds.[92] Some compounds have activities that both block carcinogens and suppress tumor formation. Many of these agents have been proposed as potential chemopreventive substances for human studies.

Role Of Aspirin In Colorectal Cancer

It has been appreciated by epidemiologists for some time that aspirin takers suffer less cancer than the rest of the population. In animal models of colorectal cancer, aspirin and nonsteroidal antiinflammatory drugs (NSAIDs) inhibit the development of tumors.[93] Furthermore, patients with FAP experience a regression of their adenomas after treatment with the NSAID sulindac.[94-96]

In 1991, an American Cancer Society–sponsored survey of more than 660,000 people revealed a significant reduction in colon cancer deaths among aspirin users, and among those who used aspirin more than 16 times per month, the relative risk was 0.60 for men and 0.58 for women.[97] Reduction in risk was even seen in people who reported aspirin use as rarely as once per month, raising interesting speculation regarding the mechanism and dose effects of this intervention. A smaller, hospital-based case-control study of colorectal cancer patients estimated that the relative risk of cancer was 0.5 (confidence interval 0.4–0.8) among aspirin users, suggested that longer duration of use was more protective, and indicated no protection for nonregular users nor those who had discontinued use more than 1 year before the study.[98] A significant reduction in adenoma recurrence (odds ratio 0.52, confidence interval 0.31–0.89) was found at the 1-year interval after initial co-

lonoscopy among consistent aspirin users but not in the group of intermittent users; this result was independent of the number of initial polyps.[99] Even more impressively, significant reductions of about 40% for deaths from cancer of the rectum, esophagus, and stomach have been reported recently from the large American Cancer Society survey.[100] The protection was greatest among long-time users (>10 years) and was not found for tumors of nondigestive organs.

The mechanism of action by which aspirin and NSAIDs protect against tumor formation in the digestive tract remains an issue of speculation and includes many possibilities.[2] The rodent model is perplexing, because prostaglandins inhibit proliferation in the rat colon[101,102] and colonic epithelial proliferation is stimulated by indomethacin or aspirin.[102,103] It cannot be assumed that the antitumor effect is necessarily related to modifications in the production of prostaglandins in the gastrointestinal tract. It has been demonstrated that cultured gastric cancer cells preferentially produce leukotrienes, whereas normal stomach tissue produces prostaglandins; that the leukotrienes act as autacoid stimulants of growth; and that prostaglandins inhibit the growth of the cancer cells.[104] There may be a change in response to eicosanoids by tissues that undergo malignant transformation, and the mechanism by which NSAIDs reduce cancer may be one that is not currently apparent.

Recommendations Regarding Diet

Although there are wide ranges in the international incidences of colorectal cancer, there is a fairly uniform, high rate of this disease in North America, Western Europe, and much of the industrialized world. Groups migrating from low-risk into high-risk regions rapidly experience an increase in the incidence of colorectal cancer. It is a reasonable conclusion that diet plays the greatest role in determining the incidence of colorectal cancer in the population. High fat intake and low fiber intake have been the most consistent associations with colorectal cancer risk. Patients who are interested in modifying their diets in hopes of reducing cancer risk might be advised to reduce caloric intake, to reduce dietary fat to less than 25% of caloric intake, to enrich the diet with fresh fruits and vegetables, and to include at least 25 g of fiber in the diet—until the perfect nutritional plan is discovered.[105]

Before the year 2000 it should be known whether any chemopreventive compounds are of benefit to high-risk groups. Because colorectal cancer strikes about 5% of the population, and because fewer than half of these persons die of the disease, it is relatively unlikely that chemopreventive agents will be recommended to the general population unless a very high degree of protection can be proven in the absence of any toxicity. However, it is possible that an agent such as aspirin, which may be taken to prevent a more common disease—such as atherosclerotic heart disease—may provide protection against colorectal neoplasia, and benefit will be derived as a fortunate side effect. However, the use of aspirin to protect against cancer is still an issue that requires validation and investigation regarding appropriate dosing and associated complications.

ETIOLOGY

Genetic Models of Multistep Carcinogenesis

Carcinogenesis in the colon and rectum was initially described in terms of the classic initiation-promotion model formulated more than four decades ago to explain carcinogenesis of the skin (see Chap. 24). According to this conceptual framework, the first step involved factors that directly damaged DNA, mutated the genome, and initiated the cells. The process was driven to completion by promotional factors that were not themselves mutagenic. It was thought that the two components of the process were strictly sequential, in that promotional factors were only effective after the administration of a genotoxic initiating agent.

This model has been greatly advanced by additional data. Colorectal neoplasia is best characterized as a multistep process that begins with genetic mutations in normal tissue that enhance proliferation and provide growth and survival advantages for affected cells. As the cells proliferate, they are susceptible to additional mutations, some of which may be lethal but certain ones of which further enhance the ability of cells to proliferate. As the most advantageous genetic changes occur, these cells clonally expand and overgrow neighboring cells. By successive waves of cellular selection,

the mutations appear to accumulate in the expanding clones. Initially, the cells retain the normal phenotype, but they are susceptible to additional genetic damage. After the accumulation of sufficient genetic damage, the neoplastic phenotype may eventually occur, and eventually, invasion and metastasis are possible.

Early Events

Many, but certainly not all, of the specific genetic events involved in colorectal carcinogenesis have been identified.[4] This has given rise to the model of sequential carcinogenesis proposed by the laboratory of Vogelstein, as illustrated in Figure 87-5. The model has been derived by detecting the genetic aberrations across the spectrum of neoplastic lesions. According to this model, point mutations and other genetic changes in genetic sequence are the initial lesions that begin to permit colorectal epithelium to escape from ordinary constraints on cell growth.[3]

The earliest identified lesion is a mutation in one allele of the *APC* (adenomatous polyposis coli) gene, which is also the locus of the germ line mutations in FAP or Gardner's syndrome (see Chap. 86).[9] This germ line mutation is present in every cell of patients with FAP, even though the manifestations of the disease are tissue-specific. In sporadically occurring adenomas, this mutation is present in the adenoma

Sporadic Cancer: Adenoma → Carcinoma

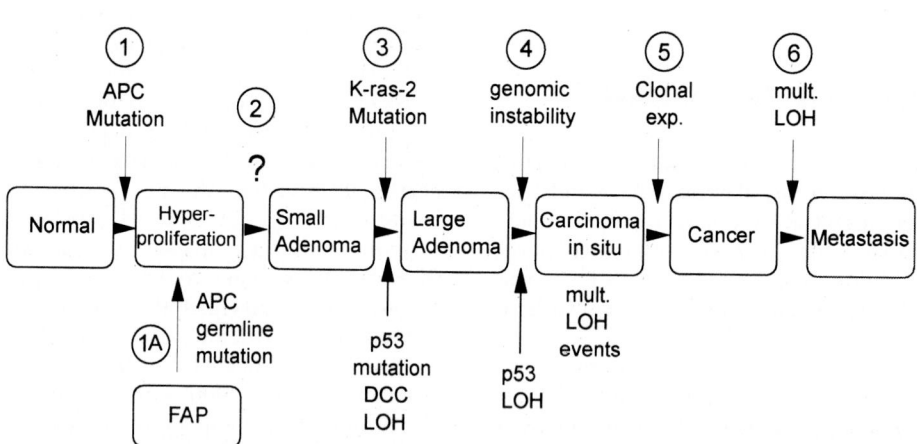

FIGURE 87-5. The proposed genetic scheme of events responsible for multistep carcinogenesis in the colon. Step 1 indicates that a mutation in the (*APC*) gene permits hyperproliferation to occur in a colonic epithelial cell. Step 1A indicates that patients with familial adenomatous polyposis (FAP) have germ-line mutations that make the entire colon hyperproliferative. The genetic mechanism that mediates the appearance of an adenoma from hyperproliferative epithelium (which is phenotypically normal) is unknown (step 2). Since most adenomas remain small, critical events occur in some of them to make them into a large adenoma (step 3) including *K-ras2* mutation, *p53* mutation, and possibly loss of heterozygosity (LOH) at the *DCC* locus. The conversion from benign to malignant neoplasia (step 4) is accompanied by the onset of genomic instability in which multiple LOH events occur. This phenomenon results in the appearance of multiple potentially malignant clones, some of which undergo clonal expansion, and which compete to become the dominate cell type in the neoplasm (step 5). LOH events continue to accumulate until a metastic phenotype develops (step 6).

but not the surrounding tissues. In this case, it represents an acquired event in a single cell which has given rise to the polyp by clonal expansion. The alterations in the *APC* gene are almost always nonsense mutations, that is, those that result in a premature stop codon and consequently the production of a truncated *APC* gene product. These mutations are present in small adenomas and are found before any other alteration that occurs in the multistep pathway. It is not known whether this mutation is sufficient for the appearance of the adenomatous polyp from hyperproliferative mucosa or whether additional lesions are required for this to occur. Furthermore, it has not been possible to identify *APC* mutations in approximately one third of colorectal adenomas, which suggests that other mechanisms may be sufficient to support the early stages of neoplasia. Many adenomatous polyps also show loss of one of the *APC* alleles, called loss of heterozygosity (LOH), suggesting a characteristic two-hit mechanism at this tumor suppressor gene locus.

The *ras* Genes and Progression of Adenomas

Many adenomas remain small and never progress beyond a benign stage. Growth and progression require additional disruption of growth control. Mutations have been identified in the *K-ras* cellular protooncogene, and this has been interpreted to be a middle-stage event that occurs in smaller adenomas and may permit them to grow larger.[3,106] The *ras* genes are highly conserved in nature; they encode for proteins located on the inner leaflet of the plasma membrane, bind guanine nucleotides, and are involved in signal transduction from the cell membrane to the nucleus.[107] Mutations located at critical positions in the gene alter the *ras* protein in such way that the signal transduction is unregulated, which leads to additional cell growth.[108] A mutation at just one of three codons—12, 13, and 61 of the *K-ras2* gene—is the mechanism by which the *ras* oncogene is activated in many colorectal neoplasms.[109] For example, in one study of human tumors, mutations of the *K-ras2* were present in 11 of 27 colorectal cancers, and in 9 of these instances, the mutation occurred at codon 12 of the gene.[110] Mutation at codon 12 was also found in 40% of 66 primary human colon cancers. The transforming mutations all occurred in the first or second of the three nucleotide positions of the codon but were not found elsewhere in the gene.[111]

K-ras mutations are present in a large percentage of adenomas. In one study, mutations were reported in no normal tissues or adenomas with only mild dysplasia, but were found in 83% of higher grade adenomas.[112] In another study using microdissected specimens, 58% of adenomas larger than 1 cm contained a *ras* gene mutation, whereas this was found in only 9% of the adenomas less than 1 cm in size.[3] *Ras* mutations have been found in 7 of 8 villous adenomas using the same method.[111] Some controversy surrounds this finding, and one laboratory has reported mutations in the field of normal-appearing tissue surrounding tumors.[106] Different results may have been related to difficulties in defining the pathology of the tissue from which the DNA was extracted. Most laboratories agree that *ras* gene mutations are less frequent in colorectal carcinomas than in adenomas, occurring

in approximately half of the cancers.[3,112,113] In spite of the fact that *ras* gene mutations are common in colorectal neoplasia, they are not universally present. Although they may facilitate the growth of small adenomas to large ones, they may not be necessary for malignant transformation, and they may be selected against in this process.[112] Furthermore, colorectal cancers with *K-ras* mutations are associated with a relatively better prognosis than those without this lesion.[113]

The *p53* Gene and Genomic Instability

Large adenomas are benign neoplasms, and despite the fact that they can occasionally grow to a size of 6 cm or more in diameter, they cannot invade the muscularis mucosae. The gene most responsible for malignant conversion appears to be the *p53* gene, which is activated by a more complex, two-hit mechanism. *p53* is a tumor suppressor gene; it serves as a cell cycle checkpoint regulator and prevents nuclear replication after injuries that are likely to damage the DNA.[114] In the presence of damaged DNA, the p53 protein level rises in the cell, and progression into the cell cycle is prevented by G_1/S arrest. The cell either repairs the damage or apoptosis (i.e., programmed cell death) ensues. Inactivation of the *p53* gene permits mutated DNA to be replicated and removes a level of restraint on abnormal cell behavior.

The mutations in *p53* are usually missense; that is, they encode for a different amino acid. They tend to occur in hotspot locations in colon cancer (codons 175, 248, and 273), and virtually all of the mutations occur in four evolutionarily conserved regions of the gene located between codons 117 and 286.[115] This region of the p53 protein is responsible for DNA binding, and oncogenic forms of the protein lose the ability to bind DNA and activate gene expression.[116] Mutations in *p53* occur in a wide range of human tumors,[117] and this is perhaps the most common and most powerful tumor-causing genetic lesion. The mutational hot spot region is where viral oncoproteins, and at least one normally expressed regulatory protein, bind and inactivate the function of *p53*.[114,115,118]

In normal cells, *p53* is expressed at very low levels, has a short half-life, and is not readily detectable. Certain mutations in the *p53* gene result in the expression of a more stable but dysfunctional p53 protein that may be detected using standard immunohistochemistry. Overexpression of p53, as evidenced by observing the protein histochemically, may be seen in some colorectal adenomas,[119] but the biologic significance of a single mutated *p53* gene is uncertain because there is still a second, normal allele present in the nucleus. A second event occurs in which the normal or wild type *p53* allele is lost, leaving the cell in the hemizygous, mutated state. This is the most common genotype associated with the malignant phenotype,[120,121] and it appears to be biologically significant, because replacement of a wild type *p53* gene suppresses the growth of cultured human colorectal cancer cells.[122] *p53* belongs to a family of genes that are responsible for restraining abnormal cell growth and are known as tumor suppressor genes. Abnormalities of these tumor suppressor genes are often seen in sporadic tumors, and germ line mutations in such genes are responsible for a genetic predisposition to cancer, as in FAP or retinoblastoma (see Chap. 24).[123]

Overexpression of the p53 protein in colorectal adenomas is more prevalent in more highly dysplastic polyps and correlates with the proliferative activity of the lesion.[119] Increased expression of p53 and loss of the wild type allele are associated with worse prognosis in colorectal cancer independently of other pathologic features.[124,125] There is evidence that loss of the wild type allele is first seen in high-grade dysplasia (i.e., carcinoma in situ) and is associated with the onset of chaotic genomic instability, in which genetic material is randomly and rapidly deleted from the nucleus, resulting in LOH.[126]

Loss of Heterozygosity

Colorectal cancers are characterized by LOH, which refers to the deletion of one chromosomal allele, at many sites throughout the tumor cell genome.[127,128] LOH is the result of genomic instability, a poorly understood process in which the nucleus can no longer symmetrically divide its chromosomes during mitosis; one daughter cell receives both copies of a genetic segment and the sister cell gets neither. Increased numbers of lost genetic loci (expressed as the fractional allelic loss) is significantly associated with worse prognosis in colorectal cancer,[128] and this is especially true if LOH occurs at specific chromosomal locations such as 17p (the locus of the p53 gene) and 18q (the locus of the deleted-in-colorectal-cancer or DCC gene).[128,129] Many of the lost genetic segments are random and may not be important for the malignant behavior of the cell, but in certain instances, LOH results in the loss of copies of tumor suppressor genes.[123] If critical growth-restraining genes are lost, the cell gains an advantage in growth and survival over other cells.

Widespread LOH events are characteristic of colorectal and other cancers, and the changing genetic background results in the generation of cellular diversity and, eventually, the metastatic phenotype with a primary tumor mass. Candidate genes have been proposed for various biological characteristics of the metastatic phenotype, such as mutations and LOH of the nm23 gene, a proposed metastasis suppressor gene,[130,131] but the metastasis genes remain a complex and incompletely understood area. As each new random combination of characteristics is generated in the unstable tumor cell genome, most provide no growth advantage or are lethal. However, after a highly advantageous genome is created by the chance deletion of tumor suppressor genes, or genes responsible for the repression of gene activation, this newly-minted cell clonally expands and overgrows all those around it.

Other Genetic Alterations

Other genetic abnormalities occurring in colorectal neoplasia may participate in multistep carcinogenesis. For example, although mutation in the myc oncogene has not been reported, this oncogene is amplified in some colon cancers.[132,133] Although amplified expression of the myc RNA has been reported in more than two thirds of primary adenocarcinomas of the colon, levels of expression do not correlate with adverse patient prognosis.[134] Hypomethylation of DNA may lead to the altered expression of genes that are neither mutated nor amplified at the genomic level. This genetic modification has

been reported in colorectal neoplasms and is found to a similar degree in benign adenomatous polyps. It appears to be one of the earlier genetic modifications in colorectal neoplasia.[135]

The cellular protooncogene src is activated by mutation, resulting in increased tyrosine kinase activity, which is associated with increased cell proliferation, similar to that described for mutated ras genes. Increased protein kinase activity of activated src is an early event in the progressive neoplastic sequence and is seen in premalignant lesions such as adenomatous polyps. The activity of the enzyme is associated with the malignant risk of the polyp.[136] Several other oncogenes are mutated or otherwise abnormally regulated in colorectal cancer, but their roles in the overall scheme of colorectal carcinogenesis remain to be elucidated.

The multistep model of neoplastic progression describes a mechanism for tumor development that begins with random mutations at critical genetic loci which permit the clonal expansion of more highly proliferative cells. These cells cross a threshold, apparently involving the p53 gene, at which genomic instability appears and generates grossly abnormal nuclear rearrangements that eventually result in highly malignant cells. However, this is not the only genetic pathway to neoplasia.

Evidence for a second genetic pathway to cancer emerged during the search for the gene for HNPCC or Lynch's syndrome. This familial colon cancer gene was found using linkage analysis techniques to link the phenotype with a specific genetic locus. This involved use of powerful genetic polymorphisms called microsatellites, which are short sequences of nucleotides (e.g., ...CACACA...) that are repeated a variable number of times throughout the human genome. Although the length of these sequences varies from person to person, they are stably replicated during mitosis. However, in HNPCC tumors, these sequences, which are interspersed more than 100,000 times throughout the genome, were found to be unstable, and replication errors frequently occurred.[10,11] Microsatellite instability was also found in nonfamilial colorectal cancers, particularly those in the proximal colon.[137] Tumors with microsatellite instability were found to have the same range of mutations in the apc, ras, and p53 genes as previously reported but did not demonstrate the chaotic nuclear disorganization produced by LOH.[11] Furthermore, tumors with microsatellite instability were more likely to be diploid and were associated with a significantly better prognosis.[11,137] Thus, it appears that a second mechanistic pathway occurs in some tumors, and that these tumors may account for some of the variable clinical outcomes that have long been observed (see Chap. 24).

Clinical Implications of Genetic Lesions

It is possible that all differences in the clinical behavior of tumors are based on variations in the appearance and accumulation of the genetic lesions found in colorectal tumors. For example, some Dukes' stage B tumors are bulky but minimally invasive, and the outcome is correspondingly better, presumably because a cellular mechanism for unregulated growth has been achieved but the genetic configuration for metastasis did not emerge. Genetic mechanisms such as ras mutation and microsatellite instability have been associated with tumors that have better patient survival. This is a reasonable explanation for the relatively better prognosis in HNPCC tumors[138] and in certain bulky but nonmetastatic cancers that can appear in the proximal colon. Alternatively, other tumors are highly aggressive early in their history and readily metastasize. The virulence of colorectal cancers has been mechanistically linked to LOH, and particularly to LOH at the *p53* locus, which occurs more commonly in the distal colon.[139]

In specialized clinical situations, such as cancers complicating ulcerative colitis, different mechanisms may be operating. These tumors are significantly less likely to have *ras* gene mutations,[140,141] but they show a high frequency of LOH, including the *p53* locus.[142,143] Although the mechanism through which these tumors have arisen may not have led to genetic lesions promoting the growth of a bulky lumenal tumor, they nevertheless may have experienced the early onset of genomic instability and, consequently, a rapidly progressive, highly malignant outcome that is directly related to the underlying biology of the tumor.

Aneuploidy

Because of the inability to identify histologic features of prognostic significance in most colorectal cancers, diagnostic approaches have been attempted to select patients at greatest risk for metastasis. Flow cytometry can be used to measure the DNA content of cell populations and to estimate the percentage of cells in different stages of the cell cycle. Resting cells are normally diploid. After the stage of new DNA synthesis is complete, the cells are briefly tetraploid, and after mitosis, they return to the diploid state. During the phase of DNA synthesis (S phase), the DNA content of a cell is transiently between the diploid and the tetraploid state. Aneuploidy is a state in which a population of cells has a stable but irregular DNA content, which appears as a spike of nondiploid, nontetraploid cells on flow cytometric analysis. Approximately 80% of solid tumors contain aneuploid populations; several studies of colon cancers have agreed that approximately 65% are aneuploid.[144,145] Furthermore, a smaller percentage (6%–19%) of adenomatous polyps are aneuploid.[145-147] Correlations between aneuploidy and state of differentiation or patient survival have been reported[148] but are on the whole inconsistent, and the studies in colorectal polyps add little to the current histopathologic classification of these lesions. Aneuploidy appears to occur early in the natural history of neoplasia (i.e., it begins to occur in larger adenomas); however, as many as 40% of malignant tumors may never become aneuploid in spite of their ability to metastasize (Fig. 87-6).[149]

Mutagenesis

It is apparent from the above discussion that colorectal cancer begins with mutations in the nuclei of colorectal epithelial cells. The human diet contains a large number of naturally occurring mutagens and substances that may be metabolized into mutagens. Most of these mutagens are toxic chemicals synthesized by plants as a primary defense against attack by bacteria, fungi, insects, and other animals. The presence of these toxic compounds is so ubiquitous that an efficient and redundant network of protective mechanisms is present throughout the gut mucosa to detoxify these compounds. In fact, the ability of the enterocyte to metabolize certain xenobiotics is amplified by their presence in the diet.[150]

The metabolic fate of procarcinogens is very complex and may involve absorption from the gut, metabolism in the liver, secretion into the bile, and additional oxidative activation in the immediate vicinity of the target organ.[151,152] There is a wide range of dietary compounds that may play a role in the initiation of carcinogenesis in the colon. The first experimental compound used to produce the laboratory model of colon cancer was cycasin, a naturally occurring glycoside extracted from cycad nuts. Hydrazines are potent carcinogens closely related to cycasin, and may be found in commercial mushrooms.[153] Bracken fern, a common plant and a major source of nutrition for foraging cattle, is a source of at least two carcinogens, quercetin and ptaquiloside.[154] Fecapentaenes, potent direct-acting mutagens of bacterial origin, have been isolated from human feces.[155] Other highly reactive lipophilic pentaenes, which spontaneously decompose and give rise to alkylating moieties, have been isolated from human feces.[156] Mutagenic quinolines have been extracted from beef, and additional compounds are generated by frying beef.[157,158] The structural analysis of these compounds can be difficult because of their highly reactive nature and tendency to spontaneously decompose.

Using the Ames' test for mutagenicity,[159] which measures the induction of mutations in a *Salmonella* species in vitro, it is possible to detect the presence of mutagens without isolating them or characterizing their structure. Two groups of Japanese individuals with different risks of colorectal cancer were studied for the presence of ether-extractable mutagens in their stool. The high-risk individuals had significantly more direct-acting mutagens in their feces than did the low-risk population.[160] However, a case-control study of the fecal mutagen fecapentaene revealed no association with colorectal cancer.[161]

In summary, mutagenesis in the colon may be produced by substances generated from an interaction between the diet, microbial flora, and colonic mucosal enzymes. It is not difficult to test for the presence of mutagenic substances in feces; however, their highly unstable and reactive nature makes them difficult to characterize structurally. The identification of several mutagenic products of microbial metabolism, together with the relative stability of the gastrointestinal flora over time,[162] suggest that it might be very difficult to eliminate all mutagens from the colonic milieu. Thus, many of the strategies aimed at reducing colon cancer accept the presence of mutagens in the colon and attempt to interfere with the interaction between carcinogens and the target tissues.

Animal Models of Colon Cancer

Much has been learned from rodent models of colonic carcinogenesis. The most commonly used model involves the administration of a member of the dimethylhydrazine (DMH)

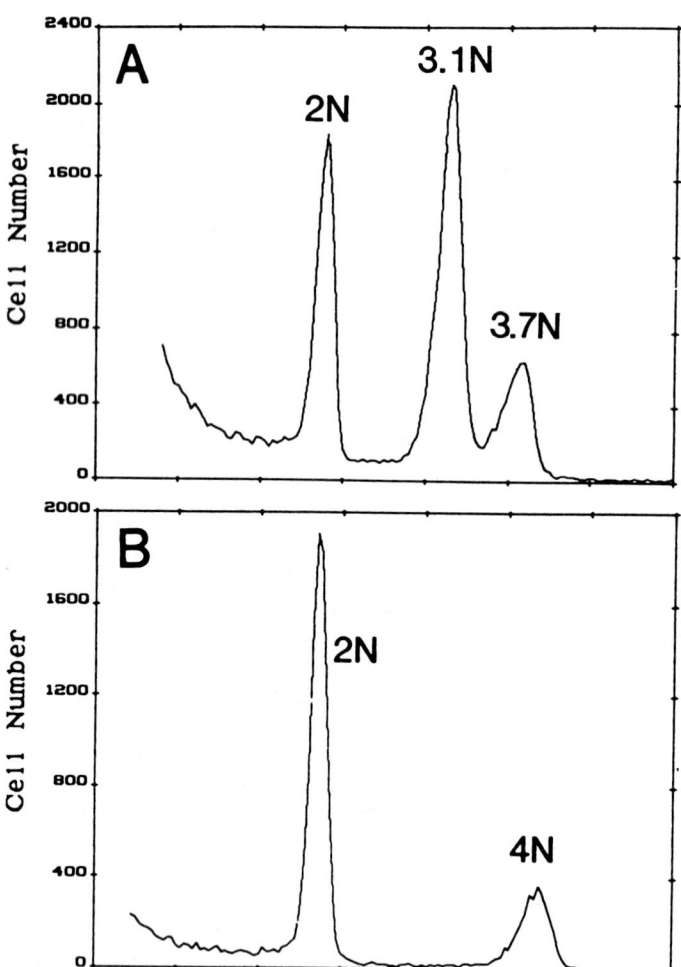

FIGURE 87-6. The DNA content of individual cells can be measured using flow cytometry and expressed in these DNA-content histograms. (**A**) A sample containing the normal cell population (2N) and two aneuploid populations with DNA contents of 3.1N and 3.7N, taken from a patient with ulcerative colitis. (**B**) A large population of normal cells (2N), and a smaller population of cells with the DNA content of 4N, indicating tetraploidy in the tumor. (From Levine DS, Rabinovitch PS, Haggitt RC, et al. Distribution of aneuploid cell populations in ulcerative colitis with dysplasia or cancer. Gastroenterology 1991;101:1198.)

family of carcinogens to rats or mice. This results in adeno-carcinomas of the colon, small intestine, and other sites, depending upon the carcinogen used, method of administration, and species of rodent. The most commonly used model involves the sequential injection of DMH into rats. DMH is an effective intestinal carcinogen whether given orally or parenterally. After absorption from the gut or subcutaneous site, DMH is taken up by the liver, where it undergoes sequential oxidations giving rise to unstable compounds that are able to methylate DNA, RNA, or proteins.[151] The value of these compounds in the rodent is that the colon is selectively, although not exclusively, affected by them. The relative specificity for the colon may be illustrated by the transposition of colon to a small intestine site or by the reverse experiment, in which a small bowel is transposed into the colon. After administration of DMH, colonic epithelium develops tumors even if transposed to a proximal site, whereas small intestine epithelium is resistant even if transposed to a distal site.[163,164] In addition, DNA damage, measured as single strand breaks, is found to occur in a organ-selective manner and in proportion to the species susceptibility to the carcinogen.[165] The neoplasms that develop in rodents are adenocarcinomas and are similar to tumors that develop in humans. In the rat, one usually observes adenocarcinomas throughout the proximal and distal large intestine,[166] although this may vary among

rat strains. In certain inbred mouse strains, the tumors occur predominantly in the distal colon, and the characteristic adenoma-carcinoma sequence is seen.[167-171]

A single dose of alkylating carcinogen (e.g., DMH) is sufficient to produce adenomas and carcinomas in mice after a latent period of approximately 4 months.[167] Oncogene activation occurs in the case of the *ras* gene by point mutations that can be produced by alkylating agents.[111,172] As has been mentioned, *ras* gene mutations appear in the middle of the overall neoplastic scheme.[3,110] Characteristic G-to-A mutations can be detected in the *K-ras* genes of colorectal tissues beginning in the 15th week of treatment with carcinogen, antedating in time the appearance of tumors, which required a latency of approximately 24 weeks.[173] This model helped to validate the sequential nature of the genetic lesions and provided additional support that the mutations found early in human colorectal carcinogenesis are the result of typical chemical carcinogenesis.

In spite of the conceptual limitations of the initiation-promotion model, these terms are frequently referred to in descriptions of the animal model. In this discussion, initiation refers to the time period during which the carcinogen or mutagen is administered, and promotion refers to any manipulation that takes place in the postinitiation period. This serves as a useful conceptual framework, because different results are obtained if one manipulates the animal during the administration of carcinogen rather than during a later time. The important point is that one can enhance or reduce tumorigenesis in experimental animals either by maneuvers that modify the generation of mutagen or by events that occur long after administration of carcinogen.

Role of Diet in Animal Carcinogenesis

The rodent model of colon carcinogenesis has been widely used for introducing dietary manipulations and observing their effects on tumor production. As previously mentioned, the epidemiologic literature suggests that fat ingestion is a key factor in the different rates of colon cancer observed around the world. There is abundant evidence in the experimental model that increasing the total dietary fat from 5% to 30% of caloric intake produces a significant increase in the number of animals that develop cancers and the number of tumors per animal.[174-177] If rats are fed a high-fat diet more than 1 month after the last injection of carcinogen, significantly more tumors are produced than if the high-fat diet is given only during the period of administration of carcinogen.[174] This suggests that a high-fat diet mediates some aspect of neoplastic progression in the postinitiation period.

The tumor-promoting effects of different types of dietary fat have been investigated. Polyunsaturated fats were initially thought to have greater tumor-enhancing effects than saturated fats for colonic as well as other tumors, such as mammary tumors. For example, a 5% corn oil diet produced a higher incidence of colonic tumors than diet containing 5% lard. However, differences between types of fat disappeared at the 20% level, at which a higher overall incidence of tumors was produced in all animals.[177] It appears that the total dose of fat is more important than the fatty acid composition. However, a diet supplemented with menhaden oil, a lipid mixture derived from fish and seals which contains high amounts of polyunsaturated fatty acids of the n-3 or ω-3 series, has been a subject of investigation because of its potential effects in preventing atherosclerosis. A diet containing 4% to 22.5% menhaden oil had no tumor-enhancing effects compared with corn oil.

Bile acids also promote the development of tumors in the rodent model. The addition of cholic acid to the diet increased the number of rodents that developed tumors, the number of tumors per animal, and the fecal excretion of secondary bile acids.[178] Enhanced tumor production may result from other maneuvers designed to increase colonic exposure to bile acids, including ileal resection,[179] cholecystectomy,[180] and distal repositioning of the papilla of Vater.[181]

Fiber is a generic term and includes a wide variety of nondigestible soluble and insoluble forms of carbohydrate (e.g., cellulose, hemicelluloses, gums, mucilages, pectins) and other substances such as lignins.[69] Bran is a heterogeneous preparation from the seed coats of cereal grains comprised of fibers and other contaminating substances, some of which may have effects on epithelial proliferation. Cellulose is a polymer of glucose found in virtually all plant tissues and is a common component of many forms of fiber.[182] Several investigators have demonstrated that purified cellulose, in doses ranging

from 4.5% to 15% of the diet, reduces tumor production in rats.[183-185] Dietary cellulose decreases mitotic indices in the colon,[186] whereas virtually opposite effects are seen with pectin, which provides no protection against tumor production.[184] Dietary histories regarding fiber intake are difficult to estimate in humans, and the data are correspondingly confusing. However, the experimental model has permitted a dissection of the issues and has clarified the fact that certain components of fiber may be protective even when others are not.

As previously mentioned, dietary fiber appears to protect against the development of colorectal cancer; however, the clinical data have not been entirely consistent. The experimental model has served to clarify this important concept. Administration of a 10% wheat bran diet inhibits tumor production and, in fact, can prevent the tumor-enhancing properties of bile salts.[187] However, the administration of a 20% wheat bran diet enhances cellular proliferation in the colon[188] and either has no effect[189] or actually increases tumor production in the rat.[190] The tumor-enhancing effect is seen only if 20% wheat bran is administered during the initiation period, whereas a reduction in benign tumors is seen if this diet is administered after the administration of the initiating agent.[190] The administration of a 14% corn bran diet increases fecal bile acid excretion and enhances tumor production, reinforcing the conclusion that not all types or doses of fiber are equally protective against colon cancer.[191] The proliferative response elicited by 20% wheat bran[188] can also be produced by a diet of 10% guar, another fiber.[192] However, two other fibers, 20% oat bran and 10% pectin, have no effect on colonic proliferation.[192]

The animal model has also permitted an exploration of factors that may modify large bowel carcinogenesis, as summarized in Table 87-3[181,190,191,193-199] and Table 87-4.[183,184,187,191,200-216] Manipulations that increase the delivery of lipid and bile acids to the colon, such as the administration of cholestyramine[193] or neomycin,[198] small intestine resection,[199] and biliary diversion to the colon,[181] all increase the number of tumors occurring in experimental animals. A large number of factors have been identified that inhibit colonic carcinogenesis, and, in some instances, inhibition is specific to either the induction phase or the promotion phase. An-

TABLE 87-3
Factors That Increase Experimental Large Bowel Cancers In Rodents

Cholestyramine
Suture material
Colitis
Butyrate
Vitamin A deficiency
Neomycin
Small intestine resection
Diversion of bile to colon
Wheat bran, 20% of diet during initiation
Corn bran, 15% of diet

Data from references 181, 190, 191, 193, 194, 195, 196, 197, 198, and 199.

Factors That Decrease Experimental Large Bowel Cancers In Rodents

Dietary fiber
    Wheat bran, 10% of diet
    Cellulose, 4.5%–9% of diet
    Lignin, 7.5% of diet
Selenium
Vitamin C
Vitamin E
Retinoic acid
β-Carotene
Epsilon-amino caproic acid
Antibiotics
Dioctylsulfosuccinate
2-Difluoromethylornithine
Indomethacin, piroxicam
β-Sitosterol
Butylated hydroxyanisole
Cabbage
Diallyl sulfide (garlic)
Disulfiram

Data from references 184, 187, 191, 193, and 200 through 216.

tioxidants such as vitamin C, vitamin E, vitamin A, butylated hydroxyaminisol (BHA), and butylated hydroxytoluene (BHT) do not prevent DNA damage, and seem to exert their protective effects during the post-induction promotional period. As previously mentioned, the vegetarian diet is rich in fiber, plant sterols such as β-sitosterol, and lignins and is simultaneously low in fat. The animal model has permitted the selective introduction of individual dietary components that are thought to modify tumor production in humans and provided insight not possible by epidemiology alone.

CLINICAL MANIFESTATIONS AND RISK FACTORS FOR COLORECTAL NEOPLASIA

Clinical Presentation

Tumors of the colon and rectum grow at a slow, somewhat unpredictable rate. It is difficult to make any estimates of growth rates because colorectal tumors are rarely left in place for observation. However, some information is available from the precolonoscopy era which suggests that approximately 11.4 years may elapse before polyps with mild atypia become malignant, although polyps containing severe dysplasia become malignant in 3.6 years.[217] Colorectal neoplasms develop cellular heterogeneity with time because of the genomic instability described earlier. As a result, some tumors grow more rapidly than others, and the rapidity of progression is far from uniform. However, colorectal neoplasms begin as adenomas and progress through stages of advancing degrees of dysplasia as they grow. Hypothetical modeling suggests that a tiny polyp requires approximately 2 to 3 years to reach 1 cm in size.[218] The period of time from the mean appearance of adenomas to the mean diagnosis of cancer in FAP is 23 years.[219,220] These estimates cannot be generalized to all neoplasms because they are based on selected lesions that have become malignant, and they fail to take into account the important consideration that many adenomas may never grow. However, these estimates serve to underscore the fact that colonic tumors grow slowly, and most are not likely to give rise to dramatic or characteristic symptoms. Therefore, one should be alerted to a change in bowel habits as a sign of distal colorectal cancer, even if the symptoms have developed over a period as long as 1 year. The presence of symptoms for up to 1 year before diagnosis seems to have no adverse effect on survival.[221] The change in bowel habits is the important clinical issue; comparing colorectal cancer patients with controls in a retrospective case-control study, no significant differences were elicited in the historical frequency of bowel movements, the presence of constipation, or the use of laxatives.[222]

As a colon cancer grows, it may give rise to one or more of four different groups of symptoms. First, the colonic lumen may be obstructed, relatively or completely, and produce corresponding symptoms. Obstruction may produce abdominal distention, pain, or, in its most extreme degree, nausea and vomiting. Most colon cancers grow as an expanding circular lesion; the traditional apple-core lesion occurs after the diameter of the tumor approaches the circumference of the bowel wall and obstructs the lumen. The colonic diameter is greatest in the cecum and ascending colon, where obstruction is much less likely to occur. The diameter is less in the transverse, descending, and sigmoid colons, which are more likely sites for obstruction. Gastrointestinal obstruction suggests the presence of a large tumor and is an ominous symptom; it is associated with a significant adverse effect on survival.[223]

Secondly, as colonic tumors expand into the bowel lumen, they tend to bleed, both because of the presence of abnormal vasculature and because of trauma from the fecal stream. Bleeding is likely to occur regardless of the location of the tumor, but it is usually not brisk. In fact, colon cancers typically lose considerably less than 6 mL of blood per day.[224] If a tumor is located near the anus, the blood may be deposited on the surface of the stool and may be grossly visible to the patient. More typically, the blood is mixed in with the stool and evades detection. Tumors in the proximal colon tend to grow larger without producing obstructive symptoms; they may bleed longer and present with iron deficiency anemia. Tumors in the sigmoid colon or rectum are more likely to produce hematochezia or give rise to a positive fecal occult bleeding test (FOBT).

The third symptom complex produced by colorectal cancer reflects the local invasive characteristics of a tumor. Obstruction and bleeding reflect complications of tumor growth into the lumen. However, an invasive tumor eventually penetrates the muscularis propria and invades adjacent tissues. This most typically produces pain, but it may produce specific symptoms depending on the organ invaded. Local invasion in the rectum can produce tenesmus, penetration in the bladder may produce urinary symptoms, growth into the bladder produces pneumaturia, the pelvic organs may be invaded and produce confusing symptoms, or a colonic perforation may occur and the patient may present with an acute abdomen. Invasion by rectal cancers of the perirectal fat may be associated with rapid extension and can produce ureteral obstruction. Invasion of other adjacent organs is less common, but the tumor may extend through the mesentery and compromise a vascular structure or, rarely, involve other visceral organs such as the small intestine or stomach by means of a malignant fistula tract. Because manifestations of local extension all indicate invasion through the muscularis propria, these manifestations are all associated with an adverse prognostic implication. In a similar way, a metastatic lesion may produce local symptoms because of its expansive or penetrating qualities. In these instances, the clinician may be drawn to the liver or bony site because of pain and later find a primary tumor in the colon that has produced a minimum of symptoms.

Finally, some tumors produce a wasting syndrome that is out of proportion to the size of the tumor, even taking into account its excessive metabolic activity. Cancer cachexia is clinically characterized by a loss of appetite, weight, and strength.[225] This is a complex disorder of metabolism that appears to be mediated by a hormone termed cachectin, or tumor necrosis factor. This peptide hormone is normally a mediator of the inflammatory response but also has profound effects on adipocyte metabolism.[226] Cancer cachexia is common in patients with any gastrointestinal malignancy, and affected patients may experience a more profound loss of subcutaneous fat than that caused by an equivalent degree of benign inflammatory disease, accounting for the characteristic look of a cancer patient.[227] This wasting occurs in spite of the fact that most patients with colorectal neoplasms do not have hypermetabolic resting energy expenditures.[228]

Colorectal neoplasia tends not to produce symptoms early in its natural history. As indicated above, three of the four symptom complexes are generally indications of advanced stages of disease. The only exception is occult gastrointestinal bleeding. If one attempts to diagnose colon cancer by evaluating patients who present with symptoms of colonic disease, the majority of those diagnosed will have advanced disease and will probably die of their cancer. Therefore, strategies developed to reduce the morbidity and mortality of colorectal cancer have attempted to detect the excess bleeding caused by the neoplasm. However, early forms of colorectal cancer lose blood at rates that are only minimally greater than normal rates of blood loss. Because the bleeding from a small carcinoma or a large adenoma is so minimal, it has been difficult to develop accurate and sensitive tests for early diagnosis.[224] This has placed additional emphasis on the improvement of tests for occult fecal blood and for the identification of subgroups of patients at greater risk for this disease.

Clinical Features of Patients at Increased Risk for Colorectal Cancer

The principal feature used to identify higher risk patients for colorectal cancer is the family history. This is not a straightforward issue, because 5% of the U.S. population develops the disease, and, depending on the number of relatives known, a sizable number of people are related to at least one person who has developed colorectal cancer. Therefore, additional information is needed to determine increased risk based on family history. Key issues are the number of affected people in a family, the age at the time of tumor development, and associated syndromic features.

There are three categories of familial colorectal cancer risk: FAP or Gardner's syndrome, and variants of this; HNPCC or Lynch's syndromes; and what might be called common variable colorectal cancer familiality, for lack of a better term.

Familial Adenomatous Polyposis or Gardner's Syndrome

The premier candidates to develop colorectal cancer are persons who inherit a germ line mutation (not to be confused with the somatic mutations that occur in sporadic tumors) at the *APC* locus and therefore have FAP or Gardner's syndrome, which are variations on a single genetic disease (see Chap. 86). These patients all develop adenomatous polyps at a median age of 16 years,[219] and virtually all of them progress to cancer, with a median age of 39 for symptomatic malignancy.[220] This represents the extreme end of the spectrum, and it serves as a paradigm of the adenoma-to-carcinoma sequence. The adenomas appear first, and, with time, one or more cancers develop from antecedent adenomas. The sequence is terminated after the colon is removed or the patient dies of a complication of the disease, so it is not possible to know whether every adenoma would enlarge or undergo malignant degeneration with time. In older patients with this disease, it appears that many or most adenomas simply remain small.

It is now possible to use genetic techniques to identify carriers of the abnormal *APC* gene even before the polyps develop in the offspring of an affected individual. Because the gene is so large, it is difficult to sequence the entire *APC* gene in each person to find the mutation, even though this is the most definitive way to make the diagnosis. Gene carriage can be identified by linkage analysis using DNA extracted from fresh lymphocytes. It usually requires at least two affected members and several other closely related members of the same family whose phenotype is established for linkage analysis. Approximately 50% of affected individuals develop their first polyps by age 16, but the reliability of estimating the likelihood of gene carriage can be increased to more than 98% using the appropriate genetic probes.[219] Newer techniques are under development to screen for the presence of the truncated APC protein.

Attenuated Adenomatous Polyposis Coli

Other families without classical FAP or Gardner's syndrome nevertheless have a genetic disease predisposing to colorectal cancer that *maps* to the *APC* locus, indicating that there is additional phenotypic variation on the FAP theme. A large Utah kindred with a high incidence of colorectal cancer was studied in detail, and 2 of 51 family members had classic characteristics of FAP. Among the rest, there was a high incidence of cancer, with an average age of 54 years, but these patients had only 2 to 40 adenomatous polyps per colon—clearly not typical FAP. On careful investigation, other stigmata of FAP were occasionally found throughout the family. Using linkage analysis (and early-stage genetic markers that have been improved since), it was possible to determine with greater than 95% likelihood which family members inherited the same *APC*-linked allele as the individuals with the FAP-like features. In the four who carried the abnormal allele, all had adenomatous polyps (at ages 17, 26, 26, and 42), and of the 15 who did not inherit this allele, 14 were free of colorectal neoplasia, and one had a polyp at age 49.[229] Abnormalities in the *APC* gene can produce a variable clinical appearance that may not look like classical FAP, and this may explain some instances of familial clusters of cancer.

Another clinical syndrome of familial risk for cancer was initially called the hereditary flat adenoma syndrome (HFAS) because of the tendency to develop a moderate number of flat adenomas, up to 100, which had a propensity to occur in the proximal colon.[230,231] Members of these families are at high risk for colorectal cancer, but the median age for development of cancer is 57 years, more than 15 years later than that typically seen in FAP or HNPCC. Although it was first thought that this was a variation of HNPCC, the trait has been genetically linked to the *APC* locus, and it appears also to be an attenuated form of FAP.[232] On careful clinical examination, other features of FAP have been found in these families, including fundic gland polyps and periampullary neoplasia.[233]

Therefore, families with an increased risk for colorectal cancer, variable numbers of colorectal adenomas, and later onset of cancer with incomplete penetrance have what has been termed attenuated adenomatous polyposis coli (AAPC).[232] It is important to recognize the incomplete expression of classical FAP and to realize that carriers of the abnormal genes can be identified by linkage analysis to the *APC* gene and by other techniques, just as in the classical forms. It is known that the virulence of the FAP phenotype can be related to the location of the mutation on the *APC* gene.[234] There is evidence that the AAPC syndromes are produced by mutations at the extreme 5' end of the *APC* gene.[234a]

Hereditary Nonpolyposis Colorectal Cancer or Lynch Syndrome

A familial colon cancer syndrome has been identified in which nearly all affected members develop cancer but with features distinct from the polyposis syndromes; this has been termed HNPCC.[235-237] This syndrome, inherited as an autosomal dominant gene that produces colon cancer two to three decades earlier than typically seen, is associated with multiple primary colonic neoplasms, both synchronous and metachronous, and has a predilection for the proximal colon. The syndrome may be divided into two variants[236]: Lynch syndrome I, which includes the early-onset colorectal cancers, and Lynch syndrome II, also called cancer family syndrome,[238] which is characterized by the early onset of carcinoma at other sites, including the endometrium, ovaries, upper urinary tract, small intestine, and stomach[239-241] (Table 87-5). These variants were reviewed by Lynch and colleagues in 1993.[237] Common tumors such as those of the lung, breast, and prostate are not more common in these HNPCC families.[239,240] The extracolonic tumors are not uniformly distributed, and they tend to cluster in certain families, underscoring the necessity to obtain detailed information on tumor development.[237,239] The

---

TABLE 87-5
Hereditary Nonpolyposis Colorectal Cancer (Lynch Syndromes)

Lynch Syndrome I
Autosomal dominant inheritance; high penetrance
Early-onset colon cancers (mean age 40 years); risk begins in the twenties
Absence of antecedent multiple polyposis
Multiple primary cancers
    Multiple synchronous primaries in 18%
    Metachronous tumors accrue in 3%–5% per year
Increased proximal tumors (60%–80% proximal to the splenic flexure)
Increased mucinous adenocarcinomas (35%–39%)

Lynch Syndrome II (Cancer Family Syndrome)
All the features of Lynch syndrome I
Increased number and early occurrence of other adenocarcinomas
    Endometrium
    Ovaries
    Renal pelvis and ureters
    Stomach
    Small intestine
    Other sites

---

majority of HNPCC families have some extracolonic cancers, most commonly in the endometrium.[241]

The Lynch syndromes were first recognized in 1895, and the index family for Lynch syndrome II was followed up in 1971 with data on 650 relatives over six generations.[238] This carefully studied family argued strongly for a genetic rather than an environmental cause of this disease, since the progeny of each of the affected members of the initial kindred continued to show this characteristic, whereas the offspring of unaffected individuals did not. HNPCC has been reported from many countries throughout North America and Europe, but its prevalence is unknown. It has been estimated that the Lynch syndromes are the most common forms of familial colon cancer and may account for approximately 5% of cases of colon cancer.[242] However, using rigorous criteria for the diagnosis, others estimate the incidence to be on the order of 2% to 3% of all colorectal cancer.[243,244] Given the small family size most typical in industrialized countries, it is difficult to establish familiality for common illnesses with variable presentations. One group of investigators demonstrated that a broad clinical definition of HNPCC could include as many as 25% of families.[245]

The principal difficulty in making this diagnosis is that the phenotype is not necessarily distinctive, and no definitive premorbid markers have been identified. Criteria for a working definition of HNPCC for clinical studies, developed by an international collaborative group, have been referred to as the Amsterdam criteria. The diagnosis is made if a family has had all of the following: three or more relatives with a verified colorectal cancer, with one person being a first-degree relative of the other two; colorectal cancer involving at least two generations; and one or more cancers diagnosed in family members younger than 50 years of age. Using data bases collected in the United States—in which the likelihood of colorectal cancer by age 74 is 0.049 for men and 0.038 for women and 7% of the diagnoses are made in persons younger than 50 years of age—the Amsterdam criteria would be met by chance alone in 0.08% of families of eight people, if all have lived to 74 years of age, and if colorectal cancer had no familial clustering.[237] Because colorectal cancers are not randomly distributed among families, however, the number of such familial clusters is much higher. It is not necessary to meet all these criteria to make the diagnosis in clinical practice, because they are stringent and may exclude small affected families.

The penetrance of the *HNPCC* gene is very high, but the age at presentation varies. Occasionally, patients develop tumors at very young ages (i.e., in their teens) and may have malignant disease before it develops in the parent, creating the erroneous initial impression of a skipped generation.[246] Therefore, in considering this extreme degree of familiality, it is important to take family histories that include grandparents, aunts and uncles, and children.

A putative locus has been identified for the Lynch syndrome gene on chromosome 2p, initially named the familial colorectal cancer gene (*FCC*), but formally termed the *COCA1* locus. Only two large families showed definite linkage to this site, and several other families did not in the first report.[10] Linkage to other putative loci, such as the *APC* gene, the *p53* gene, and the *DCC* gene, have been excluded by linkage analysis for at least some typical families.[237] The colon tumors in these kindreds were more likely to be diploid and, as described previously, demonstrated a different form of DNA alteration than did sporadic tumors.[11]

In the general population, the majority of colorectal cancers occur in the distal colon, and only 23% to 32% occur proximal to the splenic flexure; in the Lynch syndromes, 65% to 88% of the tumors occur in the proximal colon.[237,238] Significantly more mucinous carcinomas are seen in HNPCC than in control cases (35%–39% and 20%, respectively).[247] A higher proportion of poorly differentiated tumors has been reported in HNPCC, but this may be a reflection of a large number of tumors with atypical cytologic features that have been overinterpreted. In fact, patients with these tumors are diagnosed at lower Dukes' stages and have a better survival rate than controls.[237]

Although diffuse polyposis does not occur in these syndromes, these cancers develop from preexisting adenomas,[247,248] and they appear to develop through a typical adenoma-to-carcinoma pathway. In a colonoscopic screening program, 30% had polyps, and they were more likely to be multiple, large, and villous compared with those in the general population.[249,250] The prevailing opinion is that the *HNPCC* gene may predispose for rapid growth and malignant conversion in benign adenomas. In only 40% of these patients is a positive family history available before the diagnosis of the tumor, which is unfortunate because the level of suspicion of cancer is usually low in young patients.[251] These patients have an extremely high likelihood of developing metachronous colorectal tumors, with mean annual cumulative rates of approximately 3% to 5%.[251] The mean age for developing the first tumor is approximately 40 years, and cancers occurring in patients in their twenties are not unusual.[230,236,251–253] At the time of initial diagnosis, 18% have multiple synchronous tumors, so it is inappropriate to treat this syndrome

with a limited segmental colonic resection. It has been suggested that this syndrome reflects a genetic abnormality in which aggressive adenoma progression occurs, but there is as yet no insight into the mechanism.

Torre's syndrome, a rare familial condition characterized by multiple sebaceous gland neoplasms and colorectal cancer, is clinically a subset of Lynch syndrome II.[254] It has recently been suggested that multiple mandibular osteomas, similar to those found in familial adenomatous polyposis, may be found in patients with Lynch syndrome II.[255] However, this has not been confirmed by other groups, and every line of laboratory investigation indicates that HNPCC is a distinct biological entity from the FAP syndromes.[256,257]

Common Variable Familiality for Colorectal Cancer

It has long been appreciated that a positive family history of colorectal neoplasia increases an individual's risk of cancer, even in the absence of obvious Mendelian inheritance patterns or early-onset disease. Evidence obtained from international epidemiologic studies, including changes in incidence in migrating populations, indicates that environmental factors play the greatest role in colon carcinogenesis. However, within high-incidence populations, familial factors may mediate differential susceptibility to environmental risk. For example, in Israel, European-born Jews have a higher incidence of colorectal cancer than non-European born Jews. However, the relative impact of genetic factors is higher in the latter group.[258]

Family histories were obtained from death certificates in a study of 209 patients treated for colorectal cancer at a referral center. Patients with familial adenomatous polyposis were excluded. The data obtained from these records were compared with estimates derived from mortality statistics using age- and gender-matched controls. Using this approach, the number of deaths from colorectal cancer was more than three times that expected from the hypothetical matched group. Although this experimental approach has obvious weaknesses, excess numbers of deaths were not seen from cancers of the bronchus, stomach, prostate, breast, or uterus. This study also revealed that the presence of multiple synchronous neoplasms (either benign or malignant) or a prior history of carcinoma or adenomas was associated with an increased likelihood of a positive family history. Furthermore, younger patients with colorectal cancer also were more likely to have relatives with this disease.[259]

A group of 154 asymptomatic subjects with one or more first-degree relatives with colorectal cancer underwent colonoscopy in a large health maintenance organization practice to determine the value of screening on the basis of a positive family history.[260] The mean age of this group was 54 years. Eighteen percent of the patients studied had colorectal adenomas, and a significant correlation was found between age and the prevalence of adenomas (Table 87-6). The point prevalence of carcinoma in this study was zero. The overall prevalence of colorectal neoplasms was not significantly greater than the estimated incidence of colorectal neoplasms drawn from autopsy studies; however, no control group was

TABLE 87-6
Colonoscopic Findings Among 154 Asymptomatic Subjects Screened Because of a Positive Family History for Colorectal Cancer*

AGE OF SUBJECTS (y)	NEGATIVE EXAMINATION	TUBULAR ADENOMAS		VILLOUS ADENOMAS	TOTAL NO. SUBJECTS
		2–4 mm	5–9 mm		
0–39	23 (96)	1 (4)			24
40–49	24 (86)	4 (14)			28
50–59	39 (81)	7 (15)	2 (4)		48
60–69	34 (77)	6 (14)	3 (7)	1 (2)	44
70+	6 (60)	3 (30)	1 (10)		10
Total	126 (82)	21 (14)	6 (4)	1 (1)	154

* Numbers in parentheses are percentages. Likelihood of finding adenomatous polyps increases with age, but no carcinomas were diagnosed in 154 patients, and only one patient had an adenoma larger than 9 mm in diameter.

From Grossman S, Milos ML. Colonscopic screening of persons with suspected risk factors for colon cancer: I. Family history. Gastroenterology 1988;94:395.

subjected to colonoscopy. The incidence of adenomas was approximately twice as great among subjects with two affected first-degree relatives than among those with only one. Thus, although the study does not refute the role of family history in susceptibility in colon cancer, the low yield at colonoscopic screening has important implications for surveillance management. Additional support for the observation that familial risk is proportional to the number of affected relatives came from an Australian case-control study which found that the odds ratio for colorectal cancer was 1.8 for one affected first-degree relative and 5.7 for two.[261]

By screening a large number of individuals, their spouses, and first-degree relatives using a 60-cm flexible proctosigmoidoscope, a significant impact of family history was found on the prevalence of distal colorectal neoplasia.[262] The investigators used pedigree analysis to identify whether any form of Mendelian genetics would describe the inheritance seen. Their data supported dominant inheritance of a susceptibility to colorectal neoplasms in the distal colon with a gene frequency of 19% in the general population. According to their analysis, the expression of the phenotype (i.e., penetrance) among gene carriers increased with age, reaching 63% by 80 years of age. Conversely, the penetrance for the nonsusceptible genotype was estimated to be zero (i.e., nonsusceptible families would develop no polyps). The gene for this has not been identified, and risk is probably not attributable to a single gene.

This genetic model implies that a segment of the population (19%) is more susceptible to distal colonic neoplasia on a familial basis, and that many of these susceptible individuals (i.e., 63%) will develop benign neoplasms by 80 years of age. Because approximately 5% to 6% of the population as a whole develop colon cancer, it could be further speculated that additional factors, presently unknown but possibly environmental, promote the development of malignant from benign neoplasms.

Prior Polyps and Cancers

In general, autopsy studies provide estimates that approximately 30% to 40% of colons contain adenomatous polyps, the vast majority of which are less than 1 cm in diameter.[263-268] Patients with adenomatous polyps constitute the principal group identified as being at elevated risk for the development of cancer. A traditionally cited study reported that patients with adenomas had a 50% risk of developing a metachronous adenoma after 15 years of observation, with a risk of one in 12 (for men) or one in 20 (for women) for developing a cancer in that time frame.[268]

Because the prevalence of adenomas is high, attempts have been made to identify subsets at greater risk of developing cancer. It is now appreciated that not all adenomas carry the same risk of recurrence to their host. A pair of retrospective Mayo Clinic studies reported that patients who had had small adenomas removed (i.e., those smaller than 1 cm) had a diminished risk for recurrent neoplasia, and their survival rate was not reduced compared with general risk estimates established for this community.[269,270] On the other hand, those with adenomas greater than 1 cm had an increased risk for cancer of 2.7 times that estimated for the general population.[270]

In a similar vein, the relative risk for rectal cancer was found to be 0.6 for patients who had small (<1 cm) rectal adenomas removed in a British study with an average follow-up period of almost 14 years. Contrariwise, the removal of large adenomas was associated with a relative risk for rectal cancer 2.1- and 2.6-fold greater for lesions of 1 to 2 cm and lesions of more than 2 cm in size, respectively.[271] Excess risk of rectal cancer was 3.8-fold after removal of villous adenomas and 5.1-fold after removal of adenomas containing severe dysplasia (i.e., carcinoma in situ). No increased risk followed the removal of multiple lesions. Risk for colon cancer (above the reach of the rigid sigmoidoscope) was increased 3.3-, 5.0-, and 5.9-fold after the removal of severely dysplastic, villous, and large (>2 cm) lesions, respectively, and a 4.8-fold increase was seen after the removal of two or more rectal adenomas.[271] Therefore, risk estimation depends on the size, number, and histology of the index lesions, and single, small (<1 cm) adenomas probably do not predict an increased risk of recurrent neoplasia.

It is more difficult to estimate the actual incidence of metachronous cancers from the literature, and the results are influenced by the amount of colon removed during the first operation and the duration of follow-up. The best estimate is that about 5% of patients will develop a second cancer after the removal of a primary colorectal cancer.[272] It may not be possible to refine this estimate in the future because of the practice of removing all adenomas during surveillance colonoscopy of colon cancer patients.

Inflammatory Bowel Disease

Patients with chronic inflammatory bowel disease are at increased risk to develop gastrointestinal cancer. The degree of risk, however, has been a subject of debate. A British study of 624 patients at a referral center indicated that 3.5% of their patients developed colorectal cancer, which was approximately seven times as many as expected in the general population.[273] The diagnosis of cancer in this condition was made at an average age of 41 years (range 20–74 years). Relatively fewer of these cancers occurred in the rectum (22%) compared with the expected rate in the general population (38%). Thus, there are important differences in clinical presentation in the setting of inflammatory bowel disease, the most important of these being age.

The duration of inflammatory bowel disease is a critical factor in predicting the likelihood of developing adenocarcinoma of the colon.[274] A retrospective study of 267 referral patients with ulcerative colitis from New York revealed a 10% incidence of colon cancer. Cancer was more likely to occur among patients with pancolitis (13%) than among those with only left-sided disease (5%), and the latter group tended to develop cancer a decade later than the former. The incidence of colorectal cancer was less than 1% during the first decade of disease but progressively rose to 7% in the second decade, 16% in the third decade, and 53% in the fourth.

It has been suggested that the high incidence of cancer complicating ulcerative colitis may be a reflection of bias in patient selection from referral centers. A review of the clinical courses of 258 patients treated for ulcerative colitis in a private practice revealed a cancer incidence of 7% after 26 years and 11% after 32 years of disease.[275] The majority of these patients had less than universal colitis, and patients who were referred with known colon cancer were excluded from the analysis. The authors suggested that the inclusion of a relatively small number of patients referred because of cancer could produce a large impact in the apparent risk of this disease.

Geographic factors may also be important in influencing the risk of neoplasia in the setting of colitis. The incidence of cancer among children referred to a large referral center in the United States[276] was similar to that reported in Great Britain.[273] Cancer developed in 3% of the patients during the first 10 years after the onset of colitis but incidence was increased

by 20% in each of the next two decades, and was estimated to be 43% at 35 years after the onset of their disease. Contrariwise, a center receiving referrals throughout Czechoslovakia reported a cumulative cancer risk of zero at 10 years, 5% at 20 years, 15% at 30 years, and 20% at 35 years,[277] even though the incidence of colorectal cancer is high in that country.[21] Although this was a large study consisting of 959 patients, only 32% of the patients had colitis of the entire colon, and a majority of the group (60%) had been followed for less than 10 years. Thus, it is not clear whether the differences reported in the literature reflect geographic differences in the incidence of this complication or whether all of the increased risk is the result of greater extent and duration of disease.

Patients with Crohn's disease are also at increased risk for colorectal cancer; however, the incidence is lower than that reported with ulcerative colitis.[278] It is not yet possible to accurately estimate the risk of cancer in this setting; however, an excess of carcinomas of the colon, small intestine, stomach, and anus, as well as an excess of lymphomas, have been reported.[278-280]

The survival rate of patients who develop cancers in the setting of ulcerative colitis is similar to that seen for noncolitic patients.[281] This is perhaps disappointing because these patients are subjected to routine surveillance including a high index of suspicion for cancer. However, a complicating carcinoma is unlikely to produce unique symptoms early in its natural history, and these tumors may be difficult to diagnose even if viewed colonoscopically in the setting of inflammation and mucosal distortion. In addition, the natural biology of cancers in ulcerative colitis may be different from that of sporadic ones (see Chap. 24). To improve the early detection and survival from colon cancer in colitics, attempts have been made to identify early neoplastic lesions.

Dysplasia is currently the best marker for early cancer in this setting. Developing a standardized classification for dysplasia has been a major undertaking, because inflammation and attendant repair can be easily confused for early neoplasia.[282] True dysplasia is an early benign neoplastic lesion, and biologically it is analogous to adenomatous tissue. Just as it is difficult to predict the clinical behavior of a small adenoma, low-grade dysplasia is a troublesome lesion, and the predictive value for higher grades of neoplasia has been controversial.[283] Low-grade dysplasia in a biopsy may have three interpretations. First, it may reflect inflammation and be a transient change. Second, it may reflect the presence of a higher grade lesion (such as cancer) immediately adjacent to the biopsy site. Third, it may be a harbinger of a generalized problem in the colon, with additional neoplastic lesions elsewhere. Dysplasia in a plaque or elevated mass is especially worrisome and suggests the need to consider colectomy.[284] If low grades of dysplasia are found in random biopsies of flat mucosa, this is less likely to be associated with a synchronous cancer, but it is still a worrisome lesion. At this time, the management of low-grade dysplasia in ulcerative colitis is as troublesome as the management of small adenomatous polyps in the noncolitic colon. High-grade dysplasia is somewhat less ambiguous and is a worrisome finding; if it is found in a colonic mass, total colectomy should be given serious consideration. After examination of the surgical specimens, most of these colons are found to have either confirmed high-grade dysplasia (which is the equivalent of carcinoma in situ) or a frank, invasive cancer.

Colon Cancer in Patients With Nonadenomatous Polyposis Syndromes

Juvenile polyposis coli.   Juvenile polyposis coli is an entity which is frequently familial and is characterized by the development of nonneoplastic juvenile polyps in the colon. These polyps typically occur in childhood and become clinically manifest by bleeding or prolapsing. A small number of affected individuals develop colorectal cancer at an early age.[285,286] Pathologic examinations of juvenile polyps reveal that some of them contain an admixture of adenomatous epithelium.[286,287] Juvenile polyposis coli is quite distinct from familial polyposis coli, because in the former disorder juvenile polyps develop in the first decade of life, and the manifestation of the disorder may end by adulthood. In contrast, familial adenomatous polyposis consists of adenomatous polyps which first develop during adolescence. It is critical to differentiate these disorders. Juvenile polyposis is associated with a relatively low risk of cancer, in direct proportion to the adenomatous tissue present in the lesions, whereas all of the lesions in familial adenomatous polyposis are neoplastic, and colectomy is recommended for all affected patients.

Peutz-Jeghers syndrome.   Peutz-Jeghers syndrome is another autosomal dominate hereditary disease with characteristic nonneoplastic polyps and skin pigmentation. A proportion of these patients (approximately 13%) develop gastrointestinal carcinomas, and these occur at uncharacteristically early ages.[288,289] Therefore, the risk of developing colorectal cancer is substantially lower in the hamartomatosis syndromes compared with the adenomatosis syndromes, and a prophylactic colectomy is not warranted in these patients. However, all excised hamartomas should be carefully examined for evidence of adenomatous epithelium. The admixture of neoplastic tissue in these polyps suggests a risk of cancer and should prompt the initiation of routine colonoscopic surveillance.

Other Clinical Associations

Dietary history.   As mentioned in the initial section on epidemiology, one would expect to find more cancers in patients who ingest a high-fat, low-fiber, meat-rich diet, and obese, hypercholesterolemic patients would seem to be a target group for the disease. However, the diet is relatively uniform within high-risk populations, and the variation in fat intake among individuals is too minor compared with the general characteristics of the diet to make dietary history valuable for selective screening. Other features have therefore been sought to identify high-risk individuals, generally without success.

Colon cancer and cholecystectomy.   It has been suggested that patients who have undergone cholecystectomy may be at a greater risk of developing colon cancer. However, the data on this issue have been inconsistent. Cholecystectomy has been implicated as a cause for an excess of cancers among women,[290] for an increased incidence of proximal colon cancers,[291] and for an increased incidence of adenomas.[292] It has

been difficult to confirm the association between cholecystectomy and adenomatous polyps,[293,294] and other groups have suggested that the association with colon cancer is weak or absent.[295,296] Several recent studies and one meta-analysis have demonstrated no excess in the risk of either adenomas or carcinomas after cholecystectomy. It is reasonable to disregard neoplastic risk when making decisions regarding gall bladder surgery, and there is no need for extra surveillance in patients who have had this operation.[297-299]

Endocrine abnormalities.   Acromegalic patients have a threefold excess of colon cancers.[300] The role played by growth hormone has not been explored. Elevated serum gastrin levels are seen in patients with colorectal cancer,[301] and a postoperative reduction has been seen after surgery.[302] There is evidence that gastrin undergoes alternate processing in normal and neoplastic colon[303] and may function as an autocrine hormone to support the growth of tumor cells.[304]

Skin tags.   The presence of acrochordons (skin tags) suggests the simultaneous presence of colonic polyps. In a study of 94 men referred for colonoscopy, 48 had skin tags, usually located in the axilla, upper chest, or neck, and 46 did not. Among the group with skin tags, 77% had colonic polyps; in the subgroup without skin tags, 20% had colonic polyps.[305] An attempt to confirm this in an unselected group of 492 men in a primary care clinic, skin tags were found in 46% of patients. Flexible sigmoidoscopy revealed polyps in 10% of individuals with skin tags, but 8% of those without skin tags also had polyps.[306] A review of the collected studies of this issue concluded that skin tags have prognostic significance only in symptomatic patients, therefore, this finding is of little practical significance.[307] Skin tags also do not correlate with carriage of the gene for familial adenomatous polyposis.[308]

Colon cancer and *Streptococcus bovis*.   Patients with carcinoma of the colon occasionally present with septicemia or endocarditis caused by *Streptococcus bovis*.[309,310] *S bovis* may be cultured from the feces of 10% to 16% of healthy subjects, but it is significantly more prevalent in the stools of cancer patients. In a study of 29 patients with *S bovis* septicemia, 16 were found to have gastrointestinal neoplasms, and nearly half of the group did not undergo a complete diagnostic evaluation.[310] *S bovis* endocarditis has also been reported as the presenting symptom in one patient with familial adenomatous polyposis.[311] The presence of *S bovis* in the blood should prompt a complete gastrointestinal evaluation, beginning with the colon, and, if this is negative, should include an evaluation of the esophagus and the stomach. Septicemia produced by other members of the group D streptococcus family (*Streptococcus equinus*) has also been associated with colon cancer.[312]

Breath methane.   One hypothesis has implicated the role of anaerobic flora in colonic carcinogenesis. Several laboratories have reported that colon cancer patients are more likely to be breath methane excreters than the general population, presumably reflecting this difference.[313] It has been shown that the elevated methane production falls to normal after the cancer is resected, suggesting that the presence of the tumor influences methane production and that increased methane production may be a result of colon cancer rather than a reflection of a preexisting abnormality in the colonic flora.[314] Increased methane production was also reported in patients with familial polyposis and extensive ulcerative colitis in this study. Because there is a strong correlation between the methane excreter status of an individual and the status of other family members, these observations potentially have broad implications. However, breath methane measurements in more than 1000 people from South Africa from four population groups with wide differences in colon cancer risk demonstrated marked interethnic differences but no relation to cancer risk.[315] Furthermore, methane excretion is strongly affected by the use of laxatives or antibiotics and must be interpreted with caution.

Other features.   Additional risk factors for colorectal cancers have been identified, but these generally are derived from exceptional circumstances. As previously mentioned, women who have been *irradiated* for gynecologic cancer have a 2- to 3.6-fold increased risk for colorectal cancer.[29] Populations infected with *Schistosoma haematobium* may develop colon cancers in the immediate vicinity of the polyps produced by the parasite eggs.[23] Patients who have undergone an implantation of the ureter into the sigmoid colon are at risk to develop carcinomas, adenomas, or severe dysplasia in the vicinity of the *ureterosigmoidostomy*.[316] In a study of 34 such individuals, 29% had developed one of these neoplastic lesions at a mean interval of 22 years after their urinary diversion.

Bloom's syndrome is an autosomal recessive form of congenital dwarfism associated with unusual facies and hypersensitivity to sunlight.[317] This syndrome has been anecdotally associated with colorectal cancer; however, its rarity makes it difficult to document the actual incidence. The linkage of this disease with colon cancer is of interest primarily because of the high frequency of sister chromatid exchange,[317] hypersensitivity to near-ultraviolet radiation, and excessive DNA strand breakage in fibroblasts from these patients.[318]

It has been suggested that patients with *Barrett's esophagus* may be at increased risk for colonic cancer,[319,320] and one small prospective, controlled, colonoscopic study of 36 patients with Barrett's esophagus revealed three cancers and nine adenomas, two of which had severe dysplasia. The authors boldly suggested that such patients might benefit more from colonoscopic surveillance than screening of the esophagus.[321]

Patients with irritable bowel syndrome and diverticulosis[322] have no increased risk for colorectal cancer. Patients with these disorders have symptoms attracting attention to their lower gastrointestinal tracts; however, there is no need for extra surveillance for cancer among these patients.

PATHOLOGY

The overwhelming majority of colorectal cancers are adenocarcinomas, and most cancers represent malignant conversion occurring in a preexisting adenomatous lesion. As a result, a spectrum of lesions may be found, ranging from the small adenomatous neoplasm containing no more than low-grade dysplasia and no immediate ability to invade or metastasize, at one end of the spectrum, to the poorly differentiated adenocarcinoma with an unlimited capacity for local and distant spread, at the other.

Gross Pathology

Colon cancers develop within preexisting foci of adenomatous tissue. This occurs usually, but not always, in a polypoid lesion. Adenomatous change may occur in flat mucosa, and under unusual circumstances, a cancer may develop in this setting. Therefore, tiny cancers in flat mucosa are reported, but only rarely.[323–325] These represent instances in which malignant conversion occurred early in the natural history of the neoplastic lesion, and they should be considered the exception to the rule. In vitro models have demonstrated that colon carcinoma cells secrete proteases that permit destruction of adenomatous tissue and confer a growth advantage to the malignant cells, which is enhanced by the addition of a tumor promoter to the culture system.[326]

Colon cancers characteristically begin as round mass lesions, but deviations from the ideal shape occur as a result of the asymmetric sloughing of cells and the emergence of clones with rapid growth capacity (Fig. 87-7). If the resected colon is opened, a cancer typically has an elevated advancing edge, and the lumenal aspect is usually ulcerated and irregular. After the diameter of a cancer approaches the circumference of the colon, the opposite edges of the tumor converge, creating the characteristic apple-core lesion described by radiologists. This most often occurs in the sigmoid colon, which has the smallest circumference.

The older literature states that 75% of cancers are present in the rectum and sigmoid colon, making them accessible to detection by sigmoidoscopy. Numerous investigators have observed a change in the distribution of tumors over the past several decades, with a larger percentage of lesions being found in the proximal colon.[327–331] This appears to a result, in part, of the fact that proximal colonic cancers are more common among people older than 65 years of age; as the population ages, a greater number of proximal colon cancers would be expected.[327,328] There appears to be a marked decrease in rectal carcinomas, with corresponding increases in sigmoid cancers and proximal lesions.[331] However, even after correcting for age, investigators from several countries have reported a shift from a predominance of rectal tumors to those located more proximally,[328–330] and in some registries, the fall in rectal cancer has been particularly dramatic.[331]

It has been estimated that approximately one quarter of cancers may be detected with a rigid sigmoidoscope, and this may be increased to approximately two thirds by the use of the 65-cm flexible sigmoidoscope, depending on the depth of the examination (Fig. 87-8). However, a substantial proportion of lesions (at least one third) is missed with the more limited examinations, and approximately one quarter of colorectal cancers are in the cecum and ascending colon, which is the most challenging part of the colon for imaging and visualization.[332] The changing location of colon cancers has obvious implications for clinical management. Although it has not been proven, it may be that environmental factors

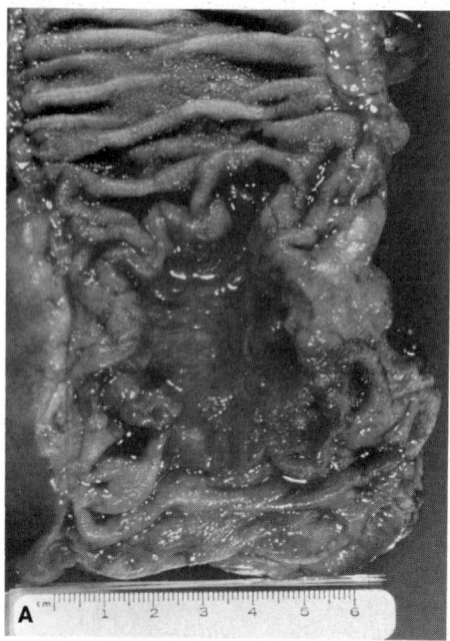 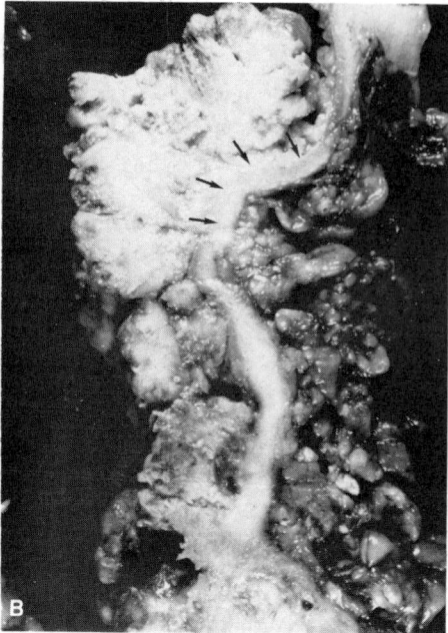

FIGURE 87-7. (**A**) A typical adenocarcinoma of the sigmoid colon has heaped-up edges and an ulcerated center as demonstrated by this en face view of the tumor. (**B**) A cross section of a Dukes' class A colon tumor demonstrates the polypoid mass (*right*) invading the white muscularis propria (*arrows*). This tumor did not infiltrate to the serosa and did not involve the regional lymph nodes, and therefore is a class A lesion with an excellent prognosis, in spite of its bulk.

are increasing the risk for colorectal cancer and that screening measures and polypectomy—which are more effective for the distal colon—have simultaneously decreased cancer incidence in the sigmoid colon and rectum.

It is not rare to find multiple primary colorectal cancers. Multiple lesions are generally divided into those that occur simultaneously (synchronous lesions) and those that occur in different time frames (metachronous lesions). Synchronous colorectal cancers occur in 3% to 6% of de novo colon cancer diagnoses.[333–335] The lesions may be either near one another or located in different portions of the colon. The incidence of multiple synchronous lesions is significantly higher in the setting of FAP or ulcerative colitis, in which it occurs in 21% and 18% of patients, respectively.[336] Synchronous adenomatous polyps are found in 36% of patients.[335] Multiple primary neoplastic lesions occur often enough that total colonoscopy is an essential part of the work-up if a neoplastic lesion is found at a more limited examination. This permits the removal of synchronous polyps and the detection of synchronous cancers, which also modifies the surgical approach.

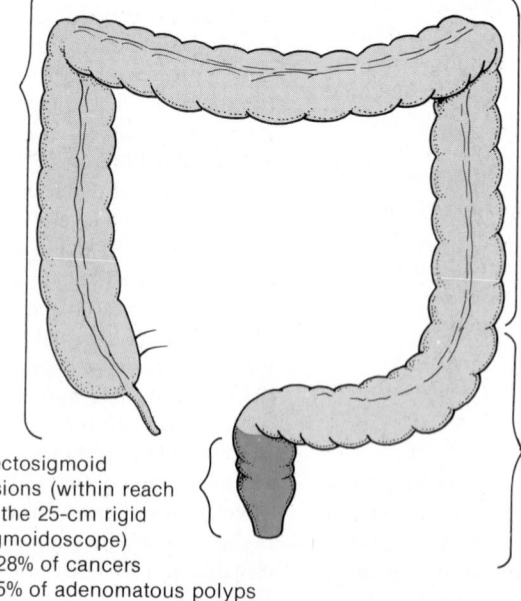

Proximal colonic lesions (above the reach of the 65-cm flexible sigmoidoscope) 36% of cancers 34% of adenomatous polyps

Distal colorectal lesions (within the reach of the 65-cm flexible sigmoidoscope) 64% of cancers 66% of adenomatous polyps

Rectosigmoid lesions (within reach of the 25-cm rigid sigmoidoscope) 28% of cancers 5% of adenomatous polyps

FIGURE 87-8. Distribution of neoplasms in the colon and rectum.

Microscopic Pathology and Tumor Staging

Most colorectal cancers are adenocarcinomas (Fig. 87-9). However, squamous cell carcinomas, adenosquamous carcinomas, lymphomas, and endocrine tumors such as carcinoids also occur in the colon. Most colonic adenocarcinomas are moderately or well differentiated tumors, and there are few morphologic features of prognostic significance among them. Approximately 20% of adenocarcinomas are poorly differentiated or undifferentiated tumors, and these two types are well known to be associated with a poorer outcome. Most adenocarcinomas secrete a small or moderate amount of mucin. Approximately 10% to 20% of tumors may be described as mucinous or colloid carcinomas on the basis of a more prodigious production of mucin. These tumors are associated with a poorer 5-year survival rate than nonmucinous tumors.[337,338]

The classification of tumor invasion was first undertaken by Dukes for rectal carcinoma.[339] The Dukes' staging has undergone many modifications, and one must define the stages precisely for purposes of discussion because there is no standard classification. A system that is perhaps a consensus of most common usage is as follows (Fig. 87-10):

Carcinoma in situ (also called high-grade dysplasia) is intramucosal carcinoma that does not penetrate the muscularis mucosae.

Stage A tumors invade through the muscularis mucosae into the submucosa but do not reach the next layer, the muscularis propria.

Stage B1 tumors invade into the muscularis propria, and B2 lesions completely penetrate the smooth muscle layer to the serosa.

Stage C lesions encompass any degree of apparent invasion but are defined by regional lymph node involvement.

Some studies subdivide Stage C lesions based upon the number of lymph nodes involved, with C1 lesions having 1 to 3 (or 4) involved, and C2 having more positive nodes.[340] The presence and number of involved lymph nodes is, however, entirely dependent on the number of nodes resected and examined pathologically, which may explain some of the inconsistencies in the literature. Stage D lesions include all those with distant metastases. There is a reasonably close relation between the histologic grade of the tumor and the stage of malignancy.[341]

The relation between advancing stage and cancer mortality has been repeatedly demonstrated.[339–342] There is no important relation between the apparent tumor size in the colonic lumen and outcome. The aggressiveness of a colorectal tumor is reflected by its ability to invade, and growth into the colonic lumen is irrelevant to this biological characteristic, except to the degree that it reflects the increasing probability that an invasive clone has had the opportunity to arise in the tumor.

In an attempt to create more uniform pathologic categories for clinical studies, the American Joint Commission on Cancer (AJCC) and the Union Internationale Contra le Cancer (UICC) have classified many tumors by a TNM system. This classification is outlined as follows:

Tis refers to carcinoma in situ, T1 indicates submucosal invasion (i.e., Dukes' stage A), T2 indicates invasion of the muscularis propria (Dukes' B1), T3 indicates invasion through the muscularis propria into the subserosa or perirectal tissues (Dukes' B2), and T4 indicates invasion into adjacent organs or tissues (sometimes referred to as stage B3).

N classes include: N0, no involved lymph nodes; N1, 1 to 3 regional lymph node metastases (as in Dukes' C1); N2, more than 3 regional lymph node metastases (Dukes' C2); and N3, a metastasis along the course of a major blood vessel.

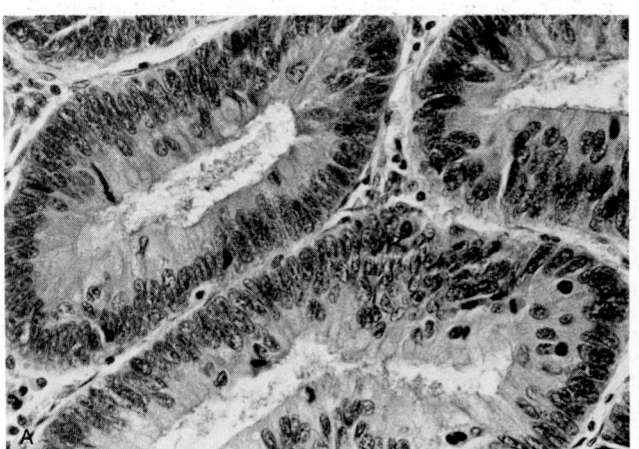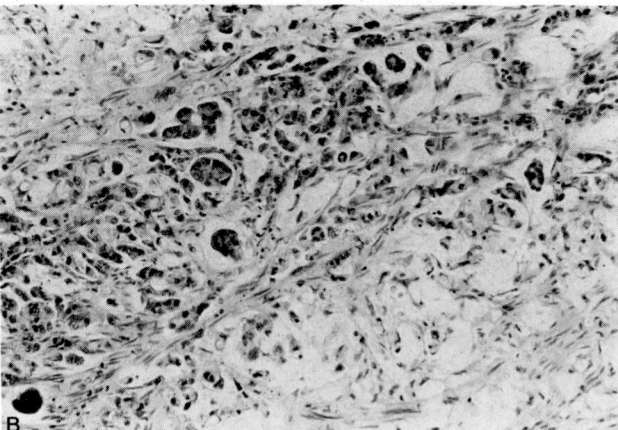

FIGURE 87-9. **(A)** A well-differentiated adenocarcinoma of the colon demonstrates the characteristic gland-like formation. In each of these glands, the nuclei are large, the chromatin is poorly condensed, and the nuclei tend to drift away from the basal lamina. Mitoses are common. **(B)** In a mucin-producing or colloid carcinoma, the cancer cells (*dark nuclei*) are suspended in pools of mucin, which is unstained in this section. The typical gland-like configuration is not seen. This microscopic appearance is associated with a more aggressive tumor.

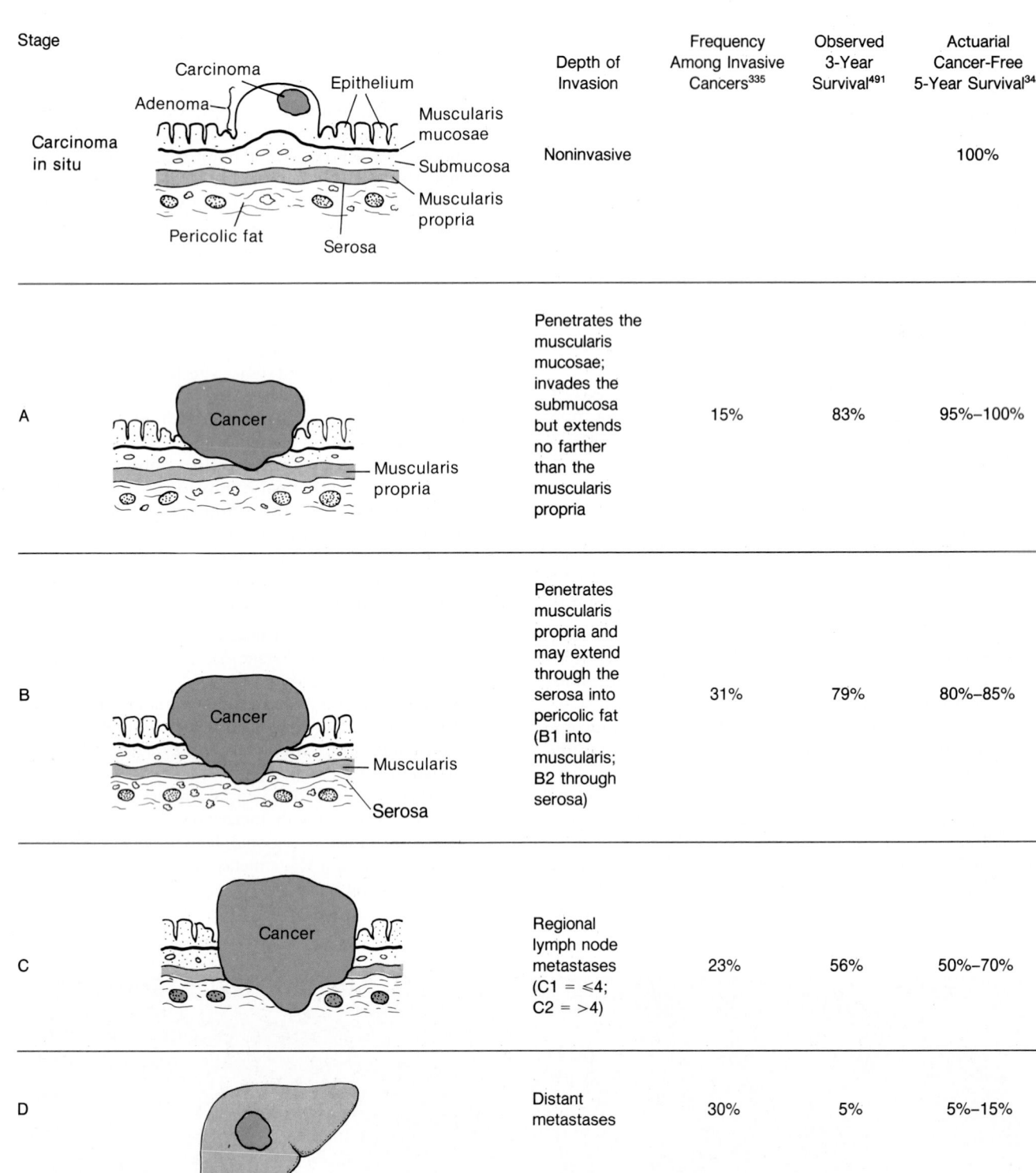

Stage		Depth of Invasion	Frequency Among Invasive Cancers[335]	Observed 3-Year Survival[491]	Actuarial Cancer-Free 5-Year Survival[342]
Carcinoma in situ		Noninvasive			100%
A		Penetrates the muscularis mucosae; invades the submucosa but extends no farther than the muscularis propria	15%	83%	95%–100%
B		Penetrates muscularis propria and may extend through the serosa into pericolic fat (B1 into muscularis; B2 through serosa)	31%	79%	80%–85%
C		Regional lymph node metastases (C1 = ≤4; C2 = >4)	23%	56%	50%–70%
D		Distant metastases	30%	5%	5%–15%

FIGURE 87-10. Numerous classifications have been proposed for colorectal cancer. Demonstrated here is the Dukes-Turnbull classification, but it is not the only classification currently in use. Of potential importance are subclassifications in classes B and C. Subclass B1 has been proposed to include invasion to the muscularis propria but not through the serosa. Subclass B2 includes tumors that penetrate the serosa to the pericolic fat but do not have regional lymph node or distant metastases. Patients with B1 lesions have a better prognosis and 5-year survival rate than patients with subtype B2 lesions. Class C lesions have been subdivided into C1, with four or fewer involved regional lymph node metastases and C2, with more than four involved regional lymph nodes. Patients with subtype C1 lesions have a better outcome than patients with C2 lesions. The observed 3-year survival and actuarial cancer-free 5-year survivals are estimated for each stage. The actuarial survival estimates reflect excessive disease-related mortality from the cancer, and the crude survival rates are considerably lower because of comorbidity.

Metastatic status is divided into M0 (no distant metastases) and M1 (metastases present).[343,344]

Table 87-7 provides estimated 5-year survival rates for rectal cancers according to Dukes', Astler-Coller, and TNM staging systems.[343]

Additional microscopic features of rectal cancers defined by Jass and colleagues have been found to correlate with survival. This classification considers the observation that the following three factors correlated best with more aggressive tumors and reduced 5-year survival: spread through the bowel wall and lymph node metastasis (as noted by all other systems); absence of lymphocytic infiltration; and an assessment of whether the invasive margin of the tumor is infiltrating (i.e., more aggressive) or expanding (i.e., less aggressive). Numerical scores were assigned to each of these features, and a high degree of correlation with outcome was found by linear regression analysis.[345]

Several groups have used flow cytometry to measure the relative DNA content, or ploidy, of colorectal cancers.[346–349] Tumors with normal DNA content are diploid, and those containing cells with abnormal DNA content are aneuploid. There has been consensus agreement that diploid and near-diploid tumors have significantly better prognoses than aneuploid tumors, and that this parameter is prognostic independent of Dukes' or other stage (up to the point of distant metastases, after which all patients do poorly). The use of flow cytometry is not yet indicated in routine clinical practice, because no prospective study has demonstrated that it can be used to direct therapeutic decision making.

TABLE 87-7
Five-Year Survival in Colon Cancer By Tumor Stage

STAGE	INVASION	FIVE-YEAR SURVIVAL FOR RECTAL CANCER (%)
Dukes		
A	(submucosal)	85
B	(perirectal tissues)	64
C	(nodal metastasis)	33
D	(distant metastasis)	
Astler-Coller		
A	(intra mucosal)	100
B1	(muscularis propria)	67
B2	(perirectal)	54
C1	(B1 + nodal metastasis)	43
C2	(B2 + nodal metastasis)	22
TNM		
0	Tis, N0, M0	100
I	T1, N0, M0	100
	T2, N0, M0	85
II	T3, N0, M0	70
	T4, N0, M0	30
III	any T, N1, M0	60
	any T, N2 or N3, M0	30
IV	any T, any M, M1	3

From Fisher ER, Sass R, Palekar A, et al. Dukes' classification revisited. Findings from the national surgical adjuvant breast and bowel projects (protocol R-01). Cancer 1989;64:2354.

Several investigators from Japan have recognized that some patients may develop early cancers of the colon that appear to arise de novo, in that they are lesions less than 1 cm in size and there is no evidence that they arose in a preexisting adenoma.[350,351] It is not yet clear how commonly carcinoma arises directly from normal colonic tissue without an early adenomatous stage or whether this variant represents the early conversion of a microadenoma to carcinoma that has been fortuitously detected as a small lesion.

One pathologic variant bears mention because of the possibility for misinterpretation. *Colitis cystica profunda* represents the displacement of mucus-secreting cells beneath the normal epithelium, usually as a result of surgery, other trauma, or inflammation. This produces an abnormal, mass-like configuration to the overlying mucosa. A biopsy reveals pools of mucus in the submucosa which may be mistaken for invasive colloid carcinoma. If this is seen in the head of an adenomatous polyp, it is referred to as pseudoinvasion.[352] This lesion may also occur at the site of a prior surgical anastomosis, and it can be a problem to correctly identify. In general, anastomotic recurrences are relatively uncommon except at the site of a resection in the rectum or at the rectosigmoid junction, where the surgeon may have taken an inadequate margin of mucosa adjacent to the tumor in an attempt to preserve the rectum. Furthermore, recurrences are likely to be histologically similar to the initial tumor. Therefore, the pathologist should carefully assess the cytologic characteristics of the cells in the biopsy if this entity is being considered.

The colonic epithelium immediately adjacent to a colon cancer is thicker than normal, is characterized by a distortion of the normal architecture, and shows an increase in sialomucin compared with normal tissues, in which sulfomucins normally predominate.[353,354] It was initially suggested that *transitional mucosa* was a field of premalignant tissue from which tumors arise. However, similar morphologic and histochemical changes are found adjacent to nonneoplastic colonic lesions[355] and lesions metastatic to the colon. The accumulated data suggest that transitional mucosa is hyperplastic epithelium that has developed in response to an adjacent tumor or other pathologic condition.[356] The presence of sialomucins in the mucosa at the margin of surgical resection predicts an anastomotic recurrence and is an adverse prognostic variable.[357]

DIFFERENTIAL DIAGNOSIS

As previously discussed, symptomatic colon cancers may present in several ways:

- as a partial or complete lower gastrointestinal obstruction
- as overt gastrointestinal bleeding (i.e., hematochezia)
- as a locally invasive or expanding tumor with invasion of the perirectal tissue, bladder, or other pelvic organs; fistulous connection with another portion of the gastrointestinal tract; or as a locally expanding metastatic lesion in the liver, bone, or other site
- less commonly, as a systemic wasting disease (i.e., cancer cachexia).

All of these symptoms carry a substantial list of possibilities in the differential diagnosis.

If a patient presents with gastrointestinal obstruction, the first step is to determine the level of the obstruction, most typically with flat plate and upright abdominal radiographs. A tumor in the cecum may obstruct the ileocecal valve and produce a selective small bowel obstruction. Alternatively, an obstructing tumor may occur at any point throughout the colon. Diseases that most commonly produce this clinical picture are tumors, diverticulitis, inflammatory masses (either in the setting of inflammatory bowel disease or an acute infectious process), postinflammatory strictures, and volvulus. A more complete differential diagnosis of lesions that may present as a colonic mass or obstruction and thereby mimic colon cancer is given in Table 87-8.

Colorectal neoplasms begin to lose blood early in their natural history, but most patients are unaware of this blood loss. Most colon cancers lose less than 10 mL of blood per day, and patients are not likely to notice this bleeding unless it is deposited on the surface of a formed stool from a lesion in the distal colon or rectum. If a patient observes bright rectal bleeding, it may represent bleeding from hemorrhoids or an anal fissure. Patients with inflammatory bowel disease commonly experience rectal bleeding, so this is not a reliable sign of early neoplasia. Bleeding from ischemic bowel disease or a diverticulum is usually more brisk than that seen from a neoplasm.

Sometimes, a locally invasive carcinoma can be difficult to differentiate from an inflammatory process, even if visualized endoscopically or surgically. A mass produced by a perforated diverticulum can be bulky and indurated, suggesting a neoplastic process, but biopsies from an inflammatory mass may not be diagnostic. Furthermore, certain entities may give rise to an ambiguous biopsy, including colitis cystica profunda, which may occur at a surgical anastomosis, and endometriosis.

DIAGNOSTIC APPROACHES TO COLON CANCER

Several distinct issues associated with the diagnosis of colorectal neoplasia overlap to some degree and are frequently confused. The first of these involves the work-up of the patient with symptoms of colonic obstruction, bleeding, or a locally invasive disease as described previously. Closely related to this is the work-up of a positive test for occult fecal bleeding in a patient without other symptoms. Finally, there is the controversial issue of screening the asymptomatic patient.

Symptomatic Patients

In the symptomatic patient, colonic disease may be strongly suspected, but cancer is only one item in the differential diagnosis. The presence of a guaiac-positive stool increases the suspicion of colonic disease, but a negative test does not exclude it.[358] These patients require either colonoscopy or a barium enema plus sigmoidoscopy to evaluate the colon. If the patient is not obstructed and there is no suspicion of perforation, the patient's colon should be cleansed and colonoscopy is the diagnostic procedure of choice. Colonoscopy is the most accurate and sensitive diagnostic modality currently available, and it permits the biopsy of suspicious mucosal lesions. The complication rate (including perforation and hemorrhage) is less than five cases per 1000 patients. This is discussed in more detail in Chapters 116 and 118.

The barium enema is a less sensitive diagnostic procedure, and removal of the administered barium is required for colonoscopic verification of any suspected lesions. Nonetheless, a barium enema may provide important complementary information not available using colonoscopy, especially if there is a colonic stricture or obstruction, or when one is dealing with an extrinsic lesion. In evaluating a patient for specific colonic symptoms, the absence of blood in the stool should not dissuade one from evaluation with colonoscopy or barium enema.

Estimating Risk For Colorectal Cancer

In determining the appropriate evaluation in a patient with symptoms that may be referable to the colon, it is helpful to focus on risk factors that make the presence of colorectal cancer more likely. Patients younger than 40 years of age are relatively unlikely to have cancer unless they have ulcerative

---

TABLE 87-8
Lesions That May Mimic Colon Cancer

Mass Lesions
Benign tumors
Diverticulitis
Inflammatory masses
   Ulcerative colitis
   Crohn's colitis
   Tuberculosis
   Amebiasis
   Fungal masses (e.g., mucor)
   Schistosomiasis
   Viral lesions (CMV, LGV)
   Cronkhite-Canada Syndrome
Fatty ileocecal valve
Colitis cystica profunda
Surgical anastomoses
Feces (x-ray diagnosis)
Solitary rectal ulcer
Endometriosis
Appendectomy stump
Lymphoid polyps/lymphoma
Carcinoid tumors
Metastatic lesions
Kaposi's sarcoma
Extrinsic compression
   Submucosal mass
   Submucosal hematoma
   Extrinsic mass

Obstructing Lesions
Strictures
   Late sequellae of inflammation
   Radiation
   Ischemic colitis
Volvulus
Extrinsic compression
   Endometriosis
   Pancreatitis

colitis, FAP, or its variants (i.e., AAPC) or come from a Lynch's syndrome kindred. At 40 years of age, the incidence of colorectal cancer begins to rise, but it remains relatively low until 50 years of age and older, when the risk rapidly accelerates. The risk of colorectal cancer continues to rise relentlessly with each decade thereafter, and age is the greatest single risk factor for colorectal cancer. Table 87-9 presents age-specific incidences of colorectal cancer.[359] Genetic factors play a special role in colorectal cancer, but the majority of patients do not have any genetic risk factors that are identifiable at this time. A more important issue to consider is a history of adenomatous polyps, because these are the precursor lesions for cancers. One should pay particular attention to patients with multiple adenomas, large adenomas, or adenomas containing villous features or carcinoma in situ.[271]

Diagnostic Work-Ups

A broad range of diagnostic studies is available to evaluate the possibility of colorectal neoplasia. First, it is important not to overlook the *visual inspection* and *digital examination* of the anus and distal rectum, even if additional studies are planned. This permits the diagnosis of anal neoplasms and the occasional adenoma or carcinoma present on the rectal side of the anal verge that can be missed on an incomplete endoscopic examination. Furthermore, stool is obtained during this procedure to test for the presence of occult bleeding.

Anoscopy and *proctoscopy* using a rigid instrument are used to examine the rectum and anus, and, additionally, therapeutic procedures may be performed using these instruments. The rigid sigmoidoscope is not used in the routine diagnosis of cancer except for special instances to evaluate the rectum. It

is painful to advance this instrument into the distal sigmoid colon, and even in the best of hands, this an insensitive test compared with flexible instruments.

Flexible fiberoptic proctosigmoidoscopy may be performed using instruments of virtually any length. Instruments measuring 35 and 60 cm are widely available, and rectosigmoid examinations may also be performed with the standard colonoscope. A rigorous preparation is not required, because an examination of the sigmoid colon and rectum is usually undertaken after cleansing enemas. No sedation is required for this, and patient acceptance of the procedure is much higher than for the rigid instrumentation. The use of the 35-cm and 65-cm instruments may be mastered by general internists and endoscopic technicians with appropriate training.

The *barium enema* is the time-honored tool for the diagnosis of polyps and cancers of the colon. The single-contrast barium examination is inadequately sensitive to exclude polyps and cancers and should be replaced by the double-contrast study. Preparation for a barium enema varies from center to center; most frequently, a clear liquid diet, combination of saline cathartics and stimulant cathartics, and cleansing enemas are requested by the radiologist. Sedating medication is not required. Approximately .03 Gy (3 rad) is radiation are delivered to the abdomen during this study, and patient acceptance is lower than it is for flexible sigmoidoscopy or colonoscopy. However, the entire colon may be examined with this technique. Overlapping loops of bowel in the sigmoid colon and the flexures are areas of particular difficulty in interpretation. The presence of extensive diverticulosis or residual fecal material can present additional diagnostic difficulties. Because of the limitations of sensitivity in the sigmoid colon and the difficulty in excluding lesions in the rectum because of the presence of an obstructing balloon, proctosigmoidoscopy is suggested as an adjunctive study to improve the sensitivity if a barium enema is selected as a diagnostic technique. The sensitivity of barium enema is directly related to the patience and diligence of the radiologist.

The *180-cm colonoscope* is the most widely used diagnostic instrument to study the colon. The entire colon can be examined in at least 90% to 95% of studies, and this approach has the highest diagnostic sensitivity of all available tests. Preparation of the colon is achieved using a nonabsorbable gastrointestinal lavage solution and does not require a liquid diet or the administration of laxatives. Intravenous sedation and analgesia are administered during the examination; therefore, the patient acceptance is very high. This is the most invasive of examinations and carries with it a small (0.1%–0.3%) incidence of severe complications such as hemorrhage and perforation, which can require surgical intervention. Perhaps the most valuable aspect of this procedure is the fact that mucosal biopsy and endoscopic polypectomy may be undertaken. Thus, definitive diagnosis and even treatment may be accomplished.

What Is The Definitive Diagnostic Test For Colorectal Neoplasia?

If the initial diagnostic procedure is a barium enema, a negative result may create a diagnostic dilemma. In a study of 97 patients who had persistent large bowel symptoms and

TABLE 87-9
Age-Specific Incidence Rates Per 10^5 Population for Cancers of the Colon and Rectum

AGE (y)	MEN	WOMEN
0–4	0.0	0.0
5–9	0.0	0.0
10–14	0.0	0.0
15–19	0.2	0.1
20–24	0.4	0.4
25–29	1.2	1.1
30–34	2.5	2.4
35–39	5.9	5.9
40–44	12.3	11.9
45–49	27.7	24.6
50–54	57.2	46.3
55–59	102.6	76.7
60–64	164.9	105.7
65–69	243.9	155.5
70–74	320.5	226.9
75–79	411.3	293.6
80–84	463.5	365.5
85+	497.6	391.5

From Eddy DM. Screening for colorectal Cancer. Ann Intern Med 1990;113: 373.

had a negative air-contrast barium enema, colonoscopy revealed 4 carcinomas and 24 adenomatous polyps not detected by the radiologic approach.[360] In a similar study of 76 patients with symptoms of colonic disease, the diagnostic evaluation began with rigid sigmoidoscopy, after which all of the patients underwent flexible sigmoidoscopy, double-contrast barium enema, and then colonoscopy. The double-contrast barium enema alone reached a final diagnosis in 67% of patients, whereas colonoscopy was successful in 91%. The addition of flexible sigmoidoscopy to double-contrast barium enema improved the diagnostic yield to 76%.[361] This suggests that colonoscopy is the preferred diagnostic procedure for the initial work-up of a patient with symptoms of colonic disease and, moreover, indicates that colonoscopy should be used to evaluate colonic symptoms or bleeding even if the air-contrast barium enema is negative. A review of 31 colon cancers overlooked on double-contrast barium enema revealed that half of the lesions were missed as a result of perceptive errors; that is, the lesions were visualized on the x-ray film, and recognized in retrospect, but could not be identified as neoplasm on the initial reading.[362] Another third of the lesions were missed because of perceptive error complicated by technical factors obscuring the lesion; the tumor was not visible even on respective viewing in 10%, and in 6% the lesion was seen but misinterpreted. In addition, almost one third of barium enemas in patients older than 65 years of age are technically inadequate because of inability of the patient to obtain a suitable preparation or inability to cooperate with the procedure.[363]

Clearly, the figures obtained are highly dependent on the skill and persistence of the radiologist and endoscopist, and it must be emphasized that some neoplastic lesions may be missed by the colonoscopist. A prospective study of tandem colonoscopy (i.e., two consecutive examinations done sequentially) on 90 patients who had a total of 221 lesions demonstrated that an experienced colonoscopist missed about 15% of neoplastic lesions less than 10 mm in size, but no lesions greater than 10 mm.[364] At this time it appears that colonoscopy will remain the gold standard for the diagnosis of colorectal neoplasia, and it would appear unlikely that any indirect approach such as radiography or sonography can approach this technique for sensitivity.

Screening for Colorectal Cancer in the Absence of Specific Symptoms

Because colorectal cancer produces few symptoms while the tumors are small and most readily curable, screening of asymptomatic individuals has been advocated. Screening for colorectal cancer can reduce the mortality from this disease. The principal issues of discussion are which screening approach is optimal, the costs of the program, and how much screening can be afforded. The approaches are discussed first in the context of screening asymptomatic individuals, and then we turn to the specialized situations of screening high-risk groups and the closely related issue of surveillance, or periodic screening in a previously screened high-risk population.

Screening Asymptomatic Individuals for Colorectal Cancer

Screening refers to testing apparently healthy people for disease. A good screening test must in some way improve the lives of those screened, by either prolonging life or improving its quality. To be effective, the test must be sensitive (i.e., it should detect all diseased individuals), must be specific (i.e., it should not subject nondiseased individuals to excessive anxiety or extra testing), and must be acceptable and affordable by those tested. At present, there are two modalities that have been evaluated for efficacy as screening tests for colorectal cancer: testing of feces for occult blood and endoscopic examination of the bowel. Both modalities are effective in reducing cancer mortality, but each has its limitations.

Fecal occult bleeding tests: technical considerations.   It has long been appreciated that colorectal neoplasms bleed early in their natural history. Hemoglobin contains peroxidase activity, which may be detected using the guaiac test. Gum guaiac is a colorless indicator that is oxidized to a pigmented quinone in the presence of peroxidase and hydrogen peroxide. The traditional bench guaiac test required the application of feces to filter paper, followed by the application of the guaiac reagent, acetic acid, and hydrogen peroxide. This was a very sensitive means of detecting fecal peroxidase activity, but it was poorly standardized and overly sensitive. Therefore, a guaiac-impregnated slide test was developed that was slightly less sensitive but more highly standardized.[365] In the laboratory, the guaiac slide test can detect hemoglobin concentrations as low as 0.12 mg/mL. In a typical 150-gram stool, the following rule of thumb may be used: each 1 mL of blood results in 1 mg of hemoglobin per gram of stool. The detection of tiny blood losses into the gastrointestinal tract seems like a simple task, but in fact, this test is fraught with complexities.

The normal gastrointestinal losses of blood may be estimated by the intravenous administration of ^{51}Cr-tagged erythrocytes, followed by measurement of the excretion of radioactivity in the stools. This has been done by several laboratories, and there is agreement that the normal losses are approximately 0.5 to 1.0 mL/day.[366,367] During its transit in the gastrointestinal tract, the blood is dispersed throughout the stool and undergoes degradation because of the presence of digestive enzymes. Moreover, there are natural inhibitors of peroxidase activity in feces.

In 1982, Macrae and colleagues reported a study that clarified the influence of diet and techniques for developing the slides on the specificity of the guaiac test (Hemoccult II in this study).[368] It had previously been noted that the guaiac test was less sensitive if the stool had dried out on the filter paper; therefore, a drop of water was often added to the back of the Hemoccult card to rehydrate the stool before development of the test. In Macrae's study, 156 normal subjects were given a diet restricted in red meat, fruits, and vegetables; none of 310 of the guaiac tests done on subjects given the low-peroxidase diet was positive, and only 2 (0.6%) of 310 were positive after rehydration of the slides. The number of falsely positive tests increased minimally (<1%) with the addition of peroxidase-containing foods to the diet; however, if the slides were rehydrated, as many as 6.6% of the tests became positive. Dietary peroxidase was principally a problem

TABLE 87-10
Bleeding From Colorectal Cancers

LOCATION OF CANCER	MEAN BLOOD LOSS (^{51}Cr-LABELED ERYTHROCYTES)	POSITIVE HEMOCCULT II TESTS*	
		Nonrehydrated	Rehydrated
Cecum, ascending colon (n = 10)	9.3 mL/d	83%	96%
Transverse and descending colon (n = 5)	1.5 mL/d	54%	54%
Sigmoid colon (n = 13)	1.9 mL/d	64%	97%
Rectum (n = 18)	1.8 mL/d	69%	93%
		69%	91%

* Hemoccult II tests performed with and without rehydration; Hemoccult II test considered positive if any of six tests positive in a 3-day test period.

From Macrae FA, St. John DJB. Relationship between patterns of bleeding and Hemoccult sensitivity in patients with colorectal cancers or adenomas. Gastroenterology 1982;82:891.

for the guaiac test after the ingestion of beef and was not present with poultry, fish, or pork.[369] The standardized guaiac test is therefore reliably negative in control subjects on restricted diets, and less than 1% of tests are falsely positive on low-peroxidase diets. However, the test becomes unreliable if performed with rehydration unless the diet is strictly regulated, diminishing the value of this maneuver.

The next critical issue in the development of a screening test was to understand how much colorectal neoplasms bleed. In a second study in 1982, Macrae and associates administered ^{51}Cr-tagged autologous erythrocytes to 46 patients with known colorectal cancer, measured fecal blood loss and correlated it with the results of Hemoccult II tests.[224] They demonstrated that the mean blood loss from a cohort of symptomatic tumors of the cecum and ascending colon was 9.3 mL/day (range, 2–28 mL/day) but was much less for lesions located distal to the hepatic flexure, from which the mean blood loss was less than 2 mL/day. This difference may have resulted from larger lesions in the proximal colon. In spite of the sensitivity of the guaiac test, a false-negative rate of 31% was encountered using this test. As indicated in Table 87-10, the false-negative rate could be reduced to 9% if the

guaiac slides were rehydrated. However, as previously mentioned, rehydration is a problem if the diet has not been strictly regulated with regard to foods containing peroxidase. As demonstrated in Table 87-11, a single guaiac test was falsely negative 50% of the time in patients with cancer. The false-negative rate fell to 31% with three consecutive days of testing, and fell to 13% after 10 days of continuous testing. The sensitivity was improved with rehydration, and the false-negative rate was only 5% after five days, but again rehydration may be accompanied by sharp loss in specificity depending on the diet.

The proportion of positive guaiac tests is closely related to the amount of blood in the stools. As illustrated in Table 87-12, the tests are usually negative if the stool hemoglobin concentration is less than 2 mL per gram of stool, and they are more likely to be positive with increasing fecal hemoglobin. Two different laboratories have demonstrated that colonic polyps may also be detected by the tests for occult bleeding, but benign lesions lose less blood, and the sensitivity of the test is much lower.[224,370] The mean blood loss from an adenomatous polyp is approximately 1.3 mL of blood per day, regardless of its location. However, polyps in the distal colon

TABLE 87-11
False-Negative Hemoccult II Tests Correlated With Duration of Testing in Patients With Known Colorectal Carcinoma*

TEST RESULT	DURATION OF TESTING (d)									
	1	2	3	4	5	6	7	8	9	10
Hemoccult false-negative rate	181/359 (50%)	117/313 (37%)	84/267 (31%)	56/222 (25%)	41/177 (23%)	28/136 (21%)	18/100 (18%)	10/68 (15%)	5/39 (13%)	2/15 (13%)
Rehydrated Hemoccult false-negative rate	80/359 (22%)	39/313 (12%)	23/267 (9%)	15/222 (7%)	9/177 (5%)	7/136 (5%)	5/100 (5%)	3/68 (4%)	2/39 (5%)	1/15 (7%)

* Proportion and percentage of tests in which patients with known colorectal cancers had falsely negative Hemoccult II tests. This demonstrates that 50% of cancers are missed by performing a single (unrehydrated) test; the false-negative rate falls to 31% after 3 days of testing and is reduced to 13% with 10 days of testing. Using the rehydrated test, the false-negative rate is only 9% with 3 days of testing, but the prohibitive rate of false-positives produced makes rehydration a maneuver of questionable value.

From Macrae FA, St. John DJB. Relationship between patterns of bleeding and Hemoccult sensitivity in patients with colorectal cancers of adenomas. Gastroenterology 1982;82:891.

TABLE 87-12
Relation Between Fecal Hemoglobin Concentration and Hemoccult II Tests in Patients With Colorectal Cancers

STOOL HEMOGLOBIN CONCENTRATION (mg Hb/g STOOL)	PROPORTION OF POSITIVE TESTS	
	HO	HO(R)
0–2	86/766 (11%)	212/758 (28%)
2–6	127/314 (40%)	213/304 (70%)
6–10	50/80 (63%)	75/80 (94%)
10–15	50/64 (78%)	60/64 (94%)
15–20	11/18 (61%)	14/18 (78%)
>20	30/58 (52%)	56/58 (97%)

HO, Hemoccult II developed without rehydration; HO(R), Hemoccult II developed with preliminary rehydration.

From Macrae FA, St. John DJB. Relationship between patterns of bleeding and Hemoccult sensitivity in patients with colorectal cancers or adenomas. Gastroenterology 1982;82:891.

(descending colon, sigmoid colon, and rectum) produce 54% positive tests, whereas those in the proximal colon produce positive tests only 17% of the time.[224] Macrae's group showed that gastrointestinal bleeding was related to polyp size (Fig. 87-11)[224]; Herzog demonstrated that a positive guaiac test is more likely if a polyp is located in the distal rather than proximal colon.[370]

Colorectal neoplasms usually add a very small amount of blood to the feces, which makes them difficult to detect using FOBTs. The standardized guaiac test is a very sensitive test and is reliably negative in healthy subjects on diets with restricted peroxidase intake. However, blood deposited in the stool is mixed throughout the stool and undergoes degradation, making it more difficult to detect with a guaiac test. Lesions located in the distal colon are usually easier to detect because the blood is deposited on the surface of the stool, where mixing and dilution are limited. The fecal hemoglobin concentration on the surface of the stool may be high enough to produce a positive test, even considering the rigors of dehydration and degradation while the guaiac cards are being mailed back to the physician. In general, maneuvers designed to increase the sensitivity of the guaiac test, such as rehydration, may increase the rate of false-positives faster than the true-positives. The guaiac-impregnated cards can be used to detect approximately two thirds of colorectal cancers and a smaller proportion of adenomatous polyps, based on both their size and location in the colon.

Numerous attempts have been made to develop a better FOBT. The manufacturers of Hemoccult II have developed a more sensitive slide test, called HemoccultSENSA (SmithKline Diagnostics, San Jose, CA), which seems to provide sensitivity similar to that seen with rehydrated Hemoccult slides. The same manufacturer has also developed an immunochemical test for fecal hemoglobin called HemeSelect. This test uses a specific antibody for human hemoglobin but is performed in the laboratory and is not a bedside test, as are the guaiac-based slide tests. The antibody-based test has the theoretical advantage of not cross-reacting with nonhuman hemoglobin, and it should also not detect bleeding from an upper gastrointestinal site because of degradation of the intact

molecule. Both HemoccultSENSA and HemeSelect are significantly more sensitive than Hemoccult II, and in one study it was reported that they detected 94% and 97%, respectively, of the symptomatic colorectal cancers, compared with 89% for Hemoccult II. However, the sensitivity for silent cancers, which are obviously more difficult to detect and are the target lesions, is uncertain (Table 87-13). The newer tests were also sensitive for adenomatous polyps greater than 1 cm in size; HemoccultSENSA was positive in 76%, HemeSelect in 60%, and Hemoccult II in 42%. The HemoccultSENSA and HemeSelect were positive in 5% and 3% of screened individuals, respectively, and most of these positive tests were not associated with colorectal neoplasia.[371] Therefore, the price for increased sensitivity is the need to perform a large number of definitive work-ups (i.e., colonoscopy) because of falsely positive tests.[371]

A quantitative test for fecal heme has been developed in the HemoQuant test.[372] This assay provides a quantitative measure of occult gastrointestinal bleeding and can detect the tiny increments of bleeding that occur in the setting of colorectal neoplasia. The test is not influenced by dietary peroxidase and should be superior to Hemoccult as a diagnostic test.[373] Unfortunately, the amount of bleeding from a variety of different lesions overlaps with that seen in colon cancer, and stool samples must be sent to the laboratory for analysis, so this is neither a simple nor a bedside test. Furthermore, it may not be as sensitive as the tests described above.[371] This is discussed in more detail in Chapter 31.

Fecal occult bleeding tests: factors modifying results. Additional factors can modify the sensitivity and specificity of the guaiac test. The Hemoccult card test has been developed so that patients could take them home, modify their diets, and collect two samples from a stool on each of three consecutive days. The cards are mailed back to the physician for developing. This technique ensures that some or all of the

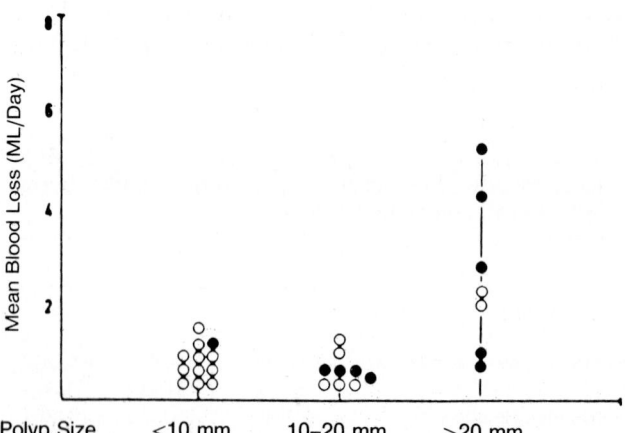

FIGURE 87-11. Mean gastrointestinal blood loss from colonic adenomatous polyps. Blood loss was determined using 51Cr-labeled erythrocytes in 28 patients with colonic adenomas. Patients with a history of overt colonic bleeding are identified by solid circles; those without are shown by open circles. (From Macrae FA, St. John DJB. Relationship between patterns of bleeding and Hemoccult sensitivity in patients with colorectal cancers or adenomas. Gastroenterology 1982;82:891.)

TABLE 87-13
Tests for Occult Fecal Bleeding

TEST	% POSITIVE (n = 1355)*	SENSITIVITY—CANCER (n = 107)	SENSITIVITY—ADENOMAS ≥1 cm (n = 45)	SENSITIVITY–ADENOMAS <1 cm (n = 36)
Hemoccult II	†	88.6%	42.2%	16.7%
HemoccultSENSA	5.0%	93.7%	60.0%	25.0%
HemeSelect	3.0%	96.2%	75.6%	36.1%
HemoQuant (>2 mg/d)	3.0%‡	64.6%	42.2%	30.6%

* 1355 Asymptomatic subjects screened with HemoccultSENSA and HemeSelect.

† Estimates are 1%–3% unrehydrated to 10% with rehydration; higher rates of positivity with unrestricted diets.

‡ Three percent of volunteers had more than 2 mg Hgb/g stool, 0% of volunteers had 3 mg Hgb/g stool (n = 106).

From St. John DJB, Young GP, Alexeyeff MA, et al. Evaluation of new occult blood tests for detection of colorectal neoplasia. Gastroenterology 1993;104:1661.

specimens will have undergone changes because of *storage*. A study using early generation Hemoccult cards, less sensitive than Hemoccult II, demonstrated that approximately 8 mg of hemoglobin per gram of stool was required to produce a positive test. After stool samples had been stored on Hemoccult cards for 4 days, the intensity of the reaction diminished, and it became negative in 8 days. Stool specimens stored in airtight containers maintained a positive reaction for 1 week. Therefore, low levels of fecal hemoglobin become undetectable the longer the delay between the collection of the stool and the development of the test.[374] Furthermore, one study reported that an inexperienced processor of Hemoccult cards can overread the result and seriously affect the outcome of a screening project.[375]

The effect of *iron* preparations on the guaiac test has been somewhat controversial. A study of 1700 guaiac tests performed in 1963 led to the conclusion that oral iron does not result in positive guaiac reactions.[376] However, a small study by Lipton and colleagues suggested that ferrous sulfate and ferrous gluconate produced false-positive reactions in more than half the ten patients tested.[377] These authors also showed that an aqueous solution of iron could produce a positive guaiac test. It has subsequently been reported by McDonnell and associates that the black pigment in stools of patients on iron supplements may have been misinterpreted as the blue color characteristic of a positive guaiac test, confirming that oral iron supplements do not produce true positive guaiac tests.[378] Furthermore, although ferrous sulfate dissolved in water produces a positive Hemoccult II test, at the pH of the stool (>6), the iron precipitates out of solution and does not produce a positive test. Ferric (Fe^{3+}) iron produces a positive guaiac reaction, but ferrous (Fe^{2+}) iron produces such a reaction only after the addition of hydrogen peroxide, which oxidizes Fe^{2+} to Fe^{3+}. The black iron pigment in stool is insoluble ferrous sulfide, and no Fe^{2+} or Fe^{3+} is elutable into water from the black stools.[378] It is unlikely that oral iron therapy contributes appreciably to false-positive guaiac reactions, and furthermore, it does not appear to cause occult gastrointestinal bleeding.[379]

Because the basis of the guaiac test is the oxidation of an indicator substance (guaiac), the presence of strong *antioxidants* could interfere with the reaction. The ingestion of 1 to 2 g/day of ascorbic acid (vitamin C) has been reported to produce a spuriously negative guaiac test.[380]

Screening Asymptomatic Populations for Occult Fecal Bleeding

Several studies are available that illustrate the benefits and limitations of screening for colon cancer. After a series of media promotions in Chicago, more than 54,000 FOBT kits were sent on request to asymptomatic individuals[381]; only 26% of the tests were completed, of which 4.4% were positive. More than one third of individuals with positive tests failed to respond to repeated inquiries for follow-up, and another 20% had an incomplete diagnostic work-up after referral to a physician. Among all those with positive tests, 5% had cancers detected, nearly two thirds of which were Dukes' stage A or B lesions. Another 30% of the patients had abnormalities other than cancer, including adenomatous polyps. Thus, compliance is an issue in a community screening program.

A large, controlled trial from Memorial Sloan-Kettering in New York is still in progress, but interim results have been published.[382,383] A cohort of patients 40 years of age or older was screened on a meat-free, high-bulk diet; the slides were not rehydrated, and there was a 4-day storage interval between slide preparation and testing. The Hemoccult tests gave a positive result in 1.7% of the group, and results were strongly age-dependent. The first-generation tests were positive in 1.0%, compared with 3.7% using the more sensitive version (Hemoccult II), which became available later. The first-generation Hemoccult slides were predictive for neoplastic lesions in 50% of patients, including 12% cancers and 38% adenomas. The more sensitive Hemoccult II slides had a predictive value of 44% for any neoplastic lesion. With rehydration, the rate of positive tests increased to 5.4%; however, the predictive value for neoplasia decreased to 19%, so this maneuver was abandoned by these investigators. In summary, modifications intended to make the test more sensitive gave a higher proportion of positive tests, found more neoplasms, and generated many more false-positive results. Although the entire group of patients were offered at least one rigid 25-cm sigmoidoscopic examination, a 43% reduction in cancer mortality was reported in the half of the group randomized to receive the FOBTs.[383] Other commercially available versions of guaiac-based FOBTs have been marketed, but each must demonstrate its sensitivity for fecal hemoglobin to be interpreted.

A large controlled, prospective trial has been reported in which the impact of screening for colon cancer was compared with the detection of colon cancer subsequent to symptoms. Hardcastle and colleagues randomized more than 20,000 patients into two groups; half were encouraged to have FOBT, and half were advised to consult their physicians if they developed colonic symptoms (Fig. 87-12).[384,385] Only 38.5% of patients offered screening returned their slides. The patients were advised to avoid red meat and vitamin C, and the slides were evaluated without rehydration. Of the group returning slides, 4.1% had a positive test, and 36% of these had neoplastic disease on air-contrast barium enema and flexible sigmoidoscopy. Of the group with a positive test, 8.5% had cancer and 28% had one or more adenomas, 30% of which were more than 2 cm in diameter. Among the 17 invasive carcinomas detected, 13 were Dukes' stage A, 2 stage B, and 2 stage C. One patient among the 4716 patients with an initial negative screen developed a stage C carcinoma of the ascending colon during the year after screening, indicating a false-negative test. Among the subjects also randomized to the screening group in the initial study,[384] who either refused the test or failed to reply, 11 developed symptomatic neoplastic disease within the following year, including 8 cancers (5 stage B and 3 stage D), and 3 patients presented with large adenomatous polyps. Among the initial 10,000 patients randomized to the screening arm, a total of 24 had cancers diagnosed; among the 10,000 control subjects, 10 patients presented with symptomatic carcinomas of the colon, 4 of which were stage B, 4 stage C, and 2 stage D. This study clearly indicated that a substantial number of cancers could be detected using the FOBT, and early-stage lesions were diagnosed (Table 87-14).[384,385]

In a follow-up study, Hardcastle and associates offered rescreening to the initial group of compliant subjects (Table 87-15).[385] They achieved 85% rescreening compliance, and 2.8% of those patients had positive tests. Of the 80 patients with positive tests, 4 (5%) had cancers, 3 of which were stage A. In the original control group of more than 10,000 unscreened patients, 7 patients presented with symptomatic colorectal cancer during the second follow-up year (in addition to the 10 detected during the first year). No tumor was stage A; 47% (8) were stage B, 35% (6) stage C, and 18% (3) stage D. This group has recently updated their study with more than 100,000 subjects, and the results are essentially unchanged.[386]

A summary of five controlled studies of screening for colon cancer is provided in Table 87-16. These controlled trials indicate that FOBTs provide a means for screening asymptomatic, average-risk patients for colorectal cancer. Asymptomatic populations have approximately 1.0% to 2.4% positive tests. If more than 1% to 2% of tests are positive, it suggests that dietary restrictions have not been adequately followed, that the clinicians have used rehydration of the guaiac test, or that a more sensitive version of the test has been used. It is recommended that beef be eliminated from the diet during the lead-in period and during the testing of feces. In addition, antiinflammatory agents and antioxidants such as vitamin C should also be avoided. Furthermore, the physician or technician should develop the slide as soon as possible, should not rehydrate the slides, and should be aware of the potential for misinterpretation of the slides in patients taking iron supplements. These measures minimize the number of false-positive FOBTs, which would increase the cost of a surveil-

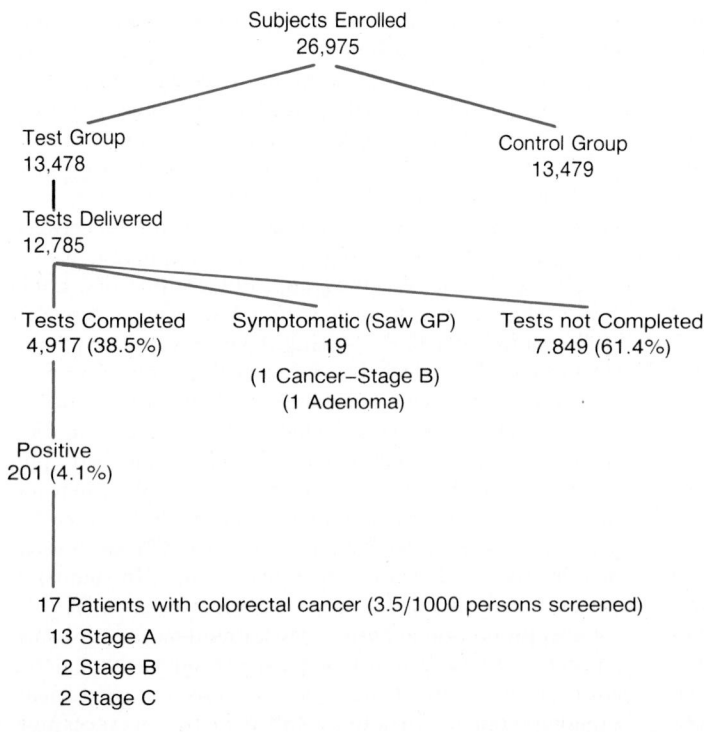

FIGURE 87-12. Distribution of subjects into surveillance group using Hemoccult II testing versus nonsurveillance groups. (From Hardcastle JD, Armitage NC, Chamberlain J, et al. Fecal occult blood screening for colorectal cancer in the general population. Results of a controlled trial. Cancer 1986;58:397.)

TABLE 87-14
Development of Colorectal Neoplasms in 20,000 Patients During First Year After Screening*

PATIENT GROUP	CARCINOMAS		ADENOMAS	
	Number	*Rate per 1000*	*Number*	*Rate per 1000*
Positive screening Hemoccult test (*n* = 77/3613)	13	3.6	42†	7.9
Negative screening Hemoccult test (*n* = 3536/3613)	1	0.3		
Offered Hemoccult test (refused or no response) (*n* = 6143)	8	1.3	3	0.5
Control group (not screened) (*n* = 10,272)	10	1.0	5	0.5

* Development of neoplasms in group described in Figure 87–12.

† In 29 patients.

From Hardcastle JD, Farrands PA, Balfour TW. Controlled trial of faecal occult blood testing in the detection of colorectal cancer. Lancet 1983;2:1.

lance program. However, by limiting the sensitivity of the test, at least one third of colorectal cancers are missed.

The studies reviewed demonstrate that early-stage cancers can be detected using FOBTs, and more recent data make the important confirmation that colorectal cancer mortality is reduced by finding these tumors. First, a case-control study was published from the Oakland Kaiser-Permanente health maintenance organization demonstrating an odds ratio of 0.69 for colorectal cancer mortality for those individuals who had had their stools screened for occult fecal blood within the previous 5 years.[387] The investigators found that the odds ratio was lowest for the first year after screening but rose to 1 (i.e., no benefit) 3 years after screening. The impact of FOBT screening therefore has a time limit.

The most important study of FOBTs was reported from the University of Minnesota and involved the use of Hemoccult cards, 83% of them rehydrated, on more than 46,000 patients studied prospectively for an average of 13 years.[388] In this three-armed study, annual FOBTs resulted in a 33% reduction of colorectal cancer mortality. This was largely achieved through stage shift, in which there was a 50% reduction in the number of Dukes' stage D tumors in the screened group, which in turn had a profound effect on survival. A number of critical issues were raised by this study.

First, a very substantial reduction in mortality was demonstrated in a large, credible, carefully controlled study, and the order of magnitude was similar to that predicted by the previous studies.[383,387] However, the use of the rehydrated Hemoccult cards raised the positivity rate among screened individuals from 2.4% (their rate without rehydration) to 9.8%, necessitating diagnostic evaluations in a large proportion of the study population. In fact, fully 38% of the annually screened group underwent at least one colonoscopy during the study. As a result, only 2.2% of those with a positive test were found to have a colorectal cancer, compared with 5.6% when the nonrehydrated tests were used briefly in the middle of the study. Although the number of adenomatous polyps removed from this group was not reported, this intervention may have added to the beneficial outcome. Finally, the large and highly significant reduction in mortality was seen only in the annually screened group. Those screened every other year experienced a nonsignificant 6% reduction in mortality, suggesting that only annual testing is effective—as predicted by the case-control study.[387] The difference between annual and biennial testing may have been to some degree artefactual, because there was an unanticipated increase in mortality in years 4 and 5 in the biennial group that confounded cumulative mortality for the next 6 years. Although one should be

TABLE 87-15
Pathologic Stage of Cancers in 20,525 Patients Followed for Two Years After Randomization to Screening or No Screening

STAGE	TEST GROUP			CONTROL GROUP (10,272)
	*Responders** (3613)*	*Nonresponders† (6640)*	*Overall (10,253)*	
Stage A	12 (60%)	2 (14%)	14 (43%)	0
Stage B	4 (20%)	7 (50%)	11 (33%)	8 (47%)
Stage C	2 (10%)	1 (7%)	3 (9%)	6 (35%)
Stage D	2 (10%)	4 (29%)	6 (15%)	3 (18%)
Total	20	14	34	17

* Responders-patients who completed the Hemoccult II fecal screening test.

† Nonresponders-patients randomized to be screened but who did not respond to request.

From Hardcastle JD, Farrands DA, Balfour TW. Controlled trial of faecal occult blood testing in the detection of colorectal cancer. Lancet 1983;2:1.

TABLE 87-16
Controlled Trials of Fecal Occult Blood Testing in Screening for Colorectal Neoplasms

LOCATION OF TRIAL	COHORT SIZE	POSITIVE FECAL OCCULT BLOOD TEST (%)	PREDICTIVE VALUE OF OCCULT BLOOD TEST FOR COLORECTAL NEOPLASMS (%)	DUKES' A OR B CANCER	
				Screened Group (%)	Unscreened Group (%)
Sweden	27,000	1.9	22	65	33
England	150,000	2.1	40	90	40
New York	22,000	1.7	30	65	33
Minnesota	48,000	2.4	31	78	35
Denmark	62,000	1.0	58	81	55

From Winawer SJ, Schottenfeld D, Flehinger BJ. Colorectal cancer screening. J Natl Cancer Inst 1991;83:243.

open to a change in this with future research, no study has yet indicated that biennial screening with FOBTs is effective in reducing mortality.

Role of Sigmoidoscopy in Screening for Colon Cancer

Screening with FOBTs has its limitations, and, as previously stated, approximately two thirds of colorectal neoplasms are within reach of the flexible sigmoidoscope. Furthermore, a large, uncontrolled observation of the effects of screening by rigid sigmoidoscopy by Gilbertsen at the University of Minnesota suggested that frequent inspection of the rectum and removal of all premalignant lesions would reduce the incidence of invasive rectal cancers to a very low number and could even eliminate the occurrence of advanced stage disease.[389] The development of flexible instruments that could reach from the anus to the cecum raised the obvious issue of how far to take the examinations and how frequently they should be repeated.

There are currently two studies that suggest a significant reduction in mortality from screening sigmoidoscopy. A case-control study from the Oakland Kaiser-Permanente program examined the use of screening sigmoidoscopy among 261 patients who died of cancer of the rectum or distal colon, compared with case-matched controls. Only 8.8% of the cancer patients had undergone screening sigmoidoscopy, compared with 24.2% of the controls. The authors estimated from this outcome that screened subjects had only 30% of the risk for fatal cancers of the rectum and distal colon, compared with the unscreened cohort. Furthermore, the data suggested that screening sigmoidoscopy may provide risk reduction for as long as 10 years. There were a similar number of fatal colon cancers above the reach of a sigmoidoscopic examination in both the screened and unscreened groups, which supported the contention that the two groups were evenly matched for colorectal cancer risk.[390]

This observation was confirmed by another retrospective case-control study from Wisconsin.[391] A history of at least a single screening sigmoidoscopy over a 10-year period of study was present in 10% of those who died of colorectal cancer but in 30% of case-controls. This group estimated that the risk of death from colorectal cancer was reduced by 79% after a single examination, and the adjusted odds ratio for death from cancer in the rectum or distal colon was 0.05. Although no systematic screening program had been instituted, no ben-

efits were observed among patients who had undergone digital examinations of the rectum or FOBTs.

No large controlled, prospective trial has been published that tests the efficacy of endoscopic screening with either sigmoidoscopy or colonoscopy. Nonetheless, there is strong and compelling evidence for a protective effect of sigmoidoscopy and, presumably, the removal of premalignant lesions. Endoscopic screening appears to bring with it a protective effect that lasts substantially longer than the 1-year protection of FOBTs. Furthermore, the magnitude of protection is substantially greater than that derived from FOBTs, presumably because one can not only detect early stage lesions but also remove premalignant lesions and interrupt neoplastic progression early in its long natural history.

Screening Recommendations for Asymptomatic Populations

The published data all indicate that mortality from colorectal cancer can be reduced either by annual FOBT programs, which provide a 33% or greater reduction, or by screening sigmoidoscopy, which provides a huge reduction, probably greater than 80%, in that portion of the bowel screened. As described above, programs that use FOBTs are complicated by the variables involved in the techniques used, the need for annual testing, and the need for follow-up colonoscopy in all those with a positive screening test. If FOBTs are used in a screening program, they should be done annually, and all positive tests must be pursued vigorously. Screening sigmoidoscopy is substantially more effective in preventing cancer mortality, but only the distal bowel is examined.

The American Cancer Society, the National Cancer Institute, and several other advisory panels have recommended that screening for colorectal cancer in average-risk individuals begin at 50 years of age and consist of annual FOBTs plus flexible sigmoidoscopy every 3 to 5 years.[392] In spite of this, these recommendations have not yet become the uniform standards of care in any community because of the costs implicit in such an ambitious program. The U.S. Office of Technology Assessment has estimated that a program of annual FOBTs plus periodic sigmoidoscopy in persons 65 to 85 years of age alone could cost 1.5 to 2.6 billion dollars annually, or $43,000 to $47,000 per year of life gained.[393] Even this may be an underestimate, but the costs of a screening program could be modified depending on who performs the tests and which ancillary charges are included in the estimates.

The recommendations made regarding screening are entirely dependent on the budgetary limitations placed on the program. The data regarding the efficacy of screening are strong and consistent, and the concept has been embraced by most reviewers.[394,395] Screened patients are significantly less likely to die of colorectal cancer or suffer morbidity related to cancer or surgery. Patients screened by endoscopic procedures appear to have even greater protection than those screened with FOBTs, in terms of both the magnitude of reduced mortality and the duration of protection provided by the examination. More screening prevents more cancer deaths but also costs more. Therefore, the real issue is how much screening can be afforded.

A compromise solution offered by one analyst from the United Kingdom (which, like the United States, has no national screening program in place) is to perform once-only sigmoidoscopy at between 55 and 60 years of age, followed by colonoscopic surveillance for those with high-risk adenomas (i.e., those >1 cm in size or with villous histology).[396] Taking into account problems with compliance and the obvious limitations of the program, it is proposed that this approach would prevent about 18% of annual colorectal cancer deaths in the United Kingdom, with a greatly reduced cost over more ambitious approaches. Although limited degrees of protection may not be acceptable to the public, either a large sum of money must be allocated to screening or some compromise will be necessary. Finally, unless funding is committed to institute such an ambitious program, there should be no legal liability for a failure to screen, in spite of the above recommendations.

Surveillance for Colorectal Cancer

Surveillance is not the same as screening. It refers to the periodic follow-up testing—usually colonoscopic—of individuals who are at high risk for colorectal cancer and who have previously had negative screening examinations. Each clinical situation should be considered individually.

Familial Adenomatous Polyposis

FAP sits at the extreme end of the spectrum for cancer risk, which makes it management less controversial. Risk is determined by being the offspring of an affected patient. The rate of new mutations in this disease is relatively high, perhaps as much as one fourth to one third of all new cases; in these instances, parents and siblings of affected patients are spared, but their children are at risk. All those who inherit the mutated *APC* gene develop polyposis of the colon and have a 50% likelihood of developing adenomatous polyps by 16 years of age[219]; these can be diagnosed by performing a limited flexible sigmoidoscopy each year, beginning in adolescence. Genetic testing by linkage analysis can be performed at referral centers from birth if blood is available from both parents and, preferably, two or more affected individuals within the family. The *APC* gene is very large, and the mutations that cause FAP are highly variable, which makes it difficult and very time-consuming to determine whether an isolated individual has a mutated gene. Also, families should be in an appropriate genetic counseling program before initiating testing, especially

if young family members are involved who may suffer psychological trauma from adverse information regarding gene carriage. Patients who develop polyps can usually wait until they have reached their full adult growth before undergoing surgery, because the incidence of cancer is quite low before 20 years of age. Sulindac may be used to inhibit polyp growth for a brief period while waiting for surgery, but its efficacy in preventing cancer is still uncertain.[96]

Families with the attenuated forms of FAP, known as AAPC, have more variable manifestations of the disease, and affected individuals tend to develop their tumors later in life than do those with the more virulent forms of the disease. These families should be screened with annual sigmoidoscopy for a much longer period of time, but they can benefit from genetic screening, because gene carriers can be identified, and those who do not carry the gene can be assured of their ordinary risk for cancer.

Hereditary Nonpolyposis Colorectal Cancer

HNPCC is more complex than FAP because there is no distinctive premalignant phenotype, and the diagnosis is often suspected only because of a strong family history. Although a putative locus for HNPCC has been mapped,[10] it is not known how inclusive this genetic locus is for genetic diagnosis, because HNPCC probably is traceable to more than one underlying genetic disorder. The gene or genes for this disorder have not yet been cloned, but progress in this area will undoubtedly modify our approach to surveillance in this disease.

Patients at risk for HNPCC develop a small number of adenomas at an early age, and these have a very high propensity to become malignant.[249,250] The majority of polyps and cancers occur above the reach of the sigmoidoscope, so the only acceptable screening technique is periodic total colonoscopy. Because the temporal relations for the progression of adenomas to carcinomas are unknown for this disease, although it is thought to be more rapid than for sporadic tumors, a cautious approach is necessary at this time. Colonoscopy is recommended, beginning at approximately 25 years of age or 5 years before the earliest colorectal cancer developed in the family, and it should be repeated every 2 years if negative. If adenomatous polyps are found, it is not unreasonable to repeat the examination in 1 year. If a cancer is found, a subtotal colectomy is the appropriate surgery, followed by careful annual sigmoidoscopic examination of the residual bowel.[138]

Positive Family History of Colorectal Cancer

After the autosomal dominantly inherited familial cancer syndromes have been ruled out, many patients remain with one or more relatives who have had colorectal cancer. Given the high rate of colorectal cancer in the United States and the fact that this disease is largely attributable to environmental influences, it follows that not all of these people are necessarily at an increased risk for cancer.

The following may be used to help target surveillance measures, but this remains an area of controversy. A family history of colorectal cancer in a first-degree relative (i.e., parents, siblings, children) increases the risk by a factor of approximately 3.5 fold.[383] As mentioned above, a large proportion of the population—nearly a third—have at least one relative with colorectal cancer, assuming the information is available and the family is large enough. It has been demonstrated that performing colonoscopy for a positive family history produces a low yield of neoplastic lesions.[260] Individuals with a single, elderly affected relative are not necessarily at increased risk of colorectal cancer, but the risk increases if there are two or more affected relatives or if the tumors have occurred in young individuals (i.e., younger than 55 years of age). Patients with any family history of cancer should enter into a routine screening program that involves annual FOBTs and periodic sigmoidoscopy, perhaps every 3 to 5 years. Patients with multiple affected family members or with first-degree relatives who developed colorectal cancer before 55 years of age need more screening, but it is not clear how much more is justified. One should perform a colonoscopic examination perhaps 5 years earlier than the earliest cancer in the family, because of the tendency for familial cancers to occur above the range of the sigmoidoscope. If this is negative for neoplasia, follow-up surveillance should consist of annual FOBTs and sigmoidoscopies every 3 to 5 years, unless the family history is more worrisome and suggests AAPC or HNPCC, in which case colonoscopy every 1 to 2 years may be necessary. Genetic screening is valuable for syndromes related to FAP (such as AAPC), and is in evolution for HNPCC; referral to a geneticist is an important option for confusing histories or worried patients.

Prior History of Adenomatous Polyps

Many patients have adenomas discovered through screening examinations, work-ups of colorectal symptoms, or other evaluations. The recommended surveillance of such patients has undergone an important change in light of new data, and a degree of restraint is appropriate for certain patients. The majority of adenomatous polyps (or flat adenomas) are small, do not produce symptoms, and have been discovered serendipitously by colonoscopy. The presence of solitary adenomas less than 1 cm in diameter does not predict an increased likelihood of recurrent neoplasia.[269,270,271] Therefore, the detection of a solitary, low-grade adenomatous polyp, especially in an elderly patient, does not mandate colonoscopic follow-up. Patients who have had more advanced lesions, such as larger adenomas (>1 cm), villoglandular or villous adenomas, multiple adenomas, or adenomas containing high-grade dysplasia, require follow-up colonoscopy.

For this group, there is no need for a repeat examination at the 1-year time interval after the colon has been cleared of lesions by a technically optimal examination. A report from the National Polyp Study Group indicated that a 3-year interval is adequate for follow-up colonoscopy.[397] This group reported that the detection of adenomas was common at the 1-year and 3-year points, with polyps found in 32% of the patients examined once and 41.7% of those examined twice during the 3 years of follow-up; however, the incidence of advanced lesions (large or higher pathologic grade) was only 3.3% in both groups, and cancers are very rare and are discovered at an early stage.[397] This again suggests that patients who have had small, solitary adenomas removed do not need colonoscopic follow-up, and those with larger lesions can wait 3 years after the colon has been cleared of lesions for follow-

up, if not longer, given the relatively small number of advanced lesions at 3 years.

Prior History of Colorectal Cancer

Follow-up colonoscopy after the resection of a cancer is frequently overdone, and the objectives of such examinations should be clear to the examiner.[398] Patients who have had sporadic cancers removed are not necessarily different from those who have had high-grade adenomas removed; the principal difference between a cancer patient and a high-grade adenoma patient is the timing of discovery of the lesion. Cancer patients need an examination of the anastomotic site within the first 3 to 6 months after surgery, and perhaps again at 1 year, but the effectiveness of this approach has never been rigorously tested. In the absence of an anastomotic recurrence, the rationale for continued colonoscopic surveillance is to remove recurrent adenomas and to detect metachronous cancers. New lesions develop through the adenoma to carcinoma sequence, which typically evolves over a period of a decade or more. Colonoscopic examination every 3 years is recommended, just as for patients with advanced adenomas.

Inflammatory Bowel Disease

Patients with ulcerative colitis are at increased risk for developing cancer. The risk is lowest in the first decade of disease, but 10% develop cancer each decade thereafter. Patients with colitis limited to the distal colon are at much lower risk. It is recommended that patients undergo screening colonoscopy after 8 to 10 years of disease, during which time all suspicious lesions should be biopsied, and biopsies should be taken from multiple regions throughout the colon. If high-grade dysplasia is found in the colon, the patient should immediately undergo repeat colonoscopy with careful inspection of the site of dysplasia and collection of multiple biopsies to exclude an adjacent cancer. Although the optimal intervals for periodic examination have not been determined, colonoscopic surveillance appears to significantly reduce colorectal cancer mortality in this setting by detecting cancers at earlier stages.[399] Barium enemas play no role in the screening for cancer in these individuals because of the abnormalities produced by inflammation and scarring. Alternatively, if the patient's disease is sufficiently severe, a colectomy should be considered at this time.[400] Such a decision should take into account the adverse effects of chronic disease as well as the risk of cancer.

Patients who have no dysplasia on multiple biopsies are at relatively low risk to develop neoplasia during the next 1 to 2 years, and these patients should undergo surveillance colonoscopy approximately every 2 years. If no dysplasia is found on follow-up colonoscopy, a longer interval between surveillance studies may be appropriate. Patients with milder disease and disease limited to the distal colon are also candidates for increased intervals between surveillance studies because of the relatively low incidence of new dysplasia among patients initially free of this abnormality. Low-grade dysplasia is more difficult to interpret, especially in the setting of acute inflammation. It is not clear whether the diagnosis of low-grade dysplasia should not increase the threshold for a consideration of colectomy; however, these patients should be studied with colonoscopy at annual intervals to detect the evolution of higher grades of neoplasia.

Patients with Crohn's disease are at increased risk to develop gastrointestinal cancer, including carcinoma of the colon. At present there is inadequate information to recommend how frequently patients with Crohn's disease of the colon should undergo routine screening colonoscopy. Crohn's colitis involving the entire colon should be considered in the same risk category as ulcerative colitis.

CLINICAL COURSE AND COMPLICATIONS

The clinical course of colorectal neoplasia includes two major considerations: first, what determines the behavior of a colon cancer, and second, if a primary tumor is removed, what determines the behavior of the rest of the colon?

Natural History of Colorectal Neoplasia

The pathologic stage of colorectal cancer is the best clinical predictor of outcome. Pathologic stage is principally a reflection of depth of invasion. Tumor diameter and total tumor mass are not strong independent predictors of clinical outcome. It is not unusual to find a large bulky tumor that neither penetrates the muscularis propria nor metastasizes, and it is also not unusual to find a small, 2- to 3-cm tumor that invades and metastasizes to distant sites. This latter situation presumably represents the temporal compression of tumor progression events resulting in the early appearance of a biologically aggressive tumor. In fact, as a group, Dukes' stage B tumors may be larger than stage C lesions.[401] The relative distribution of cancers by stage is listed in Table 87-17. Actuarial age-adjusted 5-year survival rates for colorectal cancers are approximately 99%, 85%, 67%, and 14% for stage A, B, C, and

TABLE 87-17
Distribution of Colorectal Cancer Patients by Pathologic Stage

STAGE*	ESTIMATED DISTRIBUTION†	DETECTION BY SCREENING‡
A	10%	60%
B	50% (±10%)	20%
B1	15%	
B2	35%	
C	25%	10%
C1	13%	
C2	13%	
D	15%	10%

* Pathologic stage varies by the investigator.

† These are estimates drawn from several reported studies that used differing methods to recruit and exclude patients.

‡ From Boland CR. Diagnosis and management of primary and metastatic colorectal cancers. Semin Gastrointest Dis 1992;3:33; in several large studies, 65%–90% of cancers were Stage A or B when detected by screening (see Table 87-16).

D tumors, respectively.[339] The best prognostic indicator is the depth of invasion; *crude* 5-year survival rates for modified Dukes' stage A tumors range from 81% to 84%; for stage B, 62% to 65%; for stage C, 36% to 40%; and for stage D, 0% to 3%.[402,403] Five-year survival data corrected for anticipated age-related mortality are higher. In addition to the depth of invasion, patient outcome is also related to the presence of certain genetic lesions such as LOH at tumor suppressor gene loci, and the fraction of chromosomal arms lost in colorectal cancer cells is an important independent predictor of an adverse clinical course. The outcome of the treatment of patients with colorectal cancer has been illustrated in an estimate made by August and colleagues, shown in Figure 87-13.[404]

Metastatic Disease

It is a tenet of tumor biology that cancers are relentlessly progressive. Rarely, a patient can survive for 20 or 30 years in spite of an unresected primary tumor. However, the median survival period for patients who have hepatic metastases diagnosed at the time of surgery is only 4.5 months.[405] The clinical objective is to detect colorectal tumors early in their natural histories and to intervene with appropriate surgical therapy. At present, 5-year corrected survival rates have been reported to range from 40% for all colorectal cancers[406] to 67% for patients who are candidates for potentially curative surgery for rectosigmoid tumors.[407] Approximately 25% of all these patients are diagnosed with Dukes-Turnbull's stage D tumors—that is, disease that has spread beyond the bowel and its regional lymph nodes.[341] In general, metastatic disease is disseminated when first detected and is only infrequently localized. However, a group of patients, perhaps 15% to 40%, do not have metastatic disease at the time of surgery but eventually succumb to recurrent disease within 5 years. It has been difficult to identify these patients prospectively to assess the impact of adjuvant treatment on their outcome.

It has long been appreciated that circulating tumor cells may be found in the mesenteric and systemic circulation of patients with colorectal cancer, and curiously, this is of no prognostic significance.[408] More than 80% of colorectal adenocarcinomas are well or moderately differentiated tumors, and there are few prognostic features that can be found to predict tumor recurrence in this group. Poorly differentiated and colloid (or mucinous) tumors make up the remainder of the adenocarcinomas, and the 5-year survival rate in these instances is somewhat worse than for their better differentiated counterparts.[407] As previously mentioned, the primary adverse prognostic indicators are the depth of invasion and the presence of metastasis at the time of surgery. Tumor size is not an independent predictor of outcome.[409]

Approximately three quarters of patients presenting with colorectal cancer undergo a resection that appears to be curative. The expected location of metastatic disease is related, to some extent, to the location of the primary tumor, as illustrated in Table 87-18. However, one third of these patients develop recurrent disease. Approximately 60% of this group die with recurrences in multiple sites, one quarter develop a local recurrence at the site of the primary tumor, and a small residual number develop isolated metastases in a single organ.[404] In a study of patients who underwent surgical explo-

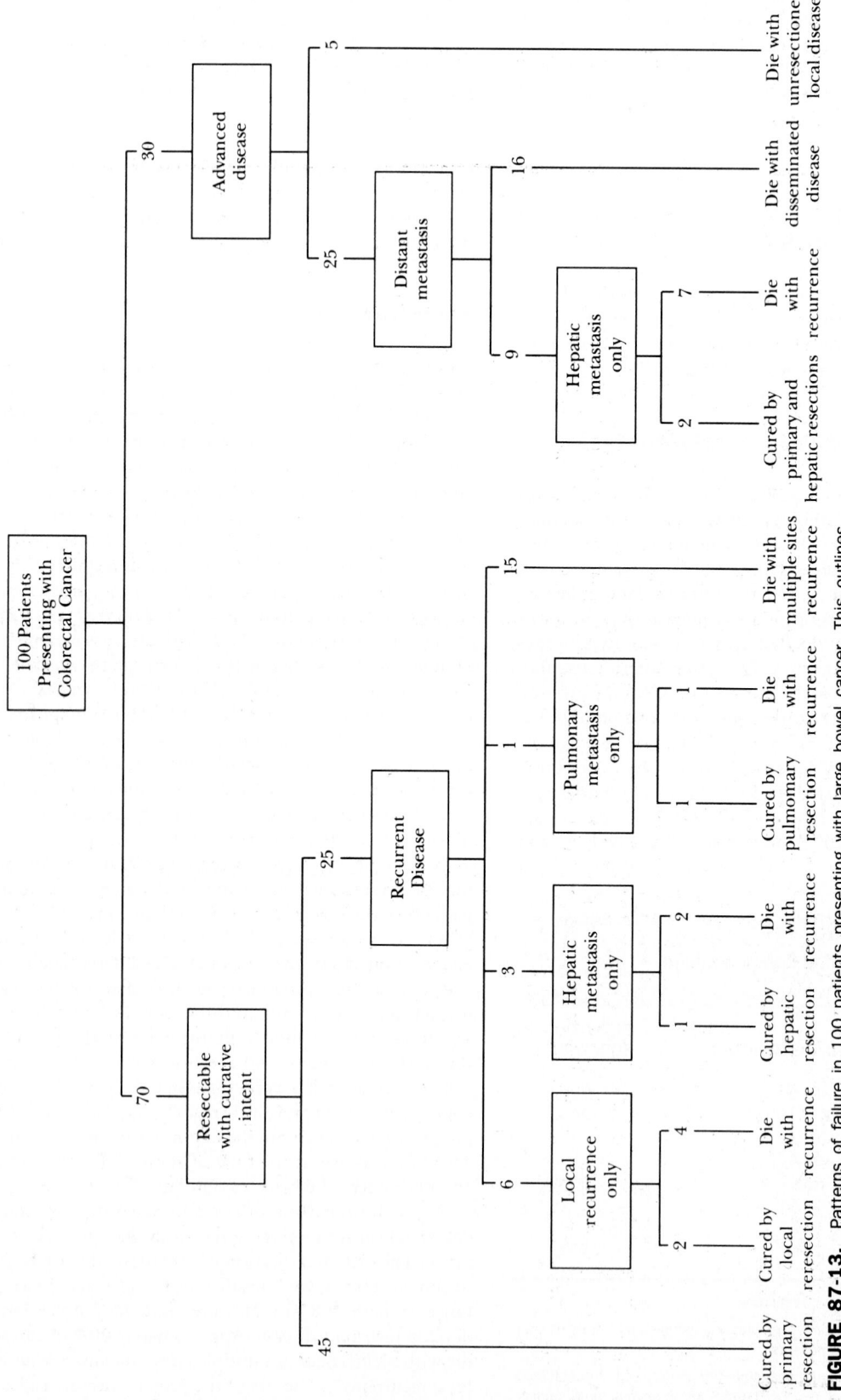

FIGURE 87-13. Patterns of failure in 100 patients presenting with large bowel cancer. This outlines the projected outcome of typical cohort of patients in which 70% appeared to be resectable for cure; 64% of that group was cured by primary resection but the other 36% experienced recurrent disease. A total of 55% either presented with advanced disease (30%) or developed postoperative recurrence (25%); approximately 11% of that group may be cured by additional surgery. (From August DA, Ottow RT, Sugarbaker PH. Clinical perspectives on human colorectal cancer metastases. Cancer Metastasis Rev 1984;3:303.)

TABLE 87-18
Distribution of Metastases From Colorectal Cancer at Autopsy

METASTATIC SITE	PRIMARY TUMOR SITE (%)		
	Right Colon	*Sigmoid Colon*	*Rectum*
Liver	67	68	48
Lung	31	43	52
Pelvis	9	27	41
Regional lymph nodes	49	57	59
Peritoneum	31	41	25
Adrenals	13	23	18
Bone	7	7	16
Brain	7	4	5

Summarized and adapted from Welch JP, Donaldson GA: The clinical correlation of an autopsy study of recurrent colorectal cancer. From Boland CR. Diagnosis and management of primary and metastatic colorectal cancer. Semin Gastrointest Dis 1992;3:33.

ration for their primary tumor, 6 (14%) of 43 had overt hepatic metastases, and the other 37 (86%) were followed at 3-month intervals for the development of recurrent disease. During 2 years of follow-up, 11 (30%) of the 37 developed overt hepatic metastases. Among these 11 patients with occult metastases, computed tomography (CT) was most sensitive in detecting silent recurrences.[410] Only one of these 11 patients with an occult hepatic metastasis survived 3 years.[411] Colorectal cancers may metastasize to sites other than the liver or regional lymph nodes, but these tend to occur with symptoms of colonic or metastatic disease.

In a study of 302 consecutive autopsies on patients with early metastatic cancer from an unknown primary site at the time of presentation, only 3.6% came from the colon or rectum.[412] Similarly, only of 3% of 62 patients who presented with cerebral metastases had a colorectal primary tumor.[413] Therefore, a colonoscopy or barium enema is a low-yield procedure in the absence of colorectal symptoms in the work-up of a metastasis of unknown origin.

TREATMENT

Treatment of Colon Cancer

Primary Surgical Treatment for Cure of Colon Cancer

Preoperative evaluation. The preoperative work-up in a patient found to have colonic cancer requires an inspection of the entire colon, preferably with colonoscopy, although an air-contrast barium enema may suffice if there is difficulty advancing the colonoscope proximal to the index lesion. Inspection of the whole colon after the discovery of an index lesion is important because of the 5% risk of a second primary cancer, which modifies the surgical approach. Additional preoperative work-up includes a CT scan of the abdomen to search for metastatic neoplastic disease, particularly in the liver. If a CT scan is performed, there is no need to perform an additional radionuclide or sonographic imaging procedure

of the liver. Radionuclide scanning with a monoclonal antibody directed against colorectal tumor antigens is now available,[414] but this does not routinely add to the information gained from a CT scan. This modality is more valuable in localizing pelvic or abdominal recurrence, which may be difficult to find on CT. A chest radiography is part of the routine preoperative evaluation, but a CT scan of the thorax is not recommended as a routine preoperative assessment. An imaging procedure of the central nervous system is also a low-yield procedure, and the cost is not commensurate with the probable benefit.

Other preoperative laboratory evaluations include a complete blood count because of the possibility of iron deficiency anemia and the need to correct this before surgery and, in the absence of metastatic disease, a measurement of carcinoembryonic antigen (CEA). The CEA should be drawn before removal of the primary tumor, because not all cancers produce this glycoprotein, and if the preoperative value is not elevated, the test is not informative in the postoperative period. If the CEA is elevated, and if the operative assessment is that all tumor has been removed, the CEA should be repeated approximately 1 month after surgery, assuming the physician and patient are prepared to undertake repeat surgery for any evidence of tumor recurrence. The upper limits of normal for plasma CEA is 5.0 ng/mL. CEA is excreted in bile, so levels are difficult to interpret in the face of biliary obstruction or hepatic dysfunction. CEA is not useful as a primary screening test because of the large number of patients with nonneoplastic conditions who have minor elevations,[415,416] and it is not useful in locating the source of metastatic lesion. Serial measurements of CEA may be of value in detecting early recurrences in the postoperative patient; however, this should not be undertaken unless the patient is prepared to accept exploratory laparotomy for an elevated result. If this course of action is unacceptable to the patient, then it may be best not to measure it.[401]

Surgery.   The primary modality for treatment for colonic cancer is surgical resection. The surgical approach is directed by the location of the tumor and the desire to remove not only wide margins of resection (a minimum of 5 cm proximal and distal to the edges of the tumor) but also regional lymph nodes. A cancer in the cecum, ascending colon, hepatic flexure, or transverse colon is treated with a right hemicolectomy, including a dissection of the mesenteric lymph nodes. Examination of the liver for gross metastatic disease helps predict the postoperative outcome. Tumors from the splenic flexure to the sigmoid colon are treated with a left hemicolectomy and primary colonic anastomosis preserving the rectum. Lesions in the sigmoid colon are treated with a segmental (low anterior) resection with an end-to-end primary colonic anastomosis. Every attempt is made to treat cancers in the rectosigmoid region with a low anterior resection, which permits the preservation of the rectum and obviates the need for colostomy. However, rectosigmoid lesions require the dissection of hypogastric lymph nodes in addition to the standard mesenteric dissection. The skill of the surgeon is an important prognostic factor that should be considered, because the operative mortality and complication rates vary significantly among surgeons.[417] Cases should be referred to surgeons with specific interest and expertise in the disease.

In general, every patient with colon cancer who is an acceptable surgical candidate should undergo resection of the primary lesions. Colonic cancers have a tendency to produce intestinal obstruction late in the clinical course, after the patient may no longer be a surgical candidate. Patients who present with obstruction are best managed with a primary resection of the tumor rather than a multistage procedure leading to delayed resection of the tumor. However, technical considerations may require tumor resection and diverting colostomy, with a delayed anastomosis. The operative mortality for colon cancer surgery is approximately 5%,[402,403,418] but it may be as high as 17% for emergency operations,[403] and has been reported to be less than 3% in one large Asian series.[419] In planning treatment, it is important to realize that this disease tends to occur in older patients with other comorbid conditions.

Cancer in an Adenomatous Polyp

A situation in which a segmental colonic resection may be avoided is that in which in situ or invasive cancer is found in a pedunculated adenomatous polyp. This is discussed in more detail in Chapter 85, but if the endoscopist and pathologist agree that the cancer has been removed, for example by snare cautery, additional surgery is not necessary.[420] An exception to this policy is the case in which poorly differentiated cancer is encountered.

Adjuvant Chemotherapy of Colon Cancer After Surgery for Apparent Cure

The postoperative prognosis for patients who undergo primary resection of colonic cancer is based on the surgical stage of disease; approximately 70% appear to have received curative surgery (i.e., all tumors Dukes' stage A, B, and C), and yet approximately one third of this group eventually develop recurrent disease. The administration of chemotherapy to patients who have undergone a complete surgical resection with curative intent is referred to adjuvant therapy, which is distinct from treating known metastatic disease.

Numerous chemotherapeutic regimens have been used in an attempt to reduce the recurrence rate of metastatic disease.[421,422] Before 1989, no regimen had been shown to improve survival in this disease. The first step forward was achieved by Laurie and colleagues, who demonstrated a significant survival benefit for the use of levamisole plus fluorouracil (5-FU) as adjuvant therapy in patients with Dukes' stage C colon cancer.[423] This benefit was confirmed in a larger study by Moertel and colleagues shortly thereafter.[424]

The first study[423] followed 401 patients with Dukes' stage B or C colorectal cancer, excluding those with stage A cancer (in which the predicted outcome is too good to justify adjuvant therapy) and those with stage D cancer (who, by definition, have advanced disease). The patients were randomized to receive either no additional therapy or 1 year of treatment with levamisole (50 mg every 8 hr for 3 days, repeated every 2 weeks) plus 5-FU (450 mg/m²/day intravenously for 5 days, followed on day 28 with single weekly injections of 450 mg/m²). Separate arms were randomized to receive only lev-

amisole or to receive no adjuvant treatment. Stage B patients were those with tumor that had invaded the serosa, pericolonic or perirectal fat, or adjacent organs by direct extension, without lymph node metastasis (stage B2 according to some classifications). Stage C patients had involvement of regional lymph nodes but no distant metastases. The median length of follow-up was longer than 7 years, and the minimum was longer than 4 years. After the data were analyzed for the entire group of patients under treatment (i.e., both stage B and stage C patients), a significant reduction (31%) in tumor recurrence rate was found for levamisole plus 5-FU, and a reduction of borderline significance (27%) was found for levamisole alone. Combination therapy also produced a delay in the time to tumor recurrence. Considering patients of both stages eligible for analysis, no improvement in survival was seen for any treatment regimen compared with controls.

The patients in the first study were then analyzed separately by tumor stage. No improvement in the recurrence interval or survival was found for patients with stage B tumors. However, a significant improvement in recurrence-free interval and survival was found in stage C tumors for the combination of levamisole plus 5-FU compared with control patients. No benefit was found for levamisole alone. The authors concluded that substantial benefits would be achieved if stage C patients were treated with adjuvant therapy.

These results were confirmed in a larger study of 1296 patients with either locally invasive (stage B2) or stage C colon cancers; rectal tumors were excluded.[424] The median time for follow-up in this larger study was 3 years. No benefit for tumor recurrence or survival was found among the patients with stage B2 disease. A 41% reduction in tumor recurrence was found in patients with stage C disease treated with levamisole plus 5-FU (p>0.0001), and the death rate was reduced 33% in this group (Fig. 87-14). No benefit was found with the use of levamisole alone. The authors concluded that adjuvant therapy with levamisole plus fluorouracil should become standard treatment for patients with stage C colon cancer. Although patients with stage B2 cancers continue to be considered for adjuvant therapy, their relatively good 5-year prognosis (77% 5-year survival rate) suggests that it may be difficult to provide significant improvement with acceptable toxicities.[425]

Patients should be advised before accepting this therapy that considerable toxicity will probably be encountered with chemotherapy. More than half of patients experienced nausea, 47% experienced diarrhea, and 17% experienced vomiting during the maintenance phase of treatment, although the side effects were described as mild in most instances.[424] Stomatitis, dermatitis, and alopecia were each observed in approximately one quarter of the patients. Mild leukopenia (2000–4000 leukocytes) was encountered in 38% of patients. A variety of neurologic symptoms were experienced by 18% of patients; these resolved after therapy was discontinued. Fully 30% of patients discontinued their therapy prematurely because of toxicity, most commonly because of nausea. Patients should be advised that substantial side effects will accompany their therapy but that significant improvement in disease-free survival may be expected for patients with stage C cancer of the colon. No benefit has been demonstrated for any treatment regimen applied to patients with stages A or B colorectal cancer.

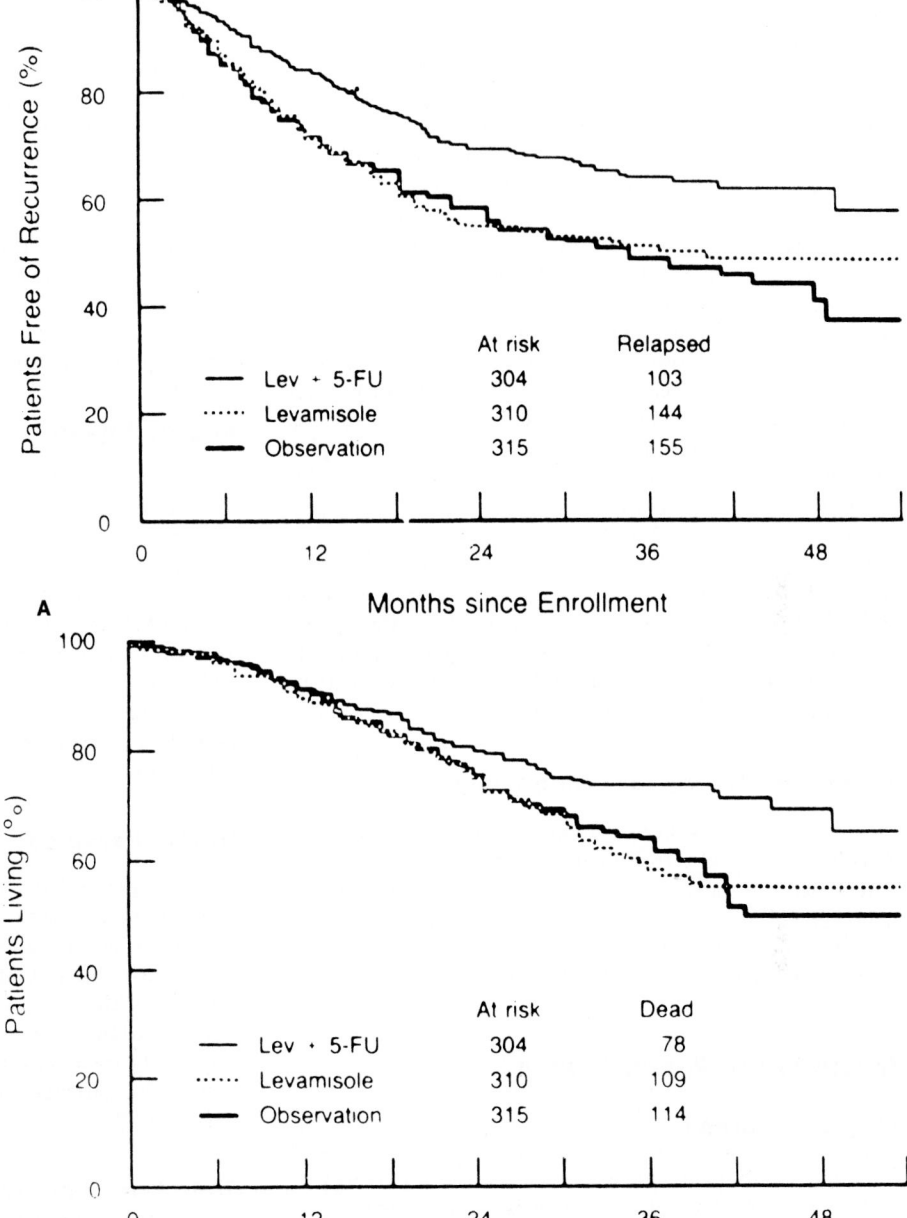

FIGURE 87-14. **(A)** Recurrence-free interval after adjuvant treatment of stage C colon cancer with levamisole (Lev) and 5-fluorouracil (5-FU). There was a significant improvement in recurrence-free status from 47% to 63% among treated patients at 42 months ($P < 0.0001$; *top*). The reduction in recurrence was greatest for sites outside the abdomen. **(B)** Survival after adjuvant treatment of stage C colon cancer with Lev and 5-FU. There was a reduction in the death rate by approximately 33% in the treated group compared with controls ($P = 0.006$; *top*). From Moertel CJ, Fleming TR, MacDonald JS, et al. Levamisole and fluorouracil for adjuvant therapy of resected colon carcinoma. N Engl J Med 1990;322: 352.)

Follow-Up of Patients After Surgical Resection

As mentioned, although approximately 70% of patients appear to have complete excision of all malignant disease, but more than one third of this group suffer later recurrences. In a small proportion of these patients, timely therapy may prolong their survival. A variety of approaches has been developed to detect early recurrences and to treat them effectively.

Colonoscopy should be performed once between postoperative months 3 and 6, and again 12 months postoperatively to detect recurrences of the primary tumor and the development of metachronous or missed synchronous tumors. Recurrences of primary tumor occur at the anastomotic site and may or may not be detectable using colonoscopic surveillance, because some occur on the serosal aspect of the bowel. Anastomotic recurrences most often develop after rectal or rectosigmoid resections, and the likelihood is strongly dependent on the Dukes' stage of the resected cancer.[426,427] The majority of these appear within 2 years of the initial operation, and 90% are heralded by persistent symptoms. It is important to diagnose local recurrences and to be aware that some of these are submucosal, because there is a 49% 5-year survival rate after resection of such disease.[426]

Measurement of serial CEA levels at 2-month intervals and CT scans at 3- to 6-month intervals have been evaluated as means for detecting early metastatic disease. There is little sense in measuring serial CEA levels unless the patient and physician are prepared to undertake additional surgery for an elevated level. CEA measurements vary among laboratories, so a reference lab with careful quality control is essential. Recurrent tumor was found at a second-look operation in 56 (93%) of 60 patients operated on solely because of serial elevations of CEA. Recurrent tumor was later identified in 3 of the remaining 4 patients, and 1 had a spurious elevation of CEA as a result of liver disease.[428] Approximately half of these patients had resectable tumor, and more than one third have had long-term disease-free survivals. Another group reported recurrent disease in 33 (89%) of 37 laparotomies performed for elevations of CEA in asymptomatic patients, with a 43% resectability rate, evenly split between local recurrences and liver metastases.[428] However, two other groups have reported that the use of serial CEA values to direct laparotomy for recurrent disease may result in long-term, disease-free survival in only 3% of a group of patients followed after colorectal surgery.[429,430] Furthermore, the cost of follow-up per resectable tumor has been estimated to be approximately $25,000, exclusive of the cost of CT scanning[431]; the added cost of the radiologic procedure, if used on all patients, could triple this cost.[432] Therefore, the willingness of the patient to undergo additional procedures and operations as well as the impact of total cost must be considered in planning an appropriate follow-up schedule, in light of the minor impact on patient outcome provided by this surveillance.

Radiation Therapy for Colon Cancer

Radiation therapy has been evaluated as an adjuvant therapy for colon cancer and as treatment for metastatic disease. There is no benefit for the use of radiation therapy as an adjunctive agent for colon cancer outside of the rectum. Adenocarcinomas of the colon tend to be relatively radioresistant, and the toxicities from abdominal radiation are considerable.

Treatment of Rectal Cancer

Surgical Therapy

The approach to the treatment of rectal carcinoma is dictated by the fact that most of this organ is located beneath the peritoneal reflection and is surrounded by perirectal fat. Any degree of invasion greater than Dukes' stage A requires a wide excision, usually consisting of a combined abdominoperineal resection and subsequent colostomy, which is not required for resections of carcinoma in the colon. Lesions located high in the rectum (>6 cm from the anus) may be treated with a low anterior resection without total proctectomy, but this approach brings with it a higher likelihood of local recurrence. Invasive cancers in the distal 6 cm of rectum are best treated with an abdominoperineal resection and hypogastric lymph node dissection. If the degree of invasion is not clear on physical examination, endorectal ultrasound may help provide important staging information.[433]

A patient with a small rectal neoplasm, even in the distal 6 cm, may refuse a proctectomy and colostomy because of the possible complications and changes in lifestyle that accompany this operation, or the patient may not be a suitable operative candidate for this procedure. In this instance, a local

excision of the tumor may be considered. The preferred lesions for this approach should be small (less than one third of the circumference of the rectum); they should be readily mobile, indicating only early or localized invasion of the submucosal tissues; and they should not be mucinous or poorly differentiated carcinomas, which carry a more ominous prognosis. Two decades ago, abdominoperineal resection was standard treatment for many rectal cancers, but surgeons with interest and expertise in this tumor are able to perform successful local resections on a growing proportion of these lesions with a sphincter-sparing operation. A study of 57 patients with distal rectal cancer treated with full-thickness local excision demonstrated an overall 5-year survival rate of 83%, and the cancer-specific mortality rate was 11%.[434]

Rectal Polyps

Pedunculated polypoid lesions in the rectum can be removed using snare polypectomy. Sessile polyps, which may create a therapeutic dilemma elsewhere in the colon, can often be treated more aggressively in the rectum, because of the additional margin of safety provided by the subperitoneal location of the rectum. As has been mentioned, transanal local excision may be elected for mobile cancers that do not penetrate the bowel wall and are not poorly differentiated adenocarcinomas, especially for the patient who is not a surgical candidate or who refuses abdominoperineal resection and colostomy.

Other Therapies

Because of the relatively encouraging outcome after local excision in patients with small rectal cancers, other nonsurgical modalities have been evaluated. Neodymium:yttrium-aluminum-garnet (Nd:YAG) laser photocoagulation has been safely applied for the removal of adenomatous polyps that cannot be removed by standard snare polypectomy.[435] Laser ablation may also be used as palliative treatment for symptomatic rectal cancers in patients who are not candidates for surgical resection.[436,437]

Radiation Therapy to Improve Operability in Rectal Carcinoma

The role of preoperative radiation therapy is sometimes overlooked in the management of rectal cancer. A retrospective review indicated that 20 (80%) of 25 patients with unresectable rectal cancer were converted into surgical candidates by preoperative radiation therapy, and 16 (80%) of 20 patients were able to undergo resection for cure. This group had 2- and 5-year survival rates of 56% and 43%, respectively.[438] Other groups have confirmed the value of preoperative radiation for rectal cancer.[439] Another study has reported that as many as 50% of patients with a fixed rectal cancer can be operated on with apparent long-term benefit after radiation therapy.[440]

A subsequent prospective study indicated that postoperative radiation therapy (or radiation therapy plus adjuvant chemotherapy) for rectal cancer prolonged survival in treated patients compared with untreated controls.[441] Additional experience in a controlled study suggests that some of the benefits achieved by preoperative radiation therapy may also be achieved using postoperative radiation.[442] Most surgeons prefer not to delay surgery for preoperative radiation, so postoperative radiation is more commonly used.

Adjuvant Therapy for Rectal Carcinoma

The incidence of local recurrence in rectal cancer is dependent on the pathologic stage; local recurrence is found in 8% of Dukes' stage A, 31% of Dukes' stage B, and 50% of Dukes' stage C patients, and the unadjusted 5-year survivals are 77%, 44%, and 23%, respectively.[427] Effective adjuvant therapy must take into account both local and systemic disease. A regimen of intravenous 5-FU given for 5 days every 10 weeks, together on alternate cycles with oral semustine (methyl-CCNU; 130 mg/m^2) on day 1 and repeated in 10-week cycles for 18 months, in combination with external beam radiotherapy for approximately 5 weeks, significantly prolonged the time to tumor recurrence, but not overall survival, in a multiinstitution study of patients with Dukes' stage B and C tumors of the rectum.[421] In another large study, patients with stage B and C rectal cancers were found to receive some benefit from chemotherapy with 5-FU, semustine, and vincristine, but improvements in survival or disease-free intervals with radiation alone were not seen.[443]

Combined postoperative adjuvant treatment consisting of chemotherapy and radiation is of benefit in patients with locally invasive (Dukes' stage B2) or Dukes' stage C rectal cancer.[444] Combined therapy consisted of an oral dose of semustine (130 mg/m^2 on day 1) plus 5-FU (300 mg/m^2 on days 1–5 and 400 mg/m^2 on days 36–40), followed by external beam radiation beginning on day 64. The radiation therapy consisted of a total of 4500 cGy and was delivered in divided doses 5 days a week for a period of 5 weeks. This form of therapy reduced pelvic recurrences by 46%, distant tumor spread by 37%, and patient deaths by 27%. Preliminary, unpublished data suggest that the use of semustine may not be necessary. Estimated 5-year recurrence rates in those patients receiving radiation only was approximately 63% and was reduced to 42% in those patients receiving the combination therapy (Fig. 87-15). Toxicity of this treatment may be considerable, as previously discussed in the context of adjuvant therapy for colon cancer. The acute side effects include bone marrow suppression and diarrhea, and late complications of radiation include proctitis, strictures, and bowel obstruction (occurring in 6.5% of all patients). It appears that combined radiation and chemotherapy is an appropriate adjuvant therapy to offer patients who have undergone apparently successful resections of Dukes' stage B2 and stage C rectal cancers. The role of semustine in this therapy remains to be elucidated; the development of late second malignancies has been associated with this agent. Gastroenterologists will be presented with the late complications after an increased number of patients are treated with this combined therapy. The role of levamisole in the treatment of rectal cancer remains to be explored.

Patients with rectal cancer who appear to be good operative candidates at the time of presentation should undergo immediate operative therapy, either abdominoperineal resection or local excision. Patients with Dukes' stage A and B1 lesions have a relatively favorable 5-year prognosis and need no further

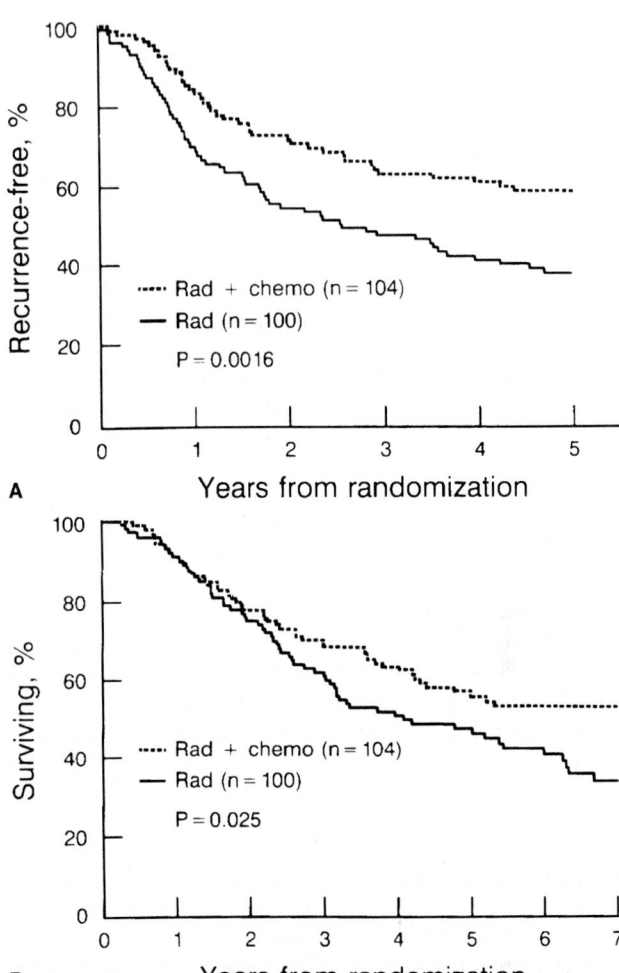

FIGURE 87-15. (**A**) Recurrence-free intervals in patients with stage B2 or C rectal cancer treated by postoperative radiation therapy with or without chemotherapy. Patients receiving chemotherapy had 34% fewer recurrences. (**B**) Survival rates in patients with stage B2 or C rectal cancer treated by postoperative radiation therapy with or without chemotherapy indicated a significant improvement in survival with adjuvant chemotherapy. (From Krook JE, Moertel TJ, Gunderson LL, et al. Effective surgical adjuvant therapy for high-risk rectal carcinoma. N Engl J Med 1991;324: 709.)

therapy. Patients with stage B2 and C lesions should undergo resection and postoperative combined adjuvant radiation and chemotherapy. Patients who appear to be inoperable at the time of presentation should first undergo radiation therapy, and then should be evaluated for the possibility that the tumor has been rendered operable.

Treatment of Metastatic Colorectal Cancer

Resection of Metastatic Disease

Anastomotic and other local recurrences of cancer may occur after resections in the colon but are more likely to occur in the pelvis after a rectal or rectosigmoid resection. Most patients with recurrences present because of symptoms, and it is reasonable to consider surgical resection of the metastatic disease.

The use of CEA measurement and CT scanning has resulted in the identification of a increasing number of patients with isolated metastatic disease in the liver. If a single hepatic metastasis or a group of lesions in a single lobe is discovered without other evidence of extrahepatic disease, surgical resection should always be considered as the primary approach, because it is the only treatment that may provide a long-term, disease-free clinical course. The median survival for an untreated solitary hepatic metastasis is approximately 10.6 months.[445] The operative mortality for this operation is less than 5% in experienced hands, and 25% to 35% of operated patients are reported to experience a five-year, disease-free survival.[445,446] Tumors recur in the liver in about one third of these patients, but a larger number of recurrences develop in extrahepatic organs. Solitary resected lesions that are smaller, have wide margins of resection, and are unassociated with extrahepatic disease are more likely to be resected for cure.[432] The limiting factor in successful resection of metastatic disease is the identification of patients who are suitable for resection, because they represent less than 5% of all patients followed after initial colonic surgery with curative intent.

The outlook is less promising for resection of isolated pulmonary metastases. In one study, only 2 of 16 patients who underwent pulmonary resection for metastatic disease from colorectal cancer survived five years, but experience with this problem remains somewhat anecdotal.[447] A more recent series of 62 patients reported 42% five-year and 22% ten-year survival rates after thoracotomy, with a mean overall survival of 24 months. A solitary pulmonary metastasis less than 3 cm in diameter should be considered for a surgical resection, but it is not yet clear what impact this has on survival and cure rates.[448,449]

Chemotherapy for Metastatic Colorectal Cancer

Less than half of all colorectal cancer patients eventually develop metastatic disease, either at a local site or in a distant organ. As mentioned above, a very small proportion of metastatic disease is amenable to surgical resection. Hence, many forms of medical therapy have been tested in an attempt to effectively manage this complication. Several systematically administered cytotoxic therapies can shrink measurable metastatic disease, but no combination of drugs appears superior to the use of 5-FU. A wide range of objective responses have been reported in the literature, but it appears that a partial response rate of 15% to 20% is a reliable estimate of efficacy. Although patients whose tumors shrink in response to 5-FU live longer than patients whose tumors are resistant to treatment, there is no evidence that a group of patients treated with chemotherapy experiences prolonged survival, nor is it possible to know whether patients whose tumors respond to treatment live longer than if they had not been treated at all.[450]

Attempts have been made to enhance the effectiveness of 5-FU for metastatic (stage D) colorectal cancer by adding leucovorin or methotrexate. Trials suggest that combined therapy may increase the number of responses, although the improvement is modest.[451–454] The added agent often enhances toxicity more than response rate, because of the inherent limitations of the antimetabolites used to treat colorectal cancer. Any claims at treatment efficacy must be documented in the setting of a prospective, controlled clinical trial. At present, systemic chemotherapy for metastatic disease is appropriately given either in a controlled clinical trial or to a patient with a *symptomatic* metastatic disease who has been informed of the limited possibilities for benefit.[455]

Chemotherapy for Localized Hepatic Metastases

More than 80% of patients who die with metastatic colorectal cancer suffer hepatic involvement, and this has prompted interest in developing effective therapies to control the growth of tumor in this organ. As mentioned, surgical resection should be considered for solitary hepatic metastases; unfortunately, these are rare. Because 95% of the blood flow to metastases is delivered by the hepatic artery, attempts have been made to intensify cytotoxic therapy while limiting systemic toxicity by administering the drug through the hepatic artery. The initial experiences with the intraarterial hepatic artery infusion chemotherapy used a percutaneous access port and reported complete disappearance of tumor in 15% of patients, 50% reduction in tumor sizes in 39%, and 25% shrinkage of tumors in another 21%.[456] Systemic drug toxicity was minimized, but a number of complications occurred, including displacement of the catheter tip and arterial thrombosis.

A totally implantable intraarterial infusion pump was introduced in 1979 in an attempt to improve the uniformity of drug delivery. A group of 93 patients were treated with hepatic arterial infusion of 5-fluorodeoxyuridine (FUDR), of whom 45% had failed prior systemic chemotherapy. Significant reductions in tumor size were seen in 83% of the patients, with a median response of 13 months, and median survival of 25 months after the diagnosis of the liver metastasis. Extrahepatic tumor did not respond to the therapy.[457] Unfortunately, the study included no control group. In a similar study, 65 patients were treated in a prospective randomized trial of surgery (if possible) plus continuous hepatic artery chemotherapy, and no significant improvement in survival was seen with FUDR.[458] In a follow-up study, toxicity was reported in more than 80% of the patients, including mucosal damage in the stomach and duodenum, cholestatic liver disease, and strictures of the bile ducts.[459] These investigators have subsequently reported the results on 162 patients after gaining additional experience with the technique and limiting the complications. Intrahepatic arterial FUDR produced a significant improvement in response compared with systemic FUDR, with response rates greater than 50%.[460] Anecdotally, some recipients of this therapy have had dramatic shrinkage of their tumors followed by several years of disease-free survival. Unfortunately, this therapy requires an operation, it still has a considerable number of serious complications, and a significant prolongation of survival has never been demonstrated. Therefore, it is difficult to recommend this therapeutic approach except in the setting of a controlled clinical trial.[461]

Immunotherapy

Because of the frustrations experienced with the described treatment modalities, innovative therapies have been proposed for the treatment of metastatic disease. These approaches are still in their developmental stages; however, dramatic anecdotal results have been reported with immunostimulant therapy. Tumor-infiltrating lymphocytes have been removed from tumors, treated in vitro with cytokines, and readministered to animals. Using a modification of this approach in human cancers, dramatic regressions of metastatic disease (largely melanomas and renal cancers) were initially reported in some patients.[462] In a follow-up study with a larger group of patients, the number of dramatic responses was considerably lower (22%), and substantial systemic toxicity was also reported.[463] This approach has not yet known to be effective for colorectal cancer. Other approaches that use tumor extracts and immunostimulants to create active tumor vaccines are under investigation.[464,465]

In a large cooperative study, 1166 patients with Dukes' stage B and C colon cancers were treated with postoperative bacillus Calmette-Guérin (BCG) therapy. Although no significant difference in disease-free survival was seen, there was a significant survival advantage in favor of the BCG-treated group.[466] The magnitude of the improved survival was modest (<10%), minor toxicities occur with the use of BCG, and additional confirmation of this form of therapy is required before it can be considered for wide application.

OTHER TUMORS OF THE LARGE INTESTINE

A variety of cancers other than adenocarcinoma also occur in the large intestine and enter into the differential diagnosis of a colonic mass discovered because of symptoms or an abnormal screening test. Lymphomas and carcinoid tumors are neoplasms that arise from cells intrinsic to the colon. Much less commonly, sarcomas may arise from the smooth muscle or adipose tissue of the submucosa. Adenoacanthomas, squamous cell carcinomas, and undifferentiated carcinomas appear to represent variant types of differentiation that may have originated from the colonic epithelium. Additionally, primary tumors from other sites may occasionally metastasize to the colon. These tumors are so rare that it is difficult to generalize regarding their clinical characteristics.

Colonic Lymphomas

Primary colonic lymphomas make up a relatively small proportion of all colonic malignancies (<0.5%) but are of importance because of the substantial differences in treatment and prognosis.[467–470] A study of 117 patients with gastrointestinal lymphoma indicated that 48 (41%) occurred in the stomach, 37 (32%) in the small intestine, 13 (11%) in the ileocecal region, 2 (2%) in the appendix, and 11 (9%) in the colon.[467] Using Rappaport's classification, 60% were diffuse histiocytic lymphomas, and the remainder were divided among multiple categories. The clinical features of ileocecal and large intestinal lymphomas are presented in Table 87-19.

TABLE 87-19
Colonic and Ileocecal Lymphomas: Clinical Features

	LOCATION OF LYMPHOMA	
	Large Intestine	*Ileocecal*
Number of patients	8	13
Average age (range) in years	58 (52–77)	37 (7–70)
Gender (M:F)	0.6:1	3.3:1
Presenting Features (%)		
Abdominal pain	50	100
Anorexia	12	23
Diarrhea	50	38
Constipation	0	7
Weight loss	12	31
Gastrointestinal bleeding	62	29
Abdominal mass	25	29
Two-Year Actuarial Survival	38%	41%

From Lewin KJ, Ranchod M, Dorfman RF. Lymphomas of the gastrointestinal tract: a study of 117 cases presenting with gastrointestinal disease. Cancer 1978;42:693.

As indicated, the symptoms are nonspecific and include abdominal pain, gastrointestinal bleeding, and constipation. Ileocecal lymphoma tends to occur in a younger group of patients than does lymphoma in the rest of the large intestine. Approximately half of gastrointestinal lymphomas have regional lymph node involvement or widespread dissemination at the time of diagnosis. The two-year actuarial survival rate was approximately 40% but was related to the stage of disease; patients with stage IE or IIE lymphomas had two-year actuarial survival rates of 82% and 71% respectively, whereas no patients with stage IV disease survived two years.

An increased likelihood of gastrointestinal lymphoma is seen in a variety of autoimmune diseases, including rheumatoid arthritis, Sjögren's syndrome, systemic lupus erythematosis, Wegener's granulomatosis, congenital immune deficiency syndromes, and acquired immunodeficiency syndrome (AIDS).[468] Patients who receive organ transplants and are treated with immunosuppressive drugs have a greatly increased likelihood of developing secondary malignancies, including gastrointestinal lymphoma. The gross and microscopic pathology of these lesions is highly variable, but they are more likely to produce single or multiple discrete lesions than diffuse colonic involvement, which may be found in approximately 10% of the cases. Although rectal lymphoma has been reported in the setting of chronic ulcerative colitis, this appears to be a very rare complication of inflammatory bowel disease.[469]

A report of eight rectal lymphomas also showed few unifying characteristics. Patients presented with a variety of symptoms, including a change in bowel habits, lower abdominal pain, and rectal bleeding, and the lesions ranged from small submucosal nodules to diffuse friable abnormalities.[471]

Treatment of colonic lymphomas has included the use of surgery, radiation, and chemotherapy. Since most colonic lymphomas are diagnosed colonoscopically, surgery can usually be avoided, but it may be considered in the case of focal disease. Most treatment regimens include chemotherapy;

however, the optimal form of treatment remains to be established.

Kaposi's Sarcoma in the Colon

Before the emergence of the AIDS epidemic, Kaposi's sarcoma was a rare neoplasm largely confined to the skin, with infrequent systemic involvement. However, it appears that Kaposi's sarcoma as a complication of AIDS includes gastrointestinal involvement in 75% of patients.[472] The stomach and duodenum are more frequently involved, but approximately one third of these patients also have colonic involvement,[472] and subcutaneous nodules and infiltrative lesions may be demonstrable using radiographic studies.[473] In a study of 50 patients with Kaposi's sarcoma, characteristic lesions were visualized using a 60-cm flexible sigmoidoscope in 28% of patients. Gastrointestinal Kaposi's sarcoma lesions are dark red macules, plaques, or nodules with the appearance of a submucosal hemorrhage, and they are recognizable to those familiar with the cutaneous lesion. These lesions are submucosal, and the biopsy confirms the visual impression in only 36% of the cases. The lesions tend to be multiple but are rarely symptomatic, and no adverse clinical sequelae of these lesions have been identified. Visceral involvement of Kaposi's sarcoma in AIDS patients is associated with a significantly poorer prognosis, and only one of nine patients followed for 2 years after the diagnosis of gastrointestinal Kaposi's sarcoma was still alive.[474]

Carcinoid Tumors of the Colon and Rectum

Carcinoid tumors are neoplasms derived from cells capable of synthesizing a wide variety of hormones and autacoids. Carcinoid tumors begin as small submucosal nodules and tend to be asymptomatic until the overproduction of a functionally active peptide produces a paraneoplastic syndrome such as flushing, wheezing, or diarrhea. Carcinoid tumors may occur anywhere throughout the gastrointestinal tract, but are most common in the appendix, ileum, and rectum, as indicated in Table 87-20. More than half occur in the appendix or ileum, and 17% may be found in the rectum. Whereas carcinoid tumors originating from the stomach or

TABLE 87-20
Distribution of 3000 Gastrointestinal Carcinoid Tumors

ORGAN	PERCENTAGE OF TOTAL	PERCENTAGE WITH METASTASIS
Stomach	3%	18%
Duodenum	1%	16%
Jejunum	2%	35%
Ileum	28%	35%
Appendix	47%	3%
Colon	2%	60%
Rectum	17%	12%

Adapted from Oloff MJ. Carcinoid tumors of the rectum. Cancer 1971;28:175.

small intestine can give rise to a variety of systemic syndromes, rectal carcinoids do not produce the carcinoid syndrome. Most are asymptomatic, and about one quarter present with rectal bleeding. In a series of rectal carcinoid tumors, 23 (61%) of 38 were less than 2 cm in diameter, only one of these was malignant, and none had distant metastases. Therefore, most carcinoid tumors are amenable to local excision. Among the 15 (39%) of 38 tumors 2 cm or more in diameter, 14 were malignant, but only one gave rise to distant metastases.[475] These larger lesions should be treated aggressively, like adenocarcinomas. Carcinoid tumors of the distal colon are often diagnosed incidentally during the biopsy of a polypoid lesion, and the key to their management is to ensure their complete removal and to consider the possibility of multiple lesions. Carcinoid tumors in the proximal colon, appendix, and ileum have a somewhat different behavior, may be locally invasive, stimulate desmoplasia in the retroperitoneal or mesentery giving rise to a variety of mechanical complications such as intestinal obstruction, and may metastasize to the liver with symptoms such as abdominal pain, cramps, diarrhea, flushing, fixed cutaneous changes, and wheezing. A carcinoid tumor confined to the intestinal tract does not produce the characteristic features of carcinoid syndrome, which is actually a manifestation of metastatic disease.[475–477]

RECENT FINDINGS

The genetic basis of the attenuated APC syndrome (AAPC) has been identified and involves premature stop codons very close to the 5′ and of the *APC* gene. Thus far, all mutations have been in one of the first three exons.[478] A molecular diagnosis of FAP can now be made on a truncated protein test.[479] This test involves the in vitro synthesis of protein from *APC* genes and is approximately 82% sensitive in FAP families. To use this assay, lymphocytes from a person known to be affected with FAP should first be tested to determine if a truncated APC protein can be detected. If so, relatives of that person can be tested by the same assay. Inasmuch as each family will have a unique mutation, the assay should first be detected in a member known to be affected and then applied to first-degree relatives. However, the test also can be used to screen individuals who might have new mutations, although a negative test would be more difficult to interpret.

Progress has been made in HNPCC. Three laboratories have detected signature mutations in the tumors in patients with HNPCC.[480–482] The nature of this mutation, called replicative errors or microsatellite instability, suggested that the germline basis of the disease might be a failure of postmitotic mutation repair. Germline mutations in four genes have been found in HNPCC families. Two laboratories have reported that a mutation in the *hMSH2* gene may produce HNPCC.[483,484] The *hMSH2* gene appears to be inactivated by mutations that cause premature truncation of the protein, similar to what has been seen in the *APC* gene; furthermore, as many as 40% of typical HNPCC families have a germline mutation detected by premature truncation assays in the *hMSH2* gene.[485] Three more genes have been found that are homologous to the yeast *MLH* gene and have been termed *hMLH1*,[486,487] *hPMS1*, and *hPMS2*.[488] Germline mutations that inactivate any one of these four mutation repair genes can produce the identical HNPCC syndrome. The site specificity of tumor development is not understood; however, it appears that inactivation of the normal allele is required as a second, somatic event to produce a neoplasm.

Allelic loss of chromosone 18q, the locus of the *DCC* gene (described previously), has a strongly negative prognostic value in patients with stage II (i.e., Dukes' stage B) colorectal cancer.[489] It has been proposed that this mutation may help identify patients with the intermediate stage of cancer who are at sufficiently high risk for recurrence that additional therapy may be indicated.

It has been documented that colonoscopic polypectomy will reduce the subsequent incidence of colorectal cancer. Through comparison with historical controls, a very substantial reduction in colorectal cancer mortality has been suggested. Follow-up colonoscopic surveillance is not required 1 year after the initial polypectomy; a 3-year interval before the first colonoscopic follow-up has an identical ability to detect early metachronous cancers.[490]

> The reader is directed to Chapter 24, Neoplasia of the Gastrointestinal Tract; Chapter 31, Approach to the Patient With Occult Gastrointestinal Bleeding; Chapter 76, Tumors and Other Neoplastic Diseases of the Small Bowel; Chapter 85, Colonic Polyps: Benign and Premalignant Neoplasms of the Colon; Chapter 86, Polyposis Syndromes; Chapter 88, Anorectal Diseases; and Chapter 116, Colonoscopy and Flexible Sigmoidoscopy.

REFERENCES

1. Thun MJ, Calle EE, Namboodiri MM, et al. Risk factors for fatal colon cancer in a large prospective study. J Natl Cancer Inst 1992;84:1491.
2. Marnett LJ. Aspirin and the potential role of prostaglandins in colon cancer. Cancer Res 1992;52:5575.
3. Vogelstein B, Fearon ER, Hamilton SR, et al. Genetic alterations during colorectal-tumor development. N Engl J Med 1988;319:525.
4. Fearon ER, Vogelstein B. A genetic model for colorectal tumorigenesis. Cell 1990;61:759.
5. Kinzler KW, Nilbert MC, Su L-K, et al. Identification of FAP locus genes from chromosome 5q21. Science 1991;253:661.
6. Nishisho I, Nakamura Y, Miyoshi Y, et al. Mutations of chromosome 5q21 genes in FAP and colorectal cancer patients. Science 1991;253:665.
7. Groden J, Thliveris A, Samowitz W, et al. Identification and characterization of the familial adenomatous polyposis coli gene. Cell 1991;66:589.
8. Joslyn G, Carlson M, Thliveris A, et al. Identification of deletion mutations and three new genes at the familial polyposis locus. Cell 1991;66:601.
9. Powell SM, Zilz N, Beazer-Barclay Y, et al. *APC* mutations occur early during colorectal tumorigenesis. Nature 1992;359:235.
10. Peltomaki P, Aaltonen LA, Sistonen P, et al. Genetic mapping of a locus predisposing to human colorectal cancer. Science 1993;260:810.
11. Aaltonen LA, Peltomaki P, Leach FS, et al. Clues to the pathogenesis of familial colorectal cancer. Science 1993;260:812.
12. Schottenfeld D. The epidemiology of cancer: an overview. Cancer 1981;47:1108.
13. Miller AB. Trends in cancer mortality and epidemiology. Cancer 1983;51:2413.
14. Doll R. General epidemiologic considerations in etiology of colorectal cancer. In: Winawer S, Schottenfeld D, and Sherlock P, eds. Colorectal cancer: prevention, epidemiology, and screening. New York: Raven, 1980:3.
15. Boring CC, Squires TS, Tong T. Cancer statistics, 1993. CA Cancer J Clin 1993;43(1):7.
16. Greenwald P. Colon cancer overview. Cancer 1992;70:1206.
17. Funkhouser E, Cole P. Declining mortality rates for cancer of the rectum in the United States: 1940–1985. Cancer 1992;70:2597.
18. Haenzel W, Kurihara M. Studies of Japanese immigrants. I. Mortality from cancer and other diseases among Japanese in the United States. J Natl Cancer Inst 1968;40:43.
19. Thind IS, Najem R, Paradiso J, et al. Cancer among blacks in Newark, New Jersey, 1970–1976. Cancer 1982;50:180.
20. Satariano WA, Swanson GM. Racial differences in cancer incidence: the significance of age-specific patterns. Cancer 1988;62:2640.
21. Parkin DM, Pisani P, Ferlay J. Estimates of the worldwide incidence of eighteen major cancers in 1985. Int J Cancer 1993;54:594.
22. Devesa SS, Silverman DT, Young JL Jr, et al. Cancer incidence and mortality trends among whites in the United States, 1947–84. J Natl Cancer Inst 1987;79:701.
23. Cheever AW. Schistosomiasis and colon cancer. Lancet 1981;1:1369.
24. Neugut AI, Jacobson JS, DeVivo I. Epidemiology of colorectal adenomatous polyps. Cancer Epidemiol Biomarkers Prev 1993;2:159.
25. Pollack ES, Nomura AMY, Heilbrun LK, et al. Prospective study of alcohol consumption and cancer. N Engl J Med 1984;310:617.
26. Sandler RS, Lyles CM, McAuliffe C, et al. Cigarette smoking, alcohol, and the risk of colorectal adenomas. Gastroenterology 1993;104:1445.
27. Enstrom JE. Colorectal cancer and beer drinking. Br J Cancer 1977;35:674.
28. Pollack ES, Nomura AMY, Heilbrum LK, et al. Prospective study of alcohol consumption and cancer. N Engl J Med 1984;310:617.
29. Sandler RS, Sandler DP. Radiation-induced cancers of the colon and rectum: assessing the risk. Gastroenterology 1983;84:51.
30. Selikoff IJ, Hammond C, Seidman H. Latency of asbestos disease among insulation workers in the United States and Canada. Cancer 1980;46:2736.
31. Levine DS. Does asbestos exposure cause gastrointestinal cancer? Dig Dis Sci 1985;30:1189.
32. Rogers AE, Longnecker MP. Dietary and nutritional influences on cancer: A review of epidemiologic and experimental data. Lab Invest 1988;59:729.
33. Ames BN. Dietary carcinogens and anticarcinogens. Oxygen radicals and degenerative diseases. Science 1983;221:1256.
34. Peters RK, Pike MC, Garabrant D, et al. The effects of diet on colon cancer. Cancer Causes Control 1992;3:457.
35. Willett WC, MacMahon B. Diet and cancer—an overview. (2 parts). N Engl J Med 1984;310:633,697.
36. Willett W. The search for the causes of breast and colon cancer. Nature 1989;338:389.
37. Armstrong B, Doll R. Environmental factors and cancer incidences and mortality in different countries with special reference to dietary practices. Int J Cancer 1975;15:617.
38. Willett WC, Stamper MJ, Colditz GA, et al. Relation of meat, fat, and fiber intake to the risk of colon cancer in a prospective study among women. N Engl J Med 1990;323:1664.
39. Stemmerman GN, Nomura AMY, Heilbrun LK, et al. Serum cholesterol and colon cancer incidence in Hawaiian Japanese men. J Natl Cancer Inst 1981;67:1179.
40. Tornberg SA, Holm L-E, Carstensen JM, et al. Risks of cancer of the colon and rectum in relation to serum cholesterol and beta-lipoprotein. N Engl J Med 1986;315:1629.
41. Bayerdorffer E, Mannes GA, Richter WO, et al. Decreased high-density lipoprotein cholesterol and increased low-density

cholesterol levels in patients with colorectal adenomas. Ann Intern Med 1993;118:481.

42. Lee I-M, Paffenbarger Jr RS. Quetelet's index and risk of colon cancer in college alumni. J Natl Cancer Inst 1992;84:1326.

43. Nomura AMY, Stemmermann GN, Chyou P-H. Prospective study of serum cholesterol levels and large-bowel cancer. J Natl Cancer Inst 1991;83:1403.

44. O'Rourke JS, Johnson A, Collins P, et al. An association between hypocholesterolaemia and colorectal carcinoma in an Irish population. Gut 1992;33:950.

45. Tornberg SA, Holm L-E, Carstensen JM, et al. Cancer incidence and cancer mortality in relation to serum cholesterol. J Natl Cancer Inst 1989;81:1917.

46. Kreger BE, Anderson KM, Schatzkin A, et al. Serum cholesterol level, body mass index, and the risk of colon cancer. Cancer 1992;70:1038.

47. Winawer SJ, Flehinger BJ, Buchalter J, et al. Declining serum cholesterol levels prior to diagnosis of colon cancer. A time-trend, case-control study. JAMA 1990;263:2083.

48. Cummings JH, Wiggins HS, Jenkins DJA, et al. Influence of diets high and low in animal fat on bowel habit, gastro-intestinal transit, fecal microflora, bile acid and fat excretion. J Clin Invest 1978;61:953.

49. Craven PA, Pfanstiel J, DeRubertis FR. Role of reactive oxygen in bile salt stimulation of colonic epithelial proliferation. J Clin Invest 1986;77:850.

50. Bull AW, Nigro ND, Golembieski WA, et al. In vivo stimulation of DNA synthesis and induction of ornithine decarboxylase in rat colon by fatty acid hydroperoxides, autoxidation products of unsaturated fatty acids. Cancer Res 1984;44:4924.

51. Bull AW, Nigro ND, Marnett LJ. Structural requirements for stimulation of colonic cell proliferation by oxidized fatty acids. Cancer Res 1988;48:1771.

52. Friedman E, Isaacson P, Rafter J, et al. Fecal diglycerides as selective endogenous mitogens for premalignant and malignant human colonic epithelial cells. Cancer Res 1989;49:544.

53. Craven PA, Pfanstiel J, DeRubertis FR. Role of activation of protein kinase C in the stimulation of colonic epithelial proliferation and reactive oxygen formation by bile acids. J Clin Invest 1987;79:532.

54. Stadler J, Stern HS, Yeung KAS, et al. Effect of high fat consumption on cell proliferation activity of colorectal mucosa and on soluble faecal bile acids. Gut 1988;29:1326.

55. Anti M, Marra G, Armelao F, et al. Effect of ω-3 fatty acids on rectal mucosal cell proliferation in subjects at risk for colon cancer. Gastroenterology 1992;103:883.

56. Hill MJ, Drasar BS, Williams REO. Faecal bile-acids and clostridia in patients with cancer of the large bowel. The Lancet 1975;1:7906.

57. Hill MJ. Bile, bacteria and bowel cancer. Gut 1983;24:871.

58. Korpela JT, Adlercreutz H, Turunen MJ. Fecal free and conjugated bile acids and neutral sterols in vegetarians, omnivores, and patients with colorectal cancer. Scand J Gastroenterol 1988;23:277.

59. Nomura AMY, Wilkins TD, Kamiyama S, et al. Fecal neutral steroids in two Japanese populations with different colon cancer risks. Cancer Res 1983;43:1910.

60. Van der Werf SDJ, Nagengast FM, Van Berge Henegouwen GP, et al. Colonic absorption of secondary bile-acids in patients with adenomatous polyps and in matched controls. Lancet 1982;1:759.

61. Burkitt DP. Epidemiology of cancer of the colon and rectum. Cancer 1971;28:3.

62. Kritchevsky D. Fiber, steroids, and cancer. Cancer Res 1983;43:2491s.

63. Dales LG, Friedman GD, Ury HK, et al. A case-control study of relationships of diet and other traits to colorectal cancer in American Blacks. Am J Epidemiol 1978;109:132.

64. Slattery ML, Sorenson AW, Mahoney AW, et al. Diet and colon cancer: assessment of risk by fiber type and food source. J Natl Cancer Inst 1988;80:1474.

65. Greenwald P, Lanza E. Role of dietary fiber in the prevention of cancer. In: De Vita VT, Hellman S, Rosenberg SA, eds.

66. Howe GR, Benito E, Castelleto R, et al. Dietary intake of fiber and decreased risk of cancers of the colon and rectum: evidence from the combined analysis of 13 case-control studies. J Natl Cancer Inst 1992;84:1887.

67. Cummings JH, Bingham SA, Heaton KW, et al. Fecal weight, colon cancer risk, and dietary intake of nonstarch polysaccharides (dietary fiber). Gastroenterology 1992;103:1783.

68. Alberts DS, Einspahr J, Rees-McGee S, et al. Effects of dietary wheat bran fiber on rectal epithelial cell proliferation in patients with resection for colorectal cancers. J Natl Cancer Inst 1990;82:1280.

69. Spiller GA, Freeman HJ. Recent advances in dietary fiber and colorectal diseases. Am J Clin Nutr 1981;34:1145.

70. Friedman E, Lightdale C, Winawer S. Effects of psyllium fiber and short-chain organic acids derived from fiber breakdown on colonic epithelial cells from high-risk patients. Cancer Lett 1988;43:121.

71. Deschner EE. Early proliferative changes in gastrointestinal neoplasia. Am J Gastroenterol 1982;77:207.

72. Terpstra OT, Van Blankenstein M, Dees J, et al. Abnormal pattern of cell proliferation in the entire colonic mucosa of patients with colon adenoma or cancer. Gastroenterology 1987;92:704.

73. Lipkin M, Uehara K, Winawer S, et al. Seventh-day Adventist vegetarians have a quiescent proliferative activity in colonic mucosa. Cancer Lett 1985;26:139.

74. Wargovich MJ, Eng VWS, Newmark HL, et al. Calcium ameliorates the toxic effect of deoxycholic acid on colonic epithelium. Carcinogenesis 1983;4:1205.

75. Bird RP, Schneider R, Stamp D, et al. Effect of dietary calcium and cholic acid on the proliferative indices of murine colonic epithelium. Carcinogenesis 1986;7:1657.

76. Newmark HL, Wargovich MJ, Bruce WR. Colon cancer and dietary fat, phosphate, and calcium: a hypothesis. J Natl Cancer Inst 1984;72:1323.

77. Lipkin M, Friedman E, Winawer SJ, et al. Colonic epithelial cell proliferation in responders and nonresponders to supplemental dietary calcium. Cancer Res 1989;49:248.

78. Lipkin M, Newmark H. Effect of added dietary calcium on colonic epithelial-cell proliferation in subjects at high risk for familial colonic cancer. N Engl J Med 1985;313:1381.

79. Rozen P, Fireman Z, Fine N, et al. Oral calcium suppresses increased rectal epithelial proliferation of persons at risk of colorectal cancer. Gut 1989;30:650.

80. Gregoire RC, Stern HS, Yeung KS, et al. Effect of calcium supplementation on mucosal cell proliferation in high risk patients for colon cancer. Gut 1989;30:376.

81. Bostick RM, Potter JD, Fosdick L, et al. Calcium and colorectal epithelial cell proliferation: a preliminary randomized, double-blinded, placebo-controlled clinical trial. J Natl Cancer Inst 1993;85:132.

82. Wargovich MJ, Isbell G, Shabot M, et al. Calcium supplementation decreases rectal epithelial cell proliferation in subjects with sporadic adenoma. Gastroenterology 1992;103:92.

83. Buset M, Lipkin M, Winawer S, et al. Inhibition of human colonic epithelial cell proliferation in vivo and in vitro by calcium. Cancer Res 1986;46:5426.

84. Schrauzer GN, White DA, Schneider CJ. Cancer mortality correlation studies. III: Statistical associations with dietary selenium intakes. Bioinorganic Chemistry 1977;7:23.

85. Willett WC, Polk BF, Underwood BA, et al. Relation of serum vitamins A and E and carotenoids to the risk of cancer. N Engl J Med 1984;310:430.

86. Willett WC, Polk BF, Morris JS, et al. Prediagnostic serum selenium and risk of cancer. Lancet 1983;2:130.

87. Longnecker MP, Martin-Moreno J-M, Knekt P, et al. Serum α-tocopherol concentration in relation to subsequent colorectal cancer: Pooled data from five cohorts. J Natl Cancer Inst 1992;84:430.

88. Paganelli GM, Biasco G, Brandi G, et al. Effect of vitamin A, C, and E supplementation on rectal cell proliferation in pa-

Important advances in oncology. Philadelphia: Lippincott, 1986:37.

tients with colorectal adenomas. J Natl Cancer Inst 1992;84:47.

89. McKeown-Eyssen G, Holloway C, Jazmaji V, et al. A randomized trial of vitamins C and E in the prevention of recurrence of colorectal polyps. Cancer Res 1988;48:4701.

90. DeCosse JJ, Miller HH, Lesser ML. Effect of wheat fiber and vitamins C and E on rectal polyps in patients with familial adenomatous polyposis. J Natl Cancer Inst 1989;81:1290.

91. Giovannucci E, Stampfer MJ, Colditz GA, et al. Folate, methionine, and alcohol intake and risk of colorectal adenoma. J Natl Cancer Inst 1993;85:875.

92. Wattenberg LW. Inhibition of carcinogenesis by minor dietary constituents. Cancer Res 1992;52:2085.

93. Pollard M. Effect of indomethacin on intestinal tumors induced in rats by the acetate derivative of dimethylnitrosamine. Science 1981;214:558.

94. Labayle D, Fischer D, Vielh P, et al. Sulindac causes regression of rectal polyps in familial adenomatous polyposis. Gastroenterology 1991;101:635.

95. Rigau J, Pique JM, Rubio E, et al. Effects of long-term sulindac therapy on colonic polyposis. Ann Intern Med 1991;115:952.

96. Giardiello FM, Hamilton SR, Krush AJ, et al. Treatment of colonic and rectal adenomas with sulindac in familial adenomatous polyposis. N Engl J Med 1993;328:1313.

97. Thun MJ, Namboodiri MM, Heath Jr. CW. Aspirin use and reduced risk of fatal colon cancer. N Engl J Med 1991;325:1593.

98. Rosenberg L, Palmer JR, Zauber AG, et al. A hypothesis: nonsteroidal anti-inflammatory drugs reduce the incidence of large-bowel cancer. J Natl Cancer Inst 1991;83:355.

99. Greenberg ER, Baron JA, Freeman Jr DH, et al. Reduced risk of large-bowel adenomas among aspirin users. J Natl Cancer Inst 1993;85:912.

100. Thun MJ, Namboodiri MM, Calle EE, et al. Aspirin use and risk of fatal cancer. Cancer Res 1993;53:1322.

101. Craven PA, Saito R, DeRubertis FR. Role of local prostaglandin synthesis in the modulation of proliferative activity of rat colonic epithelium. J Clin Invest 1983;72:1365.

102. DeRubertis FR, Craven PA, Saito R. 16,16-dimethyl prostaglandin E_2 suppresses the increases in the proliferative activity of rat colonic epithelium induced by indomethacin and aspirin. Gastroenterology 1985;89:1054.

103. Craven PA, Thornburg K, DeRubertis FR. Sustained increase in the proliferation of rat colonic mucosa during chronic treatment with aspirin. Gastroenterology 1988;94:567.

104. Shimakura S, Boland CR. Eicosanoid production by the human gastric cancer cell line AGS and its relation to cell growth. Cancer Res 1992;52:1744.

105. Wynder EL, Reddy BS, Weisburger JH. Environmental dietary factors in colorectal cancer. Some unresolved issues. Cancer 1992;70:1222.

106. Burmer GC, Loeb LA. Mutations in the K-ras2 oncogene during progressive stages of human colon carcinoma. Proc Natl Acad Sci 1989;86:2403.

107. Barbacid M. Ras genes. Ann Rev Biochem 1987;56:779.

108. Bos JL. Ras oncogenes in human cancer: a review. Cancer Res 1989;49:4682.

109. Balmain A, Brown K. Oncogene activation in chemical carcinogenesis. Adv Cancer Res 1988;51:147.

110. Bos JL, Fearon ER, Hamilton SR, et al. Prevalence of ras gene mutations in human colorectal cancers. Nature 1987;327:293.

111. Forrester K, Almoguera C, Han K, et al. Detection of high incidence of K-ras oncogenes during human colon tumorigenesis. Nature 1987;327:298.

112. Ando M, Maruyama M, Oto M, et al. Higher frequency of point mutations in the c-K-ras 2 gene in human colorectal adenomas with severe atypia than in carcinomas. Jpn J Cancer Res 1991;82:245.

113. Benhattar J, Losi L, Chaubert P, et al. Prognostic significance of K-ras mutations in colorectal carcinoma. Gastroenterology 1993;104:1044.

114. Lane DP. p53, guardian of the genome. Nature 1992;358:15.

115. Levine AJ, Momand J, Finlay CA. The p53 tumour suppressor gene. Nature 1991;351:453.

116. Kern SE, Pietenpol JA, Thiagalingam S, et al. Oncogenic forms fo p53 inhibit p53-regulated gene expression. Science 1992;256:827.

117. Nigro JM, Baker SJ, Preisinger AC, et al. Mutations in the p53 gene occur in diverse human tumour types. Nature 1989;342:705.

118. Vogelstein B, Kinzler KW. p53 function and dysfunction. Cell 1992;70:523.

119. Pignatelli M, Stamp GWH, Kafiri G, et al. Over-expression of p53 nuclear oncoprotein in colorectal adenomas. Int J Cancer 1992;50:683.

120. Baker SJ, Fearon ER, Nigro JM, et al. Chromosome 17 deletions and p53 gene mutations in colorectal carcinomas. Science 1989;244:217.

121. Baker SJ, Preisinger AC, Jessup JM, et al. p53 gene mutations occur in combination with 17p allelic deletions as late events in colorectal tumorigenesis. Cancer Res 1990;50:7717.

122. Baker SJ, Markowitz S, Fearon ER, et al. Suppression of human colorectal carcinoma cell growth by wild-type p53. Science 1990;249:912.

123. Weinberg RA. Tumor suppressor genes. Science 1991;254:1138.

124. Sun X-F, Carstensen JM, Zhang H, et al. Prognostic significance of cytoplasmic p53 oncoprotein in colorectal adenocarcinoma. Lancet 1992;340:1369.

125. Laurent-Puig P, Olschwang S, Delattre O, et al. Survival and acquired genetic alterations in colorectal cancer. Gastroenterology 1992;102:1136.

126. Boland CR, Sato J, Feinberg AP. Evidence for the role of the p53 tumor suppressor gene (TSG) in the adenoma-to-carcinoma sequence in colorectal neoplasia. Gastroenterology 1993;104:A391.

127. Vogelstein B, Fearon ER, Kern SE, et al. Allelotype of colorectal carcinomas. Science 1989;244:207.

128. Kern SE, Fearon ER, Tersmette KWF, et al. Allelic loss in colorectal carcinoma. JAMA 1989;261:3099.

129. Law DJ, Olschwang S, Monpezat J-P, et al. Concerted nonsyntenic allelic loss in human colorectal carcinoma. Science 1988;241:961.

130. Wang L, Patel U, Ghosh L, et al. Mutation in the nm23 gene is associated with metastasis in human colorectal cancer. Cancer Res 1993;53:717.

131. Cohn KH, Wang F, DeSoto-LaPaix F, Solomon WB, et al. Association of nm23-H1 allelic deletions with distant metastases in colorectal carcinoma. Lancet 1991;338:722.

132. Tsuboi K, Hirayoshi K, Takeuchi K, et al. Expression of the c-myc gene in human gastrointestinal malignancies. Biochem Biophys Res Commun 1987;146:699.

133. Alitalo K, Schwab M, Lin CC, et al. Homogeneously staining chromosomal regions contain amplified copies of an abundantly expressed cellular oncogene (c-myc) in malignant neuroendocrine cells from a human colon carcinoma. Proc Natl Acad Sci U S A 1983;80:1707.

134. Erisman MD, Litwin S, Keidan RD, et al. Noncorrelation of the expression of the c-myc oncogene in colorectal carcinoma with recurrence of disease or patient survival. Cancer Res 1988;48:1350.

135. Goelz SE, Vogelstein B, Hamilton SR, et al. Hypomethylation of DNA from benign and malignant human colon neoplasms. Science 1988;228:187.

136. Cartwright CA, Meisler AI, Eckhart W. Activation of the pp60^c-src protein kinase is an early event in colonic carcinogenesis. Proc Natl Acad Sci U S A 1990;87:558.

137. Thibodeau SN, Bren G, Schaid D. Microsatellite instability in cancer of the proximal colon. Science 1993;260:816.

138. Lynch HT, Smyrk TC, Watson P, et al. Genetics, natural history, tumor spectrum, and pathology of hereditary nonpolyposis colorectal cancer: an updated review. Gastroenterology 1993;104:1535.

139. Delattre O, Olschwang S, Law DJ, et al. Multiple genetic alterations in distal and proximal colorectal cancer. Lancet 1989;2:353.

140. Burmer GC, Levine DS, Kulander BG, et al. c-Ki-ras mutations

in chronic ulcerative colitis and sporatic colon carcinoma. Gastroenterology 1990;99:416.

141. Bell SM, Kelly SA, Hoyle JA, et al. c-Ki-*ras* gene mutations in dysplasia and carcinomas complicating ulcerative colitis. Br J Cancer 1991;64:174.

142. Burmer GC, Rabinovitch PS, Haggitt RC, et al. Neoplastic progression in ulcertive colitis: histology, DNA content, and loss of p53 allele. Gastroenterology 1992;103:1602.

143. Greenwald BD, Harpaz N, Yin J, et al. Loss of heterozygosity affecting the *p53, Rb,* and *mcc/apc* tumor suppressor gene loci in dysplastic and cancerous ulcerative colitis. Cancer Res 1992;52:741.

144. Rognum TO, Thorud E, Lund E. Survival of large bowel carcinoma patients with different DNA ploidy. Br J Cancer 1987;56:633.

145. Goh HS, Jass JR. DNA content and the adenoma-carcinoma sequence in colorectum. J Clin Pathol 1986;39:387.

146. Quirke P, Fozard JBJ, Dixon MF, et al. DNA aneuploidy in colorectal adenomas. Br J Cancer 1986;53:477.

147. Banner BF, Chacho MS, Roseman DL, et al. Multiparameter flow cytometric analysis of colon polyps. Am J Clin Pathol 1987;87:313.

148. Kokal W, Sheibani K, Terz J, et al. Tumor DNA content in the prognosis of colorectal carcinoma. JAMA 1986;255:3123.

149. Levine DS, Rabinovitch PS, Haggitt RC, et al. Distribution of aneuploid cell populations in ulcerative colitis with dysplasia or cancer. Gastroenterology 1991;101:1198.

150. Traber PG, Chianale J, Florence R, et al. Expression of cytochrome P450b and P450e genes in small intestinal mucosa of rats following treatment with phenobarbital, polyhalogenated biphenyls, and organochlorine pesticides. J Biol Chem 1988;263:9449.

151. LaMont JT, O'Gorman TA. Experimental colon cancer. Gastroenterology 1978;75:1157.

152. Miller EC, Miller JA. Searches for ultimate chemical carcinogens and their reactions with cellular macromolecules. Cancer 1981;47:2327.

153. Ames BN. Dietary carcinogens and anticarcinogens. Oxygen radicals and degenerative diseases. Science 1983;221:1256.

154. Miller EC, Miller JA. Carcinogens and mutagens that may occur in foods. Cancer 1986;58:1795.

155. Gupta I, Suzuki K, Bruce WR, et al. A model study of fecapentaenes: mutagens of bacterial origin with alkylating properties. Science 1984;225:521.

156. Hirai N, Kingston DGI, Van Tassell RL, et al. Structure elucidation of a potent mutagen from human feces. J Am Chem Soc 1982;104:6149.

157. Hargraves WA, Pariza MW. Purification and mass spectral characterization of bacterial mutagens from commercial beef extract. Cancer Res 1983;43:1467.

158. Pariza MW, Loretz LJ, Storkson JM, et al. Mutagens and modulator of mutagenesis in fried ground beef. Cancer Res 1983;43:2444s.

159. Ames BN, McCann J, Yamasaki E. Methods for detecting carcinogens and mutagens with *Salmonella* mammalian-microsome mutagenicity test. Mutat Res 1975;31:347.

160. Mower HF, Ichinotsubo D, Wang LW, et al. Fecal mutagens in two Japanese populations with different colon cancer risks. Cancer Res 1982;42:1164.

161. Shiffman MH, Van Tassell RL, Robinson A, et al. Case-control study of colorectal cancer and fecapentaene excretion. Cancer Res 1989;49:1322.

162. Simon GL, Gorbach SL. Intestinal flora and gastrointestinal function. In: Johnson LR, ed. Physiology of the gastrointestinal tract. 2nd ed. New York: Raven, 1987:1729.

163. Gennaro AR, Villanueva R, Sukonthaman Y, et al. Chemical carcinogenesis in transposed intestinal segments. Cancer Res 1973;33:536.

164. Celik C, Mittelman A, Paolini NS Jr, et al. Effects of 1,2-symmetrical dimethylhydrazine on jejunocolic transposition in Sprague-Dawley rats. Cancer Res 1981;41:2908.

165. Bolognesi C, Mariani MR, Boffa LC. Target tissue DNA damage in inbred mouse strains with different susceptibility to the colon carcinogen 1,2-dimethylhydrazine. Carcinogenesis 1988;9:1347.

166. Ward JM. Morphogenesis of chemically induced neoplasms of the colon and small intestine in rats. Lab Invest 1974;30:505.

167. Boland CR, Ahnen DJ. Binding of lectins to goblet cell mucin in malignant and premalignant colonic epithelium in the CF-1 mouse. Gastroenterology 1985;89:127.

168. Deschner EE, Long FC. Colonic neoplasms in mice produced with six injections of 1,2-dimethylhydrazine. Oncology 1977;34:255.

169. Deschner EE, Long FC, Hakissian M, et al. Differential susceptibility of AKR, C57BL/6J, and CF1 mice to 1,2-dimethylhydrazine-induced colonic tumor formation predicted by proliferative characteristics of colonic epithelial cells. J Natl Cancer Inst 1983;70:279.

170. Deschner EE, Long FC, Hakissian M, et al. Differential susceptibility of inbred mouse strains forecast by acute colonic proliferative response to methylazoxymethanol. J Natl Cancer Inst 1984;72:195.

171. Diwan BA, Meier H, Blackman KE, et al. Genetic differences in the induction of colorectal tumors by 1,2-dimethylhydrazine in inbred mice. J Natl Cancer Inst 1977;59:455.

172. Yuspa SH, Poirier MC. Chemical carcinogenesis: from animal models to molecular models in one decade. Adv Cancer Res 1988;50:25.

173. Jacoby RF, Lior X, Teng B-B, et al. Mutations in the K-*ras* oncogene induced by 1,2-dimethylhydrazine in preneoplastic and neoplastic rat colonic mucosa. J Clin Invest 1991;87:624.

174. Bull AW, Soullier BK, Wilson PS, et al. Promotion of azoxymethane-induced intestinal cancer by high-fat diet in rats. Cancer Res 1979;39:4956.

175. Hogan ML, Shamsuddin AM. Large intestinal carcinogenesis. I. Promotional effect of dietary fatty acid isomers in the rat model. J Natl Cancer Inst 1984;73:1293.

176. Reddy BS, Ohmori T. Effect of intestinal microflora and dietary fat on 3,2'-dimethyl-4-aminobiphenyl-induced colon carcinogenesis in F344 rats. Cancer Res 1981;41:1363.

177. Reddy BS. Dietary fat and its relationship to large bowel cancer. Cancer Res 1981;41:3700.

178. Cohen BI, Raicht RF. Effects of bile acids on colon carcinogenesis in rats treated with carcinogens. Cancer Res 1981;41:3759.

179. Oscarson JEA, Veen HF, Ross JS, et al. Ileal resection potentiates 1,2-dimethylhydrazine-induced colonic carcinogenesis. Ann Surg 1979;189:503.

180. Rodriguez PM, Cruz NI, Gonzalez CI, et al. The effect of a high fat diet on the incidence of colonic cancer after cholecystectomy in mice. Cancer 1988;62:727.

181. Williamson RCN, Bauer FLR, Ross JS, et al. Enhanced colonic carcinogenesis with azoxymethane in rats after pancreaticobiliary diversion to mid small bowel. Gastroenterology 1979;76:1386.

182. Cummings JH. Cellulose and the human gut. Gut 1984;25:805.

183. Freeman HJ, Spiller GA, Kim YS. A double-blind study on the effect of purified cellulose dietary fiber on 1,2-dimethylhydrazine-induced rat colonic neoplasia. Cancer Res 1978;38:2912.

184. Freeman HJ, Spiller GA, Kim YS. A double-blind study on the effects of differing purified cellulose and pectin fiber diets on 1,2-dimethylhydrazine-induced rat colonic neoplasia. Cancer Res 1980;40:2661.

185. Prizont R. Absence of large bowel tumors in rats injected with 1,2-dimethylhydrazine and fed high dietary cellulose. Dig Dis Sci 1987;32:1418.

186. Cameron IL, Ord VA, Hunter KE, et al. Suppression of a carcinogen (1,2-dimethylhydrazine dihydrochloride)-induced increase in mitotic activity in the colonic crypts of rats by addition of dietary cellulose. Cancer Res 1989;49:991.

187. Calvert RJ, Klurfeld DM, Subramaniam S, et al. Reduction of colonic carcinogenesis by wheat bran independent of fecal bile acid concentration. J Natl Cancer Inst 1987;79:875.

188. Jacobs LR, White FA. Modulation of mucosal cell proliferation

in the intestine of rats fed a wheat bran diet. Am J Clin Nutr 1983;37:945.

189. Tatsuta M, Iishi H, Yamamura H, et al. Inhibition by tetragastrin of experimental carcinogenesis in rat colon: effect of wheat bran consumption. Int J Cancer 1988;41:239.

190. Jacobs LR. Enhancement of rat colon carcinogenesis by wheat bran consumption during the stage of 1,2-dimethylhydrazine administration. Cancer Res 1983;43:4057.

191. Reddy BS, Maeura Y, Wayman M. Effect of dietary corn bran and autohydrolyzed lignin on 3,2'-dimethyl-4-aminobiphenyl-induced intestinal carcinogenesis in male F344 rats. J Natl Cancer Inst 1983;71:419.

192. Jacobs LR. Effects of dietary fiber on mucosal growth and cell proliferation in the small intestine of the rat: a comparison of oat bran, pectin, and guar with total fiber deprivation. Am J Clin Nutr 1983;37:954.

193. Asano T, Pollard M, Madsen DC. Effects of cholestyramine on 1,2-dimethylhydrazine-induced enteric carcinoma in germfree rats (S9124). Proc Soc Exp Biol Med 1975;150:780.

194. Calderisi RN, Freeman HJ. Differential effects of surgical suture materials in 1,2-dimethylhydrazine-induced rat intestinal neoplasia. Cancer Res 1984;44:2827.

195. Chester JF, Gaissert HA, Ross JS, et al. Augmentation of 1,2-dimethylhydrazine-induced colon cancer by experimental colitis in mice: role of dietary vitamin E. J Natl Cancer Inst 1986;76:939.

196. Freeman HJ. Effects of differing concentrations of sodium butyrate on 1,2-dimethylhydrazine-induced rat intestinal neoplasia. Gastroenterology 1986;91:596.

197. Newberne PM, Suphakarn V. Preventive role of vitamin A in colon carcinogenesis in rats. Cancer 1977;40:2553.

198. Reddy BS, Furuya K, Lowenfels A. Effect of neomycin on azoxymethane-induced colon carcinogenesis in F344 rats. J Natl Cancer Inst 1984;73:275.

199. Scudamore CH, Freeman HJ. Effects of small bowel transection, resection, or bypass in 1,2-dimethylhydrazine-induced rat intestinal neoplasia. Gastroenterology 1983;84:725.

200. Birt DF, Lawson TA, Julius AD, et al. Inhibition by dietary selenium of colon cancer induced in the rat by bis(2-oxopropyl)nitrosamine. Cancer Res 1982;42:4455.

201. Bull AW, Burd AD, Nigro ND. Effect of inhibitors of tumorigenesis on the formation of O^6-methylguanine in the colon of 1,2-dimethylhydrazine-treated rats. Cancer Res 1981;41:4938.

202. Nigro ND, Bull AW, Wilson PS, et al. Combined inhibitors of carcinogenesis: effect on azoxymethane-induced intestinal cancer in rats. J Natl Cancer Inst 1982;69:103.

203. Colacchio TA, Memoli VA. Chemoprevention of colorectal neoplasms. Ascorbic acid and β-carotene. Arch Surg 1986;121:1421.

204. Cook MG, McNamara P. Effect of dietary vitamin E on dimethylhydrazine-induced colonic tumors in mice. Cancer Res 1980;40:1329.

205. Temple NJ, Basus TK. Protective effect of β-carotene against colon tumors in mice. J Natl Cancer Inst 1987;78:1211.

206. Corassanti JG, Hobika GH, Markus G. Interference with dimethylhydrazine induction of colon tumors in mice by e-aminocaproic acid. Science 1982;206:1020.

207. Goldin BR, Gorbach SL. Effect of antibiotics on incidence of rat intestinal tumors induced by 1,2-dimethylhydrazine dihydrochloride. J Natl Cancer Inst 1981;67:877.

208. Karlin DA, O'Donnell RT, Jensen WE. Effect of dioctyl sodium sulfosuccinate feeding on rat colorectal 1,2-dimethylhydrazine carcinogenesis. J Natl Cancer Inst 1980;64:791.

209. Kingsnorth AN, King WWK, Diekema KA, et al. Inhibition of ornithine decarboxylase with 2-difluoromethylornithine: reduced incidence of dimethylhydrazine-induced colon tumors in mice. Cancer Res 1983;43:2545.

210. Zhang S-Z, Luk GD, Hamilton SR. Difluoromethylornithine-induced inhibition of growth of autochthonous experimental colonic tumors produced by azoxymethane in male F344 rats. Cancer Res 1988;48:6498.

211. Narisawa T, Sato M, Tani M, et al. Inhibition of development of methylnitrosourea-induced rat colon tumors by indomethacin treatment. Cancer Res 1981;41:1954.

212. Reddy BS, Maruyama H, Kelloff G. Dose-related inhibition of colon carcinogenesis by dietary piroxicam, a non-steroidal antiinflammatory drug, during different stages of rat colon tumor development. Cancer Res 1987;47:5340.

213. Raicht RF, Cohen BI, Fazzini EP. Protective effect of plant sterols against chemically induced colon tumors in rats. Cancer Res 1980;40:403.

214. Reddy BS, Maeura Y. Dose-response studies of the effect of dietary butylated hydroxyanisole on colon carcinogenesis induced by methylazoxymethanol acetate in female CF1 mice. J Natl Cancer Inst 1984;72:1181.

215. Temple NJ, Basu TK. Selenium and cabbage and colon carcinogenesis in mice. J Natl Cancer Inst 1987;79:1131.

216. Wargovich MJ. Diallyl sulfide, a flavor component of garlic (*Allium sativium*), inhibits dimethylhydrazine-induced colon cancer. Carcinogenesis 1987;8:487.

217. Kozuka S, Nogaki M, Ozeki T, et al. Premalignancy of the mucosal polyp in the large intestine: II. Estimation of the periods required for malignant transformation of mucosal polyps. Dis Colon Rectum 1975;18:494.

218. Carroll RLA, Klein M. How often should patients be sigmoidoscoped? A mathematical perspective. Prev Med 1980;9:741.

219. Petersen GM, Slack J, Nakamura Y. Screening guidelines and premorbid diagnosis of familial adenomatous polyposis using linkage. Gastroenterology 1991;100:1658.

220. Bussey HJR. Familial polyposis coli. Baltimore: Johns Hopkins University Press, 1975.

221. Polissar L, Sim D, Phil M, et al. Survival of colorectal cancer patients in relation to duration of symptoms and other prognostic factors. Dis Colon Rectum 1981;24:364.

222. Nakamura GJ, Schneiderman LJ, Klauber MR. Colorectal cancer and bowel habits. Cancer 1984;54:1475.

223. Steinberg SM, Barkin JS, Kaplan RS, et al. Prognostic indicators of colon tumors: the gastrointestinal tumor study group experience. Cancer 1986;57:1866.

224. Macrae FA, St. John DJB. Relationship between patterns of bleeding and Hemoccult sensitivity in patients with colorectal cancers or adenomas. Gastroenterology 1982;82:891.

225. Theologides A. Cancer cachexia. Cancer 1979;43:2004.

226. Beutler B, Cerami A. Cachectin: more than a tumor necrosis factor. N Engl J Med 1987;316:379.

227. Watson WS, Sammon AM. Body composition in cachexia resulting from malignant and non-malignant diseases. Cancer 1980;46:2041.

228. Dempsey DT, Feurer ID, Knox LS, et al. Energy expenditure in malnourished gastrointestinal cancer patients. Cancer 1984;53:1265.

229. Leppert M, Burt R, Hughes JP, et al. Genetic analysis of an inherited predisposition to colon cancer in a family with a variable number of adenomatous polyps. N Engl J Med 1990;322:904.

230. Lynch HT, Smyrk T, Lanspa SJ, et al. Flat adenomas in a colon cancer-prone kindred. J Natl Cancer Inst 1988;80:278.

231. Lynch HT, Smyrk TC, Lanspa SJ, et al. Phenotypic variation in colorectal adenoma/cancer expression in two families. Hereditary flat adenoma syndrome. Cancer 1990;66:909.

232. Spirio L, Otterud B, Stauffer D, et al. Linkage of a variant or attenuated form of adenomatous polyposis coli to the adenomatous polyposis coli (APC) locus. Am J Hum Genet 1992;51:92.

233. Lynch HT, Smyrk TC, Lanspa SJ, et al. Upper gastrointestinal manifestations in families with hereditary flat adenoma syndrome. Cancer 1993;71:2709.

234. Nagase H, Miyoshi Y, Horii A, et al. Correlation between the location of germ-line mutations in the *APC* gene and the number of colorectal polyps in familial adenomatous polyposis patients. Cancer Res 1992;52:4055.

234a. Spirio L, Olschwang S, Groden J, et al. Alleles of the *APC* gene: an attenuated form of familial polyposis. Cell 1993;75:951.

235. Lynch HT, Harris RE, Bardawil WA, et al. Management of hereditary site-specific colon cancer. Arch Surg 1977;112:170.

236. Boland CR, Troncale FJ. Familial colonic cancer without antecedent polyposis. Ann Intern Med 1984;100:700.

237. Lynch HT, Smyrk TC, Watson P, et al. Genetics, natural history, tumor spectrum, and pathology of hereditary nonpolyposis colorectal cancer: an updated review. Gastroenterology 1993;104:1535.

238. Lynch HT, Krush AJ. Cancer family "G" revisited: 1895–1970. Cancer 1971;27:1505.

239. Watson P, Lynch HT. Extracolonic cancer in hereditary nonpolyposis colorectal cancer. Cancer 1993;71:677.

240. Mecklin J-P, Jarvinen HJ. Tumor spectrum in cancer family syndrome (hereditary nonpolyposis colorectal cancer). Cancer 1991;68:1109.

241. Vasen HFA, Offerhaus GJA, Den Hartog Jager FCA, et al. The tumour spectrum in hereditary non-polyposis colorectal cancer: a study of 24 kindreds in the Netherlands. Int J Cancer 1990;46:31.

242. Mecklin J-P. Frequency of hereditary colorectal carcinoma. Gastroenterology 1987;93:1021.

243. Westlake PJ, Bryant HE, Huchcroft SA, et al. Frequency of hereditary nonpolyposis colorectal cancer in southern Alberta. Dig Dis Sci 1991;36:1441.

244. Kee F, Collins BJ. How prevalent is cancer family syndrome? Gut 1991;32:509.

245. Ponz de Leon M, Sassatelli R, Benatti P, et al. Identification of hereditary nonpolyposis colorectal cancer in the general population. The 6-year experience of a population-based registry. Cancer 1993;71:3493.

246. Menko FH, Te Meerman GJ, Sampson JR. Variable age of onset in hereditary nonpolyposis colorectal cancer: clinical implications. Gastroenterology 1993;104:946.

247. Mecklin J-P, Sipponen P, Jarvinen HJ. Histopathology of colorectal carcinomas and adenomas in cancer family syndrome. Dis Colon Rectum 1986;29:849.

248. Love RR, Morrissey JF. Colonoscopy in asymptomatic individuals with a family history of colorectal cancer. Arch Intern Med 1984;144:2209.

249. Lanspa SJ, Lynch HT, Smyrk TC, et al. Colorectal adenomas in the Lynch syndromes. Results of a colonoscopy screening program. Gastroenterology 1990;98:1117.

250. Jass JR, Stewart SM. Evolution of hereditary non-polyposis colorectal cancer. Gut 1992;33:783.

251. Mecklin J-P, Jarvinen HJ. Clinical features of colorectal carcinoma in cancer family syndrome. Dis Colon Rectum 1986;29:160.

252. Lynch HT, Watson P, Lanspa SJ, et al. Natural history of colorectal cancer in hereditary nonpolyposis colorectal cancer (Lynch Syndromes I and II). Dis Colon Rectum 1988;31:439.

253. Boland CR. Cancer family syndrome: a case report and literature review. Am J Dig Dis 1978;23:25s.

254. Lynch HT, Lynch PM, Pester J, et al. The cancer family syndrome. Rare cutaneous phenotypic linkage of Torre's syndrome. Arch Intern Med 1981;141:607.

255. Sondergaard JO, Svendsen LB, Witt IN, et al. Mandibular osteomas in the cancer family syndrome. Br J Cancer 1985;52:941.

256. Boland CR. Familial colonic cancer syndromes. West J Med 1983;139:351.

257. Markowitz JF, Aiges HW, Cunningham-Rundles S, et al. Cancer family syndrome: marker studies. Gastroenterology 1986;91:581.

258. Rozen P, Lynch HT, Figer A, et al. Familial colon cancer in the Tel-Aviv area and the influence of ethnic origin. Cancer 1987;60:2355.

259. Lovett E. Family studies in cancer of the colon and rectum. Br J Surg 1976;63:13.

260. Grossman S, Milos ML. Colonoscopic screening of persons with suspected risk factors for colon cancer. I. Family history. Gastroenterology 1988;94:395.

261. St. John DJB, McDermott FT, Hopper JL, et al. Cancer risk in relatives of patients with common colorectal cancer. Ann Intern Med 1993;118:785.

262. Cannon-Albright LA, Skolnick MH, Bishop DT, et al. Common inheritance of susceptibility to colonic adenomatous polyps and associated colorectal cancers. N Engl J Med 1988;319:533.

263. Williams AR, Balasooriya BAW, Day DW. Polyps and cancer of the large bowel: a necropsy study in Liverpool. Gut 1982;23:835.

264. Rickert RR, Auerbach O, Garfinkel L, et al. Adenomatous lesions of the large bowel: an autopsy survey. Cancer 1979;43:1847.

265. Eide TJ, Stalsberg H. Polyps of the large intestine in northern Norway. Cancer 1978;42:2839.

266. Bombi JA. Polyps of the colon in Barcelona, Spain. Cancer 1988;61:1472.

267. Clark JC, Collan Y, Eide TJ, et al. Prevalence of polyps in an autopsy series from areas with varying incidence of large bowel cancer. Int J Cancer 1985;36:179.

268. Morson BC, Bussey HJR. Magnitude of risk for cancer in patients with colorectal adenomas. Br J Surg 1985;72:S23.

269. Spencer RJ, Melton LJ III, Ready RL, et al. Treatment of small colorectal polyps: a population-based study of the risk of subsequent carcinoma. Mayo Clin Proc 1984;59:305.

270. Lotfi AM, Spencer RJ, Ilstrup DM, et al. Colorectal polyps and the risk of subsequent carcinoma. Mayo Clin Proc 1986;61:337.

271. Atkin WS, Morson BC, Cuzick J. Long-term risk of colorectal cancer after excision of rectosigmoid adenomas. N Engl J Med 1992;326:658.

272. Lockhart-Mummery HE, Heald RJ. Metachronous cancer of the large intestine. Dis Colon Rectum 1972;15:261.

273. Edwards FC, Truelove SC. The course and prognosis of ulcerative colitis. Part IV. Carcinoma of the colon. Gut 1964;5:15.

274. Greenstein AJ, Sachar DB, Smith H, et al. Cancer in universal and left-sided ulcerative colitis: factors determining risk. Gastroenterology 1979;77:290.

275. Katzka I, Brody RS, Morris E, et al. Assessment of colorectal cancer risk in patients with ulcerative colitis: experience from a private practice. Gastroenterology 1983;85:22.

276. Devroede GJ, Taylor WF, Sauer WG, et al. Cancer risk and life expectancy of children with ulcerative colitis. N Engl J Med 1971;285:17.

277. Maratka Z, Nedbal J, Kocianova J, et al. Incidence of colorectal cancer in proctocolitis: a restrospective study of 959 cases over 40 years. Gut 1985;26:43.

278. Hamilton SR. Colorectal carcinoma in patients with Crohn's disease. Gastroenterology 1985;89:398.

279. Gyde SN, Prior P, Macartney JC, et al. Malignancy in Crohn's disease. Gut 1980;21:1024.

280. Greenstein AJ, Gennuso R, Sachar DB, et al. Extraintestinal cancers in inflammatory bowel disease. Cancer 1985;56:2914.

281. Gyde SN, Prior P, Thompson H, et al. Survival of patients with colorectal cancer complicating ulcerative colitis. Gut 1984;25:228.

282. Riddell RH, Goldman H, Ransohoff DF, et al. Dysplasia in inflammatory bowel disease: standardized classification with provisional clinical applications. Hum Pathol 1983;14:931.

283. Dobbins WO III. Dysplasia and malignancy in inflammatory bowel disease. Ann Rev 1984;35:33.

284. Blackstone MO, Riddell RH, Rogers BHG, et al. Dysplasia-associated lesion or mass (DALM) detected by colonoscopy in long-standing ulcerative colitis: an indication for colectomy. Gastroenterology 1981;80:366.

285. Stemper TJ, Kent TH, Summers RW. Juvenile polyposis and gastrointestinal carcinoma. A study of a kindred. Ann Intern Med 1975;83:639.

286. Grotsky HW, Rickert RR, Smith WD, et al. Familial juvenile polyposis coli. A clinical and pathologic study of a large kindred. Gastroenterology 1982;82:494.

287. Jass JR, Williams CB, Bussey HJR, et al. Juvenile polyposis—a precancerous condition. Histopathology 1988;13:619.

288. Giardiello FM, Welsh SB, Hamilton SR, et al. Increased risk

of cancer in the Peutz-Jeghers syndrome. N Engl J Med 1987;316:1511.

289. Foley TR, McGarrity TJ, Abt AB. Peutz-Jeghers syndrome: a clinicopathologic survey of the "Harrisburg family" with a 49-year follow-up. Gastroenterology 1988;95:1535.

290. Linos DA, O'Fallon WM, Beart RW Jr, et al. Cholecystecomy and carcinoma of the colon. Lancet 1981;2:379.

291. Vernick LJ, Kuller LH. Cholecystecomy and right-sided colon cancer: an epidemiological study. Lancet 1981;2:381.

292. Mannes AG, Weinzierl M, Stellaard F, et al. Adenomas of the large intestine after cholecystecomy. Gut 1984;25:863.

293. Sandler RS, Martin ZZ, Carlton NM, et al. Adenomas of the large bowel after cholecystecomy a case-control study. Dig Dis Sci 1988;33:1178.

294. Neugut AI, Johnsen CM, Forde KA, et al. Cholecystectomy and adenomatous polyps of the colon in women. Cancer 1988;61:618.

295. Weiss NS, Daling JR, Chow WH. Cholecystectomy and the incidence of cancer of the large bowel. Cancer 1982;49:1713.

296. Adami H-O, Meirik O, Gustavsson S, et al. Colorectal cancer after cholecystectomy: absence of risk increase within 11–14 years. Gastroenterology 1983;85:859.

297. Neugut AI, Murray TI, Garbowski GC, et al. Cholecystectomy as a risk factor for colorectal adenomatous polyps and carcinoma. Cancer 1991;68:1644.

298. Ekbom A, Yuen J, Adami H-O, et al. Cholecystectomy and colorectal cancer. Gastroenterology 1993;105:142.

299. Giovannucci E, Colditz GA, Stampfer MJ. A meta-analysis of cholecystectomy and risk of colorectal cancer. Gastroenterology 1993;105:130.

300. Ron E, Gridley G, Hrubec Z, et al. Acromegaly and gastrointestinal cancer. Cancer 1991;68:1673.

301. Wong K, Beardshall K, Waters CM, et al. Postprandial hypergastrinaemia in patients with colorectal cancer. Gut 1991;32:1352.

302. Seitz J-F, Giovannini M, Gouvernet J, et al. Elevated serum gastrin levels in patients with colorectal neoplasia. J Clin Gastroenterol 1991;13:541.

303. Kochman ML, DelValle J, Dickinson CJ, et al. Post-translational processing of gastrin in neoplastic human colonic tissues. Biochem Biophys Res Comm 1992;189:1165.

304. Hoosein NM, Kiener PA, Curry RC, et al. Antiproliferative effects of gastrin receptor antagonists and antibodies to gastrin on human colon carcinoma cell lines. Cancer Res 1988;48:7179.

305. Leavitt J, Klein I, Kendricks F, et al. Skin tags: a cutaneous marker for colonic polyps. Ann Intern Med 1983;93:928.

306. Gould BE, Ellison RC, Greene HL, et al. Lack of association between skin tags and colon polyps in a primary care setting. Arch Intern Med 1988;148:1799.

307. Piette AM, Meduri B, Fritsch J, et al. Do skin tags constitute a marker for colonic polyps? Gastroenterology 1988;95:1127.

308. Luk GD, The Colon Neoplasia Work Group. Colonic polyps and acrochordons (skin tags) do not correlate in familial colonic polyposis kindreds. Ann Intern Med 1986;104:209.

309. Klein RS, Recco RA, Catalano MT, et al. Association of *Streptococcus bovis* with carcinoma of the colon. N Engl J Med 1977;297:800.

310. Klein RS, Catalano MT, Edberg ST, et al. *Streptococcus bovis* septicemia and carcinoma of the colon. Ann Intern Med 1979;91:560.

311. Marshall JB, Gerhardt DC. Polyposis coli presenting with *Streptococcus bovis* endocarditis. Am J Gastroenterol 1981;75:314.

312. Gilon D, Moses A. Carcinoma of the colon presenting as *Streptococcus equinus* bacteremia. Am J Med 1986;86:135.

313. Karlin DA, Jones RD, Stroehlein JR, et al. Breath methane excretion in patients with unresected colorectal cancer. J Natl Cancer Inst 1982;69:573.

314. Pique JM, Pallares M, Cuso E, et al. Methane production and colon cancer. Gastroenterology 1984;87:601.

315. Segal I, Walker ARP, Lord S, et al. Breath methane and large bowel cancer risk in contrasting African populations. Gut 1988;29:608.

316. Stewart M, Macrae FA, Williams CB. Neoplasia and ureterosigmoidostomy: a colonoscopy survey. Br J Surg 1982;69:414.

317. McKusick VA. Mendelian inheritance in man. 6th ed. Baltimore: Johns Hopkins University Press, 1983:625.

318. Cerutti PA. Prooxidant states and tumor promotion. Science 1985;227:375.

319. Sontag SJ, Schnell TG, Chesee G, et al. Barrett's oesophagus and colonic tumours. Lancet 1985;1:946.

320. Tripp MR, Sampliner RE, Kogan FJ, et al. Colorectal neoplasia and Barrett's oesophagus. Am J Gastroenterol 1986;81:1063.

321. Robertson DAF, Ayres RCS, Smith CL. Screening for colonic cancer in patients with Barrett's oesophagus. Br Med J 1989;298:650.

322. McCallum A, Eastwood MA, Smith AN, et al. Colonic diverticulosis in patients with colorectal cancer and in controls. Scand J Gastroenterol 1988;23:284.

323. Crawford BE, Stromeyer FW. Small nonpolypoid carcinomas of the large intestine. Cancer 1983;51:1760.

324. Shamsuddin AM, Kato YO, Kunishima N, et al. Carcinoma in situ in nonpolypoid mucosa of the large intestine: report of a case with significance in strategies for early detection. Cancer 1985;56:2849.

325. Kuramoto S, Oohara T. Minute cancers arising de novo in the human large intestine. Cancer 1988;61:829.

326. Friedman EA, Buset M, Winawer SJ. Tumor-promoter-enhanced destruction of noninvasive human benign colon tumor cells by cocultivated carcinoma cells. Digestion 1988;40:197.

327. Snyder DN, Heston JF, Meigs JW, et al. Changes in site distribution of colorectal carcinoma in Connecticut, 1940–1973. Dig Dis 1977;22:791.

328. Beart RW, Melton LJ III, Maruta M, et al. Trends in right and left-sided colon cancer. Dis Colon Rectum 1983;26:393.

329. Vukasin AP, Ballantyne GH, Flannery JT, et al. Increasing incidence of cecal and sigmoid carcinoma. Cancer 1990;66:2442.

330. Kee F, Wilson RH, Gilliland R, et al. Changing site distribution of colorectal cancer. Br Med J 1992;305:158.

331. Mamazza J, Gordon PH. The changing distribution of large intestinal cancer. Dis Colon Rectum 1982;25:558.

332. Netscher DT, Larson GM. Colon cancer: the left to right shift and its implications. Surg Gastroenterol 1983;2:13.

333. Lasser A. Synchronous primary adenocarcinomas of the colon and rectum. Dis Colon Rectum 1978;21:20.

334. Langevin JM, Nivatvongs S. The true incidence of synchronous cancer of the large bowel: a prospective study. Am J Surg 1980;147:330.

335. Chu DZJ, Giacco G, Martin RG, et al. The significance of synchronous carcinoma and polyps in the colon and rectum. Cancer 1986;57:445.

336. Greenstein AJ, Heimann TM, Sachar DB, et al. A comparison of multiple synchronous colorectal cancer in ulcerative colitis, familial polyposis coli, and de novo cancer. Ann Surg 1986;203:123.

337. Symonds DA, Vickery AL Jr. Mucinous carcinoma of the colon and rectum. Cancer 1976;37:1891.

338. Umpleby HC, Ranson DL, Williamson RCN. Peculiarities of mucinous colorectal carcinoma. Br J Surg 1985;72:715.

339. Donegan WL, DeCosse JJ. Pitfalls and controversies in the staging of colorectal cancer. In: Enker WE, ed. Carcinoma of the colon and rectum. Chicago: Year Book Medical Publishers, 1979:49.

340. Cohen AM, Tremiterra S, Candela F, et al. Prognosis of node-positive colon cancer. Cancer 1991;67:1859.

341. Newland RC, Chapuis PH, Fracs MT, et al. The relationship of survival to staging and grading of colorectal carcinoma: a prospective study of 503 cases. Cancer 1981;47:1424.

342. Turnbull RB. The no-touch isolation technique of resection. JAMA 1975;231:1181.

343. Fisher ER, Sass R, Palekar A, et al. Dukes' classification revisited. Findings from the national surgical adjuvant breast and bowel projects (protocol R-01). Cancer 1989;64:2354.

344. Cooper HS, Slemmer JR. Surgical pathology of carcinoma of the colon and rectum. Semin Oncol 1991;18:367.

345. Jass JR, Love SB, Northover JMA. A new prognostic classification of rectal cancer. Lancet 1987;1:1303.

346. Rognum TO, Lund E, Meling GI, et al. Near diploid large bowel carcinomas have better five-year survival than aneuploid ones. Cancer 1991;68:1077.

347. Jass JR, Mukawa K, Goh HS, et al. Clinical importance of DNA content in rectal cancer measured by flow cytometry. J Clin Pathol 1989;42:254.

348. Harlow SP, Eriksen BL, Poggensee L, et al. Prognostic implications of proliferative activity and DNA aneuploidy in Astler-Coller Dukes stage C colonic adenocarcinomas. Cancer Res 1991;51:2403.

349. Enker WE, Kimmel M, Cibas ES, et al. DNA/RNA content and proliferative fractions of colorectal carcinomas: a five-year prospective study relating flow cytometry to survival. J Natl Cancer Inst 1991;83:701.

350. Kuramoto S, Oohara T. Flat early cancers of large intestine. Cancer 1989;64:950.

351. Iishi H, Tatsuta M, Tsutsui S, et al. Early depressed adenocarcinomas of the large intestine. Cancer 1992;69:2406.

352. Qizilbash AH, Meghji M, Castelli M. Pseudocarcinomatous invasion in adenomas of the colon and rectum. Dis Colon Rectum 1980;23:529.

353. Dawson PA, Filipe MI. An ultrastructural and histochemical study of the mucous membrane adjacent to and remote from carcinoma of the colon. Cancer 1976;37:2388.

354. Riddell RH, Levin B. Ultrastructure of the "transitional" mucosa adjacent to large bowel carcinoma. Cancer 1977;40:2509.

355. Lanza G Jr, Altavilla G, Cavazzini L, Negrini R. Colonic mucosa adjacent to adenomas and hyperplastic polyps—a morphological and histochemical study. Histopathology 1985;9:857.

356. Boland CR, Kim YS. Transitional mucosa of the colon and tumor growth factors. Medical Hypotheses 1987;22:237.

357. Dawson PM, Habib NA, Rees HC, et al. Influence of sialomucin at the resection margin on local tumor recurrence and survival of patients with colorectal cancer: a multivariate analysis. Br J Surg 1987;74:366.

358. Ahlquist DA, Wieand HS, Moertel CG, et al. Accuracy of fecal occult blood screening for colorectal neoplasia. JAMA 1993;269:1262.

359. Eddy DM. Screening for colorectal cancer. Ann Intern Med 1990;113:373.

360. Aldridge MC, Sim AJW. Colonoscopy findings in symptomatic patients without x-ray evidence of colonic neoplasms. Lancet 1986;2:833.

361. Durdey P, Weston PMT, Williams NS. Colonoscopy or barium enema as initial investigation of colonic disease. Lancet 1987;2:549.

362. Kelvin FM, Gardiner R, Vas W, et al. Colorectal carcinoma missed on double contrast barium enema study: a problem in perception. AJR Am J Roentgenol 1981;137:307.

363. Tinetti ME, Stone L, Cooney L, et al. Inadequate barium enemas in hospitalized elderly patients: incidence and risk factors. Arch Intern Med 1989;149:2014.

364. Hixson LJ, Fennerty MB, Sampliner RE, et al. Prospective study of the frequency and size distribution of polyps missed by colonoscopy. J Natl Cancer Inst 1990;82:1769.

365. Ostrow JD, Mulvaney CA, Hansell JR, et al. Sensitivity and reproducibility of chemical tests for fecal occult blood with an emphasis on false-positive reactions. Am J Dig Dis 1973;18:930.

366. Pierson RN Jr, Holter PR, Watson RM, et al. Aspirin and gastrointestinal bleeding: chromate[51] blood loss measured by radioactive chromium. Gut 1960;1:177.

367. Cameron AD. Gastrointestinal blood loss measured by radioactive chromium. Gut 1960;1:177.

368. Macrae FA, St John DJB, Caligiore P, et al. Optimal dietary conditions for Hemoccult testing. Gastroenterology 1982;82:899.

369. Caligiore P, Macrae FA, St John DJB, et al. Peroxidase levels in food: relevance to colorectal cancer screening. Am J Clin Nutr 1982;35:1487.

370. Herzog P, Holtermuller K-H, Preiss J, et al. Fecal blood loss in patients with colonic polyps: a comparison of measurements with [51]chromium-labeled erythrocytes and with the Hemoccult test. Gastroenterology 1982;83:957.

371. St. John DJB, Young GP, Alexeyeff MA, et al. Evaluation of new occult blood tests for detection of colorectal neoplasia. Gastroenterology 1993;104:1661.

372. Ahlquist DA, McGill DB, Schwartz S, et al. Fecal blood levels in health and disease. A study using HemoQuant. N Engl J Med 1985;312:1422.

373. Ahlquist DA, McGill DB, Schwartz S, et al. HemoQuant, a new quantitative assay for fecal hemoglobin: comparison with Hemoccult. Ann Intern Med 1984;101:297.

374. Stroehlein JR, Fairbanks VF, Go VLW, et al. Hemoccult stool tests—false-negative results due to storage of specimens. Mayo Clin Proc 1976;51:548.

375. Niv Y. Fecal occult blood test—the importance of proper evaluation. J Clin Gastroenterol 1990;12(4):393.

376. Brayshaw JR, Harris F, McCurdy PR. The effect of oral iron therapy on the stool guaiac and orthotolidine reactions. Ann Intern Med 1963;59:172.

377. Lifton LJ, Kreiser J. False-positive stool occult blood tests caused by iron preparations. Gastroenterology 1982;83:860.

378. McDonnell WM, Ryan JA, Seeger DM, et al. Effect of iron on the guaiac reaction. Gastroenterology 1989;96:74.

379. Laine LA, Bentley E, Chandrasoma P. Effect of oral iron therapy on the upper gastrointestinal tract—a prospective evaluation. Dig Dis Sci 1988;33:172.

380. Jaffe RM, Kasten B, Young DS, et al. False-negative stool occult blood tests caused by ingestion of ascorbic acid (vitamin C). Ann Intern Med 1975;83:824.

381. Winchester DP, Shull JH, Scanlon EF, et al. A mass screening program for colorectal cancer using chemical testing for occult blood in the stool. Cancer 1980;45:2955.

382. Winawer SJ, Andrews M, Flehinger B, et al. Progress report on controlled trial of fecal occult blood testing for the detection of colorectal neoplasia. Cancer 1980;45:2959.

383. Winawer SJ, Schottenfeld D, Flehinger BJ. Colorectal cancer screening. J Natl Cancer Inst 1991;83:243.

384. Hardcastle JD, Farrands PA, Balfour TW. Controlled trial of faecal occult blood testing in the detection of colorectal cancer. Lancet 1983;2:1.

385. Hardcastle JD, Chir M, Armitage NC, et al. Fecal occult blood screening for colorectal cancer in the general population. Cancer 1986;58:397.

386. Hardcastle JD, Thomas WM, Chamberlain J, et al. Randomized, controlled trial of faecal occult blood screening for colorectal cancer: results for first 107,349 subjects. Lancet 1989;1:1160.

387. Selby JV, Friedman GD, Quesenberry CP Jr, et al. Effect of fecal occult blood testing on mortality from colorectal cancer. A case-control study. Ann Intern Med 1993;118:1.

388. Mandel JS, Bond JH, Church TR, et al. Reducing mortality from colorectal cancer by screening for fecal occult blood. N Engl J Med 1993;328:1365.

389. Gilbertsen VA, Nelms JM. The prevention of invasive cancer of the rectum. Cancer 1978;41:1137.

390. Selby JV, Friedman GD, Quesenberry CP Jr, et al. A case-control study of screening sigmoidoscopy and mortality from colorectal cancer. N Engl J Med 1992;326:653.

391. Newcomb PA, Norfleet RG, Storer BE, et al. Screening sigmoidoscopy and colorectal cancer mortality. J Natl Cancer Inst 1992;84:1572.

392. Levin B, Murphy GP. Revision in American Cancer Society recommendations for the early detection of colorectal cancer. CA Cancer J Clin 1992;42:296.

393. Wagner JL, Herdman RC, Wadhwa S. Cost effectiveness of colorectal cancer screening in the elderly. Ann Intern Med 1991;115:807.

394. Fleischer DE, Goldberg SB, Browning TH, et al. Detection and surveillance of colorectal cancer. JAMA 1989;261:580.

395. Ransohoff DF, Lang CA. Sigmoidoscopic screening in the 1990s. JAMA 1993;269:1278.

396. Atkin WS, Cuzick J, Northover JMA, et al. Prevention of co-

lorectal cancer by once-only sigmoidoscopy. Lancet 1993;341:736.

397. Winawer SJ, Zauber AG, O'Brien MJ, et al. Randomized comparison of surveillance intervals after colonoscopic removal of newly diagnosed adenomatous polyps. N Engl J Med 1993;328:901.

398. Ballantyne GH, Modlin IM. Postoperative follow-up for colorectal cancer: who are we kidding? J Clin Gastroenterol 1988;10:359.

399. Choi PM, Nugent FW, Schoetz DJ Jr, et al. Colonoscopic surveillance reduces mortality from colorectal cancer in ulcerative colitis. Gastroenterology 1993;105:418.

400. Rosenstock E, Farmer RG, Petras R, et al. Surveillance for colonic carcinoma in ulcerative colitis. Gastroenterology 1985;89:1342.

401. Boland CR. Diagnosis and management of primary and metastatic colorectal cancer. Semin Gastrointest Dis 1992;3:33.

402. Corman ML, Swinton NW, O'Keefe DD, et al. Colorectal carcinoma at the Lahey Clinic, 1962 to 1966. Am J Surg 1973;125:424.

403. Turunen MJ, Peltokllio P. Surgical results in 657 patients. Dis Colon Rectum 1983;26:606.

404. August DA, Ottow RT, Sugarbaker PH. Clinical perspective of human colorectal cancer metastases. Cancer Metastasis Rev 1984;3:303.

405. Bengtsson G, Carlsson G, Hafstrom L, et al. Natural history of patients with untreated liver metastases from colorectal cancer. Am J Surg 1981;141:586.

406. Enblad P, Adami H, Bergstrom R, et al. Improved survival of patients with cancers of the colon and rectum? J Natl Cancer Inst 1988;80:586.

407. Minsky BD, Mies C, Recht A, et al. Resectable adenocarcinoma of the rectosigmoid and rectum: 1. Patterns of failure and survival. Cancer 1988;61:1408.

408. Griffiths JD, McKinna JA, Rowbotham HD, et al. Carcinoma of the colon and rectum: circulating malignant cells and five-year survival. Cancer 1973;31:226.

409. Wolmark N, Cruz I, Redmond CK, et al. Tumor size and regional lymph node metastasis in colorectal cancer. Cancer 1983;51:1315.

410. Finlay IG, Meek DR, Gray HW, et al. Incidence and detection of occult hepatic metastases in colorectal carcinoma. Br Med J 1982;284:803.

411. Finlay IG, McArdle CS. Effect of occult hepatic metastases on survival after curative resection for colorectal carcinoma. Gastroenterology 1983;85:596.

412. Le Chevalier T, Cvitkovic E, Caille P, et al. Early metastatic cancer of unknown primary origin at presentation: a clinical study of 302 consecutive autopsied patients. Arch Intern Med 1988;148:2035.

413. Le Chevalier T, Smith F, Caille P, et al. Sites of primary malignancies in patients presenting with cerebral metastases: a review of 120 cases. Cancer 1985;56:880.

414. Patt YZ, Podoloff DA, Curley S, et al. Monoclonal antibody imaging in patients with colorectal cancer and increasing levels of serum carcinoembryonic antigen. Experience with ZCE-025 and IMMU-4 monoclonal antibodies and proposed directions for clinical trials. Cancer 1993;71:4293.

415. Loewenstein MS, Zamcheck N. Carcinoembryonic antigen (CEA) levels in benign gastrointestinal disease states. Cancer 1978;42:1412.

416. Fletcher RH. Carcinoembryonic antigen. Ann Intern Med 1986;104:66.

417. McArdle CS, Hole D. Impact of variability among surgeons on postoperative morbidity and mortality and ultimate survival. Br Med J 1991;302:1501.

418. Botsford TW, Aliapoulios MA, Curtis LE. Results of treatment of colorectal cancer at the Peter Bent Brigham Hospital. Am J Surg 1965;109:566.

419. Zhou X, Yu B, Shen Y. Surgical treatment and late results in 1226 cases of colorectal cancer. Dis Colon Rectum 1983;26:250.

420. Haggitt RC, Glotzbach RE, Soffer EE, et al. Prognostic factors in colorectal carcinomas arising in adenomas: implications for lesions removed by endoscopic polypectomy. Gastroenterology 1985;89:328.

421. Gastrointestinal Tumor Study Group. Adjuvant therapy of colon cancer—results of a prospectively randomized trial. N Engl J Med 1984;310:737.

422. Buyse M, Zeleniuch-Jacquotte A, Chalmers TC. Adjuvant therapy of colorectal cancer—why we still don't know. JAMA 1988;259:3571.

423. Laurie JA, Moertel CG, Fleming TR, et al. Surgical adjuvant therapy of large-bowel carcinoma: an evaluation of levamisole and the combination of levamisole and fluorouracil. J Clin Oncol 1989;7:1447.

424. Moertel CJ, Fleming TR, Macdonald JS, et al. Levamisole and fluorouracil for adjuvant therapy of resected colon carcinoma. N Engl J Med 1990;322:352.

425. Nauta R, Stablein DM, Holyoke D. Survival of patients with stage B2 colon carcinoma. The gastrointestinal tumor study group experience. Arch Surg 1989;124:180.

426. Vassilopoulos PP, Yoon JM, Ledesma EJ, et al. Treatment of recurrence of adenocarcinoma of the colon and rectum at the anastomotic site. Surg Gynecol Obstet 1981;152:777.

427. Rich T, Gunderson LL, Lew R, et al. Patterns of recurrence of rectal cancer after potentially curative surgery. Cancer 1983;52:1317.

428. Martin EW Jr, Cooperman M, Carey LC, et al. Sixty second-look procedures indicated primarily by rise in serial carcinoembryonic antigen. J Surg Res 1980;28:389.

429. Steele G Jr, Zamcheck N, Wilson R, et al. Results of CEA-initiated second-look surgery of recurrent colorectal cancer. Am J Surg 1986;139:544.

430. Deveney KE, Way LW. Follow-up of patients with colorectal cancer. Am J Surg 1984;148:717.

431. Sandler RS, Freund DA, Herbst CA, et al. Cost effectiveness of postoperative carcinoembryonic antigen monitoring in colorectal cancer. Cancer 1984;53:193.

432. Hughes KS, Rosenstein RB, Songhorabodi S, et al. Resection of the liver for colorectal carcinoma metastases—a multiinstitutional study of long-term survivors. Dis Colon Rectum 1988;31:1.

433. Hawes RH. New staging techniques. Endoscopic ultrasound. Cancer 1993;71:4207.

434. DeCosse JJ, Wong RJ, Quan SHQ, et al. Conservative treatment of invasive distal rectal cancer by local excision. Cancer 1989;63:219.

435. Mathus-Vliegen EMH, Tytgat GNJ. Nd:YAG Laser photocoagulation in colorectal adenoma—evaluation of its safety, usefulness, and efficacy. Gastroenterology 1986;90:1865.

436. Mathus-Vliegen WMH, Tytgat NJ. Laser photocoagulation in the palliation of colorectal malignancies. Cancer 1986;57:2212.

437. Brunetaud JM, Maunoury V, Ducrotte MP, et al. Palliative treatment of rectosigmoid carcinoma by laser endoscopic photoablation. Gastroenterology 1987;92:663.

438. Dosoretz DE, Gunderson LL, Hedberg S, et al. Preoperative irradiation for unresectable rectal and rectosigmoid carcinomas. Cancer 1983;52:814.

439. Higgins GA, Humphrey EW, Dwight RW, et al. Preoperative radiation and surgery for cancer of the rectum: Veterans Administration surgical oncology group trial II. Cancer 1986;58:352.

440. Pearlman NW, Stiegmann GV, Donohue RE. Extended resection of fixed rectal cancer. Cancer 1989;63:2438.

441. Gastrointestinal Tumor Study Group. Prolongation of the disease-free interval in surgically treated rectal carcinoma. N Engl J Med 1985;312:1465.

442. Mohiuddin M, Derdel J, Marks G, et al. Results of adjuvant radiation therapy in cancer of the rectum. Thomas Jefferson University Hospital experience. Cancer 1985;55:350.

443. Fisher B, Wolmark N, Rockette H, et al. Postoperative adjuvant chemotherapy or radiation therapy for rectal cancer: results from NSABP protocol R-01. J Natl Cancer Inst 1988;80:21.

444. Krook JE, Moertel CG, Gunderson LL, et al. Effective surgical adjuvant therapy for high-risk rectal carcinoma. N Engl J Med 1991;324:709.

445. Ballantyne GH, Quin J. Surgical treatment of liver metastases in patients with colorectal cancer. Cancer 1993;71:4252.

446. Nakamura S, Yokoi Y, Suzuki S, et al. Results of extensive surgery for liver metastases in colorectal carcinoma. Br J Surg 1992;79:35.

447. Morrow CE, Vassilopoulos PP, Grage TB. Surgical resection for metastatic neoplasms of the lung: experience at the University of Minnesota Hospitals. Cancer 1980;45:2981.

448. Goya T, Miyazawa N, Kondo H, et al. Surgical resection of pulmonary metastases from colorectal cancer—ten year follow-up. Cancer 1989;64:1418.

449. Turk PS, Wanebo HJ. Results of surgical treatment of non-hepatic recurrence of colorectal carcinoma. Cancer 1993;71:4267.

450. Nicholls J. Large bowel cancer. In: Stevin ML, Staquet MJ, eds. Randomized trials in cancer: a critical review by sites. New York: Raven, 1986:241.

451. Poon MA, O'Connell MJ, Moertel CG, et al. Biochemical modulation of fluorouracil: evidence of significant improvement of survival and quality of life in patients with advanced colorectal carcinoma. J Clin Oncol 1989;7:1407.

452. Petrelli N, Douglass HO, Herrera L, et al. The modulation of fluorouracil with leucovorin in metastatic colorectal carcinoma: a prospective randomized phase III trial. J Clin Oncol 1989;7:1419.

453. Valone FH, Friedman MA, Wittlinger PS, et al. Treatment of patients with advanced colorectal carcinomas with fluorouracil alone, high-dose leucovorin plus fluorouracil, or sequential methotrexate, fluorouracil, and leucovorin: a randomized trial of the Northern California Oncology Group. J Clin Oncol 1989;7:1427.

454. The Nordic Gastrointestinal Tumor Adjuvant Therapy Group. Superiority of sequential methotrexate, fluorouracil, and leucovorin to fluorouracil alone in advanced symptomatic colorectal carcinoma: a randomized trial. J Clin Oncol 1989;7:1437.

455. Vaughn DJ, Haller DG. Nonsurgical management of recurrent colorectal cancer. Cancer 1993;71:4278.

456. Oberfield RA, McCafferey JA, Polio J, et al. Prolonged and continuous percutaneous intra-arterial hepatic infusion chemotherapy in advanced metastic liver adenocarcinoma from colorectal primary. Cancer 1979;44:414.

457. Niederhuber JE, Ensminger W, Gyves J, et al. Regional chemotherapy of colorectal cancer metastatic to the liver. Cancer 1984;53:1136.

458. Kemeny MM, Goldberg DA, Browning S, et al. Experience with continuous regional chemotherapy and hepatic resection as treatment of hepatic metastases from colorectal primaries: a prospective randomized study. Cancer 1985;55:1265.

459. Kemeny N, Daly J, Oderman P, et al. Hepatic artery infusion chemotherapy in colorectal cancer. J Clin Oncol 1984;2:595.

460. Kemeny N, Daly J, Reichman B, et al. Intrahepatic or systemic infusion of fluorodeoxyuridine in patients with liver metastases from colorectal carcinoma: a randomized trial. Ann Intern Med 1987;107:459.

461. An implanted infusion pump for chemotherapy of liver metastases. The Medical Letter 1984;26:87.

462. Rosenberg SA, Lotze MT, Muul LM, et al. Observations on the systemic administration of autologous lymphokine-activated killer cells and recombinant interleukin-2 to patients with metastatic cancer. N Engl J Med 1985;313:1485.

463. Rosenberg SA, Lotze MT, Muul LM, et al. A progress report on the treatment of 157 patients with advanced cancer using lymphokine-activated killer cells and interleukin-2 or high-dose interleukin-2 alone. N Engl J Med 1987;316:889.

464. Hoover HC, Hanna MG. Active immunotherapy in colorectal cancers. Semin Surg Oncol 1989;5:436.

465. Rosenberg SA, Lotze MT, Yang JC, et al. Prospective randomized trial of high-dose interleukin-2 alone or in conjunction with lymphokine-activated killer cells for the treatment of patients with advanced cancer. J Natl Cancer Inst 1993;85:622.

466. Wolmark N, Fisher B, Rockette H, et al. Postoperative adjuvant chemotherapy or BCG for colon cancer: results from NSABP protocol C-01. J Natl Cancer Inst 1988;80:30.

467. Lewin KJ, Ranchod M, Dorfman RF. Lymphomas of the gastrointestinal tract: a study of 117 cases presenting with gastrointestinal disease. Cancer 1978;42:693.

468. Haber DA, Mayer RJ. Primary gastrointestinal lymphoma. Semin Oncol 1988;15:154.

469. Bartolo D, Goepel JR, Parsons MA. Rectal malignant lymphoma in chronic ulcerative colitis. Gut 1982;23:164.

470. Radaszkiewicz T, Dragosics B, Bauer P. Gastrointestinal malignant lymphomas of the mucosa-associated lymphoid tissue: factors relevant to prognosis. Gastroenterology 1992;102:1628.

471. Vanden Heule B, Taylor CR, Chir B, et al. Presentation of malignant lymphoma in the rectum. Cancer 1982;49:2602.

472. Saltz RK, Kurtz RC, Lightdale CJ, et al. Kaposi's sarcoma: gastrointestinal involvement correlation with skin findings and immunologic function. Dig Dis Sci 1984;29:817.

473. Wall SD, Friedman SL, Margulis AR. Gastrointestinal Kaposi's sarcoma in AIDS: radiographic manifestations. J Clin Gastroenterol 1984;6:165.

474. Friedman SL, Wright TL, Altman DF. Gastrointestinal Kaposi's sarcoma in patients with acquired immunodeficiency syndrome: endoscopic and autopsy findings. Gastroenterology 1985;89:102.

475. Orloff MJ. Carcinoid tumors of the rectum. Cancer 1971;28:175.

476. Beaton HL. Carcinoid tumors of the alimentary tract. CA Cancer J Clin 1982;32:92.

477. Godwin JD. Carcinoid tumors: an analysis of 2,837 cases. Cancer 1975;36:560.

478. Spirio L, Olschwang S, Groden J, et al. Alleles of the *APC* gene: an attenuated form of familial polyposis. Cell 1993;75:951.

479. Powell SM, Petersen GM, Krush AJ, et al. Molecular diagnosis of familial adenomatous polyposis. N Engl J Med 1993;329:1982.

480. Ionov Y, Peinado MA, Malkhosyan S, et al. Ubiquitous somatic mutations in simple repeated sequences reveal a new mechanism for colonic carcinogenesis. Nature 1993;363:558.

481. Aaltonen LA, Peltomaki P, Leach FS, et al. Clues to the pathogenesis of familial colorectal cancer. Science 1993;260:812.

482. Thibodeau SN, Bren G, Schaid D. Microsatellite instability in cancer of the proximal colon. Science 1993;260:816.

483. Fishel R, Lesco MK, Rao MRS, et al. The human mutator gene homolog *MSH2* and its association with hereditary nonpolyposis colon cancer. Cell 1993;75:1027.

484. Leach FS, Nicolaides NC, Papadopoulos N, et al. Mutations of a *mutS* homolog in hereditary nonpolyposis colorectal cancer. Cell 1993;75:1215.

485. Liu B, Parson RE, Hamilton SR, et al. *hMSH2* mutations in hereditary nonpolyposis colorectal cancer kindreds. Cancer Res 1994;54:4590.

486. Bronner CE, Baker SM, Morrison PT, et al. Mutations in the DNA mismatch repair gene homologue *hMLH1* is associated with hereditary non-polyposis colon cancer. Nature 1994;368:258.

487. Papadopoulos N, Nicolaides NC, Wei Y-F, et al. Mutation of a *mutL* homolog in hereditary colon cancer. Science 1994;263:1625.

488. Nicolaides NC, Papadopoulos N, Liu B, et al. Mutations of two *PMS* homologues in hereditary nonpolyposis colon cancer. Nature 1994;371:75.

489. Jen J, Kim H, Piantados S, et al. Allelic loss of chromosome 18q and prognosis in colorectal cancer. N Engl J Med 1994;331:214.

490. Winawer SJ, Zauber AG, Ho MH, et al. Prevention of colorectal cancer by colonoscopic polypectomy. N Engl J Med 1993;329:1977.

491. Ponz de Leon M, Sant M, Micheli A, et al. Clinical and pathological indications in colorectal cancer. Cancer 1992;69:626.

Textbook of Gastroenterology, second edition, edited by Tadataka Yamada. JB Lippincott Company, Philadelphia © 1995.

CHAPTER 88

Anorectal Diseases

Jeffrey L. Barnett   Steven E. Raper

ANORECTAL EXAMINATION

The anorectal examination is an important part of the gastrointestinal evaluation and not merely a means of obtaining stool for occult blood testing. It must be performed with particular care and thoroughness in anyone with anorectal complaints (Table 88-1). The anorectal evaluation is usually reserved for the terminal portion of the examination after the patient-physician relationship has at least been partially established. Step by step explanation, reassurance, and gentle technique help to minimize patient embarrassment and discomfort. The patient should be placed in the left lateral decubitus position with the buttocks protruding just beyond the edge of the examining table. The hips may be slightly raised with a sandbag or a folded sheet. The prone jackknife position is ideal for examination of the anorectum, although it requires a specialized examining table and places the patient in a somewhat unfamiliar position. After the patient is adequately draped and the instruments are at hand but out of

direct patient view, examination begins with inspection of the perineum. The buttocks, sacral region, and thighs are observed for signs of pilonidal disease, dermatologic conditions, and infections. The buttocks are then firmly retracted with both hands to permit inspection of the perianal region. Fistulous openings, fecal or mucus soiling, and excoriations or chronic skin changes give clues to underlying disease processes. Anal pathology such as tumors, skin tags, anal fissures, and prolapsing hemorrhoids are often best identified at this time. Lesions should be described with regard to their anatomic location. Clockface descriptions are confusing unless patient position and orientation are specified.

Digital examination begins with palpation of the perianal area. Induration, tenderness, or the cord of a fistulous tract may be appreciated. The examining finger is well lubricated and slowly, gently inserted into the anus (Fig. 88-1). Palpation begins away from the area of suspected pathology. Anesthetic lubricant may be necessary in those with painful lesions. Occasionally, adequate examination is impossible except under

TABLE 88-1
Differential Diagnosis of Primary Presenting Symptoms of Anorectal Diseases

ANORECTAL PAIN	BRIGHT RED BLEEDING	PALPABLE LUMP	INCONTINENCE (see Table 88-2)	PRURITUS (see Table 88-3)
Hemorrhoids	Hemorrhoids	Hemorrhoids	Diarrhea of any cause	Anorectal diseases
Thrombosis	Internal	External	Fecal impaction	Anorectal infection
Strangulation (internal)	External	(including skin tags)	Irritable bowel syndrome	Local irritants
Abscess	Varices	Internal	Anal pathology	Dermatologic diseases
Fistula	Proctocolitis	(prolapsed)	Rectal pathology	
Hidradenitis suppurativa	Anorectal malignancy	Anal cancer	Neurologic diseases	
Anal fissure	Anal fissure	Condyloma acuminata	Tumors	
Anal stenosis	Solitary rectal ulcer	Rectal prolapse	Cauda equina	
Solitary rectal ulcer	Rectal colitis cystica	Anal polyps	Pelvic	
Crohn's disease	profunda	Hypertrophic anal papillae	Retrorectal	
Lymphogranuloma venereum		Endometrioma	Endometriosis (perianal)	
Leukemia or lymphoma				
Pilonidal disease				
Proctalgia fugax				
Levator syndrome				
Coccygodynia				

anesthesia. External hemorrhoids, thrombosed internal hemorrhoids, fissures, and fistulous tracts should be sought. Sphincter tone and the posterior puborectalis impression should be appreciated with the patient at rest, during squeeze, and when bearing down. The presacral area, the prostate, and even the cul-de-sac region may be palpated. Anteriorly, the impression of the cervix or an indwelling tampon should not be confused with pathology. During the examination of the rectal mucosa, the presence of polyps, tumors, feces, and foreign bodies is ascertained.

Anoscopy is the best means of examining the anal canal. It need be performed only if the patient has specific anal complaints. A variety of short tubular metal or disposable instruments are available with either built-in or external light sources. A removable obturator piece is held in place to permit insertion of the lubricated scope into the anal canal. The obturator core is removed to allow inspection of the rectal mu-

cosa and, after slight withdrawal, the anal canal. Fistulous openings and anal canal lesions are noted. Internal hemorrhoids may be seen arising just above the dentate line. Their true magnitude is best appreciated if the patient bears down and the hemorrhoids are seen to bulge into the lumen. Injection or rubber band ligation is performed through the metal anoscope. Fissures and perianal lesions may be appreciated as the instrument is withdrawn to below the dentate line.

Rigid proctosigmoidoscopy is performed for full evaluation of the distal colon and rectum. The rigid instrument is particularly useful for preoperative documentation of the position of a rectal cancer, large-bite rectal biopsy specimens for diagnosis of amyloidosis or Hirschsprung's disease, removal of foreign bodies, and evaluation of the mucosa if fiberoptic equipment is unavailable. For most other indications, the flexible fiberoptic instrument is preferred (see Chap. 116).

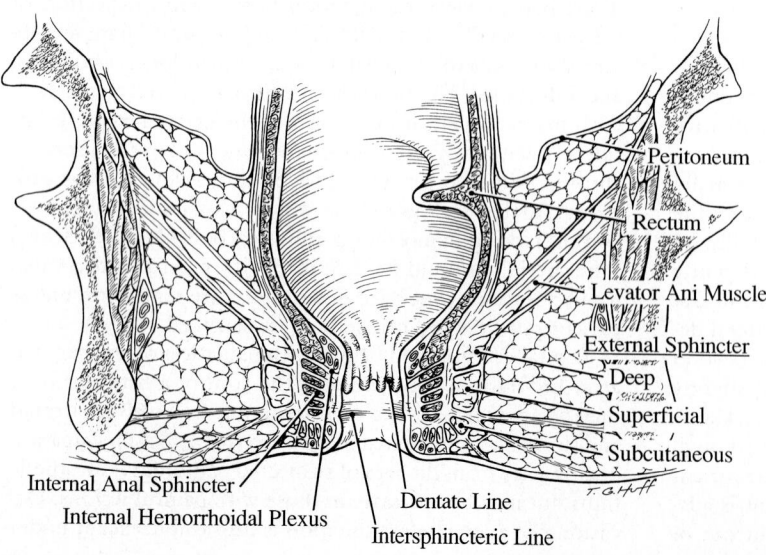

Figure 88-1. The normal anorectum.

HEMORRHOIDS

Hemorrhoids result from dilatation of the superior and inferior hemorrhoidal veins. These veins form a hemorrhoidal plexus, or cushion, in the submucosal layer of the lower rectum. Because the hemorrhoidal cushion is a normal anatomic structure, all adults are candidates for the development of symptomatic hemorrhoids. In the United States, estimates of prevalence have been as high as 50% of the adult population.[1]

Anatomic Considerations

Hemorrhoids may be either external or internal, and often both types are present in the same individual. Internal hemorrhoids arise from the superior hemorrhoidal cushion above the mucocutaneous junction of the anorectum, or dentate line. Internal hemorrhoids are lined with rectal mucosa and occur in three primary locations: right anterior, right posterior, and left lateral (Fig. 88-2). The end branches of the superior and middle hemorrhoidal arteries terminate in the submucosa above the dentate line with an anterior and posterior branch on the right and a single lateral branch on the left, corresponding to the three primary hemorrhoid locations. The right posterior and left branches give off two end branches to potentially form secondary hemorrhoids. External hemorrhoids arise from the inferior hemorrhoidal venous plexus below the mucocutaneous junction and are lined by perianal squamous epithelium. The perianal squamous epithelium of the anus contains numerous pain receptors, so that thrombosis of external hemorrhoids causes significant pain. Internal and external hemorrhoidal plexuses freely communicate to drain the lower rectum and anus. Internal and external hemorrhoids drain into the inferior vena cava through the internal pudendal veins.

Pathogenesis

The cause of hemorrhoids is not completely understood. There are three prominent theories, and various treatment regimens presume correctness of one or the other of these theories. The sliding anal lining theory is the widely held traditional view that hemorrhoids are merely enlargements of the preexisting veins of the superior and inferior hemorrhoidal plexuses. Elegant histologic studies have shown that hemorrhoids are normal features of the human anatomy. They have three important parts: the lining (rectal mucosa or anoderm), the stroma (blood vessels, smooth muscle, supporting connecting tissue), and the anchoring connective tissue (which secures the hemorrhoids to the sphincter mechanism). With age or other aggravating factors, the anchoring and supporting connective tissue deteriorates, causing the hemorrhoids to bulge and descend, leading eventually to symptoms.[2] This theory is supported by the increased incidence of hemorrhoids in patients with chronic constipation, diarrhea, pregnancy, or pelvic tumors—conditions which increase pelvic venous pressure. A second theory suggests that hemorrhoids share similarities with arteriovenous malformations. Both the bright red appearance and analysis of oxygen saturation of blood from internal hemorrhoids are more compatible with an arteriovenous anastomosis than a dilated vein.[3] This theory assumes that hemorrhoidal tissue has anatomic similarities to erectile tissue such as the corpora cavernosa.[4] Lastly, there is data to support the concept that the primary defect in the development of hemorrhoids is defective support of overlying mucosa—the hypertrophic internal anal sphincter hypothesis. Miles first tried to implicate the pecten band, or lower border of the internal anal sphincter, in the pathogenesis of hemorrhoids.[5] In certain individuals, the internal sphincter becomes hypertrophic and the anal outlet becomes functionally narrowed. At straining, the fecal bolus acts as an obturator forcing the hemorrhoidal cushions to descend through the hypertrophic sphincter, enlarge, and become symptomatic. In further support of this theory, Arabi has characterized, by means of a systematic study of anal manometry, a subgroup of hemorrhoid patients with abnormally high resting anal pressures.[6] A combined manometric and ultrasonographic study of the internal anal sphincter revealed no increase in anal sphincter thickness.[7] Hemorrhoids may then develop in response to the redundant mucosa, because the anal cushions are merely blood vessels loosely attached to smooth muscle and elastic tissue of the submucosa. Factors that increase rectal pressure include a spastic internal sphincter, chronic straining, and a gravid uterus.

Definitions

External skin tags are redundant folds of skin which arise from the anal verge. External hemorrhoids arise from the inferior hemorrhoidal plexus below the dentate line and are covered by anal squamous epithelium. Internal hemorrhoids arise from the superior hemorrhoidal plexus above the dentate line and are covered by columnar epithelium of the rectum. They may be classified according to their degree of protrusion or prolapse. First-degree hemorrhoids bulge into the lumen of the anorectal canal on anoscopy but do not protrude out of the anus. Second-degree hemorrhoids prolapse out of the anus with defecation or straining but reduce to a normal anatomic position spontaneously. Third-degree hemorrhoids prolapse out of the anus with defecation or straining and require digital reduction. Fourth-degree hemorrhoids are ir-

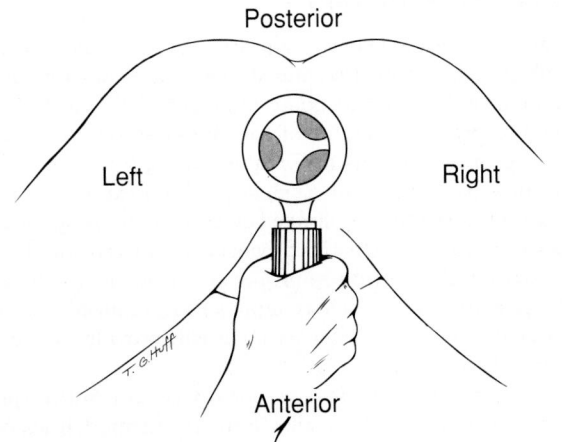

Figure 88-2. The three primary internal hemorrhoid locations: right anterior, right posterior, and left lateral.

reducible and are at risk for strangulation. The clinical presentation and recommended therapy for the various degrees of hemorrhoids are different and are discussed later. Anorectal varices are not hemorrhoids; they occur as a consequence of portal hypertension and are discussed separately in this chapter.

External Skin Tags

After thrombosis of an external hemorrhoid, the overlying skin becomes redundant, and this excess skin remains long after the underlying clot resolves. External skin tags may also arise after formal hemorrhoidectomy or de novo in cases of inflammatory bowel disease. Primary symptoms, if present, are complaints of a palpable growth near the anus and difficulty with anal hygiene. Skin tags are relatively easy to distinguish from more serious pathology such as anal cancer or condyloma acuminata by their gross appearance as normal skin and their soft, fleshy texture on palpation. Treatment is conservative whenever possible, and surgical excision is only necessary in cases of poor hygiene or patient anxiety.

External Hemorrhoids

Thrombosis of an external hemorrhoid can be an extremely painful event. Distention of overlying perianal skin and inflammation associated with the process of thrombosis may cause severe patient discomfort. Bleeding usually occurs late in the course of thrombosed external hemorrhoids after the overlying perianal skin ulcerates and the resolving, liquefied hematoma necessitates. External hemorrhoids should be distinguished from strangulated internal hemorrhoids and anorectal varices. Strangulated internal hemorrhoids tend to be larger and more circumferential, encompassing the entire anus. Anorectal varices should be considered in any patient with a history of cirrhosis or portal hypertension. The distinction is important because the therapy of anorectal varices and external hemorrhoids is quite different (see discussion elsewhere in this chapter).

Many thrombosed external hemorrhoids can be treated with warm sitz baths 2 to 3 times per day. If possible, bed rest should be prescribed to minimize additional thrombosis and swelling. Stool softening agents such as psyllium seed preparations, synthetic mucilloids, and the sodium or calcium salts of dioctyl sulfosuccinate can minimize straining at stool and prevent aggravation of the pain and thrombosis. Topical therapy with anesthetic ointments and witch hazel–impregnated pads may provide additional relief. One must temper the attribution of clinical improvements to medical therapy with the knowledge that the natural history of thrombosed external hemorrhoids is resolution after 48 to 72 hours.

If the pain is severe and the patient is seen within 48 hours of symptom onset, surgical evacuation or excision of the thrombosed external hemorrhoid should be performed. After the thrombus has organized, it cannot be evacuated. This can usually be done in the clinic setting and provides prompt relief. Simple evacuation is usually sufficient, but proponents of hemorrhoidal excision cite the potential for recurrent thrombosis and the difficulty with effective control of multiple bleeding points.

Internal Hemorrhoids

Internal hemorrhoids may be asymptomatic or associated with discomfort, pruritus ani, fecal soiling, or prolapse. Bleeding, however, is the typical complaint that brings the patient to the physician. It is described as bright red spotting on the toilet tissue or dripping into the toilet bowl. Bleeding most often occurs at the end of defecation and is separate from the stool. It does not usually occur apart from defecation. Rarely, acute severe bleeding requires transfusion and, occasionally, ongoing chronic losses cause iron deficiency anemia. However, hemorrhoids should not be considered the source of hematochezia until other potential bleeding sources in the colon and rectum have been investigated. With the possible exception of a young patient with a bleeding pattern typical of hemorrhoids, a flexible sigmoidoscopy or, if clinically appropriate, a full colonoscopy should be performed. Occult bleeding should not be attributed to hemorrhoids. Occult blood in the stool deserves a complete evaluation regardless of the presence of hemorrhoids.

Prolapse of the hemorrhoidal tissue is another common complaint. Prolapse may manifest itself anywhere along a continuum of symptoms from difficulty with anal hygiene to painful strangulation. Prolapsed tissue may also be a presenting symptom of rectal prolapse, rectal polyps, or rectal cancer. Sigmoidoscopic evaluation with biopsy of suspicious lesions should be carried out if appropriate. Anal condyloma and anal cancer are easily differentiated from prolapsing hemorrhoids, and thrombosed external hemorrhoids tend to cause pain as a presenting symptom.

All degrees of internal hemorrhoids may be associated with mild discomfort, but only strangulated hemorrhoids cause significant pain. Strangulated hemorrhoids usually possess an external and internal component and occur secondary to prolapse with subsequent lack of blood supply. Progression to gangrene with resultant infection is life-threatening and will occur if immediate surgical therapy is not instituted. In contrast to complete rectal prolapse, strangulated hemorrhoids lack concentric mucosal folds and are irreducible.

Treatment

Conservative Therapy

Dietary counseling, behavior adjustment, and topical agents are effective for most first- and second-degree hemorrhoids. A high-fiber diet and adequate fluid intake should be prescribed to promote passage of soft, bulky stools to prevent straining. Some patients may require the addition of hydrophilic bulk-forming agents such as psyllium extracts or mucilloids. Excessive and prolonged defecatory straining should be discouraged. Many patients benefit from warm sitz baths twice daily and attention to proper anal hygiene. A number of proprietary agents such as suppositories, ointments, and medicated compresses (witch hazel) usually provide astringent and anesthetic relief.

If conservative therapy does not suffice, a definitive procedure is necessary. The available treatment modalities can be broadly classified into one of two categories: those that involve loss of redundant mucosa and those that do not. In general, first- and second-degree hemorrhoids can be treated without removal of redundant hemorrhoidal tissue. Third- and fourth-degree hemorrhoids usually require a form of therapy that results in both thrombosis of the hemorrhoid and removal of redundant tissue.

Rubber Band Ligation

Barron first described a rapid, simple, effective device for the treatment of internal hemorrhoids in the office or outpatient setting.[8] In a large office-based practice, 21,000 patients were treated and 44.8% required rubber band ligation.[9] Band ligation is associated with both thrombosis of the hemorrhoid and removal of redundant mucosal tissue. By inducing submucosal scarring, development of new hemorrhoidal tissue is prevented. Rubber band ligation is a good treatment for refractory first-degree hemorrhoids as well as all second- and selected third-degree hemorrhoids. Fourth-degree hemorrhoids are not well treated by this method.

Because it is an outpatient procedure, no special preparation is needed for the majority of patients. After anorectal evaluation is performed, the anoscope is inserted and a hemorrhoidal cushion is selected for band application. No anesthetic is required if care is taken to place the band at least 0.5 cm above the dentate line. A Barron-type ligator is used to apply the elastic rubber band[10,11] (Fig. 88-3). Most authors recommend banding of only one column per session, to minimize tissue necrosis, but up to three ligations have been performed without increased morbidity.[12] Rubber band ligation allows a controlled removal of tissue rivalled only by formal hemorrhoidectomy.

Complications are rare but serious. In a series of 241 patients treated with rubber band ligation, only three required hospitalization.[13] Migration of the band onto the anoderm is associated with excruciating pain requiring immediate removal of the band. Persistent severe pain, fever, or foul-smelling rectal drainage may herald the presence of a rectal infection. A number of case reports of necrotizing infection

and death as a result of band ligation have appeared in the literature.[14,15] Mucosal slough with potential for bleeding occurs 5 to 7 days after band application, and the patient should be counseled accordingly.

Results of rubber band ligation are generally excellent, with long-term patient satisfaction of greater than 90%.[12,16,17] A drawback to the procedure is the need for repeated trips to the clinic for band application. No requirement for anesthesia and the ability to perform band ligation in the clinic setting continue to make this a popular treatment option for patients with hemorrhoids.

Injection Sclerotherapy

The use of a sclerosant solution such as sodium morrhuate or 5% phenol is an accepted treatment for first- and second-degree hemorrhoids. The sclerosant is injected with a special hemorrhoidal needle into the submucosa around, but not into, symptomatic hemorrhoids. An intense inflammatory reaction results in fixation of the mucosa to the underlying muscle. The submucosal layer in which hemorrhoids form is thus obliterated. Injection of sclerosants is a less controlled and therefore less popular technique than rubber band ligation. Known complications are mucosal slough, prostatic infection, contact hypersensitivity, and rectal infection. A recent refinement of injection sclerotherapy for hemorrhoids utilizes a flexible endoscope to inject 23.4% saline through a sclerotherapy needle into the hemorrhoidal cushion. In a small preliminary series of patients with grade I, II, or III hemorrhoids, success rates were similar to those seen with other, more conventional therapies.[18]

Cryosurgery

Special cryoprobes activated by liquid nitrogen, carbon dioxide, or nitrous oxide have been developed. When the cryoprobe is applied to a hemorrhoidal cushion, local tissue destruction is caused by freezing and subsequent necrosis. All symptomatic hemorrhoids are treated in one session. If deep freezing of the submucosal hemorrhoidal cushions does not occur, symptoms persist. Tissue damage is uncontrolled, and wound healing is accompanied by prolonged anal drainage, late bleeding, and pain.[19] Healing may not be complete for 6 to 8 weeks. Severe septic complications such as fatal meningitis have been reported.[20] Compared with rubber band ligation, patient satisfaction is less and local complications more frequent with the cryosurgical technique.[21,22]

Electrocoagulation

Electrosurgical units have been adapted for use in the outpatient therapy of internal hemorrhoids. Electrocoagulation works by inducing submucosal fibrosis.[23] Application of destructive direct electrical current is less precise than with band ligation or formal hemorrhoidectomy. Excess electrical current is grounded through the patient's body, and occasionally discharges occur that cause injury at sites distant from the area of intended tissue destruction. Heat is created around hemorrhoidal tissues, so adequate local anesthesia is required.

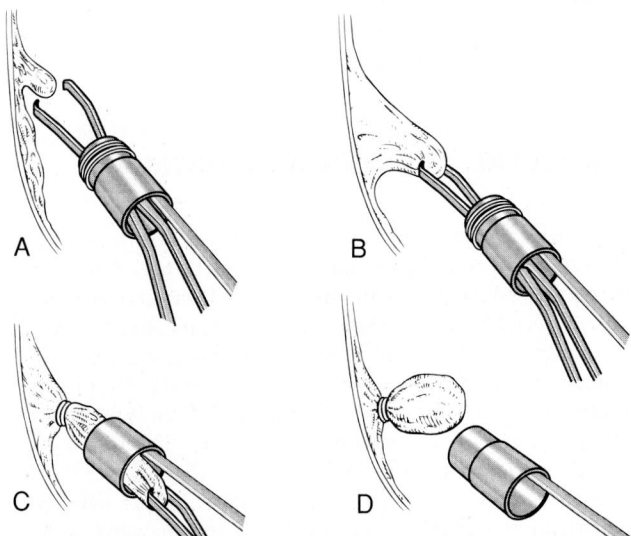

Figure 88-3. Rubber band ligation of an internal hemorrhoid.

Photocoagulation

Both infrared light and lasers have been used to treat symptomatic hemorrhoids.[24] Photocoagulation stimulates fibrosis of the submucosal layer by first causing tissue coagulation and necrosis. The application of infrared light and lasers to coagulate hemorrhoids may be performed in the outpatient setting. Advocates of photocoagulation point to the lack of electrical contact with the patient's body and a more controlled application of destructive force compared with electrofulgeration.[25] Current infrared devices are hand-held and much less expensive than laser devices. Equipment for both forms of photocoagulation is more expensive than equipment for rubber band ligation or injection sclerotherapy. In general, one hemorrhoid cushion is photocoagulated per session, so an average of 3 to 5 sessions is necessary. Results compare favorably with those of rubber band ligation and injection sclerotherapy.[26,27] Laser photocoagulation is gaining in popularity. Using a carbon dioxide laser, 1816 consecutive patients were treated with success rates approaching those of more established therapies.[28]

Hemorrhoidectomy

Surgical hemorrhoidectomy is the treatment of choice for most third-degree hemorrhoids, all fourth-degree hemorrhoids, strangulated hemorrhoids, and hemorrhoids that have persisted despite other forms of therapy. Advantages of the surgical approach include precise removal of all internal and external hemorrhoids, control of bleeding, and rapid wound healing. Disadvantages include the need for regional anesthesia, postoperative pain, risk of postoperative urinary retention, and expenses incurred from both hospitalization and lost time from work.

A number of procedures have been developed, but all incorporate three basic principles: removal of all symptomatic diseased tissue, preservation of wide intervening skin bridges to prevent anal stenosis, and avoidance of damage to the anal sphincter mechanism. Some surgeons advocate primary closure of the entire hemorrhoidectomy wound, but others close the rectal mucosal wound only to the dentate line and leave the anoderm open to allow drainage. Ferguson, using primary closure of the entire wound, reported excellent results 5 years after hemorrhoidectomy in 95% of his patients and a wound infection rate of 0.20%.[29] Similar results should be expected in the hands of any competent surgeon. Even with careful attention to perioperative fluid management, acute urinary retention requiring Foley catheterization may occur in 10% of patients.[19] The incidence of transient bacteremia may approach 8% even in uncomplicated cases.[30]

Ablation of the Internal Anal Sphincter

Two strategies have been exploited to decrease the abnormally high resting anal pressure found in some patients with hemorrhoids. Lord has advocated forceful anal dilatation under general anesthesia. He includes a rigorous protocol of daily anal dilatation for a number of weeks.[31] The procedure has the disadvantage of causing variable and uncontrolled damage to the internal and external anal sphincters with resulting fecal incontinence. Good results occur in 80% of patients, but some of the efficacy of this procedure may reflect submucosal hemorrhage and subsequent scar formation. A more controlled disruption of the internal sphincter is achieved with lateral internal sphincterotomy (see Anal Fissure). In patients with abnormally high resting anal pressures, lateral sphincterotomy achieves results as good as rubber band ligation. In patients with normal resting anal pressures, result are uniformly dismal.[6]

Anorectal Varices

Meticulous histologic study has shown that anorectal varices and hemorrhoids are unrelated.[4] Hemorrhoids have no direct connection to the portal system, and the incidence of hemorrhoids has been shown to be the same in patients with and without portal hypertension.[32,33] The distinction of anorectal varices from external hemorrhoids may be difficult. Often patients with anorectal varices have other known manifestations of portal hypertension such as esophageal varices and ascites. Anorectal varices are usually discrete, serpentine, submucosal veins. In contrast to external hemorrhoids, varices are compressible and refill rapidly. They extend from the squamous portion of the anal canal across the dentate line and into the rectum proper. In a recent prospective study, 43% of cirrhotic patients had anorectal varices.[33] In one series, 5% of patients with bleeding as a manifestation of portal hypertension bled from anorectal varices. Bleeding may occur from either the anal or rectal portion of the varix and can be massive and life-threatening.[34]

The optimal management of anorectal varices is not known. Injection sclerotherapy, cryotherapy, rubber band ligation, and hemorrhoidectomy have all been associated with torrential, occasionally fatal bleeding.[35,36] Treatment by underrunning the variceal columns with absorbable suture achieves primary control in a majority of cases and has a very low rate of morbidity.[34] Rubber band ligation has also been advocated but must be done in a controlled environment with full resuscitation capabilities.[37] Ultimately, portasystemic shunting may be required.

ANORECTAL ABSCESS AND FISTULA

Suppurative anorectal infection can be divided into two categories—anorectal abscess and anorectal fistula. Anorectal abscess may be defined as an undrained collection of perianal pus. Anorectal fistula is an abnormal communication between the anorectal canal and the perianal skin. Abscess is the acute manifestation, and fistula the chronic manifestation, of suppurative anorectal infection. In most cases, the underlying pathophysiology is thought to be the same. The treatment for each is essentially surgical, however the diagnosis and initial management may fall to any physician. Proper management requires a thorough knowledge of the anatomy of the structures of the anorectum to facilitate early diagnosis and appropriate therapy.

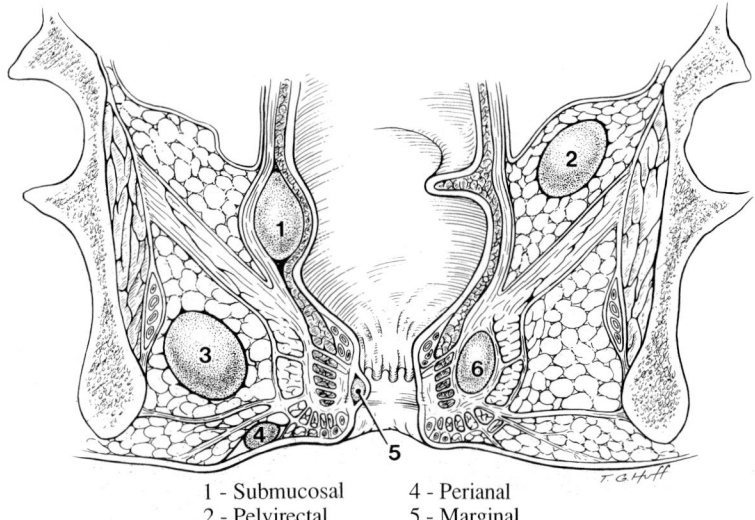

Figure 88-4. Common anatomic locations of ano-rectal abscesses.

1 - Submucosal   4 - Perianal
2 - Pelvirectal   5 - Marginal
3 - Ischiorectal   6 - Intersphincteric

Epidemiology, Etiology, and Differential Diagnosis

In a series of 1023 patients treated with anorectal abscess or fistula, the male to female ratio was 2:1. The age distribution was from 10 to 82 years, with the majority in the third and fourth decades of life. The most common associated medical diseases were hypertension, diabetes, heart disease, and inflammatory bowel disease.[38] The incidence of perirectal infection in patients with acute leukemia is approximately 8%.[39]

Current evidence suggests that infection of the anal glands is the most common cause of anorectal abscess and anorectal fistula. The most common bacterial isolates are *Escherichia coli*, *Enterococcus* species, and *Bacteroides fragilis*.[40] Histologic specimens from patients with anorectal fistula revealed infected anal glands 70% to 90% of the time. Anal glands arise from the anal canal at the level of the crypts of Morgagni. At least half of the glands are observed to penetrate into the intersphincteric space.[41] Obstruction of the anal glands may occur in the presence of trauma, anal eroticism, diarrhea, hard stools, or foreign bodies, with resultant stasis and secondary infection. This cryptoglandular origin of anorectal abscess and fistula is further supported by the fact that the primary internal orifice is found at the level of the dentate line.

Specific diseases may cause anorectal abscess and anorectal fistula in the absence of primary cryptoglandular infection. These include Crohn's disease, anorectal malignancy, tuberculosis, actinomycosis, lymphogranuloma venereum, radiation-induced proctitis, leukemia, and lymphoma. Each of these diseases should be considered during the evaluation of any patient with anorectal abscess or anorectal fistula. Other disease states that may cause a similar clinical picture and should be included in the differential diagnosis of suppurative anorectal conditions are infected presacral epidermal inclusion cysts, hidradenitis suppurativa, diverticulitis, pilonidal disease, and Bartholin's abscesses.

Anatomic Considerations

Anorectal abscesses may be classified by anatomic site of origin and potential pathways of extension (Fig. 88-4). Abscesses that are inferior to the puborectalis and levator ani muscles are classified as low intermuscular abscesses, and those that extend above these muscles are classified as high intermuscular abscesses. Low intermuscular abscesses are subclassified as perianal, submucosal, intersphincteric, or ischiorectal. High intermuscular abscesses are described as pelvirectal, retrorectal, or retrovesical. Proper surgical management is guided by correct anatomic identification of the type of anorectal abscess.

Anorectal fistulas are described based on pathogenesis of the disease (e.g., Crohn's disease, hidradenitis suppurativa) and classified according to the normal muscular anatomy of the pelvic floor. All anorectal fistulas are anatomically divided into one of four groups (Fig. 88-5). The most common type

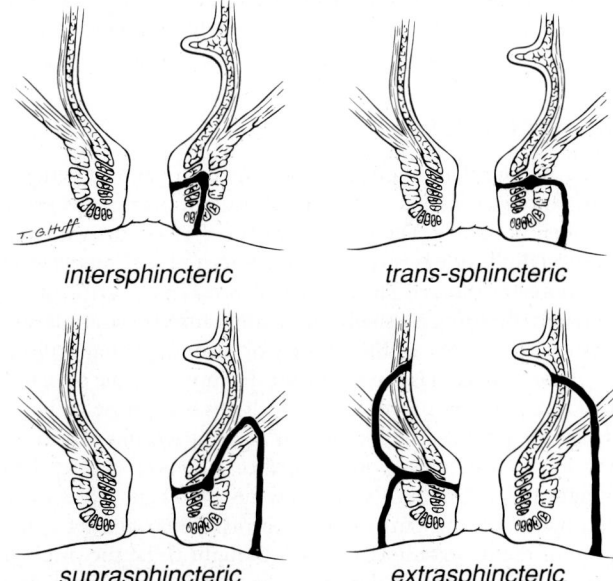

intersphincteric   *trans-sphincteric*

suprasphincteric   *extrasphincteric*

Figure 88-5. Anatomic classification of anorectal fistulas.

of anorectal fistula is the intersphincteric fistula, in which the fistula ramifies only in the areolar tissue between the internal and external anal sphincters. Transphincteric fistulas pass from the intersphincteric plane through the external sphincter and into the ischiorectal fossa. Suprasphincteric fistulas pass upward in the intersphincteric plane, over the puborectalis muscle, and into the ischiorectal fossa. Extrasphincteric fistulas pass from the perianal skin through the ischiorectal fat and levator muscles into the rectum. Division of the entire tract of either suprasphincteric or extrasphincteric fistulas results in total division of the muscles of continence.[42] Intraanal ultrasound has emerged as a modality useful in determining the position of an anorectal abscess or fistula relative to the anal sphincter complex.[43]

Clinical Manifestations

Anorectal Abscess

Acute pain and swelling are the most common complaints in the patient with anorectal abscess. Pain may occur in the absence of swelling, especially with small intersphincteric or pelvirectal abscesses. Pain is exacerbated by sitting or movement, and defecation may be actively avoided because of discomfort. Antecedent history may reveal a bout of constipation, diarrhea, or minor trauma. Constitutional symptoms include malaise and fever. The presence of foul-smelling drainage means that the abscess has necessitated, or is discharging through the primary anal orifice. Bleeding is not a primary symptom and, if present, is usually caused by an associated fissure.

Inspection of the perineum of a patient with perirectal abscess reveals the cardinal signs of inflammation: redness, heat, swelling, and tenderness. Drainage may be observed from the infected crypt orifice. An intersphincteric abscess may manifest only as localized tenderness. Rectal examination is often difficult because of pain, so evaluation under anesthesia is indicated if a complete examination is otherwise impossible. Delay in making the diagnosis of anorectal abscess leads to extension of the infection into previously uninfected spaces and also increases the subsequent risk of overwhelming sepsis.

Anorectal Fistula

Chronic, purulent drainage is the chief complaint of patients with anorectal fistula. A history of prior anorectal abscess is frequently elicited. Discomfort or pain often occurs with defecation but is not as severe as that associated with anal fissure or anorectal abscess. The perianal skin may be pruritic or excoriated. Bleeding is usually minor and caused by granulation tissue at the orifice of the primary or secondary anal orifice.

Anorectal fistulas can usually be diagnosed by the presence of a red, granular papule from which pus is expressed. Goodsall's rule predicts the location of a primary orifice based on the location of the secondary orifice; however, recent data suggests that Goodsall's rule may not be as useful as once thought.[44] The primary orifice is the fistulous opening at the level of the dentate line, which is thought to be the original site of the infected anal gland. The secondary orifice is the fistulous opening anywhere else on the perineum. Multiple

secondary openings should alert one to the possibility of either Crohn's disease or hidradenitis suppurativa. It is often possible to palpate a fistulous tract as a firm cord just beneath the perianal skin. Attempts to pass metal probes are best made in the operating room. Anoscopy and sigmoidoscopy are performed to identify the primary orifice and to determine the presence of proctocolitis.

Patients who are neutropenic as a result of hematologic malignancy are particularly susceptible to serious anorectal infection.[45] Mortality rates from anorectal infection in acute leukemics, if untreated, may be as high as 45% to 78%.[39] Early diagnosis and aggressive surgical drainage may be lifesaving in these individuals, with improvement in mortality rates to below 10%.[39] Point tenderness and poorly demarcated induration are the most frequent findings. Frequent reexamination may allow detection of an abscess if initial findings are equivocal. Because of the profound granulocytopenia, fluctuant masses are not usually seen. Necrosis and tissue breakdown may proceed quite rapidly, with extension into the genitalia and pelvis. If spontaneous drainage has already occurred, pain rapidly subsides and further surgical drainage may be postponed. *Pseudomonas aeruginosa* is a common wound isolate, and appropriate perioperative intravenous antibiotics should be administered if it is found.[46]

Treatment

Because of the risk of extension of pus into adjacent spaces and the potential for the development of necrotizing anorectal infection, the treatment of anorectal abscess is a surgical emergency. In one series, the time interval from onset of primary anorectal abscess to necrotizing anorectal infection was from .5 to 5 days, with a mortality in excess of 50%.[47] One should not temporize waiting for an abscess to point or become ripe, because the risks of necrotizing infection and extension into previously uninfected spaces rise dramatically.

In healthy patients with superficial abscesses in the perineal or ischiorectal location, drainage can be performed in the outpatient setting with local anesthesia. All other abscesses should be drained in the operating room with adequate anesthesia, lighting, and surgical instrumentation. If a primary fistula tract is identified and is not thought to encompass a large proportion of the sphincter mechanism, fistulotomy may be done in selected cases. In general, the patient should be counseled as to the possibility of persistent drainage from a retained or unidentified fistula which may require a second operation.[48] An abscess may also recur if the underlying fistula has not been definitively treated.

Antibiotics are usually not necessary, and they may temporarily mask the underlying suppurative infection and delay surgical therapy. Only in rare cases does a perianal cellulitis resolve with antibiotic therapy alone. In otherwise healthy individuals with minimal infection of the surrounding tissues, incision and drainage of the abscess is all that is required. Patients with significant underlying disease such as diabetes, acute leukemia, valvular heart disease, or extensive soft tissue infection benefit from perioperative antibiotics. The choice of antibiotics should be directed by the clinical situation and culture results but, in general, broad spectrum second- or third-generation cephalosporins are adequate. The most common wound isolates are polymicrobial with *Escherichia coli*, *Proteus vulgaris*, *Bacteroides* species, streptococci, and staphylococci predominating.[49] A high proportion of necrotizing anorectal infections contain *Clostridium* species.[47] Immunosuppressed patients often demonstrate *Pseudomonas aeruginosa*.[39]

Postoperative management consists of frequent wound inspection, warm sitz baths, attention to stool consistency, and judicious analgesia. The wound should be observed to heal from the base up so that skin bridges do not form, allowing the abscess to recur. If persistent drainage occurs, a second operation for fistulotomy is necessary. Warm baths improve hygiene and offer some symptomatic relief. Narcotic analgesics and perirectal pain both predispose to constipation, so a high-fiber diet, bulk-forming agents, or laxatives should be prescribed.

The presence of an anorectal fistula is an indication for operation. The operative approach depends on the location of the fistulous tract in relation to the sphincteric mechanism. Anorectal manometry has been used to improve the clinical and functional results of surgery for fistula in ano.[50] The basic prerequisites for successful therapy of a fistula include removal of the primary orifice, identification and opening of the entire extent of the fistula, and conservation of as much external sphincter as possible. Postoperative care is similar to that for anorectal abscess. Close inspection of the wound is needed to ensure proper healing.

Anorectal disease as a manifestation of Crohn's disease requires special consideration. In addition to standard therapy with 5-aminosalicylate derivatives and immunosuppressives, the use of metronidazole may be beneficial in the healing of perineal Crohn's disease. Unfortunately, the required long-term therapy with metronidazole is associated with several side effects, most notably paresthesias. Also, discontinuation of therapy is often associated with flaring of disease.[51] Conservative surgical techniques are usually adequate to drain abscesses, reduce inflammation, and provide relief of symptoms.[52] In one study, proctectomy—once widely practiced—was necessary in only 12% of patients with complicated perianal Crohn's disease.[53]

RECTAL PROLAPSE

Rectal prolapse is simply protrusion of the rectum through the anal orifice. Complete rectal prolapse or procidentia is the classic situation in which all layers of the rectum visibly descend through the anus. Occult rectal prolapse refers to internal intussusception of rectal tissue without visible protrusion at the anus. Mucosal prolapse is a common condition in which only distal rectal tissues and not the entire rectal circumference protrude through the anus.

Rectal prolapse in children is an uncommon problem usually seen in infancy. It may be idiopathic, associated with congenital defects such as spina bifida or myelomeningocele, or associated with cystic fibrosis. Prolapse occurs with defecation and usually reduces spontaneously. Treatment is conservative, and the condition is often self limited.

Rectal prolapse in adults occurs at least 3 to 10 times more often in women than men and is not associated with multiparity. Men may develop prolapse at any age, but in women, the peak incidence is in the sixth and seventh decades. It is associated with poor tone of the pelvic musculature, chronic straining at stool, fecal incontinence, and, sometimes, neurologic disease or traumatic damage to the pelvis.

Pathogenesis

There are two theories concerning the cause of rectal prolapse. Moschkowitz, in 1912, postulated that rectal prolapse is caused by a sliding hernia in the fascial investments of the pelvic floor.[54] Broden and Snellman suggested, after careful defecography, that the first step in prolapse was intussusception of the rectum several centimeters above the dentate line.[55] Anatomic defects that have been described with rectal prolapse include a weakened endopelvic fascia and diastasis of the levator ani, loss of the normal horizontal rectal position in the sacrum, an abnormally deep pouch of Douglas, a redundant rectosigmoid colon, and a weak anal sphincter.[56] Most authors support the view that prolapse is caused by the intussuscepting rectum and that most of the anatomic defects described occur secondarily. Weakening of the fascial attachments of the rectum to the presacral fascia allows lengthening of the rectosigmoid and its mesentery. The normal positioning of the rectum in the sacral hollow is lost. The subsequent vertical orientation of the rectum enhances the ability of the rectum to intussuscept. Chronic straining in a misguided attempt to evacuate the internally prolapsing rectal tissue only serves to exacerbate the problem. Signs of pelvic neuropathy and anal sphincter dysfunction are common in patients with rectal prolapse. Many patients complain of partial or major fecal incontinence. On manometric evaluation, incontinent patients have low basal and voluntary contraction pressures.[57] Denervation of striated musculature on electromyogram, perineal descent, and absence of the anocutaneous reflex are also common findings. The presence of disturbed sphincter function and pelvic denervation may explain the disappointingly high incidence of persistent incontinence after surgical correction of the prolapse. Manometric findings associated with a higher risk of postoperative fecal incontinence include a resting anal pressure of less than 10 mm Hg and a maximal voluntary contraction pressure of less than 50 mm Hg.[58]

Clinical Manifestations

Patients present complaining of prolapse of tissue with defecation. As the condition progresses, rectal prolapse may occur with straining or even upright posture alone. Common accompanying symptoms include straining at stool, the sensation of incomplete evacuation, tenesmus, and fecal incontinence. Protrusion of the rectum through the anus is a striking clinical sign. Complete rectal prolapse is signaled by the presence of red concentric mucosal folds with a palpable double thickness to the rectal wall tissue. The protruding rectum may extend many centimeters, and usually the lumen tip points slightly posteriorly. The patient is asked to sit and strain to produce prolapse if it is not immediately obvious. Endoscopic or barium examination is performed on all patients with rectal prolapse to exclude tumors and mucosal lesions. Sigmoidoscopy may reveal changes consistent with solitary rectal ulcer.

A voiding defecogram is the best way to identify occult prolapse (internal intussusception).

Complete rectal prolapse must be differentiated from mucosal prolapse, prolapsing internal hemorrhoids, anorectal varices, anal polyps, benign and malignant anorectal tumors, and hypertrophic anal papillae. Mucosal prolapse is characterized by a short segment of mucosa with disordered or radially arranged (not concentric) mucosal folds. Internal hemorrhoids usually have a varicose appearance and are separated into discrete cushions.

Every attempt should be made to manually reduce a persistently prolapsed rectum to avoid potential complications such as strangulation, ulceration, bleeding, and perforation. Manual reduction may be facilitated by some form of intravenous sedation. Placing granulated sugar on the prolapsed mucosa often eliminates edema and allows reduction.[59] Gangrene of the anterior rectal wall, a surgical emergency, is occasionally associated with evisceration of small bowel onto the perineum.

Treatment

Mucosal prolapse may be treated with procedures designed to remove redundant tissue and induce local fibrosis (see discussion of treatment of internal hemorrhoids). There is controversy over the appropriate treatment for occult rectal prolapse. To oversimplify, occult prolapse may be best treated surgically if fecal incontinence or chronic solitary rectal ulcer is present and conservatively if defecation difficulties or lesser symptoms predominate.[60]

To avoid complications and ongoing damage to the pelvic floor and sphincter muscles, complete rectal prolapse should be surgically corrected. Perineal muscle exercises and buttock strapping offer palliation in the patient who refuses or is unable to undergo surgery. There are many surgical options advocated for the treatment of rectal prolapse, but they can be simply summarized as follows. Management in healthy patients involves replacement of the rectum into the sacral hollow with or without resection of redundant rectosigmoid colon. The two intraabdominal operations that have been popularized in the United States are the anterior sling rectopexy (Ripstein procedure) and abdominal proctopexy with or without sigmoid resection.

Ripstein's operation involves mobilization of the rectum to the tip of the coccyx and attachment of the rectum to the presacral fascia by means of a band of nonabsorbable plastic such as Teflon or Marlex mesh. The incidence of recurrence in a large number of patients was approximately 2%, but the perioperative morbidity rate was 17%.[37] Abdominal proctopexy as a sole procedure can be performed with very acceptable recurrence rates and function. Constipation is common in patients who are continent, and continence is not assured in others. Anal manometry is helpful in predicting continence.[61] A laparoscopic approach has been used to further decrease operative morbidity.[62]

Abdominal proctopexy and sigmoid resection as a combined procedure eliminates two of the theorized causes of rectal prolapse by fixing the rectum directly to the sacral hollow by means of nonabsorbable sutures and removing the redundant sigmoid colon. Prosthetic materials such as Marlex are generally not placed in the peritoneal cavity if sigmoid resection is performed because of the risk of contamination of the mesh and resultant sepsis. In a series of 102 patients with abdominal proctopexy and sigmoid resection, 80% had good to excellent results, no mortality, and improved morbidity, compared with those treated with Ripstein's procedure.[63] Abdominal proctopexy and sigmoid resection is physiologically the most demanding procedure and should be used only in patients in good general physical condition. These procedures have continued fecal incontinence as the major postoperative complaint. Anorectal manometry may preoperatively predict those patients at risk for this troubling complication. Patients who continue to have incontinence 6 to 12 months after definitive correction of the rectal prolapse often benefit from a Parks' postanal repair or a plication sphincteroplasty.[64,65]

In the elderly or debilitated patient, a perineal or extraabdominal approach is associated with acceptable morbidity and mortality rates. Encirclement of the anus with a steel wire (Thiersch's operation) cannot be recommended. An elegant study of perineal rectosigmoidectomy for complete prolapse in 114 elderly patients demonstrated a recurrence rate of 10% with no mortality and good functional results.[66] A diverting colostomy may be also be an appropriate alternative for this group of high-risk patients.

ANAL FISSURE

Anal fissure is a painful linear ulcer in the anal canal. Primary anal fissures are usually found in young and middle-aged adults and occur equally in males and females. Primary fissures are located in the posterior midline more than 90% of the time. The remainder are found in the anterior midline. Fissures may occur secondary to an underlying disease such as inflammatory bowel disease (especially Crohn's disease), proctitis, leukemia, carcinoma, and, rarely, syphilis or tuberculosis. These lesions, in contrast to primary fissures, are usually found in a more lateral position.

Etiology

The elliptical arrangement of the anal sphincter fibers offers less muscular support to the anal canal posteriorly. This deficient support predisposes the posterior anal canal to traumatic tears during passage of a large, hard stool. Fissures may become chronic because of high resting anal sphincter tone and repeated trauma during passage of fecal boluses. Rectal distention normally causes a transient internal anal sphincter relaxation. Patients with anal fissure have an abnormal overshoot contraction following the normal relaxation. The overshoot contraction may explain the reflex spasm and pain seen after defecation. This phenomenon disappears after successful treatment of the fissure.[67] Preoperative maximal resting pressure and maximal contraction pressure are also elevated in patients with fissure.[68,69] A recent histopathologic study documented the presence of fibrosis throughout the anal sphincter in patients with anal fissure.[70]

Clinical Manifestations

Severe pain associated with scant, bright red rectal bleeding is the hallmark of anal fissure. The pain occurs during and after defecation and usually seems out of proportion to the clinical findings. Severe pain usually makes anoscopy impossible, and even digital examination is difficult without topical anesthesia. The fissure is best identified by simple inspection after spreading the buttocks. Acute fissures are small, linear tears oriented perpendicular to the dentate line in the posterior midline. Fissures located in a lateral position should prompt a search for a secondary etiology. If an acute anal fissure does not heal promptly, certain characteristic secondary features develop. The classic triad of chronic anal fissure includes the fissure, a proximal hypertrophic papilla, and a sentinel pile or fibrotic nubbin of skin found at the anal verge (Fig. 88-6).

Treatment

Stools should be softened by prescribing a high-fiber diet and adequate fluid intake. Hydrophilic bulk agents or salts of dioctyl sulfosuccinate are important aspects of therapy because many fissures are precipitated by the traumatic passage of hard, dry stools. The temporary use of topical anesthetic preparations containing agents such as benzocaine or pramoxine hydrochloride provides symptomatic relief. The use of these medications, in addition to warm sitz baths 2 to 3 times daily, acts to decrease sphincter spasm to provide additional relief. With such a conservative regimen, most acute fissures heal in 4 to 6 weeks. Occasionally, patient anxiety, severe pain, or other considerations may mitigate against such a prolonged trial of conservative therapy.

Chronic fissure usually requires some form of surgical therapy to reduce internal sphincter tone. Reduced sphincter tone permits easier passage of the fecal bolus through the anal canal. Repetitive injury is avoided so that the traumatic tear may finally heal. Lateral subcutaneous internal anal sphincterotomy best accomplishes this goal. The beneficial effects of sphincterotomy on internal sphincter spasm and healing

of anal fissure have been well documented, and surgical cure rates on the order of 95% can be expected.[67] Midline sphincterotomy with fissurectomy also offers definitive therapy for chronic anal fissure. However, in a retrospective study of 300 patients, a higher rate of postoperative complications was seen compared with the lateral sphincterotomy.[71] Also, an unfortunate complication of posterior midline sphincterotomy and fissurectomy is development of a residual keyhole deformity of the anus, which predisposes to long-term leakage of feces and mucus. Another approach to treating sphincter spasm is manual dilatation. The anus is dilated to six fingers under regional anesthesia. Manual dilatation has been shown to produce as high a rate of healing as lateral subcutaneous internal anal sphincterotomy, but because this procedure is not as controlled as sphincterotomy, the risks of incontinence or fissure recurrence have lessened the popularity of manual dilatation.[72]

ANAL STENOSIS

Anal stenosis is an abnormal narrowing of the anal canal associated with a variety of underlying diseases. Patients may complain of narrow stools, painful or resistant defecation, and bleeding from recurrent anal tears. Malignant causes of anal stenosis include anal and rectal cancer and, less commonly, transmural invasion of the anorectum by a urogenital malignancy. Common causes of benign anal stenosis are prior rectal surgery, trauma, and inflammatory bowel disease. Postsurgical stenosis of the anal canal is most often a result of injudicious excision of anal skin during hemorrhoidectomy.[73] Laxative abuse and chronic diarrhea are also associated with anal stenosis, because lack of a solid fecal bolus to intermittently dilate the anus causes hypertrophy and narrowing of the anal sphincters.[74] Other causes of anal stenosis include radiation injury, lymphogranuloma venereum, and congenital abnormalities.

Treatment is based on the severity and location of the anal stenosis. Mild strictures respond to periodic dilatation and a high-fiber diet. Severe stenosis usually requires some form of anoplasty to increase the amount of perianal skin.[75] Lateral internal sphincterotomy is often used in conjunction with anoplasty.[37] Cure rates in excess of 90% are usually seen.[73]

SOLITARY RECTAL ULCER

Solitary rectal ulcer is a chronic benign disorder related to abnormal defecation. The usual presenting symptoms are the passage of mucus and blood, altered bowel habits, anorectal pain, a feeling of incomplete evacuation, and straining at defecation. Classically at sigmoidoscopy, a shallow, discrete, 1-cm punched-out ulcer with a hyperemic margin is seen 7 to 10 cm from the anal verge on the anterior wall. However, ulcers range from 0.5 to 4 cm in diameter, are located from a few centimeters to 13 cm from the anus, and are occasionally found on the posterior wall. Furthermore, there may be multiple ulcers or no ulcer at all. Sometimes only a localized erythematous or nodular area of mucosa is noted. Characteristic histologic changes seen on biopsies taken from abnormal mucosa or ulcer margins include fibrous obliteration of the

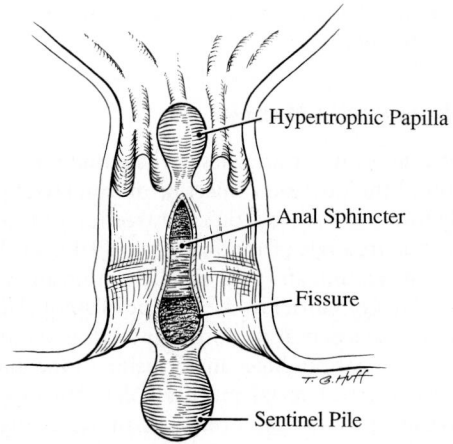

Figure 88-6. The classic triad of chronic anal fissure: hypertrophic papilla, anal fissure, and sentinel pile.

lamina propria, disorientation and thickening of the muscularis mucosa, and regenerative changes in the crypt epithelium.[76]

Pathogenesis

The pathogenesis of solitary rectal ulcer is related to prolonged straining at stool and difficulty initiating defecation. Digital evacuation is frequently practiced in these patients, but trauma caused by self-digitation is not the source of mucosal ulceration.[77] Although clinically apparent rectal prolapse through the anal orifice is only occasionally seen with solitary rectal ulcer, careful observation during sigmoidoscopy or defecography demonstrates subtle forms of mucosal prolapse during defecation in 90% of these patients.[77,78] Womack and colleagues have shown that rectal prolapse coupled with high transmural pressures during defecation is probably responsible for the mucosal trauma that causes ulceration.[78] The anterior wall mucosa 7 to 10 cm proximal to the anal margin is often the first and largest part of the intussusceptum as it descends downward into the anal canal. This corresponds to the usual location of ulceration seen clinically.

Treatment

Complications of massive bleeding, rectal stricture, and even ulcer penetration into the prostate gland have been reported but are so rare that the patient should be reassured as to the benignity of the syndrome.[79,80] Because solitary rectal ulcer is caused by repeated mechanical trauma of the prolapsing mucosa during defecation, it is appropriate to begin treatment by eliminating straining and improving bowel habits. Beneficial results should not be expected for many months, and relapses are common.[77,81] Sulfasalazine, antibiotics, and enemas of steroids or 5-aminosalicylic acid are of no use, but sucralfate retention enemas may be beneficial.[82] Symptoms refractory to conservative management may respond to surgical rectopexy (see Chap. 86).[83,84]

FECAL INCONTINENCE

Fecal incontinence is the release of rectal contents against one's wishes. It is perhaps the most embarrassing and socially disabling of all gastrointestinal problems. Prevalence rates vary, but it is clear that women, the elderly, and institutionalized persons are particularly victimized. A community-based survey of elderly women identified occasional fecal incontinence in up to 18%, the incidence rising with age.[85] More than 16% of elderly persons living in residential homes are incontinent of stool at least twice a month, and 10% are incontinent on at least a weekly basis.[86,87] The complaint of fecal incontinence is not readily volunteered because of the social stigma attached to it. Of patients presenting with complaints of diarrhea who admit to fecal incontinence on direct questioning, fewer than 50% had freely volunteered the symptom of incontinence.[88,89] Clinically, incontinence must be placed in the context of surrounding circumstances. The frequency and severity of fecal soiling in an individual with incontinence associated with urgency may simply reflect availability of a toilet. Fecal soiling in a severely mentally disabled or demented person might relate directly to a communication or recognition problem. A high prevalence of dementia in the elderly residential home population with fecal incontinence previously alluded to underscores this point.[86]

Pathophysiology

The pathophysiology of fecal incontinence must be considered in the context of normal anorectal physiology. The mechanisms of anal continence are surprising complex and poorly understood but can be simply summarized as follows.

The Anal Canal and Sphincters

The anal canal is 3 to 4 cm long and represents the distal outlet of the gut. It normally remains closed as an anteroposterior slit by tonic contractions of the surrounding musculature. Spongy vascular tissues within the canal are distensible and play a minor, fine-tuning role in fecal continence by assisting with anal closure. Minor degrees of seepage after hemorrhoidectomy may be caused by partial excision of this tissue. The circular smooth muscle layer of the rectum terminates in the thickened, rounded internal sphincter muscle. The internal sphincter is under autonomic control and is responsible for the majority of resting anal canal tone. The external sphincter is a surrounding sleeve of striated muscle that blends into the puborectalis and levator ani muscles proximally and extends to just below the internal sphincter margin distally. It is a voluntary muscle with somatic innervation from the pudendal nerve (sacral branches S2, S3, and S4). Although it is a striated muscle, the external sphincter maintains a degree of tonic neural activation and so contributes to resting anal tone (approximately 30%). However, it assumes a major role in maintaining continence by contracting in a reflex manner during times of sudden rectal distention or increased abdominal pressure (i.e., coughing, lifting). Voluntary contraction of the external sphincter approximately doubles the normal resting tone of the anal canal. Traumatic obstetric and surgical injuries, prolapsing rectal and hemorrhoidal tissues, and various neuropathic diseases are examples of processes involving the anal canal and sphincters that may cause incontinence.

The Puborectalis Muscle

The puborectalis muscle attaches to the symphysis pubis and wraps around the posterior aspect of the anorectal junction effectively forming a sling. Tonic contraction of this muscle produces an acute angle of approximately 80 degrees between the axes of the rectum and anal canal, forming an important mechanical kink or barrier to the passage of stool. The action of the puborectalis may also contribute to an as yet unproven flap-valve effect that produces an occlusion of the upper anal canal by the anterior rectal mucosa.[90] Sudden increases in intraabdominal pressure accentuate the anorectal angle to reduce transmission of pressure into the anal canal so that, in concert with the external sphincter, continence is maintained. The anorectal angle formed by the puborectalis muscle is arguably the most important structure in the preservation of gross fecal continence.[91-93] Any traumatic or neuropathic injury to this muscle causing persistent straightening of the anorectal angle leads to major fecal incontinence.

Anal Sensation

Although the rectum itself is sensitive only to stretch, the anal canal epithelium is endowed with a rich network of nerve endings sensitive to touch, pain, and temperature. Together, these sensory inputs make up an important part of so-called anal sampling, which allows differentiation between solid, liquid, and gas contents in the rectum. After material enters and distends the rectum, a transient reflex relaxation of the internal sphincter occurs (the rectoanal inhibitory reflex) to permit the rectal contents to come into contact with the sensitive anal canal mucosa. Using tactile and perhaps thermal properties, anal sampling differentiates flatus from solid or liquid stool to allow selective passage of these materials.[94] Simultaneously, the external sphincter reflexly contracts to maintain continence until voluntary contractions consciously take over. Within a short time, rectal accommodation to the new volume deactivates stretch receptors, and the sensation of urgency dissipates.

The Rectum

The motility, compliance, and sensation of the rectum are important features of fecal continence. Baseline rectal contractions are of higher frequency and amplitude than are those in the sigmoid colon. This reverse peristalsis acts as a subtle barrier to fecal flow. The rectum has the ability to accommodate different fecal volumes presented to it. This reservoir function maintains continence and allows for appropriate timing of defecation. In a similar manner, the sampling reflex and a normal call to stool depend on intact rectal sensation. Neuropathies caused by diabetes and other diseases impair rectal sensation and therefore interfere with continence.[95] Poor distensibility of the rectum in ulcerative colitis, radiation proctitis, and chronic rectal ischemia may lead to fecal urgency and incontinence.[96] Similar symptoms in those with irritable bowel syndrome are probably caused by hypersensitivity to distention and abnormal motility patterns in the rectum.

Stool Volume and Consistency

Nearly everyone has experienced fecal urgency and perhaps incontinence during an acute diarrheal illness. Large volumes of liquid stool pose a special challenge to even healthy mechanisms of continence. Some persons are incontinent of stool only if stressed with a liquid bolus; others are continent of stool but cannot retain flatus. Any disease that causes diarrhea, especially if it is associated with large volumes and rapid transit, may produce fecal incontinence.

Defecation

The process of normal defecation depends on intact mechanisms of continence. The sequence of events leading to defecation is initiated when material from the sigmoid colon enters the rectum. Rectal distention causes reflex relaxation of the internal anal sphincter, exposing the rectal contents to the anal mucosa so that sampling may occur. External sphincter contraction maintains continence until the rectum can accommodate to the bolus. After feces fills the rectum to a sufficient degree, the urge to defecate is experienced. If a conscious decision to initiate defecation is made, a squatting or sitting position is assumed. This position straightens the anorectal angle in preparation for passage of stool. If the urge is strong and the individual is exerting conscious resistance to passage of stool, simply relaxing voluntary control allows defecation to proceed. Otherwise, a Valsalva maneuver is performed to increase intraabdominal pressure and push the feces toward the anal canal. The pelvic floor descends, the rectum contracts, external sphincter activity is inhibited, and the fecal bolus is expelled out of the rectum. Stool is passed piecemeal with episodic straining or, alternatively, propulsive contractions may empty portions of the left colon in a single motion.

Clinical Manifestations

It is clinically useful to categorize fecal incontinence as either partial or major.[92] Partial incontinence is defined as minor soiling of loose stools and poor control of flatus. The elderly and those with internal sphincter deficiencies and prolapsing hemorrhoidal or rectal tissues are particularly prone to minor soiling. Fecal impaction also predisposes to partial incontinence. A rectum chronically distended with feces continuously induces internal sphincter relaxation, allowing leakage of stool in those with weakened sphincter mechanisms. Major incontinence refers to frequent loss of control of even solid stools. Neurologic diseases, traumatic injuries, and surgical damage to the puborectalis or sphincter muscles may cause major incontinence. A comprehensive list of the causes of fecal incontinence is provided in Table 88-2. Many incontinent patients have no obvious predisposing history of major trauma, anorectal disease, or neurologic disease. Careful studies using electromyography and other neurophysiologic techniques have identified striated muscle denervation damage in most of these patients with idiopathic incontinence.[97,98] Perineal descent associated with chronic straining at stool may cause stretch injury and subsequent denervation of the pudendal nerve.[99-101] Pudendal nerve injury also occurs during vaginal delivery of childbirth. Risk factors for persistent denervation are multiparity, high birth weight, forceps delivery, and third-degree perineal tears.[102] It is not surprising that more than one mechanism of continence may be disturbed in those with neuropathic incontinence.[103] Careful testing has found that motor neuropathy of the external sphincter and pelvic floor is associated with damage to the internal sphincter and a sensory deficit of the anal canal.[104,105]

An important cause of fecal incontinence not associated with pathology of the pelvic nerves or sphincter muscles is irritable bowel syndrome. The incontinence of irritable bowel syndrome commonly occurs in those with diarrhea-predominant symptoms associated with fecal urgency and cramping relieved by defecation. Physiologic or emotional stressors lead to rapid delivery of loose stools and flatus into a hypersensitive rectum. This produces occasional soiling even in the individual with an intact sphincter mechanism.

<table>
<tr><td colspan="1">

TABLE 88-2
Causes of Fecal Incontinence

</td></tr>
</table>

Diarrhea
Fecal impaction
Irritable bowel syndrome
Anal pathology
    Anal carcinoma
    Congenital abnormalities
    Protruding internal hemorrhoids
    Rectal prolapse
    Perianal infections
    Fistula
    Injury
        Surgical (e.g., hemorrhoidectomy, fistulotomy)
        Obstetrical
        Accidental trauma
Rectal pathology
    Rectal carcinoma
    Rectal ischemia
    Proctitis
        Inflammatory bowel disease
        Radiation induced
        Infectious
Neurologic diseases
    Central nervous system
        Stroke, dementia
        Toxic or metabolic disorders
        Cord injury, tumors
        Multiple sclerosis, tabes dorsalis
    Peripheral nervous system
        Diabetes, others
        Cauda equina lesions
    Idiopathic (primary neurogenic)
        Childbirth injury
        Chronic constipation
        Descending perineum
        Old age

Clinical Evaluation

After the existence of incontinence has been established, the clinical evaluation begins with an assessment as to the frequency, severity, and circumstances surrounding the incontinent episodes. Does the patient suffer from partial or major incontinence? How acute are the symptoms? Are the episodes associated with urgency, or is there no prior warning? Does incontinence occur on a background of constipation or diarrhea? Does the patient require assistance to reach the toilet? After incontinence has been characterized, detailed questions concerning childbirth, prior anorectal surgery, rectal prolapse, hemorrhoids, and straining at stool should be addressed. A history of central or peripheral nervous system diseases, diabetes mellitus, prior pelvic irradiation, or diarrheal disease should be elicited. Perianal inspection and digital examination provide clues to the cause of incontinence. Anal deformities, tumors, perianal infections, fistulas, and prolapsing hemorrhoids may be visually apparent. Absence of the anal wink (contraction of the subcutaneous portion of the external sphincter) in response to a perineal pin stroke suggests a neuropathic process. Digital examination allows a crude assessment of anal resting and voluntary squeeze tone. A rough

estimate of the anorectal angle and puborectalis function can be made by palpation of this muscle in the posterior midline at the proximal edge of the external sphincter during rest and voluntary squeeze. The presence of fecal impaction, rectal prolapse, and perineal descent can also be determined.

Clinical Testing

Several tools are available to evaluate the mechanisms of continence. The extent of investigation depends on local expertise and the patient's clinical presentation.

Anoscopy and sigmoidoscopy. Inspection of the distal colon is a minimum requirement in the evaluation of incontinence. Discovery of tumors or mucosal inflammation (infectious, ulcerative, ischemic, or radiation proctitis) directs treatment and probably eliminates the need for further evaluation.

Manometry. Sphincter function is determined by measuring resting and maximal squeeze pressures of the anal canal using balloons, miniaturized transducers, or perfused catheters. Rectal balloon inflation is performed to measure the reflex relaxation of the internal sphincter and contraction of the external sphincter muscles. Sophisticated techniques can determine spatial sphincter defects by cross-sectional mapping of the whole sphincter.[106]

Tests of rectal compliance and sensation. Estimates of rectal sensation are made by inflating a balloon in the rectum and measuring various subjective thresholds such as first volume sensed, volume producing urgency, maximum tolerated volume, and the delay in sensation.[107,108] Rectal compliance is determined by obtaining concurrent balloon volume and pressure measurements so that pressure-volume curves can be generated.

Neurophysiologic tests. External sphincter and puborectalis muscle activity can be measured using conventional concentric needle EMG or more sophisticated single-fiber EMG. These techniques measure muscular denervation and reinnervation characteristic of neuropathy and allow sphincter mapping but require considerable expertise and are uncomfortable for the patient. New research techniques can more directly characterize nerve dysfunction by measuring pudendal nerve terminal motor latencies and pudendal evoked potentials.[98,109]

Anorectal ultrasonography. Anal endosonography offers an exciting new way to image the anorectal angle and sphincter musculature with high resolution.[110–112] Muscle thickness and defects in both the internal and external sphincter can be mapped in patients with traumatic or idiopathic incontinence without radiation or the discomfort of EMG needle electrodes.

Anal sensory tests. Miniature probes can now measure thermal and electrical sensitivity of the anal canal.[94,113] Information from these novel tools may offer insights into the anal sampling reflex and anal sensory abnormalities identified in incontinent patients.[114]

Defecography. Defecography radiographically evaluates defecation by video fluoroscopic imaging during actual voiding of a simulated barium stool.[115] It is well tolerated and easy to perform. Static and dynamic measurements of the anorectal angle, pelvic floor, and puborectalis function are made during rest, squeeze, and attempted defecation. Pathology best recognized during defecation, such as perineal descent, rectal prolapse, enterocele, and rectocele, can be diagnosed, although symptoms may not correlate well with these defects.[116]

Continence testing. Several tests have been devised to challenge the integrated mechanisms of continence. These tests quantitate continence by measuring leakage of rectally infused saline or resistance to passage of a solid object.[89,117] They offer only an approximation of the clinical symptom and cannot tease out specific pathologies. However, continence tests standardize the measurement of incontinence and require no expensive equipment or particular expertise. They may be useful for comparing groups of patients or assessing an individual's response to therapy over time.

The strategy employed to evaluate fecal incontinence depends on the patient's clinical presentation, the availability of investigative tools, and the likelihood of altering future therapy. Soiling associated with an acute diarrheal illness probably requires no specific anorectal evaluation other than evaluation of the diarrhea itself. In a similar vein, the discovery of ulcerative proctitis by proctosigmoidoscopy requires no further anorectal studies, and treatment may be instituted immediately. For the majority of cases which are less clear-cut, anorectal manometry, combined with a balloon inflation estimate of rectal sensation, is an important basic diagnostic study. It also allows for future treatment in the form of anal biofeedback if necessary. Defecography is a useful adjunctive tool to dynamically assess function from a structural viewpoint. Neurophysiologic, anal sensory, and rectal compliance tests offer less clinically useful information and are primarily limited to certain investigative centers.

Treatment

Fecal incontinence often responds well to a combination of relatively simple interventions. Therapy is at least partially dependent on the underlying cause. As a first priority, diarrheal stools, if present, must be treated. Solid stools are much easier to retain than liquid stools, so this simple measure alone may eliminate all symptoms. If possible, the underlying cause of diarrhea should be corrected, but, if not, empiric therapy with fiber agents or antidiarrheals is appropriate. Loperamide and diphenoxylate are effective in producing solid stools and reducing stool frequency in those with chronic diarrhea and incontinence.[118,119] However, loperamide does this more effectively than diphenoxylate and also appears to improve continence to a standard saline load test.[119,120] Seepage of liquid stools around a fecal impaction should, of course, not be treated as diarrheal stools. Instead, the impaction must be cleared with enemas and a treatment plan for constipation instituted. Incontinent debilitated patients or those with nervous system injuries usually respond best to a bowel program of regular defecation. Such a program should take advantage of the gastrocolonic response and judiciously utilize constipating agents or enemas and suppositories as appropriate.

Fiber is useful for the frequent, low-volume, loose stools of irritable bowel syndrome but may need to be restricted for diseases with poor rectal reservoir capacity in order to decrease fecal volume. Anticholinergics should be tried to blunt the gastrocolonic response in irritable bowel syndrome patients with urgency-associated incontinence after meals. Practice of sphincter exercises several times daily to improve both the tone and the awareness of the pelvic diaphragm and sphincter muscle is a useful adjunct to treatment in the incontinent patient.

If incontinence persists despite the measures outlined and the patient is motivated, sensitive to rectal distention, and able to contract the external sphincter, anal biofeedback should be attempted.[95,121,122] This technique applies simple operant conditioning to the anal sphincter. A manometric catheter with an inflatable rectal balloon is introduced into the anorectum. A visual recording of sphincter contractions provides the biofeedback. The patient learns to associate external sphincter contraction with the appropriate visual recording by repetition and trial and error. Next, sphincter contraction in response to a perceived rectal balloon distention is taught. Finally, patients learn to contract their sphincter in response to balloon distention without the visual cues. Similar techniques can be used to gradually lower sensory thresholds to rectal distention in those with impaired rectal sensation caused by diabetes or other neuropathies.[95,107] A report of biofeedback using a simple anal plug to record external sphincter contractions argues against the need for a rectal balloon, although a recent controlled trial suggests that enhancement of rectal sensitivity is important.[123,124] Uncontrolled studies have documented an approximate 70% success rate using biofeedback therapy (defined as complete restoration of continence or at least a 75% to 90% decrease in frequency of incontinent episodes), with a follow-up period of many months.[121-123] However, a small controlled study was unable to document symptomatic or physiologic benefit using biofeedback.[125] Conditions that may predict a poor response to biofeedback therapy include severe organic lesions causing diminished rectal sensation, irritable bowel syndrome, anterior resection of the rectum, and the surgical keyhole deformity of the anal canal caused by previous surgical division of the sphincter muscle posteriorly.[121-123]

Patients with major fecal incontinence unresponsive to medical management are the most appropriate candidates for surgery. Surgical correction of rectal prolapse or third-degree hemorrhoids should be performed to improve the fecal soiling associated with these conditions. Several operations have been advocated for intractable symptoms.[126] Incontinence caused by trauma, anal surgery, or obstetric injury may respond to simple external anal sphincter repair.[127] Postanal repair (posterior proctopexy) is the procedure of choice for complex sphincter injuries or for neuropathic damage to the pelvic floor (often idiopathic) and loss of the normal anorectal angle.[92,65] More than two thirds of patients can expect good results, although reduction of the anorectal angle cannot be demonstrated.[93,128] Women with anterior sphincter defects often benefit from an anterior reefing procedure.[126] Gracilis muscle transposition (gracloplasty) is a technically demanding procedure that may benefit patients with a destroyed sphincter or congenitally poor pelvic floor development.[129] The addition of an implantable device to electrically stimulate the neoanal sphincter may offer additional benefit.[130,131] Placement of an artificial sling may be considered for those with nonreconstructable sphincters or a primary neurogenic cause for incontinence.[132] This merely offers a static mechanical barrier to fecal flow without voluntary control. Complications requiring sling removal are not unusual. Finally, as a last resort, placement of a colostomy should be considered. Substituting management of a stoma for unremitting fecal incontinence may significantly improve the quality of life for selected patients.

PRURITUS ANI

Pruritus ani is an annoying itchy sensation of the anus and perianal skin. It may be temporary or chronic, unrelenting, and difficult to treat. Pruritus is often associated with burning and soreness. Periods of intense itching vary in frequency but are characteristically most disturbing at night after daytime distractions are removed. It affects 1% to 5% of the population with a male to female predominance of 4:1.[133]

Etiology

Pruritus ani may occur as a symptom of a specific disease affecting the perianal skin or, more commonly, as an idiopathic condition possibly related to residual fecal material (Table 88-3). A number of anorectal diseases, including fissures, fistulas, and hemorrhoids, produce pruritus ani because of fecal soiling and contamination of the perianal region. These lesions make local hygiene especially difficult, and irritated, macerated skin may develop. Pruritus, discomfort, and mucus drainage are more common in hemorrhoid sufferers than in a control population and often resolve with treatment of the hemorrhoids.[134] Anal malignancies, including Bowen's disease, epidermoid cancers, and extramammary Paget's disease, may rarely present as pruritus ani and should not be discounted without careful anal inspection, even if symptoms have existed for years.[135]

Candida albicans and dermatophyte infections appear as characteristic localized erythematous rashes but may also be cultured from the perianal area even if skin lesions are not present. *Candida albicans* is more likely to be identified if random cultures are obtained, but dermatophyte infections, if present, are more likely to be associated with pruritus ani.[136] Pinworm (*Enterobius vermicularis*) causes pruritus ani that is characteristically nocturnal. Children are most commonly affected, but adults, especially those exposed to children, may occasionally become infected. The diagnosis is best made by detecting the eggs on adhesive cellophane tape applied to the perianal skin early in the morning. Scabies (*Sarcoptes scabiei*) and pubic lice (*Phthirus pubis*) can cause pruritus ani. Itching in the genital region and identification of organisms or eggs on pubic hair lead to the proper diagnosis.

Perianal bacterial infections have been implicated in pruritus ani. Separate reports have identified *Staphylococcus aureus* and erythrasma (*Corynebacterium minutissimum*) as pathogens in pruritus ani patients.[137,138] However, a controlled study has failed to provide a bacteriologic basis for this condition.[139] A number of sexually transmitted diseases have been associated

TABLE 88-3
Causes of Pruritus Ani

Anorectal Diseases and Fecal Contamination
Diarrhea
Anal incontinence
Hemorrhoids
Fissures
Fistulae
Rectal prolapse
Malignancy: Bowen's disease, epidermoid cancer, perianal Paget's disease

Infections
Fungal: candidiasis, dermatophytes
Parasitic: pinworms, scabies
Bacterial: *Staphylococcus aureus*, erythrasma
Venereal: herpes, gonococcal, syphilis, condyloma acuminatum

Local Irritants
Moisture, obesity, excessive perspiration
Soaps, hygiene products
Toilet paper: perfumed, dyed
Underwear: irritating fabrics, detergents
Anal creams, suppositories
Dietary: coffee, beer, acidic foods
Drugs: mineral oil, ascorbic acid, hydrocrotisone sodium succinate, quinidine, colchicine

Dermatologic Diseases
Psoriasis
Atopic dermatitis
Seborrheic dermatitis

Adapted from Hanno R, Murphy P. Pruritus ani: classification and management. Dermatol Clin 1987;5:81.

with pruritus ani. These include herpes simplex, gonorrhea, syphilis, condyloma acuminatum, and molluscum contagiosum.[133] Dermatologic conditions such as psoriasis that cause pruritus ani are usually apparent because of the presence of other generalized skin changes.

A variety of local irritants, allergens, and chemicals that contact the perianal skin may cause pruritus. Perfumes and dyes present in toilet paper and soaps, personal hygiene products, irritating fabrics, laundry detergents, and even well-intentioned medications in the form of topical anal creams or suppositories are examples. Clinical experience and elimination diets implicate certain dietary products such as coffee, cola, beer, tomatoes, chocolate, tea, and citrus fruits in the production of anal pruritus, although the mechanism is unknown.[140,141] Any food product that causes diarrhea in a patient may lead to pruritus simply because of frequent fecal contamination of the perianal region.

Idiopathic pruritus ani is usually caused by a combination of perianal skin fecal contamination and trauma. Not surprisingly, feces and colonic mucous secretions are irritating to perianal skin.[142,143] Acute diarrhea in an otherwise healthy person may lead to irritation of the perineum because of frequent wiping. Tiny amounts of feces repeatedly contaminate the sore perianal skin, leading to further irritation. Soon the itch-scratch cycle develops, serving to perpetuate skin trauma. Patients with chronic pruritus ani often suffer from frequent loose stools or some degree of fecal incontinence or seepage.

This hostile environment is repeatedly traumatized from vigorous wiping or scratching, and adequate healing can never occur. Pruritus is further exacerbated by inadequate perianal hygiene or excessive moisture caused by perspiration, airtight clothing, severe obesity, or a particularly deep-set anus.

Treatment

With patience and time, most causes of pruritus ani are successfully treated. Dermatologic diseases and infectious causes of pruritus ani are uncommon but, if identified, should be treated in the usual manner. Anorectal disorders that confound attempts at good perianal hygiene, such as prolapsing internal hemorrhoids or painful anal fissures, should be corrected. Fecal leakage or incontinence must be aggressively managed to avoid soiling of perianal skin. For the same reason, frequent loose stools should be minimized with antidiarrheals and fiber agents if appropriate. Foods or beverages that produce diarrhea or pruritus symptoms in a particular individual may be discontinued. Blanket recommendations to discontinue or curtail coffee, beer, citrus fruits, and other foods reported to cause pruritus ani lack firm support, but elimination diets may be appropriate in particular cases. The key to management of pruritus ani is to keep the anal area clean and dry while minimizing trauma caused by wiping and scratching.[144] The patient should be instructed to gently cleanse the anal skin with a premoistened pad or tissue after defecation. Witch hazel preparations or soothing lanolin-containing lotions are useful for this purpose. This always removes more residual feces than dry wiping alone. The area should be dried with a blow dryer or a soft tissue using a gentle dabbing, not rubbing, motion. Those with unpredictable small amounts of fecal discharge are instructed to wear a thin cotton pledget. This is barely perceptible when applied to the anus and should be changed frequently throughout the day. Excessive perspiration is corrected with application of baby powder and avoidance of tight, nonporous clothing. Irritating fabrics, greasy salves, perfumed toilet paper, hygiene products, and soaps should be avoided. A 1% hydrocortisone cream may be applied sparingly twice daily during the acute phase of pruritus ani but should not be used for longer than 2 weeks to avoid skin atrophy. Healing may be facilitated by applying a protective ointment (zinc oxide) over the antiinflammatory agent. For severe nocturnal symptoms, a nighttime dose of a systemic antipruritic such as diphenhydramine is appropriate. Long-standing, intractable pruritus ani has responded very well to intracutaneous injections of methylene blue and other agents.[145]

RECTAL FOREIGN BODIES AND TRAUMA

An astonishing hodgepodge of foreign bodies can become incarcerated in the rectum.[146] These include thermometers, enema tips, tools, bottles, light bulbs, pieces of food, and sexual devices inserted for purposes of medical treatment, concealment, assault, or, most commonly, eroticism. In an attempt to cope with an embarrassing situation, patients may claim the object was inserted to obtain relief from a particular discomfort or symptom. Occasionally, a patient presents complaining of bleeding or pain without admitting to a foreign body insertion. A directed interview and careful abdominal and rectal examination of an often sheepish patient are necessary to identify the foreign body and the potential risk of rectal trauma. Anteroposterior and lateral radiographs should be obtained to determine the object's outline and location and to detect pneumoperitoneum if present.

Nearly all objects can be removed transanally without resorting to surgery. Even if the object is easily palpable, removal under direct vision is the best way to avoid iatrogenic injury.[147] Foreign bodies may be classified by position as low-lying if in the rectal ampulla or high-lying if at or proximal to the rectosigmoid junction.[147] Small, low-lying objects are retrieved transanally using an operative anoscope. Removal of larger objects such as vibrators or rubber phalluses may require regional anesthesia, anal dilatation, and a grasping forceps. Large, bulky objects such as glass bottles and light bulbs require special care. After adequate anesthesia, several Foley catheters are inserted past the object. Air insufflation through the catheters relieves the proximal vacuum effect that may occur during attempted withdrawal. Gentle manipulation coupled with slow traction using the inflated Foley balloons successfully extricates the bulbous object in most cases. If a glass object is broken accidently during attempted removal, laparotomy is required. High-lying foreign bodies are managed using spinal anesthesia and the lithotomy position. By palpating the abdomen, the object is pushed distally and then simultaneously grasped with forceps through the sigmoidoscope to coax it into the rectal vault, from which it may be removed as a low-lying object. If the object cannot be delivered to within reach of the rigid sigmoidoscope manually or after 12 hours of observation, or if abdominal distress develops, laparotomy is indicated. Proctosigmoidoscopy should be performed after all foreign body retrievals to rule out retained objects, lacerations, hematomas, and perforation.

Other causes of rectal trauma include penetrating injuries (usually gunshot wounds), blunt trauma (motor vehicle accidents), impalement injuries (criminal assaults), homosexual activities (fist fornication), and iatrogenic injuries (endoscopy, enemas, surgical procedures).[148] Surgical management of major rectal trauma usually includes a diverting colostomy, presacral drain placement, distal rectal irrigation, and maximum preservation of sphincter musculature.[149]

ANAL CARCINOMA

Anal carcinomas are relatively rare, comprising only 1% to 2% of all colonic cancers. A variety of histologic types have been described, including squamous cell (70%–80%); basaloid, also known as transitional cell or cloacogenic (20%–30%); mucoepidermoid (1%–5%); and small cell anaplastic type (<5%).[150] All can be broadly classified as epidermoid carcinomas for purposes of clinical discussion. The mean age at presentation of patients with anal cancer is approximately 60 years.[151] Perianal and rectal carcinoma are more common in men, but the occurrence of anal canal tumors is nearly twice as common in women.[151]

Etiology

Although the cause of anal cancer is unknown, several risk factors have been identified. These tumors are strongly associated with homosexual behavior and receptive anal intercourse in men and with a history of genital warts in both sexes.[152] These data, immunohistologic studies, and polymerase chain reaction techniques suggest a causal role for human papillomavirus infection, particularly type 16.[153,154] Smoking and several other conditions have been described as primary or contributing factors (Table 88-4).

Clinical Manifestations

Bleeding, pain, and sometimes pruritus are presenting symptoms of anal cancer. However 25% of patients are symptom-free, and it is not unusual for the lesion to be discovered incidently at routine examination. Almost 2% of surgical specimens for benign anorectal disease are reported to contain previously unsuspected tumor, although a recent survey of hemorrhoidectomy specimens suggests a much lower incidence.[161,162] Rarely, a palpable metastatic inguinal lymph node is the sole presenting manifestation. Because symptoms are usually mild and nonspecific and easily confused with those of common benign anorectal lesions, the tumor is discovered late in more than 60% of patients. At presentation, 15% to 30% of patients have metastases to pelvic or inguinal lymph nodes, and 10% have distant spread to the liver or lungs.[150]

Diagnosis is made by biopsy (under anesthesia, if necessary), and the local extent of disease is determined by palpation, anoscopy, and sigmoidoscopy. Lesions originating from the anal canal tend to be undifferentiated and more aggressive, whereas those arising from the anal margin are more differentiated and less malignant.[163] A poor prognosis is portended by squamous cell tumors greater than 2 cm in size (especially those >5 cm), basaloid or anaplastic carcinomas, sphincter muscle invasion, or spread to regional pelvic or inguinal lymph nodes.[150]

Treatment

The standard therapy for small, noninfiltrating anal cancer has been wide local excision in an attempt to preserve normal anal function.[150,151] Split-thickness skin grafts may be required to cover large denuded surfaces. Large or infiltrating lesions require an abdominoperineal resection for radical excision of structures, including the sphincters, levator muscles, and rectum. Prophylactic inguinal lymph node resection is not indicated.

The advent of supervoltage radiotherapy alone or combined with surgery or chemotherapy has changed the approach to this neoplasm. Studies by Nigro and others suggest that radiotherapy (external beam or interstitial) plus chemotherapy with 5-fluorouracil and mitomycin-C causes complete tumor regression in most cases.[164–167] Subsequent abdominoperineal resection is unnecessary if follow-up biopsies document eradication of tumor. This combined approach minimizes local tumor recurrence while retaining normal anal function. The 5-year survival rate is approximately 70%.[150]

Nonepidermoid Anal Malignancies

A variety of uncommon neoplasms of the anus and perianal skin make up the nonepidermoid tumors of the anal region. *Adenocarcinoma of the anal canal* is a rare tumor often arising in anorectal fistulas.[151] This lesion may also arise from other anal glands or may be confused with distal extension of a primary rectal carcinoma. Despite radical abdominoperineal resection, recurrences are typical. *Extramammary Paget's disease* is a perianal glandular tumor that tends to spread along the epidermis and to eventually metastasize.[151] It typically appears in the seventh decade of life as an erythematous, well-demarcated eczemoid plaque with ulcerations. Wide total excision is indicated for localized disease.[168] More advanced lesions require a radical abdominoperineal resection with ipsilateral groin dissection if inguinal node involvement is seen. *Anal melanoma* accounts for 1% of all anal tumors and 1.6% of all melanomas. Typical lesions are 4 cm in diameter, nonpigmented in one third, and tend to metastasize early with 5-year survival rates of only 15%.[169] Radical resection offers no advantage over local excision and, in either case, long-term survival of a tumor thicker than 1.7 mm is rare.[170,171] *Basal cell carcinoma* of the perianal skin is a very rare lesion that produces rolled skin edges with central ulceration. The prognosis is quite good after adequate local excision or radiotherapy.[172] *Bowen's disease* is a slow-growing, cutaneous squamous cell carcinoma in situ. Lesions occur as reddish-brown scaly or crusted plaques that may resemble a patch of psoriasis or dermatitis. Simple local excision is usually curative.[173] Bowen's disease, especially of areas not exposed to sun, is reportedly associated with synchronous or metachronous neoplasms of the lung, gastrointestinal tract, and genitourinary system. The incidence may be as high as 30% to

---

TABLE 88-4
Risk Factors for Anal Carcinoma

Cigarette smoking[152,155,156]
Male homosexuality[152]
Receptive anal intercourse (men)[152]
Genital warts[152]
Condyloma acuminatum[157,158]
Other venereal diseases[152]
  Gonorrhea
  Herpes genitalis
  Chlamydia trachomatis
History of positive Papanicolaou smear[155]
Female lower genital tract tumors[159]
Renal transplant[159]
Chronic anal inflammation and scarring[150]
Crohn's disease[160]

50% within 10 years. A report by Arbesman and Ransohoff criticizes the published evidence supporting this entire association.[174]

HIDRADENITIS SUPPURATIVA

Hidradenitis suppurativa is a chronic suppurative condition of apocrine glands most often involving the axillary and inguinoperineal skin regions. Apocrine glands are activated at puberty, so the disease is not seen before adolescence and rarely occurs initially after middle age. Axillary hidradenitis suppurativa is most common, but perineal involvement is seen in nearly one third of those with the disease, especially in men.[175,176] The best recognized risk factors are obesity and acne, although perspiration and mechanical trauma to the skin and hair of the anogenital region may also predispose to perianal hidradenitis.

Pathogenesis

Occlusion, inflammation, and bacterial infection of apocrine ducts leads to abscess formation in the gland. A small, blind boil is the first manifestation of this smoldering process. Abscesses eventually enlarge and spread to infect contiguous glands. Repeated inflammation and healing may produce fibrosis and draining sinus tracts. If perineal sinus tracts are extensive, fistulas to the anus and rectum may develop. Microbiologic analysis of perineal hidradenitis suppurativa skin lesions identifies streptococci, *Staphylococcus aureus*, or, less commonly, gram-negative rods. *Streptococcus milleri* is the most common pathogen isolated, and its presence is significantly associated with disease activity.[177]

Clinical Manifestations

Perineal hidradenitis suppurativa should be suspected in the presence of tender abscess formation in the anogenital region with or without axillary disease. Early lesions may be confused with a simple inflamed epidermal or sebaceous cyst or pilonidal disease, but if recurrent abscesses and fibrosis develops, the diagnosis is apparent. Inflammatory bowel disease must be considered as a diagnostic possibility if advanced disease with fistula formation is present. Careful evaluation under anesthesia differentiates the anal fistula of hidradenitis suppurativa from that of a rectal abscess or Crohn's disease: the fistulous tract between the skin and anal canal of hidradenitis suppurativa remains superficial to the internal sphincter musculature, as opposed to the deeper penetration of the latter conditions.[178]

Perineal hidradenitis suppurativa may lead to a variety of local complications, including sinuses, fistulas, and scarring with their associated deformities. Rarely, chronic inflammation causes systemic findings of anemia or inflammatory arthritis.[176] Almost 20 cases of squamous cell carcinoma occurring in chronically infected anogenital sinuses (mean >16 years) have been reported.[179]

Treatment

Medical treatment is appropriate for early disease. Warm, wet compresses are applied, and topical and systemic antibiotics are administered on the basis of culture and bacteriologic sensitivities of draining pus. The definitive and usually necessary treatment of perianal hidradenitis suppurativa is surgical.[176,180] Recurrent draining nodules are exteriorized (unroofed), and the base is curetted and cauterized to destroy infected tissue. This allows healing and better eradication of the underlying process than repeated incision and drainage. Infected tracts must be completely excised down to fascia. Extensive disease requires total excision of the affected area and the use of skin flaps or skin grafting. A proximal diverting colostomy may be required in severe cases to allow proper perineal wound healing.

PILONIDAL DISEASE

Pilonidal ("nest of hair") disease is a common skin lesion of the internatal or gluteal cleft seen most frequently in young men. Once thought to be a congenital lesion, pilonidal abscess is now recognized to be an acquired condition of the midline coccygeal skin region, possibly induced by local stretching forces.[181] Small skin pits, probably representing enlarged hair follicles, precede development of the draining sinus or abscess. Lesions are often secondarily invaded by hair. The characteristic midline location, appearance, and lack of communication with the anorectum distinguish pilonidal disease from anorectal fistula and hidradenitis suppurativa. Acute pilonidal abscess requires incision, drainage, and hair removal.[182] A variety of surgical options exist for chronic, draining pilonidal lesions, ranging from simple excision to excision with sinus marsupialization or primary closure.[183,184] Surgical closure using flaps or Z-plasty so that suture lines avoid the midline minimizes wound disruption and recurrence.[181] Almost 40 cases of squamous cell carcinoma have been reported to arise from pilonidal sinuses, usually in those with symptomatic disease for a mean duration of 20 years.[185] This malignancy has a 44% rate of recurrence or metastasis, indicating a more aggressive course than that of squamous cell carcinoma arising from other chronically irritated skin lesions.

PROCTALGIA FUGAX AND THE LEVATOR SYNDROME

Proctalgia fugax (literally "fleeting rectal pain") is an obscure condition characterized by sudden, brief episodes of severe rectal pain. The true incidence of the disorder is unknown, although surveys of healthy people reveal attacks of rectal pain in approximately 15%.[186] Most people do not seek medical advice, probably because the pain typically lasts less than 1 minute (84%) and occurs fewer than 6 times per year (72%).[187] Modern surveys identify no consistent sexual predominance.[186,187]

Attacks are described as an intense stabbing or aching midline pain above the anus, lasting several seconds to many minutes. Pain may be variably associated with an urge to expel flatus, a desire to lie on one side with hips flexed, and, rarely, cold sweats, syncope, and priapism. Occasionally, attacks are exclusively nocturnal. Stress, fatigue, heat, cold, and sexual activity have all been reported to induce pain, but usually no clear precipitant is identified.

Not surprisingly, proctalgia fugax has been associated with the irritable bowel syndrome and a variety of psychogenic disorders. A British survey of volunteers found that proctalgia fugax sufferers were more likely to experience Manning's restrictive features of irritable bowel syndrome than those without proctalgia fugax.[188,189] A later study by the same author, however, questions this.[190] An uncontrolled study reported a high incidence of psychological disorders and functional gastrointestinal symptoms in those with proctalgia fugax.[191]

The cause of proctalgia fugax is unknown. Unsubstantiated theories include rectosigmoid intussusception, vascular migraine equivalent, accumulation of rectal gas, or spasm of the anal sphincter, rectosigmoid colon, or pelvic musculature. The diagnosis is made on the basis of a characteristic history alone. Anorectal examination and sigmoidoscopy are normal. A familial internal anal sphincter myopathy causing proctalgia fugax and difficulty with rectal evacuation has been reported.[192]

Of primary importance in the treatment of proctalgia fugax is reassurance as to the benign nature of the disorder. This advice in conjunction with treatment of irritable bowel syndrome or psychogenic disorders, if present, often suffices. A number of specific remedies have been proposed for more refractory symptoms. Their efficacy is difficult to determine given the transient nature of symptoms and the lack of even uncontrolled trials. Local therapies include rectal massage, firm manual pressure to the perineum, and application of warm soaks or baths. One author claims good results if the patient spreads the buttocks while in a knee-chest position to allow expulsion of rectal gas.[193] Pharmacologic intervention should be reserved for those with particularly frequent, severe, or disabling symptoms. Anecdotal reports claim success with a variety of drugs to reduce spasm, including amyl nitrate, sublingual nitroglycerine, salbutamol, clonidine, and diltiazem.[194–196]

The levator syndrome refers to an aching rectal pain caused by tenderness and spasm of the levator ani muscle group (ileococcygeus, pubococcygeus, and puborectalis). It is perhaps best thought of as a varient of proctalgia fugax, although the two disorders are frequently confused in the literature. The pain is more chronic, aching, and pressure-like than that of proctalgia fugax and is most commonly seen in middle-aged women.[197] Defecation, prolonged sitting, and precipitants of proctalgia fugax have been described as precipitants of levator syndrome pain. The key diagnostic finding is palpable tenderness and spasm of the levator muscles as the examining finger sweeps 180 degrees from the coccyx to the pubis posteriorly to anteriorly.[197] For unknown reasons, findings are more frequently localized to the left side. Treatment consists of variable combinations of reassurance, local heat, vigorous digital rectal massage of the levator musculature, and diazepam. In those with persistent symptoms, several groups have reported beneficial results using electrogalvanic stimulation.[198–200] This safe, painless technique apparently breaks the spasm pain cycle by delivering a high-voltage, pulsed current through a rectal probe.

MISCELLANEOUS CAUSES OF CHRONIC ANORECTAL PAIN

Coccygodynia refers to pain in the coccyx. The discomfort is sharp or aching in quality and may radiate into the rectal region or to the buttocks. Organic coccygodynia is caused by traumatic arthritis, dislocation or fracture as a result of injury, or difficult childbirth.[37] Prolonged sitting has been suggested to cause functional coccygodynia. In both cases, manipulation of the coccyx reproduces pain and muscular spasm. Many respond to symptomatic treatment with warm soaks and analgesics. Local injection of steroid with or without coccygeal manipulation is usually beneficial in those with persistent symptoms.[201] Rarely, coccygectomy is required for organic coccygodynia.

A rare genetic syndrome of familial rectal pain has been reported in a few families.[202] Afflicted members complain of an intense proctalgia shooting down the buttocks and legs, accompanied by lower limb flushing. Pain is triggered by bowel movements or other physical stimulants to the perineum. Independently occurring facial and ocular symptoms have also been described. One group has identified 12 patients with chronic idiopathic anal pain and high resting anal tone. All appeared to respond to sphincter exercises and biofeedback therapy.[203]

Unusual causes of rectal pain include cauda equina tumors, pelvic tumors, perianal endometriosis, intermittent enteroceles, and a variety of rare retrorectal tumors and cysts.[37]

> The reader is directed to Chapter 10, Motility of the Large Intestine; Chapter 78, Colon: Anatomy and Structural Anomalies; and Chapter 82, Motility Disorders of the Colon.

REFERENCES

1. Goligher JC. Surgery of the anus, rectum and colon. 5th ed. London: Bailliere Tindall, 1984.
2. Haas PA, Fox TA, Haas G. The pathogenesis of hemorrhoids. Dis Colon Rectum 1984;27:442.
3. Thulesius O, Gjores JE. Arteriovenous anastomosis in the anal region with reference to the pathogenesis and treatment of hemorrhoids. Acta Chir Scand 1973;139:476.
4. Thomson WH. The nature of hemorrhoids. Br J Surg 1975;62:542.
5. Miles WE. Observations upon internal piles. Surg Gynecol Obstet 1919;29:497.
6. Arabi Y, Alexander-Williams J, Keighley MRB. Anal pressures in hemorrhoids and anal fissure. Am J Surg 1977;134:608.
7. Sun WM, Peck RJ, Shorthouse AJ, et al. Hemorrhoids are associated not with hypertrophy of the internal anal sphincter, but with hypertension of the anal cushions. Br J Surg 1992;79:592.
8. Barron J. Office ligation treatment of hemorrhoids. Dis Colon Rectum 1963;6:109.
9. Bleday R, Pena JP, Rothenberger DA, et al. Symptomatic hemorrhoids: current incidence and complications of operative therapy. Dis Colon Rectum 1992;35:477.
10. Corman ML. Rubber band ligation of hemorrhoids. Arch Surg 1977;112:1257.
11. Nivatvongs S, Goldberg SM. An improved technique of rubber band ligation of hemorrhoids. Am J Surg 1982;144:379.
12. Khubchandani IT. A randomized comparison of single and

multiple rubber band ligations. Dis Colon Rectum 1983;26: 705.

13. Marshman D, Huber PJ Jr, Timmerman W, et al. Hemorrhoidal ligation. A review of efficacy. Dis Colon Rectum 1989;32:369.

14. O'Hara VS. Fatal clostridial infection following hemorrhoidal banding. Dis Colon Rectum 1980;23:570.

15. Russell TR, Donohue JH. Hemorrhoidal banding: a warning. Dis Colon Rectum 1985;28:291.

16. Arabi Y, Gatehouse D, Alexander-Williams J, et al. Rubber band ligation or lateral subcutaneous sphincterotomy for treatment of haemorrhoids. Br J Surg 1977;64:737.

17. Gehamy RA, Weakley FL. Internal hemorrhoidectomy by elastic ligation. Dis Colon Rectum 1974;17:347.

18. Ponsky JL, Mellinger JD, Simon IB. Endoscopic retrograde hemorrhoidal sclerotherapy using 23.4% saline: a preliminary report. Gastrointest Endosc 1991;37:155.

19. Buls JG, Goldberg SM. Modern management of hemorrhoids. Surg Clin North Am 1978;58:469.

20. Anderson J, Steger A. Fatal meningitis complicating cryosurgery for hemorrhoids. Br Med J 1984;288:826.

21. Goligher JC. Cryosurgery for hemorrhoids. Dis Colon Rectum 1976;19:213.

22. Keighley MRB, Buchmann P, Minervini S, et al. Prospective trials of minor surgical procedures and high-fibre diet for hemorrhoids. Br Med J 1979;2:967.

23. Norman DA, Newton R, Nicholas GV. Management of hemorrhoidal disease: an effective, safe, and painless outpatient approach using direct current. Gastrointest Endosc 1987;33: 176.

24. Leicester RJ, Mitchells RJ, Mann CV. Infrared coagulation: a new treatment for hemorrhoids. Dis Colon Rectum 1981;24: 602.

25. O'Connor JJ. Infrared coagulation of hemorrhoids. Practical Gastroenterology 1986;10:8.

26. Ambrose NS, Morris D, Alexander-Williams J, et al. A randomized trial of photocoagulation or injection sclerotherapy for the treatment of first- and second-degree hemorrhoids. Dis Colon Rectum 1985;28:238.

27. Johanson JF, Rimm A. Optimal nonsurgical treatment of hemorrhoids: a comparative analysis of infrared coagulation, rubber band ligation, and injection sclerotherapy. Am J Gastroenterol 1992;87:1601.

28. Iwagaki H, Higuchi Y, Fuchimoto S, et al. The laser treatment of hemorrhoids: results of a study on 1816 patients. Jpn J Surg 1989;19:658.

29. Ferguson JA, Mazier WP, Ganchrow MI, et al. The closed technique of hemorrhoidectomy. Surgery 1971;70:480.

30. Bonardi RA, Rosin JD, Stonesifer GL, et al. Bacteremias associated with routine hemorrhoidectomies. Dis Colon Rectum 1976;19:233.

31. Lord PH. A day-case procedure for the cure of third-degree haemorrhoids. Br J Surg 1969;56:747.

32. Jacobs DM, Bubrick MP, Onstad GR, et al. The relationship of hemorrhoids to portal hypertension. Dis Colon Rectum 1980;23:567.

33. Wang TF, Lee FY, Tsai YT, et al. Relationship of portal pressure, anorectal varices and hemorrhoids in cirrhotic patients. J Hepatol 1992;15:170.

34. Hosking SW, Johnson AG. Bleeding anorectal varices: a misunderstood condition. Surgery 1988;104:70.

35. Hsieh JS, Huang CJ, Huang TJ. Demonstration of rectal varices by transhepatic inferior mesenteric venography. Dis Colon Rectum 1986;29:459.

36. Keane RM, Britton DL. Massive bleeding from rectal varices following repeated injection sclerotherapy of esophageal varices. Br J Surg 1986;73:120.

37. Goldberg SM, Gordon PH, Nivatvongs S, eds. Essentials of anorectal surgery. Philadelphia: JB Lippincott, 1980.

38. Ramanujam PS, Prasad ML, Abcarian H, et al. Perianal abscesses and fistulas: a study of 1023 patients. Dis Colon Rectum 1984;27:593.

39. Barnes SG, Sattler FR, Ballard JO. Perirectal infections in acute leukemia: improved survival after incision and debridement. Ann Intern Med 1984;100:515.

40. Seow-Choen F, Hay AJ, Heard S, et al. Bacteriology of anal fistulae. Br J Surg 1992;79:27.

41. Parks AG. The pathogenesis and treatment of fistula-in-ano. Br J Surg 1961;1:483.

42. Parks AG, Gordon PH, Hardcastle JD. A classification of fistula-in-ano. Br J Surg 1976;63:1.

43. Schaarschmidt K, Willital GH. Intraanal ultrasound: a new aid in the diagnosis of pelvic processes and their relation to the sphincter complex. J Pediatr Surg 1992;27:604.

44. Cirocco WC, Reilly JC. Challenging the predictive accuracy of Goodsall's rule for anal fistulas. Dis Colon Rectum 1992;35: 537.

45. Corfitsen MT, Hansen CP, Christensen TH, et al. Anorectal abscess in immunosuppressed patients. Eur J Surg 1992;158: 51.

46. Schimpff SC, Wiernik PH, Block JB. Rectal abscesses in cancer patients. Lancet 1972;2:844.

47. Bubrick MP, Hitchcock CR. Necrotizing anorectal and perineal infections. Surgery 1979;86:655.

48. Schouten WR, van Vroonhoven TJ. Treatment of anorectal abscess with or without primary fistulectomy: results of a prospective, randomized trial. Dis Colon Rectum 1991;34:60.

49. Grace RH, Harper IA, Thompson RG. Anorectal sepsis: microbiology in relation to fistula-in-ano. Br J Surg 1982;69:401.

50. Pescatori M, Maria G, Anastasio G, et al. Anal manometry improves the outcome of surgery for fistula-in-ano. Dis Colon Rectum 1989;32:588.

51. Bernstein LH, Frank MS, Brandt LJ, et al. Healing of perineal Crohn's disease with metronidazole. Gastroenterology 1980;79: 357.

52. Williams JG, Rothenberger DA, Nemer FD, et al. Fistula-in-ano in Crohn's disease. Results of aggressive surgical treatment. Dis Colon Rectum 1991;34:378.

53. Fry RD, Shemesh EI, Kodner IJ, et al. Techniques and results in the management of anal and perianal Crohn's disease. Surg Gynecol Obstet 1989;168:42.

54. Moschowitz AV. The pathogenesis, anatomy and cure of prolapse of the rectum. Surg Gynecol Obstet 1912;15:7.

55. Broden B, Snellman B. Procidentia of the rectum studies with cineradiography: a contribution to the discussion of causative mechanism. Dis Colon Rectum 1968;11:330.

56. Goldberg SM, Gordon PH. Treatment of rectal prolapse. Clin Gastroenterol 1975;4:489.

57. Hiltunen KM, Matikainen M, Auvinen O, et al. Clinical and manometric evaluation of anal sphincter function in patients with rectal prolapse. Am J Surg 1986;151:489.

58. Williams JG, Wong WD, Jensen L, et al. Incontinence and rectal prolapse: a prospective manometric study. Dis Colon Rectum 1991;34:209.

59. Myers JO, Rothenberger DA. Sugar in the reduction of incarcerated prolapsed bowel. Report of two cases. Dis Colon Rectum 1991;34:416.

60. Lowry AC, Goldberg SM. Internal and overt rectal procidentia. Gastroenterol Clin North Am 1987;16:47.

61. Farouk R, Duthie GS, Bartolo DC, et al. Restoration of continence following rectopexy for rectal prolapse and recovery of the internal anal sphincter electromyogram. Br J Surg 1992;79: 439.

62. Berman IR. Sutureless laparoscopic rectopexy for procidentia. Technique and implications. Dis Colon Rectum 1992;35:689.

63. Watts JD, Rothenberger DA, Buls JG, et al. The management of procidentia: 30 years experience. Dis Colon Rectum 1985;28: 96.

64. Slade MS, Goldberg SM, Schottler JL, et al. Sphincteroplasty for acquired anal incontinence. Dis Colon Rectum 1977;20: 33.

65. Browning GGP, Motson RW. Anal sphincter injury: management and results of Parks sphincter repair. Ann Surg 1984;199: 351.

66. Williams JG, Rothenberger DA, Madoff RD, et al. Treatment of rectal prolapse in the elderly by perineal rectosigmoidectomy. Dis Colon Rectum 1992;35:830.

67. Nothmann BJ, Schuster MM. Internal anal sphincter derangement with anal fissures. Gastroenterology 1974;67:216.

68. Lin JK. Anal manometric studies in hemorrhoids and anal fissures. Dis Colon Rectum 1989;32:839.
69. Melange M, Colin JF, Van Wymersch T, et al. Anal fissure: correlation between symptoms and manometry before and after surgery. Int J Colorectal Dis 1992;7:108.
70. Brown AC, Sumfest JM, Rozwadowski JV. Histopathology of the internal anal sphincter in chronic anal fissure. Dis Colon Rectum 1989;32:680.
71. Abcarian H. Surgical correction of chronic anal fissure: results of lateral internal sphincterotomy vs. fissurectomy-midline sphincterotomy. Dis Colon Rectum 1980;23:31.
72. Marby M, Alexander-Williams J, Buchmann P, et al. A randomized controlled trial to compare anal dilatation with lateral subcutaneous sphincterotomy for anal fissure. Dis Colon Rectum 1979;22:308.
73. Milsom JW, Mazier WP. Classification and management of postsurgical anal stenosis. Surg Gynecol Obstet 1986;163:60.
74. Pietrusko RG. Use and abuse of laxatives. Am J Hosp Pharm 1977;34:291.
75. Corman ML, Veidenheimer MC, Coller JA. Anoplasty for anal stricture. Surg Clin North Am 1976;56:727.
76. Madigan MR, Morson BC. Solitary ulcer of the rectum. Gut 1969;10:871.
77. Ford MJ, Anderson JR, Gilmour HM, et al. Clinical spectrum of "solitary ulcer" of the rectum. Gastroenterology 1983;84:1533.
78. Womack NR, Williams NS, Holmfield JHM, et al. Pressure and prolapse—the cause of solitary rectal ulceration. Gut 1987;28:1228.
79. Alberti-Flor JJ, Halter S, Dunn DG. Solitary rectal ulcer as a cause of massive lower gastrointestinal bleeding. Gastrointest Endosc 1985;31:53.
80. Gilrane TB, Orchard JL, Al-Assaad ZA. A benign rectal ulcer penetrating into the prostate—diagnosis by prostate-specific antigen. Gastrointest Endos 1987;33:467.
81. Brandt-Gradel VVD, Huibregtse K, Tytgat GNJ. Treatment of solitary rectal ulcer syndrome with high-fiber diet and abstention of straining at defecation. Dig Dis Sci 1984;29:1005.
82. Zargar SA, Khuroo MS, Mahajan R. Sucralfate retention enemas in solitary rectal ulcer. Dis Colon Rectum 1991;34:455.
83. Keighley MRB, Shouler P. Clinical and manometric features of the solitary rectal ulcer syndrome. Dis Colon Rectum 1984;27:507.
84. Nicholls RJ, Simson JNL. Anteroposterior rectopexy in the treatment of solitary rectal ulcer syndrome without overt rectal prolapse. Br J Surg 1985;73:222.
85. Kok AL, Voorhorst FJ, Burger CW, et al. Urinary and faecal incontinence in community-residing elderly women. Age Ageing 1992;21:211.
86. Thomas TM, Ruff C, Karran O, et al. Study of the prevalence and management of patients with faecal incontinence in old people's homes. Community Med 1987;9:232.
87. Tobin GW, Brocklehurst JC. Faecal incontinence in residential homes for the elderly: prevalence, aetiology and management. Age Ageing 1986;15:41.
88. Leigh RJ, Turnberg LA. Faecal incontinence: the unvoiced symptom. Lancet 1982;1:1349.
89. Read NW, Harford WV, Schmulen AC, et al. A clinical study of patients with fecal incontinence and diarrhea. Gastroenterology 1979;76:747.
90. Bannister JJ, Gibbons C, Read NW. Preservation of faecal continence during rises in intraabdominal pressure: is there a role for the flap valve? Gut 1987;28:1242.
91. Gordon PH. The anorectum: anatomic and physiologic considerations in health and disease. Gastroenterol Clin North Am 1987;16:1.
92. Henry MM. Pathogenesis and management of fecal incontinence in the adult. Gastroenterol Clin North Am 1987;16:35.
93. Miller R, Bartolo DCC, Locke-Edmunds JC, et al. Prospective study of conservative and operative treatment for faecal incontinence. Br J Surg 1988;75:101.
94. Miller R, Bartolo DC, Roe A, et al. Anal sensation and the continence mechanism. Dis Colon Rectum 1988;31:433.
95. Wald A, Tunuguntla K. Anorectal sensorimotor dysfunction in fecal incontinence and diabetes mellitus. N Engl J Med 1984;310:1282.
96. Devroede G, Vobecky S, Masse S, et al. Ischemic fecal incontinence and rectal angina. Gastroenterology 1982;83:970.
97. Neill ME, Swash M. Increased motor unit fibre density in the external sphincter muscle in ano-rectal incontinence: a single fibre EMG study. J Neurol Neurosurg Psychiatry 1980;43:343.
98. Kiff ES, Swash M. Slowed conduction in the pudendal nerves in idiopathic (neurogenic) faecal incontinence. Br J Surg 1984;71:614.
99. Kiff ES, Barnes RPH, Swash M. Evidence of pudendal nerve neuropathy in patients with perineal descent and chronic straining at stool. Gut 1984;25:1279.
100. Jones PN, Lubowski DZ, Swash M, et al. Relation between perineal descent and pudendal nerve damage in idiopathic fecal incontinence. Int J Colorectal Dis 1987;2:93.
101. Womack NR, Morrison JFB, Williams NS. The role of pelvic floor denervation in the aetiology of idiopathic faecal incontinence. Br J Surg 1986;73:404.
102. Snooks SJ, Swash M, Henry MM, et al. Risk factors in childbirth causing damage to the pelvic floor innervation. Br J Surg 1985;72:S15.
103. Sun WM, Donnelly TC, Read NW. Utility of a combined test of anorectal manometry, electromyography, and sensation in determining the mechanism of "idiopathic" faecal incontinence. Gut 1992;33:807.
104. Lubowski DZ, Nicholls RJ, Burleigh DE, et al. Internal anal sphincter in neurogenic fecal incontinence. Gastroenterology 1988;95:997.
105. Rogers J, Henry MM, Misiewicz JJ. Combined sensory and motor deficit in primary neuropathic faecal incontinence. Gut 1988;29:5.
106. Coller JA. Clinical application of anorectal manometry. Gastroenterol Clin North Am 1987;16:17.
107. Buser WD, Miner PB. Delayed rectal sensation with fecal incontinence. Successful treatment using anorectal manometry. Gastroenterology 1986;91:1186.
108. Shouler P, Keighley RB. Changes in colorectal function in severe idiopathic chronic constipation. Gastroenterology 1986;90:414.
109. Haldeman S, Bradley WE, Bhatia NN, et al. Pudendal evoked response. Arch Neurol 1982;39:280.
110. Pittman JS, Benson JT, Sumners JE. Physiologic evaluation of the anorectum. A new ultrasound technique. Dis Colon Rectum 1990;33:476.
111. Law PJ, Kamm MA, Bartram CI. Anal endosonography in the investigation of faecal incontinence. Br J Surg 1991;78:312.
112. Cuesta MA, Meijer S, Derksen EJ, et al. Anal sphincter imaging in fecal incontinence using endosonography. Dis Colon Rectum 1992;35:59.
113. Roe AM, Bartolo DCC, Mortensen NJ. New method for assessment of anal sensation in various anorectal disorders. Br J Surg 1986;73:310.
114. Miller R, Bartolo DCC, Cervero F, et al. Anorectal temperature sensation: a comparison of normal and incontinent patients. Br J Surg 1987;74:511.
115. Ekberg O, Nylander G, Fork F. Defecography. Radiology 1985;155:45.
116. Goei R. Anorectal function in patients with defecation disorders and asymptomatic subjects: evaluation with defecography. Radiology 1990;174:121.
117. Ling L, Malmfred S, Thesleff P. Solid-sphere test for examination of anal sphincter strength. Scand J Gastroenterol 1984;19:960.
118. Harford WV, Krejs GJ, Santa CA, et al. Acute effect of diphenoxylate with atropine (Lomotil) in patients with chronic diarrhea and fecal incontinence. Gastroenterology 1980;78:440.
119. Palmer KR, Corbett CL, Holdsworth CD. Double-blind cross-over study comparing loperamide codeine and diphenoxylate in the treatment of chronic diarrhea. Gastroenterology 1980;79:1272.
120. Read M, Read NW, Barber DC, et al. Effects of loperamide on anal sphincter function in patients complaining of chronic diarrhea with fecal incontinence and urgency. Dig Dis Sci 1982;27:807.

121. Cerulli MA, Nikoomanesh P, Schuster MM. Progress in biofeedback conditioning for fecal incontinence. Gastroenterology 1979;76:742.

122. Wald A. Biofeedback therapy for fecal incontinence. Ann Intern Med 1981;95:146.

123. MacLeod JH. Management of anal incontinence by biofeedback. Gastroenterology 1987;93:291.

124. Miner PB, Donnelly TC, Read NW. Investigation of mode of action of biofeedback in treatment of fecal incontinence. Dig Dis Sci 1990;35:1291.

125. Loening-Bauke V. Efficacy of biofeedback training in improving faecal incontinence and anorectal physiologic function. Gut 1990;31:1395.

126. Stricker JW, Schoetz Jr DJ, Coller JA, et al. Surgical correction of anal incontinence. Dis Colon Rectum 1988;31:533.

127. Snooks SJ, Henry MM, Swash M. Faecal incontinence due to external anal sphincter division in childbirth is associated with damage to the innervation of the pelvic floor musculature: a double pathology. Br J Obstet Gynaecol 1985;92:824.

128. Womack NR, Morrison JF, Williams NS. Prospective study of the effects of postanal repair in neurogenic faecal incontinence. Br J Surg 1988;75:48.

129. Corman M. Gracilis muscle transportation for anal incontinence: late results. Br J Surg 1985;72:521.

130. Williams NS, Patel J, George BD, et al. Development of an electrically stimulated neoanal sphincter. Lancet 1991;338:1166.

131. Baeten CG, Konsten J, Spaans F. Dynamic graciloplasty for treatment of faecal incontinence. Lancet 1991;338:1163.

132. Christiansen J, Lorentzen M. Implantation of artificial sphincter for anal incontinence. Report of five cases. Dis Colon Rectum 1989;32:432.

133. Hanno R, Murphy P. Pruritus ani: classification and management. Dermatol Clin 1987;5:811.

134. Murie JA, Sim AW, Mackenzie I. The importance of pain, pruritus and soiling as symptoms of haemorrhoids and their response to haemorrhoidectomy or rubber band ligation. Br J Surg 1981;68:247.

135. Powell FC, Perry HO. Pruritus ani: could it be malignant? Geriatrics 1985;40:89.

136. Dodi G, Pirone E, Bettin A, et al. The mycotic flora in proctological patients with and without pruritus ani. Br J Surg 1985;72:967.

137. Baral J. Pruritus ani and staphylococcus aureus. J Am Acad Dermatol 1963;9:962.

138. Bowyer A, McColl I. Erythrasma and pruritus ani. Acta Derm Venerol (Stockh) 1971;51:444.

139. Silverman SH, Youngs DJ, Allan A, et al. The fecal microflora in pruritus ani. Dis Colon Rectum 1989;32:466.

140. Smith LE, Henrichs D, McCullah RD. Prospective studies on the etiology and treatment of pruritus ani. Am Soc Colon Rectal Surg 1982;25:358.

141. Friend WG. The cause and treatment of idiopathic pruritus ani. Dis Colon Rectum 1977;20:40.

142. Caplan RM. The irritant role of feces in the genesis of perianal itch. Gastroenterology 1966;50:19.

143. Marks MM. The influence of the intestinal pH on anal pruritus. South Med J 1968;61:1005.

144. Sullivan ES, Garnjobst WM. Pruritus ani: a practical approach. Surg Clin North Am 1978;58:505.

145. Eusebio EB, Graham J, Mody N. Treatment of intractable pruritus ani. Dis Colon Rectum 1990;33:770.

146. Busch DB, Starling JR. Rectal foreign bodies. Case reports and a comprehensive review of the world's literature. Surgery 1986;100:512.

147. Kingsley AN, Abcarian H. Colorectal foreign bodies: management update. Dis Colon Rectum 1985;28:941.

148. Abcarian H. Rectal trauma in anorectal disorders. Gastroenterol Clin North Am 1987;16:115.

149. Ivatury RR, Licata J, Gunduz Y, et al. Management options in penetrating rectal injuries. Ann Surg 1991;57:50.

150. Cummings BJ. Current management of epidermoid carcinoma of the anal canal. Gastroenterol Clin North Am 1987;16:125.

151. Adam YG, Efron G. Current concepts and controversies concerning the etiology, pathogenesis, diagnosis and treatment of malignant tumors of the anus. Surgery 1987;101:253.

152. Daling JR, Weiss NS, Hislop TG, et al. Sexual practices, sexually transmitted diseases and the incidence of anal cancer. N Engl J Med 1987;317:974.

153. Zaki SR, Judd R, Coffield LM, et al. Human papillomavirus infection and anal carcinoma. Retrospective analysis by in situ hybridization and the polymerase chain reaction. Am J Pathol 1992;140:1345.

154. Palmer JG, Scholefield JH, Coates PJ, et al. Anal cancer and human papillomaviruses. Dis Colon Rectum 1989;32:1016.

155. Holmes F, Borek D, Owen-Kummer M, et al. Anal cancer in women. Gastroenterology 1988;95:107.

156. Daling JR, Sherman KJ, Hislop TG, et al. Cigarette smoking and the risk of anogenital cancer. Am J Epidemiol 1992;135:180.

157. Butler TW, Gefter J, Kieto D, et al. Squamous-cell carcinoma of the anus in condyloma acuminatum. Dis Colon Rectum 1987;30:293.

158. Prasad ML, Abcarian H. Malignant potential of perianal condyloma acuminatum. Dis Colon Rectum 1980;23:191.

159. Penn I. Cancer of the anogenital region in renal transplant recipients. Analysis of 65 cases. Cancer 1986;58:611.

160. Slater G, Greenstein A, Aufses AH. Anal carcinoma in patients with Crohn's disease. Ann Surg 1984;199:348.

161. Grodsky L. Unsuspected anal cancer discovered after minor anorectal surgery. Dis Colon Rectum 1967;10:471.

162. Cataldo PA, MacKeigan JM. The necessity of routine pathologic evaluation of hemorrhoidectomy specimens. Surg Gynecol Obstet 1992;174:302.

163. Parks A. Squamous carcinoma of the anal canal. Ann Gastroenterol Hepatol (Paris) 1981;17:103.

164. Nigro ND. An evaluation of combined therapy for squamous cell cancer of the anal canal. Dis Colon Rectum 1984;27:763.

165. Papillon J, Montbarbon JF. Epidermal carcinoma of the anal canal. Dis Colon Rectum 1987;30:324.

166. Cummings BJ, Keane TJ, O'Sullivan B, et al. Epidermoid anal cancer: treatment by radiation alone or by radiation and 5-fluorouracil with and without mitomycin C. Int J Radiat Oncol Biol Phys 1991;21:1115.

167. Doci R, Zucali R, Bombelli L, et al. Combined chemoradiation therapy for anal cancer. A report of 56 cases. Ann Surg 1992;215:150.

168. Beck DE, Fazio VW. Perianal Paget's disease. Dis Colon Rectum 1987;30:263.

169. Weinstock MA. Epidemiology and prognosis of anorectal melanoma. Gastroenterology 1993;104:174.

170. Ward MWN, Romano G, Nicholls RJ. The surgical treatment of anorectal malignant melanoma. Br J Surg 1986;73:68.

171. Stearns Jr MW, Urmacher C, Sternberg SS, et al. Cancer of the anal canal. Curr Probl Cancer 1980;4:1.

172. Nielsen OV, Jensen SL. Basal cell carcinoma of the anus—a clinical study of 34 cases. Br J Surgery 1981;68:856.

173. Strauss RJ, Fazio VW. Bowen's disease of the anal and perianal area: A report and analysis of twelve cases. Am J Surg 1979;137:231.

174. Arbesman H, Ransohoff DF. Is Bowen's disease a predictor for the development of internal malignancy? A methodological critique of the literature. JAMA 1987;257:516.

175. Adams JD, Haisten AS. Perianal hidradenitis suppurativa. Surg Clin North Am 1972;52:467.

176. Hurley HJ. Diseases of the apocrine and eccrine sweat glands. In: Moschella SL, Hurley HJ, eds. Dermatology. Philadelphia: WB Saunders, 1985:1336.

177. Highet AS, Warren RE, Weekes AJ. Bacteriology and antibiotic treatment of perineal suppurative hidradenitis. Arch Dermatol 1988;124:1047.

178. Culp CE. Chronic hidradenitis suppurativa of the anal canal. Dis Colon Rectum 1983;26:669.

179. Williams ST, Busby RC, DeMuth RJ, et al. Perineal hidradenitis suppurativa: presentation of two unusual complications and a review. Ann Plast Surg 1991;26:456.

180. Wiltz O, Schoetz DJ Jr, Murrary JJ, et al. Perianal hidradenitis

suppurativa. The Lahey Clinic experience. Dis Colon Rectum 1990;33:731.

181. Bascom JU. Repeat pilonidal operations. Am J Surg 1987;154:118.

182. Jensen SL, Harling H. Prognosis after simple incision and drainage for a first-episode acute pilonidal abscess. Br J Surg 1988;75:60.

183. Kronborg O, Christensen K, Zimmermann-Nielsen C. Chronic pilonidal disease: a randomized trial with a complete 3-year follow up. Br J Surg 1985;72:303.

184. Solla JA, Rothenberger DA. Chronic pilonidal disease: an assessment of 150 cases. Dis Colon Rectum 1990;33:758.

185. Lineaweaver WC, Brunson MB, Smith JF, et al. Squamous carcinoma arising in a pilonidal sinus. J Surg Oncol 1984;27:239.

186. Thompson WG. Proctalgia fugax. Dig Dis Sci 1981;26:1121.

187. Panitch NM, Schofferman JA. Proctalgia fuga revisited. Gastroenterology 1975;68:106.

188. Thompson WG, Heaton KW. Proctalgia fugax. J R Coll Physicians Lond 1980;14:247.

189. Manning AP, Thompson WG, Heaton KW, et al. Towards positive diagnosis of the irritable bowel. Br Med J 1978;2:653.

190. Thompson WG. Proctalgia fugax in patients with the irritable bowel, peptic ulcer or inflammatory bowel disease. Am J Gastroenterol 1984;79:450.

191. Pilling LF, Swenson WM, Hill JR. The psychologic aspects of proctalgia fugax. Dis Colon Rectum 1972;8:372.

192. Kamm MA, Hoyle CH, Burleigh DE, et al. Hereditary internal anal sphincter myopathy causing proctalgia fugax and constipation. A newly identified condition. Gastroenterology 1991;100:805.

193. Kaufman W. Treatment of proctalgia fugax. Dig Dis Sci 1982;27:995.

194. Wright JE. Trial of inhaled salbutamol for proctalgia fugax. Lancet 1991;337:359.

195. Swain R. Case reports: oral clonidine for proctalgia fugax. Gut 1987;28:1039.

196. Boquet J, Moore N, Lhuintre JP, et al. Diltiazem for proctalgia fugax. Lancet 1986;1:1493.

197. Salvati EP. The levator syndrome and its variant. Gastroenterol Clin North Am 1987;16:71.

198. Sohn N, Weinstein MA, Robbins RD. The levator syndrome and its treatment with high-voltage electrogalvanic stimulation. Am J Surg 1982;144:580.

199. Nicosia JF, Abcarian H. Levator syndrome. A treatment that works. Dis Colon Rectum 1985;28:406.

200. Oliver GC, Rubin RJ, Salvati EP, et al. Electrogalvanic stimulation in the treatment of levator syndrome. Dis Colon Rectum 1985;28:662.

201. Wray CC, Easom S, Hoskinson J. Coccydynia. Aetiology and treatment. J Bone Joint Surg 1991;73:335.

202. Dugan RE. Familial rectal pain. Lancet 1972;1:1016.

203. Grimaud J, Bouvier M, Naudy B, et al. Manometric and radiologic investigations and biofeedback treatment of chronic idiopathic anal pain. Dis Colon Rectum 1991;34:690.

Textbook of Gastroenterology, second edition, edited by Tadataka Yamada. JB Lippincott Company, Philadelphia © 1995.

E. Pancreas

CHAPTER 89

Pancreas: Anatomy and Structural Anomalies

Michael W. Mulholland   A. R. Moossa
Rodger A. Liddle

Embryologic Development
Gross Anatomy
Surgical Exposure
Arterial Blood Supply
Venous Drainage
Lymphatic Drainage
Nerve Supply
Ductal System

Ultrastructure
Congenital Anomalies
   Agenesis or Hypoplasia of the Pancreas
   Annular Pancreas
   Heterotopic Pancreas
   Pancreas Divisum
   Congenital Cysts
   Multiple Cysts

Cross-sectional imaging techniques have greatly increased the understanding of pancreatic anatomy, and the ability to manipulate the pancreas surgically, endoscopically, and percutaneously has made it necessary for a wide variety of physicians to be familiar with pancreatic anatomic variations. The anatomy of the pancreas has been described in many standard texts, but the functional and therapeutic implications of its anatomic relations have often been underemphasized.

Diseases of the pancreas are often more difficult to manage medically or surgically than those of other abdominal viscera. The pancreas lies hidden in the deeper recesses of the retroperitoneal space of the upper abdomen, is largely protected by the lower rib cage anteriorly, and is almost completely covered by the stomach, transverse colon, and transverse mesocolon. At laparotomy, the pancreas cannot be properly visualized or palpated without extensive dissection, mobilization, and retraction.

The central position of the pancreas provides for lymphatic drainage along several major routes, namely, the splenic, hepatic, and superior mesenteric nodal systems as well as the aortocaval and other posterior abdominal wall lymphatics. Moreover, the intimate anatomic association of the pancreas with vital major vessels of the epigastrium at once limits the extent of any surgical procedure and also dictates what must be removed. Thus, when a tumor spreads a short distance to involve the superior mesenteric vein, the portal vein, or the celiac axis, it usually becomes incurable. Similarly, if the gland is removed in radical fashion, the need to excise the vessels and lymph nodes associated with it frequently makes removal of the duodenum, gallbladder, distal bile duct, spleen, upper jejunum, and part of the stomach necessary. Finally, the vascular nature of the pancreas and the adjacent organs makes it easy to understand why the most common intraoperative and postoperative complication of pancreatic resection is hemorrhage.

EMBRYOLOGIC DEVELOPMENT

The pancreas develops from two primordial outpouchings of the duodenum and is first apparent at 4 weeks' gestation. The dorsal pancreatic bud grows more rapidly than the ventral pancreas, and by the sixth week extends into the dorsal mesentery. The ventral pancreas remains smaller and is carried away from the duodenum by the development of the hepatic rudiment into the biliary system. Differential growth of the duodenum and axial rotation of the gut result in the dorsal pancreas being carried to the left and the ventral pancreas being carried to the right of the duodenum (Fig. 89-1). Migration of the distal common bile duct behind and to the left of the duodenum causes the ventral pancreas to lie below the

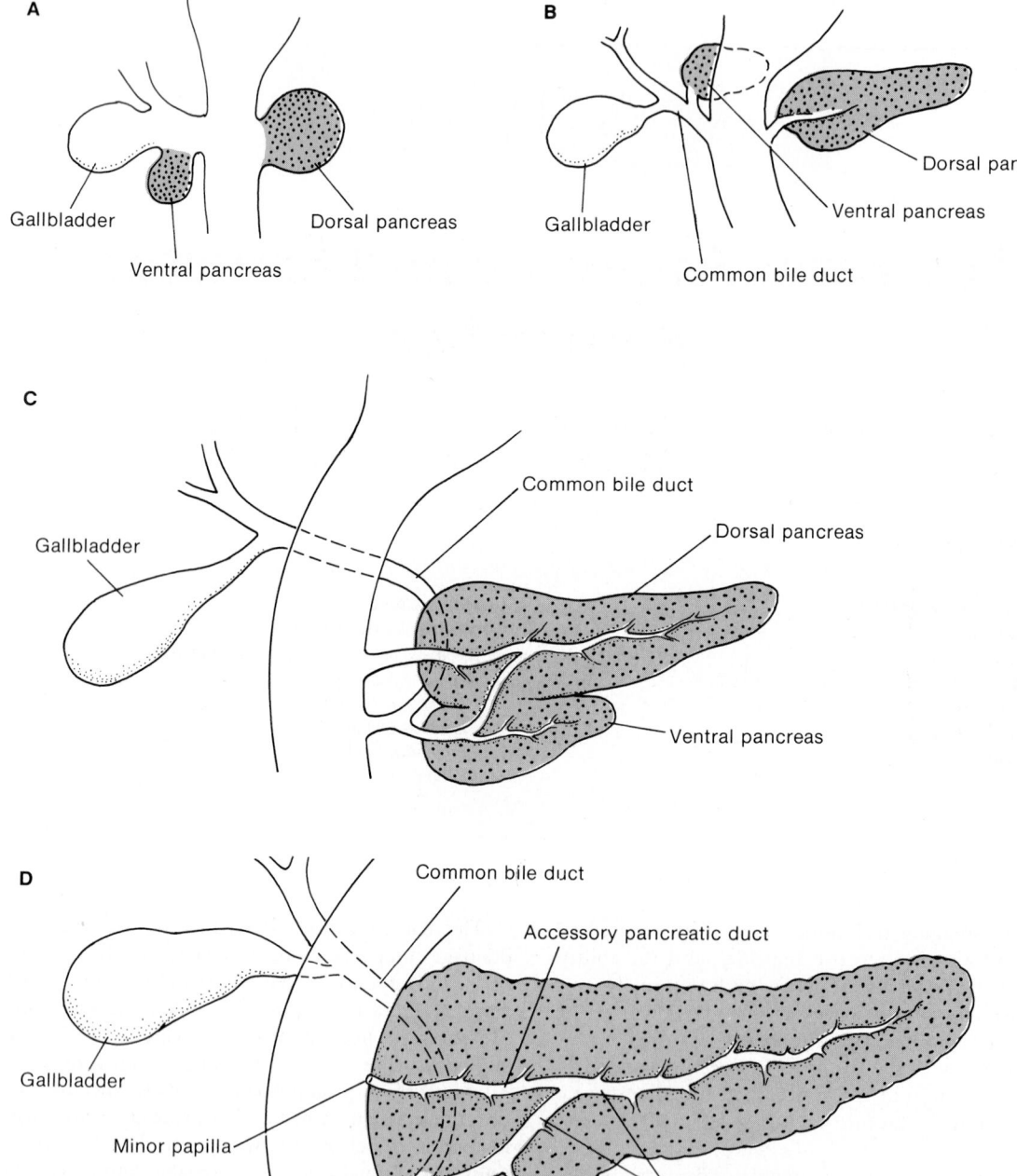

FIGURE 89-1. Embryologic development of the pancreas. The various stages of intrauterine pancreatic growth are shown at (**A**) 4 weeks, (**B**) 6 weeks, (**C**) 7 weeks, and (**D**) birth. (Adapted from Arey LB. Developmental anatomy. 7th ed. Philadelphia: WB Saunders, 1974:259.)

dorsal pancreas, forming the uncinate process of the pancreas. The common bile duct lies posterior to the dorsal pancreatic duct. Fusion of the two parts of the pancreas occurs during the seventh week of gestation. Fusion of the ventral duct with the dorsal duct results in the formation of the main pancreatic duct. The proximal end of the dorsal pancreatic duct usually does not communicate with the main duct and forms the accessory pancreatic duct.

The pancreatic acini and the first zymogen granules appear at 12 weeks' gestation. Groups of endocrine cells develop from multipotential stem cells in the ductular epithelium (nesidioblasts) at 9 weeks' gestation. Discrete islets of Langerhans can be identified at 12 weeks. Most of the islet cells develop within the tail of the pancreas and the dorsal pancreas. The first cells to produce granules are the alpha cells, soon followed by the beta and delta cells. Complete maturation of the pancreatic gland does not occur until some time after the end of gestation. The smooth muscle of the sphincter of Oddi develops independently of the duodenal musculature, and only later does it become incorporated into the duodenal wall.

Most recent evidence indicates that islet cells arise from centroacinar cells during the third month of gestation. Insulin-containing granules may be demonstrated immunocytochemically by the end of the third month. Islet cells migrate away from the acini in which they arise and move into the interlobular connective tissue. Mature islet morphology is established before birth.

GROSS ANATOMY

The pancreas is a soft, flattened, elongated gland, 12 to 20 cm long in the adult, that lies behind the peritoneum of the posterior abdominal wall and is obliquely rather than transversely oriented (Fig. 89-2; see Fig. 89-1). The pancreas has a lobular structure and, although totally invested in fine connective tissue, does not have a true fibrous capsule. The adult

gland weighs 85 to 95 g. Because of its oblique orientation, a transverse section, or computed tomography scan, does not normally pass through the entire length of the gland. The head of the pancreas is on the right side and lies within the C-shaped concavity of the duodenum at the level of the body of L2. The tail of the gland is to the left; the tail lies between the two layers of peritoneum that form the lienorenal ligament and is located at the level of the body of L1. The first portion of the duodenum is suspended in front of the head of the gland. The lesser curvature of the second part of the duodenum and the upper aspect of the third part of the duodenum intimately invest the head of the pancreas. Superiorly, the head is related to the gastroepiploic foramen and the structures that form the contents of the free border of the lesser omentum. Anteriorly, the first portion of the duodenum covers the superior part of the pancreatic head, and below this, the right side of the transverse mesocolon is attached transversely. Posteriorly, the head of the pancreas contacts the right renal hilum, both renal veins, the inferior vena cava, and the termination of the right gonadal vein as well as the right side of the aorta.[1]

The distal end of the common bile duct passes behind the upper border of the head of the pancreas. The bile duct grooves the posterior aspect of the head of the gland before passing through the substance of the head to reach the duodenal papilla of Vater. From the posterior aspect of the head, a tongue of pancreatic tissue of variable size, the uncinate process, extends to the left to occupy the concavity formed by the third and fourth part of the duodenum. The uncinate process lies anterior to the inferior vena cava and aorta and is covered superiorly and anteriorly by the superior mesenteric vessels as they emerge below the neck of the pancreas.

From the head of the pancreas, a constricted part of the gland extends toward the left and is referred to as the neck of the gland. It is 3 to 4 cm in width and joins the head of the gland to the body of the gland on the left. The pancreatic neck lies behind the posterior peritoneum of the lesser sac,

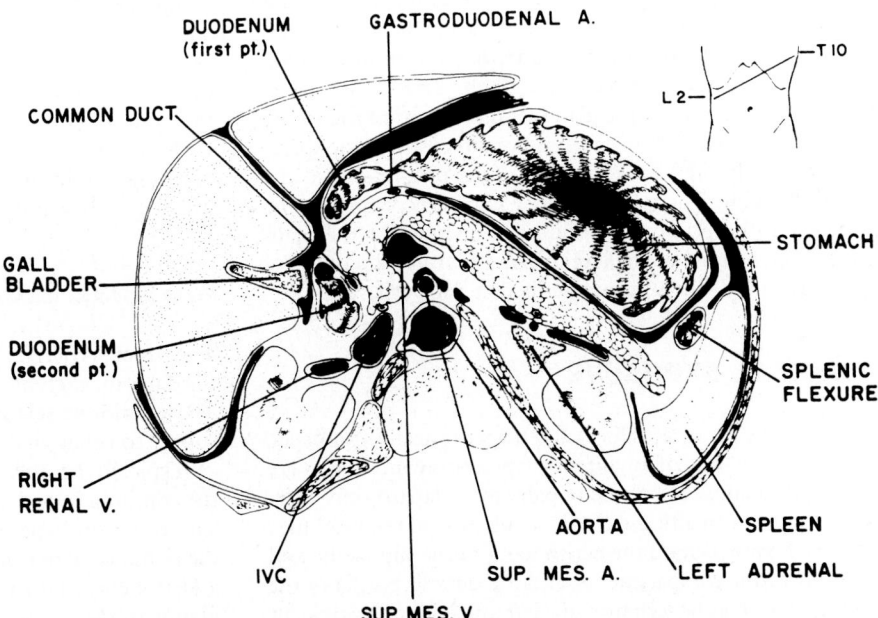

FIGURE 89-2. Oblique transverse cross section of the upper abdomen viewed from below. The section passes through the long axis of the pancreas at approximately the level indicated in the inset. The disposition and relations of structures shown approximate those seen on oblique transverse ultrasonic scanning.

its inferior border being covered by the attachments of the transverse mesocolon and the root of the small bowel mesentery. The neck of the pancreas lies anterior to and is closely related to the confluence of the superior mesenteric and splenic veins, which form the lowest part of the portal vein.

In front of the aorta in the midline, the body of the pancreas continues its retroperitoneal course toward the left side, held securely against the aorta and the posterior parietes by the posterior peritoneum of the lesser sac. The antrum and the body of the stomach contact the body of the pancreas anteriorly. Posteriorly, the left renal vein, passing between the aorta and the pancreas, is separated by the latter from the first part of the superior mesenteric artery. At a slightly higher level, elements of the celiac and superior mesenteric plexus ramify between the pancreas and the aorta. The midline part of the body of the pancreas is pushed anteriorly by the bodies of L1 and L2 and, therefore, lies closest to the anterior abdominal wall. Because of its prominence and fixity in this region, this area of the pancreas is most vulnerable to blunt abdominal injuries. In addition, a tumor in this region may be palpated as a mass that does not move with respiration and that strongly transmits the aortic pulsation. The celiac axis, surrounded by the celiac plexus, divides into its major branches between the superior border of the body of the pancreas and the crura of the diaphragm.

The body of the pancreas passes laterally, posteriorly, and slightly cephalad behind the posterior peritoneum of the lesser sac and merges imperceptibly with the tail of the gland. The exact junction of the body and tail is not discernible anatomically. The posterior relationships of the body and tail of the pancreas include the posterior attachment of the left crus of the diaphragm, the left suprarenal gland, the upper pole of the left kidney, and hilum of the spleen. The splenic vein above and the left renal vein below lie close to one another behind the body and tail of the gland.

At the upper border of the body and tail of the pancreas, the splenic artery courses to the left from its origin at the celiac axis. The transverse mesocolon is attached to the anterior part of the lower border of the gland. The splenocolic ligament attaches the splenic flexure of the colon to the hilum of the spleen and brings it adjacent to the tail of the pancreas.

There are variations in shape and disposition of the pancreas as demonstrated by pancreatography. In 57% of people, the bulk of the head of the gland is to the right of the spinal column. In about 38% of cases, it lies directly over the spine, but only rarely (5%) does the head of the pancreas lie to the left of the spine. There is a tendency in elderly people for the pancreas to be ptotic. The duodenal opening of the main pancreatic duct lies at the level of L2 to L4 in 92% of cases, but, very rarely, it has been described at a lower level.

SURGICAL EXPOSURE

Although the pancreas is located retroperitoneally, it must be approached by way of an anterior laparotomy incision. Very little of the gland can be seen or palpated at laparotomy without dissection. In a thin patient, small areas of the head may be seen directly behind the peritoneum of the supracolic and right infracolic compartments, and the inferior border of the body and tail may be seen from the left infracolic compartment

at the root of the transverse mesocolon. These limited views, however, are usually obscured by omental, mesocolic, and retroperitoneal fat. The neck of the pancreas may be felt from above by a finger passed through the gastroepiploic foramen of Winslow.

The head of the pancreas may be inspected and palpated more closely by performing two maneuvers.[2] First, the hepatic flexure of the colon is mobilized downward and medially, dividing the attachments of the transverse colon to the front of the duodenum and pancreatic head as far as the origin of the middle colic vessels. In addition, the attachments of the right side of the greater omentum to the transverse colon are divided. Thus, the lesser sac can be widely exposed on the right side of the middle colic vessels. Second, the peritoneum lateral to the second part of the duodenum is incised, and the duodenum and pancreatic head may be elevated and swept to the left by blunt dissection, exposing the right renal vein, the inferior vena cava, the right gonadal vein, the origin of the left renal vein, and the retroduodenal and retropancreatic portions of the distal common bile duct. After this mobilization (Kocher maneuver), the head of the pancreas may be palpated anteroposteriorly between the thumb and fingers. The mesenteric vessels are obscured from view by the uncinate process.

Limited visualization of the superior part of the body of the pancreas may be obtained by opening an avascular part of the lesser (gastrohepatic) omentum and retracting the lesser curvature of the stomach inferiorly. This maneuver also brings the celiac axis into view. A much more adequate visualization of the body of the pancreas may be obtained by widely opening the lesser sac. This is achieved by dividing the gastrocolic omentum at its attachment to the transverse colon. Extending this opening to the right into the subpyloric region allows visualization of the anterior aspect of the head and neck of the pancreas, especially if the right gastroepiploic vessels are ligated and divided. Extending the opening to the left and dividing the short gastric (gastrosplenic) vessels in the gastrosplenic ligament superiorly and the relatively vascular splenocolic ligament inferiorly gives complete visualization of the anterior surface of the body and tail of the pancreas. The spleen, splenic vessels, and tail of the pancreas may be mobilized medially and anteriorly en bloc, allowing inspection of the posterior aspect of the tail and body of the gland. All these surgical maneuvers may be carried out quickly and safely with little risk of damage to vital structures or troublesome bleeding. By this means, all except the region of the neck and uncinate process of the pancreas may be fully evaluated.

ARTERIAL BLOOD SUPPLY

The pancreas derives its blood supply from the celiac axis and the superior mesenteric artery (Fig. 89-3; see Color Fig. 50). These major vessels and their branches also provide the blood supply to other vital organs adjacent to the pancreas.

Typically (in 90% of people), the celiac axis divides into the common hepatic, the splenic, and the left gastric arteries. The common hepatic artery passes to the right, anterior to the portal vein, to reach the free border of the lesser omentum, and usually lies to the left of the common bile duct. After giving off the gastroduodenal artery, the hepatic artery turns

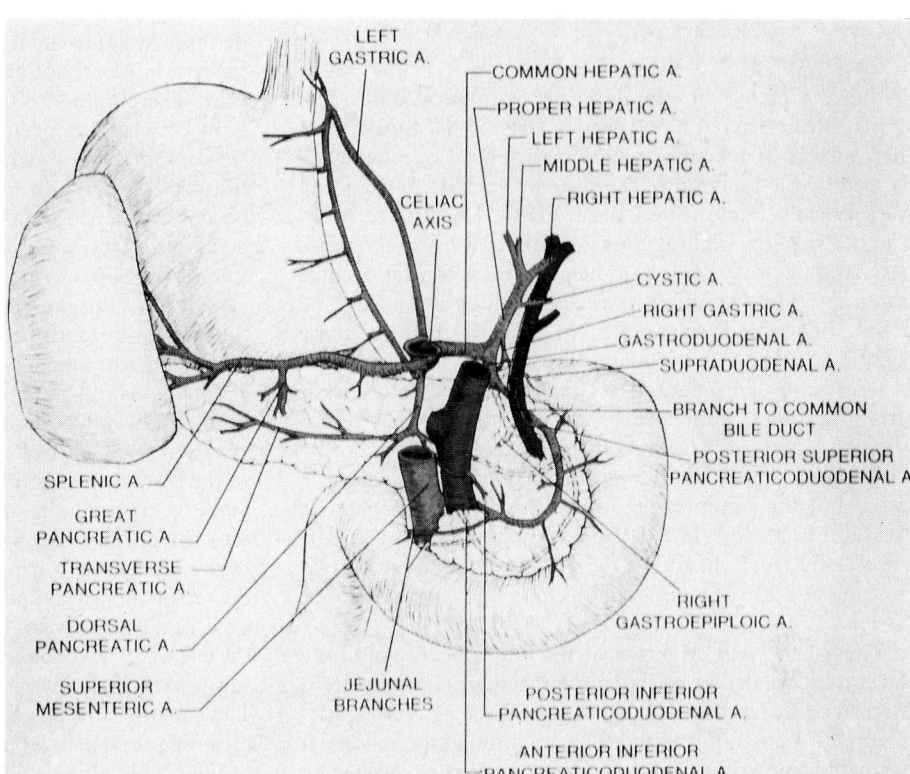

FIGURE 89-3. (See Color Fig. 50.) Blood supply of the pancreas. The pancreas, duodenum, stomach, and spleen are viewed from their posterior aspects.

upward toward the porta hepatis and divides into the left and right hepatic arteries. The middle hepatic artery, supplying the caudate lobe of the liver, is usually a branch of one of these two vessels. This arrangement of the hepatic arterial blood supply, however, occurs in only 55% of people. Replaced or accessory hepatic arteries are frequent, occurring in as many as 30% of people. The most frequent variation from normal is the right hepatic artery branching off from the superior mesenteric artery and coursing behind the uncinate process and the head of the pancreas to reach the free border of the lesser omentum.[3]

The gastroduodenal artery usually originates from the hepatic artery. The gastroduodenal artery courses from its origin behind the first part of the duodenum and, after giving off the posterior superior pancreaticoduodenal artery, lies on the anterior surface of the head of the pancreas. At the lower border of the first part of the duodenum, it branches into the right gastroepiploic artery and the anterior superior pancreaticoduodenal artery.

For the most part, the head of the pancreas and duodenum have a common blood supply—the anterior and posterior pancreaticoduodenal arcades. The anterior arcade gives off the only arteries that enter the head of the gland from its anterior aspect. This arcade is formed by the anastomosis of the anterior superior pancreaticoduodenal artery, which is a terminal branch of the gastroduodenal artery, and the anterior inferior pancreaticoduodenal artery, which is usually a branch of a common inferior pancreaticoduodenal artery, arising from the superior mesenteric artery.

The posterior pancreaticoduodenal arcade is formed by the anastomosis of the posterior superior pancreaticoduodenal artery, usually a branch of the gastroduodenal artery, and the

posterior inferior pancreaticoduodenal artery, which arises in a way analogous to the anterior pancreaticoduodenal artery. Of surgical importance is the relation of the posterior superior pancreaticoduodenal artery to the common bile duct. Typically, this vessel arises from the gastroduodenal artery and passes to the right, anterior to the common bile duct, contributing the major source of the structure's blood supply. The supraduodenal portion of the common bile duct also may be crossed anteriorly by the right hepatic artery, the right gastric artery, and the supraduodenal artery, making mobilization of the lower end of the common bile duct more difficult.

Because of the shared blood supply of the duodenum and pancreatic head, extensive interference with the pancreaticoduodenal arcades in the course of a 95% pancreatectomy may compromise the blood supply of the duodenum.[4] In addition, because the duodenojejunal flexure and the first part of the jejunum may derive their blood supply from branches of the inferior pancreaticoduodenal artery or the pancreaticoduodenal arcades, ligation of these vessels in the course of a resection may render the proximal jejunum ischemic.

The body and tail of the gland derive their blood supply chiefly from branches of the splenic artery. This vessel, the largest branch of the celiac axis (5–11 mm in diameter), courses laterally at the upper border of the pancreas; its characteristic marked tortuosity appears to be related to age, being often absent in infants and most marked in the elderly. The splenic artery gives multiple side branches to supply the neck, body, and tail of the pancreas. The termination of the splenic artery passes between the layers of the lienorenal ligament and, at the hilum of the spleen, four or five branches enter the splenic hilum separately.

The general pattern of veins draining the pancreas is the same as that of the arterial blood supply (Fig. 89-4). Blood from the pancreas drains ultimately into the portal vein, which is formed by the junction of the superior mesenteric vein and splenic vein behind the neck of the gland. The close relationship of the portal and superior mesenteric veins to the head, neck, and uncinate process of the pancreas is of vital surgical importance; in determining the resectability of a pancreatic lesion, a key step is the assessment of involvement of these veins. The portal vein originates from behind the neck of the pancreas as a continuation of the superior mesenteric vein after it becomes confluent with the splenic vein. The portal vein passes upward to the right to gain access to the free border of the lesser omentum where it lies posterior to the hepatic artery and the common bile duct. At the porta hepatis, it divides into a short, broad, right branch and a longer, narrower, left branch. In adults, the portal vein is about 8 to 10 cm long and 8 to 14 mm wide. Its average length is about 8.4 cm.[5]

The splenic vein originates at the hilum of the spleen by the confluence of five or six tributaries draining the spleen. It receives the basal brevia (short gastric veins) and left gastroepiploic veins at the hilum. It passes through the lienorenal ligament behind the tail of the pancreas and below the splenic artery and is the large, straight vein that courses to the right in contact with the posterior surface of the pancreas. It receives many tributaries from the tail, body, and neck of the gland.

Below the pancreas, the ileocolic vein passes directly, and usually without tributaries, from the ileocecal region to join the right side of the superior mesenteric vein in the midline just above the inferior border of the third part of the duo-denum. At approximately the same level on the left side, the superior mesenteric vein is joined by the jejunointermediate vein. The confluence of these three veins forms the lower limit of what has been termed the "surgical trunk" of the superior mesenteric vein. Above this point, approximately two thirds of the superior mesenteric vein lies below the inferior border of the neck of the pancreas, the remaining one third being retropancreatic. The superior jejunal vein joins the left side of the superior mesenteric vein. The middle colic vein usually joins the superior mesenteric vein immediately below the inferior border of the pancreatic neck.

The inferior mesenteric vein typically joins the splenic vein vertically behind the body of the pancreas. The latter passes horizontally and combines with the superior mesenteric vein at a right angle to form the portal vein, which turns obliquely to the right to pass into the free edge of the lesser omentum. Small veins draining the head of the pancreas pass directly into the portal vein. Similarly, small veins draining the uncinate process terminate in the right and posterior aspects of the retropancreatic superior mesenteric vein. The anterior aspects of the major veins are usually free from tributaries. From the left side, the coronary vein joins the retropancreatic portal vein and the pyloric vein joins the suprapancreatic portal vein. The superior and posterior pancreaticoduodenal veins drain into the portal vein from the right side, deep to the first part of the duodenum and opposite to the pyloric vein. The coronary, or left gastric, vein usually (60% of cases) drains into the left side of the retropancreatic portal vein, but may have a high termination well above the neck of the pancreas.

The close anatomic relationship of the splenic vein with the pancreas often leads to splenic vein occlusion in inflammatory or neoplastic diseases involving the body and tail of the gland. Retrograde venous drainage toward the splenic

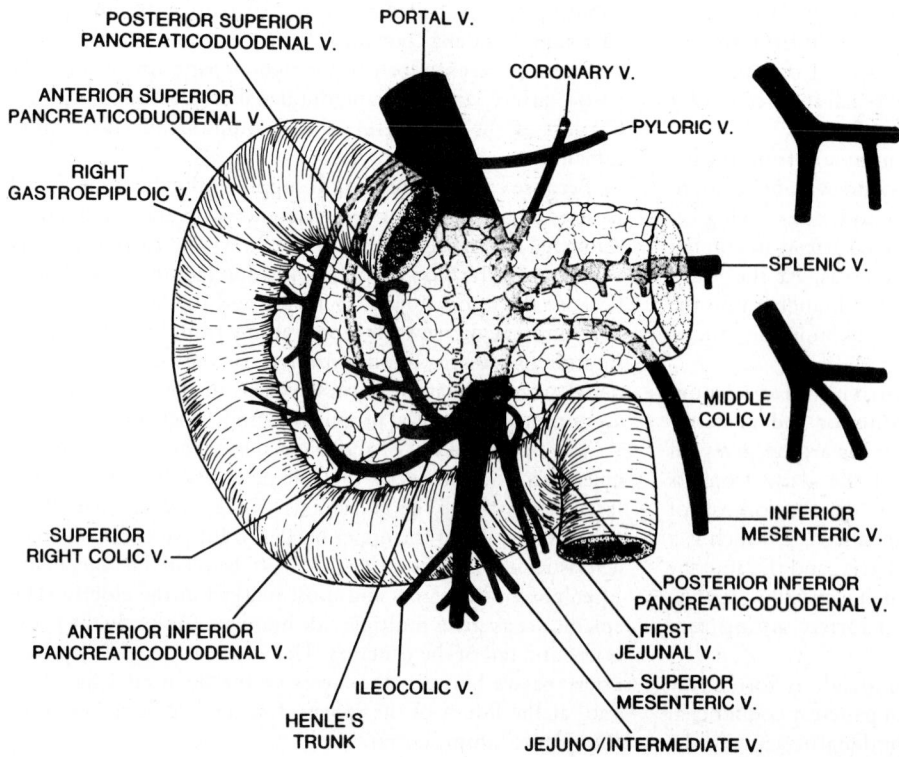

FIGURE 89-4. Venous drainage of the pancreas. The pancreas and duodenum are viewed from their anterior aspects. Insets indicate normal variations in the termination of the inferior mesenteric vein.

hilum and then by way of the short gastric veins and the left gastroepiploic vein creates the syndrome of left-sided portal hypertension and gastric varices.

LYMPHATIC DRAINAGE

The lymphatic vessels of the pancreas conform to the general pattern of deep lymphatic drainage and accompany the arterial supply (Fig. 89-5; see Color Fig. 51). The duodenum and head of the pancreas have a common lymphatic drainage, and lymph from the foregut and midgut structures, including the pancreas, liver, stomach, spleen, small bowel, and proximal large bowel, flows eventually into the celiac and superior mesenteric groups of paraaortic nodes and into the cisterna chyli.[6] The lymphatics of the tail of the pancreas pass to the splenic nodes at the hilum of the spleen, and those of the body of the pancreas pass upward to the pancreaticosplenic nodes lying along the superior border of the gland. These nodes, along with the retropancreatic nodes, drain into the celiac nodes. Lymphatics of the upper anterior part of the head of the pancreas pass through the subpyloric nodes lying behind the first part of the duodenum. Obstruction of these pancreatic lymphatic drainage pathways by tumor may result in the shunting of lymph through local collateral channels, resulting in the involvement of nodes primarily concerned with hepatic or gastric drainage. Inferiorly, the retropancreatic and antepancreatic group of nodes drain into the superior mesenteric nodes, and lymph from the latter may also pass into nodes in the root of the transverse mesocolon. The absence of fascial or retroperitoneal coverings on the posterior aspect of the pancreas allows easy communication between lymphatics of the pancreas and those of neighboring retroperitoneal tissues and organs. The lymphatic network is so rich that a thorough lymphadenectomy en bloc with a pancreatic resection frequently produces a profuse postoperative chylous leakage.[7]

NERVE SUPPLY

The sympathetic efferent innervation of the pancreas is derived from the greater, lesser, and least splanchnic nerves. The bodies of the preganglionic sympathetic neurons originate in the lateral gray matter of the thoracic spinal segments 5 through 10. After transversing the sympathetic trunks, presynaptic nerve fibers synapse with postganglionic sympathetic neurons within the celiac plexus, although there is some minor distribution to the pancreas through the hepatic and superior mesenteric plexuses. The celiac ganglion consists of two masses that lie on either side of the aorta, anterior to the crura of the diaphragm, close to the adrenal glands. The right celiac ganglion is partly covered by the inferior vena cava, and the left celiac ganglion is covered by the peritoneum of the lesser sac close to the upper border of the pancreas. The cell bodies of afferent sympathetic neurons are located in dorsal root ganglia. Afferent fibers often cross the midline in celiac ganglia before projecting centrally, so that sympathetic afferent innervation is bilateral.

The parasympathetic innervation of the pancreas is derived from the vagal nerves. The cell bodies for efferent vagal fibers are located in the medulla in the dorsal motor nucleus. Efferent fibers pass to the pancreas by way of the celiac division of the posterior vagal trunk. No synaptic connections are made within the celiac ganglia; postsynaptic neurons are located

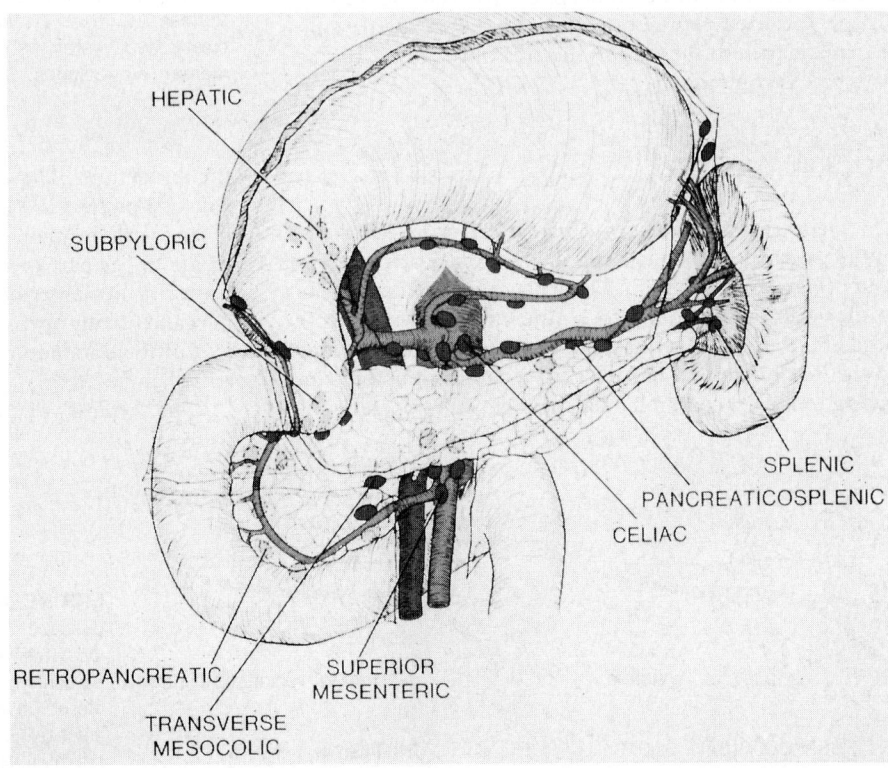

FIGURE 89-5. (See Color Fig. 51.) Lymphatic drainage of the pancreas. The pancreas is viewed from its anterior aspect. The gastrocolic ligament has been divided along the greater curvature of the stomach, which has been retracted anterosuperiorly. The transverse mesocolon has been detached from the peritoneum of the posterior abdominal wall. Labels indicate representative lymph nodes in the major regional nodal groups.

within the pancreatic parenchyma. Afferent vagal fibers also pass through the celiac ganglia; afferent cell bodies are located within the nucleus ambiguus.[8]

The ultrastructure of pancreatic innervation has been studied extensively in several animal species in addition to humans. Myelinated fibers usually are not found within the parenchyma. Intrapancreatic ganglion cells are seen within the interlobular tissues with nonmyelinated fibers passing to both exocrine and endocrine portions of the gland. The sites of nerve termination may be generally grouped as blood vessels, pancreatic acinar cells, ductal cells, and pancreatic islets. Functional correlates suggest that pancreatic nerves may modulate function of each of these pancreatic elements. In addition to the classic cholinergic and adrenergic neurons, evidence suggests that a large number of peptide-containing neurons also exist within the pancreas. Immunocytochemical methods have demonstrated the presence of fibers or cell bodies containing vasoactive intestinal polypeptide, substance P, gastrin-releasing peptide, enkephalin, galanin, neuropeptide Y, and calcitonin gene-related peptide.[9] The physiologic actions of most of these peptidergic nerves within the pancreas remain to be defined, but anatomic studies suggest that modulation of release of acetylcholine and catecholamines from autonomic nerve terminals within the pancreas may be important. Regulation of pancreas blood flow also is an important function of intrapancreatic neurons.

Pain fibers from the pancreas travel through the celiac ganglia and by way of the sympathetic splanchnic nerves and the thoracic sympathetic chain to reach the spinal root ganglia. Pain from the head of the pancreas tends to be broadly localized in the midepigastrium, and pain from the body and tail tends to be localized in the left upper quadrant. Visceral pain from the pancreas is usually sensed as a severe, constant discomfort in the epigastrium. Because the pancreas does not contact the somatically innervated parietal peritoneum, sharply localized pain does not usually occur. Radiation of pancreatic pain to the back in the area of the lower thoracic vertebrae is common.

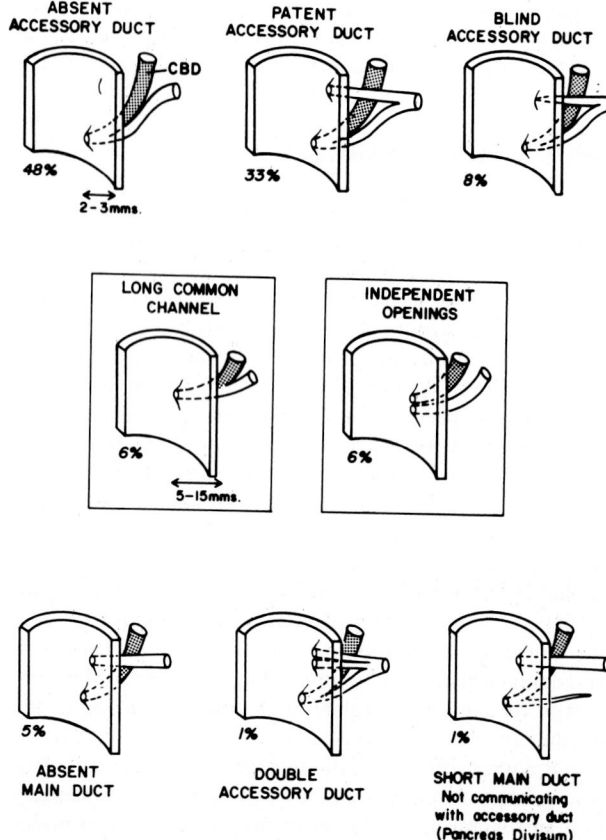

FIGURE 89-7. Variations of main and accessory pancreatic ducts, and their relation to the common bile duct (CBD) from a series of 143 postmortem preparations. Accessory duct variations and usual short common channel for CBD and main pancreatic duct (*top*); variations of CBD and main pancreatic duct terminations (*middle*); miscellaneous variations (*bottom*). (Adapted from Berman LG, Prior JT, Abramow SM, et al. A study of the pancreatic duct system in man by use of vinyl acetate casts of post mortem preparations. Surg Gynecol Obstet 1969;110:391.)

DUCTAL SYSTEM

The main pancreatic duct of Wirsung extends from the tail of the pancreas to the major duodenal papilla or ampulla of Vater (Figs. 89-6 and 89-7). The average diameter of the duct in the adult tapers from 4 to 2 mm, and it is widest in the head of the gland.[10] The main duct is close and almost parallel to the distal common bile duct for 2 to 3 mm before combining to form a common duct channel before opening into

the duodenum. The accessory pancreatic duct of Santorini, which is present in 40% to 70% of people, usually communicates with the main duct and passes transversely to the right in the upper part of the head of the pancreas. The duct of Santorini lies anterior to the intrapancreatic common bile duct and usually opens into the proximal portion of the second part of the duodenum at the minor papilla, proximal to the ampulla of Vater.

This "typical" ductal anatomy may actually be present in

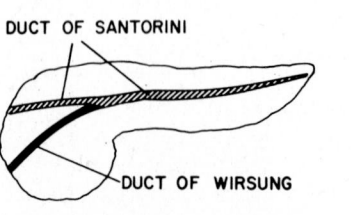

EMBRYOLOGICAL BASIS

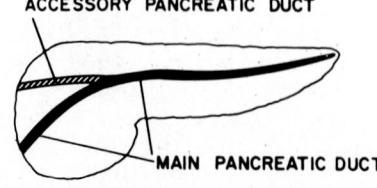

FUNCTIONAL BASIS

FIGURE 89-6. Terminology variously applied to describe the pancreatic duct system. One system indicates an understanding of ductal embryology, particularly with regard to the development of the more unusual variations (*left*). For clarity and practicality, however, the terms given on the right are preferred.

as few as 33% of people.[11] Important variations include non-patency of the accessory duct (8%), independent openings of the common bile duct and the main pancreatic duct (6%), an absent main duct (5%), and patent double accessory ducts (1%). Noncommunication between the main duct and the accessory duct, with the body and tail of the gland draining exclusively by way of the duct of Santorini, results in the anatomic variant known as *pancreas divisum,* and occurs in 2% to 6% of otherwise healthy people.

The sphincter of Oddi consists of circular smooth muscle that surrounds the common channel of the common bile duct and the main pancreatic duct at the ampulla of Vater. The muscle fibers of the sphincter of Oddi extend around the common bile duct just distal to the latter's oblique entry into the wall of the duodenum to form the choledochal sphincter. A short region of circular smooth muscle also surrounds the pancreatic duct just before its termination to form the pancreatic duct sphincter.

ULTRASTRUCTURE

The pancreas is a mixed endocrine and exocrine gland. The glandular constituents by weight are 80% exocrine tissue, 18% ductular system, and 2% endocrine tissue. The pancreas is a lobulated organ with lobular subunits composed of acini. The acini are rounded or have a short tubular form and consist of single rows of epithelial cells lying on a basal lamina. Lining the lumen of the acinus are pyramidal acinar cells and pale-staining centroacinar cells, which are unique to the pancreas. The acinar lumen connects with the intralobular ducts to form the interlobular ducts, which, in turn, coalesce to form the main pancreatic duct. Lining the ductules are columnar cells, goblet cells, and occasional argentaffin cells. The large ducts are surrounded by thick layers of connective tissue and elastic fibers.

In the resting state, the basal portion of the acinar cell contains a centrally located spherical nucleus lying within a highly basophilic cytoplasm secondary to the large number of ribosomes in the rough endoplasmic reticulum. The abundant ribosomes attest to the high protein-synthesizing capacity of the acinar cells. A clear region containing the Golgi complex separates the nucleus from numerous eosinophilic zymogen granules, each about 1 μm in diameter, lying at the apex. The acinar cell has short microvilli, averaging 0.2 μm in length, which protrude into the acinar lumen. At the apical portion, the cells are held together by tight junctions, which prevent reflux of lumenal contents. Laterally, the cells are connected by gap junctions, which permit intercellular communication.

The thin basal lamina on which the acini rest is supported by collagen fibers. A rich capillary plexus surrounds the acinus in this connective tissue and is penetrated by numerous nerve fibers, which reach the acinar cells.[12]

The endocrine portion of the pancreas consists of approximately one million islets of Langerhans. These are distributed throughout the gland but are relatively concentrated in the tail of the pancreas. The islets are about 200 μm in diameter, and each is associated with a prominent capillary plexus. The islets contain several cell types. Approximately 75% to 80% of islet cells are beta or B cells, which secrete insulin, and 10% to 20% are alpha or A cells, which contain glucagon.

Delta or D cells comprise about 5% of the islets and contain somatostatin.[13] The B cells occupy the center of the islets, whereas the perimeter is lined by A cells. D cells are dispersed in between these groups. Other peptide-secreting cells that may be associated with the islets include EC cells containing 5-hydroxytryptamine and PP cells containing pancreatic polypeptide.

CONGENITAL ANOMALIES

Agenesis or Hypoplasia of the Pancreas

Agenesis of the pancreas is a rare and, until recently, universally fatal condition.[14] Failure of the pancreas to develop may occur as an isolated anomaly or may be associated with other congenital defects, such as absence of the gallbladder.[15] Although the cause is not known, pancreatic agenesis has been associated with retarded intrauterine growth, presumably resulting from failure of the endocrine pancreas to produce insulin.[16] Partial agenesis of the pancreas results from incomplete formation of either the dorsal or ventral pancreas and has a more favorable outcome than complete agenesis. Involvement of the dorsal segment appears to be more common than involvement of the ventral pancreas. These glands possess normal exocrine and endocrine function.

Hypoplasia of the pancreas is a congenital disease involving exclusively the exocrine pancreas and has been referred to as "lipomatous pseudohypertrophy of the pancreas."[17] Pathologically, the gland appears enlarged and of normal shape but is of fatty consistency. The major pancreatic ducts are developed, and islets of Langerhans are present; however, secondary pancreatic ducts and acinar lobules are absent or underdeveloped, and fatty tissue replaces normal acinar cells.[18] The finding that the gland is of normal shape, but missing differentiated cellular components, has led investigators to postulate that embryologic development is normal in this condition. It is proposed that an intrauterine insult occurs, such as infection, causing hypoplasia of the exocrine gland.[19] Although this disease is usually diagnosed in infants, it has been reported to occur in adults.[17,18] Manifestations result from severe pancreatic exocrine insufficiency.

Annular Pancreas

Annular pancreas is an unusual complication of disturbed embryologic development in which the head of the pancreas surrounds the duodenum, often resulting in duodenal obstruction. Annular pancreas is frequently associated with other congenital defects, including Down's syndrome, Meckel's diverticulum, malrotation of the intestine, duodenal atresia and bands, intestinal webs, tracheoesophageal fistulas, imperforate anus, absence of the gallbladder, and certain types of cardiac defects.[20-24] Annular pancreas has been described in association with pancreas divisum (see Pancreas Divisum).[25] Men appear to be more commonly affected than women. The occurrence of annular pancreas is usually sporadic, although several reports describe a familial association and apparent autosomal dominant transmission.[26-28]

Typically, the annulus is a band of pancreatic tissue completely encircling the second portion of the duodenum (Fig. 89-8). The ring usually lies proximal to the major papilla, and in a few cases the annulus involves the first or third portion of the duodenum. Histologically, pancreatic tissue frequently invades the muscularis layer of the duodenum.[29]

The most popular etiologic theory suggests that the ventral pancreatic bud becomes fixed, and as the pancreas and duodenum rotate, a band of pancreatic tissue is left encircling the duodenum.[30] Supporting this theory is the report that a high concentration of pancreatic polypeptide cells, which is characteristic of the ventral pancreas, was found in annular tissue.[31] Other theories propose that hypertrophy of the dorsal and ventral ducts or ectopic pancreatic tissue causes the annulus.[32]

Over half of all cases are diagnosed in the first year of life. Severe duodenal stenosis is usually apparent within the first few days of birth. Because pancreatic tissue encircles the duodenum, causing obstruction, newborns and infants are intolerant of oral feedings and have vomiting, often of bilious material. Upper abdominal distention and visible peristalsis are often present on physical examination.[33] Although vomiting is the usual presenting symptom in children, adults often complain of postprandial colicky abdominal pain, bloating, and fullness that also may be associated with nausea and vomiting.[34–37] Upper gastrointestinal bleeding and duodenal ulcer disease occur in one third of adults, and acute pancreatitis is a commonly associated finding in this disorder.

Radiographic signs of annular pancreas are those of duodenal obstruction. Plain radiographs of the abdomen often show a "double-bubble" sign resulting from dilation of the duodenum and stomach. With high degrees of obstruction, a duodenal cutoff sign also may be seen. In infants, these findings are the only necessary radiographic tests. Radiographic findings are not specific in older children and adults, and it is usually necessary to document duodenal obstruction by upper gastrointestinal contrast studies. Constricting bands,

0.8 to 5 cm in length, around the duodenum have been detected radiographically.[38] Other signs include dilatation and reverse peristalsis of the proximal duodenum. Endoscopic evaluation of annular pancreas usually is not helpful. The mucosa usually is normal, and it is difficult to appreciate mild narrowing of the duodenum. In severe cases, concentric narrowing of the duodenum or stenosis and associated peptic ulcer disease are suggestive of the diagnosis. Endoscopic retrograde cholangiopancreatography (ERCP) has been used to visualize the ductal system in annular pancreas and is diagnostic of the disorder.[39–42] Similarly, characteristic features can be determined by computed tomography.[43]

In symptomatic patients, treatment of annular pancreas is surgical alleviation of the obstruction. Division of the annulus is not recommended because of the high incidence of pancreatitis and pancreatic fistulas complicating that procedure, and bypass of the obstructed intestinal segment is preferred.[44]

Heterotopic Pancreas

Aberrant localization of pancreatic tissue, also known as pancreatic rests or heterotopic pancreas, refers to segments of pancreatic tissue not in continuity with the main body of the pancreas. The condition is usually asymptomatic, and therefore its incidence is difficult to determine. Autopsy studies have reported frequencies ranging from 0.6% to 15%.[45,46] Seventy percent of such rests are found along the upper gastrointestinal tract; other intraabdominal locations include the gallbladder, liver, small intestine, colon, appendix, omentum, and Meckel's diverticulum.[47–49] In the stomach, pancreatic rests are found primarily in the prepyloric region along the greater curvature. Extraabdominal sites include the lung and umbilicus.[50–52] Histologically, heterotopic pancreas can contain acinar tissue, islets, and ducts, or any combination thereof. Seventy-five percent of rests are located in the submucosa of the stomach or intestine and appear as firm, yellow nodules 2 to 4 cm in diameter underlying the mucosa. These often have a central mucosal depression that may be recognized endoscopically or by radiographic contrast studies. The origin of heterotopic pancreas is not known, and it is likely that several abnormalities of embryologic development account for the locations in various sites. As pluripotential cells, pancreatic rests may represent abnormal differentiation of endodermal stem cells. Conversely, disturbances in migration of the pancreas as it rotates around the gut may account for some heterotopic locations.[53]

Heterotopic pancreas is usually an asymptomatic condition that is an incidental finding at surgery or autopsy. Symptoms attributed to this disorder include abdominal distention, epigastric pain, nausea, and vomiting.[54,55] Peptic ulcer disease and upper gastrointestinal bleeding have also been described. Because of the varied locations of pancreatic rests, involvement of other organs can occur. Pancreatitis, biliary obstruction with jaundice, intestinal obstruction, and intussusception have all been associated with heterotopic pancreas.[56–62] As a result of the combined exocrine and endocrine function of the pancreas, any pathologic change in the normal pancreas also can occur in ectopic tissue.[63] Therefore, malignant degeneration, cyst formation, and islet cell tumors also may be found in pancreatic rests.[64–68]

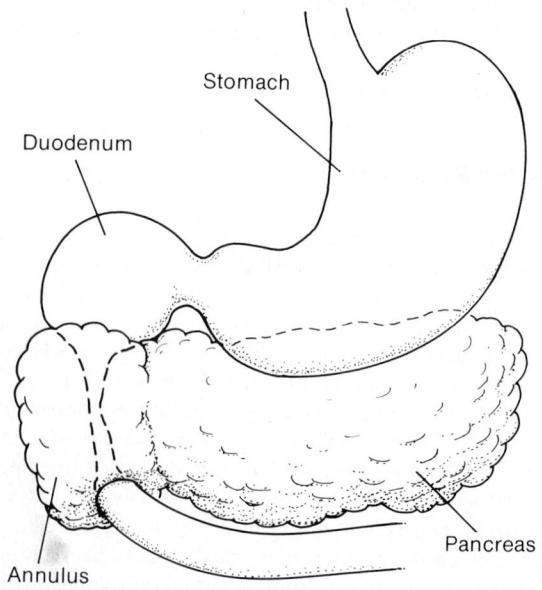

FIGURE 89-8. Annular pancreas. A band of pancreatic tissue surrounds the midportion of the duodenum.

Diagnosis of pancreatic rests involving the upper gastrointestinal tract can be made by contrast radiographs or endoscopy if submucosal nodules can be identified.[69,70] The lesions often can be confused with leiomyomas, lymphomas, or adenomatous polyps, and can be distinguished only by endoscopic biopsy.

Treatment of ectopic pancreatic tissue is indicated only for those who have significant symptoms or complications, such as recurrent upper gastrointestinal bleeding, biliary or intestinal obstruction, or malignant degeneration. Definitive treatment is surgical removal of the ectopic tissue. Asymptomatic people with incidental discovery of heterotopic pancreas do not require further evaluation or treatment.[63] If unsuspected pancreatic rests are found at the time of surgery, excision prevents the possible complication of malignant degeneration and eliminates confusion if subsequent symptoms develop.[63,71]

Pancreas Divisum

Pancreas divisum is the most common anomaly of the pancreas. Pancreas divisum is caused by failure of the ducts of the dorsal and ventral anlagen to fuse during embryologic development. Normally, the proximal one third of the dorsal pancreatic duct regresses as it fuses with the ventral duct, forming the main pancreatic duct. In pancreas divisum, the ventral duct of Wirsung empties into the duodenum through the major papilla but drains only a small portion of the pancreas. Secretions from the tail, body, neck, and remainder of the head of the pancreas drain into the duodenum through the minor papilla by way of a persistent duct of Santorini. In 2% to 3% of cases in which the ducts do not fuse, the ventral duct may not be demonstrable. Normally, drainage of the pancreas can occur by either duct, depending on fusion of the two ductal systems and the degree of patency of each. Most pancreatic drainage is through the duct of Wirsung, and although some drainage occurs through the duct of San-

torini, this volume is relatively small. Occasionally, the duct of Santorini ends blindly in the duodenal wall.

Although pancreas divisum is a long-recognized entity, only with the advent of ERCP has its clinical significance become apparent. In autopsy series, pancreas divisum has an incidence of 5% to 10%[72]; as an ERCP finding its incidence is 4%.[73-75] In a series of patients with pancreatitis, however, there was a 16% incidence of pancreas divisum, and the incidence of the abnormality increased to 25% in idiopathic pancreatitis.[73] Therefore, it appears as though pancreas divisum is associated with pancreatitis. It has been postulated that pancreatitis may result from a combination of pancreas divisum and stenosis at the level of the papilla. As a congenital defect, clinical manifestations of pancreas divisum may occur at any age, but are uncommon in childhood. Symptoms may be mild with only occasional epigastric pain occurring postprandially, but more often episodes of severe acute pancreatitis occur. Chronic pancreatitis may also develop, with all of its associated sequelae. Changes in the pancreatic ducts characteristic of chronic pancreatitis may be detected on ERCP.

Pancreas divisum is diagnosed by pancreatography (Fig. 89-9). On ERCP, the major papilla is often difficult to cannulate, but on injection with contrast fluid, the duct of Wirsung appears shortened and of small diameter. There is rapid filling of small accessory ducts, and too much contrast can be injected before it is realized that the duct of Wirsung is not in communication with the main pancreatic duct. As a result, the patient may experience sudden pain, and pancreatitis of the ventral pancreas can develop. What appears as an abrupt cutoff of the duct of Wirsung must not be confused with a mass lesion such as a malignancy or pancreatic pseudocyst. The delicate nature of the accessory ducts on the pancreatogram are helpful indicators of pancreas divisum. If possible, the accessory papilla should be cannulated. This should reveal a duct of Santorini running the entire length of the pancreas that is not in communication with the duct of Wirsung. If stenosis of the papilla is not demonstrated radiographically, it has been recommended that manometric studies

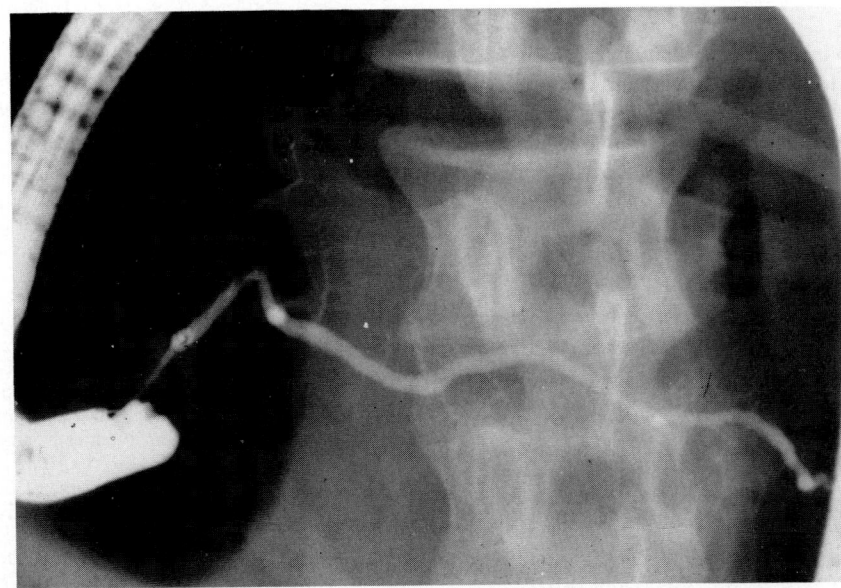

FIGURE 89-9. Pancreas divisum. An endoscopic retrograde pancreatogram performed through the accessory papilla shows the dorsal duct in pancreas divisum. (Courtesy of Peter B. Cotton, M.D., Durham, NC.)

be performed to determine the degree of patency of the papilla for use in determining future therapy.[76-78]

Those patients with mild symptoms can be managed conservatively. Patients with recurrent episodes of pancreatitis or chronic pain require intervention to alleviate papillary or ductal stenosis. Endoscopic sphincterotomy of the minor papilla usually has not been successful because of the difficult and often inaccessible location of the papilla.[73] Surgical transduodenal sphincteroplasty has been useful in some patients.[76,78] In cases in which sphincterotomy has failed or the ductal involvement is more extensive, direct ductal drainage or resection of the involved pancreas is necessary.[79,80]

Congenital Cysts

Cysts of the pancreas are distinguished from more common pseudocysts by the presence of an epithelial lining. Pseudocysts often follow bouts of acute pancreatitis, with trauma being a major precipitant. Identification of true columnar or cuboidal epithelium in congenital cysts may be difficult, and it is not always possible to distinguish a congenital cyst from a pancreatic pseudocyst. In cysts located in the peripancreatic space, identification of pancreatic enzymes in the cyst fluid is helpful in determining that it is of pancreatic origin; however, not all pancreatic cysts contain fluid rich in pancreatic enzymes. Solitary congenital cysts are rare.[81] They are more commonly diagnosed in early childhood but may remain asymptomatic and undetected into adulthood. Although other congenital anomalies have been reported with pancreatic cysts, these are more often isolated defects.[82]

The most common presentation of a solitary pancreatic cyst is as an abdominal mass. This may be associated with abdominal pain or complications resulting from expanding size, such as gastroduodenal obstruction. Encroachment on the intrapancreatic or extrapancreatic common bile duct may cause biliary obstruction.[83] Subcutaneous fat necrosis and osteolytic lesions secondary to pancreatic enzymes leaking into the circulation from a developmental pancreatic cyst have been described.[84]

The presence of a pancreatic cyst may be suggested by a plain radiograph of the abdomen or an upper gastrointestinal radiographic series demonstrating a mass displacing a portion of the stomach, duodenum, or colon. The best diagnostic test is abdominal ultrasound, which demonstrates a fluid-filled cystic lesion in the pancreas. Although computed tomography and angiography can be used to identify a pancreatic cyst, these tests usually are unnecessary. In considering the differential diagnosis, it is important to consider other possible cystic lesions of the pancreas, including pancreatic pseudocysts, cystadenomas, and cystadenocarcinoma.

Symptomatic pancreatic cysts should be removed whenever possible. This can be done by enucleation of the cyst, if it is located in the body or tail of the pancreas, or resection of the cyst with adjacent pancreatic tissue, if it is confined to the distal pancreas. If the location of the cyst precludes either of these approaches, such as a cyst in the head of the pancreas, drainage into the stomach or jejunum can be performed. With surgical drainage of the cyst, pathologic examination should be done to exclude malignancy.

Multiple Cysts

Multiple congenital pancreatic cysts are rare and are usually associated with other congenital anomalies. In particular, polycystic kidney disease and cystic fibrosis are frequently associated with pancreatic cysts. Other clinical syndromes involving multiple pancreatic cysts include von Hippel-Lindau syndrome, Ivemark's syndrome, and Bruber's syndrome, in which cysts of the lung, liver, and central nervous system are also found.[85,86] Many of the associated anomalies are lethal, although patients may have no symptoms referable to the pancreatic cysts. Because of the numerous cysts and the involvement of several organ systems, no treatment is necessary unless specific symptoms or a particular complication such as infection of a cyst dictates surgical excision or drainage.

The reader is directed to Chapter 15, Pancreatic Secretion; and Chapter 94, Hereditary Diseases of the Pancreas.

REFERENCES

1. Mackie CR, Moossa AR. Surgical anatomy of the pancreas. In: Moossa AR, ed. Tumors of the pancreas. Baltimore: Williams & Wilkins, 1980:1.
2. Silen W. Surgical anatomy of the pancreas. Surg Clin North Am 1964;44:1253.
3. Braasch JW, Gray BN. Technique of radical pancreaticoduodenectomy with consideration for hepatic arterial relationships. Surg Clin North Am 1976;56:631.
4. Mackie CR, Lu CT, Noble HG, et al. Prospective evaluation of angiography in the diagnosis and management of patients suspected of having pancreatic cancer. Ann Surg 1979;189:11.
5. Douglass BE, Baggenstoss AH, Hollinshead WH. The anatomy of the portal vein and its tributaries. Surg Gynecol Obstet 1950;91:562.
6. Evans BP, Ochsner A. The gross anatomy of the lymphatics of the human pancreas. Surgery 1954;36:177.
7. Dodd GD. Lymphiography in diseases of the liver and pancreas. Radiol Clin North Am 1970;8:69.
8. Valenzuela JE, Wiener K, Saad C. Cholinergic stimulation of human pancreatic secretion. Dig Dis Sci 1986;31:615.
9. Holst JJ. Peptidergic mechanisms of the pancreas. Arch Int Pharmacodyn Ther 1990;303:252.
10. Berman LG, Prior JT, Abramow SM, et al. A study of the pancreatic duct system in man by use of vinyl acetate casts of post mortem preparations. Surg Gynecol Obstet 1969;110:391.
11. Kreel L. Pancreatic duct calibre and variations on autopsy pancreatography. In: Anacker H, ed. Efficiency and limits of radiologic examinations of the pancreas. Acton, MA: Publishing Sciences Group, 1975:214.
12. Bonner-Weir S, Orci L. New perspectives on the microvasculature of the islets of Langerhans in the rat. Diabetes 1982;31:883.
13. Alumets J, Hakanson R, Sundler F. Ontogeny of endocrine cells in porcine gut and pancreas. Gastroenterology 1983;85:1359.
14. Howard CP, Go VL, Infante AJ, et al. Long-term survival in a case of functional pancreatic agenesis. J Pediatr 1980;97:786.
15. Mehes K, Vamos K, Goda M. Agenesis of pancreas and gallbladder in an infant of incest. Acta Paediatr Acad Sci Hung 1976;17:175.
16. Lemons JA, Ridenour R, Orsini EN. Congenital absence of the pancreas and intrauterine growth retardation. Pediatrics 1979;64:255.
17. Beresford OD, Owen TK. Lipomatous pseudohypertrophy of the pancreas. J Clin Pathol 1957;10:63.

18. Bodian M. Fibrocystic disease of the pancreas. New York: Grune & Stratton, 1953.
19. Lumb G, Beautyman W. Hypoplasia of the exocrine tissue of the pancreas. J Pathol Bacteriol 1952;64:679.
20. Kiernan PD, ReMine SG, Kiernan PC, ReMine WH. Annular pancreas: Mayo Clinic experience from 1957 to 1976 with review of the literature. Arch Surg 1980;115:46.
21. Heij HA, Niessen GH. Annular pancreas associated with congenital absence of the gallbladder. J Pediatr Surg 1987;22:1033.
22. Salonen IS. Congenital obstruction: a review of the literature and a clinical study of 66 patients, including a histo-pathological study of annular pancreas and a follow-up study of 36 survivors. Acta Paediatr Scand 1978;272:1.
23. Stanley P, Law BS, Young LW. Down's syndrome, duodenal stenosis/annular pancreas, and a stack of coins. Am J Dis Child 1988;142:459.
24. Milunsky A, Fisher JH. Annular pancreas in Down's syndrome. Lancet 1968;2:575.
25. Lehman GA, O'Connor KW. Coexistence of annular pancreas and pancreas divisum: ERCP diagnosis. Gastrointest Endosc 1985;31:25.
26. Poindexter MH, Hall GH, Leigh JE. Report of a case of annular pancreas of the newborn in two consecutive siblings. Pediatrics 1971;48:148.
27. MacFadyen UM, Young ID. Annular pancreas in mother and son. Am J Med Genet 1987;27:987.
28. Jackson GL, Apostolides P. Autosomal dominant inheritance of annular pancreas. Am J Med Genet 1978;1:319.
29. Sternberg A, Zelikovski A, Abu-Dalu J, Urca I. Fibromuscular annular pancreas: a variant of pancreatic malformation? Int Surg 1978;63:170.
30. O'Rahilly R, Muller F. A model of the pancreas to illustrate development. Acta Anat 1978;103:380.
31. Sessa F, Fiocca R, Tenti P, et al. Pancreatic polypeptide rich tissue in the annular pancreas: a distinctive feature of ventral primordium derivatives. Virchows Arch [A] 1983;399:227.
32. Newman BM, Lebenthal E. Congenital abnormalities of the exocrine pancreas. In: Go VLW, Gardner JD, Brooks FP, et al, eds. The exocrine pancreas: biology, pathobiology, and diseases. New York: Raven Press, 1986:773.
33. Merrill JR, Raffensperger JG. Pediatric annular pancreas: twenty years' experience. J Pediatr Surg 1976;11:921.
34. Liebman WM. Recurrent abdominal pain: apparent association with annular pancreas. Am J Gastroenterol 1979;71:522.
35. Lloyd-Jones W, Mountain JC, Warren KW. Annular pancreas in the adult. Ann Surg 1972;176:163.
36. MacGregor AM, Green BJ, Stern MA. Symptomatic annular pancreas in the adult. Br J Surg 1969;176:163.
37. Beachley MC, Lankau CA Jr. Symptomatic adult annular pancreas. Am J Dig Dis 1973;18:513.
38. Lieber A, Schaefer JW, Belin RP. Hypotonic duodenography: diagnosis of annular pancreas in an adult. JAMA 1968;203:425.
39. Glazer GM, Margulis AR. Annular pancreas: etiology and diagnosis using endoscopic retrograde cholangiopancreatography. Radiology 1979;133:303.
40. Clifford KM. Annular pancreas diagnosed by endoscopic retrograde pancreatography (ERCP). Br J Radiol 1980;53:593.
41. Dharmsathaporn K, Burrel M, Dobbins J. Diagnosis of annular pancreas with endoscopic retrograde cholangiopancreatography. Gastroenterology 1979;77:1109.
42. Chevillotte G, Sahel J, Raillat A, Sarles H. Annular pancreas: report of one case associated with acute pancreatitis and diagnosed by endoscopic retrograde pancreatography. Dig Dis Sci 1984;29:75.
43. Inamoto K, Ishikawa Y, Itoh N. CT demonstration of annular pancreas: case report. Gastrointest Radiol 1983;8:143.
44. Thomford NR, Knight PR, Pace WG, Madura JA. Annular pancreas in the adult: selection of operation. Ann Surg 1972;176:159.
45. Barbosa JJ, Dockerty MB, Waugh JM. Pancreatic heterotopia. Surg Gynecol Obstet 1946;82:527.
46. Feldman M, Weinberg T. Aberrant pancreas: a cause of duodenal syndrome. JAMA 1952;148:893.
47. Busard JM, Walters W. Heterotopic pancreatic tissue. Arch Surg 1950;60:674.
48. Wolloch Y. Heterotopic pancreatic tissue in the gallbladder. Acta Chir Scand 1986;152:557.
49. Curd HH. A histologic study of Meckel's diverticulum. Arch Surg 1936:32:506.
50. Beskin CA. Intralobar enteric sequestration of the lung containing aberrant pancreas. J Thorac Cardiovasc Surg 1961;41:314.
51. Jaschke W, Aleksic M, Aleksci D. Heterotopic pancreatic tissue in a bronchogenic cyst: diagnosis and therapy. Thorac Cardiovasc Surg 1982;30:58.
52. Caberwal D, Kogan SJ, Levitt SB. Ectopic pancreas presenting as an umbilical mass. J Pediatr Surg 1977;12:593.
53. Gray SW, Skandalakis JE. Embryology for surgeons: the embryological basis for the treatment of congenital defects. Philadelphia: WB Saunders, 1972:263.
54. Armstrong CP, King PM, Dixon JM, Macleod IB. The clinical significance of heterotopic pancreas in the gastrointestinal tract. Br J Surg 1981;63:384.
55. Abrahams JI. Heterotopic pancreas simulating peptic ulceration. Arch Surg 1966;93:589.
56. Qizilbash AH. Acute pancreatitis occurring in heterotopic pancreatic tissue in the gallbladder. Can J Surg 1976;19:413.
57. Laughlin EH, Keown ME, Jackson JE. Heterotopic pancreas obstructing the ampulla of Vater. Arch Surg 1983;118:979.
58. O'Reilly DJ, Craig RM, Lorenzo G, Yokoo H. Heterotopic pancreas mimicking carcinoma of the head of the pancreas: a rare cause of obstructive jaundice. J Clin Gastroenterol 1983;5:165.
59. Weber CM, Zito PF, Becker SM. Heterotopic pancreas: an unusual cause of obstruction of the common bile duct. Am J Gastroenterol 1968;49:153.
60. Anseline P, Grundfest S, Carey W, Weiss R. Pancreatic heterotopia: a rare cause of bowel obstruction. Surgery 1981;90:110.
61. Carleton CC, Ackerbaum R. Intussusception secondary to aberrant pancreas in a child. JAMA 1976;236:1047.
62. Sabini AM, Baden JP, Norman JD, Martin JR. Heterotopic pancreatic tissue in the common bile duct or ampulla of Vater. Am Surg 1970;36:662.
63. Dolan RV, Remine WH, Dockerty MB. The fate of heterotopic pancreatic tissue: a study of 212 cases. Arch Surg 1974;109:762.
64. Claudon M, Verain AL, Bigard MA, et al. Cyst formation in gastric heterotopic pancreas: a report of two cases. Radiology 1988;169:659.
65. Hickman DM, Frey CF, Carson JWW. Adenocarcinoma arising in gastric heterotopic pancreas. West J Med 1981;135:57.
66. Tanimura A, Yamamoto H, Shibata H, Sano E. Carcinoma in heterotopic gastric pancreas. Acta Pathol Jpn 1979;29:251.
67. Tomita T, Kanabe S. Islet tissue in the heterotopic pancreas. Arch Pathol Lab Med 1983;107:469.
68. Hara M, Tsutsumi Y. Immunohistochemical studies of endocrine cells in heterotopic pancreas. Virchows Arch [A] 1986;408:385.
69. Lai EC, Tompkins KR. Heterotopic pancreas: review of a 26 year experience. Am J Surg 1986;151:697.
70. DeBord JR, Majarakis JD, Nyhus LM. An unusual case of heterotopic pancreas of the stomach. Am J Surg 1981;141:269.
71. Rohrmann CA Jr, Delaney JH Jr, Protell RL. Heterotopic pancreas diagnosed by cannulation and duct study. AJR 1977;128:1044.
72. Dawson W, Langman J. An anatomical-radiological study on pancreatic duct pattern in man. Anat Rec 1961;39:59.
73. Cotton PB. Congenital anomaly of pancreas divisum as cause of obstructive pain and pancreatitis. Cut 1980;21:105.
74. Cotton PB, Kizu M. Malfusion of dorsal and ventral pancreas: a cause of pancreatitis (abstract)? Gut 1977;18:400.
75. Gregg JA. Pancreas divisum: its association with pancreatitis. Am J Surg 1977;134:539.
76. Gregg JA, Monaco AP, McDermott WV. Pancreas divisum: results of surgical intervention. Am J Surg 1983;145:488.
77. Gregg J, Solomon J, Clark G. Pancreas divisum and its asso-

ciation with choledochal sphincter stenosis. Am J Surg 1984;147:367.

78. Warshaw AL, Richter J, Schapiro RH. The cause and treatment of pancreatitis associated with pancreas divisum. Ann Surg 1983;198:443.

79. Ingram NP, Knight M. Pancreas divisum: relief of symptoms following drainage of the dorsal duct. Br J Clin Pract 1982;36:69.

80. Blair AJ, Russell CG, Cotton PB. Resection for pancreatitis in patients with pancreas divisum. Ann Surg 1984;200:590.

81. Mares AJ, Hirsch M. Congenital cysts of the head of the pancreas. J Pediatr Surg 1977;12:547.

82. DeLange C, Janssen TAE. Large solitary pancreatic cyst and other developmental errors in a premature infant. Am J Dis Child 1948;75:587.

83. Kalani BP, Broadhead RL, Bhargav RK. Giant congenital pancreatic cyst in a child. Ann Trop Paediatr 1982;2:47.

84. Hollingworth P, Isaacs D, Bydder G. Recurrent osteolytic lesions and subcutaneous fat necrosis in association with a developmental pancreatic cyst. Arch Dis Child 1979;54:790.

85. Strayer DS, Kissane JM. Dysplasia of the kidneys, liver, and pancreas: report of a variant of Ivemark's syndrome. Hum Pathol 1979;10:228.

86. Hori A, Orthner H, Kohlschutter A, et al. CNS dysplasia in dysencephalia splanchnocystica (Gruber's syndrome). Acta Neuropathol (Berl) 1980;51:93.

Textbook of Gastroenterology, second edition, edited by Tadataka Yamada. JB Lippincott Company, Philadelphia © 1995.

CHAPTER 90

Acute Pancreatitis

Fred Sanford Gorelick

Acute pancreatitis is a clinical syndrome defined by a discrete episode of abdominal pain and elevations in serum enzyme levels. It involves inflammation of the pancreas with varying amounts of injury to adjacent and distant organs. In the United States, more than 80% of the cases are related to biliary stones or alcohol use. Although there are many factors that may precipitate acute pancreatitis, it is rare for any but alcohol to lead to chronic pancreatitis.

The first reports of pancreatitis may date to the 1700s, but the first systematic analysis of pancreatitis was published by Reginald Fitz in 1889.[1] In this landmark study, the clinical and pathologic findings in 53 patients were presented. His analysis of the patterns of abdominal pain, fever, and jaundice, along with physical findings, established the criteria for diagnosing pancreatitis. Etiologic factors such as gallstones, alcohol, penetrating ulcers, and trauma were mentioned. Pancreatic pseudocyst, splenic vein thrombosis, disseminated fat necrosis, and abscess were also described. Fitz's report established the framework for studies and treatments of pancreatitis that have spanned a hundred years.

INCIDENCE

The incidence of acute pancreatitis ranges from 1 to 5/10,000 per year. This value is approximate and may vary widely among populations for several reasons. First, histologic confirmation of pancreatitis is unavailable in most patients and the diagnosis must rely on clinical assessment, biochemical tests, and radiologic evaluations, which are limited in their sensitivity and specificity. Second, the incidence of precipitating factors such as alcoholism and gallstones varies among populations. Finally, some patient groups may be systematically excluded; for example, those with mild disease may not come to a hospital.

CLASSIFICATION

Acute pancreatitis may be classified by pathology, etiology, and clinical presentation and course. The existence of various groupings reflects the different goals of such classifications. Some are useful in establishing a differential diagnosis or understanding disease mechanisms, and others may provide prognostic information or guide intervention.

A sensible classification system based on a number of clinical parameters has been described by Bradley.[2] The most important feature of this classification is that it defines a common nomenclature for describing acute pancreatitis. It separates pancreatitis into mild and severe disease based on physiologic findings, laboratory values, and radiologic imaging, which are discussed in this chapter. *Mild pancreatitis* is not associated with organ dysfunction or complications, and recovery is uneventful. *Severe pancreatitis* is associated with decreased function of the pancreas, local and systemic complications, and a complicated recovery. Bradley's classification makes several important distinctions by defining pancreatic fluid collections and pseudocysts, and separating infected pancreatic necrosis from pancreatic abscesses. This classification does not provide the criteria for establishing prognosis early in the patient's

course, as discussed later in this chapter (see section on Assessment), but does provide a clear framework for discussing acute pancreatitis using a defined set of terms.

PATHOLOGY

Two morphologic classifications are recognized: acute interstitial, and acute hemorrhagic pancreatitis. Although mortality is much more likely with the latter type, either may be fatal.

Interstitial

The gross architecture of the gland is preserved, but it is edematous. Hemorrhage is absent. Interstitial edema and inflammatory cells within the parenchyma are prominent. Detailed morphologic studies of pancreatic tissue are available from a limited number of cases of acute pancreatitis. Disruption of the normal acinar cell architecture is common and may contribute to characteristically reduced enzyme secretion. For example, zymogen granules are displaced from their fusion site in the apical domain of the cell and become dispersed throughout the cell, and the apical membrane appears contracted and microvilli disappear.[3] Zymogen granules fuse with each other instead of the apical membrane. Similar to animal models of pancreatitis,[4,5] a distinct form of cell necrosis is observed in which the apical domain of the acinar cell is shed into the lumen, resulting in intact zymogen granules within the lumen.[6] This pattern of partial cell necrosis may allow the acinus to regenerate rapidly after injury.[7]

Hemorrhagic

Macroscopically, marked tissue necrosis and hemorrhage are apparent. Surrounding areas of fat necrosis are also prominent. These are chalky areas of dead adipose tissue that are found within the peripancreatic tissue and throughout the abdomen. Large hematomas often are located in the retroperitoneal space. The microscopic appearance of the pancreas parallels the gross changes, with marked fat and pancreatic necrosis. Vascular inflammation and thrombosis are common.

PATHOPHYSIOLOGY

Activation of Pancreatic Zymogens

The cellular mechanisms that initiate acute pancreatitis have been long debated. The premature activation of pancreatic enzymes may play an important role in the initiation of pancreatitis. Active pancreatic enzymes have been detected within the pancreas in experimental[8] and clinical pancreatitis.[9] This premature activation may be the first step in a process that leads to pancreatic autodigestion and induces other forms of pancreatic injury.

Although this premature zymogen activation may take place within pancreatic ducts or the interstitial space, observations have implicated the acinar cell as the site of enzyme activation.[10–13] Two mechanisms have been proposed to account for intracellular activation of trypsinogen and the zymogen cascade: trypsinogen autoactivation, and trypsinogen activation by the lysosomal enzyme cathepsin B. Although considerably less active than trypsin, trypsinogen has autocatalytic activity with an acidic pH optimum.[14] Cathepsin B has the ability to activate trypsinogen with an acidic pH optimum. Further, even under basal conditions, some cathepsin B is found in the secretory compartment.[15,16] There is evidence that limited proteolysis of zymogens may take place within the acinar cell (Fig. 90-1). Exposure of isolated pancreatic acini to high doses of cholecystokinin in vitro, a treatment known to cause pancreatitis, results in the limited proteolysis of several zymogens.[12] The proteolytic products correspond to active enzyme forms. This proteolysis appears to require a low pH compartment; protease inhibitor studies favor the mechanism of trypsinogen autoactivation over cathepsin B as the pathway initiating proteolysis. Indeed, lysosomal enzymes such as cathepsin B may have a protective role and degrade active enzymes.[11] A variety of insults may use intracellular zymogen activation as a final common pathway to initiate pancreatitis.

Inhibition of Secretion

A feature common to cellular models of zymogen activation and pancreatitis is the inhibition of enzyme secretion.[3] This decreased secretion undoubtedly reflects blockage of secretion from the apical membrane region of the acinar cell. Interruption of acinar cell second messenger pathways[17] and its cytoskeleton may play a role in blocking secretion.[18] Such inhibition may prohibit secretion of enzymes that become active within the acinar cell. Studies suggest that in addition to intracellular zymogen activation, retention of active enzymes within the acinar cell is required to initiate pancreatitis.[19]

Protective Mechanisms

The acinar cell has evolved a number of cellular mechanisms to limit the effects of zymogens activated within the acinar cell. Potentially active enzymes are packaged within a secretory granule membrane that is impermeable to proteins. Lability of the zymogen granule membrane is reported in models of pancreatitis and may allow enzymes to be released into the cell.[20] Enzyme inhibitors, such as pancreatic trypsin inhibitor, are packaged together with trypsinogen in the secretory granule.[21] Although these inhibitors are efficient, the zymogen granule contains quantities sufficient to inhibit only a small portion of activated zymogen. Thus, large-scale zymogen activation might easily overwhelm the cellular protease inhibitors. Relative deficiencies of the pancreatic trypsin inhibitor have been found in some forms of recurrent pancreatitis.[22]

Consequences of Enzyme Activation

The potential consequences of zymogen activation are manifold (Fig. 90-2), and include damaging local effects, attack on other tissues, or activation of additional pathways. The importance of thinking about the steps in acute pancreatitis, especially the latter ones such as neutrophil recruitment, platelet activation, and formation of free radicals, lies in the potential to target future therapeutic interventions.

Undoubtedly, active digestive enzymes attack normal tissue structures; however, potent enzyme inhibitors are present in circulation and play an important role in limiting tissue damage. The major serum protease inhibitors include α_2-macroglobulin, α_1-antitrypsin, antichymotrypsin, inter-α-trypsin inhibitor, and C1 esterase inhibitor. After these inhibitors bind to enzymes, the complex is cleared by the reticuloendothelial system. Decreased amounts of circulating protease inhibitors and delayed clearance of serum protease-inhibitor complexes by the reticuloendothelial system have been associated with more severe forms of pancreatitis.[23]

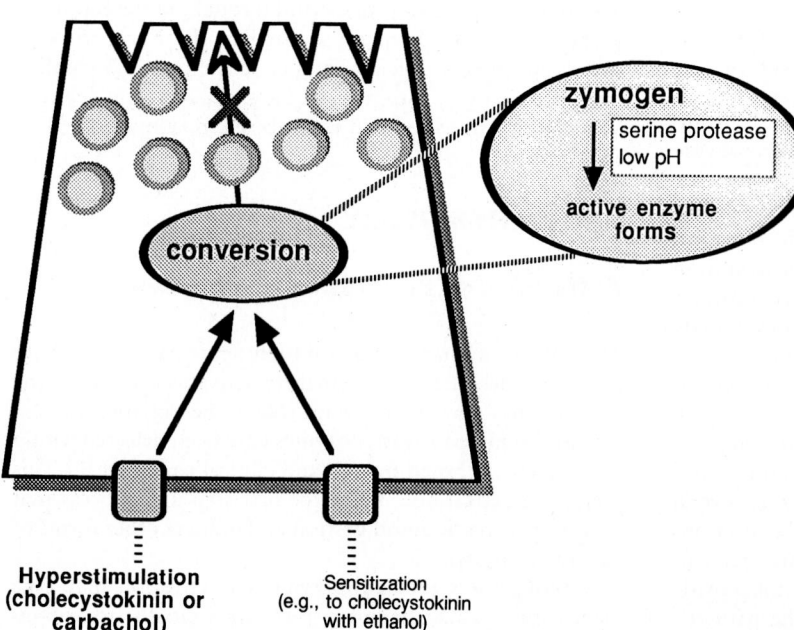

FIGURE 90-1. Potential intracellular initiating events in acute pancreatitis. Both intracellular activation of pancreatic zymogens and retention of active enzymes probably are required to initiate pancreatic autodigestion and pancreatitis. These events may be a stereotypical response to many forms of injury, including high doses of neurohumoral agents such as cholecystokinin. Some agents such as ethanol may promote intracellular activation by sensitizing the cell to cholecystokinin. Intracellular proteolysis may be initiated by a decrease in pH or other ionic changes along the secretory pathway, which promotes the activation of trypsinogen through its autoactivation or the action of the lysosomal protease cathepsin B. An alternative role for the lysosomal proteases in the secretory granule may be the degradation of activated enzymes.

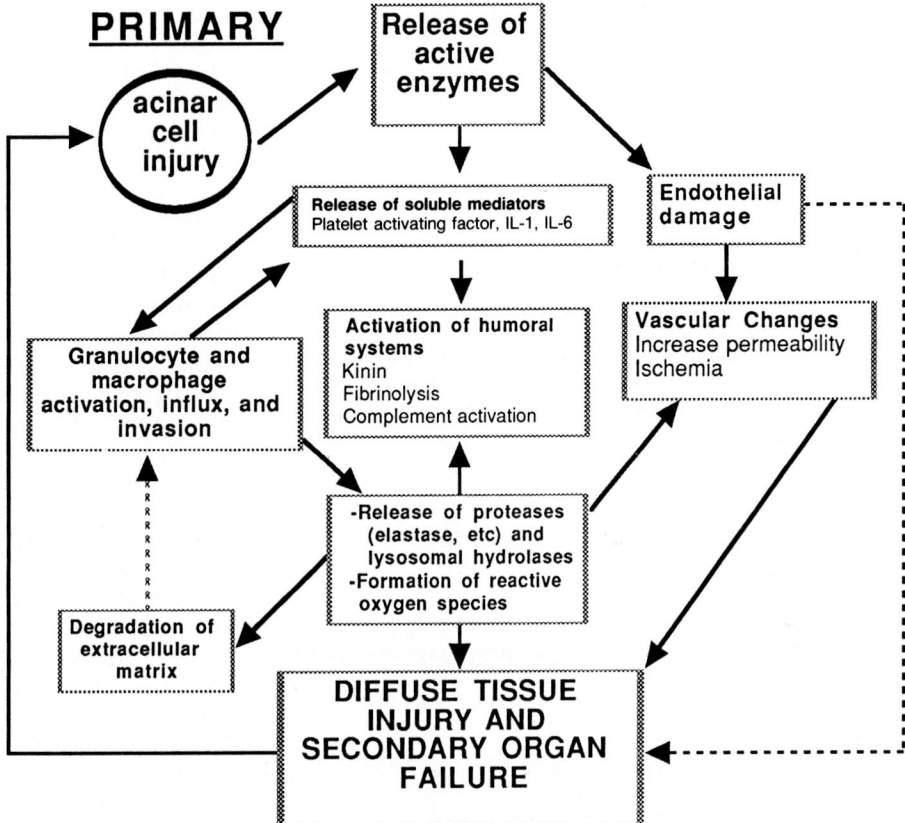

PRIMARY

FIGURE 90-2. Potential mechanisms of cellular and tissue injury in acute pancreatitis. (IL, interlukin; PAF, platelet activating factor; adapted from Lerch MM, Adler G. Acute pancreatitis. Current Opinion in Gastroenterology 1992;8:817.)

Another major event in acute pancreatitis is the recruitment of inflammatory cells into pancreatic blood vessels and later into the pancreatic parenchyma. Trypsin activation of the alternate complement pathway may play a role in neutrophil recruitment.[24] The influx of inflammatory cells may be so great as to form white cell emboli and plug small blood vessels. Fibrinolysis and complement activation correlates with disease severity.[25] Although vascular damage and ischemia have been predicted to play an important role in many forms of acute pancreatitis, this has yet to be proven.[26] The release of kinins makes capillary walls permeable and promotes tissue edema.

Oxygen free radicals have been implicated in a number of experimental models of pancreatitis, including that induced by cerulein[27] and taurocholate.[28] Free radical generation correlates with both decreased pancreatic protein and nonprotein sulfhydryl groups,[29] and the severity of pancreatic injury.[28] Free radical damage may involve both abnormal peroxidation and depletion of thiol donors such as glutathione. Attempts to prevent pancreatic injury using free radical scavengers have been only partially successful in experimental models, and are largely untested clinically.

EXPERIMENTAL MODELS

Animals models of acute pancreatitis have been developed to aid in the understanding of the disease and evaluate potential therapy.[30,31] Most models induce an injury that closely resembles interstitial pancreatitis, but models of severe hemorrhagic pancreatitis have been established.[32–34] A common shortcoming of studies that evaluate therapy for acute pancreatitis is timing of intervention; most treat at or before the onset of pancreatitis in a time frame that would not be clinically feasible.[35]

Hyperstimulation

One hundred years ago, Mouret observed that excessive cholinergic stimulation was associated with pancreatic injury.[36] Mouret speculated that the activation of trypsin might play an important role in this injury. In subsequent experimental models, infusions of the cholecystokinin analog, cerulein, were shown to generate pancreatic injury in a time- and dose-dependent manner.[11] A similar injury has been induced by exposing isolated perfused pancreas to high doses of cerulein.[37] Although the initiating events in hyperstimulation pancreatitis are thought to be related to those outlined in Figure 90-1, this remains to be proven.

Pathologic changes within the first hour of hyperstimulation include inhibition of secretion into the pancreatic duct, pancreatic edema, and margination of neutrophils.[6] Within 3 to 6 hours, inflammatory cells invade the interstitium and vacuoles form within acinar cells.[6,38]

Other

A number of other forms of experimental pancreatitis have been developed and reviewed.[30] Those relating to obstruction are discussed in the section on Gallstones. The diet-induced model is based on the observation by Lombardi, Rao, and associates that, when fed to young female mice, a choline-deficient diet supplemented with the synthetic amino acid analog of methionine, DL-ethionine, induced a fatal hemorrhagic pancreatitis.[39,40] One possibility raised by the diet model is that abnormal metabolites may contribute to pancreatitis under certain conditions such as refeeding.

SPECIFIC ETIOLOGIES

It is important to review the differential diagnosis of acute pancreatitis in each patient (Table 90-1). Many patients have an easily identifiable and remediable process such as gallstones. Less common causes should be considered in those with recurrent bouts but no gallstones.

Structural

Gallstones

Although gallstones are etiologically linked to pancreatitis, this condition develops in only a small percentage of patients with gallstones. For example, in a cohort from Minnesota

---

TABLE 90-1
Etiology of Pancreatitis

Structural
Gallstones or microlithiasis
Sphincter of Oddi spasm or stenosis
Pancreas divisum
Traumatic

Toxins
Alcohol
Drugs and other agents

Infectious
Viral
Bacterial
Parasitic

Metabolic
Hyperlipidemia
Hypercalcemia

Vascular
Atherosclerosis
Vasculitis

Other Specific Etiologies
Coronary bypass
Cystic fibrosis
Fibrocalculous (tropical)
Iatrogenic
Inflammatory bowel disease
Neoplasia
Peptic ulcer

Miscellaneous
Congenital
Idiopathic
Refeeding
Childhood

---

with gallstones, the incidence of acute pancreatitis was 0.17% per year.[41] The presence of gallstones, however, increases the relative risk for acute pancreatitis 14- to 35-fold in men and 12- to 25-fold in women.[41,42] A contributing factor that places men at greater risk may be a larger bile ductal system that favors the migration of stones into the common duct. Anomalous union of the pancreatic and biliary ducts may also predispose to pancreatitis, possibly by promoting reflux of bile into the pancreatic duct.[43,44] Metabolic factors also may increase the risk for development of pancreatitis from gallstones. For example, underlying hyperlipidemia manifest by delayed chylomicron clearance may make patients more susceptible to gallstone pancreatitis.[45]

Many models have attempted to reproduce the pancreatitis generated by stones obstructing the ampulla. Almost a century ago, Opie put forth the "common channel theory," that a gallstone at the papilla would obstruct the common opening of the pancreatic and bile duct and allow reflux of bile into the pancreatic duct. Several observations have challenged that theory: patients without a common channel can have gallstone pancreatitis[46]; and retrograde flow of bile into the pancreatic duct at physiologic pressures does not induce pancreatitis.[47,48] Although addition of increased intraductal pressure to bile infusion results in severe pancreatitis, pressures of such magnitude are not thought to occur under physiologic conditions. In general, obstruction of the pancreatic duct alone in animal models has not generated pancreatitis. In the American opossum, however, pancreatic duct obstruction alone generates acute pancreatitis.[33] This observation raises the possibility that pancreatic duct obstruction alone may be sufficient to cause gallstone pancreatitis.

It seems likely that most biliary pancreatitis is precipitated by the transient or persistent obstruction of the papilla by a stone. When patients are selected on the basis of hyperbilirubinemia and pancreatitis, stone recovery from the stool has been reported in 30% to 85%.[49] Stone passage in most patients with gallstone pancreatitis probably occurs on the day of the attack. Thus, the delay in stool collection after an attack and detection methods that miss small stones may account for low recovery rates.

If gallstones predispose to acute pancreatitis, removal of the stones should decrease this risk. In Minnesota, cholecystectomy in patients without a history of acute pancreatitis reduced the risk for the subsequent development of pancreatitis at least 10- to 20-fold.[41] Despite the increased risks for development of acute pancreatitis in those with gallstones and the success of cholecystectomy in decreasing the risk, the incidence of the disease is too low to warrant prophylactic cholecystectomy in the patient without symptomatic gallstones.[41]

Microlithiasis

The requirement for ultrasonography clearly to identify gallstones for diagnosing gallstone pancreatitis may be too stringent a criterion. Examination of patients with idiopathic recurrent pancreatitis has provided compelling evidence that diminutive gallstones, referred to as microlithiasis, may cause recurrent bouts of pancreatitis.[50,51] Microlithiasis was identified by examining the bile obtained during endoscopic retrograde cholangiopancreatography (ERCP) for crystals (cholesterol monohydrate, calcium bilirubinate, or calcium carbonate), or by observing amorphous shifting debris (sludge) within the gallbladder using ultrasonography (Fig. 90-3). Several forms of treatment have been used. Patients with cholesterol crystals have received ursodeoxycholic acid; others, cholecystectomy or endoscopic papillotomy alone. Each form of intervention has been reported to reduce the frequency of attacks by at least two thirds. These observations suggest that microlithiasis should be considered a causative factor in patients with recurrent bouts of idiopathic pancreatitis.

Stenosis and Spasm of the Sphincter of Oddi

The sphincter of Oddi is a complex muscular structure that regulates the flow of pancreatic secretions and bile into the duodenum. Acting indirectly through inhibitory neural pathways, cholecystokinin causes the sphincter to relax. When the innervation to the sphincter is interrupted, cholecystokinin may act directly on the sphincter and cause contraction.[52]

This paradoxic response may occur after biliary tract surgery, vagotomy, or gastric resection.[52] The sphincter may also obstruct pancreatic or biliary flow because it is scarred.[53]

Diagnosis of sphincter of Oddi dysfunction is hampered by a lack of specific and reproducible endoscopic or manometric criteria. In the absence of such criteria, abnormal biliary or pancreatic enzymes during an attack are required to make the diagnosis. Dilation of the common duct (>12 mm by ERCP) and its delayed drainage after ERCP have been used as endoscopic criteria.[54] Manometric criteria include a resting sphincter pressure more than 40 mm Hg above duodenal pressure,[55] and a paradoxic response to exogenous cholecystokinin.[52] Manometric abnormalities may be limited to the biliary or pancreatic segments of the sphincter.[56,57] Although some consider manometry the gold standard for diagnosing sphincter of Oddi dysfunction, such studies are technically difficult to perform, have provided conflicting results,[54] and may cause pancreatitis.[58] A potential alternative to these invasive tests are noninvasive tests that measure the rate of emptying of radionuclide from the biliary tract to detect sphincter of Oddi dysfunction.[59] Pretreatment with cholecystokinin may

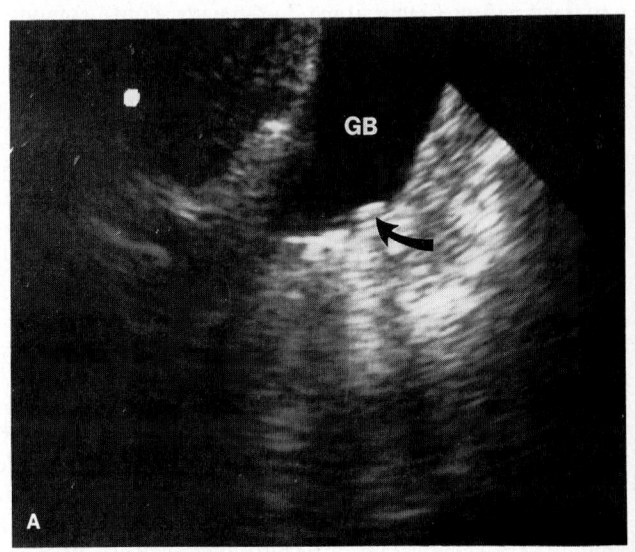

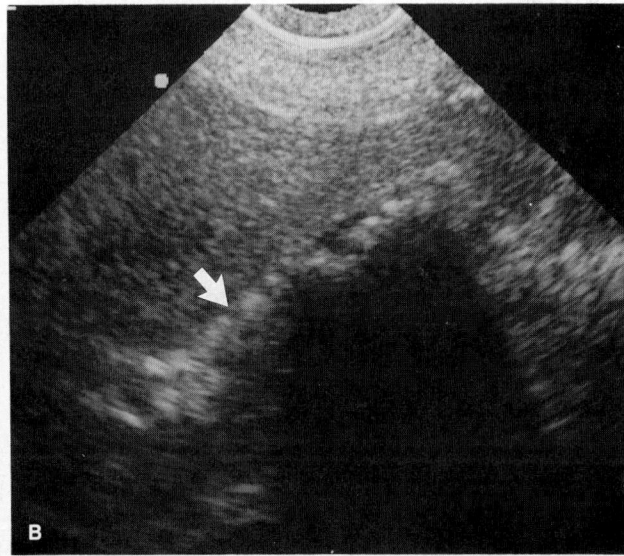

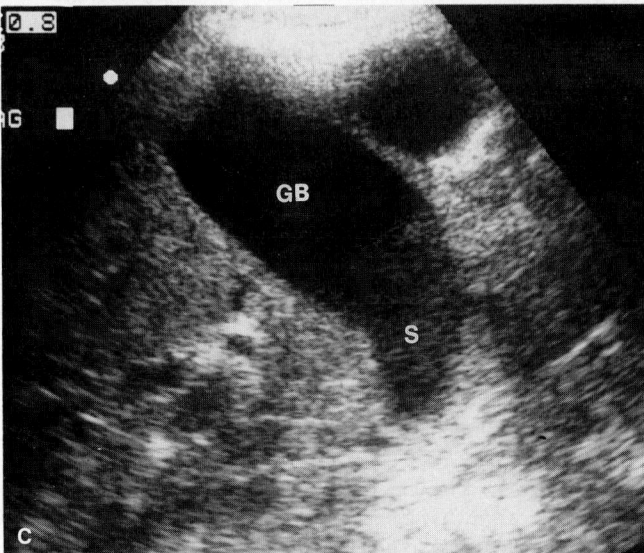

FIGURE 90-3. Ultrasonography demonstrates cholelithiasis. **(A)** Gallbladder (GB) with single gallstone (*arrow*) and acoustic shadowing (*arrowheads*). **(B)** Contracted gallbladder filled with stones (*arrow*) and having a large acoustic shadow. **(C)** Microlithiasis: the lower third of this gallbladder (GB) is filled with amorphous sludge (s). (Courtesy of Caroline Taylor, M.D., West Haven, CT.)

increase the sensitivity of the test.[59] The diagnostic role for this noninvasive test of sphincter function will be defined by future studies. Because nitrates and calcium channel blockers also cause sphincter of Oddi relaxation, the clinical response to these agents may be used as a diagnostic aid.[60]

The treatment of sphincter of Oddi dysfunction or stenosis is endoscopic or surgical papillotomy.[55,61] Although some patients respond to nitrates or calcium channel blockers, relief is usually short lived. Endoscopic papillotomy is used as the primary therapy, but the high incidence of pancreatitis and perforation in some series[62,63] should direct the clinician to use care in selecting patients for such intervention. Patients who have restenosis after repeated endoscopic papillotomy should be considered for operative sphincteroplasty.

Pancreas Divisum

During development, the dorsal and ventral buds of the pancreatic duct fuse. The opening of the ventral duct forms the major drainage of the pancreas (duct of Wirsung) and the remnant opening of the dorsal bud forms the minor drainage channel (duct of Santorini). When fusion between the two ducts is partial or absent, the duct of Santorini becomes the major drainage channel. This congenital anomaly is known as pancreas divisum, and may cause pancreatitis.[64]

The relationship of pancreas divisum to pancreatitis is unclear. Pancreas divisum is a common anatomic abnormality; autopsy series report an incidence of about 7%. The incidence assessed by ERCP ranges from 0.3%[65] to 8%.[66] This variability is likely the result of differences in the patient populations and definition of the anomaly. For example, some studies include only patients with a complete separation between the dorsal and ventral ducts. Although earlier studies estimated that pancreas divisum can be found in about 25% of patients with unexplained recurrent pancreatitis, many subsequent studies have not confirmed this association.[67] Proponents of the pathologic association have suggested that resistance to the flow of secretions through the duct of Santorini causes ductal hypertension and pancreatitis. Studies of experimental pancreatitis have shown that obstruction of the pancreatic duct alone may result in pancreatitis.[68] It is likely that a small number of patients with pancreas divisum experience recurrent pancreatitis related to obstruction at the duct of Santorini. The difficulty, however, is in identifying this group of patients.

Several rules should be followed in considering intervention for pancreas divisum.[64,69] First, an anomaly should be considered clinically significant only when it is associated with recurrent, proven pancreatitis. Second, all other causes of pancreatitis should be excluded. Finally, there should be proof of obstruction at the duct of Santorini such as dilation of the dorsal duct and elevated sphincter pressures. A noninvasive functional test of obstruction uses ultrasonography to detect pathologic dilation of the main pancreatic duct in response to secretin. This test has been reported to identify patients with pancreatitis secondary to ductal obstruction by at least one group,[69] but not confirmed by another.[70] Early reports suggest that the clinical response to placing a temporary endoscopic stent into the minor papilla may help identify those patients who would benefit from sphincterotomy.[71] Minor duct sphincterotomy has been used with some success,[72] but such intervention needs to be evaluated prospectively in ran-

domized studies. Because diagnostic tests are still being evaluated and endoscopic sphincterotomy is difficult in patients with pancreas divisum, it is probably worthwhile to refer patients with pancreas divisum and recurrent idiopathic pancreatitis to centers with a specific interest in this process.

Rarely, annular pancreas, duodenal diverticulum, ectopic pancreatic tissue, and duodenal duplication cysts may cause pancreatitis.

Trauma

The rise in violence in our society has been paralleled by an increased incidence of traumatic pancreatitis. Next to penetrating injury, blunt trauma sustained in motor vehicle accidents is now an important cause of traumatic pancreatitis. Infrequent causes include percutaneous pancreatic biopsy, abdominal surgery, and even renal lithotripsy.[73] The symptoms of pancreatic trauma may be difficult to elicit in the severely ill patient and suspected only by the location of the injury. On occasion, recurrent bouts of pancreatitis may develop months to years after injury. The midpancreatic duct, as it crosses the vertebral column, is particularly susceptible to fracture from blunt trauma. In the acute setting, computed tomography (CT) is useful in detecting a disrupted pancreatic duct, focal pancreatitis, and pancreatic necrosis. Similarly, ERCP has been used to demonstrate persistent duct disruption, ductal stricture, and focal pancreatitis. Traumatic pancreatitis has been treated with stenting of the disrupted duct[74] or, most commonly, by pancreatic resection or drainage.

Toxins

Alcohol

Alcoholic pancreatitis may present as an acute bout of pancreatitis. Although past experience has suggested that these episodes are invariably associated with established, chronic, underlying pancreatic damage, this may not be the case. In one series of patients who died of acute alcoholic pancreatitis, almost 40% demonstrated little histologic evidence of chronic pancreatitis.[75] The incidence of pancreatitis is surprisingly low in alcoholic patients. Dreiling and Koller reported that for 100 alcoholic patients, pancreatitis develops in only 5%, cirrhosis in 15%, both in 1%, and neither in 80%.[76] These data indicate that in addition to the amount of alcohol ingested, unknown factors affect a person's susceptibility to injury.

Several major physiologic mechanisms may contribute to the development of alcoholic pancreatitis, including abnormal sphincter of Oddi spasm or relaxation, obstruction of small ductules by proteinaceous plugs, and direct toxic and metabolic effects.[77]

Alcohol has been reported to have variable effects on the pressure at the sphincter of Oddi.[77,78] Alcohol has also been found to stimulate pancreatic secretion through cholinergic pathways.[79] Some have proposed that the combination of sphincter of Oddi spasm and stimulated secretion is responsible for pancreatitis. The pharmacologic doses of ethanol used in many of these studies, however, leave the importance of these effects in question.

Ethanol may change the composition of proteins secreted by the pancreas, resulting in the formation of protein plugs within small pancreatic ductules. These plugs are indistinguishable from those found early in the course of cystic fibrosis, which raises the possibility that these two diseases somehow may be linked. The protein plugs may obstruct small pancreatic ducts and promote pancreatitis. Increased viscosity and elevated protein concentrations found in pancreatic secretions from alcoholic patients are likely to contribute to plug formation.[22] By forming a rigid, insoluble protein structure, specific secretory proteins such as lithostathine[80] (formerly "stone protein") and glycoprotein-2[81,82] are very likely to contribute to the formation of these protein plugs and to stone formation. Of note, glycoprotein-2 is closely related to the principal constituent of renal tubular casts, Tamm-Horsfall protein .

Ethanol also may change the amounts of potentially damaging proteases in pancreatic secretion. For example, increased amounts of lysosomal enzymes and an increased trypsinogen : pancreatic trypsin inhibitor ratio have been reported in pancreatic juice from alcoholic patients.

Ethanol has a number of direct and indirect toxic effects.[83] Although the pancreas has little ability to metabolize alcohol, it is possible that a metabolite of ethanol, acetaldehyde, may reach the pancreas from the liver. Alcohol changes systemic and pancreatic lipid metabolism. One of the first effects of ethanol is the accumulation of lipid droplets within the acinar cell. Acute ethanol has been found to enhance de novo pancreatic triglyceride synthesis and alter membrane fluidity and integrity.[84] Fragile pancreatic lysosomes develop in ethanol-fed rats.[85] Ethanol may affect cellular signaling.[77] Previous discussions have emphasized the ability of pancreatic hyperstimulation by cholecystokinin to cause pancreatitis. Further, by augmenting pancreatic injury, cholecystokinin appears to play a role in many forms of pancreatitis.[86,87] In preliminary studies, ethanol has been found dramatically to sensitize the acinar cell to cholecystokinin-stimulated intracellular zymogen proteolysis.[88] The relevance of these findings is that a combination of moderately elevated cholecystokinin levels and ethanol may result in pancreatic "hyperstimulation," zymogen activation, and autodigestion (see Fig. 90-1). The observation that ethanol potentiated experimental pancreatitis induced by cerulein hyperstimulation,[89] and may contribute to enzyme activation,[90] supports this hypothesis.

Ethanol may have systemic effects that promote the development of pancreatitis. Ethanol can precipitate and contribute to hyperlipidemia, a known risk factor for development of pancreatitis. Diets, especially those rich in fat, may contribute to the deleterious effects of alcohol. Chronic alcoholics have diminished reticuloendothelial function and delayed clearance of protease-inhibitor complexes. Finally, inherited factors such as deficiencies in protease inhibitors may predispose to alcoholic pancreatitis.[77]

Drugs

A variety of drugs have been associated with pancreatitis. It is useful to mention those agents that have been unquestionably linked to pancreatitis and cause severe injury, drugs that are widely used but may have a low incidence of pancreatitis,

and those for which the relationship to pancreatitis is in question[91,92] (Table 90-2).

Several immunosuppressants are clearly linked to pancreatitis. The most common are azathioprine and its major metabolite, 6-mercaptopurine.[93] In one series of 396 patients, pancreatitis was induced in 3.3%. Symptoms developed in all patients within the first month of therapy. Rechallenge with either azathioprine or 6-mercaptopurine was invariably associated with a rapid recurrence of pancreatitis. Furthermore, attempts to desensitize with slowly increasing doses of 6-mercaptopurine always led to recurrent pancreatitis.

Severe bouts of pancreatitis are associated with acquired immunodeficiency syndrome (AIDS) therapy. Trimethoprim-sulfamethoxazole is given for treatment as well as prophylaxis for *Pneumocystis carinii* infection. This agent has clearly been demonstrated to precipitate pancreatitis, albeit uncommonly.[94] Pentamidine has been given intravenously and by aerosol for *Pneumocystis carinii* infection. A few years after its introduction, intravenous pentamidine was reported to cause severe and even fatal pancreatitis. To minimize its toxicity and still deliver high doses to the lung, aerosolized pentamidine replaced the parenteral form. Unfortunately, even aerosolized pentamidine accumulates in the pancreas and causes pancreatitis.[95] The most serious form of pancreatitis in patients with AIDS is that caused by the antiviral agent, 2',3'-dideoxyinosine (ddI).[96] Reports suggests that ddI may induce clinical pancreatitis in more than 20% of patients and cause asymptomatic elevations in serum amylase in an additional 40%.[97] The onset of ddI-associated pancreatitis is typically delayed for several months after the initiation of therapy. Although the mechanism of ddI-induced pancreatitis is unknown,[98] patients having a previous history of pancreatitis and those with advanced infection seem to be at the highest risk for this complication. Decreasing the dose of ddI may reduce the incidence of this serious complication.

Antiinflammatory agents and antibiotics are also reported to cause pancreatitis. Included are sulfasalazine and, in a small

TABLE 90-2 Drug-Induced Pancreatitis		
STRONG ASSOCIATION	**WEAK ASSOCIATION**	**RELATIONSHIP UNCERTAIN**
Asparaginase	Acetominophen*	Aminosalicylic acid
Azathioprine	Estrogens†	Cimetidine
6-Mercaptopurine	Ergotamine*	Corticosteroids
2',3'-Dideoxyinosine	Furosemide	Cyclosporine
Pentamidine	Isotretinoin†	Erythromycin
	Sulfonamides	Methyldopa
	Sulfasalazine	Metolazone
	Thiazide diuretics	Octreotide
	Tetracycline‡	Piroxicam
	Valproic acid	Zalcitabine

* Overdose.

† Related to dose and generation of hyperlipidemia.

‡ When taken by patients with fatty liver of pregnancy.

Adapted from Marshall JB. Acute pancreatitis: a review with an emphasis on new developments. Arch Intern Med 1993;153:1185; and Underwood TW, Frye CB. Drug-induced pancreatitis. Clin Pharm 1993;12:440.

number of patients, oral 5-aminosalicylic acid.[99,100] Reports of corticosteroids and corticotropin causing pancreatitis are difficult to interpret because most patients have other factors that predispose to pancreatitis. It is probable that corticosteroids may directly precipitate pancreatitis, but this appears to be an extremely rare event. Rare cases of pancreatitis secondary to acetaminophen overdose[101] and sulindac-related pancreatitis are reported.[102] The rare (~2%) but severe (~50% mortality) pancreatitis associated with renal or liver transplantation may be linked to drug therapy or to infection.[103] Tetracycline has been linked to pancreatitis in patients with fatty degeneration of the liver, particularly during pregnancy. Although symptoms usually develop within weeks, they have been reported after 2 years of medication. Rarely, tetracycline may precipitate pancreatitis in the absence of underlying liver disease.[104]

The incidence of pancreatitis from thiazide diuretics or furosemide is very low, but their widespread use makes them important precipitating factors.[105] A few agents induce metabolic abnormalities that predispose to pancreatitis. For example, therapy with estrogens or the retinoid derivative, isotretinoin,[106] are associated with a dose-dependent increase in triglycerides and pancreatitis. Valproic acid–induced pancreatitis is not uncommon in the young patients that receive this medication, but tends to be mild.

Agents that overstimulate neural pathways may cause acute pancreatitis. In animal models, neural stimulation can initiate pancreatitis or augment that caused by other agents. Parathion, an alkylphosphate cholinesterase inhibitor, is a widely applied agricultural insecticide. Injury may be induced by ingestion or absorption of parathion through the skin. Almost 50% of patients with toxic exposure to this agent will exhibit biochemical evidence of pancreatitis. Although parathion-induced pancreatitis is usually mild, fatal hemorrhagic pancreatitis has been reported.[107] A similar form of pancreatitis may be induced by the venom of the scorpions *Tityus trinitatis* and *Tityus serrulatus*, found in Trinidad and Brazil, respectively. The toxic polypeptides in tityustoxin have been characterized; they act through cholinergic pathways and are potent stimulants of pancreatic secretion in vitro and induce pancreatitis in animals.[108] Pancreatitis from tityustoxin may result from its stimulation of pancreatic secretion, induction of sphincter of Oddi spasm, and changes in blood flow. Decreases in blood flow account for the ischemic pancreatitis and hepatitis associated with ergotamine poisoning.[109]

Infectious

Viral

The most common viral infections that involve the pancreas are mumps and Coxsackie B virus. These are self-limiting and probably account for many of the single bouts of pancreatitis. Viral hepatitis and fulminant hepatitis, especially hepatitis B, has been associated with pancreatitis.

The high frequency of pancreatic abnormalities in AIDS deserves comment. Hyperamylasemia has been reported in up to 40% of hospital admissions for AIDS.[110] Clinical pancreatitis, however, probably occurs in less than 10% of all patients with AIDS and less than 2% of those not receiving toxic medications. Unless pancreatitis is associated with medications, it usually is mild. In addition to drugs (see section on Drugs), at least three pathologic processes contribute to pancreatitis in patients with AIDS:

1. The human immunodeficiency virus (HIV) may infect the pancreas.[111] This involvement may be responsible for the elevated serum amylase that sometime precedes the clinical onset of AIDS; however, HIV infection alone seems rarely to lead to severe pancreatitis.
2. Opportunistic infections may involve the pancreas. Most infections are caused by cytomegalovirus. In the remainder, cryptococcus, *Toxoplasma gondii*, *Mycobacterium tuberculosis*, and *Candida* species have been reported.[112,113] Similar to primary HIV infection, it is unusual for these opportunistic infections to produce severe pancreatitis.
3. Pancreatic neoplasms develop in about 5% of patients with AIDS. Kaposi's sarcoma and lymphoma are the most common and are usually accompanied by disseminated disease.[113] Pancreatitis, however, is not a common manifestation of this tumor involvement.

Bacterial and Parasitic

The list of bacteria associated with acute pancreatitis includes *Salmonella* species, *Shigella* species, *Campylobacter* species, hemorrhagic *Escherichia coli*, *Legionella* species, *Leptospira* species, and even *Brucella* species.[114-116] Pancreatitis associated with these infections is most likely secondary to released toxins. Usually, acute pancreatitis is not the primary manifestation of these infections. Direct involvement of the pancreas with parasites may commonly precipitate pancreatitis in some populations. Almost 15% of cases of biliary pancreatitis in a series from the Orient could be ascribed to *Ascaris lumbricoides* infection.[117]

Metabolic

Hyperlipidemia

Although hyperlipidemia may result from a bout of pancreatitis, hyperlipidemia may also precipitate acute pancreatitis.[118] The breakdown products of triglycerides are responsible for inducing pancreatitis. When lipase in the pancreatic capillary bed acts on the high levels of triglycerides in the serum, toxic free fatty acids are generated.[118] The endothelial lining of small pancreatic blood vessels is the first site of injury. Damage of small blood vessels leads to recruitment of inflammatory cells and thrombosis. This predicted mechanism is consistent with the clinical observation that the earliest injury in hyperlipidemia-associated pancreatitis is located at small pancreatic blood vessels.

Although triglyceride levels greater than 2000 to 3000 mg/dL usually are required for development of pancreatitis, a few patients seem to manifest this condition when serum levels are only 500 mg/dL. In addition to patients with primary hyperlipidemia (chylomicrons), elevated triglycerides may result from therapy with estrogen or the retinoid derivative, isotretinoin.[106] Typically, estrogen-related pancreatitis occurs within the first months on medication. Patients who are obese, and have underlying glucose intolerance or hypertriglyceridemia, are at greater risk. Isotretinoin, an agent used to treat severe acne, causes dose-dependent hypertriglyceridemia. Pancreatitis from this agent usually develops within the first month of therapy. Discontinuing medications that increase serum triglycerides or therapies that lower serum triglycerides relieves the bouts of pancreatitis.

Hypercalcemia

The relationship of hypercalcemia to pancreatitis has been a topic of discussion. Experimentally, acute calcium infusion causes increased pancreatic duct permeability[119] that may lead to a nonspecific increase in serum enzymes. In animals, acute hypercalcemia may induce a very mild form of pancreatic injury.[120,121] Virtually all causes of hypercalcemia, including hyperalimentation, infusions associated with cardiac bypass, immobilization, multiple myeloma, and hyperparathyroidism have been linked to pancreatitis.[105,122] These studies indicate that hypercalcemia is associated with an increase in serum enzymes, but its role in pancreatic injury is less clear.

Vascular

Primary vascular diseases may rarely precipitate pancreatitis. Pancreatic infarcts may occur in patients with underlying arteriosclerotic vascular disease or malignant hypertension. Potent vasoconstrictors may generate ischemic pancreatic and hepatic injury.[109] Vasculitis may cause pancreatitis associated with systemic lupus erythematosus,[123] Wegner's disease,[124] and Behçet's disease.[125] Pancreatitis may respond to successful treatment of the underlying vasculitis.

Other

Fibrocalculous (Tropical)

In Africa and India and a few other countries bordering the equator, pancreatitis often presents in childhood. Although diabetes is the most common presenting feature, abdominal pain and acute pancreatitis, and malabsorption are also frequent. So common is pancreatic calcification that the diagnosis is often made by an abdominal radiograph. Despite reports implicating malnutrition with a low-fat diet, alcohol, hereditary factors, and chronic cyanide exposure as causative factors,[126] the etiology remains unknown.

Iatrogenic

Occasionally, pancreatitis is induced by invasive procedures such as surgery involving the upper abdomen and especially the spleen, lithotripsy,[127] and percutaneous pancreatic biopsy.[128] The most common iatrogenic cause, however, relates to diagnostic and therapeutic pancreatic endoscopy.

ERCP as a cause of pancreatitis.   In large series published in the 1980s, the incidence of post-ERCP pancreatitis was reported as between 0.4% and 1.2%.[129] After ERCP, serum levels of pancreatic enzymes increase within several hours in all patients regardless of the development of clinical pancre-

atitis.[130] Peak levels may not be reached for 24 hours. A number of factors may influence the development of post-ERCP pancreatitis. The number of times contrast is injected into the duct and the extent of visualization are important. Injection of quantities of contrast sufficient to opacify the pancreatic parenchyma, causing acinarization, and to opacify the kidneys, increases the risks for pancreatitis 5- to 10-fold.[63] To minimize the risk of precipitating pancreatitis, the endoscopist should limit the number of injections and carefully monitor the flow of contrast into the pancreas to prevent overfilling and an "acinar blush." One small series reported that patients having low levels of α_2-macroglobulin, a serum protease inhibitor, were at increased risk for development of pancreatitis after ERCP.[130] The use of less concentrated contrast media, antibiotics, secretin, or even somatostatin has not been shown to reduce the incidence of pancreatitis. Indeed, somatostatin has been implicated in precipitating pancreatitis,[131,132] and may acutely increase sphincter of Oddi pressure.[133] In summary, although serum enzymes increase in most patients after ERCP, pancreatitis is infrequent.

Endoscopic sphincterotomy.   Performing endoscopic sphincterotomy (ES) probably doubles the risk for pancreatitis.[63] Those with sphincter of Oddi dysfunction have twice the risk of an ES-related complication. This increased risk may be related to the small and scarred papilla often encountered in patients with sphincter of Oddi dysfunction. To perform ES on such a papilla often requires considerably more electrical energy than a routine papillotomy. Thus, surrounding tissues may be subjected to greater thermal damage. Furthermore, generation of local edema and the restricted size of the papillotomy may result in obstruction to pancreatic outflow.

A complication of ES that may be confused with pancreatitis is perforation into the lesser sac. This complication is associated with epigastric and back pain and may be diagnosed by detecting air or orally administered contrast in the lesser sac by CT. Despite some opposing views, it appears that most patients with this form of perforation can be managed nonsurgically with only nasogastric suction and broad-spectrum antibiotic coverage.[63]

Peptic Ulcer

Ulcers located at the posterior duodenal bulb may burrow into the head of the pancreas. Pancreatitis associated with duodenal ulcers is rarely severe and not associated with dramatic increases in the serum amylase. This diagnosis should be considered in patients with ulcer disease when the typical epigastric burning pain of an ulcer begins to radiate to the back and is less responsive to ulcer medications.

Coronary Artery Bypass

Surgical procedures and severe illness have been associated with elevated serum amylase levels, but the incidence of pancreatitis in these settings is unclear. In a prospective study, Rattner and colleagues reported that 32% of patients had hyperamylasemia after cardiac bypass, but only 2.7% had overt pancreatitis.[134] In a retrospective study of 4473 patients who underwent cardiopulmonary bypass, Huddy and associates[135] reported acute pancreatitis in only 0.1% of patients, all of whom died. In a similar study by Lefor and colleagues,[136] acute pancreatitis was observed in 0.44% of those undergoing bypass, with a mortality of 44%. Finally, Fernandez-del Castillo and colleagues demonstrated a direct correlation between the elevation of pancreatic enzymes and the amount of calcium administered to patients during cardiac bypass.[122] Together, these studies indicate that although elevations in pancreatic enzymes are common after cardiac bypass surgery and may relate to a nonspecific effect of calcium on pancreatic duct permeability,[119,120] overt pancreatitis is uncommon. A severe form of pancreatitis sometimes does occur after cardiac bypass, however, and may be related to pancreatic ischemia.

Neoplasia

Pancreatitis is associated with both primary pancreatic tumors and metastases. Pancreatitis has been reported in up to 10% of patients with pancreatic cancer, but it was invariably mild.[137] The incidence of pancreatitis is higher with lesions of the papilla of Vater and pancreatic head. Frequently, the symptoms of pancreatitis precede the diagnosis of pancreatic cancer by months. Metastasis from gastric cancer is said to be the most common nonpancreatic tumor associated with pancreatitis.

Inflammatory Bowel Disease

Pancreatitis encountered in patients with inflammatory bowel disease may be related to drugs, structural and inflammatory changes, or may be idiopathic in nature.[138] Virtually all medications used for the treatment of inflammatory bowel disease have been reported to precipitate pancreatitis. This list includes azothiaprine, 6-mercaptopurine, sulfasalazine, and 5-aminosalicylic acid, as discussed. Reports linking corticosteroids and metronidazole[139] to pancreatitis are rare. Patients with pancreatitis and Crohn's disease often have inflammatory bowel disease involving the duodenum. The inflammatory process may be associated with stenosis of the ampulla or a fistula into the pancreatic duct. Filling of the pancreatic duct by a barium meal indicates a pancreatic fistula. The increased incidence of gallstones in patients with Crohn's disease should always direct one to examine the biliary tract. In a small number of patients, however, no etiology is identified.[140]

Miscellaneous

The most common hereditary diseases associated with acute pancreatitis are familial pancreatitis and cystic fibrosis, and may present in childhood. Many cases of childhood pancreatitis are associated with multisystem disease such as sepsis, viral infections, hemolytic-uremic syndrome, and Reye's syndrome.[141] Blunt trauma is the single most common cause of acute pancreatitis, followed in decreasing incidence by congenital defects, metabolic diseases, and drugs. An increased incidence of pancreatitis has been reported during pregnancy and the early postpartum period.[142] The increased incidence of hypertriglyceridemia and biliary stone formation during pregnancy may contribute to this predisposition.[143] Refeeding after long periods of fasting is said to precipitate pancreatitis, but this has not been well characterized. A few patients with

possible food allergy-associated pancreatitis have been reported.[144]

In the postoperative period there is an increase in the incidence of hyperamylasemia, even after extraabdominal procedures such as cardiac bypass.[136] It appears that in many cases these increases are nonspecific and unrelated to clinically overt pancreatitis, although severe pancreatitis may ensue and is related to hypotension.[136] Greater attention, however, should be given to those who may experience pancreatic trauma during upper abdominal surgery.

Idiopathic

The number of patients having unexplained bouts of pancreatitis has diminished in large part owing to imaging and invasive tests that have evolved over the past decade.[145,146] Compelling evidence that biliary microlithiasis may cause pancreatitis will undoubtedly further decrease those assigned to the idiopathic group.[50,51]

DIAGNOSIS

The diagnosis of acute pancreatitis is almost always based on the presence of severe abdominal pain and biochemical evidence of pancreatic injury. But the clinician should be aware that the ability to make a diagnosis of acute pancreatitis is limited by a number of factors. Although the gold standard for diagnosing acute pancreatitis is a direct examination of the pancreas, this information is rarely available. The biochemical markers of pancreatic injury are nonspecific and the radiologic markers are too expensive to be used on a routine basis. Finally, an appreciable number of patients with severe acute pancreatitis may present without abdominal pain. These shortcomings lead to confusing nonpancreatic diseases with pancreatitis and to missing the diagnosis entirely. In a surprising number of patients with severe, fatal pancreatitis, the diagnosis is not made before the time of autopsy.

Diagnostic advances do not appear to have reduced the rate of fatal, undetected pancreatitis.[147] The average incidence in series published before 1980 was 45% (range, 7%–86%). For series published during the 1980s, fatal pancreatitis went undetected 22% to 42% of the time.[147] Pancreatitis went undetected for several reasons. First, the typical symptoms of pancreatitis were absent. Although respiratory failure and coma were often present, abdominal pain was infrequent and may have been masked by analgesia. Second, serum amylase levels were either not measured or obtained too late in the course of the illness to be of value. Finally, the presence of pancreatitis was missed by relying on ultrasonography to exclude the diagnosis. These studies stand as an important reminder that patients with severe pancreatitis may present with multiorgan failure rather than abdominal pain. In this setting, the diagnosis of acute pancreatitis is most reliably made by CT.

Symptoms

Pain is the most common symptom of acute pancreatitis and occurs in 95% of patients. It is often located in the epigastric and umbilical region and may radiate to the low thoracic region of the back. The pain usually does not reach its peak for 30 minutes to several hours and may last for hours to days. This deep, visceral pain is among the most severe and often leaves even the medicated patient writhing in discomfort. In some, pain will decrease when sitting and leaning forward compared to when the patient lies flat. This symptom is caused by the retroperitoneal position of the pancreas and may be produced by other retroperitoneal processes. Nausea and vomiting are present in 85% of patients and may occur without an ileus or gastric outlet obstruction. Unlike patients with ulcer disease, vomiting does not relieve pain. Although rare, pancreatitis may present with respiratory failure, confusion, or coma, and without abdominal pain.

Signs

Low-grade fevers are reported in 60% of patients, but high-grade fevers may indicate the presence of cholangitis or infected necrosis. Tachycardia and hypotension are found in up to 40% of patients and may result from enhanced vascular permeability, vasodilation, and hemorrhage. Abdominal tenderness and guarding is common, and bowel sounds are often decreased or absent. Pleural effusions are most often found on the left, but may be bilateral. Mild jaundice is not unusual, but bilirubin levels greater than 4 mg/dL suggest extrahepatic obstruction or underlying liver disease. Dark discoloration in the back or the periumbilical region may arise from any retroperitoneal hemorrhage, including hemorrhagic pancreatitis.

Laboratory Tests

Markers of Pancreatic Injury

The goals of diagnostic tests for pancreatitis are to establish the diagnosis in patients with abdominal pain and to determine the severity of the process and provide prognostic information. Clinicians should be mindful that a number of factors influence the level of serum markers. First, serum levels of pancreatic enzymes are the sum of tissue production, release into the blood stream, and clearance. Thus, in patients with renal failure, the serum amylase may increase only because the enzyme is not cleared by the kidney. Second, the enzyme activities measured may be influenced by a number of "serum factors" and may not reflect absolute enzyme levels. For example, hyperlipidemia is know erroneously to reduce routine serum amylase determinations. Third, enzymes may be produced from nonpancreatic tissues, and this may limit the specificity of serum enzyme assays. In general, the higher the enzyme level, the better the chances that one is dealing with pancreatitis. Standard enzyme assays provide no information on the severity of the pancreatitis.

Amylase.   The serum amylase level has been the biochemical standard for diagnosing acute pancreatitis. Many organs generate amylase, an activity that hydrolyzes the internal 1–4 α-linkages of starch. Because there are no circulating inhibitors of amylase activity, measurements of amylase activity in serum are reliable. Amylase may be inhibited by lactescent sera, but this effect can be eliminated by sample dilution. Although many tissues synthesize amylase, most of the serum activity originates from the pancreas (~40%) and the salivary glands (~60%). P-isoamlyase arises from the pancreas, and S-isoamlyase from the salivary glands as well as other tissues such as the fallopian tubes and lung. Pancreatic amylase enters the blood through an unknown pathway and has a serum half-life of about 2 hours. Although the major portion of serum amylase and other pancreatic enzymes is probably cleared by the reticuloendothelial system, about one fourth of serum amylase is excreted in its intact form by the kidney.

Increased serum amylase during acute pancreatitis results from both enhanced release into the blood and decreased renal clearance. Serum amylase levels increase within the first hours after the onset of pancreatitis and parallel serum lipase levels. After an attack, however, the serum amylase falls much more rapidly than lipase, and may return to normal within 24 hours.[148] Lipase levels are more reliable indicators of pancreatitis in patients who are seen several days after the onset of their illness (Fig. 90-4).

In most situations, the degree of amylase elevation is not particularly useful in distinguishing among pancreatic diseases. Amylase levels tend to be lower in patients with alcoholic pancreatitis, pancreatic cancer, or penetrating ulcers, compared to patients with gallstone disease.

The sensitivity and specificity of the total serum amylase is influenced by defining abnormal values. Cutoff values of just above the normal range have been estimated to yield a sensitivity greater than 90%, but a specificity less than 70%. If the cutoff value is increased to three times the upper limit of normal, the specificity is near 100%, but the sensitivity may fall below 60%. Nonspecific increases of onefold to twofold in the serum amylase have been reported after cigarette smoking.[149]

In an attempt to enhance the specificity of amylase measurements, amylase isoforms may be measured. P-isoamlyase is probably best used to confirm that an elevated total amylase level arises from the pancreas.[150] The clinical value of measuring P-isoamlyase may be compromised by the inability of the assay accurately to measure small amounts of this isoform. Furthermore, P-isoamlyase levels may increase in the absence of pancreatitis in patients with biliary tract disease, intestinal perforation, intestinal obstruction or ischemia, and ruptured abdominal aortic aneurysms.[150]

Diseases of the salivary glands may lead to an elevated S-isoamylase; however, S-amylase levels may increase in the absence of salivary disease in chronic alcoholics, postoperative states, lactic acidosis, in patients with anorexia nervosa and bulimia, after esophageal perforation, and in neoplasms such as pulmonary, gastric, and breast carcinoma, and myeloma.[151,152]

Macroamylasemia.   On occasion, a persistently elevated serum amylase is encountered in the absence of symptoms referable to the pancreas. A benign and uncommon condition that can lead to such an elevated serum amylase is macroamylasemia. Amylase is normally found in the bloodstream as a molecule with a molecular weight of 45 kd, but macroamylase often has a molecular weight of greater than 200 kd. The normal ratio of pancreatic to salivary amylase is maintained in macroamylasemia. The high-molecular-weight ma-

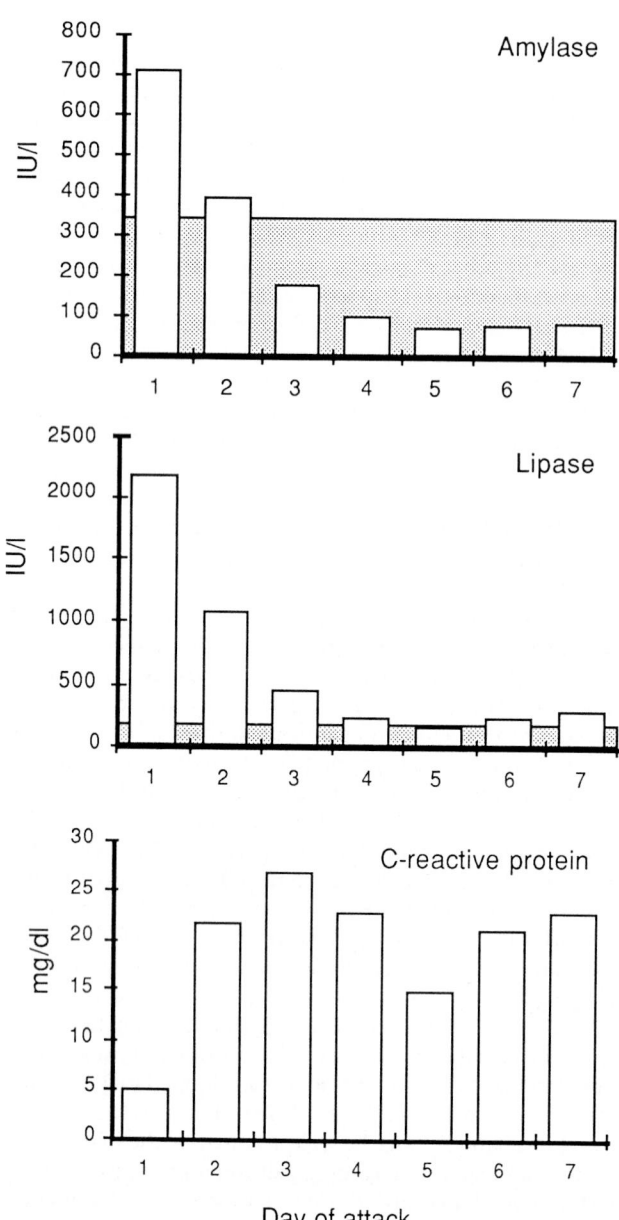

FIGURE 90-4. Serum markers of pancreatic injury. (Adapted from Kolars JC, Elis CJ, Levitt MD. Comparison of serum amylase, pancreatic isoamylase and lipase in patients with hyperamylasemia. Dig Dis Sci 1984;29:289; and Leser HG, Gross V, Scheibenboger C, et al. Evaluation of serum interleukin-6 concentration precedes acute phase response and reflects severity in acute pancreatitis. Gastroenterology 1991;101:782.)

croamylase may result from antibodies complexed to amylase or from amylase polymers.[153] Unlike normal amylase, the macroamylase complex cannot enter the renal tubule for excretion and accumulates in the serum. Several methods can be used to make the diagnosis. First, amylase-to-creatinine clearance ratios of less than 1% strongly support the diagnosis. To confirm the diagnosis in patients with a low clearance, the clinical laboratory may determine the molecular weight of the serum amylase. Alternatively, immunologic assays also may be used.[154]

Lipase. Rapid and reproducible methods for measuring serum lipase are available. Lipase activity is generated by a number of gastrointestinal tissues, including the pancreas, intestine, and liver and biliary tract, and from lingual and gastric sources. In some laboratory assays, the serum lipoprotein lipase activity is also detected.[155] The contribution of these various sources of lipase to serum lipase activity is not clear. Furthermore, the different substrates used in the various commercial assays may affect the specificity of the lipase measurement for pancreatic lipase. The least specific seems to be the Ektachem test, which has been found to have a specificity as low as 25%.[155,156] For many clinicians, the serum lipase has supplanted the amylase as the single test of choice for the diagnosis of pancreatitis. In most series,[150] it is as sensitive and more specific than the total serum amylase, and promises to improve further when the L2 pancreatic lipase is measured.[157] This enhanced specificity of the lipase compared to the amylase level also has been reported in alcoholics.[158] Because lipase levels increase in parallel to serum amylase levels, lipase is a useful early marker of pancreatitis.[150] The lipase level remains elevated longer than the amylase level, and thus may help to diagnose pancreatitis after an acute attack has passed (see Fig. 90-4). Another advantage of lipase is that levels are normal in diabetic ketoacidosis and macroamylasemia.

Other enzymes. Presumably all pancreatic enzymes are released into the blood during acute pancreatitis. Serum trypsin, chymotrypsin, elastase, ribonuclease, and phospholipase A₂ have all been reported to be elevated in acute pancreatitis, but the specificity of these tests has not been sufficiently defined. The pancreatitis-associated protein characterized by Dagorn and colleagues increases after pancreatitis and may prove to be a useful late marker of pancreatitis.[159]

Urinary enzymes. During acute pancreatitis, the renal clearance of amylase increases. Despite early claims, the increased clearance is now recognized as a nonspecific marker of renal tubular dysfunction and is observed in a variety of disease states.

Trypsinogen activation peptide. Premature activation of trypsinogen within the pancreas is thought to be an early step in pancreatitis. In the case of trypsinogen, the small peptide removed during activation is known as *trypsinogen activation peptide* (TAP). Measurement of TAP levels in the blood or urine reflects trypsin activity. The current TAP assays, however, may be too insensitive to be used as the primary test for pancreatitis.[160,161]

Inflammatory Markers

The inflammatory response is a prominent component of pancreatitis and might be expected to increase in parallel with its severity. Several serum markers have been used to quantitate the inflammatory response. *Neutrophil-specific elastase* is released by inflammatory cells and elevated serum levels are detected within the first 12 to 24 hours of pancreatitis,[162] and imaging studies demonstrate that neutrophils accumulate within the pancreas during acute pancreatitis.[163] *Interleukin-6* (IL-6), released by macrophages, also increases during the acute phases of pancreatitis.[164] Acute-phase reactants such as *C-reactive protein* are induced by IL-6 and do not increase until several days (see Fig. 90-4) after the onset of acute pancreatitis.[164] Inflammatory markers may increase during any inflammatory process, and would not be specific for pancreatitis.

Markers of Biliary Tract Involvement

Differentiation between biliary and nonbiliary forms of pancreatitis has important implications for treatment. The time course for development of biochemical and radiologic changes with biliary tract disease varies among the tests (Fig. 90-5). This consideration is particularly relevant when biliary tract obstruction is early in its course or when it is intermittent.

Stones within the common bile duct are often accompanied by an elevated bilirubin, alkaline phosphatase, and markers of acute hepatocyte injury such as the alanine (AST) or aspartate aminotransferase (ALT).[165] Marked elevations of amylase of greater than 2000 to 4000 IU/L also favor a biliary source.[166] Reports that the ratio of lipase to amylase is greater in alcoholic than in biliary pancreatitis[167] require confirmation.

One of the most critical issues in patient management is persistent choledocholithiasis. Elevations of the serum bilirubin, AST or ALT, and alkaline phosphatase are good predictors of persistent common duct stones.[165] Furthermore, when AST or similar markers of acute hepatocellular injury are elevated and fluctuate by more than 50% in a 24-hour period, it suggests intermittent biliary tract obstruction. This finding is especially helpful in patients with chronic liver dis-

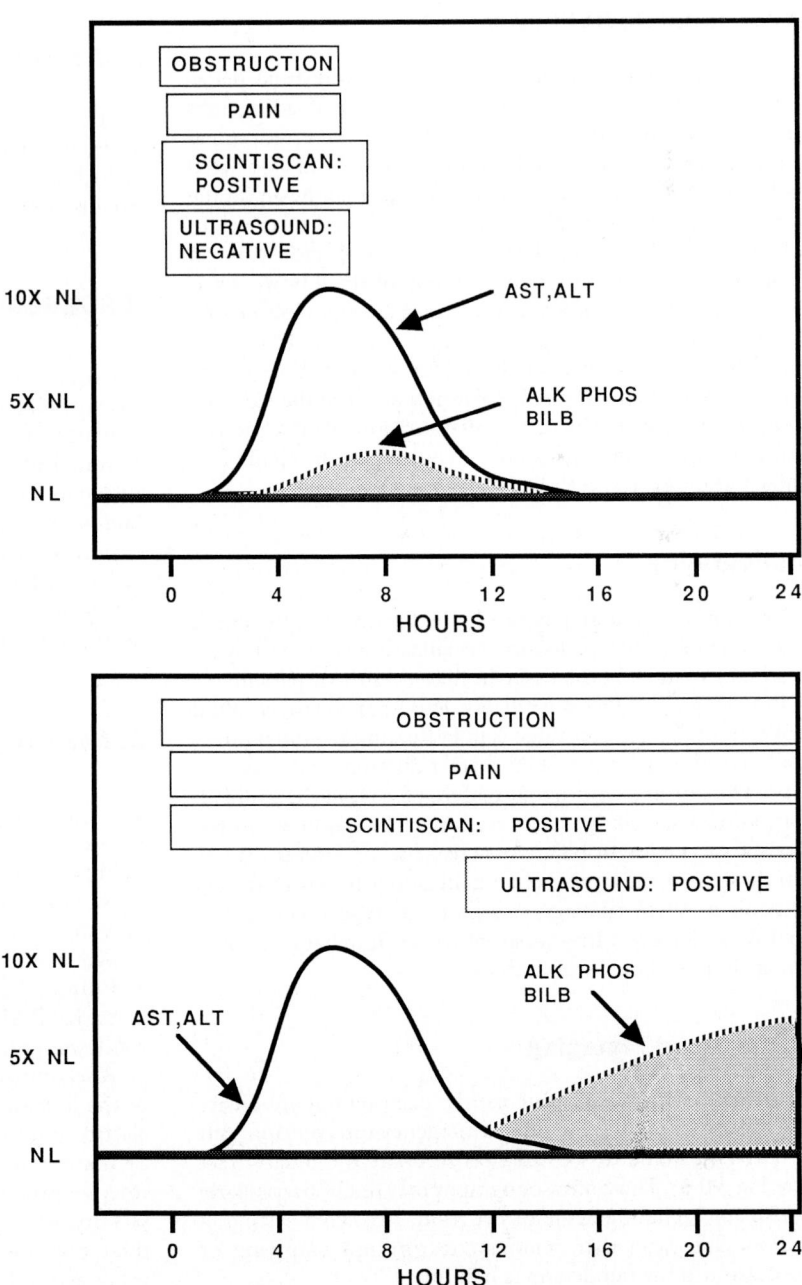

FIGURE 90-5. Usual time course of abnormalities in patients with transient (*top*) or persistent (*bottom*) biliary tract obstruction. (Courtesy of J. Dobbins, M.D., New Haven, CT.)

ease who have stable baseline elevations in AST and ALT levels.

Systemic Markers of Acute Pancreatitis

A low-grade to moderate fever is not unusual in acute pancreatitis. Persistent high fevers suggest infection. Leukocytosis is common, and severe pancreatitis has been associated with leukemoid reactions even in the absence of infection. Although measurements of methemalbumin are popular in Europe,[168] it has been found to be an insensitive marker of severe pancreatitis and is rarely used in the United States.

Imaging

Abdominal Radiographs

To exclude nonpancreatic sources such as intestinal perforation, standard and upright chest and abdominal radiographs should be performed on every patient with severe abdominal pain. A variety of radiographic findings have been associated with pancreatitis. Pleural effusions are most common on the left, but may be bilateral and rarely are limited to the right pleural space.[169] Intestinal gas patterns may demonstrate an ileus pattern or an isolated dilated loop of small bowel overlying the pancreas known as the sentinel loop. Colonic obstruction may result in air in the right and transverse colon that abruptly terminates at the splenic flexure. Loss of the psoas margins and increased separation between the stomach and colon suggest pancreatic inflammation. Pancreatic calcification or calcified gallstones may suggest an alcohol or biliary etiology, respectively.

Sonography

Although ultrasonography can be performed rapidly and at the patient's beside, pancreatic visualization is limited by intestinal gas and adipose tissue in 30% to 40% of patients.[150] Ultrasonography does not reliably detect pancreatitis or fluid collections. Its greatest value is in evaluating the biliary tract and detecting gallstones, biliary tract dilation, and cholecystitis. The shifting, amorphous material found in the gallbladder, known as "sludge," can no longer be ignored and has been associated with biliary pancreatitis.[50,51] Stones may be overlooked in the large dilated gallbladder found in fasting patients or obscured by gas, necessitating repeat sonography or ERCP. Finally, ultrasonography is an unreliable method for excluding choledocholithiasis.

Radionuclide Imaging

In patients with biliary pancreatitis, persistent acute biliary tract obstruction often requires emergency intervention. But it may take hours for obstruction to dilate the biliary tract (see Fig. 90-5). Thus, ultrasonography may not be particularly useful for excluding acute obstruction. In such a setting, a radionuclide scan that demonstrates prompt emptying of contrast into the duodenum is helpful.

Computed Tomography

CT is the optimal tool for pancreatic imaging. It is not limited by intestinal gas, or body habitus. CT may not detect up to 20% of mild cases. Cost and need to transport patients for an examination limit the routine use of CT in patients with pancreatitis. Furthermore, CT is not a satisfactory method for excluding gallstones and probably provides false-negative results 50% of the time. Its specificity for identifying gallstones, however, is near 100%. Contrast-enhanced CT is a good prognostic indicator. Patients demonstrating greater than 50% pancreatic necrosis on contrast-enhanced CT scan, especially when accompanied by extrapancreatic fluid collections with mixed densities, are at considerable risk for development of pancreatic infections.[170,171] Dynamic CT should be reserved for patients with severe pancreatitis.

Endoscopic Pancreatography

ERCP does not play a role in establishing the diagnosis of acute pancreatitis. The exceptions to this rule, patients with gallstone pancreatitis and suspected traumatic pancreatitis, are discussed elsewhere.

ASSESSMENT

There are several important reasons to establish the prognosis in acute pancreatitis. It may allow the clinician to predict the patient's course and anticipate downturns or the need for hospitalization. Prognostic information may direct the clinician to intervene using dynamic CT scanning or ERCP and endoscopic papillotomy. Finally, it allows the clinical investigator to measure the success or failure of therapeutic interventions. The tools used to measure prognosis fall into three categories: specific laboratory tests, clinical and physiologic assessment, and CT.[150,172]

Laboratory Tests

The standard laboratory tests used to diagnose pancreatitis provide little prognostic information, but several new tests hold promise for separating patients with mild disease from those with severe disease. The first is the TAP assay, an indirect measure of the amount of active trypsin. From a pathophysiologic standpoint, this is an elegant test; the more trypsin activation, the more pancreatic damage. One small study suggests that TAP levels discriminate between patients destined for development of mild or severe pancreatitis.[168]

A second group of tests provides a measure of the severity of the inflammatory response. These include the neutrophil elastase and the monokine IL-6 tests. Both are elevated within 24 hours and correlate with the severity of pancreatitis.[164] C-reactive protein is induced by IL-6 and is a late marker of severity (see Fig. 90-4). With the exception of the TAP assay, these tests measure inflammatory activity only, and can be presumed to be nonspecific.

Computed Tomography

A routine CT scan can be used to infer the presence of pancreatitis by detecting pancreatic edema and peripancreatic inflammation and fluid collections.[173] Routine CT, however, does not provide reliable information on prognosis. To provide information on the amount of tissue necrosis in acute pancreatitis, dynamic CT has been used. In this scan, rapid images are taken through the region of the pancreas before and after a bolus of intravenous contrast. A normal pancreas will demonstrate uniformly enhanced CT density, but those with necrosis exhibit regions that do not enhance after intravenous contrast. Based on the amount of the pancreas that fails to shown enhancement, the radiologist estimates the degree of pancreatic necrosis.[170] Estimates of pancreatic necrosis by dynamic CT correlate with observations made at surgery.[174] Patients with greater than 50% pancreatic necrosis have a poor prognosis. Prognostic scoring that uses routine and contrast-enhanced CT has been used to evaluate patients with pancreatitis (Table 90-3); the CT Severity Index has been shown to correlate with the Ranson criteria for assessing severity.[170] In one study, patients with CT Severity Index scores up to 2 had only 4% morbidity and no mortality, but those with scores from 7 to 10 experienced 92% morbidity and 17% mortality.[170] The most common life-threatening complication of severe necrosis is pancreatic infection. Patients with both significant pancreatic necrosis and extrapancreatic fluid collections of mixed density, lacking a well-defined margin, are at greatest risk for development of an infection. Abscesses, however, may develop within fluid collections in the absence of necrosis.[170] These distinctions may become more important as feasible approaches to preventing pancreatic abscesses are developed. In summary, the routine use of CT or dynamic CT for the evaluation of acute pancreatitis is not justified, but should be considered in patients with severe pancreatitis and intact renal function. To provide greater sensitivity, prognostic systems that use physical and laboratory measurements have been established.

TABLE 90-3
Computed Tomography Severity Index

	POINTS
Grade of Acute Pancreatitis	
A: Normal pancreas	0
B: Pancreatic enlargement	1
C: Inflammation confined to pancreas and peripancreatic fat	2
D: One peripancreatic fluid collection	3
E: Two or more fluid collections	4
Degree of Necrosis	
No necrosis	0
Necrosis of one third of pancreas	2
Necrosis of one half of pancreas	4
Necrosis of more than one half	6

Computed tomography severity index = grade points + degree of necrosis. See the text for correlation between the severity score and outcome.

Adapted from Balthazar EJ, Robinson DL, Megibow AJ, Ranson JH. Acute pancreatitis: value of CT in establishing prognosis. Radiology 1990;174:331.

TABLE 90-4
Ranson and Simplified Glasgow Prognostic Scoring Criteria

RANSON	SIMPLIFIED GLASGOW
On Admission	**Within 48 h**
Age > 55 y	Age > 55 y
WBC >16,000 mm^3	WBC >15,000 mm^3
LDH >350 IU/L	LDH >600 IU/L
Glucose >200 mg/dL	Glucose >180 mg/dL
AST >250 IU/L	Albumin <3.2 g/dL
Within 48 h	Calcium <8 mg/dL
Hematocrit decrease by >10%	Arterial PO$_2$ <60 mm Hg
Urea nitrogen increase by >5 mg/dL	Urea >45 mg/dL
Serum calcium <8 mg/dL	
Arterial PO$_2$ <60 mm Hg	
Base Deficit >4 MEq/L	
Estimated fluid sequestration >6 L	

See the text for the correlation between scores and severity.

AST, aspartate transaminase; LDH, lactate dehydrogenase; WBC, white blood cells.

Adapted from Agarwal N. Pitchumoni CS. Assessment of severity in acute pancreatitis. Am J Gastroenterol 1990; 85:356; and Marshall JB. Acute pancreatitis: a review with an emphasis on new developments. Arch Intern Med 1993;153: 1185.

Clinical and Physiologic Assessment

The criteria established by Ranson and colleagues are still the most widely applied to the assessment of acute pancreatitis.[175] Ranson's criteria (Table 90-4) are said to distinguish between patients who will have mild or severe pancreatitis 90% of the time, but are not as accurate in predicting mortality. The greatest prognostic value is derived from the Ranson criteria when applied on admission and at 48 hours. Using Ranson's criteria, patients with fewer than two signs have very low rates of morbidity (<5%) and mortality (<1%). With three to five signs, morbidity and mortality increase to approximately 30% and 5%, and with six or more signs, 90% and 20%, respectively.[175] The disadvantage of Ranson's criteria is that they require that 11 values be monitored over 48 hours of measurement. Blamey and colleagues[176] developed the Glasgow classification, which can be calculated any time within the first 48 hours of hospitalization and measures only eight parameters (see Table 90-4). The simplified Glasgow criteria appear to have prognostic accuracy similar to that of Ranson's criteria.

Although some prognostic classifications have dropped the hematocrit, base deficit, and fluid sequestration from Ranson's criteria, others have added obesity as an independent risk factor.[177] The higher risk in the obese patient may result from respiratory compromise from physical restraints, or from the provision of toxin-generating substrates (triglycerides) from peritoneal fat stores.

The most recent prognostic tool applied to acute pancreatitis is the Acute Physiology and Chronic Health Evaluation (APACHE) III criteria.[175,178,179] This system uses 14 routinely measured parameters of physiologic activity and biochemical function (Table 90-5), and generates a numerical score that depends on their deviation from the normal range. The pa-

TABLE 90-5
Measurements Required for Acute Physiology and Chronic Health Evaluation (APACHE III) Severity Assessment Prognostic Scoring Criteria*

Temperature	Serum sodium and potassium
Mean blood pressure	Serum glucose
Heart rate	Serum creatinine
Respiratory rate	Blood urea nitrogen
Oxygenation	Leukocytes
Arterial pH	Hematocrit
	Albumin
	Bilirubin

* Additional scoring factors: Age, history of severe organ system insufficiency or immunocompromise, neurologic state, and postoperative state are also scored. Each category is assigned a numerical value weighted by its deviation from the normal range. The sum of the numeric scores predicts the severity of the patient's disease.[175]

tient's age, organ insufficiency, neurologic state, and post-operative state are also weighted. The potential advantage of the APACHE is that it can be calculated instantaneously from routine measurements. Further, it can be regularly updated to follow a patient's progress. A major shortcoming of this classification is that it is complex and requires computer analysis to establish a prognostic score. Additional prospective studies are needed to established scores that provide the greatest prognostic value on admission and during the course of pancreatitis.

ACUTE TREATMENT

Fluid and Electrolyte Replacement

The cornerstone of therapy is providing supportive care. Most important is replacement of fluid, electrolyte, and colloid losses.[180] The analogy between the injury of severe pancreatitis and a burn is a useful one. Thus, albumin and other blood products may be required. Although dextrans have been used to expand intravascular volume and enhance pancreatic blood flow,[181] their use has not been widely accepted. In severely ill patients, central venous pressures should be used to monitor fluid replacement and to avoid worsening cardiopulmonary complications. Details of such treatment have been reviewed.[180]

Metabolic Abnormalities

Hyperglycemia is present in at least one fourth of patients with acute pancreatitis. It is wise to err on the side of maintaining the blood glucose level in the high range for several reasons. Limited glucagon and glycogen reserves, especially in alcoholics, diminish the ability of patients to respond to hypoglycemia. Furthermore, hyperglycemia is often transient, improving when the pancreatitis has resolved.

Serum *calcium* levels may be decreased during acute pan-

creatitis and levels below 7.5 mg/dL are associated with a poor prognosis. Factors that account for this decrease are sequestration of calcium by free fatty acids that have been generated by peritoneal fat necrosis[182]; sequestration of calcium by circulating free fatty acids; and dilution by administering calcium-poor fluids. Humoral factors such as parathyroid hormone resistance associated with hypomagnesemia, and hypersecretion of calcitonin and glucagon have been implicated in hypocalcemia, but are unlikely to play a major role. Hypocalcemia should be treated only when the patient becomes symptomatic.

Hyperlipidemia may lead to pancreatitis, accompany alcoholic pancreatitis, or be a consequence of acute pancreatitis.[118] Therapy should not be instituted for hyperlipidemia encountered during acute pancreatitis, but values should be reassayed after recovery. Only those who maintain elevated values need be considered for treatment.

Nutritional Support

Severe acute pancreatitis places metabolic demands on the patient that are similar to those seen in patients with gram-negative sepsis or severe burns. The changes include increased cardiac output, decreased peripheral resistance, increased oxygen consumption, and increased energy expenditure. The special nutritional considerations required for that small group of patients with severe and protracted pancreatitis have been reviewed.[183]

Energy expenditure is often remarkably increased in patients with severe pancreatitis.[184] This fact affects care in two ways. First, if there is any question about the severity of the patient's illness, err in the direction of providing alimentation. Second, metabolic derangement may require that the intravenous alimentation solutions be modified. Most patients in this group tolerate a glucose-based regimen with twice-weekly lipid emulsion, and have a good prognosis. In some patients, however, glucose is not tolerated despite the use of large amounts of insulin. Lipids may be used to supply up to 50% of caloric requirements in glucose-intolerant patients, but these patients have a poor prognosis compared to the glucose-tolerant group. Intravenous lipids are safe if monitored. Intravenous lipids do not stimulate pancreatic secretion, but hypertriglyceridemia may precipitate pancreatitis.[185] Patients with pancreatitis are predisposed to hypertriglyceridemia based on their underlying pancreatitis or alcoholism.[118] Furthermore, glucose intolerance and hyperglycemia are common and may also lead to hypertriglyceridemia. Based on available studies, it is prudent to use intravenous lipids, but to maintain triglyceride levels below 500 mg/dL.

Tradition holds that the patient recovering from a bout of acute pancreatitis should be started on a low-fat diet, but there is little evidence that this restriction affects recovery. This management ignores the fact that lumenal amino acids are also potent stimulants of pancreatic enzyme secretion. Probably more important than fat restriction is the subjective response of the patient to feeding. The most reliable marker for beginning feeding is hunger. Persistent elevations in serum enzymes in the absence of symptoms or evidence of a complication should not dissuade the clinician from feeding a hungry patient.

Nasogastric Suction

The use of nasogastric suction in the past was based on the unproved concept that removing the acid-dependent stimulation of the pancreas would allow the inflamed organ to rest and promote recovery. A consensus based on clinical trials suggests that the only time nasogastric suction should be used is in the patient with severe pancreatitis and an ileus.[180]

Antibiotics

The routine use of antibiotics for acute pancreatitis should be discouraged.[186] Indeed, one series found that patients with mild pancreatitis who received ampicillin fared worse than a control group. The use of antibiotics in patients with severe pancreatitis or in patients with biliary pancreatitis has not been critically evaluated, however (see section on Pancreatic Necrosis, Prevention of Infection).

Inhibition of Secretion and Enzymes

Like nasogastric suction, biochemical approaches to inhibiting pancreatic secretion with such agents as somatostatin and glucagon have not made an impact on the course of acute pancreatitis. Indeed, somatostatin has been reported to cause sphincter of Oddi spasm[133] and may even induce pancreatitis.[132] Another form of intervention has targeted the digestive enzymes that are activated during acute pancreatitis. Inhibitors of pancreatic proteases have a beneficial effect on the course of experimental pancreatitis,[35] but when administered after the onset of pancreatitis have not been shown to be beneficial in clinical trials. The relative delay in administering protease inhibitors in acute pancreatitis or their effectiveness in reaching sufficient concentrations in the pancreas may account for their lack of efficacy.

Endoscopy

In patients with peptic ulcer disease in whom mild pancreatitis develops, it is reasonable to perform an endoscopy to exclude a posterior penetrating duodenal ulcer. Upper gastrointestinal hemorrhage from erosive gastritis or duodenitis is not infrequent in patients with acute pancreatitis.

ERCP and Papillotomy in the Treatment of Pancreatitis: Emergency Treatment

Emergency ERCP is used in acute pancreatitis to remove stones that are impacted at the ampulla. But even when patients undergo ERCP soon after the onset of gallstone pancreatitis, few stones are found at the ampulla. Clinical predictors of persistent common duct stones include a dilated common bile duct, elevated bilirubin, and elevated AST and ALT levels.

Under what conditions should the clinician consider intervening with emergency ERCP? A key study by Neoptolemos and associates offers the best guidance.[187] Patients with the clinical diagnosis of acute gallstone pancreatitis were randomized to receive either emergency endoscopic papillotomy with stone removal or conservative therapy with ERCP or surgery after recovery. Patients with severe pancreatitis had fewer complications and a shorter hospital stay when managed with emergency ERCP than those treated conservatively. In patients with mild pancreatitis, outcomes were equivalent regardless of whether they underwent emergency ERCP or were managed conservatively. One report has suggested that all patients with biliary pancreatitis might benefit from emergency ERCP,[117] but this series had a high percentage of patients with biliary parasites, did not use antibiotics, and demonstrated a marginal benefit from intervention. Based on limited information, our approach is to reserve emergency ERCP and papillotomy for those patients with severe gallstone pancreatitis and cholangitis. Because cholangitis develops in less than 15% of patients with biliary pancreatitis, only a small group is considered for intervention.[188]

Elective Treatment

The management of patients with the milder forms of gallstone pancreatitis is also changing. In the past, after the resolution of pancreatitis, these patients received cholecystectomy with common duct visualization and exploration. ERCP and papillotomy now play a role in managing gallstone pancreatitis. The two major uses of ERCP are as an accompaniment to gallbladder removal to exclude and treat choledocholithiasis, and as the primary therapy. Two factors have led to these modifications of the traditional approach.

First, with the advent of laparoscopic cholecystectomy, operative pain is minimized and the hospital stay and recovery periods have been shortened. These features have made laparoscopic cholecystectomy a popular procedure. Common duct stones identified during or after laparoscopic cholecystectomy should be removed endoscopically. In patients with mild gallstone pancreatitis, ERCP need not be performed before cholecystectomy unless there is good evidence that the patient still has common duct stones. Such evidence includes a persistently dilated common bile duct, positive liver function test results, or recurrent bouts of pancreatitis.

Second, many European practitioners now assert that ERCP alone should be used as the primary therapy for choledocholithiasis, leaving the gallbladder in place after endoscopic papillotomy for choledocholithiasis. Acute cholecystitis develops in only about 15% of such patients in the 2 years after papillotomy.[189] After 2 years, the risk for development of acute cholecystitis reverts to that of the population with gallstones. This practice is followed most closely in patients who are elderly and poor operative risks, but also has been used in younger patients. A variation on this approach used in some patients with biliary pancreatitis is to perform a papillotomy even in the absence of a common duct stone. This intervention anticipates that stones that subsequently enter the common duct from the gallbladder will easily pass through an opened papilla. This contention is supported by experimental data[190]; however, too few patients have been reported to evaluate such therapy.[191]

The treatment of gallstone pancreatitis in patients with cholelithiasis and choledocholithiasis is still evolving. For those who are good operative risks, elective cholecystectomy with operative biliary tract visualization is the treatment of choice. But current practice supports the use of endoscopic papillotomy without cholecystectomy in the patient who is a poor operative risk. Future refinements in laparoscopic cholecystectomy may modify these recommendations.[192]

Emergency Surgery

There are virtually no indications to perform emergency surgery on patients with mild acute pancreatitis. In patients with severe pancreatitis, surgery has been recommended to reduce the severity of the inflammation or eliminate the cause of the disease.[193] The surgical procedures include pancreatic drainage, debridement and resection, biliary surgery, and peritoneal lavage. Although discussions can be found advocating a variety of approaches, the evidence makes it difficult to advocate any of these interventions on an emergency basis.

COMPLICATIONS

Local

Fluid Collections

Peripancreatic fluid collections probably are not uncommon among patients with pancreatitis. The major complication of such a collection is infection, which occurs in only 2% to 4% of patients with pancreatitis.[194] The chance of infection is greatest if the collection is associated with pancreatic necrosis.[170,195,196] Fluid collections may be *simple* and exhibit a uniform CT density that approximates that of water, or *complex* with multiple CT densities and poorly defined margins (Fig. 90-6). In the absence of gas within the collection, a complex density is equivalent to a *phlegmon* (a term that is now avoided because of its varied definitions), and is difficult to drain per-

cutaneously. Although some have advocated drainage for simple collections,[171] evidence demonstrating a benefit for such intervention is lacking. I believe that unless the collection is rapidly expanding or associated with clinical evidence of infection, it should be observed. Infected collections have to be drained and have been successfully treated using percutaneous catheters.[197] Because fluid collections are frequently associated with acute pancreatitis, and most resolve spontaneously, a fluid collection should be defined as a pseudocyst only if it persists for more than 4 weeks.[2]

Ascites

Several processes may contribute to the formation of ascites in acute pancreatitis. Peritoneal inflammation resulting from chemical peritonitis usually generates a small amount of fluid. Attendant chronic liver disease may contribute varying amounts of ascites. *Pancreatic ascites* refers to the presence of large amounts of fluid rich in pancreatic secretions. This form of ascites follows bouts of acute pancreatitis or abdominal trauma.[198] Pancreatic ascites produces a gradual increase in abdominal girth, and is sometimes associated with subcutaneous fat necrosis. The condition arises from a break in the pancreatic duct or drainage of pancreatic contents through a ruptured pseudocyst into the peritoneal cavity. The diagnosis should be suspected when ascites fails to respond to diuretic therapy and the serum amylase level is persistently elevated. Marked elevations in the amylase and protein concentrations above 3 g/dL are typical of pancreatic ascites.

Three forms of treatment have been used to treat massive pancreatic ascites. ERCP often can identify the site of ductal disruption or drainage into a pseudocyst. On occasion, a stent can be used to occlude the disrupted duct.[74] Alternatively, pancreatic resection may be required. Continuous infusion of somatostatin with or without prior drainage of the ascites has also been used.[198,199]

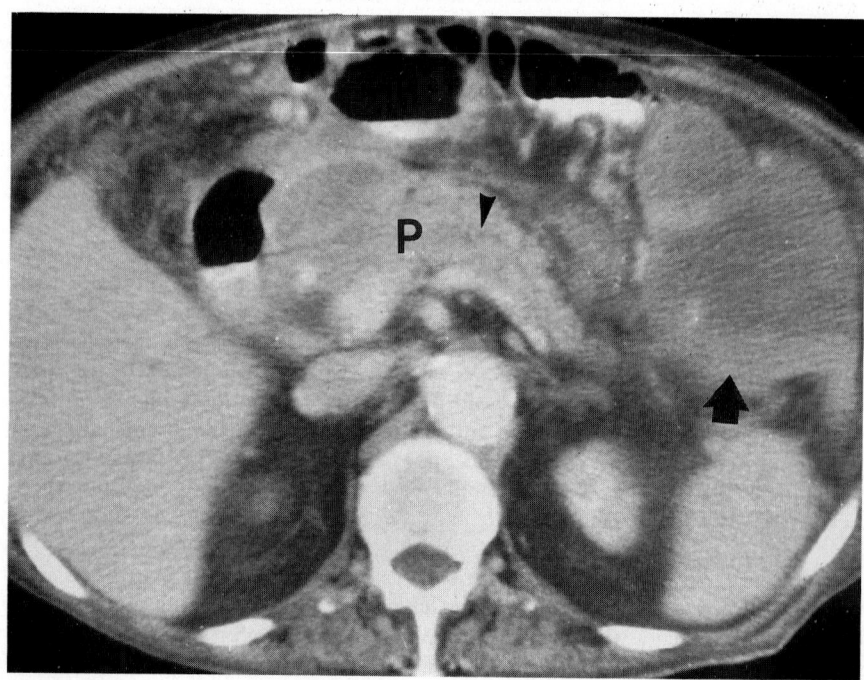

FIGURE 90-6. Fluid collection complicating acute pancreatitis. Computed tomography of pancreatitis after coronary artery bypass graft demonstrates enlargement of the pancreatic head and a mixed-attenuation fluid collection (*arrow*) contiguous with the tail of the pancreas (not shown) (*arrowhead*, pancreatic duct; courtesy of Caroline Taylor, M.D., West Haven, CT.)

Pancreatic Necrosis

Any form of acute pancreatitis may progress to severe disease and extensive pancreatic necrosis.[193,200] By estimating the amount of pancreatic necrosis, dynamic CT provides valuable prognostic information (see Table 90-3).[170] Estimates of greater than 50% necrosis, especially when accompanied by adjacent necrotic material, are associated with a high risk of death, usually due to infection.[173]

Infected Pancreatic Necrosis

The most serious outcome of pancreatic necrosis is infection. Patients with severe necrosis present the clinician with several critical management issues. First, can anything be done to avoid the life-threatening infection? Second, if infection is suspected, how should it be detected and treated? Finally, if infection is excluded, should the necrotic material be surgically debrided?

Prevention of infection.

One therapy that has been scrutinized in clinical studies has been peritoneal lavage. Past studies indicated that although it improved cardiovascular function in the short term, lavage neither prevented infectious complications nor improved survival.[201] More recently, intervention with vigorous (50 L/day) and long-term lavage was reported to eliminate pancreatic infection in patients with severe necrosis.[202] Larger, controlled studies are needed, however, before this can be accepted as a standard practice.

Broad-spectrum antibiotics have been empirically used in severe pancreatitis to prevent infection,[203] but past studies do not support such treatment.[186] Patient selection and antibiotic therapy may have influenced previous negative results. For example, antibiotics have not been used based on their ability to penetrate pancreatic tissue or target specific organisms. More recent studies demonstrated that penetration of pancreatic tissues by aminoglycosides is poor, whereas penicillins and quinolones exhibit good penetration.[204] When tissue penetration, frequency and type of bacteria, and bacterial sensitivity are weighed, the most efficacious antibiotics were ciprofloxacin, ofloxacin, and imipenem. Anaerobes play a role in pancreatic infections; metronidazole demonstrated high efficacy against anaerobes. Thus, the most appropriate regimen might include a combination of ciprofloxacin or ofloxacin with metronidazole or imipenem alone. One prospective study suggests that such prophylactic therapy might be beneficial.[205]

Clinical presentation of infection.

Pancreatic infections may be associated with biliary or alcoholic pancreatitis or occur after surgery.[195] It is convenient to divide pancreatic infections into early and late sequelae of pancreatitis. Early infections, occurring within 1 or 2 weeks after an attack, require preexistent pancreatic necrosis, peripancreatic necrosis, or a fluid collection.[196] Infected necrosis is often heralded by a sudden increase in abdominal tenderness, high fever, marked leukocytosis, and bacteremia.[202] Signs of sepsis are frequent and often accompanied by respiratory and renal failure. These early infections spread through areas of necrosis and are often poorly defined.

Late infections generate abscesses in areas of resolving necrosis or within a pseudocyst, and may not become clinically apparent until months after an attack of acute pancreatitis.[195] Abscesses present as abdominal pain with sepsis, but without evidence of pancreatitis. Pancreatic abscesses and infected pseudocysts also may be clinically indolent, presenting with poorly defined abdominal pain with or without hyperamylasemia, minimal leukocytosis, and a low-grade fever.[206] Rarely, patients with underlying chronic pancreatitis may present with pancreatic or hepatic abscesses unrelated to a bout of acute pancreatitis.[207]

Detection of infection.

Infected regions may be poorly defined as they spread through areas of necrosis or may be well defined. Although an abdominal radiograph is sometimes useful, CT usually is required to identify areas of necrosis and abnormal gas collections. Biopsy specimens from areas of suspected infection should be taken using CT-guided needle aspiration. Samples should be immediately examined by Gram's stain. Because Gram's stain alone may miss one third of the infections, culture is mandatory.[203] Polymicrobial infections are usual and carry a poor prognosis; monomicrobial infections are uncommon, but are more successfully treated.[208] Gram-negative enteric and anaerobic organisms are most common,[209] but a high incidence of *Candida* organisms has been reported in patients who received prophylactic antibiotics.[203]

Treatment of infection.

The treatment of infectious complications depends on the pattern of infection. Infections occurring early in the course of pancreatitis are found in necrotic pancreas or a phlegmon and are usually poorly demarcated. Immediate surgical debridement of such infected tissues is mandatory.[196] This treatment reduces mortality from virtually 100% to 15%.[203,209] Depending on the anatomic location of the infected tissue, a retroperitoneal approach may be appropriate.[211] Well demarcated uniloculated abscesses and infected pseudocysts have been successfully drained using percutaneous catheters.[194] Multiloculated abscesses and poorly defined areas of infection are probably best approached surgically.[211,212] Somatostatin has been used to diminish the drainage from fistulas that often follow percutaneous drainage.[213]

Treatment of sterile pancreatic necrosis.

Mortality rates of 0% to 38% are reported for sterile necrosis.[177,203,214] Factors that correlate with fatal outcome include a high APACHE III score on admission or a high Ranson score within the first 48 hours, shock, renal insufficiency, multiple systemic complications, and obesity.[177] The development of shock was the best predictor of a fatal outcome. The role of surgical debridement in the treatment of severe pancreatic necrosis has been a topic of discussion.[200,203,210] Although the notion that removal of necrotic tissue that might act as a nidus for infection is an attractive one, the risks of performing an extensive surgical procedure must be weighed. In a prospective study, Bradley and Allen reported that patients with sterile necrosis do well when treated without surgical drainage.[203] Despite the fact that more than half of their patients experience pulmonary or renal failure, none died. Although other studies support the nonsurgical approach to managing sterile necrosis,[177] some clinicians advocate surgical debridement and drainage.[214]

Pseudocyst

Localized collections of pancreatic secretions that lack an epithelial lining and persist for more than 4 weeks are known as pseudocysts. In the past, pseudocysts were detected indirectly by clinical suspicion, the appearance of a palpable abdominal mass, and from barium contrast studies that demonstrated a mass. The advent of pancreatic imaging by ultrasonography and CT has led to the realization that pancreatic fluid collections that may become pseudocysts are common and appear in 10% of patients with acute pancreatitis.[215] Although they form most frequently in patients with alcoholic pancreatitis, up to 30% of cases arise in gallstone pancreatitis.[216]

The most common presenting symptom of a pseudocyst is upper abdominal pain. Other symptoms referable to a pseudocyst include early satiety and nausea and vomiting secondary to compression of the stomach or gastric outlet obstruction. Pseudocysts may also enlarge rapidly and rupture, hemorrhage, generate pancreatic ascites, obstruct the biliary tract, compress the inferior vena cava, erode into surrounding structures, including the mediastinum, and become infected.[217,218]

Acute hemorrhage into a pseudocyst is rare but can be a life-threatening event. The source of the bleeding is usually a pseudoaneurysm (Fig. 90-7); venous bleeding is rare.[219,220] Diagnosis is made by CT scanning and angiography. The bleeding artery often can be treated by embolization, but sometimes requires surgical ligation and, rarely, broad surgical resection.[221] An infected abscess presents as a painful abdominal mass and may not arise for weeks to months after a bout of pancreatitis.

The risk for development of these complications varies with the size of a pseudocyst and its age. To avoid complications, which have been reported in 30% to 50% of those with persistent pseudocysts, drainage has been advocated even in asymptomatic patients. In the absence of complications, pseudocyst drainage has been restricted to those patients with persistent (>6 weeks) lesions more than 5 to 6 cm in diameter having a well formed wall that would facilitate internal drainage. In several series, patients with pseudocysts less than 6 cm and even one third of the pseudocysts more than 10 cm were managed without drainage.[215,222] At our institution, we follow asymptomatic patients with pseudocysts less than 6 cm in diameter.

The location of a pseudocyst and its relationship to the pancreatic duct can affect the approach taken for cyst drainage.[217,223] ERCP is helpful in delineating the structure of the pancreatic duct and its communication with a pseudocyst. Those associated with a normal pancreatic duct and that do not communicate are most amenable to percutaneous drainage. Pseudocysts that communicate with the duct, especially when it is strictured, often take a long time to resolve when drained percutaneously, and are best considered for internal surgical or endoscopic drainage.[224]

The percutaneous approach to pseudocyst drainage avoids the need for open surgery and has a low mortality rate. When technically possible, an transgastric approach is favored.[225] The disadvantages of percutaneous drainage, however, are the risk of introducing infection, incomplete drainage that necessitates placement of additional catheters or requires surgery, and development of an external fistula. Cysts located at the head of the pancreas have been effectively drained by inserting a prosthesis through the major or minor papilla.[226] Large pseudocysts that are closely opposed to the gastric or duodenal wall (cyst wall <1 cm from the intestinal lumen) and produce an obvious bulge have been drained by direct cystoenterostomy. To avoid vascular structures, the cyst

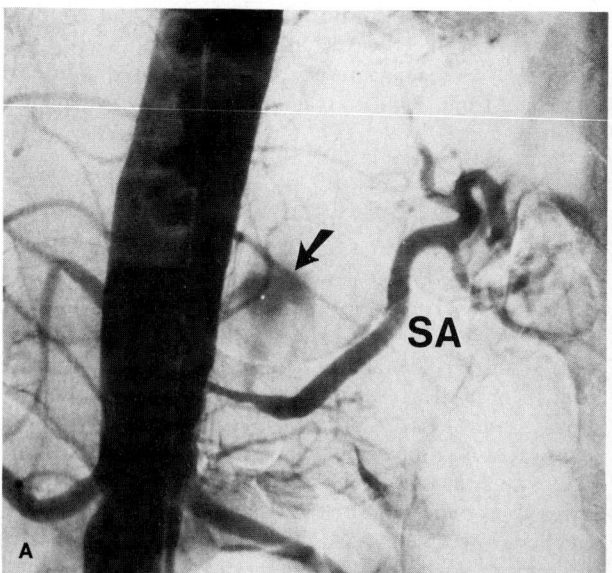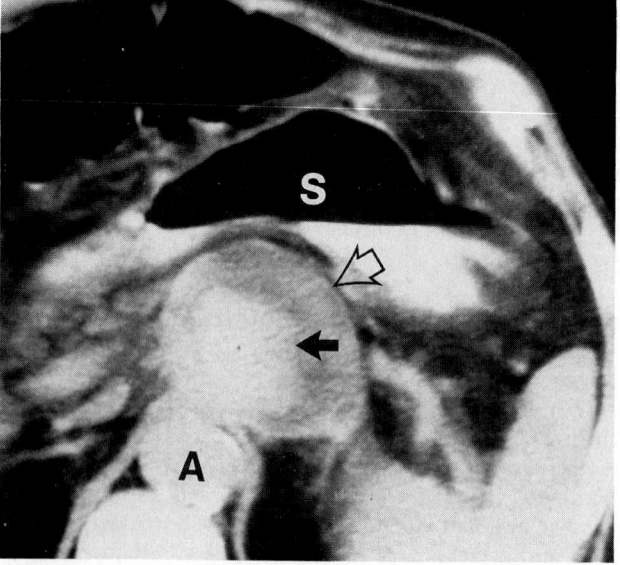

FIGURE 90-7. Pseudoaneurysm complicating acute pancreatitis. **(A)** Angiogram demonstrates pseudoaneurysm arising from the splenic artery (SA) and a jet of contrast leaking from the pseudoaneurysm (*arrow*). **(B)** Dynamic contrast-enhanced computed tomography of the same patient demonstrates the pseudoaneurysm (*open arrow*) with contrast enhancement (*black arrow*) anterior to the aorta (A) and posterior to the stomach (S). (Courtesy of Caroline Taylor, M.D., West Haven, CT.)

should be evaluated by Doppler ultrasonography and aspirated for blood before endoscopic enterostomy.

Fluid contents of a pseudocyst should be sampled for several reasons. First, a high amylase concentration within a cyst probably reflects its persistent communication with the pancreatic duct and correlates with a poor outcome for percutaneous drainage.[227] Second, the clinical symptoms from an infected pseudocyst may be indolent and suspected only after bacterial and fungal culture. Third, pseudocysts with well formed walls may not be separable from true cystic lesions of the pancreas, including cystic neoplasms.[228] Thus, amylase, carcinoembryonic antigen, and CA19-9 levels and cytology should be obtained from cystic aspirates, and biopsy of the cyst wall done if there is any consideration of malignancy.

Fistulas

Pancreatic fistulas usually arise after a bout of alcoholic pancreatitis or from pancreatic pseudocysts, but also may form after pancreatic trauma and pancreatic surgery.[229] The diagnosis should be considered in patients with pancreatic disease in whom ascites or massive pleural effusions develop. Fistulas often arise from disruption of the pancreatic duct. Anterior ductal discontinuities generate ascites, whereas those that are posterior tend to track upward through the retroperitoneal space into the mediastinum. Internal fistulas may communicate with the colon, gallbladder, and small bowel.[229] Posterior fistulas track through the esophageal or aortic hiatus or may erode through the mediastinal pleura. Fistulas within the thorax may involve the pleural space, mediastinum, and even the bronchopulmonary tree and pericardium. Fistulas to vascular structures such as the portal vein have rarely been reported, but are often associated with subcutaneous fat necrosis.[230]

The fluid from a pancreatic fistula has high protein and amylase content. The anatomy of an external fistula is best revealed by a fistulogram. Although ERCP is the most useful test for identifying an internal fistula, CT scanning may be very effective for fistulas that communicate with the thoracic cavity. Spontaneous healing is more common for cutaneous fistulas than internal fistulas. Drainage of fluid collections by thoracentesis or paracentesis helps to heal serosal discontinuities, and is recommended.[229] Decreasing pancreatic secretion with somatostatin has been reported to promote the resolution of fistulas, particularly those with cutaneous communications.[207,213] Stenting of the pancreatic duct[74] or surgical resection, however, are often required for internal fistulas.

Systemic

Specific Organ Involvement

Pulmonary. Some of the most serious complications of pancreatitis involve the lung. Abdominal pain and ascites may limit respiratory excursion. Fluid may accumulate within the pleural space and compress the lung, and the adult respiratory distress syndrome (ARDS) may restrict gas exchange. The contribution of decreased diaphragmatic movement is unclear, but may be a factor in the increased risk of a pulmonary death in those with acute pancreatitis and obesity.[177] Of greater importance are the acute pleural fluid collections that may result from sympathetic effusions or movement of pancreatic enzymes through lymphatic channels. Pancreatic-pleural fistulas may also cause pleural effusions, but it is unusual for them to form acutely. Effusions are reported in 4% to 17% of patients with acute pancreatitis; up to 50% may be associated with pseudocysts.[169] Most effusions are found on the left side or are bilateral, and most resolve spontaneously.[169] Thoracentesis is suggested only when infection is suspected or the size of the effusion results in respiratory compromise.

The most common cause of hypoxemia in acute pancreatitis is ARDS. Although high levels of triglycerides are associated with this syndrome, its pathogenesis is unclear. Histopathologic studies demonstrate capillary injury.[231] Neutrophil emboli may form and occlude small pulmonary vessels. Alveoli are often filled with protein-rich fluid. This hypoxemic state is associated with a normal wedge pressure and decreased pulmonary compliance. In patients with severe ARDS, pulmonary artery pressure monitoring and respiratory support with positive end expiratory pressure are required. Because peritoneal lavage has been demonstrated to improve pulmonary function, it should be considered if the patient is not responding to treatment.

Renal. Renal dysfunction is not unusual in acute pancreatitis, and severe dysfunction is a poor prognostic finding. Volume depletion and white cell emboli may contribute to renal failure. The kidneys may be involved by direct extension of inflammation or a pseudocyst, particularly on the left side.

Gastrointestinal hemorrhage. The proximity of the pancreas to the stomach and duodenum accounts for their frequent involvement in pancreatitis. Erosive gastritis involving the greater curvature, antrum, and duodenum are not unusual. Although these lesions rarely bleed massively, their presence may complicate urgent endoscopic papillotomy. More serious hemorrhage may arise from an abscess or pseudocyst that erodes into vascular structures. The splenic artery is often a target for the formation of such false aneurysms,[232,233] but other vascular structures may be involved.[220] Bleeding from these structures may accumulate in the retroperitoneum or result in gastrointestinal hemorrhage through the pancreatic duct.

Colon. It is not uncommon for pancreatic inflammation to extend to the transverse colon and splenic flexure.[234] Obstruction secondary to spasm and edema may cause the classic colon cutoff sign, with gas present in the right colon but absent distal to the region of obstruction in 1% to 10% of patients. Extension of pancreatic inflammation may lead to persistent colonic strictures, fistulas, or even perforation. During surgery for acute pancreatitis, especially when performed for debridement, the colon is particularly susceptible to devitalization and subsequent perforation. These complications may be avoided with new therapeutic approaches.[210] Rarely, erosion into colonic blood vessels may result in acute lower gastrointestinal hemorrhage[235] or inferior mesenteric vein thrombosis and colonic infarction.[234]

Spleen and splenic vein. The splenic vein runs along the posterior superior margin of the pancreas, and the tail of the pancreas abuts the splenic hilum. The major complications involving the spleen in acute pancreatitis are splenic vein thrombosis and extension of inflammation or a pseudocyst into the spleen. Inflammation of the splenic vein may lead to its thrombosis and subsequent splenomegaly, or to esophageal, gastric, and even colonic varices.[233] The incidence of splenic vein thrombosis is about five times greater in patients with chronic compared to acute pancreatitis. Although development of varices requires complete thrombosis, only about 50% of such patients eventually bleed.[233] Dynamic CT seems to be the favored method of diagnosis. The preferred treatment for splenic vein thrombosis is splenectomy. In the high-risk patient, splenic artery embolization may be considered. The role of splenectomy in patients with *asymptomatic* esophageal varices but without hypersplenism is unsettled; however, the high risk of bleeding leads most to recommend elective splenectomy for patients with low operative risks.

Extension of a pseudocyst, or occasionally inflammation alone, from the pancreas into the spleen may lead to a splenic hematoma and rupture. This complication is most often associated with chronic disease and may present with abdominal pain that is referred to the left shoulder, fever, and an abdominal mass. Ultrasonography or CT suggest the diagnosis. Arteriography may demonstrate splenic artery pseudoaneurysms. Although emergency splenectomy is required for splenic rupture, prophylactic splenectomy has been advocated even when splenic pseudocysts are asymptomatic.[233]

Other

Inflammatory processes within the pancreatic head may produce biliary obstruction. This form of biliary tract obstruction usually resolves unless there is underlying chronic pancreatitis with fibrosis. Clinically evident *fat necrosis* is seen in less than 1% of patients with acute pancreatitis.[236] Pancreatic enzymes have been detected in areas of fat necrosis and are presumably responsible for initiating this injury.[237] The initial injury may arise from the cleavage of adipocyte plasma membrane glycerosphingolipids by phospholipase A. Adipocyte-associated or circulating lipase activities may then enter the cell and convert triglycerides to monoglycerides and toxic free fatty acids.[237] Several clinical syndromes are associated with fat necrosis. *Cutaneous necrosis* generates widely disseminated, raised, erythematous, and tender nodules of less than 2 cm in diameter. The process is frequently associated with fever and eosinophilia.[236] The nodules typically resolve in days to weeks without residual; however, some may rupture and heal with hyperpigmentation. Fat necrosis may affect the marrow cavity and lead to vascular damage and bone infarction.[238] The typical bone lesions are frequently painless, osteolytic, develop 3 to 6 weeks after the onset of pancreatitis, and involve the ends of long bones such as the femur. Synovial pad fat necrosis may be associated with arthritis. The increased amounts of free fatty acids recovered from such joints may initiate this inflammatory process.

Severe pancreatitis is associated with confusion and coma. Multiple organ system failure often is encountered in severe pancreatitis and requires special management considerations.[239] Temporary blindness has also been experienced and

may be attributed to the retinal ischemia induced by leukocyte emboli.[240]

> The reader is directed to Chapter 36, Approach to the Patient With Acute Abdomen; Chapter 89, Pancreas: Anatomy and Structural Anomalies; Chapter 91, Chronic Pancreatitis; Chapter 94, Hereditary Diseases of the Pancreas; and Chapter 121, Ultrasonography.

REFERENCES

1. Leach SD, Gorelick FS, Modlin IM. Acute pancreatitis at its centenary: the contribution of Reginald Fitz. Ann Surg 1990;212:109.
2. Bradley EL. A clinically based classification system for acute pancreatitis. Arch Surg 1993;128:586.
3. Scheele G, Adler G, Kern H. Exocytosis occurs at the lateral plasma membrane of the pancreatic acinar cell during supramaximal secretagogue stimulation. Gastroenterology 1987;92:345.
4. Bockman DE, Boydston WR, Anderson MC. Origin of tubular complexes in human chronic pancreatitis. Am J Surg 1982;144:243.
5. Willemer S, Adler G. Histochemical and ultrastructural characteristics of tubular complexes in human acute pancreatitis. Dig Dis Sci 1989;34:46.
6. Gorelick FS, Adler G, Kern HF. Cerulein-induced pancreatitis. In: Go VLW, DiMagno EP, Gardner JD, et al, eds. The pancreas: biology, pathobiology, and disease. New York: Raven Press, 1993:501.
7. Willemer S, Elsasser HP, Kern HF, Adler G. Tubular complexes in cerulein-and oleic acid-induced pancreatitis in rats: glycoconjugate pattern, immunocytochemical, and ultrastructural findings. Pancreas 1987;2:669.
8. Yamaguchi H, Kimura T, Mimura K, Nawata H. Activation of proteases in caerulein-induced pancreatitis. Pancreas 1989;4:565.
9. Geokas MC, Rinderknecht H. Free proteolytic enzymes in pancreatic juice of patients with acute pancreatitis. Am J Dig Dis 1974;19:591.
10. Bialek R, Willemer S, Arnold R, Adler G. Evidence of intracellular activation of serine proteases in acute cerulein-induced pancreatitis in rats. Scand J Gastroenterol 1991;26:190.
11. Gorelick FS, Modlin I, Leach SD, et al. Intracellular proteolysis of pancreatic zymogens. Yale J Biol Med 1993;65:407.
12. Leach SD, Modlin IM, Scheele GA, Gorelick FS. Intracellular activation of digestive zymogens in rat pancreatic acini: stimulation by high doses of cholecystokinin. J Clin Invest 1991;87:362.
13. Steer ML, Meldolesi J. The cell biology of experimental pancreatitis. N Engl J Med 1987;316:144.
14. Kassell B, Kay J. Zymogens of proteolytic enzymes. Science 1973;180:1022.
15. Hirano T, Saluja A, Ramarao P, et al. Apical secretion of lysosomal enzymes in rabbit pancreas occurs via a secretagogue regulated pathway and is increased after pancreatic duct obstruction. J Clin Invest 1991;87:865.
16. Willemer S, Bialek R, Adler G. Localization of lysosomal and digestive enzyme in cytoplasmic vacuoles in caerulein-pancreatitis. Histochemistry 1990;94:161.
17. Powers R, Saluja AK, Houlihan MJ, Steer ML. Diminished agonist stimulated inositol triphosphate generations blocks stimulus-secretion coupling in pancreatic acini during diet-induced experimental pancreatitis. J Clin Invest 1986;77:1668.
18. O'Konski MS, Pandol SJ. Effects of caerulein on the apical cytoskeleton of the pancreatic acinar cell. J Clin Invest 1990;86:1649.
19. Grady T, Gorelick F, Modlin I, Powers R. Association of in-

tracellular zymogen and experimental pancreatitis in the rat (abstract). Pancreas 1992;7:738.

20. Saluja A, Sadamitsu H, Saluja M, et al. Subcellular redistribution of lysosomal enzymes during caerulein-induced pancreatitis. Am J Physiol 1987;253:G508.

21. Marks WH, Ohlsson K. Isolation and partial characterization of the pancreatic secretory trypsin inhibitor in the rat. Biochim Biophys Acta 1982;717:91.

22. Renner IG, Rinderknecht H, Valenzuela JE, Douglas AP. Studies of pure pancreatic secretions in chronic alcoholic subjects without pancreatic insufficiency. Scand J Gastroenterol 1980;15:241.

23. Lasson A, Ohlsson K. Protease inhibitors in acute pancreatitis: correlation between biochemical changes and clinical course. Scand J Gastroenterol 1984;19:779.

24. Roxvall L, Sennerby B, Heideman M. Activation of the complement cascade by trypsin. Biol Chem Hoppe Seyler 1991;372:273.

25. Roxvall LI, Bengtson LA, Heideman JMI. Anaphylatoxins and terminal complement complexes in pancreatitis. Arch Surg 1990;125:918.

26. Gress TM, Arnold R, Adler G. Structural alterations of pancreatic microvasculature in cerulein-induced pancreatitis in the rat. Res Exp Med 1990;190:401.

27. Neuschwander-Tetri BA, Ferrell LD, Sukhabote RJ, Grendell JH. Glutathione monoethyl ester ameliorates caerulein-induced pancreatitis in the mouse. J Clin Invest 1992;89:109.

28. Schoenberg MH, Buchler M, Baczako K, et al. The involvement of oxygen radicals in acute pancreatitis. Klin Wochenschr 1991;69:1025.

29. Dabrowski A, Chwiecko M. Oxygen radicals mediate depletion of pancreatic sulfhydryl compounds in rats with cerulein-induced acute pancreatitis. Digestion 1990;47:15.

30. Bilchik AJ, Leach SD, Zucker KA, Modlin IM. Experimental models of acute pancreatitis. J Surg Res 1990;48:639.

31. Steinberg WM, Schlesselman SE. Treatment of acute pancreatitis: comparison of animal and human studies. Gastroenterology 1987;93:1420.

32. Leli U, Saluja A, Picard L, et al. Effects of a choline-deficient ethionine-supplemented diet on phospholipase C activity in mouse pancreatic acinar cell membranes and in electropermeabilized mouse pancreatic acini. J Pharmacol Exp Ther 1990;253:847.

33. Lerch M, Saluja AK, Runzi M, et al. Pancreatic duct obstruction triggers acute necrotizing pancreatitis in the opossum. Gastroenterology 1993;104:853.

34. Niederau C, Grendell JH. Intracellular vacuoles in experimental acute pancreatitis in rats and mice are an acidified compartment. J Clin Invest 1988;81:229.

35. Suzuki M, Isaji S, Stanten R, et al. Effect of protease inhibitor FUT on acute hemorrhagic pancreatitis in mice. Int J Pancreatol 1992;11:59.

36. Mouret J. Contribution a l'etude des cellules granulaires. J Anat 1895;31:221.

37. Clemens JA, Olson J, Cameron JL. Cerulein-induced pancreatitis in the ex vitro isolated perfused canine pancreas. Surgery 1991;109:515.

38. Niederau C, Crass RA, Silver G, et al. Therapeutic regimens in acute experimental hemorrhagic pancreatitis: effects of hydration, oxygenation, peritoneal lavage, and a potent protease inhibitor. Gastroenterology 1988;95:1648.

39. Lombardi B, Ester L, Longnecker D. Acute hemorrhage pancreatis (massive necrosis) with fat necrosis induced in mice by DL-ethionine fed with a choline deficit diet. Am J Pathol 1975;79:465.

40. Rao KN, Tuma J, Lombardi B. Acute hemorrhagic pancreatic necrosis in mice: intraparenchymal activator of zymogens and other enzyme changes in pancreas and serum. Gastroenterology 1976;70:720.

41. Moreau JA, Zinsmeister AR, Melton LJ, Dimagno EP. Gallstone pancreatitis and the effect of cholecystectomy: a population-based cohort study. Mayo Clin Proc 1988;63:466.

42. Taylor TV, Rimmer S, Holt S, et al. Sex differences in gallstone pancreatitis. Ann Surg 1991;214:667.

43. Misra SP, Dwivedi M. Pancreaticobiliary ductal union. Gut 1990;31:1144.

44. Mori K, Nagakawa T, Ohta T, et al. Acute pancreatitis associated with anomalous union of the pancreaticobiliary ductal system. J Clin Gastroenterol 1991;13:673.

45. Rollan A, Guzman S, Pimentel F, Nervi F. Catabolism of chylomicron remnants in patients with previous acute pancreatitis. Gastroenterology 1990;98:1649.

46. Jones BA, Salsberg BB, Mehta MH, Bohnen JM. Common pancreaticobiliary channels and their relationship to gallstone size in gallstone pancreatitis. Ann Surg 1987;205:123.

47. Moody FG, Senninger N, Runkel N. Another challenge to the Opie myth. Gastroenterology 1993;104:927.

48. Runkel NS, Moody FG, Mueller W, et al. Experimental evidence against Opie's common channel bile reflux theory. Digestion 1992;52:67.

49. Acosta JL, Ledesma CL. Gallstone migration as a cause for acute pancreatitis. N Engl J Med 1974;290:484.

50. Lee SP, Nicholls JF, Park HZ. Biliary sludge as a cause of acute pancreatitis. N Engl J Med 1992;326:589.

51. Ros E, Navarro S, Bru C, et al. Occult microlithiasis in "idiopathic" acute pancreatitis: prevention of relapses by cholecystectomy or ursodeoxycholic acid therapy. Gastroenterology 1991;101:1701.

52. Odani K, Nimura Y, Yasui A, et al. Paradoxical response to cerulein on sphincter of Oddi in the patient with gastrectomy. Dig Dis Sci 1992;37:904.

53. Toouli J. What is sphincter of Oddi dysfunction? Gut 1989;30:753.

54. Elta GH. Sphincter of Oddi manometry in patients with possible sphincter of Oddi dysfunction. Gastroenterology 1991;101:1747.

55. Geenen JE, Hogan WJ, Dodds WJ, et al. The efficacy of endoscopic sphincterotomy after cholecystectomy in patients with sphincter-of-Oddi dysfunction. N Engl J Med 1989;320:82.

56. Meshkinpour H, Mollot M. Sphincter of Oddi dysfunction and unexplained abdominal pain: clinical and manometric study. Dig Dis Sci 1992;37:257.

57. Raddawi HM, Geenen JE, Hogan WJ, et al. Pressure measurements from biliary and pancreatic segments of sphincter of Oddi: comparison between patients with functional abdominal pain, biliary, or pancreatic disease. Dig Dis Sci 1991;36:71.

58. Sherman S, Hawes RH, Troiano FP, Lehman GA. Pancreatitis following bile duct sphincter of Oddi manometry: utility of the aspirating catheter. Gastrointest Endosc 1992;38:347.

59. Sostre S, Kalloo AN, Spiegler EJ, et al. A noninvasive test of sphincter of Oddi dysfunction in postcholecystectomy patients: the scintigraphic score [see comments]. J Nucl Med 1992;33:1216.

60. Khuroo MS, Zargar SA, Yattoo GN. Efficacy of nifedipine therapy in patients with sphincter of Oddi dysfunction: a prospective, double-blind, randomized, placebo-controlled, cross over trial. Br J Clin Pharmacol 1992;33:477.

61. Watanapa P, Williamson RC. Pancreatic sphincterotomy and sphincteroplasty. Gut 1992;33:865.

62. Fullarton GM, Murray WR. Evaluation of endoscopic sphincterotomy in sphincter of Oddi dysfunction. Endoscopy 1992;24:199.

63. Sherman S, Ruffolo TA, Hawes RH, Lehman GA. Complications of endoscopic sphincterotomy: a prospective series with emphasis on the increased risk associated with sphincter of Oddi dysfunction and nondilated bile ducts. Gastroenterology 1991;101:1068.

64. Cooperman AM, Siegel J, Hammerman H. Pancreas divisum: advocates and agnostics. J Clin Gastroenterol 1989;11:489.

65. Satterfield ST, McCarthy JH, Geenen JE. Clinical experience in 82 patients with pancreas divisum: preliminary results on manometry and endoscopic therapy. Pancreas 1988;3:248.

66. Bernard JP, Sahel J, Giovanni M, Sarles H. Pancreas divisum is a probable cause of acute pancreatitis: a report of 137 cases. Pancreas 1990;5:248.

67. Burtin P, Person B, Boyer J. Pancreas divisum and pancreatitis: a coincidental association? Endoscopy 1991;23:55.

68. Lerch MM, Saluja AK, Runzi M, et al. Pancreatic duct obstruc-

tion triggers acute necrotizing pancreatitis in the opossum [see comments]. Gastroenterology 1993;104:853.

69. Warshaw AL, Simeone JF, Schapiro RH, Flavin-Warshaw B. Evaluation and treatment of the dominant dorsal duct syndrome (pancreas divisum redefined). Am J Surg 1990;159:59.

70. Lowes JR, Lees WR, Cotton PB. Pancreatic duct dilatation after secretin stimulation in patients with pancreas divisum. Pancreas 1989;4:371.

71. Lans JI, Geenen JE, Johanson JF, Hogan WJ. Endoscopic therapy in patients with pancreas divisum and acute pancreatitis: a prospective, randomized, controlled clinical trial. Gastrointest Endosc 1992;38:430.

72. Lehman GA, Sherman S, Nisi R, Hawes RH. Pancreas divisum: results of minor papilla sphincterotomy. Gastrointest Endosc 1993;39:1.

73. Delhaye M, Vandermeeren A, Baize M, Cremer M. Extracorporeal shock-wave lithotripsy of pancreatic calculi. Gastroenterology 1992;102:610.

74. Kozarek RA, Ball TJ, Patterson DJ, et al. Endoscopic transpapillary therapy for disrupted pancreatic duct and peripancreatic fluid collections. Gastroenterology 1991;100:1362.

75. Renner JG, Savage WE, Pantoja JL, Renner VJ. Death due to acute pancreatitis; a retrospective analysis of 405 autopsy cases. Dig Dis Sci 1985;30:1005.

76. Dreiling DA, Koller M. The natural history of alcoholic pancreatitis: update 1985. Mt Sinai J Med (NY) 1985;52:340.

77. Singh M, Simsek H. Ethanol and the pancreas. Gastroenterology 1990;98:1051.

78. Guelrud M, Mendoza S, Rossiter G, et al. Effect of local instillation of alcohol on sphincter of Oddi motor activity: combined ERCP and manometry study [see comments]. Gastrointest Endosc 1991;37:428.

79. Gronroos JM, Aho HJ, Nevalainen TJ. Cholinergic hypothesis of alcoholic pancreatitis. Dig Dis 1992;10:38.

80. Sarles H, Dagorn JC, Giorgi D, Bernard JP. Renaming pancreatic stone protein as "lithostathine" (letter). Gastroenterology 1990;99:900.

81. Fukuoka S-I, Freedman SD, Yu H, et al. GP2/THP gene family encodes self-binding GP1-linked proteins in apical vesicular membranes of pancreas and kidney. Proc Natl Acad Sci USA 1992;89:1189.

82. Hoops TC, Rindler MJ. Isolation of the cDNA encoding glycoprotein-2 (G-P2), the major zymogen granule membrane protein: homology to uromodulin/Tamm-Horsfall protein. J Biol Chem 1991;266:4257.

83. Harvey MH, Cates MC, Reber HA. Possible mechanisms of acute pancreatitis induced by ethanol. Am J Surg 1988;155:49.

84. Hoek JB, Thomas AP, Rooney TA, et al. Ethanol and signal transduction in the liver. FASEB J 1992;6:2386.

85. Wilson JS, Apte MV, Thomas MC, et al. Effects of ethanol, acetaldehyde and cholesterol esters on pancreatic lysosomes. Gut 1992;33:1099.

86. Bilchik AJ, Zucker KA, Adrian TE, Modlin IM. Amelioration of cholinergic-induced pancreatitis with a selective cholecystokinin receptor antagonist. Arch Surg 1990;125:1546.

87. Modlin I, Bilchik A, Zucker K, et al. Cholecystokinin augmentation of "surgical" pancreatitis. Arch Surg 1988;124:574.

88. Katz M, Carangelo R, Modlin I, et al. Ethanol sensitizes acinar cells to the effects of cholecystokinin on intracellular zymogen proteolysis (abstract). Gastroenterology 1993;104:A311.

89. Quon MG, Kugelmas M, Wisner JR Jr, et al. Chronic alcohol consumption intensifies caerulein-induced acute pancreatitis in the rat. Int J Pancreatol 1992;12:31.

90. Singh M. Effect of chronic ethanol feeding on factors leading to inappropriate intrapancreatic zymogen activation in the rat. Digestion 1992;53:114.

91. Marshall JB. Acute pancreatitis: a review with an emphasis on new developments. Arch Intern Med 1993;153:1185.

92. Underwood TW, Frye CB. Drug-induced pancreatitis. Clin Pharm 1993;12:440.

93. Present DH, Meltzer SJ, Krumholz MP, et al. 6-Mercaptopurine in the management of inflammatory bowel disease: short- and long-term toxicity. Ann Intern Med 1989;111:641.

94. Bartels RH, Van der Spek JA, Oosten HR. Acute pancreatitis due to sulfamethoxazole-trimethoprim. South Med J 1992;85:1006.

95. Murphy RL, Noskin GA, Ehrenpreis ED. Acute pancreatitis associated with aerosolized pentamidine. Am J Med 1990;88:553N.

96. Connolly KJ, Allan JD, Fitch H, et al. Phase I study of 2′-3′-dideoxyinosine administered orally twice daily to patients with AIDS or AIDS-related complex and hematologic intolerance to zidovudine. Am J Med 1991;91:471.

97. Maxson CJ, Greenfield SM, Turner JL. Acute pancreatitis as a common complication of 2′,3′-dideoxyinosine therapy in the acquired immunodeficiency syndrome. Am J Gastroenterol 1992;87:708.

98. Grady T, Saluja AK, Steer ML, et al. In vivo and in vitro effects of the azidothymidine analog dideoxyinosine on the exocrine pancreas of the rat. J Pharmacol Exp Ther 1992;262:445.

99. Erdkamp F, Houben M, Ackerman E, et al. Pancreatitis induced by mesalamine. Neth J Med 1992;41:71.

100. Sachedina B, Saibil F, Cohen LB, Whittey J. Acute pancreatitis due to 5-aminosalicylate. Ann Intern Med 1989;110:490.

101. Mofenson HC, Caraccio TR, Nawaz H, Steckler G. Acetaminophen induced pancreatitis. J Toxicol Clin Toxicol 1991;29:223.

102. Sugerman HJ. Sulindac-induced acute pancreatitis mimicking gallstone pancreatitis. Am Surg 1989;55:536.

103. Alexander JA, Demetrius AJ, Gavaler JS, et al. Pancreatitis following liver transplantation. Transplantation 1988;45:1062.

104. Nicolau DP, Mengedoht DE, Kline JJ. Tetracycline-induced pancreatitis. Am J Gastroenterol 1991;86:1669.

105. Anderson PE, Ellis GG Jr, Austin SM. Case report: metolazone-associated hypercalcemia and acute pancreatitis. Am J Med Sci 1991;302:235.

106. McCarter TL, Chen YK. Marked hyperlipidemia and pancreatitis associated with isotretinoin therapy. Am J Gastroenterol 1992;87:1855.

107. Lankisch PG, Muller CH, Niederstadt H, Brand A. Painless acute pancreatitis subsequent to anticholinesterase insecticide (parathion) intoxication. Am J Gastroenterol 1990;85:872.

108. Possani LD, Martin BM, Fletcher MD, Fletcher PL. Discharge effect on pancreatic exocrine secretion produced by toxins purified from *Tityus serrultus* scorpion venom. J Biol Chem 1991;266:3178.

109. Deviere J, Reuse C, Askenasi R. Ischemic pancreatitis and hepatitis secondary to ergotamine poisoning. J Clin Gastroenterol 1987;9:350.

110. Murthy UK, Degregorio F, Oates RP, Blair DC. Hyperamylasemia in patients with the acquired immunodeficiency syndrome. Am J Gastroenterol 1992;87:332.

111. Bonacini M. Pancreatic involvement in human immunodeficiency virus infection. J Clin Gastroenterol 1991;13:58.

112. Cappell MS, Javeed M. Pancreatic abscess due to mycobacterial infection associated with the acquired immunodeficiency syndrome. J Clin Gastroenterol 1990;12:423.

113. Schwartz MS, Brandt LJ. The spectrum of pancreatic disorders in patients with the acquired immune deficiency syndrome. Am J Gastroenterol 1989;84:459.

114. Al-Awadhi NZ, Ashkenani F, Khalaf ES. Acute pancreatitis associated with brucellosis. Am J Gastroenterol 1989;84:1570.

115. Edwards CN, Evarard COR. Hyperamylasemia and pancreatitis in leptospirosis. Am J Gastroenterol 1991;86:1665.

116. Renner F, Nimeth C, Demmelbauer N. High frequency of concomitant pancreatitis in salmonella enteritis. Lancet 1991;337:1611.

117. Fan S-T, Lai ECS, Mok FPT, et al. Early treatment of acute biliary pancreatitis by endoscopic papillotomy. N Engl J Med 1993;328:228.

118. Toskes PP. Hyperlipidemic pancreatitis. Gastroenterol Clin North Am 1990;19:783.

119. Cates MC, Singh SM, Peick AL, et al. Acute hypercalcemia, pancreatic duct permeability, and pancreatitis in cats. Surgery 1988;104:137.

120. Frick TW, Spycher MA, Heitz PU, et al. Hypercalcaemia and pancreatic ultrastructure in cats. Eur J Surg 1992;158:289.

121. Frick TW, Spycher MA, Heitz PU, et al. Ultrastructure of the guinea pig pancreas in acute hypercalcemia. Pancreas 1992;7: 287.

122. Fernandez-Del Castillo C, Harringer W, Warshaw AL, et al. Risk factors for pancreatic cellular injury after cardiopulmonary bypass [see comments]. N Engl J Med 1991;325:382.

123. Eaker EY, Toskes PP. Systemic lupus erythematosus presenting initially with acute pancreatitis and a review of the literature. Am J Med Sci 1989;297:38.

124. Kemp JA, Arora S, Fawaz K. Recurrent acute pancreatitis as a manifestation of Wegener's granulomatosis. Dig Dis Sci 1990;35:912.

125. Le Thi Huong D, Wechsler B, Dell'Isola B, et al. Acute pancreatitis in Behcet's disease. Dig Dis Sci 1992;37:1452.

126. Pitchumoni CS, Jain NK, Lowenfels AB, Dimagno EP. Chronic cyanide poisoning: unifying concept for alcoholic and tropical pancreatitis. Pancreas 1988;3:220.

127. Mullen KD, Hoofnagle JH, Jones EA. Shock wave-induced pancreatic trauma. Am J Gastroenterol 1991;86:630.

128. Smith EH. Complications of percutaneous abdominal fine-needle biopsy: review. Radiology 1991;178:253.

129. Cotton PB, Lehman G, Vennes J, et al. Endoscopic sphincterotomy complications and their management: an attempt at consensus. Gastrointest Endosc 1991;37:383.

130. Conn M, Goldenberg A, Concepcion L, Mandeli J. The effect of ERCP on circulating pancreatic enzymes and pancreatic protease inhibitors. Am J Gastroenterol 1991;86:1011.

131. Fredrenrich A, Sosset C, Bernard JL, et al. Acute pancreatitis after short-term octreotide. Lancet 1991;338:52.

132. Gradon JD, Schulman RH, Chapnick EK, Sepkowitz DV. Octreotide-induced acute pancreatitis in a patient with acquired immunodeficiency syndrome. South Med J 1991;84:1410.

133. Binmoeller KF, Dumas R, Harris AG, Delmont JP. Effect of somatostatin analog octreotide on human sphincter of Oddi. Dig Dis Sci 1992;37:773.

134. Rattner DW, Gu ZY, Vlahakes GJ, Warshaw AL. Hyperamylasemia after cardiac surgery: incidence, significance, and management. Ann Surg 1989;209:279.

135. Huddy SP, Joyce WP, Pepper JR. Gastrointestinal complications in 4473 patients who underwent cardiopulmonary bypass surgery. Br J Surg 1991;78:293.

136. Lefor AT, Vuocolo P, Parker FB Jr, Sillin LF. Pancreatic complications following cardiopulmonary bypass: factors influencing mortality. Arch Surg 1992;127:1225.

137. Kohler H, Lankisch PG. Acute pancreatitis and hyperamylasaemia in pancreatic carcinoma. Pancreas 1987;2:117.

138. Hegnhoj J, Hansen CP, Rannem T, et al. Pancreatic function in Crohn's disease. Gut 1990;31:1076.

139. Friedman GD, Selby JV. How often does metronidazole induce pancreatitis? Gastroenterology 1990;98:1702.

140. Matsumoto T, Matsui T, Iida M, et al. Acute pancreatitis as a complication of Crohn's disease. Am J Gastroenterol 1989;84: 804.

141. Weizman Z, Durie PR. Acute pancreatitis in childhood. J Pediatr 1988;113:24.

142. Block P, Kelly TR. Management of gallstone pancreatitis during pregnancy and the postpartum period. Surg Gynecol Obstet 1989;168:426.

143. De Chalain TM, Michell WL, Berger GM. Hyperlipidemia, pregnancy and pancreatitis. Surg Gynecol Obstet 1988;167: 469.

144. Matteo A, Sarles H. Is food allergy a cause of acute pancreatitis? Pancreas 1990;5:234.

145. Carey LC. Recurrent acute pancreatitis—rarely idiopathic: 1989 Du Pont lecture. Can J Surg 1990;33:107.

146. Grendell JH. Idiopathic acute pancreatitis. Gastroenterol Clin North Am 1990;19:843.

147. Lankisch PG, Schirren CA, Kunze E. Undetected fatal acute pancreatitis: why is the disease so frequently overlooked? Am J Gastroenterol 1991;86:322.

148. Kolars JC, Elis CJ, Levitt MD. Comparison of serum amylase, pancreatic isoamylase and lipase in patients with hyperamylasemia. Dig Dis Sci 1984;29:289.

149. Dubick MA, Conteas CN, Billy HT, et al. Raised serum concentrations of pancreatic enzymes in cigarette smokers. Gut 1987;28:330.

150. Agarwal N, Pitchumoni CS, Sivaprasad AV. Evaluating tests for acute pancreatitis. Am J Gastroenterol 1990;85:356.

151. Hata H, Matsuzaki H, Tanaka K, et al. Ectopic production of salivary-type amylase by a IgA-lambda-type multiple myeloma. Cancer 1988;62:1511.

152. Kramer MR, Saldana MJ, Cepero RJ, Pitchenik AE. High amylase levels in neoplasm-related pleural effusion. Ann Intern Med 1989;110:567.

153. Kleinman DS, O'Brien JF. Macroamylase. Mayo Clin Proc 1986;61:669.

154. Novis BH, Bornman PC, Girdwood AW, Marks IN. Endoscopic manometry of the pancreatic duct and sphincter zone in patients with chronic pancreatitis. Dig Dis Sci 1985;30:225.

155. Panteghini M, Pagani F, Bonora R, et al. Diagnostic value of four assays for lipase determination in serum: a comparative reevaluation. Clin Biochem 1991;24:497.

156. Tetrault GA. Lipase activity in serum measured with Ektachem is often measured in non-pancreatic disorders. Clin Chem 1991;37:447.

157. Lott JA, Lu CJ. Lipase isoforms and amylase isoenzymes: assays and application in the diagnosis of acute pancreatitis. Clin Chem 1991;37:361.

158. Gumaste V, Dave P, Sereny G. Serum lipase: a better test to diagnose acute alcoholic pancreatitis. Am J Med 1992;92:239.

159. Keim V, Iovanna JL, Orelle B, et al. A novel exocrine protein associated with pancreas transplantation in humans. Gastroenterology 1992;103:248.

160. Fernandez-Del Castillo C, Schmidt J, Rattner DW, et al. Generation and possible significance of trypsinogen activation peptides in experimental acute pancreatitis in the rat. Pancreas 1992;7:263.

161. Grudgeon AM, Heath DI, Hurley P, et al. Trypsinogen activation peptides in the early prediction of severity of acute pancreatitis. Lancet 1990;1:4.

162. Dominguez-Munoz JE, Carballo F, Garcia MJ, et al. Clinical usefulness of polymorphonuclear elastase: predicting the severity of acute pancreatitis: a multicenter study. Br J Surg 1991;78: 1230.

163. Scholmerich J, Schumichem C, Lausen M, et al. Scintigraphic assessment of leukocyte infiltration in acute pancreatitis using technetium-hexamethyl propylene amine oxine as leukocyte label. Dig Dis Sci 1991;36:65.

164. Leser HG, Gross V, Scheibenbogen C, et al. Evaluation of serum interleukin-6 concentration precedes acute phase response and reflects severity in acute pancreatitis. Gastroenterology 1991;101:782.

165. Neoptolemos JP, London N, Bailey I, et al. The role of clinical and biochemical criteria and endoscopic retrograde cholangio-pancreatography in the urgent diagnosis of common bile duct stones in acute pancreatitis. Surgery 1986;10:732.

166. Millat B, Fingerhut A, Gayral F, et al. Predictability of clinicobiochemical scoring systems for early identification of severe gallstone-associated pancreatitis. Am J Surg 1992;164:32.

167. Gumaste VV, Dave PB, Weissman D, Messer J. Lipase/amylase ratio: a new index that distinguishes acute episodes of alcoholic from nonalcoholic acute pancreatitis. Gastroenterology 1991;101:1361.

168. Lankisch PG, Schirren CA, Otto J. Methemalbumin in acute pancreatitis: an evaluation of its prognostic value and comparison with multiple prognostic parameters. Am J Gastroenterol 1989;84:1391.

169. Gumaste V, Singh V, Dave P. Significance of pleural effusion in patients with acute pancreatitis. Am J Gastroenterol 1992;87: 871.

170. Balthazar EJ, Robinson DL, Megibow AJ, Ranson JH. Acute pancreatitis: value of CT in establishing prognosis. Radiology 1990;174:331.

171. Lee MJ, Rattner DW, Legemate DA, et al. Acute complicated pancreatitis: redefining the role of interventional radiology. Radiology 1992;183:171.

172. Banks PA. Predictors of severity in acute pancreatitis. Pancreas 1991;6(Suppl 1):S7.

173. Balthazar EJ, Chako AC. Computerized tomography in acute gastrointestinal disorders. Am J Gastroenterol 1990;85:1445.

174. Johnson CD, Stephens DH, Sarr MG. CT of acute pancreatitis: correlation between lack of contrast enhancement and pancreatic necrosis. AJR 1991;156:93.

175. Agarwal N, Pitchumoni CS. Assessment of severity in acute pancreatitis. Am J Gastroenterol 1991;86:1385.

176. Blamey SL, Imrie CW, O'Neil J, et al. Prognostic factors in acute pancreatitis. Gut 1984;25:1340.

177. Karimgani I, Porter KA, Langevin RE, Banks PA. Prognostic factors in sterile pancreatic necrosis. Gastroenterology 1992;103:1636.

178. Knaus WA, Wagner DP, Draper EA, et al. The APACHE III prognostic system: risk prediction of hospital mortality for critically ill hospitalized adults. Chest 1991;100:1619.

179. Wilson C, Heath DI, Imrie CW. Prediction of outcome in acute pancreatitis: a comparative study of APACHE II, clinical assessment and multiple factor scoring systems. Br J Surg 1990;77:1260.

180. Reynaert MS, Dugernier TH, Kestens PJ. Current therapeutic strategies in severe acute pancreatitis. Intensive Care Med 1990;16:352.

181. Klar E, Herfarth C, Messmer K. Therapeutic effect of isovolemic hemodilution with dextran 60 on the impairment of pancreatic microcirculation in acute biliary pancreatitis. Ann Surg 1990;211:346.

182. Stewart AF, Longo W, Kreutter D, et al. Hypocalcemia associated with calcium-soap formation in a patient with a pancreatic fistula. N Engl J Med 1986;315:496.

183. Pisters PW, Ranson JH. Nutritional support for acute pancreatitis. Surg Gynecol Obstet 1992;175:275.

184. Cerra FB. Hypermetabolism, organ failure, and metabolic support. Surgery 1987;101:1.

185. Leibowitz AB, O'Sullivan P, Iberti TJ. Intravenous fat emulsions and the pancreas: a review. Mt Sinai J Med (NY) 1992;59:38.

186. Bradley EL. Antibiotics in acute pancreatitis: current status and future directions. Am J Surg 1989;158:472.

187. Neoptolemos JP, Carr-Locke DL, London NJ, et al. Controlled trial of urgent endoscopic retrograde cholangiopancreatography and endoscopic sphincterotomy versus conservative treatment for acute pancreatitis due to gallstones. Lancet 1988;2:979.

188. Neoptolemos JP, Carr-Locke DL, London N, et al. ERCP findings and the role of endoscopic sphincterotomy in acute gallstone pancreatitis. Br J Surg 1988;75:954.

189. Davidson BR, Neoptolemos JP, Carr-Locke DL. Endoscopic sphincterotomy for common bile calculi in patients with gall bladder in situ considered unfit for surgery. Gut 1988;29:114.

190. Hutton SW, Sievert CE, Vennes JA, et al. Spontaneous passage of glass beads from the canine gallbladder: facilitation by sphincterotomy. Gastroenterology 1988;94:1031.

191. May GR, Shaffer EH. Should elective endoscopic sphincterotomy replace cholecystectomy for the treatment of high-risk patients with pancreatitis? J Clin Gastroenterol 1991;13:125.

192. Moreira VF, Sanroman AL. Endoscopic sphincterotomy and gallstone pancreatitis: some answers and more fuel for the flames. J Clin Gastroenterol 1992;14:85.

193. Ranson JH. The role of surgery in the management of acute pancreatitis. Ann Surg 1990;311:382.

194. Feig BW, Pomerantz RA, Vogelzang R, et al. Treatment of peripancreatic fluid collections in patients with complicated acute pancreatitis. Surg Gynecol Obstet 1992;175:429.

195. Fedorak IJ, Ko TC, Djuricin G, et al. Secondary pancreatic infections: are they distinct clinical entities? Surgery 1992;112:824.

196. Lumsden A, Bradley EL. Secondary pancreatic infections. Surg Gynecol Obstet 1990;170:459.

197. Freeny PC, Lewis GP, Traverson LW, Ryan JA. Infected pancreatic fluid collections: percutaneous catheter drainage. Radiology 1988;167:435.

198. Parekh D, Segal I. Pancreatic ascites and effusion: risk factors for failure of conservative therapy and the role of octreotide. Arch Surg 1992;127:707.

199. Gislason H, Gronbech JE, Soreide O. Pancreatic ascites: treatment by continuous somatostatin infusion. Am J Gastroenterol 1991;86:519.

200. Bitter R, Block S, Buchler M, Beger HG. Pancreatic abscess and infected pancreatic necrosis: different local septic complications in acute pancreatitis. Dig Dis Sci 1987;32:1082.

201. Mayer AD, McMahon MJ, Corfield AP, et al. Controlled clinical trial of peritoneal lavage for the treatment of severe acute pancreatitis. N Engl J Med 1985;312:399.

202. Ranson JHC, Berman RS. Long peritoneal lavage decreases pancreatic sepsis in acute pancreatitis. Ann Surg 1990;211:708.

203. Bradley EL, Allen K. A prospective longitudinal study of observation versus surgical intervention in the management of necrotizing pancreatitis. Am J Surg 1991;161:19.

204. Buchler M, Malfertheiner P, Frieb H, et al. Human pancreatic tissue concentration of bactericidal antibiotics. Gastroenterology 1992;103:1902.

205. Pederzoli P, Bassi C, Vesentini S, Campedelli A. A randomized multicenter clinical trial of antibiotic prophylaxis of septic complications in acute necrotizing pancreatitis with imipenem. Surg Gynecol Obstet 1993;176:480.

206. Fink AS, Hiatt JR, Pitt HA, et al. Indolent presentation of pancreatic abscess: experience with 100 cases. Arch Surg 1988;123:1067.

207. Ammann R, Munch R, Largiader F, et al. Pancreatic and hepatic abscesses: a late complication in 10 patients with chronic pancreatitis. Gastroenterology 1992;103:560.

208. Hurley JE, Vargish T. Early diagnosis and outcome of pancreatic abscesses in pancreatitis. Am Surg 1987;53:29.

209. Stanten R, Frey CF. Comprehensive management of acute necrotizing pancreatitis and pancreatic abscess. Arch Surg 1990;125:1269.

210. Van Vyve EL, Reynaert MS, Lengele BG, et al. Retroperitoneal laparostomy: a surgical treatment of pancreatic abscesses after an acute necrotizing pancreatitis. Surgery 1992;111:369.

211. Martin FM, Rossi RL, Munson JL, et al. Management of pancreatic fistulas. Arch Surg 1989;124:571.

212. Rotman N, Mathieu D, Anglade MC, Fagniez PL. Failure of percutaneous drainage of pancreatic abscesses complicating severe acute pancreatitis. Surg Gynecol Obstet 1992;174:141.

213. Saari A, Schröder T, Kivilaakso E, et al. Treatment of pancreatic fistulas with somatostatin and total parenteral nutrition. Scand J Gastroenterol 1989;24:859.

214. Rattner DW, Legermate DA, Lee MJ, et al. Early surgical debridement of symptomatic pancreatic necrosis is beneficial irrespective of infection. Am J Surg 1992;163:105.

215. Yeo CJ, Bastidas JA, Lynch-Nyhan A, et al. The natural history of pancreatic pseudocysts documented by computed tomography. Surg Gynecol Obstet 1990;170:411.

216. Imrie CW, Buist LJ, Shearer MG. Importance of cause in the outcome of pancreatic pseudocysts. Am J Surg 1988;156:159.

217. Jones DR, Vaughan RA, Timberlake GA. Pancreatic pseudocyst: diagnosis and management. South Med J 1992;85:729.

218. Williams KJ, Fabian TC. Pancreatic pseudocyst: recommendations for operative and nonoperative management. Am Surg 1992;58:199.

219. El Hamel A, Parc R, Adda G, et al. Bleeding pseudocysts and pseudoaneurysms in chronic pancreatitis. Br J Surg 1991;78:1059.

220. Fernandez-Cruz L, Pera M, Vilella A, et al. *Hemosuccus pancreaticus* from a pseudoaneurysm of the hepatic artery proper in a patient with a pancreatic pseudocyst. Hepatogastroenterology 1992;39:149.

221. Bender JS, Levison MA. Massive hemorrhage associated with pancreatic pseudocyst: successful treatment by pancreaticoduodenectomy. Am Surg 1991;57:653.

222. Vitas GJ, Sarr MG. Selected management of pancreatic pseudocysts: operative versus expectant management. Surgery 1992;111:123.

223. Ahearne PM, Baillie JM, Cotton PB, et al. An endoscopic retrograde cholangiopancreatography (ERCP)-based algorithm for the management of pancreatic pseudocysts. Am J Surg 1992;163:111.

224. Criado E, De Stefano AA, Weiner TM, Jaques PF. Long term

results of percutaneous catheter drainage of pancreatic pseu-docysts. Surg Gynecol Obstet 1992;175:293.

225. Grosso M, Gandini G, Cassinis MC, et al. Percutaneous treat-ment (including pseudocystogastrostomy) of 74 pancreatic pseudocysts. Radiology 1989;173:493.

226. Dohmoto M, Rupp KD. Endoscopic drainage of pancreatic pseudocysts. Surg Endosc 1992;6:118.

227. Duvnjak M, Vucelic B, Rotkvic I, et al. Assessment of value of pancreatic pseudocyst amylase concentration in the treatment of pancreatic pseudocysts by percutaneous evacuation. JCU 1992;20:183.

228. Ros PR, Hamrick-Turner JE, Chiechi MV, et al. Cystic masses of the pancreas. Radiographics 1992;12:673.

229. Lipsett PA, Cameron JL. Internal pancreatic fistula. Am J Surg 1992;163:216.

230. Willis SM, Brewer TG. Pancreatic duct–portal vein fistula. Gas-troenterology 1989;97:1025.

231. Willemer S, Feddersen CO, Karges W, Adler G. Lung injury in acute experimental pancreatitis in rats. I. Morphological studies. Int J Pancreatol 1991;8:305.

232. De Filippi VJ, Vargish T, Block GE. Massive gastrointestinal hemorrhage in pancreatitis secondary to visceral artery aneu-rysms. Am Surg 1992;58:618.

233. Lankisch PC. The spleen in inflammatory pancreatic disease. Gastroenterology 1990;98:509.

234. Aldridge MC, Francis ND, Glazer G, Dudley HA. Colonic complications of severe acute pancreatitis. Br J Surg 1989;76:362.

235. Santos JC Jr, Feres O, Rocha JJ, Aracava MM. Massive lower gastrointestinal hemorrhage caused by pseudocyst of the pan-creas ruptured into the colon: report of two cases. Dis Colon Rectum 1992;35:75.

236. Dhawan SS, Herbst JS, Fields KW. Tender nodules on the legs. Subcutaneous fat necrosis associated pancreatitis. Arch Der-matol 1991;127:249.

237. Dhawan SS, Jimenez-Asosta F. Subcutaneous fat necrosis as-sociated with pancreatitis: histochemical and electron micro-scopic findings. Am J Gastroenterol 1990;85:1025.

238. Haller J, Greenway G, Resnick D, et al. Intraosseous fat necrosis associated with acute pancreatitis: MR imaging. Radiology 1989;173:193.

239. McFadden DW. Organ failure and multiple organ system failure in pancreatitis. Pancreas 1991;6(Suppl 1):S37.

240. Pitchumoni CS, Agarwal N, Jain NK. Systemic complications of acute pancreatitis. Am J Gastroenterol 1988;83:597.

Textbook of Gastroenterology, second edition, edited by Tadataka Yamada. JB Lippincott Company, Philadelphia © 1995.

CHAPTER 91

Chronic Pancreatitis

Chung Owyang   Michael D. Levitt

CLASSIFICATION

The terminology surrounding the classification of inflammatory disease of the pancreas is confusing and based on both clinical and morphologic criteria. Over the last three decades, multiple classifications have been proposed. Differentiation by etiology allows for the prediction of responsible factors for pancreatitis but gives little information on potential overlapping pathophysiologic mechanisms. Clinical and pathologic classifications by themselves have prognostic implications, with fulminant or hemorrhagic pancreatitis having a poor prognosis and edematous pancreatitis being associated with a good prognosis, but only in a minority of patients is histologic information ever obtained, and clinical classifications are not helpful pathophysiologically. In 1963, a symposium on pancreatitis was held in Marseilles in which a clinical classification of pancreatitis was proposed, and this classification has since been widely used.[1] According to the Marseilles classification, pancreatitis can be divided into acute and chronic, with both types having relapsing and nonrelapsing varieties. The essential difference between acute and chronic pancreatitis is the presence of permanent and progressive morphologic or functional damage in the latter. Both subtypes are further classified into relapsing and nonrelapsing varieties depending on their clinical presentation. In acute pancreatitis, if the primary causes or factors are eliminated, clinical and morphologic restitution of the pancreas occurs. On the other hand, in the chronic form, anatomic or functional pancreatic damage remains even after the primary causes are eliminated.

The major drawback of the Marseilles classification is the frequent inability to distinguish acute and chronic forms of the disease based on clinical presentation. This prompted two subsequent international symposia in 1983[2] and 1984[3] to discuss the classification of pancreatitis. Some minor modifications of the original Marseilles classification were proposed. The classification of pancreatitis should be reduced to include only acute and chronic forms because it is frequently difficult to distinguish between recurrent acute pancreatitis and recurrent attacks of chronic pancreatitis, and several years' follow-up may be needed. Accordingly, chronic pancreatitis is defined as an inflammatory disease of the pancreas characterized by persistent and often progressive lesions, whereas lesions of acute pancreatitis regress when the cause is suppressed or removed. In an addendum, it was recognized that alcohol-induced pancreatitis may present acutely, and it is not inevitably progressive.

The second symposium of Marseilles[2] also proposed to distinguish obstructive chronic pancreatitis from other forms of chronic pancreatitis. Obstructive chronic pancreatitis is characterized by dilatation of the ductal system, diffuse atrophy of the acinar parenchyma, and uniform fibrosis. In contrast to other forms of chronic pancreatitis, intraductal plugs or stones usually are rare or absent, and both structural and functional changes may improve when the obstruction is relieved. Based on morphology, biochemistry, molecular biology, and epidemiology, Sarles has recently reclassified chronic pancreatitis into four groups.[4] The first and largest group, lithogenic pancreatitis (chronic calcifying pancreatitis), consists of five subgroups of stones: hereditary pancreatitis, transparent stones, nutritional pancreatitis, hypercalcemia,

pancreatitis, and pure calcium stones. The other three groups include obstructive pancreatitis due to obstruction of pancreatic ducts preceding the onset of pancreatitis, with uniform distribution of the lesions caudal to the obstruction; inflammatory pancreatitis, which is characterized by diffuse fibrosis and the destruction of exocrine parenchyma with infiltration of mononuclear cells; and pancreatic fibrosis, characterized by silent, diffuse perilobular fibrosis.

INCIDENCE AND PREVALENCE

The prevalence of chronic pancreatitis in autopsy materials ranges from 0.04%[5] to 5%.[6] Epidemiologic studies based on clinical data are few. Most epidemiologic data are obtained either from retrospective studies[7-9] or by calculation from data given in clinical material.[10,11] The only prospective study on the incidence and prevalence of chronic pancreatitis was performed in Copenhagen in 1978 and 1979.[12] It showed an incidence of 8.2 new cases per 100,000 inhabitants per year, and a prevalence of 26.4 cases per 100,000 inhabitants. The epidemiologic studies clearly demonstrate that there is enormous difference in incidence rates between different areas. Alcohol consumption is considered to be the major factor in the development of chronic pancreatitis. This may well explain the low incidence (rate) of chronic pancreatitis in Japan, which has traditionally a very low alcohol intake. However, Switzerland has a substantially higher alcohol consumption than observed in Denmark,[13] but the incidence of chronic pancreatitis is lower in Switzerland than in Denmark. The reason for this discrepancy is unknown. Environmental or hereditary factors may influence susceptibility to alcohol-induced pancreatitis. Alternatively, this may be related to regional differences in diagnostic criteria for chronic pancreatitis. Thus, figures for frequency of chronic pancreatitis differ markedly from one center to another. Most likely, this does not reflect a real difference in frequency but points strongly to regional differences in patient selection and diagnostic criteria. Valid and comparable figures for incidence and prevalence of chronic pancreatitis are pending careful, prospective, epidemiologic studies based on uniformly accepted diagnostic criteria.

ETIOLOGY

Alcohol in Western societies (70%–80%) and malnutrition worldwide represent the major etiologies of chronic pancreatitis.[14,15] In addition, metabolic and mechanical disturbances as well as hereditary disposition have been implicated (Table 91-1).

Alcohol

Alcohol consumption is the major cause of chronic pancreatitis. In Western societies, approximately 70% of cases are caused by alcohol.[16] The incidence of pancreatitis found at autopsy in alcoholics is as high as 45%—50 times the rate in nondrinking controls.[17] There is a linear relationship between the logarithm of the risk for development of chronic pancreatitis and the mean daily consumption of alcohol.[18] Further-

TABLE 91-1
Etiology of Chronic Pancreatitis

Alcohol, 70%
Idiopathic (including tropical), 20%
Other, 10%
    Hereditary
    Hyperparathyroidism
    Hypertriglyceridemia
    Obstruction
    Trauma

more, it has been demonstrated that the risk for abstainers is lower than the risk for people drinking a low quantity of alcohol (i.e., 1–20 g/day). Therefore, it appears that there is no statistical threshold for alcohol toxicity but a continuous spectrum of individual thresholds. This makes it difficult to distinguish between low-threshold alcohol-induced pancreatitis and idiopathic pancreatitis. The duration of alcohol consumption is also important. For the same daily intake, the risk increased with duration.[19] On the other hand, the type of alcohol beverages and the pattern of drinking (weekend vs. daily users) have no influence on the risk for development of chronic pancreatitis.[20] This concept, however, has been challenged.[21]

In general, prolonged alcohol intake is required to produce symptomatic chronic pancreatitis (6–12 years), although the length of time required for histologic damage in humans is unknown.[22] A study of Kondo and associates[23] emphasizes that alcohol requires other factors to induce chronic pancreatitis. They reported that the aberrant pancreas may not be susceptible to alcoholic pancreatitis. Anatomic differences in the aberrant pancreas such as innervation and different ductal drainage may explain the lack of damage after chronic alcohol ingestion. In addition, dietary factors may play a significant role. Both experimental and epidemiologic studies indicate the risk for alcohol-induced pancreatitis is higher in people with high-fat, high-protein diets. Experimentally, focal lesions of chronic pancreatitis developed in more than 50% of rats that ingested alcohol for 20 to 30 months.[24] The pancreatic juice of these rats contained higher protein concentrations than controls, a condition that appears similar to chronic pancreatitis in humans. In separate studies, Tsukamoto and colleagues[25] show that in rats with low dietary intake of corn oil fat, chronic alcohol intoxication produced only mild pancreatic injury. Severe focal lesions of chronic pancreatitis, however, were observed in rats fed higher amounts of fat, which resulted in striking potentiation of alcohol-induced pancreatic injury. Observations from these experimental studies were supported by clinical and epidemiologic studies. It has been observed in many European countries that alcoholics consuming a high-fat, high-protein diet are predisposed to chronic pancreatitis.[5,26–28] Sarles noted that the risk was less with average consumption of fat but was increased by both high (>100 g) and low (<85 g) fat intake.[18] Furthermore, the effects of alcohol, protein, and fat consumption appear to be additive. This may explain why chronic pancreatitis is more commonly observed in patients who drink more alcohol and eat more protein and fat than controls.[19] Observations

made in Europe, however, are not confirmed by studies reported from the United States and Australia.[29–31] It appears that whereas a high-fat or high-protein diet may predispose to pancreatitis, such a diet is not a prerequisite for development of pancreatitis in chronic alcoholics. Differences in genetic predisposition and quantity of alcohol and type of fat consumed by various populations may explain some of these conflicting observations.

The mechanisms by which alcohol produces chronic pancreatitis are not known. A report from Sweden[21] suggests that the type of alcohol is also important. In this report, increasing consumption of distilled liquors was related to the increasing incidence of chronic pancreatitis, but the consumption of beer and wine was not. Inferences about the pathophysiologic basis of alcohol-induced progressive pancreatic inflammation can be made from the alcohol's effects on pancreatic secretion and the known pathologic changes described by Sarles and others. Chronic alcoholism causes an increase in basal secretion of proteases, amylase, and lipase and a decrease in trypsin inhibitor in rats.[32] Furthermore, an increased responsiveness of the pancreas to cholecystokinin (CCK) stimulation has been reported in dogs[33] and humans.[34] In addition to the perturbation in the content and secretion of pancreatic enzymes, chronic alcohol consumption also causes perturbation in the lysosomal enzymes; acid phosphatase was increased in cell fractions, and cathepsin B was increased in the mitochondrial-lysosomal fraction and the zymogen granule fractions of the pancreas from alcohol-fed rats.[35] Therefore, it is conceivable that alcohol produces pancreatitis by interfering with the intracellular transport and discharge of digestive enzyme, causing colocalization of digestive and lysosomal hydrolases, a condition conducive to the initiation of autodigestion. The augmented responsiveness of the exocrine pancreas may account for the high-protein, low-bicarbonate, and low-volume pancreatic secretory output after chronic alcohol consumption.[36] Theoretically, protein precipitates would be formed, particularly in low–flow-rate areas such as the secondary pancreatic ducts. This may explain the frequent involvement of the secondary duct with relative sparing of the main pancreatic duct in early stages of chronic pancreatitis.

The discovery of a pancreatic stone protein (lithostatin) found in pancreatic juice and calculi has generated considerable interest, because this protein is capable of inhibiting the formation of insoluble calcium salts in a supersaturated milieu.[37,38] Lithostatin has been found to be decreased in the pancreatic juice of patients with alcoholic pancreatitis and in some patients with nonalcoholic chronic pancreatitis.[39] Hence, it is conceivable that a deficiency of lithostatin may play an important role in the development of pancreatic calcification.[37] The importance of this protein remains unclear, however, because not all studies have shown a reduction in lithostatin in pancreatic juice from patients with chronic pancreatitis.[40]

In addition to hypersecretion of protein, viscosity of pancreatic juice is enhanced in chronic pancreatitis because of a higher concentration of hexosamine.[41] There is a correlation between the concentrations of protein, hydrolytic enzymes, hexosamine, and viscosity.[41] Hyperviscosity of pancreatic juice may result in decreased flow and contribute to protein precipitation in chronic pancreatitis. Therefore, it appears that chronic alcoholism results in a number of changes in the pancreatic juice that create a conducive environment for the formation of intraductal protein plugs that block small ductules in a random fashion. Ductal blockade produces progressive structural abnormalities in the ducts and acinar tissue. In time, calcium is complexed to protein plugs, initially in small ductules and eventually in the main pancreatic duct. Progressive blockade results in injury and destruction of pancreatic tissue.[42]

Tropical (Nutritional) Pancreatitis

Tropical chronic pancreatitis, one of the major nutritional forms of chronic pancreatitis, is an important disease among juveniles and young adults in some Afro-Asian countries (Indonesia, southern India, and tropical Africa).[43-46] The natural history of tropical chronic pancreatitis is succinctly summarized by Gee Varghese[46] as "recurrent abdominal pain in childhood, diabetes around puberty and death at the prime of life." Abdominal pain characterizes the onset of tropical pancreatitis. The onset of diabetes typically occurs a few years after the onset of abdominal pain. Diabetes is characteristically brittle, with marked fluctuations of blood glucose. At this time, abdominal radiographs invariably show diffuse pancreatic calculi. Microscopically, dilation of the ducts, pancreatic lithiasis, chronic inflammatory cell infiltration, and atrophy of the pancreatic parenchyma are seen.

The etiology of tropical pancreatitis is not clearly understood, although the common denominator appears to be malnutrition in most cases.[47] More recent evidence suggests that other factors such as toxic products in certain nutritional components (cassava) may be more important.[48,49] Cassava is consumed in large quantities by most poor people in many Afro-Asian countries. It contains 65 mg of toxic glycoside per 100 g. When glycosides react with gastric hydrochloric acid, hydrocyanic acid is liberated. The enzyme rhodanase acts on hydrocyanic acid, leading to thiocyanate production in the presence of adequate amounts of methionine and cystine. Cyanogens impair a number of enzymes, including superoxide dismutase, an important scavenger of free radicals, which are proposed to cause cell injury.[50,51] Associated nutritional deficiencies, such as deficiencies of zinc, copper, and selenium, which are common in malnutrition, interfere with detoxification of cyanogens. Thus, the pathogenesis of tropical pancreatitis may be partly explained by micronutrient-antioxidant deficiencies and unopposed free radical injury secondary to dietary cyanogens.

Hereditary Pancreatitis

The clinical picture of hereditary pancreatitis was well described by Comfort and Steinberg.[52] Since then, many similar cases have been reported from different areas of the world (United States, Ireland, France, and New Zealand). Typically, hereditary chronic pancreatitis appears in childhood at a mean age of 10 to 12 years. The disease is inherited through an autosomal dominant gene of incomplete penetrance. The incidence is approximately equal in both sexes,[53] and there is no evidence that the disease is coupled to specific human leukocyte antigen haplotypes.[54]

In addition to the typical hereditary form described by Comfort and Steinberg, which begins at a young age, familial aggregations of two or three cases with attacks beginning in the third or fourth decade[55] have been reported. This suggests that there may be different forms of hereditary transmission.

The clinical picture of hereditary pancreatitis differs little from that of nonhereditary pancreatitis.[53] Patients frequently experience recurrent attacks of severe upper abdominal pain. Overt diabetes develops 8 to 10 years after the onset of pain in 20% of cases, and gross steatorrhea in 15% to 20%. The diagnosis of hereditary pancreatitis should be suspected if several family members have pancreatitis in the absence of alcohol consumption or other causes of chronic pancreatitis.

Hyperparathyroidism

Calcified chronic pancreatitis occurs in untreated hyperparathyroidism. Surveys suggest that the incidence is decreasing, and is no greater than 1% to 2%.[56] A likely explanation is that serum calcium is measured routinely in virtually all patients who undergo a medical checkup, and, as a result, hyperparathyroidism does not remain undiscovered and untreated for many years.

The pathogenesis of pancreatitis in hyperparathyroidism is presumed to be related to the effect of hypercalcemia. Acute hypercalcemia is a potent stimulus of human pancreatic enzyme secretion.[57,58] Furthermore, chronic hypercalcemia causes a significant increase in pancreatic calcium secretion in patients with hyperparathyroidism[59] and in experimental animals.[60] This results in precipitation of intraductal calcium in pancreatic juices. Moreover, chronic hypercalcemia causes a decrease in the diffusion barrier between the pancreatic interstitial compartment and the ductular system, resulting in excessive diffusion of calcium into the pancreatic juices.[60] These events may damage the pancreas and promote the development of calcified chronic pancreatitis.

Obstruction

Obstruction of the main pancreatic duct by tumors, benign vaterian stenosis,[61] scars (e.g., from traumatic pancreatitis), and pseudocysts[62] can lead to a distinct form of chronic pancreatitis known as obstructive chronic pancreatitis. This is characterized by acinar atrophy and fibrosis and dilation of the ductal system. In contrast to alcohol-induced chronic pancreatitis, intraductal plugs or stones are very rare in obstructive chronic pancreatitis, and both structural and functional changes may improve when obstruction is relieved.[61] The regression of fibrotic lesions may be explained by the finding that fibrosis in experimental obstructive pancreatitis consists of fractions of collagen with short half-lives (fibronectin, laminin, collagen III, and procollagen III) rather than the long-lived fraction collagen I.[63]

Trauma

Trauma to the abdomen or back may be clinically insignificant and still produce significant pancreatic injury leading to chronic pancreatitis. The pathogenesis may follow that of the obstructive type, but inflammation and pseudocysts develop frequently. Recognition of trauma as the cause for chronic pancreatitis is important because most cases are associated with severe ductal disruption, which responds poorly to medical treatment, yet results of surgical correction (particularly partial pancreatectomy) have been excellent.[64,65]

Pancreas Divisum

Pancreas divisum is the most common congenital abnormality of the pancreas (4%–11%).[66,67] Fusion of the dorsal and ventral pancreatic ducts is absent or incomplete, and drainage of the major portion of the pancreas occurs through the minor papilla. The clinical significance of pancreas divisum is unknown, although considerable controversy surrounds this issue. Several reports suggest that incidence of pancreatitis is increased in subjects with pancreas divisum. Cotton reported that the incidence of pancreas divisum in patients with idiopathic pancreatitis undergoing endoscopic retrograde cholangiopancreatography (ERCP) was 25.6%, whereas only 3.6% of patients with biliary disease undergoing ERCP had pancreas divisum.[68] Similarly, Sahel and colleagues noted that the incidence of pancreas divisum among patients with acute pancreatitis was 21%.[69] This was much higher than a 5% incidence of pancreas divisum among all patients undergoing ERCP. Richter also reported a 19% incidence of pancreas divisum in patients with idiopathic pancreatitis compared to an overall 5% incidence of pancreas divisum in patients undergoing ERCP.[70] These observations suggest that pancreas divisum might be an important cause of disease in patients with idiopathic pancreatitis. It has been hypothesized that the opening of the lesser papilla might be too small to permit free flow of pancreatic juice into the duodenum, and, as a result, pancreas divisum might cause a form of obstructive pancreatitis.

The clinical significance of pancreas divisum has been disputed. Delhaye and associates reported the results of a study in Belgium involving 6324 patients undergoing ERCP for biliopancreatic complaints, and noted that the incidence of pancreas divisum was similar in patients with chronic pancreatitis (6.4%), acute pancreatitis (7.5%), and nonpancreatic disease (5.5%).[71] Similar results have been reported by Sugawa and colleagues,[72] who noted a 2.7% incidence of pancreas divisum among 1529 patients undergoing ERCP. There was no increase in incidence of pancreas divisum among patients with idiopathic pancreatitis or people with unexplained upper abdominal pain. More recently, Burtin and colleagues[73] reported a 5.9% prevalence of pancreatic divisum in more than 1000 patients undergoing ERCP. The proportion of patients with pancreas divisum was similar among patients with and without pancreatitis. Thus, the results reported by Burtin and colleagues,[73] Delhaye and associates,[71] and Sugawa and colleagues[72] contradict the earlier studies by Cotton,[68] Sahel and colleagues[69] and Richter,[70] which indicated an increased incidence of pancreas divisum among patients with pancreatitis. It is possible that the results from earlier studies[68–70] might be biased by patient selection. Patients with pancreas divisum and patients with idiopathic pancreatitis are likely to be referred to centers with exceptional endoscopic skills, and, as a result, the incidence of pancreas divisum may appear to be increased, whereas such an increase is not present in a more random sampling of patients.

Idiopathic Pancreatitis

The major form of nonalcoholic chronic pancreatitis in North America and Europe is the idiopathic type (10%–40%). Epidemiology and clinical studies suggest that idiopathic chronic pancreatitis may be divided into two distinct groups: a juvenile type with onset of symptomatic disease at a median age of 18 years, and a senile type with an incidence peak at 60 years of age. In juvenile chronic pancreatitis, abdominal pain dominates the clinical picture at initial presentation, whereas in senile groups, painless disease is frequent and most patients present with exocrine insufficiency, diabetes, and pancreatic calcification.[74] It has been suggested that the senile form might be caused by arteriosclerosis[75]; however, firm evidence to implicate vascular insufficiency as a cause for chronic pancreatitis is lacking.

CLINICAL PRESENTATION

Pain

The presenting symptom of most patients with chronic pancreatitis is abdominal pain. The pain usually is epigastric, dull rather than sharp, and constant rather than colicky. Although the pain may radiate to both upper quadrants and occasionally to the lower quadrants, a characteristic feature is radiation directly through to the back. The pain is partially relieved by sitting with the trunk bent forward or lying prone; the supine posture aggravates the discomfort. It may take the form of attacks of several days' duration with intervening pain-free intervals, or may be nearly constant, particularly in the elderly. The almost instantaneous aggravation of pain by food ingestion is characteristic of chronic pancreatitis or carcinoma of the pancreas, and this symptom always should raise the suspicion of pancreatic disease. Although food ingestion may aggravate the pain of other abdominal conditions (i.e., irritable bowel syndrome), there is usually a much greater interval between the meal and the discomfort than is the case with pancreatic disease. Ingestion of alcohol also may aggravate the pain, although a sizable fraction of patients claim that the pain develops after 12 to 24 hours of abstinence.[76]

Pain in chronic pancreatitis may continue, diminish, or disappear completely. Several reports have suggested that pain may disappear as the severity of pancreatitis increases.[77–79] According to Ammann, pain disappears coincident with the appearance of calcifications, steatorrhea, and diabetes, which occurs 5 to 18 years after the onset of chronic pancreatitis.[79]

Chronic pancreatitis is painless or relatively painless (i.e., insufficient pain to require medical evaluation) in about 15% of patients.[80] Idiopathic pancreatitis is more likely to be painless than the alcoholic variety.

Weight Loss

Nausea, vomiting, anorexia, and weight loss are common in chronic pancreatitis. The major cause of weight loss is decreased caloric intake owing to fear of aggravation of the abdominal pain, although malabsorption or uncontrolled diabetes also may play a role. Marked weight loss is relatively unusual in other painful abdominal conditions such as peptic ulcer or irritable bowel syndrome, and the combination of chronic upper abdominal pain and rapid loss of weight always should suggest the possibility of pancreatic disease.

Malabsorption

Diarrhea, steatorrhea, and azotorrhea occur when exocrine secretion of pancreatic enzymes is insufficient to maintain normal digestion. Although most attention has been directed to the malabsorption of fat and protein in this condition, studies using breath H_2 excretion also have demonstrated malabsorption of starch.[81,82]

Because malabsorption does not occur until enzyme secretion is reduced to less than 10%[83,84] of normal, diarrhea and steatorrhea occur relatively late in the course of chronic pancreatitis. As a rule, fecal weight is less in pancreatic malabsorption than in other conditions with comparable steatorrhea. This relatively low fecal weight reflects a lesser quantity of fecal water, and patients may pass bulky, formed stool as opposed to the frank watery diarrhea observed in other conditions. The relatively low fecal water in pancreatic insufficiency probably results from the better absorption of some carbohydrates, such as disaccharides, that occurs in conditions with mucosal pathology, such as celiac sprue. Occasionally, the patient observes that gross oil leaks from the rectum or floats as an "oil slick" on the surface of water in the toilet bowl. If ingestion of mineral oil is excluded, this finding usually is indicative of pancreatic steatorrhea.

For a given degree of steatorrhea, the absorption of fat-soluble vitamins (A, D, E, and K) is much better in pancreatic insufficiency than in celiac sprue.[85] Marked deficiency of these vitamins seldom is observed in pancreatic insufficiency, and presumably this reflects the relative unimportance of lipolysis for the absorption of these compounds. The body stores of these vitamins, however, have been shown to be reduced in a large fraction of patients with chronic pancreatitis, although clinical manifestations of the deficiencies are quite rare.[86]

Pancreatic Diabetes

Although glucose intolerance is common early in the course of chronic pancreatitis, clinically evident diabetes occurs relatively late in the disease. Endocrine insufficiency eventually occurs in 60% of patients with chronic pancreatitis. In most patients, the diagnosis of chronic pancreatitis is established long before the development of symptomatic hyperglycemia; however, the occasional patient with relatively painless pancreatitis may present initially with diabetes. Ketoacidosis and diabetic nephropathy are relatively uncommon in this form of diabetes. For a given duration of diabetes, however, retinopathy and neuropathy are thought to occur with a frequency similar to that in idiopathic diabetes mellitus.[87]

Other Clinical Features

Other clinical presentations of chronic pancreatitis include jaundice secondary to common bile duct compression by the pancreas; ascites or pleural effusion due to leak of pancreatic secretions from a ruptured duct or pseudocyst; painful nodules, usually over the lower extremities, resulting from fat necrosis; and, rarely, a polyarthritis of the small joints of the hands.

In the United States, at least 70% of chronic pancreatitis is attributed to prolonged, heavy ingestion of ethanol, whereas the bulk of the remaining 30% is idiopathic. Thus, historic information concerning length and duration of ethanol ingestion is critical in all suspected cases of chronic pancreatitis. In contrast, gallstone disease virtually never is the cause of chronic pancreatitis. A family history of pancreatitis or chronic abdominal pain of unknown origin may suggest the diagnosis of familial pancreatitis.

The physical examination usually is of limited assistance in the diagnosis of chronic pancreatitis. There is epigastric tenderness during the painful episodes (and sometimes during periods of remission). Tenderness ranges from mild to marked, but involuntary guarding and rebound are unusual. The physical signs characteristically are trivial relative to the intensity of the patient's complaints. Complications of chronic pancreatitis, such as pseudocysts, ascites, or pleural effusions, may be detected on physical examination.

PATHOMECHANISM OF SYMPTOMS

Abdominal pain and malabsorption are the major symptoms of chronic pancreatitis. The pathophysiologic processes responsible for the development of these symptoms are discussed in the following sections.

Pain

The mechanisms of pain in chronic pancreatitis are unclear. Possible causes include inflammation of the pancreas, increased intrapancreatic pressure, neural inflammation, and extrapancreatic causes such as common bile duct stenosis and duodenal stenosis.

Acute inflammation of the pancreas during a relapsing attack of chronic pancreatitis or peripancreatic inflammation involving the duodenum and retroperitoneum may cause pain. Clinical and experimental evidence, however, suggests that pain may be related to increased intraductal pressure secondary to continued pancreatic secretion in the face of ductal obstruction caused by strictures or intraductal stones. Several clinical studies showed that pain relief correlates with the development of pancreatic insufficiency in patients with alcohol-induced chronic pancreatitis. For example, Ammann and colleagues noted that most patients with chronic calcific pancreatitis eventually became pain free and the onset of relief was clearly associated with decreased pancreatic secretion.[77] A similar observation was made by Girdwood, who reported that 31% of patients with painless pancreatitis had severe pancreatic insufficiency, compared with 3% who had painful pancreatitis.[78] These observations suggest that decreased secretion may reduce intraductal pressure and relieve pain. Measurements of intraductal pressure have been made in patients without pancreatic disease and those with ductal abnormalities. Among patients without pancreatic disease, intraductal pressure has been found to be 7 mm Hg by direct puncture at surgery in one patient[88] and 10 to 16 mm Hg by ERCP among 33 patients without pancreatic disease.[89-91] By comparison, in 59 patients with a dilated duct, intraductal pressure measured by direct puncture at surgery ranged from 18 to 48 mm Hg.[88,89,92] In one study,[89] all 19 patients with a dilated main pancreatic duct with elevated intraductal pressure had prompt relief of pain after decompression surgery. Pancreatic tissue pressure also appears to be elevated among patients with chronic pancreatitis with a dilated pancreatic duct and those with pseudocyst. The pressure ranged between 17 and 21 mm Hg,[88] compared to 3 to 11 mm Hg in patients with a normal pancreas.[93] The pancreatic tissue pressure normalized after decompression of the duct or cyst, and this resulted in pain relief in 12 of the 14 patients. Hence, these observations support the thesis that pain in chronic pancreatitis is related to increased intraductal and pancreatic tissue pressure.

Intrapancreatic neural inflammation is another factor that may play an important role in the genesis of pain in chronic pancreatitis. Morphologic studies indicate that pancreatic nerves appear to be larger and more numerous in chronic pancreatitis.[94] The organization of intraneural organelles such as microtubules is disrupted. Most significantly, however, there is an alteration in the perineurial sheath that ordinarily shields nerves from surrounding connective tissue.[94] The damaged perineurium allows penetration of biologically active materials from the surrounding extracellular matrix, and pain may result from the continual stimulation of the sensory fibers by noxious substances. In this regard, immunohistologic studies have shown that the amount of neurotransmitters such as substance P is increased in afferent pancreatic nerves in chronic pancreatitis.[95] There is also evidence that eosinophils are increased in the perineural space among patients with recent alcohol consumption.[96] It is conceivable that degranulation of these eosinophils might be a factor in the generation of pain.

Peripancreatic inflammation involving the duodenum and retroperitoneum may cause pain. Extension of active inflammation of the pancreatic tissue within the wall of the duo-

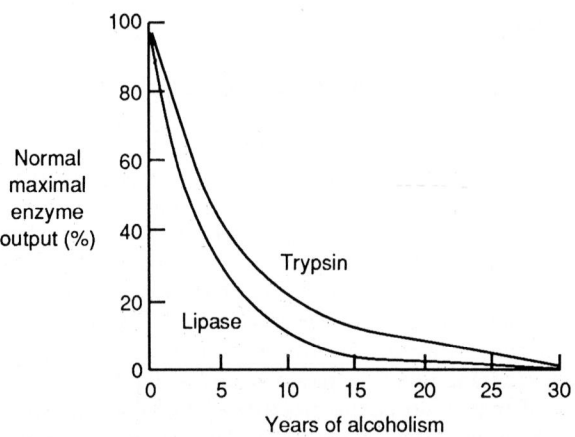

FIGURE 91-2. Relation between reductions in enzyme output and years of alcoholism in patients with alcoholic pancreatitis. (Adapted from DiMagno EP, Malagelada JR, Go VLW. Relationship between alcoholism and pancreatic insufficiency. NY Acad Sci 1975;252:200.)

denum may result in extensive fibrosis and stenosis of the descending duodenum.[97] Peripancreatic inflammation may cause stenosis of the distal common bile duct, and this has been noted to be associated with severe abdominal pain. Pain may also result from continued inflammation of the head of the pancreas.[97] Thus, it is likely that pain in chronic pancreatitis is multifactorial. Depending on the etiologic factors, structure, alteration, severity of the disease, and degree of pancreatic insufficiency, different factors may predominate in the genesis of pain. A study correlating pancreatic pathologic condition and symptoms found that intermittent attacks of pain resulted from recurrent tissue necrosis, whereas chronic pain appeared to be secondary to segmental distention behind obstructed ducts.[98]

Malabsorption

There is a 10-fold reserve for exocrine pancreatic enzyme secretion. Malabsorption occurs only after the capacity for enzyme secretion is reduced by more than 90%[83] (Fig. 91-1). In chronic pancreatitis secondary to alcoholism, it usually takes 10 to 20 years for severe pancreatic insufficiency to develop, but lipase secretion decreases more rapidly than secretion of proteolytic enzymes[84] (Fig. 91-2). Hence, steatorrhea is often an earlier and more severe problem than azotorrhea. The importance of colipase in fat malabsorption in adult patients is unknown, although colipase appears to be an important factor in children because steatorrhea and colipase correlate better than lipase and steatorrhea.[99]

Concurrent with the reduction of pancreatic enzyme secretion, there is also decreased bicarbonate secretion in patients with severe chronic pancreatitis. Not infrequently, the duodenal pH may fall to 4 or less[100,101] 90 minutes after eating. The abnormally low duodenal pH (<4) reduces lipid digestion by inactivating pancreatic enzymes and precipitating bile acids. These factors are important to consider in the treatment of pancreatic steatorrhea.

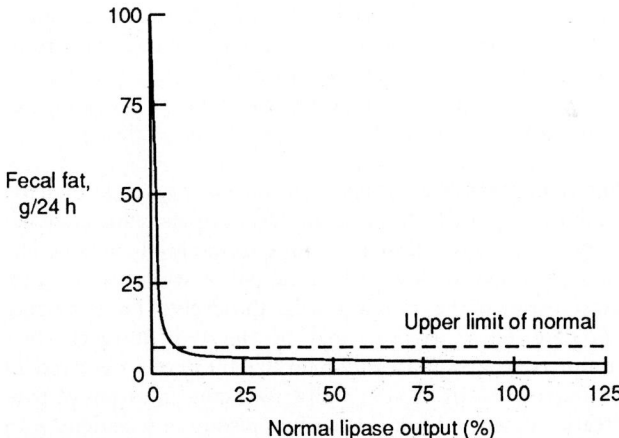

FIGURE 91-1. Relation between steatorrhea and lipase output. Steatorrhea does not occur until lipase output is reduced below 10% of normal. (Adapted from DiMagno EP, Go VLW, Summerskill WHJ. Relations between pancreatic enzyme outputs and malabsorption in severe pancreatic insufficiency. N Engl J Med 1973;288:813.)

DIAGNOSIS

Overview of Diagnostic Approaches

The diagnosis of chronic pancreatitis usually is suggested by historical information and then confirmed by radiography or laboratory tests. Over the years, an enormous number and variety of tests have been developed for the diagnosis of pancreatitis (Table 91-2). Many of these tests have not been adequately evaluated, and their true sensitivity and specificity are unknown. This section reviews many of the proposed tests for chronic pancreatitis; most are of limited clinical value. An understanding of the rationale underlying the test, however, often provides an insight into the physiologic alterations that occur in chronic pancreatitis. The diagnosis of chronic pancreatitis often can be made on the basis of history and relatively simple radiographic tests. Only the rare patient requires extensive and complicated testing. Thus, the work-up should be tailored to the individual patient.

Laboratory Evaluation

Routine Laboratory Findings

Routine blood studies usually are not helpful in making the diagnosis of chronic pancreatitis. Leukocytosis may be observed during acute exacerbations.

The anemia frequently associated with malabsorption secondary to celiac disease seldom is present in patients with pancreatic malabsorption. Although patients with chronic pancreatitis commonly have an abnormal Schilling's test result owing to the inability normally to digest R protein, megaloblastic anemia is rare.[102] Fat-soluble vitamin deficiency states (hypocalcemia, hypoprothrombinemia) seldom are observed in association with the steatorrhea of chronic pancreatitis, in contrast to their frequent occurrence in celiac sprue.

Compression of the common duct by a fibrotic process in the pancreas not infrequently leads to varying degree of cho-

---

TABLE 91-2
Tests for Chronic Pancreatitis

I. Measurement of pancreatic products in blood
   A. Enzymes
   B. Pancreatic polypeptide
II. Measurement of pancreatic exocrine secretions
   A. Direct measurement
      1. Enzymes
      2. Bicarbonates
   B. Indirect measurement
      1. Bentiromide test
      2. Dual Schilling's test
      3. Fecal chymotrypsin concentration
      4. [^{14}C]olein absorption
III. Imaging techniques
   A. Plain film radiography of abdomen
   B. Ultrasonography
   C. Computed tomography
   D. Endoscopic retrograde choliangiopancreatography

---

lestasis.[103] Alkaline phosphatase elevation in the absence of jaundice or other symptoms is the most common manifestation. Clinical jaundice results from more severe compression. Although liver disease is extremely common in alcoholics, this condition usually does not take the form of relatively pure cholestasis. The finding of cholestatic liver function in patients with pancreatitis requires extensive radiologic testing, usually culminating in ERCP to establish that the biliary obstruction results from chronic pancreatitis.

Specific Tests for the Diagnosis of Chronic Pancreatitis

The multiple tests available for the diagnosis of chronic pancreatitis can be separated into chemical measurements of pancreatic function and radiologic procedures that provide information on pancreatic structure.

Several factors make it difficult to determine accurately the true sensitivity and specificity of these tests. First, biopsies of the pancreas usually are not obtained in patients with possible chronic pancreatitis, and most series report patients that have not been followed for a period sufficient to establish the presence or absence of this condition with certainty. Thus, in most early or questionable cases, there is no histologic gold standard that can be used to determine the accuracy of the more indirect chemical or radiologic tests. Second, the sensitivity of the various diagnostic tests depends on the extent of the pancreatic damage. In long-standing disease with marked functional and anatomic alterations, virtually all proposed tests are positive. The sensitivity of the tests falls dramatically in early or mild chronic pancreatitis, however. The apparent sensitivity and specificity of the various tests also depend on the composition of subjects used to establish the normal range. For example, patients with a variety of disease states such as diabetes mellitus,[104] celiac sprue,[105] and cirrhosis[106] may have subnormal pancreatic secretion of enzymes. If such patients are used to establish the normal range, the lower limits of normal are reduced and the sensitivity of the test for chronic pancreatitis drops accordingly. If the normal range is established with healthy controls, the specificity of a low secretion is reduced. Thus, although claims are made with regard to the sensitivity and specificity of tests for chronic pancreatitis, these claims have to be interpreted in light of the types of patients composing the pancreatitis groups as well as the subjects used to establish the normal range.

Serum pancreatic enzymes. In contrast to attacks of acute pancreatitis, in which the serum level of pancreatic enzymes is almost always elevated, serum enzyme levels may be elevated, normal, or low in chronic pancreatitis. In an acute exacerbation of the chronic process, the levels of these enzymes (amylase, lipase, trypsin) may be elevated; however, their serum concentrations seldom reach the levels observed in acute pancreatitis. A very high serum concentration of pancreatic enzymes during a painful episode in a patient with very advanced chronic pancreatitis should raise the possibility that some other abdominal process such as gut perforation or infarction is responsible for the pain. A number of investigators have examined the possibility that the finding of a subnormal serum concentration of pancreatic enzymes could be a valuable diagnostic indicator of chronic pancreatitis. Enzymes studied include pancreatic isoamylase,[107] lipase,[108] trypsin,[109] and elastase.[110] Total serum amylase usually is maintained within the normal range owing to amylase secretion by the salivary glands. Although patients with end-stage chronic pancreatitis characteristically have low serum levels of these enzymes, the diagnosis usually is obvious on clinical grounds. Patients with mild to moderate degrees of pancreatic dysfunction often have normal or elevated serum enzyme concentrations. Thus, these tests have little value other than to establish that the patient has severe pancreatic insufficiency. Provocative tests such as a CCK infusion in an attempt to increase serum enzyme levels once were popular but have been shown to be unreliable.[111] Similarly, measurement of the urinary excretion of pancreatic enzymes seems to add little to the simpler serum measurements.

Plasma concentration of pancreatic polypeptide. Pancreatic polypeptide (PP) is found in high concentration in the endocrine cells as well as the exocrine tissue of the pancreas. Protein ingestion and CCK administration normally induce secretion of this peptide. A subnormal rise in plasma PP after stimulation with a protein-rich meal or secretin infusion has been used as an indicator of chronic pancreatitis.[112,113] As is the case with pancreatic enzymes, reduced plasma levels of PP frequently are observed in advanced stages of chronic pancreatitis; however, patients with mild to moderate degrees of pancreatic damage have a normal PP response.[113] One study indicated that an impaired PP response to a Lundh meal was as sensitive an indicator of chronic pancreatitis as was the finding of increased fecal fat.[114]

Tests of pancreatic exocrine function. These tests can be divided into those that directly assess pancreatic exocrine function (e.g., measurements of enzyme or bicarbonate secretion) or those that test some secondary effect of impaired enzyme secretion (e.g., malabsorption of a compound that requires pancreatic digestion for normal absorption).

Direct tests of pancreatic exocrine secretion. Because the basal secretory rate of the pancreas is highly variable, meaningful direct measurements of pancreatic secretion must be carried out in the stimulated state. Varying doses of secretin or CCK have been used for this purpose as well as a standard meal (the Lundh test).

Early studies used simple drainage of the intestine at the ligament of Trietz to obtain pancreatic secretions. Because this technique does not recover all lumenal fluid passing the collection site, more recent studies have used a constant perfusion of a nonabsorbable marker such as polyethylene glycol into the duodenal bulb. Measurements of the concentration of this marker passing the distal collection site permit assessment of the rate at which fluid passes this site, and makes it possible to quantitate the rate at which pancreatic secretory components pass this site.[83] A factor that may confound the accuracy of this technique is reflux of pancreatic secretions into the stomach, where the enzymes are irreversibly denatured by gastric acid. Some investigators have attempted to correct for this phenomenon by measuring the quantity of a duodenally infused marker that is recovered from the stomach. Finally, it has been demonstrated that pancreatic enzymes are rapidly denatured in the intestinal lumen owing to the action

of the pancreatic proteases.[115] Thus, despite the best of techniques, it is possible that pancreatic secretory studies do not provide an absolutely accurate assessment of exocrine secretion.

It is apparent from these considerations that direct measurement of pancreatic secretion is a relatively complicated procedure. In addition, each laboratory must establish its own normal range, and the time and effort required for each individual test frequently has led to the establishment of normal limits based on an inadequate number of subjects. With the advent of new radiologic techniques, the popularity of this test has waned and accurate measurements of pancreatic secretion are obtained at a relatively limited number of centers.

A wide variety of pancreatic juice components have been assessed under a bewildering array of stimulatory techniques in an attempt to find the most sensitive and specific indicator of chronic pancreatitis. Some of the secretory components that have been measured include the concentration or output of bicarbonate, amylase, lipase, and trypsin. Although claims have been made for the superiority of one of these measurements over another, comparative studies suggest all of them tend to be equally depressed in chronic pancreatitis and there is no clear-cut advantage of one measurement over another. Similarly, none of these measurements appears to be able to differentiate chronic pancreatitis from carcinoma of the pancreas. Collection of pure pancreatic juice by way of cannulation of the ampulla of Vater during ERCP apparently adds little to the accuracy of the test.[116]

Stimulation of pancreatic secretion has been produced over a wide range of doses and dosing schedules using secretin,[117] CCK,[118] cerulein,[119] and bombesin,[120] singly or in combination. Although it is difficult to compare the results of different studies, there appears to be no clear-cut advantage of one stimulatory technique over another. The relative value of direct stimulation of the pancreas with secretin-CCK versus indirect stimulation by Lundh's meal also is somewhat controversial, although most comparative studies suggest that direct stimulation is superior.[121,122]

For many years, the finding of a subnormal pancreatic secretion of enzymes or bicarbonate in aspirated duodenal contents was considered to be the most sensitive test for chronic pancreatitis, and, if pancreatic carcinoma could be excluded, a low secretion was assumed to be diagnostic of chronic pancreatitis. As noted, however, pathologic confirmation of early pancreatitis was seldom obtained in these studies. With the development of new radiologic procedures, particularly ERCP, it has become apparent that pancreatic secretion may be normal in a sizable fraction of patients with radiologic evidence of chronic pancreatitis.[123,124] Values for the sensitivity of the test range from 70% to 95%[125–127] depending on the patient population studied and the number of analyses performed on the pancreatic juice. If multiple components of pancreatic secretion are assessed, sensitivity for chronic pancreatitis increases but specificity decreases.[119] Patients with a variety of conditions, including diabetes mellitus,[104] hepatic cirrhosis,[106] Billroth II gastrectomy,[128] and celiac sprue,[105] may have diminished pancreatic secretory output with no clinical or radiologic evidence of chronic pancreatitis.

Indirect tests of pancreatic exocrine secretion. The complexity and patient discomfort involved in the direct measurement of pancreatic secretory capacity have led to a variety of simpler tests that indirectly assess the secretion of pancreatic enzymes. Most of these tests measure the absorption of some compound that first requires digestion by pancreatic enzymes. Because clinically detectable malabsorption of nutrients does not occur until pancreatic enzyme secretion has diminished to less than 10% of normal, it is axiomatic that indirect tests of pancreatic function will not be able to detect early chronic pancreatitis and, thus, will have very poor sensitivity.

The chronologic history of virtually all indirect tests of pancreatic function has taken the following pattern. The newly developed test is applied to patients with end-stage chronic pancreatitis and to otherwise healthy controls, and is found to have excellent sensitivity and specificity for the diagnosis of chronic pancreatitis. Subsequent investigators use the test in patients with less severe chronic pancreatitis and with conditions that might simulate chronic pancreatitis (i.e., malabsorption states) and find that the sensitivity and specificity are much less than advertised. Although the sensitivity of the tests cannot be improved, a variety of modifications have been developed to enhance specificity. The end result is a somewhat complex test that has little, if any, clinical utility.

The bentiromide test involves ingestion of *N*-benzoyl-L-tyrosyl-*p*- aminobenzoic acid (NBT), a tripeptide that is digested by chymotrypsin with the release of paraaminobenzoic acid (PABA).[129,130] Free PABA is absorbed in the small bowel and excreted by the kidney; the quantity excreted in urine is used as a measure of pancreatic exocrine function. As seems to be the case with virtually every pancreatic function study, innumerable variations of the basic test (i.e., dosage alterations, length of urine collection, various forms of stimulation of pancreatic secretion) have been evaluated in an attempt to improve specificity, without appreciable success.

The sensitivity of the bentiromide test varies with the extent of damage to the exocrine pancreas, with sensitivity as high as 100%[131] reported with very severe disease and as low as 40% to 50% with minor damage.[132,133] The specificity of this test is far from perfect. Reduced PABA excretion has been reported to occur commonly in diabetes mellitus,[134] renal insufficiency,[135] liver diseases,[135] and for malabsorption states other than pancreatic insufficiency, including celiac sprue,[136] Crohn's disease,[137] and postgastrectomy states.[135] The low excretion in malabsorptive states other than pancreatic insufficiency apparently results from failure to absorb the free PABA that has been split from the parent compound. These conditions can be separated from pancreatic insufficiency by testing the patient's ability to absorb free PABA in a subsequent test[131] or by simultaneously administering free [14C]PABA along with NBT-PABA and measuring the urinary excretion of the labeled and unlabeled PABA.[138]

Because sensitivity of the NBT-PABA test is limited, the results of this measurement are helpful primarily when the test is positive (and other forms of malabsorption have been excluded). Thus, it appears that the major role of this test is not in diagnosis of chronic pancreatitis but rather in determining the extent of the pancreatic insufficiency present in patients with known chronic pancreatitis.

The demonstration that vitamin B_{12} is malabsorbed in patients with pancreatic insufficiency owing to their inability to degrade R protein[139] provided the rationale for a test for chronic pancreatitis. In this test, the subject ingests both

[57Co]cobalamin bound to intrinsic factor and [58Co]cobalamin bound to R protein, plus excess intrinsic factor and a cobalamin analog that saturates all empty R protein binding sites.[140] Theoretically, the patient with pancreatic insufficiency should absorb the cobalamin bound to intrinsic factor much more efficiently than that bound to R protein. All other subjects should absorb both forms of cobalamin equally. Although the initial paper describing this technique reported excellent sensitivity and specificity for chronic pancreatitis, a subsequent paper found very poor sensitivity.[141]

The diagnosis of pancreatic insufficiency by way of measurements of fecal chymotrypsin was first described 40 years ago,[142] and a number of subsequent reports have evaluated the sensitivity and specificity of various modifications of the initial technique. The major advantage of this method is that it is rapid and simple. The far more cumbersome measurement of total fecal chymotrypsin output in timed fecal collections appears to offer little advantage over the much simpler measurement of chymotrypsin concentration in a random fecal sample.[142] Reports of sensitivity of the test range from 45%[143] to 100%,[144] depending on the extent of pancreatic damage in the study population. Specificity ranges from 49%[145] to 90%,[146] with false- positive results reported for malabsorptive conditions such as celiac sprue, damage secondary to Crohn's disease, and postgastrectomy states.[146,147]

Patients with appreciable chronic pancreatitis malabsorb fat when ingested in the form of triglyceride, and a number of indirect tests have been developed to assess such malabsorption. Most of these tests involve the feeding of [14C]olein. Hydrolysis of the triglyceride and absorption of [14C]oleate lead to the production and pulmonary excretion of $^{14}CO_2$. Measurement of breath $^{14}CO_2$ excretion can be used as a simple measure of the normality of the hydrolysis of the labeled triglyceride.[148] Unfortunately, the test is negative in a high percentage of patients with early chronic pancreatitis, and false-positive results are observed in many malabsorption states other than chronic pancreatitis.[149] A number of modifications of the basic test have been devised in an attempt to differentiate between the low $^{14}CO_2$ excretion observed in chronic pancreatitis and that of other conditions. Some of these modifications include repetition of the test with orally administered pancreatic enzymes,[149] subsequent testing with [14C]oleate, or simultaneous administration of [14C]olein and [3H]oleate.[150] In the latter test, the relative absorption rates of the two forms of labeled oleate are assessed by measuring [14C] and [3H] concentrations in serum several hours after ingestion of the labeled lipids. In theory, the oleate in the triglyceride should be absorbed more slowly than the free oleate in patients with pancreatic insufficiency, whereas absorption of the two oleates should be similar in other forms of malabsorption.

Imaging studies. The demonstration of diffuse, speckled calcification of the pancreas on a plain film of the abdomen is diagnostic of chronic pancreatitis. Although the sensitivity of this finding is limited (perhaps 30%–40%), a plain film of the abdomen should be the first diagnostic test used when attempting to establish the diagnosis of chronic pancreatitis because a positive finding obviates the need for additional testing.

The development over the past 15 years of ultrasound,

computed tomography (CT), and ERCP has made it possible to assess routinely the gross structure of the pancreas. These tests all have excellent specificity and reasonably good sensitivity. Of major importance is the ability of these imaging procedures to differentiate between carcinoma of the pancreas and chronic pancreatitis. As a result, imaging techniques have largely supplanted tests of pancreatic function in the work-up of the patient with possible chronic pancreatitis.

Ultrasound is the simplest and least expensive of the three imaging techniques. Findings on ultrasound that correlate with marked pancreatic changes on ERCP include dilation of the main pancreatic duct to greater than 4 mm, large (>1 cm) cavities, and calcifications.[151] Findings associated with less severe changes on ERCP include dilation of the duct up to, but not exceeding 4 mm, small cavities, reduction in echogenicity or echogenic foci in the parenchyma, and an irregular contour to the gland.[151] When a satisfactory ultrasound examination is obtained, the reported sensitivity of this test for chronic pancreatitis is of the order of 70% and the specificity is quite high, roughly 90%.[152-155] The finding of chronic pancreatitis on ultrasound usually requires no additional confirmatory testing.

CT is 10% to 20% more sensitive than ultrasound for the diagnosis of chronic pancreatitis[154-156]; these two techniques have roughly comparable specificity. CT is more expensive than ultrasonography and involves exposure to ionizing radiation. Therefore, in the work-up for chronic pancreatitis, CT usually should be limited to patients who have negative or unsatisfactory ultrasound examinations. The most common diagnostic findings of chronic pancreatitis on CT include duct dilation, calcifications, and cystic lesions.[157-159] Less common diagnostic findings include enlargement or atrophy of the pancreas and heterogeneous density of the parenchyma. This imaging technique is particularly helpful in the differentiation of chronic pancreatitis from carcinoma of the pancreas. The dilated duct system resulting from carcinoma tends to be smooth or beaded, in contrast to the irregular, calcified ducts that are typical of chronic pancreatitis. The sensitivity of CT

for the diagnosis of chronic pancreatitis is in the neighborhood of 80%, whereas the specificity is roughly 90%.[154,160,161] In addition to ultrasound and CT, magnetic resonance imaging has been used more recently to evaluate pancreatic structure. This technique may show abnormalities in chronic pancreatitis, but it appears to have limited value in the diagnostic work-up of patients with pancreatic disease.[162]

ERCP commonly is considered to be the most sensitive and specific test available for the diagnosis of chronic pancreatitis, and this technique has become the gold standard against which all other tests are evaluated. In the absence of histologic confirmation of disease in most patients, it is difficult to speak with complete certainty about the diagnostic accuracy of ERCP (because ERCP is the gold standard). Most authorities, however, believe that the sensitivity and specificity of ERCP approach 90% and 100%, respectively.[161,163,164]

The most commonly used classification of ERCP changes in chronic pancreatitis was developed by Kasugai and associates.[165] In minimal pancreatitis, the changes are limited to the branches and fine ducts, which show dilation and irregularity (Fig. 91-3). There is considerable observer variation in the detection of these minor changes, and differentiation of normal from abnormal is not always clear. Because minor ductal dilation and intraductal calculi may be observed in healthy elderly subjects, it may be difficult to differentiate early chronic pancreatitis from normal senile changes.[166] Moderate pancreatitis is characterized by the additional finding of dilation, tortuosity, and stenosis of the main pancreatic duct (Fig. 91-4). Advanced pancreatitis has the additional findings of cyst formation and contraction of the pancreas (Fig. 91-5). Pancreatic carcinoma usually can be readily distinguished from chronic pancreatitis in that there is a single strictured region in malignant obstruction, in contrast to the multiple stenoses, irregular branching ducts, and intraductular calculi observed in chronic pancreatitis.

In general, there is a good correlation between the changes observed on ERCP and measurements of pancreatic secretory capacity. An occasional patient, however, may have markedly

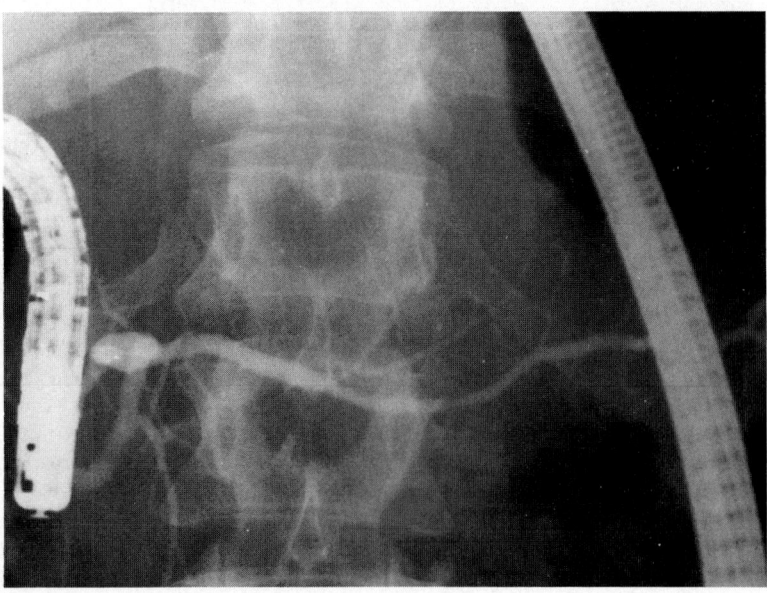

FIGURE 91-3. ERCP study shows minimal changes consistent with chronic pancreatitis. The main duct is slightly irregular, and the branches are slightly dilated. These findings are not diagnostic.

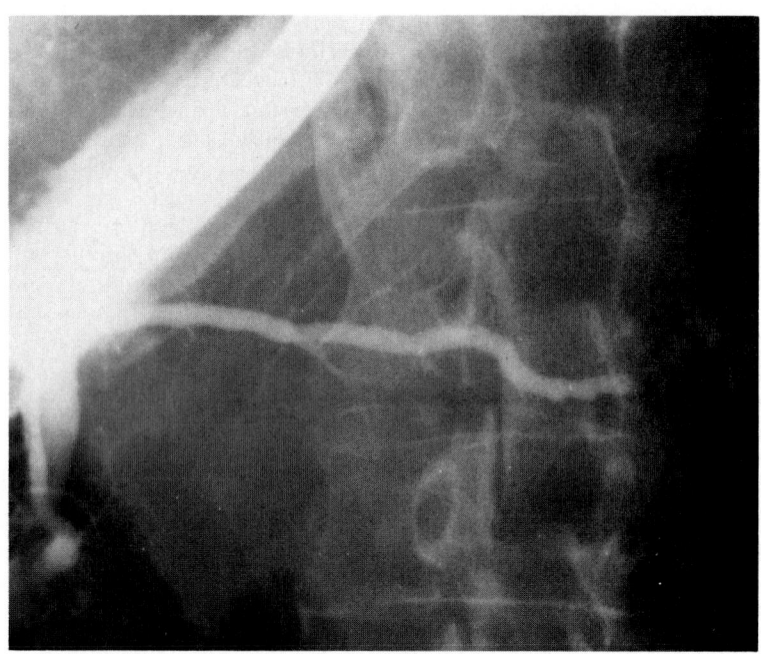

FIGURE 91-4. ERCP study shows changes of moderate pancreatitis. The main duct is irregular and dilated, and there is a pseudocyst in the tail of the pancreas.

diminished secretory function with seemingly minor changes on ERCP. Patients with minor abnormalities on ERCP often have normal secretory function.

Because ERCP is an expensive procedure and has a low, but not insignificant, rate of associated complications, this test ordinarily should be reserved for the rare patient with chronic pancreatitis in whom the diagnosis cannot be clearly established by way of other imaging techniques.

Although chronic pancreatitis and carcinoma of the pancreas usually can be reliably distinguished based on imaging studies, in an occasional patient, this differentiation may be difficult.[167,168] Attempts to use serum or pancreatic juice tumor markers, such as CA19-9, to differentiate benign from malignant pancreatic processes have not been very impressive,[168] and it is usually necessary to make a tissue diagnosis. Although laparotomy with open biopsy was required in the past, percutaneous fine-needle aspiration biopsy now makes it possible to obtain a histologic diagnosis in a very high percentage of patients with pancreatic carcinoma. Under CT or ultrasonographic guidance, a small-gauge needle is inserted into the pancreatic mass and aspirated material is examined for the presence of malignant cells. The reported specificity of this test approaches 100%, and the sensitivity is 80% to 90%.[169]

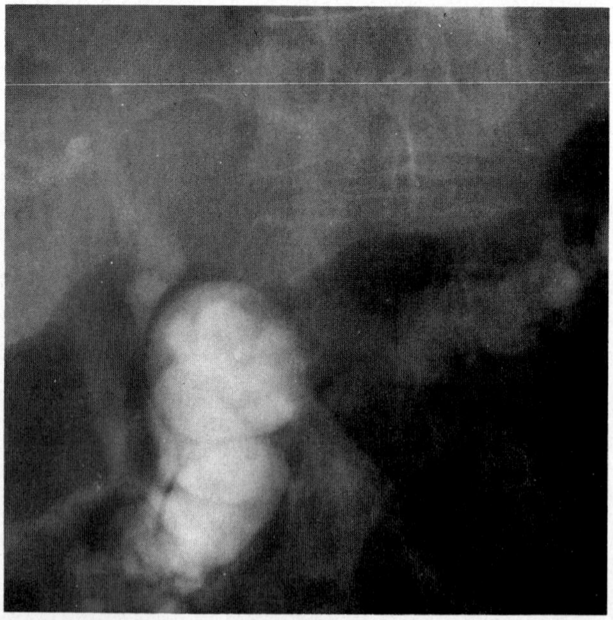

Rational Use of Tests in the Diagnosis of Chronic Pancreatitis

The evaluation should begin with a plain film of the abdomen. The finding of pancreatic calcification is virtually diagnostic of chronic pancreatitis, and no further testing is required. If calcifications are not present, the next test should be ultrasound. Once again, if this test demonstrates findings indicative of chronic pancreatitis, further procedures are not necessary. If the ultrasound examination is nondiagnostic, CT is indicated only if there is a high degree of clinical suspicion of chronic pancreatitis. Only a small percentage of patients with chronic pancreatitis have negative ultrasound and CT findings. Thus, ERCP should be reserved for those patients in whom the diagnosis of chronic pancreatitis is thought to be very likely on clinical grounds or for patients in whom ultrasound, CT, or fine-needle biopsy have not been able to differentiate between carcinoma of the pancreas and chronic pancreatitis. The tendency to perform the gamut of imaging procedures on every patient with abdominal pain in an attempt to diagnose chronic pancreatitis should be avoided. In most patients, a negative ultrasound examination, although not 100% accurate, is sufficient to exclude tentatively the diagnosis of chronic pancreatitis. Tests that either directly or indirectly

FIGURE 91-5. ERCP study shows changes of advanced chronic pancreatitis. There are massive cystic dilatations of the main duct and its branches.

assess the functional capacity of the pancreas appear to have little utility in the evaluation of chronic pancreatitis.

COMPLICATIONS

Pseudocyst

A pseudocyst is a collection of pancreatic juice outside the normal boundaries of the ductal system that is enclosed by a fibrous tissue membrane. It is the most common complication of chronic pancreatitis, occurring in up to 25% of cases in some series.[170] Most chronic pseudocysts occur in patients with chronic alcoholic pancreatitis,[171] and they are found more commonly in the body of the pancreas than in the head or tail.[171]

Little is known about the mechanism responsible for the initial formation of pancreatic pseudocysts. They probably result from rupture of a pancreatic duct, activation of interstitial pancreatic juices, necrosis of the surrounding parenchyma, escape of the pancreatic juice into the lesser sac, and reaction of local mesothelial cells to wall off the collection by a fibrous membrane. Once initiated, expansion of the embryonic pseudocyst continues until the surrounding tissue pressure equals pancreatic secretory pressure, which is usually elevated in chronic obstructive pancreatitis. Although not conclusively demonstrated, some evidence exists to suggest that pancreatic juice contained within a pseudocyst can exchange with plasma. If so, this may represent a mechanism responsible for resorption of immature pseudocysts and spontaneous resolution of chronic pseudocysts.

Pain is the major symptom of pancreatic pseudocyst. Pseudocyst should be suspected in a patient with stable chronic pancreatitis who experiences worsening of abdominal pain. Abdominal ultrasonography is most frequently used in the diagnosis and management of pseudocysts. It is best used as a serial monitor of pseudocyst size in those patients in whom definitive drainage is delayed. CT has emerged as the single most accurate method of diagnosing pancreatic pseudocyst.[172] In addition to its high accuracy rate, it is capable of providing structural details such as the size of the common duct or pancreatic duct. This has important bearing on the choice of an operative approach. In the presence of dilation of either or both the common bile duct and pancreatic duct, drainage of the pseudocyst alone is rarely sufficient.[173] Although some surgeons have advocated ERCP for all patients with pseudocysts,[174,175] others have not found routine preoperative pancreatography desirable for fear of secondary infection, which may occur in up to 25% of cases.[175] It is generally agreed, however, that patients with suspected concomitant common duct obstruction should undergo ERCP before surgical drainage.

In contrast to acute pseudocysts, chronic pseudocysts, especially those larger than 6 cm, almost never resolve spontaneously.[176,177] On the other hand, they also do not carry the same risk of serious complications as acute pseudocysts. In a study involving 75 patients with chronic pancreatitis and pseudocyst, approximately half of the patients could be managed conservatively.[178] Only one pseudocyst-related complication occurred in this group, and there was no mortality. According to this study, indications for operative management include persistent abdominal pain, enlargement, or complications of pseudocyst.

Effective treatment of pseudocyst include excision and internal or external drainage. Surgical excision provides definitive treatment and is feasible when the cyst is localized to the tail of the pancreas. In most cases, however, internal drainage is the treatment of choice. Pseudocysts that are more than 6 weeks old usually have a mature cyst wall that permits internal drainage, where the cyst is anastomosed to the stomach (cystogastrostomy), duodenum (cystoduodenostomy), or jejunum (cystojejunostomy). The fluid in the pseudocyst drains into the gastrointestinal tract and the cyst cavity collapses and becomes obliterated, usually within 1 week. There also have been reports of endoscopic drainage for the treatment of pseudocyst in chronic pancreatitis.[179,180] A pseudocyst that indents the stomach or duodenum can be punctured transendoscopically using electrocautery or lasers to create a fistulous tract between the pseudocyst and the stomach or duodenum. Cremer and colleagues reported a success rate of 96% for endoscopic cystoduodenostomy and 100% for endoscopic cystogastrostomy in 33 patients with chronic pancreatitis.[179] No significant complications were observed after successful endoscopic cystoduodenostomy, and the two complications of endoscopic cystogastrostomy were gastric hemorrhage and iatrogenic pseudocyst infection. To decrease the risks of bleeding and perforation, the use of endosonography-guided drainage of pancreatic pseudocyst has been reported.[181] Potentially, the precise sonographic definition of the cyst and local anatomy at the time of endoscopic drainage may improve the safety of endoscopic drainage. The results, however, are too preliminary for adequate evaluation.

External drainage usually is used for patients with infected pseudocysts or those in whom the wall of the pseudocysts is not mature enough to hold sutures. Drainage is achieved by surgical placement of a large catheter in the pseudocyst, and the fluid drains externally through the abdominal wall. This form of treatment usually is safe, but is associated with a higher recurrence rate compared to internal drainage.[182]

CT-guided percutaneous transabdominal catheter drainage of chronic pseudocysts has gained popularity and is considered by some as a preferred alternative to surgical treatment in the management of pancreatic pseudocysts. Van Sonnenberg and colleagues reported a 90% success rate in the percutaneous drainage of 101 pancreatic pseudocysts.[183] The mean duration of drainage was 20 days. There was no mortality, and the only major complication was superinfection in four cases. Adams and Anderson, in a retrospective study, also found that percutaneous catheter drainage was as effective as internal drainage in the management of pseudocyst, although drain tract infection was as high as 48%.[184] In a long-term retrospective study of 42 patients undergoing percutaneous catheter drainage, however, Criado and associates reported that in 9 patients the pseudocysts failed to resolve, and 7 recurred after initial resolution.[185] Hence, the effectiveness of percutaneous drainage in the management of pseudocysts remains to be established.

Somatostatin is a potent inhibitor of pancreatic secretion, and therefore may be useful in the treatment of pancreatic pseudocyst. Gullo and associates reported that 2 weeks' treatment with octreotide, a long-acting somatostatin analog, resulted in a 42% reduction in size of the pseudocysts in 4 of

7 patients.[186] In addition, octreotide also appears to be effective in decreasing persistent catheter drainage from chronic pseudocyst.[187,188] Therefore, patients with pancreatic pseudocyst resistant to drainage should be offered a course of octreotide before surgery is contemplated.

Pancreatic Ascites

The incidence of pancreatic ascites in chronic pancreatitis is usually considered to be less than 1%. It occurs as a consequence of persistent leakage of pancreatic juice from a pseudocyst or the pancreatic duct. Fifteen percent of patients with a pseudocyst may have pancreatic ascites.[189] On the other hand, 60% of patients with pancreatic ascites have pseudocysts.[190,191] Pancreatic ascites occurs typically in alcoholic patients with cirrhosis, who may complain of mild to moderate abdominal pain because of distention. The diagnosis is often erroneously attributed to decompensated cirrhosis; however, paracenteses reveals elevation of pancreatic enzyme levels and a high total protein or albumin level. These findings are diagnostic.

Most patients need surgery. A period of 2 to 3 weeks of observation and medical treatment is warranted. During this period, the patients are given nothing (orally) and placed on parenteral nutrition to improve their nutritional status. Suppression of pancreatic secretion by agents such as octreotide may be tried (100–250 μg subcutaneously every 4 hours). With this regimen, the ascites may resolve spontaneously in up to one third of patients, and surgery can be avoided. For patients who require an operation, ERCP should be performed to identify the precise site of the leak.

Pancreatic Fistula

External pancreatic fistula as a complication of chronic pancreatitis is rare. It occurs most commonly after operative or percutaneous drainage of a pseudocyst. It also may follow pancreatic biopsy or arise from a leaky pancreatic anastomosis. Clinically, pancreatic fistula should be suspected when clear fluid drains from a cutaneous orifice, and the diagnosis is confirmed when the amylase content of the fluid is found to be elevated. Treatment is conservative and consists of fluid and electrolyte replacement, nutritional support, and eradication of infection if present. Somatostatin, which suppresses pancreatic secretion and decreases the volume of fistula drainage, may be used. During the course of therapy, a fistulogram should be obtained when the tract is well formed. If there is ductal obstruction between the site of the leak and the duodenum, surgical repair may be necessary. Most of the fistulas, however, close spontaneously.

Splenic Vein Thrombosis

Splenic vein thrombosis with extrahepatic portal hypertension is a well known complication of chronic pancreatitis.[192] Because the splenic vein courses along the posterior surface of the pancreas, thrombosis may occur as a result of peripancreatic inflammation associated with acute attacks or with pseudocyst formation and extension. Rosch and Herfort[193] found occlusion of the splenic vein in approximately 4% of cases of chronic pancreatitis studied with splenoportography. Almost all patients had some impingement on the splenic vein. Varices involving the esophagus, stomach, duodenum, and colon have been described with resultant hemorrhage. Accurate diagnosis is important, because splenectomy is curative and portosystemic shunting is not required.[193] This entity should be suspected in any patient with varices, particularly gastric varices without esophageal varices, and a history of pancreatitis. Acute thrombosis may be associated with acute splenic enlargement and may suggest the diagnosis. Celiac angiography with careful venous phase radiographs may demonstrate the varices and the absence of the splenic vein.

TREATMENT

Treatment of chronic pancreatitis is mainly aimed at the control of pain and the correction of malabsorption with adequate pancreatic enzyme replacement.

Control of Pain

Avoidance of Alcohol

A long-held clinical aphorism is that avoiding alcohol ingestion decreases the frequency and severity of abdominal pain in chronic alcoholic pancreatitis. Trapnell reported that 75% of his patients with chronic alcoholic pancreatitis experienced pain relief when they stopped drinking.[194] This observation may be explained by the stimulatory effect of alcohol on pancreatic secretion.[195] The relationship between alcohol and pain in chronic pancreatitis, however, is controversial. Bornman and colleagues[195] noted that half of their patients with painful pancreatitis and half of their patients with painless pancreatitis continued to drink. Similar observations were made by Marks and associates.[196] These findings call into question whether continued alcohol ingestion is related to pain. It is conceivable that pancreatic pain is related to exocrine pancreatic secretion. In patients who maintain significant exocrine secretory function, pain may be provoked by alcohol, which acts as a secretagogue. In patients whose exocrine secretion is drastically reduced, alcohol no longer plays a role in the mechanism of pain. Further studies are needed to clarify the role of alcohol in pain production.

Analgesics

Analgesics remain the main method for pain control in chronic pancreatitis. Initially, nonnarcotic analgesics, such as salicylates or acetaminophen, should be used. Preferably, these analgesics should be given before meals to prevent postprandial exacerbation of pain. Drug doses should be individualized, and the lowest effective dose should be used. As the severity of pain increases, the dose strength or frequency of these simpler analgesics should be increased before switching to narcotics. In severe cases, however, opiate analgesics are required, and they should not be withheld for fear of narcotic addiction.

Celiac Plexus Block

Percutaneous radiologically or sonographically guided celiac ganglion alcohol injection has been used for control of pancreatic pain. This technique has been helpful in patients who have severe pancreatic pain secondary to pancreatic cancer.[197,198] In small, uncontrolled series of patients with chronic pancreatitis with debilitating pain, this procedure has produced mixed results. The occasional benefits almost never last for more than a few months,[199] and repeated treatment may not be as effective.

Enzyme Therapy

Much interest has been generated by a series of observations suggesting that the intralumenal action of pancreatic proteases plays an important role in regulating pancreatic enzyme secretion. The underlying concept of feedback regulation of the pancreas is based primarily on studies in rats that showed that diversion of pancreatic juice from the duodenum stimulates CCK release and pancreatic enzyme secretion.[200,201] On the other hand, intraduodenal administration of trypsin or chymotrypsin inhibits the release of CCK and pancreatic enzyme secretion. This protease-sensitive feedback mechanism was first reported to occur in humans in 1977.[202] Subsequently, several groups of investigators confirmed that intestinal administration of trypsin or chymotrypsin inhibits pancreatic enzyme secretion.[202-206] Thus, it is conceivable that in patients with chronic pancreatitis, decreased enzyme secretion may result in the hyperstimulation of the pancreas by elevated plasma CCK levels, with resultant pain. Some,[207-209] but not all[210,211] studies reported elevated plasma CCK levels in patients with chronic pancreatitis. It has been proposed that effective enzyme replacement therapy should reduce pancreatic stimulation, decrease intraductal pressure, and diminish pain. This hypothesis was tested in several clinical studies. In a double-blinded, crossover study, Isaksson and Ihse[212] reported pain relief in 15 of 19 patients with chronic pancreatitis. There was a 30% reduction in pain intensity and a significant decrease in the frequency of pain attacks in patients on active enzymes. Slaff and colleagues[203] studied 20 patients with painful chronic pancreatitis in a double-blinded, crossover study. Pain reduction was observed in 9 patients with mild to moderate pancreatic insufficiency, whereas only 2 of 11 with severe insufficiency responded to the treatment with enzyme replacement. Most of the "good" responders were women with idiopathic chronic pancreatitis, whereas most of the "poor" responders were men with alcohol-induced chronic pancreatitis. Favorable response was also reported by Ramo and associates,[213] who showed significant pain relief after self-administration (ad libitum) of an enzyme preparation, compared to administration of the regular dose in 10 patients with painful chronic pancreatitis. These three double-blinded studies[203,212,213] demonstrated good results by enzyme treatment in 73% (36 of 49) of the patients evaluated. A double blinded, 4-week crossover study from Denmark, however, showed that oral administration of two capsules of Pancrease with each meal did not significantly control pain compared to placebo.[214] Non–enteric-coated preparations, however, were used in the three studies that showed good results, whereas an enteric-coated preparation was used in the Danish study. Thus, it appears that non–enteric-coated preparations are more effective than enteric-coated ones. This may be because enteric-coated preparations usually deliver the enzymes to sites distal to the duodenum, where feedback inhibition of pancreatic secretion by proteases occurs.[215]

Endoscopic Therapy

Endoscopic therapy has been used for control of pain in chronic pancreatitis, with the aim of alleviating obstruction of flow caused by ductal strictures, stones, or papillary stenosis. Ductal strictures are sometimes treated by balloons or dilating catheters, but in most cases dilation is followed by stent placement across the stricture. Technical success in reported studies ranges from 70% to 100%, and pain improvement occurs in 55% to 100% of patients during a follow-up of 2 to 69 months.[216-220] In several, the stents were removed because of frequent clogging after 4 to 6 months. In addition, aggravation or ductographic changes may develop during the stent treatment.[221,222] These usually are mild and reversible in most patients.

Endoscopic techniques also have been used for the removal of pancreatic stones in chronic pancreatitis. In different series, pancreatic duct stones were removed after endoscopic sphincterotomy in 27% to 100% of patients.[218,220,223,224] In some cases, stone removal was facilitated by fragmentation with extracorporeal shock wave lithotripsy, with clinical improvement observed in 50% to 80% of cases in which the stones were successfully removed.[218,224] Inherent in these various therapies is the belief that stones are themselves causing symptoms by intensifying obstruction and that their removal will improve pancreatic flow and thereby reduce symptoms. On the other hand, it is also possible that pancreatic stones form as a result of pancreatic stricture and abnormal pancreatic juice protein, and have little to do with pain. None of the studies on endoscopic treatment of chronic pancreatitis is controlled, and no valid comparisons have been made among medical, surgical, and endoscopic treatments. These procedures should therefore be considered experimental and performed only in patients entered into prospective, randomized trials.

In one study, minor papilla endoscopic sphincterotomy was performed in 52 patients with pancreas divisum who had either chronic abdominal pain, acute recurrent pancreatitis, or chronic pancreatitis.[225] Among the three groups of patients, only those with acute recurrent pancreatitis benefited from the endoscopic procedure. This suggests that minor papilla sphincterotomy should be avoided in patients with pancreatic divisum and chronic pancreatitis.

Surgical Treatment

After all medical measures have failed to relieve pain, surgery should be considered. The type of surgery is selected according to the perceived mechanism for the pain. When the main pancreatic duct is dilated, it is assumed that there is pancreatic duct obstruction and that pancreatic duct hypertension is the cause of pain. On the other hand, if there is no ductal dilation, pain may result from diffuse parenchymal disease or blockage of small side ducts by stones, protein plugs, or scars. Relief of major duct obstruction should not affect this type of pain.

Therefore, the type of surgery should be chosen according to the severity of pain, ductal morphology, and the extent of parenchymal disease. Patients who have ductal dilation have a 70% to 80% chance of obtaining pain relief with either a partial resection with pancreaticojejunostomy or lateral pancreaticojejunostomy (modified Puestow's procedure).[196,197] The modified Puestow's pancreaticojejunostomy is particularly suitable for patients who have ductal obstruction and dilation. It is a safe and effective operation, with a morbidity of less than 5%, mortality less than 2%, and effective pain relief on the order of 80%.[226,227] On the other hand, for patients with moderate to severe parenchymal disease and no ductal dilation, partial pancreatic resection should be considered. Ninety-five percent distal resection is recommended for patients with diffuse parenchymal disease,[196] whereas local resection of major site of involvement may be sufficient for those with regional parenchymal disease.[196] Overall, 50% of these patients have had satisfactory results.

In patients undergoing a near-total pancreatectomy, islet cell autotransplantation by infusion of islet cell preparations into the portal system may prevent diabetes.[228–230] Islets from the resected pancreas can be isolated by mechanical disruption and collagenase digestion of the dispersed tissue, and injected into the portal vein. Using this method, Farney and colleagues reported that 9 of 22 patients with intraportal islet autografts were insulin independent for at least several months after surgery.[230] This method appears promising, although the major limitation is related to the availability of islets in the fibrotic glands. It is hoped that improved islet isolation procedures will improve results.

Summary of Treatment Approach for Control of Pain

We recommend the following approach to treat pain of chronic pancreatitis: When a patient first presents with pain or shows a different pain pattern, we determine if there is an anatomic reason for the occurrence of or a change in pain. The occurrence of pseudocyst, phlegmon, obstruction, and peptic ulcer is ruled out by appropriate tests. Patients are advised to stop all alcohol ingestion and to use salicylate or acetaminophen as needed. We also recommend the use of enzyme (e.g., eight tablets of Viokase with each meal), especially in patients with non–alcohol-induced chronic pancreatitis. If pain continues, narcotics may be needed. After all medical measures have failed, we recommend surgery; some centers, however, may consider celiac plexus block before surgery.

Management of Pancreatic Insufficiency

At first glance, treating malabsorption secondary to pancreatic insufficiency might appear to be relatively easy. It would seem that simple oral replacement of pancreatic enzymes would be efficacious. Unfortunately, complete correction of steatorrhea is rarely accomplished. This is related to insufficient amounts of enzyme in oral supplements and acid pepsin inactivation of pancreatic enzymes.

The maximal postprandial delivery of pancreatic lipase is approximately 140,000 IU/hour for 4 hours after meals.[83]

It has been shown that malabsorption does not occur if more than 5% of the normal maximal enzyme output is delivered to the duodenum. To meet this requirement, 28,000 IU of lipase should be delivered during a 4-hour postprandial period. Pancreatic supplements are highly variable in enzyme activity, with lipase content ranging from 0 to 8000 IU per tablet.[100,231,232] Therefore, if the clinician uses a commercially available preparation containing 3500 IU per tablet of lipase, then under the best of circumstances at least eight tablets or capsules must be taken per meal to abolish malabsorption. Smaller amounts of enzymes may reduce steatorrhea but not abolish it. Therefore, the clinician should choose those commercial enzyme preparations that have been shown to contain higher lipase activity, and ensure that sufficient amounts have been used (Table 91-3).

Another important factor to consider is acid pepsin inactivation of pancreatic enzymes. When duodenal samples were examined for lipase and trypsin activity, less than 8% of ingested lipase and less than 22% of ingested trypsin was recovered, regardless of the dosing schedule used (either prandial or hourly dosing). To eliminate steatorrhea in pancreatic insufficiency, a large number of tablets is necessary. Hyperuricosuria[233] and kidney stones have been associated with such high dosing of pancreatic supplements secondary to their high purine content, and therefore this high dosing schedule may not be clinically justified. The relatively low delivery of lipase into the proximal small bowel compared to the delivery of trypsin with routine treatment schedules may explain the relative impossibility of completely correcting steatorrhea in pancreatic insufficiency, as well as the usual correction of azotorrhea.

Preventing acid peptic neutralization of enzyme supplements by coating capsules with acid-resistant and alkali-sensitive materials or by using antacids has produced mixed results.[234,235] In most studies, there has been little success with oral antacids or enteric coating with regard to clinical improvement or alleviating steatorrhea. Antacids increase gastric secretion, and dilution of enzyme concentrations below critical levels may explain the relative ineffectiveness of antacids.[235] Enteric coating is effective only if pancreatic enzymes are delivered into the duodenum with ingested food from the stomach and adequate intraduodenal dissolution occurs. Because emptying of large tablets from the stomach may be different from that of typical antral contents, and duodenal and gastric pH have been shown to be low (<4) for prolonged times in many patients with pancreatic insufficiency,[236,237] enteric coating may not be an effective improvement over oral pancreatic supplements alone.

Pancrease (pancreatin coated with a pH-dependent polymer) is another improvement in pancreatic enzyme supplements.[238] Because this supplement is stable at an acidic pH (<4) and dissolves at a pH greater than 5, it is most effective (i.e., better than standard tablets alone) in patients who maintain acidic pH levels in the stomach postprandially. This maneuver delivers pancreatic enzymes to the upper small bowel intact, whereas standard supplements are irreversibly inactivated. In several studies, the mean reduction of steatorrhea with the use of Pancrease is not better than that with Viokase given with meals.[235,239] Normally, in chronic pancreatitis, the gastric pH increases to above 5 in the early postprandial period and then decreases to less than 4. It is likely

TABLE 91-3
Commercial Pancreatic Enzyme Preparations

PREPARATION	TYPE	CONTENT (Units)		
		Lipase	Amylase	Protease
Cotazyme	C	8000	30,000	30,000
Cotazyme-S	ECMS	5000	20,000	20,000
Creon 10	ECMS	10,000	33,200	37,500
Creon 25	ECMS	25,000	74,700	62,500
Ilozyme	UCT	11,000	30,000	30,000
Ku-zyme HP	ECMS	8000	30,000	30,000
Pancrease	ECMS	4000	20,000	25,000
Pancrease MT-4	ECMT	4000	12,000	12,000
Pancrease MT-10	ECMT	10,000	30,000	30,000
Pancrease MT-16	ECMT	16,000	48,000	48,000
Protilase	ECMS	4000	20,000	25,000
Viokase	UCT	8000	30,000	30,000
Viokase	P	16,800	70,000	70,000
Zymase	ECMS	12,000	24,000	24,000

C, capsule; ECMS, enteric-coated microspheres encased in a cellulose capsule; ECMT, enteric-coated microtablets encased in a cellulose capsule; UCT, uncoated tablet; P, powder.

Adapted from Berardi RR, Dunn-Kucharski VA. Pancreatitis and cholelithiasis. In: DiPiro JT, Talbert RL, Hayes PE, et al, eds. Pharmacotherapy: a pathophysiologic approach. Norwalk, CT: Appleton & Lange, 1993:614.

that, under these circumstances, pancreatin initially will be liberated from its enteric coat, but its enzyme activity will be irreversibly inactivated when the intragastric pH falls to less than 4. Conversely, if gastric and duodenal pH remain low (<4) throughout the postprandial period, the enteric coat of Pancrease remains intact as it traverses the upper gastrointestinal tract, and pancreatin is liberated en masse only as it reaches the jejunum, where intralumenal pH is greater than 5. This may explain the effectiveness of Pancrease in abolishing steatorrhea in some patients who secrete more acid and presumably can maintain an acidified upper small intestine for a prolonged period of time.

A major criterion for determining the efficacy of enteric-coated enzyme preparations is the size of the microspheres, which influences the timing of enzyme delivery to the intestine. It has been shown that microspheres with a diameter of approximately 1.4 mm appear to mix with chyme most thoroughly and are emptied from the stomach at the same rate as food; large spheres remain in the stomach after food has been emptied into the small bowel and are less effective in correcting malabsorption in chronic pancreatitis.[240] Some commercially marketed microspheres of pancreatin empty too slowly to be effective in digestion of food. This may explain why some enteric-coated preparations are not effective in correcting pancreatic steatorrhea. Therefore, an ideal pancreatic enzyme capsule preparation should contain a high concentration of lipase to maximize fat digestion, and a high concentration of proteases to evoke the negative feedback mechanism for pain control; be enteric coated to avoid destruction by gastric acid; and contain microspheres of approximately 1.4 mm in diameter to allow efficient delivery of enzyme to the small bowel.

H_2 receptor antagonists decrease acid production, pepsin activity, and gastric secretory volume simultaneously and should optimize pancreatic enzyme concentrations.[235,241] Duodenal lipase and trypsin activities are consistently in-

creased with concomitant Viokase and H_2 receptor antagonist treatment. Cimetidine should be considered only in patients who do not respond to standard oral pancreatic supplements because of lifelong increased cost and potential unknown long-term side effects. It has been shown that omeprazole further reduces fecal fat excretion in patients with cystic fibrosis receiving enzyme replacement for pancreatic insufficiency.[242] Therefore, in patients in whom H_2 receptor antagonist fails to abolish steatorrhea, use of omeprazole should be considered.

We recommend the following approach to treat patients with pancreatic insufficiency. It is critical that sufficient amounts of enzyme tablets be given (e.g., eight tablets of Viokase with each meal) to abolish azotorrhea and significantly reduce steatorrhea. Most patients on this regimen achieve satisfactory nutritional status and become relatively asymptomatic. In some of the symptomatic patients, the number of tablets given prandially can be increased or the amount of dietary fat reduced. These measures usually are effective in alleviating symptoms. In occasional patients, the use of Pancrease may be necessary. The addition of H_2 receptor antagonist or omeprazole should be reserved for those patients who are resistant to these maneuvers and who have documented acidic duodenal pH levels, because of cost considerations as well as potential long-term side effects. If all of these measures are ineffective, documentation of diagnosis (by pancreatic function testing) and exclusion of other contributing causes (celiac sprue, terminal ileal disease, or bacterial overgrowth) must be done.

The reader is directed to Chapter 15, Pancreatic Secretion; Chapter 34, Approach to the Patient With Abdominal Pain; Chapter 38, Approach to the Patient With Diarrhea; Chapter

REFERENCES

1. Sarles H. Pancreatitis symposium. Basel: S. Karger, 1965.
2. Cotton PB, Sarner M. International workshop on pancreatitis. In: Gyr KE, Singer MV, Sarles H, eds. Pancreatitis: concepts and classification. Amsterdam: Elsevier, 1984:239.
3. Gyr KE, Singer MV, Sarles H. Revised classification of pancreatitis. In: Gyr KE, Singer MV, Sarles H, eds. Pancreatitis: concepts and classification, Amsterdam: Elsevier, 1984:xxiii.
4. Sarles H. Definition and classifications of pancreatitis. Pancreas 1991;6:470.
5. Sarles H. An international survey on nutrition and pancreatitis. Digestion 1973;9:389.
6. Skyhoj Olsen T. The incidence and clinical relevance of chronic inflammation in the pancreas in autopsy material. Acta Pathol Microbiol Scand 1978;86:361.
7. O'Sullivan JN, Nobrega FT, Morlock CG, et al. Acute and chronic pancreatitis in Rochester, Minnesota 1940 to 1969. Gastroenterology 1972;62:373.
8. Nyboe Andersen N, Thorsgaard Pedersen N, et al. Incidence of alcoholic chronic pancreatitis in Copenhagen. Scand J Gastroenterol 1982;17:247.
9. Schmidt DN. Apparent risk factors for acute and chronic pancreatitis in Stockholm county: spirituous but not wine and beer. In: Ebbehoj N, Thorsgaard N, eds. Pancreas in focus. Copenhagen: Meda, 1989:197.
10. Haemmerli UP, Hefti ML, Schmid M. Chronic pancreatitis in Zurich 1958 through 1962. Bibl Gastroenterol 1962;7:58.
11. Müller-Wieland K. Analyse der klinik der chronischen pankreatitis. Z Klin Med 1965;158:371.
12. Copenhagen Pancreatic Study. An interim report from a prospective epidemiological multicenter study. Scand J Gastroenterol 1981;16:305.
13. Wornig H. Incidence and prevalence of chronic pancreatitis. In: Beger HG, Büchler M, Ditschuneit H, Malfertheiner P, eds. Chronic pancreatitis. Berlin: Springer-Verlag, 1990:8.
14. James O, Agnew JE, Bouchier IAD, et al. Chronic pancreatitis in England: a changing picture. Br Med J 1974;2:34.
15. Gallo L, Fontana G, Labo G. Proceedings of the fifth World Congress of Gastroenterology. Mexico City, 1974:535.
16. Worning H. Chronic pancreatitis: pathogenesis, natural history and conservative treatment. Clin Gastroenterol 1984;13:871.
17. Clark E. Pancreatitis in acute and chronic alcoholism. Am J Dig Dis 1942;9:428.
18. Durbec JP, Sarles H. Multicenter survey of the etiology of pancreatic disease: relationship between the relative risk of developing chronic pancreatitis and alcohol, protein and lipid consumption. Digestion 1978;18:337.
19. Durbec JP, Bidart JM, Sarles H. Interaction between alcohol and other foodstuffs: epidemiological aspects. In: Symposium International Alcohol et Tractus Digestif, Collogues: INSERM 1980;95:33.
20. Sarles H, Cros RC, Bidart JM. A multicenter inquiry into the etiology of pancreatic diseases. Digestion 1979;19:110.
21. Schmidt DN. Apparent risk factors for chronic and acute pancreatitis in Stockholm County. Int J Pancreatol 1991;8:45.
22. Goebell H, Bode CH, Bastian R, et al. Klinisch asymptomatische funktion sstorüngen des exokrinen pankreas bei chronischen alkoholikern. Dtsch Med Wochenschr 1970;95:808.
23. Kondo T, Hayakawa T, Shibata T, et al. Aberrant pancreas is not susceptible to alcoholic pancreatitis. Int J Pancreatol 1991;8:245.
24. Sarles H, Figarella C, Clemente F. The interaction of ethanol, dietary lipids and proteins on the rat pancreas: pancreatic enzymes. Digestion 1971;4:13.
25. Tsukamoto H, Towner SJ, Yu GSM, et al. Potentiation of ethanol-induced pancreatic injury by dietary fat: induction of chronic pancreatitis by alcohol in rats. Am J Pathol 1988;131:246.
26. Pitchumoni CS. Role of nutrition in chronic pancreatitis. In: Berger HG, Büchler M, Ditschuneit H, Malfertleiner P, eds. Chronic pancreatitis. Berlin: Springer-Verlag, 1990:15.
27. Gastard J, Joubaud F, Farbos T, et al. Etiology and course of primary chronic pancreatitis in Western France. Digestion 1973;9:416.
28. Goebell H, Hotz H. Nutritional aspects of chronic pancreatitis in Germany. Biol Gastroenterol (Paris) 1975;8:365.
29. Pitchumoni CS, Sonnenshein M, Candido FM, et al. Nutrition in the pathogenesis of alcoholic pancreatitis. Am J Clin Nutr 1980;33:631.
30. Wilson JS, Bernstein L, McDonald C, et al. Diet and drinking habits in relation to the development of alcoholic pancreatitis. Gut 1985;26:882.
31. Mezey E, Kolman C, Mae Diehl A, et al. Alcohol and dietary intake in the development of chronic pancreatitis and liver disease in alcoholism. Am J Clin Nutr 1988;48:148.
32. Singh M, LaSure MM, Bockman DE. Pancreatic acinar cell function and morphology in rats chronically fed an ethanol diet. Gastroenterology 1982;82:425.
33. Sarles H, Tiscornia O, Palasciano G, et al. Effects of chronic intragastric ethanol administration on canine exocrine pancreatic secretion. Scand J Gastroenterol 1973;8:85.
34. Renner IG, Rinderknecht H, Valenzuela JE, et al. Studies of pure pancreatic secretions in chronic alcoholic subjects without pancreatic insufficiency. Scand J Gastroenterol 1980;15:241.
35. Singh M. Alcoholic pancreatitis in rats fed ethanol in a nutritionally adequate liquid diet. Int J Pancreatol 1987;2:311.
36. Sahel J, Sarles H. Modifications of pure human pancreatic juice induced by chronic alcohol consumption. Dig Dis Sci 1979;24:897.
37. Sarles H, Barnard JP, Chonson C. Pathogenesis and epidemiology of chronic pancreatitis. Annu Rev Med 1989;40:453.
38. Yamedera K, Moriyama T, Makino I. Identification of immunoreactive pancreatic stone protein in pancreatic stone, pancreatic tissue and pancreatic juice. Pancreas 1990;5:255.
39. Multigner L, Sarles H, Lombardo D, DeCaro A. Pancreatic stone protein. I. Implications in stone formation during the course of chronic pancreatitis. Gastroenterology 1985;89:381.
40. Schmiegel W, Burchert M, Kalthoff H, et al. Immunochemical characterization and quantitative distribution of pancreatic stone protein in sera and pancreatic secretions in pancreatic disorders. Gastroenterology 1990;99:1421.
41. Harada H, Takeda M, Yabe H, et al. The hexosamine concentration and output in human pure pancreatic juice in chronic pancreatitis. Gastroenterol Jpn 1980;15:520.
42. Singn M, Simsek H. Ethanol and the pancreas: current status. Gastroenterology 1990;98:1051.
43. Zuidema PJ. Cirrhosis and disseminated calcification of the pancreas in patients with malnutrition. Trop Geogr Med 1959;11:70.
44. Shaper AG. Chronic pancreatic disease and protein malnutrition. Lancet 1960;1:1223.
45. Gee Varghese PJ, Pitchumoni CS. Pancreatic diabetes in Kerala: based on a clinico-pathological study of 325 diabetic patients with pancreatic calculi. In: Patel JC, Talvalcar NG, eds. Proceedings of the World Congress on Diabetes in the Tropics. Bombay: Diabetic Association of India, 1966:223.
46. Gee Varghese PJ. Calcific pancreatitis: causes and mechanisms in the tropics compared with those in the subtropics. St. Joseph's Trivandrum 1986.
47. Pitchumoni CS, Schelle G, Lee PC, et al. Effects of nutrition on the exocrine pancreas. In: Go VLW, Gardner JD, Brooks

FP, et al, eds. The exocrine pancreas: biology, pathophysiology and diseases. New York: Raven Press, 1986:387.

48. Pitchumoni CS. Special problems of tropical pancreatitis. Clin Gastroenterol 1984;13:541.

49. Narendranathan M. Chronic calcific pancreatitis of the tropics. Trop Gastroenterol 1981;2:40.

50. Braganza JM. Pancreatic disease: a causality of hepatic "detoxification"? Lancet 1983;2:1000.

51. Pitchumoni CS, Jain NK, Lowenfels AF, et al. Chronic cyanide poisoning: unifying concept for alcoholic and tropical pancreatitis. Pancreas 1988;3:220.

52. Comfort MW, Steinberg AG. Pedigree of a family with hereditary chronic relapsing pancreatitis. Gastroenterology 1952;21:54.

53. Gross JB. Hereditary pancreatitis. In: Go VLW, Gardner JD, Brooks FP, et al, eds. The exocrine pancreas: biology, pathophysiology and diseases. New York: Raven Press, 1986:829.

54. Layer P, Balzer K, Goebell H. Hereditary pancreatitis: presentation of another family. Hepatogastroenterology 1985;32:31.

55. Sarles H, Camatte R. Etiopathogenesis of pancreas. Recent Advances in Gastroenterology 1966:4:282.

56. Bess MA, Edis AJ, Van Heerden JA. Hyperparathyroidism and pancreatitis: chance or causal association? JAMA 1980;243:246.

57. Goebell H, Steffen C, Baltzel G, et al. Stimulation of pancreatic secretion of enzymes by acute hypercalcemia in man. Eur J Clin Invest 1973;3:98.

58. Layer P, Hotz J, Eysselein VE, et al. The effects of acute hypercalcemia on exocrine pancreatic secretion in the cat. Gastroenterology 1985;88:1168.

59. Goebell H, Horn HD, Bode C, et al. Primarer Hyperparathyreoidismus und exokrine Pankreasfunktion: Storungen der Enzym- und Elektrolytsekretion im Duodenalsaft. Klin Wochenschr 1970;48:810.

60. Layer P, Hotz J, Schmitz-Moormann HP, et al. Effects of experimental chronic hypercalcemia on feline exocrine pancreatic secretion. Gastroenterology 1982;82:309.

61. Sarles H, Sarles JC, Camatte R, et al. Observation on 205 confirmed cases of acute pancreatitis, recurring pancreatitis and chronic pancreatitis. Gut 1965;6:545.

62. Laugier R, Camatte R, Sarles H. Chronic upstream pancreatitis following the healing of a pseudocyst after acute pancreatitis. Am J Surg 1983;146:551.

63. Uscanga L, Kennedy RH, Grimaud JA, et al. Immunolocalisation des collagenes de al laminine et fibronectine dans la matrice conjonctive du pancreas normal et dans la pancreatite obstructive du rat. Gastroenterol Clin Biol 1984;8:20A.

64. Warren KW, Wagner RB. Long term results of nonpenetrating pancreatic trauma. Lahey Clin Found Bull 1967;16:217.

65. Othersen HV, Moore FT, Boles ET. Traumatic pancreatitis and pseudocysts in childhood. J Trauma 1968;8:535.

66. Reinhoff WF, Pickrell KL. Pancreatitis: an anatomical study of the pancreatic and extrahepatic biliary systems. Arch Surg 1946;51:205.

67. Berman LG, Prior JT, Abranow SW, et al. A study of pancreatic duct system in man by the use of vinyl acetate casts of postmortem preparations. Surg Gynecol Obstet 1960;110:391.

68. Cotton PB. Congenital anomaly of pancreas divisum as cause of obstructive pain and pancreatitis. Gut 1980;21:105.

69. Sahel J, Cros RC, Bourry J, et al. Clinicopathological conditions associated with pancreas divisum. Digestion 1982;23:1.

70. Richter JM. Association of pancreas divisum and pancreatitis and its treatment by sphincteroplasty of the accessory ampulla. Gastroenterology 1981;81:1104.

71. Delhaye M, Engelholm L, Cremer M. Pancreas divisum: congenital anatomic variant or anomaly? Gastroenterology 1985;89:951.

72. Sugawa C, Walt AJ, Nunez DC, et al. Pancreas divisum: is it a normal anatomic variant? Am J Surg 1987;153:62.

73. Burtin P, Person B, Charneau J, Boyer J. Pancreas divisum and pancreatitis: a coincidental association. Endoscopy 1991;23:55.

74. Layer P, Kalthoff L, Clain JE, et al. Nonalcoholic chronic pancreatitis: two diseases? Dig Dis Sci 1985;30:980.

75. Ammann RW, Sulser H. Die "senile" chronische Pankreatitis: eine neue nosologische Einheit? Schweiz Med Wochenschr 1976;106:429.

76. DiMagno EP, Clain JE. Chronic pancreatitis. In: Go VLW, Gardner JD, Brooks FP, et al, eds. The exocrine pancreas: biology, pathobiology, and diseases. New York: Raven Press, 1986:541.

77. Ammann RW, Akovbiantz A, Largiader F, et al. Course and outcome of chronic pancreatitis: longitudinal study of a mixed medical-surgical series of 245 patients. Gastroenterology 1984;86:820.

78. Girdwood AH. Does progressive pancreatic insufficiency limit pain in calcific pancreatitis with duct stricture or continued alcohol insult? J Clin Gastroenterol 1981;3:241.

79. Ammann RW. A critical appraisal of interventional therapy in chronic pancreatitis. Endoscopy 1991;23:191.

80. Kalthoff L, Layer P, Clain JE, et al. The course of alcoholic and nonalcoholic chronic pancreatitis. Dig Dis Sci 1984;29:953.

81. Maackie R, Levine AS, Levitt MD. Malabsorption of starch in pancreatic insufficiency (abstract). Gastroenterology 1981;80:1220.

82. Jain NK, Patel VP, Agarwal N, et al. A comparative study of bentinomide test (BT) vs rice flour breath hydrogen test (RFBHT) in the detection of exocrine pancreatic insufficiency (EPI). Gastroenterology 1985;88:1429.

83. DiMagno EP, Go VLW, Summerskill WHJ. Relations between pancreatic enzyme outputs and malabsorption in severe pancreatic insufficiency. N Engl J Med 1973;288:813.

84. DiMagno EP, Malagelada JR, Go VLW. Relationship between alcoholism and pancreatic insufficiency. Ann NY Acad Sci 1975;252:200.

85. Evans WB, Wollaeger EE. Incidence and severity of nutritional deficiency states in chronic exocrine pancreatic insufficiency: comparison with nontropical sprue. Am J Dig Dis 1966;11:594.

86. Twersky Y, Bank S. Nutritional deficiencies in chronic pancreatitis. Gastroenterol Clin North Am 1989;18:543.

87. Covet C, Genton P, Pointel JP, et al. Prevalence of retinopathy is similar in diabetes mellitus secondary to chronic pancreatitis with or without pancreatectomy and in idiopathic diabetes mellitus. Diabetes Care 1985;8:323.

88. Ebbehoj N, Borly L, Madsen P, et al. Pancreatic tissue pressure and pain in chronic pancreatitis. Pancreas 1986;1:556.

89. Bradley EL III. Pancreatic duct pressure in chronic pancreatitis. Am J Surg 1982;144:313.

90. Okazaki K, Yamamoto Y, Kagiyama S, et al. Pressure of papillary sphincter zone and pancreatic main duct in patients with alcoholic and idiopathic chronic pancreatitis. Int J Pancreatol 1988;3:457.

91. Staritz M, zum Büschenfelde KHM. Elevated pressure in the dorsal part of pancreas divisum, the cause of chronic pancreatitis? Pancreas 1988;3:108.

92. Madsen P, Winkler K. The intraductal pancreatic pressure in chronic obstructive pancreatitis. Scand J Gastroenterol 1982;17:553.

93. Ebbehoj N, Svendsen LB, Madsen P. Pancreatic tissue pressure: techniques and pathophysiologic aspects. Scand J Gastroenterol 1984;19:1066.

94. Bockman DE, Büchler M, Malfertheiner P, et al. Analysis of nerves in chronic pancreatitis. Gastroenterology 1988;94:1459.

95. Büchler M, Weihe E. Distribution of neurotransmitters in afferent human pancreatic nerves. Digestion 1988;38:8.

96. Keith RG, Keshavjee SH, Kerenyi NR. Neuropathology of chronic pancreatitis in humans. Can J Surg 1985;28:207.

97. Makrauer FL, Antonioli DA, Banks PA. Duodenal stenosis in chronic pancreatitis: clinicopathological correlations. Dig Dis Sci 1982;27:525.

98. Kloppel G. Pathology of chronic pancreatitis and pancreatic pain. Acta Chir Scand 1990;156:261.

99. Gaskin KJ, Durie PR, Lee L, et al. Colipase and lipase secretion in childhood-onset pancreatic insufficiency. Gastroenterology 1984;86:1.

100. DiMagno EP, Malagelada JR, Go VLW, et al. Fate of orally

ingested enzymes in pancreatic insufficiency: comparison of two dosage schedules. N Engl J Med 1977;296:1318.

101. Dutta SK, Russell RM, Iber FL. Influence of exocrine pancreatic insufficiency on the intraluminal pH of the proximal small intestine. Dig Dis Sci 1979;24:529.

102. Lankisch PG, Manthey G, Otto J, et al. Exocrine pancreatic function in insulin-dependent diabetes mellitus. Digestion 1982;25:211.

103. Regan PT, DiMagno EP. Exocrine pancreatic insufficiency in celiac sprue: a cause of treatment failure. Gastroenterology 1980;78:484.

104. Renner IG, Rinderknecht H, Wisner JR. Pancreatic secretion after secretin and cholecystokinin stimulation in chronic alcoholics with and without cirrhosis. Dig Dis Sci 1983;28:1089.

105. Toskes PP, Hansell J, Cerda J, et al. Vitamin B$_{12}$ malabsorption in chronic pancreatic insufficiency: studies suggesting the presence of a pancreatic "intrinsic factor." N Engl J Med 1971;284:627.

106. Scott J, Summerfield A, Elias E, et al. Pancreatitis: a cause of cholestasis. Gut 1977;18:196.

107. Skude G, Eriksson S. Serum isoamylases in chronic pancreatitis. Scand J Gastroenterol 1976;11:525.

108. Lesi C, Melzi-Deril GU, Pavesi F, et al. Clinical significance of serum pancreatic enzymes in the quiescent phase of chronic pancreatitis. Clin Biochem 1985;18:235.

109. Koop H, Lankisch PG, Stoeckmann F, et al. Trypsin radioimmunoassay in the diagnosis of chronic pancreatitis. Digestion 1980;20:151.

110. Del Favero G, Fabric C, Plebani M, et al. Serum elastase in chronic pancreatic disease. Klin Wochenschr 1985;63:603.

111. Otte M, Thurmayr R, Thurmayr GR, et al. Diagnostic value of the provocative test with secretin and cholecystokinin/pancreozymin. Scand J Gastroenterol [Suppl] 1976;11:88.

112. Owyang C, Scarpello JH, Vinik AI. Correlation between pancreatic enzyme secretion and plasma concentration of human pancreatic polypeptide in health and in chronic pancreatitis. Gastroenterology 1982;83:55.

113. Adrian TE, Besterman HS, Mallinson CN, et al. Impaired pancreatic polypeptide release in chronic pancreatitis with steatorrhoea. Gut 1979;10:98.

114. Imrie CW, Devine B, McKenzie J. The assessment of chronic pancreatitis. Int J Pancreatol 1989;5:11.

115. Thiruvengadam R, DiMagno EP. Inactivation of human lipase by proteases. Am J Physiol 1988;255:G476.

116. Denyer ME, Cotton PB. Pure pancreatic juice studies in normal subjects and patients with chronic pancreatitis. Gut 1979;20:89.

117. Dreiling DA, Hollander F. Studies in pancreatic function. 1. Preliminary series of clinical studies with the secretin test. Gastroenterology 1948;11:714.

118. Burton P, Evans DG, Harper AA, et al. A test of pancreatic function in man based on the analysis of duodenal contents after administration of secretine and pancreozymin. Gut 1960;1:111.

119. Gullo L, Costa PL, Fontana G, et al. Investigation of exocrine pancreatic function by continuous infusion of cerulein and secretin in normal subjects and in chronic pancreatitis. Digestion 1976;14:97.

120. Basso N, Giri S, Improta G, et al. External pancreatic secretion after bombesin infusion in man. Gut 1975;16:994.

121. Moeller DD, Dunn GD, Klotz AP. Comparison of the pancreozymin-secretin test and Lundh test meal. Am J Dig Dis 1972;17:799.

122. Gyr K, Agrawal NM, Felsenfeld O, et al. Comparison study of secretin and Lundh tests. Am J Dig Dis 1975;20:506.

123. Girdwood AH, Hatfield ARW, Bornman PC, et al. Structure and function in noncalcific pancreatitis. Dig Dis Sci 1984;29:721.

124. Malfertheiner P, Buchler M. Correlation of imaging and function in chronic pancreatitis. Radiol Clin North Am 1989;27:51.

125. Dreiling DA. Pancreatic secretory testing in 1974: symposium on diagnosis of pancreatic disease. Gut 1975;16:53.

126. Kay G, Hine P, Braganza J. The pancreolauryl test: a method

127. Braganza JM, Rao JJ. Disproportionate reduction in tryptic response to endogenous compared with exogenous stimulation in chronic pancreatitis. Br Med J 1978;2:392.

128. Forell MM, Stahlheber M, Otte M, et al. Erkrankungen der Verdauungsorgane und ihr Einfluss auf die Verdauungssekretion. Dtsch Med Wochenschr 1969;94:1097.

129. Imondi AR, Stradley RP, Wolgemuth RL. Synthetic peptides in the diagnosis of exocrine pancreatic insufficiency in animals. Gut 1972;13:726.

130. Yamato CH, Kinoshita K. Hydrolysis and metabolism of N-benzoyl-L-tyrosyl-p-aminobenzoic acid in normal and pancreatic duct-ligated animals. J Pharmacol Exp Ther 1978;206:468.

131. Mitchell CJ, Humphrey CS, Bullen AW, et al. Improved diagnostic accuracy of a modified oral pancreatic function test. Scand J Gastroenterol 1979;14:737.

132. Cavallini G, Piubello W, Brocco G, et al. Reliability of the Bz-Ty-PABA and the pancreolauryl test in the assessment of exocrine pancreatic function. Digestion 1983;27:129.

133. Ammann RW, Buhler H, Pei P. Comparative diagnostic accuracy of four tubeless pancreatic function tests in chronic pancreatitis. Scan J Gastroenterol 1982;17:997.

134. Imamura K, Miyazawa T, Abe Y, et al. Evaluation of new pancreatic function test (PFT) for determination of pancreatic function in pancreatic diseases. In: Masuda M, ed. Pancreatic function diagnostant. New York: Igaku-Shoin, 1980:47.

135. Gyr K. The use of BT-PABA in pancreatic diseases: a 5 years' experience from Switzerland. In: Masuda M, ed. Pancreatic function diagnostant. New York: Igaku-Shoin, 1980;38.

136. Arvanitakis C, Greenberger NJ. Diagnosis of pancreatic disease by a synthetic peptide: a new test of exocrine pancreatic function. Lancet 1976;1:663.

137. Freise J, Hofmann R. Zur Spezifitaet des Peptid-Paba-Tests. Z Gastroenterol 1979;17:310.

138. Tanner AR, Fisher D, Smith CL. An evaluation of the one-day NBT-PABA/^{114}C-PABA in the assessment of pancreatic exocrine insufficiency. Digestion 1984;29:42.

139. Allen RH, Seetharam B, Pedell E, et al. Effect of proteolytic enzymes on the binding of cobalamin to R protein and intrinsic factor: in vitro evidence that a failure to partially degrade R protein is responsible for cobalamin malabsorption in pancreatic insufficiency. J Clin Invest 1978;61:47.

140. Brugge WR, Goff JS, Allen NC, et al. Development of a dual label Schilling test for pancreatic exocrine function based on the differential absorption of cobalamin bound to intrinsic factor and R protein. Gastroenterology 1980;78:937.

141. Leung JWC, Frost RA, Burgess R, et al. Modified dual label Schilling test for pancreatic exocrine function. Clin Chim Acta 1988;174:93.

142. Haverback BJ, Dyce BJ, Gutentag PJ. Measurement of trypsin and chymotrypsin in stool: a diagnostic test for pancreatic exocrine function. Gastroenterology 1963;44:588.

143. Stock KP, Schenk J, Schmack B, et al. Funktions-"Screening" des exokrinen Pankreas: FDL-NBT-PABA-Test, Stuhl-Chymotrypsinbestimmung im Vergleich mit dem Sekretin-Pankreozymin-Test. Dtsch Med Wochenschr 1981;106:983.

144. Muller L, Wisniewski ZS, Hansky J. The measurement of faecal chymotrypsin: a screening test for pancreatic exocrine insufficiency. Aust Ann Med 1970;19:47.

145. Niederau C, Strueder E, Thienhaus R. Labordiagnostik bei Pankreaserkrankungen. Z Allg Med 1980;56:1238.

146. Dyck W, Ammann R. Quantitative determination of fecal chymotrypsin as a screening test for pancreatic exocrine insufficiency. Am J Dig Dis 1965;10:530.

147. Schneider R, Duerr HK, Bode JCH. Diagnostische Wertigkeit der Bestimmung von Chymotrypsin im Stuhl für die Erfassung einer exokrinen Pankreasinsuffizienz. Dtsch Med Wochenschr 1974;99:1449.

148. Schwabe AD, Cozzetto FJ, Bennett LR, et al. Estimation of fat absorption by monitoring of expired radioactive carbon dioxide after feeding a radioactive fat. Gastroenterology 1962;42:285.

149. Goff JS. Two-stage triolein breath test differentiates pancreatic

insufficiency from other causes of malabsorption. Gastroenterology 1982;83:44.

150. Pederson NT. Estimation of assimilation of simultaneously ingested ^{14}C- triolein and ^{3}H-oleic acid as a test of pancreatic digestive function. Scand J Gastroenterol 1984;19:161.

151. Jones SN, Lees WR, Frost RA. Diagnosis and grading of chronic pancreatitis by morphological criteria derived by ultrasound and pancreatography. Clin Radiol 1988;39:43.

152. Kunzmann A, Bowie JD, Rochester D. Texture patterns in pancreatic sonograms. Gastrointest Radiol 1979;4:353.

153. Cotton PB, Denyer ME, Kreel L, et al. Comparative clinical impact of endoscopic pancreatography, grey-scale ultrasonography, and computed tomography (EMI scanning) in pancreatic disease: preliminary report. Gut 1978;19:679.

154. Gmelin E, Weiss HD, Fuchs HD, et al. Vergleich der diagnostischen Treffsicherheit von Ultraschall, Computertomographie und ERCP bei der chronischen Pankreatitis und beim Pankreaskarzinon. ROFO Fortschr Geb Rontgenstr Nuklearmed 1981;134:136.

155. Hessel SJ, Siegelman SS, McNeil BJ, et al. A prospective evaluation of computed tomography and ultrasound of the pancreas. Radiology 1982;143:129.

156. Swobodnik W, Meyer W, Brecht-Kraus D, et al. Ultrasound, computed tomography and endoscopic retrograde cholangiopancreatography in the morphologic diagnosis of pancreatic disease. Klin Wochenschr 1983;61:291.

157. Karasawa E, Goldberg HI, Moss AA, et al. CT pancreatogram in carcinoma of the pancreas and chronic pancreatitis. Radiology 1983;148:489.

158. Isherwood I, Fawett HA. Computed tomography of the pancreas. In: Howat HT, Sarles H, eds. The exocrine pancreas. Philadelphia: WB Saunders, 1979;227.

159. Berland LL, Lawson TL, Foley WD, et al. Computed tomography of the normal and abnormal pancreatic duct:correlation with pancreatic ductography. Radiology 1981;141:715.

160. Foley WD, Stewart ET, Lawson I, et al. Computed tomography, ultrasonography, and endoscopic retrograde cholangio-pancreatography in the diagnosis of pancreatic disease: a comparative study. Gastrointest Radiol 1980;5:29.

161. Moss AA, Federle M, Shapiro HA, et al. The combined use of computed tomography and endoscopic retrograde cholangiopancreatography in the assessment of suspected pancreatic neoplasm: a blind clinical evaluation. Radiology 1980;134:159.

162. Semelka RC, Shoenut JP, Koreker MA, et al. Chronic pancreatitis: MR imaging features before and after administration of gadopentetate dimeglumine. J Magnet Reson Imaging 1993;3:79.

163. Braganza JM, Hunt LP, Warwick F. Relationship between pancreatic exocrine function and ductal morphology in chronic pancreatitis. Gastroenterology 1982;82:1341.

164. Caletti G, Brocchi E, Agostini D, et al. Sensitivity of endoscopic retrograde pancreatography in chronic pancreatitis. Br J Surg 1982;69:507.

165. Kasugai T, Kuno N, Kizu M. Manometric endoscopic retrograde pancreatocholangiography: techniques, significance, and evaluation. Am J Dig Dis 1974;19:485.

166. Ammann RW. Chronic pancreatitis in the elderly. Gastroenterol Clin North Am 1990;19:905.

167. Carter DC. Cancer of the head of the pancreas or chronic pancreatitis?: a diagnostic dilemma. Surgery 1992;111:602.

168. DelMaschio A, Vanzulli A, Sironi S, et al. Pancreatic cancer versus chronic pancreatitis: diagnosis with CA19-9 assessment, US, CT and CT-guided fine-needle biopsy. Radiology 1991;178:95.

169. Itoh K, Yamanaka T, Kasahara K, et al. Definitive diagnosis of pancreatic carcinoma with percutaneous fine needle aspiration biopsy under ultrasonic guidance. Am J Gastroenterol 1979;71:469.

170. Aranha GV, Prinz RA, Esguerra AC, et al. The nature and course of cystic pancreatic lesions diagnosed by ultrasound. Arch Surg 1983;118:486.

171. Bradley EL, Austin H. Multiple pancreatic pseudocysts: the principle of internal cystocystostomy in surgical management. Surgery 1982;92:111.

172. Williford ME, Foster WL, Halvorsen RA, et al. Pancreatic pseudocyst: comparative evaluation by sonography and computed tomography. Am J Radiol 1983;140:53.

173. Munn JS, Aranha GV, Greenlee HB, et al. Simultaneous treatment of chronic pancreatitis and pancreatic pseudocyst. Arch Surg 1987;122:662.

174. Sugawa C, Walt AJ. Endoscopic retrograde pancreatography in the surgery of pancreatic pseudocysts. Surgery 1979;86:639.

175. O'Connor M, Kolars J, Ansel H, et al. Preoperative endoscopic retrograde cholangiopancreatography in the surgical management of pancreatic pseudocysts. Am J Surg 1986;151:18.

176. Bradley EL, Clements JL, Gonzalez AC. The natural history of pancreatic pseudocysts: a unified concept of management. Am J Surg 1979;137:135.

177. Imrie CW, Buist LJ, Shearer MG. Importance of cause in the outcome of pancreatic pseudocysts. Am J Surg 1988;156:159.

178. Yeo CJ, Bastidas JA, Lynch-Nyhan A, et al. The natural history of pancreatic pseudocysts documented by computed tomography. Surg Gynecol Obstet 1990;170:411.

179. Cremer M, Deviere J, Engelholm L. Endoscopic management of cysts and pseudocysts in chronic pancreatitis: long term follow-up after 7 years of experience. Gastrointest Endosc 1989;35:1.

180. Kozarek AA, Ball TJ, Patterson DJ, et al. Endoscopic transpapillary therapy for disrupted pancreatic duct and peripancreatic fluid collections. Gastroenterology 1991;100:1362.

181. Grimm H, Binmoeller KF, Soehendra N. Endosonography-guided drainage of a pancreatic pseudocyst. Gastrointest Endosc 1992;38:170.

182. Shatney CH, Lillehei RC. Surgical treatment of pancreatic pseudocysts. Ann Surg 1979;189:386.

183. Van Sonnenberg E, Wittich GR, Casola G, et al. Percutaneous drainage of infected and noninfected pancreatic pseudocysts: experience in 101 cases. Radiology 1989;170:757.

184. Adams DB, Anderson MC. Percutaneous catheter drainage compared with internal drainage in the management of pancreatic pseudocyst. Ann Surg 1992;215:571.

185. Criado E, DeStefano AA, Weiner TM, Jaques PF. Long term results of percutaneous catheter drainage of pancreatic pseudocysts. Surg Gynecol Obstet 1992;175:293.

186. Gullo L, Barbara L. Treatment of pancreatic pseudocysts with octreotide. Lancet 1991;338:540.

187. Barkin JS, Reiner DK, Deutch E. Sandostatin for control of catheter drainage of pancreatic pseudocyst. Pancreas 1991;6:245.

188. Monali GA, Braverman DZ, Shemesh D, et al. Successful treatment of pancreatic pseudocyst with a somatostatin analogue and catheter drainage. Am J Gastroenterol 1991;86:515.

189. Sankaran S, Walt AJ. The natural and unnatural history of pancreatic pseudocysts. Br J Surg 1975;62:37.

190. Castle LAM, Terblanche J. Pancreatic ascites and pleural effusion. Aust NZ J Surg 1978;48:290.

191. Donowitz M, Herstein MD, Spiro HM. Pancreatic ascites. Medicine 1974;53:183.

192. Salam AA, Warren WD, Tyras DH. Splenic vein thrombosis: a diagnosable and curable form of portal hypertension. Surgery 1973;74:961.

193. Rosche J, Herfort K. Contribution of splenoportography to the diagnosis of disease of the pancreas. Acta Med Scand 1961;171:251.

194. Trapnell JE. Chronic relapsing pancreatitis: a review of 64 cases. Br J Surg 1979;66:471.

195. Bornman PC, Marks IN, Girdwood AH, et al. Is pancreatic duct obstruction or stricture a major cause of pain in calcific pancreatitis? Br J Surg 1980;67:425.

196. Marks IN, Girdwood AH, Banks S, et al. The prognosis of alcohol-induced calcified pancreatitis. S Afr Med J 1980;57:640.

197. Haber H, Alltree M, Lambie RS. The treatment of severe pancreatic pain. Middle East J Anaesthesiol 1979;5:213.

198. Bengtsson M, Lofstrom JB. Nerve block in pancreatic pain. Acta Chir Scand 1990;156:285.

199. Leung JWC, Aveling W, Bowen-Wright M, et al. Celiac plexus

block for pain control in pancreatic cancer and chronic pancreatitis. Gut 1982;23:A451.

200. Green GM, Lyman RL. Feedback regulation of pancreatic enzyme secretion as a mechanism for trypsin inhibitor-induced hypersecretion in rats. Proc Soc Exp Biol Med 1972;140:6.

201. Louie DS, May D, Miller P, et al. Cholecystokinin mediates feedback regulation of pancreatic enzyme secretion in rats. Am J Physiol 1986;250:G252.

202. Ihse I, Lilja P, Lundquist I. Feedback regulation of pancreatic enzyme secretion by intestinal trypsin in man. Digestion 1977;15:303.

203. Slaff J, Jacobson D, Tillman CR, et al. Protease-specific suppression of pancreatic exocrine secretion. Gastroenterology 1984;87:44.

204. Owyang C, Louie D, Tatum D. Feedback regulation of pancreatic enzyme secretion. J Clin Invest 1986;77:2042.

205. Calan J, Bojarski JC, Spriner CJ. Raw soya-bean flour increases cholecystokinin release in man. Br J Nutr 1987;58:175.

206. Liener JE, Goodale RL, Deshmukh A, et al. Effect of a trypsin inhibitor from soya-beans (Bowman-Birk) on the secretory activity of the human pancreas. Gastroenterology 1988;94:419.

207. Schafmayer A, Becker HD, Werner M, et al. Plasma cholecystokinin levels in patients with chronic pancreatitis. Digestion 1985;32:136.

208. Slaff JI, Wolfe MM, Toskes PP. Elevated fasting cholecystokinin levels in pancreatic exocrine impairment: evidence to support feedback regulation. J Lab Clin Med 1985;105:282.

209. Gomez Cerezo J, Codocer R, Fernandez Callo P, et al. Basal and postprandial cholecystokinin values in chronic pancreatitis with and without abdominal pain. Digestion 1991;48:134.

210. Funakoshi A, Nakano I, Shinozake H, et al. Low plasma cholecystokinin response after ingestion of a test meal in patients with chronic pancreatitis. Am J Gastroenterol 1985;80:937.

211. Jansen JMBJ, Jebbink MCW, Mulders HJA, Lamers CBHW. Effect of pancreatic enzyme supplementation on postprandial plasma cholecystokinin secretion in patients with pancreatic insufficiency. Regul Pept 1989;25:333.

212. Isaksson G, Ihse I. Pain reduction by an oral pancreatic enzyme preparation in chronic pancreatitis. Dig Dis Sci 1983;28:97.

213. Ramo DJ, Puolakkainen PA, Seppalo K, et al. Self-administration of enzyme substitution in the treatment of exocrine pancreatic insufficiency. Scand J Gastroenterol 1989;24:688.

214. Halgreen H, Pedersen NT, Worning H. Symptomatic effect of pancreatic enzyme therapy in patients with chronic pancreatitis. Scand J Gastroenterol 1986;21:104.

215. Toskes PP. Medical therapy of chronic pancreatitis. Semin Gastrointest Dis 1991;2:188.

216. McCarthy J, Geenen JE, Hogan WJ. Preliminary experience with endoscopic stent placement in benign pancreatic disease. Gastrointest Endosc 1988;84:16.

217. Kozarek RA, Patterson DJ, Ball TS, Traverso LW. Endoscopic placement of pancreatic stents and drains in the management of pancreatitis. Ann Surg 1989;209:261.

218. Grimm H, Meyer WH, Nam VCH, Soehendra N. New modalities for treating chronic pancreatitis. Endoscopy 1989;21:70.

219. Huibregtse K, Scheider B, Vrij AA, Tytgat GNJ. Endoscopic pancreatic drainage in chronic pancreatitis. Gastrointest Endosc 1988;34:9.

220. Siegel JH, Pullano WJ, Safrany L. Endoscopic sphincterotomy for acquired pancreatitis: effective long-term management. Gastrointest Endosc 1989;35:168.

221. Derfus GA, Geenen JE, Hogan WJ. Effect of endoscopic pancreatic duct stent placement on pancreatic ductal morphology. Gastrointest Endosc 1990;36:206.

222. Kozarek RA. Pancreatic stents can induce ductal changes consistent with chronic pancreatitis. Gastrointest Endosc 1990;36:93.

223. Fuji T, Amaro R, Ohmura T, et al. Endoscopic pancreatic sphincterotomy technique and evaluation. Endoscopy 1989;21:27.

224. Sauerbruch T, Holl J, Sackmann M, Paumgartner G. Extracorporeal shock wave lithotripsy of pancreatic stones. Gut 1989;80:1406.

225. Lehman GA, Sherman S, Nisi R, Hawes RH. Pancreatic divisum: results of minor papilla sphincterotomy. Gastrointest Endosc 1993;39:1.

226. Warshaw AL. Conservation of pancreatic tissue by combined gastric, biliary, and pancreatic duct drainage for pain from chronic pancreatitis. Am J Surg 1985;149:563.

227. Morrow CE, Cohen JI, Sutherland DER, et al. Chronic pancreatitis: long-term surgical results of pancreatic duct drainage, pancreatic secretion, and near total pancreatectomy and islet autotransplantation. Surgery 1984;96:608.

228. Najarian JS, Sutherland DER, Baumgartner D, et al. Total or near total pancreatectomy and islet autotransplantation for treatment of chronic pancreatitis. Ann Surg 1980;192:526.

229. Hinshaw DB, Jolley WB, Hinshaw DB, et al. Islet autotransplantation after pancreatectomy for chronic pancreatitis with a new method of islet preparation. Am J Surg 1981;142:118.

230. Farney AC, Najarian JS, Nakhleh RE, et al. Autotransplantation of dispersed pancreatic islet tissue combined with total or near total pancreatectomy for treatment of chronic pancreatitis. Surgery 1991;110:427.

231. Graham DY. Enzyme replacement therapy of exocrine pancreatic insufficiency in man: relation between in vitro enzyme activities and in vivo potency in commercial pancreatic extracts. N Engl J Med 1977;296:1314.

232. Whitehead AM. Study to compare the enzyme activity acid resistance and dissolution characteristics of currently available pancreatic enzyme preparations. Pharm Weekbl [Sci] 1988;10:12.

233. Stapleton FB, Kenedy J, Nousia-Arvanitakis S, et al. Hyperuricosuria due to high dose pancreatic extract therapy in cystic fibrosis. N Engl J Med 1976;295:246.

234. DiMagno EP. Medical treatment of pancreatic insufficiency. Mayo Clin Proc 1979;54:435.

235. Regan PT, Malagelada JR, DiMagno EP, et al. Comparative effects of antacids, cimetidine, and enteric coating on the therapeutic response to oral enzymes in severe pancreatic insufficiency. N Engl J Med 1977;297:854.

236. Benn A, Cooke WT. Intraluminal pH of duodenum and jejunum in fasting subjects with normal and abnormal gastric or pancreatic function. Scand J Gastroenterol 1971;6:313.

237. Dutta SK, Russell RM, Iber FL. Influence of exocrine pancreatic insufficiency on the intraluminal pH of the proximal small intestine. Dig Dis Sci 1979;24:529.

238. Graham DY. An enteric coated pancreatic enzyme preparation that works. Dig Dis Sci 1979;24:906.

239. Dutta SK, Rubin J, Harvey J. Comparative evaluation of the therapeutic efficacy of a pH-sensitive enteric coated pancreatic enzyme preparation with conventional pancreatic enzyme therapy in the treatment of exocrine pancreatic insufficiency. Gastroenterology 1983;84:476.

240. Meyer JH, Elashoff J, Porter-Fink V, et al. Human postprandial gastric emptying of 1–3 millimeter spheres. Gastroenterology 1988;94:1315.

241. Regan PT, Malagelada JR, DiMagno EP, et al. Rationale for the use of cimetidine in pancreatic insufficiency. Mayo Clin Proc 1978;53:79.

242. Heijerman HG, Lamers CB, Bakker W. Omeprazole enhances the efficacy of pancreatin (pancrease) in cystic fibrosis. Ann Intern Med 1991;114:200.

243. Berardi RR, Dunn-Kucharski VA. Pancreatitis and cholelithiasis. In: DiPiro JT, Talbert RL, Hayes PE, et al, eds. Pharmacotherapy: a pathophysiologic approach. Norwalk, CT: Appleton & Lange, 1993:614.

Textbook of Gastroenterology, second edition, edited by Tadataka Yamada. JB Lippincott Company, Philadelphia © 1995.

CHAPTER 92

Pancreatic Adenocarcinoma

Eugene P. DiMagno

Ductal Adenocarcinoma
  Incidence and Natural History
  Risk Factors
  Experimental Models and Molecular Biology
  Pathology
  Clinical Manifestations
  Diagnostic Investigations
  Treatment

Less Common Exocrine Pancreatic Tumors
  Mucinous Cystadenocarcinoma
  Giant Cell Tumors
  Acinar Cell Tumor
  Pancreaticoblastoma
  Solid and Papillary Epithelial Neoplasm
  Mucin-Producing Pancreatic Cancer or Mucinous Ductal
    Ecstasis

DUCTAL ADENOCARCINOMA

Ductal pancreatic carcinoma has a poor prognosis. At the time of diagnosis, 90% of the tumors cannot be resected. Diagnosis of the tumor occurs late because signs and symptoms are nonspecific and occur after advanced disease is present. A simple, reliable screening test is not available to diagnose small asymptomatic tumors in populations of high-risk patients. In this milieu, a major emphasis has been placed on earlier diagnosis with tumor markers and imaging techniques and on investigation of potential causes, to prevent the disease or identify it early enough to improve survival. In addition, chemotherapeutic regimens and improved techniques of radiation therapy for pancreatic cancer continue to be developed to treat patients with nonresectable tumors.

Most pancreatic adenocarcinomas are moderately well differentiated, mucinous carcinomas arising from the cuboidal epithelium of the pancreatic duct (Table 92-1). Hence, in this chapter most of the discussion is centered on this tumor, but the more unusual tumors, such as acinar cell, giant cell, epidermoid carcinoma, adenoacanthoma, sarcoma, cystadenocarcinoma, solid and papillary epithelial neoplasms, and mucinous ductal ectasia, are discussed briefly, particularly because some of these tumors have a different natural history from that of mucinous ductal adenocarcinoma.

Incidence and Natural History

The incidence and mortality of adenocarcinoma of the pancreatic ducts are gradually increasing, predominantly in women.[1] From 1935 to 1985, the incidence has increased from less than 5 per 100,000 to between 11 and 12 per 100,000 in men, and slightly less in women[2] (Fig. 92-1). Unfortunately, the survival of patients with resectable tumors (10% 5-year survival rate) has not improved,[1,2] and is similar regardless of whether a total pancreatectomy or a Whipple procedure is performed (Fig. 92-2). Survival is not related to the histologic grade or the presence of metastatic lesions (Fig. 92-3). Patients with nonresectable tumors who have been treated with biliary bypass surgery survive no more than 4 years, and only 10% survived as long as 2 years[3] (Fig. 92-4). The 5-year survival rate for pancreatic cancer in the United States for the period 1979 to 1984 is 3% for Caucasians and 5% for African Americans,[2] the lowest for all cancers.

Risk Factors

Table 92-2 summarizes the risk factors for pancreatic cancer. Patients with ductal adenocarcinoma of the pancreas have common demographic variables. Eighty percent of pancreatic cancers occur between the ages of 60 and 80 years, and the disease is unusual in people younger than the age of 40 years. Pancreatic cancer occurs more commonly in men, and in urban areas. In young patients (younger than 40 years), the disease occurs more commonly in women.

Diabetes and pancreatitis predispose to pancreatic cancer. Patients with diabetes mellitus have a twofold to threefold risk for development of pancreatic cancer.[4-6] About 20% of patients with pancreatic cancer have diabetes mellitus or an abnormal glucose tolerance test result more than 2 years before the diagnosis of pancreatic cancer.[7] In diabetics, pancreatic cancer is more common in women.[5] In most patients, how-

TABLE 92-1
Primary Malignant Neoplasms
of the Nonendocrine Pancreas

NEOPLASM

Duct (Ductule Cell Origin) (573; 88%)
Duct cell carcinoma (494)
Giant cell carcinoma (27)
Giant cell carcinoma, osteoclastoid type (1)
Adenosquamous carcinoma (20)
Adenosquamous (spindle cell) carcinoma
Microadenocarcinoma (solid microglandular) (16)
Mucinous (colloid) carcinoma (9)
Cystadenocarcinoma, mucinous (5)
Papillary cyst tumor (1)
Mucinous-carcinoid carcinoma
Carcinoid
Oncocytic carcinoid
Oncocytic carcinoma
Oat cell carcinoma
Ciliated cell carcinoma

Acinar Cell Origin (8; 1.2%)
Acinar cell carcinoma (7)
Acinar cell cystadenocarcinoma (1)

Mixed Cell Type (1; 0.2%)
Duct–islet cell (1)
Duct–islet acinar cell
Acinar–islet cell
Carcinoid–islet cell

Connective Tissue Origin (4; 0.6%)
Leiomyosarcoma (1)
Malignant fibrous histiocytoma (1)
Malignant hemangiopericytoma (1)
Osteogenic sarcoma (1)
Fibrosarcoma
Rhabdomyosarcoma
Malignant neurilemoma
Liposarcoma

Uncertain Histogenesis (59; 9.2%)
Pancreaticoblastoma, simple type
Pancreaticoblastoma, mixed type (1)
Unclassified (58)
   Large cell (50)
   Small cell (7)
   Clear cell (1)

Malignant Lymphoma (?)
Histiocytic
Plasmacytoma

Data were obtained from 500,000 surgical specimens and 13,882 autopsies performed at Memorial Hospital, New York, New York. In the study, 821 patients were listed as having pancreas (nonislet) cancer; adequate clinical and pathologic material was available for study in 645 patients. Diagnoses without (numbers) indicate that such a cancer did not occur in the Memorial Hospital patients during the years of the review (1949–1978), but has been reported in literature or was seen by the authors subsequent to 1978.

Adapted from references 53 and 54.

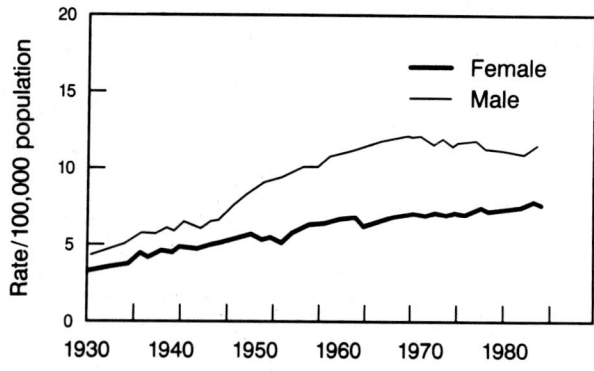

*Adjusted 1970 U.S. Census

FIGURE 92-1. Age-adjusted cancer death rates for selected sites for women and men from 1930–1985. (Adapted from Silverberg E, Lubera JA. Cancer statistics 1988. CA 1988;38:5.)

the relative risk for development of pancreatic cancer was 9.5. The cumulative risk increased steadily; at 10 and 20 years it was 1.8% and 4.0%, respectively, and was independent of gender, country, and type of pancreatitis. A fivefold risk for development of pancreatic cancer has been reported in patients with hereditary pancreatitis.[9] In one review, it was reported that the incidence of pancreatic cancer was 5% in 304 patients with hereditary pancreatitis.[10]

The association of other conditions with pancreatic cancer is less clear. The claim that gastrectomy or cholecystectomy increase the risk for pancreatic cancer has not been supported in two cohort studies.[11,12]

Reflux of bile[13] and duodenal contents, perhaps containing carcinogens, into the pancreatic duct has been postulated to cause pancreatic cancer and is related to anatomic relations among the common bile duct, pancreatic duct, and duodenum. In the dog, an animal that has separate openings for the main pancreatic duct and bile duct, less than 1% of total duodenal volume flow refluxes into the pancreatic duct post-

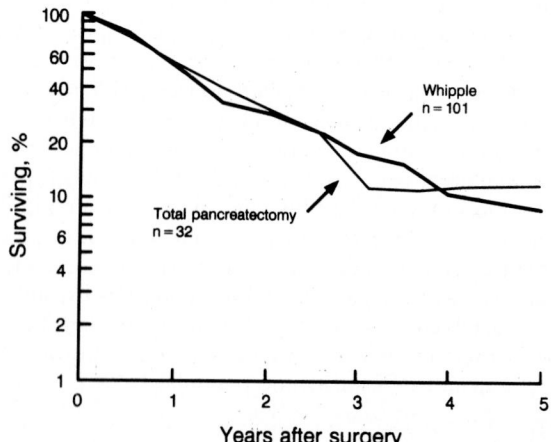

FIGURE 92-2. Actual survival rates after Whipple operation and total pancreatectomy for ductal carcinoma of the pancreas. (From Edis AJ, Kieman PD, Taylor WF. Attempted curative resection of ductal carcinoma of the pancreas: review of Mayo Clinic experience, 1951–1975. Mayo Clin Proc 1980;55:531.)

ever, diabetes does not precede the onset of pancreatic cancer. In these patients, pancreatic cancer may cause diabetes.[7]

Patients with chronic pancreatitis have an increased risk for development of pancreatic cancer. In a multicenter, historical cohort of over 1500 patients with chronic pancreatitis,[8]

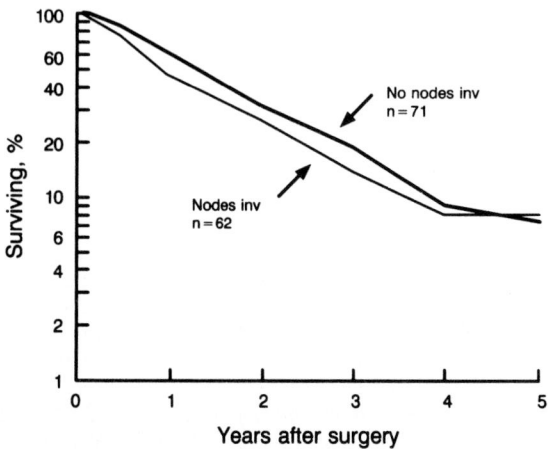

FIGURE 92-3. Effect of node status on survival after radical resection of ductal carcinoma of the head of the pancreas. (From Edis AJ, Kieman PD, Taylor WF. Attempted curative resection of ductal carcinoma of the pancreas: review of Mayo Clinic experience, 1951–1975. Mayo Clin Proc 1980;55:531.)

TABLE 92-2
Risk Factors for Pancreatic Cancer

Advanced age
Men older than 40 years of age
Urban location
Diabetes mellitus
Hereditary pancreatitis
Smoking
High-fat diet
Occupational exposure to carcinogens (chemical, petroleum
  industries)
(?) Pancreaticobiliary anatomy

prandially. In humans, similar anatomy is associated with papillary epithelial hyperplasia, perhaps a premalignant lesion of the pancreas[14] (Fig. 92-5). Because mechanisms for preventing reflux are essentially competent in experimental animals with completely separate bile ducts and main pancreatic duct openings into the duodenum, an alternative mechanism to explain this association is that the lack of a common channel might retard the flow of pancreatic secretion at the opening of the pancreatic duct into the duodenum, resulting in prolonged contact time between carcinogens and ductal cells. This hypothesis has not been experimentally tested.

Environmental factors also may be associated with pancreatic cancer. Industrial carcinogens incriminated as causing pancreatic cancer include methylnitrosourethane, acetominofluorene, methylcholanthrene, paradimethyl aminobenzene, benzidine, β-naphthylamine coal tar derivatives,[15,16] and coke.[17] In one study, chemists who were members of the American Chemical Society had an excess of cancer deaths, and 50% of these cancer-related deaths were the result of malignant lymphomas and pancreatic cancer.[18] In other studies,

however, no increased risk was related to a specific occupation,[19,20] and no excess of pancreatic cancer was found among chemists working at the DuPont Company.[21] A diet high in fat and cholesterol increases the risk for development of pancreatic cancer compared to a low-cholesterol, low-fat diet.[6,22,23] There is a direct correlation between pancreatic cancer mortality and the ingestion of fat[6] (Fig. 92-6). In animal models of pancreatic carcinogenesis, high-fat diets rich in linoleic acid (corn, safflower, sunflower oils) act as tumor promoters, but oleic acid (olive oil) and eicosapentaenoic acid (fish, marine mammals) do not.[24]

Cigarette smoking, but not alcohol and coffee consumption, definitely increases the risk for development of pancreatic cancer. In three case-control studies[6,25,26] and in two large cohort studies,[27,28] the relative risks for cigarette smokers compared with nonsmokers ranged from 1.4 to 2.3, and the age at onset in smokers is 10 years younger. The relationship between alcohol use and pancreatic cancer is weak and inconsistent. In one case-control study[29] and one population study,[30] there was an association between alcohol consumption and pancreatic cancer, but no association was found in two other case-control studies.[6,26] Moderate alcohol consumption, particularly of wine, has a protective effect for pancreatic cancer.[19] Overall, there are no conclusive data to indicate that there is a definite association between drinking coffee and development of pancreatic cancer. Two studies have shown a strong association between coffee consumption

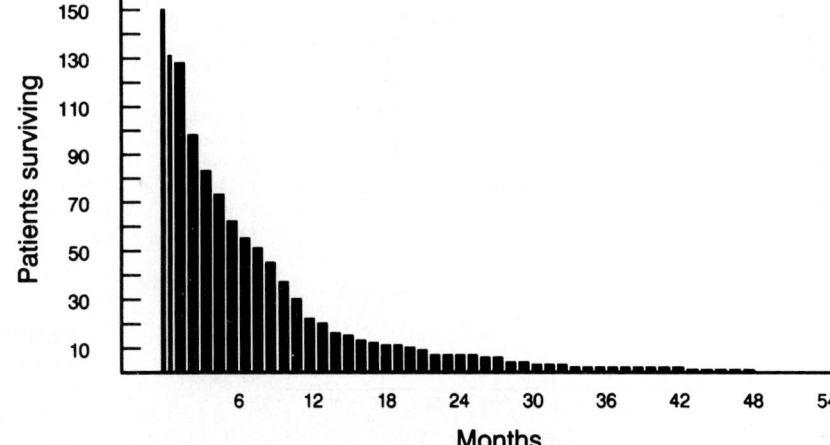

FIGURE 92-4. Survival rates after biliary bypass procedure for ductal adenocarcinoma of the pancreas. (From van Heerden JA, Heath PM, Alden CR. Biliary bypass for ductal adenocarcinoma of the pancreas: Mayo Clinic experience, 1970–1975. Mayo Clin Proc 1980;55:537.)

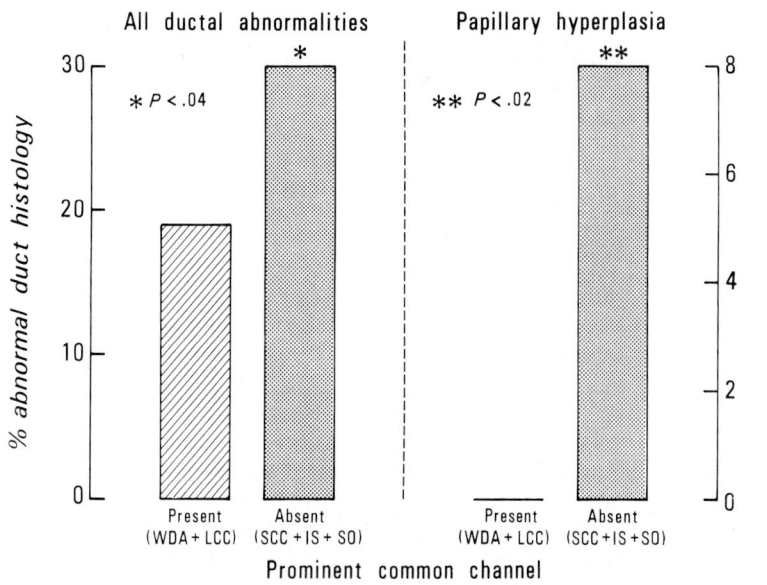

FIGURE 92-5. Relations between ductal histologic status and the presence or absence of a prominent common channel. A prominent common channel is defined as either well-delineated ampulla (WDA) or long common channel (LCC). An absent prominent common channel is defined as a short common channel (SCC), interposed septum (IS), or separate openings (SO) of the bile duct and pancreatic duct into duodenum. (From DiMagno EP, Shorter RG, Taylor WF, Go VLW. Relationships between pancreaticobiliary ductal anatomy and pancreatic ductal and parenchymal histology. Cancer 1982;49:361.)

and pancreatic cancer,[19,26] but these data have been challenged.[30-32] Cohort studies do not show a significant association of coffee with pancreatic cancer.[33-35]

In summary, the incidence of pancreatic cancer perhaps can be reduced by eliminating cigarette smoking, avoiding potentially toxic chemicals, and eating a prudent diet low in cholesterol and fat and containing olive oil and fish as the main sources of fat. The association of pancreatic cancer with other environmental factors is weak, and no other specific measures can be strongly recommended.

Experimental Models and Molecular Biology

Animal models for the study of pancreatic carcinogenesis[36] include nitrosamine-induced ductal adenocarcinoma in Syrian hamsters,[37] azaserine-induced acinar cell carcinoma in rats,[38]

in vitro models of pancreatic carcinogenesis,[39] transplantable pancreatic cancers,[40] and transgenic mouse models[41] (introduction into the germ line of the pancreatic elastase–simian virus 40 gene constructs).

A major objection is that most models are acinar cell models, whereas 90% of human pancreatic cancers are ductal cell in origin. Even the ductal cell tumor nitrosamine Syrian hamster model has a variable histogenesis because lesions involve acini, islets, and ducts. Nevertheless, animal models have provided clues to the etiology of ductal adenocarcinoma and a better understanding of tumorigenesis. For example, diets high in fat, protein, or both[42,43] enhance pancreatic ductal cancers in the golden hamster and azaserine-induced acinar cell carcinomas in rats. Continued development of animal models, particularly transgenic models, may provide answers to the questions of cell lineage and malignant transformation of pancreatic cells, as well as aid in the development of preventive measures, markers for early detection, and agents to treat the disease.[44]

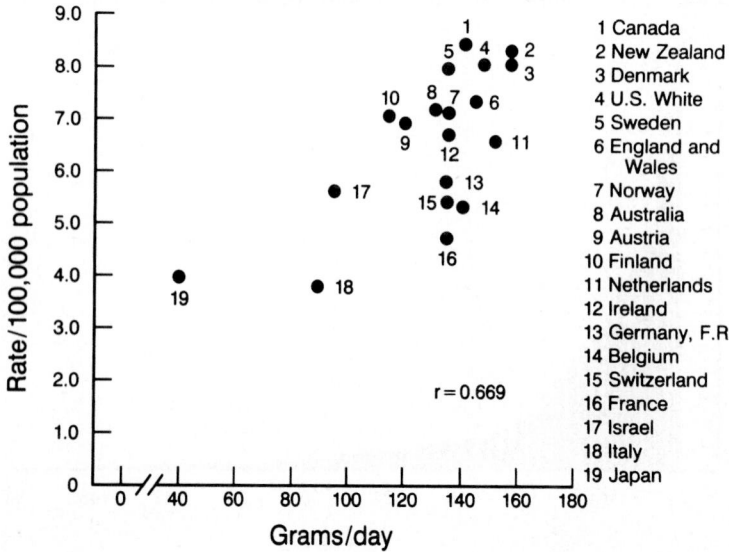

FIGURE 92-6. Relation between pancreatic cancer mortality rates and total fat intake. (From Wynder EL, Mabuchi K, Maruchi N, Fortner JG. Epidemiology of cancer of the pancreas. J Natl Cancer Inst 1973;50:645.)

Knowledge of the molecular biology of pancreatic cancer is advancing rapidly and should yield new and successful strategies to diagnose and treat this disease. The most common abnormalities in human cancer, including pancreatic cancer, appear to be deletions and mutations that can occur in many codons of the *p53* gene.[45] p53 is a nuclear protein that inhibits abnormal cellular proliferation. Mutations of the gene result in altered protein structure and loss of suppressor function. In addition, the mutated p53 nuclear protein accumulates in neoplastic tissue owing to a prolonged half-life.[45,46]

A high proportion of pancreatic cancers also have mutations in the *K-ras* gene.[47] In contrast to *p53*, the mutation of *K-ras* occurs in codon 12.[48,49] This gene likely is involved in cancer growth. The pathways regulated by the epidermal growth factor receptor[50,51] or the ERBB2 receptor also are altered, but their role in pathogenesis of pancreatic cancer is uncertain.[52]

Pathology

There are 30 different morphologic varieties of pancreatic carcinoma (see Table 92-1).[53] Approximately 90% of tumors are of ductal origin, and 75% of the total number of tumors are classic ductal cell mucin-producing adenocarcinomas. Seventeen percent of the total number of tumors are less common but well recognized ductal forms of pancreatic cancer. Of these less common ductal tumors, special note should be made of papillary cystic tumors, which are responsible for the slight increase in pancreatic tumors in young women. Among the 10% of nonductal tumors, most are of connective tissue origin, primarily sarcomas, pancreatoblastomas, which occur primarily in children, and rare primary malignant lymphomas.

Ductal cell adenocarcinoma predominantly occurs in the head of the gland (60%–70%), and most arise in the part of the head of the pancreas derived from the dorsal pancreas anlage close to the intrapancreatic portion of the common bile duct.[54] The remaining tumors of the head of the pancreas arise in the central pancreatic head behind the ampulla of Vater or in the uncinate pancreas close to the ventral pancreatic duct. The three sites of tumors of the head of the pancreas are associated with different early features of malignancy; tumors that arise in the dorsal pancreas obstruct the common bile duct and cause jaundice, whereas tumors arising near the ampulla of Vater or uncinate pancreas obstruct the main pancreatic duct and cause pancreatic insufficiency and obstructive chronic pancreatitis.

Tumors of the head of the pancreas are relatively large when first diagnosed. Even tumors that are resected have a median diameter of 2.5 to 3.5 cm, and at autopsy most tumors are 5 to 6 cm in diameter. Tumors of the body and tail of the pancreas are larger (5–7 cm) when discovered because they are detected later than tumors of the head of the pancreas.[55] Histologically, the tumor consists of well differentiated to poorly differentiated, duct-like glands that are embedded in a dense network of fibrous tissue.

Most commonly, the tumor extends to the retroperitoneal spaces behind the pancreas, envelopes and fixes the vessels, and microscopically invades peripancreatic fat, lymph channels, and perineural areas. In advanced disease, cancers of the head may invade the duodenum, stomach, peritoneum, and gallbladder, whereas carcinomas of the body and tail may invade the liver, peritoneum, spleen, stomach, and left adrenal gland.

Carcinomas of the body or tail of the pancreas may spread or metastasize to unusual locations and result in bizarre clinical manifestations. Patients have been reported to have had metastases to the iris and testes[56]; to both temporal bones, giving rise to sudden and profound hearing loss[57]; and to the distal esophagus, either by direct extension or by spread to the lymph nodes in the posterior mediastinum, giving rise to dysphagia.[58] A more common, but still unusual presentation of cancer of the body or tail of the pancreas is variceal hemorrhage secondary to portal hypertension due to occlusion of the splenic vein by direct extension of the tumor.

Clinical Manifestations

The signs and symptoms of pancreatic cancer are nonspecific (Table 92-3). A variety of nonpancreatic diseases as well as pancreatitis may cause features identical to those experienced by patients with pancreatic cancer. Only 40% of 70 patients who had signs and symptoms suggestive of pancreatic cancer (e.g., abdominal pain, weight loss, or jaundice) had pancreatic cancer.[59] These signs and symptoms do not accurately discriminate pancreatic cancer from pancreatitis, nonpancreatic intraabdominal neoplasms (e.g., lymphomas, cancers of the small intestine), or even functional gastrointestinal disorders. Most patients with pancreatic cancer, however, have abdominal pain and weight loss, and most patients with carcinoma in the head of the gland have jaundice.

TABLE 92-3
Presenting Features of Pancreatic Cancer

FEATURE	% PATIENTS
Head	
Weight loss	92
Jaundice	82
Pain	72
Anorexia	64
Dark urine	63
Light stools	62
Nausea	45
Vomiting	35
Weakness	35
Pruritus	24
Body and Tail	
Weight loss	100
Pain	87
Weakness	43
Nausea	43
Vomiting	37
Anorexia	33
Constipation	27
Food intolerance	7
Jaundice	7

Adapted from Howard JM, Jordan CL Jr. Cancer of the pancreas. Curr Probl Cancer 1977;2:1.

Pain

In up to 90% of patients,[60] pain occurs during the course of pancreatic cancer and in 79% of patients, pain is the presenting symptom.[61] Pain is present in either the abdomen, back, or both in 35%, 8%, and 36% of patients, respectively. Abdominal pain occurs most frequently in the epigastrium (46%), but it may occur in the left (13%) or right (18%) abdomen. Lower abdominal pain occurs in 11% of patients and is the only presentation of pain in 3% of patients.[60]

The pain may be vague and nonspecific and be present up to 3 months before jaundice occurs.[62] Thus, early in the course of the disease pain commonly is ignored by both patients and physicians. If a careful history is taken, however, it is often possible to elicit features suggestive of an organic and, more specifically, a retroperitoneal visceral origin of the pain. Visceral pain is mediated by unmyelinated C fibers. It is often described as constant, poorly localized, disagreeable, aversive, and causing night awakening. It is relieved by bending forward, lying on the side and drawing the knees toward the chest. Crouching on all fours on the bed or floor also may provide pain relief. The pain may be increased by lying supine, and occasionally eating causes or exacerbates pain. Postprandial pain presumably is caused by intraductal secretory pressure behind a completely or partially obstructed pancreatic duct.

Somatic pain also occurs in pancreatic cancer and is characterized as sharp, well localized pain of short duration. It is referred from the pancreas and is finally mediated by thinly myelinated A delta fibers of the intercostal thoracic and lumbar nerves. By electrically stimulating the pancreas of humans during elective surgery,[63] it was surmised that lesions in the head of the pancreas produce pain in the epigastrium and to the right of midline, mediated by the right splanchnic nerves through the right sympathetic ganglia over the sixth to eleventh thoracic nerves. Cancer of the body of the pancreas produces pain in the epigastrium and left posterior intercostal spaces mediated by the left splanchnic nerves and sympathetic ganglia from the sixth thoracic to the first lumbar nerves. Somatic pain can be alleviated by blockade of the appropriate thoracic or lumbar nerves.

It is not certain why pancreatic cancer produces pain arising from the pancreas. Both mechanical compression by the expanding mass of tumor and invasion of the perineural spaces likely release bradykinin or prostaglandins, substances that

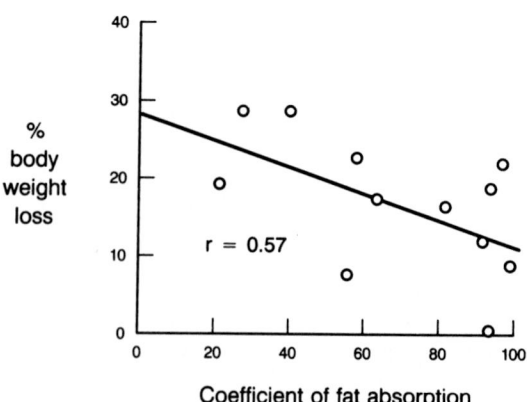

FIGURE 92-8. Relation of weight loss to fat absorption in pancreatic cancer. (Data from Perez MM, Newcomer AD, Moertel CG, et al. Assessment of weight loss, food intake, fat metabolism, malabsorption, and treatment of pancreatic insufficiency in pancreatic cancer. Cancer 1983;52:346.)

stimulate nociceptors that cause pain. This hypothesis is credible because aspirin and other nonsteroidal analgesics (inhibitors of prostaglandin formation from arachidonic acid) relieve pain in some patients.[64]

In the early stages of pancreatic cancer, pain arises from the pancreas by the previously described mechanisms. Later pain arises from a variety of anatomic sites, including an obstructed biliary tract or duodenum, lymph nodes, the retroperitoneum, and peritoneum, and may be associated with ascites. Diagnostic procedures (percutaneous aspiration biopsy, endoscopic retrograde cholangiopancreatography [ERCP]) or treatment (surgery, radiation therapy, chemotherapy) may also cause pain.

Jaundice

Jaundice is a presenting symptom in 80% to 90% of patients with cancer of the head of the pancreas and in 6% to 13% with carcinomas of the tail of the gland.[65,66] In patients with cancer of the tail of the pancreas, jaundice usually is the result of hepatic metastasis, with obstruction of the extrahepatic bile duct at the porta hepatis by lymphadenopathy secondary to metastases. The clinical aphorism that painless jaundice indicates pancreatic cancer should be discarded. Painless jaundice rarely if ever occurs in pancreatic cancer. Eliciting a careful history from jaundiced patients with pancreatic cancer reveals that all have pain.

Weight Loss

Weight loss of more than 10% ideal body weight is almost universal in patients with pancreatic cancer.[59,67] Weight loss approximates 18% of body weight and is caused by malabsorption, decreased calorie consumption, or both (Fig. 92-7). Weight loss, however, correlates with malabsorption (Fig. 92-8), but not calorie consumption.

It is likely that malabsorption plays a major role in weight loss in carcinomas of the head of the pancreas, but even in these patients, decreased food intake plays a role. Overall, if careful measurements are made, 50% of patients with cancer

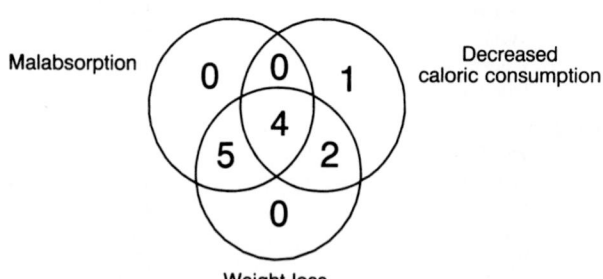

FIGURE 92-7. Malabsorption, decreased caloric consumption, and weight loss occur in patients with pancreatic cancer. (Data from Perez MM, Newcomer AD, Moertel CG, et al. Assessment of weight loss, food intake, fat metabolism, malabsorption, and treatment of pancreatic insufficiency in pancreatic cancer. Cancer 1983;52:346.)

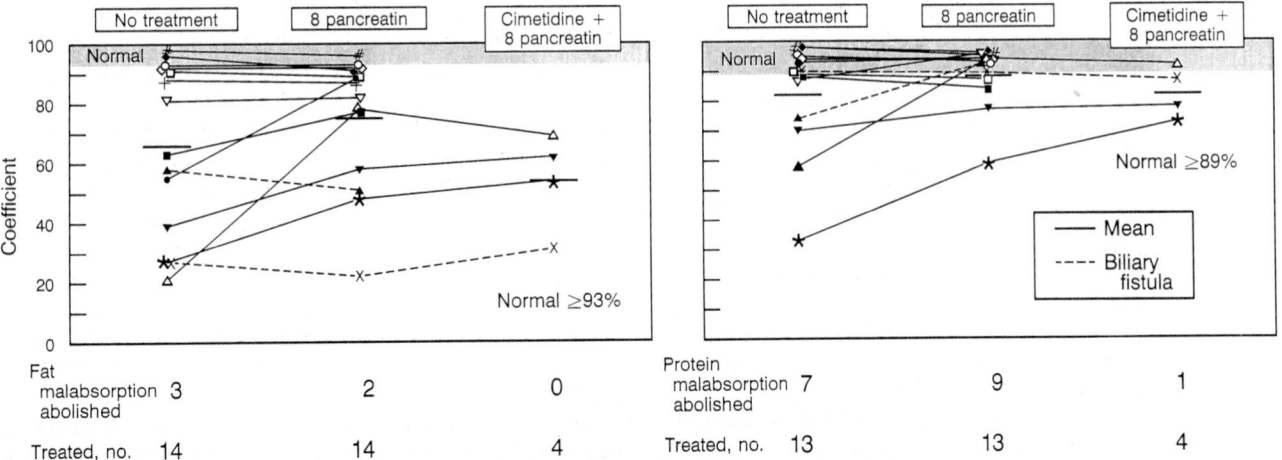

FIGURE 92-9. Coefficient of fat (*left*) and protein (*right*) absorption in patients with pancreatic cancer with no treatment and when receiving pancreatic extract. In one patient who had severe steatorrhea and did not improve with pancreatin, a biliary cutaneous fistula developed between the time of no treatment and administration of pancreatin (dashed line). (Data from Perez MM, Newcomer AD, Moertel CG, et al. Assessment of weight loss, food intake, fat metabolism, malabsorption, and treatment of pancreatic insufficiency in pancreatic cancer. Cancer 1983;52:346.)

of the pancreas will be found to have decreased consumption of calories,[67] and in patients with cancers of the body and tail, decreased food intake is a major contribution to weight loss. Fat malabsorption is more frequent (75%) and more severe than protein malabsorption (50%; Fig. 92-9). To my knowledge, no studies have been done to investigate carbohydrate malabsorption, but it probably occurs.

The major reason for malabsorption is reduced pancreatic secretion caused by tumor obstruction of the pancreatic duct. Decreased secretion of volume of fluid, bicarbonate, lipase, and trypsin from the pancreas[68] (Fig. 92-10) is not detectable until more than 60% of the total length of the pancreatic duct is obstructed. Thus, 40% of the gland proximal to the obstruction of the main duct (head of the gland) in patients with pancreatic cancer can secrete volume of fluid, bicarbonate, and enzymes at rates similar to those of healthy subjects. This finding may be the result of functional hyperplasia proximal to the obstruction. In animals, however, pancreatic en-

zyme secretion decreases before obstruction of the pancreatic duct.[69] Although carcinogenesis rather than obstruction may reduce pancreatic secretion, in experimental animal models it is difficult to separate the direct effects of the carcinogens on pancreatic secretion from those of carcinogenesis.

Diabetes Mellitus

There is a significant association between diabetes and pancreatic cancer, but the cause of the association and whether diabetes is a risk factor for pancreatic cancer has been controversial. The conclusion of a recent case control study was that diabetes in patients with pancreatic cancer is caused by the tumor.[70] Forty percent of patients with pancreatic cancer had concomitant diagnoses of cancer and diabetes, and in 16%, diabetes was diagnosed within 2 years before the diagnosis of cancer. There was no association between diabetes existing more than 3 years prior to the cancer diagnosis and the cancer. The association between diabetes and pancreatic cancer is the result of marked insulin resistance, probably secondary to increased levels of islet amyloid polypeptide (IAPP),[20a] a hormone secreted by beta cells that reduces insulin sensitivity in vivo and glycogen synthesis in vitro. Although resection of the tumor reduces IAPP levels, the source of the increased IAPP levels is mainly from islets in the noncancerous portion of the pancreas. The diabetes in most patients with pancreatic cancer is non–insulin-dependent. Consequently, manifestations of diabetes such as hyperphagia, polydipsia, and polyuria are rarely presenting features of pancreatic cancer.

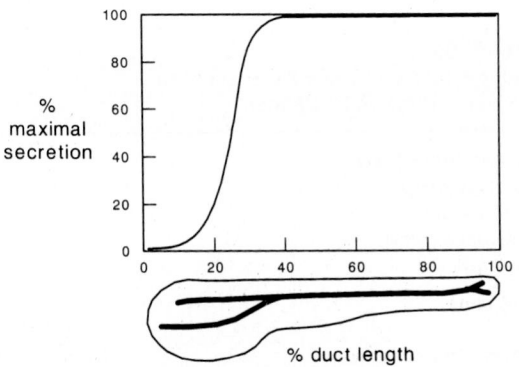

FIGURE 92-10. Relation of pancreatic enzyme secretion to the location of the ductal tumors. (Data from DiMagno EP, Malagelada J-R, Go VLW. The relationship between pancreatic ductal obstruction and pancreatic secretion in man. Mayo Clin Proc 1979;54:157.)

Other Clinical Features

Alterations in the character of the stools and stool habit occur commonly. Sixty-two percent of patients with cancer of the head of the pancreas may note light-colored stools,[66] but some patients with cancer in the head of the pancreas and up to 27% of patients with cancers of the tail of the gland may complain of constipation.[66] Patients with severe pancreatic insufficiency and gross steatorrhea have only slightly increased fecal weight, and not all have diarrhea.[71] Therefore, patients may have a relatively normal stool pattern (no diarrhea) or even constipation and yet have significant malabsorption that requires treatment with pancreatic enzymes.

Nonspecific signs and symptoms occur frequently, such as nausea, vomiting, weakness, and anorexia (30% to 36% of patients with cancers of the head or body and tail). Rare findings (<5% of patients) include superficial thrombophlebitis, gastrointestinal bleeding, psychiatric disturbance, and features related to diabetes mellitus. Gastrointestinal hemorrhage may occur as a late manifestation of direct invasion of the tumor into the stomach, duodenum, or colon. Bleeding varices may arise from direct invasion or compression of the splenic or portal vein by tumor, or secondary to obstructive pancreatitis caused by the tumor.

Depression usually is not a major problem, but depression and emotional lability as measured by the Minnesota Multiphasic Personality Inventory may occur in as many as 76% of patients with pancreatic cancer, compared with 20% of patients with other neoplasms.[72] It is unclear, however, whether these features are directly related to the pancreatic cancer or occur secondary to the chronic illness produced by the cancer.[73]

Physical Findings

At presentation, patients with pancreatic cancer of the head and patients with cancers of the body and tail of the gland have different findings. Hepatomegaly and jaundice are present in more than 80% of patients with cancer of the head of the pancreas.[65,66,74] Jaundice begins as scleral icterus and progresses to involve the skin. Pruritus may be a prominent symptom in some patients and leads to persistent scratching, which produces excoriation and lichenification. In contrast, patients with cancer of the body and tail of the pancreas may have abdominal tenderness and pain, but hepatomegaly and jaundice are present less than 30% of the time.

Courvoisier's sign (palpable gallbladder) is present in 30% of patients with carcinomas of the head of the pancreas. In carcinoma of the head or body and tail, an abdominal mass and ascites occur in less than 20% of patients. Ascites may be a sign of portal hypertension secondary to compression or occlusion of the portal or splenic vein by the tumor, and in this case may be accompanied by splenomegaly. Peripheral edema also may occur in association with ascites. An abdominal bruit is occasionally heard if the tumor compresses the aorta or splenic artery.

Diagnostic Investigations

Routine Clinical Tests

The mean values of some routine laboratory tests are statistically different in patients with pancreatic cancer compared to patients with pancreatitis, other cancers, or benign gastrointestinal disorders. A significant overlap of the values among these patient groups, however, limits the usefulness of the tests. Patients with pancreatic disease have higher values

for serum lipase, amylase, and glucose compared with other patients; however, these tests do not distinguish between pancreatic cancer and pancreatitis.[75] Levels of alkaline phosphatase, aspartate aminotransferase, and bilirubin are elevated in patients with pancreatic cancer, but these tests lack specificity in excluding benign hepatic disorders. Nevertheless, a battery of tests (Table 92-4) is recommended in patients suspected of having pancreatic cancer, including evaluation of pancreatic enzymes and radiography of the abdomen and chest.

If the enzyme levels are elevated, the suspicion of pancreatic disease increases, but further special tests are needed to make the diagnosis. Nonspecific findings such as bony lesions, pleural effusion, or ascites seen on chest and abdominal radiographs may indicate pancreatitis or pancreatic cancer. If pancreatic calcifications are seen on the abdominal films, a diagnosis of chronic pancreatitis can be made with 95% confidence. Pancreatic cancer, however, can develop in patients with calcific chronic pancreatitis, especially those with hereditary pancreatitis. Primary adenocarcinomas of the pancreas almost never calcify, but 10% of benign cystadenomas are characterized by a typical sunburst calcification,[76,77] and cavernous lymphangiomas of the pancreas may calcify.[78] Disappearance of calcifications of the pancreas has been reported to be a sign of pancreatic cancer, but it is a rare phenomenon.[79,80] Obvious pulmonary or bony metastases are diagnostic of metastatic cancer. If metastases are found, many physicians opt to perform no other diagnostic tests; others who are more aggressive obtain special tests to find the primary tumor.

Immunologic Tests

None of the available tumor markers is sensitive or specific enough to be used routinely in cancer screening or diagnosis.[81] These markers include hormones such as total thyroxine, insulin, gastrin, parathyroid hormone, and calcitonin; immunoglobulins (IgA, IgG, IgM); α-fetoprotein, pancreatic oncofetal antigen, and carcinoembryonic antigen (CEA).[75] Elevated CEA levels are present in up to 85% of patients with cancer of the pancreas. Unfortunately, 65% of patients with other cancers and 46% of patients with benign diseases also

---

TABLE 92-4
Routine Tests for Patients Suspected of Having Pancreatic Cancer

Blood and Urine Tests
Hematology group
Chemistry group
Total serum amylase*
Urinary amylase†

Radiographs
Chest
Abdominal for calcification

---

* Chosen because routinely available; if lipase or pancreatic isoamylase are available, they may be preferable.

† Measured because elevated for longer periods of time than total serum amylase.

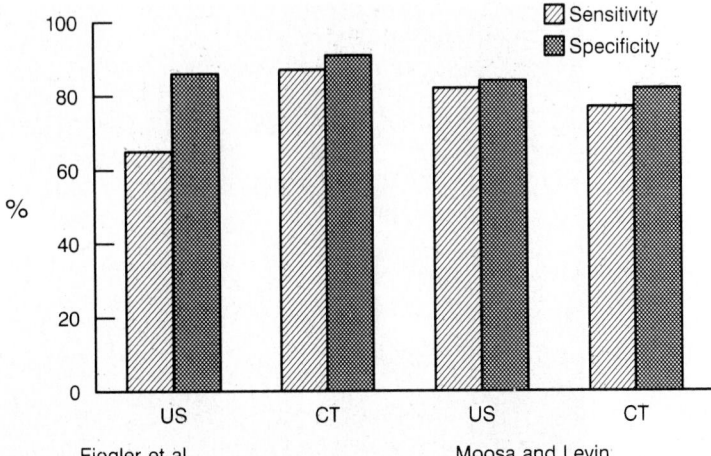

FIGURE 92-11. Sensitivity and specificity of ultrasonography (US) and computed tomography (CT) in diagnosis of pancreatic cancer. (Data from Fiegler W, Claussen C. Hedde JP. Comparison of computed tomography, automated multisector scanner [CTO-SON] and conventional ultrasound in pancreatic disease. ROFO 1984;140: 50; and Moossa AR, Levin B. Collaborative studies in the diagnosis of pancreatic cancer. Semin Oncol 1979;6: 298.)

have elevated CEA levels.[82–85] So far, antigens, including non–cross-reacting antigen (NCA), α_2-glycoprotein, β_2-microglobulin, CA 19-9, and DU-PAN-2 monoclonal antibodies have not proven to be clinically useful.

Some of the tumor markers have promise but require further testing. The leukocyte adherence inhibition test predicts the presence of cancer accurately in 80% of patients. Galactosyltransferase has a sensitivity of 67% for detection of pancreatic cancer.[86] When this test is combined with ultrasound, ERCP, or computed tomography (CT), the sensitivities of the combined tests are 80% to 100%.[86] A number of groups, including mine, have prospectively evaluated mouse hybridoma-generated monoclonal antibodies CA 19-9 and CA 125. In a study of more than 5000 patients,[87] CA 19-9 was positive in 100% of resectable lesions, whereas it was positive in only 53% of patients with advanced pancreatic cancer. It is also positive, however, in the presence of other neoplasms of the gastrointestinal tract such as gastric cancer, and has a false-positive rate of 11% in patients with pancreatitis and 2% in healthy subjects. Both CA 19-9 and CA 125 had approximately the same sensitivity, about 75%, which is somewhat better than that of CEA, which ranges from 25% to 62%.[88]

Use of tumor markers (CA 19-9, CA-50, DU-PAN-2, 47D10, SPAN-1, RA 96, PCAA, and Pa A) is summarized in a National Cancer Institute Tumor Marker Conference report.[81] Serum markers "might be helpful in confirming a diagnosis of pancreatic cancer and, in some instances, would be helpful in distinguishing benign from malignant pancreatic disease. However, their lack of tumor specificity and pancreas organ specificity made these serum markers unreliable for diagnosis when used by themselves."[81] Nevertheless, investigators continue to search for an inexpensive, sensitive, and specific marker to identify early pancreatic cancers.

Imaging Tests

The cornerstone for the diagnosis of pancreatic cancer is tests to image the pancreas, which include ultrasonography, CT scanning, ERCP, and ultrasonographic or CT-guided transcutaneous pancreatic biopsy. Radiolabeled selenium pancreatic scanning, thermography, and arteriography are no longer widely used because they are nonspecific, insensitive, and too expensive, respectively.

The sensitivity and specificity for ultrasonography and CT scanning are similar (80%) for the detection of a pancreatic mass or cancer[59,89–92] (Fig. 92-11). Because ultrasonography is less expensive and does not expose the patient to ionizing radiation, it should be used as the first special imaging test to diagnose pancreatic cancer (Fig. 92-12). When ultrasonography fails for technical reasons (10%), or if the diagnosis is uncertain (approximately 20%), CT scanning should be the next step (Fig. 92-13).

ERCP has a sensitivity and specificity of 90%[59,90] for the diagnosis of pancreatic cancer. Frequent abnormalities of ERCP in pancreatic cancer are pancreatic duct obstruction and encasement of the pancreatic duct. If the tumor is in the head of the gland, contiguous involvement of both the pancreatic and bile ducts may produce the double-duct sign, which indicates obstruction of the common bile duct and pancreatic duct (Fig. 92-14). In pancreatic cancer, the common duct obstruction is abrupt; in chronic pancreatitis, parenchymal fibrosis may cause obstruction of the distal common bile duct, but the narrowing is tapered. A tumor located in the parenchyma of the pancreas may be seen by forcing contrast media

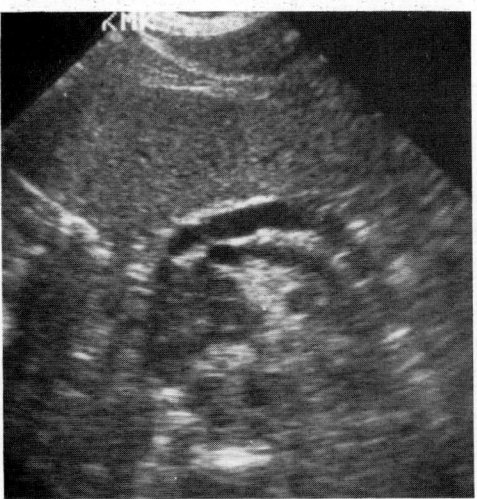

FIGURE 92-12. Ultrasonography of cancer of the head of the pancreas (hypoechoic mass) associated with dilated pancreatic duct.

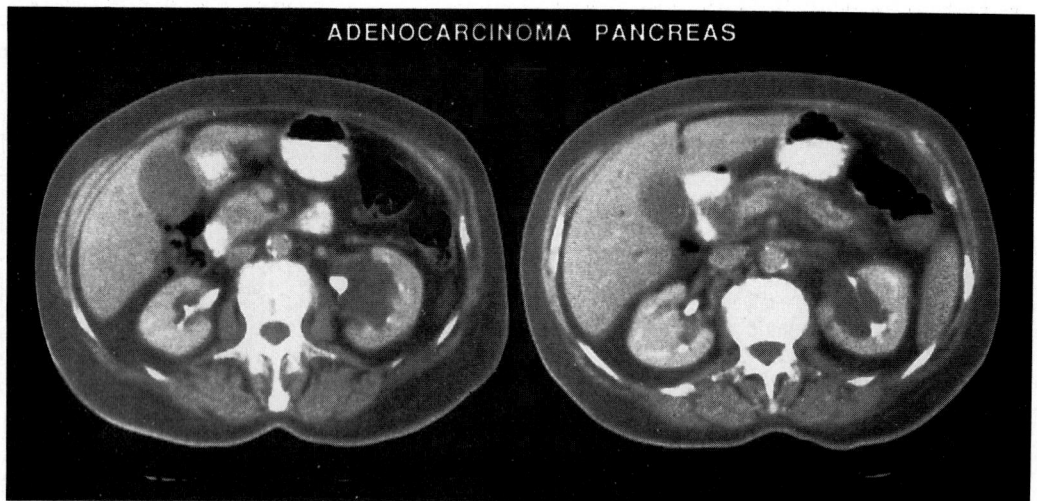

FIGURE 92-13. Computed tomography of pancreatic cancer shows a mass in the head of the pancreas (*left*) causing obstruction and dilation of the pancreatic duct (*right*).

into the entire collection system (acinarization), but this technique may cause acute pancreatitis. Filling of a tumor cavity during ERCP is a rare sign of pancreatic cancer.

Ultrasonographic or CT-guided percutaneous pancreatic biopsies have 90% sensitivity in diagnosing pancreatic cancer.[93,94] These procedures, however, are not indicated in patients who have resectable lesions, in which no metastases are detected and there is no extension of the tumor beyond the confines of the pancreas.

Newer imaging tests, such as endoscopic ultrasonography (EUS)[95] and magnetic resonance imaging, are not any more sensitive or specific than ultrasonography or CT scanning. Positron emission tomography has been evaluated in a few patients, but its accuracy in diagnosis is unknown, and it is expensive and not readily available. Availability of EUS is increasing. It is doubtful that it will be a major diagnostic test of pancreatic cancer, but it may be useful to stage tumors.

Function Tests

Secretin, cholecystokinin, or a combination of these hormones used to stimulate the pancreas after the patient is intubated have a sensitivity and specificity between 80% and 90%.[59]

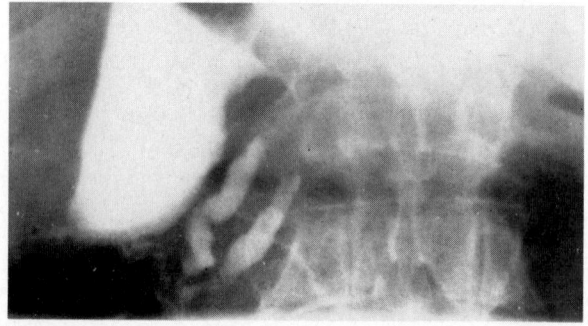

FIGURE 92-14. Endoscopic retrograde cholangiopancreatogram with double duct sign: abrupt cutoff of the bile and pancreatic ducts is secondary to cancer of the head of the pancreas.

Low outputs of pancreatic enzymes occur in 90% of patients with cancer of the pancreatic head and 70% of patients with cancer of the body and the tail of the gland.[96] Use of invasive pancreatic function tests to detect pancreatic cancer has declined sharply, however, because of the emergence of sensitive and specific imaging tests. Noninvasive tests of pancreatic function are simpler and less expensive than invasive tests, but they are not as reproducible and are too insensitive or nonspecific for use in the diagnosis of pancreatic cancer.[97] They include measurement of undigested food in stool or diminished products of digestion in breath; products of synthetic compounds that are hydrolyzed by intralumenal pancreatic enzymes, absorbed by the gut, and appear in blood and urine; and hormones that are decreased in the fasting state or after stimulation with hormones.

Staging

There is an increasing use of relatively accurate tests for preoperative staging of pancreatic cancers. Laparoscopy correctly identifies 85% of unresectable tumors.[98] The accuracy of EUS for T staging is 92%, and 74% for N staging.[99] In comparison to ultrasound, CT, and angiography, EUS is more sensitive for detecting portal vein involvement and lymph node metastasis.[100]

Summary of Diagnostic Approach

The first step in diagnosing pancreatic cancer is to recognize the patients who have a strong possibility of having the disease by their symptoms. Next, a routine battery of tests is performed that includes chemistry and hematology groups, chest and abdominal roentgenograms, and serum and urine pancreatic enzymes (Fig. 92-15).

Pancreatic disease has been identified with 90% sensitivity and specificity by a combination of ultrasonography, ERCP, and a pancreatic function test that requires gastrointestinal intubation and cholecystokinin stimulation[59] (Fig. 92-16). In the past, in patients suspected of having pancreatic cancer,

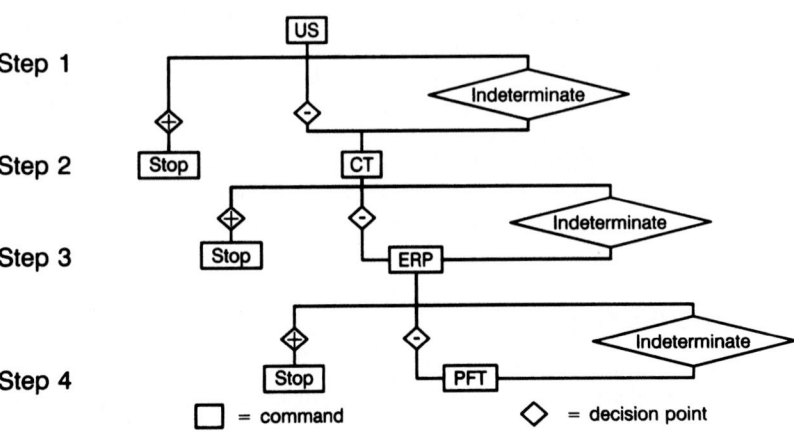

Step 1

Step 2

Step 3

Step 4

US
Indeterminate
Stop
CT
Stop
ERP
Indeterminate
Stop
PFT
Indeterminate
☐ = command   ◇ = decision point

FIGURE 92-15. Algorithm to diagnose pancreatic cancer if ultrasound (US), computed tomography (CT), endoscopic retrograde pancreatography (ERP), and pancreatic function test (PFT) are available. (From DiMagno EP. Overview: biology and diagnosis of pancreatic cancer. In: Levin B, ed. Annual clinical conference on cancer. Vol 30. Gastrointestinal cancer: current approaches to diagnosis and treatment. Houston: University of Texas Press, 1988:299.)

ultrasonography was recommended first because, in contrast to the other tests, it does not require ionizing radiation, is more widely available, is not invasive, and has the same sensitivity and specificity as CT scanning. If the results are negative or indeterminate, a CT scan should be done next, followed by ERCP. The pancreatic function test rarely is needed. This sequence of tests should identify pancreatic disease and make the differentiation between pancreatitis and cancer in 90% of patients[59] (see Fig. 92-16).

If diagnosis of pancreatitis is not apparent and no metastases are seen, a CT scan is done first. This test is usually the only additional test needed to make the diagnosis and to stage pancreatic cancer. Other tests that may be needed are ultrasonography or an ERCP. Thus, CT is the most time-saving and cost-effective test to use. If the cancer is deemed resectable, laparoscopy or EUS should be considered to determine if there is peritoneal seeding, small liver metastases, vascular invasion, or lymph node metastases.

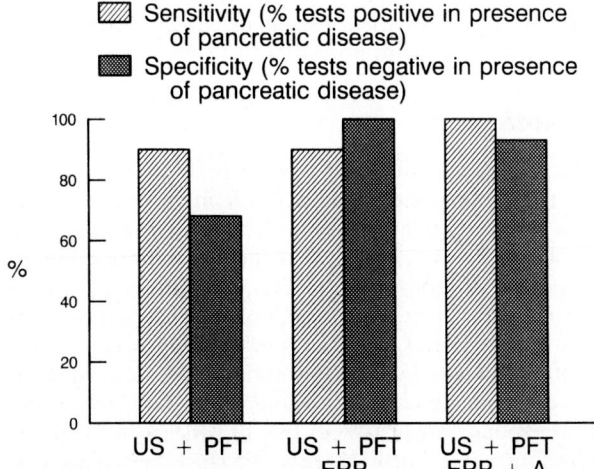

FIGURE 92-16. Sensitivity and specificity of combinations of tests in diagnosing pancreatic disease. (A, visceral arteriography; ERP, endoscopic retrograde pancreatography; PFT, pancreatic function test; US, ultrasound; from DiMagno EP, Malagelada J-R, Taylor WF, Go VLW. A prospective comparison of current diagnostic tests in pancreatic cancer. N Engl J Med 1977;297:737.)

Treatment

Surgery

Surgery provides the only chance for a cure. Unfortunately, as noted previously, only approximately 10% of patients with ductal cancer have resectable tumors.[2]

Pancreaticoduodenectomy, or Whipple's procedure, is the surgical treatment of choice for carcinomas of the head of the pancreas. High operative mortality rates up to 21%[101] have been associated with this procedure, mainly because of anastomotic leakage and hemorrhage at the pancreaticojejunostomy. In experienced hands, however, the mortality has been reported to be as low as 2% to 5%,[102–104] and the procedure offers the only realistic hope for cure.

Total pancreatectomy has been advocated by some because it offers the following theoretical advantages over Whipple's procedure: Removal of the entire pancreas ensures that multiple foci of carcinoma, which are present in 16% to 37% of pancreases, will not be the cause of recurrence; the operation eliminates the possibility of spread of the cancer by direct extension, intraductal seeding, and lymphatic dissemination; and total pancreatectomy eliminates the danger of an anastomotic leak from a pancreaticojejunostomy. There is no definite evidence, however, that total pancreatectomy is superior to Whipple's procedure in terms of operative mortality, postoperative complications, or survival. This position is supported by at least two studies that showed lymph node involvement does not affect 5-year survival[105,106] (see Fig. 92-3). Others found that lymph node involvement profoundly affects 5-year survival rates.[107,108] Perhaps the reason for this discrepancy is the size of the tumor at operation. Tsuchiya and associates reported that patients in Japan with tumors less than 2 cm in diameter treated with Whipple's procedure have a 37% 5- and 10-year survival.[109] These data from Japan are encouraging and support the hypothesis that early pancreatic cancer is curable by pancreaticoduodenectomy. Unfortunately, at this time most pancreatic tumors in patients in the United States are larger than 2 cm. Other operations that have been used include the regional pancreatectomy proposed by Fortner[110] and the pylorus-preserving pancreaticoduodenal resection.[111] The former procedure has been used when the major vessels are invaded by tumor and involves the reconstruction of one or more of these vessels by anastomosis or with grafts. This radical operation has not gained acceptance because it is attended by high mortality and morbidity and no increase in survival compared with the conventional Whipple's operation. The pylorus-preserving operation is used mainly in the surgical treatment of benign pancreatic disease and cancers of the lower duodenum and ampulla rather than as surgical treatment of pancreatic cancer because it may compromise the chance of complete removal of cancer from surgical margins.

Palliative Surgery

Palliative procedures by definition are performed to relieve symptoms of biliary or duodenal obstruction, or both, and pain.

Biliary obstruction. To relieve biliary obstruction, cholecystojejunostomy is the internal drainage procedure of choice unless the cystic duct enters the common duct close to the tumor, in which case a choledochojejunostomy should be performed. An alternative to palliative surgical treatment of biliary tract obstruction is placement of stents in the biliary tree by percutaneous combined radiologic and endoscopic methods, or by endoscopy alone. The endoscopic placement is the established method for the temporary relief of jaundice.[112] In a controlled trial of percutaneous versus endoscopic stenting in patients with malignant obstruction, patients who were randomized to the endoscopic method had greater relief of jaundice (81% vs. 61%) and lower 30-day mortality (15% vs. 3%).[113] The higher mortality after percutaneous stent placement was associated with hemorrhage and bile leaks secondary to liver puncture.

Endoscopic stenting is as successful as surgical decompression of biliary tract obstruction. In retrospective studies it appears that the 30-day mortality is 8% to 30% for surgical and 10% for endoscopic methods.[112,114,115] A major problem in these comparisons, however, is that low-risk patients may be selected for surgery, whereas high-risk patients receive stenting.[116,117] Endoscopic stenting, however, may be associated with late morbidity. In a retrospective study, recurrent jaundice occurred in almost 40% of patients and the median interval to recurrent jaundice was 154 days.[112] A major cause of recurrent jaundice is clogging of the endoprosthesis, which occurred in approximately 20% of the patients, mostly as a terminal event. Duodenal obstruction also occurs in 5% to 15% of patients.[112,118]

In a preliminary retrospective study, Dowsett and colleagues[118] reported that 85% of 403 patients with pancreatic cancer treated with endoscopic stenting had successful drainage, 2% of patients had major complications, 2% had procedure-related mortality, and 5% had late surgery for duodenal obstruction. This same group reported preliminary results of a prospective, randomized trial to compare surgical bypass and endoscopic stenting in patients with malignant obstructive jaundice.[119] Endoscopic stenting and surgical bypass were equally successful in relieving jaundice (94% with each procedure), but endoscopic stenting had lower morbidity (23% vs. 43%), procedure-related mortality (0% vs. 10%), and 30-day mortality (15% vs. 6%). There was no statistical difference in overall survival (life table), and stenting was associated with increases in late morbidity. Duodenal obstruc-

tion (14% vs. 3%) and recurrent jaundice (17% vs. 3%) occurred more frequently with endoscopic stenting. It appears that the size of the endoscopic stent (3.3 mm [10 Fr] vs. 3.96 mm [12 Fr]) does not affect the rate of stent change or the overall complication rates, but large stents are more difficult to place.[120] In a prospective, randomized trial, the Middlesex group was able successfully to place 12 Fr stents in 51%, whereas 10 Fr stents were placed successfully in 98% of patients.[111]

Obviously, patients who are at high surgical risk or have short life expectancy (1–3 months) should undergo endoscopic stent placement. A double bypass procedure, however, should be done if a nonresectable tumor is found at surgery or patients have a nonresectable tumor by diagnostic tests but have an expected life expectancy of 6 to 7 months.

Duodenal obstruction. Complete duodenal obstruction is uncommon in patients with pancreatic cancer; it usually occurs by invasion of the third or fourth part of the duodenum in 5% to 15% of patients—usually as a preterminal event.[112,118] Incomplete or functional obstruction occurs in 40% to 60% of patients. Unappreciated is the finding that abnormal gastric emptying occurs in up to 60% of patients who have no evidence of gastroduodenal obstruction.[121] These data suggest that all patients undergoing surgery who are found to have a nonresectable tumor should have a gastrojejunostomy performed. A prophylactic gastrojejunostomy during the initial operation should be strongly considered if postoperative chemotherapy or radiation therapy is to be undertaken, because a second operation after such therapy is hazardous. Many surgeons, however, advocate a gastrojejunostomy only when obstruction is present or imminent, and have challenged the concept of a prophylactic gastroenterostomy.[122]

In symptomatic patients who have not had a gastroenterostomy and in whom gastric stasis develops without organic obstruction, a combination of a cholinergic agent (bethanechol, 25 mg three times day) and a prokinetic agent (metoclopramide, 10 mg four times a day) might enhance gastric emptying. Metoclopramide has been used successfully to alleviate symptoms of gastroparesis in patients with delayed gastric emptying due to neoplasm.[123]

Chemotherapy

Neither single nor combined agents have been shown to prolong life or enhance the quality of life in patients with pancreatic cancer. Single agents that have been tested and have been shown to have an effect in reducing tumor size, but not survival, are 5-fluorouracil, (5-FU), mitomycin C, streptozotocin, doxorubicin, epirubicin, ifosfamide, semustine, and high-dose methotrexate. Dactinomycin, doxorubicin, carmustine, standard-dose methotrexate, cisplatin, melphalan, and L-asparaginase have no obvious effect. 5-FU produces a partial response rate in 10% to 15% of patients and a median survival time of less than 20 weeks.[124] The other agents (e.g., mitomycin C) have either similar or less effect. High-dose methotrexate and ifosfamide are toxic and not used. In contrast to early reports, the FAM protocol (5-FU, doxorubicin, and mitomycin C) in a large study of 144 patients has been shown to be no better than treatment with 5-FU alone.[125] Similarly, FAMM$_c$ (5-FU, doxorubicin, mitomycin C, and semustine) and SMF (streptozotocin, mitomycin C, and 5-FU) have not produced significantly different results than treatment with 5-FU alone.[126]

There is little role for the routine clinical use of chemotherapy in patients with nonresectable pancreatic cancer. Even enthusiastic chemotherapists[127] allow that chemotherapy prolongs life in only 30% of patients, and prolongation of life is 4 to 5 months in half the patients and 2 to 4 months in the rest, and virtually no 5-year survivors have been reported. It is of vital importance to continue investigation of chemotherapy; patients undergoing chemotherapy should be in prospective, randomized trials.

Radiation Treatment

Randomized trials have demonstrated that the combination of 5-FU and radiation therapy or SMF and radiation therapy improves survival compared with radiation therapy or chemotherapy alone.[128] Improvements in radiation treatment include the addition of intraoperative electron beam radiation (4500–5500 cGy)[129] and ^{125}I implants (120–210 cGy).[130] Although these modalities may limit local progression of the tumor, there has been no significant change in survival compared with extended external beam therapy alone because of the inability to control liver and peritoneal metastases.

Management of Malabsorption

When fat and protein malabsorption occur, pancreatic enzyme replacement should be instituted. One regimen for pancreatic enzyme replacement is ingestion of eight tablets of Viokase with meals containing 25 g of fat.[68] Two tablets are ingested immediately after the patient eats a few bites of the meal, two tablets at the end of the meal, and the remaining four tablets interspersed during the meal.[130–132] Common mistakes that are made in prescribing and implementing enzyme replacement therapy include failure to provide sufficient lipase, patients ingesting the tablets before meals, and failure to provide enzyme replacement with snacks.

The amount of enzyme replacement recommended is the amount of lipase theoretically needed to abolish steatorrhea. In pancreatic insufficiency,[133] we found that steatorrhea occurs when lipase delivery is below 10% of normal and that steatorrhea is abolished when peak postprandial duodenal lipase concentrations are greater than 5% of normal.[131] In severe pancreatic insufficiency,[130–132] at least 30,000 IU of lipase must be ingested to achieve these postprandial levels. This amount of lipase abolishes steatorrhea if at least 7500 IU of lipase is emptied from the stomach per hour postprandially, and if no inactivation of lipase activity occurs. These assumptions are not usually met in the clinical situation because lipase is inactivated by gastric acid. In most patients, however, steatorrhea is significantly improved, but not abolished. Whether enteric-coated microencapsulated preparations that allegedly have more lipase activity than standard pancreatin (e.g., Viokase) alleviate steatorrhea more frequently than Viokase has not been investigated. They nevertheless should be tried if malabsorption is not improved by pancreatin. The addition of H_2 blockers (cimetidine) did not improve steatorrhea in a small number of patients with pancreatic cancer (see Fig. 92-9).

Control of Pain

Most patients with pain caused by pancreatic cancer can be successfully managed by drug therapy if the following principles are kept in mind: Prescribe analgesics on a regular basis; if narcotic analgesics are needed, use adequate doses; and use adjuvant drugs when necessary.

In patients with mild to moderate pain, the drugs of choice are aspirin, acetaminophen, and nonsteroidal antiinflammatory drugs (Table 92-5). If one drug of this class does not provide significant relief, try another. Eventually, if this group of drugs fails to relieve pain, opioid analgesics should be used.

TABLE 92-5
Dose Ranges of Commonly Used Oral Analgesics

DRUG	MILD TO MODERATE PAIN (mg)*	SEVERE PAIN (mg)†
Non-narcotics		
Aspirin	650‡	
Choline magnesium trisalicylate (Trilisate)	1500–300	
Acetaminophen	650‡	
Ibuprofen (Motrin)	200–400	
Fenoprofen (Nalfon)	200–400	
Diflunisal (Dolobid)	500–1000	
Naproxen (Naprosyn)	250–500	
Morphine-like Agonists		
Morphine		60
Codeine	32–65†	200+
Oxycodone	5–10‡	30
Levorphanol (Levo-Dromoran)		4
Hydromorphone (Dilaudid)		7.5
Meperidine (Demerol)	50–100†	300+
Propoxyphine hydrochloride (Darvon)	65–130	
Propoxyphene napsylate (Darvon-N)	50	
Oxymorphone (Numorphan)		10
Methadone (Dolophine)		20
Mixed Agonist–Antagonists		
Pentazocine (Talwin)	50	60
Partial Agonists		
Buprenorphine (Temgesic SL)		0.8

SL, sublingual.

* For these equianalgesic doses, the time of peak analgesia ranges from 1.5 to 2 h and the duration from 4 to 6 h. Oxycodone and meperidine are shorter acting (3–5 h) and diflunisal and naproxen are longer acting (8–12 h).

† Based on single-dose studies in which an intramuscular dose of each drug listed was compared with morphine to establish the relative potency. Oral doses are those recommended when changing from a parenteral to an oral route. For patients without prior narcotic exposure, the recommended oral starting dose is 30 mg for morphine, 5 mg for methadone, 2 mg for levorphanol, and 4 mg for hydromorphone.

‡ These are the recommended starting doses from which the optimal dose for each patient is determined by titration, and the maximal dose limited by adverse effects.

Adapted from Foley KM. Pain syndromes and pharmacologic management of pancreatic cancer pain. Journal of Pain and Symptom Management 1988;3: 176.

Opioid analgesics, in contrast to nonopioid analgesics, do not have a "ceiling" effect; the loss of pain is linear as the dose is increased on a logarithmic scale until unconsciousness supervenes. Thus, the dose of opioid is governed by side effects and sensitivity to the drugs. Unfortunately, elderly patients (the population of patients with pancreatic cancer) are more sensitive to loss of mental function and to constipation. Thus, it is wise to begin treatment with half the recommended dose (see Table 92-5) and the dosing schedule should be based on plasma half-life.

In patients with severe pain, if an opioid drug is no longer effective or produces side effects, another opioid should be substituted at half the equianalgesic dose (see Table 92-5). Before deciding a particular drug regimen is ineffective, the drug must be given at regular intervals at appropriate doses. Most patients remain at a stable dose of opioid. Escalation of the dose usually signals progression of disease and occurs most commonly in terminally ill patients. Concern regarding drug addiction and drug dependence in patients with progressive pancreatic cancer is inappropriate. Enough drug must be given to keep patients comfortable.

The most important side effects that limit increasing the dose are sedation and drowsiness. If these symptoms are not desirable, they may be managed by decreasing the dose and using more frequent dosing intervals, or switching to another drug. Nausea and vomiting due to opioid drugs are best treated by switching to another drug or using an antiemetic. Chlorpromazine, haloperidol, or cyclizine have been used in the past, but metoclopramide has been used successfully in patients being treated with opioids. There have been no controlled studies to investigate the appropriate treatment of constipation arising from use of opioids, but a regimen of anthraquinone derivatives, especially senna compounds, has been reported to be effective in preventing narcotic-induced constipation in patients with cancer.[134] One half of a Senokot tablet is alleged to reverse the constipating effect of 60 mg of codeine or the equivalent dose of another opioid.

Most patients can be successfully managed with aspirin and the combination of aspirin and codeine. The combinations of an opioid plus an antihistamine (100 mg hydroxyzine intramuscularly) or an opioid plus an amphetamine (10 mg dextroamphetamine intramuscularly) have been advised by some authorities.[135] Combinations such as an opioid plus a benzodiazepine or an opioid plus a phenothiazine increase sedation but not analgesia.[136]

Most patients should be managed by oral regimens, but a few require subcutaneous or intramuscular medications. The subcutaneous route is less painful and preferred. The intravenous route should be avoided. One innovation has been the development of patient-controlled analgesia.[137] With this method, a small battery-operated pump is used to deliver opiate subcutaneously. Injections are given by the patient, who obtains a dose by pressing a button. Pumps are programmed with safeguards to prevent overdose. An even newer innovation is the development of epidural administration of narcotics, which produces analgesia with low doses of narcotics and, consequently, few side effects.[137] Although neither of these techniques has been approved for general use, these methods may be extremely beneficial in treating patients in severe pain secondary to advanced pancreatic cancer.

The use of neurolytic celiac plexus block has greatly sim-plified the treatment of pain in patients with pancreatic cancer. Alcohol injection into the ganglion either intraoperatively or transcutaneously, using biplane radiographs or CT scans, affords pain relief in most patients. In three series of 20,[138] 28,[139] and 13[140] patients, 92% had complete pain relief. In a single large series of 100 patients (97 with pancreatic cancer and 3 with chronic pancreatitis),[141] 60, 34, and 6 patients had marked, good, and ineffective analgesia, respectively. We find that celiac plexus block is a very effective means to control pain, and the method is attended by few serious complications. In the studies referred to here (total 161 patients), 2 patients had serious neurologic complications and 2 patients had transient radicular pain that improved. Paraplegia has been reported to have developed in an additional patient after a celiac plexus block with phenol.[142]

LESS COMMON EXOCRINE PANCREATIC TUMORS

Mucinous Cystadenocarcinoma

Formerly, mucinous cystic pancreatic neoplasms were divided into mucinous cystadenoma and mucinous cystadenocarcinoma. Both these lesions, however, should be considered malignant neoplasms because there have been numerous reports of supposedly benign mucinous cystadenomas recurring and metastasizing,[143,144] and when they are carefully examined, foci of malignant transformation may be seen.

The tumors are large, bulky, unilobular or multilobulated cysts containing mucin and are usually larger than 5 cm in diameter. Peripheral curvilinear calcifications of the fibrous capsule may occur. The cysts are lined with mucinous columnar epithelium that forms papillary projections and may contain foci of atypical or invasive adenocarcinoma.

Microcystic cystadenomas, by contrast, have no malignant potential. The multiple cysts of this condition are less than 1 to 2 cm in diameter. The cysts contain glycogen-rich fluid, and one third have a central scar with a stellate "sunburst" calcification. Women are more commonly afflicted; the mean age at diagnosis is 65 years.

Mucinous cystic neoplasms occur more commonly in women (6 : 1 female-to-male ratio) and present between the ages of 40 and 60 years as epigastric pain or discomfort. Because the pain may simulate chronic pancreatitis, and a cystic lesion is found on imaging tests, it may be considered a pancreatic pseudocyst and drained. Differentiation of cystadenoma from a pancreatic pseudocyst secondary to chronic pancreatitis may be difficult with imaging tests. The absence of historic features that may give rise to benign pancreatic disease such as trauma, previous pancreatitis, alcohol, and biliary tract diseases, however, should raise the suspicion of a cystic neoplasm. In a Mayo Clinic series of 45 patients with cystadenoma, the mean age at onset was 55 years.[145] Pain, weight loss, and nausea and vomiting occurred in 56%, 40%, and 25% of patients, respectively. Jaundice was uncommon because most cystadenomas arise in the body and tail of the pancreas. Even a tumor that originates in the head of the gland may not be associated with jaundice because fistulas between the biliary tract, cyst, and the gut may spontaneously arise that drain the biliary tract and prevent jaundice from occurring.

Although the diagnosis of a cystic neoplasm can be suggested by CT scanning or ultrasonography, a definite diagnosis can be made only by pathologic confirmation. Because of the possible confusion between a pseudocyst and a cystic neoplasm, biopsy samples of the wall of all suspected pseudocysts should be obtained before a drainage procedure.

Although mucinous cystic neoplasms are large and bulky and may reach sizes as large as 30 cm in diameter, they should be resected because the outcome is very favorable. In comparison to usual ductal carcinomas, 5-year survival rates may be as high as 50%.

Giant Cell Tumors

Giant cell tumors have a variety of morphologic features, but are characterized by the presence of bizarre giant cells and sarcomatoid cells supported by minimal fibrous tissue. Four distinct histologic types have been identified: spindle cell, malignant giant cell, pleomorphic, and anaplastic tumors.[146] All patients with these tumors have a poor prognosis. Most giant cell tumors have a worse prognosis (median survival of 2 months) than the common ductal carcinoma, and in one series,[147] all pleomorphic cancers had metastases at the time of diagnosis.

Occasional giant cell tumors are associated with prolonged survival, however. For example, one patient had only a biopsy performed and lived 10 months, whereas another patient underwent a total pancreatectomy and lived at least 15 years.[146] It has been reported that these patients with giant cell tumors and prolonged survival have, in addition to large pleomorphic and spindle cells, benign-appearing osteoblast-like cells.

Acinar Cell Tumor

Acinar cell carcinomas are uncommon and characterized by acinar arrangements supported by minimal fibrous stroma. Although the tumor cells contain no stainable amylase, zymogen granules are identifiable by electron microscopy,[148] and some patients may have elevated serum lipase levels and associated nonsuppurative panniculitis of the extremities and bone marrow, and manifest subcutaneous nodules and polyarthritis.[149] These tumors usually occur in the elderly and are rare in children.[150]

Pancreaticoblastoma

Another rare tumor, pancreaticoblastoma, occurs almost exclusively in children (15 months to 17 years of age).[151,152] This tumor may be encapsulated and have a relatively benign course or be a poorly defined, nonencapsulated tumor with a bad prognosis because it spreads into adjacent organs and recurs after resection. Pancreaticoblastoma has two general histologic types and may arise from the ventral or dorsal anlage of the pancreas. The encapsulated form[151] is composed of a distinct organoid pattern that contains squamous corpuscles and acinar cells with zymogen granules, whereas the undifferentiated, nonencapsulated form consists of primitive epithelium and mesenchyme.

Diagnosis of this rare tumor is important because it may have a favorable outcome and should be approached with aggressive surgery. For example, Horie and associates reported that 8 of 13 children with the encapsulated pancreaticoblastoma were living 6 months to 16 years after operation.[151,152]

Solid and Papillary Epithelial Neoplasm

Solid and papillary epithelial tumors are uncommon and arise from the epithelium of small ducts.[153] Grossly, the lesion averages 10 cm in size and usually occur in the pancreatic tail. A variable amount of hemorrhage and liquefaction necrosis occurs, resulting in pseudopapillae and cysts. This tumor's morphologic variability has given rise to other names, including papillary and epithelial carcinoma and papillary and cystic neoplasm.

This tumor is a distinct clinical entity, different from other pancreatic tumors that it might superficially resemble, such as cystadenocarcinoma or nonfunctioning islet cell tumors. It occurs almost entirely in young women who seek medical attention because of abdominal pain and an enlarging abdominal mass. Although CT scanning or ultrasound images may suggest a serous cystadenoma (microcystic), mucinous cystadenocarcinoma, nonfunctioning islet cell carcinoma, or ductal carcinoma, the presence of blood within the cyst and the lack of metastases should suggest the possibility of a solid and papillary epithelial neoplasm.[154] Resection of the tumor usually is associated with an excellent prognosis.[155]

Mucin-Producing Pancreatic Cancer or Mucinous Ductal Ectasis

This entity was originally described by Ohashi and Takagi.[156] There is debate whether the lesion is part of the spectrum of mucinous adenocarcinoma. Warshaw[157] suggests the term "mucinous ductal ectasis," whereas Yamada and colleagues prefer "mucin-producing cystic tumor."[158] The latter claim that 50% of the lesions arise from and are confined to the main duct; the rest arise from branch ducts and develop into mucinous cystic neoplasms.

Clinically,[159] patients may have chronic pancreatic pain from chronic pancreatitis that can occur secondary to obstruction of the pancreatic duct by intraductal tumor growth. Acute pancreatic or biliary (colic) pain can occur because of obstruction of the pancreatic or bile duct by globules of mucus. The most striking finding is the observation of globs of mucus emanating from the sphincter of Oddi at the time of ERCP.[159] Approximately half of the lesions show papillary malignant changes, but even these tumors have a better prognosis than usual ductal adenocarcinomas.[160] The natural history of benign papillary lesions is not known, but conventional wisdom is to treat by pancreatectomy.

The reader is directed to Chapter 91, Chronic Pancreatitis; Chapter 117, Endoscopic Retrograde Cholangiopancreatography, Endoscopic Sphincterotomy and Stone Removal, and Endoscopic Biliary and Pancreatic Drainage; Chapter 121, Ultrasonography; and Chapter 123, Applications of Computed Tomography to the Gastrointestinal Tract.

REFERENCES

1. Riela A, Zinsmeister AR, Melton LJ, et al. Increasing incidence of pancreatic cancer among women in Olmsted County, Minnesota, 1940 through 1988. Mayo Clin Proc 1992;67:839.
2. Silverberg E, Lubera JA. Cancer statistics 1988. CA 1988;38:5.
3. van Heerden JA, Heath PM, Alden CR. Biliary bypass for ductal adenocarcinoma of the pancreas: Mayo Clinic experience, 1970–1975. Mayo Clin Proc 1980;55:537.
4. Gordis L, Gold EB. Epidemiology and etiology of pancreatic cancer. In: Go VLW, DiMagno EP, Gardner JD, et al, eds. The pancreas: biology, pathobiology and diseases. New York: Raven Press, 1993:837.
5. Kessler II. A genetic relationship between diabetes and cancer. Lancet 1970;1:218.
6. Wynder EL, Mabuchi K, Maruchi N, Fortner JG. Epidemiology of cancer of the pancreas. J Natl Cancer Inst 1973;50:645.
7. Schwartz SS, Seidler A, Moossa AR, et al. Prospective study of glucose tolerance, insulin, C-peptide and glucagon responses in patients with pancreatic carcinoma. Am J Dig Dis 1978;23:1107.
8. Lowenfels AB, Maisonneuve P, Cavillini G, et al, and the International Pancreatitis Study Group. Pancreatitis and the risk of pancreatic cancer. N Engl J Med 1993;328:1433.
9. Castlemen B, Scully R, McNeely BU. Case records of the Massachusetts General Hospital: case 25-1972. N Engl J Med 1972;1286:1353.
10. Gross JB. Hereditary pancreatitis. In: Go VLW, Gardner JD, Brooks FP, et al, eds. The exocrine pancreas: biology, pathobiology and diseases. New York: Raven Press, 1986:193.
11. Maringhini A, Thiruvengadam R, Melton LJ, et al. Pancreatic cancer risk following gastric surgery. Cancer 1987;60:245.
12. Maringhini A, Moreau JA, Melton LJ, et al. Gallstones, gallbladder cancer and other gastrointestinal malignancies. Ann Intern Med 1987;107:30.
13. Hendricks JC, DiMagno EP, Dozois RR, Go VLW. Reflux of duodenal contents into the pancreatic duct of dogs. J Lab Clin Med 1980;96:912.
14. DiMagno EP, Shorter RG, Taylor WF, Go VLW. Relationships between pancreaticobiliary ductal anatomy and pancreatic ductal and parenchymal histology. Cancer 1982;49:361.
15. Turner HM, Grace HG. An investigation into cancer mortality among males in certain Sheffield trades. Journal of Hygiene 1938;38:90.
16. Mancuso TF, El-Attar AA. A cohort study of workers exposed to betanaphthylamine and benzidine. J Occup Med 1967;9:277.
17. Redmond CK, Strobino BR, Cypress RH. Cancer experience among coke by-product workers. Ann NY Acad Sci 1976;271:102.
18. Li FP, Fraumeni JF Jr, Mantel N, Miller RW. Cancer mortality among chemists. J Natl Cancer Inst 1969;43:1159.
19. Gold EB, Gordis L, Diener M, et al. Diet and other risk factors for cancer of the pancreas. Cancer 1985;55:460.
20. Mack TM, Paganini-Hill A. Epidemiology of pancreas cancer in Los Angeles. Cancer 1981;47:1474.
21. Hoar KS, Pell SA. A retrospective cohort study of mortality and cancer incidence among chemists. J Occup Med 1981;23:485.
22. Wynder EL. An epidemiological evaluation of the causes of cancer of the pancreas. Cancer Res 1975;35:2228.
23. Segi M, Kurihara M, Matsuyama T. Cancer mortality for selected sites in 24 countries: no. 5, 1964–1965. Sendai, Japan: Department of Public Health, Tohoku University School of Medicine, 1969.
24. Cohen LA. Diet and cancer. Sci Am 1987;257:42.
25. Lin RS, Kessler II. A multifactorial model for pancreatic cancer in man: epidemiologic evidence. JAMA 1981;245:147.
26. MacMahon B, Yen S, Trichopoulos D, et al. Coffee and cancer of the pancreas. N Engl J Med 1981;304:630.
27. Doll R, Peto R. Mortality in relation to smoking: 20 years' observations of male British doctors. Br Med J 1981;245:147.
28. Kahn HA. The Dorn study of smoking and mortality among

U.S. veterans: report on eight and one-half years of observation. Natl Cancer Inst Monogr 1966;19:1.
29. Durbec JP, Cheviollotte G, Bidart JM, et al. Diet, alcohol, tobacco and risk of cancer of the pancreas: a case-control study. Br J Cancer 1983;47:463.
30. Feinstein AR, Horwitz RI, Spitzer MD, Bottista RM. Coffee and pancreatic cancer: the problems of etiologic science and epidemiologic case control research. JAMA 1981;246:957.
31. Goldstein HR. No associations found between coffee and cancer of the pancreas (letter). N Engl J Med 1982;306:947.
32. Jick H, Dinan BJ. Coffee and pancreatic cancer (letter). Lancet 1982;2:92.
33. Heuch I, Kvale G, Jacobsen BK, Bjelke E. Use of alcohol, tobacco and coffee, and risk of pancreatic cancer. Br J Cancer 1983;48:637.
34. Nomura A, Stemmermann GN, et al. Coffee and pancreatic cancer. Lancet 1981;2:415.
35. Whittemore AS, Paffenbarger RS Jr, Anderson K, Halpern J. Early precursors of pancreatic cancer in college men. J Chronic Dis 1983;36:251.
36. Scarpelli DG, Reddy JK, Longnecker DS, eds. Experimental pancreatic carcinogenesis. Boca Raton, FL: CRC Press, 1987.
37. Pour P, Krüger FW, Althoff J, et al. A new approach for induction of pancreatic neoplasms. Cancer Res 1975;35;2259.
38. Longnecker DS, Crawford BG. Hyperplastic nodules and adenomas of exocrine pancreas in azaserine-treated rats. J Natl Cancer Inst 1974;53:573.
39. Parsa I, Marsh W H. An in vitro model of pancreatic carcinoma: morphology and in vivo growth. Am J Pathol 1976;84:469.
40. Scarpelli D G, Rao M S. Transplantable ductal adenocarcinoma of the Syrian hamster pancreas. Cancer Res 1979;39:452.
41. Ornitz DM, Hammer RE, Messing A, et al. Pancreatic neoplasm induced by SV40 T-antigen expression in acinar cells of transgenic mice. Science 1987;236:188.
42. Birt DF, Pour PM. Pancreatic cancer enhancement in the hamster model by diets high in fat and/or protein. In: Scarpelli DG, Reddy JK, Longnecker DS, eds. Experimental pancreatic carcinogenesis. Boca Raton, FL: CRC Press, 1987:175.
43. Roebuck BD. Enhancement of pancreatic carcinogenesis in the rat by dietary fats. In: Scarpelli DG, Reddy JK, Longnecker DS, eds. Experimental pancreatic carcinogenesis. Boca Raton, FL: CRC Press, 1987:187.
44. Chang B, Gutman P. Chemotherapy of pancreatic adenocarcinoma: initial report on two transplantable models in the Syrian hamster. Cancer Res 1982;42:2666.
45. Vogelstein B, Kinzler D. p53 function and dysfunction. Cell 1992;70:523.
46. Finlay CA, Hinds PW, Tan TH et al. Activating mutations for transformation by p53 produce a gene product that forms an hsc70-p53 complex with an altered half life. Mol Cell Biol 1988;8:351.
47. Almoguera C, Shibata D, Forrester D, et al. Most human carcinomas of the human exocrine pancreas contain mutant c-k-ras genes. Cell 1988;53:549.
48. Bsos JL. KRAS codon 12 mutations occur very frequently in pancreatic adenocarcinomas. Nucleic Acids Res 1988;16:7773.
49. Gruenwald K, Lyons J, Frohlich A, et al. High frequency of K-ras codon 12 mutations in pancreatic adenocarcinomas. Int J Cancer 1989;43:1037.
50. Korc M, Meltzer P, Trent J. Enhanced expression of epidermal growth factor receptor correlates with the alterations of chromosome 7 in human pancreatic cancer. Proc Natl Acad Sci USA 1986;83:5141.
51. Korc M, Chandrasekar B, Yamanaka Y, et al. Overexpression of the epidermal growth factor receptor in human pancreatic cancer is associated with concomitant increases in the levels of epidermal growth and transforming growth factor alpha. J Clin Invest 1992;90:1352.
52. Hall PA, Hughes CDM, Staddon SL, et al. The c-erbB-2 proto-oncogene in human pancreatic cancer. J Pathol 1990;161:195.
53. Cubilla AL, Fitzgerald PJ. Tumors of the exocrine pancreas.

In: Atlas of tumor pathology. 2nd series. Washington, DC: Armed Forces Institute of Pathology, 1984:fasc. 19.

54. Cubilla AL, Fitzgerald PJ. Pancreas cancer. 1. Duct adenocarcinoma: a clinical pathologic study of 380 patients. Pathol Annu 1978;13(Pt. 1):241.

55. Kloeppel G, Fitzgerald PJ. Pathology of nonendocrine pancreatic tumors. In: Go VLW, Gardner JD, Brooks FP, et al, eds. The exocrine pancreas: biology, pathobiology and diseases. New York: Raven Press, 1986:649.

56. Barsky D. Unusual tumor of the iris: a rare initial clinical manifestation of metastatic adenocarcinoma of the tail of the pancreas. Ann Ophthalmol 1978;10:1539.

57. Igaraski M, Card GG, Johnson PE, et al. Bilateral sudden hearing loss and metastatic pancreatic adenocarcinoma. Arch Otolaryngol 1979;105:196.

58. Joffe N. Right-angled narrowing of the distal oesophagus secondary to carcinoma of the tail of the pancreas. Clin Radiol 1979;30:33.

59. DiMagno EP, Malagelada J-R, Taylor WP, Go VLW. A prospective comparison of current diagnostic tests in pancreatic cancer. N Engl J Med 1977;297:737.

60. Gambill EE. Pancreatic and ampullar carcinoma: diagnosis and prognosis in relationship to symptoms, physical findings, and elapse of time as observed in 255 patients. South Med J 1970;63:1119.

61. Kalser MH, Barkin J, MacIntyre JJ, et al. Pancreatic cancer: assessment of prognosis by clinical presentation. Cancer 1985;56:397.

62. Douglas HO, Holyoke ED. Pancreatic cancer: initial treatment as the determinant of survival. JAMA 1974;229:793.

63. Briss WR, Burch B, Martin M, et al. Localization of referred pancreatic pain induced by electrical stimulation. Gastroenterology 1950;16:317.

64. Chapman CR. Pain related to cancer treatment. Journal of Pain and Symptom Management 1988;3:188.

65. Gullick HD. Carcinoma of the pancreas: a review of 100 cases. Medicine (Baltimore) 1959;38:47.

66. Howard JM, Jordan CL, Jr. Cancer of the pancreas. Curr Probl Cancer 1977;2:1.

67. Perez MM, Newcomer AD, Moertel CG, et al. Assessment of weight loss, food intake, fat metabolism, malabsorption, and treatment of pancreatic insufficiency in pancreatic cancer. Cancer 1983;52:346.

68. DiMagno EP, Malagelada J-R, Go VLW. The relationships between pancreatic ductal obstruction and pancreatic secretion in man. Mayo Clin Proc 1979;54:157.

69. Helgeson AS, Lawson T, Pour P. Exocrine pancreatic secretion in the Syrian golden hamster, *Mesocrietus auratus*. III. Effects of carcinogen administration and development of pancreatic cancer. Comp Biochem Physiol 1984;77(C):191.

70. Gullo L, Pezzilli R, Morselli-Labate AM. Diabetes and the risk of pancreatic cancer. Italian Pancreatic Cancer Study Group. New Engl J Med 1994;331:81.

70a. Permert J, Larsson J, Westermark GT, et al. Islet amyloid polypeptide in patients with pancreatic cancer and diabetes. New Engl J Med 1994;330:313.

71. Regan PT, Malagelada J-R, DiMagno EP, et al. Comparative effects of antacids, cimetidine, and enteric coating on the therapeutic response to oral enzymes in severe pancreatic insufficiency. N Engl J Med 1977;297:854.

72. Fras I, Litin EM, Pearson JS. Comparison of psychiatric symptoms in carcinoma of the pancreas with those in some other intra-abdominal neoplasms. Am J Psychiatry 1967;123:1553.

73. Holland JC, Korzun AH, Tross S, et al. Comparative psychological disturbance in patients with pancreatic and gastric cancer. Am J Psychiatry 1986;143:982.

74. Moertel CG. Exocrine pancreas. In: Holland JF, Frei E III, eds. Cancer medicine. Philadelphia: Lea & Febiger, 1973:1559.

75. Go VL, Taylor WF, DiMagno EP. Efforts at early diagnosis of pancreatic cancer: the Mayo Clinic experience. Cancer 1981;3:1698.

76. Piper CE, Remine WH, Priestly Jr. Pancreatic cystadenoma: report of 20 cases. JAMA 1962;180:648.

77. Freeney PC, Weinstein CJ, Taft DA, Allen FH. Cystic neoplasms of the pancreas: new angiographic and ultrasonographic findings. AJR 1978;131:795.

78. Dodds WJ, Margolin FR, Goldberg HI. Cavernous lymphangioma of the pancreas. Radiol Clin Biol 1969;38:267.

79. Baltaxe HA, Leslie EV. Vanishing pancreatic calcifications. AJR 1967;99:642.

80. Tucker DH, Moore IB. Vanishing pancreatic calcification in chronic pancreatitis. N Engl J Med 1963;268:31.

81. Metzgar RS, Asch HL. Antigens of human pancreatic adenocarcinomas: their role in diagnosis and therapy. Pancreas 1988;3:352.

82. Holyoke ED, Douglass HO, Goldrosen MH, Chu PM. Tumor markers in pancreatic cancer. Semin Oncol 1979;6:3.

83. Klavins JV. Tumor markers of pancreatic carcinoma. Cancer 1981;47:1597.

84. Moossa AR, Levin B. Collaborative studies in the diagnosis of pancreatic cancer. Semin Oncol 1979;6:298.

85. Zamcheck N, Martin EW. Factors controlling the circulating CEA levels in pancreatic cancer. Cancer 1981;47:1620.

86. Podolsky DK, McPhee MS, Alpert E, et al. Galactosyltransferase isoenzyme II in the detection of pancreatic cancer: comparison with radiologic, endoscopic, and serologic tests. N Engl J Med 1981;304:1313.

87. Ritts R Jr, Jacobsen D, Ilstrup D, et al. A prospective evaluation of MoAb CA 19-9 to detect GI cancer in a high risk clinic population. Cancer Detect Prev 1984;7:525.

88. Ritts R Jr, Klug T, Jacobsen D, et al. Multiple tumor marker tests enhance sensitivity of pancreatic carcinoma detection. Cancer Detect Prev 1984;7:459.

89. Fitzgerald PJ, Fortner JG, Watson RC, et al. The value of diagnostic aids in detecting pancreas cancer. Cancer 1978;41:868.

90. Moossa AR, Levin B. The diagnosis of "early" pancreatic cancer: the University of Chicago experience. Cancer 1981;47:1688.

91. Gowland M, Kalantzis N, Warwick F, Braganza J. Relative efficiency and predictive value of ultrasonography and endoscopic retrograde pancreatography in diagnosis of pancreatic disease. Lancet 1981;2:190.

92. Faintuch J, Levin B. Clinical presentation and diagnosis of exocrine tumors of the pancreas. In: Go VLW, Gardner JD, Brooks FP, et al, eds. The exocrine pancreas: biology, pathobiology and diseases. New York: Raven Press, 1986:193.

93. Ferrucci JF Jr, Wittenberg J. CT biopsy of abdominal tumors: aids for lesion localization. Radiology 1978;129:739.

94. Yeh H. Percutaneous fine needle aspiration biopsy of intraabdominal lesions with ultrasound guidance. Am J Gastroenterol 1981;75:148.

95. DiMagno EP, Regan PT, Clain JE, et al. Human endoscopic ultrasonography. Gastroenterology 1982;83:824.

96. DiMagno EP, Malagelada J-R, Moertel CG, et al. Prospective evaluation of the pancreatic secretion of immunoreactive carcinoembryonic antigen, enzyme, and bicarbonate in patients suspected of having pancreatic cancer. Gastroenterology 1977;73:457.

97. DiMagno EP. Diagnosis of chronic pancreatitis: are noninvasive tests of exocrine pancreatic function sensitive and specific? Gastroenterology 1982;83:143.

98. Warshaw AL, Gu Z, Wittenberg J, Waltman AC. Preoperative staging and assessment of resectability of pancreatic cancer. Arch Surg 1990;125:230.

99. Tio TL, Tytgat GN, Cikot RJ, et al. Ampullopancreatic carcinoma: preoperative TNM classification with endosonography. Radiology 1990;175:455.

100. Rösch T, Braig C, Gain T, et al. Staging of pancreatic and ampullary carcinoma by endoscopic ultrasonography: comparison with conventional sonography, computed tomography, and angiography. Gastroenterology 1992;102:188.

101. Shapiro TM. Adenocarcinoma of the pancreas: a statistical analysis of biliary bypass vs Whipple resection in good risk patients. Ann Surg 1975;182:715.

102. Trede M. The surgical treatment of pancreatic carcinoma. Surgery 1985;97:28.

103. Grace PA, Pitt HA, Tomkins RK, et al. Decreased morbidity

and mortality after pancreatoduodenectomy. Am J Surg 1986;151:141.

104. Braasch JW, Deziel DJ, Rossi RL, et al. Pyloric and gastric preserving pancreatic resection: experience with 87 patients. Surgery 1986;204:411.

105. Edis AJ, Kiernan PD, Taylor WF. Attempted curative resection of ductal carcinoma of the pancreas: review of Mayo Clinic experience 1951–1975. Mayo Clin Proc 1980;55:351.

106. Connolly MM, Dawson PJ, Michelassi F, et al. Survival in 1001 patients with carcinoma of the pancreas. Ann Surg 1987;206:366.

107. Crist DW, Sitzmann JW, Cameron JL. Improved hospital morbidity, mortality, and survival following the Whipple procedure. Ann Surg 1987;206:358.

108. Brooks JR, Culebras JM. Cancer of the pancreas: palliative operation, Whipple procedure, or total pancreatectomy. Am J Surg 1976;131:516.

109. Tsuchiya R, Noda T, Harad N, et al. Collective review of small carcinomas of the pancreas. Ann Surg 1986;203:77.

110. Fortner JG. Surgical principles for pancreatic cancer: regional, total and subtotal pancreatectomy. Cancer 1981;47:1712.

111. Traverso LW, Longmire WPJ. Preservation of the pylorus in pancreatoduodenectomy. Surg Gynecol Obstet 1978;146:959.

112. Huibregtse K, Katon RM, Coene PP, Tytgat GNJ. Endoscopic palliative treatment in pancreatic cancer. Gastrointest Endosc 1986;32:334.

113. Speer AG, Cotton PB, Russell RC, et al. Randomised trial of endoscopic versus percutaneous stent insertion in malignant obstructive jaundice. Lancet 1987;2:57.

114. Leung JWC, Emery R, Cotton PB, et al. Management of malignant obstructive jaundice at The Middlesex Hospital. Br J Surg 1983;70:584.

115. Sarr MG, Cameron JL. Surgical management of unresectable carcinoma of the pancreas. Surgery 1982;91:123.

116. Cotton PB. Endoscopic management of bile duct stones (apples and oranges). Gut 1984;25:587.

117. Cotton PB. Endoscopic biliary stents: trick or treatment? Gastrointest Endosc 1986;32:364.

118. Dowsett JR, Williams SJ, Hatfield ARW, et al. Does stent diameter matter in the endoscopic palliation of malignant biliary obstruction?: a randomized trial of 10 FG versus 12 FG endoprosthesis. Gastroenterology 1989;96:A128.

119. Dowsett JF, Russell RCG, Hatfield ARW, et al. Malignant obstructive jaundice: a prospective randomized trial of by-pass surgery versus endoscopic stenting. Gastroenterology 1989;96:A128.

120. Dowsett JF, Williams SJ, Hatfield ARW, et al. Endoscopic management of low biliary obstruction due to unresectable primary pancreaticobiliary malignancy: a review of 463 consecutive cases. Gastroenterology 1989;96:A129.

121. Barkin JS, Goldberg RI, Sfakianakis GN, Levi J. Pancreatic carcinoma is associated with delayed gastric emptying. Dig Dis Sci 1986;31:265.

122. Schantz S, Schickler W, Evans TK, Coffey RS. Palliative gastroenterostomy for pancreatic cancer. Am J Surg 1984;147:793.

123. Shivshanker K, Bennett RW, Haynie TP. Tumor-associated gastroparesis: correction with metoclopramide. Am J Surg 1983;145:221.

124. Moertel CG, Engstrom P, Lavin PT, et al. Chemotherapy of gastric and pancreatic carcinoma. Surgery 1979;85:509.

125. Cullinan SA, Moertel CG, Fleming TR, et al. Comparison of three chemotherapeutic regimens in the treatment of advanced pancreatic and gastric carcinoma. JAMA 1985;253:2061.

126. Karlin DA, Stroehlein JR, Bennetts RW, et al. Phase I–II study of the combination of 5-FU, doxorubicin, mitomycin, and semustine (FAMMc) in the treatment of adenocarcinoma of the stomach, gastroesophageal junction, and pancreas. Cancer Treat Rep 1982;66:1613.

127. Mallison C. Cytotoxic chemotherapy in pancreatic exocrine cancer. In: Preece PE, Cuschieri A, Rosin RD, eds. Cancer of the bile ducts and pancreas. Philadelphia: WB Saunders, 1989:209.

128. Gastrointestinal Tumor Study Group. Treatment of locally unresectable carcinoma of the pancreas: comparison of combined-modality therapy (chemotherapy plus radiotherapy) to chemotherapy alone. J Natl Cancer Inst 1988;80:751.

129. Roldan GE, Gunderson LL, Nagorney DM, et al. External beam versus intraoperative and external beam irradiation for locally advanced pancreatic cancer. Cancer 1988;6:1110.

130. DiMagno EP, Malagelada J-R, Go VLW, Moertel CG. Fate of orally ingested enzymes in pancreatic insufficiency: comparison of two dosage schedules. N Engl J Med 1977;296:1318.

131. Regan PT, Malagelada J-R, DiMagno EP, et al. Comparative effects of antacids, cimetidine, and enteric coating on the therapeutic response to oral enzymes in severe pancreatic insufficiency. N Engl J Med 1977;297:854.

132. DiMagno EP. Medical treatment of pancreatic insufficiency. Mayo Clin Proc 1979;54:435.

133. DiMagno EP, Go VLW, Summerskill WHJ. Relations between pancreatic enzyme outputs and malabsorption in severe pancreatic insufficiency. N Engl J Med 1973;288:813.

134. Maguire LG, Yon JL, Miller E. Prevention of narcotic induced constipation. N Engl J Med 1981;305:1651.

135. Foley KM. Pain syndromes and pharmacologic management of pancreatic cancer pain. Journal of Pain and Symptom Management 1988;3:176.

136. Foley KM, Inturrisi CE. Analgesic drug therapy in cancer pain: principles and practice. Med Clin North Am 1987;71:207.

137. Oliver DJ. The use of syringe driver in terminal care. Br J Clin Pharmacol 1985;20:515.

138. Moore DC, Bush WH, Burnett LL. Coeliac plexus block: a roentgenographic, anatomic study of technique and spread of solution in patients and corpses. Anesth Analg 1981;60:369.

139. Ischia S, Luzzani A, Ischia A, Faggion S. A new approach to the neurolytic block of the coeliac plexus: the transaortic technique. Pain 1983;16:333.

140. Leung JWC, Bowen-Wright M, Aveling W, et al. Coeliac plexus block for pain in pancreatic cancer and chronic pancreatitis. Br J Surg 1983;70:730.

141. Thompson GE, Moore DC, Bridenbaugh LD, Artin RY. Abdominal pain and alcohol coeliac plexus block. Anesth Analg 1977;56:1.

142. Galizea EJ, Lahiri SK. Paraplegia following coeliac plexus block with phenol. Br J Anaesth 1974;46:539.

143. Compagno J, Oertel JE. Mucinous cystic neoplasms of the pancreas with overt and latent malignancy (cystadenocarcinoma and cystadenoma): a clinicopathologic study of 41 cases. Am J Clin Pathol 1978;69:573.

144. Cullen PK, ReMine WH, Dahlin DC. A clinicopathological study of cystadenocarcinoma of the pancreas. Surg Gynecol Obstet 1963;117:189.

145. Hodgkinson DJ, ReMine WH, Weiland LH. Pancreatic cystadenoma: a clinicopathologic study of 45 cases. Arch Surg 1978;113:512.

146. Alguacil-Garcia A, Weiland LH. The histologic spectrum, prognosis, and histogenesis of the sarcomatoid carcinoma of the pancreas. Cancer 1977;39:1181.

147. Tschang TP, Garza-Garza R, Kissane JM. Pleomorphic carcinoma of the pancreas: an analysis of 15 cases. Cancer 1977;39:2114.

148. Burns WA, Matthews MJ, Hamosh M, et al. Lipase secreting acinar cell carcinoma of the pancreas with polyarthropathy: a light and electron microscopic, histochemical and biochemical study. Cancer 1974;33:1002.

149. Robertson JC, Ecles GM. Syndrome associated with pancreatic acinar cell carcinoma. Br J Med 1970;2:709.

150. Osborne BM, Culbert SJ, Cangir A, Mackay B. Acinar cell carcinoma of the pancreas in a 9-year-old child: case report with electron microscopic observations. South Med J 1977;70:370.

151. Horie A, Yano Y, Kotoo Y, et al. Morphogenesis of pancreatoblastoma, infantile carcinoma of the pancreas: report of two cases. Cancer 1977;39:247.

152. Horie A, Haratake J, Jimi A, et al. Pancreatoblastoma in Japan, with differential diagnosis from papillary cystic tumor (duc-

tuloacinar adenoma) of the pancreas. Acta Pathol Jpn 1987;37:
47.

153. Compagno J, Oertel JE, Kremzar M. Solid and papillary epithelial neoplasms of the pancreas: probably a small duct origin. A clinicopathologic study of 52 cases (abstract). Lab Invest 1979;40:248.

154. Friedman AC, Lichtenstein JE, Fishman EK, et al. Solid and papillary epithelial neoplasm of the pancreas. Radiology 1985;155:333.

155. Sanfey H, Mendelsohn G, Cameron JL. Solid and papillary neoplasm of the pancreas: a potentially curable surgical lesion. Ann Surg 1983;197:272.

156. Ohashi K, Takagi K. ERCP and imaging diagnosis of pancreatic cancer. Gastroenterol Endosc 1980;77:1493.

157. Warshaw AL. Mucinous cystic tumors and mucinous ductal ectasia of the pancreas. Gastrointest Endosc 1991;37:199.

158. Yamada M, Kozuka S, Yamao K, et al. Mucin-producing tumor of the pancreas. Cancer 1991;68:159.

159. Nickl NJ, Lawson JM, Cotton PB. Mucinous pancreatic tumors: ERCP findings. Gastrointest Endosc 1991;37:133.

160. Itoh S, Ishiguchi T, Ishigaki T, et al. Mucin-producing pancreatic tumor: CT findings and histopathologic correlation. Radiology 1992;183:81.

Textbook of Gastroenterology, second edition, edited by Tadataka Yamada. JB Lippincott Company, Philadelphia © 1995.

CHAPTER 93

Endocrine Neoplasms of the Pancreas

Robert T. Jensen   Jeffrey A. Norton

Epidemiology
Pathology
Clinical Features and Diagnosis
   Insulinoma
   VIPoma
   Glucagonoma
   Somatostatinoma
   GRFoma

PPoma and Nonfunctioning Islet Cell Tumor
Other Tumors
Tumor Localization
Treatment
   Nonmetastatic Disease
   Metastatic Disease

Endocrine tumors of the pancreas are classified according to the type of clinical syndrome present (Table 93-1). In general, they share a number of common features, including various aspects of pathology, natural history, and considerations in treatment, localization studies, and treatment of metastatic tumors. In each case, except for the PPoma syndrome (tumors secreting pancreatic polypeptide [PP]) or nonfunctioning pancreatic endocrine tumors, the principal clinical manifestations of the endocrine tumor are the result of the extensive release of hormones by the tumor into the circulation. Each of the various hormones released in the different syndromes occur naturally and are important in mediating various physiologic processes (see Chap. 2). In the pancreatic endocrine tumor syndromes, however, these hormones are not under normal physiologic regulation and are released autonomously by the tumor. Even though these tumors usually are slow growing in many cases, effective therapy requires treatment of both the effect of autonomous hormone overproduction as well as treatment directed at the tumor itself. In this chapter, the common features of these tumors are discussed together, and the distinctive features separately. Gastrinoma was discussed in Chapter 62 and, in general, is not dealt with.

EPIDEMIOLOGY

Pancreatic endocrine tumors are uncommon, having a prevalence of less than 10 per million population.[1] In some older series, insulinomas were reported to be the most common pancreatic endocrine tumor, with an incidence in various series of 0.8 to 0.9 per million population per year, whereas gastrinomas were reported to occur in 0.1 to 0.4 per million per year.[2–4] In a more recent large series,[5] however, gastrinomas were as common as insulinomas (one to three new cases per

TABLE 93-1
Endocrine Tumors of the Pancreas

TUMOR	SYNDROME	SIGNS OR SYMPTOMS	LOCATION	HORMONE CAUSING SYNDROME
Gastrinoma	Zollinger-Ellison	Abdominal pain Diarrhea Esophageal symptoms	Pancreas—60% Duodenum—30% Other—10%	Gastrin
Insulinoma	Insulinoma	Hypoglycemic symptoms	Pancreas	Insulin
Glucagonoma	Glucagonoma	Rash, anemia Diabetes or glucose intolerance Weight loss Thromboembolic disease	Pancreas	Glucagon
VIPoma	Verner-Morrison Pancreatic cholera WDHA	Severe watery diarrhea Hypokalemia	Pancreas—90% Other—10% (neural, adrenal, periganglionic tissue)	VIP
Somatostatinoma	Somatostatinoma	Diabetes mellitus Cholelithiasis Diarrhea Steatorrhea	Pancreas—56% Duodenum/jejunum—44%	Somatostatin
GRFoma	GRFoma	Acromegaly	Pancreas—30% Lung—54% Jejunum—7% Other—13% (adrenal, foregut, retroperitoneum)	GRF
PPoma	PPoma	Weight loss Abdominal mass Occasionally asymptomatic Hepatomegaly	Pancreas	None (PP released, but no known symptoms due to hypersecretion)
Nonfunctioning	Nonfunctioning pancreatic endocrine tumor	Same as PPoma	Pancreas	None

GRF, growth hormone-releasing factor; PP, pancreatic polypeptide; VIP, vasoactive intestinal polypeptide; WDHA, watery diarrhea, hypokalemia, and achlorhydria.

year per million population), which is more frequent than in older studies.[3,4] The remaining endocrine tumors occur in less than 0.2 per million per year.[2] Approximately 100 cases of glucagonoma have been reported worldwide,[6] and 27 cases of pancreatic and 21 of intestinal somatostatinomas[7]; the numbers of cases of VIPomas (tumors that secrete vasoactive intestinal polypeptide [VIP]), GRFomas (tumors that secrete growth hormone-releasing factor [GRF]), or PPomas are unclear. The best data on the relative frequency of these tumors are from Ireland, where, at a major referral unit between 1970 and 1983, there was an average incidence of 3.6 cases of neuroendocrine tumors per million population per year.[2] Insulinomas were approximately as common as the combination of PPomas and nonfunctioning tumors, twice as common as gastrinomas, 8 times as common as VIPomas, and 17 times as common as glucagonomas.[2] Somatostatinomas were rare, with no cases reported.[2] In this series, the combined incidence of all pancreatic endocrine tumors was approximately equal to that of carcinoid tumors. In autopsy studies, it has been reported that nonfunctioning endocrine pancreatic tumors occur in 1% of all subjects; however, in less than 1 of 1000 cases was a functioning pancreatic endocrine tumor thought to occur.[8] In surgical studies, nonfunctioning pancreatic endocrine tumors are reported to comprise 15% to 21% of all

pancreatic endocrine tumors removed,[9–11] and in a large pathology series to account for 36% of all pancreatic endocrine tumors.[12]

PATHOLOGY

The pancreatic endocrine tumors share a number of pathologic features. The tumors are thought to originate from cells that are part of the diffuse neuroendocrine cell system.[12,13] These cells share cytochemical properties, and these tumors, together with carcinoid tumors, medullary carcinoma of the thyroid, melanomas, and pheochromocytomas[12–15] have been called APUDomas (an acronym for amine precursor uptake and decarboxylation).[12–15] The tumors are composed of monotonous sheets of small round cells with uniform nuclei and cytoplasm (Fig. 93-1). Mitotic figures are uncommon. Ultrastructurally, the tumors demonstrate electron-dense granules that contain various peptides, amines, neuron-specific enolase, synaptophysin, and chromogranin A and C.[12,15,16] Pancreatic endocrine tumors are frequently multihormonal when examined by immunocytochemical studies.[12,17–25] In various series, more than 50% of all pancreatic endocrine tumors contain more than one hormone by immunocytochemistry.[12,17–25] In in-

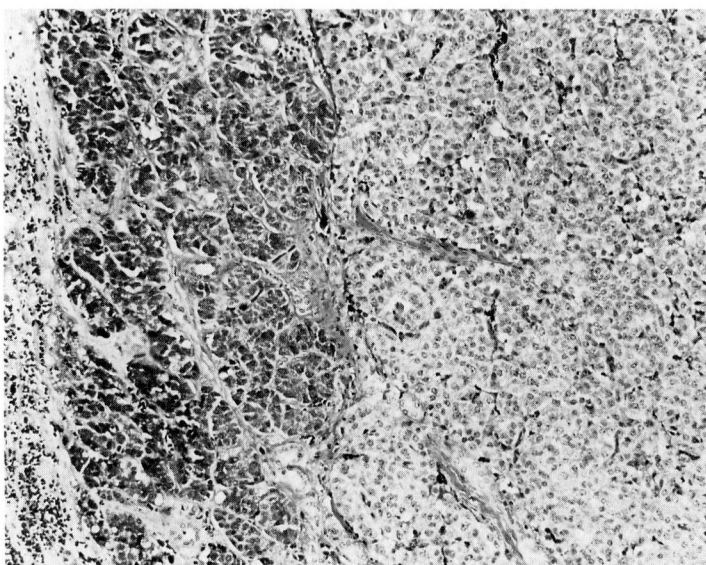

FIGURE 93-1. Photomicrograph of an insulinoma (*right*) demonstrates a typical histologic pattern seen in pancreatic endocrine tumors, with monotonous sheets of small round cells with uniform nuclei and cytoplasm. The tumor is well marginated and interfaces with the normal pancreas (*left*) by a distinct margin. (Hematoxylin and eosin stain; original magnification × 125.)

sulinomas, for example, glucagon has been identified by immunocytochemical methods in 0% to 44%, somatostatin in 0% to 18%, gastrin in 3% to 11%, PP in 18% to 39%, and corticotropin-like immunoreactivity in 11%.[15,21-23] Particularly common are PP cells, which have been identified in 22% to 39% of insulinomas, 0% to 67% of glucagonomas, and 50% to 75% of VIPomas.[21-23] In some cases, numerous hormones are released into the circulation, whereas in others only one peptide may be detectable.[22,24,25] It is not apparent why patients with a given pancreatic endocrine syndrome present with a syndrome characteristic of hypersecretion of only one of these peptides, despite the tumor containing multiple peptides. Possible explanations include that only one of the peptides produced is released, only one is released in sufficient quantity to cause symptoms, only one peptide produced is biologically active, or all the peptides are released but some have antagonistic physiologic actions.

Because patients with pancreatic endocrine tumor syndromes are now living longer with increasingly effective therapy, the development of a secondary symptomatic pancreatic endocrine syndrome may become increasingly common.[24,25] One study suggests that a secondary symptomatic pancreatic endocrine syndrome is common, occurring in 7.5% of patients with a mean follow-up of 19 months,[24] whereas another study suggests it is uncommon, occurring in only 2% of patients with gastrinoma followed for a mean of 11 years.[25] Because of the frequent presence of multiple peptides by immunocytochemistry in the pancreatic endocrine tumor, it has become increasingly difficult, if not impossible in most cases, to determine by immunocytochemistry which of the hormones found in the tumor is clinically important.[12,15,20] Therefore, those producing clinical syndromes must be classified by the type of clinical syndrome and the causative hormone, not by immunocytochemical distinctions.[20]

In general, histologic classification of pancreatic endocrine tumors has failed to predict the growth pattern of the tumor or determine whether it is malignant.[12,15,16,20] Furthermore, there was no definite correlation between the histologic pattern and the type of clinical syndrome the tumor was associated with.[15,16,18,20,26] In addition to multiple peptide production, pancreatic endocrine tumors frequently express the α-chain and less frequently the β-chain of human chorionic gonadotropin,[27-31] or chromogranin A,[20,32,33] and it has been proposed that their expression correlates with malignancy. Malignancy, however, can be unequivocally established only in those patients who are demonstrated to have metastatic tumor spread to lymph nodes or the liver, gross invasion or infiltration into adjacent organs, or clear blood vessel invasion.[12,15,20,31] Because of this, it is not completely established what percentage of pancreatic endocrine tumors are malignant. The benign nature can be established only by long-term follow-up. In general, 5% to 10% of insulinomas are reported as malignant, whereas in various series 50% to 90% of the other tumors are reported as malignant.[7,15,19,20,26]

The size of the tumor usually is not related to the severity of the hormonally induced symptoms; in general, however, there is a correlation of size with the occurrence of malignancy.[12,26] Whereas insulinomas, like gastrinomas, usually are small (<2 cm), glucagonomas and the other pancreatic endocrine tumors are larger at the time of detection (frequently >5 cm).[7,20,26,34] Most of the primary pancreatic endocrine tumors are solitary and encapsulated when not associated with the multiple endocrine neoplasia (MEN) type I syndrome.[12] When metastatic spread occurs, it is usually to regional lymph nodes first and later to the liver. Late in the course of the disease, metastases to bone also may occur.[35]

Pancreatic endocrine tumors may occur either in a nonfamilial form (sporadic) or in a familial form associated with MEN I syndrome. MEN I or Wermer's syndrome is an autosomal dominant disorder characterized by tumors or hyperplasia of multiple endocrine organs, with hypercalcemia secondary to hyperparathyroidism being the most common abnormality, occurring in 97% of patients.[36-39] Functional islet cell tumors of the pancreas are the second most frequent abnormality and are found in 80% of patients with MEN I. The incidence of gastrinomas, insulinomas, glucagonomas, and VIPomas in MEN I is 54%, 21%, 3%, and 1%, respectively.[37-39] Pituitary and adrenal cortical adenomas also occur but are much less common.[37,38] In MEN I, the chromosome defect is reported to be on chromosome 11.[39,40] Two patients have been described from MEN I kindreds with insulinomas, and the insulinomas showed the constitutional gene defect as well as a deletion in the corresponding position of the other chromosome 11.[39] Similar defects exist in other pancreatic endocrine tumors in MEN I.[41] The chromosomal results with insulinomas in patients with MEN I are in contrast to a study[41] in patients with sporadic pancreatic endocrine tumors that demonstrated that, even when malignant, sporadic tumors do not develop homozygous inactivation of the MEN I gene.[41] The exact percentage of patients with pancreatic endocrine tumors who have MEN I syndrome varies in different series, from less than 5% to 25%.[20,42] The recognition that the pancreatic endocrine tumor can be part of the MEN I syndrome is important because multiple pancreatic tumors are frequently present.[12,20,34,43] Furthermore, screening of family members for various features of the syndrome is indicated.[20,39]

Almost all insulinomas occur in the pancreas (see Table 93-1) or are attached to it,[44] although rarely an aberrant insulinoma may be found in carcinoid tumors of the duodenum, ileum, or lung.[44] Multiple insulinomas occur in only 10% of cases, and in these patients the presence of MEN I should be suspected.[26] Glucagonomas occur almost entirely within the pancreas, usually in the pancreatic body and tail.[12,26,45] In contrast to insulinomas or gastrinomas, most glucagonomas are large (5-10 cm) at the time of diagnosis.[26] VIPomas in adults are almost all pancreatic in location (i.e., >90%); however, occasionally the VIPoma syndrome is reported in association with a pheochromocytoma or carcinoid tumor of the intestine.[39,46] In children, the VIPoma syndrome is often the result of a ganglioneuroma or ganglioneuroblastoma.[47,48] VIPomas usually are large tumors.[46] Somatostatinomas, similar to gastrinomas, frequently are found in extrapancreatic locations (see Table 93-1).[7,20,39] In a review of 48 primary somatostatinomas, 56% were in the pancreas, usually in the pancreatic head, and 44% were in the small intestine (duodenum or jejunum). Similar to glucagonomas or VIPomas, somatostatinomas tended to be large (mean size of 5 cm).[49] Nonfunctioning pancreatic endocrine tumors and PPomas occur in the pancreas, and are usually larger than 5 cm in diameter.[12,39] Other, less common functioning endocrine tumors such as those associated with acromegaly (GRFomas),[50,51] paraneoplastic hypercalcemia,[52,53] or Cushing's syndrome[54-56] are usually large tumors within the pancreas.

In addition to the MEN I syndrome, studies have reported pancreatic endocrine tumors in patients with von Recklinghausen's disease,[57-59] von Hippel-Lindau disease,[60] and tuberous sclerosis.[61] In a number of patients with von Recklinghausen's disease, duodenal somatostatinomas are reported,[57,58] as well as Zollinger-Ellison syndrome.[59] In von Hippel-Lindau syndrome in one series,[60] 17% of the patients had pancreatic endocrine tumors of which three were adenomas and three carcinomas, but only one was associated with a clinical endocrine syndrome (an insulinoma). Two patients with tuberous sclerosis were reported with insulinoma, and one with a nonfunctioning pancreatic endocrine tumor.[61]

CLINICAL FEATURES AND DIAGNOSIS

In each pancreatic endocrine syndrome except PPomas and nonfunctioning islet cell tumors, early symptoms are caused by the excessive hormone release, whereas late symptoms are primarily the result of the metastatic spread of the tumor per se (cachexia, pain, bleeding).

Insulinoma

Insulinomas are endocrine tumors that originate in the pancreas, secrete excessive amounts of insulin, and cause a distinct syndrome characterized by symptoms due to hypoglycemia.

Insulinomas rarely occur in adolescence.[62] The average age of presentation in most series is between 40 and 50 years, with 60% of the insulinomas occurring in women.[26,63-66]

The clinical manifestations of insulinomas are caused by the hypoglycemia secondary to the tumor's excessive and unregulated insulin secretion. The symptoms are typically associated with fasting; the attacks characteristically occur before breakfast, when a meal is delayed, or hours postprandially. Most patients have symptoms of central nervous system dysfunction secondary to hypoglycemia (neuroglycopenic symptoms) that include headaches, confusion, lightheadedness, visual disturbances, irrational behavior, drowsiness, or even confusion resulting in coma. Patients with insulinomas misdiagnosed as psychiatric or neurologic problems have been reported.[64] Most patients also have symptoms due to catecholamine excess secondary to the hypoglycemia, such as sweating, tremor, palpitations, and irritability.[26,63-65] The average time from onset of symptoms to diagnosis is 3 years, although some studies suggest this gap is decreasing.[63,66]

The presence of an insulinoma should be suspected in all patients with hypoglycemia, especially patients with a history of fasting hypoglycemia or with a family history of MEN I. Fasting hypoglycemia can be mediated by a number of different conditions[26,67-70] (Table 93-2). It should be remembered that insulinoma is only one cause of fasting hypoglycemia, and other causes also should be suspected, such as inadvertent or deliberate administration of insulin, ingestion of oral hypoglycemia agents, alcoholism with severe liver disease or malnutrition, or other extrapancreatic tumors (see Table 93-2). The diagnosis of insulinoma requires the demonstration of hypoglycemia combined with an inappropriate elevation of plasma insulin concentration and ultimately a pancreatic endocrine tumor.

The most reliable test for hypoglycemia is a fast up to 72 hours in the hospital (with free access to water).[26,70] Blood glucose should be monitored at regular intervals (2-4 hours) and more frequently if blood sugar decreases to below 50 mg/dL. Samples also should be obtained for serum insulin values. If at any point the patient becomes symptomatic before administering glucose, repeat serum insulin and glucose levels should be obtained. The test is terminated for neuroglycopenic symptoms or for persistent glucose levels below 40 mg/dL. Over 90% of insulinomas reported have been detected in this fashion, and hypoglycemia develops in 70% to 80% of patients during the first 24 hours of fasting.[26,39,63-66] In healthy, nonobese subjects, serum insulin concentrations decrease to less than 6 μU/mL when blood glucose decreases to 40 mg/dL

TABLE 93-2
Causes of Fasting Hypoglycemia

Mediated by endogenous insulin or insulin-like factors
  Insulinoma
  Spontaneous autoimmune antiinsulin antibody syndrome
  Autoantibodies to insulin receptor
  Noninsulin tumor-associated hypoglycemia
Reduced hepatic glucose output
  Deficient gluconeogenesis or glycogen storage
  Hormonal deficiencies (e.g., adrenal insufficiency)
  Enzymatic defects (e.g., glucose-6-phosphatase deficiency)
  Ethanol consumption and poor nutrition
  Diffuse liver disease
Drugs or other pharmacologic causes
  Sulfonylureas or biguanides
  Insulin administration
  Ingestion of ackee fruits (hypoglycin)
  Other drugs (aspirin, pentamidine)

Modified from Boden G. Insulinomas and glucagonomas. Gastroenterol Clin North Am 1989;18:831; and Comi R, Gorden P, Doppman JL. Insulinoma. In: Go VLW, Di Magno EP, Gardner JD, et al, eds. The pancreas: biology, pathobiology and disease. 2nd ed. New York: Raven Press. 1993:979.

or less, and the ratio of serum insulin to glucose remains less than 0.3 (in mg/dL).[26,39,66,69,70] The test is considered positive for insulinoma if serum insulin concentrations remain constant or increase during hypoglycemia (blood sugar <50 mg/dL) or insulin : glucose ratio is more than 0.3.[26,70] In the small percentage of patients with a negative test (i.e., serum insulin concentration decreases to <6 μU/mL with hypoglycemia) in whom insulinoma is still suspected, additional tests such as various provocative tests may have to be used.[26,69,70,71]

The diagnosis of insulinoma can be difficult because an inappropriately elevated serum insulin concentration associated with hypoglycemia can be observed in a number of different conditions (see Table 93-2). Besides insulinomas, β-cell hyperplasia or nesidioblastosis, factitious or inadvertent administration of excessive insulin or oral hypoglycemia agents, and autoantibodies against insulin or the insulin receptor can also cause those findings (see Table 93-2).[26,70,72] β-cell hyperplasia or nesidioblastosis, consisting of a proliferation of insulin-producing cells, is a leading cause of hyperinsulinism in newborns and has also been reported occasionally in adults.[70,72] Of these varying causes of hypoglycemia and hyperinsulinemia (see Table 93-2), surreptitious use of insulin or sulfonylureas is the most difficult to distinguish from true insulinoma.[69,70,73] To differentiate these conditions, a combination of studies consisting of the determination of serum concentrations of proinsulin, C-peptide, antibodies to insulin, and sulfonylurea needs to be done.[69,70]

Insulin is synthesized as proinsulin, which consists of a single-chain molecule containing both a 21–amino-acid α-chain and a 30–amino-acid β-chain connected by a 33–amino-acid connecting peptide (C-peptide).[74,75] Insulin and C-peptide are liberated in equimolar amounts, and because proinsulin or its intermediate also are found in granules, proinsulin also is detected in the serum with insulin.[70,74,75] In otherwise healthy subjects, less than 25% of the serum insulin is proinsulin, whereas serum proinsulin has been re-

ported to be elevated (i.e. >25%) in 90% to 100% of patients with insulinoma.[69,70,75,76] In insulinoma, the characteristic findings are a normal or elevated serum concentration of C-peptide, antibodies to insulin are not present, and sulfonylurea is not detected in the blood.[69] In a typical patient surreptitiously using insulin, the C-peptide level is decreased, the proinsulin level is normal or decreased, antibodies to insulin usually are present, and serum sulfonylurea determinations are negative.[69,70] In patients with surreptitious use of sulfonylureas, the serum concentration of proinsulin usually is normal, antibodies to insulin are not present, and sulfonylurea is detected in the serum or the urine.[69,70]

VIPoma

The VIPoma syndrome is caused by an endocrine tumor usually located in the pancreas that secretes excessive amounts of VIP, which causes a distinct syndrome characterized by fasting, large-volume diarrhea, hypokalemia, and hypochlorhydria (Table 93-3).

The VIPoma syndrome is also called the Verner-Morrison syndrome because of its original description by these two investigators in two patients with profuse, watery diarrhea, hypokalemia, and dehydration with a non–β-cell pancreatic islet cell tumor.[77] It has also been termed pancreatic cholera[78] and the WDHA syndrome[79] (for the watery diarrhea, hypokalemia, and achlorhydria that develop in some patients).[48,80] Although the diarrhea may be episodic or intermittent early in the presentation, characteristically the diarrhea is large in volume (>1 L/day), secretory in nature, and persists during fasting (see Table 93-2).[80,81] The diarrhea fluid frequently is described as having the appearance of weak tea. An increased net secretion of sodium and chloride into the small intestine has been demonstrated in these patients.[82,83] The sum of fecal sodium and potassium concentrations multiplied by two will equal the osmolality, and thus there is no osmotic gap.[84] Steatorrhea or abdominal cramping pain usually are not considered to develop in these patients, but some studies suggest these may be more common than reported previously.[85–87] Hypokalemia is present in almost all patients (see Table 93-3),[81,87,88] and is the result of the large losses of potassium in the diarrhea fluid. Hypochlorhydria rather than achlorhydria is found in 76% of patients with VIPoma syndrome (see Table 93-3).[81,87–89] This has been attributed to the inhibitory effect of VIP on

TABLE 93-3
Clinical Features of the VIPoma Syndrome

SIGN OR SYMPTOM	FREQUENCY (%)
Secretory diarrhea	100
Hypokalemia	90–100
Hypochlorhydria	76
Hyperglycemia	25–50
Hypercalcemia	25–50
Flushing	20
Dilated, atonic gallbladder	Unknown

Data from references 87 through 89.

gastric acid secretion.[81,90] Flushing is seen in 20% of patients with the VIPoma syndrome,[87] and has been attributed to the vasodilatory effects of VIP (see Table 93-3).[81,91] The fact that prolonged infusion with VIP in humans results in a gradual decrease in the flushing suggests the development of tachyphylaxis.[92] This phenomenon has been used to explain why only a minority of patients exhibit flushing.[81] Hyperglycemia is noted in 25% to 50% of patients with VIPomas,[93] and it has been attributed[81] to the glycogenolytic effect of VIP on the liver (see Table 93-3).[94] Hypercalcemia also is reported in 25% to 76% of patients with VIPoma[81,95]; however, the mechanism of this in most cases is not established. Although VIP has been shown to have osteolytic activity in bone,[80,81] this mechanism has not been established as the cause of the hypercalcemia. Five percent of patients[42] have VIPoma as part of the MEN I syndrome, and in these patients hypercalcemia is secondary to the hyperparathyroidism that is a part of this syndrome.[33–39] This explains the hypercalcemia in only a few patients, however.

In addition to VIP, a number of substances,[81,96] including secretin,[93] gastric inhibitory polypeptide,[97] PP,[98] and prostaglandins,[99] have been implicated in the diarrheogenic secretion in these patients. Controversy arose in early studies as to whether VIP was the sole cause of the diarrhea in WDHA syndrome because different investigators did not find elevated VIP levels in all patients, and exogenous VIP infusions for 1 or 2 hours did not cause diarrhea in humans.[92,100,101] In more recent studies, however, only VIP has been found to be elevated consistently in patients with the WDHA syndrome.[46,81,95,96,102,103] Furthermore, continuous infusion of VIP for 10 hours in otherwise healthy subjects to achieve plasma VIP concentrations similar to those seen in patients with WDHA syndrome produced profuse, watery diarrhea by 6 to 7 hours.[102,104] The diarrhea produced in these patients is similar to that seen in patients with WDHA syndrome. The ability of VIP to cause intestinal secretion is consistent with its known mechanism of action. VIP has been shown to cause net chloride secretion associated with increased short-circuit current, to bind to specific receptors on intestinal epithelial cells, and to activate adenylate cyclase and increase cyclic adenosine monophosphate in intestinal cells.[105,106] Some observations, however, suggest that VIP may not be the sole mediator of the WDHA syndrome in every case.[80] Occasional patients with the WDHA syndrome have normal plasma concentrations of VIP.[81] Another peptide, peptide histidine isoleucine (PHI),[107] is a 27–amino-acid peptide originally isolated from porcine intestine. The mammalian equivalent to PHI is peptide histidine methionine, and elevated concentrations of PHI-like immunoreactivity and VIP have been found in the plasma of patients with WDHA syndrome.[108–110] Tumor tissue obtained from patients with the WDHA syndrome also demonstrated PHI-like immunoreactivity, which was produced by the same cells as VIP.[108–110] Furthermore, the RNA from a WDHA tumor demonstrated that VIP and PHI sequences are in the same gene.[110] PHI infusions also caused intestinal secretion, although PHI was 32-fold less potent than VIP,[111] and therefore, even though PHI was reported to coexist in 22 of 24 VIPomas,[108] it seems unlikely, because of the low potency, to be contributing to the diarrheal state.

The definitive diagnosis of VIPoma requires the establishment of a secretory diarrhea, demonstration of elevated serum concentrations of VIP, and identification of a pancreatic endocrine tumor. The likely possibility that VIPoma and not some other cause is responsible for the diarrhea may be suggested by measuring the stool volume.[112] In 80% of patients with VIPomas, the stool output is greater than 3 L/day,[89] and when the stool output is less than 700 mL/day the diagnosis of VIPoma is unlikely.[113] In addition, the diarrhea persists during fasting[81,113] and the sum of the concentration of stool sodium and potassium multiplied by two equals the isotonicity.[84]

A number of diseases or conditions can produce chronic secretory diarrheas of this volume, and need to be differentiated from VIPomas. These include Zollinger-Ellison syndrome,[80,114] and the surreptitious use of laxatives, or the pseudopancreatic cholera syndrome.[46,115–119] The serum gastrin concentration is elevated in patients with Zollinger-Ellison syndrome but not in patients with VIPoma. Furthermore, with effective treatment of gastric hypersecretion, the diarrhea stops in patients with Zollinger-Ellison syndrome.[20,120]

To differentiate patients with VIPoma from those with pseudopancreatic cholera syndrome or laxative abuse, a reliable VIP radioimmunoassay is required.[46,81,113] The normal fasting plasma VIP concentration in a number of laboratories is 0 to 190 pg/mL.[46,81,95] It is best that the fasting plasma VIP concentration be determined at the time when diarrhea is present, because between diarrhea periods in an occasional patient with VIPoma, VIP levels may be normal.[80,81] The mean concentration of plasma VIP in one series of 29 patients with the VIPoma syndrome was 956 pg/mL, with a range of 225 to 1850 pg/mL.[80,81] In another series[121] of 52 VIPomas, the mean value was 702 pg/mL, with a range of 159 to 2530 pg/mL. Originally it was reported that in a number of patients with VIPomas, plasma VIP concentrations were not elevated.[101] Furthermore, in a number of patients without VIPomas, some of whom have diseases that cause diarrhea,[101,102] plasma VIP concentrations were reported to be elevated. In most subsequent studies, however, plasma VIP was found to be consistently elevated in patients with VIPomas, and not in patients with other conditions such as laxative abuse.[46,80,81,87,95–97]

Glucagonoma

Glucagonomas are endocrine tumors of the pancreas that secrete excessive amounts of glucagon and cause a distinct syndrome characterized by dermatitis, glucose intolerance, weight loss, and anemia (Table 93-4).

The first description of what became known as the glucagonoma syndrome was reported in 1942[122] in a patient with a skin rash associated with pancreatic cancer. McGavran and colleagues reported in 1966 the first well described case of a patient with the glucagonoma syndrome.[123] The patient had elevated immunoreactive glucagon in plasma, diabetes mellitus, a skin rash, and a pancreatic endocrine tumor. In 1973, Wilkinson[124] introduced the term "necrolytic migratory erythema" for the skin rash associated with pancreatic tumors. Mallinson and colleagues in 1974[125] specifically established the association of glucagonoma with skin rash when they reported nine cases with the clinical glucagonoma syndrome consisting of dermatitis, diabetes mellitus, unexplained weight

TABLE 93-4
Clinical Features of the Glucagonoma Syndrome

SIGN OR SYMPTOM	FREQUENCY (%)
Dermatitis (migratory necrolytic erythema)	68–84
Hypoaminoacidemia	80–90
Glucose intolerance or diabetes mellitus	84–85
Weight loss	66–96
Anemia	85
Diarrhea	15
Thromboembolism	12–24
Glossitis	14
Psychiatric disturbance	Uncommon

Data from references 6, 127, and 130.

loss, hypoaminoacidemia, anemia, and a glucagon-producing tumor of the pancreas.

The incidence for the glucagonoma syndrome peaks from 50 to 60 years of age, and the syndrome has not been described in children.[6,26] Necrolytic migratory erythema, the characteristic skin rash associated with the glucagonoma syndrome, is present in most cases (see Table 93-4).[124,126–130] The skin lesion starts as an annular erythema at intertriginous and periorificial sites. It is normally found on the buttock, groin, perineum, and thighs. The erythema subsequently becomes raised and the central parts form superficial bullae. The top of the bullous lesion frequently detaches, leaving eroded areas that become crusted (Fig. 93-2; see Color Fig. 52). Lesions frequently become confluent. The extent and severity of the lesions may wax and wane. Healing in 2 or 3 weeks results in hyperpigmentation (see Fig. 93-2). Histologically, early skin lesions demonstrate a superficial spongiosis and necrosis and subcutaneous blister formation.[124,126,127,129–131] The pathogenic mechanism by which the glucagonoma syndrome produces this characteristic skin rash is unclear. It is not established that the skin rash is associated with the hyperglucagonemia because numerous patients have been given large doses of glucagon for long periods of time without exhibiting the characteristic rash.[126] Glucagon-induced hypoaminoacidemia may be one mechanism because correction of hypoaminoacidemia has been shown to correct the dermatitis without changing plasma glucagon concentrations.[126,131–133] The resemblance of the lesions to those seen with zinc deficiency has resulted in trials of therapy with zinc, with some responses.[134] Resolution of the rash, however, has been reported after simple hydration with glucose and saline[126,135]; therefore, it is not established that either hypoaminoacidemia or zinc deficiency are necessarily causative in all patients. A number of other clinical features are also characteristic of the glucagonoma syndrome (see Table 93-4). Angular cheilitis (see Fig. 93-2) is a common feature, as is nail dystrophy and thinning of the hair. A painful glossitis develops in some patients (see Table 93-4).

Hypoaminoacidemia occurs in most patients and, as originally pointed out by Mallinson and colleagues, the levels may vary with the intensity of the disease.[125,126] The hypoaminoacidemia is thought to be secondary to the hyperglucagonemia because glucagon infusions have been demon-

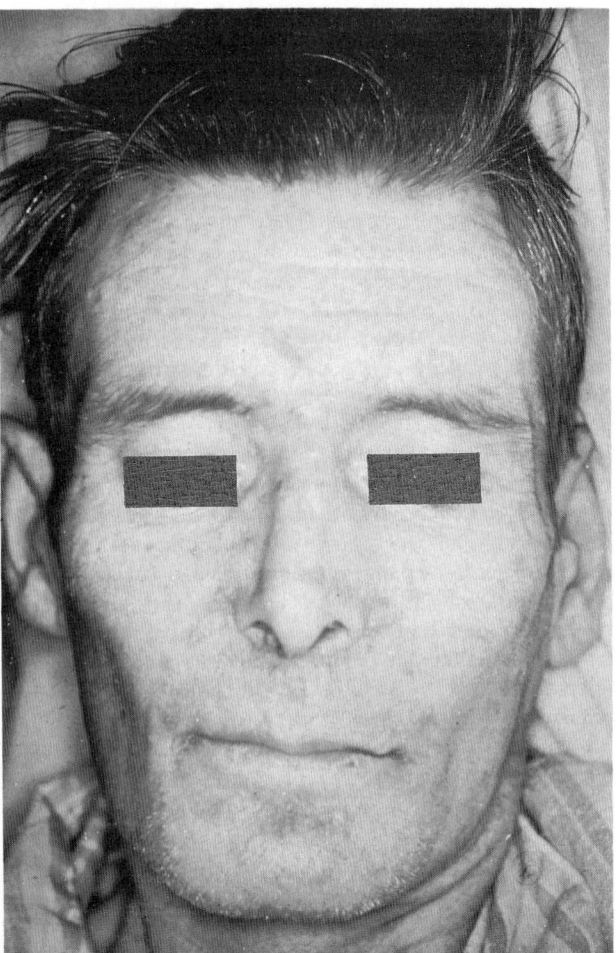

FIGURE 93-2. (See Color Fig. 52.) Migratory necrolytic erythema involving the face in a patient with metastatic glucagonoma. These typical skin lesions usually start on the extremities or on intertriginous or periorificial sites. The lesions initially are erythematous and scaly, later become raised and bullous, and finally become crusty, as is evident in this patient. Healing results in hyperpigmentation. Angular cheilitis, a common feature in patients with glucagonoma, is also present in a mild form in this patient. The patient also demonstrates loss of the buccal fat pad and temporal muscle wasting, indicative of the generalized wasting these patients characteristically undergo.

strated to have a controlling influence on amino acid metabolism by altering gluconeogenesis.[126,136,137] It has been demonstrated in humans that glucagon deficiency caused by either suppression with somatostatin or total pancreatectomy increases plasma amino acid concentrations.[138–141] On the other hand, the administration of glucagon decreases plasma amino acid concentrations.[139,140] A metabolic study using stable isotopes in a patient with glucagonoma with weight loss, hyperglycemia, and hypoaminoacidemia[142] found a 50% increase in amino acid catabolism, a 15% increase in whole body lipolysis, and a 15% increase in hepatic glucose production; energy expenditure, as well as rate of protein breakdown, were normal. It was proposed[142] that these small alterations over the long term, in conjunction with a negative energy balance, might explain the weight loss, hypoaminoacidemia, and hyperglycemia.

Diabetes mellitus and glucose intolerance are among the most frequent findings in patients with the glucagonoma syndrome (see Table 93-4).[6,126,130,140] Because of the effect of glucagon on glucose regulation, diabetes mellitus might be expected to be a constant feature of the glucagonoma syndrome, but it is not uniformly present (see Table 93-4).[6,126,127,130,140] Despite hyperglucagonemia, a number of patients with the glucagonoma syndrome do not have diabetes mellitus or glucose intolerance.[127,130] Diabetes mellitus or even glucose intolerance is a much less constant feature of the syndrome than is hypoaminoacidemia.[140] The relation of the hyperglucagonemia to the diabetes mellitus or glucose intolerance remains unclear. Glucagon levels in patients with glucagonomas do not correlate well with the degree of glucose intolerance.[26,126,127,130] Furthermore, various treatments have resulted in definite changes in plasma glucagon concentrations but have not produced correlated changes in blood glucose. For example, tumor resection and normalization of blood glucose have not resulted in the correction of the glucose intolerance.[26,126] Kahn and associates infused a somatostatin analog to depress plasma glucagon levels in a patient with glucagonoma, but no effect on blood glucose level was observed.[141] In some patients, however, removal of the glucagon-producing tumor has improved glucose tolerance.[125,126,140] Whether or not glucagon causes glucose intolerance appears to depend to a large degree on the patient's insulin reserve. If it is intact, hyperglucagonemia is present without glucose intolerance.[26,126]

Weight loss is a common feature in patients with the glucagonoma syndrome, and it may be profound (see Table 93-4).[6,26,126,127,130] Weight loss is prominent in patients with small tumors as well as in those with metastatic tumor, suggesting that cachexia is a consequence of the catabolic actions of glucagon.[126] This is supported by a study in which a patient's weight loss was reversed after being given the long-acting somatostatin analog, octreotide (SMS 201-995), which reduced the plasma glucagon concentration to a near-normal range.[143]

Thromboembolic phenomena are more common in patients with the glucagonoma syndrome (see Table 93-4).[6,26,126,127,130] Both deep vein thrombus and pulmonary emboli have been reported to occur in a significant number of cases, and have been the cause of death in some patients.[6,26,126,127,130] Glucagon is not known to affect coagulation parameters; however, the pathophysiologic process of the thromboembolic events in glucagonoma has not been systematically studied. A normochromic, normocytic anemia is also a frequent finding in patients with glucagonomas (see Table 93-4).[26,126,127] Serum iron, serum vitamin B_{12}, and serum folate concentrations usually are normal, and the anemia does not respond to therapy with any of these agents. It does respond to resection of the tumor, however.[126,143-145] Further evidence that the anemia may be caused by glucagon excess is that prolonged therapy with a long-acting glucagon preparation decreased erythropoiesis in rats and mice.[145] Psychiatric disturbances, particularly depression, have been reported in a number of patients with the glucagonoma syndrome; however, the exact frequency or even whether they are more common in patients with glucagonoma has not been established (see Table 93-4).[122,124,126]

Glucagonoma is usually suspected in patients with chronic, unexplained, and therapy-resistant dermatitis, elevated sedimentation rates associated with glucose intolerance, thromboembolic phenomena, or the MEN I syndrome (see Table 93-4). Diagnosis rests on demonstrating a pathologic elevation of the plasma glucagon concentration. In almost all patients with glucagonoma, the plasma glucagon concentration is elevated (>150 pg/mL),[126,127] with a mean value of 2110 ± 334 pg/mL (±1 SEM) in 23 patients with proven glucagonoma in one study; the highest value in a patient without glucagonoma was 409 ± 29 pg/mL. It has been suggested that a plasma glucagon concentration of more than 1000 pg/mL is diagnostic of glucagonoma,[26] because almost all patients with glucagonomas have this degree of elevation. In one study,[146] 3 of 7 patients had plasma glucagon levels in excess of 1000 pg/mL, and the authors point out that the level roughly correlated with tumor size; therefore, if the disease is diagnosed earlier, the plasma glucagon level may be lower. Other conditions associated with increased plasma glucagon concentrations include renal insufficiency, hepatic insufficiency, severe stress (trauma, exercise, diabetic ketoacidosis), prolonged fast, and familial hyperglucagonemia.[26,127,147,148] In general, these latter conditions do not demonstrate plasma glucagon elevations in the range seen with glucagonoma.[26,127,131] For the occasional patient with glucagonoma with a fasting plasma glucagon concentration less than 1000 pg/mL, which may overlap with levels in other conditions, there is no proven provocative test that will clearly distinguish these conditions.[26] Usually, however, these non-glucagonoma conditions can be excluded on clinical grounds.

Somatostatinoma

Somatostatinomas are endocrine tumors of the pancreas or intestine that secrete excessive amounts of somatostatin, which causes a distinct syndrome characterized by diabetes mellitus, gallbladder disease, diarrhea, and steatorrhea (Table 93-5).

In 1977, the first two cases of somatostatinomas were independently reported.[149,150] On the basis of these reports and the known actions of somatostatin, it was proposed that the clinical somatostatinoma syndrome consisted of mild diabetes mellitus, gallbladder disease, weight loss, and anemia.[151] Diarrhea, steatorrhea, and hypochlorhydria became

TABLE 93-5
Clinical Features of the Somatostatinoma Syndrome

SIGN OR SYMPTOM	FREQUENCY (%)	
	Pancreatic (n = 27)	Intestinal (n = 21)
Diabetes mellitus	95	21
Gallbladder disease	94	43
Diarrhea	92	38
Steatorrhea	83	12
Hypochlorhydria	86	17
Weight loss	90	69

Adapted from Vinik AI, Strodel WE, Eckhauser FE, et al. Somatostatinomas, PPomas and neurotensinomas. Semin Oncol 1987;14:263; and Vinik AI, Moattari AR. Treatment of endocrine tumors. Endocr Clin North Am 1989;18:483.

additional features as other cases were described (see Table 93-5).[49,152,153]

Somatostatin is a tetradecapeptide originally isolated and purified from ovine hypothalamic tissue.[154,155] It inhibits the release of almost all other hormones, and has direct effects on a number of gastrointestinal functions, including potent inhibition of basal and pentagastrin- or meal-stimulated acid secretion, cholecystokinin-stimulated pancreatic enzyme secretion, and intestinal absorption of amino acids.[155–157] A number of studies have suggested that somatostatin has a paracrine effect on antral gastrin release.[155] Somatostatin also has marked effects on gut motility and transit time.[155]

The mean age of patients with pancreatic somatostatinomas or intestinal somatostatinomas is 50 years, with a range of 30 to 84 years.[7,158] There is a 2 : 1 predominance of women among patients with pancreatic somatostatinomas, whereas 60% of patients with intestinal somatostatinoma are men.[7]

Initial symptoms most commonly seen in patients with somatostatinomas are diabetes, gallbladder disease, and diarrhea with steatorrhea (see Table 93-5).[7,49,152,158,159] Diabetes mellitus or glucose intolerance was reported to occur in 63% of patients in one study,[49] 55% of patients in another,[7] and 62% in a third review of cases.[159] Diabetes mellitus, however, occurred in 96% of the patients with pancreatic somatostatinomas and in only 21% of those with intestinal somatostatinomas (see Table 93-5).[7,158] The diabetes is usually mild, and severe hypoglycemia or ketosis, although reported, are uncommon.[153,160,161] The development of diabetes mellitus or glucose intolerance is secondary to the ability of somatostatin to inhibit insulin and glucagon release[7] and to the replacement of functional islet tissue by tumor.[49] This latter factor may explain why diabetes mellitus is more common in patients with pancreatic than intestinal somatostatinomas (see Table 93-5).[7]

Gallbladder disease (cholelithiasis) was reported in 65% of patients in one series[49] and in 70% in another study.[7] It was reported in 94% of patients with pancreatic and 43% of patients with intestinal somatostatinomas (see Table 93-5).[7] The high incidence of gallbladder disease in patients with somatostatinoma and its lack in patients with other islet cell tumors suggest a causative association between the gallbladder disease and somatostatinoma. This conclusion is supported by the finding of a massively dilated gallbladder in 2 patients with somatostatinoma, 1 of whom showed no evidence of cholelithiases or other pathology.[160,161] Furthermore, infusions of somatostatin into otherwise healthy subjects inhibit gallbladder emptying.[155,162]

Diarrhea and steatorrhea were reported in 35% of patients in one study,[49] and diarrhea in 68% and steatorrhea in 52% of patients in another study.[7] The diarrhea characteristically consists of 3 to 10 foul-smelling stools per day, and the steatorrhea varies from 20 to 76 g per day.[7,49] Diarrhea and steatorrhea are much less common in patients with intestinal rather than pancreatic somatostatinomas (see Table 93-5).[7,158] In some, but not all cases, the severity of the diarrhea and steatorrhea correlates with the size and degree of metastatic spread of the tumor, and improves with tumor resection.[49] Somatostatin has been shown to inhibit pancreatic enzyme and fluid secretion as well as gallbladder motility.[155,162] In addition, somatostatin also inhibits intestinal absorption of lipid,[163] D-xylose, vitamin B$_{12}$, and folate.[164] These biologic

actions of somatostatin may be responsible for the maldigestion, steatorrhea, and diarrhea observed in these patients.[49] The fact that patients with intestinal somatostatinomas have less diarrhea or steatorrhea has been attributed to their lower plasma somatostatin levels or the lack of local effects of the somatostatinoma within the pancreas (see Table 93-5).[7]

Hypochlorhydria was found in 33% of patients in one study[49] and in 53% of patients in another study.[7] Hypochlorhydria occurred in 86% of patients with pancreatic and 17% of patients with intestinal somatostatinomas (see Table 93-5).[7] Infusion of somatostatin has been shown to inhibit gastric secretion, as well as basal and food-stimulated gastrin release, in healthy subjects.[155] As with the glucagonoma syndrome, weight loss is reported to be common in patients with somatostatinomas. The weight loss may be secondary to the diarrhea and malabsorption. Other, less common features reported in patients with somatostatinoma include the occurrence of various associated endocrine disorders. In one study, four patients were reported to have hypoglycemic episodes with normal or elevated plasma insulin concentrations, and were diagnosed as having insulinomas.[49] In two patients with elevated plasma insulin concentrations, the tumors did not contain increased amounts of insulin, only somatostatin. Tumor tissue was not available from the other two cases; however, immunocytochemical studies demonstrated mostly D cells (somatostatin-producing cells), with some β cells (insulin-producing cells) in one patient, and 20% to 30% D cells with 30% to 40% β cells in another patient.[49]

In most studies, somatostatinomas have been found more or less by accident.[49] In most cases, the tumor is found at the time of exploratory laparotomy for cholecystectomy or during various imaging studies (computed tomography [CT] scan, upper gastrointestinal radiography, ultrasound) or during endoscopic studies. These imaging studies are performed because of complaints of abdominal pain, bleeding, or diarrhea in most cases. Once discovered, the tumors are identified as somatostatinomas by demonstrating elevated tissue concentrations of somatostatin, increased numbers of D cells by immunocytochemistry, or increased plasma concentrations of somatostatin-like immunoreactivity (SLI). In one review,[159] of the 11 patients with somatostatinoma who had a plasma somatostatin level measured, it was reported to be elevated in all but one patient. In the future, it is likely that the syndrome will be diagnosed earlier because of the increased clinical awareness of the somatostatinoma syndrome (see Table 93-5) and the greater availability of reliable assays for the determination of SLI in blood. These assays currently are complicated by the need for extraction of the plasma, and are not widely available.

The diagnosis of somatostatinoma at a time when plasma SLI concentrations are only marginally elevated and the tumor has not yet metastasized requires the development of reliable provocative tests. Tolbutamide and arginine have been reported to stimulate plasma SLI increases[49,165,166]; however, arginine is a well established stimulant for normal D cells and thus is unlikely to differentiate normal from supranormal secretion.[49] Furthermore, although tolbutamide stimulates SLI increases in animals,[165] it is reported not to cause changes in plasma SLI concentrations in healthy human volunteers.[167] Until an adequate provocative test is developed, if somatostatinoma is to be diagnosed earlier, it may be necessary to determine plasma SLI concentrations in all patients with diabetes mellitus without a family history, or in all patients with unexplained diarrhea[152]

GRFoma

GRFomas are endocrine tumors that frequently originate in the pancreas and secrete excessive amounts of GRF, which causes acromegaly.

GRFomas were described in 1982.[168,169] GRF is a 44–amino-acid peptide originally isolated from human pancreatic endocrine tumors that caused acromegaly, and is structurally similar to VIP.[168,170] In one immunocytochemical study[171] of pancreatic endocrine tumors, 4 of 9 (44%) contained GRF-like immunoreactivity, although only 1 patient had acromegaly. In another study,[172] 6 of 24 (25%) pancreatic endocrine tumors, of which 16 were associated with various clinical syndromes (insulinoma, 8; gastrinoma, 5; VIPoma, 2; and Cushing's syndrome, 1), were found to have GRF-immunoreactive material, but no patient had clinical acromegaly. Subsequently, a number of cases (GRFomas) have been described.[50,51,173–177] In one review[50] of 30 cases of GRFoma from the literature, 30% of the GRFomas were in the pancreas, 54% were lung tumors, 7% jejunal endocrine tumors, and 12% were from other sites, including adrenal gland, foregut, and retroperitoneum. The patients were 15 to 60 years old, with a median age of 54 years. The most common symptoms were those consistent with the diagnosis of acromegaly. The patients usually have a large pancreatic tumor (>6 cm) and in 30% of cases it is metastatic at the time of diagnosis. Forty percent of the patients with pancreatic GRFomas have associated Zollinger-Ellison syndrome, and one third of the patients had associated MEN I syndrome.

GRFomas usually are suspected in a patient with acromegaly and an elevated growth hormone level, with hepatic metastases or abdominal complaints.[50,51,168–170,173–177] Pancreatic endocrine tumors that are GRFomas are often associated with a gastrinoma and Zollinger-Ellison syndrome. Therefore, any patient with peptic ulcer symptoms, diarrhea, or symptoms suggestive of chronic esophageal reflux who presents with acromegalic features should be suspected of having a GRFoma. Furthermore, pancreatic GRFomas have occurred in a number of patients with the MEN I syndrome. Any patient with acromegaly with hyperparathyroidism or a family history of MEN I also should be suspected of having a GRFoma.[50,173,174] The diagnosis is confirmed by performing a plasma assay for GRF.[50,51,175,176]

PPoma and Nonfunctioning Islet Cell Tumor

PPomas and nonfunctioning pancreatic endocrine tumors are endocrine tumors that originate in the pancreas and secrete excessive amounts of PP (PPoma), or secrete no peptides (nonfunctioning) and cause clinical symptoms secondary to the tumor per se.

Nonfunctioning pancreatic endocrine tumors resemble PPomas but differ from the functional pancreatic endocrine tumors in their clinical presentation in that their symptoms

are entirely caused by the tumor per se, and not by any secreted products.[7,12,178] Nonfunctioning pancreatic endocrine tumors and PPomas are frequently diagnosed after the patient presents with symptoms or signs of metastatic tumor in the liver (cachexia, abdominal pain, hepatomegaly), and a liver biopsy is performed that reveals metastatic endocrine tumor. Infusion of PP into animals has been shown to have numerous effects, including inhibition of pancreatic secretion, a relaxant effect on the gallbladder, weak inhibition of pentagastrin-stimulated acid secretion, and various stimulating effects on gastrointestinal motility.[179] It is unclear why patients with pancreatic endocrine tumors with very high plasma concentrations of PP do not have symptoms secondary to the increased PP per se. Typically, the patient with a PPoma or nonfunctioning pancreatic endocrine tumor is 40 to 60 years of age.[7,178,180] In one study, 36% of patients with nonfunctioning pancreatic endocrine tumors presented with abdominal pain and 28% with jaundice; 16% of the patients were asymptomatic, and tumors were found incidentally at surgery; and the remaining patients presented with a variety of symptoms due to tumor mass.[180] In most series,[4,178,180,181] but not all,[182] most patients with PPomas or nonfunctioning pancreatic endocrine tumors have metastatic disease at the time of diagnosis.

Nonfunctioning pancreatic endocrine tumors or PPomas usually cannot be differentiated from any other malignant tumor of the pancreas before histologic studies. In one series, the diagnosis of a nonfunctioning pancreatic endocrine tumor or PPoma was not made in a single patient before surgery.[178] Furthermore, 20% of the patients were asymptomatic, and the tumors were found incidentally during other operative procedures.[178] Any patient with a long survival (>5 years) previously diagnosed as having metastatic pancreatic adenocarcinoma should be suspected of having in fact a nonfunctioning islet cell tumor or PPoma. Typically, these tumors are large when diagnosed (>5 cm) and almost all are malignant (70%–92%).[7,12,178,180] Nonfunctioning pancreatic endocrine tumors are differentiated from PPomas on the results of the plasma PP assay. Of patients with pancreatic endocrine tumors not associated with any clinical syndrome, which therefore would be classified clinically as nonfunctioning, 50% to 75% have raised fasting plasma levels of PP, and the tumors can be classified as PPomas.[7] There are no data suggesting that PPomas or nonfunctioning pancreatic endocrine tumors differ in biologic behavior or in treatment options.[39,181] Recognizing the tumor as a PPoma may be clinically important, however, in that plasma PP levels may be used to monitor the resulting therapies such as surgical resection or chemotherapy.

Other Tumors

Cushing's syndrome associated with a pancreatic endocrine tumor that secretes corticotropin is usually[54,56,150,183–187] recognized in patients with another symptomatic pancreatic endocrine syndrome. Cushing's syndrome occurs in 19% of patients with MEN I and Zollinger-Ellison syndrome and is caused by pituitary production of corticotropin; the disease in these patients is usually mild.[54] Cushing's syndrome has also been reported in a number of cases of sporadic Zollinger-Ellison syndrome,[54–56,158,183–187] and in one prospective study[54] was reported to be present in 5% of all cases. In patients with the sporadic form of Zollinger-Ellison syndrome, the symptoms of Cushing's syndrome are severe, usually occurring with metastatic disease, and the Cushing's syndrome is the result of ectopic production of corticotropin.[54] These patients usually respond poorly to chemotherapy and have a poor prognosis.[54] Cushing's syndrome as a clinical manifestation related solely to a pancreatic endocrine tumor is rare.[188]

Paraneoplastic hypercalcemia due to a pancreatic endocrine tumor releasing parathyroid hormone (PTH) or a PTH-like immunoreactive material and causing hyperparathyroidism has been reported rarely.[52,53,189] Paraneoplastic hypercalcemia associated with a pancreatic endocrine tumor that was not caused by the release of PTH or a PTH-like immunoreactive material, but by the release by the tumor of an unknown hypercalcemic substance that mimics the action of PTH, also has been reported rarely.[11,190] In most,[52,53,189,191,192] but not all[191] cases of paraneoplastic hypercalcemia with a pancreatic endocrine tumor,[52,53,189,191,192] the tumor was metastatic to the liver at the time of diagnosis.

It has been proposed that there is a neurotensinoma syndrome associated with pancreatic endocrine tumors.[7,193-198] Neurotensin is a 13–amino-acid peptide first extracted from bovine brain and subsequently isolated from the human gastrointestinal tract.[199] Neurotensin has a number of pharmacologic effects, including causing hypotension, tachycardia, and cyanosis, stimulating pancreatic protein and bicarbonate secretion, affecting intestinal motility, and stimulating jejunal and ileal fluid and electrolyte secretion.[199] The clinical features described in patients with neurotensinomas with pancreatic endocrine tumor include diarrhea with hypokalemia, weight loss, and, in some cases, diabetes, cyanosis, hypotension, and flushing.[7] Of the 6 cases included in one review,[7] 3 were cured by tumor resection and the remainder responded to streptozotocin treatment.[7,193-198] Others[25,193] have raised the question of whether a specific neurotensinoma syndrome actually exists. In one study[193] of 180 patients with functional pancreatic endocrine tumors, an elevated plasma neurotensin level was found in 6 patients with VIPomas, and the clinical symptoms in those patients did not differ from those in patients without an elevated plasma neurotensin level. In a second study,[25] 19% of patients with Zollinger-Ellison syndrome were found to have an elevated plasma neurotensin level, and their symptoms did not differ from those in patients without an elevated plasma neurotensin level. Therefore, it is not apparent that a distinct neurotensinoma syndrome exists.

TUMOR LOCALIZATION

The techniques used for tumor localization and the rationale for using various localization methods are similar for all the pancreatic endocrine tumors. Once the particular type of pancreatic endocrine tumor is established by the proper radioimmunoassays and functional studies, tumor localization studies need to be undertaken for a number of reasons. The only possible long-term cure of these syndromes is by surgical excision. In all cases except insulinoma, most, if not all of these tumors may demonstrate malignancy if followed long enough, and therefore if metastatic spread is not present at the time of diagnosis, an attempt should be made to cure

these patients surgically. Gastrinomas and insulinomas frequently present as small tumors. As much as 50% of those endocrine tumors that frequently occur extrapancreatically, such as gastrinomas,[20,39,200-202] and 10% to 20% of endocrine tumors that occur almost entirely within the pancreas, such as insulinomas,[26,66,203] are not found at surgery. Therefore, detailed localization studies may help the surgeon in finding the tumor. The tumor frequently can be multiple, with multifocal tumors reported to occur in 10% of insulinomas[26,70] and in up to 50% of some pancreatic endocrine tumors such as gastrinomas.[20,200,204] Although the other pancreatic endocrine tumors usually are reported as single adenoma,[7,26] there have been relatively few well studied cases. Furthermore, except for insulinoma, the other pancreatic endocrine tumors frequently are diagnosed only after metastatic spread to the liver has occurred[7,20,26,39,49,126,131]; therefore, if careful imaging studies are done, the extent of the tumor may be established and unnecessary surgery prevented.

Abdominal ultrasound,[20,39,205-211] CT scan (Figs. 93-3 through 93-5),[20,39,208-217] selective abdominal angiography (Figs. 93-6 and 93-7),[20,39,201,207,209,211-214,218,219] selective venous sampling for hormones from portal venous tributaries using a transhepatic approach (i.e., portal venous sampling [PVS]; Fig. 93-8),[20,39,125,210-212,219,224] magnetic resonance imaging (MRI; see Figs. 93-4 and 93-5),[217,225,226] intraoperative ultrasonography (Fig. 93-9),[211,217,227-229] hepatic venous sampling for hormones after intraarterial injection of secretin (gastrinomas) or calcium (insulinomas; see Fig. 93-8),[230-232] endoscopic ultrasound (Fig. 93-10),[233-236] and radiolabeled somatostatin scanning[237] all have been reported to be useful for localizing pancreatic endocrine tumors. Small islet cell tumors (<2 cm) have proven the most difficult to localize. Table 93-6 summarizes the results of studies on the ability of the various modalities to localize insulinomas, which are characteristically small (<2 cm) at the time of clinical presentation. Ultrasound localizes 10% to 39% of insulinomas, CT scanning 17% to 40%, selective abdominal angiography 35% to 90%, PVS for insulin 77% to 90%, intraoperative ultra-

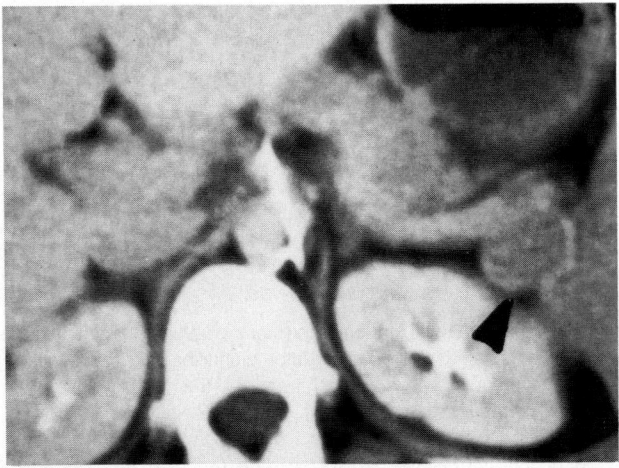

FIGURE 93-3. Computed tomographic (CT) scan in a patient with an insulinoma. The insulinoma is in the pancreatic tail (*arrow*). The splenic vein courses around the tumor. CT scan with intravenous contrast localizes 17% to 40% of insulinomas.

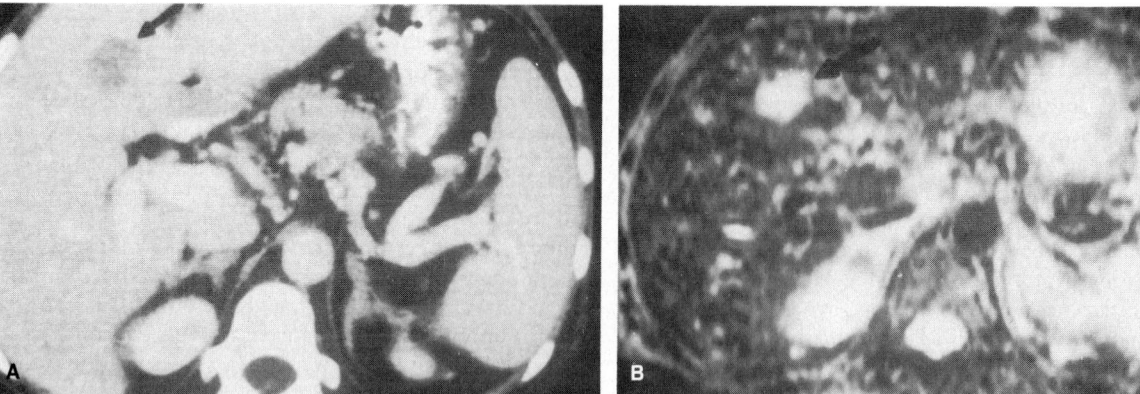

FIGURE 93-4. (**A**) Computed tomographic (CT) scan and (**B**) a T2-weighted MR image in a patient with a metastatic ACTH-producing pancreatic endocrine tumor metastatic to the liver. The CT scan demonstrates a solitary metastasis in the left lobe of the liver (*arrow*), which is faintly seen; whereas on the T2-weighted MR image, the metastasis (*arrow*) is clearly seen in the medial segment of the left lobe of the liver. Metastases from pancreatic endocrine tumors often are much more easily identified on MR images, because the tumor has a characteristically bright appearance on the T2-weighted images.

sound 90% to 94%, endoscopic ultrasound 79% to 100%, hepatic venous sampling for insulin after calcium injection 100%, and radiolabeled somatostatin scanning 50%. Similar data are not available with other pancreatic endocrine tumors. However, because VIPomas, GRFomas, and glucagonomas are almost entirely intrapancreatic, it is likely that results similar to those with insulinomas of similar size will be obtained. For somatostatinomas, which frequently are extrapancreatic, it is likely that results similar to those obtained with gastrinomas will be found. Results for localization of gastrinomas with ultrasound and CT scan are similar to those listed in Table 93-6 for insulinoma; however, angiography finds 33%

to 86% of primary gastrinomas,[20,39,218,219] selective venous sampling for gastrin 73%,[221] and intraoperative ultrasound 83%.[229] Prospective studies of patients with pancreatic endocrine tumors have demonstrated that MRI sensitivity has markedly improved over the last 5 years with the use of short inversion recovery sequences, dynamic gadolinium enhancement, and fat suppression.[217,225,226] For detecting metastatic disease to the liver, one study[226] demonstrated that MRI was more sensitive than ultrasound, CT, or angiography, and is now the imaging procedure of choice (see Fig. 93-4). For primary pancreatic endocrine tumors, the role of MRI is still unclear, with one study[226] demonstrating it has a low sensi-

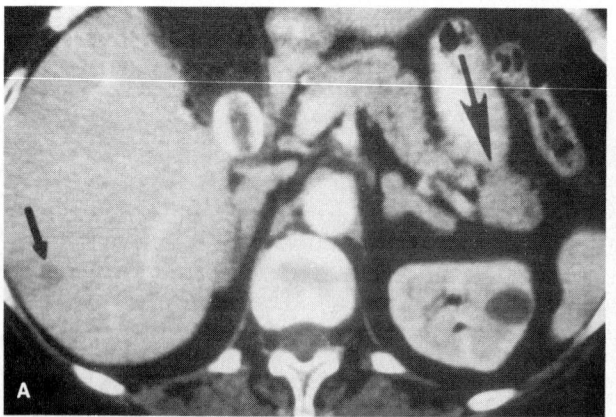
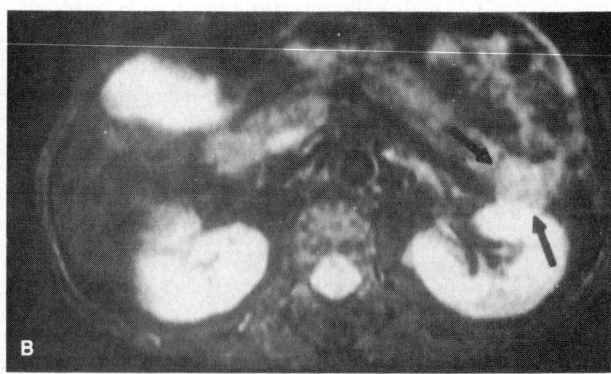

FIGURE 93-5. (**A**) Computed tomographic (CT) scan and (**B**) a T2-weighted MR image in a patient with a pancreatic endocrine tumor producing pancreatic polypeptide (PPoma) and a hepatic cyst. The CT scan demonstrates a primary tumor in the pancreatic tail (*large arrow*) and a cystic lesion in the right lobe of the liver (*small arrow*). In the T2-weighted MR image, the PPoma is seen as a bright lesion in the pancreatic tail (*arrows*) and the lesion in the right lobe of the liver is not seen, suggesting it is not a hepatic metastasis. At surgery, the lesion in the liver was found to be a simple cyst, and the lesion in the tail of the pancreas was a PPoma. For primary pancreatic endocrine tumors in large comparative studies, MR imaging is equally sensitive to CT scan and ultrasonography (20%–30%), whereas selective angiography is more sensitive, identifying 50% to 70% of lesions. For metastatic lesions to the liver, MR imaging is more sensitive than CT scanning.

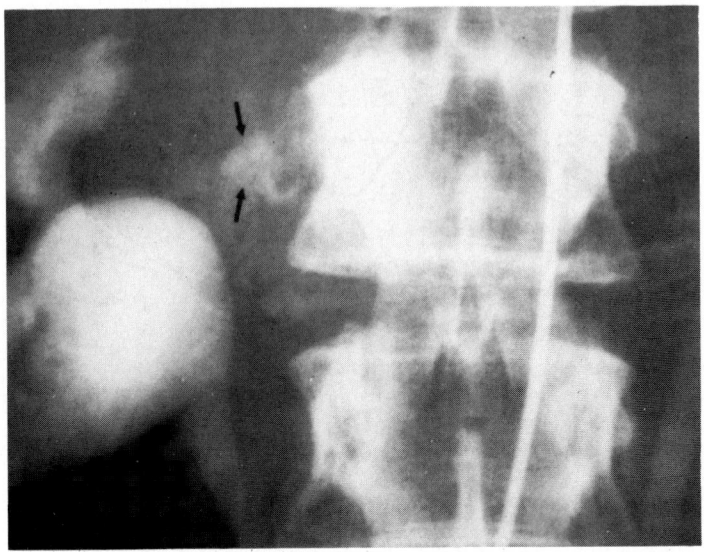

FIGURE 93-6. Selective angiographic localization of the pancreatic endocrine tumor in a patient with insulinoma. The insulinoma is localized in the pancreatic head by a selective celiac artery injection. Insulinomas, as other pancreatic endocrine tumors, are characteristically hypervascular, as demonstrated in the insulinoma in this patient, and are seen by selective angiography in 35% to 90% of all patients with insulinomas.

tivity (22%), equal to that of ultrasound and CT scanning, but significantly less than that of angiography, whereas another study[217] demonstrated that MRI with gadolinium enhancement and fat suppression detected 91% of all primary pancreatic endocrine tumors. The difference between the results of the two studies might lie in the size of primary tumors,

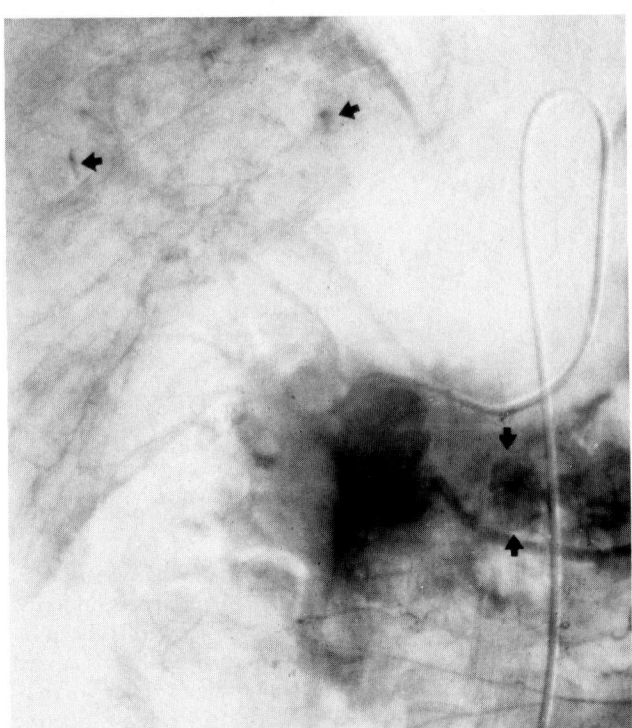

FIGURE 93-7. Selective common hepatic artery injection in a patient with metastatic insulinoma. The primary insulinoma is demonstrated in the pancreatic head (*arrows*), and two hepatic metastases are located in the liver (*arrows*). In only 10% to 15% of patients with insulinomas are the tumors malignant, and selective angiography demonstrates the metastatic spread to the liver in over 90% of these patients.

because in the latter study[217] 90% of the tumors were at least 2 cm in diameter. The results for the ability of ultrasound, CT, MRI, and selective angiography to detect pancreatic endocrine tumor have been shown to depend on the size of the tumor.[216,218,225,226] For example, using any of the imaging modalities (ultrasound, CT, selective angiography, or MRI), less than 10% of tumors smaller than 1 cm, 30% to 40% of tumors 1 to 3 cm, and 70% to 80% of tumors larger than 3 cm were detected. Therefore, most VIPomas, glucagonomas, and somatostatinomas, which usually are clinically suspected only when the tumor is large (frequently >4 cm), will be detected. One study[229] suggests the combination of PVS for localizing the hormone gradient and intraoperative ultrasound at surgery increases the ability at the time of surgery to localize pancreatic endocrine tumors that were not detected by standard imaging studies. In a subsequent prospective study[227] of patients with occult insulinomas that were not imaged by ultrasound, CT, or angiography, tumors were found at surgery in 92% of the patients using the combined localization results of PVS and intraoperative ultrasound at surgery. In this study,[227] the use of intraoperative ultrasound at surgery identified twice as many insulinomas as palpation alone. These studies demonstrate that for endocrine tumors that occur almost entirely within the pancreas (insulinomas, VIPomas, glucagonomas, GRFomas), this combination allows tumors to be found in almost all patients with negative preoperative imaging studies.[229] The functional localization of an insulinoma is shown in Figure 93-8, and the use of intraoperative ultrasound to localize an insulinoma in Figure 93-9. In contrast, in patients in whom the tumors are frequently extrapancreatic (gastrinomas, somatostatinomas), these techniques have proven less useful, and led to a change in surgical management in only 10% of all patients.[221,229] Pancreatic endocrine tumors are typically hypervascular tumors, as is demonstrated in Figure 93-6 in a patient with an insulinoma, and therefore, in almost all studies, the best single imaging modality to localize the primary tumor is selective angiography.[20,39,200,207,209,212,218] Furthermore, this hypervascularity makes it possible to detect some tumors with the use of intravenous contrast material at the time of the CT scan (see

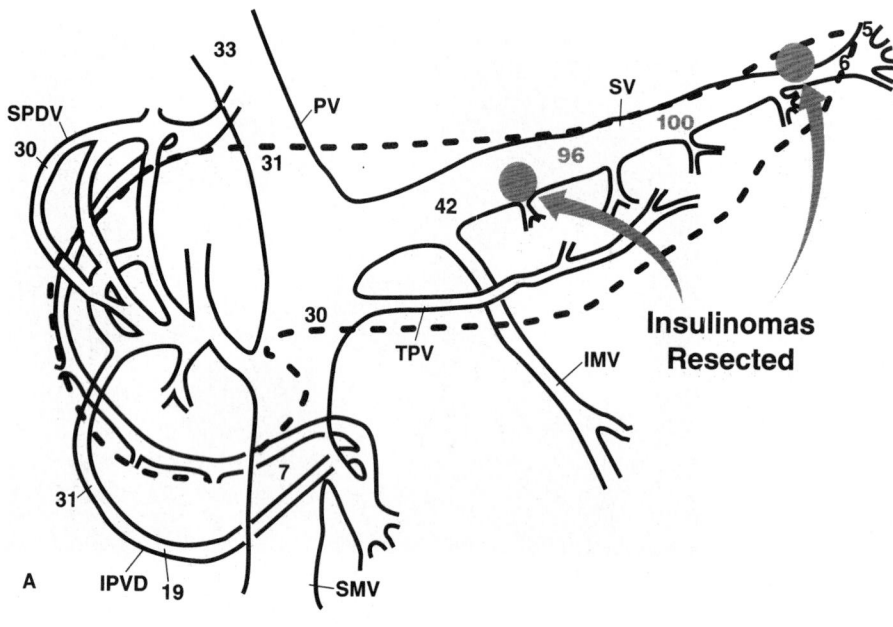

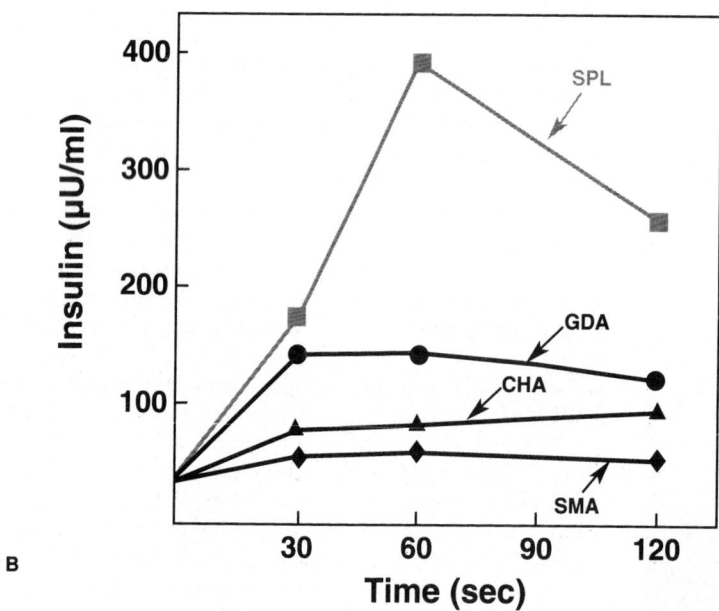

FIGURE 93-8. Functional location of an insulinoma can be achieved by **(A)** selective venous sampling for insulin from portal venous tributaries, or **(B)** selective hepatic venous sampling for insulin after intraarterial calcium injections in a patient with multiple insulinomas in the setting of MEN-I. **(A)** A sampling catheter was passed across the liver and venous samples obtained from the indicated locations, and simultaneous peripheral venous samples were obtained and assayed for insulin concentration. The average peripheral venous insulin concentration was 46 μU/mL, and an increase to 100 μU/mL is seen in the splenic vein, suggesting a tumor in the pancreatic tract. (IMV, inferior mesenteric vein; IPDV, inferior pancreaticoduodenal vein; PV, portal vein; SMV, superior mesenteric vein; SPDV, superior pancreaticoduodenal vein; SV, splenic vein; TPV, transverse pancreatic vein.) **(B)** Calcium gluconate (0.01–0.025 mEq Ca^{2+}/kg) was selectively injected into the indicated arteries and hepatic venous samples obtained before injection and at 30, 60 and 120 seconds postinjection and analyzed for insulin concentration. There was a marked increase after the splenic artery injection (SPL), whereas after injection into the gastroduodenal artery (GDA), common hepatic artery (CHA), and superior mesenteric artery (SMA), there was a much smaller increase. Two insulinomas **(A,** arrows) were found in the pancreatic tail at surgery, which is in the area localized by the PVS sampling as well as the area supplied by the splenic artery. There is much less experience with the intraarterial calcium method, but in a preliminary study,[230] it was as sensitive as PVS, has the advantage of requiring less expertise, and can be done at the time of angiography, and therefore a separate procedure is not required.

Fig. 93-3) or to detect small hepatic metastases on angiography (see Fig. 93-7).

The three more recent techniques of endoscopic ultrasound, somatostatin receptor imaging, and hepatic venous sampling for insulin gradients after intraarterial injection of calcium, may prove useful for detecting more pancreatic endocrine tumors than are found using the localization procedures reviewed in the preceding paragraph. Endoscopic ultrasound is reported to detect from 79% to 100%[233–235] of primary pancreatic endocrine tumors; however, its sensitivity for small tumors (<0.5 cm) and extrapancreatic tumors such as duodenal gastrinomas or somatostatinomas is not established.[236] Figure 93-10 provides an example of the detection by endoscopic ultrasound of an insulinoma that was not detected by other imaging procedures. Many neuroendocrine tumors possess somatostatin receptors,[239] and it has been reported that pancreatic endocrine tumors can be visualized using a radiolabeled analog of octreotide (^{125}I-Tyr[3]-octreotide).[238,239] In one study,[237] 50% of the pancreatic endocrine tumors were localized using this procedure, but it is not established whether it has greater sensitivity than the other imaging procedures for localizing the primary tumors. Studies have demonstrated that, in localizing gastrinomas functionally, hepatic venous sampling for gastrin gradients after selective intraarterial injection of secretin was more sensitive, required less expertise and had lower morbidity than PVS.[232]

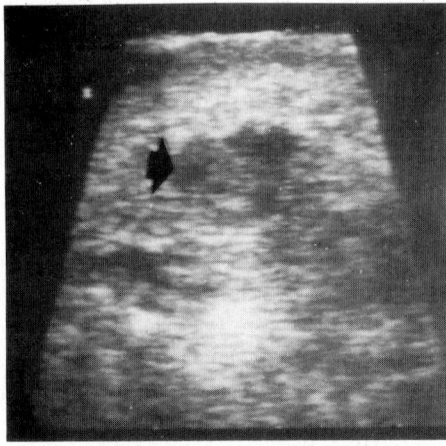

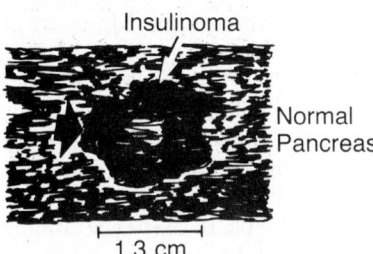

Insulinoma

Normal Pancreas

1.3 cm

FIGURE 93-9. Intraoperative ultrasonographic localization of an insulinoma. The *top* is an intraoperative ultrasound image of the insulinoma (*arrow*). The image was taken with a 10-MHz transducer. The *bottom* is a diagram of the ultrasound picture of the tumor (*arrow*). A 1.3-cm, nonpalpable insulinoma was found at surgery in the pancreatic head. In this patient, the use of intraoperative ultrasonography guided the successful enucleation of this tumor, which could not be identified at surgery by any other means.

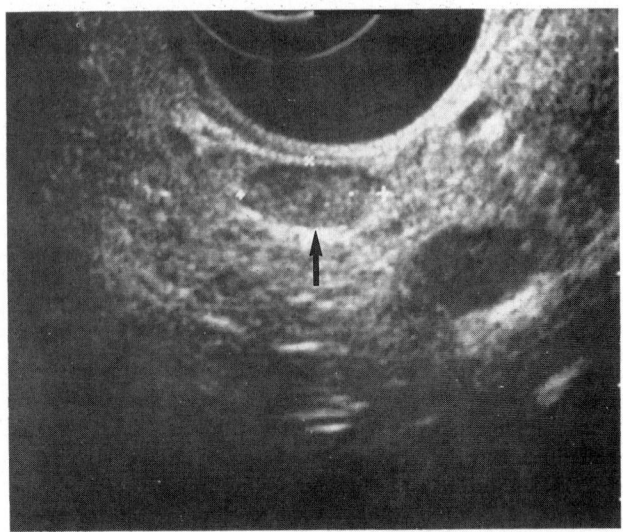

FIGURE 93-10. Endoscopic ultrasonography in a patient with an insulinoma. This image of the head of the pancreas was taken using a 12-MHz probe at the level of the duodenal bulb. It shows a 1.3- by 0.7-cm, sharply demarcated, relatively hypoechoic nodule (*arrow*), which was an insulinoma that was later enucleated at surgery. The splenic vein is seen below the tumor in the 5-o'clock position. The patient was a 29-year-old woman with clinical history and laboratory values diagnostic of insulinoma, but with negative dynamic computed tomographic and selective angiography studies. (Courtesy of Charles J. Lightdale, M.D., New York, NY.)

A similar procedure has been developed for localizing insulinomas[230] using calcium gluconate (0.01–0.025 mEq Ca^{2+}/kg). In this study,[230] all four insulinomas were localized using this procedure, suggesting it may replace PVS because of its greater simplicity and less morbidity. A typical result is shown in Figure 93-8, in which a much larger increase in insulin concentration in the hepatic vein is seen after splenic arterial injection than following injection of calcium into the other arteries that perfuse various other portions of the pancreas. At surgery, an insulinoma was found in the pancreatic tail in the area supplied by this artery.

For hepatic metastases from pancreatic endocrine tumors, ultrasound and CT scanning detect 14% to 20%[20,205–207,213,214] and 35% to 74%,[20,200,213–216] respectively. In one study,[226] MRI had a sensitivity of 83%. Selective angiography detects 33% to 86% of all hepatic metastases,[20,200,202,207,213,214, 218,219,226,235–238] which typically are hypervascular (see Fig. 93-5). In one study, the combination of CT and selective angiography detected 98% of all hepatic metastases[218]; however, in a more recent study,[226] MRI alone detected more hepatic metastases than angiography. For localizing hepatic metastases, MRI is the best initial procedure,[226] and if it is negative, then a combination of these procedures allows almost all patients with hepatic metastases to be identified pre-

TABLE 93-6
Studies Assessing the Ability of Various Modalities to Localize Insulinomas

LOCALIZING MODALITY	SUCCESSFUL LOCALIZATION (%)	REFERENCES
Ultrasonography	10–39	205–207, 209, 211, 224
CT	17–40	206, 207, 209, 211, 212, 215, 224
MRI	25–100	211, 217, 224
Selective angiography	35–90	207, 209, 211, 212, 219, 224
Selective portal venous sampling for insulin	77–90	21, 209, 211, 219, 222, 224, 227
Hepatic venous sampling for insulin after intraarterial calcium	100	230
Intraoperative ultrasonography	90–94	211, 212, 224, 228, 229
Endoscopic ultrasonography	79–100	233–235
Radiolabeled somatostatin scanning	50	237

operatively, thus avoiding unnecessary surgery. Bone metastases have been described in up to 12% of patients with advanced pancreatic endocrine tumors with metastases to the liver.[35] Somatostatin receptor imaging may be particularly useful for detecting bone metastases because in one study[237] in a number of patients with pancreatic endocrine tumors, unsuspected bone metastases were detected.

TREATMENT

All patients with functioning pancreatic endocrine tumors have two problems that are interrelated but often have to be dealt with separately. Acutely, the symptoms due to excess hormone secretion must be controlled, and ultimately the tumor itself must be dealt with. Although excision of the pancreatic endocrine tumor would solve both clinical problems, this frequently is not possible because there is metastatic disease at time of diagnosis or, occasionally, the pancreatic endocrine tumor cannot be found at surgery. Furthermore, the clinical condition of the patient may have deteriorated because of complications of the excess hormone state, necessitating treatment before surgery.

Despite the increased ability to control the symptoms of hormone excess with various medical therapies, a number of factors suggest that all patients with islet cell tumors should be considered for possible surgical resection of the tumor. First, whereas only 10% of insulinomas are reported as malignant, at least 50% of all the other pancreatic endocrine tumors are considered malignant, and in many cases this percentage or higher have metastases at the time of diagnosis. For example, in some older studies up to 90% of all gastrinomas found were malignant.[20,240] Furthermore, although in some studies large tumors are more likely to be malignant,[26] it is not established that metastases do not occur with small tumors; therefore, the fact that no tumor is found on the initial imaging studies or that the tumor is small does not establish that metastatic disease will not occur. Although a number of patients with metastatic glucagonomas,[26,126] gastrinomas,[20,184,241,242] and somatostatinomas[6,49] have been reported to have long-term survivals, detailed studies with pancreatic endocrine tumors such as gastrinoma, in which there has been very effective therapy for gastric hypersecretion for more than 15 years, suggest that the long-term prognosis is much worse in patients with advanced disease than originally thought.[20,39,243–245] Studies demonstrate that survival is directly related to tumor extent. In patients with no tumors found at the time of surgery, the 5- or 10-year survival was 90% to 100%.[20,39,243–245] In patients with complete tumor resection, the 5- or 10-year survival also was 90% to 100%. In patients whose tumors are incompletely resected or who have a postoperative recurrence, the 5-year survival varied from 14% to 76%, and 10-year survival was 20%. In patients with unresectable pancreatic endocrine tumor such as gastrinoma metastatic to the liver, the 5-year survival was 20% to 75%, and 10-year survival in one study was 30%.[20,39,243–245] These data suggest that once metastatic disease occurs, the prognosis is significantly decreased. Furthermore, because therapy for advanced disease is in many cases only partially effective,[20,39,200] it is important to attempt to resect the pancreatic endocrine tumor while it still is localized. Unlike with gastrinoma, the

long-term medical therapy of the other various pancreatic endocrine tumors is not well established, and it is not known whether all patients will continue to respond to medical treatment. Last, the long-term toxicity of most medical therapies except that for gastrinoma is not well established.

Nonmetastatic Disease

Medical

General considerations.   The initial management of patients with insulinomas and the long-term management of those patients with insulinomas who are not surgically cured, is directed at controlling the hypoglycemia. The simplest form of nonsurgical control is dietary management. Frequent, small meals may alleviate symptoms.[70] In severe cases, intravenous glucose combined with various drug therapies may be required. In general, 10% dextrose should be avoided because of the electrolyte imbalances generated by the combination of elevated serum concentrations of glucose and hyperinsulinemia.[70] Some investigators have used slowly absorbed nutrients to maintain normal blood sugar levels before surgery. This may be preferable to diazoxide administration because of reports of sudden hypotension in some patients receiving diazoxide before surgery.[246] Diazoxide (150–800 mg/day), however, has been used successfully to manage patients with insulinoma before surgery as well as in long-term treatment. Diazoxide is a benzothiadiazide that has a plasma half-life of 28 hours and a peak hyperglycemic effect 12 hours after an oral dose or 4 hours after an intravenous dose. Its hyperglycemic action is attributed to direct inhibition of insulin release by adrenergic stimulation and by enhancement of glycogenolysis.[26,158] The main side effects of diazoxide are sodium retention and gastrointestinal symptoms such as nausea.[26,70,158] Sodium retention can be minimized by administration of diazoxide with a diuretic and restricting sodium intake. The gastrointestinal side effects can be decreased by taking the drug with meals.[26,70] Diazoxide is primarily excreted by the kidneys and is known to displace various protein-bound drugs and increase their free concentrations in the serum.[70] Diazoxide therapy should be initiated with low doses and increased to a maximum of 600 to 800 mg/day in two or three divided doses as tolerated or until symptoms are controlled. In general, approximately 60% of patients respond.[26,70] The calcium channel blockers verapamil[158,247,248] and diphenylhydantoin[158,249] also have been used with some success to control hypoglycemia in some patients when diazoxide has failed. The long-acting somatostatin analog, octreotide, has been shown to be effective in 32% of patients with insulinoma (Table 93-7) for the acute and long-term control of hypoglycemia[158,250,251]; this is discussed in more detail in the next section.

In the initial management of patients with VIPomas, the most important issue is to replace the large volumes of fluid and electrolytes lost, and correct the hypokalemia and acidosis. This is particularly important because a common acute cause of death in these patients is renal failure associated with hypokalemia and hypokalemic nephropathy.[81] In the past, drug therapy included the use of high doses of prednisone (60–

TABLE 93-7
Effect of the Long-Acting Somatostatin Analog Octreotide in Patients
With Pancreatic Endocrine Tumors

	TUMOR TYPE*			
	Insulinoma	VIPoma	Glucagonoma	GRFoma
Patients treated (n)	48	29	16	8
Symptoms improved (%)	31	86	81	100
Marker hormone level reduced (%)	41	86	75	100
Dose range (µg/day)	50–1500	100–450	100–2250	100–1500
Patients treated >1 mo (n)	10	26	14	8
Decrease in tumor size (%)	4/18 (22)	0/14 (0)	0/14 (0)	1/6 (16)

* Gastrinomas were not included because they are discussed in Chapter 62.

Data are from references 276, 283, 295, 312–317, and other individual case reports from 1989–1993.

100 mg/day),[80,81,251,252] which decreases diarrhea in most patients,[81] and the use of clonidine,[253] angiotensin II,[254] norepinephrine,[254,255] indomethacin,[256,257] lithium carbonate,[258] phenothiazines,[259,260] propranolol,[261] metoclopramide,[262] lidamidine,[263] and loperamide,[263] all of which decreased diarrhea in a small number of patients. These agents primarily enhanced sodium absorption in the proximal small intestine or inhibited intestinal secretion.[80,81] More recent studies demonstrate that the long-acting somatostatin analog, octreotide, is the drug of choice, and controls diarrhea in 86% of all patients with VIPomas (see Table 93-7).

In patients with glucagonoma, the rash, migratory necrolytic erythema, may be severe. Some studies suggest that correction of hypoaminoacidemia with parenteral amino acids and normalization of plasma amino acid levels improves the rash.[132,133] Another study, however, noted disappearance of the rash after surgical resection of the glucagonoma but not dietary normalization of plasma amino acids.[135] The somatostatin analog, octreotide,[250,264,265] induces remission of the rash (see Table 93-7) and other components of the glucagonoma syndrome, and is discussed in the next section.

Medical therapy with octreotide. Somatostatin has been shown to inhibit the release of a number of hormones in both animals and in human volunteers, as well as to have direct actions on a number of target organs, including inhibition of gastric and pancreatic secretion, intestinal absorption, and gastrointestinal motility.[155–157] Administration of natural somatostatin by continuous infusion to a number of patients with functioning pancreatic endocrine tumors demonstrated symptomatic improvement in VIPomas,[250,265–268] insulinomas,[265,269–271] gastrinomas,[269,272] and glucagonomas.[273–275] Natural somatostatin, however, has a very short half-life (2–3 minutes)[276] and, therefore, has limited therapeutic efficacy because it has to be given by continuous intravenous infusion.

A long-acting synthetic octapeptide analog of somatostatin, octreotide acetate (SMS-201-995, Sandostatin), has been developed[277–279] that enables a new approach to these patients. Octreotide has a half-life (100 minutes) 33 times longer than somatostatin, and thus can be administered two to four times a day.[265,278,279] In the rat, it was 70-fold more potent than somatostatin in inhibiting growth hormone re-

lease, 3-fold more potent than native somatostatin in inhibiting insulin release, 23-fold more potent in inhibiting glucagon release, and 80-fold more potent than native somatostatin in inhibiting acid secretion.[278,279] Octreotide usually is started at a dose of 50 to 150 µg subcutaneously, two or three times a day, by self-administration, and the dose increased if not effective. Doses up to 750 µg three times a day have been used in patients with the carcinoid syndrome and pancreatic endocrine tumors (see Table 93-7).[250,265] There have been reports of small numbers of cases in which intermittent subcutaneous administration of octreotide was ineffective or only partially effective, and continuous infusion of octreotide was more effective.[176,295,317] It remains unclear as to what percentage of patients with symptomatic pancreatic endocrine tumors remain responsive to octreotide over the long term (i.e., >1 year), primarily because of the limited number of patients treated for long periods of time. One study[274] reported 7 such patients treated for a median period of 20 months (range, 13–54 months) in which octreotide was initially effective in all. Symptoms worsened and plasma hormone concentrations rose over a median period of 5 months after therapy was begun, and were initially reversed by increasing the octreotide dose. After a median of 13 months (range, 5–34 months), symptoms returned and were no longer responsive to higher doses of octreotide.

In 48 patients with insulinoma, some symptoms were improved in 31% and plasma insulin concentrations decreased in 41% (see Table 93-7); however, 65% of the patients received octreotide for less than 1 week because most went to curative surgery. Reduction in hypoglycemia attacks was noted only occasionally.[278,280,281] Octreotide was given for more than 1 month in 10 patients (see Table 93-7). Therefore, in short-term studies octreotide appears to benefit 30% of patients with insulinoma, but the true percentage of patients with insulinomas that continue to respond to octreotide is not clear.[39,250] In general, insulinomas appear to be less responsive to octreotide than glucagonomas, VIPomas, gastrinomas, or GRFomas. Data suggest that some insulinomas may lack somatostatin receptors, partially explaining the failure of a significant number of patients to respond to octreotide.[228,239,282] There have been reports of patients with insulinomas deteriorating when treated with octreotide[295,313]; therefore, it is recommended that octreotide therapy be initiated only in the hospital for patients with insulinomas.

Octreotide improved diarrhea in 25 of 29 patients with VIPomas, and plasma VIP concentrations decreased in 86% of patients (see Table 93-7).[250] Tumor size was evaluated in 26 patients with VIPomas and a decrease in size occurred in 4 (see Table 93-7).[250] All patients demonstrated a decrease in diarrhea within the first 24 hours, but in 3 patients the effect lasted only a few days.[265,284,285] Octreotide was given for more than 1 month in 90% of the patients and remained effective for more than 6 months in 50% of all patients.[250] Some patients, however, had decreased responsiveness to octreotide with time, and the dose had to be increased.[250] There was a decrease in the VIP plasma level in 89% of patients with octreotide treatment, although in many cases it did not return to within the normal range.[250,286]

In 16 patients with glucagonoma, octreotide improved the skin rash in all of the 13 patients tested, and reduced plasma glucagon concentrations in 75% of patients (see Table 93-7).[143,250,265,287–290] Weight loss, pain, and diarrhea improved in patients with these symptoms, but octreotide had little effect on diabetes mellitus[143,287,314] and tumor size.[250] Decreases in plasma glucagon concentration did not always parallel improvements in the rash.[250,288] Octreotide was administered for more than 1 month in 88% of patients and remained effective for more than 6 months in 75% of all patients[250]; in 1 case,[288] octreotide was administered for 33 months with continued effectiveness.

Octreotide also has been effective in reducing symptoms of growth hormone excess and GRF plasma concentrations in patients with GRFomas.[176,177,250,291–293] In all 8 patients reported with GRFomas, octreotide improved symptoms and reduced the GRF levels, although in one study[176] continuous infusion was required. Three of the 4 patients received treatment with octreotide for more than 6 months (see Table 93-7).[250,293] In 4 patients with PPomas or nonfunctioning islet cell tumors,[276,284,285] octreotide was reported to improve symptoms of fatigue and abdominal pain in 2; however, octreotide had no effect on tumor size in any patient.[250]

Long-term treatment with octreotide entails a number of unresolved issues.[39,250] Many patients require increasing doses of octreotide with time, and some patients require very high doses.[250,294] In a small number of patients, when the octreotide was stopped and restarted, the symptoms were controlled at a lower dose,[250] whereas other patients did not respond. Furthermore, it is unclear why intermittent subcutaneous injections are not effective in some cases, whereas continuous low-dose subcutaneous infusions are effective. Octreotide reduces the ectopic release of hormone and decreases tumor size in a small percentage of patients.[250] This is discussed in more detail in the section on Other Treatments of Metastatic Disease; however, it is not established that the dose of octreotide is the same for both effects. An additional unresolved issue is that there is not always a close correlation between changes in plasma levels of the marker hormone and symptomatic improvement.[250] For example, in some patients with VIPomas, treatment with octreotide completely stops the diarrhea, yet plasma VIP levels remain elevated in ranges above those that cause diarrhea in otherwise healthy subjects.[286] One study[296] provides evidence that this discrepancy may be the result of multiple forms of immunoreactive plasma VIP being

released. After treatment with octreotide, the biologically active native form may not be released, and the VIP-immunoreactive peptides identified are probably VIP fragments that are not biologically active.

Side effects have been recorded in approximately 50% of patients treated with octreotide, but have rarely been serious enough to stop therapy.[250,264,279] Most patients experience only some pain or discomfort at the subcutaneous injection site. Occasional postprandial hyperglycemia has been reported.[250,264,267] The most common other side effects are gastrointestinal, including nausea, vomiting, constipation, crampy abdominal pain, and diarrhea, which may improve with time.[250] Steatorrhea occurs in many patients. At low doses of octreotide, steatorrhea is usually mild and transient[297]; however, at high doses gross steatorrhea can occur.[285,298] Of particular concern are reports of the development of cholelithiasis or gallbladder sludge in patients on octreotide.[299] Occasionally, patients have been reported to have hyperglycemia[294,300] or a rebound effect after the drug was stopped.[285,301,302]

Surgical

All patients with pancreatic endocrine tumors should undergo exploratory laparotomy for possible cure.[39] Exceptions are patients with unresectable metastatic disease or those rare ones whose symptoms are well controlled by medical management yet also have a concurrent medical problem that would make the risks of surgery prohibitive. It is particularly important that the surgery be done only by a surgeon with experience in operating on patients with pancreatic endocrine tumors.[20,70] Even very experienced general surgeons and many endocrine surgeons have little experience with these rare tumors, and therefore frequently miss small tumors or perform unnecessary major resections.

As outlined previously, before surgery all patients should undergo localization studies, including endoscopic ultrasound if an experienced endoscopist is available, detailed imaging studies (CT scan, MRI, ultrasound, selective angiography), and, if localization is still unclear, functional localization studies (PVS, selective hormone sampling of portal venous tributaries) or, for insulinomas, calcium infusion with hepatic venous sampling. It is unknown whether a calcium infusion with hepatic venous hormonal sampling is also useful in localizing other, rarer functional pancreatic endocrine tumors such as VIPomas or glucagonomas. Even if localization studies are negative, provided metastatic disease or a prohibitive concurrent illness are not present, the patient should undergo exploratory laparotomy.[39]

The surgical approach has been reviewed,[39,203,213,244,303,304] and is guided by tumor location. At exploration, the liver should be carefully examined for evidence of metastatic disease. In the case of endocrine tumors that are frequently extrapancreatic in location, the entire abdomen, and especially the proximal small intestine, should be carefully explored to locate extrapancreatic tumors.[39,203,213,244,303,304] An extended Kocher's maneuver should be performed to allow thorough examination of the pancreatic head area. The entire pancreas must be carefully explored, even if one pancreatic endocrine tumor is found, because there are multiple tumors in 10% of patients with insulinoma.[70] Although this also is true with some islet cell tumors such as gastrinomas,[20,39] in most other pancreatic endocrine tumors (VIPoma, glucagonoma, somatostatinoma, PPoma, GRFoma), a single tumor usually is found. There are relatively few cases that have been carefully investigated, however. A detailed exploration for multiple endocrine tumors is particularly important in those patients with MEN I syndrome, because a number of studies have shown that they are likely to have multiple pancreatic endocrine tumors.[20,39,43,305] Isolated small insulinomas should be removed by enucleation because they are rarely malignant. Isolated noninsulinoma pancreatic endocrine tumors in the pancreatic body or tail should be removed en bloc by distal pancreatectomy because they are occasionally malignant.[213] Pancreatic head and proximal pancreatic body tumors require enucleation with careful dissection to avoid damage to the main pancreatic duct and attendant morbidity. If at surgery an isolated hepatic metastasis is found that can be removed without increased risk, then it should be excised with negative margins.[39,213] Aggressive surgery such as a proximal cephalic pancreaticoduodenectomy (Whipple procedure) is not indicated because it has not been established that the increased risk of morbidity does not outweigh the potential benefit.[20,39] Pneumococcal vaccine (Pneumovax) should be administered before surgery to lower the risk of postsplenectomy sepsis.

The use of intraoperative ultrasound may be helpful and is recommended.[20,39,248,249,303,304] This technique identifies a certain number of pancreatic endocrine tumors that would not otherwise be found (see Fig. 93-9).[20,39,248,249,303] Furthermore, in some pancreatic endocrine tumors in which malignancy was not apparent from palpation, intraoperative ultrasound established malignancy, allowing the appropriate resection to be done.[229]

In patients with insulinomas, there have been occasional reports of hypoglycemia during surgical manipulation of the tumor; the artificial pancreas (Biostator) has documented an increased glucose requirement during resection of insulinoma.[306,308] A number of centers document successful tumor removal by demonstrating rebound hyperglycemia.[308] One study, however, has shown that rebound hyperglycemia did not occur in 23% of patients with successful tumor excision,[309] and we do not recommend its use.

It has been reported in 5 cases[310] that serial measurements of serum insulin concentrations during surgery are helpful in establishing whether the insulinoma was successfully removed. Nevertheless, there is no established method that confirms complete resection of all tumors immediately after surgery; therefore, it is important that a thorough search for additional tumors be done in all patients, and that the pathologist carefully review all biopsy specimens or excised tissue for evidence of a pancreatic endocrine tumor.

In most studies, 75% to 95% of patients with insulinomas are cured by surgery.[26,70,203,209–213,311] With glucagonomas, there have been a number of reports of successful excision of the tumor,[39,126,220,317–324] and in many cases follow-up has been long enough to suggest cure. At least 50% to 75% of the patients with glucagonomas had metastases at the time of diagnosis, however, and a significant additional percentage had metastases at the time of surgery.[126,203,317] A number of cases of glucagonomas have shown recurrence during long-term following-up, despite what initially appeared to be complete resection of all tumor.[126,129,323] Therefore, the true

long-term cure rate is not established. With VIPomas, somatostatinomas, GRFomas, and PPomas, many patients present with metastatic disease, and the exact percentage of patients cured by surgical excision of the tumor has not been adequately studied.[39]

If the patient is found to have more extensive disease with either local invasion or metastases at or before surgery, then the question of debulking surgery often arises. This issue is covered in the section on Treatment, Metastatic Disease.

Metastatic Disease

Metastatic pancreatic endocrine tumors have been characterized as slow growing.[241,242] In one study[322] involving 85 patients with various functional pancreatic endocrine tumors, none of the patients without metastatic disease died (follow-up, 3–18 years; median, 8 years). Of the 41 patients with metastatic disease, however, 66% died from tumor progression, with overall 5- and 10-year survival rates of 54% and 28%, respectively. In patients with metastatic disease but not to the liver (primarily to the lymph nodes),[322] the 5-year survival was significantly better (90%; $P <0.001$) than in those with hepatic metastases at diagnosis (23%). The 5- and 10-year survival rates[322] for patients with malignant insulinomas were 50% and 50%, for gastrinomas, 47% and 18%, and for VIPomas, 88% and 25%, respectively.[322] The natural histories of metastatic VIPomas, glucagonomas, somatostatinomas, or insulinomas are not completely clear because until recently effective therapy for the excess hormone state did not exist in most cases, and patients frequently died of resulting complications. With the availability of the long-acting somatostatin analog, octreotide, however, this may change. As with gastrinomas, for which effective therapy has existed for more than 20 years,[20,200,241] it is likely that with each of the pancreatic endocrine tumors long-term mortality will be increasingly determined by the growth of the tumor, as was evident in the study mentioned earlier.[322] For example, with gastrinoma, the overall survival rate after total gastrectomy is 42% at 5 years and 30% at 10 years.[20,325–327] Of patients with metastatic disease who subsequently died, however, 50% to 70% of the deaths were secondary to tumor progression.[20,204,242,325] In patients with gastrinoma with metastatic disease, the 5-year survival ranged between 20% to 75% in different studies, and the 10-year survival ranged between 20% to 30%.[242,244,245,326,327] There are no data to suggest that the other metastatic pancreatic endocrine tumors will differ in their natural histories from gastrinoma, and the study of survival in patients with other pancreatic endocrine tumors[322] reviewed earlier in fact suggests a similar natural history. This conclusion is further supported by the fact that similar percentages of patients with each noninsulinoma pancreatic endocrine tumor have metastatic or malignant disease (56% to 60%), suggesting that the malignancy potentials and perhaps growth patterns are similar.[7,26,81,126] Therefore, most authorities agree that treat-ment directed at metastatic disease is indicated. Disagreement occurs over the type of therapy, the efficacy of the therapy, and when therapy should begin. Chemotherapy,[20,39,200,328–340,342,345–347] possible debulking surgery,[20,39,241,245,354] hepatic arterial embolization (for functional tumors metastatic to the liver with or without chemotherapy),[333,352,353] interferon,[316,344,348-351] and the use of the long-acting somatostatin analog, octreotide,[250,316,341,343] all have been reported to have positive effects on metastatic pancreatic endocrine tumor growth. Each is considered in the following sections.

Chemotherapy

A number of different chemotherapeutic regimens have been evaluated in patients with metastatic pancreatic endocrine tumors (Table 93-8). Because of the rare occurrence of pancreatic endocrine tumors, they have been considered together as a group in most studies of chemotherapy, or as other cases included in series with metastatic carcinoid tumors.[20,39,334,340,346,347,358] Although some studies[330,334,340] reported no difference in responsiveness to chemotherapeutic agents between different types of pancreatic endocrine tumors, it has been pointed out that the sample size of the various tumors included in these studies was too small to establish that each type of pancreatic endocrine tumor responds equally to chemotherapy.[20,39,339] In fact, some clinical observations suggest there may be significant differences in responsiveness. For example, in some studies, as high as 90% of metastatic VIPomas are reported to respond to streptozotocin, frequently with a complete response.[81] In contrast, in two prospective studies, only 5%[337] and 40%[339] of patients with metastatic gastrinoma that increased in size before treatment responded to streptozotocin plus 5-fluorouracil with or without doxorubicin, and in no case was there a complete response. Furthermore, as many as 93% of metastatic glucagonomas are reported to respond to dacarbazine, including several complete remissions,[39,329,356-361] whereas in other pancreatic endocrine tumors, dacarbazine has a low response rate (i.e., 6%; see Table 93-8).

In almost all studies, streptozotocin is used either alone or in combination with 5-fluorouracil or doxorubicin.[39] Streptozotocin, a nitrourea antibiotic,[362] was originally observed to induce diabetes mellitus in preclinical toxicology

TABLE 93-8
Drug Therapy of Metastatic Pancreatic Endocrine Tumors

AGENT	PATIENTS (Number)	OBJECTIVE RESPONSE	YEAR REPORTED	REFERENCE
STZ	52	26 (50%)	1973	334
	41	14 (34%)	1980	328
	16	10 (62%)	1986	329
	17	7 (41%)	1987	330
5-FU	12	3 (25%)	1981	345
DOX	20	4 (20%)	1982	331
CZT	13	7 (53%)	1983	332
	33	10 (30%)	1992	340
DTIC	16	1 (6%)	1983, 1987	114, 333
Tubercidin	6	2 (33%)	1987	333
Methyl CCNU	5	1 (20%)	1981	345
CZT + 5-FU	44	14 (32%)	1992	340
STZ + 5-FU	5	1 (20%)	1974	380
	40	25 (63%)	1980	334
	10	8 (80%)	1987	329
	30	19 (63%)	1989	316
	22	1 (5%)	1991	337
	33	15 (45%)	1992	340
STZ or STZ + 5-FU	45	19 (42%)	1986	335
STZ + DOX	5	1 (20%)	1987	333
	14	3 (21%)	1988	338
	36	25 (69%)	1992	340
Etoposide + Cisplatin	14	2 (14%)	1991	342
STZ + 5-FU + DOX	10	4 (40%)	1988	339
	30	6 (20%)	1992	322
STZ + 5-FU + Tubercidin	10	10 (100%)	1981	345
Octreotide (SMS-201-995)	66	8 (12%)	1989	341
	10	0 (0%)	1989	316
	52	23 (44%)	1992	343
Interferon	21*	1 (4%)	1986, 1989	316, 348
	11†	0 (0%)	1993	344
5-FU + DOX + Cisplatin	5	1 (20%)	1991	346

CZT, chlorozotocin; DOX, doxorubicin; DTIC, dacarbazine; 5-FU, 5-fluorouracil; STZ, streptozotocin.

* Decrease in tumor size in 4% of patients, stable disease in 50%; 23% had decrease in tumor markers ≥50%.

† Decrease in tumor size in no patients and stable disease in 3 (27%).

studies.[363] The first report of its clinical effectiveness in a pancreatic endocrine tumor was in 1968,[364] and subsequently there have been a number of case reports and trials involving this agent (see Table 93-8). In various series, streptozotocin alone is reported to cause objective remissions in 34% to 62% of pancreatic endocrine tumors, and tubercidin, doxorubicin, and dacarbazine in 6% to 33% (see Table 93-8). Chlorozotocin, a chloroethyl analog of streptozotocin, was reviewed in 1976.[365] Compared to streptozotocin, chlorozotocin was reported to have only mild to moderate gastrointestinal toxicity, with myelosuppression the dose-limiting side effect.[366,367] Furthermore, it had the practical advantage of having to be administered in only a single intravenous dose during each course of chemotherapy. Chlorozotocin alone in two studies had a response rate of 30% to 53%, which is similar to that of streptozotocin alone (see Table 93-8). Streptozotocin with 5-fluorouracil or doxorubicin or both has been reported to cause objective responses in 5% to 80% of patients, with a mean response rate of 43% among the different reports (see Table 93-8). The agents of choice for metastatic pancreatic endocrine tumors are combined streptozotocin and doxorubicin.[39,340] This recommendation is based on a comparative study[340] of streptozotocin and doxorubicin versus streptozotocin plus 5-fluorouracil or chlorozotocin in 105 patients with metastatic pancreatic endocrine tumors. Streptozotocin and doxorubicin had a 69% response rate, which was significantly higher than the 45% response rate with streptozotocin and 5-fluorouracil or 30% response rate with chlorozotocin alone. Furthermore, streptozotocin[340] plus doxorubicin had a significant advantage in terms of survival ($P = 0.0004$). A previous prospective study[334] done by the Eastern Cooperative Oncology Group also had demonstrated the superiority of double-agent therapy over streptozotocin alone, with streptozotocin plus 5-fluorouracil having a response rate of 63%, compared to 40% with streptozotocin alone, in patients with metastatic pancreatic endocrine tumors. It is not clear why the response rate in some more recent prospective studies[337,339] is significantly lower than the response rate reported in these two studies. In two prospective studies of streptozotocin with 5-fluorouracil with or without doxorubicin in patients with gastrinomas metastatic to the liver, response rates of 5% and 40% were reported.[337,339] In neither study were there any complete responders, and in one study there was no difference in survival between responders and nonresponders.[339] It is not clear whether this difference in response rates from those previously reported is the result of differences in the tumors themselves or of differences in extent of metastatic disease.

The use of both streptozotocin and chlorozotocin is associated with significant side effects. In prospective studies, 74% to 100% of patients experienced nausea and vomiting, and in 20% to 40%, renal toxicity with increased serum creatinine, proteinuria, or both developed. These side effects were reversible in most cases, although chronic renal failure can develop in a significant percentage (7%).[340] Serum creatinine and urine protein must be assessed before each cycle of chemotherapy.[334,339]

Other chemotherapy agents besides those discussed here have been used occasionally in patients with metastatic pancreatic endocrine tumors. Etoposide, actinomycin, or cisplatin have been used in a few cases, but usually have been ineffective.[39]

Other Treatments of Metastatic Disease

Because of the toxicity and relatively poor response rates of chemotherapy in patients with extensive metastatic pancreatic endocrine tumors, other agents have been investigated. Human leukocyte interferon has been reported to be effective in controlling symptoms in a number of patients with pancreatic endocrine tumors and carcinoid tumors.[39,348,351] In one study,[348] 17 of 22 (77%) patients with various pancreatic endocrine tumors were reported to respond by either a decrease in tumor markers or tumor size, with a mean duration of follow-up of 8.5 months (range, 2–36 months). Among these, 7 of 7 (100%) patients with VIPomas responded with a decrease in tumor size or serum VIP concentration, whereas 6 of 9 (66%) patients with nonfunctioning tumors or PPomas responded, as did the 1 patient with somatostatinoma. One patient with insulinoma did not respond. Although only 6 of 22 (27%) patients[348] demonstrated a decrease in tumor size, each of these patients had failed chemotherapy. Therefore, this study[348] suggested that human leukocyte interferon may be of value in patients with pancreatic endocrine tumors who fail chemotherapy.[39] More recent studies demonstrated no effect of recombinant interferon-α in 2 patients with VIPoma,[351] and in 11 patients with gastrinoma metastatic to the liver that increased in size before treatment,[344] interferon-α treatment did not result in a decrease in tumor size in any patient. In this study,[344] the tumor stopped increasing in size in 3 patients; however, it is unclear in what percentage of untreated tumors this occurs. In studies of patients with metastatic carcinoid tumors, which resemble pancreatic endocrine tumors in growth rate, histologic pattern, and malignant potential, similar results with interferon on tumor size are reported.[368–370] In three studies with human leukocyte interferon,[368–370] response rates for reduction in tumor size were 11%, 15%, and 14%, and in four series[312,369,371,372] with interferon-α, objective decrease in tumor size occurred in 0%, 0%, 10%, and 20%, including one study in which 24 million units per day of interferon were used. These studies suggest that as a primary tumoricidal agent, interferon is minimally effective.

A number of studies in animals have demonstrated that somatostatin analogs can inhibit the growth of various tumors.[373,374] Hormonal therapy with the long-acting somatostatin analog, octreotide, has been reported to cause a decrease in tumor size in 12% of patients with pancreatic endocrine tumors in one review of cases reported up to 1988 (see Table 93-8).[341] In a review of 62 cases with sufficient data to determine change in tumor size with octreotide treatment (see Table 93-7), only 4 patients (6%) had a decrease in tumor size. This percentage agrees with the data from the German Sandostatin Study Group,[348] in which patients with metastatic gastroenteropancreatic endocrine tumors are treated with up to 1500 μg/day of octreotide. For patients monitored at least 3 months, 4% had a decrease in tumor size and 54% stable disease. Many patients, however, reported symptomatic improvement despite a lack of decrease in tumor size (see Table 93-7). These results demonstrate that octreotide alone, like interferon, has minimal tumoricidal activity in pancreatic endocrine tumors. They do not rule out a possible role of octreotide in preventing progression of the disease, if this can be proven to increase survival.

Hepatic artery embolization with or without postocclusion chemotherapy (streptozotocin, Adriamycin, 5-fluorouracil, or dacarbazine) has been used successfully in patients with various pancreatic endocrine tumors.[333,352,353,361,375-378] Because the liver derives only 20% to 25% of its blood supply from the hepatic artery and 75% to 80% from the portal vein,[377] and because most pancreatic endocrine tumors are vascular with an arterial supply, hepatic artery embolization can be used to treat metastatic disease to the liver if the portal vein is patent. One study reports that 80% to 90% of patients demonstrate symptomatic improvement[376]; in another study of 7 patients with various metastatic pancreatic endocrine tumors, hepatic artery occlusion led to complete symptomatic improvement in 14%.[333] With the improvement in symptoms there was a parallel regression of hepatic metastases. In another study in which hepatic artery occlusion was combined with chemotherapy,[333,379] 64% had a complete response in symptoms, 18% had a 75% to 100% improvement, and 9% had a 50% to 75% improvement. The improvement was longer lasting when the hepatic artery ligation was combined with chemotherapy than with hepatic artery occlusion alone.[333,379] This procedure is not without significant side effects, with 2 of 14 patients dying from complications of the procedure in one study.[352] In the literature,[376] the mortality overall for this procedure is less than 3%, but pain develops in almost 100%, and fever and leukocytosis are seen in at least 50% of patients. Furthermore, in patients with gastrinoma, metastases to bone have been reported in 12% of patients with hepatic metastases,[35] suggesting that procedures such as embolization directed at the liver may be of limited value in controlling metastatic spread in patients with extensive disease. In a patient with a hormonal syndrome that cannot be controlled by other therapies, however, this procedure may be helpful. In some studies, hepatic artery embolization has been combined with treatment with human interferon-α[380,381] in patients with metastatic carcinoid tumors, which closely resemble pancreatic endocrine tumors in responsiveness and histologic features. One year after treatment, 5 of 7 patients (71%) continued to demonstrate a decrease in metastatic disease in the liver, whereas with interferon-α alone (n = 10), only 10% demonstrated a decrease.[380] In another study[381] involving 36 patients with metastatic carcinoid tumors, interferon alone resulted in a 24% response rate (decrease in 5-hydroxyindoleacetic acid secretion) and the survival rate was 40% after 5 years. In contrast,[381] with interferon and hepatic artery embolization, the response rate was 60% and the 5-year survival rate 75%. Similar studies have not been done in patients with metastatic pancreatic endocrine tumors; however, because of the similarity in these tumors, if the extended survival in patients with metastatic carcinoid tumors is the result of inhibiting tumor progression, then this regimen also may be effective in patients with pancreatic endocrine tumors.

Systematic removal of all resectable tumor (i.e., debulking surgery) may prolong the life expectancy of some patients with some functional pancreatic endocrine tumors.[20,39,220,241,245,354] Systematic removal of all resectable disease has been reported to help control symptoms in patients with glucagonomas,[26,126] VIPomas,[80,81] and somatostatinomas,[203] leading to the suggestion that resection should be performed if extensive tumor is identified at the time of surgery and resection can be done without increased risk. Two studies

using such an approach were reported, one involving 17 patients with potentially resectable metastatic pancreatic endocrine tumors,[354] and the other 37 patients with metastatic neuroendocrine tumors (24 carcinoid, 13 pancreatic endocrine tumors).[355] In the first study,[354] in 80% of cases the tumor was completely excised at surgery, and survival was 79% at 5 years with a mean follow-up of 3 years. In this study, patients who had extensive metastatic disease even postresection had a 5-year survival of 28%, equal to that of patients with inoperable tumors, whereas patients with limited metastatic disease at surgery had a significantly prolonged survival ($P = 0.019$). In the other study,[355] which was a retrospective review of patients with neuroendocrine tumors undergoing hepatic resection, 50% of resections resulted in cure with no gross residual disease, and 90% of patients with symptomatic endocrinopathies obtained complete relief. The conclusion of both of these studies[354,355] was that resection of metastatic disease should be considered in selected patients with metastatic neuroendocrine tumors. It is important to remember that these patients represent only a very small proportion (9% in one study,[355] 5% in the other[354]) of all patients with pancreatic endocrine tumors with metastatic disease. Furthermore, this approach has not been systematically evaluated, and it remains unclear whether patients identified with metastatic disease by preoperative localization studies and whose symptoms are well controlled by medical management will benefit in the long term from debulking surgery.

Most experts agree that chemotherapy, hormonal therapy, or interferon are indicated only in patients with extensive metastatic disease (usually to the liver),[20,39,200,329,335] and are not indicated for treatment of the primary tumor when surgery is not curative. There is no agreement, however, about when chemotherapy, hormonal therapy, or interferon should be started.[20,39,200] Some groups recommend treatment only when symptoms develop due to the pancreatic endocrine tumor,[334] whereas others recommend treatment only when the tumor is demonstrated to be increasing in size.[20,39,339]

The reader is directed to Chapter 2, Gastrointestinal Hormones; Chapter 38, Approach to the Patient With Diarrhea; and Chapter 62, Zollinger-Ellison Syndrome.

REFERENCES

1. Moldow RE, Connelly RR. Epidemiology of pancreatic cancer in Connecticut. Gastroenterology 1968;55:677.
2. Buchanan KD, Johnston CF, O'Hare MMT, et al. Neuroendocrine tumors: a European view. Am J Med 1986;81:14.
3. Koulie H, White TT. Pancreatic islet cell tumors and hyperplasia: experience in 14 Seattle hospitals. Ann Surg 1972;125:326.
4. Stadil F, Stage JG. The Zollinger-Ellison syndrome. Clin Endocrinol Metab 1979;9:433.
5. Ericksson B, Oberg K, Skogeid B. Neuroendocrine pancreatic tumors: clinical findings in a prospective study of 84 patients. Acta Oncol 1989;28:273.
6. Guillausseau PJ, Guillausseau C, Villet R, et al. Les glucagonomas: aspect cliniques, biologiques, anatomo-pathologiques et therapeutiques (revue general de 130 cas). Gastroenterol Clin Biol 1982;6:1029.
7. Vinik AI, Strodel WE, Eckhauser FE, et al. Somatostatinomas, PPomas and neurotensinomas. Semin Oncol 1987;14:263.

8. Weil C. Gastroenteropancreatic endocrine tumors. Klin Wochenschr 1985; 63:433.
9. Dent RB, van Heerden JA, Weiland LH. Nonfunctioning islet cell tumors. Ann Surg 1981;193:185.
10. Broder LE, Carter SK. Pancreatic islet cell carcinoma: clinical features of 52 patients. Ann Intern Med 1973;79:101.
11. Broughan TA, Leslie JD, Soto JM, Hermann RE. Pancreatic islet cell tumors. Surgery 1986;99:671.
12. Koppel G, Heitz PU. Pancreatic endocrine tumors. Pathol Res Pract 1988;183:155.
13. Bolandi RP. The neurocrestopathies: a unifying concept of disease arising from neural crest maldevelopment. Hum Pathol 1970;5:409.
14. Pearse HGE. The APUD concept and hormone production. Clin Endocrinol Metab 1980;9:211.
15. Heitz PU, Kasper M, Polak JM, Koppel G. Pancreatic endocrine tumors. Hum Pathol 1982;13:263.
16. Solcia E, Capella C. Fiocca R, et al. The gastroenteropancreatic system and related tumors. Gastroenterol Clin North Am 1989;18:671.
17. Alumets J, Falkmer S, Hakanson R, et al. Neurohormonal peptides in endocrine tumors of the pancreas, stomach and upper small intestine: an immunohistochemical study of 27 cases. Ultrastruct Pathol 1983;5;55.
18. Mukai K, Greider MH, Grotting JL, Rosai J. Retrospective study of 77 pancreatic endocrine tumors using the immunoperoxidase method. Am J Surg Pathol 1982;6:387.
19. Creutzfeldt W. Endocrine tumors of the pancreas. In: Volk BW, Arquilla ER, eds. The diabetic pancreas. New York: Plenum, 1985:543.
20. Jensen RT, Gardner JD. Gastrinoma. In: Go VLW, DiMagno EP, Gardner JD, et al, eds. The pancreas: biology, pathobiology and diseases. 2nd ed. New York: Raven Press, 1993:931.
21. Owyang C, Go VLW. Multiple hormone secreting tumors of the gastrointestinal tract. In: Glass GBJ, ed. Gastrointestinal hormones. New York: Raven Press, 1980:741.
22. Creutzfeldt W, Arnold R, Frerichs H. Insulinomas and gastrinomas. In: Bloom SR, ed. Gut hormones. New York: Churchill-Livingstone, 1978:589.
23. Larrson JI, Grimelius L, Hakanson R, et al. Mixed endocrine pancreatic tumors producing several peptide hormones. Am J Pathol 1975;79:271.
24. Wynick D, Williams SJ, Bloom SR. Symptomatic secondary hormone syndromes in patients with malignant pancreatic endocrine tumors. N Engl J Med 1988;319:605.
25. Chiang HC, O'Dorisio TM, Maton PN, et al. Multiple hormone elevations in patients with Zollinger-Ellison syndrome: preoperative study of clinical significance and development of a secondary pancreatic endocrine tumor syndrome. Gastroenterology 1990;99:1565.
26. Boden G. Insulinomas and glucagonomas. Gastroenterol Clin North Am 1989;18:831.
27. Greider MH, Rosai J, McGuigan JE. The human pancreatic islet cells and their tumors: ulcerogenic and diarrheogenic tumors. Cancer 1974;33:1423.
28. Kahn R, Rosen SW, Weintraub BD, et al. Ectopic production of chorionic gonadotropin and its subunits by islet cell tumors. N Engl J Med 1977;297:565.
29. Oberg K, Wide L. hCG and hCG subunits as tumor markers in patients with endocrine pancreatic tumors and carcinoma. Acta Endocrinol 1981;98:256.
30. Heitz PhU, Kasper M, Kloppel G, et al. Glycoprotein-hormone alpha-chain production by pancreatic endocrine tumors: a specific marker for malignancy. Immunocytochemical analysis of tumors of 155 patients. Cancer 1983;51:277.
31. Bardram L, Agner T, Hagen C. Levels of alpha subunits of gonadotropin can be increased in patients with malignant tumors and apparently benign disease. Acta Endocrinol (Copenh) 1988;118:135.
32. O'Connor DT, Deftos LJ. Secretion of chromogranin A by peptide-producing endocrine neoplasms. N Engl J Med 1986;314:1145.
33. Sobol RE, Memoli V, Deftos LJ. Hormone-negative chromogranin A-positive endocrine tumors. N Engl J Med 1989;320:444.
34. Donow C, Pipeleers-Marichal M, Stamm B, et al. Pathologie das insulinomas und das gastrinoms. Dtsch Med Wochenschr 1990;115:1386.
35. Barton JC, Hirschowitz BI, Maton PN, Jensen RT. Bone metastases in malignant gastrinoma. Gastroenterology 1986;91: 1179.
36. Wermer P. Endocrine adenomatosis: peptic ulcer in a large kindred. Am J Med 1963;35:205
37. Ballard HS, Frame B, Hartsock RT. Familial endocrine adenoma-peptic ulcer disease. Medicine 1984;43:481.
38. Eberle F, Grun R. Multiple endocrine neoplasia type-I. Adv Intern Med Pediatr 1981;5:76.
39. Norton JA, Levin B, Jensen RT. Cancer of the endocrine system. In: DeVita VT, Hellman S, Rosenberg SA, eds. Cancer: principles and practice of oncology. vol. 2. 4th ed. Philadelphia: JB Lippincott 1993:1333.
40. Larsson C, Skogsend B, Oberg K, et al. Multiple endocrine neoplasm type I genes map to chromosome 11 and is lost in insulinoma. Nature 1988;322:85.
41. Bale AE, Norton JA, Wang FL, et al. Allelic loss on chromosome 11 in hereditary and sporadic tumors related to familial endocrine neoplasia type 1. Cancer Res 1991;51:1154.
42. Welbourne RB, Wood SM, Polak JM, Bloom SR. Pancreatic endocrine tumors. In: Bloom SR, Polak JM, eds. Gut hormones. 2nd ed. New York: Churchill-Livingstone, 1981:547.
43. Thompson NW, Lloyd RV, Nishiyama, et al. MEN-I pancreas: a histological and immunohistochemical study. World J Surg 1984;8:561.
44. Stefanini P, Carboni M, Patrassi N, Basoli A. Beta-islet cell tumors of the pancreas: results of a study on 1,067 cases. Surgery 1974;75:597.
45. Ruttmann E, Kloppel G, Bommer G, et al. Pancreatic glucagonoma with and without syndrome: immunocytochemical study of 5 tumor cases and review of the literature. Virchows Arch [A] 1980;388:51.
46. Capella C, Polak JM, Butta R, et al. Morphologic patterns and diagnostic criteria of VIP-producing endocrine tumors: a histologic, histochemical, ultrastructural and biochemical study of 32 cases. Cancer 1983;52:1860.
47. Bloom SR. VIP and watery diarrhea VI. In: Bloom SR, ed. Gut hormones. New York: Churchill-Livingstone, 1978:583.
48. Long RG, Bryant MG, Mitchell SJ, et al. Clinicopathological study of pancreatic and ganglioneuroblastoma tumors secreting vasoactive intestinal polypeptide (Vipomas). Br Med J 1981;282:1767.
49. Boden G, Shimoyama R. Somatostatinoma. In: Cohen S, Soloway RD, eds. Hormone-producing tumors of the gastrointestinal tract. New York: Churchill-Livingstone, 1985:85.
50. Sano T, Asa SL, Kovacs K. Growth hormone-producing tumors: clinical, biochemical and morphological manifestations. Endocrinol Rev 1989;9:357.
51. Faglia G, Arosio M, Bazzoni N. Ectopic acromegaly. Endocrinol Metab Clin North Am 1992;21:575.
52. Bresler L, Boissel P, Conroy T, Grosdidier J. Pancreatic islet cell carcinoma with hypercalcemia: complete remission 5 years after surgical excision and chemotherapy. Am J Gastroenterol 1991;86:635.
53. Arps H, Dietel M, Schulz A, et al. Pancreatic endocrine carcinoma with ectopic PTH-production and paraneoplastic hypercalcaemia. Virchows Arch [A] 1986;408:497.
54. Maton PN, Gardner JD, Jensen RT. Cushing's syndrome in patients with the Zollinger-Ellison syndrome. N Engl J Med 1986;315:1.
55. Melmed S, Yamashita S, Kovacz K, et al. Cushing's syndrome due to ectopic proopiomelanocortin gene expression by islet cell carcinoma of the pancreas. Cancer 1987;59:772.
56. Heitz PhU, Kloppel G, Polak JM, Staub J-J. Ectopic hormone production by endocrine tumors: localization of hormones at the cellular level by immunocytochemistry. Cancer 1981;48: 2029.
57. Burke AP, Sobin LH, Shekitka KM, et al. Somatostatin-producing duodenal carcinoids in patients with von Reckling-

hausen's neurofibromatosis: a predilection for black patients. Cancer 1990;65:1591.

58. Ohtsuki Y, Sonobe H, Mizobuchi T, et al. Duodenal carcinoid (somatostatinoma) combined with von Recklinghausen's disease: a case report and review of the literature. Acta Pathol Jpn 1989;39:141.

59. Chagnon JP, Barge J, Hienin D, Blanc D. Von Recklinghausen's disease with digestive localizations associated with gastric acid hypersecretion suggesting Zollinger-Ellison syndrome. Gastroenterol Clin Biol 1985;9:65.

60. Binkovitz LA, Johnson CD, Stephens DH. Islet cell tumors in von Hippel-Lindau disease: increased prevalence and relationship to multiple endocrine neoplasia. AJR 1990;155:501.

61. Davoren PM, Epstein MT. Insulinoma complicating tuberous sclerosis. J Neurol Neurosurg Psychiatry 1992;55:1509.

62. Stanley CA, Baker L. Hyperinsulinism in infants and children: diagnosis and therapy. Adv Pediatr 1976;23:315.

63. Galbut DL, Markowitz AM. Insulinoma: diagnosis, surgical management and long term follow-up. Am J Surg 1980;139:682.

64. Glickman MH, Hart MJ, White TT. Insulinoma in Seattle: 39 cases in 30 years. Am J Surg 1980;140:119.

65. Le Quesne P, Nabarro JD, Kurtz A, Zweig S. The management of insulin tumors of the pancreas. Br J Surg 1979;66:373.

66. Service FJ, Dale AJ, Elveback LR, Jiang N. Insulinoma: clinical and diagnostic features of 60 consecutive cases. Mayo Clin Proc 1976;51:417.

67. Fajans SS, Floyd JC. Fasting hypoglycemia in adults. N Engl J Med 1976;294:766.

68. Kahn CR. The riddle of tumor hypoglycemia revisited. Clin Endocrinol Metab 1980;9:335.

69. Grunberger G, Weiner JL, Silverman R, et al. Factitious hypoglycemia due to surreptitious administration of insulin: diagnosis, treatment and long-term follow-up. Ann Intern Med 1988;108:252.

70. Comi R, Gorden P, Doppman JL. Insulinoma. In: Go VLW, DiMagno EP, Gardner JD, et al, eds. The pancreas: biology, pathobiology and disease. 2nd ed. New York: Raven Press, 1993:979.

71. Sjoberg RT, Kidel GS. Case report. A glucose-responsive insulinoma: implications for the diagnosis of insulin secreting tumors. Am J Med Sci 1992;304:164.

72. Harness JK, Geelboed GW, Thompson NW, et al. Nesidioblastosis in adults: a surgical dilemma. Arch Surg 1981;116:575.

73. Alberti KGMM, Oxbury J, Higgins G. Factitious hypoglycemia: chlorpropamide self administration by a non-diabetic. Br Med J 1972;1:87.

74. Moller PE, Flier JS. Insulin resistance: mechanisms, syndromes and implications. N Engl J Med 1991;325:938.

75. Robbins DC, Tager HS, Rubenstein AH. The biologic and clinical importance of proinsulin. N Engl J Med 1984;310:165.

76. Marks V, Teale JD. Tumors producing hypoglycemia. Diabetes Metab Rev 1991;7:79.

77. Verner JV, Morrison AB. Islet cell tumor and a syndrome of refractory watery diarrhea and hypokalemia. Am J Med 1958;29:529.

78. Matsumoto KK, Peter JB, Schultze RG, et al. Watery diarrhea and hypokalemia associated with pancreatic islet cell adenoma. Gastroenterology 1967;52:695.

79. Marks IN, Bank S, Louw JH. Islet cell tumor of the pancreas with reversible watery diarrhea and achlorhydria. Gastroenterology 1967;52:695.

80. O'Dorisio TM, Mekhjian HS. VIPoma syndrome. In: Cohen S, Soloway RD, eds. Hormone producing tumors of the pancreas. New York: Churchill-Livingstone, 1985:101.

81. O'Dorisio TM, Mekhjian HS, Gaginella TS. Medical therapy of VIPomas. Endocrinol Metab Clin North Am 1989;18:545.

82. Krejs GJ, Walsh JJ, Morawski BA, et al. Intractable diarrhea: intestinal perfusion studies and plasma VIP concentrations in patients with pancreatic cholera syndrome and surreptitious ingestion of laxatives and diuretics. Am J Dig Dis 1977;22:280.

83. Rambaud JR, Modiglianni R, Matuchansky C, et al. Pancreatic cholera: studies on tumoral secretion and pathophysiology of diarrhea. Gastroenterology 1975;69:110.

84. Krejs GJ. VIPoma syndrome. Am J Med 1987;82(Suppl 5B):37.

85. Bloom SR, Polak JM. Glucagonomas, VIPomas and somatostatinomas. Clin Endocrinol Metab 1980;9:285.

86. Long RG, Mitchell SJ, Bryant MG, et al. Clinicopathological study of pancreatic and neuron VIPomas. Gut 1979;20:A939.

87. Bloom SR, Long RG, Bryant MG, et al. Clinical, biochemical and pathological studies on 62 VIPomas. Gastroenterology 1980;78:1143.

88. Verner JV, Morrison AB. Non-B islet tumors and the syndrome of watery diarrhea, hypokalemia and hypochlorhydria. Clin Gastroenterol 1974;3:595.

89. Verner JV, Morrison AB. Endocrine pancreatic islet disease with diarrhea: report of a case due to diffuse hyperplasia of non beta islet tissue with a review of 54 additional cases. Arch Intern Med 1974;133:492.

90. Holm-Bentzen M, Schulta A, Fahrenkrug J, et al. Effect of VIP on gastric acid secretion in man. Hepatogastroenterology 1980;27(Suppl):126.

91. Domschke S, Domschke W, Bloom SR, et al. Vasoactive intestinal peptide in man: pharmacokinetics, metabolic and circulatory effects. Gut 1978;29:1049.

92. Modlin IM, Bloom SR, Mitchell SJ. Experimental evidence for vasoactive intestinal peptide as the cause of the watery diarrhea syndrome. Gastroenterology 1978;75:1051.

93. Schmitt MG, Soergel KH, Hensley GT, Chey WY. Watery diarrhea associated with pancreatic islet cell tumors. Gastroenterology 1975;69:206.

94. Go VLW, Korinek JK. Effect of vasoactive intestinal polypeptide on hepatic glucose release. In: Said SI, ed. Vasoactive intestinal peptide. New York: Raven Press, 1982:231.

95. Bloom SR, Polak JM, Pearse AGE. Vasoactive intestinal peptide and the watery-diarrhea syndrome. Lancet 1973;2:14.

96. Bloom SR, Polak JM. VIP measurement in distinguishing Verner-Morrison syndrome. Clin Endocrinol 1976;5(Suppl):223s.

97. Elias E, Bloom SR, Welbourn RB, et al. Pancreatic cholera due to production of gastric inhibitory polypeptide. Lancet 1972;2:791.

98. Tomita T, Kimmel JR, Friesen SR, Mantz FA. Pancreatic polypeptide cell hyperplasia with and without watery diarrhea syndrome. J Surg Oncol 1980;14:11.

99. Jaffe BM, Kondon S. Prostaglandins E and F in endocrine diarrheogenic syndromes. Ann Surg 1976:184:516.

100. Said SI, Falcoona GR. Elevated plasma and tissue levels of vasoactive intestinal polypeptide in the watery-diarrhea syndrome due to pancreatic, bronchogenic and other tumors. N Engl J Med 1975;193:155.

101. Gardner JD, McCarthy DM. VIP and watery diarrhea. I. Arguments against VIP being the cause of the watery diarrhea syndrome. In: Bloom SR, ed. Gut hormones. New York: Churchill-Livingstone, 1978:570.

102. Krejs GJ, Kane MG, O'Dorisio TM. VIP and the pancreatic cholera syndrome. N Engl J Med 1984;310:1465.

103. Bloom SR. Vasoactive intestinal peptide, the major mediator of the WDHA (pancreatic cholera) syndrome: value of measurement in diagnosis and treatment. Am J Dig Dis 1978;23:373.

104. Kane MG, O'Dorisio TM, Krejs GJ. Production of secretory diarrhea by intravenous infusion of vasoactive intestinal peptide. N Engl J Med 1983;309:1482.

105. Laburthe M, Amironoff B. Peptide receptors in intestinal epithelium. In: Makhlouf GM, ed. Handbook of physiology. Section 6. The gastrointestinal tract. Vol. II. Neural and endocrine biology. New York: Raven Press, 1989:215.

106. Donowitz M, Welsh MJ. Regulation of mammalian small intestinal electrolyte secretion. In: Johnson LR, ed. Physiology of the gastrointestinal tract. 2nd ed. New York: Raven Press, 1987:1351.

107. Tatemoto K, Mutt V. Isolation of the intestinal peptide porcine PHI(PHI 1-27)l, a new member of the glucagon secretin family. Proc Natl Acad Sci U S A 1981;78:6603.

108. Bloom SR, Christofides ND, Yiangan T, et al. Peptide histidine isoleucine (PHI) and Verner-Morrison syndrome. Gut 1983;24: 473.

109. Bloom SR, Christofides ND, Delamarter J, et al. Diarrhea in VIPoma patients associated with cosecretion of a second active peptide (peptide histidine isoleucine) explained by single coding gene. Lancet 1983;2:1163.

110. Christofides ND, Yiangou Y, Blank MA, et al. Are peptide histidine isoleucine and vasoactive intestinal peptide co-synthesized in the same pro-hormone? Lancet 1982;2:1398.

111. Krejs GJ. Comparison of the effect of VIP and PHI on water and ion movement in the canine jejunum in vivo. Gastroenterol Clin Biol 1984;8:868.

112. Matseche JW, Phillips SF. Chronic diarrhea: a practical approach. Med Clin North Am 1978;62:141.

113. Mekhjian HS, O'Dorisio TM. VIPoma syndrome. Semin Oncol 1987;14:282.

114. Jensen RT, Gardner JD, Raufman J-P, et al. Zollinger-Ellison syndrome: current concepts and management. Ann Intern Med 1983;98:59.

115. Morris AI, Turnberg LA. Surreptitious laxative abuse. Gastroenterology 1979;77:780.

116. Read NW, Read MG, Krejs GJ, et al. A report of five patients with large volume secretory diarrhea but no evidence of endocrine tumor or laxative abuse. Dig Dis Sci 1982;27:193.

117. Read WN, Krejs G, Read MG, et al. Chronic diarrhea of unknown origin. Gastroenterology 1980;78:264.

118. Fahrenkrug J, Schafflitzky de Muckadell OB. Verner-Morrison syndrome and vasoactive intestinal polypeptide (VIP). Scand J Gastroenterol 1979;14:57.

119. Ebeid AM, Murray PD, Fisher JE. Vasoactive intestinal peptide and the water diarrhea syndrome. Ann Surg 1978;187:411.

120. Jensen RT, Maton PN. Zollinger-Ellison syndrome. In: Gustavsson S, Kumar D, Graham DY, eds. The stomach. London: Churchill-Livingstone, 1992:341.

121. Long RG, Bryant MG, Mitchell SJ, et al. Clinicopathological study of pancreatic and ganglioneuroblastoma tumors secreting vasoactive intestinal peptide (VIPomas). Br Med J 1981;282: 1767.

122. Becker SW, Kahn D, Rothman S. Cutaneous manifestations of internal malignant tumors. Arch Derm Syphilis 1942;45: 1069.

123. McGavran MH, Unger RH, Recant L, et al. A glucagon-secreting alpha-cell carcinoma of the pancreas. N Engl J Med 1966;274:1408.

124. Wilkinson DS. Necrolytic migratory erythema with carcinoma of the pancreas. Trans St John's Hosp Dermatol Soc 1973;59: 244.

125. Mallinson CN, Bloom SR, Warin AP, et al. A glucagonoma syndrome. Lancet 1974;2:1.

126. Holst JJ. Glucagon-producing tumors. In: Cohen S, Soloway D, eds. Hormone producing tumors of the gastrointestinal tract. New York: Churchill-Livingstone, 1985:57.

127. Leichter SB. Clinical and metabolic aspects of glucagonoma. Medicine 1980;59:100.

128. Kasper CB. Necrolytic migratory erythema: unresolved problems in diagnosis and pathogenesis. A case report and review of the literature. Cutis 1992;49:120.

129. Kahan RS, Perez-Figaredo MRA, Neimanis A. Necrolytic migratory erythema: distinctive dermatosis of the glucagonoma syndrome. Arch Dermatol 1977;113:792.

130. Stacpoole PW. The glucagonoma syndrome: clinical features, diagnosis, and treatment. Endocr Rev 1981;2:347.

131. Holst JJ. Glucagonomas. In: Bloom SR, ed. Gut hormones. New York: Churchill-Livingstone, 1978:599.

132. Norton JA, Kahn CR, Schiebinger R, et al. Amino acid deficiency and the skin rash associated with glucagonoma syndrome. Ann Intern Med 1979;91:213.

133. Shepard ME, Raimer SS, Tyring SK, Smith EB. Treatment of necrolytic migratory erythema in glucagonoma syndrome. J Am Acad Dermatol 1991;25:925.

134. Tasman-Jones C, Kay RG. Zinc deficiency and skin lesions. N Engl J Med 1975;293:830.

135. Marynick SP, Fagadau WR, Duncan LA. Malignant glucagonoma syndrome response to chemotherapy. Ann Intern Med 1980;93:453.

136. Wolfe BM, Culebras JM, Aoki TT, et al. The effects of glucagon on protein metabolism in normal man. Surgery 1979;86:248.

137. Brodan V, Brodanova M, Andel M, Kuhn E. The effect of glucagon on free plasma amino acids in cirrhotics and healthy controls. Acta Hepatogastroenterol 1978;25;23.

138. Boden G, Master RW, Rezvani T, et al. Glucagon deficiency and hyperaminoacidemia after total pancreatectomy. J Clin Invest 1980;65:706.

139. Boden G, Rezvani I, Owen OE. Effects of glucagon on plasma amino acids. J Clin Invest 1984;73:785.

140. Holst JJ, Helland S, Ingemansson S, et al. Functional studies in patients with glucagonoma syndrome. Diabetologia 1979;17: 151.

141. Kahn D, Bhatena SJ, Recant L, Rivier J. Use of somatostatin and somatostatin analogs in a patient with a glucagonoma. J Clin Endocrinol Metab 1981:53;543.

142. Klein S, Jahoor F, Baba H, Townsend CM Jr, et al. In vivo assessment of the metabolic alterations in glucagonoma syndrome. Metabolism 1992;41:1171.

143. Boden G, Ryan IG, Eisenschmid BL, et al. Treatment of inoperable glucagonoma with the long-acting somatostatin analogue SMS 201-995. N Engl J Med 1986;314:1686.

144. Kessinger A, Lemon HM, Foley JF. The glucagonoma syndrome and its management. J Surg Oncol 1977;9:419.

145. Naets JP, Guns M. Inhibitory effect of glucagon on erythropoiesis. Blood 1980;55:9.

146. Edrey JA, Hoffman S, Thompson JS, Kessinger A. Glucagonoma is an underdiagnosed clinical entity. Am J Surg 1990;160:625.

147. Boden G, Owen OE. Familial hyperglucagonemia an autosomal dominant disorder. N Engl J Med 1977;296:534.

148. Palmer JP, Werner PL, Benson JW, et al. Dominant inheritance of large molecular weight immunoreactive glucagon. J Clin Invest 1978;61:763.

149. Ganda PO, Weir GC, Soeldner JS, et al. Somatostatinoma: a somatostatin-containing tumor of the endocrine pancreas. N Engl J Med 1977;296:963.

150. Larsson LI, Hirsch MA, Holst J, et al. Pancreatic somatostatinoma: clinical features and physiologic implications. Lancet 1977;1:666.

151. Unger RH. Somatostatinoma. N Engl J Med 1977;296:998.

152. Krejs GJ, Orci L, Conlon M, et al. Somatostatinoma syndrome (biochemical, morphological, and clinical features). N Engl J Med 1979;301:285.

153. Schusdziarra V, Grube D, Seifert H, et al. Somatostatinoma syndrome: clinical, morphological and metabolic features and therapeutic aspects. Klin Wochenschr 1983;61:681.

154. Burgus R, Ling N, Butcher M, et al. Primary structure of somatostatin, a hypothalamic peptide that inhibits the secretion of pituitary hormone. Proc Natl Acad Sci U S A 1973;70:684.

155. Yamada T, Chiba T. Somatostatin. In: Makhlouf GM, ed. Handbook of physiology. Section 6. The gastrointestinal tract. Vol. II. Neural and endocrine biology. New York: Raven Press, 1989:431.

156. Boden G, Sivitz MC, Owen OE. Somatostatin suppresses secretin and pancreatic exocrine secretion. Science 1975;190:163.

157. Bloom SR, Mortimer CH, Thorner MO, et al. Inhibition of gastrin and gastric acid secretion by growth hormone release inhibiting hormone. Lancet 1974;2:1106.

158. Vinik AI, Moattari AR. Treatment of endocrine tumors. Endocrinol Metab Clin North Am 1989;18:483.

159. Konomi K, Chijiiwa K, Katsato T, Yamaguchi K. Pancreatic somatostatinoma: a case report and review of the literature. J Surg Oncol 1990; 43:259.

160. Wright J, Abolfathi A, Penman E, et al. Pancreatic somatostatinoma presenting with hypoglycemia. Clin Endocrinol 1980;12:603.

161. Axelrod L, Bush MA, Hirsch HJ, et al. Malignant somatostatinoma: clinical features and metabolite studies. J Clin Endocrinol Metab 1981;52:886.

162. Levin G, Malmud L, Rock E, et al. Effects of somatostatin on gallbladder emptying in man. Clin Res 1983;31:285.

163. Schusdziarra V, Zynar E, Rouiller D, et al. Splanchnic somato-

statin: a hormonal regulator of nutrient homeostasis. Science 1980;207:530.

164. Galmiche JP, Chayvialle JA, Dubois PM, et al. Calcitonin-producing pancreatic somatostatinoma. Gastroenterology 1980;78:1577.

165. Samols E, Weir GC, Ramseur R, et al. Modulation of pancreatic somatostatin by adrenergic and cholinergic agonism and by hyper- and hypoglycemic sulfonamides. Metabolism 1978;27:1219.

166. Boden G, Baile CA, McLaughlin CL, et al. Effects of starvation and obesity on somatostatin, insulin and glucagon release from an isolated perfused organ system. Am J Physiol 1981;241:E215.

167. Pipeleers D, Couturier E, Gepts W, et al. Five cases of somatostatinoma: clinical heterogeneity and diagnostic usefulness of basal and tolbutamide-induced hypersomatostatinemia. J Clin Endocrinol Metab 1983;56:1236.

168. Rivier J, Spress J, Thorner M, Vale W. Characterization of a growth-hormone releasing factor from a human pancreatic islet cell tumor. Nature 1982;300:276.

169. Thorner MO, Perryman RL, Cronin MJ, et al. Somatotroph hyperplasia. J Clin Invest 1982;70:965.

170. Guillemin R, Brazeau P, Bohlem R, et al. Growth hormone-releasing factor from a human pancreatic tumor causing acromegaly. Science 1982;218:585.

171. Bostwick DG, Quan R, Hoffman AR, et al. Growth-hormone-releasing factor immunoreactivity in human endocrine tumors. Am J Pathol 1984;117:167.

172. Dayal Y, Lin HD, Tallberg K, et al. Immunocytochemical demonstration of growth hormone-releasing factor in gastrointestinal and pancreatic endocrine tumors. Am J Clin Pathol 1986;85:13.

173. Ch'ng JLC, Christofides ND, Kraenzlin et al. Growth hormone secretion dynamics in a patient with ectopic growth hormone-releasing factor production. Am J Med 1985;79:135.

174. Berger G, Trouillas J, Bloch B, et al. Multihormonal carcinoid tumor of the pancreas. Cancer 1983;54:2097.

175. Wilson DM, Ceda GP, Bostwick DG, et al. Acromegaly and Zollinger-Ellison syndrome secondary to an islet cell tumor: characterization and quantification of plasma and tumor human growth-releasing factor. J Clin Endocrinol Metab 1984;59:1002.

176. Moller DE, Moses AC, Jones K, et al. Octreotide suppresses both growth hormone (GH) and GH-releasing hormone (GHRH) in acromegaly due to ectopic GHRH secretion. J Clin Endocrin Metab 1989;68:499.

177. Von Werder K, Losa M, Stalla FK, et al. Long-term treatment of a metastasizing GRFoma with a somatostatin analogue (SMS 201-995) in a girl with gigantism. Scand J Gastroenterol 1986;21:238.

178. Kent RB, van Heerden JA, Weiland LH. Nonfunctioning islet cell tumors. Ann Surg 1981;193:185.

179. Taylor IL. Pancreatic polypeptide family: pancreatic polypeptide neuropeptide Y and peptide YY. In: Makhlouf GM, ed. Handbook of physiology. Section 6. The gastrointestinal tract. Vol. II. Neural and endocrine biology. Bethesda, MD: American Physiological Society, 1989:475.

180. Eckhauser FE, Cheung PS, Vinik A, et al. Nonfunctioning malignant neuroendocrine tumors of the pancreas. Surgery 1986;100:978.

181. Von Katesh S, Ordonoz NG, Ajani J, et al. Islet cell carcinoma of the pancreas: a study of 98 patients. Cancer 1990;65:354.

182. Lin TH, Zhu Y, Lui QL, et al. Nonfunctioning pancreatic endocrine tumors: an immunohistochemical and electron microscopic analysis of 26 cases. Pathol Res Pract 1992;188:191.

183. Geokas MC, Chun JY, Dinan JJ, Beck IT. Islet-cell carcinoma (Zollinger-Ellison syndrome) with fulminating adrenocortical hyperfunction and hypokalemia. Can Med Assoc J 1965;93:137.

184. Law DH, Liddle GW, Scott HW Jr, Tauber SD. Ectopic production of multiple hormones (ACTH, MSH and gastrin) by a single malignant tumor. N Engl J Med 1965;273:292.

185. Friesen SR. The development of endocrinopathies in the pro-

186. Asa SL, Kovacs K, Killinger DW, et al. Pancreatic islet cell carcinoma producing gastrin, ACTH, a-endorphin, somatostatin and calcitonin. Am J Gastroenterol 1980;74:30.

187. Lyons DF, Eisen BR, Clark MR, et al. Concurrent Cushing's and Zollinger-Ellison syndromes in a patient with islet cell carcinoma: case report and review of the literature. Am J Med 1984;76:729.

188. Clark ES, Carney JA. Pancreatic islet cell tumor associated with Cushing's syndrome. Am J Surg Pathol 1984;8:917.

189. Palmieri GMA, Nordquist RE, Omenn GS. Immunochemical localization of parathyroid hormone in cancer tissue from patients with ectopic hyperparathyroidism. J Clin Invest 1974;53:1726.

190. Vair DB, Boudreau SF, Reid EL. Pancreatic islet-cell neoplasia with secretion of a parathormone-like substance and hypercalcemia. Can J Surg 1987;30:108.

191. Rasbach DA, Hammond JM. Pancreatic islet cell carcinoma with hypercalcemia: primary hyperparathyroidism or hormonal hypercalcemia of malignancy. Am J Med 1985;78:337.

192. Cryer PhE, Hill GJ. Pancreatic islet cell carcinoma with hypercalcemia and hypergastrinemia. Cancer 1976;38:2217.

193. Blackburn AM, Bryant MG, Adrian TE, et al. Pancreatic tumours produce neurotensin. J Clin Endocrinol Metab 1981;52:820.

194. Gutniak M, Rosenqvist U, Grimelius L. Report on a patient with watery diarrhea syndrome caused by a pancreatic tumour containing neurotensin, enkephalin and calcitonin. Acta Med Scand 1980;208:95.

195. Feurle GE, Helmstaedter V, Tischbirek K, et al. A multihormonal tumor of the pancreas producing neurotensin. Dig Dis Sci 1981;26:1125.

196. Wood JR, Wood SM, Lee YC. Neurotensin-secreting carcinoma of the bronchus. Postgrad Med J 1983;59:46.

197. Shulkes A, Boden R, Cook I, et al. Characterization of a pancreatic tumor containing vasoactive intestinal peptide, neurotensin and pancreatic polypeptide. J Clin Endocrinol Metab 1984;58:41.

198. Maier W, Schumacher A, Etzrodt H, et al. A neurotensinoma of the head of the pancreas: demonstration by ultrasound and computed tomography. Eur J Radiol 1982;2:125.

199. Ferris GF. Neurotensin. In: Makhlouf GM, ed. Handbook of physiology. Section 6. The gastrointestinal tract. Vol. II. Neural and endocrine biology. Bethesda, MD: American Physiological Society, 1989:559.

200. Wolfe MM, Jensen RT. Zollinger-Ellison syndrome. N Engl J Med 1987;317:1206.

201. Deveney CW, Deveney KS, Stark D, et al. Resection of gastrinomas. Ann Surg 1983;198:546.

202. Richardson CT, Peters MN, Feldman M, et al. Treatment of Zollinger-Ellison syndrome with exploratory laparotomy, proximal gastric vagotomy, and H₂-receptor antagonists: a prospective study. Gastroenterology 1985;89:357.

203. McFadden D, Jaffe BN. Surgical approaches to endocrine-producing tumors of the gastrointestinal tract. In: Cohen S, Soloway RD, eds. Hormone producing tumors of the gastrointestinal tract. New York: Churchill-Livingstone, 1985:139.

204. Hofmann JW, Fox PS, Wilson SD. Duodenal wall tumors and the Zollinger-Ellison syndrome. Arch Surg 1973;107:334.

205. Shawker TH, Doppman JL, Dunnick NR, McCarthy DM. Ultrasound investigation of pancreatic islet cell tumors. J Ultrasound Med 1982;1:193.

206. Hancke S. Localization of hormone-producing gastrointestinal tumors by ultrasonic scanning. Scand J Gastroenterol 1979;53:115.

207. Dunnick NR, Long JA Jr, Krudy AG, et al. Localizing insulinomas with combined radiographic methods. AJR 1980;135:747.

208. London JF, Shawker TH, Doppman JL, et al. Prospective assessment of abdominal ultrasound in patients with Zollinger-Ellison syndrome. Radiology 1991;178:763.

209. Rothmund M, Angelini L, Brunt M, et al. Surgery for benign

insulinoma: an international review. World J Surg 1990;14: 393.

210. van Heerden JA, Grant CS, Czako PF, Carboneau JW. Occult functioning insulinomas: which localizing studies are indicated. Surgery 1992;112:1012.

211. Doherty GM, Doppman JL, Shawker TH, et al. Results of a prospective strategy to diagnose, localize and resect insulinomas. Surgery 1991;110:989.

212. Pasieka JL, McLeod MK, Thompson NW, Burrey RE. Surgical approach to insulinomas assessing the need for preoperative localization. Arch Surg 1992;127:442.

213. Norton JA, Collen MJ, Gardner JD, et al. Prospective study of gastrinoma localization and resection in patients with Zollinger-Ellison syndrome. Ann Surg 1986;204:468.

214. Krudy AG, Doppman JL, Jensen RT, et al. Localization of islet cell tumors by dynamic CT: comparison with plain CT, arteriography, sonography, and venous sampling. AJR 1984;143: 585.

215. Dunnick NR, Doppman JL, Mills SR, McCarthy DM. Computed tomographic detection of nonbeta pancreatic islet cell tumors. Radiology 1980;135:117.

216. Wank SA, Doppman JL, Miller DL, et al. Prospective study of the ability of computerized axial tomography to localize gastrinomas in patients with Zollinger-Ellison syndrome. Gastroenterology 1987;92:905.

217. Semelka RC, Cumming MJ, Shoenut JP, et al. Islet cell tumors: comparison of dynamic contrast-enhanced CT and MR imaging with dynamic gadolinium enhancement and fat suppression. Radiology 1993;186:800.

218. Maton PN, Miller DL, Doppman JL, et al. The role of selective angiography in the management of patients with Zollinger-Ellison syndrome. Gastroenterology 1987;92:913.

219. Roche A, Raisonnier A, Gillon-Savouret MC. Pancreatic venous sampling and arteriography in localizing insulinomas and gastrinomas: procedure and results in 55 cases. Radiology 1982;145:621.

220. Ingemansson S, Holst J, Larsson LI, Lunderquist A. Localization of glucagonoma by catheterization of the pancreatic veins and with glucagon assay. Surg Gynecol Obstet 1977;145:504.

221. Cherner JA, Doppman JL, Norton JA, et al. Selective venous sampling for gastrin to localize gastrinomas: a prospective assessment. Ann Intern Med 1986;105:841.

222. Reichardt W, Ingemasson S. Selective vein catheterization for hormone assay in endocrine tumors of the pancreas. Acta Radiol 1982;21:177.

223. Miller DL, Doppman JL, Metz DC, et al. Zollinger-Ellison syndrome: technique, results and complications of portal-venous sampling. Radiology 1992;182:235.

224. Vinik AI, Delbridge L, Moaltari R, et al. Transhepatic portal vein catheterization for localization of insulinomas: a ten year experience. Surgery 1991;109:1.

225. Frucht H, Doppman JL, Norton JA, et al. Gastrinomas: comparison of MR Imaging (MRI) with CT, angiography and US. Radiology 1989;171:713.

226. Pisegna JR, Doppman JD, Norton JA, et al. Prospective comparative study of the ability of MR imaging and other imaging modalities to localize tumors in patients with Zollinger-Ellison syndrome. Dig Dis Sci 1993;38:1318.

227. Norton JA, Shawker TH, Doppman JL, et al. Localization and surgical treatment of occult insulinomas. Surgery 1990;212: 615.

228. Charboneau WJ, James EM, Van Heerden JA, et al. Intraoperative realtime ultrasonographic localization of pancreatic insulinoma: initial experience. J Ultrasound Med 1983;2:251.

229. Norton JA, Cromack PT, Shawker TH, et al. Intraoperative ultrasonographic localization of islet cell tumors: a prospective comparison to palpation. Ann Surg 1988;207:160.

230. Doppman JL, Miller DL, Chang R, et al. Insulinomas: localization with selective intraarterial injection of calcium. Radiology 1991;178:237.

231. Imamura M, Takashi MP, Isoke Y, et al. Curative resection of multiple gastrinomas aided by selective arterial secretin injection and intraoperative secretin test. Ann Surg 1989;210:710.

232. Thom AK, Norton JA, Doppman JL, et al. Prospective study of the use of intraarterial secretin injection and portal venous sampling to localize duodenal gastrinomas. Surgery 1992;112: 1002.

233. Rosch T, Lightdale CJ, Bolet JF, et al. Localization of pancreatic endocrine tumors by endoscopic ultrasonography. N Engl J Med 1992;326:1721.

234. Lightdale CJ, Bolet JF, Woodruff JM, Brennan MF. Localization of endocrine tumors of the pancreas with endoscopic ultrasonography. Cancer 1991;68:1815.

235. Glover JR, Shorvon PJ, Lees WR. Endoscopic ultrasound for localization of islet cell tumors. Gut 1992;33:108.

236. Doppman JL. Pancreatic endocrine tumors: the search goes on. N Engl J Med 1992;326:1770.

237. Lamberts SWJ, Bakker WH, Reubi J-C, Krenning EP. Somatostatin-receptor imaging in the localization of endocrine tumors. N Engl J Med 1990;323:1246.

238. Patel YC. Somatostatin-receptor imaging for the detection of tumors. N Engl J Med 1990;323:1274.

239. Reubi J-C, Kvols L, Krenning E, Lamberts SWJ. Distribution of somatostatin receptors in normal and tumor tissue. Metabolism 1990;39(Suppl 2):78.

240. Creutzfeldt W, Arnold R, Creutzfeldt C, Track NS. Pathomorphological, biochemical and diagnostic aspects of gastrinomas (Zollinger-Ellison syndrome). Hum Pathol 1975;6:47.

241. Zollinger RM, Ellison EC, Fabri PJ, et al. Primary peptic ulceration of the jejunum associated with islet cell tumors: twenty-five-year appraisal. Ann Surg 1980;192:422.

242. Zollinger RM, Martin EW, Carey LC, et al. Observations on the postoperative tumor growth behavior of certain islet cell tumors. Ann Surg 1976;184:525.

243. Stabile BE, Passaro E Jr. Benign and malignant gastrinoma. Am J Surg 1985;149:144.

244. Norton JA, Doppman JL, Jensen RT. Curative resection in patients with Zollinger-Ellison syndrome: results of a 10-year prospective study. Ann Surg 1992;215:8.

245. Norton JA, Sugerbaker DH, Doppman JL, et al. Aggressive resection of metastatic disease in selected patients with malignant gastrinoma. Ann Surg 1986;203:352.

246. Burch PG, McLeskey CH. Anesthesia for patients with insulinoma treatment with oral diazoxide. Anesthesia 1981;55:472.

247. DeMarinis L, Barbarino A. Calcium antagonists and hormone release. I. Effects of verapamil on insulin release in normal subjects and patients with islet-cell tumor. Metabolism 1980;29: 599.

248. Murakami K, Taniguchi H, Kobayshhi T, et al. Suppression of insulin release by calcium antagonist in human insulinoma in vivo and in vitro: its possible role for clinical use. Kobe J Med Sci 1979;25:237.

249. Hofeldt FD, Dippe SE, Levin SR, et al. Effects of diphenylhydantoin upon glucose-induced insulin secretion in three patients with insulinoma. Diabetes 1974;23:192.

250. Maton PN, Gardner JD, Jensen RT. Use of long-acting somatostatin analogue SMS 201-995 in patients with pancreatic islet cell tumors. Dig Dis Sci 1989;34:285.

251. Wynick D, Bloom SR. Clinical review 23: the use of long-acting somatostatin analog octreotide in the treatment of gut neuroendocrine tumors. J Clin Endocrinol Metab 1991;73:1.

252. Charney AN, Donowitz M. Prevention and reversal of cholera enterotoxin-induced intestinal secretion by methyl prednisolone induction of Na$^+$/K$^+$-ATPase. J Clin Invest 1976;57:1506.

253. McArthur KE, Anderson DS, Durbin TE, et al. Clonidine and lidamidine to inhibit watery diarrhea in a patient with lung cancer. Ann Intern Med 1982;96:323.

254. Rao MB, O'Dorisio TM, George JM, et al. Angiotensin II and nor-epinephrine antagonize the effect of vasoactive intestinal peptide on rat ileum and colon. Peptides 1984;5:291.

255. Field M, McColl I. Ion transport in rabbit ileal mucosa. III. Effects of catecholamines. Am J Physiol 1973;225:852.

256. Jaffe BM, Kopen DF, DeSchryver-Kecskemeti K, et al. Indomethacin-responsive pancreatic cholera. N Engl J Med 1977;297:817.

257. Alburquerque RH, Owens CWI, Bloom SR. A study of vaso-

active intestinal polypeptide (VIP) stimulated intestinal fluid secretion in rat and its inhibition by indomethacin. Experientia 1979;35:1496.

258. Pandol SJ, Korman LY, McCarthy DM, et al. Beneficial effects of oral lithium carbonate in the treatment of pancreatic cholera syndrome. N Engl J Med 1980;302:1403.

259. Donowitz M, Elta G, Bloom SR, et al. Trifluoroperazine reversal of secretory diarrhea in pancreatic cholera. Ann Intern Med 1980;93:283.

260. Smith PL, Field M. In vitro antisecretory effects of trifluoroperazine and other neuroleptics in rabbit and human small intestine. Gastroenterology 1980;78:1545.

261. Powell DW, Field M. Pharmacological approaches to treatment of secretory diarrhea. In: Field M, Fordtran JS, Schultz SG, eds. Secretory diarrhea. Baltimore: Waverly Press, 1980:187.

262. Long RG, Bryant MG, Yuille PM, et al. Mixed pancreatic adenoma with symptoms of excess vasoactive intestinal polypeptide and insulin: improvement of diarrhea with metoclopramide. Gut 1981;22:505.

263. Yamashiro Y, Yamamoto K, Sato M. Loperamide therapy in a child with VIPoma-associated diarrhea. Lancet 1982;1:1413.

264. Katz MD, Erstad BL. Octreotide, a new somatostatin analogue. Clin Pharm 1989;8:255.

265. Dunne MJ, Elton R, Fletcher T, et al. Sandostatin and gastropancreatic endocrine tumors: therapeutic characteristics. In: O'Dorisio TM, ed. Sandostatin in the treatment of GEP endocrine tumors. Berlin: Springer-Verlag, 1989:93.

266. Long RG, Barnes AJ, Adrian TE, et al. Suppression of pancreatic endocrine tumor secretion by long-acting somatostatin analogue. Lancet 1979;2:764.

267. Lemon JR, Sircus W, Bloom SR, et al. Investigation of a recurrent VIPoma. Gut 1975;16:821.

268. Ruskone A, Rene E, Chayvialle JA, et al. Effect of somatostatin on diarrhea and on small intestinal water and electrolyte transport in a patient with pancreatic cholera. Dig Dis Sci 1982;27:459.

269. Crunow RT, Carey RM, Taylor A, Johanson A, Murad F. Somatostatin inhibition of insulin and gastrin hypersecretion in pancreatic islet-cell carcinoma. N Engl J Med 1975;292:1385.

270. Christensen SE, Hansen AP, Lundbaek K, et al. Somatostatin and insulinoma. Lancet 1975;1:1426.

271. Efendic S, Lins PE, Sigurdsson G, et al. Effect of somatostatin on basal and glucose-induced insulin release in five patients with hyperinsulinaemia. Acta Endocrinol (Copenh) 1976;81:525.

272. Fallucia F, Delle-Fave G, Giangrande L, et al. Effect of somatostatin on gastrin, insulin and glucagon secretion in two patients with Zollinger-Ellison syndrome. J Endocrinol Invest 1981;4:481.

273. Sohier J, Jeanmougin M, Lombrail P, Passa P. Rapid improvement of skin lesions in glucagonomas with intravenous somatostatin infusion. Lancet 1980;1:40.

274. Wynick D, Anderson JV, Williams SJ, Bloom SR. Resistance of metastatic pancreatic endocrine tumors after long-term treatment with the somatostatin analogue octreotide (SMS-201-995). Clin Endocrinol 1989;30:385.

275. Elsberg L, Glenthoj A. Effect of somatostatin in necrolytic migratory erythema of glucagonoma. Acta Med Scand 1985;218:245.

276. Sheppard M, Shapiro B, Pimstone B, et al. Metabolic clearance and plasma half-disappearance of exogenous somatostatin in man. J Clin Endocrinol Metab 1979;48:50.

277. Bauer W, Briner U, Doepfner W, et al. A very potent and selective octapeptide of somatostatin with prolonged actions. Life Sci 1982;31:113.

278. Vinik A, Tsai S-T, Moattari AR, et al. Somatostatin analogue (SMS 201-995) in the management of gastroenteropancreatic tumors and diarrhea syndromes. Am J Med 1986;81:23.

279. Kutz K, Nuesch E, Rosenthaler J. Pharmacokinetics of SMS 201-995 in healthy subjects. Scand J Gastroenterol 1986;21:65.

280. Osei KW, O'Dorisio TM. Malignant insulinoma: effects of a somatostatin analog (compound SMS 201-995) on serum glucose growth, and gastroenteropancreatic hormones. Ann Intern Med 1985;103:223.

281. Kaloustian E. Controle metabolique d'un insulinime par un agoniste d'action prolongee de la somatostatine. Presse Med 1986;15:1882.

282. Verschoor L, Uitterlinden P, Lamberts SWJ, del Pozo E. On the use of a new somatostatin analogue in the treatment of hypoglycemia in patients with insulinoma. Clin Endocrinol 1986;25:555.

283. Lamberts SWJ, Hofland LJ, von Koetsveld PM, et al. Parallel in vivo and in vitro detection of functional somatostatin receptors in human endocrine pancreatic tumors: consequence with regards to diagnosis, localization and therapy. J Clin Endocrinol Metab 1990;71:566.

284. Koelz A, Kraenzlin M, Gyr K, et al. Escape of the response to a long-acting somatostatin analogue (SMS 201-995) in patients with VIPoma. Gastroenterology 1987;92:527.

285. Kvols LK, Buck M, Moertel CG, et al. Treatment of metastatic islet cell carcinoma with a somatostatin analogue (SMS 201-995). Ann Intern Med 1987;107:162.

286. Maton PN, O'Dorisio TM, Howe BA, et al. Effect of a long-acting somatostatin analogue (SMS 201-995) in a patient with pancreatic cholera. N Engl J Med 1985;312:17.

287. Altimiri AF, Bhoopalam N, O'Dorisio TM, et al. Use of a somatostatin analog (SMS 201-995) in the glucagonoma syndrome. Surgery 1986;100:989.

288. Rosenbaum A, Flourie B, Chagnon S, et al. Octreotide (SMS 201-995) in the treatment of metastatic glucagonoma: report of one case and review of the literature. Digestion 1989;42:116.

289. Santangelo WC, Unger RH, Orci L, et al. Somatostatin-induced remission of necrolytic migratory erythema without changes in plasma glucagon concentrations. Pancreas 1986;1:464.

290. Souquet JC, Chayvaille J-A, Sassolas G, Partensky C. Biological and clinical efficacy of a long-acting somatostatin analogue (SMS 201-995) in secreting APUDomas (abstract). Can J Physiol Pharmacol 1986;64.

291. Lamberts SWJ. Non-pituitary actions of somatostatin: a review on the therapeutic role of SMS 201-995 (Sandostatin). Acta Endocrinol [Suppl] (Copenh) 1986;276:41.

292. Wilson DM, Hoffman AR. Reduction of pituitary size by the somatostatin analogue SMS 201-995 in a patient with an islet cell tumour secreting growth hormone releasing factor. Acta Endocrinol (Copenh) 1986;113:23.

293. Melmed S, Ziel FH, Braunstein GD, et al. Medical management of acromegaly due to ectopic production of growth hormone-releasing hormone by a carcinoid tumor. J Clin Endocrinol Metab 1988;67:395.

294. Anderson J, Bloom SR. Neuroendocrine tumours of the gut: long-term therapy with the somatostatin analogue SMS 201-995. Scand J Gastroenterol 1986;21:115.

295. Glaser B, Rosler A, Halperin Y. Chronic treatment of a benign insulinoma using the long-acting somatostatin analogue SMS 201-995. Isr J Med Sci 1990;26:16.

296. Maton PN, O'Dorisio TM, O'Dorisio MS, et al. Successful therapy of pancreatic cholera with long acting somatostatin analogue SMS 201-995. Scand J Gastroenterol 1986;119:181.

297. Schrezenmeir J, Plewe G, Sturmer W, et al. Treatment of APUDomas with the long-acting somatostatin analogue SMS 201-995: investigations of therapeutic use and digestive side effects. Scand J Gastroenterol 1986;21:223.

298. Richter G, Stockmann F, Lembcke B, et al. Short-term administration of the somatostatin analogue SMS 201-995 in patients with carcinoid syndrome. Scand J Gastroenterol 1986;21:193.

299. Comi R. Pharmacology and use in pituitary tumors. In: Gorden P, moderator. Somatostatin and somatostatin analogue (SMS 201-995) in treatment of hormone-secreting tumors of the pituitary and gastrointestinal tract and non-neoplastic diseases of the gut. Ann Intern Med 1989;110:36.

300. Shepherd JJ, Senator GB. Regression of liver metastases in patients with gastrin-secreting tumor treated with SMS 201-995. Lancet 1986;2:574.

301. Edwards C, Cann PA, Read NW, Holdsworth CD. Effect of

two new antisecretory drugs on fluid and electrolyte transport in a patient with secretory diarrhea. Gut 1986;27:581.

302. Edwards CA, Cann PA, Read NW, Holdsworth CD. The effect of somatostatin analogue SMS 201-995 on fluid and electrolyte transport in a patient with secretory diarrhea. Scand J Gastroenterol 1986;21:259.

303. Norton JA, Doherty GM, Fraker DL. Surgery of endocrine tumors of the pancreas. In: Go VLW, DiMagno EP, Gardner JD, et al, eds. The pancreas: biology, pathobiology and diseases. 2nd ed. New York: Raven Press 1993:1009.

304. Norton JA, Jensen RT. Unresolved surgical issues in the management of patients with the Zollinger-Ellison syndrome. World J Surg 1991;15:151.

305. Kloppel G, Willemar S, Stamm B, et al. Pancreatic lesions and hormonal profile in pancreatic tumors in multiple endocrine neoplasia type I. Cancer 1986;57:1820.

306. Massi-Benedetti M, Noy G, Johnson IDA, et al. Glucose controlled insulin infusion system (Biostator) application during surgery for a presumed pancreatic microinsulinoma. Diabetes Metab 1981;7:41.

307. Schwartz SS, Horwitz DL, Zehfus G, et al. Continuous monitoring and control of plasma glucose during operation for removal of insulinomas. Surgery 1979;85:702.

308. Karam JH, Lorenzi M, Young CW, et al. Feedback-controlled dextrose infusion during surgical management of insulinomas. Am J Med 1979;66:675.

309. Tutt GO Jr, Edis AJ, Service FJ, van Herrden JA. Plasma glucose monitoring during operation for insulinoma: a critical reappraisal. Surgery 1980;88:351.

310. Krantz AJ, Hale PJ, Baddeley RM, et al. Intraoperative blood glucose and serum insulin concentration in the surgical management of insulinoma. Postgrad Med J 1990;66:24.

311. Menogaux F, Schmitt G, Mercadier M, Chigot J-P. Pancreatic insulinomas. Am J Surg 1993;165:243.

312. Creutzfeldt W, Bartsch HH, Jacaboschke U, Stockmann F. Treatment of gastrointestinal endocrine tumors with interferon-α and octreotide. Acta Oncol 1991;30:529.

313. Buchanan KD, Collins JSA, Varghese A, et al. Sandostatin and the Belfast experience. Digestion 1990;45(Suppl 1):11.

314. Blanchin M, Deidier AJ, Chaunet-Riffaud D, Chayvaille JA. Utilisation de l'octreotide dans les tumeurs endocrines digestives: etude Francaise multicentrique. Presse Med 1992;21:697.

315. Timmer R, Koningsberger JC, Erkelens DW, et al. No effect of the long-acting somatostatin analogue octreotide in patients with insulinoma. Neth J Med 1991;38:199.

316. Oberg K, Eriksson B. Medical treatment of neuroendocrine gut and pancreatic tumors. Acta Oncol 1989;28:425.

317. Hercot O, Legmann P, Humbert M, et al. Diagnostic du glucagonom: interet du scanner, de l'echographie et de l'arteriographie. A propos de deux observations et revue de la litterature. J Radiol 1989;70:309.

318. Binnick AN, Spencer SK, Landon Dennison W, Horton ES. Glucagonoma syndrome: report of two cases and literature review. Arch Dermatol 1977;113:749.

319. Higgins GA, Recant L, Fischmann AB. The glucagonomas syndrome: surgically cured diabetes. Am J Surg 1979;137:142.

320. von Schenck H, Thorell JI, Berg J, et al. Metabolic studies and glucagon gel filtrate pattern before and after surgery in a case of glucagonoma syndrome. Acta Med Sci 1979;205:155.

321. Jensen RT. Endocrine tumors of the pancreas. In: Yamada T, ed. Textbook of gastroenterology. Philadelphia: JB Lippincott, 1991:1912.

322. Grama D, Eriksson B, Martensson H, et al. Clinical characteristics, treatment and survival in patients with pancreatic tumors causing endocrine hormonal syndromes. World J Surg 1992;16:632.

323. Lefebvre J, Lelievre G, Galle-Furnari MA, et al. Glucagonoma avec acidocetose diabetique: une observation. Diabetes Metab (Paris) 1982;8:191.

324. Reyes-Govea J, Holm A, Aldrete JS. Response of glucagonoma to surgical excision and chemotherapy: report of two cases and review of the literature. Am Surg 1989;55:523.

325. Thompson JC, Lewis BG, Weiner I, et al. The role of surgery in the Zollinger-Ellison syndrome. Am Surg 1983;197:594.

326. Mignon M, Ruszniewski R, Haffar S, et al. Current approach to the management of tumoral process in patients with gastrinoma. World J Surg 1986;10:702.

327. Bonfils S, Landor JH, Mignon M, Hervoir P. Results of surgical management in 92 consecutive patients with Zollinger-Ellison syndrome. Ann Surg 1981;194:692.

328. Broder LE, Carter SK. Pancreatic islet cell carcinoma. II. Results of therapy with streptozotocin in 52 patients. Ann Intern Med 1973;79:108.

329. Kvols LK, Buck M. Chemotherapy of the metastatic carcinoid and islet cell tumors: a review. Am J Med 1987;82:77.

330. Buchanan KD, O'Hare MMT, Russel CJF, et al. Factors involved in the responsiveness of gastrointestinal apudomas to streptozotocin. Dig Dis Sci 1986;31:551S.

331. Moertel CG, Lavin PT, Hahn RG. Phase II trial of doxorubicin for advanced islet cell carcinoma. Cancer Treat Rep 1982;66:1567.

332. Bukowski RM, McCracken JD, Balcerzak SP, et al. Phase II study of chlorozotocin in islet cell carcinoma. Cancer Chemother Pharmacol 1983;11:48.

333. Moertel CG. An odyssey in the land of small tumors. J Clin Oncol 1987;5:1503.

334. Moertel CG, Hanley JA, Johnson LA. Streptozotocin alone compared with streptozotocin plus fluorouracil in the treatment of advanced islet-cell carcinoma. N Engl J Med 1980;303:1189.

335. Bonfils S, Ruszniewski P, Haffar S, Laucournet H. Chemotherapy of hepatic metastases (HM) in Zollinger-Ellison syndrome (ZES): report of a multicentric analysis. Dig Dis Sci 1986;31:WS51.

336. Kelsen DG, Cheng E, Kemeny N, et al. Streptozotocin and adriamycin in the treatment of APUD tumors (carcinoid, islet cell and medullary thyroid). Proc Am Assoc Cancer Res 1982;23:433.

337. Ruszniewski PH, Hochlaf S, Rougier P, Mignon M. Chimiotherapie intraveineuse par streptozotocine et 5-fluoro-uracile des metastases hepatiques du syndrome de Zollinger-Ellison: etude prospective multicentrique chez 21 patients. Gastroenterol Clin Biol 1991;15:393.

338. Frame J, Kelsen D, Kemeny N, et al. A phase II trial of streptozotocin and adriamycin in advanced APUD tumors. Am J Oncol 1988;11:490.

339. Von Schrenck T, Howard JM, Doppman JL, et al. Prospective study of chemotherapy in patients with metastatic gastrinoma. Gastroenterology 1988;94:1326.

340. Moertel CG, Lefkopoulo M, Lipsitz S, et al. Streptozotocin-doxorubicin, streptozotocin-fluorouracil, or chlorozotocin in the treatment of advanced islet-cell carcinoma. N Engl J Med 1992;326:519.

341. Maton PN. Octreotide and islet cell tumors. Gastroenterol Clin North Am 1989;18:897.

342. Moertel CG, Kvols LK, O'Connell MJ, Rubin J. Treatment of neuroendocrine carcinomas with combined etoposide and cisplatin. Cancer 1991;68:227.

343. Arnold R, Neuhaus C, Rolwage M, Trautmann MF. The German Sandostatin Study Group. Metabolism 1992;41(Suppl 2):116.

344. Pisegna JR, Slimak GG, Doppman JL, et al. An evaluation of human recombinant alpha interferon in patients with metastatic gastrinoma. Gastroenterology 1993;105:1179.

345. Bodley GP, Bedekian AY, Valdiviesco M, et al. Chemotherapeutic management of hepatobillary pancreatic cancer. In: Stroehlean JR, Romsdahl MM, eds. Gastrointestinal cancer. New York: Raven Press, 1981:279.

346. Rougier P, Oliviera J, Ducreaux M, et al. Metastatic carcinoid and islet cell tumors of the pancreas: a phase II trial of the efficacy of combination chemotherapy with 5-fluorouracil, doxorubicin and cisplatin. Eur J Cancer 1991;27:1380.

347. Bukowski RM, Tangen C, Lee R, et al. Phase II trial of chlorozotocin and fluorouracil in islet cell carcinoma: a Southwest Oncology Group study. J Clin Oncol 1992;10:1914.

348. Erickson B, Oberg K, Alm G, et al. Treatment of malignant

endocrine pancreatic tumors with human leucocyte interferon. Lancet 1986;2:1307.

349. Oberg K, Ericksson B, Norheim I. Interferon treatment of neuroendocrine gut tumors. J Clin Oncol 1987;6:80.

350. Oberg K, Lindstron H, Alm G, Lundquist G. Successful treatment of therapy-resistant pancreatic cholera with human leukocyte interferon. Lancet 1985;1:725.

351. Anderson JV, Bloom SR. Treatment of malignant endocrine tumors with human leukocyte interferon. Lancet 1987;1:97.

352. Carrasco CH, Chuang, VP, Wallace S. APUDoma metastatic to the liver: treatment by hepatic artery embolization. Radiology 1983;149:79.

353. Maton PN, Camilleri M, Griffin G, et al. Role of hepatic arterial embolization in the carcinoid syndrome. Br Med J 1983;287: 932.

354. Carty SE, Jensen RT, Norton JA. Prospective study of aggressive resection of metastatic pancreatic endocrine tumors. Surgery 1992;112:1024.

355. McEntee GP, Nagorney DM, Kvols LK, et al. Cytoreductive hepatic surgery for neuroendocrine tumors. Surgery 1990;108: 1091.

356. Kessinger A, Lemon HM, Foley JF. The glucagonoma syndrome and its management. J Surg Oncol 1977;9:419.

357. Strauss GM, Weitzman SA, Aoki TT. Dimethyltriazenomidazole carboxamide therapy of malignant glucagonomas. Ann Intern Med 1979;90:57.

358. Duncan LA, Marynick SP. Glucagonoma and dacarbazine. Ann Intern Med 1982;97:930.

359. Prinz RA, Budrinath K, Banerji M, et al. Operations and chemotherapeutic management of malignant glucagon producing tumors. Surgery 1981;90:713.

360. Awrich AE, Peetz M, Fletcher WS. Dimethyltriazenomidazole carboxamide therapy of islet cell carcinomas of the pancreas. J Surg Oncol 1981;17:321.

361. Kurose T, Seino Y, Ishida LT, et al. Successful treatment of metastatic gastrinoma with dacarbazine. Lancet 1984;1:621.

362. Herr RR, Jahnke HK, Argoudelis AD. The structure of streptozotocin. J Am Chem Soc 1967;98:4808.

363. Rakieten N, Rakieten ML, Nadkani MV. Studies of the diabetogenic action of streptozotocin (NSC-37917). Cancer Chemother Rep 1969;29:91.

364. Murray-Lyon IM, Eddelston ALWF, Williams R, et al. Treatment of multiple hormone producing malignant islet cell tumor with streptozotocin. Lancet 1968;2:895.

365. Johnson TP, McCaleb GS, Montgomery JA. Synthesis of chlorozotocin, the 2-chloroethyl analogue of the anti-cancer antibiotic streptozotocin. J Med Chem 1975;18:104.

366. Hoth P, Woolley P, Green D, et al. Phase I studies on chlorozotocin. Clin Pharmacol Ther 1978;23:712.

367. Kovach JS, Moertel CS, Schutt AJ, et al. A phase I study of chlorozotocin. Cancer 1979;43:2189.

368. Oberg K, Eriksson B, Norheim I. Interferon treatment of neuroendocrine gut tumors. J Clin Oncol 1987;6:80.

369. Norbin A, Lindblom A, Mansson B, Sundberg M. Interferon treatment in patients with malignant carcinoids. Acta Oncol 1989;28:445.

370. Valimaki M, Harvinen H, Salmela P, et al. Is the treatment of metastatic carcinoid tumor with interferon not as successful as suggested? Cancer 1991;67:547.

371. Moertel CG, Rubin J, Kvols LK. Therapy of metastatic carcinoid tumor and the malignant carcinoid syndrome with recombinant leucocyte A interferon. J Clin Oncol 1989;7:865.

372. Doberauer C, Niecterle N, Klobe O, et al. Zur behandlung das metastatasserten karzoids van ileum und cecum mit arkombinatem interferon alpha. Oncologie 1987;10:340.

373. Redding TW, Schally AV. Inhibition of growth of pancreatic carcinomas in animal models by analogs of hypothalamic hormones. Proc Natl Acad Sci U S A 1984;84:248.

374. Kvols LK, Moertel CG, O'Connell MJ. Treatment of the malignant carcinoid syndrome: evaluation of a long-acting somatostatin analogue. N Engl J Med 1986;315:663.

375. Ajani JA, Carrasco H, Charnsangevej C, et al. Islet cell tumors metastatic to the liver: effective palliation by sequential hepatic artery embolization. Ann Intern Med 1988;108:340.

376. Marlink RG, Lokich JJ, Robins JR, Clouse ME. Hepatic arterial embolization for metastatic hormone-secreting tumors. Cancer 1990;65:2227.

377. Valette PJ, Souquet JC. Pancreatic islet cell tumors metastatic to the liver: treatment by hepatic artery chemo-embolization. Horm Res 1989;32:77.

378. Nesovic M, Civic J, Radojkovic S, et al. Improvement of metastatic endocrine tumors of the pancreas by hepatic artery embolization. J Endocrinol Invest 1992;15:543.

379. Moertel CG, May GR, Martin JK, et al. Sequential hepatic artery occlusion and chemotherapy for metastatic islet carcinoid tumor and islet cell carcinoma. Proc Am Soc Clin Oncol 1985;4:80.

380. Fox PS, Hofmann JW, Wilson SD, DeCosse JJ. Surgical management of the Zollinger-Ellison syndrome. Surg Clin North Am 1974;54:395.

381. Hanssen LE, Schrumpf E, Kolbenstvedt AN, et al. Treatment of malignant metastatic midgut carcinoid tumors with recombinant human-2b interferon with or without hepatic artery embolization. Scand J Gastroenterol 1989;24:787.

382. Hanssen LE, Schrumpf E, Jacobsen MB, et al. Extended experience with recombinant-2b interferon with or without hepatic artery embolization in the treatment of midgut carcinoid tumors: a preliminary report. Acta Oncol 1991;40:523.

Textbook of Gastroenterology, second edition, edited by Tadataka Yamada. JB Lippincott Company, Philadelphia © 1995.

CHAPTER 94

Hereditary Diseases of the Pancreas

Rodger A. Liddle

CYSTIC FIBROSIS

Epidemiology

Cystic fibrosis is the most common hereditary disease involving the exocrine pancreas. It is estimated that cystic fibrosis affects 1 in every 2500 live births in the Caucasian population, and although the disease occurs in all racial and ethnic groups, it appears less frequently in nonwhites.[1,2] The inheritance pattern of cystic fibrosis is autosomal recessive, with a gene frequency of approximately 5% among individuals of northern European extraction.[3,4] However, significant numbers of affected individuals are found in southern Europe, in the Ashkenazi Jewish population, and among African Americans.[5] Male and female children are affected equally.

Heterozygotes who carry one normal cystic fibrosis allele and one mutant allele are asymptomatic but are denoted as gene carriers. The child of two carriers has a one-in-four chance of inheriting one mutant allele from each parent and therefore being affected with cystic fibrosis. There are more than 30,000 persons with cystic fibrosis in the United States, and it has been estimated that 3.3% of the white population in the United States or more than 7 million people are carriers of the cystic fibrosis gene.[6]

During the past two decades, advances in the diagnosis and treatment of individuals with cystic fibrosis has led to improved survival. The median survival time for patients with cystic fibrosis is now 29 years, and it is not uncommon for patients to live into the fifth decade.

Pathophysiology

Electrophysiologic studies of airway epithelial cells demonstrated selective chloride channels on the apical surface. These channels are normally under the regulation of the second messenger cyclic adenosine monophosphate (cAMP) and are opened by agents such as epinephrine that increase intracellular cAMP levels. In contrast, cAMP is not able to elicit chloride channel activity in epithelial cells from patients with cystic fibrosis. This regulation does not occur even though there is appropriate activation of protein kinase A by cAMP. A signature of cystic fibrosis affected epithelial cells is defective activation of a cAMP-dependent chloride channel.[7]

The defect in membrane permeability to chloride ion in cystic fibrosis affects many epithelial cells, including sweat duct cells, where it is responsible for defective sodium absorption. In these cells, efflux of chloride is necessary for activation of a chloride-bicarbonate exchanger that promotes NaCl absorption.[8] It is by this mechanism that children with cystic fibrosis have excessive salt loss from sweat glands. The abnormality in salt transport has been the basis for measurements of sodium and chloride in sweat as the standard diagnostic test for cystic fibrosis.[1]

Considerable insights into the pathophysiology of cystic fibrosis have occurred since 1989, when the gene responsible for the disease was identified using positional cloning techniques.[9-11] This cystic fibrosis gene encodes a 1480–amino acid protein that, because of the initial ambiguity about its exact function, was named cystic fibrosis transmembrane conductance regulator (CFTR). Proof that the cloned gene was responsible for cystic fibrosis was born out by demonstration that mutations of the gene differentiated normal from affected individuals. A 3–base pair deletion in exon 10 of the gene, which results in the loss of a single amino acid, phenylalanine, at codon 508 (hence the name, ΔF_{508}) was found in individuals with cystic fibrosis. This mutation accounted for approximately 70% of the mutant alleles in patients with cystic fibrosis, and all homozygous patients with this mutation have cystic fibrosis.[11,12] Cystic fibrosis is caused by mutation of the gene encoding CFTR. Mutations at different regions of the gene can also cause cystic fibrosis but are much less common than the ΔF_{508} mutation.

The evidence supports the concept that CFTR normally functions as a cAMP-regulated chloride channel in epithelial cells of tissues that are affected in cystic fibrosis and that chloride transport across the apical membrane is defective in epithelial cells from sweat glands and respiratory tissues in patients with cystic fibrosis.[8,13–16] Although it was reasonable to speculate that the gene for CFTR encoded a chloride channel based on the chloride transport properties of cystic fibrosis affected cells, the gene sequence revealed that the structure of the protein shared greatest sequence homology with a superfamily of nucleotide-binding transport proteins that were not known to have channel properties.[17] Moreover, the predicted structure of CFTR did not resemble other recently cloned chloride channels.[18,19] Several studies were required to prove that CFTR was actually a chloride channel. It has been demonstrated that CFTR cDNA, when introduced into cells that do not normally express the protein or exhibit endogenous chloride channel activity, conferred cAMP-regulated chloride channel activity and that CFTR cDNA containing the ΔF_{508} mutation did not confer this activity.[20–22] Site-directed mutagenesis of the cystic fibrosis gene has been shown to alter cAMP-regulated chloride conductance.[23] Reconstitution of purified recombinant CFTR into planar lipid bilayers was shown to exhibit regulated chloride channel activity that closely resembled that found in native epithelial cells.[24] These studies demonstrated that CFTR functions as a chloride channel.

The protein product predicted from the cDNA sequence appears to have two membrane regions, each made up of six membrane-spanning domains and two nucleotide-binding folds (Fig. 94-1). The ΔF_{508} mutation, and most of the other mutations seen in cystic fibrosis, are found in the first nucleotide-binding fold. In addition to these regions, there is a highly charged cytoplasmic regulatory domain in which are located multiple potential substrate phosphorylation sites for protein kinase A.[10]

A working model for the regulation of CFTR has been devised. In the absence of phosphorylation of the regulatory domain, the channel is closed. On stimulation with cAMP, protein kinase A phosphorylates one or more serine residues in the regulatory domain. The CFTR channel can then bind ATP at the sites of the nucleotide binding folds. Cleavage of ATP is thought to induce a conformational change that opens the chloride channel.[12]

The pancreas in humans expresses the highest amounts of CFTR messenger RNA of any tissue in the body. Normally, CFTR is located in the cell membrane on the apical surface

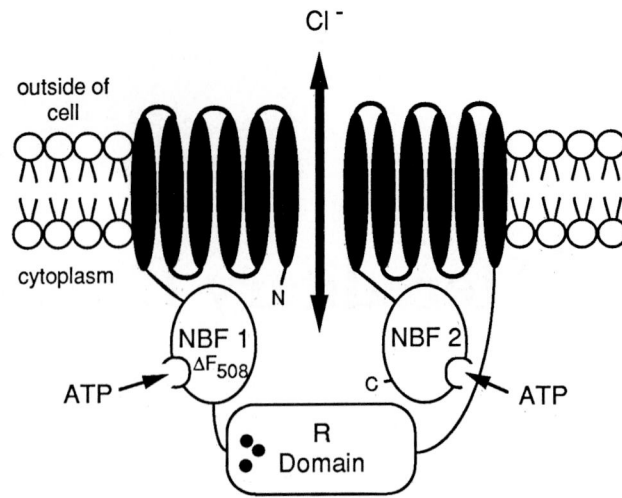

FIGURE 94-1. A model of the structure of the cystic fibrosis transmembrane conductance regulator (CFTR). Based on the cDNA sequence of the gene, CFTR is composed of two membrane regions, each composed of six membrane-spanning domains. Most of the protein is intracellular and contains two nucleotide-binding folds (NBF), which bind ATP, and a regulatory (R) domain, which possesses a cluster of sites for phosphorylation by cAMP-activated protein kinase A (●). The most common cystic fibrosis–causing mutation (ΔF_{508}) is located in the first nucleotide-binding fold.

of ductal epithelial cells.[25,26] A proposed model for CFTR in pancreatic exocrine secretion is provided in Figure 94-2. Stimulation of the duct cell through mechanisms that increase intracellular concentrations of cAMP causes the chloride channel to open, allowing chloride to flow into the lumen of the duct. This increase in intralumenal chloride activates the chloride-bicarbonate exchanger that also is located on the apical surface of the pancreatic duct cell. CFTR enhances bicarbonate, sodium, and water movement from the cell into the lumen of the duct. In cystic fibrosis, a defect in the function of CFTR results in a net reduction of fluid movement across the ductular epithelium leading to thick, less hydrated pancreatic secretions. These protein-rich secretions become inspissated, leading to obstruction of pancreatic ducts ultimately causing destruction and fibrosis of the gland.[27]

The evidence indicates that there is a defect in transport of the ΔF_{508} mutant form of CFTR to the cell surface, causing CFTR to be absent from the apical membrane.[28,29] The precise mechanisms that are involved in intracellular trafficking of CFTR and how this is disturbed in mutant forms of the protein are under investigation. Whether other abnormalities in the regulation of CFTR also contribute to the defect in chloride channel regulation in other mutations remains to be determined.

Genetically engineered mice created by homologous recombination to have defective *CFTR* genes have been described by several groups of investigators and may serve as animal models of cystic fibrosis.[30–32] All strains of homozygous *CFTR*-deficient mice displayed abnormal epithelial cell chloride conductance that is characteristic of cystic fibrosis in humans. They also demonstrated tissue damage similar in many ways to that seen in human cystic fibrosis. In some strains,

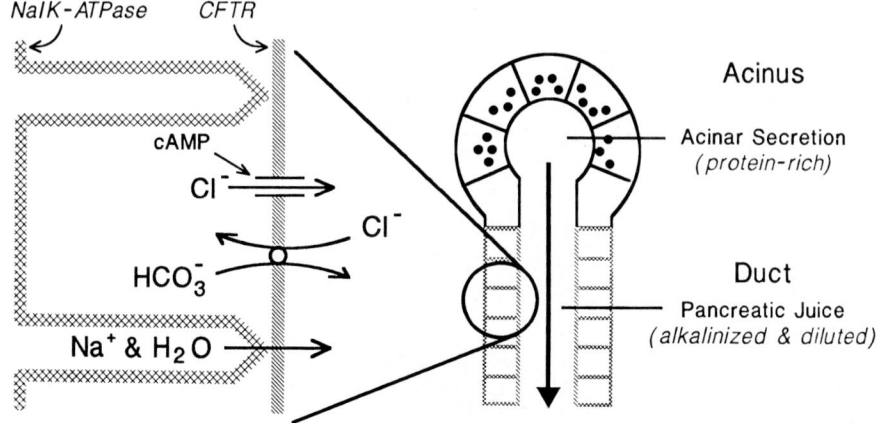

FIGURE 94-2. A proposed model for cystic fibrosis transmembrane conductance regulator (CFTR) in pancreatic exocrine secretion. CFTR is located on the apical surface of the pancreatic duct cell, where it functions as a cAMP-dependent chloride channel. On stimulation by cAMP, CFTR opens and allows chloride to flow into the lumen of the duct. This increase in chloride permits Cl^--HCO_3^- exchange on the apical surface of the ductal cell, resulting in net fluid secretion and alkalinization of pancreatic juice. In cystic fibrosis, the failure of the CFTR chloride channel to open could lead to defective dilution and alkalinization of pancreatic juice, causing inspissation of secretions and ultimately producing ductal obstruction. (From Marino CR, Matovcik LM, Gorelick FS, Cohn JA. Localization of the cystic fibrosis transmembrane conductance regulator in pancreas. J Clin Invest 1991;88:712.)

animals died young because of malabsorption of intestinal nutrients and intestinal blockage that resembled meconium ileus. These models reinforce the pivotal role that CFTR plays in the pathogenesis of cystic fibrosis and promise to be useful in understanding the pathophysiology of the disease.

Pathologic Features

The pathologic features of cystic fibrosis result from abnormalities in exocrine secretion and include increased viscosity of exocrine secretions and increased electrolyte concentration in sweat and saliva. The first comprehensive description of the disease used the term *cystic fibrosis of the pancreas* to indicate the pathologic changes that occurred with inspissation of proteinaceous plugs within small pancreatic ducts.[33] However, pathologic changes are found in exocrine glands throughout the body, resulting in impaired pancreatic exocrine secretion, focal biliary cirrhosis, obstructive pulmonary disease, and obstructive lesions of the ductal system in the male genital tract. Intrauterine growth retardation and other abnormalities in fetal development occur with high frequency in cases of cystic fibrosis.[34] These include intestinal stenosis, congenital inguinal hernias, cryptorchidism, hydrocele, omphalocele, and meconium ileus.[35,36]

Two types of pathologic exocrine involvement have been described.[37] In pancreatic acini, intestinal glands, intrahepatic bile ducts, gallbladder, prostate, and salivary glands, precipitation of exocrine secretions form concretions within the ducts. In mucous glands of the upper respiratory tract and Brunner's glands of the duodenum, there is distention and dilatation of the ducts, perhaps from hypersecretion of the glands, and a notable absence of obstructing concretions (Fig. 94-3).

The pancreas in a patient with cystic fibrosis may appear normal, but more often, it is small, firm, and irregular in shape and may contain cysts. Although pancreatic lesions may not be apparent in some cases, regardless of age, there generally is a direct correlation between age and severity of pathologic findings.[38] The earliest changes are deposition of eosinophilic concretions within the pancreatic ductules. Involvement of larger ductules leads to dilatation from obstruction of exocrine secretion. Acinar disruption follows, and enzymes may leak into the intracellular space and initiate autodigestion of the pancreas. As the disease progresses, cysts develop, and pancreatic lobules are replaced by fat and fibrous tissue. With long-standing disease, it is often difficult to differentiate cystic fibrosis from other chronic diseases of the pancreas. Histologically, islets remain among the fibrous strands, but with severe disease, insulin production is diminished, and diabetes mellitus results.

Clinical Features

Historically, cystic fibrosis has been recognized as a clinical triad involving abnormalities of the sweat gland, respiratory epithelium, and exocrine pancreas. Even though chronic pulmonary disease is the major cause of mortality in cystic fibrosis, gastrointestinal manifestations of this disease also lead to significant morbidity.

More than 80% of patients with cystic fibrosis have pancreatic insufficiency at the time of diagnosis, and even more have partial impairment in enzyme secretion.[39] Before an abnormality in enzyme output becomes apparent, a reduction in fluid and bicarbonate secretion in response to a provocative stimulus may be seen.[40,41] Pancreatic secretions have a reduced water content and are viscous. Early in the course of the dis-

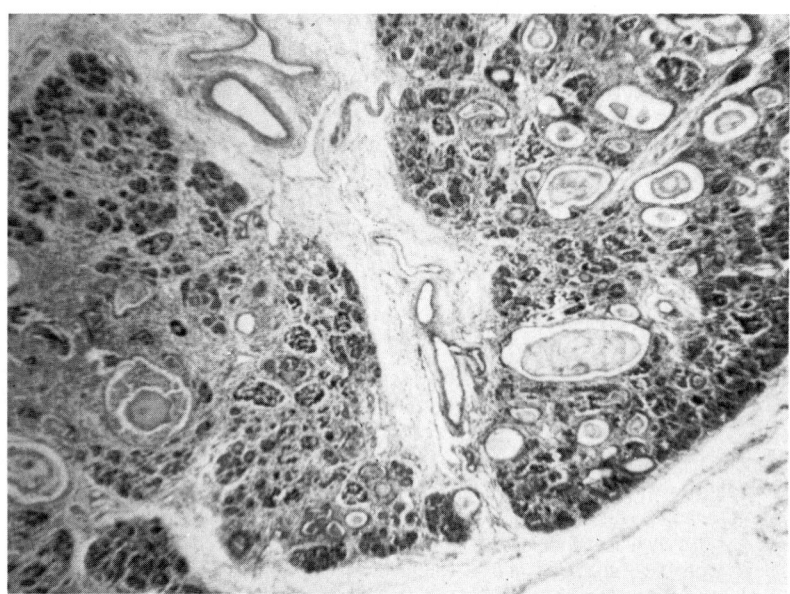

FIGURE 94-3. Photomicrograph of a histologic section of the pancreas from a patient with cystic fibrosis. Notice the fibrotic band and the numerous concretions within the pancreatic ducts. (Courtesy of William D. Bradford, M.D., Durham, NC.)

ease, basal enzyme output may be absent, but the pancreas can respond to a meal or exogenous cholecystokinin and secretin. As the disease progresses, even stimulated exocrine secretions become severely reduced. As a result of exocrine pancreatic insufficiency, malabsorption with steatorrhea and creatotorrhea occurs.

These manifestations become apparent by 2 years of age in 80% of patients. Infants often fail to gain weight despite a vigorous appetite. Within the first 6 months, infants have watery stools, and it is not until later in the first year that typical bulky, foul, greasy stools become evident. Fat malabsorption may lead to deficiencies of fat-soluble vitamins and occasionally to essential fatty acid deficiencies. Vitamin B_{12} deficiency may occur, and in rare circumstances, hemorrhagic complications may result from vitamin K deficiency. Because of malabsorption, hypoproteinemia with edema may occur and a "pot belly" is a typical physical finding. Confirmation of the diagnosis of cystic fibrosis may be difficult in such patients because of the likelihood of a false-negative sweat chloride test in the presence of edema.[42] However, with the cloning of the cystic fibrosis gene, it is possible to identify the disease at the genetic level in many patients.

The variable clinical course in patients with cystic fibrosis can be attributed in part to specific genotypes at the locus of the cystic fibrosis gene.[43] Patients with pancreatic insufficiency are likely to have two severe mutant *CFTR* alleles, such as ΔF_{508} or other mutations, and those patients without pancreatic insufficiency have at least one of the less common alleles that results in a milder phenotype.[44] The correlation between genotype and phenotype is more apparent for the severity of pancreatic disease than it is for other tissues affected by cystic fibrosis, such as pulmonary insufficiency.

Among the 15% of patients who do not have clinical pancreatic exocrine insufficiency, a small group appears to develop recurrent episodes of acute pancreatitis.[45] Symptoms of abdominal pain and clinical features of pancreatitis have been reported for children older than 7 years of age and young adults without other etiologic factors for pancreatitis. Al-

though few of these patients have been studied, endoscopic retrograde cholangiopancreatography (ERCP) findings have ranged from normal to obstruction and dilatation of the pancreatic duct. Whether recurrent pancreatitis contributes to subsequent pancreatic insufficiency is not established.

Meconium ileus occurs in 15% of infants with cystic fibrosis and becomes apparent within 1 to 2 days after birth.[46] The condition is thought to result from reduced water content of meconium, causing it to become impacted within the bowel. Intestinal crypt epithelial cells have been shown to have an apical membrane chloride channel and a chloride-bicarbonate exchanger similar to that identified in the pancreas.[47] It is likely that a defect in lumenal electrolyte and fluid transport contributes to thickened and viscous intestinal contents. Localization of CFTR to intestinal crypt cells also suggests that the physiologic defect in pancreas and intestine may have a similar basis in cystic fibrosis.[48] As a consequence, infants with meconium ileus quickly develop abdominal distention, often with visible or palpable loops of small bowel in the right lower quadrant, delayed passage of meconium, and bilious vomiting. Complications such as volvulus and small bowel atresia may be associated with peritonitis. Abdominal radiographs reveal dilatation of the small bowel and a paucity of air in the colon. The diagnosis can be confirmed by a scan after a barium enema on which a microcolon and obstructing mass in the ileum are identified.[49]

In uncomplicated cases, it is possible to alleviate the obstruction with N-acetylcysteine, Hypaque, or Gastrograffin enemas.[50-52] In cases involving volvulus, small bowel atresia, or peritonitis, surgery is necessary, and the mortality rate for complicated cases may be as high as 30%.[53] Because cystic fibrosis accounts for 30% of cases of intestinal obstruction in infants, it is imperative that sweat chloride tests be performed in all infants presenting with such disorders.

Older patients are also at risk for distal small bowel obstruction, which has been referred to as *meconium ileus equivalent*.[54] The term is actually a misnomer, because obstruction is the result of inspissation of partially digested food from viscous secretions and the lack of pancreatic digestive enzymes rather than true meconium. Obstruction may be partial or complete and may be complicated by volvulus or intussusception.[55] Oral and rectal administration of N-acetylcysteine have been useful in relieving the obstruction.[54,56] The condition is more common in patients who originally had true meconium ileus, and prevention of later obstruction can be achieved by increasing oral enzyme replacement and the use of stool softeners or cathartics.

Rectal prolapse occurs in approximately 20% of patients with cystic fibrosis, and cystic fibrosis is the leading cause of rectal prolapse in childhood in the United States.[57] Frequent passage of large bulky stools, severe coughing from respiratory complications of cystic fibrosis, and perhaps poor perineal muscle tone from relative malnutrition all contribute to rectal prolapse. The condition rarely occurs after 5 years of age and generally responds to dietary therapy with addition of pancreatic supplements. Surgical correction is usually unnecessary. However, because of the frequent association with cystic fibrosis, children presenting with rectal prolapse should have sweat chloride tests performed.

Intussusception occurs in as many as 1% of patients with cystic fibrosis and develops only in those with pancreatic insufficiency.[55] It results from inspissated stool in the distal ileum and cecum that serves as a lead point for intussusception. Although surgery may be required for alleviation of the obstruction, Gastrograffin enemas usually provide adequate therapy.

Diabetes mellitus develops in approximately 1% of children and as many as 13% of adults with cystic fibrosis.[58,59] Early in cystic fibrosis, beta cells of the islets of Langerhans appear normal, but with progression of the disease, the exocrine tissue is replaced by fibrosis and fatty tissue, and there is a gradual diminution in the number of islets. This decrease is believed to result from disruption of normal islets by pancreatic autodigestion.

Approximately 5% of patients with cystic fibrosis develop clinically apparent liver disease.[60,61] Histologically, focal accumulation of mucus in the area of the porta hepatis with periportal inflammation, fibrosis, bile duct proliferation, and cholestasis has been described in infants. These lesions may result from a primary defect in bile duct secretory function. Focal biliary cirrhosis characterized by eosinophilic inspissations within bile ducts, periportal fibrosis and inflammation, and bile duct proliferation have been found more frequently in older children and adults.[60] This lesion may progress to form regenerative nodules and resemble postnecrotic cirrhosis.[61] Clinical manifestations of liver involvement include neonatal jaundice, hypersplenism, bleeding from esophageal varices, and hepatocellular failure. The most prominent laboratory abnormality is elevated alkaline phosphatase. It is important to exclude other underlying conditions, such as drug toxicity, that could contribute to hepatic failure; otherwise, therapy is supportive. Portosystemic shunting is reserved for complications of variceal hemorrhage.

Disease of the biliary tract occurs in approximately 50% of patients with cystic fibrosis. The gallbladder is small and mucus-filled cysts are found within the epithelial lining.[60] Increased fecal loss of bile acids and a reduced bile salt pool have been demonstrated in cystic fibrosis.[62,63] Consequently, lithogenic bile exists.[64] Gallstones occur in 12% of patients,

although many patients never develop biliary symptoms.[65] It has not been established whether treatment of asymptomatic gallstones in this condition is indicated.

Diagnosis

Cystic fibrosis should be suspected in infants slow to gain weight and those who have evidence of malabsorption. Diarrheal stools may be difficult to appreciate in infancy, and only after 6 months of life do typical bulky, foul-smelling, and greasy stools become apparent. A high index of suspicion is needed to make the diagnosis early. Conditions associated with cystic fibrosis such as meconium ileus, pulmonary disease, hepatobiliary disease, hypoproteinemia, edema, and failure to thrive should alert the physician to the possibility.

The primary test to confirm the diagnosis is measurement of sweat electrolytes. Sodium and chloride levels are elevated in the sweat in 99% of patients with cystic fibrosis.[58] Because the test itself is demanding to perform and there is considerable variability among laboratories, it is important that the test is performed with reliability. False-positive tests have been reported for a variety of diseases, including adrenal insufficiency, nephrogenic diabetes insipidus, congestive heart failure, edema, fever, dehydration, and malnutrition.[66] Diuretic therapy can also alter test results. Normally, the sodium concentration in sweat is greater than the chloride concentration, but in cystic fibrosis, this ratio is reversed. Sodium and chloride levels of greater than 77 and 74 mmol/L, respectively, are consistent with the diagnosis.[67] Laboratory tests that are often obtained in evaluation of malabsorption include microscopic examination of stool revealing fat globules and undigested meat fibers, which indicate pancreatic insufficiency. The diagnosis of steatorrhea is confirmed by an abnormal 72-hour fecal fat test.

Radiographic evaluation is usually unnecessary for patients with cystic fibrosis, but contrast studies of the bowel may show thickened intestinal folds and dilution of barium. An ultrasound scan of the pancreas is nonspecific, but a small, irregularly echogenic gland is often found in patients with severe pancreatic involvement.[68] ERCP studies reveal a spectrum of findings, ranging from normal ductal anatomy to severe obstruction and dilatation of the pancreatic ducts.

Because pancreatic insufficiency is not a universal feature of cystic fibrosis, measurement of pancreatic enzyme secretion is usually unnecessary. However, for the patients for whom the sweat test is equivocal and the diagnosis is in doubt, a pancreatic stimulation test with cholecystokinin and secretin can be helpful.[67]

With the identification of the cystic fibrosis gene, chromosomal analysis can be used for fetal screening to diagnose cystic fibrosis in those in whom one of the more common mutations is the cause. Such analysis was initially thought to be straightforward because the mutation ΔF_{508} accounted for 70% of the mutant chromosomes. However, the prospects for screening became much more complicated when it was found that the remaining non-ΔF_{508} cystic fibrosis chromosomes harbor a large number of different mutations. Over 60 additional different mutations have been identified, and there is significant population variation for each of these mutations. The known mutations account for about 85% of the cystic fibrosis chromosomes.[5] Although genetic analysis may be useful in most cases of cystic fibrosis, it does not offer a perfect screening method.

Treatment and Prospects for Gene Therapy

The most striking gastrointestinal manifestation of cystic fibrosis and that which occurs earliest is failure to thrive. This results primarily from malnutrition but is complicated by recurrent pulmonary infections.

Treatment of malnutrition rests on adequate replacement of pancreatic enzymes to facilitate digestion and absorption and to ensure adequate caloric and vitamin intake. Pancreatic enzyme supplements are the mainstay of treatment. Taken with meals, enzyme replacement should prevent maldigestion and malabsorption of ingested nutrients, thereby reducing steatorrhea. However, normal digestion and absorption are rarely achieved.

Several problems arise with oral administration of pancreatic enzymes. First, acid and pepsin inactivate ingested enzymes. A pH less than 4 destroys lipase activity, and trypsin is inhibited below a pH of 3.5. Second, patients with cystic fibrosis are characteristically hypersecretors of gastric acid, which compounds the difficulty with acid inactivation of orally administered enzymes.[69] Third, the reduced pancreatic bicarbonate output does not provide a duodenal pH high enough to allow normal enzyme activity even if it did survive transit through the stomach.

To circumvent these problems, it is common to administer more enzyme orally than would be needed if all reached the duodenum intact. Six to eight tablets with each meal are generally sufficient, but the formulation of the pancreatic supplement is important and co-administration of an agent to neutralize gastric acid or suppress acid production is often necessary. It has been demonstrated that less than 22% of the enzymatic activity of ingested trypsin and 8% of lipase can be recovered from the distal duodenum.[70,71]

Efforts have been made to devise schemes that would deliver adequate pancreatic enzyme activity to the upper small intestine. Enteric coating of tablets to protect against acid degradation in the stomach has not been successful because of a lack of pancreatic bicarbonate in the duodenum, which is needed to dissolve the enteric coating. However, capsules or enteric coated microspheres of similar preparations have been more effective.[71,72] To neutralize gastric acid, administration of antacids or bicarbonate together with pancreatic supplements improves fat digestion and reduces steatorrhea.[73,74] Large amounts of bicarbonate, however, may not be tolerated by pediatric patients. Magnesium- or calcium-containing antacids are not as beneficial as could be expected based on their acid neutralizing capabilities. This probably results from calcium binding to fatty acids liberated by lipase to form insoluble calcium-fatty acid soaps.[75] Addition of H_2-blocking agents have been very useful in improving maldigestion in patients with cystic fibrosis and other types of pancreatic insufficiency.[73,76] Because there is an inverse relation between gastric acid secretion and response to pancreatic enzyme therapy, effective treatment with H_2 blockers offers distinct advantages.[77]

In an attempt to bypass the requirements of pancreatic enzymes for digestion, placing patients on diets containing protein hydrolysates, glucose polymers, and medium chain triglycerides has demonstrated improvement in weight and other clinical scores of nutrition.[78–80] However, such dietary restriction is generally not well tolerated. It is important to balance the caloric requirements of patients with cystic fibrosis, which has been estimated to be 130% of the RDA for a healthy person of the same age and sex, with their ability to tolerate dietary fat. Because fat provides over two times the number of calories as protein or carbohydrate, it is an efficient way to provide the necessary extra calories. In addition, one reason that cystic fibrosis patients are prone to essential fatty acid deficiency is that they burn essential fatty acids as a source of calories.[81] To provide dietary essential fatty acids and adequate calories, patients should be placed on balanced diets with about 40% of calories in the form of fat.[82] Pancreatic supplements are used as needed. When adequate caloric intake cannot be maintained even with proper nutritional counseling, nocturnal tube feeding, parenteral nutrition, or enterostomy feeding may be employed.

Deficiencies of the fat-soluble vitamins, A, D, E, and K and the respective clinical signs of deficiency have all been demonstrated in cystic fibrosis. Supplemental vitamins should be provided. The water-soluble vitamins are readily absorbed with the exception of B_{12}, whose absorption depends on pancreatic enzymes to cleave B_{12} from R-protein, allowing B_{12} to be absorbed in the ileum. With adequate pancreatic enzyme replacement, supplemental B_{12} is usually unnecessary.

Because heterozygotes who possess 50% of the normal CFTR protein do not suffer from cystic fibrosis, introduction of the *CFTR* gene into a sufficient number of the correct cells in patients with cystic fibrosis should correct the disease. The cloning of the *CFTR* gene and the successful transfer of this gene into cells with subsequent restoration of proper chloride channel activity supports the concept that gene therapy may be achieved for the treatment of cystic fibrosis.[12] The use of attenuated viral vectors has led to the successful gene transfer of *CFTR* cDNA into cystic fibrosis airway cells with correction of the defect in chloride transport.[83] In vivo transfer of human *CFTR* genes into rat tracheal epithelial cells and in intrahepatic biliary epithelial cells has been accomplished using replication-deficient recombinant adenovirus vectors.[84,85] Stable transgene expression of *CFTR* in human bronchial epithelia using similar vectors has set the stage for treating cystic fibrosis by somatic gene transfer.[86] Although many questions need to be answered concerning this technology, such as the best cells to treat, how long expression can be expected to last, and the possible adverse effects of *CFTR* overexpression or the use of viral vectors themselves, gene therapy has the potential to become an important treatment modality for patients with cystic fibrosis.

HEREDITARY PANCREATITIS

Hereditary pancreatitis refers to a familial syndrome characterized by recurrent episodes of pancreatitis that develop in early childhood and continue throughout life. It has only been since 1952, when pancreatitis was ascribed to a kindred, that the disease has been recognized.[87] Since then, numerous reports from around the world have described an inherited predisposition to pancreatitis, but the incidence of hereditary pancreatitis among the general population is difficult to estimate. Of the patients with pancreatitis seen in referral centers, it is estimated that 5% to 10% have the hereditary type of disease.[88,89]

Although hereditary pancreatitis can develop at any age, it commonly is revealed in childhood. Several reports describe a mean age of onset of 10 years, and it is thought to be the most common cause of pancreatitis in childhood.[88,90] The disease occurs equally in males and females and is not unique to any race. The pattern of inheritance is autosomal dominant, and the penetrance rate of the gene for hereditary pancreatitis is estimated to be 80%.[91,92] No distinctive chromosomal abnormalities have been described. The exact nature of the defect causing hereditary pancreatitis is unknown. No distinctive pancreatic anomalies or biochemical defects have been reported. However, one group found that the concentration of a "pancreatic stone protein" is decreased in chronic calcific pancreatitis.[93] This phosphoprotein with a molecular weight of 14,017 is produced in pancreatic acinar cells and secreted into the duct, where it is thought to inhibit precipitation of calcium carbonate in the pancreatic duct, preventing pancreatic stone formation.[94] Although occurring in other forms of chronic pancreatitis, low amounts of this protein have been described in patients with hereditary pancreatitis. The importance of this protein in the development of chronic pancreatitis remains to be determined.

The clinical features are similar to those seen with chronic relapsing pancreatitis from other causes. Affected individuals typically have prolonged attacks of severe epigastric abdominal pain that radiates to the back, although 4% to 5% of patients may remain pain free. Pain is improved by flexing the hips, and it is remarkable that many patients describe other family members with abdominal pain assuming a similar posture. Periods of clinical remission often increase with age, and it is not uncommon for older patients to have years between attacks.

Laboratory tests such as elevations in serum amylase and lipase are useful in diagnosing acute attacks of pancreatitis but are not to be relied on solely for confirmation of the disease. However, several radiographic features may be helpful. It has been reported that gallstones are less common in hereditary pancreatitis.[95] With recurrent attacks and with a longer duration of illness, calcification in the pancreas develops. However, in hereditary pancreatitis calculi larger than those typically seen in chronic pancreatitis and occurring in the major pancreatic ducts have been described (Fig. 94-4).[96] Because the central portions of these stones are less radiopaque, they appear as "bulls' eyes." In a patient suspected of having hereditary pancreatitis, consistent laboratory and radiographic findings together with a family history of pancreatitis in the absence of other known etiologic factors such as alcohol ingestion, gallstones, or drug toxicity, the diagnosis is usually not in doubt.

The metabolic complications of long-standing hereditary pancreatitis are typical of chronic pancreatitis and include pancreatic exocrine insufficiency with malabsorption and diabetes mellitus. Pancreatic pseudocysts are common, and with recurrent attacks of pancreatitis, vascular complications such as thrombosis of the splenic or portal vein with subsequent

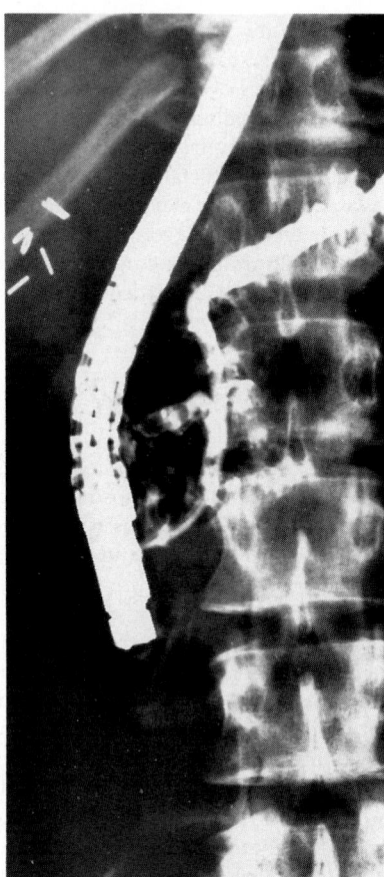

FIGURE 94-4. An endoscopic retrograde pancreatogram in a patient with hereditary pancreatitis. Notice the irregular contour of the pancreatic duct and numerous filling defects within the duct caused by protein plugs and pancreatic stones. (Courtesy of Peter B. Cotton, M.D., Durham, NC.)

formation of gastroesophageal varices and hemorrhage may occur. Pancreatic ascites and pleural effusions may develop with an acute attack or with recurrent inflammatory episodes. Edema or scarring of the head of the pancreas may encroach on the common bile duct, causing biliary obstruction and jaundice.

Treatment of acute episodes of pancreatitis is to maintain fluid and electrolyte balance, provide pain relief, and "rest" the pancreas. Severe or prolonged bouts of pancreatitis may require parenteral nutrition, especially in the face of complications such as acute pseudocyst development. With recurrent attacks, it is important to watch for the development of glucose intolerance, because diabetes mellitus occurs in 25% of patients with long-standing disease.[95]

Abdominal pain from chronic pancreatitis may be amenable to treatment with pancreatic enzyme supplementation in an attempt to decrease the stimulus for pancreatic exocrine secretion.[97] It has been reported that such therapy is useful even in the absence of overt malabsorption. As pancreatic insufficiency develops, it becomes necessary to institute pancreatic enzyme replacement to prevent malabsorption. Surgical intervention is required for treatment of refractory pain or pseudocysts that become infected or do not resolve. Endoscopic sphincterotomy may be useful in selected cases in which obstruction of the pancreatic duct may be relieved.

An increased incidence of ductal pancreatic carcinoma has been associated with hereditary pancreatitis. The combined estimated incidence from several series approaches 5%.[88,90,98,99] Because neoplastic tissue is ductal in origin, it is hypothesized that metaplasia and neoplasia may result from continued irritation by intraductal calculi or recurrent inflammation.[88] It is not clear whether ultrasound or computerized tomography scanning is useful for monitoring patients at risk for pancreatic carcinoma.[88]

α_1-ANTITRYPSIN DEFICIENCY

α_1-Antitrypsin is a 394–amino acid glycoprotein synthesized in the liver that inhibits neutrophil lysosomal elastase activity. Deficiency of α_1-antitrypsin has been associated with a clinical syndrome of emphysema in adults and liver disease in neonates. Some patients with pancreatitis and abnormally low α_1-antitrypsin levels have been reported.[100,101]

α_1-Antitrypsin deficiency is inherited autosomally through two co-dominant alleles for which the gene has been identified on human chromosome 14.[102] The disease is characterized by serum α_1-antitrypsin levels of less than 35% of normal (normal range, 150–350 mg/dL). Although originally described for its ability to inhibit trypsin, α_1-antitrypsin actually inhibits a class of serine proteases. More than 30 biochemical variants of α_1-antitrypsin have been described, of which the types abbreviated M, S, and Z are the most common. Serum α_1-antitrypsin levels are highest in the phenotype MM and lowest in ZZ.[103] The prevalence of type Z homozygotes is as high as 0.06 in northern Europe, slightly less common in other Caucasian populations, and is rare in black and Asian populations.[104,105] The most striking feature of α_1-antitrypsin deficiency is its association with emphysema, which is thought to result from unopposed damage from neutrophil proteases, particularly elastase.

Severe pulmonary dysfunction may occur as early as 30 years of age. Neonatal hepatitis occurs in a minority of patients with α_1-antitrypsin deficiency. However, when it does occur, the major features are hepatocellular damage and jaundice, which can be dramatic. Development of cirrhosis later in childhood is a frequent complication, and reports indicate that it may appear even in adulthood.[106–112]

Two studies suggest that α_1-antitrypsin deficiency may be associated with pancreatitis. In a survey of 110 patients with chronic pancreatitis in South Africa, patients had lower serum α_1-antitrypsin levels and a preponderance of the MZ phenotype compared with either of two groups of control subjects.[100] In a smaller group of 15 patients with chronic pancreatitis, low α_1-antitrypsin levels were also found, but α_1-antitrypsin phenotyping was not performed.[101] Although in both of these studies most patients had alcohol-induced chronic pancreatitis, the low α_1-antitrypsin levels and high frequency of MZ phenotypes suggest that α_1-antitrypsin deficiency may predispose patients to chronic pancreatitis. One study reported elevated α_1-antitrypsin levels in 23 patients with acute pancreatitis.[113] Because α_1-antitrypsin is an acute-phase reactive protein, the discrepant findings between acute and chronic pancreatitis are difficult to decipher. It is not established whether α_1-antitrypsin deficiency is a cause of pancreatitis, but it seems logical that abnormally low levels of a circulating protease inhibitor could have a permissive effect on protease-mediated damage of the pancreas.

SHWACHMAN'S SYNDROME

Shwachman's syndrome is the second most common cause of pancreatic insufficiency in children. It is a familial syndrome characterized by pancreatic exocrine insufficiency, neutropenia, metaphyseal dysostosis, short stature, and eczema.[114,115] Pancytopenia, diabetes mellitus, and Hirschsprung's disease are less commonly associated findings. The syndrome was initially described in 1964, and since that time, there have been more than 100 cases reported. The estimated incidence is 1 in every 20,000 live births, and there is no sexual predominance.[116]

The inheritance pattern is autosomal recessive. The disorder is usually apparent during infancy and is manifest by failure to thrive and bulky, greasy, foul-smelling stools due to steatorrhea. Secretion of all pancreatic enzymes is deficient, even with secretin and cholecystokinin stimulation. The pancreas usually is small, and acinar tissue is replaced by fat, although islets are found.[117] Fatty pancreatic tissue may produce a distinctive appearance on computed tomography scans.[118]

Several hematologic abnormalities have been described. Neutropenia, which is usually cyclic in nature, is common and is a necessary component for making the diagnosis. However, constant neutropenia can also be seen. Thrombocytopenia occurs in approximately 70% of patients, and anemia occurs in 50%.[165] Elevated levels of fetal hemoglobin occur in 45% of patients and may be an indicator of an increased risk for malignancy.[119]

Bone abnormalities appear later in childhood, and the most common, metaphyseal dysostosis, occurs in 10 to 15% of patients. The femur, tibia, and ribs are most commonly involved.[120,121]

The diagnosis is suspected in any infant with evidence of pancreatic insufficiency. After pancreatic insufficiency has been confirmed, the diagnosis of Shwachman's syndrome is established with a negative sweat chloride test to rule out cystic fibrosis and demonstration of neutropenia. Neutropenia may not be easily recognized, because the period of neutropenic cycling may be as short as 1 to 2 days.[122] The total neutrophil count should be carefully monitored before excluding the diagnosis. The absolute neutropenia and a defect in neutrophil mobility predisposes these patients to infection.

When pancreatic insufficiency is discovered, patients should be treated with pancreatic enzyme replacement. Adequate therapy should reduce steatorrhea and restore normal growth. A diet in which fat is replaced with medium-chain triglycerides, oligomers of glucose in place of starch, and supplementation with fat-soluble vitamins may also be helpful. Patients should be watched closely for the development of infection, because this is the main cause of mortality among patients with this syndrome.

The symptoms in many patients improve as they grow older, and it is remarkable that fat absorption may actually normalize over time.[120] The mechanism for this improvement is not yet understood, although one study observed a marginal increase in pancreatic lipase secretion.[123]

JOHANSON-BLIZZARD SYNDROME

A syndrome of congenital malabsorption, aplasia of the alae nasi, deafness, hypothyroidism, dwarfism, and absent permanent teeth was first described by Johanson and Blizzard in 1971.[124] Genitourinary, anorectal, and cardiac anomalies and mental retardation are sometimes associated with the syndrome.[125,126] More than 20 patients have been reported, but because of the rarity of the disorder, much of the pathophysiology remains unknown, and the findings of only two autopsies have been described.[126,127] The disease appears to be inherited in an autosomal recessive manner.[128]

Pancreatic insufficiency is a universal feature of this disorder. Pathologically, normal pancreatic tissue is replaced by fat, and there is a paucity of islets, although disturbances in glucose tolerance have not been described.[126,127] Deficient production of pancreatic enzymes is associated with malabsorption and steatorrhea and may lead to malnutrition if not corrected.

The syndrome is still not clearly defined, but it is important that malabsorption be looked for and pancreatic insufficiency must be considered in infants or children with multiple congenital defects and failure to thrive.

SIDEROBLASTIC ANEMIA AND PANCREATIC INSUFFICIENCY

A syndrome of sideroblastic anemia and pancreatic insufficiency was reported in 1976, when four patients were characterized.[129] Two of the four patients also had splenic atrophy. Pancreatic bicarbonate, amylase, and lipase secretion were low in the patients in whom these parameters were measured. On pathologic examination, atrophy of the pancreas with fibrosis and deficient acinar tissue was found. All patients had malabsorption and evidence of pancreatic exocrine insufficiency. Other congenital anomalies were not described, and in the absence of subsequent reports, the incidence and pathophysiologic basis of the syndrome remain unknown.

ISOLATED PANCREATIC ENZYME DEFICIENCIES

Lipase Deficiency

An isolated deficiency of pancreatic lipase was described in four patients in 1964, and subsequent reports confirmed and further characterized the disease.[130–133] Only lipase is involved; other pancreatic enzymes exist in variable amounts. Patients experience profound steatorrhea but do not have creatorrhea and do not experience malnutrition or growth retardation. The steatorrhea occurs early in life and is usually severe, with greasy, foul-smelling stools, often containing oil droplets. Profound nutritional deficiencies do not accompany this dis-

order. It may be that gastric and lingual lipase, phospholipase A_2, and bacterial lipolysis provide intralumenal lipase activity that partially compensates for the deficiency of pancreatic lipase and prevents essential fatty acid deficiency and growth failure.[132,134]

The cause of this disorder is unknown, although it appears to be inherited in an autosomal recessive manner.[130] Studies have indicated that there is complete absence of immunologically detectable lipase in the pancreas.[135] The diagnosis is suspected in children with steatorrhea and is confirmed by demonstrating abnormally low or absent lipase but normal trypsin and amylase activity in duodenal juice after stimulation with cholecystokinin and secretin.

Treatment is based on the use of pancreatic enzyme supplements and modification of the diet to replace long-chain fatty acids with medium-chain fatty acids. This latter treatment obviates the need for endogenous pancreatic lipase.

Colipase Deficiency

An isolated deficiency of pancreatic colipase has been reported in two brothers.[136] Both presented with steatorrhea in childhood but had no other associated abnormalities. They were found to have normal amylase, chymotrypsin, lipase, and bile salt concentrations by pancreatic function testing, but they malabsorbed fat. Fat balance studies and ^{14}C-triolein breath test results were restored toward normal with the administration of purified colipase.

Deficiencies of lipase and colipase without other enzyme abnormalities have been described, although this condition is exceedingly rare.[137] In the affected patient, fat absorption was 50% of normal and improved with pancreatic enzyme replacement.

Amylase Deficiency

An isolated deficiency of pancreatic amylase has been reported, but because pancreatic amylase content may continue to increase over the first year of life, eventually reaching normal levels, it is important to differentiate delayed amylase expression from an inherited and persistent defect in amylase.[138–140] Because some patients presenting with fermentative diarrhea and failure to thrive originally had deficient duodenal amylase levels but were found to have normal levels later in life, the existence of amylase deficiency as an isolated disorder has come into question.

Lerner and colleagues established rigid criteria for the diagnosis of congenital isolated amylase deficiency.[134] These include age greater than 1 year, clinical intolerance of starch-containing food, low amylase but normal lipase and trypsinogen concentrations in duodenal fluid with cholecystokinin-secretin stimulation, and pH in duodenal fluid, normal histology and brush, abnormal starch loading test, improvement with starch-free diet, and negative sweat chloride test to exclude cystic fibrosis. Using these criteria, it should be possible to determine if patients with suspected amylase deficiency have an isolated inherited defect or simply a delay in maturation of amylase expression.

Trypsinogen Deficiency

Three infants with isolated trypsinogen deficiency have been reported.[141-143] The condition was associated with growth failure, hypoproteinemia, edema, and anemia. In duodenal fluid, trypsin, chymotrypsin, and carboxypeptidase activity were absent but were restored to normal with addition of trypsin. Clinical manifestations improved with feeding a pre-digested protein supplement. Because activation of trypsinogen to the active enzyme, trypsin, by enterokinase is necessary for initiating the pancreatic enzyme activation cascade in the intestine, it may be difficult to differentiate trypsinogen deficiency from a defect of enterokinase.

Enterokinase Deficiency

Congenital enterokinase deficiency has been reported, and since its demonstration in siblings, it has been considered a familial disease, but too few cases prevent determination of its genetics.[144-150] The disease is revealed in infancy, and affected patients have malabsorption with creatorrhea, hypoproteinemia, edema, and growth retardation. Fifty percent of patients experience vomiting. Because enterokinase is necessary for activation of trypsin and subsequent activation of other proenzymes, the manifestations of enterokinase deficiency are similar to those of trypsin deficiency.

Examination of duodenal juice reveals very low trypsin levels but normal amylase and lipase levels. Addition of enterokinase restores trypsin activity. Patients have normal brush border enzymes, normal intestinal histology, and negative sweat chloride tests. In considering the diagnosis of congenital enterokinase deficiency, it is important to exclude secondary causes of low enterokinase activity, such as celiac disease, which involves atrophy of the small intestinal mucosa and can produce similar manifestations. The diagnosis is confirmed by demonstrating low levels of duodenal trypsin activity but normal amylase and lipase levels with cholecystokinin-secretin testing and activation of trypsin activity with addition of exogenous enterokinase. A negative sweat chloride test and normal intestinal histology are also necessary.

In treating such patients, the need for endogenous enterokinase can be bypassed by administration of trypsin, which is contained in pancreatic supplements. This treatment reverses the growth failure and restores other clinical parameters to normal. Elemental dietary supplements or protein hydrolysates may also be useful.

The reader is referred to Chapter 15, Pancreatic Secretion; Chapter 89, Pancreas: Anatomy and Structural Anomalies; Chapter 90, Acute Pancreatitis; and Chapter 91, Chronic Pancreatitis.

REFERENCES

1. Di Sant'Agnese P, Talamo RC. Pathogenesis and physiopathology of CF of the pancreas: fibrocystic disease of the pancreas (mucoviscidosis). N Engl J Med 1967;1287:
2. Steinberg AG, Brown DC. On incidence of CF of pancreas. Am J Hum Genet 1960;12:416.
3. Wood R, Boat T, Doershuk C. Cystic fibrosis. Am Rev Respir Dis 1976;113:833.
4. Danks DM, Allen J, Anderson CM. A genetic study of fibrocystic disease of the pancreas. Ann Hum Genet 1965;28:323.
5. Tsui L-C, Buchwald M. Biochemical and molecular genetics of cystic fibrosis. Adv Hum Genet 1991;20:153.
6. FitzSimmons SC. The changing epidemiology of cystic fibrosis. J Pediatr 1993;122:1.
7. Welsh MJ. Abnormal regulation of ion channels in cystic fibrosis epithelia. FASEB J 1990;4:2718.
8. Quinton PM. Chloride impermeability in cystic fibrosis. Nature 1983;301:421.
9. Rommens JM, Iannuzzi MC, Kerem B, et al. Identification of the cystic fibrosis gene: chromosome walking and jumping. Science 1989;245:1059.
10. Riordan JR, Rommens JM, Kerem B-S, et al. Identification of the cystic fibrosis gene: chromosome walking and jumping. Science 1989;245:1066.
11. Kerem B-S, Rommens JM, Buchanan JA, et al. Identification of the cystic fibrosis gene: genetic analysis. Science 1989;245:1073.
12. Collins FS. Cystic fibrosis: molecular biology and therapeutic implications. Science 1992;256:774.
13. Welsh MJ, Lieddke CM. Chloride and potassium channels in cystic fibrosis airway epithelia. Nature 1986;322:467.
14. Frizzell FA, Rechkemmer G, Shoemaker RL. Altered regulation of airway epithelial cell chloride channels in cystic fibrosis. Science 1986;233:558.
15. Quinton PM, Bijman J. Higher potentials due to decreased chloride absorption in the sweat glands of patients with cystic fibrosis. N Engl J Med 1983;308:1185.
16. Yankaskas JR, Knowles MR, Gatzy J, et al. Persistency of abnormal chloride ion permeability in cystic fibrosis nasal epithelial cells in heterologous culture. Lancet 1985;1:954.
17. Hyde SC, Emsley PS, Hartshorn MJ, et al. Structural model of ATP-binding proteins associated with cystic fibrosis, multidrug resistance and bacterial transport. Nature 1990;346:362.
18. Valdiva HH, Dubinsky WP, Coronado R. Reconstitution and phosphorylation of chloride channels from airway epithelium membranes. Science 1988;242:1441.
19. Landry DW, Akabas MH, Redhead C, et al. Purification and reconstitution of chloride channels from kidney and trachea. Science 1989;244:1469.
20. Anderson MP, Rich DP, Gregory RJ, et al. Generation of cAMP-activated chloride currents by expression of CFTR. Science 1991;251:679.
21. Kartner N, Hanrahan JW, Jensen TJ, et al. Expression of the cystic fibrosis gene in non-epithelial invertebrate cells produces a regulated anion conductance. Cell 1991;64:681.
22. Berger HA, Anderson MP, Gregory RJ, et al. Identification and regulation of the cystic fibrosis transmembrane conductance regulator-generated chloride channel. J Clin Invest 1991;88:1422.
23. Anderson MP, Gregory RJ, Thompson S, et al. Demonstration that CFTR is a chloride channel by alteration of its anion selectivity. Science 1991;253:202.
24. Bear CE, Li C, Kartner N, et al. Purification and functional reconstitution of the cystic fibrosis transmembrane conductance regulator (CFTR). Cell 1992;68:808.
25. Marino CR, Matovcik LM, Gorelick FS, et al. Localization of the cystic fibrosis transmembrane conductance regulator in pancreas. J Clin Invest 1991;88:712.
26. Cohn JA, Melhus O, Page LJ, et al. CFTR: development of high-affinity antibodies and localization in sweat gland. Biochem Biophys Res Commun 1991;181:36.
27. Marino CR, Gorelick FS. Scientific advances in cystic fibrosis. Gastroenterology 1992;103:681.
28. Denning GM, Ostedgaard LS, Welsh MJ. Abnormal localization of cystic fibrosis transmembrane conductance regulator in primary cultures of cystic fibrosis airway epithelia. J Cell Biol 1992;118:551.
29. Kartner N, Augustinas O, Jensen TJ, et al. Mislocalization of

ΔF508 CFTR in cystic fibrosis sweat gland. Nature Genet 1992;2: 13.

30. Clarke LL, Grubb BR, Gabriel SE, et al. Defective epithelial chloride transport in a gene-targeted mouse model of cystic fibrosis. Science 1992;257:1125.

31. Colledge WH, Ratcliff R, Foster D, et al. Cystic fibrosis mouse with intestinal obstruction. Lancet 1992;340:680.

32. Dorin JR, Dickinson P, Alton EWF, et al. Cystic fibrosis in the mouse by targeted insertional mutagenesis. Nature 1992;359: 211.

33. Anderson DH. Cystic fibrosis of the pancreas and its relation to celiac disease: a clinical and pathological study. Am J Dis Child 1938;56:344.

34. Boyer RH. Low birth weight in fibrocystic disease of the pancreas. Pediatrics 1955;16:778.

35. Oppenheimer E, Esterly J. Cystic fibrosis of the pancreas. Morphologic findings in infants with and without diagnostic pancreatic lesions. Arch Pathol Lab Med 1973;96:149.

36. Holsclaw DS, Shwachman H. Increased incidence of inguinal hernia, hydrocele, and undescended testicle in males with cystic fibrosis. Pediatrics 1971;48:442.

37. Anderson DH. Pathology of cystic fibrosis. Ann N Y Acad Sci 1962;95:500.

38. Oppenheimer EHS, Esterly JR. Pathology of cystic fibrosis: review of the literature and comparison with 146 autopsied cases. Perspect Pediatr Pathol 1975;2:241.

39. Shwachman H. Gastrointestinal manifestation of cystic fibrosis. Pediatr Clin North Am 1975;22:787.

40. Rick W. Pancreatic exocrine functions in cystic fibrosis of the pancreas. Med Welt 1963;113:819.

41. Hadorn B, Zoppi G, Shmerling DH, et al. Quantitative assessment of exocrine pancreas function in infants and children. J Pediatr 1968;73:39.

42. Maclean W, Tripp R. Cystic fibrosis with edema and falsely negative sweat test. J Pediatr 1973;83:86.

43. Kerem E, Corey M, Kerem B, et al. The relation between genotype and phenotype in cystic fibrosis-analysis of the most common mutation (ΔF$_{508}$). N Engl J Med 1990;323:1517.

44. Kristidis P, Bozon D, Corey M, et al. Genetic determination of exocrine pancreatic function in cystic fibrosis. Am J Hum Genet 1992;50:1178.

45. Shwachman H, Lebenthal E, Khaw KT. Recurrent acute pancreatitis in patients with cystic fibrosis with normal pancreatic enzymes. Pediatrics 1975;55:86.

46. Donnison A, Shwachman H, Gross R. A review of 164 children with meconium ileus seen at the Children's Hospital Center, Boston, MA. Pediatrics 1966;37:833.

47. Berschneider HM, Knowles MR, Azizkhan RG, et al. Altered intestinal chloride transport in cystic fibrosis. FASEB J 1988;2: 2625.

48. Crawford I, Maloney PC, Zeitlin PL, et al. Immunocytochemical localization of the cystic fibrosis gene product CFTR. Proc Natl Acad Sci U S A 1991;88:9262.

49. Byrk D. Meconium ileus: demonstration of the meconium mass on barium enema study. AJR Am J Roentgenol 1965;95:214.

50. Shaw A. Safety of N-acetylcysteine in treatment of meconium obstruction of the newborn. J Pediatr Surg 1969;4:119.

51. French R, McAlister W, Ternberg J, et al. Meconium ileus relieved by the 40 percent water-soluble contrast enemas. Radiology 1970;94:341.

52. Noblett H. Treatment of uncomplicated meconium ileus by gastrogafin enema: a preliminary report. J Pediatr Surg 1969;4: 190.

53. MPartin J, Dickson J, Swain V. Maconium ileus, immediate and long term survival. Arch Dis Child 1972;47:207.

54. Matseshe J, Go V, Dimagno E. Meconium ileus equivalent complicating cystic fibrosis in postneonatal children and young adults. Gastroenterology 1977;72:732.

55. Holsclaw DS, Rocmans C, Shwachman H. Intussusception in patients with cystic fibrosis . Pediatrics 1971;48:51.

56. Lillibridge C, Docter J, Eidelman S. Oral administration of n-acetyl cysteine in the prophylaxis of 'meconium ileus equivalent'. J Pediatr 1967;71:887.

57. Kulczycki L, Shwachman H. Studies in cystic fibrosis of the pancreas: occurrence of rectal prolapse. N Engl J Med 1958; 259:409.

58. Shwachman H. Cystic fibrosis. Curr Probl Pediatr 1978;8:1.

59. Swachman H, Kowalski M, Khaw KT. Cystic fibrosis: a new outlook, 70 patients above 25 years of age. Medicine (Baltimore) 1977;56:24.

60. Oppenheimer E, Esterly J. Hepatic changes in young infants with cystic fibrosis: possible relation to focal biliary cirrhosis. J Pediatr 1975;86:683.

61. Stern R, Stevens D, Boat T, et al. Symptomatic hepatic disease in cystic fibrosis. Incidence, course, and outcome of portal systematic shunting. Gastroenterology 1976;70:645.

62. Weber A, Roy C, Morin C, et al. Malabsorption of bile acids in children with cystic fibrosis. N Engl J Med 1973;289:1001.

63. Watkins JB, Tercyak Am, Szczepanik P, et al. Bile salt kinetics in cystic fibrosis: influence of pancreatic enzyme replacement. Gastroenterology 1977;73:1023.

64. Roy CC, Weber AM, Morin CL, et al. Abnormal biliary lipid composition in cystic fibrosis. N Engl J Med 1977;297:1307.

65. L'Heureux P, Isenberg JN, Sharp H, et al. Gallbladder disease in cystic fibrosis. AJR Am J Roentgenol 1977;297:1301.

66. Rosenfeld R, Spiegelblatt L, Chicoine R. False positive sweat test, malnutrition and the Mauriac syndrome. J Pediatr 1979;94: 240.

67. Swachman H, Mahmoodian A, Neff RK. The sweat test: sodium and chloride values. J Pediatr 1981;98:576.

68. Spehl-Robberecht M, Baran D, Dab I, et al. Ultrasonic study of pancreas in cystic fibrosis. Ann Radiol 1981;98:576.

69. Cox KL, Isenberg JN, Ament ME. Gastric acid hypersecretion in cystic fibrosis. J Pediatr Gastroenterol Nutr 1982;1:559.

70. Dimagno EP, Malagelda JM, Go VL, et al. Fate of orally ingested enzymes in pancreatic insufficiency. Comparison of two dosage schedules. N Engl J Med 1977;296:1318.

71. Graham DY. An enteric-coated pancreatic enzyme preparation that works. Dig Dis Sci 1979;24:906.

72. Regan PT, Malagelada JR, Dimagno EP, et al. Comparative effects of antacids, cimetidine and enteric coating on the therapeutic response to oral enzymes in severe pancreatic insufficiency. N Engl J Med 1977;297:854.

73. Gow R, Bradbear R, Francis P, et al. Comparative study of varying regiments to improve steatorrhea and creatorrhea in cystic fibrosis: effectiveness of an entericcoated preparation with and without anatacids and cimetidine. Lancet 1981;2:1071.

74. Nassif EG, Younoszai MK, Weinberger MM, et al. Comparative effects of antacids, enteric coating, and bile salts on the efficacy of oral pancreatic enzyme therapy in cystic fibrosis. J Pediatr 1981;98:320.

75. Graham DY, Sackman JW. Mechanism of increase in steatorrhea with calcium and magnesioum in exocrine pancreatic insufficiency: an animal model. Gastroenterology 1982;83:343.

76. Cox K, Isenberg J, Osher A, et al. The effect of cimetidine in maldigestion in cystic fibrosis. J Pediatr 1979;94:488.

77. Graham DY. Enzyme replacement therapy of exocrine pancreas insufficiency in man: relation between in vitro enzyme activities and in vitro potency in commercial pancreatic extracts . N Engl J Med 1977;296:1314.

78. Allen JD, Milner J, Moss D. Therapeutic use of an artificial diet. Lancet 1970;1:785.

79. Berry HK, Kellogg FW, Hunt MM, et al. Dietary supplement and nutrition in children with cystic fibrosis. Am J Dis Child 1975;129:165.

80. Pencharz PB. Energy intakes and low-fat diets in children with cystic fibrosis. J Pediatr Gastroenterol Nutr 1983;2:400.

81. Kraemer R, Rudeberg A, Hadorn B, et al. Relative underweight in cystic fibrosis and its prognostic value. Acta Paediatr Scand 1978;10:742.

82. Lebenthal E, Lerner A, Heitlinger L. The pancreas in cystic fibrosis. In: Go VLW, ed. The exocrine pancreas: biology, pathobiology, and diseases. New York: Raven Press, 1986;783.

83. Rich DP, Anderson MP, Gregory RJ, et al. Expression of cystic fibrosis transmembrane conductance regulator corrects defective chloride channel regulation in cystic fibrosis airway epithelial cells. Nature 1990;347:358.

84. Rosenfeld MA, Yoshimura K, Trapnell BC, et al. In vivo transfer

of the human cystic fibrosis transmembrane conductance regulator gene to the airway epithelium. Cell 1992;68:143.

85. Yang Y, Raper SE, Cohn JA, et al. An approach for treating the hepatobiliary disease of cystic fibrosis by somatic gene transfer. Proc Natl Acad Sci U S A 1993;90:4601.

86. Engelhardt JF, Yang Y, Stratford-Perricaudet LD, et al. Direct gene transfer of human CFTR into human bronchial epithelia of xenografts with E1 deleted adenoviruses. Nature Genet 1993;4:27.

87. Comfort MW, Steinberg AG. Pedigree of a family with hereditary chronic relapsing pancreatitis. Gastroenterology 1952;21:54.

88. Gross JB, Jones JD. Hereditary pancreatitis: analysis of experience to May 1969. In: Beck IT, Sinclair DG, eds. The exocrine pancreas. London: J & A Churchill, 1971;247.

89. Copenhagen pancreatitis study group. Copenhagen pancreatitis study: an interim report from a prospective epidemiological multicentre study. Scand J Gastroenterol 1981;16:305.

90. Kattwinkel J, Lapey A, di Sant'Agnese PA, et al. Hereditary pancreatitis: three new kindreds and critical review of the literature. Pediatrics 1973;51:55.

91. Sibert J. A British family with hereditary pancreatitis. Gut 1975;16:81.

92. Sibert JR. Hereditary pancreatitis in England and Wales. J Med Genet 1978;15:189.

93. Multigner L, Sarles H, Lombardo D, et al. Pancreatic stone protein. II. Implication in stone formation during the course of chronic calcific pancreatitis. Gastroenterology 1985;89:387.

94. Giorgi D, Bernard JP, De Caro A, et al. Pancreatic stone protein. I. Evidence that it is encoded by a pancreatic mesenger ribonucleic acid. Gastroenterology 1985;89:381.

95. Gross JB. Hereditary pancreatitis. In: Go VLW, ed. The exocrine pancreas: biology, pathobiology, and diseases. New York: Raven Press, 1986;829.

96. Perrault J, Gross JB, King JE. Endoscopic retrograde cholangioscopy in familial pancreatitis. Gastroenterology 1976;71:138.

97. Slaff J, Jacobson D, Tillman CR, et al. Protease-specific suppression of pancreatic exocrine secretion. Gastroenterology 1984;87:44.

98. Foster GS, Galdabini JJ. Recurrent abnormal pain and pancreatic calcification with recent jaundice. N Engl J Med 1984;87:44.

99. Girard RM, Dube S, Archambault AP. Hereditary pancreatitis: report of an affected Canadian kindred and review of the disease. Can Med Assoc J 1981;125:526.

100. Novis BH, Bank S, Young GO, et al. Chronic pancreatitis and alpha-1-antitrypsin. Lancet 1975;2:748.

101. Mihas AA, Hirschowitz BI. Alpha-1-antitrypsin and chronic pancreatitis. Lancet 1976;2:1032.

102. Brantly M, Nukiwa T, Crystal RG. Molecular basis of alpha-1-antitrypsin deficiency. Am J Med 1988;84:13.

103. Lieberman H, Gaidulis L, Garoutte B, et al. Identification and characteristics of the common alpha-1-antitrypsin phenotypes. Chest 1972;62:557.

104. Sveger T. Liver disease in alpha-1-antitrypsin deficiency detected by screening of 200,000 infants. N Engl J Med 1976;294:1316.

105. Lieberman J, Gaidulis L, Roberts L. Racial distribution of alpha-1-antitrypsin variants among junior high school students. Am Rev Respir Dis 1976;114:1194.

106. Sharp HL, Bridges RA, Krivit W, et al. Cirrhosis associated with alpha-1-antitrypsin deficiency: a previously unrecognised inherited disorder. J Lab Clin Med 1969;73:934.

107. Eriksson S. Liver disease in alpha-1-antitrypsin deficiency. Gastroenterology 1985;20:907.

108. Sveger T. Prospective study of children with alpha-1-antitrypsin deficiency: eight-year follow-up. J Pediatr 1984;104:91.

109. Nukiwa T, Brantly M, Garver R, et al. Evaluation of "at risk" alpha-1-antitrypsin genotype SZ with synthetic oligonucleotide gene probes. J Clin Invest 1986;77:528.

110. Berg NO, Erikkson S. Liver disease in adults with alpha-1-antitrypsin deficiency. N Engl J Med 1972;287:1264.

111. Cox DW, Smyth S. Risk for liver disease in adults with alpha-1-antitrypsin deficiency. Am J Med 1983;74:221.

112. Erikkson S, Carlson J, Velez R. Risk for cirrhosis and primary liver cancer in alpha-1-antitrypsin deficiency. N Engl J Med 1986;314:736.

113. Mero M, Sandholm M. Alpha-1-antitrypsin and total trypsin-inhibitor capacity in acute pancreatitis. Ann Chir Gynaecol 1979;68:39.

114. Shwachman H, Diamond LK, Oski FA, et al. The syndrome of pancreatic insufficiency and bone marrow dysfunction. Pediatrics 1964;65:645.

115. Shmerling DA, Prader A, Hitzig WH, et al. The syndrome of exocrine pancreatic insufficiency, neutropenia, metaphyseal dysostosis and dwarfism. Helv Paediatr Acta 1969;24:547.

116. Silverman A, Roy CC. Exocrine pancreatic insufficiency. In: Silverman A, Roy CC, eds. Pediatric clinical gastroenterology. St. Louis: CV Mosby, 1983;837.

117. Bodian M, Sheldon W, Lightwood R. Congenital hypoplasia of the exocrine pancreas. Acta Paediatr 1964;53:282.

118. Kurdziel JC, Dondelinger R. Fatty infiltration of the pancreas in Shwachman's syndrome: computed tomography demonstration. Eur J Radiol 1984;4:202.

119. Aggett PT, Cavanagh Npc, Matthew DJ, et al. Shwachman's syndrome. a review of 21 cases. Arch Dis Child 1980;55:331.

120. Burke V, Colebatch JH, Anderson CM, et al. Association of pancreatic insufficiency in chronic neutropenia in childhood. Arch Dis Child 1967;42:147.

121. Stanley P, Stucliff J. Metaphyseal chondrodysplasia with dwarfism, pancreatic insufficiency, and neutropenias. Pediatr Radiol 1973;1:119.

122. Aggett PJ, Harries JT, Harvey BAM, et al. An inherited defect in neutrophil mobility in Shwachman syndrome. J Pediatr 1979;94:391.

123. Hill RE, Durie PR, Gaskin KJ, et al. Steatorrhea and pancreatic insufficiency in Shwachman syndrome. Gastroenterology 1982;83:22.

124. Johanson A, Blizzard R. A syndrome of congenital aplasia of the alae nasi, deafness, hypothyroidism, dwarfism, absent permanent teeth, and malabsorption. J Pediatr 1971;79:982.

125. Moeschler JB, Lubinsky ML. Johanson-Blizzard syndrome with normal intelligence. Am J Med Genet 1985;22:69.

126. Moeschler JB, Polak MJ, Jenkins JJ3d, et al. The Johanson-Blizzard syndromes: a second report of full autopsy findings. Am J Med Genet 1987;26:133.

127. Daentl DL, Frias JL, Gilbert EF, et al. The Johanson-Blizzard Syndrome: case report and autopsy findings. Am J Med Genet 1979;3:129.

128. Schusseim A, Choi SJ, Silverberg M. Exocrine pancreatic insufficiency with congenital anomalies. J Pediatr 1976;89:782.

129. Pearson HA, Lobel JS, Kocoshis SA, et al. A new syndrome of refractory sideoblastic anemia with vacuolization of marrow precursors and exocrine pancreatic dysfunction. J Pediatr 1979;95:976.

130. Sheldon W. Congenital pancreatic lipase deficiency. Arch Dis Child 1964;39:268.

131. Muller DP, McCollum JP, Trompeter RS, et al. Proceedings: studies on the mechanism of fat absorption in congenital isolated lipase pancreatique. Gut 1975;16:838.

132. Figarella C, De Caro A, Leupold D, et al. Congenital pancreatic lipase deficiency. J Pediatr 1980;96:412.

133. Rey J, Frezal J, Royer P, et al. Absence congenitale de lipase pancreatique. Arch Fr Pediatr 1966;23:5.

134. Lerner A, Heitlinger LA, Lebenthal E. Hereditary abnormalities of pancreatic function. In: Go VLW, ed. The exocrine pancreas: biology, pathobiology, and diseases. New York: Raven Press, 1986;819.

135. Figarella C, Negri GA, Sarles H. Presence of colipase in congenital pancreatic lipase deficiency. Biochim Biophys Acta 1972;280:205.

136. Hildebrand H, Borgstrom B, Bekassy A, et al. Isolated colipase deficiency in two brothers. Gut 1982;23:243.

137. Ghishan FK, Moran JR, Durie PR, et al. Isolated congenital lipase-colipase deficiency. Gastroenterology 1984;86:1580.

138. Lowe C, May DC. Selective pancreatic deficiency: absent amylase, diminished trypsin, and normal lipase. Am J Dis Child 1951;82:459.

139. Hadorn B. The exocrine pancreas. In: Anderson CM, Burke V,

eds. Pediatric gastroenterology. Oxford: Blackwell Scientific Publications, 1975;289.

140. Lillibridge CB, Townes PL. Physiological deficiency of pancreatic amylase in infancy: a factor in iatrogenic diarrhea. J Pediatr 1973;82:279.

141. Townes PL. Trypsinogen deficiency disease. J Pediatr 1965;66:275.

142. Townes PL, Bryson MF, Miller G. Further observations on trypsinogen deficiency disease. Report of a second case. J Pediatr 1967;71:220.

143. Morris MD, Fisher DA. Trypsinogen deficiency disease. Am J Dis Child 1967;114:203.

144. Hadorn D, Tarlow MJ, Lloyd JK, et al. Intestinal enterokinase deficiency. Lancet 1969;1:812.

145. Tarlow MJ, Hadorn B, Arthurton MW, et al. Intestinal enterokinase deficiency. A newly recognized disorder of protein digestion. Arch Dis Child 1970;45:651.

146. Polonovski C, Laplane R, Alison F, et al. Pseudo-deficit en tryspsinogene par deficit congenital en enterokinase. Etude clinique. Arch Fr Pediatr 1970;27:677.

147. Lebenthal E, Antonowicz I, Shwachman H. Enterokinase and trypsin activities in pancreatic insufficiency and diseases of the small intestine. Gastroenterology 1976;70:508.

148. Ghishan FK, Lee PC, Lebenthal E, et al. Isolated congenital enterokinase deficiency. Recent findings and review of the literature. Gastroenterology 1983;85:727.

149. Haworth JC, Gourly B, Hadorn B, et al. Malabsoption and growth failure due to intestinal enterokinase deficiency. J Pediatr 1971;78:481.

150. Haworth JC, Hadorn B, Gourly B, et al. Intestinal enterokinase deficiency. Occurence in two sibs and age dependency of clinical expression. Arch Dis Child 1975;50:277.

Textbook of Gastroenterology, second edition, edited by Tadataka Yamada. JB Lippincott Company, Philadelphia © 1995.

F. Gallbladder and Biliary Tree

CHAPTER 95

Gallbladder and Biliary Tree: Anatomy and Structural Anomalies

Carlos A. Pellegrini   Quan-Yang Duh

Anatomy
  Gallbladder
  Hepatic Hilum
  Cystic Duct
  Hepatoduodenal Ligament
  Common Bile Duct

Embryology
Congenital Variations and Malformations
  Gallbladder and Cystic Duct
  Common Bile Duct and Hepatic Ducts
  Biliary Atresia, Hypoplasia, and Stenosis
  Choledochal Cyst

In the past, thorough knowledge of biliary tract anatomy was essential only to the surgeon. Detailed descriptions of the biliary ducts and their relation to the arteries and veins at the porta hepatis were found only in surgical textbooks. With advancing knowledge of the pathophysiology of biliary tract disease and with the advent and popularization of diagnostic radiology, therapeutic endoscopy, and interventional radiology, an understanding of biliary tract anatomy became essential to gastroenterologists, radiologists, and others involved in the diagnosis and treatment of biliary tract disease. Because structural anomalies are frequent, it is also important to know the common anatomic variations. These anomalies are generally related to variations that occur during the early stages of gestation and can be better interpreted with some background on the embryology of the biliary tract.

This chapter discusses the anatomy of the biliary tract from a clinician's point of view. Emphasis is placed on anatomic aspects that have clinical relevance. Embryology and devel-

opment are briefly outlined to understand common congenital malformations and the commonly found anatomic variants that are relevant to the interpretation of diagnostic procedures and to the performance of interventions on the biliary tract.

ANATOMY

Gallbladder

The gallbladder usually lies in a depression on the inferior surface of the liver at the boundary between the right and left lobes, an area known as the gallbladder bed (Fig. 95-1). This interface between the gallbladder and the liver usually contains some loose connective tissue that is traversed by small lymphatics, veins, and sometimes small accessory bile ducts. These structures have important clinical implications. For example, the lymphatic connection allows easy spread of gallbladder

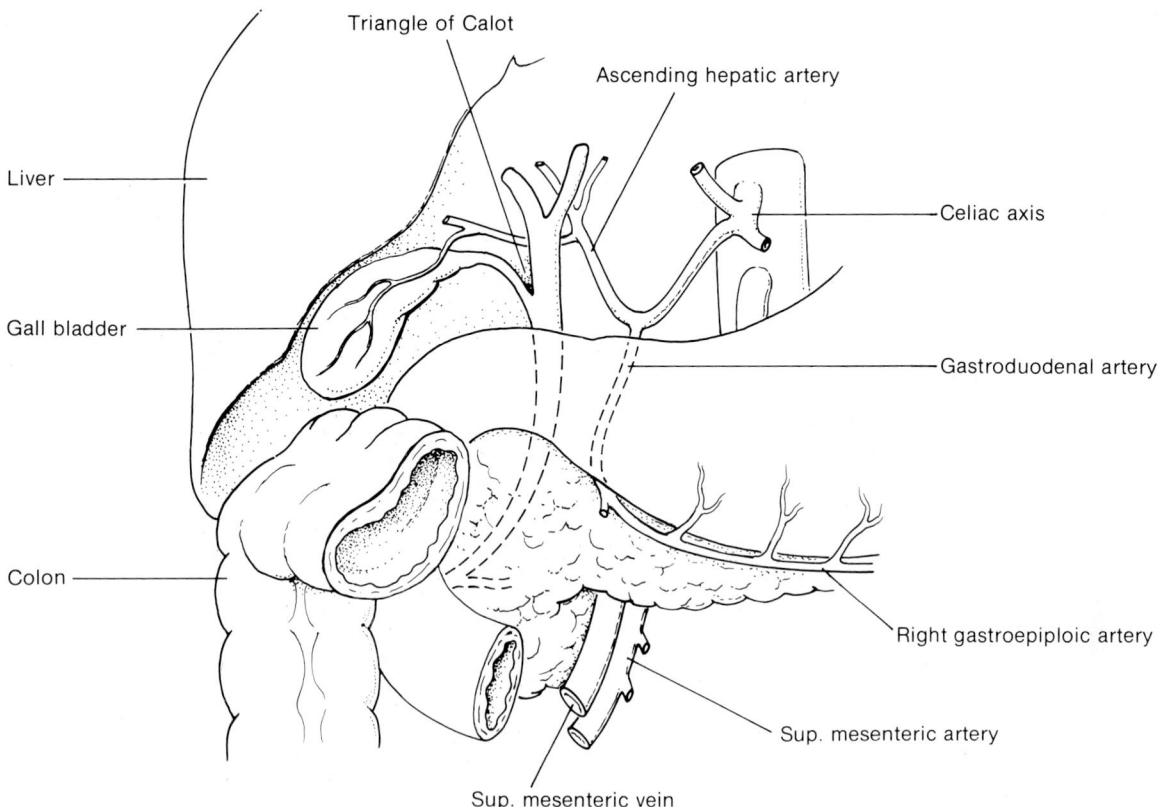

FIGURE 95-1. Relation of the gallbladder and the extrahepatic biliary tract to the liver, duodenum, colon, and pancreas.

infection or cancer into the adjacent liver parenchyma—hence the need to remove the liver portion of the gallbladder bed in patients with carcinoma of the gallbladder. The presence of bile ducts explains the occasional biliary leak after cholecystectomy if these channels have not been adequately ligated.

The area of gallbladder not attached to the liver is covered by the peritoneum and is in intimate contact with the duodenum, head of the pancreas, and hepatic flexure of the colon (see Fig. 95-1). Sometimes, the peritoneum completely covers the gallbladder, which is suspended from the liver by a mesentery, creating a "floating gallbladder." The pear-shaped gallbladder has four anatomic areas: the fundus, the body, the infundibulum, and the neck.[1]

Fundus

The fundus of the gallbladder is a rounded, blind end that usually protrudes 0.5 to 1 cm beyond the free edge of the liver. It is projected into the anterior abdominal wall at the junction of the right lateral border of the rectus abdominis muscle and the ninth costal cartilage, where it contacts the anterior peritoneum. The position of the fundus varies with respect to the abdominal wall in relation to the size of the liver and gallbladder. When the gallbladder is inflamed, as in patients with acute cholecystitis, the fundus becomes palpable and tender. Because of its contact with the anterior peritoneum, the pain is referred to the entire dermatome, and rebound, which is a sign of peritoneal inflammation, may be

elicited. However, obstruction of the biliary tract distal to the cystic duct causes dilation of the gallbladder without inflammation. The gallbladder is palpable but not tender. This is usually seen in patients with neoplastic obstruction; in most patients with obstruction due to choledocholithiasis, the scarred gallbladder wall precludes dilation of the organ. A palpable, nontender gallbladder fundus in a patient with jaundice, known as Courvoisier's sign, should raise the suspicion of tumor.[2]

Phrygian cap deformity of the gallbladder is a congenitally kinked fundus that has no pathologic significance.

Body

The body is the largest part of the gallbladder. One side of the body is usually attached to the liver at the gallbladder bed. The other side of the body, its free surface, is covered by peritoneum. This area is in direct contact with the first portion of the duodenum and the hepatic flexure of the colon (see Fig. 95-1). Inflammation from gallstones can cause a fistula between the gallbladder and the duodenum or between the gallbladder and the colon. Fistulas are usually seen in patients with acute cholecystitis in whom a large stone produces inflammation and eventually necrosis of the gallbladder wall. Because inflammation brings adjacent organs together, the stone may erode into the duodenum or colon. The resulting cholecystoduodenal or cholecystoenteric fistula "cures" the acute cholecystitis. In these patients, air in the gallbladder is revealed on abdominal films. These large stones then migrate through the intestine, where, because of their size, they may become impacted, causing "gallstone ileus."

Infundibulum

The infundibulum is the transitional area between the body and neck of the gallbladder. It is attached to the duodenum by the cholecystoduodenal ligament, which is an avascular peritoneal fold derived from the inferior margin of the right free border of the hepatoduodenal ligament. Hartmann's pouch is a shallow diverticulum on the inferior surface of the infundibulum near the undersurface of the cystic duct. Gallstones can impact and become trapped in Hartmann's pouch, causing obstruction of the cystic duct and acute cholecystitis. The inflammatory process in Hartmann's pouch sometimes produces obstruction of the common bile duct, a condition called the Mirizzi syndrome.[3] Inflammatory adhesions of the infundibulum to the cystic or common bile duct make cholecystectomy difficult and increase the risk of injury of the common bile duct.

Neck

The neck of the gallbladder is a short, 5- to 7-mm transitional area between the infundibulum and the cystic duct. The S-shaped neck is located in the deepest part of the cystic fossa. When performing an open cholecystectomy, most surgeons begin at the fundus and dissect toward the neck of the gallbladder to avoid injuring the structure within the triangle of Calot. When performing a laparoscopic cholecystectomy, surgeons begin the dissection at the neck of the gallbladder and the cystic duct and work toward the fundus; traction on the fundus is required to retract the liver during the laparoscopic operation.

Arterial Supply

The arterial supply of the gallbladder usually is from a single cystic artery originating from the proximal right hepatic artery.[4] The cystic artery generally runs posterior to the common bile duct, superior to the cystic duct, and then divides into two branches close to the neck of the gallbladder. One branch runs along the peritoneal surface, and the other runs between the gallbladder and the liver (see Fig. 95-1).

Variations of the origin and course of the cystic artery are common. It may arise from the left hepatic artery, the common hepatic artery, an aberrant right hepatic artery off the superior mesentery artery, or directly from one of the branches of the celiac artery or the superior mesentery artery. Two cystic arteries are found in 12% of cases. The cystic artery may be short or long and can be confused with the right hepatic artery during operations. It can run anterior or posterior to the common bile duct. Because of the unpredictable origin and course of this artery, it is ill advised to ligate it as the first step in a cholecystectomy. The gallbladder neck and the cystic duct should all be well dissected, and the cystic artery or its branches should be identified as they enter the gallbladder before they are ligated to avoid injury to the right hepatic artery.

The cystic artery is an end artery; it does not anastomose with other vessels that can provide alternative flow in case the origin of the artery is occluded. This makes the gallbladder more vulnerable to ischemia. It may explain gallbladder necrosis during acalculous cholecystitis and after hepatic artery ligation, chemoembolization, or chemoinfusion used in the treatment of liver tumors.

Veins and Lymphatics

There is no major cystic vein. The venous drainage of the gallbladder is by way of multiple small veins from the superior surface of the gallbladder directly into the liver or toward the cystic duct, where they join the venous radicals from the common bile duct and eventually the portal system. This venous net is barely developed in normal subjects. However, in patients with portal hypertension, these channels enlarge substantially. Removal of the gallbladder from its liver bed can cause fatal hemorrhage in these patients. Similarly, in patients with acutely inflamed gallbladders, engorgement of these veins can cause troublesome bleeding.

The lymphatic drainage of the gallbladder, which parallels that of the venous drainage, is by way of multiple small lymphatics from the superior surface of the gallbladder directly into the liver or toward the cystic duct and into the lymph nodes overlying the cystic duct.

Nerves

The gallbladder is innervated by sympathetic and parasympathetic nervous systems. Sympathetic innervation travels by way of the celiac plexus, hepatic plexus, and eventually with the hepatic artery and the portal vein to the gallbladder. Visceral pain caused by stretching or inflammation of the gallbladder and the extrahepatic biliary duct is conducted through the sympathetic fibers.

This pain is frequently referred to the epigastric or right subcostal areas and sometimes to the right scapular region. The parasympathetic nerves are branches of both vagi. The anterior vagus branches leave the main trunk proximal to the gastroesophageal junction and reach the portal arch by way of the gastrohepatic ligament (Fig. 95-2). Although gallbladder contraction is primarily mediated by cholecystokinin and secretin, gallbladder innervation, especially parasympathetic innervation, is thought to play a role in gallbladder motility as well.[5]

Histology

The gallbladder has four layers: mucosa, muscularis, a perimuscularis connective tissue layer, and the serosa. The mucosa has many folds that increase the contact surface between the cell and bile, which facilitates water absorption by the gallbladder mucosa. The basal surface of the gallbladder epithelium is in contact with a lamina propria that consists of loose connective tissue, elastic fibers, blood vessels, and lymphocytes. The muscularis is relatively well developed and receives its blood supply from a vascular net intimately attached to its outer margin. Outside this vascular net and immediately below the serosal layer, there is an almost avascular connective tissue layer that provides the plane of dissection during cholecystectomy. Near the neck of the gallbladder, the epithelium enters the lamina propria, forming glands with wide lumens. These glands secrete mucus.

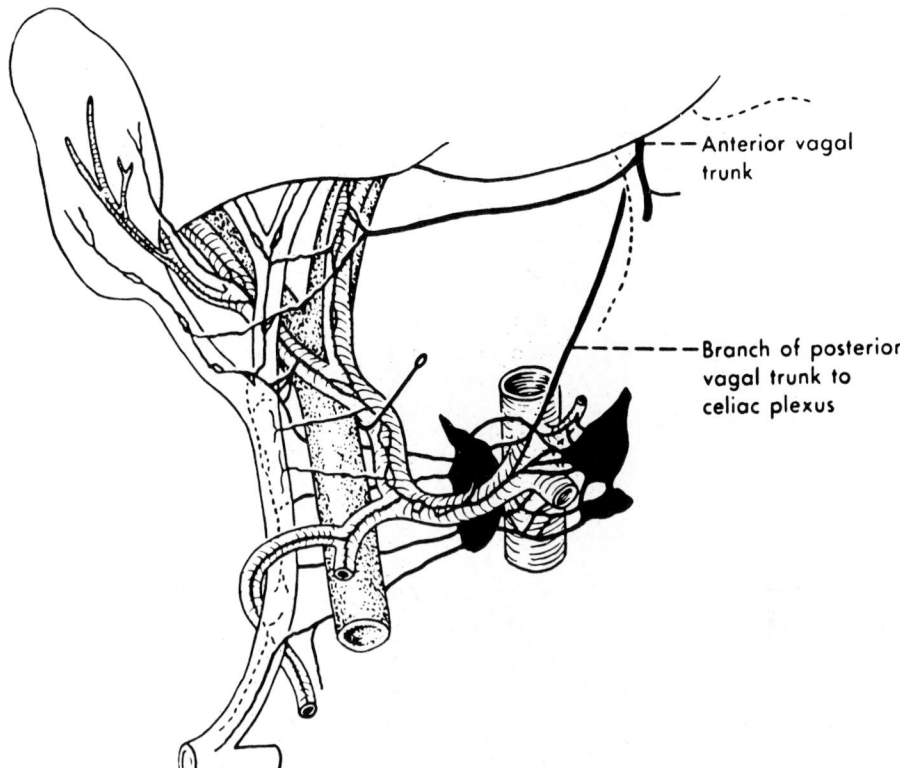

— Anterior vagal trunk

— Branch of posterior vagal trunk to celiac plexus

FIGURE 95-2. Schematic representation of the innervation of the gallbladder and extrahepatic biliary tract. The nerves originate from both vagi and from the celiac axis. They reach the biliary tract, traveling along the walls of the hepatic artery, except for the direct vagal branches of the anterior vagus, which cross through the gastrohepatic ligament.

At the electron microscopic level, the structure of the gallbladder epithelium is well suited to its physiologic function of bile concentration (Fig. 95-3). The apical surface of the gallbladder cell contains numerous microvilli. Numerous mitochondria are present, as in any tissue involved in active ion transport. The nuclei are located in the basal third of the columnar cell. The Golgi complex is well developed and found mostly between the nucleus and the apical membrane. Immediately below the lumenal surface of the epithelium, adjoining cells are tightly bound together by junctional complexes and associated tonofilaments (see Fig. 95-3). These complexes, called tight junctions, separate the paracellular space from the gallbladder lumen. During active bile concentration, the basolateral intercellular spaces are dilated by electrolytes and water. In the resting stage, the lateral cellular spaces are collapsed, and the microvilli are markedly interdigitated.[6]

Hepatic Hilum

The anatomy of the intrahepatic bile ducts follows the anatomy of the liver. Bile is secreted by the hepatocytes into the biliary canaliculi. The canaliculi drain into the true biliary ductules. The biliary ductules unite to form the segmental bile ducts.

The segmental bile ducts coalesce to form the right and left hepatic ducts. In 95% of cases, the left and right hepatic ducts join outside the liver, just below the porta hepatis, to form the common hepatic duct (Fig. 95-4). In 5% of cases they join inside the liver. The lengths of the right and left hepatic ducts vary from 0.5 to 2.5 cm. The left hepatic duct

is usually longer than the right, runs parallel to the undersurface of the liver, and because it is more superficial, is easier to dissect. It may be used to decompress the biliary tract in cases of neoplastic obstruction at the hilum. The right hepatic duct may sometimes not exist. This is important when trying to interpret x-ray films, define pathology in this area, or plan an operation. Occasionally, the right and left hepatic ducts do not join until the cystic duct has joined the right hepatic duct; in that case, there is no common hepatic duct.

The hepatic duct of the right anterior segment deserves special attention. In 20% of cases, the right anterior and right posterior hepatic ducts do not join to form the right hepatic duct. Instead, the right posterior hepatic duct joins the left hepatic duct proximally, and the right anterior hepatic duct joins it distally. This anatomic arrangement may be interpreted at first glance as if the right posterior duct is the right hepatic duct. This may lead to misinterpretations of transhepatic or endoscopic cholangiograms and may be a cause of serious injury during cholecystectomy because the right anterior (lower) duct is taken to be the cystic duct or an accessory duct and divided during cholecystectomy.

On the left side, the left medial and lateral segmental ducts join to form the left hepatic duct. In 20% of patients, two or three segmental ducts may drain the medial or lateral segment of the liver. The length of the common hepatic duct varies from 2 to 6.5 cm. It joins the cystic duct to form the common bile duct.

Strong fibrous tissue in the porta hepatis binds the hepatic ducts to the adjacent hepatic arteries and portal vein. Because of this fibrous sheath, the relation of the upper biliary ductal system to the porta hepatis remains constant despite inflammation or scarring. This constant anatomic association helps

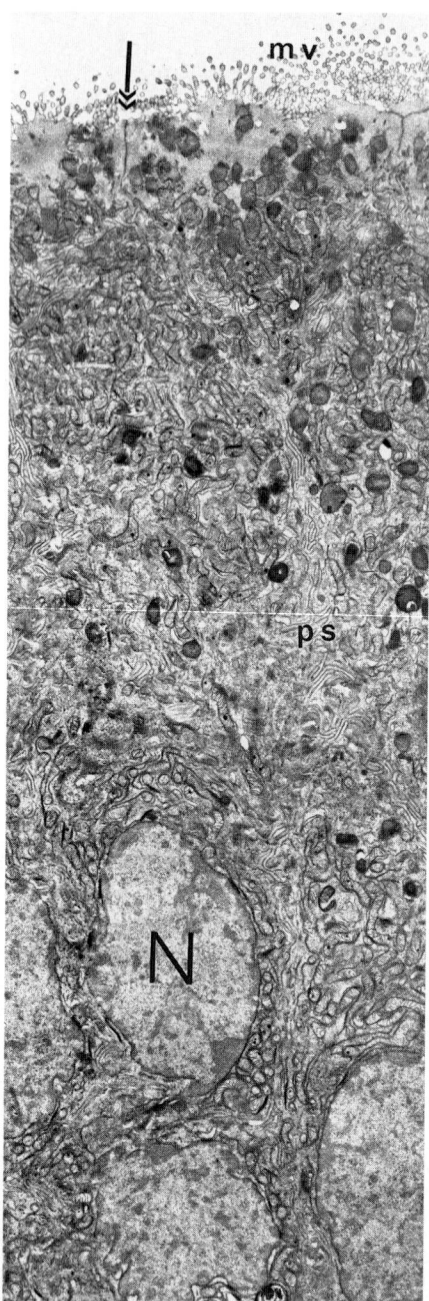

FIGURE 95-3. Electron microscopic view of a gallbladder cell. This columnar cell has the nucleus (N) in the lower third. The cytoplasm, rich in mitochondria, separates the nucleus from its apical membrane. Notice the abundant microvilli (mv) of the apical membrane and the tight junctions (*arrow*) that seal off the paracellular space. The lateral membranes of two adjacent cells interdigitate to form the paracellular space (ps), which is thought to play an important role in the process of fluid absorption. (Courtesy of A. Jones, M.D.)

the surgeon to identify the upper biliary tree, especially during reoperations.

The course of the right hepatic artery varies in relation to the right hepatic duct and the common bile duct. Usually, the right hepatic artery crosses from left to right posterior to the right hepatic duct and just superior to the junction of the

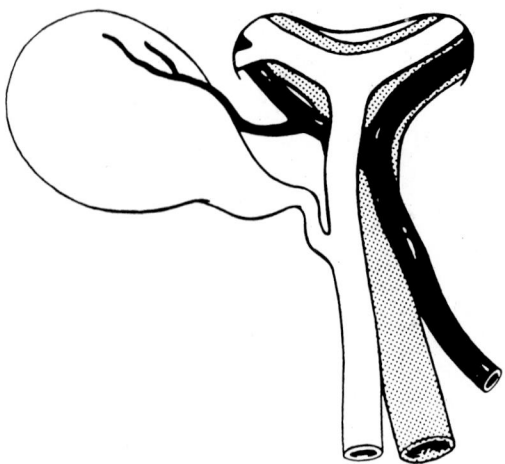

FIGURE 95-4. Schematic representation of the hilum of the liver. The right anterior and posterior hepatic ducts join to form the right hepatic duct. This duct and the left duct join outside the liver capsule to form the common hepatic duct. The left duct is usually longer and more superficial than the right. The triangle of Calot, with the right hepatic artery and the cystic artery, are also clearly displayed. (From Lindner H. Embryology and anatomy of the biliary tree. In: Way LW, Pellegrini CA, eds. Surgery of the gallbladder and bile ducts. Philadelphia: WB Saunders, 1987.)

left and right hepatic ducts (see Fig. 95-4). Occasionally, it passes anterior to the right hepatic duct or the common bile duct. The common hepatic duct is crossed anteriorly by the right hepatic artery or the cystic artery in 30% of patients. Because of this variable anatomy and its proximity to the cystic artery, the right hepatic artery can be confused with the cystic artery and may be injured during surgery.

The portal vein is the most constant element of the porta hepatis. It originates at the junction of the splenic vein and the superior mesenteric vein, behind the head of the pancreas. It runs as the most posterior element of the triad until it reaches the liver, dividing into the right and left branches (Fig. 95-5 and see Fig. 95-4).

The triangle of Calot (see Fig. 95-1) is an imaginary triangle bounded on the left by the common bile duct, on the right by the cystic duct, and superiorly by the hilum of the liver. Many important structures run through this triangle: the cystic artery, right hepatic artery, 95% of the accessory right hepatic artery, and 90% of accessory bile ducts. Understanding of these relations is important, because these structures can easily be injured during cholecystectomy.

Successful laparoscopic cholecystectomy depends on careful dissection of the triangle of Calot and identifying these structures before ligation. Caudad traction on the gallbladder neck tends to open up the angle between the cystic duct and the common duct and facilitate the dissection of the triangle of Calot.

Cystic Duct

The cystic duct connects the neck of the gallbladder to the common hepatic duct. It is 0.1 to 0.4 cm in diameter and 0.5 to 8 cm long. The course of the cystic duct and its entrance into the common hepatic duct vary. The cystic duct in about 70% of patients enters the common hepatic duct directly, but

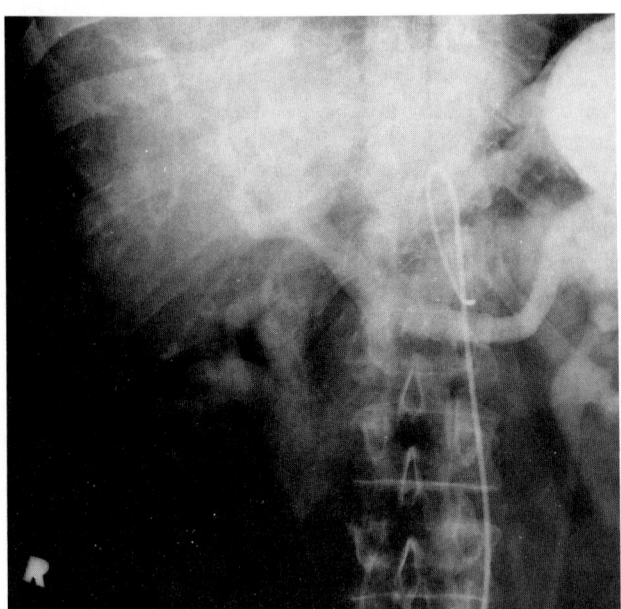

FIGURE 95-5. Venous phase of a splenic angiogram demonstrates the splenic vein, part of the superior mesenteric vein, and the main portal vein and its branches.

sometimes, it runs parallel to or spirals around the common hepatic duct before entering it. The cystic duct usually enters the right side of the common hepatic duct, but it can course dorsally and enter the posterior or left side of the common hepatic duct. A long cystic duct may run parallel to the common hepatic duct for as long as 6 cm, closely adherent to the common hepatic duct, and enter it after passing behind the first portion of the duodenum. This explains why the gallbladder may not be dilated in patients with tumors of the pancreas, because a low insertion of the cystic duct avoids early invasion. Although ideally the entire cystic duct should be removed during cholecystectomy, a long cystic duct running parallel to the common bile duct or one that inserts low is best left undisturbed. This prevents common duct injury. Occasionally, the cystic duct enters the right hepatic duct, and there is no common hepatic duct.

Spiral valves of Heister are crescent-shaped folds of the cystic duct mucosa that project into the lumen, spanning the entire length of the cystic duct. These valves prevent excessive distention or collapse of the gallbladder. They may block the passage of gallstones into the common bile duct.

The cystic artery is usually a branch of the right hepatic artery. The right hepatic artery runs superior and to the left of the cystic duct in the triangle of Calot (see Figs. 95-1 and 95-4). The cystic artery originates from the right hepatic artery, close to the cystic duct. The cystic artery usually is superior or posterior to the cystic duct. In about 5% of patients, the cystic artery is inferior to the cystic duct, outside of the triangle of Calot.

Hepatoduodenal Ligament

The common bile duct, with the hepatic artery and the portal vein, run closely associated in the hepatoduodenal ligament (see Fig. 95-4). The hepatoduodenal ligament, also called the hepatic pedicle, is the anterior border of the foramen of Winslow (i.e., epiploic foramen) and is the right free border of the hepatogastric ligament. Posterior to the hepatogastric ligament is the lesser sac. The foramen of Winslow connects the greater and the lesser peritoneal cavities. The anterior border is the hepatoduodenal ligament, containing the common bile duct, common hepatic artery, portal vein, and their branches. The posterior border is the posterior peritoneum covering the inferior vena cava. The superior border is the inferior layer of the coronary ligament of the liver. The inferior border is the proximal portion of the first segment of the duodenum.

This anatomic setting allows easy control and compression of all the elements of the hepatic pedicle. If this is needed, the left thumb is placed anterior to the hepatoduodenal ligament; the index and the long fingers are put through the foramen of Winslow and are placed posteriorly into the lesser sac. This Pringle's maneuver rapidly occludes the blood supply to the liver and is useful for controlling major liver hemorrhage.

In the hepatoduodenal ligament, the hepatic artery runs to the left of the common bile duct anterior to the portal vein. The hepatic artery originates from the celiac axis in the retroperitoneum and descends in the inferior border of the foramen of Winslow toward the duodenum (Fig. 95-6). When reaching the top of the duodenal bulb, it gives origin to the gastroduodenal artery and then curves upward, running along the left side of the common bile duct, anterior to the portal vein, to reach the porta hepatis and divides itself into the right and left hepatic arteries. Occasionally, this bifurcation is low, in which case the right hepatic artery may be confused with the cystic artery.

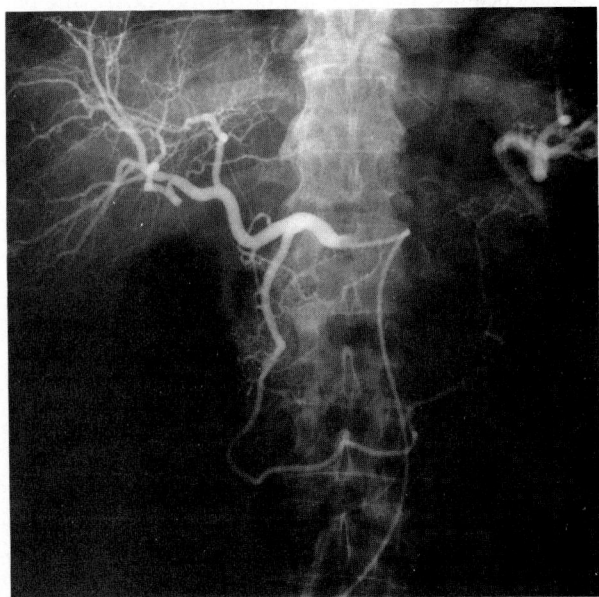

FIGURE 95-6. Normal hepatic angiogram. The common hepatic artery gives off the gastroduodenal artery, which courses downward and then gives off the right gastroepiploic artery. The common hepatic artery goes up toward the hilum and gives off the right and left hepatic arteries. The anastomosis between the right and left gastroepiploics along the greater curvature of the stomach provides retrograde filing of the splenic artery.

Although each lobe of the liver has its own artery, there are innumerable communications between them. Soon after occlusion of one of the arteries, these communications open and the alternate artery supplies the ischemic lobe. The common hepatic artery ascends inside the hepatoduodenal ligament and gives rise to the right gastric artery. In about 15% of patients, the common hepatic artery or the right hepatic artery arises from the superior mesentery artery instead of the celiac axis. The course of the left hepatic artery is more constant; it runs to the left of the bile duct in 95% of patients (see Fig. 95-4). The left hepatic artery may originate from the left gastric or splenic artery.

The splenic vein and the superior mesentery vein join behind the neck of the pancreas to form the portal vein. The inferior mesentery vein enters the splenic vein or the superior mesenteric vein or the junction of the two. The portal vein then runs posterior to the common bile duct and the common hepatic artery in the hepatoduodenal ligament (see Fig. 94-4). As it ascends in the hepatoduodenal ligament, the portal vein receives tributaries from the coronary vein, the superior pancreaticoduodenal vein, and the pyloric vein.

Common Bile Duct

The common bile duct is 5 to 17 cm long, depending on where the right and left hepatic ducts join. Its diameter varies from 0.3 to 1.5 cm but is normally about 0.9 to 1.1 cm, although it can become markedly distended by biliary obstruction.

The common bile duct contains scanty smooth muscle arranged in a circular fashion. It has a fibroareolar coat. The lumen is lined by columnar epithelium that is continuous with that of the gallbladder and the other extrahepatic bile ducts.

The common bile duct is divided into four segments: supraduodenal, retroduodenal, pancreatic, and intraduodenal.[6-8]

Supraduodenal Segment

The supraduodenal segment of the common bile duct is about 2.5 cm long. It lies in the hepatoduodenal ligament, to the right of the ascending common hepatic artery and anterior to the portal vein. Stones in this segment of the common bile duct can be palpated between the left index finger in the epiploic foramen and the thumb anteriorly. During common bile duct exploration, choledochostomy and T-tube placement should be done in the lower-most portion of this segment of the common bile duct. This prevents injury to higher structures, and if a stricture results, it is easier to repair.

Retroduodenal Segment

The retroduodenal segment of the common bile duct is posterior to the first portion of the duodenum and is about 2.5 to 4.5 cm long. Because of the close association between this segment of common bile duct and the first portion of the duodenum, the common bile duct can be involved in inflammation caused by a posterior duodenal ulcer or it can be injured during antrectomy.

A Kocher maneuver is necessary for the operative exposure of the retroduodenal segment of the common bile duct. This is done by incising the peritoneum lateral to the duodenal sweep, dissecting in the avascular plane, and then rolling the descending portion of the duodenum and the head of the pancreas medially and to the left.

Many arterial branches are close to the retroduodenal segment of the common bile duct and may cause hemorrhage during mobilization of this portion of the biliary tract. For example, the gastroduodenal artery lies just to the left of this segment of the common bile duct and is close to it, especially at the inferior margin of the first portion of the duodenum (see Fig. 95-1). While attempting to suture-ligate the gastroduodenal artery in a patient with bleeding duodenal ulcer, the surgeon should recognize this configuration to prevent injury to the bile duct. The middle colic artery arises from the superior mesenteric artery just inferior to the pylorus in a fold of the transverse mesocolon and can be injured during mobilization of the retroduodenal common bile duct. Occasionally, a supraduodenal artery of Wilkie may cross the common bile duct anteriorly near the superior border of the first portion of the duodenum. The posterosuperior pancreaticoduodenal artery also crosses the retroduodenal common bile duct anteriorly.

Pancreatic Segment

The pancreatic segment of the common bile duct is about 2 to 3 cm long (Fig. 95-7). It can be retropancreatic or intrapancreatic, depending on the lining of the common duct behind the pancreatic head.[9,10] This is best explained by the embryology. During gestational development of the biliary tract,

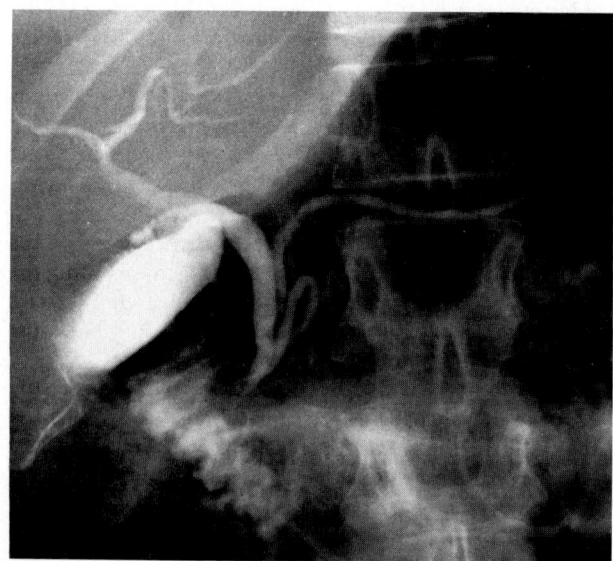

FIGURE 95-7. Normal endoscopic cholangiogram. Notice the proximity of the terminal pancreatic duct to the intrapancreatic portion of the common bile duct. The cystic duct is slightly above the gallbladder neck. The common hepatic duct is filled, as are the right and left branches. Because it is impossible to see the bifurcation of the right duct, which is usually very short, the clinician should be suspicious of an occlusion (e.g., stone, tumor) of one of the branches of this duct.

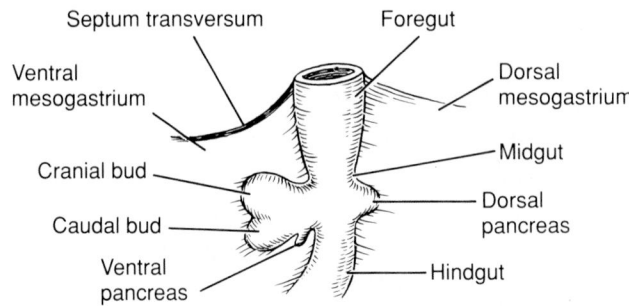

FIGURE 95-8. At the 3-mm stage of the embryo, the ventral bud enters the mesogastrium and soon divides into a cranial and a caudal bud. A smaller caudad bud represents the origin of the ventral pancreas.

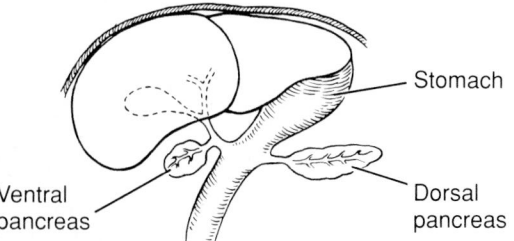

FIGURE 95-10. When the embryo reaches 7 mm, the right and left lobe of the liver occupy the position under the septum transversum. The ventral pancreas and the extrahepatic biliary tract are visible. As the ventral pancreas rotates to reach the dorsal pancreas, it pulls the lower end of the common bile duct with it.

the ventral pancreatic bulb rotates 180 degrees to join the dorsal pancreatic anlage (Figs. 95-8 through 95-11). Cancer, pancreatitis, or pseudocysts involving the head of the pancreas readily obstruct this segment of the common bile duct and cause jaundice.

As the common bile duct descends through the pancreatic head, it follows the left border of the descending duodenum and then turns to the right to enter the posteromedial surface of the descending portion of the duodenum (see Fig. 95-7). The inferior vena cava lies just posterior to this segment of bile duct. The superior pancreaticoduodenal branch of the gastroduodenal artery may cross the superior portion of this segment anteriorly or posteriorly. The pancreaticoduodenal vein runs on the left border of this segment. These vessels can be injured during dissection of the pancreatic segment of the common bile duct.

Intraduodenal Segment

The intraduodenal segment of the common bile duct lies posterior and superior to the main pancreatic duct and is about 2 cm long (see Fig. 95-7). It enters the duodenum tangentially, piercing the smooth muscle layer early, and for most of its course, it lies in a submucosal position.[11–13] This configuration allows the surgeon to create an ample opening when doing a sphincteroplasty, converting it into a true internal choledochoduodenostomy. The normal opening of the common

bile duct in the duodenum is about 7 cm distal to the pylorus, in the posteromedial wall, caudad to the crossing of the duodenum by the transverse mesocolon.[14]

This segment of common bile duct is closely associated with the main pancreatic duct (see Fig. 95-7). After running parallel for 0.2 to 1 cm, the two ducts may join outside the duodenum, or they can form a common channel as they course through the duodenal wall. In these cases, a single ostium is identified on the major duodenal papilla during endoscopy. In 20% of patients, the septum between the two ducts persists, there is no common channel, and the two ducts empty into the duodenum through two separate ostia.

The diameter of the common bile duct usually narrows substantially, to about 0.6 cm or less, in the intraduodenal segment. This explains why common bile duct stones tend to lodge there and cause biliary and pancreatic duct obstruction.

Ampulla of Vater

The lumens of the common bile duct and the main pancreatic duct usually join to form the ampulla of Vater (Fig. 95-12). In about 30% of patients, these ducts drain separately into the duodenum (in which case there is no ampulla), or the ampulla of Vater is so short (<2 mm) that it is almost non-existent.[13,14] Usually, the common bile duct narrows before it joins the pancreatic duct to form the ampulla, and the am-

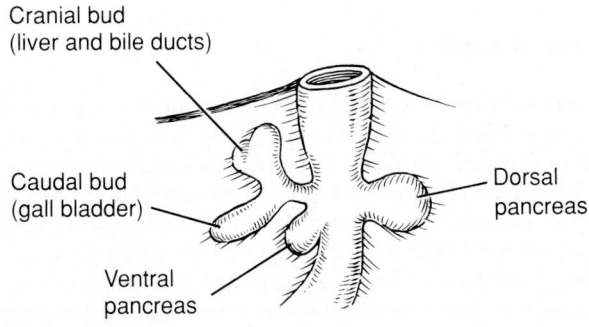

FIGURE 95-9. As the embryo reaches 5 mm, the cranial bud, which will form the liver and intrahepatic biliary tract, moves toward the septum transversum, pulling the caudal bud, which will form the gallbladder and extrahepatic bile ducts.

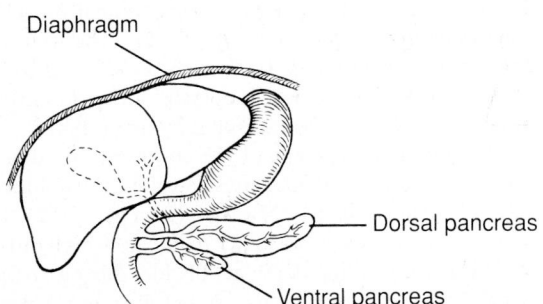

FIGURE 95-11. At the 12-mm embryonic stage, the ventral pancreas has rotated, and the anatomic relations between the bile ducts and the gastrointestinal tract have assumed their mature form.

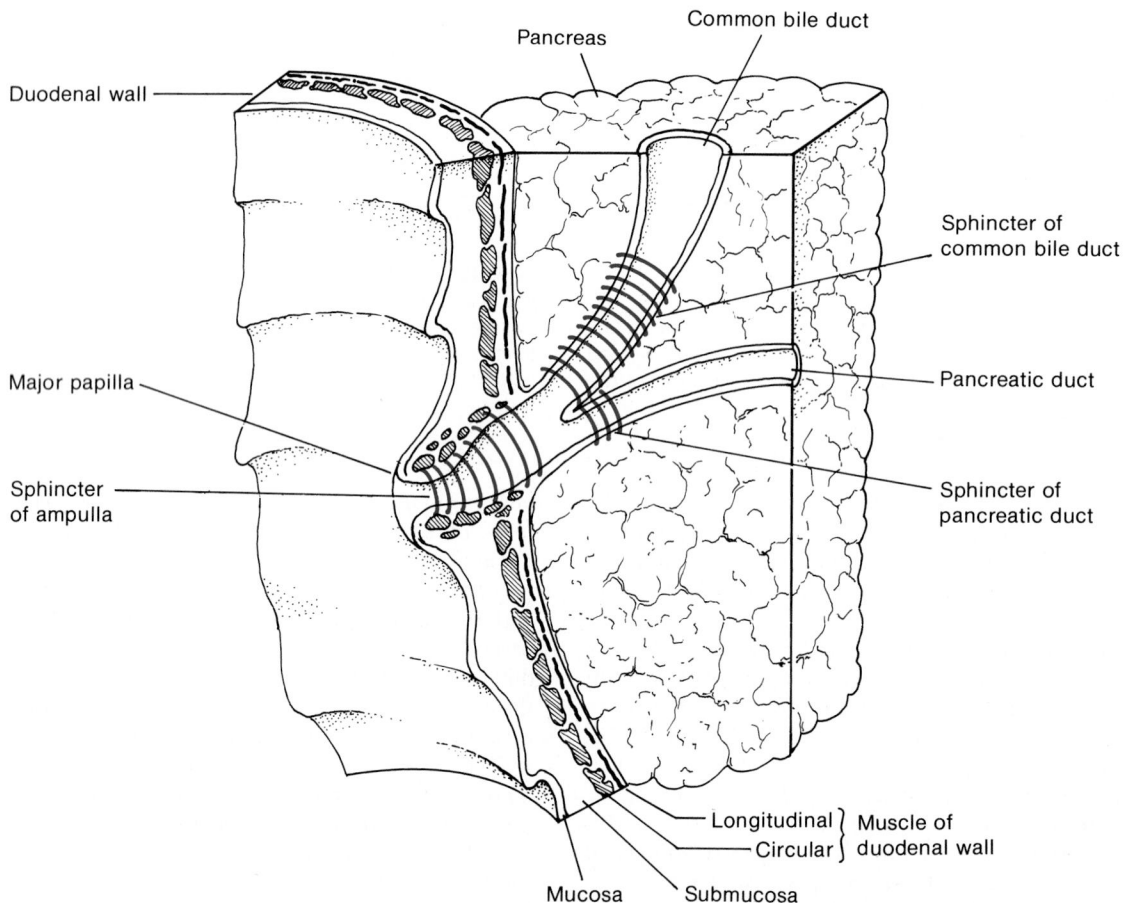

FIGURE 95-12. The muscular apparatus at the terminal end of the common bile duct. The bile duct is closely associated with the pancreatic duct, and they both enter the medial wall of the duodenum tangentially. Each duct has its own sphincter, which is poorly developed in the pancreatic duct.

pulla narrows before it enters the duodenum. These narrowings are the sites where common duct stones may lodge and cause biliary or pancreatic obstruction. They are also the sites of injury when the duct is explored by instruments that are introduced through a choledochotomy into the duodenum.

Sphincter of Oddi

The intraduodenal segment of the common bile duct and the ampulla of Vater are surrounded by a smooth muscle sheath. This complex system of circular and longitudinal muscle is called the sphincter of Oddi (see Fig. 95-12).[6] The sphincter of Oddi develops from the muscles of the bile duct and not those of the duodenum, because it operates independently of the duodenal musculature as measured by manometry.

The intraduodenal segment of the common bile duct is wrapped in a sheath of circular muscle called the sphincter choledochus or the sphincter of Boyden (see Fig. 95-12). The tone of this sphincter keeps resistance to bile flow high during fasting. This permits filling of the gallbladder during fasting. The distal main pancreatic duct sometimes has a short sphincter called the sphincter pancreaticus. The muscles of the sphincter choledochus and the sphincter pancreaticus usually interlace in a figure-of-eight fashion.

The sheath of smooth muscle surrounding the ampulla is

called the sphincter of the ampulla; it is a continuation of the sphincter of Boyden. If there is no ampulla, the distal sphincter is called the sphincter of the papilla.

During endoscopic sphincterotomy (e.g., to relieve distal common duct obstruction from a common duct stone, the sphincter of Oddi is divided by electrocautery. Optimal sphincterotomy releases the narrowing of the sphincter of Oddi and stays within the intraduodenal segment of the common bile duct.

Arterial Supply

The arterial supply of the common bile duct is segmental. The supraduodenal segment of the common bile duct, the common hepatic duct, and the distal right hepatic duct receive small arterial branches from the cystic artery (Fig. 95-13). The retroduodenal segment of the common bile duct receives small arterial branches from the posterosuperior pancreaticoduodenal artery. The pancreatic and intraduodenal segments of the common bile duct are supplied by both pancreaticoduodenal arcades. Because of the segmental nature of the arterial blood supply, the common bile duct is susceptible to ischemic injury during operations and the subsequent development of strictures.

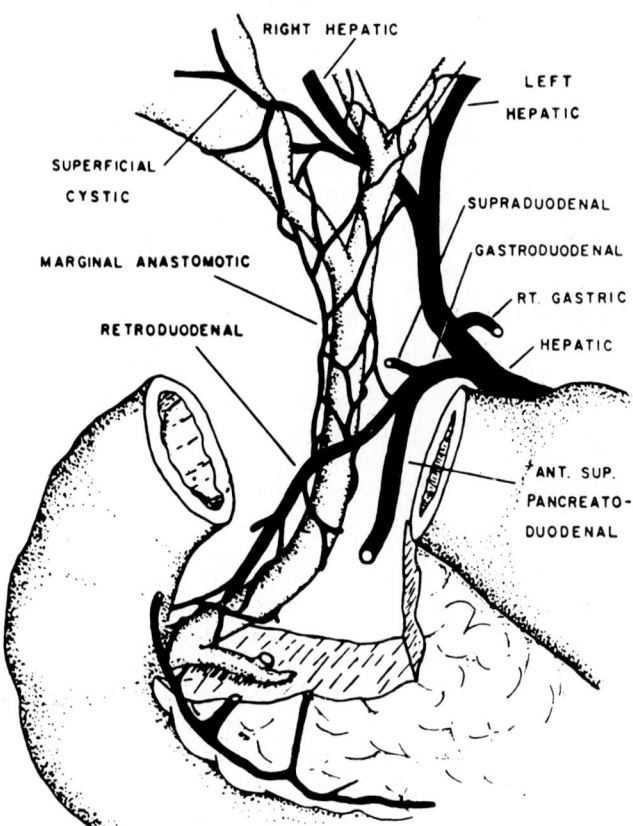

FIGURE 95-13. The extrahepatic biliary tract is supplied by a rich vascular net of vessels from the hepatic and gastroduodenal arteries. The relation between the hepatic arteries and the extrahepatic biliary tree is evident.

Venous and Lymphatic Drainage

In the proximal common bile duct, the venous drainage follows the surface of the common bile duct, hepatic ducts, and cystic duct and enters the liver directly. In the remaining portion of the common bile duct, the venous drainage is through small radicals draining into the portal vein. On the anterior surface of the supraduodenal common bile duct, a vein is frequently present that may bleed during dissection of the common bile duct or at choledochostomy.

Most of the lymphatic drainage of the common bile duct flows superiorly into the lymph nodes along the common bile duct and then into the lymph nodes in the porta hepatis. Some lymphatic drainage is through the deep pancreatic group of lymph nodes near the origin of the superior mesentery artery. Eventually, all lymphatic drainage of the common bile duct reaches the celiac lymph nodes.

EMBRYOLOGY

The biliary tract begins to develop at about the fifth week of gestation. It originates from the primitive gastrointestinal tract, just distal to the junction of the foregut and the midgut, as a ventral diverticulum (see Fig. 95-8).[14] This sacculation grows into the ventral mesogastrium and eventually gives rise to both lobes of the liver; the intrahepatic and extrahepatic

biliary tree, including the gallbladder, the cystic duct, and the common bile duct; and the ventral pancreas. The ventral pancreas ultimately becomes the posterior part of the head and the uncinate process of the pancreas. Concurrent with the development of the ventral diverticulum, a dorsal diverticulum appears, at about the same level. It grows into the posterior mesogastrium. This diverticulum gives rise to the dorsal pancreas, which becomes the anterior portion of the head of the pancreas and its body and tail.

The anatomy of the liver and biliary tract and many congenital malformations can be better understood by following the development and growth of the ventral diverticulum. Shortly after it develops, this diverticulum advances superiorly and anteriorly and divides into two buds: a cranial bud (i.e., future liver and intrahepatic ducts) and a caudal bud (i.e., future gallbladder and cystic duct). The base of the diverticulum eventually becomes the common bile duct (see Figs. 95-9 through 95-11). From this more proximal area, another small bud develops and grows inferiorly. This bud develops into the ventral pancreas.

As the cranial bud advances superiorly toward the septum transversum (i.e., future diaphragm), it divides into two smaller buds. These buds grow, and by the time they reach the undersurface of the septum, they become the right and left lobes of the liver (see Fig. 95-10). As the cranial bud advances upward, it carries the caudal bud in its undersurface (see Fig. 95-11). This explains why the gallbladder and cystic duct develop on the undersurface of the liver.

As these buds are advancing, the small appendix at the base of the ventral diverticulum, called the ventral pancreatic bud, rotates from right to left. After the rotation has completed approximately 180 degrees, it meets the dorsal pancreas, with which it fuses. Because the common bile duct is attached to the ventral pancreatic head, this rotation brings the distal common bile duct to the posteromedial side of the duodenal wall, and its most distal portion is buried between the ventral and dorsal pancreas (see Fig. 95-11).

The developing buds of the ventral diverticulum are originally composed of a solid cord of endodermal cells with no lumen. Vacuolization begins at about the seventh week of gestation, and within 1 week, an open lumen is formed in the gallbladder, cystic duct, common bile duct, and hepatic ducts. By the third month of gestation, the liver begins to secrete bile that flows through the newly canalized biliary tree into the duodenum.

CONGENITAL VARIATIONS AND MALFORMATIONS

Gallbladder and Cystic Duct

Duplication, in various degrees, of the gallbladder bud of the ventral diverticulum can cause a bilobed, cleft, or double gallbladder.[9]

Lack of development of the gallbladder bud or failure of vacuolization causes congenital absence of the gallbladder. This is frequently associated with atresia of one or more segments of the extrahepatic biliary ducts. Similarly, abnormal development of the gallbladder bud can cause congenital absence of the cystic duct. In this case, the neck of the gallbladder is interposed between the common hepatic duct and the common bile duct. If such a gallbladder were to be completely excised, it would leave a gap between the hepatic duct and the common bile duct. Failure to recognize this anomaly during cholecystectomy has led to resection of the entire distal common bile duct, which was taken to be the cystic duct arising from the gallbladder. The key to preventing injury to the biliary tree is identification of the communication of the gallbladder superiorly with the hepatic duct. When an anomalous bile duct is encountered during an operation on the biliary tract, the duct should not be divided without proper identification of all surrounding structures. This may be accomplished by a more extensive dissection or by intraoperative cholangiography.

Incomplete vacuolization of the solid endodermal cord can result in a septated gallbladder, gallbladder diverticulum, abnormal valves of Heister, or congenital stricture of the gallbladder or cystic duct.

Abnormal migration of the caudal bud of the ventral diverticulum during gestation causes an anomalous position of the gallbladder. For example, if the caudal bud advances more than the cranial bud, it tends to bury itself on the cranial bud, creating an "intrahepatic gallbladder." Most of these gallbladders are recognized preoperatively by ultrasonography. Cholecystectomy is slightly more difficult in this case, but the surgeon should always find the avascular plane between the two lobes of the liver, used by the advancing caudal bud where it buried itself into the liver parenchyma. When the caudal bud lags behind the cranial bud, the result is a "floating gallbladder." The gallbladder is then completely covered with peritoneum and suspended from the undersurface of the liver by a mesentery to the gallbladder or the cystic duct. The floating gallbladder is at higher risk for torsion, but cholecystectomy is relatively easy. Gallbladders located in the abdominal wall, falciform ligament, or retroperitoneum have been reported. The important aspect of this particular anomaly is that, because the caudal bud always remains attached to the ventral diverticulum, no matter where the gallbladder is located, the cystic duct inevitably joins the common bile duct in a relatively normal position.

Common Bile Duct and Hepatic Ducts

Accessory Extrahepatic Biliary Duct

True accessory extrahepatic biliary ducts result from the development of an extra bud from the primary biliary anlage. They are more common on the right side of the biliary tree and may drain into the gallbladder, cystic duct, right and left hepatic duct, or the common bile duct. Pseudoaccessory extrahepatic biliary ducts occur when normal biliary ducts from the right anterior segment of the liver join the right posterior segmental duct or the left hepatic duct extrahepatically.

When in doubt, a cholangiogram should be obtained to clarify the anatomy to prevent injury during cholecystectomy.

Duplication of Common Bile Duct

Completely duplicated common bile ducts are rare. When they occur, one duct drains the right lobe and the other duct drains the left lobe of the liver. These ducts open separately into the duodenum.[10] Duplication of the lower third of the common bile duct is even less common.

Biliary Atresia, Hypoplasia, and Stenosis

Biliary atresia is defined as obliteration of the intrahepatic or extrahepatic bile ducts (Fig. 93-14; see Color Fig. 53). Indirect evidence suggests that the ducts originally existed but were destroyed by a process that remains unknown.

There are two types of biliary atresia: intrahepatic and extrahepatic. In intrahepatic biliary atresia, the extrahepatic ducts are patent, but the liver has no intrahepatic bile ducts. In some patients, the parenchyma of the liver contains a few ducts. This incomplete form of atresia is known as intrahepatic biliary hypoplasia. Intrahepatic biliary atresia is usually an isolated defect but has been associated with congenital rubella, trisomy of chromosomes 17 and 18, or α_1-antitrypsin deficiency, and it may be familial.[15-17]

Extrahepatic biliary atresia (see Fig. 93-14; see Color Fig. 53) is characterized by destruction of part or all of the extrahepatic ducts. The common bile duct and the gallbladder are replaced by dense fibrotic strands and an inflammatory reaction. Extrahepatic biliary atresia almost invariably extends into the intrahepatic biliary tree. These patients have an atretic gallbladder, usually a fibrous remnant, and the green-brown liver is nodular and fibrotic. Bile capillaries and cholangioles proliferate, and progressive fibrosis typically develops in the periportal areas during the course of the disease.[18-20] Three-dimensional reconstructions of the bile duct-like channels from liver biopsies and resected extrahepatic atretic ducts show a lack of arborization of normal-diameter ducts. Instead, interconnecting ductules form a labyrinth of blind channels.

Extrahepatic biliary hypoplasia refers to a condition in which the hepatoduodenal ligament contains channels of various sizes lined by bile duct epithelium surrounded by fibrosis and chronic inflammation. The bile ducts between the liver and the duodenum are narrow, thickened, and fibrotic. There

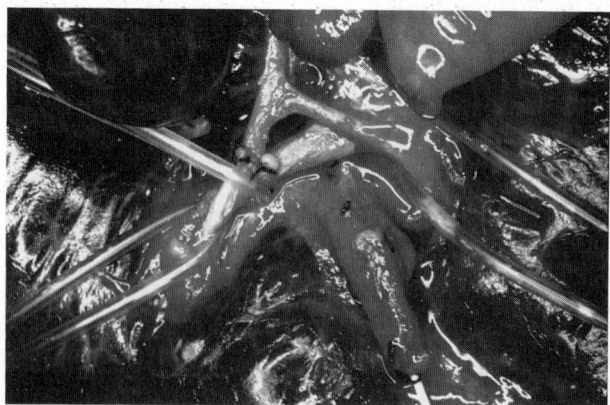

FIGURE 95-14. (See Color Fig. 53.) The liver hilum in a patient with biliary atresia. The common hepatic artery is surrounded by a tape. The right and left hepatic arteries are well dissected at the hilum of the liver. The portal vein, which is surrounded by a tape, has been dissected and is visible behind the artery. The dissection is complete, and there is no extrahepatic biliary tract. (Courtesy of Michael Harrison, M.D.)

may be multiple areas of stenosis or atresia in any segment of the extrahepatic biliary duct. This anomaly may evolve into full-blown extrahepatic biliary atresia if progressive fibrosis ensues. Hypoplasia of the intrahepatic or extrahepatic biliary system is thought by some to represent an interval stage in the evolution of biliary atresia.

There are competing hypotheses about the pathogenesis of biliary stenosis and atresia. These include incomplete vacuolization of the solid cord of endodermal cells; fetal hepatic or hepatoductal infection, such as hepatitis, causing inflammation and scarring; ischemic injury due to abnormal vascular patterns or compression by abnormal bands on the vessels supplying the duct; damage from liver or bile duct toxins; and an association of anomalies.

Failure of recanalization of the bile ducts during intrauterine development, although a tempting theory, is unlikely to be the cause of biliary atresia. Most infants who eventually develop biliary atresia are only mildly jaundiced at the time of birth and frequently have bile-stained meconium, suggesting that there is some patency of bile ducts at that time. Although biliary atresia may be congenital, the bile duct obliteration is not evident until several weeks after birth.

Familial factors probably contribute to the development of biliary atresia. For example, trisomy of chromosomes 17 and 18 has been associated with it, and congenital heart disease and other malformations have also been described in these patients.[21-23]

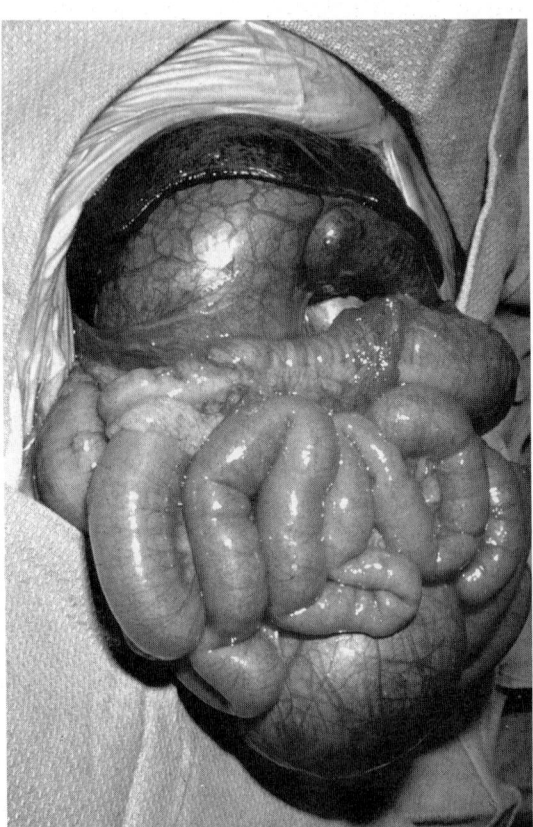

FIGURE 95-16. (See Color Fig. 55.) The liver is visible above the choledochal cyst and the intestine below. (Courtesy of Michael Harrison, M.D.)

A possible cause of biliary atresia is the excretion of a bile duct toxin by the liver.[24] Experimentally, lithocholate fed to pregnant hamsters produces an injury similar to biliary atresia.[25] It is possible that infants with biliary atresia have an inborn metabolic defect that results in the formation of a toxic bile salt or an inability to detoxify some other hepatotoxin. This theory would explain the postnatal delayed onset of biliary atresia after an initial period of normal bile flow.

Choledochal Cyst

Choledochal cyst is an anomaly characterized by saccular dilation of the extrahepatic biliary tract. It is four times more common among females and has a higher incidence among Japanese and other Asians.[26]

Three types of cysts have been described: type I, the most common form, is characterized by a fusiform dilation of the common bile duct (Figs. 95-14 through 95-16; see Color Figs. 53–55).[27] The hepatic duct proximal to the cyst is often normal (see Figs. 95-15 and 95-16; see Color Figs. 54 and 55). The cystic duct usually joins the hepatic duct above or at the margin of the cyst (see Fig. 93-15; see Color Fig. 54). The lower end of the cyst usually communicates with the distal common bile duct by a tiny opening that sometimes is difficult to identify on cholangiograms. Type II is a diverticular outpouching of the common bile duct that looks like a gallblad-

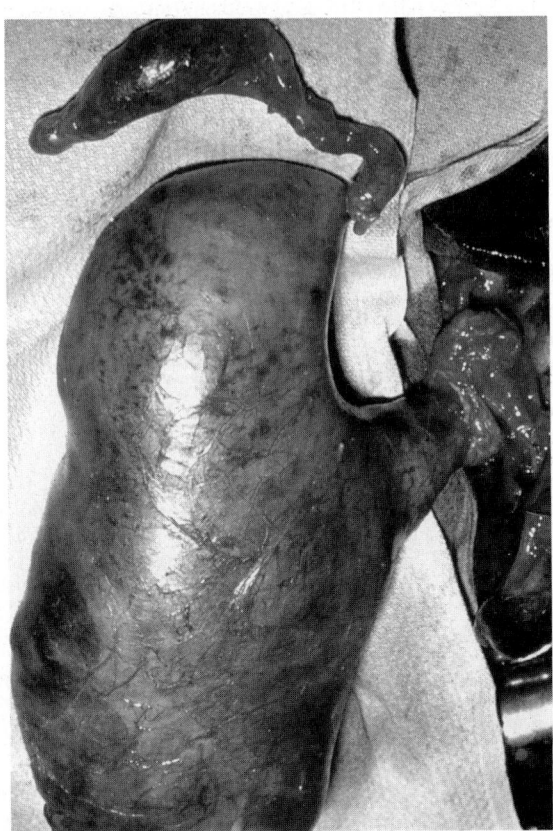

FIGURE 95-15. (See Color Fig. 54.) A giant choledochal cyst is seen outside the abdomen; the normal gallbladder and cystic duct are attached to its top portion. (Courtesy of Michael Harrison, M.D.)

der, and type III is a small saccular dilation of the distal common bile duct.

Many theories have been proposed to account for the development of choledochal cysts, but the cause is not clear. Among the more generally accepted theories are those attributing choledochal cysts to pancreatic reflux and distal obstruction of the bile duct.[28–32] Proposers of the former suggest that an abnormal pancreatic biliary duct junction results in the formation of a common channel into which pancreatic enzyme secretions are discharged. This theory is supported by the fact that, in 95% of patients with choledochal cysts, the pancreatic duct and common bile duct join to form a common channel 1.5 to 2 cm superior to the ampulla of Vater and immediately distal to the cystic swelling. According to this theory, the wall of the bile duct, weakened by enzymatic destruction and inflammation, becomes dilated and subsequently becomes cystic. The fact that a common channel is not seen in all patients with choledochal cysts and that a common channel is seen in many normal individuals casts doubts on the validity of this theory.

Ito and colleagues proposed that choledochal cysts occur from narrowing of the distal bile duct caused by failure of recanalization of this portion of the duct during intrauterine development.[33,34] They believe the narrowing leads to proximal dilation. In line with Ito's explanation, others have proposed that choledochal cysts result from a valve-like obstruction of the common duct. Repeated ascending infections of the lower common bile duct could lead to stenosis and obstruction in these patients. However, it is likely that many factors contribute to the formation of choledochal cysts and that the cysts themselves are a component of a broader malformation of the pancreatobiliary system. For example, type I choledochal cysts may be associated with intrahepatic biliary duct dilation (i.e., Caroli's disease). Recognition and appropriate early treatment of this congenital defect are critical because of the risk of severe cholangitis and adenocarcinoma (about 10%) if the cyst is left unattended.[27,35,36]

The reader is directed to Chapter 96, Gallstones; Chapter 97, Diseases of the Biliary Tree; Chapter 98, Tumors of the Biliary Tree; and Chapter 99, Postcholecystectomy Syndrome.

REFERENCES

1. Gross CM, ed. Gray's anatomy (American version). 29th ed. Philadelphia: Lea & Febiger, 1974.
2. Pellegrini CA. Pathophysiology of biliary obstruction. In: Way LW, Pellegrini CA, eds. Surgery of the gallbladder and bile ducts. Philadelphia: WB Saunders, 1987.
3. Mirizzi PL. Sindrome del conducto hepatico. J Int Chir 1948;8:731.
4. Hollinshead HW. The liver and the gallbladder. In: Anatomy for surgeons. 3rd ed. Philadelphia: Harper and Row, 1982.
5. Shaffer EA. The effects of vagotomy on gallbladder function and bile composition in man. Ann Surg 1982;195:413.
6. Mueller JC, Jones AL, Long JA. Topographic and subcellular anatomy of the guinea pig gallbladder. Gastroenterology 1972;63:856.
7. Boyden EA. Humoral vs. neural regulation of the extrahepatic biliary tract. Minn Med 1953;36:720.
8. Dowdy GS Jr, Waldron GW, Brown WG. Surgical anatomy of the pancreatico-biliary ductal system. Arch Surg 1962;84:229.
9. Anson BJ, McVay CB. Surgical anatomy. 2nd ed. Philadelphia: WB Saunders, 1971:597.
10. Hicken NF, Coray QB, Franz B. Anatomic variations of the extrahepatic biliary system as seen by cholangiographic studies. Surg Gynecol Obstet 1949;88:577.
11. Keddie NC, Taylor AW, Sykes PA. The termination of the common bile duct. Br J Surg 1974;61:623.
12. Lindner HH, Pena VA, Ruggieri RA. A clinical and anatomical study of anomalous termination of the common bile duct into the duodenum. Ann Surg 1976;184:626.
13. Schulenberg CAR. Anomalies of the biliary tract as demonstrated by operative cholangiography. Med Pr 1970;16:351.
14. Lindner HH. Embryology and anatomy of the biliary tree. In: Way LW, Pellegrini CA, eds. Surgery of the gallbladder and bile ducts. 1st ed. Philadelphia: WB Saunders, 1987:3.
15. Sass-Kortsak A, Bowden DM, Brown RJK. Congenital intrahepatic biliary atresia. Pediatrics 1956;17:383.
16. Strauss L, Bernstein J. Neonatal hepatitis in congenital rubella. Arch Pathol 1968;86:317.
17. Odievre ZM, Martin JP, Hadchonal M, et al. Alpha-1 antitrypsin deficiency and liver disease in children: phenotypes, manifestations and prognosis. Pediatrics 1976;57:226.
18. Bennett DE. Problems in neonatal obstructive jaundice. Pediatrics 1964;3:375.
19. Haas JE. Bile duct and liver pathology in biliary atresia. World J Surg 1978;1:561.
20. Kasai M, Yakovac WC, Koope CE. Liver in congenital biliary atresia and neonatal hepatitis. Arch Pathol 1962;74:152.
21. Mowat AP, Psacharopoulos HT, Williams R. Extrahepatic biliary atresia versus neonatal hepatitis. Review of 137 prospectively investigated infants. Arch Dis Child 1976;51:763.
22. Riockham PP. Neonatal biliary obstruction. In: Rickham PP, Johnston JH, eds. Neonatal surgery. New York: Appleton-Century-Crofts, 1978:152.
23. Chandra RS. Biliary atresia and other structural anomalies in congenital polysplenia syndrome. J Pediatr 1974;85:649.
24. Palmer AK, Heywood R. Pathological changes in the rhesus fetus associated with the oral administration of chenodeoxycholic acid. Toxicology 1974;2:239.
25. Silverberg M, Salomon L, Ehrlich JC. The hepatotoxic effects of lithocholic acid in the newborn hamster. Gastroenterology 1971;60:753.
26. Yamaguchi M. Congenital choledochal cyst. Analysis of 1,433 patients in the Japanese literature. Am J Surg 1980;140:653.
27. Todani T, Watanabe Y, Narusue M, et al. Congenital bile duct cysts. Classification, operative procedures and review of thirty-seven cases including cancer arising from choledochal cyst. Am J Surg 1977;134:263.
28. Carima E, Akita H. Congenital biliary tract dilatation and anomalous junction of the pancreatico-biliary ductal system. J Pediatr Surg 1979;14:9.
29. Kimura K, Tsugawa C, Ogawa K, et al. Choledochal cysts. Etiological considerations and surgical management in 22 cases. Arch Surg 1978;113:159.
30. Okada A, Oguchi Y, Kmata S, et al. Common channel syndrome—Diagnosis with endoscopic retrograde cholangiopancreatography and surgical management. Surgery 1983;93:634.
31. Ono J, Sakoda K, Akita H. Surgical aspect of cystic dilatation of the bile duct. An anomalous junction of the pancreaticobiliary tract in adults. Ann Surg 1982;195:203.
32. Sterling JA. The common channel for bile and pancreatic ducts. Surg Gynecol Obstet 1954;98:420.
33. Ito T, Ando H, Nagaya M, et al. Congenital dilatation of the common bile duct in children: the etiologic significance of the narrow segment distal to the dilated common bile duct. Z Kinderchir 1984;39:40.
34. Wong KC, Lister J. Human fetal development of the hepato-pancreatic duct junction—a possible explanation of congenital dilatation of the biliary tract. J Pediatr Surg 1981;16:139.
35. Fonkalsrud EW, Boles ET. Choledochal cysts in infancy and childhood. Surg Gynecol Obstet 1965;121:733.
36. Babbitt DP. Congenital choledochal cysts: new etiological concept based on anomalous relationships of the common bile duct and pancreatic bulb. Ann Radiol 1969;12:231.

Textbook of Gastroenterology, second edition, edited by Tadataka Yamada. JB Lippincott Company, Philadelphia © 1995.

CHAPTER 96

Gallstones

Sum Ping Lee   Rahul Kuver

Autopsy studies of Egyptian and Chinese mummies have shown that gallbladder stones have existed for more than 35 centuries. Gallstones have remained the most prevalent disease affecting the biliary system. Approximately 20 million Americans have gallstones, and 500,000 cholecystectomies are performed annually in the United States.[1] Gallstone-related symptoms and complications are among the most common gastroenterologic disorders requiring hospitalization, at an estimated annual cost of five billion dollars.[2,3] During the past two decades, there have been major advances in the understanding of the pathogenesis of gallstones, and there has been a proliferation of novel methods of treating gallstones. This chapter summarizes the features of this condition and the evolving treatment modalities.

EPIDEMIOLOGY

Gallstones are classified as cholesterol stones and pigment stones. In the United States, as in most Western countries, more than 75% of gallstones are the cholesterol type. There is a striking variation in the prevalence of gallstones in different countries and among various ethnic groups in the same country. Epidemiologic and case-control studies implicate genetic and lifestyle factors in accounting for this wide variation in prevalence of gallstones. Gallstone prevalence also varies with age and sex.

Because the disease is nonfatal and often asymptomatic, the diagnosis of gallbladder stones is not always made before death. This leads to difficulties in accurately determining the true prevalence of gallstones. Autopsy studies correlating with clinical information suggest that approximately two thirds of the population with gallstones are asymptomatic.[4] The methods used to measure gallstone prevalence include autopsy studies, determination of cholecystectomy rates, and screening ultrasonography. Later screening ultrasonography studies have confirmed earlier epidemiologic data on gallstone prevalence obtained from autopsy studies.[5] A screening ultrasound survey in Denmark showed new gallstone formation in 3% of the population older than 40 years of age in each 5-year period.[6]

International Variation in Prevalence of Gallstones

The wide scatter in gallstone prevalence among different nations and ethnic groups is strong evidence that genetic factors are involved in the formation of gallstones. Those with the highest rates of gallstone formation are the Pima Indians of North America, Chileans, and Caucasians in the United States.[4,7,8] Next are the populations of Sweden, Germany, and Austria, followed by New Zealand, England, Norway, Ireland, and Greece.[9–17] At the bottom of this list are the Asian populations in Singapore and Thailand.[18,19] In these studies, the ratio of women to men with gallstones has ranged from 0.8 to 3.0, with most showing a ratio of approximately 2.0. The prevalence among both sexes increases with age.[20]

The type of gallstone also varies among cultures. In developed countries, cholesterol gallstones are most common and usually occur in the gallbladder. In Africa and Asia, where the prevalence of gallstones is low, pigment gallstones are most common, and stones also can be found in the bile ducts.[21]

Temporal Variation in Prevalence of Gallstones

Progressive increases in the rate of gallstones during this century support a role for lifestyle and dietary factors in the pathogenesis of gallstones. Cholecystectomy rates partially reflect the provision of medical services, and autopsy gallstone rates may vary among populations within a country during a given period of time. Nevertheless, several studies have shown increases in the prevalence of gallstones over time.[11,16,22-25] In Japan, postwar westernization has provided an example of the interplay between lifestyle and disease. Since the late 1940s, the prevalence of gallstones in Tokyo has more than doubled.[23] Moreover, there has been a change from pigment to cholesterol gallstones. In Saudi Arabia over a 10-year period, the frequency of cholecystectomy has increased sharply, a rise not matched by the increase in population, use of medical services, or number of other surgical procedures. A shift to a more western diet has been suggested as a possible explanation.[26] Prospective studies, such as the Rome Group for Epidemiology and Prevention of Cholelithiasis (GREPCO) study of Italian civil servants and the population study of the town of Sermione, Italy, should help clarify these factors.[27-29]

ETIOLOGY

Pathogenesis of Cholesterol Gallstones

The total body pool of cholesterol is supplied by de novo synthesis from acetyl-coenzyme A (acyl-CoA) and dietary absorption.[30,31] Cholesterol is used to generate steroid and lipoprotein products. Most of this pool is solubilized and secreted unmodified in bile or converted to various bile acids. Approximately 20% of the cholesterol secreted in bile comes from new hepatic synthesis.[32-34] The remainder originates from a preformed pool within the liver.[35,36] Important contributors into this pool include hydrolysis of cholesteryl ester stores, dietary sources in the form of chylomicrons, and direct hepatic and extrahepatic synthesis of the high-density lipoprotein (HDL), low-density lipoprotein, and very-low-density lipoprotein. These import and export fluxes are tightly regulated so that total hepatic cholesterol is maintained without significant losses or gains.[37,38] The association with serum cholesterol levels is not straightforward; although links between the risk of gallstones and decreased HDL cholesterol and increased serum triglyceride levels have been reported, no such association was found for total serum cholesterol levels.[39]

Various defective metabolic states can disrupt this regulatory balance, resulting in absolute biliary cholesterol hypersecretion or relative bile acid hyposecretion. Both of these defects can coexist, as in the case of the Pima Indians.[40]

Several mechanisms may be operative in biliary cholesterol hypersecretion.[41-53] Clinical situations associated with excessive secretion of biliary cholesterol include obesity, aging, drug effects, and hormonal manipulation.[54] For example, progesterone and clofibrate are potent inhibitors of hepatic acyl-CoA cholesterol acyltransferase (ACAT). Hepatocyte membranes harbor the large pool of free cholesterol, and the size of this pool is regulated by the extent of cholesterol esterification. As ACAT esterifies cholesterol, its inhibition can lead to increased availability of free or unesterified cholesterol for secretion into bile. Lovastatin, an inhibitor of hepatic cholesterol synthesis, inhibits gallstone formation in an animal model.[55] Table 96-1 summarizes some of these examples and the proposed underlying pathogenesis in these cases.

Alternatively, biliary supersaturation may occur in the setting of relative bile acid hyposecretion (Table 96-2).[56-63] A diminished bile acid pool and secretion rate may result from excessive intestinal losses or decreased production. In nonobese patients with cholesterol gallstones, cholic acid and

---

TABLE 96-1
Risk Factors Associated With Cholesterol Hypersecretion in Bile

CLINICAL EXAMPLES	PATHOGENESIS
Obesity, hyperlipoproteinemia	Increased hydroxymethylglutaryl-coenzyme A activity leading to increased mevalonic acid and cholesterol synthesis
Progesterone, oral contraceptives, clofibrate	Inhibition of hepatic acyl-coenzyme A cholesterol acyltransferase activity leading to decreased conversion of cholesterol to cholesteryl ester stores
Estrogens	Increased lipoprotein receptors B and E leading to increased hepatic cholesterol uptake; inhibited synthesis of chenodeoxycholic acid
Selected nonobese Caucasians	Reduced activity of 7α-hydroxylase leading to a defect in enzymatic conversion of cholesterol to bile acids; increased enterohepatic cycling of bile acids, leading to increased biliary deoxycholate levels
Age	Age-related decrease (?) in 7α-hydroxylase activity
Marked weight reduction	Mobilization of tissue cholesterol

TABLE 96-2
Risk Factors Associated With Relative Bile Acid Hyposecretion

CLINICAL EXAMPLES	PATHOGENESIS
Ileal Disease, bypass, or resection	Impaired bile acid absorption or excessive losses
Cerebrotendinous xanthomatosis	Inherited 26-hydroxylase deficiency leading to incomplete oxidation of the cholesterol side chain and decreased bile acid production
Congenital 12-hydroxylase deficiency	Decreased cholate and deoxycholate synthesis
Selected nonobese Caucasians	Excessive feedback suppression of bile acid synthesis leading to a decreased pool, hepatic return, and secretion
Primary biliary cirrhosis	Decreased bile acid secretion
Chronic cholestasis	

chenodeoxycholic acid pools are reduced, and deoxycholic acid is often increased in bile.[58,64] Conversion of cholic acid to deoxycholic acid, possibly from increased 7α-hydroxylation in the small intestine or colonic bacterial action, may account for these changes.[65] With an expanded deoxycholate pool in bile, the biliary secretion of cholesterol rises.[66]

Cholesterol Solubilization

Free cholesterol is virtually insoluble in aqueous solution. Bile acids, because of their unique amphipathic properties, are able to solubilize cholesterol with phospholipids in the form of mixed micelles.[67-69] Phase equilibrium diagrams can be constructed to characterize cholesterol solubility in a defined milieu of various lipid concentrations. Using these data, the cholesterol saturation index (CSI) can be calculated.[70] CSI refers to the ratio of the actual amount of cholesterol in a given bile sample to the maximal cholesterol micellar-holding capacity of that sample as determined by in vitro experimentation. Bile that has a CSI greater than 1 is considered supersaturated. Supersaturated bile that does not form cholesterol crystals is called metastable.[71]

In addition to classic micelle packaging, cholesterol is solubilized with phospholipid (principally phosphatidylcholine) as unilamellar vesicles that range in size from 40 to 75 nm.[72-77] These vesicles are thought to be assembled within the hepatocyte and are then transported to the region of the canaliculus.[78] Hepatocyte biliary lipid secretion is inhibited by colchicine and vinblastine, agents that affect microtubule function.[79] Collectively, these lipid vesicles comprise a separate and distinct carriage system that probably represents the major mode of cholesterol transport from the liver cell.[80]

Bile acid secretion is the primary driving force behind the biliary secretion of cholesterol and phospholipid.[81,82] As bile acids are actively secreted against a gradient across the canalicular membrane, they induce the subsequent secretion of cholesterol-phospholipid vesicles into bile. Hydrophobic bile acids are more effective in provoking lipid secretion, although the maximum rate of biliary lipid secretion is similar for all bile acids.[80] Within the canaliculus, the bile acid concentration rises, reaching and exceeding a micellar concentration that allows adsorption onto vesicles and conversion to mixed micellar carriers. This interchange continues in a dynamic fashion within the ductules, ducts, and gallbladder.[83] The relative

percentage of cholesterol transported in the micellar fraction compared with the vesicular fraction can vary dramatically, depending on the physiologic conditions, such as bile acid concentration, total lipid concentration, and degree of cholesterol saturation. For example, at low bile acid secretion rates, as occur in the fasting state, the predominant form of cholesterol carriage in hepatic bile is vesicular.[72,74,77] Conversely, the higher bile acid concentration in the gallbladder favors a shift toward micelle formation (Figs. 96-1 and 96-2).[72,74]

Nucleation of Cholesterol Crystals

An early and indispensable step in cholesterol gallstone formation is nucleation, which is the critical emergence of solid cholesterol crystals from saturated bile. Antecedent vesicular fusion and aggregation may be crucial, if not mandatory, for crystal generation. Nucleation of crystals results in a diminution of vesicular cholesterol while having no affect on micellar cholesterol.[72] Under video-enhanced microscopy, crystals appeared to originate from aggregated vesicles.[84-86]

Vesicles in bile do not represent an homogeneous population. Gallbladder bile vesicles are likely to participate in nucleation; vesicles in hepatic bile are much more stable and resistant to nucleation.[72] The discrepancy in their behavior partly is caused by the difference in their relative cholesterol-to-phospholipid content. Vesicles that have increased ratios of cholesterol to phospholipid aggregate, fuse, and nucleate more readily.[85,87] The concentrated bile acids within the gallbladder may preferentially remove vesicular phospholipid over cholesterol during the dynamic shift to the micellar phase. In doing so, the remaining vesicles are relatively cholesterol-enriched and nucleation prone. Conversely, hepatic vesicles have lower cholesterol-to-phospholipid contents and are therefore more stable.

Many people secrete supersaturated bile without developing gallstones.[88,89] Gallbladder bile taken from patients with cholesterol stones nucleates more rapidly than equally saturated bile from controls. Taken together, these observations indicate that factors other than cholesterol supersaturation must be involved in nucleation. Considerable efforts have been exerted in identifying specific nucleating factors. Biliary proteins have generated the most attention, because total biliary protein content is increased in bile with cholesterol crystals

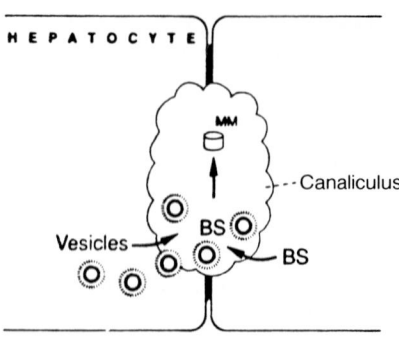 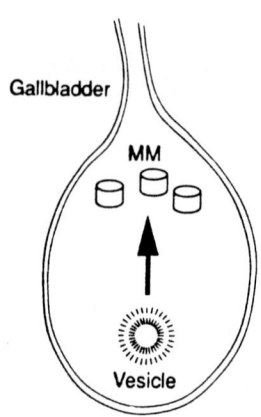

FIGURE 96-1. Schematic representation of biliary lipid secretion. At the level of the hepatocyte, vesicles of cholesterol and phospholipids are secreted through the bile canaliculus. Bile salts (BS) are also secreted, probably by a different and independent mechanism. Inside the bile canaliculus, when bile salts reach a concentration above the critical micellar concentration, mixed micelles (MM) of bile salts, cholesterol, and phospholipids are formed. In the gallbladder, as bile is being further concentrated, more mixed micelles form and more vesicles are converted into mixed micelles. Unlike the vesicles in the hepatic bile, in which there are abundant phospholipids, the vesicles in the gallbladder can be depleted of phospholipids and relatively enriched with cholesterol, because mixed micelles, when they solubilize vesicular lipids, transfer more phopholipid than cholesterol. The resultant vesicles in the gallbladder may then be unstable and susceptible to nucleation.

compared with samples without crystals.[90] Prospective agents can be evaluated by examining their effects on nucleation time assays. These assays are performed by noting the time at which cholesterol crystals are first detected when observing native or model bile daily under polarizing microscopy.[91,92] The cholesterol nucleation time was longer in bile from patients with solitary stones than in bile from patients with multiple stones, even though the CSI was not significantly different between these two groups.[93]

Burnstein and colleagues provided the first major evidence for a potent pronucleating agent in bile.[94] A small-molecular-weight glycoprotein in bile binds to concanavalin A and exhibits promoting abilities.[95] This fraction contains phospholipase C, which is also postulated to be a promoter.[96] Hepatic bile from patients with cholesterol gallstones contained proteins associated with vesicles; when purified, these vesicles

had potent cholesterol-nucleating activity.[97] Immunoglobulins in bile may act as pronucleating agents.[98] A small, pigment-associated, anionic protein appears to be important in the regulation of calcium salts and in cholesterol precipitation in bile.[99-102] Certain gallbladder protein fractions and the apolipoproteins AI and AII inhibit in vitro nucleation assays.[103]

An advance has been the introduction of an assay that detects crystal growth using spectrometric methods.[104] Using this assay, a 42- kd biliary glycoprotein was isolated that displayed concentration-dependent cholesterol-crystallization promoting activity.[105] Glycosylation of this protein is extensive (37%), and deglycosylation inactivated its promoting activity. This biliary glycoprotein may be a form of α_1-acid glycoprotein.[106]

A biliary glycoprotein heterodimer that showed inhibitory

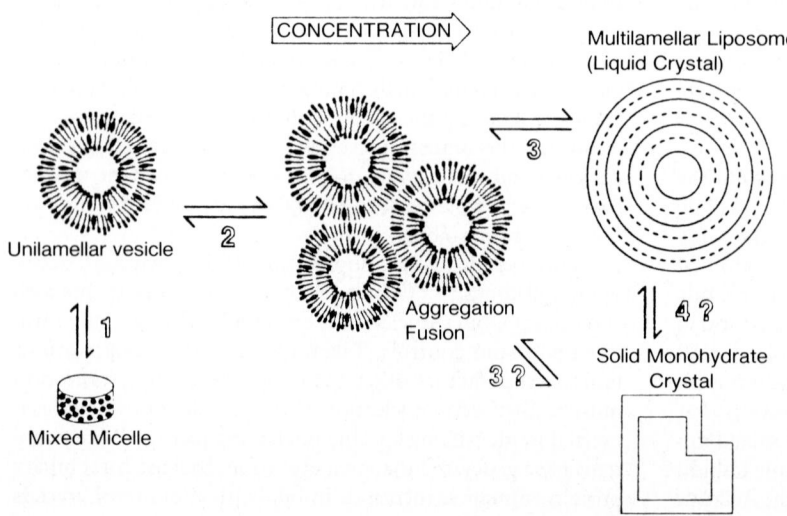

FIGURE 96-2. Schematic representation of cholesterol nucleation. In bile, cholesterol exists in two soluble forms: vesicles and mixed micelles. These forms are in dynamic equilibrium (1), depending on the total bile salt concentration and total lipid density of the bile sample. With concentration, the vesicles may be depleted of phospholipid and enriched with cholesterol. This results in a tendency for the vesicles to aggregate and fuse (2). Pronucleators may also cause vesicular fusion. The fused vesicle is a transitional form and leads to the formation of liquid crystals or multilamellar liposomes (3). Cholesterol can separate from the liquid to solid crystalline form by a process known as nucleation (4). Whether fused vesicles can nucleate into solid cholesterol monohydrate crystals is unclear.

activity in normal bile using the crystal growth assay was isolated.[107] Glycosylation also appears to be important for activity, because deglycosylation abolishes inhibition of crystal growth. This glycoprotein belongs to the cytokeratin family of proteins.[108] Taken together, these studies highlight the intensity of investigation in the field of biliary cholesterol-nucleating and -antinucleating factors.[109]

Calcium complexes are also important.[110] These complexes interfere with bile acid dissolution therapy by precipitating residual stone material.[111] Calcium salts are present in the central matrices in many, if not all, cholesterol stones according to electron probe and x-ray diffraction analyses.[112] Precipitation of calcium bilirubinate, carbonate, or phosphate may serve as potential nidi for cholesterol crystallization.[113,114] Free and total calcium increased in the bile in obese patients who developed gallstones during weight reduction.[115] Ceftriaxone was associated with an increase in total calcium concentration in the gallbladder, representing binding of free calcium ions to ceftriaxone.[116]

Role of the Gallbladder

The importance of the gallbladder in the pathogenesis of cholesterol gallstones cannot be overstated. Cholecystectomy essentially cures the patient of recurrent de novo cholesterol stone formation. Gallbladder mucosal function plays an important role in this pathogenic process. Sodium and chloride ion fluxes are altered in an animal model of lithogenesis.[117] A defect in the usual acidification of gallbladder bile in gallstone patients has been reported, and this finding is significant because the precipitation of calcium salts is favored at higher pH.[118,119] A subsequent study, however, showed that biliary acidification and ionized calcium concentrations were comparable in patients with cholesterol stones, those with pigment stones, and normal controls.[120]

Disturbances of cholesterol metabolism in gallbladder epithelium that might contribute to high cholesterol content have not been detected. Hydroxymethylglutaryl-CoA reductase activity, governing cholesterol synthesis, is lower in the gallbladder mucosa than in hepatic tissue, and the ACAT activity in the gallbladder mucosa catalyzing the esterification of cholesterol is several times higher than in the liver.[121]

Mucin is a high-molecular-weight glycoprotein that is the major organic constituent of gallbladder mucus. It consists of a polypeptide core to which multiple oligosaccharide side chains are attached. These peptide cores also contain hydrophobic domains that bind pigment, cholesterol, and phospholipid.[122,123] Mucin is a pronucleator.[124] It may also provide an architectural framework for crystal growth and stone formation.[125] Using a cholesterol-fed animal model of lithogenesis, gallbladder epithelial mucin hypersecretion and gelation were shown to precede the appearance of solid cholesterol crystals.[126,127] Mucus hypersecretion before stone formation appears to be an universal antecedent in a diverse number of animal models of lithogenesis. This secretory response can be inhibited by the administration of large doses of oral aspirin, an observation confirmed in the human gallbladder.[128] Aspirin ingestion can completely abolish subsequent formation of cholesterol crystals and gallstones.[129] Using a commercial lithogenic diet, suppression of mucin secretion was not reproduced in the prairie dog gallbladder.[130]

Inhibition of prostaglandin production with indomethacin did not prevent mucin hypersecretion in this animal.[131] Although prostaglandin activity may play a role in the pathogenesis of mucin hypersecretion, the role of other factors awaits study.[132–134] The gallbladder can also secrete in response to gastrointestinal peptides such as secretin, assisting the emptying of precipitate.[135] The successful growth of gallbladder epithelial cells in culture should facilitate this area of investigation.[136,137]

In addition to epithelial cell function, gallbladder motility is of vital importance. Cholecystic stasis is a risk factor in lithogenesis. Extended bile storage time enables mucin gels to accumulate. The physical nature of these gels may interfere with mechanical emptying. Increased cholesterol nucleation and crystal growth as well as enzymatic and nonenzymatic hydrolysis of bilirubin conjugates could occur, resulting in an increased supply of unconjugated bilirubin products, which are less soluble and more susceptible to precipitate with calcium.

A defect in gallbladder contractility has been documented in a lithogenic animal model before cholesterol stone formation.[138,139] In humans, prolonged total parenteral nutrition (TPN) induces gallbladder hypomotility and profound stasis.[140,141] This sets the stage for subsequent biliary sludge and possible stone development. High spinal cord injury is linked to gallbladder stasis.[142] Pregnancy and the use of oral contraceptives are also associated with impaired emptying and cholelithiasis. Real-time ultrasonography in pregnancy demonstrates decreased emptying rates, higher fasting volumes, and increased residual volumes after contractions. Similar but less pronounced effects can be seen with the use of oral contraceptives. Decreased gallbladder sensitivity to cholecystokinin in the early stages of gallstone formation has been observed in an animal model.[143] Erythromycin, acting as a motilin agonist, decreases fasting and postprandial gallbladder volume in normal persons and in patients with gallstone disease.[144] Hormonal influences and prostaglandins are postulated mediators of gallbladder contractility.

Biliary Sludge

Precipitates in bile have been called by many names—bile gravel, microcrystalline disease, microliths, bile sand, minilithiasis, and biliary sludge. Sludge is best diagnosed by microscopic examination of a fresh sample of gallbladder bile.[145] Sludge also can be seen ultrasonographically as echogenic material that layers in the dependent portion of the gallbladder and produces low-amplitude echoes without postacoustic shadowing.[146,147] In certain clinical conditions, sludge is a risk factor for the subsequent development of cholelithiasis.

Biochemically, sludge is composed of calcium bilirubinate granules and cholesterol monohydrate crystals embedded within a mucous gel. Ceftriaxone precipitates as a calcium salt that appears ultrasonographically as sludge.[148] These calcium precipitates, in conjunction with cholesterol crystals 50 μm or more in diameter, produce the characteristic ultrasonic echoes in sludge, and the deformable mucin gel accounts for its unique layering and flow characteristics.[147]

In a prospective study of patients receiving prolonged TPN, 6% of the patients developed sludge during the initial 3 weeks. By 4 to 6 weeks, 50% of the patients had sludge, and after 6 weeks, its appearance was universal.[149] In following this group of sludge formers, stones developed in 43%. Significantly, the reinstitution of oral feedings resulted in sludge resolution in all the patients by the end of 4 weeks. Although stasis was undoubtedly the major factor in sludge genesis, these patients represented a medically ill population with attendant complicating metabolic derangements.

Gallbladder sludge may also appear spontaneously in selected individuals. The clinical outcome of a group of patients who presented with upper abdominal pain and had the presence of sludge documented on initial ultrasound examination was examined.[147] In approximately 18%, the sludge resolved over a 2-year period. It had a disappearing and reappearing course in about 60%. Gallstones also developed in 14%. This collective cohort may represent de novo cholesterol stone formers who have been detected at an early stage. In contrast, the patients on TPN may be a more heterogeneous group in which stasis so dominates that virtually everyone develops sludge and approximately one half eventually form stones.

One scenario of cholesterol lithogenesis begins first as a defective alteration in the hepatic handling of biliary lipids. This results in cholesterol supersaturation of bile. Perhaps through the action of chemical mediators, gallbladder mucin hypersecretion and stasis develop. As the bile is progressively concentrated, the residual vesicular fraction becomes relatively cholesterol enriched. These vesicles aggregate, fuse, and produce crystals when the balance of the opposing promoting and inhibitory factors favors nucleation. The crystals formed are retained within the gallbladder, where they grow and conglomerate with mucin glycoprotein and other constituents such as calcium and bilirubin pigments. Continued stasis and impaired emptying of the viscoelastic mucin gels and embedded precipitates lead to macroscopic stone formation.

Pathogenesis of Pigment Gallstones

Chemical Composition and Chemical Associations

Pigment gallstones are subclassified into brown and black types, which differ in morphology, chemical composition, pathogenesis, and correlating clinical features (Table 96-3). Unlike its role in cholesterol gallstones, ethnic origin is not an important determinant of pigment gallstones. Black pigment stones can occur in persons with no predisposing factors. In the United States, black pigment gallstones are found in the gallbladder and are not associated with bacterial infection.

TABLE 96-3
Clinical Associations and Compositions of Black and Brown Pigment Gallstones

CHARACTERISTICS	BLACK	BROWN
Color	Black	Brown-orange-yellow
Size	0.3–0.6 cm	0.5–2 cm
Consistency	Amorphous, powdery, solid	Soft, laminated, muddy
Anatomic location	Gallbladder	Gallbladder and bile ducts
Geography	West and Asia	Mostly Asia
Diet	High-protein diet	Low-protein diet
Disease associations	Hemolysis, cirrhosis, "healthy" persons	Cholangitis, ova, parasites, sutures
Bile cultures	Usually sterile	Infected (*E. coli, Bacteroides,* ova, parasites)
Recurrent stones	Uncommon	Frequent
Radiologic calcification	Diffuse (up to 70% of stones radiopaque)	Usually radiolucent, slightly calcified
Principal components	Pigment polymer, calcium phosphate, calcium carbonate	Calcium bilirubinate, calcium soaps of fatty acids, cholesterol
Etiology	Increased excretion or hydrolysis of conjugated bilirubin	Bacterial hydrolysis of conjugated to unconjugated bilirubin
Bile pigment—total major form	40 (10–90)* Insoluble polymer	50 (28–79)* Calcium bilirubinate
Calcium	15 (3–40)	5 (3–9)
Calcium salts		
Carbonate	13 (0–65)	None
Phosphate	5 (0–32)	<1
Palmitate + stearate	1 (0–3)	23 (11–67)
Cholesterol (unesterified)	3 (1–13)	10 (2–28)
Organic matrix (glycoproteins, mucins, carbohydrates)	24 (10–73)	12 (0–30)

* Values are given as a percentage of dry weight of the stone and are means, with ranges in parentheses.

Adapted from Ostrow, J. D. The etiology of pigmented gallstones. Hepatology 1984;4:215s; and Leuschner U, Guldutuna S, and Hellstern A. Etiology, pathogenesis and therapy of pigment gallstones. Dig Dis 1991;9:282.

Factors associated with the formation of black pigment stones include chronic hemolysis (e.g., sickle cell disease), hereditary spherocytosis, thalassemia, and cardiac valvular prosthesis.[150-152] It is also associated with cirrhosis, long-term TPN, and advancing age.[153,154] Black pigment stones seldom coexist with cholesterol stones in the same gallbladder. A calcium-regulatory protein that may act as a mediator of calcium precipitation has been isolated from black pigment stones.[155]

In Asia, brown pigment stones are often found in the bile ducts and are strongly associated with bacterial infection.[156] There is a high incidence of infection with *Escherichia coli*, with the presence of bacteria within stones easily demonstrated.[157-160] Biliary secretory IgA is decreased.[161] Infected bile exhibits high bacterial β-glucuronidase activity, and this increased activity is associated with the presence of a juxtapapillary duodenal diverticulum.[162,163]

Deconjugation of Bilirubin

Bilirubin, a tetrapyrrol like cholesterol, is insoluble in water. In bile, bilirubin is secreted after glucuronidation, mainly as the diglucuronide (75%–80%), but also as the monoglucuronide (20%), with only a small amount of unconjugated bilirubin (3%). Because black and brown pigment stones contain calcium salts of bilirubin, the pathogenesis of pigment stones revolves around the deconjugation and precipitation of bilirubin.

In patients with chronic hemolysis, there is a tenfold increase in the excretion of conjugated bilirubin in the hepatic bile.[164] Bile acid mixed micelles and an acidic milieu promote bilirubin solubilization. The role of biliary β-glucuronidase in the pathogenesis of pigment gallstones has been controversial. Debate centers on the origin of the enzyme, its pH optimum, and substrate specificity. Although the hypothesis that bacterial β-glucuronidase hydrolysis of conjugated bilirubin into insoluble bilirubin fits with infection-related brown pigment stones, it does not seem to be relevant to black pigment gallstones.[165] β-Glucuronidase activity in uninfected bile has been demonstrated, providing support that enzymatic hydrolysis by β-glucuronidase (probably of epithelial cell origin) can take place without bacterial infection.[166,167] This requires another risk factor, gallbladder stasis, to be operative for precipitates of calcium bilirubinate to form.[168] Prolonged TPN has been shown to result in the formation of gallbladder sludge and black pigment stones.[149,169] Stasis, similar to the scenario described for cholesterol nucleation, can provide an opportunity for nonenzymatic hydrolysis of bilirubin diglucuronide.[170]

The gallbladder may play other contributory roles in the formation of pigment gallstones. Hepatic bile is supersaturated with calcium carbonate. The gallbladder epithelium can secrete hydrogen ion and acidify bile, resulting in calcium carbonate being undersaturated in gallbladder bile. Calcium homeostasis is intimately linked to black and brown pigment gallstones, because both kinds contain predominantly calcium bilirubinate. The inability of an inflamed gallbladder to acidify bile may be a contributing factor in producing pigment gallstones. Black and brown pigment gallstones contain a matrix of mucous glycoprotein that is secreted by the gallbladder epithelium into bile and binds to bilirubin and other hydrophobic lipids.[122]

A working hypothesis can be made of pigment gallstone formation. There is an increased excretion of bilirubin, and gallbladder stasis allows the hydrolysis of bilirubin. The inability to acidify bile by the gallbladder mucosa perturbs calcium and bilirubin solubility, and mucus secreted by the gallbladder epithelium buffers and lowers the acidity, enabling calcium carbonate, phosphate, and bilirubin to come out of solution. A complex of calcium with unconjugated bilirubin can form. For reasons poorly understood, the calcium bilirubinate in brown pigment stones remains in the monomeric form, but it undergoes significant cross-linking to become polymeric and crystalline in black pigment stones.

CLINICAL MANIFESTATIONS

Biliary Colic

Approximately one third of patients with gallstones present with clinical symptoms or complications of gallstone disease. Biliary colic is the main complaint in 70% to 80% of symptomatic patients. This is a visceral pain from tonic spasm resulting from transient obstruction of the cystic duct by a stone.[171] Implicit in the term *biliary colic* is the fact that the gallbladder mucosa does not show features of acute inflammation. The pain of biliary colic is thought to be caused by functional spasms around the obstructed cystic duct; acute cholecystitis pain is caused by gallbladder wall inflammation.

Although no pattern of abdominal pain is pathognomonic for a specific disorder, biliary pain often has specific characteristics. The pain is episodic and severe, and it is located in the epigastrium or less frequently in the right upper quadrant, left upper quadrant, the precordium, and the lower abdomen.[172,173] The pain may be precipitated by eating a large meal, but no individual dietary component is found to be a lone culprit. Pain often develops without any precipitating events.

Typically, the pain has a sudden onset, rises steeply in intensity over a 15-minute interval to a steady plateau lasting as long as 3 hours. Resolution of pain is slower than its rise. Pain lasting more than 6 hours should raise the suspicion of cholecystitis. The pain may radiate to the interscapular region or, rarely, to the right shoulder tip. Vomiting and sweating are not uncommon. The patient is usually restless and unable to find a comfortable position. Residual tenderness in the upper abdomen may persist after an attack. A diurnal rhythm, with peak pain at midnight, has been reported.[174] The interval between attacks is unpredictable and may last weeks, months, or years.

True biliary colic should be differentiated from nonspecific dyspepsia. Flatulence, pyrosis, aerophagia, vague abdominal discomfort, and fatty food intolerance are common complaints of many patients, regardless of whether they have cholelithiasis.[175,176] Whether gallstone patients experience increased distress from fatty foods is difficult to prove. Studies using blinded test meals have shown no correlation of fat content with symptoms. Moreover, quantitative ultrasonography has failed to demonstrate differences in fractional emptying of the gallbladder in response to various test meals.

The differentiation of true biliary pain from nonspecific abdominal symptoms has significant bearing on the success of a recommendation to treat gallstone disease. For example, a cholecystectomy done for gallstone-induced biliary colic is usually curative, but the result is far from gratifying if it is done for patients with cholelithiasis and nonspecific dyspepsia.[177-180] Many of these nonspecific symptoms remain after cholecystectomy or later recur. It is worthwhile to emphasize prevalent misunderstandings about biliary pain. First, biliary colic is a steady pain and not one that is intermittent with fluctuating intensity. Biliary colic is a misnomer, because the pain is not colicky. Second, the site of pain is primarily in the epigastrium. It is inappropriate to interpret pain located other than in the right upper quadrant as atypical of gallstone symptoms. Third, fat intolerance is not a feature of biliary colic. Despite the availability of many organ-imaging techniques to demonstrate the presence of gallstones, clinical judgment ultimately determines the relation of cholelithiasis to the patient's complaint.

Acute Cholecystitis

By far the most common cause of acute cholecystitis is obstruction of the cystic duct by gallstones, resulting in acute inflammation of the organ. Approximately 90% of cases are associated with cholelithiasis. In addition to the mechanical effect of distention, hydrolysis of biliary lipids such as lecithin and reabsorption of bile salts may also play a role.[181,182] Prostaglandins and other chemical mediators are involved in the evolution of inflammation.[183] Prostaglandin inhibitors such as indomethacin, when given intravenously, rapidly decrease intralumenal gallbladder pressure and the pain produced by acute cholecystitis.[184] Although it is not uncommon to find bacteria in the gallbladder bile of patients with acute cholecystitis, this is probably a secondary event.[185,186] Secondary bacterial infection can progress to empyema with or without perforation.

Acute cholecystitis can present as an acalculous disorder. Acalculous cholecystitis represents 5% to 10% of the patients with acute cholecystitis and may be increasing in frequency.[187,188] This entity is distinct from gallstone-related disease in that it usually occurs in the setting of major surgery, critical illness, extensive trauma, or burn-related injury. The patients tend to be predominantly male and older than 50 years of age.[189] Many of them are on TPN, and bile inspissation or sludge formation may occur. The pathogenesis probably involves some combination of stasis, chemical inflammation, and ischemia. Hypotension and sympathetic vasoconstriction may predispose the patient to ischemic injury as well.

Complications in acalculous cholecystitis progress more fulminantly than in calculous cholecystitis.[187,188] For this reason, it is important to suspect and pursue an early diagnosis. One retrospective study revealed that 70% of patients with acalculous cholecystitis had gangrene, empyema, or perforation of the gallbladder evident at the time of surgical exploration.[190] This increased complication rate occurring in the setting of advanced age and other illnesses contributes to the higher mortality rate associated with this disorder.

Rare causes of acute cholecystitis include specific infections, such as *Salmonella* infection.[191] This organism can colonize the gallbladder epithelium without eliciting inflammation, creating a carrier state. Cytomegalovirus and cryptosporidia can infect the biliary system and produce cholecystitis and cholangitis in severely immunocompromised patients, such as those with acquired immunodeficiency syndrome or after bone marrow transplantation.[192,193]

Most patients with acute calculous cholecystitis have had previous attacks of biliary pain. The pain of acute cholecystitis typically lasts longer than 3 hours and, at the end of 3 hours, shifts from the epigastrium to the right upper quadrant, with the emergence of localized tenderness. With time, the intensity of pain may diminish, but the tenderness increases. Vomiting is a common symptom. The sequence of clinical features represents visceral pain of ductal impaction by stones, proceeding to inflammation of the gallbladder with parietal pain. A low-grade fever of 99°F to 101°F is common, but hyperpyrexia is uncommon.

In elderly patients, pain and fever may be absent, and localized tenderness may be the only presenting sign. On physical examination, Murphy's sign may be present. This is an abrupt arrest in inspiration secondary to the pain elicited during direct palpation of the right upper quadrant. In 30% to 40% of patients, the gallbladder and perhaps adherent omentum can be perceived as a palpable mass. Jaundice occurs in approximately 15% of patients with acute cholecystitis, even without choledocholithiasis and obstruction. The pathogenesis may involve edema, swelling, and compression around the level of the impacted and inflamed cystic duct.

Chronic Cholecystitis

Patients with chronic cholecystitis usually have gallstones and have had repeated attacks of biliary pain or acute cholecystitis. This results in a thickened and fibrotic gallbladder, which on histologic examination show evaginated mucosal pouches (i.e., Rokitansky-Aschoff sinuses). It is uncommon for the gallbladder to be palpable during an attack of pain. The patient may have fewer symptoms referable to the gallbladder but may present with associated complications such as recurrent pancreatitis, choledocholithiasis, and cholangitis. Approximately 15% of patients with gallstones have concomitant stones in the common bile duct, which can lead to cholangitis and pancreatitis.

Choledocholithiasis and Cholangitis

When gallstones pass into the common bile duct from the gallbladder, they can proceed to the duodenum if the stone is small. More commonly, they remain in the common bile duct and give rise to complications. Stones in the common duct usually have the same composition as those in the gallbladder, although some are softer and more brownish because of deposits of calcium bilirubinate and other calcium salts, including fatty acid complexes, as a result of bacterial deconjugation of bilirubin and hydrolysis of phospholipids.[151] Whether clinically overt or not, common duct stones are frequently associated with infected bile.

One of the important features of choledocholithiasis is obstructive or "surgical" jaundice. There are many causes of obstructive jaundice, which must be differentiated from hepatocytic or "medical" jaundice. Obstruction of the passage of bile results in jaundice and pruritus. The pathogenesis of pruritus is unclear, although retention of bile salts with irritation of sensory nerve endings has been proposed as a mechanism. Sometimes the itching can be intense and be the predominant or incapacitating symptom. With biliary obstruction, bile and its pigments cannot enter the intestine, and the feces may be hypocholic or acholic. Light-colored or clay-colored stool is uncommon in bile duct obstruction resulting from gallstones because the obstruction is rarely complete. Clay-colored stool is more commonly observed in malignant strictures involving the common bile duct.

Obstruction of the common bile duct also gives rise to an increased pressure reflected retrograde from the site of blockage. The normal pressure in the common bile duct is 10 to 15 cm H_2O; with obstruction, the pressure can rise to above 40 cm H_2O.[194-196] This distends the biliary duct and transmits the pressure upstream, stopping bile flow and causing the reflux of bile from the canaliculus into the sinusoids. Dilatation of the extrahepatic and intrahepatic bile ducts is a valuable sign of common bile duct obstruction. This is best seen using ultrasonography or computed tomography (CT) scan. Clinically, this may only be manifested by mild hepatomegaly and right upper quadrant tenderness during an attack of cholangitis.

Unlike malignant obstruction of the common bile duct, a palpable and nontender gallbladder due to cholelithiasis is uncommon, because the obstruction is usually incomplete and the common duct stone comes from the gallbladder, which itself is likely to be a victim of chronic cholecystitis, with fibrosis and scarring rendering the organ nondistensible. The exceptions to this rule (i.e., Courvoisier's law) are substantial, with false-positive and -negative results, and should not be relied on heavily in making a clinical judgment.

With prolonged obstruction, secondary hepatic parenchymal damage sets in. This, in conjunction with increased fibrogenesis induced by bile duct obstruction, results in secondary biliary cirrhosis. The propensity for developing cirrhosis varies with the completeness and the duration of obstruction. The average time for choledocholithiasis to result in secondary biliary cirrhosis is about 5 years.[197] Patients can present with hepatic failure or portal hypertension. Patients with incomplete obstruction more commonly present with variceal bleeding, and those with complete obstruction present with hepatic decompensation.[198] Even if the patient has cirrhosis, every effort should be made to relieve the obstruction. A proportion of patients can improve remarkably after removal of obstruction; reversal of portal hypertension and secondary biliary cirrhosis have been reported.[199,200]

A common complication of choledocholithiasis is cholangitis. For bacterial infection to occur, obstruction or bile stasis always exists, although obstruction is not always associated with overt bacterial infection. For example, cholangitis is extremely common in choledocholithiasis, not uncommon in sclerosing cholangitis, and relatively uncommon (10%–15%) in malignant bile duct strictures.

The typical clinical picture, occurring in 70% of cases, consists of biliary pain, jaundice, and chills and rigors (i.e.,

Charcot's triad). Pain, usually the characteristic biliary pain involving the central upper abdomen, occurs in 90% of patients. The chills and fever due to bacteremia occur in 95% of patients. Clinical jaundice is present in 80% of cases. Clinical signs are nonspecific, with mild hepatomegaly, tenderness, and occasionally rebound tenderness.[201] Depending on the progress of the illness, endotoxemia with shock or multiple liver abscesses may result with hypotension, mental confusion, and renal failure as preterminal events. For many patients, cholangitis is a short and self-limited illness complicating choledocholithiasis or sclerosing cholangitis.

Blood cultures are often positive and reflect the organisms infecting the bile ducts. The most commonly found organisms are *E coli*, *Klebsiella*, *Pseudomonas*, and enterococci, with a 15% contribution by anaerobes.[202-204]

Acute pancreatitis may be precipitated by the passage of stones or sludge in the common bile duct, and sludge or microscopic stones may account for a significant proportion of cases of idiopathic pancreatitis.[145,205]

DIFFERENTIAL DIAGNOSIS

Clinical Signs and Symptoms

The clinical symptoms and signs of biliary tract disorders are not highly specific and can be closely mimicked by several intraabdominal and extraabdominal disorders. The patient's history, physical findings, laboratory data, and biliary tract imaging studies should be carefully examined. Because gallstones are found commonly and may coexist with other disorders, the finding of gallstones does not exclude other diseases contributing to or complicating the patient's clinical picture.

Pain arising from different organs in the abdomen may be confused with biliary colic. Gastroduodenitis with or without ulcers often produces nonspecific pain in the epigastrium. Lesions of the upper gastrointestinal tract can be diagnosed by barium x-ray studies or by endoscopy. Esophageal symptoms are often retrosternal and related to eating or regurgitation. Dysmotility-associated symptoms can be precipitated by extremes of temperature. Manometric measurements, pH monitoring, or an acid infusion test may be helpful. Renal pain from a stone or infection can be unilateral and right sided and not uncommonly felt at the anterior aspect of the abdomen instead of the costovertebral angle. Urinalysis and ultrasonography can aid in these diagnoses.

Colonic pain due to functional spasm (e.g., irritable bowel syndrome) should be differentiated from biliary colic. Unlike the constant nature of biliary pain, irritable bowel syndrome produces a true colicky pain. Although it is essentially a diagnosis of exclusion, certain features are highly suggestive, including an absence of symptoms during sleep, alteration in bowel habits (e.g., diarrhea, constipation), and lack of systemic toxicity. Colonic diverticulitis and carcinomas may present with pain exacerbated by eating and may mimic biliary symptoms. Other causes of upper abdominal pain that can be confused with biliary colic include angina pectoris, dissecting (or partially dissected) aortic aneurysm, spinal neuralgia, pleuritis, pericarditis, and uncommon metabolic disorders such a Cl esterase inhibitor deficiency (i.e., hereditary angioedema) and acute intermittent porphyria.

In addition to pain, patients with acute cholecystitis usually present with symptoms and signs of local inflammation (e.g., right upper quadrant mass, tenderness) and systemic toxicity (e.g., fever, leukocytosis). The differential diagnosis includes other causes of intraabdominal inflammation or infection. Acute appendicitis can cause a difficult diagnostic problem. The periumbilical pain shifting to the right lower quadrant with the presence of an inflamed mass may be confused with biliary colic associated with an inflamed gallbladder. A gallbladder can be low lying or an appendix can be subhepatic. Fever and leukocytosis are shared by both. Ultrasonography is usually able to identify whether the acutely inflamed organ is the gallbladder or the appendix. Biliary scintigraphy is also helpful.

It may be difficult to differentiate acute pancreatitis from cholecystitis because the two conditions produce tenderness in an overlapping area. Although acute cholecystitis alone can be associated with hyperamylasemia, pancreatitis often has higher enzyme levels. Biliary scintiscan and organ-imaging techniques such as ultrasound and CT scans are helpful diagnostically. Acute pancreatitis can be caused by gallstones, and cholecystitis and pancreatitis therefore may coexist.

Perforated peptic ulcer usually produces more dramatic pain and peritoneal signs. Plain abdominal x-ray films often show free intraabdominal air. If free air cannot be visualized and ulcer perforation is still suspected, an urgent Gastrograffin study should demonstrate the perforation.

Diagnostic Studies

Laboratory Tests

In uncomplicated biliary colic, there are usually no accompanying changes in hematologic and biochemical tests. In acute cholecystitis, leukocytosis with a "left shift" is usually observed. However, this is a nonspecific response and does not differentiate acute cholecystitis from other intraabdominal infections. The amylase level may be elevated because of transient obstruction of the pancreatic duct by a common duct stone. Edema and inflammation of the gallbladder can partially obstruct the common bile duct, causing mild elevation of the serum transaminases and alkaline phosphatase. Elevation of serum bilirubin can also be associated with the enzyme level changes, especially if the common hepatic duct or common bile duct is involved in the inflammatory reaction because of impaction of the cystic duct. Bilirubin elevation is proportional to the degree of obstruction. Alkaline phosphatase, however, is produced by bile canalicular and ductular cells, and its elevation does not depend on the magnitude or cause of obstruction.

Abdominal pain, fever, and jaundice are often the presenting features of choledocholithiasis. In such case, the bilirubin level is usually between 2 and 10 mg/dL, and the alkaline phosphatase level is less than five times normal. If the level of bilirubin is above 15 mg/dL, a neoplastic obstruction should be strongly suspected. If ductal dilatation is documented by ultrasonography or CT scans, a cholangiogram should be obtained to define the cause and level of obstruction.

Radiologic Studies

Plain abdominal films are often performed. They are rarely useful in biliary colic, because only 13% to 17% of gallstones contain sufficient calcium to be radiopaque. In acute cholecystitis, x-ray films are obtained to exclude other intraabdominal causes of abdominal pain associated with fever and leukocytosis, such as perforated ulcer or intestinal obstruction. Occasionally, when emphysematous cholecystitis is present, intramural gas outlining the gallbladder can be seen, but this is better shown using ultrasonography.

Ultrasonography has high specificity and sensitivity for the diagnosis of gallstones and should be a routine examination for confirmation or exclusion of gallstone disease. Findings include thickening of the gallbladder wall (>2 mm), intramural gas, and a pericholecystic collection of fluid. The latter two suggest active gallbladder inflammation or infection. The significance of the finding of sludge in the gallbladder is less clear. Sludge is common in extrahepatic biliary obstruction. In the absence of distal obstruction, sludge can be associated with abdominal pain (i.e., biliary colic), acute cholecystitis, or pancreatitis and should be regarded as part of the spectrum of gallstone disease.[146,147] Ultrasound scans may indicate dilatation of intrahepatic or extrahepatic bile ducts, highly suggestive of distal obstruction. However, with choledocholithiasis, the absence of sonographic demonstration of a stone does not exclude such a diagnosis.[206,207]

Hepatobiliary scintigraphy can confirm or exclude the diagnosis of acute cholecystitis with a high degree of sensitivity and specificity. After a 2- to 4-hour fast, the patient is given an intravenous injection of a ^{99m}Tc-labeled iminodiacetic acid derivative (IDA agent), which is excreted into the bile ducts and is sequentially imaged under a gamma camera. Several ^{99m}Tc-IDA compounds have been developed and differ with respect to their degree of hepatic uptake and time to reach a peak concentration in the bile.

In a normal study, images of the gallbladder, common bile duct, and small bowel appear by 30 to 45 minutes (Fig. 96-3). A normal ^{99m}Tc-IDA scan virtually rules out the diagnosis of acute cholecystitis in a patient who presents with abdominal pain. False-negative studies can occur for patients with acalculous cholecystitis. However, this is a relatively rare occurrence, because the gallbladders of most patients with this entity cannot be visualized, partly because of the edema and inflammatory changes of the cystic duct.

Failure to image the gallbladder by 90 minutes despite adequate views of the liver, common bile duct, and small bowel strongly suggests acute obstructive disease (Fig. 96-4). False positives can result from nonfasting or prolonged fasting states. Long-term fasting in a patient on TPN can lead to gallbladder stasis and poor filling. Chronic alcoholism and chronic cholecystitis are other causes of false-positive results. Delayed repeat scanning after 4 or more hours decreases the false-positive rate and provides sensitivity and specificity values of approximately 97% and 90%, respectively. Administration of low-dose morphine to augment biliary images at 1 hour may obviate the need for delayed repeat scans in certain cir-

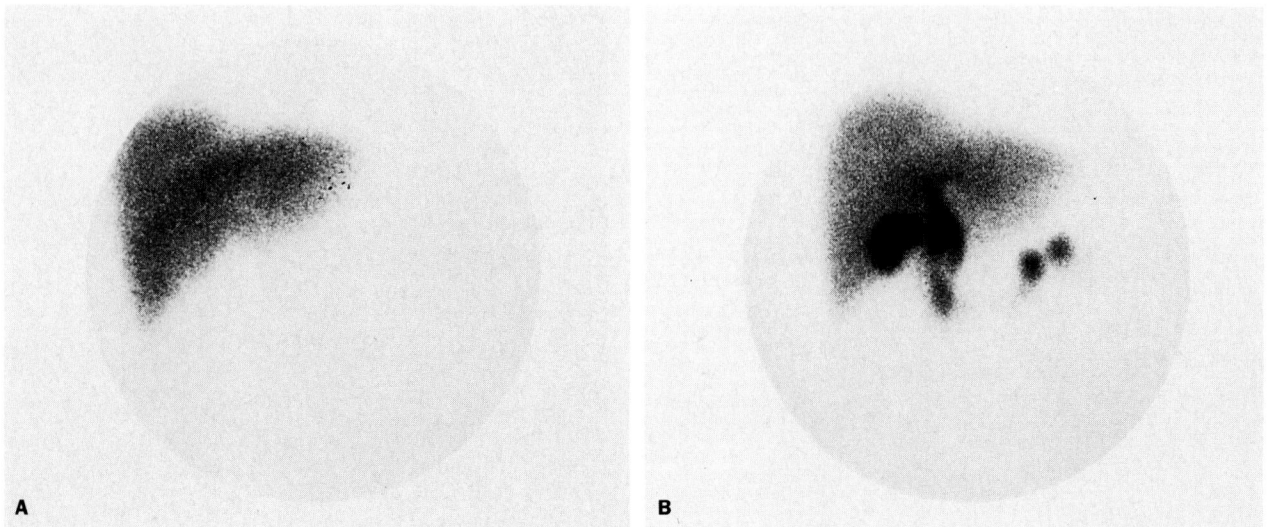

FIGURE 96-3. ⁹⁹Tc-iminodiacetic acid scintigraphy, normal result. **(A)** Homogeneous hepatic uptake occurs within 5 minutes. **(B)** At 15 minutes, the gallbladder, common bile duct, and some small bowel can be seen. (Courtesy of Arnold Jacobson, M.D.).

cumstances. There is evidence that morphine enhances filling of the cystic duct by increasing common bile duct pressure by means of contraction of the sphincter of Oddi. Cholescintigraphy cannot provide anatomic information and cannot directly identify gallstones.

Oral cholecystography is seldom employed as a primary diagnostic test for the detection of gallstones or acute cholecystitis. However, there has been a resurgence in the use of the oral cholecystogram for the selection of patients for nonsurgical treatment of gallstone disease, such as lithotripsy or bile acid dissolution therapy. The study involves the administration of oral contrast tablets such as iopanoic acid the night before. The contrast is absorbed in the small bowel,

conjugated in the liver, excreted into the canaliculi, and concentrated within the gallbladder (Figs. 96-5 and 96-6). Extrabiliary conditions such as gastric retention, pancreatitis, small bowel diseases, hepatic dysfunction, or prolonged fasting can all lead to gallbladder nonvisualization in the absence of primary disease.[208–210] Inadequate gallbladder visualization can occur in 15% to 50% of patients given a single dose of contrast. For this reason, some radiologists use two consecutive doses of contrast the evening before the study. The chief advantage of oral cholecystography over ultrasound is its ability to assess the patency of the cystic duct and gallbladder function. Moreover, the size and number of stones present and whether they are calcified can be accurately determined.

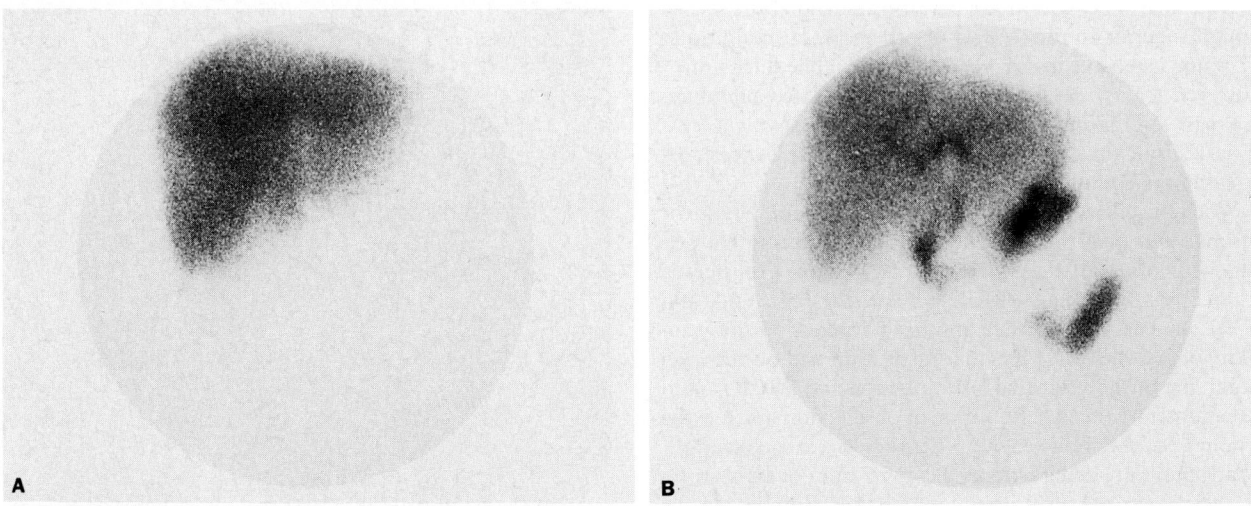

FIGURE 96-4. ⁹⁹Tc-iminodiacetic acid scintigraphy, abnormal result. **(A)** The 5-minute scan demonstrates normal liver uptake. **(B)** Failure to visualize the gallbladder by 90 minutes with adequate imaging of the liver, common duct, and small bowel is consistent with the diagnosis of acute cholecystitis. (Courtesy of Arnold Jacobson, M.D., Seattle, WA.)

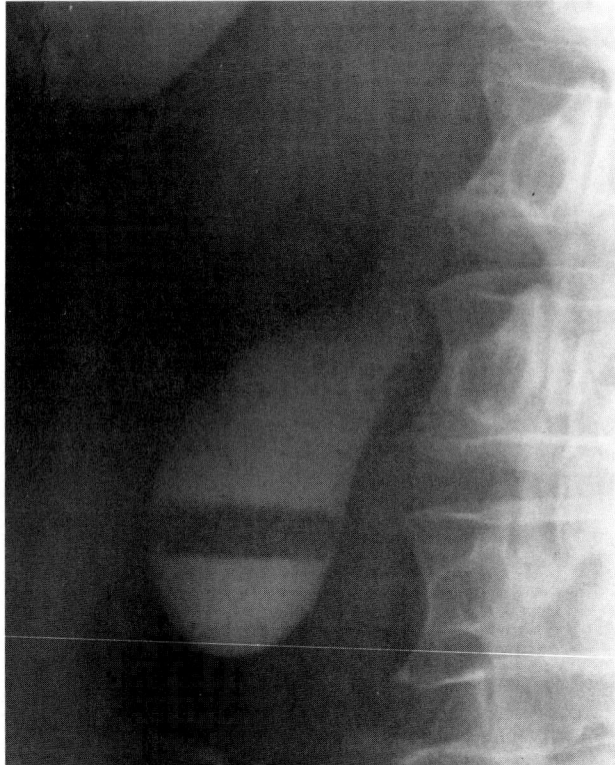

FIGURE 96-5. Oral cholecystogram with the patient in the upright position shows multiple floating gallstones layered within the gallbladder.

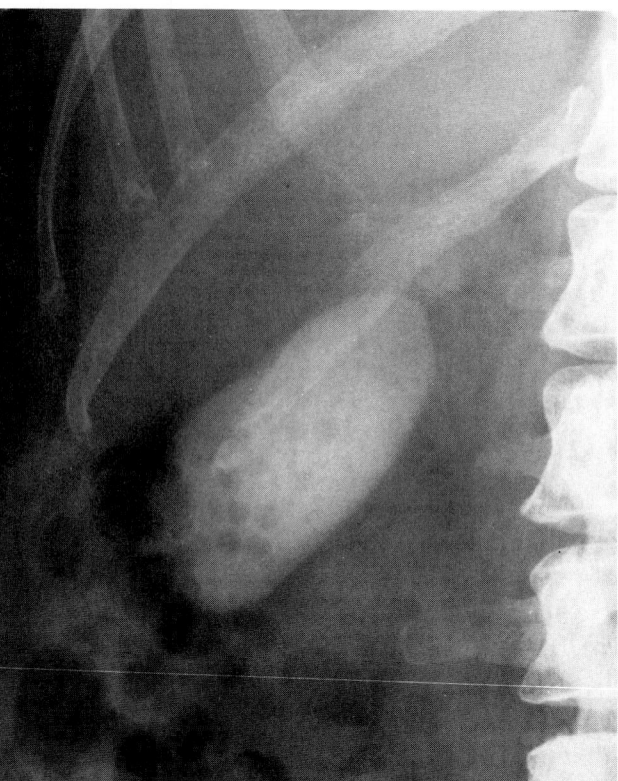

FIGURE 96-6. Several small stones are seen within an opacified gallbladder by oral cholecystography.

Intravenous cholangiography is rarely used except if liver function is normal, endoscopic retrograde cholangiopancreatography (ERCP) is technically unattainable, and percutaneous transhepatic cholangiography is undesirable. It can be combined with tomography to show the extrahepatic bile ducts.

CT can also be used in the detection of cholelithiasis. Although superior to ultrasound in other clinical conditions, CT is not as reliable in diagnosing common bile duct stones. However, CT is useful in demonstrating dilated bile ducts and mass lesions and can be considered the test of choice if clinical suspicion of a tumor (e.g., pancreatic cancer) obstructing the common bile duct is strong.

When the biliary system has to be visualized for diagnostic reasons or to plan therapy, cholangiography through a percutaneous transhepatic puncture or by way of a retrograde endoscopic route (e.g., ERCP) is required (Figs. 96-7 and 96-8). The selection of either approach depends on the availability of facilities at a particular institution and on the level and nature of the suspected lesion. In general, ERCP is used to demonstrate the lower limit of an obstruction and has the advantage of the ability to sample tissue. Percutaneous transhepatic puncture demonstrates the upper limit of an obstructive lesion or a proximal obstruction better. Both tests have a risk of introducing infection in the presence of obstruction. With the availability of many tests, the challenge to the clinician is to avoid using unnecessary or redundant investigations, which can be costly.

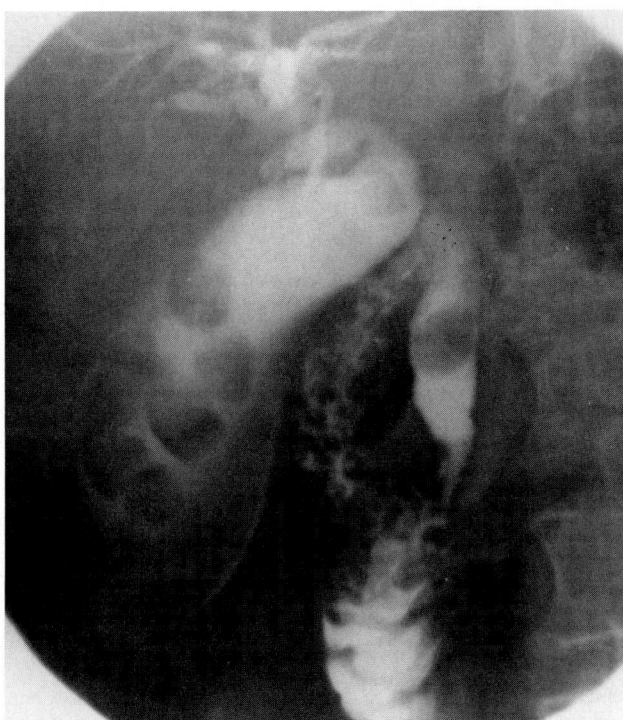

FIGURE 96-7. Endoscopic retrograde cholangiogram shows stones within the gallbladder and common duct.

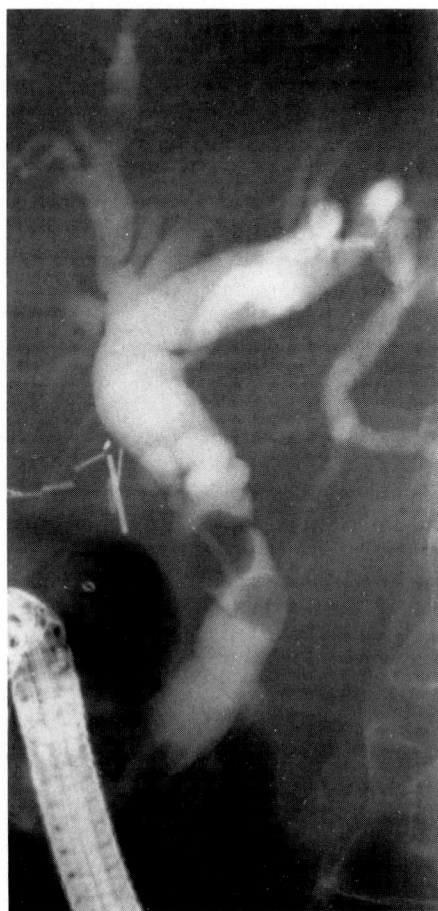

FIGURE 96-8. Endoscopic retrograde cholangiopancreatography shows a stone within a dilated common duct, with an inflated balloon catheter proximal to it. The surgical clips mark the site of a previous cholecystectomy.

CLINICAL COURSE AND COMPLICATIONS

Natural History of Asymptomatic Gallstones

It is estimated that 60% to 80% of all gallstones are asymptomatic at a given time.[28,29] The rate with which gallstones develop varies. In Pima Indians, the progression from cholesterol supersaturated bile to formation of gallstones occurs in 5 to 10 years.[211] In patients on TPN or obese persons with rapid weight loss, the interval can be weeks. When gallstones do form, the risk factors giving rise to symptoms are unknown. However, the propensity of asymptomatic stones to give rise to pain and complications is relatively small. In contrast, once gallstones start to cause biliary-specific symptoms, the risk of continuing problems is relatively high.

Studies by Wenckert and Robertson[212] and Lund[213] followed a total of 1307 patients with gallstones as long as 20 years and concluded that 50% of patients remained asymptomatic, 30% had biliary colic, and 20% had complications. Such data have been cited by advocates of prophylactic cholecystectomy for all patients found to have gallstones, re-

gardless of the severity of their symptoms. However, these patients, although asymptomatic at the time of entry to the follow-up study, had previously been hospitalized for symptoms related to gallbladder disease.

Gracie and colleagues followed a cohort of 123 asymptomatic persons with gallstones found by oral cholecystography, which opacified the gallbladder in 108 persons (88%).[214] These 110 men and 13 women (average age, 54 years) were followed for 11 to 24 years. New-onset biliary pain developed at a rate of 2% per year for the first 5 years, but the cumulative incidence plotted against time plateaued such that, at 10 years, the total incidence was 15%, and at 15 and 20 years, it was 18%. Three patients (2%) developed complications, all preceded by repeated attacks of biliary colic, and all had uneventful cholecystectomies. No deaths related to gallbladder disease occurred in this group of patients with asymptomatic gallstones.

A 20-year population-based survey of mortality in Pima Indians with and without gallstones was reported. The overall death rate was higher in those with a history of gallstones, with an age- and sex-adjusted death rate ratio of 1.9. The death rate attributed to malignancies was 6.6 times higher in those with gallstones. Among the 20 fatal malignancies in patients with gallstones, 11 were gastrointestinal tract cancers, six of which were malignancies of the gallbladder or bile ducts.[215]

This study highlights the question of whether a link between gallstones and malignancies exists. A statistical association between colon cancer and gallstones has been reported, although this more likely represents selection bias because patients with colon cancer have a greater likelihood of having their gallbladders evaluated.[216] Higher rates of gallbladder carcinoma or carcinoma of the extrahepatic bile ducts in patients with gallstones have been found in an autopsy series and in a case-control study.[217,218] This issue deserves further study.

Natural History of Symptomatic Gallstones

Once an episode of biliary colic has occurred, there is a high risk of repeated attacks of pain. Cohort studies that followed symptomatic gallstone patients indicated that 58% to 72% of patients continued to have symptoms and complications.[213,219,220] More than 90% of complications, such as cholecystitis, are preceded by attacks of pain. Gallstone-involved cholangitis and pancreatitis also usually occurred in patients with a history of biliary colic. The most serious complications are gangrene and perforation of the gallbladder. These occur in about 10% of cases of acute cholecystitis. Acalculous cholecystitis alone accounts for as many as 40% of gallbladder perforations.

When the gallbladder is perforated, the outcome depends on the anatomic relation with the neighboring structures. It can localize to form an abscess; it can be a free perforation with peritonitis; or it can communicate with another hollow viscus as a fistula.

A localized perforation with confined spillage sealed off by omentum wrapping around the inflamed organ and by firmly adherent adjacent viscera is the most common form of perforation. A pericholecystic abscess is formed. This should be suspected when acute cholecystitis is slow to resolve, especially with a second episode of elevation in temperature, right-sided abdominal pain, and the appearance of a right upper abdominal mass. Ultrasonography and CT may show the pericholecystic abscess, but this is not dependable, and the diagnosis should be made with a high degree of clinical suspicion and should be confirmed at surgery. This is especially so in elderly patients or patients on long-term steroid treatment in whom pyrexia and the local inflammatory response may be minimal.

In 1% to 2% of perforations, especially in the fundus of the gallbladder, free perforation occurs and is associated with a mortality rate of at least 30%. Bile and purulent peritonitis are almost always associated with persistent or progressive abdominal pain. When the suspicion is raised, no test can establish the diagnosis without further delaying intervention and causing additional tissue injury. Antibiotics should be given and emergency surgery performed.

When the gallbladder perforates into the adjacent intestine, an attack of acute cholecystitis often subsides. The inflamed organ is decompressed with this spontaneous drainage. The duodenum, hepatic flexure of the colon, stomach, and the jejunum are the sites of the cholecystoenteric fistula, in descending order of frequency. If the gallstones are completely discharged and the stones are small enough to pass rectally, an uncomplicated cholecystoenteric fistula results. However, if stones are still present in the gallbladder or in the common bile duct, chronic symptoms arise.

When a fistula develops and the gallstone is too large to travel through the intestine, it causes obstruction. In such cases, the diameter of the stone is greater than 2.5 cm and the site of obstruction is usually in the small intestine, with the ileocecal valve being the most common site. Gallstone ileus sometimes has a prior history of acute cholecystitis, but most of the stones erode slowly through the gallbladder, and especially in the elderly, symptoms may be minimal. Gallstone ileus should always be considered in a patient older than 65 years of age with intestinal obstruction.[221,222] Plain abdominal x-ray films may show air in the biliary tree, and barium studies often reveal the site of communication. Oral cholecystograms do not opacify the gallbladder. Ultrasound scans can detect remnant or migrated air in the biliary tree but not the site of the fistula. CT scans are less useful in detecting gallstones and fistulas, although they may show air in the biliary tree.

TREATMENT

Because gallstones are common and not everyone with them suffers, the treatment of gallstones should consider the patient's symptoms. For asymptomatic gallstones, before active treatment is instituted, the following ideas should be considered. What is the propensity with which new-onset symptoms emerge from the group of asymptomatic patients? If symptoms develop, what is the risk of these evolving to complications, and what is the risk of morbidity and mortality from such complications? What is the risk of prophylactic treatment, such as elective cholecystectomy? What are the short- and long-term costs of prophylactic treatment compared with no or delayed treatment?

The fractional and cumulative risk of developing symptoms is not great (2%–4%/year; <20% up to 20 years). Complications develop after the emergence of symptoms. Neither the evolution to complications after the onset of symptoms nor their treatment carries a mortality rate higher than the similar subsets of patients with established or chronic symptoms. There is no disadvantage in terms of morbidity or mortality in not treating the patient prophylactically. Open cholecystectomy is a safe procedure with a mortality rate of 0.1% to 0.2%.[223,224] The surgical mortality rate of 0.9% to 1.8% is higher for patients older than 60 years of age.[225,226] When the common bile duct is explored, the mortality rate is approximately two to three times higher.

Risk-benefit analyses of elective cholecystectomy have shown no advantage to aggressive prophylactic cholecystectomy for asymptomatic gallstone patients. This is significant considering the number of persons with asymptomatic gallstones, because the cost of screening and prophylactic treatment would be overwhelming.

In certain subsets of patients, it may be prudent to make exceptions and proceed with a prophylactic cholecystectomy. These groups include children with gallstones, patients with sickle cell disease and gallstones, and the morbidly obese.[227,228] In the latter group, a cholecystectomy is recommended at the time of gastric bypass if the primary operation is indicated.[229] Patients who are on large doses of corticosteroids on a long-term basis often have subdued symptoms of pain or fever, even when acute cholecystitis or perforation is imminent. Sepsis is common and difficult to control. A calcified or "porcelain" gallbladder is associated with a higher risk of cancer.[230,231] There is also agreement that if gallstones are associated with choledocholithiasis, even when they are not producing symptoms, surgery should be performed. This is reinforced by postmortem studies, which showed, even in asymptomatic patients, ductal stones contributed significantly to death.[232,233]

Patients with diabetes mellitus have an increased operative risk with elective and emergency cholecystectomy, largely because of concomitant cardiovascular disease.[234,235] Prophylactic cholecystectomy in diabetic persons is not recommended.

Symptomatic gallstones should be treated. The treatment options are to operate, to dissolve, or to fragment symptomatic gallstones.

Surgical Treatment

Cholecystectomy is the only definitive treatment. Elective cholecystectomy is usually simple, safe, and curative; is indicated for most patients with symptoms; and is the first and most overriding choice when complications ensue. For example, in recurrent acute cholecystitis or cholangitis, there must be compelling reason not to select surgery as the treatment of choice. Nonsurgical modalities of treatment are still experimental.

Not all cholecystectomies are done for cholelithiasis. For example, it may be part of a more formidable operation for pancreatic cancer or bypass of a malignant obstruction. Reports of surgical mortality for cholecystectomy that fail to differentiate the indication for the operation overestimate the mortality rate for cholecystectomy for gallstone disease. The published gross mortality rates for cholecystectomy have been reviewed.[223–225] Age is not a contraindication to surgery, but increased risks are encountered in patients with cardiovascular disease and cirrhosis of the liver. Open cholecystectomy has been performed in pregnant patients without fetal loss.[236] Cholecystectomy relieves true biliary colic. The long-term response of dyspepsia to such an operation is unpredictable, and therefore nonspecific abdominal symptoms are not an adequate justification for surgery.

Laparoscopic Cholecystectomy

In 1901, Georg Kelling reported laparoscopic examination of the abdominal cavity using a cystoscope in a dog in a procedure he called celioscopy.[237] Experience in humans with the procedure was sporadic, although technical advances, such as the Veress needle for inducing pneumoperitoneum that was introduced in 1938 and is still in use today, accumulated.[238] Laparoscopic techniques were first routinely incorporated into surgical practice by gynecologists, and it wasn't until the introduction of videolaparoscopy in the 1980s that general surgeons began to use the technique to perform cholecystectomies.[239]

Laparoscopic cholecystectomy was first performed in France in 1987.[240,241] In subsequent years, the procedure has gained remarkably rapid widespread use and acceptance in Europe and the United States, and it has become the standard of care for the treatment of acute and chronic cholecystitis. Results for more than 5000 patients have been published (Table 96-4).[242] There have been few randomized, controlled trials comparing laparoscopic with open cholecystectomy.[243] This has resulted in part from the rapid acceptance of the procedure by patients and physicians. Retrospective comparative studies have shown that laparoscopic cholecystomy produced fewer complications, shorter hospital stays, more rapid returns to normal activities and work, and minimal use of postoperative analgesia.[244,245]

The technique involves general anesthesia with endotracheal intubation. Instruments for open laparotomy are kept close at hand. A pneumoperitoneum is established, and the laparoscope with video camera attached is inserted through an umbilical incision. Accessory trocars and cannulas are inserted through separate sites. The gallbladder, cystic duct, and artery are identified. An intraoperative cholangiogram can be performed by cannulation of the gallbladder or the cystic duct; this allows the detection of common bile duct stones and delineation of the ductal anatomy. The blood supply to the gallbladder is identified and controlled, and then the cystic duct is ligated. The gallbladder is dissected from the underlying liver bed, using electrocautery or laser energy. The gallbladder is removed through the incision site, and the stones may need to be mechanically crushed within the gallbladder before removal. Stones spilled into the peritoneal cavity are retrieved.[246,247]

Greater experience with the technique has led to successful outcomes in a variety of patients. The primary indication for laparoscopic cholecystectomy is identical to that for open cholecystectomy: symptomatic cholelithiasis. Absolute contraindications include an inability to tolerate general anesthesia, scarring or inflammation that precludes access to gall-bladder using the transperitoneal approach, diffuse peritonitis, and pregnancy. The procedure has been successfully performed in anticoagulated patients, obese patients, and children.[248–250]

Examination of the results of the trial with the largest number of patients illustrates the pertinent features of the procedure. An analysis of 1518 laparoscopic cholecystectomies performed at academic and private hospitals was published.[251] In 4.7% of the patients, the procedure was converted to open cholecystectomy, most often because of difficulties in identifying anatomy secondary to inflammation or to bile duct injury.

Complications, defined as any problem that resulted in delayed discharge, undesired change in therapy, readmission, biliary injury or leakage, infection, hemorrhage, or conversion to open cholecystectomy, occurred in 5.1% of cases overall, with superficial wound infection the most common. Injuries to the common bile duct or the hepatic duct occurred at a rate of 0.5%; significantly, the rate of bile duct injury was higher early in a given surgeon's experience with the procedure. This latter finding has been borne out by a similar experience in other groups, illustrating the steep learning curve associated with the procedure. The mean hospital stay was 1.2 days, with a range of 6 hours to 30 days.

Of the 1518 patients undergoing laparoscopic cholecystectomies, 96.5% had ultrasound examinations before surgery to document cholelithiasis, and preoperative cholangiography was performed in 4.2% of patients. Laser dissection was used in 29% of cases, with electrocautery used in the remainder. Intraoperative cholangiography was used routinely by some surgeons and selectively or not at all by others. Intraoperative cholangiograms were obtained in 29.3% of patients, with a failure rate of 23.3%. One patient died.

These results bring up certain issues that merit further elaboration. Although laparoscopic cholecystectomy has been performed successfully in acute cholecystitis, this group of patients has a higher incidence of common bile duct stones, and the procedure is technically more difficult and often lasts longer.[252] Intraoperative cholangiograms may be more difficult to obtain in this setting.

There is debate about the frequency of operative cholangiography. Some argue for routine operative cholangiography to look for unsuspected common bile duct stones and to identify ductal anatomy, anomalies, and injuries. The discovery of bile duct injuries at the primary operation with immediate repair is imperative. Variant anatomy can be clarified before cystic duct ligation.[253–255] The use of fluoroscopy in conjunction with cholangiography can save time when compared with traditional intraoperative cholangiographic methods.[256] Others argue for a more selective approach. Preoperative clinical and ultrasonographic assessment can be used to predict the likelihood of common duct stones. A history of jaundice or pancreatitis, dilated common bile ducts on ultrasound, and elevated levels of bilirubin, aspartate aminotransferase, or alkaline phosphatase can be used as an indication for preoperative ERCP with sphincterotomy to clear the common bile duct if stones are found. Routine preoperative ERCP, however, is not justifiable. Minimally elevated liver function tests or a mildly dilated common bile duct can be evaluated with an intraoperative cholangiogram.[244,257,258] A third approach, reported in Europe, uses routine preoperative intra-

TABLE 96-4
Laparoscopic Cholecystectomy: Summary of Selected Results

REFERENCE	NUMBER OF PATIENTS	PATIENTS (%) WITH COMPLICATIONS	BILE DUCT INJURIES	CHOLANGIOGRAMS*				NUMBER OF DEATHS	CONVERSION TO LAPAROTOMY (%)
				PREOPERATIVE IVC	PREOPERATIVE ERCP	INTRAOPERATIVE	POSTOPERATIVE ERCP		
325	160	10 (6)	0	0			3 (0)*	0	7 (4)
326	100	4 (4)	1	0		8 (0)*	2 (1)*	0	4 (4)
327	60	3 (5)	0	0				0	0
241	39	2 (6)	0	100 (0)*				0	4 (11)
328	100	2 (2)	2	0	2 (1)*	31 (2)*	2 (2)*	0	5 (5)
251	1518	78 (5)	7	0	64 (10)*	443*	14 (14)*	1	72 (5)
329	195	7 (4)	2	0	10 (5)*	129 (2)*	1 (0)*	0	3 (2)
244	280	8 (3)	0	0	18*	150 (19)*	3 (3)*	0	14 (5)
330	162	3 (2)	0	0	43 (10)*	76 (4)*	2 (1)*	0	2 (1)
331	270	11 (4)	1	0		140*		0	26 (10)
332	210	7 (3)	0	1	27 (0)*	1 (0)*	1 (1)*	0	4 (2)
333	155	4 (3)	1	0	2 (2)*	45 (2)*	3 (0)*	0	8 (5)
253	364		1	0	20 (8)*	150 (6)*	15 (9)*	0	20 (5)
334	375	2 (0.5)	2	0		141 (5)*	6 (6)*	1	20 (5)
259	100	2 (2)	1	100 (9)*	9 (8)*	52 (1)*	1 (0)*	0	0
257	200	11 (6)	0	0	5 (3)*	39 (0)*	7 (5)*	0	5 (3)
Total	4288	154 (4)	18 (0.4%)	201	200	1405	57	2 (0.05%)	194 (5)

ERCP, endoscopic retrograde cholangiopancreatography; IVC, intravenous cholangiogram.

* Number of cholangiograms demonstrating common bile duct stones.

Adapted from Holohan TV. Laparoscopic cholecystectomy. Lancet 1991;338:801.

venous cholangiography; this procedure is seldom used in the United States.[259]

If unsuspected choledocholithiasis is discovered intraoperatively, several options are available. The surgeon may convert to an open procedure and carry out a common bile duct exploration. Laparoscopic transcystic bile duct exploration uses guidewires, catheters, and dilators to remove common duct stones. Endoscopic transcystic bile duct exploration involves direct visualization of the common bile duct stone with a flexible laparoscopic choledochoscope.[260] Laparoscopic transcystic lithotripsy can be used to apply shock waves to the common duct stone, with subsequent removal of fragments with a basket.[261] An ERCP with sphincterotomy may be performed postoperatively. The modalities of therapy in this area are evolving rapidly, and it is not yet clear which of these techniques will prove most efficacious and cost effective.

A serious direct complication of laparoscopic cholecystectomy is injury to the common bile or hepatic ducts. This may result from misidentification of the common duct for the cystic duct, resection of part of the common and hepatic ducts, and associated right hepatic arterial injury. Excessive use of cautery or laser in the region of the common duct can result in biliary strictures.[262] In one report, five of six biliary duct injuries were attributed to the use of laser in dissecting the area of Calot's triangle.[263] However, other reports have not substantiated this association. Some reports have indicated that the rate of bile duct injury with laparoscopic cholecystectomy is significantly greater than that reported for open cholecystectomy. In one report, 17 (2.9%) of 597 patients sustained bile duct injury, with 7 of these patients requiring surgery for repair of those injuries.[264] In contrast, biliary tract injuries are estimated to occur in 0.25% to 0.5% of open cholecystectomies.[265]

Conversion to an open cholecystectomy should be undertaken if inadequate visualization of the operative field due to hemorrhage, inflammation, or variant anatomy is encountered. This represents sound surgical judgment, and may prevent a complication from occurring. Risk factors for bile duct injury include scarring from prior surgery, acute cholecystitis, and obesity; in these patients, especially, there should be a low threshold for conversion to open cholecystectomy.[266]

Bile duct injury leads to two clinical manifestations: bile leakage into the peritoneum, with resulting bile peritonitis and abdominal pain, and biliary obstruction due to partial or complete hepatic or common duct ligation or to late onset stricture. Patients can present 3 to 7 days after surgery with fever, abdominal pain, anorexia, ileus, ascites, nausea, or jaundice. Cholescintigraphy using ^{99m}Tc-IDA can be used to diagnose bile leakage and may show activity in the right paracolic gutter.[267,268] ERCP can be used to make the diagnosis; endoscopic stent insertion with prophylactic stent replacement can be performed for common bile duct strictures.[269] Surgical repair may be necessary in some patients.[270]

The observation that most serious complications occur early in a surgeon's experience with the procedure highlights the importance of proper training and credentialing. Training involving hands-on animal laboratories, preceptorships, and a probationary period have been suggested as elements of a thorough training program.[271] Training in laparoscopic techniques is being incorporated in surgical residency programs.[272]

The cost effectiveness of laparoscopy has been examined. Although the direct operating room and recovery room costs were higher for laparoscopic cholecystectomy, the shortened length of hospital stay led to a net savings.[273,274] Not all such studies have demonstrated a cost savings, however.[244]

Laparoscopic cholecystectomy is a technically better and improved way of removing the gallbladder in uncomplicated cholelithiasis. Although it may be a technical improvement compared with an open operation, laparoscopic cholecystectomy should not alter the indications for removing a gallbladder containing stones. In complicated cases, including infection and obstructive jaundice, adjunctive procedures such as ERCP must be considered. The surgeon should readily convert a laparoscopic operation to an open procedure. A conversion should never be viewed as a failure.

Endoscopic Treatment

Stones may be removed from the common bile duct by means of ERCP with sphincterotomy. In the postoperative period, endoscopic and radiographic techniques may be used to extract stones through a T-tube tract. Transhepatic stone extraction using a choledochoscope can be used. In all of these modalities, the gallbladder is left in situ, allowing the possibility of recurrent stone formation.

Medical Dissolution

Oral Bile Acid Litholysis

Two bile acids, chenodeoxycholic acid ($3\alpha,7\alpha$-dihydrocholanoic acid; CDCA) and its 7β epimer ($3\alpha,7\beta$ dihydroxycholanoic acid), ursodeoxycholic acid (UDCA), have been used.[275-291] The mechanism of action of these two bile acids in gallstone dissolution is the secretion of undersaturated hepatic bile, not an increased absolute amount of bile acid secreted into bile. The biologic effect of administration of CDCA and UDCA includes suppression of de novo hepatic cholesterol synthesis by inhibiting hydroxymethylglutaryl-CoA reductase and by enhancing the activity of 7α-hydroxylase, which leads to an increase in the synthesis of bile acid.[292-294] Intestinal absorption or reabsorption of cholesterol is down-regulated.[295] By at least one of these mechanisms, unsaturated bile is secreted and cholesterol gallstones dissolved.

The proper selection of patients is a main factor affecting the success of bile acid therapy. The selection criteria include gallstones predominantly consisting of cholesterol; pigment stones or calcified stones are excluded. Small stones that are buoyant in an oral cholecystogram examination have a 90% chance of dissolution. Stones should have a large surface area in relation to the mass, and those with a diameter larger than 1.5 cm are not suitable. Because the teratogenic effect of bile acids is unknown, pregnant women or women unprotected from pregnancy should be excluded. The gallbladder should opacify and empty in response to a fatty meal or cholecystokinin infusion. Obesity, hyperlipidemia, and liver disease are contraindications to CDCA therapy.

When partial dissolution is classified as a therapeutic success, the success rate is 60% to 70%. The use of CDCA is accompanied by several side effects. Elevation of serum aminotransferases up to two times the upper limits of normal occurs in 15% to 19% of patients. However, no clinical evidence of serious or permanent liver damage has been reported. CDCA increases total serum cholesterol in some patients. The increase is in the low-density lipoprotein. This can be worrisome, because a proportion of patients with gallstones are already obese, and further increases in serum lipids can potentially increase the risk of atherosclerotic cardiovascular disease. Another frequently encountered side effect of CDCA is watery diarrhea, which occurs in 50% of patients receiving 750 mg/day. Diarrhea usually decreases or stops after reduction of the dose.

UDCA is the major bile acid in Himalayan black bear bile. It can dissolve gallstones with a success rate comparable to CDCA. When reported trials are analyzed, UDCA dissolution tends to be faster and has a higher incidence of successful complete dissolution. The patient selection criteria are similar to those of CDCA, except that obese persons and patients with liver disease are not excluded. UDCA is much more hydrophilic than CDCA. This accounts for the difference in mechanism of gallstone dissolution and in the striking differences in side effects. UDCA is a remarkably safe compound. The side effects caused by CDCA have not been found with UDCA, which has been shown to improve symptoms of cholestasis and biochemical tests in patients with chronic liver diseases, such as primary biliary cirrhosis, chronic active hepatitis, and sclerosing cholangitis.[296-298] UDCA is used in the range of 8 to 12 mg/kg/day. Because of the improved efficacy and safety profile, UDCA has superseded CDCA in cases for which oral bile acids are considered. The use of oral bile acids has been reviewed.[299]

Contact Solvents

When gallstones can be accessed by a catheter, solvents can be delivered directly to dissolve the stones. Several cholesterol solvents are available, although none is a simple, safe, and effective method of treating gallstones. Cholic acid and mono-octanoin have been used to dissolve gallstones, especially cholesterol gallstones in the common bile duct.

The treatment procedure requires several weeks and is associated with substantial side effects. Mono-octanoin, a monoglyceride, has a high in-vitro capacity to dissolve cholesterol.[300] Its clinical use, however, is limited by its high viscosity and low efficiency. It usually takes 1 to 3 weeks to achieve successful dissolution, and the results have not always been consistent.[301] D-Limonene, a terpene extract from plants, has been shown to be effective and safe in dissolving gallstones and retained bile duct stones.[302] N-acetylcysteine can dissolve cholesterol gallstones in an in vitro system.[303]

Methyl tetrabutyl ether (MTBE) is an aliphatic ether that was developed as an octane enhancer for gasoline and is used as an organic solvent in chromatography systems.[304] To dissolve gallstones, a percutaneous transhepatic puncture is made into the gallbladder. A catheter is inserted into the lumen of the gallbladder, and MTBE is introduced and withdrawn from the catheter.[305-307] A microcomputer-assisted pump can be used to ensure the solvent does not leak out to the duodenum by way of the cystic duct. Dissolution can be achieved within a few hours.[308] In well-selected patients and in specialized centers, this method is effective (90% success rate) and safe. Complications include those caused by the gallbladder catheterization procedure (e.g., hemoperitoneum, bile leak) and side effects of the solvent if the MTBE drains into the duodenum (e.g., hemolytic anemia, erosive or hemorrhagic duodenitis, aspiration pneumonia, somnolence). Cholesterol gallstones without a thick calcified rim (<3 mm) and with a diameter less than 2 cm are suitable selections. Calcified or pigment gallstones, cirrhosis of the liver with portal hypertension, and coagulopathy are contraindications to MTBE dissolution. MTBE dissolution therapy remains an experimental procedure performed in specialized centers.

Extracorporeal Shock Wave Lithotripsy

Energy generated externally can be directed to fragment gallstones. This method of treatment combines two approaches: oral bile acid therapy using UCDA and fragmentation of gallstones. Extracorporeal shock wave lithotripsy (ESWL) requires accurate localization of the gallstones within the gallbladder, usually achieved by three-dimensional ultrasonography. This spatial localization is fed into a computer, which directs the energy to focus sharply on the gallstone. The source of energy varies with different manufacturers and includes spark gap–generated and piezoelectric energy. The energy waves travel through a transmission medium, which is usually a water jacket close to the body wall. The energy waves, traveling in phases of compression and rarefaction, converge on the gallstone without causing tissue damage because no acoustic impedance occurs. Acoustic impedance and differential tensile forces develop, causing surface disintegration or cavitation.

Fragmentation of a gallstone into small fragments (<3 mm) results from successful ESWL. These fragments can be discharged into the duodenum spontaneously or, because there is a marked increase in surface area in relation to the same mass of gallstone, can be rapidly dissolved by UDCA. Depending on the type of lithotriptor, it takes one to several sessions of ESWL before optimal fragmentation can be achieved. UDCA, usually given before and concurrently with ESWL, is continued for several months until stones are completely absent in the gallbladder by ultrasound examination.[309]

If patients are properly selected, ESWL is effective and safe. Outpatient treatment has been reported.[310] Early reports indicated a promising success rate of more than 90% with single, small cholesterol stones.[311-313] However, larger stones and multiple stones have a lower fragmentation rate of 34% to 71%.[314] Selection criteria of patients for ESWL are similar to those listed for oral bile acid therapy. The best results are obtained with small, single stones, probably because it is more difficult to focus the energy waves sharply when multiple gallstones are present.[315]

About 20% of patients developed biliary colic for several weeks after ESWL (25% of these patients required cholecystectomy), and 1% had pancreatitis.[311-314] The shock waves may produce local discomfort, petechiae or bruising, transient noncontraction of the gallbladder, and microscopic hematuria. When ESWL was followed by elective cholecystectomy, edema, tissue damage in the gallbladder, and intrahepatic and perinephric hematomas were found. Despite these findings, patients seemed to do well clinically. Problematic common

TABLE 96-5
Therapeutic Options for Symptomatic Gallbladder Stones

THERAPY	CANDIDATES	STONE CLEARANCE (%)	MORTALITY (%)	DISADVANTAGES
Laparoscopic cholecystectomy	Normal GB-wall, no prior abd surgery	100	<1	Invasive, general anesthesia, bile duct injury
Oral bile acids	Floating radiolucent stones, <5 mm in diameter, patent cystic duct	80–90	0	Delayed stone clearance, no immediate alleviation of symptoms, stone recurrence
ESWL with oral bile acids	Solitary radiolucent stones up to 20 mm in diameter, patent cystic duct	70–90	<0.1	
Contact dissolution with MTBE	Radiolucent stones, GB attached to liver, patent cystic duct	50–90	Series too small	Invasive bile leakage (5%), stone recurrence

ESWL, extracorporeal shock wave lithotripsy; GB, gallbladder.
From Sauerbruch T, Paumgartner G. Gallbladder stones: management. Lancet 1991;338:1121.

bile duct stones that may not be cleared by ERCP with sphincterotomy may be amenable to a combined approach using ESWL.[316]

Rational Approach to Treating Symptomatic Gallstones

Surgery remains the definitive curative method of gallstone treatment. The advent of laparoscopic cholecystectomy and its widespread acceptance has revolutionized surgical treatment of gallstones. Laparoscopic cholecystectomy has come to be regarded as the treatment of choice for symptomatic gallstones, and for patients unable or unwilling to pursue this route, nonsurgical methods are available (Table 96-5).

The results of clinical efficacy of a nonsurgical treatment are usually the product of well-conducted clinical trials of well-selected patients with strict admission protocols. If stringent selection criteria are adhered to, the proportion of gallstone patients suitable for nonsurgical treatment may be limited. Although each regimen has minor variations, the proportion of patients satisfying all the selection prerequisites is at most 25%. Relaxing the patient selection criteria may be accompanied by a decrease in efficacy.

When stones are removed and the gallbladder is left behind, stones may recur. With oral bile acid therapy, the cumulative recurrence rate is about 15% in 2 years and 50% in 10 years.[317–322] Patients who have multiple stones have higher recurrence rates than those with single stones. There is no general agreement on whether a low fat, high-fiber diet or low-dose UDCA can protect against recurrence.[322–324] Although the long-term recurrence rate after MTBE dissolution and ESWL is not yet known, it is likely to be comparable to that observed with oral bile acids. One of the major challenges of nonsurgical treatment modalities of gallstones is preventing recurrence. Cholecystectomy is curative for gallbladder stones.

No formal comparison can yet be made between surgical and nonsurgical treatment, even with strictly selected patients in strictly executed clinical studies. Surgery has a high immediate cost and a low long-term cost, but nonsurgical means of treatment may have a low immediate cost but higher long-term cost because of recurrent or persistent disease. In the process of selecting patients for nonsurgical treatment, a diagnosis of gallstones by ultrasonography is insufficient. The physician must perform oral cholecystography to ascertain gallbladder concentrating and contractile function and a CT scan to predict chemical composition. Regular monitoring by ultrasonography during nonsurgical treatment may be necessary. These additional tests increase cost.

In approaching a patient with symptomatic gallstones, an elective cholecystectomy remains the gold standard. However, for those who cannot or will not have surgery, there are other alternatives. One of the nonsurgical methods may be selected if the patient satisfies all the criteria and if expertise is available.

> The reader is directed to Chapter 34, Approach to the Patient With Abdominal Pain; Chapter 95, Gallbladder and Biliary Tree: Anatomy and Structural Anomalies; Chapter 97, Diseases of the Biliary Tree; Chapter 99, Postcholecystectomy Syndrome; Chapter 117, Endoscopic Retrograde Cholangiopancreatography, Endoscopic Sphincterotomy and Stone Removal, and Endoscopic Biliary and Pancreatic Drainage; Chapter 121, Ultrasonography; Chapter 126, Applications of Radionuclide Imaging in Gastroenterology; and Chapter 129, Laparoscopy.

REFERENCES

1. Ingelfinger FJ. Digestive disease as a national problem: V. Gallstones. Gastroenterology 1968;55:102.
2. Almy TP. Prevalence and significance of digestive disease. Gastroenterology 1975;68:1351.
3. Diehl AK. Epidemiology and natural history of gallstone disease. Gastroenterol Clin North Am 1991;20:1.
4. Sampliner RE, Bennett PH, Comers LJ, et al. Gallbladder disease in Pima Indians. Demonstration of high prevalence and early onset by cholecystography. N Engl J Med 1970;283:1358.
5. Hopper KD, Landis JR, Meilstrup JW, et al. The prevalence of asymptomatic gallstones in the general population. Invest Radiol 1991;26:939.
6. Jensen KH, Jorgensen T. Incidence of gallstones in a Danish population. Gastroenterology 1991;100:790.
7. Martinovic I, Guerra C, Larach G. Incidencia de litiasis biliar

en material de autopsias y analisis de composicion de los calculos. Rev Med Chil 1972;100:1320.

8. Newman HG, Northrup JD. The autopsy incidence of gallstones. Int Abstr Surg 1959;109:1.
9. Lindstrom CG. Frequency of gallstone disease in a well-defined Swedish population. A prospective necropsy study. Scand J Gastroenterol 1977;12:341.
10. Rodewald H. Zur Pathologie der Gallenblase. II: Uber die Haufigkeit der Gallensteine. Zentralbl Allgem Pathol 1957;96:301.
11. Salzer GM, Olbrich E, Kutschera H. Zur Epidemiologie der Cholelithiasis. Acta Hepatogastroenterol 1970;17:65.
12. Doouss TW, Castleden WM. Gallstones and carcinoma of the large bowel. N Z Med J 1973;77:162.
13. Horn G. Observations on the aetiology of cholelithiasis. Br Med J 1956;2:732.
14. Torvik A, Hoivik B. Gallstones in an autopsy series. Incidence, complications and correlations with carcinoma of the gall bladder. Acta Chir Scand 1960;120:168.
15. Hogan J, Lonergan M, Holland PDJ. The incidence of cholelithiasis in an autopsy series. J Ir Med Assoc 1977;70:608.
16. Kalos A, Dalidou A, Kordosis T, et al. The incidence of gallstones in Greece: an autopsy study. Acta Hepatogastroenterol 1977;24:20.
17. Koutselinis A, Boukis D, Kalapothaki V, et al. Postmortem study of the prevalence of gallstones in Athens. Digestion 1975;13:304.
18. Huang WS. Cholelithiasis in Singapore. Gut 1970;11:141.
19. Stitnimankarn T. The necropsy incidence of gallstones in Thailand. Am J Med Sci 1960;240:349.
20. Heaton KW, Braddon FEM, Mountford RA, et al. Symptomatic and silent gall-stones in the community. Gut 1991;32:316.
21. Miayake H. Gallstones in Orient and Occident. In: Proceedings of the Third World Congress on Gastroenterology. Tokyo, 1966;4:148.
22. Ehrstrom R. The prevalence of gallstones and the standard of living in Finland 1836–1939. Nord Med 1942;14:1559.
23. Kameda H. Gallstones. Compositions, structural characteristics and geographical distribution. In: Proceedings of the Third World Congress on Gastroenterology. Tokyo, 1966;4:117.
24. Bateson MC, Bouchier IAD. Prevalence of gallstones in Dundee: a necropsy study. Br Med J 1975;4:427.
25. Acalovschi M, Dumitrascu D, Caluser I, et al. Comparative prevalence of gallstone disease at 100-year interval in a large Romanian town, a necropsy study. Dig Dis Sci 1987;32:354.
26. Tamimi TM, Wosornu L, Al-khozaim A, et al. Increased cholecystectomy rates in Saudi Arabia. Lancet 1990;336:1235.
27. Rome Group for Epidemiology and Prevention of Cholelithiasis (GREPCO). The epidemiology of gallstone disease in Rome, Italy. Part 1. Prevalence data in men. Hepatology 1988;8:904.
28. Rome Group for the Epidemiology and Prevention of Cholelithiasis (GREPCO). Prevalence of gallstone disease in an Italian adult female population. Am J Epidemiol 1984;119:796.
29. Barbara L, Sama C, Labate AMM, et al. A population study on the prevalence of gallstone disease: the Sermione Study. Hepatology 1987;7:913.
30. Dietschy JM, Spady DK. Measurement of rates of cholesterol synthesis using tritiated water. J Lipid Res 1984;25:1469.
31. Strange EF, Dietschy JM. Cholesterol absorption and metabolism by the intestinal epithelium. In: Danielsson H, Sjoval J, eds. Sterols and bile acids. New York: Elsevier, 1985;121.
32. Long TT, Jakoi L, Stevens R, et al. The sources of rat biliary cholesterol and bile acid. J Lipid Res 1978;19:872.
33. Turley SD, Dietschy JM. The contribution of newly synthesized cholesterol to biliary cholesterol to biliary cholesterol in the rat. J Biol Chem 1981;256:2438.
34. Robins SJ, Brunengraber H. Origin of biliary cholesterol and lecithin in the rat: contribution of new synthesis and preformed hepatic stores. J Lipid Res 1982;23:604.
35. Schwartz CC, Berman M, Vlahcevic ZR, et al. Multicompartmental analysis of cholesterol metabolism in man. Characterization of the hepatic bile acid and biliary cholesterol precursor sites. J Clin Invest 1978;61:408.
36. Stone BG, Erickson SK, Craig WY, et al. Regulation of rat biliary cholesterol secretion by agents that alter intrahepatic cholesterol metabolism. Evidence for a distinct biliary precursor pool. J Clin Invest 1985;76:1773.
37. Nervi FO, Dietschy JM. Ability of six different lipoprotein reactions to regulate the rate of hepatic cholesterol-genesis in vivo. J Biol Chem 1975;250:8704.
38. Turley SD, Dietschy JM. Regulation of biliary cholesterol output in the rat: dissociation from the rate of hepatic cholesterol synthesis, the size of the hepatic cholesteryl ester pool, and the hepatic uptake of chylomicron cholesterol. J Lipid Res 1979;20:923.
39. Thijs C, Knipschild P, Brombacher P. Serum lipids and gallstones: a case-control study. Gastroenterology 1990;99:843.
40. Grundy SM, Metzger AL, Alder RD. Mechanisms of lithogenic bile formation in American Indian women with cholesterol gallstones. J Clin Invest 1972;51:3026.
41. Bennion LJ, Grund SM. Effects of obesity and caloric intake on biliary lipid metabolism in man. J Clin Invest 1975;56:996.
42. Nisell K, Angelin B, Liljequist L, et al. Biliary lipid output and bile acid kinetics in cholesterol gallstone disease. Evidence for an increased hepatic secretion of cholesterol in Swedish patients. Gastroenterology 1985;287:293.
43. Ahlberg J, Angelin B, Bjorkhem L, et al. Hepatic cholesterol metabolism of normo- and hyperlipidemic patients with cholesterol gallstones. J Lipid Res 1979;20:107115.
44. Balasubramaniam S, Venkatesan S, Mitropoulos A, et al. The sub-microsomal localization of acyl-coenzyme A-cholesterol acyltransferase and its substrate, and of cholesterol esters in rat liver. Biochem J 1978;174:863.
45. Lichtenstein AH, Brecher P. Properties of acyl Co-A:cholesterol acyltransferase in rat liver microsomes. J Biol Chem 1980;255:9098.
46. Erickson SK, Cooper AD. Acyl coenzyme A:cholesterol acyltransferase in human liver: in vivo detection and some characteristics of the enzyme. Metabolism 1980;29:991.
47. Nervi FO, Del Pozo R, Covarrubias CF, et al. The effect of progesterone on the regulatory mechanisms of biliary cholesterol secretion in the rat. Hepatology 1983;3:360.
48. Kern F Jr, Everson GT. Contraceptive steroids increase cholesterol in bile: mechanisms of action. J Lipid Res 1987;28:828.
49. Grundy SM, Ahrens EH Jr, Salen G, et al. Mechanism of action of clofibrate on cholesterol metabolism in patients with hyperlipidemia. J Lipid Res 1972;13:531.
50. Leiss O, Meyer-Krahmer K, Von Bergmann K. Biliary lipid secretion in patients with heterozygous familial hypercholesterolemia and combined hyperlipidemia. Influence of benzabibrate and fenofibrate. J Lipid Res 1986;27:713.
51. Leiss O, Von Bergmann K, Gnasso A, et al. Effect of gemfibrozil on biliary lipid metabolism in normolipidemic subjects. Metabolism 1985;34:74.
52. Einarrson K, Nilsell K, Liejd B, et al. Influence of age on secretion of cholesterol and synthesis of bile acids by the liver. N Engl J Med 1985;313:277.
53. Myant NB, Mitropoulas KA. Cholesterol 7-alpha-hydroxylase. J Lipid Res 1977;18:135.
54. Everson GT, McKinley C, Kerf F Jr. Mechanisms of gallstone formation in women. Effects of exogenous estrogen (Premarin) and dietary cholesterol on hepatic lipid metabolism. J Clin Invest 1991;87:237.
55. Saunders KD, Cates JA, Abedin MZ, et al. Lovastatin inhibits gallstone formation in the cholesterol-fed prairie dog. Ann Surg 1991;214:149.
56. Bell CC, Vlahcevic ZR, Prazich J, et al. Evidence that a diminished bile acid pool precedes the formation of cholesterol gallstones in man. Surg Gynecol Obstet 1973;136:961.
57. Shaffer EA, Small DM. Biliary lipid secretion in cholesterol gallstone disease: the effect of cholecystectomy and obesity. J Clin Invest 1977;59:828.
58. Reuben A, Maton PN, Murphy GM, et al. Biliary lipid secretion in obese and nonobese individuals with and without gallstones. Clin Sci (Colch) 1985;69:71.
59. Oftebro H, Bjorkhem I, Stormer FC, et al. Cerebrotendinous xanthomatosis: defective liver mitochondrial hydroxylation of chenodeoxycholic acid precursors. J Lipid Res 1981;22:632.

60. Iser JH, Dowling RH, Murphy GM, et al. Congenital bile salt deficiency associated with 28 years of intractable constipation. In: Paumgartner G, Stiehl A, eds. Bile acid metabolism in health and disease. Lancaster, UK: MTP Press, 1977;231.

61. Kesaniemi YA, Salaspuro MP, Vuoristo M, et al. Biliary lipid secretion in chronic cholestatic liver disease. Gut 1982;23:931.

62. Sherlock S, Scheuer PJS. The presentation of 100 patients with primary biliary cirrhosis. N Engl J Med 1973;289:674.

63. Baker AL, Kaplan MM, Norton RA, et al. Gallstones in inflammatory bowel disease. Am J Dig Dis 1974;19:109.

64. Marcus SN, Heaton KW. Deoxycholic acid and the pathogenesis of gallstones. Gut 1988;29:522.

65. Berr F, Pratschke E, Fischer S, et al. Disorders of bile acid metabolism in cholesterol gallstone disease. J Clin Invest 1992;90:859.

66. Caruli N, Loria P, Bertolotti M, et al. Effects of acute changes of bile acid pool composition on biliary lipid secretion. J Clin Invest 1984;74:614.

67. Admirand WH, Small DM. The physico-chemical basis of cholesterol gallstone formation in man. J Clin Invest 1968;47:1043.

68. Thomas PJ, Hofmann AF. A simple calculation of lithogenic index of bile: expressing biliary lipid composition on rectangular coordinates. Gastroenterology 1973;65:698.

69. Carey MC, Small DM. Physical-chemistry of cholesterol solubility in bile. Relationship to gallstone formation and dissolution in man. J Clin Invest 1978;61:998.

70. Carey MC. Critical tables for calculating the cholesterol saturation of native bile. J Lipid Res 1978;19:945.

71. Holzbach RT. Metastability behavior of supersaturated bile. Hepatology 1984;4:155S.

72. Lee SP, Park HZ, Madani H, et al. Partial characterization of a non-micellar system of cholesterol solubilization in bile. Am J Physiol 1987;252:G374.

73. Mazer NA, Schurtenberger P, Carey MC, et al. Quasi-elastic light scattering studies of native hepatic bile from the dog: comparison with aggregative behavior of model biliary lipid systems. Biochemistry 1984;23:1994.

74. Pattinson NR, Chapman BA. Distribution of biliary cholesterol between mixed micelles and nonmicelles in relation to fasting and feeding in humans. Gastroenterology 1986;91:697.

75. Somjen GJ, Gilat T. A non-micellar mode of cholesterol transport in human bile. FEBS Lett 1983;156:265.

76. Somjen GH, Gilat T. Contribution of vesicular and micellar carriers to cholesterol transport in human bile. J Lipid Res 1985;26:699.

77. Ulloa N, Garrido J, Nervi F. Ultracentrifugal isolation of vesicular carriers of biliary cholesterol in native human and rat bile. Hepatology 1987;7:235.

78. Coleman R. Biochemistry of bile secretion. Biochem J 1987;244:249.

79. Crawford JM, Berken CA, Gollan JL. Role of the hepatocyte microtubular system in the excretion of bile salts and biliary lipid: implications for intracellular vesicular transport. J Lipid Res 1988;29:144.

80. Coleman R, Rahman K. Lipid flow in bile formation. Biochim Biophys Acta 1992;1125:113.

81. Wagner Cl, Trotman BW, Soloway RD. Kinetic analysis of biliary lipid excretion in man and dog. J Clin Invest 1976;16:133.

82. Northfield TC, Hofmann AF. Biliary lipid output during three meals and an overnight fast. 1. Relationship to bile acid pool size and cholesterol saturation of bile in gallstone and control subjects. Gut 1975;16:1.

83. Little TE, Lee SP, Madani H, et al. Interconversions of lipid aggregates in rat and model bile. Am J Physiol 1991;23:G70.

84. Kibe A, Dudley MA, Halpern Z, et al. Factors affecting cholesterol monohydrate crystal nucleation time in model systems of supersaturated bile. J Lipid Res 1985;26:1102.

85. Halpern Z, Dudley MA, Lynn MP, et al. Vesicle aggregation in model systems of bile: relation to crystal nucleation and lipid composition of the vesicular phase. J Lipid Res 1986;27:295.

86. Halpern Z, Dudley MA, Kibe A, et al. Rapid vesicle formation and aggregation in abnormal human biles. A time-lapse video-enhanced contrast microscopy study. Gastroenterology 1986;90:875.

87. Harvey PR, Somjen G, Lichtenberg MS, et al. Nucleation of cholesterol from vesicles isolated from bile of patients with and without cholesterol gallstones. Biochim Biophys Acta 1987;921:198.

88. Holzbach RT, Marsh M, Olszewski M, et al. Cholesterol solubility in bile: evidence that supersaturated bile is frequent in healthy man. J Clin Invest 1973;52:1467.

89. Small DM. Cholesterol nucleation and growth in gallstone formation. N Engl J Med 1980;302:1305.

90. Jungst D, Lang T, Von Ritter C, et al. Role of high total protein in gallbladder bile in the formation of cholesterol gallstones. Gastroenterology 1991;100:1724.

91. Marks JW, Broomfield P, Bonorris GG, et al. Factors affecting the measurement of cholesterol nucleation in human gallbladder and duodenal bile. Gastroenterology 1991;101:214.

92. Holan KR, Holzbach RT, Hermann RE, et al. Nucleation time: a key factor in the pathogenesis of cholesterol gallstone disease. Gastroenterology 1979;77:611.

93. Jungst D, Lang T, Von Ritter C, et al. Cholesterol nucleation time in gallbladder bile of patients with solitary or multiple cholesterol gallstones. Hepatology 1992;15:804.

94. Burnstein MJ, Ilson RG, Petrunka CN, et al. Evidence for a potent nucleating factor in the gallbladder bile of patients with cholesterol gallstones. Gastroenterology 1983;85:801.

95. Groen AK, Stout JPJ, Drapers AG, et al. Cholesterol nucleation influencing activity in T-tube bile. Hepatology 1988;8:347.

96. Pattinson NR, Willis KE. Effect of phospholipase C on cholesterol solubilization in model bile. Gastroenterology 1991;101:1339.

97. Miquel JF, Rigotti A, Rojas E, et al. Isolation and purification of human biliary vesicles with potent cholesterol-nucleation-promoting activity. Clin Sci 1992;82:175.

98. Harvey PRC, Upadhya GA, Strasberg SM. Immunoglobulins as nucleating proteins in the gallbladder bile of patients with cholesterol gallstones. J Biol Chem 1991;266:13996.

99. Martigne M, Domingo N, Lafont H, et al. Purification of the human anionic polypeptide fraction of the apo-bile lipoprotein complex by zonal ultracentrifugation. Lipids 1985;20:884.

100. Martigne M, Domingo N, Lechene de la Porte P, et al. Identification and localization of the apoprotein fraction of the bile lipoprotein complex in human gallstones. Scand J Gastroenterol 1988;23:731.

101. Shimuzu S, Sabsay B, Veis A, et al. Isolation of an acidic protein from cholesterol gallstones which inhibits the precipitation of calcium carbonate in vitro. J Clin Invest 1989;84:1990.

102. Kestell MF, Sekijima J, Lee SP, et al. A calcium-binding protein in bile and gallstones. Hepatology 1992;16:1315.

103. Kibe A, Holzbach RT, LaRusso NF, et al. Inhibition of cholesterol crystal formation by apolipoproteins in super-saturated model bile. Science 1984;225:514.

104. Busch N, Tokumo H, Holzbach RT. A sensitive method for determination of cholesterol crystal growth using model solutions of supersaturated bile. J Lipid Res 1990;31:1903.

105. Abei M, Kawczak P, Nuutinen H, et al. Isolation and characterization of a cholesterol crystallization promoter from human bile. Gastroenterology 1993;104:539.

106. Abei M, Kawczak P, Nuutinen H, et al. Identification of the 42 kD biliary cholesterol crystallization-promoting glycoprotein as alpha-1-acid glycoprotein. Gastroenterology 1992;102:A770.

107. Ohya T, Schwarzendrobe J, Busch N, et al. Isolation of a human biliary glycoprotein inhibitor of cholesterol crystallization. Gastroenterology 1993;104:527.

108. Schwarzendrube J, Nuutinen H, Abei M, et al. Amino acid sequence and immunological localization of a unique human 120 kD dimeric crystal growth-inhibiting biliary glycoprotein. Gastroenterology 1992;102:A882.

109. Harvey PRC, Strasberg SM. Will the real cholesterol-nucleating and -antinucleating proteins please stand up? Gastroenterology 1993;104:646.

110. Moore EW. Biliary calcium and gallstone formation. Hepatology 1990;12:206S.

111. Frabboni R, Bazzoli F, Mazzella G, et al. Acquired gallstone calcification during cholelitholytic treatment with chemodeoxycholic, ursodeoxycholic and taurodeoxycholic acids (abstract). Hepatology 1985;5:1004.

112. Been JM, Bills PM, Lewis D. Microstructure of gallstones. Gastroenterology 1979;76:548.

113. Moore EW. The role of calcium in the pathogenesis of gallstones: Ca^{++} electrode studies of model bile salt solutions and other biologic systems. Hepatology 1984;4:2285.

114. Williamson BWA, Anderson JL, Percy-Robb IW. Cholesterol gallstone pathogenesis: morphology of cholesterol nucleation on calcium salt crystals. Gut 1985;26:A561.

115. Shiffman ML, Sugerman JH, Kellum JM, et al. Changes in gallbladder bile composition following gallstone formation and weight reduction. Gastroenterology 1992;103:214.

116. Perdum PP, Shiffman ML, Moore EW. In vivo studies of biliary ceftriaxone excretion and solubility in guinea pig hepatic bile. J Lab Clin Med 1992;120:604.

117. Saunders KD, Strichartz SD, Abedin MZ, et al. Altered Na^+ and Cl^- flux during diet-induced mixed gallstone formation in the prairie dog. Dig Dis Sci 1992;37:109.

118. Shiffman ML, Moore EW. Acidification of gallbladder bile is defective in patients with all types of gallstones: a selective defect. Gastroenterology 1988;94:A591.

119. Knyrim K, Vakil N. Bile composition, microspheroliths, antinucleating activity, and gallstone calcification. Gastroenterology 1992;103:552.

120. Magnuson TH, Lillemoe KD, Zarkin BA, et al. Patients with uncomplicated cholelithiasis acidify bile normally. Dig Dis Sci 1992;37:1517.

121. Sahlin S, Ahlberg J, Reihner E, et al. Cholesterol metabolism in human gallbladder mucosa: relationship to cholesterol gallstone disease and effects of chenodeoxycholic acid and ursodeoxycholic acid treatment. Hepatology 1992;16:320.

122. Smith BF. Human gallbladder mucin binds biliary lipids and promotes cholesterol crystal nucleation in model bile. J Lipid Res 1987;28:1088.

123. Smith BF. Gallbladder mucin as a pronucleating agent for cholesterol monohydrate crystals in bile. Hepatology 1990;11:183S.

124. Levy PF, Smith BF, LaMont JT. Human gallbladder mucin accelerates nucleation of cholesterol in artificial bile. Gastroenterology 1984;87:270.

125. Smith BF, LaMont JT. Identification of gallbladder mucin-bilirubin complex in human cholesterol gallstone matrix. Effects of reducing agents on in vitro dissolution of matrix and intact gallstones. J Clin Invest 1985;76:439.

126. Lee SP, LaMont JT, Carey MC. The role of gallbladder mucus hypersecretion in the evolution of cholesterol gallstones: studies in the prairie dog. J Clin Invest 1981;67:1712.

127. Lee SP. Hypersecretion of mucus glycoprotein by the gallbladder epithelium in experimental cholelithiasis. Pathology 1981;134:199.

128. Rhodes M, Allen A, Lennard TWJ. Mucus glycoprotein biosynthesis in the human gallbladder: inhibition by aspirin. Gut 1992;33:1109.

129. Lee SP, Carey MC, LaMont JT. Aspirin prevention of cholesterol gallstone formation in prairie dogs. Science 1981;211:1429.

130. Cohen BI, Mosbach EH, Ayyad N, et al. Aspirin does not inhibit cholesterol cholelithiasis in two established animal models. Gastroenterology 1991;101:1109.

131. O'Leary DP, LaMorte WW, Scott TE, et al. Inhibition of prostaglandin synthesis fails to prevent gallbladder mucin hypersecretion in the cholesterol-fed prairie dog. Gastroenterology 1991;101:812.

132. LaMorte WW, LaMont JT, Hale W, et al. Gallbladder prostaglandin and lysophospholipids as mediators of mucin secretion during cholelithiasis. Am J Physiol 1986;251:G701.

133. Marks JW, Bonorris GG, Albers G, et al. The sequence of biliary events preceding the formation of gallstones in humans. Gastroenterology 1992;103:566.

134. Marks JW, Bonorris GG, Schoenfield LJ. Roles of deoxycholate and arachidonate in pathogenesis of cholesterol gallstones in obese patients during rapid loss of weight. Dig Dis and Sci 1991;36:957.

135. Igimi H, Yamamoto F, Lee SP. Gallbladder mucosal function: studies in absorption and secretion in humans and in dog gallbladder epithelium. Am J Physiol 1992;263:G69.

136. Ishii M, Vroman B, LaRusso NF. Isolation and morphologic characterization of bile duct epithelial cells from normal rat liver. Gastroenterology 1989;97:1236.

137. Oda D, Lee SP, Hayashi A. Long-term culture and partial characterization of dog gallbladder epithelial cells. Lab Invest 1991;64:682.

138. Doty JE, Pitt HA, Kuckenbecker SL, et al. Impaired gallbladder emptying before gallstone formation in the prairie dog. Gastroenterology 1983;85:168.

139. Li YF, Moody FG, Weisbrodt NW, et al. Gallbladder contractility and mucus secretion after cholesterol feeding in the prairie dog. Surgery 1986;100:900.

140. Cano N, Cicero F, Ranieri F, et al. Ultrasonographic study of gallbladder motility during total parenteral nutrition. Gastroenterology 1986;91:313.

141. Doty FE, Pitt HA, Porter-Fink V, et al. Cholecystokinin prophylaxis of parenteral nutrition-induced gallbladder disease. Ann Surg 1985;201:76.

142. Apstein MD, Dalecki-Chipperfield K. Spinal cord injury is a risk factor for gallstone disease. Gastroenterology 1987;92:966.

143. Poston GJ, Singh P, Draviam E, et al. Early stages of gallstone formation in guinea pig are associated with decreased biliary sensitivity to cholecystokinin. Dig Dis Sci 1992;37:1236.

144. Catnach SM, Fairclough PD, Trembath RC, et al. Effect of oral erythromycin on gallbladder motility in normal subjects and subjects with gallstones. Gastroenterology 1992;102:2071.

145. Lee SP, Nicholls JF, Park HZ. Biliary sludge as a cause of acute pancreatitis. N Engl J Med 1992;326:589.

146. Lee SP, Nicholls JF. Nature and composition of biliary sludge. Gastroenterology 1986;90:677.

147. Lee SP, Maher K, Nicholls JF. Origin and fate of biliary sludge. Gastroenterology 1988;94:170.

148. Schaad UB, Tschappeler H, Lentze MJ. Transient formation of precipitations in the gallbladder associated with ceftriaxone therapy. Pediatr Infect Dis J 1986;5:708.

149. Messing B, Dories C, Kunstlinger F, et al. Does total parenteral nutrition induce gallbladder sludge formation and lithiasis? Gastroenterology 1983;84:1012.

150. Schull SD, Wagner CI, Trotman BW, et al. Factors affecting bilirubin excretion in patients with cholesterol or pigment gallstones. Gastroenterology 1977;72:625.

151. Soloway RD, Trotman BW, Maddrey WC, et al. Pigment gallstone composition in patients with hemolysis or infection/stasis. Dig Dis Sci 1978;31:454.

152. Goodhard GL, Levison ME, Trotman BW, et al. Pigment vs. cholesterol cholelithiasis. Bacteriology of gallbladder stone, bile, and tissue correlated with biliary lipid analysis. Am J Dig Dis 1978;23:877.

153. Conte D, Barisani D, Mandelli C, et al. Cholelithiasis in cirrhosis: analysis of 500 cases. Am J Gastroenterol 1991;86:1629.

154. Trotman BW, Soloway RD. Pigment vs cholesterol cholelithiasis: clinical and epidemiological aspects. Am J Dig Dis 1975;20:735.

155. Ikido M, Shimizu S, Ostrow JD, et al. Isolation of a calcium-regulatory protein from black pigment gallstones: similarity with a protein from cholesterol gallstones. Hepatology 1992;15:1079.

156. Nagase M, Tanimura H, Setoyama M, et al. Present features of gallstones in Japan. A collective review of 2144 cases. Am J Surg 1987;135:788.

157. Tabata M, Nakayama F. Bacteria and gallstones. Etiological significance. Dig Dis Sci 1981;26:218.

158. Cetta, F. The role of bacteria in pigment gallstones disease. Ann Surg 1991;213:315.

159. Stewart L, Smith AL, Pelligrini CA, et al. Pigment gallstones form as a composite of bacterial microcolonies and pigment solids. Ann Surg 1987;206:242.

160. Speer AG, Cotton PB, Rode J, et al. Biliary stent blockage with

bacterial biofilm. A light and electron microscopy study. Ann Intern Med 1988;128:546.

161. Yio XY, Jin BW, Yin FZ, et al. Bile secretory immunoglobulin A in biliary infection and cholelithiasis. Gastroenterology 1992;102:1000.

162. Cetta F. Bile infection documented as initial event in the pathogenesis of brown pigment biliary stones. Hepatology 1986;6:482.

163. Skar V, Skar G, Bratlie J, et al. Beta-glucoronidase activity in bile of gallstones patients both with and without duodenal diverticula. Scand J Gastroenterol 1989;24:205.

164. Shull SD, Wagner CI, Trotman BW, et al. Factors affecting bilirubin excretion in patients with cholesterol or pigment gallstones. Gastroenterology 1977;72:625.

165. Maki T. Pathogenesis of calcium bilirubinate gallstones: role of E. coli, beta-glucuronidase, and coagulation by inorganic ions, polyelectrolytes and agitation. Ann Surg 1966;164:90.

166. Ho YC, Ho KJ. Human beta-glucoronidase. Measurement of its activity in gallbladder bile devoid of intrinsic interference. Dig Dis Sci 1988;33:435.

167. Boonyapisit ST, Trotman BW, Ostrow JD. Unconjugated bilirubin and the hydrolysis of conjugated bilirubin in gallbladder bile of patients with cholelithiasis. Gastroenterology 1978;74:70.

168. Holzbach RT. Gallbladder stasis: consequence of long-term parenteral hyperalimentation and risk factor for cholelithiasis. Gastroenterology 1983;84:1055.

169. Bolondi L, Bortolotti M, Santi V, et al. Gallbladder sludge formation during prolonged fasting after gastrointestinal tract surgery. Gut 1985;26:734.

170. Spivak W, DiVenuto D, Yuey W. Non-enzymic hydrolysis of bilirubin mono- and diglucuronide to unconjugated bilirubin in model and native bile systems. Biochem J 1987;242:323.

171. Sullivan FJ, Eaton SB Jr, Ferrucci JT Jr, et al. Cholangiographic manifestations of acute biliary colic. N Engl J Med 1973;288:33.

172. French EB, Robb WAT. Biliary and renal colic. Br Med J 1963;3:135.

173. Gunn A, Keddie N. Some clinical observations on patients with gallstones. Lancet 1972;2:7771.

174. Rigas B, Torosis J, McDougall CJ, et al. The circadian rhythm of biliary colic. J Clin Gastroenterol 1990;12:409.

175. Mogadam M, Albarelli J, Ahmed SW, et al. Gallbladder dynamics in response to various meals: is dietary fat restriction necessary in the management of gallstones? Am J Gastroenterol 1984;79:745.

176. Johnson AG. Cholecystectomy and gallstone dyspepsia. Clinical and physiological study of a symptom complex. Ann R Coll Surg Engl 1975;56:69.

177. Kingston RD, Windsor WO. Flatulent dyspepsia in patients with gallstones undergoing cholecystectomy. Br J Surg 1975;62:231.

178. Price WH. Gall-bladder dyspepsia. Br Med J 1963;2:138.

179. Rhind JA, Watson L. Gallstone dyspepsia. Br Med J 1968;1:32.

180. Ros E. Zambow D. Post cholecystectomy symptoms. A prospective study of gallstone patients before and two years after surgery. Gut 1987;28:1500.

181. Sjodahl R. On the development of primary acute cholecystitis. Scand J Gastroenterol 1983;18:577.

182. Neiderhiser D, Thornell E, Bjorck S, et al. The effect of lysophosphatidylcholine on gallbladder function in the cat. J Lab Clin Med 1983;101:699.

183. Jivegard L, Thornell E, Svanvik J. Pathophysiology of acute obstructive cholecystitis: implications for non-operative management. Br J Surg 1987;74:1084.

184. Thornell E. Mechanisms in the development of acute cholecystitis and biliary pain. A study on the role of prostaglandins and the effects of indomethacin. Scand J Gastroenterol 1982;17(Suppl):76.

185. Claesson BEB, Holmlund DEW, Matzsch TW. Biliary microflora in acute cholecystitis and the clinical implications. Acta Chir Scand 1984;150:229.

186. Claesson BEB, Holmlund DEW, Matzsch TW. Microflora of the gallbladder related to duration of acute cholecystitis. Surg Gynecol Obstet 1986;162:531.

187. Howard R. Acute acalculous cholecystitis. Am J Surg 1981;141:194.

188. Glenn F. Acute acalculous cholecystitis. Ann Surg 1979;189:458.

189. Orlando R, Gleason E, Drezner A. Acute cholecystitis in the critically ill patient. Am J Surg 1983;145:472.

190. Johndon L. The importance of early diagnosis of acute acalculous cholecystitis. Surg Gynecol Obstet 1987;164:197.

191. Machemer WL, Fuge WW, Mendez FL. Typhoid cholecystitis. Surgery 1952;31:738.

192. Kavin H, Jonas RB, Chowdhury L, et al. Acalculous cholecystitis and cytomegalovirus infection in the acquired immunodeficiency syndrome. Ann Intern Med 1986;104:53.

193. Blumberg RS, Kelsey P, Perrone T, et al. Cytomegalovirus and cryptosporidium-associated acalculous gangrenous cholecystitis. Am J Med 1984;76:1118.

194. Jonson G, Sundman L. Bile and dry matter output at elevated liver secretion pressure. Acta Chir Scand 1964;128:153.

195. Strasberg SM, Dorn BC, Redinger RN, et al. Effects of alteration of biliary pressure on bile composition—a method for study: primate biliary physiology V. Gastroenterology 1971;61:357.

196. Strasberg SM, Dorn BC, Small DM, et al. The effect of biliary tract pressure on bile flow, bile salt secretion, and bile salt synthesis in the primate. Surgery 1971;70:140.

197. Scobie BA, Summerskill WHJ. Hepatic cirrhosis secondary to obstruction of the biliary system. Am J Dig Dis 1965;10:134.

198. Adson MA, Wychulis AR. Portal hypertension in secondary biliary cirrhosis. Arch Surg 1968;96:604.

199. Weinbren K, Hadjis NS, Blumgart LH. Structural aspects of the liver in patients with biliary disease and portal hypertension. J Clin Pathol 1985;38:1013.

200. Yeong ML, Nicholson GI, Lee SP. Regression of biliary cirrhosis following choledochal cyst drainage. Gastroenterology 1982;82:332.

201. Boey JH, Way LW. Acute cholangitis. Ann Surg 1980;191:264.

202. Thompson JE Jr, Tompkins RK, Longmire WP Jr. Factors in management of acute cholangitis. Ann Surg 1982;195:137.

203. Shimada K, Noro T, Inamatsu T, et al. Bacteriology of acute obstructive suppurative cholangitis of the aged. J Clin Microbiol 1981;14:522.

204. Finegold SM. Anaerobes in biliary tract infection. Arch Intern Med 1979;139:1338.

205. Ros E, Navarro S, Bru C, et al. Occult microlithiasis in "idiopathic" acute pancreatitis: prevention of relapses by cholecystectomy or ursodeoxycholic acid therapy. Gastroenterology 1991;101:1701.

206. Muhletaler CA, Gerlock AJ Jr, Fleischer AC. Diagnosis of obstructive jaundice with nondilated bile ducts. AJR Am J Roentgenol 1980;134:1149.

207. Gross BH, Harter LP, Gore RM, et al. Ultrasonic evaluation of common bile duct stones: prospective comparison with endoscopic retrograde cholangiopancreatography. Radiology 1983;145:471.

208. Low-Beer T, Heaton K, Roylance J. Oral cholecystography in patients with small bowel disease. Br J Radiol 1972;45:427.

209. Zboralski F, Amberg J. Cholecystocholestasis: a cause of cholecystographic error. Am J Dig Dis 1962;7:339.

210. Mujahed Z, Evans J, Whalen J. The nonopacified gallbladder on oral cholecystography. Radiology 1974;112:1.

211. Bennion LJ, Knowler WC, Mott DM, et al. Development of lithogenic bile during puberty in Pima Indians. N Engl J Med 1979;300:873.

212. Wenckert A, Robertson B. The natural course of gallstone disease: eleven year review of 781 nonoperated cases. Gastroenterology 1966;101:171.

213. Lund J. Surgical indication in cholelithiasis: prophylactic cholecystectomy elucidated on the basis of long-term follow-up on 526 non-operated cases. Ann Surg 1960;151:153.

214. Gracie WA, Ransohoff DF. The natural history of silent gallstones. N Engl J Med 1982;307:798.

215. Grimaldi CH, Nelson RG, Pettitt DJ, et al. Increased mortality

with gallstone disease: results of a 20 year population-based survey in Pima Indians. Ann Intern Med 1993;118:185.

216. Linos DA, O'Fallon WM, Thistle JL, et al. Cholelithiasis and carcinoma of the colon. Cancer 1982;50:1015.

217. Kimura W, Shimada H, Kuroda A, et al. Carcinoma of the gallbladder and extrahepatic bile duct in autopsy cases of the aged, with special reference to its relationship to gallstones. Am J Gastroenterol 1989;84:386.

218. Lowenfels AB, Lindstrom CG, Conway MJ, et al. Gallstones and risk of gallbladder cancer. J Natl Cancer Inst 1985;75:77.

219. Gomand L, Vandenbroucke J, DeGroot J. De natuurlijke evolutie van colelilthiase. Tijdschr Gastroenterol 1966;9:594.

220. Ralson DE, Smith LA. The natural history of cholelithiasis: a 15 to 30-year followup of 116 patients. Minn Med 1965;48:327.

221. Heuman R, Sjodahl R, Wetterfors J. Gallstone ileus: an analysis of 120 patients. World J Surg 1980;4:595.

222. Kurtz RJ, Heimann TM, Kurtz AB. Gallstone ileus: a diagnostic problem. Am J Surg 1983:146;314.

223. MacLean LD, Goldstein M, MacDonald JE, et al. Results of cholecystectomy in 1000 consecutive patients. Can J Surg 1975;18:459.

224. Seltzer MH, Steiger E, Rosato FE. Mortality following cholecystectomy. Surg Gynecol Obstet 1970;130:64.

225. McSherry CK, Glenn F. The incidence and causes of death following surgery for nonmalignant biliary tract disease. Ann Surg 1980;191:271.

226. Morgenstern L, Wong L, Berci G. Twelve hundred open cholecystectomies before the laparoscopic era. Arch Surg 1992: 127:400.

227. Pokorny WJ, Saleem M, O'Gorman RB, et al. Cholelithiasis and cholecystitis in childhood. Am J Surg 1984;148:742.

228. Ware R, Filston HC, Schultz WH, et al. Elective cholecystectomy in children with sickle hemoglobinopathies: successful outcome using a preoperative transfusion regimen. Ann Surg 1988;208:17.

229. Amaral JF, Thompson WR. Gallbladder disease in the morbidly obese. Am J Surg 1985;149:551.

230. Polk HC Jr. Carcinoma and the calcified gallbladder. Gastroenterology 1966;50:582.

231. Ashur H, Siegal B, Oland Y, et al. Calcified gallbladder (porcelain gallbladder). Arch Surg 1978;113:594.

232. Bateson MC, Bouchier IAD. Prevalence of gall stones in Dundee: necropsy study. Br Med J 1975;4:4271.

233. Bateson MC. Gallbladder disease and cholecystectomy rate are independently variable. Lancet 1984;2:621.

234. Sandler RS, Maule WF, Baltus ME. Factors associated with postoperative complications in diabetes after biliary tract surgery. Gastroenterology 1986;91:157.

235. Ransohoff DF, Miller GL, Forsythe SB, et al. Outcome of acute cholecystitis in patients with diabetes mellitus. Ann Intern Med 1987;106:829.

236. McKellar DP, Anderson CT, Boynton CJ, et al. Cholecystectomy during pregnancy without fetal loss. Surg Gynecol Obstet 1992;174:465.

237. Kelling G. Uber Oesophagosckopie, gastroskopie und koelioskopie. Munch Med Wochenschr 1901:49:12.

238. Veress J. Neues instrument zur ausfuhrung vos brust-oder bauchpunktionen und pneumothoraxbehandlung. Dtsch Med Wochenschr 1938;41:1480.

239. Stellato TA. History of laparoscopic surgery. In: MacFadyen BV, Ponsky JL, eds. Laparoscopy for the general surgeon. Surgical Clinics of North America 1992:72:997.

240. Dubois F, Berthelot G, Levard H. Cholecystectomie par coelioscopie. Presse Med 1989:18:980.

241. Dubois F, Icard P, Berthelot G, et al. Coelioscopic cholecystectomy: preliminary report of 36 cases. Ann Surg 1990:211:60.

242. Holohan TV. Laparoscopic cholecystectomy. Lancet 1991:338:801.

243. Barkun JS, Barkun AN, Sampalis JS, et al. Randomised controlled trial of laparoscopic versus mini cholecystectomy. Lancet 1992;340:1116.

244. Stoker ME, Vose J, O'Mara P, et al. Laparoscopic cholecystec-

tomy: a clinical and financial analysis of 280 operations. Arch Surg 1992;127:589.

245. Glinatsis MT, Griffith JP, McMahon MJ. Open vs. laparoscopic cholecystectomy: a retrospective comparative study. J Laparoendosc Surg 1992;2:81.

246. Zucker KA, Bailey RW, Flowers J. Laparoscopic management of acute and chronic cholecystitis. In: MacFadyen BV, Ponsky JL, eds. Laparoscopy for the general surgeon. Surgical Clinics of North America 1992:72:1045.

247. Donohue JH, Grant CS, Farnell MB. Laparoscopic cholecystectomy: operative technique. Mayo Clin Proc 1992;67:441.

248. Fitzgerald SD, Bailey PV, Liebscher GJ, et al. Laparoscopic cholecystectomy in anticoagulated patients. Surg Endosc 1991;5:166.

249. Schirmer BD, Dix J, Edge SB, et al. Laparoscopic cholecystectomy in the obese patient. Ann Surg 1992;216:146.

250. Moir CR, Donohue JH, van Heerden JA. Laparoscopic cholecystectomy in children: initial experience and recommendations. J Pediatr Surg 1992;27:1066.

251. The Southern Surgeons Club. A prospective analysis of 1518 laparoscopic cholecystectomies. New Engl J Med 1991;324:1073.

252. Phillips EH, Carroll BJ, Bello JM, et al. Laparoscopic cholecystectomy in acute cholecystitis. Am Surg 1992;58:273.

253. Flowers JL, Zucker KA, Graham SM, et al. Laparoscopic cholangiography—results and indications. Ann Surg 1992;215:209.

254. Cantwell DV. Routine cholangiography during laparoscopic cholecystectomy. Arch Surg 1992;127:483.

255. Berci G. Intra-operative cholangiography during laparoscopic cholecystectomy. Aust N Z J Surg 1992;62:151.

256. Berci G. Biliary ductal anatomy and anomalies. In: MacFadyen BV, Ponsky JL, eds. Laparoscopy for the general surgeon. Surgical Clinics of North America 1992:72:1069.

257. Donohue JH, Farnell MB, Grant CS, et al. Laparoscopic cholecystectomy: early Mayo Clinic experience. Mayo Clin Proc 1992;67:449.

258. Gillams A, Russell RCG, Cheslyn-Curtis S, et al. Can cholangiography be safely abandoned in laparoscopic cholecystectomy? Ann R Coll Surg Engl 1992;74:248.

259. Joyce WP, Keane R, Burke GJ, et al. Identification of bile duct stones in patients undergoing laparoscopic cholecystectomy. Br J Surg 1991;78:1174.

260. Carroll BJ, Phillips EH, Daykhovsky L, et al. Laparoscopic choledoscopy: an effective approach to the common duct. J Laparoendosc Surg 1992;2:15.

261. Hunter JG, Soper NJ. Laparoscopic management of bile duct stones. In: MacFadyen BV, Ponsky JL, eds. Laparoscopy for the general surgeon. Surgical Clinics of North America 1992: 72:1077.

262. Davidoff AM, Pappas TN, Murray EA, et al. Mechanisms of major biliary injury during laparoscopic cholecystectomy. Ann Surg 1992;215:196.

263. Moossa AR, Easter DW, Van Sonnenberg E, et al. Laparoscopic injuries to the bile duct. Ann Surg 1992;215:203.

264. Kozarek R, Gannan R, Baerg R, et al. Bile leak after laparoscopic cholecystectomy. Arch Intern Med 1992;152:1040.

265. Moosa AR, Mayer AD, Stabile B. Iatrogenic injuries to the bile duct. Arch Surg 1990;125:1028.

266. Rossi RL, Schirmer WJ, Braasch JW, et al. Laparoscopic bile duct injuries. Arch Surg 1992;127:596.

267. Lawrence SK, Delbeke D. Bile leak after laparoscopic cholecystectomy. AJR Am J Roentgenol 1992;158:1385.

268. Pasmans HLM, Go PMHYH, Gouma DJ, et al. Scintigraphic diagnosis of bile leakage after laparoscopic cholecystectomy. Clin Nucl Med 1992;17:697.

269. Weber J, Adamek HE, Riemann JF. Endoscopic stent placement and clip removal for common bile duct stricture after laparoscopic cholecystectomy. Gastrointest Endosc 1992;38:181.

270. Wootton FT, Hoffman BJ, Marsh WH, et al. Biliary complications following laparoscopic cholecystectomy. Gastrointest Endosc 1992;38:183.

271. Asbun HJ, Reddick EJ. Credentialing in laparoscopic surgery: a survey of physicians. J Laparoendosc Surg 1992;2:27.

272. Dent TL. Training, credentialing, and evaluation in laparoscopic

surgery. In: MacFadyen BV, Ponsky JL, eds. Laparoscopy for the general surgeon. Surgical Clinics of North America 1992: 72:1003.

273. Schirmer BD and Dix J. Cost effectiveness of laparoscopic cholecystectomy. J Laparoendosc Surg 1992;2:145.

274. McIntyre RC, Zoeter MA, Weil KC, et al. A comparison of outcome and cost of open vs. laparoscopic cholecystectomy. J Laparoendosc Surg 1992;2:143.

275. Danzinger RG, Hofmann AF, Schoenfield LJ, et al. Dissolution of cholesterol gallstones by chenodeoxycholic acid. N Engl J Med 1972;268:1.

276. Bell DG, Whitney B, Dowling RH. Gallstone dissolution in man using chenodeoxycholic acid. Lancet 1972;11:1213.

277. Fromm H, Eschler A, Tollner D, et al. In vivo dissolving of gallstones: the effect of chenodeoxycholic acid. Dtsch Med Wechenschr 1975;100:1619.

278. Weis HJ, Holtermuller KH, Gilsdorf P. Gallstone dissolution with chenodeoxycholic acid: a clinical study. Klin Wochenschr 1980;58:313.

279. Schoenfield JL, Lachin JM, The Steering Committee and the National Cooperative Gallstone Study Group. Chenodiol (chenodoxycholic acid) for dissolution of gallstones. The National Cooperative Gallstone Study: a controlled trial of efficacy and safety. Ann Intern Med 1981;95:257.

280. Nakagawa S, Makino I, Ishizaki T, et al. Dissolution of cholesterol gallstones by ursodeoxycholic acid. Lancet 1977;2:367.

281. Stiehl A, Czygan P, Kommerell B, et al. Ursodeoxycholic acid versus chenodeoxycholic acid. Comparison of their effects on bile acid and bile lipid composition in patients with cholesterol gallstones. Gastroenterology 1978;75:1016.

282. Makino I, Nakagawa S. Changes in biliary lipid and biliary bile acid composition in patients after administration of ursodeoxycholic acid. J Lipid Res 1978;19:723.

283. Tokyo Cooperative Gallstone Study Group. Efficacy and indications of ursodeoxycholic acid treatment for dissolving gallstones. A multicenter double-blind trial. Gastroenterology 1980;78:542.

284. Stiehl A, Raedsch R, Czygan P, et al. Effects of biliary bile acid composition on biliary cholesterol saturation in gallstone patients treated with chenodeoxycholic acid and/or ursodeoxycholilc acid. Gastroenterology 1980;79:1192.

285. Salen G, Colalillo A, Verga D, et al. Effect of high and low doses of ursodeoxycholic acid on gallstone dissolution in humans. Gastroenterology 1980;78:1412.

286. Tint GS, Salen G, Colalillo A. Ursodeoxycholic acid: a safe and effective agent for dissolving gallstones. Ann Intern Med 1982;97:351.

287. Thistle JL, LaRusso NF, Hofmann AF, et al. Differing effects of ursodeoxycholic or chenodeoxycholic acid on biliary cholesterol saturation and bile acid metabolism in man. A dose response study. Dig Dis Sci 1982;27:161.

288. Bachrach WH, Hofmann AF. Ursodeoxycholic acid in the treatment of cholesterol cholelithiasis. Dig Dis Sci 1982;27: 161.

289. Roda E, Bazzoli F, Labate AMM, et al. Ursodeoxycholic acid vs chenodeoxycholic acid as cholesterol gallstone-dissolving agents: a comparative randomized study. Hepatology 1982;2: 804.

290. Podda M, Zuin M, Dioguardi MG, et al. A combination of chenodeoxycholic acid and ursodeoxycholic acid is more effective than either alone in reducing biliary cholesterol saturation. Hepatology 1982;2:334.

291. Roehrkasse R, Fromm H, Malavolta M, et al. Gallstone dissolution treatment with a combination of chenodeoxycholic and ursodeoxycholic acids. Studies of safety, efficacy and effects on bile lithogenicity, bile acid pool, and serum lipids. Dig Dis Sci 1986;31:1032.

292. Von Bergmann K, Epple-Gutsfeld M, Leiss O. Differences in the effects of chenodeoxycholic and ursodeoxycholic acids on biliary lipids secretion and bile acid synthesis in patients with gallstones. Gastroenterology 1984;87:136.

293. Nilsell K, Angelin B, Leijd B, et al. Comparative effects of ursodeoxycholic acid and chenodeoxycholic acid on bile acid kinetics and biliary lipid secretion in man: evidence for different modes of action on bile acid synthesis. Gastroenterology 1983;85:1248.

294. Danzinger RG, Hofmann AF, Thistle JL, et al. Effect of oral chenodeoxycholic acid on bile acid kinetics and biliary lipid composition in women with cholelithiasis. J Clin Invest 1973;52:2809.

295. LaRusso NF, Thistle JL. Effect of litholytic bile acids on cholesterol absorption in gallstone patients. Gastroenterology 1983;84:265.

296. Poupon R, Chretien Y, Poupon RE, et al. Is ursodeoxycholic acid an effective treatment for primary biliary cirrhosis? Lancet 1987;1:834.

297. Leuschner U, Leuschner M, Sieratzki J, et al. Gallstone dissolution with ursodeoxycholic acid in patients with chronic active hepatitis and two year follow up. Dig Dis Sci 1985;30:642.

298. Senior JR, Batta AK, Arora R, et al. Ursodeoxycholic acid treatment produces marked clinical and biochemical amelioration of primary sclerosing cholangitis. Gastroenterology 1989;96: A641.

299. Peine CJ. Gallstone-dissolving agents. Gastroenterol Clin North Am 1992;21:715.

300. Thistle JL, Carlson G, Hofmann AF, et al. Monooctanoin, a dissolution agent for retained cholesterol bile duct stones: physical properties and clinical application. Gastroenterology 1981;78:1016.

301. Pitt HA, McFaddan DW, Gadacz TR. Agents for gallstone dissolution. Am J Surg 1987;153:233.

302. Igimi H, Tanura R, Toraishi K, et al. Medical dissolution of gallstones: clinical experience of D-limonene as a simple, safe, and effective solvent. Dig Dis Sci 1991;36:200.

303. Niu N, Smith BF. Addition of N-acetylcysteine to aqueous model bile systems accelerates dissolution of cholesterol gallstones. Gastroenterology 1990;98:454.

304. Little CJ, Dale AD, Wheatley JA, et al. Methyl tertiary butyl ether: a new chromatographic eluent. J Chromatogr 1979;169: 381.

305. Allen MJ, Borody TJ, Bugliosi TF, et al. Rapid dissolution of gallstones by methyl tert-butyl ether. N Engl J Med 1986;312: 217.

306. Thistle JL, Nelson PE, May GR. Dissolution of cholesterol gallbladder stones using methyl tert-butyl ether. Gastroenterology 1986;90:1775.

307. Thistle JL, May GR, Bender CE, et al. Dissolution of cholesterol gallbladder stones by methyl tert-butyl ether administered by percutaneous transhepatic cathether. N Engl J Med 1989;320: 633.

308. McCullough JE, Lesma A, Thistle JL. A rapid stirring automatic pump system for dissolving gallstones using methyl tert-butyl ether (MTBE): in vitro comparison with the manual syringe method. Gastroenterology 1989;96:A629.

309. Schoenfield LJ, Berci G, Carnovale RL, et al. The effect of urosodiol on the efficacy and safety of extracorporeal shock-wave lithotripsy of gallstones. N Engl J Med 1990;323:1239.

310. Albert MB, Fromm H, Borstelmann R, et al. Successful outpatient treatment of gallstones with piezoelectric lithotripsy. Ann Intern Med 1990;113:164.

311. Sauerbruch T, Delius M, Paumgartner G, et al. Fragmentation of gallstones by extracorporeal shock-waves. N Engl J Med 1986;314:818.

312. Sackmann M, Weber W, Delius M. Extracorporeal shock-wave lithotripsy of gallstones without general anesthesia: first clinical experience. Ann Intern Med 1987;107:347.

313. Sackmann M, Delius M, Sauerbruch T, et al. Shock-wave lithotripsy of gallbladder stones. The first 175 patients. N Engl J Med 1988;318:393.

314. Ponchon T, Barkun AN, Pujol B, et al. Gallstone disappearance after extracorporeal lithotripsy and oral bile acid dissolution. Gastroenterology 1989;97:457.

315. Sackmann M, Pauletzki J, Sauerbruch T, et al. The Munich gallbladder lithotripsy study. Ann Intern Med 1991;114: 290.

316. Harz C, Henkel TO, Kohrmann KU, et al. Extracorporeal shock-wave lithotripsy and endoscopy: combined therapy for problematic bile duct stones. Surg Endosc 1991;5:196.

317. Ruppin DC, Dowling RH. Is recurrence inevitable after gallstone dissolution by bile acid treatment? Lancet 1982;1:183.

318. Dowling RH, Gleeson D, Ruppin DC, et al. Gallstone recurrence and post-dissolution management. In: Paumgartner G, Stiehl A, Gerok W, eds. Enterohepatic circulation of bile acids and sterol metabolism. Falk symposium, 1985. Lancaster, UK: MTP Press 1985;361.

319. Somerville KW, Rose DH, Bell GD, et al. Gallstone dissolution and recurrence: are we being misled? Br Med J 1982;284:1295.

320. O'Donnell LDJ, Heaton KW. Recurrence and re-recurrence of gallstones after medical dissolution: a long-term follow up. Gut 1988;29:655.

321. Gleeson D, Ruppin RC, The British Gallstone Study Group. Discrepancies between cholecystography and ultrasonography in the detection of recurrent stones. J Hepatol 1985;1:597.

322. Villanova N, Bazzoli F, Frabboni R, et al. Gallstone recurrence after successful oral bile acid treatment: a follow-up study and evaluation of post-dissolution treatment. Gastroenterology 1987;92:1789.

323. Williams CN. Prevention of cholelithiasis: intervention on risk factors. In: Capocaccia LK, Ricci G, Angelico F, Angelico M, Attili AF, eds. Epidemiology and prevention of gallstone disease. Boston: MTP Press, 1984;210.

324. Hood KA, Gallstone prevention: post-dissolution trials. In: Northfield T, Jazrani R, Zentler-Munro P, eds. Bile acids in health and disease. Lancaster, UK: Kluwer Academic Publishers, 1988;171.

325. Gadacz TR, Talamini MA, Lillemoe KD, et al. Laparoscopic cholecystectomy. Surg Clin North Am 1990;76:1249.

326. Peters JH, Ellison EC, Innes JT, et al. Safety and efficacy of laparoscopic cholecystectomy. A prospective analysis of 100 initial patients. Ann Surg 1991;213:3.

327. Dion Y-M, Morin J. Laparoscopic cholecystectomy: a report of 60 cases. Can J Surg 1990;33:483.

328. Zucker KA, Bailey RW, Gadacz TR, et al. Laparoscopic guided cholecystectomy. Am J Surg 1991;161:36.

329. Hershman MJ, Rosin RD. Laparoscopic laser cholecystectomy: our first 200 patients. Ann R Coll Surg Engl 1992;74:242.

330. Martin IG, Holdsworth PJ, Asker J, et al. Laparoscopic cholecystectomy as a routine procedure for gallstones: results of an "all-comers" policy. Br J Surg 1992;79:807.

331. Schirmer BD, Dix J, Edge SB, et al. Laparoscopic cholecystectomy in the obese patient. Ann Surg 1992;216:146.

332. Scott ADN, McMillan L, Greville AC, et al. Laparoscopic laser cholecystectomy: results of the technique in 210 patients. Ann R Coll Surg Engl 1992;74:237.

333. Rees BI, Williams HR. Laparoscopic cholecystectomy: the first 155 patients. Ann R Coll Surg Engl 1992;74:233.

334. Bailey RW, Zucker KA, Flowers JL, et al. Laparoscopic cholecystectomy: experience with 375 consecutive patients. Ann Surg 1991;214:531.

Textbook of Gastroenterology, second edition, edited by Tadataka Yamada. JB Lippincott Company, Philadelphia © 1995.

CHAPTER 97

Diseases of the Biliary Tree

Shelly Chi-Loo Lu   Neil Kaplowitz

Biliary tract disorders include calculi, infections, and fibrocystic diseases. Various pathologic processes can obstruct the biliary tract, leading to cholangitis, stone formation, and secondary biliary cirrhosis. Although the mainstay of treatment for biliary tract disorders has been surgical, management has shifted toward nonoperative management. This chapter covers the major benign diseases of the biliary tract, emphasizing calculus diseases, fibrocystic diseases, and sclerosing cholangitis. Other important causes of bile duct obstruction, such as biliary stricture, pancreatic diseases, papillary stenosis, hemobilia, and causes of biliary fistula are discussed. Since the first edition of this chapter, two areas of study have expanded: laparoscopic cholecystectomy, with its effects on biliary tract disease, and biliary tract disease associated with the acquired immunodeficiency syndrome (AIDS). These areas are also covered in this chapter. Other chapters in the book cover biliary tract dysmotility and malignancy.

CALCULUS DISEASES OF THE BILE DUCTS

Stones in the bile ducts can be classified as primary duct stones, which form de novo in the ducts, and secondary duct stones, which result from the passage of gallbladder stones through the cystic duct. They can be further subdivided into common bile duct stones and intrahepatic duct stones, which are situated proximal to the origin of the common hepatic duct. The epidemiology, pathogenesis, composition, and clinical course of stones in these two locations differ greatly. The prevalence and perhaps cause of primary duct stones vary dramatically according to the geographic location. The epidemiology and pathogenesis of primary and secondary duct stones are discussed first, followed by their clinical presentations, diagnostic studies, and management. Special mention is made of the primary duct stones seen predominantly in Asia, which comprise the distinct clinical syndrome of Oriental cholangiohepatitis or recurrent pyogenic cholangitis.

Choledocholithiasis

Pathogenesis

Secondary duct stones.   More than 500,000 cholecystectomies are performed in the United States each year, making this the most common elective abdominal operation. The common bile duct (CBD) is explored in roughly 25% of these cases, and concomitant calculi are found in 60% of these explorations, which means that concomitant choledocholithiasis is found in at least 12% to 15% of the cholecystectomies. Despite several technologic advances in biliary tract surgery, 3% to 5% of patients who have had CBD exploration, or roughly 1% of all patients having undergone cholecystectomy, are found to have a retained stone in the CBD in the immediate postoperative period.[1-3]

The prevalence of choledocholithiasis increases in older age groups. In patients younger than 59 years of age, the prevalence of concomitant common duct stones removed at cholecystectomy was 4% to 6.7%, but the rate increased to 13% to 18% for those 60 to 79 years of age and to 33.3% for those older than 80 years of age.[1]

In the Western world, 70% to 80% of gallbladder stones are cholesterol stones, and 20% to 30% are pigment stones. Approximately 55% to 70% of common duct stones are cholesterol stones.[4,5] In Western countries, most of the common duct stones are secondary stones. Several lines of evidence support this. First, when stones are found in the CBD and gallbladder at the time of surgery, the CBD stones are similar in chemical composition to gallbladder stones.[4,5] Cholesterol stones in the gallbladder and the common duct differed very little. Pigment stones in the common duct and gallbladder of the same patient differed more than the cholesterol stone pairs. Pigment stones of the CBD tended to contain more bilirubin and less residue than their gallbladder counterparts. Second, only 10% to 20% of patients with common duct stones have no stones in their gallbladders.[6]

Primary duct stones.   Formation of stones in the bile duct de novo is supported by several observations. First, 20 of 47 symptomatic patients with congenitally absent gallbladders had CBD stones.[7] Second, in cholecystectomized animals, stones form proximal to experimental strictures of the CBD, and in humans, benign and malignant strictures of the bile duct frequently result in sludge and stones proximal to the obstruction.[8] The chemical composition of primary duct stones, which are mostly calcium bilirubinate with a cholesterol content of less than 25%, is very different from that of the predominant type of gallbladder stones.

The true incidence of primary duct stones in the West is difficult to ascertain because of tremendous disagreement about diagnostic criteria. In 1924, Aschoff proposed that primary duct stones could be differentiated morphologically.[9] They are light brown, greenish brown, or black; "earthy" and soft; frequently laminated; and easily crushed to form "biliary mud." These are frequently referred to as brown pigment stones or bile pigment calcium stones, in contrast to the black stones, which are hard and brittle, almost structureless, and originate from the gallbladder. Brown stones consist mainly of calcium bilirubinate, with little cholesterol, and always contain calcium palmitate, but black stones mainly contain bilirubin polymers, usually calcium carbonate or phosphate, seldom cholesterol, and never calcium palmitate.

Using only morphologic criteria, Madden reported that 56% of the CBD stones are primary.[6] However, morphologic criteria alone may be unreliable. More than one half of the common duct stones were found at the time of initial operation for cholecystectomy. Many of these stones could have originated in the gallbladder and grown in the CBD to give the appearance of a primary stone. If the gallbladder is still in place or only recently has been removed, the origin of the duct stone is impossible to discern.

Saharia and colleagues, using strict criteria for the diagnosis of primary duct stones, found only a 4% prevalence of primary duct stones in 758 patients undergoing common duct exploration.[10] Their criteria consisted of a 2-year asymptomatic period after cholecystectomy, common duct stones with the morphologic appearance of primary duct stones, and absence of a long cystic duct remnant or biliary stricture from the previous surgery. Even though only 1 of 30 patients with primary duct stones had ampullary stenosis, all but 3 had dilated CBDs, often out of proportion to mildly abnormal serum bilirubin levels. The mean interval between cholecystectomy and diagnosis of common duct stones was 12 years (range, 2–36 years). Most gastroenterologists would accept that, if common duct stone is found within 1 or possibly 2 years after a cholecystectomy, it is more likely to be a retained gallbladder stone (i.e., secondary stone). A common duct stone found more than 1 to 2 years after cholecystectomy is usually considered to be a primary common duct stone.[11] This distinction is important, because the clinical course, prognosis, and management may differ.

Although the pathogenesis of primary duct stone formation remains unknown, several factors seem to play major roles under certain circumstances, including stasis, bacterial or parasitic infections, diet, foreign material in the duct, and juxtapapillary diverticula.

Experimental obstruction and stasis result in stone formation in animals.[7] In humans with benign or malignant strictures, sludge and stones frequently occur proximal to strictures.

In examining the role of bacteria in the pathogenesis of primary duct stones, Tabata and Nakayama cultured bile aerobically and anaerobically from 200 consecutive gallstone cases.[12] They found the prevalence of positive culture ($>10^5$ colony-forming units/mL bile) depended on the type of stone and the location of the stone. For stones localized to the gallbladder, only 5% of cases with black stones and 15% of cases with cholesterol stones were culture positive, but 80% of cases with brown stones were positive. For stones in the CBD, 100% of cases with brown stones were culture positive, and 74% of cases with cholesterol stones were culture positive. More than two organisms commonly were found in cases of brown stones.

The most common organisms isolated were *Escherichia coli*, *Klebsiella*, and other enteric gram-negative organisms. Anaerobes such as *Bacteroides* and *Clostridium* were also frequently isolated. These anaerobes possess β-glucuronidase activity like *E coli*. The investigators suggest that bacteria play a major role in the pathogenesis of brown stones. Bilirubin is excreted in bile mainly as diglucuronide and partly as monoglucuronide.[13] These molecules are subsequently transformed to unconjugated bilirubin by β-glucuronidase and combine with calcium to form calcium bilirubinate, which precipitates in aqueous media. Tissue lysosomal β-glucuronidase activity occurs in bile, but the optimal pH for its activity is 4.2. Bacterial β-glucuronidase has an optimal pH of 7.0, and the pH in bile is 6.25 to 8.10. It is therefore likely that bacterial β-glucuronidase activity leads to formation of unconjugated bilirubin, which later forms bile pigment calcium stones.

The association of biliary infection with primary common duct stones has been found by other investigators.[14–16] Lygidakis found that 73% of cases with primary duct stones had bile that was culture positive, compared with only 16% of cases with secondary stones.[15,16] He also observed positive cultures were significantly associated with the number of previous biliary tract interventions, diameter of the CBD (35%–100% positive in cases with >1.5–5-cm CBD diameter), increasing age, and duration of symptoms. Anaerobes were more likely to be cultured in those with primary duct stones.

The association between bacteria and brown stones is impressive but cannot prove a cause-and-effect association. Bacterial infection may result from common duct stones and bile

stasis. This is supported by the high prevalence of positive cultures in some reports of secondary duct stones. However, one report documented bile infection by *E coli* preceded rather than followed brown stone formation.[17] Another report showed that bacteria were observed only within brown pigment stones but not black pigment or cholesterol stones.[18] This type of evidence lends more support to the pathogenic role that bacteria play in primary, but not secondary, duct stones.

The association of parasitic infection and primary duct stones has been made predominantly in Asia. However, a report from South Africa documented that 13 of 13,500 patients (<0.001%) who underwent abdominal ultrasound examination had intrahepatic calculi.[19] None of the patients had travelled to the Far East, and all ate a predominantly Western diet. Only 1 of the 13 patients had evidence of gallbladder stones. All except 1 patient had documented *Ascaris* infection, implicating ascariasis as the etiologic factor in intrahepatic duct stones formation in these patients. Roundworm elements were reported in as many as 55% to 70% of patients with intrahepatic brown stones in series from Southeast Asia just after World War II.[20] Although worms of the biliary tree may cause obstruction and infection leading to calcium bilirubinate precipitation, roundworm infestation occurs worldwide and is epidemic in underdeveloped countries, but intrahepatic duct stones rarely occur outside Southeast Asia. This suggests that additional factors contribute to the high prevalence of cholangiohepatitis in Asia.

Dietary factors can be important. Bilirubin is excreted in bile as diglucuronide and monoglucuronide, which may then be subjected to breakdown by β-glucuronidase to glucuronic acid and free bilirubin. Inhibitors of β-glucuronidase, such as glucaro-1:4-lactone (measured as glucaric acid), free bilirubin, glucuronic acid, and Cu^{2+}, occur in bile.[21,22] The primary inhibitor appears to be glucaro-1:4-lactone; the levels of the other inhibitors in normal bile are too low to exert any appreciable effect. Glucaro-1:4-lactone is a degradation product of hepatic metabolism of glucuronic acid. The level of glucaro-1:4-lactone was lowered in animals fed diets low in protein and fat.[20] *E coli* has been shown to metabolize glucaric acid into glycerate and pyruvate.[23] Perhaps protein and fat malnutrition leads to bile low in glucaric acid and high in β-glucuronidase activity. A diet low in fat and protein may promote bile stasis because of decreased cholecystokinin release, which normally relaxes the sphincter of Oddi. *E coli* infection in the bile can further worsen this imbalance by degrading the glucaric acid present and by providing its own β-glucuronidase activity. All of these factors may contribute to formation of calcium bilirubinate (Fig. 97-1).

Indirect support for dietary factors in the pathogenesis of primary duct stones comes from studies in Asia, especially Japan, where the prevalence of calcium bilirubinate stones among patients with stones before World War II and the ensuing 10 years was 60% to 80%. After 1953, the prevalence of cholesterol gallstones rose, and that of calcium bilirubinate stones decreased.[20,24] From 1972 to 1974, cholesterol gallstones accounted for 85% of stones in Japan. From 1975 to 1978, the prevalence of intrahepatic stones found in patients undergoing biliary surgery at 40 hospitals in western Japan was only 3.03%, and the prevalence was much higher in rural hospitals than in urban hospitals (4.97% versus 1.5%).[24] All

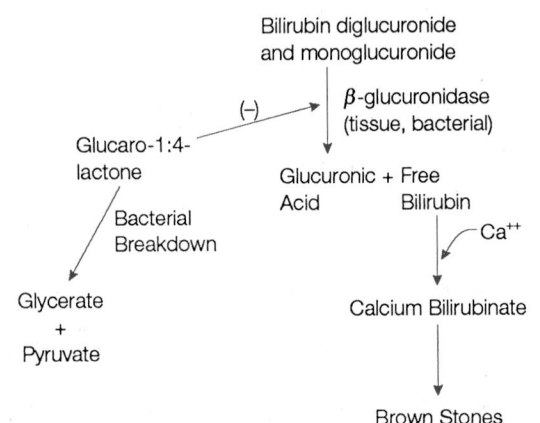

FIGURE 97-1. Proposed mechanisms of brown stone formation.

of these changes coincided with dietary changes that took place in Japan. The average daily protein intake increased from 65 to 78 g and fat intake from 16 to 48.7 g between 1949 and 1971.[20] Parasites were virtually eradicated after 1965, which may have contributed to the decreased prevalence of brown stones.[24]

Foreign material in the bile duct can be a factor in stone formation. In at least two series, 30% of recurrent stones in the CBD after cholecystectomy contained unabsorbable suture material in the center of the stone.[5,25] This could have served as a nidus for stone growth. Nonabsorbable suture material should be avoided in surgical procedures in the vicinity of the CBD.

The association of juxtapapillary diverticula and common duct stones has been observed by several researchers.[26-29] The prevalence of duodenal diverticula varies from 3% to 22% in autopsy series and 18.8% to 23% among patients who underwent endoscopic retrograde cholangiopancreatography (ERCP).[26,28] Ninety percent of duodenal diverticula occur on the medial wall of the duodenum, and two thirds are juxtapapillary. The ampulla may be adjacent to the diverticulum or may empty into it. In an ERCP study of stone recurrence after cholecystectomy, 88% of patients with juxtapapillary diverticula had recurrent common duct stones, but only 32% of patients without diverticula had recurrent common duct stones. The stones were much more likely to be pigmented and to be recurrent stones after cholecystectomy. In another study, 59% of patients with recurrent duct stones found 3 or more years after cholecystectomy had diverticula, but only 13% with stone-free ducts had diverticula.[28] Manometric studies found significantly lower sphincter of Oddi (SOD) pressures in patients with juxtapapillary diverticula. Theoretically, bacterial overgrowth in the diverticula may colonize the bile duct. These observations strongly support the association of juxtapapillary diverticula and common duct stones. How the diverticula develop in the first place and whether they predispose to the formation of duct stones is only speculative.

Two other findings associated with common duct stones are low entry of the cystic duct (<3.5 cm from the ampulla) and abnormal motor activity of the SOD.[29,30] Toouli and co-workers found no difference in the CBD pressure, SOD basal

pressure, SOD phasic wave amplitude, frequency and duration, or percentage of simultaneous SOD contractions between patients with common duct stones and normal controls. The only significant difference was the direction of SOD pressure wave propagation. In controls, $60 \pm 4\%$ of wave sequences were antegrade, and $26 \pm 3\%$ were retrograde. In patients with common duct stones, $18 \pm 5\%$ of wave sequences were antegrade, and $53 \pm 9\%$ were retrograde. It is unclear whether this abnormal motility pattern contributes to the cause of common duct stones or is a secondary effect of the common duct stones.

Primary intraductal cholesterol stones are rare. One report correlated their presence with regional loss of the anitnucleating factor, apo A-I, as determined by immunohistochemistry of hepatocytes and ductal epithelium.[31] No such loss was seen in uninvolved segments of liver or in cases of intraductal pigment stones. It remains to be seen if this is cause or effect.

Clinical Manifestations

Natural history. The natural history of choledocholithiasis is unpredictable. CBD stones may be asymptomatic for many years, or may, without warning, precipitate biliary colic, jaundice, cholangitis, or pancreatitis.[32] Millbourn reported the natural history of CBD stones in 1941, before the era of antibiotics, in 38 patients who refused surgery or were considered surgically unfit.[33] In the follow-up period of 6 months to 13 years, 17 (45%) patients remained asymptomatic, and 21 (55%) developed complications such as biliary colic, jaundice, and cholangitis.

Clinical presentation. The clinical manifestations of choledocholithiasis range from no signs or symptoms to acute suppurative cholangitis. The most common presentation is its unanticipated discovery at cholecystectomy.[1] Between 2% and 10% of patients undergoing routine cholecystectomy have unsuspected common duct stones.[34] Stones in these cases were found by the surgeon by palpating the stone in the CBD or observing an intraductal filling defect on the operative cholangiogram.

Patients with choledocholithiasis may present with biliary colic. The biliary colic caused by a stone in the common duct is clinically indistinguishable from that caused by a stone in the cystic duct. This visceral-type pain is caused by sudden obstruction in the bile duct, producing increased intralumenal pressure and distention. Typically, the pain is felt in the right upper quadrant or epigastrium, with frequent radiation to the interscapular area, but the site may vary. The term *colic* is a misnomer, because the pain is constant in nature; it is unassociated with position and typically lasts 30 minutes to several hours. Nausea and vomiting commonly occur during an attack. Discrete attacks can occur at any time of the day or night and at unpredictable intervals. Food ingestion does not specifically precipitate an attack.

One well-known complication that can occur during passage of gallstones through the ampulla is gallstone pancreatitis. This cause of pancreatitis is supported by reports of finding gallstones in the stools in 84% to 94% of patients with gallstones within 8 days after an attack of pancreatitis.[35-37] The size of gallstones recovered from the stools ranged from 1 to 12 mm, and there was no relation between stone size and severity of the pancreatitis.[36] Although gallstones may produce pancreatitis through their ball-valve action at the ampulla, this condition rarely occurs. Impacted ampullary calculi are found in only 5% to 8% of patients with gallstone pancreatitis.[38,39] Gallstone passage does not always lead to pancreatitis. In one report, 12% of gallstone patients with stones in the stools suffered no pancreatitis.[36] The reason that gallstone pancreatitis develops in some but not others is unknown. The pathogenesis of gallstone pancreatitis is discussed in detail in Chapter 90.

If the stone obstructs the bile duct for long enough and the bile becomes infected, acute cholangitis ensues. The classic triad of Charcot—fever, chills, and jaundice—occurs in only 50% to 75% of patients with acute cholangitis.[1,40,41] Peritoneal signs are infrequent in the absence of concomitant cholecystitis. Between 70% and 80% of patients with cholangitis respond to antibiotics and supportive therapy, allowing time for a complete diagnostic evaluation before definitive operation.[2,42] A few patients deteriorate despite maximal supportive therapy. Refractory sepsis manifested by hypotension and mental confusion in a patient with Charcot's triad constitutes Reynold's pentad.[1] Fortunately, all five of these features affect fewer than 10% of patients with acute suppurative cholangitis.[42]

If a stone obstructs the CBD without superinfection, asymptomatic jaundice may ensue. If obstruction persists for 4 to 5 years before the diagnosis is made and therapy is instituted, biliary cirrhosis often develops. Lindenauer and Child found an 8% incidence of biliary cirrhosis in patients operated on for choledocholithiasis.[43] These patients may present with liver failure or portal hypertension as manifestations of long-term complications from choledocholithiasis.

Laboratory Findings

Laboratory results usually reflect the degree of biliary obstruction, but they may be normal despite several common duct calculi.[44] Sometimes, a mildly elevated alkaline phosphatase level is the first clue to the presence of choledocholithiasis in an asymptomatic patient. Serum bilirubin is elevated in 50% to 72% of symptomatic patients with choledocholithiasis. The bilirubin level is usually in the range of 2 to 14 mg/dL.[41,45] There is no correlation between the duration of jaundice and the peak bilirubin level.[45] Alkaline phosphatase levels are also often elevated, but usually not more than five times above normal values. Higher levels usually denote malignant obstruction.[45] Elevated aminotransferase levels up to three to five times normal are common and occasionally rise as high as in hepatitis. Typically these elevated aminotransferase levels rapidly return toward normal and seem to reflect the release of hepatic enzymes in response to acute obstruction. The improvement of aminotransferase and bilirubin does not necessarily mean that the obstruction has been relieved.[41]

Diagnosis

The diagnosis of bile duct calculi is challenging and important because of its implications for management. The CBD is explored in about 25% of cholecystectomies. The rate of negative CBD exploration results is 30% to 50%.[1] McSherry reported

a 0.5% mortality rate for cholecystectomy, 2.4% mortality rate for a negative choledochotomy, and 3.9% mortality rate for choledocholithotomy.[46] In young, healthy patients, a negative CBD exploration adds no significant increase to the mortality rate.[46] The 30-day mortality rate for good-risk patients younger than 60 years of age is less than 1.5%. With increasing age and associated medical problems, the overall risk for patients older than 65 years of age is 5%. With each added decade of age, risk increases.[47]

To decrease the rate of negative common duct exploration, investigators have examined various parameters to predict the presence of bile duct stones that would provide a specific indication for common duct exploration. Fever, biliary colic, number and size of gallstones, history of jaundice or pancreatitis, and presence or history of acute cholecystitis were found to be of no value in predicting the presence of bile duct stones found at surgery.[1,48–51] During surgery, common duct stones are found as frequently in patients with acute cholecystitis as in those with chronic cholecystitis.[49–51] The only clinical finding that predicts the presence of a common duct stone is jaundice with cholangitis (i.e., Charcot's triad). Approximately 95% of patients with Charcot's triad were found to have common duct stones.[34,52] However, most patients with CBD stones do not present with Charcot's triad.

Dilatation of the CBD has been reported to predict the presence of bile duct stones; one study found 69% of patients with CBD more than 13 mm in diameter had CBD stones.[48] This was not confirmed by other investigators.[51] As many as one third of patients with CBD stones have nondilated bile ducts.[53,54] The diameter of a bile duct depends on the imaging study used. In one study comparing different radiologic methods in the same patients, the upper limit of normal for the extrahepatic bile duct measured at its widest point was 4 mm for ultrasound, 7.5 mm for intravenous cholangiography, and 10.5 mm for endoscopic retrograde cholangiography (ERC) and percutaneous transhepatic cholangiography (PTC).[55]

The bilirubin level may be of discriminatory value. Mild jaundice is common in cholangitis and cholecystitis, but many patients with a bilirubin level above 6.7 mg/dL had stones in the CBD.[52]

Because clinical findings are inadequate to establish the presence of choledocholithiasis in most patients with gallstone disease, imaging techniques are required for more accurate assessment. The imaging techniques that have been used in the diagnosis of bile duct stones include intravenous cholangiography, ultrasound, computed tomography (CT) scan, and ERC. Intravenous cholangiography is of no value in the diagnosis of choledocholithiasis. In a report that evaluated 128 intravenous cholangiography studies, only 55% were technically adequate. In verified analysis of adequate cholangiograms, the diagnostic error rate was 40%, largely due to missed stones.[56]

Although the ability to detect gallbladder stones and to measure duct diameter by ultrasound is excellent, the same technique is only able to detect 10% to 18% of instances of common duct stones in patients subsequently proven to have them. In jaundiced patients, this figure rises to 33% (Fig. 97-2).[53,57–59] CT scan appears to be superior to ultrasound in the detection of CBD stones, with a 50% to 90% sensitivity.[54,57]

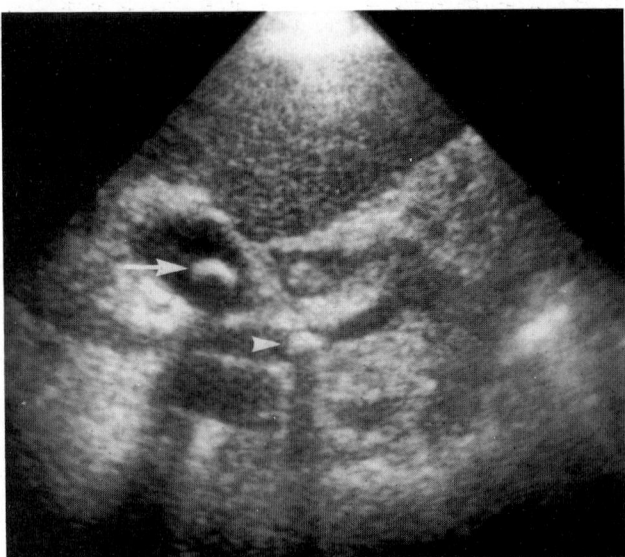

FIGURE 97-2. Secondary duct calculus. Gallbladder (*arrow*) and common bile duct (*arrowhead*) calculi presenting as echogenic foci with characteristic acoustical shadowing are seen on this ultrasound sector scan.

The role for ERC or PTC in the diagnosis of choledocholithiasis is mainly in those patients suspected of having CBD stones, but noninvasive tests (i.e., ultrasound or CT scan) failed to detect them. These procedures are also useful in the treatment of choledocholithiasis. In the case of a nondilated bile duct, ERC is preferred over PTC because of a higher success rate. In cases of dilated ducts, the success rates of PTC and ERC are comparable at 90% (Fig. 97-3). PTC should be avoided in cases of active cholangitis. The local availability of these techniques and the specific nature of each patient's presentation are the most important factors in selecting the preferred technique. However, in a poor operative risk, ERC may be preferred because it can be combined with therapeutic procedures such as sphincterotomy, stone removal, or stenting.

Diagnosis at operation.   Two main goals of the biliary tract surgeon are to decrease the frequency of unnecessary CBD exploration and to decrease the frequency of retained CBD stones. The incidence of retained CBD stones seems to be related to the number of stones found in the duct; the more stones found, the higher is the incidence of stone retention.[60]

A major advance in biliary tract surgery was the introduction of preexploratory operative cholangiography by Marizzi in 1932.[61] This procedure is routinely used in cholecystectomy and has reduced the frequency of unnecessary CBD explorations by as much as 90% and increased the detection of unsuspected stones.[1,34,51] The false-negative rate for operative cholangiography has ranged from zero to 8%, with a false-positive rate of 11% to 38%.[34,51] One of the most accurate findings in the diagnosis of choledocholithiasis is palpable stones in the bile duct. When stones are palpated in the CBD, common duct exploration yields stones in about 90% of patients.[1,34] Another major advance was the reintroduction of choledochoscopy in the 1970s. This adds an additional 15 to

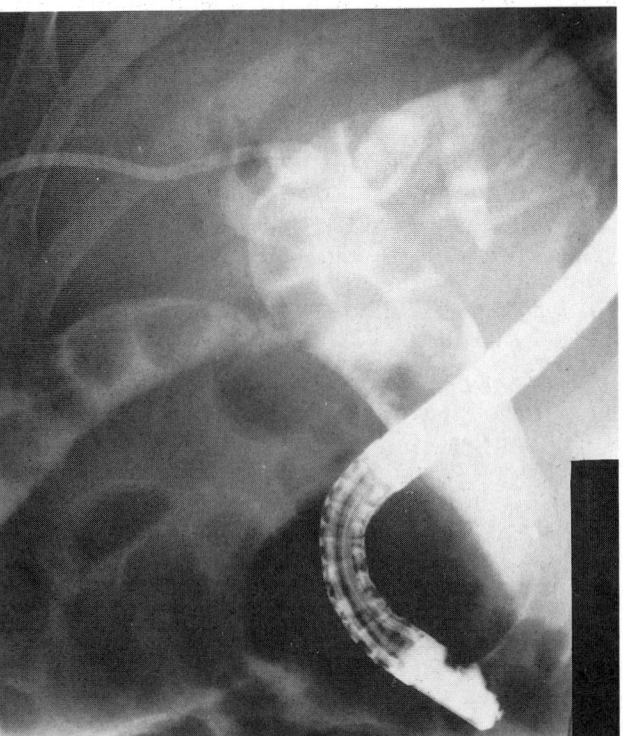

FIGURE 97-3. Common duct calculi with gallbladder in situ. Endoscopic retrograde cholangiogram shows a dilated common bile duct with multiple filling defects and a gallbladder that also has multiple filling defects. This patient had multiple stones in the common duct and gallbladder. A pigtail catheter had been placed percutaneous and transhepatically for drainage. (Courtesy of Hartley Cohen, M.D., Los Angeles, CA.)

20 minutes to operative times but causes no additional complications for most patients.[62] Routine use of postexploratory choledochoscopy has detected residual stones in 14% to 24% of patients.[1,62,63] In patients with stones found during bile duct exploration, choledochoscopy detected additional stones in one third; in patients with negative duct exploration results, choledochoscopy found stones in 7%.[62] We recommend operative cholangiography for all patients undergoing gallbladder surgery and additional choledochoscopy for patients undergoing CBD exploration. With these advances, the incidence of retained stones has decreased from 10% to 15% to a rate of 1% to 4% after CBD exploration.[1,2,62,63]

Another technique employed by some to improve diagnostic accuracy is operative manometry, combining pressure and flow measurements in the CBD with operative cholangiography. White and Bordley reported a 100% diagnostic accuracy rate and 1% incidence of recurrent stones at 6 to 8 years of follow-up.[64]

Treatment

Any treatment for bile duct stones needs to consider whether the gallbladder or a T-tube is present and consider the age and other surgical risks of the patient.

In Western countries, most calculi found in the CBD during cholecystectomy are cholesterol gallstones formed in the gallbladder and passed into the biliary tree. In most instances, the calculi are few, and cholecystectomy, CBD exploration, and removal of duct calculi suffice as treatment. Surgery should be the treatment of choice in young, good-risk patients who present with complications of duct stones, such as pancreatitis or cholangitis. Most patients with gallstone pancreatitis pass their stones. The initial therapy can be medical, followed by early elective surgery. For patients who do not respond within the first 24 to 48 hours, most gastroenterologists advocate urgent surgery for good-risk patients.[2] Several risk factors are associated with an increased mortality rate for biliary tract surgery:

> Presence of malignancy (20% versus 3.5% mortality rate for benign disease)
> Increasing age (16% mortality rate for those older than 60 versus 1.2% for those younger than 60 years of age)
> Anemia (hematocrit <30%).
> Leukocytosis (leukocyte count >10,000 mm³)
> Creatinine level higher than 1.3 mg/dL
> Albumin level less than 3.0 g/dL
> Bilirubin level more than 10 mg/dL
> Alkaline phosphatase level more than 100 IUL.[65]

For patients with two or fewer risk factors, no operative mortality was reported; for those with three to four risk factors, the mortality rate was 4% to 7%. Patients with five risk factors had an associated mortality rate of 44%, those with six risk factors had a mortality rate of 67%, and those with seven or eight risk factors had a 100% mortality rate.[65] Because of the higher mortality rates reported in cases of obstructive jaundice, several physicians recommended preoperative percutaneous biliary drainage. However, no benefit or worsening of operative mortality was found in several controlled trials.[2,66,67]

Patients with cholangitis should be initially treated with antibiotics, such as aminoglycosides and third-generation cephalosporins, that cover the common enteric gram-negative, gram-positive, and anaerobic bacteria. Most patients respond to this therapy, allowing time for elective surgery. About one third of patients presenting with suppurative cholangitis at the University of California at Los Angeles (UCLA) have required urgent operation within the first 24 to 72 hours after hospitalization. The operative mortality rate was 5% for those with common duct stones. The mortality rate correlated with the failure to respond to antibiotics.[2]

What about patients with gallbladder in situ who are older or have many operative risk factors? The best approach in this group of patients appears to be endoscopic papillotomy (ECP). The first endoscopic sphincterotomies of the papilla of Vater were performed simultaneously in 1973 by Japanese and German endoscopists.[68] Some investigators feel that a common duct stone is an indication for ECP only when the patient is older than 50 years of age or has many surgical risk factors. The reason they would not recommend ECP in younger patients is that the long-term effects of sphincterotomy are unknown. It may adversely affect the bile composition and destroy the barrier function of the papilla against bacterial infection from the intestine.[68,69] Contraindications to ECP include all of those to endoscopy and the presence of long strictures in the distal CBD. ECP is ineffective if the abnormality is restricted to the proximal bile ducts or if the stones are too large (>2.5 cm) for mechanical retrieval.

The success rate of ECP for patients with intact stomachs is 80% to 95% and 50% for patients with Billroth II anastomosis.[59,68–73] However, a success rate as high as 92% for patients with Billroth II anastomosis was reported with use of a 30-30 papillotome or by creating a suprapapillary fistulotomy.[74] About 89% of the patients with successful ECPs are cleared of bile duct stones (i.e., 55% passed spontaneously, 34% required some type of mechanical extraction). Failures are usually the result of stones being too large or impacted. Since 1984, at least 11 reports have shown that performing ECP in patients with gallbladders in situ is safe.[71–75] The incidence of subsequent cholecystitis and biliary tract complications range from 5% to 30% during a mean follow-up period of 2 to 4 years.[71,72,75] Recurrent symptoms developed in patients who also had gallbladder stones or originally had nonvisualized gallbladders but not in those who only had common duct stones.[72,74] These results argue for definitive surgery in good-risk patients. CBD stones recurred in 2.5% to 6% of patients.[68,72]

The rates of complications from ECP have been low; the worldwide rates since 1980 are 6% to 10% for morbidity and 0.6% to 1% for mortality. The complications include bleeding, pancreatitis, cholangitis, and perforation. Nevertheless, ECP compares favorably with the operative mortality rate of 5% to 10% in patients older than 60 years of age undergoing common duct exploration.[69]

ECP with biliary drainage and stone extraction is preferred over surgery for high-risk patients who failed conservative therapies for acute cholangitis or pancreatitis; the mortality rate has been 4.7% to 10% with ECP, compared with 17% to 40% with urgent surgery.[76–78] The use of urgent ERCP with ECP (<72 hours after admission) in severe acute cholangitis and acute gallstone pancreatitis was addressed in two randomized controlled trials.[78,79] Lai and colleagues compared urgent endoscopic biliary drainage followed by definitive treatment with urgent surgery for severe acute cholangitis due to CBD stones.[78] They found lower complication (14 of 41 versus 27 of 41) and mortality (4 of 41 versus 13 of 41) rates for the group randomized to endoscopic biliary drainage. Neoptolemos and colleagues studied 121 patients with acute gallstone pancreatitis who were randomized to receive conventional therapy or to undergo urgent ERCP with ECP.[79] Patients were stratified by the predicted severity of their attack using the modified Glasgow system. They found that ERCP could be safely performed and that ECP reduced major complications, especially in the group that had severe attacks (54% complication rate in the conventional group versus 18% in the ECP group); the overall mortality rate was 18% for the conventional group and 4% for the ECP group.

Some have proposed that preoperative ECP lowers the mortality rate of cholecystectomy with common duct exploration. However, three studies randomizing patients to preoperative ECP or surgery found no benefit, and one study found more complications in those undergoing preoperative ECP.[73,74,80] In a large multivariate analysis of the preoperative risk factors of patients with CBD stones, 248 underwent surgery and 190 underwent ECP, 77 of whom subsequently also had surgery. The analysis showed that the significant risk factors in those undergoing surgery were the serum bilirubin level, the use of preoperative ECP, and the presence of medical risk factors, such as any cardiovascular or respiratory condition requiring long-term drug therapy, diabetes mellitus requiring therapy, any medical condition requiring long-term steroids, any major psychiatric disorder, or central nervous system disturbance.[81] However, the significant risk factors for patients undergoing ECP were only the serum bilirubin and albumin, but not medical risk factors. The major implications of this analysis are that ECP is preferred over surgery in high-risk patients and that good-risk patients should be treated by surgery alone without routine preoperative ECP.

Since 1990, laparoscopic cholecystectomy has revolutionized the surgical approach to patients with symptomatic gallbladder stones. It has rapidly superseded all other forms of therapy. Early experience with laparoscopic cholecystectomy indicates that it compares favorably with traditional open cholecystectomy, with the major advantages of minimal morbidity, shorter hospital stay, earlier return to work, and a better cosmetic result.[82–84] A controversial area is the optimal approach to patients with CBD stones. Some have advocated preoperative ERCP and ECP. The problem with preoperative ERCP in patients suspected of having CBD stones on clinical grounds alone is that only 16% to 50% proved to have stones.[82,84] The yield of finding CBD stones on ERCP is better in patients with dilated bile duct and hyperbilirubinemia.[84] Other physicians prefer preoperative cholangiography with the options of converting to immediate open cholecystectomy with choledochotomy, laparoscopic transcystic exploration and stone extraction, or subsequent endoscopic sphincterotomy and stone removal in the early postoperative period or simply observation.[82,84,85] Further work is needed to define the optimal approach to common duct stones in patients undergoing laparoscopic cholecystectomy.

At least 1% to 4% of patients have retained common duct stones after cholecystectomy and common duct exploration. Sometimes, stones cannot be removed during surgery. These retained stones are usually found on T-tube cholangiograms performed postoperatively. Previously, the best approach in these cases has been percutaneous stone extraction through the T-tube tract 4 to 6 weeks after surgery, which is a time when the sinus tract of the indwelling T-tube has matured. There are attractive alternatives, including endoscopic extraction, dissolution, and fragmentation.[60] Reports have shown that performing ECP with the T-tube in situ has been especially successful for stones distal to the T-tube.[86,87] One retrospective analysis of a large number of patients showed comparable success and complication rates for the percutaneous and the endoscopic approaches.[87] Approaches using dissolution with methyl-tertbutyl ether (MTBE) and monoctanoin have also been reported. Janssen and colleagues reported good results using high-flow, high-temperature monoctanoin therapy as the treatment for retained ductal stones.[88] Successful dissolution has been achieved safely within 24 hours, reducing length of hospital stay and health care costs. This encouraging result awaits more data and experience from other centers. The advantage with ECP and dissolution therapy is that treatment can begin immediately after the operation once a lack of extravasation is proved on a postoperative cholangiogram.

Several methods of percutaneous extraction have been described, and most use a steerable catheter and stone basket under fluoroscopic control or choledochoscopy.[90–92] Use of tunable dye laser delivered through a T-tube tract choledo-

choscope also showed encouraging results.[89] Approximately 95% of the retained stones can be successfully removed, sometimes requiring multiple sessions.[90–92] Failure occurs if the T-tube tract is too small or tortuous or if the stone is too large, impacted, or not crushable. Complication rates in expert hands are 4% to 5%, and mortality rates are 1% to 2%. The most common complications are fever and sinus tract leak.[92] This compares favorably to the 3% to 28% mortality rates for reexploration of the CBD.[87,90]

Patients who present with duct stones months to years after cholecystectomy can first be managed with endoscopic sphincterotomy and mechanical extraction. Several other nonsurgical approaches are available for these difficult cases, including oral dissolution, instillation of solvents into the biliary tree, extracorporeal shock wave lithotripsy (ESWL), laser, and electrohydraulic lithotripsy. Other than the use of oral dissolution and monoctanoin, the methods are still experimental. Both chenodeoxycholic and ursodeoxycholic acids can dissolve bile duct stones provided that they contain mostly cholesterol. In one study, patients with common duct stones without cholangitis were randomized to ursodeoxycholic acid (12 mg/kg/day) or placebo for 24 months. Seven of 14 patients randomized to ursodeoxycholic acid had complete stone disappearance, but none of those randomized to placebo had any change in stone size.[93] However, an unreliable test—intravenous cholangiography—was used to follow these patients' progress. Nevertheless, the low response rates and the long duration of treatment limit its use in patients with bile duct stones.

The chemicals that have been directly infused into the biliary tree in an attempt to dissolve duct stones include heparin, sodium cholate, monoctanoin, clofibrate, and MTBE. The effect of heparin is probably a result of flushing rather than actual stone dissolution.[94] Sodium cholate infusion was ineffective and had high complication rates. Similarly, monoctanoin has generally fallen out of use because of the long time it requires for response (1–2 weeks), and it only has a 54% success rate.[59,95,96] An in vitro study showed 91% of stones with a cholesterol content of more than 40% dissolved within 5 days with monoctanoin; stones with high cholesterol contents probably have higher and faster response rates in vivo. However, Janssen and colleagues did have good results with monoctanoin using a high-flow and high-temperature delivery method.[88,95]

MTBE has received much attention because of rapid dissolution of cholesterol stones.[97] Unlike treating stones in the gallbladder, the use of MTBE in duct stones is more precarious. If significant overflow of MTBE into the duodenum occurs, sedation, duodenitis, and hemolysis can result. Reports of MTBE in treating duct stones have included the use of a device to occlude the distal CBD and frequent aspirations to minimize overflow.[98,99] Report of a collaborative study of MTBE dissolution therapy for CBD stones from nine U.K. centers showed that MTBE treatment was successful in only 12 of 33 patients.[100] However, another report showed 10 of 12 patients treated with MTBE were cleared of their CBD stones; three spontaneously cleared, but seven required endoscopic extraction.[101] In the latter group, the cholangiographic appearance did not change after MTBE. The investigators thought that MTBE "softened" the stones, facilitating subsequent stone removal.

The use of ESWL for CBD stones was pioneered by German investigators.[102,103] Shock waves are high-pressure waves generated outside the body and focused on the stone by hemi-ellipsoidal reflectors. Coupling of the human body to shock waves can be achieved by positioning the body in a water bath or over a water cushion. In treating common duct stones, shock waves enter posteriorly to avoid intestinal gas. A nasobiliary or percutaneous catheter delivers contrast. Positioning and monitoring are done by fluoroscopy. In a prospective, uncontrolled, multicenter trial, 113 patients who failed ECP were treated.[103] Stone disintegration was achieved in 103 patients (91%), and complete stone clearance from the bile duct was obtained in 97 patients (86%) after a median of 4 days after the procedure. The in-hospital mortality rate was 1.8%. The main determinant for failure was size of the common duct stone; those that failed had a 30 ± 13 mm average stone diameter, compared with a diameter of 22 ± 7 mm for the successful cases.

Many other reports have appeared since 1986 on the use of ESWL in treating CBD stones. The results are generally the same, with success rates of complete stone clearance near 80%, although most patients required additional ERCP or percutaneous extraction of stone fragments.[74,104] This is quite remarkable considering the large diameters of stones being treated. Even more appealing is the report of successful treatment using piezoelectric (essentially painless) machines.[105] The major drawback with this technology is the lack of Food and Drug Administration approval.

Other experimental approaches require direct contact with the stones. These include electrohydraulic, ultrasound, and tunable dye laser lithotripsy applied endoscopically.[69,106,107] It is too early to tell what roles these will play in the treatment of bile duct stones. Approximately 90% of stones that cannot be removed by ECP can be treated by one or a combination of these methods.

If bile duct stones cannot be extracted endoscopically, a nasobiliary tube can be placed as a temporizing measure. This prevents stone impaction and allows drainage until more definitive therapy is instituted. Moreover, the drain permits infusion of chemicals for stone dissolution, allows for repeat ERCP, and enables contrast delivery during ESWL. In elderly and high-risk patients with nonextractable stones, long-term internal stenting is a good palliative measure.[74,108] Although stent clogging often develops within months (earlier with 7-F than 10-F stents), long-term drainage is maintained because the stent prevents stone impaction. Patency of the prosthesis is therefore not critical, and stent changes are generally not required unless the stent spontaneously migrates out of the duct.[74] Reports of using long-term internal stenting for nonextractable CBD stones in 280 patient from 1984 to 1992 showed an excellent rate of establishing biliary drainage (~100%), with complication rates of 0% to 33% during a median follow-up of 13 to 39 months.[108] Patients with gallbladders in situ and in whom sphincterotomy was not carried out had higher complication rates.[108] Sphincterotomy may be considered a prerequisite in all patients in whom an endoprosthesis is inserted as long-term treatment.

Surgery still plays an important role for those who fail the nonsurgical approaches and for those who develop recurrent bile duct stones. Approximately 20% of patients who undergo reoperation for residual stones redevelop choledocholithia-sis.[10,93,94] Some type of surgical drainage procedure (e.g., choledochoenteric anastomosis) is indicated for patients presenting with recurrent biliary calculi. A drainage procedure is recommended at any operation if distal bile duct patency is compromised by benign stricture and if stones cannot be removed. Some surgeons would not perform a drainage procedure at the first reoperation unless too many stones or a high-grade ampullary obstruction are found or if the patient is at high reoperative risk. Most would perform a drainage procedure with the second reoperation.[1,2,70] A step-by-step multidisciplinary approach to the management of CBD calculi is suggested in a subsequent section (Fig. 97-4).

Oriental Cholangiohepatitis

Even though most gallstones are formed in the gallbladder and most duct stones originated from the gallbladder, it was speculated centuries ago that another type of stone, known as a liver stone or intrahepatic stone, was completely different in its location, consistency, number, and behavior from choledocholithiasis of gallbladder origin. According to Rufanov, isolated cases of liver stones were described in the 16th and 17th centuries.[109] The largest collective review of material up to 1890, reported by Courvoisier, consisted of 50 cases.[110] The prevalence of intrahepatic stones in Western countries has been low, ranging from 0.6% (5 of 768 in a prospective necropsy study) to 2.4% of all cases of biliary lithiasis and are rarely primary.[111-114] This contrasts with Southeast Asia, where the prevalence was as high as 50% to 80% of all gallstone cases before 1958 and has decreased dramatically in certain areas such as Japan, Hong Kong, and Taiwan as hygiene and diet have improved.[20,24] An overall prevalence of 10% in Southeast Asia, with variations among different countries has been reported: 53.5% in Taiwan, 4.6% in Japan, 3.1% in Hong Kong, and 1.7% in Singapore.[115]

The syndrome commonly referred to as Oriental cholangiohepatitis, recurrent pyogenic cholangitis, or biliary obstruction syndrome was first described in Hong Kong by Digby in 1930.[116] This syndrome is characterized by intrahepatic pigment stone formation with recurrent exacerbations and remissions of abdominal pain frequently associated with jaundice, chills, and fever. This syndrome has been endemic to certain Southeast Asian societies such as China, Hong Kong, Taiwan, Korea, Japan, and Malaysia. It has received increasing attention in the United States because of the large number of immigrants from those endemic countries.[117-121] This syndrome has been so common in Taiwan and Hong Kong that reports from 1962 claimed it to be the third commonest cause of acute abdominal surgeries in Hong Kong.[122]

Clinical Features

The clinical features of Oriental cholangiohepatitis clearly differentiate it from gallstones seen in the West (Table 97-1).

Oriental cholangiohepatitis is seen in younger patients than patients with choledocholithiasis in the West. Eighty-six percent of patients present before 50 years of age.[110] Both sexes are equally affected. Malnutrition and lower socioeconomic class are associated with a higher incidence of this syndrome.[24,110] The relation of parasites to this syndrome is dis-

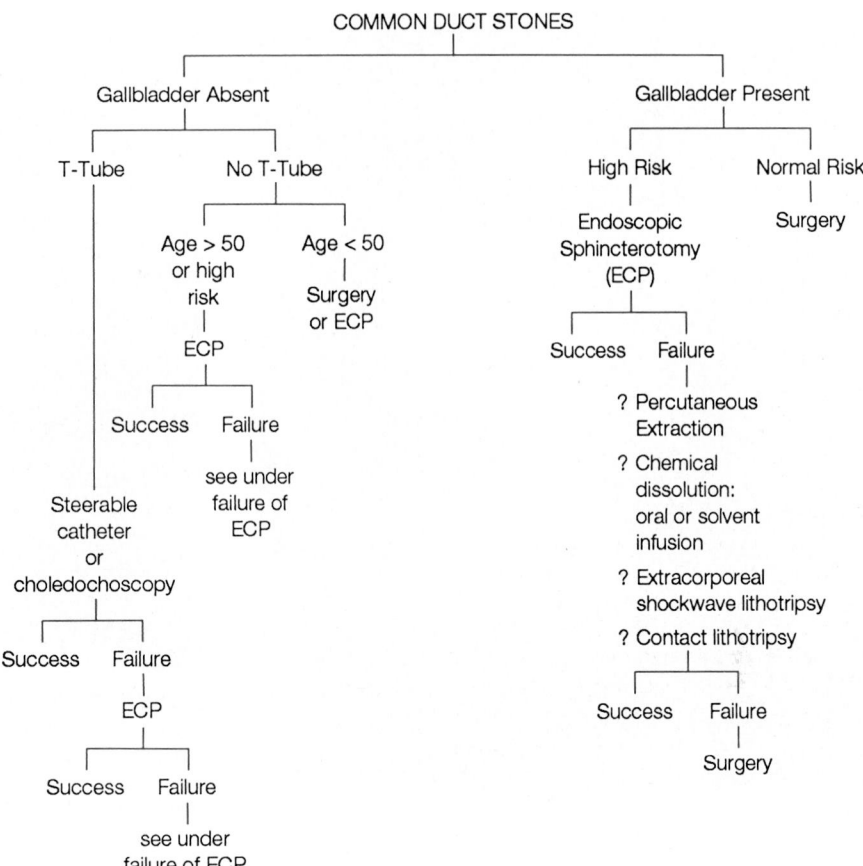

FIGURE 97-4. Multidisciplinary approach to the management of patients with common bile duct stones.

puted. About 25% of patients with this syndrome have *Clonorchis sinensis* ova in their stool, and 13% to 20% have ascariasis (Fig. 97-5).[123,124] Elements of these parasites have also been found in the center of 40% to 60% of stones.[20,125] However, the incidence of Oriental cholangitis has been high in Taiwan, where *C sinensis* infestation is rare, and the distribution of ascariasis is worldwide but Oriental cholangiohepatitis is not.[117]

The most common clinical presentation is that of Charcot's triad.[110,117,118,124] A typical attack starts with fever, shaking chills, and right upper quadrant abdominal pain. Jaundice appears 1 to 2 days later. Usually, it takes 1 to 2 weeks for a

moderate attack and longer for a more severe attack to subside spontaneously.[110] If the attack is severe, patients can be in septic shock, and death is imminent unless an operation is performed. The interval between attacks varies from once a week to once in more than a year, although 29% in one series reported more than one attack per month.[110] In addition to the usual signs of cholangitis, 19% had hepatomegaly, and 9% had palpable gallbladder.[110] Laboratory results only reflect the severity of the infection and the degree of biliary obstruction.

The typical clinical course is that of recurrent attacks. Reoperation has been common, with low surgical cure rates from

TABLE 97-1
Oriental Cholangiohepatitis and Secondary Duct Stones in the West

CHARACTERISTIC	ORIENTAL CHOLANGIOHEPATITIS	SEDONDARY DUCT STONES IN THE WEST
Age	Young and middle-aged	Rare in people <40 y
Gender	Females = males	Females > males
Socioeconomic status	Low income	General population
Nutritional status	Undernourished	Often obese
Stone composition	Calcium bilirubinate	Cholesterol
Stones in gallbladder	33%	Almost all
Radiology	Intrahepatic duct stones, duct dilation, strictures (esp. the left duct)	Stones in gallbladder and extrahepatic ducts
Prognosis	Poor, stone recurrence rates very high, reoperations common	Excellent with surgery

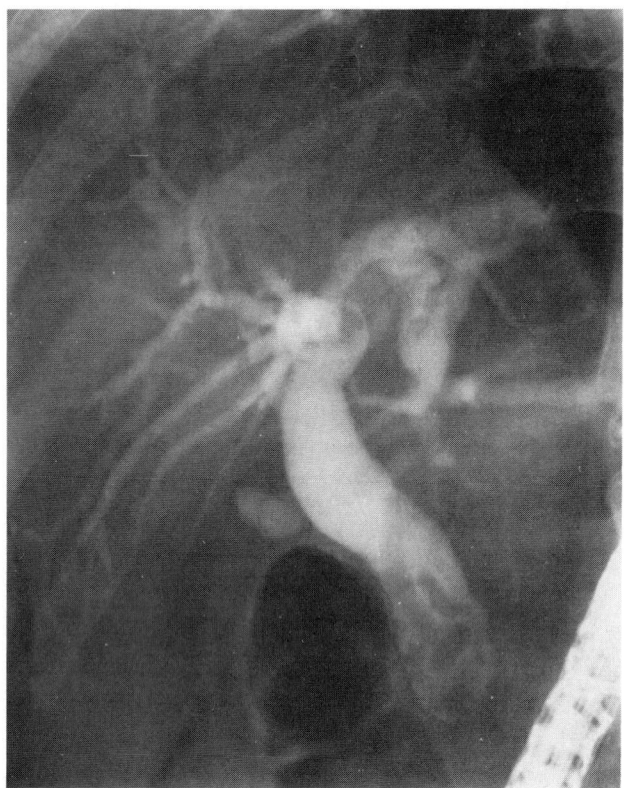

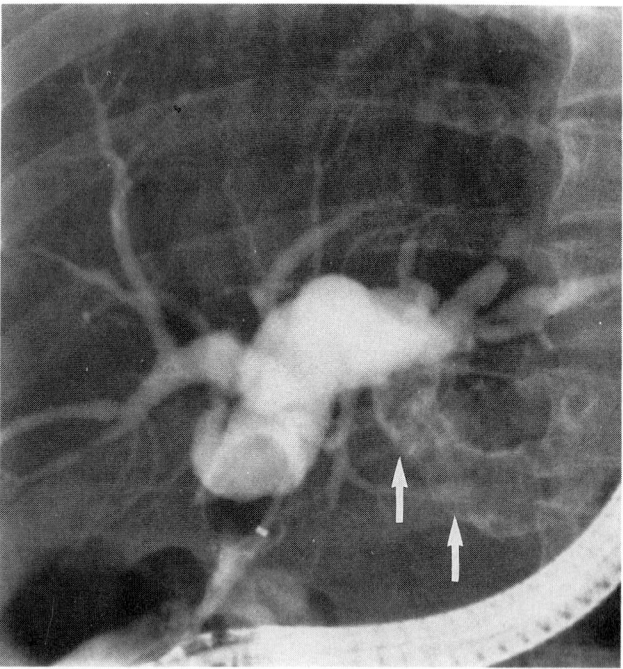

FIGURE 97-5. Biliary ascariasis. Endoscopic retrograde cholangiogram of a patient who presented with cholangitis. The common bile duct is dilated, with multiple worm-like filling defects distally. These were later found to be ascaris. (Courtesy of Hartley Cohen, M.D., Los Angeles, CA.)

FIGURE 97-6. Oriental cholangiohepatitis. The patient had choledochoduodenostomy performed a few years before presenting with cholangitis. With the aid of a balloon catheter, the endoscopic retrograde cholangiogram shows a dilated common duct and intrahepatic ducts. The left hepatic duct is especially dilated, with multiple filling defects representing pigment stones (*arrows*). The left hepatic duct is preferentially involved in Oriental cholangiohepatitis. (Courtesy of Hartley Cohen, M.D., Los Angeles, CA.)

the first operation.[110,119,126] With progressive disease secondary biliary cirrhosis can result. Some patients have died of complications of cirrhosis instead of cholangitis.

Diagnosis

In Southeast Asia, where this is a common condition, the diagnosis is readily made on clinical grounds alone. To plan surgical management, knowledge of the degree of biliary involvement and distribution of stones is crucial. Because the stones are radiolucent, plain films of the abdomen are useless. Ultrasound is also problematic because of poor visualization of the dilated intrahepatic ducts, which are often filled with echogenic sludge. Some have found CT scan to be more useful than ultrasound.[121] Since the availability of PTC in the late 1960s and ERC in the early 1970s, the anatomic involvement has been clearly delineated.

Several features are distinctive. About 35% of patients have biliary strictures.[121,125] Hilar strictures involving the left hepatic duct are found most frequently, followed by strictures of the common hepatic duct.[115] Stones are seen in 80% of cases, most commonly in intrahepatic and extrahepatic ducts.[123] The left hepatic duct is involved in 90% of cases. If only the intrahepatic ducts are involved, the ratio of involvement of left to right hepatic duct is 6 : 1 (Fig. 97-6).[115,121,125–127]

The most significant operative findings are liver congestion and an enlarged gallbladder. Even though the gallbladder was often edematous and dilated, only 15% to 33% contained gallstones—usually the same type as in the duct.[110,121–124] Chronic acalculous cholecystitis has been reported in as many as 40% of these patients.[124] Other common findings include ectasia of the lower or upper biliary tract, thickening of the bile ducts, hepatic abscess, hepatic fibrosis, and atrophy.[110,124,125] The disease affects the left lobe of the liver more severely than the right in 75% of cases. Another distinctive feature is the sphincter of Oddi, which is invariably patulous and loose, allowing easy passage of a No. 11 or 12 Bakes dilator.[110]

Histologically, there is increased fibrous tissue in the portal tracts, especially around the bile ducts and portal radicles. Proliferation of bile ducts is always found, and inflammatory cellular infiltrates extend from the portal tracts well into the liver parenchyma, accompanied by local hepatocellular necrosis. More severe cases have suppuration and abscess formation. The extrahepatic and intrahepatic ducts are dilated and strictured and may contain calculi, debris (e.g., bile pigments, shed epithelial cells, mixed exudates), and sometimes frank pus. The calculi are composed almost entirely of bile pigment. They are invariably friable. Usually, the black and green stones are formed, and the brown and yellow are amorphous and muddy.[110,123,125] The bile from these patients invariably grows enteric gram-negative organisms and frequently anaerobes as well.[119,123,124]

Pathogenesis

The theories regarding the formation of intrahepatic duct stones seen in this syndrome were outlined in the section on primary duct stones. Because foreigners living in endemic areas are not more likely to have this syndrome, genetic and ethnic factors have been suggested. However, some reports showed that the proportion of intrahepatic duct stones in all gallstone cases undergoing surgery varies among different countries in Southeast Asia: 30% to 50% in Taiwan, 4% to 6% in Japan, 3% to 15% in Hong Kong, and 1% to 27% in Singapore.[115,128] The groups in each country forming intrahepatic duct stones show no consistent ethnic pattern. This argues against ethnic factors playing a significant role in the pathogenesis.

The pathogenesis is probably multifactorial. Parasitic infection of the biliary tract can lead to fibrosis of the duct, stricture formation, bile stasis, and pyogenic cholangitis.[129,130] Protein malnutrition and parasitic infestation can lead to bile stasis, which promotes bacterial infection in the bile. Diminished levels of glucaro-1:4-lactone in bile (an inhibitor of β-glucuronidase) associated with protein malnutrition, along with increased β-glucuronidase activity from the bacteria, leads to the increased breakdown of bilirubin glucuronide to bilirubin and glucuronic acid. Free bilirubin combines with calcium and precipitates as calcium bilirubinate stones (see Fig. 97-1). The left hepatic duct may be preferentially involved because it courses horizontally in relation to the common hepatic duct and therefore forms a more acute angle at its junction and traps stones.[115]

Treatment

The goals of treatment are to eliminate painful attacks, eradicate parasites if they are found, halt progression of the disease, and prevent complications.

The primary treatment is surgical. The principles outlined by surgeons in Southeast Asia are to remove as many stones as possible, achieve adequate drainage of all stenotic or obstructed biliary ducts to permit residual stones to enter the intestinal tract, excise tissue from the liver as needed when stone removal and ductal drainage cannot be directly achieved, and perform cholecystectomy in all patients.[125,127] Some physicians have advocated hepatic lobectomy if severe atrophy or fibrosis of liver parenchyma or multiple intrahepatic strictures are found that cannot be managed by nonoperative techniques.[125,126,131]

The mortality rate within 1 month of surgery is 4% to 10%.[125–127] Two variables correlate strongly with mortality rates. The first is the length of prior illness: less than 5 years' duration, 5.6%; 5 to 10 years, 12.5%; and 10 to 20 years, 27.3%. The second is the number of previous biliary tract operative procedures: initial or second, 9%; third, 15%; and fourth or more, 40%.[127] Reoperation was required in 75% of patients who only had hepatotomy but in 24% of patients who had bilioenteric anastomosis or sphincteroplasty. Hepatic resection had the lowest failure rate (4.2%).[126] In patients with unresectable strictures of the intrahepatic ducts or with a failed previous bilioenteric anastomosis, many surgeons favor a Roux-en-Y choledochojejunostomy, with the end of the loop left in the subcutaneous tissue of the abdominal wall to allow later access for endoscopic or radiologic interventions.[119,128]

In some reports, as many as one third of the patients after the initial surgery still had residual stones.[127] These patients fare poorly unless the stones are removed. Several percutaneous approaches have been described using choledochoscopy several weeks postoperatively.[120,128,132] These are 75% to 94% successful in removing intrahepatic stones and usually require multiple sessions. Some patients with severe recurrent disease have had to undergo stone extraction every 3 to 4 months. All patients require antibiotic prophylaxis for these procedures. For stones confined to the CBD, endoscopic sphincterotomy was successful in 88%, and stone removal was achieved in 92% of patients.[133] Solvents such as monoctanoin or MTBE are ineffective, because these stones are bilirubinate stones. Leuschner reported using EDTA to dissolve intrahepatic duct stones with limited success.[134] However, EDTA can cause chemical cholangitis. ESWL, laser lithotripsy, and electrohydraulic lithotripsy are new methods on the horizon.

BILIARY CYSTS

Cystic dilatations can occur throughout the biliary system. Most commonly seen are cystic dilatations of the CBD (i.e., choledochal cysts), but cystic dilatations involving the intrahepatic ducts alone (i.e., Caroli's disease) or in combination with other cystic abnormalities of the extrahepatic ducts are being increasingly recognized. The terminology and classification are tremendously confused. The term *choledochal cyst* has commonly referred to all cystic abnormalities of the biliary tree. This term is probably best restricted to only cystic abnormalities of the CBD. Despite the many variations of these cystic abnormalities, there are underlying features that unify them.

Historic Aspects

Although biliary cysts are uncommon, they have intrigued physicians during the past century, as evidenced by the hundreds of reports in the literature. Newer diagnostic tools have also increased their recognition. Vatero is often credited with the first report of a choledochal cyst in 1723, but the first well-documented case was reported by Douglas in 1852.[135,136] By 1909, Lavenson had collected 28 cases.[137] Classic case reviews were reported by Tsardakas and Robnett in 1956 (232 cases),[138] Alonso-Lej and colleagues in 1959 (403 cases),[139] and Flanigan in 1975 (955 cases).[140] In 1980, Yamaguchi analyzed 1433 cases of biliary cysts reported in the Japanese literature.[141] The world literature contains over 3000 cases.[142]

Epidemiology

The incidence of biliary cysts is much higher in Japan, where one half to two thirds of all reported cases have originated.[139–144] Biliary cysts accounted for 1 in 1000 admissions to the Kobe Children's Hospital, in sharp contrast to 1 in 13,000 in the United States, 1 in 15,000 in Australia, and 1 in 26,000 in a London hospital.[142,145–147] The incidence is much higher among women, with a female to male ratio of 3 or 4 : 1. Between 40% and 60% of patients were diagnosed before 10 years of age, 52% to 76% before 20 years of age, and 83% to 90% before 30 years of age.[139–145] This is mainly a disease of children and young adults.

Classification

The classic review by Alonso-Lej and colleagues described three basic forms of biliary cysts.[139] Type I cysts, the most common type, are cystic dilatations of the CBD. The terminal CBD is frequently narrowed. Type II cysts are CBD diverticula. Type III cysts are distal CBD choledochoceles, most often within the duodenal wall. Subsequent recognition of more diffuse and variable forms of biliary cysts led to modifications of the original proposal by Alonso-Lej.[148,149] Todani and associates proposed the most complete and practical classification that recognizes five types of bile ducts cysts (Fig. 97-7).[148]

> Type I cysts occur commonly and include choledochal cysts in a narrow sense; segmental choledochal dilatations; and diffuse or cylindrical dilatations. Seventy-five percent to 85% of cases are type I.[140,141,144]
>
> Type II or diverticulum cysts are found anywhere in the extrahepatic ducts and make up 2% to 3% of reported cases.[140,141,144]

Type III or choledochocele cysts, also rare, represent 1.4% to 5.6% of reported cases.[140,141,144] In 1989, Sarris and Tsang reviewed 48 cases in the English literature and proposed a further anatomic classification of choledochoceles (Fig. 97-8).[150] In type A, the ampulla opens into the choledochocele, which communicates with the duodenum through another small opening. Type A choledochoceles can be further subclassified into A_1, in which the pancreatic and CBD share a common opening into the cyst (33% of cases); A_2, in which the openings are distinct (4% of cases); and A_3, in which the choledochocele is small and entirely intramural (25% of cases). In type B, the ampulla opens directly into the duodenum, with the choledochocele communicating only with the distal CBD (21% of cases). This scheme is useful because of important therapeutic implications.

Type IV cysts are also subclassified. Type IVA multiple cysts in the intrahepatic and extrahepatic ducts account for 18% to 20% of reported cases.[141,144] Type IVA cysts are further classified into four sub-subtypes depending on the shape of the intrahepatic and extrahepatic ductal dilatation, which may be cystic or cylindrical. In cystic dilatation, the width of the duct is at least one third or greater than the length of dilatation, but in cylindrical dilatation, the width is less than one third. Four possible combinations of dilatation of the extrahepatic and intrahepatic ducts are cystic-cylindrical, cystic-cystic, cylindrical-cystic, and cylindrical-cylindrical. Cystic dilatation of the intrahepatic duct is the most common of

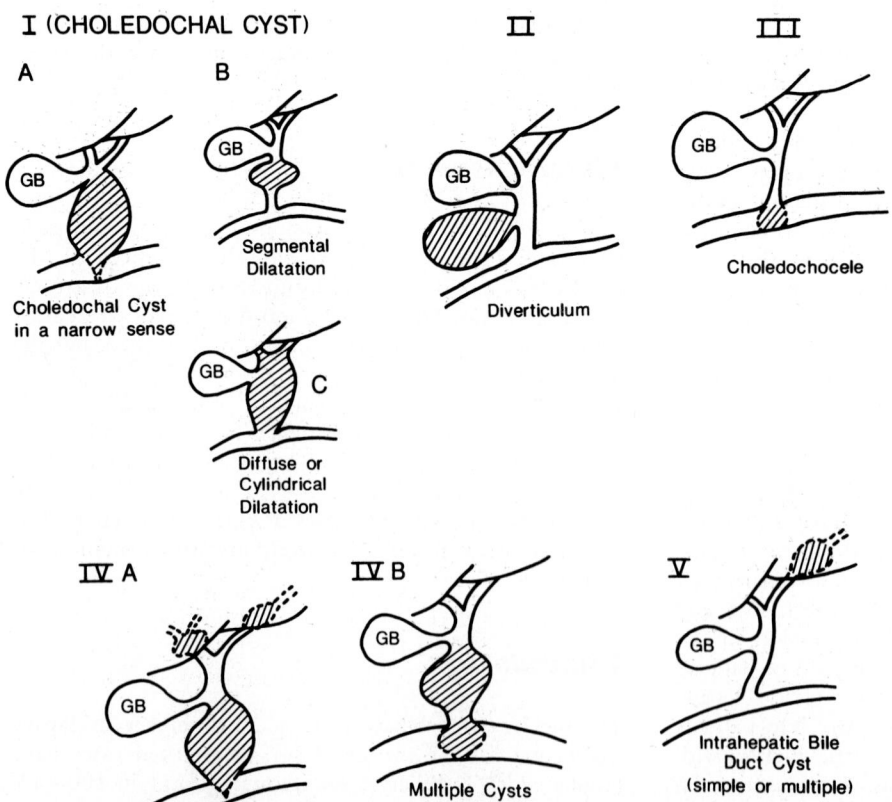

FIGURE 97-7. Todani's classification of biliary cysts is based on location. Hatched areas represent cystic dilatations.

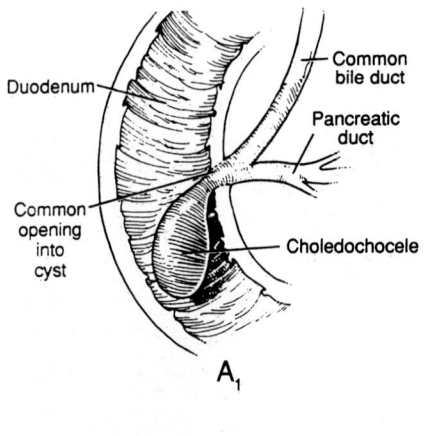
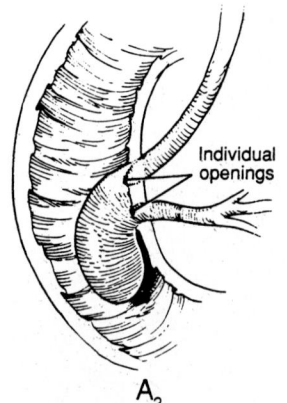
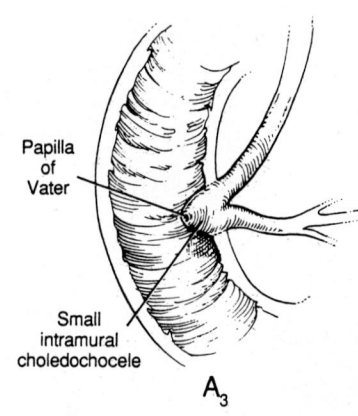
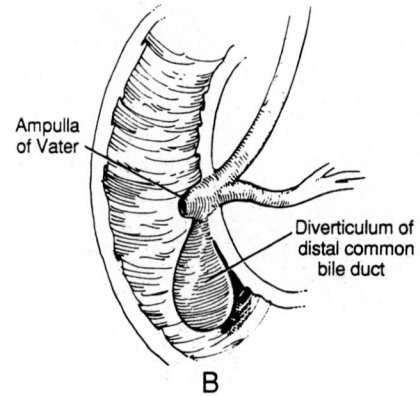

FIGURE 97-8. Proposed subclassification of choledochoceles (i.e., type III biliary cyst). In type A, the ampulla opens into the choledochocele, which communicates with the duodenum through another small opening. Type A is subclassified into A_1, in which the pancreatic and common bile duct share a common opening into the cyst (33% of cases); A_2, in which the openings are distinct (4% of cases); and A_3, in which the choledochocele is small and entirely intramural (25% of cases). In type B, the ampulla opens directly into the duodenum, with the choledochocele communicating with the distal common bile duct (21% of cases). (From Kaplowitz N, ed. Liver and biliary diseases, Baltimore: Williams & Wilkins, 1992.)

the subtypes.[151] Type IVB multiple cysts occur only in the extrahepatic duct and are much less common.

Type V intrahepatic bile duct cyst (single or multiple) are also quite rare.

Types I through III correspond to Alonso-Lej's classification, except for further subdivisions of type I. Type V bile duct cysts are thought by many to be synonymous with Caroli's disease as originally described. Serena and colleagues proposed a type VI biliary cyst, which is cystic dilatation of the cystic duct with otherwise normal intrahepatic and extrahepatic ductal systems.[152]

Anatomically based classification is of great practical importance in planning surgical management. Other classifications emphasize clinical presentation rather than ductal anatomy. For example, patients with type I cysts (i.e., choledochal cysts) have two presentations. One presentation is the infantile form in which symptoms occur early in life, characterized by obstructive jaundice and a clinical picture indistinguishable from biliary atresia. Portal hypertension and cirrhosis are frequently associated.[143,153] These infants often have distal common duct atresia caused by a primary anatomic malformation or by a secondary inflammatory stenosis. The other presentation, the noninfantile form, occurs usually after 2 years of age, with abdominal pain, abdominal mass, cholangitis, and intermittent jaundice. The degree of jaundice is much less than with the infantile form. Cirrhosis and portal hypertension are uncommon. This type of classification may reflect different pathogenesis of the choledochal cysts.

Pathogenesis

The cause of biliary cysts has been disputed. The major debate concerns whether cysts are congenital or acquired.

Many early investigators, including Douglas and Alonzo-Lej, favored the congenital malformation theory.[154] One congenital theory presented by Yotuyanagi in 1936 was an unequal proliferation of epithelial cells when the embryogenic biliary ducts are still solid. Such abnormal embryogenesis may occur throughout the entire developing biliary tree. If cellular proliferation is more active proximally than distally during epithelial occlusion, the biliary tree after canalization will be abnormally dilated proximally and normal or somewhat stenotic distally.[156] Several observations support this theory. First, biliary cysts appear in all age groups, and antenatal diagnosis has been reported as early as 15 weeks' gestation, making a congenital origin likely. In addition, many cysts fail to shrink significantly after decompressive surgery, supporting the concept of inherently abnormal ductal wall development.[143,157]

Of the theories proposing acquired cysts, that of Babbitt and associates has received the most attention.[158] They proposed that choledochal cysts develop because of an anomalous arrangement of the distal pancreaticobiliary tree. In all 7 of their patients with choledochal cysts, they found the CBD entered the pancreatic duct at a right angle at an abnormally long distance (>2 cm) from the ampulla of Vater (Fig. 97-9). This abnormal anatomy impaired normal sphincteric function at the pancreaticobiliary junction. Because the max-

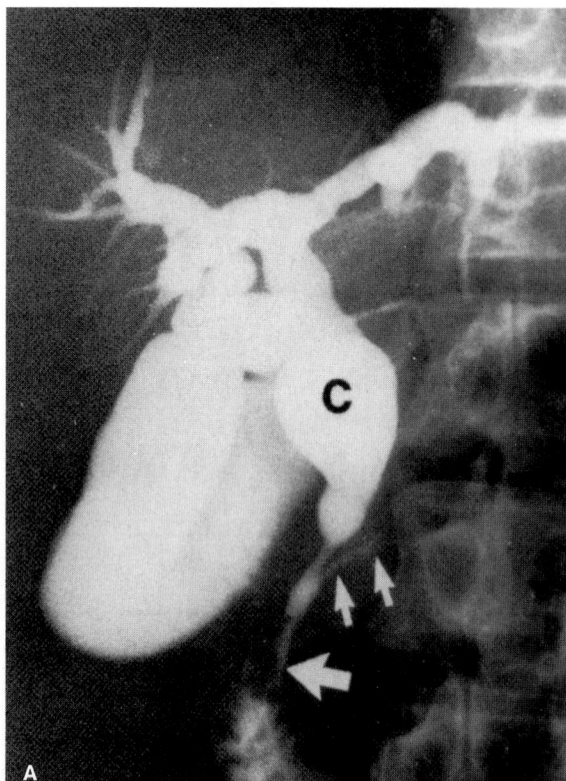
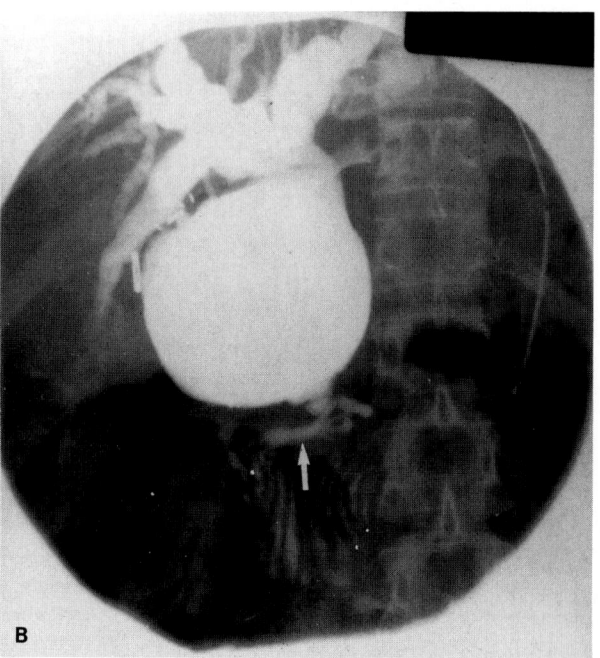

FIGURE 97-9. Choledochal cyst and anomalous ductal relations. (**A**) Cystic enlargement of the common bile duct (C), with associated dilatation of the common hepatic and intrahepatic ducts. The abnormal junction of the pancreatic duct (*small arrows*) and common bile duct and long common channel (*large arrow*) is displayed. (**B**) A large cyst involves the common hepatic and common bile duct, accompanied by intrahepatic ductal dilatation. A long common channel (*arrow*) results from the abnormally high junction with the pancreatic duct.

imal secretory pressure of the pancreas is 30 to 50 cm H_2O and that of the liver is 25 to 30 cm H_2O, pancreatic juice flows into the bile duct in the absence of a sphincter mechanism.[159] This anomaly can result in recurrent cholangitis, edema, fibrosis, and obstruction of the bile ducts, and it explains the high levels of amylase that are frequently found in the cyst fluid.[145] Kato and colleagues demonstrated that pancreatic juice in the CBDs of animals with an anomalous arrangement can cause cystic dilatation of the CBD.[160] Although amylase has been found in the cyst fluid, this enzyme probably does not play a pathogenetic role. Amylase is not detectable in the duodenal fluid of newborns and infants, but trypsin activity is the same in newborns and older children.[161] These digestive enzymes may adversely affect an already weakened bile duct wall.

The association of anomalous pancreaticobiliary ductal anatomy with choledochal cysts was first observed by Taybi in 1967.[162] In most studies, this anomaly occurs in 65% to 80% of patients with choledochal cysts.[154,163–166] However, when Kato and colleagues investigated the clinical significance of anomalous pancreaticobiliary union, they found that 9 (3%) of 300 consecutive adult patients who underwent ERCP for symptoms suggestive of pancreaticobiliary tract disease had the anomaly.[167] Three of the 9 patients had biliary cysts: one type I, one type II, and one type IVA. Five (55.6%) of the 9 patients had biliary malignancies: four carcinomas of the gall-

bladder and one carcinoma of the choledochus. Conversely, 18 (6.2%) of 291 patients without the anomaly had biliary malignancies. Seven (78%) of 9 patients with the anomaly had abnormal pancreatograms, contrasted with 37% of patients without the anomaly. Anomalous pancreaticobiliary union is associated with biliary cysts, biliary malignancies, and abnormal pancreatic ducts. This anomaly alone cannot be the only pathogenetic factor of biliary cysts because as many as 60% of biliary cysts lack the anomaly and not all patients with the anomaly have biliary cysts.

Many investigators, including Alonso-Lej, Saito, and Ishida, emphasized that cystic dilatation results from a combination of two factors: segmental weakness of the duct wall and distal obstruction.[139,168] The weakness of the wall and the distal obstruction may be congenital or acquired. Several animal experiments support the importance of distal obstruction.[143,169–171] Ligation of the distal CBD in adult rabbits, rats, and dogs gives rise to diffuse dilation of the intrahepatic and extrahepatic ducts. Similar distal CBD ligation in puppies and infant rats produces cystic dilatation of the extrahepatic ducts. This also occurs in neonatal lambs.[171] After CBD ligation, all six studied lambs developed choledochal cysts, and all four adult sheep developed isolated dilatation of the gallbladder.

The etiologic importance of these distal ductal abnormalities is unclear. The animal experiments cannot be extrapolated with certainty to humans. The distal obstruction theory also would not explain solely intrahepatic duct cysts. Not all choledochal cysts have demonstrable distal obstruction.

The infantile form of choledochal cysts appears in some cases to result from an obliterative process similar to that producing biliary atresia. Twenty-four (13%) of 188 patients with biliary cysts were also found to have biliary atresia.[172] However, well-documented cases of acquired biliary cysts in adults have appeared, including seven attributed to recurrent attacks of pancreatitis.[140,173,174] Two observations suggest other factors may be involved. One is the finding of abnormal sphincter of Oddi pressure in patients with choledochal cysts.[175,176] The other, based on study of a single case, is diminished postganglionic cholinergic activity in the distal, narrow portion of a choledochal cyst, compared with the dilated portion of the cyst and normal CBDs.[177] This suggests a pathogenesis similar to that of Hirschsprung's disease, in which physiologic obstruction of the colon and dilatation results from an abnormal distal muscle segment.

It appears that several factors may be important in the pathogenesis of biliary cysts that encompass a spectrum of lesions. The precise mechanisms for each type of biliary cyst remain uncertain.

Clinical Presentation

Type I or Choledochal Cysts

Patients with choledochal cysts present with two typical clinical constellations determined mostly by the patient's age at presentation.[143,144,149,153,164,178–180] In infancy, jaundice with or without acholic stools is the most common finding, occurring in as many as 80% of patients.[142–144,149,181,182] The presentation is often indistinguishable from biliary atresia, which is sometimes associated with choledochal cysts.[170,172] Pain may or may not be a factor, but vomiting and failure to thrive have been reported in as many as 50% of patients.[142,143,181] Hepatomegaly is often found, and 30% to 60% of patients have a palpable abdominal mass.[142,143,181] The mass is usually in the right hypochondrium. Typically, it is soft, elastic, round, mobile laterally, and may follow the movements of the diaphragm.[139,149] The classic clinical triad of pain, jaundice, and a palpable abdominal mass has been found only in 11% to 63% of large series.[142,143,181–183] Frequently, biliary cirrhosis and portal hypertension complicate the management of these patients.[144,172,184]

The noninfantile form (>2 years) covers a wide age range, with the oldest patient reported in the eighth decade.[149,155,159] Asymptomatic patients have been described.[159,185] Chronic and intermittent pain appears to be the most common presenting symptom, reported in 50% to 96% of patients.[141,144,164,178] Intermittent jaundice and recurrent cholangitis is also common, reported in 34% to 55%. Abdominal mass is much less common; it occurs in about 10% to 20% of cases. The classic triad of pain, jaundice, and a palpable mass has been reported in 3% to 13% of patients.[141,164,178] Cirrhosis and portal hypertension are less often encountered than the infantile form. Recurrent pancreatitis has been reported only in the noninfantile form, although some studies stress the rarity of this complication.[178,180,186,187] One study

pointed out that the diagnosis of pancreatitis in many of these patients was made on the basis of symptoms such as epigastric pain, nausea, vomiting, and fever accompanied by hyperamylasemia, even though definite evidence of pancreatitis was rarely observed at the time of operation.[188] At the time of bouts, these patients showed slight elevation of serum bilirubin levels and an increase in the degree of the choledochal dilatation, possibly caused by biliary obstruction. The terms *fictitious pancreatitis* or *pseudopancreatitis* have been applied to these patients.[188] One possible explanation is that amylase in the biliary tract has ready access to the blood stream. This would also explain why hyperamylasemia is almost never observed in patients younger than 1 year of age with choledochal cysts, because the amylase levels are usually very low in bile because acinar growth of the pancreas is not complete until 1 to 2 years of age.[188]

The other presentation that has been reported only in patients older than 10 years of age is that of carcinoma associated with choledochal cysts.[189]

Type II or Diverticulum Cysts

More than 50 cases of type II or diverticulum cysts have been reported in the world literature, representing 2% to 3% of large series.[140,141,190,191] Presenting symptoms generally reflect the compression of nearby structures by the cyst.

Type III or Choledochocele Cysts

The term *choledochocele* was coined by Wheeler in his 1940 report of a patient he had operated on 25 years earlier.[192] Only about 72 cases have been reported.[140,141,193–195] More than 73% of reported patients were older than 20 years of age, unlike type I cysts, which are found in 60% of the patients younger than 10 years of age.[193,194,196] There is also less female preponderance, with a female to male ratio of 1.4 : 1.[196] Common presenting symptoms include pain and obstructive jaundice. Abdominal mass is not found. Pancreatitis is much more common in choledochocele than in any other type of biliary cyst and is reported in 30% to 70% of these patients, presumably caused by reflux of bile or obstruction.[197] Stones in the cele or the CBD are also much more common, reported in 25% to 35% of these patients, in contrast to only 8% in type I cysts.[141,192–205] Rarely, intestinal (duodenal-jejunal) intussusception may be the presenting feature of choledochocele.[195]

Type IV and V Cysts or Caroli's Disease

Vachel and Stevens are generally credited with the earliest description of a case of cystic dilatation of the intrahepatic bile ducts in 1906.[206] The syndrome carries this eponym because of Caroli's paper in 1958, in which he reported a case and gave a lucid description of the clinical characteristics of the syndrome.[207] Caroli and coworkers originally described this disease as a congenital malformation of intrahepatic bile ducts, characterized by segmental cystic dilatation of the intrahepatic ducts; increased incidence of biliary lithiasis, cholangitis, and liver abscesses; absence of cirrhosis and portal hypertension; and association of renal tubular ectasia or similar renal cystic disease.

After the first report, Caroli recognized that two distinct disease entities are associated with intrahepatic duct cysts: the simple type, which was his original description, and the periportal fibrosis type.[208] The simple type is associated with medullary sponge kidney in 60% to 80% of the cases.[209] The periportal fibrosis type was first described by Grumbach.[209] In addition to intrahepatic cystic dilatation, congenital hepatic fibrosis, cirrhosis, portal hypertension, and esophageal varices are frequently seen. Hepatic function is usually well preserved in the periportal fibrosis type; the major clinical manifestations are recurrent cholangitis, liver abscess formation, and portal hypertension. Renal cystic lesions also frequently occur.[209]

Some patients classified as type V according to Todani's scheme appear to belong to the simple form of Caroli's disease. It is now apparent that Caroli's disease, including the simple and periportal-fibrosis types, represents only part of the spectrum of cystic disease of the intrahepatic ducts. In an excellent review by Barros and associates of 46 well-documented cases with hepatic histopathology and biliary tree studies available, only 13% of patients had the simple type.[210] Thirty-five percent had the periportal-fibrosis type, 22% had intrahepatic and extrahepatic cystic dilation (i.e., type IV A of Todani's classification), and 30% had all three abnormalities: cystic dilatation of the intrahepatic, extrahepatic bile ducts, and congenital hepatic fibrosis. This frequent coexistence of intrahepatic duct cysts with extrahepatic duct cysts was reported by numerous other investigators; except for Flanigan's report of 3%, others reported a 19% to 66% incidence of intrahepatic duct cysts in cases of extrahepatic duct cysts.[140,141,211–213]

The term *congenital hepatic fibrosis* refers to a unique congenital liver histology characterized by bland portal fibrosis, hyperproliferation of interlobular bile ducts within the portal areas with variable shapes and sizes of bile ducts, and preservation of normal lobular architecture.[210] This is indistinguishable from the congenital hepatic fibrosis described by Kerr and colleagues in 1961 in a group of patients with the hepatic histology of congenital hepatic fibrosis, portal hypertension, and presence of renal cysts (predominantly medullary).[214] The prevalence of biliary cysts in patients with congenital hepatic fibrosis probably has been underestimated, because most patients did not have cholangiographic studies performed. Of 15 cases of congenital hepatic fibrosis collected by de Ferron and associates until 1961, only 2 had x-ray studies of the biliary tree, and both had cystic dilatations. Boquien and colleagues performed intraoperative cholangiograms in 5 patients with congenital hepatic fibrosis, and all 5 had intrahepatic biliary dilatations.[210]

The aforementioned forms of intrahepatic biliary cystic disease should be differentiated from polycystic liver disease because of significant dissimilarities. Polycystic liver disease is an autosomal dominant genetic defect, but the manner of inheritance of Caroli's disease remains poorly defined.[209,215] Caroli's disease occurs in siblings but not in subsequent generations; polycystic liver cysts are large, contain serous fluid, and do not communicate with the biliary tree. Caroli's disease cysts communicate with the biliary tree. Portal hypertension is rare in polycystic liver disease. The prognosis for polycystic liver disease patients is determined by the effect of cystic disease on the kidneys and not the liver.[216] The incidence of

malignant transformation in the intrahepatic parenchymal cysts of polycystic liver disease is 1.3%, compared with 7% in Caroli's disease.[209,217]

Until 1984, 162 cases of Caroli's disease had been reported.[209,217] Males and females are equally involved, unlike the female predominance in choledochal cysts.[209,218] Symptoms usually appear in early adult life, with recurrent episodes of fever, chills, and abdominal pain due to cholangitis. More than 80% of patients present before 30 years of age.[209,219] Biliary lithiasis is found in 34% of these patients, which may predispose to recurrent cholangitis.[210] Occasionally, the disease is diagnosed later in life, with the sequelae of portal hypertension, most commonly bleeding esophageal varices.[209]

Diagnosis

Diagnosis of biliary cysts requires a high index of suspicion. In early series, biliary cysts were rarely correctly diagnosed preoperatively. The frequency of correct preoperative diagnosis in some series has ranged from 27% to 80%.[140,141,144,168] A correct preoperative diagnosis is important, because it was shown in older series to lower the operative mortality rate from 56.6% in undiagnosed cases to 30.5% in diagnosed cases.[138] The major reason for missed diagnosis is that biliary cysts are usually not included in the differential diagnosis of obstructive jaundice. Most patients do not present with the classic triad of pain, jaundice, and abdominal mass. Biochemical tests only reflect the degree of biliary obstruction and infection. Correct diagnosis depends on the use of imaging studies.

Ultrasonography is the best screening method for type I, II, IV, and V cysts.[142–144,153,182,220–225] Four cases of antenatal diagnosis of choledochal cyst by means of ultrasonography have been reported since 1980.[157,226] The earliest was at 15 weeks of gestation. This was most valuable in planning early surgical management of these patients.[226] When a choledochal cyst is suspected on prenatal ultrasonography, repeat ultrasonography is indicated immediately after birth so that expeditious treatment can be provided. The major drawback to ultrasonography is that it provides little anatomic or functional information.[222,227]

Intravenous radionuclide cholescintigraphy with ^{131}I-rose Bengal was used to diagnose choledochal cysts in 1970 by William and coworkers.[227] Since then, hepatobiliary scintigraphy has been advocated as a sensitive, noninvasive tool for the diagnosis of choledochal cyst. Since 1975, ^{99m}Tc-labeled agents such as pyridoxylideneglutamate or N-(2,6-dimethylphenylcarbamoylmethyl) iminodiacetic acid (HIDA) have replaced iodine-labeled complexes for liver and biliary tract studies because of better image quality, lower radiation dose, and more rapid biliary excretion than with the earlier agents.[227] This technique is useful for all except type III cysts.[227–231] The characteristic findings are biliary tract dilatation and tracer retention after 24 hours.[227,228] It provides information about excretory patterns and has therefore been recommended by many for postoperative patient follow-up.[153,181,182,229] One report claims scintigraphy suggested the correct diagnosis in 83% of patients.[227] However, the findings are not specific and cannot exclude partial biliary tract obstruction.[228]

Ultrasonography and scintigraphy are complementary and provide a sound basis for preoperative diagnosis in patients younger than 2 years of age. For older patients, CT has been advocated by some to be superior to ultrasound.[228,229,232,233] Magnetic resonance imaging has also been shown to be useful in cases for which CT examinations were inadequate.[234] The best detailed examinations are PTC and ERCP. PTC is especially useful in defining complex anatomic cysts of the intrahepatic ducts, but ERCP provides the best visualization of the distal portion of the biliary tree, especially the relation of the biliary and pancreatic ducts.[143,178,193,204,205,232,235–239]

ERCP is especially useful in the diagnosis of type III cysts (i.e., choledochoceles). The typical features are the "clubbed" appearance of the distal CBD and a round, cyst-like, contrast-filled structure in the terminal CBD, which often protrudes into the duodenal lumen. Emptying of contrast material is often delayed. Choledochoceles are easily differentiated from duodenal diverticula and duodenal duplication cysts by filling during cholangiography but not during upper gastrointestinal contrast studies (Fig. 97-10). Duodenal diverticula fill on upper gastrointestinal series but not on cholangiography. Duplication cysts do not fill with either method.[193,201,205]

Oral cholecystography and intravenous cholangiography are of no use in diagnosing biliary cysts.[141,144,236] Other non-specific findings include a mass displacing the gas shadows on plain abdominal radiographs and displacement of antrum, usually anteroinferiorly and to the left, on upper gastrointestinal series.[144,181]

The definitive diagnosis of biliary cyst and its classification is secured by intraoperative cholangiography at the time of operative intervention. Delineation of the precise anatomy is critical in preventing injury especially to the pancreatic duct because of the high frequency of the anomalous union and in providing the best operative management possible.[143]

Pathology

Giant choledochal cysts have been described. The largest one reported was 13 L.[139] The wall of the cyst is usually thickened because of productive fibrosis and inflammation. Histologically, dense connective tissue, fibrocollagenous and sometimes with smooth muscle and elastic elements, are seen. There is no epithelial lining, but islets of cylindrical or columnar epithelium may be preserved.[139,144,184] Choledochoceles are covered by duodenal mucosa externally but the internal surface is variably lined by duodenal, biliary, or enteric epithelium.[199,202,203,237]

The liver biopsy is abnormal in 60% of patients with biliary cysts, demonstrating biliary cirrhosis, portal fibrosis, or evidence of biliary atresia, although in newborn patients with biliary cysts histology is usually normal or shows mild bile duct proliferation consistent with biliary obstruction.[144,154]

Treatment

Biliary cyst treatment is surgical. Medical therapy was associated with a 97% mortality rate.[138,240] Death was caused by cyst rupture with secondary peritonitis, cholangitis, or liver cirrhosis with secondary complications.

During the past 30 years, the surgical management of biliary cysts has changed dramatically. Aspiration and external drainage of choledochal cysts were previously employed to decompress cysts and to decrease obstruction and infection. However, because external drainage alone was shown to have a 65% mortality rate and does not correct the underlying pathophysiology, it is no longer applied as definitive therapy. External drainage is still a valid initial procedure in a poor-

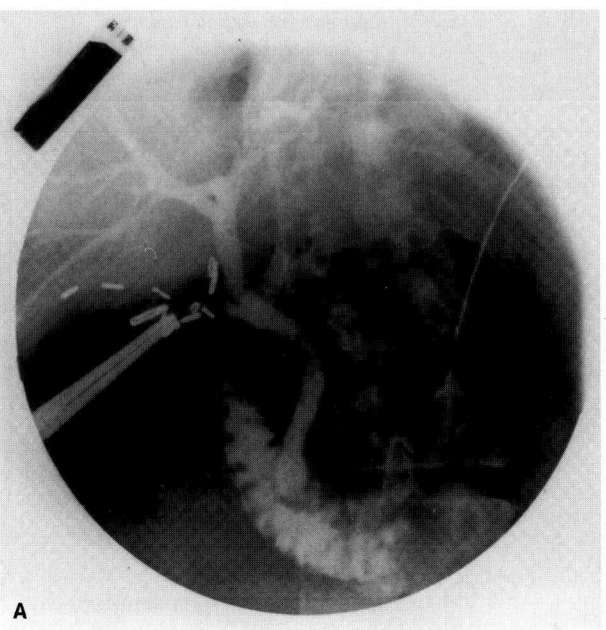
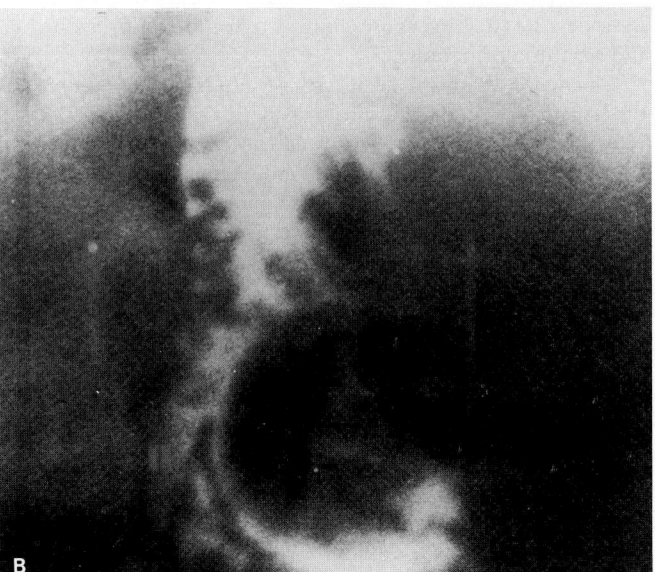

FIGURE 97-10. Choledochocele, type III cyst. **(A)** Cholangiography reveals a club-shaped enlargement of the distal common bile duct bulging into the duodenum. **(B)** Upper GI series reveals a smoothly rounded filling defect in the second portion of the duodenum.

risk patient, but should be followed with a definitive procedure when the patient's condition permits.[138,140,141]

Internal drainage procedures, such as choledochoduodenostomy and Roux-en-Y choledochojejunostomy, have been widely employed, especially in Western countries.[143,172,241] Japanese investigators have been using primary excision of the cyst as definitive treatment since the late 1960s.[148] Cyst excision was first carried out by McWhorter in 1922, but it was slowly adopted in the West because of a high operative mortality rate of 15% to 40% in early reports.[139,242] Reports since the early 1970s have shown a steady decline in the operative mortality rate for total choledochal cyst excision to 0% to 7%, figures not significantly different from that of internal drainage procedures.[140,143,183,243]

There are three major drawbacks to internal drainage procedures compared with cyst excision. First, the morbidity rate is much higher, 10%% to 50% with internal drainage procedures, compared with 2% to 8% with cyst excision.[140,172,183,241,243–245] The usual complications are recurrent pain, jaundice, stricture formation, and cholangitis. These appear to be more common after choledochoduodenostomy than after Roux-en-Y choledochojejunostomy.[143,172] The second drawback is the need for reoperation because of the high complication rate. In large series, 13% to 34% of patients have required reoperations after internal drainage, but a 0% to 4% reoperation rate was reported after cyst excision.[140,172,243] The third drawback is the risk of malignant transformation. The overall incidence of biliary tract cancer is 2.5% among patients with choledochal cyst, about 20 times greater than the general population.[143,246] In the literature up to 1976, 12 of 24 cases of biliary carcinoma associated with biliary cysts developed a mean of 4 years after an internal drainage procedure.[246] Patients who develop biliary carcinoma after excision of choledochal cyst are extremely rare; only three were reported up to 1984.[247] The fundamental reason for poor outcome after internal drainage is that diseased tissue remains and is used for biliary reconstruction. The cyst wall is inherently inflamed and fibrous, precluding normal healing. Biliary stasis persists and predisposes to recurrent cholangitis, stone, and stricture formation.

The major disadvantage of cyst excision is risk of injury to the hepatic artery, portal vein, or pancreatic duct. In 1978, Lilly described a technique for total choledochal excision in which he left intact the muscular and fibrous posterior wall of the cyst overlying the portal vein and hepatic artery, while excising all the "mucosa" or lining of the cyst.[244] This was followed by Roux-en-Y choledochojejunostomy. This technique lessens the risk of injury to the vital porta hepatis structures. Total excision of choledochal cysts with biliary tract reconstruction using an interposed jejunal segment has been advocated as an alternative to the more classic Roux-en-Y choledochojejunostomy.[248,249] This eliminates the risk of peptic ulcer disease, fat malabsorption, and reflux of intestinal contents.[248,249]

The aforementioned techniques are applicable for choledochal cysts (i.e., types I and IV cysts involving the CBD). Type II cysts should be excised. Treatment for type III cysts depends on the anatomy (see Fig. 97-4). Sarris and Tsang recommend excision of the duodenal lumenal portion of the cyst, leaving the medial portion containing the ampulla intact as the preferred treatment in most cases of type IIIA cysts

(i.e., A_1 and A_2).[150] Transduodenal sphincteroplasty and ERCP with papillotomy have been advocated as treatment for type IIIA$_3$ cysts. Type IIIB cysts should be treated by excision and sphincteroplasty. The malignant potential of choledochocele appears to be very low; only two cases have been reported.[196,197]

Intrahepatic cyst (i.e., type IVA, V) treatment depends on the degree of involvement. When segmental cystic disease is confined to one lobe (more often the left lobe), then lobectomy is usually curative.[217,218,250–253] If both lobes are involved, some have advocated establishing a permanent-access hepaticojejunostomy after partial hepatectomy to allow easy biliary tree access when necessary.[251,252] It is uncertain how effective this approach will be. If extrahepatic cysts coexist with intrahepatic cysts (type IVA), they should be excised as previously described. The cylindrical but not the cystic subtype of the intrahepatic dilatation has been reported to regress after excision of the extrahepatic cyst.[151]

Chronic antibiotic therapy in multilobar Caroli's disease may have some benefit. Ultimately, if attacks of cholangitis are frequent and quality of life poor, hepatic transplantation may be a therapeutic option. A summary of the recommended surgical treatment is listed in Table 97-2. Cholecystectomy should be performed at the time of cyst excision because continuous free bile flow minimizes the risk of reflux and cholangitis and because the gallbladder has shown clinical and histologic evidence of cholecystitis in patients in whom sec-

---

TABLE 97-2
Suggested Treatment According to Type of Biliary Cyst

TYPE OF BILIARY CYST	SUGGESTED TREATMENT
Type I	
A	Cyst excision with Roux-en-Y hepaticojejunostomy or jejunal interposition hepaticoduodenostomy
B	
C	Choledochojejunostomy, sphincteroplasty if excision is impossible
Type II	Excision
Type III	
A_1	Excision
A_2	
A_3	Sphincteroplasty or endoscopic retrograde cholangiopancreatography with papillotomy
III B	Excision and sphincteroplasty
Type IV	
A	Extrahepatic cyst excision with biliary reconstruction as in IA, IB; lobectomy if intrahepatic cyst is confined to one lobe, permanent access hepaticojejunostomy if intrahepatic cysts are diffuse (?); transplantation may be indicated in these cases
B	Cyst excision as in IA, IB
Type V	Hepatic resection for localized disease, permanent access hepaticojejunostomy for diffuse disease (?); transplantation may be an option

ondary operations have been necessary and the gallbladder appears to be predisposed to malignant change in patients with biliary cysts.[3]

Clinical Course and Complications

Complications of biliary cysts include recurrent cholangitis before treatment and after internal drainage procedures, stone formation, stenosis and stricture, pancreatitis, biliary cirrhosis, portal hypertension due to cirrhosis or portal vein thrombosis, liver abscess, especially in Caroli's disease, and cyst rupture.[140,144,149,172] Pregnancy can precipitate or aggravate symptoms of choledochal cyst, specifically cyst rupture. Twenty-six cases have been reported to rupture during pregnancy or labor.[140,144,254] It has been recommended that pregnant women with symptomatic choledochal cyst should avoid labor by having cesarean sections as soon as the fetus is mature.[254]

If definitive surgical procedure is successful, the prognosis is generally excellent. Reversal of cirrhosis has even been reported.[255]

The most feared complication is malignancy.[245,256–260] Flanigan in 1976 reviewed 24 cases of biliary carcinoma associated with biliary cysts.[246] Todani reported 277 cases of carcinomas associated with biliary cysts: 42 developing after internal drainage procedures and 235 recognized at the time of diagnosis of biliary cysts.[256] Carcinoma afflicts predominantly adults. The youngest patient with carcinoma during initial choledochal cyst surgery was 10 years of age.[256] The mean age for detecting carcinoma after enteric drainage was 35 years, with a mean interval of 10 years after the enteric drainage procedure.[256] The mean age for detecting carcinoma at the initial surgery for biliary cyst was 50 years; this is two decades earlier than the mean age for bile duct carcinoma in the general population.[256] Even though the overall incidence of biliary carcinoma in association with biliary cysts is 2.5%, it is actually 14% to 18% in the adult patients (>20 years).[143,189,256] In contrast, the overall incidence of biliary carcinoma is 0.012% to 0.48% in the general population.[144] The female to male ratio is 2.5 : 1, slightly less than that seen in choledochal cyst.

Carcinomas occur not only in the cyst wall; the remainder of the hepatobiliary and pancreatic tree can be affected. Of 154 cases of carcinoma in cases of biliary cysts, only 58% were actually in the cyst wall, 40% were gallbladder, 1.3% were pancreatic, and 0.6% were intrahepatic carcinomas.[256]

The pathogenesis of malignant change in biliary cysts is unknown. Stones are not thought to be important because they are found only in 13.8% of patients (Fig. 97-11).[256] Cancer of the gallbladder appears to be especially common in patients with biliary cysts. The high prevalence of malignant change in the gallbladder has been seen particularly in association with the presence of anomalous pancreaticobiliary ductal union, with reports of 57% to 77% in Japanese series.[261,262] Kimura and associates proposed that regurgitation of pancreatic juice may be an important factor in these patients.[261] Favoring such a hypothesis, Iwai and colleagues found higher amylase levels in the gallbladder than in the choledochal cyst in patients with the fusiform type of choledochal dilatation.[166]

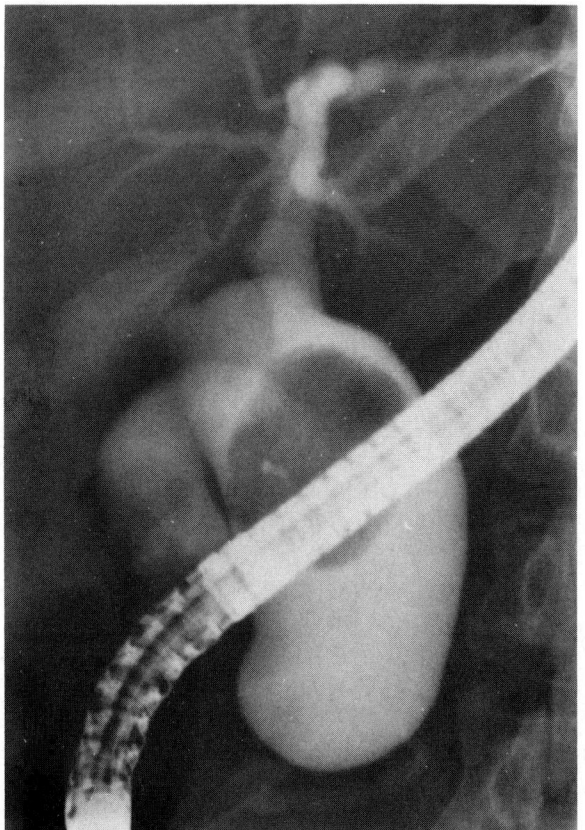

FIGURE 97-11. Choledochal cyst, type IA. Endoscopic retrograde cholangiogram shows cystic dilatation of the common bile duct with a very large filling defect due to a calculus. Stones are uncommon complications of biliary cysts, reported in only 13.8% of cases. (Courtesy of Hartley Cohen, M.D., Los Angeles, CA.)

Adenocarcinoma is the most common type, constituting 70% to 84% of all types. Other histologic types are squamous (4%–9%) and undifferentiated or anaplastic (7%–21%), and one case of small cell carcinoma was reported.[246,256,263]

Isolated intrahepatic cysts (i.e., Caroli's disease) are also associated with a higher incidence of carcinoma. Overall, 7% of patients with Caroli's disease were found to have cholangiocarcinoma, with no female predominance.[209] The average age at the time of diagnosis of carcinoma was 51 years.[209]

The prognosis of carcinoma related to biliary cysts is dismal. Almost all patients die soon after diagnosis.[209,256] One preventive therapy is total cyst excision during the initial operation. However, cyst excision does not completely eliminate the future risk of carcinoma, because the rest of the pancreaticobiliary tree appears to also be predisposed to malignant change.

SCLEROSING CHOLANGITIS

Sclerosing cholangitis encompasses a wide spectrum of pathologic processes causing bile duct injury characterized by inflammation, fibrosis, thickening, and stricture formation. Primary sclerosing cholangitis (PSC) refers to bile duct injury not attributable to other causes, but secondary sclerosing cholangitis describes the same type of bile duct injury from a known cause. Although different causes can produce the same final bile duct injury, the clinical course and treatment may differ.

History

Delbet first described the syndrome of PSC in 1924.[264] Before 1980, PSC was a medical and surgical curiosity; less than 100 cases appeared in the world literature before 1970.[265,266] Since the advent of ERCP in 1974, the number of new cases diagnosed each year has doubled at the Mayo Clinic.[266] In 1980, reviews from the Mayo Clinic and the Royal Free Hospital in London ignited tremendous interest.[266,267] Increased awareness of PSC and widespread availability of ERCP have led to increased detection of PSC and knowledge of the pathogenesis, clinical, radiographic, and histologic features and treatment of this disorder.

Classification

A practical approach is to classify sclerosing cholangitis into primary and secondary types, and subdivide the former into those associated or unassociated with other diseases.[268] Table 97-3 summarizes this approach.

The following diagnostic criteria for PSC are accepted by most investigators:

Diffuse or segmental narrowing or irregularity of the biliary system.
Exclusion of possible causes of sclerosing cholangitis such as:
Previous biliary tract surgery, although some would not include simple cholecystectomy in that category.[265–267,271,272]
Bile duct stones, possibly excluding stones thought to be secondary to stasis from PSC.[271]
Toxic agents (see Table 97-3).
Congenital biliary tract abnormalities.
Bile duct carcinoma.

TABLE 97-3
Classification of Sclerosing Cholangitis

Primary Sclerosing Cholangitis (unknown cause):
Associated with other diseases, such as ulcerative colitis
Unassociated with other diseases

Secondary Sclerosing Cholangitis (known or suspected causes):
Operative trauma
Bile duct stones
Cholangiocarcinoma
Toxic agents: formaldehyde, 20% NaCl injection of hepatic echinococcal cysts, absolute ethanol
Histiocytosis X
Chronic pancreatitis
Ischemia from liver allograft rejection, hepatic arterial infusion of floxuridine, operative trauma (?)

TABLE 97-4
Disorders Associated With Primary Sclerosing Cholangitis

DISORDER	FREQUENCY (%)
Inflammatory bowel disease	
Ulcerative colitis[273]	50–75
Crohn's disease	Rare
Fibrosing diseases	Rare
Reidel's thyroiditis[266,279]	
Retroperitoneal or mediastinal fibrosis[279,280]	
Sicca complex[268,290]	
Immunodeficiency syndromes	Rare
Familial immunodeficiency syndrome[281]	
Angioimmunoblastic lymphadenopathy[282]	
Hyperimmunoglobulin M immunodeficiency[283]	
Acquired immunodeficiency syndrome[284–287]	
Miscellaneous disorders	
Recurrent pancreatitis[266,268]	4–25
Celiac disease[288]	
Thrombotic events related to lupus anticoagulant[289]	
Diabetes mellitus[268,288]	
Rheumatoid arthritis[268]	
Sarcoidosis[268]	

Associated Disorders

PSC is associated with many disorders (Table 97-4). The most common is chronic ulcerative colitis, which occurs in 50% to 75% of PSC patients.[266–268,273] Conversely, the incidence of PSC among patients with chronic ulcerative colitis is 3% to 5%.[274–276] Usually, the colonic disease precedes the diagnosis of PSC, but PSC can occur before ulcerative colitis becomes clinically evident.[274] The activity or duration of colitis is unrelated to the disease activity of PSC.[266,267,274] The entire colon is affected in patients with PSC and ulcerative colitis.[275,276] The colonic disease is usually mild when PSC is diagnosed, and some patients may have had prior colectomy.[266–268] Cholangiographic studies have shown that PSC is present or ultimately develops in most patients with chronic ulcerative colitis who manifest a cholestatic liver enzyme pattern.[277]

Whether coexistence of inflammatory bowel disease affects the presentation and outcome of patients with PSC has been investigated. Rabinovitz and associates found that presence of inflammatory bowel disease is related to the gender distribution and disease location.[278] Specifically, gender difference was found only in patients with ulcerative colitis, and combined intrahepatic and extrahepatic bile duct involvement was found more frequently in patients with inflammatory bowel disease than in those without (81.5% versus 46.2%). Involvement of the extrahepatic bile ducts alone was more frequent in patients without inflammatory bowel disease (38.4% versus 7.4%). Response to liver transplantation and risk of bile duct cancer were not significantly affected by the presence of inflammatory bowel disease.

The rest of the disorders listed in Table 97-4 are all uncommonly associated with PSC, except for two: AIDS and pancreatitis.[284-287] The relation between pancreatitis and PSC is confusing. Of the patients with PSC, 4% to 22% had acute or chronic pancreatitis.[266,271] A syndrome complex of PSC, chronic pancreatitis, and Sjögren's syndrome had been reported in four cases up to 1984.[290] In those cases, the same pathologic process seemed to cause the injury to multiple organs.

The prevalence of abnormal pancreatograms for patients with PSC has ranged from 7.5% to 77%.[291-294] The usual abnormalities on pancreatography are side branch irregularities, although the main pancreatic duct can also be markedly irregular Abnormal pancreatograms are not unique to PSC.[294] Among biliary diseases, they are even more common in PSC and are found in 60% of patients with cholangiocarcinoma.[291,294] It has been suggested without proof that these pancreatogram abnormalities possibly resulted from cholestasis rather than any specific pathologic process leading to cholestasis. In one prospective study, 56% of 41 patients with primary biliary cirrhosis (PBC) and 36% of 22 patients with PSC had elevated serum isoamylase levels. Only the PBC patients had diminished duodenal juice flow rate and trypsin output after secretin-pancreozymin stimulation. Pancreatic involvement in PBC is closely associated with Sjögren's syndrome, which is much more common in PBC than in PSC.[290,291] This may explain why pancreatic involvement is more common with PBC. The mechanism of pancreatic injury may be different in cases associated with Sjögren's syndrome.

Chronic calcific pancreatitis can cause distal CBD stenosis.[295] About 10% of alcoholic pancreatitis patients have distal common duct stenosis manifested by greater than twofold elevated levels of alkaline phosphatase for more than 4 weeks.[295] Progressive disease can lead to diffuse stricturing of the intrapancreatic portion of the bile duct. Rarely, especially if untreated, this chronic obstruction may lead to diffuse secondary sclerosing cholangitis. Pancreatitis and sclerosing cholangitis may develop secondary to a common pathologic process (associated with Sjögren's syndrome); abnormal pancreatograms may be secondary to cholestasis, and rarely, sclerosing cholangitis may result from chronic pancreatitis.

Two other conditions that can mimic PSC deserve mentioning: patients with extrahepatic portal venous obstruction or metastatic cancer of the liver.[296-298] In the former case, the cholangiographic changes are most noticeable in the left hepatic duct and its branches. These are possibly caused by choledochal varices causing indentations on the bile duct. Jaundice secondary to the obstruction of the bile duct by enlarged choledochal varices occurs rarely. In the latter case, it has been suggested that compression or invasion of intrahepatic bile ducts by the tumors and periductal inflammation or fibrosis secondary to obstruction of bile flow contribute to the cholangiographic changes.

Pathogenesis

Primary Sclerosing Cholangitis

The cause of PSC is unknown, but several factors have been proposed to play etiologic roles.

Portal bacteremia. Because of the close association with ulcerative colitis, some researchers have proposed that portal bacteremia or the absorption of various toxins from the inflamed colon may cause PSC.[273] However portal bacteremia occurs rarely in patients with ulcerative colitis, the two disease activities are unrelated, and PSC has developed years after proctocolectomy.[299]

Viral infections. Hepatitis A and B do not cause PSC.[266] Cytomegalovirus (CMV) and rubella can cause an obliterative cholangitis of the intrahepatic ducts in the fetus but the histologic picture differs from PSC.[273,300] There has been a resurgence of interest in the role of CMV in PSC, largely because of a preliminary report from Mason and colleagues which showed CMV DNA in all 7 PSC livers and in only 5 of 20 controls.[301] However, Mehal and associates used a very sensitive polymerase chain reaction-based assay and found that 29 of 30 PSC liver biopsy specimens were negative for CMV.[302] Although this does not exclude a role for CMV as a trigger for an autoimmune process before the development of clinical disease, it does rule out any significant viral replication and reactivation being responsible during the progression of PSC.

Reovirus type 3 is associated with neonatal biliary atresia, but neither the prevalence nor the titer of antibody to reovirus type 3 differ between patients with PSC and normal controls.[303,304]

Copper. Abnormal copper metabolism occurs in almost all patients with PSC.[305] This probably results from cholestasis rather than causes PSC, because D-penicillamine treatment has failed to halt disease progression despite satisfactory cupriuresis.[306]

Genetics. Two lines of evidence suggest a genetic component to PSC. First is the familial occurrence of PSC and chronic ulcerative colitis, and second is the association of PSC with certain human leukocyte histocompatibility antigens (HLA)—specifically B8 and DR3.[307] HLA-B8 occurs in 60% of PSC patients, compared with 25% of normal controls.[308] HLA-DR3 was found in 9 of 12 PSC patients (75%), 8 of whom also had HLA-B8.[309,310] An even more striking association with HLA-DRw52a has not been confirmed.[311]

Immune system alterations. Even though serologic markers such as antimitochondrial, smooth muscle, and nuclear antibodies are typically absent, accumulating evidence supports immune system abnormalities causing PSC.[266,267,271,312] First, HLA-B8 and DR3, the two haplotypes closely associated with PSC, are also frequently associated with other autoimmune diseases.[273,288] Lymphocytes from 8 of 10 patients with PSC were sensitized to an antigen in the protein fraction of human gallbladder bile, as shown by a leukocyte migration inhibition test.[313] However, this also occurred in most patients with PBC and in 7 of 27 patients with chronic active hepatitis.[312]

Autoantibodies have also been found in patients with PSC. Studies of these autoantibodies occurring in sera of patients with inflammatory bowel disease and PSC on liver sections showed an antibody reacting exclusively with nuclei of cells infiltrating the portal tract.[314] Chapman and colleagues described two distinct autoantibodies: anticolon and antiportal tract antibodies.[314] Fifteen (62.5%) of 24 patients with PSC and chronic ulcerative colitis had anticolon antibody, but only

17% of chronic ulcerative colitis patients, and none of the PSC patients had anticolon antibody. Overall, 50% of PSC patients had antibodies to some antigen in obstructed portal tracts, which was closely associated with HLA-B8. None of the normal controls, patients with inflammatory bowel disease (IBD) or patients with extrahepatic obstruction had antiportal tract antibody.[314]

After this report, the "antigen" in obstructed portal tracts was localized to the nuclei of neutrophils.[315] Because of the reactivity of the antibody mainly in the perinuclear area of neutrophils, the antibody was called pANCA. The frequency of pANCA in patients with IBD has been reported to be 68% to 83% in patients with ulcerative colitis and 13% to 27% in patients with Crohn's disease.[316–319] The same immunofluorescence pattern has also been observed in as many as 88% of patients with PSC if they also have chronic ulcerative colitis and 40% to 80% if they do not have chronic ulcerative colitis.[317–319]

There are many clinical entities for which antineutrophilic antibodies are described; one of the most well-known is Wegener's granulomatosis.[317] In the case of Wegener's granulomatosis, the immunofluorescence pattern is granular, diffuse cytoplasmic, distinct from that seen in IBD and PSC. In IBD, the frequency of pANCA appears to depend on the method used for antibody detection; much higher frequencies were obtained if the neutrophils were fixed with ethanol than with methanol.[317,318] The method of fixation did not alter the frequency of pANCA in patients with PSC, indicating that the PSC-specific antigen was not affected by these methods, but the antigen related to IBD may be destroyed or not accessible after fixation by methanol.[318]

The etiologic and possible pathogenetic role of pANCA remains unclear. Seibold and associates, used an immunoblot system with sonified neutrophils as antigen and found that 82% of sera from patients with PSC reacted with as many as five different antigenic determinants, but only 12% of sera from patients with Crohn's disease and 11% of sera with ulcerative colitis reacted with one of the determinants, suggesting that different antigens are involved in pANCA reaction.[319] The shared antigenic determinant between PSC and ulcerative colitis, two frequently associated disorders, does raise the question of whether it may reflect a common pathogenetic link between the two.

Circulating immune complexes in the serum and in bile occur in most patients with PSC.[320,321] The high levels of circulating immune complexes in patients with PSC is likely to be associated with activation of complement through the classic pathway, because C3d and C4d were also elevated.[322] Elevated IgM levels in serum and bile also occur, as well as increased complement metabolism.[312,321,323]

T lymphocytes have been histologically identified in proximity to the destruction of bile ducts.[324] A causative role for these lymphocytes in the bile duct lesions has been suggested by reports of increased expression of the leukocyte adhesion molecule, intercellular adhesion molecule-1 (ICAM-1), on biliary epithelium and increased level of ICAM-1 in the circulation in patients with PSC and PBC.[325,326] ICAM-1 is a member of the integrin family of leukocyte adhesion molecules that mediates leukocyte adherence to target structures and to other immune cells. Normal bile ducts do not express ICAM-1; expression of ICAM-1 is strongly associated with

bile duct damage.[325] Increased expression of ICAM-1 might enhance cell-mediated damage to bile ducts in PBC and PSC by allowing T cells to interact with major histocompatibility complex antigens expressed on the biliary epithelium. Whether ICAM-1 expression is an early event in the pathogenesis of bile duct damage or a secondary response to inflammation is unknown. Enhanced autoreactivity of suppressor or cytotoxic T lymphocytes from peripheral blood also occurs.[327]

All of these studies support a strong association of altered immune function with PSC. PSC may be an autoimmune disease in individuals with an underlying genetic predisposition.[321] The exact pathogenesis still remains to be elucidated.

Secondary Sclerosing Cholangitis

Table 97-3 lists some of the known causes of sclerosing cholangitis. Their mechanisms of injury differ. For instance, sclerosing cholangitis developing within a few months after the injection of a scolicidal solution (i.e., 2% formaldehyde, 20% sodium chloride or alcohol) for the treatment of hydatid disease most likely directly results from the toxicity of these agents on bile duct epithelium (caustic sclerosing cholangitis).[328] Supporting this, only the part of the biliary tree in contact with these agents is affected. However, the sclerosing cholangitis developing in 17% to 56% of patients receiving hepatic arterial infusion of floxuridine (FUDR) is more likely related to ischemia rather than intrinsic toxicity of FUDR.[329,330] This complication of FUDR occurs only after hepatic intraarterial administration.[331] The bifurcation of the common hepatic duct is almost always involved, and the distal CBD is often spared.[329] The lower bile duct derives its arterial supply from gastroduodenal and mesenteric branches, which are isolated from drug injection. This may explain the usual sparing of the lower bile duct. Ludwig and colleagues found obstructive arteriopathy and portal venopathy in the hilus of the liver of a patient who developed liver failure from FUDR-induced sclerosing cholangitis.[330] Similar changes were found in a liver allograft from a patient with severe occlusive rejection arteriopathy.[330]

The concept of ischemic cholangiopathy has also been applied to the pathogenesis of postoperative strictures.[332] Such lesions can result from damage to small arteries paralleling the CBD. Chronic and mild ischemia may result in duct fibrosis and sclerosing cholangitis, but acute and severe ischemia may result in duct necrosis.[330,333]

Three patients with histiocytosis X and sclerosing cholangitis were reported by Thompson and associates.[334] The biliary lesion may have resulted from histiocytosis X.

Clinical Manifestations

PSC affects mostly young men. Two thirds of the patients are younger than 45 years of age.[267,269] The male to female ratio is 2 : 1.[266,267,269,272] Between 50% and 75% of patients have chronic ulcerative colitis. The natural history, clinical presentation, and laboratory, radiographic and histologic features are unchanged by the presence of chronic ulcerative colitis. Pediatric cases have been described.[335–337] Sisto and colleagues reviewed 78 pediatric cases of sclerosing cholangitis in 1987 and found 47% were associated with IBD, 10% with a variety of immunodeficiency syndromes, and 15% with histiocytosis X.[336]

Natural History

The natural history of PSC varies but most often is one of slow progression, perhaps over decades, leading to portal hypertension and death from liver failure. Earlier data from the Mayo Clinic and the Royal Free Hospital in London suggested 33% to 40% of patients with PSC die within 5 to 7 years of diagnosis, based on actuarial survival data previously reported.[266,267,338] Previous reports suggested that a poorly defined subset of asymptomatic patients do not progress.[272,339] Survival analysis from a large number of asymptomatic PSC patients showed that most asymptomatic patients had evidence of disease progression and their survival rate was worse than expected when compared with age-, sex-, and race-specific survival rates for a population from the same area.[340] Several studies also investigated the natural history and prognostic variables in PSC.[340-342] The largest up-to-date analysis includes 426 patients from five centers with median follow-up of 3 years.[342] In that study, Cox proportional hazard regression modeling was used to identify clinical variables most important in predicting survival.[342] The resulting model was assessed by applying methods of statistical cross-validation and quantifying the model's reliability by estimating confidence intervals for predicting survival probabilities. In this model, multivariate analysis revealed the independent variables most useful in predicting survival of patients with PSC to be serum bilirubin concentration, histologic stage on liver biopsy, age, and the presence or absence of splenomegaly. A mathematical model to predict survival of patients with PSC defined the risk score (R) as $R = (0.535 \times \log_e$ bilirubin in mg/dL) + $(0.486 \times$ histologic stage) + $(0.041 \times$ age in years) + 0.705 (if splenomegaly is present).

The 1- and 5-year survival probabilities for low-risk (R = 2.35–2.46) patients were 0.98 and 0.91 to 0.92; moderate-risk (R = 4.25–4.31) patients were 0.88 to 0.89 and 0.54 to 0.56; and high-risk (R = 5.23–5.42) patients were 0.68 to 0.73 and 0.15 to 0.21, respectively. Although the model still requires improvement and prospective validation, it will be extremely helpful in the management of patients with PSC, especially in the timing of liver transplantation.

Clinical Presentations

PSC usually begins insidiously, making the onset of the disease difficult to determine. Most patients suffer symptoms for an average of 2 years before diagnosis.[269,273] The most common symptom complex is that of progressive fatigue and pruritus, followed by jaundice.[266,269,272,312]

Clinical evidence of cholangitis is uncommon without previous bile duct reconstructive surgery.[269,272,343] Symptoms of cholangitis in a patient with PSC who has not had bile duct surgery may indicate the presence of a complication, such as a bile duct stone or bile duct carcinoma.[269] Totally asymptomatic patients with PSC are more frequently diagnosed because of increased awareness, ready availability of ERCP, and use of the automated chemistry panel.[272,339] Patients with chronic ulcerative colitis are often referred for ERCP with asymptomatic elevations of serum alkaline phosphatase. Even with symptoms, the physical examination may be normal in as many as one half of the patients.[266,272] The most common physical findings include hepatosplenomegaly and jaundice.[266,272]

Laboratory Evaluations

Serum biochemical profiles usually indicate cholestasis; the alkaline phosphatase concentration is elevated in 95% to 98% of cases.[266,268,272,343] The level may fluctuate widely; normal levels of alkaline phosphatase in symptomatic patients have been described.[344] Most often, alkaline phosphatase levels are at least twofold elevated and out of proportion to the serum bilirubin level.[268,269] Most patients have mildly increased serum transaminase levels.[269]

Serum antimitochondrial antibody, rheumatoid factor, smooth muscle antibody, and antinuclear antibody assays are negative in more than 90% of cases.[266,268,272,312] Increased levels of circulating immune complexes and IgM occur in 80% and 50% of patients, respectively.[267,268,320] Antineutrophilic antibody with a distinct perinuclear pattern (pANCA) has been reported in 80% to 85% of patients with PSC.[317-319]

Copper metabolism is abnormal in patients with PSC. The hepatic and urine copper levels are often as elevated as in patients with PBC or Wilson's disease.[305] Serum copper and ceruloplasmin levels are elevated in 49% and 71% of patients with PSC, respectively, but are unrelated to the histologic stage of the liver disease; however, hepatic and urine copper levels correlate with progression of the histologic stage of the liver disease.[305]

Radiologic Features

Cholangiographic findings are the most useful diagnostic features. ERCP is preferred because PTC is more difficult to perform in the presence of stricturing and fibrosis of intrahepatic ducts. Earlier studies emphasized the extrahepatic location of the ductal changes in PSC.[266,267,271] Some studies indicate the intrahepatic ducts are almost always involved, often to a greater degree than the extrahepatic ducts.[293,343,345] The hepatic duct bifurcation appears to be preferentially affected.[343] Cholangiography typically shows multifocal strictures involving intrahepatic and extrahepatic bile ducts. These strictures are diffusely distributed, short (1–2 cm) and annular, alternating with normal or slightly dilated segments to produce a beaded appearance (Fig. 97-12). Very short (1–2 mm), band-like strictures, mostly in extrahepatic ducts, occur in 21% of patients. Diverticulum-like outpouchings occur in 27% of patients. The band-like strictures and diverticulum-like outpouchings are specific findings for PSC.[293] Diffuse strictures occur in as many as 31% of patients with PBC and 10% of patients with cholangiocarcinoma.[293] In the cases of PBC, only intrahepatic ducts are involved, and band strictures or diverticula are absent.

Differentiating cholangiocarcinoma from PSC can be difficult, and in 10% of cases of bile duct carcinoma, the carcinoma is diffuse and sclerosing, mimicking PSC.[293] In extensive PSC, the duct margins become grossly nodular, irregular, and shaggy.[274] Abnormal cystic and pancreatic ducts also occur frequently.[291-294,345]

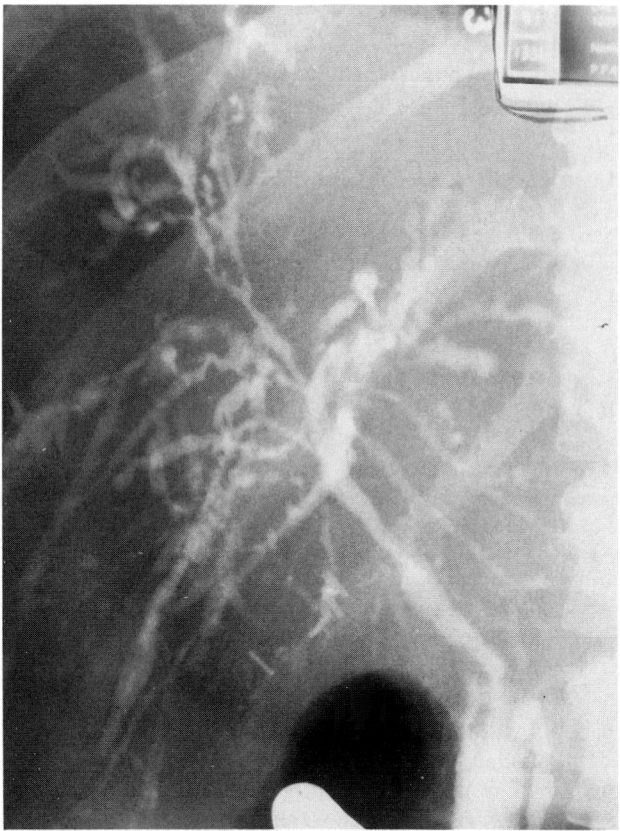

FIGURE 97-12. Cholangiographic findings in primary sclerosing cholangitis. Multifocal strictures involve intra- and extrahepatic bile ducts. These strictures are diffusely distributed, short (1–2 cm), and annular, alternating with normal or slightly dilated segments to produce a beaded appearance. (Courtesy of Hartley Cohen, M.D., Los Angeles, CA.)

Different radiographic procedures have various utilities in PSC. Ultrasound has limited use in PSC, because ducts are not dilated in most cases.[346] Hepatobiliary scintigraphy has been advocated as a noninvasive and sensitive method for the diagnosis of PSC.[347] Cholescintigraphy with ^{99m}Tc-labeled IDA analogs shows multiple persistent "hot spots" caused by stasis within segmentally dilated ducts, corresponding to beading seen on cholangiography. The advantage of scintigraphy is that it is a functional study, measuring regional clearance of the isotope. It can be repeated serially to follow patients.[347] Abnormalities on CT highly suggestive of PSC consist of focal discontinuous areas of minimal intrahepatic biliary dilation without mass lesions.[348,349] None of these noninvasive studies can replace ERCP for definitive diagnosis.

Pathology

Almost all patients with PSC have nonspecific histologic abnormalities on liver biopsy.[268,269,350] Liver biopsies are diagnostic in only 36% to 38%. Ludwig and associates developed a histologic staging system for PSC.[267,272,350] PSC begins with portal tract enlargement with increased connective tissue, edema, and interlobular duct proliferation (stage I). Later, tongues of connective tissue grow into the periportal paren-

chyma (stage II) with minimal accompanying inflammation. This leads to fibrous septa formation and bridging necrosis (stage III). Fibrosis spreads further to liver parenchyma, and biliary cirrhosis develops (stage IV).

Secondary biliary cirrhosis was found on liver biopsy in 30% of patients at the time of diagnosis of PSC.[266] Later, cholestasis and accumulation of copper-protein complexes increase. Fibrous-obliterative cholangitis, which occurs in the early stage, is pathognomonic. Another pathognomonic morphologic feature is macroscopic intrahepatic cholangiectases with duct obliteration.[351] The reported incidence of fibrous-obliterative cholangitis in needle biopsies range from 12% to 40%, and they were largely confined to medium-sized portal areas, but loss of bile ducts was the most conspicuous feature in small portal tracts.[352] Granulomatous cholangitis occurs in as many as 8% of cases with PSC, but it is much more common in PBC (71% of cases).[312]

The extrahepatic bile ducts appear as thickened cords with marked lumenal narrowing. The wall may be eight times normal thickness, with monotonous layers of connective tissue and chronic inflammation.[268] The gallbladder is frequently abnormal with chronic inflammation and fibrosis.[353] Lymphadenopathy, fibrosis, and inflammatory adhesions may also be prominent in the porta hepatis.

Pericholangitis describes a morphologic feature of PBC, extrahepatic biliary obstruction, or certain infectious diseases.[354] After Mistilis described similar morphologic changes in patients with chronic ulcerative colitis in 1965, this term became a clinical diagnosis for poorly defined chronic hepatitis and cholangitis related to chronic ulcerative colitis.[354,355] The relation of this condition to PSC and chronic active hepatitis in patients with chronic ulcerative colitis became so obscure that the International Association for the Study of the Liver omitted it from standard nomenclature in 1976.[356] Nevertheless, the group at the Mayo Clinic defined pericholangitis as "small-duct primary sclerosing cholangitis."[354] It refers to PSC-like small duct changes but without large duct PSC. They found 35% of patients with chronic ulcerative colitis and hepatobiliary disease had pericholangitis, and some eventually developed large duct PSC. PSC represents a spectrum, with persistent small duct PSC at one end and symptomatic, cholangiographically confirmed, large duct PSC at the other. Progressive hepatic fibrosis and cirrhosis has been described secondary to the small duct disease alone and may account for some of the cases of cirrhosis or "chronic active hepatitis" in association with chronic ulcerative colitis.[354]

Clinical Course and Complications

The clinical course of PSC can be variable, but it is slowly progressive in most patients. Rarely, the biliary lesions reverse.[270,357] Complications may be related to cholestasis, specifically pruritus and fat-soluble vitamin deficiencies, or to the underlying disease, specifically cholangitis, dominant strictures, duct stone formation, and cholangiocarcinoma.[273]

The incidence of cholangiocarcinoma in patients with chronic ulcerative colitis ranges from 0.4% to 1.4% and from 7% to 15% in patients with PSC.[273,358,359] Both are markedly higher than the reported incidence of 0.0008% to 0.5% in the general population.[358,359] The mean age at diagnosis of bile duct carcinoma in patients with chronic ulcerative colitis was 42 years, compared with 66 years of age for the general population. The mean duration of chronic ulcerative colitis before the diagnosis of carcinoma was 21 years. Chronic ulcerative colitis involves usually the entire colon but colonic disease activity does not correlate with the risk for bile duct carcinoma. Many patients developed bile duct carcinoma years after colectomy.[358]

The belief that cholangiocarcinoma develops only with preexisting PSC is supported by the presence of tumor-free PSC, distant from the carcinomatous areas; the presence of carcinoma in situ in areas of fibrous cholangitis; the multicentric origins of the tumors; and the documentation of hepatobiliary disease for an average of 4 years before the diagnosis of bile duct carcinoma.[359] Cholangiographic findings suggesting malignant degeneration include marked ductal dilatation, rapidly progressive stricture formation or dilatation, and presence of associated polypoid masses (>1 cm in diameter).[360,361] The mean survival after the diagnosis of cholangiocarcinoma was 11.8 months.[358]

Management

Management of PSC is a real challenge, given the array of potential complications and the absence of effective specific therapy. Opinions regarding treating asymptomatic patients differ; some advocate observation, and others advocate therapy as part of a randomized trial.[272,338] Because most asymptomatic patients with PSC have progressive disease, investigators now favor entering asymptomatic patients into drug trials. PSC management consists of measures directed against cholestatic liver disease, against the complications of PSC and against disease progression.

Treatment of Cholestasis

Pruritus and fat-soluble vitamin deficiencies are the two most commonly encountered problems. Vitamin A deficiency occurs in as many as 50% of patients with PSC, especially in those with jaundice or steatorrhea.[273] Other fat-soluble vitamins such as D, K, and E can also be deficient. A combined deficiency of two or three vitamins may occur in 30% of patients with PSC.[362] Bone biopsies from patients with PSC have shown osteoporosis rather than osteomalacia.[273] Despite absence of osteomalacia, treatment with vitamin D and calcium is recommended if serum levels are low.

Treatments for pruritus have included cholestyramine, activated charcoal, phenobarbital, plasma perfusion over charcoal-coated glass beads, and ursodeoxycholic acid.[273,363–367] In one report, cholestyramine ameliorated the underlying disease; symptoms recurred, and liver tests deteriorated when cholestyramine was discontinued but returned to normal after readministration.[363] Plasma perfusion has given inconsistent results and has not been widely used.

Treatment of Complications

Complications of PSC include cholangitis, dominant strictures, duct stone formation, and cholangiocarcinoma. Surgical manipulation of the biliary tract usually precedes cholangitis.[269] Patients with recurrent episodes of cholangitis without dominant stricture formation should receive broad-spectrum antibiotics as needed. Some have advocated prophylactic antibiotics for patients with frequent episodes of cholangitis, but the efficacy of this approach has not been demonstrated.[273]

Rapid worsening of symptoms and the hepatic biochemical profile may signal the development of dominant strictures or cholangiocarcinoma. Cholangiography is indicated to diagnose a treatable dominant stricture. This stricture can be approached percutaneously or endoscopically, and balloon dilation of the stricture can dramatically improve some patients.[273,368] If balloon dilation is insufficient, endoscopic or percutaneous endoprosthetic placement to bridge the stricture may be successful.[368–370] Advocates have suggested that balloon dilatation of dominant strictures may improve the natural history of the underlying hepatobiliary disease. However, long-term follow-up has not been reported, and multiple procedures may be necessary to achieve the desired results. Because these procedures are not without risk and offer uncertain benefits to asymptomatic patients, they should only be used for symptomatic relief of jaundice or pruritus.[268,273]

The management of cholangiocarcinoma superimposed on PSC is evolving. If the cholangiocarcinoma is resectable and the patient is not a candidate for liver transplantation, surgical resection seems reasonable. Alternatively, if the cholangiocarcinoma is not resectable or if the patient has advanced liver disease, orthotopic liver transplantation may be considered.

Treatment of Underlying Hepatobiliary Disease

Medical therapy

Numerous approaches with various drug therapies alone or in combination have been tried. Only one prospective, randomized, controlled trial reports such an approach; most of the others include small numbers of patients or uncontrolled case reports. The agents tried so far are immunosuppressants, cupruretic agents, antifibrogenic agents, and oral bile acid therapy.

Immunosuppressive agents. Corticosteroids have been used topically and systemically in several small studies in PSC.[270,371–373] Three small uncontrolled trials showed benefit from corticosteroids; however, one small controlled trial of nasobiliary lavage with corticosteroids showed deterioration.[270,371–373] Short-term, low-dose infusion did not lead to cholangiographic or biochemical improvement but was associated with biliary sepsis in 2 of 7 patients receiving steroids.

Azathioprine has been used in a few small studies without proven efficacy.[268,273] Cyclosporine is being investigated for therapeutic efficacy in a variety of autoimmune diseases, but a pilot study at the Mayo Clinic does not look promising for PSC (NF LaRusso, personal communication). Low-dose methotrexate was symptomatically and histologically effective in 2 patients.[374] The same group of investigators have extended this observation to 10 patients.[375] The results of controlled trials are awaited.

Cupruretic agents. A prospective, randomized double-blind trial with D-penicillamine showed no beneficial effect on disease progression within 36 months or on overall survival.[306] Major side effects caused permanent discontinuation of penicillamine in 21% of patients.

Antifibrogenic agents. Colchicine with prednisone showed encouraging results in a small uncontrolled study; however, more patients with longer follow-up did not confirm the initial improvements.[376,377]

Oral bile aacid therapy. Ursodeoxycholic acid has received increasing attention for treating PSC.[365-367] Preliminary data from three centers suggest ursodeoxycholic acid relieves symptoms and improves biochemical profiles. A key advantage is the safety of this drug. However, subsequent controlled trials, one published and two in preliminary form, yielded conflicting results.[378-380] There is no clear evidence that ursodeoxycholic acid halts progression of the underlying disease.

Surgical therapy

Three surgical procedures have been advocated for PSC: proctocolectomy, biliary tract reconstructive procedures, and orthotopic liver transplantation.

Proctocolectomy. Because of the association of PSC with chronic ulcerative colitis, proctocolectomy was suggested to control the hepatobiliary disease.[381] A prospective study from the Mayo Clinic showed no effect of proctocolectomy on the course of PSC.[382] This is not surprising, because PSC can develop many years after proctocolectomy in patients with prior chronic ulcerative colitis.[266-268] Proctocolectomy failed to show any benefit for hepatobiliary disease, and patients with advanced liver disease suffered considerable morbidity. In one series, 10 (53%) of 19 patients developed peristomal varices 12 to 133 months after proctocolectomy.[383] Seven of the 10 patients had recurrent bleeding requiring repeated blood transfusions. In contrast, ileoanal anastomosis was not associated with perirectal bleeding.[383] Proctocolectomy is not recommended as a means of controlling PSC; ileoanal anastomosis may be a preferred procedure in patients with chronic ulcerative colitis and advanced hepatobiliary disease but should be reserved for treatment of the bowel disease when indicated, not the biliary disease.

Biliary tract reconstructive procedures. Surgeons at the UCLA Medical Center and the Johns Hopkins Hospital have advocated aggressive surgical management of patients with PSC.[384,385] Pitt and colleagues proposed that patients with PSC who had a major area of extrahepatic blockage or primary involvement of the extrahepatic bile ducts should undergo hepaticoenteric or choledochoenteric anastomosis.[384] Thirteen (77%) of 17 patients managed this way had good to excellent results after surgery. Eighty-two percent were alive a mean of 52 months after operation and 65 months after diagnosis. Cholecystectomy was recommended as part of the operation.[384]

Cameron and colleagues have recommended extrahepatic biliary tree resection with long-term transhepatic Silastic stents.[385] They found cirrhosis influenced short- and long-term outcome. Two of the 5 cirrhotic patients died after surgery, and only 1 survived 5 years. In comparison, 24 of the 25 noncirrhotic patients survived surgery, and the actuarial 5-year survival rate for this subgroup was 77%. Moreover, 2 of the surviving patients have undergone successful liver transplantation. Their recommendation was that patients with severe hilar or extrahepatic stricturing, persistent jaundice or cholangitis, and no cirrhosis should be considered for biliary reconstruction and long-term transhepatic stenting. They think that this policy does not preclude but may postpone or avoid the need for liver transplantation.[385]

Other groups do not advocate this aggressive surgical approach to PSC.[265,267,386-388] They argue that previous biliary tract reconstructive surgery increases complications from subsequent orthotopic liver transplantation without good evidence that it is better than nonsurgical approaches in alleviating symptoms or improving survival. Moreover, infectious complications are greater after biliary tract surgery.[265,267]

The Mayo Clinic and other groups recommend biliary reconstructive surgery for patients with PSC if carcinoma cannot be excluded, for symptomatic duct stones that cannot be extracted during endoscopic papillotomy, and for dominant strictures unresponsive to endoscopic or percutaneous balloon dilation.[265,267]

Liver transplantation. With the increasing availability and improving survival rates, liver transplantation is becoming the therapy of choice for patients with any form of advanced liver disease, including PSC. PSC is the third most common indication for orthotopic liver transplantation in adults.[387] The results of 55 consecutive liver transplantations for PSC from 1980 to 1986 showed 1- and 2-year actuarial survival rates of 71% and 57%, respectively.[387] The 1-year actuarial survival rates have been reported to be up to 88%.[388] The issues of whether liver transplantation can prolong survival in patients with PSC and how to optimize the timing of liver transplantation were addressed in a one review.[389] Overall, it appears that liver transplantation improves survival in PSC patients for a wide spectrum of risk levels. Studies have also shown that patients with higher-risk scores have an increased risk of dying related to liver transplantation. Although many factors enter into the timing of liver transplantation, evidence is growing that having patients undergo transplantation a little earlier in the course of the disease rather than waiting until the patients have experienced life-threatening complications or are on life-support measures can improve survival during the early period after liver transplantation.

Two additional questions in patients with PSC undergoing liver transplantations are whether those with chronic ulcerative colitis under immunosuppression are at increased risk for developing colonic malignancy and whether PSC will recur in the transplanted liver. A Pittsburgh study followed 36 patients with PSC associated with chronic ulcerative colitis who underwent liver transplantation. Two of these patients were found to have colorectal carcinoma 11 and 21 months after transplantation.[390] Both patients had histories of chronic ulcerative colitis for 17 years or longer and negative pretransplant colorectal examinations. It is unclear whether lesions were missed preoperatively or that malignant transformation was stimulated by immunosuppression or other conditions of transplantation. Whether proctocolectomy should be considered prophylactically in patients who have had ulcerative colitis for more than 15 years undergoing liver transplantation for PSC is an unresolved issue.

One study found that 6 of 39 liver allografts from patients with PSC had intrahepatic bile duct strictures and beading compatible with PSC.[391] None of 36 liver allografts from patients with PBC had intrahepatic bile duct strictures. Because strictures can develop from chronic allograft rejection and ischemia, long-term follow-up is needed to confirm these findings.

Future Cholangitis Research

Sclerosing cholangitis represents the consequence of multiple different injurious factors on the bile ducts. In the past few years, major advances have been made in understanding the pathogenesis and defining treatments of PSC. Much more remains to be learned about the immunologic abnormalities and how they may possibly lead to PSC. Reports of treatment with ursodeoxycholic acid in PSC are exciting and may further illuminate the pathogenesis of this disorder.

MISCELLANEOUS CAUSES OF BILE DUCT OBSTRUCTION

Causes of bile duct obstruction appear in Table 97-5. The most common causes are stones and strictures. Parasites that invade the biliary tree and accompany hemobilia or hemorrhage into the biliary tract can cause obstruction. *Ascaris lumbricoides* is the most common parasite to do both.[114,392] Nine

---

TABLE 97-5
Causes of Obstruction of the Biliary Tract

Intrinsic Causes
Stones
Stenosis and strictures (localized)
  Papillary stenosis
  Duct strictures due to trauma, stones, parasites, chronic
    pancreatitis, necrotizing cholangitis, cystic fibrosis
Diffuse strictures due to sclerosing cholangitis
Abnormal anatomy-biliary atresia, biliary cysts
Infection
  Parasitic: *Ascaris lumbricoides, Clonorchis sinensis,*
    Opisthorchis felineus and *viverrini, Fasciola hepatica* and
    gigantica, echinococcus
  Fungal: candidal fungal balls
  Bacterial: tuberculosis
Tumors
  Primary: cholangiocarcinoma, other primary malignancies of the
    bile duct, ampullary carcinoma
  Metastatic
Hemobilia
  Traumatic: iatrogenic (e.g., PTC, liver biopsy), blunt and
    penetrating injury to the liver
  Nontraumatic: stones, tumors, aneurysms, parasites

Extrinsic Causes
Pancreatic: carcinoma, acute and chronic pancreatitis, pancreatic
  pseudocyst, abscess
Enlarged porta hepatis: enlarged lymph nodes from malignancies or
  adjacent inflammation
Mass lesions in the liver: tumor, cyst, abscess
Enlarged renal mass
Hepatic artery aneurysm
Duodenal disorders: diverticuli, Crohn's, villous adenoma,
  eosinophilic gastroenteritis

---

percent of hepatic echinococcal cysts rupture into the biliary tract and can cause obstruction.[393]

Another unusual infectious cause of bile duct obstruction is a candidal fungal ball.[394] Invariably patients with biliary candidiasis are immunocompromised or are receiving broad-spectrum antibiotics and have disseminated fungal infection.[394]

Other than stones, biliary cysts, and sclerosing cholangitis, three important causes of biliary tract obstruction are biliary stricture, papillary stenosis, and hemobilia.

Biliary Stricture

Benign biliary stricture is the most common serious "benign" disease of the biliary tract and, if left untreated, can lead to recurrent cholangitis and secondary biliary cirrhosis.[395,396] In most large series, 90% of benign biliary strictures follow operative trauma.[395,396] These strictures are invariably extrahepatic, distal to the cystic duct. Strictures proximal to the cystic duct are usually malignant.[397,398] Pancreatitis causes 8.5% of benign biliary strictures, and external trauma is responsible for 1.7%.[396] Other nontraumatic causes include choledocholithiasis, parasitic infestation, pericholedochal abscess, and congenital lesions associated with choledochal cysts. Rare causes include vascular rings, cystic fibrosis, and even tuberculosis.[395,399,409] Among patients with cystic fibrosis, 96% of those with associated liver disease had strictures in the distal CBD on cholangiography, but none without liver disease had stricture in the duct.[409]

Biliary Strictures Due to Operative Trauma

Most biliary strictures occur after injury to the bile duct during the course of an operation. Usually, the procedure is a cholecystectomy with or without exploration of the CBD, but injuries have followed procedures on the liver, portal vein, pancreas, or stomach and may occur posttraumatically or be secondary to an inflammatory process. Postoperative bile duct strictures can occur at the site of a biliary-enteric anastomosis done for reconstruction.[400,401] As laparoscopic cholecystectomy has rapidly become the procedure of choice for removal of the gallbladder, the most significant complication related to the procedure, bile duct injury, which occurs with an overall incidence of 0.2% (this rate is most likely an underestimate and is clearly higher with inexperienced surgeons), becomes an increasingly challenging problem to the clinician.[402,403]

The major problems with iatrogenic bile duct injuries are that more than three quarters of these cases go unrecognized at the operations during which they occur, and reoperation has been a necessity in most cases.[401] Although the injury typically occurs in the segment of bile duct between the cystic duct junction and the bifurcation of the common hepatic duct, the ducts above the bifurcation have also been injured in a number of the cases, especially the right hepatic duct.[401] In addition to factors such as misplacement of clips, excessive use of cautery, and failure to recognize congenital anomalies, the importance of ischemia of the bile duct in the formation of postoperative strictures has been emphasized.[400] Excessive dissection around the bile duct during cholecystectomy or bile duct anastomosis may divide or injure the major arteries of the bile duct. Ischemia may then contribute to fibrosis and stricture formation during healing.

Most patients with benign postoperative bile duct strictures present soon after the initial operation. About 10% are suspected within the first week after surgery, 70% are identified within the first 6 months, and 80% are reported within 1 year.[400] In the remaining patients, presentation may be delayed for many years after the initial operation. The timing of presentation often dictates the mode of presentation.

Patients that present within days to weeks of initial operation often present in one of two ways.[400,401] The more common presentation is progressive jaundice with abnormal liver function tests due to high-grade obstruction. At times, biliary sepsis can supervene. A second mode of presentation relates to the leakage of bile from the injured bile duct. Bilious drainage from operatively placed drains or through the wound after cholecystectomy is abnormal and undoubtedly represents some form of bile duct injury. In patients without drains, or in whom the drains have been removed, the bile may leak freely into the peritoneal cavity or loculate, often as a perihepatic collection. The free accumulation of bile in the peritoneal cavity may result in biliary ascites or bile peritonitis.

The presentation of patients with postoperative bile duct strictures months to years after the initial operation most frequently is associated with episodes of cholangitis. Less commonly, patients present with painless jaundice and no evidence of sepsis. There are also patients with delayed diagnosis presenting with advanced biliary cirrhosis and portal hypertension.

Diagnosis requires imaging studies. Ultrasonography and CT are helpful in demonstrating biliary dilatation, but definition of the biliary anatomy requires cholangiography. Transhepatic cholangiography is generally more valuable than ERC in defining the anatomy and allowing transhepatic catheters to be placed for drainage. In cases of bile leakage and complications that are recognized soon after surgery, radionuclide hepatobiliary scintigraphy has been extremely useful.[403]

Treatment generally requires reoperation, usually Roux-en-Y hepaticojejunostomy.[400,401] For the elderly or poor surgical candidates, balloon dilatation has been advocated with the placement of stents and expandable metallic biliary endoprostheses.[404]

Biliary Stricture Due to Pancreatic Causes

In 1886, Riedel described bile duct obstruction resulting from benign pancreatic disease.[405] The distal CBD runs in a groove on the posterior surface of the pancreas before entering the duodenum, and it is not surprising that pancreatic disease may affect the bile duct.[405,406] The primary abnormality of the pancreas determines the type of duct involvement and whether the involvement is transient or permanent. Mass tumors and cysts of the pancreas cause extrinsic compression of the CBD. Acute and chronic pancreatitis also can produce distal CBD stenosis. Obstruction caused by acute or relapsing pancreatitis (e.g., edema) and pancreatic pseudocyst (Fig 97-13) is transient, but that caused by malignant tumors and chronic pan-

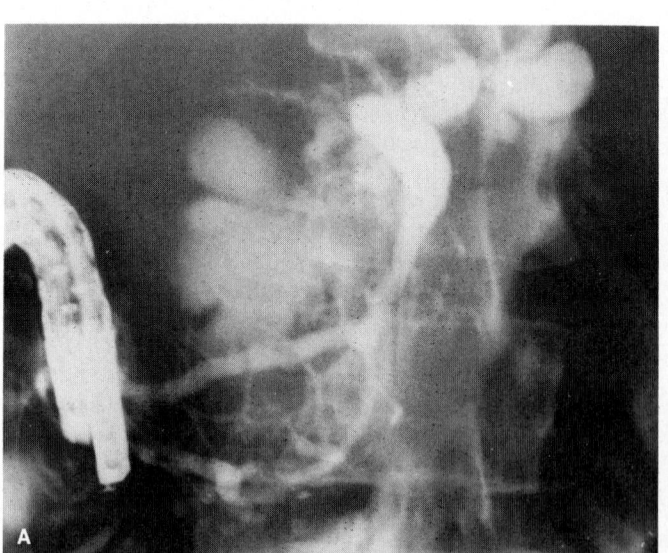
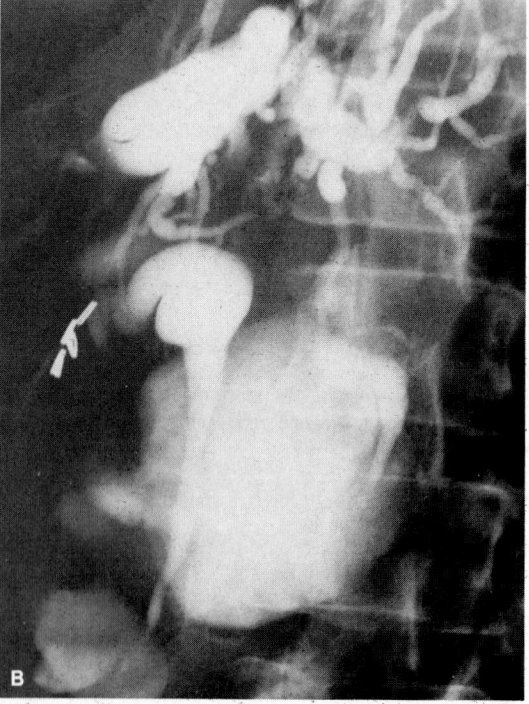

FIGURE 97-13. Endoscopic retrograde cholangiopancreatography in a patient with history of recurrent pancreatitis and progressive jaundice. (**A**) Pancreatography showed the pancreatic duct to be dilated, tortuous, and irregular, with dye extravasation into a large cavity. (**B**) Cholangiography in the same patient subsequently showed the distal common bile duct to be compressed externally by a large dye-filled structure, with dilatation of the proximal and intrahepatic ducts. The large dye-filled structure was a pancreatic pseudocyst. (Courtesy of Hartley Cohen, M.D., Los Angeles, CA.)

creatitis (i.e., fibrosis) is permanent. The prevalence of chronic CBD stenosis due to chronic alcoholic pancreatitis ranges from 4% to 10%.[295,405,406] However, in a subset of patients with alkaline phosphatase levels persistently greater than twice normal for at least 4 weeks, the prevalence of CBD stenosis was 100%.[405] The prevalence of CBD stenosis was also high (62%) among patients with chronic pancreatitis who were surgically treated. These were usually treated for pain; only 15% underwent surgery for obstructive jaundice.[407] This is a complication of severe and advanced chronic pancreatitis.

Clinically, no historical feature separates patients with from those without CBD stenosis. A history suggesting bile duct obstruction is rare.[405] Physical examination is generally not helpful. The most characteristic biochemical feature is an elevated alkaline phosphatase level that is out of proportion to the bilirubin level. Ninety-four percent of patients had this.[405,406] Eighty-six percent of patients have bilirubin elevation, but it is not progressive, and a rising and falling pattern is common.[406] Persistent, low-grade hyperbilirubinemia identifies cases at risk for rapid progression to biliary cirrhosis.[405] Seventy-eight percent of patients have mild to moderately elevated transaminase levels, and 47% of patients have elevated amylase levels.[406]

The most useful diagnostic test is cholangiography by PTC or ERCP.[405–407] A long, smooth, gradual tapering of the distal CBD is most characteristic.[406]

Histologically, features of extrahepatic biliary obstruction appear in 44% to 79% of patients.[407,408] Importantly, secondary biliary cirrhosis appeared in 29% and was shown to develop within 6 months to 1 year in some cases, despite a lack of clinical symptoms of jaundice or cholangitis.[408]

Most physicians recommend surgical decompression when CBD stenosis is caused by chronic pancreatitis, even without symptoms.[405,406] Without surgery, cholangitis, stone formation, and secondary biliary cirrhosis may complicate longstanding biliary tract obstruction. Choledochoduodenostomy and Roux-en-Y choledochojejunostomy are preferred. Sphincteroplasty has been unsuccessful in most series, primarily because of the length of the distal CBD stricture.[405,406] Preoperative evaluation should include ultrasound and ERCP to exclude pseudocysts and other pancreatic abnormalities that may require surgical intervention. Some advocate liver biopsy using the presence of periductal fibrosis or progression toward secondary biliary cirrhosis as indication for surgery. This approach should be reserved for the rare case with normal serum alkaline phosphatase.

Papillary Stenosis

Papillary stenosis (PS) is a clinical syndrome characterized by biliary colic without gallstones.[410] Most patients with PS are middle-aged women; many have had cholecystectomies. The most frequent presenting complaint is biliary colic, but pancreatitis can recur.[410] This syndrome can be a result of organic stenosis or functional obstruction, and differentiation is frequently difficult. In this section, only organic stenosis is discussed. Functional stenosis (i.e., biliary dyskinesia) is discussed in Chapter 99.

The incidence of PS varies between 0.04% and 0.12% in postmortem studies.[67] The diagnosis of PS was made in 363

(2.7%) of 13,000 diagnostic ERCPs at five gastroenterologic centers in the Federal Republic of Germany.[67] Sixty-one percent of the cases were associated with choledocholithiasis, 7% with surgical manipulation, 14% with papillary carcinoma, and 1% with juxtapapillary duodenal diverticula.[67]

Even though most cases result from stones or traumatic choledochal instrumentation, cases of idiopathic PS have been reported and are called primary PS.[410] Heterotopic pancreatic tissue in the ampulla has occasionally been implicated in the development of PS.[411]

Pathologic changes of the papilla cover a wide spectrum, including edema with acute inflammatory cell infiltration, chronic inflammation with lymphocytes and plasma cell infiltration, hyperplasia of the tubular glands, adenomyosis, granulomatous inflammatory changes, and submucosal fibrosis.[410] Despite this wide spectrum, the changes correlate poorly with clinical disease. Acute inflammatory changes and distortions of glandular architecture may be found in normal persons older than 50 years of age.[412] Inflammation or fibrosis was found in 5% of biopsies from a control group of 31 patients without biliary tract disease in another report.[413]

The criteria for diagnosing PS have been controversial.[410,414] Several investigators defined stenosis at the papilla of Vater as a narrowing preventing easy passage of a No. 3 Bakes dilator from the CBD into the duodenum.[415,416] Other investigators, using the same size probe, have found a variable incidence of PS that range from 2.5% to 58%.[410] Instead of passing a 3-mm metallic dilator, Griffith recommended calibrating the papilla by passing a 10-F (3.3-mm) soft rubber urethral catheter.[414] PS is suspected if the catheter cannot be passed into the duodenum.

Current practice emphasizes nonoperative diagnosis. Cholescintigraphy can noninvasively diagnose stenosis, but it cannot differentiate organic from functional stenosis.[417] Provocative tests combining agents producing spasm of the sphincter (e.g., morphine) with drugs increasing biliary and pancreatic secretion (e.g., neostigmine, secretin) enjoyed early popularity.[410] A positive result reproduced the abdominal pain and elevated the serum aminotransferases, amylase, or lipase. The morphine-neostigmine (Nardi) test fell into disrepute because later studies showed no relation between a positive result and biliary or pancreatic disease.[410] Ultrasonography has been used in combination with agents that stimulate biliary or pancreatic secretion to measure changes in the size of the CBD and pancreatic duct.[418] Warshaw and associates found that the pancreatic duct dilated in response to secretin in 83% of 12 symptomatic patients surgically diagnosed with PS. Comparable dilatation occurred in 14% of 14 controls without suspected ampullary disease and in none of 10 patients with no stenosis at surgery.[418]

Other investigators have recommended ERCP to diagnose PS. An inability to cannulate the ampulla and pain during contrast injection were thought to indicate PS but are of no proven value because surgical findings correlated poorly.[410] Certain cholangiographic findings suggest PS narrowed distal (intraduodenal) CBD segment, dilated CBD or pancreatic duct, and delayed contrast drainage from the biliary (>45 minutes) or pancreatic ducts (>10 minutes). However, several factors influence the duration of opacification, including the gallbladder's presence, the patient's position, and concomitantly administered drugs. ERCP cannot be quantified.[410] The most useful diagnostic tool is ERCP with manometry.[410,419] The basal SOD pressure is elevated in patients with PS but not in patients with CBD stones or postcholecystectomy. The basal pancreatic duct sphincter pressure is elevated in both patients with CBD stones and those with PS.[419] However, elevated basal SOD pressure does not differentiate organically caused from functionally caused PS. Pharmacologic attempts to make this differentiation have met with some success. The sphincter normally relaxes with cholecystokinin, glucagon, glyceryl trinitrate and hyoscine butylbromide. Failure of sphincter relaxation suggests a fixed structural stenosis.[410]

Before ECP, surgery was the treatment of choice. Ten percent of ECPs attempted were performed to treat PS, with a success rate as high as 96%.[67,420] The complication and mortality rates after ECP are twofold higher in patients with PS (without CBD stones) than in patients with CBD stones.[67] The incidence of recurrent stenosis after ECP is 11.5%.[67]

Patients with PS and recurrent pancreatitis do not respond well to ECP or to classic transduodenal sphincterotomy, presumably because neither treatment transects the pancreatic sphincter.[410] Several investigators have recommended balloon dilatation of the pancreatic sphincter after ECP; long-term follow-up is not yet available to assess efficacy.[410]

Hemobilia

In 1654, Francis Glisson described hemorrhage through the biliary tract caused by a pathologic communication between bile ducts and blood vessels.[392] Sandblom first described it in the modern era (1948) and proposed the term *hemobilia*.[421] In 1972, Sandblom reviewed 550 patients in the world literature with symptomatic hemobilia.[422] The source of bleeding was within the liver in 50%, the gallbladder in 25% and the extrahepatic biliary tree, including the pancreas, in 25%.[422] Causes of hemobilia were traumatic in 50% and nontraumatic in 50% in the literature up to 1972. The traumatic causes included blunt and penetrating trauma of the liver and iatrogenic causes (e.g., liver biopsy, operative trauma). The nontraumatic causes included inflammatory conditions, such as parasites (28%), gallstones (10%), aneurysm (7%), and tumor (5%). Cases of spontaneous hemobilia have been reported in 1 patient with hemophilia and in 1 with cirrhosis that originated from within the liver.[423,424] In the Western world, trauma is much more common, but in Asia, where the prevalence of parasitic infestation of the biliary tract and recurrent pyogenic cholangiohepatitis is high, inflammatory causes are common.[392,422] Trauma is the cause of hemobilia in most young men, but gallstones are the most common cause in elderly women.[422]

Since Sandblom's classic review in 1972, the use of diagnostic and therapeutic invasive procedures involving the hepatobiliary tract have increased. A review of the literature then showed an increasing proportion of the cases of hemobilia being iatrogenic in origin.[425–427] The latest review of the world literature from 1981 to 1985 showed that 50% of cases were traumatic (i.e., 19% accidental and 41% iatrogenic), 10% were inflammatory, 9% were due to gallstones, 7% were due to tumors, and 15% were attributed to vascular lesions.[426] The differential diagnosis for these vascular lesions include aneurysmal disease of the hepatic artery or portal vein or vasculitis.[433] Most often, the vascular lesion is caused by hepatic artery aneurysm, which is most often a result of atherosclerosis, trauma, or infection.[427] Portal hypertension has traditionally been cited as a vascular cause of hemobilia, but only five cases of spontaneous hemobilia from the portal circulation have been reported, and all but one originated from extrahepatic sources.[424] Portal hypertension is more likely to be a predisposing factor for bleeding after trauma rather than a primary cause of hemobilia. Hemobilia from vascular sources tends to be massive and life threatening.

The iatrogenic causes of hemobilia include liver biopsy, PTC, percutaneous transhepatic biliary drainage (PTBD), endoprosthesis placement, operative trauma, and anticoagulant use.[425,434] The risk of hemobilia is 4% after PTC using an 18-gauge needle.[425] The risk is 3% to 14% with PTBD.[432,433] Bleeding dyscrasias, portal hypertension, and complete obstruction of the bile duct increase the risk further.[432,434]

Hemobilia can complicate endoprostheses and chemotherapeutic hepatic artery catheters. As many as 22% of patients in one series of hepatic artery catheter infusion of FUDR suffered hemobilia.[432] Hemobilia rarely complicates percutaneous liver biopsies and hepatobiliary surgery.[425]

The degree of hemorrhage varies widely. Profuse hemobilia is rare, but occult bleeding is more common, especially after an attack of biliary colic due to gallstones or choledocholithiasis.[435] The fate of blood in the biliary tract depends on the rate of bleeding and bile flow.[436] Sandblom and colleagues demonstrated in a model of the biliary tract that, when blood was injected rapidly, as in major hemorrhage, the blood mixes with the bile and forms mushy clots; when injected slowly, as in minor hemobilia, it does not mix but flows immiscibly into the bottom of the system where it forms a solid, pure clot, producing a cast of the lumen. These pure clots remain stable, but the mixed clots dissolve with a rapidity proportionate to their bile content.[436] Clot stability also reflects the rate of bile flow; dissolution is rapid with flowing bile because of increased exposure to the fibrinolytic capacity of the bile. However, when the clot is protected from bile flow, by diversion (e.g., T-tube drainage) or by total obstruction, the clot may remain unaltered for a long time. A similar situation occurs when the rate of a continuous hemorrhage exceeds that of fibrinolysis.[432] The passage of blood into the biliary tree is the result of two principal, often associated mechanisms: rupture of a dissecting central liver hematoma into the biliary tract or an arteriobiliary fistula with or without associated intrahepatic hematomas, false aneurysms, or arterioportal fistulas.[425]

The symptoms of hemobilia form a classic triad: gastrointestinal hemorrhage (90%) presenting with melena, hematochezia or hematemesis in equal frequency, biliary colic (70%), and jaundice (60%).[392,425] Hemobilia should be considered whenever gastrointestinal hemorrhage coexists with signs of biliary tract disorder.

The period between the initial lesion and the clinical expression of hemobilia may vary from several hours to years.[392,425] Hemobilia is detected a mean of 4 days after liver biopsy and 3 to 4 weeks after liver injuries and operative trauma.[425] However, more than 1 year may pass between trauma and the onset of hemobilia.[392] After hemobilia starts, it tends to recur periodically in attacks.[392,425] Bile and its fibrinolytic activity causes this slow "healing."[392,436]

After hemobilia is suspected, upper gastrointestinal endoscopy should be performed to exclude other causes of bleeding. Occasionally, blood comes from the ampulla.[425,434] Ultrasound or CT scans are needed to look for intrahepatic fluid collections and to evaluate pancreatic causes.[425,434] Arteriography provides diagnostic and topographic data and often therapeutic options.[425]

Bleeding may cease spontaneously (e.g., after a percutaneous catheter is removed, after liver biopsy), but this is unusual.[425] Treatment options include partial hepatectomy, hepatic arterial ligation, or selective arteriographic embolization.[425,428,429] The review by Curet and colleagues included 25 patients treated by embolization and 3 others treated by other endovascular methods; 24 patients had satisfactory results.[425] Two patients died of hepatic insufficiency 72 hours after embolization. The researchers recommended embolization as the preferred therapy, but hepatectomy is necessary for those with associated hepatic devitalization.[425] Most investigators now feel that angiographic embolization is the preferred treatment for hemobilia originating from intrahepatic sites, with success rates above 95% for controlling bleeding.[427-431,433] In the instances of hemobilia originating from extrahepatic sites, surgical therapy is preferred.[427,433] In emergent cases of massive hemobilia where surgery might carry high risk of mortality and morbidity, angiographic embolization should be considered first.[429] Surgery is considered if there are no facilities for embolization, embolization fails to control the bleeding, or there is associated hepatic devitalization. The mortality rate ranges from 10 to 20%.[427,434] The prognosis for full recovery is excellent after successful treatment.[434]

BILIARY FISTULA

Fistulous connections can occur between the biliary tract and various structures, including the enteric tract, bronchial tree, skin and blood vessels. They can develop as a complication of chronic cholelithiasis (i.e., biliary enteric fistula) or infection such as liver abscess or hydatid disease (i.e., bronchobiliary, biliary cutaneous, bilioportal fistulas). They can also result from abdominal or operative trauma (i.e., biliary cutaneous fistulas).

Spontaneous Biliary Enteric Fistula

Spontaneous biliary-enteric fistula is seen in 0.5% to 5% of patients undergoing biliary tract surgery.[437,438] Spontaneous biliary enteric fistulas are produced by gallstones (90%), peptic ulcer disease (6%), and malignancy or trauma (4%).[438] The most common communication is cholecystoduodenal (61% to 77%), followed by cholecystocolonic (14% to 17%) and cholecystogastric (6%).[438,439] Fistulous communication between the CBD and the enteric tract as a result of gallstones is much more unusual. A patient with agenesis of the gallbladder with choledocholithiasis had a choledochocolonic fistula.[437] Even though most choledochoduodenal fistulas are caused by penetrating peptic ulcer, those located in the parapapillary area are more likely to be caused by stones. One study found 80 (96%) of 83 parapapillary choledochoduodenal fistulas were caused by stones.[440]

Biliary enteric fistulas have two distinct clinical manifestations: nonobstructive and obstructive.[438] Both are more common among women, with a female to male ratio of 2 to 3 : 1.[439] The average age is 60 years for the nonobstructive type and 68 years for the obstructive type.[438,439]

Symptoms are generally nonspecific in the nonobstructive type, and the diagnosis usually is made during cholecystectomy as an incidental finding on intraoperative cholangiogram.[438,439,441] Sequelae of these fistulas include ascending cholangitis if the colon is involved, weight loss, malabsorption, and rarely, bleeding.[438] The incidence of gallbladder carcinoma is 14% to 15% in patients with biliary enteric fistula, compared with 0.8% to 0.9% in other patients undergoing biliary tract surgery.[438,439]

Clinical manifestations of the obstructive type are those of mechanical bowel obstruction, acute and complete or recurrent and incomplete, lasting for weeks to months.[438] A history of previous biliary tract disease is less frequently found (20%–30%).[438,439] The gallstone usually must be larger than 2.5 cm in diameter to cause gallstone ileus.[438] The most common site for stone impaction is distal ileum (63%–85%), followed by jejunum (10%–26%) and rarely, the duodenum, colon, or rectum (5%).[438,439]

The most useful diagnostic tests are plain film of the abdomen and barium studies.[438,439] Air in the biliary tract, seen in 30% of biliary enteric fistula, is not diagnostic. One study found only 5 of 20 cases of pneumobilia had biliary enteric fistulas.[438-440] Reflux of contrast media into the biliary tree during a barium study of the bowel is most suggestive. Visualization of an ectopic radiopaque stone that varies in location is also diagnostic, but this was seen only in 3% of patients.[439]

The treatment for biliary enteric fistula is surgical. Gallstone ileus may recur in 10%, and treatment is indicated after the diagnosis.[438,439] The recommended treatment is cholecystectomy, excision of the fistula, CBD exploration, and operative cholangiography.[439] The mortality rate was high (10% to 20%) in the earlier surgical literature but decreased to 3% by the late 1970s.[354,357,439]

Biliary Fistula Due to Operative Trauma

Injury to the bile duct during cholecystectomy can result in bile duct strictures and fistulas. Approximately one third of these patients present early in the postoperative period with a cutaneous biliary fistula or an internal biliary-peritoneal fistula resulting in peritonitis or abscess.[442] Usually, the bile duct injury is not recognized during surgery. One study included 123 patients who developed biliary stricture after cholecystectomy; 12 (10%) also had cutaneous biliary fistulas.[442] Most of these patients required surgical repair. Some of these patients have been treated successfully by endoscopically placed nasobiliary tubes or endoprostheses to divert the bile drainage away from the fistulous tract.[443,444] Endoscopic embolization of external biliary fistula have been reported to work well in patients in whom the fistula had not closed after usual conservative treatment.[445]

Bronchobiliary Fistula

Most bronchobiliary fistulas are congenital or follow thoracoabdominal trauma.[446] The role of hepatic infection has also been emphasized. The incidence of bronchobiliary fistula was 4% of 453 cases of pyogenic liver abscess and 10.5% of 3608 cases of subphrenic abscesses.[446] Almost all patients presented with biloptysis (i.e., bile in the sputum) and other respiratory symptoms, and most also had cholangitis, jaundice, or sepsis.[446] Diagnosis can be made by fistulogram if an external tract is provided by ERCP or PTC; the diagnosis also can be made using cholescintigraphy.[447,448] Treatment is surgical.

Other Biliary Fistulas

Fistulous communication between the biliary tract and the vascular system is fortunately uncommon, but it can be catastrophic. Most commonly, it results from trauma, iatrogenic causes, or infection. Arterial and venous systems can be involved.[449,450] Clinical manifestations include hemobilia and even bile pulmonary embolism when the fistulous communication is between the biliary tree and the hepatic venous system.[451] Biliobiliary fistula (i.e., fistula between the accessory biliary tract, gallbladder and cystic duct, and the main biliary tract) rarely has developed as a complication of gallstones.[452] It can develop as a complication of Mirizzi's syndrome, in which a stone impacted in the cystic duct or neck of the gallbladder compresses and obstructs the common hepatic duct.[453,454] If untreated, the stone may eventually erode into the CBD and create a biliobiliary fistula. Awareness of this possibility is important, because a classic cholecystectomy in a patient with this fistula carries a high risk of injury to the right hepatic duct, the common hepatic duct, or the CBD.

BILIARY TRACT DISEASE ASSOCIATED WITH ACQUIRED IMMUNODEFICIENCY SYNDROME

Since the first recognition of the AIDS in 1981, most organ systems have been affected by the human immunodeficiency virus (HIV) itself or secondary opportunistic infections or neoplasms. Biliary tract disease associated with AIDS was first reported in 1983 with reports of human cryptosporidial infection of the bile ducts associated with biliary tract obstruction.[456,457] Since then, AIDS-associated cholangiopathy has been increasingly recognized, with pathology ranging from acalculous cholecystitis to papillary stenosis to sclerosing cholangitis.[284-287,456-466] More often than not, these lesions occur concomitantly.

Clinical Spectrum

A review by Cello of 40 patients with AIDS-associated cholangiopathy revealed that there are four different but related forms of HIV-associated cholangiopathy: papillary stenosis, sclerosing cholangitis, combined papillary stenosis with intrahepatic and extrahepatic sclerosing cholangitis, and long,

extrahepatic bile duct strictures (>1–2 cm) in patients without other potential causes for strictures.[458] The combination of papillary stenosis and sclerosing cholangitis has been found in more than one half of these patients, and the remaining forms are less frequently encountered.

The mean age of patients with AIDS-associated cholangiopathy was 36 years, and they had the diagnosis of AIDS for ~1 year.[458] Clinically, these patients usually present with right upper quadrant or epigastric abdominal pain (84% to 88%), fever (65%), and evidence of cholestasis (80%, mostly elevated alkaline phosphatase level in the 700 IU/L range). Usually, the serum bilirubin is normal or only minimally elevated.[458-466] However, these features did not differentiate patients who subsequently were confirmed to have cholangiopathy from those who did not on ERCP.[458] The only features that differentiated these two groups of patients with identical clinical presentation were abnormal ultrasound and CT findings, namely dilated intrahepatic or extrahepatic bile ducts.[458] This point is important in the diagnosis of AIDS-associated cholangiopathy. Among patients confirmed to have abnormal bile ducts on ERCP, 28 of 38 also had abnormal ultrasound, and 12 of 17 had abnormal CT scans; among patients found to have normal bile ducts on ERCP, only 1 of 10 and none of 9 had abnormal ultrasound and CT examinations, respectively.[458]

Pathogenesis

The pathogenesis of AIDS-associated cholangiopathy is unclear. Most investigators favor "infectious" causes due to opportunistic agents such as CMV, *Cryptosporidium,* and even HIV.[458,463,464] Evidence suggests that the sclerosing cholangitis seen in AIDS has a different pathogenesis from that seen in association with ulcerative colitis. In PSC associated with ulcerative colitis, the inflammatory cell infiltrates surrounding the diseased bile ducts are rich in T4 lymphocytes, the subpopulation specifically depleted in AIDS patients.[285]

CMV infection is commonly associated with HIV infection. More than 90% of patients with AIDS have evidence of CMV in autopsy series, and 50% or more have CMV viremia.[464] Among AIDS patients with evidence of extrahepatic CMV infection at autopsy, 5% to 44% also have hepatic CMV inclusions.[464] In a review of AIDS patients with CMV, patients with CMV end-organ disease (e.g., retinitis, colitis, esophagitis, gastritis) or those with CMV viremia were much more likely to develop cholestatic liver enzyme abnormalities than those without (33% versus 11%).[464] About one third of these patients with cholestatic liver enzyme abnormalities were confirmed to have abnormal bile ducts. In addition to the association of severe CMV infection with AIDS-associated cholangiopathy, CMV has been identified in gallbladder epithelium and the ampulla of Vater further supporting its etiologic role. However, ganciclovir therapy did not alter the course of cholangiopathy in patients treated for CMV, although the biliary drug level may have been insufficient.[464] Clearly, until effective therapy is available to eradicate CMV in the biliary tract, a pathogenic causal relationship is difficult to prove.

Similar to CMV, *Cryptosporidium* is also common among AIDS patients and has been suggested to play an etiologic role in AIDS-associated cholangiopathy. A retrospective study by Teixidor and associates found 13 well-documented cases of biliary cryptosporidiosis. *Cryptosporidium* was found on histologic examination of the biliary system in the absence of concomitant CMV in most these patients.[463] The presence of *Cryptosporidium* organisms in the biliary system was always associated with histologic evidence of moderate to severe inflammatory changes. Some of these patients were found to have papillary stenosis with bile duct dilatation. The basic problem of proving causal relationship is the same as with CMV, namely, lack of effective therapy.

The argument against an infectious cause had been that as many as 50% of patients with AIDS-associated cholangiopathy did not have identifiable opportunistic agents.[458,466-468] Another intestinal microsporidia, *Enterocytozoon bieneusi*, which has been implicated in as many as 30% of cases of unexplained diarrhea in AIDS patients, was also identified in patients with AIDS-associated cholangiopathy.[466-468] The role of *E bieneusi* in AIDS-associated cholangiopathy was evaluated in a prospective study of 8 patients who were referred for evaluation of unexplained AIDS-associated cholangiopathy.[468] All 8 were found to have biliary microsporidiosis. Intraepithelial plasmodia and spores of *E bieneusi* were found in 1 patient. The importance of finding intraepithelial presence of the parasite is in confirming its invasive nature. Empirical antiprotozoal chemotherapy with metronidazole had no clinical benefit with respect to cholestasis, in contrast to its efficacy in microsporidiosis of the small intestine.

Besides these infectious agents, neoplastic lesions have also been documented in the biliary tract of AIDS patients and could account for some cases of AIDS-associated cholangiopathy. Both lymphoma and Kaposi's sarcoma have been implicated.[458]

Although there is a strong association of opportunistic infectious agents with AIDS-associated cholangiopathy, the exact pathogenesis may be multifactorial. The role of immunosuppression, HIV itself, and genetic predisposition remain to be better defined.

Diagnosis

Clinical presentation alone is not sufficient to diagnose AIDS-associated cholangiopathy. In AIDS patients who present with abdominal pain, fever, and cholestasis, ultrasonography or CT examinations should be obtained.[458,465,469-471] These examinations provide information on whether the bile ducts are dilated and on the liver parenchyma and adjacent pancreas. If bile ducts are dilated, ERCP is recommended for cholangiographic diagnosis, histologic and culture examination, and therapeutic options. The cholangiographic appearance of AIDS-associated cholangiopathy differ from that of PSC. In AIDS-associated cholangiopathy, the mucosal pattern is often beaded, suggesting intramural submucosal infiltration and edema.[458] The left ductal system is disproportionately more severely involved with intrahepatic ducts having irregular sacculations often containing probable intraductal debris or shredded sloughed mucosa. The ducts are markedly irregular, and there is a pruning of the smaller intrahepatic bile ducts. The CBD is often irregularly strictured and rarely exceeds 4 to 5 mm in diameter. In contrast, in PSC, the entire CBD tends to be involved and there is usually no "beading." There are rare dilated segments, no intraductal debris, but an associated paucity of intrahepatic bile ducts. The combination of sclerosing cholangitis and papillary stenosis affects more than 50% of patients with AIDS-associated cholangiopathy.

Treatment

Patients that present with abdominal pain and documented papillary stenosis should undergo ECP. In the review by Cello, these patients benefited from ECP in terms of improvement in pain scores.[458] However, there was no substantial change in serum alkaline phosphatase, bilirubin, or transaminase levels. This may not be surprising because these laboratory abnormalities also existed in patients without cholangiopathy. In a few patients who underwent repeat ERCP evaluation after sphincterotomy, progressive intrahepatic sclerosing cholangitis has been observed.[458] Other than sphincterotomy, there have been a few attempts with balloon dilatation or stent placement. The long-term results are unknown. If Kaposi's sarcoma or lymphoma is found on biopsy of the biliary tract, then appropriate chemotherapy should be considered. In light of the strong association of AIDS-associated cholangiopathy with CMV, cryptosporidiosis, and microsporidiosis, the hope is that the cholangiopathy might respond to effective chemotherapeutic agents against these infections.

The reader is directed to Chapter 11, Motility of the Biliary Tree; Chapter 41, Approach to the Patient With Jaundice; Chapter 42, Approach to the Patient With Abnormal Liver Chemistries; Chapter 96, Gallstones; Chapter 99, Postcholecystectomy Syndrome; Chapter 117, Endoscopic Retrograde Cholangiopancreatography, Endoscopic Sphincterotomy and Stone Removal, and Endoscopic Biliary and Pancreatic Drainage; Chapter 121, Ultrasonography; Chapter 123, Applications of Computed Tomography to the Gastrointestinal Tract; and Chapter 128, Interventional Radiology.

REFERENCES

1. DenBesten L, Doty JE. Pathogenesis and management of choleolithiasis. Surg Clin North Am 1981;61:893.
2. Tompkins RK, Doty JE. Modern management of biliary tract stone disease. Adv Surg 1987;20:279.
3. Dayton MT, Contor R, Tompkins RK. Incidence of complications with operative choledochoscopy. Am J Surg 1984;147:139.
4. Berhoft RA, Pellegrini CA, Motson RW, et al. Composition and morpholopic and clinical features of common duct stones. Am J Surg 1984;148:77.
5. Whiting MJ, Watts JM. Chemical composition of common bile duct stones. Br J Surg 1986;73:229.
6. Madden JL. Common duct stones: their origin and surgical management. Surg Clin North Am 1973;53:1095.
7. Gerwig WH, Countryman LK, Gomez AC. Congenital absence of the gallbladder and cystic duct. Ann Surg 1961;153:113.
8. Imamoglu K, Perry JF, Wangesteen OH. Experimental production of gallstones by incomplete stricture of the terminal common bile duct. Surgery 1957;42:623.
9. Aschoff L. Lectures in pathology. New York: Paul B Hoeber, 1924.

10. Saharia PC, Zuidema GD, Cameron JL. Primary common duct stones. Ann Surg 1977;185:598.

11. Glenn F. Post cholecystectomy choledocholithiasis. Surg Gynecol Obstet 1972;134:249.

12. Tabata M, Nakayama F. Bacteria and gallstones. Etiological significance. Dig Dis Sci 1981;26:218.

13. Ostrow JD, Murphy NM. Isolation and properties of conjugated bilirubin from bile. Biochem J 1970;120:311.

14. Goodhart GL, Levison ME, Trotman BW, et al. Pigment vs cholesterol cholelithiasis. Bacteriology of gallbladder stones, bile and tissue correlation with biliary lipid analysis. Am J Dig Dis 1978;23:877.

15. Lygidakis NJ. Incidence and significance of primary stones of the common bile duct in choledocholithiasis. Surg Gynecol Obstet 1983;157:434.

16. Lygidakis NJ. Incidence of bile infection in patients with choledocholithiasis. Am J Gastroenterol 1982;77:12.

17. Cetta F. The role of bacteria in pigment gallstone disease. Ann Surg 1991;213:315.

18. Kaufman HS, Magnuson TH, Lillemoe KD, et al. The role of bacteria in gallbladder and common duct stone formation. Ann Surg 1989;209:584.

19. Schulman A. Non-western patterns of biliary stones and the role of ascariasis. Radiology 1987;162:425.

20. Matsushiro T, Suzuki N, Sato T, et al. Effects of diet on glucaric acid concentration in bile and the formation of calcium bilirubinate gallstones. Gastroenterology 1977;72:630.

21. Matsushiro T. Identification of glucaro-1,4-lactone in bile as an essential factor in inhibitory effect of bile upon bacterial B-glucuronidase activity. Tohoku J Exp Med 1965;85:330.

22. Matsushiro T. Effects of known constituents of bile on the activity of bacterial B-glucuronidase. Tohoku J Exp Med 1965;85:210.

23. Blumenthal HJ, Fish DC. Bacterial conversion of D-glucarate to glycerate and pyruvate. Biochem Biophys Res Commun 1963;11:239.

24. Nagase M, Hikasa Y, Soloway RD, et al. Gallstones in western Japan. Factors affecting the prevalence of intrahepatic gallstones. Gastroenterology 1980;78:684.

25. Wosiewitz V. Schenk J, Sabinski F, et al. Investigations on common bile duct stones. Digestion 1983;26:43.

26. Lotveit T. Duodenal diverticula and gallstone disease. J Oslo City Hosp 1982;32:67.

27. Lotveit T, Osnes M, Larsen S. Recurrent biliary calculi. Duodenal diverticula as a predisposing factor. Ann Surg 1982;196:30.

28. Kennedy RH, Thompson MH. Are duodenal diverticula associated with choledocholithiasis? Gut 1988;29:1003.

29. Bornman PC, Kottler RE, Terblanche J, et al. Does low entry of cystic duct predispose to stones in the common bile duct? Br Med J 1988;297:31.

30. Toouli J, Geenen JE, Hogan WJ, et al. Sphincter of oddi motor activity: a comparison between patients with common bile duct stones and controls. Gastroenterology 1982;82:111.

31. Ohta T, Nagakawa T, Takeda T, et al. Histological evaluation of the intrahepatic biliary tree in intrahepatic cholesterol stones, including immunohistochemical staining against apolipoprotein A1. Hepatology 1993;17:531.

32. Way LW. Retained common duct stones. Surg Clin North Am 1973;53:1139.

33. Millbourn E. Klinische studien uber die choledocholithiasis. Acta Chir Scand 1941;86(suppl 65).

34. Rubin JR, Beal JM. Diagnosis of choledocholithiasis. Surg Gynecol Obstet 1983;156:16.

35. Acosta JM, Ledsesma CL. Gallstone migration as a cause of acute pancreatitis. N Engl J Med 1974;290:484.

36. Kelly TR. Gallstone pancreatitis: pathophysiology. Surgery 1976;80:488.

37. Dworken HJ. Recent experience with spontaneously disappearing gallstones. Gastroenterology 1960;38:76.

38. Opie EL. The etiology of acute hemorrhagic pancreatitis. Bull Johns Hopkins Hosp 1901;12:182.

39. Kelly TR. Gallstone pancreatitis. Arch Surg 1974;109:294.

40. Saik RP, Greenberg AG, Farris JM, et al. Spectrum of cholangitis. Am J Surg 1975;130:143.

41. Anciaux ML, Pelletier G, Attali P, et al. Prospective study clinical and biochemical features of symptomatic choledocholithiasis. Dig Dis Sci 1986;31:449.

42. Boey JH, Way LW. Acute cholangitis. Ann Surg 1980;191:264.

43. Lindenauer SM, Child CG III. Disturbances of liver function in biliary tract disease. Surg Gynecol Obstet 1966;123:1205.

44. Heiss, FW, Rossi RL, Scholz FJ, et al. Common bile duct calculi 1. Surgical therapy. Postgrad Med 1984;75:88.

45. Pelligrini CA, Thomas MJ, Way LW. Bilirubin and alkaline phosphatase valves before and after surgery for bilirubin obstruction. Am J Surg 1982;143:67.

46. McSherry CK, Glenn F. The incidence and causes of death following surgery for nonmalignant biliary tract disease. Ann Surg 1980;191:271.

47. Zimmon DS. The management of common duct stones. Adv Intern Med 1986;31:379.

48. Reiss R, Deutsch AA, Nudelman I, et al. Statistical value of various clinical parameters in predicting the presence of choledochal stones. Surg Gynecol Obstet 1984;159:273.

49. Coelho JCU, Buffara M, Pozzobon CE, et al. Incidence of common bile duct stones in patients with acute and chronic cholecystitis. Surg Gynecol Obstet 1984;158:76.

50. Stryker SJ, Beal JM. Acute cholecystitis and common-duct calculi. Arch Surg 1983;118:1063.

51. Frazee RC, van Heerden JA. Cholecystectomy with concomitant exploration of the common bile duct. Surg Gynecol Obstet 1989;168:513.

52. Way LW, Admirand WH, Dunphy JE. Management of choledocholithiasis. Ann Surg 1972;176:347.

53. Cronan JJ, Mueller PR, et al. Prospective diagnosis of choledocholithiasis. Radiology 1983;146:467.

54. Baron RL. Common bile duct stones: reassessment of criteria for CT diagnosis. Radiology 1987;162:419.

55. Niederau C, Sonnenberg A, Mueller J. Comparison of the extrahepatic bile duct size measured by ultrasound and by different radiographic methods. Gastroenterology 1984;87:615.

56. Goodman MW, Ansel HJ, Vennes JA, et al. Is intravenous cholangiography still useful? Gastroenterology 1980;79:642.

57. Mitchell SE, Clark RA. A comparison of computed tomography and sonography in choledocholithiasis. AJR Am J Roentgenol 1984;142:729.

58. Gross BH, Harter LP, Gore RM, et al. Ultrasonic evaluation of common bile duct stones: prospective comparison with endoscopic retrograde cholangiography. Radiology 1983;146:471.

59. Johnson AG, Hosking SW. Appraisal of the management of bile duct stones. Br J Surg 1987;74:555.

60. Gadacz TR. Reoperation versus alternatives in retained biliary calculi. Surg Clin North Am 1991;71:93.

61. Marizzi PL. Cholangiographic durante les operaciones de las vias biliares. Bol Trab Soc Cir Buenos Aires 1932;16:1133.

62. Rattner DW, Warshaw AL. Impact of choledochoscopy on the management of choledocholithiasis. Experience with 499 common duct explorations at the Massachussetts General Hospital. Ann Surg 1981;194:76.

63. King ML, String ST. Extent of choledochoscopic utilization in common bile duct exploration. Am J Surg 1983;146:322.

64. White TT, Bordley J. One percent incidence of recurrent gallstones six to eight years after manometric cholangiography. Ann Surg 1978;188:562.

65. Pitt HA, Cameron JL, Postier RG, et al. Factors affecting mortality in biliary tract surgery. Am J Surg 1981;141:66.

66. Pitt HA, Gomes AS, Lois JF, et al. Does percutaneous biliary drainage reduce operative risk or increase hospital cost? Ann Surg 1985;201:545.

67. McPherson GAD, Benjamin IS, Hodgson HJF, et al. Pre-operative percutaneous transhepatic biliary drainage: the results of a controlled trial. Br J Surg 1984;71:371.

68. Classen M. Endoscopic papillotomy—new indications, short and long term results. Clin Gastroenterol 1986;15:457.

69. Leuschner U. Endoscopic therapy of biliary calculi. Clin Gastroenterol 1986;15:333.

70. Allen B, Shapiro H, Way LW. Management of recurrent and residual common duct stones. Am J Surg 1981;142:41.

71. Cotton PB, Vallon AG, Duodenoscopic sphincterotomy for removal of bile duct stones in patients with gallbladders. Surgery 1982;91:628.

72. Tanaka M, Ikeda S, Yoshimoto H, et al. The long-term fate of the gallbladder after endoscopic sphincterotomy. Am J Surg 1987;154:505.

73. Neoptolemos JP, Carr-Locke DL, Fossard DP. Prospective randomized study of preoperative endoscopic sphincterotomy versus surgery alone for common bile duct stones. Br Med J 1987;294:470.

74. Sherman S, Hawes RH, Lehman GA. Management of bile duct stones. Semin Liver Dis 1990;10:205.

75. Surick BG, Ghazi A. Endoscopic papillotomy while the gallbladder is in situ. Am Surg 1992;58:657.

76. Leung JWC, Sung JJY, Chung SCS, et al. Urgent endoscopic drainage for acute suppurative cholangitis. Lancet 1989;1:1307.

77. Sievert W, Vakil NB. Emergencies of the biliary tract. Gastroenterol Clin North Am 1989;17:245.

78. Lai ECS, Mok FPT, Tan ESY, et al. Endoscopic biliary drainage for severe acute cholangitis. N Engl J Med 1992;326:1582.

79. Neoptolemos JP, London NJ, Carr-Locke DL, et al. Controlled trial of urgent endoscopic retrograde cholangiopancreatography and endoscopic sphincterotomy versus conservative treatment for acute pancreatitis due to gallstones. Lancet 1988;2:979.

80. Stiegmann GV, Goff JS, Mansour A, et al. Precholecystectomy endoscopic cholangiography and stone removal is not superior to cholecystectomy, cholangiography, and common duct exploration. Am J Surg 1992;163:227.

81. Neoptolemos JP, Shaw DE, Carr-Locke DL. A multivariate analysis of preoperative risk factors in patients with common bile duct stones. Ann Surg 1989;209:157.

82. The Southern Surgeons Club. A prospective analysis of 1518 laparoscopic cholecystectomies. N Engl J Med 1991;324:1073.

83. Soper NJ, Stockmann PT, Dunnegan DL, et al. Laparoscopic cholecystectomy. The new "gold standard"? Arch Surg 1992;127:917.

84. McEntee G, Grace PA, Bouchier-Hayes D. Laparoscopic cholecystectomy and the common bile duct. Br J Surg 1991;78:385.

85. Hunter JG, Soper NJ. Laparoscopic management of bile duct stones. Surg Clin North Am 1992;72:1077.

86. Tandon RK, Nijhawan S, Arora A. Management of retained common bile duct stones in patients with T-tube in situ: role of endoscopic sphincterotomy. Am J Gastroenterol 1990;85:1126.

87. Nussinson E, Cairns SR, Vaira D, et al. A 10 year single centre experience of percutaneous and endoscopic extraction of bile duct stones with a T-tube in situ. Gut 1991;32:1040.

88. Janssen D, Bommarito A, Lathrop J. A new technique for the rapid dissolution of retained ductal gallstone with monoctanoin in T-tube patients. Am Surg 1992;58:141.

89. Joseph LG, Birkett DH. Laser lithotripsy for the management of retained stones. Arch Surg 1992;127:603.

90. Jakimowicz JJ. Mak B, Carol EJ, et al. Post-operative choledochoscopy. A five year experience. Arch Surg 1983;118:810.

91. Clouse ME, Stokes KR, Lee RGL, et al. Bile duct stones: percutaneous transhepatic removal. Radiology 1986;160:525.

92. Burhenne HJ. Percutaneous extraction of retained biliary tract stones: 661 patients. AJR Am J Roentgenol 1980;134:888.

93. Salvioli H, Salati R, Lugli R, et al. Medical treatment of biliary duct stones: effect of ursodeoxycholic acid administration. Gut 1983;24:609.

94. Girard R, Legros G. Retained and recurrent bile duct stones. Surgical or nonsurgical removal? Ann Surg 1981;193:150.

95. Sharp KW, Gadacz TR. Selection of patients for dissolution of retained common duct stones with mono-octanoin. Ann Surg 1982;196:137.

96. Palmer KR, Hofman AF. Intraductal mono-octanoin for the direct dissolution of bile duct stones: experience in 343 patients. Gut 1986;27:196.

97. Thistle JL, May GR, Bender CE, et al. Dissolution of cholesterol gallbladder stones by methyl tert-butyl ether administererd by percutaneous transhepatic catheter. N Engl J Med 1989;320:633.

98. Brandon JC, Teplick SK, Haskin PH, et al. Common bile duct calculi: updated experience with dissolution with methyl tertiary butyl ether (MTBE). Radiology 1988;166:665.

99. Murray WR, Laferia G, Fullarton GM. Choledocholithiasis in vivo stone dissolution using methyl tertiary butyl ether (MTBE) Gut 1988;29:143.

100. Neoptolemos JP, Hall C, Murray WR, et al. How good is methyl tert-butyl ether (MTBE) for common bile duct (CBD) stone dissolution? Gut 1989;30:A736 (abstract).

101. Kaye GL, Summerfield JA, McIntyre N, et al. Methyl tert butyl ether dissolution therapy for common bile duct stones. J Hepatol 1990;10:337.

102. Paumgartner G. Fragmentation of gallstones by extracorporeal shock waves. Semin Liver Dis 1987;7:317.

103. Sauerbruch T, Stern M. Fragmentation of bile duct stones by extracorporeal shock waves. Gastroenterology 1989;96:146.

104. Staritz M, Rambow A, Grosse A, et al. Electromagnetically generated extracorporeal shockwaves for fragmentation of extra- and intrahepatic bile duct stones: indications, success and problems during a 15 months clinical experience. Gut 1990;31:222.

105. Weber J, Esser M, Riemann JF. Successful piezoelectric lithotripsy of a common duct stone. Endoscopy 1989;21:145.

106. Mo LR, Hwang MH, Yueh SK, et al. Percutaneous transhepatic choledochoscopic electrohydraulic lithotripsy (PTCS-EHL) of common bile duct stones. Gastrointest Endosc 1988;34:122.

107. Kozarek RA, Low DE, Ball TJ. Tunable dye laser lithotripsy: in vitro studies and in vivo treatment of choledocholithiasis. Gastrointest Endosc 1988;34:418.

108. Peters R, Macmathuna P, Lombard M, et al. Management of common bile duct stones with a biliary endoprosthesis. Report on 40 cases. Gut 1992;33:1412.

109. Rufanov IG. Liver stones. Ann Surg 1936;103:321.

110. Wen CC. Lee HC. Intrahepatic stones. A clinical study. Ann Surg 1972;175:166.

111. Lindstrom CG. Frequency of gallstone disease in a well-defined Swedish population. A prospective necropsy study in Malmo. Scand J Gastroenterol 1977;12:341.

112. Simi M, Loriga P, Basoli A, et al. Intrahepatic lithiasis. Study of thirty-six cases and review of the literature. Am J Surg 1979;137:317.

113. Fagarasanu I. La lithiase intrahepatique. J Chir 1973;105:59.

114. Grassi G. La litiasi intraepatica. Atti accad Lancisiana 1973;17:276.

115. Nakayama F. Soloway RD, Nakama T, et al. Hepatolithiasis in East Asia. Retrospective study. Dig Dis Sci 1986;31:21.

116. Digby KH. Common duct stones of liver origin. Br J Surg 1930;17:578.

117. Yellin AE, Donovan AJ. Biliary lithiasis and helminthiasis. Am J Surg 1981;142:128.

118. Turner WW, Cramer CR. Rercurrent Oriental cholangiohepatitis. Surgery 1983;93:397.

119. Carmona RH, Crass RA, Lim RC Jr, et al. Oriental Cholangitis. Am J Surg 1984;148:117.

120. Kerlan RK Jr, Pogany AC, Goldberg HI, et al. Radiologic intervention in Oriental cholangiohepatitis. AJR Am J Roentgenol 1985;145:809.

121. Van Sonnenberg E, Casola G, Cubberley DA, et al. Oriental cholangiohepatitis: diagnostic imaging and interventional management. AJR Am J Roentgenol 1986;146:327.

122. Stock FE, Fung JHY. Oriental cholangiohepatitis. Surgery 1962;84:409.

123. Lam SK, Wong KP, Chan PKW, et al. Recurrent pyogenic cholangitis: a study by endoscopic retrograde cholangiography. Gastroenterology 1978;74:1196.

124. Seel DJ, Park YK. Oriental infestational cholangitis. Am J Surg 1983;146:366.

125. Chen HH, Zhang WH, Wang SS. Twenty-two year experience with the diagnosis and treatment of intrahepatic calculi. Surg Gynecol Obstet 1984;159:519.

126. Choi TK, Ong GB. The surgical management of primary intrahepatic stones. Br J Surg 1982;69:86.

127. Sato T, Suzuki N, Takahashi W, et al. Surgical management of intrahepatic gallstones. Ann Surg 1980;192:28.

128. Choi TK, Fok M, Lee M Jr, et al. Postoperative flexible choledochoscopy for residual primary intrahepatic stones. Ann Surg 1986;203:260.

129. Khuroo MS, Zargar SA. Biliary ascariasis. A common cause of biliary and pancreatic disease in an endemic area. Gastroenterology 1985;88:418.

130. Louw JH. Abdominal complications of ascariasis. Surgical Rounds 1981;April:54.

131. Nagase M, Tanimura H, Takenaka M, et al. Trreatment of intrahepatic gallstones. Arch Jpn Chir 1978;47:467.

132. Hwang MH, Yang JC, Lee SA. Choledochofiberoscopy in the post operative management of intrahepatic stones. Am J Surg 1980;139:860.

133. Lam SK. A Study of endoscopic sphincterotomy in recurrent pyogenic cholangitis. Br J Surg 1984;71:262.

134. Leuschner U, Baumgartel H. Chemical dissolution of common bile duct stones in intrahepatic calculi. In: Okuda K, Nakayama F, Wong J, eds. Biological research. New York: Alan R Liss, 1984:193.

135. Vatero A. Dissertation in Auguralis medica proes. Diss qua scirrhris viscerum disseret c.s. exlerus. (University Library, Edinburgh). 1723;70:19.

136. Douglas AH. Case of dilatation of the common bile duct. Monthly J Med Sc (London) 1852;14:97.

137. Laverson RS. Cysts of the common bile duct. Am J Med Sci 1909;137:563.

138. Tsardakas E, Robnett AH. Congenital cystic dilatation of the common bile duct; report of 3 cases, analysis of 57 cases and review of the literature. Arch Surg 1956;72:311.

139. Alonso-Lej F, Rever W Jr, Pessagno DJ. Congenital choledochal cyst, with a report of 2 and an analysis of 94 cases. Int Abstr Surg 1959;108:1.

140. Flanigan DP. Biliary cysts. Ann Surg 1975;182:635.

141. Yamaguchi M. Congenital choledochal cyst. Analysis of 1,433 patients in the Japanese literature. Am J Surg 1980;140:653.

142. Tan KC, Howard ER. Choledochal cyst: a 14 year surgical experience with 36 patients. Br J Surg 1988;75:892.

143. Ryckman FC, Noseworthy J. Neonatal cholestatic conditions requiring surgical reconstruction. Semin Liver Dis 1987;7:134.

144. Crittenden SL, McKinley MJ. Choledochal cyst-clinical features and classification. Am J Gastroenterol 1985;80:643.

145. Kimura K, Tsugawa C, Ogawa K, et al. Choledochal cyst. Etiological considerations and surgical management in 22 cases. Arch Surg 1978;113:159.

146. Hays DM, Goodman GN, Snyder WH, et al. Congenital cyctic dilation of the common bile duct. Arch Surg 1969;98:457.

147. Jones PG, Smith ED, Clarke M, et al. Choledochal cysts: experience with radical excision. J Pediatr Surg 1971;6:112.

148. Todani T, Watanabe Y, Narusue M, et al. Congenital bile duct cysts. Classification, operative procedures, and review of 37 cases including cancer arising from choledochal cysts. Am J Surg 1977;134:263.

149. Olbourne NA, Choledochal cysts—a review of the cystic anomalies of the biliary tree. Ann R Coll Surg Engl 1975;56:26.

150. Sarris GE, Tsang D. Choledochocele: case report, literature review, and a proposed classification. Surgery 1989;105:408.

151. Thambi Dorai CR, Visvanathan R, McAll GLG. Type IVa choledochal cysts: surgical management and literature review. Aust N Z J Surg 1991;61:505.

152. Serena SAF, Linares ES, Goepfert RH. Cystic dilatation of the cystic duct: a new type of biliary cyst. Surgery 1991;109:320.

153. O'Neill JA, Templeton JM, Schnaufer L, et al, Recent experience with choledochal cyst. Ann Surg 1986;205:533.

154. O'Neill JA. Choledochal cyst. Curr Probl Surg 1992;29:371.

155. Orenstein SR, Whitington PF. Choledochal cyst resulting in congenital cirrhosis. Am J Dis Child 1982;136:1025.

156. Yotuyanagi S. Contribution to etiology and pathology of idiopathic cystic dilatation of the common bile duct, with a report of three cases. Gann (Tokyo) 1936;30:601.

157. Schroeder D, Smith L, Prain HC. Antenatal diagnosis of choledochal cyst at 15 weeks' gestation: etiologic implications and management. J Pediatr Surg 1989;24:936.

158. Babbitt DP. Congenital choledochal cyst: new etiologic concept based on anomalous relationships of common bile duct and pancreatic duct. Ann Radiol 1969;12:231.

159. Vanderpool D, Lane BW, Winter JW, et al. Choledochal cysts. Surg Gynecol Obstet 1988;167:447.

160. Kato T, Hebiguchi T, Matsuda K, et al. Action of pancreatic juice on the bile duct. Pathogenesis of congenital choledochal cyst. J Pediatr Surg 1981;16:146.

161. Lebenthal E, Lee PC. Development of functional response in human exocrine pancreas. Pediatrics 1980;66:556.

162. Taybi H. Roentgenology of the biliary tract in children. Alimentary tract roentgenology. Vol 2. St. Louis: CV Mosby, 1967:1099.

163. Ono J, Sakoda K, Akita M. Surgical aspects of cyctic dilatation of the bile duct. Ann Surg 1982;195:203.

164. Kimura K, Ohto M, Ono T, et al. Congenital cystic dilatation of the common bile duct. Relationship to anomalous pancreaticobiliary ductal union. AJR Am J Roentgenol 1977;128:571.

165. Jona J, Babbitt D, Starshak R, et al. Anatomic observations and etiologic and surgical considerations in choledochal cyst. J Pediatr Surg 1979;14:315.

166. Iwai N, Yanagihara J, Tokiwa K, et al. Congenital choledochal dilatation with emphasis on pathophysiology of the biliary tract. Ann Surg 1992;215:27.

167. Kato O, Hattori K, Suzuki T, et al. Clinical significance of anomalous pancreaticobiliary union. Gastrointest Endosc 1983;29:94.

168. Saito S, Ishida M. Congenital choledochal cyst (cystic dilatation of the common bile duct). Prog Pediatr Surg 1974;6:63.

169. Kato T, Asakura Y, Kasai M. An attempt to produce choledochal cyst in puppies. J Pediatr Surg 1974;9:509.

170. Miyano T, Suruga K, Chen SC. A clinicopathologic study of choledochal cyst. World J Surg 1980;4:231.

171. Spitz L. Experimental production of cystic dilatation of the common bile duct in neonatal lambs. J Pediatr Surg 1977;12:39.

172. Kim SH. Choledochal cyst: survey by the surgical section of the American Academy of Pediatrics. J Pediatr Surg 1981;16:402.

173. Kozloff L, Joseph WL. Cystic dilation of the common bile duct in adults. Med Ann DC 1973;42:595.

174. Ng WD, Chan YT, Fung H. Recurrent pancreatitis contributing to choledochal cyst formation. Br J Surg 1987;74:206.

175. Iwai N, Tokiwa K, Tsuto T, et al. Biliary manometry in choledochal cyst with abnormal choledocho pancreatico ductal junction. J Pediatr Surg 1986;21:873.

176. Ponce J, Garriques V, Sala T, et al. Endoscopic biliary manometry in patients with suspected sphincter of Oddi dysfunction and in patients with cystic dilatation of the bile ducts. Dig Dis Sci 1989;34:367.

177. Kusunoki M, Yamamura T, Takahashi T, et al. Choledochal cyst. Its possible autonomic involvement in the bile duct. Arch Surg 1987;122:997.

178. Nagorney DM, McIlrath DC, Adson MA. Choledochal cysts in adults: clinical management. Surgery 1984;96:656.

179. Muto Y, Uchimura M, Tsuchiya R. Cystic dilations of the bile ducts in the adult. Chir Gastroenterol 1978;12:65.

180. Rattner DW, Schapiro RH, Warshaw AL. Abnormalities of the pancreatic and biliary ducts in adult patients with choledochal cysts. Arch Surg 1983;118:1068.

181. Bass EM, Cremin BJ. Choledochal cysts: a clilnical and radiological evaluation of 21 cases. Pediatr Radiol 1976;5:81.

182. Kobayshi A, Ohbe Y. Choledochal cysts in infancy and childhood. Arch Dis Child 1977;52:121.

183. Joseph VT. Surgical techniques and long-term results in the treatment of choledochal cyst. J Pediatr Surg 1990;25:782.

184. Suruga K. Clinical and pathological study on choledochocyst. Jpn J Surg 1973;3:199.

185. Ramage AA, Tedesco FJ, Schuman BM. Asymptomatic choledochal cyst. Am J Gastroenterol 1985;80:816.

186. Lygidakis NJ. Cystic dilation of the common bile duct. Surg Gynecol Obstet 1985;160:115.

187. Altman MS, Halls JM, Douglas AP, et al. Choledochal cyst presenting as acute pancreatitis. Am J Gastroenterol 1978;70: 514.

188. Todani T, Urushihara N, Watanabe Y, et al. Pseudopancreatitis in choledochal cyst in children: intraoperative study of amylase levels in the serum. J Pediatr Surg 1990;25:303.

189. Voyles CR, Smadja C, Shands WC, et al. Carcinoma in choledochal cysts. Age-related incidence. Arch Surg 1983;118:986.

190. Kostiainen S, Paakkonen M, Merikoski Y. Diverticulum of the common bile duct. Acta Chir Scand 1983;149:531.

191. Coyle KA, Bradley III EL. Cholangiocarcinoma developing after simple excision of a Type II choledochal cyst. South Med J 1992;85:540.

192. Wheeler WI de C. An unusual case of obstruction to the common bile duct (choledochocele?) Br J Surg 1940;27:446.

193. De Lange E, Slutsky VS, Shaffer HA Jr, et al. Choledochocele: a rare form of choledochal cyst. South Med J 1988;81:265.

194. Kagiyama S, Okazaki K, Yamamoto Y, et al. Anatomic variants of choledochocele and manometric measurements of pressure in the cele and the orifice zone. Am J Gastroenterol 1987;82: 641.

195. Ramos A, Castello J, Pinto I. Intestinal intussusception as a presenting feature of choledochocele. Gastrointest Radiol 1990;15:211.

196. Ozawa K, Yamada T, Matumoto Y, et al. Carcinoma arising in a choledochocele. Cancer 1980;45:195.

197. Martin RF, Biber BP, Bosco JJ, et al. Symptomatic choledochoceles in adults. Endoscopic retrograde cholangiopancreatography recognition and management. Arch Surg 1992;127:536.

198. Cohen F. Bernstein JR. Choledochocele presenting with jaundice. Dig Dis Sci 1981;26:667.

199. Brunton FJ, Bamforth J. Intraluminal diverticulum of the duodenum and choledochocele. Gut 1972;13:207.

200. Greene FL, Brown JJ, Rubinstein P, et al. Choledochocele and recurrent pancreatitis. Diagnosis and surgical management. Am J Surg 1985;149:306.

201. Venu RP, Geenen JE, Hogan WJ, et al. Role of endoscopic retrograde cholangiopancreatography in the diagnosis and treatment of choledochocele. Gastroenterology 1984;87:1144.

202. Goldberg PB, Long WB, Oleaga JA, et al. Choledochocele as a cause of recurrent pancreatitis. Gastroenterology 1980;78: 1041.

203. Hart MJ, White TT. Choledochocele associated with acute hemorrhapic pancreatitis. West J Med 1980;133:340.

204. Jones B. Choledochocele demonstrated on percutaneous cholangiography: a patient with acute fulminant pancreatitis. Gastrointest Radiol 1977;2:145.

205. Scholz FJ, Carrera GF, Larsen CR. The coledochocele: correlation of radiological, clinical and pathologic findings. Radiology 1976;118:25.

206. Vachel HR, Stevens WM. Case of intrahepatic calculi. Br Med J 1906;1:434.

207. Caroli J, Soupalt R, Kossakowski J, et al. La dilatation polykystique congenitale des voies biliaires intrahepatiques. Essai del classification. Sem Hop Paris 1958;34:488.

208. Caroli J. Diseases of the intrahepatic biliary tree. Clin Gastroenterol 1973;2:147.

209. Dayton MT, Longmire WP, Tompkins RK. Caroli's disease: a premalignant condition? Am J Surg 1983;145:41.

210. Barros JL, Polo JR, Sanabia J, et al. Congenital cystic dilatation of the intrahepatic bile ducts (Caroli's disease): report of a case and review of the literature. Surgery 1979;85:589.

211. Tsuchida Y, Ishida M. Dilatation of the intrahepatic bile ducts in congenital cystic dilatation of the common bile duct. Surgery 1971;69:776.

212. Glenn F, McSherry CK. Congenital segmental cystic dilatation of the common bile ductal system. Ann Surg 1973;177:705.

213. Yue, PCK. Choledochal cyst: a review of 18 cases. Br J Surg 1974;61:896.

214. Kerr DNS, Harrison CV, Sherlock S, et al. Congenital hepatic fibrosis. Q J Med 1961;30:91.

215. Newman SL, Lindahl JA, Morse PA, et al. Caroli's disease: new diagnostic and therapeutic approaches. South Med J 1986;79: 1587.

216. Foulk WT. Congenital malformation of the intrahepatic biliary tree in the adult. Gastroenterology 1970;58:253.

217. Nagasue N. Successful treatment of Caroli's disease by hepatic resection. Report of six patients. Ann Surg 1984;200:718.

218. Mercadier M, Chigot JP, Clot JP, et al. Caroli's disease. World J Surg 1984;8:22.

219. Schrumpf E, Bergan A, Blomhoff JP, et al. Partial hepatectomy in Caroli's disease. Scand J Gastroenterol 1981;16:581.

220. Fleischer AC, Born ML, Kirchner SG, et al. Complementary use of ^{99m}Tc-HIDA and upper abdominal sonography in diagnosing a choledochal cyst. South Med J 1980;73:1651.

221. Glass IA, Buschi AJ, Brenbridge NA. Choledochal cyst: sonographic evaluation of an unusual case. South Med J 1980;73: 1391.

222. Morgan CL, Trought WS, Oddson TA, et al. Ultrasonography in the diagnosis of a type I choledochal cyst. South Med J 1980;73:1389.

223. Richardson JD, Grant EG, Barth KA, et al. Type II choledochal cyst: diagnosis using real-time sonography. J Ultrasound Med 1984;3:37.

224. Kangarloo H, Sarti DA, Sample WF, et al. Ultrasonographic spectrum of choledochal cysts in children. Pediatr Radiol 1980;9:15.

225. Marchal GJ, Desmet VJ, Proesmans WC, et al. Caroli's disease: high-frequency US and pathologic findings. Radiology 1986;158:507.

226. Howell CG, Templeton JM, Weiner S, et al. Antenatal diagnosis and early surgery for choledochal cyst. J Pediatr Surg 1983;18: 387.

227. Huang MJ, Liaw YF. Intravenous cholescintigraphy using Tc-99m labeled agents in the diagnosis of choledochal cyst. J Nucl Med 1982;23:113.

228. Moreno AJ, Parker AL, Spicer MJ, et al. Scintigraphic and radiographic findings in Caroli's disease. Am J Gastroenterol 1984;79:299.

229. Cabrera J, Quintero E, Bruguera M, et al. Diagnosis of Caroli's disease by technetium-99m DISIDA cholescintigraphy. Report of 3 cases. Clinical Nucl Med 1985;10:478.

230. DiPietro MA, Taylor KJW. Imaging of idiopathic biliary duct dilatation. J Clin Gastroenterol 1980;2:299.

231. Sty JR, Sullivan P, Wagner R, et al. Hepatic Scintigraphy in Caroli's disease. Radiology 1978;127:732.

232. Araki T, Itai Y, Tasaka A. CT of choledochal cyst. AJR 1980;135: 729.

233. Pollack M, Shirkhoda A, Charnsangavej C. Computed tomography of choledochocele. J Comput Assist Tomogr 1985;9: 360.

234. Ystgaard B, Myrvold HE, Nilsen G. Magnetic resonance imaging in preoperative assessment of choledochal cysts. Eur J Surg 1992;158:567.

235. Thatcher BS, Sivak MV Jr, Hermann RE, et al. ERCP in evaluation and diagnosis of choledochal cyst: report of 5 cases. Gastrointest Endosc 1986;32:27.

236. Shemesh E, Czerniak A, Klein E, et al. The role of endoscopic retrograde cholangiopancreatogrphy in the diagnosis and treatment of adult choledochal cyst. Surg Gynecol Obstet 1988;167: 423.

237. Zimmon DS, Falkenstein DB, Manno BV, et al. Choledochocele: radiologic diagnosis and endoscopic management. Gastrointest Radiol 1978;3:349.

238. Shammaa MH, Najjar FB, Rizk AGK. Congenital cystic dilatation of the intrahepatic biliary ducts (Caroli's disease). Transhepatic cholangiography and ultrasonic diagnosis. Hepato-gastroenterol 1982;29:15.

239. Missavage AE, Sugawa C. Caroli's disease: role of endoscopic retrograde cholangiography. Am J Gastroenterol 1983;78:815.

240. Attar S, Obeid S. Congenital cyst of the common bile duct-review of the literature and a report of 2 cases. Ann Surg 1955;142:289.

241. Takiff H, Stone M, Fonkalsrud EW. Choledochal cysts: results of primary surgery and need for reoperation in young patients. Am J Surg 1985;150:141.

242. McWhorter GL, Congenital cystic dilatation of the common bile duct. Arch Surg 1924;8:604.

243. Powell CS, Sawyers JL, Reynolds VH. Management of adult choledochal cysts. Ann Surg 1981;193:666.

244. Lilly JR. Total excision of choledochal cyst. Surg Gynecol Obstet 1978;146:254.

245. Lopez RR, Pinson CW, Campell JR, et al. Variation in the management based on type of choledochal cyst. Am J Surg 1991;161:612.

246. Flanigan DP. Biliary carcinoma associated with biliary cysts. Cancer 1977;40:880.

247. Yoshikawa K, Yoshida K, Shirai Y, et al. A case of carcinoma arising in t47 intrapancreatic terminal choledochus 12 years after primary excision of a giant choledochal cyst. Am J Gastroenterol 1986;81:378.

248. Okada A, Nakamura T, Okumura K, et al. Surgical treatment of congenital dilatation of bile duct (choledochal cyst) with technical considerations. Surgery 1987;101:238.

249. Rao KLN, Mitra SK, Kochhler R, et al. Jejunal interposition hepaticoduodenostomy for choledochal cyst. Am J Gastroenterol 1987;82:1042.

250. Ramond MJ, Huguet C, Danan G, et al. Partial hepatectomy in the treatment of Caroli's disease. Report of a case and review of the literature. Dig Dis Sci 1984;29:367.

251. Aeberhard P. Surgical management of Caroli's disease involving both lobes of the liver. Br J Surg 1985;72:651.

252. Barker EM, Kallideen JM. Caroli's disease: successful management using permanent access hepaticojejunostomy. Br J Surg 1985;72:641.

253. Todani T, Narusue M, Watanabe Y, et al. Management of congenital choledochal cyst with intrahepatic involvement. Ann Surg 1978;187:272.

254. Binstock M, Sondak VK, Herd J, et al. Adenocarcinoma in a choledochal cyst during pregnancy: a case report and guidelines for management. Surgery 1988;103:588.

255. Yeong ML, Nicholson GI, Lee SP. Regression of biliary cirrhosis following choledochal cyst drainage. Gastroenterology 1982;82:332.

256. Todani T, Watanabe Y, Toki A, et al. Carcinoma related to choledochal cyst with internal drainage operations. Surg Gynecol Obstet 1987;164:61.

257. Kozuka S, Tsubone M, Hachisuka K. Evolution of carcinoma in the extrahepatic bile ducts. Cancer 1984;54:65.

258. Montana MA, Rohrmann CA. Cholangiocarcinoma in a choledochal cyst: preoperative diagnosis. AJR 1986;147:516.

259. Bloustein PA. Association of carcinoma with congenital cystic conditions of the liver and bile ducts. Am J Gastroenterol 1977;67:40.

260. Phinney PR, Austin GE, Kadell BM. Cholangiocarcinoma arising in Caroli's disease. Arch Patho Lab Med 1981;105:194.

261. Kimura K, Ohto M, Saisho H, et al. Association of gallbladder carcinoma and anomalous pancreaticobiliary ductal union. Gastroenterology 1985;89:1258.

262. Misra SP, Dwivedi M. Pancreaticobiliary ductal union. Gut 1990;31:1144.

263. Duggan DB, Anderson B, Gordon LP. Small cell carcinoma of the pancreas in association with a choledochal cyst: immunohistochemical characterization and complete response to combination chemotherapy. Medical and Pediatr. Oncology 1989;17:506.

264. Delbet P. Retrecissement du choledoque: cholecysto-duodenostomie. Bull Mem Soc Natl Chir 1924;50:1144.

265. White TT, Hart MJ. Primary sclerosing cholangitis. Am J Surg 1987;153:439.

266. Wiesner, RH, LaRusso NF. Clinicopathologic features of the syndrome of primary sclerosing cholangitis. Gastroenterology 1980;79:200.

267. Chapman RWG, Arborgh BAM, Rhodes JM, et al. Primary sclerosing cholangitis: a review of its clinical features, cholangiography, and hepatic histology. Gut 1980;21:870.

268. Lillemoe KD, Pitt, HA, Cameron JL. Sclerosing cholangitis. Adv Surg 1987;21:65.

269. LaRusso NE, Wiesner RH, Ludwig J, et al. Primary sclerosing cholangitis. N Engl J Med 1984;310:899.

270. Myers RN, Cooper JH, Padis N. Primary sclerosing cholangitis: complete gross and histologic reversal after long-term steroid therapy. Am J Gastroenterol 1970;53:527.

271. Thompson HH, Pitt HA, Tomkins RK, et al. Primary sclerosing cholangitis. A heterogenous disease. Ann Surg 1982;196:127.

272. Helzberg JH, Petersen JM, Boyer JL. Improved survival with primary sclerosing cholangitis. Gastroenterology 1987;92:1869.

273. Lindor KD, Wiesner RH, LaRusso NF. Recent advances in the management of primary sclerosing cholangitis. Sem in Liver Dis, 1987;7:322.

274. Williams SM, Harned RK. Hepatobiliary complications of inflammatory bowel disease. Radiol Clin North Am 1987;25:175.

275. Schrumpf E, Elgio K, Fausa O, et al. Sclerosing cholangitis in ulcerative colitis. Scand J Gastroenterol 1980;15:689.

276. Olsson R, Danielsoon A, Jarnerot G, et al. Prevalence of primary sclerosing cholangitis in patients with ulcerative colitis. Gastroenterology 1991;100:1319.

277. Keeffee EB. Primary sclerosing cholangitis in ulcerative colitis. Ann Intern Med 1985;103:305.

278. Rabinovitz M, Gavaler JS, Schade RR, et al. Does primary sclerosing cholangitis occurring in association with inflammatory bowel disease differ from that occurring in the absence of inflammatory bowel disease? A study of sixty-six subjects. Hepatology 1990;11:7.

279. Comings DE, Skubi KB, VanEyes J, et al. Familial multifocal fibrosclerosis. Findings suggesting that retroperitoneal fibrosis, sclerosing cholangitis, Riedel's thyroiditis and psuedotumor of the orbit may be different manifestations of a single disease. Ann Intern Med 1967;66:884.

280. Thompson BW, Reed RC. Sclerosing cholangitis and other intraabdominal fibroses. Am J Surg 1874;128:777.

281. Record CO, Shilkin KB, Eddleston ALWF, et al. Intrahepatic sclerosing cholangitis associated with a familial immunodeficiency syndrome. Lancet 1973;2:18.

282. Bass NM, Chapman RW, O'Reilly A, et al. Primary sclerosing cholangitis associated with angioimmunoblastic lymphadenopathy. Gastroenterology 1983;85:420.

283. DiPalma JA, Strobel CT, Farrow JG. Primary sclerosing cholangitis associated with hyperimmunoglobulin M immunodeficiency (dysgammaglobulinemia). Gastroenterology 1986;91:464.

284. Margulis SJ, Honig CL, Soave R, et al. Biliary tract obstruction in the acquired immunodeficiency syndrome. Ann Intern Med 1986;105:207.

285. Roulot D, Valla D, Brun-Vezinet F, et al. Cholangitis in the acquired immunodeficiency syndrome: report of two cases and review of the literature. Gut 1987;28:1653.

286. Viteri Al, Greene JF Jr. Bile duct abnormalities in the acquired immune deficiency syndrome. Gastroenterology 1987;92:2014.

287. Schneiderman DJ. Hepatobiliary abnormalities of AIDS. Gastroenterol Clin North Am 1988;17:615.

288. Hay JE, Wiesner RH, Shorter RG, et al. Primary sclerosing cholangitis and celiac disease. Ann Intern Med 1988;1090:713.

289. Kirby DF, Bile AT, Rosen ST, et al. Primary sclerosing cholangitis in the presence of a lupus anticoagulant. Am J Med 1986;81:1077.

290. Montefusco PP, Geiss AC, Bronzo RL, et al. Sclerosing cholangitis, chronic pancreatitis and Sjogren's syndrome: a syndrome complex. Am J Surg 1984;147:822.

291. Epstein O, Chapman RWG, Lake-Bakaar G, et al. The pancreas in primary biliary cirrhosis and primary sclerosing cholangitis. Gastroenterology 1982;83:1177.

292. Borkje B, Vetvik K, Odegaard S, et al. Chronic pancreatitis in patients with sclerosing cholangitis and ulcerative colitis. Scand J Gastroenterol 1985;20:539.

293. MacCarty RL, LaRusso NF, Wiesner RH, et al. Primary sclerosing cholangitis: findings on cholangiography and pancreatography. Radiology 1983;149:39.

294. Palmer KR, Cotton PB, Chapman M. Pancreatogram in cholestasis. Gut 1984;25:424.

295. Afroudakis A, Kaplowitz N. Extrahepatic obstruction in chronic alcoholic pancreatitis. Alcoholism: clinical and experimental research 1981;5:110.

296. Dilawari JB, Chawla YK. Pseudosclerosing cholangitis in extrahepatic portal venous obstruction. Gut 1992;33:272.

297. Khuroo M, Yattoo G, Zargar S et al. Biliary abnormalities with extrahepatic portal venous obstruction. Hepatology 1993;17:807.

298. Vilgrain V, Erlinger S, Belghiti J, et al. Cholangiographic appearance simulating sclerosing cholangitis in metastatic adenocarcinoma of the liver. Gastroenterology 1990;99:850.

299. Palmer KR, Duerden BI, Holdsworth CD. Bacteriological and endotoxin studies in cases of ulcerative colitis submitted to surgery. Gut 1980;21:851.

300. Finegold MJ, Carpenter RJ. Obliterative cholangitis due to cytomegalovirus: a possible precursor of paucity of intrahepatic bile ducts. Hum Pathol 1982;13:662.

301. Mason AL, Rosen G, White H, et al. Detection of cytomegalovirus (CMV) DNA in the liver of patients with PSC by the polymerase chain reaction. Hepatology 1991;14:91A.

302. Mehal WZ, Hattersley AT, Chapman RW, and Fleming KA. A survey of cytomegalovirus (CMV) DNA in primary sclerosing cholangitis (PSC) liver tissues using a sensitive polymerase chain reaction (PCR) based assay. J Hepatol 1992;15:396.

303. Bangaru B, Borecki R, Glaser JH, et al. Comparative studies of biliary atresia in the human newborn and reovirus-induced cholangitis in weanling mice. Lab Invest 1980;43:456.

304. Minuk GY, Paul RW, Lee PWK. The prevalence of antibodies to reovirus type 3 in adults with idiopathic cholestatic liver disease. J Med Virol 1985;16:55.

305. Gross JB Jr, Ludwig J, Wiesner RH, et al. Abnormalities in tests of copper metabolism in primary sclerosing cholangitis. Gastroenterology 1985;89:272.

306. LaRusso NF, Wiesner RH, Ludwig J, et al. Prospective trial of penicillamine in primary sclerosing cholangitis. Gastroenterology 1988;95:1036.

307. Quigley EMM, LaRusso NF, Ludwig J, et al. Familial occurrence of primary sclerosing cholangitis and ulcerative colitis. Gastroenterology 1983;85:1160.

308. Chapman RWG, Varghese Z, Gual R, et al. Close association between HLA-B8 and primary sclerosing cholangitis. Gut 1981;22:A871.

309. Chapman RW, Kelly PMA, Heryet A, et al. Expression of HLA-DR antigens on bile duct epithelium in primary sclerosing cholangitis. Gut 1988;29:422.

310. Shepherd HA, Selby WS, Chapman RW, et al. Ulcerative colitis and persistent liver dysfunction. Q J Med 1983;52:503.

311. Prochazka EJ, Terasaki PI, Park MS, et al. Association of primary sclerosing cholangitis with HLA-DRw52a. N Engl J Med 1990;322:1842.

312. Wiesner RH, LaRusso NF, Ludwig J, et al. Comparison of the clinicopathologic features of primary sclerosing cholangitis and primary biliary cirrhosis. Gastroenterology 1985;88:108.

313. McFarlane IG, Wojcicka BM, Tsantoula DC, et al. Leukocyte migration inhibition in response to biliary cirrhosis, sclerosing cholangitis, and other chronic liver disease. Gastroenterology 1979;76:1333.

314. Chapman RW, Cottone M, Selby WS, et al. Serum auto-antibodies, ulcerative colitis and primary sclerosing cholangitis. Gut 1986;27:86.

315. Snook JA, Chapman RW, Fleming K, et al. Anti-neutrophil nuclear antibody in ulcerative colitis, Crohn's disease and primary sclerosing cholangitis. Clin Exp Immunol 1989;76:30.

316. Saxon A, Shanahan F, Landers C, et al. A distinct subset of antineutrophil cytoplasmic antibodies is associated with inflammatory bowel disease. J Allergy Clin Immunol 1990;86:202.

317. Duerr RH, Targan SR, Landers CJ, et al. Neutrophil cytoplasmic antibodies: a link between primary sclerosing cholangitis and ulcerative colitis. Gastroenterology 1991;100:1385.

318. Klein R, Eisenburg J, Weber P, et al. Significance and specificity of antibodies to neutrophils detected by Western blotting for the serological diagnosis of primary sclerosing cholangitis. Hepatology 1991;14:1147.

319. Seibold F, Weber P, Klein R, et al. Clinical significance of antibodies against neutrophils in patients with inflammatory bowel disease and primary sclerosing cholangitis. Gut 1992;33:657.

320. Bodenheimer HC, LaRusso NF, Thayer WR Jr, et al. Elevated circulating immune complexes in primary sclerosing cholangitis. Hepatology 1983;3:150.

321. Alberti-Flor J, Medina M, Jeffers L, et al. Elevated levels of immunoglobulins and immune complexes in the bile of patients with primary sclerosing cholangitis. Am J Gastroenterol 1986;81:325.

322. Senaldi G, Donaldson PT, Magrin S, et al. Activation of the complement system in primary sclerosing cholangitis. Gastroenterology 1989;97:1430.

323. Brinch L, Teisberg P, Schrumpf E, et al. The in vivo metabolism of C3 in hepatobiliary disease associated with ulcerative colitis. Scand J Gastroenterol 1982;17:523.

324. Whiteside TL, Lasky S, Si L, et al. Immunologic analysis of mononuclear cells in liver tissues and blood of patients with primary sclerosing cholangitis. Hepatology 1985;5:468.

325. Adams DH, Hubscher SG, Shaw J, et al. Increased expression of intercellular adhesion molecule-1 on bile ducts in primary biliary cirrhosis and primary sclerosing cholangitis. Hepatology 1991;14:426.

326. Adams, DH, Mainolfi E, Burra P, et al. Detection of circulating intercellular adhesion molecule-1 in chronic liver diseases. Hepatology 1992;16:810.

327. Lindor K, Wiesner R, LaRusso NF, et al. Enhanced autoreactivity of T-lymphocytes in primary sclerosing cholangitis. Hepatology 1987;7:884.

328. Belghiti J, Benhamou J-P, Houry S, et al. Caustic sclerosing cholangitis. A complication of the surgical treatment of hydatid disease of the liver. Arch Surg 1986;121:1162.

329. Kemeny MM, Battifora H, Blayney DW, et al. Sclerosing cholangitis after continuous hepatic artery infusion of FUDR. Ann Surg 1985;202:176.

330. Ludwig J, Kim CH, Wiesner RH, et al. Floxuridine-induced sclerosing cholangitis: an ischemic cholangiopathy? Hepatology 1989;9:215.

331. Kemeny N, Daly J, Reichman B, et al. Intrahepatic or systemic infusion of fluorodeoxyuridine in patients with liver metastases from colorectal carcinoma. A randomized trial. Ann Intern Med 1987;107:459.

332. Terblanche M, Allison HF, Northover JMA. An ischemic basis for biliary strictures. Surgery 1983;94:52.

333. Makuuchi M, Sukigara M, Mori T, et al. Bile duct necrosis: complication of transcatheter hepatic arterial embolization. Radiology 1985;156:331.

334. Thompson HH, Pitt HA, Lewin KJ, et al. Sclerosing cholangitis and histiocytosis X. Gut 1984;25:526.

335. Johnson DA, Cattau EL Jr, Hancock JE. Pediatric primary sclerosing cholangitis. Dig Dis Sci 1986;31:773.

336. Sisto A, Feldman P, Garel L, et al. Primary sclerosing cholangitis in children: study of five cases and review of the literature. Pediatrics 1987;80:918.

337. El-Shabrawi M, Wlkinson ML, Portmann B, et al. Primary sclerosing cholangitis in childhood. Gastroenterology 1987;92:1226.

338. LaRusso NF, Wiesner RH, Ludwig J. Is primary sclerosing cholangitis a bad disease? Gasteroenterology 1987;92:2031.

339. Chapman RWG, Burroughs AK, Bass NM, et al. Long-standing asymptomatic primary sclerosing cholangitis. Report of three cases. Dig Dis Sci 1981;26:778.

340. Porayko MK, Wiesner RH, LaRusso NF, et al. Patients with asymptomatic primary sclerosing cholangitis frequently have progressive disease. Gastroenterology 1990;98:1594.

341. Farrant JM, Hayllar KM, Wilkinson ML, et al. Natural history and prognostic variables in primary sclerosing cholangitis. Gastroenterology 1991;100:1710.

342. Dickson ER, Murtaugh PA, Wiesner RH, et al. Primary sclerosing cholangitis: refinement and validation of survival models. Gastroenterology 1992;103:1893.

343. Cameron JL, Gayler BW, Sanfey H, et al. Sclerosing cholangtitis. Anatomical distribution of obstructive lesions. Ann Surg 1984;200:54.

344. Cooper JF, Brand EJ. Symptomatic sclerosing cholangitis in patients with a normal alkaline phospatase: two case reports

and a review of the literature. Am J Gastroenterol 1988;83: 308.

345. Chen LY, Goldberg HI. Sclerosing cholangitis: broad spectrum of radiographic features. Gastrointest Radiol 1984;9:39.

346. Williams LF Jr, Schoetz DJ Jr. Primary sclerosing cholangitis. Surg Clin North Am 1981;61:951.

347. Rodman CA, Keefe EB, Lieberman DA, et al. Diagnosis of sclerosing cholangitis with technetium 99m-labeled iminodiacetic acid planar and single photon emission computed tomographic scintigraphy. Gastroenterology 1987;92:777.

348. Ament AE, Haaga JR, Wiedermann SD, et al. Primary sclerosing cholangitis: CT findings. J Comput Assist Tomogr 1983;7:795.

349. Rahn NH, Koehler RE, Weyman PJ, et al. CT appearance of sclerosing cholangitis. AJR Am J Roentgenol 1983;141:549.

350. Ludwig J, Barham SS, LaRusso NF, et al. Morphologic features of chronic hepatitis associated with primary sclerosing cholangitis and chronic ulcerative colitis. Hepatology 1981;1:632.

351. Ludwig J, MacCarty RL, LaRusso NF, et al. Intrahepatic cholangiectases and large-duct obliteration in primary sclerosing cholangitis. Hepatology 1986;6:560.

352. Harrison RF, Hubscher SG. The spectrum of bile duct lesions in end-stage primary sclerosing cholangitis. Histopathology 1991;19:321.

353. Brandt DJ, MacCarty RL, Charboneau JW, et al. Gallbladder disease in patients with primary sclerosing cholangitis. AJR Am J Roentgenol 1988;150:571.

354. Wee A, Ludwig J. Pericholangitis in chronic ulcerative colitis: primary sclerosing cholangitis of the small bile ducts. Ann Intern Med 1985;102:581.

355. Mistilis SP. Pericholangitis and ulcerative colitis: I. pathology, etiology, and pathogenesis. Ann Intern Med 1965;63:1.

356. Leevy CM, Popper H, Sherlock S. Diseases of the liver and biliary tract: standardization of nomenclature, diagnostic criteria methodology. Fogarty Int Center Proc 1976;22:1.

357. Wood RAB, Cuschieri A. Is sclerosing cholangitis complicating ulcerative colitis a reversible condition? Lancet 1980;2:716.

358. Mir-Madjlessi SH, Farmer RG, Sivak Jr, MV. Bile duct carcinoma in patients with ulcerative colitis. Relationship to sclerosing cholangitis: report of six cases and review of the literature. Dig Dis Sci 1987;32:145.

359. Wee A, Ludwig J, Coffey R Jr, et al. Hepatobiliary carcinoma associated with primary sclerosing cholangitis and chronic ulcerative colitis. Hum Pathol 1985;16:719.

360. Gluskin LE, Payne JA. Cystic dilatation as a radiographic sign of cholangiocarcinoma complicating sclerosing cholangitis. Am J Gastroenterol 1983;78:661.

361. MacCarty RL, La Russo NF, May GR, et al. Cholangiocarcinoma complicating primary sclerosing cholangitis: cholangiographic appearance. Radiology 1985;156:43.

362. Munoz SJ, Heubi JE, Maddrey WC. Status of lipid soluble vitamins in primary sclerosing cholangitis. Gastroenterology 1989;96:A636.

363. Polter DE, Gruhl V, Eigenbrodt EH, et al. Beneficial effect of cholestyramine in sclerosing cholangitis. Gastroenterology 1980;79:326.

364. Lauterburg BH, Taswell HF, Pineda AA, et al. Treatment of pruritus of cholestasis by plasma perfusion through USP-charcoal coated glass beads. Lancet 1980;2:53.

365. O'Brien C, Senior JR, Batta AK, et al. Ursodeoxycholic acid treatment produces marked clinical and biochemical amelioration of primary sclerosing cholangitis. Gastroenterology 1989;96:A640.

366. Stiehl A, Raedsch R, Theilmann L, et al. The effect of ursodeoxycholic acid on primary sclerosing cholangitis. Gastroenterology 1989;96:A664.

367. Chazouilleres O, Poupon R, Capron JP, et al. Is ursodeoxycholic acid an effective treatment for primary sclerosing cholangitis? Gastroenterology 1989;96:A583.

368. Johnson GK, Geenen JE, Venu RP, et al. Endoscopic treatment of biliary duct strictures in sclerosing cholangitis: follow-up assessment of a new therapeutic approach. Gastrointest Endosc 1987;33:9.

369. Kerlan RK Jr, LaBerge JM, Goldberg HI, et al. Interventional

370. Krige JEJ, Terblanche J, Harries-Jones EP, et al. Primary sclerosing cholangitis: biliary drainage and duct dilatation. Br J Surg 1987;74:54.

371. Allison MC, Burroughs AK, Noone P, et al. Biliary lavage with corticosteroids in primary sclerosing cholangitis. A clinical, cholangiographic and bacteriological study. J Hepatol 1986;3: 118.

372. Grijm R, Huibregtse K, Bartelsman J, et al. Therapeutic investigations in primary sclerosing cholangitis. Dig Dis Sci 1986;31: 792.

373. Burgert SL, Brown BP, Kirkpatrick RB, et al. Positive corticosteroid response in early primary sclerosing cholangitis. Gastroenterology 1984;86:1037.

374. Kaplan MM, Arora S, Pincus SH. Primary sclerosing cholangitis and low-dose oral pulse methotrexate therapy. Clinical and histologic response. Ann Intern Med 1987;106:231.

375. Knox TA, Kaplan MM. Treatment of primary sclerosing cholangitis with oral methotrexate. Am J Gastroenterol 1991;86: 546.

376. LaRusso NF, Wiesner RH, Beaver SJ. Combined antifibrogenic and immunosuppressive therapy in primary sclerosing cholangitis. Gastroenterology 1987;92:1493.

377. Lindor KD, Wiesner RH, Colwell LJ, et al. The combination of prednisone and colchicine in patients with primary sclerosing cholangitis. Am J Gastroenterol 1991;85:57.

378. Beuers U, Spengler U, Kruis W, et al. Ursodeoxycholic acid for treatment of primary sclerosing cholangitis: a placebo-controlled trial. Hepatology 1992;16:707.

379. Van Thiel DH, Wright HI, Gavaler JS. Ursodeoxycholic acid (UDCA) therapy for primary sclerosing cholangitis: preliminary report of a randomized controlled trial. Hepatology 1992;16: 62A.

380. Lo SK, Hermann R, Chapman RW, et al. Ursodeoxycholic acid in primary sclerosing cholangitis: a double-blind placebo controlled trial. Hepatology 1992;16:92A.

381. Olsson R, Hulten L. Concurrence of ulcerative colitis and chronic active hepatitis, clinical courses and results of colectomy. Scand J Gastroenterol 1975;10:331.

382. Cangemi JR, Wiesner RH, Beaver SJ, et al. Effect of proctocolectomy for chronic ulcerative colitis on the natural history of primary sclerosing cholangitis. Gastroenterology 1989;96: 790.

383. Wiesner RH, LaRusso NF, Dozois RR, et al. Peristomal varices after proctocolectomy in patients with primary sclerosing cholangitis. Gastroenterology 1986;90:316.

384. Pitt HA, Thompson HH, Tompkins RK, et al. Primary sclerosing cholangitis: results of an aggresive surgical approach. Ann Surg 1982;196:259.

385. Carmeron JL, Pitt HA, Zinner MJ, et al. Resection of hepatic duct bifurcation and transhepatic stenting for sclerosing cholangitis. Ann Surg 207:614.

386. Thompson JS, Wood RP, Burnett DA, et al. The role of nontransplant procedures for sclerosing cholangitis. Am J Surg 1988;156:506.

387. Marsh JW Jr, Iwatsuki S, Makowka L, et al. Orthotopic liver transplantation for primary sclerosing cholangitis. Ann Surg 1988;207:21.

388. Martin FM, Rossi RL, Nugent FW, et al. Surgical aspects of sclerosing cholangitis. Ann Surg 1990;212:551.

389. Weisner RH, Porayko MK, Dickson ER, et al. Selection and timing of liver transplantation in primary biliary cirrhosis and primary sclerosing cholangitis. Ann Surg 1990;212:551.

390. Higashi H, Yanaga K, Marsh JW, et al. Development of colon cancer after liver transplantation for primary sclerosing cholangitis associated with ulcerative colitis. Hepatology 1990;11: 477.

391. Hunter EB, Wiesner RH, MacCarty RL, et al. Does primary sclerosing cholangitis recur after liver transplantation? Gastroenterology 1989;96:A610.

392. Sandblom P, Mirkovitch V. Hemobilia: some salient features and their causes. Surg Clin North Am 1977;57:397.

393. Little JM. Hydatid disease at Royal Prince Alfred Hospital, 1964 to 1974. Med J Aust 1976;1:903.
394. Ho F, Snape WJ Jr, Venegas R, et al. Choledochal fungal ball. An unusual cause of biliary obstruction. Dig Dis Sci 1988;33:1030.
395. Goldberg HJ, Doman DB. Vascular ring—an unusual cause of benign biliary stricture. Gastrointest Endosc 1988;34:347.
396. Way LW, Bernhoft RA, Thomas MJ. Biliary stricture. Surg Clin North Am 1981;61:963.
397. Silvis SE, Ansel HJ. Endoscopic retrograde cholangiography: application in biliary tract disease. In: Berk JE, ed. Bockus gastroenterology. 4th ed. Philadelphia: WB Saunders, 1985:3449.
398. Mercadier M, Fingerhut A. Strictures of the intrahepatic bile ducts. World J Surg 1984;8:15.
399. Tan ST, Ng IOL, Choi TK, et al. Tuberculosis of the bile duct: a rare cause of biliary stricture. Am J Gastroenterol 1989;84:413.
400. Lillemoe KD, Pitt HA, Cameron JL. Postoperative bile duct strictures. Surg Clin North Am 1990;70:1355.
401. Roslyn JJ, Tompkins RK. Reoperation for biliary strictures. Surg Clin North Am 1991;71:109.
402. Davidoff AM, Pappas TN, Murray EA, et al. Mechanisms of major biliary injury during laparoscopic cholecystectomy. Ann Surg 1992;215:196.
403. Trerotola SO, Savader SJ, Lund GB, et al. Biliary tract complications following laparoscopic cholecystectomy: imaging and intervention. Radiology 1992;184:195.
404. Yoshioka T, Sakaguchi H, Yoshimura H, et al. Expandable metallic biliary endoprostheses: preliminary clinical evaluation. Radiology 1990;177:253.
405. Littenberg G, Afroudakis A, Kaplowitz N. Common bile duct stenosis from chronic pancreatitis: a clinical and pathologic spectrum. Medicine 1979;58:385.
406. Aranha GV, Prinz RA, Freeark RJ, et al. The spectrum of biliary tract obstruction from chronic pancreatitis. Arch Surg 1984;119:595.
407. Wilson C. Auld CD, Schlinkert R, et al. Hepatobiliary complications in chronic pancreatitis. Gut 1989;30:520.
408. Afroudakis A, Kaplowitz N. Liver histopathology in chronic common bile duct stenosis due to chronic alcoholic pancreatitis. Hepatology 1981;1:65.
409. Gaskin KJ, Waters DLM, Howman-Giles R, et al. Liver disease and common bile duct stenosis in cystic fibrosis. N Engl J Med 1988;318:340.
410. Guelrud M. Papillary stenosis. Endoscopy 1988;20:193.
411. Weber CM, Zito PF, Becker SM. Heterotopic pancreas: an unusual cause of obstruction of the common bile duct. Am J Gastroenterol 1968;49:153.
412. Fernandez-Cruz L, Pera C. Involutive pathology of the sphincterian system of Oddi. Bull Soc Int Chir 1971;30:490.
413. Grage TB, Lober PH, Imamoglu K, et al. Stenosis of the sphincter of Oddi. A clinicopathologic review of 50 cases. Surgery 1960;48:304.
414. Griffith CA. Diagnosis of papillary stenosis by calibration. Follow-up 15 to 25 years after sphincteroplasty. Am J Surg 1982;143:717.
415. Trommald JP, Seabrook DB. Benign fibrosis of sphincter of Oddi: report of 8 cases. West J Surg Obstet Gynecol 1950;58:89.
416. Braasch JW, McCann JC. Normal luminal size of choledochoduodenal junction as determined by probe at choledochostomy. Surgery 1967;62:258.
417. Pace RF, Chamberlain MJ, Passi RB. Diagnosing papillary stenosis by technetium-99m HIDA scanning. Can J Surg 1983;26:191.
418. Warshaw AL, Simeone J, Schapiro RH, et al. Objective evaluation of ampullary stenosis with ultrasonography and pancreatic stimulation. Am J Surg 1985;149:65.
419. Gregg JA, Carr-Locke DL. Endoscopic pancreatic and biliary manometry in pancreatic, biliary, and papillary disease, and after endoscopic sphincterotomy and surgical sphincteroplasty. Gut 1984;25:1247.
420. Kawai K, Nakajima M. Present status and complications of EST in Japan. Endoscopy 1983;15:169.
421. Sandblom P. Hemorrhage into the biliary tract following trauma—"traumatic hemobilia." J Surg 1948;24:571.
422. Sandblom P. Hemobilia. Springfield, IL: Charles C Thomas, 1972.
423. Garrigues V, del Val A, Ponce J, et al. Hemobilia and hemophilia. Ann Intern Med 1988;109:345.
424. Merrell SW, Gilbertson JJ, Albo D Jr, et al. Atraumatic hemobilia arising from a cirrhotic liver. Surgery 1989;106:105.
425. Curet P, Baumer R, Roche A, et al. Hepatic hemobilia of traumatic or iatrogenic origin: recent advances in diagnosis and therapy, review of the literature from 1976 to 1981. World J Surg 1984;8:2.
426. Yoshida J, Donahue PE, Nyhus LM. Hemobilia: review of recent experience with a worldwide problem. Am J Gastroenterol 1987;82:448.
427. Stauffer JT, Weinman MD, Bynum TD. Hemobilia in a patient with multiple hepatic artery aneurysms: a case report and review of the literature. Am J Gastroenterol 1989;84:59.
428. Uflacker R, Mourao GS, Piske RL, et al. Hemobilia: transcatheter occlusive therapy and long-term follow-up. Cardiovasc Intervent Radiol. 1989;12:136.
429. Okazaki M, Ono H, Higashihara H, et al. Angiographic management of massive hemobilia due to iatrogenic trauma. Gastrointest Radiol 1991;16:205.
430. Lygidakis NJ, Damtsios OG. Iatrogenic hemobilia: how to approach it. Hepatogastroenterol 1991;38:454.
431. Czerniak A, Thompson JN, Hemingway AP, et al. Hemobilia. A disease in evolution. Arch Surg 1988;123:718.
432. Sandblom P. Iatrogenic hemobilia. Am J Surg 1986;151:754.
433. Merrell SW, Schneider PD. Hemobilia—evolution of current diagnosis and treatment. West J Med 1991;155:621.
434. Goodnight JE Jr, Blaisdell FW. Hemobilia. Surg Clin North Am 1981;61:973.
435. Floyd WN Jr. Radiologic aspects of hemobilia. South Med J 1981;74:829.
436. Sandblom P, Saegesser F, Mirkovitch V. Hepatic hemobilia: hemorrhage from the intrahepatic biliary tract, a review. World J Surg 1984;8:41.
437. Bose SM, Sastry RA. Agenesis of gallbladder with choledochal-colonic fistula. Am J Gastroenterol 1983;78:34.
438. Piedad OH, Wels PB. Spontaneous internal biliary fistula, obstructive and nonobstructive types: twenty-year review of 55 cases. Ann Surg 1972;175:75.
439. Glenn F. Biliary enteric fistula. Surg Gynecol Obstet 1981;153:527.
440. Tanaka M, Ikeda S. Parapapillary choledochoduodenal fistula: an analysis of 83 consecutive patients diagnosed at ERCP. Gastrointest Endosc 1983;29:89.
441. LeBlanc KA, Barr LH, Rush BM. Spontaneous biliary enteric fistulas. South Med J 1983;76:1249.
442. Czerniak A, Benjamin IS, Blumgart LH. The management of fistulas of the biliary tract after injury to the bile duct during cholecystectomy. Surg Gynecol Obstet 1988;167:33.
443. Sauerbruch T, Weinzierl M, Holl J, et al. Treatment of postoperative bile fistulas by internal endoscopic biliary drainage. Gastroenterology 1986;90:1998.
444. Ponchon T, Gallez J, Valette P, et al. Endoscopic treatment of biliary tract fistulas. Gastrointest Endosc 1989;35:490.
445. Krige JEJ, Bornman PC, Beningfield SJ, et al. Endoscopic embolization of external biliary fistulae. Br J Surg 1990;77;581.
446. Gugenheim J, Ciardullo M, Traynor O, et al. Bronchobiliary fistulas in adult. Ann Surg 1988;207:90.
447. Savitch I, Kew MC, Levin J. Demonstration of a biliary-bronchial fistula using Tc-99m p-butyl IDA imaging. Clin Nucl Med 1983;8:139.
448. Blue PW, Versteeg J, Cole FN, et al. Bronchobiliary fistula. Demonstration with Tc-99m PIPIDA imaging. Clin Nucl Med 1983;8:272.
449. Stauffer JT, Weinman MD, Bynum TE. Hemobilia in a patient with multiple hepatic artery aneurysms: a case report and review of the literature. Am J Gastroenterol 1989;84:59.
450. Lugagne PM, Lacaine F, Bonnel D, et al. Bilioportal fistula as a complication of choledochoduodenostomy. Surgery 1988;103:125.

451. Peven DR, Yokoo H. Bile pulmonary embolism: report of a case and review of the literature. Am J Gastroenterol 1983;78:830.

452. Rao PSV, Tandon RK, Kapur BML. Biliobiliary fistula: review of nine cases. Am J Gastroenterol 1988;83:652.

453. Csendes A, Diaz JC, Burdiles P, et al. Mirizzi syndrome and cholecystobiliary fistula: a unifying classification. Br J Surg 1989;76:1139.

454. Mishra MC, Vashishtha S, Tandon R. Biliobiliary fistula: preoperative diagnosis and management implications. Surgery 1990;108:835.

455. Pitlik S, Fainstein V, Garza D, et al. Human cryptosporidiosis: spectrum of disease: report of six cases and review of the literature. Arch Intern Med 1983;143:2269.

456. Guard LA, Stein SA, Clearly KA, et al. Human cryptosporidiosis in the acquired immune deficiency syndrome. Arch Pathol Lab Med 1983;107:562.

457. Cello JP. Human immunodeficiency virus-associated biliary tract disease. Semin Liv Dis 1992;12:213.

458. Burt AD, Scott G, Shiach CR, et al. Acquired immunodeficiency syndrome in a patient with no known risk factors: a pathological study. J Clin Pathol 1984;37:471.

459. Schneiderman DJ, Cello JP, Laing FC. Papillary stenosis and sclerosing cholangitis in the acquired immunodeficiency syndrome. Ann Intern Med 1987;106:546.

460. Dowsett JF, Miller R, Davidson R, et al. Sclerosing cholangitis in acquired immunodeficiency syndrome. Case reports and review of the literature. Scand J Gastroenterol 1988;23:1267.

461. Cello JP. Acquired immunodeficiency syndrome cholangiopathy: spectrum of disease. Am J Med 1989;86:539.

462. Teixidor HS, Godwin TA, Ramirez EA. Cryptosporidiosis of the biliary tract in AIDS. Radiology 1991;180:51.

463. Jacobson MA, Cello JP, Sande MA. Cholestasis and disseminated cytomegalovirus disease in patients with the acquired immunodeficiency syndrome. Am J Med 1988;84:218.

464. Bonacini M. Hepatobiliary complications in patients with human immunodeficiency virus infection. Am J Med 1992;92:404.

465. Beaugerie L, Teilhac M, Deluol A, et al. Cholangiopathy associated with Microsporidia infection of the common bile duct mucosa in a patient with HIV infection. Ann Intern Med 1992;117:401.

466. Pol S, Romana C, Richard S, et al. *Enterocytozoon bieneusi* infection in acquired immunodeficiency syndrome-related sclerosing cholangitis. Gastroenterology 1992;102:1778.

467. Pol S, Romana CA, Richard S, et al. Microsporidia infection in patients with the human immunodeficiency virus and unexplained cholangitis. N Engl J Med 1993;328:95.

468. McCarty M, Choudhri AH, Helbert M, et al. Radiological features of AIDS related cholangitis. Clin Radiol 1989;40:582.

469. Grumbach K, Coleman BG, Gal AA, et al. Hepatic and biliary tract abnormalities in patients with AIDS. Sonographic-pathologic correlation. J Ultrasound Med 1989;8:247.

470. Urbain D, Jeanmart J, Lemone M, et al. Cholestasis in patients with the acquired immune deficiency syndrome: comparison between ultrasonographic and cholangiographic findings. Am J Gastroenterol 1991;86:574.

Textbook of Gastroenterology, second edition, edited by Tadataka Yamada. JB Lippincott Company, Philadelphia © 1995.

CHAPTER 98

Tumors of the Biliary Tree

Courtney M. Townsend, Jr

Carcinoma of the Gallbladder	Carcinoma of the Bile Ducts
Incidence	Incidence
Etiology	Etiology
Pathology	Pathology
Clinical Manifestations	Clinical Manifestations
Diagnosis	Diagnosis
Treatment	Treatment

Benign and malignant tumors of the biliary tract, gallbladder, and bile ducts are uncommon or rare neoplasms. Carcinomas of the gallbladder and extrahepatic bile ducts account for fewer than 2% of all malignant neoplasms in the United States. There are striking differences between gallbladder cancer and bile duct cancer. Gallbladder cancers are three times more common in women than in men, but there is no gender difference for bile duct cancers. Eighty percent or more of gallbladder cancers are associated with stone disease, but fewer than 20% of bile duct cancers are associated with stones. The racial and geographic differences observed among populations and groups at high risk for developing gallbladder cancer are not found for bile duct cancer.

CARCINOMA OF THE GALLBLADDER

Carcinoma of the gallbladder is the fifth most common malignancy of the gastrointestinal tract.[1] The mortality of gallbladder cancer is related to stage, and mortality is inversely related to cholecystectomy rates.[2] Despite all that has been written about this subject, the survival of patients with gallbladder cancers has not changed in the past 80 years.

No prospective studies have evaluated significant numbers of patients to allow definitive conclusions to be made about the natural history or treatment of gallbladder cancer. However, cancers arising from gallbladder mucosa appear to behave in a fashion similar to other adenocarcinomas of the gastrointestinal tract; premalignant to invasive malignant changes can be found, metastatic spread occurs by lymphatic and vascular routes, diagnosis is often delayed, and survival is related to stage. Most reports have covered the experience of single institutions for 15 to 30 years, and the series are usually composed of fewer than 100 patients. A few reports are collective reviews of smaller series. Definitive statements regarding the cause of gallbladder cancer cannot be made, but there are striking racial, genetic, and environmental differences in the incidence of gallbladder cancer.

Incidence

Population groups with the highest incidence of gallbladder cancer include Native Americans, Hispanic-American women, and Latin-American women, Japanese women in Japan, African Zimbabwian women, European immigrant women in Israel, and northern Europeans. Low rates of gallbladder cancer occur among Nigerians, New Zealand Maoris, and Chinese natives and immigrants.[3] Cancer of the gallbladder is a disease of the elderly, with the greatest incidence occurring after 65 years of age. It is three times more common in women than in men, and it is more common in whites than in blacks. In the United States, gallbladder cancer is the most common gastrointestinal malignancy in Native Americans.[1] In contrast to the United States, gallbladder cancer is the fourth leading cause of all cancer deaths in Chile; mortality from gallbladder cancer (5.2%) in Chile is the highest in the world.[4]

Genetic differences are exceedingly important. In North America, the highest incidence of gallbladder cancer occurs among Native Americans and Mexican Americans. In North and South America, gallbladder cancer is related to Indian rather than Spanish heritage, because the incidence of gallbladder cancer in Spain, Cuba, and Puerto Rico is low. However, these differences may be the result of environmental, genetic, or biologic factors.

Etiology

Etiologic factors that appear to be important for the development of gallbladder cancer include genetic characteristics, gallstone disease, bile composition, calcification of the gallbladder wall, congenital biliary cysts, some infections, environmental carcinogens, and drugs. Geographic differences may reflect racial and genetic differences, although cultural differences possibly play a role.

Gallstone disease is associated with gallbladder cancer. Overall, the incidence of gallbladder cancer in patients with gallstone disease ranges between 0.5% and 3%.[5] Gallstones have been found in gallbladders involved with cancer in about 70% to 90% of patients. The role that gallstones play assumes great importance, but the mechanism is unknown. Duration of gallstones, patient age, size of gallstones, and possible carcinogenic effects of gallstones, such as from the chemical composition or bacteria within the stones, may be important.[6]

Most of the studies of the relation of gallstones to gallbladder cancer have come from operative or autopsy studies; however, Maringhini and colleagues conducted a prospective cohort study of patients with gallstones in Rochester, Minnesota.[7] They found that gallstones did increase the risk for gallbladder cancer, but the actual incidence was very low (9 per 10,000 per person-years), and the absolute number of cases of gallbladder cancer (5 of 2583 persons) in this population was low.

It appears that the duration of gallstones is a crucial factor for the development of cancer. Patients who have had gallstones longer than 40 years have a significantly higher incidence of developing gallbladder cancer than those who have had gallstones for a shorter time. Glenn and Hays suggested that 1% of patients older than 65 years of age with gallstones would develop gallbladder cancer.[8] This more likely reflects the duration of stone disease rather than an effect of age. However, the possibility of cancer is not an indication for cholecystectomy in a patient with asymptomatic stones. In many countries, gallbladder cancer is unknown, which is probably related to the rate of cholecystectomies performed for asymptomatic gallstones or early in the course of patients with symptomatic stones.

Little is known about the pathophysiology of gallbladder cancer in patients with gallstone disease. It may be that chronic irritation of gallbladder mucosa by stones followed by repeated episodes of epithelial repair over a period of years leads to malignant transformation. Specific components of the stones or bile may act as cocarcinogens. Possible carcinogens that have been identified include elements of stones, types of bile, and certain chemical carcinogens. Despite these associations in humans, no clear etiologic agent has been found. The chemical composition of stones may be related to development of gallbladder cancer. Cholesterol stones are the most common type associated with gallbladder cancer. Bile acids can act as cocarcinogens, and there is a chemical similarity to the known carcinogen, methylcholanthrene.[9]

Abnormalities of the composition of bile in patients with gallbladder cancer may be primary or secondary.[3] The mechanisms by which abnormal bile induces gallbladder cancer are unknown. Possible causes include genetic differences in hepatic synthesis of bile components or gallbladder function, dietary influences on bile acid composition, and environmental exposure or bacterial overgrowth that alters bile composition.

It has been proposed that mixture of bile and gastrointestinal contents or pancreatic juice plays a role in development of gallbladder cancer. This possibility was raised because the incidence of cancer in choledochal cysts after cystoenteric drainage is 20 times that of cancer of bile ducts without cysts; fewer than 25% of the patients are found to have stones. Abnormalities of the distal common bile duct also have been associated with gallbladder cancer.[10,11]

Other factors have been associated with gallbladder cancer, including partial or complete calcification of the gallbladder wall (cancer is found in 25% of porcelain gallbladders), *Salmonella typhi* carriage, and exposure to toxic environmental factors in the automotive, rubber, textile, and metal industries.[9,12]

An interesting association between previous gastric operations and gallbladder cancer was found by Caygill and colleagues.[13] They studied more than 4000 patients who had undergone gastric operations for peptic ulcer disease 25 years previously. Beyond 20 years after the surgery, the incidence of gallbladder cancer was increased 15.8-fold among patients with gastric ulcers but not significantly increased among patients with duodenal ulcers. This association was limited to gallbladder cancer and was not related to bile duct cancer.

Pathology

The pathology of tumors of the gallbladder and bile ducts has been reviewed by Albores-Saavedra and Henson, and this section summarizes their findings.[9]

Benign epithelial or mesenchymal tumors of the gallbladder are not thought to be premalignant lesions. Benign epithelial tumors include adenomas and mixed tumors. Adenomas may be tubular, papillary, or mixed. One third are multiple, and fewer than 50% are associated with stones. No clear adenoma-to-carcinoma sequence has been demonstrated for gallbladder adenomas, unlike the sequence found in the colon.

Other changes in gallbladder epithelium that do not have malignant potential include adenomatous hyperplasia, primary papillary hyperplasia, and cholesterol polyps or inflammatory polyps. Adenomatous hyperplasia may be diffuse or localized. More than 40% of benign tumors of the gallbladder result from adenomatous hyperplasia. A localized lesion that is characteristically single and almost always found in the fundus of the gallbladder may be called adenomyoma. Benign mesenchymal tumors are rare and include leiomyoma, hemangioma, and lipoma.

Premalignant lesions are associated with gallbladder cancer. It is thought that chronic inflammation may play a role in development of premalignant lesions. There is a progression from dysplasia to carcinoma in situ to invasive cancer in the gallbladder epithelium.

Two types of metaplasia, intestinal and squamous, have been found in patients with gallbladder cancer. The relation of intestinal metaplasia to subsequent development of gallbladder cancer has not been determined. Squamous metaplasia, in which squamous epithelium replaces the normal gallbladder epithelium, is a rare premalignant lesion that has been found with squamous cell cancer of the gallbladder. Cholecystitis follicularis, a rare type of inflammation, has been reported in a few cases of gallbladder cancer, but its premalignant potential is unclear.

The classification of malignant lesions of the gallbladder

TABLE 98-1
Malignant Neoplasms of the Gallbladder

Malignant Epithelial Tumors
Adenocarcinoma
Squamous cell carcinoma
Adenosquamous carcinoma
Oat cell carcinoma
Others

Malignant Mesenchymal Tumors
Embryonal rhabdomyosarcoma
Leiomyosarcoma
Malignant fibrous histiocytoma

Miscellaneous
Carcinosarcoma
Carcinoid
Lymphoma
Melanoma
Others

is shown in Table 98-1. Sixty percent of cancers of the gallbladder are found in the fundus, 30% in the body, and 10% in the neck. They may be isolated or involve the entire gallbladder through intramural spread, analogous to linitis plastica of the stomach.

Most malignant neoplasms of the gallbladder are adenocarcinomas, which behave in a manner similar to adenocarcinomas arising from other epithelial tissues. They originate as mucosal lesions, and as growth progresses, they invade the wall of the gallbladder. The anatomy of the gallbladder wall partly explains the advanced stage of disease at which most patients with gallbladder cancer present. The lack of a well-defined muscularis leads to early entry of invasive gallbladder cancer into the perimuscular connective tissue. Lymphatic, neural, and hematogenous invasion occurs earlier with gallbladder cancer than with cancers of the gut.

Gallbladder cancer frequently extends beyond the gallbladder to involve the liver and the extrahepatic biliary tree. Most patients with liver involvement have direct extension of the disease; fewer than 10% of patients have liver metastasis without full-thickness invasion of the gallbladder wall. Lymph node metastasis to the cystic, pericholedochal, peripancreatic, and celiac nodes occurs early; more than 50% of patients are found to have lymph node metastases at the time of diagnosis. Direct invasion of the duodenum and the colon also occur. Intraperitoneal spread, Krukenberg's tumors (i.e., ovarian metastases), and hematogenous dissemination occur.

A uniform staging system for gallbladder cancer has not been widely applied. Nevin and colleagues developed the first clinically useful staging system.[14] The TNM system, described by the American Joint Committee on Cancer, is the preferred staging system for all cancers, including gallbladder cancer.[15] This system is based on the extent of tumor (T) at the primary site and presence or absence of regional lymph node (N) or distant metastases (M).

Gallbladder cancers are staged by surgical exploration. The system is based on the extent of invasion of the gallbladder wall, invasion into the liver, the number of adjacent organs invaded by tumor, and presence of lymph node or distant metastases. Survival of patients with gallbladder cancer is related to stage and histologic type of cancer. Most of the long-term survivors have been patients with well-differentiated tumors that were minimally invasive and usually found incidentally after cholecystectomy (Fig. 98-1).

Clinical Manifestations

Signs and symptoms of gallbladder cancer are nonspecific and mimic symptoms of cholelithiasis and cholecystitis. Lack of specific signs and symptoms explains the delay in diagnosis of most patients with gallbladder cancer. Pain is the most common initial complaint. The pattern of the pain is nonspecific; it may be dull and aching, colicky, sharp, constant or intermittent, and it may or may not radiate to the back. Other symptoms include nausea, vomiting, anorexia, and weight loss. There is often jaundice, hepatomegaly, a palpable mass, or ascites. Jaundice develops in 30% to 60% of patients and is a poor prognostic sign because it is caused by extension of the tumor beyond the gallbladder, with obstruction of the extrahepatic bile ducts; 85% of patients with jaundice have unresectable tumors.[5] The patients may also have obstruction of the duodenum or colon. Malignant cholecystoenteric fistula may be the first indication of gallbladder cancer.

Diagnosis

Laboratory findings are not diagnostic but are related to abnormalities associated with bile duct obstruction. Patients frequently have increased alkaline phosphatase and bilirubin levels. Blood levels of carcinoembryonic antigen (CEA) or CA-19, another tumor marker, may also be elevated. These findings are not diagnostic because they may have other causes.

Diagnostic techniques include oral cholecystography, ultrasonography, computed tomography scan, and possibly a magnetic resonance scan. The most widely employed diagnostic study for biliary tract disease is ultrasound. The findings on ultrasonography that are suggestive, but not diagnostic, of gallbladder cancer include thickening of the wall, a mass projecting into the lumen, calcification of the gallbladder, multiple masses or a fixed mass in the gallbladder, a mass extending into the liver, or an extracholecystic mass. Only 8% to 16% of patients with gallbladder cancer have correct preoperative diagnoses.[5]

Treatment

Eighty percent of patients with gallbladder cancer are found to have unresectable disease at the time of operation. The correct preoperative diagnosis is uncommon; almost all patients are operated on for a presumptive diagnosis of chronic cholecystitis. Of patients who are operated on and are found to have gallbladder cancer, 60% to 80% are dead 1 year after surgery; the median survival time is 5.2 months.[16] Five-year survival rates range between 1% and 6%. However, in certain patients, surgical resection can provide cure. Between 15% and 25% of patients have early gallbladder cancer (stage I) that is usually found incidentally at the time of cholecystectomy, and this group comprises most of the patients who are cured. Advanced age should not deter resection.[17]

The extent of surgical resection is still a point of controversy. It is not clear that extensive surgical resection provides

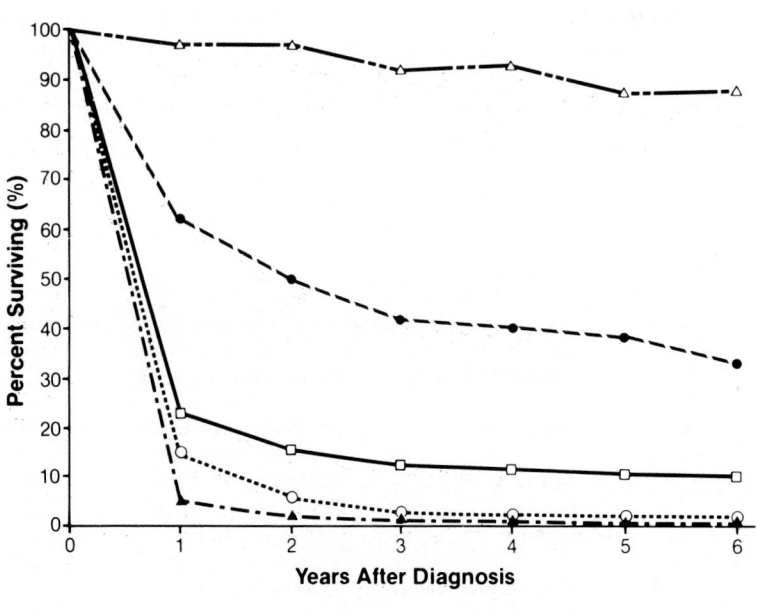

FIGURE 98-1. Gallbladder cancer survival rates by stage in all races and genders from 1973 to 1981. (From Albores-Saavedra J, Henson DE. Tumors of the gallbladder and extrahepatic bile ducts. Atlas of tumor pathology. Washington DC: Armed Forces Institute of Pathology, 1986:110.)

improved survival. Radical cholecystectomy is defined as cholecystectomy plus a wedge excision of the liver (i.e., gallbladder fossa) and regional lymphadenectomy. Recommendations for radical surgical procedures beyond simple cholecystectomy are based on small numbers of patients. Ouchi and colleagues found that 7 patients with stage I or II cancers survived 5 years after radical cholecystectomy, but 4 patients treated by cholecystectomy alone did not.[18] There are no data from prospective trials with large numbers of patients to suggest that radical resections significantly improve survival.

Right hepatic lobectomy or trisegmentectomy are radical operations but may not provide radical disease-free margins because of the extent of tumor and are rarely indicated for gallbladder cancer. Patients with stage I cancers can be cured by cholecystectomy; some patients with stage II and early stage III cancers may be cured by radical cholecystectomy; but patients with more advanced cancers are not cured even with extended resections. Extensive resection for early-stage tumors is not required, and advanced tumors are not cured by extensive resection. Survival is related to extent of disease at the time of diagnosis rather than the extent of resection.

If gallbladder cancer is grossly apparent at the time of operation, survival is limited; if cancer is found only on opening the specimen or by microscopic examination, survival is good. The finding of incidental cancer in a cholecystectomy specimen raises a difficult question for management. If incidental gallbladder cancer is found after cholecystectomy, the question of reoperation and radical cholecystectomy is raised, and the data from reported series do not provide a definitive answer.[5,19–23] However, the consensus appears to be that reoperation is not required for stage I patients, it should be performed for stage II patients and stage III patients with minimal liver invasion, and it provides no additional benefit for stage III or IV patients.

Chemotherapy is experimental and is not very helpful. Although some gallbladder cancers may be radiosensitive, radiation therapy provides little survival benefit because of the extent of tumor at the time of diagnosis. Palliation of jaundice has been reported, and intraoperative irradiation may be beneficial.[24,25] Although these types of treatments should be considered, their role has not been defined.

CARCINOMA OF THE BILE DUCTS

Incidence

Cancers of the bile ducts are less common than tumors of the gallbladder. The incidence of bile duct cancers is difficult to determine precisely because, in most cancer registries, reports of incidence and survival statistics from these cancers are usually included with liver and gallbladder cancers.[26]

There are striking differences between cancer of the extrahepatic bile duct and cancer of the gallbladder (Table 98-2). Cancer of the bile duct is somewhat more common in males, fewer than 20% of cases are associated with stone disease, the median age of patients is about 10 years younger, and no racial or geographic differences in incidence and mortality are found. The diagnosis of these tumors is often difficult. As many as 20% of patients have had prior biliary tract operations without a definitive diagnosis having being made. No specific etiologic agent has been identified for bile duct cancer, but there are certain important associations.

Etiology

Cancers may arise in the intrahepatic or extrahepatic bile ducts. There is no association of bile duct cancer with cirrhosis. However, differences in anatomic distribution may be associated with specific etiologic agents. Most intrahepatic bile duct cancers occur in China and South East Asia and are associated with chronic infestation with liver flukes.[27] Other conditions associated with cancer of the bile duct include primary sclerosing cholangitis (PSC), chronic ulcerative colitis, and congenital anomalies. The most commonly reported congenital anomaly associated with bile duct cancer is Caroli's disease, which may be considered a premalignant lesion.[28] No convincing evidence has linked carcinogens or drugs to bile duct cancers.

Patients with chronic ulcerative colitis have an increased incidence of bile duct cancer, but the cause of hepatobiliary disease in these patients is unknown. Several characteristics of patients with chronic ulcerative colitis who develop bile

---

TABLE 98-2
Comparison of Gallbladder and Bile Duct Cancer

CHARACTERISTICS	GALLBLADDER CANCER	BILE DUCT CANCER
Distribution	Worldwide; high incidence in Mexico, India, Israel	Worldwide; high incidence in Southeast Asia
Age	Middle to old	Old
Gender	Female	Both
Etiology	Stones	Liver flukes, inflammatory bowel disease, congenital anomalies
Precancerous changes	Inflammation	Adenomatous hyperplasia
Histologic type	Adenocarcinoma	Adenocarcinoma
Marker	Carcinoembryonic antigen	Carcinoembryonic antigen
Course and death	Carcinomatosis	Obstruction, sepsis, carcinomatosis

Adapted from Anthony PP, In: Preece PC, Cuscheri A, Rosin RD, eds. Cancer of the bile ducts and pancreas. Philadelphia: WB Saunders, 1989:4.

duct cancer are not found in patients who develop bile duct cancer not associated with ulcerative colitis; these include a younger age, absence of gallstones, and a long history (>15 years) of severe pancolitis.[29] Ritchie and associates estimated that these tumors occur 10 times more frequently in patients with chronic ulcerative colitis than in the general population.[29]

In the past, it was thought that chronic ulcerative colitis caused bile duct cancers, but the modern consensus is that PSC predisposes patients with chronic ulcerative colitis to bile duct cancers.[30] PSC is a disease of unknown cause that is characterized by inexorably progressive inflammation and fibrosis of the intrahepatic and extrahepatic bile ducts, which invariably leads to obliteration of the bile ducts. Secondary biliary cirrhosis is the end result.

PSC can create a diagnostic and therapeutic dilemma and may obscure the diagnosis of bile duct cancer. Five of 55 patients undergoing orthotopic liver transplantation for PSC were found to have unrecognized cholangiocarcinoma in the recipients' livers after removal.[31] LaRusso and colleagues have emphasized that the radiographic diagnosis of PSC is based on demonstration of multifocal strictures associated with irregularity and tortuosity of extrahepatic and intrahepatic bile ducts.[32,33] Although in some patients PSC may present a difficult diagnostic problem, PSC occurs primarily in young men (75%); more than two thirds are younger than 45 years of age at the time of diagnosis.[29,30]

There is no evidence that proctocolectomy has any beneficial effect on the course of PSC in patients with chronic ulcerative colitis, and proctocolectomy therefore has no protective effect against subsequent development of bile duct cancer.[34] Bile duct cancer may occur years after total proctocolectomy. Endoscopic retrograde cholangiopancreatography (ERCP) by no means ensures that the diagnosis of PSC without bile duct cancer can be made. This is a diagnostic problem for patients with end-stage PSC who are referred for transplantation. Cholangiocarcinoma may be masked by PSC. Patients with cholangiocarcinoma appear to have worse survival than patients with other types of malignancies undergoing orthotopic liver transplantation.[35]

Choledochal cysts or other cystic disease of the biliary tract (e.g., Caroli's disease) is associated with a high incidence of subsequent bile duct cancer. The treatment of choice for choledochal cysts is complete excision, not drainage.

Pathology

Benign and malignant tumors occur in the bile ducts. Benign tumors are uncommon, and most information about them comes from case reports. The most common benign tumor of the bile duct is an adenoma. Adenomas may be single, multiple, tubular, papillary, or mixed. Histologically, adenomas of the bile ducts are no different from those of the gallbladder. One fourth of the tumors occur in the proximal bile ducts. Tumors may recur after local resection. Multicentricity has been reported but is not common. Cystadenoma and granular cell tumors are rare benign tumors of the extrahepatic bile ducts. Cystadenomas are similar to and may coexist with cystadenomas of the liver and pancreas.[36] Granular cell tumors are unusual, occur most commonly in black women, and may be associated with granular cell tumors at

other sites.[37,38] The malignant potential of these lesions is unknown. Reported benign mesenchymal tumors include fibromas, lipomas, leiomyomas, and neurilemomas.

Most benign tumors are found because the patients present with jaundice resulting from obstruction by the tumor. No radiographic or ultrasonographic characteristics allow preoperative diagnosis of benign bile duct tumors. The diagnosis is made at operation, and treatment by complete local resection is usually successful. Occasionally, because of anatomic location, incomplete excision is necessary, and the tumor may recur.

Papillomatosis is a rare condition in which multiple papillary lesions involving a large amount of the bile duct mucosa may be encountered. Because malignant transformation or progression to invasive carcinoma has been reported, papillomatosis of the bile duct mucosa should be considered a premalignant lesion.[39,40] This lesion should be treated by complete excision if possible; if not, regrowth is common.

Malignant tumors of the bile duct include malignant epithelial tumors and malignant mesenchymal tumors.[9] Because few sarcomas of the bile ducts have been reported, definitive information is not available on treatment or prognosis.

Bile duct cancer can be categorized by anatomic location. The tumors may occur in intrahepatic ducts (i.e., cholangiocarcinoma), at the confluence of the right and left hepatic duct (i.e., Klatskin tumor), or anywhere in the extrahepatic bile duct below the confluence. Tompkins and associates reported that the distribution of extrahepatic bile duct cancers is 49% in the upper third, 25% in the middle third, 19% in the lower third of the duct; 7% of these cancers were diffuse.[41] Altemeier and colleagues found that bile duct tumors arising at the confluence of the hepatic ducts had an insidious course and could be mistaken for benign strictures.[42]

In 1965, Klatskin called attention to distinctive features of bile duct cancer that arose at the confluence of the right and left hepatic ducts.[43] He observed that patients with these tumors had classic initial symptoms of extrahepatic biliary obstruction and that, because of the unusual location, the tumor was often overlooked, even at operation. The tumors grossly and microscopically resembled localized scars, and the tumors tended to be smaller and remained sharply localized. They seldom metastasized, and patients ultimately died from hepatocellular failure or cholangitis.

Grossly, the bile duct cancers can be divided into three types: polypoid or nodular masses, sclerosing, and diffusely infiltrating. Some cancers may present as only a thickening of the bile duct wall, which appears to be involved in dense fibrous scar. Polypoid or papillary cancers have the best prognosis. Histologic classification of adenocarcinomas of the bile duct include well-differentiated, pleomorphic giant cell, adenosquamous, oat cell, and colloid carcinoma.

The sequence of dysplasia to invasive bile duct cancer has been described.[44,45] Davis and associates found that dysplastic epithelium and cancers express cytoplasmic staining for CEA, but normal epithelium does not.[46] There have been no reports of the extent of dysplastic epithelium within the intrahepatic bile ducts in patients with bile duct cancer. Because dysplasia progresses to carcinoma, these studies are desperately needed. Bile duct cancers have a tendency to spread along the bile duct. The longitudinal extent of cancers along the bile duct is often difficult to determine by gross examination. Shimada and colleagues examined 29 cases by histologic examination after resection and found that the mean distance of microscopic invasion beyond the gross margin was 16.8 mm toward the liver and 6.5 mm toward the duodenum.[47]

Histologic diagnosis of malignant bile duct cancers may be difficult at times. Very-well-differentiated cancers with little invasion are difficult to differentiate from the bile duct involved in scar formation. As Albores-Saavedra and Henson observed, cancers arising in the proximal segment of the extrahepatic bile ducts tend to be better differentiated with more sclerotic stroma that contains chronic inflammatory cells.[9] Bile duct cancers may be difficult to differentiate from PSC. Perineural invasion (i.e., malignant cells within nerve sheaths), a prominent feature of bile duct cancers, is not present in PSC and is the single most important diagnostic criterion of malignancy. Other problems in differential diagnosis occur with cancers of the lower bile duct that involve the ampulla, duodenum, and pancreas. Because all of these sites may give rise to malignant tumors with similar characteristics, it may be difficult to conclusively determine site of origin. Important points to be considered are that bile duct cancers do not often metastasize widely, unlike pancreatic cancers.

Bile duct cancers usually spread by direct extension to involve adjacent organs and tissues. Proximal cancers may directly invade the liver. Cancers in the common bile duct or cystic duct may directly invade the gallbladder. Regional lymph node metastases are common, but isolated liver metastases or distant metastases usually are not found. Most patients who die of bile duct cancer do so from progressive hepatic failure. The extent of cancer or stage at the time of diagnosis is the most important determinant of prognosis. A TNM staging system of extrahepatic bile duct cancer (excluding intrahepatic bile duct cancers and cancers of the ampulla of Vater) has been developed.[15] However, this staging classification has not been widely used, and most reports do not include staging information.

Clinical Manifestations

Symptoms of bile duct cancer are nonspecific gastrointestinal complaints that include nausea, vomiting, anorexia, and weight loss. Pain is rare without stones. Painless jaundice is the most prominent sign and is the usual presentation of patients with bile duct cancers. Bilirubin and alkaline phosphatase are usually elevated. There are no specific laboratory abnormalities for bile duct cancers. A diagnostic dilemma may occur if the physician is faced with a jaundiced patient with bile duct stricture who has gallstones. The level of bilirubin elevation may aid in the differential diagnosis. Patients with gallstones rarely have bilirubin levels over 8 mg/dL, but bilirubin levels greater than 12 mg/dL are usually found in patients with malignant obstructions.

Diagnosis

Ultrasonography is the most important initial diagnostic test for anyone who presents with jaundice. The finding of dilated intrahepatic bile ducts with normal distal ductal system in the absence of stones is highly suggestive of extrahepatic bile

duct cancer. Ultrasonography may also provide information about the portal vein and may demonstrate enlarged lymph nodes. Unfortunately, many cases are not so clear-cut. Endoscopic ultrasonography may help to determine the extent of tumor involvement.[48]

The definitive diagnostic test is percutaneous transhepatic cholangiography performed with a fine needle (Fig. 98-2). This allows precise definition of the anatomic location and extent of the obstructing lesion. It also allows collection of bile for cytologic examination and can be used as a guide for fine-needle aspiration of a mass for cytologic examination. Cholangiography may aid in determining whether the cancer is resectable. Bilateral involvement of the secondary branches of the intrahepatic bile ducts or multiple areas (bilobar) of intrahepatic involvement preclude curative resection. The length of the stricture of the extrahepatic bile duct is not helpful in determining resectability. ERCP is less useful in evaluating patients with bile duct cancers. It can define only the anatomy of the bile ducts distal to the point of obstruction and provides no information on proximal bile duct anatomy or extent of the cancer. However, ERCP is required to make the diagnosis of PSC.

All patients without cholangiographic evidence of unresectable cancer should have preoperative hepatic arteriography and careful study of the portal vein, particularly with hilar bile duct cancers. The information obtained from these studies is vital for determining resectability. The portal venous system is more difficult to delineate than the hepatic arterial system, but the use of digital subtraction angiography or injection of contrast into the splenic and superior mesenteric arteries or transhepatic portal venography may provide excellent visualization of the portal vein and its branches. Obstruction of the main portal vein or of one of the major portal venous branches in the porta hepatis usually means unresectability.[49]

Blumgart described the indicators of unresectable bile duct cancers: intrahepatic bile duct spread, involvement of the main trunk of the portal vein, involvement of both branches of the portal vein or bilateral involvement of the hepatic artery and portal vein, or a combination of vascular involvement on one side of the liver with extensive cholangiographic involvement on the other.[50] Information obtained from cholangiography and hepatic arteriography allows determination of extent of the tumor, which may determine resectability, and allows assessment of the size of the lobes of the liver. Lobar atrophy is important to recognize, because drainage of that segment would not relieve jaundice.

The disadvantage of biliary drainage before operation has been firmly established. Most patients with bile duct cancer do not have infected bile, although as many as 30% may have bacteria at the time of diagnosis.[51] It is important to obtain cultures at the time of percutaneous cholangiography so that patients with infected bile can be identified and antibiotic sensitivity of the bacteria can be determined. Indwelling foreign bodies in the form of percutaneous or endoprosthetic drainage catheters significantly increase the incidence of infected bile. The role of preoperative biliary decompression, percutaneously or using an endoprosthesis, should no longer be controversial. Three prospective, randomized trials have shown conclusively that preoperative biliary decompression does not decrease operative morbidity or mortality.[52–54] These studies have shown that infectious complications and bile leak

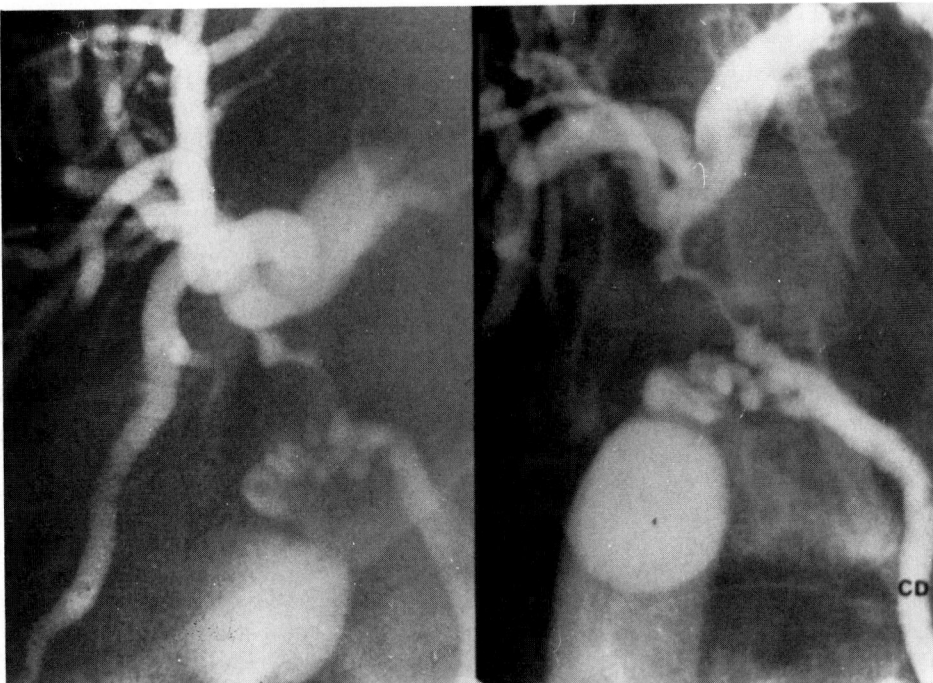

FIGURE 98-2. Cholangiogram shows Klatskin's tumor. The intrahepatic bile ducts are dilated, and the size of the common bile duct (CD) is normal.

are significantly increased in patients with prolonged preoperative biliary drainage. The inflammatory reaction to the catheter within and around the bile ducts increases the difficulty of an already difficult surgical operation. There is no place for preoperative biliary decompression in the management of patients with bile duct cancers.

Treatment

The two objectives in treatment of patients with bile duct cancers are to cure the patient of tumor and to relieve bile duct obstruction by establishing biliary-enteric drainage to prevent hepatic failure. To accomplish both these goals, resection is required. In patients with unresectable cancers, palliative decompression of the bile ducts should be performed to restore biliary-enteric bile flow.

Resections may be local or extensive; the extent of resection is usually dictated by the site of origin of the bile duct cancer. Because of the different types of resection required, it is useful to describe the treatment options by anatomic site: intrahepatic cancers, cancers that arise at the confluence of the bile ducts (i.e., Klatskin tumor), cancers that involve the midportion of the bile ducts, and cancers in the distal bile duct. Intrahepatic cancers require hepatic resection. Local resection alone or combined with hepatic resection can be employed for Klatskin tumors. For middle duct cancers, complete excision of the extrahepatic bile duct, cholecystectomy, and regional lymphadenectomy, followed by hepaticojejunostomy is the procedure of choice. For distal bile duct cancers, pancreaticoduodenal resection, with preservation of the pylorus, is employed.

With systematic preoperative diagnostic evaluation, proper diagnosis should be made, resectability should be determined, and optimal treatment for each patient should be carried out.

However, the final determination of resectability is made by surgical exploration. All patients who do not have unequivocal cholangiographic or arteriographic evidence of unresectable cancer and whose general condition is fit should undergo operative exploration with the intent to cure.

Treatment of Klatskin tumors is curative or palliative. Curative treatment is defined as complete extirpation of tumor with tumor-free margins that are verified histologically. Because most local resections do not provide adequate tumor-free margins, they should be considered palliative. Patients with histologically verified tumor-free margins live significantly longer than patients with tumor at the resection margin.[55–57] The median survival of patients with tumor-free margin is 3 to 3.4 years, compared with a median survival of 1 to 1.2 years for patients with disease at the resection margins. Three factors are responsible for local recurrence: the intimate association of the bile ducts with hepatic parenchyma, hepatic artery, and portal vein; microscopic extension of tumor along the bile duct beyond gross tumor margin; and epithelial dysplasia. The latter two factors have been inadequately studied.

Only by careful analysis of the extent of microscopic tumor invasion and epithelial dysplasia will we ever be able to determine if certain resections are possible. Unfortunately, no prospective randomized trials have compared different forms of treatment, curative or palliative, because these are uncommon lesions, and most reports extend over long periods with small numbers of patients. Because of the anatomic location of Klatskin tumors, the cancers of most patients are unresectable.[45] The operative mortality rate for local resections is low (range, 0%–3%); the operative mortality rate for hepatic resection is about 11% (range, 0%–22%). In Blumgart's series of 48 patients, 27 patients had a mean survival times of 16 months, with 6 living beyond 3 years, 5 beyond 5 years, and 3 beyond 10 years.[45] Eight of 10 patients with a mean survival of 66 months had undergone major hepatic resection. Others have reported similar results in small series of patients.[50,51,58–63] Overall, for patients who have had Klatskin tumors resected, a 30% 3-year survival rate and a 12% 5-year survival rate can be anticipated, although Iida and associates report a 29.8% 5-year survival rate for 23 patients treated by hepatic resection.[64] Patients who have their cancers resected live longer than those whose tumors are not resected (Fig. 98-3).

Cancers that involve the middle of the bile ducts are treated by resection and biliary-enteric anastomosis. Tompkins and colleagues have reported no operative mortality and a 12% 5-year survival rate for patients with midduct cancers.[38] In contrast, cancers of the lower third of the bile duct require pancreatoduodenectomy (i.e., Whipple operation) for treatment, and the operative mortality rate for these patients was reported as 6%, with a 28% 5-year survival rate.[38] Langer and associates have shown that papillary tumor type, absence of lymph node metastases, and tumor-free margins are the most important determinations of prolonged survival, regardless of anatomic location.[53]

The objectives of palliative treatment are to relieve jaundice and to restore bile flow into the intestine. Palliation can be performed by direct surgical anastomosis of an intestinal loop to a dilated duct proximal to the obstruction or by external or internal intubation of the bile duct. Biliary drainage relieves symptomatic jaundice and improves the metabolic status of the patient for the few months of remaining life. If there is obstruction of the confluence of the ducts, jaundice may be relieved by biliary-enteric anastomosis to the bile duct draining segment III of the left liver, using the technique described by Bismuth and Corlette, or by operative or percutaneous intubation techniques.[65] Assessment of results for patients who have been surgically bypassed and those who have been bypassed by intubation is difficult. Any form of intubation leads to an increased incidence of cholangitis.

The highest rates of successful relief of jaundice and lowest incidence of cholangitis are achieved with biliary-enteric anastomosis, compared with intubation techniques, regardless of location of the tumor.[53,56,66–72] The 30-day mortality rates and lengths of survival are similar. Success rates for relief of jaundice of 73% to 75% and rates of cholangitis of 13% to 26% have been reported for surgical bypass, compared with 50% to 60% and 26% to 56%, respectively, for intubation. The 30-day operative mortality rate is between 7% and 15%, compared with 30-day mortality rates of 14% to 20% after intubation. Unless patients have significant associated diseases, extensive tumor metastases, or obstruction of intrahepatic ducts with atrophy of the left liver so that segment III bypass could not be considered, all patients with Klatskin tumors should undergo operation.

The U-tube technique, popularized by Terblanche, employs a special tube inserted through a choledochotomy below the tumor and passed through the tumor and out through the surface of the liver and the anterior abdominal wall.[73] The lower limb of the tube is also brought out through the abdominal wall. Appropriately placed side holes in the tube allow bile to drain into the gut. This type of tube can be changed at intervals if obstruction from encrustations occurs and may also be used to deliver internal radiation therapy (i.e., brachytherapy). An alternative form of palliative intubation is internal drainage by percutaneous transhepatic placement of an external tube or an endoprosthesis.[61,63] Palliative intubation is not without problems. The 30-day mortality ranges between 20% and 30%, and survival averages between 3 and 6 months.

For patients who are not operative candidates, percutaneous or endoscopic intubation techniques may be employed. In patients with hilar tumors, endoscopic intubation is successful in only 42% to 55%, of patients compared with the 80% to 100% success rates for percutaneous transhepatic intubation.[61,62]

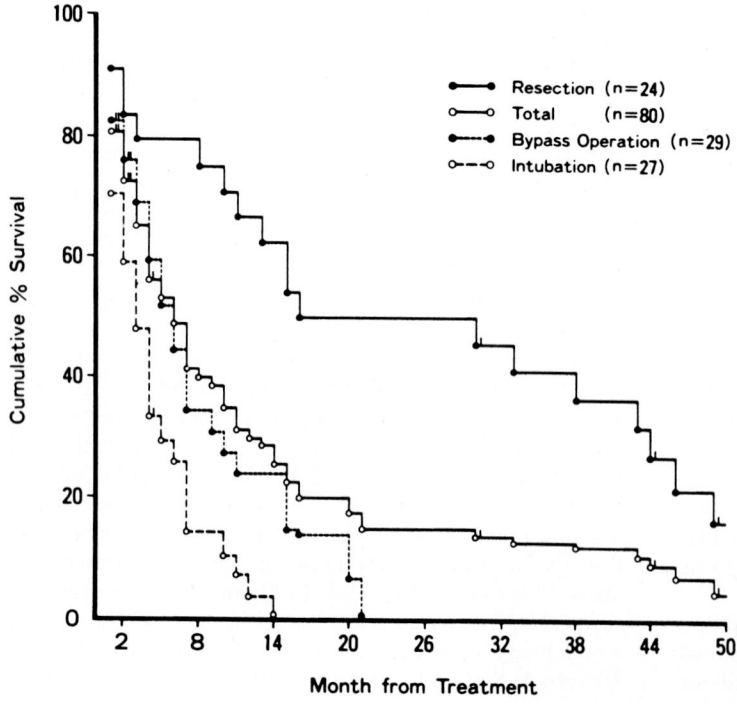

FIGURE 98-3. Cumulative survival curves for patients with bile duct cancer. (From Miyazaki K, Nagafuchi K, Nakayama F. Bypass procedure for bile duct cancer. World J Surg 1988;12:64.)

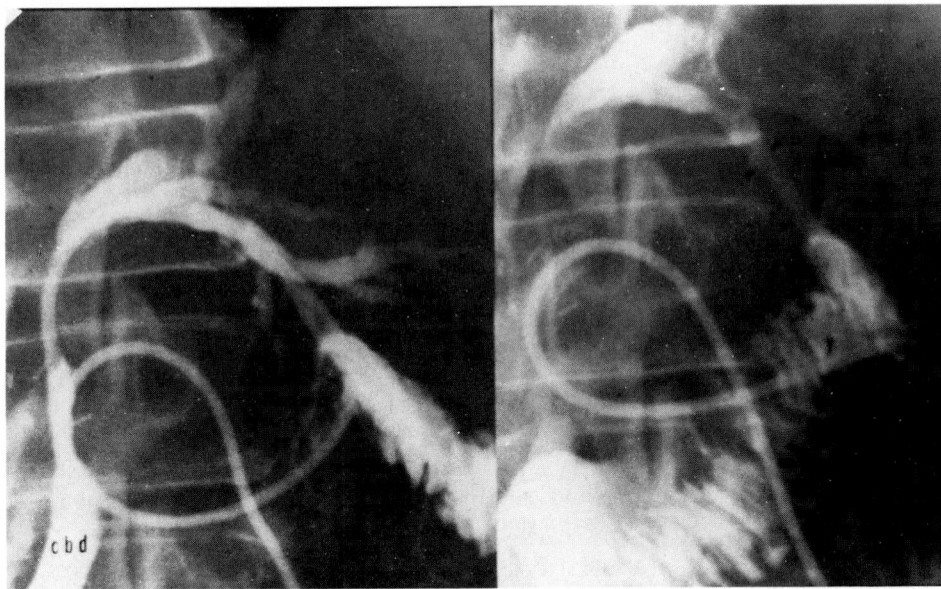

FIGURE 98-4. A catheter was placed through the anastamosis for brachy therapy (left panel). After removal of the catheter, the common bile duct (CBD; right panel, *arrows*) can be seen.

For patients in whom curative resection is impossible, palliative radiation therapy has been employed. In patients without metastatic disease, external beam irradiation significantly prolongs survival. Intraoperative radiotherapy may also be helpful.[74–76] The most successful techniques of radiotherapy employ a combination of brachytherapy with external beam irradiation. Hayes and colleagues reported that 24 patients treated in a nonrandomized study with this combination of radiation therapy had a significantly prolonged survival (12.8 months versus 2.0 months) compared with patients who received only palliative radiation therapy.[77] They found that complications, including cholangitis, hemorrhage, abscess, and gastrointestinal ulceration, were more common in patients treated using this technique for definitive radiation therapy but that recurrent biliary obstruction was prevented. Others have shown that this form of radiation therapy may provide significant palliation.[78–80] Figure 98-4 shows the radiograph of a patient with an unresectable Klatskin tumor treated by a segment III hepaticojejunostomy and brachytherapy combined with external radiation therapy. The role of adjuvant brachytherapy after resection or brachytherapy for palliation of unresectable disease has yet to be determined. Intraoperative radiation therapy may also be useful.[44,81]

Chemotherapy for bile duct cancer has not provided significant prolongation of survival. Oberfield and Rossi reviewed published studies, which included 97 patients treated by a variety of chemotherapeutic agents alone or in combination.[82] Partial responses occurred in 29% of patients without significant prolongation of survival.

Hepatic transplantation may provide long-term survival for patients with bile duct cancer, although not all reports agree.[32,58,83] Hepatic transplantation is limited to patients with unresectable bile duct cancers without evidence of extrahepatic spread.

Treatment of cancer of the extraheptic bile ducts is entering an era of new optimism based on the development over the last 15 years of significant experience with management of these uncommon cancers. As with all other cancers, complete removal offers the only chance for survival. Because preoperative preparation techniques, operative and postoperative care, and surgical techniques have improved significantly, operative mortality has decreased progressively, and long-term patient survival has increased. Despite these advances, significant improvement in survival will continue to elude us until techniques for early detection are developed.

The location of the cancer in the bile duct is the single most important determinant of resectability and potential for cure. Twenty percent to 30% of proximal bile duct tumors can be resected, but 60% to 70% of cancers arising from the distal two thirds of the bile duct are resectable. For patients in whom resection is not possible, operative biliary-enteric bypass, with restoration of bile flow, offers the best form of long-term palliation. This may result in relief of jaundice and prevention of cholangitis and hepatic failure.

New techniques in radiation therapy and new approaches to chemotherapy must be evaluated to determine their role in treatment of patients with unresectable bile duct cancers. Hepatic transplantation may offer a significant opportunity for cure of patients with otherwise unresectable bile duct cancers.

> The reader is directed to Chapter 95, Gallbladder and Biliary Tree: Anatomy and Structural Anomalies; Chapter 97, Diseases of the Biliary Tree; and Chapter 117, Endoscopic Retrograde Cholangiopancreatography, Endoscopic Sphincterotomy and Stone Removal, and Endoscopic Biliary and Pancreatic Drainage.

REFERENCES

1. Silverberg E, Lubera JA. Cancer statistics, 1989. CA 1989; 39:3.
2. Diehl AK, Beral V. Cholecystectomy and changing mortality from gallbladder cancer. Lancet 1981;2:187.

3. Strom BL, Nelson WL, Henson DE, et al. Carcinoma of the gallbladder. In: Cohen S, Soloway RD, eds. Gallstones. New York: Churchill Livingstone, 1985:275.

4. Nervi F, Duarte I, Gomez G, et al. Frequency of gallbladder cancer in Chile, a high-risk area. Int J Cancer 1988;41:657.

5. Piehler JM, Crichlow RW. Primary carcinoma of the gallbladder. Surg Gynecol Obstet 1978;147:929.

6. Diehl AK. Gallstone size and the risk of gallbladder cancer. JAMA 1983;250:2323.

7. Maringhini A, Moreau JA, Melton LJ, et al. Gallstones, gallbladder cancer, and other gastrointestinal malignancies. An epidemiologic study in Rochester, Minnesota. Ann Intern Med 1987;107:30.

8. Glenn F, Hays DM. The scope of radical surgery in the treatment of malignant tumors of the extrahepatic biliary tract. Surg Gynecol Obstet 1954;99:529.

9. Albores-Saavedra J, Henson DE, eds. Tumors of the gallbladder and extrahepatic bile ducts. Atlas of tumor pathology, 2nd series. Washington: Armed Forces Institute of Pathology, 1986.

10. Nagata E, Sakai K, Kinoshita H, Kobayashi Y. The relation between carcinoma of the gallbladder and an anomalous connection between the choledochus and the pancreatic duct. Ann Surg 1985;202:182.

11. Misra SP, Gulati P, Thorat VK, et al. Pancreaticobiliary ductal union in biliary diseases. An endoscopic retrograde cholangiopancreatographic study. Gastroenterology 1989;96:907.

12. Neugut AI, Wylie P, Brandt-Rauf PW. Occupational cancers of the gastrointestinal tract. II. Pancreas, liver, and biliary tract. Occup Med 1987;2:137.

13. Caygill C, Hill M, Kirkham J, Northfield TC. Increased risk of biliary tract cancer following gastric surgery. Br J Cancer 1988;57:434.

14. Nevin JE, Moran TJ, Kay S, King R. Carcinoma of the gallbladder. Staging, treatment and prognosis. Cancer 1976;37:141.

15. Beahrs OH, Henson DE, Hutter RVP, Myers MH, eds. Manual for staging of cancer. 3rd ed. Philadelphia: JB Lippincott, 1988.

16. Do Carmo M, Perpetuo O, Valdivieso M, et al. Natural history study of gallbladder cancer. A review of 36 years experience at M.D. Anderson Hospital and Tumor Institute. Cancer 1978;42:330.

17. Saunders K, Tompkins R, Longmire W Jr, Roslyn J. Bile duct carcinoma in the elderly. Arch Surg 1991;126:1186.

18. Ouchi K, Owada Y, Matsuno S, Sato T. Prognostic factors in the surgical treatment of gallbladder carcinoma. Surgery 1987;101:731.

19. Morrow CE, Sutherland DER, Florack G, et al. Primary gallbladder carcinoma: significance of subserosal lesions and results of aggressive surgical treatment and adjuvant chemotherapy. Surgery 1983;94:709.

20. Roberts JW, Daugherty SF. Primary carcinoma of the gallbladder. Surg Clin North Am 1986;66:743.

21. Wanebo HJ, Castle WN, Fechner RE. Is carcinoma of the gallbladder a curable lesion? Ann Surg 1982;195:624.

22. Ram MD. Carcinoma of the gallbladder. Surg Gynecol Obstet 1971;132:1044.

23. Tsunoda T, Tsuchiya R, Harada N, et al. The surgical treatment for carcinoma of the gallbladder—rationale of the second-look operation for inapparent carcinoma. Jpn J Surg 1987;17:478.

24. Todoroki T, Iwasaki Y, Orii K, et al. Resection combined with intraoperative radiation therapy (IORT) for stage IV (TNM) gallbladder carcinoma. World J Surg 1991;15:357.

25. Busse PM, Cady B, Bothe A Jr, et al. Intraoperative radiation therapy for carcinoma of the gallbladder. World J Surg 1991;15:352.

26. Cancer facts and figures. Atlanta: American Cancer Society, 1990:8.

27. Kurathong S, Lerdverasirikul P, Wongpaitoon V, et al. *Opisthorchis viverrini* infection and cholangiocarcinoma. Gastroenterology 1985;89:151.

28. Dayton MT, Longmire WP, Tompkins RK. Caroli's disease: a premalignant condition? Am J Surg 1983;145:41.

29. Ritchie JK, Allan RN, Macartney J, et al. Biliary tract carcinoma associated with ulcerative colitis. Q J Med 1974;43:263.

30. Ross AP, Braasch JW. Ulcerative colitis and carcinoma of the proximal bile ducts. Gut 1973;14:94.

31. Marsh JW Jr, Iwatsuki S, Makowka L, et al. Orthotopic liver transplantation for primary sclerosing cholangitis. Ann Surg 1988;207:21.

32. LaRusso NF, Wiesner RH, Ludwig J, MacCarty RL. Primary sclerosing cholangitis. N Engl J Med 1984;310:899.

33. Wiesner RH, Grambsch PM, Dickson ER, et al. Primary sclerosing cholangitis: natural history, prognostic factors and survival analysis. Hepatology 1989;10:430.

34. Cangemi JR, Wiesner RH, Beaver SJ, et al. Effect of proctocolectomy for chronic ulcerative colitis on the natural history of primary sclerosing cholangitis. Gastroenterology 1989;96:790.

35. O'Grady JG, Polson RJ, Rolles K, et al. Liver transplantation for malignant disease. Ann Surg 1988;207:373.

36. Keech MK. Cystadenomata of the pancreas and intrahepatic bile ducts. Gastroenterology 1951;19:568.

37. Assor D. Granular cell myoblastoma involving the common bile duct. Am J Surg 1979;137:674.

38. Manstein ME, McBrearty FX, Pellechia PE, Paskin DL. Granular cell tumor of the common bile duct. Dig Dis Sci 1981;26:938.

39. Helpap B. Malignant papillomatosis of the intrahepatic bile ducts. Acta Hepatogastroenterol 1977;24:419.

40. Neumann RD, LiVolsi VA, Rosenthal NS, et al. Adenocarcinoma in biliary papillomatosis. Gastroenterology 1976;70:779.

41. Tompkins RK, Thomas D, Wile A, Longmire WP Jr. Prognostic factors in bile duct carcinoma. Analysis of 96 cases. Ann Surg 1981;194:447.

42. Altemeier WA, Gall EA, Zinninger MM, Hoxworth PI. Sclerosing carcinoma of the major intrahepatic bile ducts. Arch Surg 1957;75:450.

43. Klatskin G. Adenocarcinoma of the hepatic duct at its bifurcation within the porta hepatis. An unusual tumor with distinctive clinical and pathological features. Am J Med 1965;38:241.

44. Laitio M. Carcinoma of extrahepatic bile ducts. A histopathologic study. Pathol Res Pract 1983;178:67.

45. Kurashina M, Kozuka S, Nakasima N, et al. Relationship of intrahepatic bile duct hyperplasia to cholangiocellular carcinoma. Cancer 1988;61:2469.

46. Davis RI, Sloan JM, Hood JM, Maxwell P. Carcinoma of the extrahepatic biliary tract: a clinicopathological and immunohistochemical study. Histopathology 1988;12:623.

47. Shimada H, Niimoto S, Matsuba A, et al. The infiltration of bile duct carcinoma along the bile duct wall. Int Surg 1988;73:87.

48. Tio TL, Cheng J, Wijers OB, et al. Endosonographic TNM stating of extrahepatic bile duct cancer: comparison with pathological staging. Gastroenterology 1991;100:1351.

49. Burchart F. Klatskin tumours. Acta Chir Scand [Suppl] 1988;541:63.

50. Blumgart LH. Cancer of the bile ducts. In: Blumgart LH, ed. Surgery of the liver and biliary tract. New York: Churchill Livingstone, 1988:829.

51. McPherson GAD, Blenkharn JI, Nathanson B, et al. Significance of bacteria in external biliary drainage systems: a possible role for antisepsis. J Clin Surg 1982;1:22.

52. Hatfield ARW, Terblanche J, Fataar S, et al. Preoperative external biliary drainage in obstructive jaundice. A prospective controlled clinical trial. Lancet 1982;2:896.

53. McPherson GAD, Benjamin IS, Hodgson HJF, et al. Pre-operative percutaneous transhepatic biliary drainage: the results of a controlled trial. Br J Surg 1984;71:371.

54. Pitt HA, Gomes AS, Lois JF, et al. Does preoperative percutaneous biliary drainage reduce operative risk or increase hospital cost? Ann Surg 1985;201:545.

55. Pinson CW, Rossi RL. Extended right hepatic lobectomy, left hepatic lobectomy, and skeltonization resection for proximal bile duct cancer. World J Surg 1988;12:52.

56. Iwasaki Y, Okamura T, Ozaki A, et al. Surgical treatment for carcinoma at the confluence of the major hepatic ducts. Surg Gynecol Obstet 1986;162:457.

57. Bengmark S, Ekberg H, Evander A, et al. Major liver resection for hilar cholangiocarcinoma. Ann Surg 1988;207:120.

58. Langer JC, Langer B, Taylor BR, et al. Carcinoma of the extrahepatic bile ducts: results of an aggressive surgical approach. Surgery 1985;98:752.

59. Skoog V, Thoren L. Carcinoma of the junction of the main hepatic ducts. Acta Chir Scand 1982;148:411.

60. Tsuzuki T, Ogata Y, Iida S, et al. Carcinoma of the bifurcation of the hepatic ducts. Arch Surg 1983;118:1147.

61. Bismuth H, Castaing D, Traynor O. Resection or palliation: priority of surgery in the treatment of hilar cancer. World J Surg 1988;12:39.

62. White TT. Skeletization resection and central hepatic resection in the treatment of bile duct cancer. World J Surg 1988;12:48.

63. Pichlmayr R, Ringe B, Lauchart W, et al. Radical resection and liver grafting as the two main components of surgical strategy in the treatment of proximal bile duct cancer. World J Surg 1988;12:68.

64. Iida S, Tsuzuki T, Ogata Y, et al. The long-term survival of patients with carcinoma of the main hepatic duct junction. Cancer 1987;60:1612.

65. Bismuth H, Corlette MB. Intrahepatic cholangioenteric anastomosis in carcinoma of the hilus of the liver. Surg Gynecol Obstet 1975;140:170.

66. Gibson RN, Yeung E, Hadjis N, et al. Percutaneous transhepatic endoprostheses for hilar cholangiocarcinoma. Am J Surg 1988;156:363.

67. Lameris JS, Stoker J, Dees J, Nix GAJJ, Van Blankenstein M, Jeekel J. Non-surgical palliative treatment of patients with malignant biliary obstruction—the place of endoscopic and percutaneous drainage. Clin Radiol 1987;38:603.

68. Cameron JL, Gayler BW, Zuidema GD. The use of Silastic transhepatic stents in benign and malignant biliary strictures. Ann Surg 1978;188:552.

69. Blumgart LH, Benjamin IS, Hadjis NS, Beazley R. Surgical approaches to cholangiocarcinoma at confluence of hepatic ducts. Lancet 1984;1:66.

70. Miyazaki K, Nagafuchi K, Nakayama F. Bypass procedure for bile duct cancer. World J Surg 1988;12:64.

71. Ottow RT, August DA, Sugarbaker PH. Treatment of proximal biliary tract carcinoma: an overview of techniques and results. Surgery 1985;97:251.

72. Malangoni MA, McCoy DM, Richardson JD, Flint LM. Effective palliation of malignant biliary duct obstruction. Ann Surg 1985;201:554.

73. Terblanche J, Saunders SG, Louw JW. Prolonged palliation in carcinoma of the main hepatic duct junction. Surgery 1972;71:720.

74. Grove MK, Hermann RE, Vogt DP, Broughan TA. Role of radiation after operative palliation in cancer of the proximal bile ducts. Am J Surg 1991;161:454.

75. Busse PM, Stone MD, Sheldon TA, et al. Intraoperative radiation therapy for biliary tract carcinoma: results of a 5-year experience. Surgery 1989;105:724.

76. Wolkov HB, Graves GM, Won M, et al. Intraoperative radiation therapy of extrahepatic biliary carcinoma: a report of RTOG-8506. Am J Clin Oncol 1992;15:323.

77. Hayes JK Jr, Sapozink MD, Miller FJ. Definitive radiation therapy in bile duct carcinoma. Int J Radiat Oncol Biol Phys 1988;15:735.

78. Gibby DG, Hanks JB, Wanebow JH, et al. Bile duct carcinoma. Diagnosis and treatment. Ann Surg 1985;202:139.

79. Jones RS, Chitwood WF, Heaston DK, Herskovic AM. The combined use of percutaneous transhepatic drainage and irradiation for carcinoma of the extrahepatic bile ducts. Contemp Surg 1983;22:59.

80. Meyers WC, Jones RS. Internal radiation for bile duct cancer. World J Surg 1988;12:99.

81. Deziel DJ, Kiel KD, Kramer TS, et al. Intraoperative radiation therapy in biliary tract cancer. Am Surg 1988;54:402.

82. Oberfield RA, Rossi RL. The role of chemotherapy in the treatment of bile duct cancer. World J Surg 1988;12:105.

83. Ringe B, Wittekind C, Bechstein WO, et al. The role of liver transplantation in hepatobiliary malignancy. A retrospective analysis of 95 patients with particular regard to tumor stage and recurrence. Ann Surg 1989;209:88.

Textbook of Gastroenterology, second edition, edited by Tadataka Yamada. JB Lippincott Company, Philadelphia © 1995.

CHAPTER 99

Postcholecystectomy Syndrome

Rama P. Venu   Joseph E. Geenen

Cholecystectomy is associated with an excellent therapeutic outcome.[1] A few patients, however, continue to have a variety of gastrointestinal symptoms. The term used to describe this condition, *postcholecystectomy syndrome* (PCS), is a misnomer because the event of cholecystectomy has almost nothing to do with the symptom complex seen in most of these patients. It is doubtful that PCS represents a specific clinical entity.[2]

The reported incidence of PCS varies widely. Approximately 20% to 40% of patients who have had a cholecystectomy complain of abdominal pain or dyspepsia.[2] In most of these patients, symptoms may be mild and transient, but severe and disabling symptoms persist in 2% to 10% of patients.[3-5]

Despite voluminous reports published in the past three decades, PCS continues to haunt the patient and the physician. Our lack of understanding about this clinical syndrome stems chiefly from the gross discrepancy in the accepted criteria of definition, diagnostic evaluation, and management of PCS. The emergence of endoscopic retrograde cholangiopancreatography (ERCP) and sphincter of Oddi (SO) manometry has contributed significantly to the identification of patients with definite biliary tract disorders among the patients with PCS. It has also rekindled interest in the pathophysiology of SO dysfunction. Ambiguous and ill-defined as it may be, clinicians have learned to live with the clinical entity of PCS, necessitating a comprehensive review.

CLASSIFICATION

Patients with PCS form a heterogeneous group with a spectrum of signs and symptoms. Although few patients have symptoms attributable to problems related to cholecystectomy, many may have symptoms unrelated to biliary tract surgery. For systematic evaluation, patients with symptoms attributable to PCS can be classified into three groups: those with symptoms of nonbiliary tract origin, those with symptoms of functional gastrointestinal disorders with or without psychiatric problems, and those with symptoms of biliary tract origin.

Some patients with PCS may have symptoms originating from the esophagus, stomach, intestine, or pancreas. In these patients with symptoms of nonbiliary tract origin, cholelithiasis happens to be an "innocent bystander," and cholecystectomy has been performed because of a clinical suspicion that symptoms were related to the gallstones. These patients continue to have abdominal pain, heartburn, vomiting, and other signs and symptoms. Careful history, physical examination, laboratory studies, and simple investigations such as esophagogram, upper gastrointestinal or endoscopic evaluation, ultrasonography, or a computed tomography (CT) scan may identify the cause of their symptoms.

Some symptoms are related to functional gastrointestinal disorders with or without psychiatric problems. This group constitutes the largest number of patients with PCS. In many of these patients, an exhaustive work-up fails to reveal any discernible abnormality. Some of these patients may have irritable bowel syndrome, diverticulosis of the colon, or other motility disorders of the gastrointestinal tract. A careful questioning may elicit a history of alternating constipation and diarrhea or abdominal bloating in most of these patients in addition to abdominal pain. Many may be suffering from psychiatric illness as well.

Some symptoms originate in the biliary tract. A relatively small number of patients with PCS may have abnormalities confined to the biliary tract. In this situation, appropriate therapeutic intervention can result in satisfactory clinical outcome. Various abnormalities identified in this group include retained common bile duct stone, common bile duct stricture, papillary tumors, cystic duct remnant, and SO dysfunction.[6-8]

CLINICAL MANIFESTATIONS

Patients with PCS characteristically present with abdominal pain. The onset of pain may occur at any time after cholecystectomy. It is usually postprandial and located in the epigastrium or right upper quadrant of the abdomen radiating to the shoulder blade. The pain is usually sharp, lasting for several hours. The onset of pain may be associated with nausea, vomiting, or both. In patients with biliary tract obstruction, fluctuating jaundice may have accompanying fever or chills. Periodicity of pain, awakening the patient from sleep, heartburn, and water brash are indications of peptic ulcer disease or gastroesophageal reflux disease. Belching, flatulence, abdominal bloating, and intolerance to fatty meals and foods such as pork, eggs, ice cream, or cabbage are symptoms rarely associated with cholelithiasis, and predictably, these annoying symptoms persist in many patients with PCS.[9] Patients presenting with abdominal pain who have undergone cholecystectomy and had no evidence of gallstones are more likely to remain symptomatic. A careful review of the surgical pathology report is helpful in identifying this group of patients.

There is a paucity of abnormal findings on physical examination of patients with PCS, and nonspecific abdominal tenderness is commonly the only finding. Laboratory studies may show transient elevation of liver function tests such as bilirubin, alkaline phosphatase, or transaminase. Repeated laboratory studies are desirable to demonstrate these abnormalities in many patients, because a single evaluation may be entirely normal. The physician must rely on several investigations for patients suffering from PCS. The diagnostic work-up for PCS should include, besides a history and physical examination, laboratory studies such as liver function tests, esophagogram, upper endoscopic evaluation, and barium enema examination. In selected cases, an ultrasound study or CT scan of the abdomen may be indicated. ERCP plays an important role in identifying patients with PCS related to biliary duct disorders. Because pain of nonbiliary tract origin and functional gastrointestinal disorder are discussed elsewhere in this text, this chapter focuses on the hepatobiliary causes of PCS. These causes include bile duct stones, bile duct strictures, cystic duct remnants, retained gallbladder, and SO dysfunction.

HEPATOBILIARY CAUSES OF POSTCHOLECYSTECTOMY SYNDROME

Common Bile Duct Stones

Residual or recurrent stones in the common bile duct may cause biliary colic, jaundice, fever, or chills as a result of intermittent biliary tract obstruction. The incidence of common bile duct stones in patients with PCS varies from 1% to 6%.[10,11] An increased incidence of common bile duct stones has been reported in patients who have had common bile duct exploration along with cholecystectomy.[12] The reported incidence of residual stones among patients who had intraoperative cholangiography, choledochoscopy, or both is 1% to 4%.

Intraoperative cholangiography and choledochoscopy have invariably led to a decrease in the incidence of common bile duct stones after cholecystectomy.[13–16] Most patients with residual common bile duct stones remain symptom free for many years. Symptoms related to common bile duct stones in the immediate postoperative period are observed in fewer than 25% of patients with residual common bile duct stones.[17]

ERCP is the diagnostic modality of choice to demonstrate the stones in these patients (Fig. 99-1). Besides diagnosing common bile duct stones, ERCP enables appropriate therapeutic intervention, such as endoscopic sphincterotomy and stone extraction (see Chap. 117).

Cystic Duct Remnant

A long cystic duct remnant left behind during cholecystectomy has been implicated as the source of pain in a minority of patients with PCS. It has been proposed that the preservation of the tortuous upper portion of the cystic duct with its Heister's valves and the ensuing inflammatory changes within the ductal structure may provide a suitable environment for stone formation. Migration of these stones into the duodenum by way of the common bile duct and the sphincter choledochus may precipitate biliary colic.[18]

A cystic duct stump can be demonstrated using ultrasonography, hepatobiliary scintigraphy, intraoperative cystic duct cholangiography, T-tube cholangiography, or ERCP. The

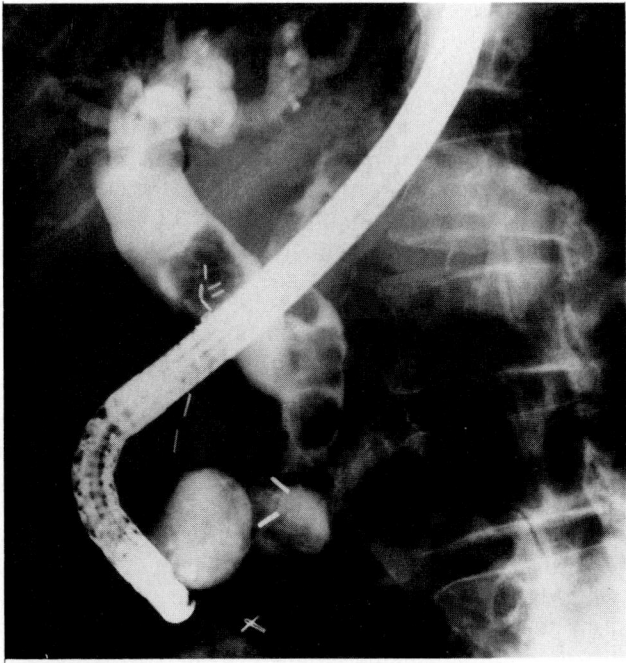

FIGURE 99-1. Endoscopic cholangiogram of patient presenting with postcholecystectomy pain demonstrates multiple common bile duct stones.

incidence of cystic duct stump depends on the technique used; ERCP, by far, remains the most reliable investigative modality. ERCP can demonstrate a cystic duct remnant in 56% to 72% of patients who had undergone cholecystectomy.[19] Many reports indicate a satisfactory outcome after operative removal of cystic duct stumps without any structural abnormality.[20,21] Others have found no appreciable difference in the frequency of cystic duct remnants between symptomatic and asymptomatic subjects.[19] It seems unlikely that the cystic duct remnant causes discernible symptoms in postcholecystectomy patients.[22] Stones in the cystic duct remnant may cause abdominal pain or biliary colic. The incidence of cystic duct stones varies, and for one of the larger series, Bodvall and Overgaard reported a 22% incidence of stones in 452 patients with gallbladder or cystic duct remnant.[23]

Two other abnormalities associated with a cystic duct remnant may cause abdominal pain: amputation neuroma and suture granuloma.[24] The incidence of neuromas varies from 30% to 45% in various series. Similar to common bile duct stones, stones in the cystic duct can be best demonstrated by ERCP. They can be removed using a Dormia basket or balloon catheter after endoscopic sphincterotomy, especially in patients with a rather wide cystic duct stump.

Bile Duct Strictures

Inadvertent injury to the bile duct during surgery constitutes the most common cause for bile duct strictures. Trauma or instrumental injury during laparoscopic cholecystectomy is becoming another important cause for bile duct stricture.[25] The incidence of postoperative strictures varies from 5% to 15%.[26] Characteristically, these patients may remain symptom free for several months after the operation. Commonly observed symptoms resulting from bile duct strictures include intermittent fever, chills, and jaundice. These symptoms are attributable to recurrent cholangitis related to sludge or small gallstones proximal to the stricture. Endoscopic retrograde cholangiography is extremely valuable in demonstrating bile duct strictures (Fig. 99-2). During ERCP, dilation of the stricture can be accomplished using a Gruntzig balloon followed by endoprosthesis placement. These newer endoscopic treatments provide a nonoperative alternative and seem to be beneficial for most patients. For more detailed discussion of biliary stricture, see Chapter 97.

Tumors of the Papilla

Benign or malignant tumors involving the bile duct can mimic symptoms related to cholelithiasis. Occasionally, cholelithiasis occurs with the neoplasm. A patient with periampullary neoplasm may present with biliary colic or jaundice.[27] Benign tumors, such as cystadenoma of the bile duct and tubular or villous adenoma of the papilla, and structural abnormalities, such as a choledochocele, may be overlooked at the time of surgery and may be responsible for PCS. A choledochocele represents a prolapse of the intramural segment of the common bile duct, which can cause biliary colic, jaundice, or pancreatitis.[28] The diagnosis of this rather rare disorder is made almost exclusively by ERCP. A cystic, contrast-filled structure seen at the termination of the common bile duct is

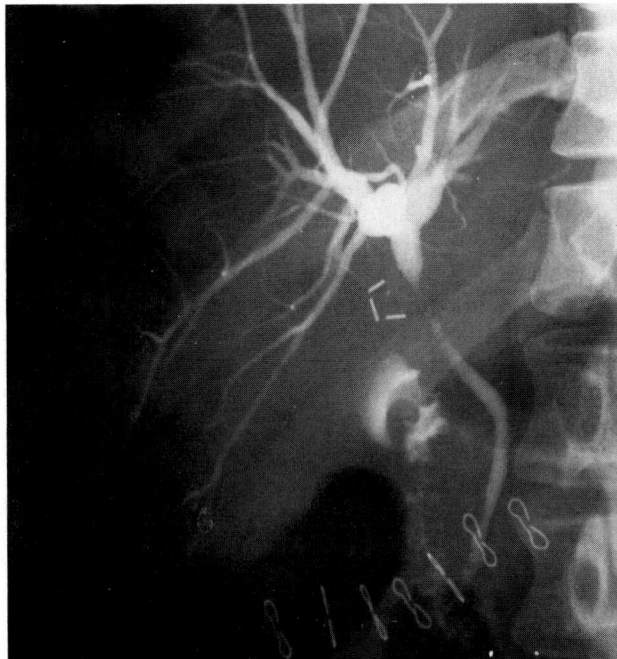

FIGURE 99-2. Cholangiogram shows a postsurgical stricture involving the common hepatic duct. Notice the mild dilatation of the bile ducts above the stricture.

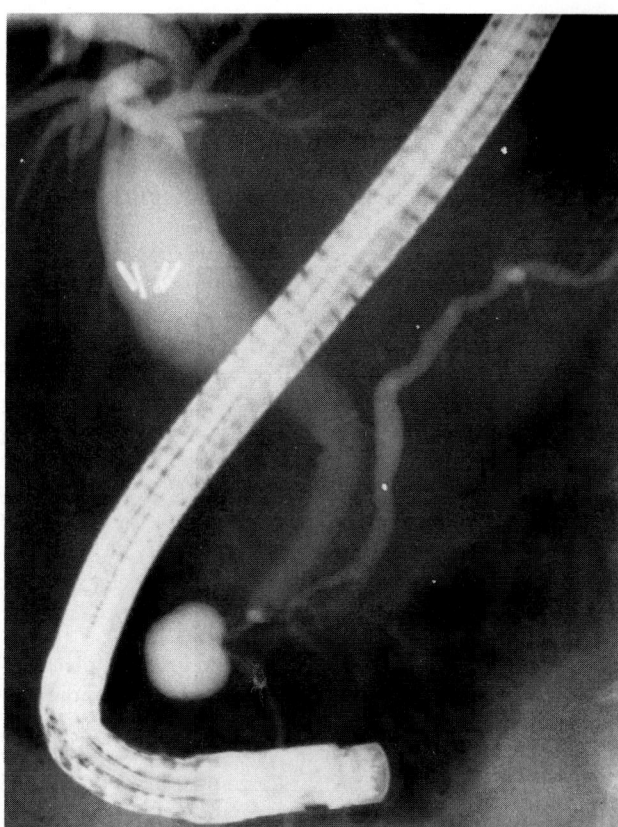

FIGURE 99-3. A choledochocele demonstrated during endoscopic retrograde cholangiopancreatography. This patient underwent cholecystectomy and presented with recurrent abdominal pain and mild jaundice. The rounded, contrast-filled cystic structure represents a choledochocele.

the characteristic radiographic finding of a choledochocele (Fig. 99-3).

Disorders Involving the Sphincter of Oddi

Structural or functional disorders involving the sphincter choledochus may impede bile flow. This ill-defined clinical syndrome, referred to as SO dysfunction, is a rare cause of PCS. Symptoms associated with SO dysfunction bear a monotonous similarity to those seen among patients with other hepatobiliary causes of PCS. Patients with SO dysfunction usually present with intermittent upper abdominal pain, nausea, vomiting, and transiently elevated liver function tests. However, SO dysfunction can be differentiated from other biliary tract abnormalities by ERCP. Fatty-meal ultrasonography, hepatobiliary scintigraphy, postsecretin ultrasonography, and SO manometry have been useful in identifying patients with this rare clinical disorder. SO manometry seems to be the most promising technique, and an elevated basal SO pressure offers a useful criterion for selecting patients with SO dysfunction. Endoscopic sphincterotomy in this situation has been associated with a favorable therapeutic outcome. A more complete discussion of SO dysfunction follows.

DYSFUNCTION OF THE SPHINCTER OF ODDI

SO dysfunction is a structural or functional disorder involving the sphincter choledochus, causing a variety of signs and symptoms resulting from an impedance to transsphincteric bile flow. A confusing array of terms, such as hypertonic

sphincter, sphincterismus, dystonia, and dysenergia, has been used to describe this disorder, which gives vivid testimony to the ambiguities surrounding this rare clinical entity. For practical reasons, SO dysfunction seems to be an attractive nomenclature.

True SO dysfunction is an uncommon clinical entity, accounting for only 1% to 10% of patients who may develop symptoms after cholecystectomy.[29] About 10% to 20% of patients with idiopathic, recurrent pancreatitis may have SO dysfunction.[30] From early on, an impedance to biliary flow at the level of the SO has been hypothesized as the mechanism for the pathogenesis of SO dysfunction. A review of surgical literature provides a detailed histologic description of narrow or stenosed ampulla and papillary orifice in many of these patients.[31,32] Many astute surgeons place great emphasis on the inability to pass a small-caliber dilator or probe through the papillary orifice as the most reliable evidence for papillary stenosis.

Careful pathologic studies of surgically obtained papillae from these patients also revealed a variety of abnormalities, from chronic inflammation to severe fibrosis.[31-33] In many patients, such severe cicatrization may be the result of chronic irritation from migrating common bile duct stones, peripapillary diverticula, or instrumentation during surgery. Tumors involving the ampulla and papillary orifice may also lead to papillary stenosis.[34] In a few patients, papillary stenosis may result from an abnormality arising primarily from the distal common bile duct or peripapillary region. Histologic examination of specimens from these patients reveals hyperplasia of the mucosal glands that penetrate into the sphincteric muscles—a condition often designated as adenomyosis of the papilla.[35] Besides these structural abnormalities, SO dysfunction may also result from a motility abnormality involving the SO. This condition is often called SO dyskinesia, biliary dyskinesia, or SO motor dysfunction. Based on the pathogenic mechanism, SO dysfunction can be broadly classified into two entities, papillary stenosis and SO dyskinesia. In contrast to the information on papillary stenosis, few histologic data are available for patients with SO motor dysfunction.

Historic Perspective

Evidence for a specialized group of smooth muscle fibers at the distal choledochus was established at the turn of the 17th century. However, information regarding the dynamic nature of this structure came a century later with the pioneering studies of Ruggero Oddi.[36] Subsequently, Meltzer, a pupil of Oddi, proposed that intermittent biliary tract obstruction and jaundice may result from abnormal motor activity of the sphincter.[37] Histologic evidence for stenosis of the choledochoduodenal junction and papillary orifice was mentioned by Del Valle and Donovan as early as 1926.[38] The introduction of perioperative cholangiography by Pablo Mirizzi provided the first opportunity to visualize the motor activity of the sphincter choledochus radiographically. The cholangiographic studies gave early glimpses of the dynamics of the SO.[39]

Two important developments, ERCP and SO manometry, have been extremely helpful in the study of PCS and SO dysfunction. The advent of SO manometry in the 1980s opened a new era in the understanding of SO motor dysfunction. A variety of motility abnormalities have been identified, and some progress has been made in treating this rare clinical disorder.

Anatomy and Physiology

The hepatic ducts emerge from the liver at the porta hepatis and unite to form the common hepatic duct. The cystic duct joins the common hepatic duct to give rise to the common bile duct. The distal segment of the common bile duct courses obliquely downward, passing through the substance of the head of the pancreas. The terminal end of the common bile duct and the pancreatic duct traverse the duodenal wall as they approach their intestinal exodus at the papilla of Vater. The intramural segment of the common bile duct is narrow and tapered. Its length varies from 2 to 8 mm.

The anatomy of the distal choledochus and sphincter as we understand it is largely based on painstaking autopsy studies by Boyden.[40,41] A variable length of the distal choledochus and the pancreatic duct are invested with circular and longitudinal smooth muscle fibers that interdigitate with the extraampullary muscle fibers of the duodenal wall to form the SO. This conglomeration of nonstriated muscle fibers contributes to the bulk of the major duodenal papilla. Boyden has described three discrete areas of muscle thickness at the distal choledochus. These minisphincters are called sphincter

papillae, sphincter pancreaticus, and sphincter choledochus. However, only one sphincter is identifiable by manometric studies in humans.

Bile secreted by the hepatocyte is delivered into the canaliculi. The canalicular bile flows into the intrahepatic ducts and finds its way to the extrahepatic ducts. Biliary flow through this rather closed, low-pressure, low-flow system is a complex phenomenon largely influenced by gallbladder motor activity and SO motor activity. Although the association of these two components seems to be complementary, the intricate details of their function still need to be elucidated. Almost two thirds of hepatic bile enters the gallbladder during periods of fasting.[42] Periodic contractions of the gallbladder take place in concert with migrating myoelectrical activity.[43] After a meal, the gallbladder contracts, emptying 50% or more of its contents.[44] Simultaneously, resistance within the zone of the SO decreases, facilitating bile flow into the duodenum. Conversely, gallbladder filling occurs when a small negative pressure gradient develops across the cystic duct region during simultaneous relaxation of the gallbladder and increased resistance to bile flow at the SO.[45] Despite the seemingly close anatomic relation between the sphincter and the duodenum, the SO behaves as an independent motor unit, as is substantiated by embryologic and electromyographic studies.

How does the SO orchestrate biliary flow? The early experimental studies showed that the SO offers a resistance to biliary flow. However, subsequent studies revealed that the sphincter had a propulsive role as well. Later elaborate studies conducted using the opossum sphincter have been helpful in explaining the seemingly contradictory roles of the sphincter proper.[46] The extraduodenal location of the opossum sphincter makes it a suitable model for studying sphincter motor activity without recording artifacts related to duodenal musculature. A high-pressure zone is located at the distal end of the choledochus. This zone extends over a length of 4 to 6 mm constituting the SO zone, with a basal tone or pressure 5 mm above the common bile duct pressure. Superimposed on this resting tone, rhythmic phasic wave contractions occur at a frequency of two to five per minute.

Simultaneous cineradiography, transsphincteric flow, and electromyographic recordings from the opossum sphincter have demonstrated the influence of phasic wave contractions on bile flow into the duodenum. Antegrade contractions initiated at the junction of the common bile duct and SO milk the bile duct contents into the duodenum. During SO phasic contractions or sphincteric systole, bile flow ceases from the bile duct to the sphincteric segment. After sphincter systole, relaxation of the sphincter or sphincter diastole takes place, and bile passively flows from the common bile duct into the sphincter segment. The next sequence of phasic wave contractions strips the bile into the duodenum, and the cycle repeats itself with sequential emptying of the common bile duct.

Experimental data suggest that the major physiologic role of the sphincter lies in regulation of emptying of bile. Cholecystokinin (CCK) octapeptide and nitrites decrease the resistance offered by the sphincter, demonstrating the possible role of SO on biliary drainage.[47]

The physiologic process regulating SO motor function is a complex phenomenon and is less well understood. Histochemical studies of the sphincter muscle from cats and dogs have demonstrated adrenergic and cholinergic neurons in the

SO segment. Several peptides, such as CCK, gastrin, secretin, and enkephalins, have also been identified in the neurons of the sphincter. Vagal transection in dogs has decreased the resistance of transsphincteric flow, indicating a cholinergic influence to the basal sphincter tone. Similarly, intravenous administration of atropine has resulted in decreased phasic contraction frequency and amplitude.

Several peptides affect the SO motor activity. CCK octapeptide inhibited phasic wave contractions in humans and in certain animals. When the animal is pretreated with tetrodotoxin, a neurotoxin that inhibits neurotransmission, CCK octapeptide produced a stimulation of phasic wave contractions.[48] This observation is remarkably similar to the response of the lower esophageal sphincter to CCK octapeptide. CCK seems to have a direct stimulatory effect that is overridden by an indirect inhibitory effect.

SO manometry has demonstrated the influence of several enteric hormones on the human SO. Intravenous administration of glucagon reduced basal pressure and markedly inhibited phasic wave contractions. This pharmacologic effect of glucagon is routinely used to accomplish SO relaxation and duodenal aperistalsis before cannulation and instrumentation of the papilla of Vater during diagnostic and therapeutic ERCP. Pentagastrin increases SO motor activity. Secretin appears initially to increase SO phasic wave amplitude and frequency, followed within minutes by a profound inhibition of SO motor activity.[49]

The human SO is exquisitely sensitive to morphine. Morphine sulfate in very low doses (0.05 µg/kg) stimulates the phasic wave contractions.[50] This stimulatory effect of morphine was less pronounced when persons were pretreated with naloxone, an opiate antagonist.

This confusing array of observations gleaned from laboratory studies suggests a multifactorial control mechanism of the SO, which is a superbly adaptive structure with occlusive and propulsive influence on bile flow. A more detailed discussion on the anatomy and physiology of the SO is presented in Chapter 11.

Clinical Features

SO dysfunction is more prevalent among middle-aged women. The reasons for this female predilection are not clear. Most patients presenting with SO dysfunction have been subjected to cholecystectomy with or without any evidence of cholelithiasis. However, SO dysfunction has been reported in patients with intact gallbladders.[51] Although it is reasonable to assume that SO dysfunction may occur in patients with an intact gallbladder, there are several practical difficulties in diagnosing SO dysfunction in this situation. Minute stones in the gallbladder, which may escape detection by conventional tests, may cause signs and symptoms similar to SO dysfunction. Similarly, gallbladder dyskinesia, another ill-defined entity, cannot be easily differentiated from SO dysfunction.

Abdominal pain is the single most common presenting symptom in persons with SO dysfunction. The pain is sharp, usually postprandial, and located in the epigastrium or right upper quadrant of the abdomen. It may last for several hours and may radiate to the back or shoulder blade. The pain may be associated with nausea or emesis or both. Jaundice, fever, and chills, the characteristic symptoms associated with biliary

tract obstruction, are uncommon symptoms of SO dysfunction. For most patients, physical examination may be completely normal. Less commonly, nonspecific abdominal tenderness may be elicited.

Laboratory studies characteristically reveal transient elevation in liver function studies of bilirubin, alkaline phosphatase, and transaminase. These elevations are modest, usually less than two or three times the normal values. Because transient elevation of liver function tests is more characteristic of SO dysfunction, it may be helpful to perform multiple laboratory studies, especially when the patient is symptomatic, to diagnose SO dysfunction accurately.

The commonly employed diagnostic investigations such as abdominal sonography, CT scan of the abdomen, or barium studies of the gastrointestinal tract may reveal no discernible abnormalities in SO dysfunction. It is often difficult if not impossible to differentiate papillary stenosis from SO dyskinesia on the basis of clinical history, laboratory studies, and other routine investigations. However, abnormal findings such as jaundice and elevated liver function tests are more frequently seen in patients with papillary stenosis. Dilatation of biliary ducts demonstrated by ultrasonography or CT scan seems to be more commonly observed in patients with papillary stenosis than those with with SO dyskinesia.

Diagnostic Investigations

Endoscopic Retrograde Cholangiopancreatography

ERCP plays a major role in the evaluation of patients with SO dysfunction. By delineating anatomic details of the biliary tree, biliary tract disorders such as choledochocele, choledocholithiasis, bile duct stricture or tumor can be excluded.

Although SO dysfunction has no characteristic radiographic findings, ERCP may reveal several cholangiographic findings that may suggest SO dysfunction. These cholangiographic criteria are based on anecdotal data and not on well established clinical studies. They include a dilated common bile duct (>12 mm) (Fig. 99-4) and delayed contrast drainage (>45 minutes) from the common bile duct to the duodenum.

The dilatation of the common bile duct results from intermittent or persistent obstruction to biliary flow at the SO zone. It has been our observation that dilatation of the bile duct and delay of contrast drainage is more prevalent in patients with papillary stenosis than with SO dyskinesia. Several investigators have observed that such dilatation of the bile duct and delayed contrast drainage are more useful findings in the diagnosis of SO dysfunction than manometric abnormalities. However, we think that, although these indirect findings may be helpful, they may be virtually absent in a significant number of patients, particularly in those with SO dyskinesia. Therefore, ERCP manometry becomes an integral part in the complete evaluation of patients suspected to have SO dysfunction.

Biliary Manometry

SO manometry is performed using a water-perfused, 200-cm-long, triple-lumen, polyethylene catheter with an outer diameter of 1.7 mm and a lumenal diameter of 0.5 mm.[49] The

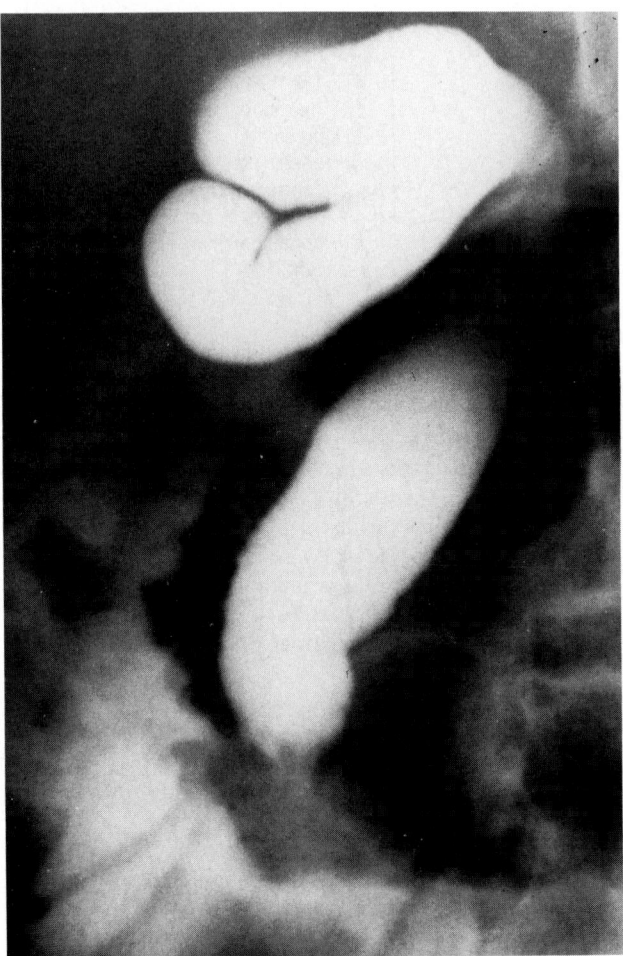

FIGURE 99-4. Roentgenograms taken during endoscopic retrograde cholangiopancreatography of a patient with papillary stenosis. Notice the markedly dilated common bile duct, which did not drain the contrast even after 60 minutes.

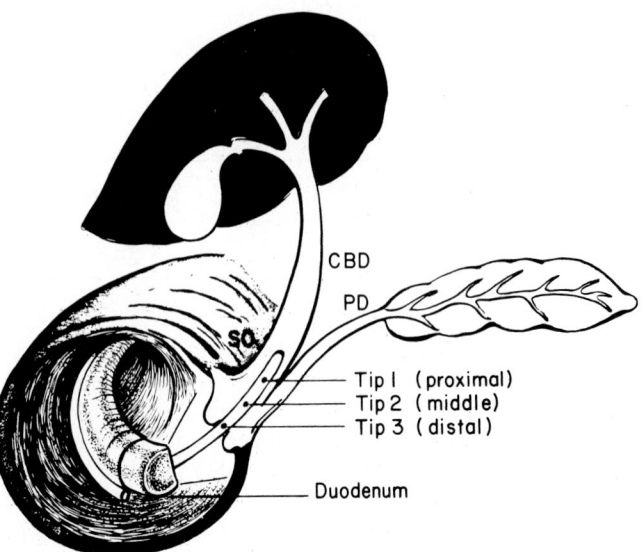

FIGURE 99-5. Human sphincter of Oddi (SO) manometry technique. Notice the manometry catheter protruding from the duodenoscope stationed at the SO zone.

lateral recording orifices are spaced 2 mm apart, with the most distal orifice located 5 mm from the catheter tip. The perfusion is accomplished by a minimally compliant hydraulic capillary system with a flow rate of 0.25 mL/minute. For manometric studies, the catheter is inserted through the biopsy channel of the duodenoscope until it exits into the duodenum. Recording orifices are maintained freely in the duodenal lumen, and the duodenal pressure is recorded. The catheter is advanced into the common bile duct. The baseline pressure of the common bile duct is recorded for 2 to 3 minutes. The manometry catheter is slowly withdrawn across the SO zone in 2- to 3-mm increments. Recordings are performed at each station for 1 to 2 minutes. The catheter is subsequently stationed within the sphincter zone so that all three orifices record phasic and basal SO pressure for 3 to 6 minutes (Fig. 99-5).

For accuracy and reproducibility, the pull-through procedures are repeated two to three times. The mean basal SO pressure is averaged from the maximal basal pressure recorded by all three catheter orifices during a minimum of two sphincteric pull-throughs. Basal SO pressure values greater than 40 mm Hg above intraduodenal pressure are considered to be abnormal. The index value of 40 mm Hg represents two standard deviations above the mean.[52] However, the manometric

criteria may vary from institution to institution. Investigators have reported basal pressure values of 15 to 25 mm Hg as their normal value.[53,54] These variations could be related to the difference in standardization technique rather than variations in the patient population.

Superimposed on the basal tone, high-amplitude phasic wave contractions occur at a mean frequency of 4 ± 0.5 per minute (Fig. 99-6). Phasic wave contractions measured 150 ± 60 mm Hg in amplitude and 4.3 ± 0.5 seconds in duration. Using the triple-lumen catheter, these phasic waves are recorded over a 4- to 6-mm segment of the distal choledochus or SO zone. The propagation of the phasic waves is directed in an antegrade fashion in most patients. A phasic wave appears in the most proximal segment, followed by sequential phasic waves in a caudad direction. However, 17% of phasic wave contractions in normal persons could be simultaneous and 10% could be retrograde.[55]

ERCP manometry has identified several well-defined abnormalities among patients with suspected SO dysfunction. These patients presented with typical abdominal pain, transient elevations of liver function test results, and absence of structural abnormalities of the biliary tract. Many patients had dilated common bile ducts and delayed biliary drainage.

One abnormality detected is increased SO basal pressure. Elevation in SO basal pressure has been observed in some patients with suspected SO dysfunction (Fig. 99-7). This is the most common manometric abnormality reported by many investigators.[56–59] Successful therapeutic outcome has also been reported for these patients after endoscopic sphincterotomy. The elevated basal pressure observed in some of these patients may be abolished by intravenous administration of CCK or glucagon. In some patients, a consistent decrease in the basal pressure has been reported after amyl nitrite inhalation. These observations suggest that the underlying mechanism of SO dysfunction in many of these patients is a dyskinesia rather than papillary stenosis. A lack of response to spasmolytics is indicative of papillary stenosis.

A paradoxical response to CCK octapeptide is seen in few

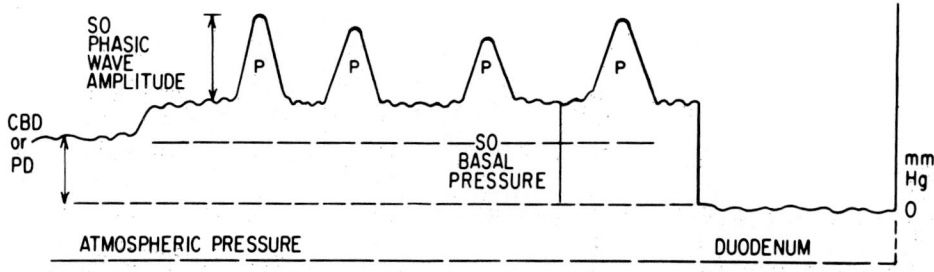

FIGURE 99-6. Normal sphincter of Oddi (SO) manometry tracing. The basal SO pressure is 5 mm Hg above the common bile duct pressure. Superimposed on the basal pressure phasic wave (P), contractions occur at a frequency of 3 to 5 per minute. The duodenal pressure is assumed to be zero.

patients. Intravenous administration of CCK octapeptide has two major effects on SO dynamics: a decrease in SO basal pressure and abolition of phasic wave contractions (Fig. 99-8). In some patients with SO dysfunction, CCK octapeptide causes a paradoxical increase in basal SO pressure (see Fig. 99-8).[60,61] A similar paradoxical response to CCK has been shown in the denervated feline SO. Paradoxical SO contraction response suggests a defect in inhibitory innervation of the SO, which subsequently unmasks a direct stimulatory effect of CCK on smooth muscle fibers.

Other patients have retrograde propagation of phasic wave contractions. Although phasic wave contractions may have retrograde sequence in 10% of normal phasic contractions, an increased frequency (>50%) of retrograde propagation occurs in a subgroup of patients with suspected SO dysfunction (Fig. 99-9). Retrograde propagation of phasic contraction waves may impede biliary flow and produce subtle biliary obstruction.

Some patients may have an increased frequency of phasic wave activity, called tachyoddia. The normal human sphincter demonstrates phasic wave contractions at a frequency of 2 to 4 per minute. Tachyoddia has been a rarely observed type of SO dysfunction (Fig. 99-10).[62]

Besides these motility abnormalities, other rare manometric abnormalities have been observed in patients with suspected SO dysfunction. These include prolonged or irregular phasic waves and decreased SO basal sphincter tone. The significance of these rare derangements is unknown.

Although SO manometry remains the gold standard for SO dysfunction, the technique of SO manometry is not with-

out problems. ERCP manometry is a difficult endoscopic procedure to master and is successful in only 75% of patients. SO manometry may be associated with acute pancreatitis in about 5% of patients.

Not all investigators agree that manometry study helps in identifying patients with SO dysfunction. Controversy exists about the reproducibility, sensitivity, and specificity of SO motility studies. The role of SO motility, especially in patients with possible type III SO dysfunction remains highly controversial, because only 15% to 30% of such patients have identifiable manometric abnormalities.[63,64]

Provocative Tests

A noninvasive test for SO dysfunction employing intramuscular administration of morphine sulfate and Prostigmin has been used for several years. Both these agents cause sphincter spasm, leading to biliary colic and elevated liver function tests in patients with suspected SO dysfunction.[65] However, some reports have shown that the morphine-Prostigmin test is inaccurate and unreliable in selecting patients with SO dysfunction.[66,67]

Secretin Ultrasonography

A change in the caliber of the pancreatic duct or the common bile duct after administration of intravenous secretin is a useful diagnostic tool for papillary stenosis or SO dysfunction. Secretin, an enteric hormone, is a potent secretagogue that causes voluminous exocrine pancreatic secretion. Intravenous

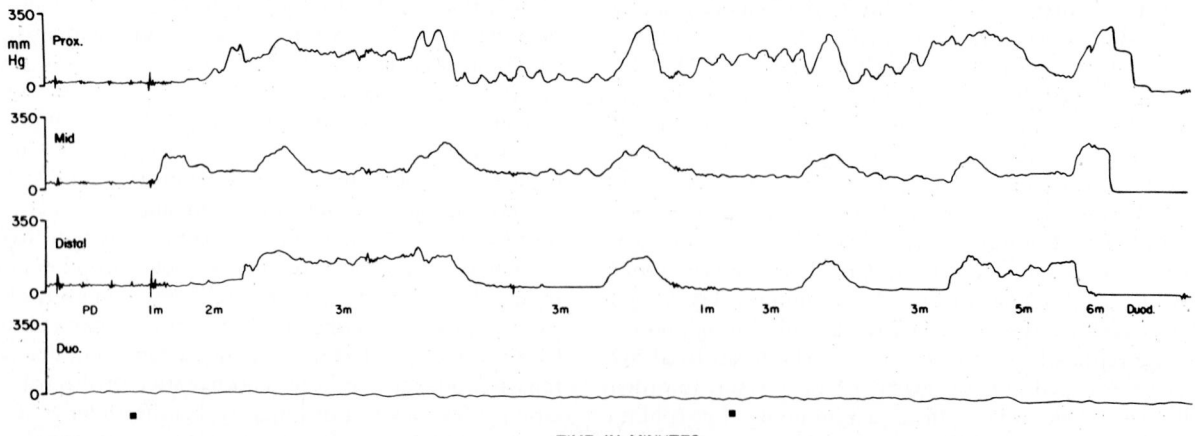

FIGURE 99-7. Manometry tracing shows elevated basal pressure. Basal pressure measured from the tracing between the phasic contraction waves is above 100 mm Hg. The upper limit of normal is 40 mm Hg.

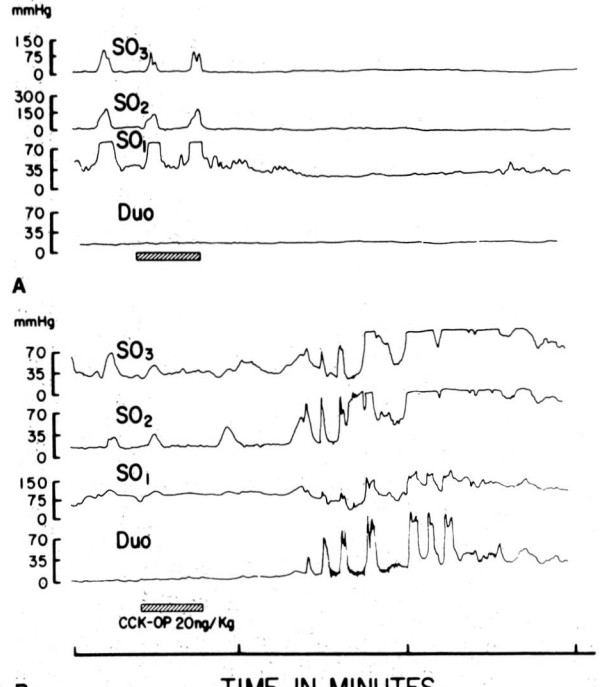

A

B   TIME IN MINUTES

FIGURE 99-8. Normal and paradoxical response of the sphincter of Oddi (SO) to cholecystokinin-octapeptide. **(A)** Normal response of the SO phasic waves. **(B)** In a paradoxical response, the SO basal pressure is increased, and there is an increased frequency of phasic wave contractions.

administration of secretin causes increased basal tone in the human SO. The generous amount of pancreatic secretion coupled with increased basal tone of the sphincter results in distention of the pancreatic duct in normal persons. In patients with papillary stenosis, this effect is more pronounced, resulting in an increased diameter of the pancreatic duct. The test consists of obtaining baseline ultrasonography of the pancreatic duct to determine its diameter. An increase in the diameter of the main pancreatic duct of 1 to 2 mm after secretin infusion is considered to be a positive test.[68] A successful

therapeutic outcome has been reported for many patients who have had a positive secretin ultrasonography test, supporting the specificity of this test.

Fatty-Meal Ultrasonography

Fatty-meal ultrasonography is a noninvasive test using the technique of ultrasonography to identify patients with SO dysfunction. It is assumed that a fatty meal results in endogenous release of CCK, which enhances biliary flow. In SO dyskinesia, the impedance of biliary flow at the sphincteric level leads to distention of the bile duct. The test consists of measuring the baseline diameter of the common bile duct and administering Lipomul at 1.5 mL/kg. The diameter of the common bile duct is measured by ultrasonography every 15 minutes for the next 60 minutes. In normal persons, the caliber of the common bile duct remains unchanged or shows an insignificant change of about 1 mm; in patients with SO dysfunction, the diameter of the common bile duct is increased by greater than 2 mm after Lipomul. In a study of 47 patients with suspected partial bile duct obstruction, including 9 patients with SO dysfunction, fatty-meal ultrasonography yielded results with 100% specificity and 74% sensitivity.[69] ERCP examination and SO manometry formed the gold standard for determining partial bile duct obstruction. An improved sensitivity would be more desirable; nevertheless, a positive fatty-meal ultrasound test seems to help in the selection of patients with true sphincteric dysfunction.

Quantitative Hepatobiliary Scintigraphy

During the past several years, quantitative hepatobiliary scintigraphy (QHS) has been reported to be a useful, noninvasive, diagnostic study for detecting patients with partial bile duct obstruction resulting from structural disorders or SO dysfunction. QHS is performed after a minimum fast of of 4 hours. After intravenous administration of 5 mCi of ^{99m}Tc-diisopropylphenylcarbamoylmethyl aminoacetic acid, counts over the abdomen were recorded for 90 minutes. Isotope distribution curves were generated for the liver, hepatic hilum, and common bile duct. In one report, the most sensitive in-

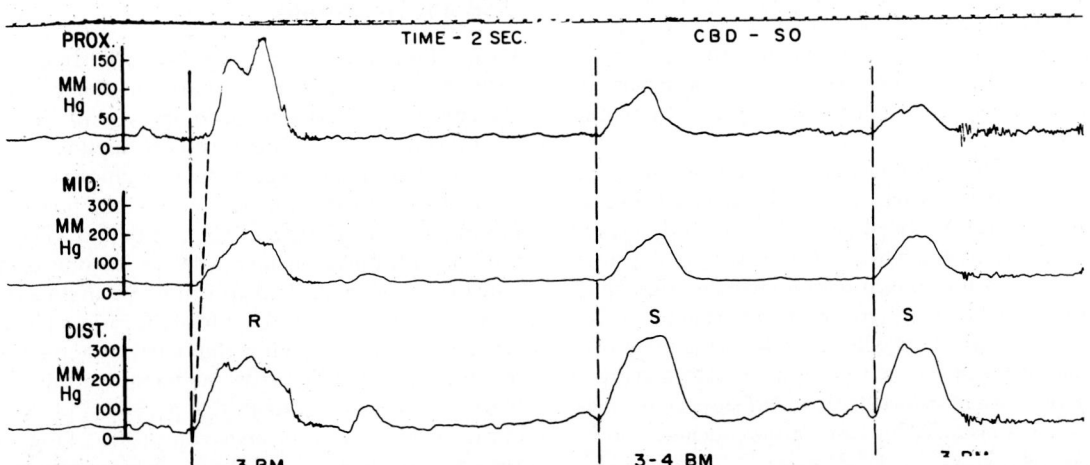

FIGURE 99-9. Retrograde propagation of phasic waves. This sphincter of Oddi manometry tracing demonstrates the phasic wave contractions beginning in the distal tip and propogated in a retrograde fashion.

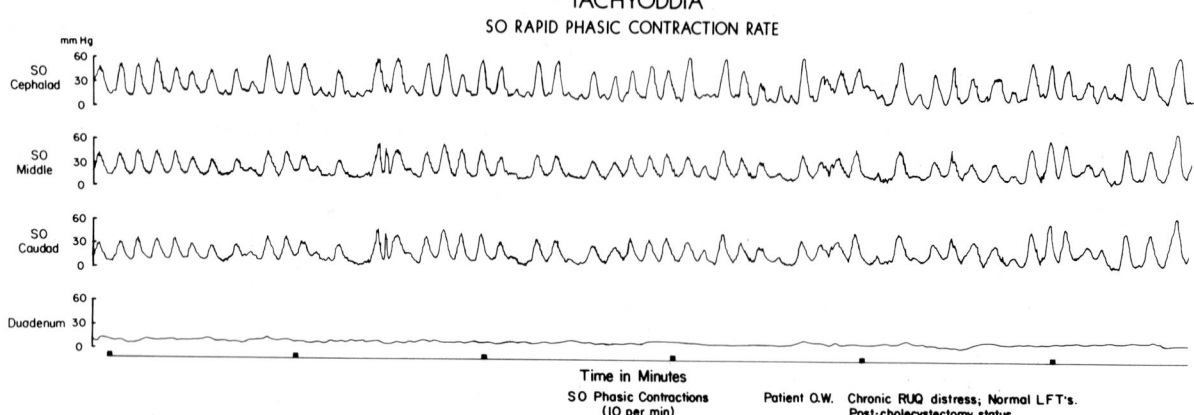

FIGURE 99-10. Increased frequency of phasic wave contractions or tachyoddia. The phasic wave frequency is more than 10 per minute.

dicator for a positive test was a 45-minute isotope clearance of less than 63%.[70,71] ERCP and SO manometry were used as the gold standard to characterize partial bile duct obstruction clearly. Modification of QHS using morphine sulfate and CCK to provoke sphincter spasm or to enhance biliary flow have been reported to be useful in the diagnosis of SO dysfunction.[72,73] QHS alone had a 67% sensitivity for identifying patients with partial bile duct obstruction; when combined with fatty-meal ultrasonography, the sensitivity improved to 80%. Although this study was not limited to patients with SO dysfunction, there were enough patients with SO dysfunction to grant serious consideration for this noninvasive diagnostic technique.

Overview of the Diagnostic Approach

Several diagnostic tests are available for identifying patients with SO dysfunction. The patient's history and physical examination are usually not very helpful. Laboratory studies such as determination of liver function tests may demonstrate transient elevation in alkaline phosphatase, transaminase, or bilirubin, especially when patients are symptomatic. Ultrasonography or CT scan of the abdomen may reveal dilatation of the bile duct. ERCP may demonstrate a dilated bile duct and delayed contrast drainage, which can be somewhat helpful. Although several noninvasive techniques, such as secretin and fatty-meal ultrasonography and QHS, have been helpful, their clinical use is still undefined, awaiting more elaborate studies.

Biliary manometry demonstrates several well-defined manometric abnormalities in patients with suspected SO dysfunction. An elevated SO basal pressure is the only manometric abnormality on the basis of which major therapeutic decisions have been undertaken with a favorable outcome. ERCP manometry, however, remains a cumbersome procedure and is not always successful. Its role in the diagnosis and treatment of SO dysfunction is not universally accepted.

Based on our current knowledge, patients suspected of SO dysfunction can be classified into three groups: definite, probable, and possible.

In the definite category, patients have biliary-type pain and abnormal liver function tests (i.e., transaminase and alkaline phosphatase twice the normal value) documented on two or

more occasions. ERCP examination revealed dilated common bile duct (>12 mm) and delayed drainage of contrast (>45 minutes). The underlying mechanism for SO dysfunction in these patients appears to be a structural alteration or stenosis rather than a functional disorder or sphincteric spasm. Although SO manometry may be helpful in this situation, it may not be essential.

In the probable category, patients have biliary-type pain but only one or two of the previously listed criteria (e.g., abnormal liver function tests, delayed drainage, dilated common bile duct). The cause of SO dysfunction in these patients may be structural or functional. Manometric pressure measurements of the SO are especially useful in this category of patients.

In the possible category, patients present with biliary pain as the exclusive clinical finding. Other objective findings are lacking for this group of patients. SO manometry is essential for the diagnosis, and the underlying mechanism is almost exclusively a functional disorder.

Management

Medical Treatment

Because the impedance to biliary flow in SO dysfunction seems to be the result of abnormal motor function of the sphincter choledochus, several pharmacologic agents that can cause smooth muscle relaxation have been used to treat patients with SO dysfunction. Agents such as glucagon, atropine, or amyl nitrite normalize the elevated SO basal pressure observed in some patients during ERCP manometry. These observations provide the rationale for the use of some of these spasmolytics in the medical treatment of SO dysfunction.

Sublingual nitroglycerin, one of the earliest pharmacologic agents tried, relieves pain within a few minutes, probably by relaxing the SO.[74] Similarly, nifedipine, a calcium-channel blocker, reduces abnormally high pressure and the symptoms of patients with postcholecystectomy pain.[75] Progesterone has been reported to alleviate pain in some patients, probably by causing relaxation of the sphincter muscles.[76] Bile acid substitutes and pancreatic enzyme preparations, when taken continuously, have been effective in reducing dyskinesia symptoms.[77] However, prostaglandin inhibitors were ineffective in the management of SO dysfunction in a series of 65 patients.

Despite these isolated encouraging reports, pharmacologic therapy generally has not been very successful. No long-term studies of medical therapy for SO dysfunction are available. However, it is customary to use analgesics and antispasmodics, sometimes in combination with tranquilizers, as the first-line treatment for SO dysfunction.

Surgical Treatment

Relatively high success rates have been achieved with surgical therapy.[78-81] Sphincterotomy, sphincteroplasty, and septectomy are the commonly employed surgical therapies for SO dysfunction. Although operative procedures are considered to be more exact and reliable to ensure adequate incision of the sphincter muscle, they are usually associated with somewhat higher complication rates than endoscopic therapy.

Endoscopic Therapy

Because the smooth muscle constituting the SO is the nidus for dysmotility in SO dysfunction, systematic severance of this structure by endoscopic sphincterotomy seems to be ideal. Manometric studies have demonstrated abolition of phasic wave contractions and the choledochoduodenal pressure gradient in postsphincterotomy patients.[82] The basal SO pressure becomes almost negligible after endoscopic sphincterotomy.

The technique of endoscopic sphincterotomy has greatly improved since its introduction more than two decades ago. Although the mortality and morbidity rates associated with endoscopic sphincterotomy are comparable to those for the operative approach, it is more cost-effective than surgery. However, endoscopic sphincterotomy for patients with SO dysfunction is associated with slightly increased complication rates compared with patients with common bile duct stones. Several reports indicate a successful therapeutic outcome in patients with SO dysfunction after endoscopic sphincterotomy.[83-86]

The efficacy of endoscopic sphincterotomy in patients with SO dysfunction was evaluated in a prospective, double-blind study.[86] Forty-seven patients, all of whom had elevated liver function tests and biliary-type pain after cholecystectomy, were randomly assigned to sphincterotomy group (23 patients) or nonsphincterotomy sham group (24 patients). Endoscopic sphincterotomy resulted in improvement of pain scores at 1-year follow-up for 10 of 11 patients with elevated SO pressure. There was improvement in only 3 of 12 patients with elevated SO pressure who underwent sham treatment or no sphincterotomy. Patients with normal pressure and abdominal pain remain unchanged, regardless of the type of treatment. After 1 year, endoscopic sphincterotomy was performed in 12 symptomatic patients who had undergone the sham procedure or no sphincterotomy. Seven of these patients had elevated SO pressure, and five had normal SO pressure. Forty patients were followed for 4 years. Of the 23 patients with elevated pressure, 17 patients remained symptom free. For patients with normal SO pressure, endoscopic sphincterotomy was no more beneficial than sham therapy. Endoscopic sphincterotomy for SO dysfunction is associated with a success rate of 50% to 75%.

The reader is directed to Chapter 2, Gastrointestinal Hormones; Chapter 11, Motility of the Biliary Tree; Chapter 34, Approach to the Patient With Abdominal Pain; Chapter 41, Approach to the Patient With Jaundice: Chapter 42, Approach to the Patient With Abnormal Liver Chemistries; Chapter 95, Gallbladder and Biliary Tree: Anatomy and Structural Anomalies: Chapter 96, Gallstones; Chapter 97, Diseases of the Biliary Tree; Chapter 98, Tumors of the Biliary Tree; Chapter 117, Endoscopic Retrograde Cholangiopancreatography, Endoscopic Sphincterotomy and Stone Removal, and Endoscopic Biliary and Pancreatic Drainage; and Chapter 121, Ultrasonography.

REFERENCES

1. McSherry CK, Glenn F. The incidence and cause of death following surgery for nonmalignant biliary tract disease. Ann Surg 1980;191:271.
2. Burnett W, Shields R. Symptoms after cholecystectomy. Lancet 1958;1:923.
3. Bodvall B. The postcholecystectomy syndromes. Clin Gastroenterol 1973;2:103.
4. Schofield GE, MacLeod RG. Sequelae of cholecystectomy. Br J Surg 1966;53:1042.
5. Collins PG. Post surgical disorders. Part I: functional disorders following surgery of biliary tract. Clin Gastroenterol 1977;6:689.
6. Tondelli P, Gyr K. Post surgical syndrome. Clin Gastroenterol 1982;12:231.
7. Christiansen J, Schmidt A. The postcholecystectomy syndrome. Acta Chir Scand 1971;137:789.
8. Glenn F, Whitsell JC. The surgical treatment of cystic duct remnants. Surg Gynecol Obstet 1961;113:711.
9. Hinkel CL, Moller GA. Correlation of symptoms, age, sex and habitus with cholecystographic findings in 1000 consecutive examinations. Gastroenterology 1957;32:807.
10. Colchock BP, McManns JE. Experiences with 1356 cases of cholecystitis and cholelithiasis. Surg Gynecol Obstet 1955;101:161.
11. Bartlett MK, Quinby WC Sr. Surgery of the biliary tract. Secondary operations on the common duct. N Engl J Med 1957;256:11.
12. Larson RE, Hodgson JR, Priestly JT. The early and long-term results of 500 consecutive explorations of the common duct. Surg Gynecol Obstet 166;122:744.
13. Farhar GJ, Pearson RN. Transcystic duct operative cholangiography. Am J Surg 1976;131:228.
14. Bartlett MK, Warshaw AL, Ottinger LW. The removal of biliary duct stones. Surg Clin North Am 1974;54:599.
15. Kappes SK, Adams MB, Wilson SD. Intraoperative biliary endoscopy. Arch Surg 1982;117:603.
16. Shore JM, Berci G, Morgenstern L. The value of biliary endoscopy. Surg Gynecol Obstet 1985;140:601.
17. Glenn F, McSherry CK. Secondary operations for symptoms following biliary tract surgery. Surg Gynecol Obstet 1965;121:979.
18. Garlock JM, Hurwitt ES. The cystic duct stump syndrome. Surgery 1951;29:833.
19. Aarimad M, Makela P. The cystic duct stump and postcholecystectomy syndrome. Ann Chir Gynecol 1981;70:297.
20. Corrente RF. Retained cystic duct stump. R I Med J 1970;53:95.
21. Larmi TKI, Fock G. Cystic duct remnant. A cause of biliary distress following cholecystectomy. Acta Chir Scand 1957;114:361.
22. Womack KW, Crider RL. The persistence of symptoms following cholecystectomy. Ann Surg 1947;126:31.
23. Bodvall B, Overgaard B. Cystic duct remnant after cholecystectomy incidence studied by cholegraphy in 500 cases and significance in 103 reoperations. Ann Surg 1966;163:382.
24. Moody FG. Postcholecystectomy syndromes. Surg Annu 1987;19:205.
25. Way LW, Bernhoft RA, Thomas MJ. Biliary stricture. Surg Clin North Am 1981;61:963.

26. Manoukian AV, Schmalz MJ, Geenen JE, Venu RP, Johnson GK. Post-laparoscopic cholecystectomy problems: "minimally invasive" ERCP therapy. Gastrointest Endosc 1992;38;2:250.

27. Venu RP, Geenen JE. Diagnosis and treatment of diseases of the papilla. Clin Gastroenterol 1986;15:439.

28. Venu RP, Geenen JE, Hogan WJ, et al. Role of endoscopic retrograde cholangiopancreatography in the diagnosis and treatment of choledochocele. Gastroenterology 1984;87:1144.

29. Bar-Meir S, Halpern H, Bardan E, et al. Frequency of papillary dysfunction among cholecystectomized patients. Hepatology 1984;4:328.

30. Venu RP, Geenen JE, Hogan WJ, Stone J, Johnson GK, Soergel KH. Idiopathic recurrent pancreatitis—an approach to diagnosis and treatment. Dig Dis Sci 1989;341:56.

31. Acosta JM, Civantos F, Nardi GL, et al. Fibrosis of the papilla of Vater. Surg Gynecol Obstet 1967;124:784.

32. Acosta JM, Nardi GL. Papillitis. Arch Surg 1966;92:354.

33. Moody FG, Beckner JM, Potts JR. Transduodenal sphincteroplasty and transpapillary septectomy for postcholecystectomy pain. Ann Surg 1983;197:627.

34. Weiss W. Juxtapapillary diverticula. In: Classen M, Geenen J, Kawai K, eds. The papilla Vateri and its diseases. New York: Verlag Gerhard Witzstrock, 1979:28.

35. Hess W. Die stinosen der papilla Vateri. Acta Chir 1968;3:81.

36. Oddi R. D'une disposition a sphincter speciale de l'ouvesture du canal choledoque. Arch Ital Biol 1887;8:317.

37. Meltzer SJ. Disturbance of law of contrary innervation as a pathogenetic factor in the diseases of the bile ducts and gallbladder. Am J Med Sci 1917;153:469.

38. Del Valle D, Donovan R. Coledoco-odditis escleroretractil. Arch Argent Enf App Digest 1926;4:1.

39. Caroli J, Porcher P, Pequignot G, Delattre M. Contributions of cineradiography to study the function of human biliary tree. Am J Dig Dis 1960;5:677.

40. Boyden EA. Anatomy of the choledochoduodenal junction in man. Surg Gynecol Obstet 1957;106:647.

41. Boyden EA. The sphincter of Oddi in man and certain representative mammals. Surgery 1937;1:25.

42. Krishnamurthy GT, Bobba VR, Kington E. Radionuclide ejection fraction of the human gallbladder. Gastroenterology 1981;80:482.

43. Itoh Z, Takahashi I. Periodic contractions of the canine gallbladder during the interdigestive state. Am J Physiol 1981;240:6183.

44. Everson GT, Braverman DZ, Johnson ML, et al. A critical evaluation of real time ultrasonography for the study of gallbladder volume and contraction. Gastroenterology 1980;79:40.

45. Ryan JP. Motility of the gallbladder and biliary tree. In: Johnson LR, eds. Physiology of the gastrointestinal tract. New York: Raven Press, 1981:473.

46. Toouli J, Dodds JW, Honda R, et al. Motor function of the opossum sphincter of Oddi. J Clin Invest 1983;71:208.

47. Toouli J, Hogan WJ, Geenen JE, et al. Action of cholecystokinin-octapeptide on sphincter of Oddi basal pressure and phasic wave activity in humans. Surgery 1982;92:497.

48. Behar J, Biancani P. Effect of cholecystokinin-octapeptide in the feline sphincter of Oddi and gallbladder. J Clin Invest 1980;66:1231.

49. Honda R, Toouli J, Dodds WJ, et al. Effect of enteric hormones on sphincter of Oddi and gastrointestinal myoelectric activity in fasted conscious opossum. Gastroenterology 1983;84:1.

50. Geenen JE, Hogan WJ, Dodds WJ. Intraluminal pressure recording from the human sphincter of Oddi. Gastroenterology 1980;78:317.

51. Venu RP, Geenen JE, Hogan WJ, et al. Patients with biliary-type pain and a normal-appearing gallbladder: where is the problem? Gastroenterology 1992;102:4:A266.

52. Geenen JE, Hogan WJ, Toouli J, et al.. A prospective randomized study of the efficacy of endoscopic sphincterotomy for patients with presumptive sphincter of Oddi dysfunction. Gastroenterology 1984;86:1086.

53. Thatcher BS, Sivak MV, Tedesco FJ. Endoscopic sphincterotomy for suspected dysfunction of the sphincter of Oddi. Gastrointest Endosc 1987;33:91.

54. Steinberg WM. Sphincter of Oddi dysfunction: a clinical controversy. Gastroenterology 1988;95:1409.

55. Geenen JE, Hogan WJ. Endoscopic access to the papilla of Vater. International workshop on endoscopy. Endoscopy 1980;Suppl: 47.

56. Hogan WJ, Geenen JE. Biliary dyskinesia. Endoscopy 1988;20: 179.

57. Bar-Meir S, Geenen JE, Hogan WJ, et al. Biliary and pancreatic duct pressures measured by ERCP manometry in patients with suspected papillary stenosis. Dig Dis Sci 1979;24:209.

58. Meshkinpour H. Bile duct dyskinesia: a clinical and manometric study. Gastroenterology 1984;87:759.

59. Toouli J. Manometric disorders in patients with suspected sphincter of Oddi dysfunction. Gastroenterology 1985;88:1243.

60. Hogan WJ, Geenen JE, Dodds WJ, et al. Paradoxical motor response to cholecystokinin (CCK-OP) in patients with suspected sphincter of Oddi dyskinesia. Gastroenterology 1983;84:1189.

61. Rolny P, Arleback A, Funch-Jensen P, et al. Paradoxical response of sphincter of Oddi to intravenous injection of cholecystokinin or ceruletide. Manometric findings and results of treatment in biliary dyskinesia. Gut 1986;27:1507.

62. Hogan WJ, Geenen JE, Venu R, et al. Abnormally rapid phasic wave contractions of the human sphincter of Oddi (tachyoddia). Gastroenterology 1983;84:1189.

63. Elta GH. Sphincter of Oddi manometry in patients with a possible sphincter of Oddi dysfunction. Gastroenterology 1991;101: 1748.

64. Thun EA, Scicchi TA, No J, Roberts-Thompson IC, Toouli J. Reproducibility of endoscopic sphincter of Oddi manometry. Dig Dis Sci 1991;36:1401.

65. Nardi GL, Acosta JM. Papillitis as a cause of pancreatitis and abdominal pain. Role of evocative test, operative pancreatography and histological evaluation. Ann Surg 1966;164:611.

66. LoGuidice JA, Geenen JE, Hogan WJ, et al. Efficacy of the morphine-prostigmine test for evaluating patients with suspected papillary stenosis. Dig Dis Sci 1979;24:455.

67. Steinberg WM, Salvago RF, Tosker PP. The morphine-prostigmine provocative tests—is it useful for making clinical decisions? Gastroenterology 1980;78:728.

68. Warshaw AL, Simeone J, Schapiro RH, et al. Objective evaluation of ampullary stenosis with ultrasonography and pancreatic stimulation. Am J Surg 1985;149:65.

69. Darweesh R, Dodds WJ, Hogan WJ, et al. Fatty meal sonography for evaluating patients with suspected partial common bile duct obstruction. AJR 1988;151:63.

70. Darweesh R, Dodds WJ, Hogan WJ, et al. Efficacy of quantitative hepatobiliary scintigraphy and fatty-meal sonography for detecting partial common bile duct obstruction. Gastroenterology 1987;92:1363.

71. Collins JS, Dodds WJ, Geenen JE, et al. Efficacy of quantitative hepatobiliary scintigraphy (QHS) for evaluating a large series of patients with suspected partial common bile duct obstruction. Gut 1988;29:A1458.

72. Fig LM, Wahl RL, Stewart RE, Schapiro B. Morphine augmented hepatobiliary scintigraphy in the severely ill; caution is in order. Radiology 1990;175:467.

73. Sostre S, Kallo AN, Spegler EJ, et al. A noninvasive test of sphincter of Oddi dysfunction in postcholecystectomy patients; a scintigraphic score. J Nucl Med 1992;33:1216.

74. Bar-Meir S, Halpern Z, Bardan E. Nitrate therapy in patients with papillary dysfunction. Am J Gastroenterol 1983;78:94.

75. Guelrud M, Medoza S, Rossiter G, et al. Effect of nifedipine on sphincter of Oddi motor function in humans. Studies in healthy volunteers and in patients with biliary dyskinesia. Gastroenterology 1987;92:1418.

76. Lasson A, Fonk FT, Tragardh B, Zederfeldt B. The postcholecystectomy syndrome. Bile ducts as pain trigger zone. Scand J Gastroenterol 1988;23:265.

77. Lasson A. The postcholecystectomy syndrome. Diagnostic and therapeutic strategy. Scand J Gastroenterol 1987;22:897.

78. Moody FG, Berenson MM, McClosky D. Transampullary septectomy for postcholecystectomy pain. Ann Surg 1977;1986: 415.

79. Jones SA, Steedman RA, Keller TB, et al. Transduodenal sphinc-

teroplasty (not sphincterotomy) for biliary and pancreatic disease. Am J Surg 1969;118:292.

80. Strom PR, Stone HH. Technique for transduodenal sphincteroplasty. Surgery 1982;92:546.

81. Antrum RM, Hall R. Transduodenal sphincteroplasty; Analysis of 118 consecutive cases. Br J Surg 1984;71:446.

82. Geenen JE, Hogan WJ, Dodds WJ, et al. Long-term results of endoscopic sphincterotomy for treating patients with sphincter of Oddi dysfunction. A prospective study. Gastroenterology 1987;92:1401.

83. Classen M. Endoscopic papillotomy—new indications, short and long-term results. Clin Gastroenterol 1986;15:457.

84. Roberts-Thompson IC, Toouli J. Is endoscopic sphincterotomy for disabling biliary-type pain after cholecystectomy effective? Gastrointest Endosc 1985;31:370.

85. Neoptolemos JP, Bailey IS, Carr-Locke DL. Sphincter of Oddi dysfunction: results of treatment by endoscopic sphincterotomy. Br J Surg 1988;75:454.

86. Geenen JE, Hogan WJ, Dodds WJ, et al. The efficacy of endoscopic sphincterotomy after cholecystectomy in patients with sphincter of Oddi dysfunction. N Engl J Med 1989;320:82.

Textbook of Gastroenterology, second edition, edited by Tadataka Yamada. JB Lippincott Company, Philadelphia © 1995.

G. Abdominal Cavity

CHAPTER 100

Abdominal Cavity: Anatomy, Structural Anomalies, and Hernias

Frank G. Moody   Ricard Calabuig

EMBRYOLOGY OF THE ABDOMINAL CAVITY

The abdominal or peritoneal cavity appears in the early stages of embryonic development as the caudal part of the celomic cavity. It contains the digestive tube, an endodermal structure in communication with the yolk sac by the vitelline duct. The association of the tube with the duct defines three digestive segments: foregut, proximal to the vitelline duct; hindgut, distal to the duct; and midgut, where the duct emerges. The upper gastrointestinal tract originates from the foregut; the small bowel and the right and transverse colon from the midgut; and the left colon, sigmoid, and rectum from the hindgut. The embryonic digestive tube is attached to the abdominal walls by mesodermic bands. Two bands are in the foregut:

the ventral and the dorsal mesogastrium. The midgut and the hindgut have only one dorsal band.[1]

During the embryonic development, the foregut rotates 90 degrees clockwise in a transverse plane (Fig. 100-1), the midgut rotates 270 degrees counterclockwise in an antero-posterior plane (Fig. 100-2), and the hindgut remains in a posterior left position.

During the migratory process of the abdominal organs, the mesodermic bands elongate and create the abdominal ligaments, the mesenterium, and the greater and lesser omenta. The dorsal mesogastrium of the foregut develops to a larger extent than its ventral counterpart, folding to the left. The spleen, formed in it, is positioned in the left side, and the dorsal pancreas is situated posteriorly. The space within the mesogastrial fold becomes the lesser sac.

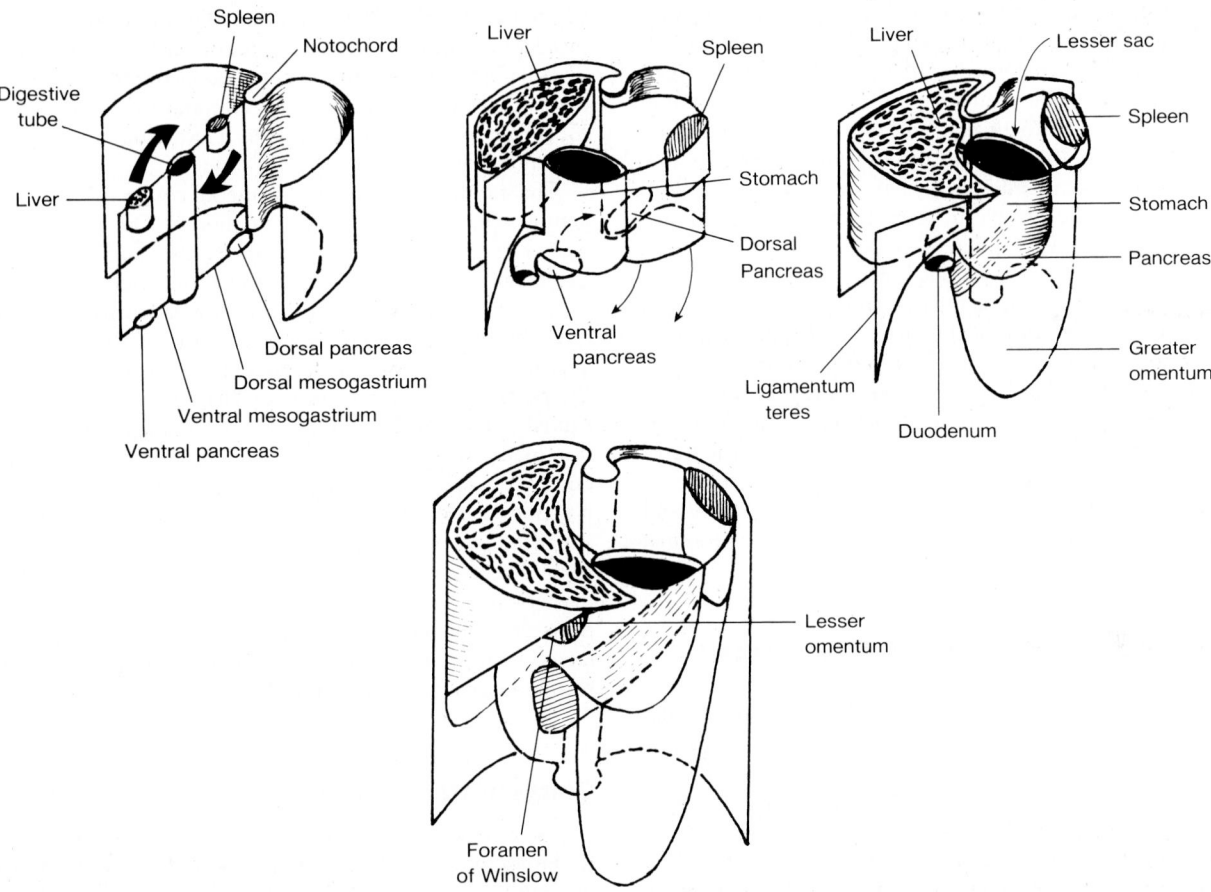

FIGURE 100-1. Embryonic development of the foregut. The organs of the upper gastrointestinal tract rotate 90 degrees clockwise in a transverse plane. Originally, ventral structures like the liver and ventral pancreas are situated to the right, and posterior organs such as the spleen, dorsal pancreas, and dorsal aspect of the future stomach are positioned to the left side of the abdominal cavity. The dorsal mesogastrium elongates and folds to the left to form the greater omentum.

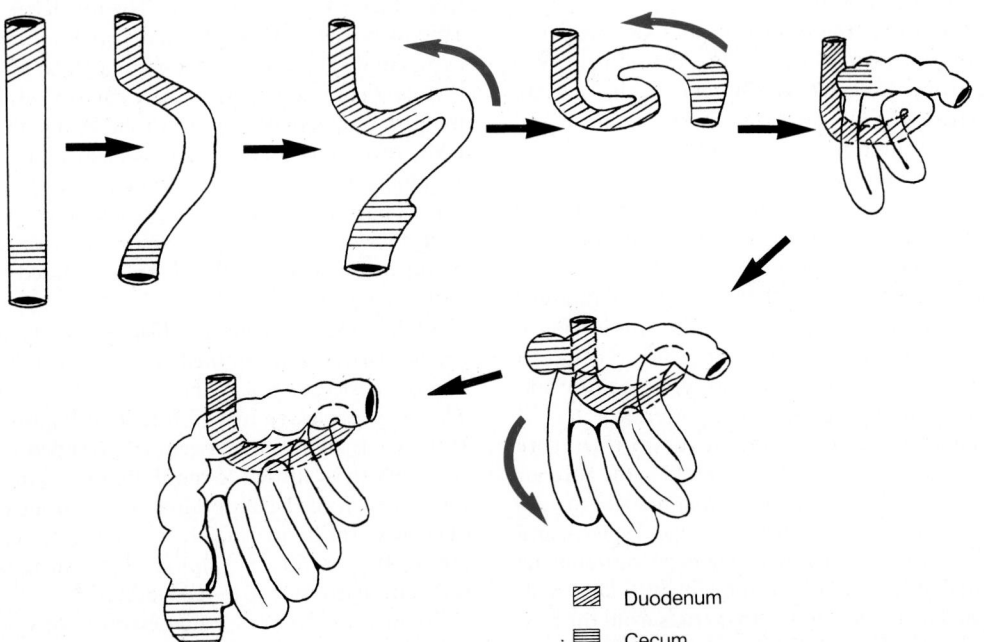

Duodenum

Cecum

FIGURE 100-2. Embryonic development of the midgut. The small intestine and right colon rotate 270 degrees counterclockwise in an anteroposterior plane until the cecum is situated in the lower right area of the peritoneal cavity.

As the dorsal mesogastrium continues to enlarge, it forms the greater omentum, which hangs anteriorly and extends free to the pelvis. The liver develops in the ventral mesogastrium. In the adult, the remnants of the ventral mesogastrium are the ligaments of the liver, coronary, falciform and teres, and the gastrohepatic ligament or lesser omentum. The umbilical vein enters the abdominal cavity through the umbilical ring and follows the ligamentum teres to end in the left branch of the portal vein. The midgut elongates and rotates during its development, and the dorsal mesodermic attachment elongates and folds, forming the mesentery. The final position of the posterior insertion of the mesentery is diagonal, from the left upper quadrant to the right lower quadrant.

The right colon adheres to the posterolateral abdominal wall and becomes retroperitoneal; the rest of the midgut is intraperitoneal. The hindgut elongates to connect the transverse colon with the anal canal. The left colon is retroperitoneal, but on reaching the pelvis, the mesocolon widens and the sigmoid is intraperitoneal. The colon leaves the abdominal cavity in the minor pelvis as the rectum.[2,3]

ANATOMY OF THE ABDOMINAL CAVITY

The limits of the abdominal cavity in the adult are the diaphragm superiorly, the abdominal walls laterally, and the pelvis inferiorly. The peritoneum is a layer of endoderm that covers the walls and organs of the abdominal cavity. The pancreas, part of the duodenum, right and left colon, and rectum are retroperitoneal and covered by peritoneum only over their anterior aspect. The intraperitoneal organs are supported by thickened bands of peritoneum: the gastrohepatic (or lesser omentum), gastrosplenic, gastrocolic, splenorenal, and splenocolic ligaments. The liver is suspended also by the falciform and coronary ligaments to the diaphragm, as well as the ligamentum teres, with the remnant of the umbilical vein, to the anterior abdominal wall.[1]

The final disposition of the embryonic mesodermic bands defines the abdominal compartments. The abdominal cavity has three compartments: lesser sac, supramesocolic, and inframesocolic. The lesser sac is limited by the stomach and gastrocolic ligament anteriorly, spleen, splenorenal, and gastrosplenic ligaments on the left side and by the pancreas and duodenum posteriorly. The right side is occupied by the liver and the lesser omentum. The superior and inferior limits are the diaphragm and the mesocolon, respectively.

The lesser sac communicates with the rest of the abdominal cavity through the foramen of Winslow. The boundaries of the foramen are the liver superiorly, hepatic pedicle (i.e., portal vein, hepatic artery, and bile duct) anteriorly, duodenum and pancreas inferiorly, and retroperitoneum posteriorly.

The supramesocolic and inframesocolic compartments are separated by the transverse mesocolon, inserted in the anterior aspect of duodenum and pancreas. The supramesocolon contains stomach and duodenum, pancreas, liver and spleen, and the lesser sac. The inframesocolic compartment contains the intestine, of variable length among individuals.[4] The small bowel is supported by the mesentery that arises from the posterior abdominal wall, obliquely from the left upper quadrant to the right iliac fossa. The colon is attached to the retroperitoneum of the right and left sides of the abdominal cavity

by the parietocolic peritoneum. In addition to the transverse mesocolon, the transverse colon is also suspended by the gastrocolic ligament and the splenocolic ligament. The area between the colon and the inferior margin of the liver is called Morison's pouch and constitutes a potential site for fluid accumulation.

The inferior limit of the peritoneum covers the pelvic urogenital organs and the inguinal region.[2,3] The most inferior part of the peritoneum between the rectum and the uterus in the female or the bladder in the male is the pouch of Douglas.

The inguinal region is a fusiform area identified superomedially by the arch of the aponeurosis of the transversus abdominis muscle and inferolaterally by the upper ramus of the pubis and the psoas muscle. The area is crossed by the caudal margin of the aponeurosis of the major obliquus abdominis muscle, the inguinal ligament along its major axis, and by the epigastric vessels along its minor axis.[5] This disposition defines four parts in the inguinal region: lateral-superior, lateral-inferior, medial-superior, and medial-inferior.[6] The vas deferens, spermatic artery and vein, and cremasteric muscle form the content of the inguinal canal, which transverses the inguinal region from the internal ring, in the lateral-superior area, to the external inguinal ring, a slit in the medial insertion of the major obliquus aponeurosis.

Congenital Anomalies

In the embryo, the celomic cavity is too small to accommodate the intestines, and they are normally located in the cord. After the 10th week, they become intraabdominal. Omphalocele is a failure in growth of the celomic walls before the 10th week, with a large herniation of viscera into the base of the umbilical cord. Gastroschisis is a similar anomaly, but the peritoneal sac has ruptured in utero and the abdominal viscera are in free contact with the exterior. The incidence is 1 in 3200 to 10,000 births, with slight male predominance. Associated congenital anomalies are found in 30% to 50% of newborns; the most common is incomplete rotation and fixation of the midgut. Omphalocele is part of the Beckwith-Wiedemann or EMG (exomphalos, macroglossia, and gigantism) syndrome, an anomaly characterized by somatic and visceral overgrowth. The diagnosis can be made prenatally by ultrasound or at birth by examination of the neonate, with the finding of a defect in the abdominal wall and extruded viscera, with or without a peritoneal sac.

Omphalocele and gastroschisis are neonatal surgical emergencies that require immediate treatment to prevent dehydration, desiccation of the herniated viscera, sepsis, and death. The sac is protected by painting it with antiseptic solutions. If the sac is absent, the viscera are wrapped in a sheet of silicone, which is sutured to the abdominal wall to serve as a sac until growth of the abdominal wall is sufficient to allow reduction of the hernia and closure of the defect. The mortality rate is 40% to 50%.[7] Amnion inversion repair may offer a safer alternative for high-risk patients.[8]

Remnants of the omphalomesenteric or vitelline ducts that fail to atrophy may lead to interim drainage of fluid from the umbilicus or an inflammatory mass in an infected cyst beneath the midline of the lower abdomen. Persistence of these remnants, including a Meckel's diverticulum, may serve as a point of volvulus of the small intestine.

Congenital Diaphragmatic Hernias

The diaphragm appears in the third week of life as a septum transversum that separates the thorax from the abdomen. It originates ventrally and extends dorsally, leaving a partial thoracoabdominal communication at both sides of the spine in the lumbar area. Pleuroperitoneal folds separate both cavities, with the left side closing later than the right side. The adult diaphragm has two weak areas on each side, the sternocostal area and the lumbocostal area. The former lies between the muscular fibers of the sternal and costal parts of the diaphragm. The lumbocostal area is a defect in the posterior growth of the diaphragm. Anteromedial diaphragmatic hernias of Morgagni are through the diaphragm. Posterolateral diaphragmatic hernias of Bochdalek are between the diaphragm and the lumbar muscles.

Congenital hernias of the diaphragm appear in 1 of 2200 births. They have been reported in 8% of autopsies of infants with other anomalies and in 1.4% of all neonatal deaths.

Anterior hernias contain stomach, colon, or omentum. This type of hernia is usually small and does not tend to cause major symptoms. The diagnosis can be established with a chest radiograph showing an air shadow lateral to the xiphoid. Posterolateral hernias are large, associated with hypoplasia of the ipsilateral lung, and often incompatible with life.[5] The symptoms result from pulmonary abnormalities, mediastinal displacement, and intestinal obstruction. The newborn presents with acute respiratory distress. The heart and mediastinum are displaced, usually to the right, and the abdomen may be scaphoid. Respiratory sounds are absent on the affected side, heart sounds may be audible in the right chest, and intestinal peristalsis is present in the left side of the thorax. Nausea and vomiting are common. Smaller hernias are better tolerated and often present in older children as recurrent respiratory difficulties, particularly after meals. The diagnosis is easily made with a chest radiograph showing multiple air-fluid levels in the left thorax, displacement of the mediastinum, and loss of the sharp diaphragmatic line separating the abdomen from the thorax (Fig. 100-3). A radiologic study using water-soluble contrast can show that the digestive organs are positioned abnormally in the thorax.[9]

The complications of congenital diaphragmatic hernias are respiratory and intestinal. Lung hypoplasia leads to acute respiratory distress and is the main cause of death in these patients. Alterations in the intestinal transit cause chronic malnutrition and failure to thrive. Bowel obstruction and strangulation are common complications, with extremely poor possibility of survival.

Congenital hernias should be surgically corrected. Anterior hernias are easily reduced and repaired with minimal morbidity and mortality. The outcome of posterolateral hernias depends on the age of the patient, associated malformations, and most important, the degree of lung hypoplasia. The mortality rate for posterolateral hernias reaches 50% for patients operated on the first week of life, but the rate rapidly decreases to 10% after the first month as lung maturity improves. The use of

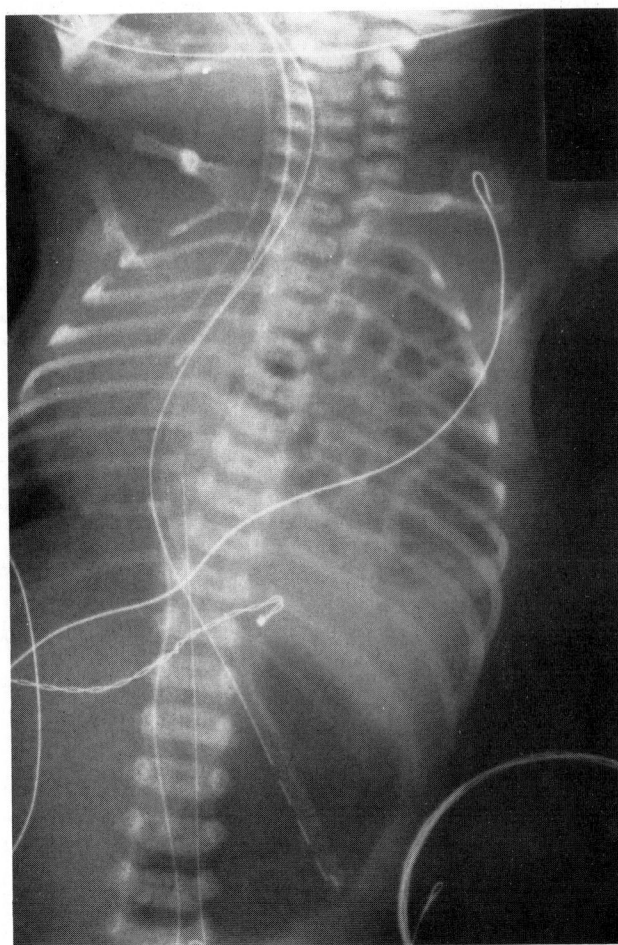

FIGURE 100-3. Chest radiograph of a child with congenital diaphragmatic hernia. The mediastinum is displaced to the right by intestinal loops in the left side of the thorax.

extracorporeal membrane oxygenation may enable further improvement in these statistics.

Umbilical Hernias in the Infant

The herniation of intraabdominal viscera through the umbilicus is an umbilical hernia. It is caused by a congenitally large umbilical ring or one that has been distended by high intraabdominal pressures.

Congenital umbilical hernias are more common in black and male infants. The incidence is related to the age of the neonate, reaching 20% in premature infants. Predisposing conditions are Down's syndrome, gargoylism, amaurotic family idiocy, cretinism, Beckwith-Wiedemann syndrome, and diseases increasing intraabdominal pressure. This type of hernia tends to reduce and heal spontaneously, and strangulation is reported in only 5% of patients. For this reason, umbilical hernias should not be operated on before the patient is 3 years of age unless specific symptoms, large defects, incarceration, or strangulation occur. The practice of adhesive strapping of the umbilicus must be abandoned because it may cause ulceration of the skin and no benefit has been observed. After

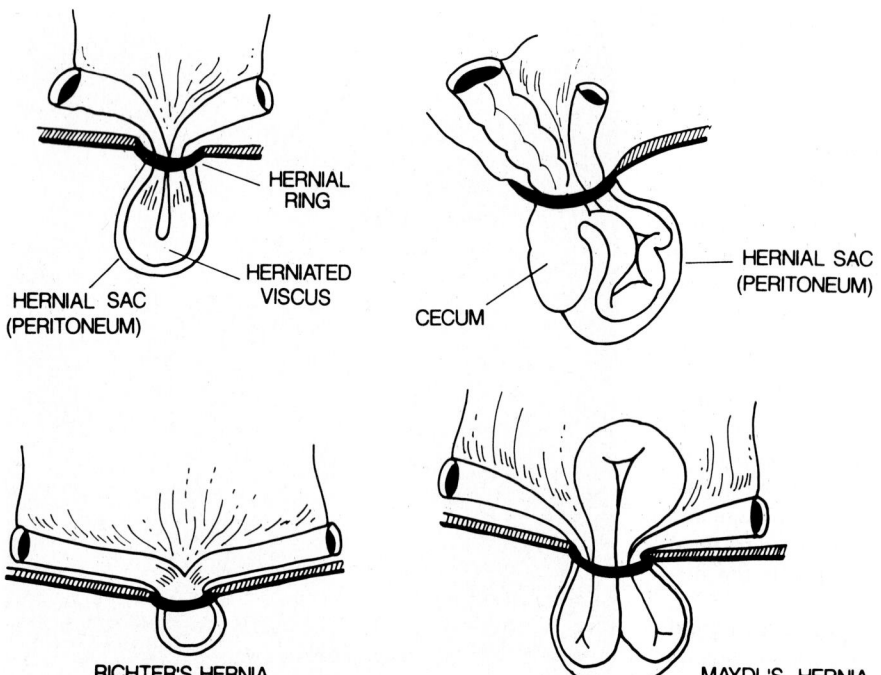

HERNIAL RING

HERNIATED VISCUS

HERNIAL SAC (PERITONEUM)

CECUM

HERNIAL SAC (PERITONEUM)

RICHTER'S HERNIA

MAYDL'S HERNIA

FIGURE 100-4. Different types of intestinal hernias.

the child reaches 3 to 4 years of age, no improvement is expected, and surgical correction is indicated.

HERNIATION IN THE ADULT

"Hernia is a protrusion of any viscus from its proper cavity" (Sir Astley Cooper, 1804). Hernias are composed of a herniated viscus, hernial sac, and hernial ring. The ring is the orifice through which the herniated viscus finds its way to the abnormal location. The hernial sac is the internal wall of the hernia, constituted by peritoneum. A prehernial lipoma often develops from the peritoneal fat corresponding to the hernial sac.

The type of hernias depends on the location of the herniated viscus. It is *external* when it passes through the abdominal, and it is *internal* when the viscus is abnormally located in an intraabdominal space. A diaphragmatic hernia is the herniation of an organ through the diaphragm into the thorax. All intraperitoneal structures can undergo herniation, but intestinal hernias are the most common. A segment of bowel can be totally or only partially herniated (Fig. 100-4).

A partial herniation occurs when only the lateral wall of the bowel is outside the abdominal cavity. This type of herniation is called a Richter's hernia. A herniation of two adjacent loops of bowel through the same hernial ring is called a Maydl's hernia. It constitutes a potentially dangerous situation because the middle loop, which lies in the abdominal cavity, has a tendency to perforate intraabdominally and cause peritonitis if strangulation occurs. A sliding hernia is the herniation of a partially retroperitoneal viscus as part of the wall of the hernial sac.

Mechanical characteristics define three types of herniation: reducible, incarcerated, and strangulated. A hernia is *reducible* when herniation occurs intermittently and returns to the ab-

dominal cavity spontaneously or by external manipulation. An *incarcerated hernia* cannot be reversed, because of its anatomic configuration or because of adhesions to other structures. A hernia, reducible or incarcerated, becomes *strangulated* when the blood supply to the herniated viscus is compromised. This transforms the hernia into a life-threatening situation that requires emergency treatment.

Epidemiology

Hernias are common and account for 10% to 15% of all the procedures in a surgical practice.[5] Of all hernias, 90% are umbilical, incisional, and in the groin (Table 100-1). Indirect

TABLE 100-1
Epidemiology of Groin Hernias*

TYPE	OCCURRENCE
Inguinal	80%
Indirect	60%
Direct	30%
Both	10%
Femoral	5%
Inguinal and femoral	2%
With a sliding component	12%
Sigmoid	8%
Cecum	4%
Maydl's hernia	2%

* Groin hernias account for 85% of all hernias.

Adapted from Ponka JL, Hernias of the abdominal wall. Philadelphia: WB Saunders, 1980, and Nyhus LM, Condon RE, eds. Hernia. Philadelphia: JB Lippincott, 1978.

inguinal hernias are the most common, followed by direct inguinal herniation. Umbilical hernias account for 8% of hernias. Incisional hernias develop after 3% to 5% of all abdominal operations, and they represent 7% of external hernias. Internal hernias are uncommon. In autopsy studies, they have been found in 0.5% of the population. Retroanastomotic hernias are more common, but their true incidence is unknown. They are an important source of iatrogenic pathology.

The incidence of different types of herniation is usually characteristic of gender. Inguinal hernias are reported to be 10 to 25 times more common in males. In 12% of male patients, the hernia is bilateral. Femoral hernias are 2 to 5 times more common in female patients. Umbilical hernias have a male to female ratio of 1 : 3 and are closely related to obesity.[6]

The principal complications of hernias are strangulation and small bowel obstruction. Groin hernias undergo strangulation in 3% to 7% of affected patients, in contrast to femoral and umbilical hernias, for which the rate is 20% to 30%. However, groin hernias still account for a significant number of patients because of the prevalence of indirect inguinal hernias.[6] Hernias rank third as a cause of small bowel obstruction (15%), after adhesions and neoplasms. Of all hernia-related cases of small bowel obstruction, 28% may be attributed to internal hernias and 72% to external hernias. The hernias that are the most common causes of bowel obstruction are inguinal (26%), incisional (21%), femoral (9%), and umbilical (8%).

Epigastric Hernias

Epigastric hernias occur in the midline of the abdominal wall between the umbilicus and the xiphoid. They affect as much as 5% of the population and are often asymptomatic. The hernia transverses a congenital weakness in the linea alba, is usually small, and contains incarcerated preperitoneal fat. Symptoms range from a small, painless nodule inferior to the xiphoid to an acute small bowel obstruction. Epigastric pain on exertion, relieved by reclining, is pathognomonic. The pain may be intense and episodic and therefore difficult to ascribe to a cause. Diagnosis is easy in large epigastric hernias, in which a mass recognizable as intestine in the midline is evident. Small hernias containing preperitoneal fat can be extremely difficult to diagnose, particularly in obese persons. The linea alba must be palpated very carefully while looking for an exquisitely tender spot. Slight elevations of the abdominal surface can sometimes be seen in the area, and pain should increase on exertion or as the patient raises the head from the examining table. Care should be taken to look for multiple hernias, which are reported for 20% of cases.[5] Surgical treatment is indicated.

Umbilical Hernias

Umbilical hernia in the adult occurs in multiparas and in patients with cirrhosis of the liver with ascites. The diagnosis is self-evident in large umbilical hernias with a visible mass of herniated bowel. Abdominal radiographs can demonstrate an intestinal loop outside the abdominal wall. Incarceration of intestine or omentum is common, and strangulation occurs in 20% to 30% of cases, particularly if the umbilical ring is small.

The most feared complication is ulceration and perforation of a large umbilical hernia in a cirrhotic patient with ascites. Forty-two percent of patients with cirrhosis of the liver and ascites have umbilical hernias.[11] Hernial rupture occurs after 2 years of ascites, on average, and is complicated by peritonitis in 23% (frequently by *Staphylococcus aureus*) and renal failure in 11%. The mortality rate is 33% for patients with spontaneous rupture and rises to 60% to 80% for patients not undergoing surgical treatment.

The rule in umbilical hernias of the adult is surgical treatment. Cirrhotic patients with ascites present a particular problem. Control of the ascites and prevention of the complications of an umbilical hernia are mandatory. Any sign increasing the likelihood of perforation, such as ulceration of the skin over the hernia, must be considered as a life-threatening situation demanding aggressive treatment of the ascites. If perforation and loss of ascitic fluid occurs, the patient needs hospital admission, antibiotic treatment specifically for gram-positive microorganisms, and fluid and electrolyte therapy. Surgical treatment without control of the ascites is doomed to immediate recurrence of the hernia and the leak of ascites. Closure of the skin defect with or without herniorrhaphy is the treatment of choice. A simultaneous peritoneovenous shunt may be necessary for control of the ascites.[12,13]

Groin Hernias

Hernias of the groin account for 85% of all hernias, and they constitute a particular problem because of their frequency and the anatomy of the region. Although many variations of herniation are possible, only three types of groin hernia are clinically relevant: inguinal indirect herniation through the internal inguinal ring into the inguinal canal; inguinal direct herniation superior to the inguinal ligament but not through the inguinal canal; and femoral herniation inferior to the inguinal ligament and medial to the epigastric artery and vein (Fig. 100-5). Ileum, omentum, or both are the typical herniated viscera. Sliding hernias involving the colon and bladder are common. A special type of an inguinal indirect hernia containing a Meckel's diverticulum is the Littre's hernia.

The main symptom of groin hernia is a mass in the inguinal area that appears intermittently after activities that increase intraabdominal pressure and disappears on relaxation or manual manipulation. Occasionally, the patient is able to relate the appearance of the mass to a particularly straining event. Pain is seldom severe and only some discomfort may be experienced. Local constant pain suggests incarceration, and colicky abdominal pain is indicative of strangulation.

The diagnosis of hernias of the groin is based on clinical examination. The patient can help by pointing out the area of maximal discomfort. In indirect hernias, it generally corresponds to the internal inguinal ring, and in direct hernias, it lies somewhat more medially. In femoral hernias, pain is more inferior in the groin.

Palpation must always be performed with the patient in the standing and in the decubitus positions, and both sides of the groin and scrotum must be examined. To perform a digital examination, the index finger is introduced into the

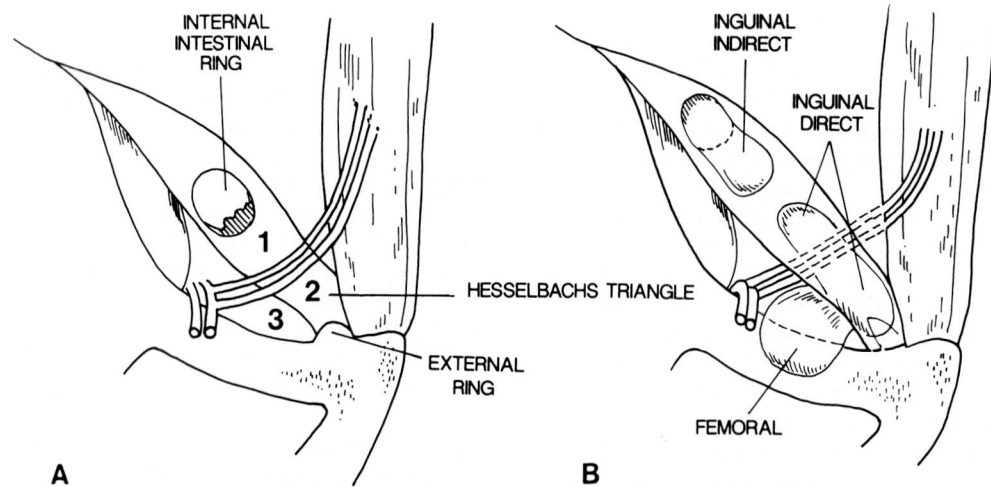

FIGURE 100-5. (**A**) Schematic anatomy of the right inguinal region, showing the spaces where hernias commonly occur; inguinal spaces (1, 2), femoral space (3), and space of Hesselbach (4). (**B**) The most common groin hernias are inguinal, or superior to the inguinal ligament, and femoral, or inferior to the inguinal ligament.

inguinal canal through the external inguinal ring by depressing the skin in the area (Fig. 100-6) If the finger is introduced far enough, the internal ring is palpated, and an indirect hernia is felt exiting the ring. When the finger is introduced in the inguinal canal, direct hernias press the finger laterally instead of at the fingertip. The relation to the epigastric artery is determined by palpating its pulsation. In femoral hernias, the digital examination of the inguinal canal is normal, but careful palpation of the groin below the inguinal ligament demonstrates the femoral mass, particularly in the area near the origin of the vena saphena magna.

The differential diagnosis must consider inguinal lipomas, tumors, lymphadenitis, abscesses, cysts, endometriosis, hydrocele, saphenous varix, and varicocele. The most common diagnostic problem is differentiating femoral hernia from lymphadenitis of the deep inguinal nodes. The main complication of groin hernias is strangulation and small bowel obstruction. Direct hernias almost never strangulate. Five percent of indirect hernias and 20% to 30% of femoral hernias strangulate and present as an emergency. Laparoscopy provides a way to identify the site of herniation and to see the bowel that may be trapped within it.[14]

Surgical correction is the proper treatment of inguinal and femoral hernias. The use of a truss is seldom indicated but can be of help in the occasional patient who is a poor surgical risk. The surgical technique involves the reduction of the hernia, excision of the sac, and closure of the hernial ring. Surgery can be carried out under general or local anesthesia. Under general anesthesia the patient is more relaxed and the repair is technically easier. Local anesthesia is preferred by some surgeons because it has less risk of urinary, cardiovascular, and respiratory complications. The hospital stay is shorter with local anesthesia, and in some centers, hernia repair is performed as an outpatient procedure.

Pelvic Hernias

The intestine can herniate in the floor of the abdominal cavity through the obturator foramen, the greater or lesser sciatic foramina, and through the perineal muscles. Sciatic and per-

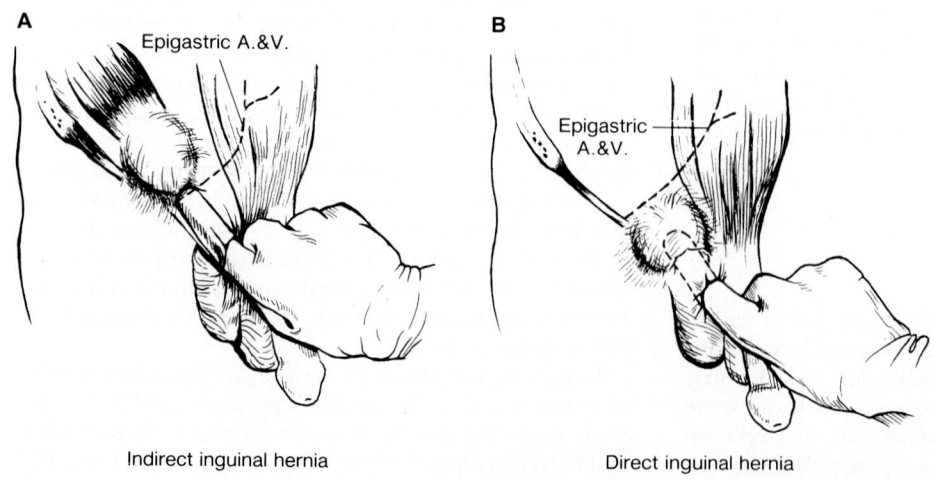

FIGURE 100-6. Digital examination of inguinal hernias. With the finger in the inguinal canal, (**A**) indirect hernias are palpated at the fingertip, and (**B**) direct hernias are palpated by pressing the finger laterally.

ineal hernias are exceedingly rare, and fewer than 100 patients have been reported in the literature.

The most common of these rare hernias is the obturator hernia. The obturator foramen is the largest foramen in the body, but all except a small area is closed by the obturator membrane. The obturator canal begins in the pelvis, traverses the defect in the obturator membrane, and ends in the obturator region in the thigh. Through this canal pass the obturator artery, vein, and nerve. Herniation occurs when the intestine and peritoneal sac enter the obturator canal. Approximately 500 cases of obturator hernia have been reported. It is five to six times more common in females, and appears after the sixth decade of life and on the right side. The sac usually contains ileum, and in 50% of the patients, the hernia is a Richter type. The typical presentation of obturator hernia is acute intestinal obstruction. A history of transient attacks of obstruction is common.

The diagnosis of obturator hernia is made at laparotomy. However, if the possibility of obturator hernia is considered, the diagnosis can be made preoperatively by knowledge of two characteristic signs or symptoms. First, it is a deep hernia, and it is seldom palpable in the thigh. However, it may be palpated on vaginal or anal examination as a soft, tender, anterolateral, fluctuating mass incarcerated in the obturator canal (Fig. 100-7). Second, the Howship-Romberg sign is present in 50% of patients and is pathognomonic of obturator hernia. This sign is pain in the medial surface of the thigh, radiating to the knee and occasionally to the hip. Flexion of the thigh ameliorates the pain, while extension, adduction, or medial rotation exacerbates it.[15] On radiologic studies, an abnormal gas shadow may be observed in the region of the obturator foramen. Several cases of incarcerated obturator hernia have been diagnosed by computed tomography of the pelvis.[16,17] Treatment is surgical.

Lumbar Hernias

The posterior abdominal wall has two naturally weak areas in the superior and inferior lumbar triangles. The superior triangle of Grynfelt-Lesshaft, also called lumbocostoabdominal triangle, is the most common site for lumbar herniation. It is limited by the 12th rib, the posterior border of the internal oblique, and the anterior border of the sacrospinalis. The inferior triangle of Petit or lumboiliac abdominal triangle is limited by the iliac crest, the anterior border of the latissimus dorsi, and the posterior border of the external oblique muscle.

Lumbar hernias can be congenital or acquired. Congenital hernias are exceedingly rare. Acquired lumbar hernias are caused by trauma to the flank or rib, by iliac crest fractures, and by removal of a fragment of iliac crest for bone grafting.[5] It is more common in males and on the left lumbar region. Symptoms range from none to a painful node in the lumbar area. Traction of viscera can cause abdominal pain referred to the back or to the pelvis. The differential diagnosis must consider abscess, hematoma, and soft tissue tumors. Abscesses and hematomas are more tender. Irreducibility and absence of a trauma antecedent raise the suspicion of tumors. Surgical repair of lumbar hernias is always advocated because their normal evolution is that of a progression in size.

Spigelian Hernias

A Spigelian hernia is a spontaneous abdominal defect lateral to the rectus abdominis, with the protrusion passing through the external oblique fascia.[18] It is a rare condition. Only 300 cases have been reported, all with the herniation below the arcuate line of Douglas. Spigelian hernias appear in elderly patients, and they are often small and difficult to diagnose because of the usual obesity of the patient.

Local pain or discomfort, increased by straining and coughing, is common. If irreducible, they can be easily confused with abdominal wall tumors. Radiologically, an abnormal gas shadow may be seen within the abdominal wall. Contrast studies can show the bowel lumen outside the abdominal cavity. Ultrasound is a useful tool in the diagnosis of small masses in the lateral abdominal wall. The relevance of Spigelian hernia resides in the awareness of its possibility when dealing with bizarre abdominal pains of a difficult diagnosis. Surgical repair is mandatory, and the results are excellent.

Traumatic Hernias of the Diaphragm

Lesions of the diaphragm result from penetrating or blunt trauma. The most common injury is a large tear of the diaphragm from the esophageal hiatus to the left costal attachments. The herniated viscera are the stomach, spleen, colon, and left lobe of the liver. Traumatic herniation of the diaphragm occurs in two phases. The first is immediately after

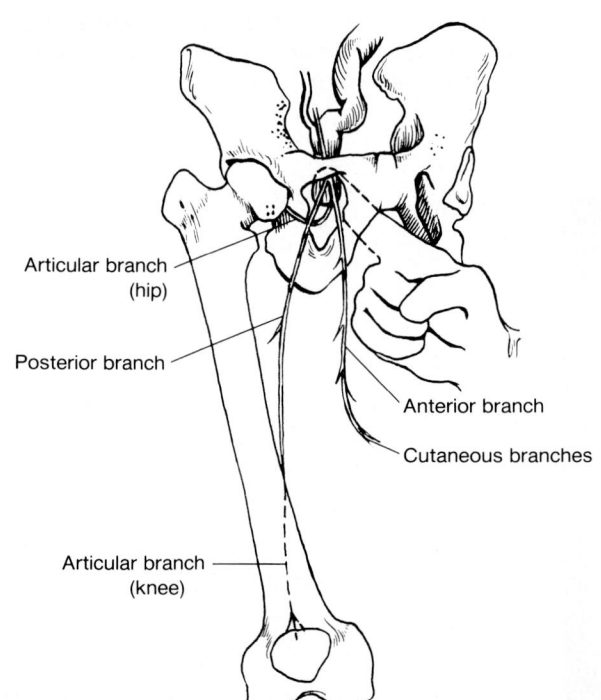

FIGURE 100-7. Rectal or vaginal palpation of the obturator foramen may confirm the existence of an obturator hernia. (Adapted from Nyhus LM, Condon RE, eds. Hernia. Philadelphia: JB Lippincott, 1978.)

Articular branch (hip)

Posterior branch

Anterior branch

Cutaneous branches

Articular branch (knee)

the trauma the diaphragm is injured, but no viscus is herniated. This phase may be accompanied by quadrant pain referred to the left shoulder and scapular area. The second phase is the herniation of abdominal viscera, which may lead to nausea and vomiting. Retching and inability to vomit raise the suspicion of an incarcerated stomach. Central abdominal pain, diaphoresis, and general discomfort result from traction of blood vessels and mesentery. Respiratory distress can appear in large hernias from lung compression and mediastinal deviation. In some patients, symptoms can be mild, and the hernia remains undiagnosed for years.[19]

The diagnosis of traumatic diaphragmatic hernia is made with a chest radiograph, with or without contrast medium, and visualization of the abdominal viscera in the thorax (Fig. 100-8). A normal radiograph does not exclude traumatic hernia, because its appearance can be delayed by days. Fluoroscopy is helpful in the evaluation of diaphragmatic excursions. Ultrasound and CT scan can detect viscera abnormally located in the thorax. The principal complication is intestinal obstruction, often involving the intraabdominal viscera more than the intrathoracic.

Wounds of the diaphragm require immediate surgical repair. Herniation can increase at any time, and a previously stable patient can rapidly develop acute respiratory distress, strangulation of the hernia contents, or compromise of the blood supply to the entrapped viscera.

INTERNAL HERNIAS

An internal hernia is the protrusion of an intraperitoneal viscus into a compartment within the abdominal cavity. The hernial ring is a natural foramen or defect of the peritoneal layers, and the hernial sac is generally nonexistent. The fossae and spaces where hernias potentially can occur are many, but herniation is rare. Internal herniation has been reported only in 0.2% to 0.9% of examinations of cadavers. In a review of 467 patients, paraduodenal hernias were the most common (53%), followed by pericecal (13%), foramen of Winslow (8%), pelvic and supravesical (7%), and intersigmoid (6%) hernias.[20]

Internal hernias have similar symptoms, regardless of their location. The herniation is often intermittent and causes recurrent postprandial attacks of small bowel obstruction, with nausea, vomiting, and colicky abdominal pain. The patient is totally asymptomatic between episodes.[21] Acute small bowel obstruction is the most common complication, and in 0.5% to 3% of patients, it is caused by an internal hernia. Strangulation is a feared complication that carries a mortality rate of 50% despite appropriate surgical treatment.

The diagnosis is often incidental, because many hernias are small and asymptomatic. The diagnosis of symptomatic hernias is made by radiologic examination or at laparotomy. Radiologic studies of the abdomen must include views of the patient in lateral and erect positions and can show abnormalities in the location and distribution of the abdominal gas pattern. The features of internal hernias in intestinal studies with barium contrast are disturbances in the arrangements of bowel loops, sacculation, segmental dilatation, stasis, and fixation of the herniated loops.[22] Reversed peristalsis is a sign of obstruction to the intestinal transit. Arteriography is helpful for the differential diagnosis of internal hernias. The arteriographic findings can show displacement of the blood vessels and, most important, reversal of their course.[23] Intraabdominal masses and tumors instead show stretching of the vessels, and thrombotic lesions show a stop in their course.

The differential diagnosis must consider intestinal volvulus, adhesions, and tumors. The treatment of internal hernias is surgical, with reduction of the herniated viscus and correction of associated anatomic defects.

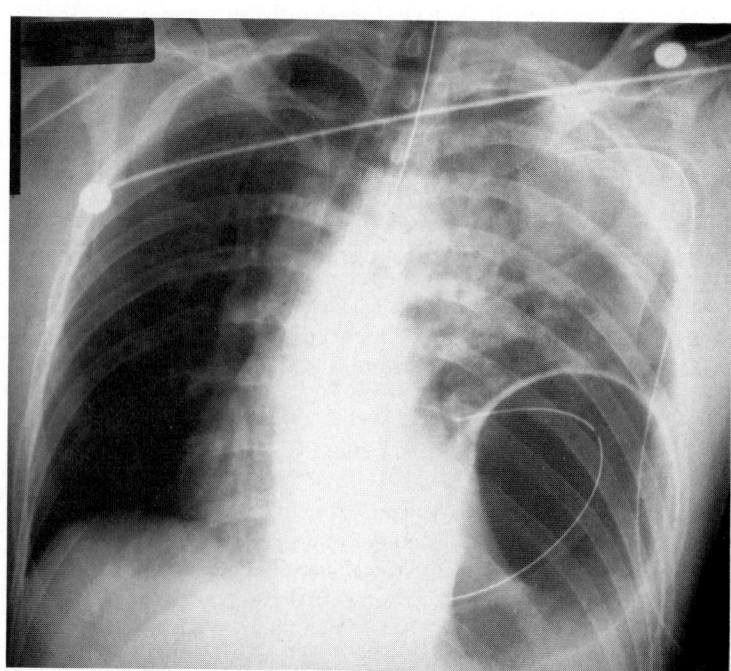

FIGURE 100-8. Traumatic hernia of the diaphragm. The diaphragmatic line on the left side has disappeared, and the gastric fundus is in the left thoracic space.

Paraduodenal Hernias

Moynihan described nine paraduodenal fossae in 1889. Of those, only the fossae of Landzert and of Waldeyer are clinically relevant. The left paraduodenal fossa of Landzert is a peritoneal pocket lateral to the fourth duodenal segment and posterior to the inferior mesenteric vein and left colic artery. The right mesentericoparietal fossa of Waldeyer is deep to the superior mesenteric artery and inferior to the third duodenal segment. Seventy-five percent of paraduodenal hernias occur in the left fossa and 25% in the right fossa.[24]

Paraduodenal hernias are thought to originate from a defect in the rotation of the midgut. A left hernia results from a rotation of the midgut dorsally to the colic branches of the inferior mesenteric artery instead of ventrally, invaginating into the mesocolon. A right hernia is formed by the incomplete rotation of the midgut, which remains in the right side of the abdomen and is trapped in a sac of which the anterior wall is the mesocolon with the right branches of the superior mesenteric artery. The cecum remains in a high position and attached to the right abdominal wall by the bands of Ladd, a thickening of the parietocolic peritoneum.[25]

Radiographs of paraduodenal hernias show encapsulation of the small bowel with stasis of the herniated loops.[26] Left large hernias displace the stomach superiorly and the left colon inferomedially. Right large hernias displace the right colon anteriorly. Erect views of the abdomen show the ovoid hernial mass with a convex inferior border and no small bowel in the pelvis. Lateral views demonstrate the abnormally posterior location of the small bowel. Arteriography is useful in the diagnosis. In left hernias, the jejunal vessels are redirected medially and posteriorly, and the superior mesenteric artery is in normal position. In right hernias, the jejunal arteries arise normally from the superior mesenteric artery, but they are reversed, behind their original vessel, toward the right.

Hernias of the Foramen of Winslow

Herniation through the foramen of Winslow into the lesser sac is facilitated by a large foramen and abnormal mobility of the colon. The small intestine is involved in 70% of cases, and the cecum and ascending colon in 25%. Radiologically, a gas-distended loop of bowel can be seen in the lesser sac. Contrast radiographs show the stomach and colon to be displaced anteriorly. Lateral views demonstrate small bowel loops in an epigastric posterior location. Usually, there are associated signs of small bowel obstruction.[27]

Pericecal Hernias

Four peritoneal fossae have been described in the appendicocecal mesentery: ileocolic, retrocecal, ileocecal, and paricecal.[20] Only the ileocecal fossa, as the site for 13% of internal hernias, is relevant. In most cases, the ileum passes through defects in the cecal mesentery and occupies the right paracolic gutter. Clinically, it manifests as right lower quadrant intermittent pain with or without recurrent small bowel obstruction.

Intersigmoid Hernias

The intersigmoid fossa, a peritoneal pocket between the two sigmoid loops, is found in 65% of cadavers. The incarceration of small bowel in the fossa is a rare phenomenon in a usually reducible hernia. The diagnosis is made by noticing ileal retrograde filling during a barium enema.[27]

Transmesenteric and Transomental Hernias

Approximately 5% to 10% of internal hernias occur through defects in the mesenterium, and 1% to 4% occur in the omentum. Transmesenteric hernias are the most common in children, accounting for 35% of internal hernias in this group of patients. Usually, they present through defects 2 to 5 cm long in the mesenterium of the first jejunal loop. Prenatal intestinal ischemic accidents have been postulated as a possible cause.[6] The area of the defect is often associated with an atretic segment of intestine. The herniated bowel can also volvulate and has a particular tendency to strangulate. The radiographic appearance is usually that of an acute small bowel obstruction.[28]

IATROGENIC HERNIAS

Iatrogenic hernias result from the creation of weak areas and abnormal foramina in the abdominal cavity. Herniation may be further facilitated by the abnormal anatomy after some surgical procedures. Seventy-five percent of iatrogenic hernias manifest in the first postoperative year.

Retroanastomotic Hernias

A retroanastomotic hernia (i.e., internal hernia) is the herniation of intestine through a mesenteric space left open in the course of an anastomosis. The classic case is herniation after a Billroth II operation through the space between the gastrojejunostomy, which is anterior, and the posterior aspect of the abdominal cavity. However, the bowel can also herniate through defects in the mesentery and mesocolon after intestinal resections.[29] Retroanastomotic hernias are frequently acute and cause intestinal obstruction. If necessary, a barium meal can define the location and type of obstruction caused by the hernia.[26] Immediate surgical treatment is mandatory on diagnosis.

Incisional Hernias

Incisional hernias (i.e., external hernias) constitute approximately 2% of all hernias. They occur after 2% to 5% of all abdominal operations.[6] The cause is multifactorial. Technical factors include defective suture of the abdominal muscles, drains exteriorized through the wound, and the type of abdominal incision. Vertical laparotomies follow the tension lines of the abdomen and damage the rectus abdominis innervation.[30] Multiple incisions from several operations aggravate the weakness of the abdominal wall. The infraumbilical area is more susceptible to incisional hernia.

Associated diseases increasing intraabdominal pressure and subjecting the wound to stress in the early postoperative period govern many incisional hernias. Coagulation defects facilitate hematomas in the wound. Infections, anemia, and malnutrition may contribute. More than 50% of patients with incisional hernias have a history of wound infection, and 30% of infected laparotomy wounds are followed by herniation.

The diagnosis of incisional hernia is evident on inspection of the abdominal scar and hernial mass. The hernial ring can be palpated. It is often wide, with the margins of the rectus abdominis far apart. Incisional hernias incarcerate but do not tend to strangulate. Operative repair is generally indicated.

The reader is directed to Chapter 34, Approach to the Patient With Abdominal Pain; Chapter 36, Approach to the Patient With Acute Abdomen; Chapter 37, Approach to the Patient With Ileus and Obstruction; Chapter 43, Approach to the Patient With Ascites; Chapter 53, Esophagus: Anatomy and Structural Anomalies; Chapter 59, Stomach: Anatomy and Structural Anomalies; Chapter 68, Small Intestine: Anatomy and Structural Anomalies; Chapter 78, Colon: Anatomy and Structural Anomalies; Chapter 101, Intraabdominal Abscesses and Fistulas; Chapter 102, Diseases of the Mesentery and Omentum; Chapter 103, Diseases of the Peritoneum; Chapter 104, Diseases of the Retroperitoneum; and Chapter 140, Exploratory Laparotomy.

REFERENCES

1. Clemente C, ed. Gray's anatomy of the human body. Philadelphia: Lea & Febiger, 1985.
2. O'Rahilly R. Anatomy. A regional study of the human structure. Philadelphia: WB Saunders, 1986.
3. Joseph J. A textbook of regional anatomy. Baltimore: University Park Press, 1982.
4. Underhill RML. Intestinal length in man. Br Med J 195;2:1243.
5. Ponka JL. Hernias of the abdominal wall. Philadelphia: WB Saunders, 1980.
6. Nyhus LM, Condon RE, eds. Hernia. 3rd ed. Philadelphia: JB Lippincott, 1989.
7. Schier VF, Schier S, Stute MP, et al. Postoperative findings from 193 cases of gastroschisis and omphalocele. Zentralbl Chir 1988;223:225.
8. Yokomori K, Ohkura M, Kitano Y, et al. Advantages and pitfalls of amnion inversion repair for the treatment of large unruptured omphalocele: results of 22 cases. J Pediatr Surg 1992;27:882.
9. Ghahremani GG, Meyers MA. Hernias. In: Teplick JE, Haskins ME, eds. Surgical radiology. Vol I. Philadelphia: WB Saunders, 1981:287.
10. Mulcha P. Small intestinal obstruction. Surg Clin North Am 1987;67:597.
11. Kirkpatrick S, Schubert T. Umbilical hernia rupture in cirrhotics with ascites. Dig Dis Sci 1988;33:762.
12. Bunt TB, Mohr JB. Ruptured umbilical hernia in cirrhotic patients: management with peritoneovenous shunting and herniorrhaphy. Southern Med J 1985;78:755.
13. O'Connor M, Allen JI, Schwartz ML. Peritoneovenous shunt therapy for leaking ascites in the cirrhotic patient. Ann Surg 1984;200:66.
14. Binderow SR, Klapper AS, Bufalini B. Hernioscopy: laparoscopy via an inguinal hernia sac. J Laparoendosc Surg 1992;2:229.
15. Young A, Hudson DA, Krige JEJ. Strangulated obturator hernia: can mortality be reduced? South Med J 1988;81:1117.
16. Cubillo E. Obturator hernia diagnosed by computed tomography. AJR 1983;140:735.
17. Meziane MA, Fishman EK, Siegelman SS. Computed tomographic diagnosis of obturator foramen hernia. Gastrointest Radiol 1983;8:375.
18. Spangen L. Spigelian hernia. Acta Chir Scand 1976;462 (Suppl):3.
19. Feliciano DV, Cruse PA, Mattox KL, et al. Delayed diagnosis of injuries to the diaphragm after penetrating wounds. J Trauma 1988;28:1135.
20. Hansmann GH, Morton SA. Intraabdominal hernia: report of a case and review of the literature. Arch Surg 1939;39:973.
21. Turley K. Right paraduodenal hernia. A source of chronic abdominal pain in he adult. Arch Surg 1979;114:1072.
22. Williams AJ. Roentgen diagnosis of intraabdominal hernia. An evaluation of the roentgen findings. Radiology 1952;59:817.
23. Cohen AM, Patel S. Arteriographic findings in congenital transmesenteric internal hernia. AJR 1979;133:541.
24. Berardi RS. Paraduodenal hernias. Surg Gynecol Obstet 1981;152:99.
25. Willwerth BM, Zollinger RM, Izant RJ. Congenital mesocolic (paraduodenal) hernia. Embryologic basis for repair. Am J Surg 1974;128:358.
26. Meyers MA. Paraduodenal hernias. Radiologic and arteriographic diagnosis. Radiology 1970;95:29.
27. Ghahremani GG. Internal abdominal hernias. Surg Clin North Am 1984;64:393.
28. Ghahremani GG, Meyers MA. Internal abdominal hernias. Curr Probl Radiol 1975;5:1.
29. Ghahremani GG, Meyers MA. Iatrogenic abdominal hernias. In: Meyers MA, Ghahremani GG, eds. Iatrogenic gastrointestinal complications. New York: Springer-Verlag, 1981:269.
30. Naraynsingh V, Ariyanayagam D. Rectus repair for midline ventral abdominal wall hernia. Br J Surg 1993;80:614.

Textbook of Gastroenterology, second edition, edited by Tadataka Yamada. JB Lippincott Company, Philadelphia © 1995.

CHAPTER 101

Intraabdominal Abscesses and Fistulas

Thomas D. Kimbrough

Despite the development of better imaging techniques, more potent antibiotics, and alternatives to surgical treatment, intraabdominal abscesses and fistulas continue to result in significant morbidity, with reported mortality rates ranging from 10% to 30%.[1,2] Although the presence of one does not require that of the other, the two entities frequently coexist.

This chapter discusses the cause, clinical manifestations, diagnosis, and treatment of each. Liver and pancreas abscesses as well as biliary and pancreatic fistulas are discussed elsewhere in this book. Abscesses and fistulas associated with inflammatory bowel disease are mentioned in this chapter but are covered in more detail elsewhere.

ABSCESSES

Epidemiology

Abscesses are defined as collections of fluid containing necrotic debris, leukocytes, and bacteria. Their incidence varies greatly among different patient populations, types of injuries, primary illnesses, and comorbidities. The chance of abscess development depends on the underlying disease process and other factors, including extent of bacterial contamination, competence of the patient's immune system, and the presence or absence of foreign material. Overall, the incidence seems to be decreasing, probably because of general advances in medical care. Paradoxically, these improvements in care have resulted in the survival of critically injured and ill patients long enough to develop abscesses. Some seriously ill patients who would previously have died earlier in their illness now live long enough to develop this complication.

Intraabdominal abscesses are usually the result of operative complications, trauma, perforations of enteric viscera, pancreatic and biliary disease, and infections of the genitourinary tract.[3] Goins and colleagues emphasized the importance of blunt trauma as a cause for intraabdominal abscesses in a report in 1990.[4] Of 325 patients who underwent laparotomy for blunt trauma, 15 developed 40 abscesses. Factors associated with an increased chance of abscess formation included blunt injuries to the pancreas and kidneys and increasing severity of injury.[4] Others report similar rates (6%–8%) of abscess development after blunt and penetrating trauma.[5,6] In an often-cited article published in 1973, Altemeier and associates reported 540 abscesses in 501 patients. Forty-four percent of the abscesses that were intraperitoneal were located in the right lower quadrant, reflecting the importance of appendicitis as a causative factor in the series.[3]

A review of published reports shows that the underlying cause varies according to the population examined. After excluding abscesses associated with the primary operation for acute appendicitis and perforated peptic ulcers, Fry and associates observed that 40% of the abscesses in their series were in trauma patients. Operative technical errors such as anastomotic leaks were the next largest group and accounted for 17.5%.[2] Later reports show complications after abdominal surgery to be a more common etiologic agent.[7,8]

Etiology

Abscesses result from the localization of infectious processes in the peritoneal cavity, its organs, or the retroperitoneum. Possible sources of bacterial contamination include exogenous organisms introduced by penetrating trauma, hematogenous seeding of abdominal tissues from adjacent or distant infections, or perforations of the gastrointestinal tract. Contamination by any source can be cleared by host defense mechanisms, cause diffuse infection, or localize into an abscess or abscesses. Which outcome results and its eventual effect on the host depends on multiple factors, including the source and size of the bacterial inoculum, the nature of the peritoneal response, and host immune function. If the contamination is overwhelming, the patient may die rapidly. If the contamination is treated promptly and effectively, the episode may be resolved with no adverse sequelae.

If host defenses are unable to clear the contamination, areas of bacterial sequestration may result. Because the mechanisms involved in sequestration can protect bacteria from host leukocytes and administered antibiotics, the walling-off process can lead to bacterial proliferation and abscess development. Other responses attendant to the typical initiating injury or infection can act as adjuvants that facilitate abscess formation. The difficulty of producing intraabdominal abscesses in animal models with pure cultures of single bacterial species point out the efficiencies of normal mammalian defense mechanisms in preventing peritoneal infection and the great importance of adjuvant factors in the development of an abscess. Animal studies have shown that hemoglobin, mucin, bile, and urine can act in an adjuvant fashion and increase mortality when bacteria are injected into the peritoneal cavity. In most clinical settings, contamination of the peritoneal cavity introduces bacterial organisms and some or all of these established adjuvants.

Peritoneal inflammation by any mechanism causes the transudation of protein-rich fluid, complement production, and leukocyte attraction and activation. These are all protective mechanisms, but they can also have undesirable effects. For example, the activation of tissue thromboplastin results in the formation of fibrin, which has a tendency to trap bacteria and prevent their absorption into local lymphatics. These substances promote bacterial proliferation, impair lymphatic clearance of bacteria from the peritoneum, and inhibit their phagocytosis by neutrophils.

The frequent presence of multiple species of bacteria in the clinical conditions preceding abscess development allows synergism, especially between aerobic and anaerobic organisms. Aerobic bacteria promote the growth of anaerobic ones by consuming available oxygen and creating more favorable growth conditions. Some anaerobic bacteria interfere with effective phagocytosis of bacteria by host neutrophils, promoting proliferation of aerobic and anaerobic species.[9]

The source of contamination determines the bacteria most likely to be cultured from an abscess, and because the source is frequently the gastrointestinal tract, enteric bacteria predominate (Table 101-1). Those most frequently isolated include gram-negative facultative organisms such as *Escherichia coli*, *Klebsiella*, *Enterobacter*, *Proteus*, and *Pseudomonas* species. The most common pathogenic anaerobic organism is *Bacteroides fragilis*, and anaerobic bacteria can be cultured in over 90% of abscesses with proper technique.

The nature of the bacterial contamination to a great extent depends on the site of perforation and associated conditions locally and systemically. For example, there are normally few bacteria present in the stomach because the acidic pH destroys those introduced. However, the increase in pH associated with the presence of food, antiulcer medications, and diseases as-

TABLE 101-1
Bacteria Commonly Isolated From Abscesses

ISOLATED ORGANISMS	POSITIVE CULTURES*
Aerobic and Facultative Isolates	
Escherichia coli	57
α-Hemolytic *Streptococcus*	15
Group D *Streptococcus*	9
Klebsiella pneumoniae	8
γ-Hemolytic *Streptococcus*	7
Pseudomonas aeruginosa	4
Anaerobic Isolates	
Bacteroides fragilis	47
Clostridium species	12
Peptostreptococcus species	7
Clostridium perfringens	6
Peptostreptococcus magnus	6

* Aerobic and anaerobic organisms cultured from 83 intraabdominal abscesses.
From Brook I. A 12 year study of aerobic and anaerobic bacteria in intraabdominal and postsurgical abdominal wound infections. Surg Gynecol Obstet 1989;169:387.

sociated with gastric achlorhydria is associated with an incremental increase in the number of viable gastric organisms. Bacterial counts in the small bowel range from 10^4 in its proximal portions to 10^8 distally. Greater bacterial proliferation is prevented by the constant peristaltic sweeping activity. When this is disrupted by an ileus or mechanical obstruction, rapid increases in small bowel bacterial counts result, with the attendant increased morbidity and mortality in the event of perforation. Bacterial concentrations in the colon range from 10^9 to 10^{12}, and as with the small bowel, the count increases greatly when normal clearance mechanisms are impaired.

The process that causes the contamination and its acuity influences the location and development of abscesses. The complexity and shape of the abdominal cavity provide many spaces in which contaminated fluid can collect and become sequestered. Abscesses can develop almost anywhere in the abdominal cavity. Several factors influence the eventual location. For example, initially localized peritoneal inflammatory processes such as appendicitis and diverticulitis cause adherence of adjacent loops of small bowel and omentum that attempt to wall off the area from the rest of the abdomen. If perforation occurs after the area is walled off, a localized abscess results. If perforation occurs before the area is isolated, diffuse peritoneal contamination may occur with the development of generalized peritonitis and possible abscess formation far from the initial site of perforation. Diffuse contamination is more likely in cases of acute contamination without a preexisting period of localized inflammation.

When generalized peritonitis occurs, fluid tends to accumulate in those portions of the abdominal cavity that are dependent in a recumbent patient. These include the subdiaphragmatic, infrahepatic, and pelvic spaces. The mechanics of respiration result in a cephalic migration of peritoneal fluid under normal circumstances. This may be helpful in a teleologic sense, because it tends to move bacteria and debris toward the lymphatic openings in the diaphragmatic perito-neum. This phenomenon may also contribute to the relative high incidence of subphrenic abscesses in many series.

The architectural arrangement of the abdominal cavity in-fluences abscess sites in ways other than gravity-related de-pendence. The transverse colon and omentum divide the peritoneal cavity into cephalad and caudad compartments, and abscesses tend to localize to one side of the the transverse colon or the other. The falciform ligament divides the upper peritoneal space into right and left and similarly localizes ab-scesses to one side or the other of the upper abdomen. The folding of loops of small bowel and mesentery one on another can result in interloop abscesses if bacteria become sequestered between them.

Clinical Manifestations

Classically, patients with an intraabdominal abscess complain of intermittent fever, abdominal pain, anorexia, and malaise. Febrile episodes are usually intermittent and spiking. Maximal temperatures are commonly greater than 102°F, and chills may precede the onset of fever. Abdominal pain may be lo-calized to the region of the abscess or may be generalized, vague, and nonspecific. Subphrenic abscesses can cause shoulder pain and hiccups from diaphragmatic irritation. If the abscess is close to the urinary bladder, the patient may experience urgency or frequency of urination. Proximity to the colon or rectum may induce diarrhea or tenesmus. An-orexia is a common accompanying symptom. Many patients with intraabdominal abscesses manifest a persistent inability to tolerate a diet and do not"feel well." The signs and symp-toms of abdominal abscesses vary widely. Symptoms are often vague, and any or all of the preceding symptoms may be absent.

Physical findings also can be quite variable. A patient with a chronic, well-localized abscess may present with point ten-derness and a palpable mass. Another patient's presentation may be that of advanced sepsis with obtundation, fever, and hypotension. Most patients with intraabdominal abscesses look sick. They are lethargic and sometimes confused. Physical examination may reveal otherwise unexplained tachycardia and tachypnea. Bowel sounds may be diminished or com-pletely absent. Abdominal distention usually accompanies di-minished motility. Careful palpation may reveal localized tenderness or even a tender mass when the abscess is near or abuts the abdominal wall. Pelvic abscesses can sometimes be palpated during rectal or vaginal examinations. With many abscesses, the physical findings are insufficient to allow more than consideration of the diagnosis.

For the critically ill patient, diagnosis by history and phys-ical findings can be even more difficult. The improved care of critically injured and ill patients has resulted in their survival long enough to develop complications such as abscesses. These patients are often on ventilators, in an altered mental state, on extensive antimicrobial therapy, and sometimes on potent immunosuppressives. All of these things can mask the clinical signs of an intraabdominal abscess and delay its recognition. If the underlying abscess remains unidentified and untreated, the clinical picture can progress to full-blown sepsis. Diagnosis

and treatment at this point in the process typically have poor results.

Clinicians must maintain a high index of suspicion for all patients at risk for abscess development. The possibility should be entertained for any patient who is not making the pro-gression to recovery as expected and who has suffered an injury or illness that could lead to abscess development. After the diagnosis is considered, it should be further evaluated by ap-propriate means. This often means using one of the imaging studies discussed in the next section.

Differential Diagnosis and Diagnostic Studies

The nonspecific and general nature of the symptoms asso-ciated with intraabdominal abscesses allow varied set of po-tential differential diagnoses. Viral infections can produce fe-ver and leukocytosis and may be associated with abdominal pain, tenderness, nausea, and vomiting. Lower thoracic and retroperitoneal inflammatory processes such as pneumonia, pleurisy, empyema, and pyelonephritis may produce signs and symptoms that are referred to the abdomen.

Inflammatory processes of the peritoneum or abdominal viscera may be impossible to differentiate from an intraab-dominal abscess. A phlegmon is a bacterial cellulitis without a localized fluid collection and therefore not amenable to drainage. The associated edema and neighboring dilated bowel can make differentiation of this lesion from an abscess difficult. To further complicate the diagnosis, some diseases such as Crohn's disease and diverticulitis can start as acute inflam-matory processes and evolve into abscess formation. The dif-ferentiation of one from the other requires diligence, persis-tence, further diagnostic studies, and sometimes laparotomy.

There are no specifically diagnostic clinical laboratory tests. The most helpful is a complete blood count. Patients with abscesses often have mild anemia and an elevated leukocyte count. Tests of liver function, particularly serum bilirubin, may be abnormal because of the deleterious effect of bacter-emia and septicemia on hepatocellular function. Abscesses in and around the pancreas can cause an elevated amylase levels. The identification of typical enteric organisms in positive blood cultures strongly suggests the presence of an intraab-dominal abscess.

Plain radiographs are seldom diagnostic but can support the diagnosis. Chest radiographs may show pleural effusions, an elevated diaphragm, and adjacent atelectasis on the side opposite a subphrenic abscess. Plain abdominal films can re-veal air-fluid levels, gas bubbles outside the intestinal tract, displacement of viscera from their normal location, and an abnormal mass. However, the most frequent finding on ab-dominal films is a relative excess of intralumenal bowel gas. Clinical evaluation, laboratory tests, and conventional radio-graphs of the chest and abdomen can establish the diagnosis of intraabdominal abscess in less than one half of patients.[11] More sophisticated and more expensive imaging techniques usually are necessary to make the diagnosis, establish abscess location, and guide therapy.

The more sophisticated imaging techniques used for iden-tifying and localizing abscesses include computed tomography (CT), ultrasonography, and nuclear scans. Magnetic resonance imaging has not shown resolution capabilities any better than CT for this problem. If the combination of history, physical examination, and plain radiographs do not readily lead to the diagnosis, the imaging test of choice is CT, followed by ultrasonography. Most clinicians use nuclear scans infrequently as a primary tool. The scans are reported to be helpful at times in complex and complicated cases. Negative imaging studies in patients harboring intraabdominal abscesses occur. Exploratory laparotomy is the final diagnostic procedure and should be considered despite equivocal or even negative studies in patients thought clinically likely to have an abscess.

The steady advances in CT technology have resulted in its present ability to diagnose more than 90% of intraabdominal abscesses.[12,13] In addition to greater sensitivity, CT has several advantages over other methods. It is much less dependent on technician skill than ultrasonography. Complete evaluation of the abdomen and pelvis can be completed by this method faster than any other, which is an important consideration in the often critically ill patients who are the target of such concerns. The images obtained are more easily interpreted and understood by clinicians. The disadvantages include its relatively high cost; the required use of ionizing radiation; difficulty at times in differentiating other fluid collections, especially hematomas, bowel loops, and phlegmons, from abscesses; interference from metal clips left at surgery; and transport of the patient for the procedure.

Abscesses visualized by CT appear as well-defined fluid collection (Fig. 101-1). Contrast is often given in the gut and intravenously to differentiate normal from abnormal structures, such as a loop of bowel containing fluid and air bubbles from an abscess. CT is the best method for visualizing abscesses in the subdiaphragmatic, retroperitoneal, and midabdominal areas. Although still accurate and useful, CT imaging can be complicated by loops of small bowel in the lower abdomen and pelvis.

Ultrasonography can be an effective tool in the diagnosis of intraabdominal abscesses, particularly if history and physical examination allow localization of the suspected abscess to a specific portion of the abdomen. It is most useful in the evaluation of the right upper quadrant, retroperitoneum, and pelvis. Its overall accuracy ranges from 57% to 96% in published reports.[14,15]

Ultrasonography is noninvasive and does not require ionizing radiation; it is relatively inexpensive and supplies immediate anatomic results; and it can be used at the patient's bedside. Because air in tissues or within loops of bowel interfere with transmission of the ultrasound wave, its usefulness can be severely limited by the presence of an ileus. Unfortunately, this is a frequent occurrence in this patient population. Another factor that sometimes hampers its usefulness is that the quality of ultrasound scans depends on the technical expertise of the person performing the scan. Abdominal wounds, stomas, and dressings can render it difficult or impossible to obtain a good study.

Radionuclide imaging techniques can be divided into two general categories. In one type, an administered radiolabeled compound is taken up by a normal organ or organs, subsequently visualized with a gamma camera, and abscess cavities identified by the presence of "cold spots" where evidence of the radioactive label would ordinarily be expected. The other type depends on the attraction of radiolabeled leukocytes to the site of the abscess. The former method is used most frequently for assessing solid organs, primarily the liver, spleen, and kidneys. The latter method has been used most often in the attempted detection of suspected intraabdominal abscesses of an unknown location.

Two agents are primarily used, gallium 67 and indium 111. Gallium binds to neutrophils, which localize in abscesses and in fresh surgical scars, colostomy and drain sites, and fracture sites. This plus the fact that gallium is phagocytized by the reticuloendothelial system and excreted into the gut

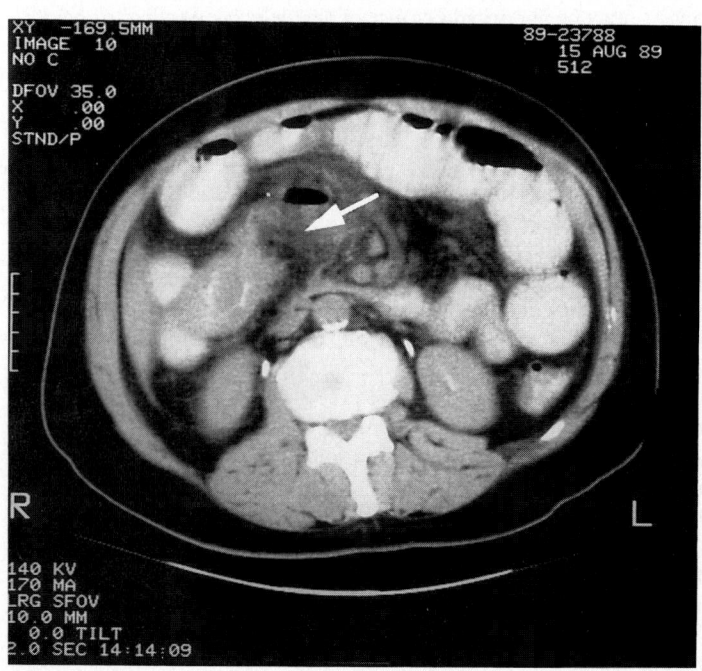

FIGURE 101-1. Pericolonic abscess associated with carcinoma of the hepatic flexure of the colon. Abscesses appear as well-defined fluid collections on CT scans, and an air-fluid level (*arrow*) is evident.

adds considerable interference to the detection of abscesses. Indium has the advantage over gallium of not being excreted into the gut or concentrated in the reticuloendothelial system, eliminating some sources of interference. The localization of neutrophils labeled with indium or gallium into fresh operative sites and inflamed peritoneum limit their usefulness in patients who have recently undergone surgery. The accuracy of gallium scans varies from 60% to 95%, and that of indium was 93% in a study of 163 patients reported by Carroll.[11,15]

The disadvantages associated with interpretation, the time required to complete the study, and the requirement for injection of radioactive materials has caused both types of nuclear scans to be supplanted by CT, although some physicians still find them useful in special circumstances. For example, Wheeler and associates, in a study of 24 patients with severe relapses of Crohn's disease poorly responsive to conventional steroid treatment, found indium 111 scans to be more accurate than ultrasound and as sensitive as CT in identifying abscesses. They felt that the modality was especially helpful in differentiating an abscess from active inflammation alone.[16]

Clinical Course and Complications

The clinical course of a patient with an intraabdominal abscess is influenced by multiple factors, including the age and previous condition of the patient; the cause, location, duration and extent of the abscess; and the response to treatment. Drainage is the key; virtually all patients with undrained abscesses die. Ochsner and DeBakey, in a 1938 review of the literature, found the mortality rate from undrained abscesses to be 90%.[17]

Other factors have important effects on morbidity and mortality. For example, Altemeier reported the mortality rate for diverticular abscesses in patients with an average age of 74 years to be 21%, and abscesses from appendicitis that occurred in a much younger population had a mortality rate of only 2%.[3] Fry and colleagues found that the factors most commonly associated with mortality were the presence of organ failure, recurrent or persistent abscess, age over 50 years, and multiple abscesses. It was their conclusion that most deaths were the result of a failure of host defense mechanisms and inadequate drainage.[2]

The primary complication of an untreated or ineffectively treated abscess is persistent sepsis leading eventually to septic shock and death. The greater the time between onset and effective treatment, the greater is the mortality. The persistent bacteremia and the systemic inflammatory response that results can lead to the systemic inflammatory response syndrome, with resultant compromise and failure of organ systems not directly involved. Once this develops, treatment is difficult, and the mortality rate is in excess of 50%.

Less draconian but significant complications can occur. Secondary abscesses can develop by direct extension or hematogenous spread. The development of secondary hepatic abscesses as a result of portal system dissemination of bacteria from an appendiceal abscess is seldom seen now. Intraabdominal abscesses can lead to bowel obstruction and enteric fistula. The proximity of an abscess to blood vessels may predispose the patient to hemorrhage by direct erosion or more commonly as a complication of methods used to drain or treat the abscess.

The chance of any of these complications developing increases with the time the abscess is untreated, emphasizing the great importance of considering the possibility of abscess in patients with a predisposing history, obtaining appropriate studies to confirm its existence and location, and instituting prompt and effective treatment. Emphasis of these principles has resulted in a reduction in the mortality rate to about 20% in the 1980s.[18-20]

Therapy

The mainstay of treatment of intraabdominal abscesses is drainage. Antibiotics are an important adjuvant therapy, but drainage is primary. This bears repeating, because placing antibiotic administration before drainage in importance is a common mistake of students and young physicians in training. Although there are a few exceptions to this rule, they are rare. Abscesses should be drained as soon as is possible. Until recently, this meant surgical drainage; however, percutaneous drainage guided by imaging methods has replaced surgery in most cases.[21,22]

Successful percutaneous drainage requires first that the abscess location be identified accurately. There must be a safe route for catheter insertion. Abscesses surrounded by loops of bowel often cannot be safely drained by the percutaneous route. Multiple abscesses or complex loculated abscesses are relative contraindications to percutaneous drainage. The abscess contents must be sufficiently liquid to permit drainage through the catheters available for this approach. Abscesses containing thick viscous fluid or infected hematomas usually must be drained operatively. The failure of percutaneous drainage to resolve symptoms should prompt further imaging studies and may ultimately require another attempt at drainage percutaneously or surgically.

Most intraabdominal abscesses are drained percutaneously. In 1991, Brolin and associates reported that 90 (76%) of 119 patients who had had abdominal abscesses over the preceding 8 years had successful resolutions with this technique.[22] A review of 83 patients treated by percutaneous drainage (42 patients) or operation (41 patients) and matched for age, abscess location, and cause found no differences in morbidity or mortality, demonstrating that percutaneous drainage is as effective as surgical treatment.[23] In a retrospective review, Deveney and associates found that mortality and initial success rates were similar in patients undergoing percutaneous or surgical drainage. Others have repeated similar findings, although most studies are retrospective (Table 101-2). They concluded that timely localization and effective drainage were more important factors in obtaining a good outcome than the drainage method used.[8]

Brolin reported that the factors significantly related to failure of percutaneous drainage were patients older than 60 years of age and pancreatic abscesses.[22] Malangoni and colleagues and Gerzof and associates reported that percutaneous drainage was less likely to be successful and mortality greater in older patients and for complex abscesses.[7,25] For these reasons, they recommended that complex abscesses be treated surgically,

TABLE 101-2
Results of Percutaneous and Surgical Drainage of Intraabdominal Abscesses

INVESTIGATION	DRAINAGE	NO. OF PATIENTS/ NO. OF ABSCESSES	SUCCESS OF DRAINAGE (%)	DURATION OF DRAINAGE (DAYS)	COMPLICATIONS (%)	MORTALITY (%)
Johnson et al, 1981	PD	27/27	89.0	17	4.0	11.0
	SD	43/43	79.0	29	16.0	26.0
Aeder et al, 1983	PD	10/13	69.0		31.0	23.0
	SD	31/32			47.0	37.0
Haslaz and van Sonnenberg, 1983	PD	11/15			27.3	9.1
	SD	19/29			18.1	10.3
Brolin et al, 1984	PD	24/24	91.7	11.7	8.3	0
	SD	24/24	87.5	21.2	20.8	12.5
Glass and Cohn, 1984	PD	15/15	47.0		6.0	
	SD	44/44	88.0		27.0	
Olak et al, 1986	PD	27/27	70.3	30.8	40.7	11.0
	SD	27/27	85.2	15.9	29.6	7.4
Deveney et al, 1988	PD	29/29	72.0	36		21.0
	SD	37/37	78.0	33		22.0
Truetner et al, 1989	PD	27/30	93.3	7.4	3.3	3.7
	SD	38/43	95.3	6.8	0	2.6

PD, percutaneous drainage, SD, surgical drainage.

From Farthmann EH, Schoffel U. Principles and limitations of operative management of intraabdominal infections. World J Surg 1990;14:210.

particularly those with associated necrotic tissue, malignancy, or enteric fistula. They advised that simple abscesses accessible percutaneously should be drained by this method, because it is as effective and less physiologically disruptive than surgery.[7]

As in the development of many new treatments, the indications for percutaneous drainage have been expanded as more experience has been gained and physicians applying it have become more adept in its use.

It should not be surprising that others who are less conservative have reported success with percutaneous drainage of complex abscesses and even those associated with biliary, enteric, and urinary fistulas.[6,26,27] Even in patients who will ultimately require operation, percutaneous drainage can be an effective temporizing measure if it achieves sufficient resolution or control of infection to allow correction of fluid and electrolyte deficits, restoration of nitrogen balance, and general improvement in the overall condition to the point that surgery can be performed under better conditions.[28]

Abscesses that abut a surface that allows easy and convenient surgical drainage should be drained surgically. Examples include abscesses that are palpable and lie next to the abdominal wall, rectum, or vagina. Deep-seated abscesses in which percutaneous drainage is impossible or unsuccessful warrant exploration of the abdominal cavity in the operating room. When possible, such operations should be conducted in such a way to avoid contamination of previously uninvolved portions of the abdominal cavity.

The primary goal of treatment is complete drainage by the least invasive means possible. If effective drainage is accomplished, complete resolution of the abscess will result. Failure of the patient to improve indicates that this has not been achieved or that other abscesses or complications exist. Patients drained by either method who do not respond but in-

stead show signs of continuing sepsis such as persistent leukocytosis or fever more than 4 days after attempted drainage should be restudied with CT or ultrasound, and repeat percutaneous drainage or laparotomy should be considered.

Antibiotic therapy is an adjunct to primary treatment (i.e., drainage) of intraabdominal abscesses. Antibiotic therapy should accompany but not delay drainage of the abscess. In many cases, the choice of antibiotic must be made before knowing the exact nature of the infecting organisms. Because most abdominal abscesses are populated by two or three types of bacteria, empiric antibiotic therapy must begin with agents that are likely to be effective against those most commonly found. The patient's history can sometimes be helpful in directing preliminary antibiotic therapy, but in most cases, the mixed cultures of gram-negative aerobes, anaerobes, and gram-positive aerobes dictate broad-spectrum coverage.

Commonly used and appropriate regimens include an aminoglycoside for gram-negative coverage plus clindamycin or metronidazole for anaerobes. When aminoglycosides are used, pharmacokinetic monitoring should be used to determine the appropriate dosage of these potentially toxic drugs. The monobactam aztreonam is an effective substitute for aminoglycosides. Concern about the presence of enterococcus prompts the addition of penicillin or ampicillin. Of the plethora of cephalosporins available, those most frequently used in this setting are single agents with broad coverage, including effectiveness against *Bacteroides*, such as cefotetan or cefoxitin. A relatively new β-lactam antibiotic, imipenem, has a broad spectrum of coverage and has been proven useful in the treatment of critically patients. However, the emergence of resistant organisms, especially *Pseudomonas*, has been a problem when it is used alone.

The duration of antibiotic treatment should be determined

by the patient's condition and the results of bacteriologic studies. Stone and colleagues found that, on the discontinuation of antibiotic therapy, sepsis was least likely to recur if the patient was afebrile and the leukocyte count and differential count were normal. If the granulocyte count was greater than 80%, there was an 83% incidence of recurrent infection.[29] If infection is persistent, the physician should suspect the presence of ischemic tissue, a foreign body, or an enteric fistula, all of which may prevent or delay the normal healing process after the abscess is drained. In addition to effective drainage and appropriate antibiotic therapy, other important therapeutic modalities include maintenance of adequate nutrition (preferably by the enteral route), fluid and electrolyte balance, and support of respiratory function.

Evidence that persistent sepsis has myriad and profound deleterious effects on the entire body continues to accumulate. The development of multiple organ failure seems to be intimately associated with septicemia, poor tissue perfusion, altered gut motility and permeability, and deranged metabolism. Although all the answers are not yet available, maintenance of adequate nutrition, adequate tissue perfusion and oxygenation, appropriate antibiotics, and eradication by timely drainage provide the best chance for success in the treatment of abdominal abscesses. Successful treatment requires first considering the possibility of abscess existence and then timely acquisition of diagnostic studies.

FISTULAS

Fistulas are abnormal communications between the lumen of a hollow organ and another hollow organ or the skin. A variety of fistulas can originate form abdominal organs, including the gastrointestinal tract, the biliary or pancreatic ducts, and the various tubes and organs composing the urinary tract. Fistulas are generally classified by their site of origin and termination (e.g., enterovesical, colocutaneous), by the amount of drainage, and sometimes by cause. This chapter discusses the more common gastrointestinal fistulas.

Etiology

Gastrointestinal fistulas develop as a consequence of several factors (Table 101-3), including complications of surgery, radiation therapy, inflammatory bowel disease, trauma, and

---

TABLE 101-3
Etiologic Classification of Enteric Fistulas

Congenital	**Inflammatory**
Tracheoesophageal fistula	Crohn's disease
Patent vitellin duct	Adjacent abscess
Postoperative	**Postirradiation**
Inadvertent injury	Spontaneous
Failure of anastomosis	Postoperative
Proximity of drain	
	Malignant
Posttraumatic	Adherence of tumor to adjacent bowel
Direct injury	or abdominal wall with subsequent
Open abdominal wound	neurosis of tumor

---

malignancy. All involve some type of breakdown or alteration of normal intestinal wall structure. Most enteric fistulas develop as a result of complications after surgery. Those that arise spontaneously are associated most commonly with cancer, radiation-damaged bowel, Crohn's disease, and diverticulitis. Rarely, fistulas develop when abscesses erode into adjacent bowel. More typically, the hole in the gut precedes and is the cause of the abscess. The increasing use of prosthetic meshes to permit closure of large abdominal wall defects or reconstruction of the pelvic floor has resulted in recent reports of enterocutaneous fistulas presumed to be the result of direct erosion by mesh through the wall of adjacent bowel.[30,31]

Clinical Manifestations

The clinical manifestations of a gastrointestinal fistula depend to some extent on cause, but the two most common modes of presentation are the appearance of enteric drainage through the skin or the signs and symptoms of an intraabdominal abscess. Once established, the quality and quantity of drainage determine other symptoms. The major clinical problems associated with fistulas are fluid and electrolyte derangements, sepsis, and malnutrition.

High-output fistulas (>500 mL/day) involving the proximal gut can cause significant fluid and electrolyte abnormalities. The loss of the alkaline fluid of the duodenum and proximal jejunum can induce a significant metabolic acidosis. In contrast, gastric fistulas can result in a hypochloremic, hypokalemic alkalosis through the loss of chloride and hydrogen ions in the fistula fluid itself and the loss of potassium in the urine as part of renal physiologic response to the metabolic alkalosis and loss of hydrogen. The high fluid losses often associated with proximal gut fistulas can result in dehydration and oliguria severe enough to cause hypotension, damage renal function, and threaten life if uncorrected. The fluid output from such fistulas can cause excoriation of the skin surrounding the fistula's external opening by activated digestive enzymes. The often inconvenient location of external fistula openings in surgical wounds, skin folds, and other sites on the abdominal wall that are difficult to protect can make prevention of extensive inflammation and even skin loss a formidable challenge.

Sepsis usually is the result of abdominal abscesses or infection resulting from the violation of the integrity of the abdominal cavity attendant to fistula development. The signs, symptoms, and sequelae of abscesses are discussed extensively in the preceding section. Many gastrointestinal fistulas are associated with incompletely drained abscesses, and until they are adequately treated, successful resolution of the fistula itself will be unsuccessful.

Malnutrition, defined as a loss of at least 10% of usual body weight, affects most patients with fistulas. Several factors can contribute, including protein and nutrient losses from the fistula itself, the decrease in appetite and food intake generally associated with any illness, and the increased energy demands attendant to illness, particularly those with infectious complications. In a 1964 article, Chapman and associates reported that malnutrition was the most important factor influencing mortality of their 58 patients with fistulas. For those judged to be undernourished, the mortality rate was 58%, and for those considered adequately nourished, it was only 16%.[32]

The clinical manifestations of some specific fistulas bear mentioning. Although most perianal fistulas are the consequence of local inflammation and abscess formation in the perianal crypts, the presence of multiple, recurrent, and complex perianal fistulas should alert clinicians to the possibility of Crohn's disease. Similarly, recurrence or persistence of adequately treated urinary tract infections can indicate the presence of an enterovesical fistula. Pneumaturia is pathognomonic of such fistulas, which are usually a complication of diverticulitis and less commonly of Crohn's disease or a malignancy. Diarrhea and malnutrition can be the mode of clinical presentation of internal abdominal fistulas that result in the bypass of significant sections of the gut and deliver of large amounts of watery fluid to the distal bowel.

Differential Diagnosis and Diagnostic Studies

Most fistulas that terminate on skin are readily apparent and not prone to confusion with other entities. Occasionally, one might be confused with a draining sinus tract from a chronic abscess in the abdominal cavity; however, continuing drainage and the presence of obviously enteric contents usually make the diagnosis clear. Confusion is easily dispelled with appropriate diagnostic studies. In this case, careful injection of appropriate radiologic contrast material down the tract in question under fluoroscopy usually demonstrates a fistula and any organ of origin.

Fistulas terminating in locations other than skin may be more difficult to differentiate and diagnose from the patient's history and physical findings. Enterovesical fistulas can mimic chronic cystitis, and differentiation from other causes can be difficult in the absence of pneumaturia. Urine cultures that grow multiple different enteric organisms suggest the possibility. Contrast studies of the small or large bowel may demonstrate disease that could cause such a fistula but usually do not demonstrate the fistula itself. The diagnostic study that is most helpful in establishing the existence of a fistula in such circumstances is cystoscopy.

Fistulas from one part of the gastrointestinal tract to another are generally manifested by symptoms from associated conditions. As is sometimes the case in medicine, the primary problem associated with failure to make the correct diagnosis in such cases is failure to consider the possibility. Once the prospect is entertained, contrast studies usually demonstrate the fistula.

Other purposes of diagnostic studies are to determine the fistula's site of origin, establish its length and degree of complexity, and detect any underlying etiologic factors such as malignancy, foreign material, or inflammatory bowel disease. Potential radiographic studies include injection of the fistula tract with contrast material (i.e., fistulogram), upper and lower gastrointestinal contrast studies, ultrasound, and CT. In the case of enterocutaneous fistulas, the fistulogram is the best radiographic study to confirm its presence and often determine the segment of bowel involved (Fig. 101-2). When a fistula

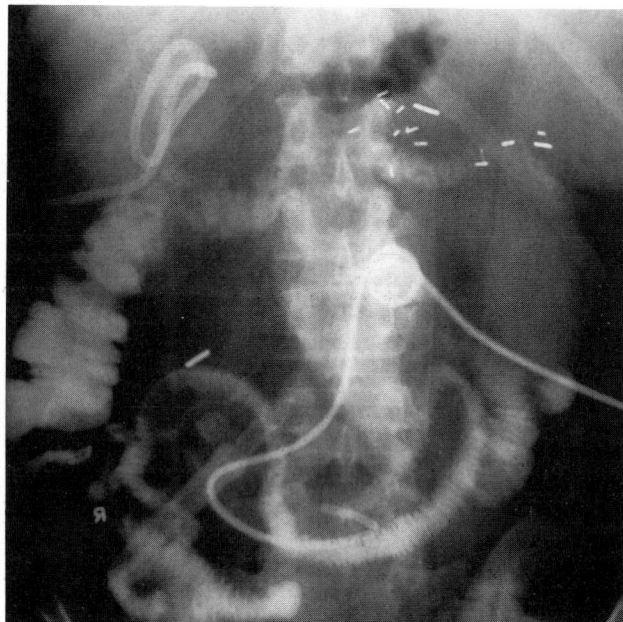

FIGURE 101-2. A fistulogram indicates an enterocutaneous fistula involving the small bowel after drainage of a pancreatic abscess.

is suspected but cannot be diagnosed radiographically, a slurry of charcoal administered orally may result in visible particles in the fistula drainage, confirming the diagnosis. Endoscopy is not often helpful, except to diagnose disease at the enteric fistula site, as with colon cancer.

Therapy

Patients with fistulas often have multiple problems that require prompt diagnosis and the establishment of treatment priorities. The goals of enterocutaneous fistula treatment are correction of electrolyte and acid-base irregularities, adequate drainage of associated abscesses or prevention of their development by the pooling of fluid along the tract, protection of the skin from damage from fistula fluid, delivery of adequate nutrition with repletion of existing deficits, diminution of the amount of drainage, and assessment of the cause and underlying conditions for determining the best method to achieve closure.

Correction of fluid and electrolyte deficits and imbalances is the first priority. Rehydration should be accomplished expeditiously, even while the exact nature and degree of the deficits is being determined. Significant aberrations of electrolytes and acid-base status can result from some fistulas. For a high-output fistula, maintenance of electrolyte and acid-base balance may require daily adjustments of replacement fluids and sometimes even the direct measurement of the electrolyte composition in fistula fluid.

When signs and symptoms of infection are present, a poorly drained fistula with a coexisting abscess should be suspected and appropriate diagnostic studies obtained. Soeters and colleagues, in an extensive review of 404 fistula patients treated over a 30-year span, concluded that the major determinant of mortality in the latest period studied was uncontrolled sepsis.[33] Associated abscesses should be adequately drained. Effective drainage of the fistula tract should be achieved to prevent pooling of fluid along its course. This can usually be achieved with sump drains. The position of the drain can be confirmed by a fistulogram. This step ensures establishment of optimal drainage and helps prevent placement of drain tips so close to the bowel opening that they impede spontaneous healing. In addition to preventing septic complications, establishment of adequate drainage permits collection of fistula output, with measurement of total volume and electrolyte content. These measures can greatly facilitate correction and maintenance of fluid and electrolyte balance.

Depending on its source, fistula drainage can be quite damaging to the skin. This is especially true of those arising from the proximal small bowel or pancreatic and biliary ducts. Fistulas from these sites can contain significant amounts of activated enzymes and bile acids that are extremely caustic to skin and other tissues. Protection of the skin from their deleterious effects can sometimes be a vexing problem. Using protective substances, such as those used for stoma appliances, is often necessary. Depending on the fistula exit site (e.g., open wound, near a large skin fold), the success in maintaining a good seal between such an appliance and the skin can be impossible with commonly available material. The help of an experienced stoma nurse or skin care team can be invaluable in designing a solution to such difficult cases.

Before the development of total parenteral nutrition, patients with enterocutaneous fistulas often died from complications related to starvation. Nutritional repletion and maintenance is essential to proper care of a patient with an enterocutaneous fistula. The best route of feeding must be determined on an individual basis. No prospective, randomized studies have compared the effects of enteral or parenteral nutrition on clinical outcome in patients with fistulas.

Rombeau and Rolandelli reviewed many studies examining nutrition and fistulas.[34] They found that enteral feeding routes are tolerated in selected patients with gastrointestinal fistulas, and in such cases, it can achieve results similar to those obtained with parenteral routes. If enteral routes are feasible, elemental diets have not been shown to offer an advantage over cheaper, standard polymeric diets. Studies comparing feeding parenterally with conventional oral intake to the amount possible show a higher rate of spontaneous closure with parenteral feeding. This probably reflects an inability to achieve an adequate intake in those fed orally.

Most fistulas that respond to such conservative therapy, including parenteral feedings, do so within 4 to 6 weeks. Traditionally, enteral feeding has been eschewed in patients with small bowel fistulas, because this route of feeding often increases fistula output. Given the recent spate of experimental and clinical data suggesting advantages of enteral over parenteral feeding, especially with regard to infectious complications, enteral feeding should probably not be abandoned until a trial has shown it impractical. Experimental data showing gut atrophy in the absence of nutrient stimulation and the potential effects of such atrophy on the healing of gut fistulas raises largely unanswered questions regarding the effects of the feeding route on spontaneous closure. The same is true for the effects of specific gut-directed food sources (e.g.,

glutamine) and intestinal growth factors. The best advice is to feed enterally when possible. Most patients with distal small bowel and colonic fistulas can be fed by this route with no adverse effects.

Levy and associates reported successfully feeding 85% of 335 patients with high-output fistulas of the jejunum and ileum.[35] Others have fed enterally through tubes placed distal to proximal small bowel fistulas and had spontaneous closure of the fistula. If enteral feeding is unsuccessful or not possible, parenteral alimentation is necessary and is capable of restoring and maintaining adequate nutrition with significant rates of spontaneous closure.

Decreasing fistula output is important in achieving spontaneous closure. Putting the bowel at rest decreases gastrointestinal secretions and should promote healing, but the potentially negative aspects of stopping enteral intake may outweigh a slight decrease in fistula output. As fistula output increases, the putative beneficial effect of stopping enteral intake would seem to increase relative to the perceived benefits of enteral feedings, if stopping enteral intake has the desired effect on fistula output.

Attention has focused on the use of somatostatin as treatment for pancreatic and gastrointestinal fistulas. Retrospective reports and nonrandomized, prospective studies indicate that somatostatin is effective in reducing the volume of intestinal secretion and fistula output, possibly promoting spontaneous closure of the fistula.[36-39] Torres and colleagues have reported a prospective, randomized study in 40 patients who recieved either TPN by itself or TPN with somatostatin.[40] Rates of spontaneous closure were similar (~83%), but in those receiving somatostatin, the fistulas healed an average of 7 days earlier.[40]

Nonoperative treatment should continue until normal fluid balance and nutritional status have been achieved. Once these supportive measures have been instituted, attention should be turned to selecting optimal definitive treatment. In selecting a course of therapy, diagnostic studies of the fistula tract can be of immense value.

Spontaneous closure rates for gastrointestinal fistulas in patients on parenteral nutrition range from 29% to 70%. This variability may reflect differences in patient populations. Nonetheless, a significant number of fistulas close spontaneously, with supportive management only.[41,42] Factors at the gut end of the fistula that preclude success with conservative treatment are malignancy, inflammatory bowel disease, foreign bodies, undrained or poorly drained abscesses, obstruction of the gastrointestinal tract distally, disruption of more than 50% of the bowel wall, and a fistula tract less than 2.5 cm from the skin. Patients with these conditions require correction of the complicating factor before conservative treatment can be successful, or they will need surgery. Additional factors unfavorable to spontaneous closure are age over 65 years, fistula output over 500 mL/day, chronicity, and site. The sites that have been shown to be less favorable for spontaneous closure are the distal small bowel and colon.

In the absence of obvious contraindications to conservative therapy, it should be continued for 4 to 6 weeks. A fistula that persists after 4 to 6 weeks is unlikely to close spontaneously and surgical treatment should be considered. Before surgical repair is attempted, the patient should be in optimal medical and nutritional condition.

The reader is directed to Chapter 26, The Gastrointestinal Microflora; Chapter 36, Approach to the Patient With Acute Abdomen; Chapter 79, Inflammatory Bowel Disease; Chapter 83, Diverticulitis; Chapter 90, Acute Pancreatitis; Chapter 102, Diseases of the Mesentery and Omentum; Chapter 103, Diseases of the Peritoneum; Chapter 104, Diseases of the Retroperitoneum; Chapter 120, Cross-Sectional Anatomy; Chapter 121, Ultrasonography; Chapter 122, Endoscopic Ultrasonography; Chapter 123, Applications of Computed Tomography to the Gastrointestinal Tract; Chapter 126, Applications of Radionuclide Imaging in Gastroenterology; Chapter 128, Interventional Radiology; Chapter 131, Microbiologic Studies; and Chapter 140, Exploratory Laparotomy.

REFERENCES

1. Fields TC, Pickleman J. Intraabdominal abscess unassociated with prior operation. Arch Surg 1985;120:821.
2. Fry DE, Garrison RN, Heitsch RC, et al. Determinants of death in patients with intraabdominal abscess. Surgery 1980;88:517.
3. Altemeier WA, Culbertson WR, Fullen WD, et al. Intra-abdominal abscesses. Am J Surg 1973;4125:70.
4. Goins WA, Rodriguez A, Joshi M, et al. Intra-abdominal abscess after blunt abdominal trauma. Ann Surg 1990;212:60.
5. Ivatury RR, Zubowski R, Psarras P, et al. Intra-abdominal abscess after penetrating abdominal trauma. J Trauma 1988;28:1238.
6. Stylianos S, Martin EC, Strker PM, et al. Percutaneous drainage of intra-abdominal abscesses following abdominal trauma. J Trauma 1989;29:584.
7. Malangoni MA, Shumate CF, Thomas HA, et al. Factors influencing the treatment of intra-abdominal abscesses. Am J Surg 1990;159:167.
8. Deveney CW, Lurie K, Deveney KE. Improved treatment of intra-abdominal abscess. Arch Surg 1988;123:1126.
9. Styrt B, Gorbach SL. Recent developments in the understanding of the pathogenesis and treatment of anaerobic infections. N Engl J Med 1989;321:241.
10. Brook I. A 12 year study of aerobic and anaerobic bacteria in intra-abdominal and postsurgical abdominal wound infections. Surg Gynecol Obstet 1989;169:387.
11. Carroll B, Silverman PM, Goodwin DA, et al. Ultrasonography and indium 111 white blood cell scanning for the detection of intraabdominal abscesses. Ultrasound 1981;140:155.
12. Koehler PR, Moss AA. Diagnosis of intra-abdominal and pelvic abscesses by computerized tomography. JAMA 1980;244:49.
13. Porter JA, Loughry CW, Cook AJ. Use of the computerized tomographic scan in the diagnosis and treatment of abscesses. Am J Surg 1985;150:257.
14. Norton L, Eule J, Burdick D. Accuracy of techniques to detect intraperitoneal abscess. Surgery 1978;84:370.
15. Dobrin PB, Gully PH, Greenlee HB, et al. Radiologic diagnosis of an intra-abdominal abscess. Arch Surg 1986;121:41.
16. Wheeler JG, Slack NF, Duncan A, et al. The diagnosis of intra-abdominal abscesses in patients with severe Crohn's disease. Q J Med 1992;82:159.
17. Ochsner A, Debakey M. Subphrenic abscess. Surg Gynecol Obstet 1938;66:426.
18. Lurie K, Plzak L, Deveney CW. Intra-abdominal abscess in the 1980s. Surg Clin North Am 1987;67:621.
19. Sanjay S, Kellum JJ, O'Leary MP, et al. Improved localization and survival in patients with intraabdominal abscesses. Am J Surg 1986;145:136.
20. Warshaw AL, Gongliang J. Improved survival in patients with pancreatic abscess. Ann Surg 1985;202:418.
21. Van Sonnenberg E, Ferrucci JT, Mueller PR, et al. Percutaneous radiographically guided catheter drainage of abdominal abscesses. JAMA 1982;247:190.
22. Brolin RE, Flancbaum L, Ercoli FR, et al. Limitations of percutaneous catheter drainage of abdominal abscesses. Surg Gynecol Obstet 1991;173:203.
23. Hemming A, Davis NL, Robins RE. Surgical versus percutaneous drainage of intra-abdominal abscesses. Am J Surg 1991;161:593.
24. Farthmann EH, Schoffel U. Principles and limitations of operative management of intraabdominal infections. World J Surg 1990;14:210.
25. Gerzof SG, Johnson WC, Robbins AH, et al. Expanded criteria for percutaneous abscess drainage. Arch Surg 1985;120:227.
26. Lameris JS, Bruining HA, Jeekel J. Ultrasound-guided percutaneous drainage of intraabdominal abscesses. Br J Surg 1987;74:620.
27. Ercoli FR, Milgrim LM, Nosher JL, et al. Percutaneous catheter drainage of abscesses associated with enteric fistulae. Am Surg 1988;54:45.
28. Van Sonnenberg E, Wing VW, Casola G, et al. Temporizing effect of percutaneous drainage of complicated abscesses in critically ill patients. AJR Am J Roentgenol 1984;142:821.
29. Stone HH, Bourneuf AA, Stinson LD. Reliability of criteria for predicting persistent or recurrent sepsis. Arch Surg 1985;120:175.
30. Patsner B, Mann WJ, Chalas E, et al. Intestinal complications associated with use of the Dexon Mesh Sling in gynecologic oncology patients. Gynecol Oncol 1990;38:146.
31. Greene MA, Mullins RJ, Malangoni MA, et al. Laparotomy wound closure with absorbable polyglycolic acid mesh. Surg Gynecol Obstet 1993;174:214.
32. Chapman R, Foran R, Dunphy JE. Management of intestinal fistulas. Am J Surg 1964;108:157.
33. Soeters PB, Ebeid AM, Fischer JE. Review of 404 patients with gastrointestinal fistulas. Ann Surg 1979;190:189.
34. Rombeau JL, Rolandelli RH. Enteral and parenteral nutrition in patients with enteric fistulas and short bowel syndrome. Surg Clin North Am 1987;67:551.
35. Levy E, Frileux P, Cugnenc PH, et al. High-output external fistulae of the small bowel: management with continuous enteral nutrition. Br J Surg 1989;76:676.
36. Nubiola P, Badia JM, Martinez-Rodenas F, et al. Treatment of 27 postoperative enterocutaneous fistulas with the long half-life somatostatin analogue SMS 201-995. Ann Surg 1989;210:56.
37. Spiliotis J, Vagenas K, Panagopoulos K, et al. Treatment of enterocutaneous fistulas with TPN and somatostatin, compared with patients who received TPN only. Br J Clin Pract 1990;44:616.
38. Rosenberg L, Brown RA. Sandostatin in the management of nonendocrine gastrointestinal and pancreatic disorders: a preliminary study. Can J Surg 1991;34:223.
39. Borison DI, Bloom AD, Pritchard TJ. Treatment of enterocutaneous and colocutaneous fistulas with early surgery or somatostatin analog. Dis Colon Rectum 1992;35:625.
40. Torres AJ, Landa JI, Azcoita MM, et al. Somatostatin in the management of gastrointestinal fistulas: a multicenter trial. Arch Surg 1992;127:97.
41. LaBerge JM, Kerlan RK, Gordon RL, et al. Nonoperative treatment of enteric fistulas: results in 53 patients. J Vasc Interv Radiol 1993;3:353.
42. Schuster MR, Crummy AB, Wojtowycz MM, et al. Abdominal abscesses associated with enteric fistulas: percutaneous management. J Vasc Interv Radiol 1992;3:359.

Textbook of Gastroenterology, second edition, edited by Tadataka Yamada. JB Lippincott Company, Philadelphia © 1995.

CHAPTER 102

Diseases of the Mesentery and Omentum

R. Daniel Beauchamp

Embryology, Anatomy, and Physiology	Solid Tumors of the Omentum and Mesentery
Mesenteric Panniculitis and Retractile Mesenteritis	Omental Vascular Accident
Mesenteric Fibromatosis	Granulomatous Infection
Mesenteric and Omental Cysts	Surgical Uses of the Omentum

The mesentery or omentum may become involved in a variety of disease processes, most of which originate in adjacent visceral organs. This chapter discusses several diseases that primarily or prominently involve the omentum, mesentery, or both mesenchymal structures (Table 102-1). The discussion does not include mesenteric vascular diseases, which are discussed elsewhere.

EMBRYOLOGY, ANATOMY, AND PHYSIOLOGY

As the peritoneal cavity develops, the splanchnic mesoderm covers the developing gut. The ventral mesentery is mostly resorbed, except for the portion that forms the gastrohepatic omentum. The greater omentum develops from the dorsal mesogastrium. It extends from the greater curvature of the stomach caudally to fuse with the transverse colon and mesocolon. At birth, the omentum is composed of a double layer of fused peritoneum, with lymphatic and blood vessels running between the layers. As development proceeds, the omentum becomes laden with fat. The arterial circulation usually comes from the right and left gastroepiploic arteries.

The midgut acquires a dorsal mesentery as it lengthens during the fifth week of development. The midgut forms a loop that is extruded into the umbilical cord, and the superior mesenteric artery extends to the apex of this loop. During subsequent midgut development, the gut returns to the abdominal cavity and undergoes counterclockwise rotation about the origin of the superior mesenteric artery to achieve the normal adult anatomic configuration by the twelfth week of development, although fixation may not be completed until birth. The mesenteries of the ascending and descending colon fuse with the posterior body wall, and the small bowel mesentery elongates to extend from the transverse mesocolon superiorly to the ileocecal junction inferiorly.[1]

The omentum and mesentery are rich in lymphatics and blood vessels. They provide a major source of macrophages and lymphocytes to aid in removal of foreign material or infection in the abdominal cavity. The small bowel mesentery contains the lymphatic and vascular network responsible for transporting all of the nutrients absorbed from the small bowel.

MESENTERIC PANNICULITIS AND RETRACTILE MESENTERITIS

Mesenteric panniculitis is a nonspecific inflammatory process involving the adipose tissue of the mesentery. This includes a spectrum of diseases, from inflammatory to fibrotic lesions, which have been called mesenteric panniculitis and retractile mesenteritis, respectively. Numerous synonyms have been used for describing these conditions, including primary liposclerosis, lipogranuloma, isolated lipodystrophy, and mesenteric Weber-Christian disease. The cause may be trauma, infection, or ischemia, but it is often unknown. Panniculitis can be a part of the generalized Weber-Christian disease, but this disease is probably unrelated to isolated mesenteritis.[2,3]

The gross pathologic findings are a diffusely thickened and rubbery mesentery, usually as a solid mass in the root of the mesentery or as several masses stuck to each other. This represents excessive growth of normal fat, with subsequent degeneration, fat necrosis, and xanthogranulomatous inflammation with lipid-laden macrophages, infiltration with histiocytes, lymphocytes, and occasional foreign body giant cells, leading to fibrotic scarring and calcification.[4] Histologically, the differentiation must be made between fat necrosis, Whipple's disease, and lymphoma.

Patients with this condition generally present in late adulthood, with the average age of 53 years. The male to female ratio is 1.8 : 1. The clinical complaints are nonspecific, and

---

TABLE 102-1
Classification of Mesenteric and Omental Diseases

MESENTERIC DISEASES	OMENTAL DISEASES
Primary Mesenteric Inflammatory Diseases	***Mass Lesions***
Mesenteric panniculitis	Primary tumors and cysts
Retractile mesenteritis	Metastatic disease
Mesenteric Cysts	Vascular Lesions Damaging Blood Supply
Embryonic and developmental cysts	Torsion
Traumatic or acquired cysts	Primary
Neoplastic cysts	Secondary: hernia, adhesion, tumor
Infective and degenerative cysts	Infarction
	Primary
	Secondary: torsion, incarceration in hernia
Mesenteric Tumors	***Inflammatory Lesions***
Benign Tumors	Adhesion and inflammation caused by peritonitis
Lipoma	
Hemangioma	
Leiomyoma	
Ganglioneuroma	
Malignant tumors	
Leiomyosarcoma	
Liposarcoma	
Rhabdomyosarcoma	
Metastatic disease	
Mesenteric fibromatosis	
Mesenteric Vascular Diseases	
Acute	
Chronic	

---

the symptoms can include cramping abdominal pain, which may be local or generalized; weight loss; nausea and vomiting; and low-grade fever. A patient with this condition occasionally presents with an acute abdomen. Forty percent are discovered as an incidental mass at examination or laparotomy, and 60% are palpable masses.[4] Transmission of aortic pulsations to the anterior abdominal wall, suggesting an abdominal aortic aneurysm, has been reported.[2,5]

Radiographic findings include displacement of intestinal segments and extrinsic compression of the bowel. Angiography may reveal nonspecific stretching of the vasa recta and vascular encasement. The computed tomography (CT) findings include an inhomogeneous, low-density mass.

Some cases of mesenteric panniculitis progress to chronic stages and become retractile mesenteritis. With retractile mesenteritis, there is a thickened mesentery that is fibrotic and retracted, and it may have pale gray, opalescent plaques. There may also be mesenteric pseudocysts from fat necrosis. A dense collagen and fibrous tissue proliferation has less fat necrosis and inflammation than is seen with mesenteric panniculitis. Rarely, there is involvement of the colonic mesentery, and fewer than 5% of patients have retroperitoneal involvement. Symptoms are continuous abdominal pain, fever, and weight loss. Some patients develop small bowel obstruction, mesenteric thrombosis, lymphatic obstruction with ascites, steatorrhea, or protein-losing enteropathy.

The prognosis for mesenteric panniculitis is usually excellent but depends on underlying disease processes. These patients should have biopsies, and if necessary, they should have colostomies or surgery to bypass obstructed intestines. Resection is usually not possible and should not be attempted.

Death from mesenteric panniculitis is rare. Soergel and Hensley reported 1 patient who died of mesenteric vein obstruction. In one large series Kipfer and colleagues reported that 31 (66%) of 47 patients were alive an average of 11 years after diagnosis.[6,7] Eight of the 16 deaths were from malignant neoplasm (4 from lymphoma), and 6 patients died of nonmalignant causes (i.e., myocardial infarction and cerebral vascular accident). Of the 23 patients who presented with pain, only 3 continued to have symptoms beyond 2 years. Of 9 patients who presented with an unresectable mass, 3 were unchanged as long as 11 years later, and in 6 patients, the masses disappeared. In patients with symptomatic progressive sclerosing or retractile mesenteritis, dramatic responses have been reported after treatment with prednisone and azathioprine or with cyclophosphamide.[8,9] Experience with these immunosuppressive agents is too small to determine their efficacy in this usually self-limiting disease.

MESENTERIC FIBROMATOSIS

Mesenteric fibromatosis, also called mesenteric desmoid, is a benign, noninflammatory fibromatous proliferation arising from the mesentery. Desmoids are nonmetastasizing, locally invasive, benign, fibrous tissue masses that arise in the musculoaponeurotic structures throughout the body. Intraabdominal desmoids may occur in the mesentery or the pelvic walls. Grossly, desmoid has an ill-defined margin, lacks encapsulation, and infiltrates into surrounding muscle and fascial planes. Histologically, mature uniform fibroblasts are seen peripherally. Mitotic figures are infrequent and atypical mitoses are extremely rare. The central regions are densely collagenous.[10]

Mesenteric fibromatosis occurs spontaneously or in association with familial polyposis (i.e., in about 3% of cases of familial polyposis coli).[11] About one half of familial polyposis coli patients who develop mesenteric fibrosis have other manifestations of Gardner's syndrome, such as extraabdominal desmoid, epidermoid or sebaceous cysts, osteomas, lipomas, or subcutaneous fibromas. The annual incidence in the general population in Scandinavian countries is between 2 and 4.3 cases per million persons.[12,13] Mesenteric fibromatosis affects 14% to 17% of patients with Gardner's syndrome.[14,15]

Approximately 8% of all desmoid tumors are mesenteric, and the remainder occur in the subcutaneous tissue of the abdominal wall (49%) or extraabdominal tissues (43%).[13] Desmoid tumors are often associated with a previous trauma, such as a previous operation, which may be an important initiating factor in some cases. Other cases have no association with previous trauma.[16] Some cases of desmoid tumor have been associated with estrogen therapy.[17]

Radiographic features are nonspecific. By ultrasound, the desmoid tumor appears to be a solid mass, and CT scan shows a nonenhancing mass with soft tissue density.

Mesenteric fibromatosis may present as an asymptomatic abdominal mass on physical examination or a mesenteric mass at laparotomy. The lesion can be mistaken for metastatic adenocarcinoma, especially in patients with familial polyposis coli.

Symptoms of intestinal obstruction are the most common complaint. Aggressive mesenteric desmoids can become infiltrative and can involve mesenteric vessels, leading to intestinal perforation. At laparotomy, desmoids are found to involve the mesentery of the small bowel or transverse mesocolon, and the most common site is the base of the small mesentery.[18,19] These lesions can be difficult to differentiate from low-grade sarcoma and can lead to misdiagnosis at operation and extensive small bowel resection.

Wide local excision, if possible, is the treatment of choice, but complete excision of the lesion in symptomatic patients may be difficult because of involvement of the root of the mesentery. In some cases, intestinal bypass is necessary for palliation. Recurrence of these lesions is common if resection is incomplete.

Several medical treatments have been tried and reported to be successful, but because these are rare tumors, the reported series are small, and definitive therapeutic efficacy has not been established for any agent. There are anecdotal reports of successful treatment with prostaglandin inhibitors (i.e., sulindac or indomethacin) and antiestrogens (e.g., tamoxifen) alone and in combination.[20,21] In a prospective therapeutic trial of 7 familial polyposis patients with desmoid tumors who were treated with indomethacin, sulindac, or tamoxifen as single agents or in combination, only 1 patient demonstrated a favorable response to treatment, and that patient presented with minimal tumor burden.[22] Cytotoxic chemotherapy has not proven effective in the treatment of these lesions.[23]

Although high-dose radiation therapy may be effective in controlling extraabdominal desmoid tumors, the risk of radiation injury to the gut limits its use for intraabdominal desmoid, as successful radiation therapy requires doses above 60 Gy.[24,25]

MESENTERIC AND OMENTAL CYSTS

Mesenteric and omental cysts are uncommon lesions, with an incidence of 1 case for every 30,000 to 100,000 persons.[26-28] The terms *mesenteric cysts* and *omental cysts* describe the topographic location and gross appearance, but they do not indicate the histologic diagnosis.[29]

Lymphangiomas (Fig. 102-1) are characteristically found in children (mean age, 6.2–10 years), are frequently large, and almost always symptomatic, usually with abdominal distention, pain, or vomiting.[29,30] Lymphangiomas are most often located in the small bowel mesentery but occasionally may be found in the mesocolon or the omentum.

Histologically, the diagnosis of cystic lymphangioma can be made if most of the following criteria can be met: flat endothelial lining, small lymphatic spaces present in the cyst wall, abundant lymphoid tissue in the cyst wall, presence of foam cells containing lipoid material, and smooth muscle in the cyst wall.[30-32] However, nonlymphangiomatous mesenteric cysts may have cuboidal or columnar lining cells or even an absent lining. They lack smooth muscle or lymphatic elements in their walls. These cysts include nonpancreatic pseudocysts, enteric cysts, and mesothelial cysts. The overall mean age of presentation of these nonlymphangiomatous mesenteric cysts is 44 years.[30] As many as one third of the nonlymphangiomatous cysts may be located in the omentum, and only 25% are symptomatic. The mean diameter of cystic lymphangiomas tends to be greater than other mesenteric cysts, but there may be considerable overlap in size.

Plain radiographs often demonstrate a mass displacing bowel gas and may demonstrate proximal dilatation of the bowel. Ultrasonography, CT, and MRI may demonstrate the multilocular or unilocular nature of the cysts, which may have homogeneous or inhomogeneous contents (Figs. 102-2 and 102-3). Of the three imaging modalities, ultrasonography probably yields the most information for the least expense.

The definitive diagnosis and treatment of these lesions is surgical resection. Percutaneous aspiration and biopsy are not warranted, because they are not likely to provide a definitive diagnosis and may lead to infection of the cyst. Total excision of the cystic lesion requires resection of adjacent attached abdominal organs (usually segments of small bowel) in 50% to 74% of cases of cystic lymphangioma, but most other types of mesenteric cysts can be simply excised.[29,30]

Included in the differential diagnosis of these lesions are cystic teratomas, cystic smooth muscle tumors, and cystic mesothelioma. Cystic teratomas of the mesentery can be differentiated from other mesenteric and omental cysts by the presence of peripheral calcification and accumulation of fat.[33] Cystic mesotheliomas arise from the peritoneum and, like cystic lymphangiomas, are often multilocular. Unlike lymphangiomas, the cystic mesotheliomas occur mostly in adult women (mean age, 41 years), they tend to recur and often require multiple operations for treatment.[31,34]

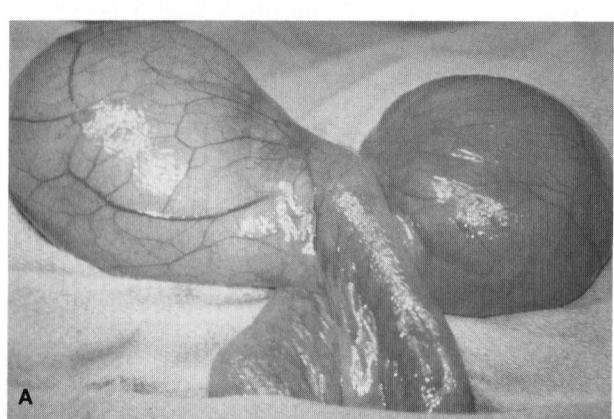
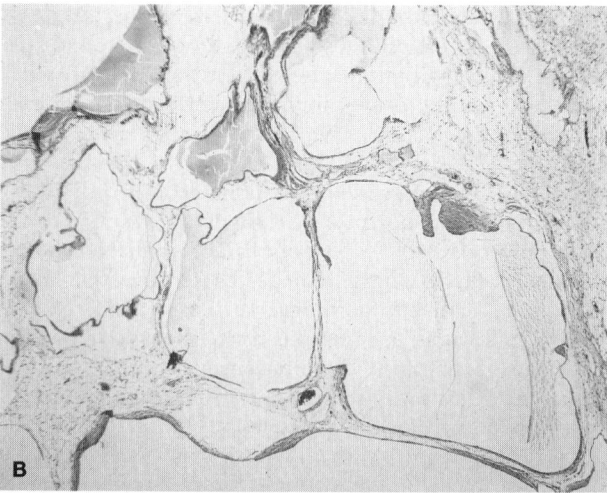

FIGURE 102-1. Gross and microscopic appearance of a lymphangioma. (**A**) A large, bilobed lymph-angioma of the mesentery is adhered to a loop of small bowel. (**B**) Multiple, thin-walled, cystic spaces are lined with endothelial cells and contain lymph. (H & E stain; original magnification ×25; from Ros PR, Olmsted WW, Moser RP Jr, et al. Mesenteric and omental cysts: histologic classification with imaging correlation. Radiology 1987;164:327.)

SOLID TUMORS OF THE OMENTUM AND MESENTERY

By far the most common types of tumors that involve the omentum and mesentery are malignant tumors that arise from intraabdominal viscera, such as the ovaries, stomach, colon, or pancreas, and secondarily involve the omentum or mesentery through metastasis or direct invasive extension. Primary tumors of the omentum and mesentery may arise from any of the cellular elements that comprise these tissues.

Primary solid tumors of the omentum are exceedingly rare. Stout and colleagues reported only 24 primary solid tumors of the omentum over a 55-year period at the Columbia University College of Physicians and Surgeons.[35] Of these 24 tu-

mors, 18 were benign. Leiomyoma is the most common omental tumor. Other benign tumors include hemangiopericytoma, neurofibroma, lipoma, and myxoma. In Stout's series of the 24 primary omental tumors, there were six sarcomas, three of which were leiomyosarcomas, and there was one fibrosarcoma, one liposarcoma, and one rhabdomyosarcoma. All benign and malignant solid primary omental tumors occurred in adults, except for one neurofibroma in the omentum of a 5-year-old child.[35]

Primary tumors can also arise from the mesentery. The types of mesenteric tumors reflect the cells of origin in the mesentery. These tumors include lipomas, xanthogranulomas, hemangiopericytomas, leiomyomas, and neurofibromas. Malignant tumors can include the malignant counterparts of the

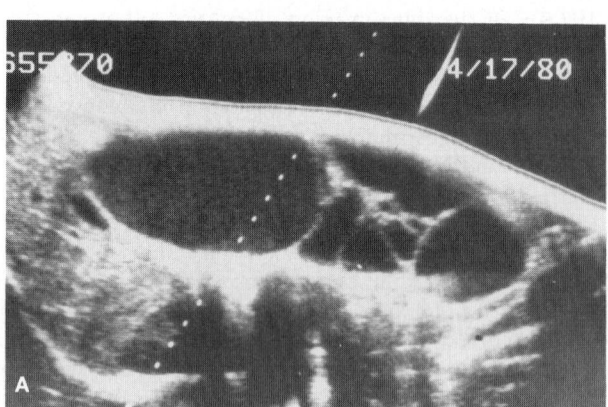
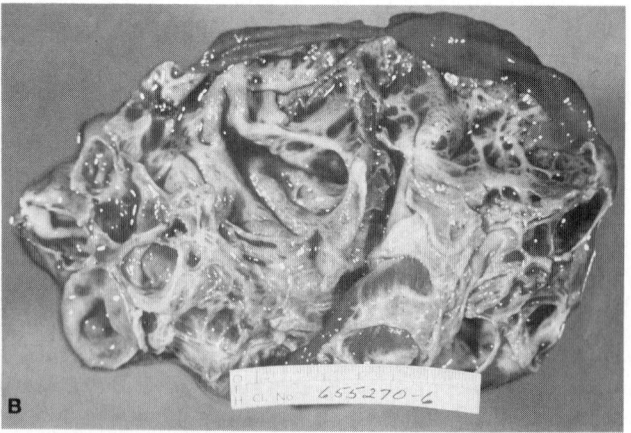

FIGURE 102-2. Sonographic appearance of a lymphangioma with a gross specimen correlation. (**A**) As in this sagittal section of the right abdomen, the loculi of a lymphangioma can be anechoic and contain echogenic debris and fluid-fluid levels (*arrows*). (**B**) The corresponding gross specimen demonstrates the multilocular nature of a lymphangioma and the different kinds of fluid contained in the loculi, ranging from hemorrhagic (*arrows*) to serous (*arrowhead*). (From Ros PR, Olmsted WW, Moser RP Jr, et al. Mesenteric and omental cysts: histologic classification with imaging correlation. Radiology 1987;164:327.)

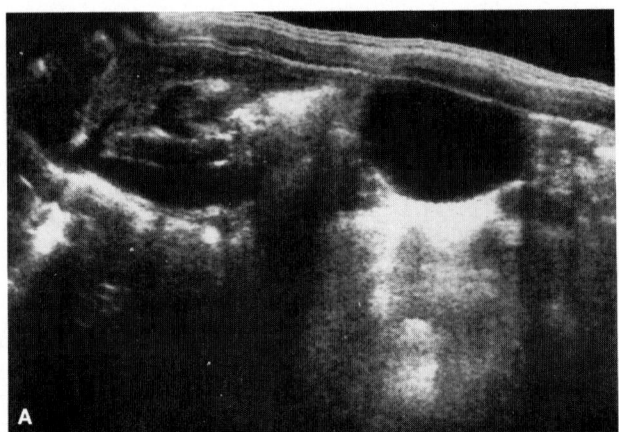

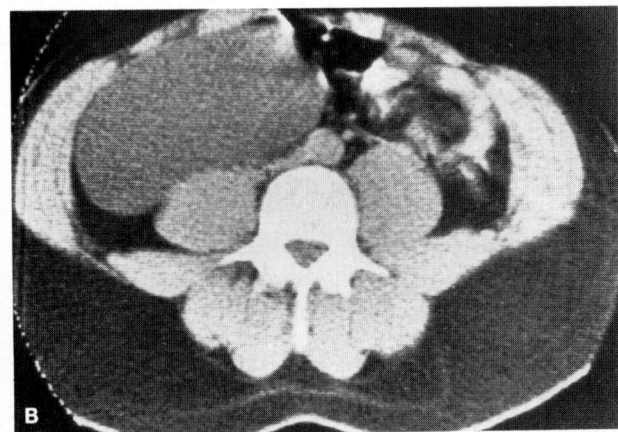

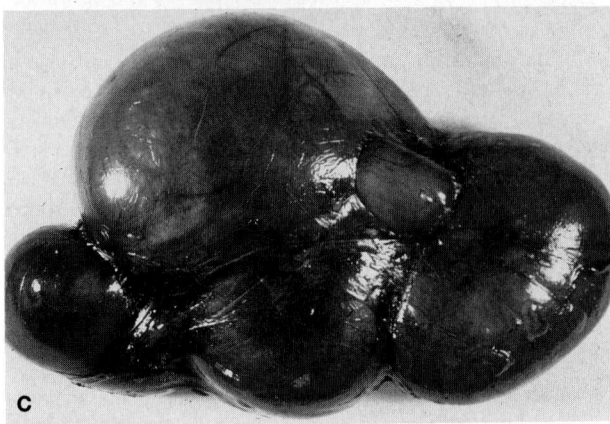

FIGURE 102-3. Sonographic and CT appearance of a mesothelial cyst with a pathologic correlation. (**A**) A longitudinal abdominal sonogram (sagittal section, to the right of the midline) reveals an anechoic mass with acoustic enhancement. The anterior location suggests an omental location. (**B**) A CT scan of another patient demonstrates a fluid-filled mass in the right lower abdomen. There is no discernible wall. (**C**) Specimen corresponding to **B** shows an elongated, thin-walled cyst. (From Ros PR, Olmsted WW, Moser RP Jr, et al. Mesenteric and omental cysts: histologic classification with imaging correlation. Radiology 1987;164:327.)

benign tumors, but leiomyosarcoma is the most common, followed by liposarcoma and rhabdomyosarcoma.[18] Mesenteric fibromatosis or mesenteric desmoid occurs more commonly than these tumors and is discussed in a different section.

Another type of tumor that can involve the mesentery, omentum, or retroperitoneum is inflammatory fibrosarcoma, which is composed of fibroblasts, plasma cells, and histiocytes. Inflammatory fibrosarcoma has been reported under a variety of names, such as inflammatory pseudotumor, plasma cell granuloma, myofibroblastoma, and omental-mesenteric myxoid hamartoma. Inflammatory fibrosarcoma may be a more accurate designation because these tumors are locally aggressive, can metastasize, and can lead to death. Inflammatory fibrosarcomas can occur at any age, but the mean age is 15 years.[36]

The most consistent presenting feature of omental and mesenteric tumors is a palpable abdominal mass that is often movable, often associated with pain, and sometimes associated with ascites or vomiting.[18,35,37] Plain abdominal x-ray films and gastrointestinal contrast studies often reveal displacement of the gut and aid in excluding the intestine as the origin of the tumor. Angiography is sometimes useful in determining whether the mass is extrinsic to the mesentery and thereby displacing the mesenteric vessels as a unit. Intrinsic mesenteric lesions may exhibit vascular encasement or distraction and separation of the blood vessels.[38] A CT scan often reveals the location of the mass within the mesentery or omentum and can exclude other organs as the origin of the mass.

The treatment of primary omental and mesenteric tumors

is surgical excision, if possible. The malignant tumors of the mesentery and omentum spread by local invasion and by peritoneal implantation and kill by involvement of vital abdominal organs. Unlike the desmoid tumors that may regress or resolve spontaneously, primary tumors of the omentum and mesentery should be treated as though they were potentially malignant. As many as 50% of lipomatous, histiocytic, or leiomyomatous tumors of the mesentery are malignant, as are approximately 25% of the omental tumors.[18,35,39]

Metastatic tumors of the mesentery are more common than primary mesenteric tumors and are usually the result of enlarged lymphomatous or carcinomatous lymph nodes. Malignant midgut carcinoid tumors often metastasize or spread directly to the mesentery. Among a series of 51 patients who underwent operation for midgut carcinoid, 84% had microscopically visible mesenteric lymph nodes or metastases.[40] More than one half of the patients had pronounced fibrosis causing mesenteric shortening, angulation, and fixation of the bowel. This fibrotic reaction often results in bowel obstruction and at times intestinal infarction due to venous or arterial occlusion.[40-42] Although serotonin (5-HT) has been proposed as a potential cause of this fibroblastic reaction, it has been found that carcinoid tumor cells express multiple peptide growth factors, such as fibroblast growth factor, platelet-derived growth factor, transforming growth factor-α, and transforming growth factor-β, that could promote the fibroblastic response.[43]

Surgical palliation of patients with metastatic carcinoid is warranted because of the indolent behavior of these tumors.

It is uncommon to accomplish curative resection, but significant symptomatic relief may be achieved. Surgery should always be considered in patients with symptoms of bowel obstruction or ischemia.[44,45]

OMENTAL VASCULAR ACCIDENT

Spontaneous primary vascular accidents, such as torsion, infarction, or hemorrhage, of the omentum are unusual causes of abdominal distress, although it is not uncommon for omental torsion and infarction to occur as a complication of hernia. Patients with primary vascular accidents of the greater omentum present with progressive abdominal pain, usually on the right side, that is often misdiagnosed as acute appendicitis or cholecystitis. The diagnosis is usually made at laparotomy.

Omental torsion occurs when the caudal free end of the omentum twists around a more proximal pivotal point. The twisting restricts venous return, causing the distal free end to become congested and edematous with hemorrhagic extravasation into the interstitial tissue and peritoneal cavity, producing aseptic peritonitis. Eventually, venous and arterial thrombosis occur, leading to hemorrhagic infarction. At laparotomy, characteristic serosanguineous ascites is found.

Etiologic factors in the development of omental torsion include anatomic variations such as bifid omentum, obesity, and vascular anomalies. Events that cause displacement of the omentum have been proposed as precipitating factors and include trauma to the abdomen, violent exercise, coughing, straining, hyperperistalsis, and acute changes in body position.[46,47] Omental infarction in the absence of torsion may be the result of embolism from the heart or aorta, may be caused by occlusive vascular disease, or may be spontaneous.[46,48,49]

The clinical features are similar regardless of the type of omental vascular accident. Typically, there is sudden onset of abdominal pain that may be generalized but is more frequently localized to the right abdomen. Other symptoms include nausea, vomiting, and anorexia. There may be a low-grade fever and moderate elevation of the leukocyte count to a range of 12,000 to 15,000/mm^3. A mobile, tender abdominal mass, often in the right side of the abdomen, has been reported in as many as one third of the patients with omental torsion.[50] This important sign can be obscured by excessive abdominal tenderness and guarding or obesity.

Most of these patients are operated on with a presumptive diagnosis of acute appendicitis or, less frequently, acute cholecystitis. At operation, serosanguineous fluid is found within the peritoneal cavity. There may be a mild inflammatory reaction in adjacent tissues, and the involved omentum may become adherent to adjacent intraabdominal structures. The treatment is resection of the involved omentum, and recovery is usually rapid and complete.[47,50]

GRANULOMATOUS INFECTION

The omentum and mesentery may be involved in infectious granulomatous diseases such as tuberculosis or mycoses, which may have a clinical presentation similar to metastatic malig-

nancy, lymphoma, or inflammatory bowel disease. CT imaging may reveal diffuse lymphadenopathy, thickening, and nodularity of the omentum and infiltration of the mesentery, liver, spleen and adrenal gland.[51,52] Biopsy for histologic analysis, stains for fungi and acid-fast bacillus testing, and appropriate microbiologic cultures are important for making the proper diagnosis of these potentially treatable infections.[53]

SURGICAL USES OF THE OMENTUM

The rich vascular and lymphatic supply of the omentum and its relative mobility and capability to wall off infection have led to its use in numerous operative situations.[54] The omentum has been used as a protective wrapping for intestinal anastomoses. It is often used as a patch for closure of perforated duodenal ulcer.

The omentum has been used to bolster esophageal and intestinal suture lines after liver resection or hepatic or splenic trauma. The omentum has been used as a viable hemostatic packing material. Reconstruction of the chest wall after sternal wound infection and dehiscence requires well-vascularized tissue to fill the large dead space of the wound, which promotes subsequent closure. The omentum fulfills this requirement and can be covered with skin graft.

> The reader is directed to Chapter 36, Approach to the Patient With Acute Abdomen; Chapter 68, Small Intestine: Anatomy and Structural Anomalies; Chapter 78, Colon: Anatomy and Structural Anomalies; Chapter 100, Abdominal Cavity: Anatomy, Structural Anomalies, and Hernias; Chapter 101, Intraabdominal Abscesses and Fistulas; Chapter 103, Diseases of the Peritoneum; Chapter 104, Diseases of the Retroperitoneum; Chapter 112, Mesenteric Vascular Insufficiency; Chapter 120, Cross-Sectional Anatomy; Chapter 123, Applications of Computed Tomography to the Gastrointestinal Tract; Chapter 127, Angiography; Chapter 129, Laparoscopy; and Chapter 140, Exploratory Laparotomy.

REFERENCES

1. Williams PL, Warwick R, eds. Embryology. In: Gray's anatomy. 36th British ed. Philadelphia: WB Saunders, 1980:200.
2. Grossman LA, Kaplan JH, Preuss HJ, et al. Mesenteric panniculitis. JAMA 1963;183:318.
3. Mitchinson MJ. Systemic idiopathic fibrosis and systemic Weber-Christian disease. J Clin Pathol 1965;18:645.
4. Durst AL, Freund H, Rosenmann E, et al. Mesenteric panniculitis: review of the literature and presentation of cases. Surgery 1977;81:203.
5. Gayliss H, Isaacson C, Decker GAG. Mesenteric panniculitis presenting as abdominal aortic aneurysm. Surgery 1973;74:626.
6. Soergel KH, Hensley GT. Fatal mesenteric panniculitis. Gastroenterology 1966;51:529.
7. Kipfer RE, Moertel CG, Dahlin DC. Mesenteric lipodystrophy. Ann Intern Med 1974;80:582.
8. Tytgat GN, Roozendaal K, Winter W, et al. Successful treatment of a patient with retractile mesenteritis with prednisone and azathioprine. Gastroenterology 1980;79:352.
9. Bush RW, Hammar SP Jr, Rudolph RH. Sclerosing mesenteritis. Response to cyclophosphamide. Arch Intern Med 1986;146:503.
10. Cotran RS, Kumar V, Robbins SL, eds. The musculoskeletal

system. In: Robbins pathologic basis of disease. 4th ed. Philadelphia: WB Saunders, 1989:1315.

11. Simpson RD, Harrison EG Jr, Mayo CW. Mesenteric fibromatosis in familial polyposis. A variant of Gardner's syndrome. Cancer 1964;17:526.

12. Dahn I, Jonsson N, Lundh G. Desmoid tumors. A series of 33 cases. Acta Chir Scand 1963;126:305.

13. Reitamo JJ, Hayry P, Nykyri E, et al. The desmoid tumor. I. Incidence, sex, age and anatomical distribution in the Finnish population. Am J Clin Pathol 1982;77:665.

14. Shiffman MA. Familial multiple polyposis associated with soft-tissue and hard-tissue tumors. JAMA 1962;179:514.

15. Naylor EW, Gardner EJ, Richards RC. Desmoid tumors and mesenteric fibromatosis in Gardner's syndrome. Arch Surg 1979;114:1181.

16. Suarez V, Hall C. Mesenteric fibromatosis. Br J Surg 1985;72:976.

17. Svanvik J, Knutsson F, Jansson R, et al. Desmoid tumour in the abdominal wall after treatment with high dose oestradiol for prostatic cancer. Acta Chir Scand 1982;148:301.

18. Yannopoulos K, Stout AP. Primary solid tumors of the mesentery. Cancer 1963;16:914.

19. Shepherd JA. Familial polyposis of the colon with associated connective tissue tumours. J R Coll Surg 1958;4:31.

20. Belliveau P, Graham AM. Mesenteric desmoid tumor in Gardner's syndrome treated by sulindac. Dis Colon Rectum 1984;27:53.

21. Waddell WR, Gerner RE, Reich MP. Nonsteroidal antiinflammatory drugs and tamoxifen for desmoid tumors and carcinoma of the stomach. J Surg Oncol 1983;22:197.

22. Klein WA, Miller HH, Anderson M, et al. The use of indomethacin, sulindac, and tamoxifen for the treatment of desmoid tumors associated with familial polyposis. Cancer 1987;60:2863.

23. Richards RC, Rogers SW, Gardner EJ. Spontaneous mesenteric fibromatosis in Gardner's syndrome. Cancer 1981;47:597.

24. Kiel KD, Suit HD. Radiation therapy in the treatment of aggressive fibromatoses (desmoid tumors). Cancer 1984;54:2051.

25. Greenberg HM, Goebel R, Weichselbaum RR, et al. Radiation therapy in the treatment of aggressive fibromatoses. Int J Radiat Oncol Biol Phys 1981;7:305.

26. Sprague NF Jr. Mesenteric cysts. Am Surg 1960;26:42.

27. Vanek VW, Phillips AK. Retroperitoneal, mesenteric, and omental cysts. Arch Surg 1984;119:838.

28. Walker AR, Putnam TC. Omental, mesenteric, and retroperitoneal cysts. A clinical study of 33 new cases. Ann Surg 1973;178:13.

29. Ros PR, Olmsted WW, Moser RP Jr, et al. Mesenteric and omental cysts: histologic classification with imaging correlation. Radiology 1987;164:327.

30. Takiff H, Calabria R, Yin L, et al. Mesenteric cysts and intraabdominal cystic lymphangiomas. Arch Surg 1985;120:1266.

31. Carpenter HA, Lancaster JR, Lee RA. Multilocular cysts of the peritoneum. Mayo Clin Proc 1982;57:634.

32. Harrow BR. Retroperitoneal lymphatic cyst (cystic lymphangioma). J Urol 1957;77:82.

33. Bowen B, Ros PR, McCarthy MJ, et al. Gastrointestinal teratomas: CT and US appearance with pathologic correlation. Radiology 1987;162:431.

34. Katsube Y, Mukai K, Silverberg SG. Cystic mesothelioma of the peritoneum. A report of five cases and review of the literature. Cancer 1982;50:1615.

35. Stout AP, Hendry J, Purdie FJ. Primary solid tumors of the great omentum. Cancer 1963;16:231.

36. Meis JM, Enzinger FM. Inflammatory fibrosarcoma of the mesentery and retroperitoneum. Am J Surg Pathol 1991;15:1146.

37. Weinberger HA, Ahmed MS. Mesenchymal solid tumors of the omentum and mesentery: report of four cases. Surgery 1977;82:754.

38. Diamond AB, Meng CH, Golden RR. Arteriography of unusual mass lesions of the mesentery. Radiology 1974;110:547.

39. Hashimoto H, Tsuneyoshi M, Enjoji M. Malignant smooth muscle tumors of the retroperitoneum and mesentery: a clinicopathologic analysis of 44 cases. J Surg Oncol 1985;28:177.

40. Makridis C, Oberg K, Juhlin C, et al. Surgical treatment of midgut carcinoid tumors. World J Surg 1990;14:377.

41. Eckhauser FE, Argenta LC, Strodel WE, et al. Mesenteric angiopathy, intestinal gangrene, and midgut carcinoids. Surgery 1981;90:720.

42. Warner TF, O'Reilly G, Lee GAM. Mesenteric occlusive lesion and ileal carcinoids. Cancer 1979;44:758.

43. Beauchamp RD, Coffey RJ Jr, Lyons RM, et al. Human carcinoid cell production of paracrine growth factors that can stimulate fibroblast and endothelial cell growth. Cancer Res 1991;51:5253.

44. Eckhauser FE, Knol JA. Invited commentary. World J Surg 1990;14:384.

45. Moertel CG. Treatment of the carcinoid tumor and the malignant carcinoid syndrome. J Clin Oncol 1983;1:727.

46. Leitner MJ, Jordan CG, Spinner MH, et al. Torsion, infarction and hemorrhage of the omentum as a cause of acute abdominal distress. Ann Surg 1952;135:103.

47. Adams JT. Primary torsion of the omentum. Am J Surg 1973;126:102.

48. Epstein LI, Lempke RE. Primary idiopathic segmental infarction of the greater omentum: case report and collective review of the literature. Ann Surg 1968;167:437.

49. Crofoot DD. Spontaneous segmental infarction of the greater omentum. Am J Surg 1980;139:262.

50. Mainzer RA, Simoes A. Primary idiopathic torsion of the omentum. Arch Surg 1964;88:974.

51. Denath FM. Abdominal tuberculosis in children: CT findings. Gastrointest Radiol 1990;15:303.

52. Alterman DD, Cho KC. Histoplasmosis involving the omentum in an AIDS patient: CT demonstration. J Comput Assist Tomogr 1988;12:664.

53. Bhansali SK. Abdominal tuberculosis. Experiences with 300 cases. Am J Gastroenterol 1977;67:324.

54. Samson R, Pasternak BM. Current status of surgery of the omentum. Surg Gynecol Obstet 1979;149:437.

Textbook of Gastroenterology, second edition, edited by Tadataka Yamada. JB Lippincott Company, Philadelphia © 1995.

CHAPTER 103

Diseases of the Peritoneum

B. Mark Evers

EMBRYOLOGY, ANATOMY, AND PHYSIOLOGY

The peritoneum is the mesothelial lining of the peritoneal cavity and its contained viscera. Embryologically, it develops from the primitive coelom which is formed by a splitting of the lateral mesoderm into somatic and splanchnic layers.[1] The parietal peritoneum, derived from the somatic layer, lines the abdominal cavity, diaphragm, and pelvis. The visceral peritoneum, from the splanchnic layer, covers the intraperitoneal organs and forms the mesenteries by which they are suspended.

The peritoneum and mesentery are supplied mainly by the splanchnic blood vessels and, to a lesser extent, by branches of the lower intercostal, lumbar, and iliac arteries. Differences arise in the innervation of the visceral and parietal peritoneum which lead to different perceptions of painful stimuli. The visceral peritoneum receives afferent innervation from the autonomic nervous system and responds primarily to traction and pressure; painful stimuli are perceived as a poorly localized, dull pain. In contrast, the parietal peritoneum is innervated by both somatic and visceral afferent nerves; noxious stimuli are perceived as a localized, sharp pain with rebound tenderness.

The peritoneum, with a total surface area of approximately 2 m², serves as a bidirectional dialysis membrane through which the passage of both large- and small-molecular-weight solutes is accomplished predominantly by simple passive diffusion.[2,3] Factors that can alter absorption include intraabdominal pressure, temperature, pH, increased portal pressure, lymphatic blockade, and scarring of the peritoneum.[4,5]

PERITONITIS

Peritonitis involves a local or generalized inflammation of the parietal and visceral peritoneum. With the development of broader-spectrum antibiotics, newer anesthetic techniques and modern pre- and postoperative monitoring in the intensive care unit, the mortality from peritonitis has been greatly reduced; however, despite these advances, peritonitis remains a formidable challenge confronting physicians.

Peritonitis can be classified as either primary or secondary. Primary peritonitis is less common and involves a spontaneous infection of preexisting ascites in the absence of any obvious intraabdominal source.[6,7] The spectrum of bacteria causing this syndrome and the patient population primarily affected have changed during the last decade. Spontaneous bacterial peritonitis is now more common in adults than in children and shows no differential gender incidence. The group most commonly affected, formerly children with nephrosis, is now adults with cirrhosis. Whereas gram-positive organisms formerly caused the majority of these infections, gram-negative enteric bacteria now account for 60% to 80% of organisms in ascitic fluid cultures, with *Escherichia coli* and *Klebsiella pneumoniae* being the most common species. Primary peritonitis is discussed in Chapter 43.

Secondary peritonitis is caused by diseases of or injury to

the intraabdominal organs. Acute suppurative peritonitis, granulomatous peritonitis, and chemical (aseptic) peritonitis belong to this category and are discussed in this chapter.

Acute Suppurative Peritonitis

Etiology

Spillage of intestinal contents into the peritoneal cavity as a result of primary intraabdominal disease (e.g., perforated peptic ulcer, appendicitis, diverticulitis, perforated carcinoma), penetrating trauma, or iatrogenic perforation after instrumentation or radiologic procedures is the usual cause of acute suppurative peritonitis.[8,9]

Clinical Manifestations

Abdominal pain, which may be sudden in onset if associated with a perforated viscus, is the predominant symptom.[10] Characteristically, patients with peritonitis lie supine with knees flexed and with frequent and limited intercostal respirations. Examination of the abdomen of a patient with generalized peritonitis reveals distention and bowel sounds that are either hypoactive or absent. Of the physical findings of peritonitis, tenderness and muscle guarding are the most important. Tenderness is often maximal over the organ in which the process originated; however, as the inflammation spreads, tenderness may be present over the entire extent of the peritoneum. Rebound tenderness, defined as the sudden and severe pain produced with the release of the hand after deep abdominal palpation, is often described as a useful adjunct in the diagnosis of the acute abdomen. This test, however, elicits no more information than that obtained from a careful and gentle examination of the abdomen and, furthermore, may cause unexpected and undue pain to the patient. Symptoms associated with acute suppurative peritonitis include anorexia, nausea that is often accompanied by vomiting, fever (38°–40°C), and signs of hypovolemia (e.g., tachycardia, dry mucous membranes, hypotension). Typical diagnostic findings in patients with acute peritonitis include a leukocytosis, often with an increased number of bands in the differential count. Roentgenographic findings are usually nonspecific, with evidence of a paralytic ileus of both the small bowel and colon in some patients. Free air under the diaphragm may be seen in an upright chest radiograph if a ruptured viscus is the cause (Fig. 103-1). Generally, the diagnosis of acute suppurative peritonitis is based on clinical manifestations and a thorough physical examination; laboratory and radiologic procedures serve mainly in a confirmatory role.

Clinical Course and Complications

Usually, suppurative peritonitis has an abrupt onset and a relatively short course with a rapid progression. Mortality results from fluid shifts and systemic endotoxin that may cause hypovolemia and septic shock. Early diagnosis with prompt surgical intervention and aggressive pre- and postoperative management is essential to reduce the morbidity and mortality

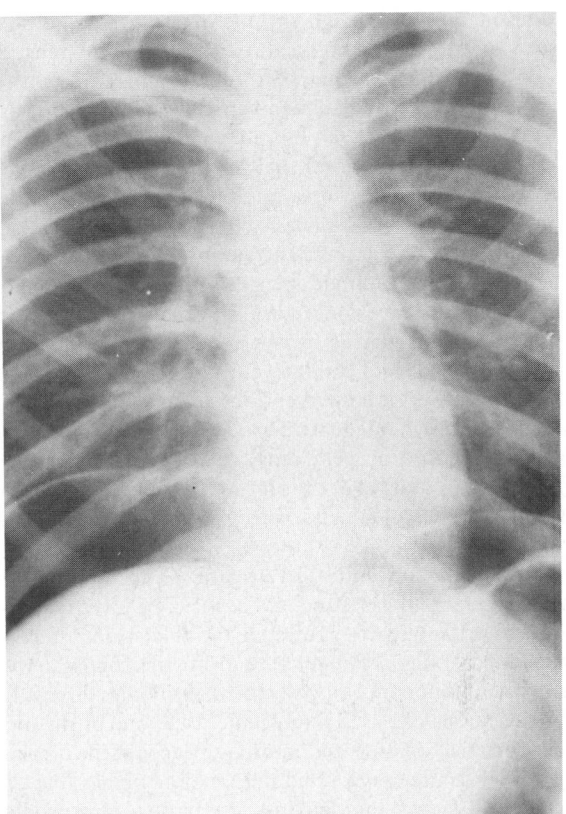

FIGURE 103-1. Upright chest film demonstrates free air under both diaphragms after perforation of a duodenal ulcer. (Courtesy of Charles J. Fagan, M.D., Galveston, TX.)

from multiple organ system failure that results from untreated peritonitis.[11-14]

Treatment

The hallmarks of treatment include resuscitation with intravenous fluids to restore normal physiology, broad-spectrum antibiotics, and operative management to control the source of peritoneal contamination and irrigate the peritoneal cavity.

Resuscitation involves aggressive administration of isotonic crystalloid fluids (e.g., Ringer's lactate) to correct hypovolemia and electrolyte imbalances. Careful monitoring of the response to rapid fluid resuscitation is necessary, particularly if large fluid volumes are required or the patient has impaired cardiac reserve. Monitoring usually entails frequent assessment of vital signs, hourly measurement of urine output, and frequent determination of central venous pressure or, preferably, placement of a Swan-Ganz catheter for pulmonary capillary wedge and pulmonary artery pressure determinations. Oxygen may be administered to overcome the mild hypoxemia that is commonly present, and nasogastric intubation is required to decompress the stomach.

Antibiotics play an important, albeit adjuvant, role in the management of patients with peritonitis. To be effective in the treatment of peritonitis, antibiotic therapy must be initiated before and continued during and after surgical therapy.

In addition, broad-spectrum antimicrobial therapy should be directed toward both aerobic and anaerobic pathogens. An aminoglycoside (e.g., gentamicin, tobramycin, amikacin), in combination with either clindamycin or metronidazole, provides coverage for most aerobic and anaerobic organisms encountered in the gastrointestinal tract.[15–17] Because of concerns about toxic effects, most notably nephrotoxicity, third-generation cephalosporins, newer broad-spectrum penicillins, and a new class of β-lactam antibiotics called carbapenems are being evaluated as single agents for treatment of bacterial peritonitis. Prospective randomized clinical trials indicate that these single agents may be as effective as the combination of an aminoglycoside and clindamycin.[18,19]

Expeditious surgical intervention remains the mainstay of treatment. After an adequate period to assure resuscitation, laparotomy should be performed to copiously irrigate the peritoneal cavity and repair the rupture. Aerobic and anaerobic cultures should be obtained to ensure appropriate antibiotic coverage.

Novel agents are under investigation and may become clinically useful in the treatment of sepsis. One investigational therapy has attempted to neutralize the deleterious effects of lipopolysaccharides (LPS) released from the bacterial wall, using either monoclonal or polyclonal antibodies directed to different regions of the LPS molecule. LPS, one of the most potent bacterial toxins, is an important trigger of the cytokine cascade. The acute exaggerated release of cytokines (e.g., tumor necrosis factor, interleukins, interferons) may produce many of the hemodynamic manifestations of septic shock; chronic production leads to tissue wasting and cachexia. Two anti-LPS monoclonal antibodies are being studied: HA-1A, a human monoclonal antibody directed against the lipid A domain of LPS,[20] and E5, a newly developed murine monoclonal IgM antibody.[21] Initial prospective randomized trials have suggested some efficacy with this treatment.[20,21] Other areas of active research include strategies to neutralize the effects of cytokines using either neutralizing antibodies or specific cytokine-receptor antagonists.[22,23] A receptor antagonist to interleukin-1 (IL-1ra) has been developed and has proven useful in experimental models of shock and cachexia.[24,25] Finally, responses elicited by cytokines appear mediated by secondary agents (e.g., eicosanoids, nitric oxide) acting at the effector sites. A competitive inhibitor of nitric oxide, N^G-methyl-L-arginine, protects against the hypotensive effects of tumor necrosis factor in a canine model, which suggests that the effect of this cytokine on hemodynamic stability may be mediated through nitric oxide and further suggests a potential clinical use of nitric oxide inhibitors in the treatment of sepsis.[26]

Granulomatous Peritonitis

Etiology

Granulomatous peritonitis is a disease process characterized by peritoneal inflammation that is associated with formation of granulomas and an increased incidence of adhesions. The disease most commonly associated with granulomatous peritonitis is tuberculosis.[27] Other, less common causes include fungal (e.g., *Candida*, histoplasma), amebic, and parasitic infections.[28–30] Iatrogenic causes of granulomatous peritonitis also occur, usually related to the presence of glove lubricants (e.g., talc, cornstarch) or cellulose fibers from gauze, surgical drapes, or gowns within the peritoneum.[31]

Tuberculous Peritonitis

Epidemiology. After years of a decreasing incidence of tuberculosis, there has been a general reemergence of this disease secondary to an increase in the cases of acquired immunodeficiency syndrome (AIDS) and an increase in the number of immigrants.[32–36] Since 1985, cases of tuberculosis have increased 18% nationwide, with the highest increases occurring in certain highly populated areas of the country. Particularly disturbing is the recent appearance of multidrug-resistant strains of tuberculosis.[34–37] In addition to patients with AIDS, other groups at high risk include poorly nourished, debilitated patients and those with cirrhosis.

Etiology. Tuberculous peritonitis is a form of abdominal tuberculosis that can involve the omentum, intestinal tract, liver, spleen, or female genital tract in addition to the parietal and visceral peritoneum. The overall incidence of abdominal tuberculosis in the United States is approximately 0.5% to 1% of all cases of tuberculosis.[32] Tuberculous peritonitis is usually associated with a primary focus of tuberculosis elsewhere. This primary focus is usually the lung; however, only about one third of cases have clinical or radiographic evidence of pulmonary tuberculosis. The pathologic organism, *Mycobacterium tuberculosis*, can gain entry to the peritoneal cavity by one of three mechanisms: transmurally from diseased bowel, from tuberculous salpingitis, or, more commonly, by hematogenous spread from a pulmonary focus.[32–34]

Clinical manifestations. Generally, the onset is quite insidious, with more than 70% of patients having had symptoms for more than 4 months before definitive diagnosis. The most common symptoms are constitutional and include fever, anorexia, weakness, malaise, and weight loss. Abdominal distention caused either by ascites or by partial obstruction may be present. On examination, the abdomen is diffusely tender in a majority of patients; however, the classic doughy abdomen is rarely found. Tuberculous peritonitis should be suspected in high-risk or immunocompromised patients with ascites, fever, unexplained generalized symptoms, and diffuse abdominal pain or tenderness.[32–34]

Differential diagnosis and diagnostic studies. Routine laboratory and radiographic studies are rarely diagnostic. A normal leukocyte count is present in most patients, and anemia is only variably found. Tuberculin skin tests are usually positive in patients with tuberculous peritonitis; however, a negative result is of no help in excluding the disease. Chest radiographs are abnormal in 80% of patients and include findings of pleural effusions or pulmonary infiltrates. Radiographs of the abdomen are seldom of benefit; however, a computerized tomography (CT) scan may be useful in identifying thickened bowel and ascites (Fig. 103-2). Examination of the peritoneal fluid may prove useful (see

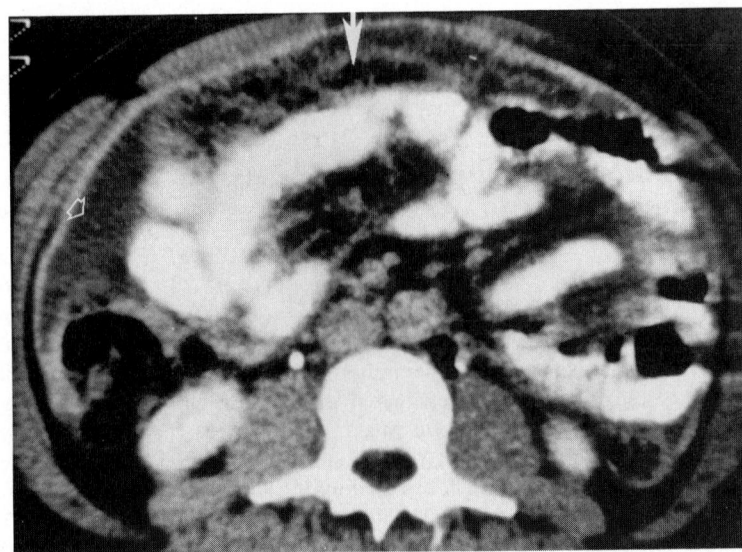

FIGURE 103-2. Computed tomography scan demonstrates ascites (*open arrow*) and small bowel thickening (*closed arrow*) in a patient with tuberculous peritonitis. (Courtesy of Charles J. Fagan, M.D., Galveston, TX.)

Chap. 43). In patients with tuberculous peritonitis, the protein content characteristically exceeds 3.0 g/dL, and glucose concentration is below 30 mg/dL in more than 80%. Most patients have a leukocyte count higher than 250 cells/mm^3 and a relative lymphocytic pleocytosis. Acid-fast stains are rarely positive unless at least 1 L of ascitic fluid is obtained, concentrated by centrifugation, and then examined. To further compound the diagnostic problem, bacterial cultures of *M tuberculosis* often require 4 to 6 weeks of incubation. For these reasons, much attention has been given to the development of a rapid diagnostic test for tuberculosis. The most promising approach involves amplification and detection using the polymerase chain reaction (PCR) procedure. Although not in widespread use, this procedure requires approximately 24 to 48 hours and can detect as few as 10 to 100 bacilli in a sample.[34-38]

The diagnosis of tuberculous peritonitis is often suggested by findings at laparoscopy or laparotomy. Tuberculous peritonitis is characterized by stalactite-like fibrinous masses from the parietal peritoneum and, in addition, the peritoneum may be studded with small granulomas.

The differential diagnosis of tuberculous peritonitis is variable, depending on the acuteness of the symptoms. In patients with a prolonged history, tuberculous peritonitis is most commonly confused with Crohn's disease or carcinoma. In patients presenting acutely, the differential diagnosis must include such entities as acute appendicitis, cholecystitis, perforated ulcer, and salpingitis.

In summary, the diagnosis of tuberculous peritonitis is often difficult to make and requires an initial suspicion based on the clinical presentation (i.e., fever, anorexia, and abdominal pain) in combination with findings of a nonexudative ascites. It is crucial that a suspected diagnosis be confirmed by open or laparoscopic-assisted biopsy before committing the patient to a long-term treatment regimen with multiagent therapy.

Clinical course and therapy. Before the advent of chemotherapy, the mortality from tuberculous peritonitis was as high as 60%; now, the disease is, for the most part, readily curable with the available agents. Therapy with isoniazid in combination with one or two additional drugs for 18 to 24 months is the treatment of choice. Although it has not proven experimentally, corticosteroids for 2 to 3 months may be beneficial in preventing the formation of dense fibrous adhesions which could lead to bowel obstruction. The most worrisome feature of the resurgence of tuberculosis has been the recent outbreaks of multidrug-resistant isolates that often fail to respond to both isoniazid and rifampin, the two cornerstone antituberculosis drugs.[33-37]

Chemical (Aseptic) Peritonitis

Etiology

Peritoneal inflammation can result from spillage of irritant materials that are initially sterile; with time, secondary bacterial contamination occurs with signs and symptoms similar to those of acute suppurative peritonitis. Most of the substances that cause a chemical peritonitis are capable of acting as adjuvants to promote the growth of bacterial contaminants. These agents include bile, usually resulting from open or laparoscopic biliary tract operations without adequate external drainage, from inadvertent injury to the biliary tract, or from external trauma[39-41]; urine, from intraperitoneal bladder rupture[42]; and chyle, which occurs secondary to injuries of large lymphatic vessels during operations on retroperitoneal organs.[43] In addition, spillage of barium sulfate, secondary to perforation of the gastrointestinal tract from diagnostic procedures, results in a severe peritoneal irritation, and, in combination with accompanying enteric bacteria, poses a lethal threat to the patient.[44,45]

Treatment

The same principles that apply to the management of acute suppurative peritonitis also apply to the treatment of chemical peritonitis. Adequate intravenous fluids to replace the peritoneal fluid sequestration and antibiotics are followed by laparotomy to irrigate the abdomen and control the source of the peritoneal contamination.

Peritonitis as a Complication of Chronic Peritoneal Dialysis

Etiology

Continuous ambulatory peritoneal dialysis (CAPD) has gained increasing acceptance as an efficacious and cost-effective alternative to chronic hemodialysis in patients with end-stage renal disease. It is estimated that, in the United States alone, approximately one fourth of the more than 100,000 dialysis patients use CAPD. Despite its obvious advantages, the most common complication of CAPD is infectious peritonitis resulting from bacterial contamination of the peritoneal cavity.[46,47] Even with better patient education regarding sterile techniques and proper cleaning around the catheter site, peritonitis in this group of patients is the major source of morbidity and the largest single cause of patient failure on CAPD. Although the incidence of peritonitis varies with the institution, peritonitis as a complication of CAPD averages 1.4 episodes per patient-year of treatment.[46,47]

Epidemiology

The most frequent portals of entry for bacteria in CAPD patients include the exit site of the dialysis catheter and the tunnel through which the catheter traverses the abdominal wall. This usually occurs as a result in a break in aseptic technique with secondary contamination. Other possibilities for contamination include hematogenous or lymphatic dissemination from a septic focus originating from the patient. In contrast to other types of peritonitis, CAPD-related peritonitis is usually caused by a single organism, in the majority of cases by gram-positive cocci (*Staphylococcus epidermidis, Staphylococcus aureus, Streptococci* and *Enterococci* organisms).[46-48] Gram-negative bacteria account for approximately 25% of all cases of CAPD peritonitis, with the most common being *Escherichia coli* and *Pseudomonas aeruginosa*. The presence of anaerobic organisms or a mixed flora should raise suspicion of an intestinal perforation or other intraabdominal disease as the cause of peritonitis. Fungal peritonitis is relatively uncommon but remains the most serious type of infective peritonitis in CAPD patients because of treatment difficulties.[49] At least 20 different fungal species have been cultured; however, *Candida albicans* and *Candida tropicalis* remain the most common.

Clinical Manifestations

The severity of symptoms is dependent on the infecting organism; however, the signs and symptoms in the majority of patients with CAPD peritonitis are clinically less severe than those in patients with suppurative peritonitis. Some cases may even be asymptomatic and detected only by the presence of a cloudy effluent. The predominant symptom found in patients is a diffuse abdominal pain, usually associated with a low-grade fever and leukocytosis. Other symptoms may include hyperhydration, diarrhea, hypotension, and pressure pain above the catheter tunnel. Characteristically, a turbid dialysis effluent is found in nearly all cases of CAPD peritonitis.

Diagnosis

The diagnosis of CAPD peritonitis is based on both clinical and laboratory findings.[46,47] The clinical diagnosis should be based on the presence of two of three criteria: abdominal pain or tenderness, a turbid dialysate containing more than 100 neutrophils/mm³, and a positive culture from the peritoneal fluid. Even if the patient's history and examination are consistent with the diagnosis of peritonitis, it is essential that the dialysate be evaluated to confirm the diagnosis and identify the causative organisms. In some centers, the use of bacteria-concentrating techniques has yielded positive cultures in more than 90% of cases.[50]

Therapy and Clinical Course

Seventy percent to 80% of patients with CAPD peritonitis can be successfully treated on an outpatient basis without hospitalization or interruption of dialysis.[46,47,51] CAPD peritonitis is most effectively treated by intraperitoneal administration of antibiotics. The initial choice of antibiotics should be broad enough to cover the most common pathogens causing CAPD peritonitis and then changed according to susceptibility testing. Vancomycin, cephalosporins, and aminoglycosides are the agents most commonly used to treat CAPD-associated peritonitis. In addition to antibiotics, heparin is also added to the dialysis bag to reduce fibrin formation and, thereby, the incidence of postinfective adhesions. Indications for catheter removal include persistence of peritonitis after 4 to 5 days of treatment and the presence of fungal or tuberculous peritonitis, fecal peritonitis, or severe skin infection at the catheter site.

Peritonitis in the Immunocompromised Host

Incidence and Etiology

The AIDS epidemic and increasing use of immunosuppressive therapy for cancer, autoimmune disease, and multiple organ transplantation procedures have combined to greatly increase the incidence of opportunistic infections of the gastrointestinal tract.[52,53] In 1990, there were more than one million people in the United States infected with the human immunodeficiency virus (HIV) and approximately 155,000 cases of AIDS; estimates at that time predicted 390,000 to 480,000 cases of AIDS by the year 1993.[52,54]

Diagnosis

The differential diagnosis of abdominal pain in AIDS is quite broad and involves both AIDS- and non-AIDS-related disorders[52-54] (see Chap. 105). Perforation of the small bowel or colon secondary to cytomegalovirus enteritis is a frequent cause of peritonitis in AIDS patients.[55] Other organisms reported to cause peritonitis in these patients include *Mycobacterium avium-intracellulare, M tuberculosis, Cryptococcus neoformans* and *Strongyloides* organisms.

Clinical Manifestations and Treatment

Immunocompromised patients with peritonitis usually present with severe abdominal pain as the predominant symptom, like patients with suppurative peritonitis. Principles of management include emergent laparotomy and resection of the involved portion of bowel, intravenous fluid resuscitation, and broad-spectrum antibiotics.

PRIMARY MESOTHELIOMA

Incidence and Etiology

Primary mesotheliomas, arising from mesenchymal and epithelial components, are rare; the reported incidence in the United States is only 2.2 cases per million population.[56,57] Of these, only 20% to 40% occur in the peritoneum, with the majority of these tumors originating from the pleura. Malignant mesothelioma is linked to exposure to asbestos, and there is a strong association with occupations that require workers to handle or work in proximity to asbestos, such as those in the textile, insulation, building, demolition, and shipyard industries.[56,57] There is a latency period of 20 to 40 years from significant asbestos exposure to development of mesothelioma; two thirds of the patients are diagnosed at 45 to 64 years of age. The incidence of mesothelioma peaked in 1984 and is now declining, probably secondary to increased public awareness regarding asbestos exposure. Although asbestos is the predominant cause of this disease, other etiologic agencies may also be associated with primary mesothelioma, including use of the angiographic contrast material Thorotrast (thorium dioxide) and radiation exposure.

Clinical Manifestations

The clinical presentation is nonspecific, with the predominant complaint being abdominal pain present in the epigastrium or right upper quadrant. Other symptoms include nausea and vomiting, malaise, fever, weight loss, diarrhea, and anemia. Ascites is the most common physical finding and occurs in 90% of patients. Peritoneal mesotheliomas can produce and secrete a variety of ectopic hormones, including antidiuretic hormone, growth hormone, and insulin-like factors, which can produce associated paraneoplastic syndromes with symptoms of hypoglycemia, hyponatremia, thrombocytosis, and increased production of fibrin-degradation products.[56]

Differential Diagnosis and Diagnostic Studies

Malignant mesothelioma is a difficult malignancy to diagnose early.[56–58] Mesotheliomas are generally firm, white tumors that present as individual nodules studding the peritoneal surface and tend to spread over the surface of the intraabdominal organs, eventually encasing the viscera. Ultrasound and CT studies can suggest the diagnosis, demonstrate the extent of tumor, and also aid in directed biopsy of suspicious lesions (Fig. 103-3); however, in most cases, the diagnosis is confirmed after diagnostic laparoscopy or laparotomy.

Microscopic and immunohistochemical studies are available to aid in the diagnosis. The typical analysis of a suspected mesothelioma should include electron microscopy, periodic acid-Schiff (PAS) stain, Alcian blue stain to detect hyaluronic acid, and an anti-carcinoembryonic antigen (anti-CEA) an-

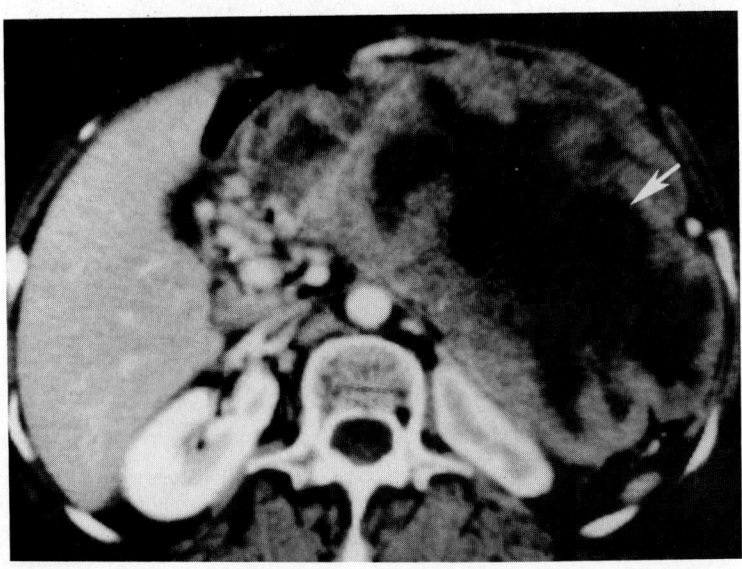

FIGURE 103-3. Computed tomography scan demonstrates diffuse mesenteric and peritoneal involvement of a soft tissue mass (*arrow*) causing displacement of intraabdominal organs in a patient with peritoneal mesothelioma. (Courtesy of Charles J. Fagan, M.D., Galveston, TX.)

tibody stain. Mesotheliomas lack intracellular mucin on PAS stains, should produce negative results on anti-CEA antibody stain, and often stain positively for hyaluronic acid. In contrast, adenocarcinomas often stain positively for mucin and CEA and do not contain hyaluronic acid. Well-characterized monoclonal and polyclonal antibodies hold great promise for improving the diagnostic accuracy.[57–59] New antibodies reactive to keratin, vimentin, lectins, and intermediate filaments are now available. In addition, antibodies raised against proteins isolated from mesothelioma cells have been isolated. The results have not been totally consistent; however, these markers remain to be widely tested.[59] Additional molecular studies that may serve as useful adjuncts to the diagnosis include the identification of high levels of the platelet-derived growth factor (PDGF) β-chain in malignant mesotheliomas.[59]

Less common primary peritoneal neoplasms that should be included in the differential diagnosis include benign papillary mesotheliomas, benign fibrous mesothelioma, adenomatoid tumors, and multicystic peritoneal mesothelioma.[60]

Treatment and Prognosis

Therapy for mesothelioma has proven disappointing, mainly as a result of the advanced stage of the disease at diagnosis and the local aggressiveness of the tumor. Rarely can surgery be performed for a curative resection; rather, laparotomy serves to establish a tissue diagnosis and perform palliative procedures such as bypassing obstructive lesions or tumor debulking. Chemotherapy offers little improvement in overall patient survival. Doxorubicin, alone or in combination with other antineoplastic agents, achieves the best, albeit minimal, response. Radiation therapy has been used in combination with intracavitary instillation of various chemotherapeutic agents or with systemic chemotherapy but with only minimal success.

Future directions for the management of mesothelioma include the use of interleukin-2 and interferon-γ, both of which have shown promise in limited trials of patients with pleural mesothelioma. In addition, the finding of alterations in chromosome 3 and in the tumor suppressor gene, *p53*, suggests that gene therapy may, in the future, be a possibility.[57–59]

The prognosis for mesothelioma of the peritoneum is poor. Death usually occurs within 1 year of the diagnosis from progressive gastrointestinal tract obstruction and debility.

PSEUDOMYXOMA PERITONEI

Incidence and Etiology

Pseudomyxoma peritonei is a rare condition manifested by diffuse, gelatinous implants of the peritoneal cavity and omentum arising from mucinous neoplasms of either the appendix or ovary.[61–63] The reported incidence of pseudomyxoma peritonei is approximately 2 in 10,000 laparotomies.

Clinical Features and Diagnosis

Women between the 45 and 55 years of age make up approximately 75% of patients with pseudomyxoma peritonei. Patients often present with an increasing abdominal girth secondary to mucinous ascites or intestinal obstruction.

Histologically, pseudomyxoma peritonei is characterized by a benign appearance with simple columnar epithelium containing mucin-filled vacuoles. Certain features noted on sonography or CT scan are characteristic for this disease. Sonographic findings include multiple intraperitoneal multilocular cysts and ascitic septation. A characteristic CT finding of pseudomyxoma peritonei is scalloping of the hepatic and bowel margins secondary to extrinsic compression by ascitic spaces containing gelatinous material (Fig. 103-4).

Treatment and Prognosis

Pseudomyxoma peritonei is a low-grade malignancy which rarely metastasizes or invades contiguous viscera. The treatment of pseudomyxoma peritonei is primarily surgical, with aggressive debulking of all intraabdominal tumor and omentectomy.[64] In addition, because of the usual involvement of both the appendix and the ovaries, it is recommended that appendectomy and bilateral oophorectomy be performed in all patients. Repeat laparotomies are indicated for recurrent disease. Chemotherapy and radiation treatment are of little benefit. Long-term survival is approximately 54% at 5 years, with death occurring usually as a result of extensive peritoneal disease and intestinal obstruction.

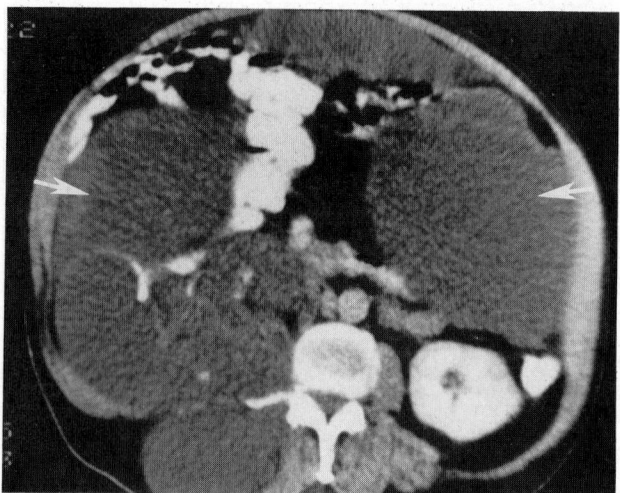

FIGURE 103-4. Computed tomography scan demonstrates large gelatinous masses (*arrows*) in a patient with pseudomyxoma peritonei. (Courtesy of Charles J. Fagan, M.D., Galveston, TX.)

The reader is directed to Chapter 36, Approach to the Patient With Acute Abdomen; Chapter 37, Approach to the Patient With Ileus and Obstruction; Chapter 43, Approach to the Patient With Ascites; Chapter 61, Acid-Peptic Disorders; Chapter 71, Chronic Infections of the Small Intestine; Chapter 83, Diverticulitis; Chapter 100, Abdominal Cavity: Anatomy, Structural

Anomalies, and Hernias; Chapter 101, Intraabdominal Abscesses and Fistulas; Chapter 102, Diseases of the Mesentery and Omentum; Chapter 104, Diseases of the Retroperitoneum; Chapter 123, Applications of Computed Tomography to the Gastrointestinal Tract; Chapter 129, Laparoscopy; and Chapter 131, Microbiologic Studies.

REFERENCES

1. Moore K. The developing human. 4th ed. Philadelphia: WB Saunders, 1988.
2. Aune S. Transperitoneal exchange. IV. The effect of transperitoneal fluid transport on the transfer of solutes. Scand J Gastroent 1970;5:241.
3. Shear L, Swartz C, Shinaberger JA, et al. Kinetics of peritoneal fluid absorption in adult man. N Engl J Med 1965;272:123.
4. Berndt WO, Gosselin RE. Differential changes in permeability of mesentery to rubidium and phosphate. Am J Physiol 1962;202:761.
5. Shear L, Castellot JJ, Shinaberger JH, et al. Enhancement of peritoneal fluid absorption by dehydration, mercaptomerin, and vasopressin. J Pharm Exp Ther 1966;154:289.
6. Cuthbert JA. Spontaneous bacterial peritonitis. J Gastroenterol Hepatol 1990;5:438.
7. Garcia-Tsao G. Spontaneous bacterial peritonitis. Gastroenterol Clin North Am 1992;21:257.
8. Maddaus MA, Ahrenholz D, Simmons RL. The biology of peritonitis and implications for treatment. Surg Clin North Am 1981;68:431.
9. Crawford E, Ellis H. Generalised peritonitis—the changing spectrum. A report of 100 consecutive cases. Br J Clin Pract 1985;39:177.
10. Nichols RL. Intraabdominal infections: an overview. Rev Infect Dis 1985;7(Suppl 4):709.
11. Bohnen J, Boulanger M, Meakins JL, et al. Prognosis in generalized peritonitis. Relation to cause and risk factors. Arch Surg 1983;118:285.
12. Baue AE. Multiple, progressive, or sequential systems failure. Arch Surg 1975;110:779.
13. Fry DE, Pearlstein L, Fulton RL, et al. Multiple system organ failure. The role of uncontrolled infection. Arch Surg 1980;115:136.
14. Pine RW, Wertz MJ, Lennard ES, et al. Determinants of organ malfunction or death in patients with intra-abdominal sepsis. Arch Surg 1983;118:242.
15. Nichols RL. Management of intra-abdominal sepsis. Am J Med 1986;80(Suppl 6B):204.
16. Dunn DL, Simmons RL. The role of anaerobic bacteria in intraabdominal infections. Rev Infect Dis 1984;6(Suppl 1):S139.
17. Ho JL, Barza M. Role of aminoglycoside antibiotics in the treatment of intra-abdominal infection. Antimicrob Agents Chemother 1987;31:485.
18. Malangoni MA, Condon RE, Spiegel CA, et al. Treatment of intra-abdominal infections is appropriate with single-agent or combination antibiotic therapy. Surgery 1985;98:648.
19. DiPiro JT, Mansberger JA, Davis JB Jr. Therapy review. Current concepts in clinical therapeutics: intra-abdominal infections. Clin Pharm 1986;5:34.
20. Zeigler EJ, Fisher CJ, Sprung CL, et al. Treatment of gram-negative bacteremia and septic shock with HA-1A human monoclonal antibody against endotoxin. N Engl J Med 1991;324:429.
21. Greenman RL, Schein RMH, Martin MA, et al. A controlled clinical trial of E5 murine monoclonal IgM antibody to endotoxin in the treatment of gram-negative sepsis. JAMA 1991;266:1097.
22. Tracey KJ, Fong Y, Hesse DG, et al. Anti-cachectin/TNF monoclonal antibodies prevent septic shock during lethal bacteraemia. Nature 1987;330:662.
23. Himmler A, Maurer-Fogy I, Krönke M, et al. Molecular cloning and expression of human and rat tumor necrosis factor receptor chain (p60) and its soluble derivative, tumor necrosis factor-binding protein. DNA Cell Biol 1990;9:705.
24. McIntyre KW, Stepan GJ, Kolinsky KD, et al. Inhibition of interleukin 1 (IL-1) binding and bioactivity in vitro and modulation of acute inflammation in vivo by IL-1 receptor antagonist and anti-IL-1 receptor monoclonal antibody. J Exp Med 1991;173:931.
25. Gershenwald JE, Fong Y, Fahey TJ III, et al. Interleukin 1 receptor blockade attenuates the host inflammatory response. Proc Natl Acad Sci U S A 1990;87:4966.
26. Kilbourn RG, Gross SS, Jubran A, et al. N^G-Methyl-L-arginine inhibits tumor necrosis factor-induced hypotension: implications for the involvement of nitric oxide. Proc Natl Acad Sci U S A 1990;87:3629.
27. Cromartie RS III. Tuberculous peritonitis. Surg Gynecol Obstet 1977;144:876.
28. Solomkin JS, Flohr AB, Quie PG, et al. The role of *Candida* in intraperitoneal infections. Surgery 1980;88:524.
29. Monga NK, Sood S, Kaushik SP, et al. Amebic peritonitis. Am J Gastroenterol 1976;66:366.
30. Lintermans JP. Fatal peritonitis, an unusual complication of *Strongyloides stercoralis* infestation. Clin Pediatr (Phila) 1975;14:974.
31. Tinker MA, Burdman D, Deysine M, et al. Granulomatous peritonitis due to cellulose fibers from disposable surgical fabrics: laboratory investigation and clinical implications. Ann Surg 1974;180:831.
32. Gentile DA, Ross CB. Tuberculous peritonitis. Case report and review of the literature. J Tenn Med Assoc 1987;80:469.
33. Hopewell PC. Impact of human immunodeficiency virus infection on the epidemiology, clinical features, management, and control of tuberculosis. Clin Infect Dis 1992;15:540.
34. Weissler JC. Southwestern internal medicine conference: tuberculosis—immunopathogenesis and therapy. Am J Med Sci 1993;305:52.
35. Bloom BR, Murray CJL. Tuberculosis: commentary on a reemergent killer. Science 1992;257:1055.
36. Farley TA. AIDS and multidrug-resistant tuberculosis: an epidemic transforms an old disease. J La State Med Soc 1992;144:357.
37. Davidson PT, Le HQ. Drug treatment of tuberculosis—1992. Drugs 1992;43:651.
38. Young DB, Cole ST. Leprosy, tuberculosis and the new genetics. J Bacteriol 1993;175:1.
39. Dinner M. Biliary peritonitis due to idiopathic perforation of the common bile duct. S Afr J Surg 1975;13:207.
40. Ruben RA, Chopra S. Bile peritonitis after liver biopsy: nonsurgical management of a patient with an acute abdomen. A case report with review of the literature. Am J Gastroenterol 1987;82:265.
41. Larmi TKI, Kairaluoma MI, Junila J, et al. Perforation of the gallbladder. A retrospective comparative study of cases from 1946–1956 and 1969–1980. Acta Chir Scand 1984;150:557.
42. Garfinkle SE, Chiu GW, Cohen SE, et al. Spontaneous perforation of the neurogenic urinary bladder. West J Med 1976;124:64.
43. Krizek TJ, Davis JH. Acute chylous peritonitis. Arch Surg 1965;91:253.
44. Grobmyer AJ III, Keplan RA, Peterson CM, et al. Barium peritonitis. Am Surg 1984;50:116.
45. Yamamura M, Nishi M, Furubayashi H, et al. Barium peritonitis. Report of a case and review of the literature. Dis Colon Rectum 1985;28:347.
46. Saklayen MG. CAPD peritonitis. Incidence, pathogens, diagnosis, and management. Med Clin North Am 1990;74:997.
47. Spencer RC. Infections in continuous ambulatory peritoneal dialysis. J Med Microbiol 1988;27:1.
48. Von Graevenitz A, Amsterdam D. Microbiological aspects of peritonitis associated with continuous ambulatory peritoneal dialysis. Clin Microbiol Rev 1992;5:36.
49. Cheng IKP, Fang G-X, Chan T-M, et al. Fungal peritonitis com-

plicating peritoneal dialysis: report of 27 cases and review of treatment. Q J Med 1989;71:407.

50. Vas SI. Microbiologic aspects of chronic ambulatory peritoneal dialysis. Kidney Int 1983;23:83.

51. Horton MW, Deeter RG, Sherman RA. Treatment of peritonitis in patients undergoing continuous ambulatory peritoneal dialysis. Clin Pharm 1990;9:102.

52. Williams RA, Wilson SE. Gastrointestinal disorders requiring surgical treatment in patients with AIDS. Compr Ther 1992;18:9.

53. Wall SD, Jones B. Gastrointestinal tract in the immunocompromised host: opportunistic infections and other complications. Radiology 1992;185:327.

54. Davidson T, Allen-Mersh TG, Miles AJG, et al. Emergency laparotomy in patients with AIDS. Br J Surg 1991;78:924.

55. Wilcox CM, Forsmark CE, Darragh TM, et al. Cytomegalovirus peritonitis in a patient with acquired immunodeficiency syndrome. Dig Dis Sci 1992;37:1288.

56. Asensio JA, Goldblatt P, Thomford NR. Primary malignant peritoneal mesothelioma. Arch Surg 1990;125:1477.

57. Roggli VL, Kolbeck J, Sanfilippo F, et al. Pathology of human mesothelioma. Etiologic and diagnostic considerations. Pathol Annu 1987;22:91.

58. Vogelzang NJ. Malignant mesothelioma: diagnostic and management strategies for 1992. Sem Oncol 1992;19(S11):64.

59. Sheibani K, Esteban JM, Bailey A, et al. Immunopathologic and molecular studies as an aid to the diagnosis of malignant mesothelioma. Hum Pathol 1992;23:107.

60. Daya D, McCaughey WTE. Pathology of the peritoneum: a review of selected topics. Semin Diagn Pathol 1991;8:277.

61. Toro DH, Reyes LI, Velazquez J. *Pseudomyxoma peritonei*: case report and review of the literature. Bol Asoc Med P R 1990;82:355.

62. Smith JW, Kemeny N, Caldwell C, et al. *Pseudomyxoma peritonei* of appendiceal origin. Cancer 1992;70:396.

63. Talerman A. Ovarian pathology. Curr Opin Obstet Gynecol 1992;4:608.

64. Mann WJ, Wagner J, Chumas J, et al. The management of *Pseudomyxoma peritonei*. Cancer 1990;66:1636.

Textbook of Gastroenterology, second edition, edited by Tadataka Yamada. JB Lippincott Company, Philadelphia © 1995.

CHAPTER 104

Diseases of the Retroperitoneum

Frank G. Moody   Norbert S. F. Runkel

Anatomic Structures
Fluid Collections
 Lymphoceles
 Gastrointestinal Secretions
Retroperitoneal Bleeding
 Trauma
 Ruptured Aneurysm
Retroperitoneal Fibrosis
 Etiology and Epidemiology
 Clinical Manifestations
 Differential Diagnosis and Diagnostic Studies

 Therapy
 Retroperitoneal Inflammation and Necrosis
Retroperitoneal Infections
 Pyogenic Infections
 Fungal Infections
 Actinomycosis and Nocardiosis
Retroperitoneal Neoplasms
 Etiology
 Clinical Manifestation
 Differential Diagnosis and Diagnostic Studies
 Therapy

ANATOMIC STRUCTURES

The retroperitoneum is the space behind the abdominal cavity extending from the posterior peritoneum and the mesenteries to the spinal column and the psoas, quadratus lumborum, and transversus abdominis muscles. It extends from the diaphragm down to the peritoneal reflection, where it continues as the extraperitoneal pelvic space. The retroperitoneum is divided into the anterior compartment, containing the pancreas, duodenal loop, and the ascending and descending colon, and the posterior compartment, containing the perinephric space with kidneys and adrenal glands and an extensive network of vessels, lymphatics, and neural structures. The retroperitoneum is an important structure for surgeons and gastroenterologists.

The retroperitoneum is involved in many gastrointestinal diseases, such as Crohn's disease and pancreatitis. Primary retroperitoneal diseases such as neoplasm and fibrosis may also affect retroperitoneal and intraabdominal structures. Retroperitoneal diseases usually present as a mass (Table 104-1), which in the past required surgical exploration. Modern diagnostic techniques, however, allow correct diagnosis without the need of surgery or before surgery. This chapter discusses the differential diagnosis and therapy of retroperitoneal masses with this concept in mind.

TABLE 104-1
Differential Diagnosis of Retroperitoneal Masses

Fluid collections
Lymph
Duodenal succus
Pancreatic juice
Bile
Urine

Hematoma
Spontaneous hemorrhage
Traumatic hemorrhage

Fat Necrosis
Acute necrotizing pancreatitis

Abscess
Primary
Secondary: extension from abdomen, kidney, vertebra

Neoplasm
Benign
    Cyst
    Benign soft tissue tumor
Malignant
    Sarcoma
    Germ cell–derived neoplasm
    Lymphoma
    Lymph node metastases

Aortic Aneurysm

Retroperitoneal Fibrosis

FLUID COLLECTIONS

Lymphoceles

Lymphoceles are collections of lymph within a closed space. They occur within the retroperitoneum during injuries or operations that interrupt the lymph channels traversing the posterior aspects of the pelvis and abdominal cavity.[1] Injury to the cisterna chyli, for example, may lead to a retroperitoneal collection. Renal and whole organ pancreatic transplantation, with placement of the organ in the flanks, may also be associated with accumulations of lymph after dissection of the recipient's iliac vessels. These collections can be readily identified and differentiated from blood, but not urine, by a computed tomography (CT) scan. Percutaneous aspiration or drainage can identify the nature of the collection and establish its bacteriologic profile and the need for more aggressive management.

Blood and fluids from the duodenum, biliary tract, pancreas, and urinary tract may leak into the retroperitoneum, forming fluid collections as large as 2 to 3 L. The most important causes are traumatic or iatrogenic injuries of structures that reside within the retroperitoneum. The therapeutic effort is directed toward the drainage of the collection and identification of the point of leakage or injury of the involved organ. Percutaneous catheter drainage with CT or ultrasonographic guidance offers a safe and effective means to achieve this end. Surgical intervention for repair is then carried out at an appropriate time.

Gastrointestinal Secretions

Duodenal Succus

Injuries to the duodenum are relatively uncommon and represent fewer than 5% of all abdominal trauma cases. Other causes of duodenal injury include sphincterotomy and perforation of a peptic ulcer or diverticulum. Traumatic duodenal perforations are usually detected and repaired at the initial exploratory laparotomy; a Whipple resection is reserved for extensive injuries to the pancreas, ampulla, or common bile duct.[2] The onset of symptoms from nontraumatic duodenal injuries may be delayed; the pain is uncharacteristic, vague, and often points to the back. The diagnosis is made with an upper gastrointestinal constraint Gastrograffin study. A CT scan may differentiate a duodenal hematoma from full-thickness perforation of the duodenal wall.[3] Conservative management is most successful if initiated early. Operative therapy is necessary for retroperitoneal infection after duodenal fluid leakage.[4]

Pancreatic Juice

Injury of the pancreatic ducts is caused by acute and chronic pancreatitis, abdominal trauma, and pancreatic surgery. Collections due to pancreatitis may be resorbed if the underlying inflammation subsides, but persisting collections result in pseudocyst formation. Pancreatic trauma is uncommon and is usually combined with additional injuries that are identified at the initial exploratory laparotomy.[5] The critical distinction of the presence or absence of ductal injury is crucial, and preoperative or intraoperative pancreatography may be helpful in making this determination.[6] Drainage procedures are performed for small ductal injuries. Major pancreatic lacerations with duct injuries require partial pancreatic resections.

Bile

Injuries of the distal common bile duct with retroperitoneal bile collection are rare. The main causes are abdominal trauma and endoscopic or surgical duct manipulation. Isolated distal bile duct injuries with bile leakage require primary repair or the less preferable T-tube drainage and secondary repair. Most traumatic injuries to the distal common bile duct are combined with pancreatic and duodenal injuries, and a Whipple procedure is recommended.[7]

Urine

Major trauma is the leading cause of injuries to the collecting system of the kidney, causing urine extravasation into the perinephric space. CT scanning or intravenous urography is the primary diagnostic step. Avulsion of the entire renal collecting system usually necessitates nephrectomy, but lacerations of the renal pelvis and avulsion of the ureteropelvic junction can usually be repaired.[8] Injuries to the ureter are caused by instrumentation, surgery, and penetrating trauma rather than by blunt trauma. In this case, immediate suture repair is mandatory. Proximal injuries require additional stenting and proximal diversion by nephrostomy. Stenting is also advisable for more complex injuries of the middle and distal ureter.[9] If the diagnosis of ureteral injury is delayed and hydronephrosis or urosepsis has developed, definitive repair is performed at a later stage after temporary nephrostomy.

RETROPERITONEAL BLEEDING

Trauma

The major cause of retroperitoneal bleeding is traumatic vessel injury associated with pelvic or vertebral fractures or with avulsion of the vascular pedicle of a kidney. Other causes include anticoagulation therapy, spontaneous hemorrhage into an adrenal gland or retroperitoneal tumor, acute pancreatitis, ruptured aortic aneurysm, and ruptured uteroovarian veins during pregnancy. The clinical course and outcome depend on the intensity of the bleeding. If the bleeding is self-limited, the hemorrhage may appear to be a retroperitoneal vascular injury.[10]

Emergency surgery is mandatory in all cases of massive or persistent bleeding, and for ruptured aortic aneurysms, hemorrhage during pregnancy, and penetrating wounds.[11] The late outcome of retroperitoneal hematomas is resorption, liquefaction, or fibrosis with calcification.

Ruptured Aneurysm

Etiology and Epidemiology

Abdominal aortic aneurysms have been found in almost 2% of postmortem examinations. Most are of atherosclerotic origin. Sometimes, a unique inflammatory reaction surrounds the external calcified layer (i.e., inflammatory aneurysms). Mycotic aneurysms are rare. They are caused by bacterial or fungal infection of the arterial wall after episodes of bacteremia, trauma, or direct extension of an infectious focus.[12] Most aneurysms involve the segment of the aorta between the takeoff of the renal arteries and the bifurcation, but they may include the iliac vessels. Suprarenal abdominal aneurysms are often part of thoracoabdominal aortic dilatations.

Clinical Manifestations

Most abdominal aneurysms remain asymptomatic until rupture ensues. Rupture is characterized by severe back pain with signs of acute retroperitoneal bleeding. Physical examination may reveal a tender, pulsatile mass. Other complications include claudication of the legs due to repeated embolization and back pain due to distention. Abdominal discomfort, tenderness, and ureteral obstruction are indicative of inflammatory aneurysms.[13] Mycotic aneurysms present as tender, enlarging masses.

Differential Diagnosis and Diagnostic Studies

Ultrasound is extremely useful in screening abdominal aneurysms. It provides information about their size and the presence of retroperitoneal hematoma or inflammation. An ultrasound examination helps to confirm the diagnosis of rupture in the emergency room. CT scanning is equally effective but more expensive and time consuming. A chest radiograph is obtained to exclude a thoracic aortic aneurysm. Preoperative aortography is necessary only if visceral, renal, or peripheral vascular disease is suspected.

Therapy

Symptoms and complications are related to aneurysm size. At the time of initial presentation, only 5% of aneurysms smaller than 5 cm have complications, compared with almost 30% of those larger than 7 cm.[14] Elective surgery is recommended for all aneurysms larger than 5 to 6 cm and for smaller ones that enlarge on sequential ultrasound examinations.

The infrarenal aorta is replaced with a synthetic tubular or bifurcate graft. Symptomatic aneurysms have an impending risk of rupture and should be repaired urgently. If rupture has already occurred, prompt laparotomy to control bleeding is the only chance for survival.[15] The high mortality rate of 40% after emergency repair contrasts vividly with a 2% mortality rate after elective surgery. Postoperative complications include myocardial infarction, stroke, renal failure, bleeding, and ischemic colitis after the sacrifice of the inferior mesenteric artery.

RETROPERITONEAL FIBROSIS

Etiology and Epidemiology

Retroperitoneal fibrosis is a chronic inflammatory process characterized by progressive fibrosis of connective and adipose tissue. It originates in the lower retroperitoneum and spreads bilaterally toward the renal hilus, encircling the vessels and ureters. The cause remains unknown in about 75% of cases. Studies indicate that idiopathic retroperitoneal fibrosis may be caused by an allergic reaction to insoluble lipids that leak through atherosclerotic arterial walls.[16] Serotonin and methysergide may induce retroperitoneal fibrosis. The disease typically affects middle-aged patients, with a male to female ratio of 2 : 1. Most patients are hypertensive. Secondary retroperitoneal fibrosis usually remains a localized and nonprogressive disease (Table 104-2).

Clinical Manifestations

Uncharacteristic abdominal or back pain is the most frequent presenting symptom. Other complaints include anorexia, fatigue, and fever. Ureteral obstruction causes hydronephrosis, pyelonephritis, and progressive renal failure. Anuria is the presenting symptom in 10% of patients. Rarely, symptoms may develop from stenosis of the biliary tract (e.g., jaundice), lymphatics (e.g., edema, enteropathy), veins (e.g., portal hypertension, peripheral thrombosis), and arteries (e.g., intermittent claudication).

Differential Diagnosis and Diagnostic Studies

The physical and laboratory findings are not specific. An abdominal or pelvic mass is palpable in 15% of patients. Pyelography typically shows medial displacement and segmental

---

TABLE 104-2
Causes of Retroperitoneal Fibrosis

Primary
Idiopathic
In conjunction with other fibrotic processes (e.g., mediastinal
   fibrosis, mesenteric fibrosis, sclerosing cholangitis, orbital
   pseudotumor)
Drug-associated (e.g., methysergide, LSD)
Paraneoplastic (e.g., sarcoma, Hodgkin's disease, carcinoid tumor)

Secondary
Radiotherpay
Retroperitoneal infection
Retroperitoneal fluid collection of hematoma
Inflammatory abdominal aortic aneurysm

---

narrowing of one or both ureters at the level of the fifth lumbar vertebra and proximal dilatation. A CT scan usually identifies the extent of the fibrotic plaque.

Therapy

Progression may be slowed by steroid therapy in the earlier stages of the disease or in combination with surgery.[17] Obstructive uropathy is treated by operative ureterolysis or renal autotransplantation into the pelvis. Acute obstruction or urosepsis requires preoperative ureteral indwelling catheterization or nephrostomy. The long-term prognosis is good, because the course of the disease is normally slow.[18] Spontaneous regression is occasionally observed, particularly in the drug-induced fibrosis after discontinuation of methysergide intake.

Retroperitoneal Inflammation and Necrosis

Noninfectious inflammation in the retroperitoneal space is found in retroperitoneal fibrosis, inflammatory aortic aneurysms, fluid collections, or tumors. Severe retroperitoneal inflammation and necrosis are typical findings of acute pancreatitis (see Chap. 90).[19] In mild forms, edema and fat necrosis are limited to the peripancreatic vicinity. In severe pancreatitis, inflammation and necrosis spread to the left and, less frequently, to the right pararenal spaces, the mesenteric roots, both paracolic gutters, and paraaortically into the lower retroperitoneum. Serial CT scanning is the method of choice to follow these changes; CT-guided aspiration detects secondary infection, which occurs in about 40% of cases.[20] The initial management is conservative, but major pancreatic necrosis requires necrosectomy, lavage, and drainage.

RETROPERITONEAL INFECTIONS

Primary bacterial infections of the retroperitoneum are rare, but secondary infections occur frequently and originate from the abdominal organs, urinary tract, and vertebral column. Infections in the retroperitoneum are less dramatic than those localized in the abdominal cavity and are therefore discovered late, when abscess formation is complete. Retroperitoneal abscesses are most commonly located in the anterior compartment, resulting from appendicitis, acute pancreatitis, penetrating duodenal ulcer, perforating colonic carcinoma and diverticulitis, and Crohn's ileocolitis. Abscesses of the anterior compartment can extend into the posterior compartment; only perinephric abscesses usually remain confined to their space.

The psoas abscess, although located in the iliopsoas muscle outside the retroperitoneal space (i.e., retrofascial abscess), usually is considered a retroperitoneal abscess. A psoas abscess may be primary, as is the *Staphylococcus aureus* abscess in children, or it may be secondary because of extension of an intraabdominal or vertebral infection (Fig. 104-1). Psoas ab-

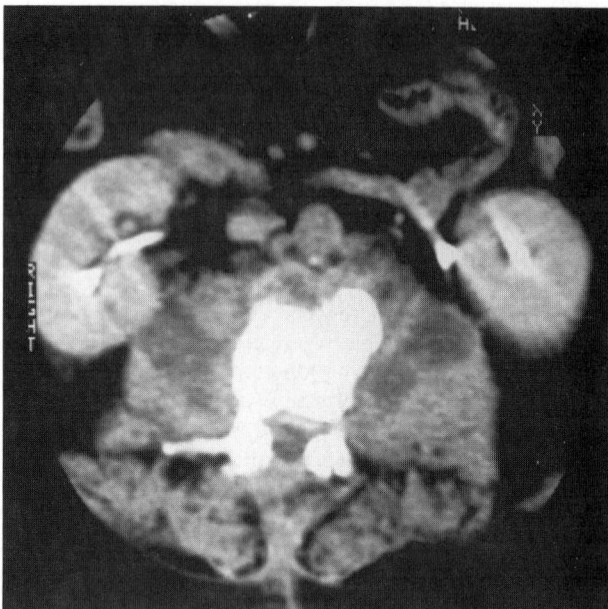

FIGURE 104-1. Computed tomographic scan discloses a bilateral psoas abscess, which developed after lumbar surgery. Transcutaneous catheter drainage was successful.

scesses secondary to intraabdominal infections are usually caused by mixed enteric organisms.[20] Crohn's disease is the most frequent cause, followed by appendicitis, colonic diverticulitis, and cancer.

Abscesses in the retroperitoneum present with fever, malaise, abdominal discomfort, and pain in the flank, back, or thigh. Fever, leukocytosis, and a retroperitoneal mass are the leading clinical findings. CT scanning is more effective than sonography in assessing the site and extent of retroperitoneal and psoas abscesses. Preoperative needle aspiration of the collection may allow bacteriologic studies to adjust antibiotic therapy before surgery.

Operative drainage under broad antibiotic coverage is the treatment of choice. Generally, retroperitoneal and secondary psoas abscesses require a transabdominal approach with resection of the involved bowel.[22,23] Percutaneous catheter drainage is successful in selected patients with a well-defined abscess of low viscosity.

Pyogenic Infections

A quarter of all extrapulmonary active tuberculosis affects the retroperitoneum as renal, adrenal, and spinal tuberculosis with psoas abscess and retroperitoneal lymphadenitis.[24] These sites are seeded at the time of the initial dissemination, and the organisms persist until some shift in the host-organism equilibrium causes the bacteria to proliferate. Renal tuberculosis originates in the cortex and then spreads into the medulla, causing papillary necrosis and cavitation. The lower urinary tract and the male reproductive organs are frequently involved. The symptoms include dysuria, urinary frequency, hematuria, and occasional flank pain. The diagnosis is suggested by pyelography and abnormal urinalysis (e.g., sterile pyuria).

Chemotherapy is usually highly effective. Because the clinical features of tuberculous lymphadenitis are nonspecific, surgery is often necessary to provide diagnostic material for bacteriologic and histologic analyses. Although chemotherapy is usually successful, resolution of nodal enlargement may be delayed for months. Tuberculosis of the spine with a secondary cold psoas abscess requires incision and drainage in combination with chemotherapy.

Fungal Infections

Fungal infections of the retroperitoneum are caused by pathogenic and opportunistic fungi. Pathogenic fungi disseminate from a primary pulmonary focus. The adrenals are the most frequently involved organs in disseminated histoplasmosis. The characteristic CT findings are bilateral, symmetric adrenal enlargement with focal hemorrhage, necrosis, and cavitation.[24] The caseous necrosis eventually results in Addison's disease, which is fatal if untreated. Similarly, the adrenals are also susceptible to generalized paracoccidioidomycosis and blastomycosis, which may also affect the kidneys.[25] Fungal dissemination into the retroperitoneal space rarely occurs in generalized coccidioidomycosis in the form of renal or psoas abscesses. Opportunistic fungi (e.g., *Candida, Aspergillus, Cryptococcus*) may spread to the retroperitoneum during generalized dissemination in patients with altered immune response, such as acquired immunodeficiency syndrome, imbalance of normal fungal and bacterial flora, and disruption of physiologic barriers.[26]

The kidneys and adrenals are the primary target organs in the retroperitoneum. The standard therapy for all forms of systemic mycosis is amphotericin B. The initial dosage of 10 to 20 mg daily is slowly increased until 0.6 mg/kg body weight/day and blood levels of 0.5 to 3.5 μg/mL are obtained. A total course consists of 1 to 4 g. Clinical cure is achieved in most patients with pathogenic fungal infections who can tolerate the drug and complete the course. The prognosis for opportunistic fungal infections depends almost entirely on the patient's status. If the underlying disease is not corrected, the fungal infection is usually fatal despite systemic antimycotic therapy.

Actinomycosis and Nocardiosis

Actinomycosis of the retroperitoneum may be caused by perforation of the appendix or colon. The disease is characterized by formation of chronic abscesses, with multiple sinus tracts exuding "sulfur granules" and direct spread to neighboring structures, including the vertebra. Unless draining sinuses to the skin develop, actinomycosis is rarely diagnosed before exploratory laparotomy. Incision and drainage is combined with 500,000 to 20 million units of penicillin daily for 4 to 12 weeks.[27]

Retroperitoneal infections with *Nocardia* are secondary to dissemination from a pulmonary focus.[28] The kidney is the primary site for infection. The infection is characterized by multiple abscess formations with little fibrosis and scarring and no sinus tracts. Retroperitoneal nocardiosis affects mostly immunocompromised patients. The most widely accepted treatment regimen consists of the combination of 800 to 1250 mg of sulfamethoxazole and 160 to 220 mg of trimethoprim twice daily for 3 to 4 months.

RETROPERITONEAL NEOPLASMS

Etiology

Primary neoplasms of the retroperitoneum are derived from soft tissue, lymphoid tissue, or germ cells (Table 104-3). Most are malignant, and most of these are sarcomas, particularly liposarcomas, leiomyosarcomas, and malignant fibrous histiocytomas. Sarcomas constitute less than 1% of all malignant tumors, and only 15% of these are located in the retroperitoneum.[29] Approximately 500 new cases are diagnosed annually in the United States. Rhabdomyosarcomas, neuroblastomas, ganglioneuroblastomas, and teratomas tend to occur in children. Sarcomas are classified as well differentiated with a potential for distant metastases (grade 1) or high grade (grades 2 and 3).[30]

The retroperitoneum is a common site for secondary neoplasms, particularly lymphatic metastasis from primary neoplasms of the abdominal cavity, the lower extremities, and the genitourinary system. Lymphomas of the retroperitoneum are not uncommon. The non-Hodgkin's lymphomas more frequently develop in this region and usually indicate widespread disease. Hodgkin's lymphomas often involve the spleen first, and then spread to the hilar and eventually to the paraaortic lymph nodes.

Clinical Manifestation

Retroperitoneal neoplasms present late or are incidental findings during clinical or sonographic examination. Larger lesions may cause fatigue and abdominal discomfort, radiating pain to the back and thigh, and symptoms from compression of lymphatics, veins, and urinary tract. Most sarcomas have no discernible spread to distant sites at the time of detection.

Differential Diagnosis and Diagnostic Studies

Because of the variable presentation, the initial radiologic evaluation usually includes contrast studies of the gastrointestinal and urinary tract. If a retroperitoneal tumor is suspected (Fig. 104-2), CT, contrast-enhanced CT, or nuclear

---

TABLE 104-3
Classification of Primary Retroperitoneal Neoplasm by Histogenesis

NEOPLASM	BENIGN	MALIGNANT
Soft Tissue		
Fibrous tissue	Fibroma	Fibrosarcoma
Adipose tissue	Lipoma	Liposarcoma
Smooth muscle	Leiomyoma	Leiomyosarcoma
Striated muscle	Rhabdomyoma	Rhabdomyosarcoma
Histiocytes	Fibrous histiocytoma	Malignant fibrous histiocytoma
Blood or lymph vessels	Hemangioma	Angiosarcoma
	Lymphangioma	Lymphangiosarcoma
	Hemangiopericytoma	Hemangiopericytoma
Nervous system		
Supportive tissue	Neurilemoma	Malignant schwannoma
	Neurofibroma	
Sympathetic ganglia	Ganglioneurinoma	Sympathicobalstoma (i.e., neuroblastoma)
Paraganglionic cells	Pheochromocytoma	Malignant pheochromocytoma
	Paraganglioma	Malignant paraganglioma
Undifferentiated	Myxoma	Myxoma
Mesenchyme	Mesenchymoma	Malignant mesenchymoma
Germ Cell	Teratoma	Malignant teratoma
		Seminoma
		Embryonal carcinoma
Lymphoid Tissue		Malignant lymphoma
		Non-Hodgkin's type
		Hodgkin's type
Uncertain	Undifferentiated	
Cysts	Lymphatic, dermoid	
	Teratomatous, mesocolic	

Modified from Arlen M, Marcove RC. Surgical management of soft tissue sarcomas. Philadelphia: WB Saunders, 1987.

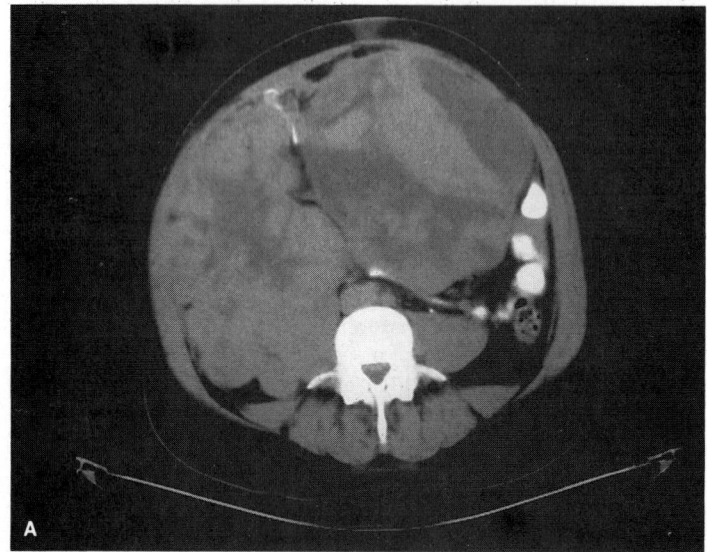

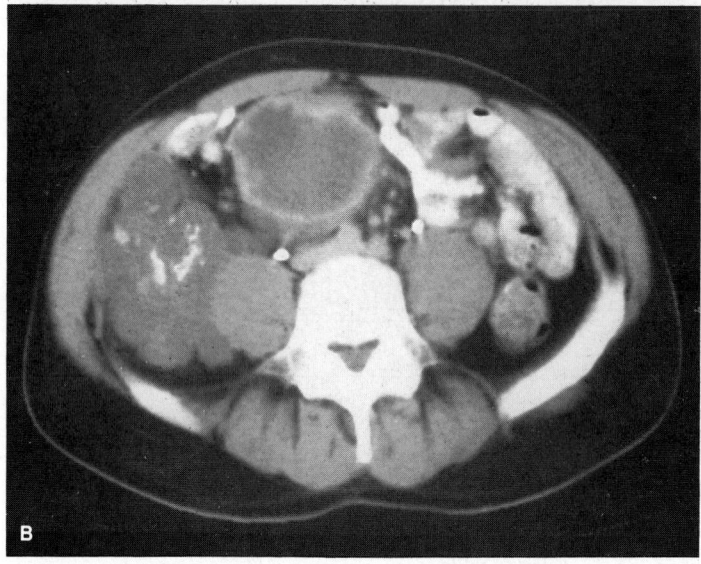

FIGURE 104-2. (A) Computed tomographic scan of the abdomen shows a large, inhomogeneous sarcoma occupying the abdominal cavity and probably invading the right psoas muscle. (B) After chemotherapy, the tumor size decreased markedly, leaving a residual soft tissue mass on the right side, with internal calcification and a cystic mass in the midline of the abdomen.

magnetic resonance imaging is essential to determine its site of origin and gross morphology; however, the diagnosis of invasion of adjacent organs requires the angiographic demonstration of neovascularity from the feeding arteries of those organs.[31] The histopathologic type can be determined with percutaneous needle biopsy in up to 80% of cases, but only surgery can provide an accurate stating and classification. The exact histologic diagnosis is particularly important for lymphomas, and the largest and most accessible lymph node is chosen for diagnostic biopsy. In Hodgkin's disease, staging laparotomy, splenectomy, and extensive retroperitoneal lymph node biopsies are standard diagnostic procedures.

Therapy

The treatment of choice for retroperitoneal tumors is a one-stage en bloc resection of the tumor mass and the involved surrounding structures.[29] Complete excision is possible in most patients with benign tumors but only in one half of the

patients with malignant tumors. Patients with large, symptomatic sarcomas may benefit from debulking procedures. About 50% of the tumors recur within 3 years, even after complete removal. Recurrence occurs locally in 30%, in the lungs in almost 20%, and simultaneously at multiple sites in almost 50% of patients.

The 3-year survival rates of resected grade 1, 2, and 3 tumors are 100%, 87%, and 28%, respectively.[32] Adjuvant radiotherapy and chemotherapy are given to most patients with high-grade sarcomas, but the response is generally poor.[33] Retroperitoneal lymphomas should be resected if they are localized, because this contributes to long-term disease-free survival.[34] Patients with retroperitoneal lymphomas undergo standard regimens of chemotherapy and radiotherapy.

The reader is directed to Chapter 36, Approach to the Patient With Acute Abdomen; Chapter 46, Approach to Gastrointestinal Problems in the Immunocompromised Patient; Chapter 71,

REFERENCES

1. Garrett HE Jr, Richardson JW, Howard HS, et al. Retroperitoneal lymphocele after abdominal aortic surgery. J Vasc Surg 1989;10:245.
2. Buck JR, Sorensen VJ, Fath JJ, et al. Severe pancreaticoduodenal injuries: the effectiveness of pyloric exclusion with vagotomy. Am Surg 1992;58:557.
3. Kunin JR, Dorobkin M, Ellis JH, et al. Duodenal injuries caused by blunt abdominal trauma: value of CT in differentiating perforation from hematoma. AJR Am J Roentgenol 1993;160:1221.
4. Harker L, Hutton L, Passi RB. Radiologic findings of retroperitoneal perforation after sphincterotomy. J Can Assoc Radiol 1986;37:169.
5. Heimansohn DA, Canal DF, McCarthy MC, et al. The role of pancreaticoduodenectomy in the management of traumatic injuries to the pancreas and duodenum. Am Surg 1990;56:511.
6. Sukul K, Lont HE, Johannes EJ. Management of pancreatic injuries. Hepatogastroenterology 1992;39:447.
7. Burgess P, Fulton RL. Gallbladder and extrahepatic biliary duct injury following abdominal trauma. Injury 1992;23:413.
8. Guerriero WG. Etiology, classification and management of renal trauma. Surg Clin North Am 1988;68:1071.
9. Toporoff B, Sclafani S, Scalea T, et al. Percutaneous antegrade ureteral stenting as an adjunct for treatment of complicated ureteral injuries. J Trauma 1992;32:534.
10. Gordon RL, Fast A, Amer H, et al. Control of massive retroperitoneal bleeding associated with pelvic fractures by angiographic embolization. Isr J Med Sci 1983;19:185.
11. Holting T, Buhr HJ, Richter GM, et al. Diagnosis and treatment of retroperitoneal hematoma in multiple trauma patients. Arch Orthop Trauma Surg 1992;116:323.
12. Gomes MN, Choyke PL, Wallace RB. Infected aortic aneurysms. A changing entity. Ann Surg 1992;215:435.
13. Tennant WG, Hartnell GG, Baird RN, et al. Inflammatory aortic aneurysms: characteristic appearance on magnetic resonance imaging. Eur J Vasc Surg 1992;6:399.
14. Kaufman JA, Bettmann MA. Prognosis of abdominal aortic aneurysms: a population-based study. Invest Radiol 1991;26:612.
15. Mannick JA, Whittemore AD. Management of ruptured os symptomatic abdominal aortic aneurysms. Surg Clin North Am 1988;68:377.
16. Bullock N. Idiopathic retroperitoneal fibrosis. Br Med J 1988;297:240.
17. Higgins PM, Bennet-Jones DN, Naish PF, et al. Non-operative management of retroperitoneal fibrosis. Br J Surg 1988;75:573.
18. Hem E, Mathisen W. Retroperitoneal fibrosis. Eur Urol 1984;10:43.
19. Nordback I, Lauslahti K. Clinical pathology of acute necrotizing pancreatitis. J Clin Pathol 1986;39:68.
20. Beger HG. Surgery in acute pancreatitis. Hepatogastroenterology 1991;38:92.
21. Ricci MA, Rose FB, Meyer KK. Pyrogenic psoas abscess: worldwide variation in etiology. World J Surg 1986;10:834.
22. Walsh TR, Reilly JR, Hanley E, et al. Changing etiology of iliopsoas abscess. Am J Surg 1992;163:413.
23. Bradley EL III. A fifteen year experience with open drainage for infected pancreatic necrosis. Surg Gynecol Obstet 1993;177:215.
24. Alvarez S, McCabe WR. Extrapulmonary tuberculosis revisited: a review of experience at Boston City and other hospitals. Medicine (Baltimore) 1984;63:25.
25. Wilson DA, Muchmore HG, Tisdal RG, et al. Histoplasmosis of the adrenal glands studied by CT. Radiology 1984;150:779.
26. Rippon JW. Medical mycology: the pathogenic fungi and the pathogenic actinomycetes. Philadelphia: WB Saunders, 1988.
27. Axelrod FB, Fonda JN, Bradley EL III. Retroperitoneal actinomycosis: a rare manifestation of an uncommon disease. South Med J 1982;75:1156.
28. Stevens DA. Clinical and clinical laboratory aspects of nocardial infection. J Hyg 1983;91:377.
29. Jaques DP, Coit DG, Hajdu SI, et al. Management of primary and recurrent soft-tissue sarcoma of the retroperitoneum. Ann Surg 1990;212:51.
30. Leyvraz S, Costa J. Histological diagnosis and grading of soft-tissue sarcomas. Semin Surg Oncol 1988;4:3.
31. Davidson AJ, Hartmann DS. Imaging strategies for tumors of the kidney, adrenal gland, and retroperitoneum. CA Cancer J Clin 1987;37:151.
32. Potter DA, Glenn J, Kinsella T, et al. Patterns of recurrence in patients with high-grade soft-tissue sarcomas. J Clin Oncol 1985;3:353.
33. Glenn J, Sindelar WF, Kinsella T, et al. Results of multimodal therapy of resectable soft-tissue sarcomas of the retroperitoneum. Surgery 1985;97:316.
34. Mentzer SJ, Osteen RT, Pappas TN, et al. Surgical therapy of localized abdominal non-Hodgkin's lymphomas. Surgery 1988;103:609.

Textbook of Gastroenterology, second edition, edited by Tadataka Yamada. JB Lippincott Company, Philadelphia © 1995.

H. Miscellaneous

CHAPTER 105

Gastrointestinal Complications of the Acquired Immunodeficiency Syndrome

Donald P. Kotler

Etiology and Pathogenesis	*Neoplastic Diseases*
Complications and Concomitant Diseases	*Hepatobiliary Diseases*
Diseases of the Oral Cavity and Esophagus	*Pancreatic Diseases*
Gastric Diseases	*Gastrointestinal Emergencies*
Primary Intestinal Diseases	**Symptom Diagnosis**
Intestinal Disease Secondary to Systemic Infections	**Nutritional Considerations**
Anorectal Diseases	

Throughout evolution, the maintenance of an effective barrier against the external environment has been an important task of the body's defense systems. Nowhere is this more evident than in the mucous membranes that line the interfaces between sterile internal and contaminated external environments. All mucous membranes have specialized functions, such as nutrient absorption by the villus epithelium or gas exchange by pulmonary epithelium, requiring intimate contact between the epithelium and the external environment. The conflicting needs of maintaining close communication while remaining a barrier to the outer world promoted the evolution of complex immunologic and nonimmunologic defense mechanisms. Intestinal injury and dysfunction should be an expected result of immune deficiency. Immune function and dysfunction in the intestine are considered in detail in Chapters 5, 46, and 110.

The aims of this chapter are to catalog and describe the major intestinal complications in acquired immunodeficiency syndrome (AIDS); to demonstrate their relation to specific immune deficits; to outline their diagnosis and treatment; to

discuss symptom diagnosis in AIDS; and to introduce the nutritional management of patients with AIDS.

ETIOLOGY AND PATHOGENESIS

The first descriptions of groups of homosexual men presenting with complications indicating an acquired deficiency of immune function were published in 1981.[1,2] Early observations suggested that an infectious agent was responsible for the illness, and reports from several laboratories almost simultaneously identified a retrovirus in infected patients. The agent was subsequently named the human immunodeficiency virus type 1 (HIV-1), which is a member of the family of lentiviruses, the classic slow viruses.[3,4]

Retroviruses are RNA viruses that contain reverse transcriptase, an enzyme that transcribes DNA from RNA. Retroviruses produce chronic degenerative diseases in many animal species, including several animal models of immune deficiency. These viruses exist in the host in latent form, in which DNA is integrated into the host genome, or as a productive infection, in which RNA replication and viral assembly occur. The number of cells with replicating virus at any time is low compared with the number of latently infected cells. This fact may account for the protracted course of lentiviral diseases and for the fact that the immune response, no matter how vigorous, is unable to clear the infection completely.

Several cellular reservoirs for HIV have been identified. The CD4+ lymphocyte (i.e., helper T lymphocyte) was the first infected cell type identified. It is vulnerable to infection by virtue of having a high density of CD4 receptors on the cell membrane. The receptor, which is involved in antigen recognition in association with the major histocompatibility antigen II system, also is the attachment site for HIV.[5] Other cell types expressing CD4, including macrophages, dendritic cells, and a variety of neural cells, can be infected by HIV. Different isolates of HIV have distinct cellular tropisms that occur as a result of heterogeneity in the structure of the viral envelope protein.[5] Changes in the structure of the viral envelope that occur during the course of an infection may alter the cell tropism of the virus and promote disease progression. These changes also may diminish the effectiveness of the immune response to the infection.

There are several reports documenting HIV in the gastrointestinal tract. In situ hybridization studies demonstrated HIV-1 RNA in lymphocytes and macrophages in the lamina propria in as many as one half of intestinal mucosal biopsies from HIV-infected individuals.[6] Other studies have shown HIV DNA in intestinal cells, including the epithelium.[7,8] HIV core antigen (p24) also has been found by immunohistochemical methods in intestinal epithelial cells, intraepithelial lymphocytes, and lamina propria mononuclear cells.[9,10] Several studies have shown the ability of experimental cell lines to be productively infected with HIV.[11,12] In feline and simian models, mucosal infection by retroviruses producing immune deficiency associated with severe diarrhea and wasting were demonstrated by molecular and immunohistochemical techniques.[13] However, definitive electron microscopic evidence of HIV viral particles in epithelial or other cells in intestinal biopsies in HIV-infected patients is lacking. It is possible that the presence of HIV antigens in epithelial cells is a result of phagocytosis and antigen presentation, which is a known property of epithelial cells.[14] The determination that epithelia in the intestine or elsewhere can be productively infected by HIV would be an extremely important finding, with great implications for understanding the pathogenesis of AIDS and the transmission of HIV infection.

The steps leading from HIV infection to immune deficiency are poorly understood.[15] Factors leading to progressive disease include antigenic variation in HIV related to a relatively high rate of mutation, especially in the genes coding for envelope proteins.[16] Such mutations may affect viral tropism, intrinsic virulence, or the effectiveness of the immune response and anti-HIV therapies.

Active systemic humoral and cell-mediated immune responses to HIV occur in asymptomatically infected people[17-19] Evidence of a systemic inflammatory process may be demonstrated by elevated serum concentrations of acute-phase reactants such as β_2-microglobulin and neopterin.[20,21] It is possible that the virus periodically escapes from immune control and proliferates rapidly until effective immunologic control is reestablished. Evidence of immune dysfunction may be detected long before clinical progression to AIDS occurs. The immune system is forced repetitively to respond to new HIV antigens as its overall function is declining. Disease progression in asymptomatically infected people can be predicted by the finding of persistently elevated concentrations of acute-phase reactants accompanied by falling titers of antibody to HIV p24 antigen and the presence of free p24 in the serum.[22] The associations between these surrogate markers and disease progression are approximate and are not sufficiently sensitive for easy clinical application.

The immune dysfunction in AIDS is related to several aspects of the disease process.[23] The most important is a depletion of CD4+ helper T cells. These cells are the coordinators for integrated immune function.[24] A loss of T-cell help blunts the antibody response to foreign antigens; diminishes the intensity of delayed hypersensitivity reactions to viral, mycobacterial, and fungal infection; impairs the process of immune surveillance against neoplasms; and diminishes macrophage functions, such as cytotoxic activity. Clinical evidence for all of these problems may be seen in AIDS.

Other aspects of the disease process may exacerbate the problems caused by the loss of T cells. Destruction of dendritic cells by HIV impairs the ability to present antigen and initiate immune reactions. Damage to thymic epithelium and thymocytes, which has been reported in AIDS, inhibits the development of immune competence, especially in neonates.[25,26] Immune dysregulation with the synthesis of autoantibodies, including antilymphocyte antibodies, also exacerbates the problem.

Mucosal immunity in AIDS has received little attention. It is likely that homologous defects occur in the mucosal and systemic immune systems. Studies of mucosal lymphocyte subpopulations have demonstrated equivalent decreases in the population of helper T cells in patients with AIDS-related complex and with AIDS.[27] Secretory immune deficiency was demonstrated by finding a depletion of IgA-containing plasma cells in rectal and jejunal biopsies from AIDS patients and a decrease in salivary IgA secretion.[28] Abnormal regulation of the IgA system is implied by the findings of elevated serum IgA concentrations, IgA in serum immune complexes, and an IgA rheumatoid factor in serum samples from AIDS patients.[29,30] Evidence of specific anti-HIV activity of lamina propria lymphocytes has been reported, although its variation with disease progression is ambiguous.[31] The co-localization of specific anti-HIV immune processes and productive HIV infection to the intestine would imply the presence of an ongoing immune reaction. Evidence for such a process has been reported.

COMPLICATIONS AND CONCOMITANT DISEASES

Gastrointestinal symptoms are common in patients with AIDS. Clinical observations have demonstrated a wide variety of infections and other diseases (Table 105-1). In this section, the reported complications of AIDS are classified as those causing diseases of the oral cavity and esophagus, gastric diseases, primary intestinal diseases, enterocolitis secondary to systemic infections, anorectal diseases, neoplastic diseases,

TABLE 105-1
Treatment of Specific Infections in AIDS

ORGANISM	INDUCTION THERAPY*	MAINTENANCE THERAPY
Cryptosporidium sp	Paromomycin 500 mg PO qid† Azithromycin, 900–1800 mg OD	Paromomycin, 500 mg PO qid†
Microsporidium sp	Albendazole, 400 mg bid†	
Isospora belli	Pyrimethamine, 25 mg/d, + sulfadiazine, 1 g qid, + leukovorin, 5 mg/d	Pyrimethamine, 25 mg/d
Giardia lamblia	Quinacrine, 100 mg tid × 7 d, or metronidazole, 750 tid × 7 d, or metronidazole, 250 tid × 21 d,	Repeat course if necessary
Salmonella sp	Trimethoprim-sulfamethoxazole double strength, 1 tablet bid,‡ or ampicillin, 500 mg qid, or ciprofloxacin, 500 mg bid,	Often necessary
Shigella sp	Trimethoprim-sulfamethoxazole, 1 tablet bid, or ampicillin, 500 mg qid,	Often necessary
Campylobacter sp	Erythromycin, 500 mg qid, or tetracycline, 500 mg qid, or gentamicin, 150 mg q 8 h IV	
Mycobacterium tuberculosis	Isoniazid, 300 mg, ethambutal, 15 mg/kg, rifampin, 300 mg, and pyridoxine, 50 mg × 9 mo	Isoniazid, 300 mg
Mycobacterium avium complex (MAC)	Multiple treatment regimens are being tried, using a variety of antibiotics with antituberculosis activity. Several of the drugs have good in vitro activity against MAC, including clarithromycin, 1 g bid, clofazimine, 150 mg OD†, amikacin, 7.5 mg/kg q 12 h, ciprofloxacin, 500–750 mg bid, ethambutal, 25 mg/kg, rifampin, 300 mg	
Clostridium difficile	Vancomycin, 125 mg qid, or metronidazole, 250 qid	Repeat course or cholestyramine, 4 g qid
Cytomeglavorius	Ganciclovir, 5 mg/kg IVSS bid† × 14 d	Ganciclovir, 6 mg/kg 5 times/wk
Herpes simplex	Acyclovir, 400 mg 4 times/d, or acyclovir, 5 mg/kg q 8 h IV	Acyclovir, 200 mg tid

* The dosages have been simplified for this table. Standard texts or guidelines should be consulted if necessary before initiating therapy.

† Experimental therapy or non-FDA approved indication.

‡ Parenteral therapy is indicated in the event of bacteremia.

hepatic diseases, pancreatic diseases, and gastrointestinal emergencies.

Diseases of the Oral Cavity and Esophagus

Candidiasis

Oral candidiasis is the most commonly encountered complication in HIV-seropositive patients. Early clinical observations associated the occurrence of thrush, not related to antibiotic usage or other known immune deficiency, with an increased risk of progression to AIDS within 6 months.[32] The disease is caused by *Candida albicans* in most cases. Candidiasis in AIDS takes a different clinical form than in other immunodeficiency states, such as uncontrolled diabetes mellitus or drug-induced leukopenia. In AIDS, the disease is predominantly mucosal in location: septicemia and disseminated infection are distinctly uncommon. The reason is unclear, although neutrophil function in AIDS may be normal, unlike that in other conditions conducive to *Candida* septicemia. Disseminated candidiasis in AIDS usually is associated with drug-induced neutropenia.

Clinically, the infection appears as erosions or as whitish plaques on the gingiva, palate, hypopharynx, or esophagus. The oral cavity or the esophagus may be infected without involvement of the other area. The infection typically is more extensive on the esophageal than on the tracheal side of the epiglottis. The gastric and duodenal mucosae are not involved grossly or microscopically. Esophageal erosions with or without exudate can be seen radiologically. Symptoms generally mirror the extent of involvement. The most common complaints are sore throat and odynophagia, sometimes with choking, or a mild to moderate substernal discomfort after swallowing. The differential diagnosis of oral candidiasis includes mucus hypersecretion resulting from chronic sinusitis and excessive postnasal drip, and oral hairy leukoplakia.

The diagnosis usually is made by inspection. A presumptive diagnosis can be made with great reliability using barium studies. At endoscopy, scattered to confluent plaques are seen. Histopathology of biopsy or brush cytology specimens is characteristic, with pseudohyphae visible on periodic acid-Schiff or Gomori methenamine silver stains. The diagnosis also can be made using transnasal brush cytology if contamination by oral contents can be avoided. In high-risk cases, presumptive therapy without formal diagnosis is allowable.

Topical therapies for oral candidiasis include 500,000 U

of nystatin administered four to six times per day or clotrimazole troches (Mycelex) taken four times per day. Systemic therapy usually is preferred to topical therapy for the treatment of esophageal candidiasis. The mainstays of therapy are imidazole derivatives, such as ketoconazole, fluconazole, and itraconazole; miconazole and clotrimazole are less effective. Treatment is suppressive, and infection recurs unless maintenance suppressive therapy is given.

Potential toxicities of therapy include liver dysfunction, which has been associated with ketoconazole but not with fluconazole or itraconazole. All imidazoles may promote adrenal insufficiency, an effect related to a drug-induced inhibition of steroidogenesis rather than to adrenal injury. Resistant symptoms despite therapy may be related to infection by organisms other than *C albicans*, although candidiasis resistant to ketoconazole has been seen. *Torulopsis glabrata* also has been found, and it may be resistant to all drugs except amphotericin. Drug interactions with rifampin or others could lead to rapid drug metabolism and decreased effectiveness. Ketoconazole requires an acid milieu for absorption, and resistant candidiasis has been associated with hypochlorhydria.[33] Drug administration with an acidic liquid may improve its effectiveness. Amphotericin has been used in refractory esophageal candidiasis, which occurs in less than 10% of cases. Doses of 20 mg or less, given intravenously, are all that is needed. For maintenance, once or twice weekly dosings usually are sufficient.

The physician should be cautious about relying solely on the diagnosis of candidiasis as the cause for oral or esophageal symptoms. Neurologic impairment can cause pharyngeal dysfunction with choking and aspiration, with and without candidiasis. Serious esophageal pathology, such as cytomegalovirus (CMV) esophagitis, may be masked by *Candida*. Further evaluation after successful therapy of candidiasis is indicated if symptoms do not resolve completely. Esophageal candidiasis is discussed in Chapter 56.

Oral Hairy Leukoplakia

Oral hairy leukoplakia is a lesion that has been mistakenly identified as candidiasis. It is a whitish, verrucous excrescence occurring mainly along the sides of the tongue.[34] The degree of involvement may vary. The lesion produces few symptoms. Epstein-Barr virus has been found in the lesions by molecular hybridization studies and electron microscopic examinations. A few studies also have shown coexisting infection with specific serotypes of human papillomavirus.

The diagnosis is made by inspection. If clinically indicated, a biopsy can rule out other lesions or identify Epstein-Barr virus in tissue. Therapy with acyclovir (2–3 g/day in divided doses) leads to clearance of the lesion.[35]

Esophageal Ulcers

Painful ulcers of the oral cavity, hypopharynx, or esophagus have been seen in many patients. The lesions may remit and recur, and they can cause significant impairment of food intake. Viral causes include the herpesviruses, herpes simplex virus (HSV), CMV, and varicella zoster. The ulcers produce severe, acute odynophagia without dysphagia. On examination, multiple, shallow, coalescing ulcers are found, which

may progress to a single, large, shallow ulcer. Characteristic viral inclusions are seen in the epithelial layer in HSV infections and in endothelial cells and other stromal cells in CMV ulcers. It is unclear whether CMV is the cause of all ulcers in which it is found. Some investigators think that CMV can superinfect ulcers originating from other causes. Resolution occurs in response to high-dose oral or parenteral acyclovir for HSV ulcers and with parenteral ganciclovir or foscarnet therapy for CMV ulcers (see Table 105-1). Maintenance therapy usually is required to avoid recurrences.

HIV has been associated with large "idiopathic" ulcers seen in severely immunosuppressed patients.[36,37] Transient ulcers have been seen as part of the primary illness associated with seroconversion.[38] Electron microscopic studies have identified viral particles suggestive of HIV in these ulcers. The role of HIV in the pathogenesis and persistence of the ulcer is unknown. These ulcers cause severe odynophagia and spontaneous substernal pain. In some patients, the pain is positional and increases with bending or twisting of the torso. The pain also may radiate to the back. Barium studies show single or multiple deep ulcers with undermined edges. Sinus tracts may be identified. Endoscopically, the lesions are differentiated by their large size and by the extensive undermining of the mucosa. Mucosal bridging may be found, with an impression on radiograph of a double-barreled esophagus. Occasionally, multiple interconnecting ulcers are observed and produce a cobblestone appearance. The lesion is highly inflamed, with cell necrosis, granulation tissue, neutrophils, and eosinophils seen on histologic examination.

Several reports have documented symptomatic relief and ulcer healing with systemic or intralesional corticosteroids.[38-40] Despite potential problems related to worsening immune suppression with steroid therapy, treatment has been given with relative safety. Treatment must be prolonged, because the ulcers may take several months to reepithelialize. Often, a submucosal defect remains after healing, leading to an erroneous radiologic impression of ulcer persistence.

Mycobacterial causes of esophageal ulcers include *Mycobacterium tuberculosis* and *Mycobacterium avium* complex (MAC). These infections represent spread of disease from subcarinal or mediastinal nodes. Prior mediastinal tuberculosis probably is the underlying cause of the traction diverticula (unrelated to AIDS) seen in the past. The ulcer presents as odynophagia, although bleeding tracheoesophageal fistulas have been reported. Radiologically and endoscopically, the lesion may present as an ulcer or as a sinus tract. The infection responds to typical antituberculous regimens (see Table 105-1), although an esophageal stricture may be a late complication.

Fungal ulcers of the esophagus are uncommon but have been associated with histoplasmosis, coccidiomycosis, and blastomycosis. Fungal ulcers occur by secondary spread from lymph nodes in the mediastinum and are not primary infections. They present as nonspecific ulcers causing odynophagia and dysphagia. If untreated, the lesions may fistulize. The diagnosis can be suspected by ascertaining a history of residence in an endemic area. The Caribbean islands, Central America, and South America contain areas endemic for fungal infection. Radiologically and endoscopically, the lesions are similar to those of tuberculous esophagitis. The differential diagnosis can be made on biopsy with special stains or culture.

These infections respond to intravenous amphotericin therapy, at usual total doses of up to 2 g, followed by maintenance therapy. Studies have shown that itraconazole has excellent clinical activity against histoplasmosis for acute treatment and maintenance. This represents a significant advance in therapy for this infection.

Other Oral and Gastroesophageal Lesions

Kaposi's sarcoma (KS) or lymphoma in patients with AIDS may produce symptoms such as impaired mastication, choking, or dysphagia. Symptoms occur as a result of anatomic distortion from the mass or because of ulceration and inflammation. These lesions may respond to a variety of therapies.

Periodontitis is a common complication of AIDS, although it is not unexpected in patients because of the degree of illness. However, acute necrotizing ulcerative gingivitis is a very dramatic lesion.[41] These are focal, destructive processes of uncertain origin that cause marked discomfort and difficulty in maintaining adequate oral intake. The relation to idiopathic esophageal ulcers is unknown. No successful therapies have been reported.

Gastric Diseases

Gastric involvement in HIV-infected individuals and AIDS patients has received little attention despite the common occurrence of dyspepsia, other gastric symptoms, and eating disorders. Although the stomach is uncommonly the primary site of disease, it may be involved by disseminated infections such as CMV, MAC, and fungus, or tumors such as KS, lymphoma, and adenocarcinoma.

Peptic ulcer disease is not a commonly reported problem in AIDS patients. The results of early studies demonstrated that hypochlorhydria may be present in as many as one third to one half of AIDS patients but may not be present in HIV-infected non-AIDS patients.[42-44] Decreased secretion of intrinsic factor also may contribute to the frequent finding of low serum vitamin B_{12} concentrations. Achlorhydria may alter the absorption of drugs such as ketoconazole and promote increased bacterial colony counts in the stomach and upper small intestine, with potentially adverse effects on nutrient absorption.[33]

Other sources of dyspepsia have been reported, including gastritis caused by *Helicobacter pylori*.[45] The incidence of *H pylori* infection in HIV-infected individuals is no higher and may be lower than in noninfected populations, possibly because of the more frequent use of broad-spectrum antibiotics in HIV-infected persons. Some medications, such as nonsteroidal antiinflammatory agents, promote gastric ulceration and produce dyspepsia. Dyspepsia is caused by a low-grade pancreatitis in some patients and may precede the development of biliary tract disease in others.

The clinical symptoms associated with gastric disease can be nonspecific. The presence of weight loss or fever implies a serious complication, such as a systemic infection or ulcerating tumor. Diagnosis can be reached by imaging procedures or endoscopic examination. The relative risks and benefits are the same as in the non–HIV-infected individual. In general,

the pathologic findings uncovered during evaluation are sufficient to explain the presenting signs and symptoms.

The treatment of dyspeptic complications depends on their exact nature. Symptomatic *H pylori* in an AIDS patient is treated in a standard fashion. Diagnosis of infection with an organism such as CMV implies disseminated disease and is an indication for systemic antiinfective therapy. Widespread or ulcerating KS or lymphoma is an indication for systemic chemotherapy. The treatment regimen should ensure sufficient caloric intake.

Primary Intestinal Diseases

Alteration in bowel habits, particularly diarrhea, is a common symptom in HIV-infected individuals and may occur in more than one half of patients at some point during the disease course. An increasing number of infectious complications have been identified, although a substantial proportion of patients have symptoms that remain unexplained after evaluation. The intestinal complications in AIDS can be subdivided into infections that normally produce intestinal injury and infections in which the gastrointestinal tract is affected secondarily, as part of disease dissemination.

Cryptosporidiosis

Cryptosporidiosis in AIDS has received wide attention because of its persistence and debilitating nature. The illness is caused by the protozoan *Cryptosporidium*, a member of the family of coccidia that also includes *Pneumocystis carinii* and *Toxoplasma gondii* (see Chap. 106).[46] In my experience, cryptosporidiosis accounts for about 10% of the cases of chronic diarrhea in patients with AIDS. The important processes of normal immunity to these organisms and the relation between cryptosporidiosis and a specific immune deficit in AIDS also are unknown. Cases of chronic intestinal cryptosporidiosis have been reported in agammaglobulinemic patients without AIDS, suggesting that the associated B-cell deficiency is responsible.[47]

The disease affects immunocompetent and immunodeficient people. The clinical illness associated with cryptosporidiosis is self-limited in most immunocompetent patients, although there may be prolonged shedding of cysts. The infection is associated with prolonged diarrhea and wasting in most affected AIDS patients, although a small percentage of patients undergo spontaneous remission. Endoscopically, the involved mucosa may be reddened and may be covered with a mucoid exudate. The major histologic findings in the small intestine are partial villus atrophy and crypt hyperplasia associated with marked acute and chronic inflammation (Fig. 105-1). The lesion is diffuse in the small intestine and causes a sprue-like pattern on barium radiograph (Fig. 105-2). In the colon, crypt epithelial cell damage associated with cryptitis may be focal or diffuse (see Fig. 105-1).

There is considerable variation in the location of cryptosporidiosis in AIDS. Most patients have diffuse small intestine disease without or with mild colonic involvement. A subset of these patients have a severe diarrheal syndrome. A smaller percentage of patients have a *Cryptosporidium*-related colitis

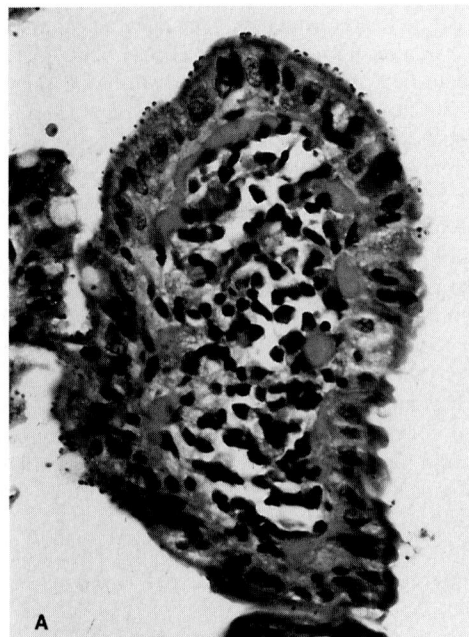
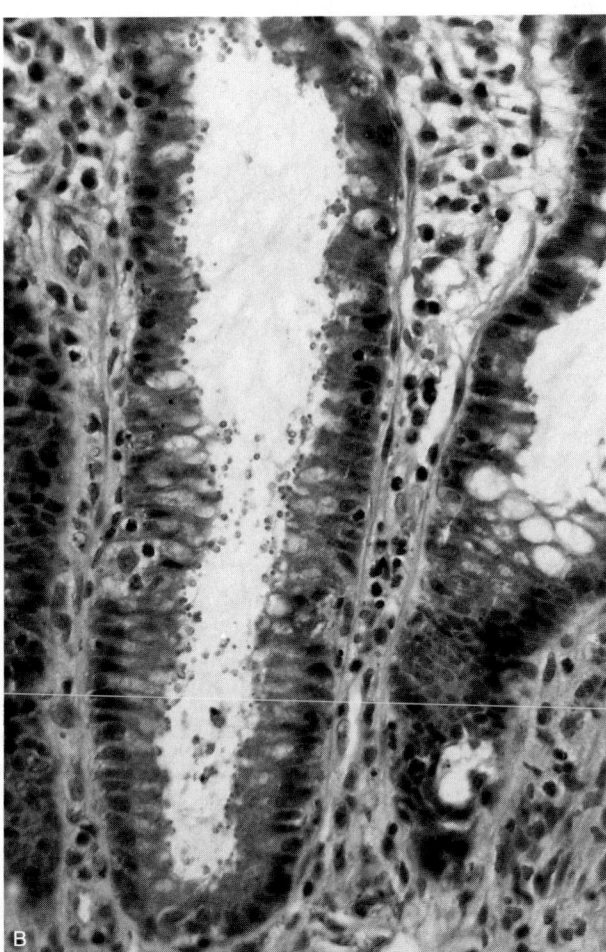

FIGURE 105-1. Intestinal cryptosporidiosis. **(A)** Intestinal villus, demonstrating cryptosporidial forms near and beneath the brush border membrane. (Original magnification ×400.) **(B)** Colonic crypt with cryptosporidia in the crypt lumen.

with no clinical or laboratory evidence of jejunal disease.[48] In some patients, the disease extends to the bile ducts and gallbladder. Attacks of acalculous cholecystitis or cholangitis have been observed. A few patients have been reported with *Cryptosporidium* in other locations, such as the stomach, esophagus, nasal mucosa, and bronchi, or with tissue invasion beyond the epithelial basement membrane.

The diagnosis of cryptosporidiosis can be made by stool examination. The most reliable stain is a modified Kinyoun stain. The yield is increased using methods to concentrate the oocysts.[49] The diagnosis also can be made by biopsy. The organisms are readily apparent on routine stains, although an acid-fast stain may enhance the ease of recognition.

There is no known effective therapy for cryptosporidiosis. Drug therapies for the disease have been disappointing. Some patients have improved greatly during treatment with paromomycin (Humatin), although others have had no response. Experimental trials of letrazuril (Janssen) and azithromycin (Zithromax, Pfizer) are ongoing (see Table 105-1). The macrolide spiramycin (Rovomycin) has been clinically helpful in a few patients. The report of successful therapy with hyperimmune bovine colostrum to treat cryptosporidiosis in an agammaglobulinemic child sparked interest in the use of biologicals to treat the disease in patients with AIDS.[50] Parenteral hydration with electrolyte repletion and parenteral nutritional support have been employed, and clinical stabilization has allowed prolonged survival outside of the hospital.

Treatment of the diarrhea may be difficult and varies according to whether the major disease localization is in the small intestine or colon. Diet modification may be helpful in patients with clinically mild disease. A lactose-free, low-fat diet with calorie-rich fluid supplements containing extra protein may be well tolerated. Standard formulas containing substantial quantities of long-chain fatty acids and high concentrations of sugar often cause bloating and worsen the diarrhea. Hydrophilic bulking agents usually are unhelpful. Opiates such as diphenoxylate, paregoric, or tincture of opium may be effective, although the dose required sometimes causes excessive sedation.

A subset of patients with AIDS have a severe diarrheal illness, with fluid losses of 6 to 12 L/day. Rapid volume depletion with azotemia occurs commonly, and hypokalemia may be severe. The disease resembles cholera clinically, although secretory enterotoxins have not been reported to be associated with *Cryptosporidium* infection. Partial success has been obtained using indomethacin or the phenothiazines, chlorpromazine, or trifluoperazine (Stelazine). These compounds inhibit chloride secretion such as that induced by cholera toxin. Reports of successful therapy with a somatostatin analog have been published.[51] Despite these approaches,

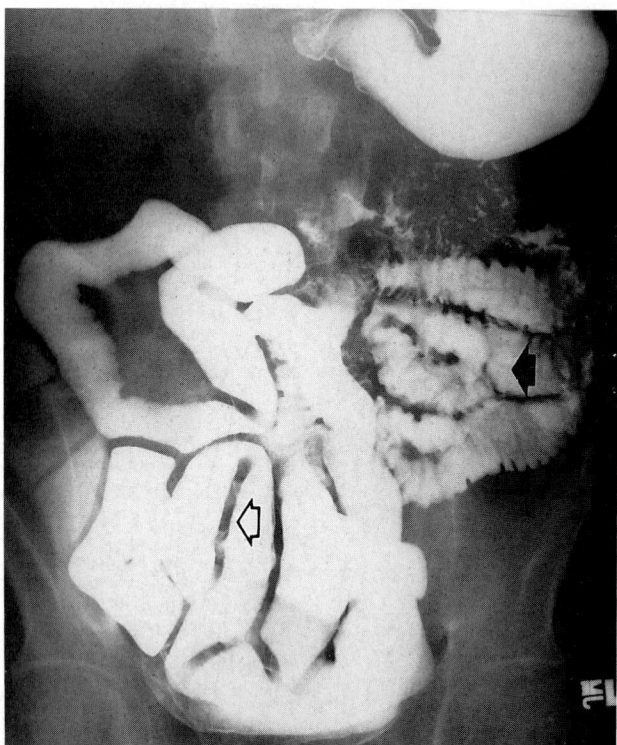

FIGURE 105-2. A radiograph of the small intestine after barium swallow shows diffuse abnormalities, with thickening of the mucosal folds in the upper intestine (*solid arrow*) and loss of markings in the ileum (*open arrow*).

parenteral fluids often are required to maintain a normal state of hydration.

Microsporidiosis

Microsporidia are protozoa only recently recognized to infect humans, although they are known to cause disease in other animals.[52] Two species causing microsporidiosis have been identified on intestinal biopsy: *Enterocytozoon bieneusi* and *Septata intestinalis*.[53,54] The infection is recognized with increasing frequency and may be responsible for as many as one third of cases of persistent diarrhea and weight loss in patients with AIDS.[55] Diagnosis is difficult because of the small size of the organisms and poor staining characteristics using routine stains. For this reason, electron microscopy has been required for diagnosis.

Clinically, infection with Microsporida resembles infection with *Cryptosporidium*, other diffuse small intestine diseases, or short bowel syndrome. The patients affected usually have severe immunodeficiency, with peripheral blood CD4+ lymphocyte counts lower than 50 cells/mm³. The infection is limited to the small intestine in most cases, although microsporidiosis has been associated with gallbladder and biliary tract disease. Endoscopically, the small intestine mucosa ranges from normal to a diffuse erythema with a mucoid exudate. Microscopically, partial villus atrophy and crypt hyperplasia are the rule. Prominent cytopathic changes in villus epithelial cells, especially in the upper villus, is a clue to the diagnosis (Fig. 105-3). The supranuclear region may contain

a globular inclusion, which deforms the nucleus and may have a cat's eye appearance (see Fig. 105-3). This inclusion has been identified from ultrastructural studies as the meront.[53] Five to 20 spores are found in cells with or without meronts. These spores can be seen to erupt through the brush border membrane into the lumen. The loss of cytoplasm leads to nuclear fragmentation, which is seen as basophilic debris in the affected areas.

Although *E bieneusi* infection is limited to enterocytes, *S intestinalis* can produce invasive and disseminated disease.[56] Microsporidia spores can be found in epithelial cells in the urinary sediment. Autopsy studies have also localized the organism to the kidney and the liver.

Little is known of the life cycle of the organism or of the epidemiology of the infection. The pathogenic process and the relation to immune deficiency are probably similar to those in cryptosporidiosis. Intestinal microsporidiosis was found to be associated with partial villus atrophy in the jejunum, decreased specific activities of intestinal disaccharidases, and xylose malabsorption, implying a pathogenic role for this organism.[57]

In the past, diagnosis of microsporidiosis required small intestine biopsy and electron microscopy. Later studies demonstrated an ability to detect microsporidial organisms using light microscopic techniques. Spores may be detected in stool samples or intestinal aspirates using a modified trichrome stain.[58] Light microscopic confirmation in mucosal biopsies can be obtained using touch preparations and a diluted Giemsa stain or by tissue Gram's stain, chromotrope 2R trichrome stain, or Giemsa stain. The use of these techniques undoubtedly will lead to an increased number of diagnoses of this organism.

There is no known effective therapy, and patients later shown to have microsporidiosis have been treated with a variety of antibiotics without success. Patients may respond symptomatically to treatment with metronidazole, paromomycin, or trimethoprim-sulfamethoxazole, although histologic evidence of intestinal injury and nutrient malabsorption persist. Studies using albendazole for *E bieneusi* infection are ongoing, although persistent infection has been seen.[59] Albendazole (SmithKline Beecham) appears to be effective therapy for *S intestinalis* infection and results in a complete clinical response.[60] Nutritional therapy is based on diet modification to decrease the fat and lactose content. Elemental diets may be well tolerated, but their efficacy in maintaining or repleting body mass has not been established. Parenteral nutritional therapy has been used in some patients and can result in nutritional repletion.

Microsporidial organisms comprise an important and newly recognized pathogen. The organism may be a significant cause of enteric disease in patients with AIDS, in the United States and elsewhere, and in infectious diarrhea in general. Additional studies are needed to enhance the diagnostic and therapeutic armamentarium against the organism.

Isosporiasis

Isospora belli is another coccidium that causes chronic infections in AIDS patients.[61] The organism has been reported to occur frequently in Africa and Haiti, and a few cases have been seen in New York City. *Isospora* is a small intestine

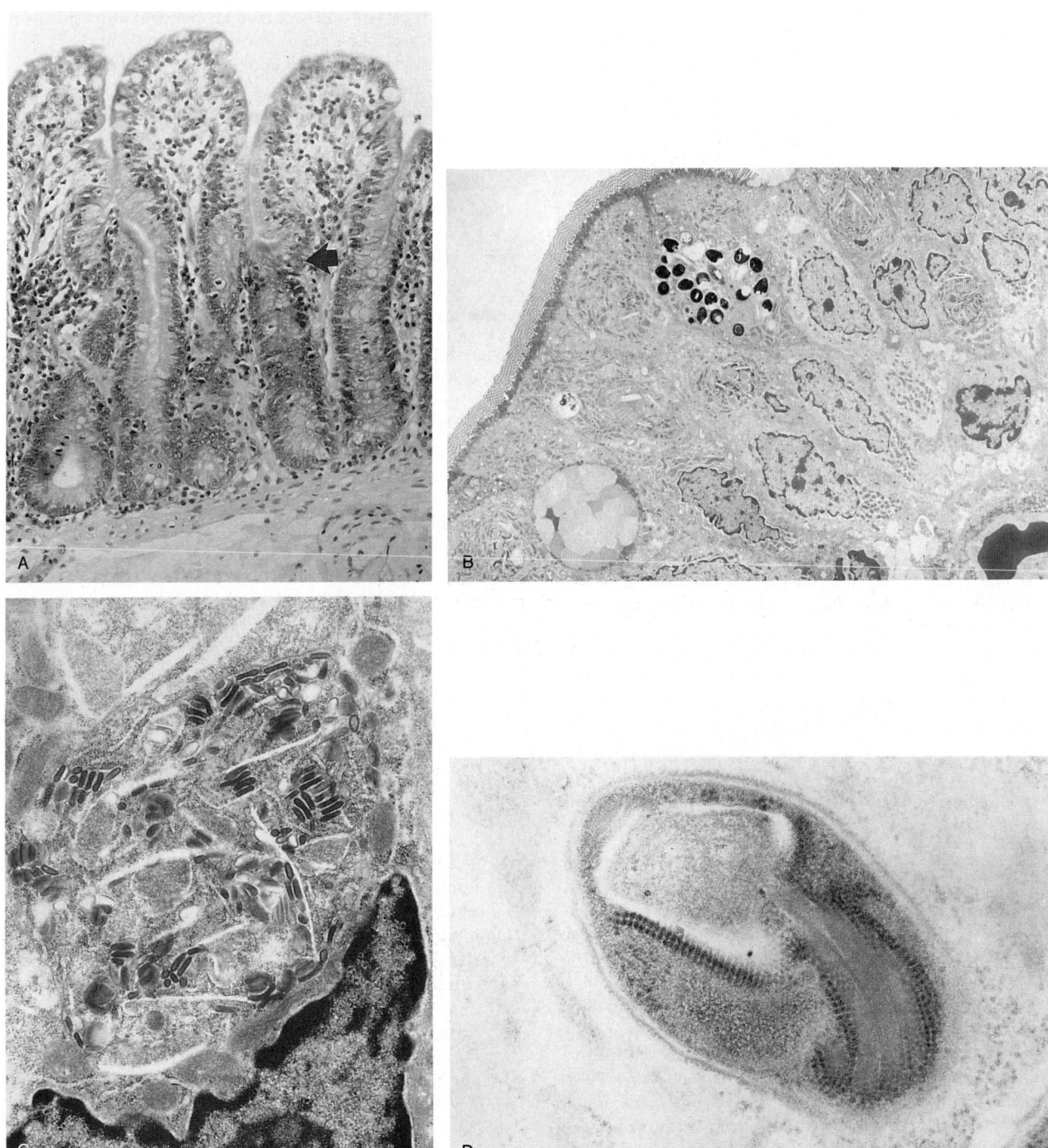

FIGURE 105-3. (**A**) Light micrograph of a jejunal biopsy specimen from a patient with microsporidiosis. Partial villus atrophy with crypt hyperplasia is seen with a crypt-villus ratio greater than 1. The arrow points to the villus-crypt junction. (**B**) The low-power electron micrograph demonstrates meronts in the apical cytoplasm and developing spores. Epithelial cell morphologic characteristics, such as microvilli, are preserved at this stage of infection. (Original magnification ×5000.) (**C**) A developing meront is located in the supernuclear region and indents the nucleus. The artifactual clefts are characteristic and can be seen on light and electron microscopy. (Original magnification ×16,000.) (**D**) A mature spore has a coiled polar filament. (Original magnification ×29,000; courtesy of Jan M. Orenstein, M.D., Ph.D., Washington, DC.)

pathogen, and infection results in tissue injury and nutrient malabsorption by mechanisms similar to those in cryptosporidiosis and microsporidiosis. The disease may rarely be disseminated. The diagnosis can be made by stool examination, using the same concentration and staining methods that are used for cryptosporidiosis. The organism also can be detected by small intestine biopsy, although electron microscopy may be necessary for definitive identification.

Isospora is sensitive to antimicrobial therapy (see Table 105-1). Trimethoprim-sulfamethoxazole usually brings prompt relief of diarrhea and weight gain. Pyrimethamine plus folinic acid also may be effective. Clinical recurrence is common after discontinuation of therapy; therefore, patients usually require repeated courses or chronic therapy. Successful long-term suppression of symptoms also can be accomplished by chronic treatment with trimethoprim.

Enteropathogenic Bacterial Infection

A syndrome of chronic diarrhea and malabsorption has been recognized and associated with epithelial cell damage caused by adherent bacteria.[62] The bacteria produce an attaching and effacing lesion on the microvilli of the superficial epithelium. These ultrastructural findings have been associated with chronic protracted enteropathy in infants and are caused in immunocompetent individuals by bacteria expressing a specific pilus-associated virulence factor. It is unclear whether the same mechanism applies in AIDS patients or whether the immunodeficiency renders the mucosa vulnerable to "nonpathogens." Treatment with broad-spectrum antibiotics may produce clinical improvement. The role of chronic enteropathogenic (i.e., enteroadherent) bacterial infections in causing unexplained diarrhea in AIDS requires further investigation.

Giardiasis

Enteric infection with *Giardia lamblia* is an important problem in many parts of the world but probably is not an important pathogen in patients with AIDS. The diagnosis of giardiasis was made commonly in sexually active homosexual men during the 1970s and early 1980s, and the infection was thought to be a frequent cause of the "gay bowel syndrome." The infection is acquired during ingestion of cysts in contaminated water or through sexual activity with oral-anal contact. The trophozoites, which live in the intestinal lumen, have a lectin on their surface that binds to a receptor on the epithelial cell brush border. The organism elicits a strong immune response which includes elements of the B-cell and T-cell systems. However, the infection may not be eradicated completely because of specific alterations in relevant giardial antigens.[63]

Giardiasis is not a common cause of acute diarrhea in patients with AIDS. Cysts have been identified by stool examination in some cases, and organisms have been seen on intestinal biopsy in very few cases. Small intestine structure in these cases was normal. The lack of intestinal injury is consistent with the hypothesis that small intestine injury in giardiasis is mediated by cytotoxic T cells.[64] In the absence of intestinal injury, *Giardia* may affect nutrient absorption by

local damaging effects on brush border proteins, bile salt deconjugation in the lumen, or other mechanisms.

The diagnosis can be made by examination of stool specimens or intestinal aspirates, or by small intestine biopsy. Drug therapy is indicated if cysts or trophozoites are found in symptomatic patients, although suspicion of other causes should remain high. Therapy with quinacrine or metronidazole at various doses is indicated (see Table 105-1). A course of antibiotic therapy may be repeated if clinical symptoms are not improved, but the patient also should be evaluated for other pathogens.

Bacterial Enteritides

Bacterial enteritides in AIDS have distinctive features. There are many reports of infection with species of *Salmonella*, *Shigella*, or *Campylobacter* in HIV-infected patients with or without AIDS.[65-67] It is unclear whether the incidence is increased compared with that in the surrounding population, although enhanced susceptibility could be related to decreased gastric acid secretion in AIDS.[33] Classic studies have demonstrated the relation between gastric acidity and the infective dose of various enteric pathogens.[68]

Bacterial enteritides in AIDS often are associated with bacteremia and a chronic, relapsing course. The presentation often is that of enteric fever, with clinical features reminiscent of the classical reports of typhoid fever.[69] There is persistent fever, abdominal distention, and a diarrheal syndrome varying from ileocolitis to proctocolitis. The diagnosis is straightforward with routine evaluation. Blood cultures should be part of the workup of suspected infectious diarrhea with fever in an HIV-infected patient. Patients respond to antibiotic therapy with parenteral agents.

An unusual feature of bacterial enteritides in AIDS is the tendency for clinical or microbiologic relapse after antibiotics are discontinued. Because many enteric bacterial pathogens are intracellular pathogens, it is possible that disease recurrence is a function of impaired intracellular macrophage killing resulting from deficient T-cell help. Furthermore, this intracellular reservoir may offer the organisms protection against certain antibiotics. Newer antibiotics such as ciprofloxacin can penetrate macrophages and are bacteriocidal to intracellular organisms.[70] Further studies are needed to determine whether complete eradication of the enteric bacterial pathogens in AIDS is possible or whether chronic therapy will continue to be needed.

Antibotic-Associated Colitis

Antibotic-associated colitis, related to elaboration of *Clostridium difficile* toxin (see Chap. 84), has been demonstrated in several AIDS patients with acute diarrheal syndromes. AIDS patients are particularly vulnerable to this complication, because they often receive prolonged courses of antibiotics (e.g., clindamycin for the treatment of cerebral toxoplasmosis). The clinical syndrome produced by *C difficile* toxin is similar in AIDS and non-AIDS patients and is an acute colitis. Suspicion should be raised by the clinical situation and diagnosis confirmed by stool toxin assay. Treatment with vancomycin is as effective in AIDS patients as in non-AIDS patients (see Table 105-1). A less expensive alternative is metronidazole. Residual symptoms can be managed with oral cholestyramine (Questran), which binds the bacterial toxin. Surveillance against recurrent colitis may be necessary in patients who require chronic antibiotic therapy.

Intestinal Disease Secondary to Systemic Infections

Cytomegalovirus Infection

CMV has long been known to be an enteric pathogen, although premortem recognition was rare in the past. Isolated reports described the characteristic viral inclusions in cells in the bases of chronic nonhealing ulcers, at the sites of otherwise unexplained intestinal perforations, in a few cases of toxic megacolon associated with ulcerative colitis, and in patients receiving immunosuppressive therapy. Clinical observations and autopsy series demonstrate that disseminated CMV infection is a frequent complication in AIDS and that progressive disease produces wasting and local symptoms.[71] The gastrointestinal tract may be involved focally or diffusely in this process.

CMV is a member of the herpesvirus family.[72] Serologic prevalence rates are high in the general population and extremely high in people from groups at high risk for contracting AIDS. CMV infects many cell types, including epithelial cells in mucous membranes. For this reason, CMV may be shed in the body's secretions. Sexually promiscuous persons are probably infected with multiple strains of the virus.

After initial infection, the virus disseminates to multiple cellular reservoirs. The primary viral infection is not a significant clinical illness in most cases, although a mononucleosis-like syndrome has been observed. After primary infection, the disease enters a latent phase that is lifelong in most immunocompetent people. In the HIV-infected patient with diminished T-cell function, repeated episodes of viral reactivation occur, as demonstrated by virus shedding and the reappearance of anti-CMV IgM antibodies in the serum. The reactivations become more frequent and prolonged over time, until persistent reactivation occurs and leads to tissue injury.

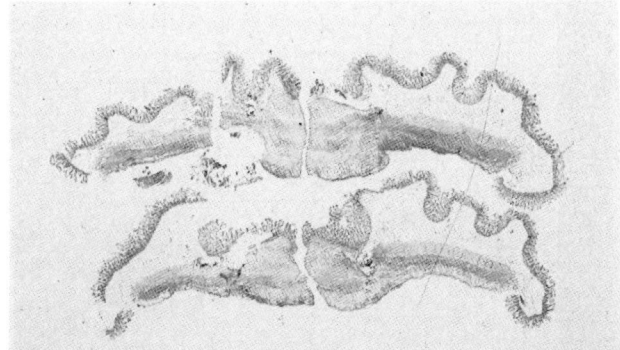

FIGURE 105-4. The whole-mount preparation of resected ileum demonstrates a discrete transmural ulceration. Characteristic cytomegalovirus inclusions were found in the inflamed areas, in other areas of the intestine, and in the retina. (From Yamada T, Alpers DA, Owyang C, et al. Atlas of gastroenterology. Philadelphia: JB Lippincott, 1992:381.)

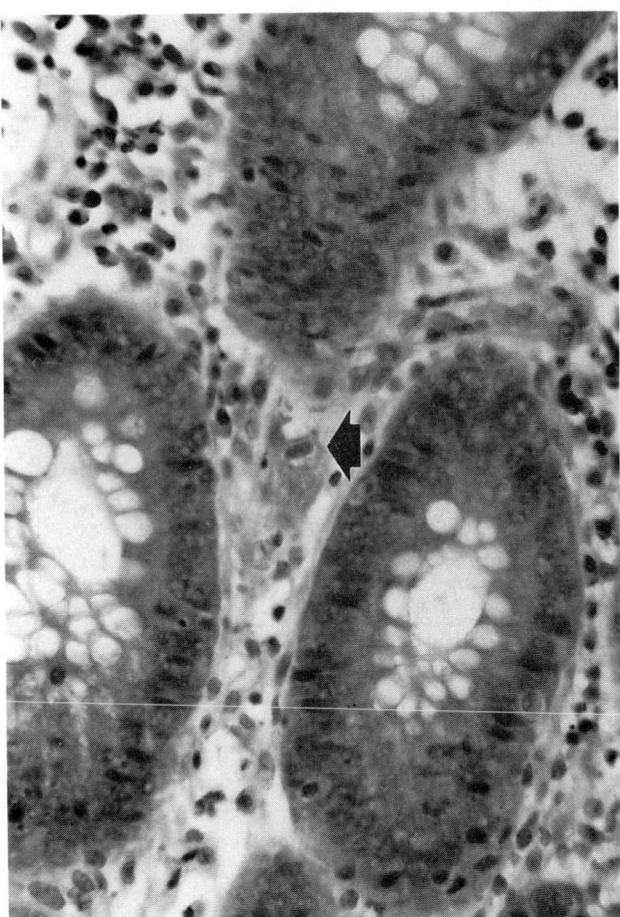

FIGURE 105-5. A colonic biopsy specimen shows a characteristic intranuclear inclusion of cytomegalovirus infection (*arrow*). The intranuclear inclusion is surrounded by a clear space, which differentiates this inclusion as one caused by cytomegalovirus. (Original magnification ×200.)

At autopsy, CMV inclusions may be found in many organs, especially the adrenal glands, lungs, and gastrointestinal tract.

Several gastrointestinal syndromes have been associated with CMV, including esophageal ulcers, esophagitis, gastritis, isolated intestinal ulcers, terminal ileitis, spontaneous intestinal perforation, and focal or diffuse colitis. The clinical syndromes are diagnosed based on the usual evaluation of presenting signs and symptoms. The endoscopic pathology varies with location. Esophageal ulcers tend to be shallow and broad with rounded edges. CMV gastritis appears as aphthous ulcers or focal areas of inflammation with central erosion. These lesions may appear as intramucosal masses. The small intestine is involved less frequently, although CMV duodenitis and ileitis have been seen.[73] Focal, deep ulcers in the small intestine with perforation have been reported (Fig. 105-4).

The colonic picture of CMV is quite variable. The mucosa can appear normal, but it is more likely to be affected by variable degrees of focal erythema or petechial hemorrhage. Occasionally, fine vesicles or erosions can be seen. In more advanced cases, scattered ulcers are visible.

The hallmark of CMV infection on histologic examination is the viral inclusion (Fig. 105-5). The most characteristic form is an intranuclear inclusion, which often is surrounded by a halo, producing an "owl-eyed" appearance. There may be cytoplasmic inclusions. Most inclusion bodies are found in vascular endothelial cells. Epithelial cell inclusions also may be seen, especially in the stomach. In areas of severe inflammation, such as an ulcer bed, many cell types may demonstrate viral inclusions. The diagnosis of an inclusion body caused by CMV usually is straightforward. For inclusions that are rare or atypical, immunohistologic or in situ hybridization techniques developed for clinical use may be helpful. These techniques have confirmed the accuracy of diagnosis by experienced clinical pathologists and are not needed on a routine basis.

There are several agents undergoing clinical trials that are able to inhibit CMV replication. The most widely studied is ganciclovir, which is structurally related to acyclovir.[74] Several studies have demonstrated clinical benefit from ganciclovir therapy in patients with gastrointestinal disease caused by CMV, including clinical stabilization, repletion of body mass, and prolonged survival.[75-78] As presently formulated, ganciclovir must be administered intravenously. Treatment is given by an induction phase (5 mg/kg every 12 hours for 14 days), followed by maintenance treatment (6 mg/kg 5 times per week) to prevent disease recurrence (see Table 105-1). Because the drug has hematologic toxic effects, the most relevant of which is neutropenia, blood counts must be followed. In most cases, a chronic indwelling catheter must be placed. Despite the potential problems, patients receiving ganciclovir have been followed as outpatients for more than 3 years with reasonable comfort and good functional performance.

Foscarnet is an antiviral agent that is active against CMV and HIV, and evidence of clinical benefit has been reported.[79] Like ganciclovir, the drug must be given by intravenous infusion. Further development of treatment regimens is expected.

The indications for anti-CMV therapy are unsettled.[80] In the case of gastrointestinal disease, histopathologic evidence of infection (i.e., tissue injury and local viral replication in inclusions) represents a risk of serious local disease or widespread reactivation with wasting, justifying therapy. This standard is based on the premise of thorough direct gastrointestinal evaluation and tissue sampling. The indications for treatment based on the results of viral cultures or serologies are less clear, because asymptomatic viral shedding may occur without detectable tissue damage, and serologic evidence of viral infection is extremely common and not specific for tissue injury. The potential use of antiviral agents in patients with idiopathic wasting, especially if accompanied by CMV viremia, requires further study, as does their use as prophylactic agents.

Mycobacterial Infections

Mycobacterial infection is a frequent cause of intestinal disease in AIDS.[81] *M tuberculosis* is not a common clinical problem in the lumenal gastrointestinal tract in AIDS, although the intestine is infected in other instances of miliary tuberculosis. However, MAC is a common cause of gastrointestinal disease in AIDS. MAC is an atypical *Mycobacterium* related to the type that causes cervical adenitis with fistula formation (i.e., scrofula). The infection probably is acquired through the ingestion of contaminated water. The organisms that enter the body are phagocytosed by macrophages, which then are unable to lyse the organism, probably because of the loss of a T-lymphocyte factor, presumably interferon-γ. Several studies have shown that monocytes from AIDS patients are capable of responding to interferon-γ and lysing mycobacteria or protozoa in vitro.[82]

Clinical disease results from infiltration of infected macrophages into tissue compartments and from the effects of cytokines released by the macrophages. The abdominal viscera often are involved by the infection. Organomegaly is associated with retroperitoneal and mesenteric lymphadenopathy. The enlarged nodes are especially prominent on computed tomography (CT) examinations but must be differentiated from other infections and neoplasms (Fig. 105-6). Occasionally, nodes undergo liquefaction necrosis and produce a mycobacterial peritonitis. Liquefaction can be detected as a lucent node on the CT scan. Diagnosis is important, because the clinical presentation may mimic an acute abdominal crisis.

The lumenal gastrointestinal tract also is involved by MAC. Massive thickening of the proximal intestine may occur (Fig.

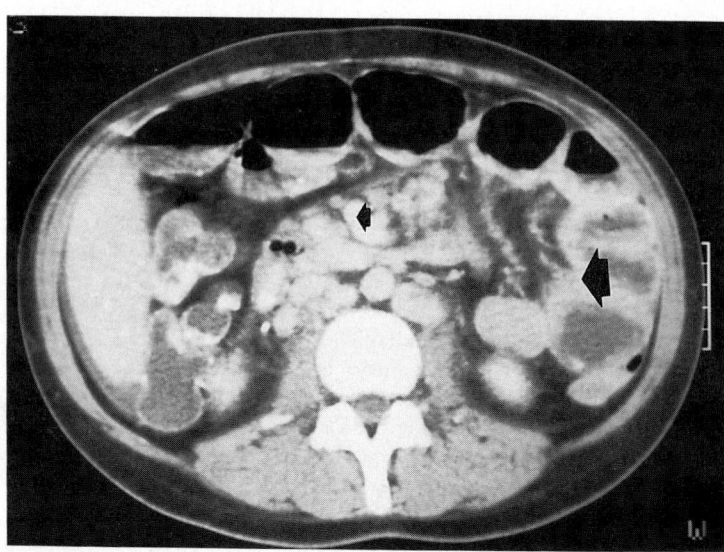

FIGURE 105-6. The CT scan of the abdomen of a patient with *Mycobacterium avium-intracellulare* infection demonstrates enlarged mesenteric nodes (*small arrow*) and thickening of the bowel wall (*large arrow*).

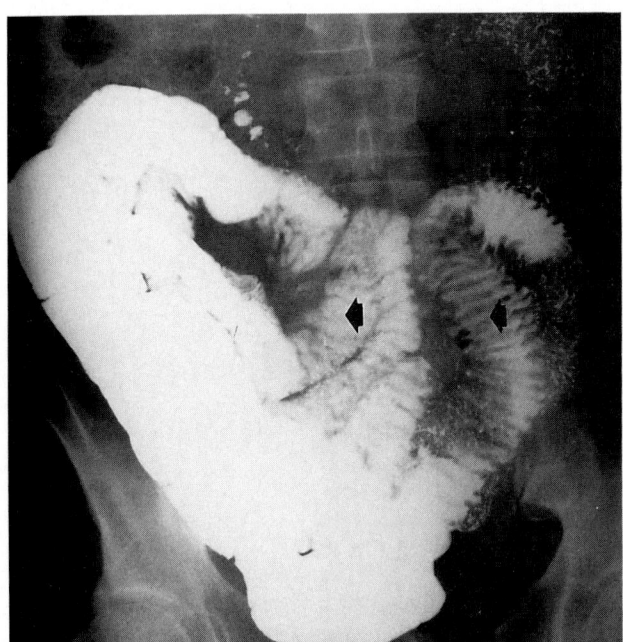

FIGURE 105-7. A radiograph of the small intestine in a patient with *Mycobacterium avium-intracellulare* (MAI) infection demonstrates thickened folds in the middle and distal jejunum (*arrow*), which were confirmed by biopsy to be caused by MAI.

105-7). Small intestine biopsy reveals infiltration of the lamina propria by macrophages containing large numbers of acid-fast bacilli (Fig. 105-8). The macrophages may appear fibrillar because of the intracellular tubercle bacilli. In severe cases, the overlying villi may be deformed.

The clinical presentation of MAC is characterized by diarrhea, fever, anorexia, and progressive wasting. The fevers often are preceded by rigors and followed by sweats. They are responsive to therapy with prostaglandin synthetase inhibitors such as indomethacin. The pathophysiology of gastrointestinal dysfunction is the same as occurs in Whipple's disease and is related to abnormal infiltration of macrophages and an in-

tramucosal block in lymphatic flow, which leads to fat malabsorption and exudative enteropathy.[83] The absorption of sugars, amino acids, and other nutrients also is adversely affected. Most patients also have abnormal liver function tests with cholestatic features. Malnutrition results from a combination of anorexia and metabolic derangements associated with the febrile illnesses and a variable degree of malabsorption.

The diagnosis of mycobacterial infection is made by culture or histology. Stool smears may demonstrate acid-fast bacilli, but a specific correlation with tissue localization has not been made. However, these patients should be considered at high risk for disseminated infection and should be evaluated and treated accordingly. Blood culture, using a special transport medium (i.e., Dupont isolator), is sensitive and often can detect bacteremia before the development of clinical symptoms. Histologic demonstration of acid-fast bacilli in intestinal or liver tissue is straightforward. Molecular hybridization techniques are being developed to allow species identification using tissue sections.

The treatment of *M tuberculosis* in AIDS and non-AIDS patients generally is similar. The organism usually is responsive to antimicrobial therapy, and multidrug regimens are used. The optimal length of treatment needed is unknown. Some clinicians continue antituberculosis therapy indefinitely.

The therapy for MAC is evolving. Early studies with single- or two-drug regimens were unsuccessful, and later studies showed that a substantial proportion of patients may respond clinically, with significant decreases in the bacterial colony counts in peripheral blood. Several drugs have in vitro efficacy against MAC, including the macrolide clarithromycin (Biaxin), ethambutol (Myambutal), mycobutin (Rifabutin), and clofazimine (Lamprene). Other drugs with in vivo or in vitro efficacy include amikacin, ciprofloxacin, cycloserine, and ethionamide. The response to these multidrug regimens is slow, and the disease does not always respond to therapy, although there are many instances of clinical stabilization, disease regression, and prolonged survival. Therapy for this complication is suppressive and palliative. The use of exogenously administered interferon-γ is being evaluated. Improved treatment modalities are needed for MAC.

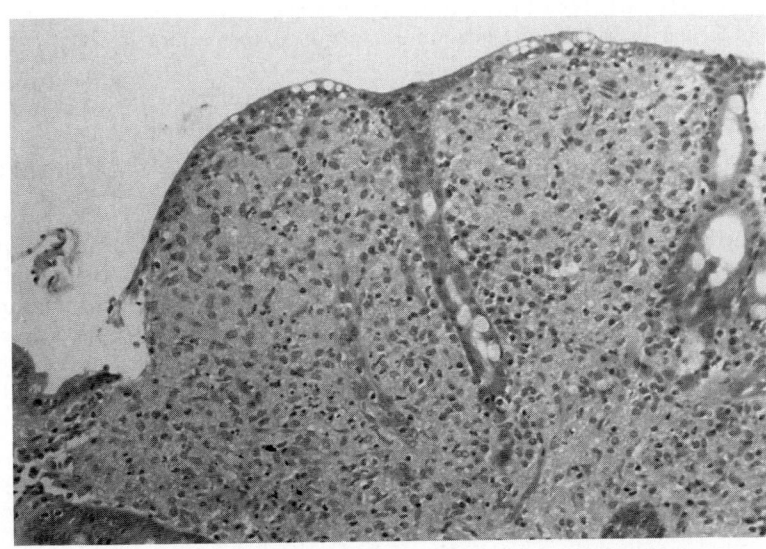

FIGURE 105-8. A small intestine biopsy specimen shows a massive infiltration of the lamina propria by foamy macrophages, which have spread diffusely, causing distortion of the villus architecture. (Original magnification ×200.)

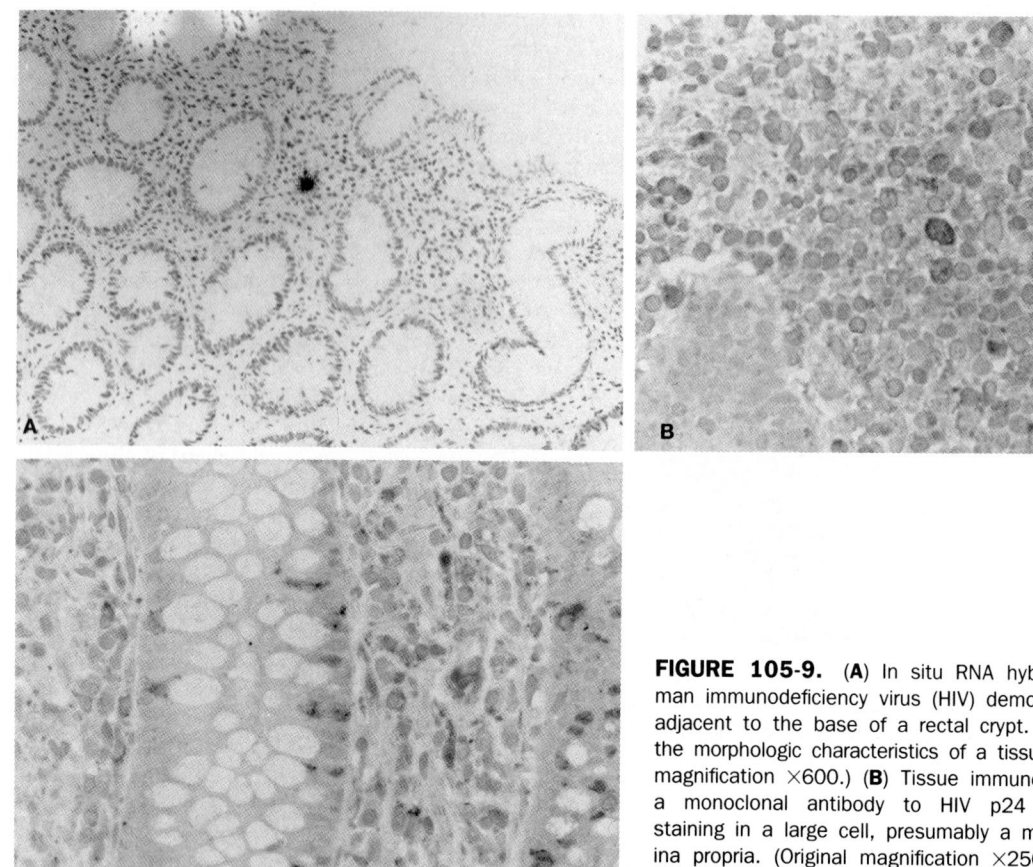

FIGURE 105-9. (**A**) In situ RNA hybridization study for human immunodeficiency virus (HIV) demonstrates a staining cell adjacent to the base of a rectal crypt. The cell's nucleus had the morphologic characteristics of a tissue macrophage. (Original magnification ×600.) (**B**) Tissue immunoperoxidase stain using a monoclonal antibody to HIV p24 antigen demonstrates staining in a large cell, presumably a macrophage, in the lamina propria. (Original magnification ×250.) (**C**) Staining of epithelial cells (*arrows*) by monoclonal anti-p24 antibody. (Original magnification ×400.)

Human Immunodeficiency Virus Infection

There are several reasons to suspect that HIV plays a role in intestinal disease. Many cellular reservoirs for HIV are found in the gut, including CD4+ lymphocytes, macrophages, dendritic cells, and epithelial cells. The intestinal mucosa also is an important site of HIV entry into the body. Unexplained gastrointestinal symptoms are prevalent in HIV-infected patients. HIV has been localized to the intestinal mucosa by molecular hybridization and immunohistologic techniques (Fig. 105-9).

The associations among HIV infection, clinical symptoms, and pathologic findings in the intestines are unclear. Intestinal injury could occur as a direct result of virus-induced cytopathology, as an indirect effect of anti-HIV immunity, or as a result of a systemic inflammatory process.[84] Focal crypt epithelial necrosis (i.e., apoptosis) has been seen in the gastrointestinal tracts of HIV-infected patients.[85]

The role of HIV in producing intestinal disease was studied prospectively in HIV-infected persons with or without AIDS.[86,87] Most AIDS patients with diarrhea had identifiable enteric pathogens, compared with a minor percentage of HIV-infected individuals without AIDS. The symptom of altered bowel habits occurred independently of enteric infections. Rectal mucosal histology varied with clinical disease stage. Mucosal histology could be classified as abnormal in a majority of cases; abnormalities did not correlate with the presence of pathogens but did correlate with altered bowel habits. Expression of HIV-associated antigens and HIV RNA varied with disease stage and were highest in non-AIDS persons with altered bowel habits but no enteric pathogens. HIV expression correlated with altered bowel habits and histologic mucosal abnormalities. Altered cytokine expression also has been demonstrated in these patients.[88] These results imply an association of chronic mucosal inflammation with HIV production. Other studies also have correlated the expression of HIV with chronic colitis.[89] The pathogenic significance of these associations remains undetermined.

Fungal Infection

The lumenal gastrointestinal tract, liver, spleen, and mesenteric lymph nodes may be involved by fungus infection such as histoplasmosis or coccidioidomycosis. Systemic fungal infections in AIDS are serious, rapidly progressive diseases and produce multisystem failure in the absence of vigorous therapy. The diseases represent reactivation from latency and are associated with widespread dissemination. They are associated with decreased appetite, nausea and vomiting, diffuse abdominal pain, organomegaly, and abnormal liver function tests. The disease manifests as a chronic febrile illness. Suspicion should be aroused by a history of residence in an endemic area. The diagnosis is made by culture or examination with special stains of tissue samples, including liver. Treatment with antifungal agents must be continued for months and perhaps indefinitely.

Anorectal Diseases

Chronic Ulcerative Perianal Herpes Simplex Virus Infection

HSV infection is a common problem in patients at risk for developing AIDS. In immunocompetent patients, viral reactivations are manifested as the transient appearance of vesicles. The major clinical form of HSV in AIDS is a chronic perineal ulcer that is painful, shallow, and slowly spreading. It may be found in the anal canal, perianal skin, or other sites in the perineum. Another common symptom of perianal herpes is difficulty in evacuation. Herpetic proctitis does not accompany the perineal ulcer.

The diagnosis is made by inspection. HSV can be isolated readily from a swab culture. Biopsies usually are unnecessary. If done, they may show the viral inclusion of HSV in skin epithelial cells. Perineal HSV is treated with intravenous acyclovir (5 mg/kg every 8 hours) or orally (400 mg four times daily). Topical therapy is insufficient for this lesion. The lesions usually heal completely. Oral acyclovir therapy should be continued indefinitely to prevent disease recurrence (see Table 105-1).

Squamous Cell Cancer

Squamous cell cancer of the anus has been associated with male homosexuality.[90] Several cases of squamous cell cancer of the anus in AIDS patients also have been seen. The lesion is probably related to infection by oncogenic strains of human papillomavirus. In AIDS, impaired immune surveillance may be a cofactor for the clinical expression of the tumor. Squamous cell cancer in AIDS can be a devastating disease, with widespread local involvement and distant metastases.

Anal Ulcers

Deep, painful ulcers of the anal canal, sometimes including rectal mucosa or perianal skin, are distressing complications in AIDS and cause considerable suffering. In most cases, evaluation fails to uncover offending agents, and biopsy shows only granulation tissue. A possible association of this lesion with HIV infection has not been confirmed. The lesion is resistant to all therapies except corticosteroid therapy; which can be administered locally. Intestinal diversion has been required in several cases.

Neoplastic Diseases

Kaposi's Sarcoma

KS was the first complication that brought patients with AIDS to the attention of the Centers for Disease Control in 1981.[91] Since its original description by Moritz Kaposi in 1872, it had been known to be an uncommon disease of elderly Jewish or Italian men. The disease usually was limited to the skin of

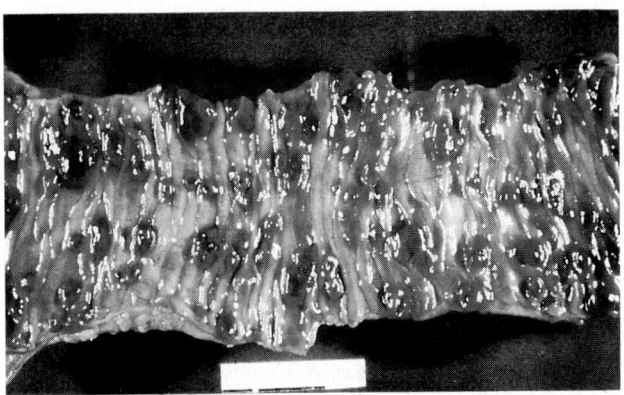

FIGURE 105-10. Autopsy presentation of bulky lesions of Kaposi's sarcoma in the small intestine. This patient had a partial obstruction and later had an acute hemorrhage from the lesions.

the lower extremities, although visceral dissemination eventually occurred in about 10% of cases. An endemic form of KS, often involving lymph nodes, also was seen in Africa. The association of KS and immune deficiency was highlighted by the reported cases of KS after organ transplantation and successful control by decreasing the intensity of immunosuppression. The cell of origin of this tumor is an endothelial cell, based on immunohistologic studies using antibodies to factor VIII. The demonstration of an angiogenesis factor released from T cells infected with HIV and from KS-associated cells suggests that the lesion may have hyperplastic properties distinct from those of the usual cancer and could be multifocal in origin rather than metastatic.[92]

KS is a common complication in AIDS. Although the lesion is pathologically identical to that seen in classic KS, the distribution and clinical course differ in patients with AIDS. Cofactors in addition to immune deficiency must be responsible, because the complication is much more prevalent in homosexual men than in intravenous drug abusers. The disease has visceral dissemination at the time of diagnosis in more than 50% of cases. Lesions relevant to the gastrointestinal tract include bulky lesions of the gingiva or palate that interfere with mastication, lesions in the hypopharynx that affect swallowing, lesions of the stomach or intestine that obstruct lumenal flow, lymphatic obstruction with exudative enteropathy, and gastrointestinal bleeding in far advanced cases. In most cases, the gastrointestinal disease is clinically silent for most or all of the clinical course.

The diagnosis of KS is made by inspection, with biopsy in noncharacteristic cases. Several researchers have suggested that yields from endoscopic biopsies are low because of the submucosal location of the lesion.[93] However, most biopsies are positive in patients with large KS lesions (Fig. 105-10). The key histologic feature is the presence of spindle cells, representing the abnormal vascular proliferation, with trapped red blood cells in the stroma. The tumor may be treated by local or systemic therapy. Laser excision using a CO_2 laser has been used successfully in oral and pharyngeal lesions,* and ablation of lesions in the esophagus, stomach, and colon has been

---

* Pollack G, personal communication, March 1989.

performed using a Nd:YAG laser.† This therapy is recommended for patients with obstructive lesions. Laser therapy also may be effective in bleeding lesions, as may sclerotherapy. The lesion also is responsive to radiation therapy, although radiation-induced xerostomia and anal strictures are distressing long-term complications. KS is sensitive to chemotherapy. Combinations of doxorubicin, bleomycin, and vincristine are effective in patients able to tolerate the therapy and are indicated for progressive disease.

Lymphoma

An unusually high incidence of high-grade B-cell lymphomas was noticed in young men at about the time that AIDS first was recognized. Many patients with lymphoma subsequently were shown to be infected with HIV.[94] Lymphoma is the second most common neoplasm in AIDS. It typically is extranodal; the most common locations are the brain and the gastrointestinal tract. Most lymphomas are B-cell lymphomas and include small and large cell types, with smaller subgroups of patients having Burkitt's lymphoma, Hodgkin's disease, and other forms.

The role of viral infection in lymphomagenesis is controversial. Epstein-Barr virus (EBV) has been implicated in Burkitt's lymphoma occurring in patients with and without AIDS.[95] The EBV genome also has been demonstrated in the Reed-Sternberg cell found in Hodgkin's disease.[96] However, most other lymphomas in AIDS patients do not contain detectable quantities of the EBV genome.‡ Other viruses, including HIV, also can infect and transform B cells.[97] The human T-lymphotropic virus type I has been associated with T-cell lymphoma or leukemia in AIDS and non-AIDS patients. Whatever the precise cause, malignant lymphoproliferation in HIV infection is promoted by the loss of immune surveillance resulting from the T-cell deficiency. Benign and malignant forms of lymphoproliferation are found in patients receiving immunosuppressive therapy after organ transplantation.

Most intestinal lymphomas in AIDS are biologically aggressive. They often are found in the mesentery with extension into retroperitoneum and viscera (Fig. 105-11). However, they may have unusual presentations, such as in the base of a chronic anal ulcer. Intestinal wall lymphomas may lead to obstruction, intussusception, or perforation.

The diagnosis is based on biopsy results. If biopsies are performed in patients suspected of having lymphoma, tissue should be frozen in case studies of cell markers are needed. Fine-needle aspiration of abdominal nodes with sonographic or CT guidance may give the correct diagnosis, although the small yield of cells usually precludes cell marker studies.

Lymphoma in AIDS is treated with combination chemotherapy. Complete remissions have been documented in patients in whom the lymphoma is the first recognized complication of the disease. The response is poorer in AIDS patients who have had many disease complications before the development of lymphoma, because they are unable to tolerate aggressive chemotherapy.

---

† Winkler WP, personal communication, May 1989.

‡ Subar M, personal communication, June 1989.

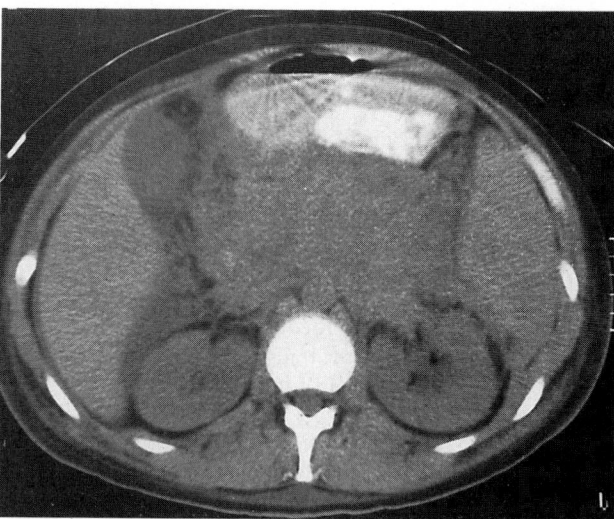

FIGURE 105-11. A CT scan of the abdomen of a patient with B-cell lymphoma demonstrates an amorphous mass in the mesentery that is invading the left renal pelvis and displacing the abdominal viscera anteriorly. Free fluid also is detected by the scan.

Other Cancers

Scattered reports suggest that the rates of malignancies other than KS and lymphoma also are increased in patients with AIDS. Diagnoses of carcinomas of the stomach, cervix, esophagus, colon, anus, and prostate have been made in young adults infected with HIV who do not fit any other clinical pattern for early expression of tumor. These tumors typically are biologically aggressive and do not respond well to therapy.

Hepatobiliary Diseases

Liver dysfunction occurs commonly in AIDS and may be related to previous hepatic diseases such as viral or alcoholic hepatitis, specific complications of the immune deficiency, or toxicity from drug therapy.[98] There are three distinct clinical syndromes of AIDS-related hepatobiliary disease: diffuse hepatocellular injury, granulomatous hepatitis, and sclerosing cholangitis. Anecdotal reports suggest that a syndrome similar to primary biliary cirrhosis also may develop. Many patients with abnormal liver function tests have macrovesicular or microvesicular fatty infiltration or other nonspecific changes.

Diffuse Hepatitis

Diffuse hepatitis is uncommon in patients with AIDS. Many patients exposed to HIV have had prior exposure to hepatitis B. Acute hepatitis B infection usually is mild in HIV-seropositive people, because hepatocyte injury is produced by the immune reaction and not by the virus. A relatively high percentage of HIV-infected persons have circulating hepatitis B surface antigen and e antigen. However, there is no evidence that immune deficiency causes a reactivation of prior hepatitis B. Autoimmune chronic active hepatitis also is a clinically mild syndrome in HIV-seropositive people. Because hepatocyte injury as a direct result of viral or other cytopathology is unaffected by the immune deficiency, delta hepatitis and drug-induced hepatitis are as severe in HIV-seropositive as in HIV-seronegative people.[99] Chronic hepatitis C infection also occurs in HIV-infected individuals, and there is evidence that HIV infection is associated with more rapid progression to liver failure.[100]

Granulomatous Hepatitis

Granulomatous hepatitis in AIDS occurs as a result of mycobacterial or fungal diseases or other causes. Fever is prominent and usually associated with rigors and sweats, anorexia, weight loss, and progressive debilitation. Liver function tests demonstrate elevations in the levels of alkaline phosphatase and γ-glutamyl transpeptidase, which rise progressively over time. The indication for a biopsy to diagnose granulomatous hepatitis is the progressive rise, not the absolute level, of these enzymes. The total bilirubin level usually is within normal limits, although the conjugated fraction may be elevated. The aminotransferases are mildly elevated, and hypoalbuminemia is evident. Liver biopsy reveals focal collections of histiocytes, which may be organized into poorly formed granulomas that are scattered throughout the parenchyma. Giant cells are seen only rarely.

The responsible organism often can be identified by special stains on biopsy. Acid-fast stains usually disclose large numbers of organisms, especially in cases of MAC. This observation differs from the usual rarity of acid-fast bacilli in granulomas from non-AIDS–related tuberculosis.[101] Because tuberculosis cannot be differentiated from MAC by biopsy alone, culture of a liver specimen also should be done, and therapy should be based on clinical judgment until results are known. Histoplasmosis and coccidioidomycosis can be diagnosed with great certainty by biopsy using specific histologic stains. However, an aliquot of the biopsy specimen also should be cultured for fungus.

Sclerosing Cholangitis

A syndrome of sclerosing cholangitis affects AIDS patients.[102] The disease in AIDS bears a striking resemblance to the non-AIDS variety (see Chap. 97), although the disease in AIDS may be more rapidly progressive. The cause and pathogenesis of sclerosing cholangitis in AIDS are as obscure as they are in the non-AIDS variety. Some patients have been shown to have biliary involvement with protozoa, namely cryptosporidiosis and microsporidiosis. Other patients have been shown to have CMV infection of the liver and biliary tree. In other patients, no etiologic agent can be identified.

Patients with sclerosing cholangitis present with nonspecific abdominal complaints. There are progressive abnormalities in the liver function tests; pruritus may or may not be present. On physical examination, the liver is mildly enlarged. Ultrasound examination is normal or shows some dilated bile ducts. Endoscopic retrograde cholangiography demonstrates multiple areas of narrowing and dilatation of the intrahepatic and extrahepatic ducts (Fig. 105-12). The mucosal surface of bile ducts appears ulcerated in many cases. Examination of bile and pancreatic juice may reveal bacterial overgrowth, viruses, or *Cryptosporidium*. Attempts have been made to treat this complication by sphincterotomy, during endoscopic ret-

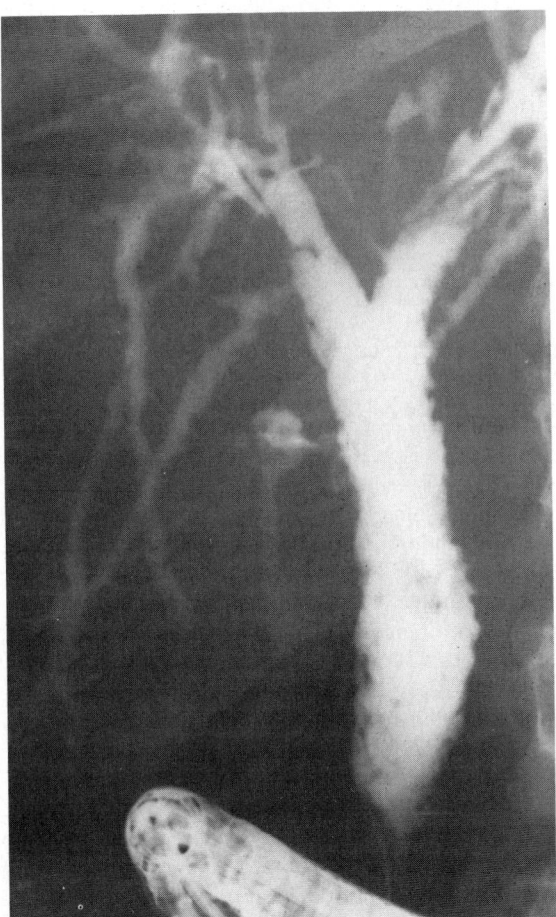

FIGURE 105-12. An endoscopic retrograde cholangiogram demonstrates diffuse ulceration in the intra- and extrahepatic bile ducts in a patient with AIDS-associated sclerosing cholangitis.

rograde cholangipancreatography or at laparotomy. The short-term results are variable, and the long-term results are poor. Attempts at operative decompression are not indicated unless there is a strong suspicion that a single stricture is responsible for the obstruction. Other patients have been treated for CMV infection with ganciclovir, without any effect on the course of the biliary disease. In a few patients, long-term follow-up has shown progressive jaundice and liver failure.

Pancreatic Diseases

Pancreatic diseases have received little attention in the study of AIDS.[103] Pancreatic involvement often is not recognized premortem. The pancreas may be affected as part of a systemic complication such as CMV, MAC, herpes zoster, fungal infection, or KS or other lymphoma or as a toxic complication of a medication. The most common clinical presentation is acute pancreatitis. The disease, which is clinically mild in most cases, is associated with abdominal pain, nausea, vomiting, and elevations of serum amylase and lipase concentrations. In some cases, a medication such as trimethoprim-sulfamethoxazole or pentamidine can be implicated, but often no etiologic agent can be found. The antiretroviral agent dideoxyinosine (ddI or Videx, Bristol Myers) has been associated with the development of pancreatitis, which may be severe.[104] Intravenous pentamidine therapy for *Pneumocystis* pneumonia also has been associated with hypoglycemia caused by selective damage to beta cells in the islets of Langerhans.[105] A few patients have become insulin-requiring diabetics after pentamidine therapy. Hyperlipidemic pancreatitis has been observed in a patient receiving intravenous lipids for nutritional support. There is no evidence of chronic pancreatitis or pancreatic insufficiency occurring as a result of AIDS.

Gastrointestinal Emergencies

Acute Abdomen

Abdominal pain is an important symptom in AIDS patients. The major enteric pathogens such as *Cryptosporidium*, CMV, *Salmonella*, and *Shigella* cause abdominal cramps, not pain. Severe acute abdominal pain often is a sign of a significant pathologic process, such as a perforated viscus. The clinical signs of abdominal tenderness, guarding, and rebound have the same significance in AIDS patients as in immunocompetent patients. AIDS patients may develop peritonitis for the same reasons as patients without AIDS or for reasons specific to AIDS. The diagnoses of cholecystitis or appendicitis are based on the usual clinical criteria.

Special causes of abdominal pain or surgical abdomen in AIDS patients include intestinal perforation of a CMV ulcer and perforation associated with lymphoma. Appendiceal obstruction with perforation from KS has been reported. Other clinical syndromes mimicking an acute abdomen include mycobacterial peritonitis, massive splenomegaly with splenic infarcts, and intussusception of a mass lesion such as lymphoma, KS, or areas of lymphoid hyperplasia.

Many centers have approached the question of laparotomy in AIDS patients with caution. Early clinical observations indicated substantial short- and long-term postoperative mortality, although the deaths appeared to be related to progression of underlying disease rather than the surgery itself. Other studies showed that specific subgroups of patients, such as patients undergoing splenectomy for refractory thrombocytopenia, had an acceptable postoperative mortality. Further experience has shown that, with the appropriate indication and clinical status, laparotomy can be clinically beneficial.

Gastrointestinal Hemorrhage

Gastrointestinal hemorrhage is not a common problem in AIDS. However, if it occurs, gastrointestinal bleeding may be life threatening.[106] Many causes of gastrointestinal bleeding associated with complications of AIDS have been reported, including localized solitary ulcers in the esophagus or bowel, bleeding duodenal or gastric ulcers with or without associated use of nonsteroidal antiinflammatory agents, and extensive mucosal KS, which is a late or terminal event. Extremely debilitated patients may develop deep anal fissures with hemorrhage. The proper management of gastrointestinal bleeding depends on the precise cause and is related to local therapeutic expertise. Techniques that have been used successfully include injection sclerotherapy of bleeding lesions of KS and angiographic embolization of a bleeding ulcer in the terminal ileum.

The proper management of gastrointestinal bleeding in an AIDS patient probably is not different from that for an immunocompetent patient.

SYMPTOM DIAGNOSIS

Specific recommendations for the evaluation of gastrointestinal symptoms in HIV-seropositive patients are unavailable, because the relevant clinical background about intestinal pathogens in AIDS has not been completely described and because of the diverse levels of sophistication of the clinical units that evaluate such patients. However, general principles can be discussed. Although a substantial proportion of patients have clinical syndromes without identifiable causes and others have only untreatable infections, diagnostic evaluation is indicated because an increasing number of these agents are responsive to specific treatments, and successful therapy is associated with clinical improvement. Supportive therapies may bring clinical benefits even in the absence of cure. Because AIDS patients may be infected with several agents simultaneously, a thorough evaluation is required, even after a single infection has been discovered. The following section is a distillation of clinical experience with AIDS patients with gastrointestinal symptoms and is intended to help streamline the diagnostic evaluations undertaken.

Persistent hiccups usually are associated with central nervous system lesions, such as toxoplasmosis or lymphoma, or with infiltrating diseases on either side of the diaphragm, such as lymphoma or MAC. Treatment with chlorpromazine or similar agents may be effective.

Oral and oropharyngeal complaints are most commonly related to candidiasis or hairy leukoplakia. These disorders may be grossly indistinguishable and may coexist; a response to antifungal therapy favors the former, and a response to acyclovir therapy favors the latter diagnosis. Biopsy or diagnostic electron microscopy rarely is needed.

Many AIDS patients complain of dry mouth or altered taste perception. These symptoms, especially the latter, may be related to a specific medication, although a Sjögren's-like syndrome in AIDS has been reported.[107] Dry mouth also may be related to nasal congestion with mouth breathing or mucus hypersecretion with postnasal drip.

Odynophagia may be a result of viral ulcerations or erosions, after esophageal candidiasis is treated or ruled out. Because the shaggy appearance of the esophageal mucosa on radiography is characteristic but not specific for candidiasis, culture, biopsy, and brushings for cytologic analysis may be needed, especially if symptoms do not respond to treatment.

Dysphagia is caused by esophageal narrowing by infiltrating masses such as KS or lymphoma, esophageal strictures related to ulcers, or muscle spasm associated with inflammatory disorders. True persistent dysphagia is not caused by uncomplicated esophageal candidiasis.

Dyspepsia often results from a specific medication, but epigastric discomfort also may be caused by mucosal ulcerations from CMV or lymphoma. *H pylori* also has been found in some patients. The syndrome suggests bile reflux gastritis or esophagitis in many cases, and the symptoms may respond to prokinetic agents. Duodenal ulcers are distinctly uncommon in AIDS patients.

The most common cause of nausea and vomiting in patients with AIDS is sensitivity to a medication. Antimycobacterial medications are an especially frequent cause for nausea. Persistent vomiting also has been seen in patients with expanding CNS lesions, severe intestinal injury and biliary infestation by *Cryptosporidium*, disseminated mycobacteriosis, and intestinal obstruction from KS or lymphoma. Parasitic infestation causing labyrinthitis and troublesome vertigo has been reported.

Diarrhea is an exceedingly common gastrointestinal symptom in AIDS and occurs with distinct clinical patterns (Table 105-2). The clinical features of diarrhea usually can be explained by the localization and severity of the underlying pathology. In most patients, the diarrhea can be classified as being small bowel (i.e., enteropathic) or colonic in origin, although some patients have features of both types.

Enteropathic diarrhea occurs because of malabsorption and results from primary small intestine diseases such as cryptosporidiosis. There are 3 to 10 bowel movements per day, and they occur at irregular intervals but especially at night or in the early morning. Some of the bowel movements are of large volume, indicating normal compliance in the colon, and others are of small volume. Occasionally, formed stool is passed. The bowel movements are nonbloody and are not associated with tenesmus, although there may be a sense of urgency. Stool volumes are decreased by fasting but may not be abolished. Patients often have no fever and a good appetite.

Patients with colitis have a different clinical presentation. There are multiple unformed or mucoid bowel movements of small volume, which occur at regular intervals throughout the day and night. The small volume indicates decreased rectal compliance caused by the inflammation. Patients often have fever, weakness, and anorexia. There may be abdominal tenderness, and the stool contains occult blood. The most common causes of colitis in AIDS are infection with CMV, *Salmonella*, *Shigella*, and *Campylobacter* and colitis associated with *C difficile* toxin. A significant percentage of patients with colitic symptoms, especially patients with AIDS-related complex, have no identifiable cause, suggesting that the colitis could be related to the HIV infection.

NUTRITIONAL CONSIDERATIONS

Protein-energy malnutrition is a common complication in AIDS. One of the diagnostic criteria for AIDS established by the Centers for Disease Control is HIV seropositivity with wasting, defined as a loss of more than 10% of body weight over 2 months without obvious cause after evaluation.[108] The development of protein-energy malnutrition in AIDS is multifactorial and includes poor food intake, small intestine injury with nutrient malabsorption, and chronic systemic infections with fevers and hypermetabolism.[109]

In a cross-sectional study, AIDS patients had significant depletion of body cell mass and variable depletion of body fat compared with homosexual and heterosexual controls.[110] There was hypoalbuminemia and increased extracellular water content in the AIDS group. Longitudinal studies demonstrated progressive body mass depletion. The relation between malnutrition and survival in patients dying of a wasting illness was examined by analyzing body cell mass depletion as a function of time before death, and a progressive depletion of body cell mass was found.[111] After extrapolation to the time of death, there was a loss of body weight to one third of that below ideal and a loss of body cell mass of almost one half of estimated premorbid values. The degree of depletion observed is similar to that seen in historical precedents of death from starvation, such as occurred in the Warsaw ghetto in 1943. These results imply that death from wasting in AIDS may be related to the magnitude rather than the cause of tissue depletion.

Progressive wasting is not a constant feature of AIDS but results from complications that may be definable and treatable. This was demonstrated in a group of clinically stable AIDS patients who maintained body mass over a 6-week follow-up period.[112] However, several studies have shown that metabolic alterations, such as elevated resting metabolic rate and fasting serum triglycerides, may occur early in the disease course.[113,114] Specific associations have been made between metabolic and immunologic alterations, such as the correlation of fasting hypertriglyceridemia with circulating levels of interferon-α.[115]

An important question in nutritional support is the po-

TABLE 105-2
Clinical Differentiation between Small Intestine and Colonic Types of Diarrhea

CHARACTERISTIC	SMALL INTESTINE TYPE	COLONIC TYPE
Frequency	3–8 times/d	3–30 times/d
Volume	Variable, often large	Small
Intervals*	Variable	Regular
Formed Stools (?)	Rarely	Never
Blood in Stools	No	Occult
Urgency	Yes	No
Tenesmus	No	Sometimes
Fever	No	Yes
Debiliation	Mild, Moderate	Moderate to severe
Appetite	Fair to good	Fair to poor
Pathophysiology	Malabsorption	Inflammation

* Refers to regularity or lack of regularity in bowel movements during the day.

tential for successful body mass repletion. Studies have shown that proper use of enteral or parenteral modes of nutritional support may be associated with body cell mass repletion.[116,117] Weight gain may be associated with the use of AZT (Retrovir), an antiviral agent that inhibits HIV replication.[118] Successful treatment of CMV colitis with ganciclovir also was associated with repletion of body cell mass.[76]

The provision of nutritional support should be based on the precise nutritional problem. Appetite stimulants can be tried after appropriate work-up.[119] Enteral nutrition is sufficient therapy for patients whose major problem is impaired ingestion or swallowing of food, but long-term parenteral nutrition may be indicated for patients with severe uncorrectable malabsorption. Patients with serious systemic infections typically do not respond well to nutritional therapy unless the underlying infection is brought under control. However, a temporizing period of parenteral nutritional support may be indicated.

A national task force on nutrition in AIDS has been created, and an initial set of guidelines on nutritional support have been published.[120] Several general recommendations were made. Patients should be counseled as early as possible concerning good nutritional practices and the importance of maintaining nutritional balance. Body weight should be monitored closely, and the development of weight loss should prompt an investigation as to the cause. Ad libitum oral food intake is the first choice for providing nutrition, but if this is not sufficient, enteral nutritional therapy, by volitional or nonvolitional means, should be used. Although temporary support by partial parenteral nutrition may be indicated for a variety of reasons, long-term parenteral therapy should be used only if enteral therapy is not feasible or successful.

The decision to provide nutritional support for an AIDS patient may be an emotionally charged issue because of the ultimately fatal nature of the disease and the costs of providing the support. Formal cost-benefit and cost-effectiveness analyses have not been performed for AIDS. Although the costs of nutritional support can be identified and calculated, the ability of nutritional therapy to allow patients to exist outside of the hospital rather than as inpatients or to lead productive lives is a potential benefit and cost savings that has not been quantitated.

The general indications for providing specialized nutritional support are the same in AIDS as in any other disease: progressive weight loss occurring in the clinical context of an illness that is otherwise manageable and the potential for prolonged or improved survival with nutritional support. Indications for exclusion are the inability to stabilize an acute illness and no potential for prolonged survival.

The enteral route is the preferred site of nutrient delivery if nutritional support is needed. It is important to remember that fat malabsorption is common in AIDS, even in patients without diarrhea.[109] For some patients who may not tolerate the standard enteral formulas, switching to a fat-reduced or elemental diet may be beneficial. A convenient way to administer chronic enteral feedings is through a percutaneous endoscopic gastrostomy tube, which reduces the morbidity of gastrostomy tube placement. Opiates or other antidiarrheals can be added to the nutrient formula. Small amounts of bulk-forming agents also can be added if the solution does not become too concentrated and clog the feeding tube. Pro-

spective longitudinal studies have demonstrated that feeding through a percutaneous endoscopic gastrostomy tube may be associated with body cell mass repletion in AIDS patients.[117]

Parenteral nutritional support can be given as partial or total parenteral nutrition. Partial parenteral nutrition can be given by peripheral vein and is intended only for short-term application of 10 days or less. The primary calorie substrate is lipid, and no more than about 1300 kcal/day can be administered. Long-term parenteral support is provided by total parenteral nutrition (TPN). Glucose is the primary caloric substrate in TPN, although lipid emulsions can supply up to 30% of calories. Studies have documented body cell mass repletion in AIDS patients with malabsorption syndromes who were treated with TPN.[116] The use of intravenous lipid emulsions may have to be limited, because many AIDS patients have baseline hypertriglyceridemia that may be related to increased triglyceride synthesis and reduced triglyceride clearance.

Malnutrition in AIDS is a complex process, and the approach to nutritional therapy should be based on knowledge of the underlying disorder. Effective nutritional therapy can enhance the quality of life and the length of survival for AIDS patients, as it does for patients with other chronic diseases.

Acknowledgment

This work was supported in part by grant AI 21414 from the National Institutes of Health.

The reader is referred to Chapter 5, The Immune System; Chapter 46, Approach to Gastrointestinal Problems in the Immunocompromised Patient; Chapter 56, Esophageal Infections; Chapter 70, Small Intestine: Infections With Common Bacterial and Viral Pathogens; Chapter 71, Chronic Infections of the Small Intestine; Chapter 84, Bacterial Infections of the Colon; Chapter 106, Parasitic Diseases: Protozoa; Chapter 107, Parasitic Diseases: Helminths; Chapter 109, Gastrointestinal Manifestations of Systemic Diseases; Chapter 130, Endoscopic Mucosal Biopsy; and Chapter 131, Microbiologic Studies.

REFERENCES

1. Gottlieb MS, Schroff R, Schanker HM, et al. *Pneumocystis carinii* pneumonia and mucosal candidiasis in previously healthy homosexual men: evidence of a newly acquired cellular immunodeficiency. N Engl J Med 1981;305:1425.
2. Siegel FP, Lopez C, Hammer GS, et al. Severe acquired immunodeficiency in male homosexuals manifested by chronic perianal ulcerative herpes simplex lesions. N Engl J Med 1981;305:1439.
3. Kaslow RS, Phair JP, Friedman HB, et al. Infection with the human immunodeficiency virus: clinical manifestations and their relationship to immune deficiency. Ann Intern Med 1987;107:474.
4. Nathanson N, Georgsson G, Palsson PA, et al. Experimental visna in Icelandic sheep: the prototype lentviral infection. Rev Infect Dis 1985;7:75.
5. Ho DD, Pomerantz RJ, Kaplan JC. Pathogenesis of infection with human immunodeficiency virus. N Engl J Med 1987;317:278.
6. Fox CH, Kotler DP, Tierney AR, et al. Detection of HIV-1 RNA in intestinal lamina propria of patients with AIDS and gastrointestinal disease. J Infect Dis 1989;159:467.

7. Nelson JA, Wiley CA, Reynolds-Kohler C, et al. Human immunodeficiency virus detected in bowel epithelium from patients with gastrointestinal symptoms. Lancet 1988;2:259.

8. Mathijs JM, Hing M, Grierson J, et al. HIV infection of rectal mucosa. Lancet 1988;1:1111.

9. Kotler DP, Reka S, Borcich A, Cronin W. Detection, localization and quantitation of HIV-associated antigens in intestinal biopsies from HIV-infected patients. Am J Pathol 1991;139:823.

10. Rene E, Jarry A, Brousse N, et al. Demonstration of HIV infection of the gut in AIDS patients: relation with symptoms and other digestive infection. Gastroenterology 1988;94:373A.

11. Adachi A, Koenig S, Gendelman HE, et al. Productive, persistent infection of human colorectal cell lines with human immunodeficiency virus. J Virol 1987;61:209.

12. Yahi N, Fantini J, Chermann JC. Infection of HIV-1 and HIV-2 through the luminal and serosal sides of polarized human intestinal epithelial cells. AIDS 1992;6:335.

13. Hoover EA, Mullins JI, Quackenbush SL, et al. Experimental transmission and pathogenesis of immunodeficiency syndrome in cats. Blood 1987;70,1880.

14. Cerf-Bensussan N, Quaroni A, Kurnick JT, Bhan AK. Intraepithelial lymphocytes modulate Ia expression by intestinal epithelial cells. J Immunol 1984;132:2244.

15. Fauci AS. AIDS: immunopathogenic mechanisms and research strategies. Clin Res 1987;35:503.

16. Dougherty JP, Temin HM. Determination of the rate of base pair substitution and insertion mutations in retrovirus replication. J Virol 1988;62:2817.

17. Wahren B, Morpheldt-Mansson L, Biberfield G, et al. Characteristics of the specific cell-mediated immune response in human immunodeficeincy virus infection. J Virol 1987;61:2017.

18. Walker BD, Chakrabarti S, Moss B, et al. HIV-specific cytotoxic T lymphocytes in seropositive individuals. Nature 1987;328:345.

19. Rook AH, Lane HC, Folks T, et al. Sera from HTLV-III/LAV antibody positive individuals mediate antibody dependent cellular cytotoxicity against HTLV-III/LAV infected T cells. J Immunol 1987;138:1064.

20. Grieco MH, Reddy MM, Kothari HB, et al. Elevated β_2-microglobulin and lysozyme levels in patients with acquired immune deficiency syndrome. Clin Immunol Immunopathol 1984;32:174.

21. Lambin P, Desjobert H, Debbia M, et al. Serum neopterin and β-2-microglobulin in anti-HIV positive blood donors. Lancet 1986;2:1216.

22. Allain J-P, Laurian Y, Payl DA, et al. Long term evaluation of HIV antigen and antibodies to p24 and gp41 in patients with hemophilia: potential clinical importance. N Engl J Med 1987;317:1114.

23. Seligmann M, Chess L, Fahey JL, et al. AIDS—an immunologic reevaluation. N Engl J Med 1984;11:1286.

24. Nossal GJV. Current concepts: immunology—the basic components of the immune system. N Engl J Med 1987;316:1320.

25. Schnittman SM, Denning SM, Greenhoouse JJ, et al. Evidence for susceptibility of intrathymic T-cell precursors and their progeny carrying T-cell antigen receptor phenotypes TCR alpha/beta+ and TCR gamma/delta+ to human immunodeficiency virus infection. A mechanism for CD4+ (T4) lymphocyte depletion. Proc Natl Acad Sci U S A 1990;87:7727.

26. Savino W, Dardenne M, Marche C, et al. Thymic epithelium in AIDS: an immunohistologic study. Am J Pathol 1986;122:302.

27. Rodgers VD, Fassett R, Kagnoff MF. Abnormalities in intestinal mucosal T cells in homosexual populations including those with the lymphadenopathy syndrome and acquired immunodeficiency syndrome. Gastroenterology 1986;90:552.

28. Kotler DP, Tierney AR, Scholes JV. Intestinal plasma cell alterations in the acquired immunodeficiency syndrome. Dig Dis Sci 1987;32:129.

29. Jackson S, Dawson LM, Kotler DP. IgA$_1$ is the major immunoglobulin component of immune complexes in the acquired immune deficiency syndrome. J Clin Immunol 1988;8:64.

30. Jackson S, Tarkowski A, Collins JE, et al. Occurence of polymeric immunoglobulin A1 rheumatoid factor in the acquired immune deficiency syndrome. J Clin Immunol 1988;9:390.

31. DiMassimo AM, Placido R, Bach S, et al. Cytotoxic activity of intestinal lamina propria lymphocytes on human immunodeficiency virus (HIV) infected cells. Immunology 1992;76:117.

32. Klein RS, Harris CA, Small CB, et al. Oral candidiasis in high risk patients as the initial manifestation of the acquired immunodeficiency syndrome. N Engl J Med 1984;311:354.

33. Lake-Bakaar G, Quadros E, Beidas S, et al. Gastric secretory failure in patients with the acquired immunodeficiency syndrome (AIDS). Ann Intern Med 1988;1:502.

34. Greenspan JS, Greenspan D, Lennette ET, et al. Replication of Epstein-Barr virus within the epithelial cells of oral "hairy" leukoplakia, an AIDS-associated lesion. N Engl J Med 1985;313:1564.

35. Friedman-Kein AE. Viral origin of hairy leukoplakia. Lancet 1986;2:694.

36. Kotler DP, Wilson CS, Haroutounian G, Fox CH. Detection of HIV-1 RNA in solitary esophageal ulcers in two patients with the acquired immunodeficiency syndrome. Am J Gastroenterol 1989;84:313.

37. Kotler DP, Reka S, Orenstein JM, Fox CH. Chronic idiopathic esophageal ulceration in the acquired immunodeficiency syndrome: characterization and treatment with corticosteroids. J Clin Gastroenterol 1992;15:284.

38. Rabeneck L, Popovic M, Gartner S, et al. Acute HIV infection presenting with painful swallowing and esophageal ulcers. JAMA 1990;263:2318.

39. Wilcox CM, Schwartz DA. A pilot study of oral corticosteroid therapy for idiopathic esophageal ulcerations associated with human immunodeficiency virus infection. Am J Med 1992;93:131.

40. Bach MC, Valenti AJ, Howell DA, Smith TJ. Odynophagia from aphthous ulcers of the pharynx and esophagus in the acquired immunodeficiency syndrome. Ann Intern Med 1988;109:338.

41. Winkler JR, Murray PA. Peridontal disease, a potential oral expression of AIDS may be a rapidly progressive peridontitis. Calif Dent Assoc J 1987;15:20.

42. Lake-Bakaar G, Tom W, Lake-Bekaar D, et al. Gastropathy and ketoconazole malabsorption in the acquired immunodeficiency syndrome. Ann Intern Med 1988;109:471.

43. Herzlich BC, Schiano TD, Moussa Z, et al. Decreased intrinsic factor secretion in AIDS: relation to parietal cell acid secretory capacity and vitamin B$_{12}$ malabsorption. Am J Gastroenterol 1992;87:1781-8.

44. Shaffer RT, LaHatte LJ, Kelly JW, et al. Gastric acid secretion in HIV-1 infection. Am J Gastroenterol 1992;87:1777.

45. Battan R, Raviglione M, Palagiarro A, et al. *Helicobacter pylori* infection in patients with acquired immune deficiency syndrome. Am J Gastroenterol 1990;85:1576.

46. Levine ND. A newly revised classification of the protozoa. J Protozool 1980;27:37.

47. Sloper KS, Dourmashkin RR, Bird RB, et al. Case report: chronic malabsorption due to cryptosporidiosis in a child with immunoglobulin deficiency. Gut 1982;23:80.

48. Clayton FC, Heller TH, Reka S, Kotler DP. Variation in the distribution of cryptosporidiosis in AIDS. Am J Clin Pathol (in press).

49. Casemore DP, Armstrong M, Sands RL. Laboratory diagnosis of cryptosporidiosis. J Clin Pathol 1985;38:1337.

50. Tzipori S, Roberton D, Chapman C. Remission of diarrhoea due to cryptosporidiosis in an immunodeficient child treated with hyperimmune bovine colostrum. Br Med J 1986;293:1276.

51. Cello JP, Grendell JH, Basuk P, et al. Effect of octreotide in refractory AIDS-associated diarrhea. Ann Intern Med 1991;115:705.

52. Canning EU, Lom J. The microsporidia of vertebrates. New York: Academic Press, 1986.

53. Orenstein J, Chiang J, Steinberg W, et al. Intestinal microsporidiosis as a cause of diarrhea in HIV-infected patients: a report of 20 cases. Hum Pathol 1990;21:475.

54. Cali A, Kotler DP, Orenstein JM. *Septata intestinalis* N.G., N.SP., an intestinal microsporidian associated with chronic

diarrhea and dissemination in AIDS patients. J Eukaryot Microbiol 1993;40:101.

55. Orenstein JM. Microsporidiosis in the acquired immunodeficiency syndrome. J Parasitol 1991;77:843.

56. Orenstein JM, Dieterich DT, Kotler DP. Systemic dissemination by a newly recognized microsporidia species in the acquired immunodeficiency syndrome. AIDS 1992;6:1143.

57. Kotler DP, Reka S, Chow K, Orenstein JM. Effects of enteric parasitoses and HIV infection upon small intestinal structure and function in patients with AIDS. J Clin Gastroenterol 1993;16:10.

58. Weber R, Bryan RT, Owen RL, et al. Improved light microscopical detection of microsporidia spores in stool and duodenal samples. N Engl J Med 1992;326:161.

59. Dieterich DT, Lew EA, Kotler DP, et al. Treatment with albendazole for intestinal disease due to *Enterocytozoon bieneusi* in patients with AIDS. J Infect Dis 1994;169:173.

60. Orenstein JM, Dieterich DT, Kotler DP. Albendazole as a treatment for intestinal and disseminated microsporidiosis due to *Septata intestinalis* in AIDS patients. AIDS Suppl 1994;7:540.

61. DeHovitz JA, Pape JW, Boncy M, Johnson WD Jr. Clinical manifestation of *Isospora belli* infection in patients with the acquired immunodeficiency syndrome. N Engl J Med 1986;315:87.

62. Kotler DP, Orenstein JM. Diarrhea and malabsorption due to enterocyte-adherent bacterial infection in a patient with AIDS. Ann Intern Med 1993;119:127.

63. Nash TE, Agrawal A, Adam RD, Conrad JT, Merritt JW Jr. Antigenic variation in *Giardia lamblia*. J Immunol 1988;141:636.

64. Stevens D, Frank D, Mahmoud AAF. Thymus dependency of host resistance to *Giardia muris* infection in nude mice. J Immunol 1978;120:680.

65. Smith PD, Macher AM, Bookman MA, et al. *Salmonella typhimurium* enteritis and bacteremia in the acquired immunodeficiency syndrome. Ann Intern Med 1985;102:207.

66. Baskin DH, Lax JD, Barenberg D. *Shigella* bacteremia in patients with acquired immune deficiency. Am J Gastroenterol 1987;82:338.

67. Pasternak J, Bolivar R, Hopfer RL, et al. Bacteremia caused by *Campylobacter*-like organisms in two male homosexuals. Ann Intern Med 1984;101:339.

68. Hornick RB, Musik SI, Wenzel R, et al. The Broad St. pump revisited: response of volunteers to ingested cholera vibrios. Bull N Y Acad Med 1971;47:1181.

69. Oster W. Typhoid fever. In: Osler W, ed. The principles and practice of medicine. New York: D Appleton, 1892:2.

70. Easmon CSF, Crane JP. Uptake of ciprofloxacin by macrophages. J Clin Pathol 1985;38:442.

71. Reichert CM, O'Leary TJ, Levens DL, et al. Autopsy pathology in the acquired immune deficiency syndrome. Am J Pathol 1983;112:357.

72. Weller TH. The cytomegalovirus: ubiquitous agents with protean clinical manifestations. N Engl J Med 1971;285:203.

73. Kotler DP, Baer JW, Scholes JV. Isolated ileitis due to cytomegalovirus in a patient with AIDS. Gastrointest Endosc 1991;37:571.

74. Koretz SH, Buhles WC, Brewin A, et al. Treatment of serious cytomegalovirus infections using 9-(1,3-dihydroxy-2-propoxymethyl) guanine in patients with AIDS and other immunodeficiencies. N Engl J Med 1986;314:801.

75. Chachoua A, Dieterich D, Krasinski K, et al. 9-(1,3-Dihydroxy-2-propoxymethyl)guanine in the treatment of cytomegalovirus gastrointestinal disease with the acquired immunodeficiency syndrome. Ann Intern Med 1987;107:133.

76. Kotler DP, Tierney AR, Altilio D, et al. Body mass repletion during ganciclovir therapy of cytomegalovirus infections in patients with the acquired immunodeficiency syndrome. Arch Intern Med 1989;149:901.

77. Kotler DP, Culpepper-Morgan J, Tierney AR, Klein EB. Treatment of disseminated cytomegalovirus infection with 9-(1,3-dihydroxy-2-propoxymethyl)guanine: evidence of prolonged survival in patients with the acquired immunodeficiency syndrome. AIDS Research 1987;2:299.

78. Dieterich DT, Kotler DP, Busch D, et al. Ganciclovir treatment of cytomegalovirus colitis in AIDS: a randomized, double-blind, placebo-controlled multicenter trial. J Infect Dis 1992;167:278.

79. Weber JN, Thom S, Barrison I, et al. Cytomegalovirus colitis and esophageal ulceration in the context of AIDS: clinical manifestations and preliminary report of treatment with foscarnet. Gut 1987;28:482.

80. Culpepper-Morgan J, Kotler DP, Tierney AR, Scholes JV. Evaluation of diagnostic criteria for disseminated cytomegalovirus infection in the acquired immune deficiency syndrome. Am J Gastroenterol 1987;82:1264.

81. Young LS, Interlied CB, Berlin OG, Gottlieb MS. Mycobacterial infections in AIDS patients, with an emphasis on the *Mycobacterium avium* complex. Rev Infect Dis 1986;8:1024.

82. Johnson JL, Shiratsuchi H, Toba H, Elner JJ. Preservation of monocyte effector functions against *Mycobacterium avium intracellulare* in patients with AIDS. Infect Immun 1991;59:3639.

83. Roth RI, Owen RL, Keren DF, Volberding PA. Intestinal infection with *Mycobacterium avium* in acquired immunodeficiency syndrome (AIDS): histological and clinical comparison with Whipple's disease. Dig Dis Sci 1985;30:497.

84. Elson CO, Reilly RW, Rosenberg IH. Small intestinal injury in the graft versus host reaction: an innocent bystander phenomenon. Gastroenterology 1977;72:886.

85. Kotler DP, Weaver SC, Terzakis JA. Ultrastructural features of epithelial cell degeneration in rectal crypts of patients with AIDS. Am J Surg Pathol 1986;10:531.

86. Kotler DP, Reka S, Clayton FC. Intestinal mucosal inflammation associated with human immunodeficiency virus infection. Dig Dis Sci 1993;38:1119.

87. Clayton F, Cronin WJ, Reka S, et al. Rectal mucosal histopathology in HIV infection varies with disease stage and HIV protein content. Gastroenterology 1992;103:919.

88. Reka S, Kotler DP. Detection and localization of HIV RNA and TNF mRNA in rectal biopsies from patients with AIDS. Cytokine 1993;5:305.

89. Hing M, Goldschmidt C, Mathijs JM, et al. Chronic colitis associated with human immunodeficiency virus infection. Med J Aust 1992;156:683.

90. Hill SA, Coghill SB. Human papillomavirus in squamous cell carcinoma of anus. Lancet 1986;2:1333.

91. Friedman-Kien AE, Laubenstein LJ, Rubinstein PI, et al. Disseminated Kaposi's sarcoma in homosexual men. Ann Intern Med 1982;96:693.

92. Nakamura S, Salahuddin SZ, Biberfeld P, et al. Kaposi's sarcoma cells: long-term culture with growth factor from retrovirus-infected CD4+ T cells. Science 1988;242:426.

93. Friedman SL, Wright TL, Altman DF. Gastrointestinal Kaposi's sarcoma in patients with acquired immunodeficiency syndrome: endoscopic and autopsy findings. Gastroenterology 1985;98:102.

94. Ziegler JL, Beckstead JA, Volberding PA, et al: Non-Hodgkin's lymphoma in 90 homosexual men: relation to generalized lymphadenopathy and the acquired immunodeficiency syndrome. N Engl J Med 1984;311:565.

95. Petersen JM, Tubbs RR, Savage RA, et al. Small noncleaved B cell Burkitt-like lymphoma with chromosome t(8;14) translocation and Epstein-Barr virus nuclear-associated antigen in a homosexual man with acquired immune deficiency syndrome. Am J Med 1985;78:141.

96. Weiss LM, Movahed LA, Warnke RA, Sklar J. Detection of Epstein-Barr viral genomes in Reed-Sternberg cells of Hodgkin's disease. N Engl J Med 1989;320:502.

97. Schnittman SM, Lane HC, Higgins SE, et al. Direct polyclonal activation of human B lymphocytes by acquired immune deficiency syndrome. Science 1986;233:1084.

98. Cappell MS. Hepatobiliary manifestations of the acquired immunodeficiency syndrome. Am J Gastroenterol 1992;86:1.

99. Novick DM, Farci P, Croxson TS, et al. Effect of human immunodeficiency virus on the increased severity of liver disease associated with delta hepatitis. Gastroenterology 1988;94:578A.

100. Martin P, DiBisceglie AM, Kassianides C, et al. Rapidly progressive non-A, non-B hepatitis in patients with human im-

munodeficiency virus infection. Gastroenterology 1989;97: 1559.

101. Harrington PT, Gutierrez JJ, Ramirez-Ronda CH, et al. Granulomatous hepatitis. Rev Infect Dis 1982;4:638.

102. Schneiderman DJ, Cello JP, Laing FC. Papillary stenosis and sclerosing cholangitis in the acquired immunodeficiency syndrome. Ann Intern Med 1987;106:546.

103. Marche C, Zoubi D, Michon C. Les lesions hepatiques, biliaires et pancreatiques au cours de l'infection par LAV-HTLVIII. Ann Pathol 1986;6:287.

104. Seidlin M, Lambert JS, Dolin R, Valentine FT. Pancreatitis and pancreatic dysfunction in patients taking dideoxyinosine. AIDS 1992;6:831.

105. Bouchard P, Sai P, Reach G, et al. Diabetes mellitus following pentamidine-induced hypoglycemia in humans. Diabetes 1982;31:40.

106. Parente F, Cernuschi M, Valsecchi L, et al. Acute upper gastrointestinal bleeding in patients with AIDS: a relatively uncommon condition associated with reduced survival. J Br Soc Gastroenterol 1991;32:987.

107. Gordon J, Golbus J, Kurtides E. Chronic lymphadenopathy and Sjögren's syndrome in a homosexual man. N Engl J Med 1984;311:1441.

108. Revision of the CDC surveillance case definition for acquired immunodeficiency syndrome. MMWR Morb Mortal Wkly Rep 1987;36:3.

109. Kotler DP, Gaetz HP, Klein EB, et al. Enteropathy associated with the acquired immunodeficiency syndrome. Ann Intern Med 1984;101:421.

110. Kotler DP, Wang J, Pierson R. Studies of body composition in patients with the acquired immunodeficiency syndrome. Am J Clin Nutr 1985;42:1255.

111. Kotler DP, Tierney AR, Wang J, Pierson RN Jr. The magnitude of body cell mass depletion determines the timing of death from wasting in AIDS. Am J Clin Nutr 1989;50:444.

112. Kotler DP, Tierney AR, Brenner SK, et al. Preservation of short-term energy balance in clinically stable patients with AIDS. Am J Clin Nutr 1990;52:7.

113. Hommes M, Romijn JA, Godfried MH, et al. Increased resting energy expenditure in human immuodeficiency virus-infected men. Metabolism 1990;39:1186.

114. Grunfeld C, Kotler DP, Hamadeh R, et al. Hypertriglyceridemia in the acquired immunodeficiency syndrome. Am J Med 1989;86:27.

115. Grunfeld C, Kotler DP, Shigenga JK, et al. Circulating interferon alpha levels and hypertriglyceridemia in the acquired immunodeficiency syndrome. Am J Med 1991;90:154.

116. Kotler DP, Tierney AR, Culpepper-Morgan JA, et al. Effect of home total parenteral nutrition upon body composition in AIDS. J Parenter Enteral Nutr 1990;14:454.

117. Kotler DP, Tierney AR, Ferraro R, et al. Effect of enteral feeding upon body cell mass in AIDS. Am J Clin Nutr 199153:149.

118. Yarchoan R, Weinhold KJ, Lyerly HK, et al. Administration of 3'azido-3'deoxythymidine, an inhibitor of HTLV-III/LAV replication, to patients with AIDS or AIDS-related complex. Lancet 1986;1:575.

119. Von Roenn JH, Murphy RL, Weber KM, et al. Megesterol acetate for treatment of cachexia associated with human immunodeficiency virus infection. Ann Intern Med 1988;109: 840.

120. Winick M and the National Task Force on Nutrition in AIDS. Guidelines on nutritional support in AIDS. Nutrition 1989;5: 390.

Textbook of Gastroenterology, second edition, edited by Tadataka Yamada. JB Lippincott Company, Philadelphia © 1995.

CHAPTER 106

Parasitic Diseases: Protozoa

David R. Hill   William A. Petri, Jr.   Richard L. Guerrant

Entamoeba histolytica (AMEBIASIS)

The cytolytic protozoan parasite *Entamoeba histolytica* is the cause of amebiasis. Human disease from infection with *E histolytica* includes asymptomatic colonization, invasive colitis, liver abscess, intestinal perforation, and peritonitis. Amebae were first isolated from the stool of patients with cholera by the surgeon Timothy Lewis in 1869, although association of dysentery with liver abscess had been noted 40 years earlier by James Annesley in his monographs on the prevalent diseases of India. The potential for amebae to cause colitis was demonstrated by F. Losch in St. Petersburg, Russia, in 1874. The understanding of the pathogenesis of amebiasis was greatly advanced by Robert Koch, who performed autopsies on two patients with dysentery and liver abscess and observed amebae at the base of colonic ulcers and in capillaries near the liver abscesses. Councilman and Lafleur reviewed 14 cases of amebiasis from Baltimore at the turn of the century. They described the flask-shaped amebic ulcer in the colon and introduced the terms *amebic dysentery* and *amebic liver abscess*. Quinke and Roos identified the cyst of *E histolytica* as the infective form at about the same time. Antiamebic therapy was introduced by Leonard Rogers in Calcutta in 1912, who treated three patients with emetine. The axenic (free of associated microorganisms) culture of *E histolytica* was accomplished by Diamond in 1961.[1]

There are other enteric amebae, mostly nonpathogenic, that must be distinguished from *E histolytica*. *Entamoeba gingivalis* is found only in the mouths of those with poor dental hygiene. It has no identified cyst form. It can be confused with *E histolytica* in the sputum of patients with suspected amebic lung abscess. *Entamoeba hartmanni* is a commensal organism with morphology identical to that of *E histolytica*, but with smaller cyst and trophozoite sizes. *Entamoeba coli* is also a nonpathogenic protozoan whose cysts contain up to eight nuclei. *Entamoeba polecki* has uninucleate cysts and infects pigs and monkeys in the tropics, but rarely causes human disease. *Dientamoeba fragilis* does not have a cyst form, and its trophozoites are recognizable because they are binucleate. *D fragilis* can cause a prolonged or inflammatory diarrhea. *Endolimax nana* and *Iodamoeba butschlii* are nonpathogenic commensals of the large bowel; both trophozoite forms are smaller than *E histolytica*, with sluggish motility. *I butschlii* cysts contain a large glycogen vacuole that stains with iodine.[1]

The life cycle of *E histolytica* consists of the infective cyst and the potentially tissue-invasive trophozoite. Infection begins with the ingestion of fecally contaminated material containing *E histolytica* cysts. The cysts are resistant to gastric acidity. Excystation occurs in the large or small bowel, where the cysts' four nuclei divide before cytoplasmic division occurs to form eight trophozoites. The trophozoites colonize the large bowel, produce cysts, and in a minority of infected people invade the colonic epithelium to initiate intestinal and extraintestinal amebiasis. Amebic cysts are never found within invaded tissue.[1]

Epidemiology

Amebiasis is a common worldwide parasitic infection with a prevalence in 1984 of 500 million infected people, with 40 to 50 million cases of colitis or abscess resulting in 40,000 to 110,000 deaths annually. *E histolytica* is surpassed only by malaria and schistosomiasis as a leading parasitic cause of death. Primates and humans are the only known reservoirs of *E histolytica*, and there are no known arthropod vectors. If an antiamebic vaccine that prevented colonization of the large bowel could be developed, it would be theoretically possible to eliminate *E histolytica* as a cause of human infection.

The parasite's distribution is worldwide, although the preponderance of morbidity and mortality is experienced in Central and South America, Africa, and India. An increased severity of illness is seen in malnourished people, the very young and old, pregnant women, and patients receiving corticosteroids. For example, invasive amebiasis in 85 malnourished, hospitalized patients in Dhaka, Bangladesh, was most common in children 2 to 3 years of age and in adults older than 40 years of age, with an overall 29% case fatality rate despite hospitalization and antiamebic chemotherapy.[2]

Epidemiologic studies have identified groups at increased risk for amebic infection in developed nations where amebiasis is uncommon in the general population (Table 106-1).

Pathogenesis and Immunology

Ingestion of *E histolytica* cysts initiates amebic infection. After excystation to the trophozoite, large bowel colonization occurs. In the minority of patients, colonization is followed by the disruption of intestinal mucosal barriers, leading to the trophozoite's adherence to and subsequent contact-dependent lysis of the intestinal epithelial cells. Colonization and virulence may be influenced by the strain of *E histolytica* ("pathogenic zymodemes"), interactions with the colonic bacterial flora, resistance to complement-mediated lysis, and host factors, including age, malnutrition, and corticosteroid therapy. *E histolytica* contains several acid, thiol-dependent, and neutral proteases as well as collagenases that may be involved in the disruption of the protective intestinal mucosal barriers. Amebic production of an extracellular enterotoxin may be responsible for the mucosal inflammation without ulceration that occurs before amebic attachment to the colonic epithelium. Lysates of *E histolytica* contain enterotoxins and cytotoxins as well as serotonin; however, none of these has been shown to be released from intact trophozoites in the large bowel.

Adherence of *E histolytica* to the intestinal surface initiates the host tissue lysis for which the organism is named. Amebae kill mammalian cells in culture in a contact-dependent manner.[3] The contact between amebae and target cells in vitro is mediated by an amebic galactose or *N*-acetyl-D-galactosamine

---

TABLE 106-1
Groups at Increased Risk for *Entamoeba histolytica* Infection in Developed Nations

Immigrants from endemic areas
Long-term visitors to endemic areas
Promiscuous male homosexuals
Patients with the acquired immunodeficiency syndrome
Institutionalized people

binding adherence lectin.[4,5] Blockade of the adherence lectin with galactose prevents amebic adherence to and lysis of target cells. Human colonic mucin contains galactose-terminal glycoproteins, which, in vitro, are high-affinity ligands for the amebic adherence lectin.[6] These colonic mucin glycoproteins probably represent an in vivo receptor for amebic attachment and may serve as a protective barrier to protect the intestinal epithelial cells from amebic contact-mediated lysis. An early event in target cell lysis is an increase in the target cell intracellular calcium.[7] Cytolytic activity requires the maintenance of an acid pH in amebic intracellular vesicles, is enhanced by phorbol esters, and may involve an amebic pore-forming protein.[1,8–10,11]

The migration of amebae from colonic lesions to the liver is probably by way of the portal vein. Areas of amebic invasion in the colon and liver contain amorphous eosinophilic debris as a result of the tissue lysis by the amebae and lack an exuberant inflammatory response, perhaps because of the trophozoites' ability to lyse neutrophils and monocytes.[12,13]

Humoral and cell-mediated immune responses have been documented in patients recovering from invasive *E histolytica* infection. The parasite's adherence lectin is the major antigen recognized by the immune sera of patients with amebic liver abscess or amebic colitis. Although nonimmune T cells and macrophages are lysed by the amebae, immune T lymphocytes or interferon-γ–activated macrophages have the ability to kill trophozoites in vitro. Recurrence of invasive amebiasis after cure of amebic liver abscess or invasive colitis is unusual. Of 1021 patients with amebic liver abscess in Mexico City followed for 5 years, only 3 (0.29%) had a second abscess.

Clinical Presentation

The recognized clinical presentations of amebiasis are listed in Table 106-2. The variety of clinical manifestations from *E histolytica* infection may be partly responsible for the not infrequent failure of physicians in developed countries to diagnose amebiasis.

TABLE 106-2
Clinical Manifestations of *Entamoeba histolytica* Infection

Intestinal Disease
Noninvasive intestinal colonization
Diarrhea in patients with the acquired immunodeficiency syndrome
Acute amebic rectocolitis
Chronic nondysenteric intestinal amebiasis
Ameboma
Toxic megacolon
Amebic peritonitis secondary to perforation
Amebic strictures

Extraintestinal Disease
Liver abscess, rarely with direct extension to thorax, pericardium, or
   peritoneum
Brain abscess
Cutaneous amebiasis
Venereal infection

Intestinal Disease

In most patients infected with *E histolytica*, amebic colitis or liver abscess do not develop. These colonized patients may note occasional abdominal colic or a change in bowel habits, or they may be asymptomatic. *Noninvasive colonization* with *E histolytica* is confirmed by the lack of trophozoites containing ingested erythrocytes, the lack of blood in the stool, and normal-appearing mucosa on colonoscopy. Most of these patients remain asymptomatic without treatment, and over a period of months the infection clears; however, in a small percentage of colonized patients followed for months to years, invasive amebiasis subsequently develops.

E histolytica infection is a *sexually transmitted disease* in male homosexuals. Amebic infection has been associated with oral-anal contact and multiple sexual partners. Up to one third of urban homosexual men have been found to harbor *E histolytica*. Gastrointestinal symptoms have been common complaints in these patients but have not been correlated with the presence of *E histolytica* infection. *E histolytica* isolates from homosexual men have been determined by isoenzyme analysis to belong to "nonpathogenic zymodemes" or strains. It has been recommended that *E histolytica* isolates belonging to nonpathogenic zymodemes be reclassified as *E dispar* because of genetic evidence that they are a distinct species.[14,15]

Patients with *acute amebic rectocolitis* complain of 1 to 3 weeks of a gradually increasing frequency of grossly bloody diarrheal bowel movements with abdominal pain and tenderness. Constitutional symptoms are mild, and many patients continue to work and retain their appetites. Only about one fifth of patients will have had more than 4 weeks of illness. Diarrhea and dysentery are seen in virtually all patients, whereas fever is present in only one third. Weight loss is common. Fecal leukocytes may not be present in the stool, but virtually all patients' stools will be heme positive. The mortality from uncomplicated amebic colitis was less than 1% in a 20-year series of 3013 adults from South Africa.[16] In contrast, a mortality rate of 29% was seen in malnourished patients from Bangladesh.[2]

Chronic nondysenteric intestinal amebiasis has been mistakenly diagnosed as ulcerative colitis, with subsequently disastrous complications from steroid administration. One third of a series of 159 patients from Pakistan with chronic amebiasis had more than 5 years of abdominal pain, flatulence, intermittent diarrhea, mucus in stools, and weight loss. All 159 patients had *E histolytica* present in the stool, and 77% had ulcers containing amebae demonstrated by colonoscopy. Physicians in developed nations must be alert for the chronic presentation of intestinal amebiasis. One third of patients with amebic colitis seen in central Virginia had more than 1 year of symptoms.

An *ameboma* can present as a tender, palpable abdominal mass. It is a segmented mass of granulation tissue in the cecum or ascending colon that occurs in 0.5% to 1.5% of patients with amebic colitis. Amebic dysentery was present in two thirds of patients with amebomas at the time of diagnosis. Amebomas can appear as single or multiple "apple core" lesions on barium enema. The diagnosis is established by colonoscopy with biopsy, and the ameboma responds to antiamebic chemotherapy without surgery.

Toxic megacolon is an unusual but severe complication of

amebic colitis that occurs more commonly in patients who inappropriately receive corticosteroids and in patients who acquire their infection by way of colonic irrigation therapy. The colon is markedly distended, and intramural gas is present. Colectomy is frequently required.

Amebic peritonitis from intestinal perforation has been reported to have a mortality of 40% to 75% that is probably caused by the concurrent bacterial peritonitis that results from colonic perforation. The onset of peritonitis is often insidious because of slow leakage through the severely diseased colon. Acute perforation was clinically recognizable in only 6 of 39 deaths from amebic peritonitis. The onset of amebic peritonitis can be suspected when increased abdominal distention and ileus occur, with clinical deterioration of the patient.

Amebic strictures in the large bowel occur in less than 1% of patients with amebic dysentery. *E histolytica* has been identified in the granulation tissue, and the strictures respond to antiamebic therapy. Strictures have been seen with or without concurrent amebic dysentery.

Extraintestinal Disease

Amebic liver abscess develops in about 10% of patients who have had invasive amebiasis. At the time of diagnosis of the liver abscess, only a minority of patients have amebic dysentery or *E histolytica* identified in their stools. Most patients will have had dysentery within the last year, which is a useful historical point for distinguishing them from patients with bacterial liver abscesses. Amebic liver abscess occurs predominately in male patients, can occur at any age, and presents acutely or chronically. Of patients with less than 10 days of symptoms, 85% had fever and abdominal pain; in those with a more chronic (2–12 weeks) presentation, hepatomegaly and weight loss were present in two thirds. Acute presentations were associated with multiple amebic abscesses. Not surprisingly, point tenderness over the liver is a common finding. Hepatomegaly is present in half of the patients, and peritoneal signs or jaundice are unusual.[17,18]

Direct extension of an amebic liver abscess into the thorax is the usual route for infection of the lung, with hematogenous infection rare. Atelectasis, elevation of the right hemidiaphragm, and serous pleural effusion occur in up to 75% of patients with amebic liver abscess and do not by themselves represent primary pulmonary disease. Peritonitis from rupture of the liver abscess into the peritoneum has a lower mortality than peritonitis from a perforated colon because there usually is not concurrent bacterial peritonitis. Amebic pericarditis is a rare complication from direct extension of an amebic liver abscess. Other rare manifestations of extraintestinal amebiasis include cutaneous amebiasis (perianally or from an enterocutaneous fistula), amebic brain abscess, and amebic ulcerations of the penis and cervix.

Differential Diagnosis and Diagnostic Studies

Intestinal Infection

The differential diagnosis of bloody diarrhea includes inflammatory bowel disease, ischemic colitis, and infectious causes of diarrhea, including, in addition to amebiasis, *Salmonella* sp, *Shigella* sp, *Campylobacter* sp, invasive *Escherichia coli*, and enterohemorrhagic *E coli*, especially strain O157:H7.

To make the diagnosis of intestinal amebiasis, three separate stool specimens should be examined. The stool examination should include a wet preparation performed within 30 minutes of passage to look for motile trophozoites that may contain ingested red blood cells (Fig. 106-1) and a formalin–ethyl acetate concentration step to identify cysts (Fig. 106-2). Enzyme-linked immunosorbent assays (ELISA) to detect trophozoites and cysts using antiamebic monoclonal and polyclonal antibodies specific for pathogenic *E histolytica* appear promising but are not yet commercially available.[19] Barium, bismuth, kaolin compounds, magnesium hydroxide, castor oil, and hypertonic or soap suds enemas all interfere

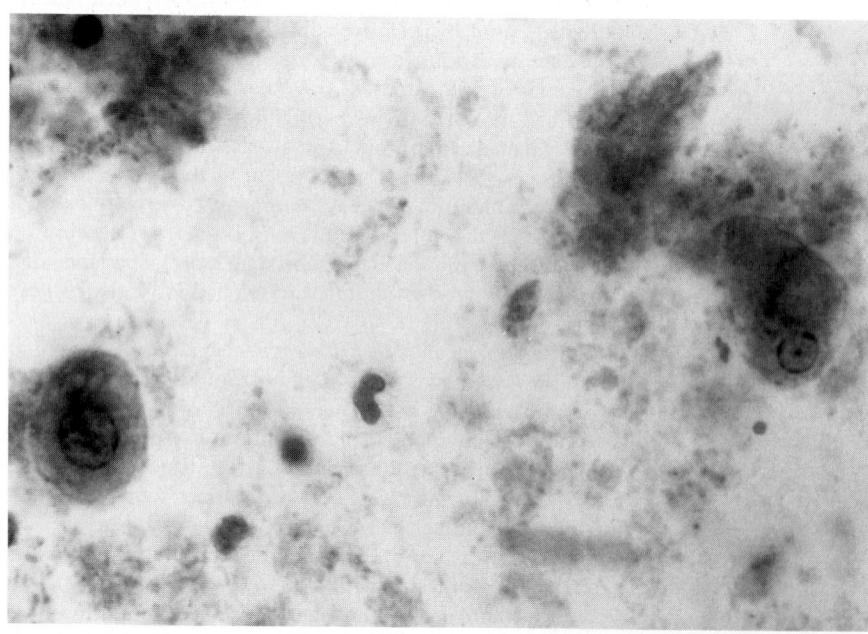

FIGURE 106-1. *Entamoeba histolytica* trophozoites in stool. (Trichrome stain; courtesy of Centers for Disease Control and Prevention, Atlanta, GA.)

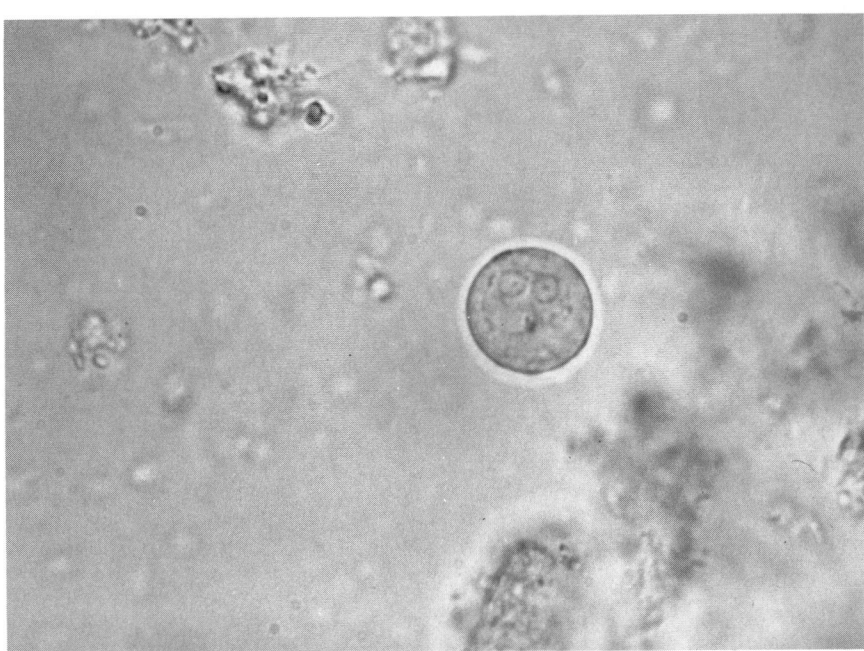

FIGURE 106-2. *Entamoeba histolytica* cyst from stool stained with iodine. (Courtesy of Centers for Disease Control and Prevention, Atlanta, GA.)

with the ability to detect *E histolytica* in stool. Culture of *E histolytica* from stool has not proved to be practical in a clinical laboratory setting.

Colonoscopy is preferable to sigmoidoscopy because patients may have disease isolated to the cecum or ascending colon. Cathartics or enemas should not be used to prepare patients because these interfere with identification of the parasite. The colonic mucosa appears hemorrhagic, and amebic ulcers frequently appear as shallow-based, discrete ulcers with raised edges. Wet preparations can be made to look for motile trophozoites from material aspirated or scraped with a pipette from the base of these ulcers. Biopsy specimens should be taken from the edge of ulcers, and special stains such as periodic acid-Schiff should be used to highlight the amebae. Serologic tests for antiamebic antibody are an important part of the diagnosis of amebiasis because amebae may be missed even with biopsy of the colonic ulcers. The indirect hemagglutination assay (IHA) is positive in up to 88% of patients with amebic dysentery, 99% of patients with amebic liver abscess, and only 5% of the general population in developed nations.[20] The IHA remains positive for years after the treatment of invasive amebiasis; therefore, it is not useful for distinguishing past from present infection. Barium enemas do not serve to differentiate amebiasis from other ulcerative diseases of the colon, and interfere with the identification of *E histolytica* in the stool.

Liver Abscess

The diagnosis of an *E histolytica* liver abscess is frequently a diagnosis of exclusion because patients with amebic liver abscess rarely have concurrent amebic dysentery and amebae are difficult to visualize in aspirates (Fig. 106-3). If an aspirate of a liver abscess is negative for bacteria and the serum is positive for *E histolytica* antibody by IHA, then the liver abscess is normally considered amebic in origin. In endemic areas, however, 5% to 30% of the population is IHA positive from previous amebic disease, and other diseases such as hepatocellular carcinoma and echinococcal cysts can mimic the appearance of a liver abscess on ultrasound or abdominal computed tomography. An antigen test indicating the presence of current invasive *E histolytica* infection would be a valuable diagnostic tool, but is unavailable.

A febrile patient with right upper quadrant abdominal pain is more likely to have an amebic liver abscess when he or she is from a group at high risk for amebic infection (see Table 106-1) and has had dysentery within the last year. An ultrasound study of the hepatobiliary system should be obtained quickly to rule out acute cholecystitis.[21] The IHA for antiamebic antibodies is positive in up to 99% of patients with an amebic liver abscess but may initially be negative in the first week of illness. Aspiration of an amebic liver abscess may be required diagnostically if it is not possible to distinguish on clinical grounds a pyogenic from an amebic abscess. Aspiration of an echinococcal cyst should be avoided because it can be complicated by anaphylaxis if cyst contents spill.

Treatment and Prevention

Asymptomatic cyst passers in highly endemic areas need not be treated because of the likelihood of reinfection. In developed nations with little risk of reinfection, treatment eliminates the potential risk of future invasive disease and prevents the spread of infection. Lumenal agents with little systemic absorption, such as diloxanide furoate, iodoquinol, or paromomycin, minimize side effects while maximizing drug delivery to the amebic cysts and trophozoites in the lumen of the colon. Metronidazole, because of its high systemic uptake, requires 10 days of oral treatment to be highly effective in the elimination of colonic colonization.

Metronidazole is the drug of choice for invasive colonic

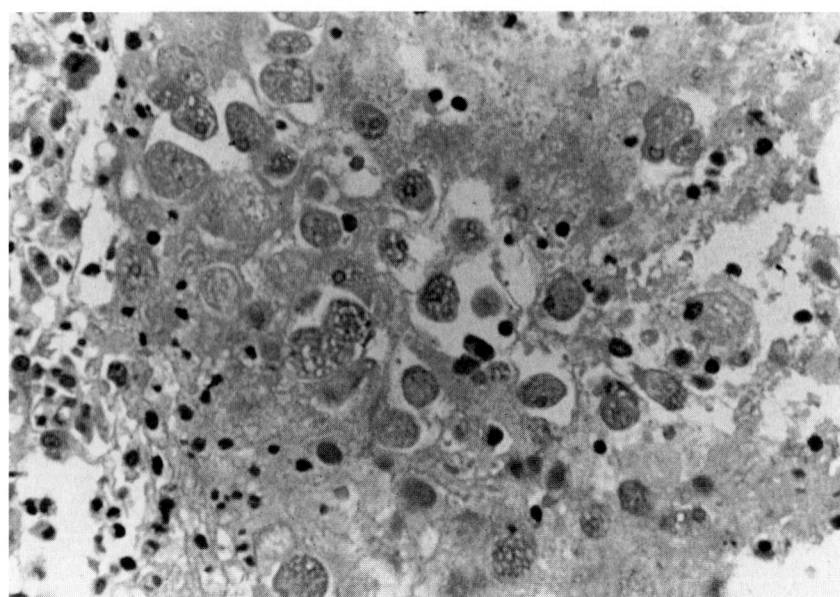

FIGURE 106-3. *Entamoeba histolytica* in liver abscess. (Hematoxylin and eosin stain.)

disease or liver abscess; a poorly absorbed agent should be added to eliminate *E histolytica* in the lumen of the colon. Most patients respond to metronidazole within 3 to 5 days. Needle aspiration of an amebic liver abscess usually is not necessary for successful treatment, and surgical resection in intestinal disease is technically difficult and usually not recommended except when unavoidable (e.g., toxic megacolon). Second-line drugs for invasive amebiasis include the ipecac alkaloids emetine and dehydroemetine, which must be given intravenously and have frequent cardiovascular side effects, and chloroquine, which is sometimes added to metronidazole therapy if an initial clinical response is not seen.[22]

Prevention of amebiasis requires the interruption of the fecal-oral spread of the cyst. Patients should be advised of the risks of travel to endemic areas and of sexual activity that promotes fecal-oral contamination. Pending the availability of a vaccine or the financial resources to improve public sanitation in the developing world, *E histolytica* will remain an important worldwide cause of morbidity and mortality.

Giardia lamblia

Giardia lamblia was discovered by van Leeuwenhoek in the late 1600s, and until the 1960s was thought to be a harmless commensal. Its association with symptomatic diarrhea and malabsorption in children and with disease after water-borne outbreaks, travel, and experimental human infection has clearly established its pathogenicity. Giardiasis is an important cause of endemic and epidemic diarrhea throughout the world, and *G lamblia* is the leading infectious agent identified in water-borne outbreaks of diarrhea in the United States.

The genus *Giardia* belongs to the class Zoomastigophorea, the order Diplomonadida, and the family Hexamitidae. It is one of the most primitive of all eukaryotes.[23] Although *Giardia* has been traditionally separated into species by morphology and host range, it now can be grouped on the basis of antigens, isoenzymes, and DNA patterns.[23–25] Its genetic

structure also is being determined.[23] Information from these studies indicates that several different species exist. The species that infects humans is designated *G lamblia* (also called *intestinalis* or *duodenalis*). Differences between isolates of a given species and antigenic variation of individual isolates have been documented in experimental human and animal infection.[26–28]

There are two stages to the life cycle of *G lamblia*: the trophozoite and the cyst. The trophozoite measures 9 to 21 μm by 5 to 15 μm (Fig. 106-4*A*), and has a convex dorsal surface and a flat ventral surface containing the disk. Four pairs of posteriorly directed flagella are involved in parasite movement. The disk cytoskeleton is composed of a clockwise spiral array of microtubules that contain important antigens.[23,29] The protozoan has two nuclei, each with a prominent central karyosome, which create the characteristic face-like image on stained preparations. Tight collections of microtubules called median bodies are placed transversely in a claw-like manner in *G lamblia* and may be helpful in species differentiation.

G lamblia is the only *Giardia* species that has been cultured successfully in vitro. Growth is enhanced by low oxygen tension, biliary lipids, intestinal mucus, and epithelial cells, in keeping with the predilection of *Giardia* to colonize the upper small bowel.[23,30] The trophozoite divides by longitudinal binary fission and has a doubling time in culture of 9 to 12 hours. It is an aerotolerant anaerobe; metabolizes glucose to ethanol, acetate, and CO_2; lacks mitochondria; and scavenges phospholipids, fatty acids, cholesterol, and pyrimidines from the environment.[23]

After exposure to secondary bile salts, a neutral pH, and other intestinal factors, *G lamblia* trophozoites encyst to form smooth, oval-shaped, thin-walled cysts measuring 8 to 12 μm long and 7 to 10 μm wide (Fig. 106-4*B*).[23,31] This encystation process has been accomplished in vitro.[31] It is the cyst form that is orally ingested, because trophozoites would be readily killed by stomach acid. As the cyst matures, a single trophozoite division may occur.

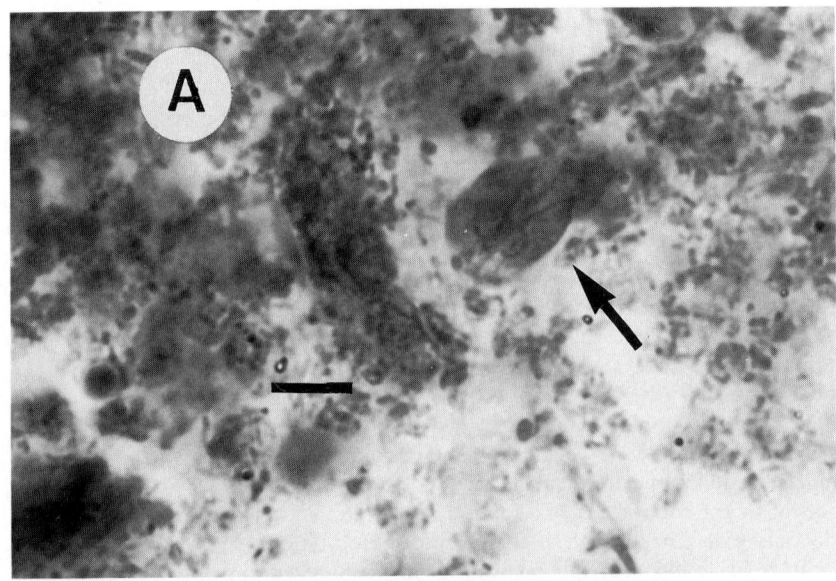

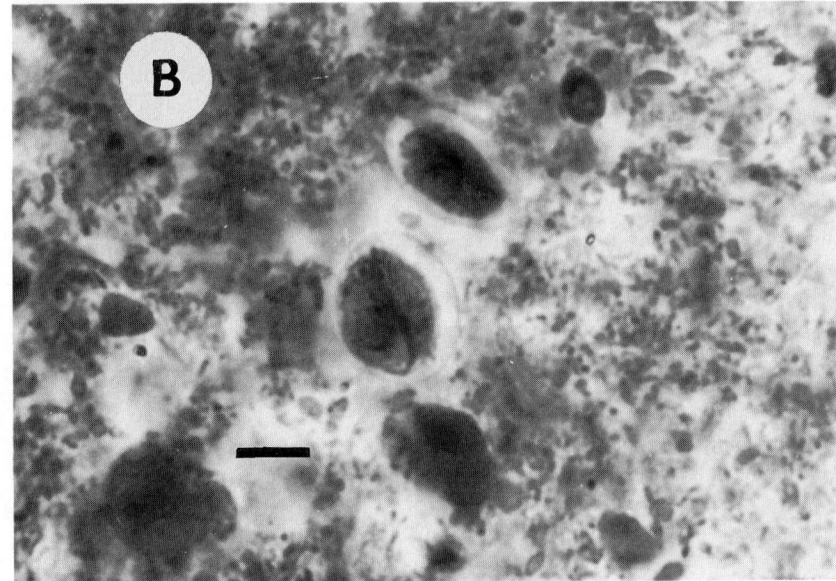

FIGURE 106-4. (**A**) Trichrome stain of a *Giardia lamblia* trophozoite. Two nuclei can be seen with prominent central karyosomes. (**B**) A *G lamblia* cyst is seen in a trichrome stain of fecal material. The cyst is smooth walled, and the trophozoite within it has separated from the wall, leaving a clear space. The transversely placed median bodies are also seen. (Bar = 10 μm.)

Epidemiology

G lamblia is prevalent throughout the world. In the United States, *Giardia* is the most commonly identified intestinal parasite, with isolation rates in some areas as high as 20%. In the developing world, *Giardia* is one of the first enteric pathogens to infect infants, with peak prevalence rates of 15% to 20% occurring in children younger than 10 years of age.[32-34]

Studies indicate that *G lamblia*-type parasites can infect many mammalian species, including humans, sheep, beavers, cattle, dogs, and cats.[23,24,35-37] Whether these species are important reservoirs for human infection remains unclear[38,39]; however, the determination that beavers were the source of human infection in at least one water-borne outbreak of giardiasis suggests they may be.[40]

Water is the most frequent mode of transmission of *Giardia*, indicating the ease by which public water supplies may become fecally contaminated, and the ability of cysts to survive well in this medium.[41] In the United States, *G lamblia* has been the most commonly identified pathogen in outbreaks of water-borne diarrheal illness, and has affected over 23,500 people.[42] Many outbreaks have occurred in the mountainous regions of the Northeast, Northwest, and Rocky Mountains of the United States and British Columbia in Canada.[40,42,43] Common to most of these has been the use of surface water that has been inadequately purified by lack of treatment with flocculation, sedimentation, and filtration, in addition to chlorination.[44] Contaminated water may also be a problem for hikers to wilderness areas and for the international traveler.

Person-to-person transmission is the second most commonly identified mode of acquisition and may account for many of the sporadic cases. It occurs in groups that may exhibit poor fecal-oral hygiene: small children in day care centers, sexually active male homosexuals, and people in custodial institutions. In children younger than 3 years old in day care centers, the prevalence of *Giardia* cyst passage may be as high as 20% to 50%.[45] Many of these children are symptomatic and can spread disease to family members and within their community. Food has been documented as a source of *Giardia* in commercial food establishments, corporate office settings, and within small groups. This indicates that food is a more common vehicle for disease transmission than is recognized.[46–48]

Pathogenesis and Immunology

The disease giardiasis is the result of a complex interaction of *Giardia* with the host, with the outcome related to the strain of *Giardia* ingested and to the host's immune response to the parasite. After ingestion of as few as 10 to 25 cysts there is excystation after exposure to gastric acid and pancreatic enzymes, and subsequent trophozoite colonization and multiplication in the upper small bowel. *Giardia* trophozoites adhere to gut enterocytes by a suction or clasping action of the ventral disk, or through specific receptor-ligand binding.[49]

It is likely that several mechanisms contribute to the pathogenesis of giardiasis. Some of these are related to the parasite itself and its direct effect on the gut; others may relate to the response of the host to infestation with *Giardia*. First, those mechanisms relating to the parasite itself are outlined. Electron microscopy has demonstrated damage to the brush border,[50] and documentation of deficiencies of brush border enzymes, especially lactase,[51] support this idea. Mucosal invasion is probably a rare event for this predominantly lumenal parasite. Simultaneous colonization of the small bowel with *Giardia* and enterobacteriaceae or yeast may contribute to malabsorption in some patients by the deconjugation of bile salts. In mice infected with *Giardia muris*, there is increased epithelial cell turnover in the crypt region, potentially changing the bowel's absorptive capacity.[52] No enterotoxins have been identified for *Giardia*.

Experimental studies in animals and epidemiologic studies in humans have shown that partially protective immunity to *Giardia* develops.[32,53–55] The prevalence of *Giardia* in areas endemic for the parasite is higher in younger age groups and decreases with increasing age.[32] In addition to playing a protective role, the immune response may also contribute to clearance of *Giardia* by the production of secretory antibodies, and to disease by initiating an inflammatory response.[56]

The components of *Giardia* immunity are humoral, cellular, and macrophage mediated.[56,57] The humoral response is manifested by the development of systemic antibodies in patients with *Giardia*. Antibody measurements have been useful in seroprevalence studies and in the recognition of *Giardia* antigens.[23,32,54,57–59] Serum may also be lethal for *G lamblia* trophozoites. Because *Giardia* is confined to the lumen of the gastrointestinal tract, secretory immunoglobulins are likely to play the most important role in immunity. Elevation of gut immunoglobulins has been documented during human *Giardia* infection, as has elevation of systemic IgA antibody.[58,60–62] In the mouse intestine, IgA secretion correlates temporally with clearance of *Giardia*, and its absence is associated with failure to resolve infection.[63] It most likely acts by binding to trophozoites and inhibiting a critical adherence step.[57]

Cellular immunity coordinates the antibody response through helper T-cell enhancement of anti-*Giardia* secretory

IgA production.[64] Also, other lymphocyte populations may engage in specific anti-*Giardia* cytotoxicity. Although partially protective immunity and clearance are beneficial effects of the host immune response, a potentially deleterious effect is gut inflammation. Athymic, T-cell–deficient mice are unable to clear *Giardia* until they are reconstituted with lymphoid cells.[65] Reconstitution is associated with the development of intestinal histologic abnormalities paralleling the changes seen in some humans with giardiasis; these include sprue-like lesions with marked flattening of the villi, crypt hypertrophy, and a dense mononuclear cell infiltration of the submucosa.[60,66,67] Finally, any immune response is likely to be initiated when antigen is taken up and processed by macrophages residing in Peyer's patches.[68,69]

Human milk is cytotoxic to *Giardia* trophozoites; cytotoxicity occurs when free fatty acids are released from milk triglycerides by the action of bile salt-stimulated lipase.[70] Both human and animal breast milk contain anti-*Giardia* antibodies, and breast-feeding may protect infants from infection.[71]

Conditions that predispose patients to giardiasis include common variable immunodeficiency and the more severe X-linked agammaglobulinemia in children.[72] These patients have symptomatic disease with prolonged diarrhea, malabsorption, and severe classic changes on small bowel biopsy, as well as nodular lymphoid hyperplasia. With anti-*Giardia* therapy, their symptoms and pathologic changes improve. It remains unclear if (selective) IgA deficiency is a predisposing factor. Susceptibility to giardiasis has also been seen in patients with previous gastric surgery and reduced gastric acidity. Patients with the acquired immunodeficiency syndrome (AIDS) may have an increased risk of giardiasis because of achlorhydria and more frequent infections with fecal-oral pathogens. Disease does not appear to be more severe than that in normal hosts, but the immune responses to the parasite are impaired in these patients.[73,74]

Clinical Presentation

Infection with *G lamblia* includes asymptomatic cyst passage, acute, self-limited diarrhea, and a chronic syndrome of diarrhea, malabsorption, and weight loss. After ingestion of *G lamblia* cysts, there is an incubation period of 1 to 2 weeks before the onset of symptoms. Approximately half of those ingesting cysts have diarrhea, a small number become asymptomatic cyst passers, and the remainder do not become infected. Asymptomatic children in day care centers may pass cysts for as long as 6 months.[45] Symptomatic giardiasis (Table 106-3) is characterized by the acute onset of diarrhea, abdominal cramps, bloating, and flatulence with malaise, nausea, anorexia, and sulfuric belching. Vomiting, fever, and tenesmus are infrequent. Initially, stools may be profuse and watery but later are commonly greasy, foul smelling, and may float. Gross blood, pus, and mucus usually are absent, and, if examined microscopically, the stool is free of polymorphonuclear cells.

Important clinical features are the prolonged duration of diarrhea and weight loss. At presentation, most patients have been symptomatic for more than a week. Weight loss of about 4.5 kg occurs more than 50% of the time. Symptoms may resolve spontaneously after 3 or 4 days, but most patients

TABLE 106-3
Symptoms of Giardiasis

	PERCENTAGE OF INFECTED PATIENTS	RANGE
Diarrhea	90	64–100
Malaise	86	72–97
Flatulence	75	35–97
Foul-smelling, greasy stools	75	57–87
Abdominal cramps	71	44–85
Bloating	71	42–97
Nausea	69	59–79
Anorexia	66	41–82
Weight loss	66	56–76
Vomiting	23	11–36
Fever	15	0–24
Constipation	13	0–26
Urticaria	10	5–14

Adapted with permission from Hill DR. Giardiasis. In: Mandell GR, Douglas RG, Bennett J, eds. Principles and practice of infectious diseases. New York: Churchill-Livingstone, 1990:2113.

will remain symptomatic for several weeks. Rarely, a reactive polyarticular arthritis occurs. Biliary tract and gastric infection have been documented. The latter is associated with achlorhydria.[75]

Patients who continue on to chronic diarrhea have profound malaise, lassitude, occasional headache, and diffuse abdominal and epigastric discomfort, often exacerbated by eating. Periods of diarrhea may be interrupted by periods of constipation or normal bowel habits. The syndrome may wax and wane over months until therapy or spontaneous resolution.

Various degrees of malabsorption may be present. Giardiasis may present in children as failure to thrive or as a sprue-like illness.[67,76] Malabsorption of fat, vitamins A and B_{12}, protein, and D-xylose has been documented.[76,77] Lactose deficiency occurs in 20% to 40% of patients with post-*Giardia* lactose intolerance, sometimes persisting for several weeks after treatment. This may be confused with relapse or reinfection, and should be ruled out before retreatment is considered.

The role of chronic giardiasis in the impairment of growth and development of children in the developing world has generated much interest.[77–79] A possible deleterious effect on growth suggests the need to treat recurrent disease[33,77,78]; however, reinfection occurs so rapidly in areas of poor sanitation that repeated therapy is impractical.[32,79] Many children also are simultaneously infected with other bacterial, viral, or parasitic agents, making it difficult to interpret the role that *Giardia* plays in their illness. Until more information is obtained, it seems reasonable to treat only symptomatic children in these situations.

Differential Diagnosis and Diagnostic Studies

The differential diagnosis of giardiasis includes diarrhea due to other parasites such as *Cryptosporidium*, *Dientamoeba fragilis*, and mild cases of infection with *E histolytica* and the newly described protozoa, the microsporidia and *Cyclospora*.[80,81] Infections with enteric viruses and noninvasive bacteria are also part of the differential diagnosis, although these agents usually cause disease of shorter duration. Syndromes of malabsorption such as tropical sprue, gluten-sensitive enteropathy, and lactose intolerance also should be considered. Irritable bowel syndrome may mimic giardiasis. A careful history, physical examination, and specific laboratory studies are usually sufficient to confirm giardiasis. The white blood cell count should be normal and eosinophilia absent. Barium studies are nonspecific and may demonstrate upper small bowel thickening and increased transit time, but also may interfere with the examination of stools.

For patients with a history of recent travel to an endemic area, or the presence in the home of children who attend day care centers, or an active homosexual lifestyle, the diagnosis of giardiasis becomes more likely. The traditional method of diagnosis is a stool examination for trophozoites or cysts.[82,83] Newer antigen detection assays are important additions to diagnosis, especially when *Giardia* is the exclusive agent being sought (e.g., in outbreaks, in screening children in day care, or in testing for cure).[84,85] For the stool ova and parasite examination, a saline wet mount of fresh liquid stool may detect motile trophozoites (see Fig. 106-4A). More often, however, the stool is semiformed, and trophozoites are not found. In these cases, cysts may be detected in fresh stool by iodine staining or after preservation in formalin or polyvinyl alcohol and subsequent trichrome or iron hematoxylin staining (see Fig. 106-4B).[86] Formalin-ether or zinc sulfate flotation concentration techniques may increase the yield. *Giardia* should be identified 50% to 70% of the time after one stool and as high as 90% of the time after three stools.[82] Occasionally, passage of parasites in the stool may follow the development of symptoms by a few days. Purging does not increase the yield.

There are two available antigen detection assays: an ELISA of a 65-kd *Giardia* glycoprotein probably of cyst wall origin (ProSpecT/*Giardia* Assay; Alexon Inc., Mountain View, CA);[84] and a combination assay that identifies *Giardia* and *Cryptosporidium* by immunofluorescence (Meriflor; Meridian Diagnostics, Inc., Cincinnati, OH).[85] Both assays have excellent sensitivity and specificity.

Careful examination of stool by microscopy and the new antigen assays have made sampling of duodenal contents less necessary for diagnosis. In particularly difficult cases, however, one of three methods may be used: the string test (Entero-Test; HDC Corporation, San Jose, CA),[87] duodenal aspiration, and duodenal biopsy. After the patient swallows the Entero-Test string, it is allowed to remain for 4 to 6 hours or overnight while the patient is fasting. The string is then removed and the bile-stained mucus stripped off and examined for trophozoites. The duodenal aspirate can be cultured for small bowel overgrowth as well as examined for *Giardia*. Biopsies and touch preparations require Giemsa staining and a careful search for trophozoites. Small bowel biopsy may demonstrate the classic sprue-like lesions of giardiasis, or may be negative. Biopsy also may demonstrate lesions not caused by giardiasis, which may be particularly helpful in evaluating malabsorption syndromes.

Testing for systemic anti-*Giardia* antibody, although not widely available, has been useful in seroepidemiologic studies throughout the world.[32,54,58] IgG antibodies remain elevated for long periods of time, making them less helpful diagnostically in areas endemic for giardiasis. Serum anti-*Giardia* IgM, however, may be useful in distinguishing current from past giardiasis.[88] Detection of parasite nucleic acid has been performed in experimental situations.

Treatment and Prevention

The routine isolation, culture, and susceptibility testing of *Giardia* have been difficult, with wide variation in results.[23,83] Most information on drug efficacy, therefore, relies on clinical experience (Table 106-4).[82,89,90] Although the acridine dye quinacrine has been considered by some to be the drug of choice, it is no longer manufactured in the United States. This leaves metronidazole as the major agent available for therapy. Quinacrine has had an efficacy of approximately 90%, although it is often poorly tolerated, especially in children. The most common side effects are nausea, vomiting, and abdominal cramping. Yellow discoloration of the skin, urine, and sclerae can occur occasionally, and exfoliative dermatitis and toxic psychosis are rare side effects. Metronidazole, a nitroimidazole, has never been approved for use in giardiasis in the United States, but has an efficacy in the range of 80% to 95%. It usually is better tolerated in the pediatric age group. Although concerns about potential carcinogenicity make its routine use in children debatable, this risk has never been documented in humans.[91] The side effects of metronidazole are a metallic taste in the mouth, nausea, dizziness, headache, and, rarely, reversible neutropenia. Taken with alcohol, it can produce a disulfiram-like effect. High-dose, short-course regimens have lower efficacy rates and may be poorly tolerated. Furazolidone, a nitrofuran, has been advocated as an alternative drug in the pediatric age group because of its availability in liquid suspension form.[92] It can have gastrointestinal side effects, turn urine brown, and cause mild hemolysis in G6PD-deficient patients. Another nitroimidazole not available in the United States, tinidazole, has shown excellent efficacy (approximately 90%) when given in a single 2-g dose for adults.[93] For patients who fail one drug course or relapse, a second course of the same drug or a switch to a drug from a different class usually is effective. In rare patients, combination therapy may be necessary.[94]

Pregnant women should be carefully evaluated if they need treatment because drug therapy may in theory be associated with toxicity.[83] If adequate hydration and nutrition can be maintained, treatment may be delayed until after delivery or at least until after the first trimester. If a pregnant woman requires treatment, an oral, poorly absorbed aminoglycoside, paromomycin, may be tried initially; its efficacy, however, is only 60% to 70%.[83,95,96] Metronidazole may be given after the first trimester, at which time it appears to be safe.[96,97] High-dose regimens should not be used.

Treatment of the otherwise healthy, well nourished, asymptomatic cyst passer, adult or child, is controversial. If there is a low likelihood of reinfection, treatment is often recommended, particularly to decrease transmission to others. This would be important for food handlers. Management of endemic foci of *Giardia* in day care centers is particularly challenging. Because of the difficulty in preventing the spread of fecal-oral pathogens, and the potential side effects of treatment regimens, some recommend that only symptomatic children be treated.[45,98] All infected children, however, may bring *Giardia* home to family members and can contribute to high rates of infection in communities.[47,99] Therefore, if strict hand washing and treatment of symptomatic children fail to control an outbreak of diarrhea, then consideration can be given to treating all infected children.[100]

The prevention of giardiasis includes adequate purification of drinking water and good personal hygiene. Although chlorination alone is sufficient to kill *G lamblia* cysts, water temperature, clarity, pH, and contact time may alter its efficacy.[44,101] Thus, in addition to chlorination, public water should be treated by flocculation, sedimentation, and filtration. For the traveler to the back country or to developing areas, water should be brought to a boil for 10 minutes, and longer at higher elevations. Treatment of small volumes of water by halogenation also usually is effective. Chlorine-based preparations include Halazone, 5 tablets/L/30 minutes, and chlorine bleach, 4% to 6%, 4 drops/quart; iodine-based preparations include Potable Agua, 1 tablet/L/30 minutes, and saturated crystalline iodine, 12.5 mL/L/30 minutes.[101] Personal filtration devices remove *Giardia* cysts if their pore size is no larger than 2 μm. Venereal transmission of *Giardia* can be decreased by avoidance of oral-anal and oral-genital sex. There is no immunoprophylactic or chemoprophylactic strategy for giardiasis.

Cryptosporidium SPECIES

Long recognized by veterinarians as a potential parasitic cause of diarrhea, *Cryptosporidium* has attracted significant medical attention only since 1982 with the advent of the severe, life-threatening, cholera-like diarrhea it causes in patients with AIDS. Before that, there had been only a half dozen isolated case reports of *Cryptosporidium* causing diarrhea, mostly in immunocompromised patients. *Cryptosporidium* was first described in the gastric epithelium of asymptomatic laboratory mice in 1907 by Tyzzer (and possibly in 1895 by J. J. Clark).[102,103] This parasite attracted little attention until 1955, when Slavin noted diarrhea with cryptosporidiosis in poultry.[104] Interest increased when Panciera and colleagues noted bovine diarrhea with *Cryptosporidium* infections in 1971.[105] Human cases were recognized only anecdotally in healthy and immunocompromised children from 1976 until 1982,

TABLE 106-4
Treatment of Giardiasis

DRUG	DOSAGE Adult	Pediatric
Quinacrine	100 mg tid × 5–7 d	2 mg/kg tid × 7 d
Metronidazole	250 mg tid × 7 d	5 mg/kg tid × 7 d
Furazolidone	100 mg qid × 7–10 d	2 mg/kg qid × 10 d
Paromomycin	25–30 mg/kg/d in 3 doses × 5–10 d	

when the severe diarrhea in patients with AIDS was reported.[106,107] *Cryptosporidium* is now documented as a widespread and difficult water-borne pathogen that may cause large outbreaks of self-limiting, subacute diarrhea (much like giardiasis) in otherwise healthy people, as well as persistent diarrhea often in association with malnutrition among children in tropical, developing areas. It also causes diarrhea in children in day care centers and in veterinary and health care workers and travelers of all ages.[107-109]

The *Cryptosporidium* parasite is a 2- to 6-μm sporozoan protozoan relative of *Toxoplasma*, *Isospora*, and *Sarcocystis* (the other "true coccidia"; Fig. 106-5).[103,107,109] A single species, *Cryptosporidium parvum*, is thought to be the primary mammalian intestinal pathogen infecting calves, piglets, foals, mice, and goats, as well as humans.[103] Other probably distinct species include *Cryptosporidium muris* (causes asymptomatic gastric infections in rodents), and *Cryptosporidium baileyi* and *Cryptosporidium meleagridis* (infect the gastrointestinal and respiratory tracts of birds).[103,110,111] Unlike *Isospora* and the animal *Eimeria*, *Cryptosporidium* completes its life cycle in a superficial parasitophorous vacuole confined to the microvillous region of the bowel mucosal epithelial cells. There they develop into sporulated oocysts that are infectious when shed in the stools, and are the characteristic diagnostic form seen on modified acid-fast stain (Fig. 106-6; see Fig. 106-5).

Epidemiology

Despite the more severe, life-threatening diarrhea seen in immunosuppressed patients, the more common form of cryptosporidiosis is a self-limited diarrhea in immunocompetent hosts.[108-113] In more than 36,000 patients with diarrhea, 2.1% were positive for *Cryptosporidium* in 16 reports from Europe, North America, and Australia, and 8.0% were positive in 14 reports from Asia, Africa, and Latin America (Table 106-5).[109,111,113-116] In a compilation of data from 78 reports of over 130,000 immunocompetent cases and 6000 controls by Adal and colleagues,[117] *Cryptosporidium* was seen in 2.1% to 6.1% of symptomatic cases from developed and developing countries, respectively, and in 0.15% to 1.5% of controls. Similar rates from 22 studies of human immunodeficiency virus-infected people with diarrhea showed 14% to 24% for developed and developing countries, respectively.[117] In young children, rates tend to be higher than in other immunocompetent people. Risk factors include weaning, crowding, summer and autumn months, contact with infected patients or animals, housing in institutions such as day care centers or hospitals, and use of contaminated water. Infections tend to occur early in life, especially in developing countries, where they are a major cause of persistent diarrhea.[118,119]

The reservoir of *Cryptosporidium* infections appears to be in animals. Transmission of *C parvum* has been documented between several mammals and humans.[103,108,110] Infections in young domestic calves, piglets, goats, and lambs are important veterinary problems and may be zoonotic sources for human disease, with the vehicle being contaminated surface water that drains into drinking water supplies. Increasingly impressive data suggest, however, that person-to-person spread is a major means of transmission, especially in hospitals, day care centers, and families. Rates of infection in day care centers may reach as high as 50%, with significant secondary spread in family contacts.[120,121] Up to 31% of hospital personnel exposed to an infected patient may acquire *Cryptosporidium* infections.[122]

The tiny, hardy oocysts of *Cryptosporidium* may be very difficult to kill and may survive in cold water for over 12 months. Large water-borne outbreaks have been reported in Wisconsin, Texas, Georgia, and England.[123-125] It is thought that cattle contaminated some of these water supplies, with the infectious oocysts surviving chlorination that eradicated detectable fecal coliforms.

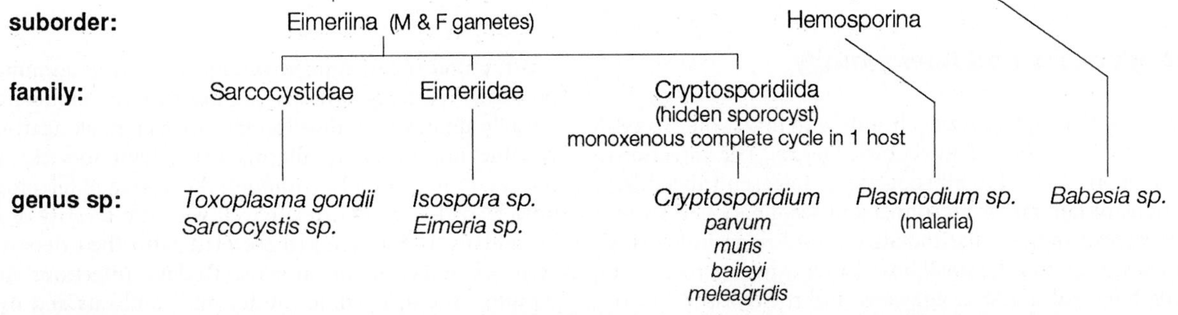

FIGURE 106-5. Taxonomy of *Cryptosporidium*. (Adapted from references 103, 107, and 109.)

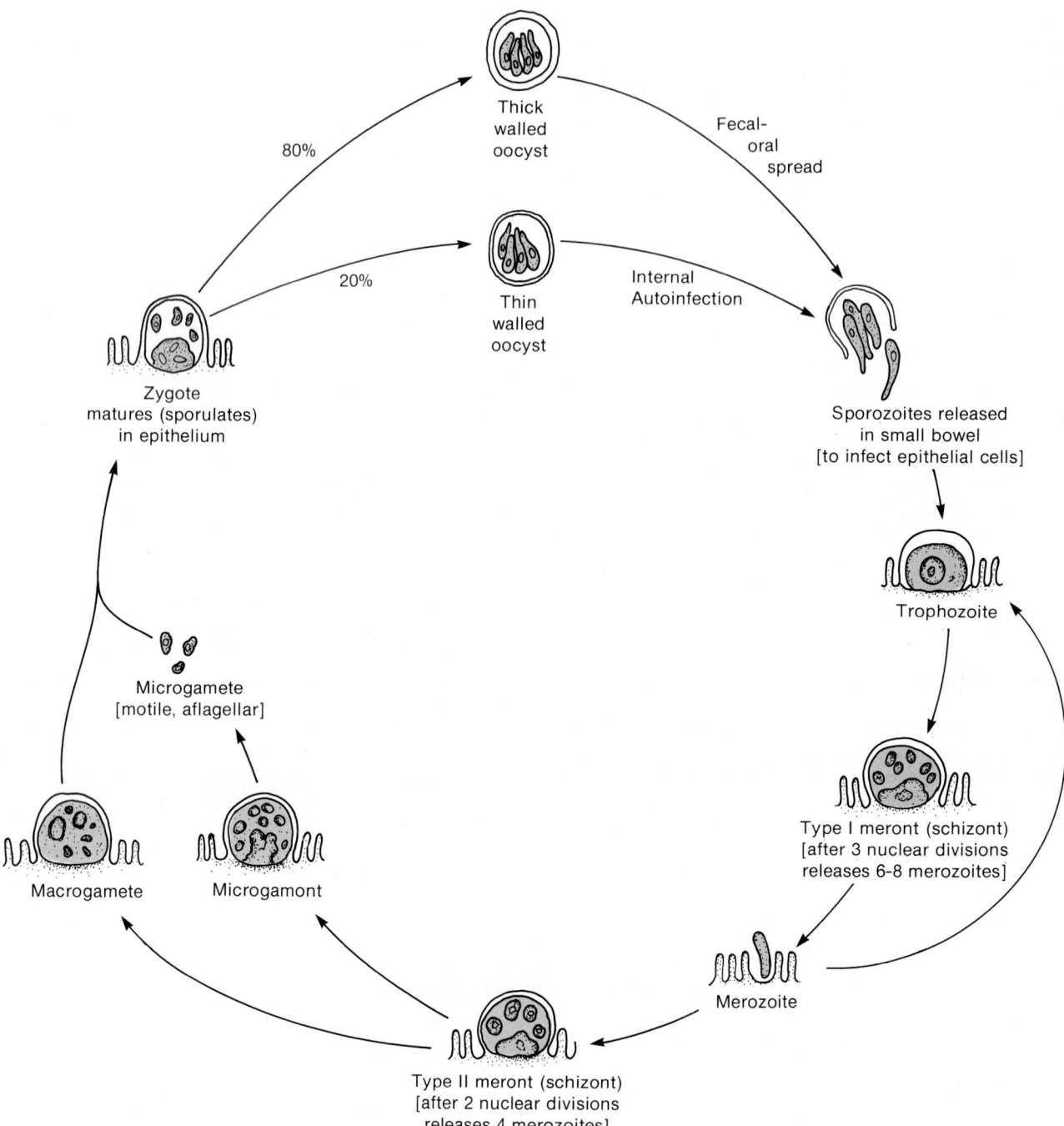

FIGURE 106-6. Life cycle of *Cryptosporidium*.

Pathogenesis and Immunology

Infection with *Cryptosporidium* begins with ingestion of a relatively small number of infectious oocysts. The infectious dose is reportedly 100 to 500 oocysts for mice, and anecdotal infections of laboratory personnel and secondary person-to-person spread suggest that the infectious dose in humans is low. These excyst in the small bowel after exposure to gastric acidity, bile, and digestive enzymes, and the released sporozoites infect the mucosal epithelium, usually leaving the ul-

trastructural architecture intact. Particularly in immunocompromised patients, villous architecture is moderately to severely abnormal, with villous atrophy, crypt elongation, and variable infiltration of plasma cells, lymphocytes, macrophages, or neutrophils. Although the degree of histologic abnormality does not correlate well with the severity of illness in humans, it does tend to correlate with the extent and severity of infection in animals. Rodent infections may be symptomatic in athymic (nude) mice and rats and in killer lymphocyte-depleted (beige) mice, suggesting that the ab-

TABLE 106-5

Frequencies of Positive Stool Examinations for *Crytosporidium* Organisms in People With Sporadic Diarrhea and Asymptomatic Controls in Developed and Developing Countries[109,111,113]

	NUMBER OF PATIENTS WITH DIARRHEA	POSITIVE MEDIAN (RANGE)	NUMBER OF ASYMPTOMATIC CONTROLS	POSITIVE MEAN (RANGE)
Developed countries (from 16 reports from Europe, North America, Australia)	32,636	2.1% (0.1%–9.1%)	589	0.2% (0%–1%)
Developing countries (from 14 reports from Asia, Africa, Latin America)	4301	8.0% (3.2%–16.7%)	928	0.8% (0%–5.9%)

normal pathology is not dependent on T lymphocytes or on natural killer cells.[126–128] Indeed, the prolonged infections in athymic rodents and in immunocompromised patients (especially patients with AIDS) suggest that helper T-cell immunity is critical to the control of *Cryptosporidium* infections.[126–129]

Cryptosporidium infections may cause either malabsorptive or secretory diarrhea by unclear mechanisms. An enterotoxin is suggested by the severe watery diarrhea, but studies have failed to confirm preliminary reports of a secretory enterotoxin.[130,131] A potential role of neurohumoral or inflammatory mediators remains to be clarified.[132] Fat, D-xylose, and vitamin B_{12} malabsorption, and protein-losing enteropathy as measured by fecal α_1-antitrypsin, have been noted in infected patients with AIDS, and lactase deficiency has been described in infected calves.[127,133–135] The capacity of this parasite to disrupt the brush border epithelium by virtue of its localized, superficial microvillus attachment and electron-dense "feeder organelle" may be the mechanism whereby it reduces brush border enzymes or delivers an unidentified "toxic" product to the epithelial cell, inducing fluid and electrolyte secretion.[136,137]

Clinical Presentation

The clinical presentation of cryptosporidiosis is greatly influenced by the immune status of the host. It is a common infection in otherwise healthy children, especially in tropical, developing areas, and in travelers, day care workers, parents, hospital personnel, veterinarians, and those exposed to contaminated water, as well as in immunocompromised patients (with AIDS or agammaglobulinemia, or those undergoing chemotherapy). By far the most common symptom in both otherwise healthy and impaired hosts is watery, noninflammatory diarrhea.

In the otherwise healthy host, the illness is characterized by self-limited diarrhea, crampy abdominal pain, anorexia, malaise, occasional myalgias, weight loss, and low-grade fever (<39°C).[107,109] Although the life cycle can be completed in vitro in as little as 3 days, the incubation period is usually about 1 week, with a range of 3 to 14 days. The illness closely mimics that seen with giardiasis (with which coinfections are not uncommon, suggesting common exposures and epidemiology). Diarrhea typically lasts 10 to 14 days, although one quarter of illnesses in previously healthy people may last more

than 1 month.[112,138] Of epidemiologic importance, infectious oocysts usually are shed for 1 week *after* symptoms have resolved, and may persist for several weeks.[138]

In the immunocompromised host, *Cryptosporidium* infections may cause severe, cholera-like diarrhea that may exceed 17 L/day and often contributes to malnutrition or death (see Chap. 105). Biopsy or autopsy findings have documented *Cryptosporidium* infection of the epithelium in every portion of the gastrointestinal tract from the pharynx to the rectum. Biliary tract colonization is not uncommon in patients with AIDS, and it may cause cholecystitis.[109] It has occasionally been seen in the bronchial epithelium, presumably arriving there after regurgitation of infectious oocysts. Infections may persist to death or may resolve after withdrawal of immunosuppressive chemotherapy.

Differential Diagnosis and Diagnostic Studies

In the otherwise healthy host, particularly those with likely exposure to contaminated surface water, or to children or infected patients, other causes of watery, noninflammatory diarrhea must be excluded, including giardiasis, enterotoxigenic *E coli*, rotavirus, Norwalk-like virus, occasionally *Strongyloides stercoralis*, and, rarely, *Isospora belli* infections. A history of food, travel, day care, hospital, laboratory, animal, antibiotic, or contaminated water exposures provides helpful clues to the diagnosis. Most food poisoning syndromes are shorter in duration, and *Clostridium difficile*, *Shigella* sp, *Salmonella* sp, and *Campylobacter* sp infections are usually more inflammatory, with a greater likelihood of fever, and blood or numerous leukocytes in the stool.

The clinical presentation in immunocompromised hosts must be distinguished from rotavirus, adenovirus, Coxsackie virus, *Isospora*, microsporidia mycobacterial, cytomegalovirus, *Salmonella* sp, cytotoxic *C difficile*, and other infections that commonly cause diarrhea in immunosuppressed patients. Because several of these agents may require specific therapy, a diagnostic evaluation is important not only for the patient but also for epidemiologic purposes of control.

The diagnosis of cryptosporidiosis has included several approaches. The most convenient and widely used method is the modified acid-fast stain of unconcentrated or concentrated fecal specimens.[139] A characteristic red staining of oocysts is seen in the stool of most patients with acute symptomatic infections, with or without concentration by formalin-ether or Sheather's sucrose flotation methods. Intestinal biopsy adds little to proper stool examinations and may be negative when stool oocysts are present. The acid-fast characteristic of *Cryptosporidium* oocysts also allows use of fluorescence microscopy after auramine staining. Direct immunofluorescence staining using fluorescein-labeled oocyst antibody (including an IgG1 monoclonal antibody) may add sensitivity by detecting smaller numbers of oocysts in asymptomatic carriers or in contaminated water supplies. The monoclonal antibody also adds specificity and is commercially available in conjunction with a different fluorescence antibody to *G lamblia* (Meridian Diagnostics).[85,140] An antigen capture ELISA also has been developed (LMD Laboratories, Carlsbad, CA) that is reasonably specific, but less sensitive than direct examination using an acid-fast stain with human diarrheal specimens.[141]

Elevated serum IgM or IgG antibody titers can be detected by immunofluorescent antibody or ELISA methods in 95% to 100% of patients at presentation, or within 2 weeks of onset of acute cryptosporidiosis. Detectable IgG titers are present in over 50% of adults in serosurveys, suggesting that infections are common and that IgG titers persist for long periods.[142]

Treatment and Prevention

Although an extensive list of more than 80 antimicrobial and antiparasitic agents has been studied, no effective chemotherapy is available to treat cryptosporidiosis. Despite initial promise, bovine transfer factor, diloxanide furoate, furazolidone, quinine plus clindamycin, amprolium, and interleukin-2 have failed to eradicate this organism.[143] α-Difluoromethylornithine, although active against a related organism, *Eimeria*, has toxicity that outweighs demonstrated benefit. The macrolide antibiotic spiramycin (available from Rhone-Poulenc Pharmaceuticals, Montreal, Quebec, Canada) is still under study, with conflicting reports on its efficacy.[144] Hyperimmune bovine colostrum or immunoglobulin concentrate has given symptomatic relief in immunocompromised patients, without eradication of the infection.[145] Sulfadimethoxine has shown promise in a dexamethasone-treated rat model of cryptosporidiosis, and may warrant further study in humans. Data suggest that paromomycin is at least transiently effective at reducing symptoms and oocyst shedding in immunocompromised subjects and in animal models, although relapses may occur when the drug is discontinued.[146,147] Azithromycin has also shown some promise in animal and preliminary human studies.[148]

Prevention of cryptosporidiosis poses as many challenges as its chemotherapy. This hardy protozoan oocyst survives most disinfectants and may remain viable in cold water for more than 12 months. The most effective methods of killing this organism are freezing, heating to over 65°C, 10% formol saline, 5% ammonia (for 18 hours), and commercial bleach. Careful hand washing is important in preventing spread in hospitals and day care centers, and contaminated water should be avoided when traveling to endemic areas.[103] Infected people often continue to shed infectious oocysts for 1 to 2 weeks or more after their symptoms resolve.[138]

OTHER ENTERIC PROTOZOA

Cyclospora *Species*

Initially called "large *Cryptosporidium*" or cyanobacterium-like bodies, large, 8- to 9-μm autofluorescent organisms were identified in association with subacute, often protracted diarrhea in travelers in Nepal and among hospital personnel in Chicago.[149-153] It has been suggested that this organism, also seen in children with diarrhea in Peru, is a new sporozoan protozoan parasite, *Cyclospora*.[81] The continued emergence of reports of this parasite in stool samples, or jejunal aspirates and biopsies in travelers, in water-borne outbreaks, and in children with endemic diarrhea in tropical areas all suggest that this parasite should be sought in these settings using an acid-fast stain.[81,154]

Isospora belli

I belli is a coccidian protozoan that causes a prolonged syndrome of diarrhea and weight loss in human immunodeficiency virus-infected people, other immunocompromised patients, and, rarely, in travelers (see Chaps. 105 and 110). It has most frequently been described in patients with AIDS from Haiti, in whom it may be responsible for 15% of cases of diarrhea.[155] Other regions of risk are tropical areas of the developing world; disease is increasingly being described in immigrants to temperate areas.[156] *Isospora* is probably transmitted by environmental contamination. Once ingested, the sporulated oocysts excyst in the small intestine, where invasion of the intestinal epithelium occurs. Asexual reproduction produces merozoites that invade other epithelial cells or form gametes that sexually replicate to produce infective oocysts.

Clinically, *Isospora* infection causes illness similar to that with *Cryptosporidium*. Crampy abdominal pain and nausea are common, and there may be a prolonged syndrome of diarrhea (as long as 6 months if not treated). Weight loss is common, fever and vomiting are uncommon. *Isospora* oocysts can be detected in the stool by modified Kinyon acid-fast stain demonstrating ovoid-shaped, thin-walled cysts 20 to 30 μm in length and 12 to 14 μm in width (Figs. 106-7 and 106-8). Intracellular parasites should be detected on small bowel biopsy. Unlike cryptosporidiosis, there is effective treatment for *Isospora* infection: trimethoprim-sulfamethoxazole given for 10 days. Patients with AIDS, however, may relapse and require either a second course of treatment or prolonged suppressive therapy.[157] For sulfonamide-intolerant patients, pyrimethamine alone may be an effective alternative.[158]

Blastocystis hominis

Blastocystis hominis is an intestinal protozoan commonly detected in the stool. It remains controversial whether it is a cause of diarrhea.[159] The parasite is a strict anaerobe, lacks a cell wall, and varies in diameter from 4 to 15 μm. It usually undergoes division by binary fission.[160] In the developed world the prevalence of *Blastocystis* is 5% to 10%, and in the developing world 20% or more.

Studies examining the role of *Blastocystis* as a cause of diarrhea indicate that it is frequently detected in both asymptom-

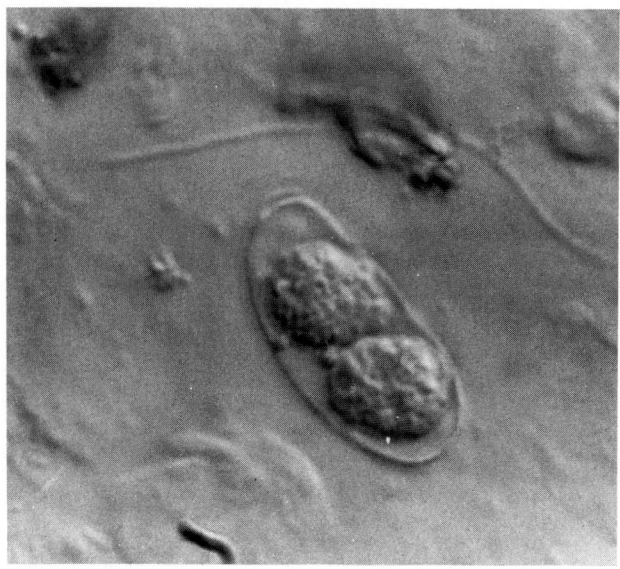

FIGURE 106-7. *Isospora belli* sporulated oocyst from stool. (Nomarski image.)

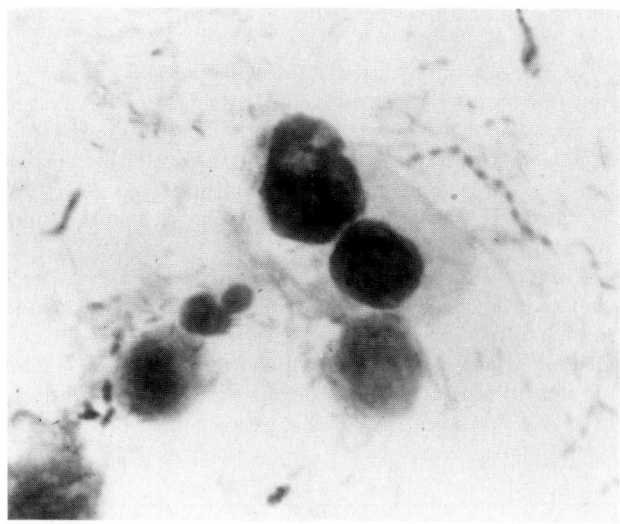

FIGURE 106-8. *Isospora belli* speculated oocyst from stool. (Modified acid-fast stain.)

atic and symptomatic patients, it is commonly associated with other intestinal pathogens, and treatment does not always correlate with improvement of symptoms or eradication of the parasite.[161-166] Nevertheless, *Blastocystis* infection may be the cause of illness in patients in whom a careful search for other viral, bacterial, or parasitic organisms is negative. Symptoms attributed to it include diarrhea, abdominal pain, anorexia, weight loss, and flatulence. The parasite is detected by a wet mount or trichrome stain of fresh or concentrated stool specimens. Although a criteria of more than five organisms per high-powered field has been used to distinguish clinically significant infections, both symptomatic and asymptomatic patients can excrete more or less than this number.[160,162,166] Metronidazole and iodoquinol have been used for therapy with variable success.

Microsporidia

Microsporidian protozoa of several genera have been recognized as causing widespread infection in patients with AIDS (see Chap. 105).[167] The parasite can also chronically and latently infect mammals. Microsporidian infections, predominantly those of *Enterocytozoon bieneusi* and possibly *Septata intestinalis*, most frequently cause persistent diarrhea in patients with AIDS. Although initially requiring intestinal biopsy and electron microscopy for diagnosis, improved stains and perhaps fluorescence antibody and other methods are being developed, and hold promise for improved diagnosis of microsporidial infection with fecal specimens.[168]

Balantidium coli

Balantidium coli is a ciliate protozoan that can cause ulcerations of the rectosigmoid colon with secondary bacteremia or dysentery. Extraintestinal spread has not been described. It is a rare cause of diarrhea in the United States.

Trypanosoma cruzi *(Chagas' Disease)*

Trypanosoma cruzi is mentioned in this chapter because of the gastrointestinal manifestations of chronic Chagas' disease. The megaesophagus and megacolon that result from *T cruzi* infection are covered more extensively in the chapters on esophageal and colonic dysfunction (Chaps. 54 and 82). *T cruzi* infection is spread by the bite of the reduvid bug in Central and South America. The reduvid insects become infected by ingesting blood containing trypomastigotes from infected animals or humans. *T cruzi* differentiates into epimastigotes and then infective metacyclic trypomastigotes in the intestinal tract of the insect. Insect feces that contain trypomastigotes contaminate mucous membranes or puncture sites during the time of feeding and are the means by which a new human host is infected.

Epidemiologic studies indicate that several million people in Latin America are infected with this parasite, resulting in thousands of deaths annually. In the United States, increased numbers of cases have occurred secondary to the entry of immigrants from Mexico, Central America, and South America. As examples, 5% of Central American immigrants tested in Washington, DC were positive for *T cruzi*, and 1 of every 1000 prospective blood donors in Los Angeles was found to be infected with the parasite.[169,170] The effect of this changing epidemiology has been seen in a small number of transfusion-associated cases, some of which have resulted in fulminant disease when the recipient was immunocompromised.[171]

The acute infection is usually asymptomatic; however, children and, less frequently, adults may show symptoms of unilateral periorbital edema at the site of the reduvid bite (Romaña's sign), fever, adenopathy, hepatosplenomegaly, and constitutional symptoms. A few patients may have severe myocarditis. Chronic disease occurs many years after infection and is primarily manifested by cardiac or gastrointestinal disease. The pathogenesis of infection is multifactoral and involves host genetics, parasite-derived factors, and autoimmune responses.[172] Slow destruction of both the myocardium itself and its conduction system results in arrhythmias, myocarditis, and cardiomyopathy.

In the gastrointestinal tract, esophageal and colonic abnormalities are most common, and in their extreme can result in megaesophagus and megacolon.[172-174] A progressive loss of innervation in both the esophagus and colon because of neuronal destruction, along with abnormal responses to gut hormones, result in symptoms of dysphagia, regurgitation, and constipation.

Diagnosis of Chagas' disease can be made in an appropriate clinical setting by detecting parasites in Giemsa-stained blood smears, cultivating the organisms in specialized medium, performing xenodiagnosis with reduvid bugs, or using one of the new serologic tests. Unfortunately, in chronic disease, chemotherapy is not useful and patients must be managed symptomatically.

> The reader is directed to Chapter 26, The Gastrointestinal Microflora; Chapter 38, Approach to the Patient With Diarrhea; Chapter 39, Approach to the Patient With Constipation; Chapter 46, Approach to Gastrointestinal Problems in the Immunocompromised Patient; Chapter 54, Motility Disorders of the Esophagus; Chapter 70, Small Intestine: Infections With Common Bacterial and Viral Pathogens; Chapter 71, Chronic Infections of the Small Intestine; Chapter 82, Motility Disorders of the Colon; Chapter 84, Bacterial Infections of the Colon; Chapter 105, Gastrointestinal Complications of the Acquired Immunodeficiency Syndrome; Chapter 110, Gastrointestinal Manifestations of Immunologic Disorders; Chapter 116, Colonoscopy and Flexible Sigmoidoscopy; Chapter 130, Endoscopic Mucosal Biopsy; and Chapter 131, Microbiologic Studies.

REFERENCES

1. Ravdin JI, Petri WA Jr. *Entamoeba histolytica*. In: Mandell GL, Douglas RG Jr, Bennett JR, eds. Principles and practice of infectious disease. New York: Churchill-Livingstone, 1990:2036.
2. Wanke CA, Butler T, Islam M. Epidemiologic and clinical features of invasive amebiasis in Bangladesh. Am J Trop Med Hyg 1988;38:335.
3. Ravdin JI, Croft BY, Guerrant RL. Cytopathogenic mechanisms of *Entamoeba histolytica*. J Exp Med 1980;152:377.
4. Ravdin JI, Guerrant RL. The role of adherence in cytopathogenic mechanisms of *Entamoeba histolytica*: study with mammalian tissue culture cells and human red blood cells. J Clin Invest 1980;68:1305.
5. Petri WA Jr, Smith RD, Schlesinger PH, et al. Isolation of the galactose binding adherence lectin of *Entamoeba histolytica*. J Clin Invest 1987;80:1238.
6. Chadee K, Petri WA Jr, Innes DJ, Ravdin JI. Rat and human colonic mucins bind to and inhibit the adherence lectin of *Entamoeba histolytica*. J Clin Invest 1987;80:1245.
7. Ravdin JI, Sperelakis N, Guerrant RL. Effect of ion channel inhibitors on the cytopathogenicity of *Entamoeba histolytica*. J Infect Dis 1983;147:217.
8. Long-Krug SA, Fischer KJ, Hysmith RM, et al. Phospholipase A enzymes of *Entamoeba histolytica*: description and subcellular localization. J Infect Dis 1985;152:536.
9. Weikel CS, Sando J, Ravdin JI. Phorbol ester binding activity and promotion of cytolytic activity in *Entamoeba histolytica*. Clin Res 1986;34:537A.
10. Young JDE, Young TM, Lu LP, et al. Characterization of a membrane pore-forming protein from *Entamoeba histolytica*. Exp Med 1982;156:1677.
11. Dodson JM, Petri WA Jr. Pore formation and cytolysis by *Entamoeba histolytica*. Parasitology Today 1994;10:7.
12. Guerrant RL, Brush J, Ravdin JI, et al. The interaction between *Entamoeba histolytica* and human polymorphonuclear leukocytes. J Infect Dis 1981;143:83.
13. Salata RA, Pearson RD, Ravdin JI. The interaction of human leukocytes and *Entamoeba histolytica*: killing of virulent amebae by the activated macrophage. J Clin Invest 1985;76:491.
14. Krogstad DJ. Isoenzyme patterns and pathogenicity in amebic infection. N Engl J Med 1986;315:390.
15. Diamond LS, Clark CG. A redescription of *Entamoeba histolytica* Schaudinn, 1903 (Emended Walker, 1911) separating it from *Entamoeba dispar* Brumpt, 1925. J Eukaryot Microbiol 1993;40:340.
16. Adams EB, MacLeod IN. Invasive amebiasis. I. Amebic dysentery and its complications. Medicine 1977;56:315.
17. Adams EB, MacLeod IN. Invasive amebiasis. II. Amebic liver abscess and its complications. Medicine 1977;56:325.
18. Katzenstein D, Rickerson V, Braude A. New concepts of amebic liver abscess derived from hepatic imaging, serodiagnosis and hepatic enzymes in 67 consecutive cases in San Diego. Medicine 1982;61:237.
19. Haque R, Kress K, Wood S, et al. Diagnosis of pathogenic *Entamoeba histolytica* infection using a stool ELISA based on monoclonal antibodies to the galactose-specific adhesin. J Infect Dis 1993;167:247.
20. Kagan IG. Serologic diagnosis of parasitic diseases. N Engl J Med 1970;282:685.
21. Ralls PW, Quinn MF, Boswell WD, et al. Patterns of resolution in successfully treated hepatic amebic abscess: sonographic evaluation. Radiology 1983;149:541.
22. Drugs for parasitic infections. Med Lett Drug Ther 1993;35:111.
23. Adam RD. The biology of *Giardia* spp. Microbiol Rev 1991;55:706.
24. Nash TE, Keister DB. Differences in excretory-secretory products and surface antigens among 19 isolates of *Giardia*. J Infect Dis 1985;152:1166.
25. Campbell SR, van Keulen H, Erlandsen SL, et al. *Giardia* sp.: comparison of electrophoretic karyotypes. Exp Parasitol 1990;71:470.
26. Nash TE, Herrington DA, Losonsky GA, et al. Experimental human infections with *Giardia lamblia*. J Infect Dis 1987;156:974.
27. Visvesvara GS, Dickerson JW, Healy GR. Variable infectivity of human-derived *Giardia lamblia* cysts for Mongolian gerbils (*Meriones unguiculatus*). J Clin Microbiol 1988;26:837.
28. Nash TE, Herrington DA, Levine MM, et al. Antigenic variation of *Giardia lamblia* in experimental human infections. J Immunol 1990;144:4362.
29. Peattie DA. The giardins of *Giardia lamblia*: genes and proteins with promise. Parasitology Today 1990;6:52.
30. Gault MJ, Gillin FD, Zenian AJ. *Giardia lamblia*: stimulation of growth by human intestinal mucus and epithelial cells in serumfree medium. Exp Parasitol 1987;64:29.
31. Gillin FD, Boucher SE, Reiner DS. *Giardia lamblia*: the roles of bile, lactic acid, and pH in completion of the life cycle in vitro. Exp Parasitol 1989;69:164.
32. Gilman RH, Brown KH, Visvesvara GS, et al. Epidemiology and serology of *Giardia lamblia* in a developing country: Bangladesh. Trans R Soc Trop Med Hyg 1985;79:469.
33. Farthing MJG, Mata L, Urrutia JJ, et al. Natural history of *Giardia* infection of infants and children in rural Guatemala and its impact on physical growth. Am J Clin Nutr 1986;43:395.
34. Gilman RH, Marquis GS, Miranda E, et al. Rapid reinfection by *Giardia lamblia* after treatment in a hyperendemic third world community. Lancet 1988;1:343.
35. Erlandsen SL, Sherlock LA, Januschka M, et al. Cross-species transmission of *Giardia* spp.: inoculation of beavers and muskrats with cysts of human, beaver, mouse, and muskrat origin. Appl Environ Microbiol 1988;54:2777.
36. Buret A, denHollander N, Wallis PM, et al. Zoonotic potential

of giardiasis in domestic ruminants. J Infect Dis 1991;162:231.

37. Capon AG, Upcroft JA, Boreham PFL, et al. Similarities of *Giardia* antigens derived from human and animal sources. Int J Parasitol 1989;19:91.

38. Castor SB, Lindqvist KB. Canine giardiasis in Sweden: no evidence of infectivity to man. Trans R Soc Trop Med Hyg 1990;84:249.

39. Bemrick WJ, Erlandsen SL. Giardiasis: is it really a zoonosis? Parasitology Today 1988;4:69.

40. Issac-Renton JL, Cordeiro C, Sarafis K, Shahriari H. Characterization of *Giardia duodenalis* isolates from a waterborne outbreak. J Infect Dis 1993;167:431.

41. deRegnier DP, Cole L, Schupp DG, et al. Viability of *Giardia* cysts suspended in lake, river, and tap water. Appl Environ Microbiol 1989;55:1223.

42. Craun GF. Waterborne giardiasis in the United States 1965–1984. Lancet 1986;2:513.

43. Birkhead G, Vogt RL. Epidemiologic surveillance for endemic *Giardia lamblia* infection in Vermont: the roles of waterborne and person-to-person transmission. Am J Epidemiol 1989;129:762.

44. Jakubowski W. Purple burps and the filtration of drinking water supplies (editorial). Am J Public Health 1988;78:123.

45. Pickering LK, Woodward WE, DuPont HL, Sullivan P. Occurrence of *Giardia lamblia* in children in day care centers. J Pediatr 1984;104:522.

46. Mintz ED, Hudson-Wragg M, Mshar P, et al. Foodborne giardiasis in a corporate office setting. J Infect Dis 1993;167:250.

47. White KE, Hedberg CW, Edmonson LM, et al. An outbreak of giardiasis in a nursing home with evidence for multiple modes of transmission. J Infect Dis 1989;160:298.

48. Quick R, Paugh K, Addiss D, et al. Restaurant-associated outbreak of giardiasis. J Infect Dis 1992;166:673.

49. Ward HD, Lev BI, Kane AV, et al: Identification and characterization of taglin, a mannose-6-phosphate binding, trypsin-activated lectin from *Giardia lamblia*. Biochemistry 1987;26:8669.

50. Balazs M, Szaltocky E. Electron microscopic examination of the mucosa of the small intestine in infection due to *Giardia lamblia*. Pathol Res Pract 1978;163:251.

51. Welsh JD, Poley JR, Hensley J, et al. Intestinal disaccharidase and alkaline phosphatase activity in giardiasis. J Pediatr Gastroenterol Nutr 1984;3:37.

52. Buret A, Gall DG, Nation PN, Olson ME. Intestinal protozoa and epithelial cell kinetics, structure and function. Parasitology Today 1990;6:375.

53. Roberts-Thomson IC, Stevens DP, Mahmoud AAF, et al. Giardiasis in the mouse: an animal model. Gastroenterology 1976;71:57.

54. Miotti PPG, Gilman RH, Santosham M, et al. Age-related rate of seropositivity of antibody to *Giardia lamblia* in four diverse populations. J Clin Microbiol 1986;24:972.

55. Istre GP, Dunlop TS, Gaspard GB, et al. Waterborne giardiasis at a mountain resort: evidence for acquired immunity. Am J Public Health 1984;74:602.

56. denHollander N, Riley D, Befus D. Immunology of giardiasis. Parasitology Today 1988;4:124.

57. Heyworth MF. Immunology of *Giardia* and *Cryptosporidium* infections. J Infect Dis 1992;166:465.

58. Ljungström I, Castor B. Immune response to *Giardia lamblia* in a water-borne outbreak of giardiasis in Sweden. J Med Microbiol 1992;36:347.

59. Reiner DS, Gillin FD. Human secretory and serum antibodies recognize environmentally induced antigens of *Giardia lamblia*. Infect Immun 1992;60:637.

60. Ridley MJ, Ridley DS. Serum antibodies and jejunal histology in giardiasis. J Clin Pathol 1976;29:30.

61. Char S, Cervallos AM, Yamson P, et al. Impaired IgA response to *Giardia* heat shock antigen in children with persistent diarrhoea and giardiasis. Gut 1993;34:38.

62. Birkhead G, Janoff EN, Vogt RL, et al. Elevated levels of immunoglobulin A to *Giardia lamblia* during a waterborne outbreak of gastroenteritis. J Clin Microbiol 1989;27:1707.

63. Underdown BJ, Skea DL, Loney GM, et al. Murine giardiasis and mucosal immunity: a model for the study of immunity to intestinal protozoan parasites. Monogr Allergy 1988;24:287.

64. Heyworth MF, Carlson JR, Ermak TH. Clearance of *Giardia muris* infection requires helper/inducer T lymphocytes. J Exp Med 1987;165:1743.

65. Roberts-Thomson IC, Mitchell GF. Giardiasis in mice. I. Prolonged infections in certain mouse strains and hypothymic (nude) mice. Gastroenterology 1978;75:42.

66. Duncombe VM, Bolin TD, Davis AE, et al. Histopathology in giardiasis: a correlation with diarrhea. Aust N Z J Med 1978;8:392.

67. Hjelt K, Paerregaard A, Krasilnikoff PA. Giardiasis causing chronic diarrhoea in suburban Copenhagen: incidence, physical growth, clinical symptoms and small intestinal abnormality. Acta Paediatr 1992;81:881.

68. Hill DR, Pohl R. Ingestion of *Giardia lamblia* trophozoites by murine Peyer's patch macrophages. Infect Immun 1990;58:3202.

69. Hill DR. Lymphocyte proliferation in Peyer's patches of *Giardia muris* infected mice. Infect Immun 1990;58:2683.

70. Reiner DS, Wang CS, Gillin FD. Human milk kills *Giardia lamblia* by generating toxic lipolytic products. J Infect Dis 1986;154:825.

71. Morrow AL, Reves RR, West MS, et al. Protection against infection with *Giardia lamblia* by breast feeding in a cohort of Mexican infants. J Pediatr 1992;121:363.

72. LoGalbo PR, Sampson HA, Buckley RH. Symptomatic giardiasis in three patients with X-linked agammaglobulinemia. J Pediatr 1982;101:78.

73. Janoff EN, Smith PD, Blaser MJ. Acute antibody responses to *Giardia lamblia* are depressed in patients with AIDS. J Infect Dis 1988;157:798.

74. Smith PD, Lane HC, Gill VJ, et al. Intestinal infections in patients with the acquired immunodeficiency syndrome (AIDS): etiology and response to therapy. Ann Intern Med 1988;108:328.

75. Doglioni C, De Boni M, Cielo R, et al. Gastric giardiasis. J Clin Pathol 1992;45:964.

76. Burke JA. Giardiasis in childhood. Am J Dis Child 1975;129:1304.

77. Solomons NW. Giardiasis: nutritional implications. Rev Infect Dis 1982;4:859.

78. Gupta MC, Urrutia JJ. Effect of periodic antiascaris and antigiardia treatment on nutritional status of preschool children. Am J Clin Nutr 1982;36:79.

79. Sullivan PS, DuPont HL, Arafat RR, et al. Illness and reservoirs associated with *Giardia lamblia* infection in rural Egypt: the case against treatment in developing world environments of high endemicity. Am J Epidemiol 1988;127:1272.

80. Weber R, Bryan RT, Owen RL, et al. Improved light microscopical detection of microsporidia spores in stool and duodenal aspirates. N Engl J Med 1992;326:161.

81. Ortega YR, Sterling CR, Gilman RH, et al. Cyclospora species: a new protozoan pathogen of humans. N Engl J Med 1993;328:1308.

82. Wolfe MS. Giardiasis. Clin Microbiol Rev 1992;5:93.

83. Hill DR. Giardiasis: issues in management and treatment. Infect Dis Clin North Am 1993;7:503.

84. Addiss DG, Mathews HM, Stewart JM, et al. Evaluation of a commercially available enzyme-linked immunosorbent assay for *Giardia lamblia* antigen in stool. J Clin Microbiol 1991;29:1137.

85. Garcia LS, Shum AC, Bruckner DA. Evaluation of a new monoclonal antibody combination reagent for direct fluorescence detection of *Giardia* cysts and *Cryptosporidium* oocysts in human fecal specimens. J Clin Microbiol 1992;30:3255.

86. Thornton SA, West AH, DuPont HL, Pickering LK. Comparison of methods for identification of *Giardia lamblia*. Am J Clin Pathol 1983;80:858.

87. Goka AKJ, Rolston DDK, Mathan VI, et al. The relative merits of faecal and duodenal juice microscopy in the diagnosis of giardiasis. Trans R Soc Trop Med Hyg 1990;84:66.

88. Sullivan PB, Neale G, Cevallos AM, et al. Evaluation of specific

serum anti-*Giardia* IgM antibody response in diagnosis in children. Trans R Soc Trop Med Hyg 1991;85:748.

89. Davidson RA. Issues in clinical parasitology: the treatment of giardiasis. Am J Gastroenterol 1984;79:256.
90. Lerman SJ, Walker RA. Treatment of giardiasis: literature review and recommendations. Clin Pediatr 1982;21:409.
91. Beard CM, Noller KL, O'Fallon WM, et al. Cancer after exposure to metronidazole. Mayo Clin Proc 1988;63:147.
92. Murphy TV, Nelson JD. Five vs. ten days' therapy with furazolidone for giardiasis. Am J Dis Child 1983;137:267.
93. Speelman P. Single-dose tinidazole for the treatment of giardiasis. Antimicrob Agents Chemother 1985;27:227.
94. Taylor GD, Wenman WM, Tyrrell DLJ. Combined metronidazole and quinacrine hydrochloride therapy for chronic giardiasis. Can Med Assoc J 1987;136:1179.
95. Kreutner AK, Del Bene VE, Amstey MS. Giardiasis in pregnancy. Am J Obstet Gynecol 1981;140:895.
96. Rotblatt MD. Giardiasis and amebiasis in pregnancy. Drug Intell Clin Pharm 1983;17:187.
97. Briggs GG, Freeman RK, Yaffe SJ. Metronidazole. In: Briggs GG, Freeman RK, Yaffe SJ, eds. Drugs in pregnancy and lactation. 3rd ed. Baltimore: Williams & Wilkins, 1990:430.
98. Ish-Horowicz M, Korman SH, Shapiro M, et al. Asymptomatic giardiasis in children. Pediatr Infect Dis J 1989;8:773.
99. Dennis DT, Smith RP, Welch JJ, et al. Endemic giardiasis in New Hampshire: A case-control study of environmental risks. J Infect Dis 1993;167:1391.
100. Bartlett AV, Englender SJ, Jarvis BA, et al. Controlled trial of *Giardia lamblia*: control strategies in day care centers. Am J Public Health 1991;81:1001.
101. Ongerth JE, Johnson RL, MacDonald SC, et al. Backcountry water treatment to prevent giardiasis. Am J Public Health 1989;79:1633.
102. Tyzzer EE. A sporozoan found in the peptic glands of the common mouse. Proc Soc Exp Biol Med 1907;5:12.
103. Current WL. The biology of *Cryptosporidium*. ASM News 1988;54:605.
104. Slavin D. *Cryptosporidium* meleagridis (sp. Nov.). J Comp Pathol 1955;65:262.
105. Panciera RJ, Thomassen R, Garner FM. Cryptosporidial infection in a calf. Vet Pathol 1971;8:479.
106. Centers for Disease Control. *Cryptosporidium*: assessment of chemotherapy of males with acquired immunodeficiency syndrome (AIDS). MMWR 1982;31:589.
107. Navin TR, Juranek DD. Cryptosporidiosis: clinical, epidemiologic, and parasitologic review. Rev Infect Dis 1984;6:313.
108. Current WL, Reese NC, Ernst JV, et al. Human cryptosporidiosis in immunocompetent and immunodeficient persons. N Engl J Med 1983;308:1252.
109. Soave R, Armstrong D. Cryptosporidium and cryptosporidiosis. Rev Infect Dis 1986;8:1012.
110. Tzipori S. Cryptosporidiosis in animals and humans. Microbiol Rev 1983;47:84.
111. Fayer R, Ungar BLP. Cryptosporidium spp. and cryptosporidiosis. Microbiol Rev 1986;50:458.
112. Wolfson JS, Richter JM, Waldron MA, et al. Cryptosporidiosis in immunocompetent patients. N Engl J Med 1985;312:1278.
113. Janoff EN, Reller LB. Cryptosporidium species, a protean protozoan. J Clin Microbiol 1987;25:967.
114. Mata L, Bolanos H, Pizarro D, Vives M. Cryptosporidiosis in children from some highland Costa Rican rural and urban areas. Am J Trop Med Hyg 1984;33:24.
115. Weikel CS, Johnston LI, de Souza MA, Guerrant RL. Cryptosporidiosis in northeastern Brazil: association with sporadic diarrhea. J Infect Dis 1985;151:963.
116. Hojlyin N, Molbak K, Jepsen S. Cryptosporidium spp., a frequent cause of diarrhea in Liberian children. J Clin Microbiol 1986;23:1109.
117. Adal KA, Sterling CR, Guerrant RL, *Cryptosporidium* and related species. In: Blaser MJ, Smith PD, Ravdin JI, et al, eds. Infections of the gastrointestinal tract. New York: Raven Press, 1994.
118. Newman RD, Zu S-X, Wuhib R, et al. Household epidemiology of *Cryptosporidium parvum* infection in an urban community in Northeast Brazil. Am Intern Med 1994;120:500.

119. Fang G, Lima AAM, Martins CC, et al. Etiology and epidemiology of persistent diarrhea in northeastern Brazil: a hospital-based prospective case control study. J Pediatr Gastroenterol Nutr 1994 (in press).
120. Alpert G, Bell LM, Kirkpatrick CE, et al. Outbreak of cryptosporidiosis in a day care center. Pediatrics 1986;77:152.
121. Crawford FG, Vermund SH, Ma JY, Dedielbaum RJ. Asymptomatic cryptosporidiosis in a New York City day care center. Pediatr Infect Dis J 1988;7:806.
122. Koch KL, Phillips DJ, Aber RC, Current WL. Cryptosporidiosis in hospital personnel. Ann Intern Med 1985;102:593.
123. D'Antonio RG, Winn RE, Taylor JP, et al. A waterborne outbreak of cryptosporidiosis in normal hosts. Ann Intern Med 1985;103:886.
124. Smith HV, Girdwood RWA, Patterson WJ, et al. Waterborne outbreak of cryptosporidiosis. Lancet 1988;1:1484.
125. Hayes EB, Matt TD, O'Brien TR, et al. Large community outbreak of cryptosporidiosis due to contamination of a filtered public water supply. N Engl J Med 1989;320:1372.
126. Heine J, Moon HW, Woodmansee DB. Persistent *Cryptosporidium* infection in congenitally athymic (nude) mice. Infect Immun 1984;43:856.
127. Moon HW, Pohlenz JFL, Woodmansee DB, et al. Intestinal cryptosporidiosis: pathogenesis and immunity. Microecol Ther 1985;15:102.
128. Gardner AC, Key JH, Roche JK, et al. Symptomatic cryptosporidiosis: an immunocompromised rat model of infection. Clin Res 1989;37:428A.
129. Weikel CS, Gaynes BN, Roche JK. Diarrhoeal diseases in the immunocompromised patient. In: Guerrant RL, ed. Baillière's clinical tropical medicine and communicable diseases. London: Baillière Tindall, 1988:401.
130. Garza DH, Fedorak RN, Soave R, et al. Enterotoxin-like activity in cultured cryptosporidia: role in diarrhea. Gastroenterology 1986;90:1424.
131. Guerrant RL, Petri WA, Weikel CS. Parasitic causes of diarrhea: an overview. In: Lebenthal E, Duffey M, eds. Pathophysiology of secretory diarrhea. New York: Raven Press, 1990:273.
132. Musch MW, Miller RJ, Field M, Siegel MI. Stimulation of colonic secretion by lipoxygenase metabolites of arachidonic acid. Science 1982;217:1255.
133. Modigliani R, Bories C, Charpentier YL, et al. Diarrhoea and malabsorption in acquired immune deficiency syndrome: a study of four cases with special emphasis on opportunistic protozoan infestations. Gut 1985;26:179.
134. Koch KL, Shankey V, Weinstein GS, et al. Cryptosporidiosis in a patient with hemophilia, common variable hypogammaglobulinemia, and the acquired immunodeficiency syndrome. Ann Intern Med 1983;99:337.
135. Petras RE, Carey WD, Alanis A. Cryptosporidial enteritis in a homosexual male with an acquired immunodeficiency syndrome. Cleve Clin Q 1983;50:41.
136. Current WL, Reese NC. A comparison of endogenous development of three isolates of *Cryptosporidium* in suckling mice. J Protozool 1986;33:98.
137. Vetterling JM, Takeuchi A, Madden PA. Ultrastructure of *Cryptosporidium wrairi* from the guinea pig. J Protozool 1971;18:218.
138. Jokipii L, Jokipii MM. Timing of symptoms and oocyst excretion in human cryptosporidiosis. N Engl J Med 1986;315:1643.
139. Ma P, Soave R. Three step stool examinations for cryptosporidiosis in 10 homosexual men with protracted watery diarrhea. J Infect Dis 1983;147:824.
140. Arrowood MJ, Sterling CR. Comparison of conventional staining methods and monoclonal antibody-based methods for *Cryptosporidium* oocyst detection. J Clin Microbiol 1989;27:1490.
141. Newman RD, Jaeger KL, Wuhib R, et al. Evaluation of an antigen capture enzyme-linked immunosorbent assay for detection of *Cryptosporidium* oocysts. J Clin Microbiol 1993;31:2080.
142. Ungar BLA, Soave R, Fayer R, Nash TE. Enzyme immunoassay detection of immunoglobulin M and G antibodies to *Cryptosporidium* in immunocompetent and immunocompromised persons. J Infect Dis 1986;153:570.

143. Lourie E, Borkowsky W, Klesius PH, et al. Treatment of cryptosporidiosis with oral bovine transfer factor. Clin Immunol Immunopathol 1987;44:329.

144. Wittenberg DF, Miller NM, Van Den Ende J. Spiramycin is not effective in treating *Cryptosporidium* diarrhea in infants: results of a double-blind randomized trial. J Infect Dis 1989;159:131.

145. Tzipori S, Roberton D, Cooper DA, White L. Chronic cryptosporidial diarrhoea and hyperimmune cow colostrum. Lancet 1987;2:344.

146. Armitage K, Flanigan T, Carey J, et al. Treatment of cryptosporidiosis with paromomycin: a report of five cases. Arch Intern Med 1992;152:2497.

147. Fichtenbaum CJ, Ritchie DJ, Powderly WJ. Use of paromomycin for treatment of cryptosporidiosis in patients with AIDS. Clin Infect Dis 1993;16:298.

148. Sperber SJ, Gornish N. New macrolide antibiotics. Ann Intern Med 1992;117:533.

149. Soave R, Dubey JP, Ramos LJ, Tummings M. A new intestinal pathogen? Clin Res 1986;34:533A.

150. Long EG, Ebrahimzadeh A, White EH, et al. Alga associated with diarrhea in patients with acquired immunodeficiency syndrome and in travelers. J Clin Microbiol 1990;28:1101.

151. Long EG, White EH, Carmichael WW, et al. Morphologic and staining characteristics of a cynobacterium-like organism associated with diarrhea. J Infect Dis 1991;164:199.

152. Centers for Disease Control. Outbreaks of diarrheal illness associate with cyanobacteria (blue green algae)-like bodies: Chicago and Nepal, 1989 and 1990. MMWR 1991;40:325.

153. Shlim DR, Cohen MT, Eaton M, et al. An alga-like organism associated with an outbreak of prolonged diarrhea among foreigners in Nepal. Am J Trop Med Hyg 1991;45:3.

154. Bendall RP, Lucas S, Moody A, et al. Diarrhoea associated with cyanobacteria-like bodies: a new coccidian enteritis of man. Lancet 1993;341:590.

155. DeHovitz JA, Pape JW, Boncy M, Johnson WD. Clinical manifestations and therapy of *Isospora belli* infection in patients with the acquired immunodeficiency syndrome. N Engl J Med 1986;315:87.

156. Sorvillo F, Lieb L, Iwakoshi K, Waterman SH. *Isospora belli* and the acquired immunodeficiency syndrome (letter). N Engl J Med 1990;322:131.

157. Pape JW, Verdier RI, Johnson WD. Treatment and prophylaxis of *Isospora belli* infection in patients with the acquired immunodeficiency syndrome. N Engl J Med 1989;320:1044.

158. Weiss LM, Perlman DC, Sherman J, et al. *Isospora belli* infection: treatment with pyrimethamine. Ann Intern Med 1988;109:474.

159. *Blastocystis hominis*: commensal or pathogen? (editorial). Lancet 1991;337:5521.

160. Zierdt CH. *Blastocystis hominis*: past and future. Clin Microbiol Rev 1991;4:61.

161. Senay H, MacPherson D. *Blastocystis hominis*: epidemiology and natural history. J Infect Dis 1990;162:987.

162. Udkow MP, Markell EK. *Blastocystis hominis*: prevalence in asymptomatic versus symptomatic hosts. J Infect Dis 1993;168:242.

163. Miller RA, Minshe BH. *Blastocystis hominis*: an organism in search of a disease. Rev Infect Dis 1988;10:930.

164. Grossman I, Weiss LM, Simon D, et al. *Blastocystis hominis* in hospital employees. Am J Gastroenterol 1992;87:729.

165. O'Gorman MA, Orenstein SR, Proujansky R, et al. Prevalence and characteristics of *Blastocystis hominis* infection in children. Clin Pediatr 1993;32:91.

166. Kain KC, Noble MA, Freeman HJ, Barteluk RL. Epidemiology and clinical features associated with *Blastocystis hominis* infection. Diagn Microbiol Infect Dis 1987;8:235.

167. Shattuck JA. Human microsporidiosis and AIDS. Rev Infect Dis 1989;11:203.

168. Weber R, Bryan RT, Owen RL, et al. Improved light microscopic detection of microsporidia spores in stool and duodenal aspirates. N Engl J Med 1992;326:161.

169. Kirchhoff LV, Gam AA, Gilliam FC. American trypanosomiasis (Chagas' disease) in Central American immigrants. Am J Med 1987;82:915.

170. Kerndt PR, Waskin HA, Kirchhoff LV, et al. Prevalence of antibody to *Trypanosoma cruzi* among blood donors in Los Angeles, California. Transfusion 1991;31:814.

171. Grant IH, Gold JWM, Wittner M, et al. Transfusion-associated acute Chagas' disease acquired in the United States. Ann Intern Med 1989;111:849.

172. Tanowitz HB, Kirchhoff LV, Simon D, et al. Chagas' disease. Clin Microbiol Rev 1992;5:400.

173. Koeberle F. Chagas' disease and Chagas' syndromes: the pathology of American trypanosomiasis. Adv Parasitol 1968;6:63.

174. Tanowitz HB, Simon D, Grumprecht JP, et al. Gastrointestinal manifestations of Chagas' disease. In: Rustgi VK, ed. Gastrointestinal infections in the tropics. Basel: S. Karger, 1990:56.

Textbook of Gastroenterology, second edition, edited
by Tadataka Yamada. JB Lippincott Company,
Philadelphia © 1995.

CHAPTER 107

Parasitic Diseases: Helminths

Richard D. Pearson

Intestinal Nematodes
    Trichuris trichiura *(Whipworm)*
    Enterobius vermicularis *(Pinworm)*
    Capillaria philippinensis
    Trichostrongylus *Species*
    Ascaris lumbricoides
    Trichinella spiralis
    Hookworms
    Strongyloides stercoralis
    Intestinal Nematodes of Animals That Infect Humans
Cestodes (Tapeworms)

    Taenia saginat
    Taenia solium
    Diphyllobothrium latum
    Hymenolepis nana
    *Echinococcosis (*Echinococcus granulosus *and*
        Echinococcus multilocularis*)*
Trematodes
    Schistosomiasis
    Liver Flukes
    Intestinal Flukes

Intestinal helminths are prevalent throughout the world in areas where sanitation and public health measures are poor. Although many of those infested are asymptomatic, the impact of helminthic infections on health and childhood development in endemic areas can be substantial. In industrialized countries, *Enterobius vermicularis*, the pinworm, is common among children, and other intestinal helminths are encountered among immigrants, returning travelers, and occasionally local residents.

The pathogenic intestinal helminths (Table 107-1) are divided into the roundworms (Nemathelminthes of the class Nematoda) and the flatworms (Platyhelminthes), which are subdivided into the Cestoda, or tapeworms, and the Trematoda, or flukes.[1-4] This classification system is useful clinically because members of these groups tend to have similar life cycles, metabolic pathways, and susceptibilities to chemotherapeutic agents.

The degree to which intestinal helminths compromise health depends on multiple factors, including their genetically determined pathogenicity and the nutritional status and immune responses of their hosts. In general, tissue damage and disease correlate with the magnitude of the parasite load, although there are instances in which a single worm or limited number of worms or larvae produce life-threatening disease. Helminths typically have complex life cycles and cannot multiply in their human hosts; the degree of infection, therefore, depends on the magnitude of the infecting inoculum. Exceptions are *Strongyloides stercoralis*, *Capillaria philippinensis*, and *Hymenolepis nana*, in which autoinfection can result in large

parasite burdens and persistent infection. Adult helminths also have finite life spans. Most of the common intestinal nematodes die after several years, although a few of the intestinal flukes, such as *Clonorchis sinensis*, can survive for more than 30 years.

Exposure in an endemic area along with clinical evidence of disease should alert the clinician to the possibility of an intestinal helminthic infection. Eosinophilia may be present, but it is neither a sensitive nor a specific measure of infection. A species-specific diagnosis usually depends on identification of adult worms, larvae, or ova in stool or tissue. Serologic tests provide presumptive evidence of infection. A number of excellent drugs are available for the treatment of helminthic infections (Table 107-2).[5,6]

INTESTINAL NEMATODES

Intestinal nematodes, or roundworms (see Table 107-1), are prevalent in areas of the world where indiscriminate defecation occurs. It is not uncommon for most residents in a rural area to be infected with more than one species. Children tend to have the highest worm burdens. The life cycles of the intestinal nematodes vary, but they can be divided into three general patterns. In the case of *Trichuris trichiura* and *E vermicularis*, infection follows ingestion of ova, which excyst and then develop within the confines of the gastrointestinal tract. After ingestion of *Ascaris lumbricoides* ova, excystation occurs in the gastrointestinal tract, and larvae invade the intestinal wall,

TABLE 107-1
Helminthic Infections Involving the Human Gastrointestinal Tract

Intestinal Nematodes (Roundworms)

Infection confined to the gastrointestinal tract
- Trichuris trichiura
- Enterobius vermicularis
- Capillaria philippinensis
- Trichostrongylus species

Infection begins in the gastrointestinal tract; larvae invade other organs, adults reside in the gastrointestinal tract
- Ascaris lumbricoides
- Trichinella spiralis

Larvae invade the skin and enter the systemic circulation; adults are confined to the gastrointestinal tract
- Hookworms (Ancylostoma duodenale, Necator americanus)
- Strongyloides stercoralis

Intestinal nematodes of animals that can infect humans
- Cutaneous larva migrans (Ancylostoma braziliense, Ancylostoma caninum, and others)
- Visceral larva migrans (Toxocara canis, Toxocara cati, and others)
- Anisakiasis (Anisakis sp and others)
- Angiostrongylus costaricensis

Cestodes (Tapeworms)

Taenia saginata
Taenia solium
Diphylobothrium latum
Hymenolepis nana
Echinococcosis (Echinococcus granulosus, Echinococcus multilocularis)

Trematodes (Flukes)

Schistosomiasis (Schistosoma mansoni, Schistosoma japonicum, Schistosoma haematobium)
Liver flukes (Clonorchis sinensis, Opisthorchis viverrini, Fasciola hepatica)
Intestinal flukes (Fasciolopsis buski, Heterophyes heterophyes, Metagonimus yokogawai, Echinostoma species, Nanophyetus salmincola)

---

pass through the venous system to the lungs, migrate into the alveoli, ascend to the pharynx, and are then swallowed, reaching maturity in the intestinal tract. The hookworms and *S stercoralis* invade the skin, pass through the venous system to the lungs, and then follow a pattern of migration comparable to that of *Ascaris*. The clinical manifestations of these helminthic infections usually depend on the organ systems involved. In addition, children in Kenya have had improved growth rates after receiving treatment for hookworms, *T trichiura*, and *A lumbricoides* infections.[7]

Trichuris trichiura (Whipworm)

The whipworm, *T trichiura*, is prevalent in the tropics.[4] Humans become infected when they ingest embryonated eggs. After excystation, larvae penetrate the intestinal mucosa with their thread-like anterior ends, molt, mature, and reattach as adults to the mucosa of the cecum or wall of the colon (Fig. 107-1; see Color Fig. 56). Mature female worms release 2000

to 6000 eggs (Fig. 107-2) per day into the feces. Maturation requires a period of 10 to 14 days in the soil. About 3 months elapse between the ingestion of eggs and the production of ova by mature whipworms. Adults persist in the colon for several years.

Epidemiology

T trichiura has a worldwide distribution. Various *Trichuris* species infect different animals, but only *T trichiura* infects humans. Ova require warm, moist, shaded soil for development. Infection is most frequent in areas without latrines and in communities where untreated human fecal material is used for fertilizer. The severity of infestation usually varies within a community. People with heavy infections are more likely to show manifestations of disease.

Clinical Manifestations

Mild *T trichiura* infections are often asymptomatic.[8] Heavy infections are most common in children between 2 and 10 years of age, and may be associated with frequent, bloody, mucoid stools, anemia, and growth retardation.[9] Rectal prolapse is a rare but potentially serious consequence of heavy infection (see Fig. 107-1 and see Color Fig. 56). Colonic obstruction and perforation also have been reported.[10,11] Eosinophilia is frequently present and may accompany even light infection.

Diagnosis, Treatment, and Prevention

The diagnosis of trichuriasis is confirmed by identifying ova in the stool or adult worms in the colonic mucosa. Mebendazole is the recommended therapy (see Table 107-2).[5,6] Albendazole,[12] which is not yet licensed in the United States, is also effective and has been used in single-dose regimens for mass treatment in endemic communities.[7] *T trichiura* infection can be prevented by adequate sanitary disposal of human feces, hand washing before meals, and proper preparation of food.

Enterobius vermicularis (Pinworm)

E vermicularis is endemic in both temperate and tropical climates.[13,14] It is most frequently encountered among school-aged children living in areas of high population density. People become infected when they ingest ova. The ova hatch in the upper small bowel. Larvae mature as they migrate to the ileum. Adults live 7 weeks (males) to 13 weeks (females). The earliest that eggs appear in the stool is 5 weeks. An infected person may harbor anywhere from a few to several hundred adult pinworms.

At the time of oviposition, the adult female (Fig. 107-3; see Color Fig. 57) migrates out through the anus to lay her eggs on the perianal or perineal skin. Eggs (Fig. 107-4; see Color Fig. 58) are expelled by uterine contraction or death and disintegration of the adult worm, or disruption of the worm during scratching. The shell of the ova consists of a thick outer albuminous layer, which plays a role in adherence to objects in the environment.

TABLE 107-2
Drugs for Treatment of Helminthic Infections

INFECTION	DRUG	ADULT DOSAGE
Roundworms		
Angiostrongylus costaricensis	Thiabendazole*†	25 mg/kg tid × 3 d (max. 3 g/day)
	OR surgical intervention	
Anisakiasis	Surgical or endoscopic removal	
Ascaris lumbricoides	Mebendazole	100 mg bid × 3 d
	OR Pyrantel pamoate	11 mg/kg once (max. 1 g)
	OR Albendazole‡	400 mg once
Capillaria philippinensis	Mebendazole†	200 mg bid × 20d
	OR Albendazole‡	200 mg bid × 10 d
	OR Thiabendazole*	25 mg/kg/d in 2 doses × 30 d
Enterobius vermicularis (pinworm)	Pyrantel pamoate	A single dose of 11 mg/kg (max. 1g); repeat in 2 wk
	OR Mebendazole	A single dose of 100 mg; repeat in 2 wk
	OR Albendazole‡	400 mg once; repeat in 2 weeks
Hookworms		
(*Ancylostoma duodenate, Necator americanus*)	Mebendazole	100 mg bid × 3 d
	OR Pyrantel pamoate*	11 mg/kg (max. 1 g) × 3 d
	OR Albendazole‡	400 mg once
Strongyloides stercoralis	Thiabendazole¶	25 mg/kg bid (max. 3 g/d) × 2 d
	OR Ivermectin	200 mg/kg/d × 1–2 d
Trichnella spiralis	Mebendazole* plus steroids for severe symptoms	200–400 mg tid × 3 d, then 400–500 mg tid × 10 d
Trichostrongylus species	Pyrantel pamoate*	11 mg/kg once (max. 1 g)
	Mebendazole*	100 mg bid × 3 d
	OR Albendazole‡	400 mg once
Trichuris trichiura (whipworm)	Mebendazole	100 mg bid × 3 d
	OR Albendazole‡	400 g once (×3 d for heavy infections)
Visceral larva migrans	Diethylcarbamazine*	2 mg/kg tid × 7–10 d
	OR Albendazole	400 mg bid × 3–5 d
	OR Mebendazole*·‖ ‖	100–200 mg bid × 5 d
Flukes		
Clonorchis sinensis (Chinese liver fluke)	Praziquantel	25 mg/kg tid × 1 d
Fasciola hepatica (sheep liver fluke)	Bithionol§	30–50 mg/kg on alternate days × 10–15 doses
Fasciolopsis buski (intestinal fluke)	Praziquantel*	25 mg/kg tid × 1 d
	OR Niclosamide*	A single dose of 4 tablets (2 g), chewed thoroughly
Heterophyes heterophyes (intestinal fluke)	Praziquantel*	25 mg/kg tid × 1 d
Metagonimus yokogawai (intestinal fluke)	Praziquantel*	25 mg/kg tid × 1 d
Nanophyetus salmincola	Praziquantel*	20 mg/kg tid × 1 d
Opisthorchis viverrini (liver fluke)	Praziquantel*	25 mg/kg tid × 1 d
Paragonimus westermani (lung fluke)	Praziquantel*	25 mg/kg tid × 2 d
	OR Bithionol§	30–50 mg/kg on alternate days × 10–15 doses
Schistosoma species:		
S *haematobium*	Praziquantel	20 mg/kg bid × 1 d
S *japonicum*	Praziquantel	20 mg/kg tid × 1 d
S *mansoni*	Praziquantel	20 mg/kg bid × 1 d
	OR Oxamniquine‖	15 mg/kg once‖
S *mekongi*	Praziquantel	20 mg/kg tid × 1 d
Tapeworms (Adult or Intestinal Stage)		
Diphyllobothrium latum (fish), *Taenia saginata* (beef), *Taenia solium* (pork), *Dipylidium caninum* (dog)	Praziquantel*	10–20 mg/kg once
	OR Niclosamide#	A single dose of 4 tablets (2 g) chewed thoroughly
Hymenolepis nana (dwarf tapeworm)	Praziquantel*	25 mg/kg once
	OR Niclosamide	A single daily dose of 4 tablets (2 g), chewed thoroughly, then 2 tablets daily × 6 d

(continued)

TABLE 107-2.   *(Continued)*

INFECTION	DRUG	ADULT DOSAGE
Tapeworms (Larval or Tissue Stage)		
Echinococcus granulosus	Albendazole‡**	400 mg bid × 28 d, repeated as necessary
	OR Surgical resection	
Echinococcus multilocularis	Surgical resection††	
Cysticercus cellulosae (cysticercosis)‡‡	Praziquantel*	50 mg/kg/d in 3 divided doses × 15 d
	OR Albendazole‡	15 mg/kg/d in 3 divided doses × 28 d, repeated as necessary

* An approved drug, but considered investigational for this condition by the U.S. Food and Drug Administration.

† Effectiveness documented only in animals.

‡ Investigational. Available in the United States from SmithKline Beckman, the manufacturer.

§ In the U.S. this drug is available from the CDC Drug Service, Centers for Disease Control, Atlanta, Georgia 30333, telephone 404-639-3670 (evenings, weekends, and holidays 404-639-2888).

‖ Neuropsychiatric disturbances and seizures have been reported in some patients (Stokvis H, Bauer AGC, Stuiver PC, et al. Seizures associated with oxamniquine therapy. Am J Trop Med Hyg 1986;35:330). In East Africa the dose should be increased to 30 mg/kg/d, and in Egypt and South Africa, 30 mg/kg/d × 2 d Contraindicated in pregnancy.

¶ In disseminated strongyloidiasis, thiabendazole therapy should be continued for at least 5 days.

Niclosamide is effective for the treatment of *T solium,* but because it causes distintegration of segments and release of viable eggs, its use creates a theoretic risk of causing cysticercosis. Some physicians recommend that it be followed in 3 or 4 hours by a purge.

** With a fatty meal to enhance absorption. Some patients may benefit from or require surgical resection of cyst. (From Tompkins RK. Management of echinococcal cysts. Mayo Clin Proc 1991;66:1281.)

†† Surgical excision is the only reliable means of treatment, although some reports have suggested the use of albendazole or mebendazole (WIlson JF, Rausch RL, McMahon BJ, et al. Albendazole therapy in alveolar hydatid disease: a report of favorable results in two patients after short-term therpay. Am J Trop Med Hyg 1987;37:162; and Davis A, Pawlowski ZS, Dixon H. Multicentre clinical trials of benzimidazolecarbamates in human echinococcosis. Bull WHO 1986;64:383.)

‡‡ Corticosteroids should be given for 2 to 3 days before and during praziquantel therapy. Any cysticercoidal drug may cause irreparable damage when used to treat ocular or spinal cysts, even when corticosteroids are used. (From Drugs for parasitic infections. Med Lett Drugs Ther 1993;35:111.)

§§ Albendazole or flubendazole may also be effective.

‖‖ One report of a cure using 1 g tid for 21 days has been published. (From Bekhti A. Mebendazole in toxocariasis. Ann Intern Med 1984;100:463.)

From Drugs for parasitic infections. Med Lett Drugs Ther 1993;35:111.

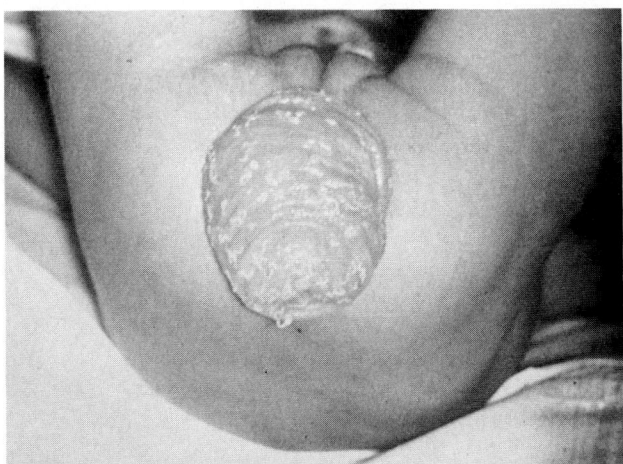

FIGURE 107-1. (See Color Fig. 56.) *Trichuris trichiura* associated with rectal prolapse in a child. Adult *T. trichiura* are seen as white threads on the mucosal surface. (From Smith JW, et al. Intestinal helminths. Atlas of diagnostic medical parasitology series. Chicago: American Society of Clinical Pathologists, 1984.)

Epidemiology

E vermicularis can infect all ages, but it is most prevalent among children 5 to 10 years of age.[14-16] Poor personal hygiene and exposure to infected peers in school are contributing factors. As many as 30% of elementary school students in the United States may be infected, although a report based on laboratory surveillance in New York City suggested that the number of cases has decreased.[17] Enterobiasis has also been reported among male homosexuals, who probably become infected through anilingus.

Clinical Manifestations

The most important consequence of *E vermicularis* infection is irritation of the perianal or perineal skin,[13-15] although many of those infected are asymptomatic. Scratching, self-induced trauma to the skin, and, in some, a secondary bacterial dermatitis can result. Vulvovaginitis sometimes develops in prepubertal girls when adult pinworms migrate to the vagina.[18] It has been postulated that perineal irritation, with concomitant scratching, can result in secondary enuresis[19] or introital

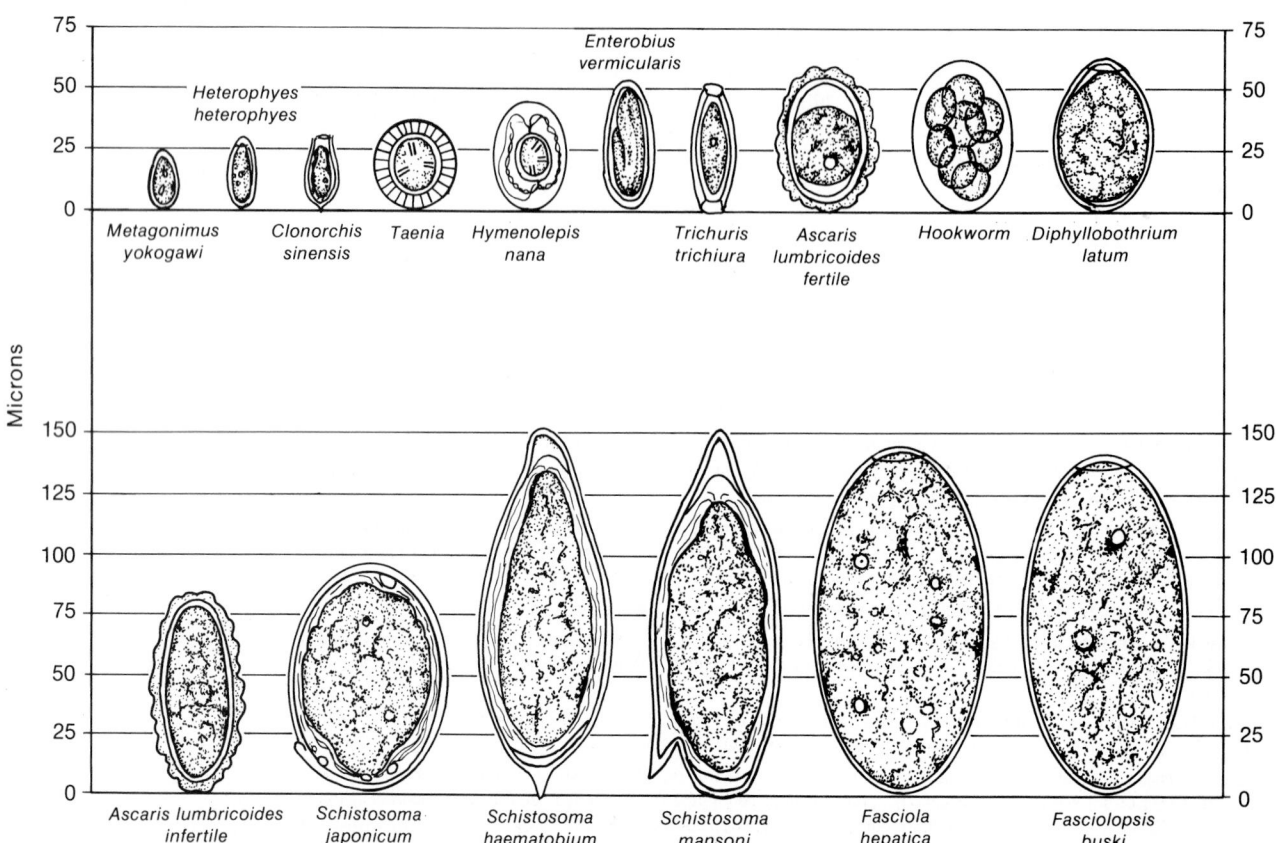

FIGURE 107-2. Relative sizes and shapes of helminth ova. (Adapted from Smith JW, et al. Intestinal helminths. Atlas of diagnostic medical parasitology series. Chicago: American Society of Clinical Pathologists, 1984.)

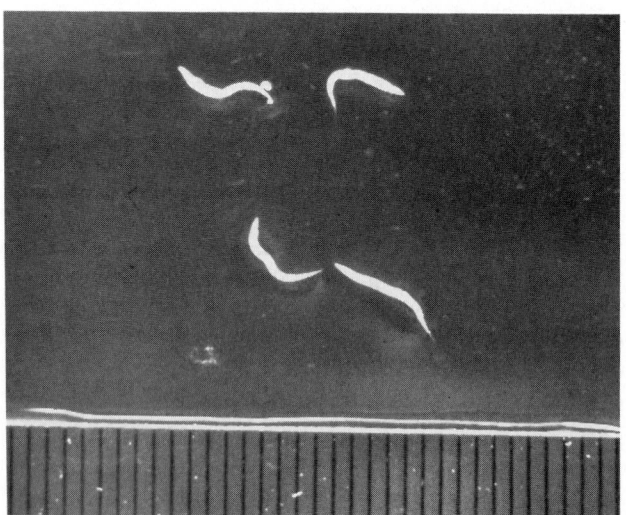

FIGURE 107-3. (See Color Fig. 57.) Adult female *Enterobius vermicularis* (pinworms) may be found on the perianal skin or occasionally on the surface of stools. Adult female pinworms are 8 to 13 mm in length and 0.3 to 0.5 mm wide. (The scale is in millimeters; from Smith JW, et al. Intestinal helminths. Atlas of diagnostic medical parasitology series. Chicago: American Society of Clinical Pathologists, 1984.)

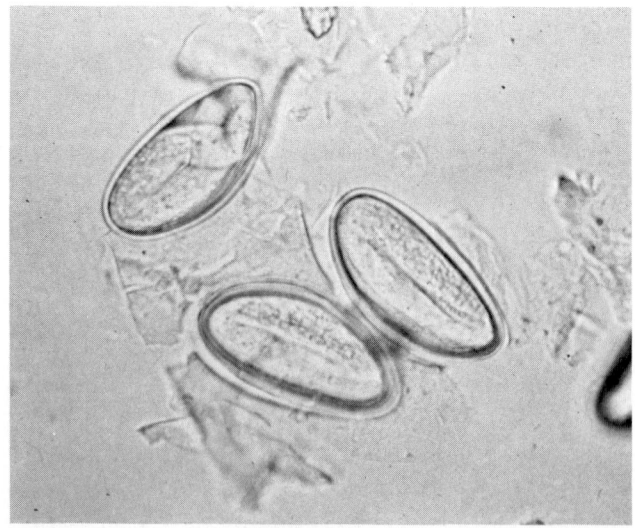

FIGURE 107-4. (See Color Fig. 58.) A cluster of typical embryonated eggs of *Enterobius vermicularis* is seen in a cellulose-tape preparation. Each ova contains an infective larva. Ova are 56 to 58 μm by 27 to 29 μm. (From Smith JW, et al. Intestinal helminths. Atlas of diagnostic medical parasitology series. Chicago: American Society of Clinical Pathologists, 1984.)

colonization with coliforms, which might predispose to the development of urinary tract infection in girls.[20] Adult pinworms are occasionally found in the appendix after surgical excision, but they do not appear to cause acute appendicitis.

On rare occasions, adult female pinworms reach the peritoneum by traversing the female genital tract or migrating through a perforation in the bowel associated with appendicitis, diverticulitis, or intestinal malignancy.[21,22] Granulomatous reactions to dead worms or eggs can result in small peritoneal nodules, which grossly may be confused with metastatic carcinoma. Granulomatous inflammation in response to worms or eggs has been observed in the vulva, vaginal wall, cervix, endometrium, salpinx, and ovaries, as well as in the liver and epididymis.[23]

Diagnosis, Treatment, and Prevention

The diagnosis of enterobiasis is made by finding ova or pinlike adult female worms on the perianal skin (see Figs. 107-3 and 107-4; see Color Figs. 57 and 58). The most successful approach uses a strip of transparent tape that is held with the adhesive side out affixed to a tongue depressor.[14] When a person first arises in the morning, the buttocks are spread and the tape is pressed against the perianal skin several times. The strip is then transferred to a microscope slide with adhesive side down. Eggs are prominent at low power. A single smear detects approximately 50% of those infected. Ninety percent of those infected can be detected with three swabs. Routine stool examination for ova and parasites is positive in only 10% to 15% of cases. On rare occasions, ova are found in vaginal smears treated with Papanicolaou's stain or in the urine sediment.

E vermicularis is susceptible to a number of anthelmintic drugs (see Table 107-2). Spread of *E vermicularis* can be reduced by hand washing and by treating infected children. Because the home environment is often contaminated with viable ova, it is advisable to launder clothes and linen, to vacuum around beds, curtains, and other potentially contaminated areas, and to cover food to avoid dust-borne eggs. Anthelmintic treatment of the entire household may be necessary to interrupt transmission.

Capillaria philippinensis

C philippinensis, a small intestinal nematode, is a cause of severe diarrhea and malabsorption[24] among residents in localized areas of the Philippines and Thailand. Cases have also been reported from Indonesia, Japan, Taiwan, Egypt, and Iran.[25] Infection follows ingestion of raw freshwater fish, the intermediate host, that contain infectious larvae. Fish-eating birds are the usual definitive hosts.

The adults of *C philippinensis* invade the epithelium and lamina propria of the small intestine of their human hosts.[24] Inflammatory changes develop in the lamina propria and are associated with chronic diarrhea, abdominal pain, borborygmus, constitutional symptoms, malabsorption, and weight loss. Ova are released into the lumen. Some are passed in the stool, whereas others excyst in the intestine and result in autoinfection. Deaths have occurred as a result of malnutrition,

electrolyte imbalance, or secondary infections in debilitated patients.

The diagnosis of *C philippinensis* is made by finding characteristic ova, larvae, or adult worms in the stool. Multiple stool examinations often are required because the ova are shed in low numbers or sporadically. Mebendazole (see Table 107-2), albendazole, or flubendazole and supportive care with fluid, electrolyte, and nutritional replacement are necessary. Thorough cooking of fish prevents infection.

Trichostrongylus Species

Trichostrongylus sp are common parasites of herbivorous animals.[4,8] They have been reported from many areas of the world, but human infections appear to be most prevalent in the Middle East and Asia. Ova are passed in the feces of animals, hatch in 1 or 2 days under favorable conditions, and pass through three free-living stages before becoming infective in approximately 3 days. Human infection usually occurs when larvae are ingested in contaminated food or water, although larva can invade through the skin. Larval migration through the lungs is not necessary for maturation. Adult worms reside in the duodenum or upper jejunum with their heads embedded in the mucosa.

Most human infections are asymptomatic or mild, but epigastric pain, diarrhea, and flatulence have been observed. Rarely, anemia and emaciation are prominent. Eosinophilia is present in a minority of cases. The diagnosis is made by identifying *Trichostrongylus* ova, which are larger and more pointed on the ends than hookworm ova, in the stool. Pyrantel pamoate, mebendazole, or albendazole can be used for treatment (see Table 107-2). Potentially contaminated vegetables should be cooked thoroughly and water boiled before ingestion in endemic areas.

Ascaris lumbricoides

A lumbricoides is the most prevalent and the largest of the intestinal nematodes that infect humans; it is the one that truly looks like a "worm." Female ascarids produce a prodigious number of ova (see Fig. 107-2)—200,000 each day. Fertilized eggs develop in moist, warm, shaded soil. After ingestion in contaminated food or water, eggs hatch in the duodenum. Larvae subsequently penetrate the intestinal wall, enter the venous circulation, and migrate to the lungs. They break into the alveoli, ascend to the trachea, are swallowed, and complete their development in the small intestine. The time from ingestion of ova to the production of eggs by mature females is 10 to 12 weeks.

Epidemiology

An estimated 1.2 billion people are infected with *Ascaris* worldwide.[26] Only cold, arid climates are spared. Transmission of *Ascaris* is continuous in the tropics and intermittent in temperate areas. Only a small proportion of the population, usually children younger than 10 years of age, harbor a large number of worms at any given time.[27]

Clinical Manifestations

The clinical manifestations of ascariasis can be divided into those associated with migration of larvae through the lungs and those associated with adult worms in the gastrointestinal tract.[26] Migrating larvae in the lungs can elicit pulmonary hypersensitivity reactions, including bronchospasm, hypersecretion of mucus, and bronchiolar inflammation. Sputum may contain Charcot-Leyden crystals and, on occasion, larvae. The presence of eosinophilia with pulmonary infiltrates leads to the clinical diagnosis of Löffler's syndrome. Urticaria and other manifestations of hypersensitivity also may be present during the pulmonary phase. *Ascaris* antigens are among the most potent allergens. Hypersensitivity reactions have been a major problem for investigators working with *Ascaris* in vitro.

Accurate characterization of the gastrointestinal manifestations of *Ascaris* infection is confounded by the high frequency of concurrent infestations with other intestinal parasites and enteropathogenic bacteria. Patients harboring *Ascaris* have reported abdominal pain, nausea, anorexia, and diarrhea, but it has been difficult to determine how frequently *Ascaris* is responsible for these symptoms. The impact of heavy *Ascaris* infections on nutritional status has been debated,[28,29] but children infected with *Ascaris* and other common intestinal nematodes in Kenya demonstrated improved growth rates after treatment.[7]

The most serious complications with *Ascaris* occur when adult worms migrate out of the intestine or when a large number become intertwined to form a bolus, causing partial or complete intestinal obstruction (Fig. 107-5; see Color Fig. 59)[26,30] In the latter instance, nausea, vomiting, abdominal pain, and, occasionally, a palpable mass may result. The presentation may mimic an acute abdomen. Intestinal obstruction has been estimated to occur in 2 per 1000 *Ascaris*-infected children per year.[30] Rarely, a mass of worms results in intussusception or volvulus of the small bowel. Bowel perforations

with peritonitis and localized abscesses have been reported, but the role of *Ascaris* in these cases remains uncertain. Intestinal obstruction has also been attributed to adhesions caused by extraintestinal *Ascaris*.

On occasion, adult *Ascaris* migrate to the oropharynx, much to the consternation of the host, or they may enter the common bile duct, producing obstruction with biliary colic. The latter may be complicated by acute cholecystitis, ascending bacterial cholangitis, secondary liver abscess, perforation of the bile duct resulting in bile peritonitis, intrahepatic or bile duct calculi, or acute pancreatitis.[31]

Diagnosis, Treatment, and Prevention

The diagnosis is made by identifying embryonated or unembryonated ova in feces (see Fig. 107-2). On occasion, migrating adult worms, which range from 10 to 35 cm in length, are found in feces, are detected radiographically in the gastrointestinal tract or sonographically in the bile duct, or emerge from the oropharynx or nose.

Several drugs are available for the treatment of *Ascaris* (see Table 107-2). Therapy for the complications of *Ascaris* depends on the organs involved. Intestinal obstruction may require surgery, but some patients are successfully treated with rehydration and anthelmintic medications administered by nasogastric tube. Conservative therapy is appropriate for uncomplicated biliary colic due to *Ascaris*. Obstruction of the common bile duct may require surgery or endoscopic removal of dead worms after anthelmintic chemotherapy.

In principle, ascariasis can be prevented by sanitary disposal of human feces and good personal hygiene. In practice, this is difficult to achieve. *Ascaris* eggs are relatively stable in the environment and can persist for years. Community-based mass treatment programs are effective for the short term, but treatment must be repeated periodically.[27]

Trichinella spiralis

Trichinella spiralis is widespread among carnivorous animals.[32] Humans become infected when they ingest inadequately cooked meat containing infective larvae.[32-36] The encysted larvae are released in the small intestine and molt four times within 36 hours to become adults. After mating, females remain embedded in the mucosa. In approximately 5 days, viviparous females begin to deposit larvae, which invade the mucosa, enter the lymphatics or bloodstream, and ultimately encyst in skeletal muscle cells. They remain there until ingested by another carnivore or until their death from senescence after several years. A single female worm produces approximately 1500 larvae during her life.

Epidemiology

Approximately 50 cases of trichinosis occur in the United States each year. Most are related to ingestion of pork or sausage from domestic, garbage-fed pigs, but infection can also result from inadequately cooked wild boar, bear, walrus, horse, or other meat.[32-36] Cases of trichinosis are usually sporadic, but small outbreaks are not uncommon; some occur in returning travelers.[35]

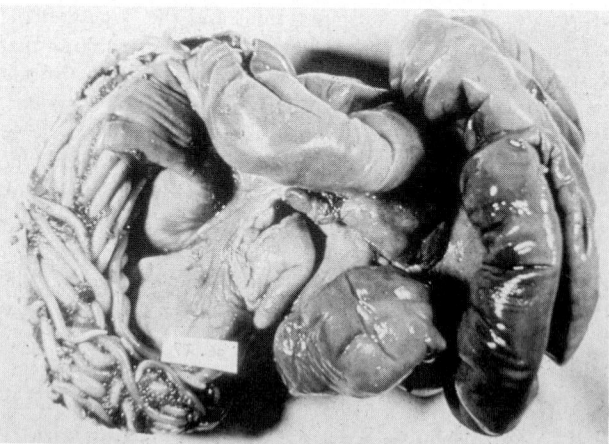

FIGURE 107-5. (See Color Fig. 59.) Intestinal obstruction caused by a mass of adult *Ascaris lumbricoides* is seen in this autopsy specimen. Intestinal obstruction is an unusual complication of heavy *Ascaris* infection. (From Smith JW, et al. Intestinal helminths. Atlas of diagnostic medical parasitology series. Chicago: American Society of Clinical Pathologists, 1984.)

Clinical Manifestations

During the initial, intestinal phase of trichinosis, nausea, vomiting, abdominal pain, or diarrhea occur as the result of larval invasion of the intestinal mucosa. The systemic phase, which typically begins 1 to 3 weeks after ingestion of contaminated meat, is characterized by fever, myalgias, facial or periorbital edema, headache, conjunctivitis, and occasionally a rash.[32-36] Extraocular muscles are frequently affected. Cardiac or central nervous system involvement with meningoencephalitis is rare but potentially fatal. Trichinosis among the native Inuit of northern Canada differs in that prolonged diarrhea is the dominant symptom in infections in previously sensitized people.[36]

Diagnosis, Treatment, and Prevention

The diagnosis of trichinosis is suggested by the constellation of fever, myalgia, eosinophilia, and a history of eating raw, or inadequately cooked, potentially contaminated meat. Creatine phosphokinase is elevated in approximately half of the cases. The clinical diagnosis is eventually confirmed by serologic evidence, either a positive bentonite flocculation test, indirect immunofluorescence test, or ELISA, but anti-*Trichinella* antibodies are usually not detectable until the third week of infection or later.[32] The diagnosis can be confirmed parasitologically by muscle biopsy, but that is seldom necessary.

Mebendazole is recommended for the treatment of trichinosis, along with corticosteroids when symptoms are severe (see Table 107-2).[5,37] Bed rest and nonsteroidal antiinflammatory agents are used for symptomatic relief of fever and myalgias.

Trichinosis can be prevented by cooking pork or other potentially contaminated meat to at least 76.6°C (170°F). Meat less than 6 inches thick can be rendered safe if frozen at −15°C (5°F) for 20 days, unless it is infected with *Trichinella* isolates from the arctic.[32,36]

Hookworms

Hookworm disease is caused by *Ancylostoma duodenale*, *Necator americanus*, and, in restricted geographic areas, *Ancylostoma ceylonicum*. Adult hookworms are small, creamy white nematodes.[4,38-40] The anterior portion of *N americanus* is sharply curved in the direction opposite the curve of the body, resulting in a hook-like appearance.

Adult hookworms anchor themselves in the mucosa of the small intestine and secrete an anticoagulant that facilitates the flow of blood.[41] They periodically change their location. Bleeding from the site of attachment contributes to the total blood loss. *N americanus* results in the loss of approximately 0.03 mL/day per adult hookworm, and *A duodenale* 0.15 to 0.26 mL/day.[42,43] Ova (see Fig. 107-2) are excreted in feces and excyst in the soil, liberating rhabditiform larvae, which feed actively on organic debris and bacteria. They increase in size and molt twice to become infectious filariform larvae, which migrate in response to pressure, carbon dioxide, or warmth and invade the epidermis through fissures or hair follicles, most commonly between the toes or on the dorsum of the feet. Infection may also be acquired through the interdi-

gital spaces of the hands. Invading larvae exsheath as they enter the host, and pass through the venous circulation to the lungs. There they break out of the alveoli, ascend to the respiratory tract, reach the pharynx, and are swallowed. Although invasion is principally through the skin, filariform larvae of *A duodenale* are occasionally ingested and complete their life cycle entirely in the gut.

Epidemiology

A duodenale and *N americanus* are widely distributed in tropical and subtropical Asia and Africa. *A duodenale* is also found in the Middle East, North Africa, and southern Europe. *N americanus* is the predominant species in the New World, but there are focal sites of *A duodenale* in the Caribbean islands and in Central and South America. Human infection with *A ceylonicum* has been reported in the Philippines and in Calcutta, India. *N americanus* infections were once common in the southeastern part of the United States, but treatment and control measures resulted in a drop in prevalence from 37% in 1914 to 4% by 1965.[44] Iron deficiency anemia due to hookworms is now exceedingly rare among residents of the United States.

Hookworm infections are limited to areas where the climate allows development of larvae in the soil. Larvae are readily killed by desiccation or freezing. Several factors favor the spread of hookworm infection. Poor sanitation is central to transmission. A population that does not wear shoes is at obvious risk. Cultural differences in attitude toward human excrement are also very important. Heavy infections have been caused by the use of human feces as fertilizer in China. In contrast, infections tend to be light in India where Hindu culture limits the use of human feces as manure.

Clinical Manifestations

The clinical manifestations of hookworm infection correlate with the life cycle of the organism and the intensity of infection.[38-40] Penetration of the skin by filariform larvae may produce a papular eruption with intense pruritus, vesiculation, and local edema ("ground itch" or "dew itch"). As larvae pass through the lung, they may elicit a hypersensitivity reaction with cough, wheezing, infiltrates on chest radiograph, and eosinophilia (Löffler's syndrome).

Epigastric pain, flatulence, and abdominal tenderness accompany the early intestinal phase of infection in some. Humans experimentally infected with *N americanus*[45] experienced abdominal pain and flatulence 35 to 40 days after exposure to filariform larvae; eosinophilia peaked between 38 and 64 days; and eggs first appeared in the stool during the sixth week. At times, abdominal pain was severe enough to suggest peptic ulcer disease and was occasionally accompanied by diarrhea with mucus or blood in the stool. In young children with very heavy primary hookworm infections, massive invasion by filariform larvae can result in acute gastrointestinal hemorrhage, a condition that is rare but potentially life threatening.[46]

The hallmark of chronic hookworm disease is iron deficiency anemia.[38-40,47] The parasite burden, the infecting species of hookworm, and the iron requirements, iron reserves, and diet of the host are important variables. In areas of high iron intake and bioavailability, even heavy hookworm infections may not produce anemia. Hypoalbuminemia is often present and generally correlates with the degree of anemia.[48] Hookworm disease with severe anemia is particularly important in young children, stunting growth and intellectual development, and during pregnancy, causing increased maternal and neonatal mortality.[48]

Diagnosis, Treatment, and Prevention

Hookworm disease should be considered in any person from an endemic area who presents with iron deficiency anemia. Eosinophilia frequently accompanies hookworm infection.[49] Direct fecal examination for ova is adequate to detect clinically significant infections. It is not easy or necessary to differentiate between the eggs of *N americanus* and *A duodenale*. Hookworm ova may hatch in stool specimens that have been allowed to stand, and occasionally it is necessary to differentiate the rhabditiform larvae of hookworms from those of *S stercoralis*. Hookworm larvae have a long buccal tube, in contrast to the short buccal tube of *S stercoralis*.

The treatment of hookworm disease includes iron repletion as well as anthelmintic therapy (see Table 107-2).[50] During pregnancy, iron deficiency anemia is treated with ferrous sulfate alone, and anthelmintic therapy, which is potentially teratogenic, is administered after delivery. The transmission of hookworm infection can theoretically be interrupted by sanitary disposal of human feces, use of footwear, and treatment of infected people.

Strongyloides stercoralis

S stercoralis is an important intestinal pathogen that can produce life-threatening hyperinfection in immunocompromised hosts.[51–53] *Strongyloides fülleborni*, primarily a pathogen of infrahuman primates, is recognized as a cause of human strongyloidiasis in Papua–New Guinea and Africa.[54]

Like the hookworms, *S stercoralis* enters the skin from fecally contaminated soil, migrates through the venous circulation to the lungs, penetrates alveoli, and ultimately reaches the small bowel.[4] Adults reside in the superficial mucosa of the duodenum or jejunum and release ova into the lumen. The ova hatch quickly, releasing rhabditiform larvae. Autoinfection occurs when rhabditiform larvae convert to filariform larvae in the gut or on the skin. Filariform larvae can penetrate the intestinal mucosa or perianal skin to reach the venous circulation and then go on to complete the life cycle. *Strongyloides* infections often persist for decades because of low levels of autoinfection.[55–58] The conversion of rhabditiform to filariform larvae seems to be enhanced in immunosuppressed people, in whom life-threatening hyperinfection may develop.[51–53] Unlike other intestinal nematodes, the entire life cycle of *S stercoralis* can also occur completely in the soil after larvae are passed in the feces.

Epidemiology

S stercoralis is endemic in tropical areas of Africa, Asia, and Latin America as well as the southern part of the United States and in Eastern Europe. Prevalence rates of 3% to 21% have been reported from Nigeria and as high as 2.5% in some areas of eastern Tennessee.[59,60] Many U.S. military personnel who were infected in Southeast Asia during World War II or the Vietnam War have remained infected for years.[55–58]

Clinical Manifestations

Most people are asymptomatic at the time of cutaneous larval penetration, although some manifest a maculopapular rash or linear urticaria called "larva currens."[61] Larva currens can also be seen on the buttocks as a consequence of external autoinfection. The pulmonary phase of strongyloidiasis is usually asymptomatic, but cough, shortness of breath, wheezing, fever, transient pulmonary infiltrates, and eosinophilia may occur.[62]

After *S stercoralis* reaches the gut, it can produce nonspecific, aching epigastric or diffuse abdominal pain or diarrhea.[63,64] Eosinophilia is common. With heavy infections of the upper small bowel, vomiting, malabsorption, steatorrhea, and weight loss may occur.[65–67] Rarely, functional obstruction develops as a consequence of edema of the small bowel. Of note, approximately one third of chronically infected World War II veterans were asymptomatic, whereas the other two thirds experienced recurrent urticaria (larva currens) or gastrointestinal or pulmonary symptoms years after leaving endemic areas.

S stercoralis can produce life-threatening hyperinfection in people with suppressed cell-mediated immunity. The syndrome had been most commonly associated with renal transplantation, malignancies (especially lymphoma and leukemia), and corticosteroid therapy. Hyperinfection has also been reported in people with protein-calorie malnutrition, lepromatous leprosy, and other chronic debilitating infections. Surprisingly, it has not been frequently associated with human immunodeficiency virus infection.[68]

Strongyloides hyperinfection is characterized by multisystem disease. Gastrointestinal and pulmonary symptoms are usually severe. Concurrent polymicrobial bacterial infections result as a consequence of bacteria on the surface of invading filariform larvae; sepsis, meningitis, peritonitis, or endocarditis occur in 45% of cases. The mortality rate with hyperinfection exceeds 50%.

Diagnosis, Treatment, and Prevention

The diagnosis is made by identifying larvae (Fig. 107-6; see Color Fig. 60) in stool or in aspirates or biopsy samples of the small intestine. Baermann's funnel and agar plate methods increase the sensitivity of stool examination.[69] In people with the hyperinfection syndrome, larvae may also be found in sputum or tissue. Several serologic tests, including ELISA, have been developed and provide presumptive evidence of infection. Eosinophilia is often present in immunocompetent patients with strongyloidiasis, but it may be absent in the immunocompromised host.

Thiabendazole has been the treatment of choice for strongyloidiasis (see Table 107-2),[5,6,70,71] but side effects are frequent. Ivermectin and albendazole are alternatives. Because these drugs cannot be administered parenterally, administration by way of a nasogastric tube is necessary in people unable to take the drug orally. Prevention of strongyloidiasis depends

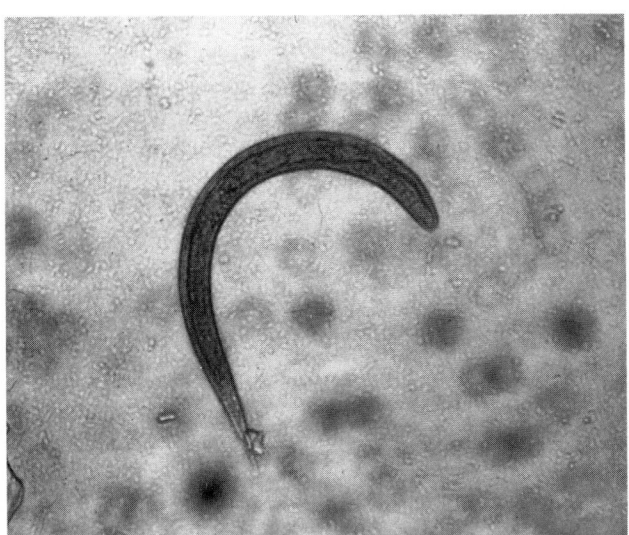

FIGURE 107-6. (See Color Fig. 60.) *Strongyloides stercoralis* rhabditiform larva 225 mm by 16 mm in size was found in the stool of a patient who had epigastric pain and eosinophilia. (Courtesy of Richard L. Guerrant, M.D., Charlottesville, VA.)

on improved standards of living and personal hygiene. It is advisable to screen transplant recipients and others receiving immunosuppressive therapy who have been exposed to *S stercoralis*.

Intestinal Nematodes of Animals That Infect Humans

Cutaneous Larva Migrans

Cutaneous larva migrans, also known as creeping eruption, is a distinctive form of dermatitis characterized by serpiginous, papulovesicular, erythematous, pruritic lesions.[72] It is typically a consequence of migrating larvae of intestinal nematodes of animals that cannot complete their life cycles in humans. Hookworms of dogs and cats, primarily *Ancylostoma braziliense* and, less commonly, *Ancylostoma caninum* or other nematodes, are responsible. Cutaneous larva migrans is prevalent in many tropical and subtropical areas of the Caribbean, Africa, and South America. It is encountered in North America along the Gulf and southern Atlantic coasts. Infection is acquired when people, often travelers to tropical areas, come in contact with infected soil in playgrounds, beaches, or crawl spaces under houses. Topical thiabendazole is the treatment of choice (see Table 107-2). Oral albendazole is an alternative.

Visceral Larva Migrans

Visceral larva migrans is a systemic syndrome resulting from invasion of human organs by larvae of the dog and cat ascarids, *Toxocara canis* and *Toxocara cati*,[73] and other nematodes of animals. Infection follows ingestion of ova originating in animal feces. The syndrome is most commonly seen in children with a history of pica, but on occasion it is seen in adults.[74]

Larvae are released and penetrate the intestine, but because these helminths are unable to complete their life cycle in humans, they wander through various organs. *Toxocara* sp are common throughout tropical and temperate zones.

The clinical course of visceral larva migrans is highly variable, ranging from no symptoms to fever, cough, abdominal pain, and urticarial skin rash. Physical examination may reveal hepatomegaly, pneumonitis, dermatitis, or ocular involvement. Eosinophilia is common and may be pronounced. The characteristic pathologic lesion consists of a granulomatous inflammatory response with eosinophils.

The triad of eosinophilia, hepatomegaly, and hypergammaglobulinemia suggests visceral larva migrans. An ELISA is available to detect anti-*Toxocara* antibodies. High levels of isohemagglutinins against AB blood group antigens also are frequently observed. Thiabendazole or diethylcarbamazine can be used for treatment (see Table 107-2). Control measures include worming dogs, covering sandboxes, and preventing promiscuous defecation of dogs in areas where children play.

Anisakiasis

Anisakiasis is caused by members of the family Anisakidae, which are pathogens of fish, including cod, herring, salmon, mackerel, Pacific pollock, Pacific red snapper, and squid.[75,76] Anisakine larvae normally reside in the viscera of fish, but they migrate to muscle if fish are not promptly filleted after being caught. Anisakiasis occurs after contaminated fish or squid are eaten raw or are inadequately cooked. Symptoms develop when larvae attempt to invade the human stomach, small intestine or colon. A severe, local inflammatory response results at the site of attempted penetration. Although eosinophils are prominent in the local inflammatory response, eosinophilia is usually absent.

Anisakiasis is common in Japan and Europe, areas where fish is consumed raw. A few cases have been reported in the United States, but there is concern that this may change as sushi becomes more popular. Anisakine larvae are prevalent in susceptible types of fish along the California coast and in the northern Atlantic Ocean.

Few if any symptoms develop when anisakine larvae remain in the lumen of the human bowel, but the presentation can be dramatic when mucosal invasion occurs. In acute gastric anisakiasis, severe abdominal pain, nausea, vomiting, and occasionally gastric bleeding may develop within 12 to 24 hours of ingesting contaminated fish.[77] In intestinal anisakiasis, symptoms mimicking acute appendicitis, regional enteritis, small bowel obstruction, or perforation begin several days after the ingestion of fish. Local inflammation and edema may appear as lumenal narrowing, thumbprinting, or a mass lesion radiographically, and may be confused with a neoplasm.

The diagnosis of anisakiasis is often made at endoscopy, and worms have been successfully extracted by biopsy forceps from the stomach and duodenum.[77] Surgical resection is occasionally necessary to relieve intestinal obstruction, to repair a perforation of the bowel, or to rule out malignancy, but many patients can be managed conservatively. Anisakiasis can be prevented by filleting freshly caught fish before larvae have a chance to penetrate muscle, by cooking fish to 60°C (140°F) for at least 10 minutes, or by freezing for 24 hours at −20°C (−4°F).[76]

Angiostrongylus costaricensis

Angiostrongylus costaricensis is found in rodents from California[78] to South America; human disease is most often observed in children in Central America. Adult *A costaricensis* typically reside in mesenteric arteries in the ileocecal region of rodents but occasionally infect the same site in humans. The eggs are released and hatch in the arteries. Larvae migrate through the intestinal wall, are passed in the feces, and invade slugs. Humans presumably become infected by ingesting slug-infested vegetation.

Adult worms and ova elicit a granulomatous arteritis with eosinophilic infiltration in the ileocecal region that can also result in arteritis, thrombosis, local infarction, and bowel perforation. The clinical manifestations vary from a visceral larva migrans-like syndrome to those of an acute abdomen. Nausea, vomiting, right lower quadrant pain, and fever are common. A right lower quadrant mass may be palpable, suggesting acute appendicitis or malignancy, and radiographic studies may document a mass lesion in the ileocecal region. Eosinophilia and leukocytosis are common. Neither ova nor larvae are found in the stool. Surgery is often necessary, and the diagnosis is typically made when adult worms or ova are identified in surgical specimens. Thiabendazole has been used for treatment, but there are no data on its efficacy. Cooking slug-infested vegetables and hand washing reduce the risk of infection.

CESTODES (TAPEWORMS)

The important pathogenic cestodes are *Diphyllobothrium latum* (fish tapeworm), *H nana* (dwarf tapeworm), *Taenia solium* (pork tapeworm), *Taenia saginata* (beef tapeworm), *Echinococcus granulosus*, and *Echinococcus multilocularis*. Cestodes have complex life cycles, living as adults in the gastrointestinal tract of their definitive mammalian hosts and as solid or bladder larvae in tissues of vertebrate or invertebrate intermediate hosts. Adult tapeworms are ribbon-like, with a scolex at the

anterior end that is responsible for attachment in the small intestine. A neck region connects the scolex to the strobila, a chain of progressively developing segments known as proglottids. The number of proglottids ranges from 3 to 4000 depending on the cestode species, and the total length of adult cestodes varies from several millimeters in the case of *E granulosus* to several meters in the case of *T saginata*.[1]

Humans are the definitive host for *T saginata*, *T solium*, *H nana*, and *D latum*. On rare occasions, humans serve as the definitive host for *Hymenolepis diminuta*, which is primarily a parasite of rats and mice, and *Dipylidium caninum*, the dog tapeworm. Both of the latter infections are uncommon, light, and usually of little consequence. Humans serve as intermediate hosts for *E granulosus*, *E multilocularis*, as well as *T solium*. In general, adult tapeworms produce little evidence of disease in their human hosts, but *D latum* can result in vitamin B_{12} deficiency. In contrast, cestode larvae can produce severe, life-threatening disease when humans serve as the intermediate host.

Taenia saginata

The beef tapeworm, *T saginata*, is renowned for its length (4–6 m; Fig. 107-7; see Color Fig. 61) and the occasional finding of strobila up to several feet in length in the stool.[79] Humans become infected when they ingest beef or meat from other herbivores, such as camels, that contains the bladder or cysticercus stage. As the meat is digested, the cysticercus breaks down, releasing a scolex that usually attaches in the upper jejunum of humans. Development of the worm is followed by the appearance of proglottids and ova in the stool. Cattle become infected when they ingest ova from human feces. Larvae are released in the intestine of the cow, penetrate the mucosa, and find their way to muscle, where they mature to form cysticerci, completing the cycle.

Although nonspecific symptoms such as abdominal discomfort, epigastric pain, nervousness, vertigo, nausea, vomiting, diarrhea, and weight loss have been attributed to *T saginata*, most people are asymptomatic. There is usually no evidence of weight loss or malnutrition. The diagnosis of *Taenia* infection is made by finding ova or proglottids in the stool. The ova of *T saginata* are indistinguishable from those of *T solium* (see Fig, 107-2), and a species-specific diagnosis requires identification of the rectangular proglottids of *T saginata* (Fig. 107-8; see Color Fig. 62). Niclosamide is the treatment of choice (see Table 107-2).[80]

Taenia solium

Humans can serve as the definitive host or as an intermediate host for the pork tapeworm, *T solium*.[79] Infection is common in areas of Latin America, Africa, and Asia where hogs are raised. People become infected when they ingest inadequately cooked pork containing infective cysts known as cysticerci cellulosae, which release scoleces in the small intestine. Adult worms usually cause few if any symptoms, although a number of nonspecific gastrointestinal complaints have been attributed to them. Eosinophilia may be present. Mature proglottids and ova of *T solium* are released in the stool. Hogs, the normal intermediate host, become infected when they ingest ova.

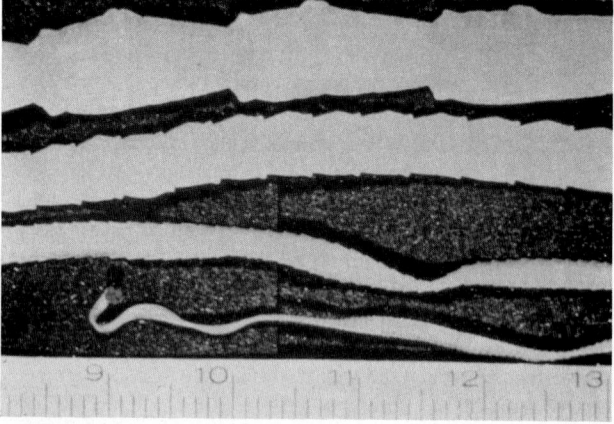

FIGURE 107-7. (See Color Fig. 61.) *Taenia saginata.* The scolex with its four suckers is seen (*lower left*). Mature proglottids are found at the distal end of the worm. (From Smith JW, et al. Intestinal helminths. Atlas of diagnostic medical parasitology series. Chicago: American Society of Clinical Pathologists, 1984.)

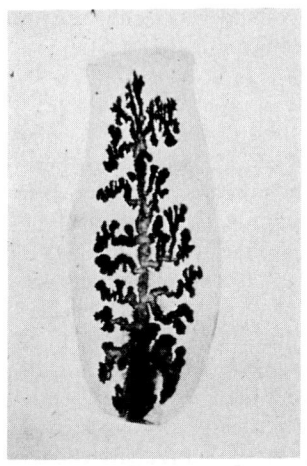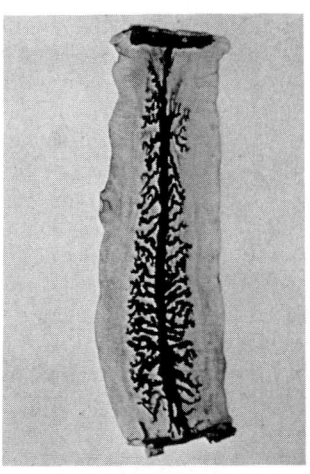

FIGURE 107-8. (See Color Fig. 62.) India ink–injected proglottids of *Taenia saginata* (*right*) and *Taenia solium* (*left*). Proglottids of *T saginata* have more lateral uterine branches than those of *T solium*. (From Smith JW, et al. Intestinal helminths. Atlas of diagnostic medical parasitology series. Chicago: American Society of Clinical Pathologists, 1984.)

The major risk with *T solium* is cysticercosis,[79] which develops when humans ingest ova or, theoretically, if internal autoinfection occurs in people harboring adult worms. Ova excyst in the intestine. Larvae invade and disseminate to form cysticerci in the brain, subcutaneous tissue, skeletal muscle, eye, or other organs. Neurocysticercosis is a potentially life-threatening complication. It is prevalent in many Latin American countries and is encountered in the United State among immigrants from endemic areas as well as travelers. Autochthonous cases of neurocysticercosis have occurred in the United States among contacts of tapeworm carriers.[81]

Intestinal infection is diagnosed by finding *Taenia* ova (see Fig. 107-2) or proglottids (see Fig. 107-8 and see Color Fig. 62) in the stool. The diagnosis of cysticercosis usually is made on the basis of a history of exposure in an endemic area, the clinical presentation, and typical computed tomographic or magnetic resonance findings. Antibodies are detectable in serum or cerebrospinal fluid in many, but not all, people.

Either niclosamide or praziquantel can be used to treat intestinal *T solium* infection (see Table 107-2). Niclosamide is effective, but it causes disintegration of the adult worm,[80,82] raising the theoretic possibility of autoinfection. Praziquantel is active against larvae as well as adult worms, but it is more expensive. Many physicians recommend a purge after therapy to expedite expulsion of proglottids, but there are no data to prove that it is necessary.[82]

Praziquantel and albendazole have proved effective in the treatment of symptomatic, parenchymal neurocysticercosis.[83,84] Most physicians use corticosteroids concurrently to prevent cerebral edema, which may develop secondary to release of parasite antigens.

Infection with *T solium* can be prevented by proper disposal of human feces, treatment of infected people, inspection of pork, and thorough cooking of pork to at least 50°C before it is eaten. Freezing pork below −12°C is an effective way to kill cysticerci, but they can remain viable for as long as 2 months in meat frozen at 0°C to −2°C.[85]

Diphyllobothrium latum

The fish tapeworm, *D latum*, is known for its ability to compete successfully with its human host for vitamin B_{12}.[86] The parasite has a complex life cycle. Ova are passed in human feces. Free-swimming coracidia are released in fresh water and infect small crustaceans (copepods). When infected copepods are ingested by freshwater fish, procercoid larvae are released and penetrate into the body of the fish. Humans become infected when they ingest raw or inadequately cooked fish, including pike, salmon, trout, whitefish, or turbot. *D latum* is endemic in regions of northern Europe, northern Asia, northern North America, and temperate areas of South America. Urban Jewish homemakers who prepare gefilte fish have become infected when they sample the raw fish as condiments are added.

A number of minor gastrointestinal complaints have been associated with *D latum*,[87] but most infected people are asymptomatic. Some present with macrocytic anemia due to vitamin B_{12} deficiency, but anemia was not observed in a recent series of Finns with *D latum* infection. The diagnosis is made by identifying ova or the typical broad, rectangular proglottids in the stool. Treatment is with niclosamide (see Table 107-2).[80] Thorough cooking or freezing of fish (−10°C for 24 hours) prevents infection.

Hymenolepis nana

The dwarf tapeworm, *H nana*, is the most prevalent of the cestodes that infect humans. As many as 20 million people are infected worldwide. *H nana* has been diagnosed among immigrants to the United States from a number of endemic areas, including Southeast Asia. Natural hosts include humans, mice, and rats.

Infection with *H nana* follows ingestion of ova (see Fig. 107-2). Transmission is often hand-to-mouth, particularly among children, or by ingestion of fecally contaminated food or water. An oncosphere is liberated from each ova in the intestine. It penetrates a villus and develops into a cercocystis. At maturity, the cercocystis ruptures, releasing a scolex, which becomes anchored in the small intestine. Some eggs are passed in the stool; others excyst in the lumen of the small intestine and invade villi to produce internal autoinfection.

Light *H nana* infections are usually asymptomatic or associated with vague abdominal complaints; heavy infections can produce loss of appetite, abdominal pain with or without diarrhea, anorexia, flatulence, or weight loss.[88] The diagnosis is made by identifying eggs in the feces (see Fig. 107-2). Praziquantel is the treatment of choice (see Table 107-2).[83,84] Person-to-person spread of *H nana* can be interrupted by improved sanitation.

Echinococcosis (Echinococcus granulosus *and* Echinococcus multilocularis)

E granulosus resides as an adult worm in the intestine of canines, the definitive hosts, and as a hydatid cyst in sheep, humans, or other mammals.[89] *E granulosus* is found in areas where dogs, sheep, and humans live in close proximity under conditions of poor sanitation. Infection is endemic in areas of Australia, New Zealand, North Africa, the Middle East, and South America. Scattered autochthonous cases have been reported from the western part of the United States. In some areas of Canada, moose and caribou serve as intermediate hosts, and the wolf is the predominant definitive host.

Humans become infected with *E granulosus* when they ingest ova. Transmission is often hand-to-mouth from the fur of infected dogs or by way of fecally contaminated food or water. Ova excyst in the human intestine and the larvae invade the intestinal mucosa and then disseminate through the lymphatics and circulation to various organs. Approximately two thirds of the cysts develop in the liver (Fig. 107-9; see Color Fig. 63), one fifth in the lung, and the remainder in bone, brain, muscle, eye, heart, or other organs. The typical *E granulosus* cyst is unilocular and contains an external hyaline cuticula, an inner germinal membrane with brood capsules, protoscoleces, which are known as "hydatid sand," and daughter cysts that are replicas of the mother cyst.

The natural history of *E granulosus* cysts in humans has not been fully defined. Hydatid cysts grow slowly, and most people remain asymptomatic for prolonged periods of time. Tissue damage is usually secondary to pressure from an enlarging hydatid cyst or to rupture of a cyst into the biliary tract, peritoneum, or lung. Rarely, obstructive jaundice results.[90] Spillage of cyst material can result in anaphylaxis or seeding of the peritoneal surface. Rupture into the biliary tract may present as ascending cholangitis.[91] Cysts outside the liver often pose diagnostic dilemmas. The radiologic findings may be suggestive of neoplasm, particularly when cysts occur in the testes, urinary bladder, retroperitoneum, heart, or eye.

The diagnosis of *E granulosus* is based on a history of exposure in an endemic area and identification of a typical hydatid cyst by computed tomography, magnetic resonance imaging, or ultrasound. Various serologic tests can be used to detect antibodies, but antibodies are not detectable in all cases.[92]

Surgical excision remains one approach to treatment.[93] Historically, physicians avoided percutaneous needle aspiration because of the theoretical risk of leakage of cyst contents into the peritoneal cavity with the potential for anaphylaxis or implantation of germinal membrane. Some reports, however, suggest that percutaneous aspiration and drainage of hydatid liver cysts may be safe.[94,95] A scolicide should be injected into the cyst at the time of surgery or percutaneous drainage; a 20% solution of sodium chloride is safe and effective. Injection of formalin has produced sclerosing cholangitis and death.[96] Treatment with high doses of mebendazole or albendazole before surgery has been advocated to reduce the risk of peritoneal implants.[97] Suppressive chemotherapy is used to treat inoperable cysts; albendazole at high doses for prolonged periods of time is recommended.[98]

Progress has been made in controlling transmission of *E granulosus* in endemic sheep-raising areas. The parasite has a low reproductive rate in its domestic life cycle, and it is thought to be relatively unstable and potentially susceptible to eradication.[99]

E multilocularis, which is found in northern regions of North America and Asia, has a life cycle analogous to that of *E granulosus*. Foxes, sled dogs, and other canines serve as definitive hosts; mice and voles are natural intermediate hosts. Humans become infected by eating wild plants contaminated with canine feces or by hand-to-mouth spread from the fur of infected dogs.

In humans, *E multilocularis* is typically found as an alveolar hepatic cyst—a spongy mass with a jelly-like matrix. These cysts resemble neoplasms in their ability to spread locally and metastasize. The initial symptoms of *E multilocularis* are often vague. Hepatomegaly, abdominal pain, obstructive jaundice, and invasion of contiguous structures follow.[100]

The diagnosis is based on the history of exposure in an endemic area and ultrasonographic, computed tomographic, or magnetic resonance findings. A negative serologic test does not exclude the diagnosis, but the presence of antibodies against *Echinococcus*-specific antigen 5 has a high degree of specificity.[101] Although antibodies against antigen 5 have also been observed in patients with cysticercosis, the two diseases can usually be differentiated on clinical grounds.

Albendazole is now recommended for the treatment of *E granulosus* infection, but some patients may benefit from or require surgical resection of cysts. Surgery is the only reliable means of treating *E multilocularis* infection. Mebendazole or albendazole have been used in inoperable cases (see Table 107-2).[5,98] Echinococcosis can be prevented by avoiding uncooked, potentially contaminated wild fruits, by worming sled dogs, and by washing hands after exposure to potentially infected animals.

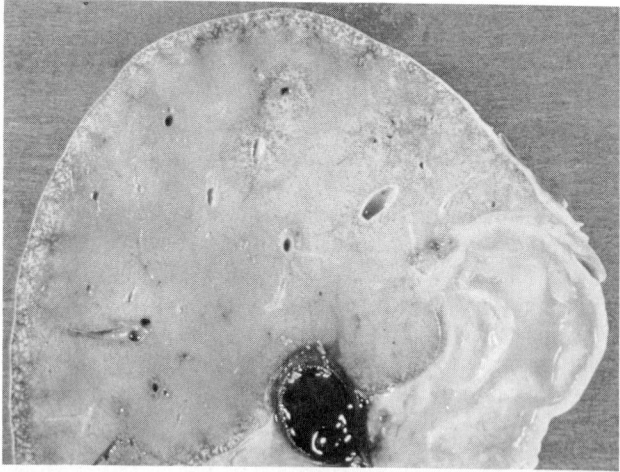

FIGURE 107-9. (See Color Fig. 63.) *Echinococcus granulosus* (hydatid) liver cysts have well defined capsules, each with an irregular lining. These capsules contain a semiopaque, tan liquid with hydatid sand composed of protoscoleces, each of which can mature to one adult worm. (From Smith JW, et al. Intestinal helminths. Atlas of diagnostic medical parasitology series. Chicago: American Society of Clinical Pathologists, 1984.)

TREMATODES

Schistosoma species, which are blood flukes, are among the most prevalent of the trematodes that infect humans. *Schistosoma mansoni* and *Schistosoma japonicum* are major causes of gastrointestinal pathology. Less prevalent are *Schistosoma intercalatum* and *Schistosoma mekongi*. The latter is closely related to *S japonicum*. *Schistosoma haematobium* primarily affects the urinary tract, although it too on occasion involves the bowel. Other pathogenic trematodes live in the biliary tract or the lumen of the small intestine. They include the liver flukes *C sinensis*, *Opisthorchis viverrini*, and *Fasciola hepatica*, and the intestinal flukes, which include *Fasciolopsis buski*, *Heterophyes heterophyes*, and *Metagonimus yokogawai*. These trematodes have complex life cycles that involve vertebrate and invertebrate hosts.[102]

Schistosomiasis

Schistosoma species have a complex life cycle. The delicate adult worms live as pairs within venules in their definitive human host (Fig. 107-10; see Color Fig. 64). The female spends her life in the gynecophoric canal of the male. From 300 eggs in the case of *S mansoni* to 3500 in the case of *S japonicum* are passed into the venules daily. Lytic enzymes produced by the ova allow penetration of the wall of the vessel and permit ova to reach the lumen of the intestine. The ova are excreted in the stool. Miracidia are released when ova hatch in fresh water. The next phase of infection begins when miracidia penetrate snails of the appropriate genera. After development in the snail, fork-tailed cercariae emerge. They enter human skin when contact is made during bathing, fishing, or other water-related activities.

The tails of the cercariae are lost when they enter the skin, and the resulting schistosomulae make their way through the vasculature to the portal circulation. After approximately 3 weeks, *S mansoni* migrates primarily to the superior mesenteric veins and *S japonicum* to the inferior mesenteric veins. Adult worms can live as long as 30 years in humans.[103]

Epidemiology

S mansoni is widespread in Africa and is also endemic in multiple areas of Latin America. Scattered foci are present in the Middle East. *S intercalatum*, only relatively recently identified,

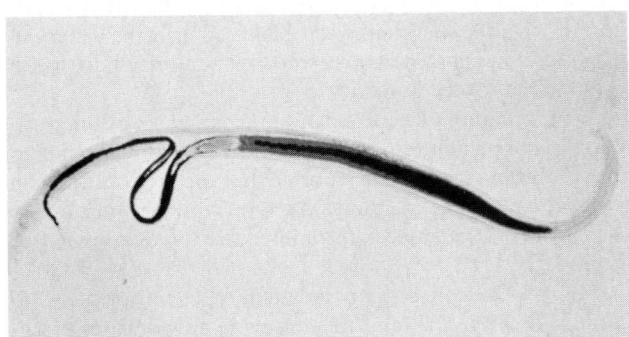

FIGURE 107-10. (See Color Fig. 64.) *Schistosoma mansoni*, adult worm pair. The long, slender female is protruding from the gynecophoral canal of the larger male worm. *S mansoni* pairs such as these usually reside in the mesenteric plexus in the distribution of the superior mesenteric vein. (Carmine stain; from Smith JW, et al. Intestinal helminths. Atlas of diagnostic medical parasitology series. Chicago: American Society of Clinical Pathologists, 1984.)

is encountered in areas of Western and Central Africa. *S japonicum* is endemic in the Far East, China, coastal river valleys in Japan, numerous islands in the Philippines, and Indochina. The prevalence of disease in China has decreased dramatically as a result of labor-intensive efforts to limit the reproduction of snails.[104] *S mekongi* is found along the Mekong River in Indochina.

Clinical Manifestations

Invasion of skin by cercariae of these *Schistosoma* species is usually asymptomatic, but a mild pruritic dermatitis may result. Acute schistosomiasis, or Katayama fever, was initially described among people with primary *S japonicum* infection, but it can occur with *S mansoni* and other *Schistosoma* sp.[105] The time from invasion by cercariae to onset of symptoms ranges from 6 to 8 weeks for *S japonicum* to 3 to 8 weeks for *S mansoni*, and coincides with the onset of egg production. Katayama fever is a serum sickness-like syndrome characterized by fever, malaise, urticaria, abdominal discomfort, diarrhea, weight loss, cough, mild hepatosplenomegaly, lymphadenopathy, and eosinophilia. Symptoms can persist for as long as several months.

Chronic schistosomiasis develops as a consequence of the inflammatory response elicited by schistosome eggs that are deposited in the intestine, are carried to the liver by way of the portal circulation, or reach the lungs or other sites by way of the systemic circulation. The degree of pathology depends on the worm burden and the host's immune response to eggs. Intestinal disease is characterized by congestion, hypertrophy, and ulceration of the mucosa. Those infected may experience abdominal pain, diarrhea, and bloody stools. Intestinal polyps and strictures may result late in disease.[106]

Eggs that are swept to the liver elicit a granulomatous inflammatory response. "Symmers'" periportal fibrosis of varying severity develops in infected people and can progress to severe "pipe-stem" portal fibrosis with presinusoidal portal hypertension.[107] Hepatomegaly and splenomegaly are common in people with heavy infection. The pathology in the liver is predominantly mesenchymal, and the parenchyma and liver function usually are preserved until late in the disease. Heavy infections have been associated with growth retardation in children. Bleeding from esophageal varices and ascites develops late in hepatosplenic schistosomiasis.

Portosystemic anastomoses also allow shunting of eggs to the pulmonary vasculature, where granulomas followed by fibrosis may result in chronic obliterative arteritis, pulmonary hypertension, and eventually cor pulmonale.[108] Granulomatous responses to eggs are occasionally observed in other organs, including the gallbladder, where they have been associated with cholecystitis and cholelithiasis. *S mansoni* eggs have been found in the spinal cord,[109,110] and *S japonicum* eggs have been found in the central nervous system.[111] In some patients, *S mansoni* infection is associated with immune complex glomerulonephritis and occasionally results in the nephrotic syndrome. This complication is rare with *S japonicum*.

S haematobium resides primarily in venules of the vesical plexus, but on occasion it too involves the gastrointestinal tract. *S haematobium* has been found in association with acute appendicitis, although its role in the pathogenesis is uncertain,[112,113] and it has been reported as a cause of asymptomatic appendiceal calcification.[114]

Diagnosis, Treatment, and Prevention

The diagnosis of schistosomiasis is confirmed by identifying ova in feces or biopsy material. Direct smears of stool are of relatively low sensitivity; Kato thick smears using 20 to 50 mg of fecal material are more sensitive.[115] Diffuse or patchy mucosal hyperemia, friability, and occasionally schistosomal polyps may be observed at colonoscopy.[116] A rectal biopsy may be necessary to document light infections. Ultrasonography has been widely used to assess hepatosplenic involvement and responses to chemotherapy.[117,118] Several serologic assays are available and provide suggestive evidence of schistosomiasis,[119] but they are of no help in determining the magnitude or duration of infection.

Praziquantel is recommended for treatment of all *Schistosoma* species (see Table 107-2).[5,6] It is effective in killing the parasite, and has been associated with decreased periportal fibrosis, hepatomegaly, and splenomegaly,[117,118] but treatment does not reverse all of the effects of severe, chronic schistosomiasis.

Oxamniquine is a therapeutic alternative for *S mansoni.* Portal hypertension with bleeding esophageal varices may require endoscopic sclerotherapy or surgical decompression.[120,121] Control measures in endemic areas include improved sanitation, avoidance of fresh water, use of molluscacides,[104] and mass treatment programs. Despite these efforts, schistosomiasis remains prevalent in many areas of the world. There is reason to hope that vaccine will eventually become available.[122]

Liver Flukes

The liver flukes *C sinensis* and *O viverrini* are found in Japan, China, Indochina, South Korea, and Taiwan among those who eat uncooked fish.[123] It has been estimated that 6 to 7 million people are infected in northeastern Thailand alone. Adult liver flukes live in the biliary tract. Eggs are released into the bile and passed in the stool. Snails are the first intermediate host, and freshwater fish are the second. Humans become infected when they eat raw or incompletely cooked fish. Liver flukes have life spans of 10 to 30 years. In the United States, *C sinensis* and *O viverrini* are encountered among immigrants from Southeast Asia.

Slight liver enlargement and tenderness may be observed at the onset of infection. The major pathologic changes of chronic infection are in the bile ducts. Initially there is desquamation of the biliary epithelium, followed by hyperplasia and eventually adenomatous proliferation. Fibrosis and stricture of the bile ducts may follow.

The precise relationship of infection to gastrointestinal symptoms is uncertain. Light infections are usually symptomless. In heavy infections, dyspepsia, abdominal discomfort or pain, anorexia, hepatomegaly, icterus, edema, and diarrhea may occur. Pyogenic cholangitis, cholelithiasis, chronic cholecystitis, pancreatitis, and cholangiocarcinoma are potential long-term complications.[124,125]

The diagnosis is confirmed by identifying ova in the stool or bile (see Fig. 107-2). Ultrasonographic examination may reveal liver enlargement; dilation, sludge, and thickening of the wall of the gallbladder, dilation of intrahepatic bile ducts, or evidence of cholangiocarcinoma.[126] Endoscopic retrograde cholangiopancreatography may show small, irregular filling defects in the common bile duct, tortuosity and irregular dilation of the intrahepatic ducts, or blunting of the terminal branches of the biliary tree.[127] Praziquantel is the only drug that is active against these flukes (see Table 107-2).

F hepatica, which is responsible for "liver rot" in sheep and other herbivorous mammals, including humans, is cosmopolitan in sheep- and cattle-raising areas of the world. Snails are intermediate hosts. Humans become infected when they eat wild watercress contaminated with encysted metacercariae. Larvae excyst in the small intestine, penetrate the gut wall, migrate through the peritoneal cavity, and enter the liver through the capsule. Larvae may wander through the human liver for periods of 6 to 9 weeks before finally penetrating into the bile ducts, where they spend their adult lives. Infected people frequently experience fever, hepatomegaly, right upper quadrant pain, weight loss, anemia, eosinophilia, and diarrhea, but not all infections are symptomatic. The diagnosis is made by identifying ova in bile, duodenal aspirates, or stool. Serologic assays provide presumptive evidence of infection. Multiple low-density areas may be observed in the liver by computed tomography. The recommended treatment is bithionol (see Table 107-2)[5,6,128]; therapeutic failures have been reported with praziquantel.

On rare occasion, *Dicrocoelium dendriticum,* a liver fluke of sheep and cattle, is isolated from humans who have ingested field ants, the second intermediate host. Most infections are asymptomatic, but hepatobiliary disease and eosinophilia have been reported.

Intestinal Flukes

The intestinal fluke *F buski* has as its definitive hosts humans, hogs, and occasionally dogs. It is endemic in Asia. The adult flukes attach to the mucosa of the upper small intestine and release ova into the feces. Snails serve as the intermediate hosts. Cercariae encyst on water plants such as the water caltrop, water hyacinth, water chestnut, or water bamboo, which are ingested raw by humans.

Inflammation, ulceration, and mucosal abscesses may develop in the small intestine. Epigastric pain, nausea, and diarrhea of varying severity are reported, but many people remain asymptomatic. The diagnosis is made by identifying ova in the stool. Praziquantel is recommended for treatment (see Table 107-2).[5,6]

Many species of the trematode family, Heterophyidae, including *H heterophyes* and *M yokogawai,* are parasites of humans and other fish-eating mammals. The first intermediate hosts are snails, and the second intermediate hosts are freshwater or brackish-water fish. Humans become infected by eating raw or inadequately cooked fish. *H heterophyes* is encountered in the Middle East and the Orient. It does relatively little damage to the intestine. Colicky pain, abdominal tenderness, and diarrhea are experienced by some, particularly those with heavy infections. Eosinophilia may be present. One case of *Heterophyes* infection was reported in the United States in a woman who ate sushi imported from the Orient.[129] *M yokogawai* is found primarily in the Far East where it has infected American travelers, causing diarrhea.[130] *M yokogawai* on rare occasions is associated with the formation of egg-related granuloma at distant foci such as the heart or central nervous system. The diagnosis of these infections is made by finding ova in the feces. Praziquantel is the treatment of choice (see Table 107-2).[5,6] Infection can be prevented by eating only thoroughly cooked fish.

On rare occasions, people living in the Pacific Northwest or Siberia become infected with *Nanophyetus salmincola* when they ingest raw or inadequately cooked salmonid fish. Abdominal pain, diarrhea, nausea, and vomiting may result, along with eosinophilia.[131] Praziquantel has been used for therapy (see Table 107-2). Infection with one of many *Echinostoma* species may occur after ingestion of raw, infected snails, fish, or amphibians, but symptoms, when present, are usually mild.[132]

The reader is directed to Chapter 36, Approach to the Patient With Acute Abdomen; Chapter 37, Approach to the Patient With Ileus and Obstruction; Chapter 38, Approach to the Patient With Diarrhea; Chapter 46, Approach to Gastrointestinal Problems in the Immunocompromised Patient; Chapter 51, Advice to Travelers; Chapter 105, Gastrointestinal Complications of the Acquired Immunodeficiency Syndrome; Chapter 106, Parasitic Diseases: Protozoa; Chapter 130, Endoscopic Mucosal Biopsy; and Chapter 131, Microbiologic Studies.

REFERENCES

1. Levine ND. Nematode parasites of domestic animals and man. Minneapolis: Burgess, 1968.
2. Burt DRR. Platyhelminthes and parasitism: an introduction to parasitology. New York: American Elsevier, 1970.
3. Erasmus DA. The biology of trematodes. New York: Crane, Russak, 1972.
4. Strickland GT, ed. Hunter's tropical medicine. 7th ed. Philadelphia: WB Saunders, 1991.
5. Drugs for parasitic infections. Med Lett Drugs Ther 1993;35: 111.
6. Pearson RD. Antiparasitic agents. In: Mandell GL, Bennett JE, Dolan R, eds. Principles and practice of infectious diseases. 3rd ed. New York: Churchill-Livingstone, 1990:398.
7. Stephenson LS, Latham MC, Kurz KM, et al. Treatment with a single dose of albendazole improves growth of Kenyan school children with hookworm, *Trichuris trichiura*, and *Ascaris lumbricoides* infections. Am J Trop Med Hyg 1989;41:78.
8. Wolfe MS. Oxyuris, trichostrongylus and trichuris. Clin Gastroenterol 1978;7:201.
9. MacDonald TT, Choy M-Y, Spencer T, et al. Histopathology and immunocytochemistry of the caecum in children with *Trichuris* dysentery syndrome. J Clin Pathol 1991;44:194.
10. Gilman RH, Chong TH, David C, et al. The adverse consequences of heavy *Trichuris* infection. Trans R Soc Trop Med Hyg 1983;77:432.
11. Fishman JA, Perrone TL. Colonic obstruction and perforation due to *Trichuris trichiura*. Am J Med 1984;77:154.
12. Ramalingam S, Sinniah B, Krishnan U. Albendazole, an effective single dose broad spectrum anthelmintic drug. Am J Trop Med Hyg 1983;32:984.
13. Cram EB. Studies on oxyuriasis. XXVIII. Summary and conclusions. Am J Dis Child 1943;65:46.
14. Jones JE. Pinworms. Am Fam Physician 1988;38:159.
15. Weller TH, Sorenson CW. Enterobiasis: its incidence and symptomatology in a group of 505 children. N Engl J Med 1941;224:143.
16. Wagner ED, Eby WC. Pinworm prevalence in California elementary school children, and diagnostic methods. Am J Trop Med Hyg 1983;32:998.
17. Vermund SH, MacLeod S. Is pinworm a vanishing infection?: laboratory surveillance in a New York City medical center from 1971 to 1986. Am J Dis Child 1988;142:566.
18. Paradise JE, Campos JM, Friedman HM, et al. Vulvovaginitis in premenarcheal girls: clinical features and diagnostic evaluation. Pediatrics 1982;70:193.
19. Sachdev YV, Howards SS. Enterobius vermicularis and secondary enuresis. J Urol 1975;113:143.
20. Kropp KA, Cichocki A, Bansal NK. *Enterobius vermicularis* (pinworms), introital bacteriology and recurrent urinary tract infection in children. J Urol 1978;120:480.
21. Symmers WSC. Pathology of oxyuriasis. Arch Pathol Lab Med 1950;50:475.
22. Pearson RD, Irons RP Sr, Irons RP Jr. Chronic pelvic peritonitis due to the pinworm *Enterobius vermicularis*. JAMA 1981;245: 1340.
23. Sun T, Schwartz NS, Sewell C, et al. *Enterobius* egg granuloma of the vulva and peritoneum: a review of the literature. Am J Trop Med Hyg 1991;45:249.
24. Cross JH. Intestinal capillariasis. Clin Microbiol Rev 1992;5: 120.
25. Hoghooghi-Rad N, Maraghi S, Narenj-Zadeh A. *Capillaria philippinensis* infection in Khoozestan Province, Iran: case report. Am J Trop Med Hyg 1987;37:135.
26. Pawlowski ZS. Ascariasis: host-pathogen biology. Rev Infect Dis 1982;4:806.
27. Hall A, Anwar KS, Tomkins AM. Intensity of reinfection with *Ascaris lumbricoides* and its implications for parasite control. Lancet 1992;339:1253.
28. Schultz MG. Ascariasis: nutritional implications. Rev Infect Dis 1982;4:815.
29. Stephenson LS. Ascariasis. In: Stephenson LS, portions with Holland C, eds. The impact of helminth infections on human nutrition: schistosomes and soil-transmitted helminths. London and New York: Taylor & Francis, 1987:89.
30. Blumenthal DS, Schultz MG. Incidence of intestinal obstruction in children infected with *Ascaris lumbricoides*. Am J Trop Med Hyg 1975;24:801.
31. Khuroo MS, Zarqar SA, Mahajan R. Hepatobiliary and pancreatic ascariasis in India. Lancet 1990;335:1503.
32. Campbell WC, ed. *Trichinella* and trichinosis. New York: Plenum Press, 1983.
33. Petri WA Jr, Holsinger JR, Pearson RD. Common-source outbreak of trichinosis associated with eating raw home-butchered pork. South Med J 1988;81:1056.
34. Schmitt N, Bownmer EJ, Simon PC, et al. Trichinosis from bear meat and adulterated pork products: a major outbreak in British Columbia. Can Med Assoc J 1972;107:1087.
35. Bailey TM, Schantz PM. Trends in the incidence and transmission patterns of trichinosis in the United States: comparisons of the periods 1975–1981 and 1982–1986. Rev Infect Dis 1990;12:5.
36. MacLean JD, Poirier L, Gyorkos TW, et al. Epidemiology and serologic definition of primary and secondary trichinosis in the Arctic. J Infect Dis 1992;165:908.
37. McCracken RO, Taylor DD. Mebendazole therapy of parenteral trichinellosis. Science 1980;207:1220.
38. Gilman RH. Hookworm disease: host-pathogen biology. Rev Infect Dis 1982;4:824.
39. Miller TA. Hookworm infection in man. Adv Parasitol 1979;17: 315.
40. Gilles HM, Williams EJW, Ball PAJ. Hookworm infection and anaemia: an epidemiological, clinical, and laboratory study. Q J Med 1964;33:1.
41. Hotez PJ, Cerami A. Secretion of a proteolytic anticoagulant by *Ancylostoma* hookworms. J Exp Med 1983;157:1594.
42. Farid Z, Nichols JH, Bassily S, et al. Blood loss in pure *Ancy-*

lostoma duodenale infection in Egyptian farmers. Am J Trop Med Hyg 1965;14:375.

43. Martinez-Torres C, Ojeda A, Roche M, et al. Hookworm infection and intestinal blood loss. Trans R Soc Trop Med Hyg 1967;61:373.

44. Fulmer HS, Huempfner HR. Intestinal helminths in eastern Kentucky: a survey in three rural counties. Am J Trop Med Hyg 1965;14:269.

45. Maxwell C, Hussain R, Nutman TB, et al. The clinical and immunologic responses of normal human volunteers to low dose hookworm (*Necator americanus*) infection. Am J Trop Med Hyg 1987;37:126.

46. Riva H, Escamilla DG, Frati AC. Acute massive intestinal bleeding caused by hookworm. JAMA 1981;246:68.

47. Roche M, Layrisse M. The nature and causes of "hookworm anemia." Am J Trop Med Hyg 1966;15:1030.

48. Variyam EP, Banwell JG. Hookworm disease: nutritional implications. Rev Infect Dis 1982;4:830.

49. Nutman TB, Ottesen EA, Ieng S, et al. Eosinophilia in Southeast Asian refugees: evaluation at a referral center. J Infect Dis 1987;155:309.

50. Holzer BR, Frey FJ. Differential efficacy of mebendazole and albendazole against *Necator americanus* but not for *Trichuris trichiura* infestations. Eur J Clin Pharmacol 1987;32:635.

51. Scowden EB, Schaffner W, Stone WJ. Overwhelming strongyloidiasis: an unappreciated opportunistic infection. Medicine 1978;57:527.

52. Morgan JS, Schaffner W, Stone WJ. Opportunistic strongyloidiasis in renal transplant recipients. Transplantation 1986;42:518.

53. Igra-Siegman Y, Kapila R, Sen P, et al. Syndrome of hyperinfection with *Strongyloides stercoralis*. Rev Infect Dis 1981;3:397.

54. Hira PR, Patel BG. Human strongyloidiasis due to the primate species *Strongyloides fulleborni*. Trop Geogr Med 1980;32:23.

55. Gill GV, Bell DR. *Strongyloides stercoralis* infection in former Far East prisoners of war. Br Med J 1979;2:572.

56. Grove DI. Strongyloidiasis in allied ex-prisoners of war in Southeast Asia. Br Med J 1980;280:598.

57. Pelletier LL Jr. Chronic strongyloidiasis in World War II Far East ex-prisoners of war. Am J Trop Med Hyg 1984;33:55.

58. Pelletier LL Jr, Gabre-Kidan T. Chronic strongyloidiasis in Vietnam veterans. Am J Med 1985;78:139.

59. Berk SL, Verghese A, Alvarez S, et al. Clinical and epidemiologic features of strongyloidiasis: a prospective study in rural Tennessee. Arch Intern Med 1987;147:1257.

60. Walzer PD, Milder JE, Banwell JG, et al. Epidemiologic features of *Strongyloides stercoralis* infection in an endemic area of the United States. Am J Trop Med Hyg 1982;31:313.

61. Smith JD, Goette DK, Odom RB. Larva currens: cutaneous strongyloidiasis. Arch Dermatol 1976;112:1161.

62. Milder JE, Walzer PD, Kilgore G, et al. Clinical features of *Strongyloides stercoralis* infection in an endemic area of the United States. Gastroenterology. 1981;80:1481.

63. Berry AJ, Long EG, Smith JH, et al. Chronic relapsing colitis due to *Strongyloides stercoralis*. Am J Trop Med Hyg 1983;32:1289.

64. Paola D, Dias LB, Silva JR. Enteritis due to *Strongyloides stercoralis*: a report of 5 fatal cases. Am J Dig Dis 1962;7:1086.

65. Bartholomew C, Butler AK, Bhaskar AG, et al. Pseudo-obstruction and a sprue-like syndrome from strongyloidiasis. Postgrad Med J 1977;53:139.

66. Milner PF, Irvine RA, Barton CJ, et al. Intestinal malabsorption in *Strongyloides stercoralis* infestation. Gut 1965;6:574.

67. Yoeli M, Most H, Berman HH, et al. II. The clinical picture and pathology of a massive *Strongyloides* infection in a child. Trans R Soc Trop Med Hyg 1963;57:346.

68. Petithory JC, Derouin F. AIDS and strongyloidiasis in Africa. Lancet 1987;1:921.

69. Lima JP, Delgado PG. Diagnosis of strongyloidiasis: importance of Baermann's method. Am J Dig Dis 1961;6:899.

70. Grove DI. Treatment of strongyloidiasis with thiabendazole: an analysis of toxicity and effectiveness. Trans R Soc Trop Med Hyg 1982;76:114.

71. Schumaker JD, Band JD, Lensmeyer GL, et al. Thiabendazole treatment of severe strongyloidiasis in a hemodialysed patient. Ann Intern Med 1978;89:644.

72. Herbener D, Borak J. Cutaneous larva migrans in northern climates. Am J Emerg Med 1988;6:462.

73. Gillespie SH. Human toxocariasis. J Appl Bacteriol 1987;63:473.

74. Glickman LT, Magnaval J-F, Domanski LM, et al. Visceral larva migrans in French adults: a new disease syndrome? Am J Epidemiol 1987;125:1019.

75. Kwee HG, Sautter RL. Anisakiasis. Am Fam Physician 1987;36(2):137.

76. Smith JW, Wootten R. Anisakis and anisakiasis. Adv Parasitol 1978;16:93.

77. Hsiu J-G, Gamsey AJ, Ives CE, et al. Gastric anisakiasis: report of a case with clinical, endoscopic, and histological findings. Am J Gastroenterol 1986;81:1185.

78. Hulbert TV, Larsen RA, Chandrasoma PT. Abdominal angiostrongyliasis mimicking acute appendicitis and Meckel's diverticulum: report of a case in the United States and review. Clin Infect Dis 1992;14:836.

79. Despommier DD. Tapeworm infection: the long and the short of it. N Engl J Med 1992;327:727.

80. Pearson RD, Hewlett EL. Niclosamide for the treatment of tapeworm infections. Ann Intern Med 1985;102:550.

81. Schantz PM, Moore AC, Munoz JL, et al. Neurocysticercosis in an orthodox Jewish community in New York City. N Engl J Med 1992;327:692.

82. Richards F Jr, Schantz PM. Treatment of *Taenia solium* infections. Lancet 1985;1:1264.

83. Pearson RD, Wilson ME. Role of praziquantel in the treatment of helminthic diseases. Internal Medicine for the Specialist 1986;7:183.

84. King CH, Mahmoud AAF. Drugs five years later: praziquantel. Ann Intern Med 1989;110:290.

85. Sotelo J, Rosas N, Palencia G. Freezing of infested pork muscle kills cysticerci. JAMA 1986;256:893.

86. Von Bonsdorff B. Diphyllobothriasis in man. London: Academic Press, 1977.

87. Saarni M, Nyberg W, Grasbeck R, et al. Symptoms in carriers of *Diphyllobothrium latum* and in non-infected controls. Acta Med Scand 1963;173:147.

88. Biagi F, Lopez R, Viso J. Analysis of symptoms and signs related with intestinal parasitosis in 5,215 cases. Prog Drug Res 1975;19:10.

89. Man, dogs and hydatid disease (editorial). Lancet 1987;1:21.

90. Brannath J, Bartscher U. Echinococcosis of bile duct as a rare cause of obstructive jaundice. Dtsch Med Wochenschr 1987;112:16.

91. Van Steenbergen W, Fevery J, Broeckhaert L, et al. Hepatic echinococcosis ruptured into the biliary tract: clinical, radiological and therapeutical features during five episodes of spontaneous biliary rupture in three patients with hepatic hydatidosis. J Hepatol 1987;4:133.

92. Allerberger F, Roberts G, Dierich MP, et al. Serodiagnosis of echinococcosis: evaluation of two reference laboratories. Trop Med Parasitol 1991;42:109.

93. Langer B. Surgical treatment of hydatid disease of the liver. Br J Surg 1987;74:237.

94. Brett PM, Fond A, Bretagnolle M, et al. Percutaneous aspiration and drainage of hydatid cysts in the liver. Radiology 1988;168:617.

95. Filice C, Di Perri G, Strosselli M, et al. Parasitologic findings in percutaneous drainage of human hydatid liver cysts. J Infect Dis 1990;161:1290.

96. Russo A, Giannone G, Virgilio C. Sclerosing cholangitis following removal of an echinococcus cyst. Endoscopy 1987;19:178.

97. Sayek I, Cakmakci M. The effect of prophylactic mebendazole in experimental peritoneal hydatidosis. Surg Gynecol Obstet 1986;163:351.

98. Davis A, Pawlowski ZS, Dixon H. Multicentre clinical trials of benzimidazolecarbamates in human echinococcosis. Bull WHO 1986;64:383.

99. Gemmell MA, Lawson JR, Roberts MG. Control of echino-

coccosis/hydatidosis: present status of worldwide progress. Bull WHO 1986;64:333.

100. Wilson JF, Rausch RL. Alveolar hydatid disease: a review of clinical features of 33 indigenous cases of *Echinococcus multilocularis* infection in Alaskan Eskimos. Am J Trop Med Hyg 1980;29:1340.

101. Hira PR, Bahr GM, Shweiki HM, et al. An enzyme-linked immunosorbent assay using an arc 5 antigen for the diagnosis of cystic hydatid disease. Ann Trop Med Parasitol 1990;84:157.

102. Shoop WL. Trematode transmission patterns. J Parasitol 1988;74:46.

103. Cook GC, Bryceson ADM. Longstanding infection with *Schistosoma mansoni*. Lancet 1980;1:127.

104. Conrad F. Schistosomiasis eradication in China. Science 1988;239:1079.

105. Farid Z, Trabolsi B, Hafez A. Acute schistosomiasis mansoni (Katayama syndrome). Ann Trop Med Parasitol 1986;80:563.

106. Cheever AW, Kamel IA, Elwi AM, et al. *Schistosoma mansoni* and *S. haematobium* infections in Egypt. III. Extrahepatic pathology. Am J Trop Med Hyg 1987;27:55.

107. Kamel IA, Elwi AM, Cheever AW, et al. *Schistosoma mansoni* and *S. haematobium* infections in Egypt. IV. Hepatic lesions. Am J Trop Med Hyg 1978;27:939.

108. Andrade ZA, Andrade SG. Pathogenesis of schistosomal pulmonary arteritis. Am J Trop Med Hyg 1970;19:305.

109. Cosnett JE, Van Dellen JR. Schistosomiasis (bilharzia) of the spinal cord: case reports and clinical profile. Q J Med 1986;61:1113.

110. Suchet I, Klein C, Horwitz T, et al. Spinal cord schistosomiasis: a case report and review of the literature. Paraplegia 1987;25:491.

111. Watt G, Adapon B, Long GW, et al. Praziquantel in treatment of cerebral schistosomiasis. Lancet 1986;2:529.

112. Al-Kraida A, Giangreco A, Shaikh MU, et al. Appendicitis and schistosomiasis. Br J Surg 1988;75:58.

113. Duvie SOA, Diffang C, Guirguis MN. The effects of *Schistosoma haematobium* infestation on the vermiform appendix: the Nigerian experience. J Trop Med Hyg 1987;90:13.

114. Fataar S, Satyanath S. The radiographic evaluation of appendiceal calcification due to schistosomiasis. Am J Trop Med Hyg 1986;35:1157.

115. Peters PA, El Alamy M, Warren KS, et al. Quick Kato smear for field quantification of *Schistosoma mansoni* eggs. Am J Trop Med Hyg 1980;29:217.

116. Radhakrishnan S, Nakib BA, Shaikh H, et al. The value of colonoscopy in schistosomal, tuberculous, and amebic colitis: two years experience. Dis Colon Rectum 1986;29:891.

117. Ohmae H, Tanaka M, Hayashi M, et al. Improvement of ultrasonographic and serologic changes in *Schistosoma japonicum*-infected patients after treatment with praziquantel. Am J Trop Med Hyg 1992;46:99.

118. Doehring-Schwerdtfeger E, Abdel-Rahim IM, Kardoff R, et al. Ultrasonographical investigation of periportal fibrosis in children with *Schistosoma mansoni* infection: reversibility of morbidity twenty-three months after treatment with praziquantel. Am J Trop Med Hyg 1992;46:409.

119. Maddison SE. The present status of serodiagnosis and seroepidemiology of schistosomiasis. Diagn Microbiol Infect Dis 1987;7:93.

120. Sakai P, Boaventura S, Ishioka S, et al. Sclerotheraphy of bleeding esophageal varices in schistosomiasis: comparative study in patients with and without previous surgery for portal hypertension. Endoscopy 1990;22:5.

121. Silva LC, Strauss E, Gayotto LCC, et al. A randomized trial for the study of the elective surgical treatment of portal hypertension in mansonic schistosomiasis. Ann Surg 1986;204:148.

122. Sher A, James SL, Correa-Oliveira R, et al. Schistosome vaccines: current progress and future prospects. Parasitology 1989;98(Suppl):S61.

123. Upatham ES, Viyanant V, Kurathong S, et al. Relationships between prevalence and intensity of *Opisthorchis viverrini* infection and clinical symptoms and signs in a rural community in north-east Thailand. Bull WHO 1984;62:451.

124. Belamaric J. Intrahepatic bile duct carcinoma of the liver and *C. sinensis* infection in Hong Kong. Cancer 1973;31:468.

125. Kurathong S, Lerdverasirikul P, Wongpaitoo V, et al. *Opisthorchis viverrini* infection and cholangiocarcinoma: a prospective, case-controlled study. Gastroenterology 1985;89:151.

126. Lim JH, Ko YT, DH Lee, et al. Clonorchiasis: sonographic findings in 59 proved cases. AJR 1989;152:761.

127. Leung JW, JY Sung, SC Chung, et al. Hepatic clonorchiasis: a study by endoscopic retrograde cholangiopancreatography. Gastrointest Endosc 1989;35:226.

128. Bacq Y, Besnier JM, Duong TH. Successful treatment of acute fascioliasis with bithionol. Hepatology 1991;14:1066.

129. Adams KO, Jungkind DL, Bergquist EJ, et al. Intestinal fluke infection as a result of eating sushi. Am J Clin Pathol 1986;86:688.

130. Goldsmith RS. Chronic diarrhea in returning travelers: intestinal parasite infection with the fluke *Metagonimus yokogawai*. South Med J 1978;71:1513.

131. Eastburn RL, Fritsche TR, Terhune CA Jr. Human intestinal infection with *Nanophyetus salmincola* from salmonid fishes. Am J Trop Med Hyg 1987;36:586.

132. Huffman JE, Fried B. Echinostoma and echinostomiasis. Adv Parasitol 1990;29:215.

Textbook of Gastroenterology, second edition, edited
by Tadataka Yamada. JB Lippincott Company,
Philadelphia © 1995.

CHAPTER 108

Gastrointestinal Manifestations of Specific Genetic Disorders

Maren Scheuner   Huiying Yang   Jerome I. Rotter

Genetic Disorders With Prominent Gastrointestinal Presentations
Malabsorption Disorders
  Defects in Carbohydrate Metabolism
  Defects in Amino Acid Transport
  Disorders of Electrolyte Absorption
  Intestinal Defects in Protein Absorption
  Intestinal Defects in Lipid Absorption
  Exocrine Pancreas Abnormalities
  Disorders of Vitamin and Mineral Assimilation
Chronic Diarrhea Syndromes Not Characterized by Malabsorption
Recurrent Gastrointestinal Bleeding Syndromes
  Neurofibromatosis
  Osler-Weber-Rendu Syndrome
  Klippel-Trenaunay-Weber Syndrome
  Blue Rubber Bleb Nevus Syndrome
  Ehlers-Danlos Syndrome
  Pseudoxanthoma Elasticum
  Cutis Laxa Type I
  Syndromes Characterized by Macrocephaly, Multiple
    Lipomas, and Hemangiomas
  Hermansky-Pudlak Syndrome
Intestinal Motility or Pseudoobstruction Disorders

  Visceral Myopathy Syndromes
  Duchenne's Muscular Dystrophy
  Myotonic Dystrophy
  Kearns-Sayre Syndrome
  Visceral Neuropathy Syndromes
  Hirschsprung's Disease
  Familial Achalasia and Diffuse Esophageal Spasm
  Familial Dysautonomia
Mechanical Obstruction and Malformation Syndromes
Chronic Abdominal Pain Syndromes
  Familial Mediterranean Fever
  Fabry's Disease
  Hereditary Angioneurotic Edema
  Hereditary Fructose Intolerance
  Hereditary Pancreatitis Syndromes
Gastrointestinal Neoplasm Syndromes
Common Gastrointestinal Disorders With Complex Genetic Causes
Pernicious Anemia and Atrophic Gastritis
Gluten-Sensitive Enteropathy
Inflammatory Bowel Disease
Gallstones

Genetics and environment play important roles in the development of gastrointestinal (GI) diseases. An interaction between a genetic susceptibility and an environmental trigger is probably necessary for disease expression, and the contribution of each factor appears to depend on the specific disease.

A family history may demonstrate a particular pattern of inheritance (e.g., autosomal dominant, autosomal recessive, X-linked, mitochondrial) that reveals a discrete genetic component for a GI disease with a predictable effect on disease manifestation within that family. More formal genetic epidemiologic studies (e.g., adoption, twin, spouse, linkage and association) are required to recognize the more complex genetic contribution of other GI diseases. These patterns of inheritance and genetic epidemiologic methods are delineated in Chapter 49.

Basic genetic principles are important tools for the modern clinician working in a field in which preventive strategies are emphasized. With an understanding of the genetic mechanisms of a GI disorder and its associated manifestations, a clinician is better equipped to provide accurate diagnostic, prognostic, and therapeutic measures to his patients and their family members at risk. Preventive programs for patients and their at-risk relatives can be recommended. Examples include serial colonoscopy screening in familial polyposis coli pedigrees and the institution of colchicine to prevent renal amyloidosis in patients with familial Mediterranean fever.

This chapter is organized into two parts. The first reviews the known genetic syndromes that can present with GI manifestations. Most of these are single-gene disorders that follow distinct mendelian patterns of inheritance, and most have additional manifestations in other organ systems. Although many of these syndromes present early in life (e.g., inborn errors of malabsorption), others primarily present in adulthood (e.g., dominant colon cancer syndromes).

The second part of this chapter reviews the significant genetic contribution to some common GI problems, such as inflammatory bowel disease and gallstones. These disorders usually present in adulthood. Single-gene disorders may be responsible in some instances, but most are caused by complex genetic and environmental interactions (see Chap. 49).

The pathophysiology, diagnosis, and treatment for the common mendelian (e.g., lactose intolerance) and complex, nonmendelian GI diseases (e.g., inflammatory bowel disease) mentioned in this chapter are covered elsewhere in this text and are not fully addressed here unless genetics plays a primary role, as in the case of genetic marker studies for diagnostic or counseling purposes in cases of cystic fibrosis.

Genetic Disorders With Prominent Gastrointestinal Presentations

MALABSORPTION DISORDERS

There are many genetic syndromes that involve defects of intestinal absorption (Table 108-1). Most of these are disorders of the brush border enzymes or transport proteins that transfer sugars, amino acids, electrolytes, lipids, vitamins, and minerals from the lumen of the gut to the circulation. These disorders may involve a singular, specific function, such as lactase deficiency, or they may cause a more general malabsorptive defect, such as Hartnup disease. The other large group of genetic malabsorption syndromes involves disorders of the exocrine pancreas. The most common of these is cystic fibrosis, followed in frequency by the Schwachman-Bodian syndrome and the much rarer Johanson-Blizzard syndrome.

Defects in Carbohydrate Metabolism

Congenital Lactase Deficiency

Patients with congenital lactase deficiency (i.e., disaccharide intolerance II) present with watery diarrhea, usually after the first feeding of breast milk. Lactase appears to be absent in the duodenal mucosa of affected infants. The duodenum is otherwise histologically and enzymatically normal.[1] The missing enzyme has lactase and phlorizin hydrolase activity.

The complete DNA sequence of human lactase-phlorizin hydrolase has been reported and mapped to chromosome 2.[2,3] The late consequences of congenital lactase deficiency are not fully known, but it has been speculated that affected persons may have a lower incidence of cardiovascular disease because they avoid dairy products, similar to fructose-intolerant persons who avoid fruits and have fewer caries.[4]

Adult Lactase Deficiency

In most mammals, lactase activity peaks in the newborn period. Shortly thereafter, it can diminish to about 10% of maximal activity, which is the usual activity found in adults with lactase deficiency (i.e., disaccharide intolerance III). Three fourths or more non-Caucasian adults are lactase deficient. Among Caucasians, the prevalence of lactase deficiency ranges from 5% to 30% in adults, depending on the specific ethnic group (see Chap. 73).[5,6]

Affected members of ethnic groups with a greater than 50% prevalence of late-onset lactase deficiency (i.e., hypolactasia) present between the ages of 1 and 5 years with diarrhea and crampy abdominal pain after the ingestion of lactose-containing foods. In Caucasians destined to have hypolactasia, symptoms usually do not appear until later, at approximately age 13. The diagnosis can be made by assaying oligosaccharidase activity from a peroral biopsy or by noninvasive techniques of oral lactose tolerance tests or breath tests.[5–7]

Studies designed to explain the differences in adult lactase activities in different ethnic groups have shown that human lactase activity is independent of lactose intake; it appears clear that the differences are genetic. It has been suggested that persistence of lactase function is the abnormal state, parallel to the persistence of fetal hemoglobin.[8] The lactase enzymes in adults and infants are identical.[9] No difference has been detected in the sequence of the lactase-phlorizin hydrolase gene in adults with high or low levels of lactase activity.[10] Crossed immunoelectrophoresis of small intestine biopsies of adults with hypolactasia have shown that the molecular defect is a decreased amount of active brush border lactase protein.[6,7]

The developmental pattern of lactase expression is probably regulated at the level of gene expression.[11] Two phenotypes have been described: phenotype I is characterized by a decrease in mRNA coding for lactase-phlorizin hydrolase; phenotype II is characterized by abnormal posttranslational processing of lactase-phlorizin hydrolase, with retention of the molecule in the endoplasmic reticulum.[12]

The inheritance pattern of hypolactasia is autosomal recessive.[13] Although it could be expected that only siblings would be affected in families, the parents and offspring are commonly affected. As discussed in Chapter 49 under autosomal recessive inheritance, this finding is the result of the inordinately high prevalence of the gene for hypolactasia in the population. This sometimes results in an affected homozygote marrying a heterozygous carrier; on average, half the offspring are affected in such matings.

Trying to determine why lactase deficiency is the rule among human populations (and lactase persistence the exception) has yielded interesting speculations.[5,6] There is little evidence that suggests large segments of the population of the world depend on milk for nutrition. However, milk contains a substantial amount of calcium, and lactose appears to increase intestinal calcium absorption; populations receiving low ultraviolet radiation or insufficient dietary vitamin D may have been protected against rickets by the maintenance of intestinal lactase.

(text continues on p. 2386)

TABLE 108-1
Genetic Disorders of Intestinal Malabsorption

CONDITION	INHERITANCE PATTERN	GASTROINTESTINAL MANIFESTATIONS	OTHER FEATURES AND COMMENTS
Defects in Carbohydrate Absorption			
Congenital lactase deficiency (disaccharide intolerance II)	AR	Watery diarrhea within the first 10 days of life	Possibly less cardiovascular disease due to avoidance of dairy products
Adult lactase deficiency or hypolactasia (disaccharide intolerance III)	AR	Abdominal pain, bloating, diarrhea after lactose ingestion	Present in >75% of non-Caucasians and about 20% of Caucasians
Congenital lactose intolerance	?AD	Vomiting and diarrhea	Failure to thrive, dehydration, renal tubular acidosis, disacchariduria, aminoaciduria, liver damage, cataracts, and brain damage
Sucrase-isomaltase deficiency (disaccharide intolerance I)	AR	Variable symptoms, from severe diarrhea in infancy to stomach upset in adults after sucrose ingestion	Starch well tolerated
Glucose-galactose malabsorption	AR	Bloating, abdominal pain, and diarrhea after ingestion of most carbohydrates	Mild defect in renal tubular absorption of glucose
Fanconi's syndrome with intestinal malabsorption and galactose intolerance	AR	Poor appetite, generalized malabsorption	Impaired galactose metabolism, normal glucose absorption, slow weight gain, retarded psychomotor development, and abnormal renal tubular function
Trehalase deficiency	AR	Diarrhea and vomiting after ingestion of trehalose-containing foods (e.g., insects, mushrooms)	Rare in American Caucasians, found in 10%–15% of Greenland Eskimos
Defects in Amino Acid Transport			
Iminoglycinuria	AR	None	A membrane transport defect causing excess excretion of proline, hydroxyproline, and glycine—of no clinical consequence; frequency among Caucasians, 1 in 15,000
Hartnup's disease	AR	None	Intermittent, red, scaly, pellagra-like rash after sun exposure; cerebellar ataxia, psychiatric disorders, low or subnormal intelligence, massive aminoaciduria of neutral and aromatic amino acids; U.S. incidence of 5 per 100,000
Cystinuria	AR	None	Renal tubule and intestinal epithelium transport abnormalities of all dibasic amino acids; nephrolithiasis due to insolubility of cystine in urine; U.S. incidence of 1 in 15,000
Lysinuric protein intolerance (dibasic aminoaciduria I and II)	AR	Vomiting and diarrhea after ingestion of cow's milk	Hyperammonemia, failure to thrive, organomegaly, mental retardation, lens opacities, elastic skin, and sparse hair
Blue diaper syndrome	AR	None	Hypercalcemia, nephrocalcinosis, and indicanuria due to intestinal tryptophan transport defect
Oasthouse syndrome	AR	Diarrhea	White hair, hyperpnea, seizures, mental retardation, and an odor of an oasthouse (i.e., kiln for drying hops)
Lowe oculocerebrorenal syndrome	XLR	None	Cataracts, mental retardation, vitamin D–resistant rickets, glaucoma, generalized aminoaciduria and organic aciduria; death from renal failure; impaired intestinal and

(continued)

TABLE 108-1. *(Continued)*

CONDITION	INHERITANCE PATTERN	GASTROINTESTINAL MANIFESTATIONS	OTHER FEATURES AND COMMENTS
			renal absorption of lysine and arginine; mapped to Xq; carrier detection possible
Lysine intolerance	AR	Episodic vomiting, rigidity	Coma in infancy relieved by low-protein diet; hyperammonemia and high lysine and arginine levels, apparently due to defective L-lysine: NAD-oxidoreductase activity in liver
Lysine malabsorption syndrome	?AR	Impaired intestinal absorption of lysine	Physical and mental retardation; hyperlysinuria and hypolysinemia, probably due to lysine transport defect
Glutamate-aspartate transport defect	?AR	None	Defective intestinal and renal transport of glutamic and aspartic acids, leading to moderate hyperprolinemia and hypoglycemia
Disorders of Electrolyte Absorption			
Congenital chloride diarrhea	AR	Voluminous, chloride-containing, watery stools	Polyhydramnios, premature birth, hypochloremia, hypokalemia, metabolic alkalosis, growth retardation
Congenital sodium diarrhea	AR	Voluminous, sodium- and bicarbonate-containing stools	Polyhydramnios, premature birth
Microvillus inclusion disease	AR	Severe, watery diarrhea	No polyhydramnios or premature birth
18-Oxidation defects of aldosterone	AR	Vomiting, intestinal salt wasting	Dehydration, hypernatremia, and hypokalemia; deficiencies of 18-hydroxylase and 18-hydroxysteroid dehydrogenase
Congenital adrenal hyperplasia	AR	Intestinal salt wasting	Deficiency in any one of several enzymes in cortisol synthesis; virilization, renal salt losing, or hypertension
Hypomagnesemia	AR	Primary intestinal malabsorption of magnesium	Hypomagnesemia, hypocalcemia, seizures, and tetany in newborn period
Defects in Intestinal Protein Absorption			
Intestinal lymphangiectasia	AD	Intestinal loss of protein, dilated lymphatic spaces in small bowel and partial villous atrophy	Neonatal edema, high incidence of stillbirth, congenital malformations, lymphopenia, hypogammaglobulinemia, skin anergy, dysproteinemia, leg edema and ulcers in males
Aplasia cutis congenita with intestinal lymphangiectasia	AR	Intestinal loss of protein	Aplasia cutis congenita of the vertex, nonpitting limb edema, hypoproteinemia, lymphopenia
Protein-losing enteropathy	AR	Diarrhea, abdominal pain, ascites, intestinal loss of protein	Edema, growth retardation, clubbing, hypoproteinemia, iron-deficiency anemia, no lymphopenia; hepatic vein stenosis can lead to Budd-Chiari syndrome
Epidermolysis bullosa letalis with pyloric atresia	AR	GI symptoms may dominate the clinical picture; pyloric atresia, diarrhea, and protein-losing enteropathy	Bilateral pyelonephrosis due to stenosis at the uterovesical junctions; prenatal diagnosis by ultrasound, demonstrating dermal-epidermal separation at the lamina lucida in the fetal skin

(continued)

TABLE 108-1. *(Continued)*

CONDITION	INHERITANCE PATTERN	GASTROINTESTINAL MANIFESTATIONS	OTHER FEATURES AND COMMENTS
Vascular hyalinosis	AR	Diarrhea, rectal bleeding, malabsorption, protein-losing enteropathy	Progressive hyalinosis of the capillaries, arterioles and small veins of the GI tract, kidneys, and brain; poikiloderma and graying of the hair in the twenties
Hereditary lymphedema	AD	Loss of albumin through the intestines	Severe edema below the waist; onset at birth; paucity of lymph nodes above the inguinal ligaments; distinct from hereditary lymphedema II, which has onset at puberty
Defects in Fat Absorption			
Familial amyloidosis polyneuropathy type 1	AD	Abnormal GI motility with resultant bacterial overgrowth and malabsorption of bile acids; initial constipation followed by bouts of diarrhea	Progressive sensorimotor neuropathy beginning in the lower extremities; orthostatic hypotension, and impotence
Abetalipoproteinemia	AR	Steatorrhea with malabsorption of fat, poor weight gain, impaired absorption of fat-soluble vitamins	Beginning in the second decade: peripheral neuropathy, cerebellar ataxia, atypical retinitis pigmentosa, mild to moderate anemia, and acanthocytes; coagulopathy and low serum lipid values
Anderson's disease	AR	Steatorrhea with malabsorption of fat	Growth retardation; low serum lipid values
Familial hypobetalipoproteinemia	AD	Mild fat malabsorption	Low serum levels of low-density lipoprotein and high-density lipoproteins; normal triglycerides
Wolman's disease	AR	Intestinal malabsorption	Death usually in infancy; tissue accumulation of cholesterol esters and triglycerides in liver, adrenals, spleen, lymph nodes, bone marrow, small intestines, lungs, and thymus; prenatal diagnosis made by amniocytes demonstrating enzyme deficiency
Cholesterol ester storage disease	AR	Intestinal malabsorption	Similar to Wolman's disease, with later onset and milder symptoms
Wolman's disease with hypolipoproteinemia and acanthocytosis	AR	Intestinal malabsorption	Similar to Wolman's disease; also features hypolipoproteinemia and acanthocytosis
Storm's syndrome	AD	Fat malabsorption	Early, progressive, calcific cardiac valvular disease; loss of eyebrows and eyelashes; premature thinning and graying of hair; taut skin over hands and face
Groll-Hirschowitz syndrome	?AR	Diminished gastric motility due to a vagal nerve abnormality; multiple diverticula with jejunoileal ulceration; malabsorption of fat and intestinal loss of protein	Progressive sensory neuropathy; nerve deafness with onset in first three decades
Glucose-stimulated secretory diarrhea with common variable immunodeficiency	AD	Severe, watery diarrhea; malabsorption of fat, bile acids, vitamin B_{12} and xylose	Combined immunodeficiency syndrome; perfusion studies show glucose-stimulated secretion of water, sodium, and chloride in the jejunum and ileum, with normal transport for bicarbonate and mannitol

(continued)

TABLE 108-1.   *(Continued)*

CONDITION	INHERITANCE PATTERN	GASTROINTESTINAL MANIFESTATIONS	OTHER FEATURES AND COMMENTS
Exocrine Pancreas Abnormalities			
Cystic fibrosis	AR	Intestinal malabsorption, steatorrhea	Thickened secretions, respiratory infections; maps to chromosome 7
Shwachman-Bodian syndrome	AR	Steatorrhea, intestinal malabsorption	Incidence of 1 in 250,000 births; poor growth, recurrent respiratory infections, moderate dwarfism with dysplastic metaphyseal changes
Johanson-Blizzard syndrome	AR	Intestinal malabsorption	Aplasia or hypoplasia of the nasal alae, upswept frontal hair, widely spaced teeth, congenital deafness, hypothyroidism, postnatal growth retardation, mental retardation, midline ectodermal scalp defects, absent permanent teeth, and genitourinary and anorectal abnormalities; insulin-requiring diabetes in adulthood
Cartilage-hair hypoplasia (metaphyseal chondrodysplasia, McKusick type)	AR	Intestinal malabsorption, Hirschsprung's disease	Dwarfing syndrome with radiographic changes called metaphyseal dysostosis; fine, sparse, light-colored hair; anemia, susceptibility to chicken pox, and malignancies
Asphyxiating thoracic dystrophy (Jeune's syndrome)	AR	Intestinal malabsorption	Skeletal dysplasia with marked involvement of the rib cage causing asphyxia; polydactyly, chronic nephritis, cystic changes of liver, kidneys, and pancreas
Pearson's marrow-pancreas syndrome	mt	Intestinal malabsorption	Refractory anemia requiring transfusion; thrombocytopenia, neutropenia, and hepatic dysfunction
Lipase or colipase deficiency	AR	Steatorrhea with malabsorption of fat-soluble vitamins	Stature is within normal limits; responds to exogenous administration of lipase or colipase
Trypsinogen deficiency	AR	Diarrhea	Failure to thrive, edema, hypoproteinemia with normal sweat electrolytes, imperforate anus; gene mapped to 7q
Enterokinase deficiency	AR	Diarrhea	Similar to trypsinogen deficiency; favorable response with pancreatic enzyme replacement
Congenital pancreatic hypoplasia	AR	Diarrhea	Exocrine and endocrine insufficiency, intrauterine growth retardation, and early-onset insulin-dependent diabetes
Cystinosis	AR	Diarrhea	Intralysosomal storage of cystine, leading to pancreatic exocrine and endocrine insufficiency in long-term survivors; corneal deposits with photophobia and corneal erosions, ovarian failure, hypothyroidism, confusion, short-term memory loss, cerebral atrophy, Fanconi syndrome, and renal failure; myopathy and CNS involvement; prenatal diagnosis by studies of cystine uptake and retention by chorionic villi. Heterozygotes have six times the normal free cystine concentration.

(continued)

TABLE 108-1.   *(Continued)*

CONDITION	INHERITANCE PATTERN	GASTROINTESTINAL MANIFESTATIONS	OTHER FEATURES AND COMMENTS
Disorders of Vitamin and Mineral Assimilation			
Imerslund-Gräsbeck syndrome	AR	Malabsorption of vitamin B_{12} not corrected with exogenous intrinsic factor	Chronic, relapsing megaloblastic anemia; no antibodies to intrinsic factor or gastric parietal cells; proteinuria and malformations of the urinary tract
Folic acid transport defect	AR	Malabsorption of folic acid	Defect in transport of folic acid into CNS, causing seizures; mental retardation and movement disorder; megaloblastic anemia corrected by parenteral administration of folic acid
Pseudo–vitamin D deficiency	AR	Defective calcium absorption	Several subtypes; responds to large doses of vitamin D; rickets and short stature, myopathy, hypocalcemia, and hypophosphatemia; distinct from X-linked vitamin D–resistant rickets
Familial isolated deficiency of vitamin E	AR	No evidence of fat malabsorption; selective defect in vitamin E absorption	Ataxia, areflexia, loss of proprioception; increased serum lipids, xanthelasmata, and xanthomas of the Achilles tendon; neurologic symptoms may improve with administration of vitamin E. Heterozygotes may manifest tendinous xanthomata and elevated serum cholesterol levels.
Menkes' syndrome (kinky hair disease)	XLR	Defective intestinal copper absorption	Light-colored, kinky hair, growth retardation, severe neurologic impairment, metaphyseal changes, tortuosity of vessels, bladder diverticula; low serum copper and ceruloplasmin levels
X-linked cutis laxa (occipital horn syndrome)	XLR	Defective copper absorption	Occipital bony prominences; short, broad clavicles, fused carpal bones, hooked nose, long philtrum, multiple bladder diverticula, varicosities, inguinal hernias, joint laxity; low serum copper and ceruloplasmin levels
Hereditary iron-handling disorder	?AR	Selective iron malabsorption	Microcytic anemia unresponsive to oral iron therapy, partial response to intramuscular iron dextran
Acrodermatitis enteropathica	AR	Intermittent diarrhea due to zinc malabsorption	Bullous dermatitis, failure to thrive; alopecia of scalp, eyebrows, and eyelashes; thymic hypoplasia; improvement with zinc supplementation

AD, autosomal dominant; AR, autosomal recessive; CNS, central nervous system; mt, mitochondrial; NAD, nicotinamide adenine dinucleotide; U.S., United States; XLR, X-linked recessive.

Congenital Lactose Intolerance

Congenital lactose intolerance is distinct from congenital lactase deficiency. It is a more serious disorder and can be fatal unless diagnosed promptly. It is characterized by vomiting, failure to thrive, dehydration, renal tubular acidosis, disacchariduria, aminoaciduria, liver damage, cataracts, and brain damage. Intestinal lactase is present in normal amounts, and the disease phenotype is thought to be caused by the abnormal absorption of lactose. It was observed that the lactose absorption in this disorder occurs in the stomach rather than the duodenum.[14] Lactose may be toxic to the liver and brain, analogous to the toxicity of galactose-1-phosphate in galactosemia. Treatment consists of avoiding lactose. The disorder spontaneously resolves between 12 and 18 months of age. The inheritance pattern is thought to be autosomal dominant.

Sucrose-Isomaltose Malabsorption

Patients with the sucrose-isomaltose malabsorption disorder, also known as sucrase-α-dextrinase deficiency (see Chap. 73), can present with a wide variety of symptoms, from severe diarrhea in infancy to occasional stomach upset in adults.[7,15] The disorder affects 0.2% of North Americans and 10% of Greenland Eskimos. Symptoms are similar to those of lactase deficiency, except that they are evoked by table sugar and not by milk. Starch is well tolerated. Symptoms begin with the ingestion of sweetened foods and fruits. The diagnosis is made using the same techniques as used in lactase deficiency. Tolerance to the offending sugars increases with age. Ingesting live yeast, preferably on a full stomach, can ameliorate the symptoms after sucrose ingestion. Fresh bakers' yeast has sucrase activity.

Attempts to elucidate the nature of the defect have shown that the isomaltase part of the sucrase-isomaltase complex is labile in the absence of sucrase, suggesting that the primary defect is in the sucrase, with secondary effects on isomaltase. Several investigators have demonstrated a defect in intracellular processing of the enzyme.[16,17] Three abnormalities have been described: the enzyme accumulates in the endoplasmic reticulum, the transport of the enzyme complex is blocked in the Golgi, and a catalytically altered enzyme is transported to the cell surface.[18] These findings illustrate the heterogeneity of even a relatively uncommon, single-gene disorder.

The disease is inherited as an autosomal recessive trait. In general, homozygotes have severe enzyme deficiency with symptoms throughout life, but heterozygotes have intermediate enzymatic activity with no symptoms in adulthood but may have mild symptoms as infants. The sucrase-isomaltase gene has been localized to chromosome 3q, and linkage to chromosome 3q has been demonstrated in families with sucrase-isomaltase deficiency, indicating the sucrase-isomaltase gene is the disease gene.[19,20]

Glucose-Galactose Malabsorption

Intestinal monosaccharide transport deficiency presents clinically indistinguishably from intestinal disaccharidase deficiency.[7] In glucose-galactose malabsorption, diarrhea and dehydration occur after ingestion of almost any carbohydrate, because virtually all contain at least one of these sugars. The diagnosis is suggested by examination of stools, which are acidic and contain glucose and galactose. It can be differentiated from disaccharidase deficiency because there is no significant rise in plasma glucose in the course of a glucose-galactose oral tolerance test. Patients who have been carefully evaluated have also been found to have a mild defect in renal tubular reabsorption of glucose; they excrete 250 to 1000 mg/dL glucose in the urine. Treatment consists of substituting fructose for other carbohydrates in the diet.

The underlying abnormality is in the transport mechanism in the small intestine; the mucosa is unable to take up glucose and galactose. As with sucrase-isomaltase deficiency, tolerance to the offending sugars improves with age. The inheritance is autosomal recessive. The glucose-galactose transporter gene (SGLT1) has been mapped to chromosome 22.[21] Turk and colleagues identified a point mutation in the SGLT1 gene and established that this protein may be primarily responsible for the glucose and galactose transport defect.[22]

Trehalase Deficiency

Trehalase deficiency is rare in Caucasian Americans but is found in 10% to 15% of Greenland Eskimos.[23] The symptoms include diarrhea and vomiting after ingestion of trehalose-containing foods. Trehalose is a disaccharide found in insects and mushrooms.

Defects in Amino Acid Transport

Proteins are normally absorbed by two major mechanisms. One involves transport of liberated free amino acids by group-specific sodium-dependent amino acid transport systems, and the other involves uptake of unhydrolyzed peptides by means independent of the specific entry mechanisms. There are at least three major group-specific active transport systems: monoamino monocarboxylic (neutral) amino acids; dibasic amino acids and cystine; and dicarboxylic (acidic) amino acids. The genetic disorders of amino acid absorption involve deficiencies in one or more of these transport mechanisms.[24]

Iminoglycinuria

Iminoglycinuria consists of five subtypes. All are benign inborn errors of imino acid (i.e., proline and hydroxyproline) and glycine absorption in the kidneys, and two of the subtypes also involve the intestine.[25] In most cases, iminoglycinuria has been discovered during investigations carried out for other purposes. The diversity of clinical abnormalities in probands with familial iminoglycinuria suggests that there is probably no direct relation between the inherited disorder and the accompanying illness, and no treatment is necessary.

When any of the three amino acids is given orally, excretion of the other two increases, indicating a group-specific membrane transport defect. Heterogeneity in the disorder is suggested by several lines of evidence, including the fact that some homozygotes show no proline transport defect. Obligate heterozygotes may be hyperglycinuric or not. At least four alleles for the disorder are known, but it is not known whether they are all at the same locus. The condition is inherited in an autosomal recessive pattern and occurs most often in Ashkenazi Jews. The frequency of affected persons among Caucasians is about 1 in 15,000, giving a heterozygote frequency of about 2%.

The existence of an autosomal dominant form of glycinuria with oxalate urolithiasis has been postulated. This type of disorder occurs more often in Ashkenazi Jews than in other groups, and it is probably a particular heterozygote form of iminoglycinuria that predisposes some persons to urolithiasis.

Hartnup's Disease

Hartnup's disease is a rare disorder with an incidence of 5 cases per 100,000 members of the population, as observed in a Massachusetts urine screening program. The disorder produces virtually no symptoms or signs in more than 90% of affected persons. In those with symptoms, the onset occurs in childhood with an intermittent, red, scaly, pellagra-like rash after sun exposure and attacks of cerebellar ataxia, sometimes accompanied by psychiatric disorders. Some persons have low-normal or subnormal intelligence.

The single constant feature and the only diagnostic test is massive aminoaciduria involving a group of neutral and aromatic monoamino monocarboxylic amino acids that share a common renal reabsorption mechanism in the proximal tubule.[26] Patients also have diminished capacity for jejunal absorption of these amino acids because of a transport defect at the brush border. This results in the retention of the amino acids in the intestine for abnormally long periods, allowing intestinal bacteria to convert them into dipeptide decomposition products, some of which are absorbed. A subgroup of patients with Hartnup's disease has been identified in whom intestinal absorption is normal and the patients are clinically normal. There is inadequate nicotinamide synthesis because of diminished tryptophan absorption, causing pellagra. The formation of decomposition products that are toxic to the central nervous system, coupled to pellagra, produces the cerebellar and psychiatric manifestations. A general nutritional deficiency results from the diminished availability of essential amino acids. Patients are treated by the administration of nicotinamide.

Although the disorder is autosomal recessive, the fact that only a small group of patients have the typical manifestations has prompted the theory that other genes may affect the clinical outcome.[27]

Cystinuria

Cystinuria is an autosomal recessive disorder characterized by cystine, lysine, ornithine, and arginine transport abnormalities in the renal tubule and intestinal epithelium.[28] The clinical manifestations are confined to nephrolithiasis resulting from the insolubility of cystine in the urine.

Three types of cystinuria have been recognized. Urinary stones form in all three types, and investigation of the stones leads to the diagnosis. The stones are radiopaque and are present as hexagonal cystine crystals in the urine. Treatment is directed at reducing the concentration of cystine in urine by increasing urine volume, increasing solubility by alkalinization, and as a last alternative, reducing free cystine excretion by administration of D-penicillamine.

Classification of the three types of cystinuria has been accomplished by evaluating the excretion rates of amino acids in obligate heterozygotes. In type I, heterozygotes excrete no excess amino acids. Excretion of as much as twice the normal amount characterizes type III heterozygotes, and type II is assigned to those heterozygotes who excrete 9 to 15 times the normal amount, which is still less than the amount necessary for the formation of stones.

Although cystinuria is a relatively rare disease in most populations, it is thought to have an incidence of 1 in 2500 among Israeli Jews of Libyan origin. The incidence in the United States, based on the screening of newborns, is 1 in 15,000. The second and third decades of life are the peak times for expression of the disorder. It affects male patients more severely than it does females, although the disorder occurs equally in both sexes.

Lysinuric Protein Intolerance

Lysinuric protein intolerance, also known as dibasic aminoaciduria II, is characterized by abnormal transport of dibasic amino acids across the basolateral membranes of intestinal and renal tubular cells.[29] Its onset is in infancy, when cow's milk or cow's milk formula is introduced. It is associated with vomiting, diarrhea, failure to thrive, severe growth retardation, hepatosplenomegaly, and mental retardation. Lens opacities are common, the skin may be elastic, and the joints may be hyperextensible. The hair of many patients is sparse and brittle. Affected infants show a markedly diminished rise in plasma levels of arginine, lysine, and ornithine after an oral protein load, indicating malabsorption of these amino acids. In addition, reduced tubular reabsorption of these same amino acids occurs in the kidney. Analysis of plasma amino acids indicates subnormal levels of arginine, lysine, ornithine, leucine, and tyrosine. Serine and citrulline levels are normal, and glutamine and alanine levels may be markedly increased. Lysinuria occurs.

The diagnosis is based on the finding of dibasic aminoaciduria without cystinuria, impaired intestinal absorption of basic amino acids, and protein intolerance. Hyperammonemia is the result of deficient hepatic uptake of the amino acids, which produces a deficiency of some intermediate products of the urea cycle. Treatment consists of protein restriction with citrulline and lysine supplements. Some of the abnormalities resolve on this therapy.

The disorder is autosomal recessive, and consanguinity is common. Some heterozygotes manifest partial intestinal malabsorption after an oral protein load. Affected male siblings, 32 and 36 years of age, presented in adult life with hyperammonemic coma due to lysinuric protein intolerance. They were presumably homozygotes, but they had normal intellect and were in good health because of an unconscious, self-imposed avoidance of dietary protein.[30]

Blue Diaper Syndrome

Blue diaper syndrome is a rare, probably autosomal recessive disorder of tryptophan malabsorption.[24] Unlike the previously described abnormalities, the kidney is apparently unaffected. The unabsorbed tryptophan is converted to indoles in the intestine by bacteria. The indoles are absorbed and converted in the liver to indican, which, when oxidized, becomes indigo blue in the urine. Infants present with failure to thrive, recurrent fever, infections, irritability, and constipation in addition to the bluish discoloration of the diapers. Hypercalcemia and nephrocalcinosis also occur because of increased absorption of calcium. Included in the differential diagnosis is the blue-green discoloration that can occur from a pigment elaborated by *Pseudomonas aeruginosa*.[31]

Oasthouse Disease

Oasthouse syndrome is an autosomal recessive condition of methionine absorption, so named because affected patients excrete urine containing α-hydroxybutyric acid, a product of bacterial metabolism of methionine that has the odor of an oast house, a kiln for drying hops.[24] The clinical features include white hair, hyperpnea, convulsions, diarrhea, and mental retardation. A methionine-free diet improves the symptoms.

Disorders of Electrolyte Absorption

There are four well-described genetic causes of electrolyte and water malabsorption in the intestine: microvillus inclusion disease, congenital chloride diarrhea, congenital sodium diarrhea, and disorders of aldosterone metabolism causing significant salt wasting.[32]

Microvillus Inclusion Disease

Microvillus inclusion disease is an autosomal recessive disorder involving the brush border membrane that results in severe congenital fluid and electrolyte malabsorption. This disorder may represent the most common cause of severe refractory diarrhea in the newborn period.[33] Unlike sodium and chloride diarrheas, polyhydramnios is not seen prenatally. Microvillus inclusion disease may result from defective brush border assembly and differentiation or from an error of intracellular transport. Localization of the cytoplasmic inclusions to the microvillus membrane in villus cells is revealed by electron microscope examination.[33–35] Rectal biopsy was proposed as a dependable and easy method for early diagnosis. Therapies such as octreotide, clonidine, and epidermal growth factor have had limited success. It has been suggested that the only therapy to reduce fluid losses may be enterectomy.[36] Survival is unusual after 2 years of age. Small bowel transplantation may become the best available treatment (see Chap. 73).

Congenital Chloride Diarrhea

Congenital chloride diarrhea is an autosomal recessive disorder that may present in utero with polyhydramnios, presumably because of diarrhea. The infant may be born prematurely with a distended abdomen. Voluminous, watery stools containing large amounts of chloride are produced, leading to hypochloridemia, hypokalemia, and metabolic alkalosis.[37] With later presentation or with inadequate replacement therapy, weight and height gains are affected. Adult manifestations of this disease have been described in a 31-year-old man. He had had watery diarrhea since birth. He had required 18 hospital admissions for dehydration and electrolyte abnormalities. As an adult, additional, unexplained features included glucose intolerance, gout, proteinuria, and mild renal function impairment.[38] These features may or may not have been attributable to his underlying disorder of chloride malabsorption.

The diagnosis is made by measuring the chloride content of the stools and by the characteristic serum electrolyte changes. Treatment consists of administering prostaglandin inhibitors (primarily indomethacin) and potassium chloride. The secretory diarrhea in this condition results from a deficiency in intestinal brush border chloride-bicarbonate exchange (see Chap. 73).

Congenital Sodium Diarrhea

Congenital sodium diarrhea presents similarly to congenital chloride diarrhea with polyhydramnios, premature birth, and voluminous, watery stools in the first days of life. The diagnosis is based on stool electrolyte measurement, which reveals excess sodium and bicarbonate. Treatment consists of replacement of sodium and bicarbonate. Perfusion studies show that the jejunum is in a net secretory state, with intact hexose transport but with abnormal intestinal sodium-hydrogen exchange activity. The inheritance pattern is probably autosomal recessive.

Intestinal Defects in Protein Absorption

There are many genetic syndromes that feature selective protein malabsorption. Most of these involve abnormalities of the intestinal lymphatic system and include intestinal lymphangiectasia, protein-losing enteropathy, and vascular hyalinosis. A rare association of protein-losing enteropathy with neurofibromatosis has been described.[39] This patient had massive protein loss from a localized segment of small intestine with possible neurofibromatosis involvement of the mesenteric vessels. Table 108-1 lists additional disorders.

Intestinal Defects in Lipid Absorption

There are several important genetic disorders that may present in adulthood that have lipid malabsorption as a clinical manifestation. Many are caused by inborn errors of apolipoprotein or lipid metabolism. Familial amyloidosis polyneuropathy is also an important disorder with onset in adulthood that may present with lipid malabsorption. The clinical features common to most of these syndromes are caused by the deficiency of fat-soluble vitamins. Neurologic symptoms may be present because of a deficiency of vitamin E, and a coagulopathy may be caused by vitamin K deficiency.

Familial Amyloidosis Polyneuropathy

The amyloid protein in familial amyloidosis polyneuropathy type 1 is composed of abnormal transthyretin molecules; transthyretin is a plasma protein that transports thyroid- and retinol-binding proteins. Systemic deposition of this abnormal protein causes a progressive sensorimotor neuropathy that begins in the lower limbs. The autonomic nervous system may also be involved, causing orthostatic hypotension, impotence, and abnormal GI motility. There is initial constipation followed by bouts of diarrhea. Malabsorption of bile acids is common and appears to be the result of GI motility dysfunction from the autonomic neuropathy, with resultant bacterial overgrowth, rather than from the amyloid deposits in the intestinal mucosa.[40]

This is an autosomal dominant trait that can be presymptomatically diagnosed with a restriction enzyme that recognizes the mutation site in the transthyretin gene on chromosome 18.[41]

Abetalipoproteinemia

The principal GI symptom of abetalipoproteinemia is malabsorption of fat, often beginning in infancy with steatorrhea and poor weight gain. The disorder is often misdiagnosed as celiac disease. Impaired absorption of fat-soluble vitamins is responsible for many of the clinical features. Histopathologic analysis of the small bowel shows normally formed villi with lipid-engorged enterocytes. Treatment consists of avoidance of fat and the administration of fat-soluble vitamins.

The neurologic symptoms usually begin in the second decade and include peripheral neuropathy and cerebellar ataxia. Patients also complain of decreased night vision and color vision, caused by an atypical retinitis pigmentosa. There is a mild to moderate anemia, usually with hemolysis. Most circulating red cells are acanthocytes. There may be an iron or folate deficiency because of malabsorption. There is usually a coagulopathy due to decreased vitamin K stores. The total cholesterol values are in the range of 20 to 50 mg/dL, and triglyceride values are also very low, with little postprandial increase. There are no chylomicrons, very-low-density lipoproteins, low-density lipoproteins, or apolipoprotein B particles, the major structural apolipoprotein for these lipids.[42]

Abetalipoproteinemia is an autosomal recessive disorder. Heterozygotes have no symptoms and have normal plasma lipids. The genetic defect does not involve the apolipoprotein B gene itself. There seems to be a defect in the ability of the liver and intestines to assemble or secrete apolipoprotein B. Patients with abetalipoproteinemia lack a microsomal triglyceride transfer protein that mediates the intracellular transport of membrane-associated lipids.[43]

Anderson's Disease

Patients with Anderson's disease have malabsorption of fat with steatorrhea and growth retardation, but acanthocytosis and the neuroocular symptoms of abetalipoproteinemia are lacking. Low-density lipoprotein particles are present in the plasma, but there is a failure of chylomicron formation. Enterocytes from intestinal biopsies show numerous fat droplets, and monoclonal antibody staining reveals the presence of apolipoprotein B48, the form produced by the intestine. Defective glycosylation of apolipoprotein B48 has been observed, which may underlie the absence of formation and secretion of chylomicrons.[44] Anderson's disease is not linked to the apolipoprotein B gene locus.[45]

Familial Hypobetalipoproteinemia

Several investigators have described familial cases of hypobetalipoproteinemia due to truncated versions of the normal apolipoprotein B100 molecule. For example, Steinberg and colleagues described a family with a truncated apolipoprotein B, called apolipoprotein B37.[46] These individuals have low levels of low-density lipoproteins, normal amounts of triglycerides, low levels of high-density lipoproteins, mild fat malabsorption, and a defect in chylomicron clearance. There were no reports of neuroocular abnormalities.

Wolman's Disease and Cholesterol Ester Storage Disease

Wolman's disease is a severe congenital disorder, with death usually occurring in infancy. Cholesterol esters and triglycerides accumulate in the liver, adrenal, spleen, lymph nodes, bone marrow, small intestine, lungs, and thymus because of lysosomal acid lipase deficiency. Death is thought to be the result of intestinal malabsorption.[47]

Cholesterol ester storage disease is a later-onset disorder with milder manifestations. It also involves lysosomal acid lipase deficiency and may be allelic with Wolman's disease.

Prenatal diagnosis has been performed by demonstration of deficient enzyme activity in cultured amniocytes.[48] The lysosomal acid lipase gene has been mapped to chromosome 10.[49]

Exocrine Pancreas Abnormalities

Defects in protein and fat absorption are more commonly caused by abnormalities of the exocrine pancreas. Examples include deficiencies of specific pancreatic exocrine enzymes, cystic fibrosis, the Shwachman-Bodian syndrome, and the Johanson-Blizzard syndrome. Table 108-1 has a list of genetic syndromes manifesting with exocrine pancreas insufficiency.

Cystic Fibrosis

Cystic fibrosis (CF) is the most common lethal autosomal recessive disorder in the Caucasian population, occurring with a frequency of about 1 in 2500 births. The disorder is characterized by viscous secretions and dysfunction of multiple exocrine glands, leading to pancreatic insufficiency, malabsorption, chronic pulmonary infection with emphysema, and a high chloride concentration in sweat (see Chap. 94).[50]

The GI manifestations of CF are reviewed here. Because of the life-threatening nature of the pulmonary complications of CF, less emphasis is paid to the GI complications. However, their importance is underscored by the fact that CF is the leading cause of malabsorption in children. More than one third of patients with CF survive to adulthood and develop many of the GI complications with time.[51-54]

Almost 90% of patients with CF have pancreatic insufficiency leading to achylia. Most are born with insufficiency and require enzyme replacement therapy by their first birthdays. Because the pancreatic secretions are abnormal, the pancreatic ducts become plugged, leading to destruction of distal ducts. Proximal to these clogged ducts, autodigestion and inflammation lead to fibrosis and ultimately to exocrine insufficiency. The result is malabsorption, primarily of fats, which causes malnutrition; susceptibility to hemorrhage due to lack of vitamin K, tetany due to hypocalcemia from losses in the stool, and neurologic problems due to vitamin E deficiency. Treatment consists of pancreatic enzyme replacement. Untreated patients may absorb an excess of iron and develop hemosiderosis of the liver. The patients are also at risk of developing vitamin B_{12} deficiency. The islets of Langerhans may become secondarily affected by fibrosis of the pancreas, leading to glucose intolerance or clinical diabetes that is similar to noninsulin-dependent diabetes in approximately 50% of patients with CF.

Approximately 25% to 30% of CF patients develop focal biliary cirrhosis. In 2% to 5% of these, multilobular biliary cirrhosis with portal hypertension may develop. Thick secretions plug the bile ducts, leading to inflammation and fibrosis. There usually is a history of pancreatic insufficiency in these cases.[55]

The earliest clinical manifestation of CF is often meconium ileus, occurring in approximately 10% to 15% of patients.

This is thought to be caused by the lack of fluid in the small intestine because of a lack of pancreatic secretion or defective intestinal epithelial secretion. Gastrografin enema or oral N-acetylcysteine may resolve the obstruction; if not, surgery is necessary. A similar abnormality occurring later in life, called the distal intestinal obstruction syndrome, may occur in 10% to 20% of CF patients, causing symptoms of colicky pain and constipation.[55] These symptoms may be relieved with Golytely, mineral oil, an increase in pancreatic enzymes or N-acetylcysteine. Rectal prolapse occurs in approximately one fourth of patients before 2 years of age, but it usually does not occur in patients receiving pancreatic enzyme replacement therapy. The mechanism for the prolapse is unknown.[53]

The gene responsible for CF has been localized to chromosome 7q using reverse genetics techniques.[56] The putative protein for the CF gene has been called the cystic fibrosis transmembrane regulator (*CFTR*), and it has been demonstrated that the CFTR product forms a cAMP-regulated chloride channel.[57] More than 100 mutations have been described in CF, and all the known CF mutations combined account for approximately 85% of all mutant chromosomes.[58] The most common mutation is δF508, a deletion of the amino acid residue phenylalanine at codon 508, occurring in 70% of CF patients. The F508 deletion is located near an apparent binding site for ATP, and it may interfere with the phosphorylation of the CF protein or with some other need for energy provided by ATP. Most of the non-δF508 mutations are relatively rare, affecting less than 1% to 10% of CF patients.[59] Some *CFTR* genotypes are associated with pancreatic sufficiency or insufficiency, suggesting that the genotype at the *CFTR* locus is responsible for susceptibility to pancreatic insufficiency. δF508 and the common Ashkenazi Jewish mutation, W1282X, are examples of pancreatic insufficiency alleles.[60]

Shwachman-Bodian Syndrome

The Shwachman-Bodian syndrome, also called congenital lipomatosis of the pancreas, is the second most frequent pancreatic cause of malabsorption in childhood, with an incidence of 1 in 250,000 births. Symptoms include poor growth, intestinal malabsorption, steatorrhea, and recurrent respiratory infections. Dysplastic changes in the metaphyses of long bones lead to a moderate dwarfism. Patients may suffer from a pancytopenia and are at risk for hematologic malignancies. The pancreatic enzyme replacement required in infancy may not be necessary later.[61] The inheritance pattern is autosomal recessive.

Johanson-Blizzard Syndrome

In addition to pancreatic insufficiency causing malabsorption, Johanson-Blizzard syndrome features aplasia or hypoplasia of the nasal alae, upswept frontal hair, widely spaced teeth, congenital deafness, hypothyroidism, postnatal growth retardation, mental retardation, midline ectodermal scalp defects, and absent permanent teeth. Genitourinary and anorectal abnormalities have also been described. Autopsy findings have shown almost complete replacement of the pancreas with fat and a paucity of islet cells. Death usually occurs in childhood from malabsorption-related complications. Survival to adult-

hood is rare but possible if continuous enzyme replacement is instituted. Insulin-requiring diabetes is a feature in adulthood, similar to the situation for CF patients, presumably because of the loss of beta cells.[61] The inheritance pattern is autosomal recessive.

Cartilage-Hair Hypoplasia

Cartilage-hair hypoplasia (i.e., metaphyseal chondrodysplasia, McKusick type) is a dwarfing syndrome with radiologic changes called metaphyseal dysostosis. The clinical features include fine, sparse, light-colored hair, anemia, malabsorption due to pancreatic insufficiency, Hirschsprung's disease, and a susceptibility to chicken pox. Malignancies may be more frequent in patients with this disorder.[62]

Asphyxiating Thoracic Dystrophy

Asphyxiating thoracic dystrophy, also called Jeune syndrome, is a skeletal dysplasia that usually has a fatal outcome in the newborn period because involvement of the rib cage causes asphyxia. Milder cases allow survival to adulthood. In addition to short stature, other features include polydactyly, chronic nephritis, and malabsorption because of pancreatic insufficiency.[63] Cystic changes occur in the kidney, liver, and pancreas. This syndrome shares clinical features seen in two other genetic syndromes, Ellis–van Creveld and renal-hepatic-pancreatic dysplasia. It may be that these syndromes form part of a disease spectrum rather than being distinct disorders.[64]

Disorders of Vitamin and Mineral Assimilation

Imerslund-Gräsbeck Syndrome

Imerslund-Gräsbeck syndrome is a disorder of chronic relapsing megaloblastic anemia due to malabsorption of vitamin B_{12}, which is not corrected with exogenous intrinsic factor. No antibodies to intrinsic factor or gastric parietal cells are detected. The defect appears to be located between the attachment of B_{12} to the surface of the ileal cell and the binding to transcobalamin II. In some cases, the defect is a selective failure of intrinsic factor secretion; in others, it may be the absence of an ileal receptor; and in others, the defect is unknown. Associated features include proteinuria and malformations of the urinary tract. This syndrome should be differentiated from intrinsic factor deficiency and transcobalamin II deficiency.[65,66]

Menkes' Syndrome

Menkes' syndrome, also called kinky hair disease, is an X-linked recessive disorder of copper metabolism, caused by a defect in the intestinal absorption of copper.[67] This affects many of the copper-dependent enzymes in the body, producing a particular phenotype. The characteristic features of this disorder include light-colored, kinky hair, growth retardation, severe neurologic impairment with focal cerebral and cerebellar degeneration, changes in the metaphyses of the long bones, tortuosity of vessels, and bladder diverticula. Most patients die between 6 months and 3 years of age. Milder cases, presumably allelic forms of the disease, have survived to adolescence. Low serum copper levels in the appropriate clinical setting is a simple and reliable diagnostic method. Heterozygotes may be detected by the finding of pili torti (i.e., kinky hair). The gene for Menkes' syndrome has been mapped to the long arm of the X chromosome.[68]

X-Linked Cutis Laxa

X-linked cutis laxa, also called occipital horn syndrome, may be an allelic variant of Menkes' syndrome. The disorder is characterized by occipital bony prominences called occipital horns and by short broad clavicles, fused carpal bones, a hooked nose and long philtrum, multiple large diverticula of the bladder, varicosities, inguinal hernias, joint laxity, and diarrhea. Serum levels of copper and ceruloplasmin are low, similar to the findings in patients with Menkes' syndrome.[69]

Acrodermatitis Enteropathica

Acrodermatitis enteropathica is an autosomal recessive disorder of zinc malabsorption. It is characterized by intermittent diarrhea and dermatitis and a failure to thrive. Additional features include alopecia of the scalp, eyebrows, and eyelashes. The findings at autopsy include islet cell hyperplasia, absence of the thymus, and absence of germinal centers with plasmacytosis of the lymph nodes and spleen. The laboratory findings include low serum levels of zinc and alkaline phosphatase (i.e., a zinc metalloenzyme) and diminished urinary zinc excretion. Oral zinc therapy has been successful in ameliorating symptoms.[70] This disorder is usually diagnosed by low serum zinc levels; however, variant cases with normal serum levels have been described. Ultrastructural abnormalities of the Paneth's cells of the small intestine (i.e., cells that usually contain high concentrations of zinc) or a trial of oral zinc supplementation with good clinical response may provide evidence for the diagnosis in these variant cases.[71]

CHRONIC DIARRHEA SYNDROMES NOT CHARACTERIZED BY MALABSORPTION

There are several genetic disorders featuring chronic, recurrent diarrhea that are not associated with a specific malabsorption syndrome. Many of the inherited immunodeficiency disorders involving T-cell antigens, T-cell antigen receptors, B cells, and immunoglobulin and complement deficiencies are characterized by a chronic diarrhea. Inherited colitis syndromes, neurologic disorders, and endocrinopathies may also feature chronic or recurrent diarrhea as a common manifestation. Many of the polyposis syndromes may present with complaints of chronic diarrhea. Table 108-2 reviews the disorders that may be more commonly encountered by the clinician.

RECURRENT GASTROINTESTINAL BLEEDING SYNDROMES

In the evaluation of recurrent acute or occult GI hemorrhage, a variety of genetic disorders should be considered (Table 108-3). These include disorders of structural abnormalities, such as the polyposis syndromes (e.g., Peutz-Jeghers syndrome, Gardner's syndrome); vascular abnormalities, such as those that occur in vascular malformation syndromes and connective tissue disorders (e.g., Osler-Weber-Rendu syndrome, Ehlers-Danlos syndrome); and disorders of the hematologic system that may involve platelets, clotting factors, or abnormalities in fibrinolysis. The polyposis syndromes are reviewed in Chapters 49 and 86.

Many of the structural and vascular abnormality syndromes that cause GI bleeding belong to a group of disorders called the phakomatoses, including neurofibromatosis, basal cell nevus syndrome, Gardner's syndrome, Klippel-Trenaunay-Weber syndrome, Osler-Weber-Rendu syndrome, and Peutz-Jeghers syndrome. *Phakos* means spots, and these disorders are characterized by their spotty or patchy lesions. Other common features include a major vascular component to some lesions, involvement of the skin and central nervous system, and an autosomal dominant inheritance pattern with a high mutation rate.[72] Occasionally, two of these disorders occur in the same person, which is probably more than a coincidence. One possible explanation is that these lesions have a common embryologic origin and are derived from abnormal neural crest development.[73]

There are many genetic hematologic disorders that predispose the patient to GI bleeding. Deficiencies of the clotting factors may result in a bleeding diathesis. Von Willebrand's disease and combined deficiency of factor VII and VIII are autosomal dominant disorders that may present with recurrent GI bleeding.[4] The most common factor deficiency is factor VIII deficiency, better known as hemophilia A, an X-linked condition occurring with a frequency of 1 in 10,000.[74] This disorder usually presents with hemarthroses that result in a chronic arthropathy, deep muscle hematomas, frank hematuria, and spontaneous intracranial bleeds. GI bleeding is not a common complication.

Abnormalities in fibrinolysis may also predispose affected individuals to bleeding. Deficiencies of the anti-clotting factors, protein C, protein S, and antithrombin III, can cause portal vein thrombosis, which can be complicated by ruptured esophageal varices.[75]

There are several genetic disorders relating to platelet number or function. Glanzmann's thrombasthenia (i.e., platelet glycoprotein IIb-IIIa deficiency) is an autosomal recessive bleeding diathesis with deficient clot retraction and abnormal platelet morphology. Mucosal bleeding is typical and gingival bleeding, epistaxis, and laryngeal bleeding are common features.[76] There is an autosomal dominant form of Glanzmann's thrombasthenia with similar features. Bernard-Soulier's syndrome (i.e., platelet glycoprotein Ib deficiency) is an autosomal recessive bleeding disorder characterized by unusually large platelets and a prolonged bleeding time. The platelet membrane is abnormal and lacks a receptor, glycoprotein Ib, involved in the adhesion of platelets to subendothelium and von Willebrand's factor; patients are susceptible to mucosal bleeding.[77] Thromboxane synthase deficiency, leading to platelet aggregation abnormalities, is inherited as an autosomal recessive trait and may present with petechiae, bruising, epistaxis, hematuria, or massive GI bleeding. The Hermansky-Pudlak syndrome is also characterized by abnormal platelets and is discussed in a later section of this chapter.

TABLE 108-2
Diarrhea Syndromes

CONDITION	INHERITANCE PATTERN	GASTROINTESTINAL MANIFESTATIONS	OTHER FEATURES AND COMMENTS
Immunodeficiency Syndromes			
T3 T-cell antigen deficiency	AD	Nonspecific malabsorption	
T-cell antigen receptor deficiency, zeta subunit	AD	Anorexia, diarrhea; small bowel shows absence of villi	Failure to thrive, pneumonia
Bare lymphocyte syndrome (BLS)	AR	Severe, persistent diarrhea	A member of the severe combined immunodeficiency syndromes (SCID); mucocutaneous candidiasis, interstitial pneumonitis, and bacterial infections. In BLS type 1, the defect is the lack of HLA class I molecules. In type 2, there is a lack of HLA class I and II molecules. BLS maps to chromosome 19p and seems to involve defects that affect gene expression.
Agammaglobulinemia, Swiss type, X-linked severe combined immunodeficiency disease	XLR	Chronic diarrhea	Susceptibility to infections, thymic hypoplasia, and severe thrush
IgA and IgG2 deficiency	AD	Nonspecific malabsorption	Infections, atopy, autoimmune disorders; association with HLA-B8; stronger association with neutral amino acids at the 57 position of HLA-DQ beta chain
Kappa light chain deficiency	AD	Diarrhea	Recurrent respiratory infections
Deficiency of complement component 5	AD	Intractable diarrhea	General seborrheic dermatitis, recurrent local and systemic infections (gram negative), and marked wasting
Wiskott-Aldrich syndrome	XLR	Bloody diarrhea	Eczema, thrombocytopenia, susceptibility to infections; death by age 10; lymphoreticular malignancies. Therapy consists of bone marrow transplant. Carriers have a defect in platelet oxidative phosphorylation. Frequency is 4 per million male births; prenatal diagnosis possible with closely linked DNA markers
Hereditary mucoepithelial dysplasia	AD	Diarrhea in infancy; esophageal stenosis or webs	Periorofacial flat, red mucosal lesions, follicular keratosis, photophobia, and nystagmus in infancy; keratitis, pannus, and cataracts; fibrocystic lung disease and cor pulmonale in adulthood; nonscarring alopecia; vaginal, oral, or urinary PAP smears show large immature cells containing vacuoles and strand-shaped inclusions. Mild mucocutaneous candidiasis, increased susceptibility to bacterial infection, possibly hypoadrenocorticism
Colitis Syndromes			
Lethal cutaneous photosensitivity and colitis	AR	Severe colitis, refractory diarrhea	Early cutaneous photosensitivity; skin lesions are erythematous and vesicular
Enterocolitis	AR	Bloody diarrhea	Death within a few weeks
Hermansky-Pudlak syndrome	AR	Inflammatory bowel disease, usually in Puerto Ricans	Oculocutaneous albinism with bleeding tendency, restrictive lung disease,

(continued)

TABLE 108-2. *(Continued)*

CONDITION	INHERITANCE PATTERN	GASTROINTESTINAL MANIFESTATIONS	OTHER FEATURES AND COMMENTS
			pigmented reticular cells, defect in platelet ADP release, causing prolonged bleeding time and defective platelet aggregation
Neuropathy Syndromes			
Charcot-Marie-Tooth disease	AD, AR, or XLR	Chronic diarrhea, nausea and vomiting	Begins with a motor and sensory neuropathy involving the distribution of the peroneal nerve; loss of reflexes and trophic changes may occur; pes cavus is common; linkage to chromosome 1, 17 and X established (genetic heterogeneity)
Fatal neonatal radiculoneuropathy	AR	Chronic diarrhea	Prenatal polyhydramnios, floppy infant, distal muscle weakness, areflexia, opisthotonic posturing, autonomic instability
Endocrinopathy Syndromes			
Multiple endocrine neoplasia type 1	AD	Severe peptic ulcer disease and chronic diarrhea secondary to gastrinomas	Pituitary, parathyroid, and pancreatic adenomas; bronchial and duodenal carcinoid; malignant schwannomas
Polyglandular autoimmune syndrome type 1	AR	Diarrhea	Triad of Addison's disease, hypoparathyroidism, and chronic mucocutaneous candidiasis; frequently associated with chronic active hepatitis, pernicious anemia and primary hypogonadism; IDDM and thyroid disease are infrequent; no HLA association
IDDM–secretory diarrhea syndrome	XLR	Severe secretory diarrhea	Newborn presentation of brittle IDDM; death in infancy from septicemia, malnutrition, and poor diabetes control
X-linked diarrhea, polyendocrinopathy, fatal infection syndrome	?XLR	Intractable diarrhea	Eczema, hemolytic anemia, diabetes or thyroid autoimmunity, increased susceptibility to viral infections
Miscellaneous Syndromes			
Systemic infantile hyalinosis	AR	Diarrhea in infancy	Early thickening and focal nodularity of the skin, causing reduced mobility and joint contractures; gum hypertrophy and osteoporosis, failure to thrive, and recurrent infections. Histopathology shows deposits of hyaline in the skin, muscle, GI tract, and endocrine glands.
Rapadilino's syndrome	AR	Diarrhea	Radial and patellar aplasia or hypoplasia, absence of thumbs, dislocation of joints, long face with narrow palpebral fissures, long slender nose, small chin, unusual ears, cleft or high-arched palate, small stature, normal intelligence
Hyperphosphatemia, polyuria, and seizures	?AR	Vomiting, diarrhea due to hyperphosphatemia	Seizures, intermittent polyuria and hyperphosphatemia occurring together or separately; irritability, anorexia, high-pitched cry, carpopedal spasm, and overt tetany secondary to hyperphosphatemia
Dutch-type periodic fever	AR	Diarrhea during attacks; otherwise	Recurrent attacks of fever, headache,

(continued)

TABLE 108-2.   *(Continued)*

CONDITION	INHERITANCE PATTERN	GASTROINTESTINAL MANIFESTATIONS	OTHER FEATURES AND COMMENTS
Aspartylglycosaminuria	AR	minimal abdominal symptoms; no serositis Diarrhea in infancy	and swollen glands; leukocyte count of 10,000–20,000 cells/µL A lysosomal disorder caused by deficiency of *N*-aspartyl-*β*-glucosaminidase; sagging skin of the cheeks, broad nose and face, short neck, cranial asymmetry, scoliosis, hyperactivity, severe mental retardation, vacuolated lymphocytes, and frequent infections
Fatal infantile diarrhea with abnormal hair	?AR	Severe diarrhea preceded by excoriated buttocks	Large, low-set, simple ears; flat nasal bridge, large mouth, and wooly, easily removed hair; hepatic fibrosis, hemosiderosis, and islet cell hyperplasia; increased serum galactose. Consider Menkes syndrome in differential diagnosis.
Erythroderma desquamativa of Leiner	?AR	Severe diarrhea	Susceptibility to infection, lymphatic hypoplasia, and increase in reticular cells of the lymph nodes

AD, autosomal dominant; AR, autosomal recessive; BLS, bare lymphocyte syndrome; HLA, human leukocyte antigen; IDDM, insulin-dependent diabetes mellitus; PAP, Papanicolaou; SCID, severe combined immunodeficiency; XLR, X-linked recessive.

Neurofibromatosis

There are several types of neurofibromatosis (NF): NF type 1 (NF1), NF type 2 (NF2), and atypical types.[78] NF1 and NF3, otherwise known as familial intestinal neurofibromatosis, can be associated with GI hemorrhage because of ulceration of neurofibromas in the lumen of the bowel. Additional characteristics of NF1 include multiple café au lait macules of the skin, multiple neurofibromas or plexiform neurofibromas, axillary or inguinal freckling, optic gliomas, multiple Lisch nodules (i.e., iris hamartomas), and bony dysplasia of the sphenoid or long bones. NF1 is an autosomal dominant disorder, with a frequency of 1 case per 4000 persons. Genetic linkage studies have localized the *NF1* gene to chromosome 17q, and cloning and characterization of the mutant gene has been achieved.[79] NF3 only has intestinal neurofibromas and none of the other features seen in NF1. It is not clear if NF3 is allelic with NF1 or if it is a separate genetic disease.[80]

Osler-Weber-Rendu Syndrome

Osler-Weber-Rendu syndrome, also called hereditary hemorrhagic telangiectasia (HHT), is an autosomal dominant disorder of high penetrance characterized by mucocutaneous telangiectases. The usual presenting feature is epistaxis occurring at puberty. The cutaneous telangiectases appear much later, usually between 5 and 20 years of age. Blood loss from the mucosal lesions in the gut can be chronic or acute. Larger vessel involvement is common. Pulmonary arteriovenous malformations occur in approximately 15% to 20% of cases and can lead to embolic complications or high-output cardiac failure. Arteriovenous malformations occur less often in the cerebral and hepatic vessels.[81] Genetic linkage studies initially suggested an association between the HLA region on chromosome 6 and HHT.[82] However, later linkage analysis in two large, multigeneration HHT pedigrees established significant linkage with markers on chromosome 9q.[83]

Klippel-Trenaunay-Weber Syndrome

The Klippel-Trenaunay-Weber syndrome is a presumably autosomal dominant disorder that features varicose veins and large, cutaneous hemangiomas with hypertrophy of the underlying bones and soft tissues.[84] Diffuse cavernous hemangiomas of the colon are found in 1% to 12.5% of patients and can sometimes cause significant GI bleeding. Partial colectomy and endoscopic laser ablation of residual abnormal colonic mucosa has been successful in the management of this complication.[85]

Blue Rubber Bleb Nevus Syndrome

The blue rubber bleb nevus syndrome is an autosomal dominant disorder characterized by the presence of bladder-like hemangiomatous skin lesions that are easily compressible, refill quickly, and have the look and feel of rubber nipples. The most common sites for involvement are the trunk and upper extremities, but the mucosa of the nasopharynx and GI tract, particularly the small bowel, can also be affected. Bleeding is an important complication of these lesions. Nocturnal pain and regional hyperhidrosis may also be features of this disorder.[86]

TABLE 108-3
Recurrent Gastrointestinal Bleeding Syndromes

CONDITION	INHERITANCE PATTERN	GASTROINTESTINAL MANIFESTATIONS	OTHER FEATURES AND COMMENTS
Polyposis syndromes		See Chapter 86	
Neurofibromatosis type 1 (NF1)	AD	GI bleeding secondary to ulceration of intestinal neurofibromata	Multiple café au lait macules, neurofibromas, axillary and inguinal freckling, multiple Lisch nodules, optic gliomas, bony dysplasia of the sphenoid and long bones; associated neoplasms include pheochromocytoma, meningiomas, and malignant degeneration of neurofibromas
Neurofibromatosis type 3 (NF3)	AD	GI bleeding due to ulceration of intestinal neurofibromas	None of the other features seen in NF1
Multiple endocrine neoplasia type 1	AD	GI bleeding due to peptic ulcer disease secondary to gastrinomas	Triad of pancreatic (i.e., insulinomas and gastroinomas), parathyroid, and pituitary adenomas; disease gene located on chromosome 11q
Muir-Torre syndrome	AD	GI bleeding secondary to multiple primary carcinomas of the colon, duodenum, and larynx	Keratoacanthomata of the face; multiple sebaceous tumors
Macrocephaly, multiple lipomas and hemangiomata	AD	Multiple visceral hemangiomata and intestinal hamartomas predipose to GI bleeding	Macrocephaly, pseudopapilledema, multiple hemangiomas involving the skin; males may have hyperpigmented macules on the penis
Cutis laxa type 1	AR	Diverticula of the GI tract that are susceptible to bleeding (X-linked cutis laxa also features GI diverticula)	Diaphragmatic and other hernias, diverticula of the urinary tract, and pulmonary emphysema
Small intestinal diverticulosis	AR	Small bowel diverticula and ulcerative colitis predispose to GI bleeding	Possible increase in autoimmune disorders, including rheumatoid arthritis, thyroiditis, and nonviral hepatitis
Diverticulosis of bowel, hernia, and retinal detachment	AR	Diverticula of large or small bowel	Femoral or inguinal hernias, diverticula of bladder, myopia, strabismus, and retinal detachment
Williams' syndrome	AD	Risk for GI bleeding due to diverticulosis; constipation	Supravalvular aortic stenosis, peripheral pulmonary artery stenosis, elfin face, dental abnormalities, infantile hypercalcemia, growth and mental deficiency; estimated frequency of 1 in 10,000
Ehlers-Danlos syndrome	AD, AR	Bowel and large vessel rupture, more common in type IV	Type I: soft, extensible skin; lax joints, easy bruisability, atrophic scarring, hernias, and premature birth. Type IV caused by type III collagen defect, thin, translucent skin; localized to chromosome 2q
Pseudoxanthama elasticum	AR	Abnormal vasculature causes GI and urinary tract bleeding; hematemesis is common	Pseudoxanthomatous changes of the skin of the flexural areas; angioid streaks of the retina
Osler-Weber-Rendu (hereditary hemorrhagic telangiectasia)	AD	Mucocutaneous telangiectases with acute or chronic blood loss	Epistaxis, cutaneous telangiectatias, arteriovenous malformations in the lung, liver, and brain
Klippel-Trenaunay-Weber syndrome	?AD	Diffuse cavernous hemangiomas of the colon causing GI bleeding	Varicose veins, large cutaneous hemangiomas with hypertrophy of underlying soft tissues and bone
Blue rubber bleb nevus syndrome	AD	Hemangiomas of the nasopharynx and GI tract	Hemangiomatous skin lesions of the trunk and upper extremities

(continued)

TABLE 108-3.   *(Continued)*

CONDITION	INHERITANCE PATTERN	GASTROINTESTINAL MANIFESTATIONS	OTHER FEATURES AND COMMENTS
Idiopathic colonic varices	AD	GI bleeding from colonic varices in the absence of portal hypertension	
Hermansky-Pudlak syndrome	AR	Inflammatory bowel disease and defective platelet aggregation predispose to GI bleeding	Partial albinism, restrictive lung disease; common in Puerto Ricans
Cutaneous photosensitivity and colitis	?AR	GI bleeding secondary to severe colitis; refractory diarrhea	Early cutaneous photosensitivity, causing erythematous, vesicular lesions of the skin

AD, autosomal dominant; AR, autosomal recessive; XLR, X-linked recessive.

Ehlers-Danlos Syndrome

Connective tissue disorders in which the integrity of structural tissues is impaired may predispose patients to GI bleeding. The Ehlers-Danlos syndrome is a heterogenous group of connective tissue disorders affecting the skin, ligaments, joints, blood vessels, and internal organs. There are at least 10 subtypes of Ehlers-Danlos syndrome. The classic form, known as Ehlers-Danlos syndrome type I, is characterized by soft, velvety, hyperextensible skin, lax joints, easy bruisability, atrophic scarring, venous varicosities, hernia, and prematurity due to rupture of fetal membranes. GI bleeding due to bowel and arterial rupture is not a usual manifestation but may occur.[87] Linkage analysis in a large Ehlers-Danlos syndrome type I kindred excluded collagen types I and III as candidate genes.[88] Ehlers-Danlos syndrome type IV is more commonly associated with bowel and large vessel rupture. The affected persons have very thin, fragile skin and tissues; tight skin over the fingers, face, and ears; and hyperextensible distal interphalangeal joints. A defect in type III collagen is responsible for the phenotype. The type III collagen gene maps to chromosome 2q.[89] Ehlers-Danlos syndrome type IV may be inherited as an autosomal dominant or recessive trait.

Pseudoxanthoma Elasticum

Pseudoxanthoma elasticum primarily affects the skin of the neck, axillae, and other flexural areas; the Bruch's membrane of the eye, resulting in angioid streaks on fundoscopic examination; and the arteries, producing GI and urinary tract hemorrhage, precocious calcification, and occlusive vascular changes.[90] Recurrent, severe hematemesis was the presenting feature of one of the first reported cases.

Hematemesis is much more common than melena; superficial hemorrhages and erosions may be seen in the stomach. Bleeding tends to occur as early as the first decade of life, before the skin and eye changes are evident. Pregnant women are more susceptible to bleeding.

The diagnosis is made on the basis of clinical examination. At least four subtypes are thought to exist: two autosomal dominant and two autosomal recessive forms.[90] The dominant type I is characterized by peau d'orange skin, severe vascular complications, and severe choroiditis. The dominant type II is more common than type I and is characterized by macular or focal changes in the skin, which is very stretchy, and by myopia, a high-arched palate, blue sclerae, and loose jointedness. The recessive type I is similar to the dominant type I and is much more common than the recessive type II, which is characterized by generalized skin changes with no ocular or vascular abnormalities.

Cutis Laxa Type I

Cutis laxa type I is an autosomal recessive disorder characterized by abnormalities of the elastic tissue. Two forms of type I cutis laxa have been described.[91] The first features diaphragmatic and other hernias; diverticula of the GI and urinary tract, which are susceptible to bleeding; and pulmonary emphysema, which may lead to cor pulmonale. Death usually occurs in the first year of life. The second form is less severe and is characterized by prenatal and postnatal growth deficiency, large fontanels with delayed closure, congenital hip dislocation, and lax joints. Diminished elastin production has been verified in these patients, and quantitation reveals decreased elastin mRNA, perhaps caused by decreased rates of transcription or degradation of unstable transcripts.[92] A dominant form of cutis laxa does not have the visceral manifestations characteristic of the recessive forms. X-linked cutis laxa is discussed in the vitamin and mineral malabsorption section of this chapter. It also features diverticular disease of the GI tract, increasing the possible risk for GI hemorrhage.

Syndromes Characterized by Macrocephaly, Multiple Lipomas, and Hemangiomas

A collection of several syndromes, including Bannayan-Zonana syndrome, Riley-Smith syndrome, and Ruvalcaba-Myhre-Smith syndrome, with similar features may represent different allelic mutations or genetic heterogeneity.[93,94] Typical features include macrocephaly, pseudopapilledema, multiple lipomas, multiple hemangiomas involving the skin and viscera, and intestinal hamartomatous polyposis. The latter two features create a susceptibility to GI hemorrhage. Males may have hyperpigmented macules on the penis. High birth weight and length is typical, but growth levels off at 6 to 7 years of age. There is delayed motor development, and problems with incoordination are lifelong. Intelligence may be subnormal. Seizures may result from intracranial hemorrhage due to arteriovenous malformations. Arteriovenous malformations may also lead to extremity overgrowth, necessitating amputation. The inheritance pattern is autosomal dominant.

Hermansky-Pudlak Syndrome

Hermansky-Pudlak syndrome occurs most frequently in Puerto Rico, where the prevalence is 1 case in 2000.[95,96] It is a storage disorder of a ceroid-like substance and is associated with characteristic features of partial albinism, restrictive lung disease, and a platelet abnormality. There is a deficiency of the granule storage pool in platelets, causing defective ADP release, which leads to a prolonged bleeding time and defective platelet aggregation. Inflammatory bowel disease with an onset between the ages of 12 and 30 years is also common in the Puerto Rican patients.[97] The combination of inflammatory bowel disease and defective platelets contribute to the occurrence of GI bleeding in these patients. The inheritance pattern is autosomal recessive.

INTESTINAL MOTILITY OR PSEUDO OBSTRUCTION DISORDERS

Intestinal pseudoobstruction may result from intrinsic enteric myopathies and neuropathies or from generalized muscular and neurologic disorders. This section reviews the genetic disorders that feature abnormal intestinal motility or pseudo-obstruction in each of these categories (Table 108-4).

Intestinal pseudoobstruction is suggested clinically by recurrent signs and symptoms of intestinal obstruction in the absence of mechanical obstruction, as proven by appropriate radiologic, endoscopic, or surgical investigations. The presence and severity of complications depend on the age of the patient (i.e., infant or adult), primary site of involvement, and degree of functional impairment. In the adult, a long-standing history of symptoms suggesting GI motility dysfunction, such as dysphagia, early satiety, and constipation or diarrhea, may precede the onset of acute symptoms. Patients usually present in the second to fourth decades of life with complaints of abdominal pain, distention, and sometimes vomiting. Malnutrition is common and results from decreased food intake, impaired digestion, or malabsorption. Infants with these disorders usually present with acute, severe obstructive symptoms of abdominal pain and distention after feeding. Reflux esophagitis and aspiration pneumonia due to impaired gastroesophageal motility is also common in infants.

After mechanical obstruction has been ruled out, diagnostic studies to evaluate pseudo-obstruction include esophageal and intestinal manometry, gastric emptying studies, and full-thickness biopsy with silver stains. Esophageal manometry shows aperistalsis and incomplete relaxation of the lower esophageal sphincter. Intestinal manometry usually shows a hypomotile pattern. Gastric emptying studies show a delay for solids and a variable pattern for liquids. Silver stains delineate neuropathic from myopathic forms. Detection of sub-

clinically affected family members at risk can be accomplished with these diagnostic techniques.[98]

Visceral Myopathy Syndromes

Clinical GI manifestations of the visceral myopathic and neuropathic forms of intestinal pseudo-obstruction are similar. In the myopathic form, there may be other evidence of myopathy, such as megacystis, vesicoureteral reflux, ophthalmoplegia, ptosis, and small intestine diverticulosis. The pathogenetic mechanisms of the GI manifestations include degenerative changes and thinning of intestinal smooth muscle, especially of the longitudinal layers; the enteric neurons are normal. A mitochondrial myopathy associated with intestinal pseudo-obstruction due to a visceral myopathy has been described.[99] It may be that some forms of visceral myopathy are mitochondrial myopathies. Diagnosis of a mitochondrial myopathy can be made by a Gomori trichome–stained skeletal muscle biopsy, which shows the characteristic ragged, red fibers. There have been no reports of a mitochondrial DNA mutation responsible for intestinal pseudo-obstruction.[100] The reported familial cases have followed an autosomal dominant or recessive mode of inheritance, and they lack the maternal pattern of transmission seen with mitochondrial DNA mutations. If a mitochondrial myopathy is involved, it is likely that the disease gene responsible in most cases resides in the nucleus.

Duchenne's Muscular Dystrophy

Duchenne's muscular dystrophy is an X-linked disorder characterized by skeletal muscle degeneration causing atrophy and weakness.[101] The incidence in male births is about 1 in 3500. The onset of symptoms usually begins before the patient is 5 years of age, with progressive symptoms of muscle weakness, toe walking, and difficulty rising from a chair and climbing stairs. Affected boys have a waddling gait, and pseudohypertrophy of the calves is typical. By 11 years of age, most are confined to a wheelchair; they then develop joint contractures and scoliosis. Death usually occurs in the late teens or early twenties from respiratory infections or heart failure. Laboratory studies show elevated serum levels of aldolase, lactate dehydrogenase, and creatine kinase. GI symptoms are also common and include abdominal pain and distention, delayed gastric emptying, acute gastric dilatation, and chronic intestinal pseudo-obstruction.[102] The disease gene responsible for Duchenne's muscular dystrophy has been localized and cloned.[103] The gene product is a protein found in skeletal muscle called dystrophin, which is lacking in affected boys and deficient in female carriers.

Myotonic Dystrophy

Myotonic dystrophy is an autosomal dominant disorder that features abnormalities of delayed muscular relaxation, facial weakness and muscle atrophy, ptosis, cataracts, gonadal atrophy, cardiac conduction abnormalities, and male pattern baldness.[104] There are significant GI complications caused by

(text continues on p. 2402)

TABLE 108-4
Intestinal Motility and Pseudo-Obstruction Disorders

CONDITION	INHERITANCE PATTERN	GASTROINTESTINAL MANIFESTATIONS	OTHER FEATURES AND COMMENTS
Visceral Myopathies			
Visceral myopathy with megaduodenum or megacystitis	AD	Intermittent abdominal pain, distention, vomiting, constipation, and diarrhea, usually presenting in the first to second decade	Megacystitis occurs without obstruction but with vesicoureteral reflux, predisposing to urinary tract infections; diagnosis often made in adults. Family study can prevent unnecessary diagnostic surgery for symptomatic relatives.
Visceral myopathy with external ophthalmoplegia	?AR, ?mt	Chronic diarrhea, abdominal distention and pain, dilated duodenum and jejunum with diverticulosis	Ptosis, ophthalmoplegia, proximal muscle weakness and atrophy; mitochondrial myopathy may accompany or be responsible for disorder; usually adult onset
Megacystitis–microcolon–intestinal hypoperistalsis syndrome	AR	Microcolon and dilated small intestine with symptoms of obstruction; abdominal distention and bilious vomiting	Symptom onset in infancy; marked dilatation of the bladder, hydronephrosis, external appearance of prune belly, multiple cardiac rhabdomyomata; 4:1 female preponderance, possibly due to increased severity in males; prenatal diagnosis by ultrasound identifying distended GI tract and bladder; death usual by 3 y from malnutrition of sepsis
Hereditary internal anal sphincter myopathy	AD	Severe anal pain, constipation	Onset 3rd to 5th decades; noncompliant, thickened internal anal sphincter
Duchenne's muscular dystrophy	XLR	Bloating, abdominal fullness, delayed gastric emptying, acute gastric dilatation, chronic intestinal pseudo-obstruction	Skeletal muscle degeneration, causing severe debilitating weakness due to deficiency of the gene product dystrophin
Myotonic dystrophy	AD	Problems with swallowing, aspiration, and constipation; more severe complications occur with congenital myotonic dystrophy with gastroparesis, subacute obstruction, megacolon, and constipation	Delayed muscular relaxation, ptosis, cataract, gonadal atrophy, cardiac, conduction defects, and male pattern baldness; disease gene localized to chromosome 19p; maternal transmission associated with more severe phenotype of congenital myotonic dystrophy with mental retardation, neonatal hypotonia, and facial diplegia
Oculopharyngeal muscular dystrophy	AD, rarely AR	Dysphagia	Ptosis; weakness and wasting of facial, neck, and distal limb muscles; mitochondrial abnormalities seen on electron microscopy
Kearns-Sayre syndrome	mt (deletions)	Swallowing difficulties	Progressive external ophthalmoplegia, pigmentary retinopathy, cardiac conduction defects due to cytochrome C oxidase deficiency; deletions in the mitochondrial DNA responsible for the phenotype; all reported cases are sporadic
Visceral Neuropathies			
Deficiency of argyrophil myenteric plexus	AR	Intermittent abdominal pain, distention and vomiting, functional intestinal obstruction; short, small intestine; malrotation and pyloric hypertrophy	Ataxia, abnormal pupillary reflexes, dysarthria, absent deep tendon reflexes, peripheral neuropathy and autonomic neuropathy; eosinophilic

(continued)

TABLE 108-4.   *(Continued)*

CONDITION	INHERITANCE PATTERN	GASTROINTESTINAL MANIFESTATIONS	OTHER FEATURES AND COMMENTS
		due to failure of the development of the myenteric plexus	nuclear inclusions in the myenteric neurons, brain, spinal cord, and celiac plexus ganglia
Microcolon	?AR	Obstruction, abdominal distention, vomiting	Aganglionosis of the entire colon and distal small intestine leads to microcolon; may be secondary to congenital atresia or mechanical obstruction (e.g., meconium ileus).
Hirschsprung's disease	?AD multifactorial	Aganglionic megacolon with constipation and abdominal distention	Risks to family members increases with severity and number of female relatives affected
Hirschsprung's disease, microcephaly, and iris coloboma	?AR	Aganglionic megacolon	Microcephaly, hypertelorism, iris coloboma, submucous cleft palate, short stature, learning problems; similar features described in chromosome deletion syndromes; high-resolution karyotype recommended
Hirschsprung's disease with bilateral bicolored irides	?AR	Aganglionic megacolon	Heterochromia, two distinct colors present in the same iris
Hirschsprung's disease with polydactyly, renal agenesis, and deafness	?AR	Aganglionic megacolon	Polydactyly, unilateral renal agenesis, hypertelorism, and congenital deafness
Hirschsprung's disease with ulnar polydactyly, polysyndactyly of big toes, and ventricular septal defect	?AR	Aganglionic megacolon	Ulnar polydactyly, polysyndactyly of big toes, and ventricular septal defect
Hirschsprung's disease with hypoplastic nails and dysmorphic facial features	?AR	Aganglionic megacolon	Hypoplastic nails, minor dysmorphic facial features, bilateral hydronephrosis, imperforate anus, inguinal hernia; death in infancy
Hirschsprung's disease and Ondine's curse	?AR, ?AD	Short segment and total colonic aganglionosis	Idiopathic, congenital hypoventilation; possible abnormality of the neural crest
13q-syndrome	Chromosomal	Aganglionc megacolon	Growth deficiency, microcephaly, mental deficiency, abnormal facies with prominent nasal bridge, hypertelorism, ptosis, epicanthal folds, microphthalmia, colobomas, retinoblastoma, prominent maxilla, prominent, slanting, low-set ears, micrognathia, hypoplastic or aplastic thumbs, cardiac defects, club feet, hypospadius, cryptorchidism
Down's syndrome	Chromosomal	Aganglionic megacolon in 5.9% of cases	Hypotonia, protruding tongue, joint laxity, short stature, mental retardation, speckling of irides (i.e., Brushfield's spots), small ears, flat facial profile, upslanted palpebral fissures, small ears, redundant neck skin, single transverse palmar crease, 5th finger clinodactyly, hypothyroidism; leukemia in 1% of cases
Cartilage-hair hypoplasia (metaphyseal chondrodysplasia, McKusick's type)	AR	Megacolon with constipation	Dwarfing syndrome with radiographic changes called metaphyseal dysostosis; fine, sparse, light-colored hair; anemia; susceptibility to chicken pox and malignancies
Waardenburg-Shah syndrome	AR	Intestinal obstruction with dilated	White forelock, white eyebrows and

(continued)

TABLE 108-4. *(Continued)*

CONDITION	INHERITANCE PATTERN	GASTROINTESTINAL MANIFESTATIONS	OTHER FEATURES AND COMMENTS
Waardenburg's syndrome	AD	proximal ileum, collapse of distal ileum and colon Short segment aganglionosis megacolon	eyelashes, isochromia irides (i.e., mosaic pattern in light brown irides) Dystopia canthorum, broad nasal root, white forelock, white skin patches, deafness. This and the above syndrome may represent a single dominant gene with pleiotropic effects. A more severe phenotype exists in homozygotes.
Familial achalasia and diffuse esophageal spasm	?Multifactorial, ?AR	Retrosternal discomfort, progressive dysphagia, intermittent regurgitation, diverticulosis of the esophagus	Severity varies in family members. HLA studies suggest an immunogenetic mechanism in the pathogenesis of this disorder.
Achalasia-microcephaly syndrome	?AR	Onset of dysphagia and regurgitation due to achalasia in early childhood	Microcephaly and mental deficiency
Congenital deafness with vitiligo and achalasia	AR	Dysphagia and regurgitation due to achalasia	Deafness, short stature, and vitiligo; variable expressivity; some family members with only vitiligo and achalasia
Groll-Hirschowitz syndrome	AR	Dysphagia, nausea, diverticula of the small bowel	Cachexia; protein and fat malabsorption, progressive sensory neuropathy, tachycardia, and abnormal GI motility secondary to vagus nerve involvement; progressive nerve deafness, with neurologic deficit ascribed to a process of demyelinization
Polip's syndrome	?AR, ?mt	Severe GI dysmotility due to visceral neuropathy with chronic malabsorption and malnutrition	Progressive sensorimotor peripheral neuropathy, cranial neuropathy (i.e., external ophthalmoplegia and deafness), abnormal cerebral and cerebellar white matter, endoneural fibrosis and demyelination, ragged red fibers in skeletal muscles, partial defect of cytochrome C oxidase
Familial dysautonomia (Riley-Day syndrome)	AR	Dysphagia, emesis, and aspiration pneumonia	Failure to thrive, dehydration secondary to GI manifestations, autonomic instability
Hereditary coproporphyria	AD	Nausea, vomiting, abdominal pain and distention, constipation due to an autonomic neuropathy	Pruritic skin blisters, weakness and paresthesias of the extremities due to a peripheral neuropathy, elevated fecal coproporphyrins with normal erythrocyte uro-1-synthase and δ-aminolevulinic acid dehydratase
Multiple endocrine neoplasia type IIb	AD	Chronic constipation with megacolon or diarrhea, frequently developing before the endocrine neoplasms	Neuromas from lips to rectum; prominent lips, nodular tongue, thickened eyelids, medullary thyroid carcinoma, pheochromocytoma, marfanoid habitus
Optiz G syndrome	AD	Esophageal dysmotility and laryngeal tracheal clefts causing swallowing difficulties; imperforate anus	Mild to moderate mental deficiency, hypertelorism, widow's peak, hypospadius, cryptorchidism, bifid scrotum, and hernias

AD, autosomal dominant; AR, autosomal recessive; mt, mitochondrial; XLR, X-linked recessive.

abnormal functioning at all levels of the GI tract, from the pharynx to the anal sphincters. This effect is the result of degenerative changes in smooth muscle and fatty infiltration, causing problems with swallowing, aspiration, and constipation.[105] The disease gene has been localized to chromosome 19p and involves a trinucleotide repeat.[106,107] Expansion of the repeat can occur in subsequent generations, providing a molecular basis for the clinical phenomenon of anticipation (i.e., earlier clinical onset of disease in subsequent generations) in this disorder. The more severe phenotype of congenital myotonic dystrophy only occurs with alleles of maternal origin.[108] The congenital form features mental retardation, hypotonia, facial diplegia, gastroparesis, subacute intestinal obstruction, megacolon and constipation.

Kearns-Sayre Syndrome

Kearns-Sayre syndrome is caused by mutations in the mitochondrial genome. The disorder is characterized by progressive external ophthalmoplegia, pigmentary retinopathy, cardiomyopathy, and cardiac conduction defects; weakness of facial, trunk, and extremity muscles; and deafness, small stature, electroencephalographic changes, and increased cerebrospinal fluid protein.[109] The GI symptoms relate to the pharyngeal muscle weakness experienced by affected individuals, causing swallowing difficulties and dysphagia.[110] The mitochondrial mutations characteristic of this disorder are deletions ranging in size from 2.0 to 7.0 kilobases.[111]

Visceral Neuropathy Syndromes

The visceral neuropathic forms of intestinal pseudo-obstruction are characterized by abnormal pupillary reflexes, ataxia, and dysarthria; peripheral nervous system abnormalities, including absent deep tendon reflexes and impaired vibratory and position sense; and autonomic neurologic abnormalities such as inappropriate blood pressure responses to phenylephrine, Valsalva maneuver, upright posture, and lack of sweating on warming. One type is also associated with basal ganglia calcification and mental retardation. Histologic sections of tissues stained with a silver stain reveal degenerative changes of myenteric plexus neurons.

Hirschsprung's Disease

Hirschsprung's disease is probably a multifactorial disorder that usually occurs as an isolated congenital anomaly but may be a syndromic association of several genetic conditions (see Table 108-4). With isolated Hirschsprung's disease, the risk to family members increases with severity (i.e., length of GI tract involved) and the number of affected relatives, especially female relatives. Empiric risk estimates are 7.2% for the siblings of affected females and 2.6% for the siblings of affected males.[112] Complex segregation analysis of data on 487 cases and their families demonstrated mendelian inheritance patterns when the length of affected bowel was considered.[113] Cases with aganglionosis beyond the sigmoid colon had a mode of inheritance that was compatible with an autosomal dominant trait with incomplete penetrance. Cases with aganglionosis no more proximal than the sigmoid colon had in-

heritance patterns consistent with multifactorial inheritance or autosomal recessive inheritance with very low penetrance. Linkage studies have localized at least one of the genes responsible for Hirschsprung's disease to chromosome 10q in several multigeneration families with isolated, nonsyndromic disease.[114,115]

Familial Achalasia and Diffuse Esophageal Spasm

Familial occurrence of achalasia has been reported in several families without a distinct inheritance pattern, which may suggest multifactorial inheritance.[116] The cause of achalasia is unknown. The disorder involves the esophagus, causing symptoms of progressive dysphagia, retrosternal discomfort, and intermittent regurgitation. Diverticulosis of the esophagus may also occur. The severity of the disorder may vary among family members. Esophageal ganglion cells and dorsal motorneurons of the vagal nucleus are decreased, and there is the wallerian degeneration of the vagus nerve. An autoimmune response may explain these findings. HLA association studies were carried out, and a positive association with HLA allele DQw1 with a relative risk of 4.2 was observed in the Caucasian population and a relative risk of 3.6 in the African-American population. DRw53 was found to be reduced among Caucasians, with a relative risk of 0.23.[117]

Familial Dysautonomia

Familial dysautonomia, also called Riley-Day syndrome, is an autosomal recessive disorder involving the autonomic nervous system. It is most prevalent in the Ashkenazi Jewish population, with an incidence of about 1 in 3500.[118] It is characterized by symptoms of autonomic instability, including lack of tearing, emotional lability, paroxysmal hypertension, increased sweating, cold hands and feet, corneal anesthesia, red blotching of the skin, and drooling. The GI manifestations include oropharyngeal incoordination, abnormal esophageal motility, and decreased lower esophageal sphincter pressure, prolonged gastric emptying, and gastroesophageal reflux, all of which result in dysphagia, emesis, and aspiration pneumonia. Affected individuals are reluctant to eat and suffer from dehydration and failure to thrive.[119] Fundoplication and gastrostomy has been beneficial in the management of these cases.[120] Diagnosis is determined by a lack of axon flare after intradermal injection of histamine, absence of fungiform papillae on the tongue, miosis of the pupil after instillation of methacholine chloride (2.5%), absent deep tendon reflexes, and diminished tear flow.[121] Linkage studies have localized the disease gene for Riley-Day syndrome to chromosome 9q.[122]

MECHANICAL OBSTRUCTION AND MALFORMATION SYNDROMES

Most genetic disorders that cause mechanical obstruction are related to congenital malformations, and in general, they have more importance in the pediatric population than they do for adults.[4] A common genetic cause for mechanical obstruction that is not caused by malformation is meconium ileus, seen in 10% to 15% of cystic fibrosis patients. The anatomic site or sites of malformation in these syndromes is usually restricted to derivatives of the embryologic foregut, midgut, and hindgut. In a rostral to caudal distribution, Table 108-5 reviews genetic malformation syndromes that may present with symptoms secondary to a mechanical obstruction.

CHRONIC ABDOMINAL PAIN SYNDROMES

There are many genetic syndromes that can present with recurrent bouts of abdominal pain, including familial Mediterranean fever (FMF), Fabry's disease, hereditary angioneurotic edema, hereditary fructose intolerance, and the hereditary pancreatitis syndromes (Table 108-6). Although these syndromes (except for FMF) are relatively rare, making the correct diagnosis in a patient may prevent them from having unnecessary and invasive procedures and may similarly benefit their family members.

Familial Mediterranean Fever

Familial Mediterranean fever (FMF) is an autosomal recessive disorder with protean manifestations and an obscure cause.[123,124] The clinical disorder of FMF has a frequency of approximately 1 in 2400 in Israel, a country in which it has been studied intensively.[123] One half of the patients are of Sephardic Jewish descent, about 20% are Armenian, 20% are Turkish or Arabic, and the remainder are Italian, Greek, or Ashkenazi Jews. The disease occurs rarely in northern Europeans. Approximately 50% of the patients do not have a positive family history.

The manifestations usually appear during childhood or adolescence and are characterized by brief episodic febrile attacks, recurring in varying intervals and associated with painful inflammation involving a variety of serosal surfaces, including the abdomen, chest, joints, and skin, lending the alternative name of recurrent familial polyserositis. Attacks last typically for 1 to 2 days and occur once or twice each month. The natural history of the attacks can vary considerably, even in an individual patient. The clinical features include fever, abdominal pain, and signs of peritonitis in most patients. Because the peritonitis is nonspecific, other acute febrile conditions must be considered, such as appendicitis, cholecystitis, pancreatitis, and intestinal obstruction. Common but less constant features include pleuritic pain, mild arthritis of the large joints, and a transient erysipelas-like skin lesion on the lower extremities. In 1% of patients, meningitis also occurs. When arthritis occurs, it is an episodic monarthritis or oligoarthritis of the large joints, mimicking oligoarthritic forms of juvenile rheumatoid arthritis. The attacks usually last days to weeks but may last for months and are associated with radiographic changes of periarticular osteopenia without erosions.

Laboratory test results are nonspecific during the attacks of pain and fever. The leukocyte count averages 16,000 cells/μL but may be as high as 40,000 cells/μL. The erythrocyte sedimentation rate increases, as do other acute-phase reactants. Albuminuria and microscopic hematuria also occur. Radiographic studies may show bowel edema and air-fluid levels in the small bowel, causing confusion with obstruction. The diagnosis is made in patients with the appropriate ethnic background, who have typical, self-limited, and recurrent attacks of fever and abdominal pain.

The most severe feature of this disease is the progressive accumulation of a specific protein known as amyloid fibrillar protein AA in the kidney, which manifests clinically as a nephropathy. There is considerable ethnic variation in the incidence of amyloidosis in FMF. Amyloidosis occurs least frequently in Armenians with the disorder, even though FMF occurs most commonly in Armenians (1 in 400). Amyloidosis occurs commonly in non-Ashkenazi Jews (1 in 2400) and is most common in Moroccan Jews in Israel (up to 30%). In some patients, the amyloid develops before any other clinical sign. The genetic or environmental factors that account for these differences in the incidence of amyloidosis are not clear.[125] The amyloidosis appears to be a phenomenon secondary to the periodic inflammation, because its occurrence is reduced by colchicine therapy.

Colchicine (0.6 mg), administered orally two to three times per day, is an effective treatment in the prevention of the acute febrile attacks of the disease. A very-low-fat diet (20 g/day) may also prevent the attacks.[126] Colchicine does not allay symptoms if taken during attacks. Some patients use it intermittently to forestall attacks when they recognize that one is imminent.

The cause of FMF is unknown. It seems to involve a genetically determined defect in the regulation of inflammatory responses. Research into the cause of FMF has included studies of suppressor T cells, leukocyte chemotaxis, lysosome release from neutrophils, and immune globulins, all without a definitive identification of the pathophysiologic defect.[127] Complement component C5a was found to be decreased to a level less than 10% of controls in the peritoneal fluid of five FMF patients.[128] The proposed hypothesis was that a deficiency in the inhibitory activity of C5a in the inflammatory response in synovial and other fluids may play an important role in the pathogenesis of the characteristic recurrent attacks in FMF. Proof of this hypothesis awaits cloning of the C5a inhibitor gene.

The FMF susceptibility gene has been mapped to chromosome 16p, making presymptomatic screening using linkage analysis in at-risk family members possible.[129] Although clinical heterogeneity exists, as reflected by the different prevalence rates of renal amyloid in different ethnic groups, there is no evidence for locus heterogeneity, because the FMF gene is linked to the same locus in the non-Ashkenazi Jewish and Armenian populations.[130]

Fabry's Disease

Fabry's disease, also called diffuse angiokeratoma, is an X-linked recessive lysosomal storage disorder due to a deficiency of α-galactosidase.[131] Deposition of lipoid material in several tissues is responsible for the characteristic findings, which include attacks of pain in the abdomen and extremities (probably due to lipid changes in ganglion cells of the autonomic nervous system), vascular lesions in the fundi of the eye and the kidney, corneal opacities, a hypertrophic cardiomyopathy, and characteristic skin lesions of a vascular nature called angiok-

TABLE 108-5
Mechanical Obstruction and Malformation Syndromes

CONDITION	INHERITANCE PATTERN	GASTROINTESTINAL MANIFESTATIONS	OTHER FEATURES AND COMMENTS
VATER association	Sporadic	Tracheoesophageal fistula with esophageal atresia and anal atresia	Vertebral defects; radial, renal, and cardiac abnormalities
Hiatal hernia and congenital short esophagus	?AD	Gastroesophageal reflux, esophagitis	
Galloway's syndrome	AR	Reflux with vomiting of feedings from birth	Microcephaly, large ears, nephrotic syndrome, renal microcystic dysplasia and focal glomerulosclerosis; death by age 3 y
Tracheoesophageal fistula with or without esophageal atresia	?Multifactorial	Aspiration, dysphagia	
Leiomyoma of vulva and esophagus	AD	Dysphagia due to an obstructing lesion (e.g., leiomyoma)	Vulvar lesions, clitoromegaly due to leiomyoma involvement at its base
Abnormal hands, feet, short palpebral fissures, microcephaly and esophageal or duodenal atresia	AD	Polyhydramnios, duodenal atresia secondary to annular pancreas, tracheoesophageal fistula	Microcephaly, upslanting, short palpebral fissures, fifth finger clinodactyly, syndactyly of fourth and fifth toes
Familial short rib syndrome, Beemer's type	?AD	Pyloric stenosis, short bowel, malrotation	Short stature, short ribs, severe respiratory failure, hydrops
Epidermolysis bullosa dystrophica, Hallopeau-Siemens type	AR	Mucosal surfaces may be involved with bullae, leading to esophageal stricture and perforation	Destructive bullae develop on hands, feet, elbows, and knees, with secondary joint contractures; conjunctiva and cornea may be involved due to excessive collagenase activity; disease gene maps to chromosome 11q
Epidermolysis bullosa letalis with pyloric atresia	AR	Membranous diaphragmatic obstruction at the pyloris, diarrhea, protein-losing gastroenteropathy	Bilateral stenosis at the uterovesical junction, causing hydronephrosis; prenatal diagnosis by demonstration of dermal-epidermal separation at the lamina lucida level in fetal skin
Pyloric atresia	AR	Dysphagia	Congenital pyloric atresia due to reduction of the pylorus to a fibrous band or obstruction from a membranous diaphragm
Pyloric stenosis	AD, multifactorial	Projectile vomiting at about 1 month of age	Recurrence risk of about 10% for male relatives and 2% for females; male predominance
Smith-Lemli-Opitz syndrome	AR	Vomiting secondary to pyloric stenosis	Dysmorphic facial features, microcephaly, mental retardation, hypotonia, hypospadius, syndactyly of second and third toes
Familial intrathoracic gastric volvulus	AD	Sharp, epigastric discomfort, occult blood loss, liquid dysphagia	
Duodenal atresia	AR	Bilious vomiting	May be seen in Down's syndrome (5.9% of cases)
Annular pancreas	AD	GI obstruction with vomiting due to duodenal stenosis	
Jejunal atresia	AR	Abdominal pain and distention	Agenesis of the mesentery leading to distal small bowel coming straight off cecum and twisting around the marginal artery, creating an apple-peel appearance seen at surgery; primary abnormality may be obliteration of the superior mesenteric artery
Volvulus of midgut	?AD	Abdominal pain, distention, and constipation	Present in infancy or early childhood; atresia of the ascending colon may be present

(continued)

TABLE 108-5.   *(Continued)*

CONDITION	INHERITANCE PATTERN	GASTROINTESTINAL MANIFESTATIONS	OTHER FEATURES AND COMMENTS
Fryns' syndrome	AR	Duodenal atresia, pyloric hyperplasia, malrotation and common mesentery in about 50% of patients	Diaphragmatic defects, lung hypoplasia, cleft lip and palate, cardiac defects, renal cysts, urinary tract malformation, distal limb hypoplasia, hypoplastic external genitalia, Dandy-Walker brain anomaly, agenesis of the corpus callosum
Miller's syndrome	?AR	Migdut malrotation, gastric volvulus	Postaxial and preaxial ray defects; renal anomalies
Multiple intestinal atresia	AR	Multiple atretic lesions from stomach to anus	Intraluminal calcifications seen on radiographs
Cornelia de Lange's syndrome	Unknown	Intestinal atresia in a minority of patients	Hirsutism, synophrys, broad nasal root, micrognathnia, malformed ears, abnormal hands, congenital heart disease, severe mental retardation; 2–5% recurrence risk
Anosacral anomalies	?AR	Imperforate anus	Anterior sacral meningocele, anal canal duplication cyst
Imperforate anus	?AR, ?XLR	Imperforate or ectopic anus	Rectovaginal fistula, hypospadias, hearing loss
Townes-Brocks syndrome	AD	Imperforate anus	Triphalangeal thumbs and other anomalies of the hands and feet, mild sensorineural deafness, lop ears, renal anomalies
Cat-eye syndrome	Chromosomal	Imperforate anus	Vertical pupil due to iris coloboma, periauricular tags or fistulas, cardiac and urinary tract abnormalities, mental deficiency; extra chromosomal material, probably a derived dicentric chromosome 22
Optiz G syndrome	AD	Imperforate anus, pharyngeal incoordination with regurgitation	Mild to moderate mental deficiency, hypertelorism, widow's peak, hypospadias, cryptorchidism, bifid scrotum, hernias
Reiger's syndrome	AD	Anal stenosis	Iris coloboma, broad nasal root, umbilical malformation, glaucoma
Schinzel's syndrome	?AD	Anal atresia and pyloric stenosis	Abnormalities of the fourth and fifth fingers, hypoplastic ulna, small penis, delayed puberty, obesity

AD, autosomal dominant; AR, autosomal recessive; XLR, X-linked recessive.

eratoma. Symptoms may present in adulthood, and death usually occurs after renal failure. Female heterozygotes may have renal insufficiency and proteinuria, but they almost never have skin lesions. α-Galactosidase activity is deficient in the leukocytes of male patients, and carrier females can be identified because of decreased activity.[132] Several mutations in the α-galactosidase gene (*GLA*) on the X chromosome in patients with Fabry's disease have provided the definitive evidence to indicate that this is the gene for Fabry's disease.[133]

Hereditary Angioneurotic Edema

Hereditary angioneurotic edema is an autosomal dominant disorder that affects the respiratory and GI tracts.[134] Symptoms of choking occur because of edema of the airways. This can be precipitated by acts of trauma, such as tracheal intubation. The GI symptoms include abdominal pain, nausea, vomiting, and diarrhea. Barium studies during an acute attack show bowel wall edema. Associated findings include an increased incidence of autoimmune disorders.

Deficiency of C1 esterase inhibitor is the underlying pathophysiologic defect in these patients. This protein regulates the first component of complement (C1) by inhibition of the proteolytic activity of its subcomponents C1r and C1s, preventing activation of C4 and C2 by C1s and inhibiting other serine proteases, including plasmin, kallikrein, and the coagulation factors XIa and XIIa.[135] Low levels of C4 and normal levels of C1 are characteristic of hereditary angioneurotic edema. These low levels of C4 are responsible for the increased incidence of systemic lupus erythematosus, glomerulonephritis, and vasculitis among these patients. Het-

TABLE 108-6
Chronic or Recurrent Abdominal Pain Syndromes

CONDITION	INHERITANCE PATTERN	GASTROINTESTINAL MANIFESTATIONS	OTHER FEATURES AND COMMENTS
Familial Mediterranean fever	AR	Recurrent bouts of abdominal pain	Recurrent fever, pain in chest and joints due to a serositis; elevated leukocyte count, erythrocyte sedimentation rate, renal amyloidosis; mapped to chromosome 16p
Fabry's disease	XLR	Abdominal pain	A lysosomal storage disease due to α-galactosidase deficiency; accumulation of lipoid material in the skin, corneas, vessels, kidneys, heart, and ganglion cells of the autonomic nervous system; skin lesions called angiokeratoma characteristic but non-specific
Hereditary angioneurotic edema	AD	Abdominal pain	Choking, laryngeal edema; C1 esterase inhibitor deficiency is underlying defect; androgens useful in prophylaxis against attacks; mapped to chromosome 11p
Hereditary fructose intolerance	AR	Abdominal pain, vomiting after fructose ingestion	Kidney and liver damage, growth retardation, coma and death on chronic exposure to fructose; caused by aldolase B deficiency; mapped to chromosome 9q
Hereditary pancreatitis	AD	Severe abdominal pain	Fever, elevation of serum amylase, pancreatic insufficiency, diabetes, pseudocyst; hemorrhagic pleural effusions and portal or splenic vein thrombosis possible
Deficiency of pancreatic stone protein (PSP)	AD	Chronic calcifying pancreatitis	PSP inhibits $CaCO_3$ crystal growth; PSP gene maps to chromosome 2p
Familial hypertrophy of the sphincter of Oddi	AD	Chronic pancreatitis	Rare but a surgically correctable cause of pancreatitis
Pancreatitis, sclerosing cholangitis and sicca complex	AR	Pancreatitis	Dry eyes and mouth; HLA-DR3 associated with primary sclerosing cholangitis
Lipoprotein lipase deficiency	AR	Recurrent attacks of abdominal pain, chronic pancreatitis	Massive hyperchylomicronemia on a normal diet; hepatosplenomegaly, eruptive xanthomas, lactescent plasma; early atherosclerosis not a feature; heterozygotes show slight hyperlipemia, maps to chromosome 8p
Apolipoprotein C-II deficiency	AR	Chronic pancreatitis	A necessary cofactor for lipoprotein lipase; clinically and biochemically similar to lipoprotein lipase deficiency except xanthomas and hepatosplenomegaly are less common
Glycogen storage disease type 1 (Von Gierke's disease)	AR	Chronic pancreatitis due to hyperlipidemia	Defect in glucose-6-phosphatase; hypoglycemia, lacticacidemia and ketonemia; hyperlipidemia causing xanthomata; hyperuricemia causing gout, hepatosplenomegaly, hepatic adenomas, which may undergo malignant degeneration; renal insufficiency and proteinuria. Dietary therapy consists of continuous nocturnal infusions and frequent administration of raw cornstarch; survival to adulthood is usual.
Homocystinuria (cystathionine β-synthase deficiency)	AR	Pancreatitis with pseudocyst formation	Marfanoid habitus, ectopia lentis, osteoporosis, arterial and venous thromboembolic events, elevated urine methionine and homocystine

AD, autosomal dominant; AR, autosomal recessive; XLR, X-linked recessive.

erozygotes have about 10% to 20% of the normal levels of C1 inhibitor rather than the expected 50%, possibly because of complex formation of the activated C1 inhibitor and activated C1 or because of increased catabolism of the protein.[136] Androgens are effective in stimulating increased synthesis of C1 inhibitor from the normal allele and are useful for prophylaxis against attacks. Concentrates of C1 inhibitor are useful in acute attacks.[137]

The C1 inhibitor gene has been localized to chromosome 11p.[138] Two clinically indistinguishable types of hereditary angioneurotic edema are described. Type 1 patients have a deletion of the C1 inhibitor gene or a truncated transcript, and type 2 patients have a single base substitution.

Hereditary Fructose Intolerance

Hereditary fructose intolerance (HFI) is an autosomal recessive disorder caused by a deficiency of aldolase B (i.e., fructose-1-phosphate aldolase). This enzyme is expressed in tissues that metabolize fructose: the liver, kidney, and small intestine. It catalyzes the reversible cleavage of fructose-1-phosphate into dihydroxyacetone phosphate and glyceraldehyde. After fructose, sorbitol, or sucrose ingestion, patients with HFI present with severe abdominal pain, vomiting, and hypoglycemia. Liver and kidney damage, growth retardation, coma, and even death may result from chronic ingestion of fructose. Most patients with HFI learn to avoid fructose-containing foods. Problems arise when they are unable to avoid them, as during infancy, or if given intravenous infusions containing fructose or sorbitol, a practice used in some European countries.[139] Intravenous fructose loading tests and measurement of aldolase B activity in liver biopsy specimens are methods used for the diagnosis of HFI.

The aldolase B gene (*ALDOB*) has been localized to chromosome 9q. It consists of 9 exons that code for 363 amino acids. At least 10 mutations have been described; three missense mutations of A149P, A147D, and N334K account for 87% of alleles in the European HFI population and 68% in the North American population.[140] The A149P mutation is the most common and widespread, accounting for 58% of HFI alleles in Europe and 55% in North America. Linkage studies suggest that the A149P allele arose once during evolution and spread through the mechanism of genetic drift, rather than occurring several times in different populations. Testing for the common mutations with amplified DNA specimens against a panel of allele-specific oligonucleotides would be an appropriate initial diagnostic approach that could identify most patients in a noninvasive manner.

Hereditary Pancreatitis Syndromes

Hereditary pancreatitis is a genetic disorder that is similar clinically to nonfamilial chronic pancreatitis. It is characterized by steatorrhea and recurrent attacks of severe abdominal pain, fever, and marked elevation of serum amylase levels. The elevated amylase level differentiates the disorder from FMF. The mean age at onset is 13 years. Between 5% and 10% of affected persons have pancreatic insufficiency, diabetes,

and pseudocysts. As in nonsyndromic pancreatitis, the attacks can be precipitated by emotional stress, alcohol, or a diet rich in fat. The disorder is autosomal dominant with 80% penetrance.[141]

Genetic syndromes involving obstruction of the pancreatic duct, such as secretory pancreatic stone protein deficiency, familial hypertrophy of the sphincter of Oddi or sclerosing cholangitis, pancreatitis, and sicca complex, can present as cases of familial or recurrent pancreatitis. Recurrent pancreatitis due to a submucosal ampullary tumor has also been described in a patient with neurofibromatosis.[142] Cases of hereditary or recurrent pancreatitis may be caused by genetic disorders of triglyceride metabolism, leading to hypertriglyceridemia, such as lipoprotein lipase deficiency, apolipoprotein C-II deficiency, and familial hypertriglyceridemia (see Table 108-6).

GASTROINTESTINAL NEOPLASM SYNDROMES

An exciting and important contribution of genetics to oncology and gastroenterology has been the realization that there is a strong heritable component to many GI malignancies. The significance of this finding is the possibility of presymptomatic screening and early treatment for prevention of malignancy in at-risk relatives of affected individuals. The clinical features of GI malignancies and familial polyposis are covered in many other chapters of this volume. Genetic syndromes that are associated with increased risks for GI tract neoplasms are listed in Table 108-7.

Common Gastrointestinal Disorders With Complex Genetic Causes

In addition to the many single mendelian inherited genetic disorders with GI manifestations previously reviewed in this chapter, there are several common GI disorders whose genetic susceptibilities are inherited in a more complex mode. These disorders include pernicious anemia, celiac disease, inflammatory bowel disease, gallstone disease, peptic ulcer, and colon cancer. Colon cancer and the genetics of peptic ulcer are reviewed in Chapters 86, 87, and 49. The remaining four groups of diseases are discussed in this section.

Common diseases often show familial aggregation caused by genetic factors or the combination of genetic and environmental factors. They also exhibit associations with certain genetic markers. Studies of family aggregation, twin data, subclinical markers, and genetic markers have been essential in demonstrating the importance of genetic determinants in the development of these common diseases.

PERNICIOUS ANEMIA AND ATROPHIC GASTRITIS

Pernicious anemia is characterized by megaloblastic anemia caused by an atrophic gastropathy that leads to deficient intrinsic factor secretion and eventual vitamin B_{12} deficiency. Vitamin B_{12} is a compound required for normal hematopoiesis

and functioning of the central nervous system. To be absorbed, it must attach to a specific carrier protein called intrinsic factor, which comes from the gastric parietal cells. The complex of intrinsic factor and B_{12} is taken up by receptors in the ileum, where the vitamin B_{12} attaches to another carrier protein called transcobalamin II, which enters the bloodstream.[143-145]

The importance of vitamin B_{12} derives from its role as a cofactor in two reactions: the synthesis of methionine from homocystine and the conversion of methylmalonic acid to succinic acid. An inadequate supply of methionine leads to inadequate formate formation, which is necessary for the methylation of deoxyuridine to form thymidine.

Almost all causes of vitamin B_{12} deficiency have a genetic basis. They include impaired vitamin B_{12} absorption due to a lack of normal intrinsic factor, impaired absorption in the ileum, or impaired transport mechanisms for the ileum to the bloodstream.[143-145] The vitamin B_{12} deficiency results in a failure of the marrow cells to respond properly to folic acid, and immature and abnormal red cells are produced, resulting in a characteristic morphologic pattern called megaloblastic anemia.

The most common cause of pernicious anemia is a familial type of atrophic gastritis of the fundic gland mucosa of the stomach.[143,146] This type A atrophic gastritis is differentiated

TABLE 108-7
Intestinal Neoplasm Syndromes

CONDITION	INHERITANCE PATTERN	GASTROINTESTINAL MANIFESTATIONS	OTHER FEATURES AND COMMENTS
Keratosis palmaris et plantaris with esophageal cancer	AD	Esophageal cancer	Palms and soles are diffusely hyperkeratotic; onset in first year of life; low serum vitamin A level in some cases; distinct from keratosis palmaris et plantaris familiaris because of the esophageal cancer association
Dyskeratosis congenita	XLR, AD	Leukoplakia of the oral mucosa and sometimes of anal mucosa	Cutaneous pigmentation, continuous lacrimation due to atresia of the lacrimal ducts, nail dystrophy, testicular atrophy, thrombocytopenia and anemia, opportunistic infections
Neurofibromatosis type 1 (NF1)	AD	Malignant degeneration of intestinal neurofibromas, duodenal carcinoid containing somatostatin	Multiple café au lait macules, neurofibromas, axillary and inguinal feckling, multiple Lisch nodules, optic gliomas, bony dysplasia of the sphenoid and long bones; associated neoplasms include pheochromocytoma, meningiomas and malignant degeneration of neurofibromas
Neurofibromatosis type 3 (NF3)	AD	Malignant degeneration of intestinal neurofibromas	None of the other features seen in NF1
Carney's triad	?AD	Gastric leiomyosarcomas	Pulmonary chondromas and paraganglionomas; all cases are sporadic
Basal cell nevus syndrome (Gorlin-Goltz syndrome)	AD	Hamartomas of the stomach	Many basal cell nevi usually appear at puberty, rarely at birth. Basal cell nevi may develop at sites of therapeutic amounts of ionizing radiation. Associated neoplasms include medulloblastoma, astrocytoma, and ovarian fibroma. Other features include mild prognathism, lateral displacement of the inner canthi, frontal and biparietal bossing, odontogenic keratocysts of the jaw, kyphoscoliosis, abnormal cervical spine, calcified falx cerebri, short fourth metacarpal, and palmar and plantar pits
Cowden's syndrome	AD	Hamartomatous polyps of the intestines	Multiple hamartomas of the skin, mucous membranes, breast, and thyroid; verrucous skin lesions of the face and limbs; papules of the gingiva and buccal mucosa, multiple facial trichilemmomas, macrocephaly; females have high frequency of breast cancer
Cronkhite-Canada syndrome	?AD	Intestinal polyposis	Diffuse skin hyperpigmentation, alopecia, fingernail changes; all cases sporadic with no proof of genetic basis; possible phenocopy for the genetic polyposis syndromes
Multiple lipomatosis	AD	Gastrointestinal lipomas	Multiple subcutaneous lipomas, cytogenetic abnormalities within the lipomas is common. If chromosome 12q13-q14 is involved, there is a tendency for malignant degeneration.
Multiple endocrine neoplasia type 1 (MEN1)	AD	Severe peptic ulcer disease due to Zollinger-Ellison syndrome secondary to gastrinoma; duodenal carcinoid in some cases	Triad of pancreatic (i.e., insulinomas, gastrinomas), parathyroid, and pituitary adenomas; intrafamilial uniformity of tumor types usual; MEN2 lacks pancreatic adenomas and has pheochromocytomas; MEN1 disease gene localized to chromosome 11q
Multiple endocrine neoplasia type 3 (MEN3 or MEN2b)	?AD	Multiple true neuromas throughout the GI tract; megacolon and colonic diverticulosis common; duodenal carcinoid in some cases	Hypertrophy of lips and thickened eyelids from neuroma, pheochromocytoma, medullary thyroid cancer; prophylactic thyroidectomy indicated; no parathyroid disease; disease gene is localized to chromosome 10
Intestinal carcinoid	?AD	Familial incidences of appendiceal and ileal carcinoid reported	Duodenal carcinoid seen in MEN1, MEN3, and NF1
Pancreatic carcinoma	?AR	Pancreatic acinar carcinoma	No history of pancreatitis or tumors at other sites
Von-Hippel-Lindau disease	AD	Pancreatic cysts and pancreatic carcinoma	Cardinal features are angiomata of the retina and hemangioblastoma of the cerebellum. Other features include hypertension due to pheochromocytoma; hypernephroma-like renal tumors; polycyethemia due

(continued)

TABLE 108-7. *(Continued)*

CONDITION	INHERITANCE PATTERN	GASTROINTESTINAL MANIFESTATIONS	OTHER FEATURES AND COMMENTS
			to renal tumor or cerebellar hemangioblastoma; hemangiomas of the spinal cord, lungs, and adrenals; cysts of the pancreas, liver, and kidneys; and epididymal cystadenomas. The gene has been mapped to chromosome 3p, and direct mutational analysis is available in about 15% of cases.
Ataxia-telangiectasia (AT)	AR	Pancreatic carcinoma	Progressive cerebellar ataxia; telangiectases, especially of the conjunctiva; susceptibility to sinopulmonary infection, oculomotor apraxia; strong predisposition to malignancy, especially leukemias. Heterozygotes for AT are also at an increased risk for malignancy. Women heterozygotes exposed to certain types of ionizing radiation are at increased risk for breast cancer. The disease gene maps to chromosome 11q.
Muir-Torre syndrome	AD	Multiple, primary, carcinomata of the colon, duodenum, and larynx	Keratoacanthomata of the face, multiple sebaceous tumors

AD, autosomal dominant; AR, autosomal recessive; XLR, X-linked recessive.

by primary involvement of the fundic gland mucosa with essential sparing of the gastric antrum. It is commonly accompanied by evidence of immunologic derangements, such as the presence of autoantibodies against the parietal cell and intrinsic factor in sera and gastric juice.[143,147] In addition to humoral antibody in sera and gastric juice, cell-mediated immunity directed against intrinsic factor can be demonstrated in most pernicious anemia patients.[143] The destruction of parietal cells by the inflammatory process results in a lack of acid secretion and impaired intrinsic factor production. The autoantibodies can also directly interfere with intrinsic factor production or binding. There is less binding of intrinsic factor with dietary vitamin B_{12} in the stomach. As a consequence, less intrinsic factor–B_{12} complex presents to the specific receptors in the terminal ileum, absorption is impaired, and vitamin B deficiency results.

The incidence of pernicious anemia is age related; most cases occur after 40 years of age. The prevalence of pernicious anemia has been estimated to be 127 cases for 100,000 members of the population in the United Kingdom, Denmark, and Sweden. Adequate data are not available elsewhere, but it seems to be most common among persons of Northern European descent. About 20% to 30% of pernicious anemia patients have a positive family history of the disease.[143] Relatives of patients with pernicious anemia may have a 20-fold increased risk of developing the disease compared with the general population.[143] Besides the increased familial aggregation of clinical pernicious anemia, further evidence for a genetic component to the severe atrophic gastritis is the increased frequency in relatives of subclinical abnormalities such as parietal cell antibodies, atrophic gastritis on biopsy, low or absent gastric acid secretion, an elevated serum gastrin level, a low serum pepsinogen I level, and a low serum pepsinogen I : II ratio.[148,149]

The familial aggregation of the type A atrophic gastritis is most consistent with a dominant inheritance pattern.[150] The association of pernicious anemia with HLA is less strong than for other autoimmune disorders. It has been reported that the HLA-DR2 and possibly DR5 are associated with pernicious anemia.[151,152]

The clinical implications of the genetic nature of pernicious anemia or atrophic gastritis are twofold. First, the affected person is at risk for other autoimmune disorders, most commonly autoimmune thyroid disease.[143,146,147] Second, the first-degree relatives are at risk for autoimmune thyroid disease and atrophic gastritis. Relatives can be screened by endoscopic biopsy, assessment of gastric acid secretion, or measurement of serum gastrin, pepsinogen I, and pepsinogen II.[148] Because the type A gastritis of pernicious anemia affects primarily the oxyntic gland mucosa of the gastric fundus and spares the antrum, the serum pepsinogen I level, which reflects the chief cell mass, is usually greatly reduced. However, because the antrum is spared, the serum pepsinogen II level, which originates from cells in the fundus and antrum, is maintained. In addition, lack of acid results in lack of inhibitory feedback to the G cells of the antrum and therefore in a rise in serum gastrin levels. The serum pepsinogen I : II ratio has the greatest screening efficiency for atrophic gastritis, but the serum gastrin and pepsinogen I levels may be used as well.[148] These tests may be used to determine which family members have atrophic gastritis, and these persons should have their serum vitamin B_{12} levels measured to detect the earliest deficiencies and to determine when they should be treated.

Other genetically determined causes of vitamin B_{12} deficiency occur much earlier in life. A lack of vitamin B_{12} absorption occurs in cases of congenital intrinsic factor deficiency because of the absence of intrinsic factor or presence of a biologically inert intrinsic factor and in cases of congenital selective vitamin B_{12} malabsorption (i.e., Imerslund-Grasbeck syndrome), apparently because of a defect in the ileal receptor for intrinsic factor–B_{12} complex.

These syndromes are autosomal recessive in their inheritance pattern, and none is accompanied by atrophic gastritis.

In congenital intrinsic factor deficiency, children develop

normally for a year and then show clinical stigmata of megaloblastic anemia, with irritability, constipation or diarrhea, pallor, anorexia, organomegaly, and diminished deep tendon reflexes.[145,153] Vitamin B_{12} levels are very low. The clinical signs return to normal with the administration of intrinsic factor orally or vitamin B_{12} parenterally. Congenital intrinsic factor deficiency due to the production of biologically inert intrinsic factor is clinically similar to congenital intrinsic factor deficiency.

Patients with Imerslund-Gräsbeck syndrome present at any time between 2 and 15 years of age with pallor, weakness, irritability, vomiting, pyrexia, glossitis, and constipation.[144,154,155] Megaloblastic anemia, leukopenia, and thrombocytopenia are found. Serum vitamin B_{12} levels are very low, and folic acid levels are usually normal. Investigation reveals impaired intestinal absorption of vitamin B_{12} that is not corrected by the addition of more intrinsic factor.[145] More than 90% of patients also have proteinuria that is not correctable by the administration of parenteral vitamin B_{12}. The treatment consists of monthly intramuscular doses of 250 μg of hydroxocobalamin or intramuscular doses every 2 to 3 months of 1000 μg of hydroxycobalamin. Because mental retardation may ensue from delay or lack of treatment, the siblings of an affected person should be screened.

GLUTEN-SENSITIVE ENTEROPATHY

Celiac disease or gluten-sensitive enteropathy (GSE) is a small intestinal malabsorptive disorder caused by atrophy of the small intestinal villi associated with gluten ingestion. GSE is a state of abnormal immunity to gluten and related prolamins that appears restricted to genetically predisposed individuals.[156] From a number of studies, it has become apparent that 50% to 60% of individuals with this condition may be clinically asymptomatic or latent. The term *gluten sensitivity* has been suggested, to embrace all persons with typical and atypical presentations, all cases of dermatitis herpetiformis (i.e., skin lesions associated with GSE), and those with latent disease.[157] The concept of clinically silent celiac disease is important in the genetic studies of the disease, because the identification of all individuals with disease susceptibility genes is necessary to determine the penetrance of the disease susceptibility gene(s) and to understand the mode of inheritance. Celiac disease occurs largely in Caucasians, with an especially high incidence among those of Irish descent. The incidence is 1 in 1000 to 2000 in Great Britain, 1 in 1000 in Sweden and Norway, and as much as 1 in 600 in Western Ireland.[158]

This disorder has a strong familial aggregation.[159] Reported estimates of the prevalence of celiac disease in first-degree relatives vary from 2%[160] to more than 20%,[161,162] with most ranging between 10% and 12%. The large variation observed in these estimates conceivably results from genetic and environmental heterogeneity among populations and from the differences among the studies, including variations in the sampling schemes (i.e. which relatives are investigated and how they were selected), in the screening procedures (i.e., whether clinical, hematologic, biochemical, and immunologic screening procedures or intestinal biopsy were used), and in diagnostic criteria. Familial aggregation has also been demonstrated for subclinical features, including measurements of circulating antigliadin and antiendomysial antibodies,[163] intestinal permeability,[164] and intestinal biopsy.[159]

The dramatic familial aggregation and the reported high concordance rate (approximately 70%) among monozygotic twins supports the concept that celiac disease is a heritable disorder.[165] For two decades, it has been recognized that celiac disease occurs much more frequently in individuals having certain HLA alleles. The concordance rate among HLA-identical siblings is about 30%, suggesting that a substantial part of the genetic susceptibility maps to the HLA gene complex.[166] However, the different concordance rate between monozygotic twins and HLA identical siblings indicate that other genes, unlinked to HLA, may be required for the development of the disease.[167-169] The mode of inheritance in the HLA region is not fully understood, even though dominant and recessive have been proposed.[170,171] This is probably a result of the underlying complexity of the interactions of different HLA class II gene products.

Initially, celiac disease was observed to be associated with the HLA class I, B locus marker B8, as defined by serologic results.[172] Later, it was recognized that celiac disease had a stronger association with the class II D region marker, HLA-DR3. The association with B8 appeared to primarily reflect strong linkage disequilibrium between the allele that encodes HLA-B8 and the allele that encodes HLA-DR3. (B8 and DR3 are found on the same chromosomes in the population more frequently than just by chance alone. Persons who have DR3 often have B8). The association between celiac disease and DR3 has been found in all studied populations.[173] An association of HLA-DR7 with celiac disease has been observed if it is in conjunction with HLA-DR3 or HLA-DR5.[166] An analytic review of the data indicates that, in all populations studied, most celiac disease patients have DR3 or are heterozygous for DR5/DR7, and only a few (<10%) are neither DR3 nor DR5/DR7.[174]

Further advances have shown that HLA-DQ2, an HLA class II molecule at the nearby DQ locus in linkage disequilibrium with DR3 and DR7, has an even stronger association with celiac disease.[175] Sequencing of HLA-DQ genes has shown that the DR3-DQ2 haplotype (i.e., a haplotype is one set of markers on one chromosome) carries the *DQA1*0501* and *DQB1*0201* alleles (i.e., alleles determined at the DNA level).[176,177] The DR5-DQ7 haplotype carries the *DQA1*0501* and *DQB1*0301* alleles,[178] and the DR7-DQ2 haplotype carries the *DQA1*0201* and *DQB1*0201* alleles.[179,180] It has been suggested that celiac disease is primarily associated with a particular HLA-DQ $\alpha\beta$ heterodimer, DQ($\alpha 1*0501$, $\beta 1*0201$), that is encoded in the *cis* position on the same chromosome, such as DR3-DQ2, or in the *trans* position on opposite chromosomes, such as DR5-DQ7/DR7-DQ2 (Table 108-8).[174,181] This heterodimer hypothesis was tested by generating alloreactive T-cell clones.[182] These T-cell clones recognized the DQ($\alpha 1*0501$, $\beta 1*0201$) molecule when encoded by cells carrying the *DQA1*0501* and *DQB1*0201* genes in *cis* position (i.e., DR3-DQ2) or in trans position (i.e., DR5-DQ7/DR7-DQ2). Later, similar findings were made using gliadin-reactive T cells.[183]

However, only a small proportion of the individuals who have the appropriate HLA-DQ($\alpha 1*0501$, $\beta 1*0201$) molecule

TABLE 108-8
DQ(α1*0501, β1*0201) Heterodimer Associated With Gluten-Sensitive Enteropathy Encoded in *cis* or in *trans* Positions of the HLA-DQ Molecule

ENCODED IN *cis*			ENCODED IN *trans*		
β DQB1	α DQA1	Class II Haplotype	β DQB1	α DQA1	Class II Haplotype
0201	**0501**	DR3-DQ2	0301	**0501**	DR5-DQ7
			0201	0201	DR7-DQ2

develop celiac disease. This suggests that non-HLA genes contribute to the development of the disease. The observation of discordant twin pairs also suggests a role of environmental factors, although stochastic variation in the immune system is an alternative explanation for discordant twins with autoimmune diseases.

Although the response of the small intestine biopsy specimen to gluten withdrawal and challenge is the gold standard for diagnosis, the presence of the DQ(α1*0501, β1*0201) molecule may serve as a additional supporting diagnostic marker. Such HLA typing can be used as the first step in screening potential at-risk relatives, because the risk of celiac disease in relatives of patients is correlated with the sharing of specific HLA alleles.[184] As reviewed by Strober,[159] based on the observed data[166] and estimated risks,[184] the risk of a sibling of a celiac patient having celiac disease is about 10%. However, if the sibling is HLA identical with the celiac patient (i.e., shares both HLA haplotypes from each of the two chromosomes), the risk increases to at least 30%. If the sibling is totally HLA nonidentical (i.e., has no HLA haplotypes in common), the risk is 1% or less. If the sibling shares one HLA haplotype but has HLA-DR3 in the unshared haplotype, the risk may approach that of full identity (30%). With non-HLA-DR3 in the unshared haplotype, the risk falls to low levels (<5%).

Although more such families studies are needed, especially with HLA molecular typing, the differential risks among relatives with various HLA types warrant the use of HLA typing to determine which family members should undergo examination for the presence of subclinical disease. HLA-identical siblings of patients and relatives of celiac disease patients who have the DQ(α1*0501, β1*0201) molecule should perhaps be studied vigorously (e.g., with jejunal biopsy), and other asymptomatic relatives may only need to be followed by screening of serum antibodies. Besides allowing treatment of subclinical malabsorption, early detection and treatment of celiac disease in asymptomatic individuals may be beneficial in reducing the incidence of malignancies in these patients.[185]

INFLAMMATORY BOWEL DISEASE

There is ample evidence that the inflammatory bowel diseases (IBD), which include Crohn's disease and ulcerative colitis, are in large part determined by genetic predispositions. The supporting lines of evidence include ethnic differences in disease frequency, familial aggregation, an increased monozygotic twin concordance rate compared with that in dizygotic twins, the existence of genetic syndromes that feature IBD, and associations between IBD and genetic markers.[186,187]

There are large differences in IBD frequency among various ethnic groups. Although environmental and genetic explanations may appear equally plausible, an important finding is the repeated observations that the incidence in the Jewish population is consistently higher than the rates for other ethnic groups in the same geographic locations.[188] That the Jewish and non-Jewish differences occur across different periods and different geographic areas strongly suggests the existence of a genetic predisposition as the most parsimonious explanation.[189]

Familial aggregation is clearly increased in IBD, although the data fit no simple mendelian pattern of inheritance (Table 108-9). There is an approximate 10- to 30-fold increase in the disease prevalence among siblings compared with community-wide prevalence.[189,190] The rate of ulcerative colitis is increased among the relatives of ulcerative colitis patients, and Crohn's disease is increased among the relatives of Crohn's disease patients. However, the two diseases do exist in the same family with a frequency higher than that explained by chance alone, suggesting an etiologic association between ulcerative colitis and Crohn's disease.[191] It has been observed that a positive family history is somewhat more likely among Crohn's disease patients than among ulcerative colitis patients[186,189] and that the relatives of Crohn's disease patients have a higher risk for IBD than those of ulcerative colitis patients.[191,192] This suggests that Crohn's disease is to some degree more often familial than ulcerative colitis and may indicate a more important role for genetic predisposition in this form of IBD.

The aggregated twin data indicate that there is a higher concordance rate for monozygotic twins than for dizygotic twins in Crohn's disease and ulcerative colitis. The higher concordance rate in monozygotic twins than in dizygotic twins supports the argument that genetic factors are an important component in the development of IBD. Although familial aggregation can be the result of environmental factors alone, the increased monozygotic twin concordance rates, the rarity of IBD concordance in spouses,[189] and the numerous instances of affected relatives whose disease onset is completely separated geographically and temporally from other affected family members[193] argue for a major genetic component to disease susceptibility.

TABLE 108-9
Inferences Regarding Inflammatory Bowel Disease Family Aggregation

EVIDENCE	INFERENCE
IBD exhibits familial aggregation	Increased risk factors within families
Twin concordance, MZ > DZ; no increase in spouses	Genetic factors responsible for familial aggregation
Positive family history in CD > UC; twin concordance; CD > UC	CD more genetic or more deterministic; UC may be more stochastic and may be more immunologic
Each form occurs in families of other	Some genetic aspects of CD and UC are shared
No mixed IBD (UC and CD) MZ twin pairs	Some genetic aspects of CD and UC are distinct
Familial risks are much greater than expected under polygenic model	Genetic susceptibility not polygenic
Familial risks in Jews > familial risks in neighboring non-Jews	Genetic susceptibility not simple mendelian pattern
Non-Jewish families have proportionally more mixed IBD than Jewish families	Mixed IBD not a simple overlap, but possibly a different disease (i.e., genetic heterogeneity)
Clinical features concordant in CD families	Genetic heterogeneity within CD
Greatly increased risks to offspring when both parents have IBD	Limited number of disease genes
DZ twin concordance rate equals sibling risk	Environmental factors are probably macroenvironmental

CD, Crohn's disease; DZ, dizygotic; IBD, inflammatory bowel disease; MZ, monozygotic; UC, ulcerative colitis.

IBD is also associated with three well-defined genetic syndromes: Turner syndrome, which results from the lack of all or part of one of the X chromosomes; the autosomal recessive Hermansky-Pudlak syndrome, which manifests as oculocutaneous albinism with a defect in the second phase of platelet aggregation, producing a bleeding diathesis and ceroid-like pigment accumulation; and the glycogen storage disease type 1b, which generates neutropenia and abnormal neutrophil function.[186,194,195] IBD has been less dramatically associated with several rare syndromes involving immunodeficiency (Table 108-10).[186] Studies of rare syndromes associated with IBD suggest that a variety of immunodeficiency states, autoimmune diseases, and miscellaneous genetic syndromes appear to increase the risk for IBD. Studies of elements of the immune pathways may be useful in understanding the etiopathogenesis of some forms of IBD.

One approach used to identify genes for IBD is the study of subclinical markers, which are pathophysiologic abnormalities found in patients and in their relatives. The best-studied subclinical markers have been antineutrophil cytoplasmic antibodies (ANCAs) in ulcerative colitis and intestinal permeability in Crohn's disease. Intestinal permeability has

TABLE 108-10
Genetic Syndromes With Inflammatory Bowel Disease

Turner's syndrome
Hermansky-Pudlak syndrome
Glycogen storage disease type Ib
Immunodeficiency disorders
    Secretory immunoglobulin deficiency
    Agammaglobulinemia or hypogammaglobulinemia
    Selective IgA deficiency
    Chediak-Higashi syndrome
    Deficiency of C2
    Hereditary angioedema

been examined in several family studies of Crohn's patients, and the summary data suggest abnormalities in a subset of at-risk relatives.[196,197]

ANCAs were first observed as an important marker in Wegener granulomatosis in 1985. In 1990, a distinct ANCA subset was found to be associated with ulcerative colitis.[198] The prevalence of positive ANCA results for patients with ulcerative colitis ranges from 50% to 86%.[189] This ulcerative colitis–associated ANCA has a perinuclear immunofluorescence binding pattern that is different from other ANCAs, such as the granular cytoplasmic pattern in Wegener's granulomatosis and the nuclear staining in systemic lupus erythematosus. There has not been any detectable difference in the level of ANCA binding between ulcerative colitis patients with rectosigmoid disease and those with pancolitis or between patients with active disease and those with inactive colitis.[198,199] ANCAs have also been found in patients with ulcerative colitis after colectomy. This antibody is highly specific for ulcerative colitis compared with other forms of colitis, including that of Crohn's colitis.[200] ANCAs are more commonly found in the clinically healthy relatives of ulcerative colitis patients than in environmentally and ethnically matched controls.[201]

The cumulative observations of constancy, specificity, and increased prevalence in unaffected relatives suggest that ANCAs are not simply an epiphenomenon related to active colonic inflammation. These data suggest that the presence of ANCAs in patients with ulcerative colitis may reflect a fundamental disturbance of immune regulation. The ulcerative colitis–specific antibody has a familial distribution; the relatives of ANCA-positive ulcerative colitis patients are more likely to have the ANCA than the relatives of ANCA-negative ulcerative colitis patients.[201] This familial distribution of ANCA has been investigated using genetic markers.[202]

Genetic marker studies provide one approach to identifying the genes that predispose to IBD. Because of the immunogenic feature of the disease, HLA class II genes are considered to be the primary candidates for the genetic studies of IBD because they are crucial in antigen recognition, fundamental to the immune response, and associated with various autoimmune diseases. Although there is still a relative lack of studies of the HLA class II (i.e., DR, DQ, and DP) region, some interesting results emerge when the data are reviewed in aggregate. In the Japanese, all available studies show a significant association of HLA-DR2 with ulcerative colitis.[189] In Caucasians, an increased incidence of DR2 among ulcerative colitis patients was observed in most studies, with a significant association observed in the most recent ethnically matched case-control study conducted with a combination of serologic and molecular methods.[203] The consistent, significant DR2 association in the Japanese is of interest. If there is genetic etiologic heterogeneity within ulcerative colitis, it would be expected that heterogeneity is minimized in a more homogeneous population such as the Japanese. The limited sample size in some of the Caucasian studies and population heterogeneity may also explain the inconsistent results from studies of the Caucasian population. Besides the positive association with DR2, ulcerative colitis was also found to be negatively associated with DR4 in the ethnically matched study[203] and in the Japanese studies.[204,205]

Even within ulcerative colitis patients from the same ethnic background, there is genetic heterogeneity in the HLA class II associations stratified by the presence or absence of ANCA. The positive association for DR2 and ulcerative colitis and the negative association for DR4 and ulcerative colitis were mainly contributed by the ulcerative colitis patients with ANCAs.[202] The familial distribution of ANCA appears to be determined in a significant fashion by the gene variation in the HLA class II region.

For Crohn's disease, a dramatic increase in DR4 has been reported in the Japanese population, and less dramatic increases of DR4 were found in some Caucasian populations.[189] Using a combination of molecular and serologic techniques and carefully selected ethnically matched controls, an increased frequency of the DR1-DQ5 combination was observed.[203] The DR1-DQ5 haplotype association was further identified by a specific suballele of DQ5(DQB1*0501). Investigators in Pittsburgh independently reported a positive association of DQ5 with CD, further supporting this specific HLA class II gene association with Crohn's disease.[206] If these results hold, the associated HLA class II gene (i.e., DR1/DQ5 or DR4) itself is unlikely to be the disease susceptibility gene, but the results indicate that the disease susceptibility gene is in linkage disequilibrium with other, more specific IBD susceptibility genes within the HLA complex.

The HLA antigens may not be specific enough to detect distinct differences between IBD patients and control groups. Further molecular studies of the associations of ulcerative colitis with DR2 and Crohn's disease with DR4 or DR1-DQ5 are needed to identify the specific suballeles associated with these diseases.

The polygenic or multifactorial model of inheritance appears incompatible with the available family data, and a major gene contribution has been suggested in ulcerative colitis and Crohn's disease (see Table 108-9).[189] However, with available familial empiric risk data, mendelian single-gene models for IBD in general and for ulcerative colitis and Crohn's disease individually also can be rejected. The clearest evidence is the observation of significantly different lifetime familial risks for IBD overall and for ulcerative colitis and Crohn's disease individually between relatives of Jewish patients and relatives of non-Jewish patients.[191] The most likely and workable model for IBD genetic susceptibility is that of genetic heterogeneity.[207-209] The concept of genetic heterogeneity considers IBD as several etiologically and genetically distinct diseases presenting a similar clinical picture rather than as a single disease. The HLA class II association data support this model, because ulcerative colitis and Crohn's disease have distinct HLA class II associations. Even ulcerative colitis patients with ANCAs have different HLA associations than patients without these antibodies.

For counseling purposes, the available empiric risk estimates from several studies suggest that the risk of developing IBD for siblings is between 2% and 5%, the risk for parents is between 1% and 5%, and the risk for offspring is between 1% and 4%.[189] When a modified life table approach is used to calculate lifetime empiric risks for IBD, the results suggest that the lifetime risks for siblings and offspring of developing IBD may be as high as 8% to 9% among Jews[191,192] and 4% among non-Jews.[191] The knowledge obtained from subclinical marker (e.g., ANCAs) and genetic marker (e.g., HLA class II genes) studies will probably provide the basis for new therapies, leading to methods of cure and prevention for these debilitating GI diseases.

GALLSTONES

Gallstone disease is an excellent example of a genetically heterogeneous disorder. Although most gallstones are composed of bile supersaturated with cholesterol, some are caused by excess cholesterol and others by undersecretion of bile acids. One of the important lines of evidence suggesting the importance of genetic factors in gallstone disease has been the large variations in incidence among ethnic groups; the rate of gallstone disease is especially high in Mexican Americans and Native Americans.[210-212] In a comprehensive epidemiologic study, Mexican Americans were found to be at increased risk of gallstone disease even when other risk factors, such as age, education, skin fold measures, diabetes, impaired glucose tolerance, and oral contraceptive usage, were controlled in multiple logistic regression analysis.[212]

Familial aggregation of gallstone disease has been observed in many populations.[213,214] One difficulty in assessing the role of genetic factors in such a common disease is that there is a fairly high likelihood that the relative of a patient could be affected by chance alone or by family-shared environmental factors (e.g., diet) and not because of a genetic factor. However, well-controlled studies comparing siblings and spouses of affected patients have shown that there is familial clustering of the disease that is probably caused by genetic factors; siblings are affected much more commonly than the spouses of the same sex.[214,215] Further supportive evidence for genetic factors is provided by a Danish study of twin pairs surviving to the age of 40, which showed concordance for 14 of 25 monozygotic pairs but concordance for only 6 of 40 pairs of like-sexed dizygotic twins.[215]

Genetic studies of gallstone disease have encountered the problem of silent disease. Necropsy studies have shown that about half of the cases of gallstone disease are unrecognized during life, and clinical studies alone underestimate the degree of family aggregation. Studies using oral cholecystography have shown that the incidence of silent gallstones is also increased among family members.[216]. Studies of biliary lipid composition in siblings and twins further indicate that the contributing factors to gallstone formation, such as molar percentage of biliary cholesterol, bile acid composition, cholesterol synthesis, and bile cholesterol saturation, are under significant genetic control.[217,218]

There are a limited number of genetic marker studies in gallstone disease. ABO blood groups are associated with various diseases and with metabolic processes, including cholesterol metabolism.[219] In an ABO blood group and gallstone study, although there seemed to be no overall association with any specific ABO allele, symptomatic gallstone disease patients with blood group A had more stones with less than 25% cholesterol or with no cholesterol than patients with other blood groups.[220] The incidence of cholesterol stones (49%) in group A patients was lower than the average of cholesterol stones observed in Western countries (70%–80% of all symptomatic gallstones). The significance of this observation needs to be evaluated.

The incidence of HLA-A19 was increased among patients with cholesterol gallstones and with a family history of the disease, but it was not increased among patients with non-cholesterol gallstones or those without a family history of disease.[221] It was shown that apolipoprotein E polymorphism affects the cholesterol content of gallstones. The median cholesterol content of the gallstones was higher in the apolipoprotein E4 category than in the E3 and E2 groups of patients.[222] It was suggested that the presence of the E4 allele appeared to lead to promoting nucleation. The potential clinical application of these findings is that the knowledge of the E4 phenotype could be useful in determining whether a patient is a candidate for gallstone dissolution, because patients with high gallstone cholesterol content are particularly responsive to such therapy.

Acknowledgments

Supported in part by an NIH Program Project grant (DK46737), grants from the Stuart Foundations and the Crohn's and Colitis Foundation of America, and the Board of Governors' Chair in Medical Genetics.

The reader is directed to Chapter 49, Genetic Counseling for Gastrointestinal Patients; Chapter 72, Celiac Disease; Chapter 73, Disorders of Epithelial Transport in the Small Intestine; Chapter 79, Inflammatory Bowel Disease; Chapter 86, Polyposis Syndromes; and Chapter 94, Hereditary Diseases of the Pancreas.

REFERENCES

1. Levin B, Abraham JM, Burgess EA, Wallis PG. Congenital lactose malabsorption. Arch Dis Child 1970;45:173.
2. Mantei N, Villa M, Enzler T, et al. Complete primary structure of human and rabbit lactase-phlorizin hydrolase: implication for biosynthesis, membrane anchoring and evolution of the enzyme. EMBO J 1988;7:2705.
3. Kruse TA, Bolund L, Grzeschik K-H, et al. The human lactase-phlorizin hydrolase gene is located on chromosome 2. FEBS Lett 1988;240:123.
4. McKusick VA. Mendelian inheritance in man—catalogs of autosomal dominant, autosomal recessive, and X-linked phenotypes. 10th ed. Baltimore: Johns Hopkins University Press, 1992.
5. Paige DM, Bayless TM, eds. Lactose digestion. Clinical and nutritional implications. Baltimore: Johns Hopkins University Press, 1981.
6. Flatz G. The genetic polymorphism of lactase activity in adult humans. In: Scriver CR, Beaudet AL, Sly WS, Valle D, eds. The metabolic basis of inherited disease. 6th ed. New York: McGraw-Hill, 1989:2999.
7. Harries JT. Disorders of carbohydrate absorption. Clin Gastroenterol 1982;11:17.
8. Rahimi AG, Delbruck H, Haeckel R, Gaedde HW, Flatz G. Persistence of high intestinal lactase activity (lactose tolerance) in Afghanistan. Hum Genet 1976;34:57.
9. Potter J, Ho M-W, Bolton H, Furth AJ, Swallow DM, Griffiths B. Human lactase and the molecular basis of lactase persistence. Biochem Genet 1985;23:423.
10. Boll W, Wagner P, Mantei N. Structure of the chromosomal gene and cDNAs coding for lactase-phlorizin hydrolase in humans with adult-type hypolactasia or persistence of lactase. Am J Hum Genet 1991;48:889.
11. Montgomery RK, Buller HA, Rings EHHM, Grand RJ. Lactose intolerance and the genetic regulation of intestinal lactase-phlorizin hydrolase. FASEB J 1991;5:2824.
12. Lorenzsonn V, Lloyd M, Olsen WA. Immunocytochemical heterogeneity of lactase-phlorizin hydrolase in adult lactase deficiency. Gastroenterology 993;105:51.
13. Sahi T. Genetics and epidemiology of hypolactasia. In: Rotter JI, Samloff IM, Rimoin DL, eds. Genetics and heterogeneity of common gastrointestinal disorders. New York: Academic Press, 1980:215.
14. Russo G, Milica F, Mazzone D, Santonocito B. Congenital lactose intolerance of gastrogen origin associated with cataracts. Acta Paediatr Scand 1974;63:457.
15. Semenza G, Auricchio S. Small-intestinal disaccharidases. In: Scriver CR, Beaudet AL, Sly WS, Valle D, eds. The metabolic basis of inherited disease. 6th ed. New York: McGraw-Hill, 1989:2975.
16. Hauri H-P, Roth J, Sterchi EE, Lentze MJ. Transport to cell surface of intestinal sucrase-isomaltase is blocked in the Golgi apparatus in a patient with congenital sucrase-isomaltase deficiency. Proc Natl Acad Sci U S A 1985;82:4423.
17. Lloyd ML, Olsen WA. A study of the molecular pathology of sucrase-isomaltase deficiency: a defect in the intracellular processing of the enzyme. N Engl J Med 1987;316:438.
18. Naim HY, Roth J, Sterchi EE, et al. Sucrase-isomaltase deficiency in humans: different mutations disrupt intracellular transport, processing and function of an intestinal brush border enzyme. J Clin Invest 1988;82:667.
19. Davis MB, Green FR, West LF, Kearney A, Povey S, Swallow DM. Mapping of the gene encoding human sucrase-isomaltase (SI) to chromosome 3q25-26 (abstract). Cytogenet Cell Genet 1987;46:604.
20. Swallow DM, Islam I, Attwood J, et al. Analyses of linkage between SI (sucrase-isomaltase) and markers on chromosome 3 (abstract). Cytogenet Cell Genet 1991;58:1881.
21. Hediger MA, Coady MJ, Mohandas T, Shapiro HJ, Wright EM. The human Na/glucose cotransporter gene is located on chromosome 22 (abstract). FASEB J 1988;2:A1021.
22. Turk E, Zabel B, Mundlos S, Dyer J, Wright EM. Glucose/galactose malabsorption caused by a defect in the Na+/glucose cotransporter. Nature 1991;350:354.
23. McNair A, Gudmand-Hoyer E, Jarnum S, Orrild L. Sucrose malabsorption in Greenland. Br Med J 1972;2:19.
24. Silk DBA. Disorders of nitrogen absorption. Clin Gastroenterol 1982;11:47.
25. Scriver CR. Familial renal iminoglycinuria. In: Scriver CR, Beaudet AL, Sly WS, Valle D, eds. The metabolic basis of inherited disease. 6th ed. New York: McGraw-Hill, 1989:2529.

26. Levy HL. Hartnup disorder. In: Scriver CR, Beaudet AL, Sly WS, Valle D, eds. The metabolic basis of inherited disease. 6th ed. New York: McGraw-Hill, 1989:2515.

27. Scriver CR, Mahon B, Levy HL, et al. The Hartnup phenotype: mendelian transport disorder, multifactorial disease. Am J Hum Genet 1987;40:401.

28. Segal S, Thier SO. Cystinurias. In: Scriver CR, Beaudet AL, Sly WS, Valle D, eds. The metabolic basis of inherited disease. 6th ed. New York: McGraw-Hill, 1989:2479.

29. Simell O. Lysinuric protein intolerance and other cationic aminoacidurias. In: Scriver CR, Beaudet AL, Sly WS, Valle D, eds. The metabolic basis of inherited disease. 6th ed. New York: McGraw-Hill, 1989:2497.

30. Shaw PJ, Dale G, Bates D. Familial lysinuric protein intolerance presenting as coma in two adult siblings. J Neurol Neurosurg Psychiatry 1989;52:648.

31. Libit SA, Ulstrom RA, Doeden D. Fecal *Pseudomonas aeruginosa* as a cause of the blue diaper syndrome. J Pediatr 1972;81:546.

32. Milla PJ. Disorders of electrolyte absorption. Clin Gastroenterol 1982;11:31.

33. Cutz E, Rhoads JM, Drumm B, Sherman PM, Durie PR, Fostner GG. Microvillus inclusion disease: an inherited defect of brush-border assembly and differentiation. N Engl J Med 1989;320:646.

34. Davidson GP, Cutz E, Hamilton JR, Gall DG. Familial enteropathy: a syndrome of protracted diarrhea from birth, failure to thrive, hypoplastic villus atrophy. Gastroenterology 1978;75:783.

35. Phillips AD, Jenkins P, Raafat F, Walker-Smith JA. Congenital microvillus atrophy: specific diagnostic features. Arch Dis Child 1985;60:135.

36. Rhoads JM, Volger RC, Lacey SR, et al. Microvillus inclusion disease: in vitro jejunal electrolyte transport. Gastroenterology 1991;100:811.

37. Homberg C, Perheentupa J, Launiala K. Colonic electrolyte transport in health and in congenital chloride diarrhea. J Clin Invest 1975;56:302.

38. Gorden P, Levitin, H. Congenital alkalosis with diarrhea: a sequel to Darrow's original description. Ann Intern Med 1973;78:876.

39. Tatemichi M, Nagata H, Morinaga S, Kaneda S. Protein-losing enteropathy caused by mesenteric vascular involvement of neurofibromatosis. Dig Dis Sci 1993;38:1549.

40. Suhr O, Danielsson A, Steen L. Bile acid malabsorption caused by gastrointestinal motility dysfunction? An investigation of gastrointestinal disturbances in familial amyloidosis with polyneuropathy. Scand J Gastroenterol 1992;27:201.

41. Wallace MR, Dwulet FE, Williams EC, Conneally PM, Benson MD. Identification of a new hereditary amyloidosis prealbumin variant, Tyr-77, and detection of the gene by DNA analysis. J Clin Invest 1988;81:189.

42. Rader DJ, Brewer HB Jr. Abetalipoproteinemia: new insights into lipoprotein assembly and vitamin E metabolism from a rare genetic disease. JAMA 1993;270:865.

43. Wetterau JR, Aggerbeck LP, Bouma ME, et al. Absence of microsomal triglyceride transfer protein in individuals with abetalipoproteinemia. Science 1992;258:999.

44. Levy E, Marcel Y, Deckelbaum RJ, et al. Intestinal apoB synthesis, lipids and lipoproteins in chylomicron retention disease. J Lipid Res 1987;28:1263.

45. Pessah M, Benlian P, Beucler I, et al. Anderson's disease: genetic exclusion of the apolipoprotein-B gene in two families. J Clin Invest 1991;87:367.

46. Steinberg D, Grundy SM, Mok HYI, et al. Metabolic studies in an unusual case of asymptomatic familial hypobetalipoproteinemia with hypoalphalipoproteinemia and fasting chylomicronemia. J Clin Invest 1979;64:292.

47. Wolman M Sterk VV, Gatt S, Frenkel M. Primary family xanthomatosis with involvement and calcification of the adrenals: report of two more cases in siblings of a previously described infant. Pediatrics 1961;28:742.

48. Desai PK, Astrin KH, Thung SN, et al. Cholesteryl ester storage disease: pathologic changes in an affected fetus. Am J Med Genet 1987;26:689.

49. Koch G, Lalley PA, McAvoy M, Shows TB. Assignment of LIPA, associated with human acid lipase deficiency to human chromosome 10 and comparative assignment to mouse chromosome 19. Somatic Cell Genet 1981;7:345.

50. Tizzano EF, Buchwald M. Cystic fibrosis: beyond the gene to therapy. J Pediatr 1992;120:337.

51. Lloyd-Still JD. Textbook of cystic fibrosis. Boston: John Wright, 1983.

52. Taussig LM. Cystic fibrosis. New York: Thieme-Stratton, 1984.

53. Zentler-Munro PL. Cystic fibrosis—a gastroenterological cornucopia. Gut 1987;28:1531.

54. Shepherd RW, Cleghorn GJ. Cystic fibrosis: nutritional and intestinal disorders. Boca Raton: CRC Press, 1989.

55. Park RW, Grand RJ. Gastrointestinal manifestations of cystic fibrosis: a review. Gastroenterology 1981;81:1143.

56. Rommens JM, Ianuzzi MC, Kerem B, et al. Identification of the cystic fibrosis gene: chromosome walking and jumping. Science 1989;245:1059.

57. Anderson MP, Gregory RJ, Thompson S, et al. Demonstration that CFTR is a chloride channel by alteration of its anion selectivity. Science 1991;253:202.

58. Tsui LC, Buchwald M. Biochemical and molecular genetics of cystic fibrosis. Adv Hum Genet 1991;20:153.

59. Cystic Fibrosis Genetic Analysis Consortium. Worldwide survey of the deltaF508 mutation: report from the Cystic Fibrosis Genetic Analysis Consortium. Am J Hum Genet 1990;47:354.

60. Kristidis P, Bozon D, Corey M, et al. Genetic determination of exocrine pancreatic function in cystic fibrosis. Am J Hum Genet 1992;50:1178.

61. Trellis D, Clouse R. Johanson-Blizzard syndrome, progression of pancreatic involvement in adulthood. Dig Dis Sci 1991;36:365.

62. Burke V, Colebatch JH, Anderson CM, Simons MJ. Association of pancreatic insufficiency and chronic neutropenia in childhood. Arch Dis Child 1967;42:147.

63. Karjoo M, Koop CE, Cornfield D, Holtzapple PG. Pancreatic exocrine enzyme deficiency associated with asphyxiating thoracic dystrophy. Arch Dis Child 1973;48:143.

64. Brueton LA, Dillon MJ, Winter RM. Ellis-van Creveld syndrome, Jeune syndrome, and renal-hepatic-pancreatic dysplasia: separate entities or disease spectrum? J Med Genet 1990;27:252.

65. MacKenzie, IL Donaldson RM, Trier JS, Mathan VI. Ileal mucosa in familial selective vitamin B$_{12}$ malabsorption. N Engl J Med 1972;286:1021.

66. Broch H, Imerslund O, Monn E, Hovig T, Seip M. Imerslund-Grasbeck anemia: a long-term follow-up study. Acta Paediatr Scand 1984;73:248.

67. Menkes JH. Kinky hair disease. Pediatrics 1972;50:181.

68. Verga V, Hall BK, Wang S, Johnson S, Higgins JV, Glover TW. Localization of the translocation breakpoint in a female with Menkes syndrome to Xq13.2-q13.3 proximal to PGK-1. Am J Hum Genet 1991;48;1133.

69. Kaitila I, Peltonen L, Kuivaniemi H, Palotie A, Elo J, Kivirikko KI. A skeletal and connective tissue disorder associated with lysyl hydroxylase deficiency and abnormal copper metabolism. In: Papadatos CJ, Bartsocas CS, eds. Skeletal dysplasias. New York: Alan R Liss, 1982:307.

70. Nelder KH, Hambridge KM. Zinc therapy of acrodermatitis enteropathica. N Engl J Med 1975;292:879.

71. Mack D, Koletzko B, Cunnane S, Cutz E, Griffiths A. Acrodermatitis enterpathica with normal serum zinc levels: diagnostic value of small bowel biopsy and essential fatty acid determination. Gut 1989;30:1426.

72. Ricccardi VM. The phakomatoses. In: Emery AH, Rimoin DL, eds. Principles and practice of medical genetics. 2nd ed. New York: Churchill Livingstone, 1990:435.

73. Bolande RP. The neurocristopathies: a unifying concept of disease arising in neural crest maldevelopment. Hum Pathol 1974;5:109.

74. Ludlam CA. Congenital disorders of haemostasis. In: Emery AH, Rimoin DL, eds. Principles and practice of medical genetics. 2nd ed. New York: Churchill Livingstone, 1990:1371.

75. Valla D, Denninger M-H, Delvigne J-M, Rueff B, Benhamou

J-P. Portal vein thrombosis with ruptured oesophageal varicies as presenting manifestations of hereditary protein C deficiency. Gut 1988;29:856.

76. Awidi AS. Increased incidence of Glanzmann's thrombasthenia in Jordan as compared with Scandinavia. Scand J Haematol 1983;30:218.

77. Hagen I, Nurden A, Bjerrum OJ, Solum NO, Caen J. Immunochemical evidence for protein abnormalities from patients with Glanzmann's thrombasthenia and Bernard-Soulier syndrome. J Clin Invest 1980;65:722.

78. National Institutes of Health. Consensus Development Conference on Neurofibromatosis Report. Neurofibromatosis 1988;1:172.

79. Wallace MR, Marchuk DA, Andersen LB, et al. Type 1 neurofibromatosis gene: identification of a large transcript disrupted in three NF1 patients. Science 1990;249:181.

80. Heimann R, Verhest A, Verschraegen J, Grosjean W, Draps JP, Hecht F. Hereditary intestinal neurofibromatosis. 1. A distinctive genetic disease. Neurofibromatosis 1988;1:26.

81. Porteous MEM, Burn J, Proctor SJ. Hereditary hemorrhagic telangiectasia: a clinical analysis. J Med Genet 1992;29:527.

82. Sensi A, Abbasciano V, Balboni A, Levato F, Baricordi OR. Hereditary hemorrhagic telangiectasia (HHT) and HLA. Tissue Antigens 1986;28:275.

83. McDonald M, Papenberg K, Ghosh S, et al. Genetic linkage of hereditary hemorrhagic telangiectasia to markers on 9q (abstract). Am J Hum Genet 1993;53(Suppl 3):140.

84. Viljoen DL. Klippel-Trenaunay-Weber syndrome (angio-osteohypertrophy syndrome). J Med Genet 1988;25:250.

85. Myers BM. Treatment of colonic bleeding in Klippel-Trenaunay syndrome with combined partial colectomy and endoscopic laser. Dig Dis Sci 1993;38:1351.

86. Berlyne GM, Berlyne N. Anaemia due to "blue-rubber-bleb" naevus disease. Lancet 1960;2:1275.

87. Schofield PF, MacDonald N, Clegg JF. Familial spontaneous rupture of the colon: report of two cases. Dis Colon Rectum 1970;13:394.

88. Sokolov BP, Prytkov AN, Tromp G, Knowlton RG, Prockop DJ. Exclusion of COL1A1, COL1A2, and COL3A1 genes as candidate genes for Ehlers-Danlos syndrome type I in one large family. Hum Genet 1991;88:125.

89. Emanuel BS, Cannizzaro LA, Seyer JM, Myers JC. Human alpha-1(III) and alpha-2(V) procollagen genes are located on the long arm of chromosome 2. Proc Natl Acad Sci U S A 1985;82:3385.

90. Goodman RM. Pseudoxanthoma elasticum and related disorders. In: Emery AH, Rimoin DL, eds. Principles and practice of medical genetics. 2nd ed. New York: Churchill Livingstone, 1990:1083.

91. Agha A, Sakati NO, Higginbottom MC, Jones KL Jr, Bay C, Nyhan WL. Two forms of cutis laxa presenting in the newborn period. Acta Paediatr Scand 1978;67:775.

92. Olsen DR, Fazio MJ, Shamban AT, Rosenbloom J, Uitto J. Cutis laxa: reduced elastin gene expression in skin fibroblast cultures as determined by hybridization with a homologous cDNA and an exon 1-specific oligonucleotide. J Biol Chem 1988;263:6465.

93. Cohen MM Jr. Bannayan-Riley-Ruvalcaba syndrome: renaming three formerly recognized syndromes as one etiologic entity (letter). Am J Med Genet 1990;35:291.

94. Dvir M, Beer S, Aladjem M. Heredofamilial syndrome of mesodermal hamartomas, macrocephaly, and pseudopapilledema. Pediatrics 1988;81:287.

95. Witkop CJ Jr, Quevedo WC Jr, Fitzpatrick TB, King RA. Albinism. In: Scriver CR, Beaudet AL, Sly WS, Valle D, eds. The metabolic basis of inherited disease. 6th ed. New York: McGraw-Hill, 1989:2905.

96. Shanahan F, Randolph L, King R, et al. Hermansky-Pudlak syndrome: an immunologic assessment of 15 cases. Am J Med 1988;85:823.

97. Schinella RA, Greco MA, Cobert BL, Denmark LW, Cox RP. Hermansky-Pudlak syndrome with granulomatous colitis. Ann Intern Med 1980;92:20.

98. Mayer EA, Schuffler MD, Rotter JI, Hanna P, Mogard M. A familial visceral neuropathy with autosomal dominant transmission. Gastroenterology 1986;91:1528.

99. Veronique LI, Hostein J, Romero NB, et al. Chronic intestinal pseudo-obstruction with myopathy and ophthalmoplegia: a muscular biochemical study of a mitochondrial disorder. Dig Dis Sci 1992;37:456.

100. Lowsky R, Davidson G, Wolman S, Jeejeebhoy KN, Hegele RA. Familial visceral myopathy associated with a mitochondrial myopathy. Gut 1993;34:279.

101. Emery AEH. The muscular dystrophies. In: Emery AH, Rimoin DL, eds. Principles and practice of medical genetics. 2nd ed. New York: Churchill Livingstone, 1990:539.

102. Barohn RJ, Levine EJ, Olson JO, Mendell JR. Gastric hypomotility in Duchenne's muscular dystrophy. N Engl J Med 1988;319:15.

103. Koenig M, Hoffman EP, Bertelson CJ, Monaco AP, Feener C, Kunkel LM. Complete cloning of the Duchenne muscular dystrophy (DMD) cDNA and preliminary genomic organization of the DMD genes in normal and affected individuals. Cell 1987;50:509.

104. Harper PS. Myotonic dystrophy and related disorders. In: Emery AH, Rimoin DL, eds. Principles and practice of medical genetics. 2nd ed. New York: Churchill Livingstone, 1990:579.

105. Eckardt VF, Nix W. The anal sphincter in patients with myotonic muscular dystrophy. Gastroenterology 1991;100:424.

106. Buxton J, Shelbourne P, Davies J, et al. Detection of an unstable fragment of DNA specific to individuals with myotonic dystrophy. Nature 1992;355:547.

107. Aslanidis C, Jansen G, Amemiya C, et al. Cloning of the essential myotonic dystrophy region and mapping of the putative defect. Nature 1992;355:548.

108. Redman JB, Fenwick RG Jr, Fu Y-H, Pizzuti A, Caskey T. Relationship between parental trinucleotide GCT repeat length and severity of myotonic dystrophy in offspring. JAMA 1993;269:1960.

109. Kearns TP. Eternal ophthalmoplegia, pigmentary degeneration of the retina, and cardiomyopathy: a newly recognized syndrome. Trans Ophthal Soc U K 1965;63:559.

110. Shaker R, Kupla JI, Kidder TM, Arndorfer RC, Hofmann C. Manometric characteristics of cervical dysphagia in a patient with the Kearns-Sayre syndrome. Gastroenterology 1992;103:1328.

111. Zeviani M, Moraes CT, DiMauro S, et al. Deletions of mitochondrial DNA in Kearns-Sayre syndrome. Neurology 1988;38:139.

112. Passarge E. Genetic heterogeneity and recurrence risk of congenital intestinal aganglionosis. Birth Defects 1972;2:63.

113. Badner JA, Sieber WK, Garver KL, Chakravarti A. A genetic study of Hirschsprung disease. Am J Hum Genet 1990;46:568.

114. Lyonnet S, Bolino A, Pelet A, et al. A gene for Hirschsprung disease maps to the proximal long arm of chromosome 10. Nature genetics 1993;4:346.

115. Angrist M, Kauffman E, Slaugenhaupt SA, et al. A gene for Hirschsprung disease (megacolon) in the pericentromeric region of human chromosome 10. Nature Genetics 1993;4:351.

116. Frieling T, Berges W, Borchard F, Lubke HJ, Enck P, Wienbeck M. Familial occurrence of achalasia and diffuse spasm of the oesophagus. Gut 1988;29:1595.

117. Wong RKH, Maydonovitch CL, Metz SJ, Baker JR Jr. Significant DQw1 association in achalasia. Dig Dis Sci 1989;34:349.

118. Axelrod F. Autonomic and sensory disorders. In: Emery AH, Rimoin DL, eds. Principles and practice of medical genetics. 2nd ed. New York: Churchhill Livingstone, 1990:397.

119. Linde LM, Westover JL. Esophageal and gastric abnormalities in dysautonomia. Pediatrics 1962;29:303.

120. Axelrod FB, Gouge TH, Ginsburg HB, Bangaru BS, Hazzi C. Fundoplication and gastrostomy in familial dysautonomia. J Pediatr 1991;118:388.

121. Axelrod FB, Porges RF, Sein ME. Neonatal recognition of familial dysautonomia. J Pediatr 1987;110:946.

122. Blumenfeld A, Slaugenhaupt SA, Axelrod FB, et al. Localization of the gene for familial dysautonomia on chromosome 9 and definition of DNA markers for genetic diagnosis. Nature Genetics 1993;4:160.

123. Eliakim M, Levy M, Ehrenfeld M. Recurrent polyserositis. Amsterdam: Elsevier, 1981.
124. Schwabe AD, Peters RS. Familial Mediterranean fever in Armenians. Analysis of 100 cases. Medicine (Baltimore) 1974;53:453.
125. Shohat M, Shohat T, Rotter JI, et al. Serum amyloid A and P protein genes in familial Mediterranean fever. Genomics 1990;8:83.
126. Mellinkoff SM, Schwabe AD, Lawrence JS. A dietary treatment for familial Mediterranean fever. Arch Intern Med 1961;108:80.
127. Shohat M, Korenberg JI, Schwabe AD, Rotter JI. Hypothesis: familial Mediterranean fever—a genetic disorder of the lipocortin family? Am J Med Genet 1989;34:163.
128. Matzner Y, Brzezinski A. C5a-inhibitor deficiency in peritoneal fluids from patients with familial Mediterranean fever. N Engl J Med 1984;311:283.
129. Pras E, Aksentijevich I, Gruberg L, et al. Mapping of a gene causing familial Mediterranean fever to the short arm of chromosome 16. N Engl J Med 1992;326:1509.
130. Shohat M, Bu X, Shohat T, et al. The gene for familial Mediterranean fever in both Armenians and non-Ashkenazi Jews is linked to the alpha-globin complex on 16p: evidence for locus homogeneity. Am J Hum Genet 1992;51:1349.
131. Patel V, Watanabe I, Zeman W. Deficiency of alpha-L-fucosidase. Science 1972;176:426.
132. Kint JA. Fabry's disease: alpha-galactosidase deficiency. Science 1970;167:1268.
133. Bernstein HS, Bishop DF, Astrin KH, et al. Fabry disease: six gene rearrangements and an exonic point mutation in the alpha-galactosidase gene. J Clin Invest 1989;83:1390.
134. Osler W. Hereditary angioneurotic oedema. Am J Med Sci 1888;95:362.
135. Davis AE III, Whitehead AS, Harrison RA, et al. Human inhibitor of the first component of complement, C1: characterization of cDNA clones and localization of the gene to chromosome 11. Proc Natl Acad Sci U S A 1986;83:3161.
136. Quastel M, Harrison R, Cicardi M, Alper CA, Rosen FS. Behavior in vivo of normal and dysfunctional C1 inhibitor in normal subjects and patients with hereditary angioneurotic edema. J Clin Invest 1983;71:1041.
137. Cicardi M, Bergamaschini L, Marasini B, Boccassini G, Tucci A, Agostoni A. Hereditary angioedema: an appraisal of 104 cases. Am J Med Sci 1982;284:2.
138. Bock SC, Skriver K, Nielsen E, et al. Human C1 inhibitor: primary structure, cDNA cloning, and chromosomal localization. Biochemistry 1986;25:4292.
139. Collins J. Metabolic disease, time for fructose solutions to go. Lancet 1993;341:600.
140. Brooks CC, Tolan DR. Association of the widespread A149P hereditary fructose intolerance mutation with newly identified sequence polymorphisms in the aldolase B gene. Am J Hum Genet 1993;52:835.
141. Sibert JR. Hereditary pancreatitis in England and Wales. J Med Genet 1978;15:189.
142. Kahrilas PJ, Hogan WJ, Geenen JE, Stewart ET, Dodds WJ, Årndorfer RC. Chronic recurrent pancreatitis secondary to a submucosal ampullary tumor in a patient with neurofibromatosis. Dig Dis Sci 1987;32:102.
143. Chanarin I. The megaloblastic anaemias. 3rd ed. Oxford: Blackwell Scientific, 1990.
144. Chanarin I. Disorders of vitamin absorption. Clin Gastroenterol 1982;11:73.
145. Fenton WA, Rosenberg LE. Inherited disorders of cobalamin transport and metabolism. In: Scriver CR, Beaudet AL, Sly WS, Valle D, eds. The metabolic basis of inherited disease. 6th ed. New York: McGraw-Hill, 1989:2065.
146. Kass L. Pernicious anemia. Philadelphia: WB Saunders, 1976.
147. Irvine WJ. Autoimmune atrophic gastritis. In: Rotter JI, Samloff IM, Rimoin DL, eds. Genetics and heterogeneity of common gastrointestinal disorders. New York: Academic Press, 1980:149.
148. Samloff IM, Varis K, Ihamaki T, Siurala M, Rotter JI. Relationships among serum pepsinogen I, serum pepsinogen II, and gastric mucosal histology. A study in relatives of patients with pernicious anemia. Gastroenterology 1982;83:204.
149. Varis K, Samloff IM, Tiilikainen A, et al. Gastritis in first-degree relatives of pernicious anemia, gastric cancer patients, and controls. In: Rotter JI, Samloff IM, Rimoin DL. Genetics and heterogeneity of common gastrointestinal disorders. New York: Academic Press, 1980:177.
150. Kekki M, Siurala M, Varis K, Sipponen P, Sistonen P, Nevanlinna HR. Classification principles and genetics of chronic gastritis. Scand J Gastroenterol 1987;22(Suppl 141):1.
151. Ungar B, Mathews JD, Tait BD, Cowling DC. HLA-DR patterns in pernicious anaemia. Br Med J 1981;1:768.
152. Van den Berg-Loonen EM, Hilterman TCM, Bins M, Nijnhuis LE, Engelfriet CP. Increased incidence of HLA-DR2 in patients with pernicious anemia. Tissue Antigens 1982;19:158.
153. Carmel R. Gastric juice in congenital pernicious anemia contains no immunoreactive intrinsic factor molecule: study of three kindreds with variable ages at presentation, including a patient first diagnosed in adulthood. Am J Hum Genet 1983;35:67.
154. Imerslund O. Idiopathic chronic megaloblastic anemia in children. Acta Pediatr Scand 1960;49(Suppl 119):1.
155. Grasbeck R, Gordin R, Kantero I, Kuhlback B. Selective vitamin B$_{12}$ malabsorption and proteinuria in young people. A syndrome. Acta Med Scand 1960;167:289.
156. Kagnoff MF. Genetic basis of coeliac disease: role of the HLA genes. In: Marsh MN, ed. Coeliac disease. Oxford, England: Blackwell Scientific, 1992:215.
157. Marsh MN. Gluten sensitivity and latency: can patterns of intestinal antibody secretion define the great "silent majority"? Gastroenterology 1993;104:1550.
158. McConnell RB, ed. The genetics of coeliac disease. Lancaster, UK: MTP Press, 1981.
159. Strober W. Gluten-sensitive enteropathy. In: King RA, Rotter JI, Motulsky AG, eds. The genetic basis of common diseases. New York: Oxford University Press, 1992:279.
160. Stenhammar L, Brandt A, Wagermark J. A family study of coeliac disease. Acta Paediatr Scand 1982;71:625.
161. Stokes PL, Asquith P, Cooke WT. Genetics of coeliac disease. Clin Gastroenterol 1973;2:547.
162. McKenna R, Stevens FM, McNicholl B, Scholz S, Albert E, McCarthy CF. Family and population studies of HLA and coeliac disease in the west of Ireland. Tissue Antigens 1983;22:175.
163. Corazza G, Valentini RA, Frisoni M, et al. Gliadin immune reactivity is associated with overt and latent enteropathy in relatives of celiac patients. Gastroenterology 1992;103:1517.
164. Van Elburn RM, Uil JJ, Mulder CJJ, Heymans HSA. Intestinal permeability in patients with coeliac disease and relatives of patients with coeliac disease. Gut 1993;34:354.
165. Polanco I, Biemond I, van Leeuwen A, et al. Gluten sensitive enteropathy in Spain: genetic and environmental factors. In: McConnell RB, ed. The genetics of coeliac disease. Lancaster, UK: MTB Press, 1981:211.
166. Mearin ML, Biemond I, Peña AS, et al. HLA-DR phenotypes in Spanish coeliac children: their contribution to the understanding of the genetics of the disease. Gut 1983;24:532.
167. Greenberg DA, Rotter JI. Two locus models for gluten sensitive enteropathy: population genetic considerations. Am J Med Genet 1981;8:205.
168. Risch N. Assessing the role of HLA-linked and unlinked determinants of disease. Am J Hum Genet 1987;40:1.
169. Rotter JI, Landaw EM. Measuring the genetic contribution of a single locus to a multilocus disease. Clin Genet 1984;26:529.
170. Hernandez JL, Michalski JP, McCombs CC, McCarthy CF, Stevens FM, Elston RC. Evidence for a dominant gene mechanism underlying coeliac disease in the west of Ireland. Genet Epidemiol 1991;8:13.
171. Greenberg DA, Hodge SE, Rotter JI. Evidence for recessive and against dominant inheritance at the HLA "linked" locus in coeliac disease. Am J Hum Genet 1982;34:263.
172. Falchuk ZM, Rogentine GN, Strober W. Predominance of histocompatibility antigen HLA-8 in patients with gluten-sensitive enteropathy. J Clin Invest 1972;51:1602.

173. Tiwari JL, Terasaki PI. HLA and disease associations. New York: Springer-Verlag, 1985.
174. Sollid LM, Thorsby E. HLA susceptibility genes in celiac disease: genetic mapping and role in pathogenesis. Gastroenterology 1993;105:910.
175. Tosi R, Vismara D, Tanigaki N, et al. Evidence that celiac disease is primarily associated with a DC locus allelic specificity. Clin Immunol Immunopathol 1983;28:395.
176. Schenning L, Larhammar D, Bill P, et al. Both a and b chains of HLA-DC class II histocompatibility antigens display extensive polymorphism in their amino-terminal domains. EMBO J 1984;3:447.
177. Boss JM, Strominger JL. Cloning and sequence analysis of the human major histocompatibility complex gene DC-3b. Proc Natl Acad Sci U S A 1984;81:5199.
178. Schiffenbauer J, Didier DK, Klearman M, et al. Complete sequence of the HLA DQa and HLA DQb cDNA from a DR5/DQw3 cell line. J Immunol 1987;139:228.
179. Chang H-C, Moriuchi T, Silver J. The heavy chain of human B-cell alloantigen HLA-DS has a variable N-terminal region and a constant immunoglobulin-like region. Nature 1983;305:813.
180. Karr RW, Gregersen PK, Obata F, et al. Analysis of DRb and DQb chain cDNA clones from a DR7 haplotype. J Immunol 1986;137:2886.
181. Sollid LM, Markussen G, Ek J, Gjerde H, Vartdal F, Thorsby E. Evidence for a primary association of celiac disease to a particular HLA-DQ a/b heterodimer. J Exp Med 1989;169:345.
182. Lundin KEA, Sollid LM, Qvigstad E, Markussen G, Gjertsen HA, Ek J, Thorsby E. T lymphocyte recognition of a celiac disease-associated cis- or trans-encoded HLA-DQ a/b-heterodimer. J Immunol 1990;145:136.
183. Lundin KEA, Scott H, Hansen T, et al. Gliadin-specific, HLA-DQ(a1*0501,b1*0201) restricted T cells from the small intestinal mucosa of celiac disease patients. J Exp Med 1993;178:187.
184. Lin HJ, Rotter JI, Conte WJ. Use of HLA marker associations and HLA haplotype linkage to estimate disease risks in families with gluten-sensitive enteropathy. Clin Genet 1985;28:185.
185. Holmes GKT, Prior P, Lane MR, Pope D, Allan RN. Malignancy in coeliac disease—effect of a gluten free diet. Gut 1989;30:333.
186. Yang H, Rotter JI. The genetics of inflammatory bowel disease: genetic predispositions, disease markers, and genetic heterogeneity. In: Targan SR, Shanahan SR, eds. Inflammatory bowel disease: from bench to bedside. Baltimore: Williams & Wilkins, 1994:32.
187. McConnell RB, Vadheim CM. Inflammatory bowel disease. In: King RA, Rotter JI, Motulsky AG, eds. The genetic basis of common diseases. New York: Oxford University Press, 1992.
188. Rotter JI, Yang H, Shohat T. Genetic complexities of inflammatory bowel disease and its distribution among the Jewish people. In: Bonne-Tamir B, Adam A, eds. Genetic diversity among Jews: diseases and markers at the DNA level. New York: Oxford University Press, 1992:395.
189. Yang H, Rotter JI. Genetic aspects of idiopathic inflammatory bowel disease. In: Kirsner JB, ed. Inflammatory bowel disease. 4th ed. Philadelphia: Lea & Febiger (in press).
190. Orholm M, Munkholm P, Langholz E, Nielsen OH, Sorensen TIA, Binder V. Familial occurrence of inflammatory bowel disease. N Engl J Med 1991;324:84.
191. Yang H, McElree C, Roth M-P, Shanahan F, Targan SR, Rotter JI. Familial empiric risks for inflammatory bowel disease: differences between Jews and non-Jews. Gut 1993;34:517.
192. Roth M-P, Petersen GM, McElree C, Vadheim CM, Panish JF, Rotter JI. Familial recurrence risk estimates of inflammatory bowel disease in Ashkenazi Jews. Gastroenterology 1989;96:1016.
193. Kirsner JB. Genetic aspects of inflammatory bowel disease. Clin Gastroenterol 1973;2:557.
194. Couper R, Kapelushnik J, Griffiths AM. Neutrophil dysfunction in glycogen storage disease Ib:Association with Crohn's-like colitis. Gastroenterology 1991;100:549.
195. Roe TF, Coates TD, Thomas DW, Miller JH, Gilsanz V. Brief report: treatment of chronic inflammatory bowel disease in glycogen storage disease type Ib with colony-stimulating factors. N Engl J Med 1992;326:1666.
196. Hollander D, Vadheim CM, Brettholtz E, Petersen GM, Delahunty T, Rotter JI. Increased intestinal permeability in Crohn's patients and their relatives: an etiological factor? Ann Intern Med 1986;105;883.
197. Hollander D. Permeability to Crohn's disease: altered barrier functions in healthy relatives? Gastroenterology 1993;104:1848.
198. Saxon A, Shanahan F, Landers C, Ganz T, Targan S. A subset of antineutrophil anticytoplasmic antibodies is associated with inflammatory bowel disease. J Allergy Clin Immunol 1990;86:202.
199. Cambridge G, Rampton DS, Stevens TRJ, McCarthy DA, Kamm M, Leaker B. Anti-neutrophil antibodies in inflammatory bowel disease: prevalence and diagnostic role. Gut 1992;33:668.
200. Duerr RH, Targan SR, Landers CJ, Sutherland LR, Shanahan F. Antineutrophil cytoplasmic antibodies in ulcerative colitis. Comparison with other colitides/diarrheal illnesses. Gastroenterology 1991;100:1590.
201. Shanahan F, Duerr RH, Rotter JI, et al. Neutrophil autoantibodies in ulcerative colitis: familial aggregation and genetic heterogeneity. Gastroenterology 1992;103:456.
202. Yang H, Rotter JI, Toyoda H, et al. Ulcerative colitis: a genetic heterogeneous group defined with genetic (DR2) and subclinical markers (anti-neutrophil cytoplasmic antibodies). J Clin Invest 1993;92:1080.
203. Toyoda H, Wang S-J, Yang H, et al. Distinct association of HLA class II genes with inflammatory bowel disease. Gastroenterology 1993;104:741.
204. Sugimura K, Asakura H, Mizuki N, et al. Analysis of genes within the HLA region affecting susceptibility to ulcerative colitis. Hum Immunol 1993;36:112.
205. Kobayashi K, Atoh M, Konoeda Y, Yagita H, Inoko H, Sekiguchi S. HLA-DR, DQ and T cell antigen receptor constant beta genes in Japanese patients with ulcerative colitis. Clin Exp Immunol 1990;80:400.
206. Neigut D, Proujansky R, Trucco M, Dorman JS, Kocoshis S, Carpenter AB, Ball EJ. Association of an HLA-DQB-1 genotype with Crohn's disease in children. Gastroenterology 1992;102:A671.
207. Rotter JI. Immunogenetic susceptibilities in inflammatory bowel disease. Can J Gastroenterol 1990;4:261.
208. Rotter JI, Shohat T, Vadheim CM. Is IBD a genetic disease? In: Rachmilewitz D, Zimmerman J, eds. Inflammatory bowel diseases, 1990. Dordrecht, The Netherlands: Kluwer Academic Publishers, 1990:5.
209. Rotter JI, Yang H. Delineating the major aetiological risk factors for IBD: the genetic susceptibilities. In: Scholmerich J, Kruis W, Goebell H, Hohenberger W, Gross V, eds. Inflammatory bowel diseases—pathophysiology as basis of treatment. Dordrecht, The Netherlands: Kluwer Academic Publishers, 1993:9.
210. Bennion LJ, Knowler WC. Epidemiology of gallstones. In: Rotter JI, Samloff IM, Rimoin DL, eds. Genetics and heterogeneity of common gastrointestinal disorders. New York: Academic Press, 1980:297.
211. Dieh AK, Haffner SM, Knapp JA, Hazuda HP, Stern MP. Dietary intake and the prevalence of gallbladder disease in Mexican Americans. Gastroenterology 1989;97:1527.
212. Maurer KR, Everhart JE, Knowler WC, Shawker TH, Roth HP. Risk factors for gallstone disease in the Hispanic populations of the United States. Am J Epidemiol 1990;131:836.
213. Nurnberg D, Berndt H, Pannwitz H. Familial incidence of gallstones. Dtsch Med Wochenschr 1989;114:1059.
214. Leoci C, Chiloiro M, Guerra V, Misciagna G. Genetic epidemiology of cholelithiasis: a case control study of a population. Minerva Gastroenterol Dietol 1991;37:35.
215. Van der Linder W. Genetics of cholelithiasis. In: Rotter JI, Samloff IM, Rimoin DL, eds. Genetics and heterogeneity of common gastrointestinal disorders. New York: Academic Press, 1980:313.
216. Gilat T, Feldman C, Halpern Z, Dan M, Bar-Meir S. An in-

creased familial frequency of gallstones. Gastroenterology 1983;84:242.

217. Danzinger RG, Gordon H, Schoenfield LJ, Thistle JL. Lithogenic bile in siblings of young women with cholelithiasis. Mayo Clin Proc 1972;47:762.
218. Kesaniemi YA, Koskenvuo M, Vuoristo M, Miettinen TA. Biliary lipid composition in monozygotic and dizygotic pairs of twins. Gut 1989;30:1750.
219. Whincup PH, Cook DG, Phillips AN, Shaper AG. ABO blood group and ischaemic heart disease in British men. Br Med J 1990;300:1679.
220. Juvonen T, Niemelä O. ABO blood group and gallstone disease. Br Med J 1992;305:26.
221. Papasteriades C, Al-Mahmoud I, Papageorgakis N, et al. HLA antigens in Greek patients with cholelithiasis. Dis Markers 1990;8:17.
222. Juvonen T, Kervinen K, Kairaluoma MI, Lajunen LHJ, Kesäniemi YA. Gallstone cholesterol content is related to apolipoprotein E polymorphism. Gastroenterology 1993;104:1806.

Textbook of Gastroenterology, second edition, edited by Tadataka Yamada. JB Lippincott Company, Philadelphia © 1995.

CHAPTER 109

Gastrointestinal Manifestations of Systemic Diseases

Garry A. Neil   Joel V. Weinstock

Cardiovascular Diseases
 Valvular Aortic Stenosis
 Congestive Heart Failure
 Other Cardiac Diseases
Chromosomal Abnormalities and Other Genetic Disorders
 Anderson-Fabry Disease
 Down's Syndrome
 Familial Mediterranean Fever
 Gaucher's Disease
 Hepatic Porphyrias
 Hereditary Angioedema
 Familial Hyperlipidemias
 Niemann-Pick Disease
 Tangier Disease
 Turner's Syndrome
Connective Tissue Diseases
 Ehlers-Danlos Syndrome
 Pseudoxanthoma Elasticum
 Progressive Systemic Sclerosis
 Polymyositis and Dermatomyositis
 Rheumatoid Arthritis
 Sjögren's Syndrome
 Systemic Lupus Erythematosus
 Mixed Connective Tissue Disease
 Seronegative Spondyloarthropathies
Dermatologic Diseases
 Ataxia-Telangiectasia
 Blue Rubber Bleb Nevus Syndrome

 Cowden's Syndrome
 Epidermolysis Bullosa
 Pemphigus
 Hereditary Hemorrhagic Telangiectasia
 Neurofibromatosis
 Psoriasis
 Stevens-Johnson Syndrome
 Tylosis
 Urticaria
Endocrinologic Disorders
 Acromegaly
 Addison's Disease
 Diabetes Mellitus
 Hyperparathyroidism
 Hypoparathyroidism
 Thyroid Disease
 Hyperthyroidism
 Hypothyroidism
 Pregnancy
Granulomatous Diseases
Heavy Metal Toxicity
 Lead Poisoning
 Arsenic Poisoning
 Gold
Hematologic Disorders
 Hemolytic Uremic Syndrome
 Thrombotic Thrombocytopenic Purpura
                    (continued)

Hypercoagulability
Deficits of Coagulation Factors
Platelet Defects
Plummer-Vinson-Kelly Syndrome
Sickle Cell Anemia
Hemoglobin C
Hereditary Spherocytosis
Metabolic Diseases
Systemic Amyloidosis
Capillary Leak Syndrome
Neoplastic Disorders
Hematologic Malignancies
Nonhematologic Malignancies
Neuromuscular Disorders
Brain Injuries
Dementia Syndromes
Migraine
Multiple Sclerosis
Muscular Dystrophies
Parkinsonism
Spinal Cord Transection
High Spinal Cord Lesions
Other Neuromuscular Diseases
Nutritional Disturbances
Malnutrition
Obesity
Other Factors
Complications of Organ Transplantation
Bone Marrow Transplantation
Graft-Versus-Host Disease
Renal Transplantation

Cardiac Transplantation
Blood Transfusion
Psychological Disorders
Anorexia Nervosa and Bulimia
Anxiety and Stress
Major Depression or Conversion Disorder
Munchausen's Syndrome
Schizophrenia
Pulmonary Diseases
Gastroesophageal Reflux Disease
Respiratory Failure
α_1-Antitrypsin Deficiency
Aspiration of Gastroenteric Contents
Cystic Fibrosis
Renal Disorders
Acute Renal Failure
Substance Abuse
Drug Abuse
Alcohol Consumption
Cocaine
Narcotics
Smoking
Vasculitides
Behçet's Disease
Giant Cell Arteritis
Henoch-Schönlein Purpura
Köhlmeier-Degos Disease
Polyarteritis Nodosa
Churg-Strauss Disease
Wegener's Granulomatosis
Cryoglobulinemia

Gastrointestinal symptoms or signs are frequently evident during the course of systemic diseases. In some cases, the gut or liver are targets of the disease process, whereas in others they are indirectly affected. In some cases, it is the gastrointestinal manifestations that cause the patient to seek medical attention. It is our purpose in this chapter to discuss some common systemic diseases with well recognized gastrointestinal manifestations and to highlight some of their more important effects on the digestive system.

CARDIOVASCULAR DISEASES

Valvular Aortic Stenosis

Valvular aortic stenosis is a relatively common condition affecting predominantly men in middle to late life. This condition is associated with an increased incidence of gastrointestinal bleeding,[1-3] often attributed to angiodysplasias of the gut (Heyde's syndrome).[4,5] Although 15% to 41% of patients with gastrointestinal angiodysplasias also have hemodynamically significant aortic stenosis, gastrointestinal angiodysplasias also are common in people without aortic stenosis. Thus, the validity of the association between the two conditions remains in question.[6,7]

Most angiodysplasias in patients with aortic stenosis are found in the right colon. Gastric and intestinal lesions have also been described.[8,9] Lesions identified by angiography or endoscopy can be incriminated as the bleeding source if active hemorrhage is observed. Endoscopic cautery and intestinal resection remain standard therapy for active bleeding. Endoscopic ablation and laser therapy[10] have also been suggested to ameliorate bleeding. Aortic valve replacement has resulted in the cessation of bleeding in some cases,[11-13] but the angiodysplasias may persist.[14] The use of oral contraceptives has been suggested as an effective medical alternative to surgery.[15] These latter approaches to management need validation.

Congestive Heart Failure

Congestive heart failure results from pump failure and a consequent inability to maintain tissue metabolic demands. There are many causes, including valvular heart disease, myocarditis, coronary artery disease, hypertension, anemia, and hypermetabolic states (e.g., thyrotoxicosis and sepsis). Congestion of the splanchnic venous bed is a frequent complication, leading to anorexia, nausea, and abdominal pain and distention. Rarely, venous congestion is sufficiently severe to produce ischemic injury, diarrhea, malabsorption, or protein-losing enteropathy.[16-20] A greater-than-expected frequency of peptic ulcer disease and upper gastrointestinal bleeding has also been observed.[20] Hepatic congestion secondary to right heart failure

(Fig. 109-1; see Color Fig. 65) is a relatively common cause of jaundice, right upper quadrant pain, abnormal liver enzyme levels, transudative ascites, and prolongation of the prothrombin time, which may mimic biliary tract disease or hepatitis.[21] Prolonged congestion rarely progresses to cardiac cirrhosis.[22]

The medical therapy of heart failure frequently produces gastrointestinal problems. Digoxin causes anorexia, nausea, and vomiting in many patients, particularly when levels exceed the therapeutic range.[23,24] Digoxin-associated constriction of splanchnic vessels may contribute to intestinal ischemia.[25] Quinidine and other agents used to control arrhythmias may produce nausea, anorexia, and diarrhea. Constipation or pseudoobstruction can result from diuretic-induced hypokalemia and hypomagnesemia. Severe pancreatitis has been attributed to a variety of diuretics, including thiazides, furosemide, and ethacrynic acid.[26] Oral potassium supplements have been implicated in esophagitis, ulcers, and, rarely, intestinal strictures.[27]

The differential diagnosis of many of these complaints is long, and many patients are subjected to prolonged, fruitless investigation before the actual cause is discovered. Treatment is aimed at improving cardiac function. Cardiac medications are changed or reduced when drug toxicity is suspected. Lax-

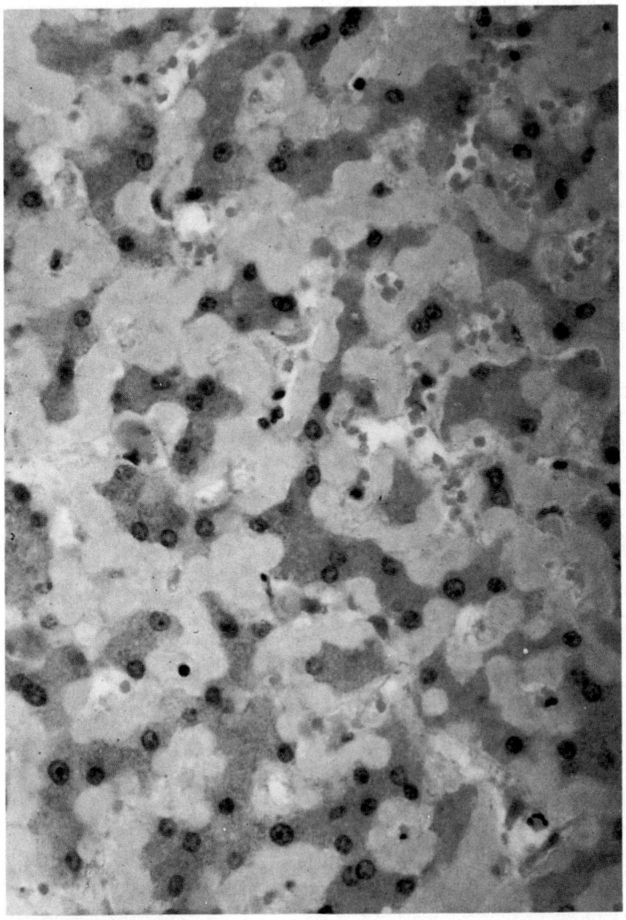

FIGURE 109-1. (See Color Fig. 65.) Hepatic congestion and cirrhosis secondary to congestive heart failure. (Hematoxylin and eosin stain; original magnification ×100.)

atives, dietary changes, and potassium and magnesium supplements are administered as required.

Other Cardiac Diseases

Other cardiac diseases associated with gastrointestinal problems include dysphagia resulting from left atrial enlargement in patients with mitral valve disease.[28] Chronic cough and recumbency contribute to gastroesophageal reflux in some patients. Embolism from atrial thrombi, cardiac myxomas, or endocarditis may result in intestinal infarction. Bacterial endocarditis is associated with septic emboli and liver abscesses. More than 600,000 cardiac surgeries are now performed each year in the United States. Complications of cardiac surgery include acid-peptic disease, cholecystitis, pancreatitis, intestinal infarction, hepatic necrosis, and others.[29,30] As in other situations, acid peptic disease after cardiac surgery correlates with age, the need for reoperation, and hypoperfusion.[31]

CHROMOSOMAL ABNORMALITIES AND OTHER GENETIC DISORDERS

Anderson-Fabry Disease

Anderson-Fabry disease, an X-linked glycosphingolipidosis, is caused by impaired function of the enzyme α-galactosidase A, and is characterized by the deposition of ceramide trihexose in the lysosomes of endothelium, nerves, and smooth muscle cells. Deposition of sphingolipid in endothelial cells is responsible for the frequently observed thrombotic and embolic sequelae, which include chronic renal failure, pain and paresthesias of the extremities, and cerebrovascular events. Gastrointestinal manifestations are present in as many as 62% of affected men and 29% of female carriers. They include episodic constipation, diarrhea, nausea and vomiting, and abdominal pain,[32] and, rarely, intestinal ischemia and perforation.[33] The cause of these symptoms is unclear but may be related, in part, to impaired gastrointestinal motility and vascular insufficiency.[34] Jejunal and rectal biopsies reveal foamy or electron-dense deposits in the vascular endothelium and unmyelinated neurons.

Down's Syndrome

Down's syndrome (chromosome 21 trisomy) is associated with gastrointestinal anomalies. Most commonly seen are duodenal stenosis and atresia. Infants present with vomiting, abdominal distention, and the "double-bubble" sign on abdominal radiography. Annular pancreas may accompany congenital duodenal obstruction. Esophageal abnormalities include tracheoesophageal fistula, esophageal stenosis, hiatal hernia, and gastroesophageal reflux. Imperforate anus, Hirschsprung's disease, and malrotation of the intestine have been described repeatedly.[35] There is a high incidence of hepatitis B infection in patients with Down's syndrome; this may result from institutional confinement combined with poor individual hygienic habits.

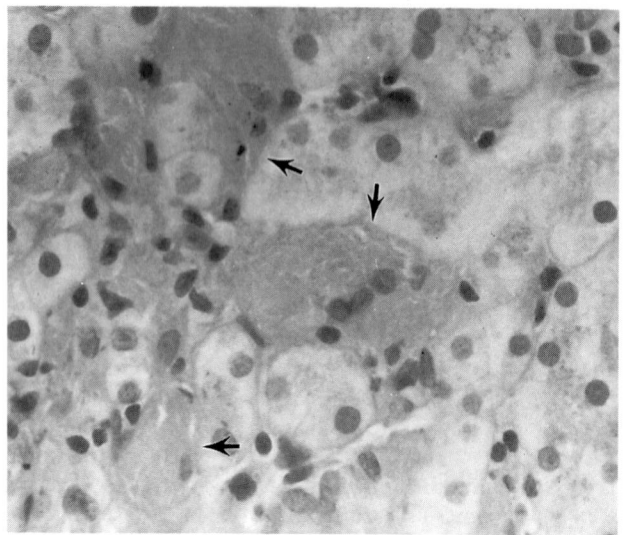

FIGURE 109-2. (See Color Fig. 66.) Gaucher's disease of the liver. Multinucleated Gaucher cells (*arrows*) are present. (Hematoxylin and eosin stain; original magnification ×400.)

Familial Mediterranean Fever

Familial Mediterranean fever (recurrent polyserositis or periodic disease) is a disease of autosomal recessive inheritance, recently mapped to chromosome 16,[36] afflicting Sephardic Jews, Armenians, and Arabs.[37-40] The target organ appears to be the blood vessel, although a specific biochemical abnormality has not yet been described. Clinical manifestations begin in childhood and include recurrent episodes of fever, synovitis, serositis, and dermatitis. Attacks are precipitated by a variety of inciting factors, including stress and infections.[38]

The diagnosis is suspected when a patient of Mediterranean extraction and a positive family history presents with recurrent episodes of abdominal pain, peritoneal signs, arthritis, fevers, and leukocytosis. The patient often has undergone previous fruitless diagnostic work-ups, including laparotomy. Frequent complications include amyloidosis, degenerative arthritis, renal vein thrombosis, and narcotic addiction.[37-41] No specific diagnostic test is available. Treatment with colchicine has been suggested to be beneficial in preventing and ameliorating acute attacks.[39,41,42]

Gaucher's Disease

Gaucher's disease is a rare inherited disease characterized by the deposition of sphingolipid in the reticuloendothelial system, including the liver and spleen.[43] It may present in adulthood with hepatosplenomegaly as a consequence of hepatic infiltration, hepatic fibrosis, or cirrhosis. Ascites or esophageal varices, which occasionally may bleed massively,[44] have been described (Fig. 109-2; see Color Fig. 66).

Hepatic Porphyrias

The hepatic porphyrias are a collection of inherited metabolic disorders of heme synthesis associated with increased urinary excretion of porphobilinogen and δ-aminolevulonic acid (Table 109-1).[45,46] With the exception of porphyria cutanea tarda, all of the hepatic porphyrias are inherited in an autosomal dominant fashion. Acute intermittent porphyria, hereditary coproporphyria, and variegate porphyria manifest with recurrent attacks of abdominal pain (probably due to an autonomic neuropathy), nausea, vomiting, constipation, disorientation, seizures, and peripheral neuropathy. Attacks may be precipitated by the administration of drugs (e.g., barbiturates, steroids, sulfonamides, and alcohol), surgery, or pregnancy.[46] The diagnosis is established by the demonstration of excessive amounts of porphobilinogen and δ-levulonic acid in the urine. Acute attacks may be ameliorated by infusion of glucose and hematin, which suppress aminolevulonic acid synthetase.[47]

TABLE 109-1
General Description of the Hepatic Porphyrias

DISORDER	NEUROPSYCHIATRIC SYMPTOMS	SKIN LESIONS	STRUCTURAL HEPATIC DISEASE	PRINCIPAL BIOCHEMICAL ABNORMALITIES*		
				Erythrocytes	*Urine*	*Feces*
Acute intermittent porphyria	+	0	0	0	↑ PBG and ALA	0
Variegate porphyria	+	+	0	0	↑ Coproporphyrin ↑ PBG and ALA	↑ Protoporphyrin and coproporphyrin
Hereditary coproporphyria	+	+	0	0	↑ Coproporphyrin ↑ PBG and ALA	↑ Coproporphyrin
Porphyria cutanea tarda	0	+	+	0	↑ Uroporphyrin	0
Protoporphyria	0	+	+	↑ Protoporphyrin	0	↑ Protoporphyrin
Secondary porphyrinuria	0	0	+	0	↑ Coproporphyrin	0

* This table does not list all the biochemical abnormalities and only serves as a guide to indicate which measurements are most critical in the evaluation of a particular porphyric disorder.

ALA, δ-aminolevulinic acid; PBG, porphobilinogen

From Bloomer JR. The hepatic porphyrias. Gastroenterology 1976;71:689.

Hereditary Angioedema

Hereditary angioedema is the most common genetic disorder of the complement system. The underlying pathophysiology is an autosomal dominantly inherited deficiency of C1 esterase. This enzyme is the sole regulator of early events in the classic complement pathway. It also assists in the regulation of the kinin and fibrinolytic cascades.[48] The characteristic swelling may be mediated by bradykinin.

The major clinical feature is recurrent, episodic, self-limited swelling of the orofacial region, extremities, and gastrointestinal tract. The swelling is often provoked by emotional stress or minor trauma. Edema in the cervical region may be life threatening if the upper airway is compromised. Colic, bloating, and nausea and vomiting secondary to enteric mucosal edema are characteristic of abdominal attacks. Abdominal tenderness may be present but peritoneal signs, jaundice, and hyperamylasemia are absent.[49] Barium studies have demonstrated "thumbprinting" and other signs of mucosal edema.[50] Treatment with synthetic androgens (e.g., danazol or methyltestosterone) increases the levels of C1 esterase inhibitor and helps to ameliorate attacks.[51] Acute abdominal attacks are treated with analgesics, antiemetics, and epinephrine as needed.[48] Premedication with fresh frozen plasma or antifibrinolytic agents (e.g., ε-amino caproic acid, tranexamic acid) should be considered before oropharyngeal manipulations such as upper endoscopy.[52]

Familial Hyperlipidemias

The familial hyperlipidemias are a collection of inherited disorders of lipid metabolism, characterized by elevated plasma lipid levels. Types I (*hyperchylomicronemia*) and V (*hyperlipoproteinemia*) are associated with recurrent episodes of pancreatitis.[53] Patients with type IV hyperlipidemia also may be subject to an increased incidence of gallstones, which can be aggravated by treatment with clofibrate.[54] It should be noted that only those disorders that predispose to high levels of triglycerides are associated with acute pancreatitis.[55,56] Hypertriglyceridemia may amplify the effect of alcohol in inducing pancreatitis.[55]

Niemann-Pick Disease

Niemann-Pick disease is a rare, inherited lipid storage disease that principally afflicts people of Jewish ancestry. The patients manifest hepatosplenomegaly and hepatic failure in infancy. Adult cases have also been reported.[57] The enzyme sphingomyelinase is absent or nonfunctional, leading to the accumulation of sphingomyelin in the lysosomes of reticuloendothelial cells.

Tangier Disease

Tangier disease (named for Tangier Island in Chesapeake Bay, where the disease was first described) is a rare autosomal recessive deficiency of plasma α-lipoprotein. Affected patients exhibit low plasma levels of cholesterol and high-density lipoproteins along with elevated plasma triglycerides. Choles-

terol is deposited in the reticuloendothelial system, leading to hepatosplenomegaly.[58] Accumulation of cholesterol results in enlarged orange or red tonsils, lymphadenopathy, peripheral neuropathy, and yellow-orange patches in the colonic mucosa.[59]

Turner's Syndrome

Turner's syndrome (X chromosome monosomy) presents with a variety of external somatic features and congenital anomalies of internal organs. The syndrome has also been associated with gastrointestinal hemorrhage due to intestinal vascular malformations.[60]

CONNECTIVE TISSUE DISEASES

Ehlers-Danlos Syndrome

Ehlers-Danlos syndrome is a collection of inherited diseases affecting collagen synthesis and manifesting excessively stretchable skin, easy bruising, and hyperextensible joints. At least eight different subtypes are described, although gastrointestinal involvement is common in only types I (gravis) and IV (arterial). Patients with Ehlers-Danlos syndrome type I have fragile, hyperelastic skin and hyperextensible joints. They often complain of bleeding gums and easy bruising after even minor trauma. Severe gastrointestinal bleeding from mucosal lesions occasionally occurs.

Ehlers-Danlos syndrome type IV is unique in that hyperelastic skin is lacking and joint hyperextensibility is much less prominent. Ecchymosis and "cigarette paper" scars are, however, common. A defect in type III collagen synthesis leads to multiple aneurysms, often involving splanchnic arteries. Thrombosis or rupture of these aneurysms results in mesenteric ischemia or intraabdominal bleeding.[61,62] Megaesophagus, small intestinal dilation,[63] and bacterial overgrowth,[64] as well as colonic hypomotility and perforation[65] have been reported.

Pseudoxanthoma Elasticum

Pseudoxanthoma elasticum is a rare inherited disorder of connective tissue synthesis with a prevalence of between 1/70,000 and 1/160,000.[66] Characteristic plaques resembling xanthomata may be seen on the skin. Degeneration of elastic fibers in visceral blood vessels results in ineffectual vasoconstriction and vessel retraction after injury, leading to a predisposition to gastrointestinal bleeding.[67,68] Gel-Foam embolization has been successful in controlling hemorrhage,[69] but infusion of vasoconstricting agents should be undertaken with caution because many patients have associated coronary artery disease,[70] and because the efficacy of such agents in this setting is in doubt.

Progressive Systemic Sclerosis

Progressive systemic sclerosis (PSS) or scleroderma is characterized by vasculitis of small arteries and fibrosis of skin and other organs. More than 50% of patients have gastrointestinal complications.[71] These include tightening of the perioral skin with restricted ability to open the mouth, inflammation of the gingivae, and impaired taste sensation, all of which may contribute to malnutrition. Esophageal involvement is present in at least 70% of patients.[72] The esophagus exhibits diminished, low-amplitude esophageal contractions (first noted in the smooth muscle but later in the skeletal muscle as well) and weakening of the lower esophageal sphincter, leading to heartburn, dysphagia, reflux esophagitis, and esophageal ulcers.[71] All patients exhibit a diminished lower esophageal sphincter response to gastrin. Gastric emptying is delayed, and acid secretion may be increased,[73] predisposing to esophageal reflux.

The small intestine is frequently involved, often exhibiting extensive gut wall fibrosis and smooth muscle atrophy. This leads to hypomotility, dilation, pseudodiverticula, and thickening of the bowel. Forty percent of patients have abnormalities of small intestinal motility.[71] Stasis, pseudoobstruction, and bacterial overgrowth may ensue and produce anorexia, abdominal distention, malabsorption, diarrhea, steatorrhea, and weight loss. The colon may also be involved, exhibiting pseudodiverticula (Fig. 109-3) and telangiectasias. Constipation, pseudoobstruction, and volvulus may develop.[74,75] Treatment with metoclopramide, other motility-enhancing drugs, and antibiotics is helpful in some patients, but parenteral nutrition is often required in advanced cases. New agents, including cisapride[76] and octreotide,[77] may benefit some patients who fail to respond to standard therapy.[76] The clinical course is variable and largely depends on the type and extent of organ involvement.[71]

Polymyositis and Dermatomyositis

Polymyositis and dermatomyositis are rheumatologic diseases characterized by inflammation of striated and, to a lesser extent, smooth muscle. A characteristic skin rash accompanies

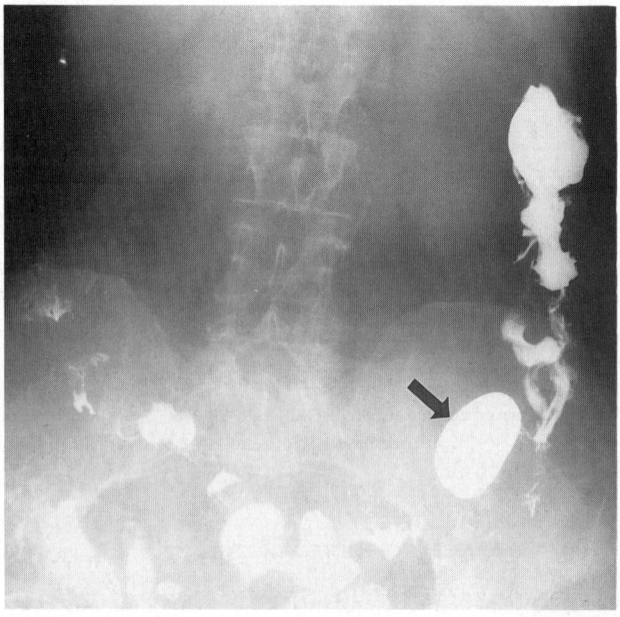

FIGURE 109-3. Wide-mouthed pseudodiverticula are present in a patient with scleroderma.

dermatomyositis. The gastrointestinal tract may be affected throughout its entire length, but the proximal esophagus is most commonly involved.[75,78] Patients may complain of dysphagia, regurgitation, and aspiration. Esophageal and gastric motility may be impaired, leading to esophageal reflux and gastric stasis.[79,80]

Small and large bowel involvement is well documented and constipation is a fairly common complaint. Colonic pseudodiverticula and pneumatosis intestinalis also may develop. Suggested contributing causes include neurologic dysfunction and diminished smooth muscle contractility as a consequence of muscle atrophy, fibrosis, or inflammation. Acute inflammation of smooth muscle may result in gut wall edema, ulceration, or even perforation.

An association of dermatomyositis and malignancy, particularly gastric cancer, has long been postulated. Cancers have been found in as many as 25% of patients,[81,82] but a true association has been questioned.[83] The need for malignancy screening in these patients is thus controversial.

Rheumatoid Arthritis

Rheumatoid arthritis is a chronic systemic disease characterized by a deforming symmetrical polyarthritis and the presence of serum rheumatoid factors. It most commonly afflicts women between the third and seventh decades of life and has a prevalence of approximately 1% in the United States.[84]

Gastrointestinal manifestations are common and protean. Involvement of the temporomandibular joint impedes chewing and may lead to nutritional impairment. Sicca syndrome is present in some patients and is accompanied by stomatitis and gingivitis. Abnormalities of esophageal motility have been described,[85] although heartburn and dysphagia are not usually prominent. Secondary amyloidosis may occur in patients with long-standing rheumatoid arthritis and may involve any portion of the gastrointestinal tract.

Vasculitis is less common than in other rheumatic diseases; however, both small and large vessels may be involved in the setting of severe arthritis, subcutaneous nodules, high titers of rheumatoid factor, and depressed serum complement levels.[86] Necrotizing vasculitis of the mesenteric vessels may result in intestinal ischemia, bleeding, and infarction.[87] Cholecystitis, appendicitis,[88] perisplenitis, splenic infarction, pancreatitis, and hepatic arteritis have also been described.[86]

The most common gastrointestinal manifestations of rheumatoid arthritis are iatrogenic. Chronic administration of salicylates and nonsteroidal antiinflammatory drugs often produces gastric erosions or gastroduodenal ulcers that in many cases are minimally symptomatic[89,90]; however, they may result in anorexia, nausea, abdominal pain, and severe gastrointestinal bleeding.[91] In most cases, duodenal ulcers heal with H_2 antagonists or barrier-enhancing drugs even if the offending drugs are continued, but interruption of antiinflammatory therapy may be necessary to allow healing of gastric ulcers.[92,93] The administration of cytoprotective agents (e.g., misoprostol) along with antiinflammatory medication should be considered in these patients because such agents have been shown to prevent gastric erosions and ulcers in this setting.[94,95] H_2 antagonists appear to be less efficacious.[89]

Therapy with methotrexate can result in hepatic fibrosis.

Hence, monitoring of liver function tests and periodic liver biopsy is indicated when this drug is used.[95] The toxic effects of gold preparations are discussed in the section on Heavy Metal Toxicity. Patients with Felty's syndrome (rheumatoid arthritis, splenomegaly, and leukopenia) exhibit a proclivity for intraabdominal sepsis for reasons that are as yet undefined.[96] Other gastrointestinal complications are similar to those of rheumatoid arthritis.

Sjögren's Syndrome

Sjögren's syndrome is characterized by *keratoconjunctivitis sicca* (dry eyes and mouth) in association with rheumatoid arthritis. Atrophy of the salivary glands leads to lack of saliva, which can, in turn, impair swallowing. In addition, as many as one third of patients show evidence of disordered esophageal motility.[97] Pancreatic acinar involvement may result in pancreatic insufficiency and steatorrhea in some patients.[98,99] There is also an association between Sjögren's syndrome and chronic liver diseases such as primary biliary cirrhosis and chronic active hepatitis.[98]

Systemic Lupus Erythematosus

Systemic lupus erythematosus (SLE) is a systemic autoimmune disease most common among young and middle-aged women. It is characterized by arthritis, myalgias, fever, rash, lymphadenopathy, renal disease, polyserositis, and central nervous system involvement. It commonly affects the gastrointestinal tract in a variety of ways. Inflammation of serosal surfaces may produce lupus peritonitis,[100,101] which usually is self-limited but may be associated with ascites. Intestinal ischemia or perforation secondary to mesenteric vasculitis can present a diagnostic conundrum for the clinician, especially because these patients often receive corticosteroid therapy that can mask symptoms. Gastritis, mucosal ulceration, and pancreatitis also occur and produce abdominal pain and nausea and vomiting. Intussusception, enteritis, and pneumatosis intestinalis may be seen. Motility disorders can lead to esophageal reflux, dysphagia, or gastric retention. Pancreatitis, sometimes severe, has been associated with SLE; the mechanisms remain obscure.[102]

Although clinically significant liver disease is uncommon in SLE, many patients have hepatomegaly and abnormal liver enzyme levels.[101] Drug-induced hepatotoxicity is probably the most common underlying cause. Abnormal liver enzyme levels and hepatocellular necrosis have been attributed to aspirin therapy, even when salicylate levels are within the therapeutic range.[103] Cessation of aspirin therapy usually results in prompt regression of this syndrome. Other drugs such as azathioprine may produce similar abnormalities. Hepatic vasculitis is another rare cause of liver disease, which in extreme cases has resulted in liver rupture.[104]

Mixed Connective Tissue Disease

Mixed connective tissue disease, or overlap syndrome, is a heterogeneous autoimmune disorder with features of lupus, scleroderma, and polymyositis. Gastrointestinal manifestations resemble those described for the aforementioned rheumatoid diseases.

Seronegative Spondyloarthropathies

The seronegative spondyloarthropathies are a collection of rheumatoid diseases including *ankylosing spondylitis*, *psoriatic arthritis*, the *reactive arthritides* (e.g., *Reiter's syndrome)*, the arthritis associated with inflammatory bowel disease, and Whipple's disease. Serum rheumatoid factor is lacking.[105] Patients with reactive arthritis frequently have an antecedent gram-negative enteric or chlamydial infection.[106] Many have chronic gastrointestinal symptoms (e.g., mild diarrhea and abdominal cramps), and most patients have endoscopic evidence of ileocolonic inflammation sometimes resembling Crohn's disease.[106,107] The significance of these findings awaits clarification. In addition to enterocolonic inflammation, many patients with reactive arthritis have recurrent oral and genital ulcers.

DERMATOLOGIC DISEASES

Ataxia-Telangiectasia

Ataxia-telangiectasia is an autosomal recessive disorder that, in the homozygote state, has many deleterious effects. This disorder is characterized by progressive ataxia, telangiectasia on the bulbar conjunctiva and on sun-exposed regions, sinopulmonary infections, immunodeficiency, and a propensity for lymphoreticular and other malignancies.[108] The patients frequently respond poorly to viral antigens, have a marked deficiency in serum IgA and IgE, and manifest defects in cell-mediated immunity.[109] Gastrointestinal disease, however, is not a prominent feature of this disorder.[110] Death at an early age has occasionally been attributed to adenocarcinoma of the stomach and colon, and intestinal lymphoma. Serum smooth muscle and anti-mitochondrial antibodies also may develop without clinically relevant disease. The patients frequently have high serum concentrations of α-fetoprotein of liver origin without evidence of liver damage.[111]

Blue Rubber Bleb Nevus Syndrome

Blue rubber bleb nevus syndrome presents with distinctive, rubbery, cutaneous angiomas. The gastrointestinal tract can be involved, resulting in intestinal bleeding.[112-114]

Cowden's Syndrome

Cowden's syndrome is a disease of autosomal dominance characterized by ectodermal, mesodermal, and endodermal hamartomatous neoplasms. Patients manifest innumerable mucocutaneous trichilemmomas that present as 1- to 3-mm verrucous or papillomatous papules. Other skin lesions, such as fibromas and lipomas, also appear. There is a strong propensity for thyroid goiter, thyroid cancer, and, in women, breast cancer. Other organ systems may be involved.[115] Multiple hamartomatous polyps of various sizes can develop from the esophagus to the colon, and have a low potential for malignant degeneration; however, they can cause chronic gastrointestinal blood loss and partial intestinal obstruction.[116,117]

Epidermolysis Bullosa

Epidermolysis bullosa is a group of diseases in which disruption of the cohesion between epidermis and dermis occurs after minor trauma. This results in formation of vesicles or bullae. *Epidermolysis bullosa lethalis* is an autosomal recessive disorder of the newborn period associated with extensive bullae formation. Early death results from dehydration and infection. Oral, anal, and esophageal blistering is common. It is also associated with congenital pyloric atresia.[118] Other forms of this entity include *epidermolysis dystrophica* of recessive inheritance, epidermolysis dystrophica of dominant inheritance, and *simple epidermolysis* of dominant inheritance. Clinically significant esophageal disease is seen only in recessive epidermolysis dystrophica. Esophageal involvement becomes less frequent if the patient survives past childhood. Odynophagia and dysphagia are common because esophageal bullae lead to erosions, ulcers, pseudodiverticula, webs, strictures, and obstruction. The esophagus may shorten, resulting in a traction hiatal hernia and gastroesophageal reflux. Difficulty with swallowing may result in severe malnutrition. In some patients, eating a soft or pureed diet may limit mechanical injury to the esophagus. Corticosteroids or phenytoin, used to inhibit the genetically altered collagenase related to the etiology of this disease, may also prove helpful in controlling esophageal bullae formation. Strictures respond to frequent dilation with inflatable balloons. Bougienage probably should be avoided because shearing forces could perpetuate the injury.[119,120]

Pemphigus

Pemphigus is a group of diseases characterized histologically by acantholysis resulting in bullae formation. The onset is usually between the fifth and seventh decade of life. Pemphigus can result from the administration of some drugs such as D-penicillamine, which is used in management of Wilson's disease. Pemphigus vulgaris can occasionally involve the esophagus, but rarely induces clinically significant disease.[121]

Hereditary Hemorrhagic Telangiectasia

Hereditary hemorrhagic telangiectasia is an autosomal dominant condition associated with the formation of telangiectasias, aneurysms, and arteriovenous malformations throughout the body. The disease frequency is 1 to 2 per 100,000, and it occurs in all races. Cutaneous telangiectasias usually appear after the second or third decade of life and are located most frequently on the face, lips, nares, tongue, ears, and hands. The most prominent clinical feature of this disease is recurrent mucosal hemorrhage from telangiectasias, precipitated by minor trauma or occurring spontaneously. Epistaxis is the most common form of bleeding, with gastrointestinal hemorrhage developing in from 10% to 40% of patients. Genitourinary, pulmonary, and intracerebral bleeding may occur. Occasionally, large vascular ectasias develop associated with mucosal hyperplasia, forming a mass lesion.[122] Hepatic vascular malformations cause arterioportal and intrahepatic portosystemic shunts. These can result in hepatomegaly, hemobilia, portal hypertension, esophageal varices, hepatic encephalopathy, bruit, cardiomegaly, and high-output congestive heart failure. Oral or systemic administration of iron frequently is required to control iron deficiency anemia resulting from bleeding. Frequent transfusions may be needed. Endoscopic coagulation of intestinal vascular malformations may effectively control life-threatening hemorrhage. When large intrahepatic arteriovenous fistulas result in high-output congestive failure, embolization of these vessels or ligation of select branches of the hepatic artery may result in improvement.[123]

Neurofibromatosis

Neurofibromatosis is a dominantly inherited disease. The gene frequency is 1 in 3000 births. Cutaneous diseases comprise café au lait spots and neurofibromas, which can rarely develop into sarcoma.[124] The gastrointestinal tract bears neurofibromas in approximately 25% of patients.[125] Rarely, the liver and gallbladder are also affected.[126,127] Neurofibromas occasionally can cause gastrointestinal bleeding and obstruction, presenting as melena and abdominal pain. Gastrointestinal leiomyomas, sarcomas, and neurogenic neoplasms also are reported.

Psoriasis

Psoriasis is not associated with gastrointestinal disease; however, difficult psoriasis is often controlled by prolonged methotrexate administration. This drug carries the risk of potentially serious hepatotoxicity, including fatty liver, hepatic fibrosis, and cirrhosis.[128,129] Serial liver biopsies are required to detect early hepatic damage because biochemical changes poorly reflect the extent of liver injury. On rare occasions, methotrexate induces colitis.[130]

Stevens-Johnson Syndrome

Stevens-Johnson syndrome is a severe hypersensitivity reaction characterized by a diffuse rash (erythema multiforme) that may progress to an exfoliative dermatitis. It is often accompanied by fever and mucositis of both the gut and the respiratory tract. Etiologic agents include drugs (e.g., sulfonamides, penicillins, anticonvulsants, nonsteroidal antiinflammatory drugs) and infectious agents. The oropharyngeal mucosa frequently exhibits erosions and mucosal sloughing, although the entire gut may be involved in severe cases. Oropharyngeal pain may be severe enough to limit oral intake. Mucosal injury may result in dysphagia, odynophagia, abdominal pain, and gastrointestinal bleeding.[131] Esophageal stricture has been reported as a sequela of the Stevens-Johnson syndrome.[132]

Management includes identification and elimination of the inciting factors, rehydration, nutritional support, antibiotics, and vigilance for respiratory embarrassment and secondary infections. It is unclear whether the use of H_2-receptor antagonists, antacids, or barrier-enhancing agents is beneficial in limiting gastrointestinal mucosal damage or in preventing bleeding. Complete recovery sometimes takes several weeks.[131–133]

Tylosis

Tylosis is a rare, autosomal dominant disorder characterized by thickening of the skin on the palms and soles (Fig. 109-4; see Color Fig. 67). The esophageal mucosa forms papillomas. Those affected have approximately a 95% probability for development of esophageal carcinoma by the age of 65 years.[134,135]

Urticaria

Urticaria is a reactive inflammatory vascular dermatosis characterized by vasodilation, increased vascular permeability, and extravasation of protein and fluids into the dermis.[136] Fluid infiltration results in characteristic peau d'orange wheals. Urticaria of less than 6 weeks' duration is usually related to inciting factors such as medications, radiographic contrast material, or food. Chronic cases are usually idiopathic. Implicated in the pathophysiology of both acute and chronic urticaria is the release of histamine and other inflammatory mediators.

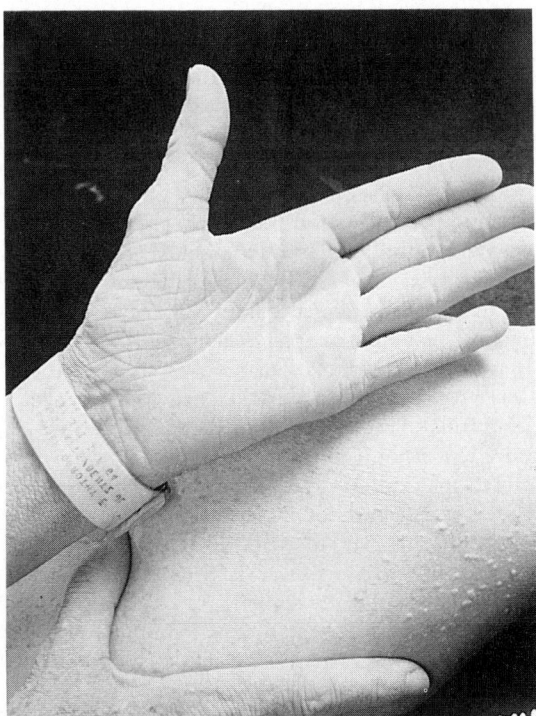

FIGURE 109-4. (See Color Fig. 67.) Hyperkeratosis of the palm and leg may be indicative of tylosis.

Gastrointestinal manifestations have been reported in a number of patients suffering from chronic urticaria. These include abdominal pain, gastroduodenitis, peptic ulcer, and enteric mucosal "hives."[137] Gastrointestinal histamine release has been postulated to account for some of these clinical features.[138]

Urticaria has been observed in the setting of systemic vasculitis. It may accompany a collagen vascular disease, a familial complement deficiency, or an infection. The extracutaneous manifestations of the vasculitis most frequently involve the joints, kidneys, and the gut. Involvement of the latter produces crampy abdominal pain, nausea and vomiting, and diarrhea. The symptoms are often transient. They may appear in concert with cutaneous urticaria and are more in keeping with mucosal edema than with ischemia.[139,140] Hypocomplementemia is frequently evident during the acute attack. Treatment with histamine blockers, corticosteroids, antimalarials, or plasma exchange has met with variable success.

ENDOCRINOLOGIC DISORDERS

Acromegaly

Acromegaly is a disorder resulting from excessive growth hormone production. Patients with acromegaly manifest enlargement of the tongue and other organs of the digestive system. These patients have a propensity for adenomatous colon polyps and perhaps colon cancer.[141]

The adrenal cortex is the source of corticosteroids. Excess circulating corticosteroids from endogenous overproduction or from exogenous administration induce Cushing's syndrome. It is still uncertain whether corticosteroid excess predisposes to the formation of peptic ulcers.

Addison's Disease

Addison's disease, which results from insufficient production of mineralosteroids and corticosteroids by the adrenals, is associated with steatorrhea. The prominent clinical features include anorexia, vomiting, weight loss, abdominal pain, apathy, hypotension, hyponatremia, and hyperkalemia. Mucosal and cutaneous pigmentation occur in primary adrenal failure. Addison's disease of autoimmune etiology is associated with gastritis, and antibodies against H^+,K^+-adenosine triphosphatase and intrinsic factor, and uncommonly achlorhydria and pernicious anemia.

Diabetes Mellitus

Diabetes mellitus is a series of metabolic diseases resulting in primary hyperglycemia and other metabolic disturbances. After one to two decades of overt disease, complications often develop that lead to appreciable morbidity and early mortality. Arteriosclerosis may result in myocardial infarct, stroke, or vascular compromise of the extremities. Other frequent complications include nephropathy with resulting renal failure, retinopathy progressing to blindness, various sensory or motor neuropathies, and susceptibility to infection.

Nausea, vomiting, anorexia, and abdominal pain are frequent accompaniments of acute diabetic acidosis. Gastritis, with a modest propensity for hemorrhage, can develop. Distention of the hepatic capsule secondary to acute fatty liver may result in acute right upper quadrant discomfort. Persistent, severe abdominal pain may signal that the diabetic acidosis is the consequence of some other serious intraabdominal process. In one series, approximately 15% of patients who died from diabetic ketoacidosis had unrecognized pancreatitis discovered at postmortem examination.[142]

Later stages of the disease commonly entail gastrointestinal symptoms of a more chronic nature. Many of the chronic symptoms are believed to result from visceral autonomic neuropathy, thought to be a consequence of a metabolic disturbance of peripheral nerves.[143]

Patients with peripheral neuropathy frequently have abnormal esophageal motor function. As demonstrated radiologically, these abnormalities include esophageal dilation, reflux, and delayed esophageal emptying. Changes demonstrated manometrically may include feeble peristaltic pressure waves that are at times multipeaked or multiphasic, increased frequency of nonperistaltic contractions, and decreased lower esophageal sphincter pressure.[144] Clinical manifestations of esophageal dysfunction, often consisting of mild pyrosis and dysphagia, are unusual.

Severe odynophagia could signify *Candida* esophagitis, which is a condition most common in patients with diabetes and other chronic debilitating diseases that lead to an immunocompromised state. Oral thrush accompanies *Candida* esophagitis in no more than 50% of patients. The endoscopic appearance of *Candida* esophagitis ranges from an erythematous, friable mucosa to complete covering of the mucosal surface with a heavy, creamy white pseudomembrane. The most common finding is that of cream-colored plaques scattered throughout the lower portion of the esophagus. The diagnosis is made through endoscopic biopsy and brushing of the inflamed esophageal mucosa.

Gastric and pyloric motor dysfunction may result in a condition termed *gastroparesis diabeticorum*. Vagal nerve impairment and alterations in gastric myoelectric activity result in gastric dilation, slow peristalsis, delayed gastric emptying, and achlorhydria. Increased pyloric resistance and small intestinal dysmotility may also contribute to retardation of transpyloric flow.[145] Symptoms, which usually occur in advanced diabetes, may include early satiety, bloating, heartburn, persistent nausea, and paroxysmal vomiting. Patients are also predisposed to the formation of gastric bezoars. Yet, most patients with diabetes with abnormalities of gastric emptying have no symptoms. The diagnosis is obtained by upper gastrointestinal series or by gastroscintiscanning using test meals to demonstrate delayed gastric emptying. Radiopaque markers also can be used.[146] Endoscopy supports the diagnosis by confirming absence of pyloric stenosis and revealing a substantial gastric residual after an overnight fast. Treatment of diabetic gastroparesis includes adequate control of blood sugar, correction of electrolyte disturbances, and administration of metoclopramide. The latter accelerates gastric emptying and is an antiemetic. Newer motility-promoting agents under study, such as cisapride, also may prove helpful. Metoclopramide[147] and other drugs that promote gastrokinesis, however, may have only a short-term beneficial effect on gastric motility

owing to tachyphylaxis. Surgery to improve gastric drainage should be contemplated only as a last resort, because success is limited.[148] Repeated, objective measurements of gastric emptying usually are not helpful because they do not discriminate well between symptomatic and asymptomatic patients, and they do not predict the response to treatment.

Diarrhea and, rarely, steatorrhea can appear, particularly in advanced disease.[149,150] The diarrhea is watery and painless. It can remit after days or months, but recurrence is frequent. The condition most likely results from damage to intestinal autonomic innervation. Occasionally, bacterial overgrowth resulting from sluggish small bowel motility is a contributing factor. The diagnosis is made by excluding the long list of other diseases, such as pancreatic insufficiency and celiac sprue, that cause similar symptoms. For instance, chronic pancreatitis can lead to combined endocrine and exocrine insufficiency of the pancreas, resulting in diarrhea secondary to steatorrhea. Also, there is a higher-than-expected incidence of celiac disease in patients with diabetes. Many patients with diabetes and celiac disease share human leukocyte antigen haplotypes, and altered immune function has been implicated in both these diseases.[151] The diarrhea is treated with good glucose control, opiates, and bulk-forming agents containing psyllium. Some patients may improve with clonidine hydrochloride, an α_2-adrenergic agonist, which possibly stimulates an increase in intestinal fluid absorption by enhancing adrenergic activity[152,153]; however, this medication may induce appreciable side effects such as hypotension. Other patients with suspected bacterial overgrowth may respond to antibiotic therapy.

Severe constipation associated with colonic motor abnormalities[154] occurs in 20% of patients with diabetes with neuropathy.[155] The onset of constipation is often insidious. Management includes the use of a variety of nonstimulant laxatives.

Fecal incontinence, usually associated with diarrhea, may develop in part from anal sphincter dysfunction and decreased rectal sensation.[155,156] Diarrhea control and biofeedback training[156] may provide complete or partial relief.

Diabetes mellitus may feature significant abdominal pain secondary to thoracic radiculopathy.[157] The pain can develop unilaterally with or without paresthesia or hypesthesia. Electromyographic examination frequently provides evidence of impairment of thoracic or lumbar nerve roots.[158] Antidepressant drugs such as amitriptyline or desipramine may help control painful diabetic neuropathy.[159] They probably work through modulation of peripheral neurotransmitter pathways.

Arteriosclerosis of large mesenteric vessels or microvascular disease can result in intestinal angina, malabsorption, diarrhea, gastrointestinal bleeding, and, ultimately, intestinal infarct. There are reports of painless infarct.[160]

Diabetes may lead to large, poorly functioning gallbladders that have a predilection for cholelithiasis.[161] Contrary to previous assumptions, patients with diabetes with acute cholecystitis may not have a substantially increased risk of complications compared with the general population.[162] Thus, the previous recommendation that patients with diabetes with silent gallstones have prophylactic cholecystectomy needs to be reconsidered.

Hepatic dysfunction also occurs. Hepatomegaly and fatty liver are frequent findings, especially in patients with poorly controlled blood sugar and obesity. A rare hepatic lesion resembling alcoholic hepatitis has been described that can result in cirrhosis.[163]

Hyperparathyroidism

Hyperparathyroidism is a disorder of calcium and phosphate metabolism. It results from excess secretion of parathyroid hormone, usually adenomatous, hyperplastic, or, rarely, carcinomatous parathyroid-like hormone, that can induce a syndrome similar to primary hyperparathyroidism. Secondary forms of the diseases can result from any condition in which there is a tendency toward hypocalcemia, such as chronic renal failure. Symptoms that are probably consequences of high serum calcium concentrations include anorexia, nausea, vomiting, constipation, and abdominal pain. Hypercalcemia induces gastric hypersecretion. Controversy still exists over whether this disease predisposes to peptic ulcer formation.[164,165] Pancreatitis can develop when hypercalcemia is moderate to severe.[166]

Hypoparathyroidism

Hypoparathyroidism, or low serum ionized calcium from whatever cause can lead to neuromuscular irritability. Gastrointestinal manifestations can include abdominal pain, intestinal tetany, diarrhea, steatorrhea, and intestinal pseudoobstruction.[167] Oral and esophageal candidiasis secondary to immune dysfunction may accompany this syndrome.

Thyroid Disease

Thyroid disease can have important gastrointestinal manifestations. Simple goiters are a common occurrence. They usually are classified as endemic or sporadic. Endemic goiters are those that occur in a large fraction of a particular population of a geographic region, usually because of a particular environmental factor such as iodine deficiency. Sporadic goiters occur in about 5% of the general population and usually are of unknown cause. Most patients with simple goiter are euthyroid and asymptomatic. If the goiter reaches a substantial size, it may cause respiratory obstruction and displacement of the esophagus, resulting in dysphagia.[168]

Hyperthyroidism

Hyperthyroidism is the clinical state induced by excessive circulating thyroid hormone. Although several disorders can induce this syndrome, 85% of the cases are a consequence of *Graves' disease*, which is probably of autoimmune etiology. The symptoms of hyperthyroidism include nervousness, palpitations, heat intolerance, excessive perspiration, fatigue, weakness, dyspnea, and eye complaints. Patients frequently experience enhanced appetite, but usually have weight loss because of their hypermetabolic state. In older patients or those with more advanced disease, anorexia, nausea, and vomiting may develop. The most common physiologic effect on the gastrointestinal system is an alteration in intestinal motility, resulting in shortened small bowel and colonic transit time.[169] This may result in mild steatorrhea[170] and increased stool frequency, but rarely frank diarrhea.[171] The gastric emptying rate usually remains normal.[172] Esophageal motility is essentially normal except for enhanced propagation velocity.[173] There is also a high incidence of gastritis and hypochlorhydria or achlorhydria.[174] Approximately 30% of patients have autoantibodies to gastric parietal cell adenosine triphosphatase, although it is unknown whether this is related to the development of gastritis and disturbances in acid secretion. Moderate to severe hyperthyroidism is occasionally associated with hepatic dysfunction. Increases in blood alkaline phosphatase, transaminases, and bilirubin have been attributed to liver injury. In some cases, passive congestion of the liver secondary to heart failure could be the underlying mechanism. Some liver diseases, such as primary biliary cirrhosis and chronic active hepatitis, have been associated with an increased incidence of the autoimmune-type thyroid diseases (Graves' or Hashimoto's type). Many of the drugs used in the treatment of thyrotoxicosis can induce serious liver damage[175]; also, drug metabolism is altered in the hyperthyroid as well as the hypothyroid state.[176]

Hypothyroidism

Hypothyroidism is the clinical syndrome resulting from deficiency of thyroid hormone. Most cases are a consequence of thyroid gland dysfunction resulting from Hashimoto's thyroiditis or therapy of hyperthyroidism. Symptoms include weakness, dry skin, swelling of the extremities, mental aberrations, coarse voice, paresthesias, arthralgias, and muscle cramps. Patients have a general decrease in metabolism, and experience anorexia and frequently moderate weight gain. Motility is slowed throughout the gastrointestinal tract. Dysphagia may develop related to delayed esophageal emptying, a consequence of weak and prolonged esophageal contractions.[177] Intestinal transit is slowed,[169] usually manifesting as constipation[171]and abdominal distention. Rarely, intestinal pseudoobstruction or megacolon results.[178,179] Equally rare is diarrhea resulting from bacterial overgrowth in the hypomotile small intestine.[180] The gallbladder also may dilate and contract poorly. Other gastrointestinal manifestations include impairment in salivary, gastric, intestinal, and pancreatic[181] secretion, and, not infrequently, achlorhydria. Ascites, usually having a high protein concentration, is a rare complication of myxedema. It can be associated with histologic changes in liver architecture suggestive of central congestive fibrosis, without congestive heart failure.[182] The ascites resolves after appropriate thyroid replacement therapy.[183] Surgery should be avoided whenever possible, because hypothyroidism predisposes to an appreciably higher surgical morbidity and mortality.[184]

Pregnancy

Pregnancy is accompanied by a variety of physiologic changes, many of which have been attributed to the effects of progesterone or β-human chorionic gonadotropin on gastrointestinal motility, and displacement of the viscera by the gravid uterus. The pathophysiology remains incompletely understood, however. Common gastrointestinal symptoms of pregnancy include altered appetite, pica, ptyalism, gingivitis, vomiting, heartburn, constipation, and hemorrhoids.

Gastroesophageal reflux occurs in about 40% of pregnancies and is worse during the third trimester. Impairment of lower esophageal sphincter tone, esophageal peristalsis, and gastrointestinal transit are probably contributory.[185] Conventional therapy with antacids, avoidance of stooping and straining, limiting the size of meals, and elevation of the head of the bed usually suffice.

Morning sickness occurs in about 60% of women during early pregnancy.[186] When extreme, the condition is termed *hyperemesis gravidarum* and can result in dehydration and malnutrition. Vomiting and retching can exacerbate esophagitis and produce Mallory-Weiss tears. Ingestion of dry foods and reassurance are often effective therapy for mild morning sickness. In difficult cases, antiemetics, rehydration, and nutritional support may be required.[187] Endoscopy can be safely performed when the diagnosis is in doubt, but gastrointestinal radiography should be avoided if possible.

Constipation is common and may relate to mechanical compression of the colon and motility disturbance, as well as to a lack of exercise. The problem is rarely severe. It is readily managed by increasing fluid intake and by administrating glycerin suppositories or nonabsorbed laxatives.[188]

Delayed emptying of the gallbladder has been reported, and the incidence of cholecystitis is slightly increased during pregnancy.[189] Hepatobiliary ultrasonography is the diagnostic modality of choice when the diagnosis of acute cholecystitis is suspected.

Although liver function is normal in pregnancy, palmar erythema and spider nevi are often observed, perhaps as a result of elevated steroid hormones. Serum alkaline phosphatase and leucine amino peptidase levels are increased, attributable to placental production. Other liver enzyme levels are normal. Jaundice is infrequent, but when it occurs it is most often the result of *benign intrahepatic cholestasis*.[190] *Toxemia* may produce prehepatic jaundice secondary to hemolysis. When disseminated intravascular coagulation complicates the course, shock and multisystem failure (including liver failure) may be present. The *HELLP syndrome* is a potentially catastrophic variant of toxemia characterized by *h*emolysis, *e*levated *l*iver enzymes, and *l*ow *p*latelets.[191] Its features suggest a thrombotic microangiopathic process, and it must be distinguished from acute fatty liver of pregnancy, hemolytic-uremic syndrome, and thrombotic thrombocytopenic purpura.[192] *Acute fatty liver of pregnancy* resembles Reye's syndrome and usually occurs in young primigravida women in the third trimester.[193] Vomiting, jaundice, encephalopathy, and acute renal failure are often present. Microvesicular fat in the central zone is seen on liver biopsy. Treatment is directed at liver and renal failure.

Splenic artery rupture is a rare but life-threatening complication of pregnancy. It presents with acute abdominal pain and shock.[194] Early delivery may be beneficial.

GRANULOMATOUS DISEASES

The granuloma is normally a protective immune mechanism that permits the host to contain and eventually destroy poorly degradable, harmful stimuli that are resistant to immune at-

tack by other means. Yet, granulomas may have deleterious effects, focally injuring organs and inducing appreciable fibrosis. They are dynamic, usually focal inflammatory processes composed of macrophages and other inflammatory cell types. Many factors such as infectious agents, silica, metals complexed to macromolecules, carrageenan, and immune complexes can evoke a granulomatous response. Granulomas form in some idiopathic conditions such as Crohn's disease, sarcoidosis, and giant cell arteritis. Even when there is a known nidus, the cause of a granuloma is not always apparent on histologic examination. Granulomas that form in response to an antigen that induces a delayed hypersensitivity reaction are called hypersensitivity granulomas. The granulomas seen in diseases such as schistosomiasis, leprosy, tuberculosis, histoplasmosis, berylliosis, and probably Crohn's disease are hypersensitivity lesions. Lesions evoked by substances that do not stimulate a hypersensitivity response are termed foreign body granulomas; examples are granulomas that develop in response to mineral oil and talc.

Many infectious and noninfectious diseases are associated with granuloma formation in the liver and intestines (Table 109-2).[195,196] Although many of these associations are undoubtedly correct, the issue is complicated by the observation that granulomas are present in from 3% to 10% of liver specimens obtained at abdominal surgery or autopsy. The etiology of a granuloma can, at times, be ascertained by identification of bacteria, ova, mineral crystals, or other agents within individual lesions, and by the distribution of the granulomas within an organ. Some granulomas may have distinctive morphology, such as the ring granuloma that usually signifies Q fever, although ring granulomas have been described in other conditions rarely.[197,198] Serologic testing, culture of the involved tissue, or clinical presentation may provide the diagnosis in other circumstances.

In industrialized societies, the etiologic factors most frequently responsible for hepatic granulomas are sarcoidosis and tuberculosis (Table 109-3). Primary biliary cirrhosis and occasionally other primary liver diseases account for many of the remaining cases. In many patients, it is not possible to identify an etiologic factor or an associated disease. Patients may be asymptomatic or present with fever, fatigue, hepatosplenomegaly, and jaundice. Biochemical tests may suggest liver dysfunction or injury. When present, serum enzyme abnormalities frequently demonstrate a disproportionate increase in alkaline phosphatase over transaminases. The process occasionally progresses to extensive hepatic fibrosis and cirrhosis.

Causes of granulomatous inflammation of the intestines are less well characterized (see Table 109-2). *Crohn's disease* and *tuberculous enteritis*, secondary to *Mycobacterium tuberculosis* infection, are the most frequent diagnoses. It can be difficult to distinguish these two entities.[199] Both diseases can have a chronic course, presenting with abdominal pain, fever, fatigue, weight loss, diarrhea, and gastrointestinal bleeding. Both have a predilection for the terminal ileum and result in intestinal strictures. The diagnosis of tuberculosis is suspected if the chest radiograph shows characteristic lesions and the tuberculin skin test is strongly positive. The lungs, however, appear normal in half the patients. Granulomatous hepatitis or ascites secondary to tubercular peritonitis supports the diagnosis. Tuberculin granulomas can have histologic features

TABLE 109-2
Some Conditions Associated With Granulomatous Inflammation of the Liver (L) and/or Intestines (I)

Infections
Bacterial
　Atpyical myocobacteria (L)
　Brucellosis (L)
　Cat scratch disease (L)
　Leprosy (L)
　Tuberculosis (L, I)
　Tularemia (L)
　Yersinia (I)
Chlamydial
　Lymphogranuloma venereum (L, I)
Fungal
　Blastomycosis (L, I)
　Coccidiodomycosis (L, I)
　Cryptococcosis (L)
　Histoplasmosis (L, I)
　Nocardiosis (L)
　Systemic candidiasis (L)
　Trichosporosis (L)
Helminthic
　Ascariasis (L)
　Capillariasis (L)
　Enterobiasis (L)
　Strongyloidiasis (L, I)
　Tongue worm (L)
　Toxocariasis (visceral larva migrans) (L)
Protozoan
　Giardiasis (L)
　Toxoplasmosis (L)
　Visceral leishmaniasis (L)
Rickettsial
　Q fever (L)
Spirochetal
　Secondary syphillis (L, I)
Viral
　Cytomegalorvirus (L)
　Mononucleosis (L)

Drug Hypersensitivity
Allopurinol (L)
Amoxicillin-clavulanic (L)
Diphenylhydantoin (L)
Halothane (L)
Hydralazine (L)
Methyldopa (L)
Nitrofurantoin (L)
Phenylbutazone (L)
Procainamide (L)
Quinidine (L)
Quinine (L)
Sulfasalazine (L)
Sulfonamides (L)
Sulfonylurea (L)

Malignancy
Hodgkin's disease (L)
Non-Hodgkin's lymphoma (L)

Metals
Barium (I)
Beryllium (L)
Copper (L)

Vasculitis
Giant cell arteritis (L)
Lupus erythematosus (L)
Polyarteritis nodosa (L)
Polymyalgia rheumatica (L)
Rheumatoid arthritis (L)
Wegener's granulomatosis (L, I)

Miscellaneous
Appendiceal granuloma (I)
Bacile Calmette-Guérin immunotherapy (L)
Crohn's disease (L, I)
Idiopathic granulomatous gastritis (I)
Idiopathic granulomatous hepatitis (L)
Immunodeficiency (L)
Jejunoileal bypass surgery (L)
Mineral oil (L, I)
Primary biliary cirrhosis (L)
Sarcoidosis (L, I)
Silica (L)
Whipple's disease (L)

distinct from those of Crohn's disease. They are frequently big lesions, tend to coalesce, and often contain giant cells that are numerous and large. Caseation, although rare in the intestine, suggests tuberculosis. Histologic staining or culture may identify acid-fast bacilli.[200]

In all forms of granulomatous inflammation, treatment usually is directed at eliminating the offending agent. Lesions that defy diagnosis or are of unknown cause present special problems. Many are asymptomatic and require no therapy. Unusual conditions like idiopathic granulomatous hepatitis frequently respond to corticosteroid administration. Sarcoidosis and Crohn's disease usually respond to immunosuppressants or antiinflammatory agents.

HEAVY METAL TOXICITY

Lead Poisoning

Lead poisoning remains a common form of heavy metal intoxication, often producing vague, nonspecific, and transient symptoms. Approximately 40,000 new cases occur yearly in the United States.[201] The diagnosis should be entertained in patients presenting with abdominal complaints and a history of occupational or environmental exposure, such as ingestion or removal of lead-based paints, manufacture of batteries or jewelry, welding, automobile radiator repair, and eating from painted dishes acquired abroad.[202] Inner-city children in major

TABLE 109-3
Etiologies of Hepatic Granulomas in Several Reported Series From Around the World

DIAGNOSIS	NUMBER WITH LISTED DIAGNOSIS IN INDICATED SERIES								TOTAL (%)
	1	2	3	4	5	6	7	8	
Sarcoidosis	15	6	92	8	28	11	217	81	395 (35)
Tuberculosis	6	13	51	34	15	5	70	30	224 (20)
Undetermined diagnosis	4	10	11	13	15	18	45	13	129 (11)
Primary biliary cirrhosis						3	59		62 (5)
Other cirrhosis						4	51		55 (5)
Schistosomiasis			9		1		19		29 (2)
Lymphomas		1		3		3	11	4	22 (2)
Brucellosis	1	1	4	1			4	8	19 (2)
Drug-induced or toxic hepatitis							13	10	13 (1)
Acute viral hepatitis							13		13 (1)
Fungal infections				3	1	6			10 (1)
Other infectious causes*	3	7		1			14	27	52 (5)
Other noninfectious causes†	3		45	1			49	6	104 (9)
Unspecified etiology			2						
Total	32	38	214	64	60	50	565	106	1129

* Including Mediterranean fever (Olmer disease), 13 cases; typhoid fever, 7; infectious mononucleosis, 5; syphilis, 5; unspecified bacterial infections, 4; unspecified viral infections, 4; leprosy, 3; toxoplasmosis, 3; cytomegalovirus, 2; lymphogranuloma, 2; actinomycosis, 1; influenza B, 1; visceral larva migrans, 1; and bacille Calmette-Guérin infection, 1.

† Including primary liver disease, 44 cases; biliary and pancreatic disorders, 17; berylliosis, 9; malignancy, 9; fatty liver; 8; chronic active hepatitis, 4; temporal arteritis, 3; regional enteritis, 2; Wegener's granulomatosis, 2; erythema nodosum, 1; eosinophilic granuloma of the lung, 1; starch granuloma of the peritoneum, 1; hypogammaglobulinemia, 1; and celiac disease, 1.

Adapted from Harrington PT, Gutierrez JT, Ramirez-Ronda CH, et al. Granulomatous hepatitis. Rev Infect Dis 1982:4:639.

metropolitan areas are particularly at risk because of lead-based paint ingestion.

Common symptoms include recurrent, severe abdominal pain (lead colic), oral ulcers, constipation, stocking-glove paresthesias, and a metallic taste in the mouth. Lead colic may be sufficiently severe to mimic an acute abdomen or an acute myocardial infarction. Physical findings include a gingival lead line (absent in edentulous patients) and peripheral neuropathy. Anemia and renal dysfunction also may be evident at the time of presentation.[202] Mild acute hepatitis that responds to chelation therapy has been described in the setting of lead intoxication.[203] Lead inhibits enzymes involved in the synthesis of heme. Secondary porphyria may result, characterized by elevated δ-aminolevulonic acid and other porphyrin metabolites in the urine.

The diagnosis of lead poisoning is best established by 72-hour urine testing after administration of calcium disodium edetate.[202,204] Blood lead levels reflect only recent exposure. Treatment of lead poisoning with chelating agents is usually successful if the diagnosis is made in time.[202] Lead colic is usually self-limited, but corticosteroids may shorten and ameliorate the acute episode.[205]

Arsenic Poisoning

Arsenic poisoning is endemic in many parts of the world, including North America, as a result of environmental contamination. Arsenic continues to enjoy wide use, particularly in the preservation of wood and the manufacture of glass and metal.[206,207] It also remains a favorite means of intentional poisoning.[208]

Acute Arsenic Poisoning

Acute arsenic poisoning results in a reversible inactivation of sulfhydryl-containing enzymes. Cellular oxidative processes are thereby blocked and tissue hypoxemia ensues.[209] Patients present with severe abdominal pain, vomiting, profuse diarrhea, malodorous ("garlicky") breath, dysphagia, hepatomegaly, jaundice, and circulatory collapse. Doses of 100 to 300 mg may be fatal.[206]

The diagnosis is made by Gutzeit's or Reinsch's test,[209] or by measuring arsenic levels in tissue sample (e.g., hair or nails). Treatment of acute poisoning consists of gastric lavage, rehydration, the use of chelators (e.g., dimercaprol or penicillamine), and hemodialysis. Medicolegal advice should be sought if intentional poisoning is suspected.

Chronic Arsenic Toxicity

Chronic arsenic toxicity is more insidious. Patients often manifest nonspecific symptoms, including weakness, nausea, diarrhea, or constipation. Macular skin pigmentation, leukoderma, palmar and plantar keratoses, pancytopenia, edema, peripheral vascular disease, neuropathy, cirrhosis, and accompanying portal hypertension may appear alone or in combination.[209,210] An association with cutaneous, hematologic, respiratory, and hepatic malignancies (especially hemangioendothelioma) has also been suggested.[210]

Gold

Gold preparations (e.g., gold sodium thimalate and auranofin) have long been used in the treatment of rheumatoid arthritis. Adverse effects include aplastic anemia, proteinuria, rash, stomatitis, and diarrhea. The latter is particularly common with auranofin, an oral preparation that increases intestinal permeability and decreases intestinal transit time.[211]

Gold-induced enterocolitis is a rare but serious complication[212] that can involve both the small and large intestine. The clinical course is protracted, with a mortality approaching 40%.[213] Endoscopy reveals an erythematous, friable, ulcerated mucosa resembling ulcerative colitis. Gold should be withdrawn as soon as the condition is recognized. Corticosteroid therapy is of uncertain benefit.[213,214]

HEMATOLOGIC DISORDERS

Hemolytic Uremic Syndrome

The hallmarks of the hemolytic uremic syndrome are hemolysis, thrombocytopenia, and acute renal failure. All age groups are affected, but the disease is most common in children. A variety of inciting factors have been associated with this disorder, especially antecedent gram-negative enteric infections such as those with *Salmonella*, *Shigella*, and *Campylobacter* sp.[215,216] Verotoxin-producing strains of *Escherichia coli*, especially serotype O157:H7, appear to be responsible for most cases in children[217,218] and probably many cases in adults. The pathophysiology is poorly understood. Endothelial cell injury (perhaps mediated by endotoxins or immune complexes) followed by intravascular coagulation, and, finally, thrombotic microangiopathy in the glomerulus and the gastrointestinal mucosa, are consistent features (Fig. 109-5; see Color Fig. 68).[219] A deficiency in prostacyclin may help to

perpetuate intravascular platelet activation and intravascular coagulation with resulting thrombocytopenia.[220] The spectrum of gastroenterologic symptoms ranges from gastroenteritis to fulminant colitis with toxic megacolon or colonic perforation, almost always preceding the development of renal failure. The disease is usually self-limited, although the course may be prolonged. There is no evidence that early treatment of the enteric infection obviates the development of hemolytic uremic syndrome.[221] Treatment centers on general support, antibiotics, and dialysis. Steroids are of doubtful benefit, but occasional reports of a beneficial effect from plasmapheresis have appeared.[222]

Thrombotic Thrombocytopenic Purpura

Thrombotic thrombocytopenic purpura closely resembles hemolytic uremic syndrome and has a similar etiology. The syndrome differs in its predilection for older people (30–40 years of age), frequent fever, and neurologic findings. In addition, thrombotic thrombocytopenic purpura is associated with acute cholecystitis.[223] The treatment is similar to that of hemolytic uremic syndrome.

Hypercoagulability

Hypercoagulability is an important cause of gastrointestinal morbidity. Oral contraceptives, pregnancy, inflammation, and surgery may lead to *diminished antithrombin levels* and a consequent propensity for venous thrombosis and embolism. *Paroxysmal nocturnal hemoglobinuria* is an acquired hemolytic disorder associated with a thrombotic diathesis. *Antithrombin III deficiency* and *protein C deficiency* are inherited (autosomal dominant) disorders associated with recurrent venous thrombosis.[224,225] In the latter diseases, affected people require lifelong therapy with warfarin to prevent vascular catastrophe. In all of these conditions, involvement of the mesenteric circulation may result in intestinal ischemia or portal hypertension on the basis of *portal vein thrombosis* or *Budd-Chiari syndrome*.

Deficits of Coagulation Factors

Deficits of coagulation factors may be inherited or acquired, and are often associated with bleeding tendencies. The best known of the inherited factor deficits is *hemophilia A*, an X-linked disorder of factor VIII synthesis. Other inherited forms include *hemophilia B*, or *Christmas disease* (factor IX deficiency), and *factor XI deficiency*. Acquired or iatrogenic coagulation factor deficiencies are commonly seen as a consequence of vitamin K deficiency, warfarin therapy, or liver disease.[226] Another cause is *disseminated intravascular coagulation*. In conditions such as SLE and cancer, circulating anticoagulants of endogenous origin can appear and interfere with normal coagulation. Gastrointestinal bleeding occurs in all of the diseases. It may be mucosal, intramural, or intraabdominal and involve virtually any part of the gastrointestinal tract. Bleeding can be spontaneous or follow trauma or surgery.

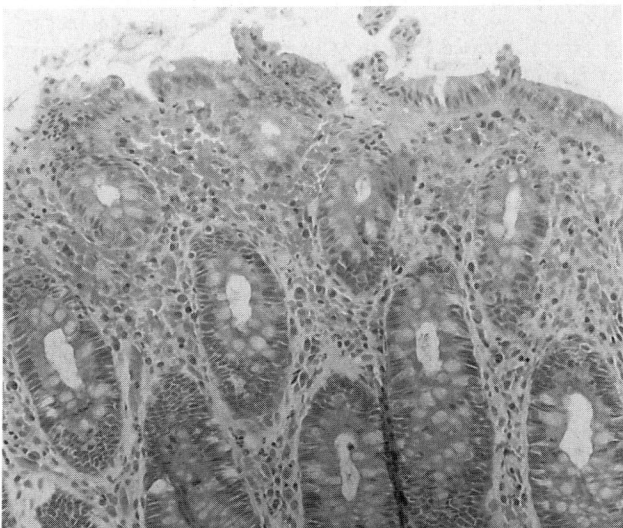

FIGURE 109-5. (See Color Fig. 68.) Colonic biopsy specimen from a patient with hemolytic uremic syndrome shows intravascular coagulation and thrombotic microangiopathy. (Hematoxylin and eosin stain; original magnification ×16.)

Platelet Defects

Platelet defects also may result in severe bleeding diatheses. *Von Willebrand's disease*, the *Bernard-Soulier syndrome*, and *Glanzman's thrombasthenia* are inherited diseases of platelet adhesion and aggregation associated with prolonged bleeding times.[226] Aspirin, nonsteroidal antiinflammatory agents, and other drugs (e.g., penicillins, cephalosporins) may interfere with platelet function by inhibiting cyclooxygenase activity and thereby prolong the bleeding time for 5 to 7 days.[227] Patients should be instructed to avoid the use of these drugs before and after elective surgery, liver biopsy, and endoscopy.

Plummer-Vinson-Kelly Syndrome

Dysphagia and iron deficiency anemia are the clinical manifestations of the Plummer-Vinson-Kelly syndrome. Middle-aged women are most commonly affected. Glossitis, dyspepsia, diarrhea, flatulence, hoarseness, and paresthesias are frequently present.[228] Poor nutrition, cheilosis, pyorrhea, koilonychia, glossitis, atrophic gastritis, and splenomegaly are also evident in many patients. An association with hypopharyngeal and esophageal cancer has been reported.[229,230]

The dysphagia is caused by the presence of hypopharyngeal or esophageal webs of squamous epithelium. Inflammation is frequently present in the submucosa and may contribute to the dysphagia by producing fibrosis. The webs usually are thin (less than 2 mm thick) and notoriously difficult to visualize radiographically and endoscopically (the endoscope may inadvertently rupture them). The optimal way to detect them is with rapid cinefluorography, in which they are visualized transiently in the lateral view when the esophagus is maximally distended.[231,232]

The significance of iron deficiency anemia with regard to the pathogenesis of Plummer-Vinson-Kelly syndrome is unknown. Hereditary factors, as well as deficiencies of riboflavin, thiamine, and pyridoxine also have been implicated in the cause of the syndrome.[228]

Therapy includes dilation of the webs and fibrous tissue to alleviate the dysphagia. Iron and vitamin supplementation is indicated. A careful endoscopic evaluation of the hypopharynx and upper esophagus also should be undertaken to exclude cancer.

Sickle Cell Anemia

Sickle cell anemia is an autosomal recessively inherited disease of hemoglobin synthesis (hemoglobin SS). Eight percent of the African-American population of the United States are heterozygotes; hence, as many as 15 of every 100,000 African Americans may be affected.[233] A broad spectrum of clinical manifestations result from the tendency for the erythrocytes to sickle under conditions of low oxygen tension and to become lodged in capillary beds. This causes widespread venous congestion, thrombosis, and microinfarction, and leads to the clinical "crisis." Abdominal pain and ileus may be seen during the acute crisis. Multiple air fluid levels evident on plain abdominal films may lead the clinician wrongly to sus-

pect intestinal obstruction.[234] Mucosal ulcers and gastrointestinal bleeding have also been reported, and may be due to splanchnic circulatory compromise.[235]

The liver and spleen are frequently involved in sickle cell anemia. In one large series, more than half of the patients exhibited jaundice (usually "prehepatic") and hepatomegaly.[236] Cholelithiasis, cholecystitis, and transfusion-related liver problems including hemosiderosis also are common.[237-239] Splenomegaly is frequent in the early stages of the disease, but "autosplenectomy" due to repeated splenic infarctions often results in a shrunken, fibrotic, or calcified spleen.

It is often difficult to distinguish a sickle cell crisis from other gastrointestinal emergencies such as cholecystitis, appendicitis, and bowel obstruction. Moreover, these intraabdominal illnesses may themselves provoke a sickle cell crisis. The absence of extraabdominal symptoms is suggestive of a primary intraabdominal cause.[240] Sickle cell crises often resolve in several days (usually less than 4 days). Hence, abdominal symptoms of long duration should raise the possibility of another diagnosis.

Hemoglobin C

Patients with hemoglobin C disease may have similar but milder attacks. In this disease, autosplenectomy is less common, and hence splenomegaly usually persists into adulthood.

Hereditary Spherocytosis

Hereditary spherocytosis is a disease of autosomal dominant inheritance characterized by small, fragile, spherical erythrocytes. Hemolysis leads to indirect hyperbilirubinemia, jaundice, and splenomegaly in infancy. Pigment gallstones may be evident even in childhood. Splenectomy has been advocated for children and young adults, but is of doubtful benefit to older, well compensated patients.[241] Relapsing pancreatitis has been described in patients with spherocytosis, and may be related to the passage of gallstones or debris.

METABOLIC DISEASES

Systemic Amyloidosis

Systemic amyloidosis is a disease process characterized by the widespread extracellular deposition of amyloid, a protein.[242,243] Small blood vessels of virtually any organ, neurolemma, and sarcolemma become encased by the insoluble, fibrillar protein.[242,244] Both primary and secondary forms of systemic amyloidosis exist. The latter is found in association with multiple myeloma and chronic infectious or inflammatory diseases, such as tuberculosis and familial Mediterranean fever. Localized forms of the disease are well described.[245-247]

The gastrointestinal tract may be involved at any site. Infiltration of the tongue results in macroglossia in as many as 20% of cases of primary amyloidosis,[242,244,245,247,248] but is uncommon in secondary forms of the disease. Esophageal involvement occurs in two thirds of patients. This weakens the lower esophageal sphincter and disturbs normal esophageal contractility. Reflux and dysphagia are the consequence.[248] Gastric infiltration produces prominent gastric folds, gastric outlet obstruction, ulcer, and bleeding.[244]

Amyloid commonly accumulates between the muscle layers of the intestine, causing coarsening of the valvulae coniventes (Fig. 109-6; see Color Fig. 69).[249,250] Mesenteric retraction and intestinal obstruction also can result from amyloid infiltration. Pseudoobstruction, possibly a consequence of nerve, muscle, and mucosal involvement, leads to stasis, bacterial overgrowth, and malabsorption in some patients. Intestinal ischemia resulting in pain, enterocolitis, bleeding, and infarction also has been reported.[245,246]

Liver and spleen infiltration causes hepatosplenomegaly, but liver failure and portal hypertension are uncommon. Ascites may result from nephrotic syndrome-induced hypoproteinemia. Pancreatic involvement has occasionally produced exocrine pancreatic insufficiency and steatorrhea.[242–245]

The diagnosis is often established by rectal biopsy, which reveals evidence of amyloid in as many as 80% of cases, providing submucosa is present in the sample.[244] Treatment of the underlying disease process may result in amyloid regression.

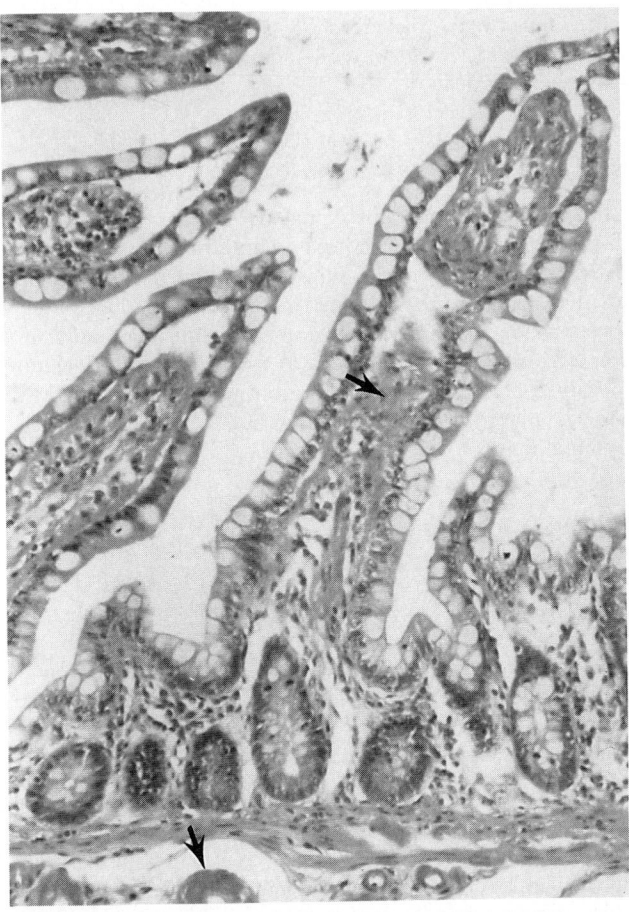

FIGURE 109-6. (See Color Fig. 69.) Amyloid infiltration of the small intestine (*arrows*). (Congo red stain; original magnification ×200.)

Capillary Leak Syndrome

Capillary leak syndrome is an episodic illness of variable severity characterized by increased small vessel permeability and fluid shifts.[251] Its association with systemic toxicity, sepsis, and administration of a number of recombinant protein medications, including interleukin-2 and GM-CSF, supports the contention that it is directly mediated by cytokines.[251,252] In addition to hemoconcentration, hypotension, and a frequently present monoclonal gammopathy, patients can experience severe nausea, vomiting, and diarrhea secondary to impaired fluid absorption in the gastrointestinal tract.[251] Therapy with aminophylline and terbutaline has been reported to ameliorate the syndrome in some patients.[253,254]

NEOPLASTIC DISORDERS

Hematologic Malignancies

Acute and Chronic Leukemias

Gastrointestinal involvement with acute and chronic leukemias is common. The gastrointestinal manifestations result chiefly from leukemic infiltration, chemotherapy, and opportunistic infection. Gingivitis is a consequence of leukemic invasion of the gums and causes oral pain and bleeding. Massively enlarged tonsils in acute lymphocytic leukemia have rarely resulted in oropharyngeal dysphagia. Leukemic infiltration of the esophagus, stomach, intestine, or colon produces mucosal or intramural lesions that may cause dysphagia, obstruction, bleeding, or enterocolitis.[255,256] Hepatosplenomegaly and portal hypertension are additional complications of leukemic infiltration. Subcapsular splenic hemorrhage and splenic rupture have been reported, particularly in acute lymphoblastic leukemia.[257]

Chemotherapy is associated with gastrointestinal manifestation. *Stomatitis* or *mucositis* frequently follow chemotherapy and are caused by a combination of epithelial cell toxicity and secondary infection. The oropharyngeal membranes are inflamed and friable. Therapy with 5-fluorouracil seems particularly toxic to the oral mucous membranes.[258] Cryotherapy,[259] topical vitamin E,[260] and sucralfate oral suspensions[261] all have been suggested to ameliorate 5-fluorouracil-related mucositis.

Nausea, vomiting, diarrhea, or constipation are ubiquitous after chemotherapy, and may exacerbate inanition. Idiopathic or pseudomembranous colitis also are commonly seen in this setting. Induction chemotherapy can induce an often fatal syndrome characterized by acute abdomen, paralytic ileus, diarrhea, and gastrointestinal bleeding.[262] This catastrophic event is often attributed to *necrotizing enterocolitis* or *typhlitis*, a severe inflammatory process usually involving the distal small bowel, cecum, or appendix (Fig. 109-7).[256,257,262] It is most often seen in the setting of postchemotherapy neutropenia, but similar lesions have been described in other immunocompromised states. Infectious agents and antineoplastic medications have been implicated in the etiology of the disease. Diarrhea (sometimes bloody), right lower quadrant pain or tenderness, nausea, and vomiting are the usual presenting features, developing over hours to many days. The differential diagnosis includes infectious colitis caused by

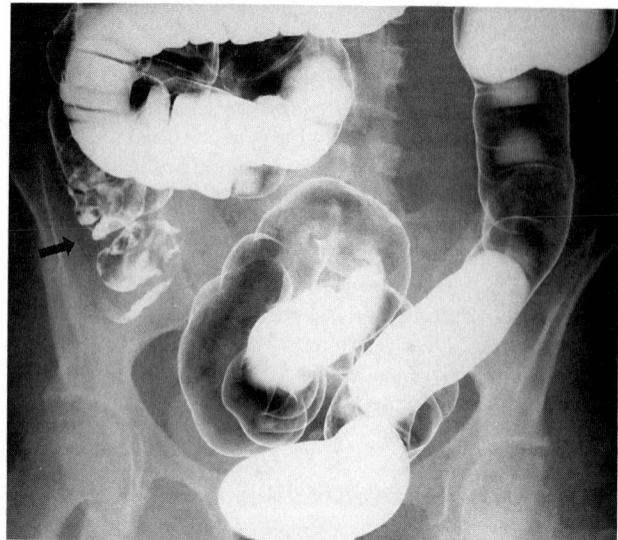

FIGURE 109-7. Typhlitis involves terminal ileum and cecum in a patient with acute myelogenous leukemia.

Clostridium difficile, cytomegalovirus, and other organisms; appendicitis; Ogilvie's syndrome; and bowel obstruction. Patients at risk must be watched closely for evidence of cecal perforation.

Like other immunocompromised hosts, neutropenic patients with cancer are subject to opportunistic infections. Pharyngitis and esophagitis attributable to *Candida*, herpesvirus, or cytomegalovirus infection may present as odynophagia, dysphagia, and upper gastrointestinal bleeding. Gastritis, enteritis, and colitis may be caused by a wide variety of fungal, viral, bacterial, and parasitic infections. Malabsorption, diarrhea, bleeding, and perforation can result. In addition to these opportunistic infections, infection with bowel flora is an important source of morbidity. Also common in this setting are stercoral ulcers, perianal and perirectal abscesses, pseudomembranous colitis, and necrotizing enterocolitis.[263]

Multiple Myeloma

Multiple myeloma results from the neoplastic proliferation of monoclonal plasma cells. Middle-aged and older people usually are affected. Osteolytic lesions of the skeleton, hypercalcemia, anemia, monoclonal gammopathy, and renal disease are characteristic findings.[264] When the gastrointestinal tract is invaded, plasmacytomas form with attendant abdominal pain, ulceration, and bleeding or obstruction. The lesions may be detected radiographically or endoscopically,[265] and sometimes must be differentiated from peptic ulcer disease. Some patients have hyperviscosity syndromes as a result of elevated serum immunoglobulin. Visceral ischemia and thrombosis may result. Angiographic studies are undertaken with caution, because administration of radiographic contrast medium may precipitate acute renal failure, especially in dehydrated patients. Amyloidosis is a well recognized complication of myeloma (see Metabolic Diseases). Involvement of the liver and spleen results in hepatosplenomegaly and, rarely, portal hypertension.[266]

Waldenström's macroglobulinemia is an IgM-secreting variant of myeloma characterized by the presence of macroglobulin (monoclonal IgM) in the serum. Osteolytic lesions are less commonly seen than in myeloma, whereas lymphadenopathy and hyperviscosity are more prominent. Massive hepatosplenomegaly results from infiltration by plasma cells. The deposition of large amounts of IgM in the intestinal lamina propria and mesenteric lymph nodes can impair absorption,[267] resulting in diarrhea and steatorrhea.

Heavy Chain Diseases

The heavy chain diseases are related neoplastic disorders of B cells. The neoplastic B cells produce abnormal monoclonal heavy chains. The disease variants are classified according to the heavy chain isotype secreted (i.e., α, γ, μ, and δ).[268]

α-Heavy chain disease (Mediterranean lymphoma) is the most common of these entities and is seen in two forms, pulmonary and enteric. The former is more common in the United States, but rarely exhibits gastrointestinal manifestations.[268] The latter is principally found in the Mediterranean region and countries where hygiene is rudimentary. Infiltration of the small intestine and abdominal lymph nodes by malignant B cells and α-heavy chains produces abdominal pain and masses, vomiting, weight loss, malabsorption, steatorrhea, and hypocalcemia.[269] Additional complications include obstruction, intussusception, and intestinal perforation. Clubbing and low-grade fever are commonly seen. *γ- and μ-Heavy chain disease* are infrequent and rarely involve the gastrointestinal tract.

Hodgkin's Disease

Clinically evident gastrointestinal involvement in Hodgkin's disease is infrequent, although a substantial proportion of patients who die from this illness are found to have hepatic involvement at autopsy (Fig. 109-8; see Color Fig. 70).[270] Presinusoidal portal hypertension can result from either increased intrahepatic blood flow as a consequence of splenomegaly, or intrahepatic infiltration with malignant cells. Rarely, enlarged mesenteric lymph nodes manifest as an abdominal mass or produce obstruction.[271]

Non-Hodgkin's Lymphoma

In contrast, as many as 10% of patients with non-Hodgkin's lymphoma have gastrointestinal tract involvement. Obstruction, bleeding, abdominal masses, and perforation are among the more frequently recognized clinical features. Invasion of the liver and spleen is frequent.[272,273] Primary small intestinal lymphoma of the Western type produces complications similar to that of α-heavy chain disease (see Chap. 76).

Polycythemia Vera

Polycythemia vera is a myeloproliferative disorder of unknown cause affecting middle-aged people and characterized by an increased red cell mass.[274] Many patients have associated thrombocytosis. The clinical features are a result of the ery-

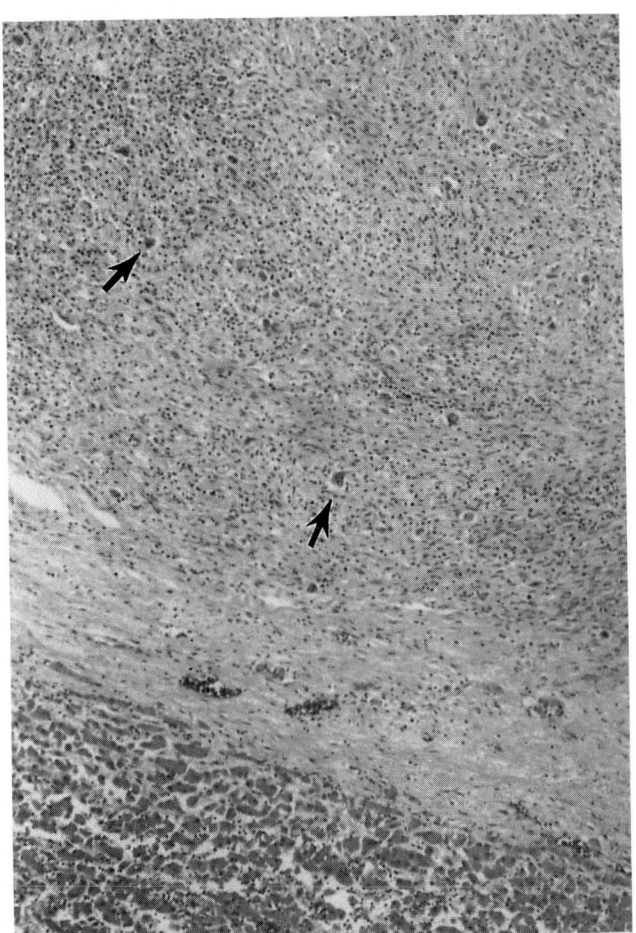

FIGURE 109-8. (See Color Fig. 70.) Hodgkin's disease infiltrating the liver. Reed-Sternberg cells are present (*arrows*). (Hematoxylin and eosin stain; original magnification ×25.)

throcytosis and hyperviscosity syndrome and include plethora, headache, vertigo, dizziness, visual disturbances, vascular ischemia, and thrombosis. Gastrointestinal manifestations include a fourfold increase in peptic ulcer disease compared with unaffected people.[275] Budd-Chiari syndrome may develop as a consequence of hepatic vein thrombosis. Splanchnic circulatory insufficiency and gastrointestinal bleeding[275] are also seen. The latter is aggravated by an accompanying deficit in platelet aggregation. Hepatosplenomegaly due to extramedullary hematopoiesis produces upper abdominal fullness in some patients. Iron deficiency-induced cheilosis and glossitis have been reported in patients treated by extensive phlebotomy.[276]

Primary or Essential Thrombocytosis

Primary or essential thrombocytosis is a myeloproliferative disorder characterized by a platelet count greater than 10^6/mm^3, but without an increase in the red cell mass.[277] This condition must be differentiated from the secondary thrombocytosis that accompanies inflammation and iron deficiency. As for polycythemia vera, platelet aggregation defects predispose to gastrointestinal bleeding or thrombosis. Hepato-

splenomegaly is evident in many patients,[278] and is caused by extramedullary hematopoiesis or Budd-Chiari syndrome.

Nonhematologic Malignancies

Malignant Melanoma

Intestinal metastasis from tumors originating in locations outside the gastrointestinal system can induce significant symptomatology. Malignant melanoma has a propensity for such behavior. As revealed in postmortem examination, the stomach is involved in 26%, the small intestine in 58%, and the colon in 26% of all cases. Liver, pancreas, and, rarely, gallbladder also can be effected. The gastrointestinal metastases are usually numerous, variable in size, and either pigmented or amelanotic. Most remain asymptomatic. When complications do arise, they include nonspecific abdominal pain, anorexia, occult or massive gastrointestinal hemorrhage, and intestinal perforation. Pain is often secondary to intussusception or obstruction. Bleeding and perforation usually result from ulceration of metastases. Jaundice can arise from extrinsic compression of the bile duct, whereas gallbladder involvement may result in cholecystitis. In appropriate circumstances, surgical intervention to alleviate significant gastrointestinal complications is warranted, because melanoma frequently permits prolonged survival.[279]

Other malignancies derived from organs such as the breast,[280] lung, and thyroid rarely metastasize to the intestines and produce symptoms. In approximately half of the patients with Kaposi's sarcoma, a frequent accompaniment of acquired immune deficiency syndrome, intraoral or intestinal involvement develops (Fig. 109-9; see Color Fig. 71).[281]

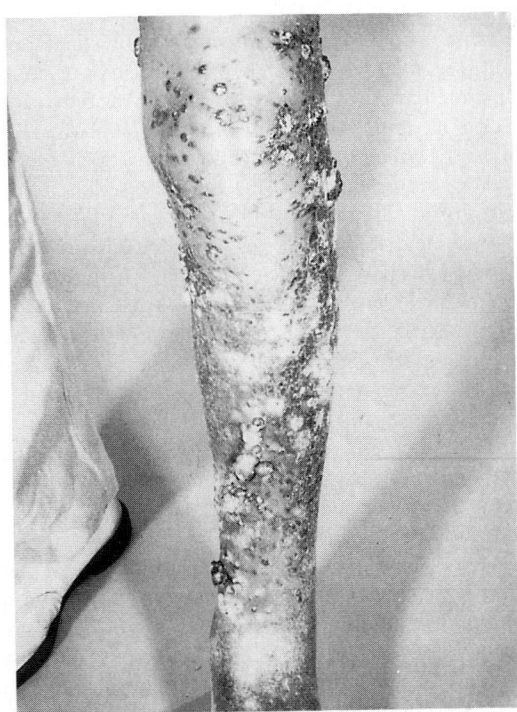

FIGURE 109-9. (See Color Fig. 71.) Kaposi's sarcoma of the lower extremities.

Ovarian Cancer

Tumors can produce gastrointestinal complications by local extension. Ovarian cancer frequently encases the abdominal viscera. Intestinal obstruction leading to malnutrition and intestinal infarction commonly causes death.[282] Other nearby tumors, such as bladder or prostate carcinoma, can infiltrate the bowel wall or destroy nearby vital vascular, lymphatic, or neuronal elements, resulting in intestinal bleeding, vascular compromise, obstruction, or pseudoobstruction. Adrenal tumors may invade the hepatic vein and induce Budd-Chiari syndrome. The chemical and radiation therapies used to control cancer also produce appreciable intestinal morbidity.

Paraneoplastic Syndromes

Paraneoplastic syndromes are disorders resulting from underlying malignancy that are not related to local extension of primary or metastatic tumor. The major clinical gastrointestinal manifestations of such syndromes include anorexia, constipation, and diarrhea.

Cancer Cachexia

Cancer cachexia is a paraneoplastic syndrome characterized by progressive involuntary weight loss, anorexia, and a variety of metabolic disturbances.[283] The syndrome may occur during early tumor development; however, it is usually associated with widely disseminated disease. The humoral factors responsible for this condition are unknown. One determinant may be tumor necrosis factor released from macrophages in response to infection, trauma, and tumors.

Constipation is a common symptom of patients with cancer. It may be a consequence of factors such as decreased physical activity, reduced fluid intake, and changes in diet. Many drugs, such as the opioids that are used to relieve pain, induce constipation. Metabolic disorders or intestinal lumenal narrowing secondary to tumor growth can also be responsible. Constipation may result from hypercalcemia related to ectopic production of parathyroid-like hormone by neoplasms. Rarely, malignancy, particularly small cell carcinoma of the lung, produces a *paraneoplastic visceral neuropathy* that results in aberrant motor activity throughout the gastrointestinal system.[284] In some cases, inflammation and degeneration of the myenteric plexus have been documented. The motor disturbances may include esophageal spasm, achalasia, or simply loss of esophageal peristalsis, gastroparesis, slow intestinal transit, and intestinal pseudoobstruction.[285] The presenting complaints are frequently dysphagia, nausea, vomiting, abdominal distention, and constipation. Some patients manifest a constellation of other neurologic disorders involving peripheral nerves and the central nervous system.

Several tumors frequently are associated with the development of chronic diarrhea and, at times, steatorrhea.[286] They release one or more of a variety of agents into the circulation that affect gastrointestinal function. Many of the tumors arise predominantly, but not exclusively, from amine precursor uptake and decarboxylation (APUD) cells in the pancreas or gastrointestinal tract. These include carcinoid tumors, gastrinomas, glucagonomas, somatostatinomas, and VIPomas. Other tumors that form from APUD cells outside the gastrointestinal system and commonly produce the syndrome include ganglioneuroblastomas, ganglioneurofibromas, medullary thyroid carcinomas, and pheochromocytomas. Unrelated tumors, such as bronchogenic carcinoma, can on occasion elicit watery diarrhea.

Multiple Endocrine Neoplasia Syndromes

Many of these tumors arise as part of the multiple endocrine neoplasia syndromes (MEN), which are dominantly inherited proliferative disorders.[287] Two main types are distinguished. *MEN I* is characterized by the combined occurrence of tumors of the pituitary gland, pancreatic islets, and parathyroid. Islet tumors may include gastrinomas, insulinomas, and, rarely, glucagonomas, VIPomas, and others. There is also a propensity for carcinoid tumors. *MEN IIA* is characterized by pheochromocytoma, medullary thyroid carcinoma, and hyperparathyroidism. *MEN IIB* is similar to type IIA, but without involvement of the parathyroid glands. It is associated with the development of ganglioneuromas throughout the gastrointestinal tract and a marfanoid habitus. Several mixed forms of these syndromes have been described.

Mastocytosis

Mastocytosis is a rare disorder of mast cell proliferation associated with diarrhea. The disease occurs in both cutaneous and systemic forms. Skin involvement is termed *urticaria pigmentosa*. In systemic mastocytosis, mast cell proliferation arises in almost any organ, including intestines and liver. Occurrence of the latter can result in portal hypertension. Common symptoms are headache, pruritus, flushing, dizziness, wheezing, and tachycardia. Gastrointestinal dysfunction develops in 25% of patients, resulting in abdominal pain, nausea, diarrhea, malabsorption, gastritis, and peptic ulcers.[288,289] Stroking cutaneous lesions or drinking alcohol may precipitate symptoms. Symptomatology is probably secondary to the release of many mast cell products such as histamine. Treatment with cromoglycate or histamine receptor antagonists provides relief in some patients.[290]

Diffuse Esophageal Leiomyomatosis

Diffuse esophageal leiomyomatosis is a rare disorder of autosomal dominance.[291] Affected family members manifest achalasia caused by leiomyomatosis of the esophagus with entrapment of ganglia. Many of these patients with achalasia also have systemic mastocytosis and intestinal leiomyomas or neurofibromas. All have urticaria pigmentosa.

NEUROMUSCULAR DISORDERS

Brain Injuries

Brain injuries secondary to *stroke*, *trauma*, *tumor*, or *surgery* affect the gastrointestinal system. Acute injury causes physiologic alterations in the gastric mucosa, which can rapidly result in erosions, ulcerations (Cushing's ulcer), and bleeding. The etiology is unknown.[292,293] Common chronic sequelae of brain injury include oropharyngeal and cricopharyngeal dysfunction manifesting as dysphagia, aspiration, and malnutrition. Anal incontinence and constipation frequently occur secondary to neuromuscular dysfunction and debilitation.

Aspirin and other antiplatelet agents are often used after transient ischemic attack to prevent stroke. Nonsteroidal antiinflammatory drugs are a leading cause of gastric and duodenal mucosal injury.

Dementia Syndromes

Dementia syndromes, such as *Alzheimer's disease* and *Huntington's disease*, feature gastrointestinal pathology similar to that encountered in other forms of chronic brain injury. Diminished recent memory and disorientation impede rapid diagnosis of common and often easily recognized medical problems. Failure to thrive may be related to an occult esophageal foreign body,[294] peptic ulcer disease, or other pathologic intraabdominal processes.

In advanced terminal neurologic diseases, ethical decisions must be made pertaining to providing or withholding enteral feedings administered by nasogastric tube or other invasive feeding procedures.[295] New techniques of enteral alimentation permit more effective, longer administration of defined enteral diets that can prolong the end stage of patients in a "vegetative state." Enteral support through feeding tubes is a form of medical treatment that is not necessarily mandatory for all patients in such a condition.[296] Percutaneous endoscopic gastrostomy is a popular method of administering enteral feeding. Jejunostomies should be avoided for tube feedings in most situations, because they have a high overall complication rate and are more difficult to use. Moreover, in patients without severe esophageal reflux, they provide no additional protection against aspiration pneumonia.

Migraine

Migraine is a periodic headache syndrome that usually begins early in life. Well defined visual, sensory, or motor dysfunctions may precede or accompany the headache. Gastrointestinal manifestations may include nausea, vomiting, abdominal pain, and diarrhea. A migraine equivalent termed *abdominal migraine* is encountered particularly in childhood.[297] The diagnostic criteria include recurrent identical attacks of usually upper abdominal pain, no abdominal symptoms between attacks, family history of migraine, and response to β-blockade or other appropriate migraine therapy. The symptoms occasionally are accompanied by headache or prodrome. Various food or chemicals may precipitate migraine episodes through allergic or idiosyncratic mechanisms.[298] The differential diagnosis of paroxysmal, repetitive pain includes the much less commonly encountered *abdominal epilepsy*, which is diagnosed by demonstration of spike and wave activity on the electroencephalogram. Abdominal epilepsy is encountered predominantly in the pediatric age group.

Multiple Sclerosis

Multiple sclerosis is a focal demyelinating neurologic disorder of the central nervous system. The condition is associated with anorectal dysfunction,[299] gastroparesis, abnormal colonic motor and myoelectrical activity,[300] and oropharyngeal motor disturbances. Patients frequently experience incontinence, nausea, vomiting, constipation, megacolon, and dysphagia.[301,302]

Muscular Dystrophies

Muscular dystrophies are inherited myopathies featuring progressive weakness and muscle wasting. They have been subclassified into a number of syndromes based on clinical and genetic evidence. Several forms have been associated with motor disturbances of the gastrointestinal system, probably related to skeletal and smooth muscle degeneration within visceral organs.

Duchenne's Muscular Dystrophy

Duchenne's muscular dystrophy is an X-linked recessive disorder that usually presents with initial proximal skeletal muscle weakness by the age of 5 years, progressing to incapacitation and death by the third decade of life. Gastrointestinal symptomatology includes nausea, vomiting, abdominal distention, and constipation. Acute gastric dilation and intestinal pseudoobstruction have been reported.[303,304] Gastric hypomotility occurs frequently in advanced disease.[305]

Myotonic Dystrophy

Myotonic dystrophy is an autosomal dominant, slowly progressive condition. The distinctive features are delayed relaxation of muscle after initial contraction, muscle wasting of a characteristic pattern, frontal baldness in men, testicular atrophy, dysarthria, and cataracts. Gastrointestinal symptoms are prominent. Weak or myotonic contractions of the tongue and pharynx can result in oropharyngeal dysphagia and aspiration. Weakness of the upper esophageal sphincter and low-amplitude esophageal peristaltic contractions are frequent motor disturbances that may manifest even during early stages of the disease.[306] Many patients with marked esophageal motor dysfunction have minor symptoms. Delayed gastric emptying, prolonged intestinal transit time, and abnormal anal sphincter function also can develop.[307-309] Symptoms such as nausea, abdominal distention and pain, ileus, diarrhea, and constipation may result.[303,310] Some authorities believe that cholelithiasis is common, possibly secondary to gallbladder muscular dysfunction and bile stasis.

Oculopharyngeal Muscular Dystrophy

Oculopharyngeal muscular dystrophy is a rare autosomal dominant disorder with ptosis and dysphagia as the cardinal features.[311] Dysphagia may present first. The oropharynx and usually the esophagus demonstrate weak contractile activity. Oropharyngeal dysphagia is accompanied by pharyngooral and pharyngonasal regurgitation, which can be partially relieved by cricopharyngeal myotomy.[312] The upper esophageal sphincter appears to function normally.

Parkinsonism

Parkinsonism is a syndrome of multiple etiologies characterized by rigidity, tremor at rest, bradykinesia, and diminished postural reflexes. Regularly observed pathologic changes include degeneration of pigmented brain stem nuclei, which contain distinctive eosinophilic intracytoplasmic inclusions termed Lewy bodies. The swallowing centers can be affected, resulting in oropharyngeal dysphagia. Esophageal disturbances may include dilation with slowed barium transit time and decreased peristalsis.[313,314] Achalasia with Lewy bodies in the esophageal myenteric plexus has been reported.[315] Constipation is a common symptom caused by reduced colonic mobility, and is aggravated by the anticholinergic effects of antiparkinsonian medications. Megacolon and pseudoobstruction may occur.

Spinal Cord Transection

Spinal cord transection results in profound neurologic deficits. Constipation and incontinence are frequent sequelae. Lost are rectal sensation, voluntary control of defecation, and normal anal sphincter function.[316] Abnormal colon compliance and motor activity are accompaniments.[317] In addition to laxatives, manual distention of the rectum is useful to induce bowel movements through stimulation of the intact defecation reflex.

High Spinal Cord Lesions

High spinal cord lesions can also impair gastric and small bowel motility.[318] This predisposes to gastric distention, esophageal reflux, and adynamic ileus.

Diagnosis of acute abdominal emergencies is rendered difficult in the setting of spinal cord lesions. The classic autonomic responses to intraabdominal disease are dependent on intact spinal reflex arcs. Pain may refer aberrantly, or be perceived as vague and nonlocalizing. Abdominal tenderness and rigidity often do not occur. Early findings may include only anorexia, fever, headache, and hypertension. An important sign is increased abdominal muscle spasticity.[319]

Other Neuromuscular Diseases

Other neuromuscular diseases have gastrointestinal manifestations. *Stiff man syndrome* consists of symmetrical, progressive stiffness and painful spasm of axial musculature. Dysphagia may develop, possibly related to muscle spasm of the cricopharyngeus and upper esophagus.[320] *Amyotrophic lateral sclerosis* and *myasthenia gravis* also feature dysfunction of the oropharynx. *Kearns-Sayre* syndrome is a rare multisystem disorder caused by mitochondrial disease with a deficiency of cytochrome *c* oxidase. It is characterized by progressive external ophthalmoplegia, cardiac conduction defects, and pigmentary retinopathy. Some patients have swallowing difficulties. Manometric findings in one patient revealed striated muscle dysfunction in the oropharynx and proximal esophagus.[321] There are other types of mitochondrial myopathies and *familial enteric neuropathies* associated with intestinal pseudoobstruction and other extraintestinal manifestations.[322,323] *Hereditary internal anal sphincter myopathy* is an autosomal dominant inherited myopathy specifically of the internal anal sphincter. Associated features are hypertrophic sphincteric

muscle with myopathic histologic changes, constipation, and proctalgia fugax.[324] Pure *dysautonomia* is a rare affliction of the adrenergic or cholinergic systems. Patients may manifest intestinal motor disturbances, including pseudoobstruction.[325]

NUTRITIONAL DISTURBANCES

Malnutrition

Malnutrition results from famine, poor dietary habits, or chronic disease. *Kwashiorkor-marasmus* syndromes are causally related to protein or protein-calorie undernutrition. Vitamin and mineral deficiencies are also commonly associated.[326] Diarrhea and infection are manifestations of the terminal illness. Malnutrition causes immunodeficiency, which renders the mucosa susceptible to bacterial overgrowth and infection by various pathogens such as parasites, toxogenic bacteria, and viruses. Atrophy of the intestinal mucosa and pancreas contribute substantially to the formation of the diarrheal state. Hepatomegaly in conjunction with fatty liver and calcific pancreatitis[327] may develop. Refeeding of extremely malnourished patients should be done gradually to permit mucosal and metabolic adaptation, and to avoid exacerbation of the diarrhea.[328] Rapid-onset refeeding with high-caloric solutions rich in carbohydrate can lead to death by precipitating severe hypophosphatemia, hypokalemia, and hypomagnesemia, and by intensifying other metabolic disturbances.[329]

Obesity

Obesity predisposes to gallstone formation, esophageal reflux, and fatty liver. Two commonly performed surgical procedures for morbid obesity are vertical banded gastroplasty and gastric bypass. Although both are partially effective in most patients, complications are common in both the early and late postoperative periods. Also, these patients are susceptible to cholecystitis, particularly during the period of rapid weight loss. Vitamin B_{12}, folate, and iron deficiencies are common.[330] Thus, surgery is considered for morbid obesity only in subjects who are well informed and motivated, and who have failed a rigorous nonsurgical program. Jejunoileal bypasses are rarely done because of the high incidence of serious liver and intestinal complications.

Other Factors

Dietary habits as well as *food and water contaminants* can predispose to gastrointestinal lesions such as esophageal, gastric, colonic, pancreatic, and liver cancer. Markedly excessive vitamin A consumption causes hepatotoxicity. Herbal medications are self-prescribed and often advertised as safe; however, agents such as germander can induce severe liver disease.[331] Reactions to foods commonly precipitate gastrointestinal symptoms like diarrhea, abdominal distention, and cramps. Acute episodes, frequently associated with vomiting and fever, are usually caused by pathogenic bacteria and their toxins. Malabsorption of select dietary carbohydrates, food allergies,[332] or other unknown mechanisms also cause acute episodes.

COMPLICATIONS OF ORGAN TRANSPLANTATION

Bone Marrow Transplantation

Gastrointestinal complications of bone marrow transplantation are common, resulting from the induction regimen (lethal doses of radiation therapy and chemotherapy), impairment of the immune system, and graft-versus-host disease.[333] The rapidly proliferating oral and gastrointestinal epithelium is highly susceptible to injury by cytotoxic drugs and radiation. It is usual for mucositis to ensue, resulting in complaints of oropharyngeal pain, nausea, vomiting, abdominal pain, diarrhea, and gastrointestinal bleeding. These symptoms usually appear within a few days of induction and resolve after 3 to 4 weeks.

Immune system dysfunction predisposes the marrow transplant recipient to life-threatening infections. Bacterial and fungal infections are more common during the initial 30 days, whereas viral and parasitic infections are observed more often after day 30.[334] Infection must be differentiated from graft-versus-host disease. Bacterial sepsis (especially due to gram-negative and anaerobic bowel flora) is frequently observed. *Candida albicans* is the most common opportunistic pathogen invading the gastrointestinal tract in marrow transplant recipients. Oropharyngeal and esophageal thrush are frequent, but the entire gut may be involved. Cytomegalovirus and herpesvirus infections are common and may involve any portion of the gastrointestinal tract. Esophageal stricture formation is a possible sequela. *C difficile* infection can cause severe and prolonged diarrhea. Pseudomembranes, which are largely composed of neutrophils, are often absent in the leukopenic patient. Parasites, including *Giardia lamblia*, *Isospora belli*, *Cryptosporidium* sp, and *Microsporidium* sp, also have been demonstrated to cause persistent diarrhea.

Graft-Versus-Host Disease

Graft-versus-host disease often complicates marrow transplantation and may be either acute (onset less than 100 days posttransplant) or chronic (onset more than 100 days posttransplant). It is much less likely to occur when syngeneic or T-cell–depleted marrow is transplanted. In this disease, donor cytotoxic T lymphocytes destroy host cells in a variety of organs, including the skin, liver, and gut.

The earliest sign is often the onset of a watery, secretory diarrhea that may contain protein. Anorexia, nausea, vomiting, and abdominal pain are frequent. Radiographic findings include thickening of the bowel wall, rapid transit time, and loss of distal small bowel mucosal folds.[335] Rectal biopsies frequently reveal single epithelial cell necrosis, crypt abscesses, and crypt obliteration. Thus, the diagnosis can be made by a sigmoidoscopy with rectal biopsy, a relatively safe and simple procedure (Fig. 109-10; see Color Fig. 72).[336] The diarrhea often improves with intensified immunosuppression. Infectious enteritis must be considered in the differential diagnosis.

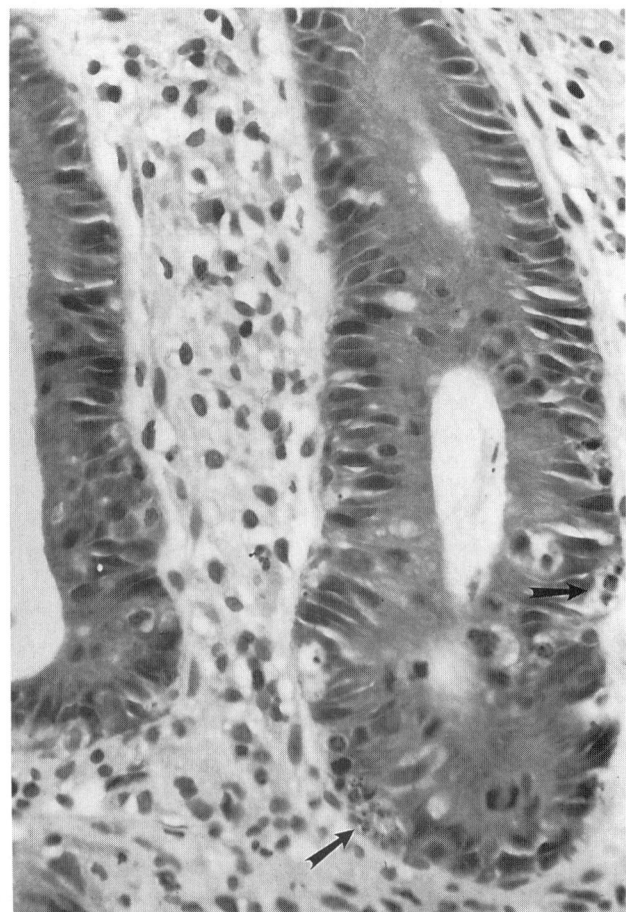

FIGURE 109-10. (See Color Fig. 72.) Rectal biopsy specimen shows crypt cell degeneration, which is the characteristic lesion of graft-versus-host disease. (Hematoxylin and eosin stain; original magnification ×100.)

Renal Transplantation

Renal transplantation is associated with gastrointestinal complications. Oral and esophageal thrush result from immunosuppression and antibiotic administration. Gastrointestinal bleeding is a frequent and life-threatening complication. It is usually secondary to gastritis (which may have a viral etiology), stress, or peptic ulcers.[337] Intestinal ischemia, diverticulitis, cytomegalovirus-induced colitis, and intraabdominal abscesses complicate the postoperative course of some patients. Severe posttransplantation pancreatitis occurs in a few patients, often resulting from azathioprine or prednisone therapy.[338] Immunosuppressive drugs are likely to dampen the symptoms and physical findings of acute intraabdominal illness, warranting increased vigilance for their appearance. Lymphomas, Kaposi's sarcoma, and other malignancies occur with a greater-than-expected frequency in chronically immunosuppressed patients.[338]

Cardiac Transplantation

Cardiac transplantation is often complicated by acute gastrointestinal problems. As in other critically ill patients, upper gastrointestinal bleeding is frequent in the postoperative period and is largely the result of hemorrhagic gastritis and peptic ulcer disease.[339] Pancreatitis develops in 20% of patients. Cholecystitis is also a significant source of postoperative morbidity.[340] Colonic ileus, bowel perforation, gastric outlet obstruction, and perirectal abscesses have been reported.[339,340]

Blood Transfusion

It is often forgotten that blood transfusion is the commonest organ transplantation procedure. A relatively rare syndrome of *graft-versus-host disease* has been described in association with transfusion of blood from first-degree relatives to immunocompromised recipients. Occasionally, immunocompetent recipients are affected. It is suggested that blood donations from first-degree relatives not be used unless the blood is first irradiated.[341]

PSYCHOLOGICAL DISORDERS

Anorexia Nervosa and Bulimia

Anorexia nervosa is an eating disorder characterized by severe voluntary weight loss, disturbed body image, and morbid fear of obesity.[342] *Bulimia* is a distinct syndrome characterized by cyclic binge eating followed by self-induced vomiting, fasting,

laxative abuse, or excessive exercising to promote weight loss.[343] The etiologies of these disorders remain unknown. Both syndromes are common and have a predilection for women of late adolescence and early adulthood. Anorexia nervosa may carry a mortality of up to 9%. The complications of anorexia nervosa are predominantly those of starvation,[344] whereas those of bulimia are the consequence of binge eating and purging (Table 109-4). Binge eating causes acute gastric dilation that can result in gastric rupture. Vomiting is associated with dental enamel erosion, esophagitis, Mallory-Weiss tears, and esophageal rupture. Although pancreatitis may occur, the hyperamylasemia in patients with eating disorders is frequently caused by increased salivary-type amylase.[345,346]

Anxiety and Stress

Anxiety and stress can alter gastrointestinal function and produce a broad range of gastrointestinal symptomatology. In some patients, emotional factors may be the etiology of or contribute to the symptomatology of globus syndrome, esophageal spasm, nutcracker esophagus, nonulcer dyspepsia, and irritable bowel syndrome.[347] The commonly held notion that stress or anxiety disorders are related to the development of peptic ulcers has not been established. It is no longer commonly held that ulcerative colitis and Crohn's disease have a close association with psychiatric illness.[348,349]

TABLE 109-4
Physical Manifestations of Anorexia Nervosa and Bulimia

MANIFESTATION	ANOREXIA NERVOSA	BULIMIA
Endocrine or metabolic	Amenorrhea Osteoporosis Euthyroid sick syndrome Decreased norepinephrine secretion Decreased somatomedin C Elevated growth hormone Decreased or erratic vasopressin secretion Abnormal temperature regulation Hypercarotenemia	Menstrual irregularities
Cardiovascular	Bradycardia Hypotension Arrhythmias	Ipecac poisoning
Renal	Increased blood urea nitrogen Decreased glomerular filtration rate Renal calculi Edema	Hypocalcemia (diuretic induced)
	Decreased gastric emptying Constipation Elevated hepatic enzymes	Acute gastric dilation, rupture Parotid englargement Dental enamel erosion Esophagitis Mallory-Weiss tears, esophageal rupture Hypokalemia (laxative induced)
Hematologic	Anemia Leukopenia Thrombocytopenia	
Pulmonary		Aspiration pneumonia

From Herzog DB, Copeland PM. Eating disorders. N Engl J Med 1985;313:297.

Major Depression or Conversion Disorder

Major depression or conversion disorder can manifest as psychogenic vomiting.[350] Also, depression is often associated with an increased frequency of gastrointestinal complaints.

Munchausen's Syndrome

Munchausen's syndrome is the repeated seeking of medical care for factitious illness. In contrast to hysteria, the symptoms are subject to "conscious" control. Patients have feigned many gastrointestinal diseases, including abdominal emergencies, hematemesis, and inflammatory bowel diseases. Satisfactory treatment of this syndrome is rare.[351]

Schizophrenia

Some patients with schizophrenia are subject to recurrent voluntary ingestion of foreign bodies such as razor blades, glass, and pins. Also, antipsychotic agents have cholinergic-blocking activity that may cause severe gastric retention, megacolon, and constipation.

PULMONARY DISEASES

Gastroesophageal Reflux Disease

Gastroesophageal reflux disease (GERD) is a common condition that may occasionally present with symptoms resembling asthma. The symptoms are thought to result from aspiration of gastric contents, although reflex bronchial constriction has been suggested as a mechanism.[352,353] Not all nocturnal exacerbations of asthma are attributable to GERD, however. Pyrosis as well as other symptoms of GERD, asthma onset in middle age, absence of coincident allergy, or eosinophilia are clues to a possible association with GERD.[353] Chronic cough and hoarseness are also sometimes caused by GERD.[354,355] When the diagnosis of GERD-associated asthma is suspected, appropriate evaluation, including endoscopy with biopsy, pH monitoring, and barium swallow, should be considered. Therapy is directed primarily at limiting reflux.[352,355]

Respiratory Failure

Respiratory failure and mechanical ventilation may be complicated by gastrointestinal bleeding from erosive gastritis and peptic ulcer disease.[356] Hypoxemia, hypotension, sepsis, and the use corticosteroids contribute to the development of these lesions. The use of antacids, H_2 antagonists, and barrier-enhancing drugs prophylactically in critically ill patients reduces the incidence of stress ulcerations[357,358] and should be considered for ventilated patients. It has been suggested, however, that raising the gastric pH might permit colonization of the stomach by gram-negative bacteria and other pathogens. This may, in turn, predispose to nosocomial pneumonia and in-testinal bacterial overgrowth. One study has shown that acidification of enteral feeding solutions reduces bacterial colonization in critically ill patients.[359] Hence, barrier-enhancing agents (e.g., sucralfate) may be considered as alternative therapy.[356] Chronic respiratory failure is also thought to be an etiologic factor in *pneumatosis intestinalis*.[360]

α_1-Antitrypsin Deficiency

α_1-Antitrypsin (AAT) deficiency is a recessively inherited condition that may cause cirrhosis, primarily in children, and chronic obstructive pulmonary disease in adults.[361] The ZZ phenotype has been associated most frequently with severe disease.[362] Adult patients can be screened effectively by serum AAT levels. Those with a level less than 80 mg/mL should undergo AAT phenotyping.[362] Liver disease is less commonly seen in adults and is associated with AAT granules in the periportal areas on liver biopsy, a finding unrelated to the severity of the liver disease.[363] Liver transplantation is an effective form of therapy for patients with severe liver disease.[364]

Aspiration of Gastroenteric Contents

Aspiration of gastroenteric contents is a common complication of enteral feeding in respiratory patients, even when these patients are ventilated. Life-threatening acute respiratory failure or pneumonia can result. Unless aspiration of gastric contents is massive, it may go undetected. Methylene blue coloration of tube-feeding solutions has been used to increase the sensitivity of detection of aspiration, but appears less sensitive than the use of glucose oxidase strips for this purpose.[365] The use of small-volume feeds, postpyloric feeding tubes, and nursing of patients in head-elevated positions may help to reduce the frequency, but does not eliminate this complication.[366]

The medical therapy of respiratory failure may result in gastrointestinal disturbances. The most commonly seen complication is theophylline toxicity, which is often associated with dyspepsia, nausea, diarrhea, and an increase in gastric acid secretion.[367] Systemic and inhaled corticosteroids, used in the management of asthma and chronic obstructive pulmonary disease, may result in oral and esophageal candidiasis. When severe, dyspepsia and candidiasis may exacerbate the often-present nutritional impairment of patients with chronic respiratory failure.

Cystic Fibrosis

Cystic fibrosis is the most common inherited disease affecting Caucasians in North America, with an incidence of about 1 per 2000. Accumulating evidence points to an underlying defect in mucosal ion and water transport. A net shift in fluid from the lumen results in viscous secretions and duct obstruction in the respiratory tract, salivary glands, pancreas, and hepatobiliary tree.[368]

The presence of viscous secretions in the intestinal lumen has important clinical consequences. Affected infants may present with *meconium ileus*, intussusception, intestinal atresia,

The presence of viscous secretions in the intestinal lumen has important clinical consequences. Affected infants may present with *meconium ileus*, intussusception, intestinal atresia, volvulus, and perforation.[369] Tenacious secretions can obstruct the distal small bowel in older children (*meconium ileus equivalent*).[370] Chronic constipation is common and may lead to rectal prolapse. Constipation is usually controllable with laxatives. Mineral oil or acetylcysteine also may be effective.[370]

Gastroesophageal reflux is a common complaint. Contributing factors are decreased saliva production, gastrointestinal hypomotility, chronic cough, and postural drainage of pulmonary secretions.[371] Standard antireflux therapy is usually effective.

Nutritional impairment is caused by pancreatic insufficiency; 90% of patients manifest steatorrhea and malabsorption of nonfat nutrients.[372] Protein-calorie malnutrition is aggravated by chronic respiratory tract infections and also may contribute to progressive lung damage. Improvement of exercise tolerance and pulmonary function can result from enteralparenteral nutritional support and pancreatic enzyme replacement, and fat-soluble vitamin supplementation.[373] Glucose intolerance is found in most adult patients, although frank diabetes mellitus develops in only 7% to 15%.[368] When present, diabetes further complicates nutritional therapy and exacerbates the proclivity to infections.

Some degree of chronic biliary obstruction is common, but progression to biliary cirrhosis and associated portal hypertension is rare. If variceal bleeding occurs, sclerotherapy or portosystemic shunting are the therapeutic modalities of choice. Administration of propranolol in an attempt to lower portal pressure may aggravate the pulmonary disease, and has not been shown to reduce the incidence of bleeding in these patients.[374] Gallstones occur at a greater-than-expected frequency. Cholecystitis and choledocholithiasis have been reported.[375]

RENAL DISORDERS

Acute Renal Failure

Acute renal failure is frequently accompanied by gastrointestinal disturbances such as anorexia, dyspepsia, nausea, vomiting, and gastrointestinal bleeding.[376] The latter is commonly caused by erosive gastritis. Poor renal and dialysis clearance requires that doses of H_2 antagonists be reduced (or the dosing interval increased), and that Mg^{++}-containing antacids be avoided because of the risk of hypermagnesemia.[377]

The uremic state is associated with a number of gastrointestinal disturbances. Dysgeusia, a metallic taste in the mouth, and fetor uremia are often noted by uremic patients. Some patients manifest a peculiar oral inflammation termed *uremic stomatitis*. Parotitis and sicca syndrome occur commonly in uremic patients, further limiting compliance with fluid restriction. These oral and gustatory complications can also exacerbate decreased nutritional intake in uremic patients. Intensified dialysis and zinc supplementation may be helpful in some patients.[378]

Renal failure is very commonly associated with anorexia,

nausea, vomiting, epigastric pain,[379] gastroduodenitis, Brunner's gland hypertrophy,[380,381] nodular duodenitis,[382] and perhaps peptic ulcer disease.[383] Gastrointestinal bleeding from hemorrhagic gastritis or angiodysplasias is well documented in renal failure.[384–389] As in other situations, estrogen-progesterone therapy has been used in an attempt to control the bleeding from angiodysplasias in renal failure, but its widespread use should await further study.[390] Peptic ulcer disease, gastritis, esophagitis, and duodenitis may be managed with H_2 antagonists or antacids, with the same caveats as noted for treatment of acute renal failure.[377]

Duodenal pseudomelanosis is an idiopathic condition in which pigmentation develops in the proximal duodenal mucosa. It is sometimes found in association with renal failure.[391] A variety of pigments have been implicated, including iron sulfide and hemosiderin (Fig. 109-11; see Color Fig. 73).[392] There are no known symptoms attributable to this syndrome.

Intestinal manifestations of uremia include abdominal pain, constipation, pseudoobstruction, and intussusception. Intestinal motility disturbances may contribute to their etiol-

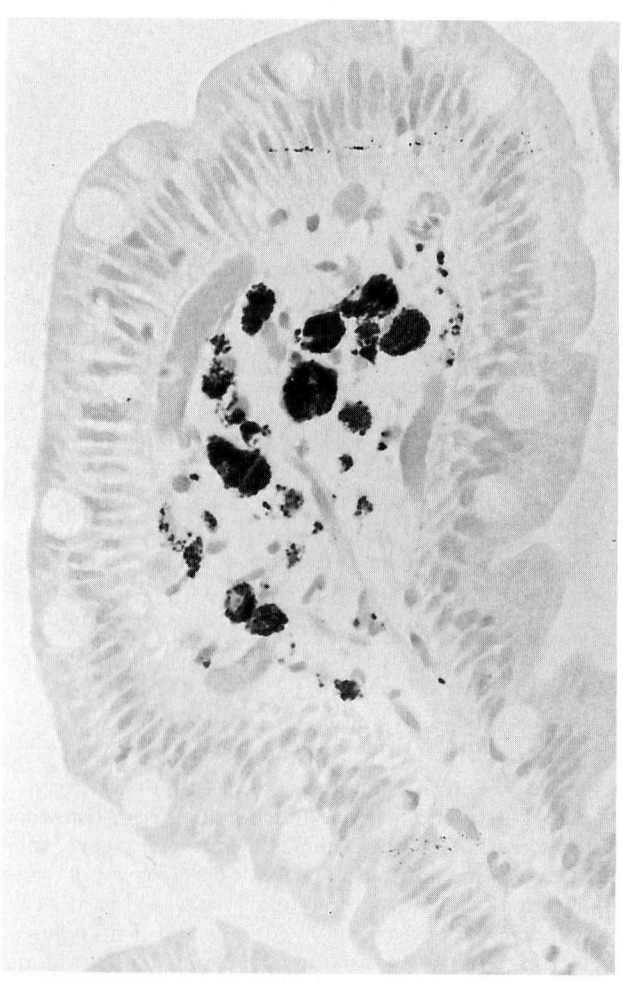

FIGURE 109-11. (See Color Fig. 73*B*.) Duodenal biopsy specimen from a patient with pseudomelanosis duodeni shows the deposition of pigment within lamina propria macrophages.

ogy. Important factors in the development of constipation include oral fluid restriction and the use of aluminum hydroxide–containing antacids. Diarrhea secondary to a variety of causes is common. Fecal impaction may result in overflow diarrhea, stercoral ulcers, and rectal bleeding. Abnormal bile acids have been reported to occur in uremia and may be associated with "uremic diarrhea."[393] Although conditions such as bacterial overgrowth and pseudomembranous colitis must be considered, the cause of most cases remains idiopathic.

Gastrointestinal hormones, including secretin, gastric inhibitory polypeptide, and cholecystokinin, may be elevated in uremic patients. Their contribution to gastrointestinal dysfunction and symptoms is uncertain.[394] Most patients exhibit some degree of hypochlorhydria and hypergastrinemia, perhaps on the basis of impaired parietal cell response to gastrin.[387]

Pancreatic exocrine insufficiency and steatorrhea have been described in uremic patients and may contribute to protein-calorie malnutrition and the wasting syndrome of chronic renal failure.[395,396] Treatment with pancreatic enzymes is effective. The incidence of *pancreatitis* in chronic renal failure is unknown. Elevation of serum amylase is common and should not necessarily be attributed to impaired renal clearance, especially if the level exceeds twice the upper limit of normal.[397]

A number of other gastrointestinal problems are found in association with renal disease. Polycystic kidney disease is associated with large colonic diverticula that are prone to perforate.[398] *Metastatic calcification* has resulted in the deposition of calcium in visceral vessels leading to intestinal ischemia, bleeding, and infarction.[399]

Dialysis is occasionally associated with gastrointestinal manifestations. Patients undergoing peritoneal dialysis are subject to bacterial peritonitis. Rarely, adherence of the catheter to omentum or bowel causes intestinal obstruction or perforation.[399] Refractory exudative ascites occurs in a few patients, particularly in those who have had previous peritoneal dialysis.[400,401] Intensive hemodialysis, fluid restriction, nephrectomy, and peritoneovenous shunting are sometimes successful in alleviating this often troublesome problem.[402] Patients undergoing chronic hemodialysis are subject to viral illnesses. Many are found to have hepatitis B surface antigen in their serum.[403] Uremia-induced immunodeficiency has been suggested as a predisposing factor. Chronic hepatitis and cirrhosis develop in some patients. Dialysis and transplant patients who have received numerous blood transfusions are at increased risk for iron overload, particularly *hemosiderosis*, which has been shown to be diagnosable by magnetic resonance imaging.[404]

SUBSTANCE ABUSE

Drug Abuse

Drug abuse can have deleterious effects on the gastrointestinal system. Alcohol profoundly influences every organ. The effects of alcohol on the body are not entirely separable from the nutritional and social consequences of alcoholism.

Alcohol Consumption

Alcohol consumption can produce dysphagia and promote esophageal reflux. It commonly enhances lower esophageal sphincter pressure, decreases the frequency of esophageal peristaltic contractions, and delays esophageal emptying. High-amplitude peristaltic contractions have also been noted (nutcracker esophagus).[405] These alterations in function can result in chest pain, esophagitis, and esophageal strictures, and may predispose to Barrett esophagus.

The capacity of alcohol to injure the gastric mucosa is well recognized. Alcohol produces acute and chronic gastritis possibly by disruption of the gastric mucosal barrier. Heavy acute ingestion can result in gastric erosions and hemorrhage. Tolerance to serious mucosal injury develops with chronic use. The relationship of alcohol to the formation of peptic ulcers is unsettled.[406]

Alcoholism may result in diarrhea and malabsorption. There are many etiologic factors. Alcohol enhances small intestinal transit, decreases brush border enzyme activity, and impairs absorption of nutrients. Chronic pancreatitis, chronic liver disease, protein-calorie malnutrition, and vitamin deficiencies are contributing factors.[407]

There are other notable deleterious effects. These include acute and chronic pancreatitis,[408] fatty liver, alcoholic hepatitis, and cirrhosis.[407,409] Epidemiologic evidence strongly suggests that alcohol or alcohol in conjunction with other factors is associated with carcinoma of the larynx, nasopharynx, esophagus, and liver. Reports linking alcohol to colonic and pancreatic cancer are more tenuous.[410–412]

Cocaine

The use of cocaine and related metabolites is widespread. Numerous psychological, neurologic, and cardiovascular complications are known.[413] Few effects on the gastrointestinal system have been reported. Anorexia and diarrhea are common. Intestinal ischemia[414] and hepatotoxicity with zone 3 necrosis[415] are rare complications. The practice of smuggling cocaine in condoms concealed in the digestive system can result in intestinal obstruction. Death can result if a bag ruptures, because the amount of cocaine in each packet usually exceeds the lethal dose. The management of ingested cocaine packets is controversial.[416]

Narcotics

Narcotic administration for abuse or for pain relief frequently results in physical dependency with resulting physical symptoms on withdrawal. These symptoms are anxiety, depression, irritability, and drug craving. Depending on the drug used, other manifestations may include perspiration, rhinorrhea, tearing, yawning, dilated pupils, myalgias, tremor, insomnia, and, rarely, convulsions. Gastrointestinal symptomatology can comprise anorexia, nausea, vomiting, and abdominal pain. Patients may feign major medical illness to obtain narcotics.[417] Narcotics slow colonic peristalsis and thus frequently induce constipation.

Parenteral administration of illicit drugs often results in

the expected complications of nonsterile conditions.[418] In the digestive system, these include viral hepatitis, cirrhosis, and hepatic abscess. The injection of contaminants such as talc can cause hepatic granulomas.

Smoking

Smoking is a major cause of gastrointestinal illness. There is an association between smoking and the development of oropharyngeal, esophageal, and pancreatic cancers. Smokers have a higher prevalence of peptic ulcer disease that is less responsive to therapy.[419] Smoking is also a risk factor for the development of Crohn's disease and for recurrence after surgical resection.[420]

VASCULITIDES

Behçet's Disease

Behçet's disease is a systemic illness of unknown etiology characterized by necrotizing vasculitis. It was originally described in people of Middle Eastern or Japanese extraction. Common manifestations include orogenital ulcerations, eye inflammation, skin lesions, arthritis, and migratory thrombophlebitis, as well as gastrointestinal tract involvement.[421-423] A curious and virtually pathognomonic sign is the development of pustules at the site of needle punctures.

Oral lesions resemble aphthous ulcers and may be single or multiple. Esophageal ulcerations are frequently seen and occasionally cause esophageal bleeding, stricture, or perforation.[424-427] Intestinal involvement can resemble Crohn's disease.[428,429] Intestinal bleeding or perforation may result. Sites of bowel involvement may be identified with an indium 111 scan.[430] Therapy with corticosteroids often ameliorates the disease. Resection of severely diseased segments of the gut may be required, but postoperative recurrence is common.[421]

Giant Cell Arteritis

Giant cell arteritis is a granulomatous disease that usually involves large or medium-sized arteries, including the aorta and the temporal arteries. Disseminated fibrinoid necrosis of smaller vessels can result in visceral ischemia, abdominal pain, nausea, anorexia, weight loss, bleeding, and perforation.[431,432]

Henoch-Schönlein Purpura

Henoch-Schönlein purpura is a syndrome characterized by systemic small vessel vasculitis. It has a peak age of onset in early childhood, but all ages may be affected. Penicillin allergy and streptococcal infection have been implicated in some cases, but the cause remains obscure. The gastrointestinal tract is involved in as many as 50% of patients. Any part of the gastrointestinal tract may be affected, but rectal involvement is said to be relatively rare.[433] Gastrointestinal symptoms include abdominal pain, vomiting, diarrhea, intestinal obstruc-

tion, or intussusception, and can precede the onset of the characteristic purpuric rash.[434] The bowel may be edematous and show evidence of submucosal or subserosal hemorrhage.[435] Radiographic findings include thickening of small bowel folds, colonic wall edema, and intussusception.[436]

Köhlmeier-Degos Disease

Köhlmeier-Degos disease (malignant atrophic papulosis) affects mainly young men. The skin develops characteristic depressed, "atrophic-appearing" lesions.[437] Vasculitis of small and medium-sized arteries may lead to renal failure, intestinal ischemia, bleeding, or perforation.[438]

Polyarteritis Nodosa

Polyarteritis nodosa is a systemic necrotizing vasculitis affecting small and medium-sized arteries of nearly every organ system, and giving rise to a wide spectrum of clinical findings. Approximately half the cases are associated with hepatitis B infection.[439] Fever, weight loss, arthralgias, subcutaneous nodules, hypertension, and peripheral neuritis are common. Gastrointestinal complaints are present in about two thirds of patients, and are usually secondary to visceral ischemia.[440] The most common clinical manifestations are epigastric pain, nausea, anorexia, mucosal ulceration, intestinal bleeding, and diarrhea.[441] Peritonitis and intraabdominal abscess may follow ischemic necrosis and perforation of the intestine.[442] Appendicitis, cholecystitis, pancreatitis, cataclysmic intraabdominal hemorrhage, bowel obstruction, and liver infarction have been reported. Pseudomembranous colitis[443] and pneumatosis intestinalis[444] also have been noted. Corticosteroid and cyclophosphamide therapy have dramatically improved the overall survival of these patients. These medications, however, may mask underlying gastrointestinal pathology or enhance the risk of bleeding from mucosal ulceration, especially if bone marrow depression leads to thrombocytopenia.[445]

Churg-Strauss Disease

Churg-Strauss disease is a systemic vasculitis that resembles polyarteritis nodosa but differs in several important respects. Granuloma formation, peripheral and tissue eosinophilia, and an association with asthma are noteworthy. Gastrointestinal manifestations, which include nausea, vomiting, gastrointestinal hemorrhage, perforation, and cholecystitis, are related to mesenteric vasculitis and are similar to those found in polyarteritis nodosa.[442]

Wegener's Granulomatosis

The clinical manifestations of Wegener's granulomatosis are diverse, but the triad of focal glomerulonephritis, vasculitis, and necrotizing granulomas usually is required to establish the diagnosis.[446] The associated vasculitis may result in intestinal or colonic ischemia, bleeding, and perforation. Massive intraabdominal hemorrhage has been reported.[447] The finding of anti-neutrophil cytoplasmic antibodies may be helpful in establishing the diagnosis.[448]

Cryoglobulinemia

Cryoglobulinemia occurs in a variety of clinical settings such as lymphoproliferative disorders, infections, and autoimmune diseases, or as an idiopathic process. Essential mixed cryoglobulinemia is the most frequently diagnosed variant and usually is characterized by the presence of immune complexes composed of monoclonal IgM specific for polyclonal IgG. These circulating immune complexes may engender a vasculitic process that involves the gut in 20% of patients.[449] The clinical features include recurrent episodes of crampy abdominal pain, enterocolitis, and, rarely, small or large bowel ischemia. The clinical presentation and the presence of radiographic "skip lesions" may lead to the erroneous diagnosis of Crohn's disease.[449]

The reader is directed to Chapter 44, Skin Lesions Associated With Gastrointestinal Diseases; Chapter 47, Approach to the Female Patient With Gastrointestinal Disease; Chapter 48, Approach to the Patient Requiring Nutritional Supplementation; and Chapter 110, Gastrointestinal Manifestations of Immunologic Disorders.

REFERENCES

1. Shbeeb I, Prager E, Love JW. The aortic valve: colonic axis. Dis Colon Rectum 1984;27:38.
2. Schoenfeld Y, Eldar M, Bedazovsky B, et al. Aortic stenosis associated with gastrointestinal bleeding: a survey of 612 patients. Am Heart J 1980;100:179.
3. Cody MC, Donovan PB, Hughes RW Jr. Idiopathic gastrointestinal bleeding and aortic stenosis. Dig Dis 1974;19:393.
4. Greenstein RJ, McElhinney AJ, Reuben D, Greenstein AJ. Colonic vascular ectasias and aortic stenosis: coincidence or causal relationship? Am J Surg 1986;151:347.
5. Meyer CT, Troncale FJ, Galloway S, Sheahan DG. Arteriovenous malformations of the bowel: an analysis of 22 cases and a review of the literature. Medicine (Baltimore) 1981;60:36.
6. Imperiale TF, Ransohoff DF. Aortic stenosis, idiopathic bleeding and angiodysplasia: is there an association? A methodologic critique of the literature. Gastroenterology 1988;95:1670.
7. Kheterpal S. Angiodysplasia: a review. J R Soc Med 1991;84:615.
8. Leimbach WN Jr, Marsidi I, Leininger NR, Needleman S. Aortic stenosis and intestinal angiodysplasia: a case of gastric involvement. West Med J 1981;135:139.
9. Gunnlaugsson O. Angiodysplasia of the stomach and duodenum. Gastrointest Endosc 1985;31:251.
10. Buchi KN. Vascular malformations of the gastrointestinal tract. Surg Clin North Am 1992;72:559.
11. Cappell MS, Lebwohl O. Cessation of recurrent bleeding from gastrointestinal angiodysplasias after aortic valve replacement. Ann Intern Med 1986;105:54.
12. Scheffer SM, Leatherman LL. Resolution of Heyde's syndrome of aortic stenosis and gastrointestinal bleeding after aortic valve replacement. Ann Thorac Surg 1986;42:477.
13. King RM, Pluth JR, Giuliani ER. The association of unexplained gastrointestinal bleeding with calcific aortic stenosis. Ann Thorac Surg 1987;44:514.
14. Love JW. The syndrome of calcific aortic stenosis and gastrointestinal bleeding: resolution following aortic valve replacement. J Thorac Cardiovasc Surg 1982;83:779.
15. Granieri R, Mazzulla JP, Yarborough GW. Estrogen-progesterone therapy for recurrent gastrointestinal bleeding secondary to gastrointestinal angiodysplasia. Am J Gastroenterol 1988;83:556.
16. Davidson JD, Waldmann TA, Goodman DG, Gordon RS Jr. Protein losing enteropathy in congestive heart failure. Lancet 1961;1:899.
17. Jones RD. Fat malabsorption in congestive cardiac failure. Br Med J 1961;1:1276.
18. Singh V, Jindal SK, Khattri HN, et al. A study of fat, D-xylose, folate mono-glutamate and vitamin B12 malabsorption in chronic congestive cardiac failure. Indian J Chest Dis Allied Sci 1977;19:105.
19. Hyde RD, Loehry CA. Folic acid malabsorption in cardiac failure. Gut 1968;9:717.
20. Kimata S. Complications of adult cases with congestive heart failure. Jpn Circ J 1986;50:324.
21. Richman SM, Delman AJ, Grob D. Alterations in indices of liver function in congestive heart failure with particular reference to serum enzymes. Am J Med 1961;30:211.
22. Dunn GD, Hayes P, Breen KS, et al. The liver in congestive heart failure: a review. Am J Med Sci 1973;265:174.
23. Moorman JR. Digitalis toxicity at Duke Hospital, 1973 to 1984. South Med J 1985;78:564.
24. Lely AH, Van Enter CHJ. Non-cardiac symptoms of digitalis intoxication. Am Heart J 1972;83:149.
25. Longhurst JC, Ross J. Extracardiac and coronary vascular effects of digitalis. J Am Coll Cardiol 1985;5:99A.
26. Eckhauser ML, Dokler M, Imbembo AL. Diuretic-associated pancreatitis: a collective review and illustrative cases. Am J Gastroenterol 1987;82:865.
27. Barloon TJ, Moore SA, Mitros FA. A case of stenotic obstruction of the jejunum secondary to slow-release potassium. Am J Gastroenterol 1986;81:192.
28. Behl PR, Holden MP. Mitral valve disease and dysphagia. Eur Heart J 1984;5:919.
29. Johnston G, Vitikainen K, Knight R, et al. Changing perspective on gastrointestinal complications in patients undergoing cardiac surgery. Am J Surg 1992;163:525.
30. Ohri SK, Desai JB, Gaer JAR, et al. Intraabdominal complications after cardiopulmonary bypass. Ann Thorac Surg 1991;52:826.
31. Rosen HR, Vlahakes GJ, Rattner DW. Fulminant peptic ulcer disease in cardiac surgical patients: pathogenesis, prevention and management. Crit Care Med 1991;20:354.
32. Sheth KJ, Werlin SL, Freeman ME, Hodach AE. Gastrointestinal structure and function in Fabry's disease. Am J Gastroenterol 1981;76:246.
33. Bryan A, Knauft RF, Burns WA. Small bowel perforation in Fabry's disease. Ann Intern Med 1977;86:315.
34. O'Brien BD, Shnitka TK, McDougall R, et al. Pathophysiologic and ultrastructural basis for intestinal symptoms in Fabry's disease. Gastroenterology 1982;82:957.
35. Buchin PJ, Levy JS, Schullinger JN. Down's syndrome and the gastrointestinal tract. J Clin Gastroenterol 1986;8:111.
36. Shohat M, Bu X, Shohat T, et al. The gene for familial Mediterranean fever in both Armenians and non-Ashkenazi Jews is linked to the alpha-globin complex on 16p: evidence for locus homogeneity. Am J Hum Genet 1992;51:1349.
37. Sohar E, Gafni J, Pras M, Heller H. Familial Mediterranean fever: a survey of 470 cases and review of the literature. Am J Med 1967;43:227.
38. Meyerhoff J. Familial Mediterranean fever: report of a large family, review of the literature and discussion of the frequency of amyloidosis. Medicine (Baltimore) 1980;59:66.
39. Zemer D, Pras M, Sohar E, et al. Colchicine in the prevention and treatment of the amyloidosis of familial Mediterranean fever. N Engl J Med 1986;314:1001.
40. McMenemy A. Whipple's disease, familial Mediterranean fever and adult-onset Still's disease. Curr Opin Rheumatol 1991;3:597.

41. Mery JP, Kenouch S. Familial Mediterranean fever-associated amyloidosis. Ren Fail 1993;15:379.

42. Levy M, Spino M, Read SE. Colchicine: a state-of-the-art review. Pharmacotherapy 1991;11:196.

43. Beutler-E. Gaucher disease. Blood Rev 1988;2:59.

44. Aderka D, Garfinkel D, Rothem A, Pinkhas J. Fatal bleeding from esophageal varices in a patient with Gaucher's disease. Am J Gastroenterol 1982;77:838.

45. Bloomer, J.R. The hepatic porphyrias: pathogenesis, manifestations and management. Gastroenterology 1976;71:689.

46. Tschudy DP, Lamon LM. Porphyrin metabolism and the porphyrias. In: Bondy PK, Rosenberg LE, eds. Metabolic control and disease. 8th ed. Philadelphia: WB Saunders, 1980:939.

47. Dhar GJ, Bossenmaier I, Petryka ZJ. Effects of hematin in hepatic porphyria: further studies. Ann Intern Med 1975;83:20.

48. Brickman CM, Hosea SW. Hereditary angioedema. Int J Dermatol 1983;22:141.

49. Weinstock LB, Kothari T, Sharma RN, Rosenfeld SI. Recurrent abdominal pain as the sole manifestation of hereditary angioedema in multiple family members. Gastroenterology 1987;93:1116.

50. Peerson KD, Buchignann JS, Shimkin PM, et al. Hereditary angioneurotic edema of the gastrointestinal tract. AJR 1972;116:256.

51. Sheffer AL, Fearon DT, Austen KF. Methyltestosterone therapy in hereditary angioedema. Ann Intern Med 1977;86:306.

52. Sheffer AL, Fearon DT, Austen KF. Tranexamic acid: preoperative prophylactic therapy for patients with hereditary angioneurotic edema. J Allergy Clin Immunol 1977;60:38.

53. Havel RJ. Approach to the patient with hyperlipidemia. Med Clin North Am 1982;66:31.

54. Ahlberg J, Angelin B, Einarsson K, et al. Biliary lipid composition in normal and hyperlipoproteinemia. Gastroenterology 1980;79:90.

55. Dominguez-Munoz JE, Malfertheiner P, Ditschuneit HH, et al. Hyperlipidemia in acute pancreatitis: relationship with etiology, onset, and severity of the disease. Int J Pancreatol 1991;10:261.

56. Thompson GR. Primary hyperlipidaemia. Br Med Bull 1990;46:986.

57. Wilson JA, Raufman JP. Hepatic failure in adult Niemann-Pick disease. Am J Med Sci 1986;292:168.

58. Dechelotte P, Kantelip B, Laguillaumie BV, et al. Tangier disease: a histological and ultrastructural study. Pathol Res Pract 1985;180:424.

59. Tarao K, Iwamura K, Fujii K, Miyake H. Japanese adult siblings with Tangier disease and statistical analysis of reported cases. Tokai J Exp Clin Med 1984;9:379.

60. Reinhart WH, Staubli M, Mordasini C, Scheurer U. Abnormalities of gut vessels in Turner's syndrome. Postgrad Med J 1983;59:122.

61. Nardone DA, Reuler JB, Girard DE. Gastrointestinal complications of Ehlers-Danlos syndrome. N Engl J Med 1979;300:863.

62. Silva R, Cogbill TH, Hansbrough JF, et al. Intestinal perforation and vascular rupture in Ehlers-Danlos syndrome. Int Surg 1986;71:48.

63. Harris RD. Small bowel dilatation in Ehlers-Danlos syndrome: an unreported gastrointestinal manifestation. Br J Radiol 1974;47:623.

64. McLean AM, Paul RE Jr, Kritzman J, Farthing MJ. Malabsorption in Marfan (Ehlers-Danlos) syndrome. J Clin Gastroenterol 1984;7:304.

65. Sigurdson E, Stern HS, Houpt J, et al. The Ehlers-Danlos syndrome and colonic perforation: report of a case and physiologic assessment of underlying motility disorder. Dis Colon Rectum 1985;28:962.

66. Altman LK, Fialkow PJ, Parker F, Sagebiel RW. Pseudoxanthoma elasticum: an underdiagnosed genetically heterogeneous disorder with protean manifestations. Arch Intern Med 1974;134:1048.

67. Kundrotas L, Novak J, Kremzier J, et al. Gastric bleeding in pseudoxanthoma elasticum. Am J Gastroenterol 1988;83:868.

68. Belli A, Cawthorne S. Visceral angiographic findings in pseudoxanthoma elasticum. Br J Radiol 1988;61:368.

69. Cunningham JR, Lippman SM, Renie WA, et al. Pseudoxanthoma elasticum: treatment of gastrointestinal hemorrhage by arterial embolization and observations on autosomal dominant inheritance. Johns Hopkins Med J 1980;147:168.

70. Athanasoulis CA. Therapeutic applications of angiography. N Engl J Med 1980;302:1117.

71. Cohen S. The gastrointestinal manifestations of scleroderma: pathogenesis and management. Gastroenterology 1980;79:155.

72. Hostein J, Fournet J. Gastrointestinal manifestations of collagen diseases. Dig Dis 1986;4:240.

73. Akesson A, Akesson B, Gustafson T, Wollhein F. Gastrointestinal function in patients with progressive systemic sclerosis. Clin Rheumatol 1985;4:441.

74. Baron M, Srolovitz H. Colonic telangiectasias in a patient with progressive systemic sclerosis. Arthritis Rheum 1986;29:195.

75. Frabach RC, Kadell BM, Nies KM, et al. Sigmoid volvulus in patients with progressive systemic sclerosis. J Rheumatol 1978;5:195.

76. McCallum RW, Prakash C, Campoli-Richards DM, Goa KL. Cisapride: a preliminary review of its pharmacodynamic and pharmacokinetic properties, and therapeutic use as a prokinetic agent in gastrointestinal motility disorders. Drugs1988;36:652.

77. Soudah HC, Hasler WL, Owyang C. Effect of octreotide on intestinal motility and bacterial overgrowth in scleroderma. N Engl J Med 1991;325:1508.

78. Kleckner FS. Dermatomyositis and its manifestations in the gastrointestinal tract. Am J Gastroenterol 1970;53:141.

79. De Meriieux P, Verity A, Clements PJ, Paulus H. Esophageal abnormalities and dysphagia in polymyositis and dermatomyositis: clinical, radiographic and pathologic features. Arthritis Rheum 1983;26:9612.

80. Horowitz M, McNeil JD, Maddern GJ, et al. Abnormalities of gastric and esophageal emptying in polymyositis and dermatomyositis. Gastroenterology 1986;90:434.

81. Okayasu I, Mizutani H, Kurihara H, Yanagisawa F. Cancer in collagen disease: a statistical analysis by reviewing the Annual of Pathological Autopsy Cases (Nippon Boken Shoho) in Japan. Cancer 1984;54:1841.

82. Talbott JH. Acute dermatomyositis-polymyositis and malignancy. Semin Arthritis Rheum 1977;6:305.

83. Lakhanpal S, Bunch TW, Ilstrup DM, Melton LJ III. Polymyositis-dermatomyositis and malignant lesions: does an association exist? Mayo Clin Proc 1986;61:645.

84. Mitchell DM, Spitz PW, Young DY, et al. Survival, prognosis, and causes of death in rheumatoid arthritis. Arthritis Rheum 1986;29:706.

85. Sun DCH, Roth SH, Mitchell CS, England DWW. Upper gastrointestinal disease in rheumatoid arthritis. Am J Dig Dis 1974;19:405.

86. Lindsay MK, Tavadia HB, Whyte AS, et al. Acute abdomen in rheumatoid arthritis due to necrotizing arteritis. Br Med J 1973;2:592.

87. Scott DGI, Bacon PA, Tribe CR. Systemic rheumatoid vasculitis: a clinical and laboratory study of 50 cases. Medicine 1981;60:288.

88. Fayaemi AO, Ali M, Baun EV. Necrotizing vasculitis of the gallbladder and the appendix: similarity in the morphology of rheumatoid arthritis and polyarteritis nodosa. Am J Gastroenterol 1977;67:608.

89. Roth S, Bennett RE, Mitchell CS, Hartman RJ. Cimetidine therapy in nonsteroidal anti-inflammatory drug gastropathy: double-blind long-term evaluation. Arch Intern Med 1987;147:1798.

90. Morris AD, Holt SD, Silvoso GR, et al. Effect of anti-inflammatory drug administration in patients with rheumatoid arthritis: an endoscopic assessment. Scand J Gastroenterol 1981;67:131.

91. Fries JF, Miller SR, Spitz PW, et al. Toward an epidemiology of gastropathy associated with nonsteroidal antiinflammatory drug use. Gastroenterology 1989;96:647.

92. Davies J, Collins A, Dixon A. The influence of cimetidine on

peptic ulcer disease in patients with arthritis taking antiinflammatory drugs. Br J Rheumatol 1986;25:54.

93. Caldwell J. Sucralfate in the relief of gastrointestinal symptoms associated with non-steroidal antiinflammatory drugs. South Med J 1985;78:938.

94. Cohen MM, McCready DR, Clark L, Sevelius H. Protection against aspirin-induced antral and duodenal damage with enoprostil. Gastroenterology 1985;88:382.

95. Nyfors A, Poulsen H. Liver biopsies from psoriatics related to methotrexate therapy. Acta Pathol Microbiol Scand 1976;84:253.

96. Dillon AM, Luthra HS, Conn DL, Ferguson RH. Parenteral gold therapy in the Felty syndrome: experience with 20 patients. Medicine 1986;65:107.

97. Tsianos EB, Chiras CD, Drosos AA, Moutsopoulos HM. Esophageal dysfunction in patients with Sjögren's syndrome. Ann Rheum Dis 1985;44:610.

98. Trevano H, Tsianos EB, Schenker S. Gastrointestinal and hepatobiliary features in Sjögren's syndrome. In: Talal H, Moutsopoulos HM, Kanan ES, eds. Sjögren's syndrome. New York: Springer-Verlag, 1987.

99. Constantopoulos S-H, Tsianos E-V, Moutsopoulos H-M. Pulmonary and gastrointestinal manifestations of Sjögren's syndrome. Rheum Dis Clin North Am 1992;18:617.

100. Jovaisas A, Kraag G. Acute gastrointestinal manifestations of systemic lupus erythematosus. Can J Surg 1987;30:185.

101. Hoffman BI, Katz WA. The gastrointestinal manifestations of systemic lupus erythematosus: a review of the literature. Semin Arthritis Rheum 1980;9:237.

102. Petri M. Pancreatitis in systemic lupus erythematosus: still in search of a mechanism (editorial). J Rheumatol 1992;19:1014.

103. Seaman WE, Ishak KG, Plotz PH. Aspirin-induced hepatotoxicity in patients with systemic lupus erythematosus. Ann Intern Med 1974;80:1.

104. Haslock I. Spontaneous rupture of the liver in systemic lupus erythematosus. Ann Rheum Dis 1974;33:482.

105. Calin A. The spondyloarthropathies. Sci Am Med 1983;9:1.

106. Mielants H, Veys EM, Cuvelier C, et al. HLA B27 related arthritis and bowel inflammation. Part 2. Ileocolonoscopy and bowel histology in patients with HLA B27 related arthritis. J Rheumatol 1985;12:294.

107. De Vos M, Cuvelier C, Mielants H, et al. Ileocolonoscopy in seronegative spondyloarthropathy. Gastroenterology 1989;96:339.

108. Waldmann TA, Misiti J, Nelson DL, Kraemer KJ. Ataxia-telangiectasia: a multisystem hereditary disease with immunodeficiency, impaired organ maturation, x-ray hypersensitive, and a high incidence of neoplasia. Ann Intern Med 1983;99:362.

109. Ament ME. Immunodeficiency syndromes and the gut. Scand J Gastroenterol 114:127, 1985;

110. Becker Y. Ataxia-telangiectasia: a recessive human genetic disorder causing immune deficiency and predisposition to cancer. Clin Immunol Newsletter 1988;9:117.

111. Ishiguro T, Taketa U, Gatti RA. Tissue oxygen of elevated alphafetoprotein in ataxia telangiectasia. Disease Markers 1986;4:293.

112. Baker AL, Kahn PC, Binder SC, Patterson JF. Gastrointestinal bleeding due to blue rubber bleb nevus syndrome. Gastroenterology 1971;61:530.

113. Jennings M, Ward P, Maddocks JL. Blue rubber bleb naevus disease: an uncommon cause of gastrointestinal tract bleeding. Gut 1988;29:1408.

114. Shahed M, Hagenmuller F, Rosch Th, et al. A 19-year-old female with blue rubber bleb nevus syndrome: endoscopic laser photocoagulation and surgical resection of gastrointestinal angiomata. Endoscopy 1990;2:54.

115. Mallory SB, Stough DB. Genodermatoses with malignant potential. Dermatol Clin 1987;5:221.

116. Carlson GJ, Nivatvongs S, Snover DC. Colorectal polyps in Cowden's disease (multiple hamartoma syndrome). Am J Surg Pathol 1984;8:763.

117. Weinstock JV, Kawanishi H. Gastrointestinal polyposis with orocutaneous hamartomas. Gastroenterology 1978;74:890.

118. Rosenbloom MS, Ratner M. Congenital pyloric atresia and epidermolysis bullosa letalis in premature siblings. J Pediatr Surg 1987;22:374.

119. Feurle GE, Weidawer H, Baldauf G, et al. Management of esophageal stenosis in recessive dystrophic epidermolysis bullosa. Gastroenterology 1984;87:13.

120. Gryboski JD, Touloukian R, Campanella RA. Gastrointestinal manifestations of epidermolysis bullosa in children. Arch Dermatol 1984;124:746.

121. Eliakim R, Goldin E, Livshin R, Okon E. Esophageal involvement in pemphigus vulgaris. Am J Gastroenterol 1988;83:155.

122. Yakshe PN, Albert F, Ragsdale B, et al. An unusual vascular lesion in a patient with hereditary hemorrhagic telangiectasia. Gastrointest Endosc 1990;36:513.

123. Peery WH. Clinic spectrum of hereditary hemorrhagic telangiectasia (Osler-Weber-Rendu disease). Am J Med 1987;82:989.

124. Hochberg FH, Dasilva AB, Galdabini J, et al. Gastrointestinal involvement in von Recklinghausen's neurofibromatosis. Neurology 1984;24:1144.

125. Riccardi VM. Von Recklinghausen neurofibromatosis. N Engl J Med 1981;305:1617.

126. Lederman SM, Martin EC, Laffey KT, Lefkowitch JH. Hepatic neurofibromatosis, malignant schwannoma, and angiosarcoma in von Recklinghausen's disease. Gastroenterology 1987;92:234.

127. Morizumi H, Sano T, Hirose T, Hizawa K. Neurofibroma of the gallbladder seen as a papillary polyp. Acta Pathol Jpn 1988;38:259.

128. Weinstein GD. Methotrexate. Ann Intern Med 1977;86:199.

129. Van De Kerkhof PCM, Hoefnagel WHL, Van Haelst UJGM, Mali JWH. Methotrexate maintenance therapy and liver damage in psoriasis. Clin Exp Dermatol 1985;10:194.

130. Atherton LD, Leib ES, Kaye MD. Toxic megacolon associated with methotrexate therapy. Gastroenterology 1984;86:1583.

131. Zweiban B, Cohen H, Chandrasoma P. Gastrointestinal involvement complicating Stevens-Johnson syndrome. Gastroenterology 1986;91:469.

132. Stein M, Thomson CK, Sawicki JE, Martel AJ. Esophageal stricture complicating Stevens-Johnson syndrome. Am J Gastroenterol 1974;62:435.

133. Crosby SS, Murray KM, Marvin JA, et al. Management of Stevens-Johnson syndrome. Clin Pharm 1986;5:682.

134. Lightdale CJ, Winawer SJ. Screening diagnosis and staging of esophageal cancer. Semin Oncol 1984;11:101.

135. Harper PS, Harper RMJ, Howel-Evans AW. Carcinoma of the esophagus with tylosis. Q J Med 1970;39:317.

136. Jorizzo JL. Classification of urticaria and the reactive inflammatory dermatoses. Dermatol Clin 1985;3:3.

137. Champion RH, Highet AS. Investigation and management of chronic urticaria and angio-edema. Clin Exp Dermatol 1982;7:291.

138. Reimann HJ, Ring J, Ultsch P, et al. Release of gastric histamine in patients with urticaria and food allergy. Agents Actions 1982;12:111.

139. Soter NA. Clinical presentations and mechanisms of necrotizing angiitis of the skin. J Invest Dermatol 1976;67:354.

140. Gammon WR. Urticarial vasculitis. Dermatol Clin 1985;3:97.

141. Klein I, Parveen G, Gavaler JS, Van Thiel DH. Colonic polyps in patients with acromegaly. Ann Intern Med 1982;97:27.

142. Hughes PD. Diabetic acidosis with acute pancreatitis. Br J Surg 1961;49:90.

143. Niakan E, Harati Y, Comstock JP. Diabetic autonomic neuropathy. Metabolism 1986;35:224.

144. Loo FD, Dodds WJ, Soergel KH, et al. Multipeaked esophageal peristaltic pressure waves in patients with diabetic neuropathy. Gastroenterology 1985;88:485.

145. Horowitz M, Edelbroek M, Fraser R, et al. Disordered gastric motor function in diabetes mellitus. Scand J Gastroenterol 1991;26:673.

146. Feldman M, Smith HJ, Simon TR. Gastric emptying of solid radiopaque markers: studies in healthy subjects and diabetic patients. Gastroenterology 1984;87:895.

147. Loo FD, Palmer DW, Soergel KH, et al. Gastric emptying in patients with diabetes mellitus. Gastroenterology 1984;86:485.

148. Roon AJ, Mason GR. Surgical management of gastroparesis diabeticorum. Calif Med 1972;116:58.

149. Feldman M, Schiller LR. Disorders of gastrointestinal motility associated with diabetes mellitus. Ann Intern Med 1983;98:378.

150. Miller LJ. Small intestinal manifestations of diabetes mellitus. Yale J Biol Med 1983;56:189.

151. Trier JS. Celiac sprue. N Engl J Med 1991;325:1709.

152. Durbin T, Rosenthal L, McArthur L, et al. Clonidine and li-damidine stimulate sodium and chloride absorption in the rabbit intestine. Gastroenterology 1982;82:1352.

153. Fedorak RN, Field M, Chang EB. Treatment of diabetic diarrhea with clonidine. Ann Intern Med 1985;102:197.

154. Battle WM, Snape WJ Jr, Alavi A, et al. Colonic dysfunction in diabetes mellitus. Gastroenterology 1980;79:1217.

155. Schiller LR, Santa Ana CA, Schmulen AC, et al. Pathogenesis of fecal incontinence in diabetes mellitus: evidence for internal-anal-sphincter dysfunction. N Engl J Med 1982;307:1666.

156. Wald A, Tununguntla K. Anorectal sensorimotor dysfunction in fecal incontinence and diabetes mellitus: modification with biofeedback therapy. N Engl J Med 1984;310:1282.

157. Longstreth GF, Newcomer AD. Abdominal pain caused by diabetic radiculopathy. Ann Intern Med 1977;86:166.

158. Streib EW, Sun SF, Paustian FF, et al. Diabetic thoracic radiculopathy: electrodiagnostic study. Muscle Nerve 1986;9:548.

159. Max MB, Lynch SA, Muir J, et al. Effects of desipramine, amitriptyline, and fluoxetine on pain in diabetic neuropathy. N Engl J Med 1992;326:1250.

160. Selby CD, Dennis MJS, Whincup PH. Painless mesenteric infarction in patient with diabetes mellitus. Diabetic Care 1987;10:259.

161. Bartoli E, Ferrari E, Saporetti N, Rossi L. Prevalence of cholelithiasis in diabetes mellitus: a cholecystosonographic study. Diagn Radiol 1987;12:43.

162. Ransohoff DF, Miller GL, Forsythe SB, Hermann RE. Outcome of acute cholecystitis in patients with diabetes mellitus. Ann Intern Med 1987;106:829.

163. Falchuk KR, Fiske SC, Haggitt RC, et al. Pericentral hepatic fibrosis and intracellular hyalin in diabetes mellitus. Gastroenterology 1980;78:535.

164. Corlew DS, Bryda SL, Bradley EL III, DiGirolamo M. Observations on the course of untreated primary hyperparathyroidism. Surgery 1985;98:1064.

165. Gardner EC Jr, Hersh T. Primary hyperparathyroidism and the gastrointestinal tract. South Med J 1981;74:197.

166. Sitges-Serra A, Alonso M, deLecea C, et al. Pancreatitis and hyperparathyroidism. Br J Surg 1988;75:158.

167. Tagbi H, Keele D. Hypoparathyroidism: a review of the literature and report of two cases in sisters, one with steatorrhea and intestinal pseudoobstruction. AJR 1962;88:432.

168. Jorgensen F, Hesse B, Gronbaek P, et al. Abnormal oesophageal function in patients with non-toxic goiter or enlarged left atrium, demonstrated by radionuclide transit measurements. Scand J Gastroenterol 1989;24:1186.

169. Shafer RB, Prentiss RA, Bond JH. Gastrointestinal transit in thyroid disease. Gastroenterology 1984;86:852.

170. Hellesen C, Friis TH, Larsen E, Pock-Steen CO. Small intestinal histology, radiology and absorption in hyperthyroidism. Scand J Gastroenterol 1969;4:169.

171. Baker JT, Harvey RF. Bowel habits in thyrotoxicosis and hypothyroidism. Br Med J 1971;1:322.

172. Miller LJ, Yang COW, Malagelada JR, et al. Gastric, pancreatic and biliary responses to meals in hyperthyroidism. Gut 1980;21:695.

173. Meshkinpour H, Afrasiabi MA, Valenta LJ. Esophageal motor function in Graves' disease. Dig Dis Sci 1979;24:159.

174. Siurala M, Julkunen H, Lamberg BA. Gastrointestinal tract in hyperthyroidism before and after treatment. Scand J Gastroenterol 1966;1:79.

175. Sheridan R. Thyroid hormones and the liver. Clin Gastroenterol 1983;12:797.

176. O'Connor P, Feely J. Clinical pharmacokinetics and endocrine disorders: therapeutic implications. Clin Pharmacokinet 1987;13:345.

177. Christensen J, Clifton J. Esophageal manometry in myxedema. Gastroenterology 1967;52:1130.

178. Solano FX, Starling RC, Levey GS. Myxedema megacolon. Arch Intern Med 1985;145:231.

179. Salerno N, Grey N. Myxedema pseudoobstruction. AJR 1978;130:175.

180. Goldin E, Wengrower D. Diarrhea in hypothyroidism: bacterial overgrowth as a possible etiology. J Clin Gastroenterol 1990;12:98.

181. Gullo L, Pezzilli R, Bellanova B, et al. Influence of the thyroid on exocrine pancreatic function. Gastroenterology 1991;100:1392.

182. Baker A, Kaplan M, Wolfe H. Central congestive fibrosis of the liver in myxedema ascites. Ann Intern Med 1972;77:927.

183. de Castro F, Bonacini M, Walden J, Schubert T. Myxedema ascites: report of two cases and review of the literature. J Clin Gastroenterol 1991;13:411.

184. Ladenson PW, Levin AA, Ridgway EC, Daniels GH. Complications of surgery in hypothyroid patients. Am J Med 1984;77:261.

185. Wald A, Van Thiel DH, Hoechstetter L, et al. Effect of pregnancy on gastrointestinal transit. Dig Dis Sci 1982;27:1015.

186. Klebanoff MA, Koslowe PA, Kaslow R, Rhoads GG. Epidemiology of vomiting in early pregnancy. Obstet Gynecol 1985;66:612.

187. Levine MG, Esser D. Total parenteral nutrition for the treatment of severe hyperemesis gravidarum: maternal nutritional effects and fetal outcome. Obstet Gynecol 1988;72:102.

188. Burgess DE. Constipation in obstetrics. In: Jones FA, Godding EW, eds. Management of constipation. Oxford, Blackwell, 1972:176.

189. Landers D, Carmona R, Crombleholme W, Lim R. Acute cholecystitis in pregnancy. Obstet Gynecol 1987;69:131.

190. Holzbach T. Jaundice in pregnancy. Am J Med 1976;61:367.

191. Weinstein L. Preeclampsia/eclampsia with hemolysis, elevated liver enzymes and thrombocytopenia. Obstet Gynecol 1985;66:657.

192. Ducroz B, Villemonteix P, Magnin G, Pourrat O. The HELLP syndrome: is this a clinical form of thrombotic microangiopathy? J Gynecol Obstet Biol Reprod (Paris) 1990;19:729.

193. Hatfield A, Stein JH, Greenberger MM, et al. Idiopathic acute fatty liver of pregnancy: death from extrahepatic manifestations. Am J Dig Dis 1972;17:617.

194. Lowry SM, O'Dea TP, Gallagher DI, Mozenter R. Splenic artery aneurysm rupture: the seventh instance of maternal and fetal survival. Obstet Gynecol 1986;67:291.

195. Weinstock JV. Immunoregulation of granulomatous inflammation in the liver and intestines. In: Marsh MN, ed. Immunopathology of the small intestine. London: John Wiley & Sons, 1987:151.

196. Harrington PT, Gutierrez JJ, Ramirez-Ronda RH, et al. Granulomatous hepatitis. Rev Infect Dis 1982;4:638.

197. Stricker BHCh, Blok APR, Babany G, Benhamou J-P. Fibrin ring granulomas and allopurinol. Gastroenterology 1989;96:1199.

198. Ponz E, Garcia-Pagan JC, Bruguera M, et al. Hepatic fibrin-ring granulomas in a patient with hepatitis A. Gastroenterology 1991;100:268.

199. Foster GS. Weekly clinicopathological exercise. N Engl J Med 1980;303:445.

200. Bhargava DK, Kushwaha AKS, Dasarathy S, et al. Endoscopic diagnosis of segmental colonic tuberculosis. Gastrointest Endosc 1992;38:571.

201. Saenger P, Rosen J, Markowitz M. Diagnostic significance of edetate disodium calcium testing in children with increased lead absorption. Am J Dis Child 1982;136:312.

202. Ibels LS, Pollock CA. Lead intoxication. Med Toxicol 1986;1:387.

203. Beattie AD, Mullin PH, Baxter RH, Moore MR. Acute lead poisoning: an individual case of hepatitis. Scott Med J 1979;24:318.

204. Pollock CA, Ibels LS. Lead intoxication in Sydney Harbour Bridge workers. Aust N Z J Med 1988;18:46.

205. Janin Y, Couinaud C, Stone A, Wise L. The "lead-induced colic" syndrome in lead intoxication. Surg Annu 1985;17:287.

206. Zaloga GP, Deal J, Spurling T, et al. Unusual manifestations of arsenic intoxication. Am J Med Sci 1985;289:210.

207. Szuler IM, Williams CN, Hindmarsh JT, Park Dincsoy H. Massive variceal hemorrhage secondary to presinusoidal portal hypertension due to arsenic poisoning. Can Med Assoc J 1979;120:168.

208. Mackell MA, Gantner GE, Poklis A, Graham M. An unsuspected arsenic poisoning murder disclosed by forensic autopsy. Am J Forensic Med Pathol 1985;6:358.

209. Schoolmeester WL, White DR. Arsenic poisoning. South Med J 1980;73:198.

210. Philipp R. Arsenic exposure: health effects and the risk of cancer. Rev Environ Health 1985;5:27.

211. Behrens R, Devereaux M, Hazleman B, et al. Investigation of auranofin-induced diarrhoea. Gut 1979;27:59.

212. Huston GJ. Gold colitis: therapy and confirmation of mucosal recovery by measurement of rectal potential differences. Postgrad Med J 1980;56:875.

213. Stein HB, Urnowitz MB. Gold-induced enterocolitis case report and literature review. J Rheumatol 1976;3:21.

214. Michet CJ, Rakela J, Luthra MD. Auranofin-associated colitis and eosinophilia. Mayo Clin Proc 1987;62:142.

215. Griffin PM, Ostroff SM, Tauxe RV, et al. Illnesses associated with *Escherichia coli* O167:H7 infections: a broad clinical spectrum. Ann Intern Med 1988;109:705.

216. Delans RJ, Biuso JD, Saba SR, Ramirez G. Hemolytic uremic syndrome after *Campylobacter*-induced diarrhea in an adult. Arch Intern Med 1984;144:1074.

217. Bitzan M, Karch H. Indirect hemagglutination assay for diagnosis of *Escherichia coli* O157 infection in patients with hemolytic-uremic syndrome. J Clin Microbiol 1992;30:1174.

218. Cleary TG. *Escherichia coli* that cause hemolytic uremic syndrome. Infect Dis Clin North Am 1992;6:163.

219. Koster F, Levine J, Walker L, et al. Hemolytic uremic syndrome after shigellosis: relation to endotoxemia and circulating immune complexes. N Engl J Med 1978;298:927.

220. Webster J, Reese AJ, Lewis PJ, et al. Prostacyclin deficiency in hemolytic uremic syndrome. Br Med J 1980;281:271.

221. Cohen MB, Giannella RA. Hemorrhagic colitis associated with *Escherichia coli* O157:H7. Adv Intern Med 1992;37:173.

222. Dennenberg T, Friedberg M, Holmberg L, et al. Combined plasmapheresis and hemodialysis treatment for severe hemolytic-uremic syndrome following *Campylobacter* colitis. Acta Paediatr Scand 1982;71:243.

223. Jacobs WA. Acute thrombotic thrombocytopenic purpura and cholecystitis. J Emerg Med 1985;2:265.

224. Schafer AI. The hypercoagulable states. Ann Intern Med 1985;102:814.

225. Clouse LJ, Comp PC. The regulation of hemostasis: the protein C system. N Engl J Med 1986;314:1298.

226. Rizza CR, Matthews JM. Clinical features of clotting factor deficiencies. In: Biggs R, Rizza CR, eds. Human blood coagulation, hemostasis and thrombosis. Boston: Blackwell, 1984: 119.

227. Roth GJ, Stanford N, Majerus PW. Acetylation of prostaglandin synthetase by aspirin. Proc Natl Acad Sci USA 1975;72: 3073.

228. Klifto EJ, Allen SK, Metzman M, et al. Plummer-Vinson syndrome: report of a case and review of the literature. J Am Osteopath Assoc 1983;83:56.

229. McNab J, Jones RF. The Paterson-Brown-Kelly syndrome: its relationship to iron deficiency and postcricoid carcinoma. J Laryngol Otol 1961;75:529.

230. Larsson LG, Sandstrom A, Westling P. Relationship of Plummer-Vinson disease to cancer of the upper alimentary tract. Cancer Res 1975;35:3308.

231. Nosher JL, Campbell WL, Seaman WB. The clinical significance of cervical esophageal and hypopharyngeal webs. Radiology 1975;117:45.

232. Nicholl F, Troiso A, Bedogni G, Conigliaro R. Radiologic and endoscopic diagnosis in Plummer-Vinson syndrome. Rays 1986;11:51.

233. Davies SC, Wonke B. The management of haemoglobinopathies. Baillieres Clin Haematol 1991;4:361.

234. Ferrone FA. The polymerization of sickle hemoglobin in solutions and cells. Experientia 1993;49:110.

235. Powars DR. Sickle cell anemia and major organ failure. Hemoglobin 1990;14:573.

236. Karayalcin G, Rosner F, Kim KY, et al. Sickle cell anemia: clinical manifestations in 100 patients and review of the literature. Am J Med Sci 1975;269:51.

237. Comer GM, Ozick LA, Sachdev RK, et al. Transfusion-related chronic liver disease in sickle cell anemia. Am J Gastroenterol 1991;86:1232.

238. Johnson CS, Omata M, Tong MJ, et al. Liver involvement in sickle cell disease. Medicine (Baltimore) 1985;64:349.

239. Omata M, Johnson CS, Tong M, Tatter D. Pathological spectrum of liver diseases in sickle cell disease. Dig Dis Sci 1986;31: 247.

240. Pollack CV Jr. Emergencies in sickle cell disease. Emerg Med Clin North Am 1993;11:365.

241. Gairdner D. Association of gallstones with acholuric jaundice in children. Arch Dis Child 1963;14:109.

242. Kyle RA, Bayrd ED. Amyloidosis: review of 236 cases. Medicine (Baltimore) 1975;54:271.

243. Cohen AS. Primary (AL) amyloidosis. Ren Fail 1993;15:429.

244. Kyle RA, Greipp PR. Amyloidosis (AL): clinical and laboratory features in 229 cases. Mayo Clin Proc 1983;58:665.

245. Chernenkoff RM, Costopoulos LB, Bain GO. Gastrointestinal manifestations of primary amyloidosis. Can Med Assoc J 1972;106:567.

246. Ectors N, Geboes K, Kerremans R, et al. Small bowel amyloidosis, pathology and diagnosis. Acta Gastroenterol Belg 1992;55: 228.

247. Tada S, Iida M, Iwashita A, et al. Endoscopic and biopsy findings of the upper digestive tract in patients with amyloidosis. Gastrointest Endosc 1990;36:10.

248. Rubinow A, Burakoff R, Cohen AS, Harris LD. Esophageal manometry in systemic amyloidosis: a study of 30 patients. Am J Med 1983;75:951.

249. Pear BL. Radiographic studies of amyloidosis. CRC Crit Rev Radiol 1972;3:425.

250. Carlson HC, Breen JF. Amyloidosis and plasma cell dyscrasias: gastrointestinal involvement. Semin Roentgenol 1986;21:128.

251. Teelucksingh S, Padfield PL, Edwards CR. Systemic capillary leak syndrome. Q J Med 1990;75:515.

252. Economou JS, Hoban M, Lee JD, et al. Production of tumor necrosis factor alpha and interferon gamma in Interleukin-2-treated melanoma patients: correlation with clinical toxicity. Cancer Immunol Immunother 1991;34:49.

253. Ewan PW, Lachmann PJ, Morice AH, Forster PJG. Treatment of systemic capillary leak syndrome. Lancet 1988;2:1496.

254. Droder RM, Kyle RA, Greipp PR. Control of systemic capillary leak syndrome with aminophylline and terbutaline. Am J Med 1992;92:523.

255. Prolla JC, Kirsner JB. The gastrointestinal lesions and complications of the leukemias. Ann Intern Med 1964;61:1084.

256. Hunter TB, Bjelland JC. Gastrointestinal complications of leukemia and its treatment. AJR 1984;142:513.

257. Hawkins JA, Mower WR, Nelson EW. Acute abdominal conditions in patients with leukemia. Am J Surg 1985;150:739.

258. McCarthy GM, Skillings JR. Orofacial complications of chemotherapy for breast cancer. Oral Surg Oral Med Oral Pathol 1992;74:172.

259. Mahood DJ, Dose AM, Loprinzi CL, et al. Inhibition of fluorouracil-induced stomatitis by oral cryotherapy. J Clin Oncol 1991;9:449.

260. Wadleigh RG, Redman RS, Graham ML, et al. Vitamin E in the treatment of chemotherapy-induced mucositis. Am J Med 1992;92:481.

261. Pfeiffer P, Madsen EL, Hansen O, May O. Effect of prophylactic sucralfate suspension on stomatitis induced by cancer chemotherapy: a randomized, double-blind cross-over study. Acta Oncol 1990;29:171.

262. Jones GT, Abramson N. Gastrointestinal necrosis in acute leu-

kemia: a complication of induction therapy. Cancer Invest 1983;1:315.

263. Alt B, Glass NR, Sollinger H. Neutropenic enterocolitis in adults. Am J Surg 1985;149:405.

264. Kapadia SB. Multiple myeloma: a clinicopathologic study of 62 consecutively autopsied cases. Medicine (Baltimore) 1980;59:380.

265. Gradishar W, Recant W, Shapiro C. Obstructing plasmacytoma of the duodenum: first manifestation of relapsed multiple myeloma. Am J Gastroenterol 1988;83:77.

266. Benson WJ, Scarffe JH, Houwen B, Crowther D. Gastrointestinal involvement with myeloma. Med Pediatr Oncol 1983;11:256.

267. Veloso FT, Fraga J, Saleiro JV. Macroglobulinemia and small intestinal disease: a case report with review of the literature. J Clin Gastroenterol 1988;10:546.

268. Seligmann M, Mihaesco E, Preudhomme JL, et al. Heavy chain diseases: current findings and concepts. Immunol Rev 1979;48:145.

269. Seligmann M, Rambuad JC. Alpha-chain disease: an immunoproliferative disease of the secretory immune system. Ann NY Acad Sci 1983;409:478.

270. Abt AB, Kirschner RH, Belliveau RF, et al. Hepatic pathology associated with Hodgkin's disease. Cancer 1974;33:1564.

271. Sherlock P, Winawer JJ, Lacher MJ, Ehrlich AN. Gastrointestinal manifestations of Hodgkin's disease. In: Lacher MJ, ed. Hodgkin's disease. New York: John Wiley & Sons, 1976:297.

272. Sherlock P. The gastrointestinal manifestations and complications of malignant lymphoma. Schweiz Med Wochenschr 1980;110:1031.

273. Mentzer SJ, Osteen RT, Pappas TN, et al. Surgical therapy of localized abdominal non-Hodgkin's lymphomas. Surgery 1988;103:609.

274. Wasserman LR. Polycythemia rubra vera: its course and treatment. Relation to myeloid metaplasia and leukemia. Bull NY Acad Med 1954;3:343.

275. Tinney WS, Hall BE, Griffin HZ. Polycythemia vera and peptic ulcer. Mayo Clin Proc 1943;18:24.

276. Calabreri P, Meyer OO. Polycythemia vera. I. Clinical and laboratory manifestations. Ann Intern Med 1959;50:1182.

277. Silverstein MK. Primary thrombocythemia. In: Williams WJ, ed. Hematology. New York: McGraw-Hill, 1983:218.

278. Wu KK. Platelet aggregability and thrombosis in patients with thrombocytosis. Ann Intern Med 1978;88:7.

279. Jorge E, Harvey HA, Simmonds MA, et al. Symptomatic malignant melanoma of the gastrointestinal tract. Ann Surg 1984;199:328.

280. Taal BG, den Hartog Jager FDA, Steinmetz R, Peterse H. The spectrum of gastrointestinal metastases of breast carcinoma. I. Stomach. Gastrointest Endosc 1992;38:130.

281. Keeney K, Abaza NA, Tidwel O, Quinn P. Oral Kaposi's sarcoma in acquired immune deficiency syndrome. J Oral Maxillofac Surg 1987;45:815.

282. Clarke-Pearson DL, DeLong ER, Chin N, et al. Intestinal obstruction in patients with ovarian cancer. Arch Surg 1988;123:42.

283. Kern KA, Norton JA. Cancer cachexia. JPEN J Parenter Enteral Nutr 1988;12:286.

284. Chinn JS, Schuffler MS. Paraneoplastic visceral neuropathy as a cause of severe gastrointestinal motor dysfunction. Gastroenterology 1988;95:1279.

285. Gerl A, Storck M, Muller-Hocker J, et al. Paraneoplastic chronic intestinal pseudoobstruction as a rare complication of bronchial carcinoid. Gut 1992;33:1000.

286. Rambaud J, Hautefeuille M, Ruskone A, Jacquenoid J. Diarrhea due to circulating agents. Clin Gastroenterol 1986;15:603.

287. Lips CJ, Vasen HF, Lamers CB. Multiple endocrine neoplasia syndromes. CRC Crit Rev Oncol Hematol 1984;2:117.

288. Fishman RS, Fleming CR, Li CY. Systemic mastocytosis with review of the gastrointestinal manifestations. Mayo Clin Proc 1979;54:51.

289. Barriere H, Dreno B, Pecquet C, et al. Systemic mastocytosis and intestinal malabsorption. Semin Hop Paris 1983;59:2925.

290. Frieri M, Alling DW, Metcalfe DD. Comparison of the therapeutic efficacy of cromolyn sodium with that of combined chlorpheniramine and cimetidine in systemic mastocytosis: results of a double-blind clinical trial. Am J Med 1985;78:9.

291. Marshall JB, Diaz-Arias AA, Bochna GS, Vogele KA. Achalasia due to diffuse esophageal leiomyomatosis and inherited as an autosomal dominant disorder. Gastroenterology 1990;98:1358.

292. Jura E. Gastrointestinal disturbances in stroke. Acta Neurol Scand 1987;76:168.

293. Griffin MR, Ray WA, Schaffner W. Nonsteroidal anti-inflammatory drug use and death from peptic ulcer in elderly persons. Ann Intern Med 1988;109:359.

294. Peters TE, Racey GL, Nahman BJ. Dental prosthesis as an unsuspected foreign body. Ann Emerg Med 1984;60:109.

295. Olins NJ. Feeding decisions for incompetent patients. J Am Geriatr Soc 1986;34:313.

296. Peck A, Cohen CE, Mulvihill MN. Long-term enteral feeding of aged demented nursing home patients. J Am Geriatr Soc 1990;38:1195.

297. Symon DNK, Russel G. Abdominal migraine: a childhood syndrome defined. Cephalalgia 1986;6:223.

298. Perkin JE, Hartje J. Diet and migraine: a review of the literature. J Am Diet Assoc 1983;83:459.

299. Anderson JT, Bradley WE. Abnormalities of detrusor and sphincter function in multiple sclerosis. Br J Urol 1976;48:193.

300. Glick ME, Meshkinpour H, Haldeman S, et al. Colonic dysfunction in multiple sclerosis. Gastroenterology 1982;83:1002.

301. Sullivan SN, Ebers GC. Gastrointestinal dysfunction in multiple sclerosis (letter). Gastroenterology 1983;84:1640.

302. Hinds JP, Eidelman BH, Wald A. Prevalence of bowel dysfunction in multiple sclerosis. Gastroenterology 1990;98:1538.

303. Nowak TV, Ionasescu V, Anuras S. Gastrointestinal manifestations of the muscular dystrophies. Gastroenterology 1982;82:800.

304. Leon SH, Schuffler MD, Kettler M, Rohrmann CA. Chronic intestinal pseudoobstruction as a complication of Duchenne's muscular dystrophy. Gastroenterology 1986;90:455.

305. Barohn RJ, Levine EJ, Olson JO, Mendell JR. Gastric hypomotility in Duchenne's muscular dystrophy. N Engl J Med 1988;319:15.

306. Echardt VF, Nix W, Kraus W, Bohl J. Esophageal motor function in patients with muscular dystrophy. Gastroenterology 1986;90:628.

307. Lemieux B, Scott H. Functional abnormalities of the anal sphincters in patients with myotonic dystrophy. Gastroenterology 1984;86:1469.

308. Nowak TV, Anuras S, Brown BP, et al. Small intestinal motility in myotonic dystrophy patients. Gastroenterology 1984;86:808.

309. Eckardt VF, Nix W. The anal sphincter in patients with myotonic muscular dystrophy. Gastroenterology 1991;100:424.

310. Dabaghi RE, Scott LD. Intestinal pseudo-obstruction in a patient with myotonic dystrophy. Tex Med 1986;82:42.

311. Duranceau AC, Beauchamp G, Jamieson GG, Barbeau A. Oropharyngeal dysphagia and oculopharyngeal muscular dystrophy. Surg Clin North Am 1983;63:825.

312. Taillefer R, Duranceau AC. Manometric and radionuclide assessment of pharyngeal emptying before and after cricopharyngeal myotomy in patients with oculopharyngeal muscular dystrophy. J Thorac Cardiovasc Surg 1988;95:868.

313. Calne DB, Shaw DG, Speirs ASD, Stern GM. Swallowing in parkinsonism. Br J Radiol 1970;43:456.

314. Logemann JA, Blonsky ER, Boshes B. Dysphagia in parkinsonism. JAMA 1975;231:69.

315. Qualman SJ, Haupt HM, Yang P, Hamilton SR. Esophageal Lewy bodies associated with ganglion cell loss in achalasia. Gastroenterology 1984;87:848.

316. Sun WM, Read NW, Donnelly TC. Anorectal function in incontinent patients with cerebrospinal disease. Gastroenterology 1990;99:1372.

317. Glick ME, Meshkinpour H, Haldman S, et al. Colonic dysfunction in patients with spinal cord injury. Gastroenterology 1984;86:287.

318. Fealey RD, Szurnszewski JH, Merrit JL, DiMagno EP. Effect of traumatic spinal cord transection on human upper gastroin-

testinal motility and gastric emptying. Gastroenterology 1984;87:69.

319. Juler GL, Eltorai IM. The acute abdomen in spinal cord injury patients. Paraplegia 1985;23:118.

320. Sulwy MJ, Baume PE, Davis E. Stiff-man syndrome presenting with complete esophageal obstruction. Am J Dig Dis 1970;15:79.

321. Shaker R, Kupla JI, Kidder TM, et al. Manometric characteristics of cervical dysphagia in a patient with the Kearns-Sayre syndrome. Gastroenterology 1992;103:1328.

322. Li V, Hostein J, Romero NB, et al. Chronic intestinal pseudoobstruction with myopathy and ophthalmoplegia: a muscular biochemical study of a mitochondrial disorder. Dig Dig Sci 1992;36:456.

323. Camilleri M, Carbone LD, Schuffler MD. Familial enteric neuropathy with pseudoobstruction. Dig Dis Sci 1991;36:1168.

324. Kamm MA, Hoyle CH, Burleigh DE, et al. Hereditary internal anal sphincter myopathy causing proctalgia fugax and constipation. Gastroenterology 1991;100:805.

325. Vassallo M, Camilleri M, Caron BL, Low PA. Gastrointestinal motor dysfunction in acquired selective cholinergic dysautonomia associated with infectious mononucleosis. Gastroenterology 1991;100:252.

326. Bhattacharyya AK. Protein-energy malnutrition (Kwashiorkor-Marasmus syndrome): terminology, classification and evolution. World Rev Nutr Diet 1986;47:80.

327. Dani R, Penna FJ, Nogueira CE. Etiology of chronic calcifying pancreatitis in Brazil: a report of 329 consecutive cases. Int J Pancreatol 1986;1:399.

328. Roediger WE. Metabolic basis of starvation diarrhea: implications for treatment. Lancet 1986;1:1082.

329. Solomon SM, Kirby DF. The refeeding syndrome: a review. JPEN J Parenter Enteral Nutr 1990;14:90.

330. Consensus Development Conference Panel. Gastrointestinal surgery for severe obesity. Ann Intern Med 1991;115:956.

331. Larrey D, Vial T, Pauwels A, et al. Hepatitis after germander administration: another instance of herbal medicine hepatotoxicity. Ann Intern Med 1992;117:129.

332. Crowe SE, Perdue MH. Gastrointestinal food hypersensitivity: basic mechanisms of pathophysiology. Gastroenterology 1992;103:1075.

333. Memoli D, Spitzer TR, Cottler Fox M, et al. Acute esophageal stricture after bone marrow transplantation. Bone Marrow Transplant 1988;3:513.

334. Wolford JL, McDonald GB. A problem-oriented approach to intestinal and liver disease after marrow transplantation. J Clin Gastroenterol 1988;10:419.

335. Schimmelpenninck M, Zwaan F. Radiographic features of small intestinal injury in human graft-versus-host disease. Gastrointest Radiol 1982;7:29.

336. Snover DC, Weisdorf SA, Vercellotti GM, et al. A histopathologic study of gastric and small intestinal graft-versus-host disease following allogeneic bone marrow transplantation. Hum Pathol 1985;16:387.

337. Meyers WC, Harris N, Steer S, et al. Alimentary tract complications after renal transplantation. Ann Surg 1979;190:535.

338. Musola R, Franzin G, Mora R, Manfino C. Prevalence of gastroduodenal lesions in uremic patients undergoing dialysis and after renal transplantation. Gastrointest Endosc 1984;30:343.

339. Steed DL, Brown B, Reilly JJ, et al. General surgical complications in heart and heart-lung transplantation. Surgery 1985;98:739.

340. Colon R, Frazier OH, Kahan BD, et al. Complications in cardiac transplant patients requiring general surgery. Surgery 1988;103:32.

341. O'Connor NT, Mackintosh P. Transfusion associated graft versus host disease in an immunocompetent patient. J Clin Pathol 1992;45:621.

342. Herzog DB, Copeland PM. Eating disorders. N Engl J Med 1985;313:295.

343. Mitchell JE, Seim HC, Colon E, Pomeroy C. Medical complications and medical management of bulimia. Ann Intern Med 1987;107:71.

344. Waldholtz BD, Andersen AE. Gastrointestinal symptoms in anorexia nervosa: a prospective study. Gastroenterology 1990;98:415.

345. Humphries LL, Adams LJ, Eckfeldt JH, et al. Hyperamylasemia in patients with eating disorders. Ann Intern Med 1987;106:50.

346. Heigh RI, Matz J, Roberts IM, et al. Atypical eating disorder masquerading as recurrent acute pancreatitis: the value of multiple pancreatic serological markers. J Clin Gastroenterol 1990;12:78.

347. Whitehead WE, Crowell MD, Robinson JC, et al. Effects of stressful life events on bowel symptoms: subjects with irritable bowel syndrome compared with subjects without bowel dysfunction. Gut 1992;33:825.

348. Clouse RE. Anxiety and gastrointestinal illness. Psychiatr Clin North Am 1988;11:399.

349. North CS, Clouse RE, Spitznagel EL, Alpers DH. The relation of ulcerative colitis to psychiatric factors. A review of findings and methods. Am J Psychiatry 1990;147:974.

350. Muraoka M, Mine K, Matsumoto K, et al. Psychogenic vomiting: the relation between patterns of vomiting and psychiatric diagnoses. Gut 1990;31:526.

351. Weekly Clinicopathology Exercise. N Engl J Med 1984;311:108.

352. Perrin-Fayolle M. Gastroesophageal reflux and chronic respiratory disease in adults: influence and results of surgical therapy. Clin Rev Allergy 1990;8:457.

353. Kozarek RA. Complications of reflux esophagitis and their medical management. Gastroenterol Clin North Am 1990;19:713.

354. Irwin RS, Zawacki JK, Curley FJ, et al. Chronic cough as the sole presenting manifestation of gastroesophageal reflux. Am Rev Respir Dis 1989;140:1294.

355. Harper PC, Bergner A, Kaye MD. Antireflux treatment for asthma. Arch Intern Med 1987;147:56.

356. Streiter RM, Lynch JP III. Complications of the ventilated patient. Clin Chest Med 1988;9:127.

357. Shuman RB, Schuster DP, Zuckerman GR. Prophylactic therapy for stress ulcer bleeding: a reappraisal. Ann Intern Med 1987;106:562.

358. Tryba M, Zevounou F, Torok M, et al. Prevention of acute stress bleeding with sucralfate, antacids or cimetidine: a controlled study with pirenzepine as a basic medication. Am J Med 1986;79:55.

359. Heyland D, Bradley C, Mandell LA. Effect of acidified enteral feedings on gastric colonization in the critically ill patient. Crit Care Med 1992;20:1388.

360. Kussin SZ, Henry C, Navarro C, et al. Gas within the wall of the stomach: report of a case and review of the literature. Dig Dis Sci 1982;27:949.

361. Fisher RL, Taylor L, Sherlock S. Alpha-1 antitrypsin deficiency in liver disease: the extent of the problem. Gastroenterology 1976;71:646.

362. Buist AS. Alpha 1-antitrypsin deficiency—diagnosis, treatment, and control: identification of patients. Lung 1990;168(Suppl):543.

363. Brind AM, Bassendine MF, Bennett MK, James OF. Alpha 1-antitrypsin granules in the liver: always important? Q J Med 1990;76:699.

364. Esquivel CO, Marino IR, Fioravanti V, Van Thiel DH. Liver transplantation for metabolic disease of the liver. Gastroenterol Clin North Am 1988;17:167.

365. Potts RG, Zaroukian MH, Guerrero PA, Baker CD. Comparison of blue dye visualization and glucose oxidase test strip methods for detecting pulmonary aspiration of enteral feedings in intubated adults. Chest 1993;103:117.

366. Korsberg TZ, Birkett DH, Hirsch EF, The Critical Care Research Team. Nutritional outcome and pneumonia in critical care patients randomized to gastric versus jejunal tube feedings. Crit Care Med 1992;20:1377.

367. Foster LJ, Trudeau WL, Goldman AL. Bronchodilator effects on gastric acid secretion. JAMA 1979;241:2613.

368. Zentler-Munro PL. Cystic fibrosis: a gastroenterological cornucopia. Gut 1987;28:1531.

369. Wheeler WB, Colten HR. Cystic fibrosis: current approach to diagnosis and management. Pediatr Rev 1988;9:241.

370. Rubinstein S, Moss R, Lewiston N. Constipation and meconium ileus equivalent in patients with cystic fibrosis. Pediatrics 1986;78:473.

371. Dab I, Malfroot A. Gastroesophageal reflux: a primary defect in cystic fibrosis? Scand J Gastroenterol [Suppl] 1988;143:125.

372. Davis PB, Di Sant'agnese PA. Diagnosis and treatment of cystic fibrosis: an update. Chest 1984;85:802.

373. Abramson SJ, Baker DH, Amodio JB, Berdon WE. Gastrointestinal manifestations of cystic fibrosis. Semin Roentgenol 1987;22:97.

374. Park RW, Grand RJ. Gastrointestinal manifestations of cystic fibrosis: a review. Gastroenterology 1981;81:1143.

375. Shwachman H. Gastrointestinal manifestations of cystic fibrosis. Pediatr Clin North Am 1975;22:787.

376. El Ghonaimy E, Barsoum R, Soliman M, et al. Serum gastrin in chronic renal failure: morphological and physiological correlations. Nephron 1985;39:86.

377. Randall RE Jr. Hypermagnesemia in renal failure: etiology and toxic manifestations. Ann Intern Med 1974;61:73.

378. Vreman HJ, Venter C, Leegwater J, et al. Taste, smell and zinc metabolism in patients with chronic renal failure. Nephron 1980;26:163.

379. Shepherd AMM, Stewart WK, Wormsley KG. Peptic ulceration in chronic renal failure. Lancet 1973;1:1357.

380. Muto S, Asano Y, Hosoda S, Miyata M. Hypochlorhydria and hypergastrinemia and their association with gastrointestinal bleeding in young patients with chronic renal failure. Nephron 1988;50:5.

381. Paimela H, Harkonen M, Karonen SL, et al. Relation between serum group II pepsinogen concentration and the degree of Brunner's gland hyperplasia in patients with chronic renal failure. Gut 1985;26:198.

382. Cassar-Pullicino VN, Davies AM, Hubscher S, Burrows F. The nodular duodenum in chronic renal failure. Clin Radiol 1990;41:326.

383. Andriulli A, Malfi B, Recchia S, et al. Patients with chronic renal failure are not at risk of developing chronic peptic ulcers. Clin Nephrol 1985;23:245.

384. Zuckerman GR, Cornette GL, Clouse RE, Harter HR. Upper gastrointestinal bleeding in patients with chronic renal failure. Ann Intern Med 1985;102:588.

385. Blackstone MO. Angiodysplasia and gastrointestinal bleeding in chronic renal failure (letter). Ann Intern Med 1985;103:805.

386. McKinney M. Gastrointestinal angiodysplasia in chronic renal failure (letter). Ann Intern Med 1985;103:960.

387. Marcuard SP, Weinstock JV. Gastrointestinal angiodysplasia in renal failure. J Clin Gastroenterol 1988;10:482.

388. Muto S, Asano Y, Hosoda S, Miyata M. Hypochlorhydria and hypergastrinemia and their association with gastrointestinal bleeding in young patients with chronic renal failure. Nephron 1988;50:5.

389. Ala-Kaila K. Upper gastrointestinal findings in chronic renal failure. Scand J Gastroenterol 1987;22:372.

390. Bronner MH, Pate MB, Cunningham JT, Marsh WH. Estrogen-progesterone therapy for bleeding gastrointestinal telangiectasias in chronic renal failure: an uncontrolled trial. Ann Intern Med 1986;105:371.

391. Gupta TP, Weinstock JV. Duodenal pseudomelanosis associated with chronic renal failure. Gastrointest Endosc 1986;32:358.

392. West B. Pseudomelanosis duodeni. J Clin Gastroenterol 1988;10:127.

393. Gordon SJ, Miller LJ, Haeffner LJ, et al. Abnormal intestinal bile acid distribution of azotemic man: a possible role in the pathogenesis of uremic diarrhea. Gut 1976;17:58.

394. Grekas DM, Raptis S, Tourkantonis AA. Plasma secretin, pancreozymin, and somatostatin-like hormone in chronic renal failure patients. Uremia Invest 1984;8:117.

395. Bartos V, Melichar J, Erben J. The function of the exocrine pancreas in chronic renal disease. Digestion 1970;3:33.

396. Sachs EF, Hurwitz FJ, Bloch HM, Milne FJ. Pancreatic exocrine hypofunction in the wasting syndrome of end-stage renal disease. Am J Gastroenterol 1983;78:170.

397. Levitt MD, Rappoport M, Cooperhead SR. The renal clearance of amylase in renal insufficiency, acute pancreatitis and macroamylasemia. Ann Intern Med 1969;71:919.

398. Scheff RT, Zuckerman G, Harter H, et al. Diverticular disease in patients with chronic renal failure due to polycystic kidney disease. Ann Intern Med 1980;92:202.

399. Cooper MM. Metastatic calcification:an unusual cause of lower intestinal hemorrhage. NY State J Med 1988;88:389.

400. Rodriguez HJ, Walls J, Slatopolsky E. Recurrent ascites following peritoneal dialysis. Arch Intern Med 1974;124:283.

401. Arismendi GS, Izard MW, Hampton WR, Maher JF. The clinical spectrum of ascites associated with maintenance dialysis. Am J Med 1976;60:46.

402. Yen MC, Stewart EE. Peritoneo-venous shunt for ascites associated with maintenance dialysis. Clin Nephrol 1977;8:446.

403. Seaworth B, Drucker J, Starling J, et al. Hepatitis B vaccines in patients with chronic renal failure before dialysis. J Infect Dis 1988;157:332.

404. Miller FH, Fisher MR, Soper W, Gore RM. MRI of hepatic iron deposition in patients with renal transplant. Gastrointest Radiol 1991;16:229.

405. Keshavarzian A, Iber FL, Ferguson J. Esophageal manometry and radionuclide emptying in chronic alcoholism. Gastroenterology 1987;92:651.

406. Burbige EJ, Lewis R Jr, Halsted CH. Alcohol and the gastrointestinal tract. Med Clin North Am 1984;68:77.

407. Malagelada JR. The pathophysiology of alcoholic pancreatitis. Pancreas 1986;1:270.

408. Singh M, Simsek H. Ethanol and the pancreas. Gastroenterology 1990;98:1051.

409. Alcohol, alcoholism and alcoholic liver disease. Semin Liver Dis 1988;8:1.

410. Driver HE, Swann PF. Alcohol and human cancer. Anticancer Res 1987;7:309.

411. Kikendall JW, Bowen PE, Burgess MB, et al. Cigarettes and alcohol as independent risk factors for colonic adenomas. Gastroenterology 1989;97:660.

412. Cope GF, Wyatt JI, Pinder IF, et al. Alcohol consumption in patients with colorectal adenomatous polyps. Gut 1991;32:70.

413. Mody CK, Miller BL, McIntyre HB, et al. Neurological complications of cocaine abuse. Neurology 1988;38:1189.

414. Yang RD, Han MW, McCarthy JH. Ischemic colitis in a crack abuser. Dig Dis Sci 1991;36:238.

415. Wanless IR, Dore S, Gopinath N, et al. Histopathology of cocaine hepatotoxicity: report of four patients. Gastroenterology 1990;98:497.

416. Sherman A, Zingler B. Successful endoscopic retrieval of a cocaine packet from the stomach. Gastrointest Endosc 1990;36:152.

417. Robison JC, Gitlin N, Morrelli HF, Mann LJ. Factitious hyperamylasuria. N Engl J Med 1982;306:1211.

418. Blank RR, Ream NW, Deleese JS. Infectious complications of illicit drug use. Int J Addict 1984;19:221.

419. Fielding JE. Smoking: health effects and control. N Engl J Med 1985;313:491.

420. Sutherland LR, Ramcharan S, Bryant H, Fick G. Effect of cigarette smoking on recurrence of Crohn's disease. Gastroenterology 1990;98:1123.

421. Griffin JW Jr, Harrison HB, Tedesco FJ, Mills LR IV. Behcet's disease with multiple sites of gastrointestinal involvement. South Med J 1982;75:1405.

422. Wilkey D, Yocum DE, Oberley TD. Budd-Chiari syndrome and renal failure in Behcet's disease: report of a case and review of the literature. Am J Med 1983;74:54.

423. Arbesfeld SJ, Kurban AK. Behcet's disease: new perspectives on an enigmatic syndrome. J Am Acad Dermatol 1988;19:767.

424. Anti M, Marra G, Rapaccini GL, et al. Esophageal involvement in Behcet's syndrome. J Clin Gastroenterol 1986;8:514.

425. Brookes GB. Pharyngeal stenosis in Behcet's syndrome: the first reported case. Arch Otolaryngol 1983;109:338.

426. Anti M, Marra G, Rapaccini GL, Fedeli G. Ulcerative esophagitis

in Behcet's syndrome (letter). Gastrointest Endosc 1985;31: 289.

427. Powderly WG, Lombard MG, Murray FE, et al. Oesophageal ulceration in Behcet's disease presenting with haemorrhage. Ir J Med Sci 1987;156:193.

428. Johnson DA, Everhart CW. Colitis in Behcet's syndrome (letter). Gastrointest Endosc 1986;32:58.

429. Stringer DA, Cleghorn GJ, Durie PR, et al. Behcet's syndrome involving the gastrointestinal tract: a diagnostic dilemma in childhood. Pediatr Radiol 1986;16:131.

430. Harre RG, Conrad GR, Seabold JE. Colonic localization of indium-111 labeled leukocytes in active Behcet's disease. Clin Nucl Med 1988;13:459.

431. Morita T, Kamimura A, Koizumi F. Disseminated visceral giant cell arteritis. Acta Pathol Jpn 1987;37:863.

432. Lie JT. Disseminated visceral giant cell arteritis: histopathologic description and differentiation from other granulomatous vasculitides. J Clin Pathol 1978;69:209.

433. Klein GL, Stafford S III. Unusual gastrointestinal manifestations of Henoch-Schonlein purpura. Am J Dis Child 1975;129: 1238.

434. Goldman LP, Lindenberg RL. Henoch-Schonlein purpura: gastrointestinal manifestations with endoscopic correlation. Am J Gastroenterol 1981;75:357.

435. Novy SB, Weaver RM, Jensen KM, O'Donnell WW. Henoch-Schonlein purpura of the colon: an unusual gastrointestinal manifestation. South Med J 1977;70:884.

436. Glasier CM, Siegel MJ, McAlister WH, Shackelford GD. Henoch-Schonlein syndrome in children: gastrointestinal manifestations. AJR 1981;136:1081.

437. Black MM. Malignant atrophic papulosis (Degos' disease). Int J Dermatol 1976;15:405.

438. Barlow RJ, Heyl T, Simson IW, Schulz EJ. Malignant atrophic

papulosis (Degos' disease): diffuse involvement of brain and bowel in an African patient. Br J Dermatol 1988;118:117.

439. Boyer TD, Jong MJ, Rakela J, Reynolds TB. Immunologic studies and clinical follow-up of HB Ag-positive polyarteritis nodosa. Am J Dig Dis 1977;22:497.

440. Harvey MH, Neoptolemos JP, Fossard DP. Abdominal polyarteritis nodosa: a possible surgical pitfall? Br J Clin Pract 1984;38:282.

441. Guillevin L, Le THD, Godeau P, et al. Clinical findings and prognosis of polyarteritis nodosa and Churg-Strauss angiitis: a study in 165 patients. Br J Rheumatol 1988;27:258.

442. Roikjaer O. Perforation and necrosis of the colon complicating polyarteritis nodosa: case report. Acta Chir Scand 1987;153: 385.

443. Lee EL, Smith HJ, Miller GL III, et al. Ischemic pseudomembranous colitis with perforation due to polyarteritis nodosa. Am J Gastroenterol 1984;79:35.

444. Buffo GC, Deitch JS. Pneumatosis intestinalis in a patient with polyarteritis nodosa. Gastrointest Radiol 1986;11:286.

445. Fauci AS, Katz P, Haynes BF, Wolff SM. Cyclophosphamide therapy of severe systemic necrotizing vasculitis. N Engl J Med 1979;301:235.

446. Godman GC, Churg J. Wegener's granulomatosis: pathology and review of the literature. Arch Pathol 1954;58:533.

447. Coward RA, Gibbons CP, Brown CB, et al. Gastrointestinal haemorrhage complicating Wegener's granulomatosis. Br Med J [Clin Res] 1985;291:865.

448. Kallenberg CG, Mulder AH, Tervaert JW. Antineutrophil cytoplasmic antibodies: a still-growing class of autoantibodies in inflammatory disorders. Am J Med 1992;93:675.

449. Baxter R, Nino-Murcia M, Bloom RJ, Kosek J. Gastrointestinal manifestations of essential mixed cryoglobulinemia. Gastrointest Radiol 1988;13:160.

Textbook of Gastroenterology, second edition, edited by Tadataka Yamada. JB Lippincott Company, Philadelphia © 1995.

CHAPTER 110

Gastrointestinal Manifestations of Immunologic Disorders

Stephan R. Targan   Fergus Shanahan

Immunodeficiency Diseases and the Gut
Classification of Immunodeficiency Disorders
   B-Lymphocyte (Antibody) Defects
   Predominantly T-Lymphocyte Defects
   Combined B- and T-Lymphocyte Defects
   Phagocytic Cell Defects
   Complement Deficiency

Immunodeficiency Secondary to Gut Disease
   Protein-Losing Enteropathy and Intestinal Lymphangiectasia
   Other Secondary Immunodeficiency States of
      Gastroenterologic Importance
Food Allergy (Hypersensitivity)
   Classification and Terminology

(continued)

IMMUNODEFICIENCY DISEASES AND THE GUT

The mucosal surface of the gastrointestinal tract is one of the principal sites where the host interacts with the environment. The surface area of the small intestine alone is equivalent to that of a tennis court, and only a single layer of intestinal epithelial cells separates the external environment from the internal milieu. Throughout life, the gastrointestinal mucosa of the healthy host is challenged repeatedly with potential environmental pathogens. In children, acute gastrointestinal infections account for approximately 5 million deaths worldwide annually.[1] It is therefore not surprising that the gut is one of the major target organs for opportunistic infections in immunodeficiency states.

Mucosal defense mechanisms include a precisely regulated mucosal immune system supported by a variety of nonimmunologic protective factors, such as gastric acidity, digestive enzymes, peristalsis, mucus secretion, and the mutually competitive interactions of the gut flora. The spectrum of gastrointestinal infections seen in patients with the acquired immunodeficiency syndrome is testimony to the critical role played by the mucosal immune system in host defense against the myriad potentially pathogenic organisms in our environment. Patients with milder, more selective forms of immunodeficiency (e.g., IgA deficiency), however, are frequently free of infectious complications. The nonimmunologic mucosal defenses, in addition to the overlapping functional reserves of the immune system, probably account for the resistance of these patients to infection.

CLASSIFICATION OF IMMUNODEFICIENCY DISORDERS

Immunodeficiency disorders are categorized into two major groups, primary and secondary. The primary immune deficiency disorders may be congenital or acquired and result from intrinsic defects in the cellular components of the immune system or their secretory products. The fundamental defect in most of these disorders has not been identified, although in many cases there appears to be a specific metabolic defect or a disorder of gene regulation.[2,3] The World Health Organization classification of primary immunodeficiency diseases lists 24 separate conditions, some of which are so rare that only a few cases have been described.[4] Those that are of particular gastroenterologic importance are discussed in the

following sections. For convenience, this heterogeneous group of conditions is discussed under the following headings: predominantly B-cell (antibody) defects, predominantly T-cell defects, combined B- and T-cell defects, phagocytic cell defects, and complement deficiency. Because of the functional and regulatory interactions between T and B cells, however, all such classifications are artificial.

Secondary immunodeficiencies are far more common than the primary disorders. Causes include protein-calorie malnutrition, protein-losing enteropathy, cancer, immune senescence with aging, and the increasingly recognized iatrogenic immunodeficiencies associated with organ transplantation and immunosuppressive agents. The most important secondary immunodeficiency disorder is the acquired immunodeficiency syndrome, which is discussed separately in Chapter 105.

B-Lymphocyte (Antibody) Defects

X-Linked (Congenital or Burton's) Hypogammaglobulinemia

This is considered the prototypic disorder for assessing the significance of primary humoral immunodeficiency.[5] It occurs in men, although rare cases of a similar clinical syndrome have been described in women. Serum levels of all immunoglobulins are less than 200 mg/dL, and there is an inability to make functional serum antibodies. An intrinsic B-cell defect with a maturation block in pre–B-cell to B-cell differentiation is present.[2,3] The pre-B cells fail to express functional IgM on the cell surface because of an inability to rearrange immunoglobulin light-chain genes. Pre-B cells are present in bone marrow in normal numbers, but circulating B cells are absent. The thymus and T-cell functions are normal. Patients usually present with recurrent pyogenic infection during infancy (after disappearance of maternal IgG) or in early childhood. The respiratory and gastrointestinal tracts are the most frequent sites of infection.[5–7] Gastrointestinal infections, although not as dominant a clinical feature as they are in common variable hypogammaglobulinemia, occur in 30% of patients.[5] These are usually infectious diarrheal episodes commonly caused by *Campylobacter* organisms.[6,7] Giardiasis has been reported to cause severe mucosal damage and steatorrhea in these patients, but it is responsive to therapy and is surprisingly uncommon.[5–10] Perirectal abscess formation and small bowel bacterial overgrowth may also occur.[5] In asymptomatic patients, rectal biopsy characteristically reveals an absence of plasma cells and a mild lamina propria neutrophil infiltrate with early crypt abscess formation.[8] This may lead to an erroneous diagnosis of chronic colitis, which is uncommon. Although cellular immunity is normal, these patients are susceptible to certain virus infections, notably hepatitis and enterovirus.[6,10] There is an increased risk of malignancy, particularly lymphomas and leukemias.[3,6,10] Treatment is with parenteral immunoglobulin replacement.

Selective IgA Deficiency

Selective IgA deficiency is the most common primary immune deficiency, with a prevalence reported as high as 1 per 500 of the population (range, 1/500–1/3000).[10,11] Its occurrence is usually sporadic, but familial cases have been reported. Most patients lack both serum and secretory IgA_1 and IgA_2. The basic defect is not known, and there may be etiologic heterogeneity as well as clinical heterogeneity.[2,3,12] Occasionally, IgA deficiency may be transient,[10] and drugs such as phenytoin, penicillamine,[10] and sulfasalazine[13] have been reported to cause reversible deficiency.

Although IgA deficiency is associated with a wide range of conditions,[12–14] mainly recurrent infections of mucosal tissues and autoimmune disorders (Table 110-1), most IgA-deficient people are asymptomatic and free of any complicating disease.[10,11] The associations with celiac disease and pernicious anemia are well established and may in part be the result of a common linkage of IgA and such diseases with human leukocyte antigen-B8/DR3.[7,15,16] In one case study, IgA deficiency with malabsorption and villous atrophy was associated with an IgG antibody to intestinal epithelial cells and a favorable response to cyclophosphamide.

When infections occur in IgA-deficient people, they are usually recurrent bacterial and viral sinopulmonary disorders; the gastrointestinal tract is seldom involved.[16] Giardiasis has been reported in IgA-deficient subjects, but unlike in panhypogammaglobulinemia, its frequency in IgA deficiency is probably the same or minimally increased in comparison with the general population.[16,17] Persistent or recurrent infections should raise the suspicion of associated immunologic defects, such as deficiencies of IgG subclasses, particularly IgG_2 and IgG_4, which have been found in some patients with IgA deficiency.[6,18] Jejunal biopsy specimens usually are morphologically normal in selective IgA deficiency. Immunofluorescence studies reveal an absence or paucity of IgA-producing cells and an increase in IgM-secreting cells. This may be an important host compensatory response because IgM, like IgA, can bind to secretory component.

There is no specific treatment for IgA deficiency. Replacement with serum IgA is futile because only locally produced IgA is transported into the lumen. Furthermore, parenteral administration of IgA-containing blood is contraindicated because of the risk of anaphylactic reactions due to the development of anti-IgA antibodies.[3]

Secretory Component Deficiency

Secretory component is a glycoprotein receptor on the basolateral surface of the mucosal epithelial cell that is essential for the transepithelial delivery of IgA and IgM from the lamina propria to the lumen. A deficiency in secretory component affects not only lumenal IgA levels but also any compensatory effects of IgM. Such a deficiency appears to be exceptionally rare. In isolated case reports, it has been associated with intestinal candidiasis and diarrhea.[19,20] Administration of IgA-rich bovine colostrum may result in symptomatic improvement.[19]

Common Variable Hypogammaglobulinemia

Common variable hypogammaglobulinemia is second to selective IgA deficiency as the most common primary immunodeficiency in adults. It appears to be a heterogeneous group of disorders in which an intrinsic defect in terminal B-lymphocyte differentiation is present in most patients.[2,3] Although alterations in T-cell function may be found in many patients, excessive suppressor T-cell activity, which was described in earlier studies, is no longer considered to account for the hypogammaglobulinemia in most patients.[2] Most cases are sporadic, but the condition can be familial.

Clinically, common variable hypogammaglobulinemia may be similar to X-linked agammaglobulinemia, but differences include the later age of onset, less severe infections, and the fact that the lymphoid tissue (tonsils, lymph nodes, and spleen) may be normal or enlarged.[3] Patients usually present in the second or third decade of life, with either recurrent respiratory tract infections (most commonly caused by pneumococci, staphylococci, and *Hemophilus influenzae*) or diarrhea and steatorrhea (Table 110-2).[21,22] Up to 60% of patients have chronic recurrent diarrhea, and two thirds of these have malabsorption.[21] Unlike in IgA deficiency, giardiasis appears to be a particularly common cause of symptoms in the panhypogammaglobulinemia of common variable hypogammaglobulinemia; thus, IgG antibodies are important in the

---

TABLE 110-1
Disorders That May Occur in Association With IgA Deficiency

Gastrointestinal Manifestations and Associations

None (usually)

Infections, especially giardiasis (may not be any more common than in general population)

Gluten-sensitive enteropathy (IgA prevalence in celiac disease is 1:50)

Pernicious anemia

Vitamin B_{12} deficiency secondary to bacterial overgrowth

Intrinsic factor deficiency

Nodular lymphoid hyperplasia

Food allergy (increased serum antibodies to food antigens but clinical disease apparently rare)

Crohn's disease (IgA deficiency prevalence reported to be 1:73)

Disaccharidase deficiencies (unproven association)

Extraintestinal Manifestations and Associations of IgA Deficiency

Non–organ-specific autoimmune disorders (e.g., collagen vascular diseases)

Atopy

Malignancy (lymphomas, carcinoma reported but extent of risk is unclear and probably low)

Risk of anaphylaxis if given IgA-containing solutions, including blood

TABLE 110-2
Disorders That May Occur in Association With Common Variable Hypogammaglobulinemia

Gastrointesinal
Giardia lamblia infection
Small bowel bacterial overgrowth
Viral gastroenteritis (e.g., rotavirus)
Infectious diarrheas (Campylobacter, Salmonella, Shigella)
Secondary diaccharidase deficiency
Pernicious anemia, atrophic gastritis, gastric carcinoma
Gluten-senstive sprue
Sprue refractory to gluten-free diet
Nodular lymphoid hyperplasia

Extraintestinal
Increased incidence of generalized lymphomas
Increased incidence of autoimmune diseases
Recurrent respiratory tract infections

defense against this parasite.[7,10,16] In contrast to immuno-competent people, giardiasis in common variable hypogammaglobulinemia may lead to extensive mucosal damage with steatorrhea and malabsorption,[23] although it is usually reversible with appropriate anti-Giardia therapy. Other parasitic infections, such as cryptosporidiosis and strongyloidiasis, may occur but are much less common; they are the cause of as many as 0.6% to 4.3% of all diarrheal illnesses in North America.[24] Another common cause of diarrhea is infection with Campylobacter species (C jejuni and C fetus), which occasionally may mimic ulcerative colitis.[7] Isolates are usually responsive to erythromycin. Bacterial overgrowth with anaerobes has also been described,[16] although it does not appear to be an important cause of symptoms in most patients.

In some patients, a sprue-like syndrome may be found on intestinal biopsy.[6–8,10] The cause is probably multifactorial, but giardiasis should always be carefully ruled out. True gluten-sensitive enteropathy has been clearly documented in common variable hypogammaglobulinemia,[7] but most case reports of this have not been well documented. Jejunal biopsy generally shows a paucity of plasma cells in the lamina propria, in contrast to the usual lesion of sprue. When the mucosa is flat, an enteropathy refractory to a gluten-free diet is likely. The cause of this is not clear, but may include chronic viral or other infections. Other intestinal inflammatory disorders that have been reported in common variable hypogammaglobulinemia include Crohn's disease and idiopathic ulcerative jejunitis.[6,10]

In one third of patients with common variable hypogammaglobulinemia, atrophic gastritis and pernicious anemia develop, with an increased risk of gastric cancer. Differences between classic pernicious anemia and the gastric atrophy of common variable hypogammaglobulinemia include the absence of mucosal plasma cells, lack of autoantibodies, involvement of the entire gastric mucosa, and normal rather than elevated serum gastrin levels.[6,16,21] Indeed, defective gastrin release in response to bombesin or food has been found to be a highly specific means of distinguishing common variable hypogammaglobulinemia from other forms of hypogammaglobulinemia.[25]

Chronic liver disease has occurred in up to 10% to 15% of patients with common variable hypogammaglobulinemia.[6,22] In many cases, this may have been caused by a non-A, non-B hepatitis acquired from prior plasma infusion; it has not been a problem with the use of licensed intravenous immunoglobulin preparations.[22] Cholelithiasis appears to be common in common variable hypogammaglobulinemia.[21] Other potential causes of hepatobiliary disease include autoimmune hepatitis, sclerosing cholangitis, and biliary cryptosporidiosis.

Nodular lymphoid hyperplasia is a common finding in common variable hypogammaglobulinemia,[7,21] but it does not occur in X-linked hypogammaglobulinemia and is rare in selective IgA deficiency. The lymphoid nodules usually involve the small intestine, but may affect the colon, rectum, and stomach. Microscopically, the nodules consist of large lymphoid follicles with germinal centers within the lamina propria. Plasma cells are either absent or markedly diminished. The lymphoid hyperplasia is thought to reflect B cells unable to undergo full differentiation to immunoglobulin-secreting plasma cells, and therefore lacking feedback regulation of proliferation.[26] Localized forms of nodular lymphoid hyperplasia may occur in apparently immunocompetent people, particularly in the large bowel. In children and adolescents, a self-limited lymphoid hyperplasia in the terminal ileum is a frequent radiologic finding.[7] Although there is an increased incidence of lymphomas in common variable hypogammaglobulinemia,[27] intestinal nodular lymphoid hyperplasia per se does not appear to be premalignant.

Miscellaneous B-Cell Defects

A variety of other syndromes associated with immunoglobulin abnormalities have been described. Gastrointestinal manifestations may occur but seldom are a dominant component of the clinical picture. Detailed reviews are available.[2,28]

Predominantly T-Lymphocyte Defects

Congenital Thymic Hypoplasia (DiGeorge's Syndrome)

This rare syndrome results from defective formation of the third and fourth pharyngeal pouches during embryogenesis. It is characterized by absent T-lymphocyte function, hypoparathyroidism, and cardiovascular abnormalities, in particular of the aortic arch. Presentation is usually with neonatal tetany or seizures. There may be unusual facies. Other structures developing at the same stage of embryogenesis also may be affected; for example, esophageal atresia may occur. Other gastrointestinal manifestations include candidiasis, chronic diarrhea, and malabsorption.[6]

Chronic Mucocutaneous Candidiasis

Chronic mucocutaneous candidiasis represents a group of clinical syndromes in which there is an increased susceptibility to chronic *Candida* infections of the mucosa, skin, and nails. Five subtypes are recognized, which vary in their mode of inheritance (autosomal recessive and sporadic), age of onset (rarely or late), and frequency of association with endocrinopathies such as Addison's disease, diabetes mellitus, hypothyroidism,[29] and hypoparathyroidism. Oropharyngeal and esophageal candidiasis may occur. Esophageal candidiasis may be present in the absence of oral lesions and may be complicated by stricture formation. Treatment with ketoconazole is usually effective, but intravenous amphotericin may be required.[6]

Combined B- and T-Lymphocyte Defects

Severe Combined Immunodeficiency Syndromes

Severe combined immunodeficiency represents a group of syndromes with distinct underlying defects characterized by profound deficiency of T- and B-lymphocyte function.[2,3,28] The pattern of inheritance may be X-linked recessive or autosomal recessive. In approximately one third of patients, the fundamental defect is an autosomal recessively inherited adenosine deaminase deficiency. In other patients, there is defective expression of major histocompatibility complex (MHC) antigens, either MHC class I or both MHC class I and class II antigens. Another variant of severe combined immunodeficiency is reticular dysgenesis, in which there is a coexisting deficiency of granulocytes. Clinically, the syndrome presents in early infancy with severe, life-threatening infections, chronic diarrhea, malabsorption, and failure to thrive. Graft-versus-host disease due to transplacentally acquired maternal lymphocytes may occur during the neonatal period. There is increased susceptibility to virus infections, including cytomegalovirus, and chronic rotavirus infection may account for the intractable diarrhea in some patients. Jejunal biopsy reveals absent plasma cells, and in some cases there is partial villous atrophy with numerous periodic acid–Schiff-positive macrophages in the lamina propria.[30] Without a bone marrow graft, the clinical course is rapidly fatal. In those cases with adenosine deaminase deficiency, enzyme replacement with irradiated erythrocytes is possible, and gene therapy may be a future possibility.[31]

Wiskott-Aldrich Syndrome

Wiskott-Aldrich syndrome is an X-linked recessive condition characterized by eczema, thrombocytopenia, and recurrent infections. There is progressive defect in T-cell function and a poor antibody response to polysaccharide antigens. Atopy with elevated IgE levels is common. Gastrointestinal manifestations include hemorrhage and chronic diarrhea. Malabsorption and nonspecific colitis may also occur. Without treatment, patients succumb to hemorrhage or the development of malignant lymphoma. Bone marrow transplantation is the treatment of choice.

Ataxia-Telangiectasia

Ataxia-telangiectasia is an autosomal recessive, multisystem disorder. There are defective DNA repair mechanisms, frequent chromosomal abnormalities, and increased sensitivity to ionizing radiation. The chromosomal location of the genetic defect responsible for this syndrome has been identified,[32] and a common molecular mechanism to link the various clinical manifestations has been proposed.[33] The most prominent clinical features are progressive cerebellar ataxia, oculocutaneous telangiectasia, chronic recurrent sinopulmonary infections, and a high incidence of malignancy. The immunodeficiency is variable and affects both cellular and humoral elements. IgA deficiency occurs in over 50% of patients and may be associated with IgG$_2$ subclass deficiency.[34] Malignancies are the most common cause of death in this condition. They usually are lymphoreticular, but adenocarcinomas may also occur. Other than malignancy, gastrointestinal complications are not common in ataxia-telangiectasia.[6] Mild abnormalities of liver function test results may be noted, and levels of α-fetoprotein are elevated.

Phagocytic Cell Defects

Intrinsic defects in neutrophils, monocytes, and macrophages include several disorders of cell locomotion, chemotaxis, killing, and metabolism.[35] Numerically, the most important and the most frequently encountered in gastroenterologic practice is chronic granulomatous disease.

Chronic Granulomatous Disease

Chronic granulomatous disease represents a group of disorders of phagocytic cell oxidative metabolism. There are several variants of the basic biochemical defect in oxidase function and more than one mode of genetic transmission.[36–38] In its classic form, inheritance is X-linked, but, more rarely, chronic granulomatous disease may be transmitted in an autosomal recessive or dominant pattern. The respiratory burst associated with stimulation of phagocytes is lacking. This results in defective microbicidal activity because of the failure to generate toxic oxygen metabolites such as hydroxyl radical and hydrogen peroxide. There is a markedly increased susceptibility to pyogenic and fungal infections. Common pathogenic organisms include staphylococci, *Serratia marcescens*, *Salmonella* species, and gram-negative enterococci. Fungal infections include *Candida* and *Aspergillus* species. There is particular susceptibility to infections with catalase-positive organisms. In such organisms, the catalase destroys the hydrogen peroxide produced by the organism. In contrast, catalase-negative organisms such as pneumococci, streptococci, and lactobacilli are not major pathogens in chronic granulomatous disease because they do not destroy their endogenous hydrogen peroxide, and thereby contribute to their own demise.[35]

The condition classically presents during infancy, although variants of the disease may present later. Every organ is vulnerable to infection, and the granulomas associated with this condition occur throughout the body.[37] Their formation is not well understood. They consist of plasma cells, lymphocytes, macrophages, and occasional multinucleated giant cells. Organisms usually are not found in these granulomas. A second type of granuloma may occur in association with fungal infections, in which hyphal elements are found in giant cells. An additional histologic feature of chronic granulomatous disease is the presence of pigmented, lipid-bearing tissue histiocytes.[39]

Hepatic and gastrointestinal disorders are a prominent feature of chronic granulomatous disease. Hepatomegaly is very common, with liver abscess formation occurring in over 30% of patients.[37] This frequently requires surgery and may be recurrent in some patients. *Staphylococcus aureus* is the most common culprit.

Gastrointestinal presentations of chronic granulomatous disease may mimic Crohn's disease. Common gastrointestinal problems include chronic gingivitis and stomatitis, perianal abscesses with fistulas, *Salmonella* gastroenteritis, diarrhea, and malabsorption.[36,37,39,40] The granulomas and pigmented histiocytes are characteristic and may be found in patients with no gastrointestinal symptoms. In some patients, the granulomatous reaction leads to stricture formation, which most commonly occurs in the gastric antrum. Although surgical treatment may be required, resolution of strictures after antibiotic therapy is well known, and aggressive antimicrobial therapy is the treatment of first choice.[41]

Complement Deficiency

Deficiency states involving the individual complement proteins are rare. In general, they are associated with a high incidence of infectious and autoimmune disorders.[42] Deficiency of C1 esterase inhibitor is the most common complement deficiency state and also the only one in which gastrointestinal symptoms are a prominent feature. A possible exception to this exclusive status is the implication of a defective C5a inhibitor protein in serosal fluid in patients with familial Mediterranean fever.[43]

Hereditary Angioedema (C1 Esterase Inhibitor Deficiency)

Hereditary angioedema is an autosomal dominant disorder caused by either a quantitative or qualitative deficiency of a regulatory inhibitor of the activated first component of complement. Clinically, it is characterized by recurrent, self-limited attacks of circumscribed, nonpitting, subepithelial edema in the skin and mucous membranes.[44] The skin lesions are painless, and, unlike in urticaria, pruritus is absent. The onset of symptoms is variable, although most patients have their first episode in childhood. A positive family history is common but not always present. Attacks may develop over hours and may last from hours to several days. They are often precipitated by minor local trauma, dental extractions, infections, and surgery. There is frequently an initial awareness of a tingling sensation in the affected area, and a faint macular or serpiginous erythema may precede the swelling. The most serious manifestation is laryngeal edema, which may lead to fatal airway obstruction. Gastrointestinal involvement is common and includes colicky abdominal pain, vomiting, and watery diarrhea. Significant intestinal fluid loss can occur and can lead to hypotension and shock. Fever and leukocytosis are notably absent. The abdomen may be tender but not rigid. Bowel sounds may be increased. Barium studies during an attack may show the "stacked coin" appearance of mucosal edema. The lesions consist primarily of circumscribed edema without inflammatory cellular infiltrates. The edematous segment of bowel can cause intussusception. When gastrointestinal symptoms precede other manifestations, or occur in isolation, the diagnosis is often delayed, and many of these patients have been subjected to unnecessary abdominal surgery.[45]

The underlying biochemical defect in hereditary angioedema exists in two forms.[46] In 85% of patients, the levels of C1 esterase inhibitor (C1-INH) are low. In the remaining 15%, the levels are normal or increased, but the inhibitor protein is functionally defective. Acquired forms of C1-INH deficiency that are clinically similar to the hereditary disorder also have been described, particularly in patients with lymphoproliferative disorders and collagen vascular diseases. The pathogenesis of angioedema is not fully understood, but the increased vascular permeability is thought to be mediated by kinins. C1-INH not only prevents autoactivation of C1 but inhibits activated Hageman factor and kallikrein. The diagnosis is confirmed by quantitative and qualitative analysis of C1-INH. In addition, levels of C4 are secondarily reduced between attacks and nearly absent during attacks. Anabolic steroids with attenuated androgenic effects, such as danazol and stanozolol, are effective in preventing attacks.

IMMUNODEFICIENCY SECONDARY TO GUT DISEASE

Protein-Losing Enteropathy and Intestinal Lymphangiectasia

Immunodeficiency due to protein loss may be a component of any severe inflammatory condition in the gastrointestinal tract; examples include protein-losing gastropathy (Menetrier's disease) and extensive Crohn's disease. The more severe cases of gastrointestinal protein loss, however, occur in the setting of primary lymphangiectasia or secondary lymphatic obstruction. Gastrointestinal protein loss is most conveniently demonstrated with the use of chromium 51-labeled albumin clearance or by measurement of stool levels of α_1-antitrypsin, which is a sensitive index of protein loss. Protein loss from the gut is nonselective, and an important diagnostic point is that hypogammaglobulinemia is always accompanied by hypoalbuminemia. The serum IgG level is usually the most severely reduced, whereas levels of IgA and IgM may be well maintained; this is because of the slower synthetic rate of IgG. The hypogammaglobulinemia is rarely severe enough to be of clinical significance. When protein loss is the result of lymphatic disorders, however, it is associated with loss of lymphocytes, particularly T cells, in addition to immunoglobulins. The resulting lymphopenia is frequently associated with skin test anergy and, rarely, with increased susceptibility to infection.[47]

Other Secondary Immunodeficiency States of Gastroenterologic Importance

Protein-calorie malnutrition leads to significant depression of cell-mediated immune function. This also may occur in association with malignancy, particularly lymphoreticular tumors. Iatrogenic immunosuppression is an increasingly common cause of secondary immunodeficiency. An example is the occurrence of reversible IgA deficiency with sulfasalazine[13] and other drugs such as penicillamine and phenytoin.[10] The increased susceptibility to *Candida* organisms and other infectious agents with corticosteroid use is well known, but corticosteroid use also is the most common cause of superinfection with *Strongyloides stercoralis*.[48] Immunosuppression in patients undergoing organ transplantation is discussed in Intestinal Manifestations of Graft-Versus-Host Disease.

FOOD ALLERGY (HYPERSENSITIVITY)

Increasing public perception of potential adverse reactions to foods and food additives in today's health-conscious society requires that physicians have a clear understanding of the true significance of food allergies. Although immunologic hypersensitivity to foodstuffs was clearly demonstrated in the 1920s and 1930s by Prausnitz and Kustner and by Brunner and Walzer, the issue of food allergy has been shrouded in controversy.[49] Misconceptions and wildly inaccurate accounts of the spectrum of food allergy in the popular press have been matched by prejudice and skepticism in the minds of some physicians who view the issue at the level of food faddism and quackery. Much confusion surrounding the subject has been created by the failure of some authors to use appropriate terminology distinguishing food allergy from other forms of adverse food reaction, and to use a methodic, objective, and unbiased approach to the investigation of potential adverse reactions to foods. Fortunately, in the 1980s, the development of several scientifically sound experimental approaches advanced our understanding of the pathogenesis of food allergy and improved diagnostic management of the problem. Reviews and recommendations by the American Academy of Allergy and National Institutes of Health[50] have clarified and standardized terminology regarding adverse reactions of foods.

Classification and Terminology

Adverse reactions to foods may be separated into two broad categories, depending on whether the immune system contributes to the abnormal reaction (Table 110-3). The terms "food allergy" and "food hypersensitivity" may be used interchangeably, but should be reserved for those reactions that have been shown to be mediated by the immune system. Food intolerance is a term that should be used to describe nonimmunologically mediated adverse reactions to food or food additives. Nonimmunologically mediated adverse reactions may closely mimic acute allergic reactions. In addition, some foods may produce adverse reactions by multiple mechanisms in different people. For example, adverse reactions to milk are common and include allergic reactions to milk proteins and, rarely, to contaminant antibiotics, or they may result from lactose intolerance or fat intolerance.

Prevalence

Food allergies, although a definite clinical entity, are uncommon.[49-51] Community surveys indicate that 20% to 40% of adults believe that they have an adverse reaction to some

TABLE 110-3
Differential Diagnosis of Adverse Reactions to Foods*

Immunologically Mediated
Early: IgE mediated
Delayed: Late-phase reactions, immune complex–mediated or cell-mediated immunity (e.g., celiac disease, most cases of cow's milk allergy)

Non–Immunologially Mediated
Idiosyncratic
    Gastrointestinal (e.g., lactase deficiency)
    Systemic (e.g., glucose 6-phosphate-dehydrogenase deficiency)
Pharmacologic (e.g., caffeine, tyramine, serotonin, alcohol, histamine)
Toxic (e.g., aflatoxins, botulism, mushroom toxins)
Infectious (e.g., salmonellosis)
Other contaminants and additives
    Antibiotics, pesticides
    Dyes (e.g., tartrazine)
    Flavorings and preservatives (e.g., monosidum glutamate [Chinese restaurant syndrome], sulfites, benzoate, nitrites, and nitrates)
Gastrointestinal disorders (e.g., peptic ulcer, cholelithiasis)
Psychological (e.g., phobias, distaste, food pseudoallergy)

* This list is intended to be representative and is not comprehensive.

food.[52] When tested objectively, using double-blinded food challenges, most complaints of possible adverse reactions to foods cannot be reproduced.[53,54] Most adverse reactions to food are probably not immunologically mediated. The prevalence of true food allergy is not known but has been estimated to be in the range of 0.3% to 7.5% of children.[55] It is more common in atopic individuals and declines with age. In adults, it is a well documented entity,[56] but is uncommon.

Immune Response to Dietary Antigens

Despite the presence of multiple immunologic and nonimmunologic defense mechanisms, small amounts of antigenic macromolecules can penetrate the gastrointestinal "mucosal barrier" and reach the systemic circulation under normal circumstances. This occurs to a greater degree in early life and in conditions causing disruption of the mucosal defenses. Uptake of antigenic material and presentation to the mucosal immune system may occur by three routes. First, the specialized microfold or M cells that overlie lymphoid follicles are adapted to sampling lumenal antigens and presenting them to the immune system. Second, the nonspecialized or surface enterocytes lining the intestine are also capable of presenting antigens, and can selectively stimulate suppressor T cells.[57] Although it remains to be conclusively shown that the enterocyte is capable of uptake and processing of antigens, the preferential stimulation of suppressor cells could be an important mechanism in preventing hypersensitivity reactions to dietary antigens. Finally, antigens that gain entry by a paracellular route can be presented to the mucosal immune system by macrophages and dendritic cells in the intestinal lamina propria.

When dietary antigen engages the immune system, there may be a local secretory IgA antibody response, but a systemic immune response rarely occurs. Most commonly, a state of immunologic tolerance develops. Oral tolerance (sometimes termed the Sulberger-Chase phenomenon) is a state of specific immunologic unresponsiveness that occurs after oral ingestion of antigen. The phenomenon is an important homeostatic mechanism regulating immune response to dietary antigens.[58] It has been known for over a century and has been reproduced and extensively investigated in laboratory animals. The immune responses that are most easily suppressed or tolerated by feeding proteins are IgE-mediated and delayed-type hypersensitivity responses. Not surprisingly, these are the major immunologic reactions mediating food allergy. Stated differently, food allergy–hypersensitivity represents a breakdown in oral tolerance. Mechanisms responsible for the induction and maintenance of oral tolerance are not fully understood, but include the actions of suppressor T cells. The liver may also play a role in down-regulating systemic immune responses to dietary antigens.[52,58]

Food Allergens

Most food hypersensitivity reactions are caused by a relatively small number of foods. Most commonly implicated are milk, eggs, nuts, fish, shellfish, soybeans, and wheat. For several of these foods, the specific allergen has been isolated and characterized. Many food allergens are heat and acid stable, are resistant to proteolysis, and most have a relatively low molecular weight (10–70 kd). Their immunogenicity may therefore be retained with food processing and digestion, and they have the appropriate size for bridging IgE on the surface of mast cells.[52,59]

Pathogenesis

There are two major categories of food allergic or hypersensitivity reaction: *immediate* (IgE-mediated, type I hypersensitivity: and *delayed* (late-phase IgE-mediated, immune complex-mediated, and cell-mediated). Immediate or IgE-mediated hypersensitivity reactions are focused on because they account for most immunologically mediated adverse reactions to foods. Delayed-type hypersensitivity is involved in the pathogenesis of gluten-sensitive enteropathy (discussed in Chapter 72).

The wheal and flare reaction that occurs in some people after intradermal injection of a food allergen is caused by the presence of food-specific IgE antibodies on the surface of cutaneous mast cells; adjacent IgE molecules are crossed-linked by the allergen and trigger degranulation of the mast cell. Experiments performed in the 1920s showed that this phenomenon could be passively transferred.[52,60] Thus, when otherwise healthy subjects were injected with serum from fish-sensitive patients, they manifested wheal and flare reactions at the injection site on ingestion of fish. In addition to demonstrating the passive transfer of a serum-sensitizing factor (now known to be IgE), these classic experiments also showed that in most healthy subjects, such antigens can reach and trigger mast cells at extragastrointestinal sites.[60] Similar re-

actions have been described in human ileal and colonic mucosa after passive sensitization followed by ingestion or direct application of the antigen.[52]

The central role of mast cell degranulation in the pathogenesis of food allergy is supported by the fact that plasma levels of histamine rise significantly in patients with cutaneous, gastrointestinal, and respiratory symptoms elicited by double-blinded, placebo-controlled food challenge, but not in patients with negative food challenges.[61,62] Evidence suggests that, in addition to having IgE to specific foods on the mast cell surface, some patients with food-induced symptoms may also produce a histamine-releasing factor spontaneously in their mononuclear cells.[63] Mast cells are abundant in the gut and are present at every level and in every layer of the gut wall (Fig. 110-1).[64] In the mucosa they require special fixation and staining procedures for identification. Extensive evidence suggests that mucosal mast cells are cytochemically and functionally distinct from their counterparts in nonmucosal tissues.[65] This may have implications for the management of food allergic reactions because intestinal mucosal mast cells are not responsive to the actions of certain antiallergic agents.[65]

Clinical Manifestations

Symptoms usually occur within minutes of ingestion but may be delayed several hours. Systemic anaphylaxis is the most serious manifestation of food hypersensitivity and may be the

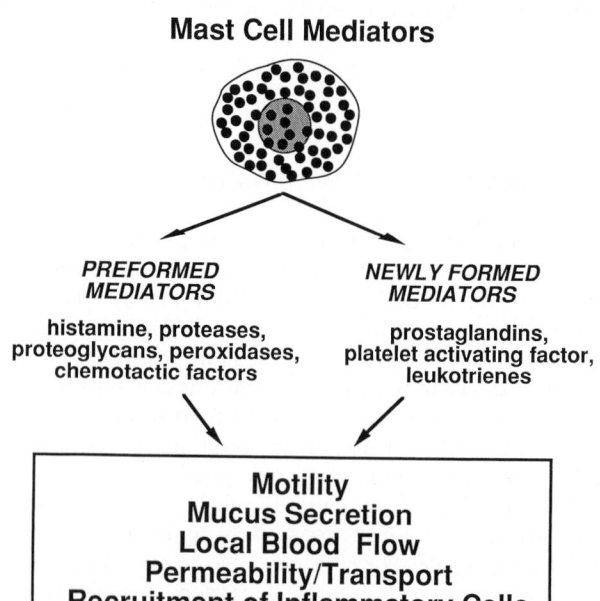

FIGURE 110-1. Mast cell mediators and potential consequences of their release. Mediator release is triggered when adjacent IgE antibodies on the surface of the mast cell are bridged by binding to an allergen. Mast cell secretion may also be stimulated by a variety of other endogenous and exogenous factors, including activated complement components (C3a and C5a), neuropeptides, bee venom, polymyxin, ionomycin, and opiates.

first presentation. Cofactors such as aspirin ingestion or exercise may have a profound effect on the clinical expression of food hypersensitivity. Postprandial, exercise-induced systemic anaphylaxis has been well documented. More common, a variety of less severe and usually transient symptoms may be experienced. The organs primarily affected are the skin (eczema, urticaria), the respiratory tract (rhinitis, asthma), and the gut.[52,64,66]

Evaluation of the Patient With Suspected Food Allergy

General Remarks

Only a small number of adult patients referred with a supposed food allergy can be demonstrated to have a reproducible, immunologically mediated adverse reaction to food. A careful and objective assessment is important not only to detect preventable disease in such patients but to offset inappropriate and potentially harmful dietary restriction in others. Although the differential diagnosis of food-related symptoms is broad (see Table 110-3), a detailed history and physical examination often indicate the correct diagnostic category to pursue. The most definitive criteria for the diagnosis of food allergy are: the demonstration that ingestion of the implicated food can reproducibly induce the patient's symptoms; and evidence that an immunologic mechanism is involved. A generalized set of diagnostic guidelines is provided in Table 110-4. In practice, however, the diagnostic approach should be individualized, and the rigor with which the clinician attempts to prove the diagnosis is influenced by several factors, such as the age of the patient, the nature and nutritional importance of the food implicated, the likely reliability of the patient's history and compliance with challenge test protocols, and the severity of the symptoms. For example, patients who are thought to be allergic to several major food groups require an accurate confirmation of the diagnosis because of the inconvenience and potential danger of malnutrition with prolonged, complicated restriction diets. In contrast, patients with only episodic symptoms triggered by uncommonly encountered or nonessential foods should be instructed to avoid such foods and do not require rigorous food challenges. For reliable patients with a clear history of objectively verifiable symptoms and signs, an open challenge may suffice. The greatest difficulty is posed by the patient with vague or subjective complaints, self-diagnosed as an adverse reaction to food. In adults, and in particular the nonatopic person, the likelihood of such symptoms being the result of food allergy is very small. Prolonged investigative evaluation beyond simple screening tests may not be appropriate or desirable for these patients.

TABLE 110-4
General Guidelines to Investigation of Adult Patients With Suspected Food Allergy

---

History of Severe Reaction or Anaphylaxis
1. Avoid implicated food
2. Do not attempt a skin test or a food challenge
3. Use in vitro test (e.g., RAST)

Less Severe Reactions With Specific Food(s) Implicated by History
1. Skin test (prick/puncture technique with fresh food or commercial extract is available)

If skin test is positive:	If skin test is negative:
2a. Elimate implicated food(s) temporarily, then perform open challenge	2b. Immediate hypersensitivity is very unlikely, but if the history is impressive, consider temporary elimination of implicated food(s) followed by open challenge
If open* challenge is negative:	If open* challenge is positive:
3a. No food restriction; observe and repeat challenge if symptoms recur	3b. Same as in 3a
If open challenge is positive:	If open challenge is positive:
4a. Eliminate guilty food, but perform double-blind, placebo-controlled oral food challenge if several foods of nutritional importance are involved or if symptoms or signs are not objectively verifiable	4b. Perform double-blind gel placebo-controlled oral food challenge

Food Allergy Claimed, But No Specific Foods or Multiple Foods Are Implicated
1. Reassess full clinical picture and consider nonimmunologic causes for symptoms (see Table 108-1)
2. If history is impressive, perform skin tests for commonly encountered foods and instruct patient to keep a food diary
3. Temporary elimination diet if specific food(s) are implicated by skin tests or diary, then proceed as in 2a
4. If specific food(s) are still not implicated and symptoms persist, consider systematic, temporary elimination diet
5. If specific food(s) are implicated, proceed as in 2a
6. If symptoms persist and specific food(s) are not implicated after systematic elimination diets, consider once again nonimmunologic causes, including a psychogenic orgin

---

* Depending on the nature of the food and the ease with which it can be camouflaged in other food preparations, a single-blinded challenge may be performed in preference to open challenge.

RAST, radioallergosorbent test.

Food challenges and skin testing with food antigens can trigger potentially serious and even fatal anaphylaxis in a small percentage of patients. Such diagnostic tests should be carried out only by experienced physicians and should be attempted only in a facility equipped to deal with serious allergic reactions.

Test Procedures

Skin tests and in vitro assays.

Little is known about delayed-type hypersensitivity reactions to food. In vitro tests for cellular immunity to food antigens and assays for food antigen-antibody complexes are under investigation and are not recommended for routine diagnostic use. For practical purposes, the demonstration that an adverse reaction to food is immunologically mediated involves the demonstration of IgE antibodies that have specificity for the implicated food allergen. Direct skin testing with the prick technique with food extract and control solution is a simple and sensitive method of detecting specific mast-cell–bound IgE antibodies.[67] If properly performed, a negative skin test means that immediate hypersensitivity to the food tested is highly unlikely. A positive test (wheal >3 mm larger in diameter than the diluent control wheal), however, merely indicates the presence of sensitizing antibodies and not necessarily the presence of clinical food hypersensitivity, which can be confirmed conclusively only by food challenge (see Table 110-4).

Skin testing should not be attempted if the clinical history indicates that there is a substantial risk of anaphylaxis; an in vitro assay for the presence of allergen-specific IgE in the serum should be used. Assays for IgE antibodies to several of the known food allergens include the commercially available radioallergosorbent test and enzyme-linked immunosorbent assay kits. Less commonly used is the basophil histamine release assay, which is performed mainly in research laboratories. There is no place for the cytotoxicity food allergy test, which is still widely advertised in the lay press. This test is based on the unsubstantiated notion that incubation of allergenic food extracts with whole blood from supposedly food-allergic subjects results in death of leukocytes. It has not been validated scientifically, and is not approved by the American Academy of Allergy.[68]

Elimination diets.

Systematic elimination of different foods and the use of a food-symptom diary may help identify foods to which a patient might be allergic. Resolution of symptoms and recurrence with reintroduction of selected foods is consistent with a diagnosis of food hypersensitivity. If multiple or several major food groups are implicated, confirmation should be obtained by controlled food challenge. The design of the diet, particularly the degree of food restriction, depends on the patient's history and the number of potential food allergens thought to be involved. Detailed discussion and examples of different elimination diets are available elsewhere.[69] Ideally, the design of the diet should involve an experienced dietitian. Reintroduction of the implicated foods should be supervised by a physician; anaphylaxis was reported in 5% of patients with atopic dermatitis during food challenge after elimination trials.[70]

The most restrictive elimination diet is an elemental diet. Elemental diets are unpleasant to take, but on a short-term basis they may be diagnostically useful in patients claiming to have allergies to multiple foods, or in cases in which the possibility of food allergy is a major concern but no specific food has been implicated by the clinical history. Persistence of symptoms on such a diet excludes food allergy from the differential diagnosis. If symptoms resolve on an elemental diet, various foods may be reintroduced in a systematic fashion.

Oral food challenge.

A double-blinded, placebo-controlled oral food challenge is the most reliable and unbiased method for determining if symptoms are related to a specific food. Like direct skin testing, however, oral food challenge is contraindicated in patients with a history of food-related anaphylaxis. Dehydrated foods are most convenient for diagnostic challenges because they can easily be disguised in a variety of vehicles or may be placed in gelatin capsules. In addition, encapsulated dried food preparations are commercially available for food challenges. Detailed guidelines for the performance of food challenges have been published.[71] Because the double-blinded, placebo-controlled food challenge is time consuming and expensive, "single-blinded" or "open" challenges are convenient initial tests in selected cases to rule out food allergy or to help identify those who require a double-blinded challenge (see Table 110-4).

Treatment and Prevention

The only acceptable treatment of food allergy is avoidance of the offending food. Patient education is the best means of ensuring good dietary compliance. Expert instruction and supervision by an experienced dietitian reduce the likelihood of inadvertent ingestion of food allergens. Drug therapy with antihistamines and corticosteroids has only a secondary role in the management of symptoms due to inadvertent ingestion of food allergens.[72] There is no evidence for a role for oral or parenteral immunotherapy (hyposensitization) with food extracts. There is some evidence to suggest that breast-feeding until the infant is 6 months old may have a protective effect against the development of food allergy.[52,64]

EOSINOPHILIC GASTROENTERITIS

Eosinophilic gastroenteritis was first recognized by Kaijser in 1937.[72] Since then, over 100 cases have been reported. The etiology of this disease is unknown, and it is likely that eosinophilic gastroenteritis is not a single entity but rather a heterogeneous collection of disorders of varied causes with similar clinicopathologic features. It affects patients of all ages and has even been described in an infant.[73]

Pathophysiology

A definitive pathologic mechanism has not been elucidated in eosinophilic gastroenteritis. Allergic phenomena, particularly food hypersensitivity, have been proposed, but the evidence for this is limited. Although food hypersensitivity (usually to milk) may be found in children with eosinophilic gastroenteritis, the response to dietary elimination is usually disappointing. Some patients have no atopic symptoms, and less than half of all patients described with eosinophilic gastroenteritis have a positive family history of allergy. Evidence for an immune pathogenesis is inconclusive.[73,74]

Clinical Manifestations

The clinical manifestations of eosinophilic gastroenteritis depend on the gastrointestinal site primarily affected and the layer of bowel wall predominantly involved. The stomach and intestine are most commonly involved, but the disease may affect any part of the gastrointestinal tract, including the colon.[73-77]

When the predominant involvement is mucosal, the condition behaves like other forms of inflammatory bowel disease, with diarrhea, cramping, postprandial nausea, vomiting, and periumbilical pain. If the eosinophilic infiltration is extensive, there may be malabsorption, weight loss, protein-losing enteropathy, blood loss, and anemia. In preadolescent patients, growth retardation can be noted. A low level of peripheral eosinophilia occurs in most cases. Stools may be positive for occult blood, although frank hematochezia is rarely seen. In addition, Charcot-Leyden crystals secondary to lumenal extrusion of eosinophils may be seen.[76] Intestinal perforation has been reported in a small number of cases of eosinophilic gastroenteritis.[78,79] Diagnosis of mucosal eosinophilic gastroenteritis is made by barium roentgenography and gastric and small bowel biopsies. A diffuse mucosal pattern with nodules or intralumenal masses and a "saw-tooth" mucosal pattern may be noted in the small bowel. A widening of small bowel segments may be seen secondary to mesenteric nodal involvement. Gastric lesions may have a "cobblestone" appearance in the antrum and thickening of mucosal folds.[74,75] Small bowel biopsies may be diagnostic, showing a diffuse infiltration of the mucosa with eosinophils. Because eosinophilic gastroenteritis may present as a patchy intestinal disease, however, multiple biopsies at different levels of the gastrointestinal tract should be performed.[76]

When eosinophilic gastroenteritis predominantly involves the muscularis layer of the intestine, the clinical presentation consists of intestinal obstruction with nausea, vomiting, pain, and abdominal distention.[74,76,80-82] Barium studies of the upper gastrointestinal tract usually demonstrate irregular narrowing of the distal antrum or small bowel.[77,83] Endoscopic mucosal biopsies may not be helpful. Occasionally, isolated infiltration of the esophageal muscles may be seen, with symptoms and manometry evaluations suggestive of achalasia.[75] Rarely, the eosinophilic infiltration is predominantly serosal and may be associated with eosinophilic ascites. Eosinophilic pleural effusions have also been described.[82]

Differential Diagnosis

Diseases that should be considered in the differential diagnosis of eosinophilic gastroenteritis fall into two categories. One category consists of diseases associated with peripheral eosin-

ophilia, in addition to mucosal eosinophilic infiltrates that may mimic idiopathic mucosal eosinophilic gastroenteritis. The most frequently encountered is the hypereosinophilic syndrome. Gastrointestinal involvement is usually diffuse in the hypereosinophilic syndrome; there is a high peripheral eosinophilia, and several other organs also are infiltrated with eosinophils. Periarteritis nodosa also may be associated with a peripheral eosinophilia, and abdominal pain and nodular masses in the stomach and small bowel may be seen on radiography. This condition may be distinguished from eosinophilic gastroenteritis by the systemic nature of the inflammatory process and the finding on mucosal biopsy of an eosinophilic infiltrate localized to the perivascular region. The nodular polypoid mucosal findings on radiography in periarteritis nodosa are secondary to ischemia and inflammation rather than eosinophilic infiltration. Intestinal parasitism is another cause of peripheral eosinophilia and gastrointestinal symptoms, including diarrhea and abdominal pain. The diagnosis is usually suggested by the clinical history and confirmed by stool analysis and examination of a duodenal aspirate. Parasites that are associated with peripheral eosinophilia include hookworm, *Ascaris*, *Strongyloides*, *Toxocara*, *Trichuris*, *Capillaria*, and *Trichinella* species. Protozoal infections such as amebiasis and giardiasis are not associated with eosinophilia. Finally, intramural collections of mature eosinophils are often seen in eosinophilic granuloma. The stomach is the most common site of involvement. These patients present with symptoms of gastric obstruction. The isolated nature of the granuloma may help distinguish this disorder. A young patient presenting with biliary and partial duodenal obstruction had eosinophilic infiltration of the duodenum, which is unusual.[84]

The second major category of diseases that may mimic eosinophilic gastroenteritis clinically and radiologically includes a variety of inflammatory and infiltrative disorders, such as gastrointestinal lymphoma, scirrhous carcinoma of the stomach, and Crohn's disease. These conditions may be associated with a mild increase in eosinophils histologically.

Treatment

There is no specific treatment for eosinophilic gastroenteritis. An attempt to identify a specific environmental or food allergen may be considered if there is a convincing history of symptoms triggered by food and if there is a strong background of atopy. In most adult patients, a specific food is not implicated, and prolonged investigation with elimination diets is not appropriate. If necessary, a trial of an elemental diet can be used quickly to eliminate a role for food hypersensitivity. Oral corticosteroids (prednisone, 20–40 mg/day) are effective in most patients. A short course of 7 to 10 days usually produces clinical remission, although repeat courses may be required. Some patients may require more prolonged treatment.[68,70-80,83] The long-term prognosis for patients with eosinophilic gastroenteritis usually is favorable, and the disease course is one of waxing and waning severity.[68,70-80,83] Occasionally, total parenteral nutrition is required to manage patients with severe disease and symptoms that are refractory to steroids. Segmental resection of the intestine has been performed with minimal success, and has been known to result in obstruction and perforation.[79]

INTESTINAL MANIFESTATIONS OF GRAFT-VERSUS-HOST DISEASE

Bone marrow transplantation is increasingly used for the treatment of a variety of disease entities.[85] Intestinal complications frequently encountered in these patients include the effects of the multistep protocol (radiation, chemotherapy, or both) used for induction before the bone marrow graft; acute and chronic graft-versus-host disease in which mature donor lymphocytes attack the recipient's tissues; and opportunistic infections (including fungal and cytomegalovirus) secondary to the immunodeficiency state associated with both the induction procedure and graft-versus-host reactions.[86,87] Some of the clinical and diagnostic characteristics that help distinguish these entities in the setting of bone marrow transplantation are listed in Table 110-5.

Intestinal Disease Secondary to Induction Protocols

Induction protocols (see Table 110-5) are quite varied and include multiple agents (both chemotherapeutic agents and high-dose radiation), all of which are capable of injuring rapidly dividing cell populations. The combination of chemotherapeutic agents and radiation produces intestinal cell necrosis. This necrosis occurs immediately during the induction, and up to 3 weeks are required before there is mucosal regeneration.[88] Anorexia, cramping, and abdominal pain, with watery diarrhea, may develop. Both the small and large intestine are damaged during this process. During healing, there is atypia of cell nuclei and regeneration of crypt cells, but the surface epithelium is normal.[89,90] This histopathologic picture is important in helping distinguish this entity from acute graft-versus-host disease or secondary viral infections. The time of onset after bone marrow transplantation, rectal biopsy, and stool cultures is the most important diagnostic test and clue

(see Table 110-5). Treatment consists of supportive measures and total parenteral nutrition.

Acute Graft-Versus-Host Disease

The onset of the syndrome of acute graft-versus-host disease usually takes place 3 to 4 weeks after bone marrow transplantation, and it consists clinically of a complex of symptoms and signs, including dermatitis, mucositis, enteritis, and hepatic dysfunction. Features that help distinguish this condition from the enteritis associated with the induction protocol include an erythematous, maculopapular skin rash over the palms, soles, and trunk, and liver test result abnormalities, including hyperbilirubinemia. The syndrome of acute graft-versus-host disease may be staged based on the degree of skin, gut, and liver damage.[87,91] A moderate to severe degree of acute graft-versus-host disease develops in 30% to 50% of patients with sustained engraftment.

Pathogenesis

There are three theories of the mechanism leading to acute graft-versus-host disease. One theory holds that graft-versus-host disease represents a form of local immunodeficiency secondary to destruction of host immune cells by donor cells. The actual destructive lesion is the result of a secondary infection.[92] A second hypothesis is that graft-versus-host disease is a form of innocent-bystander tissue damage, without a direct attack on the target epithelium. Effector lymphocytes from the donor interact with the recipient's lymphoid cells within the mucosa. This is associated with activation of cytotoxic mechanisms and release of cytotoxic factors and cytokines, which lead to destruction of the innocent bystander epithelial cells in the vicinity.[92–94] The third theory of the mechanism of graft-versus-host disease proposes direct recognition of alloantigens on the recipient epithelial cells by donor cytotoxic cells, leading to direct destruction of epithelial cells.[95,96]

TABLE 110-5
Gastrointestinal Complications of Bone Marrow Transplantation

	SECONDARY TO INDUCTION PROTOCOL	ACUTE GVHD	CHRONIC GVHD
Time onset after BMT (days)	0–20	20–80	>80
Clinical features	Anorexia, abdominal pain, diarrhea	Diarrhea (large volume), abdominal pain ± skin rash ± liver disease	Dysphagia, oral ulcers, diarrhea
Roentogenographic changes	Not helpful	Mucosal edema, mucosal ulcers, pneumatosis	Esophageal strictures and webs
Endoscopy or manometry	Nonspecific	Normal → erythema → mucosal sloughing; stomach and rectum are spared	Upper esophageal bands and webs; lower third of esophagus is spared
Histology: source and changes	Rectal: atypia of cell nuclei, crypt cell regeneration	Early → rectal; crypt cells/apoptosis Late → mucosal disintegration	Esophagus: neutrophil infiltration, basal layer necrosis
Differential diagnoses	Intestinal infection, esophagitis, early GVHD	Infection, drug effect	Peptic esophagitis, infection—Candida, herpes, CMV
Stool findings	Negative for pathogens	Negative for pathogens, cellular debris, increased protein	Negative for pathogens

BMT, bone marrow transplantation; CMV, cytomegalovirus; GVHD, graft-versus-host disease.

Clinical Manifestations

The onset or continuance of profuse, watery diarrhea 3 weeks after bone marrow transplantation is indicative of intestinal acute graft-versus-host disease. The severity of the intestinal condition usually parallels that of the skin and liver involvement, although some may have profound gastrointestinal symptoms without any gross skin or liver changes. The clinical picture, when severe, includes anorexia, vomiting, buccal mucositis, abdominal pain, intestinal bleeding, protein loss, and secondary infection (see Table 110-5). High-volume diarrhea may occur, and the amount of fluid generated is an index of extent and severity of disease activity. Extensive disease may be associated with up to 10 L of diarrheal fluid loss per day. The large amount of stool volume may lead to distention and pain. The distention of the bowel may be exacerbated by opiate analgesics, which should be used with caution.

Because many of the symptoms of graft-versus-host disease are not specific, there should be constant vigilance for other complications, particularly infections. The most common cause of gastrointestinal bleeding in these patients is esophagitis and gastric erosions. When a discrete ulcer develops, however, cytomegalovirus infection is an important consideration. Treatment of such lesions is unsatisfactory, and if bleeding is persistent, surgical resection may be required.

Differential Diagnosis

The diagnosis of acute graft-versus-host disease may be made with confidence approximately 3 weeks after bone marrow transplantation if there is evidence for a functioning graft and if there is watery diarrhea accompanied by a diffuse skin rash and jaundice (see Table 110-5). The patient who presents with gastrointestinal symptoms but without jaundice or skin rash, however, represents a much more difficult diagnostic challenge. Other diagnostic considerations include an opportunistic intestinal infection and the residual effects of the radiation and chemotherapy conditioning lasting beyond the usual 3-week period. Careful attention to detail is required, with a combination of stool examinations, barium radiographic studies, endoscopy, and histopathologic study (see Table 110-5).

Because of the nature of the intestinal injury, the stool usually contains large amounts of cellular debris and red and white blood cells. Protein loss in the stool may be sufficiently severe to lead to profound hypoalbuminemia. The absence of pathogens in the stool is important but does not necessarily rule out an infection of the midgastrointestinal tract.

Barium roentgenography may be helpful in the differential diagnosis and in establishing extent of disease. Widespread changes may occur, including mucosal and submucosal edema, pneumatosis cystoides intestinalis, and mucosal ulcerations. These radiologic findings can also be consistent with other conditions, such as cytomegalovirus enteritis and the effects of acute radiation. The acute radiologic features may return to normal, or in some cases they progress to a chronic segmental, ribbon-like appearance, usually in the small intestine.

Endoscopic appearances can be normal or can show patchy erythema or extensive mucosal sloughing. These lesions are most prominent in the ileum, cecum, and ascending colon, with relative sparing of the gastric and rectal mucosa. Histologic changes seen in biopsies from advanced or severe lesions may not be as useful diagnostically as those from early lesions. Therefore, endoscopic biopsies should be taken from intact mucosa as well as from areas involved with gross inflammation. The earliest change seen on light microscopy is necrosis of individual cells in the intestinal crypts. This characteristic finding is referred to as apoptosis (Fig. 110-2). It is diagnostic, if obtained from normal-appearing mucosa, at least 20 days after transplantation.[96] Inflammatory cells or microorganisms are not present in the adjacent mucosa. Later, the histopathologic course can progress to a total denudation of the mucosa; the apoptosis lesion is no longer evident, and changes are not specific.

Treatment

The management of acute intestinal graft-versus-host disease consists of nutritional support, maintenance of fluid and electrolyte balance, steroid and immunosuppressive treatment, and vigilance for secondary infectious complications. For patients with severe, high-volume diarrhea, subcutaneous ad-

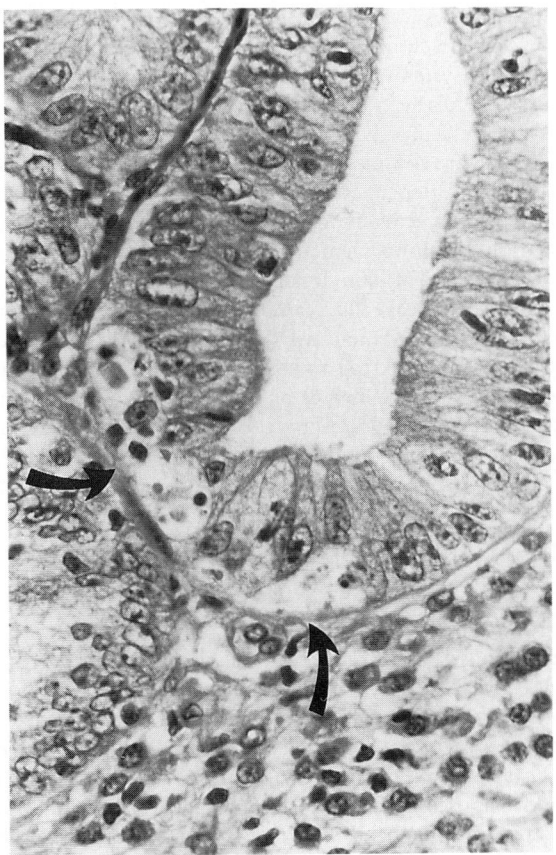

FIGURE 110-2. Rectal biopsy specimen taken after bone marrow transplantation from a patient with acute graft-versus-host disease shows apoptotic bodies (*arrows*). This necrosis of individual cells within the crypt is the first change seen on light microscopy and is characteristic of acute graft-versus-host disease if found after day 20, when damage from chemoradiation therapy has resolved.

ministration of the somatostatin analog, octreotide, may provide significant relief. To improve long-term survival, doses of prednisone ranging up to 2 mg/kg, for up to 1 to 2 weeks, may be used. Cyclosporine also may be used in combination with antithymocyte globulin or more specific anti–T-cell monoclonal antibodies.

Research has focused on the prevention of graft-versus-host disease.[94] Methods for the prior removal of mature donor T lymphocytes from the bone marrow graft have been successfully developed. These T cells mediate the graft-versus-host reaction, and their removal has resulted in a marked reduction in the incidence of the disease, but unfortunately has been associated with reduced graft survival. The future focus will probably be on selective removal of subsets of effector T cells.

Chronic Graft-Versus-Host Disease

Chronic graft-versus-host disease is a multisystem disorder that occurs 80 to 400 days after allogeneic transplantation (see Table 110-5). Most patients have had prior acute graft-versus-host disease; however, approximately one fourth of the patients with chronic graft-versus-host disease have had no clinical indications of any prior acute graft-versus-host illness. The skin, liver, and gastrointestinal tract are predominantly involved. The clinical features resemble those of sicca syndrome and systemic sclerosis. Gastrointestinal involvement occurs particularly in the oral mucosa (mucositis), esophagus, and small intestine. Esophageal symptoms of dysphagia with weight loss are common presenting gastrointestinal manifestations.[97,98] Patients with skin involvement (hyperpigmentation and scleroderma-like changes) frequently, but not always, have esophageal involvement. Esophageal disease may occur in the absence of skin lesions, however. Dysphagia with chronic esophageal reflux can lead to chronic lung disease. Small bowel involvement with chronic graft-versus-host disease can be attributed to two possible pathogenic mechanisms. The first is a patchy fibrosis of the lamina propria and submucosa; in the second, bacterial overgrowth may occur as a result of stasis and dysmotility. This latter abnormality responds to oral broad-spectrum antibiotics.

Differential Diagnosis

As with other immunosuppressed conditions, opportunistic gastrointestinal infections are a constant threat and must always be considered in the differential diagnosis. An important diagnostic challenge is the distinction between esophageal involvement with chronic graft-versus-host disease and reflux peptic disease of the esophagus. The combination of radiography, esophagoscopy, biopsy, and manometry may be required. Endoscopic lesions of chronic graft-versus-host disease can range from generalized desquamation of the upper and midesophagus to web-like, fibrous bands.[97] Manometry with pH monitoring shows a nonspecific motor abnormality and a decreased ability to clear acid from the esophagus. In contrast to peptic esophagitis, the distal esophagus is usually spared in chronic graft-versus-host disease.[98] Histologic changes within the esophagus include infiltration with neutrophils and lymphocytes and necrosis of individual cells of the basal mucosa, a picture analogous to the changes found in the skin and oral mucosa. In contrast to scleroderma, submucosal fibrosis may be found, but there are no muscle or neural abnormalities.

Treatment

In contrast to acute graft-versus-host disease, the treatment of chronic graft-versus-host disease is frequently satisfactory. Early diagnosis and drug therapy prevent much of the disability associated with this condition. Prednisone alone, or in combination with azathioprine, has been effective. Aggressive antireflux therapy is important for reducing the symptoms associated with esophageal involvement. Fibrosis tends to be progressive, however, and esophageal dilation may be required for treatment of webs and strictures.

Graft-Versus-Host Disease in Small Bowel Transplantation

An extremely new procedure in humans is small bowel transplantation. To date, only a very small number of these grafts have been tried, and with little success overall. This is a very active area of research in animal models, however, the results of which will be applied to the human situation, and will, it is hoped, lead to improved results.

Attempts are underway to define the causes of the development of graft-versus-host disease in conjunction with small bowel transplantation. One study found a correlation with the size of the small bowel transplanted and the development of graft-versus-host disease.[99] The researchers found that small grafts (including only a segment of the jejunum) decreased the intensity of graft-versus-host disease, whereas grafting the entire small bowel, jejunum, and ileum increased the mortality rate.

One investigation attempted to determine the effect of the large numbers of lymphocytes in the small bowel graft on the incidence and severity of graft-versus-host disease.[100] The researchers, using rat models, found a positive correlation between the presence of the gut-associated lymphoid tissue and the mesenteric lymph nodes in the small bowel graft for the parameters studied.

In small bowel transplantation studies using fully allogeneic rats and large animals, it was found that the prevalent phenomenon was graft rejection and *not* graft-versus-host disease.[101] When animals in this study did manifest graft-versus-host-disease, the cells found in the grafts were of recipient origin. Another study of fully allogeneic rat small bowel transplantation found that 40% had transient graft-versus-host disease (although none of the animals showed clinical signs of the disease), and that treatment with cyclosporine A led to longer life than treatment with FK506.[102] Graft-versus-host disease in MHC-mismatched rats after small bowel transplant was found by other investigators to be treatable by rapamycin, a relatively new immunosuppressant.[103]

Natural killer cells have been hypothesized to play a role in the mechanisms of graft-versus-host disease after small bowel grafts in rats. Inhibition of graft-versus-host disease using deoxyspergualin was evaluated.[104] Eight of 10 deoxyspergualin-treated rats did not have cutaneous or lethal graft-versus- host disease, although life was not prolonged in the host by this treatment.

The immune system of the intestine is distinct from the systemic immune system (which is the inducer of bone marrow transplant-related graft-versus-host disease), possessing many unique cellular elements with separately regulated immune responses.[105] The studies outlined in this section suggest that to understand the development of graft-versus-host disease resulting from small bowel transplantation, the unique nature of the systems and the cells must be defined, and must be taken into account in choosing treatment agents as well.

The reader is directed to Chapter 5, The Immune System; Chapter 46, Approach to Gastrointestinal Problems in the Immunocompromised Patient; Chapter 77, Miscellaneous Diseases of the Small Intestine; and Chapter 105, Gastrointestinal Complications of the Acquired Immunodeficiency Syndrome.

REFERENCES

1. Brogan MD. Mucosal immunity and infection. Ann Intern Med 1987;106:853.
2. Rosen FS, Cooper MD, Wedgewood RJP. The primary immunodeficiencies. N Engl J Med 1984;311:235.
3. Buckley RH. Immunodeficiency diseases. JAMA 1987;258:281.
4. Primary immunodeficiency diseases: report of a World Health Organization scientific group. Clin Immunol Immunopathol 1986;40:166.
5. Lederman HM, Winkelstien JA. X-linked agammaglobulinemia: an analysis of 96 patients. Medicine 1985;64:145.
6. Ament ME. Gastrointestinal manifestations of immunodeficiency diseases in infants, children, and adults. In: Targan S, Shanahan F, eds. Immunology and immunopathology of the liver and gastrointestinal tract. New York: Igaku-Shoin, 1989: 355.
7. Webster ADB. Immune deficiency. In: Booth CC, Neale G, eds. Disorders of the small intestine. Oxford: Blackwell, 1985: 135.
8. Ament ME, Ochs HD, Davis SD. Structure and function of the gastrointestinal tract in primary immunodeficiency syndromes: a study of 39 patients. Medicine 1973;35:227.
9. Seidman EG, Walker WA. Gastrointestinal manifestations of primary and secondary immunodeficiency states. Front Gastrointest Res 1986;13:187.
10. Doe WF. Immunodeficiency and the gastrointestinal tract. Clin Gastroenterol 1983;12:839.
11. Seggev JS, Ben-Yosef N, Meytes D. Is selective IgA deficiency associated with morbidity?: review and re-evaluation. Isr J Med Sci 1988;24:65.
12. Hanson LA, Bjorkander J, Carlsson B, et al. The heterogeneity of IgA deficiency. J Clin Immunol 1988;8:159.
13. Leickly FE, Buckley RH. Development of IgA and IgG2 subclass deficiency after sulfasalazine therapy. J Pediatr 1986;108:481.
14. Amman AJ, Hong R. Selective IgA deficiency: presentation and a review of the literature. Medicine 1971;50:223.
15. Wilton AN, Lobain TJ, Dawkins RL. Familial studies of IgA deficiency. Immunogenetics 1985;21:333.
16. Brown WR, Strober W. Immunologic diseases of the gastrointestinal tract. In: Samter M, Talmage DW, Frank MM, et al, eds. Immunological diseases. 4th ed. Boston: Little, Brown & Co., 1988:1995.
17. McCarthy DM, Katz SI, Gazze L, et al. Selective IgA deficiency associated with total villus atrophy of the small intestine and an organ-specific antiepithelial cell antibody. J Immunol 1978;120:932.
18. Oxelius V-A, Laurell A-B, Lindquist B, et al. IgG subclass in selective IgA deficiency. N Engl J Med 1981;304:1476.
19. Strober W, Krakauer R, Klaeveman HL, et al. Secretory component deficiency. N Engl J Med 1976;249:351.
20. Fisher SE, Smith WI, Rabin BS, et al. Secretory component and serum immunoglobulin A deficiencies with intestinal antibody formation and autoimmune disease: a family study. J Pediatr Gastroenterol Nutr 1982;1:35.
21. Hermens PE, Diaz-Buxon JA, Stobo JD. Idiopathic late-onset immunoglobulin deficiency. Am J Med 1976;61:221.
22. Cunningham-Rundles C. Clinical and immunologic analyses of 103 patients with common variable immunodeficiency. J Clin Immunol 1989;9:22.
23. Ament ME, Rubin CE. Relation of giardiasis to abnormal intestinal structure and function in gastrointestinal immunodeficiency syndromes. Gastroenterology 1972;62:216.
24. Kuhls TL, Greenfield RA, Mosier DA, et al. Cryptosporidiosis in adult and neonatal mice with severe combined immunodeficiency. J Comp Pathol 1992;106:399.
25. den Hartog G, van der Meer JWM, Jansen JBMJ, et al. Decreased gastrin secretion in patients with late-onset hypogammaglobulinemia. N Engl J Med 1988;318:1563.
26. Nagura H, Kohler PF, Brown WR. Immunocytochemical characterization of the lymphocytes in nodular lymphoid hyperplasia of the bowel. Lab Invest 1979;40:66.
27. Kinlen LJ, Webster ADB, Bird AG, et al. Prospective study of cancer in patients with hypogammaglobulinemia. Lancet 1985: 1;263.
28. Waldmann TA. Immunodeficiency diseases: primary and acquired. In: Samter M, Talmage DW, Frank MM, et al, eds. Immunological diseases. 4th ed. Boston: Little, Brown & Co., 1988:411.
29. Ammann AJ, Hong R. Disorders of the T-cell system. In: Stiehm ER, ed. Immunologic disorders in infants and children. Philadelphia: WB Saunders, 1989:286.
30. Horowitz S, Lorenzsonn VW, Olson WA, et al. Small intestinal disease in T-cell deficiency. J Pediatr 1974;85:457.
31. Orkin SH. Molecular genetics and potential gene therapy. Clin Immunol Immunopathol 1986;40:151.
32. Gatti RA, Izzet B, Boder E, et al. Localization of an ataxia-telangiectasia gene to chromosome 11q22-23. Nature 1988;336:557.
33. Peterson RDA, Funkhouser JD. Speculations on ataxia-telangiectasia: defective regulation of the immunoglobulin gene superfamily. Immunol Today 1989;10:313.
34. Oxelius V-A, Berkel AI, Hanson LA. IgG2 deficiency in ataxia telangiectasia. N Engl J Med 1982;306:515.
35. White CJ, Gallin JI. Phagocyte defects. Clin Immunol Immunopathol 1986;40:50.
36. Gallin JI, Buescherr ES, Seligmann BE, et al. Recent advances in chronic granulomatous disease. Ann Intern Med 1983;99: 657.
37. Tauber AI, Borregaard N, Simons E, Wright J. Chronic granulomatous disease: a syndrome of phagocyte oxidase deficiencies. Medicine 1983;62:286.
38. Ezekowitz RAB, Newberger PE. New perspectives in chronic granulomatous disease. J Clin Immunol 1988;8:419.
39. Ament ME, Ochs HD. Gastrointestinal manifestations of chronic granulomatous disease. N Engl J Med 1973;288:382.
40. Mike N, Hanel TT, Newman J, Asquith P. Granulomatous enteropathy in common variable immunodeficiency: a cause of chronic diarrhoea. Postgrad Med J 1991;67:446.
41. Mulholland MW, Delaney JP, Simmons RL. Gastrointestinal complications of chronic granulomatous disease: surgical implications. Surgery 1983;94:569.
42. Ross SC, Densen P. Complement deficiency states and infection: epidemiology, pathogenesis, and consequences of neisserial and other infections in immune deficiency. Medicine 1984;63:243.
43. Matzner Y, Brzezinski A. C5-a inhibitor deficiency in peritoneal fluid from patients with familial Mediterranean fever. N Engl J Med 1984;311:287.
44. Frank MM, Gelfand JA, Atkinson JP. Hereditary angioedema: the clinical syndrome and its management. Ann Intern Med 1976;84:580.

45. O'Regan PFB, Shanahan F, Barnes L, Lennon JR. Hereditary angioedema: a cause of abdominal pain, often missed. Ir J Med Sci 1981;150:335.

46. Davis AE. C1 inhibitor and hereditary angioneurotic edema. Annu Rev Immunol 1988;6:595.

47. Strober W. Intestinal lymphangiectasia: the prototype protein-losing enteropathy. In: Kirsner JR, Shorter RG, eds. Gastrointestinal immunity for the clinician. Orlando: Grune & Stratton, 1985:113.

48. Igra-Siegman Y, Kapila R, Seu P, et al. Syndrome of hyperinfection with *Strongyloides stercoralis*. Rev Infect Dis 1981;3:397.

49. Shanahan F. Food allergy: fact, fiction and fatality. Gastroenterology 1993;104:1229.

50. Finn R. Food allergy: fact or fiction. J R Soc Med 1992;85:560.

51. Crowe SE, MH Perdue. Gastrointestinal food hypersensitivity: basic mechanisms of pathophysiology. Gastroenterology 1992;103:1075.

52. Duerr RH, Shanahan F. Food allergy. In: Targan S, Shanahan F, eds. Immunology and immunopathology of the liver and gastrointestinal tract. New York: Igaku-Shoin, 1989:507.

53. May CD. Food allergy: material and ethereal. N Engl J Med 1980;302:1142.

54. Pearson DJ, Rix KJB, Bentley SJ. Food allergy: how much in the mind? A clinical and psychiatric study of suspected food hypersensitivity. Lancet 1983;1:1259.

55. Metcalfe DD. Food hypersensitivity. J Allergy Clin Immunol 1984;73:749.

56. Atkins FM, Steinberg SS, Metcalfe DD. Evaluation of immediate adverse reactions to foods in adults. I. Correlation of demographic, laboratory, and prick skin test data with response to controlled oral food challenge. J Allergy Clin Immunol 1985;75:348.

57. Bland P. MHC class II expression by the gut epithelium. Immunol Today 1988;9:174.

58. Mowat AM. The regulation of immune responses to dietary protein antigens. Immunol Today 1987;8:93.

59. Taylor SL, Lemanske RF, Bush RK, et al. Food allergens: structure and immunologic properties. Ann Allergy 1987;59(Part II):93.

60. Brunner M, Walzer M. Absorption of undigested proteins in human beings: the absorption of unaltered fish proteins in adults. Arch Intern Med 1928;42:172.

61. Sampson HA. IgE-mediated food intolerance. J Allergy Clin Immunol 1988;81:495.

62. Sampson HA, Jolie PL. Increased plasma histamine concentration after food challenges in children with atopic dermatitis. N Engl J Med 1984;311:372.

63. Sampson HA, Broadbent KR, Bernhisel-Broadbent J. Spontaneous release of histamine from basophils and histamine-releasing factor in patients with atopic dermatitis and food hypersensitivity. N Engl J Med 1989;321:228.

64. Sampson HA, Buckley RH, Metcalfe DD. Food allergy. JAMA 1987;258:2886.

65. Irani AMA, Schwartz LB. Mast cell heterogeneity. Clin Exp Allergy 1989;19:143.

66. Metcalfe DD. Diseases of food hypersensitivity. N Engl J Med 1989;321:255.

67. Bahna SL, Heiner DC. Cow's milk allergy pathogenesis, manifestations, diagnosis, and management. Adv Pediatr 1978;25:1.

68. Reisman RE. American Academy of Allergy position statements: controversial techniques. J Allergy Clin Immunol 1981;67:333.

69. Anderson JA, Sogn DD, eds. Adverse reactions to foods. American Academy of Allergy and Immunology Committee on Adverse Reactions to Foods, NIH Publication No. 84-2442. Bethesda, MD: National Institutes of Health, 1984.

70. David TJ. Anaphylactic shock during elimination diets for severe atopic eczema. Arch Dis Child 1984;59:983.

71. Bock SA, Sampson HA, Atkins FM, et al. Double-blind, placebo-controlled food challenge (DBPCFC) as an office procedure: a manual. J Allergy Clin Immunol 1988;82:986.

72. Kaijser R: Zur kenntnis der Allergischen Affektionen des verdauungskanals vom Standpunkt des Chirurgan aus. Arch Klin Chir 1937;188:36.

73. Peterson NE, Silverman A, Campbell JB. Eosinophilic cystitis and coexistent eosinophilic gastroenteritis in an infant. Pediatric Radiology 1989;19:484.

74. Caldwell JH, Mekhjian HS, Hurtubise PE, Beman FM. Eosinophilic gastroenteritis with obstruction. Gastroenterology 1978;74:825.

75. Zora JA, O'Connell EJ, Sachs MI, Hoffman AD. Eosinophilic gastroenteritis: a case report and review of the literature. Ann Allergy 1984;53:45.

76. Johnstone JM, Morson BC. Eosinophilic gastroenteritis. Histopathology 1978;2:335.

77. Schulman A, Morton G, Dietrich BE. Eosinophilic gastroenteritis. Clin Radiol 1980;31:101.

78. Blanco-Guerra C, Cazana JL, Villas F, et al. Ileal perforation due to eosinophilic gastroenteritis. Am J Gastroenterol 1991;86:1689.

79. Wang C-S, Hsueh S, Shi L-Y, Chen M-F. Repeated bowel resections for eosinophilic gastroenteritis with obstruction and perforation. Acta Chir Scand 1990;156:333.

80. Keshavarzian A, Saverymuttu SH, Tai PC, et al. Activated eosinophils in familial eosinophilic gastroenteritis. Gastroenterology 1985;88:1041.

81. Snyder JD, Rosenblum N, Wershil B, et al. Pyloric stenosis and eosinophilic gastroenteritis in infants. J Pediatr Gastroenterol Nutr 1987;6:543.

82. Rumans MC, Lieberman DA. Eosinophilic gastroenteritis presenting with biliary duodenal obstruction. Am J Gastroenterol 1987;82:775.

83. Cello JP. Eosinophilic gastroenteritis: a complex disease entity. Am J Med 1979;67:1097.

84. Farahvash MJ, Bastani B, Farahvash MR, Irvanlou G. Eosinophilic gastroenteritis presenting with biliary and partial duodenal obstruction. Am J Gastroenterol 1990;85:1022.

85. Trounce JQ, Tanner MS. Eosinophilic gastroenteritis. Arch Dis Child 1985;60:1186.

86. Bortin MM, Rimm AA. Increasing utilization of bone marrow transplantation. Transplantation 1986;42:229.

87. McDonald GB, Shulman HM, Sullivan KM, Spencer GD. Intestinal and hepatic complications of human bone marrow transplantation. Part I. Gastroenterology 1986;90:460.

88. Beschorner WE, Pino J, Boitnott JK, et al. Destruction of the intestinal mucosa after bone marrow transplantation and graft-versus-host disease. Am J Pathol 1980;99:369.

89. Epstein RJ, McDonald GB, Sale GE, et al. The diagnostic accuracy of the rectal biopsy in acute graft-versus-host disease: a prospective study of thirteen patients. Gastroenterology 1980;78:764.

90. Weisbrot IM, Liber AF, Gordon BS. The effects of therapeutic radiation on colonic mucosa. Cancer 1975;36:931.

91. McDonald GB, Shulman HM, Sullivan KM, Spencer GD. Intestinal and hepatic compilations of human bone marrow transplantation. Part II. Gastroenterology 1986;90:770.

92. Beschorner WE, Turnicky RP. Intestinal and hepatic manifestations of graft-versus-host disease. In: Targan S, Shanahan F, eds. Immunology and immunopathology of the liver and gastrointestinal tract. New York: Igaku-Shoin, 1989:589.

93. Shearer GM, Levy RB. Graft-versus-host associated immune suppression is activated by recognition of allogeneic murine I-A antigens. J Exp Med 1983;157:936.

94. Mason DW. Subpopulations of T-cells in the rat that mediate graft-versus-host reactions and lethal graft-versus-host disease. Adv Exp Med Biol 1982;149:545.

95. Slavin RE, Santos GW. The graft-versus-host reactions in man after bone marrow transplantation: pathology, pathogenesis, clinical features and implication. Clin Immunol Immunopathol 1973;1:472.

96. Gallucci BG, Sale GE, McDonald GB, et al. The fine structure of human rectal epithelium in acute graft-versus-host disease. Am J Surg Pathol 1982;6:293.

97. McDonald GB, Sullivan M, Schuffler MD, et al. Esophageal abnormalities in chronic graft-versus-host disease in humans. Gastroenterology 1981;80:914.

98. McDonald GB, Sullivan KM, Plumley TF. Radiographic features of esophageal involvement in chronic graft-versus-host disease. AJR 1984;142:501.
99. Pirenne J, D'Silva M, Hamoir E, et al. Influence of the length of the small bowel graft on the severity of graft versus host disease. Microsurgery 1990;11:303.
100. Pirenne J, Lardinois F, D'Silva M, et al. Relevance of mesenteric lymph nodes to graft-versus-host disease following small bowel transplantation. Transplantation 1990;50:711.
101. Murase N, Demetris AJ, Woo J, et al. Lymphocyte traffic and graft-versus-host disease after fully allogeneic small bowel transplantation. Transplant Proc 1991;23:3246.
102. de Bruin RWF, HogenEsch H, Heineman E, et al. Fulminant graft-versus-host disease after FK506 treatment in fully allogeneic small bowel transplantation. Transplant Proc 1991;23:3257.
103. Fabian MA, Denning SM, Bollinger RR. Rapamycin suppression of host-versus-graft and graft-versus-host disease in MHC-mismatched rats. Transplant Proc 1992;24:1174.
104. Tanaka S, Okada K, Uda M, et al. Mechanism of graft-versus-host disease and inhibition with deoxyspergualin on small bowel transplantation in rats. Transplant Proc 1992;24:1161.
105. Targan SR. The lamina propria: a dynamic, complex mucosal compartment. An overview. Ann NY Acad Sci 1992;664:61.

Textbook of Gastroenterology, second edition, edited by Tadataka Yamada. JB Lippincott Company, Philadelphia © 1995.

CHAPTER 111

Vascular Lesions: Ectasias, Tumors, and Malformations

Ray E. Clouse

Vascular Ectasia Disorders
  Angiodysplasia
  Gastric Antral Vascular Ectasia: The "Watermelon Stomach"
  Telangiectasia Associated With Multisystem Disease
Vascular Tumors

Hemangiomas
Multiple-Hemangioma Syndromes
Malignant Vascular Tumors
Other Vascular Lesions
  Dieulafoy's Lesion
  Miscellaneous Lesions

Vascular lesions represent important causes of gastrointestinal bleeding. Many different terms have been used to describe vascular abnormalities, resulting in a confusing nosology. Arteriovenous malformation, an encompassing term that carries no specific pathologic meaning, should be reserved for broad generalizations. A more precise vocabulary that envelopes pathologic, etiologic, and clinical implications continues to evolve. Although various classification schemes have been proposed,[1–4] none is uniformly acknowledged or consistently used. In this chapter, for convenience, lesions have been clustered into one of three categories: vascular ectasias, vascular tumors, and other vascular lesions (Table 111-1).

VASCULAR ECTASIA DISORDERS

Angiodysplasia

The term "angiodysplasia" is used to describe distinct gastrointestinal mucosal vascular ectasias that are not associated with cutaneous lesions, systemic vascular disease, or a familial syndrome (Figs. 111-1 and 111-2; see Color Figs. 74 and 75). The lesions have many similarities to those of the telangiectasias (see Telangiectasia Associated With Multisystem Disease), but angiodysplasia is not a component of a systemic, metabolic, or hereditary disease with other manifestations.[5]

TABLE 111-1
Vascular Lesions of the Gastrointestinal Tract

Vascular Ectasia Disorders
Angiodysplasia
Gastric antral vascular ectasia (i.e., "watermelon stomach")
Telangiectasia associated with multisystem disease (e.g., hereditary hemorrhagic telangiectasia, CREST syndrome, Turner's syndrome)

Vascular Tumors
Hemangiomas
Multiple-hemangioma syndromes (e.g., intestinal hemangiomatosis, universal hemangiomatosis, blue rubber bleb nevus syndrome, Klippel-Trenaunay-Weber syndrome)
Malignant vascular tumors (e.g., angiosarcoma, hemangiopericytoma, Kaposi's sarcoma)

Other Vascular Lesions
Dieulafoy's lesion
Miscellaneous (e.g., multiple phlebectasia, pseudoxanthoma elasticum, Ehlers-Danlos syndrome, other congenital vascular malformations)

CREST, calcinosis, Raynaud's phenomenon, esophageal hypomotility, sclerodactyly, telangiectasia.

Angiodysplasia received little attention before the late 1970s, but it has become clear that these localized ectatic lesions represent important causes of both upper and lower gastrointestinal bleeding.

Epidemiology

Angiodysplasia is an increasingly recognized disorder, and the prevalence appears higher than was originally suspected. Angiodysplasia of the stomach or duodenum has been found in 1% to 2% of consecutive subjects undergoing upper gastrointestinal endoscopy for a variety of indications.[6] The lesions have been detected and incriminated in up to 4% of those subjects being evaluated for upper gastrointestinal bleeding,[7-9] and in a larger percentage of patients being evaluated for unexplained anemia.[7] Angiodysplasia often is found

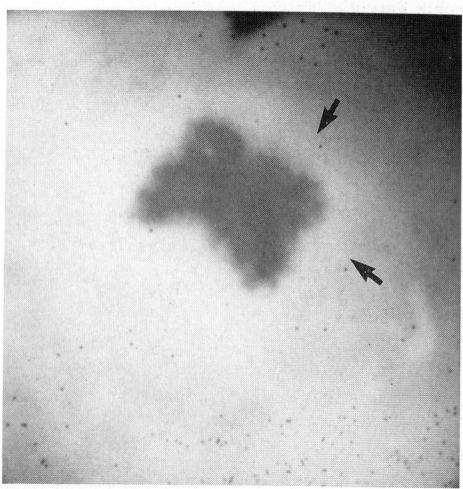

FIGURE 111-1. (See Color Fig. 74.) A well-demarcated, 3-mm, duodenal angiodysplastic lesion with fern-like margins is surrounded by a pale halo (*arrows*).

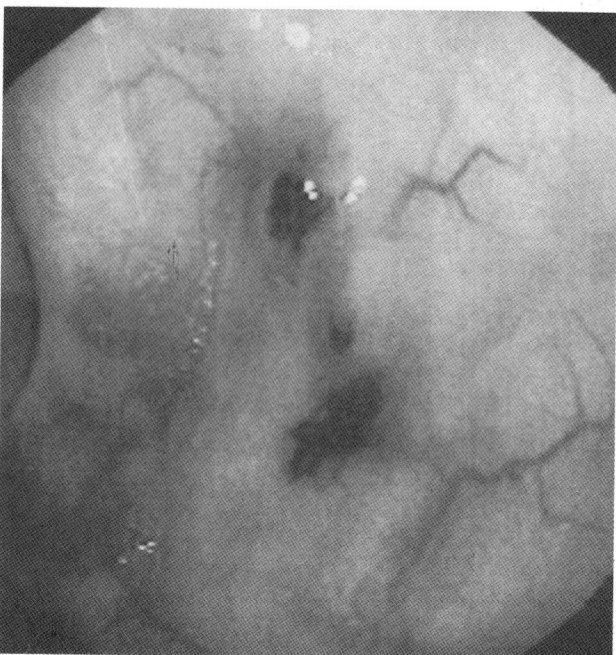

FIGURE 111-2. (See Color Fig. 75.) Three clustered angiodysplastic lesions were detected in the right colon during colonoscopic evaluation for chronic gastrointestinal bleeding. The deeper, prominent, draining vein is also apparent.

coincidentally with peptic disease or other bleeding sites during evaluation of upper gastrointestinal hemorrhage, and may be an incidental finding in over half of the cases in which the lesions are detected.[7]

Angiodysplasia is found during colonoscopy at a slightly higher rate, that is, in 3% to 6% of subjects undergoing the procedure for a variety of indications.[10,11] Colonic angiodysplasia can be an incidental finding as well in nearly half of the cases in which it is detected.[11] Despite the relatively low overall prevalence, this lesion likely represents the most frequent cause of recurrent lower gastrointestinal tract bleeding in elderly subjects.[12] Angiodysplasia is at least as important as diverticular disease as a source of lower gastrointestinal hemorrhage.[12,13]

Both the upper and lower tract lesions are typically seen in elderly patients of both genders. Although gastric and duodenal lesions occasionally have been reported in subjects in the third decade of life,[6,9] the mean age of subjects with these upper tract lesions usually exceeds 60 years.[6,8,9,14] One notable exception to this is a Indian series by Jesudason and colleagues, wherein all subjects were younger than 50 years of age at the onset of symptoms, with a mean age of 34 years.[15] Angiodysplasia of the colon typically presents no sooner than the sixth decade of life.[3,16-18] In some series, most subjects have been 70 years of age or older,[17,19] but, as with upper tract lesions, very young subjects with colonic angiodysplasia also have been described.[16]

Etiology and Pathology

The etiology of angiodysplasia remains uncertain. Because the lesions usually are found in an older population, presumably they are acquired. Two theories of etiology have been

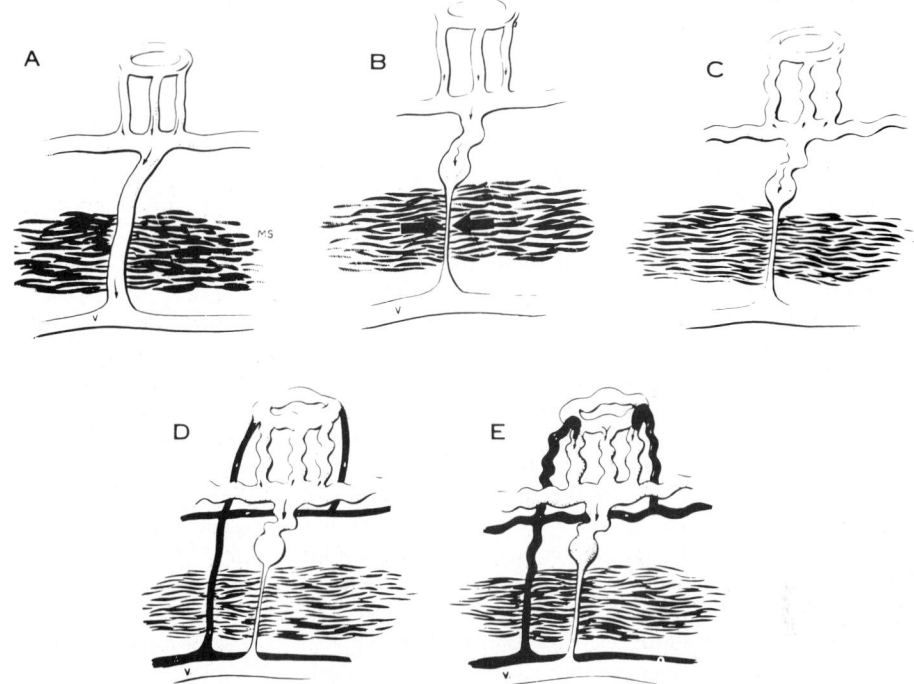

FIGURE 111-3. One proposed mechanism for the development of angiodysplasia. (**A**) The normal state of mucosal and submucosal venous drainage is partially obstructed (**B**) by muscular contraction or increased intraluminal pressure. (**C**) After repeated episodes over years, the submucosal vein becomes dilated and tortuous, and (**D**) veins and venules draining into the abnormal submucosal vessel subsequently become involved. (**E**) Ultimately, the capillary ring dilates, the precapillary sphincter becomes incompetent, and a small arteriovenous communication is present through the lesion. (From Boley SJ, Sammartano R, Adams R, et al. On the nature and etiology of vascular ectasias of the colon: degenerative lesions of aging. Gastroenterology 1977;72:650.)

popularized: The ectatic lesions are a degenerative process of aging and result from chronic, low-grade obstruction of the submucosal veins[20]; or, the lesions result from chronic mucosal ischemia.[21] Spatial clustering of lesions in the gastrointestinal tract suggests that local factors have an important role in pathogenesis regardless of which theory is correct.[22]

Boley and colleagues have been most influential in supporting the first theory for the development of angiodysplasia. By injecting resected colonic specimens with a silicone rubber compound to fill the vascular lesions, these authors have been able to demonstrate consistently certain histopathologic features (Fig. 111-3). Prominent dilated and tortuous submucosal veins are present beneath the angiodysplastic mucosal lesions,[23] and similar submucosal abnormalities also are detected beneath areas where mucosal vessels appear normal.[24] The ectasias themselves consist of dilated, distorted, thin-walled vessels lined by epithelium alone or by a small amount of smooth muscle. The dilated vessels are most consistent with dilated veins, venules, and capillaries, extend very closely to the lumenal surface, and occasionally are not even covered by surface epithelium. Dilated submucosal veins has been one of the most consistent histologic findings and may represent the earliest abnormality in colonic angiodysplasia. This histologic feature supports the theory of chronic venous obstruction in the genesis of angiodysplasia. In more developed lesions, increasing numbers of dilated and deformed vessels are found in the mucosa, nearly replacing normal architecture. Enlarged arteries and thick-walled veins are seen occasionally in large lesions and may represent the maturation of small arteriovenous fistulas resulting from the angiodysplastic changes.[20]

Whether a similar theory of venous obstruction should be proposed for lesions in the stomach and small intestine is less certain; thorough histologic evaluations have not been performed. Marked dilation of submucosal veins and capillaries

has been a consistent histopathologic feature,[15] and a maze of dilated small vessels has been found in typical gastric lesions.[8] These are similar to mucosal features of colonic angiodysplasia. Likewise, ectatic vascular channels can be found in close proximity to the gastric lumen, being covered by only a single layer of surface epithelium (Fig. 111-4).[8] Weaver and associates compared several angiodysplastic lesions from the stomach and right colon and thought that histologic features were indistinguishable between the two locations.[25]

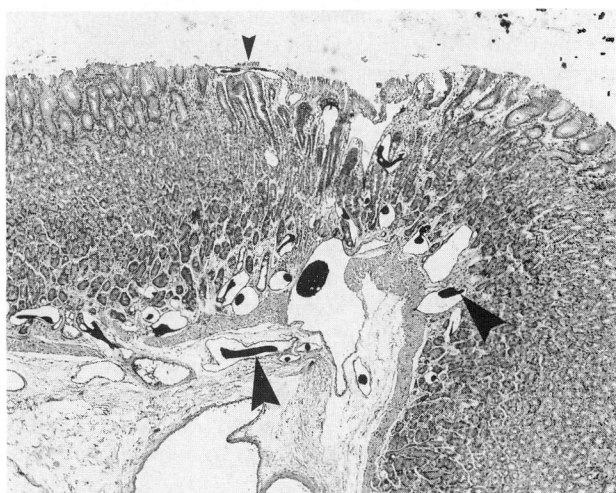

FIGURE 111-4. Gastric angiodysplasia. This surgical specimen was injected with latex (dark material in vascular channels) shortly after resection. Dilated vessels are seen in the mucosa and submucosa (*large arrows*) and immediately beneath surface epithelium (*small arrows*). (From Clouse RE, Costigan DJ, Mills BA, Zuckerman GR. Angiodysplasia as a cause of upper gastrointestinal bleeding. Arch Intern Med 1985;145:458.)

The theory that angiodysplasia may result from chronic hypoxia or hypoperfusion of the mucosa is derived mostly from clinical observation rather than histopathologic correlates. It had long been recognized that gastrointestinal bleeding was associated with aortic valvular disease, and it became apparent that angiodysplastic lesions in both the colon and upper gastrointestinal tract were in part responsible for the association.[19,21,25–27] Mucosal hypoperfusion from the cardiac disease was then postulated. Subsequent analyses indicated that only a few patients with the gastrointestinal lesions have significant valvular heart disease,[8,9,28] an observation potentially related to underrecognition of cardiac disease.[26] Thus, the importance of the cardiac finding in the development of the ectatic vascular lesions remains unclear.

It seems unlikely that hypoperfusion from cardiac disease contributes to the development of angiodysplasia. It is possible, however, that hypoperfusion or hypooxygenation from cardiac or pulmonary disease results in ischemic necrosis of an existing angiodysplastic lesion.[11,29] This seems logical but is not consistent with the observation that low cardiac output is usually a late occurrence in the course of aortic valve disease, and that the low cardiac output associated with mitral stenosis is not associated with a propensity for gastrointestinal bleeding.[30,31] Nevertheless, there is some anecdotal evidence that replacement of the aortic valve in severe aortic stenosis[30] or correction of heart failure in hypertrophic subaortic stenosis[32] halts bleeding from gastrointestinal angiodysplasia. Thus, an association between *aortic valvular disease* and bleeding from existing angiodysplasia of the gastrointestinal tract may have more credence than any theory linking valvular heart disease to development of the vascular lesions.[33]

Other disease associations have been noted with angiodysplasia, but in no case has a direct causal relationship been established. *Chronic renal failure* requiring dialysis was found with an unexpectedly high prevalence in subjects with bleeding upper gastrointestinal tract angiodysplasia,[8,34] but this has not been a consistent finding.[35,36] Coagulopathies that accompany renal failure may be responsible for any apparent association,[37] leaving renal failure with no direct etiologic role in the formation of the vascular lesions. An association of renal failure with colonic angiodysplasia has been occasionally suggested.[38] Likewise, bleeding from angiodysplastic lesions in the upper and lower gastrointestinal tract has been reported in subjects with *von Willebrand's disease.*[39,40] Angiodysplasia and von Willebrand's disease may be linked to a shared mesenchymal disorder,[40] but it seems more likely that the coagulopathy is responsible for bleeding than for development of lesions. Although an acquired form of von Willebrand's disease could explain some clinical observations linking bleeding from angiodysplasia to other medical disorders,[41] measurements usually used to diagnose this coagulation disorder (von Willebrand's antigen, factor VIII, and ristocetin cofactor) were unproductive in one prospective study of angiodysplasia patients.[42]

Clinical Manifestations

Angiodysplasia manifests only through gastrointestinal bleeding. Because lesions may be located throughout the gastrointestinal tract and because bleeding may be brisk or occult, presentation ranges from hematemesis or hematochezia to occult anemia. Despite a tendency for spatial clustering, angiodysplastic lesions often are present in more than one location within the gastrointestinal tract, and presentation may vary during a patient's clinical course. For example, angiodysplasia of the colon is found in at least 15% to 20% of subjects with upper gastrointestinal tract lesions.[8,35] In addition, gastrointestinal hemorrhage from small bowel lesions has occurred in as many as 22% of subjects in whom angiodysplasia of the colon was the presumed source of index bleeding.[43] Even within an organ region, the lesions are often multiple. Forty percent to 60% of subjects with gastric and duodenal lesions have multiple lesions found at endoscopy[8,9]; likewise, angiodysplastic lesions in the colon are more frequently multiple than not.[17,29] To diagnose and manage patients with suspected angiodysplasia, the diffuse location of lesions and the propensity for multiplicity must be taken into account.

For patients with upper tract lesions, hematemesis is a frequent occurrence, but bleeding usually is not life threatening.[6,8] In fact, presentation with hemodynamically well compensated, chronic bleeding is typical and often suggests the diagnosis.[35] Bleeding histories from patients with upper tract lesions can range from days to years.[6,8] Bleeding from colonic lesions also is most often chronic and low grade, but up to 15% of patients present with acute massive hemorrhage.[27] Tarry, melenic stools are passed in at least a quarter of patients with colonic bleeding. A similar variability in presentation is noted for small intestinal angiodysplasia. Patients with lesions in this location also have prolonged bleeding histories, some having been transfused more than 40 units before diagnosis.[14,16] Spontaneous cessation of bleeding is the rule for lesions located in any part of the gastrointestinal tract.

Differential Diagnosis and Diagnostic Studies

The lesions of angiodysplasia are most readily diagnosed by endoscopic studies. Gastric lesions typically have been described as discrete, flat, or slightly raised, 2- to 10-mm, bright red lesions (see Fig. 111-1; see Color Fig. 74). The lesions often have stellate configuration or fern-like margins.[6,8,25,34] Lesions in the proximal small intestine appear similar to those in the stomach but at times are only pin-point in size. A surrounding pale rim or "halo" often is included in the descriptions of upper tract lesions (see Fig. 111-1; see Color Fig. 74).[7] Upper tract lesions can be confused with intramucosal or submucosal hemorrhage.

The endoscopic appearance of the colonic lesions can be quite variable. They are most often discrete and small in size with scalloped or frond-like edges and a visible draining vein (see Fig. 111-2; see Color Fig. 75).[17] The lesions may be flat or slightly raised, and can be well hidden within folds.[19] Angiodysplasia may be detected anywhere in the colon, with a propensity for right colonic location (Fig. 111-5). Injected specimens reveal that these lesions are usually less than 10 mm in diameter.[29] Small lesions with a pale coloration may be encountered as incidental findings,[44,45] whereas the elevated centers of very bright lesions appear related to recent hemorrhage.[46]

Despite this typical endoscopic appearance, angiodysplasia can be confused with the ectasias associated with systemic

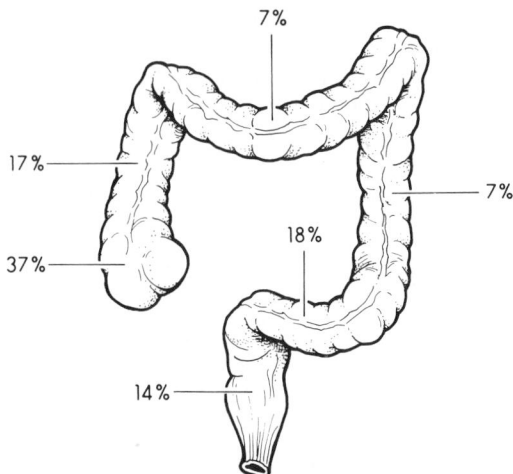

FIGURE 111-5. Distribution of colonic angiodyplastic lesions in one series of 59 patients. Over one half of the lesions were found in the cecum and ascending colon. (Data from Hochter W, Weingart J, Kuhner W, et al. Angiodysplasia in the colon and rectum: endoscopic morphology, localisation and frequency. Endoscopy 1985;17:182.)

disease. Although hereditary hemorrhagic telangiectasia (HHT) cannot be excluded by endoscopic or histologic criteria, the other characteristic extraintestinal lesions seen with HHT are not present. Likewise, the small vascular lesions seen in association with pseudoxanthoma elasticum, Ehlers-Danlos syndrome, and the CREST syndrome (i.e., calcinosis, Raynaud's phenomenon, esophageal hypomotility, sclerodactyly, and telangiectasia) may also show striking resem-

blance to angiodysplasia and can be differentiated only by the other clinical features that typify these systemic disorders.

Diagnosis of gastric and duodenal lesions is made almost exclusively by endoscopy. Celiac artery and superior mesenteric artery injections frequently fail to demonstrate these lesions, although large lesions with well formed and enlarged draining veins have been reported in the gastric antrum.[8,15,26,47] Angiography has demonstrated successfully lesions in the more distal small intestine and is very useful in this region less accessible to endoscopic evaluation.[15,48]

Colonic lesions may be detected either by angiography or colonoscopy. Colonoscopy may overdiagnose angiodysplasia, misinterpreting other discrete, red lesions as vascular ectasias.[49] Because colonoscopy is a principal tool in the evaluation of gastrointestinal hemorrhage, however, diagnosis often originates from colonoscopic examination. Comparative studies using selective angiography and colonoscopy indicate that the sensitivity of colonoscopy exceeds 80% when the lesions are located in the area examined by colonoscopy.[17,50] Most angiodysplastic lesions are located in the right colon, so it is essential that the entire colon be examined.[50] Angiography has the advantage of detecting additional angiodysplastic lesions not visualized by colonoscopy. In one series, 17% of subjects were found to have concomitant colonic and extracolonic angiodysplasia when studied by triple-vessel angiography.[51] Thus, angiography and colonoscopy can play important complementary roles.

Three angiographic signs typify angiodysplasia in any part of the intestinal tract (Fig. 111-6):

1. The most frequent sign is that of a densely opacified, dilated, and slowly emptying draining vein within the in-

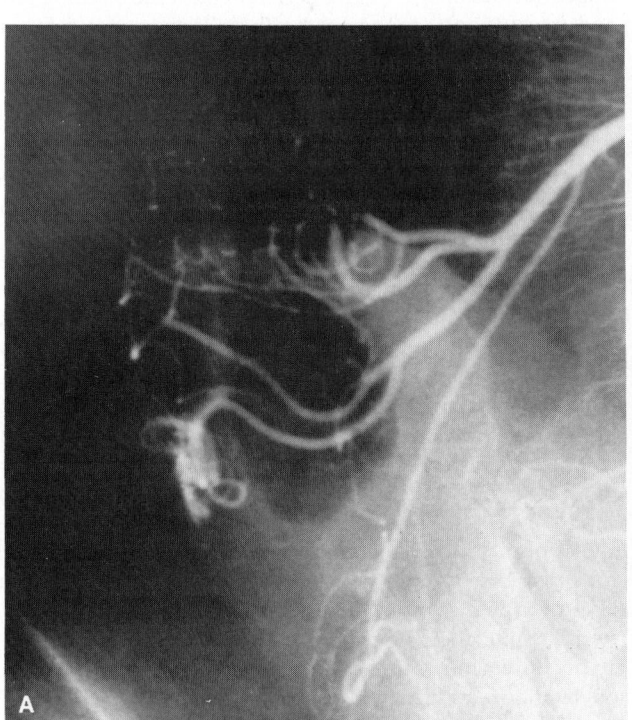
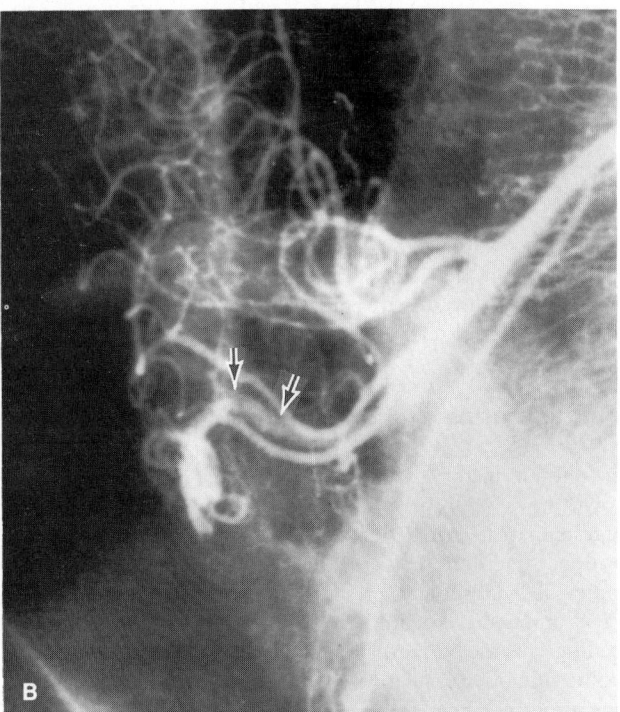

FIGURE 111-6. Mesenteric angiogram in a patient with angiodysplasia. **(A)** The vascular tuft of angiodysplasia is apparent in the cecum. **(B)** A draining vein from the same lesion becomes apparent while the injection is still in the arterial phase. (Courtesy of Daniel D. Picus, M.D., St. Louis, MO.)

testinal wall. This vein is detected in the venous phase of the study and is present in nearly all subjects with the other angiographic findings.

2. A vascular tuft may become apparent during the arterial phase of the study, representing an extension of the dilation process to the mucosal venules.

3. An early filling vein may be seen in the arterial phase, indicating a more developed arteriovenous communication through the angiodysplastic lesion.

The latter two angiographic signs are seen in 60% to 80% of the colonic lesions, but their prevalence has been recorded less systematically in other parts of the intestinal tract.[18] Although all three findings typify angiodysplasia, they occasionally also are found in other disorders, including malignancy[52]; careful interpretation is required, taking into account all clinical information. Extravasation of angiographic dye, a very useful finding in patients being evaluated for severe bleeding, is seen in only 10% to 20% of patients bleeding from colonic angiodysplasia because of the episodic nature of bleeding from these lesions.[18]

Several specialized diagnostic tests have been used in the evaluation of angiodysplastic lesions. Radionuclide scanning using technetium 99m–labeled red blood cells may be helpful in detecting and localizing active bleeding from angiodysplasia, especially when the data are reviewed on a cinematic display.[53,54] The intermittent bleeding nature of angiodysplasia has limited the utility of radionuclide studies in this disorder. Positive findings from a radionuclide study should be confirmed by colonoscopy or, in most cases, angiography if surgical resection is being planned. Angiography of resected specimens also has been used to confirm appropriate resection when preoperative studies are equivocal or unsatisfactory.[55] This form of post hoc diagnosis should be reserved for unusual cases, but was developed because of the difficulty in detecting the lesions histologically. An intralumenal formalin fixation technique on the resected specimen followed by mucosal dissection is another method for documenting correct resection.[56] Small bowel enteroscopy and intraoperative enteroscopy have both helped in the localization of distal small bowel lesions.[57-61] In addition, an angiographic catheter can be placed before surgery into the appropriate feeding vessel to the angiodysplastic lesion.[62] The surgeon can then identify the catheter during surgery and explore and resect the appropriate small bowel segment.

Clinical Course and Complications

The natural history of untreated lesions is incompletely known; however, retrospective review of bleeding histories suggests that the course remains indolent in many patients. For upper tract lesions, over a mean follow-up period of 14 months, 50% of subjects presenting initially with some form of gastrointestinal bleeding had at least one subsequent frank bleeding episode.[8] Likewise, half of subjects with bleeding colonic angiodysplasia treated only with observation and transfusion continued to have bleeding episodes over the next several years.[63] But the fact that one third to one half of subjects do *not* appear to have repeat bleeding episodes in the first 2 years after presentation with gastrointestinal hemor-

rhage must be taken into account when evaluating any therapeutic modality.

The natural history of incidental angiodysplastic lesions discovered at colonoscopy[17] remains unknown; however, because mucosal ectasias can be demonstrated in more than 25% of subjects older than 60 years of age when resected colonic specimens are injected with silicone rubber material,[29] it seems prudent to assume that these lesions remain asymptomatic through life in most patients. Supervention of a bleeding disorder or possibly a medical illness such as renal failure may precipitate bleeding from angiodysplasia in some patients.

Therapy

Gastric and duodenal angiodysplastic lesions have been managed most frequently with endoscopic obliteration techniques. Monopolar electrocautery can destroy the lesions, but frank bleeding recurs in as many as 50% of subjects (presumably from other areas of angiodysplasia), and the reduction in posttherapy transfusion requirement is not statistically superior to no specific therapy.[8,64] The multiplicity of angiodysplastic lesions undoubtedly contributes to this observation. Other obliteration techniques, such as heater probe or multipolar coagulation devices, may have more favorable results.[65] Sclerotherapy using 0.5 to 1 mL of 1.5% sodium tetradecyl sulfate also has been used successfully to obliterate upper tract lesions, but bleeding recurred in half the subjects. In each case the bleeding appeared to arise from new or previously unrecognized areas of angiodysplasia.[7] Argon and neodymium–yttrium-aluminum-garnet (Nd-YAG) lasers possibly are the most beneficial endoscopic obliteration instruments for upper tract lesions.[65-67] A reduction in both the bleeding rate and transfusion requirement has been demonstrated for at least 12 months after laser therapy. Effectiveness appears reduced in patients with more numerous angiodysplastic lesions, with coagulation disorders, and possibly in older age,[66,68] and rebleeding commonly occurs over time.[68]

Colonic lesions also have been managed by endoscopic obliteration. Monopolar electrocoagulation appears relatively safe in this setting and may help control acute bleeding episodes, but its long-term efficacy remains in question. The rebleeding rate approximates 50%, and the transfusion requirement resembles that of patients receiving no therapy.[63,64] The heater probe and the multipolar electrocoagulation probe may be more beneficial for these lesions.[69] As for the upper gastrointestinal tract lesions, endoscopic laser photocoagulation has shown promising results in controlling bleeding from colonic angiodysplasia.[70,71] Significant complications occur in up to 15% of patients and are particularly common when the Nd-YAG laser is used in the right colon.[66,70] Deeper coagulation of the vascular abnormalities may be responsible for better results (and more frequent complications) from laser therapy than from other forms of endoscopic obliteration. Despite good short-term results, the cumulative probability of remaining free of bleeding at 24 months after laser obliteration is less than 60% for patients with colonic lesions.[68]

Angiography can be used for control of acute hemorrhage from angiodysplasia, although it is seldom necessary. In some severely ill patients who are not candidates for surgical intervention, transcatheter embolization after selective cannulation of branches of the mesenteric arteries has been successfully accomplished using Gelfoam (Upjohn, Kalamazoo, MI).[72] The rate of serious complications is sufficiently high that the use of transcatheter embolization must be weighed against the risk of surgery even in the seriously ill patient.[72] Selective infusion of vasopressin is less effective than embolization as a definitive therapy because of a high rebleeding rate.[73] Angiography appears to play a more important role in the preoperative localization of small bowel lesions immediately before surgical resection, because intraoperative palpation, endoscopy, and visual inspection through multiple enterotomies are of little value in this disease.[74,75] A variety of techniques have been used, including placement of the angiographic catheter in a very distal arterial branch that feeds the angiodysplastic lesion, injection of dyes such as methylene blue, indigo carmine, or fluorescein, and even intraoperative angiography.[62,76–80]

Surgical resection is used as definitive therapy if the bleeding lesion is identified clearly with diagnostic studies. As with endoscopic obliteration techniques, however, surgical treatment may provide only short-term benefits. Partial or complete gastrectomy has been infrequently reported for the management of gastric angiodysplasia, but subsequent bleeding occurs in up to 50% of patients.[6,8,25] Surgical resection is also beneficial for some patients with colonic lesions, but is not curative for all. In one series, 8 subjects underwent surgical resection of the identified lesion, but 2 rebled within 3 months of resection.[28] In a series with longer follow-up (mean of 3.6 years), 63% of the subjects remained free of intestinal bleeding after right hemicolectomy, whereas 6 subjects (37%) had some degree of recurrent bleeding.[26] A trend toward reduced transfusion requirements has been observed in patients with angiodysplasia who have undergone surgical management.[64] This same trend, however, was seen in subjects who had undergone electrocoagulation as the only mode of therapy or who had received no specific intervention.[64] Thus, surgical resection seems most appropriate for acute management of severe hemorrhage or for the management of recurrent hemorrhage over a relatively short time period accompanied by a large transfusion requirement. Because of these clinical observations, a graduated approach to management has been recommended, using iron replacement therapy and endoscopic obliteration techniques when required, while reserving surgical intervention for particularly problematic patients.

Several other management techniques have been tried in some situations. Although the true relationship of aortic stenosis to angiodysplasia remains in question,[33] several case reports have illustrated a dramatic cessation in bleeding from angiodysplastic lesions in both the upper and lower gastrointestinal tract after aortic valve replacement.[30,81,82] One series also suggested that the failure rate from bowel resection for angiodysplasia is higher in the subset of patients with aortic stenosis (80%).[83] In that same series, aortic valve replacement effectively terminated gastrointestinal bleeding in 93% of subjects, although the presence of angiodysplasia was not established completely in most patients.[83] These observations need further documentation, but certainly aortic valve replacement with a bioprosthesis (not requiring anticoagulation) should not be delayed because of recurrent bleeding from angiodysplasia in patients with sufficiently severe aortic stenosis to require operation. In fact, valve replacement might

result in reduction or cessation of gastrointestinal blood loss. Some subjects have undergone repeat endoscopic examinations after aortic valve replacement, and the angiodysplastic lesions persist.[25,30,84]

Estrogen–progesterone therapy, previously used to treat bleeding associated with hereditary hemorrhagic telangiectasia,[85,86] also has been tried in patients with gastrointestinal bleeding from angiodysplasia. Suggested mechanisms by which hormonal therapy might affect bleeding include improvement in coagulation, alterations in the microvascular circulation, and improvements in endothelial integrity.[87] Seven patients with chronic renal failure and bleeding angiodysplastic lesions in the stomach or colon were treated with a synthetic estrogen–progesterone combination (norethynodrel and mestranol) for 4 to 28 months (mean of 12 months).[87] Bleeding ceased in all patients over the follow-up period. Likewise, estrogen–progesterone therapy was found abruptly to stop persistent gastrointestinal bleeding from angiodysplasia in 1 subject without chronic renal failure.[88] Data from a double-blinded, crossover trial using 0.05 mg ethinylestradiol and 1 mg norethisterone given daily to 10 elderly patients with gastrointestinal ectasias (6 of the patients had hereditary hemorrhagic telangiectasia) have indicated that the combination significantly reduces bleeding and transfusion requirements.[89] A subsequent cohort study of 64 patients with angiodysplasia could not show a benefit of hormonal therapy.[90] In that study, 30 patients were given 5 to 10 mg of norethynodrel with mestranol (0.075–0.15 mg) or with conjugated estrogens (0.625 mg), and the bleeding rates were compared before and after therapy and with bleeding rates of historical controls or of patients who refused therapy. Consequently, the efficacy of hormonal therapy for angiodysplasia has not been fully established. Potential side effects of hormonal therapy, such as gynecomastia, are of concern.[89] In the cohort study, vaginal bleeding, fluid retention, and a cerebrovascular accident were attributed to treatment (23% of the treated patients).[90]

One additional clinical observation deserves mention: Subjects with underlying coagulation defects tend to do poorly no matter what therapeutic maneuver is used. Poor outcomes from electrocoagulation with subsequent hemorrhage have been reported.[91] Concomitant correction or attenuation of hemostatic defects may be beneficial, and should be a component of the management program.[39]

Gastric Antral Vascular Ectasia: The "Watermelon Stomach"

Gastric antral vascular ectasia represents a discrete vascular abnormality in the distal stomach that appears distinct from other vascular ectasia disorders. This uncommon lesion has been recognized only comparatively recently. As of 1987, 43 cases compatible with the diagnosis had been described[92]; the number is slowly increasing, primarily from case reports containing few patients. The term "watermelon stomach" derives from the striking endoscopic appearance of parallel, longitudinal, red columns that traverse the gastric antrum and resemble the stripes on a watermelon (Fig. 111-7; see Color Fig. 76).[93]

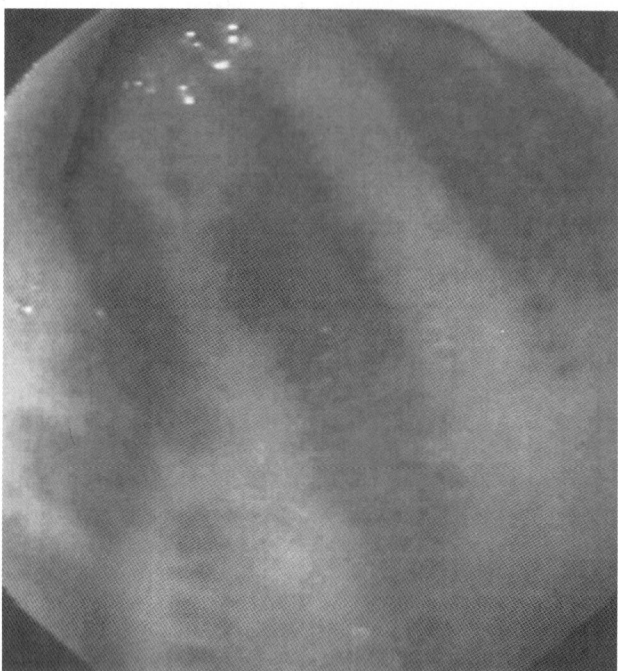

FIGURE 111-7. (See Color Fig. 76.) Gastric antral vascular ectasia was detected in a 73-year-old woman with chronic iron-deficiency anemia and occult fecal blood. Intensely red stripes (dark bands) alternate with areas of more normal mucosa, providing the watermelon appearance.

compartment (an effect that would promote the fibromuscular hyperplasia observed histologically in this lesion). Prostaglandin E_2 has vasodilator- and acid-inhibitory effects, and also may play a role in pathogenesis. Biosynthesis of this prostanoid is elevated in the antral mucosa of cirrhotic patients with antral ectasias compared with cirrhotic patients who do not have vascular abnormalities.[107] Local neurotransmitter release also may be partially responsible for the observed vasodilation. Proliferation of extraepithelial and intraepithelial neuroendocrine cells containing large quantities of 5-hydroxytryptamine and vasoactive intestinal polypeptide has been well demonstrated by immunohistochemical and electron-microscopic studies of an antral resection specimen.[108] Considering the current state of understanding, these observations simply may be epiphenomena not directly related to lesion development.

Examination of gastrectomy specimens has revealed typical and consistent findings. The mucosa appears to be mobile and loosely attached to underlying gastric muscularis propria.[93] Microscopically, the antral mucosa is hypertrophied and folded. The glands themselves are hyperplastic with irregular surface plications, and mild chronic inflammation can be detected. The more striking feature is the maze of dilated vascular channels located primarily in the submucosa, with some penetration into the mucosa (Fig. 111-8). The lesion is predominantly composed of dilated, tortuous, thin-walled veins. Focal thrombosis is observed in dilated mucosal vascular channels, and fibromuscular hyperplasia is apparent within

Epidemiology, Etiology, and Pathology

As with angiodysplasia, antral vascular ectasia is seen commonly in an older age group, with the mean age of presentation approximating 70 years.[93–95] In contradistinction to angiodysplasia, however, this disorder predominates in women (4 : 1, female : male).[92–105] The well-developed lesion with typical endoscopic appearance may be quite rare; in one series it was detected 3 times in 10,000 upper endoscopic examinations.[93] Now that endoscopists are aware of this lesion, better estimates of its prevalence will likely appear.

The etiology of gastric antral vascular ectasia is unknown. It frequently has been associated with hepatic cirrhosis (in more than one third of cases) and with achlorhydria or severe hypochlorhydria in at least 40% of cases.[92] The hypochlorhydria, at least in those with concomitant cirrhosis, usually is not accompanied by morphologic evidence of gastric atrophy.[106] Scleroderma and other connective tissue diseases probably also are present in patients with gastric antral vascular ectasia at a higher rate than would be expected by chance.[94–98] No disease association, however, has been strong enough to provide a distinct clue as to the etiology of this finding, and, in fact, several different mechanisms may be responsible for the histologic and physiologic manifestations.

Because of the hypochlorhydria, hypergastrinemia has been postulated as participating in the development of the lesion, and has been detected in as many as 75% of patients.[98] Hypergastrinemia also has been detected in a significantly higher proportion of cirrhotic patients with gastric ectasias than in those without.[99] Gastrin does have a gastric vasodilation effect and could possibly have a trophic effect on the spindle cell

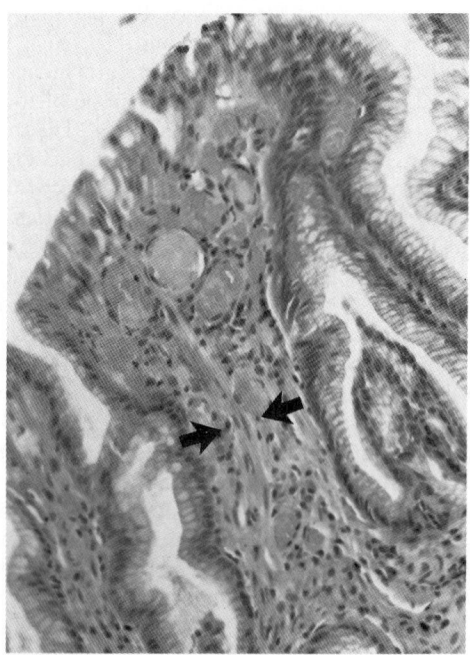

FIGURE 111-8. Endoscopic mucosal biopsy specimen from a patient with gastric antral vascular ectasia. Ectatic vascular channels are seen just beneath the surface epithelium. Spindle cell proliferation extends into the superficial mucosa in the region of the ectatic vessels (*arrows*). (From Gilliam JH III, Geisinger KR, Wu WC, et al. Endoscopic biopsy is diagnostic in gastric antral vascular ectasia: the "watermelon stomach." Dig Dis Sci 1989;34:885.)

the lamina propria.[93,95,100] The lesion itself appears to be restricted to the gastric antrum.

Clinical Manifestations and Diagnosis

Nearly all subjects with gastric antral vascular ectasia have presented with iron deficiency anemia.[92–98,102–104,109] The mean duration of anemia before diagnosis was 2 years in one series,[105] but histories exceeding 20 years have been reported.[103,105] Overt gastrointestinal bleeding with melena has been noted, but does not dominate the clinical picture. In contrast, severe iron deficiency anemia that requires repeated transfusions and is refractory to oral iron therapy is typical. In contradistinction to angiodysplasia, vascular ectasias in other parts of the gastrointestinal tract rarely have been reported in patients with this gastric lesion.[96,98]

Diagnosis is made primarily by the distinctive endoscopic appearance of this lesion. In the typical case, parallel, intensely red stripes are noted in the gastric antrum. These linear marks are on the crests of longitudinal folds and alternate with a paler, normal-appearing antral mucosa providing the striped, watermelon appearance (see Fig. 111-7; see Color Fig. 76). Visible, convoluted columns of small ectatic vessels produce the red component.[93] The ectatic vessels may on occasion have a patchy distribution in the antrum,[95] but the striped appearance is more typical.[93–95] The red linear streaks can be differentiated from an antral gastritis with a high-resolution endoscope[102] or by noting that the vascular channels blanch when compressed with a biopsy forceps.[94]

Nonspecific prominence of antral folds on an upper gastrointestinal series or thickening of the antral wall by computed tomography are the only radiographic correlates.[110] Despite the large number of vascular channels in antral vascular ectasia, angiography has not been a useful diagnostic tool.[94,96,102] The tortuous, enlarged draining veins seen in angiodysplasia are not a component of this lesion. A pattern of antral hypervascularity arising from the gastroduodenal artery has been noted on one occasion.[104]

Endoscopic biopsy can be safely performed, although a greater degree of bleeding than expected from a mucosal biopsy can occur.[93] A systematic comparison of mucosal biopsies from antral vascular ectasia and controls with other antral lesions indicates that sufficiently distinctive histopathologic features are present to allow recognition of this disorder by endoscopic biopsy alone in most cases.[100,101] Significant differences in mean vessel cross-sectional area, percentage of mucosal area occupied by vascular channels, the presence of intravascular fibrin thrombi, and presence of fibromuscular hyperplasia were found when comparing biopsies from antral vascular ectasia to the other specimens. The endoscopist should take both visual inspection and histologic results into consideration when making the diagnosis, because the biopsy findings may be insufficient in some situations.[111]

Therapy

Maintenance of normal hemoglobin with oral iron replacement therapy may be adequate in some patients, because no outcome other than gastrointestinal bleeding is recognized from this lesion. Iron replacement therapy, however, appears to be unsatisfactory in most cases. As for angiodysplasia, sur-

gical, endoscopic, and medical approaches to treatment have been used. Unlike angiodysplasia, the localized nature of antral vascular ectasia makes surgical intervention a more attractive alternative. Antrectomy with Billroth I anastomosis has been the most successfully reported therapy to date.[92] Rebleeding or recurrence of anemia is almost uniformly absent in follow-up periods of up to 2 years after resection.

Many patients with this disorder are not good surgical candidates because of age or overt concomitant medical illness. The lesion is easily approached endoscopically, and obliteration techniques, including heater probe[100,112] and Nd-YAG or argon laser therapy,[105,113–115] have been used. The value of electrocoagulation or heater probe coagulation would seem limited considering the expanse of the ectasia lesion, but all 12 patients in one series were successfully managed with the heater probe after an average of four treatment sessions.[112] Results from endoscopic laser trials are equally encouraging; an increment in hemoglobin (mean 4.0 g/dL) occurred in 12 treated subjects over a mean follow-up period of 6 months.[105] Although both argon and Nd-YAG lasers appear effective, the latter results in obliteration of the vascular lesion with fewer treatment sessions.[113] Although multiple treatment sessions will be required, sufficient data are available to indicate that endoscopic obliteration techniques should be attempted before surgical intervention in most instances. Complications are uncommonly reported,[113] but circumferential scarring with stenosis, ulceration, and hemorrhage could occur.

Information regarding medical treatment of this disorder is scant. At least temporary control of bleeding has been reported after prednisolone therapy in a small number of patients with antral vascular ectasia, possibly by reversing gastric atrophy, improving acid secretion, and reducing hypergastrinemia.[103,104,116–118] Maintenance of one patient on an estrogen–progesterone regimen (ethinylestradiol 30 µg and norethisterone 1.5 mg daily for 3 weeks per month) was accompanied by a marked reduction in blood transfusion.[118] The actual mechanism for this seemingly positive effect in management of ectasia disorders is not known, and the benefits are not fully proven. In response to the observation that serotonin-containing neuroendocrine cell proliferation may play a role in the pathogenesis of antral vascular ectasia,[108] one group offered ciproheptadine, 4 mg orally three times per day, to a single patient with this lesion.[119] Bleeding resolved and the vascular lesion partially regressed by serial endoscopic evaluation. Although encouraging, medical treatments are still at an anecdotal level, and their use should be considered secondary to the other available approaches.

Telangiectasia Associated With Multisystem Disease

Hereditary Hemorrhagic Telangiectasia

This familial disease is characterized by small vascular ectasias of skin and mucous membranes and by recurrent episodes of gastrointestinal bleeding. The disorder is known also as Osler-Weber-Rendu disease because of the initial independent descriptions of the syndrome by these authors. The gastrointestinal lesions are called telangiectasias so as to not confuse them with isolated angiodysplasia. Although the venules in telangiectasias of HHT may be thick with well-developed longitudinal muscles,[120] it is the general consensus that these vascular lesions cannot be differentiated from angiodysplastic lesions on histologic grounds.[121] The disorder is inherited in an autosomal dominant fashion.

Telangiectasias occur on the skin, on the mucous membranes, and in internal organs. Usually lesions are noted in the first few years of life, and recurrent epistaxis in childhood is characteristic. Gastrointestinal hemorrhage often does not become manifest until the fourth decade of life, and it occurs in at least 15% of patients.[122,123] Typical clinical features that help identify the patient with HHT include family history (up to 80% of patients), telangiectasias on the lips, oral and nasopharyngeal membranes, tongue, and hands (nearly all patients with gastrointestinal bleeding), and pulmonary arteriovenous fistulas (up to 20% of subjects).[18,124] When evaluating the patient with gastrointestinal bleeding from telangiectasia, a systematic skin examination must be performed to establish a diagnosis of HHT, because there is no specific relationship between the site or number of skin lesions and presence of gastrointestinal bleeding (Table 111-2).[124]

Gastrointestinal bleeding usually manifests as melena and occasionally as hematemesis.[125] Because recurrent epistaxis is so common in this patient population, melanotic stools may not be related always to gastrointestinal bleeding. Lesions may be found throughout the gastrointestinal tract, and presentation (even during the course of an individual patient) is quite variable. The endoscopic appearance of gastric and colonic lesions seen in HHT can be identical to that of angiodysplasia,[27] although HHT lesions may appear at times more nodular. Angiography has been less useful in detecting the ectatic lesions of HHT, and an aggressive endoscopic approach to diagnosis usually is necessary.[126]

The management of gastrointestinal bleeding in HHT can be very difficult owing to the multiplicity of lesions. More lesions usually are found in the upper intestinal tract than in the lower, and upper tract bleeding is the most significant problem in these patients. Endoscopic obliteration techniques

---

TABLE 111-2

Location of Telangiectasias on Skin and Mucous Membranes in a Series of Patients With Hereditary Hemorrhagic Telangiectasia

LOCATION	PERCENTAGE OF PATIENTS
Skin	
Hands or feet	67
Face	55
Chest	39
Mucous Membranes	
Nose	78
Lips	70
Tongue	62
Cheek	53
Palate	32
Conjunctiva	9

Adapted from Reilly PJ, Nostrant TT. Clinical manifestations of hereditary hemorrhagic telangiectasia. Am J Gastroenterol 1984;79:363.

---

have been used with similar results in HHT as for angiodysplasia. The most promising data have been with the use of endoscopic lasers; bleeding was successfully controlled in 9 of 10 patients with HHT over a mean follow-up period of 15 months.[127] Because of the multiplicity of lesions in this syndrome, surgery should be reserved for problematic bleeding from a site that is well localized by angiography.[128] Estrogen–progesterone therapy has been used to reduce epistaxis in this syndrome,[85,86,125] but its use for gastrointestinal hemorrhage has been limited.[89] It appears that obliteration of large or recently bleeding lesions with the endoscopic laser may have the most promise.

Other Telangiectasia Syndromes

Gastrointestinal telangiectasias are a well-recognized component of progressive systemic sclerosis and related connective tissue diseases, such as the *CREST syndrome*.[2] In this disorder, the lesions are most common on the hands, lips, face, and tongue. Gastrointestinal hemorrhage has been reported from telangiectasias in the stomach, colon, and rectum.[129,130] Clinically significant bleeding can be managed with the endoscopic obliteration techniques used in the management of angiodysplasia. Gastrointestinal telangiectasias have been detected at a low frequency in *Turner's syndrome*.[131,132] The lesions can be present throughout the intestinal tract, but may have a predilection for the small intestine. A conservative approach has been recommended because the gastrointestinal vascular lesions in Turner's syndrome tend to regress with time.[2]

VASCULAR TUMORS

Hemangiomas

Hemangiomas are hamartomatous vascular growths that can be found throughout the gastrointestinal tract. The lesions appear at birth, or shortly after birth, and then enlarge with normal organ growth. Lesions may be single or multiple and may be associated with hemangiomas in other organs or on the skin. Both histologic and clinical features can differentiate *capillary* hemangiomas from *cavernous* hemangiomas. In some cases, the histologic lesion shows a mixture of both types.

Epidemiology

Hemangiomas are uncommon. They represent only 5% to 10% of the benign neoplasms in the small intestine,[133] where they are equally distributed between the jejunum and ileum. Duodenal hemangiomas are rare.[134] Colonic hemangiomas also are uncommon, with most symptomatic tumors arising distally in the rectum and rectosigmoid.[135] Hemangiomas usually present in young men and women, often in the third decade of life. A hereditary predisposition usually is not observed, although some familial cases have been reported.

Pathology

Hemangiomas arise from submucosal vascular plexuses and present as two distinct histologic types, capillary and cavernous. The capillary lesion is uncommon, is usually solitary, and has a predilection for the small intestine, appendix, and perianal skin.[135,136] Tiny vessels, the caliber of normal capillaries, are closely packed in these small lesions into clusters separated by a scant connective tissue stroma that is deficient in elastin.[137] The vessels are lined by a well-differentiated, hyperplastic endothelium. Although the lesions are well circumscribed, they are not encapsulated.[137]

Cavernous hemangiomas have large, thin-walled vascular channels, in contrast to the capillary variety.[135,137] As with capillary hemangiomas, the endothelial lining is hyperplastic, and the sinuses are supported by scant connective tissue septa. Thrombosis within sinuses may lead to hyalinization and calcification.[2] These hemangiomas can remain polypoid (circumscribed). Alternatively, they may become expansive so as to replace the intestinal wall from serosa to mucosa, extend through as much as 20 to 30 cm of intestinal length, and encroach on the intestinal lumen (diffuse). Cavernous lesions are most frequently diffuse and located in the large intestine (70% of these are in the rectum).[135] A mixed lesion with both capillary and cavernous histologic features has been recognized in stomach, small intestine, or appendix.[135]

Although these vascular lesions are considered usually to be congenital hamartomas, independent growth characteristics, particularly of cavernous hemangiomas, suggest that hemangiomas are true neoplastic tumors.[135,137] Nevertheless, it is agreed generally that these lesions initiate as embryonic developmental errors.

Clinical Manifestations

These tumors often are discovered incidentally or because of their potential for bleeding. Bleeding from capillary lesions tends to be slow and may be occult.[136,138] In contrast, up to 90% of patients with cavernous hemangiomas have overt bleeding.[135,136,139,140] In fact, because of their large vascular channels, cavernous hemangiomas may present with brisk or massive recurrent bleeding, and death from exsanguination has occurred.[136,138,141] The bleeding history often dates back to childhood and frequently exceeds 10 years.[142]

Other clinical manifestations include pain from intussusception of polypoid tumors and symptoms of obstruction from large annular or diffuse rectal lesions.[135,136,143,144] Intramural or retroperitoneal bleeding may complicate large cavernous lesions. Impaired coagulation from thrombocytopenia and low serum fibrinogen levels also is recognized in association with hemangiomas,[145] and a microangiopathic hemolytic anemia can occur.[146] Additional lesions are detected on the lips and perianal skin and in the oral cavity in a large proportion of patients,[137,147,148] and approximately 10% of subjects have multiple intestinal tract lesions.[149-155] Intestinal hemangiomas may also be part of specific multisystem syndromes (see Multiple Hemangioma Syndromes).

Differential Diagnosis and Diagnostic Studies

Although these lesions are rare, they must be considered in the differential diagnosis of gastrointestinal bleeding. Hemangiomas in the stomach are very uncommon, but symptoms may mimic peptic disease, carcinoma,[149] or intermittent pyloric obstruction.[150] Small intestinal polypoid hemangiomas

could be confused with other, more frequent benign neoplasms of the small intestine (e.g., leiomyoma, lipoma, and adenoma), and because of the rarity of these lesions, they are misdiagnosed frequently. The colorectal lesions have been mistaken for carcinoma, internal hemorrhoids, inflammatory bowel disease, tuberculosis, and amebiasis.[137,156]

Small hemangiomas may be diagnosed most readily by endoscopic visualization, whereas the diagnosis of larger tumors often is established by mesenteric arteriography. Physical examination contributes only if the bulk of large gastric or colonic lesions is detected by abdominal examination, if a soft compressible mass is detected by digital rectal examination, or if the cutaneous manifestations mentioned previously are present. Focal calcific densities discovered on plain films of the abdomen also can be important indicators of a cavernous lesion (Fig. 111-9).[136,138] These calcific densities represent phlebolith formation in dilated sinuses, are most frequently found in the rectum, and also have been detected in large extracolonic lesions.[151] Phleboliths may be present normally in the pelvis and spleen, but those appearing in clusters and in atypical locations should alert the clinician to the possibility of a hemangioma.

Diagnosis is made most typically by endoscopic visualization and more elaborate radiologic techniques. The endoscopic appearance of rectal hemangiomas is that of a bluish or wine-colored submucosal mass resembling nodular dilated veins (that collapse with air insufflation).[136,152] Small cavernous lesions may resemble bluish-colored polyps, whereas the capillary hemangioma appears as a bright red spot or nodule on the mucosal surface (Fig. 111-10; see Color Fig. 77).[140] When lesions cannot be defined adequately by endoscopic methods, arteriography may help determine a site of active bleeding and accurately delimit the size of a hemangioma

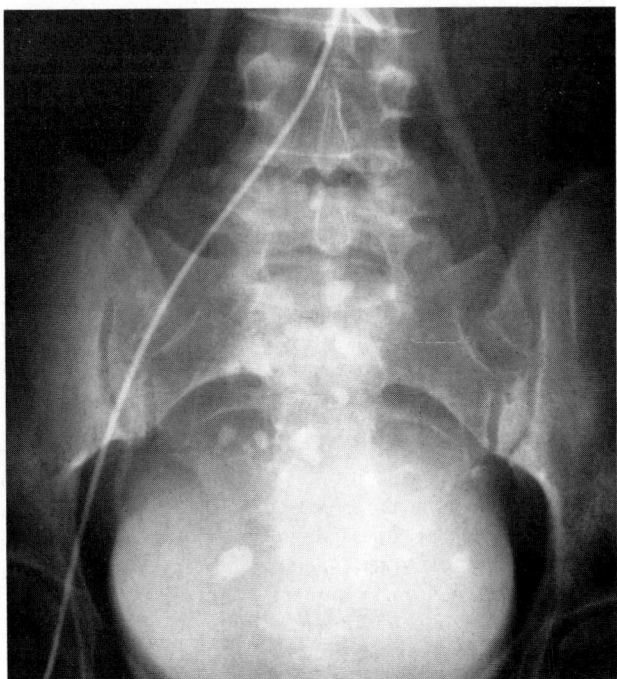

FIGURE 111-9. Scattered calcifications represent phleboliths in a large colonic cavernous hemangioma.

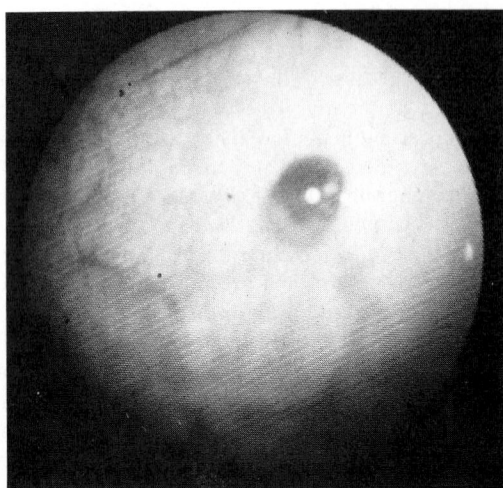

FIGURE 111-10. (See Color Fig. 77.) A 3- to 4-mm capillary hemangioma with a smooth, round appearance was detected during colonoscopy.

before surgical intervention. Arteriography is successful in identifying large cavernous lesions in two thirds of cases.[153] A puddling of contrast in the venous phase is a typical finding.[136] Computed tomography may help identify and delineate large cavernous lesions of the rectosigmoid.[153] Computed tomography also may be helpful in detecting local adherence to adjacent organs and bony structures, enhancing preoperative preparation.[153]

Therapy

These lesions usually require surgical management. Smaller polypoid lesions may be removed by local excision or fulguration, but most symptomatic or significant hemangiomas are large, cavernous, and sessile, making them unamenable to endoscopic manipulations. Although smaller lesions have been removed safely with the colonoscope, endoscopic biopsy and fulguration can result in massive hemorrhage or perforation.[152] Larger lesions present more typically with significant bleeding and require surgical intervention. A variety of procedures have been recommended, particularly for the colonic lesions.[137,157] Alternative treatments have been used in unresectable cases. These approaches include injection of sclerosants,[136,155] cryosurgery,[143] radium implantation,[152] and ablation of arterial supply,[136,152,158] but are unreliable and provide temporary control at best in most cases. Spontaneous involution of hemangiomas occurs rarely.[154]

Multiple-Hemangioma Syndromes

Multiple intestinal hemangiomas are detected in up to 10% of subjects who have these vascular tumors. *Intestinal hemangiomatosis* most often refers to cases in which many hemangiomas (at times hundreds) are detected.[159] This syndrome may present in infancy or childhood,[159] and hemangiomas can be found to involve all parts of the intestinal tract.[160] Most often these tumors are of the cavernous histologic type. Even more extensive studding of the skin, brain, and viscera with hemangiomas is seen in *universal heman-*

giomatosis or *diffuse neonatal hemangiomatosis.*[161] This syndrome is very rare and fatal in infancy in all but exceptional cases.[162]

The *blue rubber bleb nevus syndrome* is an unusual syndrome manifesting as cutaneous and intestinal cavernous hemangiomas. The condition was given this peculiar name because the cutaneous hemangiomas have the appearance and feel of rubber nipples.[163] Several to several hundred cutaneous lesions (up to 10 cm in size) are observed.[164] Although most of the cutaneous lesions have the blue, rubbery nipple appearance, larger disfiguring hemangiomas and darker, flat macules or papules also may be seen. The limbs, trunk, and face are the main sites of cutaneous involvement, and these lesions often are present at birth or appear in childhood. This syndrome usually is not a familial disorder, but several cases with familial transmission in an autosomal dominant pattern have been observed.[165] The syndrome occurs only rarely in those of African descent.[166]

Although extracutaneous lesions have been described occasionally in liver, lung, eye, central nervous system, and peritoneal cavity, gastrointestinal tract involvement with the hemangiomas of blue rubber bleb nevus syndrome is very common.[167] In fact, the original report of this disease by Gascoyen more than a century ago included gastrointestinal bleeding.[168] Lesions are found throughout the intestinal tract,[165] most commonly in the small intestine. The intestinal hemangiomas bleed readily, but bleeding usually is not brisk. A typical presentation is that of a young adult with chronic iron deficiency anemia and typical cutaneous findings. The hemangiomas also can produce intussusception. A variety of diagnostic tests, including barium studies, endoscopy, angiography, and computed tomography have been used to document and localize the gastrointestinal hemangiomas (Fig. 111-11).[167] As with other small polypoid lesions in the small

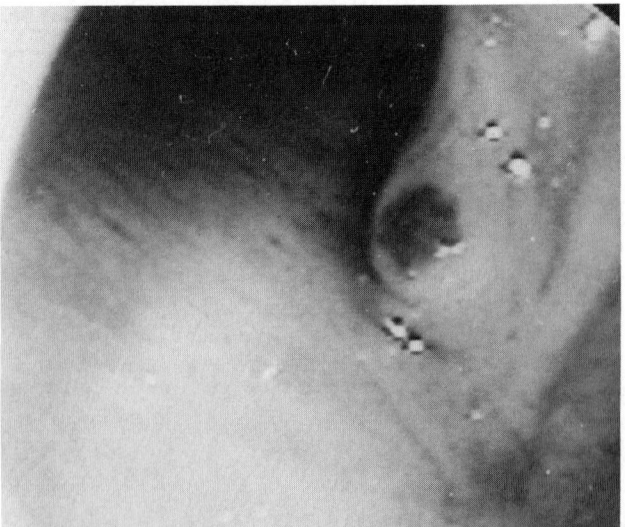

FIGURE 111-11. Polypoid lesion of blue rubber bleb nevus syndrome was detected during colonoscopy in a 26-year-old man. The nipple-like protruberances, 0.5 to 1.5 cm in size, with dark red caps, were found in the upper and lower gastrointestinal tracts. (From Gallo SH, McClave SA. Blue rubber bleb nevus syndrome: gastrointestinal involvement and its endoscopic presentation. Gastrointest Endosc 1992;38:72.)

intestine, these hemangiomas may be demonstrated more effectively by enteroclysis than by standard small bowel barium studies.[167] Because of the multiplicity of lesions in this syndrome, conservative management (e.g., iron therapy) is recommended. If bleeding is significant and the lesions are relatively confined, localized resection can be effective, but other bleeding lesions may develop subsequently. Laser coagulation of intestinal lesions has been described as an alternative or adjunct to surgical palliation for bleeding.[169,170]

Gastrointestinal hemangiomas also occasionally have been reported in association with *Klippel-Trenaunay-Weber syndrome*. Three main features characterize this unusual disorder: cutaneous hemangiomas, varicose veins, and soft tissue and bony hypertrophy of one limb.[171] This sporadic disorder of children and young adults is associated occasionally with intestinal hemangiomas.[172,173] The hemangiomas are restricted commonly to the colon and rectum, but more proximal intestinal lesions have been reported.[174] The tumors in this syndrome usually are of the cavernous histologic type.[172] Other named syndromes with cutaneous and extracutaneous hemangiomas also at times may be accompanied by gastrointestinal tract lesions.[175]

Malignant Vascular Tumors

Malignant vascular tumors of the gastrointestinal tract are extraordinarily rare. In their exhaustive review of gastrointestinal vascular tumors, Gentry and colleagues found only 16 cases over a 20-year period in the Mayo Clinic records.[176] *Angiosarcoma* is an uncommon malignancy in general, and accounts for only 2% of all soft tissue sarcomas.[177] This tumor has been found occasionally in the stomach, small intestine, and colon.[178,179] Presentation may be related to obstruction or gastrointestinal bleeding.[180] Angiosarcoma of the terminal ileum has followed irradiation for ovarian malignancies on several occasions.[180] *Epithelioid hemangioendothelioma* with malignant features also has been detected in the gastrointestinal tract.[181] This malignant counterpart of a typically benign lesion has histologic characteristics resembling those of angiosarcoma. *Hemangiopericytoma* is a rare tumor that arises from pericytes, primitive mesenchymal cells associated with capillary endothelial cells.[182] At least 50% of these tumors have malignant characteristics.[183] Although this lesion is detected most typically in the soft tissue of the trunk and extremities, hemangiopericytomas have been noted to arise at all levels of the gastrointestinal tract (small bowel being most common), resulting in obstruction, intussusception, and gastrointestinal bleeding.[184,185] *Kaposi's sarcoma* is seen in the gastrointestinal tract and can be histologically similar to angiosarcoma. This tumor is now most commonly encountered in association with the acquired immunodeficiency syndrome (see Chap. 105).

OTHER VASCULAR LESIONS

Dieulafoy's Lesion

Dieulafoy's lesion is a distinctive vascular abnormality found most commonly in the proximal stomach. The abnormality initially was named exulceratio simplex and also has been called Dieulafoy's ulcer, Dieulafoy's disease, gastric aneurysm, submucosal arterial malformation, cirsoid aneurysm, caliber persistent artery, and solitary exulceratio simplex. The disorder presents dramatically as acute and rapidly recurrent massive upper gastrointestinal hemorrhage when a small submucosal artery ruptures into the gastric lumen. The lesion is seen twice as frequently in men as in women, and the mean age of presentation is in the sixth decade of life.[186] Upper gastrointestinal hemorrhage also has been reported from Dieulafoy's lesion in an infant and in a patient as old as 93 years of age.[187,188] The lesion is uncommon, but is seen in 1% to 2% of patients presenting with massive upper gastrointestinal hemorrhage.[189,190]

Etiology and Pathology

Although a variety of pathogenic explanations have been proposed for this disorder, it generally is accepted that the principal defect is an abnormally large artery running within the submucosa.[189] The vessel itself is normal histologically but fails to reduce in caliber as the arterial branch penetrates the outer layers of the gastric wall.[191] No aneurysmal dilation is evident. Thus, the large artery may represent only a variation of normal.[186] The vessel itself may be 1 to 3 mm in diameter and usually runs a tortuous course for a variable distance through the mucosa.[186] In places, the arterial wall is in intimate contact with the mucosa, and bleeding can result from erosion of this artery even when a tiny mucosal defect (typically no more than a millimeter or two) is present (Fig. 111-12).

Some debate remains as to whether mucosal ulceration is the key event leading to gastrointestinal hemorrhage from this artery.[189] A lack of mucosal inflammatory reaction at the site of arterial rupture indicates that it is not an acid-peptic process.[189] Also, the artery lacks vasculitic changes that are associated typically with peptic ulceration. It is possible that thrombosis within the artery and subsequent necrosis of the arterial wall plays a primary role in the ultimate arterial rupture.[189] Thus, it is uncertain whether the abnormal artery in its own right has a predilection for rupture or whether chance ulceration over an otherwise innocent large-caliber artery is responsible for bleeding.

Clinical Manifestations

Massive upper gastrointestinal hemorrhage is the typical presentation from a Dieulafoy's lesion.[186,192] Repeated hemorrhages within the first week also are quite common.[186,192] Rarely have patients reported recurrent bouts of hematemesis over long periods of time preceding diagnosis.[193] Symptoms of peptic ulcer disease typically are absent, and no associated medical conditions are reported consistently. Bleeding from similar histologic lesions in the duodenum, jejunum, right colon, and rectum also has been described.[194–203] In the latter cases (colon and rectum), patients presented with massive lower gastrointestinal hemorrhage. The severity of gastrointestinal hemorrhage from Dieulafoy's lesion is so great that some form of intervention almost always is necessary. Although reduced significantly over the past two decades, the mortality rate remains approximately 25%.[186]

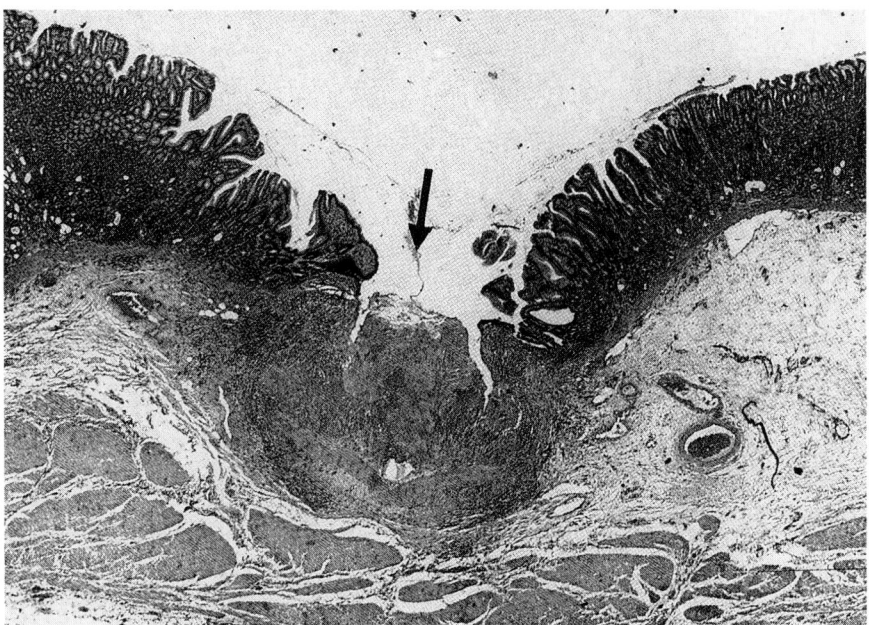

FIGURE 111-12. Pathologic appearance of Dieulafoy's lesion in the stomach. The eroded large artery with secondary thrombosis is seen just beneath a small defect in the gastric mucosa (*arrow*). (From Veldhuyzen van Zanten SJ, Bartelsman JF, Schipper ME, Tytgat GN. Recurrent massive haematemesis from Dieulafoy vascular malformations: a review of 101 cases. Gut 1986;27:213.)

Differential Diagnosis and Diagnostic Studies

The differential diagnosis for Dieulafoy's lesion includes all causes of massive upper or lower gastrointestinal hemorrhage (see Chap. 30). Diagnosis of the gastric lesion can be made by endoscopy, but repeated procedures may be necessary before the precise location is identified by active bleeding at the time of endoscopy. The endoscopist should examine carefully the proximal third of the stomach, especially around the lesser curvature and near the gastroesophageal junction, because a small erosive defect may be found surrounding a visible vessel or a projection of fibrin clot (Fig. 111-13; see Color Fig. 78). In over 80% of cases, the lesion has been detected within 6 cm of this junction and in proximity to the lesser curvature.[186] Rarely is the diagnosis made by angiography, and only then if active bleeding is detected at the time of the diagnostic procedure. Colonic lesions resembling the typical gastric vascular abnormality have been identified by angiography because bleeding may be too massive for colonoscopic visualization.[196]

Therapy

Until recently, surgery was the only effective management for Dieulafoy's lesions. The surgeon operating with this diagnosis in mind must carefully examine the stomach and duodenum for the bleeding site, particularly the upper third of the stomach along the lesser curvature. The lesion is palpable occasionally.[204] Because rebleeding has occurred after simple coagulation and ligation, a wide wedge resection of the entire area traversed by the large submucosal artery has been recommended.[186] On rare occasions more than one lesion has been detected.[205] Rebleeding that occurs in the postoperative setting (because of failure to identify the correct lesion or inadequate management of Dieulafoy's abnormality) appears to carry a poor prognosis. For adequate surgical management

of lower gastrointestinal lesions resembling the typical gastric abnormality, resection of the right colon or wide oversew of a rectal lesion has been required.[196,198]

Only since the late 1980s has consistently successful endoscopic management of gastric or duodenal Dieulafoy's lesions been reported.[190,199,203,206] In the larger series, at least 80% of patients have been managed with endoscopic coagulation attempts alone, each patient making an uncomplicated recovery.[190,203,206] Emergency endoscopy is essential to identify the precise bleeding site. In one study, control was achieved by local injection of a sclerosant agent (polidocanol injected at four sites around the vessel and then into the vessel itself) or by bipolar electrocoagulation with a similar targeting pat-

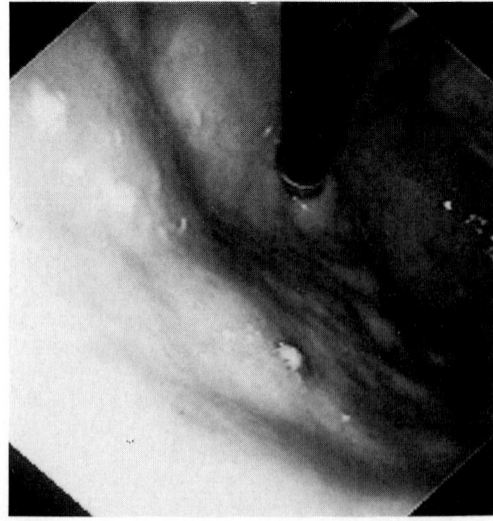

FIGURE 111-13. (See Color Fig. 78.) A fibrin plug protrudes from a Dieulafoy's lesion on the lesser curvature of the proximal stomach. The endoscope is seen in retroflexion at the esophagogastric junction.

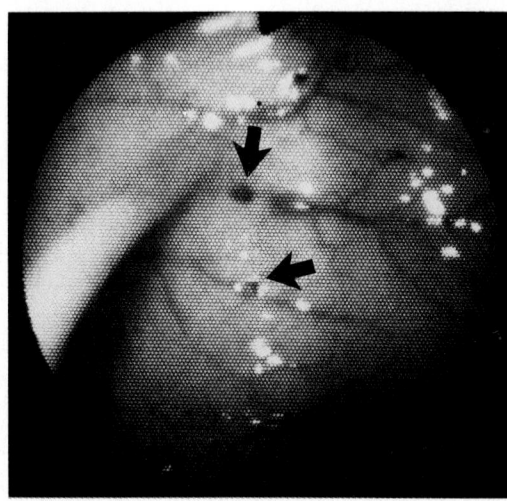

FIGURE 111-14. (See Color Fig. 79.) Small, venous varicosities consistent with the diagnosis of multiple phlebectasia are seen in the colon. The lesions in this case were 4 to 10 mm in size, with a bluish discoloration (*arrows*).

tern.[190] Heater probe coagulation after perilesional epinephrine injection for hemostasis was very effective in another report.[203] Endoscopic complications apparently are infrequent unless very aggressive or repeated coagulation attempts are necessary.[207] Based on these observations, endoscopic therapy should be considered the preferred initial treatment in most instances of upper tract bleeding, but patients should be monitored carefully for rebleeding episodes, given the natural course of these lesions.

Miscellaneous Lesions

Several other nonclassifiable gastrointestinal vascular lesions have been reported. *Multiple phlebectasia* denotes multiple nonneoplastic venous varicosities.[208] The lesions are compressible, bluish-red nodules varying in size from several millimeters to more than a centimeter in diameter (Fig. 111-14; see Color Fig. 79). Histologically, these varicosities have a normal endothelial lining and are located in the submucosa with only a thin layer of overlying mucosa.[208] The small cavernous structures arise from venous arcades[209] and have been classified with the cavernous hemangiomas by some authors. These lesions are often clustered and have been found in all parts of the intestinal tract.[208,210] Gastrointestinal hemorrhage can occur, and diagnosis in the past often has been made during surgical exploration.

Gastrointestinal bleeding also has been associated with inherited metabolic disorders such as *pseudoxanthoma elasticum* and *Ehlers-Danlos syndrome*. Although there are many manifestations of these two hereditary cutaneous diseases (see Chaps. 44 and 108), gastrointestinal hemorrhage can result from spontaneous vascular rupture in both.[211–213] Interference with constriction of submucosal vessels, thus preventing the shunting of blood away from the mucosa, may lead to severe hemorrhage from a variety of lesions in these disorders.[212–214]

The reader is directed to Chapter 22, Gastrointestinal Blood Flow; Chapter 30, Approach to the Patient With Gross Gastrointestinal Bleeding; Chapter 31, Approach to the Patient With Occult Gastrointestinal Bleeding; Chapter 44, Skin Lesions Associated With Gastrointestinal Diseases; Chapter 115, Upper Gastrointestinal Endoscopy; Chapter 116, Colonoscopy and Flexible Sigmoidoscopy; Chapter 126, Applications of Radionuclide Imaging in Gastroenterology; Chapter 127, Angiography; and Chapter 138, Endoscopic Control of Nonvariceal Upper Gastrointestinal Hemorrhage.

REFERENCES

1. Peterson WL. Stomach and duodenum. In: Rogers AI, Bernstein LH, Burnett DA, et al. Medical knowledge self-assessment program in the subspecialty of gastroenterology and hepatology. Philadelphia: American College of Physicians, 1993:48.
2. Camilleri M, Chakwick VS, Hodgson HJF. Vascular anomalies of the gastrointestinal tract. Hepatogastroenterology 1984;31:149.
3. Moore JD, Thompson NW, Appelman HD, Foley D. Arteriovenous malformations of the gastrointestinal tract. Arch Surg 1976;111:381.
4. Richardson JD. Vascular lesions of the intestines. Am J Surg 1991;161:284.
5. Athanasoulis CA, Galdabini JJ, Waltman AC, et al. Angiodysplasia of the colon: a cause of rectal bleeding. Cardiovasc Radiol 1977/1978;1:3.
6. Gunnlaugsson O. Angiodysplasia of the stomach and duodenum. Gastrointest Endosc 1985;31:251.
7. Marwick T, Kerlin P. Angiodysplasia of the upper gastrointestinal tract: clinical spectrum in 41 cases. J Clin Gastroenterol 1986;8:404.
8. Clouse RE, Costigan DJ, Mills BA, Zuckerman GR. Angiodysplasia as a cause of upper gastrointestinal bleeding. Arch Intern Med 1985;145:458.
9. Moreto M, Figa M, Ojembarrena E, Zaballa M. Vascular malformations of the stomach and duodenum: an endoscopic classification. Endoscopy 1986;18:227.
10. Hochter W, Weingart J, Kuhner W, et al. Angiodysplasia in the colon and rectum: endoscopic morphology, localisation and frequency. Endoscopy 1985;17:182.
11. Heer M, Sulser H, Hany A. Angiodysplasia of the colon: an expression of occlusive vascular disease. Hepatogastroenterology 1987;34:127.
12. Boley SJ, DiBase A, Brandt LJ, Sammartano RJ. Lower intestinal bleeding in the elderly. Am J Surg 1979;137:57.
13. Welch CE, Athanasoulis CA, Galdabini JJ. Hemorrhage from the large bowel with special reference to angiodysplasia and diverticular disease. World J Surg 1978;2:73.
14. Weaver GA, Bordley J IV, Olson JE. Management of bleeding angiodysplasia of the upper small intestine. J Clin Gastroenterol 1985;7:145.
15. Jesudason SRB, Devasia A, Mathen VI, et al. The pattern of angiodysplasia of the gastrointestinal tract in a tropical country. Surg Gynecol Obstet 1985;161:525.
16. Cavett CM, Selby JH Jr, Hamilton JL, Williamson JW. Arteriovenous malformation in chronic gastrointestinal bleeding. Ann Surg 1977;185:116.
17. Richter JM, Hedberg SE, Athanasoulis CA, Schapiro RH. Angiodysplasia: clinical presentation and colonoscopic diagnosis. Dig Dis Sci 1984;29:481.
18. Boley SJ, Brandt LJ, Mitsudo SM. Vascular lesions of the colon. Adv Intern Med 1984;29:301.
19. Boley SJ, Sammartano R, Brandt LJ, Sprayregen S. Vascular ectasias of the colon. Surg Gynecol Obstet 1979;149:353.
20. Boley SJ, Brandt LJ. Vascular ectasias of the colon: 1986. Dig Dis Sci 1986;31(9 Suppl):26S.
21. Baum S, Athanasoulis CA, Waltman AC, et al. Angiodysplasia

of the right colon: a cause of gastrointestinal bleeding. Am J Roentgenol 1977;129:789.

22. Cappell MS. Spatial clustering of simultaneous nonhereditary gastrointestinal angiodysplasia: small but significant correlation between nonhereditary colonic and upper gastrointestinal angiodysplasia. Dig Dis Sci 1992;37:1072.

23. Mitsudo SM, Boley SJ, Brandt LJ, et al. Vascular ectasias of the right colon in the elderly: a distinct pathologic entity. Hum Pathol 1979;10:585.

24. Hamoniere G, Grenier A, Lalloue C, et al. Recherches sur l'angiectasie du colon droit. Lyon Chir 1982;78:125.

25. Weaver GA, Alpern HD, Davis JS, et al. Gastrointestinal angiodysplasia associated with aortic valve disease: part of a spectrum of angiodysplasia of the gut. Gastroenterology 1979; 77:1.

26. Meyer CT, Troncale FJ, Galloway S, Sheahan DG. Arteriovenous malformations of the bowel: an analysis of 22 cases and a review of the literature. Medicine 1981;60:36.

27. Brandt LJ. Gastrointestinal disorders of the elderly. New York: Raven Press, 1984:313.

28. Tedesco FJ, Griffin JW Jr, Khan AQ. Vascular ectasia of the colon: clinical, colonoscopic, and radiographic features. J Clin Gastroenterol 1980;2:233.

29. Boley SJ, Sammartano R, Adams A, et al. On the nature and etiology of vascular ectasias of the colon: degenerative lesions of aging. Gastroenterology 1977;72:650.

30. Scheffer SM, Leatherman LL. Resolution of Heyde's syndrome of aortic stenosis and gastrointestinal bleeding after aortic valve replacement. Ann Thorac Surg 1986;42:477.

31. McNamara JJ, Austen WG. Gastrointestinal bleeding occurring in patients with acquired valvular heart disease. Arch Surg 1968;97:538.

32. Schwartz J, Rozenfeld V, Habot B. Cessation of recurrent bleeding from gastrointestinal angiodysplasia, after beta blocker treatment in a patient with hypertrophic subaortic stenosis: a case history. Angiology 1992;43:244.

33. Imperiale TF, Ransohoff DF. Aortic stenosis, idiopathic gastrointestinal bleeding, and angiodysplasia: is there an association? Gastroenterology 1988;95:1670.

34. Cunningham JT. Gastric telangiectasias in chronic hemodialysis patients: a report of six cases. Gastroenterology 1981;81:1131.

35. Cappell MS, Gupta A. Changing epidemiology of gastrointestinal angiodysplasia with increasing recognition of clinically milder cases: angiodysplasia tend to produce mild chronic gastrointestinal bleeding in a study of 47 consecutive patients admitted from 1980–1989. Am J Gastroenterol 1992;87:201.

36. Alvarez L, Puleo J, Balint JA. Investigation of gastrointestinal bleeding in patients with end stage renal disease. Am J Gastroenterol 1993;88:30.

37. Zuckerman GR, Cornette GL, Clouse RE, Harter HR. Upper gastrointestinal bleeding in patients with chronic renal failure. Ann Intern Med 1985;102:588.

38. Flynn CT, Chandran PKG. Renal failure and angiodysplasia of the colon. Ann Intern Med 1985;103:154.

39. Woodlock TJ, Francis CW, Rowe JM, et al. Prolonged remission after life-threatening gastrointestinal hemorrhage from coexistent angiodysplasia and acquired bleeding diathesis. Am J Hematol 1988;27:125.

40. Duray PH, Marcal JM Jr, LiVolsi VA, et al. Gastrointestinal angiodysplasia: a possible component of von Willebrand's disease. Hum Pathol 1984;15:539.

41. Warkentin TE, Moore JC, Morgan DG. Aortic stenosis and bleeding gastrointestinal angiodysplasia: is acquired von Willebrand's disease the link? Lancet 1992;340:35.

42. Gostout CJ, Bowie EJW, Balm R, Fischer PK. Angiodysplasia associated with von Willebrand's disease? Gastroenterology 1990;98:A172.

43. Steger AC, Galland RB, Hemingway A, et al. Gastrointestinal haemorrhage from a second source in patients with chronic angiodysplasia. Br J Surg 1987;74:726.

44. Boley SJ, Brandt LW, Franck MS. Severe lower intestinal bleeding: diagnosis and treatment. Clin Gastroenterol 1981;10:65.

45. Rogers BH. Endoscopic diagnosis and therapy of mucosal vascular abnormalities of the gastrointestinal tract occurring in elderly patients and associated with cardiac, vascular, and pulmonary disease. Gastrointest Endosc 1980;26:134.

46. Howard OM, Buchanan JD, Hunt RH. Angiodysplasia. Lancet 1981;2:1340.

47. Tung KT, Millar AB. Gastric angiodysplasia: a missed cause of gastrointestinal bleeding. Postgrad Med J 1987;63:865.

48. Iuchtman M, Zer M, Auslander L, Rabinson S. Importance of small bowel involvement in bleeding angiodysplasia. Isr J Med Sci 1986;22:828.

49. Stamm B, Heer M, Buhler H, Ammann R. Mucosal biopsy of vascular ectasia (angiodysplasia) of the large bowel detected during routine colonoscopic examination. Histopathology 1985;9:639.

50. Salem RR, Wood CB, Rees HC, et al. A comparison of colonoscopy and selective visceral angiography in the diagnosis of colonic angiodysplasia. Ann R Coll Surg Engl 1985;67:225.

51. Emanuel RB, Weiser MM, Shenoy SS, et al. Arteriovenous malformations as a cause of gastrointestinal bleeding: the importance of triple-vessel angiographic studies in diagnosis and prevention of rebleeding. J Clin Gastroenterol 1985;7:237.

52. Belli AM, Hemingway AP. Malignant "angiodysplasia." Clin Radiol 1991;44:31.

53. Maurer AH, Rodman MS, Vitti RA, et al. Gastrointestinal bleeding: improved localization with cine scintigraphy. Radiology 1992;185:187.

54. Alavi A, Dann RW, Baum S, Biery DN. Scintigraphic detection of acute gastrointestinal bleeding. Radiology 1977;124:753.

55. Aldabagh SM, Trujillo YP, Taxy JB. Utility of specimen angiography in angiodysplasia of the colon. Gastroenterology 1986;91:725.

56. Thelmo WL, Vetrano JA, Wibowo A, et al. Angiodysplasia of colon revisited: pathologic demonstration without the use of intravascular injection technique. Hum Pathol 1992;23:37.

57. Lewis BS, Waye JD. Chronic gastrointestinal bleeding of obscure origin: role of small bowel enteroscopy. Gastroenterology 1988;94:1117.

58. Szold A, Katz LB, Lewis BS. Surgical approach to occult gastrointestinal bleeding. Am J Surg 1992;163:90.

59. Gostout CJ, Schroeder KW, Burton DD. Small bowel enteroscopy: an early experience in gastrointestinal bleeding of unknown origin. Gastrointest Endosc 1991;37:5.

60. Foutch PG, Sawyer R, Sanowski RA. Push-enteroscopy for diagnosis of patients with gastrointestinal bleeding of obscure origin. Gastrointest Endosc 1990;36:337.

61. Lau WY, Wong SY, Yuen WK, Wong KK. Intraoperative enteroscopy for bleeding angiodysplasias of small intestine. Surg Gynecol Obstet 1989;168:341.

62. Reed DK, Porter LE, Zajko AB, et al. Pre- and intraoperative localization of small bowel arteriovenous malformation. J Clin Gastroenterol 1986;8:166.

63. Trudel JL, Fazio VW, Sivak MV. Colonoscopic diagnosis and treatment of arteriovenous malformations in chronic lower gastrointestinal bleeding: clinical accuracy and efficacy. Dis Colon Rectum 1988;31:107.

64. Hutcheon DF, Kabelin J, Bulkley GB, Smith GW. Effect of therapy on bleeding rates in gastrointestinal angiodysplasia. Am Surg 1987;53:6.

65. Jensen DM, Machicado GA, Kovacs TOG, et al. Bleeding colonic angiomata: diagnosis, treatment and outcome (abstract). Gastrointest Endosc 1989;35:173.

66. Rutgeerts P, Van Gompel F, Geboes K, et al. Long term results of treatment of vascular malformations of the gastrointestinal tract by neodymium YAG laser photocoagulation. Gut 1985;26: 586.

67. Bown SG, Swain CP, Storey DW, et al. Endoscopic laser treatment of vascular anomalies of the upper gastrointestinal tract. Gut 1985;26:1338.

68. Naveau S, Aubert A, Poynard T, Chaput JC. Long-term results of treatment of vascular malformations of the gastrointestinal tract by neodymium YAG laser photocoagulation. Dig Dis Sci 1990;35:821.

69. Jensen DM, Machicado GA. Bleeding colonic angioma: endoscopic coagulation and follow-up. Gastroenterology 1985;88: 1433A.

70. Buchi KN. Vascular malformations of the gastrointestinal tract. Surg Clin North Am 1992;72:559.
71. Cello JP, Grendell JH. Endoscopic laser treatment for gastrointestinal ectasias. Ann Intern Med 1986;104:352.
72. Uflacker R. Transcatheter embolization for treatment of acute lower gastrointestinal bleeding. Acta Radiol 1987;28:425.
73. Browder W, Cerise EF, Litwin MS. Impact of emergency angiography in massive lower gastrointestinal bleeding. Ann Surg 1986;204:530.
74. Hines JR, Stryker SJ, Neiman HL, et al. Intraoperative angiography intestinal angiodysplasia. Surg Gynecol Obstet 1981;152:453.
75. Netterville RE, Hardy JD, Martin RS Jr. Small bowel hemorrhage. Ann Surg 1968;167:949.
76. Crawford ES, Roehm JO Jr, McGavran MH. Jejunoileal arteriovenous malformation: localization for resection by segmental bowel staining techniques. Ann Surg 1980;191:404.
77. Bambach CP, Coupland GA, Sorby W, Roche J. Angiodysplasia of the small bowel: a method of intraoperative identification. Aust N Z J Surg 1978;48:317.
78. Athanasoulis CA, Moncure AC, Greenfield AJ, et al. Intraoperative localization of small bowel bleeding sites with combined use of angiographic methods and methylene blue injection. Surgery 1980;87:77.
79. Fazio VW, Zelas P, Weakley FL. Intraoperative angiography and the localization of bleeding from the small intestine. Surg Gynecol Obstet 1980;151:637.
80. Ohri SK, Jackson J, Desa LA, Spencer J. The intraoperative localization of the obscure bleeding site using fluorescein. J Clin Gastroenterology 1992;14:331.
81. Love JW. The syndrome of calcific aortic stenosis and gastrointestinal bleeding: resolution following aortic valve replacement. J Thorac Cardiovasc Surg 1982;83:779.
82. Cappell MS, Lebwohl O. Cessation of recurrent bleeding from gastrointestinal angiodysplasias after aortic valve replacement. Ann Intern Med 1986;105:54.
83. King RM, Pluth JR, Giuliani ER. The association of unexplained gastrointestinal bleeding with calcific aortic stenosis. Ann Thorac Surg 1987;44:514.
84. Bourdette D, Greenberg B. Twelve-year history of gastrointestinal bleeding in a patient with calcific aortic stenosis and hemorrhagic telangiectasia. Dig Dis Sci 1979;24:77.
85. Harrison DFN. Use of estrogen in treatment of familial hemorrhagic telangiectasia. Laryngoscope 1982;92:314.
86. McGee RR. Estrogen–progestogen therapy for gastrointestinal bleeding in hereditary hemorrhagic telangiectasia. South Med J 1979;72:1503.
87. Bronner MH, Pate MB, Cunningham JT, Marsh WH. Estrogen–progesterone therapy for bleeding gastrointestinal telangiectasias in chronic renal failure: an uncontrolled trial. Ann Intern Med 1986;105:371.
88. Granieri R, Mazzulla JP, Yarborough GW. Estrogen–progesterone therapy for recurrent gastrointestinal bleeding secondary to gastrointestinal angiodysplasia. Am J Gastroenterol 1988;83:556.
89. van Cutsem E, Rutgeerts P, Vantrappen G. Treatment of bleeding gastrointestinal vascular malformations with oestrogen–progesterone. Lancet 1990;335:953.
90. Lewis BS, Salomon P, Rivera-MacMurray S, et al. Does hormonal therapy have any benefit for bleeding angiodysplasia? J Clin Gastroenterol 1992;15:99.
91. Bell AJ, Mufti GJ, Oscier DG, et al. Angiodysplasia of the colon in patients with hemostatic defects: risk of secondary hemorrhage after electrocoagulation treatment. Angiology 1984;35:511.
92. Borsch G. Diffuse gastric antral vascular ectasia: the "watermelon stomach" revisited. Am J Gastroenterol 1987;82:1333.
93. Jabbari M, Cherry R, Lough JO, et al. Gastric antral vascular ectasia: the watermelon stomach. Gastroenterology 1984;87:1165.
94. Wheeler MH, Smith PM, Cotton PB, et al. Abnormal blood vessels in the gastric antrum: a case of upper-gastrointestinal bleeding. Dig Dis Sci 1979;24:155.
95. Lee FI, Costello F, Flanagan N, Vasudev KS. Diffuse antral vascular ectasia. Gastrointest Endosc 1984;30:87.
96. Gilliam JH, Geisinger KR, Wu WC, et al. The "watermelon stomach": Morphologic diagnosis by endoscopy. Gastroenterology 1985;88:1394.
97. Appel C, Weissman G, Bronzo R, et al. Gastric antral vasculopathy: a distinct clinical entity. Gastroenterology 1985;88:1308.
98. Gostout CJ, Ahlquist DA, Viggiano TR, et al. Watermelon stomach (WMS): clinical features and response to endoscopic laser therapy (abstract). Gastroenterology 1989;96:A178.
99. Quintero E, Pique JM, Bombi JA, et al. Gastric mucosal vascular ectasias causing bleeding in cirrhosis. Gastroenterology 1987;93:1054.
100. Suit PF, Petras RE, Bauer TW, Petrini JL Jr. Gastric antral vascular ectasia: a histologic and morphometric study of "the watermelon stomach." Am J Surg Pathol 1987;11:750.
101. Gilliam JH III, Geisinger KR, Wu WC, et al. Endoscopic biopsy is diagnostic in gastric antral vascular ectasia: the "watermelon stomach." Dig Dis Sci 1989;34:885.
102. Tovey FI. Gastric antral vascular ectasia: the watermelon stomach. Gastroenterology 1985;88:1293.
103. Calam J, Walker RJ. Antral vascular lesion, achlorhydria, and chronic gastrointestinal blood loss: response to steroids. Dig Dis Sci 1980;25:236.
104. Kruger R, Ryan ME, Dickson KB, Nunez JF. Diffuse vascular ectasia of the gastric antrum. Am J Gastroenterol 1987;82:421.
105. Gostout CJ, Ahlquist DA, Radford CM, et al. Endoscopic laser therapy for watermelon stomach. Gastroenterology 1989;96:1462.
106. Perez-Ayuso RM, Pique JM, Saperas E, et al. Gastric vascular ectasias in cirrhosis: association with hypoacidity not related to gastric atrophy. Scand J Gastroenterol 1989;24:1073.
107. Saperas E, Perez-Ayuso RM, Poca E, Bordas JM, et al. Increased gastric PGE2 biosynthesis in cirrhotic patients with gastric vascular ectasia. Am J Gastroenterol 1990;85:138.
108. Lowes JR, Rode J. Neuroendocrine cell proliferations in gastric antral vascular ectasia. Gastroenterology 1989;97:207.
109. Park RH, Danesh BJ, Upadhyay R, et al. Gastric antral vascular ectasia (watermelon stomach): therapeutic options. Postgrad Med J 1990;66:720.
110. Urban BA, Jones B, Fishman EK, et al. Gastric antral vascular ectasia ("watermelon stomach"): radiologic findings. Radiology 1991;178:517.
111. Saperas E, Pique JM, Perez-Ayuso R, et al. Comparison of snare and large forceps biopsies in the histologic diagnosis of gastric vascular ectasia in cirrhosis. Endoscopy 1989;21:165.
112. Petrini JL Jr, Johnston JH. Heat probe treatment for antral vascular ectasia. Gastrointest Endosc 1989;35:324.
113. Bjorkman DJ, Buchi KN. Endoscopic laser therapy of the watermelon stomach. Lasers Surg Med 1992;12:478.
114. Brennan FN, Cowen AE, Laurence BH. Successful treatment of two patients with gastric antral vascular ectasia "watermelon stomach" using endoscopic Nd-YAG laser therapy. Aust N Z J Med 1991;21:439.
115. Tsai HH, Smith J, Danesh BJ. Successful control of bleeding from gastric antral vascular ectasia (watermelon stomach) by laser photocoagulation. Gut 1991;32:93.
116. Kishi K, Kinoshite Y, Kitajima N, et al. Two cases of gastric antral vascular ectasia: response to medical treatment. Gastroenterol Jpn 1991;26:757.
117. Rawlinson WD, Barr GD, Lin BPC. Antral vascular ectasia: watermelon stomach. Med J Aust 1986;144:709.
118. Moss SF, Ghosh P, Thomas DM, et al. Gastric antral vascular ectasia: maintenance treatment with oestrogen–progesterone. Gut 1992;33:715.
119. Pina Cabral JE, Pontes JM, Toste M, et al. Watermelon stomach: treatment with a serotonin antagonist. Am J Gastroenterol 1991;86:927.
120. Martini GA. The liver in hereditary haemorrhagic telangiectasia: an inborn error of vascular structure with multiple manifestations. A reappraisal. Gut 1978;19:531.
121. Pounder DJ, Rowland R, Pieterse AS, et al. Angiodysplasias of the colon. J Clin Pathol 1982;35:824.

122. Hodgson CH, Burchell HB, Good CA, Clagett OT. Hereditary hemorrhagic telangiectasia and pulmonary arteriovenous fistula: survey of a large family. N Engl J Med 1959;261:625.

123. Driscoll JE, Rabe MA. Hemorrhagic telangiectasis of the gastrointestinal tract: an obscure source of gastrointestinal bleeding. Am Surg 1954;20:1281.

124. Reilly PJ, Nostrant TT. Clinical manifestations of hereditary hemorrhagic telangiectasia. Am J Gastroenterol 1984;79:363.

125. Smith CR Jr, Bartholomew LG, Cain JC. Hereditary hemorrhagic telangiectasia and gastrointestinal hemorrhage. Gastroenterology 1963;44:1.

126. Thompson JN, Hemingway AP, McPherson GAD, et al. Obscure gastrointestinal hemorrhage of small-bowel origin. Br Med J 1984;288:1663.

127. Gostout CJ, Bowyer BA, Ahlquist DA, et al. Mucosal vascular malformations of the gastrointestinal tract: clinical observations and results of endoscopic neodymium:yttrium-aluminum-garnet laser therapy. Mayo Clin Proc 1988;63:993.

128. Campbell EW Jr, Jewson D, Gilbert E. Angiographic identification of enteric lesions: guide to therapy in hereditary hemorrhagic telangiectasias. Arch Intern Med 1970;125:705.

129. Heald RJ, Ray JE. Vascular malformations of the intestine: an important cause of obscure gastrointestinal hemorrhage. South Med J 1974;67:33.

130. Hagihara PF, Chuang V, Griffen WO. Arteriovenous malformations of the colon. Am J Surg 1977;133:681.

131. Frame B, Dhanwada SR, Ohorodnik JM, Kwa DM. Gastrointestinal haemorrhage in Turner's syndrome: long-term follow-up with postmortem examination. Arch Intern Med 1977;137:691.

132. Rutlin E, Wisloff F, Myren J, Serck-Hanssen A. Intestinal telangiectasis in Turner's syndrome. Endoscopy 1981;13:86.

133. Lowe WC. Neoplasms of the gastrointestinal tract. Flushing, NY: Medical Examination Publishing, 1972:130.

134. Wilson JM, Melvin DB, Gray G, Thorbjarnarson B. Benign small bowel tumour. Ann Surg 1975;181:247.

135. Gentry RW, Dockerty MB, Clagett OT. Collective review: vascular malformations and vascular tumors of the gastrointestinal tract. Int Abstr Surg 1949;88:281.

136. Head HD, Baker JQ, Muir RW. Hemangioma of the colon. Am J Surg 1973;126:691.

137. Lyon DT, Mantia AG. Large-bowel hemangiomas. Dis Colon Rectum 1984;27:404.

138. Condon RE, Loyd RD. Hemangioma of the colon. Am J Surg 1968;115:720.

139. Lazarus JA, Marks MS. Benign intestinal tumors of vascular origin. Surgery 1947;22:766.

140. Allred HW. Hemangiomas of the colon, rectum, and anus. Mayo Clin Proc 1974;49:739.

141. Dachman AH, Ros PR, Shekitka KM, et al. Colorectal hemangioma: radiologic findings. Radiology 1988;167:31.

142. Rissier HL Jr. Hemangiomatosis of the intestine: discussion, review of the literature and report of two new cases. Gastroenterologia (Basel) 1960;93:357.

143. Bland KI, Abney HT, MacGregor AMC, Hawkins IF. Hemangiomatosis of the colon and anorectrum: case report and a review of the literature. Am J Surg 1974;40:626.

144. Weinstein EC, Moertel CG, Waugh JM. Intussuscepting hemangiomas of the gastro-intestinal tract: report of case and review of the literature. Ann Surg 1963;157:265.

145. Blix S, Aas K. Giant haemangioma, thrombocytopenia, fibrinogenopenia, and fibrinolytic activity. Acta Med Scand 1961;169:63.

146. Inceman S, Tangun Y. Chronic defibrination syndrome due to a giant hemangioma associated with microangiopathic hemolytic anemia. Am J Med 1969;46:997.

147. Hagood MF, Gathright JB. Hemangiomatosis of the skin and gastrointestinal tract: report of a case. Dis Colon Rectum 1975;18:141.

148. Killingback M, Coombes B, Francis P. Intestinal and cutaneous haemangiomatosis. Med J Aust 1974;1:749.

149. Flannery MG, Caster MP. Hemangioma of the stomach with a roentgenologic diagnostic point. AJR 1957;77:38.

150. Eusterman GB, Senty EG. Benign tumors of the stomach. Surg Gynecol Obst 1922;34:5.

151. Kerekes ES. Gastric hemangioma: a case report. Radiology 1963;82:468.

152. Bell GA, McKenzie AD, Emmons H. Diffuse cavernous hemangioma of the rectum: report of a case and review of the literature. Dis Colon Rectum 1972;15:377.

153. Aylward CA, Orangio GR, Lucas GW, Fazio VW. Diffuse cavernous hemangioma of the rectosigmoid-CT scan, a new diagnostic modality, and surgical management using sphincter-saving procedures: report of three cases. Dis Colon Rectum 1988;31:797.

154. Wallerstein RO. Spontaneous involution of giant hemangioma: simultaneous regression of tumor and thrombocytopenia in newborn. Am J Dis Child 1961;102:233.

155. Figliolini FJ, Cutait DE, deOliveira MR, Bastos E da S. Rectosigmoidal hemangioma: report of two cases. Dis Colon Rectum 1961;4:349.

156. Benson JM, Orlay G. Colorectal haemangioma and its relationship to haemorrhoids in childhood. Aust N Z J Surg 1991;61:537.

157. Takamatsu H, Akiyama H, Noguchi H, et al. Endorectal pull-through operation for diffuse cavernous hemangiomatosis of the sigmoid colon, rectum and anus. Eur J Pediatr Surg 1992;2:245.

158. Gabriel WB. The principles and practice of rectal surgery. Springfield, IL: Charles C Thomas, 1963:116.

159. Ibarguen E, Sharp HL, Snyder CL, et al. Hemangiomatosis of the colon and peritoneum: case report and management discussion. Clin Pediatr 1988;27:425.

160. Mellish RW. Multiple hemangiomas of the gastrointestinal tract in children. Am J Surg 1971;121:412.

161. Burman D, Mansell PW, Warin RP. Miliary haemangiomata in the newborn. Arch Dis Child 1967;42:193.

162. Latifi HR, Siegel MJ. Diffuse neonatal hemangiomatosis: CT findings in an adult. J Comput Assist Tomogr 1992;16:971.

163. Bean WB. Vascular spiders and related lesions of the skin. Springfield, IL: Charles C Thomas, 1958:178.

164. Rice JS, Fischer DS. Blue rubber bleb nevus syndrome: generalized cavernous hemangiomatosis or venous hamartoma with medulloblastoma of the cerebellum. Case report and review of the literature. Arch Dermatol 1962;86:503.

165. Berlyne GM, Berlyne N. Anaemia due to "blue rubber bleb" naevus disease. Lancet 1980;2:1275.

166. Fleischer AB Jr, Panzer SM, Wheeler CE. Blue rubber bleb nevus syndrome in a black patient: a case report. Cutis 1990;45:103.

167. Sandhu KS, Cohen H, Radin R, Buck FS. Blue rubber bleb nevus syndrome presenting with recurrences. Dig Dis Sci 1987;32:214.

168. Gascoyen M. Case of naevus involving the parotid gland and causing death from suffocation: naevi of the viscera. Trans Pathol Soc (London) 1860;11:267.

169. Shahed M, Hagenmuller F, Rosch T, et al. A 19-year-old female with blue rubber bleb nevus syndrome: endoscopic laser photocoagulation and surgical resection of gastrointestinal angiomata. Endoscopy 1990;22:54.

170. Morris L, Lynch PM, Gleason WA Jr, et al. Blue rubber bleb nevus syndrome: laser photocoagulation of colonic hemangiomas in a child with microcytic anemia. Pediatr Dermatol 1992;9:91.

171. Lindenauer SM. The Klippel-Trenaunay syndrome: varicosity, hypertrophy and haemangioma with no arteriovenous fistula. Ann Surg 1965;162:303.

172. Schmitt B, Posselt HG, Waag KL, et al. Severe hemorrhage from intestinal hemangiomatosis in Klippel-Trenaunay syndrome: pitfalls in diagnosis management. J Pediatr Gastroenterol Nutr 1986;5:155.

173. Gandolfi L, Rossi A, Stasi G, Tonti R. The Klippel-Trenaunay syndrome with colonic hemangioma. Gastrointest Endosc 1987;33:442.

174. Brown R, Ohri SK, Ghosh P, et al. Case report: jejunal vascular malformation in Klippel-Trenaunay syndrome. Clin Radiol 1991;44:134.

175. Jennings M, Ward P, Maddocks JL. Blue rubber bleb naevus

disease: an uncommon cause of gastrointestinal tract bleeding. Gut 1988;29:1408.

176. Gentry RW, Dockerty MB, Clagett OT. Vascular malformations and vascular tumors of the gastrointestinal tract. Int Abstr Surg 1949;88:281.

177. Rosenberg SA, Suit HK, Baker LH. Sarcomas of soft tissues. In: DeVita VT, Hellman S, Rosenberg SA, eds. Cancer: principles and practice of oncology. 2nd ed. Philadelphia: JB Lippincott, 1985:1243.

178. Taxy JB, Battifora H. Angiosarcoma of the gastrointestinal tract: a report of three cases. Cancer 1988;62:210.

179. Ordonez NG, del Junco GW, Ayala AG, Ahmed N. Angiosarcoma of the small intestine: an immunoperoxidase study. Am J Gastroenterol 1983;78:218.

180. Nanus DM, Kelsen D, Clark DG. Radiation-induced angiosarcoma. Cancer 1987;60:777.

181. Saito R, Bedetti CD, Caines MJ, Kramer K. Malignant epithelioid hemangioendothelioma of the colon: report of a case. Dis Colon Rectum 1987;30:707.

182. McMaster MJ, Soule EH, Ivins JC. Hemangiopericytoma: a clinicopathologic study and long-term followup of 60 patients. Cancer 1975;36:2232.

183. Backwinkel KD, Diddams JA. Hemangiopericytoma: report of a case and comprehensive review of the literature. Cancer 1970;25:896.

184. Binder SC, Wolfe HJ, Deterling RA Jr. Intra-abdominal hemangiopericytoma: report of four cases and review of the literature. Arch Surg 1973;107;536.

185. Genter B, Mir R, Strauss R, et al. Hemangiopericytoma of the colon: report of a case and review of literature. Dis Colon Rectum 1982;25:149.

186. Veldhuyzen van Zanten SJ, Bartelsmam JF, Schipper ME, Tytgat GN. Recurrent massive haematemesis from Dieulafoy vascular malformations: a review of 101 cases. Gut 1986;27:213.

187. Goldman RL. Submucosal arterial malformation ("aneurysm") of the stomach with fatal hemorrhage. Gastroenterology 1964;46:589.

188. Rossi NP, Green EW, Pike JD. Massive bleeding of the upper-gastrointestinal tract due to Dieulafoy's erosion. Arch Surg 1968;97:797.

189. Juler GL, Labitzke HG, Lamb R, Allen R. The pathogenesis of Dieulafoy's gastric erosion. Am J Gastroenterol 1984;79:195.

190. Pointner R, Schwab G, Konigsrainer A, Dietze O. Endoscopy treatment of Dieulafoy's disease. Gastroenterology 1988;94:563.

191. Molnar P, Miko T. Multiple arterial caliber persistence resulting in hematomas and fatal rupture of the gastric wall. Am J Surg Pathol 1982;6:83.

192. Mortensen NJ, Mountford RA, Davies JD, Jeans WD. Dieulafoy's disease: a distinctive arteriovenous malformation causing massive gastric haemorrhage. Br J Surg 1983;70:76.

193. Frank W. Hematemesis associated with gastric arteriosclerosis: review of the literature with case report. Gastroenterology 1946;7:231.

194. Matuchansky C, Babin P, Abadie JC, et al. Jejunal bleeding from a solitary large submucosal artery. Gastroenterology 1978;75:110.

195. Barbier P, Luder P, Triller J, et al. Colonic hemorrhage from a solitary minute ulcer. Gastroenterology 1985;88:1065.

196. Richards WO, Grove-Mahoney D, Williams LF. Hemorrhage from a Dieulafoy type ulcer of the colon: a new cause of lower gastrointestinal bleeding. Am Surg 1988;54:121.

197. Farrell JD, Bennett MK. Dieulafoy's vascular malformation as a cause of large intestinal bleeding. J Clin Pathol 1992;45:363.

198. Franko E, Chardavoyne R, Wise L. Massive rectal bleeding from a Dieulafoy's type ulcer of the rectum: a review of this unusual disease. Am J Gastroenterol 1991;86:1545.

199. Goldenberg SP, DeLuca VA Jr, Marignani P. Endoscopic treatment of Dieulafoy's lesion of the duodenum. Am J Gastroenterol 1990;85:452.

200. Vetto JT, Richman PS, Kariger K, Passaro E Jr. Cirsoid aneurysms of the jejunum: an unrecognized cause of massive gastrointestinal bleeding. Arch Surg 1989;124:1460.

201. Ma CK, Padda H, Pace EH, Szilagyi E. Submucosal arterial malformation of the colon with massive hemorrhage: report of a case. Dis Colon Rectum 1989;32:149.

202. McClave SA, Goldschmid S, Cunningham JT, Boyd WP Jr. Dieulafoy's cirsoid aneurysm of the duodenum. Dig Dis Sci 1988;33:801.

203. Stark ME, Gostout CJ, Balm RK. Clinical features and endoscopic management of Dieulafoy's disease. Gastrointest Endosc 1992;38:545.

204. Holten I, Tait N. Dieulafoy's ulcer: a palpable entity? Aust N Z J Surg 1992;62:815.

205. Sherman L, Shenoy SS, Satchidanand SK, et al. Arteriovenous malformation of the stomach. Am J Gastroenterol 1979;72:160.

206. Lin HJ, Lee FY, Tsai YT, et al. Therapeutic endoscopy for Dieulafoy's disease. J Clin Gastroenterol 1989;11:507.

207. Bedford RA, van Stolk R, Sivak MV Jr, et al. Gastric perforation after endoscopic treatment of a Dieulafoy's lesion. Am J Gastroenterol 1992;87:244.

208. Peoples JB, Kartha R, Sharif S. Multiple phlebectasia of the small intestine: case report. Am Surg 1981;47:373.

209. Wood DA. Tumors of the intestines. In: Armed Forces Institute of Pathology atlas of tumor pathology. Section 6. Part 22. Baltimore: Williams & Wilkins, 1967:44.

210. Shandalow SL. Fatal massive gastrointestinal hemorrhage due to multiple phlebectasia of the small intestine: report of a case. J Int Coll Surg 1956;25:445.

211. Flatley FJ, Atwell ME, McEvoy RK. Pseudoxanthoma elasticum with gastric hemorrhage. Arch Intern Med 1963;112:352.

212. Goodman RM, Smith EW, Paton D, et al. Pseudoxanthoma elasticum: a clinical and histopathological study. Medicine (Baltimore) 1963;42:297.

213. Beighton PH, Murdoch JL, Votteler T. Gastrointestinal complications of the Ehlers-Danlos syndrome. Gut 1969;10:1004.

214. Belli A, Cawthorne S. Visceral angiographic findings in pseudoxanthoma elasticum. Br J Radiol 1988;61;368.

Textbook of Gastroenterology, second edition, edited by Tadataka Yamada. JB Lippincott Company, Philadelphia © 1995.

CHAPTER 112

Mesenteric Vascular Insufficiency

J. Augusto Bastidas   Patrick M. Reilly
Gregory B. Bulkley

Mesenteric vascular insufficiency is a common and frequently lethal problem, whether caused by anatomic occlusion of the mesenteric macrovasculature or pathophysiologic vasospasm at the microvascular level. Despite advances in the management of the critically ill patient, a large proportion of the patients recognized with the diagnosis of overt mesenteric ischemia succumb acutely.[1] Lesser degrees of mesenteric ischemia, even when not manifested overtly as the classic clinical syndrome, may contribute to the development of systemic sepsis and the multiple organ dysfunction syndrome, a problem seen with increasing frequency in critically ill patients.[2,3] The understanding, recognition, and proper management of mesenteric vascular insufficiency have therefore become important, not only for those patients recognized to have one of the conventional syndromes of splanchnic ischemia, but also for the increasing population of patients critically ill from other diseases.

DEFINITION

A state of mesenteric vascular insufficiency exists when the blood flow to one or more gastrointestinal organs is insufficient to maintain its nutrient needs. Usually this condition is a consequence of a reduction in splanchnic blood flow, but in some cases an increased nutrient demand secondary to a severe hypermetabolic state, such as sepsis, may contribute substantially.

CLASSIFICATION

It is useful to classify mesenteric ischemia on both an anatomic and an etiologic basis. Anatomically, the clinical syndromes associated with splanchnic ischemia include not only small intestinal ischemia and ischemic colitis, but also acute erosive ("stress") gastritis, ischemic hepatitis, ischemic pancreatitis, and some forms of acalculous cholecystitis (Table 112-1). Mesenteric vascular insufficiency can also be classified on the basis of etiology (Table 112-2). It is often caused by a cessation of arterial inflow, frequently secondary to an embolus to the superior mesenteric artery (SMA) or one of its primary branches.

Chronic mesenteric arterial insufficiency may be manifest clinically as intestinal angina. This condition almost always implies global ischemia of the mesenteric vascular bed, usually due to occlusion of at least two of the three major splanchnic vessels: the celiac, superior, and inferior mesenteric (IMA) arteries. Here blood flow may be sufficient to sustain resting metabolic needs, but inadequate to meet the increased metabolic demand that follows the ingestion of a meal or, more rarely, the vascular "steal" produced by exercise of the extremities.

Venous occlusion occurs rarely,[4] usually as a result of acute thrombosis. This condition may produce a spectrum of clinical severity, ranging from an unrecognized, self-limited episode to a catastrophic event. In the latter case, major shifts of fluid into the mesenteric bed and peritoneal cavity occur, even before intestinal gangrene and sepsis develop. The result is systemic instability due to hypovolemia.

The most common form of mesenteric ischemia is strangulation obstruction of the small bowel, usually produced by an adhesive band. In most reports of patients operated on for complete small intestinal obstruction, strangulation is present in 20% to 40%.[5] Here lymphatic and then venous obstruction predominate, at least initially.

Nonocclusive mesenteric ischemia (NOMI) is a distinct clinical and pathologic entity resulting from splanchnic vasoconstriction in response to cardiogenic or hypovolemic shock, and probably other forms of severe systemic physiologic stress as well.[6] In the adult, this mesenteric vasospasm may precipitate acute mesenteric ischemia, especially when it is superimposed on a chronic, previously asymptomatic vascular occlusion. Neonatal necrotizing enterocolitis (NEC), a complex and still poorly understood condition occurring predominantly in premature infants subjected to severe physiologic stress, is probably another, unique manifestation of NOMI. Although the etiology of this condition is multifactorial, there is evidence that vasospastic intestinal ischemia may well play an important initial role.[7]

TABLE 112-1
Anatomic Classification in Splanchnic Ischemia Syndromes

ORGAN	CONDITION
Small intestine	Mesenteric ischemia
Large intestine	Ischemic colitis
Stomach	Acute erosive (i.e., stress) gastritis
Liver	Ischemic hepatitis
Pancreas	Ischemic pancreatitis
Gallbladder	Acalculous cholecystitis (some forms)

TABLE 112-2
Causes of Mesenteric Ischemia

Occlusive
Arterial
  Acute
    Global (thrombotic or embolic)
    Segmental (usually embolic)
  Chronic—intestinal angina (usually atherosclerotic)
Venous (acute thrombotic)
Strangulation (segmental, predominantly venous)

Nonocclusive
Nonocclusive mesenteric ischemia
Neonatal necrotizing enterocolitis

SPLANCHNIC HEMODYNAMICS AS RELATED TO ISCHEMIA

Vascular Elements

It is helpful to envision the mesenteric vasculature as composed of several vascular circuits coupled both in series and in parallel (Fig. 112-1).[8] The three primary parallel circuits serve the muscularis propria, the submucosa, and the mucosa, respectively. Each of these circuits is itself composed of five series-coupled components:

1. The resistance arterioles are the primary determinants of vascular resistance and thereby regulate nutrient blood flow both to the splanchnic bed as a whole and through each parallel circuit. As it is in any organ, the blood flow is proportional to the arterial (inflow) pressure and inversely proportional to the vascular resistance. Therefore, under normal conditions of stable (constant) arterial pressure, nutrient blood flow is regulated primarily by the tone of these resistance vessels.

2. Although the precapillary sphincters, located distal in the cascade to the resistance arterioles, contribute little to overall vascular resistance, they do play an important role in the regulation of transcapillary exchange, determining capillary bed patency, and thereby perfused capillary density (see Chap. 22).

3. The capillary exchange vessels allow fluid, solute, and metabolite exchange through diffusion and convection at the tissue level.

4. The postcapillary sphincters, although having little impact on total vascular resistance, greatly influence the postcapillary : precapillary resistance ratio. This ratio, which determines mean hydrostatic capillary pressure, strongly influences net fluid filtration across the proximal exchange vessels. Thus an increase in venous tone can markedly increase net fluid filtration and thereby cause edema and fluid accumulation within the lumen.

5. The tone of the distal venous capacitance vessels (venules and small collecting veins) determines the overall volume of blood sequestered within the splanchnic bed. In the resting adult, this compartment may comprise as much as

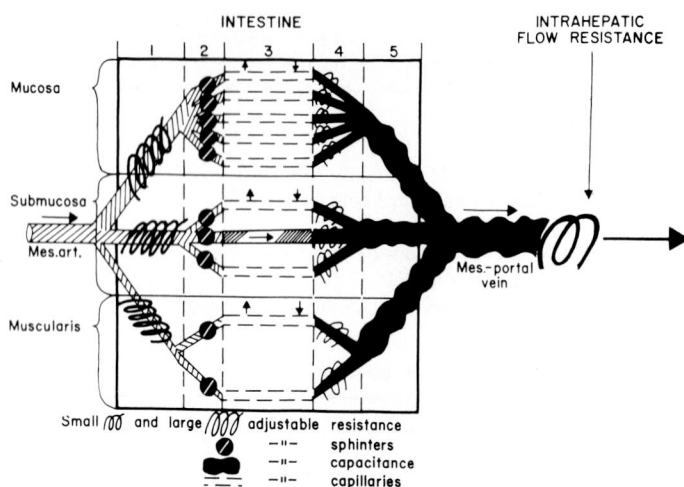

FIGURE 112-1. Microvascular anatomy of the splanchnic circulation. The fundamental anatomic arrangement of the intestinal microvasculature is in three parallel circuits serving the muscularis propria, submucosa, and mucosa, respectively. Each individual circuit is itself composed of five series-coupled components. (From Folkow B. Regional adjustments of intestinal blood flow. Gastroenterology 1967;52: 423.)

30% of the total blood volume.[9] This highly elastic compartment plays an important role in the splanchnic hemodynamic response to hypotension. For example, it is the major component of the systemic hemodynamic response to the carotid sinus reflex.[10]

Autoregulation of Blood Flow

An acute reduction of perfusion pressure within most organs is accompanied by a compensatory dilation of the resistance arterioles, which serves partially to restore tissue perfusion.[11] This phenomenon, termed *autoregulation* of blood flow, also occurs in the splanchnic vasculature, although to a somewhat lesser degree than in the brain or the kidney (Fig. 112-2).[12] This autoregulatory vasodilation is also responsible for the reactive hyperemia seen after periods of vascular occlusion or sympathetic discharge.[13] The mechanisms involved in this vasodilatory response of the precapillary arterioles include both a direct myogenic response to a reduction in perfusion pressure, as well as a metabolic response to the accumulation of local ischemic metabolites, including adenosine.[14,15]

In addition to the autoregulation of total organ blood flow, the splanchnic organs respond to reductions in perfusion pressure by redistributing blood flow within the organs themselves by adjusting the relative tone of the precapillary arterioles of adjacent parallel vascular beds (see Fig. 112-1). This

response usually favors the mucosa at the expense of the muscularis propria.[15,16]

Maintenance of Oxygen Consumption

A major factor protecting the gut from ischemic injury secondary to hypoperfusion is its ability to increase oxygen extraction (as much as sixfold) and thereby maintain oxygen consumption at or near normal levels despite substantial reductions in blood flow, and thus even after blood flow autoregulation has been overwhelmed (see Fig. 112-2).[17] This effect is the result not only of the more rapid (passive) diffusion of oxygen along a steeper concentration gradient, but also of the opening of unperfused capillary beds. The net result is an increase in perfused capillary density, which decreases the distance that oxygen must diffuse as flow is reduced. Still, below a critical level of blood flow, this capacity to increase extraction is exceeded and oxygen consumption can no longer be maintained. The capacity to maintain oxygen consumption during periods of ischemia has been found to correlate closely with the protection of the intestine from ischemic injury in experimental animals. Although this mechanism can be overwhelmed by severe ischemia, increased oxygen extraction provides an important defense against mild to moderate degrees of splanchnic ischemia, even under conditions in which the cardiac output is effectively redistributed to other organs.[12]

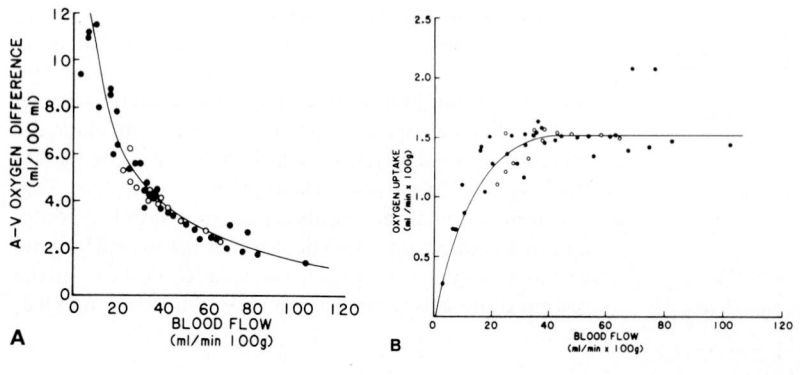

FIGURE 112-2. Maintenance of oxygen consumption shown in an isolated loop of canine colon. (**A**) As blood flow is reduced, oxygen extraction (A − VO_2 difference) increases reciprocally. (**B**) As a result, oxygen consumption (uptake) remains constant over a wide range of blood flows. Only when flow falls below a critical level does oxygen consumption fall, reflecting the fact that this homeostatic capacity has been exceeded. (From Bulkley GB, Kvietys PR, Perry MA. Effects of cardiac tamponade on colonic hemodynamics and oxygen uptake. Am J Physiol 1983;244:G605.)

Collateral Circulation

The splanchnic vascular bed is supplied with a particularly rich collateral circulation at four basic levels (Table 112-3).[18] Collateral anastomoses between the systemic and the splanchnic circulatory beds at the esophagogastric junction and in the rectum are a major source of both arterial and venous collateral blood flow.

At the esophagogastric junction, the esophageal and phrenic vessels from the systemic circulation anastomose primarily with branches of the left gastric vessels and the short gastric branches of the splenic vessels from the celiac axis of the splanchnic system. In the rectum, the branches of the superior rectal (hemorrhoidal) vessels from the splanchnic (unpaired) inferior mesenteric vessels join with branches of the middle rectal vessels from the systemic (paired) internal iliac vessels. These primary-level collaterals are important not only as a potential source of arterial nutrient inflow, but as release for venous hypertension. The consequences of this latter function include esophageal varices and hemorrhoids in patients with portal hypertension.

Within the splanchnic bed itself, at the primary level, are the collateral connections between each of the three major splanchnic vascular beds (Fig. 112-3):

1. The celiac axis communicates with the superior mesenteric vessels through the junction of the superior and inferior pancreaticoduodenal vessels (pancreaticoduodenal arcade, Fig. 112-3A).
2. The superior mesenteric vessels connect with the inferior mesenteric vessels by branches of the middle colic and the left colic vessels by way of the marginal vessels at the splenic flexure of the colon (Fig. 112-3B, C).
3. In cases of chronic ischemia, a large supplemental collateral vessel often forms by dilation of an otherwise unnamed branch in the mesentery, and in this case is known as the meandering (or "wandering") mesenteric artery.

At the secondary level, numerous collateral channels exist within the mesentery of each major vascular bed, best seen in the jejunum, and in the marginal vessels in the ileum and colon (see Fig. 112-3B, C).[19] Collateral flow through these marginal vessels is substantial, often providing the blood flow

TABLE 112-3
Splanchnic Collateral Circulation

Systemic–splanchnic collaterals
 Celiac–systemic: phrenic-esophageal vessels
 IMA–systemic: middle-inferior hemorrhoidal vessels
Primary splanchnic collaterals
 Celiac–superior mesenteric artery: pancreaticoduodenal vessels
 Superior mesenteric artery–inferior mesenteric artery: marginal vessels at splenic flexure
Secondary splanchnic collaterals
 Vascular arcades
 Marginal vessels
Tertiary splanchnic collaterals
 Intramural vessels

sufficient to maintain viability after segmental (often embolic) occlusion. Clinically, this rich collateral system is used to maintain viability of colonic grafts used for esophageal replacement.

Finally, the intramural vessels themselves provide an extremely limited degree of collateral flow distal to the marginal vessels. Although this network is a rich one, located mostly at the submucosal level, it contributes only minimally to collateral flow and will maintain blood flow only a few millimeters beyond the point of marginal vessel devascularization.[20] This tertiary level of collateral flow is important when constructing an intestinal anastomosis, ileostomy, or colostomy, where the surgical extramural devascularization of a segment more than 1 to 2 cm in length will result in either necrosis, anastomotic leakage, or later ischemic stricture. For example, strictured Brooke's ileostomy is often an indication that the surgeon who constructed it paid inadequate attention to this principle.

Under conditions of segmental ischemia, collateral blood flow itself is established and maintained primarily by the reduced vascular resistance in the ischemic segment, produced by vasodilation of the precapillary resistance vessels in the ischemic bowel segment in response to the accumulation of local metabolites. There is no measurable effect of segmental occlusion on the vascular resistance of the adjacent nonischemic bed. As a consequence, collateral flow is usually optimal without the addition of exogenous vasoactive agents.[21] Experimentally, the addition of vasodilating agents actually reduces collateral flow by preferentially dilating the adjacent (donor) vascular beds (the ischemic bed is already maximally dilated), and thereby generating a relative vascular steal phenomenon. Therefore, although the clinical use of splanchnic vasodilator agents such as papaverine may be useful for patients with intestinal ischemia caused by primary splanchnic vasospasm, there is little scientific basis for their use to treat ischemia caused by macrovascular occlusion, unless endothelial trauma, hypovolemia, or sepsis have superimposed nonocclusive vasospasm on macrovascular occlusion.

The Splanchnic Hemodynamic Response to Hypotension and Shock

The splanchnic response to systemic hypotension reflects the systemic neurohumoral response superimposed on, and largely overriding the previously mentioned local hemodynamic control mechanisms, especially with respect to the precapillary resistance vessels.

Parasympathetic and sympathetic neural systems affect ambient splanchnic precapillary and postcapillary tone. The response of the splanchnic precapillary resistance vessels to adrenergic stimulation usually is *proportional* to that of the systemic circulation.[22-28] Therefore, although adrenergic stimulation affects the "set" point of splanchnic vascular resistance, the clinically important consequence of sympathetic stimulation is a *disproportionate* increase in the tone of the postcapillary venous capacitance vessels, resulting in a substantial increase in systemic venous return (cardiac "preload"), thereby supporting the cardiac output by means of the Starling relationship in the heart.

Unlike these changes in splanchnic vascular capacitance,

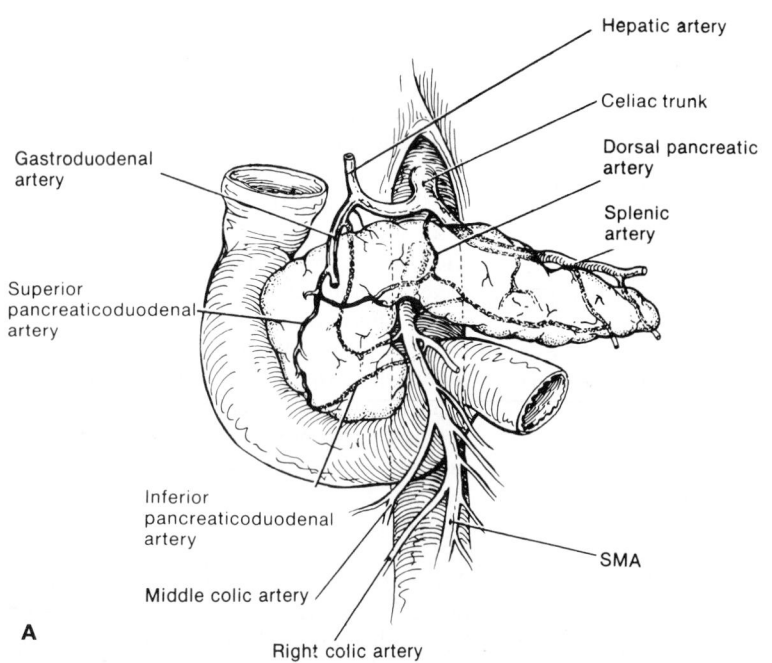

Hepatic artery

Celiac trunk

Dorsal pancreatic artery

Splenic artery

Gastroduodenal artery

Superior pancreaticoduodenal artery

Inferior pancreaticoduodenal artery

Middle colic artery

A

Right colic artery

SMA

FIGURE 112-3. Splanchnic collateral circulation. (**A**) The celiac axis and pancreaticoduodenal arcade. The major collateral conduit between the celiac axis and the superior mesenteric artery (SMA) is through the pancreaticoduodenal arcade, which also supplies the duodenal C-loop and the head of the pancreas. During acute occlusion of the SMA, collaterals from this arcade can supply as much as 50 cm of jejunum. Note that this arcade actually consists of two vessels—one anterior and one posterior—reflecting the two leaves of what is essentially the duodenal mesentery. The corresponding venous collateral drainage follows a similar but not identical pattern. (**B**) The SMA circulation. The most important vessel of the alimentary tract, the SMA arises from the aorta about 1 cm below the celiac trunk. In its course, the SMA passes through the pancreas and in front of the third portion of the duodenum before passing into the mesentery of the small intestine. (This area may be seen on a supine barium study and mistaken for a point of partial obstruction.) The first branch of the SMA is the inferior pancreaticoduodenal artery, which forms part of the pancreaticoduodenal arcade (see **A**). The middle colic and right colic arteries then arise from the SMA before the vessel arborizes into several intestinal branches. (**C**) The inferior mesenteric artery (IMA) circulation. Much smaller than the SMA, the IMA supplies the left (descending) and sigmoid colon, the rectum, and the upper anal canal. The vessel itself arises 4 cm above the aortic bifurcation. The left colic is the first branch of the IMA, extending cephalad to the splenic flexure where it gives off one branch forming the arch of Riolan, the major collateral conduit between the SMA and IMA. When this anastomosis is not well developed, the splenic flexure may be particularly vulnerable to ischemic injury. (**D**) The pelvic collateral vessels. In the pelvis, paired branches of the internal iliac arteries give rise to the paired middle and inferior rectal (hemorrhoidal) arteries. These supply the lower rectum as well as the lower anal canal and anal sphincters. They anastomose with the branches of the superior rectal (hemorrhoidal) arteries from the (unpaired) IMA, and thereby provide a major collateral conduit from the systemic to the portal circulation. (From Marston A, Pegington J. Macroscopic anatomy. In: Marston A, Bulkley GB, Fiddian-Green RG, Haglund UH, eds. Splanchnic ischemia and multiple organ failure. London: Edward Arnold, 1989:13.)

changes in splanchnic vascular resistance result in substantial alterations in the amount of nutrient blood flow, in effect redistributing blood flow away from the gut to other organs, such as the heart, brain, kidney, and skeletal muscle. Multiple mechanisms effect these changes in the splanchnic resistance vessels, including the perfusion pressure itself, adrenergic tone, and circulating humoral agents. Probably most important are the humoral mechanisms, which include a variety of circulating hormones, vasoactive peptides, and inflammatory mediators, the most important of which is the renin–angiotensin axis.[22–27,29–32] The increased sensitivity of the splanchnic vascular resistance bed to this system mediates the *disproportionate* decrease in splanchnic blood flow seen during cardiogenic

and hemorrhagic shock, a response that is *not* significantly affected by sympathetic blockade. This angiotensin-mediated selective splanchnic vasospasm is seen not only in the small intestine, but in the colon,[23] stomach,[24] and liver.[25] Thus it seems that not only nonocclusive small bowel ischemia, but ischemic colitis, acute hemorrhagic mucosal "stress" erosions of the stomach, ischemic hepatitis, and perhaps ischemic pancreatitis[33,34] and some cases of acalculous cholecystitis[35,36] are each disparate manifestations of the selective splanchnic vascular response to the activation of the renin–angiotensin axis (and perhaps, to a lesser degree, vasopressin) in response to hypotension. Each of these conditions is discussed individually later in this chapter.

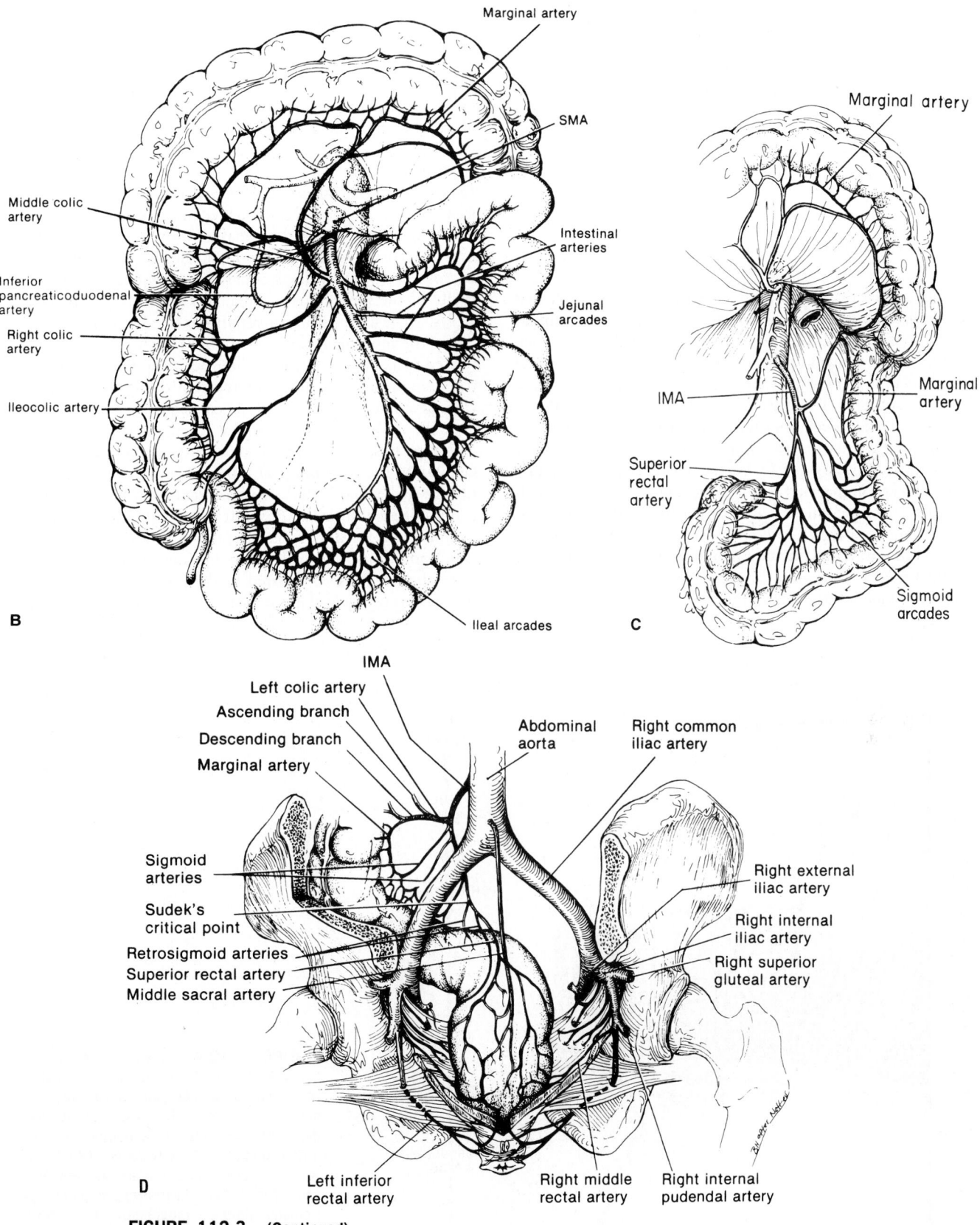

Marginal artery

SMA

Intestinal arteries

Jejunal arcades

Middle colic artery

Inferior pancreaticoduodenal artery

Right colic artery

Ileocolic artery

Ileal arcades

B

Marginal artery

IMA

Marginal artery

Superior rectal artery

Sigmoid arcades

C

IMA

Left colic artery

Ascending branch

Descending branch

Marginal artery

Abdominal aorta

Right common iliac artery

Sigmoid arteries

Sudek's critical point

Retrosigmoid arteries

Superior rectal artery

Middle sacral artery

Right external iliac artery

Right internal iliac artery

Right superior gluteal artery

Left inferior rectal artery

Right middle rectal artery

Right internal pudendal artery

D

FIGURE 112-3. (Continued)

MECHANISMS OF ISCHEMIC GUT INJURY

Ischemia (hypoxia) has long been considered the primary mechanism of splanchnic organ injury resulting from mesenteric hypoperfusion. In more recent years, a number of other mechanisms have been found also to play important roles. These include toxic oxygen metabolites, neutrophils, toxic lumenal proteases, bacteria, and toxins.

Hypoxic Injury

Hypoxia itself may significantly contribute to the injury that is seen after ischemia. In perfused segments of canine jejunum, reductions in blood flow to levels just above those at which reductions in oxygen uptake occur do not result in intestinal mucosal injury unless they are severe enough to compromise oxygen uptake.[12] These studies provide circumstantial evidence that the critical event is the impairment of oxygen consumption (hypoxia) in the underperfused vascular bed, not the reduction of flow per se. Further evidence is provided by the observation that perfusion of a segment of intestine with oxygenated saline can substantially ameliorate the injury seen in ischemic segments.[37] Although several possible mechanisms have been postulated, including increased calcium influx and cellular acidosis, the precise mechanisms whereby hypoxia leads to tissue injury remain unknown.

Gradient of Injury

With ischemia, a gradient of injury develops from the most superficial layers of the bowel wall (the villus tip) to the deeper layers (muscularis propria) as an ischemic insult progresses (Fig. 112-4).[38] The earliest manifestation is an increase in capillary permeability to large molecules.[12,39,40] Subsequently the mucosal epithelial layer allows leakage of large molecules through a normally selective barrier. More severe or prolonged ischemia produces a subepithelial edema, followed by actual shedding of epithelial cells, initially from the villus tip. Even more prolonged ischemia eventually leads to full mucosal necrosis, followed by disruption of the submucosa, and eventually of the muscularis propria, producing transmural necrosis.[38] The preferential sensitivity of the mucosa in general, and of the villus tip in particular, to ischemic injury is probably related to its distal location in the arborization of the vascular tree (Fig. 112-5).[41] The countercurrent diffusion of oxygen from arteriole to venule, with its consequent shunting away from the villus tip, may explain this sensitivity (see Chap. 22). Although the physiologic role of countercurrent exchange in facilitating the absorption of water and solutes has been seriously challenged,[42] the countercurrent diffusion of oxygen is amplified greatly at low flow rates, and is therefore probably an important factor contributing to villus injury under ischemic conditions. The explanation for increased mucosal susceptibility may also be related to the presence of high concentrations of the enzyme xanthine oxidase within the villus

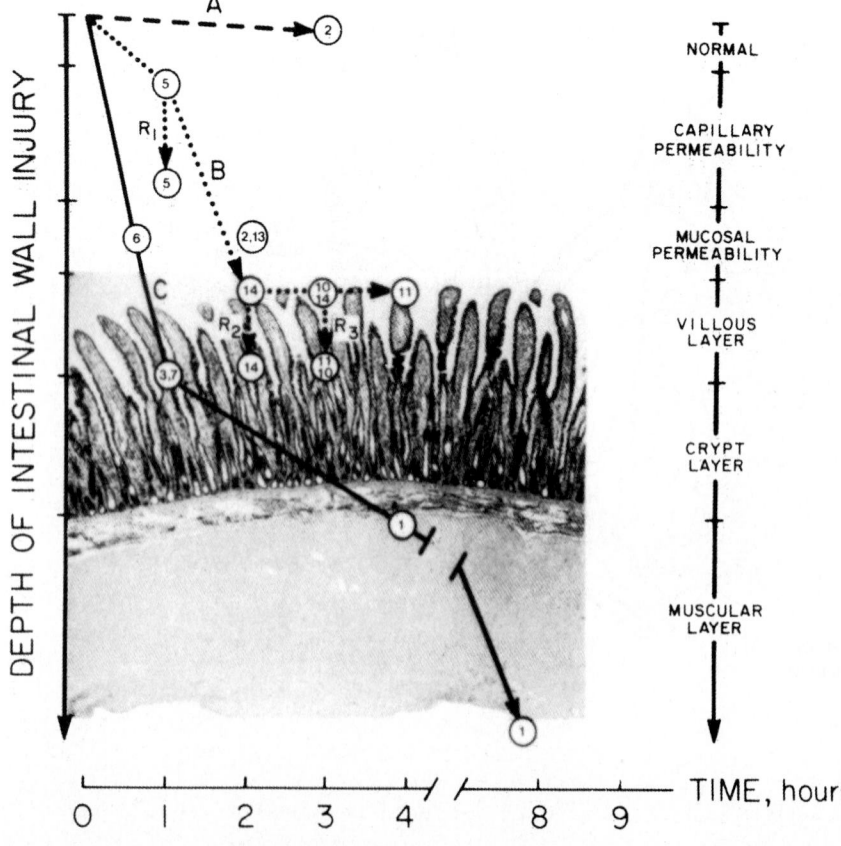

FIGURE 112-4. Gradient of injury. Lines A, B, and C represent mild, moderate, and total vascular occlusions, respectively. Numbers in circles indicate the depth of injury seen in a number of published studies.[35] Data were compiled from various species in a number of laboratories. Note that increasing degrees of ischemia produce progressive injury, from the villus tips inward, ultimately to the muscularis propria. (From Haglund U, Bulkley GB, Granger DN. On the pathophysiology of intestinal ischemic injury. Acta Chir Scand 1987;153:321.)

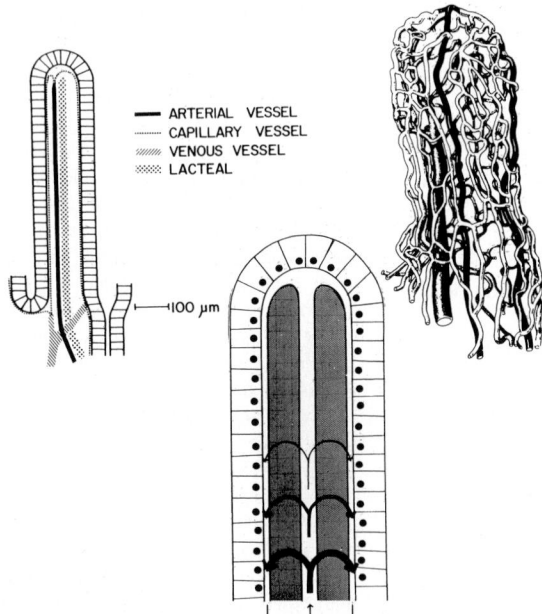

FIGURE 112-5. Villous microvascular anatomy. The villus is fundamentally a longitudinal structure, containing a central arteriole that arborizes near the villus tip to form a network of surface capillaries. Blood draining from these capillaries is collected into a central venule which runs close to the central arteriole. In the schematic diagram of the countercurrent exchange, the arteriole and venule are antiparallel, allowing the diffusion of small molecules, such as oxygen, directly from arteriole to venule, thereby shunting oxygen away from the villus tip. (From Lundgren O. Studies on blood flow distribution and countercurrent exchange in the small intestine. Acta Physiol Scand 1967;303:1.)

enterocyte (see Reperfusion Injury),[43] and the presence of digestive enzymes, toxins, and microorganisms within the lumen.

Reperfusion Injury

Although hypoxia plays a role in organ injury during hypoperfusion, much of the injury is sustained not only during the period of ischemia itself, but also during reperfusion.[44,45] The net catabolism of adenosine triphosphate during ischemia leads to increased concentrations of hypoxanthine and xanthine. Simultaneously, ischemia appears to mediate the conversion of xanthine dehydrogenase to xanthine oxidase. Unlike xanthine dehydrogenase, xanthine oxidase requires oxygen as an electron acceptor and thereby generates the superoxide free radical (O_2) in association with the oxidation of these purines to uric acid. Although oxygen is absent during ischemia, it is available suddenly and in excess at reperfusion. The superoxide generated by xanthine oxidase then triggers a classic free radical chain reaction, the cascade of events leading to injury (Fig. 112-6).[46,47] These reactive oxidants also act to arrest, trap, and activate neutrophils circulating within the microvasculature to precipitate endothelial and epithelial injury.[48-50] Studies suggest that enterocytes in the gut, and endothelial cells (which contain a great deal of xanthine oxidase) in most organs, may serve as an ubiquitous initiator of free

radical-mediated reperfusion injury by this xanthine oxidase-based endothelial cell trigger mechanism.[51]

Numerous studies have shown that the blockade of toxic oxygen metabolites significantly ameliorates postischemic injury.[44,45] In many studies, however, free radical ablation had little or no beneficial effect.[52,53] It seems that a therapeutic window exists, during which the effects of reperfusion injury outweigh the effects of ischemia, and wherein ablation of free radical mechanisms results in prevention of injury.[54] During longer periods of hypoperfusion, the ischemic component of injury far outweighs the reperfusion component, and free radical blockade has little effect.

Toxic Lumenal Factors

The primary function of the gastrointestinal tract is the digestion and absorption of ingested animal and plant tissue. To facilitate this process, a number of potent corrosive substances are secreted into the lumen. These same agents have the potential to cause both local and systemic tissue injury when the gut epithelial barrier is breached. These factors include hydrochloric acid, bile salts, bacteria, bacterial toxins, proteases, and other digestive enzyme systems (Table 112-4).

Hydrochloric Acid

The concept that toxic lumenal factors may play a role in gastrointestinal tract injury is not new. In 1855, Claude Bernard first demonstrated that the ability of the stomach to resist digestion by gastric acid was not an inherent property of living tissue, but a highly specialized function of the stomach lining.[55] Led by Davenport, numerous subsequent studies have demonstrated that the remarkable gastric mucosal barrier to what is, in fact, a million-fold concentration gradient of the hydrogen ion forms an integral part of the stomach's ability to resist autodigestion.[56] The relationship between splanchnic ischemia and mucosal integrity was first proposed by Virchow in 1853, and is now firmly based on numerous studies.[57,58] It seems clear that the gastric mucosa sustains a severe ischemic (and reperfusion) injury after a period of severe physiologic stress as a consequence of an intense and disproportionate vasoconstriction of the splanchnic resistance microvasculature (previously discussed).[24] Gastric hemorrhage, the clinical manifestation of this mucosal ulceration, usually does not appear until several days after the insult, probably reflecting the effects of the resumed secretion of gastric acid on a mucosa that has lost its barrier (protective) capability. The fact that neutralization of gastric acid can largely prevent the hemorrhage seen in this clinical syndrome is not inconsistent with this hypothesis.

Proteases

Included among the digestive enzymes are proteases, enzymes that catalyze the hydrolysis of the peptide bonds. The pancreas secretes approximately 5 to 10 g of proteases each day, mostly of the serine variety. Experimentally, ligation of the pancreatic duct or the intralumenal administration of protease inhibitors markedly attenuates the injury seen after periods of ischemia.[59-61] Moreover, intralumenal administration of the proteases trypsin or elastase aggravates such lesions. Isolation of

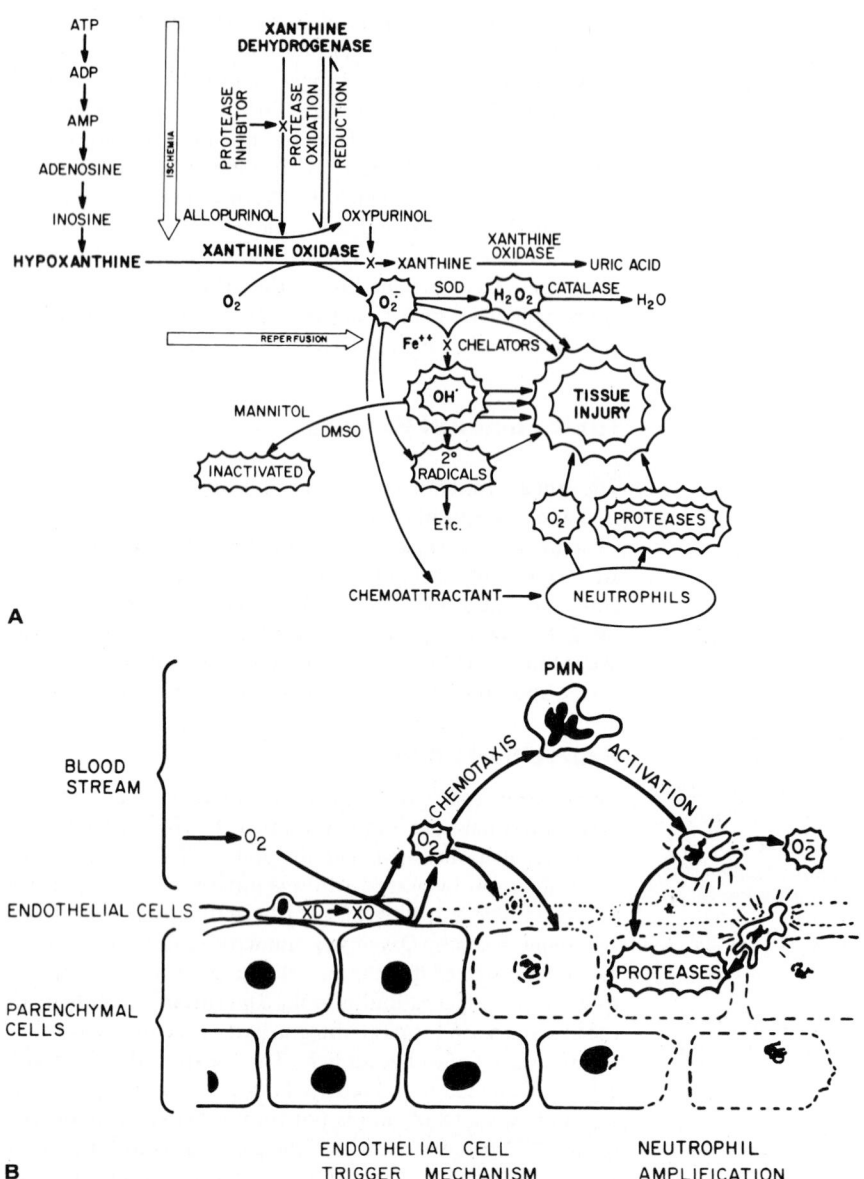

FIGURE 112-6. Proposed mechanism of oxygen free radical production. (**A**) During ischemia, the breakdown of high-energy phosphate compounds results in the accumulation of purine bases, including hypoxanthine and xanthine. At the same time, xanthine oxidoreductase is converted from a non–radical-generating form, xanthine dehydrogenase, to the superoxide radical-generating form, xanthine oxidase. At reperfusion, oxygen is reintroduced suddenly and in excess, allowing the oxidation of hypoxanthine and xanthine to uric acid, with the secondary generation of the superoxide free radical. This can then secondarily generate the highly toxic hydroxyl radical (OH*). In addition, free radical generation may lead to neutrophil accumulation and activation. Consequent tissue injury may be mediated by xanthine oxidase-generated radicals, neutrophil-generated radicals, or neutrophil proteases. (Modified from Granger DN, Hollworth ME, Parks DA. Ischemia–reperfusion injury: role of oxygen derived free radicals. Acta Physiol Scand 1986;548:97.) (**B**) Endothelial cell trigger mechanism. During ischemia, xanthine dehydrogenase (XD) is converted to xanthine oxidase (XO) in the endothelial cell. The reintroduction of oxygen at reperfusion results in the production of superoxide (O_2^-) by the mechanism detailed in (**A**). Cellular injury may occur as a direct consequence of this endothelial cell radical production or as a result of secondary neutrophil activation, which acts as an amplifier of the initial endothelial cell injury. (Modified from Raytch RE, Chuknyiska RS, Bulkley GB. The primary localization of free radical generation following anoxia/reoxygenation in isolated endothelial cells. Surgery 1987;102:122.)

the ischemic segment from the intestinal stream also protects against ischemic injury.[62] Should an ischemic insult be severe or prolonged, transmural necrosis occurs in the absence of proteases. With a less extensive ischemic insult, however, intralumenal proteases may exacerbate the initial injury.

Bacteria and Toxins

The normal human intestinal tract is colonized with large quantities of aerobic and anaerobic bacteria. The concentrations of these bacteria increase from the duodenum to the colon. The concept that these bacteria (or their products) may play a role in mucosal injury after ischemia is not novel.[63] Unfortunately, it is difficult to demonstrate definitively. It is well known that bacterial overgrowth of intestinal segments predisposes to clinical symptoms, and occasionally intestinal injury. The use of antacids, H_2 blockers, and antibiotics, common in critically ill patients, is associated with gastric and

intestinal bacterial colonization and overgrowth.[64,65] This phenomenon may contribute to the high rates of nosocomial infection seen in intensive care units. Patients with otherwise subclinical levels of mesenteric ischemia (and subsequent loss of the gut epithelial barrier) are also at an increased risk for "bacterial translocation" from the gut lumen to the gut wall, mesenteric lymph nodes, portal circulation, liver, and even the systemic circulation.[66,67] Evidence is emerging that enteral feeding, especially of glutamate, may play an important role in the prevention of pneumonia, hypermetabolism, organ failure, and perhaps even death by maintaining this gut mucosal barrier.[68]

The cell wall endotoxins of gram-negative bacteria and exotoxins of gram-positive bacteria fall into two broad categories: membrane-active toxins (e.g., phospholipases and hemolysins), and intracellularly active toxins (e.g., diphtheria toxin). Anaerobic bacteria, which are approximately a thousand times more abundant than aerobic bacteria in the oth-

TABLE 112-4
Toxic Lumenal Factors of Splanchnic Origin

LUMENAL ORIGIN	TISSUE ORIGIN
Bacteria	Vasoactive peptides
Endotoxins	Arachidonic acid metabolities
Exotoxins	Cardiotoxic factors (MDF)
Hydrochloric acid	Xanthine oxidase
Bile salts	
Proteases	
Other digestive enzymes	

MDF, myocardial depressant factors.

erwise healthy gut, predominantly produce toxins of this latter category (i.e., those that alter metabolic pathways). Stasis and ischemia promote overgrowth of these bacteria, which serve as a rich source of toxins that subsequently have easy access to ischemic mucosal segments.[69] High concentrations of endotoxin have been documented on the mucosal surface of ischemic segments of bowel.[70] Here endotoxin can act on mucosal cellular function, activate complement and coagulation pathways, and stimulate neutrophils and monocytes, which further elaborate cytokine production. The net result may be a marked inflammatory response at the local or systemic levels.

The best known and most well characterized toxin is *Clostridium difficile* endotoxin, the agent responsible for pseudomembranous colitis (see Chap. 84). A toxin from *Escherichia coli* 0157:H7 has been associated with a form of ischemic colitis.[71] Other, as yet uncharacterized, toxins may be responsible for other clinical syndromes. Further evidence implicating a role for intralumenal bacteria comes from experiments in which a portion of the colon is isolated from gastrointestinal continuity (Thiery-Vella loops). These studies demonstrated an increased survival in animals with these segments rendered ischemic compared to animals in which the ischemic segment was in intestinal continuity.[72]

Recovery After Ischemic Injury

The determining factor in tissue recovery is not tissue viability per se, but the patency of the intestinal microvasculature.[73] If ischemia is allowed to proceed long enough for microvascular injury and consequent thrombosis to occur, irreversible progressive necrosis results in the loss of the integrity of the muscularis propria and the consequent loss of bowel wall integrity. If thrombosis is prevented by pretreatment with an anticoagulant, however, the small intestine can tolerate much longer periods of complete ischemia with complete recovery. Clinically, microvascular patency is assessed using intravenous fluorescein for the intraoperative determination of postischemic bowel viability. After flow is restored, the mucosal injury caused by mild to moderate degrees of ischemia resembles a second-degree burn of the skin, and epithelial integrity can be restored through epithelial regeneration. Data suggest that mucosal cell migration contributes significantly to this mucosal reconstitution after ischemia.[74]

SYSTEMIC INFLUENCES OF INTESTINAL ISCHEMIA

Hemodynamic

At any given time, the adult splanchnic circulation contains approximately 1400 mL, or about 30% of the circulating blood volume. Thus, alterations in splanchnic blood volume distribution have a substantial systemic effect.

In shock states, the major vascular resistance response of the body as a whole is mediated in the gut.[22-27] This response is one of the primary means by which systemic blood pressure is maintained. This maintenance in "afterload" contributes to the sustenance of mean aortic pressure, compensating partially for the hypotension normally seen with hypovolemia. This selective vasospasm is largely mediated by the activation of the renin–angiotensin axis.[22-25]

Constriction of the postcapillary (venous) capacitance vessels effectively decreases the volume of blood pooled in the splanchnic bed. The result is an "autotransfusion" that increases cardiac "preload" and serves to maintain cardiac output. This hemodynamic mechanism, mediated largely by the sympathetic nervous system, serves as a first line of defense against acute hypovolemia, helping to maintain perfusion of such vital organs as the brain, heart, and kidneys at no expense to nutrient blood flow in the gut.

These splanchnic hemodynamic responses are seen in both cardiogenic and hemorrhagic shock. The events that occur in septic shock are less well understood, and more variable.

Circulating Mediators of Splanchnic Origin (Gut-Derived Toxic Factors)

Considerable attention has been focused on the role of the gastrointestinal tract in promoting and maintaining the hypermetabolic state seen in severe stress and surgical illness. Once thought a "passive" organ, the gut may play a central role in the pathophysiology of such illness. As the gut mucosal barrier fails, multiple gut-derived factors gain entry into the lymphatic, portal, and perhaps the systemic circulation (see Table 112-4).[66,67,75] The consequences may be not only systemic hemodynamic alterations, but distant, nonsplanchnic organ injury.[76,77]

Bacteria and Bacterial Toxins

As discussed, intestinal bacteria may "translocate" from the gut lumen to the bowel wall, the mesenteric lymph nodes, the liver, and to the portal and even the systemic circulation.[78-81] The initial pathophysiologic event may be the "leak" of endotoxin, rather than bacterial translocation itself.[82] In experimental studies, ileal ischemia resulted in death of rats with normal ileal flora, whereas the germ-free rats uniformly survived.[83] Some human studies have also documented portal bacteremia in as many as 30% of patients subjected to surgical stress.[77,78] Other studies have shown that portal, as well as systemic levels of endotoxin are markedly increased in critically ill animals and humans.[84-86] All of these findings give credence to the hypothesis that normal intestinal bacteria are at least associated with the lethal effects of intestinal ischemia.

Myocardial Depressant Factors

It has been recognized for some time that fluid shifts alone cannot account for the cardiovascular changes observed in patients with intestinal ischemia. One favored explanation is that humoral substances exist that may actually be "cardiotoxic." The exact nature of this humoral substance(s) remains unclear, but a great deal of work has focused on a purported "myocardial depressant factor" or factors.[87,88]

Other Gut-Derived Inflammatory Mediators

Ischemic injury can result in the systemic release of a number of inflammatory mediators that may contribute to distant organ injury. The most extensively studied model is that of adult respiratory distress syndrome, in which toxic oxygen metabolites and complement fragments (especially C'5a) have been put forward as mediators of this injury.[89]

Arachidonic acid metabolites have also been implicated in mediating systemic effects of gut ischemic injury.[90–93] It is becoming increasingly clear that local intestinal injury can generate an inflammatory response that may act systemically to cause distant organ injury.

MANAGEMENT OF SPLANCHNIC ISCHEMIA: GENERAL CONSIDERATIONS

Preoperative Diagnosis

The diagnosis of splanchnic ischemia, whether nonocclusive or occlusive, requires a high index of suspicion to identify mesenteric vascular insufficiency before the development of irreversible bowel necrosis. Clinically, intestinal ischemia often is not identified until irreversible damage to the bowel wall has occurred. The conventional image of intestinal ischemia, usually established by an indelible early clinical experience, is one of a patient with a fulminant clinical presentation of advanced mesenteric infarction. This clinical presentation, almost always associated with a rapid demise of the patient, not only reinforces a pessimistic prognostic impression, but also misleads the less experienced clinician to overlook a less dramatic clinical picture in those salvageable patients with early, reversible bowel ischemia. This observation is supported by a study of diagnostic capability in mechanical small bowel obstruction in which the *only* patients whose strangulation was recognized before surgery were those with nonviable intestinal ischemia. Not a single case of *reversible* (viable) ischemia was recognized before surgery.[5] Unless the more subtle indicators of early intestinal ischemia are recognized, there is little likelihood of a successful clinical outcome.

The triad of severe acute abdominal colic, significant preexisting cardiovascular disease, and spontaneous gastrointestinal emptying (vomiting and defecation) is helpful in identifying a patient with emerging mesenteric infarction.[94] Abdominal pain, the classic symptom associated with all forms of acute mesenteric ischemia (Table 112-5), is characteristically abrupt in onset and severe. This pain is often disproportionate to the degree of abdominal tenderness and, at first, not associated with signs of peritoneal inflammation. Although initially colicky, the pain characteristically becomes continuous, milder, and less variable in intensity as mucosal

ischemia progresses toward transmural infarction. This pain is often associated with vomiting and bowel evacuation secondary to the intense peristalsis that ischemia causes initially. Bloody diarrhea manifesting necrosis and sloughing of the intestinal mucosa may occur, but usually is seen only after several hours. The absence of blood in the stool does *not* rule out the presence of early intestinal ischemia.

Physical examination often reveals mild abdominal distention. Bowel sounds, which may be hyperactive in the early stages, become markedly decreased as an ileus develops, and finally are lost. A tender abdominal mass may develop as the extent of ischemia within an intestinal segment progresses. The presence of parietal peritonitis is a grave sign, usually indicating that progression to irreversible bowel infarction has already occurred.

Numerous laboratory tests have been advocated for the diagnosis of mesenteric ischemia (Table 112-6). Unfortunately, these tests are not only nonspecific, but, because they reflect the body's inflammatory response to de facto intestinal necrosis, they are of limited utility for the *early* recognition of *salvageable* ischemic bowel.[95] These nonspecific laboratory findings include, for example, leukocytosis, often in the range of $20,000/mm^3$ or more. Systemic metabolic acidosis and a significant base deficit are also described.[96,97] Serum phosphate,[98,99] amylase, and creatinine phosphokinase[100,101] levels may become elevated, but usually not until after mesenteric ischemia has become irreversible. As an earlier sign of mesenteric ischemia, the use of creatinine phosphokinase isoenzymes has been proposed[102]; however, the utility of this practice has not yet been established in critical studies.

Plain abdominal radiographs often demonstrate a nonspecific bowel gas pattern with a few air-filled small bowel loops.[103] The air already within the bowel lumen can be used as a contrast agent, sometimes revealing thickened bowel walls, indicating mucosal edema. This finding is suggestive of mesenteric ischemia.[104] Pneumatosis intestinalis may be seen (Fig. 112-7), but is usually a late finding. Barium studies are seldom indicated in cases of small bowel infarction, but are sometimes helpful in the diagnosis of ischemic colitis. Diagnostic angiography is often critical in confirming the diagnosis of mesenteric ischemia. This imaging modality is particularly useful in the diagnosis of arterial embolism and NOMI, as well as in the assessment of chronic mesenteric ischemia. Computed tomography[105] and magnetic resonance imaging[106] may also be of benefit, particularly in diagnosis of mesenteric venous thrombosis. Duplex ultrasound evaluation of the aorta and its visceral branches has been advocated in the assessment of both acute and chronic arterial mesenteric insufficiency.[107]

Endoscopy is used to diagnose acute erosive "stress" gastritis and is particularly useful in assessing suspected colonic ischemia. Diagnostic laparoscopy is gaining more widespread use for the evaluation of the patient suspected of having early mesenteric ischemia. Its utility and application, however, have yet to be defined precisely by clinical studies.

Preoperative Management

Preoperative management of the patient with mesenteric ischemia involves treatment of the sepsis and hemodynamic instability often associated with acute mesenteric ischemia,

TABLE 112-5
Diagnosis of Acute Intestinal Ischemia

CONDITION	CLINICAL SETTING	SYMPTOMS	PHYSICAL SIGNS	LABORATORY INDICATORS	DEFINITIVE DIAGNOSIS
Arterial thrombosis	ASCVD H/O intestinal angina Dehydration CHF	Severe pain 　Sudden onset 　Crampy → 　　continuous Nausea/vomiting	Early: 　Benign abdomen 　Hyperactive bowel sounds 　Abdominal distention 　Stool + or − for blood 　Often systemically stable	Early: None Late: 　Leukocytosis 　Acidosis	Angiogram Laparotomy
Arterial embolism	Atrial fibrillation Recent MI Recent cardioversion Cardiac 　catheterization Arteriogram	Abdominal distention Transient diarrhea Bloody stool	Late: 　Diffusely acute abdomen 　Ileus 　Sepsis 　Cardiovascular collapse	Hemoconcentration AP/CPK	
Traumatic disruption	Abdominal trauma Postoperative: 　Abdominal 　　aneurysm 　Bowel resection 　Colostomy or 　　ileostomy	Usually none	Trauma: Intraabdominal 　hemorrhage Postoperative: 　None 　Ileus, distention, or 　　sepsis	Trauma: Falling 　HCT/Hgb Postoperative: 　None 　Leukocytosis 　Acidosis	Laparotomy ± Angiogram
Strangulation obstruction	Previous abdominal 　surgery Hernia H/O congential 　defects	Signs of simple 　obstruction Severe pain Continuous pain Bloody stool	Early: 　Signs of simple 　　obstruction Late: 　Acute abdomen 　Sepsis 　Cardiovascular collapse	Early: None Late: 　Leukocytosis 　Acidosis 　AP/CPK	Laparotomy
Nonocclusive ischemia	Shock Sepsis Respiratory failure CHF Vasoconstrictor 　therapy Digitalis Recent 　cardiopulmonary 　bypass	None (obtuned) Diffuse, continuous 　pain Abdominal distention Nausea/anorexia Ileus	Early: None Late: 　Acute abdomen 　Sepsis 　Cardiovascular collapse	Early: None Late: 　Leukocytosis 　Acidosis 　AP/CPK	Angiogram ± Laparotomy (late)
Venous thrombosis	Dehydration CHF Polycythemia H/O thrombophlebitis Recent portal venous 　surgery	Subacute onset Abdominal distention Dehydration Transient diarrhea Bloody stool	Early: 　Abdominal distention 　Dehydration 　Ascites Late: 　Acute abdomen 　Sepsis 　Cardiovascular collapse	Early: 　Hemoconcentration Late: 　Leukocyosis 　Acidosis 　AP/CPK	Angiogram (venous phase) ± Laparotomy (late)
Ischemic colitis	Same as nonocclusive 　ischemia Recent aortic surgery Recent 　cardiopulmonary 　bypass	None Distention	Early: None Late: 　Acute abdomen 　Sepsis 　Cardiovascular collapse	Early: 　Hemoconcentration Late: 　Leukocytosis 　Acidosis 　AP/CPK	Sigmoidoscopy Colonoscopy

+, positive; −, negative; AP, alkaline phosphatase; ASCVD, atherosclerotic cardiovascular disease; CHF, congestive heart failure; CPK, creatine phosphokinase; HCT, hematocrit; Hgb, hemoglobin; H/O, history of; MI, Myocardial infarction.

From Bulkley GB. Mesenteric vascular occlusive disease. In: Cameron JL, ed. Current surgical therapy. vol 2. Philadelphia: BC Decker, 1986:76.

TABLE 112-6
Laboratory Tests for the Diagnosis of Mesenteric Ischemia

Blood Values
Conventional
    Leukocyte and differential blood count
    Base deficit
    Lactic acid
    Amylase
    Phosphate
    CPK (and isoenzymes)
    LDH
    Alkaline phosphatase
    ALT/AST

Experimental
    Diamine oxidase
    VIP
    N-acetyl-β-hexosaminidase

Urine
Phosphate

Peritoneal Fluid
Leukocyte count
Erythrocyte count
Phosphate
Bacteria

ALT, alanine aminotransferase; AST, aspartate aminotransferase; CPK, creatine phosphokinase; LDH, lactate dehydrogenase; VIP, vasoactive intestinal peptide.

From Reilly PM, Jones B, Bulkley GB. Noninvasive assessment of ischemic bowel syndromes. In: Ernst CB, Stanley JB, eds. Current therapy in vascular surgery. Vol 2. Philadelphia: BC Decker, 1990:721.

or the underlying shock that predisposed to NOMI. Appropriate fluid resuscitation is mandatory and usually requires central venous or pulmonary artery pressure monitoring. Monitoring of hourly urine output with an indwelling Foley catheter is mandatory. Frequently a systemic metabolic acidosis must be corrected, and a need for ventilatory support is not uncommon in these often elderly patients.

Broad-spectrum antibiotics covering both aerobic and anaerobic organisms should be administered intravenously to help control the developing sepsis. The use of antioxidants or of antibodies directed at endotoxins or cytokines has yet to be established to be of value in clinical trials. Laparotomy, although often urgently indicated, should not be undertaken until stabilization of the cardiovascular, respiratory, and acid–base status.

Intraoperative Assessment and Management

At laparotomy, the identification of frankly gangrenous bowel is usually straightforward. Lesser degrees of mesenteric ischemia may prove more challenging to the operating surgeon. Close observation for a "pink" hue and the presence of peristalsis[108] or arterial pulsations provide the basis for the standard clinical criteria of intestinal viability. In most cases,

when these signs seem to be definitive, they have proven to be reliable.[109] The use of the Doppler probe to identify pulsations on the antimesenteric border of the bowel has been used as a supplement, but false signals may be picked up from underlying bowel, and the rapid evaluation of large lengths of bowel is nearly impossible.[110] Although enthusiastically advocated by some,[111,112] controlled studies have shown that the Doppler technique may often be *less* reliable than standard clinical judgment.[113] The fluorescence pattern of the bowel wall, observed under Wood lamp (3600 nm) illumination after the intravenous injection of 1 g of sodium fluorescein, has proven to be significantly more sensitive and specific for the rapid and convenient discrimination of viable from nonviable ischemic intestine than any other method.[113,114] This technique is a useful adjunct when the standard clinical criteria are equivocal.

All nonviable bowel should be resected. When small bowel resection is required, gastrointestinal continuity can often be reestablished if the resection margin is unequivocally viable, frank peritonitis is absent, and the patient's hemodynamic and respiratory status are reasonably stable. Moreover, primary colonic anastomosis after emergent colon resection of ischemic bowel usually is not indicated. These situations are best

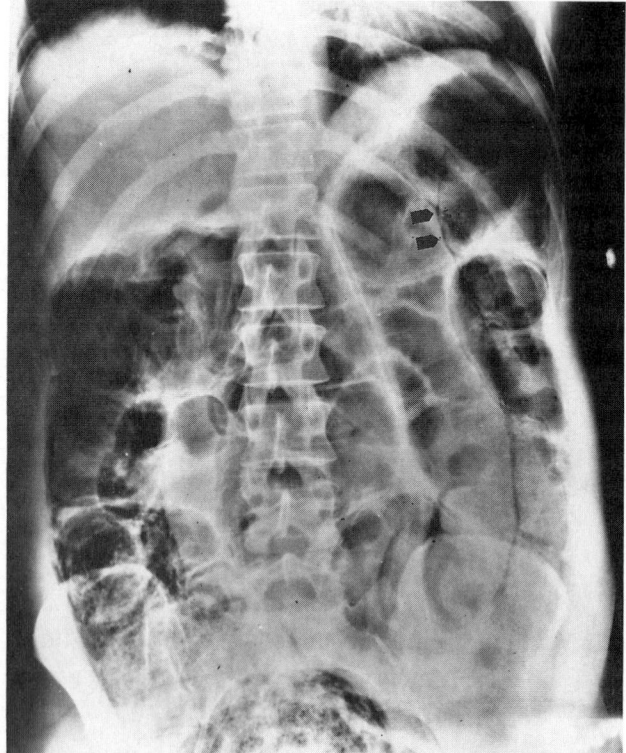

FIGURE 112-7. Pneumotosis intestinalis. In cases of acute mesenteric ischemia, the plain radiograph may show distended, air-filled loops of intestine with thickening of the bowel wall or even, as seen here, air in the bowel wall or tributaries of the superior mesenteric vein or portal vein. Unfortunately, the latter findings, although diagnostic, only appear late in the course of the disease, after irreversible transmural bowel necrosis has been sustained.

managed with appropriate ostomies, with reanastomosis planned when the patient has recovered.

Postoperative Considerations

Hemodynamic monitoring, continued fluid resuscitation, correction of acidosis, antibiotic therapy, and often ventilatory support are required through the immediate postoperative period. Anticoagulation therapy with heparin is appropriate in treating mesenteric venous thrombosis and in treating the underlying conditions (e.g., atrial thrombus) that have given rise to arterial emboli. Intravenous nutritional support should be considered early, especially in patients requiring massive bowel resection who are at risk for short gut syndrome. Enteral feeding should also be used whenever possible. The patient's clinical course can then be followed, with overall improvement expected in the first few postoperative days.

Many surgeons have advocated a second-look laparotomy at 24 to 48 hours to reevaluate the viability of bowel originally left in situ, even when the patient shows no signs of clinical deterioration. This approach is taken to define the viability of bowel that had been of questionable viability at the time of initial exploration, and therefore allows such bowel to be left unresected, at least initially. The value and timing of such an approach, however, are controversial, not supported by laboratory studies, and not established by clinical trials. In cases of mesenteric vein occlusion (in which the process of venous thrombosis may progress after surgery) or especially after surgical revascularization, this approach may be useful.[115] Nevertheless, there is no published evidence that a planned second-look laparotomy affects the mortality from acute intestinal ischemia. In one controlled laboratory study, the fluorescein technique at initial laparotomy was found to be *superior* to clinical judgment at a second-look laparotomy 24 hours later.[113]

SPLANCHNIC ISCHEMIA SYNDROMES

Strangulation Obstruction

Etiology and Pathophysiology

Strangulation obstruction involves vascular compromise of a segment of the intestine by extrinsic mechanical compression. This process may involve the small bowel (mechanical small bowel obstruction; Chap. 37), the colon (sigmoid or cecal volvulus; Chap. 37), or the stomach (paraesophageal hernia with volvulus; Chap. 67). All patients with mechanical obstruction of a hollow viscus are at risk for strangulation.

Pathophysiologically, strangulation involves compromise of both venous and arterial blood flow. Traditionally, this process has been thought to occur secondary to massive dilation of a segment of bowel with resultant increases in intralumenal pressure sufficient to impair first venous, then arterial flow. More often, however, segmental dilation produces volvulus and the resultant pinching off of the major segmental vascular supply to the involved loop, with consequent ischemia (Fig. 112-8). Sometimes a twisted segment will spon-

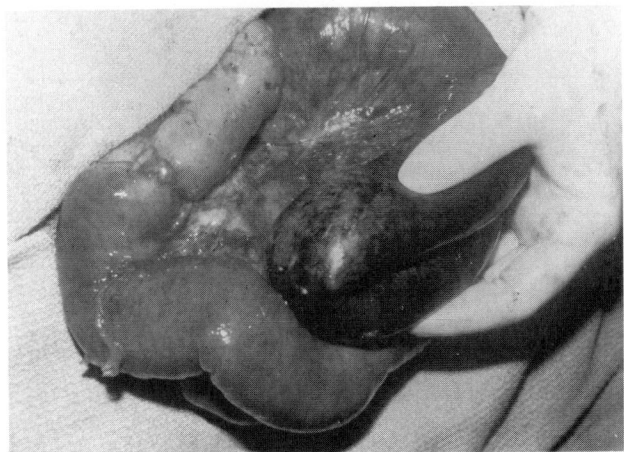

FIGURE 112-8. Strangulation obstruction. Gross appearance of strangulated, necrotic bowel in a patient who presented with small bowel obstruction. Note the abrupt line of demarcation.

taneously reduce itself, thus averting progression to frank gangrene, although once frank strangulation occurs, it rarely reduces without surgical intervention.

Epidemiology

Intestinal strangulation causes the most common and most treatable form of mesenteric vascular insufficiency. It is estimated that strangulation is present in 20% to 40% of patients operated on for small bowel obstruction.[5] Moreover, the presence of strangulation nearly doubles the 5% to 10% mortality associated with small bowel obstruction.

Clinical Features and Diagnosis

The diagnosis of bowel obstruction itself is usually straightforward. The early recognition of strangulation obstruction by clinical or laboratory means obviously would be of significant benefit in the management of these patients.[5,116] Traditional teaching has held that continuous (as opposed to colicky) pain, fever, tachycardia, physical signs of parietal peritoneal inflammation (involuntary guarding, "rebound" tenderness), leukocytosis, hyperkalemia, hyperphosphatemia, and serum enzyme elevations were discriminant signs of intestinal ischemia. Retrospective studies, however, have repeatedly found that these diagnostic criteria, alone or in combination, are not discriminant.[116] Moreover, a prospective study found that a senior clinician's best clinical judgment, based on all available clinical and laboratory information and a personal knowledge of the patient, was no better than pure chance in making this discrimination.[5] Based on this study, the clinical assessment of a patient to have simple (nonstrangulated) obstruction was associated with a 31% ± 8% chance of error (i.e., that intestinal ischemia was indeed present; Table 112-7). It is, quite simply, not possible on clinical grounds to discriminate reliably between those patients with early strangulation and those with simple obstruction.[5]

TABLE 112-7
Classic Signs of Intestinal Ischemia

SIGN	SENSITIVITY (%)	SPECIFICITY (%)	PREDICTIVE VALUE (%)
Continuous pain	27	91	67
Fever	24	70	36
Tachycardia	52	43	39
Peritoneal signs	29	97	86
Leukocytosis	81	37	47
Base deficit	75	80	75
Abdominal mass	5	87	20
Blood in stool	14	75	22

Sensitivity and Specificity of Classic Physical Signs

	NUMBER OF POSITIVE SIGNS				
	1/5	2/5	3/5	4/5	5/5
Sensitivity	95%	67%	43%	10%	0%
Specificity	0%	40%	93%	100%	100%

Experienced Clinical Judgment in Small Bowel Obstruction
(Preoperative Diagnosis of Strangulation)

Sensitivity	48%
Specificity	83%
Predictive Value	
Assessment of strangulation	67%
Assessment of no strangulation	69%

Adapted from Reilly PM, Jones B, Bulkley GB. Noninvasive assessment of ischemic bowel syndromes. In: Ernst CB, Stanely JB, eds. Current therapy in vascular surgery. Vol 2. Philadelphia: BC Decker, 1990:721.

Treatment

The treatment of strangulation obstruction is straightforward. The underlying cause of the obstruction (adhesions, hernia, carcinoma) must be surgically corrected and any segments of nonviable bowel resected. In many instances a primary anastomosis is appropriate. Occasionally, when dealing with massive intraperitoneal sepsis or the obstructed colon, an ostomy and delayed reconstruction is the more prudent choice.

Prognosis

The most important element in the management of strangulation obstruction is its prevention. Clinically, this translates into early differentiation of partial from complete intestinal obstruction, and early, prompt laparotomy for most cases shown to be complete. Mortality rates in patients with intestinal obstruction dramatically increase with the advent of bowel necrosis. Prompt laparotomy, reduction of the strangulated segment, and resection of all nonviable bowel provide the best chance of successful outcome.

Acute Mesenteric Arterial Embolus

Etiology and Pathophysiology

Acute mesenteric infarction is most often caused by an embolic or thrombotic occlusion of one or more mesenteric vessels. Arterial emboli usually originate from the heart and ac-

count for nearly 75% of cases.[117] Most emboli occur in patients in atrial fibrillation. A mural thrombus after a myocardial infarction is also a common source of peripheral emboli. The proximal aorta may also shower atheromatous plaques downstream, resulting in peripheral embolization. Emboli to the SMA comprise approximately 5% of all cases of peripheral arterial embolization.[118] The embolus usually lodges slightly distal to the origin of the SMA, thus occluding the vessel several centimeters from its origin. It is not uncommon, however, for the embolus to lodge in more distal branches, occluding the origins of the middle colic, right colic, or even smaller peripheral branches.[119] The clinical impact of such an embolic event depends not only on the anatomic site of occlusion, but also on the adequacy of preexisting collateral circulation.

Epidemiology

Typical patients at risk for mesenteric emboli are those elderly, often institutionalized people with preexisting, widespread atherosclerotic vascular disease.[120,121] They often have a history of stroke, myocardial infarction, or peripheral vascular insufficiency (Table 112-8). Patients who present with mesenteric emboli are often in and out of atrial fibrillation, have a history of recent cardioversion, or have suffered a recent large myocardial infarction.

Clinical Features

A history of an embolic event is frequently documented in patients with acute mesenteric occlusion. Evidence of other (often simultaneous) embolic sites, such as the eyegrounds, feet, or fingernails, may be present in the patient with an acute onset of abdominal pain. Vital signs usually are normal for a short time; however, intralumenal sequestration of fluids soon leads to dehydration, manifest clinically as tachycardia, decreased urine output, and even hypotension. A low-grade fever, sometimes below 38°C, may also be present.

Diagnosis

Because most patients at risk for embolic occlusion of a mesenteric vessel are elderly and have little physiologic reserve, prompt diagnosis is of paramount importance. Arteriography not only serves to confirm the diagnosis of mesenteric ischemia in the patient at risk, but also demonstrates relevant anatomy, allowing the surgeon to plan reconstructive efforts before laparotomy. For this reason, most patients should undergo arteriography before operative intervention, when it is available, without delay.[122,123]

Interpretation of the arteriogram can be difficult. Commonly complicating the arteriographic picture are preexisting atherosclerotic lesions, often including a total, previously asymptomatic occlusion of a major splanchnic vessel. The presence of prominent collateral vessels, such as a meandering mesenteric artery, can be a useful indication of the chronic nature of such occlusions. Still, the most common "positive" finding at arteriography is occlusion of the SMA at the origin of the middle colic artery (Fig. 112-9). Significant associated vasospasm and a paucity of collateral circulation may be present. This vasospasm may present difficulties in the successful

TABLE 112-8
Clinical Factors that Predispose to Mesenteric Ischemia

Arterial Occlusion
Embolism (15%–40% of cases)
    Prior embolic event
    Atrial fibrillation (recent cardioversion)
    Rheumatic heart disease
    Prosthetic valve(s)
    Recent myocardial infarction
    Recent vascular instrumentation
        Cardiac catheterization
        Angiography
        Angioplasty
Thrombosis (15%–65%)
    Known vascular disease
        Atherosclerosis
        Aortic dissection
        Vasculitis (including SLE)
    Trauma
    Hypercoaguable states
        Dehydration

Venous Thrombosis (2%–20%)
Hypercoaguable state
    Hormones or pregnancy
    Carcinoma and carcinomatosis
    Polycythemia
    Coagulopathies
    Protein S deficiency
    Protein C deficiency
    Dehydration
Venous obstruction
    Portal hypertension
    Budd-Chiari syndrome
    Carcinoma
Low splanchnic blood flow
    Congestive heart failure
    Shock
Bowel obstruction
Trauma
Sclerotherapy

Vasospasm (5%–25%)
Dehydration
Shock
Congestive failure
Pericardial tamponade
Cardiopulmonary bypass
Dialysis
Vasoconstrictive drugs
    Digitalis glycosides
    α-Adrenergic agonists
    β-Adrenergic antagonists
    Vasopressin
    Cocaine

From Reilly PM, Jones B, Bulkley BG. Noninvasive assessment of ischemic bowel syndromes. In: Ernst CB, Stanley JB, eds. Current therapy in vascular surgery. Vol 2. Philadephia: BC Decker, 1990:719.

operative management of these lesions, as is discussed in the following section.

Treatment

After the diagnosis of a mesenteric embolism has been established, prompt laparotomy is indicated. At laparotomy, several characteristic patterns of ischemia have been observed. The most common, secondary to emboli lodging in the proximal SMA but distal to the takeoff of several jejunal branches, is ischemia of most of the small bowel and proximal colon, but with sparing of the proximal jejunum. Less common is a pattern of patchy necrosis with intervening areas of intestinal viability, commonly caused by "trashing" of small emboli into the distal SMA branches. Thrombosis of the SMA, on the other hand, usually produces ischemia that involves the entire small bowel and proximal colon. In association with celiac axis, IMA occlusion, or both, the surgeon may find frank necrosis of the entire gut, from duodenum to rectum. Surgical management consists of reestablishment, if possible, of arterial inflow, accurate assessment of bowel viability, and resection of frankly ischemic segments. In the case of SMA emboli, flow is best reestablished by isolating the proximal SMA at the point where the pulsations stop, making a transverse incision in the vessel, and removing the embolus and any adjacent clot with a balloon embolectomy catheter. After the artery is cleared, it should be liberally flushed with heparinized saline. Pulsations should be evident in the distal branches of the SMA after successful embolectomy. In some cases, the infusion of a vasodilator such as papaverine is used to overcome the vasospasm that often follows embolectomy, and heparinization is often used to help prevent thrombosis secondary to endothelial trauma, as well as to treat the underlying source of the embolus.

After revascularization, nonviable bowel must be resected. Clinically, the assessment of bowel viability is usually straightforward, but may be difficult. If compromised bowel is left behind, it may act as a source of sepsis. On the other hand, unnecessary resection may lead to the development of short gut syndrome.

Prognosis

The mortality from mesenteric vascular embolic disease is high, varying from 50% to 90%.[104,119] Most patients are encountered late in the course of their disease, when severe systemic manifestations are already present, and the intestinal ischemia has progressed to frank gangrene. Nevertheless, with the availability of parenteral nutrition, resection usually should be undertaken, and parenteral nutrition begun, in an attempt to salvage the patient.[124] The most effective efforts to improve the outcome, however, are prevention, rapid diagnosis, and aggressive early treatment, whenever possible.

Acute Mesenteric Arterial Thrombosis

Etiology and Pathophysiology

Thrombotic occlusion of the mesenteric vascular supply accounts for approximately 10% to 15% of cases of acute mesenteric ischemia, although the precise differentiation between

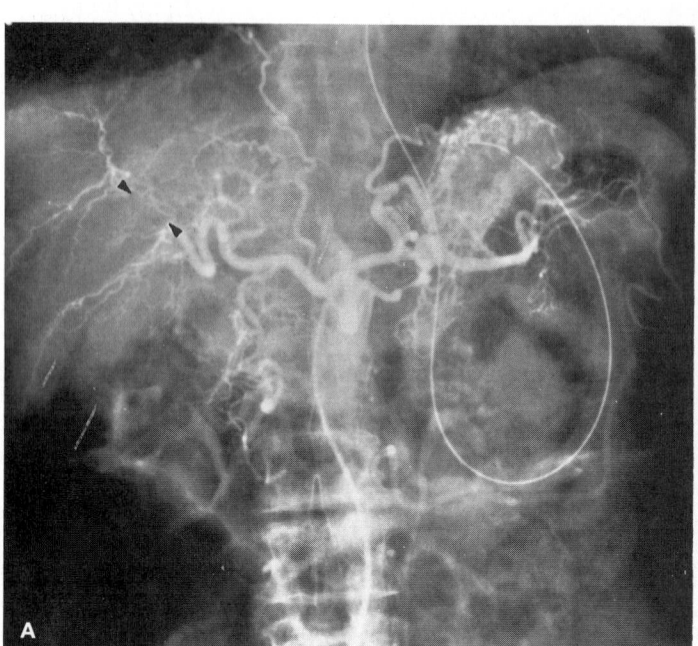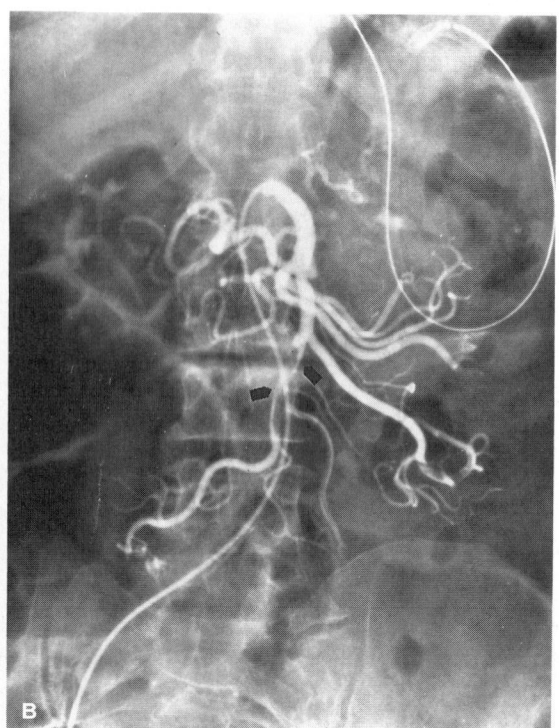

FIGURE 112-9. Visceral embolic disease. Arteriographic demonstration of splanchnic embolic disease. These two views from the same patient demonstrate emboli in two different splanchnic vessels. (**A**) Hepatic artery embolus. (**B**) Superior mesenteric artery embolus.

embolus and thrombosis is often difficult.[125] Acute mesenteric thrombosis usually occurs at the site of a preexisting atherosclerotic lesion or other anatomic abnormality (see Celiac Artery Compression). A decrease in cardiac output secondary to dehydration or hemorrhage, or after a myocardial infarction, often precedes the thrombotic episode. The clinical manifestations of arterial thrombosis, like those of embolism, depend on the presence and adequacy of collateral flow.

Epidemiology

Mesenteric arterial thrombosis frequently occurs in the setting of a low-flow state (see Table 112-8).[126] Typical patients at risk for mesenteric thrombosis are the elderly, with preexisting atherosclerotic narrowing of the origin of the SMA, patients with congestive heart failure, and those with a recent myocardial infarction. Hypercoagulable states (polycythemia vera, dehydration, postsplenectomy syndrome, carcinoma), aortic dissection, and trauma have also been associated with mesenteric arterial thrombosis.[127]

Clinical Features

Mesenteric arterial thrombosis may present in a more insidious fashion than does an acute mesenteric embolism. The pain may be more gradual in onset, and more moderate in intensity, and only variably present. Physical findings are similar to those of early embolic occlusion, with little tenderness in proportion to the pain, mild abdominal distention, and hypoactive bowel

sounds in the presence of a soft abdomen. Signs of systemic atherosclerosis, including diminished peripheral pulses or bruits, are often found. Late findings are similar to those of mesenteric infarction from embolic disease.[128]

Diagnosis

The same principles used in the diagnosis of mesenteric embolism apply to mesenteric thrombosis. Thrombotic disease, however, often presents much more insidiously. As with arterial embolic disease, laboratory tests and plain radiographs usually are of diagnostic value only after infarction has occurred. Arteriography is essential to confirm the diagnosis of mesenteric arterial thrombosis and to plan an operative approach. The occlusion is commonly present in the first portion of the SMA, with both the SMA and the celiac axis occluded. Here again the presence of large collateral vessels from the IMA and lumbar arteries may indicate chronic ischemia on which an acute process has been superimposed.

Treatment

After the diagnosis of mesenteric thrombosis has been established, prompt laparotomy usually is indicated. At laparotomy, the bowel appears ischemic for a variable distance, depending on the collateral circulation. If previous occlusion of two of the three mesenteric vessels has occurred, acute thrombosis of the remaining vessel may produce ischemia from the stomach to the rectum. As in embolic disease, surgical management consists of reestablishment of arterial inflow, assessment of bowel viability, and resection of frankly ischemic segments. In the case of SMA thrombosis, revascularization is often more difficult, usually requiring a saphenous vein bypass of the occlusive lesion. This procedure begins with mobilization of the fourth portion of the duodenum from the ligament of Treitz, allowing close approximation of the proximal SMA to the aorta. A short segment of saphenous vein is then interposed from the infrarenal aorta to a suitable portion of the SMA. Alternate sites of graft inflow include the supraceliac aorta and the right hepatic artery.[118] In many cases such a heroic effort is not indicated, either because of the irreversibility of the gastrointestinal injury, or the condition of the patient. In these patients, surgery should be confined to the resection of all nonviable bowel.

Thrombolytic therapy has also been suggested as a possible treatment for mesenteric arterial thrombosis.[129,130] Although this approach may hold some promise for the future, especially if ischemia is diagnosed promptly, the risks of bleeding and the possible release of toxic lumenal factors from the bowel lumen have limited its usefulness.

Prognosis

The mortality for mesenteric vascular thrombosis is high, averaging 70% to 90%.[125,128] Successful revascularization, however, may be associated with a good long-term outcome. The widespread availability of parenteral nutritional support has resulted in an increase in postoperative survival.

Mesenteric Venous Thrombosis

Etiology and Pathophysiology

Mesenteric venous thrombosis (MVT) may be idiopathic or evolve secondarily as a consequence of a number of particular clinical disorders. Inherited hypercoagulable disorders, including deficiency of protein S, protein C, and antithrombin III account for a large percentage of cases previously classified as idiopathic.[131,132] Secondary venous occlusion may be the result of trauma, hypercoagulable states, or intraperitoneal irritation.[133,134]

Acute thrombosis of the mesenteric veins is followed by hyperemia, edema, and subserosal hemorrhage in the affected bowel—the picture of a hemorrhagic infarct. The lumen of the bowel rapidly fills with a dark, bloody fluid. Sequestration of fluid is particularly prominent in cases of venous occlusion, and may be massive. With extensive venous occlusion, secondary thrombosis of the arterial circulation may also develop. As a result, the initial site of the occlusion, whether arterial or venous, may never be determined. Moreover, septic phlebitis secondary to inflammation (pyelophlebitis) of the portal system may develop and give rise to septic emboli to the liver.

Epidemiology

Although nearly 50% of cases of MVT are idiopathic, patients at risk can be identified (see Table 112-8). Patients with portal hypertension, dehydration, or a source of intraperitoneal sepsis (appendicitis, inflammatory bowel disease, diverticulitis) are at risk for secondary thrombosis, as are patients in a hypercoagulable state.[133-135] Reports have also described MVT as a complication of endoscopic sclerotherapy.[136]

Clinical Manifestations

Mesenteric venous thrombosis tends to be insidious in onset. The symptoms include vague abdominal pain, diarrhea (often bloody), and vomiting. Often these nonspecific symptoms are followed by circulatory collapse as hypovolemia develops. On physical examination, generalized abdominal tenderness, guarding, and distention develop later. Frank peritonitis develops only when transmural infarction or perforation have already occurred.

Diagnosis

The sometimes insidious onset of mesenteric venous thrombosis may lead to a delay in diagnosis. Laboratory tests often reveal a leukocytosis and elevated hematocrit, the latter a reflection of hemoconcentration. As with arterial occlusion, other serum markers usually change only as ischemia progresses to infarction. Plain radiographs often demonstrate dilated, fluid-filled loops of bowel. Mucosal edema may be more prominent than in arterial occlusion. The noninvasive diagnostic modalities of magnetic resonance imaging and computed tomography can sometimes provide an early diagnosis of MVT,[105,106] allowing for initiation of anticoagulation. Eventually, however, most patients show clear indications for laparotomy.

Treatment

Some cases of segmental or partial venous thrombosis are treatable with anticoagulants, particularly if an early diagnosis can be made. Once the diagnosis of frank venous infarction has been made, however, surgery is indicated. At laparotomy, the thickened, edematous bowel filled with dark, bloody fluid gives the bowel a maroon hue. The affected bowel closely resembles a strangulated loop, another condition where venous occlusion predominates. Resection should be undertaken, with care to excise areas beyond the area of gross infarction, where thrombosed veins may remain. As discussed, a second-look laparotomy is often indicated in these cases because thrombosis may well progress after surgery.[115]

After surgery, anticoagulation with heparin and subsequently warfarin should be undertaken.[137,138] This therapy is usually continued on a long-term basis. In addition, if the thrombosis is idiopathic in nature, a thorough evaluation of the patient's clotting function and family history should be performed. In some cases, a search for an occult malignancy is warranted.

Prognosis

The results of surgery for mesenteric venous thrombosis are slightly better than those for arterial occlusion. The frequent segmental nature of the occlusion probably accounts for this improved outcome. As with arterial ischemia, however, early diagnosis and prompt surgical intervention are the keys to a successful outcome.

Nonocclusive Mesenteric Ischemia

Etiology and Pathophysiology

The fundamental mechanism leading to NOMI is a selective splanchnic vasoconstriction that overwhelms the normal autoregulation of blood flow in the intestinal microvasculature.[22-27] The result is intestinal ischemia as the body redirects gut blood flow to other vital organs. Severe splanchnic vasoconstriction occurs in the setting of cardiogenic or hemorrhagic shock and other forms of severe physiologic stress. This phenomenon, characterized as the "fight-or-flight" response, was first recognized as a variation of the diving reflex of marine mammals by Cannon in the 1920s.[139] Humoral mediators, particularly angiotensin II and perhaps vasopressin, directly mediate this response (see The Splanchnic Hemodynamic Response to Hypotension and Shock).[22-27] The right colon seems to be particularly susceptible to NOMI.[140]

Epidemiology

Since the original description of NOMI in 1958, clinical awareness of this problem has grown considerably.[141] Early reports suggested that NOMI comprised about 10% to 20% of all cases of mesenteric ischemia. More recent reports, suggesting that the incidence may be as high as 50%,[142] seem improbable. This apparent increase in incidence may reflect not only an increased awareness of this clinical syndrome, but also a decreased threshold for inclusion of patients into this diagnostic category. Because most patients in circulatory shock have some reduction in splanchnic perfusion, it remains difficult to discriminate a normal homeostatic response from its pathologic extension to clinically important gut ischemia. In fact, the true incidence of NOMI is probably decreasing as pulmonary artery catheters and vasodilator agents are increasingly used to monitor and optimize systemic hemodynamics in the modern intensive care setting.[22,143]

Myocardial infarction, congestive heart failure, cardiac arrhythmias, major visceral surgery, peritonitis, chronic dialysis, hypovolemia, and shock all predispose a patient to NOMI, as do digitalis glycosides (themselves potent and selective splanchnic vasoconstrictors), vasopressors, diuretics, and cocaine abuse.[143-145]

Clinical Features

Presenting signs and symptoms of NOMI may be similar to those of acute mesenteric thrombotic disease: a gradual onset of an initially crampy, periumbilical abdominal pain, which changes to a constant, dull ache as the ischemic insult progresses. The onset is often quite subtle clinically. Moreover, many of these patients, already obtunded, may not manifest any overt symptoms, leading to a delay in diagnosis. Abdominal distention, diffuse abdominal pain, malabsorption, and maldigestion with ileus all are commonly seen in patients with NOMI. Unfortunately, these findings are nonspecific.

Diagnosis

Increased white blood cell counts and electrolyte abnormalities have been reported in up to 75% of patients with NOMI. These studies are not helpful, because they often simply reflect the severity of the underlying illness, or they indicate the presence of frank bowel necrosis. Plain abdominal radiographs usually reveal only nonspecific gas patterns.

The key to the successful management of this problem lies in a high index of suspicion, coupled with early diagnosis and treatment.[142,143] Practically, this means that when confronted with a patient with nonspecific abdominal pain and distention superimposed on a preexisting picture of critical illness, the diagnosis of mesenteric ischemia should be entertained, and angiography seriously considered.

Radiographic diagnosis of splanchnic vasospasm rests on selective superior mesenteric arteriography, usually through a transfemoral approach (Fig. 112-10). The arteriogram requires experience to interpret, and is best approached through intimate consultation between an experienced clinician and radiologist.[123] The coexistence of atherosclerotic lesions often complicates this interpretation. The typical picture involves

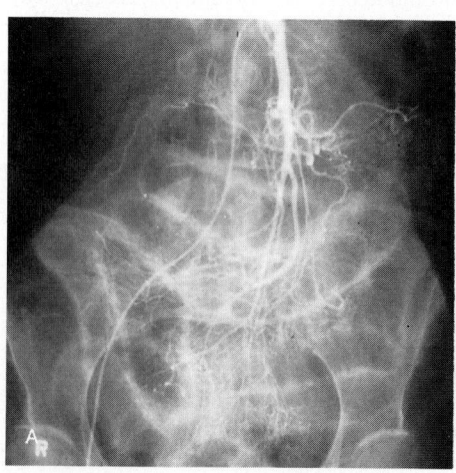
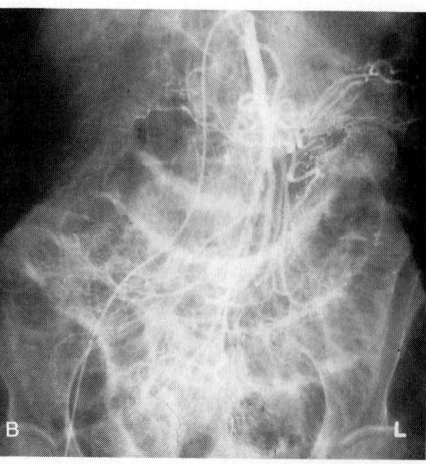

FIGURE 112-10. Nonocclusive intestinal ischemia—arteriographic findings. **(A)** On initial mesenteric arteriography of a patient with nonocclusive intestinal ischemia, vasospasm and irregularities of the celiac and superior mesenteric artery (SMA) vessels are noted. The normal arterial blush of the bowel wall is lost. **(B)** After infusion of papaverine, substantial vasodilation is seen at both the macrovascular and microvascular levels. This radiograph is compatible with a normal SMA arteriogram but is diagnostic for nonocclusive mesenteric ischemia when compared with **A.**

visible spasm of the macroscopic vessels (not the lesion responsible for the ischemia), as well as a loss of the normal arterial blush of the bowel wall microvessels. Despite the difficulty in interpretation, the arteriogram most often confirms or refutes the diagnosis, and allows specific intervention to be initiated.

Treatment

Initial management of patients suspected of having NOMI should be directed at the correction of the underlying disorders contributing to the mesenteric vasospasm.[142,146] Foremost is optimization of intravascular volume status and cardiac output. Therefore, volume resuscitation, afterload reduction, the avoidance of vasoconstricting agents (including digitalis), and sometimes selected inotropic agents form the basis for initial therapy. In addition, nasogastric suction, supplemental oxygen, and antibiotics provide further support measures. Efforts should be made to avoid any intervention that increases the activation of the renin–angiotensin axis, vasopressin secretion, or sympathetic nervous system. After the diagnosis by mesenteric arteriography, a bolus injection of tolazoline (25 mg) or papaverine (60 mg) can be given over 20 minutes. A repeat arteriogram is then performed to assess therapeutic response. Often an improvement in the vasospasm will be seen (see Fig. 112-10). After this bolus injection, a continuous infusion of papaverine (30–60 mg/hour) is administered, and the patient is transported back to the intensive care unit with the SMA catheter in place. Therapy may then be continued for 12 to 24 hours with attention given to signs of clinical improvement (decreased abdominal distention, return of gut peristalsis [bowel sounds, defecation], decreased pain, and improved sepsis control) or deterioration.

Surgery plays an important although secondary role in the management of nonocclusive ischemia. Early unnecessary laparotomy may actually worsen the splanchnic vasospasm, while delaying diagnostic and therapeutic arteriography; thus, it is important to obtain arteriograms before laparotomy. If the abdomen is opened and nonocclusive ischemic disease is recognized, the abdomen should be closed and the patient transported to the angiography suite for arteriography and vasodilator infusion. If laparotomy is to be performed, it is important that the bowel be examined at *optimal* perfusion status so that rational decisions can be made regarding viability and the consequent need for resection (Fig. 112-11). Surgery is appropriate for the evaluation and resection of frankly necrotic bowel. If a bowel resection is performed, second-look operations may be needed to assess subsequent viability, especially if the underlying hemodynamic instability persists.

Prognosis

NOMI represents a difficult clinical problem associated with a high (>90%) mortality rate, in large part because of the severity of the underlying illness. Although it has been suggested that an aggressive approach toward this problem, combined with a liberal policy toward arteriography, can result in a decrease in mortality to 50%,[142] many believe that this improvement is more apparent than real, owing to the inclu-

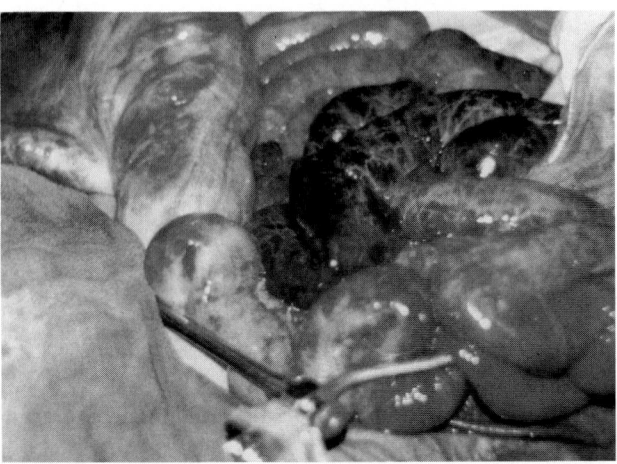

FIGURE 112-11. Nonocclusive intestinal ischemia—gross findings. Findings at laparotomy in a patient with nonocclusive mesenteric ischemia. Although the bowel wall is mottled, it remains viable. Patient had undergone angiography and vasodilator infusion, but irreversible bowel necrosis had already occurred, necessitating the subsequent laparotomy and resection.

sion of mild or even questionable cases with a better prognosis that might have resolved spontaneously in response to ongoing conventional supportive care. The refusal of advocates of this aggressive approach to randomize treatment has not helped to resolve this controversy.

Neonatal Necrotizing Enterocolitis

Etiology and Pathophysiology

NEC is a life-threatening disease occurring almost exclusively in severely stressed, premature infants. It is characterized by abdominal distention, bloody diarrhea, vomiting (with failure to feed), and clinical deterioration. The incidence of NEC has increased with the extensions of modern neonatal intensive care and the aggressive treatment of particularly premature infants.

The precise etiology of NEC is not clear, but it appears that the underlying initial insult is splanchnic vasoconstriction secondary to severe physiologic stress.[147] There appears to be a two-step pathophysiologic process: Mesenteric vasoconstriction produces ischemia, and an initial mucosal injury that probably disrupts its barrier function. This initial event is followed by a progression of this reversible mucosal lesion to transmural infarction, related to a number of other factors, including early feeding of non–breast milk formulas,[148] bacterial overgrowth (*Klebsiella* may be cultured), and probably most important, immune incompetence. Perhaps the immaturity of the premature infant's immune system allows a normally reversible lesion (epithelial necrosis) to progress, by bacterial invasion, to irreversible transmural infarction. Histologically, the intestine demonstrates ischemic necrosis with the mucosa being preferentially affected (similar to mesenteric ischemia).

Epidemiology

NEC can occur in both endemic and epidemic patterns in the same intensive care unit. Sex, race, maternal socioeconomic status, geography, and season all have no effect on the incidence of NEC.[149] It is unusual to see NEC in an infant born after 35 to 36 weeks of gestation. Prematurity, non–breast milk feeding, and severe physiologic stress, such as infant respiratory distress syndrome, are the important predisposing factors.

Clinical Features

The classic presentation of NEC is the insidious deterioration of a premature infant younger than 2 to 3 weeks of age. Abdominal distention develops, and the baby stops feeding and may manifest bloody diarrhea or Hemoccult-positive stools. The signs and symptoms of ileus or obstruction are seen. Systemic signs include apnea, bradycardia, hypothermia, and lethargy. Without treatment, the infant may progress to intestinal perforation, sepsis, acidosis, and hypotension.

Diagnosis

Laboratory tests in the diagnosis of NEC are nonspecific. A thrombocytopenia, with or without disseminated intravascular coagulation, is often noted, as are leukopenia, refractory metabolic acidosis, and hyponatremia. The diagnosis is suggested by a radiographic picture of gas in the wall of the intestine, although this finding is not always noted, especially in the unfed infant.[150] Frank pneumoperitoneum may also occur, although this finding also is not specific to NEC.

Treatment

Early diagnosis and treatment may allow successful nonoperative management in a number of cases of NEC.[151] The treatment of this disease is similar to that of NOMI in the adult, but without the use of vasodilators or angiography. Hypovolemia should be corrected, bowel rest (nasogastric decompression) instituted, and systemic antibiotics administered. Parenteral nutrition should also be started early; feeding will likely not be resumed for 10 to 14 days. Frequently such measures are sufficient to allow regeneration of the injured mucosa and prevent the secondary progression to transmural infarction. Most gastroenterologists believe surgery should be reserved for only the most severe cases, often those that have progressed to transmural infarction, with or without perforation.[152] Treatment then consists of resection of necrotic bowel, decompressive ileostomy, and delayed reconstruction.

Prognosis

With early diagnosis and proper therapy, a successful outcome can obtained in 60% to 80% of infants.[153,154] Once perforation has occurred and severe systemic signs of sepsis have developed, however, the mortality approaches 50%.

Chronic Mesenteric Ischemia (Intestinal Angina)

Etiology and Pathophysiology

Intestinal angina is the clinical syndrome of intermittent, postprandial abdominal pain that originates as a result of chronic (usually atherosclerotic) obstruction of the splanchnic arteries. It is analogous to angina pectoris and calf claudication, two more common manifestations of episodic tissue hypoxia.

True intestinal angina is an exceedingly rare clinical problem, in large part owing to the excellent collateral circulation present in the small bowel and colon.[155] When intestinal angina does occur, it almost always is the result of severe atherosclerotic narrowing of a major splanchnic vessel, associated with occlusion of one or two of the remaining vessels. Although an asymptomatic narrowing of these vessels is a common radiographic (as well as autopsy) finding,[156,157] the fully developed syndrome of intestinal angina occurs much less frequently. No relation has been noted between the degree of arterial stenosis seen postmortem and digestive symptoms during the life of the patient.[155]

Epidemiology

Patients at risk for chronic mesenteric ischemia are those with diffuse peripheral arterial disease. Therefore, patients with hypercholesterolemia and diabetes are at an increased risk. As expected, this disease is seen in the middle aged and elderly.

Clinical Features

Intestinal angina is defined by the clinical triad of postprandial pain, chronic weight loss, and sitophobia (fear of eating). These symptoms are very characteristic and essential to the diagnosis. The pain, which is crampy in nature, is analogous to that of angina pectoris. Diarrhea and constipation may also be present, the latter the consequence of anorexia. Physical examination is nonspecific except for evidence of chronic weight loss and the findings of other, associated manifestations of generalized atherosclerosis. Examination during an attack may reveal hyperperistalsis.

Diagnosis

The diagnosis is suspected when a patient presents with the typical clinical picture of emaciation with postprandial abdominal pain. Confirmation is obtained by arteriographic study, requiring biplanar studies to allow visualization of the visceral vessels. Although the precise diagnosis cannot be made on arteriographic grounds alone, the findings of severe narrowing in multiple visceral vessels with extensive collateral formation, coupled with the typical clinical picture, are sufficient to warrant treatment. Most important, however, the patient must evidence substantial weight loss, or the diagnosis is not tenable.

Duplex Doppler ultrasound imaging may play a role in the future evaluation of mesenteric flow. This noninvasive technique has been experimentally used to quantitate mesenteric blood flow, with a reported error of ±10%.[158,159] Bowel gas and obesity may be confounding factors. Unfortunately, this technology is still not fully developed and not universally available. One case report describes a provocative approach to diagnosing chronic mesenteric ischemia by measuring intralumenal pH in the small bowel after a test meal.[160]

Treatment

There is no effective medical therapy for intestinal angina. If the remaining evaluation of the patient's abdominal pain is negative, surgery is usually considered to alleviate pain and to avoid impending infarction (Fig. 112-12). Surgically, three approaches have been advocated[161]: endarterectomy, bypass grafting with either prosthetic or autogenous material, and reimplantation of distal mesenteric vessels into nondiseased aortic segments. The preferred approach is bypass grafting of the SMA with either autologous saphenous vein or prosthetic material; a clear advantage of autologous tissue has not been shown for visceral revascularization, as it has for renal and extremity revascularization. Controversy exists as to the adequacy of single-vessel bypass compared to multivessel reconstruction.

Percutaneous translumenal angioplasty has been advocated in the treatment of chronic mesenteric ischemia.[162] The risk and incidence of technical failure, however, including vessel

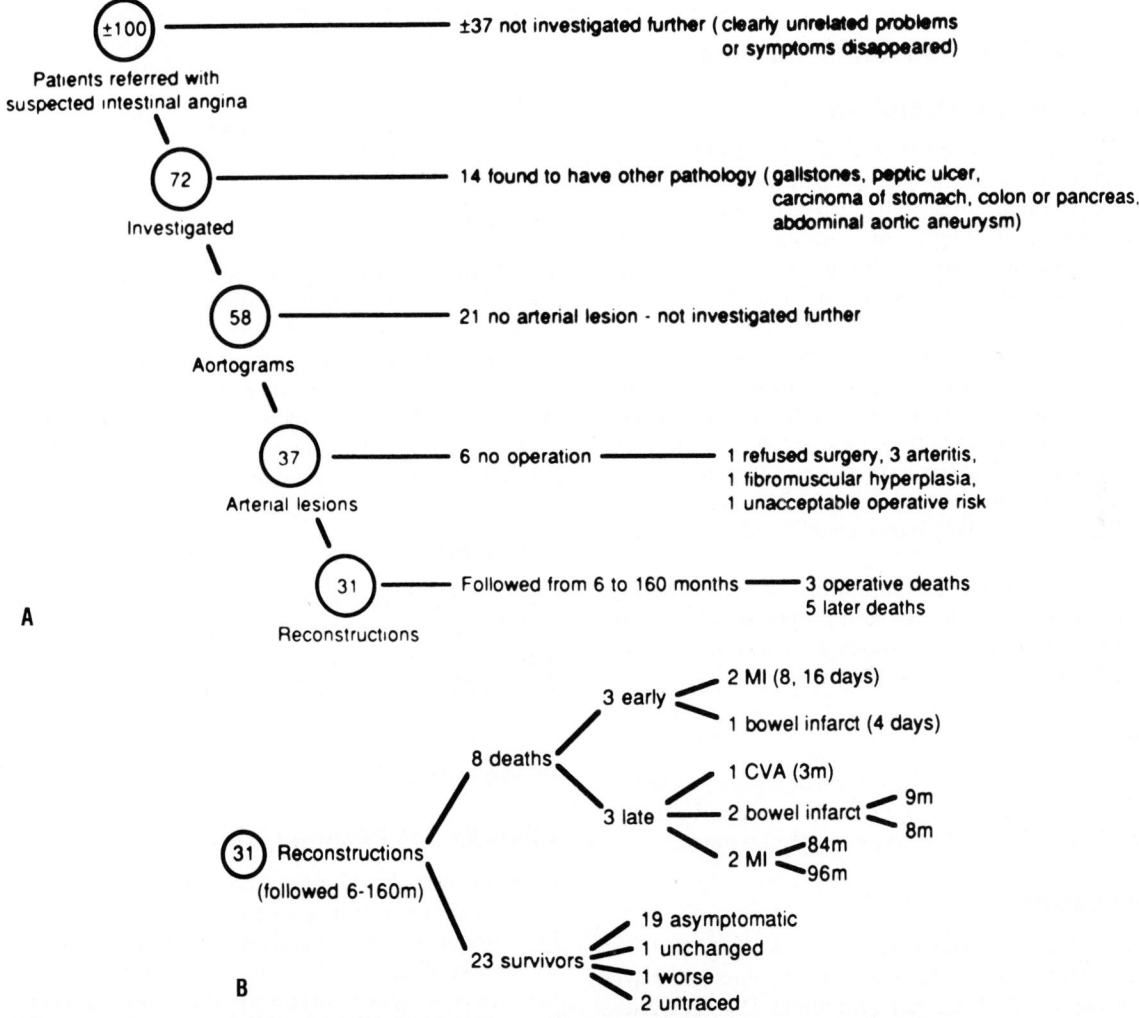

FIGURE 112-12. Evaluation of intestinal angina. (**A**) The importance of a careful history in the evaluation of a patient with suspected chronic intestinal ischemia cannot be overemphasized. Nearly one third of all patients referred for intestinal angina do not turn out to have persistent symptoms of intestinal angina. After careful selection of patients, nearly two thirds of the aortograms performed demonstrate arterial lesions. (**B**) Results of surgery for chronic intestinal ischemia. Nearly two thirds of patients revascularized benefited from surgery. The mortality rate from surgery was significant, however, reflecting both the age of the population at risk and the diffuse nature of their atherosclerotic process. (From Marston A. Chronic intestinal ischemia. In: Marston A, Bulkley GB, Fiddian-Green RG, Haglund UH, eds. Splanchnic ischemia and multiple organ failure. London: Edward Arnold, 1989:323.)

dissection, are increased in the mesenteric vasculature. For this reason, the use of angioplasty here has not yet gained widespread acceptance.

Prognosis

The natural history of untreated mesenteric angina is unknown. Although some have advocated aggressive treatment of all patients suspected of having mesenteric angina, it appears that acute small bowel ischemia ultimately goes on to develop in only a small percentage of patients. If the patients are selected carefully (see Fig. 112-12), the results of surgery, usually limited to bypass of the SMA from the infrarenal aorta, are good. Mortality rates range from 3% to 30%, and over 90% of survivors treated are relieved of their abdominal pain, gain weight, and resume normal eating habits.[161,163]

Celiac Artery Compression Syndrome

Etiology and Pathophysiology

Since the original case report from Finland in 1963 of a 57-year-old man with chronic abdominal pain and celiac stenosis,[164,165] the possibility of a "celiac artery compression syndrome" (median arcuate ligament syndrome) has generated great interest among clinicians who deal with patients with chronic abdominal pain of unexplained origin.[166–168]

As described by Harjola, the syndrome consists of chronic abdominal pain associated with celiac artery stenosis, caused by fibers of the median arcuate ligament of the diaphragm. At laparotomy, the vessel is often found to be normal, but compressed by fibrous bands from the ligament. Although it is unquestionable that subjective improvement in abdominal pain has been noted by some patients after this procedure, it is unclear whether objective parameters of blood flow actually improve.

The irritation of visceral autonomic nerves by constricting fibers of the diaphragm also has been proposed as the cause of this syndrome; however, perivascular sympathectomy or ganglionectomy is not consistently palliative.

Epidemiology

In contrast to patients with atherosclerotic disease, these patients are often younger, with a mean age at diagnosis in the fifth decade. There is a 3 : 1 predominance of women.

Clinical Features

Most patients have abdominal pain, but less than half have the classic symptoms of intestinal angina. The remainder have a variety of vague abdominal pain syndromes. Diarrhea, nausea, and vomiting are often present. Many patients relate a significant loss of weight (because of avoidance of food) in the previous months.

Diagnosis

Centers with the most experience with this syndrome report that the diagnosis is difficult, and considerable experience and judgment are necessary to achieve satisfactory therapeutic re-

sults. Central to the diagnostic process is a thorough evaluation of the gastrointestinal tract to exclude other possible intraabdominal conditions accounting for the patient's symptoms. Therefore, it is recommended that most patients should undergo an upper gastrointestinal series with small bowel follow-through, a barium enema, endoscopic retrograde cholangiopancreatography, an oral cholecystogram, intravenous urography, and abdominal computed tomography. If these studies fail to reveal significant disease, and if an experienced clinician still suspects celiac artery entrapment, arteriography may be warranted. Selective celiac arteriography should demonstrate compression of the proximal celiac artery, with lateral views revealing eccentric compression of the celiac artery with caudal displacement (Fig. 112-13). The SMA and IMA usually appear normal. There is no study, however, demonstrating a good correlation between the degree of stenosis and symptoms or therapeutic results.

Used prior to arteriography, duplex ultrasonography is a less invasive test for confirming the diagnosis of mesenteric vessel stenosis.[158] MRI also can be used to measure mesenteric blood flow in the fasted and fed states[169] and may be useful in identifying candidates for surgery.

Treatment

Successful treatment requires division of the crural fibers responsible for entrapment until the entire celiac axis, up to the trifurcation, is cleared.[168] In addition, the periceliac neural tissue on either side of the celiac axis is mobilized and excised. Intraoperative celiac artery dilation may then be accomplished in a retrograde manner by way of the splenic artery. If necessary, celiac artery reconstruction may be carried out, by resection and primary reanastomosis, or bypass grafting.

Prognosis

Optimal results may require both celiac axis decompression and dilation or reconstruction. In the hands of experienced surgeons, long-term relief of symptoms has been reported in 70% to 80% of patients.[168]

Ischemic Colitis

Etiology and Pathophysiology

Ischemic colitis has become increasingly recognized since the 1960s with the advent of aortic aneurysm surgery. A clinical spectrum of colonic ischemic disease may develop secondary to a variety of causes, including iatrogenic arterial injury, low-flow states, increased intralumenal pressure, or spontaneous thrombosis of a major arterial or venous supply to the colon.[170]

The most common cause of ischemic colitis is iatrogenic interruption of the IMA during aortic surgery. This event occurs in as many as 3% to 5% of patients undergoing aortic replacement without IMA reimplantation.[171] Colonic ischemia, however, can occur spontaneously from a variety of other causes such as atherosclerotic disease and low-flow states. Unlike small intestinal ischemia, noniatrogenic colonic ischemia rarely occurs from the abrupt occlusion of arterial inflow,

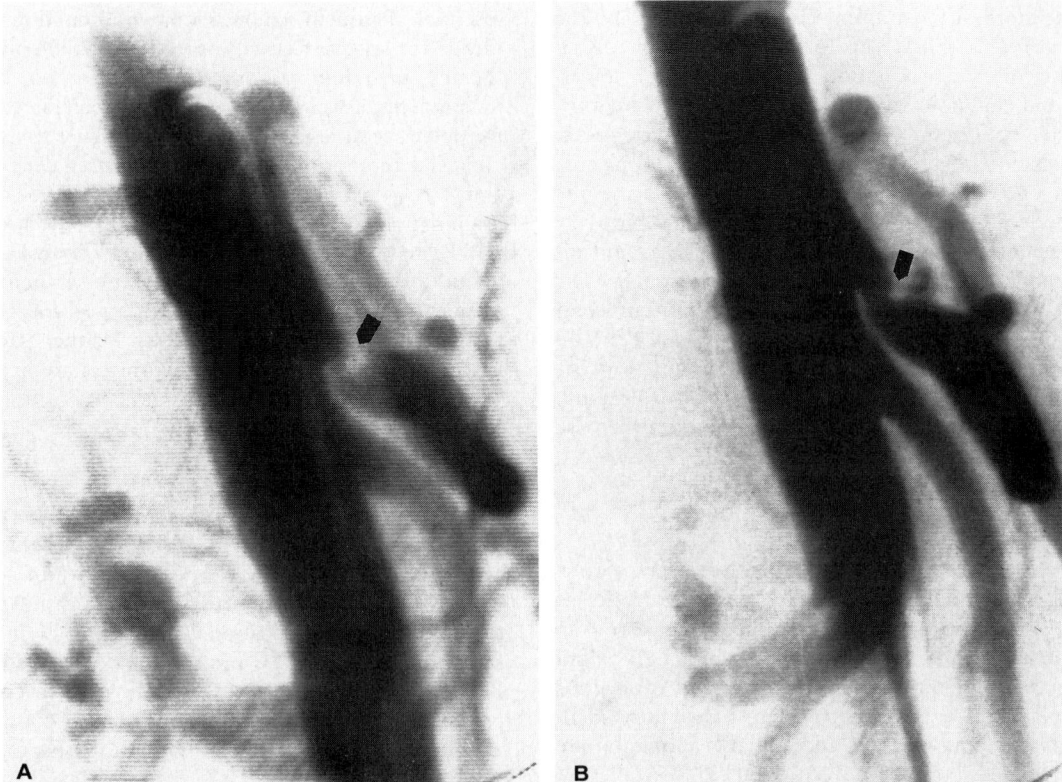

FIGURE 112-13. Celiac artery compression. Lateral views of an arteriogram of a patient with suspected celiac artery compression syndrome. **(A)** On inspiration, an area of stenosis is noted in the proximal celiac artery. **(B)** With expiration, the constriction appears to relax and the stenotic area becomes less prominent. It remains unclear and therefore controversial whether this radiographic lesion is hemodynamically significant.

but rather as the result of decreased perfusion pressure, vasoconstriction, or both. As in the small intestine, this vasoconstriction is mediated largely by the renin–angiotensin axis.[23] The distribution of injury is usually segmental, but may involve the entire colon, depending on the underlying cause. Many instances of colonic ischemia are not clinically recognized, and many do not require specific medical or surgical intervention.

Pathologically, the colon demonstrates thickening, mucosal ulceration, and stenosis. There is a gradient of injury from the mucosa to the muscularis propria.

Epidemiology

Most patients with ischemic colitis are middle aged or elderly. A history of ischemic heart disease or peripheral arterial insufficiency is often present. Patients with connective tissue disorders, diabetes, or prior colon disease are also at risk.[172] Spontaneous cases of colonic ischemia tend to occur in severely ill and compromised patients, often suffering from systemic illnesses that contribute to low-flow states. Often there is an antecedent history of lower abdominal pain that had resolved spontaneously. It may also occur in marathon runners of all ages, especially women, and cocaine abusers.[173]

Clinical Features

Colon ischemia presents in one of three basic clinical patterns.[174,175] Most commonly, patients present with crampy lower abdominal pain, classically in the left iliac fossa. Nausea, vomiting, diarrhea, and the passage of blood or mucous per rectum are frequently noted.[176] Less commonly, an acute abdominal catastrophe occurs, with obvious signs of grave illness and peritonitis as the first presenting signs. A smaller subset of patients have subclinical disease, and only present later with stricture formation.

On physical examination, the patient may have a low-grade fever and tachycardia. Most patients do not appear gravely ill. Tenderness is usually, but not invariably, noted in the left iliac fossa, and blood is often noted on rectal examination. Obtunded patients are particularly difficult to evaluate.

Diagnosis

Laboratory tests are usually nonspecific, with a mild leukocytosis the only consistent finding. The diagnosis of ischemic colitis is most easily established by flexible sigmoidoscopy.[176] Historically, clinicians were reluctant to perform endoscopy on these patients, for fear of perforation; however, by performing the examination with caution, and minimizing air insufflation, morbidity is minimized. Most commonly, the mucosa appears normal for up to 12 to 15 cm, the usual extent of the collateral circulation from the middle rectal arteries. Beyond this point the mucosa becomes edematous, hemorrhagic, friable, and ulcerated. Biopsy of this area often demonstrates nonspecific injury, but may suggest ischemic colitis if the process is acute. Chronic ischemic colitis results in hemosiderin deposition, a diagnostic finding on biopsy.

Barium enema examination may demonstrate an inflammatory lesion of the colon in a segmental distribution. Specific features include "thumbprinting" (indicative of mucosal edema; Fig. 112-14), sacculation, and narrowing of the involved segment.[177] Angiography usually is not necessary for the diagnosis of ischemic colitis, and can often be misleading: IMA occlusion is a frequent incidental finding in otherwise healthy people.

Treatment

Most cases of ischemic colitis require supportive therapy only. Maintenance of optimal cardiovascular status, avoidance of splanchnic vasoconstrictors, and provision of nasogastric decompression and systemic antibiotics covering enteric flora serve as the basis of therapy. Endogenous and exogenous causes of splanchnic vasoconstriction must also be avoided. Close observation and repeated abdominal examination are essential. Frequent colonoscopic examination provides a means for repeated visual inspection of the colon. Medical therapy, including vasodilators and glucagon, has been attempted, but its value has not been demonstrated. Indications for operative intervention include frank peritonitis, ongoing clinical deterioration, sepsis, bleeding from deep ulcerations, and, later, obstruction. In addition, if repeated endoscopic examinations demonstrate a progression of the disease, surgery is indicated. Should surgery be required, optimal management includes resection of obvious ischemic segments and exteriorization of the remaining ends of bowel (or, alternatively, formation of a Hartmann's pouch). Neither attempts at revascularization nor primary anastomosis are appropriate in this setting.

Prognosis

Many cases of colonic ischemia resolve spontaneously. A surprisingly small number of patients go on to stricture formation after the ischemic episode. The possibility of stricture formation should not be regarded as an indication for early intervention; this complication is best dealt with in the chronic state when the bowel is prepared and the surgery elective. Because of a high incidence of cardiovascular disease, those patients who require early emergent surgery continue to have a high mortality, in spite of modern intensive care.[178,179]

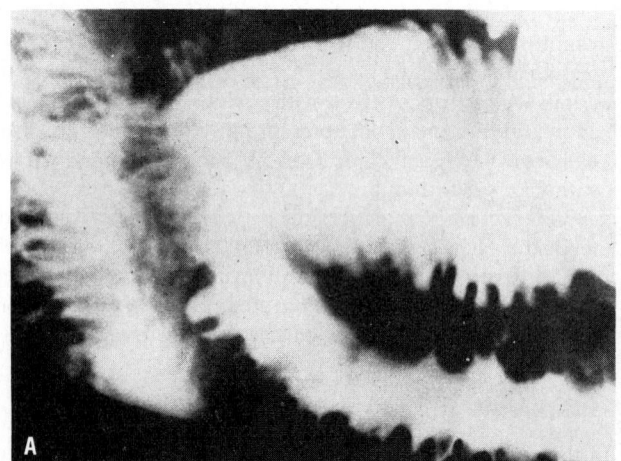
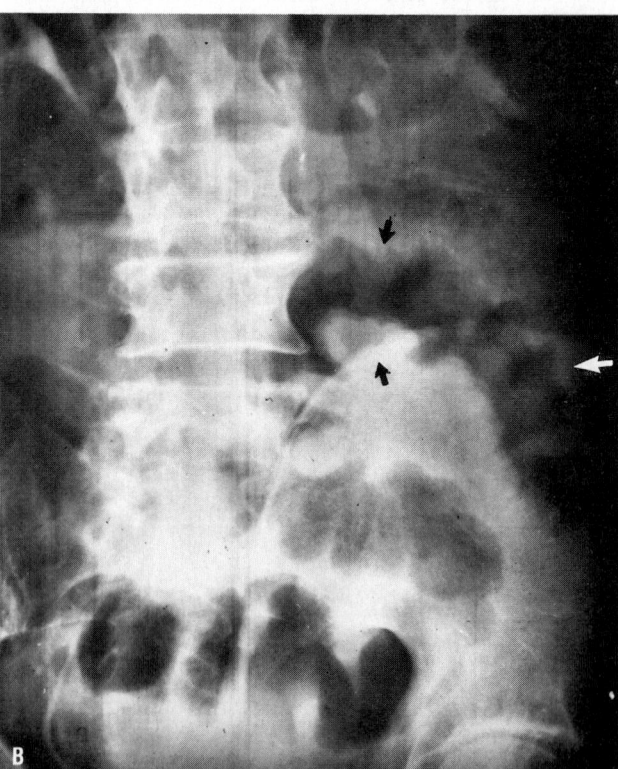

FIGURE 112-14. Thumbprinting. One of the earliest changes seen in the course of ischemic colitis is submucosal edema and sometimes hemorrhage. Radiographically, this manifests as blunt, semiopaque projections into the intestinal lumen—thumbprinting. Although well demonstrated with (**A**) luminal contrast, it can also be striking to the astute observer on the (**B**) plain abdominal radiograph, where it strongly suggests the diagnosis of ischemic colitis.

Acute Erosive Stress Gastritis

Etiology and Pathophysiology

In many patients who have suffered severe physiologic stress (hypotension, multiple trauma, major burns), acute erosions in the gastric mucosa develop, often within hours, but usually several days after the acute event (see Chap. 64).[180-182] Endoscopic surveillance of critically ill intensive care patients demonstrates that virtually 100% have some evidence of mucosal ulceration. Most of these lesions disappear within 7 to 14 days, but massive bleeding may occur if the erosions persist.[183,184]

Although the etiology of stress ulceration is multifactorial,[185] diminished gastric mucosal blood flow seems to be the primary underlying factor.[24,186,187] The exact mechanism by which this ischemia predisposes the gastric mucosa to ulceration is unknown. Toxic oxygen metabolites generated at reperfusion seem to play a role. Some prostaglandins are probably protective. The consequence of this ischemia is a loss of mucosal resistance to acid back-diffusion.[188] In addition to mucosal ischemia, intralumenal acid is required to promote the injury, and the maintenance of the intragastric pH above 4.0 has been shown to reduce the incidence of bleeding and mortality rates.

Pathologically, the earliest lesions are focal areas of hyperemia and pallor in the fundus. These progress with time to frank erosion. The antrum and duodenum may also be involved, but usually to a lesser extent.

Epidemiology

Stress ulceration occurs typically in the clinical setting of prolonged intensive care after severe trauma, hemorrhage, cardiogenic shock, major burns, or other extreme physiologic stresses. Stress ulceration should be distinguished from the mucosal injury seen after neurologic injury or drug ingestion. Cushing's ulcers occur with neurologic injury and are clinically and pathophysiologically distinct from stress ulcers. They tend to be single ulcerations occurring on the greater curvature of the stomach, and are often associated with massive acid hypersecretion or perforation. In contrast, lesions from stress ulceration are often multiple, shallow, and well demarcated, usually located in the gastric fundus with relative sparing of the antrum and duodenum. They are most often associated with bleeding rather than perforation. Curling's ulcers, associated with burn injury, seem to be pathophysiologically similar to the stress ulcers seen in nonburn patients.

Clinical Features

Although these lesions can be demonstrated endoscopically in most severely ill patients, frank clinical manifestation thereof is rare. Upper gastrointestinal bleeding is the complication of stress ulceration most feared by physicians. Although a guaiac-positive nasogastric aspirate is seen in 15% of patients in the intensive care unit,[184,189,190] clinically significant bleeding, requiring transfusion, occurs in less than 3%.[191] Typically the bleeding occurs several days into the hospital course. This course probably reflects the return of normal gastrointestinal function (acid secretion) in a patient beginning to recover from a critical illness. It is often heralded by a change in nasogastric drainage to a dark red, guaiac-positive consistency. Most episodes resolve spontaneously with adequate medical therapy (H_2 blockers, antacids, or sucralfate). Only occasionally is the bleeding persistent and life threatening, requiring more specific treatment.

Treatment

The most important aspect of treatment of this disorder is its prevention.[189] The management is progressive, including optimization of hemodynamics, saline lavage, and acid neutralization. Every effort should be made to provide adequate circulating blood volume, to prevent shock and hypotension, and to treat sepsis in an effort to prevent the gastric mucosal ischemia critical to its development. Neutralization of gastric acid with either antacids, histamine receptor blockade, or proton pump inhibitors has proven effective.[191,192] At an intragastric pH above 5.0, 99% of gastric acid is buffered and the activity of the digestive enzyme pepsin is effectively inhibited. Most patients stop bleeding with this relatively simple therapy and several studies have shown a significant decrease in the incidence of clinical bleeding with these measures.[193,194]

If bleeding continues, other nonoperative measures, including endoscopic coagulation[195,196] or arteriographic infusion of vasopressin (Pitressin), or even embolization, should be considered. An additional 80% to 90% of these patients can be controlled with these procedures. There remains, however, a very small minority of patients who fail to stop bleeding even after aggressive nonoperative management. Operative intervention carries a high mortality (30%) and should be undertaken only after all attempts at nonoperative measures fail. When unavoidable, it should not be delayed, and a total gastrectomy must be considered.

Prognosis

The prognosis of patients with this problem is poor, but related more to the underlying disease than to the gastric ulcerations themselves.[197] Over 80% are successfully controlled with conservative therapy, and a further 80% of the remainder are controlled successfully with more invasive, but nonoperative, treatment. Thus, only about 10% of patients with this problem have an otherwise altered outcome secondary to the development of stress gastric bleeding.

Ischemic Hepatitis

Etiology and Pathophysiology

Ischemic hepatitis is defined as hepatic insufficiency associated with centrilobular necrosis, which appears after a period of circulatory shock.[198-200] Also known as shock liver or posttraumatic hepatic insufficiency, this entity has quite specific histopathologic features.

The liver is unique among splanchnic organs in that it derives its blood supply from two sources that differ markedly in their relative oxygen content, but not in their response to ischemia. Approximately two thirds of the blood supply is provided by the portal circulation, which, under resting conditions, has a mixed venous oxygen saturation of 35% to 50%.[201] During shock, this drops to as low as 6% to 10%, because of increased oxygen extraction in the splanchnic bed.[202] In addition, both hepatic artery and portal vein blood flows decrease (disproportionately) in response to shock.[25] Although under normovolemic conditions, the isolated occlusion of either the hepatic artery or portal vein is associated experimentally with compensatory vasodilation in the bed of the other vessel (termed the hepatic arterial buffer response),[203] both beds are compromised in parallel during shock because this homeostatic mechanism is overwhelmed by the selective response of both vascular beds to angiotensin II.[25] As a result, the liver, a metabolically active organ with high oxygen needs under normal conditions, is ill suited to tolerate prolonged periods of shock.

Although the initiating factor in ischemic hepatitis is anoxia,[25,204] it appears that the generation of toxic oxygen metabolites at reperfusion may play an important role as well.[205] The liver is rich in xanthine oxidase, both in the hepatocyte[206] and in the vascular endothelium.[207,208] Therefore, the enzyme as well as its substrates (O_2, hypoxanthine) are in excess during reperfusion.

Epidemiology

Ischemic hepatitis was first recognized in association with cardiogenic shock and congestive failure, often after acute myocardial infarction.[198,199] As the management of patients with hemorrhagic and cardiogenic shock has improved, the appearance of unexplained hepatic insufficiency a day or two after otherwise successful management of a period of hypotension has become more common.[209]

Two major groups of patients are at risk for ischemic hepatitis: those with underlying cardiovascular disease, manifest as either cardiac failure or arrhythmias[210,211]; and those with hypotension secondary to hemorrhage, dehydration, or sepsis. The reported incidence varies widely,[199,212] but we have seen a significant elevation of bilirubin in nearly 33% of those patients who have experienced major hypotensive episodes.

Clinical Features

The clinical manifestations of ischemic hepatitis are limited to the appearance of jaundice in association with transient elevations in serum levels of transaminases after a period of hypotension. The course of ischemic liver disease can be divided into three distinct phases.[209] *Initiation* of the hepatic insult begins with hemodynamic insufficiency and ends with restoration of normal flow. During this phase, the serum enzyme levels are usually normal. *Hepatic injury* is characterized by variable elevations in the aminotransferases, alkaline phosphatase, and lactate dehydrogenase. Elevations of bilirubin usually lag 2 to 3 days behind the enzyme elevations and are rarely greater than to 5 to 10 mg/dL. These laboratory abnormalities usually resolve over a course of 1 to 2 weeks. *Hepatic recovery* usually occurs spontaneously if the underlying cause of hepatic ischemia is eliminated.

Diagnosis

Ischemic hepatitis is suspected by identifying those patients at risk in the appropriate clinical setting. The diagnosis is confirmed by finding elevations in serum levels of transaminases and bilirubin in the absence of evidence for primary hepatic or biliary disease. In some cases, ischemic hepatitis can be confused with, or even superimposed on hepatobiliary disease from other causes. This situation not only makes the diagnosis more difficult, but can substantially worsen the outcome. In most cases, biliary tract disease should be ruled out by sonography or cholangiography.

Treatment

The treatment of ischemic hepatitis is largely supportive. The most important element, as in all splanchnic ischemia syndromes, is the prevention of ischemic insults and prompt intervention when these insults occur. Important measures include avoidance of vasoconstricting agents, optimization of hydration and systemic hemodynamics and cardiac function, and maintenance of adequate oxygen saturation. Sepsis may be a comorbid factor that should be avoided or aggressively treated whenever possible.

Prognosis

Fortunately, the degree of hepatic dysfunction seen with ischemic hepatitis is usually not life threatening, making the lack of specific treatment less important. In the most severely ill patients, the liver injury usually contributes only one component to a spiral of events that terminates in multiple organ failure and death. If the patient survives, however, hepatic dysfunction usually resolves.

Acalculous Cholecystitis

Etiology and Pathophysiology

Acalculous cholecystitis is necrotic cholecystitis occurring in the absence of demonstrable gallstones.[213] It often, although not always occurs in critically ill, shocked, traumatized, or postoperative patients (see Chap. 96).[214] The etiology of acalculous cholecystitis is clearly multifactorial, but it appears that nonocclusive ischemia may play a fundamental role in a number of cases.[215] Obstruction of the cystic duct, narcotics,[216,217] and numerous other factors (thromboxane A_2, leukotrienes, platelet-activating factor, tumor necrosis factor) have also been implicated. Biliary stasis, as occurs with prolonged fasting and parenteral nutrition, most likely accounts for some cases as well.

Epidemiology

The severely ill patient is most at risk for the development of acalculous cholecystitis, as are those who have undergone emergency surgery.[218] Prolonged fasting, parenteral nutrition, ventilation with positive end expiratory pressure, and severe trauma all have been associated with this syndrome as well.[215,216]

Clinical Features

The clinical diagnosis of acalculous cholecystitis is frequently difficult. In the setting of severe illness or injury and in patients who have altered neurologic status, right upper quadrant pain and nausea are the most frequently reported symptoms. Ventilatory support, sedation, and excessive analgesia often mask otherwise obvious clinical signs. Distention, unexplained fever, loss of bowel sounds, and unexpected deterioration in the overall clinical condition are the most important clinical signs in the diagnosis of acalculous cholecystitis.[217]

Diagnosis

Leukocytosis is usually present, but is often secondary to severe underlying disease. Other laboratory values also are nonspecific.[216] Often an unexplained fever or elevated leukocyte count prompts the clinician to consider the diagnosis. Mild elevations in serum levels of bilirubin, alkaline phosphatase, and transaminases are sometimes seen. Ultrasound and computed tomography may be helpful in suggesting the diagnosis by demonstrating an enlarged gallbladder with thickened wall (6 mm) and pericholecystic fluid that may appear as a halo. Tenderness to palpation with the ultrasound probe, or the presence of a diffuse, homogeneous, nonshadowing, medium-level echogenicity indicative of pus within the gallbladder lumen all are considered "positive" findings. Using these criteria, a sensitivity of 98% has been reported for the diagnosis of acalculous cholecystitis using ultrasound.[219,220] Diagnostic percutaneous aspiration of the gallbladder also may be of some value, but remains controversial.[221] Biliary scintigraphy is less valuable because it is commonly positive in this patient population, even in the absence of cholecystitis.[222]

Treatment

Unlike acute cholecystitis for gallstone disease, there is no role for medical therapy in acalculous cholecystitis. Treatment consists of prompt cholecystectomy once the diagnosis is made. Procedures short of cholecystectomy are controversial, and many authors report higher mortality rates with cholecystostomy than with conventional cholecystectomy.[223] Delay in surgical treatment often leads to progressive gangrenous changes in the gallbladder, with eventual perforation and peritonitis.[216] When treated promptly, the mortality rate can be low (10%–15%), despite the severity of the underlying illness and the age of the patient.

Prophylaxis against acalculous cholecystitis has been supported by some studies. Regular emptying of the gallbladder, usually stimulated by a high-fat diet or the intravenous administration of cholecystokinin, has been suggested.[224] Although this approach may prove helpful to avoid stasis, those cases that are primarily related to nonocclusive ischemia will not likely be affected.

Ischemic Pancreatitis

Etiology and Pathophysiology

The splanchnic ischemia that occurs in association with shock or hypotension has been implicated in the initiation of some cases of clinical pancreatic disease.[33] This ischemic pancreatitis may be defined as acute pancreatitis developing after a period of circulatory compromise, when no other predisposing factors are found.

Many factors have been suggested in the etiology of ischemic pancreatitis, including hypovolemia, thromboembolism, splanchnic vasoconstriction secondary to pressor release, diuretics, atheroembolism, hypercalcemia, operative trauma, and electrical shock. Cardiopulmonary bypass (CPB) may predispose to pancreatitis because of low-flow, nonpulsatile perfusion, hypothermia, and venous sludging.[225,226] Although no studies have been published directly evaluating the role of vasopressors in the etiology of ischemic pancreatitis, the renin–angiotensin axis is strongly activated by the nonpulsatile perfusion of CPB that is associated most commonly with ischemic pancreatitis.

Pathologically, the most common findings are hyperemia, bruising, microscopic hemorrhage, focal necrosis, and interstitial edema—all findings that are seen commonly postmortem in the pancreas of patients who have died in shock.[227]

Epidemiology

Patients at risk for ischemic pancreatitis are those who have sustained a period of shock, and subsequently been resuscitated. Although the biochemical incidence of pancreatitis (primarily hyperamylasemia) after significant hypotension may be nearly 80%,[33] clinical manifestations of the disease are seen in far fewer patients. Moreover, patients undergoing CPB are at an increased risk for postoperative pancreatitis, with as much as 4% of the mortality seen after cardiac surgery associated with this complication.[225] Hyperamylasemia is seen in as many as half the patients subjected to CPB, but in many cases analysis of amylase isoenzymes reveals that in a significant proportion this increase is caused by elevated levels of salivary amylase.[228] Other studies show a good correlation between the total serum amylase levels and the clinical manifestations of pancreatitis.

Clinical Features

Many patients with ischemic pancreatitis are asymptomatic, and are found only at autopsy to have pancreatitis. When symptoms do occur, abdominal pain and nausea are seen most frequently. Abdominal distention and an ileus may develop, often several days after the shock insult. A low-grade fever also may be present, but is nonspecific. In rare cases, the condition may progress to fulminant pancreatitis, pancreatic necrosis, and even abscess formation.

Diagnosis

The diagnosis of ischemic pancreatitis is difficult. Hyperamylasemia is the most common laboratory finding, often first appearing 24 to 48 hours after the period of shock. An elevated amylase is not uncommon after shock, however, and is not specific for pancreatitis. The analysis of amylase isoenzymes and pancreatic lipase may be helpful. Fever and leukocytosis may also develop, and the clinician must distinguish this condition from other intraabdominal crises, such as ischemic or perforated intestine.

The routine use of new generation computed tomography,

with and without intravenous contrast, is helpful in making a diagnosis of pancreatitis. Often, the diagnosis is made at laparotomy or autopsy.

Treatment

As with pancreatitis caused by more common etiologies, treatment for ischemic pancreatitis is nonspecific and largely supportive. Bowel rest, nasogastric suction, and parenteral nutrition are probably beneficial. In severe cases, antibiotic coverage is recommended, although controlled trials in patients with more conventional forms of mild pancreatitis have failed to show a benefit from prophylactic antibiotic use.[229] As in other splanchnic ischemia syndromes, treatment should be particularly aimed at reducing potential causes of splanchnic vasoconstriction. With control of the underlying disease, most patients recover without significant sequelae.

Multiple Organ Dysfunction Syndrome

Etiology and Pathophysiology

The multiple organ dysfunction syndrome (MODS; formerly multisystem organ failure, MSOF) affects an increasing number of critically ill or injured patients. The complex includes initial tissue injury, adult respiratory distress syndrome, and hypermetabolism, followed by sequential organ failure (Table 112-9).[230] It accounts for most intensive care unit stays longer than 5 days in duration, and over 90% of the deaths in many surgical intensive care units.[231,232] Moreover, the care of patients with MODS consumes major human and financial resources.[233]

The inciting events that lead to MODS are local injury from trauma, infection, or hypoperfusion.[230] A local inflammatory response subsequently occurs, probably as a result of platelet activation, endothelial injury, the release of inflammatory mediators, and activation of the clotting cascade. As a result, the complement, coagulation, and kallikrein systems are activated, leading to the development of a hypermetabolic state, with a marked increase in oxygen consumption and,

---

TABLE 112-9
Organ Involvement in Multiple Organ Dysfunction Syndrome

Gastrointestinal Organs
Small intestine—nonocclusive musocal ischemia
Large intestine—ischemic colitis
Stomach—stress gastritis
Liver—ischemic hepatitis
Gallbladder—acalculous cholecystitis
Pancreas—ischemic pancreatitis

Nongastrointestinal Organs
Lung—adult respiratory distress syndrome
Heart—decreased myocardial contractility
Kidney—renal failure
Central nervous system—obtundation
Clotting system—disseminated intravascular coagulation
Immune system—activation of inflammatory mediators,
    immunosuppression

---

therefore, demand. Often the lung is the first organ to fail, producing a picture of adult respiratory distress syndrome, and resulting in prolonged ventilator dependence. Failure of the kidneys, immune system, gastrointestinal tract, and liver follows, resulting ultimately in cardiovascular collapse, sepsis, and death.

Controversy exists as to whether this syndrome is necessarily associated with a septic state. Although the hemodynamic and metabolic characteristics of MODS mimic those seen with sepsis of any cause, many of these patients have no identifiable septic source and are repeatedly culture negative. Even with optimal management of bacterial contamination and septic sources, a syndrome of sequential organ failure may develop and progress. Clearly, some of these patients do have an ongoing, endogenous source of sepsis, perhaps secondary to persistent bacteremia and endotoxemia from their own gastrointestinal tract.

There is accumulating evidence that the gastrointestinal tract may play a central role in the development and maintenance of this hypermetabolic state, and of the full-blown MODS syndrome. As discussed previously, the breakdown of the gastrointestinal mucosal barrier allows a portal of entry not only for bacteria, but for endotoxin and other lumenal factors that may contribute to a systemic inflammatory response and distant organ injury. Indeed, it has been suggested that maintaining the intestinal mucosal barrier by means of enteral feedings may provide a mechanism for decreased mortality in the critical care setting, whereas parenteral nutritional support may increase the incidence of bacterial translocation by promoting gut atrophy.[234,235]

Of all the proposed etiologies for MODS, ischemia–reperfusion injury to the superficial gut mucosal barrier seems the most likely. Patients subjected to circulatory shock, hypoxia, sepsis, and other initial forms of severe physiologic stress sustain a mild, nonocclusive ischemia of the gut that often does not progress to frank bowel necrosis. Although this process may not be directly recognized clinically, it may result in mucosal damage with the subsequent loss of the barrier function of the epithelium. Critically ill patients coming to autopsy are now seen to have these ischemic intestinal lesions, whereas previously these findings were often signed out as "autolysis," not being recognized as a premortem change.

After the barrier function has been lost, the translocation of bacteria, and perhaps other lumenal toxins, is facilitated. In rats subjected to hemorrhagic shock, the full sequence of events is seen, and is prevented by pretreatment with allopurinol, suggesting that free radicals, generated from xanthine oxidase at reperfusion, may play an important role.[66] It is not known whether it is the bacteria, toxins, or digestive enzymes themselves that mediate the systemic injury, or whether these agents merely trigger the release of inflammatory mediators from the gut itself, the liver, or elsewhere. In any case, the loss of this barrier function is probably the basis for the fact that the "gut is the motor of multiple organ failure."[234]

Epidemiology

Patients at risk for MODS are those who have experienced severe physiologic stress, including trauma, hemorrhage, cardiac failure, cardiopulmonary bypass, severe illness, burns, or major surgery.[236,237] An occult source of sepsis is often but not always present. Although "blind" laparotomy (or laparoscopy) has been recommended in patients showing progressive deterioration without an obvious source, this approach is not supported by definitive studies.

Clinical Features

MODS is a syndrome of progressive, sequential (rather than simultaneous) organ failure. The time course can vary from days to months and can be described in stages.[237] The initial stage is clinically similar to sepsis, with fever and leukocytosis. By the second stage, progressive organ failure becomes evident and a defect in systemic oxygen extraction is noted. In this stage, the condition accounts for a nearly 50% mortality.[238] If the disease progresses, late organ failure develops, and finally, cardiovascular collapse results in death.

Diagnosis

No laboratory or radiographic test is diagnostic of MODS. The diagnosis must be made by evaluation of the entire clinical picture, with special attention given to immunologic and pulmonary status.

Treatment

There is no specific treatment for multiple organ failure. Therapy includes supportive measures with persistent, aggressive evaluation of possible infectious sources. A number of experimental therapies are being evaluated, including nutritional, immunotherapeutic, and cardiovascular support agents. Many are being evaluated in clinical studies and may soon become available for widespread use. Nonspecific measures directed at prevention and support remain the mainstays of therapy, however.

Prognosis

Although remaining a major source of mortality in the intensive care unit, MODS has undergone a progressive reduction in mortality from nearly 90% several years ago to 35% to 40% today.[232] As an increasing number of organ systems fail, however, mortality approaches 100%.

The reader is directed to Chapter 22, Gastrointestinal Blood Flow; Chapter 30, Approach to the Patient With Gross Gastrointestinal Bleeding; Chapter 34, Approach to the Patient With Abdominal Pain; Chapter 36, Approach to the Patient With Acute Abdomen; Chapter 37, Approach to the Patient With Ileus and Obstruction; Chapter 42, Approach to the Patient With Abnormal Liver Chemistries; Chapter 59, Stomach: Anatomy and Structural Anomalies; Chapter 61, Acid-Peptic Disorders; Chapter 67, Miscellaneous Diseases of the Stomach; Chapter 68, Small Intestine: Anatomy and Structural Anomalies; Chapter 75, Short Bowel Syndrome; Chapter 78, Colon: Anatomy and Structural Anomalies; Chapter 89, Pancreas: Anatomy and Structural Anomalies; Chapter 90, Acute Pancreatitis; Chapter 96, Gallstones; Chapter 127, Angiography; and Chapter 140, Exploratory Laparotomy.

REFERENCES

1. Sachs SM, Morton JH, Schwartz SI. Acute mesenteric ischemia. Surgery 1982;92:646.
2. Marston AM. Vascular occlusion. In: Marston AM, Bulkley GB, Fiddian-Green RG, Haglund UH, eds. Splanchnic ischemia and multiple organ failure. London: Edward Arnold, 1989:51.
3. Wilmore DW, Smith RJ, O'Dwyer ST, et al. The gut: a central organ after surgical stress. Surgery 1988;104:917.
4. Grendell JH, Ocknner RK. Mesenteric venous thrombosis. Gastroenterology 1982;82:358.
5. Sarr MG, Bulkley GB, Zuidema GD. Preoperative recognition of intestinal strangulation obstruction. Am J Surg 1983;145:176.
6. Boley SJ, Sprayregan S, et al. Initial results from an aggressive surgical approach to acute mesenteric ischemia. Surgery 1977;82:848.
7. Bailey RW, Bulkley GB, et al. Pathophysiology of nonocclusive mesenteric ischemia. Surg Forum 1982;33:194.
8. Folkow B. Regional adjustments of intestinal blood flow. Gastroenterology 1967;52:423.
9. Rothe CF. Reflex control of veins and vascular capacitance. Physiol Rev 1983;63:1281.
10. Brunner MJ, Greene AS, Frankle AE, Shoukas AA. Carotid sinus baroreceptor control of splanchnic resistance and capacity. Am J Physiol 1988;255:H1305.
11. Shepherd AP, Granger DN. Metabolic regulation of the intestinal circulation. In: Shepherd AP, Granger DN, eds. Physiology of the splanchnic circulation. New York: Raven Press, 1984:38.
12. Bulkley BB, Kvietys PR, Parks DA, et al. Relationship of blood flow and oxygen consumption to ischemic injury in the canine small intestine. Gastroenterology 1985;89:852.
13. Bulkley GB, Haglund UH, Morris JB. Mesenteric blood flow and the pathophysiology of mesenteric ischemia. In: Bergan JJ, Yao ST eds. Vascular surgical emergencies. Orlando, FL: Grune & Stratton, 1987:25.
14. Sawmiller DR, Chou CC. Role of adenosine in postprandial and reactive hyperemia in canine jejunum. Am J Physiol 1992;263:G487.
15. Redfors S, Hallback DA, Haglund U, et al. Blood flow distribution, villous tissue osmolality and fluid and electrolyte transport in the cat small intestine during regional hypotension. Acta Physiol Scand 1984;121:193.
16. Lundgren O, Svanik J. Mucosal hemodynamics in the small intestine of the cat during reduced perfusion pressure. Acta Physiol Scand 1973;88:551.
17. Kvietys PR, Granger DN. Relationship between intestinal blood flow and oxygen uptake. Am J Physiol 1982;242:G202.
18. Bulkley GB, Womack WA, Downey JM, et al. Characterization of segmental collateral blood flow in the small intestine. Am J Physiol 1985;249:G228.
19. Michels NA, Padmanabhan S, Kornblith PL. Routes of collateral circulation of the gastrointestinal tract as ascertained by the dissection of 500 bodies. Int Surg 1968;49:8.
20. Lee WPA, Weiss AC, Bulkley GB. Effect of collateral circulation on intestinal viability following segmental devascularization in the rat. Am Surg 1986;52:630.
21. Bulkley BB, Womack WA, Downey JM, et al. Collateral blood flow in segmental intestinal ischemia: effects of vasoactive agents. Surgery 1986;100:157.
22. Bailey RW, Bulkley GB, Hamilton SR, et al. Protection of the small intestine from nonocclusive mesenteric ischemia injury due to cardiogenic shock. Am J Surg 1987;153:108.
23. Bailey RW, Bulkley GB, Hamilton SR, et al. Pathogenesis of nonocclusive ischemic colitis. Ann Surg 1986;203:590.
24. Bailey RW, Bulkley GB, Hamilton ST, et al. The fundamental hemodynamic mechanism underlying gastric "stress ulceration" in cardiogenic shock. Ann Surg 1987;205:597.
25. Bulkley GB, Oshima A, Bailey RW. Pathophysiology of hepatic ischemia in cardiogenic shock. Am J Surg 1986;151:87.
26. McNeill JR, Stark RD, Greenway CV. Intestinal vasoconstric-

tion after hemorrhage: roles of vasopressin and angiotensin. Am J Physiol 1970;219:1342.

27. McNeill JR, Wilcox WC, Pang CCY. Vasopressin and angiotensin: reciprocal mechanisms controlling mesenteric conductance. Am J Physiol 1977;232:H260.

28. Gershon MD, Erde SM. The nervous system of the gut. Gastroenterology 1981;80:1571.

29. Said SI. Vasoactive peptides: state of the art review. Hypertension 1983;5(Suppl 1):117.

30. Gunther S, Gimbrone MA Jr, Alexander RW. Identification and characterization of the high affinity vascular angiotensin II receptor in rat mesenteric artery. Circ Res 1980;47:278.

31. Adar R, Franklin A, Spark RF, et al. Effect of dehydration and cardiac tamponade on superior mesenteric artery flow: role of vasoactive substances. Surgery 1976;79:534.

32. Bailey RW, Oshima A, O'Roark WA, Bulkley GB. A reproducible, quantitatable, and rapidly reversible model of cardiogenic shock in swine. In: Tumbleson ME, ed. Swine in biomedical research. New York: Plenum, 1987:363.

33. Warshaw A, O'Hara P. Susceptibility of the pancreas to ischemic injury in shock. Ann Surg 1978;188:1971.

34. Clemens JA, Bulkley GB, Cameron JL. Ischemic pancreatitis. In: Marston A, Bulkley GB, Fiddian-Green RG, Haglund UH, eds. Splanchnic ischemia and multiple organ failure. London: Edward Arnold, 1989:273.

35. Flancbaum L, Majerus TC, Cox EF. Acute post-traumatic acalculous cholecystitis. Am J Surg 1985;150:252.

36. Haglund U, Arvidsson D. Acute acalculous cholecystitis. In: Marston A, Bulkley GB, Fiddian-Green RG, Haglund UH, eds. Splanchnic ischemia and multiple organ failure. London: Edward Arnold, 1989:269.

37. Haglund U, Abe T, Ahren C, et al. The intestinal mucosal lesions in shock. I. Studies on the pathogenesis. Eur Surg Res 1976;8:435.

38. Haglund U, Bulkley GB, Granger ND. On the pathophysiology of intestinal ischemic injury. Acta Chir Scand 1987;153:321.

39. Menzies IS. Transmucosal passage of inert molecules in health and disease. In: Skadhauge E, Heintzek K, eds. Intestinal absorption and secretion. London: MTP Press, 1983:527.

40. Maxton DG, Bjarnason I, et al. Lactulose, ^{51}Cr-labeled EDTA, l-rhamnose, and polyethyleneglycol 500 as probe markers for assessment in vivo of human intestinal permeability. Clin Sci 1986;71:71.

41. Lundgren O, Haglund U. The pathophysiology of the intestinal countercurrent exchanges. Life Sci 1978;23:1411.

42. Eade MN, Pybus J, Readt J. No evidence of a countercurrent multiplier in the intestinal villus of the dog. Gastroenterology 1990;98:3.

43. Parks DA, Granger DN. Xanthine oxidase: biochemistry, distribution and physiology. Acta Physiol Scand 1986;548:47.

44. Granger DN, Rutili G, McCord JM. Superoxide radicals in feline intestinal ischemia. Gastroenterology 1981;81:22.

45. Parks DA, Bulkley GB, Granger DN, et al. Ischemic injury to the cat small intestine: role of superoxide radicals. Gastroenterology 1982;82:9.

46. Parks DA, Granger DN. Ischemia-induced vascular changes: role of xanthine oxidase and hydroxyl radicals. Am J Physiol 1983;245:G285.

47. Granger DN, Hollwarth ME, Parks DA. Ischemia–reperfusion injury: role of oxygen derived free radicals. Acta Physiol Scand 1986;548:97.

48. Hernandez LA, Grisham MB, Twohig, et al. Role of neutrophils in ischemia–reperfusion induced microvascular injury. Am J Physiol 1987;253:H699.

49. Grisham MB, Hernandez LA, Granger DN. Xanthine oxidase and neutrophil infiltration in intestinal ischemia. Am J Physiol 1986;251:G567.

50. Romson JL, Hook BG, Kunkel SL, et al. Reduction of the extent of ischemic myocardial injury by neutrophil depletion in the dog. Circulation 1983;67:1016.

51. Sussman MS, Buchman TG, Bulkley GB. Mechanisms of organ injury by toxic oxygen metabolites. In: Fry DE, ed. Multiple

organ failure: pathogenesis and management. Chicago: Yearbook Medical Publishers, 1990.

52. Chambers DE, Parks DA, Patterson G, et al. Role of oxygen derived free radicals in myocardial ischemia. Fed Proc 1983;42:1093.

53. Marzella L, Jesudass RR, Manson PN, et al. Functional and structural evaluation of the vasculature of skin flaps after ischemia and reperfusion. Plast Reconstr Surg 1988;81:742.

54. Hoshino T, Maley WR, Bulkley GB, et al. Ablation of free radical-mediated reperfusion injury for the salvage of kidneys taken from non-heart-beating donors. Transplantation 1988;45:284.

55. Bernard C. Lecons de physiologie experimentale appliquee a la medicine. Paris: JB Baillies et fils, 1856:406.

56. Davenport HW. Why the stomach does not digest itself. Sci Am 1972;226:86.

57. Virchow R. Historisches Kritisches und Positives zur lehre unterliebsa Funktionen. Arch Pathol Anat 1853;5:632.

58. Harjola PT, Sivula A. A single ulceration following experimentally induced hypovolemia and hemorrhagic stasis. Ann Surg 1966;163:21.

59. Bounous G, Menard D, De Medicis E. Role of pancreatic proteases in the pathogenesis of ischemic enteropathy. Gastroenterology 1977;73:102.

60. Bounous G. Pancreatic proteases and oxygen-derived free radicals in acute ischemic enteropathy. Surgery 1986;99:192.

61. Bounous G. Acute necrosis of the intestinal mucosa. Gastroenterology 1982;82:1457.

62. Evans E, Shore RT, Carey LC, Darin JC. Effect of intestinal exclusion in *Escherichia coli* endotoxin shock. Arch Surg 1967;95:511.

63. Fine J. The intestinal circulation in shock. Gastroenterology 1967;52:454.

64. Driks MR, Craven DE, Celli BR, et al. Nosocomial pneumonia in intubated patients given sucralfate as compared with antacids or histamine type 2 blockers. N Engl J Med 1987;317:1376.

65. Hillman KM, Riordan T, O'Farrell SM. Colonization of gastric contents in critically ill patients. Crit Care Med 1982;10:444.

66. Deitch EA, Bridges W, Baker J, et al. Hemorrhagic shock-induced bacterial translocation is reduced by xanthine oxidase inhibition or inactivation. Surgery 1988;104:191.

67. Wells CL, Maddaus MA, Simmons RL. The role of the macrophage in the translocation of intestinal bacteria. Arch Surg 1987;122:48.

68. Cerra FB, Shronts EP, Konstantinides NN, et al. Enteral feeding in sepsis: a prospective randomized double blind trial. Surgery 1985;98:632.

69. Bennion RS, Wilson SE, Serota AI, Williams RA. The role of gastrointestinal microflora in the pathogenesis of complications of mesenteric ischemia. Rev Infect Dis 1984;6:(Suppl 1):S132.

70. Yale CE, Balish E. The importance of clostridia in experimental intestinal strangulation. Gastroenterology 1976;71:793.

71. Griffin PM, Olmstead LC, Petras RE. *Escherichia coli* 0157:H7-associated colitis. Gastroenterology 1990;99:142.

72. Williams RA, Wilson SE. Thiery-Vella segments applied to ischemic colon studies. J Surg Res 1979;27:214.

73. Amano H, Bulkley GB, Gorey T, et al. The role of microvascular patency in the recovery of small intestine from ischemic injury. Surg Forum 1980;31:157.

74. Park P, Haglund U. Regeneration of small bowel mucosa after intestinal ischemia. Crit Care Med 1992;20:135.

75. Deitch E, Berg RD. Endotoxin but not malnutrition promotes bacterial translocation of the gut flora in burned mice. J Trauma 1987;27:161.

76. Rutenberg SH, Schweinberg FB. The bacterial factor in traumatic shock. N Engl J Med 1959;260:214.

77. Berg RD. Translocation of indigenous bacteria from the intestinal tract. In: Hentges DJ, ed. Human intestinal microflora in health and disease. New York: Academic Press, 1983:333.

78. Schatten WE, Desprez JD, Holden WD. A bacteriologic study of portal-vein blood in man. Arch Surg 1955;71:404.

79. Ambrose NS, Johnson M, Burdon DW, Keighley MR. Incidence

of pathogenic bacteria from mesenteric lymph nodes and ileal serosa during Crohn's disease surgery. Br J Surg 1984;71:623.

80. Bennion RS, Wilson SE, Williams RA. The role of gastrointestinal microflora in the pathogenesis of complications of mesenteric ischemia. J Infect Dis 1984;119:151.

81. Bennion RS, Wilson SE, Williams RA. Early portal anaerobic bacteremia in mesenteric ischemia. Arch Surg 1984:119:151.

82. Papa M, Halperin Z, Rubinstein E, et al. The effect of ischemia of the dog's colon on transmural migration of bacteria and endotoxin. J Surg Res 1983;35: 264.

83. Yale CE, Altemeier WA. Intestinal obstruction in germ free rats. Arch Surg 1965;91:241.

84. McCartney AC, Piotrowicz BI, Edlin S, Ledingham I McA. Measurement of endotoxin in the acute phase of septic shock. Prog Clin Biol Res 1988;272:225.

85. Ramsay G, Newman PM, McCartney AC, Ledingham I McA. Endotoxaemia in multiple organ failure due to sepsis. Prog Clin Biol Res 1988;272:237.

86. McCartbet AC, Banbs JG, Clements GB, et al. Endotoxaemia in septic shock: clinical and post mortem correlations. Intensive Care Med 1983;9:117.

87. Brand ED, Lefer AM. Myocardial depressant factor in plasma from cats in irreversible post-oligemic shock. Proc Soc Exp Biol Med 1980;122:200.

88. Hinshaw LB, Archer LT, Black MR, Greenfield LJ. Myocardial performance in splanchnic arterial occlusion shock. J Surg Res 1973;15:417.

89. Ward PA, Till GO, Hatherill JR, et al. Systemic compliment activation, lung injury, and products of lipid peroxidation. J Clin Invest 1985;76:517.

90. Lefer AM. Thromboxane A_2 and leukotrienes are eicosanoid mediators of shock and ischemic disorders. Adv Shock Res 1988;9:101.

91. Lefer AM. Eicosanoids as mediators of ischemia and shock. Fed Proc 1985;44:275.

92. Tate RM, Morris HG, Schroeder WR, et al. Oxygen metabolites stimulate thromboxane production and vasoconstriction in isolated saline-perfused rabbit lungs. J Clin Invest 1984;74: 608.

93. Klausner JM, Paterson IS, Kobzik L, et al. Oxygen free radicles mediate ischemia-induced lung injury. Surgery 1989;105:192.

94. Bergan JJ, Dry L, Conn J, et al. Intestinal ischemic syndromes. Ann Surg 1969;169:120.

95. Reilly PM, Jones B, Bulkley GB. Noninvasive assessment of bowel ischemic syndromes. In: Ernst CB, Stanley JB, eds. Current therapy in vascular surgery. 2nd ed. Philadelphia: BC Decker, 1991:718.

96. Brooks DH, Carey LC. Base deficit in superior mesenteric artery occlusion, an aid to early diagnosis. Ann Surg 1973;177:352.

97. Robertson OS, Lyall AD, Macrae JG. Acid–base disturbances in mesenteric occlusion. Surg Gynecol Obstet 1969;128:15.

98. May LD, Berenson MM. Value of serum inorganic phosphate in the diagnosis of ischemic bowel disease. Am J Surg 1983;146: 266.

99. Taylor BM, Jamieson WG, Durand D. Preinfarction diagnosis of acute mesenteric ischemia by simple measurement of inorganic phosphate in body fluids. Can J Surg 1979;22:40.

100. Graeber GM, Wukich DK, et al. Changes in peripheral serum CPK and LDH in acute experimental colonic infarction. Ann Surg 1981;194:708.

101. Graeber GM, Cafferty PJ, et al. Changes in serum total creatinine phosphokinase and its isoenzymes caused by experimental ligation of the superior mesenteric artery. Ann Surg 1981;193: 499.

102. Fried MW, Murthy UK, Hassig SR, et al. Creatine kinase isoenzymes in the diagnosis of intestinal infarction. Dig Dis Sci 1991;36:1589.

103. Scott JR, Miller WT, et al. Acute mesenteric infarction. AJR 1971;113:269.

104. Tomchik FS, Wittenberg J, Ottinger LW. The roentgenographic spectrum of bowel infarction. Radiology 1970;96:249.

105. Kim JY, Ha HK, Byon JY, et al. Intestinal infarction secondary to mesenteric venous thrombosis: CT-pathologic correlation. J Comput Assist Tomogr 1993;17:382.

106. Gehl HB, Bohndor FK, Klose KC, Gunther RW. Two-dimensional MR angiography in the evaluation of abdominal veins with gradient refocussed sequences. J Comput Assist Tomogr 1990;14:619.

107. Haddad MC, Clark DC, Sharif HS, et al. MR, CT, and ultrasonography of splanchnic venous thrombosis. Gastrointest Radiol 1992;17:34.

108. Laufman H, Method H. The role of muscular spasm in recovery of strangulated intestine. Surg Gynecol Obstet 1947;85:675.

109. Gorey TF. Tests of intestinal viability. In: Marston A, ed. Vascular disease of the gut. London: Edward Arnold, 1986.

110. Gorey TF. The recovery of intestine after ischemic injury. Br J Surg 1980;67:699.

111. Wright CB, Hobson RW. Prediction of intestinal viability using Doppler ultrasound techniques. Am J Surg 1975;129:643.

112. Cooperman M, Martin EW, Keith LM, Cavey LC. Use of Doppler ultrasound in intestinal surgery. Am J Surg 1979;138: 856.

113. Bulkley G, Zuidema G, Hamilton S, et al. Intraoperative determination of small intestinal viability following ischemic injury. Ann Surg 1981;193:628.

114. Stolar CJ, Randolph JG. Evaluation of ischemic bowel viability with a fluorescent technique. J Pediatr Surg 1987;13:221.

115. Horsbrugh AG. Occlusion of the mesenteric veins. In: Hadfield J, Hobsley M, eds. Current surgical practice. Vol I. London: Edward Arnold, 1976.

116. Leffal LD, Syphax B. Clinical aids in strangulation intestinal obstruction. Am J Surg 1970;120:756.

117. Wilson C, Gupta R, Gilmour DG, Imrie CW. Acute superior mesenteric ischemia. Br J Surg 1987;74:279.

118. Mosley JG, Marston A. Acute intestinal ischemia. In: Marston A, Bulkley GB, Fiddian-Green RG, Haglund UH, eds. Splanchnic ischemia and multiple organ failure. London: Edward Arnold, 1989:279.

119. Ottinger LW. The surgical management of acute occlusion of the superior mesenteric artery. Ann Surg 1978;188:721.

120. Williams LF. Vascular insufficiency of the intestines. Gastroenterology 1971;61:757.

121. Williams CF. Mesenteric ischemia. Surg Clin North Am 1988;68:331.

122. Clark RA, Gallant TE. Acute mesenteric ischemia: angiographic spectrum. AJR 1984;142:555.

123. Siegelman SS, Sprayregen S, Boley SJ. Angiographic diagnosis of mesenteric arterial vasoconstriction. Radiology 1974;112: 533.

124. Bergqvist D, Bowald S, Eriksson I, et al. Small intestinal necrosis after aortoiliac reconstruction. Br J Surg 1986;73:28.

125. Hildebrand HD, Zierler RE. Mesenteric vascular disease. Am J Surg 1980;139:188.

126. Boley SJ, Schwartz SS, Williams LW. Vascular disorders of the intestine. New York: Appleton-Century-Crofts, 1971:657.

127. Sachs SM, Morton JH, Schwartz SI. Acute mesenteric ischemia. Surgery 1982;92:646.

128. Kwaan JH, Connolly JE. Prevention of intestinal infarction resulting from mesenteric arterial occlusive disease. Surg Gynecol Obstet 1983;157:321.

129. Flickinger EG, Johnsrude IS, Ogburn NL, et al. Local streptokinase infusion for superior mesenteric thromboembolism. AJR 1982;140:771.

130. Boley SJ, Sprayregen S, Siegelman SS, Veith FJ. Initial results from an aggressive approach to acute mesenteric ischemia. Surgery 1977;82:848.

131. Gruenberg JC, Smallbridge RC, Rosenberg RD. Inherited antithrombin III deficiency, causing mesenteric venous infarction. Am Surg 1975;181:791.

132. Kitchens CS. Evolution of our understanding of the pathophysiology of primary mesenteric venous thrombosis. Am J Surg 1992;163:346.

133. Kirschner PA. Occlusion of the mesenteric arteries and veins with infarction of the bowel. J Mt Sinai Hosp 1955;21:307.

134. Anane-Sefah JC, Blair E, Reckler S. Primary mesenteric venous occlusive disease. Surg Gynecol Obstet 1975;141:740.

135. Abdu RA, Zakhour BJ, Dallis DJ. Mesenteric venous thrombosis: 1911–1984. Surgery 1987;101:363.

136. Ashida H, Kotoura Y, Nishioka A, et al. Portal and mesenteric venous thrombosis as a complication of endoscopic sclerotherapy. Am J Gastroenterol 1989;84:306.

137. Umpleby HC. Thrombosis of the superior mesenteric vein. Br J Surg 1987;74:694.

138. Khodadadi J, Rozencwajg J, Nacasvh N, et al. Mesenteric vein thrombosis. Arch Surg 1980;115:315.

139. Cannon WB. Bodily changes in pain, hunger, fear and rage: an account of recent researches into the function of emotional excitement. New York: D. Appleton & Co, 1920.

140. Landrenean RJ, Fry WJ. The right colon as a target organ of nonocclusive mesenteric ischemia. Arch Surg 1990;125:591.

141. Ende N. Infarction of the bowel in cardiac failure. N Engl J Med 1958;258:879.

142. Boley SJ, Regan JA, Runick PA, et al. Persistent vasoconstriction: a major factor in non-occlusive mesenteric ischemia. Ann Top Surg Res 1971;3:425.

143. Gottlieb JE, Menashe PI, Cruz E. Gastrointestinal complications in critically ill patients. Am J Gastroenterol 1986;81:227.

144. Valentine RJ, Whelan TV, Meyers HF. Nonocclusive mesenteric ischemia in renal patients: recognition and prevention of intestinal gangrene. Am J Kidney Dis 1990;15:598.

145. Freudenberger DS, Cappell MS, Hutt DA. Intestinal infarction after intravenous cocaine administration. Ann Intern Med 1990;113:715.

146. Athanasoulis CA, Wittenberg J, Berenstein J, Williams F. Vasodilatory drugs in the management of non occlusive bowel ischemia. Gastroenterology 1975;68:146.

147. Bailey RW, Bulkley GB. Role of the circulation in NEC. In: Kvietys PR, Barrowman JA, Granger DN, eds. Pathophysiology of the splanchnic circulation. Boca Raton, FL: CRC Press, 1987: 141.

148. Barlow B, Santulli TV. An experimental study of acute neonatal necrotizing enterocolitis: the importance of breast milk. J Pediatr Surg 1974;7:232.

149. Kliegman RM, Hack M, Jones P, et al. Epidemiologic study of NEC among low birth weight infants. J Pediatr 1982;100:440.

150. Stone HH, Allen WB, Smith BB, et al. Infantile pneumatosis intestinalis. J Surg Res 1968;8:301.

151. Reid WD, Shannon MP. Necrotizing enterocolitis: a medical approach to treatment. Can Med Assoc J 1973;108:573.

152. Kosloske AM. Necrotizing enterocolitis in the neonate. Surg Gynecol Obstet 1979;148:259.

153. Kanto WP, Wilson R, Ricketts RR. Management and outcome of neonatal necrotizing enterocolitis. Clin Pediatr 1985;24:79.

154. Gregory JR, Campbell JR, Harrison MW, et al. Neonatal necrotizing enterocolitis: a ten year experience. Am J Surg 1981;141:562.

155. Croft RJ, Menon GP, Marston A. Does intestinal angina exist?: a critical study of obstructed visceral arteries. Br J Surg 1981;68: 316.

156. Reiner L. Mesenteric arterial insufficiency and abdominal angina. Arch Intern Med 1964;114:765.

157. Fisher DF, Fry WJ. The collateral mesenteric circulation. Surg Gynecol Obstet 1987;164: 487.

158. Moneta GL, Yeager RA, et al. Duplex ultrasound criteria for diagnosis of splanchnic artery stenosis on occlusion. J Vasc Surg 1991;14:511.

159. Jager K, Bollinger A, et al. Measurement of mesenteric blood flow by duplex scan. J Vasc Surg 1986;3:462.

160. Boley SJ, Brandt LJ, Veith FJ, et al. A new provocative test for chronic mesenteric ischemia. Am J Gastroenterol 1991;86:888.

161. Connolly JE, Kwaan JH. Management of chronic visceral ischemia. Surg Clin North Am 1982;62:345.

162. Golden DA, Ring EJ, McLean GK, Freiman DB. Percutaneous transluminal angioplasty in the treatment of abdominal angina. AJR 1982;139:247.

163. Stoney RJ, Reilly LR. Chronic visceral ischemia: an often overlooked cause of abdominal pain. Postgrad Med 1983;74:111.

164. Harjola PT, Lahtiharju A. Celiac axis syndrome: abdominal angina caused by external compression of the celiac artery. Am J Surg 1968;2:795.

165. Harjola, PR. A rare obstruction of the celiac artery: report of a case. Ann Chir Gynaecol Fenn 1963;52:547.

166. Gillespie SW, Little JM. Celiac axis compression syndrome: factors predicting a favorable outcome. Surgery 1985;98: 879.

167. Szilagyi DE, Rian RL, Elliot JP, et al. The celiac artery compression syndrome: does it exist? Surgery 1972;72:849.

168. Reilly LM, Ammar, AD, Stoney RJ, et al. Late results following operative repair for celiac artery compression syndrome. J Vasc Surg 1985;2:79.

169. Li VE, McDonnel CH, et al. Chronic mesenteric ischemia. Radiology 1994;190:175.

170. Boley SJ, Schwartz S, Lash J, et al. Reversible vascular occlusion of the colon. Surg Gynecol Obstet 1963;116:53.

171. Johnson WC. Nabseth DC. Visceral infarction following aortic surgery. Ann Surg 1974;180:312.

172. Marston A. Ischemic colitis. In: Marston A, Bulkley GB, Fiddian-Green RG, Haglund UH, eds. Splanchnic ischemia and multiple organ failure. London: Edward Arnold, 1989:301.

173. Yang RD, Han MW, McCarthy JH. Ischemic colitis in a crack abuser. Dig Dis Sci 1991;36:238.

174. Tampkins RK. Ischemic colitis. In: Cameron JL, ed. Current surgical therapy. vol. 4. St. Louis: Mosby Year Book, 1992: 186.

175. Sakai L, Keltner R, Kaminski D. Spontaneous shock-associated ischemic colitis. Am J Surg 1980;140:755.

176. Barcewitz PA, Welch JP. Ischemic colitis in young adult patients. Dis Colon Rectum 1980;123:109.

177. Reeders WAJ, Tytgat GNJ, Rosenbusch G, Gratama S. Ischaemic colitis. The Hague: Martinus Nijhoff, 1984.

178. Parish KL, Chapman WC, Williams LF. Ischemic colitis: an everchanging spectrum. Am Surg 1991;57:118.

179. Guttormson NL, Bubrick MP. Mortality from ischemic colitis. Dis Colon Rectum 1989;32:469.

180. Haglund U, Jodal M, Lundgren O. The small bowel in arterial hypotension and shock. In: Shepherd AP, Granger DN, eds. Physiology of the intestinal circulation. New York: Raven Press, 1984:305.

181. Lucas CE, Sugawa C, Riddle J, et al. Natural history and surgical dilemma of "stress" gastric bleeding. Arch Surg 1971;102:266.

182. Czaja AJ, McAlhany JC, Pruit BA. Acute gastroduodenal disease after thermal injury: an endoscopic evaluation of incidence and natural history. N Engl J Med 1974;291:925.

183. Peura DA, Johnson LF. Cimetidine for prevention and treatment of gastroduodenal mucosal lesions in patients in an intensive care unit. Ann Intern Med 1985;103:173.

184. Zinner MJ, Zuidema GS, Smith PL. The prevention of upper gastrointestinal tract bleeding in patients in an intensive care unit. Surg Gynecol Obstet 1981;153:214.

185. Silen W, Merhav A, Simson JNL. The pathophysiology of stress ulcer disease. World J Surg 1981;5:165.

186. Marrone GC, Silen W. Pathogenesis, diagnosis and treatment of acute gastric mucosal lesions. Clin Gastroenterol 1984;13: 635.

187. Knight A, Bihari D, Tinker J. Stress ulceration in the critically ill patient. Br J Hosp Med 1985;33:216.

188. Mersereau WA, Hinchey EJ. Effect of gastric acidity on gastric ulceration induced by hemorrhage in the rat, utilizing a gastric chamber technique. Gastroenterology 1973;64:1130.

189. Hastings PR, Skillman JJ, Bushnell LS, Silen W. Antacid titration in the prevention of acute gastrointestinal bleeding: a controlled randomized trial in 100 critically ill patients. N Engl J Med 1978;298:1041.

190. Schuster DP, Rowley H, Feinstein S, et al. Prospective evaluation of the risk of upper gastrointestinal bleeding after admission to a medical intensive care unit. Am J Med 1984;76:623.

191. Basso N, Bagarani M, Materia A, et al. Cimetidine and antacid prophylaxis of acute upper gastrointestinal bleeding in high risk patients. Am J Surg 1981;141:339.

192. McAlhany JC, Czaja AJ, Pruit BA. Antacid control of compli-

cations from acute gastroduodenal disease after burns. J Trauma 1976;16:645.
193. Collins R, Langman M. Treatment with histamine H_2 antagonists in acute upper gastrointestinal hemorrhage: implications of randomized trials. N Engl J Med 1985;313:660.
194. Baltas B, Dobronte Z. Randomized prospective trail of cimetidine in the treatment of acute gastrointestinal hemorrhage. Acta Chir Hung 1984;25:147.
195. Swain CP, Bown SG, Storey DW, et al. Controlled trial of argon laser photocoagulation in bleeding peptic ulcers. Lancet 1981;2: 1313.
196. Kiefhaber P, Kiefhaber K, Huber F, Nath G. Endoscopic neodymium: YAG laser coagulation in gastrointestinal hemorrhage. Endoscopy 1986;18:(Suppl 2):46.
197. Cheung LY. Pathogenesis, prophylaxis and treatment of stress gastritis. Am J Surg 1988;156:437.
198. Clarke WIW. Centrilobular hepatic necrosis following cardiac infarction. Am J Pathol 1949;26:249.
199. Ellenberg M, Osserman KE. The role of shock in the production of central liver cell necrosis. Am J Med 1951;11:170.
200. Birgens HS, Henriksen J, Matzen P, Paulsen H. The shock liver: clinical and biochemical findings in patients with centrilobular liver necrosis following cardiogenic shock. Acta Med Scand 1978;204:417.
201. McMichael J. The oxygen supply of the liver. Q J Exp Physiol 1937;27:73.
202. Smith LL, Veragut UP. The liver and shock: initiating and perpetuating factors. Prog Surg 1964;4:55.
203. Laut WW. Relationship between hepatic blood flow and overall metabolism: the hepatic arterial buffer response. Fed Proc 1983;42:1662.
204. Clarke WIW. Centrilobular hepatic necrosis following cardiac infarction. Am J Pathol 1949;26:249.
205. Adkison D, Hollwarth ME, Benoit JN, et al. Role of free radicals in ischemia–reperfusion injury to the liver. Acta Physiol Scand 1986;126:(Suppl 548):101.
206. Della Corte F, Gozzetti G, Novello F, Stirpe F. Properties of the xanthine oxidase from human liver. Biochim Biophys Acta 1969;191:164.
207. Jarasch ED, Grund C, Bruder G, et al. Localization of xanthine oxidase in mammary-gland epithelium and capillary endothelium. Cell 1981;25:67.
208. Ratych RE, Chuknyiska RS, Bulkley GB. The primary localization of free radical generation after anoxia/reoxygenation in isolated endothelial cells. Surgery 1987;102:122.
209. Champion HR, Jones RT, Trump BF, et al. A clinicopathologic study of hepatic dysfunction following shock. Surg Gynecol Obstet 1976;142:657.
210. Kaymakcaln H, Doukdourekas D, Szanto PB, Steigmann F. Congestive heart failure as cause of fulminant hepatic failure. Am J Med 1978;65:384.
211. Gibson PR, Dudley FJ. Ischemic hepatitis: clinical features and prognosis. Aust N Z J Med 1984;14:822.
212. Killip T, Payne MA. High serum transaminase activity in heart disease: circulatory failure and hepatic necrosis. Circulation 1960;21:646.
213. Glenn F. Acute cholecystitis following the surgical treatment of unrelated disease. Ann Surg 1947;126:411
214. Frazee RC, Nagorney DM, Mucha P. Acute acalculous cholecystitis. Mayo Clin Proc 1989;64:163.
215. Meissner K. Die Gallblase als Schockorgan: Beitrag zur Pathogenese der postoperitiven und der post-trumatischen Cholecystitis. Langenbecks Arch Chir 1974;336:25.
216. DuPriest RW, Khaneja SC, Cowley RA. Acute cholecystitis complicating trauma. Ann Surg 1979;189:84.
217. Howard RJ. Acute acalculous cholecystitis. Am J Surg 1981;141:194.
218. Scher KS, Sarap MD, Jaggers RL. Acute acalculous cholecystitis complicating aortic aneurysm repair. Surg Gynecol Obstet 1986;163:475.
219. Shuman WP, Rogers JV, Rudd TG, et al. Low sensitivity of sonography and cholescintigraphy in acalculous cholecystitis. AJR 1984;142:531
220. Mirvis SE, Vainright JR, Nelson AW, et al. The diagnosis of acute acalculous cholecystitis: a comparison of sonography, scintigraphy, and CT. AJR 1986;147:1171.
221. Vauthey JN, Lerut J, Martini M, et al. Indications and limitations of percutaneous cholecystostomy for acute cholecystitis. Surg Gynecol Obstet 1993; 176:49.
222. Garner WL, Marx VM, Fabri PJ. Cholescintigraphy in the critically ill. Am J Surg 1988;155:727.
223. Flancbaum L, Majerus TC, Cox EF. Acute post-traumatic acalculous cholecystitis. Am J Surg 1985;150:252.
224. Sitzmann JV, Pitt HA, Steinborn PA, et al. Cholecystokinin prevents parenteral nutrition induced biliary sludge in humans. Surg Gynecol Obstet 1990;170:25.
225. Haas G, Warshaw A, Aretz H, et al. Acute pancreatitis after cardiopulmonary bypass. Am J Surg 1985;149:508
226. Lefor AT, Vuocolo P, Parker FB, Sillin LF. Pancreatic complications following cardiopulmonary bypass. Arch Surg 1992;127:1225.
227. Gnaz-Nikulin, Nikulin A, Gaon D, et al. Pancreatic lesions in shock and their significance. J Pathol 1981;135:223.
228. Weaver DW, Busuito MJ, Bouwman DL. Hyperamylasemia following cardiopulmonary bypass: does this indicate pancreatitis? Surg Forum 1984;35:181.
229. Howes R, Zuidema GD, Cameron JL. Evaluation of prophylactic antibiotics in acute pancreatitis. J Surg Res 1975;18: 197.
230. Cerra FB. The hypermetabolism organ failure complex. World J Surg 1987;11:173.
231. Carrico CJ, Meakins J, Marshall J, et al. Multiple organ failure syndrome. Arch Surg 1986;121:196.
232. Pine RW, Wertz MJ, Lennard ES, et al. Determinants of organ malfunction or death in patients with intraabdominal sepsis. Arch Surg 1983;118:242.
233. Madoff RD, Sharpe SM, Fath JJ, et al. Prolong surgical intensive care. Arch Surg 1985;120:698.
234. Meakins JL, Marshall JC. The gut as the motor of multiple system organ failure. In: Marston A, Bulkley GB, Fiddian-Green RG, Haglund UH, eds. Splanchnic ischemia and multiple organ failure. London: Edward Arnold, 1989:339.
235. Souba WW, Smith RJ, Wilmore DW. Glutamine metabolism by the intestinal tract. JPEN J Parenter Enteral Nutr 1985;9: 608.
236. Desai MH, Herndon DN, Rutan RL, et al. Ischemic intestinal complications in patients with burns. Surg Gynecol Obstet 1991;172:257.
237. DeCamp MM, Demling RH. Posttraumatic multisystem organ failure. JAMA 1988;260:530.
238. Baue AE, Chaudry IH. Prevention of multiple system failure. Surg Clin North Am 1980;60:1167.

Textbook of Gastroenterology, second edition, edited by Tadataka Yamada. JB Lippincott Company, Philadelphia © 1995.

CHAPTER 113

Radiation Injury

Timothy T. Nostrant   John M. Robertson
Theodore S. Lawrence

Almost since the discovery of x-rays in 1895 by Wilhelm Roentgen, radiation-induced injury to the gastrointestinal tract of humans has been reported.[1-3] In the early years of radiation treatment, the development of skin hyperemia and burns imposed dose limitations that reduced both radiation complications and radiation effectiveness. The development of supervoltage techniques allowed administration of higher doses of radiation without skin injury, and this ushered in a new era of deep tissue radiation damage, including damage to the gastrointestinal tract. With improving techniques of radiation localization using tomographic fielding, radiation doses, effectiveness, and use all have increased.[4] It is estimated that up to 50% of patients with cancer will receive radiation during their treatment.[5] Radiation therapy is now a prominent part of many cancer treatment programs, particularly in combination with debulking surgery and chemotherapy—therapies that potentiate the toxic effects of radiation. Thus, despite great strides in radiation technology, radiation injury is still likely to be a significant problem for patients and hence for the gastroenterologist and radiation oncologist.

The prevalence of radiation-induced gastrointestinal injury varies, with estimated incidences of 1% to 25% of treated patients.[6-9] Much of this variability has been the result of differences in radiation technique from 1940 to 1960, and a lack of recognition of disease. Significant abdominal cramping, diarrhea, and food intolerance were disregarded by both patient and physician, whereas rarer, but more serious forms of radiation injury such as radiation proctitis and enteritis, received undue emphasis.

This chapter discusses the pathobiology, pathology, and clinical features of radiation-induced gastrointestinal injury, as well as its treatment and prevention.

RADIATION PATHOBIOLOGY

An understanding of how ionizing radiation affects the gastrointestinal tract at the cellular and organ level requires knowing a number of terms that are frequently used in radiation biology. The accepted unit of dose of radiation is the gray (Gy), which is 1 joule of energy deposited in 1 kilogram. One Gy is equal to 100 rads, the older and more widely known term. The term "centigray" (cGy), which is 0.01 Gy, is equal to the formerly used "rad." Another term often encountered is the "rem," which means the dose in rads times a quality factor. It is hard to assign a biologic effectiveness to the rem because, for the same physical dose, some forms of ionizing radiation (such as neutrons and alpha particles) can cause 10 times the biologic damage caused by the more commonly used megavoltage photons.[10,11]

Megavoltage photons used in modern radiation therapy interact with tissues chiefly through the "Compton effect," that is, high-energy electrons ejected by the photon as it passes through the body.[12] These electrons are responsible for most of the biologic effects of radiation. DNA is a target for most forms of radiation damage. High-energy electrons can damage DNA through what have been termed "direct" and "indirect" actions. Thirty percent of the DNA damage occurs as electrons interact directly with DNA. The electron also interacts with other cellular constituents (chiefly water) to generate free radicals, which indirectly inflict DNA damage.[10] Although the cell has evolved elaborate mechanisms for repairing such damage, the damage may be lethal.[13,14] On the average, radiation produces approximately 5×10^{-9} double-strand breaks per gray per base pair.[15,16] It has been estimated that a single, unrepaired double-strand DNA break can, under some conditions, kill a cell.[17]

A number of environmental factors contribute to the biologic effects of radiation on healthy and cancer cells. Among the most important is the partial pressure of oxygen at the time of irradiation. Cells that are irradiated under hypoxic conditions (particularly PO_2 <3 mm Hg) are markedly resistant to photon irradiation ("the oxygen effect"). This finding has prompted two lines of clinical research: development of hypoxic cell-sensitizing drugs that mimic oxygen by facilitating the generation of free radicals and that selectively increase the sensitivity of cancer cells because healthy cells are already well oxygenated; and use of neutrons or charged particles, forms of irradiation having a significantly smaller oxygen effect than standard photons. It is not yet clear if either of these approaches will yield an improved therapeutic index.[18,19]

In addition to oxygen status, cell cycle phase influences radiation sensitivity. Cells undergoing mitosis and entering S phase appear to be significantly more sensitive than cells in mid-S phase, although these effects may be more pronounced in rodent cells than in human tumor cells.[20] This observation has encouraged the use of cell cycle synchronizing agents such as hydroxyurea to increase the efficacy of radiation. In a randomized trial, hydroxyurea, a ribonucleotide reductase inhibitor that has no intrinsic activity against cervical cancer, improved the survival of patients treated with radiation.[21]

Radiation sensitizers such as the halopyrimidines that do not rely on tumor hypoxia are frequently used in the treatment of gastrointestinal cancers.[22-32] Fluorouracil, fluorodeoxyuridine, bromodeoxyuridine, and iododeoxyuridine are examples of such drugs. Fluorouracil used in combination with radiation improved the survival of patients with resected cancer of the rectum,[22] pancreas,[23] and esophagus.[24] Bromodeoxyuridine and iododeoxyuridine appear both to increase radiation DNA damage and decrease DNA repair.[29-32]

Another approach to improving the therapeutic index of radiation in the treatment of gastrointestinal cancers is selectively to protect healthy intestine, an approach particularly important under clinical situations in which patient positioning or small bowel exclusion procedures are not helpful, such as when there are fixed segments of small intestine or during whole-abdomen or whole-body irradiation. One such agent is WR-2721, an aminothiol that is hypothesized to be a radioprotector by virtue of scavenging free radicals. Clinical trials using WR-2721 have had mixed results.[33,34]

Although modifiers such as hypoxia, cell cycle synchronizers, sensitizers, and protectors have an important influence on the response of the tumor and the healthy intestine to irradiation, physical factors such as volume of the irradiated organ, total dose, and fraction size also are critical. The relation between complications and the maximum dose of radiation received by an organ has traditionally been expressed as the 5% (or 50%) risk of a complication by 5 years (TD 5/5 and TD 5/50, respectively) with a particular dose and volume of the organ.[35] Although this expression of complication risk is reasonably accurate for whole-organ radiation, it cannot be applied equally well to partial-organ radiation. Within the limit of these uncertainties, however, attempts have been made to estimate organ tolerance, and these are described in detail in the section Specific Organ Involvement.

PATHOLOGY

The principal effects of radiation come about through its interaction with nuclear DNA in dividing cells, halting mitosis or causing mutations or cell death.[36,37] These effects are accentuated by coadministration of chemotherapeutic agents such as doxorubicin, actinomycin D, and bleomycin.[38-40] Radiation effects are ameliorated by intrinsic DNA reparative processes, but these built-in defenses can be overcome by repeated radiation exposure.

In contrast to defenses against chemical and biologic agents, there are no structural barriers at the tissue or cellular levels to the penetration of most forms of radiation.[36] The amount of radiation injury depends on the type and quantity of radiation energy delivered. Damage is highest with alpha particles, intermediate with beta particles, and lowest with gamma radiation, including x-rays.[36,37] Deep tissue injury is most common with x-rays, however, because of their greater penetration and wider therapeutic use. Radiation damage can be divided into that associated with whole-body irradiation and that secondary to localized irradiation.

For whole-body radiation doses in excess of 500 cGy, injury follows a rather stereotypic sequence of events.[41,42] The initial phase is characterized by nausea, vomiting, and decreased gastric acid secretion. If radiation exposure is less than 150 cGy, the nausea and vomiting appears to be mediated by central nervous system stimulation and usually resolves with no sequelae.[42,43] At doses greater than 600 cGy, the initial phase resolves but is followed in 2 to 5 days by diffuse gastrointestinal mucosal destruction and loss of all cellular lines in the bone marrow.[42,43] Altered mucosal function and changes in bowel flora lead to growth of facultative organisms and loss of gastrointestinal mucosal and systemic defenses, which results in gram-negative sepsis and massive fluid and electrolyte loss into the gut wall and gastrointestinal lumen, resulting finally in death.[42,44,45] Lesser radiation exposure results in milder, more reversible damage that usually resolves over several weeks.[42-45] Therapeutic whole-body irradiation is most commonly used as a pretreatment for bone marrow transplantation, and maximal damage occurs in the small intestine.

The changes noted after localized radiation are separated into early (acute) and late (chronic) changes. In addition, late complications can be separated into chronic radiation damage and secondary carcinogenesis.[46,47]

The first recorded changes in the intestine after acute radiation exposure are loss of lamina propria lymphocytes, and microscopic damage to mucosal epithelial cells and vascular endothelial cells.[46,47] Reduced maturation and simplification of the mucosal surface with villous blunting and a decrease in crypt regenerative cells are the first visible epithelial cellular effects in the gut.[48] In the esophagus, there is loss of basal mitotic cells and extensive damage to the squamous epithelium, and there is loss of chief and parietal cells in the stomach with a resultant decrease in gastric secretion.[46] Coincident with these epithelial changes, marked submucosal edema is seen secondary to increased vascular permeability.[46-49] Superficial ulcers can be seen but are uncommon. If relatively low doses of radiation are used, all of these changes are reversible without significant sequelae.[49-51]

With increasing doses of radiation, there is persistence and extension of ulcerations with irregular dilation of small vessels (telangiectasia).[51-53] In addition, these is a marked increase in granulation tissue and collagen formation in excess of that predicted by the level of tissue damage.[51] Irregular, enlarged, atypical fibroblasts appear and are a relatively specific marker for radiation damage.[51] In most cases of severe radiation injury, endothelial inflammation coupled with vascular muscle and intimal fibroblast proliferation may lead to lumenal narrowing and thrombosis.[53] The other mesenchymal elements are radioresistant but can be damaged secondarily by infection and mucosal ischemia. The later effects of irradiation consist of progressive changes in the epithelia, resulting in atrophy, increasing fibrosis leading to stricture formation, and thrombosis causing secondary ischemic damage. Progressive ischemia and secondary infection can lead to ulceration, fistulization, and, in rare cases, perforation.

A potential late effect of radiation is the development of a secondary epithelial or stromal tumor in the gastrointestinal tract.[54-57] The short survival of patients with cancer secondary to their primary tumor limits this carcinogenic potential. Exceptions to this rule are patients with cervical, prostatic, and testicular cancers. It has been estimated that 3% of carcinomas arising in the gastrointestinal tract may be a consequence of prior irradiation, with 2.5% caused by natural or accidental radiation exposure, and 0.5% caused by cumulative diagnostic and therapeutic radiation.[57] Carcinomas develop at a similar age and in similar sites to those of naturally occurring carcinomas.[55-58] Cancer histopathology in patients with radiation-associated carcinomas is similar to those in patients with carcinomas without prior irradiation.[57,58] Carcinomas can be seen in areas devoid of significant radiation damage, but they usually lie within the field of radiation. Prominent secondary carcinomas include colorectal cancer after gynecologic irradiation and rectal cancer after prostatic irradiation. Radiation should not be implicated in a case of carcinoma unless the carcinoma occurs more than 10 years after the treatment course.[56-58]

The exact mechanisms by which radiation causes cancer are unknown.[36] There is considerable support in human and animal experimentation for direct DNA oncogenic mutations. Alternatively, mutations may promote viral protooncogene expression, which may lead to immunosuppression, thus fostering the development of secondary neoplasms.[36,37]

SPECIFIC ORGAN INVOLVEMENT

Esophagus

Esophageal radiation injury occurs primarily after radiation therapy for contiguous neoplasms of the lung, mediastinum, and thymus. Radiation damage to the esophagus consistently occurs at doses greater than 6000 cGy administered in fractions of more than 1000 cGy/week.[50,59] Mucositis, dysphagia, and odynophagia begin by the end of the second week in most patients.[59,60] The radiologic and endoscopic findings can mimic opportunistic infections, particularly candidiasis. Most patients recover if radiation treatment is interrupted for 2 to 7 days.[50,59,60] Hemorrhage and perforation do not occur during the acute phase of treatment because of intact regenerative processes.[50,59-61] Failure of primary peristalsis and poor relaxation of the lower esophageal sphincter contribute to dysphagia in these patients.[50,59,60]

Late effects are usually determined by the dose of radiation received and the length of the esophagus that is irradiated. Small segments tolerate a higher radiation dosage that longer ones. Seaman and Ackerman demonstrated development of esophageal stenosis 4 months after betatron therapy with 5000 cGy over 21 days and 7300 cGy given over 48 days.[62] These stenoses result from progressive fibrosis of the lamina propria and submucosa. Dysphagia for solids can present as long as 5 years after cessation of radiation therapy. Fistulas, sinus tracts, and ulcers are caused primarily by tumor necrosis and thus are only secondarily radiation induced. Persistent deep ulcerations can produce both tracheoesophageal fistulas with recurrent postprandial aspiration and aortoesophageal fistulas with lethal hemorrhage.[59,60] Rubin and Cassarett predicted that 1% to 5% of patients exposed to 6000 cGy, and 50% of those exposed to 7500 cGy to the esophagus would develop clinically significant radiation-induced esophageal injury in 5 years.[63]

The diagnosis of radiation-induced esophagitis is made primarily on the basis of history and exclusion of other disorders. Reflux-induced esophagitis if the damage is in the distal esophagus; pill-induced esophagitis if the ulcers are circumscribed and short; and opportunistic esophageal infections, including candidiasis, herpes simplex, and cytomegalovirus infections, particularly if severe ulcerative esophagitis is found, are common in the differential diagnosis. Nodularity, mucosal bridging, telangiectasia, and rigid esophageal narrowing with fixation at the time of barium or endoscopic study point to radiation injury. Primary and secondary neoplasms should also be excluded.[50,59,60,64] Secondary squamous cell tumors of the esophagus due to radiation are rare, and usually occur more than 10 years after the original treatment.[30,31,65] Given the small number of patients with secondary tumors and the lack of distinguishing features from the primary lesions, it is difficult to implicate radiation as the cause of the carcinoma. Some carcinomas, however, have occurred with radiation of extraesophageal nonsquamous cell neoplasia with no predisposing risk factors for esophageal carcinoma.[56]

Except for the occasional interruption of radiation treatment, a 10% reduction in the daily dose and modification of the radiation field (oblique and lateral ports) are frequently all that is necessary to diminish or eliminate significant esophageal injury.[50,59,60] Lead shielding may be helpful to decrease cricopharyngeal damage during proximal esophageal radiation. Viscous lidocaine may be used for topical anesthesia, particularly in the proximal esophagus. Prokinetic agents and calcium blockers have shown some promise as supportive treatment in the acute phase because of the known disruption in esophageal body motility in radiation-induced esophagitis.[65] Acid reduction therapy and sucralfate therapy are commonly used, but there is no proof of their efficacy.[59,60] Treatments such as indomethacin showed promise in experimental models of radiation injury, but proved ineffective in clinical trials.[66-68] The use of radioprotectants is under investigation. Agents such as WR-2721 that donate thiol compounds for hydrogen or free radical scavenging show promise in animal models but have significantly limiting side effects.[60]

Late radiation effects to the esophagus consist primarily of tight esophageal stenosis. Marked submucosal and muscular fibrosis with loss in compliance are hallmarks of these strictures. Cytologic and biopsy evaluation of these stenoses is mandatory, but interpretation can be difficult given the bizarre epithelial and lamina propria cellular changes produced by radiation, which can mimic the primary carcinoma. Cautious dilation with guidewire placement and radiologic assistance is the key to treatment at this stage. If strictures show advanced changes such as diverticula, angulation, or long, irregular segmentation, iatrogenic esophageal perforation becomes a real concern. Treatment at this advanced stage should be aimed at enteral alimentation by nasoenteric or gastrostomy tube feeding if the prognosis is guarded, or resection with or without colonic interposition if long-term survival is anticipated and the patient's clinical condition warrants it. Anastomotic leakage is relatively common with both esophagoesophageal and esophagocolonic anastomoses.[4,59,60]

Treatment of interorgan fistulization is much more difficult. Smoldering vasculitis with transmural involvement of the trachea and esophagus leads to tracheoesophageal fistula.[59,60] Direct surgical repair is rarely possible. Short midesophageal stents, particularly those with terminal balloons to hold them in place, or long stents if the fistula is more distal, may be helpful, although worsening of esophageal damage by pressure necrosis is a serious consideration. Percutaneous gastrostomy placement is the most viable alternative in the terminally ill patient with esophageal cancer if nutritional support is deemed appropriate.[59,60]

Stomach

Except for its mucosa, the stomach is relatively radioresistant.[50] The gastric mucosal response to irradiation is unique because only the differentiated cells (parietal and chief cells), and not the germinative cells, are radiosensitive. There have been rare reports of gastric damage after radiation; these usually occur when the stomach is irradiated for reasons other than primary tumors or when the stomach is in the radiation field of an extragastric neoplasm.[50,69] Symptoms after gastric irradiation also may be minimized by the large size of the gastric lumen, which attenuates radiation damage by localizing the effect to only a small portion of the stomach.[50,69,70]

Primary radiation of the stomach was used in the past to treat peptic ulcer disease in patients who were poor surgical candidates.[50] The usual dose of radiation was 1600 to 1700 cGy. Histamine-fast achlorhydria occurred in 10% and was usually transitory. Lack of treatment response occurred in 9%, and, in almost all patients restudied after 2 years, acid secretion returned to basal levels.[4,50]

The ulcerations and stenosis of gastric radiation are rarely if ever seen at doses below 4500 cGy. Gastric stenosis is most common in the antrum and cardia areas, which are naturally narrow. More extensive mural necrosis, gastric perforation, or interorgan fistula are reported, but extremely rare. With modern techniques such as dose limitation and tissue shielding, radiation damage to the stomach has been greatly reduced.[50]

Liver

The first reports of radiation liver damage appeared in the 1960s.[71,72] The largest study included 40 patients of whom 13 had clinical signs or symptoms of Budd-Chiari syndrome or obstruction of the suprahepatic veins. Symptoms included rapid weight gain, hepatic enlargement, and, occasionally, jaundice and ascites.[71,72] Because more than 3000 to 3500 cGy produced damage consistently, and this dose was considered therapeutically ineffective, radiation therapy was considered of limited value in treating hepatic solid tumors.

New technologies such as nonaxial beam planes and dose–volume histogram analysis have produced a resurgence of interest in treating hepatic solid tumors with radiation.[73] With these approaches, more than 7000 cGy can be delivered safely to small hepatic volumes. The development of bone marrow transplantation has spurred interest in limiting radiation damage to the liver. The incidence of venoocclusive disease is higher with combined chemotherapy and radiation, but is seen at lower rates with either treatment alone.[74,75]

Hepatic toxicity after irradiation usually occurs 4 to 8 weeks after completion of treatment, although it has been described as early as 2 weeks or as late as 7 months.[71,74-76] Fatigue, weight gain, increased abdominal girth, and right upper quadrant pain are commonly seen, although patients are rarely jaundiced at presentation.[77,78] Ascites is usually present but may only be detected by imaging techniques. Increased serum alkaline phosphatase with minimal increase in bilirubin and transaminases are the usual biochemical patterns. Intrahepatic neoplasia and partial biliary obstruction are the usual differential diagnoses. Computed tomography commonly shows hypodense areas in most patients receiving more than 4500 cGy.[79] Conservative treatment with salt and fluid restriction and diuretics is standard, with substantial improvement seen in 1 to 2 months. Jaundice develops in a few patients, and progressive ascites and death are commonly seen in this patient group. Overall mortality in radiation-induced liver disease is 10% to 20%.[71,72]

Allogeneic bone marrow transplantation, which is used for treatment of leukemia and aplastic anemia, requires aggressive preparation techniques, including high-dose chemotherapy and total-body irradiation.[74-76] Liver toxicity after combined treatment manifests itself 1 to 4 weeks after transplantation with at least two or more of the following symptoms: jaundice (98%), weight gain (fluid retention; 93%), right upper quadrant pain (75%), hepatomegaly (68%), ascites (51%), and encephalopathy (47%).[75] Early onset of jaundice with smaller rises in alkaline phosphatase and higher transaminases are features distinguishing this syndrome from typical radiation (alone)-induced liver disease. Overall mortality in combined modality treatment is 30% to 50%.

The structural changes seen in the liver with combined modality treatment and with radiation alone are similar to lesions seen in other forms of venoocclusive disease. Congestion of acinar zone 3 is marked. Liver size may be large or small, depending on the time of radiation and liver examination.[80] Severe sinusoidal congestion with atrophy of the liver plates is the hallmark of this reaction.[74-77] Liver cells around the hepatic veins frequently disappear. The sublobular veins show significant obstruction by fine collagen fibers; large veins such as the hepatic veins or inferior vena cava usually are unaffected. Rarely, portal vein changes, including obstruction, may be seen. Chronic radiation changes include progressive fibrosis of venous structures and central-to-portal zone bridging. In most cases, chronic radiation changes occur in asymptomatic patients.[81]

The genesis of this lesion appears to result from the pattern of radiation dosing and the combination of radiation with chemotherapy.[81] To prevent such damage, total liver irradiation is limited to 3000 cGy at 180 to 200 cGy/day, but up to 4000 cGy can be given if only one third to one half of the liver is irradiated.[82] Use of full three-dimensional volume–dose distribution analysis has shown that larger radiation doses can be directed to even smaller parts, thus minimizing significant damage to the whole liver.[35,83,84]

Chemotherapy may increase the radiosensitivity of the liver. Fluoropyrimidines do not appear to increase liver radiation damage[85]; however, serious or fatal liver disease may occur at a dose of 19.5 Gy (delivered in 1-Gy fractions) when delivered with mitomycin C.[86] Other agents such as doxorubicin, CCNU (2-chloroethyl, 3-cyclohexyl, 1-nitrosurea), pro-MACE (prednisone, methotrexate, adriamycin, cyloxan, etoposide), MOPP (nitrogen mustard, vincristine, procarbazine, and prednisone), and CHOP (cyclophosphamide, doxorubicin, vincristine, and prednisone) therapy have been associated with severe liver radiation damage at doses that did not produce significant liver damage when given alone.[87]

Small Intestine

The small intestine is the region of the gastrointestinal tract that is the most sensitive to radiation and the most thoroughly investigated. Most cases of radiation enteritis occur after radiation therapy to the mesentery, retroperitoneum, and pelvis. The lack of mobility of the distal ileum and cecum is the most important factor for intestinal damage after pelvic irradiation.[51,88,89] A decreasing order of radiation sensitivity has been claimed for the duodenum to the ileum.[90] Other factors promoting radiation injury include previous abdominal surgery (which immobilizes the bowel through adhesions); low-lying small intestinal loops; thin body habitus; cardiovascular disease, particularly mesenteric insufficiency; chemotherapy; and vasoactive medications, including digitalis.[25,88,89]

Acute injury to the small intestine after radiation is probably a regular event. The occurrence is dose dependent, with low radiation doses producing mild, reversible disease and higher doses producing more serious and potentially irreversible lesions. The percentage of patients having significant lesions is 90% in those receiving more than 3000 cGy, 40% in those receiving 1000 to 3000 cGy, and 20% in those re-

ceiving less than 1000 cGy.[47] The transient injury is explained by minimal loss of regenerating epithelium followed by replacement of damaged epithelium within 14 days after radiation exposure.[46-48]

The development of chronic radiation enteritis is highly variable. Initial studies in children showed a high association between acute and chronic damage, although this does not appear so in adults.[48,51,91] In adults, chronic radiation enteritis occurs with a mean incidence of 5.7% (0.5%–17%) of exposed patients.[48,51] The onset of symptoms is even more variable, with disease developing in most patients in 1 to 2 years, although chronic radiation enteritis may become symptomatic as late as 20 years after treatment.[92-94] Vascular injury with progression to localized ischemia is the major mechanism of intestinal injury.[95,96] Progressive intestinal fibrosis with intestinal obstruction and bacterial overgrowth, fistulization with abdominal abscess formation, recurrent genitourinary infections, and, rarely, extensive infarction with perforation are the end stages of this vascular occlusion.[95,96] Forty percent of established patients progress with further complications even if surgical resection is used.[95,96]

The clinical presentation depends on the degree and permanence of epithelial and vascular damage. Epithelial damage with associated malabsorption was thought initially to be only a consequence of acute radiation injury, and was rarely seen with chronic radiation damage.[97] Studies using objective questionnaires and testing, however, have shown permanent alteration of bowel habit in 70% and malabsorption in up to 90% of patients attending a radiation oncology clinic.[98-100] Objective abnormalities in gastrointestinal function were seen with equal frequency in those with and without symptoms. A decrease in stool consistency was the most common pattern seen. Diarrhea was multifactorial, with bile salt malabsorption (65%), bacterial overgrowth (45%), severe fat malabsorption (40%), and rapid intestinal transit (35%) incriminated as the major factors.[98,99] Lactose intolerance with lactase deficiency and abnormal small bowel biopsy specimens with villous blunting were seen in up to 20% of patients with small bowel radiation injury.[98-100]

The natural history of patients with severe radiation-induced vascular damage to the small bowel is hard to ascertain because only surgical patients or patients who have died from radiation have been extensively studied.[95,101,102] Of 70 consecutive patients presenting to a surgical oncology unit with radiation enteritis, 61 underwent surgery, with 11 dying of intestinal operation-related causes (17%).[95,101] Fifty percent of the patients who survived more than 3 months and were followed up to 12 years (median 12 months) had no recurrent symptoms, but the remainder had persistence of symptoms, new radiation complications (stricture, malabsorption and severe diarrhea, or intermittent small bowel obstruction), or both. These complications occurred more commonly in those presenting with perforation or fistula, or in those with stricture formation at initial surgery, but were rare in those patients with bleeding as their initial presentation.[95,101,102] One third of the patients with continuing problems or complications required surgery, and 50% died postsurgery. Five-year survival was 40% for the entire group, but 70% in those surviving surgery. Low 5-year survival rates and more serious and progressive disease in patients with perforation and fistula have been confirmed by others.[103,104] Small intestinal or colon obstruction, however, is not always radiation related.[104] Recurrent tumors (particularly ovarian), inflammatory strictures, and postoperative adhesions accounted for 83% of all postoperative obstructions, but for only 30% 6 months after surgery.[104]

Management of radiation enterocolitis is determined by its stage. Acute radiation damage is usually reversible and usually requires supportive treatment only. A 10% dose reduction may be enough to ameliorate symptoms without compromising tumor control.[8,9,50] Antispasmodic, bulk-forming, and antimotility agents, including opiates, have been useful during the early stages of injury, but can cause intestinal obstruction in patients with stricture formation secondary to tumor or surgery.[88,89,96] Mennie and colleagues found that buffered acetyl salicylate, a prostaglandin E synthesis inhibitor, decreased diarrhea compared to placebo.[105] Cholestyramine, which binds bile salts, has also decreased diarrhea.[98,105,106] Perforation from irradiated small bowel may not produce clinical peritonitis; high fever, tachycardia, and oliguria may be the only presenting signs.[105,107] Free air may not be seen secondary to air trapping in adhesions.[105,106] Thin contrast infusion into the small bowel may be necessary to detect perforation in patients presenting with clinical deterioration but no peritoneal signs.[106,107]

Treatment of chronic small bowel strictures and fistulas is difficult and requires a long-term commitment. The potential for multiple small bowel strictures after pelvic irradiation complicates the management greatly (Fig. 113-1). Various dietary changes, including milk and fat restriction, have been recommended.[108–110] Elemental diets are costly and have not improved status over more polymeric diets. In addition, poor protein use with elemental diets has been documented compared to short-peptide diets. Total parenteral nutrition improved clinical, immunologic, and radiologic parameters compared to a low-residue diet.[109,110] The addition of methylprednisolone enhanced the effect, but this drug must be used with caution, particularly in those presenting with perforation or fistulization.[111,112] Anecdotal reports of sulfasalazine and oral prednisolone benefiting small bowel radiation damage require confirmation in controlled studies.[113] Acute small bowel obstruction is treated with conservative measures such as nasogastric drainage and parenteral nutrition, with return to oral alimentation after the obstruction is relieved.

Surgery is used as a last resort because of the difficulty in operating in an irradiated field and the occurrence of multiple postoperative complications involving irradiated bowel loops. Surgical resection with reanastomosis is frequently complicated by breakdown of the anastomosis secondary to decreased muscle tensile strength.[114] Irradiated but not strictured small bowel has less tensile strength than normal small intestine, and an anastomosis of two segments of irradiated bowel is weaker than one containing only one segment of irradiated bowel. When repairing radiation-damaged bowel, a wide resection is recommended with 50 cm of small intestine removed before reanastomosis to exclude irradiated bowel from the proximal limb.[95,101,102] Resection is preferable to bypass procedures despite the reported decrease in operative mortality and anastomotic leakage with bypass (36% leakage and 1% mortality with resection versus 6% leakage and 10% mortality

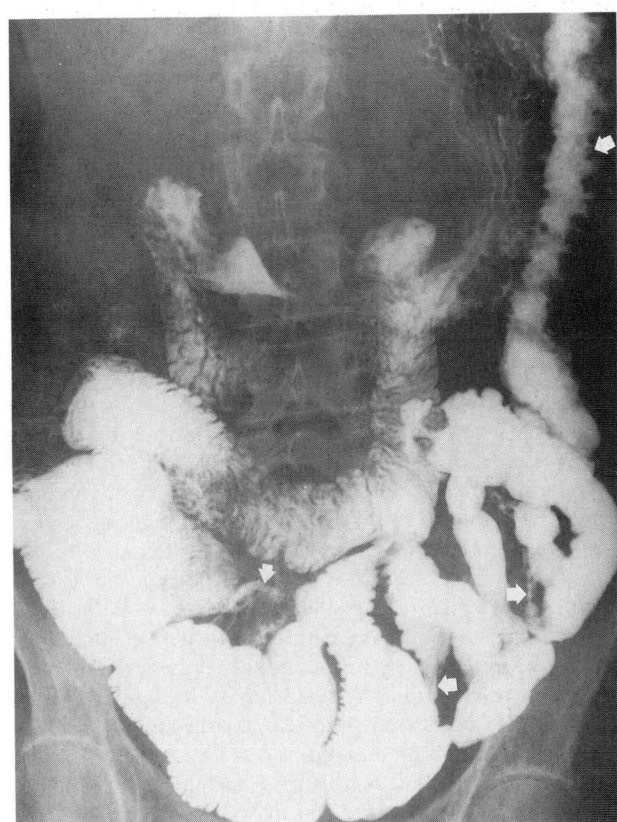

FIGURE 113-1. Radiation enteritis. Multiple strictures are present throughout both the proximal and distal small bowel (*bottom arrows*). Long segment of distal colon with nodularity and narrowing can be seen (*top arrow*). Multiple areas of small bowel dilatation are present proximal to strictured areas.

with bypass).[115] The reasons for avoiding bypass surgery are the high incidence of bacterial overgrowth, perforation, and fistulization in the bypass loop (45%).[115] Carcinoma may also occur in the bypassed segment.[95,101,102]

The management of radiation-induced fistulas is particularly difficult. Undetected synchronous carcinomatous lesions may occur, particularly with rapidly proliferating lesions such as ovarian cancer and melanoma. Direct local repair may be impossible because of pelvic matting of bowel loops secondary to extensive intraloop fistulization, and a bypass procedure may be all that is possible. Piver and Lele found that bypass combined with isolation of the fistula was safer than bypass alone.[116] In severe disease with extensive adhesions, the less surgery the better, and a diverting ostomy may be the only recourse.

Colon

Although the colon is relatively radioresistant, the incidence of colonic radiation damage is the greatest because of the high doses of radiation used for tumors in this area and the relative immobility of the rectum and sigmoid colon. Radiation damage to the rectum and sigmoid colon occurs most commonly with treatment of cancers of the cervix, uterus, prostate, urinary bladder, and testes.[117,118] Testicular tumor radiation therapy has been associated with a 16% incidence of radiation-induced damage to the transverse colon in patients receiving 3000 cGy and 37% in those receiving 6000 cGy.[119] Cervical radiation therapy is associated with a 10% incidence of large intestinal damage, with half the patients showing damage to the rectum and 75% having damage in other areas of the colon.[120] External beam radiation therapy produces more severe damage than implant treatment, most likely owing to the larger field with external radiation.[119,120] The combination of external beam radiation with radiation implants increases damage, and is frequently used with both prostate and cervical cancer treatment because of greater effectiveness.

Radiation-induced proctosigmoiditis is the most common clinically apparent form of colonic damage after pelvic irradiation, and has accounted for up to 75% of cases in some series.[92,121,122] Radiation injury of the distal colon and rectum presents in two different ways. First, in half the patients there is acute injury with primary symptoms of diarrhea and tenesmus occurring either during radiation treatment or within 6 weeks after completion.[121,122] Bleeding is rare and symptoms resolve in 2 to 6 months. Endoscopy is negative (50%) or shows only nonspecific changes.[24,67,98] The second form is chronic radiation proctosigmoiditis, which is seen in patients previously irradiated for a genitourinary malignancy (95%).[123] Rectal pain, diarrhea, and bleeding herald chronic damage. The total radiation dose delivered is linearly correlated with chronic damage. Most symptoms occur in the first 2 years, but long latent periods are possible. The latent period from

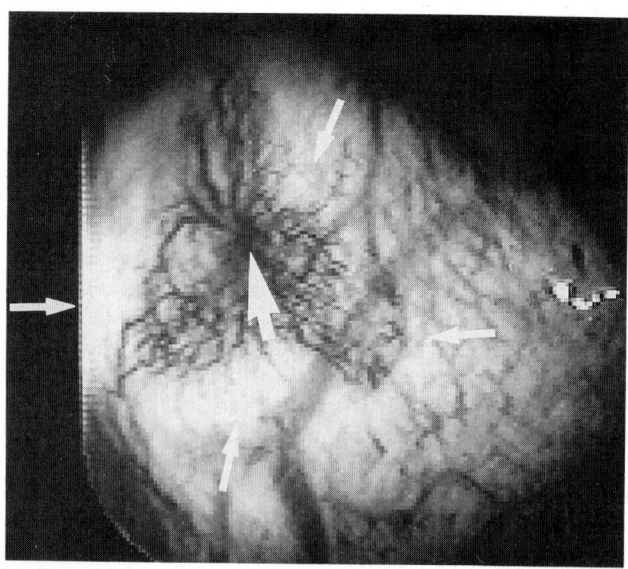

FIGURE 113-3.   Close-up of radiation proctitis with prominent telangectasia. Pallor is present surrounding very prominent central arteriole (*long arrows*), with marked arborization of capillaries (*short arrow*).

radiation to bleeding is usually 9 months. Patients with minimal bleeding alone requiring no transfusions and minimal intestinal symptoms had a high rate of spontaneous remission (70%), and only 5% required surgery. In contrast, patients requiring blood transfusions or who had significant bowel disturbance had a low spontaneous remission rate (0%–20%), required surgery (50%), and had a higher mortality rate (60% vs. 25%).[123] Radiation-induced complications accounted for 40% of deaths in this group.[123] Associated genitourinary complications such as urethral stenosis, rectovaginal fistulas, and cystitis occurred in 55% and were direct contributors to mortality in 25% of patients.[123–126] Radiologic studies discovered disease in 90% of patients with significant complications such as stenosis or fistula, but missed mucosal disease in one third of patients presenting with bleeding alone.[124] Mucosal pallor with friability and telangiectasia are seen at endoscopy (Figs. 113-2 and 113-3). Discrete ulcers are rare. Endoscopic biopsy is not useful for diagnosis because pathognomonic changes are rarely seen on mucosal biopsies.[123,124]

The management of radiation-induced colitis and proctitis and subsequent complications is difficult both diagnostically and therapeutically. Obstructive symptoms require imaging techniques coupled with endoscopic biopsies to rule out recurrent neoplasia. Barium studies of the colon are better for demonstrating fistulas and extent of radiation damage, although the radiologically normal colon may show endoscopic abnormalities. Diagnostic testing requires an individualized approach based on symptom presentation. Both radiology and endoscopy should be used to maximize diagnostic information.

Medical treatments of large bowel radiation injury are possible for rectal or colonic bleeding and for low-lying short colonic strictures. Unfortunately, medications such as sulfasalazine, steroid enemas, and both oral and 5-aminosalycilic

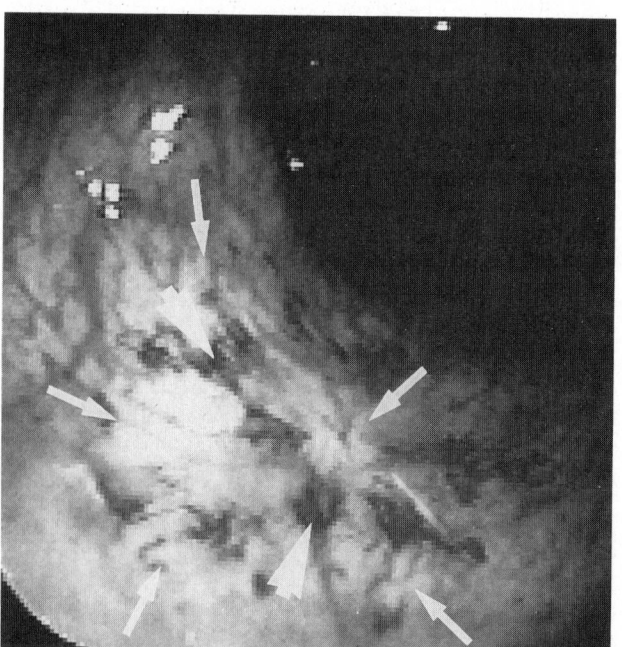

FIGURE 113-2.   Distal rectal radiation proctitis. There is an area of intense pallor (*long arrows*) and multiple telangiectasias with several ectatic vessels (*short arrows*).

acid preparations have either minimal or no effects on rectal bleeding or tenesmus.[127,128] One prospective study showed some clinical benefit when oral sulfasalazine was combined with steroid enemas, and also some benefit for sucralfate enemas alone, although response was better with sucralfate enemas.[127,128] Patient tolerance was also better with sucralfate enemas (2 g in 20 mL of tap water). Placebo-controlled trials are needed to confirm this promising result.

Cessation of rectal bleeding has been reported after multiple sessions of hyperbaric oxygen.[129] A single case of 3.6% formalin irrigation diminished rectal bleeding in a severely bleeding patient who was not an operative candidate.[130] The presumed mechanism was coagulative necrosis, similar to the effects of formalin in hemorrhagic cystitis. Placebo-controlled trials with adequate numbers are needed.

Endoscopic application of laser cautery or electrocoagulation can be effective in the treatment of localized colonic bleeding (usually rectal) in patients presenting with overt bleeding and in most patients who present with anemia. Such therapy has produced a fourfold decrease in blood transfusion requirements and hospital admissions for patients with localized radiation damage to the colon or rectum.[131,132] Argon laser ablation may offer similar effectiveness with less risk of transmural injury to the bowel, a complication of treatment reported in up to one fourth of patients with radiation proctitis treated with neodymium:yttrium-aluminum-garnet laser.[131,132] Anecdotal reports of bipolar electrocoagulation show promise, offering a more accessible, less expensive treatment modality.[133]

Radiation fibrosis may progress, often to recurrent low rectal strictures and anastomotic strictures. Mild obstructive symptoms usually can be handled with stool softeners and mineral oil enemas. Transendoscopic balloon or Savary-Guillard dilation can significantly alleviate severe obstructive symptoms in short strictures with minimal angulation.[134] Long or tortuous strictures are best handled surgically because of the risk for perforation. Such perforations after dilation can remain clinically silent for extended periods after the procedure.

Surgical management of radiation-induced strictures is usually resection followed by immediate reanastomosis.[50,58,70] Anastomotic leaks were common after surgery if only short segments of colon were removed. Ensuring that at least one limb of the anastomosis is free of radiation damage decreased anastomotic leaks from 36% to 6%.[95,107,125] Postoperative complications can be reduced by use of a proximal anastomotic site at the splenic flexure after removal of left colonic strictures, or ileotransverse anastomosis after removal of ileal or right colonic strictures. Marks and Mohiudden described no leaks for intraperitoneal anastomoses and only 4 in 52 extraperitoneal anastomoses in patients with deep pelvic radiation injuries.[126] Good functional results were seen in 86%.[126] Extensive disease with or without distal rectal or anal involvement is likely to have a poor result from surgery. Abdominoperitoneal resection may be all that is possible in up to one third of cases.[126] Satisfactory results are reported, although recurrent disease or severe urinary complications develop in 50% in follow-up (median, 18–24 months).[124-126] Presacral sympathectomy has been recommended for uncontrolled pain, but long-term results are unknown.[101,102]

PREVENTION OF RADIATION INJURY

The incidence of small bowel complications after abdominal or pelvic radiation therapy depends, in part, on the radiation dose and the volume of small bowel in the treated area. Because of this relation, a number of techniques have been developed that use the mobility of the small bowel physically to move it outside of the irradiated area. Synthetic surgical mesh,[135,136] omental slings,[136,137] and inflatable prostheses[138] all have been reported to be of value in excluding the small bowel from the pelvis, and are of greatest usefulness when pelvic radiation therapy is performed. These techniques are of particular interest for the adjuvant postoperative treatment of rectal cancer, because this patient group may be at a higher risk for small bowel complications owing to the surgery and the concurrent administration of chemotherapy.

Aside from surgical exclusion, proper radiation planning can minimize small bowel radiation.[139] Alternating the beam direction both laterally and from front to back reduces the volume of small bowel treated.[139] Preradiation contrast infusion to delineate bowel position can improve custom shielding. Bladder filling can lift the small intestine out of the pelvis. A combination of these techniques was shown to be equal to surgical exclusion.[140] More contemporary studies have shown that multiple ports and small bowel contrast in computer simulation reduced small bowel complications to 5%, which is comparable to results achieved with surgery alone.[141-143] Fixed organs such as the esophagus, liver, duodenum, ascending and descending colon, and the rectum cannot be protected by shielding techniques, and require alternative strategies.

Another possible mucosal protector is an elemental diet.[144,145] It has been speculated that elemental diets are radioprotective by virtue of reducing pancreaticobiliary secretions and improving absorption of nutrients in the intestine. Indeed, both animal studies[144,145] and small clinical trials in humans[145,146] have shown that elemental diets appear to protect the intestinal mucosa. Larger randomized trials have not been performed. Topical protection of the gastrointestinal mucosa from the fecal stream may also be achieved by administration of sucralfate during radiation.[128] Sucralfate appears to form a protective barrier over areas of denuded mucosa, shielding these areas from the effects of gastrointestinal and pancreaticobiliary secretions. In a randomized, double-blind, placebo-controlled trial of 70 patients being treated with pelvic radiation therapy (up to 64 Gy at 2 Gy/day) for bladder or prostate cancer, those receiving sucralfate during radiation therapy had statistically significant reductions in both acute and chronic side effects compared with patients receiving a placebo.[128] Overall, these data support the concept that radioprotection of the intestinal mucosa is possible, and may be beneficial in reducing acute and long-term side effects of radiation therapy, with the possibility of improving the therapeutic index.

Three-dimensional treatment planning techniques may offer safer treatment and better prediction of long-term complications.[147-150] This technique involves a three-dimensional representation of the patient constructed from a computed tomography scan of the patient in the treatment position. Normal tissue damage can be minimized by using multiple planes to deliver the radiation. Tumor volume along the treatment plane allows proper dosing to deliver maximal radiation to the maximal tumor volume. Such three-dimensional planning also allows construction of mathematical models of normal tissue complication probability, which allows preradiation prediction of complications and may improve understanding of the clinical effects of partial organ radiation.

Three-dimensional treatment planning is likely to have its greatest role in intrahepatic malignancy. A clinical trial was designed to see if total radiation dose to the liver depended on the amount of normal liver spared. Patients were treated with 30 to 36 Gy to the whole liver, or with either low-dose (45–52.8 Gy) or high-dose radiation (60–72 Gy) to the focal liver abnormalities.[149,150] Complication rates were similar, and yet treatment effects were enhanced if high-dose treatment for focal lesions was used. Information from this study is likely to spur new interest in radiation treatment for intrahepatic malignancy.

To continue to improve effectiveness without increasing complications, the radiation biologist will need to develop better techniques for three-dimensional localization of radiation treatment, coupled with better means of radioprotection for healthy tissue. The internist–gastroenterologist will still play a significant role in the management of bleeding complications and early stricture formation from radiation with laser coagulation and dilation, respectively. The surgeon will eventually handle obstructing lesions as well as extensive fistulization that are not prevented by the radiation biologist or treated effectively by the internist–gastroenterologist. Cooperation between these physician groups will decrease the incidence of these last two patient groups.

The reader is directed to Chapter 21, General Nutritional Principles; Chapter 65, Tumors of the Stomach; Chapter 87, Malignant Tumors of the Colon; and Chapter 135, Gastrointestinal Dilation.

REFERENCES

1. Walsh D. Deep tissue traumatism from roentgen ray exposure. Br Med J 1897;2:272.
2. Franz K, Orth J. Fall einer Rontgenschadingung. Berl Klin Wochenschr 1917;45:662.
3. Buie LA, Malmgren GE. Factitial proctitis. Trans Am Proctol Soc 1930;29:80.
4. Earnest DL, Trier JS. Radiation enteritis and colitis. In: Sleisenger MH, Fordtran JS, eds. Gastrointestinal disease: pathophysiology, diagnosis and management. Philadelphia: WB Saunders, 1993:1257.
5. Kinsella TJ, Bloomer WP. Tolerance of the intestine to radiation therapy. Surg Gynecol Obstet 1980;151:273.
6. Yudeleu M, Kuten A, Tatcher M, et al. Correlations of dose and time dose fraction factors (TDF) with treatment results and side effects in cancer of the uterine cervix. Gynecol Oncol 1986;23:310.
7. Kimose HH, Fischer L, Spjelenaes N, et al. Late radiation injury of the colon and rectum: surgical management and outcome. Dis Colon Rectum 1989;32:684.
8. Allen-Mersh TG, Wilson EJ, Hope-Stone HF, et al. The management of late radiation-induced rectal injury after treatment of carcinoma of the uterus. Surg Gynecol Obstet 1987;164:521.
9. Dietel M, To TB. Major intestinal complications of radiotherapy management and nutrition. Arch Surg 1987;122:1421.
10. Hall EJ. Radiobiology for the radiologist. 3rd ed. Philadelphia: JB Lippincott, 1988.
11. Awwad HK. Radiation oncology: radiobiological and physiological perspectives. In: Burendsen GW, Suit H, eds. Boston: Kluwer Academic, 1990:1.
12. Johns HE, Cunningham JR. The physics of radiology. 4th ed. Springfield, IL: Charles C Thomas, 1993:1.
13. Wallace SS, Painter RB, eds. Ionizing radiation damage to DNA: molecular aspects. Los Angeles: Wiley-Liss, 1990:69.
14. Taccioli GE, Rathbun G, Oltz E, et al. Impairment of V(D)J recombination in double strand break repair mutants. Science 1993;260:207.
15. Ager DD, Dewey WC. Calibration of pulsed field gel electrophoresis for measurement of DNA double-strand breaks. Int J Radiat Biol 1990;58:249.
16. Lawrence TS, Davis MA, Normolle DP, et al. The use of biphasic linear ramped pulsed field gel electrophoresis to quantify DNA damage based on fragment size distribution. Int J Radiat Oncol Biol Phys 1993;27:659.
17. Elkind MM. DNA damage and cell killing: cause and effect? Cancer 1985;56:2351.
18. Brown JM. Sensitizers and protectors in radiotherapy. Cancer 1985;55:2222.
19. Coleman CN. Hypoxia in tumors: a paradigm for the approach to biochemical and physiologic heterogeneity. J Natl Cancer Inst 1988;80:310.
20. Tang H-yi, Davis MA, Strickfaden SM, et al. Fluorodeoxyuridine-mediated radiosensitization of human colon cancer (HT29) cells is not caused by cell cycle redistribution. Radiat Res 1994;138(Suppl 1):S109.
21. Piver MS, Vongtama V, Emrich LJ. Hydroxyurea plus pelvic radiation versus placebo plus pelvic radiation in surgically staged stage IIIB cervical cancer. J Surg Oncol 1987;35:129.
22. Krook JE, Moertel CG, Gunderson LL, et al. Effective surgical adjuvant therapy for high-risk rectal carcinoma. N Engl J Med 1991;324:709.
23. Moertel CG, Frytak S, Hahn RG, et al. Therapy of locally unresectable pancreatic carcinoma: a randomized comparison of high dose (6000 rads) radiation alone, moderate dose radiation (4000 rads + 5-fluorouracil), and high dose radiation + 5-fluorouracil. Cancer 1991;48:1705.
24. Herskovic A, Martz K, al-Sarraf M, et al. Combined chemotherapy and radiotherapy compared with radiotherapy alone in patients with cancer of the esophagus. N Engl J Med 1992;326:1593.
25. Cummings BJ, Keane TJ, O'Sullivan B, et al. Epidermoid anal cancer: treatment by radiation alone or by radiation and 5-fluorouracil with and without mitomycin C. Int J Radiat Oncol Biol Phys 1991;21:1115.
26. Robertson JM, Lawrence TS, Dworzanin LA, et al. Treatment of primary hepatobiliary cancers with conformal radiation therapy and regional chemotherapy. J Clin Oncol 1993;11:1286.
27. Bruso CE, Shewach DS, Lawrence TS. Fluorodeoxyuridine-induced radio-sensitization and inhibition of DNA double strand break repair in human colon cancer cells. Int J Radiat Oncol Biol Phys 1990;19:1411.
28. Heimburger DK, Shewach DS, Lawrence TS. The effect of fluorodeoxyuridine on sublethal damage repair in human colon cancer cells. Int J Radiat Oncol Biol Phys 1991;21:983.
29. Kinsella TJ, Dobson PP, Mitchell JB, et al. Enhancement of x-ray induced DNA damage by pre-treatment with halogenated pyrimidine analogs. Int J Radiat Oncol Biol Phys 1987;13:733.
30. Lawrence TS, Davis MA, Maybaum J, et al. The effect of single versus double stranded substitution on halogenated pyrimidine-induced radiosensitization and DNA strand breakage in human tumor cells. Radiat Res 1991;123:192.
31. Iliakis G, Kurtzman S, Pantelias G, et al. Mechanism of radiosensitization by halogenated pyrimidines: effect of BrdU on radiation induction of DNA and chromosome damage and its correlation with cell killing. Radiat Res 1989;119:286.
32. Lawrence TS, Davis MA, McKeever PE, et al. Fluorodeoxy-

uridine-mediated modulation of iododeoxyuridine incorporation and radiosensitization in human colon cancer cells in vitro and in vivo. Cancer Res 1991;51:3900.

33. Montana GS, Anscher MS, Mansbach CM, et al. Topical application of WR-2721 to prevent radiation-induced proctosigmoiditis: a phase I/II trial. Cancer 1992;69:2826.

34. Liu T, Liu Y, He S, Zhang Z, et al. Use of radiation with or without WR-2721 in advanced rectal cancer. Cancer 1992;69:2820.

35. Emami B, Lyman J, Brown A, et al. Tolerance of normal tissue to therapeutic irradiation. Int J Radiat Oncol Biol Phys 1991;21:109.

36. Little JB. Cellular effects of ionizing radiation I and II. N Engl J Med 1968;278:308.

37. Fajardo LF, Berthrong M. Radiation injury in surgical pathology. Part I. Am J Surg Pathol 1978;2:159.

38. Hagemann RF, Concannon JP. Mechanism of intestinal radiosensitization by actinomycin D. Br J Radiol 1973;46:302.

39. Phillips TL, Fu KK. Quantification of combined radiation therapy and chemotherapy effects on critical normal tissues. Cancer 1976;37:1186.

40. Rubin P. Late effects of chemotherapy and radiation therapy. Radiat Oncol Biol Phys 1984;10:5.

41. Key CR. Studies of the acute effects of the atomic bombs. Hum Pathol 1971;2:475.

42. Dubois A, Walker RI. Prospects for management of gastrointestinal injury associated with the acute radiation syndrome. Gastroenterology 1988;95:500.

43. Danquechin E, Mueller GP, Eng RR, et al. Effect of ionizing radiation on gastric secretion and gastric motility in monkeys. Gastroenterology 1985;89:374.

44. Carpenter DO, Briggs DB, Knox AP, et al. Radiation induced emesis in the dog: effects of lesions and drugs. Radiat Res 1986;101:307.

45. Geraci JP, Jackson KL, Mariano MS. The intestinal radiation syndrome: sepsis and endotoxin. Radiat Res 1985;101:442.

46. Berthrong M, Fajardo LF. Radiation injury in surgical pathology. Part 2. Alimentary tract. Am J Surg Pathol 1981;5:153.

47. Tarpila S. Morphological and functional response of human small intestine to ionizing radiation. Scand J Gastroenterol 1971;6(Suppl 12):1.

48. Trier JS, Browning TH. Morphologic response of the mucosa of the human small intestine to x-ray exposure. J Clin Invest 1966;45:194.

49. Haboubi NY, Schofield PF, Rowland PL. The light and electron microscopic features of early and late phase radiation-induced proctitis. Am J Gastroenterol 1988;83:1140.

50. Novak JM, Collins JT, Donowitz M, et al. Effects of radiation on the human gastrointestinal tract. J Clin Gastroenterol 1979;1:9.

51. Sher ME, Bauer J. Radiation induced enteropathy. Am J Gastroenterol 1990;85:121.

52. Kirkpatrick JB. Pathogenesis of foam cell lesions in irradiated arteries. Am J Pathol 1967;50:291.

53. Hasleton PS, Carr N, Schofield PF. Vascular changes in radiation bowel disease. Histopathology 1985;9:517.

54. Sadoue M, Block M, Rossof HH, et al. Radiation carcinogenesis in man: primary neoplasms in fields of prior radiation. Cancer 1981;48:1139.

55. Sandler RS, Sandler DP. Radiation induced cancers of the colon and rectum: assessing the risk. Gastroenterology 1983;84:51.

56. Lieber MR, Winans CS, Griem ML, et al. Sarcomas arising after radiotherapy for peptic ulcer disease. Dig Dis Sci 1985;30:593.

57. Jablon S, Bailas JC III. Contribution of ionizing radiation to cancer mortality in the United States. Prev Med 1980;9:219.

58. Schottenfield D. Radiation as a risk factor in the natural history of colorectal cancer (editorial). Gastroenterology 1983;84:186.

59. Chowdan NM. Injurious effects of radiation on the esophagus. Am J Gastroenterol 1990;85:115.

60. Vanagunas A, Jacob P, Olinger E. Radiation induced esophageal injury. Am J Gastroenterol 1990;85:808.

61. Fox BW, Lajtha LG. Radiation damage and repair phenomena. Br Med Bull 1973;29:16.

62. Seaman WB, Ackerman LV. The effect of radiation on the esophagus: a clinical and histologic study of the effects produced by the betatron. Radiology 1957;68:536.

63. Rubin P, Cassarett A. A direction for clinical radiation pathology. Front Radiat Ther Oncol 1972;6:1.

64. Black WC, Ackerman LV. Carcinoma of the large intestine as a late complication of pelvic radiation. Radiother Clin Radiol 1965;16:278.

65. Goldstein HM, Rogers LF, Fletcher GH, et al. Radiological manifestations of radiation induced injury to the normal upper gastrointestinal tract. Radiology 1975;117:135.

66. Northway MG, Bennett A, Carroll B, et al. Comparative effects of antiinflammatory agents and radiotherapy on normal esophagus and tumors in animals. Gastroenterology 1980;78:1229.

67. Northway MG, Libshitz HI, Osborne BM, et al. Radiation esophagitis in the opossum: radioprotection with indomethacin. Gastroenterology 1989;78:883.

68. Nicolopoulos N, Mantidis A, Stathopoulos E, et al. Prophylactic administration of indomethacin for irradiation esophagitis. Radiother Oncol 1985;3:23.

69. Kellum JM, Jaffe BM, Calhoun T, et al. Gastric complications after radiotherapy for Hodgkin's disease and other lymphomas. Am J Surg 1977;134:314.

70. Hamilton FE. Gastric ulcer following radiation. Arch Surg 1947;55:394.

71. Ingold DK, Reed GB, Kaplan HS. Radiation hepatitis. AJR 1965;93:200.

72. Reed GB, Cox AJ. The human liver after radiation injury. Am J Pathol 1966;48:597.

73. McShan DL, Fraass BA, Lichter A. Full integration of the beam's eye view concept into computerized treatment planning. Int J Radiat Oncol Biol Phys 1990;18:1485.

74. McDonald GB, Sharma P, Matthews DE, et al. Venocclusive disease of the liver after bone marrow transplantation: incidence and predisposing factors. Hepatology 1984;4:116.

75. McDonald GB, Sharma P, Matthews DE, et al. The clinical course of 53 patients with venocclusive disease of the liver after marrow transplantation. Transplantation 1985;35:603.

76. Shulman HM, McDonald GB, Matthews DE, et al. An analysis of hepatic venocclusive disease and centrilobular hepatic degeneration following bone marrow transplantation. Gastroenterology 1980;79:1178.

77. Wharton JT, Declos L, Gallager S, et al. Radiation hepatitis induced by irradiation with the cobalt 60 moving strip technique. AJR 1973;117:73.

78. Bernard JA, Marshall GS, Neblett WN, et al. Noncirrhotic portal fibrosis after Wilms tumor therapy. Gastroenterology 1986;90:1054.

79. Unger EC, Lee JKT, Weyman PJ. CT and MRI imaging of radiation hepatitis. J Comput Assist Tomogr 1987;11:264.

80. Fajardo LF. Pathology of radiation injury. New York: Masson, 1982:88.

81. Fajardo LF, Colby TV. Pathogenesis of venocclusive liver disease after radiation. Arch Pathol Lab Med 1980;104:584.

82. Jirtle RL, Anscher MS, Alati T. Radiation sensitivity of the liver. Adv Radiol Biol 1990;14:269.

83. Lyman JT. Complication probability as assessed from dose volume histograms. Radiat Res 1985;8(Suppl):513.

84. Niemierko A, Goitein M. Calculation of normal tissue complication probability and dose volume histograms reduction schemes for tissues with a critical element architecture. Radiother Oncol 1991;20:166.

85. Rotman M, Kuruvilla AM, Choi K, et al. Response of colorectal hepatic metastases to concomitant radiotherapy and intravenous infusion of 5 fluorouracil. Int J Radiat Oncol Biol Phys 1986;12:2179.

86. McCracken JD, Weatherall TJ, Oishi N, et al. Adjuvant intrahepatic chemotherapy with mitomycin and 5 Fu with hepatic irradiation in high risk patients with carcinoma of the colon: a Southwest oncology group phase II pilot study. Cancer Treat Rep 1985;69:129.

87. Haddad E, LeBourgeois JP, Kuentz M, et al. Liver complications in lymphoma treated with combined chemotherapy and radiotherapy: preliminary results. Int J Radiat Oncol Biol Phys 1983;9:1313.

88. Mann WJ. Surgical management of radiation enteropathy. Surg Clin North Am 1991;71:977.

89. Hauer-Jensen M. Late radiation injury of the small intestine: clinical, pathophysiologic and radiobiologic aspects. Acta Oncol 1990;29:401.

90. Roswit B. Complications of radiation therapy: the alimentary tract. Roentgenology 1974;9:51.

91. Donaldson SS, Jundt S, Ricour C, et al. Radiation enteritis in children: a retrospective review, clinicopathologic correlation, and dietary management. Cancer 1975;35:1167.

92. Decosse JJ, Rhodes RS, Wentz WB, et al. The natural history and management of radiation injury of the gastrointestinal tract. Ann Surg 1969;170:369.

93. Schier J, Symmonds RE, Dahlin DC. Clinicopathologic aspects of radiation enteritis. Surg Gynecol Obstet 1964;119:1019.

94. Wellwood JM, Jackson BT. The intestinal complications of radiotherapy. Br J Surg 1973;60:814.

95. Galland RB, Spencer J. The natural history of clinically established radiation enteritis. Lancet 1985;1:1257.

96. Dencker H, Holmdahl KH, Lunderquist A, et al. Mesenteric angiography in patients with radiation injury of the bowel after pelvic irradiation. AJR 1972;114:476.

97. Greenberger NJ, Isselbacher KJ. Malabsorption following radiation injury to the gastrointestinal tract. Am J Med 1964;36:450.

98. Danielsson A, Nyhlin H, Persson H, et al. Chronic diarrhea after radiotherapy for gynaecological cancer: occurrence and etiology. Gut 1991;32:1180.

99. Miholic J, Vogelsang H, Schlappack O, et al. Small bowel function after surgery for chronic radiation enteritis. Digestion 1989;42:30.

100. Banares F, Villa S, Esteve M, et al. Acute effects of abdominopelvic irradiation on the orocecal transit time: clinical symptoms and malabsorption. Am J Gastroenterol 1991;86:1771.

101. Galland RB, Spencer J. Surgical management of radiation enteritis. Surgery 1986;99:133.

102. Harling H, Balslev IB. Long term prognosis of patients with severe radiation enteritis. Am J Surg 1988;155:517.

103. Jahnson S, Westerborn O, Gerdin B. Prognosis of surgically treated radiation induced damage to the intestine. Eur J Surg Oncol 1992;18:487.

104. Krebs HB, Goplerud DR. Mechanical intestinal obstruction in patients with gynecologic disease: a review of 368 patients. Am J Obstet Gynecol 1987;157:577.

105. Mennie AT, Dalley VM, Dinneen LC, et al. Treatment of radiation induced gastrointestinal distress with acetylsalicylate. Lancet 1975;1:942.

106. Wellwood JM, Jackson BT, Bates TD. Breakdown of small bowel anastomoses after pelvic radiotherapy. Ann R Coll Surg 1974;54:2.

107. Galland RB, Spencer J. Spontaneous postoperative perforation of previously asymptomatic irradiated bowel. Br J Surg 1985;72:285.

108. Thiel HJ, Fietkau R, Sauer R. Malnutrition and the role of nutritional support for radiation therapy patients. Recent Results Cancer Res 1988;108:205.

109. Silvain C, Besson I, Ingrand P, et al. Long term outcome of severe radiation enteritis treated by total parenteral nutrition. Dig Dis Sci 1992;37:1065.

110. Pezner R, Archambeau JO. Critical evaluation of the role of nutritional support for radiation therapy patients. Cancer 1985;55:263.

111. Beer WH, Fan A, Halstead CH. Clinical and nutritional implications of radiation enteritis. Am J Clin Nutr 1985;41:85.

112. Loiudice TA, Lang J. Treatment of radiation enteritis: a comparison study. Am J Gastroenterol 1983;78:481.

113. Goldstein F, Khoury J, Thornton JJ. Treatment of chronic radiation enteritis and colitis with salicylazosulfapyridine and systemic steroids. Am J Gastroenterol 1976;65:201.

114. Saclarides TJ, Rohrer DA, Bhattacharyya AK, et al. Effect of intraoperative radiation on the tensile strength of small bowel anastomoses. Dis Colon Rectum 1992;35:151.

115. Swan RN, Fowler WC, Buronow RC. Surgical management of radiation injury of the small intestine. Surg Obstet Gynecol 1976;142:325.

116. Piver MS, Lele S. Enterovaginal and enterocutaneous fistulae in women with gynecologic malignancies. Obstet Gynecol 1976;48:560.

117. Cosset JM, Henry-Amar JMV, Burgers EM. Late radiation effects after therapy for Hodgkin's disease. Radiother Oncol 1988;13:61.

118. Schmitz RM, Chao JH, Bartolome JS. Intestinal injuries from irradiation of carcinoma of the uterus and cervix. Surg Gynecol Obstet 1984;138:29.

119. Friedman M. Calculated risks of radiation injury of normal tissue in the treatment of cancer of the testis. In: American Cancer Society: Proceedings of the Second National Cancer Conference. New York: National Cancer Institute USPHS Federal Science Agency, 1952:390.

120. Stockbrine MF, Hancock JE, Fletcher GH. Complications in 831 patients with squamous cervical carcinoma. AJR 1970;108:293.

121. Earnest DL. Radiation proctitis. Practical Gastroenterology 1991;15(1):15.

122. Perez CA, Breaux S, Bedwineic JM, et al. Radiation therapy alone in the treatment of carcinoma of the uterine cervix. Cancer 1984;54:235.

123. Gilinsky NH, Burns DG, Barbezat GO, et al. The natural history of radiation induced proctosigmoiditis: an analysis of 88 patients. Q J Med 1983;205:40.

124. Taylor M, Johnson RJ, Eddleston B, et al. Radiological changes in the gastrointestinal and genitourinary tract following radiotherapy for carcinoma of the cervix. Clin Radiol 1990;41:165.

125. Galland RB, Spencer J. Natural history and surgical management of radiation enteritis. Br J Surg 1987;74:742.

126. Marks G, Mohiudden M. The surgical management of radiation injured intestine. Surg Clin North Am 1983;63:81.

127. Kochhar R, Patel F, Dhar A, et al. Radiation induced proctosigmoiditis: randomized trial of oral sulfasalasine and rectal steroids versus rectal sucralfate. Dig Dis Sci 1991;36:103.

128. Henriksson R, Franzen L, Littbrand B. Effects of sucralfate on acute and late bowel discomfort following radiotherapy of pelvic cancer. J Clin Oncol 1992;10:969.

129. Charneau J, Bouachour G, Person B. Severe hemorrhagic radiation proctitis advancing to gradual cessation with hyperbaric oxygen. Dig Dis Sci 1991;36:373.

130. Rubinstein E, Isben T, Rasmussen RB, et al. Formalin treatment of radiation induced hemorrhagic proctitis. Am J Gastroenterol 1986;81:44.

131. Alexander TJ, Dwyer RM. Endoscopic Nd:Yag laser treatment of severe radiation injury of the lower gastrointestinal tract: long term follow up. Gastrointest Endosc 1988;34:407.

132. Ahlquist DA, Gostout CJ, Viggiano TR, et al. Laser treatment of radiation proctitis. Mayo Clin Proc 1986;61:927.

133. Maunoury V, Brunestaud JM, Cortot A. Bipolar electrocoagulation treatment for hemorrhagic radiation injury of the lower digestive tract. Gastrointest Endosc 1991;37:492.

134. Triadafilopoulos G, Sarkisian M. Dilatation of radiation induced stricture using sequential Savary-Guillard dilators. Dis Colon Rectum 1990;33:1065.

135. Devereux DF, Kavanah MT, Feldman MI, et al. Small bowel exclusion from the pelvis by a polyglycolic acid mesh sling. J Surg Oncol 1984;26:107.

136. Kavanah MT, Feldman MI, Devereux DF, et al. New surgical approach to minimize radiation associated small bowel injury in patients with pelvic malignancies requiring surgery and high dose irradiation. Cancer 1985;56:1300.

137. Russ JE, Smoron GL, Gagnon JD. Omental transposition flap in colorectal carcinoma: adjunctive use in prevention and treatment of radiation complications. Int J Radiat Oncol Biol Phys 1984;10:55.

138. Sugarbaker PH. Pelvic displacement prosthesis to prevent small

bowel damage with pelvic irradiation. Surg Gynecol Obstet 1983;157:269.

139. Gunderson LL, Russell AH, Llewellyn HJ, et al. Treatment planning for colorectal cancer radiation and surgical techniques and value of small bowel films. Int J Radiat Oncol Biol Phys 1985;11:1379.

140. Gallagher MJ, Brereton HD, Rostock RA, et al. A prospective study of treatment techniques to minimize the volume of pelvic small bowel with reduction of acute and late effects associated with pelvic irradiation. Int J Radiat Oncol Biol Phys 1986;12:1565.

141. Vigliotti A, Rich TA, Romsdahl MM, et al. Postoperative adjuvant radiotherapy for adenocarcinoma of the rectum and rectosigmoid. Int J Radiat Oncol Biol Phys 1987;13:999.

142. Hoskins RB, Gunderson LL, Dosoretz DE, et al. Adjuvant postoperative radiotherapy in carcinoma of the rectum and rectosigmoid. Cancer 1985;55:61.

143. Duttenhaver JR, Hoskins RB, Gunderson LL, et al. Adjuvant postoperative radiation therapy in the management of adenocarcinoma of the colon. Cancer 1986;57:955.

144. Bounous G. The use of elemental diets during cancer therapy. Anticancer Res 1983;3:299.

145. Bounous G, Le Bel E, Shuster J, et al. Dietary protection during radiation therapy. Strahlentherapie 1975;149:476.

146. McArdle AH, Reid EC, Laplante MP, et al. Prophylaxis against radiation injury: the use of elemental diet prior to and during radiotherapy for invasive bladder cancer and in early postoperative feeding following radical cystectomy and ileal conduit. Arch Surg 1986;121:879.

147. Lichter AS, Sandler HM, Robertson JM, et al. Clinical experience with three-dimensional treatment planning. Semin Radiat Oncol 1992;2:257.

148. Ten Haken RK, Lawrence TS, McShan DL, et al. Technical considerations in the use of 3-D beam arrangements in the abdomen. Radiother Oncol 1991;22:19.

149. Lyman JT, Wolbarst AB. Optimization of radiation therapy. III. A method of assessing complication probabilities from dose–volume histograms. Int J Radiat Oncol Biol Phys 1987;13:103.

150. Kutcher GJ, Burman C. Calculation of complication probability factors for non-uniform normal tissue irradiation: the effective volume method. Int J Radiat Oncol Biol Phys 1989;16:1623.

PART FOUR

Diagnostic and Therapeutic Modalities in Gastroenterology

Textbook of Gastroenterology, second edition, edited by Tadataka Yamada. JB Lippincott Company, Philadelphia © 1995.

CHAPTER 114

General Considerations

Fred E. Silverstein   Eric B. Larson
Charles A. Rohrmann, Jr.

Theoretical Considerations
Use of Scientific Methods
Predictive Value of Diagnostic Tests
Evaluation of Efficacy

Practical Considerations
  Physical Principles of Imaging
  Anatomy and Pathology
Clinical Applications

THEORETICAL CONSIDERATIONS

This textbook addresses gastroenterology in its entirety by progressing beyond the consideration of specific diseases to the following section, which discusses state-of-the-art diagnostic and therapeutic procedures in gastroenterology. The gamut of procedures that are applicable to the management of patients with gastrointestinal disease is considered. The authors in this section have been asked to emphasize the theory, indications, and usefulness of these procedures as well as to address what is likely to happen in their fields in the future.

The techniques of performance are explained in brief segments, with the emphasis on the physical basis of the test or procedure, indications and contraindications, and comparative performance in terms of efficacy, specificity, sensitivity, safety, and cost. A section on cross-sectional anatomy is included to provide a review of the relations between the intestinal organs relevant to modern diagnostic testing and their application to a patient's problem.

Medical practitioners are increasingly confronted with new techniques of diagnosis, treatment, or intervention.[1] Assessing a newly introduced device, technique, or procedure involves critical analysis of its indications, accuracy, and efficacy.[2–5] Each of the following chapters presents information so that the reader can evaluate the varied aspects of each technique or method. In addition, the reader is referred to an excellent review of advances in diagnostic imaging by Black and Welch.[6] This well-written review explains the impact that increasingly accurate imaging techniques can have on estimates of disease prevalence and on assessment of response to therapy.

USE OF SCIENTIFIC METHODS

What is the usefulness of the procedure or device? In what situation is the procedure clearly indicated; when is it potentially indicated; and when is it clearly not indicated? These considerations require careful review.[7] Analytic research studies that fulfill criteria for scientific rigor are needed to judge properly the indications for a procedure. Anecdotal descriptive series of cases are usually not sufficient to assess adequately a new procedure except when a technique is unquestionably an advancement over existing technology.

Good clinical research, like all good science, requires a well-developed, clearly stated hypothesis. The experimental design will vary depending on the technique and the question to be answered, but certain aspects should remain relatively constant. In most cases a control or comparison group is required. The control group should be carefully selected based on the clinical problem and the study group. Certain potentially important factors must be described, matched in cases and controls, or adjusted for, if not evenly distributed in cases and controls, including age, sex, race in some circumstances, patient status (in the hospital or outpatient), and other factors known to be important in the clinical problem. For instance, regarding smoking in peptic ulcer disease: If a study is designed to compare active treatment to placebo control and the active and control groups are not balanced in terms of smoking history, the results may be biased by the adverse effect that smoking has on ulcer healing.

In treatment studies, randomization should be used to increase the chance that confounding factors, such as smoking, are equally distributed between control groups. Even with

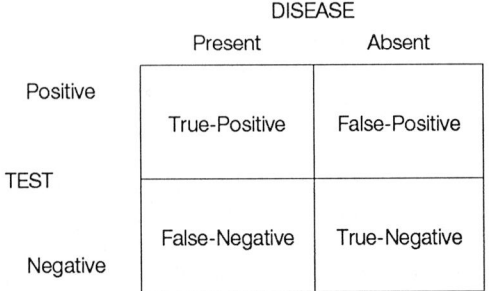

FIGURE 114-1. There are four possible test results as related to the disease state. Correct results may be true positive or true negative. Incorrect results may be false positive or false negative.

randomization, the distribution of demographic features and known confounders should be reported, and, if appropriate, adjustments should be made for maldistribution.

The methods should be clearly delineated and the techniques under evaluation carefully and consistently applied. The investigators must have informed consent for studies in humans. The randomization method should be described, and then all patients must be entered randomly. Selection bias should be minimal. For example, if 400 patients are considered but only 50 are actually selected for randomization and entry into the trial, the reader must ask whether the patients entered were a special subset, not representing the overall patient population with the disease entity. This might significantly limit the applicability of the conclusions to patient populations with this disease.

Ideally, investigators and patients should not be aware of the treatment the patient received. This requirement, called blinding, is difficult to achieve. The inadvertent biases inherent in a nonblinded study are very strong. Because the effect of this bias usually is not measurable, correct interpretation of the results from nonblinded studies is problematic. An nonblinded or uncontrolled study is useful only as pilot work, which then suggests hypotheses that can be tested in a better designed, controlled clinical trial.

The results must be presented clearly, including the mean (or median), standard deviations, and the range. The comparative results must then be analyzed by use of appropriate statistical methods. Analyses should be planned before the study is completed, and the criteria for "clinically important difference" should be established in advance.[8,9] The preestablishment of expected outcomes, especially the clinically important differences, allows for the calculation of required sample sizes and thereby improves study efficiency and precision. It is also an important part of hypothesis development.

PREDICTIVE VALUE OF DIAGNOSTIC TESTS

Establishing diagnoses is an imperfect process resulting in a probability rather than a certainty of being right. A knowledge of the possible relations between the properties of diagnostic tests and the information they yield is helpful to the practicing clinician (Fig. 114-1).[10]

Of the four possible interpretations of the test results, two are correct and two are wrong. Assessment of accuracy or "the truth" is based on an independent validation or "gold standard." Although in some cases the gold standard is relatively easy to determine, it is frequently elusive in clinical research.

The performance of a diagnostic test usually is defined by a series of parameters: sensitivity, specificity, false-negative and false-positive rates, and positive and negative predictive values (Fig. 114-2).[11]

Sensitivity is the probability of the test being positive in a patient with the disease, also called the true-positive rate. The false-negative rate is the probability of a test being negative in a patient with the disease. The *specificity* is the probability of a test being negative in patients without the disease, also called the true-negative rate. The false-positive rate is the probability of a test being positive in a patient without disease. The *positive predictive value* (+PV) is the probability of disease being present in a patient with a positive test result. The *negative predictive value* (−PV) is the probability of no disease being present in a patient with a negative test result.[12]

Usually, there is a trade-off between the sensitivity and specificity of a diagnostic test. Ideally, a test is both highly sensitive and highly specific; however, tests that are very specific frequently are not as sensitive, and tests that are very

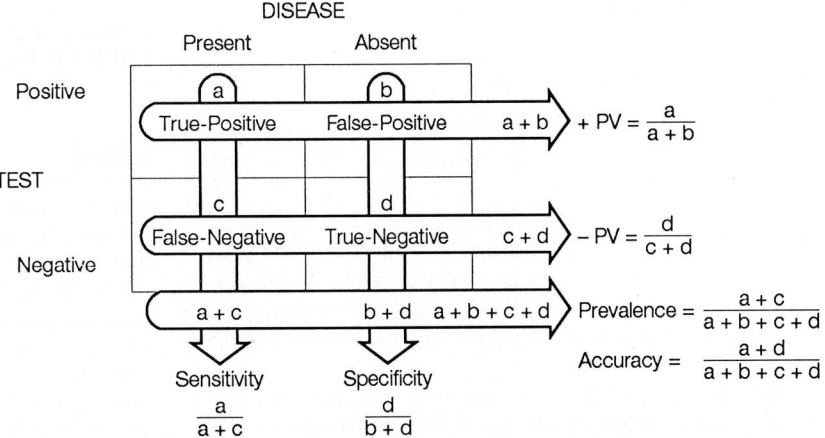

FIGURE 114-2. Diagnostic test characteristics and definitions. (PV, predictive value; from Fletcher RH, Fletcher SW, Wagner EH. Clinical epidemiology: the essentials. Baltimore: Williams & Wilkins, 1982.)

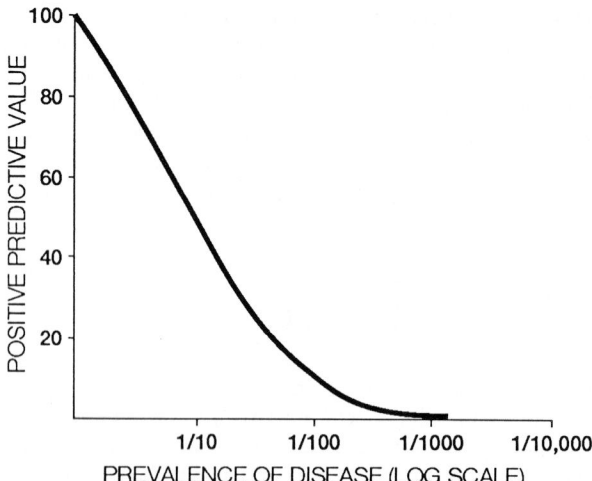

FIGURE 114-3. The relation between prevalence and positive predictive value, where sensitivity equals 90% and specificity equals 90%. (From Fletcher RH, Fletcher SW, Wagner EH. Clinical epidemiology: the essentials. Baltimore: Williams & Wilkins, 1982.)

sensitive are not as specific. The relationship between sensitivity and specificity can be mapped by use of a receiver operating characteristic curve.[13] This relationship is expressed in a figure plotting the true-positive rate (sensitivity) against the false-positive rate (1 minus specificity).[12]

Whenever a test is sensitive but not specific, the penalty is paid in terms of a relatively large number of patients with false-positive test results. The clinician searching for a serious and treatable disease may be willing to accept misleading preliminary information (false-positive) in some patients in exchange for a more sensitive test. On the other hand, it is more difficult to justify a large number of false-positive results when the diagnosis has less important therapeutic implications.

Sensitivity and specificity are properties of a test that are considered when deciding whether or not to order a test. Once the results of a test are known, however, the probability of interest is the predictive value of the test (see Fig. 114-2). The predictive value of a test is not a property of the test alone; it is determined by sensitivity, specificity of the test, and the prevalence of the disease in the population being tested. This relationship is calculated according to Bayes' theorem of probability:

Predictive value of a positive test

$$= (\text{sensitivity} \times \text{prevalance})/(\text{sensitivity} \times \text{prevalence})$$
$$+ [(1 - \text{specificity}) \times (1 - \text{prevalence})].$$

As shown in Figure 114-2, the more sensitive the test is, the better the negative predictive value—in other words, the more confident the clinician can be that a patient with a negative test result does not have the disease. On the other hand, the more specific the test is, the better the positive predictive value of the test.

The effect of prevalence on predictive value is not intuitively obvious. When a test is applied to patients with a low

likelihood of having disease, positive results even for a very specific test can be largely false-positive results. It has been shown that clinicians tend to overestimate the prevalence of disease, thereby increasing the likelihood of a false-positive result. Similarly, even for a very sensitive test, negative results when applied to patients with a high chance of having the disease are likely to be false negative (Fig. 114-3).

This is also demonstrated in Table 114-1 for an extremely common disease, prostatic carcinoma.[14] The main reason prevalence often is more important than sensitivity and specificity in determining predictive value is that prevalence commonly varies over a wider range—especially given the broad range of patients seen by most physicians.

Two final test performance characteristics are the likelihood ratio statistics. The likelihood ratio for a positive test is the likelihood of a positive result in a patient with disease divided by the probability of a positive test result in a patient who does not have the disease. This can also be represented by the sensitivity (true-positive rate) divided by 1 minus specificity, or the false-positive rate. The likelihood ratio for a negative test is the likelihood of a negative test in a patient who does have the disease divided by the likelihood of a negative test in a patient who does not have the disease. This can also be represented by the false-negative rate (1 − sensitivity) divided by the true-negative rate (specificity).

If the pretest odds of a target disorder are known and the likelihood ratio for a diagnostic test result is known, the posttest odds for the target disorder can then be calculated. Higher likelihood ratios for positive tests (>10–20) and lower likelihood ratios for negative tests (<0.2) will have a greater effect on the posttest probability of a target disorder after the test has been done, compared with intermediate values of the likelihood ratio. The likelihood ratio is an important statistic in working through decision trees.[11,15]

EVALUATION OF EFFICACY

Ideally, a new diagnostic technology will go through an orderly development and evaluation. Five levels of efficacy have been described as summarized by the Institute of Medicine.[1,16] The first two levels of evaluation are called technical and di-

TABLE 114-1
Effect of Prevalence on Predictive Value*

SETTING	PREVALENCE (CASES/100,000)	POSITIVE PREDICTIVE VALUE (%)
General population	35	0.4
Men aged 75 y or older	500	5.6
Clinically suspicious prostatic nodule	50,000	93.0

* Positive predictive value of prostatic acid phosphatase for prostatic cancer (sensitivity = 70%, specificity = 90%) in various clinical settings.

From Fletcher RM, Fletcher SW, Wagner EH. Clinical Epidemiology: the essentials. Baltimore: Williams & Wilkins, 1982:55.

agnostic efficacy. Technical efficacy refers to the ability of a test to produce the information it is designed to produce. Diagnostic efficacy, on the other hand, is the test's ability to make the diagnosis in question. Diagnostic efficacy is typically evaluated by sensitivity and specificity. Because most new tests are compared with existing tests, the third level of efficacy is comparative diagnostic efficacy. The clinician typically would like to know how a new test compares with existing tests in terms of sensitivity, specificity, costs, risks, and other parameters.

The upper levels of diagnostic efficacy involve therapeutic decision-making (level 4) and outcome efficacy (level 5), which include the assessment of whether the test affects either diagnostic decisions or the use of other techniques. A test should ideally improve patient outcomes; thus, outcome efficacy is the ultimate level in assessing new diagnostic techniques. Traditionally, most well-established diagnostic tests have fairly good information on the first four levels of efficacy. Few tests have been shown to improve outcomes in carefully documented clinical trials.

Finally, the cost and risk associated with a treatment or diagnostic test must also be considered.[2-5,7,17-19] The cost of a procedure should be considered in the broad sense and not in terms of "what the market will bear." This does not reflect the true economics of a procedure. Cost includes the resources used to produce a procedure plus expenses that are more difficult to measure, such as inconvenience, pain, lost time, and so forth. In general, the clinician makes fairly imprecise estimates of cost and risk in the decision to order a procedure for a single patient.

In the establishment of standards of practice, however, cost effectiveness and risk–benefit considerations are extremely important. For example, the decision of whether a hospital should perform a bone marrow transplantation as opposed to chemotherapy, and whether an insurance company should pay for this, may be aided by information from a cost-effectiveness analysis. Similarly, the decision to perform an angiogram, a contrast-enhanced computed tomography (CT) scan, or a magnetic resonance imaging scan may be driven by risk–benefit considerations in which the relatively lower risk of magnetic resonance imaging becomes the driving force.

PRACTICAL CONSIDERATIONS

The application of these principles to testing in gastroenterology can have a positive influence on decisions regarding selection and timing of imaging tests. In addition, physical principles of image production, patient morphology, anatomic relationships, and pathologic considerations all should influence selection and sequence of imaging tests.

It is important for the person interested in assessment of outcome to understand the concepts of lead-time bias and length bias. Lead-time bias refers to relating the time of diagnosis to the natural history of the disease. Length bias addresses the importance of how rapidly a disease progresses. Without an understanding of these concepts, the clinician can draw incorrect conclusions about the effect of diagnosis and treatment on outcome.[6]

Physical Principles of Imaging

The physical principles of image production can significantly influence the value of a test as applied to a specific patient or as used in evaluating a suspected disease process. How x-ray photons, ultrasound, or radio waves interact with tissue to influence image production, what anatomic structures are imaged by the modality, the resolution of the technique, and the ability of the image to be viewed, stored, transmitted, and compared with prior or future images, all influence the value of the modality as applied to a specific gastroenterologic problem.

As an example, CT and ultrasound can be applied to similar patient problems. The physical principles of image production, however, are quite different. CT relies on the x-ray attenuation differences of tissues, whereas ultrasound depends on the differing reflective character of the tissue to ultrasonic waves. With CT, iodinated contrast can be administered intravenously to accentuate tissue attenuation differences, and oral or rectal contrast can be used to define intestinal segments. Ultrasonography contrast agents are being introduced and may enhance diagnostic accuracy.

Ultrasound is obtained as a "real-time" evaluation, whereas CT images are static. The image quality is significantly influenced by the general patient morphology (amount of fatty tissue) and structures contiguous to the organs of interest. The ultrasound image is degraded by excess fat because fat attenuates ultrasonic waves. The CT image relies on differences in x-ray attenuation and is adversely affected by the lack of fat in a cachectic person. The CT image is accentuated by fat separating contiguous organs of similar radiographic density (Fig. 114-4). When considering only the patient's body type, CT should be applied to the person with above normal

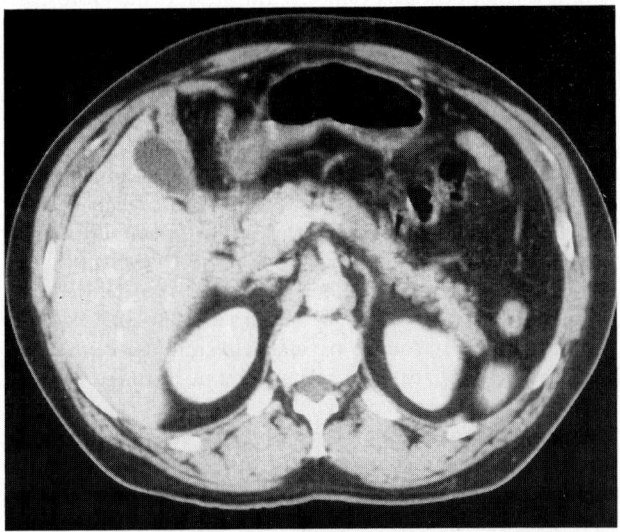

FIGURE 114-4. Abdominal computed tomogram emphasizing contribution of mesenteric and retroperitoneal fat to delineation of normal organs. The stomach, celiac axis vessels, colon, and pancreas are separated by intraabdominal fat. Intravascular contrast allows the portal vein to be distinguished from the pancreas.

adipose tissue, whereas ultrasound is best used in a patient who is thin.

The ultrasound beam is reflected by gas, calcium, and barium contrast material, whereas CT is not as adversely affected by these factors. Ultrasound is ideal for structures close to the surface, such as the gallbladder; the acuity of the sound waves diminishes with deeper penetration. Evaluating a gassy and obese patient with residual barium in the colon for a potential pancreatic mass would therefore be better done by CT rather than ultrasound.

These considerations relating to the physical bases of image production allow the physician better to understand the optimal application of a technology to a suspected disease process in a specific patient.

Anatomy and Pathology

Consideration of normal anatomy and the normal anatomic relations between the organ suspected to be diseased and its contiguous structures is of great importance in selecting the best approach to imaging. Some imaging modalities do better with certain types of tissue, whereas others do not examine these tissues as well. The nature of the tissue or organ to be examined, such as its fluid or fat content, and its relations to adjacent structures such as bone, skin, or lung affect the imaging process. The pathologic changes that occur in normal tissue with disease are also important.

For example, knowing that the target organ is solid but that the disease state involves accumulation of fluid favors the selection of an imaging modality such as ultrasound, which has great precision in differentiating solid from fluid-filled lesions.

Direct acoustic access through the liver to a target organ such as the biliary tree could influence the selection of ultrasound as the most anatomically direct, and therefore cost-effective, approach. If there is intervening bone or lung, percutaneous ultrasound is not as applicable, and CT is a better approach. An example of this is the staging of esophageal neoplasms. The esophageal wall is not visible with percutaneous ultrasound because of the intervening air-filled lung and bone surrounding the target organ; CT is a much better choice.

If the disease process is suspected to originate in the mucosa, a technique that is sensitive for detecting mucosal disease, such as endoscopy, double-contrast barium radiography, or endoscopic ultrasound, would be selected instead of CT, percutaneous ultrasound, or magnetic resonance imaging, which are less able to define mucosal abnormalities.

These factors are becoming increasingly important because the future of imaging will most certainly include the modification and refinement of available techniques as well as the introduction of new techniques. The determination of metabolic change in diseased tissue with the use of techniques such as magnetic resonance spectroscopy will allow advances in imaging for the study of physiologic function, such as that represented by hepatobiliary scintigraphy. Expansion of the knowledge base regarding the appearance of the target tissue in health and disease will be necessary to determine the application of new imaging modalities. It is also important to understand which abnormal structures are clinically significant so that the results of diagnostic tests are applied appropriately to patient management.

CLINICAL APPLICATIONS

The culmination of this decision process is the application of these diagnostic and therapeutic devices or tests to patients. Making the decision to apply any one of these requires that a series of decisions be made. Understanding the normal anatomy, the pathologic anatomy of the disease process, and the potential interaction of the available imaging techniques with the suspected process contributes to this decision process. In addition, diagnostic efficacy (sensitivity and specificity), safety, cost, availability, reproducibility of the results, and patient convenience and comfort are important. Practical considerations such as how long the test takes, how soon the patient can be scheduled, and how soon the results are available often determine imaging strategies.

Even when these factors are known, the clinician often must still make difficult decisions. The first is whether any imaging is necessary. What will be done with the information? Will it be useful for the management of the patient? Curiosity is not a sufficient reason to put a patient through any test or procedure; it must be in the patient's best interest. If the information will not affect patient management, the test should not be done.

Once it is decided that testing is indicated, the initial test should be determined by several important criteria. If there is low pretest probability of the disease for which the test is being done, the test should be inexpensive, easy, and the least invasive of those available. It should have low risk and low patient discomfort. It should be considered more of a "screening" test because the pretest probability of disease is low.[12]

Conversely, if the pretest probability of disease is high, going directly to a test with higher cost, greater invasiveness, and possibly greater risk, but one that can also potentially provide treatment for the disease process, has merit. An example of these considerations could be a patient suspected of having choledocholithiasis. In a patient with minimal symptomatology, no specific laboratory tests suggesting this disease, and no predisposing factors, a noninvasive test such as ultrasound, with its low risk and cost, would be logical to initiate the work-up.

If there is high clinical suspicion or probability of bile duct stones or if dilated bile ducts or stones are visualized on ultrasound, a more invasive and therapeutic test, such as endoscopic retrograde cholangiography with sphincterotomy, should be considered. In such a patient with high pretest probability of choledocholithiasis (prior gallstone disease, active cholangitis, or jaundice), the more invasive test with which definitive therapy is possible should be considered earlier, even though it has higher risk and cost.[13]

It is important to plan the order or sequence of tests to refine the patient's differential diagnosis. A proper sequence can prevent unnecessary delay in patient evaluation, minimize the cost of evaluation, and enhance the diagnostic potential of the examinations used. In most diagnostic evaluations, the least expensive and least invasive of the appropriate tests should be undertaken initially. When considering the radiologic evaluation, plain-film radiography and ultrasound may be the most efficacious initial investigations for many gastrointestinal conditions. More invasive and complicated tests may then follow (Table 114-2).

A diagnostic test might be inappropriate early in the management of a patient if it is not likely to answer the clinical question or if it interferes with subsequent tests. For example, barium sulfate in the gut can significantly degrade the image of many other diagnostic examinations: Barium introduces a reflective interface, causing artifactual shadows that obscure anatomy on ultrasound images; barium residue inhibits endoscopic inspection of the gut mucosa; barium can obscure radiography of important regions, making angiography, endoscopic retrograde cholangiopancreatography, and tube injections difficult; and barium can produce degradation of the CT image, only partially compensated for by newer-generation equipment and software. Therefore, in many instances the administration of barium contrast media should be withheld until all other examinations are accomplished (Table 114-3).

As competing and complementary tests become more numerous and as technology and cost-containing health care reform continue to advance, issues of test sequencing and resource management become of greater importance. To provide guidance for the diagnostic work-up and imaging of complex patient problems, several centers have instituted imaging consulting services.[20-22] These services consist of experienced clinicians and radiologists in prospective consultation to determine which imaging tests and in which sequence most effectively address the potential diagnoses. Benefits of such prospective planning of the diagnostic work-up include more appropriate and less redundant testing, diminished number of tests and time to complete the evaluation, and the consequent cost savings.[23,24] This process can therefore be a cost-effective means of accurate and time-efficient diagnosis. Table 114-4 presents some examples of clinical problems and the initial imaging procedure suggested by an imaging consultation service.

Finally, it is essential to develop a sense of when to limit the imaging evaluation. If the clinician understands the differential diagnosis, the likelihood of various diagnostic pos-

sibilities, and the specificity and sensitivity of the test used, he or she can decide when it is appropriate to stop a work-up. This is an increasing challenge in clinical medicine and gastroenterology as cost containment pressures intensify.

When has the clinician ordered sufficient studies to reduce the likelihood of significant disease being present? As the search gets more complex, the risk to the patient often increases. At some point, the risk–benefit ratio of further investigation may not support continued testing in light of the low likelihood of significant disease being present or the inability of the physician to provide effective treatment for the disease being sought by the diagnostic process.[25,26] When this

---

TABLE 114-3

Examinations Compromised by Intralumenal Barium Sulfate or Iodinated Contrast Media

Ultrasonography
Computed tomography
Angiography
Endoscopic retrograde cholangiopancreatography, percutaneous transhepatic cholangiography
Tube studies
Fistulography
Radionuclide examinations

TABLE 114-4

An Imaging Consultation Service: Examples of Clinical Problems Presented and Suggested Initial Imaging Procedures

CLINICAL PROBLEM	INITIAL IMAGING PROCEDURE
Oropharyngeal swallowing difficulty	Barium pharyngoesophagography
Dysphagia	Barium esophagography or endoscopy
Right upper quadrant pain	Ultrasonography
Epigastric pain and weight loss	Computed tomography
Suspected liver metastases	Computed tomography
Suspected liver mass	Computed tomography
Suspected liver hemangioma	Magnetic resonance imaging
Jaundice with history of gallstones	Endoscopic retrograde cholangiography
Suspected hemochromatosis	Magnetic resonance imaging
Suspected abdominal abscess	Computed tomography
Suspected Meckel's diverticulum	Technetium nuclear scintigraphy
Suspected small bowel inflammatory disease	Barium small bowel examination
Suspected small bowel mass, hemorrhage	Small bowel enterocylsis
Suspected retroperitoneal mass	Computed tomography
Suspected typhlitis, toxic colon	Abdominal plain film radiography, computed tomography
Suspected portal vein thrombosis	Duplex ultrasonography with color Doppler

---

TABLE 114-2

General Sequence of Radiologic Examinations in Patients Being Evaluated for Gastrointestinal Disease

1. Plain film radiography
2. Ultrasonography
3. Radionuclide examination
4. Computed tomography
5. Angiography
6. Direct cholangiography and pancreatography
7. Tube studies, fistulography, sinography
8. Barium sulfate or iodinated contrast examinations of the intestinal tract
9. Magnetic resonance imaging

point is reached, the best approach could be serial clinical observation or "tincture of time" coupled with sympathetic reassurance. In general, clinicians have a natural reluctance to rely on "tincture of time," but this strategy is often underused and relatively undervalued by clinicians.

It is the purpose of the chapters that follow in this textbook to provide the reader with the information necessary to assist with these decisions. When these chapters are combined with the sections on basic science, gastrointestinal disease, and the clinical approach to problem solving, it is hoped that the diagnostic process in gastroenterology will become more logical and understandable.

> The reader is directed to Chapter 120, Cross-Sectional Anatomy.

REFERENCES

1. Institute of Medicine. Assessing medical technologies. Washington, DC: National Academy Press, 1985.
2. Begg CB. Biases in the assessment of diagnostic tests. Stat Med 1987;6:411.
3. Begg CB, McNeil BJ. Assessment of radiologic tests: control of bias and other design considerations. Radiology 1988;167:565.
4. Gelfand DW, Ott DJ. Methodologic considerations in comparing imaging methods. AJR 1985;144:1117.
5. Greenes RA, Begg CB. Assessment of diagnostic technologies: methodology for unbiased estimation from samples of selectively verified patients. Invest Radiol 1985;20:751.
6. Black WC, Welch HG. Advances in diagnostic imaging and overestimations of disease prevalence and the benefits of therapy. N Engl J Med 1993;328:1237.
7. Hiatt HH. Protecting the medical commons: who is responsible? N Engl J Med 1975;293:235.
8. Cook D, Sackett DL. On the clinically important differences. ACP Journal Club 1992 Sep–Oct. Ann Intern Med 1992; 117(Suppl 2):A16.
9. Laupacis A, Sackett DL, Roberts RS. An assessment of clinically useful measures of consequences of treatment. N Engl J Med 1988;318:1728.
10. Fletcher RM, Fletcher SW, Wagner EH. Clinical epidemiology: the essentials. Baltimore: Williams & Wilkins, 1982.
11. Sackett DC, Haynes RB, Tywell P. Clinical epidemiology: a basic science for clinical medicine. Boston: Little, Brown & Co, 1985.
12. Galen RS, Gambino SR. Beyond normality: the predictive value and efficacy of medical diagnoses. New York: John Wiley & Sons, 1975.
13. McNeil BJ, Keller E, Adelstein SJ. Primer on certain elements of medical decision making. N Engl J Med 1975;293:211.
14. Watson RA, Tang DB. The predictive value of prostatic acid phosphatase as a screening test for prostatic cancer. N Engl J Med 1980;303:497.
15. Fagan TJ. Nomogram for Bayes' theorem. N Engl J Med 1975;293:257.
16. Kent DL, Larson EB. Magnetic resonance imaging of the brain and spine: is clinical efficacy established after the first decade? Ann Intern Med 1988;108:402.
17. Weinstein MC, Stason WV. Foundation of cost-effectiveness analysis for health and medical practices. N Engl J Med 1977;296:716.
18. Kent DL, Larson EB. Diagnostic technology assessments: problems and prospects. Ann Intern Med 1988;108:759.
19. Welch HG, Larson EB. Cost effectiveness of bone marrow transplantation in acute non-lymphocytic leukemia. N Engl J Med 1989;321:807.
20. Shuman WP, Heilman RS. The radiologist as consultant. JAMA 1979;242:1519.
21. Baker SR. The operation of a radiology consultation service in an acute care hospital. JAMA 1982;248:2152.
22. Seltzer SE, Beard JO, Adams DF. Radiologist as consultant: direct contact between referring clinician and radiologist before CT examination. AJR 1985;144:661.
23. Shuman WP, Heilman RS, Larson EB. DRGs and the radiologist as a consultant. AJR 1984;143:193.
24. Baker SR, Stein HD. Radiologic consultation: its application to an acute care surgical ward. AJR 1986;147:637.
25. Rogers DE. On technological restraint. Ann Intern Med 1975;134:93.
26. Larson EB. Medical technologies: restraint or discretion. J Gen Intern Med 1990;5:178.

Textbook of Gastroenterology, second edition, edited by Tadataka Yamada. JB Lippincott Company, Philadelphia © 1995.

CHAPTER 115

Upper Gastrointestinal Endoscopy

Guido N. J. Tytgat

Technical Considerations
Fiberoptic Endoscopes
Videoendoscopes
Patient Preparation and Monitoring

Passing the Endoscope
Endoscopic Examination
Disinfection of Endoscopic Equipment
(continued)

This chapter reviews the current status of upper endoscopy employed for diagnosis and treatment and the use of flexible endoscopes with fiberoptic or video systems. Diagnostic considerations include when to use endoscopy, in which situations is it useful to the patient, how to use biopsy and cytology, and some new approaches to diagnosis.[1] The use of this technology as a therapeutic approach for endoscopic hemostasis, therapy of obstructing tumors, removal of foreign bodies, and dilation of strictures is also reviewed.[2,3]

In a section that introduces the technical aspects of endoscopy, followed by an analysis of indications, limitations, and pitfalls of upper intestinal endoscopy, five areas of interest are highlighted: dysphagia, reflux-like dyspepsia, peptic ulcer disease, upper gastrointestinal bleeding, and upper gastrointestinal neoplasia. This chapter also addresses the risks and contraindications for endoscopy and other gastrointestinal tract imaging modalities to help the reader understand the cost-benefit analysis of a procedure compared with alternative diagnostic or therapeutic approaches. The final section considers speculations about endoscopy in the future and improvements in diagnostic and therapeutic modalities.

TECHNICAL CONSIDERATIONS

A variety of factors are necessary for safe and effective endoscopy. These include properly trained endoscopists; well-trained and clinically experienced assistants; high-quality, well-maintained endoscopic equipment; and a well-designed endoscopy suite containing all the necessary facilities and accessories for endoscopy and for emergency procedures that may occur during endoscopy.

It is essential to have equipment that goes to the bedside for endoscopy, especially for acutely ill patients in the intensive care unit. Adequate storage is essential for the many endo-

scopic accessories. There must be an area for endoscope disinfection and preparation of accessories for sterilization. It is critical to have an area in which to watch patients after endoscopy, especially if they have received sedation or have serious medical illnesses.

Performance of electrocautery requires that at least one state-of-the-art electrocautery unit is available. All of these electronic devices should be checked periodically for electrical safety by the hospital electrical safety team. Equipment to document the visual appearance of lesions is also important.

Fiberoptic Endoscopes

The critical part of a flexible fiberoptic endoscope is the fiber bundle that transmits a coherent image. The imaging bundle consists of several thousand thin glass fibers, 6 to 12 μm in diameter, that transmit light. Each fiber consists of an inner core of glass surrounded by an outer glass layer made of a second type of glass with a lower refractive index. Light entering the fiber reflects off the junction between these two types of glass and propagates down the fiber. A total of 10,000 to 40,000 fibers are grouped together to form the imaging bundle and generate a coherent image. The resolution of the imaging bundle depends on the diameter of the fibers. Fibers may break with excessive bending and torquing or during retraction of an accessory if the tip of the endoscope is flexed. A broken fiber appears as a black dot in the visual image.

The small image at the proximal or viewer's end of the coherent fiber bundle is enlarged with a 15$\times$ to 30$\times$ magnifying lens in the endoscope ocular. The image cannot be overly magnified because this would make individual fibers visible, interfering with image interpretation. Standard flexible fiberoptic endoscopes have a depth of focus that allows examination of objects 3 to 100 mm away from the tip. The field of view of the imaging system is up to 110 or 120 degrees. Special high-magnification endoscopes are available.

Endoscope design includes the objective lens system, which focuses the target onto the fiberoptic image bundle; the light source, which illuminates the target; a nozzle for air insufflation; a nozzle for a water jet to clean the viewing objective lens; and a suction channel, which is used to remove gas and fluids and also to pass a variety of accessories by way of the endoscope into the intestinal lumen. Side-viewing endoscopes contain these same features but have a different design that allows the examiner to look sideways; the suction or accessory channel has an elevator, which can change the position of an accessory. Most modern endoscopes can be totally submerged to facilitate the important tasks of cleaning and disinfection.

The endoscope control handle contains valves for air and water as well as suction and control knobs. These knobs are attached to wires that go down the length of the flexible insertion tube to the distal bending tip. By maneuvering these wires in an up-and-down or right-and-left direction, it is possible to turn the tip of the endoscope and inspect the entire lumen of the organ being evaluated. In most endoscopes, it is possible to turn the tip of the bending section more than 100 degrees (retroflex) to allow the inspection of surfaces such as the cardia of the stomach, which are difficult to see with the instrument in a straight position.

Upper endoscopes are designed to be torque stable. Clockwise or counterclockwise rotation of the control handle results in the same rotation of the tip. The flexibility of the insertion tube varies; often, it is more flexible distally and less flexible proximally.

It is possible to have a second viewer observe the endoscopic procedure by use of a teaching attachment. This attachment uses a beam splitter, which divides the light returning up the image bundle into a portion for the primary examiner and a portion diverted by way of a fiberoptic bundle to the teaching attachment. This causes some loss of brightness for the primary endoscopist, but, in general, the image is satisfactory.

A teaching attachment is mandatory if a lesion must be shown to a second observer. Documenting can be accomplished by attaching a 35-mm single lens reflex or instant print camera to the eyepiece. These cameras are automatically brought into focus. It is also possible to make 35- or 16-mm motion pictures or to attach a television camera to the eyepiece, allowing imaging by means of a television system and videotaping.

Videoendoscopes

Videoendoscopy, introduced in the mid-1980s, has changed the field of endoscopy. The design of the endoscope no longer includes a coherent imaging fiber bundle made of glass fibers. The image is generated electronically using a charge-coupled device (CCD) located in the tip of the endoscope. These devices are approximately 3 mm in diameter.

The first videoendoscopes used a color wheel. Green, red, or blue light was sequentially sent down the illumination bundle of the endoscope and activated the CCD at the tip. It was possible to reconstruct a color image using the three sets of images generated by the colored lights. The videoprocessor

displayed a full-color image of the gastrointestinal tract lining. Later videoendoscopes use a color chip that actually obtains the image in color on the tip of the endoscope. These devices use 30,000 to 100,000 pixels of resolution.[4]

There are several advantages inherent in videoendoscopy: the control unit is located away from the endoscopist's face, reducing the chance of contamination by way of splatter from the suction port; everyone present in the room can watch the monitor; the image can be sent outside of the room and multiple television sets can be used for simultaneous observation throughout the hospital, elsewhere in the city, or even by way of satellite to another country; for complicated procedures, the assistants can better assist the primary endoscopist because they can watch the procedure on the monitor simultaneously; and images can be easily documented and stored for teaching or clinical follow-up. Digital images can now be recorded on magneto-optical disks. These images can be recalled from a central image storage system and sent to any location in the endoscopy service. The disks can be used for image processing and for management and reliable storage of endoscopic images and information.[5,6] The video system is not sensitive to irradiation and is less sensitive to damage caused by bending and torquing than are fiberoptic imaging systems.

The most important contributions from videoendoscopy occur when the digitized image is used to provide information that cannot be obtained using standard fiberoptic endoscopes. Examples include quantitative analysis of mucosal color to estimate mucosal hemoglobin content and mucosal blood flow, examination of spontaneous or laser-induced fluorescence of target tissue, detection of injected dyes, and manipulation of the visual image to increase contrast resolution or detect structures not readily seen by a fiberoptic system.

A disadvantage of videoendoscopic systems is that it is possible to overload the CCD, which results in a white area on the screen that can interfere with the interpretation of the image. This occurs if the tip of the endoscope comes close to the target and causes a "blooming" effect. This effect may also occur during the use of lasers in the gastrointestinal tract with some videoendoscopes.

Other than the method of delivering the image, the videoendoscope is similar to a fiberoptic endoscope. The same controls are used for air, water, and suction; knobs for up-and-down and right-and-left bending of the tip; and a suction channel to remove gas and fluid and to pass a variety of accessories to the tip of the endoscope. There are also buttons on the videoendoscope control handle to activate videotaping, freeze the image, and obtain a photograph.

Patient Preparation and Monitoring

In most patients, a spray or gargle of topical anesthetic is used for topical anesthesia of the pharynx and hypopharynx just before passing the upper endoscope. Lignocaine used as a spray has improved tolerance to upper endoscopy.[7,8] Anticholinergics were used in the past to reduce secretions and motility but are rarely used today.

Most endoscopists consider proper sedation to be an essential element of endoscopy. Surveys in the United States and the United Kingdom indicate that more than 90% of endoscopists use intravenous sedation.[9,10] In considering the use of combined sedatives and narcotics, a working party report presented at the world congress in Sydney and an international forum on quality control in endoscopy urged caution in the combined use of these drugs.[11,12] The concern is that each of these drugs—benzodiazepines; opioids, such as fentanyl, nalbuphine, morphine, or pethidine; and barbiturates—has synergic effects with the others. If one is given, the dose of the second must usually be reduced to avoid respiratory depression, apnea, and a fall in blood pressure.

Midazolam is preferred by most endoscopists. If necessary, flumazenil is used to reduce profound sedation. This effect of flumazenil lasts for 45 to 60 minutes. Rather than routinely reversing the sedative effect of midazolam, the most appropriate approach is to titrate the initial dose of midazolam to avoid oversedation. This is a problem in the elderly, in whom more than 50% of endoscopic complications are thought to be caused by cardiorespiratory problems related to sedation. Prevention of complications involves careful use and titration of medication dose and patient monitoring, including pulse, blood pressure, and oximetry.

If endoscopy is essential in patients with evidence of cardiac or pulmonary disease or in the elderly, an electrocardiographic monitor and oximeter should be used.[5–13] Following the pulse and blood pressure during endoscopy is also recommended. A skilled, trained, and attentive endoscopy assistant should monitor the patient. The assistant must also be trained to assist the endoscopist in the event of an emergency, such as a cardiac arrest or respiratory depression. The endoscopist and the endoscopy assistant should periodically retrain to keep their skills in cardiopulmonary resuscitation current.[14]

Passing the Endoscope

There are two methods of passing an endoscope: the blind method and the direct vision method. The blind method involves passing the tip of the endoscope into the patient's mouth through a bite guard and advancing the tip of the endoscope to approximately 18 to 20 cm from the incisor teeth. The patient is asked to swallow, which opens the cricopharyngeal sphincter, and the tip of the endoscope is gently advanced into the proximal esophagus. This may be performed by simply bending the tip of the endoscope without placing the fingers in the patient's mouth to guide the tip. In some circumstances, one or two fingers may be used to keep the tip of the endoscope midline and guide the endoscope as it is advanced. If fingers are placed in the patient's mouth, a bite guard must be used.

The direct vision technique involves passing the endoscope through a bite guard and watching endoscopically to observe the anatomy of the hypopharynx as the tip of the instrument is advanced. The cricopharyngeus is directly visualized, and the instrument is advanced into this area. The patient is asked to swallow, and under direct vision, the tip of the instrument is passed into the proximal esophagus. This technique is in general more advisable but is especially important in patients with distortion of the hypopharyngeal anatomy (e.g., tumor, prior surgery) or with a suspected diverticulum proximally, in whom blind passage might cause inadvertent injury to the proximal esophagus or perforation of the diverticulum. The direct vision technique also allows an inspection of the hypopharyngeal anatomy.

Most experienced endoscopists prefer to hold the endoscopic controls (e.g., air, water, and suction valves; tip direction wheels) in the left hand. The right hand is used to advance the instrument and intermittently to come back to the endoscope control to turn the control wheels. Torquing the endoscope is accomplished by rotating the instrument control handle, which results in rotation of the entire shaft and tip of the endoscope.

Endoscopic Examination

The endoscopic examination is carried out under direct vision. The esophagus is studied from 20 to 40 cm. At 40 cm lies the ora serrata, which is the junction between the pearly stratified squamous mucosa and the more red gastric columnar epithelium. It is also possible to identify the level of the diaphragm by having the patient sniff. This is important for identification of a hiatal hernia. The esophagus folds can be seen to change with air distention. It is possible to see extrinsic pressure on the esophagus from adjacent structures such as the aorta and the left main stem bronchus.

With slight angulation to the left and anteriorly, the endoscope is passed into the stomach. Air is insufflated to facilitate gastroscopy. The fluid in the gastric pool is removed to improve the endoscopy and to reduce the likelihood of regurgitation and aspiration during the procedure. It is important to notice the presence of bile, food, or blood in the gastric fluid. The gastric mucosa is inspected, and observations are made about the amount of mucus, fold thickness and pliability, and the appearance of blood vessels. Normally, it is not possible to see blood vessels through the mucosa. The gastric folds begin in the upper portion of the stomach and extend down to the entrance into the antrum. With distention of the stomach, these folds often flatten.

Endoscopy of the stomach is not complete without a careful retroflexion examination in which the tip of the endoscope is bent more than 180 degrees. This allows inspection of the lesser curvature, cardia, and fundus. A lesion such as a tumor, Mallory-Weiss tear, or ulcer is often impossible to see in these areas unless the endoscope is retroflexed. Retroflexion also permits inspection of a hiatal hernia. After retroflexion, the instrument can be rotated clockwise and counterclockwise and gently moved in and out to inspect the entire area of the cardia, lesser curvature, and fundus.

The incisura angularis is a fold that marks the entrance to the antrum. The fold is located on the lesser curvature of the stomach. The mucosa in the antrum does not have rugal folds and is usually smooth. Peristalsis begins in the midbody and progresses down to the antrum; the frequency is approximately three per minute. These contractions progress to the pylorus and stop. The pylorus is usually open at rest, but as the contraction wave reaches it, it closes. It is useful to watch several contraction waves as they progress toward the pylorus to determine whether there is an area of wall that is not pliable, suggesting an inflammatory or infiltrative process. Peristalsis may be weak or absent in a heavily sedated patient.

The tip of the endoscope is placed through the pylorus into the duodenal bulb. It is sometimes necessary to create a greater curvature loop before the tip of the endoscope can progress to and through the pylorus.

With most end-viewing endoscopes, the entire surface of the duodenal bulb can be inspected. With a small-caliber endoscope, it is possible to inspect the fornices. The endoscope is passed beyond the apex of the duodenal bulb into the second portion of the duodenum (i.e., descending duodenum). Passage from the tip of the bulb into the descending duodenum is often possible under direct vision but occasionally requires looking to the right and down and advancing the instrument gently, even though it is not possible to see the lumen until the tip of the instrument enters the descending duodenum. The duodenal bulb is usually free of folds; duodenal folds begin in the descending portion of the duodenum. The endoscope is withdrawn, inspecting the mucosa of the duodenum, stomach, and esophagus. With a cooperative patient, it is often possible to inspect the larynx and hypopharynx as the instrument is withdrawn.

Disinfection of Endoscopic Equipment

The endoscopes and ancillary equipment must be cleaned carefully after each use. Endoscopes are complicated biomedical devices that contain small tubes for air, water, and suction, which also must be cleaned. If the endoscope and the channels are not correctly cleaned, debris may accumulate, which can plug channels, make subsequent cleaning more difficult, and limit access to microorganisms by the disinfecting solutions. Some parts of the endoscope can be removed and sterilized or disinfected, such as the valves for air, water, and suction, the distal tip of the endoscope, and the water containers. These should be removed and sterilized or treated with high-level disinfection between patients.

Cleaning between examinations always requires a mechanical scrubbing of the outside of the endoscope and brushing of the channels with detergent solution, followed by soaking in disinfectant solution, usually a 2% solution of glutaraldehyde. Most modern endoscopes are completely submersible in the disinfecting solution. After disinfection, the instrument must be rinsed well to remove all traces of the disinfecting solution, which may be toxic to the next patient and cause mucosal inflammation. It is also important to dry the instrument before storage to prevent the growth of bacteria, especially *Pseudomonas* in retained moisture. Automatic washing devices are available. Most of these machines include a soaking period in a disinfectant such as glutaraldehyde as part of the disinfection process.

It is becoming increasingly important to sterilize all endoscopic accessories that are to be reused between patients. A steam autoclave or ethylene oxide gas can be used to sterilize. After sterilization, the endoscope must be aerated to remove all traces of ethylene oxide, because this gas may be irritating to the next patient or to the staff. An ultrasonic cleaner may be helpful to remove debris from the interstices of devices such as biopsy forceps before sterilization.

The high-level disinfection and sterilization procedures used for fiberoptic and video endoscopes do not always produce optimal disinfection.[15] Initial mechanical cleaning of the endoscope to remove debris before disinfection is critical. If the biologic residual material is not removed, the disinfectant cannot get to the instrument surfaces to accomplish high-level disinfection. This initial mechanical cleaning may be the most important step in endoscope cleaning and disinfection. It is critical to use an effective chemical agent for high-level disinfection and that disinfection procedures follow the concept of universal precautions. Every patient should be regarded as a potential carrier of a variety of infections, including hepatitis B, hepatitis C, and human immunodeficiency virus (HIV). Procedures to disinfect these agents should be used at all times on all patients. It is not always possible to identify which patient is a carrier of these infectious agents. If accessories such as biopsy forceps are to be reused, they must be cleaned thoroughly and sterilized before use on the next patient.

Thorough mechanical cleaning and high-level disinfection eliminate infectious agents such as HIV and other viruses.[16] The definition of high-level disinfection means that all organisms are removed from the equipment, with the exception of some spores. If the instrument is cleaned mechanically before high-level disinfection with 2% glutaraldehyde for an adequate period of time, vegetative organisms that can cause infection after endoscopy and other organisms of concern such as HIV and hepatitis B virus are destroyed.

ACCESSORIES AND METHODS FOR SPECIAL APPLICATIONS

During endoscopy, to increase diagnostic information beyond the visual appearance, a variety of endoscopic accessories can be passed down the biopsy channel. These include measuring devices, biopsy forceps, cytology brushes, needles for cytologic puncture or infection therapy, Doppler probes, probes to obtain an ultrasound image, and probes capable of measuring electrical activity or the pH of fluid at the tip of the endoscope.

Biopsy Forceps

Although all biopsy forceps are similar, they vary in diameter, in whether a central spike is present to impale the tissue and thereby improve the sample size, and whether the cups are closed or fenestrated (Fig. 115-1). Gentle manipulation is required, because excessive force on the control handle can break the forceps. As with other endoscopic accessories, it is important to ensure the forceps is functioning before use.

After obtaining the biopsy specimen, the tissue is removed from the cup, often by using the tip of a toothpick. It is possible to orient this material on a mesh to improve the diagnostic quality of the specimen. The larger biopsy forceps are useful to obtain a slightly deeper specimen, which is essential for diagnosis in lymphomas involving the stomach and linitis plastica.

Most endoscopic forceps obtain mucosa and, occasionally, a small amount of submucosa. To sample more deeply into a lesion such as a submucosal tumor, needle cytology should be applied, or repetitive sampling with a large biopsy forceps should be made in the same area. Alternatively, a large-particle biopsy may be obtained using a polypectomy snare. The snare is placed over the fold or polypoid area, tightened, and gently pulled away from the wall. As the snare is pulled through the lesion, the electrosurgical current causes coagulation and prevents bleeding (Fig. 115-2; see Color Fig. 80).

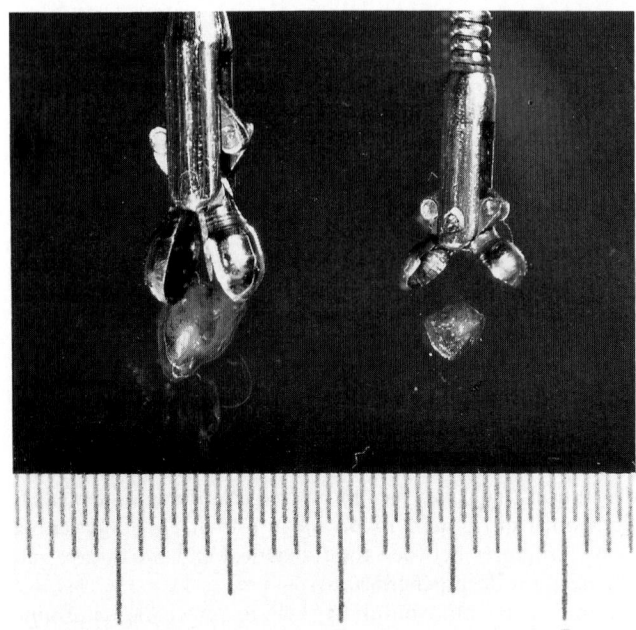

FIGURE 115-1. Standard 7-Fr (2.3-mm) and large-caliber biopsy forceps.

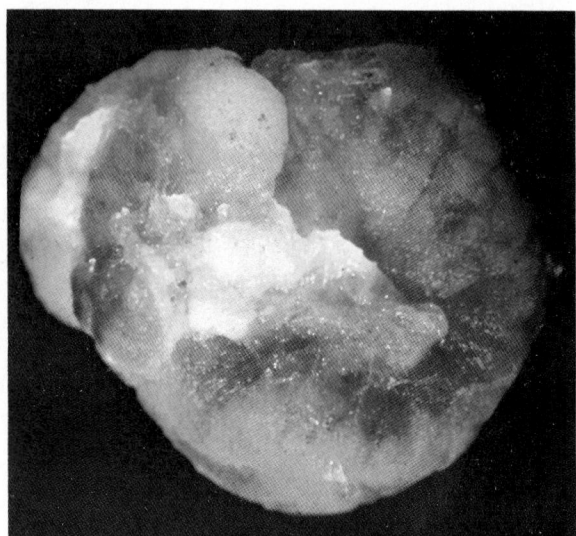

FIGURE 115-2. (See Color Fig. 80.) A big-particle biopsy specimen of a large gastric erosion was removed with an electrosurgical snare.

The lift and cut biopsy technique uses an endoscope with two channels to pass a forceps and a snare. The snare is opened, and the forceps is directed through the snare. The tissue is grasped by the forceps and pulled up into the snare. The snare can be tightened, and the tissue can be excised with electrocautery. This technique may result in unexpectedly large, deep biopsy specimens and is not recommended for the inexperienced endoscopist.

A newer technique for obtaining large samples involves turning the endoscope toward the mucosa and suctioning the mucosa into the open biopsy forceps to impale the tissue. This turn and suction or aspiration biopsy technique is associated with a more adequate size of tissue sample.[17]

Cytology Brushes

Cytology brushes are used to obtain cell samples from the surface of a lesion for cytologic study or for examination of an exudate to detect, for example, the presence of *Candida*. These brushes are often protected by a plastic overtube or sheath, which allows the examiner to advance the brush out of and pull it back into the sheath. The sheath prevents loss of material and oropharyngeal contamination of the specimen because it covers the brush as it is removed.

Specimens obtained with a sheathed cytology brush are often superior to those obtained using an unsheathed brush. These brushes are disposable or can be sterilized. Cytology brushing is especially important in areas that are inaccessible for biopsy, such as narrow strictures in the esophagus. After removal of the cytology brush from the endoscope biopsy channel, the mucus and fluid are placed on a glass slide and into Carnoy's or another appropriate fixative solution.[18,19]

Other approaches to obtaining cytologic material include salvage cytology and needle aspiration. The salvage technique uses a mucus trap, which is placed between the suction channel of the endoscope and the suction line. It is possible to aspirate the biopsy channel contents between each passage of a biopsy forceps. The 5 to 20 mL of fluid collected contains cellular debris from each of the specimens. This material can be placed in alcohol or another fixative and examined cytologically, allowing detection of malignant cells remaining in the biopsy channel.[18,19]

Material can be aspirated for cytologic examination using an endoscopic needle technique. A 4-mm-long, 23-gauge sclerotherapy needle can be placed into the target, such as a submucosal tumor or an ulcerating malignancy, to obtain cellular material from below the mucosa or below the surface exudate, adding to the diagnostic yield of biopsy and brush cytology.[20]

Measuring Devices

In many instances, it is important to know the actual size of the target, for example, to determine whether an ulcer is healing. However, the closer the tip of the endoscope is to the target, the larger the target appears. Measuring methods include using open biopsy forceps with a known distance between the tips of the biopsy cups, using a spring-type measuring probe with gradations of known length, and using a projected grid obtained by employing an argon laser that allows the examiner to see the contour of the target and make three-dimensional ulcer measurements.[21]

Measuring Mucosal Blood Flow

Mucosal blood flow is thought to be an important parameter to determine response of the body to conditions such as shock and to monitor effective ulcer healing. Several devices can be

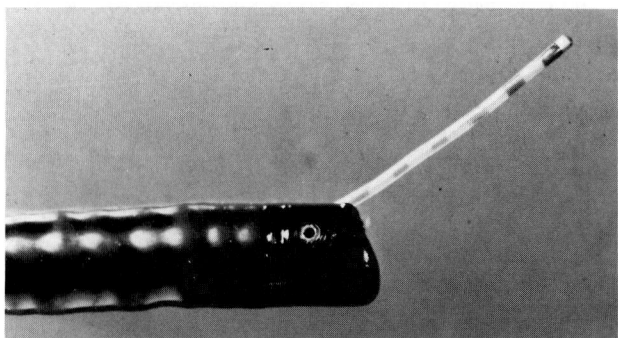

FIGURE 115-3. A doppler probe is passed through the instrumentation channel of a side-viewing endoscope.

passed down the endoscope suction channel to study blood flow and distribution. Doppler ultrasound probes passed down the biopsy channels (Fig. 115-3) can detect the flow in blood vessels below the mucosa, such as varices, or in an artery in the base of an ulcer. Doppler devices can be used before and after endoscopic hemostatic therapy, specifically with injection sclerotherapy for varices and injection or thermal therapy for an artery in the base of an ulcer. The Doppler probes have a circumferential radiating pattern (i.e., Doppler signal) and have a controllable depth of acoustic interrogation.[22-24] It is also possible to use a laser Doppler device to measure mucosal red blood cell velocity, a parameter thought to correlate with mucosal blood flow. The acoustic and laser techniques require the probe to touch the target mucosa.[25]

Reflectance spectrophotoscopy can also be achieved by passing a probe down an endoscope biopsy channel to touch the mucosa gently and measure mucosal oxygen saturation and hemoglobin concentration.[26] The videoendoscope can be used to calculate the red to green signal ratio and estimate mucosal blood hemoglobin.[27] This method assumes that hemoglobin is the predominant light-absorbing pigment in the mucosa and that the degree of absorption of light is proportional to the amount of hemoglobin present.

Endoscopic Ultrasonography

Endoscopists are limited to inspection of the mucosal surface. By combining endoscopy with ultrasound, it is possible to look below the surface at lesions of the intestinal wall and at lesions involving adjacent structures. There are two approaches to this combination of technologies. In the first approach, the endoscope has an ultrasound device built into the tip of the endoscope (Fig. 115-4). In the second approach, an endoscopic catheter is passed down the biopsy channel of the endoscope, and the examiner is able to obtain an image by moving the tip of the endoscope in and out or by rotating and creating a sector scan. Ultrasound permits analysis of the layers of the intestinal wall and of contiguous organs. By taking the ultrasound transducer adjacent to the intestinal target, it is possible to use high frequency and obtain high resolution. It is also possible to reduce problems with percutaneous ultrasound involving intestinal gas, intervening bony structures between the transducer and the target, and the need for deep penetration.

Endoscopic ultrasound may help to detect and determine the stage of an early malignancy in the intestinal tract, to stage advanced malignancy in the intestinal tract, and to guide therapy of these lesions (e.g., with endoscopic lasers), and it is useful for the differential diagnosis of lesions such as large folds, submucosal nodules, mucosal indentations, and mucosal vascular structures (Fig. 115-5).[28,29] Puncture of tissue using ultrasound guidance allows histologic and cytologic samples to be obtained from wall abnormalities and possible metastases to adjacent lymph nodes.[29]

Dye Scattering

Dye scattering (i.e., chromoendoscopy) is an in vivo technique in which dye is scattered on the mucosa to study and outline the fine detail of the target structure or to enhance the ability to detect a particular lesion.[30] The dye solution can be swallowed by the patient before endoscopy, or the dye can be sprayed against the mucosa using a catheter passed down the

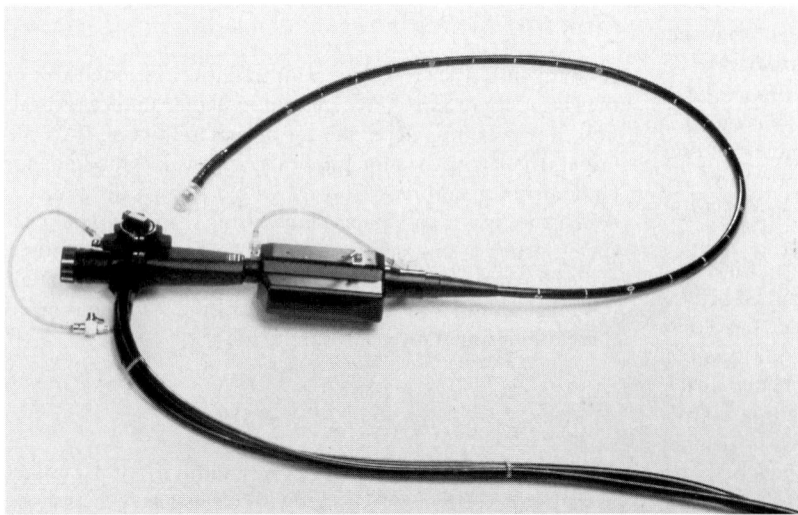

FIGURE 115-4. Instrument for endoscopic ultrasonography. The echo source is built in at the tip of the instrument. The box along the shaft contains the motor, which drives the echo for radial sector scanning.

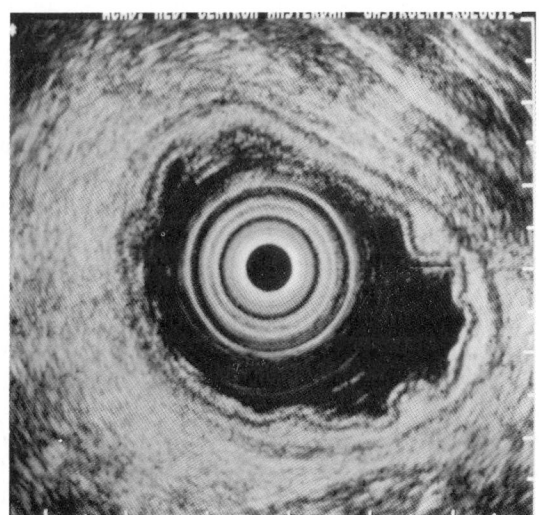

FIGURE 115-5. Endosonographic image of the five-layer structure of the gastric wall.

biopsy channel of the endoscope. If the dye is taken orally, it is important to reposition the patient to ensure that the entire gastric mucosa is coated. The dyes most often reported to be useful are 1% to 2% Lugol's solution, 1% to 2% methylene blue, 0.2% to 0.3% indigo-carmine, 1% to 2% toluidine blue, and 0.3% Congo red. Before using any of these dyes, it is necessary to reduce mucus in the stomach. This is often accomplished using a solution of dimethyl polysiloxane, sodium bicarbonate, and pronase. A 10% solution of N-acetylcysteine can be used before spraying the dye as an alternative method.[31]

Vital Staining

The dye is absorbed by epithelial cells but may also penetrate necrotic tissue. One or two minutes after spraying, the mucosa is washed with water and the surface can be observed.

Lugol's solution stains intracellular glycogen in nonkeratinized squamous epithelium. Metaplastic columnar epithelium in the esophagus or injured squamous mucosa does not stain. Esophageal cancer does not stain with Lugol's solution. Lugol's solution is not useful for detecting areas of dysplasia in squamous epithelium. Methylene blue dye detects columnar epithelium but not squamous epithelium. Congo red stains the acid-producing parietal cell mucosa; after the dye is acidified it turns from red to dark blue. Because toluidine blue stains nuclear DNA more strongly than cytoplasmic RNA, dysplastic or neoplastic cells stain blue.

It is not clear under what clinical circumstances vital staining is useful. The possibilities include looking for plaques overlying varices, studying the esophageal mucosa in patients with cancer of the head and neck, and studying esophageal mucosal abnormalities in patients who are alcoholic and smokers. This type of staining may help to delineate a neoplasm of the esophagus or to rule out a synchronous lesion or an area of dysplasia. Vital staining in the stomach may be useful in a nonhealing ulcer if early gastric cancer is suspected or to study an area of mucosal abnormality such as scarring of the mucosal surface or irregularities of the color of the

surface. Vital staining may help to detect or rule out areas of dysplasia or malignancy.

Contrast Chromoendoscopy

Dyes can be used to accentuate irregularities in mucosal architecture by accumulating in normal mucosal structures and accentuating small lesions. This is best achieved using indigo-carmine or methylene blue (Fig. 115-6; see Color Fig. 81).

Removal of Foreign Bodies

Not all ingested foreign bodies require removal, but some foreign bodies that are impacted or have sharp aspects should be removed. An immediate clinical concern is impaction of a foreign body in the esophagus or hypopharynx. Profuse salivation in a patient is considered a clinical sign of esophageal obstruction that must be addressed immediately. Experienced clinicians know that flexible endoscopes cannot remove all foreign bodies safely. An irregular, sharp object, an object with a ragged surface, or an object that is impacted in the wall (e.g., dental plate) may require a rigid esophagoscope to be passed under general anesthesia for removal of the foreign body. During removal of a foreign body, it is essential to protect the airway of the patient. An overtube provides a degree of protection of the airway by preventing dropping of the foreign body during removal, but the only way to ensure complete airway patency is to use a cuffed endotracheal tube.

Flexible endoscopes are the preferred method for foreign body removal. The exception is foreign bodies located in the hypopharynx or the area of the cricopharyngeal muscle. These foreign bodies are better removed by an ear, nose, and throat surgeon using direct laryngoscopy. However, the removal of most other foreign bodies in the esophagus, stomach, and

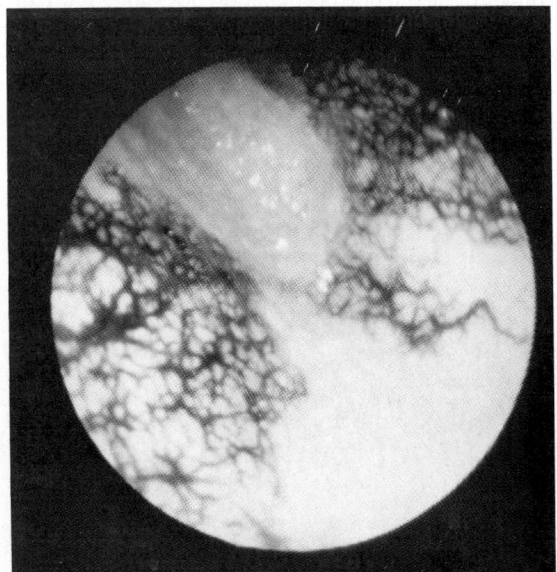

FIGURE 115-6. (See Color Fig. 81.) Methylene blue staining reveals villus atrophy as a result of gluten enteropathy.

duodenum can be accomplished by the gastrointestinal endoscopist. Open surgical removal is necessary in approximately 1% of cases. These procedures require a series of instruments that can be passed down the endoscope biopsy channel to grasp and hold the foreign bodies. These include baskets of the Dormia type, forceps for grasping the foreign body, and polypectomy snares. Most of these instruments can pass down a standard endoscope biopsy channel, which is 2.8 mm in diameter. Coins are best grasped using alligator forceps with teeth. These forceps are also useful for other types of smooth objects. If an object is irregular or soft, a variety of other devices can be used, such as baskets, snares, and graspers with three prongs.

If the foreign body is sharp, a plastic overtube can be used on the endoscope (Fig. 115-7). The endoscope can be withdrawn into the overtube while grasping the foreign body, which protects the mucosa from injury by the sharp foreign body as it is being removed. This also eliminates the possibility of dropping the foreign body in the hypopharynx, causing pulmonary aspiration of the object. The overtube is useful if the endoscope must be passed several times for removal of a foreign body, such as a piece of meat.

Most experienced endoscopists practice before attempting foreign body removal. A foreign body similar to that swallowed by the patient is manipulated with the type of instrument available to grasp the foreign body during endoscopy. This time spent in forethought and planning makes the foreign body removal safer and easier.[32]

Endoscopic Control of Upper Gastrointestinal Bleeding

Upper gastrointestinal bleeding is a commonly encountered problem in clinical medicine. Most endoscopists prefer that patients with upper gastrointestinal bleeding undergo diagnostic upper endoscopy because, for approximately 85% to 95% of these patients, a precise diagnosis of the cause of the bleeding can be obtained with endoscopy. For a few patients with massive hemorrhage, emergency surgery may be required, although it may be possible to perform the endoscopy immediately before the patient's surgery. In most bleeders, endoscopy can be performed as soon as the patient is stabilized hemodynamically. The appearance of the base of the lesion

helps to determine whether it is the bleeding source. Active bleeding with oozing or spurting is obviously helpful diagnostically, as is the presence of an adherent clot in the base of the ulcer, which is often adherent to the side of the bleeding artery. The presence of this visible vessel or a dark spot in an ulcer also suggests that this is the bleeding lesion.[33]

Bleeding lesions discovered during endoscopy can be divided into variceal and nonvariceal lesions. In a patient with bleeding varices, the esophagus and stomach are examined for varices and for portal hypertensive or congestive gastropathy. Varices are assessed by size (e.g., small, medium, large) and the presence of red color signs on the surface of the varix (e.g., red wale markings, hematocystic spots, cherry red spots).[34]

Sclerotherapy is commonly used for bleeding esophageal varices. The agent injected varies. In Europe, ethoxysclerol or polidocanol (1%) is used; in the United States, sodium morrhuate or 5% ethanolamine is used.[35] Usually, an intravariceal technique is used in which the needle is inserted into the varix and the injection is made directly into the vein (Fig. 115-8; see Color Fig. 82).[2] Limiting the length of the sclerotherapy needle to less than 5 mm reduces the likelihood of esophageal perforation. Most endoscopists limit the total volume of sclerosant to 30 mL in one sclerotherapy session. It is important that the endoscopy assistant and the endoscopist agree on instructions to be used during injection such as "needle in" and "needle out." Substantial bleeding sometimes occurs after the needle is removed from the varix; in this case, the endoscope should be advanced beyond the site of the injection to tamponade the bleeding area. Sclerotherapy sessions should usually be spaced at least 3 days apart.

Hemostasis is achieved in more than 80% of patients, with a complication rate of approximately 5%. Complications of sclerotherapy include ulceration, esophageal stricture, and rarely, perforation. Complete eradication of the varices is the goal. The endoscopist tries to accomplish eradication as quickly as possible, because most rebleeding episodes occur within the first 6 weeks of the initial bleed. Immediate hemostasis of massive variceal bleeding is possible by injecting N-butyl-2-cyanoacrylate (histoacryl), a tissue adhesive.[36,37] Isobutylcyanoacrylate is an aqueous solution that can be injected through an endoscopic catheter. It is recommended that this solution be injected intravariceally, 0.5 to 1.0 mL

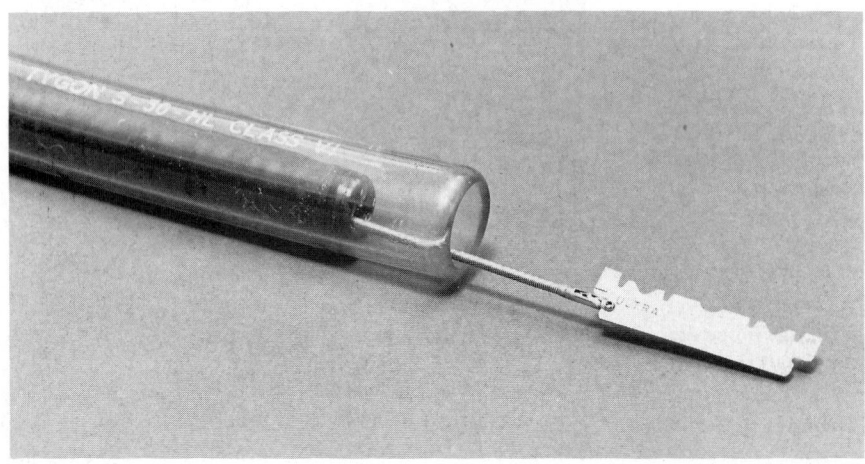

FIGURE 115-7. A plastic overtube around the endoscope allows safe retrieval of sharp or pointed foreign bodies.

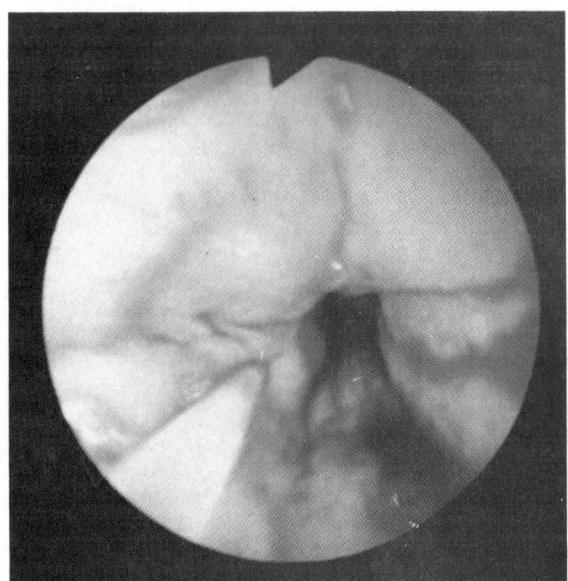

FIGURE 115-8. (See Color Fig. 82.) In the technique of endoscopic sclerotherapy, the sclerotherapy needle is inserted in the variceal structure.

per injection site, to obliterate the varix. The injection must be fairly rapid because the solution solidifies within 20 seconds in a moist environment. Typically, after several days, the adhesive and surrounding tissue slough and disappear into the lumen.

A newer type of therapy for esophageal varices is that of variceal banding or ligation. In this technique, a cylinder is attached to the endoscope tip. A varix is pulled into the cylinder at the tip of the endoscope by suction and a rubber band is placed on the base of the varix. This banded varix undergoes necrosis and sloughs. An overtube is used to allow multiple passages of the endoscope for placing bands and to protect the airway and oral pharynx.[38] Variceal banding is thought by many endoscopists to be a more reliably effective technique that is easier to apply and less prone to complications such as deep ulceration than is sclerotherapy.

For the endoscopic therapy of nonvariceal lesions, there are many potential approaches. Injection therapy using adrenaline (1:10,000) or adrenaline plus 1% ethoxysclerol directly around the bleeding artery is becoming increasingly popular and seems to be effective and safe.[39–41] The exact mechanism of action of injection therapy is unknown but may include mechanical compression of the bleeding vessel and vasoconstriction or fixation of the tissue by the sclerosant. Other techniques for controlling bleeding include electrocoagulation using monopolar probes, bipolar probes, and monopolar electrical probes with a liquid flow, referred to as electrohydrothermal probes.[42–45] The initial hemostasis rate is reported to be higher than 80% for these devices, and the overall success rate has been approximately 90%. These methods are relatively safe and cost effective. The probes may adhere to the coagulated tissue, and the problem of rebleeding also exists, but in many cases, the probe can be used again to control rebleeding.

Another approach to thermal endoscopic hemostasis is the heater probe. The tip of this device is covered with a nonad-

hering surface. The probe heats rapidly to deliver a preset number of joules of energy to the target tissue. It is thought that the optimal method of applying this probe, as with electrocautery probes, is to compress or coapt the vessel before heating. This coaptation reduces blood flow and prevents the heat sink effect of flowing blood. The hemostatic seal is better with coaptive coagulation.[46–49] A water jet is used to clear the lesion of blood before therapy.

Endoscopic hemostatic therapy can be accomplished with laser photocoagulation of bleeding lesions. The laser most often used is the neodymium:yttrium-aluminum-garnet (Nd:YAG) system. A theoretical advantage of the laser system is that no contact is made between the tip of the laser delivery catheter and the bleeding target. As with the contact probe, initial hemostatic effectiveness is approximately 90%. Laser photocoagulation can reduce the risk of rebleeding from visible vessels in the base of peptic ulcers, but with spurting arterial lesions there is a high rebleeding rate after treatment with the Nd:YAG laser.[50,51] The disadvantages of lasers are that they are expensive and are not especially portable. For these reasons, the heater probe, electrocautery probes, and injection therapy are more convenient and cost-effective endoscopic treatments for hemostasis.

A series of randomized, controlled clinical trials suggest that thermal coagulation with the heater probe and multipolar electrocoagulation probes is equally as effective as injection therapy for controlling bleeding ulcers. Injection therapy is selected for the initial therapy by some because it is inexpensive and can be performed easily even if the bleeding spot or bleeding vessel cannot be well visualized. In the case of an actively bleeding vessel on the base of a peptic ulcer, an injection of dilute adrenaline to a total of 10 to 20 mL seems to be effective. Adding a sclerosing agent is not more effective hemostatically. For a visible vessel in the base of an ulcer that is not bleeding, injection of dilute adrenaline followed by thermal coagulation or injection of a sclerosant to obliterate the bleeding vessel is recommended.

Polypectomy

If a polyp is encountered in the upper gastrointestinal tract, it should be removed so that a precise histologic diagnosis can be obtained and the symptoms caused by the polyp can be treated. Polypectomy is accomplished using a wire snare placed over the polyp and tightened at the base of the polyp. Snares of a variety of sizes and shapes are available. Shapes include a symmetric ellipse, a hexagon, and a slightly hooked configuration. After the handle is closed, the tip of the snare should retract at least 1 cm into the plastic overtube. A small snare may be used for removing small polyps. As the snare is tightened on the lesion, an electrocoagulative current is applied, alone or in combination with a cutting current, during the transection of the polyp.

The process of placing a snare on a polyp is not technically difficult. It often is difficult to decide whether the polyp is suitable for endoscopic removal. After this decision has been made and the loop has been passed over the polyp, it may be helpful to advance the plastic tube around the wire snare to the spot on the polyp at which the snare will be closed. As the loop is closed, it is possible to control where the transection occurs. As polypectomy is accomplished, the endoscopist can see a whitish discoloration on both sides of the loop, which indicates that coagulation is taking place.

Many polyps in the upper gastrointestinal tract are sessile rather than pedunculated (Fig. 115-9; see Color Fig. 83). There are two methods of removal: in a single piece or removal of multiple sections. If the polyp is to be removed in a single piece, the snare is placed over the polyp, and the wire is tightened at the junction of the base of the polyp and the wall. The polyp is gently pulled away from the wall to create a pseudopedicle, and electrical current is used to transect the polyp. Larger sessile tumors with a broad attachment can be removed, but the entire polyp is not removed in one transection. Electrosurgical current is used as each piece of polyp is snared and removed.

All portions of the polyp are removed until the area at the base of the lesion is free of polyp tissue. On occasion, these polyps are removed in several sessions. Bleeding or difficulty in visualization may mandate that the endoscopist stop after removal of several pieces of the polyp and reexamine the patient at a later date. After the area of the polypectomy is reinspected, there may be no residual polyp because of heating generated as the polypectomy snare was used to remove segments of the polyp during the first endoscopy. If tissue is left, it can be removed during the second endoscopy.[1,2,52]

The complications occurring with gastric polypectomy include hemorrhage and perforation. Because of the thickness of the gastric wall, perforation is unusual, but hemorrhage may be a significant problem.[53]

Dilation

Flexible endoscopy is playing an increasingly important role in dilating strictures. Endoscopically passed guidewires are used to guide the tip of the dilating device, especially in treating diverticula, eccentric strictures, tight or tortuous strictures (Fig. 115-10; see Color Fig. 84), and angulated strictures, such as those formed after surgical anastomosis.

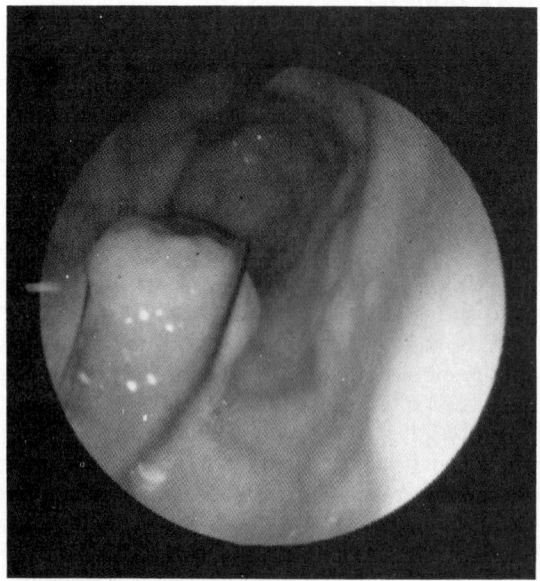

FIGURE 115-9. (See Color Fig. 83.) In polypectomy, the snare loop is positioned around the sessile, adenomatous, gastric polyp.

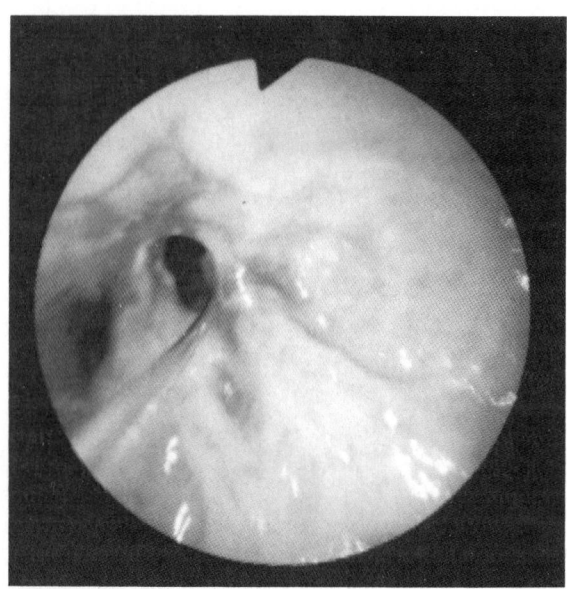

FIGURE 115-10. (See Color Fig. 84.) A guidewire has been passed through this eccentric, reflux-induced stricture.

The guidewire with a spring tip is passed by way of the endoscope. If the small-caliber endoscope can be passed through the stricture, the wire can be located below the narrowed area. If it is not possible to pass the endoscope through the stricture, the wire can be passed under direct endoscopic vision with fluoroscopic monitoring to ensure that the wire is correctly placed. The guidewire and the spring tip should remain below the area to be dilated throughout the procedure. Several different types of dilators are available, including the Savary-Gilliard and Celestin types.

Three dilators, gradually increasing in size, are passed per session, especially if there is moderate to severe resistance offered by the narrowed tissue. Repeat dilation occurs at intervals of 2 to 7 days. Usually, the last dilator used in the previous session is passed first on the next visit.[54,55] It is also possible to pass catheters with balloon tips through the biopsy channel of an endoscope to dilate strictures.[56] These balloons vary from 4 to 20 mm in diameter when fully inflated. The diameter of the balloon catheter that can be passed depends on the diameter of the channel in the endoscope. Some balloon catheters have a central channel that can be passed over a guidewire. In this case, the guidewire is passed endoscopically, the endoscope is removed, and the balloon catheter is passed over the guidewire without the endoscope in position. Fluoroscopy is used to guide the position of the balloon at the tip of the catheter.

The advantages and disadvantages of balloon dilation are discussed in Chapter 135. The direct pressure applied to the stricture in a circumferential pattern by the balloon may be an advantage compared with the shearing force created by the use of bougies. Balloons are especially useful for narrow, tortuous strictures. However, it may be difficult to keep a balloon in position if the stricture is irregular and tortuous, and the rigid stenotic segments may be difficult to dilate with balloons.

For tight fibrotic strictures less than 12 mm in diameter, the the Savary-Gilliard dilators are preferred. The safest dilation of tight strictures involves the use of a guidewire with fluoroscopic monitoring of the passage of the dilators and attention to tactile sensation by the endoscopist during the dilation. It is possible to use through-the-scope (TTS) balloon dilators in strictures that are asymmetric and 12 mm in diameter or larger. If fluoroscopy is not available and the endoscopist encounters an unexpected esophageal stricture, a TTS balloon that can be guided endoscopically may be the best method of dilating the stricture. The perforation rates for bougies are approximately 0.5%, and for balloons, the rates are 0.3% to 9.5%.[57]

Pyloric stenosis is often dilated with TTS balloons that are 3 cm long and have diameters from 9.9 to 17.8 mm (30–54 F). These balloons are best passed through a large-caliber endoscope instrument channel. It is mandatory to monitor passage of the balloon and its inflation with fluoroscopy to be certain that the waist of the balloon, representing the stricture, has been obliterated. If initial balloon dilation is not successful, dilation is often repeated with balloons passed over guidewires. In this case, the guidewire is placed into the second or third portion of the duodenum. Balloons with a diameter of 17.8 to 19.8 mm (54–60 F) are then passed over the guidewire. In 60% to 80% of patients, the dilation cures the pyloric stenosis with a low risk of complication.[58]

Stents

In some patients with cancer of the esophagus, nonsurgical palliation with stents may be the preferred method of treatment (Fig. 115-11). Endoscopy is critically important to diagnose the malignancy, evaluate the degree of narrowing, measure the length of the tumor narrowing, and determine the distance from the top of the tumor to the incisor teeth, an important factor in placing the prosthesis.

An endoscope usually cannot be passed through the lumen of a patient presenting with an obstructing tumor. In this circumstance, a guidewire is passed through the biopsy channel under endoscopic guidance. Fluoroscopy is used to follow the tip of the guidewire until it enters the stomach and is positioned on the greater curvature. The endoscope is removed, and the guidewire can be used to dilate the malignant narrowing with metal olives, balloons, or Savary-Gilliard bougies.

After the length of the stricture is determined, the prosthesis length should be long enough to include 2.5 to 3 cm proximal to the narrowing and the same distance distal to the narrowing to prevent early restenosis by tumor. Stents that can be placed in the esophagus include nonexpandable and expandable devices. The nonexpandable prosthesis can be made from inexpensive polyvinyl tubing. Usually, tubing with an outer diameter of 18.7 mm and an inner diameter of 12.5 mm is used. These devices can be obtained commercially (Fig. 115-12). These prostheses are inserted using an introducing device, which can be a balloon, a bougie, a Keymed introducer, a small-diameter endoscope, or an Amsterdam introducer that has a flexible shaft.[59,60] The prosthesis is pushed into position using a pusher tube such that the funnel on the proximal end rests on the beginning of the stenosing tumor mass. For a malignant fistula, a Wilson-Cook fistula prosthesis is used. In this device, a sponge placed circumferentially around the prosthesis expands to close the fistulous tract after a vacuum is released.

Self-expanding metal stents (e.g., Wall, Gianturoco, Ul-

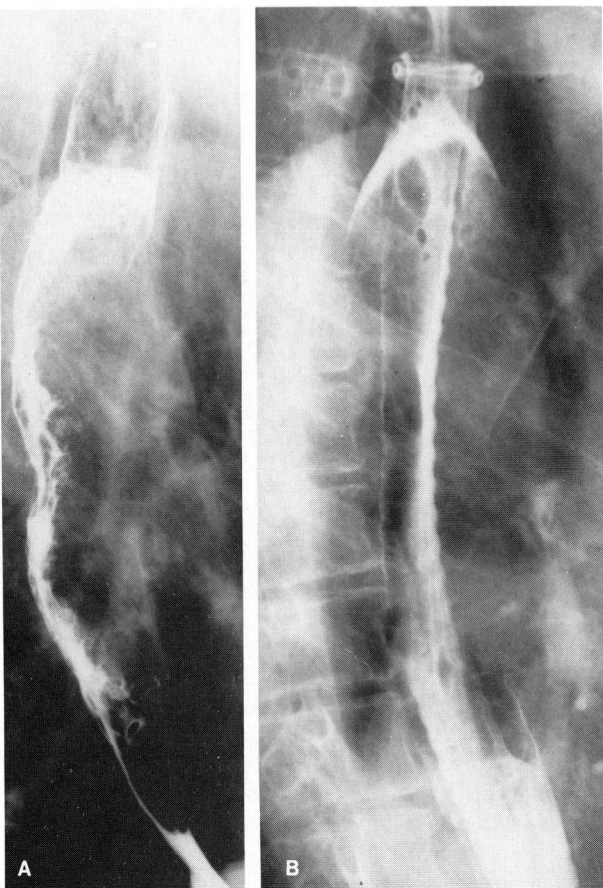

FIGURE 115-11. Esophageal carcinoma (**A**) before and (**B**) after stenting with a Tygon endoprosthesis.

traflex) have been introduced. These stents are made of thin stainless steel wire shaped with zig-zag bands or a mesh formed into a cylinder. The ends of the steel wires are soldered so that it is smooth. These devices are passed over a guidewire through the malignant narrowing, with a sheath covering the compressed stent. After the constraining sheath is released, the stent is left in place and expands. Some stent designs, such as Wall and Ultraflex stents, shorten to 40% of their original length as they assume their final shape. The expanding stents have the advantage of producing a wide lumen through the stenosing tumor mass without having to dilate the tumor before placement. However, these stents are not removable. Stents covered by a silicone membrane are being evaluated. These devices may prevent tumor ingrowth, which has been a problem in the expandable stents. If the esophageal lumen obstructs again after tumor ingrowth or if a fistula forms, a plastic stent can be inserted into the original expandable stent lumen. The self-expanding stents are expensive.

Laser Tumor Ablation

An endoscope can be used to guide an Nd:YAG laser to open a lumen obstructed by tumor. A typical laser delivery fiber is used, including a jet of gas to keep the fiber tip clean. Safety considerations for the patient, staff, and endoscopist are extremely important, including the use of appropriate filters and safety goggles.

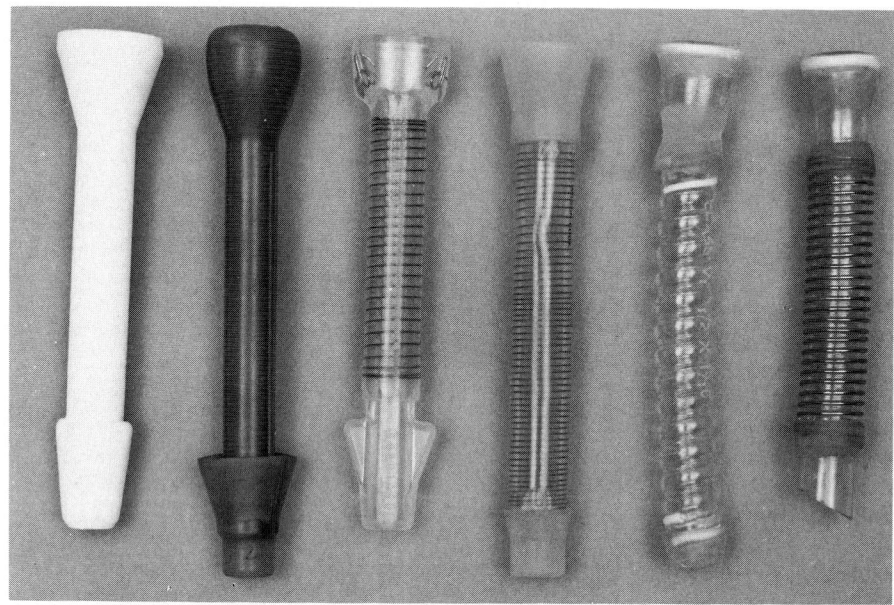

FIGURE 115-12. The endoprostheses most commonly used are (*left to right*) Key-Med, Celestin, Eska-Buess, Wilson-Cook, regular Tygon, and reinforced Tygon with metal spiral.

The goal of laser therapy is to remove tumor tissue with as small a risk of perforation as possible. The current recommendation is to start coagulating at the distal portion of the tumor so that this tissue can slough and pass down the gastrointestinal tract. This may require dilating the tumor before laser therapy.[61-65] If it is not possible to dilate the tumor, it may be necessary to begin laser coagulation at the proximal margin. This is more difficult, because it may not be clear where the lumen is, and tissue edema from tumor nodules may impair passage of the endoscope to the more distal portions of the tumor. In general, the laser is applied in a circumferential pattern for a tumor that extends around the circumference of the esophagus. To avoid evaporation and cavitation, the laser beam should not be focused on one spot for a long time. Treated areas appear necrotic and yellow-white. If the tumor does not slough spontaneously, this tissue is gently removed before further treatment with the laser.

An alternative method of applying laser photocoagulation is with contact laser probes, which use lower power. These probes have a tip made of ceramic or sapphire attached to the tip of the quartz fiber delivery system. The laser energy affects the tumor by the combined direct mechanical effect of the hot tip of the probe to the tissue and delivery of heat through photocoagulation.

For small tumors of the esophagus and stomach, photodynamic therapy may be used. A photosensitizing agent, such as a hematoporphyrin derivative, is injected intravenously and is taken up in high concentration in the area of the tumor. A light is used to activate the agent by selecting an appropriate frequency for the particular drug. This produces a cytotoxic singlet oxygen, resulting in necrosis of the tumor.[66] A dye laser is commonly used.

Local Irradiation Tumor Therapy

Cesium or iridium can be used to treat a tumor using intracavitary radiotherapy.[67] This therapy requires precise positioning of the applicator into the area of the tumor. Endoscopy is used to place a guidewire, over which the applicator is passed. Fluoroscopy documents the exact locations of guidewire, applicator, and tumor. The applicator probe is fixed in position by attachment to a face mask. The patient is transferred to the treatment area, and the position of the applicator is confirmed by fluoroscopy before passage of the radioactive compound for therapy.

Thermal Tumor Therapy

Direct heat can also be used to treat tumors for palliation. One device for this application is a bipolar device (BICAP) located on a conventional olive dilator. The bipolar electrodes are arranged as stripes around the entire circumference of the olive or a portion of the circumference. Diameters of the probes vary from 6 to 15 mm. A guidewire is passed endoscopically through the narrowed lumen, the endoscope is removed, and the tumor probe is passed over the guidewire.[68,69] It is possible to pass a small endoscope next to the BICAP shaft to observe coagulation of the proximal tumor margin. The distal tumor margin is treated by bringing the probe up into the tumor at distances appropriate to cause overlapping coagulation through the narrow tumor segment.

PATIENT PREPARATION

Before endoscopy is performed, patients should be asked about pertinent medical illnesses, previous endoscopic procedures, previous gastrointestinal surgery, and medications, especially those that may be related to gastrointestinal tract inflammation or irritation or interfere with coagulation. It is essential to know if the patient has a history of dysphagia, because this may give an indication that the person has a Zenker's diverticulum, another type of diverticulum, or a history of aspiration. Aspiration suggests a fistula in a patient with a cervical or thoracic malignancy or inflammatory disease.

The physician should know about bleeding tendencies in the patient or the patient's family and about any history of drug allergies. If there is a history of bleeding abnormalities, a clotting screen with a prothrombin time, partial thromboplastin time, platelet count, and bleeding time is indicated. If there is evidence of chronic liver disease or other hematologic disorder, it is important to check coagulation.

Diagnostic endoscopy with biopsy is usually safe in patients who are taking oral anticoagulants. The endoscope should be passed gently, using the direct vision technique. However, for a patient who is to be treated with electrocoagulation for polypectomy or hemostasis, anticoagulants should be discontinued before the endoscopic procedure and for as long as 2 weeks after the procedure to prevent delayed bleeding. Aspirin-containing compounds and other antiplatelet agents such as nonsteroidal antiinflammatory drugs and ticlopidine should be avoided for an appropriate interval (i.e., aspirin for 7–10 days; nonsteroidals for 2–3 days) before an endoscopic procedure that may involve biopsy or removal of tissue.

The patient must provide written or verbal informed consent before the procedure.

Most patients are examined and begin fasting after midnight the evening before the endoscopy. The patient should have no liquids for 4 hours before endoscopy and no solids for at least 6 to 8 hours beforehand. Patients with gastric outlet obstruction may be kept on a clear liquid diet for 24 to 48 hours, and lavage of the stomach with a large-bore tube may be necessary to remove retained stomach contents.

Medications may be given before upper endoscopic procedures to anesthetize the posterior pharynx, reduce anxiety, reduce discomfort, and diminish motility and secretions. Which medications are used depends on the clinical situation, including the patient's age, the existence of debilitating diseases, the anxiety level of the patient, the medication, and the patient's history of alcohol use. Upper gastrointestinal endoscopy is almost never performed with general anesthesia, with certain exceptions such as removal of foreign bodies in small children.

For endoscopic procedures that are expected to be brief and in which small-caliber endoscopes are used, no intravenous sedation may be necessary unless the patient is anxious. For therapeutic procedures that involve larger-diameter instruments and longer periods, the patient is usually given intravenous sedation. Physicians and endoscopy assistants must monitor the patient during the endoscopy for evidence of excessive sedation caused by the medication. Physicians and assistants should be up to date in cardiopulmonary resuscitation, and the equipment necessary for resuscitation must be immediately accessible.

After the procedures, patients must be observed as they recover from sedation. The patient should not drive for 24 hours after receiving intravenous sedation. Many units give the patient written instructions after the procedure in the event that the patient does not remember what he or she is told while still under the effect of sedation.

Bacteremia may be associated with endoscopic procedures. In a patient with a preexisting heart condition, there may be risk of developing infectious endocarditis, although this risk is small. The efficacy of antibiotic prophylaxis for endocarditis is unproven, although prophylaxis appears to be effective in patients with prosthetic valves. Prophylactic antibiotics are advised for patients with known endocarditis or prosthetic cardiac valves.[70] For gastrointestinal endoscopic procedures, the standard regimen is 2 g of ampicillin, administered intravenously or intramuscularly, plus gentamicin (1.5 mg/kg, not to exceed 80 mg), administered intravenously or intramuscularly 30 minutes before the procedure, followed by 1.5 g of amoxicillin taken orally 6 hours after the initial medication. Alternatively, the parenteral regimen may be repeated once 8 hours after the initial dose.

INDICATIONS FOR UPPER ENDOSCOPY

Endoscopy is a highly accurate method of evaluating the mucosal surface of the esophagus, stomach, and duodenum. In addition to the various indications discussed in this section, endoscopy is used to evaluate the patient with upper gastrointestinal symptoms before barium radiography is performed. This approach is referred to as primary panendoscopy. In many centers, the cost of this primary endoscopy is reduced, because it can often be performed quickly and without any sedation. However, it is still important for the endoscopist to evaluate the patient before the procedure.

Dysphagia

Dysphagia is an important symptom in gastroenterology that mandates a full evaluation, and endoscopy is critical in the evaluation of these symptoms.[71] Some endoscopists think a barium esophagogram should be performed before endoscopy, but endoscopy may be the first diagnostic test in a patient with dysphagia. In a patient whose symptoms suggest dysphagia caused by Zenker's diverticulum, it is essential to have a barium esophagogram study before endoscopy to avoid injury to the diverticulum during passage of the endoscope.

If a patient has symptoms referable to the pharynx or neck, enlarged cervical lymph nodes, or neck pain, evaluation should be done first with direct inspection of the larynx, pharynx, and nasal passages. Flexible endoscopy is of limited value in examining the pharynx and hypopharynx. It is possible to view lesions that cause dysphagia endoscopically, including reflux-induced strictures (see Fig. 115-10; see Color Fig. 84), caustic injury strictures, strictures resulting from radiation, achalasia, and benign (Fig. 115-13; see Color Fig. 85) and malignant tumors.

Esophageal Cancer

A patient often presents with esophageal cancer after the malignancy is far advanced. Advanced cancers have three morphologic appearances (Fig. 115-14; see Color Fig. 86). A tumor that is nodular and friable with a hemorrhagic surface with ulcers or erosions is referred to as *exophytic* and has a wide base. The second type of tumor, in which the lesion is an ulcer with heaped-up surrounding edges, is referred to as *ulcerative*. The third morphologic presentation is a thickened, rigid length of esophageal wall caused by infiltrating cancer, referred to as an *infiltrating* type, in which the mucosa is often nodular and appears fixed.

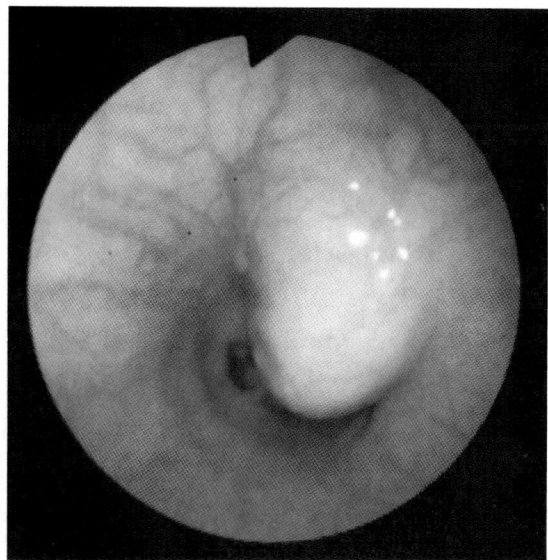

FIGURE 115-13. (See Color Fig. 85.) Esophageal leiomyoma.

The diagnosis of esophageal cancer requires multiple endoscopic biopsies. Obtaining tissue for a good histologic examination is occasionally difficult because of overlying inflammatory exudate, but in most polypoid tumors, biopsies are positive because the proximal tumor edge is visible and can be directly targeted. If the approach to the lesion is tangential, it may help to use a biopsy forceps with a central spike. An alternative is to use needle cytology. If nodular lesions are proximal to the main lesion, a biopsy should be performed, because they may represent intramural metastasis from the primary tumor.

If the lesion appears as a narrowing or stenosis, it may be difficult to obtain positive biopsy specimens. In this instance, multiple biopsies and brush cytologies may be necessary to make a precise diagnosis. There are two approaches to ob-

taining tissue from the narrowed area. The first is to use a small-diameter endoscope, which can be passed through the stenotic segment and can obtain biopsy specimens from the entire length of the stenosis. If the stenosis is too tight to permit even a small-caliber endoscope, it may be possible to obtain brush cytology samples from the narrowing and perform a biopsy at the proximal edge. The second approach is to perform dilation of the narrowed segment before performing biopsy and cytology procedures. By dilating up to a diameter of 10 mm, it is possible to pass a small-caliber endoscope through the length of the lesion and obtain biopsy specimens from the proximal and distal edges and along the length of the stenosis.

Overall, a correct diagnosis for esophageal cancer is made in more than 90% of patients if six or more biopsies are performed and if cytologic samples are examined. Multiple biopsies are especially important if there is a large amount of necrotic tumor and exudate.[72]

Reflux Esophagitis

Not all patients with esophageal reflux symptoms require endoscopy. If a patient has a chronic or intermittent symptom complex, if the symptoms are not controlled using standard antireflux measures, or if the symptoms occur at night and cause difficulty with coughing, hoarseness, and aspiration, endoscopy may be indicated. Of the patients who present with reflux symptoms, approximately one half have endoscopic evidence of mucosal injury in the distal esophagus. The purpose of endoscoping the patient is to detect this injury, to grade the severity of acid-pepsin or alkaline-induced injury, and to detect esophageal columnar metaplasia in the distal esophagus.

It is possible during endoscopy to diagnose hiatal hernia. The ora serrata or the squamocolumnar junction is identified. The level of the diaphragmatic impression must also be located, if necessary by having the patient sniff during assessment. If, during quiet observation without excessive distention of the esophagus with air, the squamocolumnar junction is more than 2 to 3 cm above the diaphragm, this condition probably represents an axial hiatal hernia. The hernia appears endoscopically to be a pouch or widening just below the mucosal junction and just above the diaphragm. After the instrument is passed into the stomach and is retroflexed, it is possible to examine the cardia from below and diagnose a hiatal hernia.

Grading of reflux mucosal injury may be accomplished by several schemes, but the modified Savary system is often used. One difference between the various rating approaches is whether equivocal changes are included. These changes include erythema, friability, and blurring of the ora serrata. To reconcile the existing systems, the system shown in Table 115-1 has been proposed: grade 0, normal; grade 1, equivocal changes; grade 2, solitary erosion; grade 3, confluent erosion; grade 4, circumferential erosion; grade 5, ulceration; grade 6, strictures. Any degree of abnormality can exist with or without a columnar segment (Fig. 115-15; see Color Fig. 87).[73]

The sentinel fold or polyp is an abnormality found in some patients with a hiatal hernia. It is a fold with a polypoid proximal margin that is located just distal to the squamocolumnar junction. There is often a small erosion or ulcer on the prox-

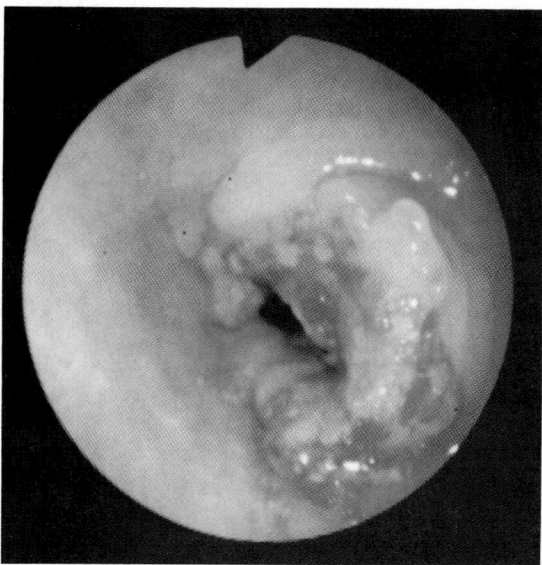

FIGURE 115-14. (See Color Fig. 86.) Esophageal carcinoma obstructs the esophagus.

TABLE 115-1
Grading of Reflux Esophagitis

GRADE	DESCRIPTION*
0	No evidence of reflux-induced damage: crisp, sharply delineated squamocolumnar junction. No evidence of friability: smooth and shiny squamous mucosa in the distal esophagus.
1	Mild, patchy or more diffuse erythema at the level of the squamocolumnar junction; slight blurring of the squamocolumnar junction; minor friability; loss of shininess of the distal squamous mucosa. Such abnormalities are equivocal and cannot be interpreted as genuinely characteristic for reflux-induced damage. There is no apparent break in the mucosa.
2	One or more discrete superficial erosions, seen as red dots or streaks, with or without adherent whitish exudate. Such linear erosions are usually small and often on top of the esophageal folds. They involve less than 10% of the mucosal surface of less than the distal 5 cm of the squamous segment of the esophagus above the gastroesophageal junction.
3	Confluent but noncircumferential erosions seen as defects that merge either longitudinally or laterally. There may be additional exudate covering the erosive defects or slough formation. Less than 50% of the overall mucosal surface of the distal 5 cm is involved.
4	Circumferential erosions or exudative lesions at the level of the squamocolumnar junction, regardless of the extent along the distal esophagus.
5	Deep ulceration anywhere along the esophagus.
6	Various degrees of stricturing, prohibiting passage of a standard (>9 mm) or small-caliber (<9 mm) endoscope.

* Grades 1 through 6 can be present with or without a segment of columnar metaplasia.

Adapted from Armstrong D, Monnier P, Nicolet M, et al. Endoscopic assessment of oesophagitis. Gullet 1990;1:63.

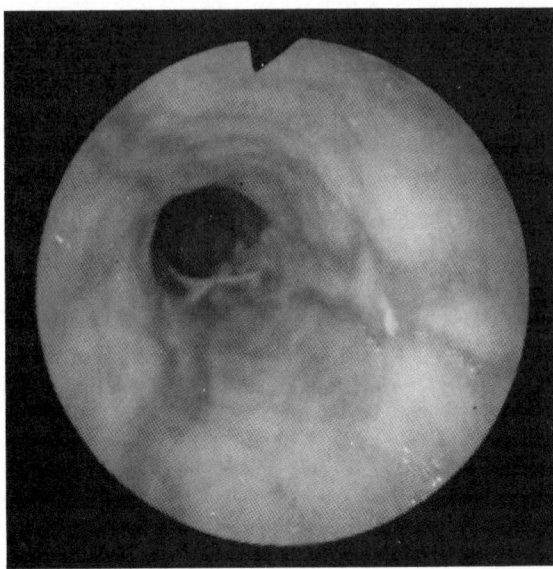

FIGURE 115-15. (See Color Fig. 87.) Reflux esophagitis, grade II, with confluent but noncircumferential erosions.

imal tip of the fold, which may be seen in a patient with a hiatal hernia and reflux.

Esophageal Columnar Metaplasia

Esophageal columnar metaplasia, also called Barrett's metaplasia, is a change in the normal appearance of the esophagus; the mucosa that is normally stratified squamous is replaced by a columnar mucosa. The normal ora serrata or squamocolumnar junction migrates proximally in the esophagus. The only way to determine the anatomic junction of the esophagus and the stomach is that this junction occurs just proximal to the gastric folds.[74] This is a useful landmark, because the distance from the incisor teeth to the proximal margin of the gastric folds does not vary and should be consistent from one endoscopy to the next.

The distance from the squamocolumnar junction to the proximal gastric folds usually is less than 2 cm. If the distance from the squamocolumnar junction to the proximal gastric folds in a hiatal hernia is longer than 2 cm, it usually means

that there is a segment of columnar metaplastic mucosa (Fig. 115-16; see Color Fig. 88). If specialized or intestinal-type columnar metaplastic epithelium is found, the examiner can then identify even a short segment of Barrett's metaplasia. The squamocolumnar junction often moves proximally; it may remain relatively linear or may be irregular with small islands of the pearly white squamous mucosa at the junction.

It is often possible to observe that the tubular esophagus is lined with a columnar epithelium that appears salmon pink instead of the normal pearly white of the squamous mucosa of the esophagus. Single or multiple ulcerations may be found in the columnar metaplastic segment.[73] Barrett's metaplasia is considered a premalignant condition of the esophagus. It is essential to diagnose early malignancies in Barrett's

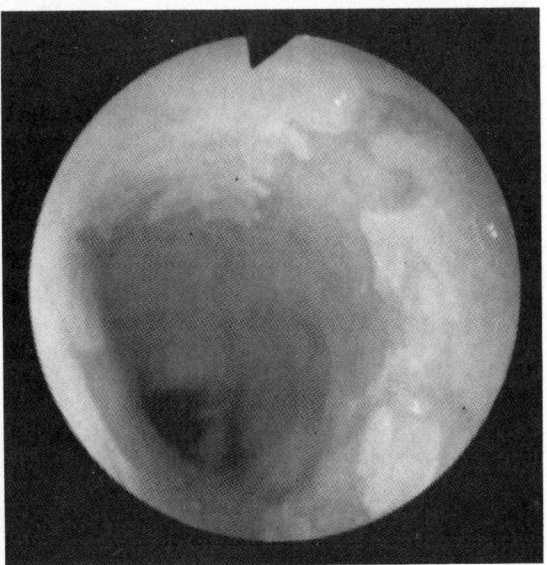

FIGURE 115-16. (See Color Fig. 88.) A columnar cell–lined esophagus, also known as Barrett's esophagus.

metaplasia to increase the likelihood of treatment for cure. One half of these areas of early tumor are virtually invisible to endoscopic inspection and require biopsies for diagnosis.[75-78]

Biopsy is not routinely performed in patients with reflux esophageal symptoms unless columnar metaplasia is suspected. In a patient with reflux esophagitis, periodic endoscopy is not required. Exceptions are patients who have not responded to therapy, especially if they have severe esophagitis; patients who are being considered for surgery; and patients who are to undergo any surgery for reflux, in whom presurgical endoscopy is indicated.

Dyspepsia

The symptom complex known as dyspepsia includes pain, burning in the epigastrium, nausea, epigastric fullness, and excessive gas. Only about 1 of 5 patients who present with these symptoms actually has a peptic ulcer. Endoscopy is a valuable tool in the evaluation of the patient with dyspepsia.

A full endoscopic work-up is indicated for patients who present with a complication of peptic ulcer or in whom dyspeptic symptoms recur rapidly after antiulcer drugs are stopped.[79] Endoscopy is often used as the first diagnostic procedure in these patients. Barium radiographs are less accurate, and if biopsy and cytology are necessary, endoscopy has to be performed after the barium radiograph.

Endoscopy is valuable in the evaluation of ulcer complications, including upper gastrointestinal bleeding and obstruction. In a patient who presents with gastric outlet obstruction, endoscopy can identify an ulcer and determine that the obstruction is not caused by another lesion. Balloon dilation can be performed under endoscopic guidance. The gastric outlet obstruction associated with ulceration may be caused by scarring or by inflammation and edema. If the patient presents with a possible perforation, endoscopy is contraindicated.

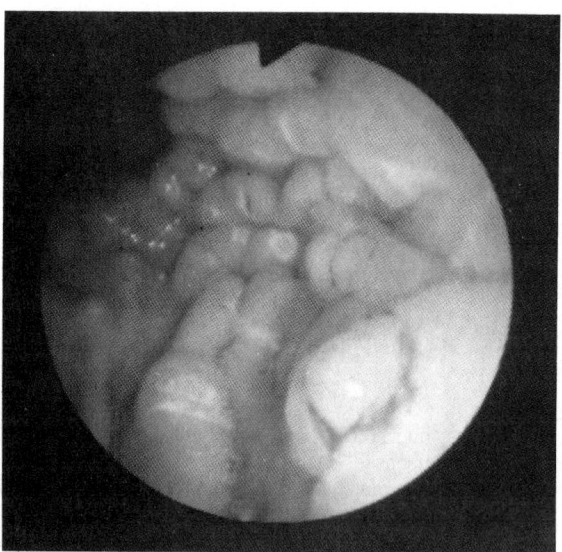

FIGURE 115-18. (See Color Fig. 90.) Endoscopic view of erosive gastritis.

The endoscopic result may be negative for patients with dyspepsia. It is possible to see abnormalities such as erythema and erosions without distinct ulceration. Some of these patients are found to have *Helicobacter pylori* infection after the area is biopsied and cultured. Gastritis may also be found in the body and fundus of the stomach (Fig. 115-17; see Color Fig. 89). Erosive gastritis may be observed in the stomachs of patients with dyspepsia. These erosions may occur anywhere in the stomach and are thought in some patients to be caused by ulcerogenic drugs (Fig. 115-18; see Color Fig. 90). The erosions typically have a white base surrounded by mucosal erythema. In evaluating a patient with dyspepsia, mucosal biopsies should be taken from the gastric antrum and the corpus.[80] Antral and some fundal biopsies should be obtained for *H pylori* culture, histologic examination, and urease testing.[81] *H pylori* is considered to be a major factor in peptic ulcer disease that is not associated with nonsteroidal antiinflammatory drugs.[81] The role of *H pylori* infection in nonulcer dyspepsia has not been determined.

Gastric Ulcers

Ulcers extend through the mucosa and the muscularis mucosae into the submucosa or the muscularis propria. Most often, these benign gastric ulcers are found close to the incisura or in the distal corpus of the stomach. The antrum just proximal to the pylorus is another common area of ulceration, especially of drug-induced ulceration. Ulcers occur in the upper portions of the stomach more commonly in elderly persons. If multiple ulcers are present, a drug-induced ulcer should be suspected.

Although occasionally a very large ulcer is discovered, most gastric ulcers have diameters less than 3 cm. Typically, an ulcer has a white base with erythematous mucosal margins. These margins are smooth and slightly raised in a benign gastric ulcer. It is important to examine the base of the ulcer to detect a sentinel clot or visible vessel and to measure the

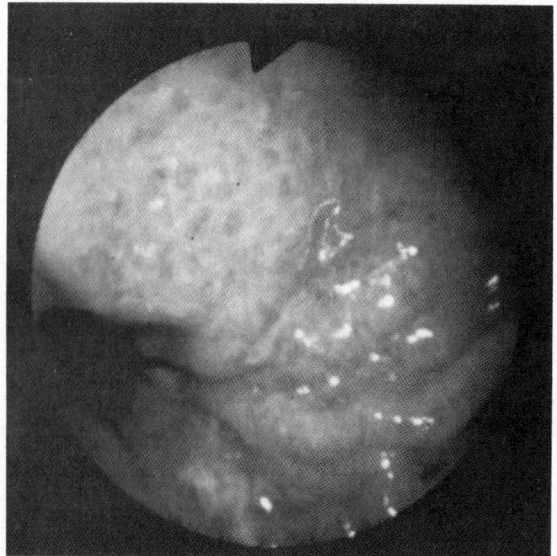

FIGURE 115-17. (See Color Fig. 89.) Endoscopy reveals gastritis with punctate erythema and swelling.

diameter of the ulcer. The folds surrounding a benign gastric ulcer usually radiate from the ulcer margin without intervening nodularity; nodularity raises the possibility of a malignant ulcer.

It is often impossible to be certain from the radiographic or endoscopic appearance that no malignancy is present in a gastric ulcer. Of those that appeared benign radiographically, 5% to 10% were found to be malignant in some studies. Endoscopy and biopsy are mandatory if the gastric ulcer radiographically appears to be indeterminate or suspicious (Fig. 115-19; see Color Fig. 91).

Under endoscopic guidance, the physician should obtain multiple biopsy specimens from the margin of a gastric ulcer.[82,83] At least six biopsy specimens should be taken from the margin of the ulcer in each quadrant. It is important to take the biopsy specimens of the ulcer margin as close to the ulcer base as possible to increase the yield if a tumor is present.[83] If the ulcer base is abnormal or appears to have nodules, a biopsy should be performed there. It may be important to follow gastric ulcers with a repeat endoscopy and multiple biopsies in certain circumstances. It is possible for a malignant ulcer to heal with therapy.

If the patient presented initially with an upper gastrointestinal bleed, endoscopy for biopsies of a gastric ulcer is often deferred until the patient is stable, so that the biopsies can be safely performed. If the endoscopic appearance of the lesion was atypical or the biopsy specimens were atypical, it may be important to repeat endoscopy and biopsy after several weeks of therapy.

Duodenal Ulcers

Endoscopy is considered more accurate than radiography in the evaluation of the duodenal bulb to detect a duodenal ulcer. Approximately 50% of duodenal ulcers are located on

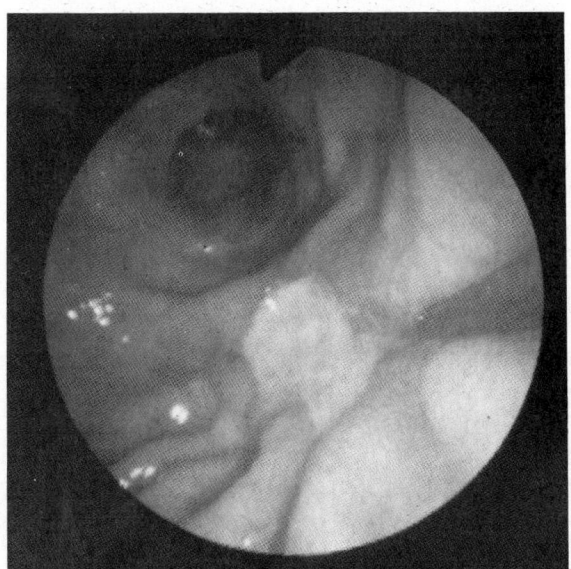

FIGURE 115-19. (See Color Fig. 91.) Atypical gastric ulceration along the greater curvature was presumably induced by nonsteroidal antiinflammatory drugs.

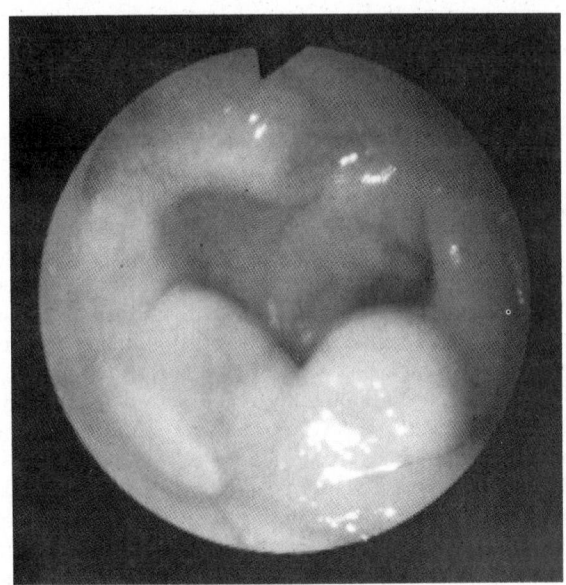

FIGURE 115-20. (See Color Fig. 92.) This deformed bulb was caused by scarring after prior ulceration and recurrent duodenal ulcer.

the anterior surface of the duodenal bulb. As with gastric ulcers, it is important to examine the base of the ulcer to detect a sentinel clot or visible vessel. A duodenal ulcer is often round and less than 1 cm in diameter. Giant ulcers in the duodenum are rare. As with gastric ulcers, the mucosa surrounding the ulcer is often red. Adjacent to the ulcer, there may be a second duodenal ulcer, duodenal erosions, or duodenal scarring from previous ulceration. As the ulcer heals, the mucosal margin remains red. Duodenal ulcers heal at a rate of several millimeters per week. If there is profound scarring from previous ulceration, there may be outpouchings of the bulb resembling diverticula (Fig. 115-20; see Color Fig. 92).

In a patient with a duodenal ulcer, an antral biopsy should be obtained to document the presence of *H pylori* infection. If appropriate, antimicrobial sensitivities can also be obtained. Almost all duodenal ulcers are positive for *H pylori*. Rare causes of duodenal ulcer include acid hypersecretion caused by gastrinoma, Crohn's disease, and nonsteroidal antiinflammatory drugs. It is not recommended that biopsies be taken directly from a duodenal ulcer unless it is in some way atypical, suggesting the presence of Crohn's disease, malignancy, or infectious or parasitic disease.

Upper Gastrointestinal Tract Bleeding

In a patient who presents with upper gastrointestinal bleeding, endoscopy is the first diagnostic procedure undertaken. Endoscopy in an acutely bleeding patient is not simple and requires a skilled examiner. It is usually possible to perform endoscopy on all patients with upper gastrointestinal bleeding unless they have torrential hemorrhage. Endoscopy provides valuable information for the diagnosis and planned therapy of the patient: whether this is an upper gastrointestinal bleed, what the lesion is, where this lesion is located, what the activity of the bleeding is, whether a vessel is visible in the base of the ulcer, whether there is an adherent clot, and if there are several potential bleeding sites, which is the likely source of the hemorrhage.[33,40,84,85]

The advent of therapeutic endoscopy has given the endoscopist the chance to change the natural history in the bleeding patient. Endoscopic hemostasis may reduce mortality. It is essential to know what lesion is bleeding to help guide therapy.[86-88] Two metanalyses of the role of endoscopic therapy and nonvariceal bleeding have demonstrated that endoscopic hemostasis is beneficial in patients with bleeding ulcers.[87,88] The benefit is only apparent in patients who are considered to be high risk, with endoscopic features including active bleeding and nonbleeding visible vessels. In these patients, endoscopic therapy reduces the rate of further bleeding, mortality, and the need for surgery.

Most endoscopists stabilize a patient presenting with upper gastrointestinal bleeding hemodynamically and then perform endoscopy. Endoscopy may be useful for localizing the general area of the bleeding, even if it is impossible to see the exact bleeding lesion because of clots. The risk of rebleeding is increased with pulsatile arterial bleeding or stigmata of recent ulcer hemorrhage, including an adherent blood clot, pigmented protuberance, flesh-colored protuberance, and flat blood spot on the ulcer base that resists vigorous rinsing with a wash catheter. After a bleeding lesion has been identified, it is possible to apply endoscopic therapy with heat (e.g., heater probe, monopolar electrocoagulation, bipolar electrocoagulation, lasers) or injection therapy (e.g., adrenaline, alcohol, sclerosants). If it appears that the patient requires surgery, endoscopy is important to detect the area of bleeding and the bleeding lesion and to help plan the appropriate surgical procedure.

Urgent early endoscopy is indicated if the patient is not stable hemodynamically, if the patient has liver disease, if the patient has rebled, or if there is a history of previous aortic-prosthetic surgery because of the possibility of aortoenteric fistula. As the role of endoscopic therapy is better understood, the timing of endoscopy may change.

Performing endoscopy in a patient with an acute upper gastrointestinal bleed is a challenge. It is critical to have well-trained assistants present to monitor the patient, set up diagnostic and therapeutic equipment, assist the endoscopist during the procedure, and suction blood and fluid from the patient's mouth during the procedure. It is imperative to watch the patient constantly during the procedure to be certain that the patient's status does not change. Monitoring pulse, blood pressure, and oxygen saturation is often useful in this clinical circumstance.

The esophagus is examined to determine whether obvious lesions are present that can account for the bleeding, such as esophageal varices or a mucosal tear. The gastric examination is performed with the instrument straight ahead and retroflexed. Before endoscopy, it is often advisable to lavage the stomach to remove clots; if a clot is still present in the stomach, most endoscopists advance the tip of the endoscope over the clot and into the antrum. If there is brisk duodenal bleeding, blood can be seen refluxing back through the pylorus into the antrum from the duodenum. The endoscope is passed through the pylorus into the duodenal bulb and down into the de-

scending duodenum. If an ulcer is encountered, its size, appearance, associated visible vessel or sentinel clot, and bleeding activity are assessed. The instrument is withdrawn into the stomach and retroflexed to examine the lesser curvature, cardia, and fundus. If blood and clots are present, the patient's position may have to be changed to allow the entire gastric mucosa to be inspected. In some instances, it is possible to follow a trail of blood up the mucosa and find the actively bleeding lesion.

The distribution of lesions varies in different areas of the world and in different patient populations. In the esophagus, the most important lesions are esophageal varices (see Fig. 115-8; see Color Fig. 82) and Mallory-Weiss tears. Other lesions include cancers, Barrett's ulcers, and severe reflux esophagitis. The most common causes of bleeding in the stomach are gastric ulcer, gastric varices (Fig. 115-21; see Color Fig. 93), vascular abnormalities such as telangiectasis (Fig. 115-22; see Color Fig. 94), gastric erosions, or hemorrhagic gastritis, often associated with stress, malignancies, or Dieulafoy's vascular lesion. In the duodenal bulb, the most common cause of bleeding is duodenal ulcer (Fig. 115-23; see Color Fig. 95). Other lesions include erosive duodenitis, often thought to be drug induced. The duodenum may also bleed from vascular abnormalities and from tumors, especially pancreatic tumors burrowing into the duodenum.

The natural history of a bleeding ulcer in the stomach and duodenum is affected by the nature of the artery underlying the lesion. Because of the proximity to large vessels, there is an increased risk of rebleeding from deep ulcers high on the lesser curvature of the stomach or in the posterior inferior wall of the duodenal bulb. Rebleeding from ulcers in these locations may be severe. If the left gastric artery is underneath a gastric ulcer or the gastroduodenal artery is underneath a duodenal ulcer, a massive hemorrhage may result, which may be difficult to control endoscopically, and sometimes even surgical control is a challenge, especially in the case of the gastroduodenal artery in a duodenal ulcer.

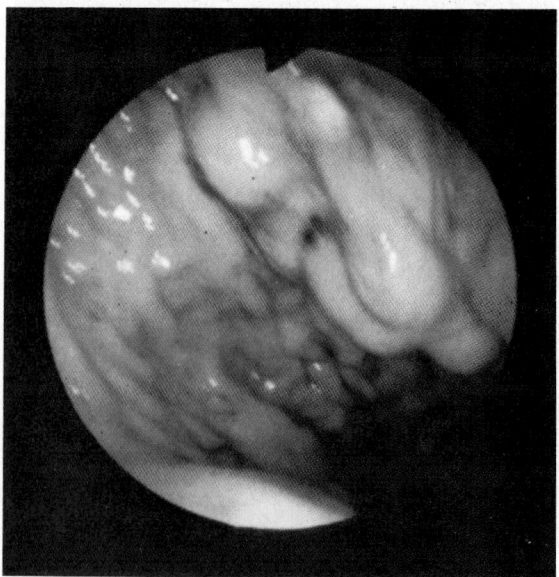

FIGURE 115-21. (See Color Fig. 93.) Gastric fundus varices.

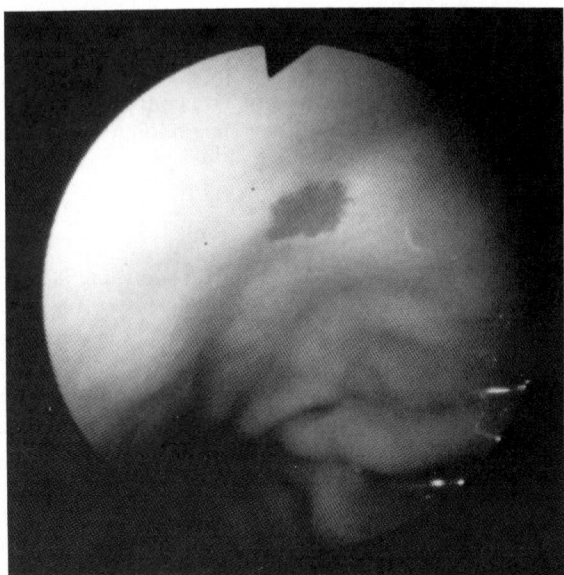

FIGURE 115-22. (See Color Fig. 94.) Gastric mucosal vascular anomaly.

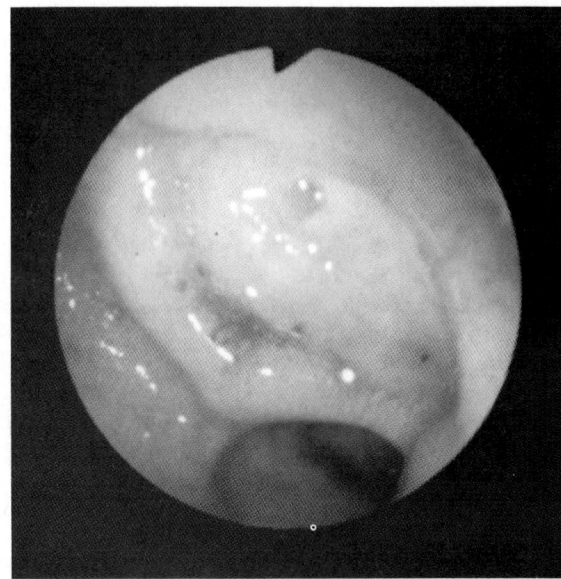

FIGURE 115-23. (See Color Fig. 95.) A vessel is visible in the base of this duodenal ulcer.

Infection of the Esophagus

Candida infection of the esophagus occurs in immunosuppressed patients and in patients who are not clearly immunocompromised, including those with conditions such as malnutrition or diabetes and patients on steroids. At endoscopy, several characteristic appearances are seen for *Candida*, including a typical white exudate, pseudomembranes, ulcers, and friable mucosa. The most accurate method of diagnosing fungal infection of the esophagus is endoscopic brushing and biopsy.[89] Brush specimens of the esophageal exudate show mycelia. Some endoscopists obtain a biopsy specimen, because the sample may show evidence of deeper tissue involvement with fungus. It is not useful to culture the exudate or the biopsy specimen, because *Candida* may be demonstrated by culture without significant mucosal infection.

In the differential diagnosis of esophageal infection in the immunocompromised host, several viral infections must be considered, including herpes simplex virus (HSV), varicella-zoster virus (VZV), and cytomegalovirus (CMV). Each of these viruses may be associated with ulcers in the esophagus, usually in patients who are immunocompromised. CMV is thought to affect the deeper, submucosal tissue, and HSV and VZV affect more superficial epithelium.

In HSV infection, vesicles are often seen as the initial lesion. As the lesion progresses, the center of the vesicle sloughs, leaving a small ulcer, the edges of which are usually raised. If these ulcers coalesce, extensive areas may be involved. The diagnosis is made by histologic examination and viral culture of brushings or biopsy specimens taken from the edge or center of the ulcers. A necrotizing esophagitis can also occur from VZV infection, especially in immunocompromised patients. As with HSV, lesions may vary from vesicles to larger lesions, and biopsy specimens and brushings are obtained for histologic analysis.

The lesions of CMV esophagitis involve the submucosa.

The typical endoscopic appearance is that of a geographic pattern ulcer, which may be large, especially in the distal esophagus.[90] Endoscopic brushing of the exudate is less useful for culturing CMV. Biopsy specimens from the center of the ulcer are often required for the diagnosis of CMV.[89] In the immunocompromised host, CMV infection may involve the mucosa and submucosa of the stomach and duodenum in addition to the esophagus.

Removal of Foreign Bodies

Foreign body ingestion occurs in all types of patients, but there is an increased incidence in children, in patients who wear dental plates, and in psychiatrically ill patients or prisoners. Most commonly, adults present with dysphagia or esophageal obstruction caused by a piece of meat or a bone, but children and psychiatrically disturbed patients ingest a variety of objects.[32] The foreign body tends to lodge in the esophagus in areas of physiologic narrowing, such as near the left main stem bronchus, aortic arch, and just above the diaphragm.[91]

In removing a foreign body, the endoscopist should ensure that the airway is not obstructed and be certain that the foreign body does not injure the lining of the gastrointestinal tract. The airway can be protected by the placement of an endotracheal tube. The mucosa can be protected, especially in the removal of sharp objects, by using an overtube to protect the intestinal lining during removal of the foreign body.[92] It is possible to remove foreign bodies with rigid and flexible endoscopes. Foreign bodies in the area of the hypopharynx and very proximal esophagus are often best removed with an open laryngoscope and grasping forceps. For other foreign bodies, flexible endoscopes are used, preferably with a large channel (2.8–3.5 mm). The larger channel allows a variety of snares, baskets, and forceps to be used to grasp the foreign body.

Any foreign object that impacts in the esophagus needs attention, including coins or batteries, which contain corrosive elements. If a radiopaque foreign body passes spontaneously into the stomach, serial abdominal flat films can be used to watch its progress through the gastrointestinal tract. A sharp object, such as an open safety pin or razor blade that remains stuck for more than 2 or 3 days, should be removed endoscopically or surgically.

A coin often lodges in the proximal esophagus just distal to the cricopharyngeal muscle. Posteroanterior and lateral radiographic views of the neck are necessary to identify the exact location of the foreign body and to determine whether the foreign body is in the esophagus or the trachea. A rigid laryngoscope and forceps can be used to remove the coin; alternatively, forceps or a snare are passed by way of a flexible endoscope. The patient can be placed in Trendelenburg's position to prevent aspiration of the coin into the trachea if an endotracheal tube is not used. Special care is required if a coin or button battery is pulled through the upper esophageal sphincter, because these foreign bodies may become dislodged from a snare or toothed forceps as they are being removed.

A foreign body such as meat is commonly encountered in adults and may totally obstruct the distal esophagus. A polypectomy snare can often be used to grasp and remove the meat. Experience has shown that after a meat bolus has been snared or placed in a basket, it is best to pull the bolus up against the tip of the endoscope as the endoscope is being withdrawn to minimize the likelihood of the bolus becoming dislodged from the snare or basket as it is being removed. If the meat fragments into smaller pieces, an overtube is necessary to reduce patient discomfort. As the endoscope is passed in and out to remove small pieces of the foreign body, the overtube protects the airway and prevents a piece of the foreign body from being dropped in the hypopharynx.

In some instances, a small-diameter endoscope can be passed next to the obstructing bolus to determine whether a stricture is present below the meat. If a stricture is found, it can be dilated with a balloon. The instrument can be withdrawn to above the bolus of meat and can be used to push the bolus of meat gently down into the patient's stomach. However, pushing a foreign body distally without knowing the cause of the obstruction should be avoided, because this can cause a perforation.

The greatest difficulty in protecting the airway occurs with sharp objects such as pins or razor blades. If a single-edged razor blade is lodged in the esophagus, an overtube should be used. The razor blade should be pulled into the overtube as it is gently removed, protecting the esophageal mucosa. An overtube is also helpful for removing a pin. If a safety pin is open in the esophagus with the sharp end of the pin pointing proximally, the best management approach is to push the pin into the stomach, rotate it, and pull it out by the hinge with the pointed portion of the pin trailing and pointing away from the endoscope. Other commonly encountered foreign bodies are small batteries. The batteries should be removed to prevent possible serious and even fatal complications if they are stuck in the esophagus. If small batteries rapidly move into the stomach, they usually pass without problems.

After a foreign body has passed the pylorus and is in the small bowel, it usually passes spontaneously. In some instances, a foreign body must be removed surgically from the stomach or from the intestinal tract beyond the stomach if endoscopic removal is not successful.[19] A radiograph should be taken immediately before attempted removal because, in many instances, the foreign body has spontaneously passed out of the stomach, and endoscopy is no longer indicated.

Caustic Injury

Caustic injury may vary from a minimal and superficial burn to severe necrosis involving the entire upper gastrointestinal tract into the duodenum. Ingestion of alkali is often more problematic than ingestion of strong acids.[93] Endoscopy allows the physician to assess the organs injured and, to some degree, determine the extent of the injury.[94,95] In most instances, endoscopy should be performed early in the patient's evaluation if the patient is stable. If there is evidence of a full-thickness injury to the intestinal tract with possible perforation, shock, or severe injury to the hypopharynx or epiglottis, endoscopy should not be performed. The examination is usually performed with a small-caliber endoscope. The recommended technique of passage is under direct vision with minimal air insufflation. If an area of severe necrosis is visualized, the endoscopy should not proceed beyond this area.

It is possible to divide the extent of the injury caused by caustics into three degrees of injury.[96] The mildest or first-degree injury is characterized by mild friability, erythema, and edema but no evidence of necrosis or ulceration. These superficial injuries often heal completely without long-term sequelae. Second-degree injuries extend into the wall and occasionally to the muscularis propria. Endoscopically, a more severe injury is seen with necrosis, ulcers, exudates, and areas of hemorrhage. These deeper injuries characteristically result in strictures of the severely injured organ, the esophagus or stomach. The most severe injury is a third-degree burn involving the full thickness of the wall. The injury is seen endoscopically as a dark exudate, with sloughing of the mucosa in addition to hemorrhage and ulceration. The organ may appear aperistaltic and dilated. This injury often leads to the late sequelae of esophageal stricture or strictures in the stomach. Third-degree burns may also be associated with injury to adjacent organs and may present with mediastinitis or peritonitis.

The purpose of early endoscopy is to determine the extent and severity of the burn. A black necrotic area with ulceration suggests an injury through the full thickness of the wall and an increased risk of perforation. In these patients, early surgical intervention must be considered before perforation occurs. If, at the initial endoscopy, an area of full-thickness injury is suspected, it is usually recommended that the endoscopy be discontinued at that point and repeated after 48 hours to determine whether these areas appear to be healing. The patient must be watched for clinical signs of perforation requiring operative intervention.

Drug-Induced Injury

Injury to the lining of the esophagus caused by medications occurs more commonly than is usually appreciated. Some medications, such as tetracycline, ascorbic acid, and iron preparations, have an acid pH and directly injure the mucosa. Tetracycline is probably the most common injurious agent to the esophagus.[97] Some medications, such as potassium preparations, are designed for slow release, and if they remain for a prolonged time in the esophagus, they can cause injury. This problem is made worse if the patient swallows the medication with a small amount of water before going to bed. In the elderly patient, a reduced amount of saliva also may contribute to the problem.[98]

Endoscopically, these patients have ulcerations of the esophagus characteristically located above areas of physiologic narrowing, where these medications tend to lodge. The injury may vary from friability and erythema to multiple clear-cut ulcerations, often seen as kissing ulcers in direct opposition to one another on the esophageal mucosa. These iatrogenic drug-induced injuries may promote esophageal stricture, especially if the medication is taken over a long period.

Mass Lesions

Endoscopy is often used to evaluate masses seen on barium radiographs in the upper gastrointestinal tract, especially in the stomach. Endoscopy provides information about the mass, including its size, whether the mucosa over the mass is involved, whether there is associated ulceration and evidence of bleeding, and whether the mass appears to be primarily in the wall of the gastrointestinal tract or caused by an adjacent extrinsic lesion. Endoscopic ultrasound may prove to be important in the evaluation of these mass lesions.

Gastric adenocarcinomas are categorized by Borrmann's classification into four types of tumors. The first type is an exophytic mass protruding into the gastric lumen. Type 2 is a protruding mass with associated ulceration. Type 3 is a diffusely infiltrating tumor, often associated with ulceration. Type 4 is an infiltrating mass without associated ulcer. Type 1 carcinomas are readily recognized and biopsied for diagnosis. These occur in the gastric body, cardia, and antrum. Type 2 lesions may be more difficult to recognize because they are less protuberant. One of the characteristic endoscopic findings is that the folds surrounding the area of ulceration do not terminate at the actual ulcer margin but are separated from the ulcer margin by areas of nodularity or by abnormal-appearing mucosa and, in some instances, depressed mucosa.

Type 3 lesions can be confused with a benign gastric ulcer. To make this distinction, at least six to eight biopsy specimens from all quadrants of the ulcer are necessary to detect carcinoma. Brush cytology may also be useful. Type 4 adenocarcinoma is often referred to as linitis plastica, with diffuse involvement of the gastric wall. This tumor may be mainly submucosal, and biopsy of the mucosal surface over the tumor may reveal relatively normal tissue. It is important to biopsy any abnormal areas of mucosa associated with these lesions, because these are most likely to be the areas in which the tumor has broken through to the surface and to produce biopsy specimens that are positive for tumor. Most endoscopists prefer using a biopsy forceps of large caliber for these biopsies or needle cytology.

Early adenocarcinoma of the stomach, if diagnosed correctly, may be associated with an excellent 5-year survival rate. The classification for early gastric cancer was defined by the Japanese Endoscopic Society. Type 1 is a small polypoid lesion. Type 2 can be elevated (2a), flat (2b), or depressed (2c). Type 3 is a lesion that presents as a gastric ulcer with an adenocarcinoma at the margin, often producing a discolored and slightly depressed area. The most common types of early gastric cancer are types 2c and 3.

The appearance of gastric lymphoma varies from nodular or polypoid to that of ulcerations surrounded by a nodular and infiltrated mucosa. A deep, volcano-like ulcer is reported, which has elevated surrounding margins. The ulcers are characteristically irregular in their margins and are associated with nodules. Exudate in the base may appear gray. Multiple biopsies often are necessary to diagnose a gastric lymphoma correctly.

In each of these lesions, endoscopic ultrasound plays a potentially important role in diagnosis, staging, guiding therapy, and determining the response to therapy.

ENDOSCOPIC SURVEILLANCE FOR PREMALIGNANT LESIONS

The incidence of neoplasia is increased in several conditions and in some postoperative circumstances in the upper gastrointestinal tract. However, well-designed controlled studies are lacking to define precisely the risk of these conditions for developing malignancy, and it is difficult to determine exactly which conditions require periodic surveillance.

Achalasia

Esophageal cancer develops in 2% to 8% of patients with untreated achalasia after more than 15 years of disease. If the patient is adequately treated with balloon dilation or a surgical myotomy, there may be a smaller increase in the risk of malignancy.[99,100] There does not seem to be a role for endoscopic surveillance in achalasia. However, any patient with achalasia who experiences a change in signs or symptoms should undergo endoscopy to determine whether a malignancy is present.

Esophageal Columnar Metaplasia

There is an increased risk of adenocarcinoma, in the range of 8% to 10%, in patients with Barrett's metaplasia. The premalignant risk does not seem to be reduced by antireflux surgery, despite the fact that this surgery may be associated with a reduction in inflammation. Most endoscopists agree that patients with columnar metaplasia should be screened endoscopically with multiple biopsies, although the exact frequency of surveillance has not been determined.[101,102] Other factors may influence the timing of endoscopic surveillance, such as flow cytometric abnormalities in the tissue or dysplasia.

Gastric Polyps

Adenomatous gastric polyps are thought to have an increased risk for containing malignancy within the polyp.[103] Hyperplastic polyps are not associated with cancer in the polyp.

However, adenomatous and hyperplastic polyps may be associated with gastric atrophy, which has been associated with gastric cancer in areas other than the polyp.

Larger adenomatous polyps seem to pose a greater risk of malignancy. It is necessary to remove the entire polyp for adequate histologic assessment for tumor, because random biopsies may miss a focal cancer. Polypectomy may also treat symptoms caused by a polyp, such as bleeding or obstruction. If a polyp is encountered, it should be removed by endoscopy or surgery. The size of the polyp, the number of polyps, and the patient's general medical condition are important factors in determining whether surgery or endoscopy should be used for treatment. Further treatment and decisions about surveillance often depend on the histologic findings. If the polyp is hyperplastic, no further surveillance endoscopy is indicated. If the patient has a limited number of small adenomatous polyps (<2 cm), endoscopic removal of the polyp is recommended. These patients are followed with surveillance endoscopy to detect recurrent polyps or the development of a carcinoma. If the polyp is adenomatous but is large and sessile, there is an increased risk of complications from endoscopic removal, and surgical therapy is often recommended. Because bleeding may occur after polypectomy, some endoscopists recommend injecting the base of the polyp with a dilute epinephrine solution before endoscopic polypectomy.

Atrophic Gastritis or Gastric Atrophy

Chronic gastritis with severe atrophy is associated with gastric adenocarcinoma (Fig. 115-24; see Color Fig. 96). An accepted hypothesis is that gastric carcinoma results from a defined histologic pathway.[104] The theory is that *H pylori* infection, especially with onset at a young age, seems to be the initiating event leading to gastric inflammation, which evolves over years to atrophy.[105] Intestinal metaplasia, especially type 3, seems to be an important step in this pathway, representing a precursor lesion.[106] Only rarely can extensive intestinal metaplasia

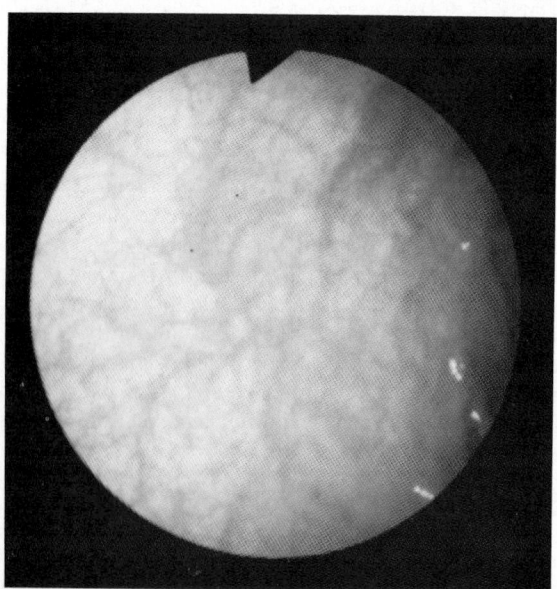

FIGURE 115-24.   (See Color Fig. 96.) Atrophic gastritis.

be identified endoscopically. Mucolysis followed by methylene blue staining may facilitate the recognition of intestinal metaplasia endoscopically and allow targeted biopsy of the lesion.

Autoimmune Gastritis and Pernicious Anemia

Several population-based studies indicate that the risk of gastric adenocarcinoma and carcinoid tumor is increased in patients with pernicious anemia, but only slightly over that of the general population. Periodic surveillance endoscopy in patients with pernicious anemia is not recommended, except in patients who have known dysplastic changes of the mucosa and in patients in Scandinavian countries.[107-111] The importance of small carcinoids and endocrine cell hyperplasia in the corpus requires further investigation.

Adenocarcinoma in the Gastric Remnant After Partial Gastrectomy

Several studies have demonstrated that patients undergoing gastric resection for benign gastric or duodenal ulcers are at increased risk for later developing dysplasia and adenocarcinoma. The reported increase in the risk of cancer ranges from 2% to 8.7%.[112-114] However, other reported series have failed to demonstrate an increased risk of carcinoma in these postoperative patients.[115]

There may be a geographic variability in the risk of gastric cancer postoperatively. In some areas of Europe, there is an increased risk of gastric carcinoma, and in these populations, the risk of cancer in the stump after gastrectomy does seem to be elevated. However, in the United States, the risk of developing gastric cancer is low, and the risk of postoperative stump cancer is also low. Overall, there does seem to be an increased risk in postgastrectomy patients, approximately twice that in nonoperated patients.[112]

Based on these studies, the risk of malignancy is not thought to be high enough to warrant routine endoscopic screening of patients who have had gastric resections. However, in countries in which the risk of postgastrectomy cancer is several times the normal incidence, the patients should be screened endoscopically, especially patients who underwent surgery before 50 years of age and if the resection was performed at least 15 years ago.[112] If endoscopy is being performed for a different indication on a patient who had gastric resection many years earlier, some endoscopists recommend taking multiple biopsy specimens from the margin of the stoma to look for evidence of dysplasia or early cancer.

RISKS AND CONTRAINDICATIONS

Endoscopic examination of the upper gastrointestinal tract by an experienced endoscopist is a safe procedure. Cardiopulmonary complications, infection, bleeding, and perforation occur only rarely. Each of these complications is thought to occur in fewer than 0.1% of patients undergoing endoscopy. The smaller-caliber endoscopes are safer.[116]

Several studies have suggested that the complication rate of endoscopy in patients who were experiencing acute gastrointestinal bleeding is higher than in patients who were electively examined. There is, however, no evidence that endoscopy exacerbates bleeding. Cardiopulmonary complications account for more than one half of endoscopy-associated deaths.[13,117] Patients who are heavily sedated may undergo oxygen desaturation. This is a risk in patients with poor saturation at baseline.

Contraindications for endoscopy include suspected perforation, an uncooperative patient, severe shock or respiratory distress, and severe injury to the hypopharynx. Patients with coagulopathies should be examined endoscopically only in life-threatening situations and if the result of the endoscopy is thought to be critical for the patient's care.

ASSESSMENT OF RESULTS

Diagnostic Endoscopy

Physicians have for years debated the relative merits of fiberoptic endoscopy and barium contrast radiography in evaluating the esophagus, stomach, and duodenum (Table 115-2).[118-124] Studies comparing these diagnostic modalities have always suffered from the problem of which technique is to be used as the standard. Even studies that are thought to best address this issue have been criticized.[123] Radiologists contend that they are able to detect important lesions of the upper gastrointestinal tract in a manner comparable to that achieved with endoscopy.[124] This includes lesions such as carcinoma of the esophagus and stomach, esophageal stricture, and large peptic ulcers.

There are some advantages to fiberoptic endoscopy. First, endoscopy allows detection of superficial mucosal lesions such as reflux esophagitis, gastritis, and duodenitis better than radiography. Endoscopy is thought to be more sensitive and specific for peptic ulcer and is therefore the standard for peptic ulcer healing trials. Endoscopy permits cytology and biopsy, making endoscopy superior to radiology for diagnosing infectious conditions such as esophagitis with *Candida* or CMV or diagnosing gastritis with *H pylori*. However, each type of diagnostic study fails to detect certain lesions, and there are clinical circumstances in which one or the other of these modalities is best or in which a combination of modalities is required.

The addition of endoscopic ultrasound expands the diagnostic usefulness of endoscopy. This is especially important in the detection and staging of lesions in the wall of the gastrointestinal tract, including malignancies of the esophagus and stomach.[29]

In upper gastrointestinal bleeding, endoscopy is the diagnostic procedure of choice. Barium radiography has a low rate of detection of the bleeding source, and the barium can interfere with subsequent endoscopy or angiography. Endoscopy offers the possibility of hemostatic therapy. Because endoscopy is thought to be more accurate, allows the endoscopist to take targeted biopsy specimens, permits brush cytology, and permits the delivery of various types of therapy, the rapid increase in use of endoscopy seems to be justified.[125-128]

Therapeutic Endoscopy

There are few well-designed clinical trials comparing endoscopic therapy with alternative modes of therapy, specifically surgery. However, the morbidity and mortality rates of endoscopic therapy are significantly lower than those associated with surgical therapy. For benign strictures of the esophagus, dilation should be performed in a nonsurgical manner, often with endoscopic guidance. Removal of foreign bodies is much safer and easier for the patient if it is achieved endoscopically. Polyps of the upper gastrointestinal tract can usually be removed with endoscopy. However, for large polyps or polyps in areas that are difficult to visualize endoscopically, surgical removal may still be important. For submucosal neoplasms, surgery is usually required.

Various modalities for endoscopic hemostasis have been tested, and several controlled trials demonstrate that these techniques can decrease the continued bleeding rate, rebleeding rate, number of patients requiring emergency surgery, and overall mortality rate. However, the comparison must also take into account the mortality thought to result from concomitant illness rather than from the bleeding lesion itself.

The role of endoscopy in variceal bleeding is more problematic. Endoscopy stops bleeding in a high percentage of patients, with an immediate lowering of morbidity and mortality compared with emergency surgery. However, long-term differences in mortality and outcome have not been clearly demonstrated.[129] There are a variety of approaches to variceal bleeding. The newer approach of esophageal banding is a valid

---

TABLE 115-2
Usefulness of Endoscopy and Radiography in the Evaluation of Dyspepsia Caused by Peptic Ulcer or Malignancy

	ENDOSCOPY		RADIOGRAPHY	
CONDITION	Sensitivity (%)	Specificity (%)	Sensitivity (%)	Specificity (%)
Gastric ulcer	85–95	90–100	44–91	93–99
Duodenal ulcer	77–99	95–100	50–73	96–99
Gastric cancer	94–100	100	50–89	95–100

Data from references 118 through 122.

alternative and is being increasingly applied. Studies are needed to identify patients best treated with sclerotherapy, β blockade, banding, shunt surgery, transjugular intraperitoneal portasystemic stent-shunt (TIPS), or liver transplantation.

TRENDS

The role of endoscopy in clinical medicine will continue to increase in the future; however, a patient presenting with dyspepsia will not undergo endoscopy, because serologic testing for *H pylori* will be used by primary care physicians. As effective eradication regimens for *H pylori* become widely available, there may also be a decrease in the incidence of peptic ulcer and possibly in associated gastric cancer in patients positive for *H pylori*.

The training of new endoscopists is important, and as part of this education, a standardization of terminology is vital, especially in the use of videoendoscopy to examine areas of inflammation. Issues such as interobserver and intraobserver variability must be considered as we examine the sensitivity and specificity of endoscopy. The use of videoendoscopy is likely to increase because it offers assessment of physiology and pathophysiology not possible with fiberoptic endoscopes (e.g., evaluation of the intestinal wall vasculature).

Ultrasound endoscopy will be used increasingly for diagnosis and for guiding therapy. The wall of the intestinal tract and the nature of the surrounding structures can be studied with ultrasound. Ultrasound can be used to guide biopsy and cytologic puncture of structures to optimize diagnostic information.

Long-term, well-designed, controlled clinical trials are important for defining the way endoscopy should be used in patients thought to be at increased risk for gastrointestinal malignancy.

> The reader is directed to Chapter 114, General Considerations; Chapter 119, Contrast Radiology; and Chapter 120, Cross-Sectional Anatomy.

REFERENCES

1. Silverstein FE, Tytgat GNJ. Atlas of gastrointestinal endoscopy. 2nd ed. New York: Gower Medical Publishing, 1991.
2. Waye J, Geenen J, Fleischer D. Techniques in therapeutic endoscopy. New York: Gower Medical Publishing, 1987.
3. Sivak MV. Gastrointestinal endoscopy. Philadelphia: WB Saunders, 1987.
4. Sivak MV. Video endoscopy. Ann Gastrointest Endosc 1988;1:115.
5. Fujino MA, Ikeda M, Yamamoto Y, et al. Development of an integrated filing system for endoscopic images. Endoscopy 1991;23:11.
6. Fujino MA, Kawai T, Morozumi A, et al. Endoscopic image manipulation: state of the art. Endoscopy 1992;24(Suppl 2):516.
7. Jameson JS, Kapadia SA, Polson RJ, et al. Is oropharyngeal anaesthesia with topical lignocaine useful in upper gastrointestinal endoscopy? Aliment Pharmacol Ther 1992;6:739.
8. Hedenbro JL, Ekolund M, Jansson D, Lindblom A. A randomized, double-blind, placebo-controlled study to evaluate topical anaesthesia of the pharynx in upper gastrointestinal endoscopy. Endoscopy 1992;24:585.
9. Keefe EB, O'Connor KW. ASGE survey of endoscopic sedation and monitoring practice. Gastrointest Endosc 1990;36:513.
10. Daneshmend TK, Bell GD, Logan FRA. Sedation for upper gastrointestinal endoscopy: results of nationwide survey. Gut 1991;32:12.
11. Benjamin S. Proceedings of the Symposium on Sedation and Monitoring in Endoscopy at the World Congress of Gastroenterology. Scan J Gastroenteral 1990;25(Suppl 179):1.
12. McCloy R. Quality control in endoscopy. New York: Springer, 1991.
13. Lieberman DA, Wuerker CK, Katon RM. Cardiopulmonary risk of esophagogastroduodenoscopy. Gastroenterology 1985;88:468.
14. Bell GD, McCloy RF, Charlton JE, et al. Recommendation for standards of sedation and patient monitoring during gastrointestinal endoscopy. Gut 1991;32:823.
15. Kaczmarek RG, Moore RM, McCrohan J, et al. Multi-state investigation of the actual disinfection/sterilization of endoscopes in health care facilities. Am J Med 1992;92:257.
16. Hanson PJV, Gor D, Clarke JR, et al. Contamination of endoscopes used in AIDS patients. Lancet 1989;2:86.
17. Levine DS, Reid BJ. Endoscopic biopsy technique for acquiring larger mucosal samples. Gastrointest Endosc 1991;37:482.
18. Winawer SJ. Tissue diagnosis in upper gastrointestinal malignancy (editorial). Gastroenterology 1982;82:379.
19. Graham DY, Spjut HJ. Salvage cytology. An alternative fiberoptic technique. Gastrointest Endosc 1979;25:137.
20. Kochhar R, Rajwanshi A, Malik AK, et al. Endoscopic fine needle aspiration biopsy of gastroesophageal malignancies. Gastrointest Endosc 1988;34:321.
21. Yamaguchi M, Okazaki Y, Yanai H, Takemoto T. Three-dimensional determination of gastric ulcer size with laser endoscopy. Endoscopy 1988;20:263.
22. McCormack T, Martin T, Smallwood RH, et al. Doppler ultrasound probe for assessment of blood-flow in oesophageal varices. Lancet 1983;1:667.
23. Martin RN, Gilbert DA, Silverstein FE, et al. An endoscopic Doppler probe for assessing intestinal vasculature. Ultrasound Med Biol 1985;11:61.
24. Kohler B, Riemann JF. Endoscopic doppler: evaluation of bleeding gastroduodenal ulcers. Scand J Gastroenterol 1991;26:666.
25. Lunde OC, Kvernebo K, Larsen S. Clinical evaluation of endoscopic laser Doppler flowmetry for measurement of human gastric blood flow. Methodological aspects. Scand J Gastroenterol 1988;23:1072.
26. Leung FW, Morishita T, Livingston EH, et al. Reflectance spectrophotometry for the assessment of gastroduodenal mucosal perfusion. Am J Physiol 1987;252:G797.
27. Tsuji S, Sato N, Kawano S, et al. Functional imaging for the analysis of the mucosal blood hemoglobin distribution using electronic endoscopy. Gastrointest Endosc 1988;34:332.
28. Tio TL, Tytgat GNJ. Atlas of transintestinal ultrasonography. Aalsmeer, The Netherlands: Mur-Kostverloren, 1986.
29. Tytgat GNJ, Fockens P. Endoscopic ultrasonography. Scand J Gastroenterol 1992;27(Suppl 192):80.
30. Ida K, Tada M. Chromoscopy. In: Sivak MV, ed. Gastrointestinal endoscopy. Philadelphia: WB Saunders, 1987:203.
31. Fennerty MB, Sampliner RE, McGee DL, et al. Intestinal metaplasia of the stomach: identification by a selective mucosal staining technique. Gastrointest Endosc 1992;38:696.
32. Webb WA. Management of foreign bodies of the upper gastrointestinal tract. Gastroenterology 1988;94:204.
33. Tytgat GNJ. Non-surgical management of upper gastro-intestinal bleeding. In: Vincent JL, ed. Update in intensive care and emergency medicine. Berlin: Springer Verlag 1986:417.
34. The North Italian Endoscopic Club for the Study and Treatment of Esophageal Varices. Prediction of the first variceal hemorrhage in patients with cirrhosis of the liver and esophageal varices. A prospective multicenter study. N Engl J Med 1988;319:983.
35. Sivak MV. Esophageal varices. In: Sivak MV, ed. Gastroenterologic endoscopy. Philadelphia: WB Saunders, 1987:342.

36. Soehendra N, Grimm H, Nam V CH, Berger B. *N*-Butyl-2-cyabo-acrylate: a supplement to endoscopic sclerotherapy. Endoscopy 1987;19:221.

37. Soehendra N, Grimm H, Maydeo A, et al. Endoscopic sclerotherapy—personal experience. Hepatogastroenterology 1991;38:220.

38. Stiegmann GV, Goff JS, Sun JH, et al. Endoscopic elastic band ligation for active variceal hemorrhage. Am Surg 1989;55:124.

39. Chung SCS, Leung JWC, Steel RJC, et al. Endoscopic injection of adrenaline for actively bleeding ulcers: a randomized trial. Br Med J 1988;1:365.

40. Chen PC, Wu C-S, Liaw Y-F. Hemostatic effect of endoscopic local injection with hypertonic saline-epinephrine solution and pure ethanol for digestive tract bleeding. Gastrointest Endosc 1986;32:319.

41. Chung SCS, Leung HT, Chan ACW. Epinephrine or epinephrine plus alcohol for injection of bleeding ulcers? Gastrointest Endosc 1992;38:231.

42. Papp JP. Electrocoagulation in upper gastrointestinal bleeding. Dig Dis Sci 1981;26:41S.

43. Laine L. Multipolar electrocoagulation in the treatment of active upper gastrointestinal hemorrhage. A prospective controlled trial. N Engl J Med 1987;316:1613.

44. Laine L. Multipolar electrocoagulation in the treatment of ulcers with non-bleeding visible vessels: a prospective, controlled trial. Ann Intern Med 1989;110:510.

45. Laine L. Multipolar electrocoagulation versus injection therapy in the treatment of bleeding peptic ulcers. Gastroenterology 1990;99:1303.

46. Johnston JH, Sones JQ, Long BW, Posey EL. Comparison of heater probe and Yag laser in endoscopic treatment of major bleeding from peptic ulcers. Gastrointest Endosc 1985;31:175.

47. Lin HJ, Lee FY, Kong WM, et al. Heat probe thermocoagulation and pure alcohol injection in massive peptic ulcer hemorrhage: a prospective, randomized controlled trial. Gut 1990;31:753.

48. Chung SCS, Leung JWC, Sung JY, et al. Injection or heat probe for bleeding ulcer. Gastroenterology 1991;100:33.

49. Choudari CP, Rajgopal C, Palmer KR. Comparison of endoscopic injection therapy versus the major peptic ulcer heater probe in haemorrhagia. Gut 1992;33:1159.

50. Swain C. Controlled trial of Nd:YAG laser photocoagulation in bleeding peptic ulcers. Lancet 1986;2:1113.

51. Kiefhaber P. Indication for endoscopic neodymium-YAG laser treatment in the gastrointestinal tract. Scand J Gastroenterol 1987;22(Suppl 139):53.

52. Waye JD. Techniques of polypectomy: hot biopsy forceps and snare polypectomy. Am J Gastroenterol 1987;82:615.

53. Hughes RW. Gastric polyps and polypectomy: rationale, technique and complications. Gastrointest Endosc 1984;30:101.

54. Boyce HW Jr. Precepts of safe esophageal dilation. Gastrointest Endosc 1977;23:215.

55. Tulman AB, Boyce HW Jr. Complications of esophageal dilatation and guidelines for their prevention. Gastrointest Endosc 1981;27:229.

56. Graham DY, Tabibian N, Schwartz JT, Smith JL. Evaluation of the effectiveness of through-the-scope balloons as dilators of benign and malignant gastrointestinal strictures. Gastrointest Endosc 1987;333:432.

57. Mühldorfer SM, Kekos G, Hahn EG, Ell C. Complications of therapeutic gastrointestinal endoscopy. Endoscopy 1992;24:276.

58. Kozarek RA, Botoman VA, Patterson DJ. Long-term follow-up in patients who have undergone balloon dilatation for gastric outlet obstruction. Gastrointest Endosc 1990;36:558.

59. Tytgat GN, Bartelsman JF, den Hartog Jager FC, et al. Upper intestinal and biliary endoprosthesis. Dig Dis Sci 1986;31:57S.

60. Tytgat GNJ, den Hartog Jager FCA, Bartelsman JFWM. Endoscopic prosthesis for advanced esophageal cancer. Endoscopy 1986;18(Suppl 3):32.

61. Lambert R, Sabben G, Chevaillon A, et al. Results of Nd:YAG laser treatment in epidermoid esophageal cancer. Lasers Surg Med 1984;3:340.

62. Fleischer D, Sivak MV. Endoscopic Nd:YAG laser therapy as a palliation for esophagogastric cancer. Parameters affecting initial outcome. Gastroenterology 1985;89:827.

63. Riemann JF, Ell C, Lux G, Demling L. Combined therapy of malignant stenosis of the upper gastrointestinal tract by means of laser beam bougienage. Endoscopy 1985;17:43.

64. Bown SG. Endoscopic laser therapy for oesophageal cancer. Endoscopy 1986;18(Suppl 3):26.

65. Mathus-Vliegen EMH, Tytgat GNJ. Laser photocoagulation in the palliative treatment of upper digestive tract tumors. Cancer 1986;57:396.

66. Bown SG. Photodynamic therapy of tumours. World J Surg 1983;7:700.

67. Rowland CG, Pogliero KM. Intracavitary irradiation in palliation of carcinoma of esophagus and cardia. Lancet 1985;2:981.

68. Johnston J, Fleischer D, Petrini J, et al. Palliative bipolar electrocoagulation therapy of obstructing esophageal cancer. Gastrointest Endosc 1987;33:349.

69. Jensen DM, Machicado GA, Randall GM. Palliation of obstructing esophageal cancer with BICAP tumor probe or YAG laser. Gastrointest Endosc 1987;33:173.

70. Dajani AS, Bisno AL, Chung KJ, et al. Prevention of bacterial endocarditis—recommendation by the American Heart Association. JAMA 1990;264:2919.

71. Tytgat GNJ, Onstenk R, Cheng J. An overview on dysphagia. Endosc Forum Dig Dis 1989;5:1.

72. Tytgat GNJ. Modern diagnostic evaluation and preoperative staging of esophageal cancer. Schweiz Med Wochenschr 1993;123:1088.

73. Tytgat GNJ, Hameeteman W, Onstenk R, Schotborg R. The spectrum of columnar-lined esophagus—Barrett's esophagus. Endoscopy 1989;21:177.

74. McClave SA, Boyce HW Jr, Gottfried MR. Early diagnosis of columnar-lined esophagus: a new endoscopic diagnostic criterion. Gastrointest Endosc 1987;33:413.

75. Dent J, Bremner CG, Collen MJ, et al. Barrett's oesophagus. J Gastroenterol Hepatol 1991;6:1.

76. Reid BJ. Barrett's esophagus and esophageal adenocarcinoma. Gastroenterol Clin North Am 1991;20:817.

77. Phillips RW, Wong RKH. Barrett's esophagus. Gastroenterol Clin North Am 1991;20:791.

78. Tytgat GNJ, Hameeteman W. The neoplastic potential of columnar-lined (Barrett's) esophagus. World J Surg 1992;26:308.

79. Health and Public Policy Committee, American College of Physicians, Philadelphia, Pennsylvania. Endoscopy in evaluation of dyspepsia. Ann Intern Med 1985;102:266.

80. Misiewicz JJ, Tytgat GNJ, Goodwin CS. The Sydney system: a new classification of gastritis. J Gastroenterol Hepatol 1991;6:207.

81. Tytgat GNJ, Noach LA, Rauws EAJ. *Helicobator pylori* infection and duodenal ulcer disease. Gastroenterol Clin North Am 1993;22:127.

82. Dekker W, Tytgat G. Diagnostic accuracy of fiberoptic endoscopy in detection of upper intestinal malignancy. Gastroenterology 1977;73:710.

83. Graham DY, Schwartz JT, Cain GO, Gyorkey F. Prospective evaluation of biopsy number in the diagnosis of esophageal and gastric carcinoma. Gastroenterology 1982;82:228.

84. Storey DW. Endoscopic prediction of recurrent bleeding in peptic ulcers. N Engl J Med 1981;305:915.

85. Foster DN, Miloszewski KJ, Laowsky MS. Stigmata of recent haemorrhage in diagnosis and prognosis of upper gastrointestinal bleeding. Br Med J 1978;1:1173.

86. Roth HP. Endoscopy: what is its role in upper gastrointestinal bleeding? Dig Dis Sci 1981;26(Suppl):1S.

87. Sacks HS, Cholmers TC, Blum AL, et al. Endoscopic hemostasis: an effective therapy for bleeding peptic ulcers. JAMA 1990;264:494.

88. Cook DJ, Guyatt GH, Salena BJ, Laine LA. Endoscopic therapy for acute nonvariceal upper gastrointestinal hemorrhage: a meta-analysis. Gastroenterology 1992;102:139.

89. McDonald GB. Esophageal diseases caused by infection, systemic illness and trauma. In: Sleisinger MH, Fordtran JS, ed. Gastrointestinal disease. Philadelphia: WB Saunders, 1989:460.

90. Kumar A, Posner G, Colby S, Nicholas A. Giant esophageal ulcer in AIDS-related complex. Gastrointest Endosc 1988;34:153.

91. Henderson CT, Engel J, Schlesinger P. Foreign body ingestion: review and suggested guidelines for management. Endoscopy 1987;19:68.

92. Cotton PB. Overtubes (sleeves) for upper gastrointestinal endoscopy. Gut 1983;24:863.

93. Gumaste VV. Clinical review of ingestion of corrosive substances by adults. Am J Gastroent 1992;87:1.

94. Sugawa C, Mullins RJ, Lucas CE, Leibold WC. The value of early endoscopy following caustic ingestion. Surg Gynecol Obstet 1981;153:553.

95. Dilawari JB, Singh S, Rao PN, Amand BS. Corrosive acid ingestion in man: a clinical and endoscopic study. Gut 1984;2:183.

96. Frank BA, Boyce HW. Caustic injury. In: Bayless TM, ed. Current therapy in gastrointestinal and liver disease. Vol 2. New York: BC Dekker, 1986:20.

97. Amendola MA, Spera TD. Doxycycline-induced esophagitis. JAMA 1985;253:1009.

98. Bott S, Prakash C, McCallum RW. Medication-induced esophageal injury: survey of the literature. Am J Gastroenterol 1987;82:758.

99. Carter R, Brewer LA. Achalasia and esophageal carcinoma. Am J Surg 1975;130:114.

100. Hawkins JR, McLaughlin JS. The association of carcinoma of the esophagus with achalasia. J Thorac Cardiovasc Surg 1975;69:355.

101. Hameeteman W, Tytgat GNJ, Houthoff HJ, van den Tweel JG. Barrett's esophagus. Development of dysplasia and adenocarcinoma. Gastroenterology 1989;96:1249.

102. Monnier PH, Fontolliet C, Savary M, Ollyo J-B. Barrett's oesophagus or columnar epithelium of the lower oesophagus. Baillieres Clin Gastroenterol 1987;1:769.

103. Kamiya T, Morishita T, Asakura H, et al. Long-term follow-up study on gastric adenoma and its relation to gastric protruded carcinoma. Cancer 1982;50:2494.

104. Correa P. A human model of gastric carcinogenesis. Cancer Res 1988;48:3554.

105. Sipponen P. *Helicobator pylori* infection—a common worldwide environmental risk factor for gastric cancer. Endoscopy 1992;24:424.

106. Craanen ME, Dekker W, Blok P, et al. Intestinal metaplasia and *Helicobator pylori*: an endoscopic biopsy of the gastric antrum. Gut 1992;33:16.

107. Sipponen P, Kekki M, Siurala M. Atrophic gastritis and intestinal metaplasia in gastric carcinoma. Cancer 1983;52:1062.

108. Stockbrugger RW, Menon GG, Beilby JOW, et al. Gastroscopic screening in 80 patients with pernicious anaemia. Gut 1983;24:1141.

109. Borch K. Epidemiologic, clinicopathologic and economic aspects of gastroscopic screening of patients with pernicious anaemia. Scand J Gastroenterol 1986;21:21.

110. Svendsen JH, Dahl C, Svendsen LB, Christiansen PM. Gastric cancer risk in achlorhydric patients. A long-term follow-up study. Scand J Gastroenterol 1986;21:16.

111. Sjöblom SM, Sipponen P, Järvinen H. Gastroscopic follow-up of pernicious anaemia patients. Gut 1993;34:28.

112. Tytgat GNJ, Offerhaus GJ, Mulder CJJ, Berg BJ. Consequences of gastric surgery for benign conditions: an overview. Hepatogastroenterology 1988;35:271.

113. Tytgat GNJ, Offerhaus JGA, van der Stadt J, Huibregtse K. Early gastric stump cancer: macroscopic and microscopic appearance. Hepatogastroenterology 1989;36:103.

114. Offerhaus GJA, Tersmette AC, Giardiello FM, et al. Evaluation of endoscopy for early detection of gastric-stump cancer. Lancet 1993;340:33.

115. Schafer LW, Larson DE, Melton LJ, et al. The risk of gastric carcinoma after surgical treatment for benign ulcer disease. N Engl J Med 1983;309:2210.

116. Shamir M, Sehuman BM. Complications of fiberoptic endoscopy. Gastrointest Endosc 1980;26:86.

117. Habr-Gama A, Waye JD. Complication and hazards of gastrointestinal endoscopy. World J Surg 1989;13:193.

118. Gelfand DW, Ott DJ, Muritz HA, et al. Radiology and endoscopy: a radiologic viewpoint. Ann Intern Med 1984;101:550.

119. Herlinger H, Glanville JL, Weel L. An evaluation of the double contrast barium meal (DCBM) against endoscopy. Clin Radiol 1977;28:307.

120. Miller-Walser R, Hess H, Würsch RG, et al. Fiberendoskopie und radiologie bei ulcus ventriculi, marojenkarzinom und hiatus hernie: Fragestellung, Zeitpunke und Aussagekraft. Schweiz Med Wochenschr 1979;109:3.

121. Brown P, Salmon PR, Burwood RJ, et al. The endoscopic, radiological, and surgical findings in chronic duodenal ulceration. Scand J Gastroenterol 1978;13:557.

122. Deschamps J-P, Allemand H, Gauffeny B, et al. Evaluation diagnostique et economique de l'endoscopic digestive haute en premiere intention dans l'exploration eoso-gastro-duodenale: resultats d'une etude prospective, en dehors des hemorragies digestives. A propos de 184 malades. Gastroenterol Clin Biol 1982;6:229.

123. Dooley CP, Larson AW, Stace NH, et al. Double-contrast barium meal and upper gastrointestinal endoscopy: a comparative study. Ann Intern Med 1984;101:538.

124. Dekker W, Op den Orth JO. Biphasic radiologic examination and endoscopy of the upper gastrointestinal tract. J Clin Gastroenterol 1988;10:461.

125. Kahn KL, Kosecoff J, Chassin MR, et al. The use and misuse of upper gastrointestinal endoscopy. Ann Intern Med 1988;109:664.

126. Morrisey JF. The problem of inappropriate endoscopy. Ann Intern Med 1988;109:605.

127. National Health Technology Advisory Panel. Usage of endoscopy in Australia 1987.

128. Statements and guidelines developed by the Standards of the Training and Practice Committee of the ASGE. Gastrointest Endosc 1988;3(Suppl):1S.

129. Lieberman DA. In the eye of the needle. A reappraisal of endoscopic sclerotherapy. J Clin Gastroenterol 1988;10:249.

130. Armstrong D, Monnier P, Nicolet M, et al. Endoscopic assessment of oesophagitis. Gullet 1990;1:63.

Textbook of Gastroenterology, second edition, edited by Tadataka Yamada. JB Lippincott Company, Philadelphia © 1995.

CHAPTER 116

Colonoscopy and Flexible Sigmoidoscopy

Christopher B. Williams   Jerome D. Waye

Flexible fiberoptic technology began to be used for visualization of the colon several years after fiberoptic gastroscopy was introduced in 1957. The first commercially available fibercolonoscope, the Overholt Coloscope American Cystoscope Makers Incorporated, or ACMI, appeared in the early 1960s.

Early flexible colonoscopes were difficult to use because of limited tip deflection and a narrow angle of view. By the late 1960s, manufacturers had improved the instrumentation, and endoscopists had developed a technique for total colonoscopy, the alpha maneuver, which depended on fluoroscopic imaging. The need for fluoroscopy and the initial reluctance of endoscopists to use sedation during colonoscopy contributed to its slow acceptance in clinical practice as compared with the rapid and widespread acceptance of fiberoptic gastroscopy.

The advent of colonoscopic snare polypectomy, which provided a major therapeutic and cancer preventive role for colonoscopy, gave a sudden impetus to its use throughout the world.[1,2] In the United States, Shinya,[3] and later, in Germany, Deyhle,[3a] introduced and taught the techniques of snare polypectomy. Further advances in instrument development and techniques of colonoscopic manipulation have made co-

lonoscopy a major imaging technique in patients with colonic disease. Total-colon diagnostic evaluation is possible in a high proportion of cases. Biopsy specimens can be taken anywhere in the colon or terminal ileum, and therapy is possible during the initial endoscopic examination.

Although colonoscopy remains a technical challenge because of the tortuosity of the colon, several factors greatly favor its use. Almost all colonic disease starts on the inner mucosal aspect, and the mucosa is insensitive to heat or biopsy. Almost all colonic neoplasms, except in colitis, project above the mucosal surface as visible polyps, even if only 1 to 2 mm in diameter. The time course of most colonic pathology is slow; therefore, early diagnosis is both feasible and worthwhile.

Despite the technical demands on the endoscopist, rigorous preparation, and some discomfort for the patient, the results of colonoscopy have made it a primary method for examining the colon. Colonoscopy often eliminates the need for a radiographic contrast examination of the large bowel and helps to avoid surgery. With increasing knowledge about the capabilities and limitations of colonoscopy, specific indications are being defined for its use as a first-line investigative technique with therapeutic options, although there are situations in which the barium enema remains the investigation of choice.

TECHNICAL CONSIDERATIONS

Instrumentation

Modern colonoscopes, whether fiberoptic or video, give a brilliant, high-resolution, color view of the mucosa through wide-angle (110–130 degrees) optics. The 20- to 30-fold magnification at 5-mm distance rivals the close-up view of a dissecting microscope, but colonoscopes provide excellent distant views as well. Tip angulation in four directions to more than 180 degrees allows angulation around most acute flexures. Retroflexion (i.e., J configuration) is possible in the proximal colon or rectum, thus minimizing the risk of missing significant lesions in capacious areas that could not be seen with older, less maneuverable instruments. The length of the instruments varies from 35- to 70-cm flexible sigmoidoscopes to the 165-cm long colonoscope. The instruments range in shaft diameter from 1-cm pediatric colonoscopes to 15- to 17-mm adult instruments. Instrumentation and suction channel sizes range from 2.7 to 4.2 mm in diameter. In most ways, a colonoscope is similar in design to a gastroscope, but it has a more flexible shaft to accommodate the various colonic bends encountered, optional CO_2 insufflation facilities are incorporated, and there often is an additional syringe water-wash attachment, which is necessary because of the greater likelihood of lens soiling. The shaft of a colonoscope must have the right combination of sufficiently springy stiffness to advance when pushed, extra flexibility near the tip to help pass acute bends, but also complete torque stability so that it responds to the forceful twisting movements that are a valuable part of colonoscopic technique. Smaller-diameter pediatric colonoscopes or standard gastroscopes, which are more maneuverable in the colons of babies and small children, also have a place in examining ileostomies and fixed or strictured adult colons.

A full range of endoscopic accessories is available for colonoscopes, including biopsy forceps, electrocoagulating hot-biopsy forceps, cytology brushes, washing and spraying catheters, sclerotherapy needles, a range of dilating balloons and bougies, and various polypectomy snares and retrieving devices. Other standard techniques can be applied to the colon with colonoscopy, such as the introduction of balloons or tubes over a guide wire. Instrumental techniques such as the heater probe or laser are as applicable to the lower gastrointestinal tract as they are to the upper gastrointestinal tract. Some endoscopists use an overtube as a splinting or stiffening device to control looping in the sigmoid colon or as a temporary stent to facilitate rapid withdrawal and reinsertion of the colonoscope.

Blind rectal ultrasound probes have been developed to assess invasion in tumors of the anorectal area. Direct-vision, ultrasound-bearing colonoscopes may have a limited role. Technologic advances allow small ultrasound probes to be passed through the colonoscope's instrument channel to enable ultrasound as desired at any point throughout the colon (e.g., before removal of sessile lesions, to check the relation of the colon wall to surrounding organs before electrocoagulation).

Cleaning and Disinfecting

The colonic lumen is laden with bacteria and potentially with pathogenic organisms, including hepatitis B virus and the AIDS virus. Although only a few cases of infection transmitted by way of contaminated colonoscopes have occurred, and no viral transmission has been reported, this is clearly a risk. Endoscopes must be rigorously disinfected to render them demonstrably noninfectious before use.[4] Colonoscopes are totally immersible and designed so that all parts, including air-water and suction channels, are accessible for thorough mechanical cleaning. The cleaning and disinfecting process includes brushing or perfusion with detergent solution before immersing and filling of all channels for a minimum of a 4- to 5-minute period in a strong bactericidal and virucidal disinfectant agent such as glutaraldehyde.[5] Assuming prior removal of organic matter, which can decrease the access of the disinfectant solution, all organisms, including AIDS and hepatitis B, are inactivated within approximately 2 minutes. Mycobacterial spores require 60 minutes or more; the rare pathogen *Cryptosporidium* is difficult to eradicate, but 10% ammonia solution is effective in rendering it inactive.

Accessories, including water bottles, should receive equally scrupulous attention. Some accessories, such as injection needles, are difficult to clean but, because they are of particular risk, they should be sterilized by autoclaving; others, such as biopsy forceps, should receive additional ultrasonic cleaning before disinfection. Use of disposable accessories is increasing. Gas-sterilizing of instruments and accessory equipment is not essential, because all common infectious bacteria and viral agents are killed by routine, commonly accepted disinfecting methods. Nonetheless, some centers recommend sterilization of all reusable accessories by autoclaving or ethylene oxide gas. Instruments used on a patient with known AIDS need not be handled differently than any other potentially infected instrument and should be subjected to rigorous mechanical cleaning and a 5- to 10-minute disinfectant soak-cycle.[6] Because of the known bacterial contamination of the large bowel, every endoscope used to explore the colon must be treated as potentially infected, including flexible sigmoidoscopes.

Well-trained nursing and ancillary staff must apply scrupulous cleaning and disinfecting methods to each instrument between examinations and also to additional instruments. An instrument cannot be properly cleaned and disinfected in less than 12 to 15 minutes, and thorough cleaning often takes longer. Consequently, for adequate cleaning and to allow for breakdowns, two to three endoscopes are required to manage a practice without exposing patients to unacceptable risk. A flexible sigmoidoscope with an integral disposable sheath has been introduced to prevent contamination of the instrument and its biopsy channels.

ANATOMIC BASIS OF COLONOSCOPY

The ease or difficulty of colonoscopy in a given patient is, to a large extent, determined during fetal development and is related to the degree to which the supporting mesenteries fuse to the posterior abdominal wall. Although the descending and ascending colon conventionally become fixed retroperitoneally in the paravertebral gutters, in about 10% to 15% of subjects they remain mobile on mesocolons identical to those that are normal for the sigmoid and transverse parts of the colon. The consequence for the endoscopist is that some colons are mobile and can loop and move around freely and unpredictably within the abdomen and are also uncontrollable by the various straightening or rotation maneuvers that are effective with conventional colonic anatomy.

It can be surprisingly difficult to orientate in the inflated rectum with its angulations formed by the infolded Houston's valves. Inexperienced endoscopists initially have difficulty in following the lumen and may tend to impact or retrovert the endoscope tip.

By about 17 cm, the colonoscope enters the narrower, extraperitoneal part of the sigmoid colon (Fig. 116-1; see Color Fig. 97); thereafter, an expert endoscopist notes whether the sigmoid colon looks and feels long and mobile or, alternatively, short and fixed. The sigmoid has frequent circular haustral infoldings, which may be very exaggerated in some patients, especially those with diverticular disease, into which the instrument tip impacts if steering is not accurate. There are no fixed anatomic landmarks between the anus and the ileocecal valve, but there are geographic clues; these clues are often helpful but may also be misleading.

In contrast to the zig-zag path of the sigmoid colon, the descending colon is usually a short, tubular segment that the instrument must traverse to reach the splenic flexure area. An acute angulation of the instrument tip at the junction of the sigmoid and descending colon may afford a clear view of the tubular descending colon, but forward progress may be im-

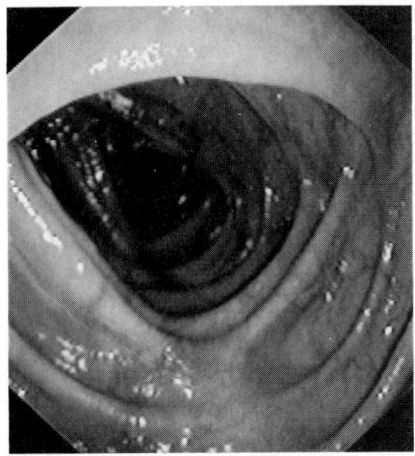

FIGURE 116-2. (See Color Fig. 98.) Transverse colon shows the characteristic triangular outline resulting from the relative thickness of the three longitudinal teniae coli. The circular muscle is much thinner.

peded by loops in the instrument caused by passage through a tortuous and convoluted sigmoid colon. When a large-volume, fluid-electrolyte oral preparation is used, the posturing by gravity of residual fluid provides useful clues to the anatomy. In the left lateral position, the descending colon is fluid-filled, whereas the sigmoid and transverse colon are dry.

The transverse colon (Fig. 116-2; see Color Fig. 98) frequently shows a triangular configuration as a result of its three longitudinal muscles, or teniae coli. The liver is a fairly predictable landmark. The flat, bluish gray surface has sharply

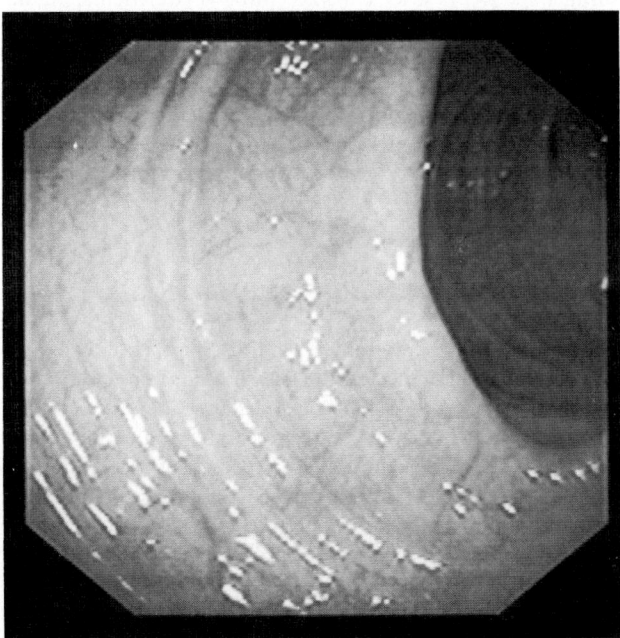

FIGURE 116-1. (See Color Fig. 97.) In the sigmoid colon, the circular outline with the light reflex over arcs of circular musculature clearly indicates the center of the lumen for close-up endoscopic steering purposes.

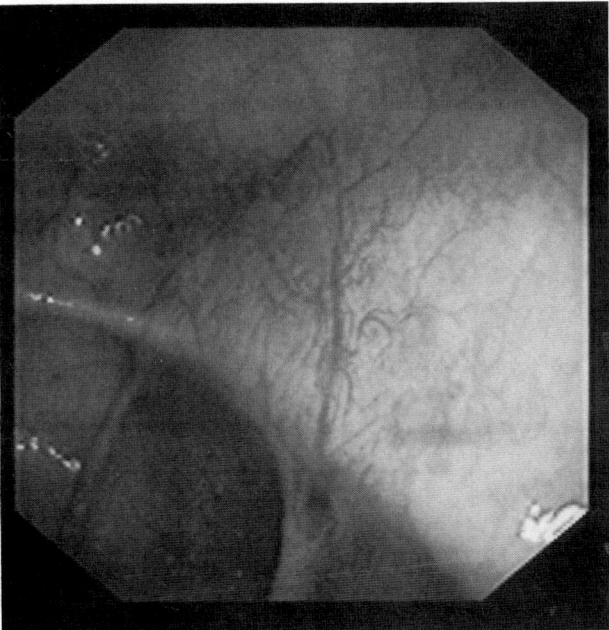

FIGURE 116-3. (See Color Fig. 99.) Hepatic flexure shows the impression of the liver. Similar discoloration can be caused by other extracolonic viscera at the splenic flexure or in the distal colon. Note the longitudinal impression of a tenia, and the transverse haustral folds.

defined edges caused by the balloon-like, air-filled colon contacting the hepatic surface (Fig. 116-3; see Color Fig. 99).

On rounding the hepatic flexure and entering the ascending colon, the superior lip of the ileocecal valve may appear in the distance as a flattening on the first circular haustral fold in the colon (Fig. 116-4; see Color Fig. 100). The upper lip may be seen as a notched bulge or may appear thickened by fat accumulation. Sometimes the opening is slit-like on the inferior side of the fold and can be seen only by retroversion of the instrument within the cecal pole. The appendiceal orifice, a less definite landmark, is seen as an unimpressive crescent-shaped slit or a circular convolution of folds at the blind saccular cecal pole, which may also have tiny red rings (Fig. 116-5; see Color Fig. 101).[7] Multiple, pale reddish, 1- to 2-mm circular halos are often seen in proximity to the appendix when using the videoendoscope. These represent lymphoid follicles.

The ileal mucosa has a granular appearance when the ileum is air-filled, and short frond-like villi are visible in pools of fluid. The granular appearance is caused by multiple light reflections from the individual villi. One- to 3-mm nodules of lymphoid tissue, sometimes aggregated into 10- to 15-mm plaques of Peyer's patches, are normal in the last few centimeters of the terminal ileum and are particularly prominent in children. By contrast, the normal colorectal mucosa is smooth and shiny, although with deflation, fine transverse innominate grooves may show, especially with surface dye spray.

Throughout the colon, a fine, interlacing, vascular pattern is visible in the mucosa through the transparent overlying epithelium. When the vascular pattern is not visible, a patho-

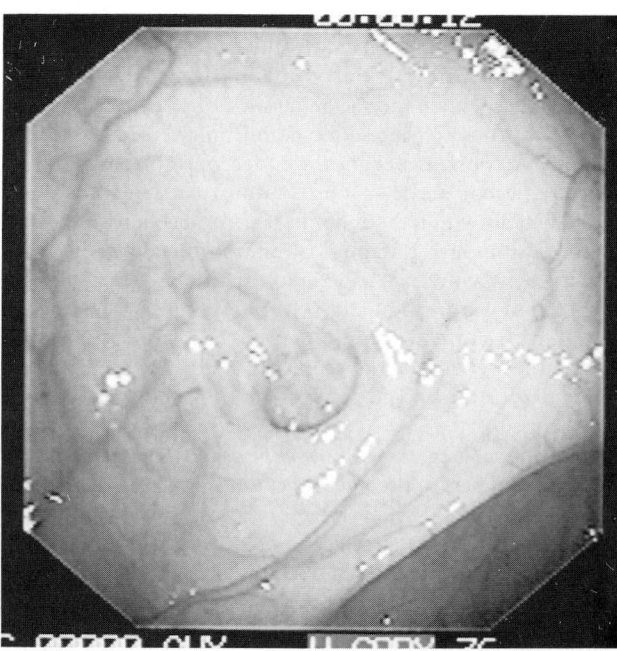

FIGURE 116-5. (See Color Fig. 101.) The appendix orifice is variable in configuration. Here, the orifice is round, but it may also be seen as a crescent-shaped slit. It is usually rather insignificant in appearance. The internal aspect remains the same after appendectomy.

logic process causing hyperemia of the epithelial mucosal vessels must be considered, but biopsies are needed to differentiate between inflammatory change and traumatic or reactive hyperemia. Opacity of the surface can also be caused by thickening that occurs after chronic colitis or by edema. In the rectum, the vascular pattern becomes more pronounced, with thickening of each vessel, and the hemorrhoidal veins may appear wide and tortuous. A U-turn (i.e., retroflexion) maneuver in the rectum affords a view of the dentate line (Fig. 116-6; see Color Fig. 102) and perianal internal hemorrhoids, but the rigid anoscope gives a superior view of this area by dilating it maximally.

Localization During Colonoscopy

The position of the colonoscope can be approximately judged by a combination of factors: the length of instrument inserted and then maximally straightened back, the amount of colon traversed, and the characteristic appearances of certain areas, including the circular, fluid-filled, descending and triangular, air-filled, transverse colon. Most instruments, but not all videoendoscopes, are bright enough to transilluminate the abdominal wall where the bowel approximates to the surface at the splenic flexure (left midaxillary line), transverse colon, or ascending colon and cecum. Fluoroscopic guidance is rarely used but can be useful in the endoscopist's learning phase and in a few difficult cases.

Alternatively, the transabdominal impression of the endoscopist's palpating fingers may be seen from within. Transillumination or visible finger palpation in the right iliac fossa,

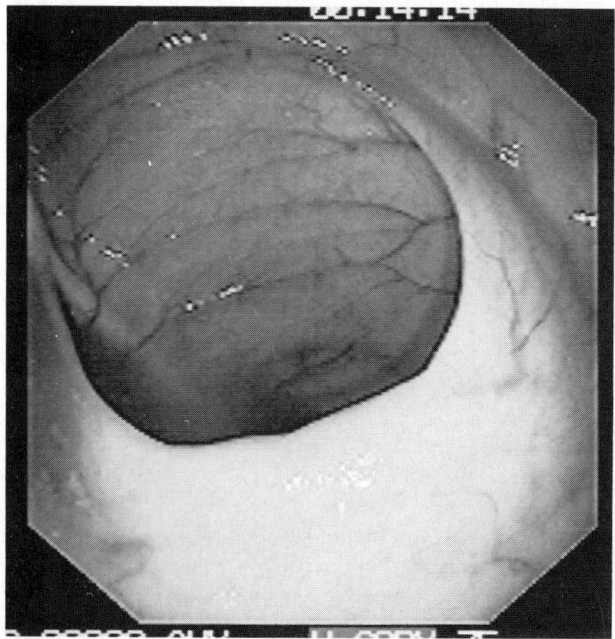

FIGURE 116-4. (See Color Fig. 100.) Ileocecal fold shows the characteristic notch on a flattened fold. The notch denotes the superior labia of the ileocecal valve. The opening is just below the notch and cannot be seen without marked angulation of the instrument tip.

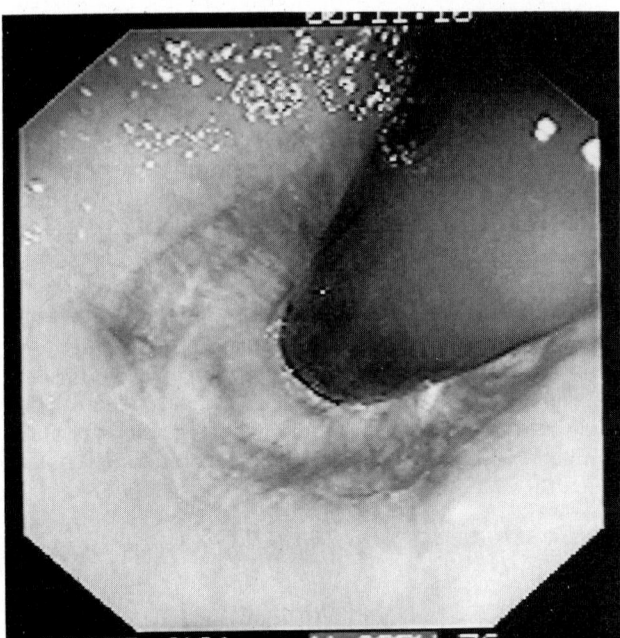

FIGURE 116-6. (See Color Fig. 102.) Retroversion of the endoscope in the rectum is a useful maneuver to find or remove small polyps in the distal part of the rectal ampulla. The dentate (pectinate) line is serpiginous at the junction of the squamous mucosa of the rectal canal (purple) and the columnar rectal mucosa.

however, does not necessarily indicate that the tip of the instrument is located in the cecum, because the instrument tip may stretch almost any portion of the colon into the right lower quadrant during colonoscopic intubation. For instance, mobile portions of the bowel, such as the sigmoid or the midpoint of the transverse colon, can be pushed toward the right iliac fossa.

All localizing judgments can be mistaken. For instance, using the length of scope inserted, in a long or mobile colon, 80 cm of shaft may be looped in the proximal sigmoid, whereas in the same patient during withdrawal, the instrument may be straightened so that the splenic flexure is 40 cm from the anus, and the hepatic flexure (or even the cecum) can be reached with 50 to 60 cm of instrument. The only definitive landmark is the ileum seen through the ileocecal valve, but even this may be difficult to locate, and the valve can be effaced after severe or long-standing inflammatory disease.

Because of the absence of absolute landmarks throughout the colon, even if the endoscopist has succeeded in total colonoscopy with identification of the ileocecal valve and cecal pole, there is the possibility of being grossly mistaken about the location of the instrument tip and the anatomic localization of pathologic finding.[8] Even an experienced endoscopist can mistake the splenic flexure for the hepatic flexure or the hepatic flexure for the cecum, and thereby mislead the surgeon as to the site of an obstructing tumor.

In the absence of fluoroscopy, any lesion seen by colonscopy can be marked with sterilized India ink injected through a long, flexible, injector needle, either for subsequent surgical localization or to enable the endoscopist to find it on a subsequent examination. A 1-mL, gray-blue, submucosal stain

of India ink remains at the injection site for years after injection.[9] It is possible to mark the proximal extent of tip progress with metal clips, but this technique is not frequently clinically useful, because the clip-marking device can only be passed through a large-channel colonoscope.[10]

BOWEL PREPARATION

Total colonoscopy is rarely possible in the unprepared colon. Patients with profuse watery diarrhea are sometimes mistakenly thought not to require preparation and are often found to have an opaque mucosal coating of fecal material that obscures adequate view of the surface. In this instance, preparation is required.

Even patients with a surgically defunctionalized bowel produce inspissated mucoid residue and require cleansing. A patient with massive colonic bleeding may effectively cleanse the colon of fecal material, but often a residual coating of blood obscures mucosal events during the colonoscopic examination.

Limited Preparation

When it is necessary to examine only the distal colon segments, an adequate preparation can consist of one or two evacuant enemas of tap water, saline, or more usually, a small-volume hypertonic phosphate or other proprietary enema, given 1 hour before the examination begins. This allows enough time for proper bowel clearance but is not so long that proximal contents move distally. Limited bowel preparation assumes normal colonic ability to empty the whole left colon rapidly by mass action. This may not happen in patients with diverticular disease or strictures, for whom even limited examination must usually be preceded by full bowel preparation.

Full Preparation

No topic in colonoscopy excites as much discussion as the ideal bowel preparation, a clear indication that present preparation regimens are not completely satisfactory. The ideal may not be attainable because of the huge variation in individual preferences and intestinal dynamics—what suits one patient nauseates or produces cramps in another or even fails to work altogether. Ideal attributes for bowel preparation include pleasant taste and avoidance of excessive volume, cramps, or the need for enemas.

Certain modifications of medication and diet are common sense before preparation. Oral iron medications must be stopped 4 to 5 days before colonscopy, because the formation of organic iron tannates in combination with dietary green-vegetable residue renders colon contents black and offensive, making them sticky and difficult to clear. Constipating agents such as codeine phosphate or loperamide should be discontinued 12 hours before colonoscopy. Aspirin and other antiplatelet drugs or anticoagulants may require discontinuation 7 days before examination to reduce the risk of immediate or delayed bleeding should polypectomy be performed.

No matter what the preparation regimen requires, in almost all of the methods, colon cleansing is enhanced by a clear or full-liquid diet for 24 to 48 hours before the examination.

Purgative Regimens

Purgative regimens, with or without enemas, are still the most commonly used form of bowel preparation. Their advantage is that the colon, after a contact laxative such as senna, castor oil, or bisacodyl, is stimulated to evacuate most of the bowel contents. Disadvantages are that the evacuation stimulus can cause severe cramping abdominal pain, that the cecal region is often poorly cleared, and that some solid residue often remains distally. Therefore, enemas are normally required to supplement the cleaning effect of the purgative, but they must be of large volume (up to 2–3 L in some cases) to reach the proximal colon. Enemas are not popular with patients and are also time-consuming for nursing staff.

Osmotic purges can be used as an alternative to enemas, either adding to or supplementing the oral purgative with up to 2 L of an agent such as magnesium salts (e.g., citrate, sulfate) or a nonabsorbed carbohydrate (e.g., mannitol, lactulose, sorbitol). Magnesium sulfate has strong purgative and osmotic effects but also an unpleasant taste, so that the milder but citrus-flavored magnesium citrate is generally preferred. A low-volume sodium phosphate preparation has been well received by patients.[11] Mannitol has been the most widely used of the carbohydrate solutions. Its sweet taste can be reduced by cooling, and the likelihood of nausea is prevented by preadministration of an oral antiemetic prokinetic agent such as domperidone or metoclopramide 30 minutes before administration. Five-percent mannitol is isotonic, and 2 L are drunk slowly over 1 hour or more. Routine use of mannitol or other carbohydrate preparations risks explosion during electrosurgical procedures, because of the production of hydrogen gas resulting from fermentation by intestinal bacteria. This risk can be effectively eliminated by insufflation of carbon dioxide during the procedure or by meticulously aspirating gas and reinsufflating air before electrosurgery. Two 45-mL aliquots of sodium phosphate taken orally the evening before and 3 hours prior to colonoscopy produce a vigorous catharsis. Cleansing enemas are not required. Fluid balance shifts, and absorption of electrolytes such as magnesium or sodium may cause deleterious effects, especially in the presence of cardiac or renal disease.

Balanced electrolyte solutions, administered in a volume of 4 L orally or by nasal tube, result in an acceptable bowel preparation. Flavored solutions are available and may increase patient compliance. Simple saline solution (0.9% sodium chloride) is effective and arguably safe for preparation of the majority of patients, but potassium losses and electrolyte fluxes can be avoided by appropriate additional ingredients. The first commercial balanced electrolyte solutions with added polyethylene glycol (PEG; e.g., Golytely, Colyte) had an unpleasantly bitter taste from the added sodium sulfate and potassium chloride which caused around 10% of patients to stop drinking the solution and thereby fail to prepare their colon adequately. Other patients can tolerate the taste but have trouble with the volume to be drunk. Newer formulations of the large-volume balanced electrolyte solutions hold the promise of improved palatability.[12] Although packaged instructions advise minimal dietary restrictions, better results can be expected from a 24-hour full liquid diet.

The regimen chosen for whole-colon preparation necessarily varies according to circumstance, patient preference, and clinical indication. Patients need to sleep and must be able to travel without fear of incontinence, so that the timing of preparation must also be adjusted according to the time of examination and travel arrangements. Frail, ill, and elderly patients may require modified preparation, sometimes on an inpatient basis if cooperation is uncertain. If obstruction is a possibility, oral preparations may be dangerous or at least should be spread out over a longer period. In almost all circumstances, a patient fit for total colonoscopy is fit for full-bowel preparation. Compromise in reducing the regimen may result in poor preparation and in only being able to perform a limited examination or a less accurate colonoscopy.

Medication

Sedation

Sedation is unnecessary for some examinations, especially those that are limited or in patients after sigmoid colon resection, or in those in whom a procedure is known to have been easy on previous occasions. An experienced endoscopist with skilled technique who already knows the patient may opt for no sedation, whereas a trainee endoscopist faced with an unfamiliar and frightened patient is wise to use it. A great deal also depends on the patient's attitudes and on local custom. Some people know that they can tolerate pain or are motivated to do so because they wish to drive or pursue normal activities after the examination; others can be hysterical or do not want to know anything about it. Endoscopists in some countries rarely sedate; those in other countries almost always do. As for bowel preparation, a skilled physician adapts to what is best for the individual patient, remembering that using less sedation makes for better patient cooperation, easier change of position, and greater safety. Using no sedation allows the patient to leave rapidly and unescorted after the procedure. However, endoscopists who never use sedation may have a lower success rate in total colonoscopy and do not usually solicit their patients' views on acceptability.

Some stretching of peritoneal attachments is inevitable, at least transiently, during colonoscopy. This causes gnawing or acute unpleasant visceral pain. Coupled with air distention and the sensation of rectal fullness simulating the desire to defecate, this can make a slow examination difficult for some patients, although others tolerate it easily.

The patient receiving conscious sedation with pethidine-meperidine and a benzodiazepine is capable of responding to painful stimuli during the colonoscopic examination. Many patients are minimally sedated, enabling them to carry on a coherent conversation during the procedure and to change position if required.

Drugs administered for sedation should be given intravenously just before the examination so that peak levels and effect occur during the few minutes required to pass the looping distal colon. Intravenous administration also results in the shortest recovery period thereafter. The unpredictable absorption and longer action of intramuscularly administered drugs make this route less suitable.

Benzodiazepines

Benzodiazepines (e.g., diazepam 3–10 mg IV, midazolam 2–5 mg IV) are used in colonoscopy, as in upper gastrointestinal endoscopy, for their calming and amnestic effects. They are administered by slow intravenous injection at the start of the procedure. Younger patients and heavy drinkers can become disinhibited or agitated by benzodiazepines, and older patients can experience hypotension or respiratory depression. Consequently, larger doses are rarely necessary or wise. It is a particular mistake to use incremental doses of benzodiazepines for pain, because they have only weak analgesic effects. If respiratory depression or collapse occurs, a benzodiazepine antagonist (e.g., flumazenil, 0.1 mg) should be immediately available and is rapidly effective.

Midazolam has a longer lag time between injection and the peak onset of action than does diazepam, a factor that tends to result in midazolam overdosage if the endoscopist relies on the patient's counting or on the absence of slurred speech to give an incremental dose. It is also more potent dose-for-dose than diazepam. The amnestic effect frequently results in failure to recall any unpleasantness during the examination and inability to remember any postprocedure advice or discussion.

Opiate Analgesics

Opiate analgesics, especially pethidine or meperidine, 25 to 75 mg IV, but also pentazocine or fentanyl, should be the mainstay of medication for colonoscopy because of their superior analgesic effect, often with a useful feeling of euphoria. If additional medication is required, opiate injections for extra analgesia can be administered. unless the patient is allergic, only prior medication with monoamine oxidase inhibitor antidepressants contraindicates the use of opiates. Lower doses of opiates should be administered to elderly patients because of their synergistic hypotensive and respiratory depressant effects coupled with benzodiazepines and an already stressful procedure. Clinical, blood pressure, and pulse oximetry monitoring may be of importance in the elderly or high-risk patient; if in doubt, the procedure can be terminated or the antagonist (naloxone, 0.2–0.4 mg IV or IM) can be given to reverse the opiate effects.

Neuroleptanalgesia

Neuroleptanalgesia (e.g., droperidol and haloperidol), the combination of a neuroleptic agent to cause central dissociation and an intravenous opiate for analgesia, is popular in France. To be effective, a dosage level is required that makes anesthesiologic supervision desirable. Because the after-effects are more drawn out than those of benzodiazepine-opiate combinations or even general anesthesia, the regimen has little attraction.

General Anesthesia

General anesthesia is rarely or never employed by skilled endoscopists. It should never be used as a cover-up for poor colonoscopic technique, because it may add to the risk of complications by removing any feedback from the patient relating to trauma from unexpected loops or adhesions and from problem electrosurgical procedures.

Antispasmodics

Antispasmodics (glucagon, 0.5–1 mg IV; hyosine-N-butyl bromide, 20–40 mg IV) may increase the difficulty of insertion by rendering the colon atonic and therefore more likely to stretch and loop, but they eradicate circular muscle spasm and may increase the accuracy of examinations for small lesions such as polyps or angiodysplasias.

Antibiotics

Antibiotics in broad-spectrum combination (e.g., ampicillin 1 g or amoxicillin 1 g, gentamicin 80 mg) are given intravenously 10 to 30 minutes before the procedure in patients who are immunosuppressed; have metal heart valve replacement, septal defects, ascites; or are receiving peritoneal dialysis.[13] Some endoscopists feel it is necessary to give full antibiotic prophylaxis whenever there is an artificial prosthesis such as hips or other joints or breast implants.[14] A logical parallel can be drawn with other major operative procedures, such as dental extraction, for which prophylactic antibiotics are routine. This is because of the transient bacteremia known to occur during the mucosal trauma of insertion, as well as rare cases of septicemia or sepsis after colonoscopy.

MONITORING DURING ENDOSCOPY

The best monitor is an alert and trained gastrointestinal endoscopy assistant who observes the patient for color, pulse, change in respiration, diaphoresis, and other pertinent signs during the procedure. Mechanical monitoring techniques, such as continuous electrocardiography, pulse oximetry, and respirometers, have not been shown to be effective in the patient receiving conscious sedation during colonoscopy, but they are, nonetheless, increasingly being used. The level of analgesia cannot be equated to patients receiving general anesthesia, who are totally reliant on the anesthesiologist for oxygen exchange.

Oxygen should be given in any patient, especially the very old or very young, in whom pulse oximetry shows repeated or prolonged desaturation or when clinical features such as pallor, sweating, and semicollapse make desaturation a possibility.

COLONOSCOPY FROM THE PATIENT'S POINT OF VIEW

Some patients fear colonoscopy, and none look forward to it, which is why most endoscopists use an intravenous sedative-analgesic injection beforehand. As a result, because the actual examination is invariably less unpleasant than the patient expects, it is usually well tolerated and even interesting when watched by the patient on monitor screen or down the sidearm attachment of the instrument. During colonoscopy, unlike gastroscopy, the patient can also converse with the endoscopist. In the minority of cases in which the procedure is traumatic because of unavoidable loops or bends, additional sedation can be given, with resulting amnesia.

Patients dislike the preparation phase most of all, including dietary modification, starvation, and, depending on the chosen regimen, the need to drink a large volume of unpleasant solution, endure cramping induced by purgatives, or submit to the indignity of enemas. Twenty-four hours of low-residue or liquid diet are generally sufficient, and, thereafter, the best bowel preparation should be short-lived and taken as near as possible to the time of examination with due allowance for sleep. Whichever of the different oral or purgative regimens is chosen, it must cause profuse, clear, fluid diarrhea. A more vigorous preparation may be required for the patient with chronic constipation or severe diverticular disease or a patient whose bowel was not properly cleansed with a previous regimen.

The intravenous medication used, usually a benzodiazepine and pethidine-meperidine, has maximum effect for about 5 minutes, during which the patient may have little memory. During the procedure, there is a feeling of distention and often the urge to defecate or pass wind, all mainly caused by the periodic stretching of the colon by the instrument rather than to actual overinflation. Pain during colonoscopy can usually be rapidly diminished or eliminated by reducing the loop or loops responsible for traction on the root of the mesentery. Normal diet, activities, and medication can usually be resumed as soon as the mild stress of the examination and the effects of medication are over. The ambulatory patient may benefit from administration of a narcotic or benzodiazepine antagonist. Sedated patients cannot drive, and most do not return to work until the next day.

COLONOSCOPY PROCEDURE

Position and Position Changes

The left lateral position is most commonly used for flexible sigmoidoscopy and colonoscopy, mainly because it gives convenient access to the perineum for insertion. However, colonoscopic examinations can be, and in some centers are, performed in other positions, including lithotomy, knee-chest/elbow and right lateral positions. Especially if a large-volume fluid preparation regimen has been used, position changes can modify both the configuration of the colon and of the air and fluid within it because of the effects of gravity. Thus, in the left lateral position, the sigmoid colon is somewhat dependent but full of air, whereas the descending colon is relatively airless but full of fluid. Rotating the patient to the right lateral position sometimes improves the configuration of the sigmoid-descending colon junction and always improves the view of the descending colon, because air rises into it and fluid runs out. Such changes of position may be useful during difficult insertions and are of particular importance for colonoscopy in the bleeding patient, because by posturing blood out of and air into the field of view, the colonoscope can be inserted even if the colon contains blood and clot. When forward progress can no longer be accomplished, a change in the patient's position will aid tip advancement in two thirds of cases.[15]

Insertion of the Endoscope and Flexible Sigmoidoscopy

Digital examination of the anorectum is used to lubricate the area generously and to palpate any lesion. A local anesthetic gel may reduce anal discomfort. The instrument tip may be directly inserted into the rectum, or the distal bending section may be supported with the forefinger, pressing the tip obliquely against the external sphincter until it relaxes. When there is rectal stenosis, fistulation, or abnormal anal sensitivity, it may be desirable to use a small-diameter pediatric instrument.

The technique for flexible sigmoidoscopy is the same as for the first part of a colonoscopy, except that it is less important to avoid looping, because the proximal colon is not to be intubated. Characteristically, there is a red-out when the instrument enters the rectum, because the tip abuts on the rectal mucosa. Simultaneous air insufflation and instrument withdrawal are required to disimpact it, and angulation or rotational movements are useful to find the rectal lumen. Movements of the instrument tip should thereafter be slow and deliberate, taking care to steer toward the lumen *before* pushing inward, so as to avoid constantly losing the view.

When the lumen cannot be seen, continuing to push the instrument shaft into the rectum stretches the sigmoid colon into unnecessary and painful loops and rarely results in tip advancement, because once it is impacted against a haustral fold, the tip tends to remain stationary while the rest of the scope flexes into a loop.

Slide-by is a term describing the appearance when the lens is against the mucosal surface and the instrument is pushed forward, so that the mucosal vessel pattern visibly slides in close-up across the lens. This maneuver should be avoided but is permissible for short distances and only when the instrument is known to be pointing in the correct direction; if tip movement stops and the mucosa blanches, additional pressure risks perforation, and the instrument must immediately be withdrawn to locate the lumen. Withdrawal and disimpaction of the tip is a routine procedure performed every time the view is lost for more than a few seconds.

Diverticular disease is often associated with thickened rings of circular muscle or fixation of the sigmoid colon by pericolic adhesions from previous inflammatory episodes. The resulting distortion and angulations can make it difficult to locate the lumen and coax the instrument through, because the tip is not free to maneuver normally. In a few cases, a small-diameter pediatric colonoscope or a standard gastroscope with the capability for greater tip deflection may allow passage through diverticular disease where the standard colonoscope cannot be passed. Despite the technical problems in intubation, endoscopic examination of diverticular disease can be clinically valuable, mainly because the distorted appearances seen on barium enema may make it impossible to exclude malignancy on radiologic grounds. Similar bowel fixation and angulation may occur after hysterectomy as a result of postoperative adhesions between the sigmoid colon and anterior aspect of the pelvic cavity.

If any pathology is seen during flexible sigmoidoscopy, a biopsy can be easily and safely performed. However, routine electrosurgery for polyp removal is contraindicated after the limited bowel preparation for flexible sigmoidoscopy because of the significant hazard of explosive gas mixtures unless CO_2 insufflation or a careful dilutional aspiration-reinsufflation technique is used.

Total Colonoscopy

It is important to understand the fundamentals of insertion technique, because they are the basis of rapid, relatively pain-free, accurate total colonoscopy. Endoscopists who experience difficulty during intubation of the proximal colon or passage around the hepatic flexure are invariably those who have not recognized the importance of straightening out the colonoscope in the distal colon before attempting the last part of the insertion. Looping in the sigmoid colon is the bugbear of the endoscopist throughout a colonoscopy but especially when it is necessary to push harder to transmit force around the curved colonoscope to reach the cecum.

During a colonoscopy, options available to the endoscopist include pushing the instrument in or pulling it out; twisting the shaft to the right or the left; insufflation or withdrawal of air; using tip controls to steer up, down, right, or left; use of abdominal pressure to reduce loops; and changes of patient position. The difference between the slow endoscopist who reaches the cecum infrequently after a traumatic examination and a fast endoscopist who examines the whole colon in 95% of patients within an average time of 10 minutes is the ability to run through the various options logically, quickly, and sequentially without repeating a nonproductive maneuver over and over again. Because some of these options need to be performed together or in a logical sequence, concentration and careful decision-making are essential.

The ease with which the instrument is inserted depends on the variable anatomy, mobility, and distensibility of the colon, requiring the skilled endoscopist continually to analyze the type of problem encountered and to use a series of logical or empiric maneuvers to coax the tip inward while avoiding excessive force or undue looping of the shaft. This includes the use of twist in one direction while simultaneously pushing or pulling, deflation of the colon to keep it short and pliable, external hand pressure to reduce loops or influence the instrument in the required direction, and even changes of patient's position so that gravity modifies both the position of colonic loops and air and fluid inside the segment being examined. Dexterously manipulating the instrument controls to keep an adequate view of direction, concentrating on visual detail to locate and find the direction when it is briefly lost, and backing off quickly if the tip impacts into a bend or fold, the endoscopist should, to some extent, *feel* when the instrument is passing freely and can be advanced or when it is becoming snarled and should be withdrawn before pushing in again. The biggest mistake of the inexperienced endoscopist is to think that a good view of the lumen is an unqualified signal to push, especially when looped in the sigmoid with a view of the descending colon; pushing often results in an expanding sigmoid loop with resultant pain but without tip progress.

Some sigmoid loops, such as the spiral alpha loop configuration that may form in the sigmoid colon, are favorable, because they allow the instrument to proceed into the de-scending colon without forming acute angulations; others, such as the N loop which more frequently occurs in the sigmoid, put the tip into an acute angulation at the descending colon junction, making this area difficult and painful to pass through. Fluoroscopy is not necessary to ascertain the presence or position of a loop, because it is apparent that a loop is forming whenever the shaft pushes in more than the tip advances. Additionally, once a loop is stretched on its mesentery, additional pushing hurts the patient. Conversely, when the colonoscope shaft runs straight, with the colon shortened or pleated over it rather than stretched, intubation can be accomplished by a light touch on the instrument with 1:1 correspondence between shaft and tip in push-pull and rotational movements. At the same time, when free of excessive loops, tip angling using the dial controls is easy and full.

A good endoscopist examining a colon with normal attachments and no excessive adhesions tries to maintain a straight instrument and a comfortable patient for most of an examination and rapidly straightens out any unavoidable loops to regain the responsiveness of the instrument whenever it is lost for more than a short period. Because of the multiple bends, folds, and twists of the large bowel, it is inevitable during a colonoscopy that the instrument will loop or start to loop on many occasions. After each advance, by pulling back and restraightening the shaft, the colon is effectively shortened and pleated over the instrument, which is progressively advanced on a three-steps-forward-and-two-steps-back basis.

It is not possible to keep the instrument straight or the patient completely comfortable all the time because of the unpredictability of the sigmoid colon. There may be a minute or two of difficulty or looping before the tip reaches the fixed retroperitoneal part of the descending colon or the splenic flexure, where the shaft can be fully straightened by pulling back with clockwise rotation to only 50 cm from the anus. Unfortunately, because of the variability of the anatomy and attachments of the sigmoid and descending colon, this first part of a colonoscopy is the most difficult part of the procedure.

Passing the splenic flexure into the transverse colon is usually easy if the sigmoid can be held straight. After maximal shaft withdrawal, the combination of gentle shaft advancement with clockwise twist maintained, simultaneous abdominal pressure over the sigmoid, and avoidance of tip overdeflection, usually allows progress into the transverse colon. Overaggressive pushing tends to reform the loop in the sigmoid, and overangulation impacts the tip into the flexure (i.e., the walking-stick effect). If, after several attempts, the tip does not advance, the instrument should be withdrawn and restraightened; rotating the patient into the right lateral position almost invariably causes the splenic flexure to drop downward, allowing the instrument to slide around to the midtransverse colon. With the patient in the right lateral position, the midtransverse colon often sags down into a rather acute bend, providing a good point at which to withdraw and restraighten the colonoscope once again and also to rotate the patient back into the left lateral position before insertion into the proximal colon.

Once the colonoscope is in the proximal transverse colon or hepatic flexure region, and thereafter in the even more capacious ascending colon, deflation is extremely helpful in advancing the instrument and shortening the distance to the ileocecal region. Aspiration of air causes the colon to deflate concentrically so that the diameter is smaller, but it also results in shortening the colon longitudinally. A few additional maneuvers may be helpful in assisting total intubation, such as rolling the patient into the prone or supine position or asking the patient to inspire to lower the diaphragm. The more difficult it is to reach up or around the hepatic flexure and down to the cecal pole, the less likely it is that simple forward pushing will work. The longer and more mobile the colon is, the more certain it is that force will generate loops that will absorb all the motive power applied, whereas with attention to technique and patience, even a redundant colon often shortens to only 50 to 60 cm at the hepatic flexure, permitting the tip to slip down the last few centimeters with ease.

Only occasionally is it necessary to consider the possibility of using fluoroscopy or accessories such as the overtube, and some endoscopists never use either. In the endoscopist's learning phase, x-ray imaging may give some insight into the problems of localization, the variability of loops, and the degree of force and twisting movements needed to reduce them. Thereafter, fluoroscopy is rarely helpful, although in an ideal situation, any endoscopist might be glad to have x-ray films available to increase the accuracy of localization of obstructing tumors or the confidence to manipulate the outsize or atypical loops that can form in patients with redundant or mobile colons. Advances in technology have recently permitted electromagnetic imaging devices to record, in real time, the three-dimensional localization of the colonoscope shaft without x-ray involvement.

A brief mention should be made of the new stiffening overtube, which is used to splint and control the sigmoid colon when conventional methods fail, to withdraw and reinsert the colonoscope for instrument exchange, or to provide for easy removal of multiple polyp specimens from the proximal colon. Split overtubes, incised lengthwise so that they can be placed over the shaft of the instrument and the split taped over with strong adhesive tape, may be added during the procedure and removed again immediately after fulfilling their purpose. The overtube does not help in passing the looped sigmoid colon and is only used when the tip is in the upper descending colon or splenic flexure region after the sigmoid loop has been straightened. In patients with anal stenosis, diverticular disease, or adhesions, overtube insertion may be impossible.

Ileocecal Region

On reaching the last few centimeters before the cecal pole, an appreciation of local anatomy is needed to find the ileocecal valve. Even experienced endoscopists can be mistaken in thinking that a capacious hepatic flexure is the cecal pole, or that tonic contraction of the ileocecal fold represents the appendiceal orifice. The appendiceal orifice is seen often merely as a crescent-shaped slit or a circular convolution of folds. Only by withdrawing the colonoscope 10 cm or so back up the ascending colon and looking for the tell-tale inward bulge of the valve on the ileocecal fold, which is the first encircling fold back from the cecal pole, can the endoscopist determine

where to angulate and enter the ileum. Even so, ileal intubation can be difficult and may require several minutes and not a little skill and patience. The anatomy is variable, and both colon and colonoscope can rotate or move during attempted insertion. Some ileocecal valves show prominent pouting lips, others are the merest slit on the reverse side of the ileocecal fold, which may require visualization by retroversion of the bending section of the colonoscope within the cecal pole.

Terminal Ileum

A skilled endoscopist can enter the terminal ileum with reasonable ease in approximately 80% of cases and can almost invariably obtain a blind forceps biopsy through the valve in the remaining patients. Failures arise mainly when deformity or scarring make angulation impossible or make the opening too narrow, but poor bowel preparation or difficulty in maneuvering if the instrument is looped can be contributory problems. Endoscopic assessment of the mucosa of the terminal ileum is straightforward. Although the polypoid lymphoid follicles that are frequently present may cause a mistaken diagnosis of Crohn's disease and cobblestoning radiologically, to the endoscopist, these nodules and the surrounding mucosa are covered with normal pink mucosa with a granular surface in air or with small villi visible underwater.

The endoscopic view of the terminal ileum is usually limited to 5 to 10 cm. There is rarely a serious indication to attempt further insertion, because ileal Crohn's disease almost invariably involves the terminal part of the ileum, other lesions such as ileal angiodysplasia are exceedingly rare, and a Meckel's diverticulum is not endoscopically accessible, because it is located 1 m proximally. If deep ileal intubation is attempted, 30 to 50 cm is usually the limit of what can be seen because of the acute angulations that occur in the small bowel.

Role of the Assistant

Colonoscopy cannot be performed by one person alone. While the endoscopist pays full attention to the endoscopic image, the endoscopic assistant monitors the patient and assists with accessories. If polyps are encountered, the snare and patient return-plate must be plugged into the electrocautery apparatus, which requires setting the proper diathermy levels and testing to ensure that all equipment is functioning properly. During the examination, additional lubricant, gloves, and abdominal pressure may be required from time to time during various phases.

A properly trained and observant gastrointestinal assistant is an absolute necessity for the proper performance of colonoscopy. The assistant's functions extend beyond the confines of the endoscopic procedures itself. The room must be set up before the procedure, endoscopic photographs must be recorded, biopsy specimens must be duly noted, and requisition forms for the histopathologist must be filled out. Supplies, equipment, and accessories must be ordered in advance, and all equipment that may possibly be necessary for the procedure must be assembled and available before the examination.

The assistant orders and prepares the necessary preendoscopic medications and is responsible for maintenance of the emergency cart, which must include antidotes for the various medications used, cardiac drugs, resuscitation equipment such as an Ambubag, endotracheal tubes and laryngoscopes, intravenous solutions, and oxygen. The cleaning, care and maintenance of all the endoscopy equipment is in the hands of the assistant, who is responsible for mechanical cleaning and disinfection procedures.

Most colonoscopists prefer to advance and withdraw the shaft of the instrument with the right hand, while the left hand manipulates the dial controls as well as the air-water and suction buttons. However, some colonoscopists prefer a two-person technique, whereby the assistant advances the instrument while the endoscopist handles the control portion of the colonoscope.

THERAPEUTIC PROCEDURES

In addition to its diagnostic capabilities, colonoscopy makes possible a range of therapeutic procedures.[16] Polypectomy is the most obvious, but electrocoagulation, laser photocoagulation, or injection therapy of vascular lesions (e.g., telangiectases, angiodysplasias, hemangiomas) are all routine. Laser photodestructions also make possible the ablation of some tumor masses and large sessile polyps if conventional surgical or snare polypectomy techniques are inappropriate.[17] Snare polypectomy, around the stalk of pedunculated polyps or in one or more sessions of piecemeal polypectomy for sessile polyps according to size, is an efficient, rapid, and relatively safe method.[18] By constricting the tissue within the closed snare wire, low electrical power is sufficient (often only 15–20 watts) for transection with very localized tissue heating. The high-frequency alternating current used causes no nerve or muscle depolarization or shock. Because the colon mucosa is insensitive to thermal injury, the patient should feel nothing during polypectomy or electrocoagulation unless full-thickness heating is occurring, which causes the patient to warn of peritoneal pain at an early stage, before actual damage has occurred. If small polyps are found, simultaneous biopsy and electrocoagulation with electrically insulated hot-biopsy forceps often can be performed. This rapid procedure ensures that a histologic specimen is obtained.[19] An alternative technique for small sessile polyps is cold resection, or cheese-wiring across the base by closing the snare in the absence of current. Snared tissue can be retrieved for pathologic analysis by aspiration through the instrument channel into a filtered suction-trap. Larger polyps can be retrieved whole using the snare loop or other grasping devices, although this may necessitate several reinsertions of the endoscope for multiple polyps.

Except for polyps with an extremely broad base, almost all polyps encountered can be removed endoscopically. Pedunculated polyps are removed with snare application around the pedicle, with sufficient visible electrocoagulation before transection. Pure coagulating current at low power is used by most endoscopists; during snare-loop tightening, this provides controlled and localized tissue heating for blood vessel obliteration.[20] Thicker stalks with increased risk of immediate or delayed bleeding can be preinjected with 1 mL of an epinephrine-sclerosant mixture to ensure hemostasis before snaring; Similarly, broad-stalked or sessile polyps can be preinjected at the base with 3 to 10 mL of saline or diluted epinephrine solution to act as a fluid safety-cushion before snare transection or piecemeal removal. Flat polyps or barely invasive colon carcinomas may be successfully resected by a strip biopsy technique, whereby the polyp is elevated by a submucosal saline injection prior to transection. If the polyp is very large and snare placement is difficult, it may be useful to remove segments sequentially until the base can be easily visualized and complete transection can be accomplished. Even very large pedunculated polyps may be removed in piecemeal fashion. Usually, polyps that cannot be removed endoscopically are those that cover a substantial area of the colonic surface (i.e., more than 25% of the circumference) or extend over two interhaustral folds.

Every effort should be made to retrieve all the resected portions of each polyp and to submit them to the pathologist for histologic evaluation. Because of the force of gravity, however, polyps have a tendency to fall into fluid pools or crevices that hide them from view, making retrieval difficult. There are various techniques for polyp retrieval. Although in clinical circumstances, only about 94% of transected colon polyps are recovered for full histopathologic interpretation, those most likely to be lost are small and of little clinical significance.

Tube placement in patients with pseudoobstruction (i.e., Ogilvie's syndrome) or postoperative ileus can be either by direct intubation through the instrumentation channel, over an endoscopically placed guide wire after withdrawal of the colonoscope,[21] or by carrying the tube up alongside the endoscope during insertion. Immediate decompression occurs, but because of the frequency with which redilation occurs, it is wise to leave the tube in situ until it is expelled spontaneously, signaling restoration of normal propulsive contractions.[22] A stiff guide wire within the tube avoids premature ejection.

Balloon dilatation is possible, usually with through-the-scope (TTS) balloons inserted under direct vision into the stricture, with or without prior guide wire placement.[23] The largest available TTS balloon is 18 mm, which gives sufficient dilation for most circumstances with minimal risk of splitting the stricture. Other techniques for stricture dilation include incision into the stricture with electrocoagulation by way of a needle-knife, the edge of a polypectomy snare, or a papillotome. These methods are only useful for relatively thin, short strictures.

A larger balloon can be passed over an endoscopically positioned guide wire with correct insertion and dilation observed either endoscopically or on fluoroscopy. Short strictures, such as those after right hemicolectomy for Crohn's disease or when postoperative complications result in localized anastomotic narrowing, respond very well to endoscopic dilatation. A single dilatation can be either permanently effective or can last 6 to 9 months, depending on the presence of any inflammatory condition likely to cause restenosis.[24]

Postoperative anastomotic stenoses may be dilated widely during the first examination, because there is usually considerable fibrosis around the anastomotic site, making the occurrence of free perforation unlikely. Strictures in inflammatory bowel disease, however, do not have the same surrounding cicatricial reaction, and the initial dilation should be limited to not greater than twice the diameter of the stricture. Frequently, the lumenal narrowing in Crohn's disease is related to active inflammation with circular muscle spasm and therefore is rarely ameliorated by attempts at endoscopic dilation techniques.

INDICATIONS

Flexible Sigmoidoscopy

Flexible sigmoidoscopy should be the procedure of first choice for examination of the rectum and sigmoid colon. It should replace rigid proctosigmoidoscopy except when used for screening examinations of the rectum on grounds of cost, expediency, and the ease of taking larger biopsy specimens.[25] The rigid proctoscope (i.e., anoscope) is preferred for assessment of hemorrhoids and anal canal pathology, which are often poorly seen with a flexible instrument.

Flexible sigmoidoscopy alone may be considered sufficient examination in patients with minor disturbance of bowel habit, obvious hemorrhoidal bleeding, or localized left iliac fossa pain. With minimal discomfort and no sedation, the rectum, sigmoid colon, and often the descending colon or splenic flexure can be examined.

Colonoscopy

Colonoscopy can be performed in any patient fit for barium enema and for a similarly wide range of indications. With the increasingly widespread availability of endoscopic skills and improvements in instrument technology, colonoscopy can often be regarded as a first-line procedure not preceded by barium enema. A prior barium enema rarely helps the endoscopist, because the configuration on x-ray films, unless the colon is seen to be excessively long, gives little indication as to how easy or difficult the colonoscopy will be. Most patients find barium enema a more unpleasant experience than colonoscopy because of the sustained inflation required in the double-contrast barium enema (DCBE)[26] and because of the sedative-analgesic medications given for colonoscopy.

High-Yield Indications

The highest diagnostic yield of endoscopic pathology is in patients with tumor, polyps, stricture, or mucosal disease diagnosed on DCBE. Colonoscopy replaces either repeat x-ray investigation or laparotomy as the means of histologic confirmation or confident exclusion of a questionable abnormality,[27] and it allows immediate therapy where appropriate.

Polyps

Nearly all polyps can be snare-resected during the procedure, and even some radiologically diagnosed carcinomas prove to be benign lesions that are manageable endoscopically.[28] The rule of thumb is that, unless there is a typical apple-core carcinoma on x-ray films, no patient should be submitted to surgery on radiologic grounds without considering colon-

oscopy. Even with an apple-core lesion on x-ray films, colonoscopy can confirm the histology of the lesion and rule out synchronous polyps and cancers.

Five percent of pedunculated or broad-based polyps removed endoscopically are found histologically to contain invasive carcinoma with malignant cells traversing the muscularis mucosa into the submucosal layer. The term *carcinoma-in-situ* to describe the biologically benign entity in which malignant cells are present only superficial to the muscularis mucosa should not be used in favor of the more innocuous term *severe dysplasia*. Surgical resection is not necessary if there is a sufficient margin between the limit of invasive carcinoma and the resection line, if the carcinoma is well or moderately well differentiated, and if there is no lymphatic or venous invasion.[29–32] There is controversy as to whether these endoscopic and histologic principles should be applied to the local removal of sessile polyps or whether surgery should be recommended unless the patient is a poor operative risk. Because malignant polyps and polypoid carcinomas tend to occur in older, frail patients, and surgery rarely yields resectable lymph nodes without evidence of distant metastases, there is an increasing tendency to use conservative endoscopic management, even in lesions failing to meet the criteria, unless the patient is an excellent surgical risk.[33] The use of India-ink tattooing makes it possible to localize a malignant polypectomy site with accuracy in the event that surgical resection is necessary or for subsequent local surveillance after an interval of 2 to 3 months before entering a normal follow-up regimen.[34]

Rectal Bleeding

Rectal bleeding, especially if sustained, dark, or mixed in the stools, is frequently caused by tumor or mucosal pathology. In the subgroup of patients with visible rectal bleeding in whom a barium enema and sigmoidoscopy are normal, about 10% of referral patients have cancer, 15% to 20% have polyps (Fig. 116-7; see Color Fig. 103), and up to 50% have some kind of a visible abnormality, including traumatized, inflamed,

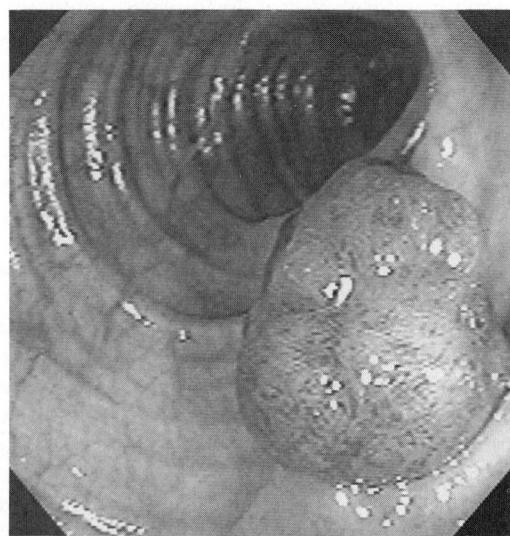

FIGURE 116-7. (See Color Fig. 103.) Smooth sessile adenoma is located in the descending colon.

or ulcerated mucosa. Blood loss, particularly in elderly persons, remains the highest-yield indication for colonoscopy. Total colonoscopy should be performed rather than DCBE in the assessment of rectal bleeding, whether overt or occult, because of the obvious bonus of color view in seeing blood, altered blood, or bleeding points, which can be flat and totally invisible on x-ray films. It may also be possible to treat the cause of bleeding endoscopically.[35]

Acute Colonic Bleeding

Acute colonic bleeding of overwhelming proportions may require surgery and perioperative bowel irrigation with on-table colonoscopy.[36] Ten percent of patients with acute colonic bleeding will have an upper gastrointestinal source, which must be considered in all instances. In most cases of acute bleeding, an attempt at conventional colonoscopy examination is indicated *before* resorting to angiography, scintigraphy, or other investigational techniques. If possible, oral or nasal tube electrolyte bowel preparation is started immediately after the patient presents, because blood coating makes localization of the bleeding site very difficult without preparation or if enemas reflux blood proximally. Colonoscopy should be started as soon as practicable, because the aim is to examine the bowel while fresh bleeding continues.[37] Changes of patient position during the examination help to maintain adequate visualization. Expertise is needed in this situation, but a cause for bleeding should be apparent in over one half of the cases, and treatment may be possible by polypectomy, electrocoagulation injection therapy, or other means.

Anemia

Anemia of the iron-deficient variety or a positive fecal occult blood test indicate colonoscopy rather than DCBE, because flat lesions such as angiodysplasia or minor inflammatory change cannot be diagnosed radiologically. Even if radiographs appear normal, endoscopy is known to find significant numbers of radiologically missed lesions such as cecal carcinomas. In anemic patients, gastroscopy and colonoscopy can be performed at the same visit. The object of endoscopy in anemic patients mainly is to rule out carcinoma or vascular anomalies (Fig. 116-8; see Color Fig. 104) with certainty; about 80% have negative examinations, but the endoscopic opinion is considerably more certain than a negative x-ray film result.

Chronic Diarrhea or Known Inflammatory Bowel Disease

Whereas diarrhea of short duration is often self-limiting and adequately investigated by simpler means, it is imperative in patients with long-standing bowel frequency to make an accurate examination with histologic or other specimens as appropriate.[38] Rectal biopsy and bacteriologic assessment diagnose or exclude etiologic factors adequately in many patients, but total colonoscopy and ileal examination complete the investigation and sampling process in one test. Chronic diarrheal illnesses may not result in any grossly visible mucosal abnormality, but biopsy should be obtained vide infra.

Often, the mucosal appearances are sufficient to make immediate assessment of the extent and type of colitis.[39] Crohn's disease, in particular, shows a rather characteristic pattern of small aphthoid (i.e., mouth ulcer–like) ulcers with intervening normal mucosa quite unlike the generalized redness of early ulcerative colitis. More advanced inflammatory disease of any type, including ulcerative colitis, Crohn's disease, tuberculosis, or amoebic colitis, can be nearly indistinguishable from each other because of the colon's limited range of responses to various diseases that affect the mucosal surface (Fig. 116-9; see Color Fig. 105).[40] Ischemic colitis has a range of appearances, from slight reddening and friability, to varying degrees of ulceration, to frank gangrene; the diagnosis is often possible by combining endoscopic assessment with the typical history of sudden onset of pain, bleeding, and diarrhea and with the perisplenic distribution.

Microscopic or Collagenous Colitis

Both forms of colitis can occur despite normal endoscopic appearances; therefore, biopsy specimens must be taken in any patient with chronic diarrhea or increased bowel frequency.[41] The normal colonic mucosa frequently harbors inflammatory cells, and great care should be taken to avoid misinterpretation and overdiagnosis of disease when none is truly present, based on the histopathologist's report of acute and chronic inflammation on biopsy specimens. Collagenous colitis is diagnosed histologically from a thickened intraepithelial collagen layer; the condition has a disputed relation to inflammatory microscopic or lymphocytic colitis.

Cancer Surveillance or Prevention

The unique tendency of the colon to precede cancer with a long period during which focal adenomatous polyp formation is visible above the normal mucosal surface gives the endoscopist the opportunity for accurate visualization, biopsy, and destruction of precancerous lesions, even at sizes of 1 to 2 mm.[42] Accuracy is possible, because color makes it easy to distinguish which small excrescences are fecal, which are air bubbles, and which are polyps. The radiologic threshold for diagnosis is higher than that of colonoscopy, both to avoid overdiagnosing artifacts, and because barium does not always coat smaller or flatter polyps. Colonoscopy is indicated for any patient at increased risk for polyp and cancer formation, including probands with first-degree relatives with colorectal cancer, the 5% of patients with an inherited genetic risk (e.g., familial adenomatous polyposis, cancer family syndrome,[43] colorectal cancer family members), patients needing first examination or follow-up after removal of known adenomas or colorectal cancer, and patients in whom there is a predisposing risk for long-term colorectal cancer (e.g., longstanding extensive ulcerative colitis,[44] previous ureteric implantation into the sigmoid colon). The exact interval between surveillance examinations is a matter of debate, varying from patients judged to be at higher risk who may be examined at yearly intervals, to the majority in whom 2- to 3-year intervals or even longer intervals may be appropriate.[45]

Surveillance examinations in extensive ulcerative colitis and possibly Crohn's colitis[46] patients normally start 8 years after onset of disease and are repeated at 1- or 2-year intervals, with

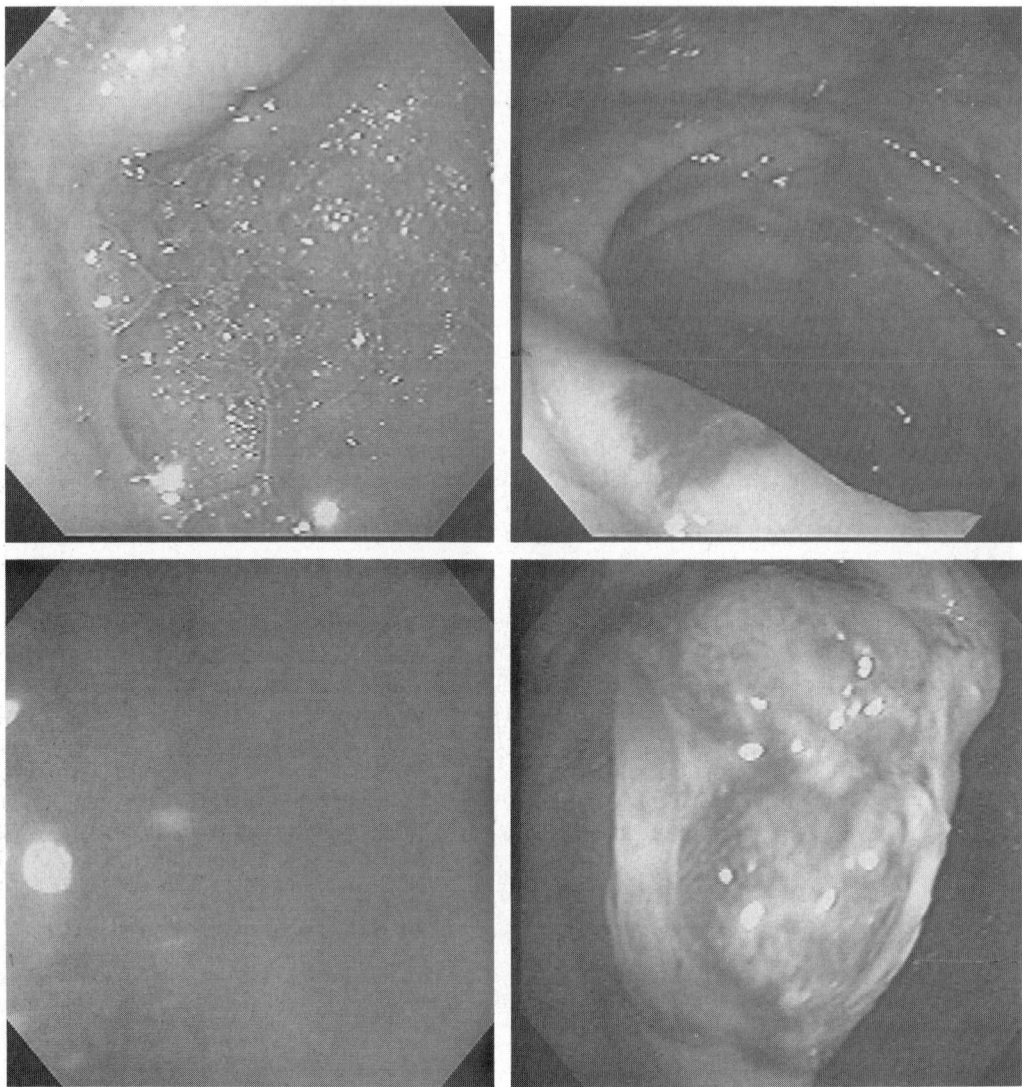

FIGURE 116-8. (See Color Fig. 104.) Dilated blood vessels characteristic of angiodysplasia are found in the right side of the colon.

10 or more biopsy specimens taken at representative sites around the colon. The endoscopist is alert for any nodular, indurated, or plaque-like lesions in the colon, but varying degrees of low- or high-grade dysplasia may be found in relatively normal-looking mucosa.

Low-Yield Indications

The particular virtues of colonoscopy, accuracy and the ability to take biopsy specimens, are irrelevant to conditions manifesting with functional symptoms such as long-standing constipation, bloating, or left iliac fossa discomfort, which can safely be investigated by x-ray examination if there is no occult or overt colonic bleeding. The colon in idiopathic or acquired megacolon and Hirschprung's disease may be almost impossible to prepare and offensive and difficult to endoscope, whereas radiology gives a perfect assessment of colon configuration. In elderly patients with symptoms suggestive of di-

verticular disease, x-ray films rapidly and easily exclude serious pathology in most cases; in the same patients, unless the endoscopist is expert, colonoscopy can be relatively slow, traumatic, and more hazardous. On the other hand, the elderly patient may be unable to cooperate with the need to retain barium, resulting in a poor radiographic examination. Bowel symptoms in patients older than 70 years of age may be better investigated by colonoscopy than barium enema.

It is possible to compromise between colonoscopy and DCBE. For instance, when skilled endoscopy is not available and colonoscopy proves unreasonably difficult, endoscopy can be abandoned, aspirating residual air as far as possible and proceeding to immediate DCBE. Using CO_2 rather than air insufflation is an advantage, because in 15 minutes, there is total absorption of residual CO_2, leaving the radiologist a nondistended bowel that is easy to fill and coat with barium.[47,48] Endoscopic biopsies can be performed safely before DCBE,[49] and in all probability, hot biopsies and snare removal of small stalked polyps may also safely precede the x-ray examination.

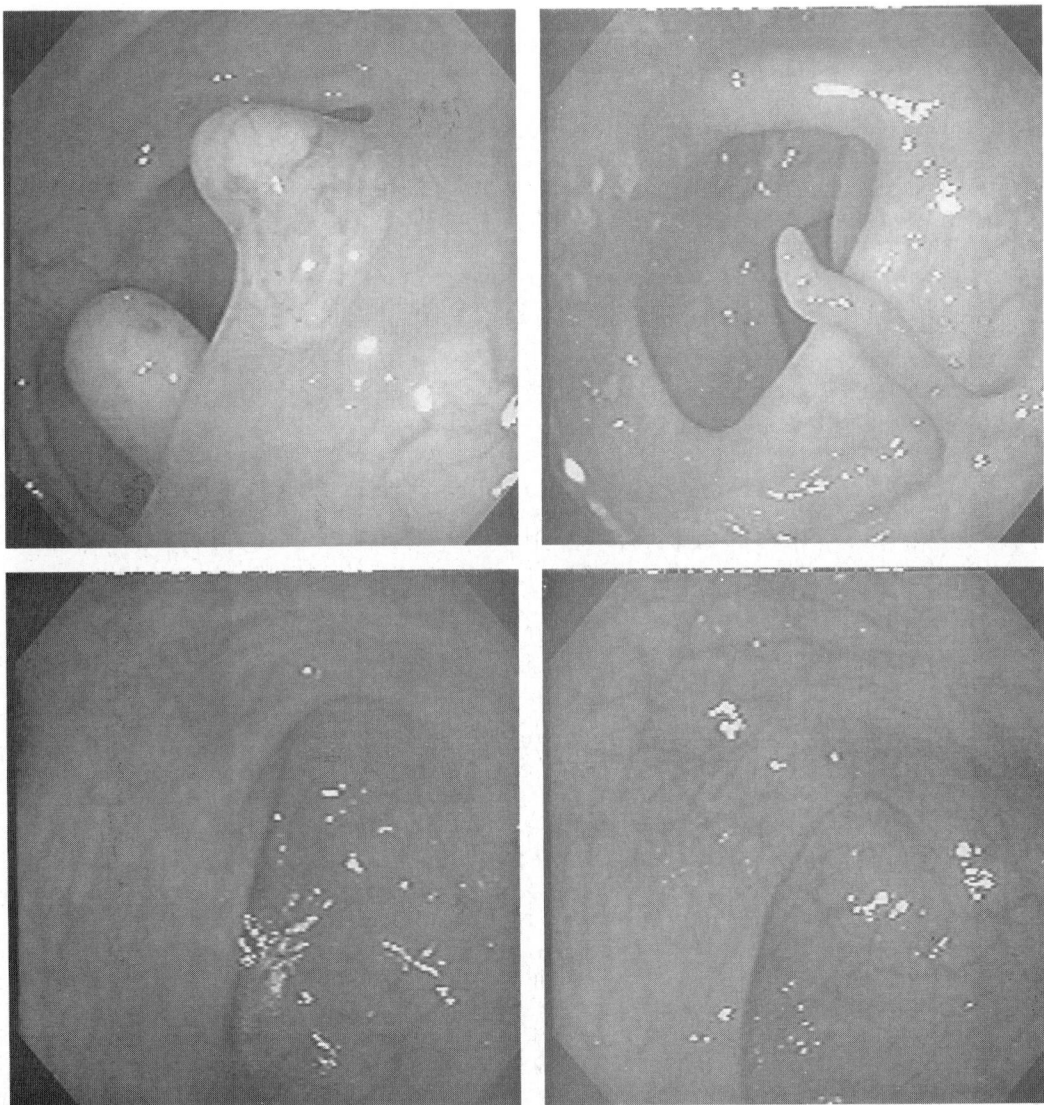

FIGURE 116-9. (See Color Fig. 105.) Filamentous inflammatory polyp in the descending colon. There is no mucosal activity related to chronic ulcerative colitis.

INTRAOPERATIVE COLONOSCOPY

The most common indication for intraoperative colonoscopy is to localize the site of a previously endoscopically resected malignant polyp. The site may heal completely in 3 weeks, leaving no external sign of its location, but it can often be endoscopically identified as a scar on the mucosal surface. Another indication is to assist the surgeon in identifying which colonic segment is the source of massive lower gastrointestinal hemorrhage. The presence of a large volume of blood can completely obscure intralumenal vision. Blood can be rapidly flushed out of the colon by a large-volume saline lavage instilled through a cecostomy.

CONTRAINDICATIONS AND RISKS

Colonoscopy is a relatively stressful physiologic experience and a strong vagal stimulus that can produce dysrhythmias,[50] minor disturbances of electrocardiographs, and a degree of hypotension; therefore, it is contraindicated for several weeks after myocardial infarction.[51]

Both the air pressure involved in distention of the colon and the unavoidable stretching during passage around loops and bends have the potential to exacerbate any existing risk of perforation. Colonoscopy is therefore contraindicated in the acute or abscess phase of diverticulitis. Severe acute episodes of ulcerative, Crohn's, ischemic, or infective colitis have generally been considered a contraindication for colonoscopy, but recent reports suggest that it is safe and may be of value in therapeutic decision-making in these situations.

Bacteremia occurs transiently during colonoscopy, which therefore should be avoided in patients with ascites or those on peritoneal dialysis.[52] In these patients and in patients with heart valve replacement, immunodepression, or immunosuppression, including sick or marasmic infants, prophylactic antibiotics should be administered.[53] An appropriate combination is given intravenously 10 to 30 minutes before the procedure and can be repeated in seriously at-risk subjects over the subsequent 24 hours.

Therapeutic maneuvers increase the hazards of colonoscopy.[54] Balloon dilatation in a sick patient may justify antibiotics. Polypectomy carries a small risk of immediate primary bleeding or of delayed secondary hemorrhage for up to 12 days after the procedure. The likelihood of delayed bleeding is especially increased in patients with a coagulopathy or in those taking anticoagulants or antiplatelet therapy. When medical conditions prohibit discontinuation of coumadin, the patient requires admission to the hospital for the substitution of heparin for oral anticoagulation. Once the prothrombin time has returned to normal levels, the heparin dosage should be stopped 4 hours before colonoscopy with polypectomy. If a clean polypectomy has been performed without bleeding, heparin may be restarted 4 hours after the procedure, and oral anticoagulants can be reinstituted 12 to 24 hours later. The patient must remain on heparin until prothrombin levels have returned to the therapeutic level. If polypectomy is associated with bleeding, an attempt should be made to withhold heparin for 8 to 12 hours, if it is considered that the patient can safely remain off anticoagulants for that period.

Polypectomy can also result in perforation by cutting through the bowel wall or by applying sufficient thermal energy to burn through and necrose the full thickness of the colon, resulting in a perforation delayed for between several minutes to a few hours after the polypectomy. Some features of a full-thickness thermal injury to the colon wall may occur 6 to 24 hours after polypectomy, known as the postpolypectomy or transmural burn syndrome, including localized pain, fever, and leukocytosis.[55] Transmural damage is localized and self-sealing when bowel loops, mesentery, omentum, or other adjacent peritoneal surfaces become adherent, so that conservative management with antibiotics and bed rest is usually sufficient.

When signs of frank perforation occur after colonoscopy, it is safest to advise immediate surgery. If only a small amount of free air is present on a postendoscopy x-ray film and the patient has no symptoms, it may be safe to treat the patient conservatively, with antibiotics but without surgery. In any event, a surgeon should always be involved in observation of the patient and in deciding whether or not surgery is indicated.[56]

Oversedation is a risk during colonoscopy, especially for inexpert endoscopists. Patients who for technical or other reasons cannot tolerate colonoscopy despite standard levels of sedative-analgesic medication may sometimes require rescheduling with an anesthesiologist present. Particularly in babies and the elderly, it is hazardous to administer large doses of benzodiazepine-opiate combinations, which can cause sudden cardiorespiratory arrest or dangerous levels of hypotension and hypoxia, which can easily pass unnoticed unless pulse oximetry is employed. Sedative-analgesic medication doses should usually be decreased in those older than 70 years of age, and appropriate antidotes, full resuscitation and monitoring equipment, and oxygen should be immediately available in the endoscopy suite.

Current morbidity and mortality rates for colonoscopy are unknown but are certainly much higher than those for barium enema. An accepted, probably pessimistic, quote is for a perforation rate of 1 in 1700 colonoscopies and mortality of 1 in 5000, with most deaths occurring after inappropriate conservative management of suspected perforation.[57]

The bleeding rate after polypectomy is around 1.5% of polypectomies but is likely to be reduced with better attention to hemostatic techniques such as the sole use of coagulating current, slow transection, stalk injection, and other methods being explored. The use of injection for immediate control of bleeding should avoid the small number of cases in which angiographic or operative intervention was necessary because of uncontrollable bleeding. Unexpected x-ray demonstration of free air in the abdominal cavity (pneumoperitoneum) of symptomless patients submitted to routine abdominal x-ray after colonoscopy has been reported.[57a] Surgeons also report the existence of hematomas, serosal splits, and manifestations of local colonic trauma in patients coming for laparotomy soon after colonoscopy. These facts serve as a reminder to all endoscopists, particularly those in the learning phase, to be cautious, to be considerate to the patient, to avoid oversedation, and to be prepared to abandon a colonoscopy that appears unreasonably traumatic.

COMPARISON WITH BARIUM ENEMA

Colonoscopy has become a procedure of first choice for most colonic investigations since instrumentation has advanced technically, allowing total colonic intubation in over 90% of cases.[58] Nonetheless, the problem in colonoscopy is in the mechanical aspects of insertion technique; the procedure is dependent on the dexterity of the operator. Endoscopic interpretation is easy because of the close-up color view backed by the ability to take pathologic specimens when necessary. However, the colonoscopist can be quite unaware of lesions in blind spots behind acute colonic bends or of submucosal or extracolonic pathology, which may be visible to the radiologist.[59] It is estimated that it is unusual to miss a polyp of 1 cm in diameter during colonoscopy.[27]

DCBE requires different skills. Whereas insertion of the liquid barium column is easy, considerable judgment and experience are needed to introduce the correct quantity of barium and air to coat and distend all parts of the colon and its mucosal surfaces adequately, and to take the necessary radiographs. Even having obtained good-quality films, the radiologist can have difficulty in interpretation. Poor preparation, convoluted bowel loops, circular muscle spasm, diverticular disease, or air bubbles may modify the view. The radiologist's assessment of fine mucosal detail, including the smallest polyps and lesser degrees of ulceration or inflammatory change, is considerably inferior to that of the endoscopist, who views intralumenal appearances directly and in full color.[60,61] Unfortunately, patients with very long and mobile colons or with advanced diverticular disease who are difficult to endoscope are also difficult for the radiologist. Barium enema can be performed following failed or difficult colonoscopy, but endoscopy is impossible in the presence of barium; it is therefore logical to attempt colonoscopy first in most circumstances, providing that each technique is equally available and that the criteria for performing primary colonoscopy are present.

Technical difficulties of colonoscopy in patients with severe constipation and megacolon make them best managed by modified barium technique, sometimes with no bowel preparation, whereas patients who have reduced mobility, rectal incontinence, prolapse, or stomas are best examined by colonoscopy because of technical difficulty in obtaining proper filling and coating with x-ray contrast material. Barium enema is particularly effective in assessing the configuration and gross morphology of the colon, especially when there are multiple strictures or fistulas that may be impassable or invisible to the endoscopist.

Barium enema films are easily stored and retrieved for review and comparison with subsequent examinations, a feature not available with colonoscopy, because there is no method for endoscopic photographic mapping of the large bowel. Watching 20 to 40 minutes of a colonoscopic videotape is a tedious task that is not likely to be a standard part of any endoscopic review.

LIMITATIONS OF COLONOSCOPY

The capability of direct colon visualization of the large bowel and great accuracy of most colonoscopic examinations have been explained. It is pertinent to mention that the endoscopist is capable of gross errors in localization and occasionally of missing large lesions. Certain areas, including the rectal ampulla and behind acute bends, flexures (especially the mobile sigmoid-descending colon junction), spastic muscle contractions, or acute haustrations, can create blind spots for the endoscopist. Adhesions or strictures can render the endoscope tip immobile and make a proper view for targeted biopsies impossible. Large polyps on long stalks can be missed by the endoscopist because they move around and may spring out of the field of view as the colonoscope is pulled back. Poor preparation and redundant or mobile colons also make the endoscopic examination less accurate.

Careful inspection for possible abnormalities is important on the way in as well as during the withdrawal phase of a colonoscopy, because the view of the stretched colon is quite different from that obtained when the bowel is shortened. Several passes may be needed to see all aspects of an angulated or convoluted area properly. There is no room for complacency by the endoscopist over the accuracy of colonoscopy, because it takes dexterity and integrity to be sure that an optimum examination has been performed. It can be assumed that 5% to 10% of the mucosal surface is not seen during colonoscopy. This explains the significant pick-up of lesions up to 5 to 10 mm in diameter during the check colonoscopies usually performed within 1 year of a previous colonoscopy and polypectomy to establish a clean colon that is free of adenomas. Careful colonoscopy can, nonetheless, claim up to 95% accuracy in detecting polypoid lesions of any size, a precision that is equalled by few other diagnostic methods. Misses of colonic neoplasm can occur in the intramucosal lesions of chronic ulcerative colitis, within strictures, or where there is submucosal involvement by extrinsic neoplasm or metastases.

Mucosal surface appearances, especially color, give a good idea of underlying pathology. The surface epithelium is normally transparent, giving a view of the underlying submucosal vessels, arteries, or veins in branching configuration or vascular pattern, which disappear into a red uniformity with hyperemia or inflammation. In inflammatory bowel disease, redness usually indicates inflammation, but because dilated vessels can persist even when the inflammation subsides, histologic confirmation is necessary. Conversely, because of the minor inflammatory change or microscopic colitis that can occur

despite normal mucosal appearance, biopsies are taken in any patient with diarrhea, even if the appearances are normal.

In addition to diagnostic difficulties, the mechanical limitations of colonoscopy are relevant. An expert manages up to 98% to 99% total colonoscopy, especially if there is no stricture or stenosing lesion to prevent insertion. Less expert endoscopists achieve only 70% to 75% total colonoscopy and are more likely to be slow, inaccurate in diagnosis and localization, and more traumatic and liable to complications. The lack of proper means of teaching colonoscopy skills limits its clinical application worldwide.

COSTS

Colonoscopy is highly cost-effective. The instrumentation involved is inexpensive compared to x-ray. A colonoscope, although seemingly expensive, should last for about 500 examinations before replacement becomes necessary. Compared to the enormous hidden costs of installation, upkeep, repair, and amortization of x-ray equipment, the capital sums involved in endoscopy are modest.

The overall cost is approximately equal if an x-ray and flexible sigmoidoscopy-first schema is compared to a colonoscopy-only approach to the investigation of patients with lower gastrointestinal symptoms. Many patients with an abnormal sigmoidoscopy or barium enema demonstrating a lesion or probable pathology will have a subsequent colonoscopy for confirmation, polypectomy, or biopsy; only a few with the colonoscopy-first approach will require a barium enema.

Because of the nature of colonoscopy, intense involvement of the physician is required at all stages of the procedure. The actual physician time involved per procedure is greater for colonoscopy than for the barium enema, during which examination films may frequently be taken by a technician.

Colonoscopic examinations rarely require repeating except for follow-up purposes. By combining diagnostic accuracy and the opportunity for immediate therapy, usually on an outpatient basis, colonoscopy represents excellent value for money.[62] Nonetheless, in many parts of the world, the widespread availability of barium enema, its low cost, low risk, and satisfactory patient acceptance will ensure that x-ray evaluation retains a major role in colonic diagnosis for years to come.

FUTURE DEVELOPMENTS

Videocolonoscopy will allow improvements in image resolution as well as potential for computer enhancement and related developments that should improve diagnostic accuracy, localization, and ease of instrument handling. Advances in bowel preparation should permit comfortable clearance in a few hours instead of the 24- to 48-hour preparations employed. Developments in safe, short-lived analgesia should make insertion easily tolerated while allowing normal activities soon afterward, such as driving or return to work. Computerized interactive teaching models will permit education in manipulative and interpretive skills without imposing an undue burden on and risk to patients during the endoscopist's early training phase.

Development of other diagnostic and therapeutic modalities will allow the endoscopist to apply miniaturized imaging probes to areas of interest and to ablate lesions more completely and safely than can be performed at present. For instance, ultrasound probes passed through the instrumentation channel help to determine the presence and depth of penetration of malignancy. With improved photosensitizing agents and laser photocoagulation or locally injected immunotherapeutic agents, colonoscopy should be able to make further inroads into territory that is currently considered the domain of the surgeon.

The reader is directed to Chapter 78, Colon: Anatomy and Structural Anomalies; Chapter 114, General Considerations; Chapter 119, Contrast Radiology; and Chapter 120, Cross-Sectional Anatomy.

REFERENCES

1. Hunt RH, Waye JD. Colonoscopy: techniques, clinical practice and colour atlas. London: Chapman & Hall, 1981:404.
2. Cotton PB, Williams CB. Practical gastrointestinal endoscopy. 3rd ed. Oxford: Blackwell Scientific, 1983.
3. Shinya H. Colonoscopy: diagnosis and treatment of colonic diseases. New York/Tokyo: Igaku Shoin, 1982:256.
3a. Deyhle P, Seuberth K, Jenny S, Demling L. Endoscopic polypectomy in the proximal colon. Endoscopy 1971;2:103.
4. Van Gossum A, Loriers M, Serruys E, Cremer M. Methods of disinfecting endoscopic material: results of an international survey. Endoscopy 1989;21(6):247.
5. Fraser VJ, Zuckerman G, Clouse RE, et al. A prospective randomized trial comparing manual and automated endoscope disinfection methods. Infect Control Hosp Epidemiol 1993;14(7):383.
6. Axon ATR. Disinfection and endoscopy—summary and recommendations. J Gastroenterol Hepatol 1991;6:1:23.
7. Fleshner PR, Ackroyd FW, Shellito PC. The freckle sign—an endoscopic feature of the cecum. Dis Colon Rectum 1990;33:836.
8. Hyman N, Waye JD. Endoscopic four quadrant tattoo for the identification of colonic lesions at surgery. Gastrointest Endosc 1991;37:56.
9. Fennerty MB, Sampliner RE, Hixson LJ, Garewal HS. Effectiveness of India ink as a long-term colonic mucosal marker. Am J Gastroenterol 1992;87(1):79.
10. Tabibian N, Michaletz PA, Scwhwartz JT. Use of endoscopically placed clip can avoid diagnostic errors in colonoscopy. Gastrointest Endosc 1988;34:262.
11. Kolts BE, Lyles WE, Achem SR, Burton L, Geller AJ, Macmath T. A comparison of the effectiveness and patient tolerance of oral sodium phosphate, castor oil, and standard electrolyte lavage for colonoscopy or sigmoidoscopy preparation. Am J Gastroenterol 1993;88(8):1218.
12. DiPalma JA, Marshall JB. Comparison of a new sulfate-free polyethylene glycol electrolyte lavage solution versus a standard solution for colonoscopy cleansing. Gastrointest Endosc 1990;36(3):285.
13. The Standards Task Force of the American Society of Colon and Rectal Surgeons. Practice parameters for antibiotic prophylaxis: supporting documentation. Dis Colon Rectum 1992;35(3):278.
14. Neu HC. Recommendations for antibiotic prophylaxis before endoscopy. Am J Gastroenterol 1989;84:1488.
15. Waye JD, Yessayan SA, Lewis BS, Fabry TL. The technique of abdominal pressure in total colonoscopy. Gastrointest Endosc 1991;37(2):147.
16. Geenen JE, Fleischer DE, Waye JD. Techniques in therapeutic endoscopy. 2nd ed. New York: Gower Medical, 1992.
17. Brunetaud JM, Maunoury V, Cochelard D, Boniface B, Cortot A, Paris JC. Endoscopic laser treatment for rectosigmoid villous adenoma: factors affecting the results. Gastroenterology 1989;97:272.
18. Walsh RM, Ackroyd FW, Shellito PC. Endoscopic resection of large sessile colorectal polyps. Gastrointest Endosc 1992;38:303.
19. Williams CB. Diathermy-biopsy: a technique for the endoscopic management of small polyps. Endoscopy 1973;5:215.
20. Van Gossum A, Cozzoli A, Adler M, Taton G, Cremer M. Colonoscopic snare polypectomy: analysis of 1485 resections comparing two types of current. Gastrointest Endosc 1992;38:472.
21. Jetmore AB, Timmcke AE, Gathright JB Jr, Hicks TC, Ray JE, Baker JW. Ogilvie's syndrome: colonoscopic decompression and analysis of predisposing factors. Dis Colon Rectum. 1992;35(12):1135.
22. Harig JM, Fumo DE, Loo FD, et al. Treatment of acute nontoxic megacolon during colonoscopy: tube placement versus simple decompression. Gastrointest Endosc 1988;34(1):23.
23. Kozarek RA. Hydrostatic balloon dilation of gastrointestinal stenoses: a national survey. Gastrointest Endosc 1986;32:15.
24. Breysem Y, Janssens JF, Coremans G, Vantrappen G, Hendrickx G, Rutgeerts P. Endoscopic balloon dilation of colonic and ileo-colonic Crohn's strictures: long-term results. Gastrointest Endosc 1992;38(2):142.
25. Winawer SJ, Flehinger BJ, Schottenfeld D, Miller DG. Screening for colorectal cancer with fecal occult blood testing and sigmoidoscopy. J. Natl Cancer Inst 1993;85(16):1311.
26. VanNess MM, Chobanian SJ, Winters C, Diehl AM, Esposito RL, Cattau EL. A study of patient acceptance of double-contrast barium enema and colonoscopy — Which procedure is preferred by patients? Arch Intern Med 1987;147:2175.
27. Hixson LJ, Fennerty MB, Sampliner RE, Garewal HS. Prospective blinded trial of the colonoscopic miss-rate of large colorectal polyps. Gastrointest Endosc 1991;37:125.
28. Shinya H, Wolff WI. Morphology, anatomic distribution and cancer potential of colonic polyps. Analysis of 7000 polyps endoscopically removed. Ann Surg 1979;190:679.
29. Haggitt RC, Glotzbach RE, Soffer EE, Wruble LD. Prognostic factors in colorectal carcinomas arising in adenomas implications for lesions removed by endoscopic polypectomy. Gastroenterology 1985;89:328.
30. Riddell RH. Hands off malignant polyps (editorial). Gastroenterology 1985;89:432.
31. Cranley JP, Petras RE, Carey WD, Paradis K, Sivak MV. When is endoscopic polypectomy adequate therapy for colonic polyps containing invasive carcinoma? Gastroenterology 1986;91:419.
32. Williams CB, Whiteway JE, Jass JR. Practical aspects of endoscopic management of malignant polyps. Endoscopy 1987;19:31.
33. Christie JP. Polypectomy or colectomy? Management of 106 consecutively encountered colorectal polyps. J Am Surg 1988;54:93.
34. Ponsky JL, King JF. Endoscopic marking of colonic lesions. Gastrointest Endosc 1975;22:42.
35. Lichtiger S, Kornbluth A, Salomon P, Waye JD. Lower gastrointestinal bleeding. In: Taylor MB, Gollan JL, Peppercorn MA, Steer ML, Wolfe MM, eds. Gastrointestinal emergencies. Baltimore: Williams & Wilkins, 1992.
36. Campbell WB, Rhodes M, Kettlewell MG. Colonoscopy following intraoperative lavage in the management of severe colonic bleeding. Ann Roy Coll Surg Engl 1985;67:290.
37. Jensen DM, Machicado GA. Diagnosis and treatment of severe hematochezia: the role of urgent colonoscopy after purge. Gastroenterology 1988;95:1569.
38. Waye J. Endoscopy in inflammatory bowel disease: indications and differential diagnosis. Med Clin North Am 1990;74:51.
39. Pera A, Caldera D, Ponti V. Colonoscopy in inflammatory bowel disease. Diagnostic accuracy and proposal of an endoscopic score. Gastroenterology 1987;92:181.
40. Modigliani R, Mary JY, Simon JF, Cortot A. Clinical, biological,

and endoscopic picture of attacks of Crohn's disease. Evolution on prednisolone. Groupe d'etude therapeutique des affections inflammatoires disgestives. Gastroenterol 1990;98:811.

41. Lee E, Schiller LR, Vendrell D, Santa Ana CA, Fordtran JS. Subepithelial collagen table thickness in colon specimens from patients with microscopic colitis and collagenous colitis. Gastroenterology 1992;103:1790.

42. Bond JH. Polyp guideline: diagnosis, treatment, and surveillance for patients with nonfamilial colorectal polyps. The Practice Parameters Committee of the American College of Gastroenterology. Ann Intern Med 1993;119(8):836.

43. Fitzgibbons RJ, Lynch HT, Stanslav GV, Watson PA. Recognition and treatment of patients with hereditary nonpolyposis colon cancer (Lynch syndromes I and II). Ann Surg 1987;206:289.

44. Choi PM, Nugent FW, Schoetz DJ Jr, Silverman ML, Haggitt RC. Colonoscopic surveillance reduces mortality from colorectal cancer in ulcerative colitis. Gastroenterology 1993;105(2):418.

45. Lashner BA, Silverstein MD, Hanauer SB. Hazard rates for dysplasia and cancer in ulcerative colitis. Results from a surveillance program. Digestive Diseases and Sciences 1989;34:1536.

46. Albert MB, Nochomovitz LE. Dysplasia and cancer surveillance in inflammatory bowel disease. Gastroenterol Clin North Am 1989;18:83.

47. Stevenson GW, Wilson JA, Wilkinson J, Norman G, Goodacre RL. Pain following colonoscopy: elimination with carbon dioxide. Gastrointest Endosc 1992;38:564.

48. Mark DG, Rex DK, Lappas, JC. Quality of air contrast barium enema performed the same day as incomplete colonoscopy with air insufflation. Gastrintest Endosc 1992;38:693.

49. Harned RK, Consigny PM, Cooper NB, Williams SM, Woltzen AJ. Barium enema examination following biopsy of the rectum or colon. Radiology 1982;145:11.

50. Jaffe PE, Fennerty MB, Sampliner RE, Hixson LJ. Preventing hypoxemia during colonoscopy. A randomized controlled trial of supplemental oxygen. J Clin Gastroenterol 1992;14(2):114.

51. McKee CC, Ragland JJ, Myers JD. An evaluation of multiple clinical variables for hypoxia during colonoscopy. Surg Gynecol Obstet 1991;173(1):37.

52. Bernard D, Tasse D, Morgan S, Wassef R. Is preoperative colonoscopy in carcinoma a realistic and valuable proposition? Can J Surg 1987;30:87.

53. Meyer GW. Prophylaxis of infective endocarditis during colonoscopy: report of a survey. Gastrointest Endosc 1981;27:58.

54. Macrae FA, Tan KG, Williams CB. Towards safer colonoscopy: a report on the complications of 5000 diagnostic or therapeutic colonoscopies. Gut 1981;24:376.

55. Christie JP, Marrazzo J. "Mini-perforation" of the colon—not all postpolypectomy perforations require laparotomy. Dis Colon Rectum 1991;34:132.

56. Kavin H, Sinicrope F, Esker AH. Management of perforation of the colon at colonoscopy. Am J Gastroenterol 1992;87:357.

57. Habr-Gama A, Waye JD. Complications and hazards of gastrointestinal endoscopy. World J Surg 1989;13:193.

57a. Ecker MD, Goldstein M, Hoexter B, Hyman RA, Naidish JB, Stein HL. Benign pneumoperitoneum after fiberoptic colonoscopy: a prospective study of 100 patients. Gastroenterology 1977;73:226.

58. Marshall JB, Barthel JS. The frequency of total colonoscopy and terminal ileal intubation in the 1990s. Gastrointest Endosc 1993;39:(4):518.

59. Glick SN, Teplick SK, Balfe DM, Levine MS, Gasparaitis AE, Maglinte DDT, Shortsleeve MJ, Brandon JC. Large colonic neoplasms missed by endoscopy. AJR Am J Roentgenol 1989;152:513.

60. Irvine EJ, O'Connor J, Frost RA, et al. Prospective comparison of double contrast barium enema plus flexible sigmoidoscopy versus colonoscopy in rectal bleeding: barium enema versus colonoscopy in rectal bleeding. Gut 1988;29:1188.

61. Fork FT. Diagnostic procedures in colorectal cancer: barium enema or colonoscopy? Or both? Eur J Surg Oncol 1987;13:147.

62. Rex DK, Weddle RA, Lehman GA, et al. Flexible sigmoidoscopy plus air contrast barium enema versus colonoscopy for suspected lower gastrointestinal bleeding. Gastroenterology 1990;98(4):855.

Textbook of Gastroenterology, second edition, edited
by Tadataka Yamada. JB Lippincott Company,
Philadelphia © 1995.

CHAPTER 117

Endoscopic Retrograde Cholangiopancreatography, Endoscopic Sphincterotomy and Stone Removal, and Endoscopic Biliary and Pancreatic Drainage

Kees Huibregtse   Michael B. Kimmey

Endoscopic Retrograde Cholangiopancreatography
   Technical Considerations
   Indications
   Contraindications and Risks
   Results
   Clinical Implications
Endoscopic Sphincterotomy and Stone Removal
   Technical Considerations
   Indications

   Contraindications and Risks
   Results
   Clinical Implications
Endoscopic Biliary and Pancreatic Drainage
   Technical Considerations
   Indications
   Contraindications and Risks
   Results
   Clinical Implications

Duodenoscopy and endoscopic cannulation of the papilla of Vater with visualization of the biliary tree and pancreatic duct was first described in 1968.[1] Many reports on endoscopic retrograde cholangiopancreatography (ERCP) followed from all over the world in the early 1970s. Within a few years, ERCP became one of the most reliable methods for diagnosing biliary and pancreatic disorders. Research reports and extensive reviews of the subject are available.[2,3]

The development of therapeutic endoscopy has greatly contributed to the widespread use of ERCP. Endoscopic sphincterotomy (ES) and gallstone extraction, first described in 1973, allowed further advances in endoscopic treatment of biliary and pancreatic disorders.[4,5] This combination of techniques has become the preferred treatment for bile duct stones after cholecystectomy and for patients with intact gallbladders who have complications of common bile duct stones.

Nasobiliary drainage was subsequently popularized to prevent stone impaction after ES and to avoid cholangitis after ERCP in patients with malignant obstructive jaundice.[6,7] An endoscopic technique for placement of internal biliary stents for the long-term relief of biliary obstruction was later described.[8] This therapeutic endoscopic approach to obstructive jaundice has since been adopted by many centers around the world.[9-13]

In this chapter, the discussion of biliary and pancreatic endoscopy is divided into three parts. Diagnostic ERCP is discussed in the first part, ES and stone removal is covered in the second part, and biliary and pancreatic drainage procedures are reviewed in the third part.

ENDOSCOPIC RETROGRADE CHOLANGIOPANCREATOGRAPHY

Technical Considerations

Patient Preparation

ERCP implies an endoscopy of the upper gastrointestinal tract. The general measures taken for endoscopy must also be taken for ERCP. Special attention is paid to complaints of dysphagia, because the esophagus is passed blindly with the side-viewing endoscope used for ERCP. The risk of perforating a Zenker's diverticulum or unsuspected esophageal stricture is increased with this type of endoscope. A history of gastric surgery or symptoms of gastric outlet obstruction should alert the endoscopist to possible technical difficulties. Duodenal obstruction and pyloric stenosis can also prevent passage of the duodenoscope to the level of the ampulla.

The procedure and its potential benefits and risks are carefully explained to the patient, and consent for the procedure is obtained. Further information on endoscopic therapeutic procedures and their surgical alternatives must be given to patients in whom endoscopic treatment is contemplated after the diagnostic ERCP.

In most centers, conscious sedation is achieved with intravenous diazepam or midazolam. Patients are medicated for the procedure while in the left lateral decubitus or prone position, before passage of the endoscope. The oropharynx is anesthetized with a topical anesthetic spray. Fentanyl or meperidine can be added in individual cases as needed. Anticholinergic agents such as atropine, hyoscine, or glucagon can be used before or during the procedure to inhibit duodenal motility.

Although antibiotic prophylaxis is not routinely given to all patients before ERCP, antibiotics are usually given to patients before endoscopic therapeutic procedures if bile duct obstruction is suspected.

Instruments

ERCP is a combined endoscopic and radiologic method. A high-performance radiographic instrument and video image intensifier is required for optimal radiologic diagnosis and to avoid complications such as inadvertent overfilling of the pancreatic duct. A side-viewing endoscope with an elevator at the end of the channel is usually used. These endoscopes are available for diagnostic purposes with channels of 2.8 or 3.2 mm. Endoscopes are available for therapeutic purposes with channels of 4.2 and 5.5 mm. Cannulation of the papilla of Vater may be easier with a forward-viewing endoscope in patients who have undergone antrectomy and Billroth II gastrojejunostomy.[14-16]

A variety of cannulation catheters is available to facilitate cannulation of the papilla of Vater. In practice, however, only two or three different catheters are used by experienced endoscopists. Catheters with a metal ball tip or a metal conical tip facilitate fluoroscopic localization and monitoring of catheter movement without contrast injection. Some catheters allow passage of a 0.89-mm (0.035-inch) guidewire, facilitating subsequent exchange of the catheter for cytology brushes, papillotomes, and biliary drainage catheters.

Water-soluble contrast materials such as diatrizoate meglumine are usually used at a concentration of 60%. Lower concentrations may be desirable for detecting small gallstones. The risk of a systemic allergic reaction from the contrast material is low because there is very little contrast absorption. In patients with known allergy to the contrast material, use of special media of lower ionic strength should further reduce any small risk of systemic reaction.[17]

Procedure

The patient is placed in the left lateral position with the left arm behind the patient's back to facilitate movement to the prone position after the endoscope is in the duodenum. The endoscope is introduced into the oropharynx and is swallowed by the patient. The esophagus is passed blindly, although the distal esophagus can be inspected in most patients. After it is passed into the stomach, the tip of the endoscope must be angled down to obtain a panoramic view of the stomach and to locate the antrum. The pylorus is passed by manipulation and further insertion of the endoscope; the endoscopist knows that the endoscope tip is in the duodenal bulb by the change in mucosal appearance and by a palpable reduction in resistance as the endoscope passes the pylorus.

The endoscope is advanced to the second part of the duodenum. The endoscope is now in a long position, stretching out along the greater gastric curvature. At this point, it is important to straighten the endoscope so that it is alongside the lesser gastric curvature. A straight endoscope allows direct and easy transmission of subtle movements of the handle and knobs of the endoscope to the tip of the instrument. This position of the endoscope is obtained by withdrawing the instrument with 45 to 90 degrees of clockwise rotation; the tip of the endoscope moves first to the proximal part of the duodenum with the papilla seen distally, and then with further withdrawal the tip advances down the duodenum, bringing the papilla into close view. In the straight position, the end of the endoscope is at approximately 60 cm from the incisors in most cases. The papilla may be located distal to this usual position in approximately 15% of cases.[18]

Attempts at cannulation of the papilla begin after the endoscope is in position. In 85% of cases, the pancreatic duct and common bile duct share a common orifice. The first step is to introduce the cannula into the papillary orifice perpendicular to the duodenal wall and directed slightly to the right. This is the optimal direction for cannulation of the pancreatic duct. Cannulation with a small change in direction of the catheter tip should be reattempted if the duct is not immediately opacified. It is better to cannulate many times with frequent changes of catheter direction than to push hard in the same direction. Forceful movements and pushing create edema, making subsequent cannulation more difficult.

Cannulation of the bile duct requires placement of the catheter in the orifice at the 11-o'clock position. The catheter is further introduced in a direction parallel to the intraduodenal segment of the bile duct. This position is sometimes obtained only by maximal elevator use and by upward deflection of the endoscope tip after the catheter tip is placed just inside the orifice. Slight changes of catheter direction should be tried if the bile duct is not opacified. Cannulation may be difficult in the presence of periampullary diverticula or invading periampullary tumors and after Billroth II gastrojejunostomy.

Radiography

A plain abdominal radiograph should be taken before the procedure with the patient supine to examine the field for obscuring old contrast material and to establish the location of soft tissue shadows and calcifications. During the procedure, radiographs are usually taken with the patient in the prone position after injection of contrast material. The pancreatic tail and the right hepatic duct are nondependent in the prone position and fill last. Overviews are taken of the ductular systems, and spot films are taken of any abnormal or suspicious findings. The constant attendance of a radiologist during the procedure is desirable and enhances the quality of the radiographic examination.

The pancreatic duct should be filled with contrast material under fluoroscopic control until the tail and the first-order side branches are visualized. Further filling and, in particular, parenchymography should be avoided to reduce the risk of acute pancreatitis. Radiographs should be taken at once, while the endoscope and the catheter are still in place, because the pancreatic duct empties rapidly.

The biliary tree is filled with contrast material until the intrahepatic bile ducts, cystic duct, and gallbladder are opacified, and appropriate films are then taken. The outflow of contrast material through the papilla may be slow. The endoscope can be removed after opacification of the biliary tree, and a complete, detailed radiographic examination is made of biliary anatomy and papillary motor function with the patient in various positions. Delayed films should also be taken to detect small gallstones.

Injection of air with the contrast material should be avoided because air bubbles can be mistaken for gallstones. Air bubbles can be differentiated from gallstones by changing the position of the patient. Air bubbles tend to move proximally and gallstones distally with the patient in the upright or the supine position.

Manometry

Manometry of the biliary and pancreatic sphincters at the time of ERCP has been used as a diagnostic tool in patients with unexplained biliary pain or pancreatitis.[19] The technique should not be used routinely at ERCP but should be reserved for specific indications. The patient is premedicated with only diazepam, because narcotics, anticholinergics, and glucagon alter sphincter measurements.

Most centers use a continuously perfused catheter, as in the technique of esophageal manometry, to make pressure recordings, although a microtransducer method has also been described.[20] The perfusion catheter is selectively passed into the bile duct to obtain pressure measurements within the duct and from the sphincter as the catheter is pulled back. All pressures are referenced to duodenal lumen pressure, which is arbitrarily designated as zero. Basal pressures within the duct and the sphincter are calculated as an average of several measurements. The frequency, amplitude, and propagation direction of sphincter contractions are also computed. Pressures obtained from the pancreatic duct and pancreatic sphincter may be different from those obtained from the bile duct, and they should be measured after selective pancreatic duct cannulation with the perfusion catheter.

Indications

The indications for ERCP can be divided into five main groups and are listed in Table 117-1. Indications for ERCP have changed since its introduction because the procedure is less invasive than originally believed and because improved imaging techniques are now available.

Acute cholangitis and acute pancreatitis were contraindi-

TABLE 117-1
Indications for Endoscopic Retrograde Cholangiopancreatography

Suspected Biliary Disorders
Jaundice or cholestasis
Post cholecystectomy complaints
Post biliary surgery complaints
Acute cholangitis
Acute biliary pancreatitis
Confirmation of lesions demonstrated by other imaging techniques

Suspected Pancreatic Disorders
Obstructive jaundice
Upper abdominal pain
Increased serum pancreatic amylase or lipase
Recent-onset diabetes mellitus
Unexplained weight loss
Steatorrhea
Unexplained gastric varices
Unexplained ascites or pleural effusion
Unexplained recurrent pancreatitis
Confirmation of lesions demonstrated by other imaging techniques

Before Therapeutic Endoscopic Procedures
Endoscopic papillotomy
Endoscopic biliary drainage
Endoscopic pancreatic drainage
Balloon dilatation of strictures

Preoperative Mapping
Chronic pancreatitis
Pancreatic pseudocysts

Additional Procedures
Collection of pure pancreatic juice or bile
Manometry of the sphincter of Oddi

cations for many years. Today, cholangitis and acute biliary pancreatitis are indications for emergency ERCP, provided that endoscopic therapeutic procedures are available at the same session. Ultrasonography has become the standard screening technique for patients with suspected biliary or pancreatic disorders. ERCP is indicated in patients with chronic pancreatitis only if ultrasonography is ambiguous, if preoperative mapping is required, or if endoscopic therapy is being considered.

The indications for sphincter of Oddi manometry are evolving and are likely to change with further experience. The greatest experience with this test is in patients with recurrent biliary pain after cholecystectomy. These patients may have a fixed stenosis at the papilla or a dynamic motility disorder of the sphincter.[21] Patients with typical biliary pain associated with elevated levels of serum liver enzymes who have a dilated common bile duct that does not readily drain after a diagnostic cholangiogram do not need manometry to predict a favorable outcome from ES. Patients who have biliary pain but whose liver enzyme levels are normal or who have bile ducts that are not dilated and drain well present more of a therapeutic dilemma. Studies of this group have suggested a beneficial response to ES in the subset of patients with an elevated basal sphincter pressure.[22] Other investigators have not found a clear correlation between the results of manometry and the results of sphincterotomy, although the patient populations studied were not strictly comparable.[23,24]

The role of sphincter of Oddi manometry in the evaluation of patients with idiopathic pancreatitis is uncertain and requires further study.[25,26] Elevated pancreatic sphincter pressures have been reported in 20% to 50% of patients with recurrent idiopathic pancreatitis.[25,26] It is not known, however, whether therapeutic intervention with endoscopic pancreatic sphincterotomy or surgical sphincteroplasty in patients with elevated sphincter pressure results in fewer recurrences of pancreatitis. Until controlled trials show a therapeutic benefit to knowing the results of pancreatic sphincter manometry, this technique should be used primarily in a clinical investigation setting.

Contraindications and Risks

The relative contraindications to diagnostic ERCP are suspected conditions that carry an increased risk of infection, such as biliary strictures and stones and pancreatic pseudocysts.[27] An ERCP should only be performed in these situations if a surgical or endoscopic drainage procedure can immediately follow the diagnostic procedure. Antibiotics should be started immediately after inadvertent filling of an obstructed biliary or pancreatic ductal system; plans for adequate biliary or pancreatic drainage should be made. Complications of ERCP and their incidence are listed in Table 117-2.

Acute pancreatitis is the most frequent complication of diagnostic ERCP. A moderate rise in serum amylase level is observed after 40% to 75% of pancreatograms.[28,29] This frequent hyperamylasemia is not accompanied by clinical symptoms and usually subsides in 1 to 2 days. An attack of clinically apparent acute pancreatitis after ERCP occurs in 0.7% to 7.4% of patients. Severe necrotizing pancreatitis is seen in approximately 0.1% of patients. Overfilling the pancreatic duct and staining the pancreatic parenchyma with contrast material is claimed to be the main causative factor in the development of acute pancreatitis, but this varies. Trauma and subsequent edema of the papilla is probably also an important causative factor. Repeated attempts at cannulation or repeated pancreatic duct cannulation and filling constitute the main risk factors for acute pancreatitis. However, acute pancreatitis has

been observed in some patients after unsuccessful cannulation of the pancreatic duct. Addition of sphincter of Oddi manometry to diagnostic ERCP increases the incidence of post-procedural pancreatitis.[21]

Cholangitis was the most frequent and severe complication of ERCP before endoscopic biliary drainage procedures became available. Cholangitis develops if the outflow of bile (and contrast material) is delayed or blocked by a stone or stricture. The causative pathogens are usually enteric gram-negative bacteria, such as *Escherichia coli*, *Klebsiella*, and anaerobes.[30] The best prevention of cholangitis is the immediate provision of unhindered bile flow. This can be achieved by ES and stone extraction or by an endoscopic biliary drainage procedure. Systemic antibiotics should be instituted at once in cases of failure to relieve the biliary obstruction. Endoscopes and ancillary equipment should be disinfected before every examination. Cases of *Pseudomonas aeruginosa* cholangitis caused by contaminated endoscopes should no longer occur.[31]

Infection of a pancreatic pseudocyst with subsequent pancreatic abscess formation should be a rare complication with careful planning. Ultrasonography done before ERCP detects most pseudocysts. An ERCP should not be performed in these patients unless surgical or endoscopic drainage of the pseudocyst is planned to immediately follow the pancreatogram.

Respiratory depression or hypotension, which are side effects of premedicating drugs, occur particularly in elderly and frail patients. Monitoring of oxygen saturation, pulse rate, and blood pressure in these patients allows early detection of complications and is therefore mandatory. Oxygen administration may be considered in the elderly.

Results

The papilla is readily identified by experienced endoscopists in more than 98% of cases. Difficulties in finding the papilla may arise in cases of large papillary tumors, duodenal stenosis, or edematous folds caused by acute pancreatitis or if the papilla is located inside a diverticulum. In patients with a Billroth II gastrojejunostomy, the success rate decreases to 60% to 85%.[14-16] A long or kinked afferent loop may prevent the endoscope from being advanced to the area of the papilla. The success rate of cannulation depends not only on the experience and persistence of the endoscopist but also on the underlying disease.[2] It is well known that cannulation of the common bile duct is easier in patients with gallstone disease than it is in patients whose distal common bile duct has been displaced or compressed by tumor.

Selective cholangiography with pancreatography is successful in only 90% to 95% of cases, even if performed by skilled endoscopists. Incision of the roof of the papilla with a diathermy knife can increase the success rate of cannulation of the common bile duct. However, this technique is more aggressive and carries a higher risk, justifying its use only if a therapeutic procedure is anticipated.

Endoscopic Findings

The distal stomach and pylorus can be inspected during passage of the duodenoscope toward the papilla. Impression of the antrum, displacement of the pylorus, and a duodenal ste-

TABLE 117-2
Complications of Endoscopic Retrograde Cholangiopancreatography

FINDING	% OF CASES
Pancreatitis	1.0
Cholangitis	0.8
Pancreatic abscess	0.3
Drug side effects	0.6
Gastrointestinal tract injury	0.2
Mortality	0.2

From Bilbao MK, Dotter CT, Lee TG, Katon RM. Complications of endoscopic retrograde cholangiopancreatography (ERCP). Gastroenterology 1976;70:314.

nosis may indicate the presence of a periampullary tumor. Pancreatic cancers may grow into the duodenal wall, and biopsy specimens from duodenal wall abnormalities may reveal the malignancy. Duodenal invasion by pancreatic cancer is usually found proximal to a normal-appearing papilla.

The minor papilla, if present, is located 1 to 2 cm proximal to the major papilla. Most duodenal diverticula are located in the descending part of the duodenum near the papilla of Vater (Fig. 117-1). Cannulation of a papilla in a diverticulum or in the mouth of a diverticulum is more demanding; however, overall success rates in experienced hands exceed 90%.[32] Peripapillary diverticula are associated with an increased prevalence of gallstones and common bile duct stones.[33]

The papilla and its region must be examined carefully before attempts at cannulation. Recent stone passage can cause a patent papillary orifice with red, edematous edges. A peripapillary fistula may be a result of spontaneous stone perforation or false passage of surgical bougies.[34] A bulging papilla may be caused by an impacted stone, an ampullary tumor, or a choledochocele. Endoscopic papillotomy is usually necessary to determine the cause of a bulging papilla.

Carcinomas of the ampulla of Vater may be seen as fleshy, friable, exophytic growths or as large ulcerative lesions at the site of the papilla. Cannulation of these tumors may be difficult because bleeding occurs if the tumor is touched with the cannula or endoscope. A bulging papilla covered with normal duodenal mucosa is found if the tumor arises from within the ampulla. Histologic proof of malignancy can be obtained in only 85% of cases, even if large snare biopsies are taken after the tumor has been exposed by ES.

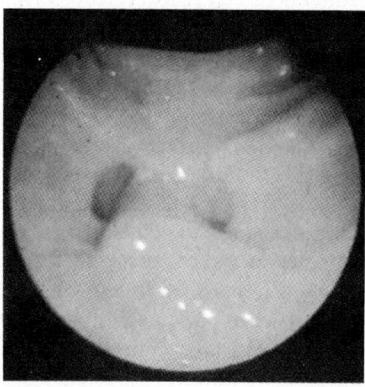

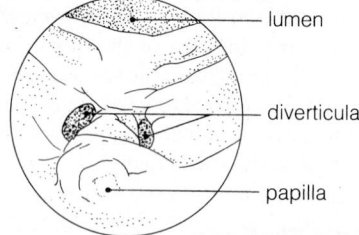

lumen

diverticula

papilla

FIGURE 117-1. The papilla of Vater is located between two juxtapapillary diverticula. (From Silverstein FE, Tytgat NJ. Atlas of gastrointestinal endoscopy. New York: Gower Medical Publishing, 1987.)

Normal Cholangiogram

A normal cholangiogram shows a common bile duct of not more than 9 mm in diameter.[35,36] The common bile duct is wider in patients after cholecystectomy.[37] The cystic duct may insert into the common bile duct anywhere along its length, from the hepatic bifurcation to the area of the papilla. A slight narrowing of the common hepatic duct at the site of the confluence is occasionally seen. Just distal to the hepatic bifurcation, vessels may cause an impression on the common hepatic duct, especially if the patient is in the prone position. The intrapancreatic portion of the distal common bile duct may show a tubular narrowing. The anatomy of the intrahepatic biliary tree varies but is considered normal if there is arborization with smooth lining and tapering of side branches. The gallbladder and cystic duct may also show anatomic variations.

Cholelithiasis

Gallstones may be found in all parts of the biliary tract and vary in number, size, and shape. Stones with an irregular shape are mostly composed of sludge; small stones are mostly solid. Cholangiography is indispensable in the investigation of patients with complications of gallstones. Gallstones can perforate through the bile duct into the duodenum or pancreatic duct, leaving a fistula. Impacted gallstones may give rise to inflammation and secondary strictures of the bile duct. The cystic duct can be considered occluded if gallbladder filling does not take place after complete filling of the intrahepatic bile ducts and after changing the position of the patient.[38] A gallstone impacted in the cystic duct with surrounding inflammation can give rise to an irregular stenosis of the common bile duct (Mirizzi's syndrome). The stenosis of the bile duct in this syndrome can mimic a malignant stricture.[39]

Cholangiography is also useful to define complications of biliary surgery. Bile duct injury occurs in 0.6% to 2.7% of patients after laparoscopic cholecystectomy.[40,41] Biliary strictures occur in 0.20% to 0.25% of patients after open biliary surgery.[41] These strictures are short and smooth, unless they are the result of extensive oversewing of a traumatized bile duct. Dilated ducts proximal to the narrowed area are found in fewer than 50% of patients. In general, differential diagnosis from a malignant stricture poses no problem.[42] Ongoing leakage is usually caused by distal obstruction from an impacted stone or stricture. Ongoing leakage and postoperative bile leaks or fistulas are easily demonstrated by ERCP. In a minority of instances, closure of a fistula is retarded or prevented by excessive sphincter of Oddi motor activity.

Benign Bile Duct Strictures

Most benign bile duct strictures are caused by surgical injury. Common bile duct strictures are also seen in as many as 60% of patients with chronic pancreatitis sufficiently severe to require surgical treatment.[43] Common bile duct strictures caused by pancreatitis are usually longer, smoothly delineated, and incomplete, in comparison with strictures produced by pancreatic cancer. Usually, the ERCP catheter can easily be advanced through a stricture caused by chronic pancreatitis but not through a stricture caused by pancreatic cancer.[44]

Pancreatography can often help differentiate these two types of biliary stricture.

Malignant Bile Duct Strictures

Bile duct carcinoma can develop at any level of the biliary tree. However, most bile duct carcinomas are located at the confluence of the left and right hepatic ducts or in the common hepatic duct. Concentric strictures, usually accompanied by a shelf or with "shouldering," are characteristic of cholangiocarcinoma. Intrahepatic bile duct dilatation proximal to a tumor at the confluence is seen in 40% to 50% of cases. Bile duct dilatation is more prominent and is found in most patients in whom the stricture is located more distally.

Cholangiocarcinoma involving the hilum of the liver may be restricted to the common hepatic duct (type I), obstruct the communication between the right and left hepatic systems (type II), or extend into the liver with involvement of second- or third-order ducts (type III).[45] Filling of the intrahepatic bile ducts with contrast material may be difficult even after deep cannulation if long, tight strictures exist. In these cases, opacification can be achieved by wedging the diagnostic cannula and guidewire in the stricture or by using a balloon occlusion catheter. High-pressure contrast injection can then usually opacify the entire intrahepatic biliary system.

Differentiation between cholangiocarcinomas and primary sclerosing cholangitis can be difficult, especially because the two diseases can coexist.[46] Brush cytology and biopsy of strictures are helpful if malignant cells are found, but negative results do not exclude malignancy.

Carcinoma of the gallbladder can cause obstructive jaundice by compression or invasion of the common hepatic duct. Cholangiography shows a tapering or irregular stricture of the common hepatic duct, which is characteristically deviated from its normal position. Gallbladder cancer may also spread into the liver with involvement of the right, left, or both hepatic ducts at the bifurcation.

Carcinoma of the pancreas is the most common cause of malignant biliary obstruction and can produce obstruction of the intrapancreatic or suprapancreatic portion of the common bile duct.[47] The obstruction may be tapered, rounded, square, or convex. The common bile duct is frequently deviated medially, and the dilated proximal part of the bile duct may show a horizontal course. Occasionally, narrowing at the bifurcation is seen because of metastatic lymph nodes. If the distal common bile duct and pancreatic ducts are stenosed (i.e., double duct sign), there is a high likelihood of pancreatic head carcinoma.[48] However, this sign is not pathognomonic, and the finding may be caused by chronic pancreatitis.[49] Pancreatic cancer occasionally develops in patients with chronic pancreatitis. Differentiating a malignant biliary stricture from a benign stricture caused by pancreatitis can be very difficult in this situation. Brush cytology of the bile duct is often not helpful in such circumstances because the pancreatic tumor has usually not invaded through the common bile duct wall.

Distal common bile duct carcinoma may be indistinguishable from invading pancreatic cancer. A normal pancreatogram and a normal intraduodenal segment of the distal common bile duct favor the diagnosis of cholangiocarcinoma. Metastases to the head of the pancreas or adjacent lymph nodes can mimic the biliary stricture seen in primary pancreatic cancer or cholangiocarcinoma.

Periampullary Carcinoma

Cancer of the ampulla of Vater usually obstructs the distal common bile duct and the pancreatic duct. The characteristic findings are a dilated bile duct and a dilated pancreatic duct together with a short, irregular stricture at the site of the papilla. Shouldering of the obstructed common bile duct is often seen. Pancreatic duct dilatation is absent if pancreatic drainage occurs through a patent Santorini duct and minor papilla.

Other Malignancies

Intrahepatic metastases are best detected with ultrasonography or computed tomography (CT). Intrahepatic duct displacement or amputation may be seen on endoscopic cholangiography. Endoscopic cholangiographic findings of multiple intrahepatic metastases may be similar to those of macronodular cirrhosis. Lymphadenopathy caused by lymph node metastasis or lymphoma produces rounded impressions in the bile duct wall.

Sclerosing Cholangitis

Sclerosing cholangitis usually produces abnormalities in the intrahepatic and extrahepatic biliary tree (Fig. 117-2).[50,51] Occasionally, only a local stricture exists, causing differential diagnostic difficulties with cholangiocarcinoma. Usually, multiple strictures and dilatations of varying lengths are seen, giving the characteristic picture of beading.[52] Diverticular outpouchings of the extrahepatic ducts are specific for sclerosing cholangitis. Sclerosing cholangitis may be indistinguishable from a diffusely spreading form of cholangiocarcinoma. Abnormalities identical to those in primary sclerosing cholangitis have also been described after irradiation, after intraarterial chemotherapy with fluorodeoxyuridine, and in the acquired immunodeficiency syndrome (AIDS).[53-60] However, in contrast to primary sclerosing cholangitis, in AIDS cholangitis there is often also papillary stenosis, which may be the only extrahepatic biliary abnormality. ES in this situation often provides good patient palliation.[60] The biliary ductal abnormalities seen in AIDS have been attributed to opportunistic infection with *Cryptosporidium*, microsporidia, or cytomegalovirus.[57,59] Pancreatography shows irregularities of the pancreatic ductal system in 20% to 70% of patients with sclerosing cholangitis.[52]

Cysts, Abscesses, and Cirrhosis

Choledochal cysts and Caroli's disease are rare. Cholangiography often shows a long common channel with insertion of the common bile duct at a right angle into the pancreatic duct more than 15 mm from the papillary orifice.[61] Cholangiography is useful in the preoperative assessment of patients with these congenital anomalies and in detecting complications such as gallstones, abscesses, and cholangiocarcinoma. Cholangiocarcinoma develops in a minority of patients with Caroli's disease and choledochal cysts.

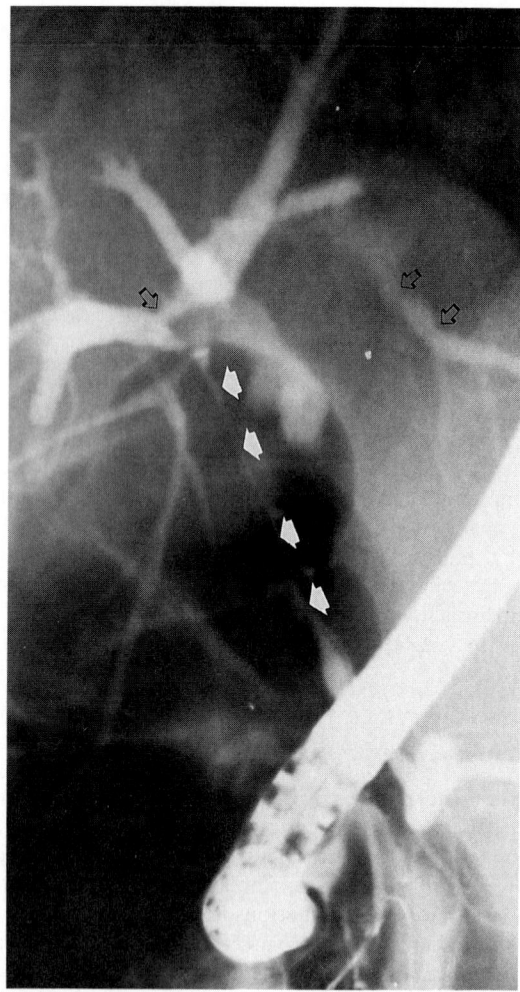

FIGURE 117-2. This patient with primary sclerosing cholangitis has a dominant extrahepatic stricture (*solid arrows*), although there are also minor changes in the intrahepatic bile ducts (*open arrows*).

Abscesses secondary to bile duct obstruction may be seen on cholangiography if they communicate with the biliary tree. Urgent biliary drainage must be implemented. Traumatic biliary fistulas can also be identified with ERCP.[62]

Echinococcal cysts may also communicate with the biliary tree and give characteristic findings.[63] Daughter cysts may be seen in the bile duct as filling defects. These cysts can be removed after ES. Worms and foreign bodies are extreme rarities and can also be removed after ES.

A paucity of intrahepatic bile ducts is seen in hepatic cirrhosis and in the vanishing bile duct syndrome after liver transplantation. Macronodular cirrhosis and polycystic liver disease can produce deviation and bile duct rarefaction; the bile ducts may take an irregular and kinked course as a result of hepatic involution and scarring.

Normal Pancreatogram

The normal pancreas is situated in the retroperitoneum and crosses the second lumbar vertebra. The course of the main pancreatic duct may be compared with the form of a pistol.

The mean length of the pancreatic duct is about 20 cm. The width of the duct gradually decreases from head to tail. The mean diameters of the duct are 4 mm in the head, 3 mm in the corpus, and 2 mm in the tail. After 40 years of age, the width of the main pancreatic duct increases significantly. Two major side branches in the pancreatic head can be observed. One, the ramus capitis inferior, leads to the uncinate process. The other, Santorini's duct, connects the main pancreatic duct with the minor papilla. The major characteristics of a normal duct include a smooth lining, absence of caliber changes, and tiny regular side branches. The shape of the pancreas varies considerably; pancreatic duct deviations without indentation or derangement of the side branches are common and have little diagnostic significance.[64]

Proper interpretation of a pancreatogram requires knowledge of the many congenital ductal anomalies. The most common variant is pancreas divisum, resulting from incomplete fusion of the dorsal and ventral anlagen (Fig. 117-3). This anomaly is seen in 4% to 6% of patients in ERCP studies.[65] Cannulation of the main papilla results in opacification of the small ventral portion. Delineation of the remainder of the pancreas requires opacification of Santorini's duct through the accessory or minor papilla. The question as to whether the pancreas divisum predisposes to pancreatic diseases is still controversial.[65,66] A rare anomaly is the annular pancreas, which may be shown by ERCP.[67]

Chronic Pancreatitis

The ductular abnormalities in chronic pancreatitis range from normal to severe destruction (Fig. 117-4). Chronic pancreatitis can be divided into three stages according to the intensity

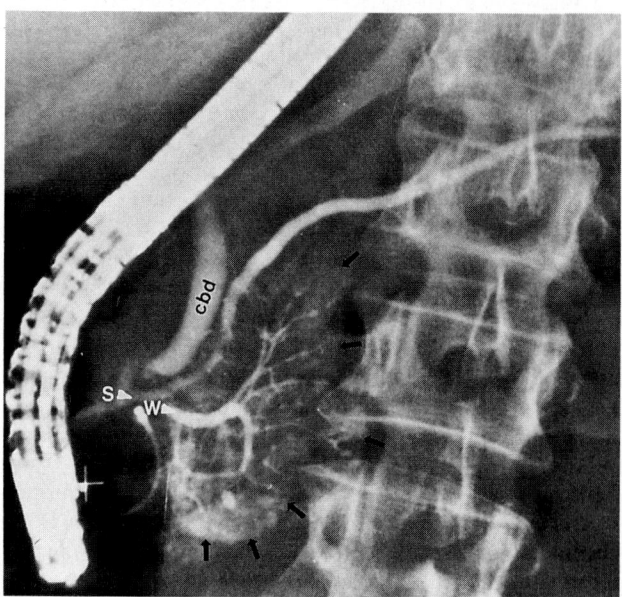

FIGURE 117-3. The dorsal and ventral pancreatic ducts in this patient with pancreas divisum have been filled with contrast medium by separately injecting the duct of Santorini (S) and the duct of Wirsung (W). Excessive contrast injection into the duct of Wirsung has resulted in acinarization, revealing the limits of the ventral pancreatic parenchyma (*arrows*). The distal common bile duct (cbd) is also seen.

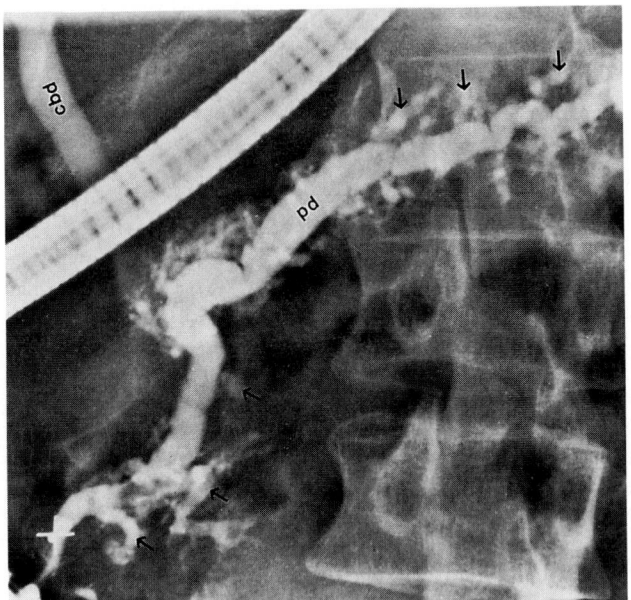

FIGURE 117-4. This pancreatogram shows changes of moderately severe chronic pancreatitis with a dilated main pancreatic duct (pd) and dilated side branches (*arrows*). The distal common bile duct (cbd) is also seen.

of these changes. In the first stage, minor irregularities of the small ducts occur as a result of inflammation and shrinkage. In the second stage, irregularities and minor caliber changes of the main duct and more pronounced alterations of the side branches are present. In the third stage, the entire ductal system is abnormal. The main duct shows areas of dilatation and stenosis. The side branches may be cystically dilated. Caliber changes with multiple strictures and dilatations form the characteristic "chain of lakes" appearance. Intraductal filling defects and calcifications may also occur. In most patients, a combination of these findings is seen.

Several classifications of ductular changes in chronic pancreatitis have been presented. A new classification was suggested during an international workshop in 1983.[68] The researchers suggested that the pancreatogram in chronic pancreatitis should be divided into normal, equivocal, mild,

moderate, and severe alterations, which are diffuse or localized (Table 117-3).

ERCP can also be useful in evaluating the patient with recurrent pain after pancreaticojejunostomy.[69]

Pancreatic Carcinoma

Pancreatograms in patients with pancreatic carcinoma can be classified into five major types: stenosis with prestenotic dilatation, complete obstruction, ductal tapering, side branch deviation, and cavity formation (Fig. 117-5). These changes are not pathognomonic but are more often found in carcinoma than in chronic pancreatitis. A normal pancreatogram may be found in 2.5% to 12.5% of cases with pancreatic carcinoma.[70] Most pancreatic tumors are located in the head of the pancreas, often also affecting the common bile duct. Concomitant distal common bile duct abnormalities are helpful in improving the overall diagnostic accuracy.

Clinical Implications

ERCP should be compared with several other diagnostic modalities to place its role in proper perspective. Comparisons must include not only diagnostic accuracy but also cost in terms of dollars and degree of patient suffering. ERCP must be considered intermediate in cost and the degree of patient discomfort. Clinical evaluation, including history and physical examination and routine laboratory tests, is considerably less expensive and easier on the patient than ERCP. Abdominal ultrasound examination is a useful screening tool for patients with jaundice and abdominal pain and is well tolerated and less expensive than ERCP. Abdominal CT scans are comparable in cost to ERCP but less invasive. The risks of these diagnostic modalities are also negligible.

The cost of percutaneous transhepatic cholangiography (PTC) approximates the cost of ERCP if hospital charges and radiologic and endoscopic professional fees are included. The risks of complications with diagnostic PTC using a skinny needle are somewhat greater than those of diagnostic ERCP. Diagnostic PTC using a skinny needle has an overall complication rate of approximately 3%, primarily resulting from sepsis, bile leakage, and intraperitoneal hemorrhage.[71] It is difficult to compare discomfort experienced by the patient

---

TABLE 117-3
Classification of Pancreatograms in Chronic Pancreatitis

PANCREATOGRAM	SIDE BRANCHES*	MAIN DUCT*
Normal	Normal	Normal
Equivocal	Less than three abnormal	Normal
Mildly abnormal	More than three abnormal	Normal
Moderately abnormal	More than three abnormal	Abnormal
Markedly abnormal	More than three abnormal	Abnormal plus one or more of the following: large cavity, obstruction, filling defects, severe dilation

* Changes may involve the entire pancreas or only a part of it.

From Axon ATR, Classen M, Cotton PB, et al. Pancreatography in chronic pancreatitis: international definitions. International workshop, Kings College, Cambridge, March 23–25, 1983. Gut 1984;25:1107.

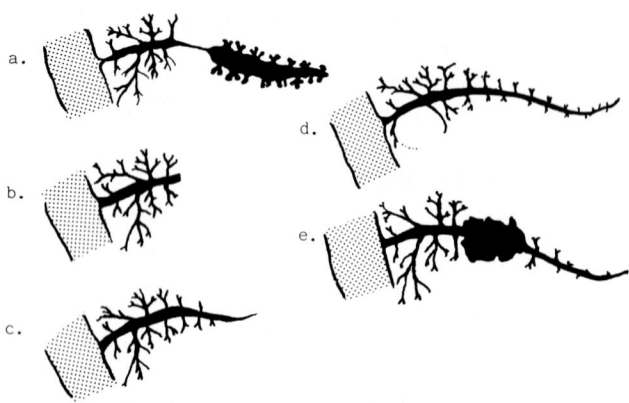

FIGURE 117-5. Pancreatograms of patients with pancreatic carcinoma help to classify five types: (**a**) ductal stenosis with prestenotic dilatation; (**b**) complete ductal obstruction; (**c**) ductal tapering; (**d**) side branch deviation; and (**e**) cavity formation.

during ERCP and PTC. The pain associated with penetrating the liver capsule is greater than that experienced with ERCP; however, the gagging and retching sometimes associated with the latter procedure is not experienced by patients undergoing PTC. ERCP allows the application of therapeutic modalities not available through PTC, as discussed in the next two sections of this chapter. In addition, ERCP enables imaging of the pancreatic duct, which is rarely possible with PTC.[72]

These diagnostic tests should also be compared for their appropriate role in the management of patients with abdominal pain, jaundice, and miscellaneous other pancreatic or biliary conditions. Patients with unexplained abdominal pain do not benefit from ERCP unless there are objective findings suggesting diseases of pancreatic or biliary origin. Chronic pancreatitis may be suggested by typical pancreatic pain along with abnormal serum amylase or lipase levels, pancreatic calcification seen on plain abdominal radiographs, or unexplained steatorrhea. Pancreatography may detect ductal changes that are not seen on ultrasound or CT.

Patients with pain suggesting a biliary origin should also have elevations of liver enzymes during pain or an abnormal ultrasound before undergoing ERCP. Partial biliary obstruction may be observed in the absence of dilated bile ducts on ultrasound. If gallstones are found in the gallbladder on ultrasound and the patient has symptoms and laboratory findings consistent with choledocholithiasis, cholangitis, or biliary pancreatitis, then ERCP should be performed despite the absence of biliary ductal dilation.

ERCP has a better defined role in the evaluation of the jaundiced patient. Patients with unexplained cholestatic jaundice should undergo ERCP even if ducts are not dilated on ultrasound. Abnormalities such as sclerosing cholangitis or anatomic bile duct obstruction in the presence of a scarred or sclerotic liver may only be detected by cholangiographic changes. Patients with ductal dilatation defined by ultrasound or CT should have ERCP only after the diagnostic and therapeutic plan has been formulated. Injection of radiographic contrast material into an obstructed biliary tree leads to cholangitis in a significant number of cases unless biliary drainage is instituted. If an operation is planned for the patient, then cholangiography should be done within 24 hours of surgery.

If nonoperative palliation is to be pursued, then it should be instituted at the same sitting as the diagnostic ERCP.

ERCP is often recommended as a diagnostic adjunct in the evaluation of the patient with unexplained weight loss or steatorrhea or recent onset of diabetes mellitus and in the preoperative mapping of the pancreatic duct in patients with chronic pancreatitis or pancreatic pseudocyst. Few studies are available comparing ERCP with other modalities in these situations. Generally, the same principles apply as outlined previously for the role of ERCP in the evaluation of abdominal pain and jaundice. If there are other clinical factors that indicate a pancreatic or biliary origin of the problem, then ERCP may be helpful. Without these factors, the diagnostic yield is low. Preoperative delineation of the pancreatic duct is often helpful to the pancreatic surgeon before pancreaticojejunostomy or cystoenterostomy. Anatomic detail provided by pancreatography cannot be provided by indirect imaging studies such as ultrasound or CT. Whether surgical outcome is changed by the knowledge obtained from the pancreatogram has not been rigorously tested.

ENDOSCOPIC SPHINCTEROTOMY AND STONE REMOVAL

Just as ERCP transformed the diagnostic approach to suspected biliary problems and jaundice, so ES or papillotomy has had a dramatic impact on the management of biliary disease in general and on the treatment of common bile duct stones in particular. Nonoperative treatment of several biliary diseases was made possible by the introduction of this technique in 1973.[4,5] The technique of ES and the technique of gallstone extraction are discussed in this section.

Technical Considerations

Patient Preparation

Patients are prepared for ES in the same way as for diagnostic ERCP. Coagulation parameters are measured or a careful bleeding history is taken before the procedure. Patients are asked to avoid taking aspirin for 1 week and taking other nonsteroidal antiinflammatory drugs for 3 days before the procedure, if possible, in an effort to reduce the risk of bleeding. Patients with known biliary obstruction are usually given antibiotics before the procedure.[73]

Instruments

The same side-viewing endoscopes used for diagnostic ERCP are also used for ES. The most widely used instrument is Erlangen's papillotome.[74] This papillotome consists of a plastic catheter with a metal wire that is partly outside the lumen of the catheter. When the wire is tightened, the tip of the catheter is bowed so that the exposed wire is brought away from the catheter. Several types of papillotomes are commercially available, all of them differing in the length of the tip in front of the wire and the length of the exposed wire. We prefer using a papillotome with a metal tip because it is easier to see during fluoroscopy (Fig. 117-6). The tip of this papillotome is 1.5 cm long, and the exposed wire measures 2 or

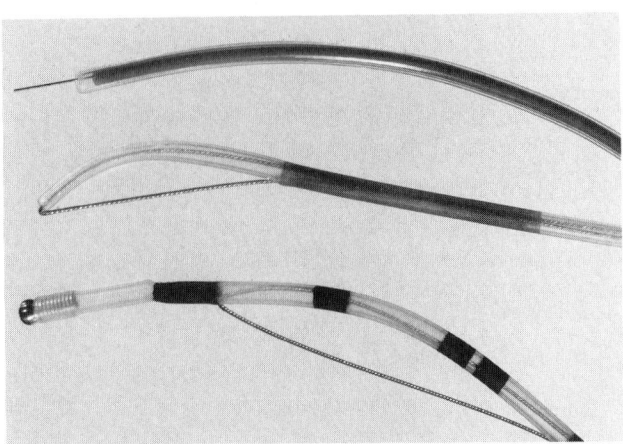

FIGURE 117-6. The three types of papillotomes are the needle knife papillotome (*top*), the precut papillotome (*middle*), and the standard Erlangen papillotome with a radiopaque metal tip (*bottom*).

3 cm. The long tip prevents slippage out of the papilla when the wire is tightened.

In cases in which a difficult cannulation of the papilla has been achieved by a diagnostic catheter, exchange for a wire-guided sphincterotome can be facilitated by first inserting a guidewire through the catheter. The catheter is then removed, and the sphincterotome is introduced over the guidewire. The guidewire is then removed and ES is performed.

Several devices are available for use in difficult situations but are not for routine use because they are associated with increased complications (see Fig. 117-6). A precut papillotome has no distal tip at all.[75] The wire starts at the tip and is 1 cm long. The precut needle knife consists of a plastic catheter with a thin, straight metal wire that can be advanced out of the catheter for not more than 5 mm.[76,77] Balloon catheters and a variety of baskets are available for stone extraction.

Procedure

A diagnostic ERCP is performed to define biliary anatomy and the pathologic process that can be treated by ES. The standard papillotome is then inserted in the common bile duct, and its position is verified using fluoroscopy. The papillotome is withdrawn until about one half to two thirds of the wire is visible in the duodenum. The wire is tightened and pushed slightly into the roof of the papilla by using the up-and-down deflecting knob of the endoscope and the elevator. The papilla is then cut stepwise by applying a combination of high-frequency cutting and coagulation current (Fig. 117-7; see Color Fig. 106). The cut should be made in the direction of the common bile duct (i.e., toward the 11-o'clock position). The length of the cut is dictated by the length of the endoscopically visible intramural bile duct and by the length needed for the situation (e.g., the size of the stone to be extracted). The cut should not be extended beyond the impression of the distal common bile duct in the duodenal wall. The sphincter can be judged to have been cut sufficiently if the tightened papillotome can be moved in and out of the common bile duct without resistance. The sphincterotomy

can also be measured by pulling an inflated balloon catheter of known size through the opening.

Precut papillotomy may be performed if cannulation with a standard papillotome fails. With the precut papillotome an initial cut of the roof of the papilla can be made after introduction of the papillotome only a few millimeters into the orifice.[75] The needle knife is used in two different ways. Some endoscopists prefer to cut an opening directly into a bulging papilla above its orifice.[78] More commonly, the needle knife is inserted into the orifice, and a cut is made in the direction of the common bile duct, using the controls of the endoscope to direct the wire.[76] The needle knife papillotome is an alternative to conventional papillotomes for ES in patients after Billroth II gastrectomy.[79,80]

Stones less than 1 cm in diameter in the distal duct are usually easily removed with a balloon catheter. Catheters with balloons ranging in size from 8 to 15 mm are available for this purpose. The catheter is advanced through the sphincterotomy and to a point above the stone using fluoroscopic monitoring. The balloon is then inflated, and the catheter is pulled to deliver the stone through the sphincterotomy. Larger stones and intrahepatic stones may be extracted more easily using a basket. Baskets of various sizes, shapes, and numbers of wires are available, but a standard wire basket of the Dormia type is used most often (Fig. 117-8). These baskets can often be directed proximally into one of the intrahepatic ducts, if needed, to capture the stone with the aid of fluoroscopy. Stones should be removed from the common bile duct immediately after ES. If the stones cannot be removed, a nasobiliary catheter (Fig. 117-9) or endoprosthesis should be left in place to avoid impaction of remaining stones in the distal duct and ensuing cholangitis.[81]

Special techniques may be required to extract stones that are larger than 15 mm in diameter or in a few special situations: stones that fill the entire ductal lumen, become impacted in the distal duct or at the sphincterotomy, lodge in the cystic duct, wedge beside a T-tube, or reside above a ductal stricture. Surgical removal of the stone must always be considered if standard endoscopic techniques fail.

Patients who are at increased risk for surgery may benefit from extraction of stone fragments after the stone is broken. Several types of fragmentation or lithotripsy are possible, including mechanical crushing with special baskets, use of intraductal electrohydraulic shock waves, firing of a tunable dye or neodymium:yttrium-aluminum-garnet (Nd:YAG) laser fiber placed directly through the endoscope channel or guided by a miniature endoscope placed into the duct, or use of extracorporeal shock waves aimed fluoroscopically with the aid of contrast material placed through a nasobiliary tube.[82-88] Dissolution therapy for common duct stones has not been very successful. Slow dissolution rates are obtained with mono-octanoin.[89] Methyl tertiary butyl ether is effective but causes duodenitis and general anesthesia if it escapes from the duct.[90]

Elderly and very-high-risk patients can be managed by placement of an endoprosthesis or stent if it is not possible to remove the stones after ES.[81] The stones are left in place, but impaction and subsequent cholangitis are prevented by the presence of the endoprosthesis (Fig. 117-10). In contrast to use of endoprostheses for draining biliary strictures, occlusion of the device usually does not require its exchange because

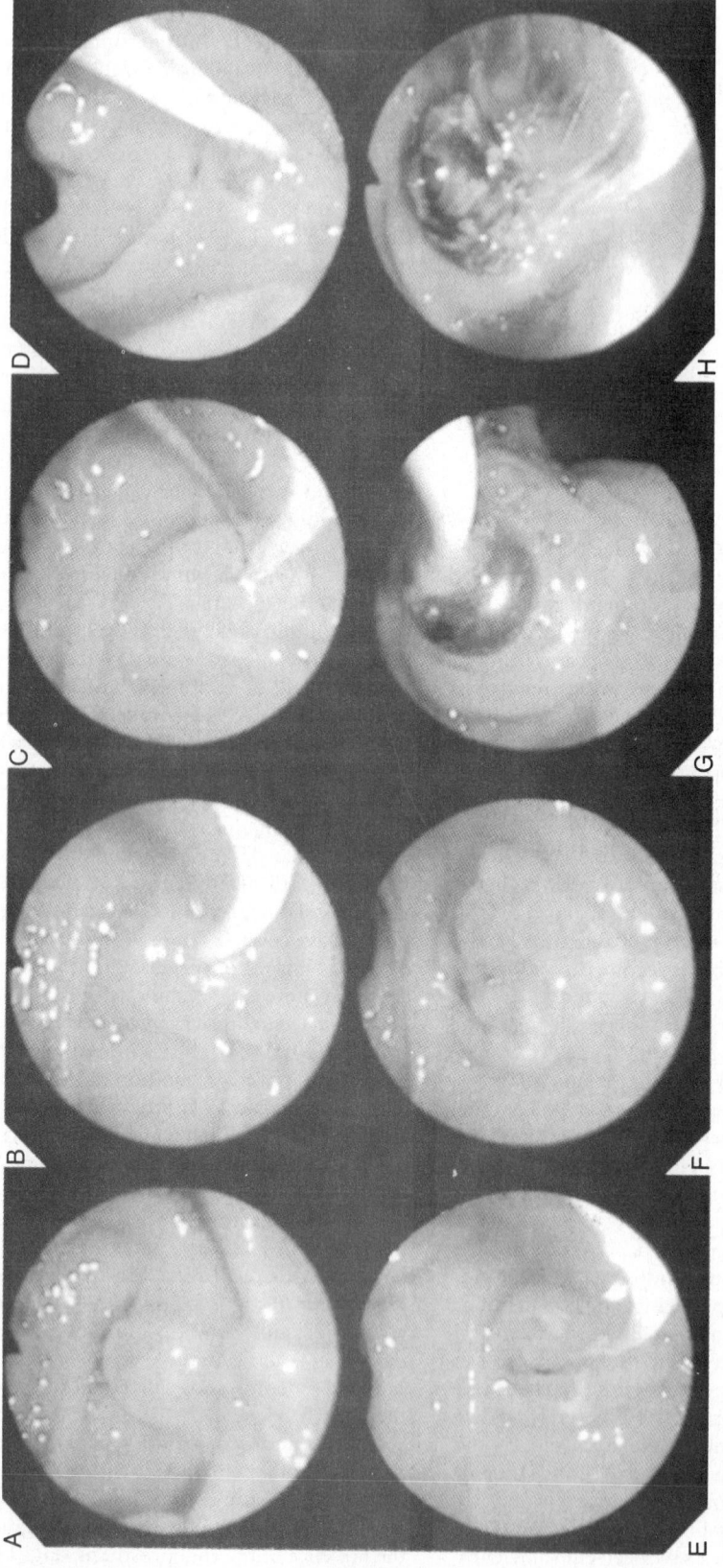

FIGURE 117-7. (See Color Fig. 106.) The sequence of endoscopic sphincterotomy and stone extraction is demonstrated. (**A**) A normal appearing papilla (**B**) is first cannulated with a diagnostic catheter. (**C**) The papillotome is introduced into the papilla, (**D**, **E**) and an incision is made using electrocautery, (**F**) leaving a completed sphincterotomy. (**G**) A balloon catheter is then used to calibrate the size of the sphincterotomy, (**H**) and the stone is pulled into the duodenum. (From Silverstein FE, Tytgat NJ. Atlas of gastrointestinal endoscopy. 2nd ed. New York: Gower Medical Publishing, 1987.)

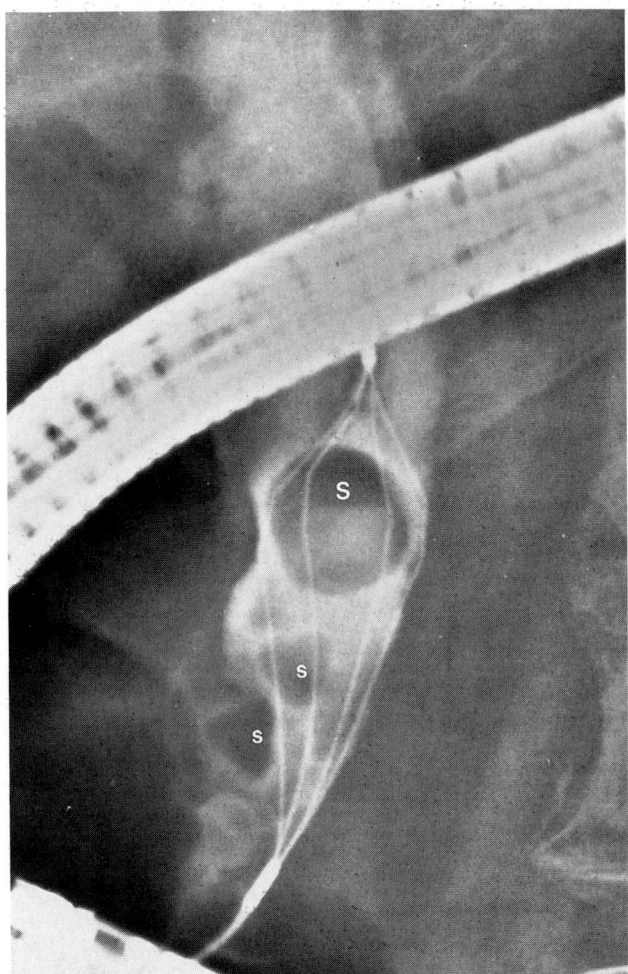

FIGURE 117-8. A Dormia stone basket has been used to capture a stone (S) that is approximately 1 cm in diameter. Two smaller stones (s) are seen in the common bile duct below the stone in the basket.

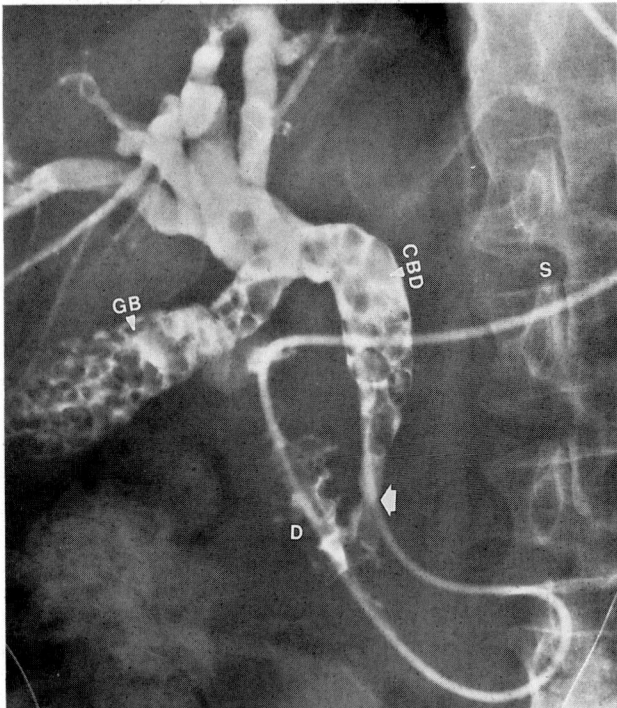

FIGURE 117-9. A nasobiliary tube has been placed to provide temporary biliary drainage in this patient with multiple small common bile duct (CBD) and gallbladder (GB) stones. The nasobiliary tube traverses the stomach (S) and forms a loop in the duodenum (D) before entering the papilla (*arrow*).

of ample room for bile flow around the endoprosthesis through the sphincterotomy.

Indications

Common Bile Duct Stones After Cholecystectomy

Choledocholithiasis after open or laparoscopic cholecystectomy is the main indication for ES. This indication is widely accepted for elderly patients, although there is some debate whether ES is also the preferred treatment in younger patients. The mortality rate of ES is 0.5% to 1% for all age groups, but the surgical treatment of common bile duct stones carries a mortality rate of less than 0.5% for younger patients and about 7% for older patients.[91,92] With the advent of laparoscopic cholecystectomy, indications have become more liberal. Most centers prefer preoperative ERCP if common bile duct stones are clinically suspected. ES and stone removal is performed if stones are found, even in young patients, in view of the difficulties in exploring the common bile duct laparos-

copically. Late complications of ES, such as ascending cholangitis, stricturing of the papillotomy, and recurrent stones, are unusual. The occurrence of late complications no longer plays a role in favoring surgical treatment of common bile duct stones in younger patients. Many patients prefer the endoscopic treatment over surgery because of the short hospitalization and the absence of general anesthesia.

Common Bile Duct Stones With the Gallbladder In Situ

ES is indicated for patients with choledocholithiasis and an intact gallbladder if they have an increased surgical risk or if they have complications, such as cholangitis or severe acute pancreatitis.[93–99] Interval cholecystectomy can then be done at a later stage, after these complications have subsided. The decision whether to proceed with cholecystectomy after ES should be based on the relative risks of complications from leaving the gallbladder in situ and those of cholecystectomy for a given patient. It is not necessary to proceed to cholecystectomy in all patients after ES. In some instances, it is appropriate to wait and see if pain or acute cholecystitis develops.

Acute Biliary Pancreatitis

Acute pancreatitis is an indication for ERCP if biliary tract stones are suspected to be the etiologic agent and if the pancreatitis is severe.[100] Complications may be reduced by ES

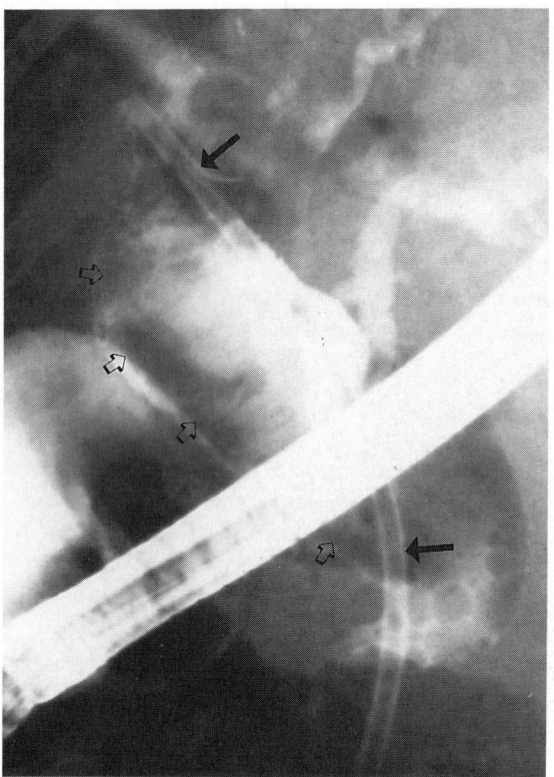

FIGURE 117-10. Acute cholangitis in this elderly patient was successfully treated by providing biliary drainage through a 10-Fr (3.3-mm) endoprosthesis (*closed arrows*) placed around a 4-cm diameter common duct stone (*open arrows*).

with stone extraction in patients with severe pancreatitis.[100] ERCP in the setting of acute pancreatitis does not appear to cause a worsening of the condition, although excessive injection of the pancreatic duct should be avoided.[101,102] If common bile duct stones are found on imaging tests in patients with acute pancreatitis, an ES is also indicated.

Patients with acute pancreatitis and cholestasis or who are suspected to have gallstones based on ultrasound or biochemical predictors should undergo ERCP without delay.[103] ES is performed, and the common duct stones are removed. Whether or not an ES should be performed in patients who have gallbladder stones without common bile duct stones is controversial. Our practice is to perform an ES in this setting if the size of the gallbladder stones and the diameter of the cystic duct are such that passage of the stones into the common duct is possible.

Acute Cholangitis

Acute cholangitis is caused by choledocholithiasis in more than 80% of cases, with other benign and malignant causes of biliary obstruction accounting for the remainder. ERCP allows diagnosis of the cause of biliary obstruction and is followed by ES for treatment. Stone extraction allows definitive treatment in most cases.[104–107] If stones cannot be removed or if a stricture exists, placement of a nasobiliary tube or endoprosthesis allows adequate drainage so that definitive

therapy for the obstruction can be accomplished after treatment of sepsis.[106]

Acute cholangitis is an indication for early ES and drainage. Approximately two thirds of patients with cholangitis respond to antibiotics and conservative therapy, allowing ES to be performed under controlled conditions.[106] However, the other one third of patients have a higher mortality rate unless obstruction is immediately relieved by ES. Hypotension may be a predictor of the one third of patients who need immediate ES.[106] Treatment of cholangitis with ES results in a lower mortality rate than surgical decompression.[107]

Bulging Papilla

A bulging papilla may be caused by a distal common bile duct stone, a papillary tumor, or a choledochocele. In most cases, a papillotomy is necessary to elucidate the cause. In general, these papillas are difficult to cannulate. If the standard papillotome cannot be inserted, the experienced endoscopist often uses the needle knife to create the sphincterotomy. If a mass is encountered, brushings and biopsy specimens can be obtained through the sphincterotomy.

Sump Syndrome

Patients with recurrent biliary pain or pancreatitis after surgical choledochoduodenostomy may have calculi or food particles occluding their common bile duct at or below the surgical anastomosis. This "sump syndrome" can be adequately treated with ES.[108]

Sphincter of Oddi Dysfunction

Recurrent right upper quadrant pain, usually in the patient who has had a cholecystectomy, has been attributed to sphincter of Oddi dysfunction. ES of the choledochal sphincter has been used in an attempt to reduce episodes of pain with variable results in these patients.[23,24] The presence of an elevated pressure in the sphincter of Oddi appears to be a better predictor of pain relief after ES than the cholangiographic findings of a dilated common bile duct or delayed drainage of contrast material.[23] Complication rates, especially perforation, appear to be approximately twice as frequent in ES treatment of sphincter of Oddi dysfunction as in treatment of common duct stones.[25] Patients without a dilated common bile duct are more likely to have a complication.[25]

Contraindications and Risks

The only strict contraindication for ES is severe coagulopathy. Juxtapapillary diverticula are often considered to be a relative contraindication, although the risk of complications is not increased if the papilla lies on the rim of the diverticulum. If the papilla lies deep within the diverticulum, the risk of perforation is increased, creating a relative contraindication to ES.

Large gallstones above a relatively narrow distal common duct segment are no longer contraindications for papillotomy. Newer techniques for dissolution, mechanical breakage, or extracorporeal lithotripsy of the common duct stones usually allow their successful removal. Gastrectomy with a Billroth II gastrojejunostomy is not a contraindication to ES, although the success rate of ES is only about 65%, even in expert hands.[79,80] Old age and poor general condition are not contraindications and do not increase the risks of ES.[91]

The rate of complications after ES varies between 4.8% and 8.4% in large series.[91,109] These complications are approximately equally divided between bleeding, perforation, cholangitis, and pancreatitis. Most of these complications can be treated conservatively, although 1% to 2% require surgical correction and 0.5% to 1.3% of patients die after ES.[91,109]

Bleeding after sphincterotomy occurs in 1.5% to 2% of cases. Most bleeding stops spontaneously, although blood transfusions are sometimes required. Torrential or continuous bleeding requires special treatment and occurs in 15% to 20% of bleeding episodes. Some patients with bleeding can be treated endoscopically by balloon tamponade, epinephrine injection, electrocoagulation, or laser coagulation if there is adequate endoscopic vision. Torrential bleeding requires immediate angiographic embolization or surgery. The sphincterotomy wound can be oversewn or the gastroduodenal artery ligated at the time of surgery.

Perforations of the choledochoduodenal angle occur in 0.6% to 1.1% of patients after ES. If the perforation is detected immediately, conservative treatment with nasoduodenal suction and antibiotics is often successful. Retroperitoneal leaks usually resolve with these conservative measures, leaving a minority of patients to eventually require abscess drainage. Intraperitoneal perforation is best managed surgically with oversewing and drainage. Most perforations occur in patients with large stones, in whom a long ES is necessary for stone removal. The advent of techniques to dissolve or to break large stones has reduced the need for long sphincterotomies. As a consequence, perforations have become less frequent.

Cholangitis after ES develops if stones are left in the common duct or if bile drainage is otherwise impaired. The frequency of cholangitis varies between 1.3% and 3.2%. This complication can be prevented by routinely inserting a nasobiliary drain or endoprosthesis if stones cannot be removed immediately after the ES. Rarely, cholangitis occurs after complete stone removal in patients with a very dilated common bile duct and a juxtapapillary diverticulum. Bile stasis in a grossly dilated bile duct is probably the cause of cholangitis in this situation.

A rise of serum amylase level after ES is seen in about 70% of patients. Clinical acute pancreatitis develops in 0.8% to 1.5% of cases. Only conservative treatment is indicated for most patients, although severe necrotizing pancreatitis occasionally develops.

In 0.5% to 1% of procedures, a stone or basket around a stone becomes impacted after ES. Although this used to be an indication for immediate surgery, impaction can usually be treated endoscopically by inserting a nasobiliary drain or endoprosthesis alongside the impacted stone. A few days later, after the edema from the ES subsides, it is often possible to remove the stone and basket endoscopically. Immediate treatment of an impacted stone basket is possible by placing the cable of a mechanical lithotriptor over the stone basket cable to cause stone fragmentation or breakage of the impacted basket wires.

Results

Successful ES can be carried out in approximately 95% of patients.[91] Complete duct clearance may be obtained in 85% to 90%. In as many as 15% of patients, immediate stone removal is difficult and a second or third endoscopy is required for complete clearance.[81,91]

During follow-up, 4% to 10% of patients develop new stones, stenosis, or both.[110] These problems can usually be treated by repeat ES. Rarely, patients continue to form new stones despite the presence of a widely patent papillary opening. Drug therapy has not been adequately studied to prevent recurrent stone formation but has not been helpful in our experience. Repeated endoscopic extractions or surgical choledochoenterostomy is then required.

Almost half of the patients who undergo ES have not undergone any previous biliary surgery. The major concern in leaving the gallbladder in situ is the risk of subsequent acute cholecystitis. Acute cholangitis and pancreatitis are unlikely after an adequate sphincterotomy has been made. The reported incidence of subsequent acute cholecystitis after ES is approximately 10% with follow-up of as long as 9 years.[93–95,111] The highest risk is seen in the first year after ES. Cystic duct obstruction at the time of ES and persistent gallbladder stones appear to be predictors of the minority of patients who have subsequent acute cholecystitis.[97,99] Some patients have passage of gallbladder stones into the duodenum after ES.[112] This may relate to the finding that sphincterotomy in the dog facilitates passage of beads from the gallbladder into the duodenum.[113] The mechanism for this may be related to a lower gallbladder resting volume and an increased gallbladder ejection fraction after sphincterotomy.[113]

Clinical Implications

ES should be compared with common bile duct exploration for safety and efficacy. Unfortunately, prospective randomized studies are scarce. Comparison of surgical and endoscopic series may be instructive; however, caution should be exercised because selection biases are inevitable in these series.[112]

Bile Duct Stones After Cholecystectomy

ES has gained the greatest acceptance, by internists and surgeons, for the removal of duct stones in patients with prior cholecystectomy.[109,114,115] Surgical and endoscopic success rates for stones smaller than 1.5 cm in diameter are comparable. Mortality rates are comparable in the young and healthy. Cost and length of hospitalization are significantly less with ES. Patients with significant underlying medical illness appear to have little increased risk associated with ES compared with young and healthy patients.[116] Surgical mortality rates are higher in patients with significant underlying medical illness, under emergency conditions, and if more than one operation is required.[92,112,116]

Acute Cholangitis

Patients with acute cholangitis are often very ill and have an increased operative risk. These patients are good candidates for ES. A retrospective study compared the outcome of patients with common bile duct stones and cholangitis who were treated surgically with the outcome of those treated with ES over the same period of time.[107] The 43 patients treated with ES were older (mean age, 75) and had more medical risk factors than the 28 patients treated surgically (mean age, 66). The 30-day mortality rate was 5% in the ES group and 21% in the surgical group ($P<0.02$). The common duct was not cleared of stones in 10% of both groups.

Acute Pancreatitis

As has been discussed, early ES may reduce the frequency of complications in patients with severe biliary pancreatitis. There are no prospective comparisons of ES with early surgery, and it is very likely that there never will be, because common bile duct exploration in patients with severe acute pancreatitis carries too high a rate of complications and death.[117]

Bile Duct Stones With Gallbladder In Situ

The role of ES in patients with intact gallbladders who do not have cholangitis or pancreatitis is controversial. ES is not justified before open cholecystectomy in average-risk patients with common bile duct stones and intact gallbladders. A prospective randomized study from the United Kingdom showed that preoperative ES followed by cholecystectomy did not reduce morbidity or mortality rates compared with cholecystectomy and common bile duct exploration.[118] There were numerically more complications in the ES group, but this did not reach statistical significance. The patients in this study were relatively young (median age, 60) and had few risk factors for complications of surgery. ES with interval cholecystectomy should be considered for patients with recent, reversible conditions (e.g., myocardial infarction, other major surgery, pregnancy). Whether other patients who are at high risk for surgery should have ES and the gallbladder left in situ depends on an assessment of specific individual risk factors and life expectancy.

The popularization of laparoscopic cholecystectomy has altered the role of ERCP before cholecystectomy. ERCP and ES are often performed before laparoscopic cholecystectomy, if stones are suspected.

ENDOSCOPIC BILIARY AND PANCREATIC DRAINAGE

Endoscopic biliary drainage through endoprostheses for obstructive jaundice has been adopted by many centers around the world since its initial description in 1979. It is now generally known what can be achieved technically and which types of patients and strictures are particularly difficult to drain.[119] The spectrum, frequency, and management of complications are appreciated. Many unanswered questions regarding the precise indications for these endoscopic procedures remain. In general, endoscopic biliary drainage is the treatment of choice for high-risk elderly and frail patients. For younger, lower-risk patients, the treatment of choice is less clear. Comparative randomized controlled studies are difficult to perform

in this setting; few data are available on which therapeutic decisions may be based.

Technical Considerations

Patient Preparation

Patients are prepared for biliary drainage procedures in much the same way as for diagnostic ERCP and ES. If it is known in advance that the patient has obstructive jaundice, antibiotics are usually given prophylactically before the procedure. Antibiotics may be unnecessary in the afebrile patient if stenting is successful, but they may reduce the risk of cholangitis developing if only partial drainage or no drainage is achieved. Coverage of gram-negative bowel flora with an aminoglycoside plus extended-spectrum penicillin or a third-generation cephalosporin is desirable.[120]

Instruments

Side-viewing endoscopes with large-bore instrumentation channels (3.7, 4.2, or 5.5 mm) are used to allow insertion of large-caliber endoprostheses. Stents and nasobiliary tubes with a diameter of 2.6 mm (8 Fr) can be placed through the 3.2-mm channel of diagnostic duodenoscopes but have a high occlusion rate. Stents and drainage tubes of various types are usually placed in position with the use of guidewires and guiding catheters.

The first endoprosthesis or stent used for transpapillary endoscopic drainage was a single pigtail 2.3-mm (7-Fr) angiographic catheter (Fig. 117-11).[8] Further experience and technical improvements led to the development of two main types of endoprosthesis: the straight Amsterdam-type endoprosthesis with side flaps to prevent migration and the double-pigtail endoprosthesis (see Fig. 117-11). These endoprostheses are available in diameters of 2.3, 3.3, 3.8, and 4.6 mm (7, 10, 11.5, and 14 Fr, respectively) and in several lengths ranging from 5 to 20 cm. The straight stent is used most often. This endoprosthesis has side flaps 2 cm from the proximal tip and 1 cm from the distal tip.

Metal self-expandable or balloon-expandable stents of various design are available. The particular advantage of these stents is their large diameter after deployment (9.9 mm, or 30 Fr), which reduces the frequency of stent occlusion.[121] Tumor ingrowth through the wire mesh or over the ends of the stent is the main cause of obstruction. The development of covered metal stents may reduce the frequency of this complication.

Many guidewires of differing diameter, length, and flexibility are available for directing guiding catheters and endoprostheses through strictures. The most frequently used guidewires are 0.97-mm (0.038-in), 0.89-mm (0.035-in), or 0.81-mm (0.032-in) Teflon-coated springs with a flexible atraumatic tip. The flexible tip can be of a fixed or adjustable length. Straight endoprostheses larger than 2.3 mm (7 Fr) are inserted over a smooth but rigid Teflon catheter that is placed over the guidewire. Some 2-mm (6-Fr) catheters of this type have a metal ring at the tip to aid fluoroscopic localization. Stents are pushed through the endoscope and then the stricture by using a stiff Teflon pusher tube.

The metal stents are also inserted over a guidewire and

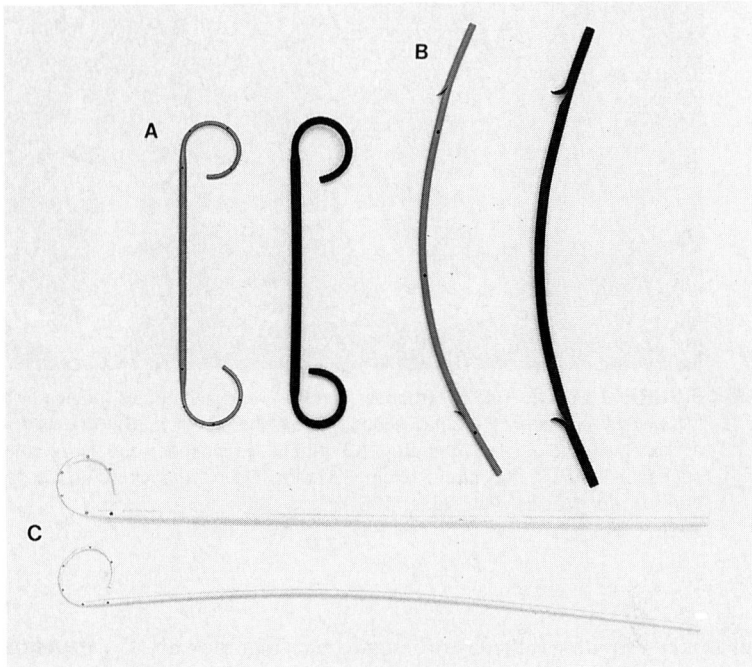

FIGURE 117-11. Three types of endoprostheses are shown. (**A**) The 7-Fr (2.3-mm) and 10-Fr (3.3-mm) double-pigtail stents. (**B**) The 7-Fr (2.3-mm) and 10-Fr (3.3-mm) straight Amsterdam stents. (**C**) The 7-Fr (2.3-mm) and 10-Fr (3.3-mm) single-pigtail stents like those used in the first endoscopic biliary drainage procedure.

after correct positioning are deployed by the gradual withdrawal of a protective covering or by inflation of a balloon to forcefully expand the stent. After deployment, the metal stents cannot be removed.

Stricture dilation is usually unnecessary for placing an endoprosthesis through distal strictures. Prior dilatation may be required, however, in more proximal, postoperative, and inflammatory strictures. Radiopaque Teflon dilating catheters with a tapered tip of gradually increasing diameter and dilating balloons of various diameters have been developed for use over a guidewire in this setting.

Stents are also available for insertion into the pancreatic duct, through the major or minor papilla. These stents are usually smaller in diameter than biliary stents, beginning with a 1.6-mm (5 Fr) outer diameter.[122] Guidewires are also smaller, with a 0.46-mm (0.018-in) diameter wire often needed in the minor papilla.

Brushes and biopsy forceps are also available for obtaining specimens from strictures for pathologic examination.[123–127] Small specimens are obtained if standard biopsy forceps are used.[123] Specimens with a higher yield are secured if larger forceps are used after sphincterotomy and before stent insertion. Alternatively, brush cytology can be accomplished by using a specially constructed brush mounted 3 cm proximal to the tip of a flexible guidewire.[127] The wire and brush assembly are advanced into a stricture from a 1.6-mm (5-Fr) catheter sleeve.

Long Teflon tubes are useful for temporary nasobiliary and nasopancreatic drainage. These tubes form a pigtail within the duct after removal of the guidewire. They vary in diameter from 1.6 to 2.6 mm (5–8 Fr) and are placed over a guidewire. A soft, larger-caliber tube is provided with these kits for exchange of the tube from mouth to nose after removal of the endoscope.

Procedure

Drainage procedures begin with a diagnostic ERCP. Preferably, the pancreatic and bile ducts should be filled to aid in diagnosis and to define the anatomy. Knowledge of the exact location and nature of the bile duct stenosis is essential before attempting endoprosthesis insertion.

A limited sphincterotomy is occasionally performed after the diagnostic study to facilitate introduction of the guiding catheter and the endoprosthesis (Fig. 117-12). The sphincterotomy facilitates exchange of the endoprosthesis in case of clogging. Many endoscopists insert 3.3- and 3.8-mm (10- and 11.5-Fr) stents without a prior sphincterotomy, now that recannulation is circumvented by the over-the-guidewire exchange of catheters.

After selective cannulation of the common bile duct, the rigid Teflon guiding catheter is inserted into the distal common bile duct. This catheter cannot easily be advanced through the stenosis in most cases. The rather blunt tip generally abuts against the stricture and inhibits easy passage through the stenosis. Forceful pushing should be avoided because of the risk of creating a false passage through the tumor. This catheter can be used to inject contrast material to facilitate guidewire manipulation.

The atraumatic, flexible-tip guidewire is placed through the guiding catheter and then manipulated through the stricture using fluoroscopy. Subsequently, the catheter is advanced over the guidewire through the stricture. After the catheter tip is introduced beyond the stricture, the endoprosthesis can be inserted over the catheter. The guidewire remains in position to further stiffen the catheter during endoprosthesis insertion.

The endoprosthesis is advanced with the help of the pusher tube to the tip of the endoscope. The length of the pusher

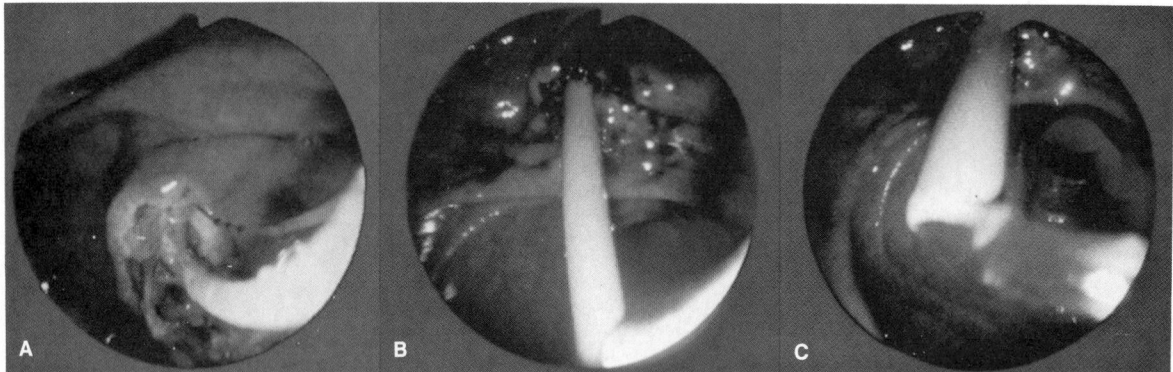

FIGURE 117-12. (**A**) Insertion of a biliary endoprosthesis begins with a diagnostic cholangiogram, followed by creation of a small endoscopic sphincterotomy. (**B**) The stent is then pushed into place over a guidewire and guiding catheter. (**C**) When the pusher tube is removed, a gush of bile enters the duodenum through the stent. (From Silverstein FE, Tytgat NJ. Atlas of gastrointestinal endoscopy. New York: Gower Medical Publishing, 1987.)

tube and the guiding catheter are designed such that the catheter emerges from the end of the pusher tube that is outside the body before the endoprosthesis reaches the tip of the endoscope. The assistant secures and withdraws the guiding catheter slightly, as the endoscopist advances the pusher tube.

The elevator bridge is opened after the endoprosthesis reaches the tip of the instrumentation channel, and the endoprosthesis is gradually pushed out of the endoscope. The whole assembly of the catheter, guidewire, pusher tube, and endoprosthesis is moved forward by advancing the pusher tube.

The endoprosthesis is moved up the duct in a stepwise fashion as the endoscopist opens and closes the elevator bridge in coordination with elevation of the endoscope tip toward the papilla. The procedure is repeated until the distal side flap reaches the papilla. The assistant can then pull the catheter and guidewire back while the endoscopist holds the endoprosthesis in position with the pusher tube (see Fig. 117-12). Leaving 1 cm of the endoprosthesis free in the duodenum allows easy retrieval in the event of clogging. After adequate drainage is seen endoscopically or fluoroscopically, the endoscope containing the pusher tube, catheter, and guidewire can be removed from the patient (see Fig. 117-12).

Small-caliber endoprostheses and nasobiliary tubes can be placed without use of a guiding catheter. Stents are loaded over the guidewire and pushed into position with a small-caliber pusher tube.

Biliary endoprostheses can also be placed endoscopically with assistance from the interventional radiologist.[128] If difficulty is encountered cannulating the papilla or in passing a guidewire through a stricture, percutaneous transhepatic drainage is undertaken. A guidewire 450 cm long is then advanced through the stricture by the radiologist and grasped by the endoscopist with a snare or basket passed through the therapeutic duodenoscope. After pulling the guidewire back through the endoscope's operating channel, the guide catheter and stent are placed in the standard fashion. Both ends of the guidewire are securely held in this technique, allowing relatively easy stent placement through even tight strictures.

Pancreatic Drainage

Placement of endoprostheses and nasopancreatic drains has been described for the treatment of symptomatic pancreatic ductal obstruction.[129–131] Drainage tubes of various sizes are placed into the pancreatic duct over a guidewire with or without a prior pancreatic sphincterotomy.[132,133] Balloon dilatation may be necessary in some cases.[134] The 1.6- and 2.3-mm (5- and 7-Fr) stents have also been placed through the minor papilla in patients with pancreas divisum.[130] Stents are placed over a 0.46-mm (0.018-in) guidewire that is placed into the dorsal pancreatic duct without a prior sphincterotomy.[130] It is also possible to extract pancreatic stones through the major papilla after sphincterotomy in some patients.[129,133,134] Experience with stenting and stone extraction in the pancreatic duct is limited; these procedures should be undertaken only by highly skilled endoscopists.

Radiography

Fluoroscopy is essential during placement of endoprostheses. Maintenance of the guidewire within the biliary or pancreatic duct system is necessary to avoid complications. Monitoring of guidewire, guide catheter, and stent position requires high-quality fluoroscopic visualization. A plain abdominal radiograph after the procedure is important to document drainage of contrast material and to establish the position of the stent in case migration is suspected at a later date.

Indications

Benign Biliary Strictures

Endoscopic biliary drainage has been used to relieve biliary obstruction in patients with benign bile duct strictures. These strictures may be the result of direct or ischemic bile duct injury that occurred during cholecystectomy or common bile duct exploration or they may be caused by sclerosing cholangitis.

Postcholecystectomy strictures. Although some patients may present within weeks after surgery, many develop symptoms years later. Most patients with these strictures present with abdominal pain; a few have jaundice, pruritus, or cholangitis.[135] Serum bilirubin and alkaline phosphatase levels are elevated in most cases, and ultrasound or CT often shows dilated intrahepatic bile ducts.

ERCP is indicated to diagnose the cause of biliary obstruction in patients with benign biliary strictures. Most strictures are smoothly marginated (Fig. 117-13A) and can be distinguished from malignant strictures based on the cholangiographic appearance, although a high suspicion of malignancy should be maintained because some benign-appearing strictures may be found to be malignant on follow-up. Most benign postoperative strictures are located near the cystic duct stump, in the common hepatic duct, or at the bifurcation.[135,136]

After diagnosis of the stricture, ES may be performed to facilitate access to the bile duct. Balloon dilatation over a guidewire to a 3.3-mm (10-F) balloon diameter is tried initially, although most strictures are observed on cholangiography to reform immediately after removal of the balloon. Some of these strictures are very tight and may not allow passage of a guidewire or a balloon. Unsuccessful guidewire passage makes safe endoscopic dilatation impossible; percutaneous transhepatic or surgical therapy should be considered in this situation. If the guidewire but not the balloon can be passed, then the use of dilating catheters of increasing size or placement of a small-caliber endoprosthesis usually allows adequate drainage.

If balloon dilatation fails, an endoprosthesis must be inserted through the stricture to achieve successful drainage.[135,136] Although comparative studies of stent size and number used is limited, our practice is to use the largest stents feasible and to insert two stents side by side whenever possible (Fig. 117-13B). This achieves the greatest bile duct diameter while the stents are in place and should allow earlier stent removal. Stents are removed at 3- to 4-month intervals to avoid stent occlusion and are replaced if interval cholangiograms show persistence of the stricture. Most patients have no stents in place by 2 years after the initial procedure.[135]

Biliary fistulas. Patients in the early postoperative period are more likely to present with persistently elevated volumes of T-tube drainage or biliary cutaneous or biliary peritoneal fistulas. Distal obstruction caused by unrecognized stones or strictures is often found. Stones should be removed after sphincterotomy. The best management for patients without stones is unclear. Some authors suggest that sphincterotomy alone is sufficient.[137,138] Others prefer to insert a nasobiliary tube without sphincterotomy.[139] We prefer to insert an endoprosthesis in most cases. This allows more time for the fistula to heal before endoprosthesis removal.[140,141]

Primary sclerosing cholangitis. Endoscopic biliary drainage has been used in a limited number of patients with primary sclerosing cholangitis.[142–146] The precise role of ERCP in the management of patients with this disease is evolving. These patients can be symptomatic with recurrent episodes of clinical

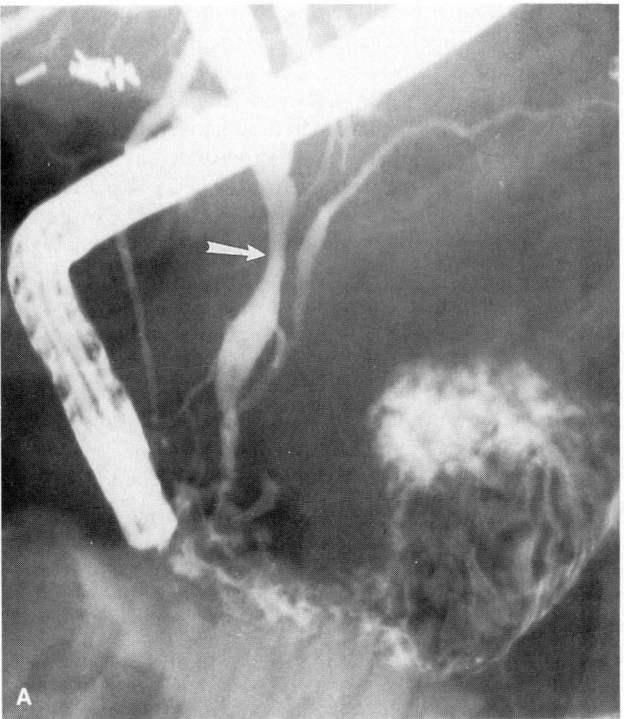
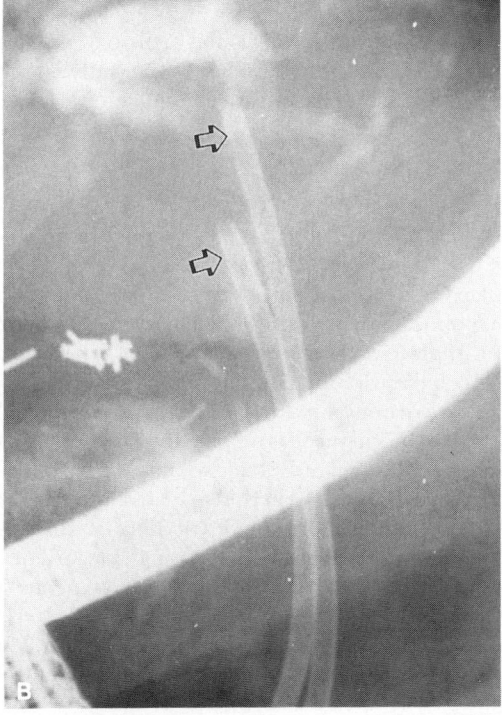

FIGURE 117-13. (**A**) A benign postcholecystectomy stricture (*arrow*) has caused abdominal pain and cholestasis in this patient. (**B**) Two 10-Fr (3.3-mm) endoprostheses (*open arrows*) have been placed to dilate the stricture and will be changed every 3 months until the cholangiograms demonstrate adequate stricture caliber.

cholangitis, but there may also be long periods before evidence of liver failure occurs. Endoscopic management should be directed toward patients who have significant symptomatic extrahepatic biliary strictures but with relatively preserved hepatic function. These patients should benefit by a reduction in the morbidity rate and in the hospitalizations required for treatment of episodes of cholangitis. Biliary reconstructive surgery can also be avoided so that subsequent hepatic transplantation remains a viable therapeutic option should signs of liver failure develop. Patients with only a few episodes of cholangitis are probably better managed with repeat courses of antibiotics so that the risks of ERCP and drainage are avoided.

The optimal method of endoscopic biliary drainage for patients with primary sclerosing cholangitis is unknown. Insertion of a nasobiliary tube for infusion of saline or corticosteroids has been reported to be beneficial in a small number of cases and deserves further evaluation.[142,143] Most studies report using a combination of balloon dilatation and endoprosthesis placement after ES.[144-146]

Endoscopic biliary drainage is also used for patients with chronic pancreatitis who have intrapancreatic biliary strictures. The natural history of these strictures is unclear; only a minority of patients with strictures have symptoms or evidence of progressive liver injury.[147,148] In one series, only 1 of 20 patients with mild degrees of biliary obstruction and bilirubin levels of 3 to 4 mg/dL required surgical biliary drainage over a mean follow-up of almost 4 years.[148] Endoprosthesis insertion is an alternative to biliary enteric bypass surgery for symptomatic patients with a limited life expectancy.

Malignant Biliary Strictures

A biliary endoprosthesis has two potential roles in patients with malignant obstructive jaundice: preoperative drainage in patients with resectable lesions and palliation in patients with unresectable tumors.

Preoperative biliary drainage

Obstruction of the biliary tract may be associated with dysfunction of multiple organs. Energy metabolism and protein synthesis may be abnormal because of hepatocyte dysfunction, anorexia, poor caloric intake, and impaired digestion and assimilation of proteins, fats, and carbohydrates. Theoretically, preoperative biliary drainage should correct these defects and result in a lower surgical mortality and morbidity rates.[149]

Preoperative percutaneous transhepatic drainage has been extensively studied. One early study found that the operative mortality rate was reduced after preoperative drainage compared with historic controls.[150] Two other studies using historic controls and three studies using concurrent but nonrandomized controls suggest that percutaneous preoperative drainage confers some benefit.[151-155] However, three prospective randomized trials have shown no benefit and have emphasized the complications of percutaneous drainage.[156-158]

Endoscopic stenting avoids some of the complications of percutaneous transhepatic drainage. Bleeding and bile leakage associated with liver puncture and the complications of external bile loss can be avoided. Patients who are managed

with internal drainage with an endoscopically placed stent can spend several weeks at home allowing hepatocellular function to recover. Whether the benefits of drainage outweigh the complications of the endoscopic procedure can only be assessed in prospective randomized trials, which are in progress.

Palliative biliary drainage

The best-evaluated role of biliary endoprostheses is the definitive palliation of obstructive jaundice caused by unresectable biliary and pancreatic malignancies. Biliary drainage in this setting is best reviewed by considering the location of the obstruction.

Ampullary carcinoma. Ampullary or papillary carcinoma is an uncommon, but not rare, cause of malignant obstructive jaundice, accounting for approximately 8% of cases of malignant biliary obstruction.[159,160] Cannulation is often difficult in cases of ampullary cancer because the orifice may be displaced to an unusual location. These tumors are extremely friable and may bleed as soon as they are probed with the cannula.

Because ampullary tumors bleed easily, it is preferable to place an endoprosthesis without a preliminary sphincterotomy if possible. However, in at least 25% of cases, a precut papillotomy must be made to obtain access to the common bile duct or to obtain a tissue specimen. After access to the bile duct is achieved, insertion of a short endoprosthesis is usually not difficult because the guidewire and guiding catheter easily traverse the soft tumor. An alternative to placement of an endoprosthesis is making a large sphincterotomy. There is an increased risk of bleeding with these sphincterotomies, and restricturing occurs in most patients after a mean interval of 7 months.[161]

Patients with ampullary carcinoma, unlike those with carcinoma of the pancreas, have a relatively good prognosis, with 5-year survival rates of 30% to 40% after resection.[162,163] Patients who have no evidence of metastatic disease and who are reasonable surgical candidates should be treated surgically with pancreaticoduodenectomy or local tumor resection. Placement of a biliary endoprosthesis for definitive palliation should be reserved for elderly patients with severe underlying disease and those with advanced or metastatic cancer.

Pancreatic carcinoma. Pancreatic cancer is the most common tumor leading to obstructive jaundice and accounts for more than 50% of such cases. Tumors growing near the papilla may distort the common bile duct and pancreatic duct, making cannulation and papillotomy difficult. Papillotomy with a needle knife may be necessary to obtain access to the common bile duct.[164] In a minority of cases, it may be difficult to pass a guidewire through the stricture because of sharp angulation or tortuosity of the duct.[164,165] Expandable metal stents have been best studied in patients with pancreatic cancer (Fig. 117-14).[121]

Middle common bile duct obstruction. Middle common bile duct obstruction is usually caused by primary bile duct carcinoma or gallbladder cancer invading the bile duct.[166] Management is similar regardless of the primary origin of the

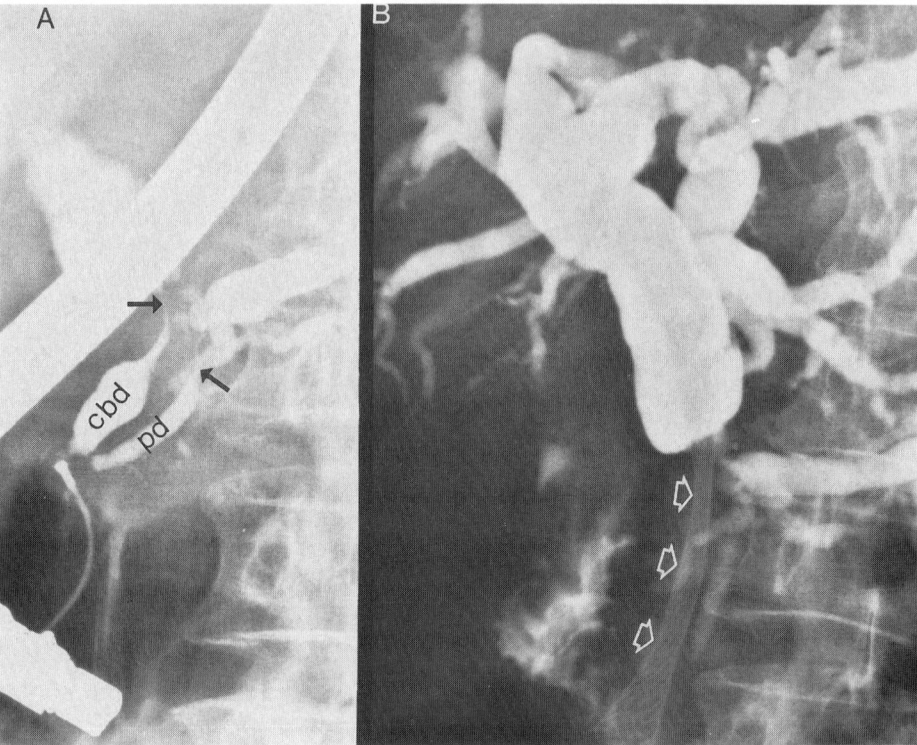

FIGURE 117-14. (**A**) The common bile duct (cbd) and pancreatic duct (pd) are obstructed (*arrows*) in this patient with pancreatic cancer. (**B**) A metal Wallstent is shown (*open arrows*) after deployment in the bile duct. The stent will expand further to the full 30-Fr (9.9-mm) diameter in 2 to 3 days.

tumor. Obstruction of the middle common duct by tumor accounts for 15% to 20% of all malignant common duct obstructions. Surgical bypass procedures are often difficult in these situations.[167] Endoscopic endoprosthesis placement is a reasonable alternative, especially in poor-risk patients or those with obvious tumor spread or recurrence after surgery.

Malignant hilar strictures. Tumors at the bifurcation of the common hepatic duct may arise from the duct or be caused by metastases from breast, colon, lung, stomach, and other malignancies.[168–170] Tumors in this location account for about 20% of cases of malignant biliary tract obstruction. Bifurcation tumors are difficult to treat by any modality. Surgical access is often limited by proximal spread of the neoplasm into the liver; only about 20% of primary biliary tumors in this location are resectable.[171,172] Cholangitis is a common complication of surgically placed U-tubes or hepaticojejunostomies. Palliative procedures are likewise difficult in patients with malignant bifurcation strictures. The technical difficulty in placing endoscopic stents depends on the extent of the stricture at the hilum.[45] Bifurcation strictures have been classified as follows: a stricture involving the common hepatic duct within 2 cm of the bifurcation but not the left or right duct is type I (Fig. 117-15A); a stricture involving left and right ducts without intrahepatic ductal involvement is type II (Fig. 117-15B); and a stricture involving the left and right hepatic ducts plus intrahepatic ducts is type III (Fig. 117-15C).[45] Type III strictures are usually associated with more extensive and often metastatic disease. As a result, stent insertion and relief of jaundice is more successful in types I and II compared with type III strictures. Survival rates for patients with type I strictures is longer.[45]

Contraindications and Risks

Early Complications

Early complications of endoprosthesis placement may be related to the preceding sphincterotomy or to endoprosthesis insertion. Complications of the sphincterotomy are generally less frequent than complications of ES for common duct stones, probably because of the small sphincterotomy size necessary for endoprosthesis insertion compared with stone removal. Bleeding is seen in 1% to 2% of patients, and pancreatitis occurs in as many as 1%, but perforation of the duodenum or bile duct is rare.

Acute cholangitis is the greatest risk of endoprosthesis insertion in frequency and in severity. Bacterial contamination of the biliary system during ERCP is unavoidable. Proper disinfection of endoscopes and ancillary equipment is mandatory but does not prevent the introduction of bacteria from the mouth and the upper gut into the obstructed biliary tract. If biliary drainage is incomplete, there is a high risk of cholangitis. Cholangitis is more frequent after drainage procedures in patients with bifurcation tumors because complete biliary drainage is often difficult.[45]

The rate of cholangitis is directly correlated with the number of attempts at prosthesis insertion before success is achieved. Repeat endoprosthesis insertion is usually tried on a day subsequent to the initial attempt. In 200 consecutive patients with pancreatic carcinoma, the overall incidence of cholangitis after endoprosthesis placement was 8%.[164] The risk of cholangitis was only 2.7% if successful insertion was achieved at the first attempt and was 23% if two or more attempts were required. It is likely that bacterial contamination

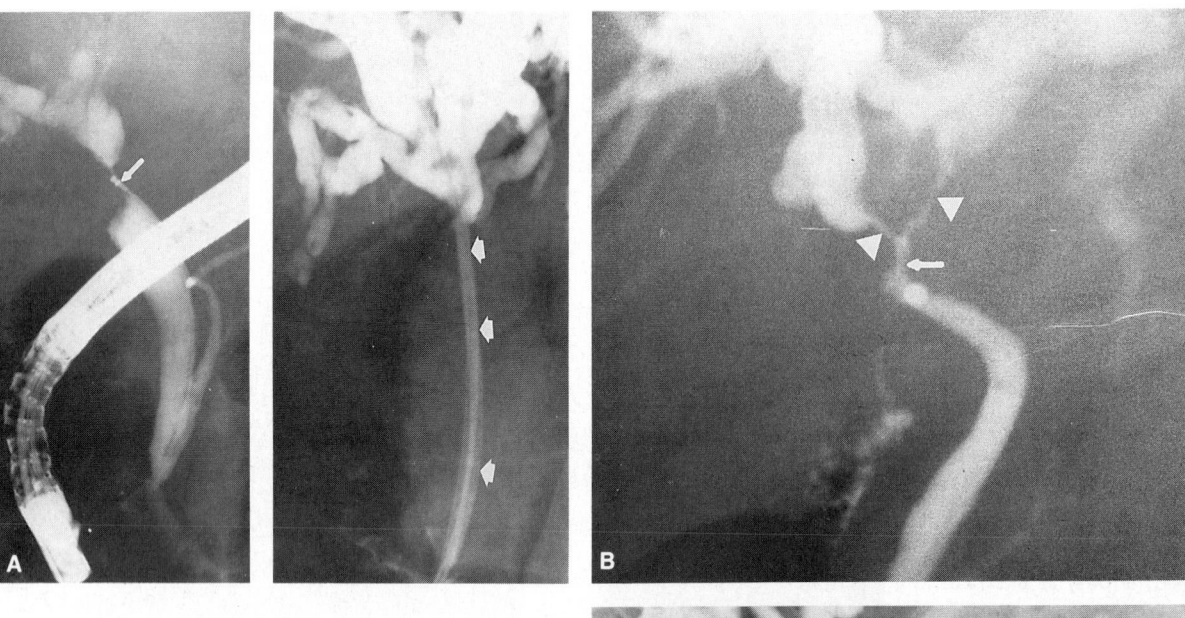

FIGURE 117-15. The strictures seen on cholangiograms of patients with malignant biliary obstruction at the hilum of the liver have been classified into three types. (**A**) Type I strictures involve the common hepatic duct within 2 cm of the bifurcation. A metal-tipped cannula (*arrow*) has been wedged into the stricture to obtain a cholangiogram before insertion of two endoprostheses (*solid arrows*). (**B**) Type II strictures involve the common hepatic duct (*arrow*) and the origins of the left and right hepatic ducts (*arrowheads*), without involvement of other branch ducts. (**C**) Type III strictures involve the major central ducts (*open arrow*) and small branch ducts (*small arrows*).

is introduced into the biliary tract during the first attempt with ensuing cholangitis 2 or more days later.

Other early complications related to endoprosthesis placement are very unusual and consist of bile duct perforation, acute cholecystitis, and early clogging of the endoprosthesis by clots or tumor fragments. The mortality rate directly related to sphincterotomy and endoprosthesis placement is 2% to 6%, with cholangitis being the main cause of death. The 30-day mortality rate for these patients, who often have advanced cancer, ranges from 10% to 30%.[45]

Late Complications

The main late complication is clogging of the endoprosthesis, which occurs in 21% to 36% of cases.[45,164,173] Clogging may occur from 8 days to more than 15 months after placement of a plastic endoprosthesis, with a mean of about 5 months. Expandable metal stents appear to last a few months more before tumor ingrowth causes occlusion.[121,174] Patients with a clogged endoprosthesis present with a flu-like syndrome, malaise, low-grade fever, or recurrence of liver function abnormalities. If this syndrome is not recognized early, frank cholangitis and jaundice occur. Prompt recognition of early symptoms should lead to immediate removal and replacement of the clogged endoprosthesis. Cleaning, brushing, and irrigation of a clogged endoprosthesis is technically possible, but repeat obstruction of the endoprosthesis quickly occurs. Replacement of a clogged endoprosthesis is usually technically simple and should require less than 30 minutes, because the preliminary sphincterotomy has already been accomplished. Cholangitis and jaundice are usually promptly relieved by stent replacement. Tumor ingrowth or clogging of an expandable metal stent is usually treated by placing a straight plastic endoprosthesis through the center of the metal one.

A clogged endoprosthesis contains inspissated bile, calculous-like debris, and proteinaceous material.[175-177] Endoprostheses removed 2 months after insertion are covered with a layer of protein, especially at the site of the side-flap holes. Bacteria are present in this layer, but it is not clear whether the proteins are produced by the bacteria or are from bile.[177,178] Clinical studies show that patency of a 3.3-mm (10-Fr) endoprosthesis is longer than that of a 2.3- or 2.6-mm (7- or 8-Fr) endoprosthesis, but apparently no further advantage is conferred by use of larger 4-mm (12-Fr) prosthesis.[173,179] Replacement stents do not remain patent as long as the original ones.[180] Other late complications are unusual and include acute cholecystitis, migration of the endoprosthesis into the more proximal bile ducts or into the bowel, and duodenal or bile duct perforation.[181]

Duodenal obstruction may occur after endoprosthesis insertion because of continued growth of the ampullary or pancreatic carcinoma. The incidence of delayed duodenal obstruction can be kept to less than 10% if surgical gastroenterostomy and biliary enteric surgical drainage is recommended to patients who have duodenal compression at the time of the initial ERCP.[164] Duodenal obstruction has been reported in 15% to 25% of patients with ampullary carcinoma treated with an endoprosthesis.[159]

Results

Benign Biliary Strictures

Dilatation of postcholecystectomy benign biliary strictures is successful in about 90% of cases.[135,136] Endoprosthesis placement is required in most cases, although balloon dilatation alone may suffice in about 20%.[135] Symptoms are relieved in most patients, with follow-up of as long as 5 years being reported.[135] Some patients have developed cholangitis as a result of clogging of the endoprosthesis, so routine changing at 3- to 4-month intervals is recommended. A few patients may also develop intrahepatic stones above an endoprosthesis, which should be removed with a basket whenever possible.

Postoperative biliary cutaneous fistulas can be controlled in most cases after biliary drainage. Most fistulas stop draining within 1 week after sphincterotomy alone, nasobiliary suction drainage, or insertion of biliary stents.[138-140]

Patients with primary sclerosing cholangitis who have dominant major bile duct strictures have fewer hospitalizations for recurrent cholangitis after biliary drainage.[146] Serum bilirubin levels are reduced after drainage, although alkaline phosphatase levels may remain elevated owing to concomitant intrahepatic disease. Complication rates are higher in patients with primary sclerosing cholangitis, with clinical cholangitis seen in 4 of 11 patients who had an endoprosthesis placed.[146]

Malignant Biliary Strictures

The diagnostic yield of biopsy specimens of malignant biliary strictures is approximately 40%.[126] Newer brush biopsy specimens may yield a positive diagnosis of malignancy in as many as 70% of cases.[127] False-positive diagnoses of malignancy from benign biliary strictures are uncommon.

Many thousands of patients with malignant obstructive jaundice have been palliated with a transpapillary endoprosthesis. The overall success rate of introduction varies between 75% and 90%. In general, success is greatest with ampullary tumors (95%-97%), followed by pancreatic and distal common duct tumors (88%-92%), with middle common bile duct and bifurcation tumors being the most difficult (75%-85%).[45,119,159,164,165] Failure of endoprosthesis placement may result from duodenal compression by tumor, inability to perform a sphincterotomy, or failure to pass a guidewire through the stricture.

Almost all patients with ampullary, pancreatic, and distal common duct tumors have a decline in bilirubin level after the proper placement of an endoprosthesis. About 90% of patients with bifurcation tumors have a drop in the bilirubin value after technically successful stenting procedures. Hospital mortality rate for patients with ampullary cancer after stenting is less than 2%, but patients with distal strictures have a hospital mortality rate of 7% to 12%.[159,164,165] The 30-day mortality rate for patients with middle common duct and bifurcation tumors ranges between 20% and 30%.[45,166]

Endoscopic placement of an endoprosthesis is the only palliative procedure needed for most patients. Median survival in this group is about 13 months for patients with ampullary cancer, 5 months for those with distal common duct strictures, and 3 to 5 months for those with middle common duct and bifurcation strictures.[45,159,164-166]

The necessity of placing an endoprosthesis into both sides of the liver in obstructing hilar tumors is controversial. In a group of 300 patients with a bifurcation tumor it was possible to insert two endoprostheses in only 25% of patients.[119] No difference in the incidence of early cholangitis or bilirubin normalization was found between patients with one endoprosthesis and patients with two endoprostheses. The only difference between the two groups was the substantially longer survival in those with two endoprostheses. This may be related to the easier insertion of two endoprostheses in patients with smaller type I lesions. Others have also reported a low risk of cholangitis with placement of only one endoprosthesis in patients with type II or type III strictures.[182]

A reduced complication rate and longer patient survival were reported by a group from Belgium after endoprostheses were inserted into both sides of the liver of patients with type II and type III hilar strictures.[45] A combined percutaneous and endoscopic procedure was required in 25% of cases in this series.[45] There were fewer cases of early cholangitis, fewer septic deaths, and a lower 30-day mortality rate for the group that received two stents. Most of the patients who received only one stent were seen in the years before the investigators began a policy of placing two stents; this raises questions regarding the role of other procedural factors in the difference between the two groups. Prospective randomized studies are required to resolve the question of whether one or two stents is best.

Pancreatic Drainage

Stent placement has been successful in achieving pancreatic drainage in more than 90% of attempts by experienced endoscopists (Fig. 117-16). However, the number of patients reported is small. A reduction in episodes of pain and acute pancreatitis was reported in 17 of 19 patients with pancreas divisum after stent placement through the minor papilla.[130] Others have reported a reduction of chronic pain and resolution of pancreatic pseudocysts in selected patients with chronic pancreatitis and dominant strictures or pancreatic stones.[129,131] Approximately half of patients with idiopathic recurrent pancreatitis and elevated pancreatic sphincter pressures may also benefit from pancreatic sphincterotomy and stent placement, although there may be an increased risk of complications, including acute pancreatitis and perforation.[129,131] Endoscopic pancreatic drainage is considered by most to still be investigational.

Clinical Implications

Benign Biliary Strictures

Patients with symptomatic benign bile duct strictures should undergo drainage procedures to relieve symptoms of pain, pruritus, and jaundice and to avoid complications such as cholangitis. The choice of drainage procedures includes biliary enteric bypass surgery, percutaneous transhepatic balloon dilatation or stenting, and endoscopic stenting.[41,183–186] There

are no controlled comparative studies of these three options; the decision of which therapeutic option to exercise in a given patient depends on several factors, including the reported success rates of individual procedures, patient age and operative risk, location of the stricture, and availability of local expertise for a specific procedure.

Surgical bypass of benign biliary strictures offers the advantage of a definitive single procedure for most patients and allows direct inspection with biopsy of suspicious areas to exclude malignancy. Unfortunately, morbidity and mortality rates are high, and approximately one fourth of patients may require another operation, usually for restricturing at the biliary enteric anastomosis.[41,183] Endoscopic stenting is not possible to treat a stricture at a choledochojejunostomy, forcing a percutaneous transhepatic dilatation or repeat surgery. For these reasons, a nonsurgical approach may be the best initial procedure, with surgery reserved for the patients who cannot be adequately drained or who have recurrences after transhepatic or endoscopic drainage. Biliary bypass surgery is best avoided in patients with primary sclerosing cholangitis; if endoscopic and percutaneous drainage procedures fail, these patients should be considered for hepatic transplantation.

The choice of endoscopic drainage or transhepatic drainage as the initial procedure usually depends on the location of the stricture. Balloon dilatation is usually not adequate for good long-term drainage, whether applied endoscopically (as discussed in this chapter) or percutaneously.[186] For most patients, an indwelling endoscopically placed biliary stent is preferable to caring for the external end of a transhepatically placed stent. Percutaneously placed internal stents are not desirable for the treatment of benign strictures because they are not easily changed after they obstruct. If possible, endoscopic stent placement should be attempted first. This approach is usually successful for strictures that are below the bifurcation. Transhepatic stenting or a combined endoscopic-

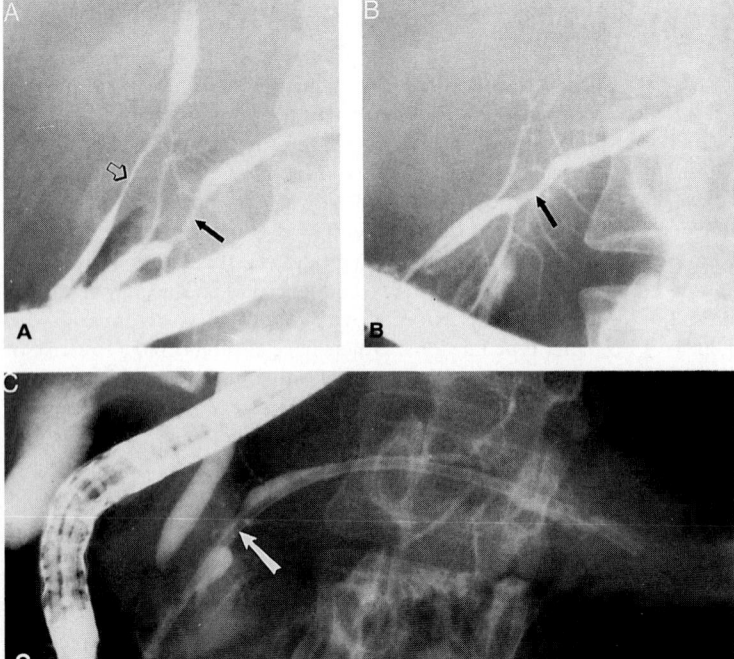

FIGURE 117-16. (**A**, **B**) Strictures of the common bile duct (*open arrow*) and pancreatic duct (*solid arrow*) are seen in a patient with chronic alcoholic pancreatitis. (**C**) A 7-Fr (2.3-mm) endoprosthesis (*arrow*) has been placed across the pancreatic duct stricture.

transhepatic approach may be required for more proximal strictures.

Malignant Biliary Strictures

Many of the principles discussed in selection of a drainage procedure for patients with benign biliary strictures also apply to patients with malignant strictures. However, more data comparing the different drainage procedures are available for malignant strictures because of their greater frequency. Randomized studies are available to help guide the choice between endoscopic or transhepatic drainage and the choice between endoscopic drainage or surgical bypass.

Patient selection for these trials affects their interpretation and should be discussed first. Patient characteristics often dictate the selection of a drainage procedure more than the success and complication rates of the procedure. Although the 5-year survival rate after pancreaticoduodenectomy for pancreatic adenocarcinoma is only 20%, young patients with evidence on imaging tests of limited disease should be offered surgery for a chance of cure.[187,188] Whether preoperative biliary drainage reduces operative morbidity and mortality rates for these patients is controversial, because retrospective and controlled trials have produced conflicting results.[150-158] Our practice is to institute drainage procedures preoperatively in patients who have clinical evidence of cholangitis or azotemia or if there is an anticipated delay of surgery for longer than 48 hours. Drainage in cases in which surgery is delayed also may avoid the development of cholangitis as a result of the retrograde cholangiogram.

Patients who have evidence of gastroduodenal obstruction on contrast studies or at the time of ERCP should also have surgery; biliary enteric bypass and gastroenterostomy can be performed at the same laparotomy, avoiding the necessity of later stent replacements for clogging. Patients who live in remote areas may also be better treated by surgical bypass to avoid the need for repeated procedures for stent exchange. Finally, patients who are moribund at the time of presentation should be allowed to die without intervention with any type of drainage procedure.

Alternatives to surgical bypass for patients with unresectable tumors have been sought in an effort to reduce operative morbidity and mortality rates and to reduce hospitalization time. The average 30-day mortality rate for biliary enteric bypass in patients with pancreatic carcinoma is approximately 20%.[188] The mortality rate is higher among patients older than 60 years of age and in those with metastases.[189]

The choice of drainage procedure in elderly patients and those with metastatic cancer is usually between endoscopic and transhepatic endoprosthesis placement because of the high surgical mortality rate. A carefully executed, randomized controlled trial has been reported of endoscopic and percutaneous stent insertion in elderly patients with malignant biliary obstruction who were not surgical candidates.[190] In this study, jaundice was relieved and a lower 30-day mortality rate was achieved in the group that was stented endoscopically. Patients stented percutaneously had a higher complication rate, primarily because of intraperitoneal bile leakage and hepatic bleeding. This study suggests that endoscopic stent insertion should be attempted first in patients with malignant

biliary obstruction who are not considered to be candidates for palliative surgery.

For the larger group of patients with unresectable cancers who require palliation but who are not high operative risks, the choice between endoscopic biliary stenting and a biliary enteric bypass operation is less clear. Two randomized trials have shown no difference in overall patient survival between endoscopically and surgically palliated groups.[191,192] A reduction in hospitalization time and in the 30-day mortality rate for patients treated with endoscopic stenting has to be weighed against the greater risk of recurrent jaundice and cholangitis from late stent occlusion and of duodenal obstruction in patients treated endoscopically.

There are currently several treatment options for the patient with malignant obstructive jaundice. The results of controlled trials provide guidance; however, caution must be exercised in generalizing to individual patients and to local therapeutic expertise. The choice of drainage procedure in individual cases should be made after discussion of the relative benefits and risks of the various procedures. Early results and late complications should be taken into consideration.

The reader is directed to Chapter 41, Approach to the Patient With Jaundice; Chapter 42, Approach to the Patient With Abnormal Liver Chemistries; Chapter 96, Gallstones; Chapter 97, Diseases of the Biliary Tree; and Chapter 98, Tumors of the Biliary Tree.

REFERENCES

1. McCune WS, Shorb PE, Moscowitz H. Endoscopic cannulation of the ampulla of Vater: a preliminary report. Ann Surg 1968;167:752.
2. Ohto M, Ono T, Tsuchiya Y, et al. Cholangiography and pancreatography. Tokyo: Igaku-Shoin, 1978.
3. Jacobson IM. ERCP—diagnostic and therapeutic applications. New York: Elsivier, 1989.
4. Classen M, Demling L. Steinextraktion aus dem Gallengang endoskopisch moglich. Med Trib 1973;27:1.
5. Kawai K, Akasaka Y, Murgkami K, et al. Endoscopic sphincterotomy of the papilla of Vater. Gastrointest Endosc 1974;20:148.
6. Cotton PB, Burney PGJ, Mason RR. Transnasal bile duct catheterisation after endoscopic sphincterotomy. Gut 1979;20:285.
7. Wurbs D, Philip J, Classen M. Experience with the long standing nasobiliary tube in biliary diseases. Endoscopy 1980;12:219.
8. Soehendra N, Reijnders-Frederix V. Palliative Gallengandrainage. Dtsch Med Wochenschr 1979;104:206.
9. Soehendra N, Reijnders-Frederix V. Palliative bile duct drainage: a new endoscopic method of introducing a transpapillary drain. Endoscopy 1980;12:8.
10. Huibregtse K, Haverkamp HJ, Tytgat GNJ. Transpapillary positioning of a large 3.2 mm biliary endoprosthesis. Endoscopy 1981;13:217.
11. Huibregtse K, Tytgat GNJ. Palliative treatment of obstructive jaundice by transpapillary introduction of large bore bile duct endoprosthesis. Gut 1982;23:371.
12. Cotton P. Duodenoscopic placement of biliary prosthesis to relieve malignant obstructive jaundice. Br J Surg 1982;69:501.
13. Kozarek RA, Sanowski RA. Nonsurgical management of extrahepatic obstructive jaundice. Ann Intern Med 1982;96:743.
14. Safrany L. Endoscopic treatment of biliary tract diseases: an international study. Lancet 1978;2:783.
15. Osnes M, Myren J. Endoscopic retrograde cholangiopancreatography (ERCP) in patients with Billroth II partial gastrectomy. Endoscopy 1975;7:227.

16. Katon RM, Bilbao MK, Parent JA, et al. ERCP in patients with gastrectomy and gastrojejunostomy (Billroth II). Gastrointest Endosc 1975;21:164.

17. Palmer FJ. The RACR survey of intravenous contrast media reactions: final report. Australas Radiol 1988;32:426.

18. Lindner HH, Pena VA, Ruggeri RA. A clinical and anatomical study of anomalous terminations of the common bile duct into the duodenum. Ann Surg 1976;184:626.

19. Gregg JA, Carr-Locke DL. Endoscopic pancreatic and biliary manometry in pancreatic, biliary and papillary disease and after sphincteroplasty. Gut 1984;25:1247.

20. Tanaka M, Ikeda S. Sphincter of Oddi manometry: comparison of microtransducer and perfusion methods. Endoscopy 1988;20:184.

21. Steinberg WM. Sphincter of Oddi dysfunction: a clinical controversy. Gastroenterology 1988;95:1409.

22. Geenen JE, Hogan WJ, Dodds WJ, et al. The efficacy of endoscopic sphincterotomy after cholecystectomy in patients with sphincter of Oddi dysfunction. N Engl J Med 1989;320:82.

23. Roberts-Thomson IC, Toouli J. Is endoscopic sphincterotomy for disabling biliary-type pain after cholecystectomy effective? Gastrointest Endosc 1985;31:370.

24. Thatcher BS, Sivak MV, Tedesco FJ, et al. Endoscopic sphincterotomy for suspected dysfunction of the sphincter of Oddi. Gastrointest Endosc 1987;33:91.

25. Toouli J, Roberts-Thomson IC, Dent J, et al. Sphincter of Oddi motility disorders in patients with idiopathic recurrent pancreatitis. Br J Surg 1986;72:859.

26. Venu RP, Geenen JE, Hogan W, et al. Idiopathic recurrent pancreatitis: an approach to diagnosis and treatment. Dig Dis Sci 1989;34:56.

27. Bilbao MK, Dotter CT, Lee TG, Katon RM. Complications of endoscopic retrograde cholangiopancreatography (ERCP). Gastroenterology 1976;70:314.

28. Hannigan BF, Keeling PWN, Slavin B, et al. Hyperamylasemia after ERCP with ionic and non-ionic contrast media [letter]. Gastrointest Endosc 1985;31:109.

29. Okuno M, Himeno S, Kurakawa M, et al. Changes in serum levels of pancreatic isoamylase, lipase, trysin and elastase 1 hr after endoscopic retrograde pancreatography. Hepatogastroenterology 1985;32:87.

30. Gigot JF, Leese T, Dereme T, et al: Acute cholangitis: multivariate analysis of risk factors. Ann Surg 1989;209:435.

31. Allen JI, Allen MO, Olson MM, et al. *Pseudomonas* infection of the biliary system resulting from use of a contaminated endoscope. Gastroenterology 1987;92:759.

32. Chang-Chien CS. Do juxtapapillary diverticula of the duodenum interfere with cannulation at endoscopic retrograde cholangiopancreatography? Gastrointest Endosc 1987;33:298.

33. Kennedy RH. Are duodenal diverticula associated with choledocholithiasis? Gut 1988;29:1003.

34. Tanaka M, Ikeda S. Parapapillary choledochoduodenal fistula: an analysis of 83 consecutive patients diagnosed at ERCP. Gastrointest Endosc 1983;29:88.

35. Meier P, Ansel H, Silvis S, et al. Comparison of ultrasound and ERCP measurements of bile duct size. Gastroenterology 1984;87:615.

36. Niederau C, Sonnenberg A, Müller J. Comparison of the extrahepatic bile duct size measured by ultrasound and by different radiographic methods. Gastroenterology 1984;87:615.

37. O'Connor HJ, Bartlett RJ, Hamilton I, et al. Bile duct calibre: the discrepancy between ultrasonic and retrograde cholangiographic measurement in the post-cholecystectomy patient. Clin Radiol 1985;36:507.

38. Rohrmann CA, Ansel JH, Protell RC, et al. The significance of the non-opacified gallbladder in the differential diagnosis of the abnormal endoscopic retrograde cholangiogram. AJR Am J Roentgenol 1979;132:191.

39. Cruz FO, Barringa P, Tocornal J, et al. Radiology of the Mirizzi syndrome: diagnostic importance of the transhepatic cholangiogram. Gastrointest Radiol 1983;8:249.

40. Deziel DJ, Millikan KW, Econonov SG, et al. Complications of laparoscopic cholecystectomy: a national survey of 4292 hospitals and an analysis of 77,604 cases. Am J Surg 1993; 165:9.

41. Pitt HA, Miyamato T, Parapatis SK, et al. Factors influencing outcome in patients with postoperative biliary strictures. Am J Surg 1982;144:14.

42. Vallon AG, Mason RR, Laurence BH, et al. Endoscopic retrograde cholangiography in postoperative bile duct strictures. Br J Radiol 1982;55:32.

43. Wilson C, Auld CD, Schliakert R, et al. Hepatobiliary complications in chronic pancreatitis. Gut 1989;30:520.

44. Aranha G, Prinz R, Freeark R, et al. The spectrum of biliary obstruction from chronic pancreatitis. Arch Surg 1984;119: 595.

45. Deviere J, Baize M, de Toeuf J, et al. Long-term follow up of patients with hilar malignant stricture treated by endoscopic internal biliary drainage. Gastrointest Endosc 1988;34:95.

46. Mir-Madjlessi SH, Farmer RG, Sivak MV. Bile duct carcinoma in patients with ulcerative colitis, relationship to sclerosing cholangitis: report of six cases and review of the literature. Dig Dis Sci 1987;32:145.

47. Freeny PC, Ball TJ. Endoscopic retrograde cholangiopancreatography (ERCP) and percutaneous transhepatic cholangiography (PTC) in the evaluation of suspected pancreatic carcinoma: diagnostic limitations and contemporary roles. Cancer 1981;47:1666.

48. Freeny PC, Bilbao MK, Katon RM, et al. Blind evaluation of endoscopic retrograde cholangiopancreatography (ERCP) in diagnosis of pancreatic carcinoma: the "double duct" and other signs. Radiology 1976;119:271.

49. Plumley TF, Rohrmann CA, Freeny PC, et al. Double duct sign reassessed: significance in ERCP. AJR Am J Roentgenol 1982;183:31.

50. Blackstone MO, Nemchausky BA. Cholangiographic abnormalities in ulcerative colitis associated pericholangitis which resemble sclerosing cholangitis. Am J Dig Dis 1978;23:579.

51. Chapman RWG, Arborgh BAM, Rhodes JM, et al. Primary sclerosing cholangitis: a review of its clinical features, cholangiography, and hepatic histology. Gut 1980;21:870.

52. MacCarty RL, LaRusso NF, Wiesner RH, et al. Primary sclerosing cholangitis: findings on cholangiography and pancreatography. Radiology 1983;149:39.

53. Martenson JA, Gunderson LL, Buskirk SJ, et al. Hepatic duct stricture after radical radiation therapy for biliary cancer: recurrence or fibrosis? Mayo Clin Proc 1986;81:530.

54. Pien EH, Zeman RK, Benjamin SB, et al. Iatrogenic sclerosing cholangitis following hepatic arterial chemotherapy infusion. Radiology 1985;156:329.

55. Shea WJ, Demas BE, Goldberg HI, et al. Sclerosing cholangitis associated with hepatic arterial FUDR chemotherapy: radiographic-histologic correlation. AJR Am J Roentgenol 1986;146: 717.

56. Haq MM, Valdes LG, Peterson DF, et al. Fibrosis of extra hepatic biliary system after continuous hepatic artery infusion of floxuridine through an implantable pump (infusaid pump). Cancer 1986;57:1281.

57. Schneiderman DJ, Cello JP, Laing FC. Papillary stenosis and sclerosing cholangitis in the acquired immunodeficiency syndrome. Ann Intern Med 1987;106:546.

58. Roulot D, Valla D, Brun-Vezinet F, et al. Cholangitis in the acquired immunodeficiency syndrome, report of two cases and review of the literature. Gut 1987;28:1653.

59. Dowsett JF, Miller R, Davidson R, et al. Sclerosing cholangitis in acquired immunodeficiency syndrome. Scand J Gastroenterol 1988;23:1267.

60. Jones B, Wall SD. Gastrointestinal disease in the immunocompromised host. Radiol Clin Nth Am 1992;30(3):555.

61. Wiedmeyer DA, Stewart ET, Dodds WJ, et al. Choledochal cyst: findings on cholangiopancreatography with emphasis on ectasia of the common channel. AJR Am J Roentgenol 1989;153:969.

62. Nelson AM. Demonstration of a traumatic biliary fistula by ERCP. Gastrointest Endosc 1984;30:315.

63. Dyrszka H, Sanghavi B. Hepatic hydatid disease: findings on

endoscopic retrograde cholangiography. Gastrointest Endosc 1983;29:248.

64. Classen M, Hellwig H, Rösch W. Anatomy of the pancreatic duct: a duodenoscopic-radiological study. Endoscopy 1973;5: 14.

65. Delhaye M, Engelholm L, Cremer M. Pancreas divisum: congenital anatomic variant or anomaly. Gastroenterology 1985;89:951.

66. Cotton PB. Congenital anomaly of pancreas divisum as a cause of obstructive pain and pancreatitis. Gut 1980;21:105.

67. Dowsett JF, Rode J, Russell RCG. Annular pancreas: a clinical, endoscopic, and immunohistochemical study. Gut 1989;30: 130.

68. Axon ATR, Classen M, Cotton PB, et al. Pancreatography in chronic pancreatitis: international definitions. International Workshop, Kings College, Cambridge, March 23–25, 1983. Gut 1984;25:1107.

69. Kugelberg C, Wehlin L, Arnesjo B, et al. Endoscopic pancreatography in evaluating results of pancreaticojejunostomy. Gut 1976;17:267.

70. Gilinsky NH, Bornman PC, Girdwood AH, et al. Diagnostic yield of endoscopic retrograde cholangiopancreatography in carcinoma of the pancreas. Br J Surg 1986;73:539.

71. Harbin WP, Mueller PR, Ferrucci JT. Transhepatic cholangiography: complications and use patterns of the fine-needle technique. Radiology 1980;135:15.

72. Ferrucci J. Mueller P. Interventional radiology of the biliary tract. Gastroenterology 1982;82:974.

73. Deviere J, Motte S, Dumonceau JM, Serruys E, Thys JP, Cremer M. Septicemia after endoscopic retrograde cholangiopancreatography. Endoscopy 1990;2:72.

74. Demling L. Endoscopic papillotomy (EPT): indications and technique. Endoscopy 1983;15:162.

75. Siegel JH. Precut papillotomy: a method to improve success of ERCP and papillotomy. Endoscopy 1981;12:130.

76. Huibregtse K, Katon RM, Tytgat GNJ. Precut papillotomy via fine-needle knife papillotome: a safe and effective technique. Gastrointest Endosc 1986;32:403.

77. Shakoor T, Hogan WJ, Geenen JE. Needle knife papillotomy— efficacy and risks. Gastrointest Endosc 1992;38:251.

78. Kozarek RA, Sanowski RA. Endoscopic choledochoduodenostomy. Gastrointest Endosc 1983;29:119.

79. Forbes A, Cotton PB. ERCP and sphincterotomy after Billroth II gastrectomy. Gut 1984;25:971.

80. Osnes M, Rosseland AR, Aabakken L. Endoscopic retrograde cholangiography and endoscopic papillotomy in patients with a previous Billroth II resection. Gut 1986;27:1193.

81. Cairns SR, Dias L, Cotton PB, et al. Additional endoscopic procedures instead of urgent surgery for retained common bile duct stones. Gut 1989;30:535.

82. Riemann JF, Seuberth K, Demling L. Clinical application of a new mechanical lithotripter for smashing common bile duct stones. Endoscopy 1982;14:226.

83. Riemann JF, Demling L. Lithotripsy of bile duct stones. Endoscopy 1983;15:191.

84. Koch H, Rösch W, Walz V. Endoscopic lithotripsy in the common bile duct. Gastrointest Endosc 1980;26:16.

85. Nishioka NS, Levins PC, Murray SC, et al. Fragmentation of biliary calculi with tunable dye lasers. Gastroenterology 1987;93:250.

86. Ell C, Lux G, Hochberger J, et al. Laser lithotripsy of common bile duct stones. Gut 1988;29:746.

87. Kozarek RA. Direct cholangioscopy and pancreatoscopy at time of endoscopic retrograde cholangiopancreatography. Am J Gastroenterol 1988;83:55.

88. Sauerbruch T, Stern M, and the Study Group for Shock-Wave Lithotripsy of Bile Duct Stones. Fragmentation of bile duct stones by extracorporeal shock waves. Gastroenterology 1989;96:146.

89. Palmer KR, Hofmann AF. Intraductal mono-octanoin for the direct dissolution of bile duct stones: experience in 343 patients. Gut 1986;196.

90. Murray WR, Laferla G, Fullarton GM. Choledocholithiasis: in vivo stone dissolution using methyl tertiary butyl ether (MTBE). Gut 1988;29:143.

91. Cotton PB, Lehman G, Vennes J, et al. Endoscopic sphincterotomy complications and their management: an attempt at consensus. Gastrointest Endosc 1991;37:383.

92. Larson RE, Hodgson JR, Priestley JT: The early and long-term results of 500 consecutive explorations of the common duct. Surg Gynecol Obstet 1966;122:744.

93. Davidson BR, Neoptolemos JP, Carr-Locke DL: Endoscopic sphincterotomy for common bile duct calculi in patients with gallbladders in situ considered unfit for surgery. Gut 1988;29: 114.

94. Escourrou J, Cordon JA, Lazarthes F, et al. Early and late complications after endoscopic sphincterotomy for biliary lithiasis with and without gallbladder "in situ." Gut 1984;25:598.

95. Neoptolemos JP, Carr-Locke DL, Fraser I, et al. The management of common bile duct calculi by endoscopic sphincterotomy in patients with gallbladder in situ. Br J Surg 1984;71:68.

96. Hawes R, Vallon AG, Holton JM, et al. Long-term follow-up after duodenoscopic sphincterotomy in patients with prior cholecystectomy. Gastrointest Endosc 1987;33:157.

97. Tanaka M, Ikeda S, Yoshimoto H, et al. The long-term fate of the gallbladder after endoscopic sphincterotomy. Am J Surg 1987;154:505.

98. Hansell DT, Millar MA, Murray WR, et al. Endoscopic sphincterotomy for bile duct stones in patients with intact gallbladder. Br J Surg 1989;76:856.

99. Worthley CS, Toouli J: Gallbladder non-filling contraindicates leaving the gallbladder in-situ after endoscopic sphincterotomy. Gastrointest Endosc 1987;33:160.

100. Neoptolemos JP, Carr-Locke DL, London NJ, et al. Controlled trial of urgent endoscopic retrograde cholangiopancreatography and endoscopic sphincterotomy versus conservative treatment for acute pancreatitis due to gallstones. Lancet 1988;2:979.

101. Neoptolemos JP, London N, Slater ND, et al. A prospective study of ERCP and endoscopic sphincterotomy in the diagnosis and treatment of gallstone acute pancreatitis. Arch Surg 1986;121:697.

102. Fan ST, Lai ECS, Mok FTP et al. Early treatment of acute biliary pancreatitis by endoscopic papillotomy. N Engl J Med 1993;4:228.

103. Neoptolemos JP, Bailey I, Shaw D, et al. The role of clinical and biochemical criteria and endoscopic retrograde cholangiopancreatography in the urgent diagnosis of common bile duct stones in acute pancreatitis. Surgery 1986;100:732.

104. Popiela T, Karcz D, Marecik J. Endoscopic sphincterotomy as a therapeutic measure in cholangitis and as prophylaxis against recurrent biliary tract stones. Endoscopy 1987;19:14.

105. Gogel HK, Runyon BA, Volpicelli NA, et al. Acute suppurative obstructive cholangitis due to stones: treatment by urgent endoscopic sphincterotomy. Gastrointest Endosc 1987;33:210.

106. Leung JWC, Chung SCS, Sung JJY, et al. Urgent endoscopic drainage for acute suppurative cholangitis. Lancet 1989;1:1307.

107. Lai ECS, Mok FPT, Tan ESY, et al. Endoscopic biliary drainage for severe acute cholangitis. N Engl J Med 1992;326:1582.

108. Marbet UA, Stalder GA, Faust H, et al. Endoscopic sphincterotomy and surgical approaches in the treatment of the "sump syndrome." Gut 1987;28:142.

109. Leese T, Neoptolemos JP, Carr-Locke DL. Successes, failures, early complications and their management following endoscopic sphincterotomy: results in 394 consecutive patients from a single center. Br J Surg 72;215:1985.

110. Seifert E. Long-term follow-up after endoscopic sphincterotomy (EST). Endoscopy 1988:20;232.

111. Cotton PB, Vallon AG: Duodenoscopic sphincterotomy for removal of bile duct stones in patients with gallbladders. Surgery 1982;91:628.

112. Cotton PB. Endoscopic management of bile duct stones: apples and oranges. Gut 1984;25:587.

113. Hutton SW, Sievert CE, Vennes JA, et al. Spontaneous passage of glass beads from the canine gallbladder: facilitation by sphincterotomy. Gastroenterology 1988;94:1031.

114. Summerfield JA: Biliary obstruction is best managed by endoscopists. Gut 1988;29:741.

115. Bouchier IAD. Non-surgical treatment of gallstones: many contenders but who will win the crown? Gut 1988;29:137.

116. Neoptolemos JP, Shaw DE, Carr-Locke DL. A multivariate analysis of preoperative risk factors in patients with common duct stones. Ann Surg 1989;209:157.

117. Kelly TR, Wagner DS. Gallstone pancreatitis: a prospective randomized trial of the timing of surgery. Surgery 1988;104:600.

118. Neoptolemos JP, Carr-Locke DL, Fossard DP. Prospective randomized study of preoperative endoscopic sphincterotomy versus surgery alone for common bile duct stones. Br Med J 1987;294:470.

119. Huibregtse K. Endoscopic biliary and pancreatic drainage. Stuttgart: Georg Thieme Verlag, 1988.

120. Gerecht WB, Henry NK, Hoffman WW, et al. Prospective randomised comparison of mezlocillin therapy alone with combined ampicillin and gentamicin therapy for patients with cholangitis. Arch Intern Med 1989;149:1279.

121. Davids PHP, Groen AK, Rauws EAJ, et al. Randomised trial of self-expanding metal stents versus polyethylene stents for distal malignant biliary obstruction. Lancet 1992;340:1488.

122. Grimm H, Meyer WH, Nam VC, et al. New modalities for treating chronic pancreatitis. Endoscopy 1989;21:70.

123. Seifert E, Urakami Y, Elster K. Duodenoscopic guided biopsy of the biliary and pancreatic duct. Endoscopy 1980;9:154.

124. Danzygier H, Phillip J, Hagenmüller F, et al. Forceps biopsy of human bile ducts: light and electron microscopical findings, clinical significance. Gastroenterology 1983;84:1132.

125. Bourgeois N, Dunham F, Verhest A, et al. Endoscopic biopsies of the papilla of Vater at the time of endoscopic sphincterotomy: difficulties in interpretation. Gastrointest Endosc 1984;30:163.

126. Aabakken L, Karesen R, Serck-Hanssen A, et al. Transpapilliary biopsies and brush cytology from the common bile duct. Endoscopy 1986;18:49.

127. Venu RP, Prabhu M, Geenen JE, et al. Improved sensitivity in the cytologic diagnosis of cholangiocarcinoma. Gastrointest Endosc 1989;35:181.

128. Robertson DAF, Hacking LN, Birch S, et al. Experience with a combined percutaneous and endoscopic approach to stent insertion in malignant obstructive jaundice. Lancet 1987;2:1449.

129. Huibregtse K, Schneider B, Vrij AA, et al. Endoscopic pancreatic drainage in chronic pancreatitis. Gastrointest Endosc 1988;34:9.

130. McCarthy J, Geenen JE, Hogan WJ. Preliminary experience with endoscopic stent placement in benign pancreatic diseases. Gastrointest Endosc 1988;34:16.

131. Kozarek RA, Patterson DJ, Ball TJ, et al. Endoscopic placement of pancreatic stents and drains in the management of pancreatitis. Ann Surg 1989;209:261.

132. Cremer M, Sugai B, Delhaye M, et al. Expandable pancreatic metal stent (Wallstent) for chronic pancreatitis: first world series (abstract). Gastroenterology 1990;98:A215.

133. Fuji T, Amano H, Ohmura R, et al. Endoscopic pancreatic sphincterotomy: technique and evaluation. Endoscopy 1989;21:27.

134. Siegel JH, Guelrud M. Endoscopic cholangiopancreatoplasty: hydrostatic balloon dilation in the bile duct and pancreas. Gastrointest Endosc 1983;29:99.

135. Geenen DJ, Geenen JE, Hogan WJ, et al. Endoscopic therapy for benign bile duct strictures. Gastrointest Endosc 1989;35:367.

136. Davids PHP, Rauws EAJ, Coene PPLO, et al. Endoscopic stenting for post-operative biliary strictures. Gastrointest Endosc 1992;38:12.

137. O'Rahilly S, Duignan JP, Lennon JR, et al. Successful treatment of a postoperative external biliary fistula by endoscopic papillotomy. Endoscopy 1983;15:68.

138. Del Olmo L, Merono E, Moreira VF, et al. Successful treatment of postoperative external biliary fistulas by endoscopic sphincterotomy. Gastrointest Endosc 1988;34:307.

139. Sauerbruch T, Weinzierl M, Holl J, Pratschke E. Treatment of postoperative bile fistulas by internal endoscopic biliary drainage. Gastroenterology 1986;90:1998.

140. Davids PHP, Rauws EAJ, Coene PPLO, et al. Postoperative bile leakage: the endoscopic management. Gut 1992;33;1118.

141. Foutch PG, Harlan JRE, Hoefer M. Endoscopic therapy for patients with a postoperative biliary leak. Gastrointest Endosc 1993;39:416.

142. Grijm R, Huibregtse K, Bartelsman J, et al. Therapeutic investigations in primary sclerosing cholangitis. Dig Dis Sci 1986;31:792.

143. Allison MC, Burroughs AK, Noone P, et al. Biliary lavage with corticosteroids in primary sclerosing cholangitis: a clinical, cholangiographic and bacteriological study. J Hepatol 1986;3:118.

144. Hamilton I, Soutar JS, Bouchier IA, et al. Short-term biliary dilatation and stenting in primary sclerosing cholangitis. J Clin Gastroenterol 1987;9:70.

145. Cotton PB, Nickl N. Endoscopic and radiologic approaches to therapy in primary sclerosing cholangitis. Seminars in liver disease 1991;11;40.

146. Johnson GK, Geenen JE, Venu RP, et al. Endoscopic treatment of symptomatic primary sclerosing cholangitis: is this the next therapeutic choice? Gastrointest Endosc 1989;35:165.

147. Petrozza J, Dutta S, Latham P, et al. Prevalence and natural history of distal common bile duct stenosis in alcoholic pancreatitis. Dig Dis Sci 1984;29:890.

148. Stahl TJ, O'Connor Allen M, et al. Partial biliary obstruction caused by chronic pancreatitis. Ann Surg 1988;207:26.

149. Gouma DJ, Coelho JC, Schlegel JF, et al. The effect of preoperative internal and external biliary drainage on mortality of jaundiced rats. Arch Surg 1987;122:731.

150. Nakayama T, Ikeda A, Okuda K. Percutaneous transhepatic drainage of the biliary tract. Gastroenterology 1978;74:554.

151. Denning DA, Ellison EC, Carey LC. Pre-operative percutaneous transhepatic biliary decompression lowers operative mortality in patients with obstructive jaundice. Am J Surg 1981;141:61.

152. Gobien RP, Stanley JH, Soucek CD, et al. Routine preoperative biliary drainage: effect on management of obstructive jaundice. Radiology 1984;152:352.

153. Gundry SR, Strodel WE, Knol JA, et al. Efficacy of preoperative biliary tract decompression in patients with obstructive jaundice. Arch Surg 1984;119:703.

154. Norlander A, Kalin B, Sundblad R. Effect of percutaneous transhepatic drainage upon liver function and postoperative mortality. Surg Gynecol Obstet 1982;155:161.

155. Takada T, Hanyu F, Kibayashi S, et al. Percutaneous transhepatic cholangial drainage: direct approach under fluoroscopic control. J Surg Oncol 1976;8:83.

156. Hatfield ARW, Tobas R, Terblanche J, et al. Pre-operative external biliary drainage in obstructive jaundice: a prospective controlled clinical trial. Lancet 1982;2:896.

157. McPherson GAD, Benjamin IS, Hodgson HJF, et al. Pre-operative percutaneous transhepatic biliary drainage: the results of a controlled trial. Br J Surg 1984;71:371.

158. Pitt HA, Gomes AS, Lois JF, et al. Does pre-operative percutaneous biliary drainage reduce operative risk or increase hospital cost? Ann Surg 1985;201:545.

159. Huibregtse K, Schneider B, Rauws E, et al. Carcinoma of the ampulla of Vater: role of endoscopic drainage. Surg Endosc 1987;1:79.

160. Gmelin E, Weiss HD. Tumours in the region of the papilla of Vater: diagnosis via endoscopy, biopsy, brush cytology, ERCP and CT scan. Eur J Radiol 1981;1:301.

161. Seyrig JAC, Liquory B, Meduri O, et al. Endoscopie dans les tumeurs de la région oddienne: possibilités diagnostiques et thérapeutiques. Gastroenterol Clin Biol 1985;9:103.

162. Warren KW, Choe DS, Plaza J, et al. Results of radical resection for periampullary carcinoma. Ann Surg 1975;181:534.

163. Makipur H, Cooperman A, Donzi JT, et al. Carcinoma of the ampulla: review of 38 cases with emphasis on treatment and prognostic factors. Ann Surg 1976;183:341.

164. Huibregtse K, Katon RM, Coene PP, et al. Endoscopic palliative treatment in pancreatic cancer. Gastrointest Endosc 1986;32:334.

165. Siegel JH, Snady H. The significance of endoscopically placed prostheses in the management of biliary obstruction due to carcinoma of the pancreas: results of non-operative decompression in 227 patients. Am J Gastroenterol 1986;81:634.
166. Huibregtse K, Schneider B, Coene PP, et al. Endoscopic palliation of jaundice in gallbladder cancer. Surg Endosc 1987;1:143.
167. Blumgart LH, Benjamin IS, Hodges NS, et al. Surgical approaches to cholangiocarcinoma at confluence of hepatic ducts. Lancet 1984;1:66.
168. Popp JW, Schapiro RH, Warshaw AL. Extrahepatic biliary obstruction caused by metastatic breast carcinoma. Ann Intern Med 1979;91:568.
169. Warshaw AL, Welch JP. Extrahepatic biliary obstruction by metastatic colon carcinoma. Ann Surg 1978;188:593.
170. Thomas JH, Pierce GE, Karlin C, et al. Extrahepatic biliary obstruction secondary to metastatic cancer. Am J Surg 1981;142:770.
171. Klatskin G. Adenocarcinoma of the hepatic duct at the bifurcation within the porta hepatis. Am J Med 1964;38:241.
172. George PA, Brown C, Foley RTE. Carcinoma of the hepatic duct junction. Br J Surg 1981;68:14.
173. Deviere J, Baize M, Buset M, et al. Complications of internal endoscopic biliary drainage. Acta Endosc 1985;30:168.
174. Carr-Locke DL, Ball TJ, Connors PJ, et al: Multicenter, randomized trial of Wallstent biliary endoprosthesis versus plastic stents. Gastrointest Endosc 1993;39:310.
175. Groen AK, Out T, Huibregtse K, et al. Characterization of the content of occluded biliary endoprostheses. Endoscopy 1987;19:57.
176. Wosiewitz U, Schrameyer B, Safrany L. Biliary sludge: its role during bile duct drainage with an endoprosthesis. Gastroenterology 1985;88:1709.
177. Speer AG, Cotton PB, Rode J, et al. Biliary stent blockage with bacterial biofilm: a light and electron microscopy study. Ann Intern Med 1988;108:546.
178. Leung JWC, Ling TKW, Kung JLS, et al. The role of bacteria in the blockage of biliary stents. Gastrointest Endosc 1988;34:19.
179. Dowsett JF, Williams SJ, Hatfield ARW, et al. Does stent diameter matter in the endoscopic palliation of malignant biliary obstruction? A randomized trial of 10FG versus 12FG endoprostheses. Gastroenterology 1989;96:A128.
180. Conn M, Speer AG, Cotton PB. Factors affecting the duration of biliary stent patency in patients with pancreatic cancer. Gastrointest Endosc 1989;35:162.
181. Cohen ME, Goldberg RI, Barkin JS, et al. Bile duct perforation: a complication of large caliber endoprosthesis. Gastrointest Endosc 1989;35:456.
182. Polydorou AA, Cairns SR, Dowsett JF, et al. Palliation of proximal malignant biliary obstruction by endoscopic endoprosthesis insertion. Gut 1991;32:685.
183. Pellegrini C, Thomas MJ, Way LW. Recurrent biliary stricture. Am J Surg 1984;147:175.
184. Martin EC, Fankucken K, Laffey J, et al. Percutaneous management of benign biliary disease. Gastrointest Radiol 1984;9:207.
185. Salomonawitz E, Castaneda-Zuniga WR, Lund I, et al. Balloon dilatation of benign biliary strictures. Radiology 1984;151:613.
186. Vogel SB, Howard RJ, Caridi J, et al. Evaluation of percutaneous transhepatic balloon dilatation of benign strictures in high-risk patients. Am J Surg 1985;149:73.
187. Lerut JP, Gianello PR, Otte JB, et al. Pancreaticoduodenal resection: surgical experience and evaluation of risk factors in 103 patients. Ann Surg 1984;199:432.
188. Warshaw AL, Swanson RS. Pancreatic cancer in 1988: possibilities and probabilities. Ann Surg 1988;208:541.
189. Pitt HA, Cameron JL, Postier RG, et al. Factors affecting mortality in biliary tract surgery. Am J Surg 1981;141:66.
190. Speer AG, Russell RC, Hatfield ARW, et al. Randomised trial of endoscopic versus percutaneous stent insertion in malignant obstructive jaundice. Lancet 1987;2:57.
191. Shepherd HA, Royle G, Ross APR, et al. Endoscopic biliary endoprosthesis in the palliation of malignant obstruction of the distal common bile duct: a randomized trial. Br J Surg 1988;75:1166.
192. Dowsett JF, Russell RCG, Hatfield ARW, et al. Malignant obstructive jaundice: a prospective randomized trial of by-pass surgery versus endoscopic stenting. Gastroenterology 1989;96:A128.

Textbook of Gastroenterology, second edition, edited by Tadataka Yamada. JB Lippincott Company, Philadelphia © 1995.

CHAPTER 118

Procedure-Related Complications

Stanley Bernard Benjamin

Types of Complications
Medication-Related Complications
Procedure-Related Complications
Reducing Complications in Gastrointestinal Endoscopy

Universal Precautions
Role of Patient Monitoring
Postprocedure Evaluation and Recognition of Complications
Preventive Maintenance

Gastrointestinal endoscopy has evolved over the last 25 years from a pure diagnostic modality to one that provides therapeutic alternatives in a wide variety of situations. It has progressed from a subspecialty of internal medicine essentially limited to the cognitive aspects of patient care to a specialty demanding the same highly evolved cognitive skills plus those required to perform surgery through an endoscope.

The modern gastroenterologist must be an astute clinician and be able to perform a wide array of diagnostic and therapeutic endoscopic interventions. To provide this comprehensive care, the endoscopist-gastroenterologist must be aware of the situations for which the procedures are indicated and the appropriate methods for these interventions; understand the appropriate timing of therapy; and be cognizant of potential complications and able to respond to them.

In many situations, the new techniques have enabled therapy that was previously unavailable, and the endoscopic methods offer a safer, more easily performed option for patients. Despite these advantages, there are risks associated with these procedures. Because of the infrequency of complications, many physicians are unprepared for them. It is essential that the endoscopist understand the potential for complications, be aware of ways to prevent them, and know appropriate methods for treating them.

Complications associated with endoscopic procedures range from those specific to individual types of procedures to the generic complications of conscious sedation, administration of intravenous contrast, or infection transmission during endoscopy. The incidence of complications must be cataloged by individual procedure and listed as major or minor, documenting whether a complication is related to instrument injury, cardiopulmonary problems, bleeding, or infection. Although it is often difficult to make exact comparisons between the available information because of variations in the methods of data collection, results from a variety of such series are surprisingly similar (Table 118-1).[1-6]

This chapter reviews the potential problems and complications associated with endoscopic procedures. In the performance of a large number of these procedures, complications are almost certain to occur, but by recognizing them and responding appropriately, morbidity and mortality can be minimized.

TYPES OF COMPLICATIONS

Medication-Related Complications

In the current practice of gastrointestinal endoscopy, almost all procedures involve the use of some premedication. This is especially true for procedures that are classified as endoscopic surgery, such as endoscopic sphincterotomy, biliary stent placement, and colonoscopic polypectomy. It is this same group of procedures that are often performed in elderly patients who have a variety of comorbid conditions that have made them high risks for standard surgical approaches. Although it is generally believed that endoscopic procedures provide a lower-risk option for their therapy, measurable risks still exist with the associated medications.

This trend toward the routine use of premedications is a phenomenon of the flexible fiberoptic era of endoscopy. In the textbook by Rudolph Schindler, one of the pioneers of the modern endoscopic era, it was emphasized that routine premedication other than atropine and small doses of barbiturates given intramuscularly before the procedure was not used, because the patient should be conscious to minimize the risks associated with the passage of a semirigid gastroscope.[7] Today, the use of intravenous medications immediately before beginning the procedure is routine, although the exact types of medications used, alone or in combination, are highly individualized. The term applied to this process is *conscious sedation*, referring to the production of sedation and amnesia by the medications used for endoscopic procedures. Conscious sedation is best defined as the production of a relaxed state with minimal anxiety and discomfort. Implied in this term is that the patient is able to independently and continuously maintain respiratory and airway control, respond to tactile stimuli, and cooperate with verbal commands. This is not anesthesia, in which elimination of nociception is the goal.

There are no data that allow us to determine which method of preparing the patient for an endoscopic procedure is the best or safest, because there are tremendous variations in patients' responses to the drugs commonly used. The physician must be aware of the spectrum of untoward responses that may occur including, reactions to topical agents, respiratory

TABLE 118-1
Incidence of Procedure-Related Complications During Gastrointestinal Endoscopy

TYPE OF PROCEDURE	COMPLICATION (%)				
	Cardiac	Perforation	Bleeding	Infection	Mortality
EGD	0.06–0.20	0.01–0.1	0–0.03	0–0.008	0.006–0.012
ERCP*	0.1–0.6	0.03	0.05–1.0	0.87–2.0	0.1–1.4
Colon					
Diagnostic	0.04	0.14–0.26	0.008–0.7		0.008–0.03
Other	0.03	0.11–0.42	0.77–2.2		0–0.1

* Wide variation in incidence is related to a series that included sphincterotomy.

EGD, esophagogastric duodenoscopy; ERCP, endoscopic retrograde cholangiopancreatography.

depression, allergic reactions, paradoxical reactions, and local reactions.

Response to Topical Agents

Although considered by some as an afterthought, the application of medications to the oropharynx during upper endoscopic procedures should be considered as a part of premedication. Although infrequent, untoward effects of such agents are possible as a direct effect of the agent, and in some situations, their use may increase the risk of aspiration.

A variety of topical agents are available for use in routine upper endoscopy. Although the likelihood of complications is small, possible untoward effects have been reported. Spray preparations have been shown to be superior to gargles or lozenges. Gargles increase the systemic absorption if this material is aspirated while gargling. It is the absorption from mucosal surfaces that result in the potential systemic complications.[8,9] Medications such as tetracaine and Xylocaine have produced altered mental status, seizures, and cardiac dysrythmias. Serious side effects and even death have been attributed to the systematic absorption of tetracaine. The least soluble and therefore the least likely to have systemic effects is benzocaine.

The use of topical anesthetics may increase the risk of aspiration during upper endoscopic procedures. This risk is minimal during routine diagnostic endoscopy but is likely to be increased during emergency endoscopy, with active hemorrhage, or during the performance of percutaneous gastrostomy when the patient is in the supine position. Studies have demonstrated no real benefit to the patient from the use of topical anesthesia, and the use of these agents during percutaneous gastrostomy and upper gastrointestinal hemorrhage should be discouraged.[10]

Respiratory Depression

The most frequent complication during procedures using premedication is respiratory depression. Medications used in gastrointestinal endoscopy are intravenous sedatives (typically benzodiazepines), often in combination with narcotic analgesics, both of which routinely produce some degree of respiratory depression as a consequence of their pharmacologic activity. However, because in the general practice of endoscopy a wide variety of medications are used in various combinations, the degree and significance of respiratory depression and hypoxemia seen during endoscopic examinations are extremely variable.

During upper gastrointestinal endoscopy, topical anesthetics are often administered, and the endoscope is placed in the mouth and hypopharynx. The relative contributions of each of these factors to the hypoxemia that is routinely seen with upper gastrointestinal endoscopy have been evaluated. Topical hypopharyngeal anesthesia alone does not appear to lower oxygen concentration, but the presence of the endoscope in the hypopharynx seems to contribute to a fall in arterial oxygen saturation. Because comparable degrees of hypoxemia are routinely seen during colonoscopy, it is logical to assume that the premedications make the largest contribution to hypoxia in patients undergoing endoscopic procedures.[11-14]

There is considerable debate among gastroenterologists about the safety of the medications used individually or in combination to provide the conscious sedation for endoscopy. The benzodiazepines have almost replaced barbiturates as the premedication for endoscopy. The combination of diazepam or midazolam with a narcotic analgesic (e.g., meperidine) given intravenously has evolved as a favorite premedication regimen.

The introduction of midazolam, a water-soluble benzodiazepine, was viewed as a significant advance or a dangerous addition to endoscopic medications. Having the advantage of rapid onset and brief duration of action with a more significant degree of amnesia, this drug had been viewed by some as overly dangerous in the endoscopic setting because of its ability to cause significant respiratory depression. The reasons for the problems related to midazolam seem to be multiple: increased sensitivity of the elderly to the respiratory depressive effects; original packaging recommendations similar to diazepam despite increased potency, which may have resulted in its administration at excessive doses; and lack of available data on drug effects in combination with narcotic analgesics.[15]

Much of the controversy regarding endoscopic medications resulted from the lack of controlled studies. Studies have shown little difference except an increased incidence of amnesia with midazolam, when used appropriately.[16,17] However, the use of medications that depress respiration carry the risk of severe hypoxemia, potentially leading to myocardial ischemia. The endoscopist must be aware of this potential and be prepared to respond appropriately, but more importantly, she or he must take precautions to minimize this risk.

The availability of medications able to reverse the effects of narcotics and benzodiazepines, such as naloxone (Narcan) and flumazenil (Mazicon), appears to add a measure of safety to conscious sedation. Neither of these drugs have agonist activity in the absence of the drugs they antagonize. Agents that cannot be reversed should be used infrequently or not at all. There are limits to the usefulness of the antagonists, and the drugs themselves may produce complications.

Anesthesiologists are extremely cautious with naloxone because of the possibility, albeit rare, of producing a generalized sympathetic discharge that may result in serious cardiovascular complications. Based on this possibility, naloxone should not be routinely used after conscious sedation but instead be reserved for medically indicated situations. In patients who are narcotic dependent, naloxone may produce a withdrawal syndrome that may be confused with other complications of endoscopy, such as generalized anxiety and abdominal pain.

The use of flumazenil, a competitive antagonist of all benzodiazepines, has two important caveats. First, flumazenil does not reverse the respiratory depression associated with benzodiazepine use, and its administration in the setting of chronic benzodiazepine use may induce seizures. Second, because as much as 11% of the adult population may be using benzodiazepines routinely, a careful history of benzodiazepine use should be a part of the routine evaluation before endoscopy. In such patients, this drug should be avoided, especially if the drug is used solely to minimize postprocedure time to return to a normal level of consciousness.[18]

TABLE 118-2
Recommendations of the American Heart Association for Endocarditis Prophylaxis

---

Endocarditis Prophylaxis Recommended
Prosthetic cardiac valves, including bioprosthetic and homograft valves
Previous bacterial endocarditis, even without heart disease
Most congenital malformations
Rheumatic and other acquired valvular dysfunction, even after valvular surgery
Hypertrophic cardiomyopathy
Mitral valve prolapse with valvular regurgitation

Standard Regimen
For genitourinary or gastrointestinal tract procedures (e.g., esophageal dilation, sclerotherapy of esophageal varices); biopsy is no longer
    considered an indication for prophylaxis
    Ampicillin (2.0 g IM or IV) plus gentamicin (1.5 mg/kg IM or IV, not to exceed 80 mg), given 0.5 to 1 hour before procedure, followed by
    amoxicillin (1.5 g PO) 6 hours after initial dose; alternatively, the parenteral regimen may be repeated once 8 hours after initial dose.

Special Regimens
Oral regimen for minor or repetitive procedures in low-risk patients:
    Amoxicillin, 3.0 g PO, 1 hour before the procedure and 1.5 g 6 hours after the initial dose.
Penicillin-allergic patients:
    Vancomycin (1.0 g IV) *slowly* over 1 hour, plus gentamicin (1.5 mg/kg IM or IV, not to exceed 80 mg) given 1 hour before procedure. May
    be repeated once 8 hours after initial dose.

From Dajani AS, Bisno AL, Chung KJ, et al. Prevention of bacterial endocarditis. Recommendations of the American Heart
Association. JAMA 1990;264:2919.

Allergic Reactions

The administration of any medication carries with it the potential for an allergic reaction. However, there is a great variation in the potential for individual medications to result in a true allergic reaction with the risk of anaphylaxis. During standard diagnostic or therapeutic endoscopy, intravenous medication is almost routinely given for the induction of conscious sedation. Although untoward responses to these medications (e.g., paradoxical reactions, abdominal pain, or respiratory depression) may be observed, these are not to be construed as allergic reactions. The incidence of true allergy to these medications is extremely small and does not represent a significant risk to the patient.

The real risk for anaphylaxis exists in situations in which other medications (e.g., antibiotics for endocarditis prophylaxis) or intravenous contrast (e.g., percutaneous transhepatic cholangiography) are used.[19,20] The use of antibiotic prophylaxis for the prevention of bacterial endocarditis or infection of an iatrogenic foreign body (e.g., prosthetic joint, vascular graft) has been the subject of considerable discussion.[21,22] The debate is fueled by a paucity of information about the cost effectiveness of prophylaxis, except with prosthetic heart valves or newly implanted vascular grafts or prostheses. Moreover, the costs and the risk of anaphylaxis with the medications that are routinely given parenterally (e.g., penicillins and their derivatives, aminoglycosides) are substantial. The standard recommendations call for antibiotics before endoscopy in patients with "significant" valvular heart disease, prosthetic valves, or vascular grafts (Table 118-2).[23] In guidelines published by the American Society of Gastrointestinal Endoscopy, antibiotic prophylaxis in most situations is not recommended (Table 118-3).[22] In practice, the endoscopist must weigh the need for prophylaxis against the risks of anaphylaxis for each patient. If antibiotics are used, the skill and the equipment necessary to respond to anaphylaxis must be available.

Of the medications routinely used for diagnostic purposes by physicians, intravenous contrast agents represent a class of compounds with a predictable risk for allergy and anaphylaxis.[20] Radiologists have long recognized the risks associated with these agents and have evaluated this problem extensively. Corticosteroid pretreatment 12 and 2 hours before exposure is thought to be effective in preventing this response.[20] Gastroenterologists use contrast agents during endoscopic retrograde cholangiopancreatography (ERCP). After the introduction of this technique, there was concern about possible allergic reactions, with anaphylaxis similar to that seen during the intravenous administration of contrast. However, a large clinical experience has shown that, although erythema and rash have been reported, anaphylaxis is not a problem.[24] The reason for this is unclear, because water-soluble contrast ad-

---

TABLE 118-3
Statement of ASGE on Antibiotic Prophylaxis for Gastrointestinal Endoscopy

---

1. The decision about whether to use antibiotic prophylaxis for gastrointestinal procedures is complicated.*
2. For patients with prosthetic valves, surgically constructed systemic-pulmonary shunts, and a previous history of endocarditis, antibiotic prophylaxis is recommended.
3. For other situations, their use is optional, and the physician's decision should be based on his or her interpretation of the existing data, specific aspects of the individual clinical setting, and discussions with the patient.

---

* A combined committee of the ASGE and the AHA convened in the fall of 1993 to resolve variations in recommendations for antibiotic prophylaxis related to gastrointestinal endoscopy.

From Infection control during gastrointestinal endoscopy, guidelines for clinical application. ASGE Publication No. 1018, Manchester MA, January 1988.

ministered during ERCP does enter the vascular compartment after injection, as shown by nephrograms during or after ERCP.

There are no recommendations requiring premedication of patients with a history of dye allergy who are scheduled to have ERCP, but many practitioners routinely administer corticosteroids or antihistamines (e.g., Benadryl, cimetidine), before the performance of ERCP because of the low risk of these medications and the desire not to have the first case of contrast allergy during ERCP. The art of medicine allows the practitioner much latitude, but there is no information available to support the requirement of such treatment. Pretreatment should follow a protocol shown to be effective for intravenous contrast.[20] The availability of nonionized contrast agents, for which the risk of anaphylaxis is decreased, may further minimize this risk, but the greater cost of these agents should be considered in making the decision.

Paradoxical Reactions

A paradoxical reaction to intravenous sedative medications refers to the development of emotional lability, restlessness, agitation, and even rage instead of the calming effect that usually ensues after their administration.[25,26] Paradoxical reactions to the medications generally used (e.g., benzodiazepines) may occur in as many as 29% of patients, and 7% of these are pronounced reactions. When patients respond in this manner, the endoscopist must decide if the patient is insufficiently sedated, oversedated, or having a paradoxical reaction. If the response is recognized as a paradoxical reaction, the administration of these medications in higher doses is not warranted, and a decision to postpone the procedure or proceed after careful observation of the patient must be made. Potential injury to the patient and the endoscopist may exist if an attempt is made to proceed when the patient is agitated. Equally important is an appreciation that these same features may be a reflection of hypoxemia, making the administration of further medication extremely dangerous.

The almost routine use of pulse oximetry has been a considerable aid in this situation. The patient who is agitated because of hypoxemia is easily detected by pulse oximetry, minimizing the risk of severe respiratory depression. In some patients, the induction of conscious sedation may be difficult. These patients, who are predominantly chronic alcoholics, may have a limited response to otherwise appropriate doses of benzodiazepines and narcotics. They may be effectively sedated by adding neuroleptic drugs, such as droperidol (Inapsine).[27]

Local Reactions

A frequent, but usually innocuous, problem encountered in endoscopy is the development of local reactions, such as erythema or phlebitis, after the insertion of an intravenous line or the administration of intravenous medications. This phenomenon is a function of the types of medications used during endoscopy, particularly diazepam, which is associated with a predictable incidence of phlebitis, especially when given in high concentration in a small vein (i.e., without a freely run-

ning intravenous solution).[28] When diazepam is given in the form of Diazamuls (available in Europe), this effect is less common, because this form of the drug is water soluble. One of the advantages of the newest benzodiazepine, midazolam, is the low incidence of venous irritation because it is water soluble. Regardless of the drug used, the risk for developing septic phlebitis mandates that intravenous medications used for sedation should not be given through a peripheral line that is left in place after the endoscopy, especially in a hospitalized patient and if diazepam is to be administered.

Procedure-Related Complications

Cardiopulmonary Complications

Cardiopulmonary complications represent a series of interrelated events that may have cardiac arrest as their final common pathway. They may be preceded by the hypoxemia seen with conscious sedation, the underlying diseases seen in an elderly population, aspiration during upper gastrointestinal endoscopy, the vagal effects of the endoscope as it negotiates the gastrointestinal tract, or the increased sympathetic tone secondary to anxiety. Although these factors can be discussed separately, they should be viewed as additive or synergistic events.

With all of these contributing factors, it is not surprising that cardiac dysrythmias are extremely frequent (33%–40%) in patients undergoing upper and lower endoscopy.[29–31] Many of these changes are seen before introduction of the endoscope, reflecting the contribution of anxiety and increased sympathetic tone. What is surprising is the rarity of serious cardiac complications during endoscopy. In the American Society of Gastrointestinal Endoscopy survey, only 16 major cardiac events were recorded in 211,410 procedures.[31] These included six myocardial infarctions, ventricular fibrillation, atrial fibrillation, and cardiac arrest. Patient age, associated chronic lung disease, and atherosclerotic disease were the major risk factors of these patients. Similar events are recorded during colonoscopy, with the major addition of an increased incidence of vagal effects related to the stretch of the colon in combination with distention of the organ by insufflated gas. In the largest retrospective review of patients undergoing endoscopy, the limited incidence of serious cardiopulmonary complications was confirmed. This Food and Drug Administration–financed and American Society for Gastrointestinal Endoscopy–coordinated study of more than 20,000 patients also demonstrated that no differences could be related to the widespread use of midazolam (Versed), which was viewed initially as more likely to induce respiratory depression.[6]

Patients with cardiac pacemakers represent a small group of patients who need particular attention. Unipolar pacemakers may be shorted out by the electrical interference from the monopolar generator. These concerns have been minimized by the changes in pacemaker design, but the endoscopist must be aware of the potential risks and the type of pacemaker and should monitor the heart rate of these patients carefully. The use of permanently implanted defibrillators adds a new dimension of concern to the use of monopolar cautery. Although the risks appear to be minimal, continuous monitoring and cardiology consultation are warranted.

Instrument Injury

Injury to the patient as a direct consequence of the endoscope is one of the most feared complications of endoscopy, and it represents the second most common cause of major morbidity.[32] Perforation reflecting transmural injury during endoscopy is in large part a function of the type of procedure being performed (see Table 118-1). Perforation during upper endoscopy is usually related to surgically altered or abnormal anatomy and has been reported for 1 of every 3300 examinations. Abnormalities of the hypopharynx or proximal esophagus, such as Zenker's diverticulum, cervical spurs, cancer, or stricture, are found in almost one half of all upper gastrointestinal perforations (Fig. 118-1). In the remaining patients, a variety of conditions, including electrosurgical procedures, biopsy of deep ulcers, and postoperative changes (e.g., Billroth II), appear to be major risk factors. These same factors in conjunction with the use of a side-viewing instrument make the incidence (3 of 1000) of perforation considerably higher during ERCP.[24]

However, colonoscopy causes the greatest concern for perforation. A combination of factors, including mechanical pressure transmitted through the scope to the antimesenteric border of the sigmoid, bowel distention with insufflated gas, abnormal anatomy, operator inexperience, and the use of monopolar cautery in the relatively thin-walled colon, make perforation a real possibility (Fig. 118-2; see Color Fig. 107).[33,34] These are likely to be free perforations into the peritoneum rather than confined to the retroperitoneum. Gas patterns on plain radiographs are usually diagnostic for the site of injury, free or confined. Risk factors for this complication include operator inexperience, adhesions, diverticular

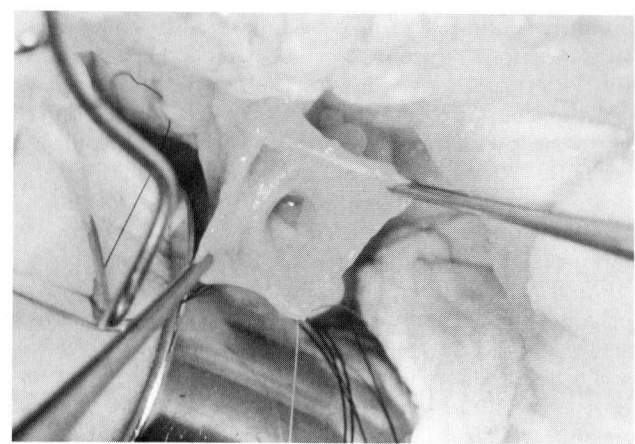

FIGURE 118-2. (See Color Fig. 107.) Operative view of a sigmoid perforation that occurred during diagnostic colonoscopy. A 15-cm segment of the antimesenteric portion of the sigmoid colon has been torn open.

disease, severe inflammation, overdistention, cautery, and use of an overtube. The risk of perforation ranges from 0.14% for diagnostic studies to 0.42% for procedures for which cautery is employed. A wide array of complications have been reported after therapeutic interventions.[32,33]

Several conditions may cause considerable confusion when patients are evaluated after endoscopy. The overinflation with air may produce a pseudoacute abdomen due to small bowel distention or the postcolonoscopy distention syndrome (Fig. 118-3).[35] As many as 1% of patients may have free intraperitoneal air after colonoscopy, and slightly more than 2% have intramural air.[36] These conditions may be difficult to sort out in terms of diagnosis and appropriate response.

Many unusual complications have been observed after endoscopy, including salivary gland enlargement, trauma to the hypopharynx, lacerated mesentery, and traumatic injury to surrounding structures, such as a ruptured spleen or liver laceration. Intraabdominal or subserosal bleeding can occur, especially in patients who are anticoagulated.

Bleeding

With few exceptions, bleeding as a complication of endoscopy occurs in the setting of therapeutic procedures. During diagnostic endoscopy, bleeding may be precipitated by inadvertently removing a clot from an ulcer or disrupting a visible vessel. Bleeding can be precipitated in patients with underlying or iatrogenic coagulation defects, especially thrombocytopenia. It appears that, although this risk is real, diagnostic procedures can be carried out with minimal risk and are justified when the information required is essential to the patients' overall management.[37] In addition to mucosal bleeding, these patients may bleed submucosally or even from the serosa. Elective procedures in the setting of such coagulation defects must be weighed carefully.

The real risk of hemorrhage during endoscopy occurs with therapeutic procedures such as esophageal variceal injection sclerotherapy (EIS), hemostatic control of bleeding ulcers, endoscopic sphincterotomy (ERS), and especially colonos-

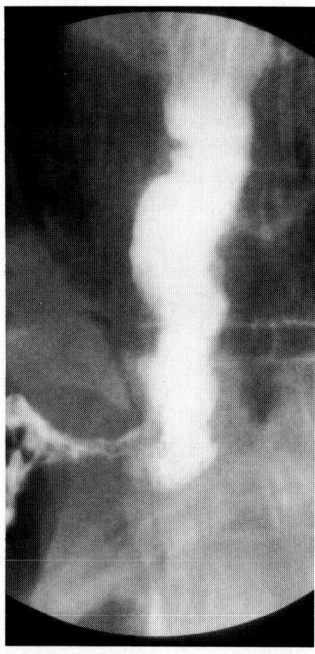

FIGURE 118-1. In a radiographic study performed after endoscopy and dilation in a patient with esophageal cancer and stricture, barium can be seen coursing into the mediastinum through a perforation.

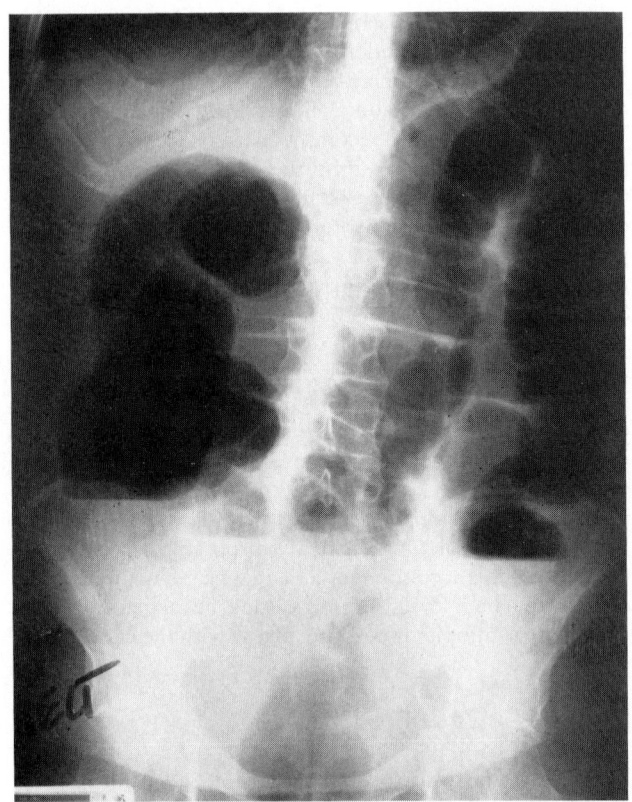

FIGURE 118-3. Postcolonoscopy distention syndrome. The patient returned to the emergency department 12 hours after an uneventful colonoscopy with abdominal pain and was unable to pass gas rectally.

copic polypectomy. Data from many studies suggest that the risk of initiating hemorrhage while treating ulcers with adherent clot (i.e., stigmata of recent hemorrhage) occurs in approximately 5% of cases.[38–40] This same risk exists when performing EIS acutely, chronically, or prophylactically.[41] Bleeding after ERS constitutes one of the major morbidities of this procedure and is reported for 0.4% to 4% of patients.[42] In all such situations, the therapeutic endoscopist must be prepared to deal appropriately with induced bleeding.

Intralumenal hemorrhage is most likely to occur after colonoscopic polypectomy, reflecting the nature and frequency with which this technique is employed. The reported incidence is between 0.77% and 2.2%.[33,34] Bleeding usually occurs immediately after the cut is made, reflecting inadequate coagulation due to techniques of cautery application or patient coagulation abnormalities (e.g., aspirin use before the procedure), but hemorrhage may occur as a delayed complication 7 to 10 days, and rarely as long as 21 days, after polypectomy. This delayed bleeding appears to be much more likely in patients who are taking Coumadin on a chronic basis. There also is concern about delayed hemorrhage after hot biopsy removal of diminutive polyps.[43]

Infection

The endoscope, the endoscopist, and even the patient may infrequently transmit disease. A variety of potential routes of infection are possible. The endoscope can carry infectious or-

ganisms into the patient from an outside source (e.g., hospital water sources used to rinse endoscopes or fill water bottles). There is concern, spurred by attitudes about acquired immunodeficiency syndrome (AIDS), about the potential for transmission of infectious material, including the human immunodeficiency virus (HIV), from one patient to another, from patient to physician, or from physician to patient.[22]

Despite the widespread application of endoscopy, only a small number of documented cases of transmission of infection from the endoscope have been reported. In a literature review, 281 documented cases were compiled.[44] These cases, most of which were reported in the early 1980s, represent bacterial contamination from inappropriately disinfected endoscopes or transmission from hospital water sources. The organisms found in these situations are disproportionately represented by *Salmonella* and *Pseudomonas* species, but other organisms such as *Helicobacter pylori* and *Clostridium difficile* have been reported. Serious clinical consequences and even death have been reported, particularly in the setting of ERCP.

In a statement by the American Society for Gastrointestinal Endoscopy, the infection risk, based on a literature review, was placed at 1 in 1.8 million endoscopies.[45] Only one case of hepatitis B virus transmission (HBV) has been documented.[46] No HIV transmission during endoscopy has been documented.

The infection risk associated with ERCP represents a problem that must be addressed by physicians performing these procedures. Data on these infections suggest that two sources are most often responsible: the inadequately or inappropriately disinfected endoscope and the rinse water used to clean the endoscope lens. The latter source can be traced to potable water in the hospital. Organisms such as *Pseudomonas*, *Klebsiella*, and *Mycobacterial* species are common to this water source and may be transmitted to the patient.

The recommendations for appropriate handling of endoscopes calls for high level disinfection, defined as the destruction of all microbes with the exception of certain bacterial spores, between patients. This requires appropriate exposure of all parts of the endoscope to a high-level disinfectant (i.e., 2% glutaraldehyde or an equivalent agent) after proper mechanical cleansing. Lipid envelope viruses, such as HIV and HBV, are readily destroyed by such exposure. Scopes should be rinsed with sterile or filtered water to prevent contamination and colonization with hospital water-borne organisms, followed by an alcohol rinse to promote drying. Preliminary results relating to the development of sheathed endoscopes that have a disposable patient contact surface have been reported. The ultimate role of such products is unknown, but they are a consequence of the widespread concern about infection transmission during endoscopy.

Although high-level disinfection is the standard for most endoscopy, this is not the case for severely immunocompromised patients, particularly those with significant leukopenia (i.e., absolute polymorphonuclear leukocyte counts <1000). For these patients, infection from *Pseudomonas* and *Strongyloides* with serious sequelae has been reported after routine endoscopy. For leukemic patients after chemotherapy, bone marrow transplant patients before engraftment, and advanced AIDS patients, sterilized equipment should be used.

Transient bacteremia originating from the patient's mucosal surfaces or intralumenal contents has been documented in a small number of individuals after endoscopic manipulation. These episodes tend to be transient, with the organisms reflecting the portion of the bowel that was manipulated.[47,48] The logical concerns are the potential for bacterial endocarditis after endoscopic procedures and the appropriate management of these patients. Guidelines published by the American Heart Association (see Table 118-2) differ significantly from the recommendations of the American Society of Gastrointestinal Endoscopy (see Table 118-3).[22,23] At the center of this dilemma is the lack of data and concern for the medicolegal consequences of not providing the expected "standard of care."

The United States Food and Drug Administration has taken over the responsibility for disinfectant solutions used for patient care activities and is in the process of evaluating and approving the many products on the market.

REDUCING COMPLICATIONS IN GASTROINTESTINAL ENDOSCOPY

Universal Precautions

The appearance of AIDS and the identification of HIV have changed the level of concern about the risks associated with medicine for patients, physicians, and associated personnel. The risk of infection has always been a concern to those involved in endoscopy. Much was written about the potential for transmission of HBV from endoscope to patient or from patient to physician. It was determined that proper disinfection between procedures mitigated these concerns. With the recognition of AIDS, many endoscopic units developed a system in which different instruments were used for AIDS patients than for non-AIDS patients. These instruments were often gas sterilized between procedures.

After the identification of HIV and our ability to test patients, it was recognized that there is a long incubation period during which transmission is possible but the patient is asymptomatic. This observation, coupled with a determination that vigorous disinfection kills the HIV virus, led to the promulgation of universal precautions for medical interventions (Table 118-4). The routine use of gas sterilization and

---

TABLE 118-4
Universal Precautions

All health care workers should *routinely* use appropriate barrier precautions to prevent skin and mucous-membrane exposure when contact with blood or any body fluids is anticipated or possible.
1. Hand washing
2. Gloves
3. Masks and protective eyewear
4. Gowns
5. Nondisposable instruments that touch mucous membranes should be sterilized *or* receive high-grade disinfection.

From Centers for Disease Control. Update: Universal precautions for prevention of transmission of human immunodeficiency virus, hepatitis B and other blood-borne pathogens in health care settings. MMWR 1988;37:377.

---

separate equipment for HIV-infected patients is not recommended; instead, all endoscopic equipment must undergo high-level disinfection between cases. A survey by the Food and Drug Administration demonstrates the alarming frequency with which such recommendations are ignored.[49] All patients are to be dealt with in the same manner. All health care workers in specific areas, including gastrointestinal endoscopy, must use barrier precautions, including gloves, gowns, and eye protection. Compliance with all aspects of universal precautions is being regulated by the Occupational Safety and Health Administration.

Other concerns about HIV risk focused on videoendoscopy and endoscopic accessories. The use of videoendoscopy scopes has many advantages, one of which is the ability of the endoscopist to be physically more distant from the patient, minimizing his or her potential contamination. Disposable accessories have also become more popular. Although these items have been thought of as reusable, many manufacturers are developing one-time-use, truly disposable accessories. If these disposable accessories are used, appropriate mechanical cleaning and high-level disinfection must be carried out before their reuse in another procedure, just as with the endoscopes.

Role of Patient Monitoring

Because the most-feared complications of endoscopy are cardiopulmonary problems, the question of monitoring often occurs. In the clinical situation, the question is frequently about the use of extracorporeal equipment for patients about to undergo endoscopy. Intense discussions reflect the medicolegal concerns, physician categories of responsibility, and a desire to hold costs in line. This confusion reflects the fact that there are no data to support the concept that "appropriate" monitoring has any beneficial effect on patient outcome. In an effort to address these issues at a time when insufficient data are available to mandate one method of monitoring over another, the American Society of Gastrointestinal Endoscopy has prepared a series of guidelines for monitoring in the setting of gastrointestinal endoscopy (Table 118-5). Objective data reflecting appropriately performed studies should be available in the near future.

Another issue is the physician's responsibility to respond to complications during endoscopy. It is mandatory that the endoscopist be in a facility where the necessary equipment is available to respond to any emergency. The endoscopist must be trained and up to date in his or her emergency medical management skills. Although this area of expertise is not fully defined, it would seem logical that a minimum of advanced cardiac life support training and certification should be required, because most major complications are related to cardiopulmonary compromise.

Postprocedure Evaluation and Recognition of Complications

Complications are inherent to the performance of any type of procedure and most are to be expected during the actual performance of the procedure. Complications occurring immediately after the procedure or even remote from the pro-

Adapted from ASGE guidelines on patient monitoring. Publication No. 1022. Boston: American Society for Gastrointestinal Endoscopy, 1989.

TABLE 118-5
American Society for Gastrointestinal Endoscopy Guidelines for Patient Monitoring During Endoscopy

1. Monitoring is one aspect of endoscopy unit policy. It should be part of the overall quality assurance program for the endoscopy unit.
2. A well-trained gastrointestinal assistant working closely with the physician who observes the patient's status during the endoscopic procedure is the most important part of the monitoring process.
3. The use of extracorporeal equipment to monitor patients may be a useful adjunct to patient surveillance, but it is never a substitute for conscientious clinical assessment.
4. Although changes in blood pressure, pulse, cardiac rhythm, and oxygen saturation do occur during endoscopy, no controlled studies address the question about whether noninvasive monitoring with extracorporeal equipment decreases the complications.
5. The amount of monitoring should be proportional to the perceived risk to the patient undergoing the procedure. It may vary from one procedure to the next.
6. The minimal clinical monitoring for all sedated patients should include the determination of heart rate, blood pressure, and respiratory rate before sedation, during the procedure, immediately after the procedure, and when the patient is released from the endoscopy area.
7. The proper role for pulse oximetry and continuous electrocardiographic monitoring during endoscopic procedures remains controversial.
8. Given the cost of the equipment and the personnel needed to use it, the decision about whether it should be used should be based on data exhibiting that such monitoring affects patient outcome. Such data do not exist.
9. However, if the individualized need of the patient indicates that more frequent assessment of cardiac rhythm or oxygen saturation will complement the clinical assessment, the use of electrocardiographic monitoring or pulse oximetry may be beneficial. (In an update of this publication universal oximetry will be recommended.)

cedure are to be expected, especially those related to surgical endoscopy. Unlike the surgical specialties in which a 30-day standard for morbidity and mortality is accepted, the time after a procedure for which the endoscopist is responsible for any complication has not been set. It is imperative that the endoscopist not ignore patient complaints or physical findings that occur, even at times remote from the procedure. The physician must always be prepared to appropriately respond to these problems.

After completion of an endoscopic procedure, the patient must be given specific instructions about problems that may be related to the procedure, how to respond to them, and when to contact the physician. Many patients, especially those who are hospitalized or ill with a variety of associated conditions, may not be able to respond. Appropriate orders must be in place to ensure that the patient is observed for possible complications and that an appropriate response is made.

Late complications of endoscopy are more likely to occur after therapeutic procedures. These complications include perforation after endoscopic hemostasis or polypectomy; transmural injury may occur several days after thermal or chemical injury. Transmural injury may occur without clinical consequence. Data from animal experiments suggest that the power settings normally used during endoscopy are sufficient to cause thermal injury that is transmural, but in most cases, no evidence of perforation develops.

The major portion of the bowel wall that provides tensile strength is the submucosa. No evidence of transmural injury or inflammation is seen even after prolonged thermal burns until 24 to 48 hours after injury, but omentum can be seen covering the injured area. This scenario is clinically manifested after colonoscopic polypectomy. Complaints of fever and pain can occur several days after polypectomy without the development of true perforation and only requiring conservative therapy. The development of pain at or during the performance of thermal therapy in the bowel wall should suggest that transmural injury has occurred and the risk of true perforation is likely to occur.

Late-onset bleeding can have two causes. First, endoscopic hemostasis may fail, and the bleeding lesion, vessel, or varix, may again rebleed. Second, effective hemostasis may be followed by rebleeding due to the evolution of the clotting process and the sloughing of the coagulum 10 to 14 days after the iatrogenic injury. This is particularly true of patients on chronic Coumadin therapy. This delayed bleeding is uncommon but must be assumed to be a complication of the procedure. For this reason, drugs that interfere with coagulation are avoided, if possible, for 10 to 14 days after endoscopic therapy that carries a risk of delayed bleeding, such as polypectomy or endoscopic hemostasis.

Preventive Maintenance

Modern gastrointestinal endoscopy is a highly sophisticated subspecialty requiring the physicians and ancillary personnel to routinely use complicated equipment to ensure maximum effectiveness and patient safety. Anyone who uses equipment in the performance of her or his work must be certain of its appropriate performance. The days when a light source and an endoscope were the only pieces of equipment used are gone.

All electric equipment used in hospitals, including electrocardiogram monitors, oximeters, oximeter units, and light sources, requires clearance by biomedical engineering. The equipment must be regularly checked for electrical safety, including current leakage ground wire resistance, power output, and general physical condition. These safety procedures should be performed and documented on a routine basis. Other aspects of preventive maintenance include routine inspection of endoscopes, ensuring that there are no sharp edges on endoscope tips that could cause bowel wall injury and that the endoscope controls for turning and top deflection (duodenoscope) work properly. This approach includes routine leak testing of all endoscopes to ensure no breaks in the outer sheath provide a difficult to clean and disinfect nidus, potentially promoting infection transmission. Scopes that fail this testing should not be used.

Special considerations are appropriate for laser use in endoscopy. Proper maintenance of equipment and certain safety precautions must be achieved to protect the endoscopic equipment, patient, physician, and ancillary staff. When fiberoptic scopes are used, the application of filters to the fiberscope or protective eyewear are standard. When chip scopes are used, these precautions are not necessary, because the laser energies are not passed through the chip scopes. The addition of special white tips to the endoscope can minimize laser damage to scope tips by reflecting the laser energy.

This concept of preventive maintenance of equipment is an accepted practice in most hospitals. The emergence of outpatient endoscopic units and in-office endoscopy removed endoscopy from the hospitals where these practices were routine. Just as standards of practice for endoscopy are unchanged regardless of the location of the procedure, preventive maintenance of all equipment must be a regular part of all endoscopic units, whether or not they are hospital based.

The reader is directed to Chapter 115, Upper Gastrointestinal Endoscopy; Chapter 116, Colonoscopy and Flexible Sigmoidoscopy; and Chapter 117, Endoscopic Retrograde Cholangiopancreatography, Endoscopic Sphincterotomy and Stone Removal, and Endoscopic Biliary and Pancreatic Drainage.

REFERENCES

1. Gilbert DA, Silverstein FE, Tedesco FJ, et al. The national ASGE survey in upper gastrointestinal bleeding. III. Endoscopy in upper gastrointestinal bleeding. Gastrointest Endosc 1981;27:94.
2. Gilbert DA, Hallstrom AP, Shaneyfelt SL, et al. The national ASGE colonoscopy survey: complications of colonoscopy. Gastrointest Endosc 1984;30:156A.
3. Carey WD. Indications, contraindications and complications of upper gastrointestinal endoscopy. In: Sivak MV Jr, ed. Gastrointestinal endoscopy. Philadelphia: WB Saunders, 1987:296.
4. Rankin GB. Indications, contraindications and complications of colonoscopy. In: Sivak MV Jr, ed. Gastrointestinal endoscopy. Philadelphia: WB Saunders, 1987:868.
5. Ferguson DK, Sivak MV Jr. Indications, contraindications and complications of ERCP. In: Sivak MV Jr, ed. Gastrointestinal endoscopy. Philadelphia: WB Saunders, 1987:581.
6. Arrowsmith JB, Gerstman BB, Fleischer DF, Benjamin SB. Results from the American Society for Gastrointestinal Endoscopy/U.S. Food and Drug Administration collaborative study on complication rates and drug use during gastrointestinal endoscopy. Gastrointest Endosc 1991;37:421.
7. Schindler R. Gastroscopy. The endoscopic study of gastric pathology. 2nd ed. New York: Hafner Publishing, 1950:98.
8. O'Donohue WJ, Moss LM, Angelillo VA. Acute methemoglobinemia induced by topical benzocaine and lidocaine. Arch Intern Med 1980;140:1508.
9. Patel D, Chopra S, Berman MD. Serious systemic toxicity resulting from the use of tetracaine for pharyngeal anesthesia in upper endoscopic procedures. Dig Dis Sci 1989;34:882.
10. Canter DS, Baldridge ET. Premedication with meperidine and diazepam for upper gastrointestinal endoscopy precludes the need for topical anesthesia. Gastrointest Endosc 1986;32:339.
11. Whorwell PJ, Smith CL, Foster KJ. Arterial blood gas tensions during upper gastrointestinal endoscopy. Gut 1976;17:797.
12. Rozen P, Oppenheim D, Ratan J, et al. Arterial oxygen tension changes in elderly patients undergoing upper gastrointestinal endoscopy. I. Possible causes. Scand J Gastroenterol 1979;14:577.
13. Rotykus PS, McDonald GB, Albert RK. Upper intestinal endoscopy induces hypoxemia in patients with obstructive pulmonary disease. Gastroenterol 1980;78:488.
14. Rozen P, Fireman Z, Gilat T. The causes of hypoxemia in elderly patients during endoscopy. Gastrointest Endosc 1982;28:243.
15. FDA's regulation of the new drug Versed. Hearings before a subcommittee on government operations. House of Representatives, One Hundredth Congress. Washington, DC: U.S. Government Printing Office, 1988:51.
16. Porro GB, Baroni S, Parente F, Lazzaroni M. Midazolam versus diazepam as premedication for upper gastrointestinal endoscopy: a randomized, double-blind crossover study. Gastrointest Endosc 1988;34:252.
17. Cole SG, Brozinsky S, Isenberg J. Midazolam, a new more potent benzodiazepine, compared to diazepam: a randomized, double-blind study of pre-endoscopic sedatives. Gastrointest Endosc 1983;29:219.
18. Bartelsman JFWM, Sars PRA, Tytgat GNJ. Flumazenil used for reversal of midazolam-induced sedation in endoscopy outpatients. Gastrointest Endosc 1990;36:S9.
19. Shorvon PJ, Eykyn SJ, Cotton PB. Gastrointestinal instrumentation, bacteremia, and endocarditis. Gut 1983;24:1078.
20. Lasser EC, Berry CL, Talner LB, et al. Pretreatment with corticosteroids to alleviate reactions to intravenous contrast material. N Engl J Med 1987;317:845.
21. Kaye D. Prophylaxis for infective endocarditis. Ann Intern Med 1986;104:419.
22. Infection control during gastrointestinal endoscopy. Guidelines for clinical application. Gastrointest Endosc 1988;34(Suppl):37.
23. Dajani AS, Bisno AL, Chung KJ, et al. Prevention of bacterial endocarditis. Recommendations of the American Heart Association. JAMA 1990;264:2919.
24. Bilboa MK, Dotter CT, Lee TG, Katon RM. Complications of endoscopic retrograde cholangiopancreatography. A study of 10,000 cases. Gastroenterology 1976;70:314.
25. Litchfield BM. Complications of intravenous diazepam adverse psychological reactions (an assessment of 16,000 cases). Anaesth Prog 1980;27:175.
26. Short TG, Forrest P, Galletly DC. Paradoxical reactions to benzodiazepines—a genetically determined phenomenon. Anaesth Intensive Care 1987;15:333.
27. Wilcox CM, Forsmark CE, Cello JP. Utility of droperidol for conscious sedation in gastrointestinal endoscopic procedures. Gastrointest Endosc 1990;36:112.
28. Langdon DC, Harlon JR, Bailey RL. Thrombophlebitis with diazepam used intravenously. JAMA 1973;223:184.
29. Fugita R, Kumura F. Arrhythmias induced by gastric endoscopic procedures. Am J Gastroenterol 1975;64:44.
30. Alam M, Schuman BM, Duvernoy WFC, et al. Continuous electrocardiographic monitoring during colonoscopy. Gastrointest Endosc 1976;22:203.
31. Prixtautz H, Biffl H, Leitner W, et al. Influence of an antiarrhythmic premedication and the development of premature ventricular contractions during fiberoptic gastroduodenoscopy. Endoscopy 1981;13:57.
32. Mandelstam P, Sugawa C, Silvis SE, et al. Complications associated with esophagogastroduodenoscopy and with esophageal dilation. Gastrointest Endosc 1976;23:16.
33. Rodgers BHG, Silvis SE, Nebel OT, et al. Complications of flexible fiberoptic colonoscopy and polypectomy. An analysis of the 1974 ASGE survey. Gastrointest Endosc 1975;22:73.
34. Fruhmorgen P, Demling L. Complications of diagnostic and therapeutic colonoscopy in the Federal Republic of Germany. Results of an inquiry. Endoscopy 1979;11:146.
35. Ramarkrisknan J. Adynamic ileus complicating colonoscopy. South Med J 1979;72:92.
36. Goldstein M, Hoexter B, et al. Benign pneumoperitoneum after fiberoptic colonoscopy: a prospective study of 100 patients. Gastroenterol 1977;73:226.
37. Chu DZ, Shivshanker K, Stroehlein JR, Nelson RS. Thrombocytopenia and gastrointestinal hemorrhage in the cancer patient: prevalence of unmasked lesions. Gastrointest Endosc 1983;29:269.
38. Krejs GJ, Little KH, Westergaard H, et al. Laser photocoagulation for the treatment of acute peptic ulcer bleeding. A randomized controlled clinical trial. N Engl J Med 1987;316:1618.

39. Kovacs TOG, Jensen DM. Endoscopic control of gastroduodenal hemorrhage. Annu Rev Med 1987;38:267.
40. Cook DJ, Guyatt GH, Salena BJ, Laine LA. Endoscopic therapy for acute nonvariceal upper gastrointestinal hemorrhage: a meta-analysis. Gastroenterology 1992;102:139.
41. Santangelo WC, Dueno Mi, Estes BL, Krejs GJ. Prophylactic sclerotherapy of large esophageal varices. N Engl J Med 1988;318:814.
42. Classen M. Endoscopic papillotomy. In: Sivak MV Jr, ed. Gastrointestinal endoscopy. Philadelphia: WB Saunders, 1987:631.
43. Wadas DD, Sanowski RA. Complications of the hot biopsy forceps technique. Gastrointest Endosc 1987;33:32.
44. Spach DH, Silverstein FE, Stamm WE. Transmission of infection by gastrointestinal endoscopy and bronchoscopy. Ann Intern Med 1993;118:117.
45. American Society for Gastrointestinal Endoscopy Technology Assessment. Transmission of infection by gastrointestinal endoscopy. 1993;39:885.
46. Birnie G, Quigley E, Clements G, et al. Case report: endoscopic transmission of hepatitis B virus. Gut 1983;24:171.
47. Doherty DE, Falko JM, Lefkovitz N, et al. *Pseudomonas aeruginosa* sepsis following retrograde cholangiopancreatography (ERCP). Dig Dis Sci 1982;27:169.
48. Classen DC, Jacobson JA, Burke JP, et al. Serious *Pseudomonas* infections associated with endoscopic retrograde cholangiopancreatography. Am J Med 1988;84:590.

Textbook of Gastroenterology, second edition, edited by Tadataka Yamada. JB Lippincott Company, Philadelphia © 1995.

CHAPTER 119

Contrast Radiology

Marc S. Levine   Stephen E. Rubesin   Hans Herlinger
Igor Laufer

Pharynx
Indications
Normal Anatomy
Technique
Abnormalities
Upper Gastrointestinal Tract
Technique
Indications
Contraindications and Risks
Abnormalities
Small Bowel

Techniques
Application of Techniques
Abnormalities
Colon
Single Versus Double Contrast
Radiology Versus Colonoscopy
Indications
Contraindications
Complications

The development of routine double-contrast techniques for examining the gastrointestinal tract has dramatically improved our ability to diagnose a variety of inflammatory and neoplastic diseases in the pharynx, esophagus, stomach, duodenum, small bowel, and colon. A major advantage of these techniques is their ability to demonstrate superficial mucosal abnormalities that cannot easily be recognized on conventional single-contrast examinations. In other cases, double-contrast studies may detect lesions that are missed or misinterpreted on endoscopy. Double-contrast radiography is also less expensive and less invasive than endoscopy. It is a valuable technique for evaluating patients with suspected gastrointestinal disease. All radiologists should strive for excellent double-contrast studies to maximize the information available from the procedure.

PHARYNX

With increased survival of the elderly, pharyngeal disorders have become an increasingly frequent problem in modern medical practice. Approximately 35% of nursing home patients have some form of swallowing dysfunction.[1] Aspiration pneumonia and choking are particularly common causes of morbidity and mortality. Pharyngeal carcinoma is another devastating disease that is frequently encountered in the elderly. Radiographic examination of the pharynx is now recognized as a valuable tool in the diagnostic work-up of this large group of patients with pharyngeal disorders. Nevertheless, diseases of the pharynx and esophagus are closely interrelated, and both structures should be evaluated radiographically in patients with swallowing dysfunction.

Indications

A radiographic examination of the pharynx is most frequently performed on patients who have difficulty swallowing. However, disorders of the pharynx also may be manifested by respiratory and speech problems. Laryngeal aspiration may lead to recurrent pneumonia, asthma, chronic bronchitis, coughing, or choking. In other patients, soft-palate insufficiency may result in nasal regurgitation or may give the voice a nasal quality. A pharyngoesophagram may be helpful in patients who have a wide spectrum of respiratory, speech, and swallowing difficulties. Barium studies are also useful in assessing pharyngeal function and morphology in patients with a history of neuromuscular disease, stroke, pharyngeal tumor, or prior head and neck surgery or radiation.

Normal Anatomy

The pharynx is a complex muscular tube suspended superiorly from the skull base and styloid process, posteriorly from the cervical spine, and anteriorly from the mandible and hyoid bone. At least 26 muscles and six cranial nerves participate in pharyngeal function.[2] The intrinsic muscles of the pharynx include an outer circular layer (i.e., superior, middle, and inferior constrictor muscles) and an inner longitudinal layer (i.e., palatopharyngeus, salpingopharyngeus, and stylopharyngeus muscles).[3]

The pharynx can be arbitrarily divided into three portions: the nasopharynx, oropharynx, and hypopharynx. The soft palate separates the nasopharynx from the oropharynx, and the pharyngoepiglottic fold separates the oropharynx from the hypopharynx. The tongue forms the anterior wall of the oropharynx (Fig. 119-1). The larynx, with its associated epiglottic, thyroid, cricoid, and arytenoid cartilages, forms the anterior wall of the hypopharynx. This laryngeal complex often protrudes into the lower hypopharynx as an apparent mass.

The mucosal surface of the pharynx is thrown into a series of folds by underlying lymphoid and muscular tissue. The vertical surface of the base of the tongue often has a nodular appearance due to the circumvallate papillae and lingual tonsil (see Fig. 119-1). Nodular lymphoid tissue or linear webs may

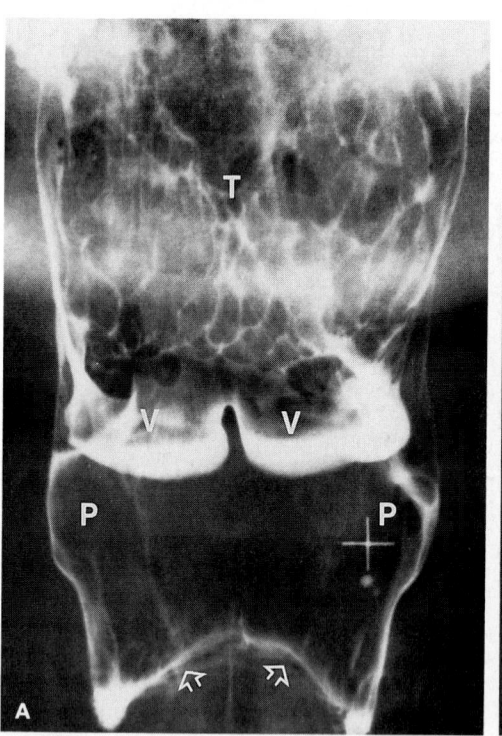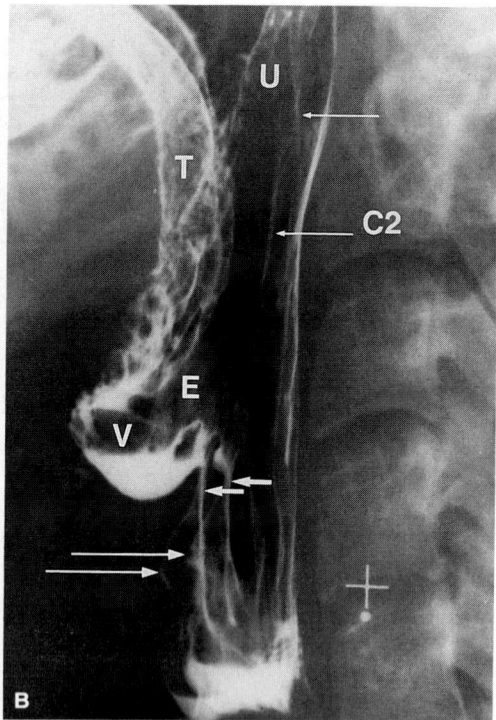

FIGURE 119-1. Normal anatomy. **(A)** Frontal view of the pharynx shows the normal appearance of vallecullae (V) and piriform sinuses (P). Notice how the base of the tongue (T) has a uniformly nodular appearance en face due to an underlying lingual tonsil. Inferiorly, the arcuate line (*open arrows*) is formed by the larynx impressing on anterior wall of lower hypopharynx. **(B)** Lateral view of the pharynx shows the base of the tongue (T), tip of the uvula (U), vallecullae (V), and epiglottis (E). Paired palatopharyngeal folds (*medium-length arrows*) overlie the palatopharyngeus muscle and form the posterior tonsillar pillar. Paired aryepiglottic folds (*short arrows*) extend inferiorly toward the muscular processes of the arytenoid cartilages. The anterior wall of the hypopharynx (piriform sinus) bulges anteriorly (*long arrows*). The C2 vertebral body is labelled for orientation. (From Rubesin SE, Glick SN. The tailored double-contrast pharyngogram. Crit Rev Diagn Imaging 1988;28:133.)

also interrupt the normally smooth surface of the valleculae. Although the anterior border of the hypopharynx usually has a smooth contour, close apposition of the longitudinal muscles of the pharynx to the overlying squamous mucosa results in longitudinal striations of the lateral and posterior walls of the hypopharynx.[3] Horizontal mucosal striations are seen in the redundant mucosa overlying the arytenoid processes and cricoid cartilages.[3]

Technique

A complete radiographic examination of the pharynx includes a cine or video pharyngoesophagram to evaluate motility and a series of spot films to evaluate morphology.[4–6] In patients with suspected foreign body, fistula, or abscess, frontal and lateral plain films of the neck should also be obtained.

The barium study is performed with a high-density barium suspension for optimal visualization of the pharynx. The patient is asked to swallow barium in frontal, lateral, and if necessary, oblique projections. A cine or video recording of each swallow permits a frame-by-frame or slow-motion analysis of the various parameters of deglutition. Movement of the tongue, soft palate, and epiglottis as well as laryngeal closure and cricopharyngeal opening are best evaluated in the lateral projection. However, symmetry of tongue motion, pharyngeal peristalsis, and epiglottic tilt are best evaluated in the frontal projection.

After individual swallows of barium, double-contrast spot films of the pharynx are obtained in frontal and lateral projections. These double-contrast views are possible because of residual high-density barium coating the pharyngeal mucosa immediately after each swallow. The spot films are obtained during suspended respiration and during a modified Valsalva maneuver or phonation to optimally distend the pharynx.[7] The frontal view is best for demonstrating the contours of the valleculae and piriform sinuses, the lateral walls of the tonsillar fossae and hypopharynx, and the superior border of the base of the tongue (see Fig. 119-1A). The lateral view is best for demonstrating the inferior border of the base of the tongue, the soft palate, the posterior pharyngeal wall, the anterior hypopharyngeal wall, the epiglottis, and the cricopharyngeus (see Fig. 119-1B).

After the pharyngeal examination has been completed, upright double-contrast and prone single-contrast views of the esophagus should also be obtained to rule out associated esophageal disease.

Abnormalities

Laryngeal Penetration and Aspiration

Laryngeal penetration occurs when barium enters the laryngeal vestibule during swallowing. Penetration may be limited to the region of the subepiglottic space or may extend as far as the true vocal cords or trachea. Laryngeal penetration occurs because of poor timing of oral and pharyngeal events associated with swallowing or pharyngeal dysmotility due to neuromuscular disorders such as amyotrophic lateral sclerosis, multiple sclerosis, or cerebrovascular accidents. Inflammatory or neoplastic diseases that restrict pharyngeal motility may also cause penetration.

Aspiration occurs when barium enters the laryngeal vestibule during normal breathing. Aspiration results from stasis and retention of pharyngeal contents because of tumor, diverticula, or neuromuscular disease in the pharynx. Aspiration may also be caused by gastroesophageal reflux or reflux of esophageal contents above an obstructing esophageal lesion, such as a stricture or carcinoma. Penetration is primarily associated with dysmotility, and aspiration is associated with stasis.

Cricopharyngeal Prominence

The pharyngoesophageal segment (PES), the radiographic equivalent of the manometrically defined upper esophageal sphincter (UES), is formed by the inferior pharyngeal constrictor muscle, cricopharyngeus, and possibly the proximal cervical esophagus.[8,9] Although the UES is tonically contracted at rest, initiation of swallowing causes the sphincter to relax ahead of the oncoming bolus. The UES also acts as part of the pharyngeal peristaltic wave, functioning in sequence with the constrictor musculature. The pharyngoesophageal segment is best evaluated on a dynamic recording of the pharynx in a lateral projection.

During swallowing, a prominent cricopharyngeus appears as a smooth, 1-cm, bar-like protrusion of the posterior pharyngeal wall into the barium column on lateral projections (Fig. 119-2). This finding may be caused by delayed opening, incomplete opening, or early closure of the cricopharyngeus. A prominent cricopharyngeus is detected on barium studies in about 5% of asymptomatic individuals.[10,11] However, some patients with this finding complain of dysphagia. In symptomatic patients, a prominent cricopharyngeus is often associated with pharyngeal paresis or occurs as a compensatory response to gastroesophageal reflux or esophageal obstruction.

Lateral Pharyngeal Pouches and Diverticula

Lateral pharyngeal pouches are transient protrusions of the lateral pharyngeal wall at sites of anatomic weakness, such as the posterior thyrohyoid membrane and tonsillar fossae after a tonsillectomy.[12] These pouches are common findings, usually occurring as normal variants in asymptomatic patients. In contrast, lateral pharyngeal diverticula are persistent protrusions from the tonsillar fossae or region of the thyrohyoid membrane. These diverticula are much less common than pharyngeal pouches, occurring primarily in individuals who have markedly elevated pharyngeal pressure, such as glassblowers and tuba players. If stasis occurs in pharyngeal pouches or diverticula, the subsequent spillage of pouch contents into the hypopharynx may result in aspiration into the larynx or tracheobronchial tree. Diverticula may also be manifested by neck masses and occasionally may be sites of ulceration or neoplasia.

Lateral pharyngeal pouches appear on frontal views as transient, hemispheric protrusions of mucosa in the upper hypopharynx above the calcified edge of the thyroid cartilage (Fig. 119-3). These pouches can be recognized on lateral views as ovoid barium collections or rings anteriorly in the upper hypopharynx just below the hyoid bone. In contrast, lateral

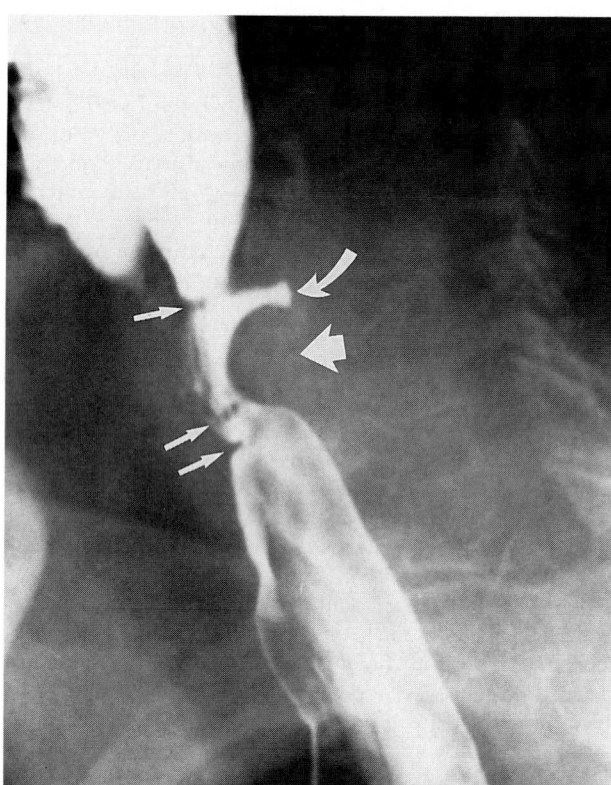

FIGURE 119-2. Incomplete opening of cricopharyngeus, manifested by posterior indentation on pharyngoesophageal segment (*large arrow*). Notice the associated webs anteriorly (*small arrows*) and pseudo-Zenker's diverticulum posteriorly (*curved arrow*) that are seen because barium is trapped above a prominent cricopharyngeus. Cricopharyngeal dysmotility is often related to underlying gastroesophageal reflux or pharyngeal paresis.

pharyngeal diverticula appear as persistent protrusions in these areas.

Zenker's Diverticulum

Zenker's diverticulum or posterior hypopharyngeal diverticulum is an acquired mucosal herniation through an area of anatomic weakness in the region of the cricopharyngeus (i.e., Killian's dehiscence). This area of anatomic weakness is located between the thyropharyngeus and cricopharyngeus or between the oblique and horizontal fibers of the cricopharyngeus.[8,9] Many patients with Zenker's diverticulum have an associated hiatal hernia or gastroesophageal reflux. Rarely, these diverticula are complicated by ulceration or malignancy.

During swallowing, Zenker's diverticulum appears radiographically as a posterior bulging of the distal pharyngeal lumen above an anteriorly protruding cricopharyngeal bar (Fig. 119-4A). At rest, the barium-filled diverticular sac often extends below the level of the cricopharyngeus posterior to the proximal cervical esophagus (Fig. 119-4B). Large diverticula may also protrude to the left or compress the cervical esophagus.

Inflammatory Conditions

Barium studies are of limited value in patients with viral, bacterial, or fungal infection of the pharynx.[13] Such patients usually have normal pharyngograms or nonspecific lymphoid hyperplasia of the palatine tonsil or base of the tongue. Occasionally, however, *Candida* or herpes pharyngitis may be manifested on double-contrast radiographs by plaques or ulcers in the pharynx, particularly in patients with acquired immunodeficiency syndrome (AIDS). Barium studies may also be helpful in a patient who has a chronic sore throat to determine whether there is underlying gastroesophageal reflux or reflux esophagitis.

Tumors

Double-contrast pharyngography has an important role in the initial detection and subsequent work-up of pharyngeal tumors. Double-contrast radiographs of the pharynx can accurately define the size, level, and extent of the lesion. The

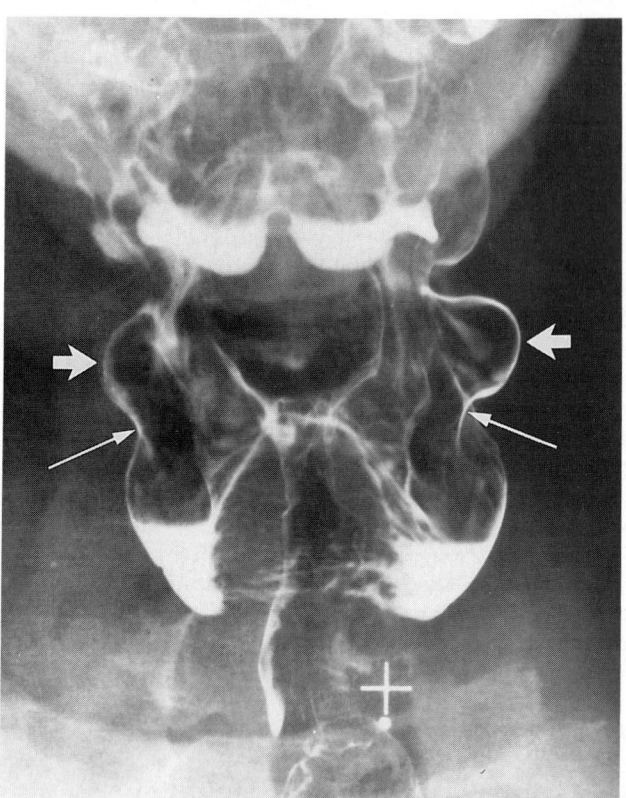

FIGURE 119-3. Lateral pharyngeal pouches (*short arrows*) are seen after a modified Valsalva maneuver. The inferior portion of the pouch represents the junction of the thyrohyoid membrane and thyroid cartilage (*long arrows*). These pouches occur as transient protrusions of hypopharyngeal wall at areas of weakness in the thyrohyoid membrane. Notice the laryngeal penetration, with barium outlining vocal cords and proximal trachea. (From Rubesin SE, Jessurun J, Robertson D, et al. Lines of the pharynx. Radiographics 1987;7:217.)

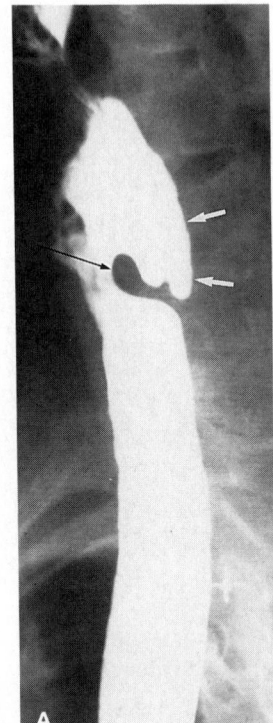
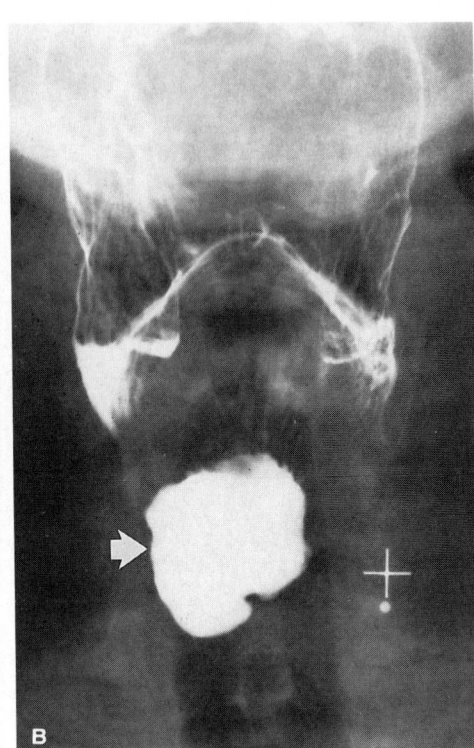

FIGURE 119-4. (**A**) Zenker's diverticulum seen as a posterior outpouching of the hypopharyngeal wall (*white arrows*) above a prominent cricopharyngeus (*black arrow*) during swallowing. (**B**) A frontal view shows retention of barium in a diverticulum (*arrow*) at completion of the swallow.

radiologic examination is particularly helpful in demonstrating regions of the pharynx (e.g., valleculae, lower hypopharynx, cricopharyngeus) that are difficult to visualize at endoscopy. It also enables detection of submucosal masses that are easily missed at endoscopy. Although its accuracy is limited in the region of the palatine tonsil, the double-contrast examination is capable of detecting more than 95% of all mucosal neoplasms in the pharynx below the level of the pharyngoepiglottic fold.[14]

Whatever the underlying histology, benign pharyngeal tumors tend to appear radiographically as smooth, sharply circumscribed, hemispheric masses en face and in profile.[15] The most common benign lesions are retention cysts of the valleculae or aryepiglottic folds.

Squamous cell carcinoma is by far the most common malignant tumor of the pharynx. With an overall 5-year survival rate of approximately 20%, this tumor has a somewhat better prognosis than esophageal carcinoma. These lesions may be manifested on double-contrast radiographs by an intralumenal mass, mucosal irregularity, or loss of distensibility (Fig. 119-5).[16] An intralumenal mass may cause asymmetry or obliteration of the normal pharyngeal contour, barium-coated lines in unusual locations, or a superimposed radiodensity. Mucosal irregularity may be manifested by an irregular, lobulated, nodular, or granular surface pattern. A loss of distensibility may be associated with fixation of pharyngeal structures by infiltrating tumor. When malignant lesions are detected in the pharynx, the esophagus should be carefully evaluated radiographically because of the increased incidence of synchronous esophageal cancers in these patients.[17]

UPPER GASTROINTESTINAL TRACT

The development of routine double-contrast techniques for examining the upper gastrointestinal tract has dramatically improved our ability to diagnose a variety of inflammatory and neoplastic diseases in the esophagus, stomach, and duodenum. Despite increasing acceptance of this technique, some investigators advocate endoscopy as the initial screening study in patients with dyspepsia or other upper gastrointestinal symptoms. Although fiberoptic endoscopy has been recognized as a highly accurate technique for examining the upper gastrointestinal tract, it is also an invasive technique with a small but measurable risk of gastric perforation or other complications. It is an expensive technique, costing three to four times more in the United States than double-contrast upper gastrointestinal examinations. Because barium studies are safer and less expensive than endoscopy, radiologic evaluation of the upper gastrointestinal tract remains a viable alternative as long as its accuracy approaches that of endoscopy for clinically significant disease. We think that a carefully performed double-contrast examination provides the best opportunity for radiology to be competitive with endoscopy as a diagnostic modality.

Technique

The routine double-contrast upper gastrointestinal examination should be performed as a biphasic study in which double-contrast and single-contrast views of the esophagus,

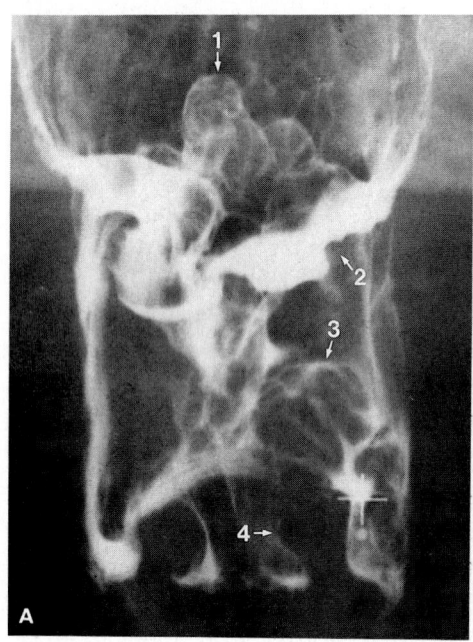 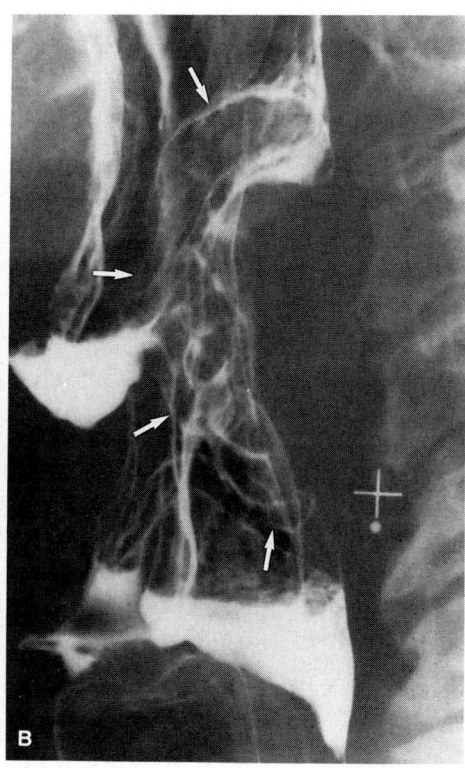

FIGURE 119-5. Pharyngeal carcinoma. (**A**) Frontal view of large supraglottic carcinoma, manifested by a lobulated mass (1) in region of epiglottis. Notice the flattened, nodular contour of the left vallecula (2), nodular appearance of the mucosa overlying the muscular process of the left arytenoid cartilage (3), and displacement of the left false vocal cord (4). There is radiographic evidence of tumor involving the epiglottis, left val-lecula, lateral pharyngeal wall, left arytenoid process, and left false vocal cord. (**B**) Lateral view from a different patient shows a large, lobulated mass (*arrows*) arising from the posterior wall of the pharynx. Notice the barium in the laryngeal vestibule, ven-tricle, and proximal trachea due to pharyngeal dysmotility result-ing from neural invasion by tu-mor. (From Rubesin SE, Glick SN. The tailored double-contrast pharyngogram. Crit Rev Dign Imaging 1988;28:133.)

stomach, and duodenum are obtained.[18] In the double-contrast portion of the study, a series of maneuvers is required to achieve adequate gaseous distention of the lumen while a thin layer of high-density barium is spread on the mucosa. The major purpose of fluoroscopy is to determine the volume of barium and gas, to assess mucosal coating, and to ensure accurate positioning and timing of spot films. The double-contrast examination is facilitated by the use of pharmacologic agents (e.g., 0.1 mg of glucagon given intravenously) to in-duce gastric hypotonia. After the double-contrast portion of the study has been completed, prone or upright single-contrast views of the esophagus, stomach, and duodenum are obtained with a low-density barium suspension and various degrees of compression to supplement the double-contrast study. Be-cause of its greater diagnostic yield, this biphasic study has been advocated as the best radiologic technique for examining the upper gastrointestinal tract.

Indications

Esophagus

In patients with reflux symptoms, barium studies have tra-ditionally been advocated to document the presence of a slid-ing hiatal hernia or gastroesophageal reflux, to detect com-plications such as strictures, and to rule out other abnormalities in the esophagus that can mimic reflux esoph-agitis. By permitting a more detailed assessment of the esoph-ageal mucosa, double-contrast radiographic techniques have made it possible to detect superficial ulceration and other changes of esophagitis before the development of deep ulcers and strictures.

Because modern medical care is prolonging the survival of patients who are immunosuppressed, infectious esophagitis has become an increasingly frequent problem. When infec-tious esophagitis is suspected on clinical grounds, double-contrast esophagography may be performed to confirm the diagnosis and differentiate the various underlying organisms. The radiologist's ability to differentiate fungal and viral esophagitis is particularly important in patients with AIDS, because some gastroenterologists are reluctant to perform en-doscopy on these individuals because of fear of contaminating their endoscopic instruments or exposing themselves to the AIDS virus. However, endoscopy is a more definitive diag-nostic test because it permits biopsy, cytology, and culture.

Dysphagia is another important indication for performing barium studies. If the sensation of dysphagia is localized to the pharynx, a careful pharyngeal examination should be ob-tained. However, some lesions involving the distal esophagus or cardia may cause referred dysphagia to the upper esophagus or pharynx. Thus, the gastric cardia and esophagus should be carefully evaluated radiographically in all patients with unex-plained pharyngeal dysphagia to rule out a distal lesion mas-querading as a pharyngeal disorder.

Stomach and Duodenum

The most common indications for performing a double-contrast examination of the stomach and duodenum include epigastric pain or discomfort, bloating, belching, early satiety, and signs or symptoms of upper gastrointestinal bleeding, such as hematemesis, melena, and guaiac-positive stool. If erosive gastritis or duodenitis, duodenal ulcers, or unequiv-ocally benign-appearing gastric ulcers are diagnosed radiographically, the patient can be treated medically without need for endoscopic intervention. If, however, the double-contrast examination demonstrates a gastric ulcer or other lesion that is equivocal or suspicious for malignancy, endoscopy and biopsy should be performed for a more definitive diagnosis. If the double-contrast examination is normal, the decision for endoscopy should be based on the severity of symptoms, age, and overall health of the patient.

Contraindications and Risks

Because oral barium sulfate is contraindicated in patients with suspected esophageal or gastric perforation, water-soluble contrast media (i.e., Gastrografin) should be employed if there are any clinical or radiographic signs of mediastinitis or peritonitis. Otherwise, the risks of the barium study are negligible. Nevertheless, a double-contrast examination may be difficult to perform on elderly or debilitated patients who cannot undergo the turning maneuvers required for this examination. These patients may be evaluated by conventional single-contrast barium studies. Similarly, single-contrast studies may be performed for patients suspected of having high-grade gastric outlet obstruction.

Abnormalities

Reflux Esophagitis

Conventional single-contrast esophagography has been considered an unreliable technique for diagnosing reflux esophagitis, with an overall sensitivity of only 50% to 75% reported in the literature. However, the use of double-contrast esophagography has increased the radiographic sensitivity to almost 90%.[19] In relatively mild reflux esophagitis, mucosal edema and inflammation may be manifested on double-contrast radiographs by a granular or finely nodular mucosa.[19] Other patients may have shallow ulcers and erosions appearing as one or more tiny collections of barium in the distal esophagus near the gastroesophageal junction (Fig. 119-6). In more severe disease, the esophagus may have a grossly irregular contour, with serrated margins and decreased distensibility due to extensive ulceration, edema, and spasm. Although other causes of esophagitis may produce similar findings, the presence of an associated hiatal hernia or gastroesophageal reflux should suggest the correct diagnosis.

Barrett's esophagus is a well-recognized complication of reflux esophagitis that is associated with a significantly increased risk of developing esophageal adenocarcinoma. Unfortunately, the classic radiologic features of Barrett's esophagus (i.e., a high esophageal stricture or ulcer or a reticular mucosal pattern) occur in only a minority of patients.[20] However, data suggest that double-contrast esophagography can be a valuable screening study for Barrett's esophagus to determine the relative need for endoscopy and biopsy in patients with reflux symptoms.[21]

Infectious Esophagitis

Esophagography has also been considered an unreliable technique for diagnosing *Candida* esophagitis, with an overall sensitivity of less than 50%.[22] With double-contrast technique,

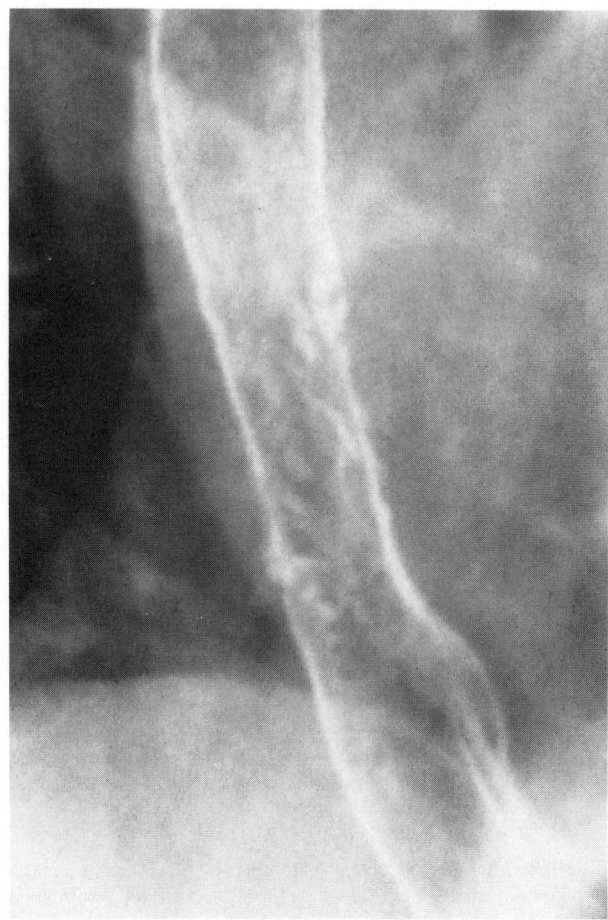

FIGURE 119-6. Reflux esophagitis with multiple areas of shallow ulceration seen en face and in profile in the distal esophagus. (From Levine MS, Rubesin SE, Herlinger H, Laufer I. Double-contrast upper GI examination: technique and interpretation. Radiology 1988;168:593.)

esophagography has a sensitivity of about 90% in diagnosing *Candida* esophagitis.[23] The major advantage of this technique is its ability to demonstrate mucosal plaques that cannot easily be recognized on conventional single-contrast studies. These discrete, plaque-like lesions tend to be longitudinally oriented, appearing on double-contrast radiographs as linear or irregular filling defects with normal intervening mucosa (Fig. 119-7A).

The worsening AIDS epidemic has led to the development of a more fulminant form of *Candida* esophagitis, manifested by a "shaggy" esophagus with a grossly irregular contour due to multiple plaques, pseudomembranes, and ulcers (Fig. 119-7B).[24] Because this degree of esophagitis rarely occurs in other immunocompromised patients, the possibility of AIDS should be suspected when a shaggy esophagus is detected on barium studies, particularly in young homosexual men.

Herpes and, less frequently, cytomegalovirus (CMV) esophagitis also occur in immunosuppressed patients with odynophagia, and these conditions should be suspected in the same clinical setting as *Candida* esophagitis. More than 50% of patients with herpes esophagitis have discrete, superficial ulcers on the esophageal mucosa that are readily detected on double-contrast radiographs (Fig. 119-8).[25] CMV esoph-

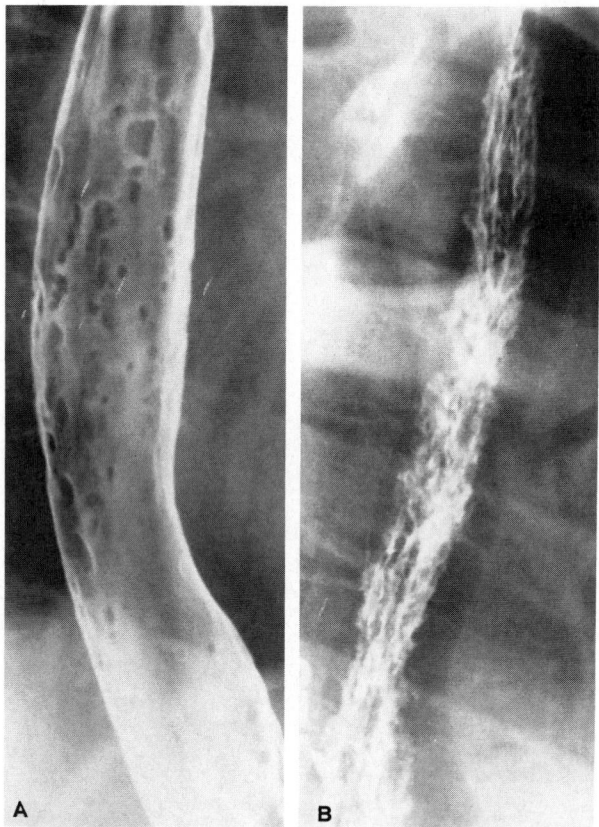

FIGURE 119-7. *Candida* esophagitis. **(A)** Double-contrast esophagram shows discrete plaque-like defects with normal intervening mucosa. This appearance is characteristic of candidiasis. (From Levine MS, Macones AJ, Laufer I. *Candida* esophagitis: accuracy of radiographic diagnosis. Radiology 1985;154: 581.) **(B)** Severe *Candida* esophagitis in AIDS patient. Notice the shaggy contour of the esophagus, caused by multiple plaques, pseudomembranes, and ulcers.

agitis, which occurs primarily in patients with AIDS, is often manifested by the development of one or more large, relatively flat ulcers in the esophagus.[24] Whatever the size or shape of the lesions, discrete ulcers on an otherwise normal mucosa suggest viral esophagitis, because in patients with candidiasis, ulceration almost always occurs on a background of diffuse plaque formation.

Human immunodeficiency virus (HIV) has been recognized as another cause of giant esophageal ulcers in HIV-positive patients with odynophagia. The lesions typically appear radiographically as giant, flat ulcers indistinguishable from those caused by CMV.[26] Because HIV-related ulcers may respond dramatically to oral steroids, endoscopy is required to differentiate HIV from CMV infection in the esophagus before initiating treatment.

Esophageal Carcinoma

Esophageal carcinoma is a deadly disease with an overall 5-year survival rate of only 5% to 10%. This dismal prognosis is primarily related to the advanced stage of the disease at the time of clinical presentation. Occasionally, esophageal cancer

may be discovered at an early stage, and unlike advanced esophageal carcinoma, early esophageal cancer is a readily curable lesion with reported 5-year survival rates approaching 90%. In Western countries, detection of these lesions is best accomplished by some form of radiologic or endoscopic surveillance of patients known to be at increased risk for developing esophageal cancer. For example, patients with Barrett's esophagus may alternate undergoing double-contrast esophagography and endoscopy at 6-month intervals, with the hope of detecting cancer or dysplasia in Barrett's mucosa at the earliest possible stage.

Early esophageal cancers classically appear on double-contrast esophagrams as protruded lesions less than 3.5 cm in diameter.[27] They may be plaque-like lesions or small, sessile polyps with smooth or slightly lobulated contours. Other superficial spreading carcinomas may be manifested radiographically by tiny coalescent nodules or plaques causing localized nodularity or granularity of the mucosa.[28] In contrast, advanced esophageal carcinomas appear as polypoid, ulcerated, or infiltrating lesions with mass effect, ulceration, or irregular narrowing of the lumen.

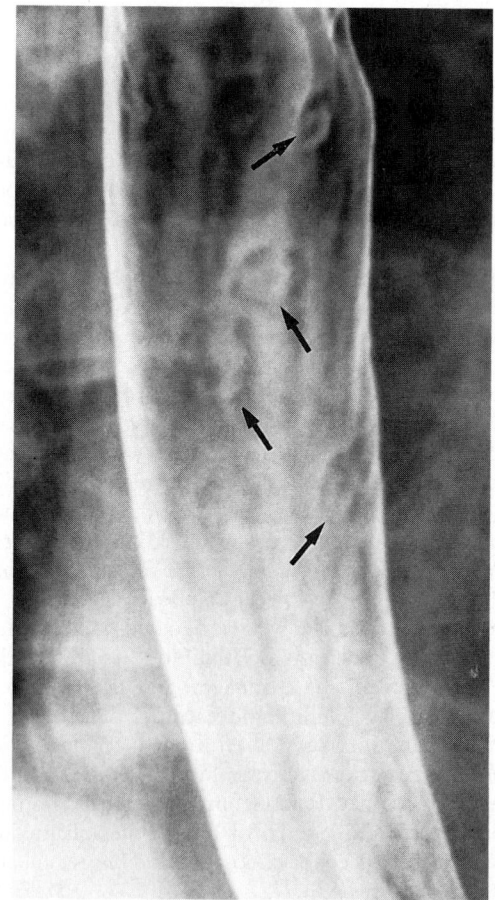

FIGURE 119-8. Herpes esophagitis with discrete superficial ulcers (*arrows*) on relatively normal background mucosa. Radiolucent halos of edematous mucosa surround the ulcers. (From Levine MS, Woldenberg R, Herlinger H, Laufer I. Opportunistic esophagitis in AIDS: radiographic diagnosis. Radiology 1987;165: 815.)

Erosive Gastritis

Gastric erosions may be classified radiographically as complete or incomplete erosions. Most patients have complete or varioliform erosions in which a punctate or slit-like collection of barium is surrounded by a radiolucent halo of edematous mucosa (Fig. 119-9A).[29] Varioliform erosions are most commonly found in the gastric antrum and are often aligned on rugal folds. In contrast, incomplete or "flat" erosions appear as dots or streaks of barium without an edematous halo. Because the surrounding mucosa is normal, incomplete erosions have been extremely difficult to detect radiographically, accounting for less than 5% of all erosions seen on double-contrast studies.

Although no etiologic significance is attributed to the shape or location of gastric erosions, aspirin and other nonsteroidal antiinflammatory drugs may produce distinctive linear or serpiginous erosions that tend to be clustered in the body of the stomach, on or near the greater curvature (Fig. 119-9B).[30] It has been postulated that these erosions result from localized mucosal injury as the dissolving tablets collect by gravity in the most dependent portion of the stomach. If recent ingestion of these drugs is confirmed, withdrawal of the offending agent should lead to a rapid clinical response.

Gastric Ulcers

In the past, some researchers have advocated endoscopy and biopsy of all radiographically diagnosed gastric ulcers to rule out cancer in these patients. However, several studies have found that virtually all gastric ulcers with an unequivocally benign appearance on double-contrast upper gastrointestinal examinations are benign lesions.[31,32] In those studies, about two thirds of all benign ulcers had a benign radiographic appearance. As a result, unnecessary endoscopy could be avoided in the initial evaluation of most gastric ulcers diagnosed on

double-contrast examinations. Instead, typically benign gastric ulcers could be followed radiographically to complete healing with no need for endoscopic intervention. Because endoscopy is a considerably more expensive procedure than double-contrast radiography, the potential financial savings are enormous.

Most gastric ulcers detected on double-contrast studies are smaller than 1 cm in diameter.[32] Although some benign ulcers are round and symmetric, others have a rod-shaped or linear appearance. Large areae gastricae are often observed surrounding the ulcer as a result of edema and inflammation of the adjacent mucosa. Almost all benign ulcers occur in the antrum or body of the stomach, and most are located on the lesser curvature or posterior wall (Fig. 119-10A).[32] Occasionally, benign gastric ulcers may be found on the greater curvature of the distal stomach. The latter ulcers are almost always caused by ingestion of aspirin or aspirin-containing compounds.[32] These aspirin-induced greater curvature ulcers have a tendency to penetrate inferiorly into the gastrocolic ligament, occasionally leading to the development of gastrocolic fistulas.[33]

Ulcer healing may be manifested radiographically by a decrease in the size of the ulcer and by a change in its shape. In most cases, ulcer healing produces a radiographically visible scar with a central pit or depression, radiating folds, or retraction of the adjacent gastric wall.[32] Although a residual depression could be mistaken for an active ulcer crater, the central portion of a reepithelialized scar sometimes can be differentiated from an active ulcer by the presence of normal areae gastricae within the scar (Fig. 119-10B).[32]

Gastric Carcinoma

Gastric carcinoma has a relatively bleak prognosis, with 5-year survival rates of only 10% to 30%. These tumors may appear radiographically as polypoid or ulcerated lesions or,

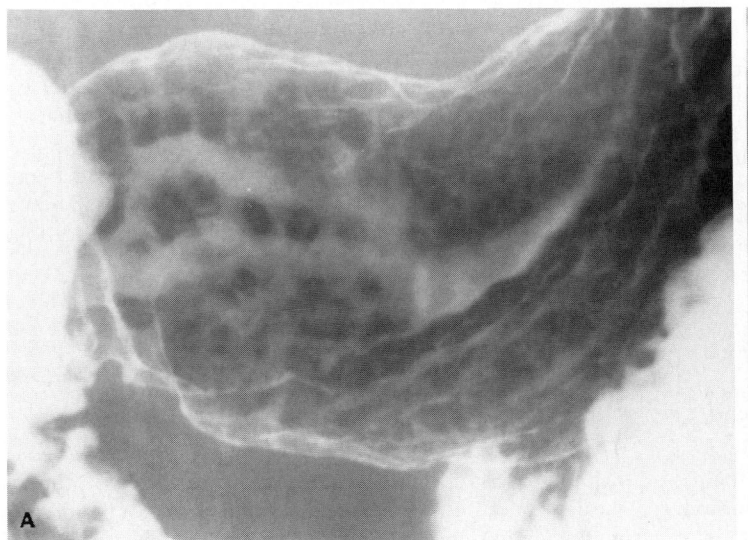 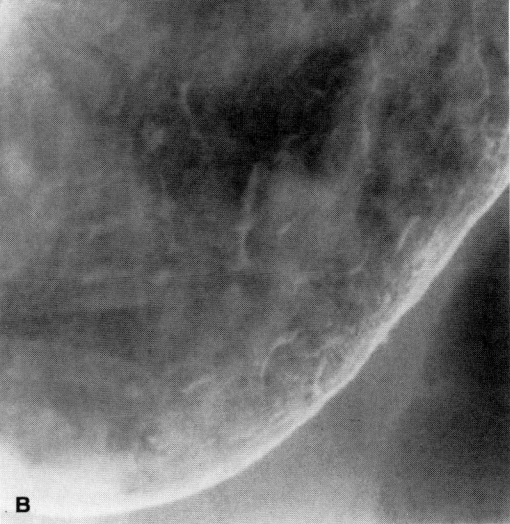

FIGURE 119-9. Erosive gastritis. **(A)** Typical varioliform erosions in the gastric antrum. The erosions are aligned on the rugal folds. **(B)** Linear and serpiginous erosions in the body of the stomach near the greater curvature are the result of recent ingestion of indomethacin.

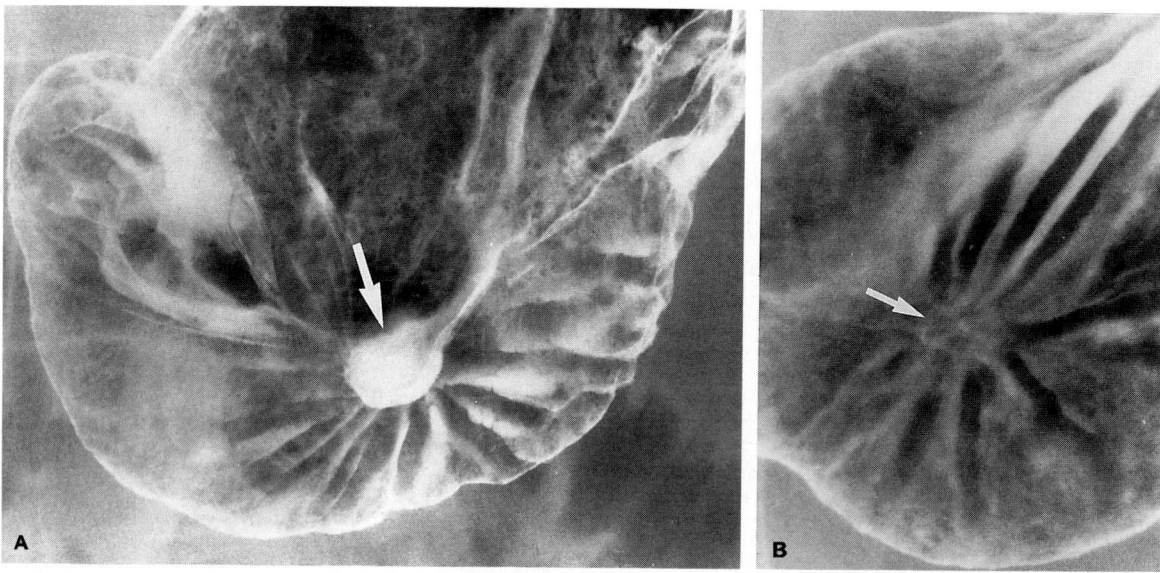

FIGURE 119-10. Benign gastric ulcer and ulcer scar in different patients. (**A**) Round, symmetric ulcer (*arrow*) on the posterior gastric wall, with smooth folds radiating to the edge of the crater. This ulcer has the typical radiologic features of a benign gastric ulcer. (**B**) Reepithelialized ulcer scar with radiating folds and normal areae gastricae (*arrow*) in the central portion of scar.

less frequently, as infiltrating lesions with diffuse narrowing of the stomach, producing a "linitis plastica" appearance. Early gastric cancer is a curable disease, with reported 5-year survival rates as high as 95%. The Japanese have developed an elaborate system for classifying these tumors based on whether they are predominantly elevated, flat, or depressed lesions. Unfortunately, most patients in the United States with gastric carcinoma already have advanced lesions at the time of clinical presentation, and early gastric cancer is unlikely to be detected on double-contrast studies or endoscopy as long as these examinations are performed predominantly on symptomatic patients.[34]

Duodenitis

Duodenitis may be manifested radiographically by thickened folds, mucosal nodules, erosions, or deformity of the bulb.[35] Duodenal erosions are detected less frequently than gastric erosions on double-contrast studies because of the difficulty in differentiating these lesions from normal mucosal pits. However, erosive duodenitis can be diagnosed when double-contrast radiographs reveal central barium collections surrounded by radiolucent halos of edematous mucosa.

Duodenal Ulcers

Unlike gastric ulcers, which occur primarily on the lesser curvature or posterior wall of the stomach, as many as 50% of duodenal ulcers are located in the anterior wall.[18] Because most double-contrast radiographs are obtained with the patient in a supine or supine oblique position, the anterior wall of the duodenum is not optimally coated with barium, and anterior wall ulcers may be missed on the double-contrast portion of the study. For this reason, double-contrast views of the duodenum should be supplemented with prone compression views obtained with a low-density barium suspension to demonstrate ulcers on the anterior wall. Thus, the biphasic technique is particularly important for evaluating the duodenum.

SMALL BOWEL

The conventional small bowel follow-through examination usually consists of a series of overhead abdominal radiographs obtained at regular intervals after ingestion of barium. With this technique, the small bowel is evaluated fluoroscopically only if the overhead radiographs appear abnormal. Because this technique is extremely unreliable in detecting pathology in the small bowel, this form of examination should have no place in modern radiologic practice. Instead, adequate evaluation of the small bowel requires more detailed methods of examination, such as the small bowel meal and small bowel enema. However, these techniques require time, effort, and interest by the radiologist. Barium studies of the small bowel should be requested only if there are legitimate indications of small bowel disease.

Techniques

Small Bowel Meal

The "dedicated" or "fluoroscopic" small bowel meal (SBM) includes overhead films but uses fluoroscopy as the primary means of examining the small bowel. Metoclopramide (20 mg) is administered orally 20 minutes before the examination to accelerate transit of barium through the stomach and small bowel. The patient then ingests 500 to 600 mL of an appropriate 35% to 40% (w/v) suspension of barium sulfate. After a brief examination of the upper gastrointestinal tract, intermittent fluoroscopy is performed until all small bowel loops have been demonstrated. Periodic spot films are obtained to document the fluoroscopic findings.

Small Bowel Enema

The small bowel enema (SBE) permits a more detailed examination of the entire small bowel.[36] The patient first receives 20 mg of oral metoclopramide to accelerate small bowel transit. The distal duodenum or proximal jejunum is then intubated, preferably with a balloon catheter to prevent reflux of contrast into the stomach. Approximately 200 to 240 mL of a 75% to 80% (w/v) suspension of barium is injected into the small bowel, followed by 1500 to 2000 mL of a 0.5% solution of methylcellulose. This is a biphasic examination that permits demonstration of the small bowel first by single-contrast and then by double-contrast technique (Fig. 119-11). The radiologist must be present throughout the examination to observe the flow of contrast through the small bowel, to assess individual small bowel loops with graded abdominal compression, and to document the fluoroscopic findings with periodic spot films. The examination is completed by obtaining an overhead radiograph of the entire small bowel.

Application of Techniques

Small Bowel Meal

The major advantage of the SBM is that it does not require intubation. Transit acceleration by oral metoclopramide is an important component of the examination, because it decreases

flocculation of barium and the time needed to perform the study. However, because acceleration is achieved by increasing small bowel peristalsis, lumenal distention is compromised by this technique.

The SBM is an appropriate examination for evaluating well-established diseases of the small bowel, such as Crohn's disease. It is also adequate for investigating pathologic processes that prevent lumenal distention, such as radiation enteritis, ischemia, and hematomas. This technique can be used to demonstrate the level and degree of small bowel obstruction, although it is less successful in determining the cause.

Small Bowel Enema

The major advantage of the SBE is that it combines transit acceleration with lumenal distention. The SBE also causes significantly less flocculation of barium than the SBM. As a result, the double-contrast images obtained on the SBE permit assessment of mucosal surface detail, even through overlapping small bowel loops. The straightening of mucosal folds that occurs with lumenal distention also permits detection of small, relatively subtle lesions. Normality becomes measurable in terms of wall thickness, fold thickness and height, and distance between folds.

The major indications for the SBE include the following:

Small bowel obstruction, particularly intermittent obstruction: SBE often permits differentiation of the various causes of obstruction.[37]

Malabsorption states: SBE may demonstrate findings of celiac disease, lymphangiectasia, Whipple's disease, or other conditions associated with malabsorption.

Crohn's disease: SBE permits delineation of the full extent

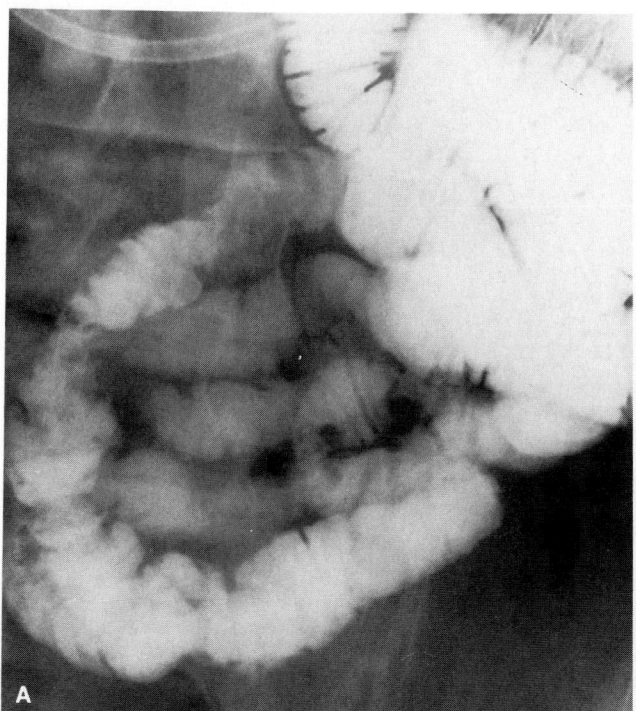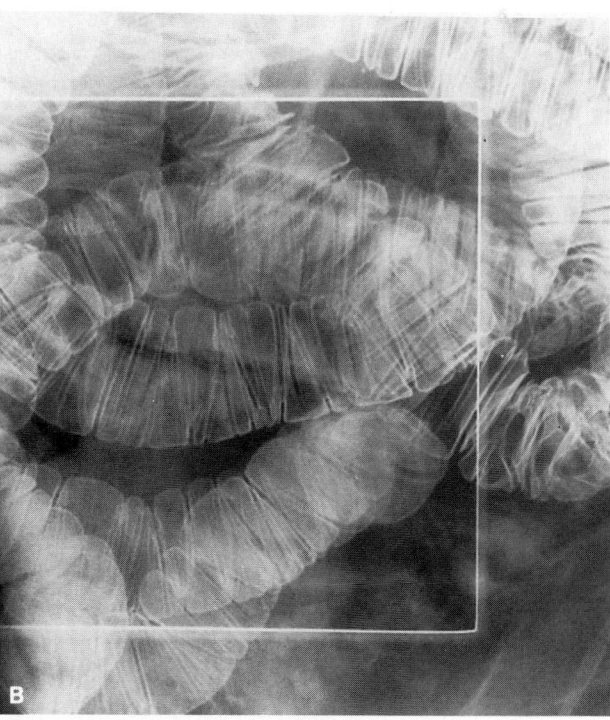

FIGURE 119-11. Normal small bowel enema. **(A)** Distal jejunum seen on a preliminary single-contrast examination. **(B)** Same jejunal loops on double-contrast examination.

of disease, including skip lesions, and can be used to detect complications such as strictures and fistulas.

Small bowel tumors, particularly primary and secondary malignancies and lymphoma.

Meckel's diverticulum: the ability to detect this abnormality is greatly improved on the SBE by increasing lumenal distention.[38]

Normality: SBE is the most reliable radiologic examination for establishing morphologic normality of the small bowel.

Abnormalities

Small Bowel Obstruction

Because of concern about the potential problem of barium inspissating above a small bowel obstruction, some surgeons prefer that a water-soluble contrast medium such as Gastrografin be used to evaluate these patients radiographically.[39] However, animal studies and clinical experience have shown that barium almost never inspissates in the small bowel.[40] High-osmolality water-soluble contrast agents tend to cause an outpouring of fluid into the obstructed small bowel lumen, diluting the contrast to such a degree that it is rarely possible to obtain a diagnostic examination. Water-soluble contrast agents should be used only to examine the small bowel in patients with suspected perforation, but barium should be used in patients with suspected obstruction. In the latter cases, the SBE is the best radiologic technique for delineating the site and cause of obstruction. If a decompression tube has already been placed in the small bowel, the SBE can be performed through the tube.

Adhesions. Adhesions account for almost 75% of small bowel obstructions. The SBE can identify features that favor obstruction by a single band, multiple bands, or extensive adhesions. Single bands are more likely to produce high-grade obstruction, closed-loop obstruction, or complications such as focal ischemia or strangulation. Multiple bands are almost always associated with adherence of the small bowel to anterior abdominal wall scars. Like extensive adhesions, they tend to produce low-grade small bowel obstruction. Because of its ability to distend the lumen, the SBE draws attention to single bands as a cause of low-grade or intermittent obstruction (Fig. 119-12), even when symptoms are minimal or absent.

Hernias. Barium studies are not required for small bowel obstructions caused by clinically evident external hernias. However, the SBE is extremely useful in detecting hernias of developmental or postsurgical origin, including peristomal, spigelian, or Richter's hernias.

Malignancy. In patients who have undergone laparotomy for abdominal malignancy, small bowel obstruction may be caused by adhesions, metastases, radiation, or residual tumor. These conditions can be differentiated by SBE in more than 80% of patients.[36] This information can facilitate surgical management by providing a preoperative choice between resection of tumor, bypass of radiation-damaged bowel, or lysis of adhesions.

Malabsorption States

Malabsorption is usually diagnosed by clinical and laboratory criteria. The purpose of barium studies is to determine the most likely cause of a clinically diagnosed malabsorption state

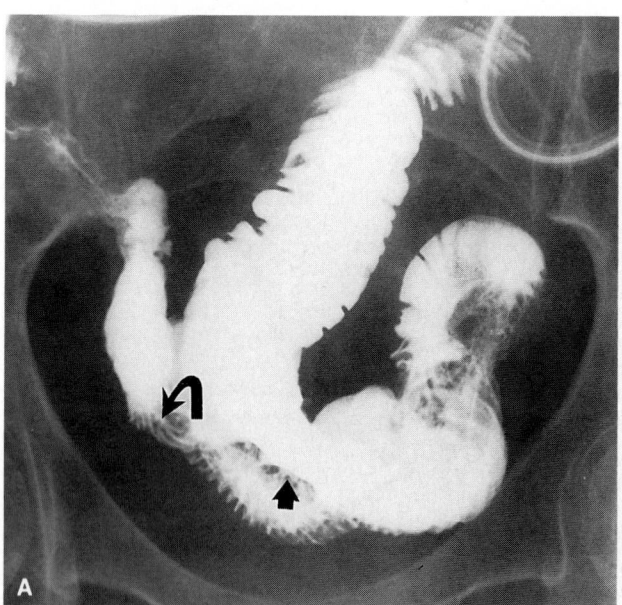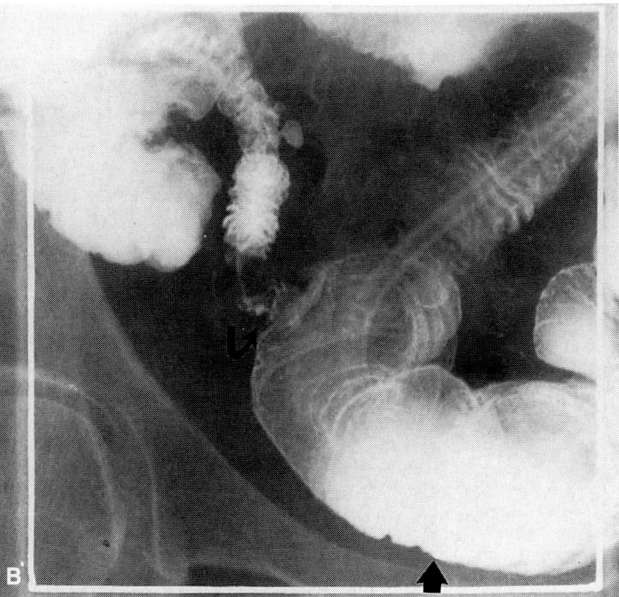

FIGURE 119-12. Small bowel enema by means of a Miller-Abbot tube shows low-grade obstruction due to an adhesive band. **(A)** The site of the obstruction is not obvious on single-contrast examination. **(B)** Lumenal distention during double-contrast examination permits diagnosis of a single-band obstruction. The position of the end of the tube (*straight arrow*) and the site of the adhesive band (*curved arrow*) are indicated.

or to document complications. In many conditions associated with malabsorption, abnormal accumulation of intralumenal fluid causes flocculation of barium on SBM. Because flocculated barium prevents accurate depiction of mucosal surface detail, the SBE is the preferred radiologic examination to accelerate transit and decrease flocculation of barium in the small bowel.

Celiac disease. The diagnosis of celiac disease must be firmly established to justify placing the patient on life-long dietary restrictions. A confident diagnosis can be made in patients who have characteristic mucosal changes on jejunal biopsy and have shown a satisfactory response to gluten withdrawal. However, about 50% of patients have atypical clinical presentations. Endoscopic biopsies are often taken from the duodenum, where interpretation may be limited by the presence of duodenitis. As a result, the diagnosis of celiac disease may first be suggested on SBE.

Although the findings on conventional barium studies are nonspecific, the SBE can demonstrate a measurably increased separation of folds in the distended proximal jejunum in patients with celiac disease (Fig. 119-13). In one study, zero to three folds per inch of jejunum were found on SBE in 73% of celiac patients but in only 2% of controls.[41] Conversely, patients with five or more folds per inch of jejunum rarely had celiac disease. Thus, abnormal separation of jejunal folds on SBE (i.e., zero to three folds per inch) suggests celiac disease.

The SBE can also detect various complications of celiac disease, including non-Hodgkin's lymphoma, ulcerative jejunoileitis, and intestinal carcinoma. Other complications, such as hyposplenism and the rare lymph node cavitation syndrome, may be detected by computed tomography (CT).

Bacterial overgrowth syndrome. Barium studies can accurately depict many structural abnormalities in the small bowel that cause stasis and subsequent bacterial overgrowth. These abnormalities include strictures, blind pouch and blind loop syndromes, jejunoileal diverticulosis, and coloenteric fistulas. Other patients with bacterial overgrowth syndrome may have chronic intestinal pseudo-obstruction due to scleroderma or other causes. Small bowel involvement by scleroderma may lead to intestinal dilatation with tightly spaced folds, producing the classic "hide-bound bowel."[42]

Intestinal lymphangiectasia. The primary and secondary forms of intestinal lymphangiectasia are manifested by nonspecific changes of fold thickening and fluid increase on conventional barium studies of the small bowel. With the SBE, it is possible to demonstrate tiny (1–3 mm) nodules that represent villi distended by dilated lacteals. Whipple's disease involving the small bowel may also be manifested by tiny nodules due to villi laden with foamy macrophages and para-aminosalicylic–positive material. A similar nodular pattern may be demonstrated in patients with macroglobulinemia, IgA deficiency, and other unusual conditions.

Crohn's Disease

Early radiologic findings of Crohn's disease in the small bowel include a coarse villous pattern of the mucosa, thickened folds, and aphthous ulcers (Fig. 119-14). The subsequent development of linear fissures and ulcers may produce a cobblestone appearance. Ulcers frequently occur on the mesenteric border of the bowel, with redundancy, pleating, and sacculation of the antimesenteric border. Advanced changes of Crohn's dis-

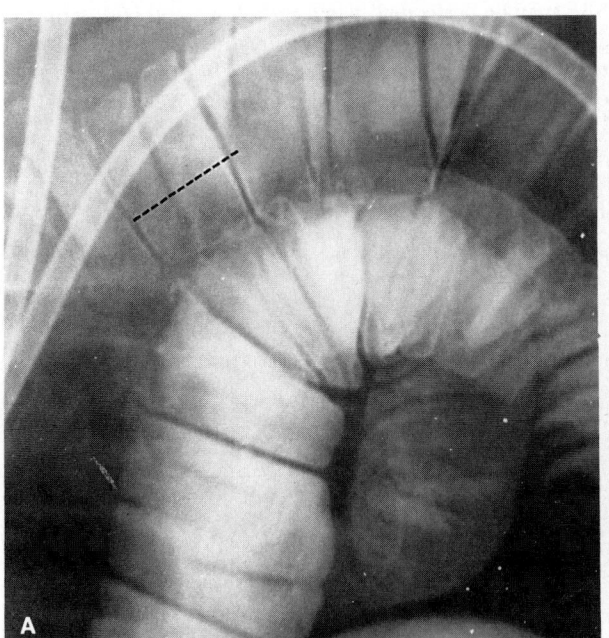 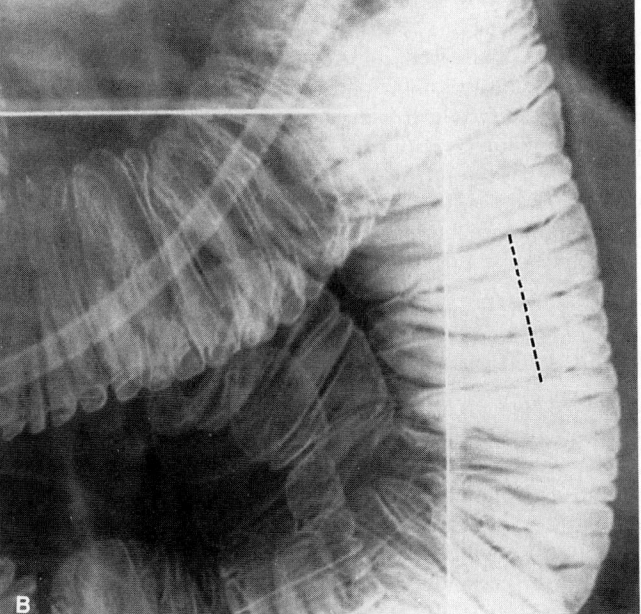

FIGURE 119-13. Diagnosis of celiac disease using a small bowel enema. **(A)** The distended proximal jejunum shows an increased separation of folds, with only three folds per inch (*dotted line*). **(B)** In comparison, the distended jejunum in a patient without celiac disease shows five folds per inch (*dotted line*).

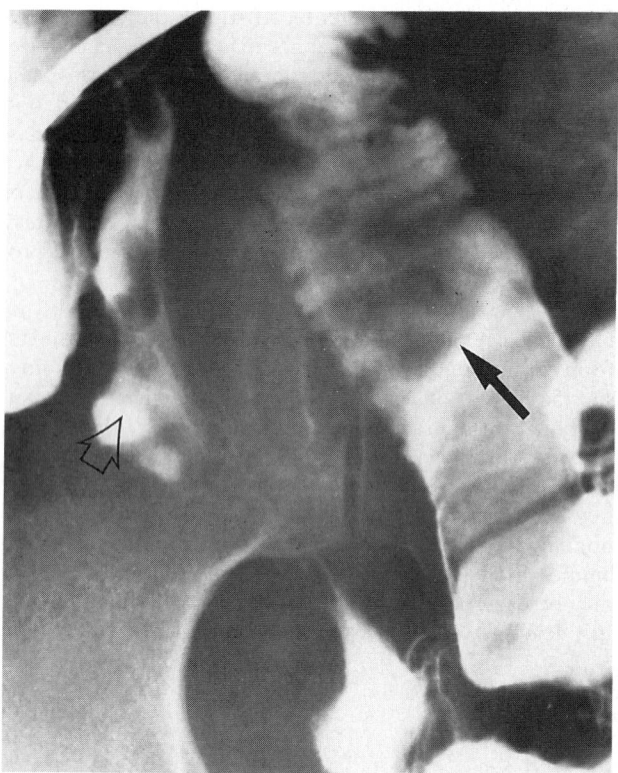

FIGURE 119-14. Advanced Crohn's disease in the terminal ileum (*open arrow*), with a more proximal segment of ileum containing thickened folds, coarse villous pattern, and aphthous ulcers (*arrow*).

ease include strictures, fistulas, inflammatory masses, and abscesses.

Many features of Crohn's disease can be demonstrated as effectively by the SBM as by the SBE. Disease of the terminal ileum is particularly well shown by combining the SBM with a peroral pneumocolon (i.e., introducing air into the rectum to distend the terminal ileum).[43] However, the SBE is the optimal radiologic examination for detecting early lesions, particularly the more proximal skip lesions. It is also a better examination for differentiating Crohn's disease from other pathologic conditions in the small bowel, such as lymphoma, tuberculosis, ischemia, metastatic disease, and adenocarcinoma.

Malignant Tumors

Adenocarcinoma. Most primary adenocarcinomas of the small bowel are advanced tumors with regional lymph node involvement at the time of clinical presentation. As a result, they most often appear radiographically as annular lesions. In the absence of obstruction, these tumors can be missed on conventional small bowel follow-through examinations, and the SBE is the best radiologic technique for diagnosing these lesions (Fig. 119-15).

Lymphoma. Primary small bowel lymphomas typically appear as cavitary lesions extending into the mesentery or as localized infiltrating lesions. In other patients with dissemi-

nated lymphoma, barium studies may demonstrate submucosal nodules of various sizes or mesenteric masses that secondarily infiltrate the bowel wall.[36] CT can be used to better delineate the extent of mesenteric and lymph node involvement.

Other malignancies. Small bowel carcinoids may be recognized on barium studies as multiple intramural lesions associated with distortion of folds and extension into the mesentery. CT may demonstrate the typical retractive changes caused by mesenteric metastatic masses. Less advanced carcinoid tumors may appear as small, submucosal nodules, most frequently in the terminal ileum. Both hematogenous and intraperitoneal-seeded metastases to the small bowel tend to occur as multiple lesions, often associated with signs of obstruction. Leiomyosarcomas may appear as excavated, exoenteric masses.

Meckel's Diverticulum

The SBE is the best radiologic technique for diagnosing Meckel's diverticulum, with an overall detection rate comparable to that found at autopsy.[38] The diverticulum arises from the antimesenteric border of the distal ileum, forming a blind sac, with a characteristic mucosal fold pattern at its site of origin. Occasionally, it is possible to identify a defect in the diverticulum due to ectopic gastric mucosa. An isotope scan may confirm the presence of gastric mucosa in the diverticulum, although this technique is less reliable in adults than in children.

Obscure Blood Loss

In patients with unexplained gastrointestinal blood loss, a SBE may be performed when radiologic and endoscopic examinations of the upper gastrointestinal tract and colon fail to demonstrate a source of bleeding. Unfortunately, the yield of the SBE in this clinical setting is relatively low. Many of

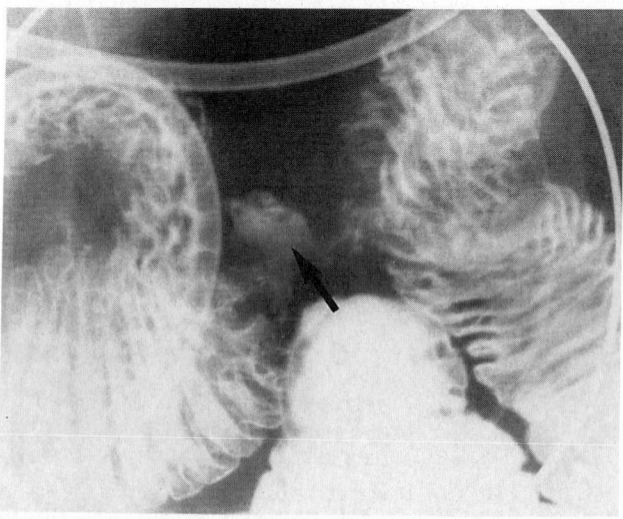

FIGURE 119-15. Annular adenocarcinoma of the proximal jejunum with a central ulceration (*arrow*).

these patients are ultimately found to have upper gastrointestinal or colonic lesions that were initially missed on barium studies or endoscopy. In almost 10% of cases, however, the SBE may demonstrate a tumor, ischemic lesion, Meckel's diverticulum, vascular malformation, or other abnormality in the small bowel to account for the patient's bleeding.[44]

COLON

For more than 70 years, the barium enema was used as the primary nonsurgical method for investigating the colon. In the past 20 years, colonoscopy has become an important diagnostic modality for evaluating the colonic mucosa and for removing polyps. Cross-sectional imaging techniques, particularly CT, have also become important for evaluating the extramucosal extent of disease. CT and ultrasound may also be used to assess bowel wall thickness. Because of its simplicity, low cost, safety, and accuracy, the barium enema remains the most widely used diagnostic technique for investigating the colon.

Single Versus Double Contrast

Radiologic examination of the colon can be performed by a single- or double-contrast technique. In single-contrast studies, the entire colon is filled with a relatively low-density barium suspension (Fig. 119-16*A*). The examination is performed under fluoroscopic control, with extensive palpation and compression of the colon as it fills. A postevacuation

radiograph is usually obtained to demonstrate additional mucosal detail. In double-contrast studies, a smaller volume of high-density barium is introduced into the colon, followed by insufflation of air. With this technique, the mucosal surface is coated by a thin layer of high-density barium, and the lumen is distended with air (Fig. 119-16*B*).

The double-contrast examination is considered to be the best radiologic technique for demonstrating fine mucosal lesions such as small polyps and the early changes of inflammatory bowel disease (IBD).[45,46] It can also better demonstrate segments of the large bowel that are inaccessible to palpation, such as the rectum and the hepatic and splenic flexures. The single-contrast barium enema is the preferred technique when careful control of the flow of barium is required. A single-contrast study should be performed in patients with suspected obstruction, diverticulitis, fistulas, or Hirschsprung's disease. This technique is also frequently used in patients who are too old or debilitated to tolerate a double-contrast study. During the past 15 years, the percentage of all barium enemas performed by double-contrast rather than single-contrast technique has increased from 20% to more than 40%.

Radiology Versus Colonoscopy

There is ongoing controversy about the relative roles of radiology and endoscopy in investigating colonic disease. In general, the choice of technique depends on the clinical setting and the relative skill and experience of the examiners. Nevertheless, it should be recognized that colonoscopy is primarily of value for detecting mucosal lesions. It should not be used

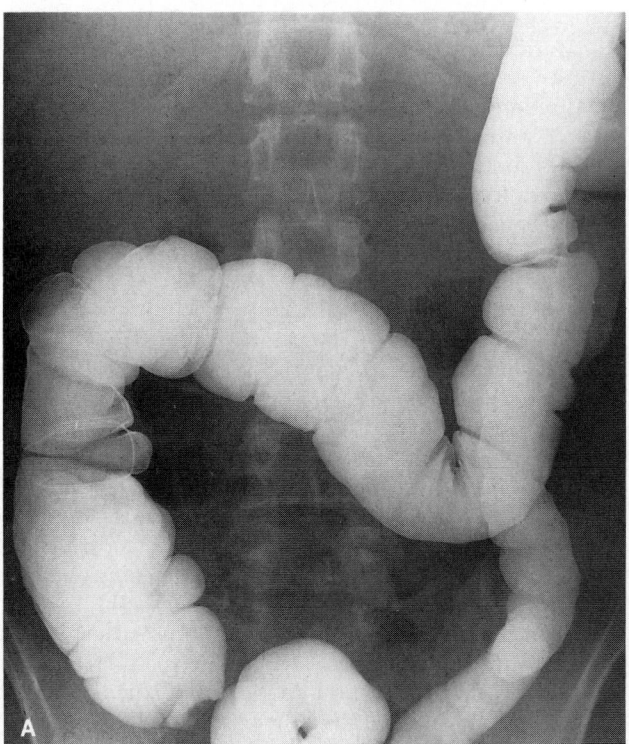
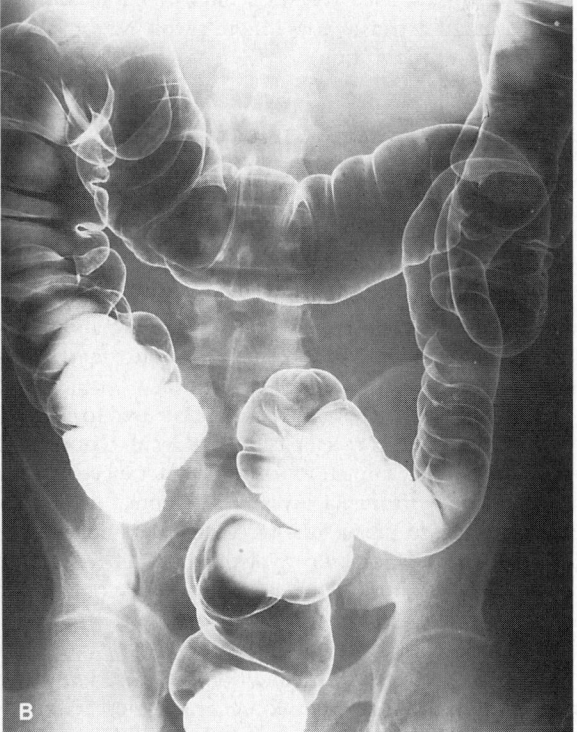

FIGURE 119-16. Normal appearances of the colon. (**A**) Single-contrast examination. (**B**) Double-contrast examination.

as the primary diagnostic modality when the patient's symptoms suggest an intramural or extrinsic lesion involving the bowel.

Colonoscopy probably is more accurate than radiology in demonstrating subtle mucosal abnormalities in the colon. When compared with high-quality, double-contrast barium enemas, this benefit applies primarily to the detection of polypoid lesions less than 1 cm in diameter and the early, preulcerative changes of IBD. However, this benefit must be balanced against the higher cost and complication rate of colonoscopy. The colonoscopist may be unsuccessful in advancing the endoscope to the cecum in 20% to 25% of patients, but the cecum is usually seen on barium enema studies.[47]

We recommend contrast examination of the colon for patients with symptoms that could be caused by diseases of the colon. This group includes patients with abdominal pain, constipation, change in bowel habit, and anemia. Colonoscopy is generally the examination of choice for the evaluation of uncertain radiologic findings, for removal or biopsy of lesions found at barium enema, and for the evaluation of patients who are at high risk for developing colorectal cancer or who are positive for fecal occult blood.

Indications

Although radiologic examination of the colon may be performed for a wide variety of indications, the most common include the following:

    Detection of colorectal polyps and cancer
    Assessment of the type, extent, and severity of IBD
    Diagnosis of diverticular disease and its complications
    Evaluation of extrinsic mass lesions involving the colon
    Evaluation of the rectum

Colorectal Polyps and Cancer

The barium enema is the mainstay of diagnosis for patients with symptomatic colorectal cancer. It is a valuable technique for diagnosing the primary lesion and for detecting synchronous carcinomas elsewhere in the colon. The double-contrast barium enema has an overall accuracy of approximately 95% in diagnosing colorectal cancer. However, there appears to be an irreducible minimum error rate of approximately 5%, primarily the result of perceptive error.[48]

The double-contrast barium enema is also used to evaluate patients who have overt rectal bleeding or occult blood in the stool on routine screening tests for colorectal cancer. In such cases, the goal is to detect invasive carcinomas and small adenomas that are precursors of colonic carcinoma (Fig. 119-17). These adenomatous polyps should be removed endoscopically to prevent the subsequent development of cancer.[49]

The double-contrast barium enema also has a role in the surveillance of patients with conditions that are known to predispose patients to the development of colorectal carcinoma. Such high-risk patients include those with a personal or family history of colon cancer or polyps and those with a history of chronic ulcerative colitis. For these high-risk groups,

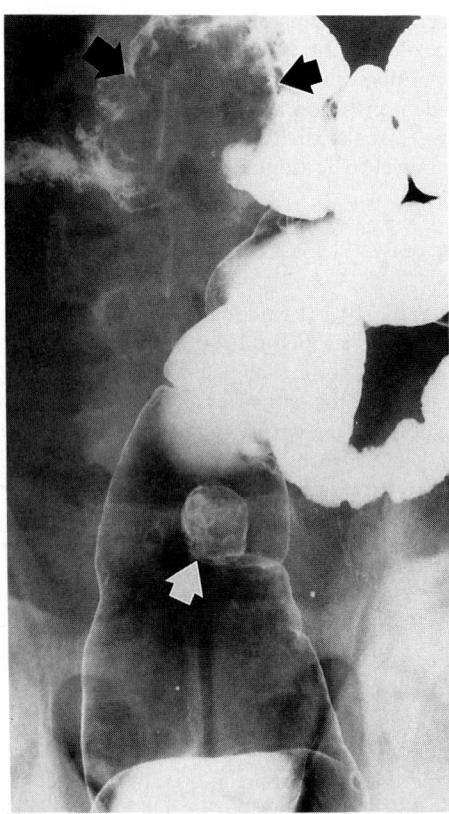

FIGURE 119-17. Example of a coexisting carcinoma and benign adenoma in the same patient. Notice the polypoid carcinoma (*black arrows*) in the transverse colon and small tubulovillous adenoma (*white arrow*) in the distal sigmoid colon.

we recommend a screening program that alternates colonoscopy and double-contrast barium enema to maximize the diagnostic yield.

Contrast examination of the colon may also have a role in the routine screening of patients for colorectal cancer. Eddy and colleagues suggested that annual fecal occult blood testing and barium enema every 5 years may be the most cost-effective way of reducing the mortality from colorectal cancer.[50]

Inflammatory Bowel Disease

Radiologic examination of the colon serves a variety of purposes in patients with known or suspected IBD. It can establish the presence of disease in patients who have not had prior sigmoidoscopy or in those who have had a negative sigmoidoscopy because the disease did not involve the rectosigmoid colon. It can also define the extent of disease in the colon. This information is particularly important in patients with ulcerative colitis, because the risk of developing carcinoma is related to the extent of colonic involvement.

Radiologic examination of the colon can differentiate ulcerative from granulomatous colitis. In typical cases, ulcerative colitis is characterized on double-contrast radiographs by a granular mucosa involving the rectum and extending proximally to a variable degree (Fig. 119-18A). In contrast, granulomatous colitis is characterized by a progression from discrete aphthous ulcers (Fig. 119-18B) to transmural disease

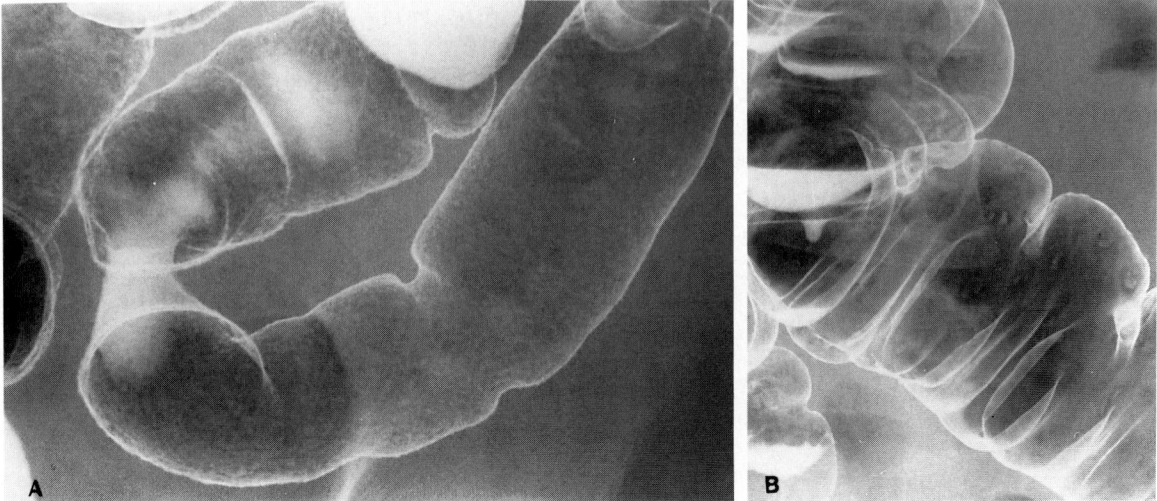

FIGURE 119-18. Early findings of inflammatory bowel disease detected by a double-contrast barium enema. (**A**) Ulcerative colitis with typical granular mucosa in sigmoid colon. (**B**) Granulomatous colitis with discrete, aphthous ulcers in the transverse colon.

with deep ulcers, fissures, fistulas, and abscesses. The rectum is often spared, and colonic involvement tends to be discontinuous and patchy.

Radiologic examination also can detect the complications of chronic ulcerative or granulomatous colitis, including the development of strictures, abscesses, fistulas, and inflammatory or postinflammatory polyps. In patients who develop colitic carcinoma, the tumor can be diagnosed, and in some cases, the development of dysplasia or "precancer" can be recognized on double-contrast studies.[51]

Diverticular Disease

Diverticular disease is one of the most common afflictions of Western society. The presence of massive diverticulosis poses a particular dilemma in interpreting double-contrast studies, because the multiplicity of ring shadows makes it difficult to differentiate diverticula from polyps. As a result, single-contrast studies may be easier to interpret than double-contrast studies in patients with severe diverticular disease.

Diverticulitis is a complication of diverticulosis in which a diverticular perforation leads to the formation of a pericolic abscess. Because barium may extravasate into the abscess, it is important to control the flow of barium into the colon in these patients, and a single-contrast barium enema is our preferred technique for diagnosing diverticulitis (Fig. 119-19). CT may also be helpful for demonstrating the extent of extracolonic abscess formation in some patients.[52]

Extrinsic Mass Lesions

In patients with abdominal or pelvic masses, the barium enema is a useful technique for determining whether the colon is displaced, compressed, or actually invaded by these lesions. The barium enema can also detect intraperitoneal seeding of the colon by metastatic tumor, inflammatory lesions, or endometriosis. In many cases, the barium study must be correlated with CT or other cross-sectional imaging modalities to determine the true extent of disease in the abdomen.

Rectum

When barium enemas were performed primarily by the single-contrast technique, the rectum was not considered to be in the province of radiology. With the use of the double-contrast technique, the rectum has become one of the simplest portions of the large bowel to evaluate radiographically.

The anatomy of the rectum, including the columns of Morgagni and the valves of Houston, can be demonstrated in exquisite detail (Fig. 119-20A).[53] Radiologic evaluation of the rectum is particularly important for the diagnosis of rectal tumors, IBD, and other unusual conditions such as the solitary rectal ulcer syndrome.[54] The double-contrast examination can

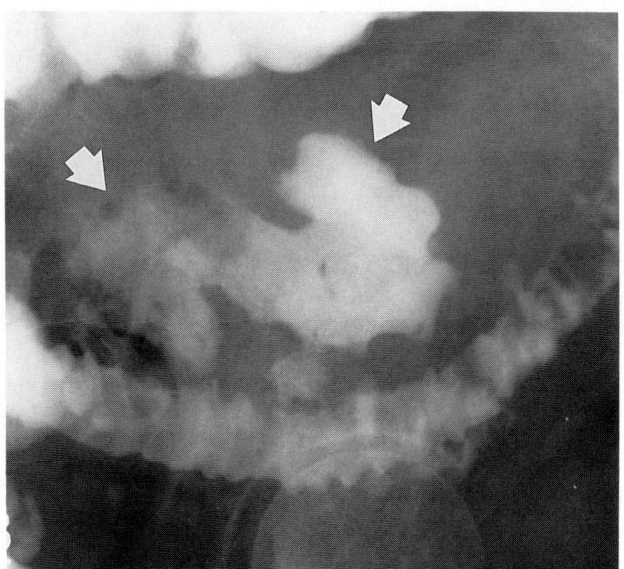

FIGURE 119-19. Diverticulitis with pericolic abscess. Barium has extravasated from a perforated diverticulum into an abscess (*arrows*). Notice the diverticula in the sigmoid colon.

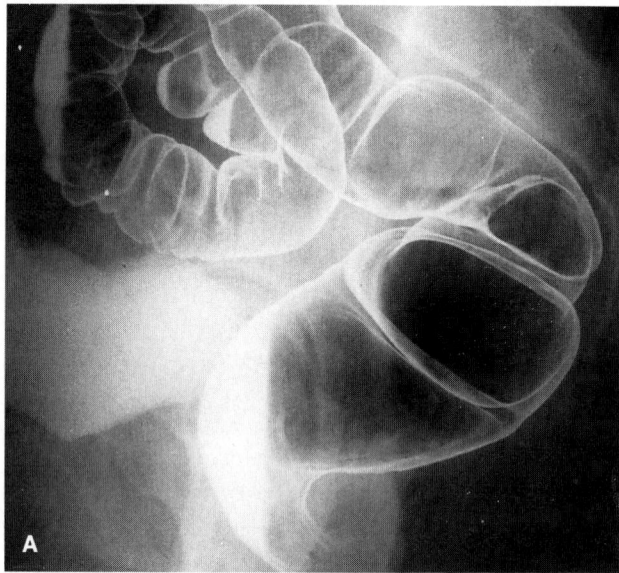
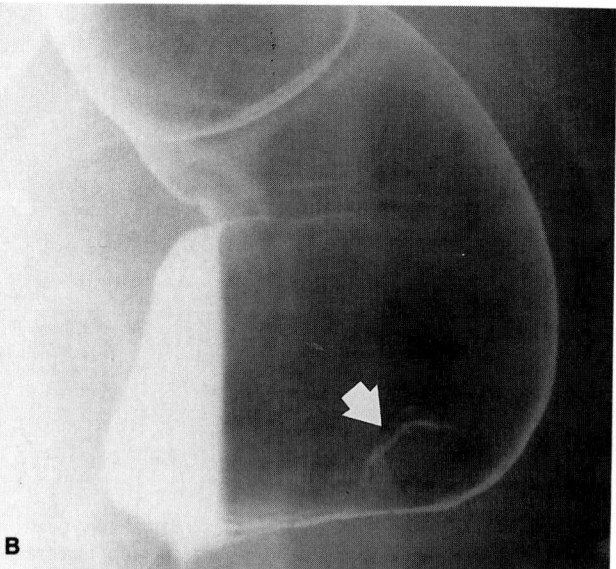

FIGURE 119-20. (A) Normal anatomy of the rectum shown on a cross-table lateral film. (B) Villous carcinoma (*arrow*) of the posterior wall of the rectum that had been missed on prior digital and proctoscopic examinations.

detect rectal carcinomas that are missed by digital rectal examination and proctoscopy (Fig. 119-20B).[55] The routine double-contrast barium enema should include a careful examination of the rectum.

Contraindications

The barium enema examination is generally a safe procedure, but there are several conditions for which the study is contraindicated or should be performed with extreme caution. These conditions include toxic megacolon, ischemic colitis, or other diseases in which the bowel wall is friable and more likely to perforate during the procedure. When a colonic perforation is suspected, the radiologic examination should be performed with water-soluble iodinated contrast material that can be reabsorbed from the peritoneal cavity if extravasation occurs.

Complications

The most feared complication of the barium enema is colonic perforation.[56] When this complication occurs, the perforation usually involves the intraperitoneal portion of the colon. Extravasated barium in the peritoneal cavity may be seen outlining loops of bowel. Surgical treatment is usually required. On some double-contrast barium enemas, a colonic perforation may be manifested only by a pneumoperitoneum without extravasation of barium into the peritoneal cavity. If these patients are aggressively treated with intravenous fluids and antibiotics, surgery may be avoided in some cases.

Retroperitoneal perforations usually result from laceration of the rectum by an inflated retention balloon on the enema tip in cases of diffuse rectal disease, such as ulcerative or radiation proctitis. In such cases, barium may be observed radiographically in the rectal wall or in the perirectal soft tissues. Because of the risk of rectal laceration, it is our practice not to inflate the retention balloon routinely. When the balloon is required in patients who have poor anal sphincter tone, it should be inflated under careful fluoroscopic control after barium has been instilled into the rectum.

Despite a few complications, the barium enema examination is a safe, simple, and relatively inexpensive procedure. It provides reliable information about the nature and extent of mucosal disease and about disease within and outside the bowel wall. Most patients undergo barium enema to rule out colonic neoplasm or IBD, and a double-contrast study is the best radiologic technique for evaluating these individuals. In other patients with suspected diverticulitis or colonic obstruction, a single-contrast barium enema should be performed. Whether single- or double-contrast technique is used, the barium enema examination has few contraindications, and the complications can be minimized by careful attention to the clinical history and examination technique. In complicated or difficult cases, correlation of the radiologic and endoscopic findings may be necessary to clarify the nature and extent of colonic disease.

> The reader is directed to Chapter 115, Upper Gastrointestinal Endoscopy; Chapter 116, Colonoscopy and Flexible Sigmoidoscopy; and Chapter 120, Cross-Sectional Anatomy.

REFERENCES

1. Donner MW, Jones BJ. The multidisciplinary approach to dysphagia. Gastrointest Radiol 1985;10:194.
2. Donner MW, Bosma JF, Robertson DL. Anatomy and physiology of the pharynx. Gastrointest Radiol 1985;10:196.

3. Rubesin SE, Jessurun J, Robertson D, et al. Lines of the pharynx. Radiographics 1987;7:217.

4. Ekberg O, Wahlgren L. Dysfunction of pharyngeal swallowing: a cineradiographic study in 854 dysphagial patients. Acta Radiol Diagn 1985;26:389.

5. Ekberg O, Nylander G. Cineradiography of the pharyngeal stage of deglutition in 250 patients with dysphagia. Br J Radiol 1982;55:258.

6. Ekberg O, Nylander G. Double-contrast examination of the pharynx. Gastrointest Radiol 1985;10:263.

7. Rubesin SE, Jones B, Donner MW. Contrast pharyngography: the importance of phonation. AJR 1987;148:269.

8. Perrott JW. Anatomical aspects of hypopharyngeal diverticula. Aust N Z J Surg 1962;31:307.

9. Zaino C, Jacobson HG, Lepow H, Ozturk C. The pharyngoesophageal sphincter. Radiology 1967;89:639.

10. Ekberg O. The cricopharyngeus revisited. Br J Radiol 1986;59:875.

11. Ekberg O, Nylander G. Cineradiography of the pharyngeal stage of deglutition in 150 individuals without dysphagia. Br J Radiol 1982;55:253.

12. Bachman AL, Seaman WB, Macken KL. Lateral pharyngeal diverticula. Radiology 1968;91:774.

13. Balfe DM, Heiken JP. Contrast evaluation of structural lesions of the pharynx. Curr Probl Diagn Radiol 1986;15:73.

14. Semenkovich JW, Balfe DM, Weyman PJ, et al. Barium pharyngography: comparison of single and double contrast. AJR 1985;144:715.

15. Bachman AL. Benign non-neoplastic conditions of the larynx and pharynx. Radiol Clin North Am 1978;16:273.

16. Rubesin SE, Glick SN. The tailored double-contrast pharyngogram. Crit Rev Diagn Imaging 1988;28:133.

17. Goldstein HM, Zornoza J. Association of squamous cell carcinoma of the head and neck with cancer of the esophagus. AJR 1978;131:791.

18. Levine MS, Rubesin SE, Herlinger H, Laufer I. Double contrast upper gastrointestinal examination: technique and interpretation. Radiology 1988;168:593.

19. Graziani L, Bearzi I, Romagnoli A, et al. Significance of diffuse granularity and nodularity of the esophageal mucosa at double-contrast radiography. Gastrointest Radiol 1985;10:1.

20. Levine MS, Kressel HY, Caroline DF, et al. Barrett esophagus: reticular pattern of the mucosa. Radiology 1983;147:663.

21. Gilchrist AM, Levine MS, Carr RF, et al. Barrett's esophagus: diagnosis by double-contrast esophagography. AJR 1988;150:97.

22. Mathieson R, Dutta SK. *Candida* esophagitis. Dig Dis Sci 1983;28:365.

23. Levine MS, Macones AJ, Laufer I. *Candida* esophagitis: accuracy of radiographic diagnosis. Radiology 1985;154:581.

24. Levine MS, Woldenberg R, Herlinger H, Laufer I. Opportunistic esophagitis in AIDS: radiographic diagnosis. Radiology 1987;165:815.

25. Levine MS, Loevner LA, Saul SH, et al. Herpes esophagitis: sensitivity of double-contrast esophagography. AJR 1988;151:57.

26. Levine MS, Loercher G, Katzka DA, et al. Giant human immunodeficiency virus-related ulcers in the esophagus. Radiology 1991;180:323.

27. Levine MS, Dillon EC, Saul SH, Laufer I. Early esophageal cancer. AJR 1986;146:507.

28. Itai Y, Kogure T, Okuyama Y, Akiyama H. Superficial esophageal carcinoma: radiological findings in double-contrast studies. Radiology 1978;126:597.

29. Laufer I, Hamilton J, Mullens JE. Demonstration of superficial gastric erosions by double contrast radiography. Gastroenterology 1975;68:387.

30. Levine MS, Verstandig A, Laufer I. Serpiginous gastric erosions caused by aspirin and other nonsteroidal antiinflammatory drugs. AJR 1986;146:31.

31. Thompson G, Somers S, Stevenson GW. Benign gastric ulcer; a reliable radiologic diagnosis? AJR 1983;143:331.

32. Levine MS, Creteur V, Kressel HY, et al. Benign gastric ulcers: diagnosis and follow-up with double contrast radiography. Radiology 1987;164:9.

33. Levine MS, Kelly MR, Laufer I, et al. Gastrocolic fistulas: the increasing role of aspirin. Radiology 1993;187:359.

34. White RM, Levine MS, Enterline HT, Laufer I. Early gastric cancer: recent experience. Radiology 1985;155:25.

35. Gelfand DW, Dale WJ, Ott DJ, et al. Duodenitis: endoscopic-radiologic correlation in 272 patients. Radiology 1985;157:577.

36. Herlinger H, Maglinte DDT. Clinical radiology of the small intestine. Philadelphia: WB Saunders, 1989.

37. Caroline DF, Herlinger H, Laufer I, et al. Small-bowel enema in the diagnosis of adhesive obstructions. AJR 1984;142:1133.

38. Maglinte DDT, Elmore MF, Isenberg M, Dolan PA. Meckel's diverticulum: radiologic demonstration by enteroclysis. AJR 1980;134:925.

39. Ellis H. Special forms of intestinal obstruction. In: Maingot R, ed. Abdominal operations. 7th ed. New York: Appleton-Century-Crofts, 1980.

40. Nelson SW, Christoforidis AJ. The use of barium sulfate suspensions in the study of suspected mechanical obstruction of the small intestine. AJR 1967;101:367.

41. Herlinger H, Maglinte DDT. Jejunal fold separation in adult celiac disease: relevance of enteroclysis. Radiology 1986;158:605.

42. Horowitz AL, Meyers MA. The "hide-bound" small bowel of scleroderma: characteristic mucosal fold pattern. AJR 1973;119:332.

43. Glick SN. Crohn's disease of the small intestine. Radiol Clin North Am 1987;25:25.

44. Herlinger H, Levine MS, Furth EE, Moonka D. Arteriovenous malformation of the small bowel diagnosed by enteroclysis. AJR 1992;159:1225.

45. Ott DJ, Gelfand DW. Colorectal tumors: pathology and detection. AJR 1978;131:691.

46. Laufer I, Mullens JE, Hamilton J. Correlation of endoscopy and double-contrast radiography in the early stages of ulcerative and granulomatous colitis. Radiology 1976;118:1.

47. Gilbert DA, Shaneyfelt SL, Silverstein FE, et al. The National ASGE colonoscopy survey—analysis of colonoscopic practices and field. Gastrointest Endosc 1983;29:188.

48. Kelvin FM, Gardiner R, Vas W, et al. Colorectal carcinoma missed on double contrast barium enema study: a problem in perception. AJR 1981;137:307.

49. Gilbertsen VA. Procto-sigmoidoscopy and polypectomy in reducing the incidence of rectal cancer. Cancer 1974;34:936.

50. Eddy DM, Nugent FW, Eddy JF, et al. Screening for colorectal cancer in a high-risk population. Gastroenterology 1987;92:682.

51. Stevenson GW, Goodacre R, Jackson R, et al. Dysplasia to carcinoma transformation in ulcerative colitis. AJR 1984;143:108.

52. Morris J, Stellato TA, Lieberman J, et al. The utility of computed tomography in colonic diverticulitis. Ann Surg 1986;204:128.

53. Laufer I. The double contrast enema: myths and misconceptions. Gastrointest Radiol 1976;1:19.

54. Levine MS, Piccolello ML, Sollenberger LC, et al. Solitary rectal ulcer syndrome: a radiologic diagnosis? Gastrointest Radiol 1986;11:187.

55. Evers K, Laufer I, Gordon RL, et al. Double-contrast enema examination for detection of rectal carcinoma. Radiology 1981;140:635.

56. Gelfand DW. Complications of gastrointestinal radiologic procedures: I. Complications of routine fluoroscopic studies. Gastrointest Radiol 1980;5:293.

Textbook of Gastroenterology, second edition, edited by Tadataka Yamada. JB Lippincott Company, Philadelphia © 1995.

CHAPTER 120

Cross-Sectional Anatomy

Lane A. Deyoe   Dennis M. Balfe

Abdominal Cavity
  Gastroesophageal Junction
  Stomach
  Liver
  Spleen
  Peritoneal Spaces

Pancreas
Duodenum
Small Intestine and Mesentery
Colon
Imaging of Abdominal Disease
Pelvic Anatomy

All medical imaging is problem-solving, and the problems confronting today's clinicians are not appreciably different from those of a century ago: "What is the diagnosis?" and "What is the overall extent of the disease?" Imaging helps to answer both of these questions.

Problems in diagnosis arise when patients present with clinical complaints that are nonspecific or confusing. Imaging in this situation is best at showing the site of disease. As an example, a patient experiencing left upper quadrant pain and fever may have unsuspected gallbladder disease. Imaging can depict the gallbladder wall and show the affected peritoneal spaces producing this unusual presentation (Fig. 120-1).

When the diagnosis is known or strongly suspected, assessing the extent of disease is important for guiding therapy. Preoperative evaluation of carcinoma is an obvious example of this kind of problem, but similar important questions arise in assessing inflammatory problems, such as evolving abscesses in granulomatous enteritis. The degree to which imaging succeeds is directly related to the correspondence between morphology and pathology. Computed tomography (CT) and all other imaging methods fail to detect metastatic lymph nodes unless they are enlarged. Cross-sectional imaging methods sensitive to abnormal physiology are being developed but are still unavailable as clinical tools.

Every radiologist has learned from experience that mastery of the full spectrum of normal variation is essential for recognition of what is abnormal. This chapter attempts to give readers an understanding of the fundamental relations of organ systems in the abdomen and pelvis, with specific attention to those observations important to solving clinical problems.

ABDOMINAL CAVITY

Gastroesophageal Junction

The anatomy of the gastroesophageal junction is difficult to display by any means but is probably easiest to understand in the transaxial projection.[1,2] The thoracic esophagus lies immediately anterior to the aorta (Fig. 120-2), traversing the diaphragm through a hiatus formed by separation of the fibers of the right crus. As the esophagus enters the abdomen, it passes to the left and anteriorly for 1 to 2 cm before joining the stomach. In its abdominal course, the esophagus lies posterior and to the left of the left lobe of the liver, anterior to the aorta, and to the right of the gastric fundus. Just inferior to its curved pathway is the superior recess of the lesser sac; perforations of the abdominal segment of the esophagus often enter that space.[3]

The diameter of the esophageal hiatus is variable and tends to expand with age. Abdominal fat and portions of the stomach commonly herniate into larger defects. Fluid accumulations, arising from pancreatitis or from massive ascites, may appear in the thorax, using the hiatus as a conduit.

Because of the complex curve of the esophagus and stomach at their junction, it is difficult to predict the radial spread of distal esophageal tumors with cross-sectional imaging techniques. A radially symmetric imaging tool, such as endoscopic ultrasound, may have promise in this region.

Stomach

The stomach takes on a variety of appearances on cross-sectional images, depending on the level and its degree of distention. Near the diaphragm, the cardia and fundus are

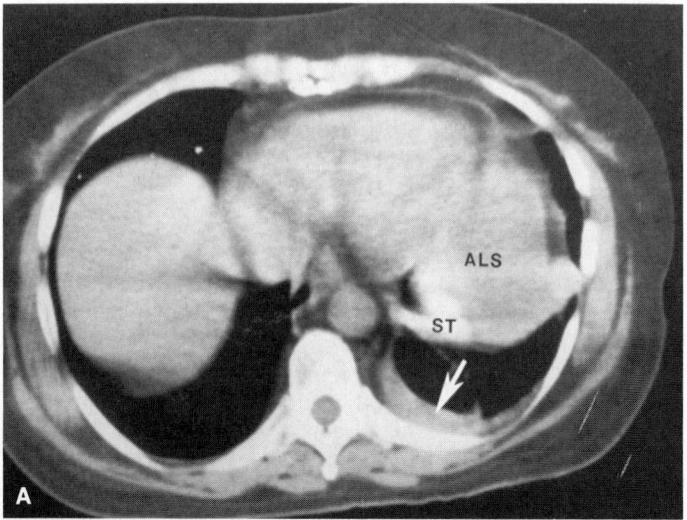

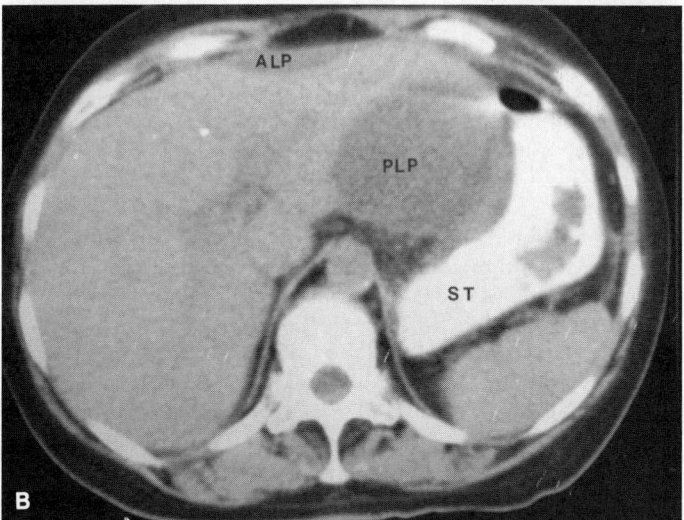

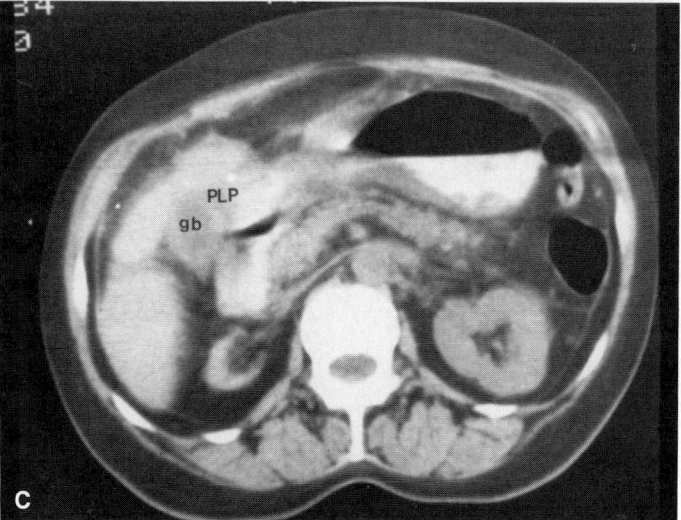

FIGURE 120-1. Anatomic depiction of a patient with a confusing clinical presentation: a 50-year-old woman with left upper quadrant pain, fever, and left pleuritic chest pain. (**A**) The CT section through the dome of the diaphragm shows an abscess (ALS) in the anterior left subphrenic space, pushing the stomach (ST) medially and posteriorly and producing a left pleural effusion (*arrow*). This was the cause of the patient's left pleuritic pain. (**B**) Three centimeters caudal to **A**, a CT section shows a large abscess (PLP) in the posterior left perihepatic space, with extension to the anterior left perihepatic space (ALP). The stomach (ST) is also seen in these sections. (**C**) Another section 4 cm caudal to **B** shows a thick-walled gallbladder (gb) with pericholecystic fluid (PLP) in the most caudal portion of the left posterior perihepatic space. The surgically proven gallbladder perforation with left peritoneal space abscess accounted for her unusual clinical presentation.

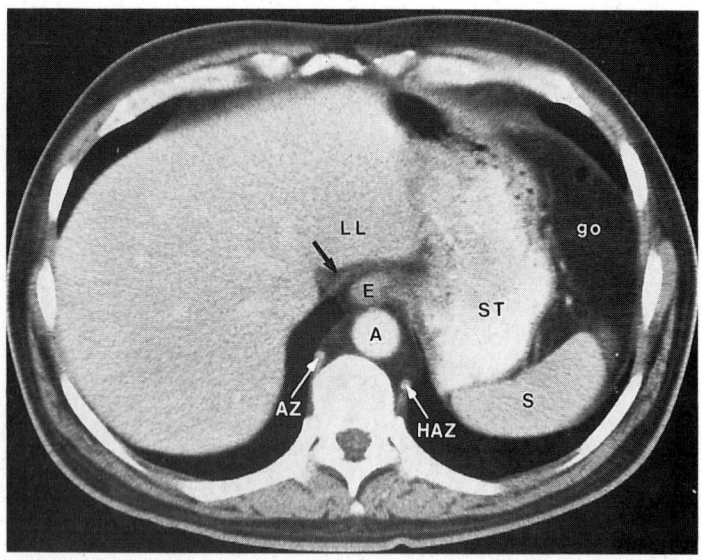

FIGURE 120-2. Gastroesophageal junction. The distal thoracic esophagus (E) lies in the posterior mediastinum, accompanied by mediastinal fat. It is anterior to the aorta (A), and to the azygos (AZ) and hemiazygos (HAZ) veins. (*Black arrow,* right crus of diaphragm; go, greater omentum; LL, left lobe of liver; S, spleen; ST, fundus of stomach.)

relatively posterior structures, bounded anteriorly by the tip of the left lobe of the liver and by the fat in the greater omentum, which usually curves lateral to the stomach as well (see Fig. 120-2). The spleen most often borders the posterolateral aspect of the stomach, and medially, the stomach abuts extraperitoneal fat. At the fissure for the ligamentum venosum, the lesser omentum connects the liver to the lesser curve.[4] On more inferior sections, the stomach turns first anteriorly and then to the right to form the body and antrum (Fig. 120-3).

The posterior wall of the stomach at these levels is the front wall of the lesser sac, and it abuts the pancreatic body and tail and the transverse mesocolon. Diverticula arising from the stomach almost always project posteriorly from the fundus, occupying a position posterior to the splenic vessels. A fluid-filled diverticulum may therefore mimic an adrenal mass.[5,6] The stomach turns posteriorly as it continues rightward, to form the pylorus at its connection with the duodenal bulb.

Cross-sectional imaging successfully depicts the thickness of the gastric wall, which should not exceed 1 cm when the stomach is well distended, and more important, it displays the extragastric spread of primary stomach tumors. Direct spread tends to occur along ligaments. Lesser curve tumors spread into the liver hilus by way of the lesser omentum (i.e., the gastrohepatic ligament), and greater curvature tumors may spread by way of the greater omentum, the gastrosplenic ligament, or the transverse mesocolon. The omentum is often involved by tumors that spread by peritoneal seeding.

On barium examination, the greater curve of the stomach shows only fixation and nodularity in cases of omental tumor spread; CT displays the extent of the tumor to better advantage.[7] The major lymph node groups that drain the stomach lie within the mesenteries also. Imaging techniques have been relatively insensitive in detecting metastatic involvement of these mesenteric nodes, chiefly because the nodes do not necessarily enlarge when they are involved with cancer.

Because the midportion of the transverse colon lies im-

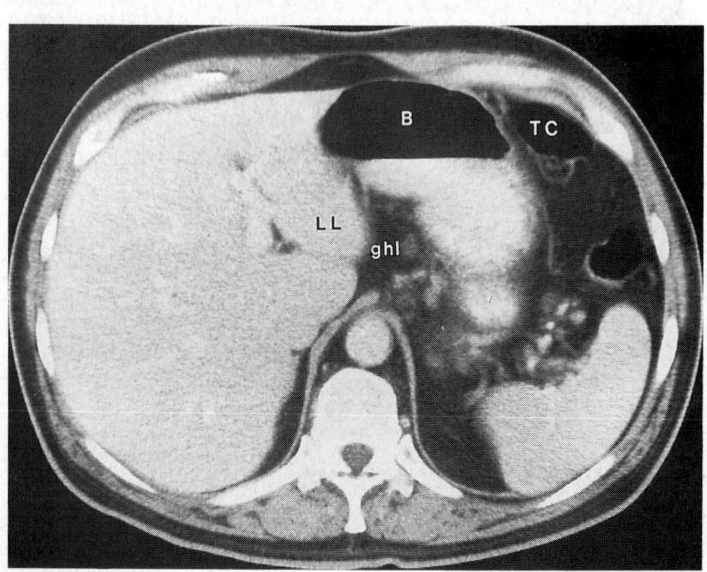

FIGURE 120-3. The gastric body (B) curves anteriorly and rightward, abutting the liver's lateral segment (LL) and arching over the gastrohepatic ligament (ghl). The transverse coion (TC) can also be seen at this level.

mediately inferior to the greater curvature of the stomach, transaxial sections cannot easily display their association; sagittal scanning by magnetic resonance (MR) imaging can define the interface much more easily.

Liver

Embryologically, the liver arises from the ventral mesogastrium and remains within that structure except for its upper posterior surface, which grows into the septum transversum.[8] The liver is connected to the anterior body wall by the ligamentum teres and falciform ligament, to the stomach by the lesser omentum, and to the diaphragm by the coronary and triangular ligaments. The hepatic region between the reflections of the coronary ligament is devoid of peritoneum and is termed the bare area. The diaphragmatic surface of the liver is smooth and featureless. The visceral surface faces predominantly downward, to the left, and medially, and it presents a series of indentations into which fit the right kidney and adrenal gland, inferior vena cava, hepatoduodenal ligament, and stomach.[9]

CT and ultrasound allow accurate interrogation of the internal architecture and identification of the vascular anatomy of the liver. Lesion detection and location is important, because patients with certain hepatic malignancies can benefit from surgical resection.[10]

Conventional hepatic segmental anatomy divides the liver into right and left lobes by the middle hepatic vein coursing in the interlobar fissure.[11,12] The right lobe is subdivided into anterior and posterior segments by the right hepatic vein. The left lobe is subdivided into medial and lateral segments by the left hepatic vein. The major hepatic veins are functionally important landmarks that guide hepatic surgery (Fig. 120-4).[13]

A more precise classification of hepatic segmental anatomy is based on the distribution of the hepatic and portal veins. The hepatic veins divide the liver longitudinally, and the portal veins divide it transversely. The result is a liver divided into eight segments (Fig. 120-5). The caudate lobe, which has a complex embryologic deviation from left and right lobes, is designated as segment 1. It is bordered posteriorly by the inferior vena cava, laterally by the ligamentum venosum, and anteriorly by the portal vein. Segments 2 (superior) and 3 (inferior) are lateral to the ligamentum teres within the left lobe. Segment 4, also known as the quadrate lobe, is medial to the ligamentum teres within the left lobe.

The middle hepatic vein and main hepatic fissure separate segment 4 (left lobe) from the right lobes. The plane of the right hepatic vein divides the right lobe into anterior and posterior segments. These are subdivided by the transverse plane formed by the right portal vein into superior and inferior segments. Segments 5 (anterior) and 6 (posterior) are the two inferior segments; segments 7 (posterior) and 8 (anterior) are the two superior segments.

Precise anatomic placement of lesions helps communicate accurate information to the surgeon for preoperative surgical planning and is useful for guiding intraoperative ultrasound assessment.

Each lobe is subdivided further by the left or right hepatic vein. Hepatic and portal veins are best seen in transaxial imaging planes; the main portal vein also is well visualized on coronal MR images. The inferior vena cava and its relation to the caudate lobe are best seen in sagittal section.

When liver diseases produce segmental or lobar hepatic atrophy, the relation of the liver and gallbladder to important external landmarks changes: the gallbladder may become superficial and rotate far posteriorly when the right lobe atrophies, presenting a hazard to percutaneous biopsy procedures. Similarly, the proximal transverse colon may occupy the space

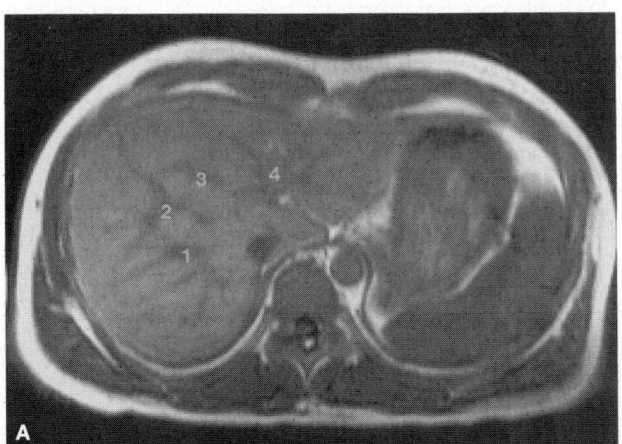 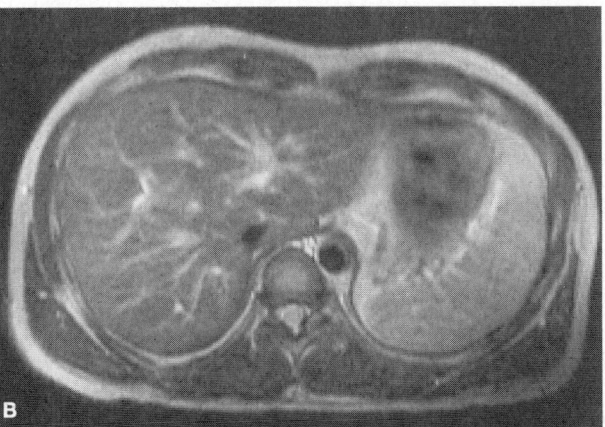

FIGURE 120-4. (A) In the T1-weighted magnetic resonance (MR) image of the upper abdomen, the normal spleen has a decreased signal intensity relative to the liver. Vessels and bile ducts have low signal intensities relative to liver parenchyma. Each hepatic segment is bounded by a hepatic vein and supplied by a central portal vein. This section also shows the right hepatic vein (1), right portal vein (2), middle hepatic vein (3), and left portal vein (4). (B) In a T2-weighted MR image at approximately the same level, the normal spleen has an increased signal intensity relative to the liver. However, in this sequence, the vessels and bile ducts have increased signal intensities relative to hepatic parenchyma.

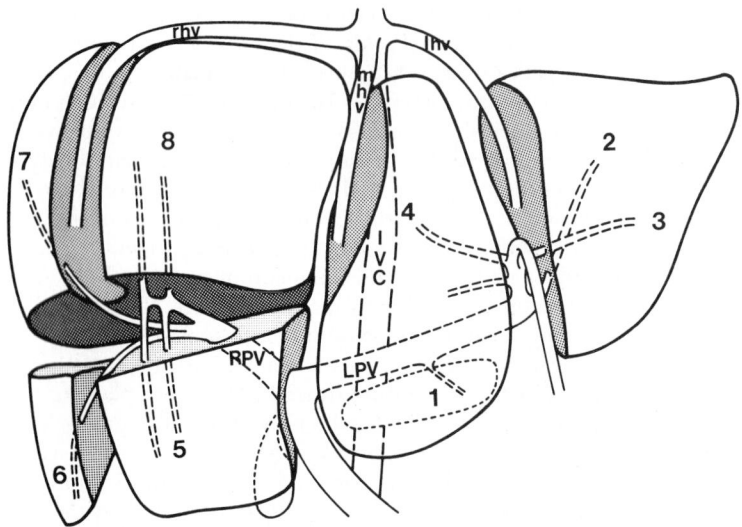

FIGURE 120-5. The diagram of the hepatic segments (1–8) shows the anatomic relations of the portal and hepatic veins. (Adapted from Lafortune M, Madore F, Patriquin H, Breton G. Segmental anatomy of the liver: a sonographic approach to the Couinaud nomenclature. Radiology 1991;181:443.)

between the diaphragm and the anterolateral surface of the liver.[14]

The lesser omentum and its contents are important structures that may be difficult to image. Abnormalities in the hepatic artery or portal vein are best assessed with Doppler ultrasound or MR, both of which are sensitive to flow phenomena and morphology. The lesser omentum is a major conduit for extrahepatic disease arising in the gallbladder, stomach, or pancreas and spreading into the liver hilus or for hepatic biliary disease spreading into the retroperitoneum.[15,16] A large group of lymphatics exist within the same pathway, between the inferior vena cava and the portal vein.[17]

Spleen

The spleen occupies a position posterior or posterolateral to the stomach. Its broadest surface is smooth and abuts the left hemidiaphragm. Its smaller visceral surface relates to the pancreatic tail at the splenic hilus, to the greater curve of the stomach (to which it is connected by the gastrosplenic ligament), and to the distal transverse colon. There is also a small nonperitonealized area on its medial inferior surface, related to the left adrenal gland and upper renal pole.[18]

The spleen is easily seen on CT and MR images of the abdomen. Administering intravenous iodinated contrast material when examining the spleen by CT is useful, but when contrast material is injected in a rapid bolus, most patients initially exhibit a heterogeneous pattern of splenic enhancement due to variable patterns of blood flow within different splenic compartments. It is important not to misinterpret this heterogeneous enhancement pattern as an indication of focal abnormality. In confusing cases, the area of interest should be rescanned 1 or more minutes after contrast material injection, at which time normal splenic parenchyma of uniform, homogeneous density will appear.

Peritoneal Spaces

The peritoneal spaces of the upper abdomen are not visible unless a fluid collection is present. However, they exert a profound effect on the distribution of such collections. In the embryo, the peritoneal spaces are bounded by the body wall laterally and anteriorly, the retroperitoneum posteriorly, and the mesenteries medially. During fetal growth, intramesenteric viscera (e.g., liver, spleen, pancreas) expand the mesenteries and undergo rotation so that the adult peritoneal spaces are considerably more complex than those of the embryo (Fig. 120-6).

The left peritoneal spaces include anterior and posterior perihepatic spaces, which surround the lateral segment of the left hepatic lobe, and anterior and posterior subphrenic spaces. The former lie between the stomach and the diaphragm and the latter between the spleen and the diaphragm.[19]

There are two portions of the right peritoneal space. The perihepatic portion follows the curve of the liver to the right of the falciform ligament posteriorly to the bare area. On caudal sections, the bare area gradually disappears, and the perihepatic space proceeds anteriorly and medially between the right hepatic lobe and the kidney. The second portion of the right peritoneal space is the lesser sac.[20] The small superior recess of the lesser sac surrounds the caudate lobe; it is continuous with the larger inferior recess, which occupies the broad space between the stomach and the pancreas.[21]

Imaging of peritoneal spaces is performed almost exclusively before draining abscesses. For this purpose, sagittal sections obtained by sonography or MR are useful in assessing left perihepatic fluid collections; the relation of the collection to the inferior tip of the left lobe is far easier to see with use of this plane (Fig. 120-7). All other collections are best imaged by transaxial sections. A path from skin to collection that does not require angulation of the needle out of a well-chosen transaxial plane can almost always be found.[22]

Pancreas

The pancreas arises from two mesenteric sources; the body and tail originate within the dorsal mesentery posterior to the spleen. This part of the mesentery rotates in a clockwise direction to fuse with the left part of the retroperitoneum. The head and uncinate process arise from a separate bud in the ventral mesentery; this portion first rotates counterclock-

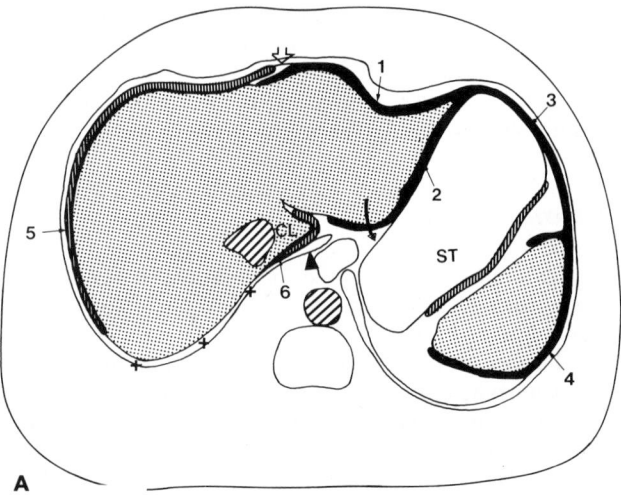 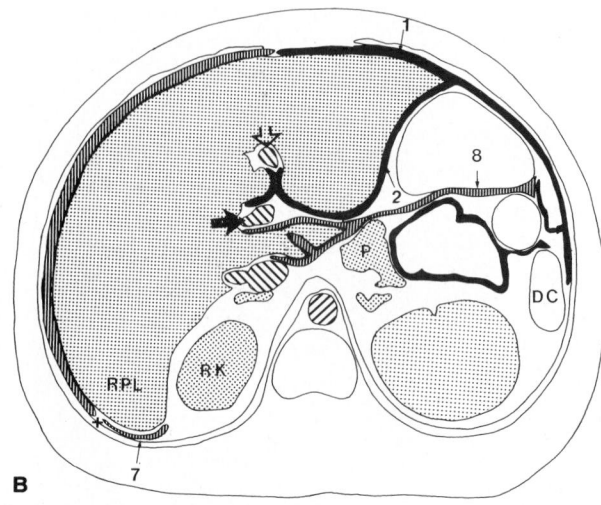

FIGURE 120-6. Peritoneal spaces. Schematic diagrams of cross-sectional anatomy: elements of the right peritoneal space are vertically hatched; elements of the left peritoneal space are solid black. (**A**) Section through the gastroesophageal junction. At this level, the left peritoneal space has four components: an anterior perihepatic space (1) to the left of the falciform ligament (*open arrow*); a posterior perihepatic space (2) along the lesser curve of the stomach (ST), limited on the right and posteriorly by the lesser omentum (*curved arrow*); an anterior subphrenic space (3) immediately anterior to the stomach; and a posterior subphrenic space (4) that almost encircles the spleen. The right peritoneal spaces include a perihepatic space (5), bounded by the right hemidiaphragm, and the superior recess of the lesser sac (6), which abuts the left surface of the caudate lobe (CL) and the right diaphragmatic crus (*arrowhead*). Between these spaces lies the bare area of the liver (+ + +), a broad, nonperitonealized zone that becomes progressively smaller as scans proceed caudally. (**B**) Four centimeters caudal to **A**, the left posterior perihepatic space (2) extends deep within the liver, abutting the left (*open arrow*) and main (*arrow*) portal vein. Fusion of the descending colon (DC) below the tip of the spleen has obliterated the perisplenic space. The right visceral space (7), or Morison pouch, lies on the posterior surface of the right lobe (RPL) and, on caudal sections, extends between the liver and right kidney (RK). The most caudal portion of the bare area (+), the triangular ligament, is revealed on this section. At this level, the inferior recess of the lesser sac (8) extends posterior to the stomach and anterior to the pancreas (P).

wise (as seen from below) with the duodenum to fuse to the right side of the retroperitoneum. The uncinate process then undergoes another counterclockwise 180-degree rotation and comes to lie medial and posterior to the rest of the pancreas, "wrapping around" the right side of the root of the small bowel mesentery. The superior mesenteric artery and vein therefore lie just posterior to the pancreatic neck. The artery is surrounded by mesenteric fat, and virtually no process except pancreatic cancer infiltrates this fat plane.[23]

Because the pancreas arises from the ventral and dorsal mesenteries, fluid collections occurring in pancreatitis can spread to affect any upper abdominal viscus. The left posterior renal fascia is commonly affected; the effusion dissects anterior to the left kidney, then splits the laminar renal fascia to produce a potentially large collection.[24] For most applications, transaxial imaging is the optimal means to image pancreatic pathology.

The pancreatic duct can be seen clearly on high-resolution CT or sonography, and either method can detect enlargement or intraductal calculi. The complex peripheral branching pattern, however, cannot be shown by any cross-sectional technique.

A long segment of the splenic vein passes immediately posterior to the pancreatic body and tail (Fig. 120-8). It is easy to understand how pancreatitis or pancreatic carcinoma could produce splenic vein occlusion resulting in short gastric and gastroepiploic collaterals. MR and contrast-enhanced CT are reliable in identifying the collateral vessels and often the splenic vein thrombus as well.

Duodenum

The duodenum spans the major landmarks of the upper abdomen, connecting stomach to jejunum, peritoneum to retroperitoneum, and the right side to the left. The duodenal bulb lies in the peritoneal cavity, just distal to the pylorus. Its lateral surface is often indented by the gallbladder; the free edge of the hepatoduodenal ligament courses posteriorly, containing the hepatic artery, portal vein, common bile duct, and several lymphatics.

The duodenum itself enters the retroperitoneum just lateral to the pancreatic head; the gastroduodenal artery lies in the fat plane that separates the two structures at this level. As it descends inferiorly, the duodenum passes anterior to the right perirenal space, often abutting the renal vein or renal pelvis. The third portion turns sharply leftward, just inferior to the left renal vein and uncinate process. It crosses anterior to the

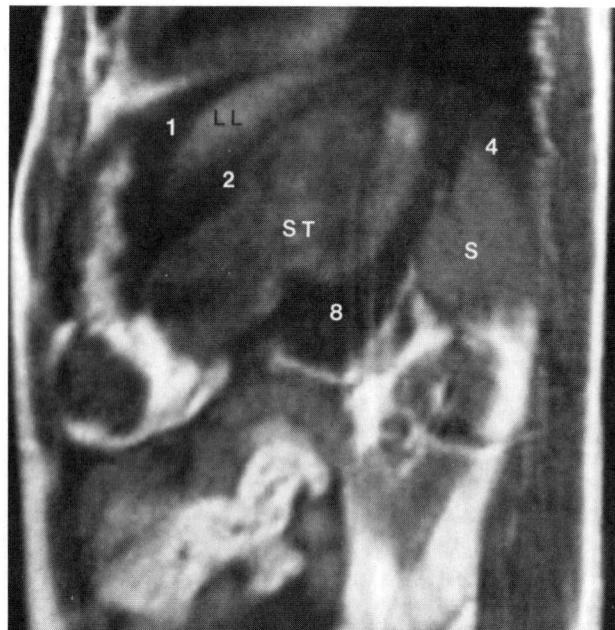

FIGURE 120-7. Malignant ascites. The sagittal magnetic resonance image through the lateral segment of the left lobe (LL) shows the anterior (1) and posterior (2) left perihepatic spaces and the posterior subphrenic space (4). There is a large collection of ascitic fluid in the inferior recess of the lesser sac (8). (S, spleen; ST, stomach.)

inferior vena cava, aorta, left ureter, and inferior mesenteric veins and posterior to the superior mesenteric vein and artery contained within the root of the small bowel mesentery.

Because of the duodenum's anatomic proximity to the perirenal spaces, duodenal processes may easily extend to involve the kidneys (usually the right), psoas muscles, and pancreas. Pancreatic processes are most likely to affect the duodenum before spreading to more distant sites.

No single imaging plane optimally displays the duodenum, but the important associations with the pancreas and perirenal spaces are generally best seen on transaxial sections.

Small Intestine and Mesentery

Small bowel loops fill most of the peritoneal cavity from the transverse mesocolon to the true pelvis. The root of the small intestine mesentery is a short (≈ 15 cm) structure identified on cross section by its contained superior mesenteric artery and vein. It originates from the undersurface of the pancreatic neck and courses to the right and inferiorly to end at the ileocecal valve. Fanning out segmentally from this central root are the leaves of the mesentery, which contain jejunal or ileal arteries and veins and accompanying lymphatics (Fig. 120-9). The mesenteric fat normally has the same CT attenuation as subcutaneous fat and contains no focal structures larger than 4 mm in diameter.[25] When adequately distended, the wall of the small bowel should not be thicker than 3 mm; plica circulares occasionally can be seen in jejunal segments but are rarely found in the ileum.

The root of the mesentery originates close to the pancreas and can be affected by pancreatic effusions. As it descends, it passes just anterior to the aorta, inferior vena cava, and right ureter. Crohn's disease involving the ileum occasionally infiltrates the perivascular fat to produce ureteral obstruction.

Colon

The abdominal portion of the colon is divided into four segments: cecum, ascending colon, transverse colon, and descending colon.

The position of the cecum is variable; it may lie within the pelvis in some individuals, particularly in women after hysterectomy. Its most common location is anteromedial to the right iliopsoas muscle, just behind the anterior abdominal wall. Loops of ileum usually occupy the space medial to the cecum, but a distended urinary bladder or, in women, the uterus or right ovary may be located near its medial surface. The appendix also courses through this space, somewhat posterior to the distal ileum. When it is retroperitoneal, the appendix may lie along the lateral border of the cecum and proximal ascending colon just anterior to the belly of the iliacus muscle.

The ascending colon begins at the ileocecal valve, which marks the end of the mesenteric root. The valve usually is easily identified as an accumulation of fat just inside the medial colonic wall at the cecocolic junction. As it ascends, the colon passes lateral to the right kidney and posterior to mesenteric ileal loops and the tip of the right lobe of the liver. Unusual locations of the ascending colon are important variants. The ascending colon may lie almost directly medial to the renal hilus, resulting in lateral displacement of the kidney.[26,27] Less commonly, the colon may lie in a retrorenal position, presenting a potential hazard in the performance of percutaneous nephrostomy.[28,29] The ascending colon terminates by turning abruptly anterior, lateral to the transverse duodenum, at which point it acquires a mesentery and becomes the transverse colon.

The root of the transverse mesocolon is the boundary that separates the peritoneal spaces of the upper abdomen from the lower. As it passes from right to left, it crosses anterior to the proximal descending duodenum; the head, body, and tail of the pancreas; the medial part of the lower pole of the spleen; and the splenorenal ligament. The transverse colon, because of its long mesentery, may occupy a variety of intraperitoneal positions. Most commonly, it lies in the anterior midabdomen, separated from the abdominal wall by the greater omentum. After the transverse colon crosses the spleen, it curves posteriorly to reenter the retroperitoneum. Laterally, the mesocolon fuses with the diaphragm at this point to form the phrenicocolic ligament, which partially seals off the perisplenic space from the left paracolic gutter.

As the colon descends, it passes anterior to the spleen's tip and anterolateral to the left kidney and perirenal fat. Branches of the inferior mesenteric artery and vein lie in its original dorsal mesentery, medial to the descending colon. Its lateral and posterior surfaces lie in continuity with the posterior pararenal space and iliacus muscle. The colon then turns medially, crossing the psoas muscle to become the sigmoid colon.

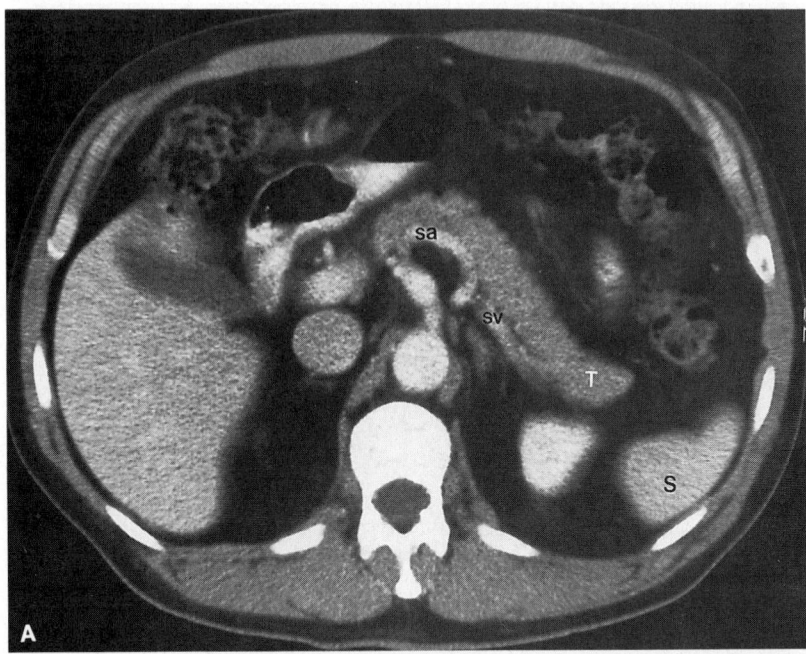

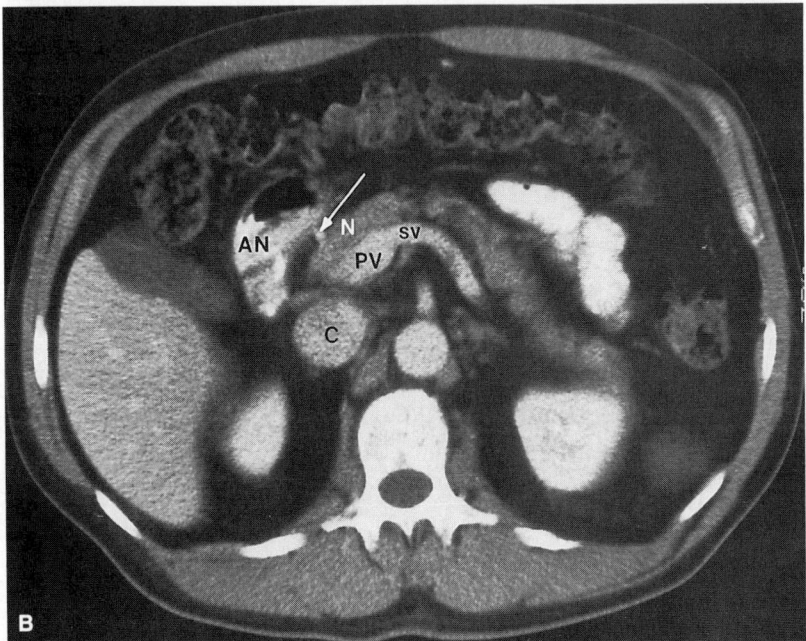

FIGURE 120-8. Position of the pancreas. (A) The pancreatic tail (T) projects posteriorly toward the hilus of the spleen (S), passing anterior to the splenic artery (sa) and vein (sv). (B) One centimeter caudal to **A**, the gastroduodenal artery (*arrow*) abuts the anterolateral aspect of the pancreatic neck (N) and the posteromedial surface of the gastric antrum (AN). (C, inferior vena cava; PV, portal vein, SV, splenic vein.)

Imaging of the colon is directed toward discovery and staging of extralumenal disease. Carcinoma of the colon may invade adjacent viscera, such as the gallbladder, duodenum, stomach, spleen, or bladder, or it may extend diffusely into the retroperitoneal fat. Appendicitis can invade and dissect along the planes of the right iliopsoas muscle, presenting as a tender mass in the upper thigh.[30] Lymph nodes follow the arterial supply of the involved colonic segment and are therefore imaged within the transverse mesocolon if the primary neoplasm arises in the transverse colon. If the primary neoplasm arises from ascending or descending segments, they are imaged within the original dorsal mesentery, part of the anterior pararenal space.[31]

The antimesenteric portion of the retroperitoneum is commonly involved in diverticulitis. Penetration of a diverticular abscess into the posterior pararenal space, from which it can extend to the diaphragm, is an occasional complication.

The proximity of colonic segments to the urinary tract at multiple sites explains many puzzling clinical circumstances.[32] Right hydronephrosis is a common sequela of appendicitis or Crohn's disease, and left colonic diverticulitis routinely produces inflammation of the bladder dome or left ureter.[33]

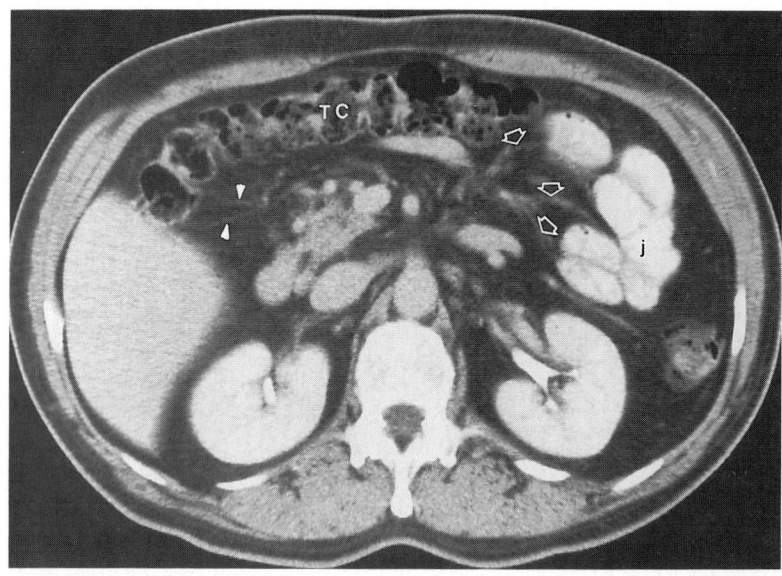

FIGURE 120-9. Small and large intestine. CT image of a section through the midabdomen shows the transverse colon (TC) occupying the anterior peritoneum, supplied by mesocolic vessels (*arrowheads*). The mesentery of the jejunum (j) with multiple jejunal vessels (*open arrows*) is well depicted.

Imaging of Abdominal Disease

The advent of cross-sectional imaging has had a major impact on the diagnosis of abdominal disease. CT provides an accurate depiction of many pathologic processes involving the abdominal parenchymal organs, the peritoneal spaces, and the retroperitoneum. Primary abnormalities of the alimentary tract are initially imaged with barium studies in most cases, but CT frequently provides important ancillary information,

particularly in patients with tumors or inflammatory processes involving the gut.

Spiral CT is a new technique that allows continuous axial scanning of the abdomen often with a single breathhold. Advantages include the ability to obtain excellent reformations in any plane desired (Fig. 120-10). Although there is some loss of spatial resolution, there is an important gain in the reduced time required to scan a large portion of the entire abdomen. Scans can be targeted to a specific vascular phase

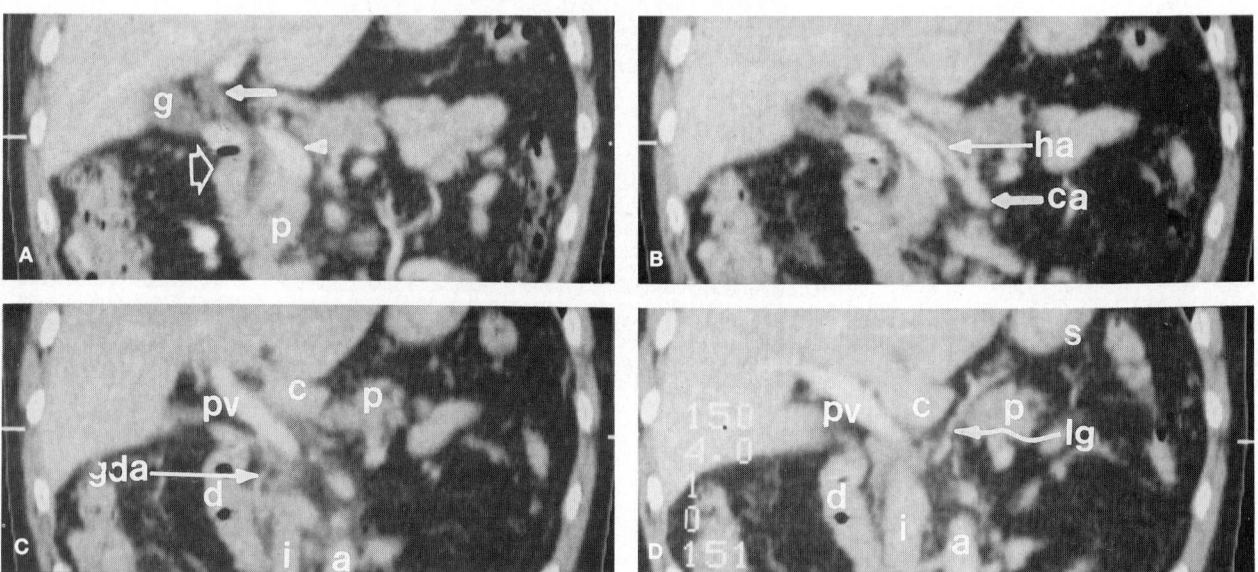

FIGURE 120-10. Coronal reformations of a spiral CT scan depict the normal anatomy in the region of the hepatoduodenal ligament. (**A**) A section through the anterior aspect of the hepatoduodenal ligament shows the common hepatic duct (*arrow*) coursing just lateral to the portal vein (*arrowhead*) and medial to the duodenum (*open arrow*). (g, gallbladder; p, pancreas.) (**B**) A section 2 mm posterior to **A** identifies the common hepatic artery (ha) as it exits the celiac trunk (ca). (**C**) A section 2 mm posterior to **B** shows the gastroduodenal artery (gda) as a branch off the common hepatic artery. (a, aorta; c, caudate lobe of the liver; i, inferior vena cava; d, duodenum; p, pancreas; pv, portal vein.) (**D**) A section 2 mm posterior to **C** shows the inferior vena cava (i) and aorta (a). The left gastric artery (lg) arises from the celiac trunk and courses upward within the gastrohepatic ligament. (c, caudate lobe of the liver; d, duodenum; pv, portal vein; p, pancreas; s, stomach.)

(e.g., arterial, capillary, venous) within a selected organ. This has been most useful in examining the liver, pancreas, and kidneys.

Ultrasound is also used extensively for diagnosing abdominal disorders, especially those involving the liver, gallbladder, and kidneys, and to a lesser extent, the pancreas, spleen, and adrenal glands.

MR imaging of the abdomen has been hampered somewhat by motion-induced artifacts caused by bowel peristalsis, respiratory motion, and blood flow. However, MR imaging is a rapidly evolving technology that is likely to improve with further development. MR imaging is comparable to CT for assessing focal hepatic abnormalities; with the development of artifact-suppression methods and MR contrast agents, it may eventually replace CT as the primary technique for imaging liver metastases.

PELVIC ANATOMY

Pelvic anatomy, taken as a whole, is somewhat complex, but from the perspective of the gastrointestinal tract, it is relatively simple. It consists primarily of the distal portions of the alimentary canal: the sigmoid colon, rectum, and anus. The cecum, appendix, and portions of the ileum may also lie within the major pelvis; however, these structures have already been described.

In the left lower quadrant of the abdominal cavity, the descending large intestine assumes a mesentery and becomes somewhat tortuous, forming the sigmoid colon. The mesentery of the sigmoid colon serves as its attachment to the posterior parietal peritoneum. The root of the sigmoid mesentery begins approximately at the level of the left sacroiliac joint, from which point it courses inferiorly and to the right, terminating at the rectosigmoid junction.

The upper part of the rectum is covered by peritoneum on its anterior and lateral surfaces; the midrectum is covered only on its anterior surface. The posterior wall of the rectum is

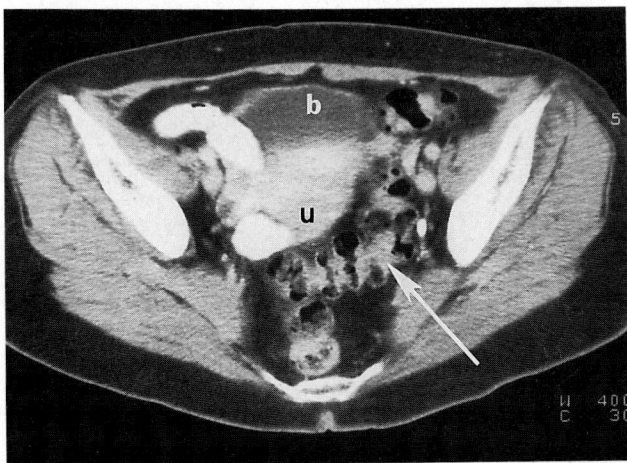

FIGURE 120-11. A transaxial CT section at the level of the pelvic inlet shows the sigmoid colon (*arrow*) passing posteriorly and to the right in proximity to the urinary bladder (b) and the uterus (u).

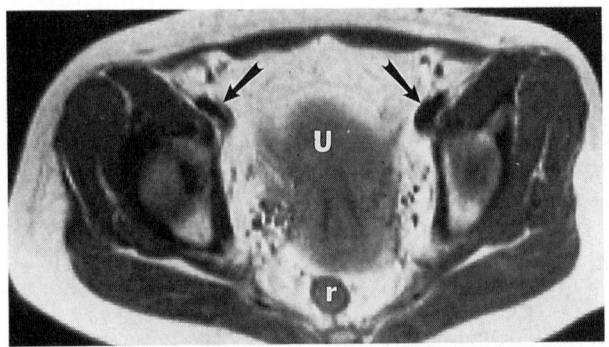

FIGURE 120-12. A T1-weighted transaxial MR scan shows the rectum (r) surrounded by perirectal fat. The uterus (u) and external iliac vessels (*black arrows*) are also seen at this level.

directly adjacent to the retroperitoneal tissue in the presacral space. About 5 cm above the pelvic diaphragm, the peritoneum on the anterior surface of the rectum reflects forward to cover the seminal vesicles and the posterosuperior surface of the bladder in men and the posterior walls of the upper vagina and uterus in women, forming the rectovesical and rectouterine pouches, respectively.

What follows is an examination of cross-sectional pelvic anatomy using CT, MR, and ultrasound images as a guide. The emphasis is on structures commonly affected by gastrointestinal disease processes.

The sigmoid colon has a variable appearance on cross-sectional images. It has two fixed points: the first, just distal to the junction of the descending colon and sigmoid colon anteromedial to the left external iliac vessels near the internal inguinal ring, and the second, just proximal to the rectosigmoid junction, where the sigmoid colon enters the perirectal fat near the sacral promontory. Although the course of the sigmoid colon is highly variable between these two points, it is most often seen on transaxial section at the level of the pelvic inlet passing posteriorly and to the right from a position anteromedial to the left iliacus muscle (Fig. 120-11). The urinary bladder, if relatively well distended, can also be seen at this level, as well as the uterus in female patients. The proximity of the sigmoid colon to the bladder accounts for the risk of enterovesical fistula formation in patients with diverticulitis, Crohn's disease, or sigmoid colon carcinoma.

At a more caudal level, the rectum is identified as being surrounded by retroperitoneal fat (Fig. 120-12). Spread of rectal neoplastic or inflammatory disease into the perirectal fat can often be appreciated on transaxial sections through this level by the use of CT or MR.[34,35] Transrectal ultrasound has also shown considerable promise for evaluating the perirectal area and the depth of rectal wall penetration by tumor in patients with rectal carcinoma. Occasionally, small branches of the superior rectal (hemorrhoidal) vessels can be appreciated on CT or MR scans. Small lymph nodes within the perirectal fat can also be seen; these are important nodal stations, representing the first sites of metastatic spread of rectal carcinoma.

In the male patient, the seminal vesicles can be identified as bilateral, oval structures that converge at the midline, situated directly posterior to the bladder and anterior to the rectum. In the female patient, the upper vagina is located just posterior to the bladder base and anterior to the rectum (Fig.

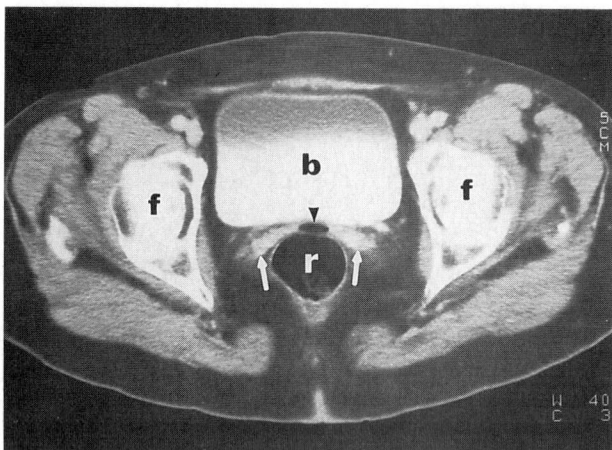

FIGURE 120-13. A transaxial CT section at the level of the femoral heads (f) shows the upper vagina between the urinary bladder (b) and the rectum (r). The vagina has a small amount of air within it (*arrowhead*). The white arrows point to the lateral fornices of the vagina.

120-13). Rectal invasion from posterior spread of cervical carcinoma can be assessed with transaxial CT or MR.

At a more caudal level (Fig. 120-14), the symphysis pubis and ischia are seen. The pectineus muscles lie just lateral to the symphysis pubis. The obturator internus muscles attach to the posterolateral aspect of the pubis and extend to the medial surface of the acetabular portion of the ileum. In men, the spermatic cord is identified at the notch between the medial border of the pectineus muscle and the lateral border of the rectus abdominis muscle. Inguinal hernias can be readily identified in this area on CT and MR scans.

The levator ani muscles are seen partially encircling the bladder and rectum (see Fig. 120-14). These muscles, along with the coccygeus muscles, form the pelvic diaphragm. The levator ani muscles that form the major portion of the pelvic diaphragm extend from one lateral pelvic wall to the other and between the pubis anteriorly and the coccyx posteriorly. They are perforated by the urethra and anal canal in males

and the urethra, vagina, and anal canal in females. The smaller coccygeus muscles arise from the ischial spines and expand to insert on the lateral borders of the lower two sacral and upper two coccygeal segments. They blend with the sacrospinous ligaments on their external surface.

Transaxial images at this level demonstrate the rectum just proximal to the anal canal, the prostate gland in males, and the urethra and lower vagina in females. The tissue outside of the levator ani muscles, bounded by the obturator internus muscles laterally and the gluteus maximus muscles posteriorly, represents fat in the ischiorectal fossa. Transaxial CT and MR sections are useful for assessing tumor spread from the rectum to adjacent structures, including the levator ani muscles, the ischiorectal fossa, and the vagina or prostate gland.

The sagittal plane that can be readily obtained with MR imaging is useful for showing the anatomic associations of the rectosigmoid with the uterus and vagina in females and the bladder, seminal vesicles, and urethra in males (Fig. 120-15). Sagittal and coronal MR sections have been useful for delineating congenital anorectal anomalies.[36] The location and development of the sphincter muscles can be estimated, and associated anomalies involving the kidneys and spine can be demonstrated.

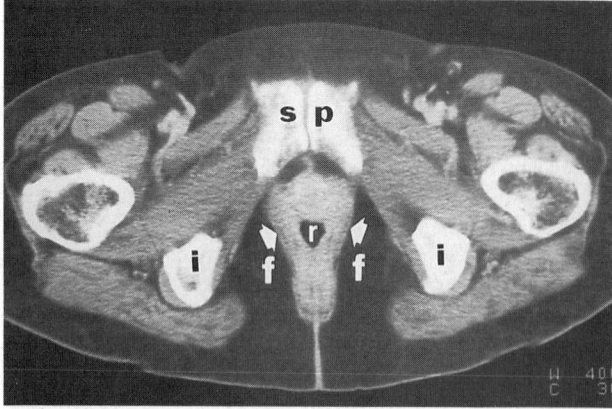

FIGURE 120-14. A transaxial CT section shows the distal rectum (r) between the V-shaped levator ani muscles (*arrows*). The fat in the ischiorectal fossa (f) is also seen at this level, as are the ischia (i) and the symphysis pubis (sp).

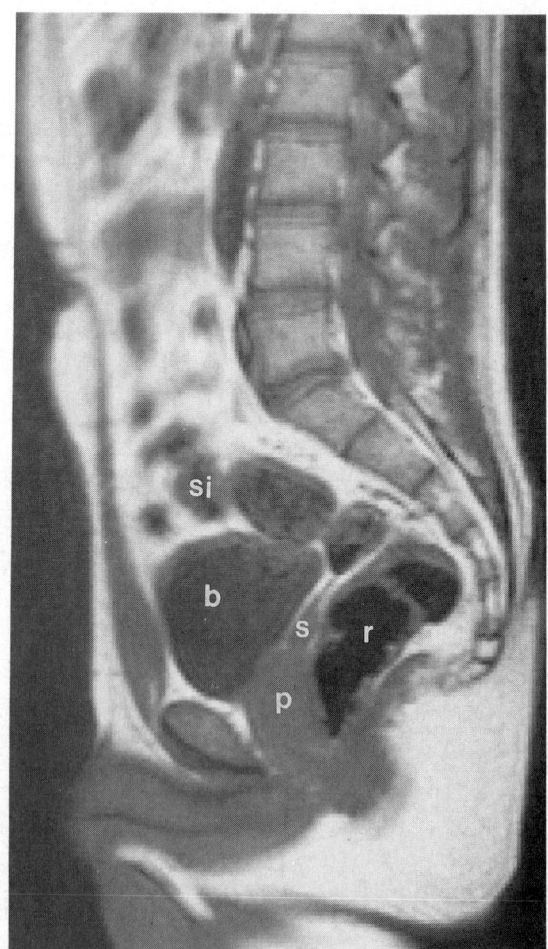

FIGURE 120-15. A sagittal T1-weighted MR image demonstrates the association of the sigmoid colon (si) and rectum (r) with the prostate gland (p), seminal vesicles (s), and bladder (b).

The advent of cross-sectional imaging techniques has enhanced our ability to evaluate gastrointestinal disease processes in the pelvis. Although mucosal abnormalities of the sigmoid colon and rectum are better visualized endoscopically or on air-contrast barium enema, the cross-sectional imaging modalities are valuable for assessing bowel wall thickening, the site and extralumenal extent of colorectal masses, and the spread of neoplastic or inflammatory abnormalities to surrounding tissues, adjacent organs, and regional lymph nodes.

CT provides a sensitive method of documenting the presence of enterovesical fistulas, and it can depict the extravesical component of the primary disease process in these cases.[37] CT is accepted as the cross-sectional imaging modality of choice for evaluating most gastrointestinal abnormalities in the pelvis. MR imaging and transrectal ultrasound have shown promise in this area, and investigations are under way to determine their roles more precisely.

The reader is directed to Chapter 53, Esophagus: Anatomy and Structural Anomalies; Chapter 59, Stomach: Anatomy and Structural Anomalies; Chapter 68, Small Intestine: Anatomy and Structural Anomalies; Chapter 78, Colon: Anatomy and Structural Anomalies; Chapter 89, Pancreas: Anatomy and Structural Anomalies; Chapter 95, Gallbladder and Biliary Tree: Anatomy and Structural Anomalies; and Chapter 100, Abdominal Cavity: Anatomy, Structural Anomalies, and Hernias.

REFERENCES

1. Marks WM, Collen PW. Gastroesophageal region: source of confusion on CT. AJR 1981;136:359.
2. Thompson WM, Halvorsen RA, Williford ME, et al. Computed tomography of the gastroesophageal junction. Radiographics 1982;2:179.
3. Allen KS, Siskind BN, Burrell MI. Perforation of distal esophagus with lesser sac extension: CT demonstration. J Comput Assist Tomogr 1986;10:612.
4. Balfe DM, Mauro MA, Koehler RE, et al. Gastrohepatic ligament: normal and pathologic CT anatomy. Radiology 1984;150:485.
5. Schwartz AN, Goiney RC, Graney DO. Gastric diverticulum simulating an adrenal mass: CT appearance and embryogenesis. AJR 1986;146:553.
6. Silverman PM. Gastric diverticulum mimicking adrenal mass: CT demonstration. J Comput Assist Tomogr 1986;10:709.
7. Cooper C, Jeffrey RB, Silverman PM, et al. Computed tomography of omental pathology. J Comput Assist Tomogr 1986;10:62.
8. Langman J. Medical embryology. 2nd ed. Baltimore: Williams & Wilkins, 1969.
9. Sexton CC, Zeman RK. Correlation of computed tomography, sonography, and gross anatomy of the liver. AJR 1983;141:7118.
10. Bismuth H, Houssin D, Castaing D. Major and minor segmentectomies "réglées" in liver surgery. World J Surg 1982;6:10.
11. Fried AM, Kreel L, Cosgrove DO. The hepatic interlobar fissure: Combined in vitro and in vivo study. AJR 1984;143:561.
12. Lafortune M, Madore F, Patriquin H, Breton G. Segmental anatomy of the liver: a sonographic approach to the Couinaud nomenclature. Radiology 1991;181:443.
13. Pagani JJ. Intrahepatic vascular territories shown by computed tomography. Radiology 1983;147:173.
14. Vogelzang RL. Acquired malposition of the colon and gallbladder in patients with cirrhosis: CT findings and clinical implications. Radiology 1989;171:739.
15. Weinstein JB, Heiken JP, Lee JKT, et al. High resolution CT of the porta hepatis and hepatoduodenal ligament. Radiographics 1986;6:55.
16. Oliphant M, Berne AS. Computed tomography of the subperitoneal space: Demonstration of direct spread of intraabdominal disease. J Comput Assist Tomogr 1982;6:1127.
17. Zirinsky K, Auh YH, Rubenstein WA, et al. The portacaval space: CT with MR correlation. Radiology 1985;156:453.
18. Vibhakar SD, Bellon EM. The bare area of the spleen: a constant CT feature of the ascitic abdomen. AJR 1984;141:953.
19. Halvorsen RA, Jones MA, Rice RP, Thompson WM. Anterior left subphrenic abscess: Characteristic plain film and CT appearance. AJR 1982;139:283.
20. Jeffrey RB, Federle MP, Goodman PC. Computed tomography of the lesser peritoneal sac. Radiology 1981;141:117.
21. Dodds WJ, Foley WD, Lawson Tl, et al. Anatomy and imaging of the lesser peritoneal sac. AJR 1985;144:567.
22. Vincent LM, Mauro MA, Mittelstaedt CA. The lesser sac and gastrohepatic recess: Sonographic appearance and differentiation of fluid collections. Radiology 1984;150:515.
23. Megibow AJ, Bosniak MA, Ambos MA, Beranbaum ER. Thickening of the celiac axis and/or superior mesenteric artery: a sign of pancreatic carcinoma on computed tomography. Radiology 1981;141:449.
24. Raptopoulos V, Kleinman PK, Marks S, et al. Renal fascial pathway: posterior extension of pancreatic effusions within the anterior pararenal space. Radiology 1986;158:367.
25. James S, Balfe DM, Lee JKT, Picus D. Small bowel disease: categorization by CT examination. AJR 1987;148:51.
26. Boijsen E, Ling G. Lateral displacement of the right kidney by the ascending colon. J Comput Assist Tomogr 1983;7:344.
27. Silverman PM, Kelvin FM, Korobkin M. Lateral displacement of the right kidney by the colon: an anatomic variation demonstrated on CT. AJR 1983;140:313.
28. Hopper KD, Sherman JL, Luethke JM, Ghaed N. The retrorenal colon in the supine and prone patient. Radiology 1987;162:443.
29. Sherman JL, Hopper KD, Greene AJ, Johns TT. The retrorenal colon on computed tomography: a normal variant. J Comput Assist Tomogr 1985;9:339.
30. Van Dyke JA, Holley HC, Anderson SD. Review of iliopsoas anatomy and pathology. Radiographics 1987;7:53.
31. Dodds WJ, Darweesh RMA, Lawson TL, et al. The retroperitoneal spaces revisited. AJR 1986;147:1155.
32. Love L, Meyers MA, Churchill RJ, Reynes CJ, et al. Computed tomography of extraperitoneal spaces. AJR 1981;136:781.
33. Feldberg MAM, Hendricks MJ, Van Waes PFGM. Role of CT in diagnosis and management of complications of diverticular disease. Gastrointest Radiol 1985;10:370.
34. Butch RJ, Stark DD, Wittenberg J, et al. Staging rectal cancer by MR and CT. AJR 1986;146:1155.
35. Grabbe E, Lierse W, Winkler R. The perirectal fascia: morphology and use in staging of rectal carcinoma. Radiology 1983;149:241.
36. Sato Y, Pringle KC, Bergman RA, et al. Congenital anorectal anomalies: MR imaging. Radiology 1988;168:157.
37. Goldman SM, Fishman EK, Gatewood OMB, et al. CT in the diagnosis of enterovesical fistulae. AJR 1985;144:1229.

Textbook of Gastroenterology, second edition, edited by Tadataka Yamada. JB Lippincott Company, Philadelphia © 1995.

CHAPTER 121

Ultrasonography

Lauren S. LoVerde   Carol A. Mittelstaedt

Ultrasonography has come a long way since its initial use as an imaging technique. With the introduction of high-resolution, real-time systems, ultrasound has become a less technically dependent study. The real-time systems allow greater flexibility with regard to scan plane and patient position, something not possible with the older articulated arm static (B-mode) systems. Some clinicians view ultrasound as simply an extension of the physical examination. If a mass is palpated, the ultrasound scan can be performed over the mass to identify the origin of the structure; often the palpable mass may be a normal structure such as a Riedel's lobe of the liver or inferior pole of the right kidney. Unlike computed tomography (CT) and magnetic resonance imaging (MRI), ultrasound can be performed rapidly, repeatedly, without radiation or contrast administration, and at the bedside of critically ill patients.

THEORETICAL CONSIDERATIONS

Diagnostic ultrasound employs the pulse-echo principle to convert electrical energy into sound waves. Materials such as ceramics and quartz within the transducer change shape in an electrical field or if mechanically stressed so that an electrical impulse generates a sound wave that is transmitted and vice versa; this is the piezoelectric effect. The returning sound waves are transformed into electrical energy with a magnitude proportional to the amplitude. The echoes transmitted to the transducer consist of a series of echoes from internal reflectors along the path of the sound beam in the body, with the earliest returning echoes from the interactions close to the transducer and the later echoes coming from correspondingly distant reflectors.

An interface occurs where two tissues of different acoustic impedance are in contact. Acoustic impedance is related to tissue density and the speed of sound in the tissues; the greater the density difference between two tissues, the stronger is the returning echo. Structures with different acoustic impedances, such as the gallbladder and liver, are much easier to differentiate than two structures with similar acoustic texture, such as the kidney and liver. If there is a large acoustic interface close to the transducer, a strong echo is generated, producing a reverberation artifact. Because this echo is so strong, it returns to the tissues again, causing additional echoes parallel to the first. From the known direction of the sound beam in the body and the measured time of arrival of its echo, the exact anatomic location of each reflector may be calculated. The transducer is repeatedly fired as it is moved across the body to build up a two-dimensional image of cross-sectional anatomy.

Sound is absorbed or scattered as it travels through the body, weakening the beam. This attenuation is caused by scatter, absorption, and reflection. Because there is little attenuation of sound traveling through a fluid-filled structure, structures distal to the cystic lesion appear to contain more echoes than neighboring areas. This is referred to as acoustic enhancement. Failure of the sound beam to pass to a structure results in acoustic shadowing, which is caused by reflection or absorption of the sound beam and which may be complete or partial. To couple the transducer to the skin, eliminating the air interface between the transducer and the skin, a gel is used with acoustic properties similar to that of skin.

The highest-frequency transducer is chosen, resulting in superior resolution, with the lower-frequency transducers allowing greater penetration. The focal zone of the transducer is that depth in the sound beam at which resolution is the highest. Resolution is the ability to differentiate two adjacent structures (interfaces). The frequency of the transducer is the number of times the wave is repeated per second as measured in cycles per second (Hz). The sound waves used in medical imaging are in the 3- to 15-MHz range (i.e., million cycles per second), which is why the term *ultrasound* is applied; the audible range of frequencies of the human ear is 20 to 16,000 Hz.

Shades of gray are used to represent the strength of the echo amplitude at the anatomic site. If the background of the ultrasound image is black, the lighter shades of gray represent higher amplitude echoes; the reverse is true if the background is white. The following terminology has evolved: anechoic, meaning echo free; hypoechoic, meaning relatively echo free; isoechoic, meaning similar in echo production to another tissue or substance; and hyperechoic, meaning very echo producing.

Ultrasound equipment employs complex transducers capable of acquiring 15 to 30 images (i.e., frames) per second; older ultrasound units used a single-element transducer, which took 5 to 20 seconds to produce an image. Two types of real-time transducers have been developed to acquire the ultrasound images automatically and repetitively: mechanically steered systems and electronically steered systems. The older units, referred to as static scanners, did have the advantage of producing a large field of view, demonstrating total cross-sectional skin surface, and it was easier for the viewer to identify the precise anatomic location of the scan plan obtained independently by the operator. With the high frame rates in the newer units, the internal patient anatomy is present in real time, and tissue may be studied temporally and spatially. Real-time ultrasound has the advantages of a rapid and complete survey, reduced examination time, and less operator scanning skill.

Doppler ultrasound units are pulsed systems capable of producing color-coded flow images in real time. With pulsed Doppler, bursts of ultrasound are emitted at a regular repetition rate into the body tissue. Until echoes from the previous pulse have ceased or significantly diminished, a new pulse is not transmitted. The pulse depth can be determined by noting the time of its flight to an interface and return. The reflected echo frequency is shifted up or down relative to the incident wave by an amount proportional to the velocity along the beam direction if the interface of the scatter is moving. The Doppler signal is converted into an audible signal, with a typical sound for veins and for patent and partially obstructed arteries. For the pulsed Doppler system to determine the spectrum of a reflected wave from many depths simultaneously in real time, extremely fast parallel processors are needed to carry out the many Fourier transformations.

Measurement of blood velocity and associated physiologic parameters with Doppler ultrasound is a powerful diagnostic technique. Doppler ultrasound measurements may be used to determine the presence of flow, determine the direction of flow, identify time-varying velocity characteristics, and detect velocity disturbances. Color-coded images are often used to display the multidimensional data, including flow magnitude, direction, and location. Color is used to encode direction, and hue is used to encode relative magnitude of flow in the image.

LIMITATIONS

The ultrasound procedure has several limitations. If the patient has a large amount of bowel gas, the sound beam is reflected, and there is inadequate penetration of the sound beam beneath that structure. Patients with ileus, acute pancreatitis, and other conditions are prone to have larger amounts of bowel gas. Abscesses containing air may reflect the ultrasound beam and escape detection. In many cases, the amount of bowel gas is unpredictable. It is difficult to examine adequately the markedly obese patient, because the depth of penetration of the sound beam is limited. A lower frequency transducer may give greater depth of penetration, but still some patients are impossible to scan. Burn patients can usually be scanned sterilely with a sterile drape over the transducer and sterile antibiotic ointment as a coupling agent. For patients scanned in the immediate postoperative period, intraabdominal air may cause a problem by reflecting the sound beam. With ostomies and incisions, the skin access may be limited, although the patient's abdomen may be scanned in a sterile fashion.

EVALUATION OF THE LIVER

Ultrasound and other imaging modalities can aid the gastroenterologist in the evaluation of liver disease. Although the liver is the largest abdominal organ, it is not easy to evaluate clinically because of its anatomic site. Hepatomegaly does not necessarily exist just because the liver edge is below the costal margin.

Technical Applications

There is no specific preparation for a liver ultrasound. However, because the liver is usually studied in conjunction with the biliary system and the pancreas, an overnight fast is beneficial; this reduces bowel gas and promotes gallbladder distention. Most liver scans are performed with the patient supine. Left lateral decubitus scans may be performed at times, enabling the examiner to evaluate lesions in the posterior and lateral portions of the right lobe of the liver. This position is also helpful if there is poor penetration of the sound beam into the posterior liver, as in patients with hepatocellular disease. As with all ultrasound examinations, the highest-frequency transducer is used that allows adequate penetration of the sound beam into the structure being studied.

Normal Anatomy

The normal adult liver is 15 to 17 cm long, with the right hepatic lobe approximately six times as large as the left. The right lobe is used for the sonographic measurement of hepatic size. The parenchyma of the normal liver is moderately echogenic with a fine, homogeneous echo texture (Fig. 121-1). The liver is similar in echo density to the spleen, more echogenic than or isoechoic with the kidney, and less echogenic than or isoechoic with the pancreas.

The anatomic landmarks dividing the liver into lobes

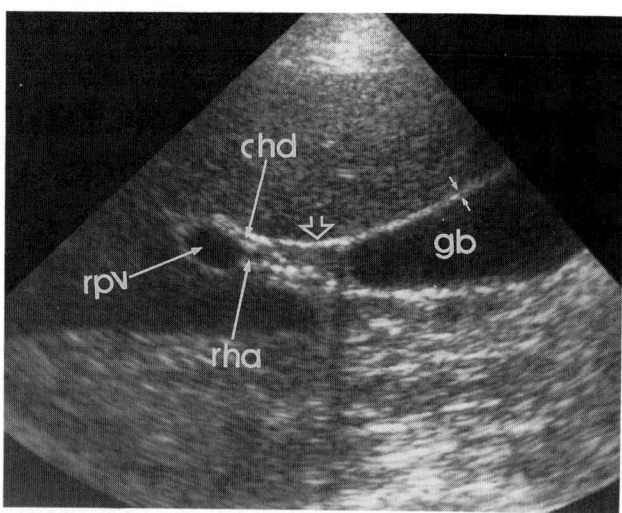

FIGURE 121-2. On a sagittal view, the normal gallbladder (gb) is seen as an anechoic structure with a thin wall (*arrows*). It is located by identifying the echogenic line of the major fissure (*open arrow*) of the liver. The internal diameter of the common hepatic duct (chd) is measured anterior to the right portal vein (rpv), near the right hepatic artery (rha).

and segments can be seen with ultrasound (Figs. 121-2 and 121-3). The ligaments and fissures are echogenic because of collagen and fat. The right and left hepatic lobes are divided by a plane intersecting the gallbladder fossa inferiorly, the inferior vena cava (IVC) posteriorly, and the middle hepatic

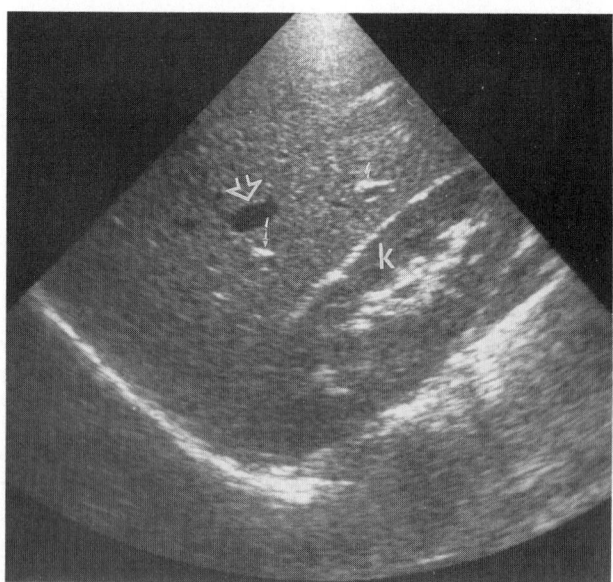

FIGURE 121-1. Parenchyma of the normal liver. Sagittal view of the right lobe of the liver demonstrates a smooth homogenous echo pattern. The portal vein radicles (*small arrows*) usually have brightly echogenic margins, and the hepatic vein radicles (*open arrow*) have less well-defined margins. The echodensities of the liver and renal (k) parenchyma are similar.

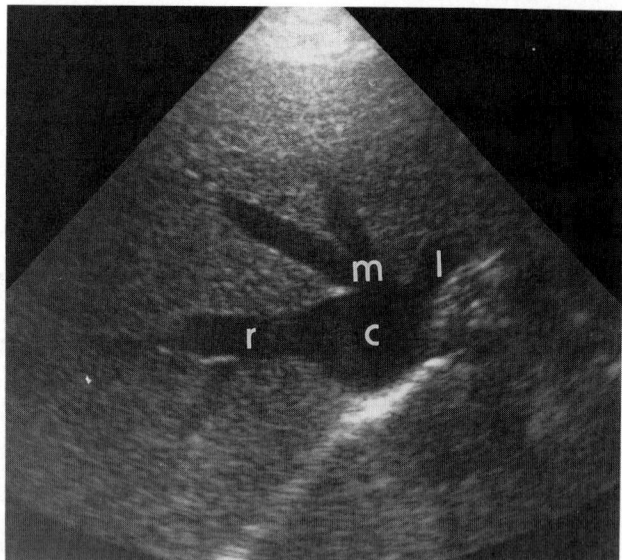

FIGURE 121-3. On a transverse scan, the right (r), middle (m), and left (l) hepatic veins of the normal liver are seen draining into the inferior vena cava (c). The left lobe is that portion of the liver medial to the middle hepatic vein. The medial segment of the left lobe is between the middle hepatic vein and the left hepatic vein, with the lateral segment medial to the left hepatic vein. The anterior segment of the right lobe is anterior to the right hepatic vein, between the right hepatic vein and the middle hepatic vein, with the posterior segment posterior to the right hepatic vein.

vein superiorly (see Fig. 121-2). The left lobe is further divided into medial and lateral segments by the falciform ligament inferiorly and the left hepatic vein superiorly (see Fig. 121-3). The right hepatic lobe is subdivided into anterior and posterior segments by the right hepatic vein. The caudate lobe is between the fissure for the ligamentum venosum and the IVC, posterior to the porta hepatis.

The portal triads can be visualized within the liver with ultrasound as lucent structures with echogenic margins caused by collagen and fat deposition around them. Portal veins can usually be differentiated from hepatic veins, because the former have highly echogenic walls, but the latter have imperceptible walls (see Fig. 121-1). Color and spectral Doppler can be used to differentiate these vascular structures from bile ducts. Within the porta hepatis, the common bile duct lies anterolateral to the portal vein and the hepatic artery anteromedial (Fig. 121-4). A transverse sonogram through the porta hepatis is one of the simplest methods for determining the presence of biliary obstruction.

Diffuse Disease

Fatty Infiltration

Fatty infiltration of the liver is associated with several diseases. Most patients with moderate or severe fatty infiltration demonstrate brightly reflective echo patterns (Fig. 121-5).[1] With generalized fatty infiltration, a pseudotumor or hypoechoic area has been described in the region of the quadrate lobe or medial segment of the left lobe. This area, which represents normal hepatic parenchyma, appears hypoechoic in contrast to the surrounding liver, which is echogenic as a result of the fatty infiltration.[2,3] At times, this fat infiltration may not be uniform, producing a patchy distribution throughout the liver.

This type of pattern appears to predominantly involve the right lobe of the liver and may pose a problem in its diagnosis.[1] With this pattern, the normal areas of the liver appear as hypoechoic focal defects.[1]

Hepatitis

Various ultrasound patterns have been associated with hepatitis.[1] With acute hepatitis, there is overall decreased echogenicity of the liver, with accentuated brightness and more extensive demonstration of the portal vein radicle walls (Fig. 121-6).[1] With chronic hepatitis, there is an overall increase in the liver echogenicity, with a decrease in the brightness and the number of portal vein radicle walls.[1]

Cirrhosis

The ultrasound findings associated with cirrhosis include increased echoes anteriorly within the liver, with decreased echoes posteriorly; liver significantly more echogenic than renal parenchyma; and small portal and venous vessels not well seen and decreased in the peripheral liver.[1] Regional changes associated with cirrhosis include caudate lobe enlargement and diminution of the right lobe (Fig. 121-7).[1] Cirrhotic livers may be separated from noncirrhotic livers by using the ratio of the transverse caudate lobe width to the transverse right lobe width. Cirrhosis is unlikely if the ratio is less than 0.6 and can be diagnosed with 99% confidence if the ratio is greater than 0.73.[1] Cirrhosis is 96% likely if the ratio is 0.65.[1] Several series report difficulty in differentiating fatty infiltration, hepatitis, and cirrhosis.[1] Ultrasound may have a limited value in the diagnosis of diffuse hepatic abnormalities unless there are gross changes in the normal pattern.[1] It may be more appropriate on ultrasound to make the diagnosis of hepatocellular disease.

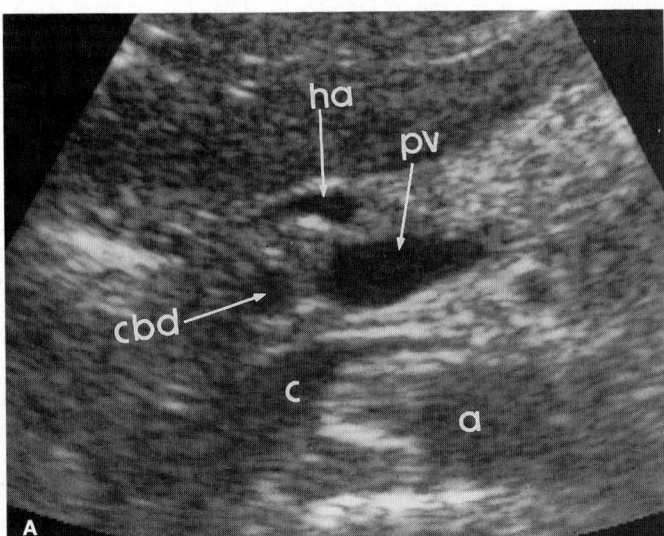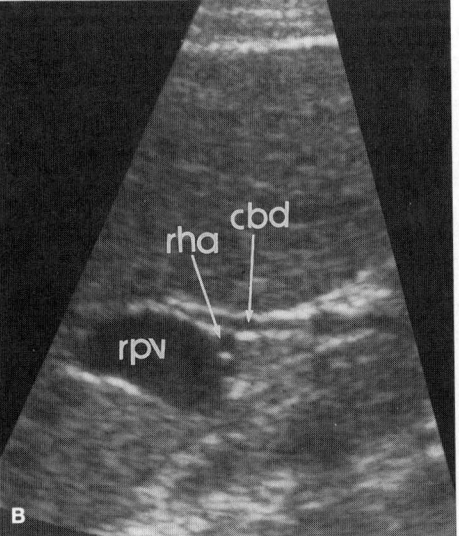

FIGURE 121-4. **(A)** The transverse view shows the relation of the common bile duct (cbd), proper hepatic artery (ha), and main portal vein (mpv) in the porta hepatis in the normal liver. The common bile duct is anterolateral to the main portal vein, with the hepatic artery more anteromedial. The aorta (a) and vena cava (c) are also seen on this scan. **(B)** The sagittal oblique view demonstrates the normal proximal common bile duct (cbd) anterior to the right hepatic artery (rha) and right portal vein (rpv).

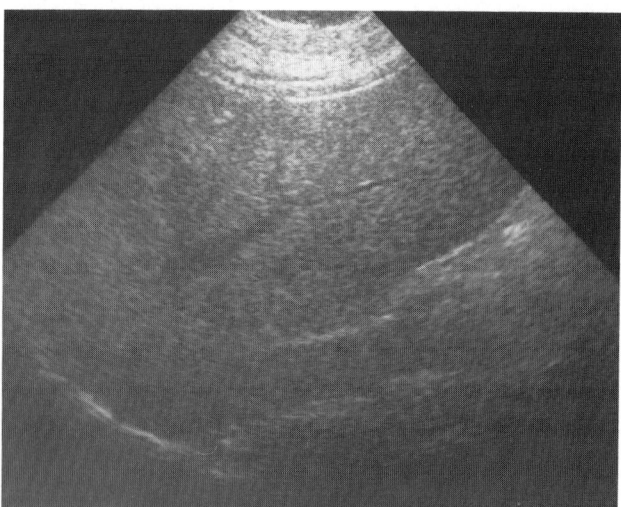

FIGURE 121-5. A sagittal view of the right lobe of the liver demonstrates a brightly echogenic liver, caused by diffuse fatty infiltration. Few internal vessels can be seen.

Vascular Abnormalities

Portal hypertension. Ultrasound evaluation for portal hypertension includes evaluation of the portal vein and its collaterals.[1] The normal portal vein, which can be identified in 97% of patients, has been found with ultrasound to measure 1.1 to 1.3 cm.[1] However, portal vein dilatation alone is not an accurate method for diagnosing portal hypertension, because it has a sensitivity of only 41.8%.[1] The sensitivity of ultrasound may be increased to 79.7% with a specificity of 100% if an evaluation of the caliber variation of the splenic and superior mesenteric veins during respiration is added.[1] Because there is a marked increase in the intrahepatic resistance in cirrhosis, there is less variation of the portal vein from respiration. The diagnosis of portal hypertension may be based on the lack of normal caliber variation (i.e., increase during

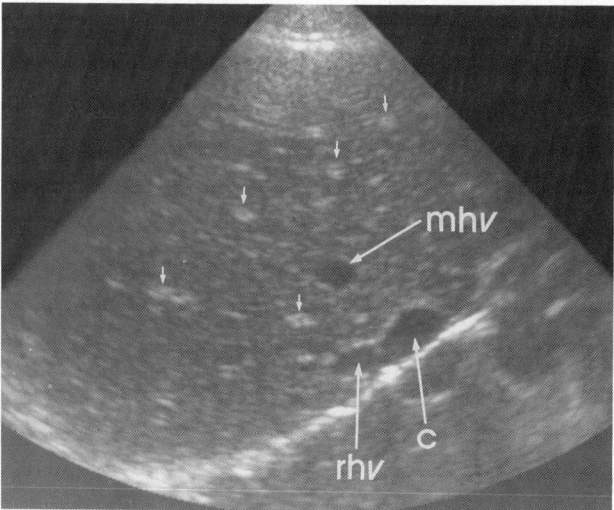

FIGURE 121-6. A transverse view of the liver demonstrates increased density (*arrows*) in a periportal location. This pattern has been described with acute hepatitis. (c, inferior vena cava; mhv, middle hepatic vein; rhv, right hepatic vein.)

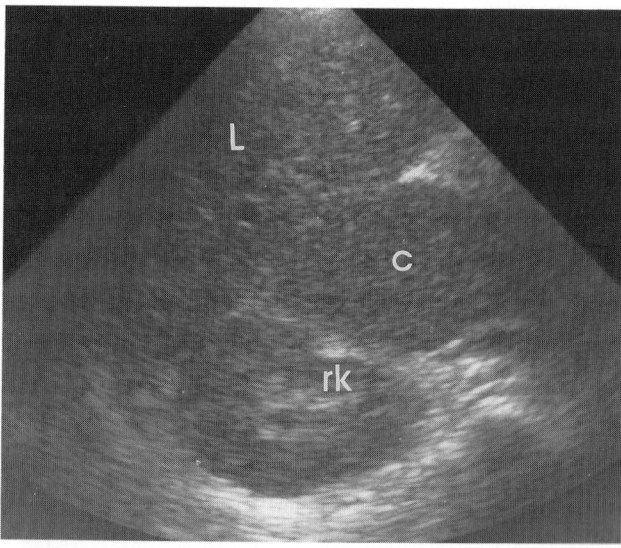

FIGURE 121-7. A transverse image shows an enlarged or hypertrophied caudate lobe (c) projecting medially, anterior to the right kidney (rk). The liver (L) was enlarged as a result of diffuse cirrhosis.

inspiration and decrease during expiration) in the superior mesenteric and splenic veins.[1]

Portosystemic venous channels associated with portal hypertension may be evaluated with ultrasound.[1] Representing closed or partially closed embryonic channels, these collaterals reopen, connecting the portal and systemic venous systems. Several collaterals can be seen with ultrasound: recanalized umbilical vein or paraumbilical vein and the splenorenal, gastrorenal, and intestinal collaterals.[1] The recanalized umbilical vein, which connects the left portal vein to the epigastric veins in the anterior abdominal wall at the level of the umbilicus, is seen in cases of portal hypertension; it decompresses the portal vein (Fig. 121-8).[1] Doppler ultrasound may be used to demonstrate flow in this collateral and the direction of flow.[1] If massive hepatopetal flow is observed in the umbilical vein that exceeds the hepatopetal flow in the portal vein, the likelihood of esophageal varices and variceal bleeding may be reduced.[4] Identification of coronary-gastroesophageal varices by ultrasound is limited by their small size in the early stage of portal hypertension.[1] The coronary vein with its gastroesophageal varices is the easiest portosystemic collateral to identify (Fig. 121-9). Coronary collaterals have been identified with a sensitivity of 80%; a 64% sensitivity has been reported with the identification of the gastroesophageal varices.[1]

In addition to identifying collaterals, duplex Doppler may be performed for the qualitative assessment of splanchnic venous hemodynamics in patients suspected of portal hypertension.[5] The splenic, superior mesenteric-portal, intrahepatic-portal, and portosystemic collaterals can be evaluated for caliber and direction of flow (Fig. 121-10).[5] This Doppler examination may establish the diagnosis of clinically significant portal hypertension with a technical success rate of 95%, although 10% of examinations are incomplete because of intestinal gas.[5] The combined use of Doppler and routine ultrasound allows the precise evaluation of the vascular anatomy in portal venous hypertension.[5]

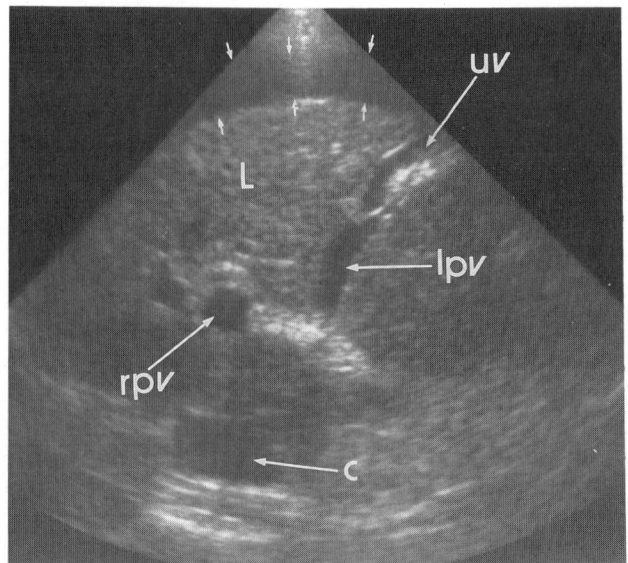

FIGURE 121-8. A sagittal oblique view of the liver, with the patient in the left lateral decubitus position, demonstrates the recanalized umbilical vein (uv) draining into the left portal vein (lpv). This patient had cirrhosis with an inhomogeneous liver echo pattern. Ascites are seen as a lucent area (*arrows*) surrounding the liver (L). (c, inferior vena cava; rpv, right portal vein.)

Besides evaluating for the presence of portal hypertension, ultrasound can be employed to study patients with surgical portosystemic shunts. The portacaval shunt is the easiest to demonstrate on ultrasound (Fig. 121-11); the mesocaval and splenorenal shunts may also be seen. Doppler ultrasound may be used to evaluate shunt patency.[1]

Portal vein obstruction.   With portal vein obstruction, ultrasound may identify the hepatic and portal veins, detect hepatic or portal venous thrombosis, and suggest the cause of the thrombosis—neoplastic or nonneoplastic determined by the

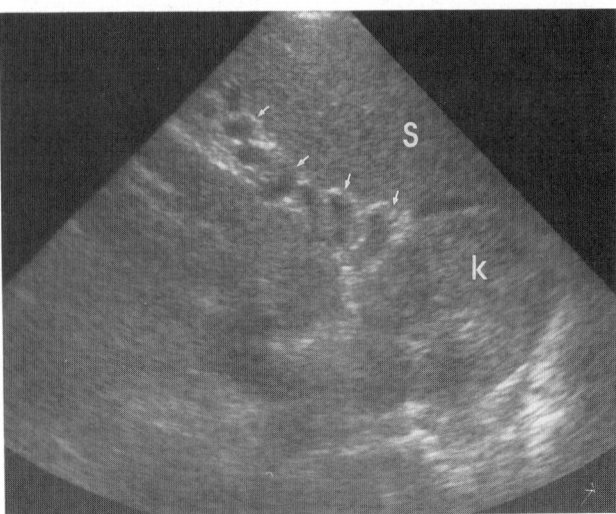

FIGURE 121-10. A transverse view of the splenic hilum demonstrates many small lucent areas (*arrows*), which represent splenic collaterals. The spleen (S) and left kidney (k) of this patient with portal hypertension are also seen on the ultrasound scan.

presence of a liver neoplasm.[1] Because the portal vein is normally seen on ultrasound in most patients, the inability to identify the portal vein is strong evidence of occlusion.[1] The ultrasound findings include presence of thrombi within the portal vein; splenic and superior mesenteric vein dilatation proximal to the point of portal vein occlusion; and many periportal collaterals (i.e., cavernous transformation) identified, with loss of the normal portal venous landmarks (Fig. 121-12).[1] If the portal vein obstruction has been present for a long time, other ultrasound findings may be demonstrated: splenomegaly, normal-appearing liver on ultrasound, and hepatopetal collaterals.[1] Doppler ultrasound may also aid in the evaluation of portal vein obstruction.

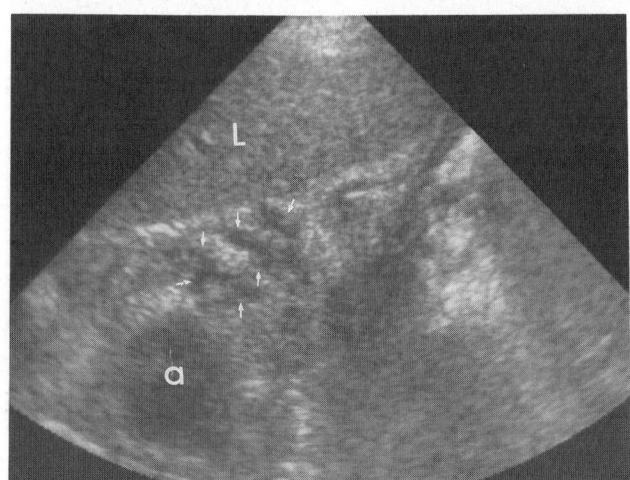

FIGURE 121-9. Portal hypertension with esophagogastric varices. The transverse view high within the abdomen shows the liver (L) and coronary-gastroesophageal collaterals as lucent structures (*arrows*) anterior to the abdominal aorta (a).

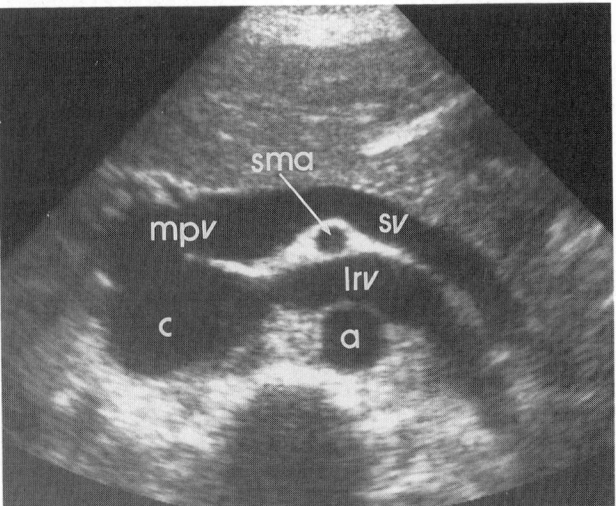

FIGURE 121-11. Portocaval shunt. On this transverse view, communication between the main portal vein (mpv) and the inferior vena cava (c) can be seen. Flow was demonstrated between the two vessels by Doppler ultrasound. (a, aorta; lrv, left renal vein; sma, superior mesenteric artery; sv, splenic vein.)

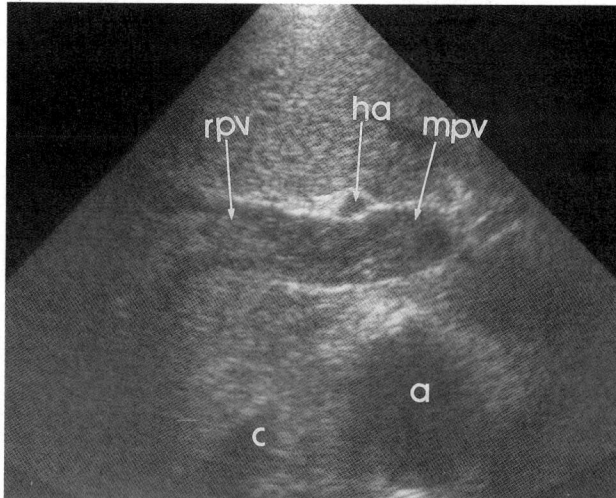

FIGURE 121-12. On a transverse view of the main (mpv) and right (rpv) portal vein, internal echoes representing thrombus are seen within the lumen. Doppler ultrasound could not demonstrate flow, consistent with the diagnosis of portal vein thrombosis. (a, aorta; c, inferior vena cava; ha, hepatic artery.)

Budd-Chiari syndrome. Budd-Chiari syndrome may be produced by occlusion of hepatic vascular channels at various levels: occlusion of the IVC with or without hepatic vein occlusion; occlusion of the major hepatic veins with or without IVC occlusion; and occlusion of the small central lobar veins.[1] The ultrasound findings associated with Budd-Chiari syndrome depend on the stage of the disease process. A large, hypoechoic caudate lobe may be identified; the hypertrophy of the caudate lobe is caused by its multiple direct connections with the IVC.[1] Ascites may be seen. A lack of flow may be demonstrated by Doppler ultrasound within the obstructed portion of the IVC.[1] Duplex and color-flow Doppler imaging are potential noninvasive methods of diagnosing patients with Budd-Chiari syndrome and evaluating them after surgery for patency and direction of flow.[6] Correlation with angiography is excellent, and color-flow Doppler can precisely define intrahepatic, portal, and IVC circulatory dynamics.[6]

Focal Abnormalities

Cysts

Nonparasitic cysts. Nonparasitic cysts appear anechoic, with well-defined borders and acoustic enhancement.[1] Included in the differential diagnosis for a lucent lesion in the liver are cyst, necrotic metastasis, echinococcal cyst, hematoma, hepatic cystadenocarcinoma, and abscess.[1] Several metastatic lesions have been described as anechoic: leiomyosarcoma of the gastrointestinal tract, colon carcinoma, embryonal cell carcinoma, testicular carcinoma, carcinoid, and melanoma.[1] The ultrasound diagnosis of a cyst is 95% to 100% accurate. An ultrasound-guided percutaneous cyst aspiration may be performed if the diagnosis is in doubt. Because definitive therapy requires surgical removal of the cyst lining or internal drainage

by marsupialization, percutaneous aspiration lacks permanent therapeutic benefit.[1]

Echinococcal cysts. Diseases formerly confined to endemic areas are spreading because of increased worldwide travel brought on by tourism and immigration.[1] Such is true with hydatid disease. Several associated ultrasound patterns have been described: discrete simple cysts, with or without calcification; multiple cysts, in which the daughter cyst appears dense early in the course; honeycomb cysts, which are fluid collections with septa; and solid-appearing cysts.[1] Ultrasound is considered the primary diagnostic modality in the evaluation of hydatid disease if the liver and other abdominal organs are affected. Although surgery is usually the treatment of choice, removal of the cyst is often difficult or incomplete with a risk of dissemination.[7] Hence, medical therapy has a distinct advantage, especially in patients at higher operative risk. Ultrasound can be used to monitor patients undergoing therapy with benzoimidazolic compounds.[7] The following changes have been seen on ultrasound with cyst degeneration: decrease in size, detachment of cyst membrane, and appearance of echogenic material in the cyst cavity.[7]

Infection

Pyogenic abscess. The main origin for the bacteria (usually *Escherichia coli*) producing a pyogenic liver abscess appears to be the biliary tree, with the following findings on ultrasound: variable size; 80% right lobe involvement; single or multiple abscesses that are round or ovoid; irregular walls with poor definition; anechoic to highly echogenic, with most less echogenic than liver; and acoustic enhancement in 50% (Fig. 121-13).[1] The marked echogenicity or acoustic shadowing may be caused by the presence of gas.[1] It sometimes may be

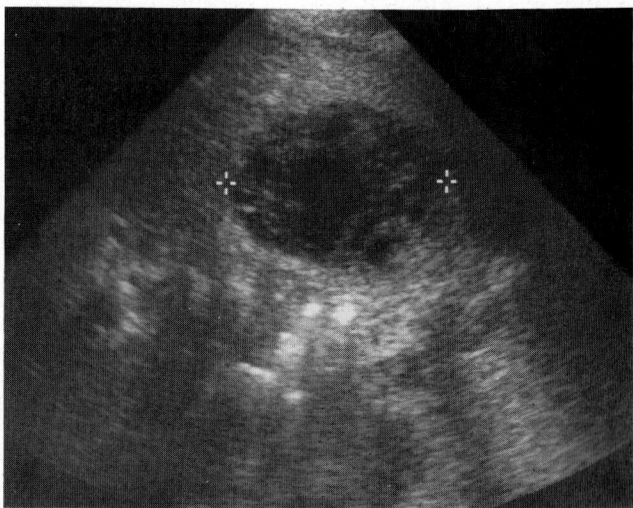

FIGURE 121-13. On a transverse view of the left lobe of the liver, a complicated cystic mass (*calipers*) is seen. Although the mass is lucent, it does contain some internal echoes. The differential diagnosis for such a lesion would have to be a hepatic abscess, hematoma, or necrotic tumor. The patient underwent catheter drainage of this pyogenic abscess.

difficult to differentiate a pyogenic from an amebic abscess on ultrasound. With ultrasound-guided percutaneous puncture, a definitive diagnosis of a pyogenic abscess may be made, and ultrasound may be used to guide catheter drainage.[1]

Amebic abscess.   The ultrasound findings of amebic abscess include poor wall definition; round or oval shape; echogenicity less than liver; location contiguous with liver capsule; and distal acoustic enhancement.[1,8] Two features that appear more prevalent in amebic abscesses than pyogenic abscesses are round or oval shapes (82%) and hypoechoic (compared with liver) lesions, which are internally homogeneous on high-gain scans (58%).[8] Ultrasound can be employed to follow the change in the amebic abscess during medical therapy; with healing, there is usually complete resolution of the ultrasound abnormality occurring in 6 weeks to 23 months.[1,9] Because the diagnosis is usually confirmed by hemagglutination titers and response to therapy, aspiration is rarely indicated. If amebic and pyogenic abscesses are indistinguishable, a diagnostic aspiration may be indicated.[8,9] However, if the ultrasound findings are coupled with clinical and laboratory data, a correct diagnosis can be made for 86% of patients with amebic abscess.[8] Therapeutic aspiration or drainage may be indicated for pyogenic superinfection and large juxtacardiac abscesses.[9]

Candidiasis.   Noncutaneous candidiasis, although uncommon, has been associated with various ultrasound patterns (in order of appearance in the disease process): wheel within a wheel; bull's-eye or target; uniformly hypoechoic lesion; and echogenic foci with variable degrees of posterior acoustic shadowing.[1,10] With the wheel within a wheel pattern, the earliest finding on ultrasound, there is a peripheral hypoechoic area with an internal echogenic area and a central hypoechoic area. The most classic ultrasound pattern described is a hypoechoic area with a central area of increased echogenicity (e.g., bull's-eye or target).[1] With the use of ultrasound-guided percutaneous aspiration, a definitive diagnosis occasionally is made, although there have been some false-negative results.[10] To monitor immunocompromised patients, ultrasound and precontrast and postcontrast CT may be performed to achieve maximal sensitivity in identifying these lesions.[10] If all imaging studies are negative and there is a strong clinical suspicion of candidiasis, an open biopsy may be indicated to make the diagnosis.[10]

Benign Neoplasms

Cavernous hemangioma.   The most common benign hepatic tumor, the cavernous hemangioma, demonstrates the following ultrasound appearance: homogeneously echogenic mass (94%); subcapsular location (70%); less than 2 cm in diameter (32%); multiple lesions (35%); round (75.5%), oval (13.5%), or lobulated (11%) shape; sharply defined borders (90%); and lesions larger than 3 cm with a polylobular contour (90%; Fig. 121-14).[1] One study followed hemangiomas on ultrasound for 1 to 6 years after the initial scans.[11] It was shown that 82% of these lesions did not change their ultrasound appearance on follow-up study.[11] After hemangiomas are visible on ultrasound in adults, they only rarely change in size or appearance. In the proper setting, a follow-up scan may

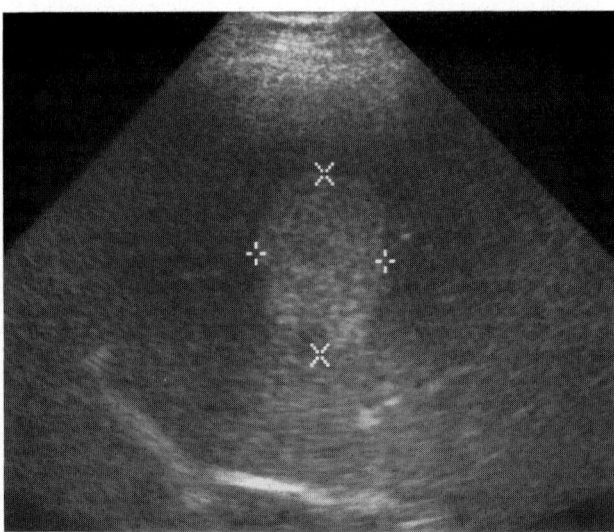

FIGURE 121-14.   A transverse view of the liver shows a well-defined, echogenic lesion (*calipers*), which measured 3 by 4 cm. This liver hemangioma demonstrated increased uptake on a tagged red blood cell liver scan, confirming the diagnosis.

be obtained to differentiate hemangioma from metastases by presence or absence of change.

For cavernous hemangiomas smaller than 1.5 cm, ultrasound has been shown to be more accurate than CT because it is difficult to evaluate the CT enhancement pattern in these small lesions.[1] Lesions smaller than 3 cm are uniformly echogenic on ultrasound because of the presence of multiple acoustic interfaces.[1] Depending on the size and circumstance, ultrasound may be combined with CT, MRI, radionuclide-tagged red blood cell study, or biopsy to make a definitive diagnosis. A percutaneous biopsy can be performed safely and can yield a specific histologic diagnosis without serious complication.[12]

Focal nodular hyperplasia.   Several characteristic ultrasound findings have been demonstrated with focal nodular hyperplasia: variable size; dense nonshadowing linear or stellate echoes representing the central scar; hypoechoic, isoechoic, or hyperechoic pattern; and frequent involvement of the right lobe.[1] Ultrasound may be combined with a radionuclide liver and spleen scan to make a definitive diagnosis; colloid uptake is usually normal in focal nodular hyperplasia.[1]

Liver cell adenoma.   As with focal nodular hyperplasia, liver cell adenomas are more common in females and are linked to oral contraceptive use. The ultrasound pattern may be similar to focal nodular hyperplasia: hypoechoic, isoechoic, or dense.[1]

Malignant Neoplasms

Hepatocellular carcinoma.   Most patients (90%) with hepatocellular carcinoma (HCC) present with hepatomegaly. The ultrasound pattern may be discrete echogenic, discrete anechoic, mixed, isoechoic, or diffuse infiltrative (Fig. 121-15). Most lesions smaller than 3 cm have a hypoechoic

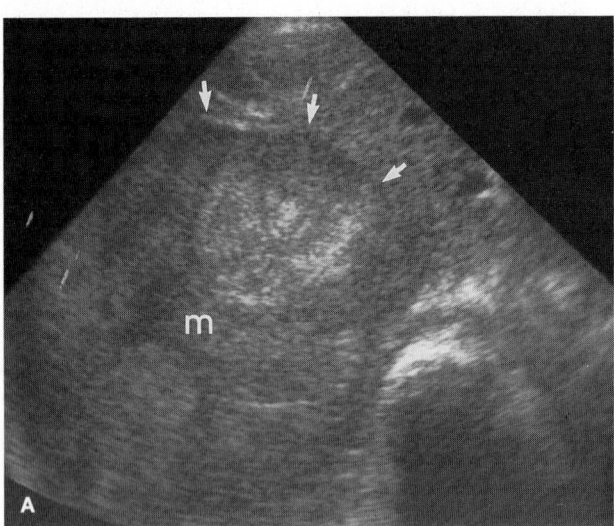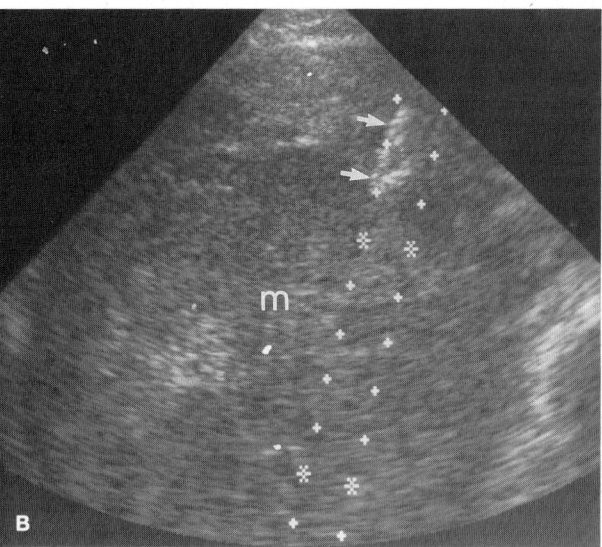

FIGURE 121-15. Hepatocellular carcinoma. **(A)** The transverse view of the right lobe of the liver demonstrates a large solid mass (m, *arrows*) within the posterior aspect. The mass has an inhomogeneous echo pattern. **(B)** A transverse view, more magnified than **A**, shows a needle (echogenic line, *arrows*) within the needle guide track during a percutaneous ultrasound-guided biopsy.

pattern.[13] Differentiation of HCC from focal fatty change, lipoma, and angiomyolipoma may be difficult if there is fatty metamorphosis in the tumor causing the carcinoma to appear echogenic.[14] HCC may be differentiated from metastatic liver lesions by several findings: a mosaic internal echo pattern (i.e., heterogeneous), posterior acoustic enhancement, and lateral shadow patterns.[13] Metastatic nodules (<10 mm) from HCC may be detected with intraoperative ultrasound.[15] However, differentiation of small nodules from regenerating cirrhotic nodules in cases associated with severe liver cirrhosis may be difficult, even with intraoperative ultrasound.[15] Ultrasound has a 90% sensitivity and 93% specificity for the detection of HCC, and it is the most sensitive method for the detection of small tumors.[1] Ultrasound can also be used to guide a percutaneous needle biopsy (see Fig. 121-15*B*).

Metastatic disease.   The most common malignant neoplasm of the liver is metastatic tumor. The more common primary origins are the gastrointestinal tract (especially colon), breast, and lung. Metastatic tumor usually causes hepatic enlargement and typically involves both lobes. Ultrasound demonstrates discrete hypoechoic, discrete echogenic, anechoic, and diffuse inhomogeneous patterns (Figs. 121-16 and 121-17).[1]

The discrete echogenic pattern is frequently seen with colon metastases (54%), with fewer instances of this pattern seen with HCC (25%).[1] As a rule, the ultrasound appearance lacks specificity in defining the primary organ. If calcification is demonstrated, cancer of the colon is the more common primary (see Fig. 121-17).[1] Other tumors that demonstrate calcification are endocrine tumors of the pancreas, leiomyosarcoma, malignant melanoma, cystadenocarcinoma of the ovary, adenocarcinoma of the stomach, lymphoma, osteosarcoma, pleural mesothelioma, neuroblastoma, and breast cancer.[1] A hypoechoic pattern is the most common pattern associated with hepatic lymphoma, although the ultrasound

appearance is not specific.[1] Diffuse and hypoechoic patterns have been seen in Hodgkin's and non-Hodgkin's lymphoma; the bull's-eye and echogenic lesions have only been associated with non-Hodgkin's lymphoma.[1] Multiple, discrete masses may be associated with leukemia. These lesions may be solid and anechoic or exhibit a bull's-eye pattern with a dense center secondary to necrosis.[1] However, because the hepatic involvement may be microscopic, the ultrasound appearance may be normal, even with diffuse metastases.

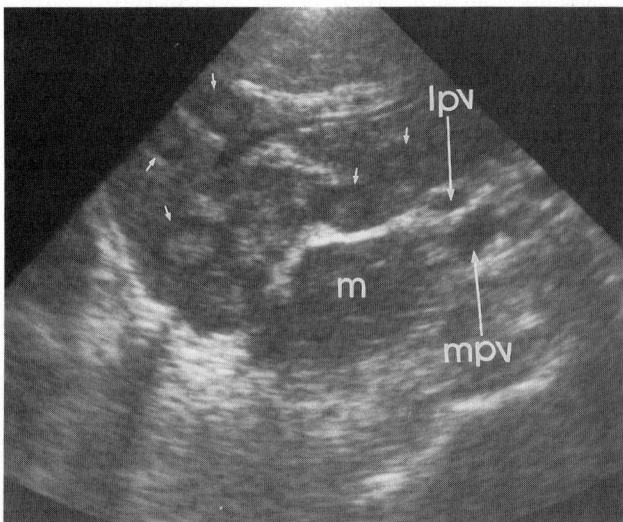

FIGURE 121-16. Metastatic carcinoma of the lung. The sagittal view of the left lobe demonstrates multiple bull's-eye lesions (*small arrows*) throughout the liver. There is a mass (m) of nodes superior to the portal vein. (lpv, left portal vein; mpv, main portal vein.)

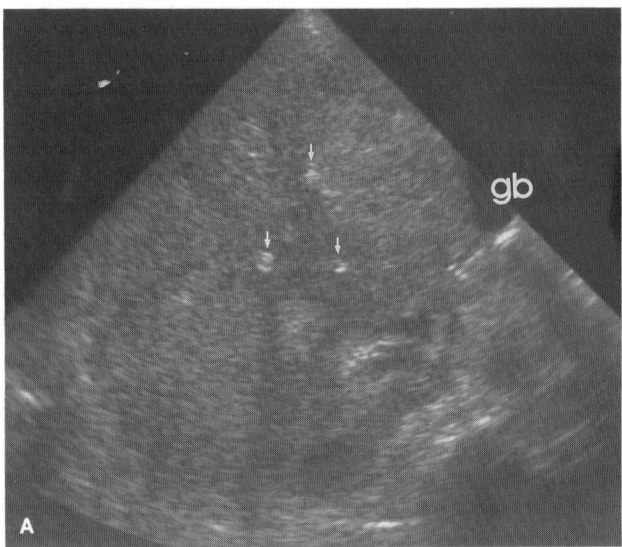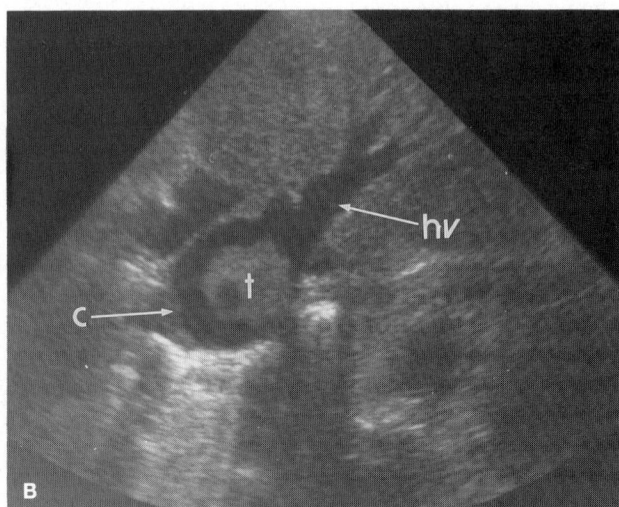

FIGURE 121-17. Metastatic, poorly differentiated adenocarcinoma. (**A**) On a transverse view of the right lobe, an inhomogeneous echo pattern is observed. Discrete lesions cannot be outlined. There are some echogenic foci (*arrows*), which represent calcification associated with posterior shadowing. (gb, gallbladder.) (**B**) The high transverse view of the inferior vena cava (c) shows a large echogenic mass (t) that is a tumor thrombus and the left hepatic vein (hv).

For patients with metastatic liver disease, ultrasound can be employed to assess the chemotherapeutic response by looking for changes in size and echo pattern.[1] Ultrasound also may be used to guide a biopsy of hepatic lesions. A greater than 90% accuracy has been reported in diagnosing malignant or benign lesions with a single pass.[1] A 91.6% cytohistologic accuracy has been reported, with a sensitivity of 92.2% and a specificity of 88.9%.[1] Ultrasound is usually the modality of choice for needle biopsy guidance provided the lesion is visualized by ultrasound (some lesions are visualized by CT) because of its simplicity and safety, and the procedure can be performed on an outpatient basis. Ultrasound can also be used to guide the intratumor injection of absolute ethanol used to treat small HCCs, other small hepatic tumors, and abdominal tumors; occasionally, there is incomplete necrosis of the tumor.[16,17]

Trauma

Hepatic hematomas may be secondary to trauma or rupture of a neoplasm such as an adenoma, metastatic choriocarcinoma, or cavernous hemangioma. With liver trauma, there may be rupture of the liver and its capsule, separation of the capsule from the liver parenchyma resulting in subcapsular hematoma, and central rupture of the liver. The liver is often evaluated initially with CT and followed serially with ultrasound.

The pattern demonstrated on ultrasound depends on the time of the trauma relative to the time of the scan, and the location and degree of injury. Most hepatic hematomas are hypoechoic with poorly defined margins, although the hematoma may initially be echogenic. Subcapsular hematomas appear as anechoic areas bordering the liver.

Transplantation

Duplex sonography and color Doppler ultrasound play important roles in the preoperative and postoperative evaluation of patients undergoing liver transplantation. The preoperative assessment involves determining the presence and direction of flow in the portal vein and the size of the vessel; this information helps predict the difficulty in performing the surgery and may preclude transplantation in some cases. A careful evaluation of the hepatic parenchyma is performed to exclude masses, because the incidence of hepatoma is significantly increased in this population. The hepatic artery, hepatic veins, IVC, biliary system, and portosystemic collaterals should be evaluated routinely in the pretransplant patient.

Postoperatively, ultrasound is performed routinely at many institutions to detect complications. The most serious of these is hepatic artery thrombosis, which is an early complication occurring in 3% to 12% of adults and 11% to 42% of children.[1,18] This is more common in children because of the smaller size of the hepatic artery. Other complications that can be assessed with ultrasound include portal vein thrombosis, IVC stenosis or thrombosis, biliary dilatation, and extrahepatic fluid collections.

Correlative Imaging

For a patient with suspected hepatic neoplasm, the physician must choose among ultrasound, CT, radionuclide imaging, or MRI as the initial diagnostic procedure. CT is thought to be most effective; ultrasound and radionuclide scan are equivalent but less effective. MRI is fast becoming a highly regarded technique for evaluating the liver. The diagnostic accuracy of ultrasound depends almost entirely on the quality of the image, which is a direct result of the skills of the physician and technologist and the capabilities of the machine.

Some investigators think CT should be the first choice for the examination of the patient with suspected liver disease because of the greater sensitivity and specificity of contrast-enhanced CT for focal lesions; the ability to detect diffuse liver abnormalities; the greater ease in standardization and interpretation; the ability to predict accurately the histology of many focal and diffuse diseases; and the greater accuracy in the detection and characterization of extrahepatic abnormalities.[1] Ultrasound may be done if CT scanning is not available, if intravenous contrast cannot be given, if there are other problems with technique, and if patients require ultrasound for other reasons. Radionuclide scanning and MRI should be reserved for solving cases of nondiagnostic ultrasound or CT studies.

Future of Liver Ultrasonography

Ultrasound "contrast" agents, such as perfluorochemicals, a class of compounds composed entirely of carbon and fluorine atoms, are being investigated. Perfluorodecalin, perfluorotripropylamine, and perfluorooctylbromide (PFOB) are known to produce increased liver echogenicity relative to kidney echogenicity in rabbits. With PFOB, an echogenic rim is seen around hepatic tumors in rabbits. During its vascular phase, PFOB enhances tissues, with the degree of enhancement related to the degree of perfusion.[19] This increased echogenicity in proportion to the degree of vascularity may allow ultrasound to be used to estimate the degree of tissue perfusion and to visualize areas of infarction and tumors.[19] These compounds or others may serve as echogenic contrast materials in the future, facilitating visualization of hepatic tumors.

Assessment of tumors with duplex and color-flow Doppler to look at their hemodynamic characteristics shows great potential.[20-23] Abnormal Doppler ultrasound signals have been detected in 94% of patients with primary malignant tumors of the liver, kidney, adrenal, or pancreas.[21] HCC exhibits a very large Doppler shift, but hemangiomas show little to no Doppler shift, and metastases appear to produce low Doppler shifts.[20] Preliminary results have shown similar success in differentiating benign from malignant pancreatic and renal masses.[22] To determine the ultimate value of this technique, particularly its sensitivity and specificity, further study is needed.

EVALUATION OF THE BILIARY SYSTEM

Ultrasound is the best initial screening test for evaluating the biliary system. The high-resolution, real-time ultrasound systems may identify the gallbladder and extrahepatic ducts in most patients, despite body habitus or clinical condition. Ultrasound also permits study of adjacent neighboring structures, such as the liver, pancreas, and other organs, at the same time.

Technical Applications

The biliary scan is performed after an overnight fast or a fast for at least 6 hours, because fasting promotes gallbladder distention, yielding better visualization of the gallbladder. For

an emergency case or critically ill patient, there is usually no problem with gallbladder visualization, because these patients are fasting. The examiner assesses focal tenderness over the gallbladder during scanning. In conjunction with the gallbladder examination, the extrahepatic ducts (i.e., common hepatic duct, common bile duct) are always identified and measured. For optimal visualization of intralumenal filling defects (e.g., stones), evaluation of the gallbladder wall, and optimal visualization of the ducts, the study is performed in various positions, including supine, left lateral decubitus, and sometimes erect and prone, and the patient may be given water to drink to improve visualization of the distal common bile duct.[24] The patient is then studied in the erect or right lateral decubitus position, which optimally positions the air and fluid in the stomach for better visualization of the duct. To enhance the visualization of ductal stones, the patient may be given a fatty meal to dilate the duct.[25]

Normal Anatomy

Most gallbladders can be visualized by ultrasound. The gallbladder is 7 to 10 cm long and 2 to 3 wide and has a capacity of 30 to 50 mL.[24] The normal gallbladder appears as an anechoic structure adjacent to and indenting the inferomedial aspect of the right lobe of the liver (see Fig. 121-2). The main lobar fissure can be seen as a linear echo density connecting the gallbladder to the area of the right or main portal vein.[24] The gallbladder wall is thin, usually less than 3 mm, even in children.[24]

The normal extrahepatic ducts may be seen routinely with ultrasound. In its supraduodenal segment, the normal common bile duct can be seen anterior to the portal vein and lateral to the hepatic artery (see Fig. 121-4A). At a higher level in the porta hepatis, the common bile duct may be seen anterior to the hepatic artery (see Fig. 121-4B). The internal diameter of the duct at this level should be 4 to 6 mm, with 7 mm as the upper limit of normal.[24] The distal common bile duct is seen as a lucency along the posterolateral margin of the pancreatic head or within the pancreatic head (Fig. 121-18). The common hepatic duct can be seen superior to the level of the gallbladder neck and cystic duct (see Fig. 121-2). If measured anterior to the right portal vein, the maximal lumenal diameter should not exceed 4 mm.[24]

Gallbladder Abnormalities

Gallstones

Stones appear echo dense, with a posterior acoustic shadow (Fig. 121-19A).[24] Stones containing more than 88% cholesterol float and create a shadow on ultrasound.[24] In 100% of cases, if a mobile echogenic structure in the gallbladder has an acoustic shadow, it is a stone. The acoustic shadow is described as a clean shadow if distinct margins are seen without reverberation echoes.[24] Reverberation echoes are seen within the shadow of stones containing calcium; stronger reverberations are seen with the more densely calcified stones. Choosing patients for chenodeoxycholic acid therapy for stone dissolution may be influenced by the ultrasound compositional

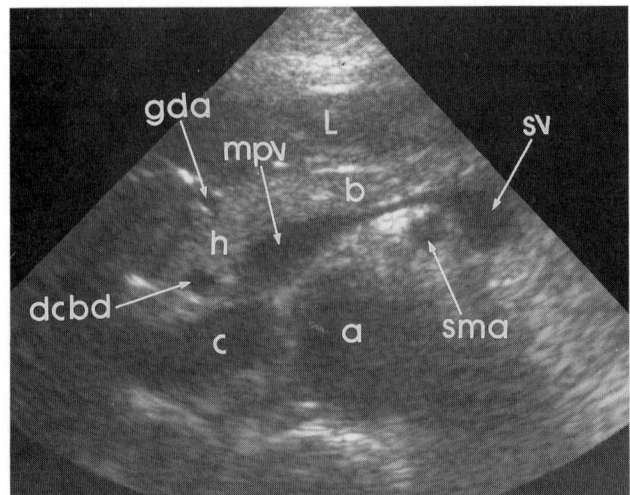

FIGURE 121-18. On this transverse view, the normal head (h) and body (b) of the pancreas can be seen along with its landmarks. (a, aorta; c, inferior vena cava; dcbd, distal common bile duct; gda, gastroduodenal artery; L, liver; mpv, main portal vein; sma, superior mesenteric artery; sv, splenic vein; from Mittelstaedt CA. Pancreas. In: General ultrasound. New York: Churchill Livingstone, 1992:371.)

analysis of stones for detection of calcification.[24] Other imaging methods such as CT may better reveal stone composition.

Contracted or nonvisualized gallbladder. The gallbladder may not be visualized in 15% to 25% of patients with stones. In such cases, it is helpful to demonstrate the double arc sign, in which two parallel arcuate echogenic lines are separated by

a thin anechoic space with distal acoustic shadowing. The proximal arc represents the near wall of the gallbladder, the anechoic space is the bile, and the distal arc is secondary to the gallbladder stones.[24]

Porcelain gallbladder. The ultrasound patterns associated with porcelain gallbladder are a hyperechoic semilunar structure with posterior acoustic shadow or variable acoustic shadowing with a biconvex curvilinear echogenic structure or irregular clumps of echoes.[24]

Sludge

Sludge represents nonshadowing, low-amplitude echoes that layer in the dependent part of the gallbladder. Sludge is mainly composed of calcium bilirubinate, with the source of echoes predominately pigment granules and lesser amounts of cholesterol crystals.[24] It is seen in patients with extrahepatic biliary obstruction, acute and chronic cholecystitis, and those undergoing fast or hyperalimentation. The common factor appears to be stasis of bile in the gallbladder. The differential diagnosis of sludge includes hemobilia, parasitic infestations, blood clot, and aggregate material. Sludge may simulate tumor-producing mass effect because of temporary clumping of highly viscous material from bile stasis.[25]

Cholecystitis

The criteria for the ultrasound diagnosis of acute cholecystitis include stones, sludge, increased wall thickness, gallbladder distention, and focal right upper quadrant pain.

Ultrasound signs: gallbladder wall. Evaluation of the gallbladder wall thickness and patterns may be helpful in the

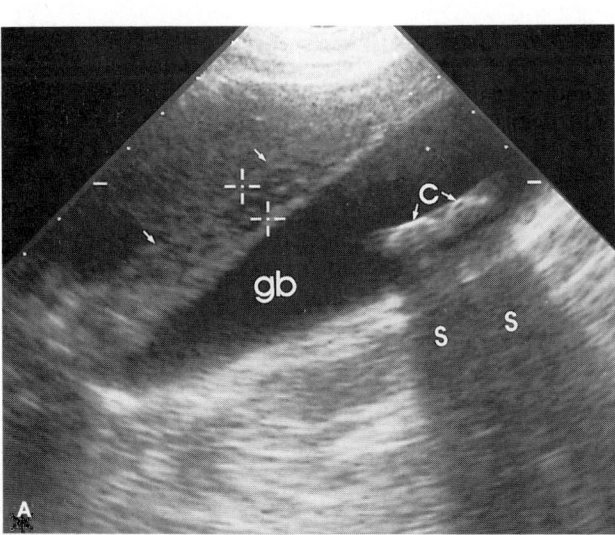
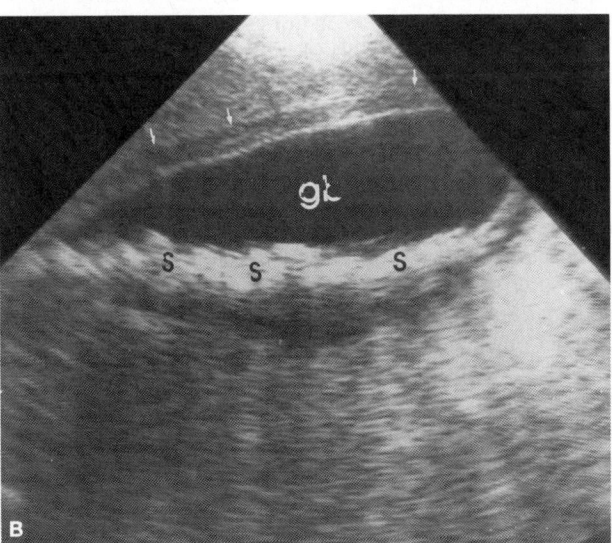

FIGURE 121-19. Acute cholecystitis with cholelithiasis. **(A)** This sagittal ultrasound scan demonstrates a gallbladder (gb) with internal calculi (c) and associated acoustic shadowing (s) with striated wall thickening (*arrows*). The width of the gallbladder wall was 9 to 12 mm. This patient had a positive Murphy's sign. **(B)** A Sagittal left lateral decubitus scan of the gallbladder (gb) demonstrates gallstones (s) with wall thickening (*arrows*). (From Mittelstaedt CA. Biliary system. In: General ultrasound. New York: Churchill Livingstone, 1992:249.)

ultrasound diagnosis of acute cholecystitis. In 95% of asymptomatic patients with no stones, the average gallbladder wall thickness is 2 mm or less, but 45% of patients with stones have a wall thickness of 3 mm or greater. With acute cholecystitis, the mean gallbladder wall thickness is 9 mm (range, 3–16 mm); in chronic cholecystitis, the mean thickness is 5 mm.[26] Increased gallbladder wall thickness is a nonspecific finding and has been reported in hepatitis, ascites, alcoholic liver disease, hypoproteinemia, hypoalbuminemia, heart failure, systemic venous hypertension, renal disease, multiple myeloma, and as a normal variant with physiologic wall thickening during partial wall contraction. In 26% of patients with acute cholecystitis, a gallbladder halo or diffuse hyporeflective wall thickening with hazy wall delineation is seen along with gallbladder distention.[24] Striated wall thickening or alternating irregular, discontinuous, lucent and echogenic bands within the wall is seen in 62% of patients with acute cholecystitis (see Fig. 121-19).[26]

Ultrasound signs: right upper quadrant pain.   In 85% of patients with acute cholecystitis, maximal tenderness is found over the gallbladder (i.e., sonographic Murphy's sign). The accuracy of this sign is reported to be 87.2%, with a sensitivity of 63%, a specificity of 93.6%, a positive predictive value of 72.5%, and a negative predictive value of 90%.[24] Ultrasound has demonstrated nonbiliary pathology in 21% of patients during screening for right upper quadrant pain.[24]

Acalculous cholecystitis.   The ultrasound findings associated with acalculous cholecystitis include an enlarged gallbladder, diffuse or focal wall thickening, focal hypoechoic regions in the wall, pericholecystic fluid, diffuse homogeneous echogenicity in the gallbladder lumen, and a positive sonographic Murphy's sign.[24] A sensitivity of 63% to 67% is reported with these criteria.[24] In one study, ultrasound had a sensitivity of 92% and a specificity of 96% in the diagnosis of acute acalculous cholecystitis using the major criteria of wall thickness of 4 mm or greater in a gallbladder distended to at least 5 cm in its long axis, with no evidence of ascites or hypoproteinemia; presence of pericholecystic fluid or subserosal edema; calculi; intramural gas; sloughed mucosal membrane; or complete lack of response to cholecystokinin (CCK).[27] Minor criteria include presence of echogenic bile (i.e., sludge); distention greater than 8 cm in long axis or 5 cm in the transverse diameter; or partial response (50% decrease in longitudinal and transverse dimensions) after CCK injection.[27] This study was considered positive if it included a minimum of two major criteria or one major with one minor criterion.

Gangrenous cholecystitis.   Ultrasound findings in gangrenous cholecystitis include diffuse, medium-to-coarse intralumenal echoes within the gallbladder that do not layer or produce acoustic shadowing.[24] In 58% of patients, there are intralumenal membranes or marked irregularities of the gallbladder wall. Additional findings may be pericholecystic fluid, thickening of the gallbladder wall, and a dilated gallbladder.[28] Although a positive sonographic Murphy's sign is often seen associated with acute cholecystitis, it is not as prevalent among patients with gangrenous cholecystitis. In one series, only 33% of patients with proven gangrenous cholecystitis had a positive Murphy's sign.[28] The absence of a positive Murphy's sign increases the possibility of gangrenous cholecystitis in patients with abdominal pain and ultrasound findings of cholecystitis.[28]

Gallbladder perforation.   The most common location for gallbladder perforation is in the fundal region. The perforation may be acute, with free perforation causing bile peritonitis; subacute (most common), with walled-off perforation causing pericholecystic abscess; and chronic, with perforation resulting in internal biliary fistulas. The ultrasound findings range from a well-defined band of low-level echoes around the gallbladder to multiple, poorly defined, hypoechoic masses surrounding an irregular, indistinct gallbladder (Fig. 121-20).[24]

Gallbladder Neoplasms

Benign neoplasm.   Papillomas and adenomas represent localized overgrowths involving the gallbladder. Adenomyomatosis, which is proliferation of the surface epithelium with gland-like formation and outpouchings of mucosa into or through the thickened muscular layer (i.e., Rokitansky-Aschoff sinuses) may be diffuse or segmental and localized.[24] Ultrasound findings include diffuse or segmental thickening of the gallbladder wall and intramural diverticula seen as anechoic or echogenic foci with or without associated acoustic shadowing or reverberation artifacts. Cholesterol polyps associated with cholesterolosis have nonshadowing single or multiple fixed echoes projecting within the lumen of the gallbladder.

Malignant neoplasm.   Gallbladder carcinoma has been associated with a spectrum of ultrasound findings, including localized thickening of the gallbladder wall; polypoid lesion with irregular borders; solid mass filling the gallbladder (most common type); and loss of the usual smooth outline of the gallbladder (Fig. 121-21).[24] The diagnosis of gallbladder carcinoma can be made with ultrasound for 84.6% of patients.

Ductal Abnormalities

Dynamic Changes

Dynamic changes of the ducts can be evaluated with ultrasound. The common hepatic duct remains the same size or decreases in caliber after a fatty meal in normal persons. If a normal-sized duct increases in size or a slightly dilated duct remains the same or increases in size, an abnormal response is indicated. However, a dilated common bile duct that does not decrease in size after a fatty meal is not specific for obstruction.[29] An increase in ductal diameter is an abnormal response; a decrease in ductal diameter is normal; and a lack of change in ductal diameter is not associated with obstruction. The ingestion of a fatty meal stimulates CCK release, which causes the gallbladder to contract, increasing the bile flow in the liver and relaxing the sphincter of Oddi.[24,29] If there is no change in ductal diameter, there is no distal obstruction to give rise to increased pressure or dilatation in the duct, and the increased flow produced by the fatty meal is balanced by the sphincter relaxation.[29] Failure of change in size after a fatty meal may be caused by loss of elasticity in the duct as a result of chronic dilatation, inflammation, or aging.[29]

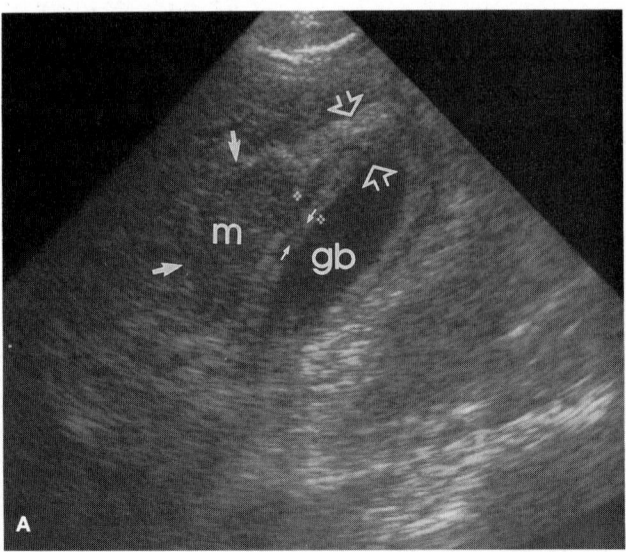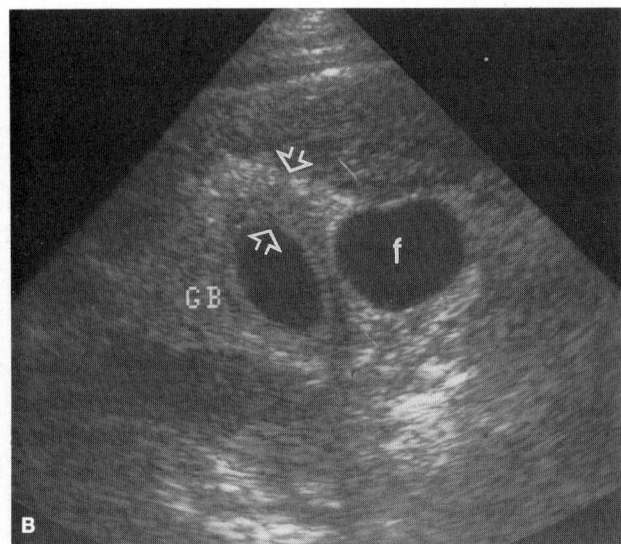

FIGURE 121-20. Gallbladder perforation. (**A**) The sagittal view shows a mass (m, *large arrows*) within the gallbladder (gb) wall and thickening (*open arrows*). There is a defect (*small arrows*) within the gallbladder wall. (**B**) The transverse view shows pericholecystic fluid (f) medial to the gallbladder. The gallbladder (GB) wall is thickened (*open arrows*). (From Mittelstaedt CA. Biliary system. In: General ultrasound. New York: Churchill Livingstone, 1992:249.)

Biliary Dilatation

Several ultrasound findings are associated with biliary system dilatation. Those seen with intrahepatic dilatation include peripheral lucencies within the liver, which demonstrate acoustic enhancement; tubular lucencies within the liver that have an antler or stellate branching pattern; and lucencies within the left lobe of the liver (Fig. 121-22A, B).[24] Doppler ultrasound may help differentiate ducts from vessels (Fig. 121-22C).[30] Findings associated with extrahepatic ductal dilatation include a common hepatic duct that is 6 mm or larger,

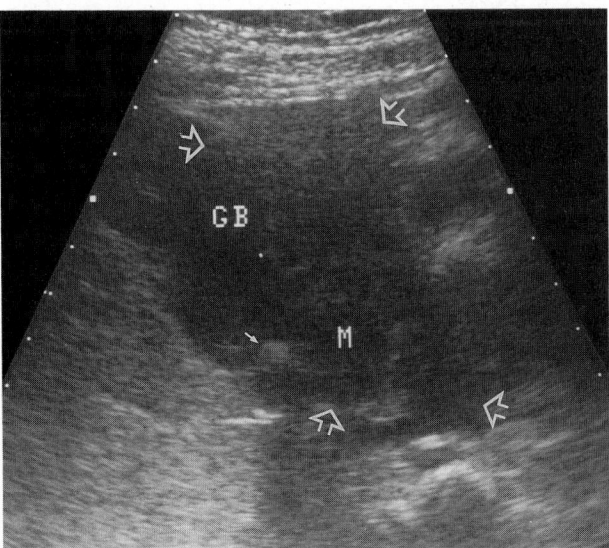

FIGURE 121-21. Gallbladder carcinoma. On a transverse view of the gallbladder, a poorly defined hypoechoic mass (M, *open arrows*) is seen medially. The internal stones (*small arrow*) were better demonstrated on other views.

as measured at a location anterior to the right portal vein, and common bile duct greater than 7 mm (see Figs. 121-4 and 121-22).[24]

Postcholecystectomy patients. There are conflicting opinions regarding the ductal size after cholecystectomy. Some report dilatation of the extrahepatic ducts, but others state that there is no evidence of common bile duct dilatation in 95% of patients.[24] Most recommend further study, such as ultrasound evaluation after a fatty meal, if the common hepatic duct is 6 mm or wider or the common bile duct is 8 mm or larger.[24] A decrease in ductal size after a fatty meal seems to indicate normal bile duct dynamics and excludes obstruction. Bile duct pathology is strongly indicated if the duct enlarges after the fatty meal.[24]

False-positive diagnosis of obstruction. One study demonstrated bile duct dilatation after laparotomy.[31] The mean diameter of the duct is seen to double postoperatively. This finding is also demonstrated in a variety of conditions of intestinal hypomotility, such as paralytic ileus resulting from surgery, abdominal or thoracic inflammatory processes, or trauma; hyperalimentation (parenteral); narcotics; or previous vagotomy. One proposed mechanism is the persistent contraction of the sphincter of Oddi, which occurs if intestinal hypomotility eliminates stimuli for CCK release.[31]

Level and cause of obstruction. If ultrasound demonstrates biliary tract dilatation, a special effort should be made to identify the level and cause of the obstruction. The most common level of obstruction is the distal common bile duct, and choledocholithiasis is the most common cause (80.5%). The suprapancreatic portion of the common bile duct is the second most common location for obstruction.[32] In cases such as this, the pancreas and distal common bile duct appear

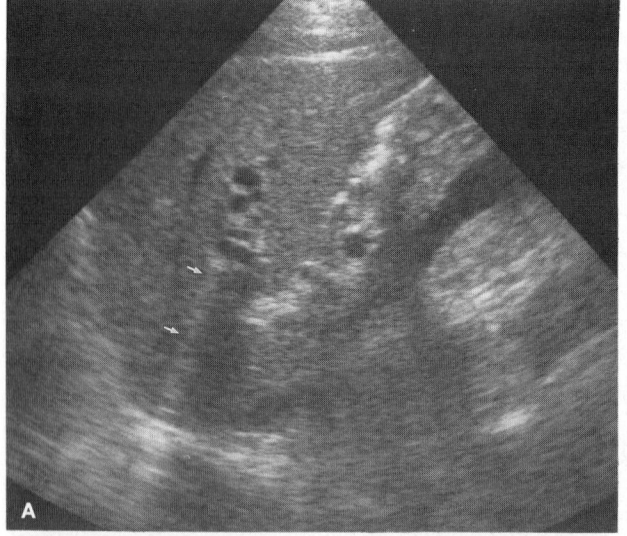

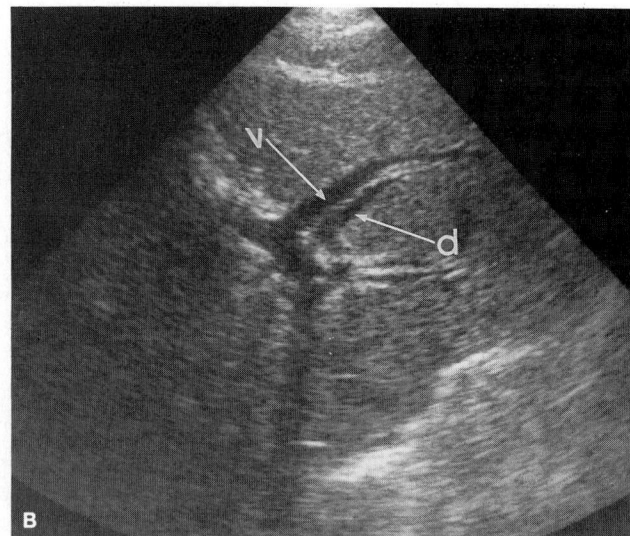

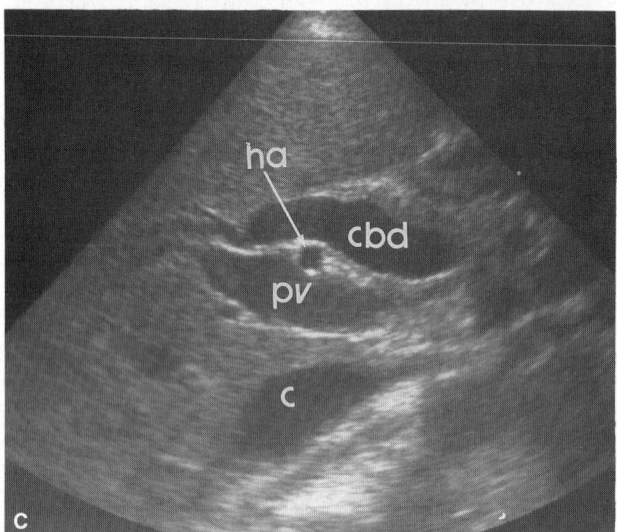

FIGURE 121-22. Dilated biliary system. (**A**) The sagittal view shows lucencies within the left lobe. There is subtle acoustic enhancement (*arrows*) beyond some of the intrahepatic ducts. (**B**) The transverse scan shows the relation of the left duct (d) to the left portal vein (v). (From Mittelstaedt CA. Biliary system. In: General ultrasound. New York: Churchill Livingstone, 1992: 249.) (**C**) A sagittal view of the porta hepatis demonstrates three lucent tubular structures, with the more anterior one measuring 14 mm. Doppler ultrasound can be used to differentiate vascular from biliary structures. The middle tubular structure was found to have an arterial wave form consistent with the hepatic artery (ha). The more anterior structure showed no flow and represented a dilated common bile duct (cbd). (c, inferior vena cava; pv, portal vein.)

normal. At the suprapancreatic level, malignancy is the most common cause, and stones are second. If the dilatation arises at the level of the porta hepatis or proximal, the cause is most often neoplasm.[32]

Choledocholithiasis

The role of ultrasound in the diagnosis of choledocholithiasis in the past was uncertain. To make a positive diagnosis, the examiner must see echogenic material within the duct; without surrounding bile, the diagnosis is difficult (Fig. 121-23). The reasons for the difficulties in the diagnosis on ultrasound include the deeper position of the common bile duct than the gallbladder; difficulty in continuously observing the stone because of interference from changing pockets of gas within overlying bowel; reflection and refraction of the beam by the curved wall of the duct; the common bile duct out of the optimal focal zone of transducer; and minute amounts of fluid surrounding stone, especially in the minimally dilated or normal-sized duct.[24] Using special techniques, such as varied patient positioning or ingesting water or a fatty meal, the

accuracy of the diagnosis of choledocholithiasis may be increased. The marked improvement in the detection of ductal stones is a result of improved imaging technology and increased diagnostic efforts, based on the recognition of subtle ultrasound signs needed to make the diagnosis.[33]

Cholangitis and Other Infections

Oriental cholangiohepatitis.   Pyogenic cholangitis or Oriental cholangiohepatitis is being seen more often in the United States because of the influx of immigrants from Southeast Asia.[24] Massively dilated ducts are demonstrated on ultrasound, with the duct often as large as 3 to 4 cm in diameter. The dilated ducts are packed with huge pigmented stones. Stones may also be seen within the gallbladder. The most frequently involved structure is the common bile duct, followed by the left and right hepatic ducts. Because of the soft mud-like consistency of the stones, ultrasound may fail to demonstrate the ductal calculi and extrahepatic dilatation.[24]

Sclerosing cholangitis.   The cause of sclerosing cholangitis is unknown but may be bacterial or metabolic alteration of

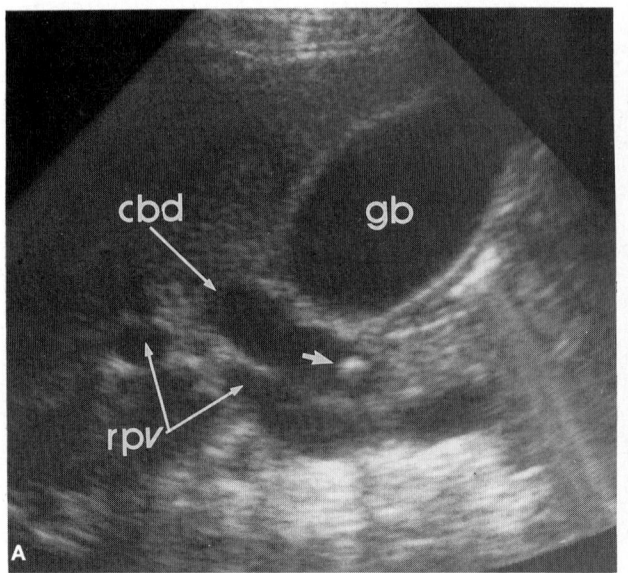

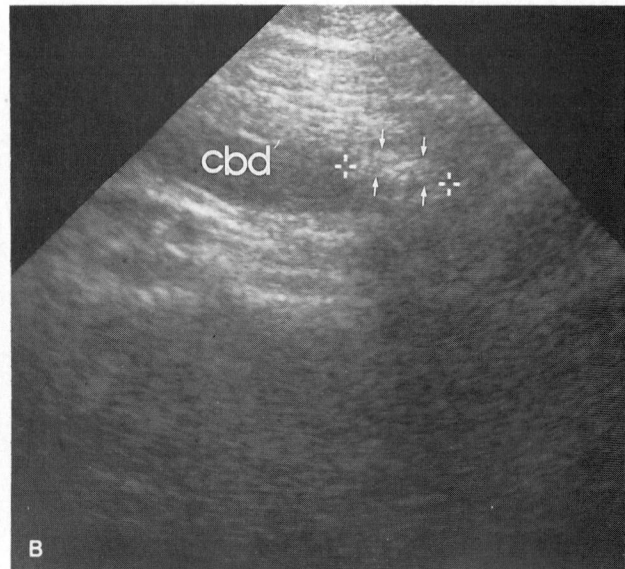

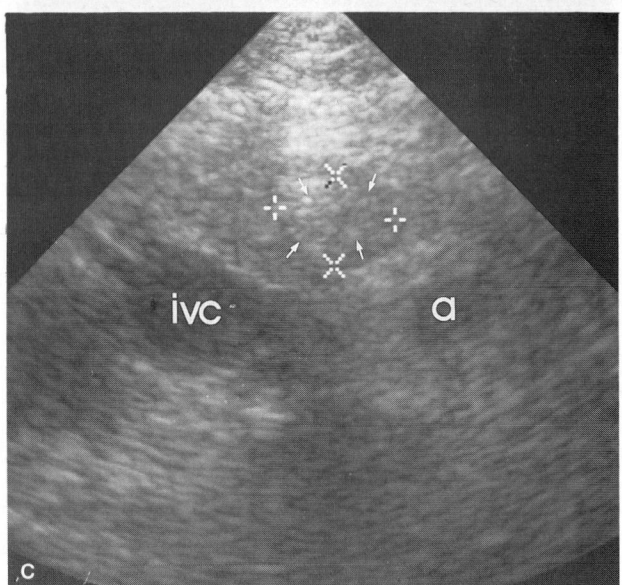

FIGURE 121-23. Choledocholithiasis. **(A)** On a sagittal view through the gallbladder (gb), an echogenic focus (*arrow*) is seen within the dilated proximal common bile duct (cbd) above the right portal vein (rpv). **(B)** Long axis view of the common bile duct (cbd) nearer the distal end reveals a 2-cm echogenic calculus (*arrows*). **(C)** A transverse scan through the pancreatic head region in the area of the distal common bile duct shows the large calculus (*arrows*) in the region of the distal common bile duct. (a, aorta; ivc, inferior vena cava.)

bile acids. Tumors, previous surgery or trauma, and passage of large gallstones with resultant strictures may cause secondary cholangitis. Marked concentric thickening of the intrahepatic and extrahepatic ducts with biliary dilatation is seen on ultrasound scans.[24]

Acquired immunodeficiency syndrome–related cholangitis. Patients with AIDS are at risk for infection of the biliary tract with a variety of opportunistic infections; the most commonly cited organisms are cytomegalovirus and *Cryptosporidium*.[34] The biliary tract abnormalities described in patients with AIDS include gallbladder wall thickening in 55%, dilated gallbladder in 18%, biliary sludge in 23%, and gallstones in 5%.[24,34] The walls of the intrahepatic and extrahepatic bile ducts may be thickened in a smooth or irregular fashion, sometimes resulting in focal areas of biliary ductal dilatation from lumenal compromise (Fig. 121-24).[35] This appearance is virtually identical to that seen with sclerosing cholangitis. However, the combination of papillary stenosis and intrahepatic ductal dilatation is unique to AIDS-related cholangitis.

Biliary Neoplasms

Primary biliary neoplasm.   In descending order of frequency, the sites of location of cholangiocarcinoma are the common bile duct (especially distal); junction of the cystic duct, common hepatic duct, and common bile duct; hepatic ducts; cystic duct; and duodenal portion of the common bile duct.[24] The ultrasound signs of cholangiocarcinoma include marked biliary obstruction with a normal pancreas; focal biliary tract stricture or abrupt termination; delineation of a mass involving bile duct; irregularly defined, coarse acoustic shadow arising from obstructive mass; contained intralumenal soft-tissue echoes; and echogenic bands across the lumen.[24] The most common appearance of intrahepatic cholangiocarcinoma on ultrasound is that of a homogeneously hyperechoic mass or masses.[36] Findings that help differentiate it from other primary intrahepatic tumors include a homogeneously echogenic or high-attenuation appearance on images, the presence of calcification, and the uncommon invasion of portal or hepatic veins.[36] An additional sign described with cholangiocarcinoma

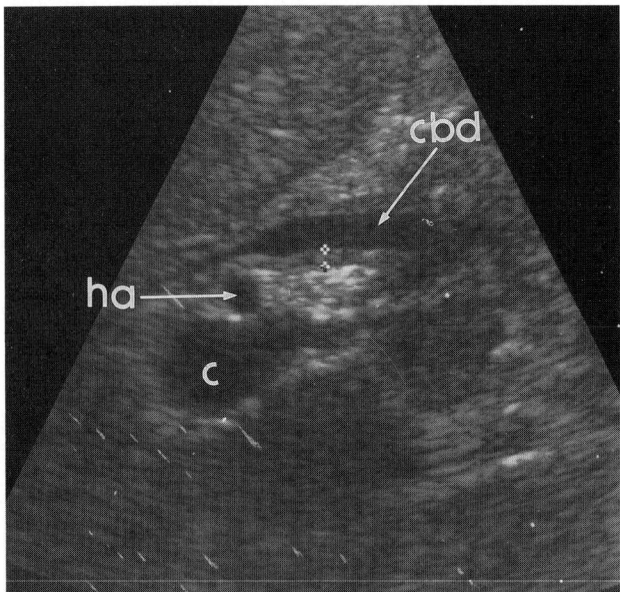

FIGURE 121-24. AIDS cholangitis. In this AIDS patient with cytomegalovirus infection and abnormal liver function tests, there is thickening (*calipers*) of the common bile duct (cbd) wall (2.5 mm), with a lumen of 4 mm. Dilated intrahepatic ducts were observed on other views. (c, inferior vena cava; ha, hepatic artery.)

is a discrepancy between the biliary tract dilatation seen on ultrasound and CT.[37] The dilatation may appear more severe on CT if there is advanced neoplastic disease spreading along the course of the biliary tree, creating the false-positive appearance of ductal dilatation as a result of its low density; this does not occur on the ultrasound study.[37]

Carcinoma arising at the hepatic duct bifurcation (i.e., Klatskin's tumor) is associated with several ultrasound findings: dilatation of the intrahepatic ducts but not of the extrahepatic ducts; nonunion of the right and left hepatic ducts; small, solid masses in the hepatic hilum; apparent intraductal mass at the confluence of the right and left intrahepatic ducts; enlarged portal lymph nodes; and hepatic metastases.[24,38] In one series, all patients demonstrated dilated intrahepatic bile ducts with a normal-sized extrahepatic biliary tree. The location of these tumors allows significant obstruction to occur before the primary tumor attains considerable size. This tumor has a worse prognosis than other cholangiocarcinomas because its location makes treatment difficult.

Cystadenoma and cystadenocarcinoma are rare biliary neoplasms.[24] On ultrasound, these lesions have a distinctive pattern: cystic multiloculated intrahepatic masses with thick, highly echogenic internal septations and papillary projections.[24] In indeterminate cases, aspiration may yield a mucinous, bile-tinged or brownish, cloudy fluid.

Metastatic disease in the biliary system. The most common cause of malignant obstruction of the biliary system is pancreatic carcinoma, which is usually seen as a relatively hypoechoic lobulated mass in the area of the pancreatic head. Less common causes include carcinoma of the ampulla of Vater,

nodal masses caused by lymphoma or other metastatic disease involving the liver hilum or peripancreatic lymph nodes, and primary biliary ductal or gallbladder carcinoma.[24] HCC may produce biliary obstruction and even produce filling defects in the proximal extrahepatic ducts.

Correlative Imaging

Ultrasound is the preferred method for the evaluation for gallstones, with most studies demonstrating an overall accuracy of 96% to 98.9%, with a sensitivity of 98%, a specificity of 93.5% to 97.7%, a false-negative rate of 2.2% to 4%, and a false-positive rate of 2.8%.[24] In diagnosing cholecystitis, ultrasound is often compared with radionuclide studies. Nuclear medicine studies have 84.7% to 88% accuracy, 90.2% to 100% specificity, 95% to 98.3% sensitivity, and a false-negative rate of 5%.[24] Diagnostic ultrasound scans have 88.1% rate of accuracy, 60.2% to 100% specificity, and 76% to 97% sensitivity.[24] A later study reported the positive predictive value for stones combined with a positive sonographic Murphy's sign (92.2%) or gallbladder wall thickening (95.2%) to be excellent for the diagnosis of acute cholecystitis.[39] The negative predictive value demonstrated with the combination of the primary and secondary signs (i.e., for no stones and negative Murphy's sign) to exclude acute cholecystitis is 95%.[39] Ultrasound can be definitive in the diagnosis of almost 80% of patients with suspected acute cholecystitis using the primary and secondary signs.[39] Striated-appearing wall thickening has a positive predictive value of 100%.

Ultrasound is the modality of choice for screening patients with jaundice. Ultrasound has an accuracy of 86% to 97% for differentiating obstructive from nonobstructive jaundice, with a predictive value of 97% in obstructive and 84% in nonobstructive cases.[24] Ultrasound has been correct regarding the level of obstruction in 91.8% to 95% of cases, designating the correct cause in 70.9% to 98%.[32,40] A primary or metastatic neoplasm can be diagnosed correctly with ultrasound in 90.5% of cases.[32] CT is more accurate in identifying the level of the obstruction and the cause, and ultrasound can be used as a screen for obstruction in jaundiced patients.

Various degrees of accuracy have been reported for the ultrasound evaluation of choledocholithiasis. Older series listed the accuracy for ultrasound at 15% to 60%. Later series reported an overall sensitivity of 75%, with 89% for proximal and 70% for distal calculi visualized with ultrasound.[24,25] CT is superior to ultrasound in diagnosing the cause of obstruction and is thought to be more effective than ultrasound in imaging for common bile duct stones. CT is effective in defining the level and cause of obstruction, and ultrasound is an excellent initial procedure for detecting biliary dilatation. CT has a sensitivity of 87%, with an overall accuracy rate of 84%.

Future of Biliary Ultrasonography

Perhaps the most difficult diagnosis with regard to the biliary system is choledocholithiasis, for the reasons described. Further changes in the real-time systems and transducer design may improve the visibility of ductal stones.

EVALUATION OF THE PANCREAS

The pancreas has been a difficult organ to image. In the past, pancreatic disease was suspected if there were indirect changes seen on plain radiographs or upper gastrointestinal series. The pancreas and its associated changes can be imaged directly with the modalities of ultrasound, CT, or MRI. Early changes can be observed, and the changes can be followed. High-resolution, real-time ultrasound can visualize the pancreas, but it remains the most difficult abdominal organ to image. To demonstrate the pancreas adequately, the examiner must be persistent, innovative, meticulous, and familiar with normal and abnormal anatomy.

Technical Applications

As with the biliary and liver scans, it is best to perform a pancreatic scan after an overnight fast or after at least a 6- to 8-hour fast. This improves visualization of the gallbladder, which is most often scanned in conjunction with the pancreas, and ensures an empty stomach and usually less bowel gas. The head, body, and tail of the pancreas are identified with the pancreatic landmarks, such as superior mesenteric vein, superior mesenteric artery, portal vein, distal common bile duct, splenic vein, IVC, aorta, and pancreatic duct. To obtain optimal visualization, the pancreas may be examined with the patient in supine, erect, or lateral decubitus positions. The patient may be given water to drink; the examiner maneuvers the patient in various positions, using the fluid-filled stomach as an acoustic window overlying the targeted portion of the pancreas.[41]

Normal Anatomy

The normal pancreas is seen as a comma-shaped structure anterior to the IVC and aorta (see Fig. 121-18). Other vascular landmarks include the splenic vein, portal vein, superior mesenteric vein and artery, and gastroduodenal artery. The distal common bile duct is seen as a lucent structure along or within the posterior aspect of the pancreatic head. The normal pancreatic texture is isoechoic or hyperechoic to that of the liver.

Acute Pancreatitis

Ultrasound can be most helpful in evaluating biliary tract disease in patients with acute pancreatitis, because many of these patients have associated stones and ductal dilatation. Only 62% of pancreases are visualized by ultrasound, but 98% are visualized by CT.[41] If complications of acute pancreatitis are suspected and if the pancreas is not visualized on ultrasound, CT is recommended.

Several characteristic ultrasound patterns are associated with acute pancreatitis. The pancreas may appear normal (29%) or have a diffuse increase in size, with loss of the normal ultrasound texture (52%) or focal enlargement (28%).[41] The pancreas develops poorly defined margins, and there may be loss of the outline of the splenic vein. Before an abnormal serum amylase level is found, the ultrasound appearance may be abnormal. However, CT more accurately defines peripancreatic thickening of surrounding fascial planes.

Hemorrhagic Pancreatitis

The ultrasound pattern seen with hemorrhagic pancreatitis depends on the age of the hemorrhage.[41] Early in the course, the pancreas may appear echogenic; with time, it becomes hypoechoic to anechoic. On CT, a similar mass may be of higher density initially, changing to lower density after a week, when it appears cystic on ultrasound scans.

Phlegmonous Pancreatitis

The pancreas appears hypoechoic on ultrasound with acoustic enhancement. The mass usually extends into the lesser sac, left anterior pararenal space, and transverse mesocolon.

Complications of Pancreatitis

Aneurysm

Occasionally, aneurysms may be a complication of acute pancreatitis. The splenic artery is more often affected; less commonly involved are the celiac artery, common hepatic artery, gastric arteries, and gastroduodenal arteries.[41] Such an aneurysm would appear anechoic on ultrasound, much like a pseudocyst. Because intrinsic pulsations may not be seen, all anechoic masses in the pancreas should be evaluated with Doppler ultrasound to exclude the possibility of an aneurysm.

Abscess

Developing secondary to the superinfection of necrotic pancreatic and retroperitoneal tissues, the pancreatic abscess appears similar on ultrasound to the appearance of acute pancreatitis or a pseudocyst.[41] It may be a hypoechoic mass with well-defined borders or a hypoechoic mass with irregular walls and internal echoes.[41] A positive diagnosis can be made only by aspiration of the pancreatic or peripancreatic fluid.

Pseudocyst

Pseudocysts are usually single and round, and they vary in size. They can develop in any part of the pancreas and cause dilatation of the pancreatic duct. They represent collections of fluid arising from loculation of inflammatory processes, necrosis, or hemorrhage. On ultrasound, a typical pseudocyst appears as an anechoic to hypoechoic mass with well-defined borders and acoustic enhancement (Fig. 121-25).[41] There may be internal septation, internal echoes, and a lack of acoustic enhancement. Ultrasound is more successful in identifying pseudocysts (50%—92%) than in identifying acute pancreatitis. The most common location for pseudocysts is in the lesser sac, followed by the anterior pararenal space. The pseudocyst may extend into the mediastinum or involve the duodenum.

Ultrasound is used to identify pseudocysts and follow these lesions over time. If indicated, ultrasound can be used to guide aspiration or drainage of a pseudocyst. The result of aspiration can differentiate the infected from the noninfected

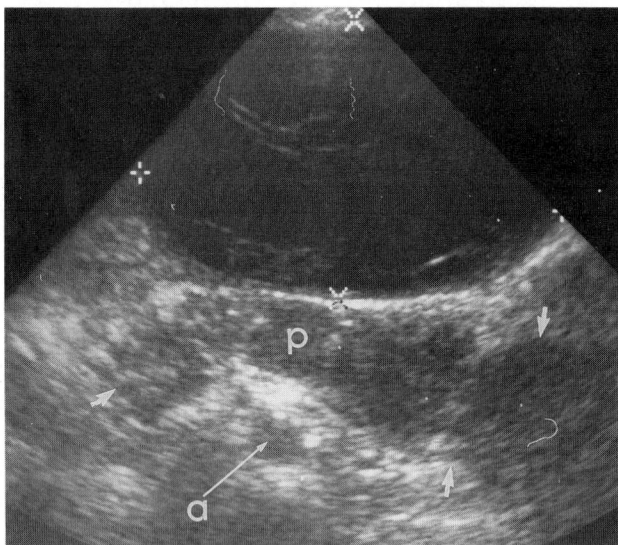

FIGURE 121-25. A transverse view through the abdomen reveals a large, complicated cystic mass (*calipers,* 7 by 11 cm) anterior to the enlarged hypoechoic pancreas (p, *arrows*) above the aorta (a). This patient had acute pancreatitis with pseudocyst formation.

pseudocyst; drainage can be curative in cases of noninfected pseudocysts.[42] Percutaneous drainage helps to stabilize the patient and can be a cure or a temporizing measure until surgery.[42] The cure rate for catheter drainage of pseudocysts is 67%.[42]

Chronic Pancreatitis

Chronic pancreatitis usually represents progressive destruction of the pancreas by repeated flare-ups of a mild or subclinical type of acute pancreatitis. This process more commonly affects alcoholics and less frequently affects patients with biliary tract disease. Calcium carbonate stones can develop in addition to pseudocysts. Several changes are identified on ultrasound. The affected pancreas becomes more echogenic with calcification (92%), ductal dilatation (41%), and an irregular outline (Figs. 121-26 and 121-27).[41] As with acute pancreatitis, there may be diffuse or focal enlargement (27%), with an irregular outline (45%). The stones appear as small echogenic areas, giving the pancreas a stippled appearance (see Fig. 121-26).[41] The exact location of the stones—ductal or glandular—can be determined by ultrasound, although endoscopic retrograde cholangiopancreatography (ERCP) is the most accurate method for investigating duct dilatation and intraductal lithiasis. Besides making the diagnosis of chronic pancreatitis, ultrasound can assess complications, including pseudocysts (in 20%), thrombosis of the splenic or portal vein, and carcinoma (4%–25%; see Fig.121-27).[41] Ultrasound may not be able to differentiate chronic pancreatitis from carcinoma, but an ultrasound-guided biopsy can make the determination.

Trauma

With acute injury, there may be contusion with edema, laceration, hemorrhage, and transection (usually occurring in the pancreatic body). Ultrasound findings associated with

trauma depend on the extent of the injury. A focal hypoechoic mass or a diffuse hypoechoic enlargement of the gland may be seen with contusion.[41] With a traumatic pseudocyst, a well-defined anechoic mass with acoustic enhancement may be identified. With rupture, fluid may be seen within the retroperitoneum or peritoneum.

Neoplasms

Adenocarcinoma

Most adenocarcinomas (60%–70%) are in the pancreatic head, with 20% to 30% in the body and 5% to 10% in the tail. The detection of this lesion on ultrasound depends on adequate visualization of the pancreas, the rate of which varies from 82% to 94%.[41] Approximately 95% of masses demonstrated within the pancreas are hypoechoic, but approximately 3% of masses may be echogenic (Fig. 121-28). Associated changes that may be identified include pancreatic ductal dilatation (18%), biliary dilatation, liver metastases, nodal metastases, portal venous system involvement, splenic vein enlargement, superior mesenteric artery displacement, and ascites.[41]

Mucin-secreting carcinomas of the pancreas can be associated with diffuse dilatation of the main pancreatic duct.[43] The dilated main pancreatic ducts may be filled with amorphous or well-defined filling defects resulting from mucin or tumor.[43] ERCP is indicated in such cases to confirm or rule out mucin-hypersecreting carcinoma of the pancreas. Masses located at the confluence of the bile duct, pancreatic duct, and duodenum are referred to as hepaticopancreatic ampullary tumors and usually range in size from 1.6 to 2 cm.[44] Findings associated with tumor in this location include an intralumenal polypoid mass in the distal part of the common bile duct and a sharply delineated mass with abrupt termination of the distal duct.[44] These have a better prognosis than other tumors that occur in this area, because jaundice is an early sign and leads

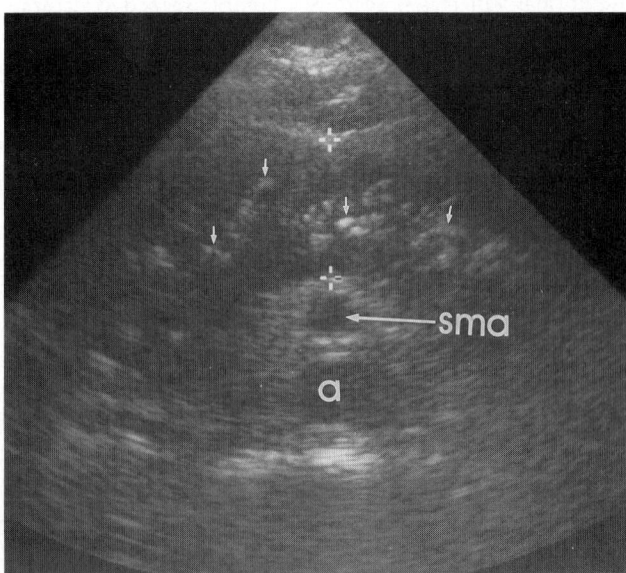

FIGURE 121-26. Chronic pancreatitis and lithiasis. On the transverse view through the body of the pancreas (*calipers*), multiple echogenic foci (*arrows*) are seen. (a, aorta; sma, superior mesenteric artery; from Mittelstaedt CA. Pancreas. In: General ultrasound. New York, Churchill Livingstone, 1992:371.)

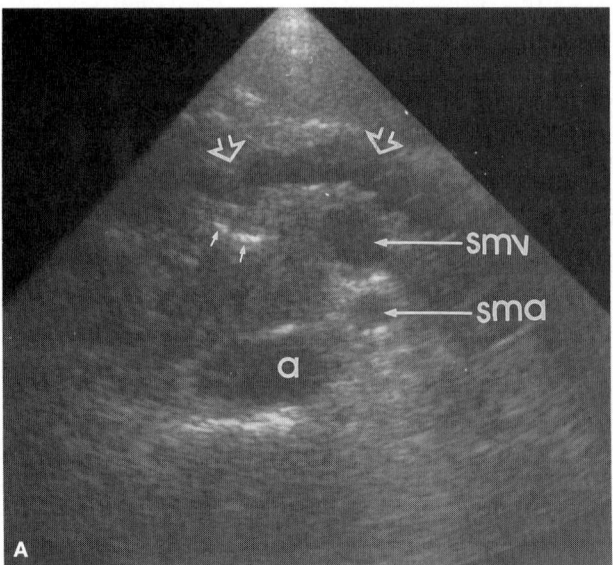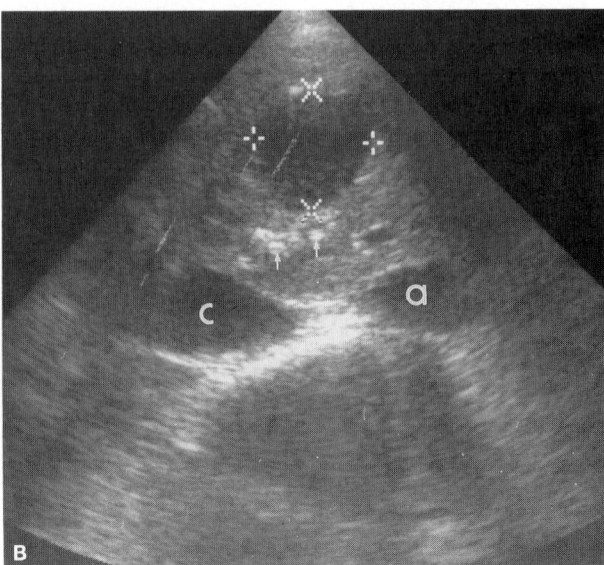

FIGURE 121-27. Lithiasis, pseudocyst, and focal enlargement in chronic pancreatitis. (**A**) The transverse scan through the body and tail region shows a dilated pancreatic duct (*open arrows,* 6 mm) with calculi (*arrows*) that represent calcification. (**B**) On the transverse scan at a lower level than **A**, a pseudocyst (*calipers*) is seen within the pancreatic head. There are echogenic foci (*arrows*) within the head, representing calculi. (a, aorta; c, inferior vena cava; sma, superior mesenteric artery; smv, superior mesenteric vein; from Mittelstaedt CA. Pancreas. In: General ultrasound. New York, Churchill Livingstone, 1992:371.)

to early diagnosis.[44] Ultrasound can contribute to improved detection and prompt treatment in these lesions.

Cystadenoma and Cystadenocarcinoma

Pancreatic cystic neoplasms have been classified pathologically as microcystic or serous adenomas and mucinous or cystic neoplasms; the latter are subdivided into mucinous or ma-crocystic cystadenoma and mucinous or macrocystic cystadenocarcinoma.[41] The ultrasound appearance of cystadenoma or carcinoma is similar to that of pseudocysts: a well-defined anechoic mass associated with acoustic enhancement.[41] There may be internal echoes, irregular margins, masses protruding into the lumen, or completely echogenic masses. The microcystic adenomas contain more than six small cysts (<2 cm) and often have central, stellate scars that are calcified.[41,45] The

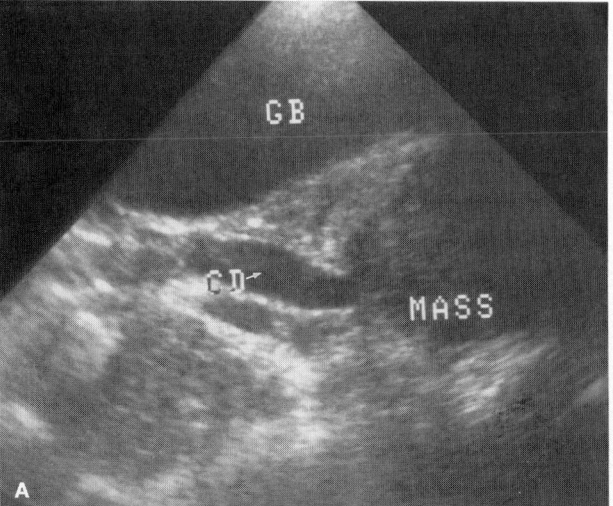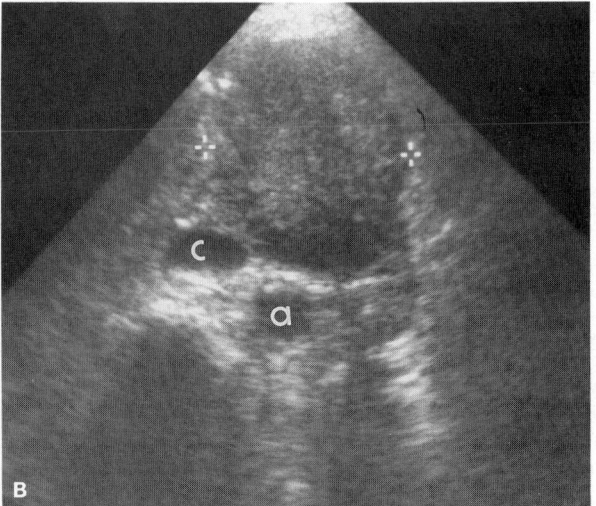

FIGURE 121-28. Pancreatic adenocarcinoma. (**A**) The sagittal scan shows the distended gallbladder (GB) with the dilated duct (CD) and a mass (MASS) near the distal end of the duct. (**B**) The transverse view shows the mass within the region of the uncinate process of the pancreas. (a, aorta; c, inferior vena cava; from Mittelstaedt CA. Biliary system. In: General ultrasound. New York: Churchill Livingstone, 1992:249.)

mucinous cystadenomas and cystadenocarcinomas contain six or fewer cysts with diameters greater than 2 cm.[45] Ultrasound is more accurate in classifying mucinous (93%) than microcystic (78%) cysts.[45]

One group of investigators reported an unusual appearance, referred to as ductectatic, for the mucinous cystadenoma and cystadenocarcinoma.[46] These cystic lesions, which are usually 3 cm in diameter and located in the uncinate process, are associated with localized cystic dilatation of a side branch of the main pancreatic duct.[46] If a cystic lesion encountered in the uncinate process is observed along with ductal dilatation, ERCP is recommended to exclude the possibility of this potentially or overtly malignant disease.

Islet Cell Carcinoma

Functional (85%) and nonfunctional (15%) islet cell tumors represent benign adenomas or malignant tumors. These can be detected with ultrasound in only 51% of cases. Functional tumors are more difficult to visualize than nonfunctional tumors, because they are smaller at presentation. If these lesions are detected with ultrasound, they appear hypoechoic, much like adenocarcinoma, although some of the larger ones appear moderately echogenic.[41] Lesions with necrotic cystic areas probably represent nonfunctional tumors, and functional tumors are more likely to be solid. In addition to identifying the primary pancreatic lesion, ultrasound can detect hepatic metastases, which are usually isodense with the liver.

Perhaps the greatest asset of ultrasound is its ability to localize these lesions intraoperatively. The combined sensitivity of intraoperative ultrasound and surgical palpation for detecting solitary insulinomas is 100%; with ultrasound only, the sensitivity is 84%.[47] If preoperative ultrasound, angiography, and CT are compared for detecting solitary insulinomas, their respective sensitivities are 61%, 54%, and 30%.[47] Intraoperative ultrasound can detect lesions that are not palpable.[47] Ultrasound is useful in detecting insulinomas and in defining the location of insulinomas relative to the pancreatic and bile ducts.[47]

Metastatic Disease

Metastatic disease affecting the pancreas is uncommon. In cases of lymphoma, a large, lumpy, hypoechoic mass may be demonstrated along with involved nodes. Direct invasion by tumors from surrounding organs (e.g., gastric, colonic, duodenal, or biliary tumors) may also appear similar to a primary pancreatic neoplasm with a hypoechoic pattern.[41]

Aspiration and Biopsy

If a focal hypoechoic mass is identified within the pancreas, a definitive diagnosis cannot be made using ultrasound alone. However, ultrasound can be employed to guide an aspiration biopsy of the mass, usually making a definitive diagnosis. A diagnosis can be made in 78% to 88.7% of pancreatic carcinomas using a fine needle.[41] A specificity of 100% has been reported, with a sensitivity of 86%.[41] The diagnostic rate can be increased to 100% by combining cytologic analysis with carcinoembryonic antigen assay.[41]

Besides guiding the sonologist for an aspiration biopsy,

ultrasound can be used to localize the pancreatic duct for percutaneous pancreatography.[48] This procedure can be used to demonstrate pancreatic duct morphology if ERCP has failed or proven nondiagnostic. The ductal system can be mapped before pancreatic surgery. Ultrasound-guided pancreatography can help differentiate carcinoma from chronic pancreatitis by assessing duct appearance.[48]

Usefulness of Ultrasound in Pancreatic Neoplasm

As the most readily available and least expensive of the imaging modalities, ultrasound is useful for detecting pancreatic tumors and assessing the extent of disease.[49] With persistent and careful technique, ultrasound assessment of the pancreas is possible in most patients. Further work-up may be required for patients considered for resection because of the low sensitivity of ultrasound in the identification of resectable disease, mainly as a result of undetected vascular involvement.

Correlative Imaging

CT is most sensitive in the evaluation of patients with acute pancreatitis because it can better visualize the fascial thickening and more accurately identify the locations and extent of associated fluid collections than other modalities.[41] CT provides good to excellent visualization of the pancreatic area in 64% of patients, compared with only 20% of patients who can be examined with ultrasound. Ultrasound is recommended as the initial examination of patients with pancreatitis to document the pancreatitis, examine the gallbladder for stones, and detect collections of fluid or other conditions that may predispose the patient to recurrent attacks.

CT and ultrasound have been compared in several studies of their ability to detect pancreatic pseudocysts. CT and ultrasound each have an accuracy of 75% to 95%. Ultrasound is recommended to screen pseudocysts because of its lower cost and availability. CT may be used to plan the surgical approach or confirm the nature of the lesion before surgery.

One investigation reported an accuracy of 96% for CT and 84% for ultrasound in detecting pancreatic cancer.[41] A positive predictive value of 84% has been reported with ultrasound, with a negative predictive value of 99%, a sensitivity of 94%, and a specificity of 96% to 99%.[41] Studies have reported CT to have a sensitivity of 87%, with a specificity of 90%. Many researchers recommend CT as the initial diagnostic imaging modality for evaluating pancreatic carcinoma. Some advocate ultrasound because it allows reliable exclusion of this disease in a noninvasive way. This is an important feature, because symptoms of this disease are common in the elderly.

Future of Pancreatic Ultrasonography

Visualization of the pancreas is often compromised by overlying bowel gas. Endoscopic ultrasound (see Chap. 122) seems to offer improved pancreatic visualization in those difficult cases. With this technique, a small transducer (i.e., linear array or sector scanner) is coupled to an endoscope, and the pancreas is scanned through the stomach. Small pancreatic tumors can be identified, and the examiner can visualize portions of the heart, aorta, spleen, liver, bile ducts, gallbladder, kidney, and gastrointestinal mucosa. The scan plane is determined by the endoscope, which sometimes makes the anatomic orientation difficult.[41]

EVALUATION OF THE GASTROINTESTINAL TRACT

Although ultrasound is not the primary method for evaluating the gastrointestinal tract, it may be the first method that alerts the physician to the possibility of an abnormality. It is often the first approach to a patient who has had a prior gastrointestinal study, because retained barium causes extensive artifact on a CT scan. Ultrasound is definitely the first diagnostic modality used in patients with palpable abdominal masses. It differentiates masses originating from a parenchymal organ or the gastrointestinal tract and can streamline the work-up of the patient if a gastrointestinal lesion is suspected by ultrasound.

Technical Applications

The examination of the gastrointestinal tract is tailored to the portion of the tract being studied. The results are better if the patient is fasting. Normal, nondistended bowel and stomach usually appear as a target or bull's-eye structure, with the lucency representing the muscular wall and the dense center representing the echogenic mucosa surrounding the lumen. To facilitate examination of stomach and duodenum, the patient may be given fluid to drink. The stomach, pylorus, and duodenum can be recognized by their locations and peristalsis. The small bowel is not usually identified with ultrasound unless the lumen is fluid filled; it is identified by its location and its valvulae conniventes. The colon can be visualized if it is fluid filled and by its location and haustral markings. In some instances, a water enema may be employed while examining with real-time ultrasound to evaluate a suspicious pelvic mass.

Normal Anatomy

The patterns that help to identify the gastrointestinal tract on ultrasound scans are related to gas, mucus, and fluid within the tract. Intralumenal air appears echogenic. The rim of lucency of the bull's-eye pattern represents the wall (i.e., intima, media, and serosa), with its periserosal fat producing the outer echogenic border of the tract wall. The thickness of the rim should not exceed 5 mm. With water distention of the gastrointestinal tract lumen, particularly the stomach, the layers of the wall can be defined (Fig. 121-29). Much of the small bowel and colon is not usually visualized by ultrasound. The fluid-filled duodenum (second portion) can be seen lateral to the pancreatic head.

Abnormalities of the Stomach

Gastric Dilatation

A palpable mass may represent a large, fluid-filled stomach that is secondary to gastric outlet obstruction from pylorospasm, inflammation, or intrinsic or extrinsic tumor or gas-

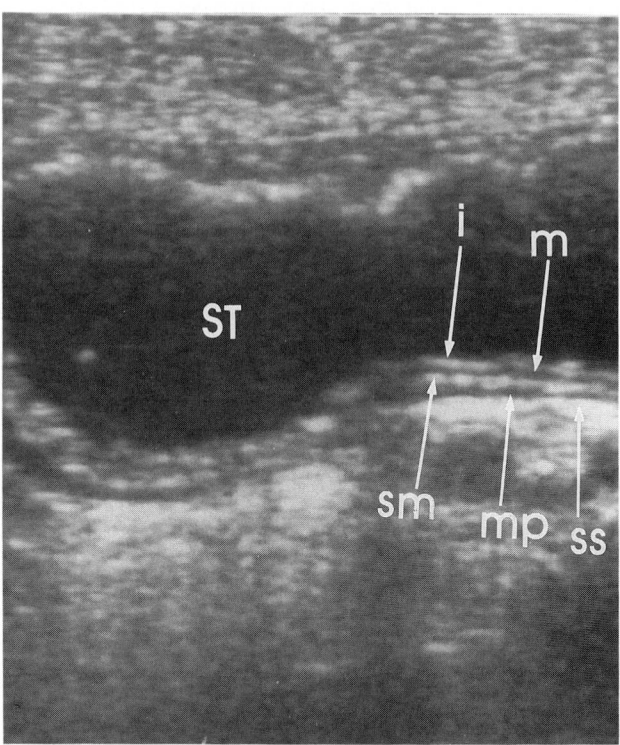

FIGURE 121-29. On the transverse view of the fluid-filled gastric antrum using a 5-MHz linear array transducer and magnification, the normal structure of the gastric wall can be seen. The five layers include the echodense interface echo (i), hypoechoic mucosa (m), echodense submucosa (sm), hypoechoic muscularis proprius (mp), and echodense subserosa, serosa, and interface echo (ss). (ST, fluid-filled stomach, from Mittelstaedt CA. Gastrointestinal tract. In: General ultrasound. New York, Churchill Livingstone, 1992:449.)

troparesis from electrolyte imbalance, diabetes, amyloidosis, neurologic disease, or medications.[50] Ultrasound can make a correct diagnosis by locating a pear-shaped cystic structure in the expected location of the stomach in the left upper quadrant and by detecting peristalsis.

Gastric Duplication

Although rare, gastric duplication of the greater curvature of the stomach occurs more frequently in females.[50] Identification may be delayed until adulthood, although the condition usually exists in infancy. With ultrasound, these lesions are seen as cystic masses with a thin inner echogenic rim (i.e., mucosa) and a wider outer hypoechoic rim (i.e., muscle layer).[50]

Gastritis and Ulcer Disease

The gastric wall thickening seen on ultrasound with some types of chronic gastritis and ulcer disease cannot be differentiated from tumor. However, ultrasound may be helpful in looking for complications associated with gastric ulcer disease. In cases of perforation, intraabdominal fluid may be seen with ultrasound. This localized fluid collection, unlike free peritoneal fluid, does not change in shape or location when the patient changes position.

Benign Tumor

Benign polypoid lesions may be identified within the stomach if there is adequate fluid distention of the stomach. As the most common tumor of the stomach, leiomyoma may be seen on ultrasound as a mass similar to carcinoma.[50] It may appear as an echogenic mass with internal cystic regions caused by necrotic areas.

Malignant Tumor

On ultrasound, a target pattern or pseudokidney structure (i.e., a description ascribed to gastrointestinal lesions) is seen with gastric carcinoma.[50] This target pattern may also be seen with lymphoma, metastatic disease, caustic gastritis, and pancreatitis involving the stomach. The wall thickening may be diffuse or localized and eccentric. There is usually significant infiltration of the mucosa and muscularis and exogastric extension if ultrasound demonstrates a mass. Ultrasound can be used to assess metastases after a gastrointestinal lesion is identified.

Lymphoma can involve the stomach as a primary gastrointestinal tumor. Typically, it appears on ultrasound scans as a relatively large, hypoechoic mass with marked thickening of the gastric wall.[50] Other signs are a spoke-wheel pattern within the target-like lymphomatous mass produced by the marked increase in thickness and height of the mucosal folds and thickened gastric folds that are hypoechoic.[50]

A large, bulky, intramural or subserosal mass is seen with leiomyosarcoma. The pattern on ultrasound is variable, although a target lesion may be seen. The mass may appear as an echo-free zone without enhancement if there is necrosis.[50] With hemorrhage, irregular echoes may be seen within a cystic mass. A leiomyosarcoma is suggested by the pattern of a solid mass anteriorly located outside a solid viscus, necrosis, and intestinal lumen or air close to the mass.

Abnormalities of the Small Bowel

Obstruction and Dilatation

With small bowel obstruction, there is dilatation of the bowel loops proximal to the site of the obstruction. If the dilated loops are filled with gas, ultrasound visualization is not possible. If the dilated loops are filled with fluid (6% of patients), they can be identified on ultrasound. They appear tubular on a long-axis view and as round echo-free masses on a transverse view.[50] With adynamic or nonobstructed ileus, the dilated bowel loops (less distended than with dynamic ileus) have normal to somewhat increased peristaltic activity. Dynamic or obstructed ileus produces more distention, with variable peristaltic activity (i.e., markedly increased to none). The level of the obstruction may be judged by the distribution of the distended fluid-filled loops, but not all fluid-filled bowel loops are associated with obstruction. They can be seen in cases of gastroenteritis and paralytic ileus.

With a closed-loop obstruction or volvulus, a single, dilated, aperistaltic loop of bowel may be seen. A U-shaped structure is seen on the longitudinal scan, and a C-shaped anechoic area with a dense center is seen on the transverse scan in cases of volvulus.[50]

After a subtotal gastrectomy in which a Billroth II anastomosis is performed for ulcer disease, afferent loop obstruction may develop because of internal herniation or a kink of the afferent loop. This abnormality is difficult to diagnose definitely before surgery. On ultrasound scans, a large, cystic structure is seen in the upper abdomen, and it may have echogenic debris in its dependent part.[50] A U-shaped configuration of an obstructed afferent duodenal loop seen in the coronal plane helps to make the diagnosis.

Hematoma

Intramural hemorrhage may occur with or without trauma or may be related to bleeding diatheses, hemophilia, anticoagulant therapy, blunt trauma, leukemia, lymphoma, Henoch-Schöenlein anaphylactoid purpura, and thrombocytopenic purpura. The duodenum is more often affected by trauma because it is fixed in position. On ultrasound, the target sign or possibly an echogenic mass may be seen.[50] Eccentric bowel wall thickening may also be seen with a hematoma.

Duplication

The most common site of duplication cysts is the ileum, and obstruction is the most common presenting symptom. On ultrasound, these lesions range from anechoic cysts to echogenic masses.[50] An echogenic inner rim representing the bowel mucosa suggests the diagnosis.

Intussusception

Although uncommon in adults, intussusception is the most common cause of obstruction in children. There is an identifiable bowel lesion at the leading point in 75% to 85% of adult cases; most lesions in the small bowel are benign, and 50% of those in the colon malignant.[50] Ultrasound is usually employed only if the patient's presentation is atypical. On ultrasound, a large target lesion is seen, with the thickened rim representing the edematous intussuscipiens and the hyperechoic center caused by the multiple interfaces of compressed mucosal and serosal surfaces of the intussusceptum.[50]

Granulomatous Enterocolitis

Crohn's disease or regional enteritis affects the small bowel, especially terminal ileum, or colon at any level and involves the entire thickness of the bowel wall with a granulomatous inflammatory reaction. A target lesion is seen on ultrasound because of the thickened bowel wall (Fig. 121-30).[50] If an abscess is present, an irregular or ill-defined, poorly echogenic mass may extend into the iliopsoas muscle, extend anteriorly into the rectus muscle, or may compress the bladder. Real-time ultrasound can differentiate mass from fluid-filled bowel by detecting peristalsis. Ultrasound can also determine whether the right ureter is significantly compromised, causing hydronephrosis.

In appendiceal phlegmon and in Crohn's disease, a combination of a thickened ileum, cecum, and appendix can be seen.[51] These two entities can be differentiated on ultrasound scans. The mural thickening and the infiltrative changes are more prominent around the appendix in appendiceal phleg-

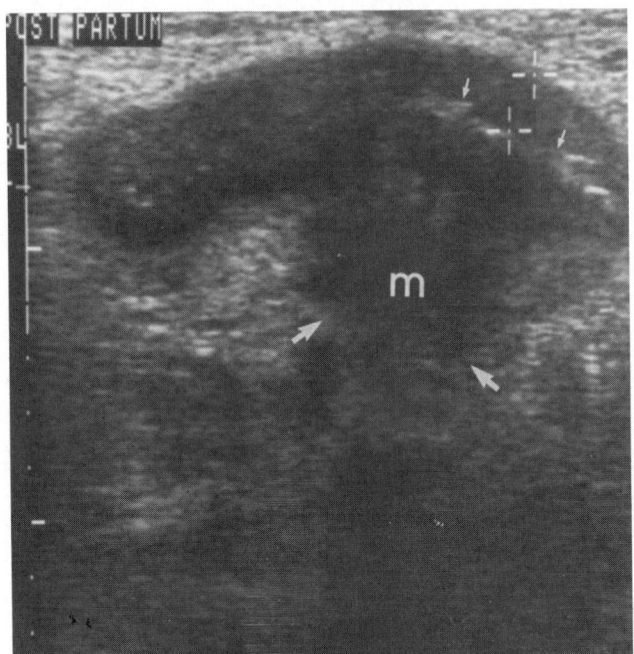

FIGURE 121-30. Crohn's disease abscess. The transverse view shows bowel wall thickening and an associated hypoechoic mass (m, *arrows*). The lumen of the affected bowel loop is echogenic (*small arrows*) because of air. The thick wall (*calipers*) can be measured between the lumen and outer surface. The linear array transducer allows better evaluation of fistula formation in the soft tissues of the abdominal wall. (From Mittelstaedt CA. Gastrointestinal tract. In: General ultrasound. New York, Churchill Livingstone, 1992:449.)

mon, and the thickening of the ileum and cecum is mild and often extrinsic.[51] The mural thickening of the ileum and cecum is severe in Crohn's disease, and the infiltrative changes around the inflamed appendix are minimal.[51] Appendicitis is an initial manifestation of Crohn's disease.[52] Primary Crohn's disease of the appendix has a favorable long-term prognosis after simple appendectomy, despite a 10% incidence of recurrence as granulomatous ileocolitis.[52] If a severely thickened ileum and cecum with a moderately thickened appendix are seen on ultrasound scans, a diagnosis of Crohn's disease should be considered and further clinical and radiologic evaluations should be done.[51]

Mesenteric Adenitis and Acute Terminal Ileitis

Mesenteric adenitis is the most frequent clinical diagnosis in patients with acute appendicitis who undergo surgery and who are found not to have appendicitis. This disease process is secondary to bacterial infection caused by *Yersinia enterocolitica*, *Campylobacter jejuni*, *Salmonella enteriditis*, and rarely, *Yersinia pseudotuberculous*.[52,53] Various degrees of mesenteric adenitis combined with an edematous, thickened terminal ileum occur in this disease process.[52] If these patients are examined with ultrasound using the graded compression technique, the only ultrasound finding consists of enlarged mesenteric lymph nodes in combination with mural thickening of the terminal ileum and cecum.[52–55] If the appendix is not visualized on ultrasound in patients suspected of acute appendicitis, and instead the examiner sees enlarged mesenteric lymph nodes and mural thickening of the terminal ileum, the diagnosis is probably mesenteric adenitis with acute terminal ileitis, and appendectomy should be avoided.[53] The most probable diagnosis is *Yersinia* or *Campylobacter* enteritis, conditions that should be treated conservatively.[55]

Tumor

Tumors involving the small bowel are rare. Lymphoma of the gastrointestinal tract is usually part of a systemic involvement, although lymphoma may originate in the gastrointestinal tract in 10% to 20% of patients. On ultrasound scans, a lymphomatous mass is usually a large irregular mass that has internal echoes because of necrosis. Various patterns have been described: large discrete mass (5–11 cm) with a target pattern; an exoenteric pattern with a large mass on the mesenteric surface of bowel; and a small anechoic mass (1–2 cm), representing subserosal nodes or mesenteric nodal involvement.[50]

Leiomyosarcoma and carcinoid are other tumors occurring in the small bowel. On an ultrasound scan of a leiomyosarcoma, a large solid mass containing necrotic areas is seen anterior to a solid viscus, with the intestinal lumen or air seen close to the mass.[50] About 73% of carcinoids are smaller than 1.5 cm and are difficult to visualize. If identified with ultrasound, the lesion has nonspecific characteristics: a well-defined hypoechoic mass with a lobulated contour and no acoustic enhancement.[50]

Abnormalities of the Appendix

Acute Appendicitis

Ultrasound can be of value in the diagnosis of acute appendicitis.[56–61] The typical target lesion may be seen in the right lower quadrant, and the normal appendix (<6 mm in diameter) can occasionally be visualized.[60] The primary criterion for the ultrasound diagnosis of acute appendicitis is visualization of a noncompressible appendix.[60] The ultrasound findings of appendicitis have been expanded to include an appendiceal diameter greater than 6 mm, muscular wall thickness greater than 3 mm, and visualization of a complex mass.[50,61] The most useful criteria in the diagnosis of acute appendicitis are an appendiceal muscle wall thickness greater than 3 mm and visualization of a complex mass separate from the adnexa in females. These criteria have a sensitivity of 68% and a specificity of 98% in making an accurate diagnosis.[61] A period of close clinical observation is probably warranted rather than early surgery in patients with a maximal outer appendiceal diameter of 6 mm or less; exceptions include compelling clinical evidence of appendicitis or multiple appendicoliths identified at ultrasound.[60] Ultrasound is recommended as a useful diagnostic study after the initial clinical screening.[61]

Ultrasound is reported to be 90% to 95% accurate, with an overall sensitivity of 80% to 89%, a specificity of 95% to 100%, a positive predictive value of 89% to 91%, and a negative predictive value of 90% to 91%.[56–59] The overall accuracy in women is 96%.[56] Ultrasound may be useful in establishing alternative diagnoses in patients with suspected acute appendicitis.[58] Ultrasound has the advantage of being able to examine other areas of the abdomen in patients with right lower quadrant pain. It has an accuracy of 70% in establishing other causes, including gynecologic disease, visceral disease, including hollow viscera, disease of liver, pancreas, or spleen, and urinary tract abnormalities.[57] Visualization of a noncompressible appendix with ultrasound appears to be a sensitive and specific method for the diagnosis of appendicitis in patients with acute right lower quadrant pain.[56]

Appendiceal Abscess

Complications of appendicitis include peritonitis, localized periappendiceal abscess, pylephlebitis with thrombosis of the portal venous drainage, liver abscess, and septicemia. The ultrasound findings reported with perforation include loculated pericecal fluid, prominent pericecal fat and circumferential loss of the submucosal layer of the appendix.[62] Most specific is the presence of loculated pericecal fluid indicating abscess.[62] A fluid collection or hypoechoic mass may be seen surrounding the appendix (Fig. 121-31). In some cases, the fluid collection or abscess may be far from the appendix, such as in the pelvis. In women, it is important to differentiate an appendiceal abscess from a tubo-ovarian abscess, twisted ovarian cyst, ruptured tubal pregnancy, or ruptured follicular or luteal ovarian cyst.[50]

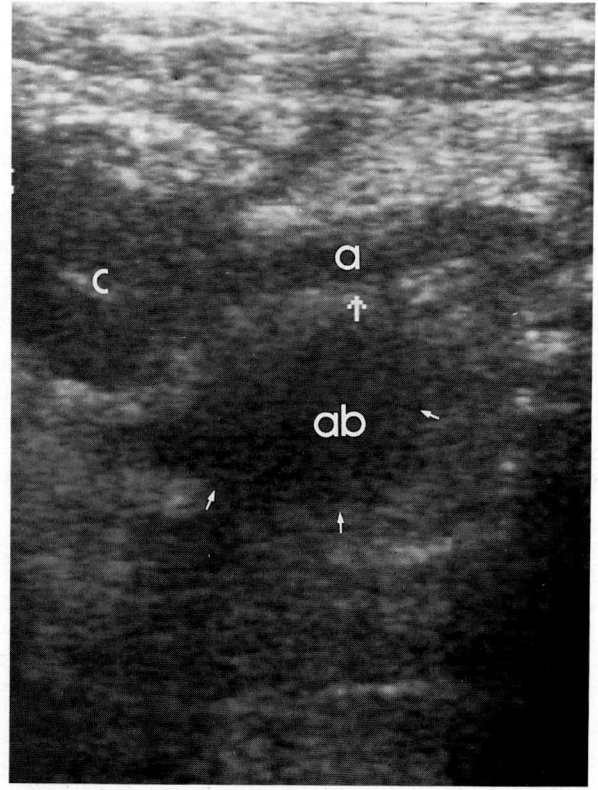

FIGURE 121-31. Appendiceal abscess. A hypoechoic mass (ab, *arrows*; 3 by 3 cm) is associated with the appendix (a), near the cecum (c).

Mucocele

Mucocele occurred in 0.25% to 0.3% of 43,000 appendectomies.[50] As a benign condition that obliterates the lumen of the appendix, it is associated with distention of the appendix by mucus. Ultrasound examination shows a well-defined, predominately cystic or hypoechoic mass, which may contain an echogenic solid area, in the right lower quadrant.[50]

Tumor

The most common carcinoma of the appendix is carcinoid (88.2%), and mucinous adenocarcinoma (8.3%) is second.[50] Ultrasound examination shows a bull's-eye lesion with an asymmetric echogenic core and an irregularly lobulated outline, with a wall thickness greater than 2 cm secondary to tumor.

Abnormalities of the Colon

Diverticular Disease

Diverticular disease is characterized by numerous saccular outpouchings in the colon; patients may not be symptomatic. In asymptomatic patients, the diverticula are not identified on ultrasound examination. If there is spasm, edema, and inflammation of the gut wall, there is improved visualization of the thickened gut segment, because inflammation of the diverticular wall accentuates the diverticulum. On ultrasound scans, these inflamed diverticula are seen as outpouchings protruding beyond the lumen of the gut into or beyond the thickened wall.[63] It is important to differentiate acute appendicitis from acute diverticulitis and other causes of acute right lower quadrant pain.

To make the diagnosis of acute diverticulitis using ultrasound, two of the following should be seen: focal gut wall thickening (>4 mm); inflamed diverticula (i.e., echogenic shadowing foci seen in outpouches of thickened colon wall or beyond pericolonic soft tissues); inflammatory changes in the pericolic fat (i.e., poorly defined zones of hypoechogenicity in pericolic fat); intramural or pericolic inflammatory mass (i.e., fluid or air in mass or abscess); and intramural fistulas.[63,64] In uncomplicated acute diverticulitis, one of the major ultrasound findings appears to be the hypoechoic round or oval focus protruding from segmentally thickened colon wall.

If there is a perforation of an inflamed diverticulum or spread of a peridiverticulitis producing a paracolic abscess, a hypoechoic to anechoic mass may be seen within the pelvis. An abscess should be suspected if a hypoechoic mass is seen and the patient is known to have diverticular disease and is symptomatic. If there is a strong suspicion of an abscess or if ultrasound is nondiagnostic, a CT scan is recommended.

Inflammatory Bowel Disease

Patients with Crohn's disease of the colon and ulcerative colitis can be assessed with ultrasound using the water-filled colon technique.[65] The criteria used to evaluate for the presence of disease and help differentiate these two processes include the width of the intestinal lumen, appearance of the haustration, thickness of the bowel wall, and presence of typical bowel stratification.[65] With Crohn's disease, several characteristics may be found: clearly thickened hypoechoic bowel wall, loss of typical wall stratification, loss of haustration, diminished compressibility, and no peristaltic motion.[65] The wall thickening in Crohn's disease may be 1.1 ± 0.3 cm, but in ulcerative colitis, the wall is increased only moderately to 0.6 ± 0.2 cm.[65] In ulcerative colitis, several symptoms and signs are observed: moderately thickened hypoechoic bowel wall, typical wall stratification, loss of haustration, diminished compressibility, and no peristaltic motion.[65] Although ultrasound cannot replace contrast radiography in diagnosing inflammatory colonic disease, it may serve as a safe and useful alternative diagnostic method for the detection, differentiation, and progression of Crohn's disease and ulcerative colitis.[65]

Tumor

Carcinoma of the colon occurs most commonly in the rectum, rectosigmoid, or sigmoid (80%), and 2.6% to 5% of cases have multiple lesions.[50] Although ultrasound is not the traditional diagnostic method for this tumor, it may detect such lesions. A tumor is suspected if the bowel wall is thickened and compressed or obliterated.[50] There is wall thickening producing the typical target pattern, with a hypoechoic oval mass containing a central echogenic area produced by lumenal air.[50]

Although more common in the small bowel, lymphoma may occur in the colon. A bull's-eye lesion or a hypoechoic mass may be seen on ultrasound. If real-time ultrasound shows a reflective pattern (because of bowel gas) or peristalsis within the mass, bowel involvement is suspected.

Transrectal Ultrasonography

Transrectal ultrasound is performed using a 4- to 7-MHz radial (axial) transducer that is inserted into the rectum.[66] The transducer is covered with a fluid-filled condom or rubber sheath to avoid contamination of the transducer and probe. The examination is performed with the patient in the left lateral decubitus or the dorsal lithotomy position after an enema. Images are obtained at 1-cm intervals from 2 cm superior to the anus to 15 cm or the maximum length of the transducer.

Although transrectal ultrasound was originally intended for evaluation of the prostate, it has been applied to the evaluation of diseases of the rectum and perirectal area.[67,68] Using transrectal ultrasound, the normal rectal wall is defined, similar to the definition of the gastric wall with fluid distention (see Fig. 121-29). Masses within 12 cm of the anus can be detected.[68] Other abnormalities can be identified, including primary and secondary rectal carcinomas, metastases, villous adenoma, leiomyosarcoma, endometriosis, sacrococcygeal teratoma, chordoma, retroperitoneal cystic hamartoma, pelvic lipomatosis, diverticulitis, and perirectal abscess.[67] It may also be useful in the ultrasound-guided biopsy of perirectal masses.[67]

Transrectal ultrasound has several applications. In assessing rectal tumors, its purpose is to improve surgical planning, to provide a prognosis in nonsurgical candidates, and to indicate which patients are suitable for local excision.[67] These rectal

tumors appear as hypoechoic masses that abruptly interrupt the normal sequence of the rectal wall layers (Fig. 121-32). It is the only imaging technique that differentiates the individual layers of the rectal wall to determine depth of invasion and that characterizes the lymph nodes.[69] Metastatic disease to the lymph nodes is more likely than inflammatory disease if the nodes are hyperechoic.[67] Because this technique can assess the depth of invasion and lymph node disease, it is an accurate method of staging rectal tumors. It can also be used to confirm and more accurately define the extent of neoplastic infiltration after recurrence. Transrectal ultrasound also may be employed to evaluate abscesses, particularly supralevator abscess. These lesions generally appear as hypoechoic masses and can be drained using transrectal ultrasound guidance.

Investigators have evaluated the staging of rectal carcinoma with transrectal ultrasound.[70] In detecting tumor extension into fat, ultrasound has been found to be 67% sensitive (53% for CT) and 77% specific (53% for CT), with a positive predictive value of 73% (56% for CT) and a negative predictive value of 72% (50% for CT).[70] In detecting lymph node infiltration, transrectal ultrasound is 50% sensitive (27% for CT), with 92% specificity (88% for CT), a positive predictive value of 68% (46% for CT), and a negative predictive value of 84% (76% for CT).[70] These data suggest that transrectal ultrasound may be more accurate than CT in the preoperative staging of rectal cancer.

Endoscopic Ultrasonography

Endoscopic ultrasound is a new technique that combines a small, high-frequency transducer with an endoscope to allow direct visualization of the gastrointestinal tract wall layers and surrounding tissues. This technique is used in the esophagus to evaluate primary and recurrent carcinoma, leiomy-

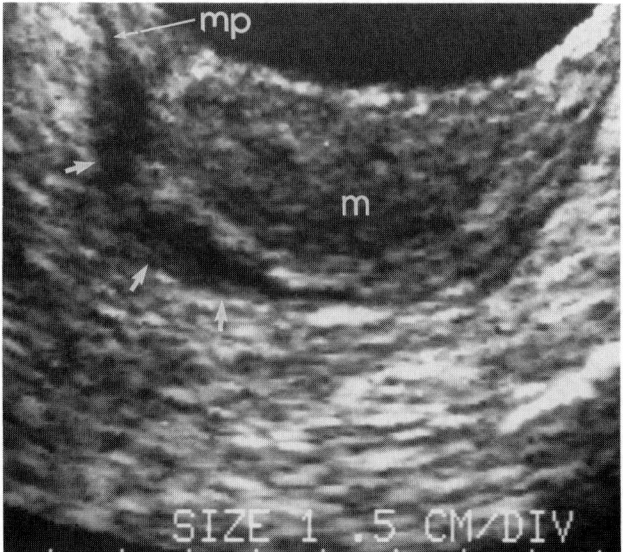

FIGURE 121-32. Rectal carcinoma. The transrectal ultrasound scan shows a solid mass (m) with disruption (*arrows*) of the muscularis propria (mp) and invasion into the perirectal fat planes.

omas, duplication cysts, and varices.[71] The stomach can be evaluated for gastritis, polyps, varices, primary and recurrent carcinoma, and lymphoma.[72] A colonoscope has been combined with ultrasound for evaluation of colon lesions, such as sessile adenomas and anastomotic recurrence of colon carcinoma.[73] For further information regarding endoscopic ultrasound, see Chapter 122.

Correlative Imaging

There have been no studies comparing the various cross-sectional imaging modalities, such as CT and ultrasound, in the evaluation of lesions of the gastrointestinal tract.

EVALUATION OF THE ABDOMINAL CAVITY

Ultrasound is an ideal diagnostic modality for evaluating intraabdominal, extraorgan pathology, because most lesions consist of fluid or fluid-containing structures or are associated with intraperitoneal fluid. These fluid collections include ascites, pus or inflammatory fluid, blood, bile and cerebrospinal fluid.

Technical Applications

There is no specific preparation for evaluation of the abdominal cavity. To evaluate for abdominal fluid collections, scans are obtained in subphrenic areas, the subhepatic space, along both pancreatic gutters, and in the pelvis. Most studies of the abdomen are tailored to the question asked and the abnormality identified.

Evaluation of Fluid Collections

Ascites

Ascites is seen as an echo-free region indenting and shaped by surrounding organs and viscera (Fig. 121-33). As little as 30 to 40 mL of fluid may be detected by ultrasound in the hepatorenal recess.[74] Detection of this fluid by ultrasound depends on amount and location. The smallest amounts of fluid are first detected around the tip of the liver, in the superior portion of the right flank, and in the pelvic cul-de-sac.

Several factors other than volume affect the distribution of the intraperitoneal fluid, including peritoneal pressure, patient position, area from which the fluid originates, the rapidity of fluid accumulation, the presence or absence of adhesions, the density of the fluid with respect to other abdominal organs, and the degree of bladder fullness.[74] If there are internal echoes, loculations or unusual distributions, matting or clumping of bowel loops, and thickening of interfaces between the fluid and neighboring structures, the examiner should suspect exudative (i.e., inflammatory or malignant) rather than transudative fluid. If a disproportionate amount of fluid is observed within the lesser sac (not typical for generalized peritoneal ascites), the physician should search for pathology

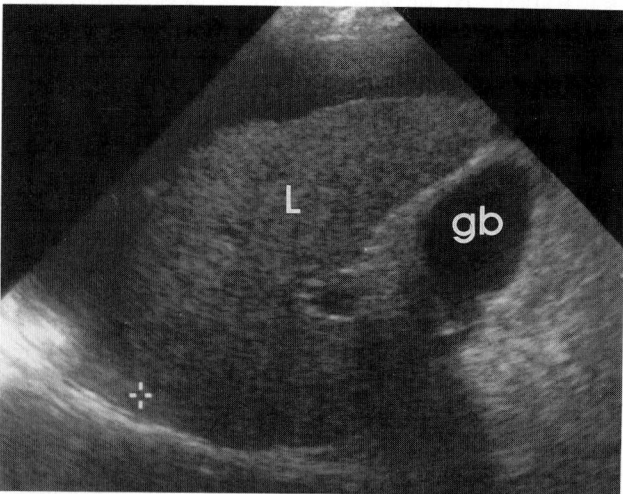

FIGURE 121-33. Ascites. The sagittal view of the right upper quadrant demonstrates free fluid (*black areas*) surrounding the liver and gallbladder (gb). The liver (L) is small as a result of cirrhosis.

in adjacent organs (e.g., acute pancreatitis, penetrating posterior gastric ulcer) or consider a malignant cause (e.g., carcinoma of the pancreas or ovary).[74] If fluid is demonstrated within the hepatorenal recess in a patient with an acute abdomen, the examiner should consider inflammatory fluid from acute cholecystitis, fluid from pancreatic autolysis, or blood from a ruptured hepatic neoplasm or ectopic gestation.

Abscess

An abscess on ultrasound may have a variety of appearances, from a cyst-like fluid to a solid pattern. The configuration of intraabdominal abscesses depends on the particular anatomic compartment in which the abscesses are localized. Searching for an abscess may be difficult with ultrasound because of its lack of specificity; the presence of incisions, drains, or ostomies; and a view obscured by bowel gas. However, ultrasound can be used to guide needle aspiration and catheter drainage.

Hematoma

The ultrasound appearance of intraabdominal, extraorgan hematomas depends on the age of the collection and the transducer frequency. Acute and old hematomas appear cystic or anechoic. Coarse echogenic lumps of material representing clot may be seen within chronic hematomas. The shape of the hematoma is determined by the location of the blood. Septations appear within 10% to 44% of hematomas.[74] Although fine-needle aspiration may be performed with ultrasound guidance, this procedure may be unsuccessful because clotted blood on ultrasound may appear anechoic, simulating fluid.

Biloma

Bilomas are extrahepatic, loculated collections of bile that develop as a complication of trauma, biliary surgery, or gallbladder neoplasm. Extravasated bile walls itself off with the formation of a sharply defined pseudocapsule. Bilomas appear echo free with acoustic enhancement, are sharply marginated, and are located in the right or middle upper abdomen in continuity with the liver or biliary structures on ultrasound. Some bilomas contain internal echoes or demonstrate a fluid-debris level. As with other fluid collections, the ultrasound appearance is not specific. A definitive diagnosis may be made with an ultrasound-guided aspiration of fluid, and ultrasound can be used to guide catheter drainage.

Omental and Mesenteric Cyst

Uncommon lesions, cysts of the mesentery and omentum may be embryologic and developmental, traumatic or acquired, neoplastic, or infective and degenerative. A mesenteric cyst, in broadest terms, is a cystic structure originating in the mesentery; omental cysts originate in the omentum. Histologically, these cysts represent lymphangiomas, nonpancreatic pseudocysts, enteric duplication cysts, mesothelial cysts, and enteric cysts.[75] On ultrasound, a unilocular or multilocular cystic structure of variable size is seen with smooth walls and without internal echoes unless there is superimposed hemorrhage or infection. This mass is easily differentiated from ascites or free intraperitoneal fluid.

Pseudomyxoma Peritonei

Arising from mucinous tumors of the appendix and ovary, pseudomyxoma peritonei is characterized by diffuse involvement of the peritoneal surfaces and omentum with gelatinous mucinous implants. On ultrasound, this abnormality may suggest only an exudative ascites, with a "nonfloating" posterior position of bowel loops.[74] Several patterns have been described on ultrasound: ascites with numerous echoes; highly echogenic masses containing scattered, numerous cystic spaces; a large, intraperitoneal, multiseptate, cystic-appearing mass; numerous, thick-walled, multiseptate, fluid-filled masses; and multiple, rounded, echo-dense masses. If echogenic bowel is surrounded by widespread homogeneous masses, intraabdominal carcinomatosis or lymphomatous involvement should be suspected.

Tumors of the Peritoneum, Mesentery, and Omentum

Peritoneal Metastases

Peritoneal metastases may develop from cellular implantation across the peritoneal cavity, or may be carried in lymph or blood. The most common primary sites are the ovary, stomach, and colon. On ultrasound scans, these peritoneal metastases may appear nodular, sheet-like, or irregular. Bowel loops may adhere to the masses.

Omental and Mesenteric Lymphoma

Involvement of the greater omentum by lymphoma results in a uniformly thick, hypoechoic, band-shaped structure that follows the convexity of the anterior and lateral abdominal wall.[74] A lobulated, confluent, anechoic mass surrounding a centrally positioned echogenic area may occur with mesenteric lymphomatous involvement. The pattern is produced by infiltration of the mesenteric leaves, encasing the superior mesenteric artery and veins. In most cases, there is paraaortic or retroperitoneal adenopathy.

Omental and Mesenteric Primary Tumor

Lymphoma and secondary tumors are the most common neoplasms involving the peritoneum and mesentery. The most common primary solid neoplasms of the mesentery are fibrous tumors; smooth muscle tumors are the most common lesions found in the greater omentum. Most of the primary tumors of the mesentery tend to be large. The mobility of the mesentery often permits large growth before symptoms other than a palpable mass are produced. On ultrasound scans, these masses move characteristically from side to side but not in the craniocaudad direction.

Mesenteric desmoids appear as well-circumscribed and predominately hypoechoic lesions, containing scattered, high-level echoes that may mimic other mesenteric lesions. With extrahepatic mesenchymal sarcomas involving the mesentery, abdominal hollow viscera, and retroperitoneal areas, the findings include hyperechoic masses intermixed with anechoic zones, hyperechoic masses with central fluid-filled zones, homogeneous hyperechoic masses, and homogeneous hypoechoic masses.[74] The ultrasound appearance of a large tumor mass with signs of necrosis should suggest the possibility of a sarcoma.

Correlative Imaging

Ultrasound is the method of choice for evaluating ascites. The overall accuracy of ultrasound in differentiating transudate from exudate fluid is 82%. The amount of intraperitoneal fluid necessary for recognition by ultrasound depends on the fluid location and the volume. As little as 30 to 40 mL of fluid can be detected in the hepatorenal recess.

Ultrasound has an accuracy as high as 96.8% in diagnosing suspected abscesses, with a sensitivity of 93% and a specificity of 98.6%.[74] A multiple-imaging approach to abscess detection is often superior to the use of any single modality. CT has a well-documented advantage compared with ultrasound in accurately detecting abscesses. Ultrasound is often preferred as the initial screening examination, because it is a rapid and flexible modality and is portable. Ultrasound is a better diagnostic modality for the upper abdomen than the lower abdomen, and the diagnostic rate is increased if clinical signs can direct the examination to a specific location or quadrant. CT may be the preferable initial modality, depending on patient habitus, suspected location of abnormality, presence of ileus, or presence of wounds and dressings. Even with the demonstration of an abnormal collection by ultrasound, CT may be needed to clarify the extent of the process and relate it to surrounding structures or to define a safe access route for aspiration biopsy or therapeutic drainage.

Despite the introduction of other imaging modalities, especially CT and MRI, ultrasound remains the initial examination in the work-up of many disorders. It is usually the initial screening modality for evaluation of the biliary system, because ultrasound can identify the gallbladder and extra-hepatic ducts in most patients despite body habitus or clinical condition, employing the newer high-resolution real-time systems. It is often the modality used to localize and characterize focal hepatic lesions and to guide aspiration or biopsy of these lesions. Some clinicians now think of ultrasound as an extension of the physical examination, because it is a rapid diagnostic modality that can be applied at the bedside or in an examining room.

> The reader is directed to Chapter 120, Cross-Sectional Anatomy, and Chapter 122, Endoscopic Ultrasonography.

REFERENCES

1. Grant EG. Liver. In: Mittelstaedt CA, ed. General ultrasound. New York: Churchill Livingstone, 1992:173.
2. Sauerbrei EE, Lopez M. Pseudotumor of the quadrate lobe in hepatic sonography: a sign of generalized fatty infiltration. AJR Am J Roentgenol 1986;147:923.
3. White EM, Simeone JF, Mueller RR, et al. Focal periportal sparing in hepatic fatty infiltration: a cause of hepatic pseudomass on ultrasound. Radiology 1987;162:57.
4. Mostbeck GH, Wittich GR, Herold C, et al. Hemodynamic significance of the paraumbilical vein in portal hypertension: assessment with duplex US. Radiology 1989;170:339.
5. Patriquin H, Lafortune M, Burns PN, Dauzat M. Duplex Doppler examination in portal hypertension: technique and anatomy. AJR Am J Roentgenol 1987;149:71.
6. Grant EG, Perella R, Tessler FN, et al. Budd-Chiari syndrome: the results of duplex and color Doppler imaging. AJR Am J Roentgenol 1989;152:377.
7. Bezzi M, Teggi A, DeRossa F, et al. Abdominal hydatid disease: US findings during medical treatment. Radiology 1987;162:91.
8. Ralls PW, Barnes PF, Radin DR, et al. Sonographic features of amebic and pyogenic liver abscesses: a blinded comparison. AJR Am J Roentgenol 1987;149:499.
9. Ralls PW, Barnes PF, Johnson MB, et al. Medical treatment of hepatic amebic abscess: rare need for percutaneous drainage. Radiology 1987;165:805.
10. Pastakia B, Shawker TH, Thaler M, et al. Hepatosplenic candidiasis: wheels within wheels. Radiology 1988;166:417.
11. Gibney RG, Hendin AP, Cooperberg PL. Sonographically detected hepatic hemangiomas: absence of change over time. AJR Am J Roentgenol 1987;149:953.
12. Cronan JJ, Esparza AR, Dorfman GS, et al. Cavernous hemangioma of the liver: role of percutaneous biopsy. Radiology 1988;166:135.
13. Yoshida T, Matsue H, Okazaki N, Yoshino M. Ultrasonographic differentiation of hepatocellular carcinoma from metastatic liver cancer. J Clin Ultrasound 1987;15:431.
14. Yoshikawa J, Matsui O, Takashima T, et al. Fatty metamorphosis in hepatocellular carcinoma: radiologic feature in 10 cases. AJR Am J Roentgenol 1988;151:717.
15. Hayashi N, Yamomota K, Tamaki N, et al. Metastatic nodules of hepatocellular carcinoma: detection with angiography, CT, and US. Radiology 1987;165:61.
16. Sheu J-C, Huang G-T, Chen D-S, et al. Small hepatocellular carcinoma: intratumor ethanol treatment using new needle and guidance systems. Radiology 1987;163:43.
17. Livraghi T, Festi D, Monti F, et al. US-guided percutaneous alcohol injection of small hepatic and abdominal tumors. Radiology 1986;161:309.
18. Morton MJ, James EM, Wiesner RH, Krom RAF. Applications of duplex ultrasonography in the liver transplant patient. Mayo Clinic Proc 1990;65:360.
19. Mattrey RF. Perfluorooctylbromide: a new contrast agent for CT, sonography, and MR imaging. AJR Am J Roentgenol 1989;152:247.
20. Taylor KJW, Ramos I, Morse SS, et al. Focal liver masses: differential diagnosis with pulsed doppler US. Radiology 1987;164:643.
21. Taylor KJW, Ramos I, Carter D, et al. Correlation of Doppler US tumor signals with neovascular morphologic features. Radiology 1988;166:57.
22. Taylor KJW, Burns PN, Carter D, Fortune K. Detection of neovascular signals in malignant tumors by pulsed Doppler US (abstract). Radiology 1986;161P:130.
23. Shimamoto K, Sakuma S, Ishigaki T, Makino N. Intratumoral blood flow: evaluation with color Doppler echography. Radiology 1987;165:683.
24. Mittelstaedt CA. Biliary system. In: Mittelstaedt CA, ed. General ultrasound. New York: Churchill Livingstone, 1992:249.
25. Dong B, Chen M. Improved sonographic visualization of choledocholithiasis. J Clin Ultrasound 1987;15:185.
26. Cohan RH, Mahony BS, Bowie JD, et al. Striated intramural gallbladder lucencies in US studies: predictions of acute cholecystitis. Radiology 1987;164:31.
27. Mirvis SE, Vainright JR, Nelson AW, et al. The diagnosis of acute acalculous cholecystitis: a comparison of sonography, scintigraphy and CT. AJR Am J Roentgenol 1986;147:1171.
28. Simeone JF, Brink JA, Mueller PR, et al. The sonographic diagnosis of acute gangrenous cholecystitis: importance of the Murphy sign. AJR Am J Roentgenol 1989;152:289.
29. Wilson SA, Gosink BB, van Sonnenberg E. Unchanged size of a dilated common bile duct after a fatty meal: results and significance. Radiology 1986;160:29.
30. Ralls PW, Mayekawa DS, Lee KP, et al. The use of color Doppler sonography to distinguish dilated intrahepatic ducts from vascular structures. AJR Am J Roentgenol 1989;152:291.
31. Raptopoulos V, Smith EH, Cummings T, et al. Bile-duct dilatation after laparotomy: a potential effect of intestinal hypomotility. AJR Am J Roentgenol 1986;147:729.
32. Laing FC, Jeffrey RB Jr, Wing VW, Nyberg DA. Biliary dilation: defining the level and cause by real-time. Radiology 1986;160:39.
33. Cronan JJ. US diagnosis of choledocholithiasis: a reappraisal. Radiology 1986;161:133.
34. Grumback K, Coleman BG, Gal AA, et al. Hepatic and biliary tract abnormalities in patients with AIDS: sonographic-pathologic correlation. J Ultrasound Med 1989;8:247.
35. Dolmatch BL, Laing FC, Federle MP, et al. AIDS-related cholangitis: radiographic findings in nine patients. Radiology 1987;163:313.
36. Ros PR, Buck JL, Goodman ZD, et al. Intrahepatic cholangiocarcinoma: radiologic-pathologic correlation. Radiology 1988;167:689.
37. Pastakia B, Shawker TH, Horvath K. Biliary neoplasm simulating dilated bile ducts. Role of computed tomography and ultrasound. J Ultrasound Med 1987;6:333.
38. Machan L, Muller NL, Cooperberg P. Sonographic diagnosis of Klatskin tumor. AJR Am J Roentgenol 1986;147:590.
39. Ralls PW, Colletti PM, Lapin SA, et al. Real-time sonography in suspected acute cholecystitis. Prospecific evaluation of primary and secondary signs. Radiology 1985;155:767.
40. Gibson RN, Yeung E, Thompson JN, et al. Bile duct obstruction: radiologic evaluation of level, cause, and tumor resectability. Radiology 1986;160:43.
41. Mittelstaedt CA. Pancreas. In: Mittelstaedt CA, ed. General ultrasound. New York: Churchill Livingstone, 1992:371.
42. Torres WE, Evert MB, Baumgartner BR, Bernardino ME. Percutaneous aspiration and drainage of pancreatic pseudocysts. AJR Am J Roentgenol 1986;147:1007.
43. Itai Y, Kokubo T, Atomi Y, et al. Mucin-hypersecreting carcinoma of the pancreas. Radiology 1987;165:51.
44. Robledo R, Prieto ML, Perez M, et al. Carcinoma of the hepaticopancreatic ampullar region: role of US. Radiology 1988;166:409.
45. Johnson CD, Stephens DH, Charboneau JW, et al. Cystic pancreatic tumors: CT and sonographic assessment. AJR Am J Roentgenol 1988;151:1133.

46. Itai Y, Ohhaski K, Nagai H, et al. "Ductectatic" mucinous cystadenoma and cystadenocarcinoma of the pancreas. Radiology 1986;161:697.
47. Galiber AK, Reading CC, Charboneau JW, et al. Localization of pancreatic insulinomas: comparison of pre- and intraoperative US with CT and angiography. Radiology 1988;166:405.
48. Lees W, Heron CW. US-guided percutaneous pancreatography: experience in 75 patients. Radiology 1987;165:809.
49. Campbell JP, Wilson SR. Pancreatic neoplasms: how useful is evaluation with US? Radiology 1988;167:341.
50. Mittelstaedt CA. Gastrointestinal Tract. In: Mittelstaedt CA, ed. General ultrasound. New York: Churchill Livingstone, 1992:449.
51. Puyluert JBC, vander Werf SDJ, Ulrish C, Weldhuizen RW. Crohn disease of the ileocecal region: US visualization of the appendix. Radiology 1988;166:741.
52. Agha FP, Ghahremani GG, Panella JS, Kaufman MW. Appendicitis as the initial manifestation of Crohn's disease: radiologic features and prognosis. AJR Am J Roentgenol 1987;149:515.
53. Puylaert JBCM. Mesenteric adenitis and acute terminal ileitis: ultrasound evaluation using graded compression. Radiology 1986;161:691.
54. Puylaert JBCM. Ultrasound of appendicitis and its differential diagnosis. New York: Springer-Verlag, 1990:63.
55. Puylaert JBCM, Lalisang RI, van der Werf SDJ, Doornbos L. *Campylobacter* ileocolitis mimicking acute appendicitis: differentiation with graded-compression US. Radiology 1988;166:737.
56. Jeffrey RB Jr, Laing FC, Lewis FR. Acute appendicitis: high resolution real-time US findings. Radiology 1987;163:11.
57. Gaensler EHL, Jeffrey RB Jr, Laing F, Townsend RR. Sonography in patients with suspected acute appendicitis: value in establishing alternative diagnosis. AJR Am J Roentgenol 1989;152:49.
58. Puylaert JBCM. Acute appendicitis: US evaluation using graded compression. Radiology 1986;158:355.
59. Abu-Yousef MM, Bleicher JJ, Maher JW, et al. High-resolution sonography of acute appendicitis. Radiology 1988;167:327.
60. Jeffrey RB Jr, Laing FC, Townsend RR. Acute appendicitis: sonographic criteria based on 250 cases. Radiology 1988;167:327.
61. Worrell JA, Drolshagen LF, Kelly TC, et al. Graded compression ultrasound in the diagnosis of appendicitis: a comparison of diagnostic criteria. J Ultrasound Med 1990;9:145.
62. Borushok KT, Jeffrey RB Jr, Laing FC, Townsend PR. Sonographic diagnosis of perforation in patients with acute appendicitis. AJR Am J Roentgenol 1990;154:275.
63. Wilson SR, Toi A. The value of sonography in the diagnosis of acute diverticulitis of the colon. AJR Am J Roentgenol 1990;154:1199.
64. Parulekar SG. Sonography of colonic diverticulitis. J Ultrasound Med 1985;4:659.
65. Limberg B. Diagnosis of acute ulcerative colitis and colonic Crohn's disease by colonic sonography. J Clin Ultrasound 1989;17:25.
66. Jochem RJ, Reading CC, Dozois RR, et al. Endorectal ultrasonographic staging of rectal carcinoma. Mayo Clin Proc 1990;65:1571.
67. St. Ville EW, Jafri SZH, Madrazo BL, et al. Endorectal sonography in the evaluation of rectal and perirectal disease. AJR Am J Roentgenol 1991;157:503.
68. Rifkin MD, Marks GJ. Transrectal US as an adjunct in the diagnosis of rectal and extrarectal tumors. Radiology 1985;157:499.
69. Hildebrandt U, Feifel G, Dhom G. The evaluation of the rectum by transrectal ultrasonography. Ultrasound Q 1988;6:167.
70. Rifkin MD, Ehrlich S, Marks G. Staging of rectal carcinoma: prospective comparison of endorectal US and CT. Radiology 1989;170:319.
71. Botet JF, Lightdale C. Endoscopic sonography of the upper gastrointestinal tract. AJR Am J Roentgenol 1991;156:63.
72. Lightdale CJ, Botet JF, Kelsen DP, et al. Diagnosis of recurrent upper gastrointestinal cancer at the surgical anastomosis by endoscopic ultrasound. Gastrointest Endosc 1989;35:407.
73. Rosch T, Lorenz R, Classen M. Endoscopic ultrasonography in the evaluation of colon and rectal disease. Gastrointest Endosc 1990;36:533.
74. Vincent LM. Peritoneal cavity and abdominal wall. In: Mittelstaedt CA, ed. General ultrasound. New York: Churchill Livingstone, 1992:589.
75. Ros PR, Olmsted WW, Moser RP Jr, et al. Mesenteric and omental cysts: histologic classification with imaging correlation. Radiology 1987;164:327.

Textbook of Gastroenterology, second edition, edited by Tadataka Yamada. JB Lippincott Company, Philadelphia © 1995.

CHAPTER 122

Endoscopic Ultrasonography

Michael B. Kimmey   Kenjiro Yasuda   Keiichi Kawai

Technical Considerations
Ultrasound Physics
Ultrasound Coupling
Echo Generation

Normal Gastrointestinal Wall Structure
Ultrasound Appearance of Extraintestinal Structures

(continued)

Gastrointestinal endoscopy has revolutionized the diagnosis and treatment of upper and lower digestive tract mucosal diseases, but evaluation of abnormalities of the walls of hollow gastrointestinal organs has been limited. Endoscopy may suggest the presence of a mass within or outside the gastrointestinal wall but cannot further elucidate the character of the mass.

Extracorporeal imaging techniques have not been useful in imaging the gastrointestinal wall. Transcutaneous ultrasound and computed tomography (CT) do not have sufficient resolution to differentiate wall abnormalities. These imaging modalities may show wall thickening but cannot differentiate the causes of increased wall thickness or evaluate the depth or localization of a specific abnormality. Magnetic resonance imaging (MRI) of the abdomen requires prolonged imaging times, producing significant motion artifacts that impair resolution.

These deficiencies in conventional imaging techniques led investigators and endoscope manufacturers to combine endoscopy with ultrasound in an effort to obtain more information about diseases of the gastrointestinal tract and other intraabdominal organs. In this chapter, the principles of ultrasound that allow its combination with endoscopy are outlined, and the types of endoscopic ultrasound (EUS) equipment are reviewed. The application of these devices to diseases of the gastrointestinal tract and the extraintestinal abdominal organs are evaluated, and particular attention is given to how EUS compares with other imaging modalities in the management of specific diseases.

The concept of using ultrasound within the lumen of the gastrointestinal tract is not new. Wild first proposed this application of ultrasound almost 40 years ago.[1,2] Technical developments were slow, and the first reported use of a combined ultrasound endoscope in a person was not until 1980.[3,4] The past decade has been one of multiple technologic advances leading to the widespread clinical use of ultrasound endoscope systems in Japan and Europe and to their progressive use in the United States.

TECHNICAL CONSIDERATIONS

Ultrasound Physics

Principles of ultrasound imaging have been outlined in Chapter 121. A few concepts that are pertinent to the combination of ultrasound with endoscopy should be emphasized. These concepts underline the potential advantages of EUS over transcutaneous ultrasound for imaging the gastrointestinal tract and adjacent organs.

Increasing the frequency of an ultrasound system results in an increased ability of the ultrasound beam to resolve tissue structure. Although resolution is improved with higher frequencies, the distance into the tissue that the beam penetrates is reduced. Skin, bone, and intestinal gas attenuate the ultrasound beam more than does soft tissue, further reducing its penetration. Conventional abdominal ultrasound imaging is performed with 3.5- to 7.5-MHz transcutaneous ultrasound systems. Higher frequencies have not been useful, because the penetration achieved with these higher frequencies does not adequately image intraabdominal structures.

Placing the ultrasound transducer next to the mucosa of the gastrointestinal tract avoids the necessity of having an ultrasound beam penetrate far into the tissue. Higher ultrasound frequencies can be used to increase resolution. EUS systems have used ultrasound frequencies between 7.5 and 20 MHz. These systems can resolve two points as close as 0.2 mm from each other in the direction of the ultrasound beam.[5,6] The ultrasound endoscope with the greatest use worldwide has frequencies of 7.5 and 12 MHz.[7]

Ultrasound Coupling

Transmitted and reflected ultrasound waves require the presence of a liquid or soft tissue medium between the ultrasound transducer and the target tissue. Air within the lumen of the gastrointestinal tract does not conduct ultrasound. EUS transducers must be placed directly against the mucosa, or a fluid medium must be between the transducer and the mucosa. Placing the transducer directly against the mucosa is the simplest of the two alternatives and is often used when extramural structures are being examined. However, this technique limits examination of the gastrointestinal wall, because echoes from structures close to the transducer are lost in the artifact produced by transducer excitation and the gastrointestinal wall layers may not be in the optimal focal zone of the transducer.

By putting water directly into the lumen or by filling a balloon around the transducer, the fluid can be used to couple the ultrasound transducer to the tissue. Water in the gastric and rectal lumen allows excellent imaging of the mucosa and adjacent structures. A water-filled balloon around the transducer is commonly used in the esophagus, duodenum, and colon because lumenal fluid moves with gravity away from the area of tissue being imaged. An echo is created where the ultrasound wave encounters the balloon. This echo combines with the first mucosal echoes when the balloon touches the intestinal wall. The balloon may also compress the gastrointestinal wall, resulting in compression of the superficial layers.[8]

Echo Generation

A knowledge of what generates echoes within tissue is helpful in interpreting EUS images. Echoes are produced when acoustic energy is reflected back to the transducer. This echo occurs when there is nonhomogeneity within a tissue and when the acoustic wave encounters a change in the acoustic impedance between adjacent tissue types.[9]

Tissue inhomogeneities are responsible for most of the echoes coming from a homogeneous organ such as the liver or pancreas. The microscopic structure of these organs determines the magnitude of the echoes. In many tissues, fat and collagen are responsible for the brightest echoes. For example, a fatty liver is more echogenic than a normal liver. Within the gastrointestinal tract, collagen and fat are found primarily in the submucosa and subserosal or mesenteric fat, probably accounting for the echogenicity of these tissue layers.

Echoes created by a change in the acoustic impedance between adjacent tissues are called interface echoes, and the amplitude of an interface echo is determined by the magnitude of the difference between the acoustic impedances of the two tissues.[9] The greatest amplitudes are seen at air-fluid and bone-fluid interfaces. The thickness or duration of the echo is produced by a factor related to the axial resolution of the ultrasound system. The interface echo thickness in most conventional imaging systems is less than 1 mm. In imaging a large area such as the liver, these interface echoes contribute little to the overall image. When imaging the gastrointestinal wall, which is normally only about 3 mm thick, interface echoes make a greater contribution to the overall appearance of the image. Interface echoes begin at a place in the image that corresponds to the location of the interface. The thickness or duration of the echo extends into the deeper tissue. If the deeper tissue is echogenic, the interface echo blends with the echoes from the deeper layer. However, if the deeper layer is echo-poor, the interface echoes obscure the echoes normally present. This effect can potentially add thickness to a superficial, echogenic tissue layer and subtract thickness from a deeper, echo-poor tissue layer.[10]

Endosonographers must be aware of artifacts that may confound accurate image interpretation. The best images are obtained when the ultrasound beam is perpendicular to the target. If the beam is tangential, the image is distorted, and wall layers may appear artifactually thickened.[9] Other artifacts can be helpful in image interpretation. When a fluid-filled structure is imaged, more ultrasound energy is transmitted through the structure, resulting in more echoes returning from its deep wall. When a structure with increased fat or collagen content is imaged, the ultrasound beam is attenuated, resulting in a shadow on the deep side of the structure. Other artifacts to be aware of include reverberation artifacts from the transducer casing and mirror image artifacts from an air and water interface.[11]

Normal Gastrointestinal Wall Structure

Early experience with EUS revealed a layered configuration in images of the normal upper and lower gastrointestinal tract. Interpretation of the anatomic counterparts to these layers on the images has evolved with further experience and as careful comparisons with histology were made. The interpretation of the basic layered structure is the same through the gastrointestinal tract.[10,12,13]

The ultrasound image of the normal gastrointestinal wall usually consists of five layers (Fig. 122-1). There are three echogenic layers separated by two echo-poor layers. The first echogenic layer, beginning at the mucosal surface, is thin and is produced by the interface between lumenal fluid or the balloon around the transducer and the mucosa. This layer varies in thickness, corresponding to the roughness or degree of irregularity in the mucosal surface. This layer is thin in the esophagus, where the squamous mucosa is smooth, and thicker in the stomach and colon, corresponding to the presence of gastric pits and colonic crypt openings.

The second layer is echo-poor and represents the remainder of the mucosa. This layer was formerly attributed to the muscularis mucosae; however, the normal muscularis mucosa is too thin to account for all of the second layer.[10,13] The muscularis mucosae is usually obscured by an echo occurring at its interface with the lamina propria so that the location of the muscularis mucosae corresponds to the most superficial part of the third (submucosal) layer. If the muscularis mucosae is thicker than the interface echo, a separate thin hypoechoic layer is seen between this interface echo and the underlying submucosal layer.[13-15]

The third ultrasound layer is the easiest layer to recognize because it is the most echogenic. This layer corresponds to the submucosa but is thicker. This is because it includes the interface between the submucosa and muscularis propria.[10] This layer may be less echogenic if edema exists.

The fourth layer is echo-poor and corresponds to the muscularis propria. The superficial part of the muscularis propria is obscured by the interface with the submucosa that contributes to the third layer.[10] In areas with a well-developed inner circular and outer longitudinal muscle component, a small

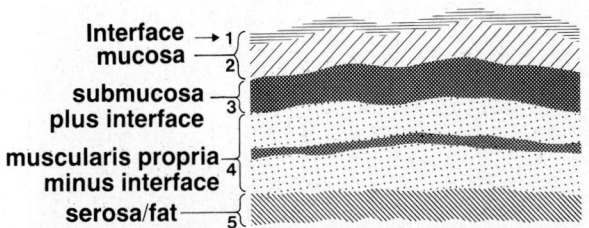

FIGURE 122-1. The layers of the normal gastrointestinal wall as seen on ultrasound images. The ultrasound image comprises echoes arising from the anatomic layers and from the acoustic interfaces between tissue layers.

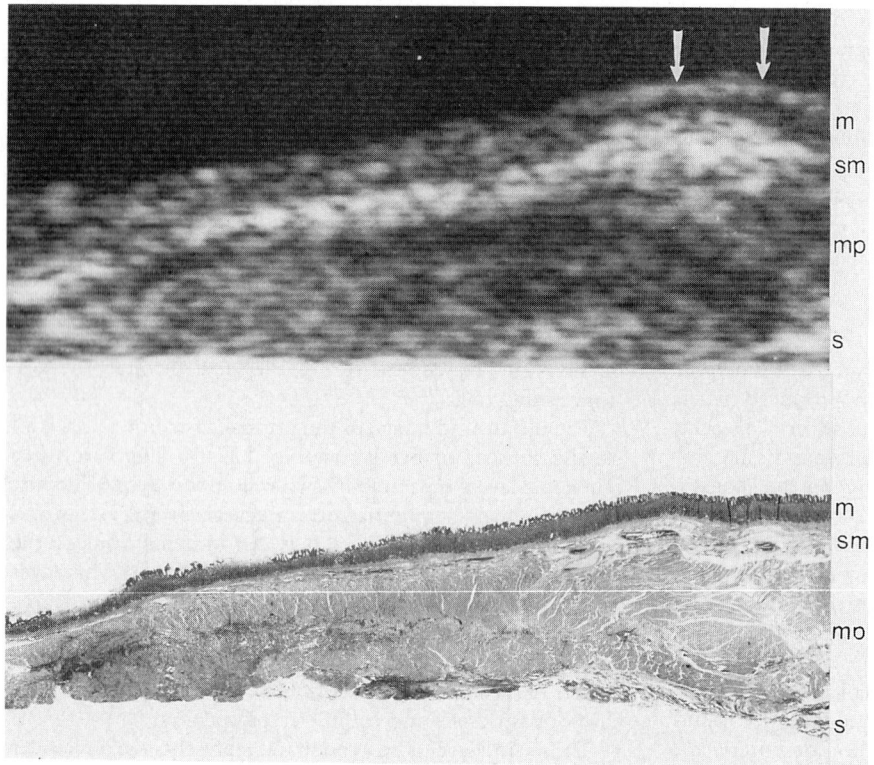

FIGURE 122-2. The ultrasound image of the normal stomach made in vitro with an 8.5-MHz ultrasound system (*top*) is shown with the histologic section (*bottom*) of precisely the same area of tissue. The first two ultrasound layers correspond to mucosa (m), with the superficial echoic line (*arrows*) caused by the interface between fluid over the tissue and the mucosal surface. Layers corresponding to submucosa (sm), muscularis propria (mp), and serosa (s) are also seen.

amount of connective tissue between the muscle layers may produce a line of echoes within the muscularis propria.[10,12]

The fifth layer is echogenic but of variable thickness. If no subserosal fat or inflammation is present, this echogenic layer corresponds to the serosa and the interface between the serosa and the surrounding tissue. The layer can be very thick in the rectum, where there is often abundant perirectal fat that is also echogenic. An example of the ultrasound image and the corresponding histology of the normal stomach is shown in

Figure 122-2. An EUS image of the gastric body made with a 10-MHz ultrasound endoscope is shown in Figure 122-3.

Some endosonographers have described as few as three layers or as many as nine layers in gastrointestinal wall ultrasound images. Low-frequency transcorporeal ultrasound imaging of the intestine in cross section reveals only three layers corresponding to wall, lumenal contents, and wall.[16] Low-frequency intralumenal transducers may also reveal only a three- or four-layered structure, probably because of inade-

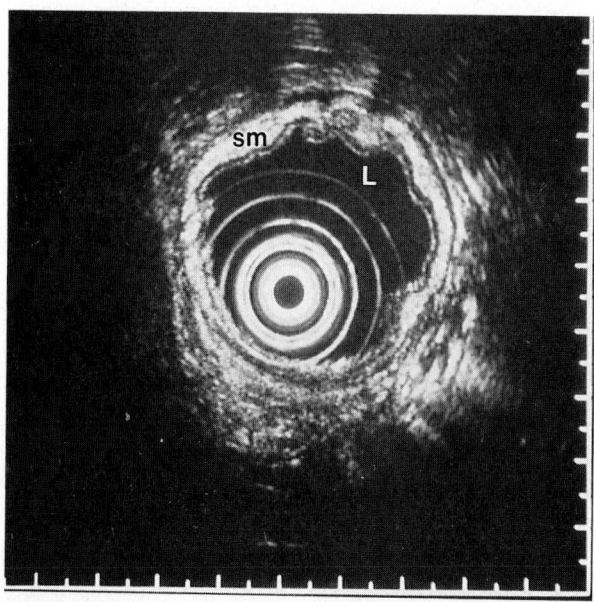

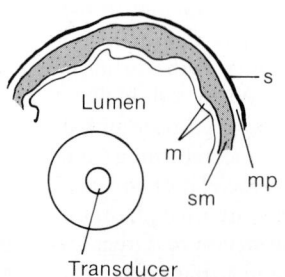

FIGURE 122-3. The ultrasound image of the normal stomach made with a 10-MHz mechanical sector scanning ultrasound endoscope is shown. All of the anatomic layers, including mucosa (m), submucosa (sm), muscularis propria (mp), and serosa with surrounding structures (s), are seen in this image made through water in the gastric lumen (L).

quate resolution.[17,18] Reports of a seven-layered structure are usually secondary to dividing the fourth layer, corresponding to the muscularis propria, into three separate layers when an echogenic line corresponding to connective tissue divides the inner circular and outer longitudinal muscle components of the muscularis propria.[12] When the second layer is also divided into three layers because of a thickened muscularis mucosae, a nine-layered wall is seen.[13]

Ultrasound Appearance of Extraintestinal Structures

The appearance of other intraabdominal organs is similar to that seen with transcorporeal ultrasound. The liver, pancreas, and spleen are homogeneous and of intermediate echogenicity (see Chap. 121). The liver can usually be differentiated from the spleen by the bright echoes adjacent to intrahepatic portal venous branches. The kidneys are easily recognized by the characteristic appearance of the urinary collecting system.

The importance of differentiating benign from malignant lymph nodes in cancer staging has encouraged study of the endosonographic appearance of these nodes.[19,20] Lymph node diameter is less important than the sonographic characteristics of the nodes. Malignant lymph nodes are usually hypoechoic, similar in echogenicity to the primary neoplasm, with sharply defined boundaries with adjacent tissue. The internal echoes from the nodes can be homogeneous or inhomogeneous. Benign nodes tend to have poorly defined boundaries with the surrounding tissue and may be hyperechoic.

Some of the newer EUS instruments have Doppler capability. This feature coupled with imaging results is called duplex Doppler. The direction of blood flow within vessels can be displayed in color. Experience with the endosonographic application of Doppler is limited, but this technology should be helpful in image interpretation by delineating retroperitoneal and other blood vessels.[21]

Instrument Types

Ultrasound endoscopes can be classified according to the type of endoscope and by the type of ultrasound system (Table 122-1). The largest worldwide experience has been obtained with a mechanical sector scan on the end of a side- or oblique-viewing endoscope.[4,5,7,22,23] Development of this instrument began in 1979 and has progressed through six generations of improvements.[7] The most recent model produces a 360-degree

radial scan by using a selectable ultrasound frequency of 7.5 or 12 MHz. The ultrasound transducer at the end of the endoscope is rotated by a motor mounted on the proximal shaft of the endoscope. Optical viewing is achieved through a forward-oblique lens mounted on the side of the endoscope 2.5 cm from the tip. A small biopsy channel allows aspiration or biopsy, but the catheter path does not coincide with the imaging plane. The transducer can be placed directly against the mucosa, or imaging can be performed through water placed in the lumen or inside a balloon covering the transducer. The limitations of this device include difficulty in orienting the ultrasound image, and the inability to pass through tight strictures. A longer forward-viewing variation of this type of instrument has been developed for use in the colon by omitting a 30-degree sector of the ultrasound image to allow passage of fiber bundles to the endoscope tip.[24]

An electronic curved-array ultrasound endoscope is being increasingly used in the United States and throughout the world.[25-27] The ultrasound array is mounted along the long axis of the tip of a forward-oblique–viewing endoscope. The array of transducer elements is slightly convex to the endoscope, and their signals are processed electronically to produce a 100-degree sector scan that is aligned with the endoscopic image. Switchable ultrasound frequencies of 5 and 7.5 MHz are available. Potential advantages of this system include color Doppler capability and the ability to follow needle catheters into a target using ultrasound guidance.[28]

A linear array of ultrasound elements attached to the side of forward-viewing endoscopes have been used but are not commercially available in the United States.[3,29-32] These instruments vary in ultrasound frequency between 5 and 8 MHz, producing a rectilinear image approximately 3 cm wide and 6 cm deep. Electronic complexity and difficult endoscopic maneuverability imposed by the long, rigid endoscope tip have limited the widespread use of these instruments.

Another method of combining ultrasound and endoscopy is to place an ultrasound probe through a rigid endoscope or down conventional or video endoscopes.[6,33-39] The first probes studied produced only an A-mode ultrasound tracing.[33,34] The amplitude of returning echoes could be analyzed to measure rectal wall thickness and to differentiate cystic from solid masses, but a conventional ultrasound image was not available. The newer probes contain an ultrasound transducer element that rotates or is mechanically moved in a linear direction along the gastrointestinal wall.[36-39] These probes vary in frequency from 7.5 to 20 MHz, producing high-resolution images with limited tissue penetration. These systems may prove to be useful for imaging endoscopically visible abnormalities or for use within the pancreatic or bile ducts but are unlikely to be useful for imaging extraintestinal organs such as the pancreas.

Other ultrasound systems designed for use within the gastrointestinal tract do not have an optical system. Ultrasound imaging is performed after blind insertion into the esophagus or rectum. Transesophageal ultrasound probes are primarily used by cardiologists for imaging the heart.[40] Most of these systems use electronic phased arrays with ultrasound frequencies of 3.5 to 7 MHz. The probes have flexible shafts with bidirectional tip-bending controls like an endoscope but have no fiber bundles. A 7.5-MHz mechanical sector transducer on a flexible shaft without endoscopic optics has also

TABLE 122-1
Comparison of Endoscopic Ultrasound Systems

CHARACTERISTIC	SECTOR SCAN	LINEAR ARRAY	CURVED ARRAY
Frequency	7.5 & 12 MHz	5–8 MHz	5 & 7.5 MHz
Penetration	10 cm	10 cm	10 cm
Resolution	0.2 mm	0.3 mm	0.3 mm
Diameter	12 mm	12 mm	11.5 mm

been used to image esophageal strictures that do not allow passage of larger caliber ultrasound endoscopes.[41,42] Transrectal probes have been used for imaging the prostate, bladder, uterus, and rectum. These probes are linear array or mechanical sector scanners with ultrasound frequencies of 3.5 to 7 MHz.[12,18,43] Most of these systems do not possess an optical system and are rigid, limiting imaging to the rectum.

Ultrasound has also been combined with laparoscopes for use in imaging the liver from within the peritoneal cavity.[44,45] Rigid probes with an ultrasound transducer mounted on the end are placed through the trocar during laparoscopy. A 10-MHz mechanical sector scanner and a 7.5-MHz linear array have been described.[45] Imaging is performed with optical guidance after the probe is placed on the liver surface.

Imaging Technique

Detailed descriptions of imaging techniques and the proper positioning of an ultrasound endoscope have been published.[22,23,46–48] Patients are prepared for the procedure as they would be for a standard upper endoscopy. After an overnight fast, topical anesthesia to the oropharynx and intravenous sedation are administered. Anticholinergic agents may be administered to reduce intestinal motility.

A preliminary standard endoscopy is often performed first because limited endoscopic views are obtained with oblique-

viewing ultrasound instruments.[5] The ultrasound endoscope is then passed blindly through the mouth and into the stomach. The endoscope is directed to the area of clinical interest by use of a combination of endoscopic views and the ultrasound image. Esophageal imaging is accomplished by withdrawing the instrument to the position of interest. The distance markers on the insertion tube are used as a guide. The water-filled balloon method is used for imaging the esophagus, or the transducer can be placed directly against the esophageal mucosa.

The ultrasound endoscope is visually directed into the duodenal bulb and descending duodenum for imaging of the ampulla of Vater, pancreatic head, distal common bile duct, gallbladder, right lobe of the liver, and retroperitoneal lymph nodes. Passage out of the stomach is accomplished with the same technique that is used with side-viewing duodenoscopes for endoscopic retrograde cholangiopancreatography (ERCP). Duodenal distortion by tumor or ulcer disease can make passage into the descending duodenum difficult. The water-filled balloon method is most commonly used in the duodenum, although mucosal polypoid structures may be better imaged by placing water in the duodenal lumen. Ultrasound visualization of the common bile and pancreatic ducts, aorta, inferior vena cava, and portal vein are important landmarks to guide imaging in the duodenum (Fig. 122-4*A, C*).

Imaging from within the stomach is also directed by prior knowledge of the area of clinical interest. Lesions of the gastric

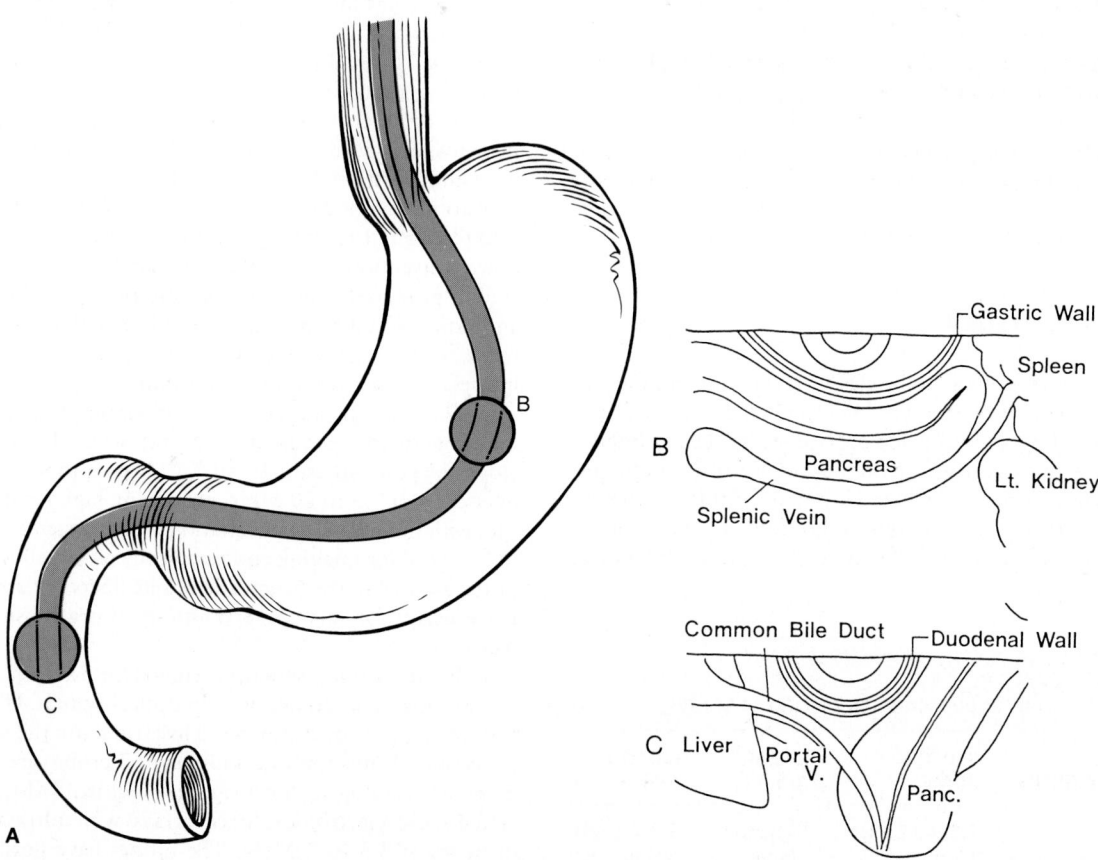

FIGURE 122-4. (**A**) The position of the ultrasound endoscope when imaging from the stomach (B) and the duodenum (C) is shown. The relative positions of the abdominal organs to the ultrasound transducer when it is (**B**) in the stomach and (**C**) when it is in the duodenum are also diagrammed.

wall are first identified with endoscopic vision. The ultrasound transducer is then directed over the abnormality. Water is placed through the endoscope's channel into the lumen for most imaging in the stomach. Artifacts caused by mucus and bubbles can be reduced by using simethicone and *N*-acetyl cysteine.[49] The patient may need to be turned to allow gravitation of water to the area of interest. The water-filled balloon method may also be used.

The body of the pancreas is imaged through the antrum and body of the stomach. The pancreatic tail can be imaged through the fundus of the stomach. Pancreatic imaging is aided by identifying the superior mesenteric artery and vein and the splenic vein posterior to the pancreas and by following the course of the pancreatic duct (see Fig. 122-4*A*, *B*). The spleen and left lobe of the liver can also be imaged through the gastric fundus.

The technique of transrectal ultrasound is described in detail elsewhere.[12] In most cases, the probe is inserted blindly until resistance is encountered at an obstructing neoplasm or at the rectosigmoid junction. Imaging is accomplished through a water-filled balloon as the probe is withdrawn. Areas of particular interest within the rectum can also be scanned by infusing water into the lumen.

Optimal performance of EUS requires specific training and substantial experience. The degree of difficulty of EUS is comparable to that of therapeutic ERCP.[50] Attendance of EUS courses, and study of cross-sectional anatomy and EUS atlases are helpful but should be supplemented by supervised, hands-on training.[22,51-53]

ENDOSCOPIC ULTRASONOGRAPHY OF THE UPPER GASTROINTESTINAL TRACT

Focal Intramural and Extramural Mass Lesions

Focal abnormalities of the upper gastrointestinal wall are often suspected based on results of radiographic contrast and endoscopic examinations. Barium x-ray films may reveal a smooth, rounded defect impinging on the lumen, or the endoscopist may encounter a bulge covered with normal mucosa. The clinical significance of these masses can be difficult to ascertain but may be facilitated by knowing whether the mass is intramural or extramural and whether it is benign or malignant. EUS can be useful in defining the location of the mass and can assist in obtaining a biopsy specimen to determine whether it is malignant.[54]

Intramural masses arise from a well-defined ultrasound layer that corresponds to one of the histologic layers of the gastrointestinal wall.[55-61] Extramural masses may compress the outer echogenic layer of the gut wall or, if malignant, may disrupt normal layer structure. The results of EUS examinations of 139 patients with suspected intramural or extramural masses of the esophagus, stomach, and duodenum have been reported.[55] EUS correctly identified the mass as intramural (80 cases) or extramural (59 cases) in every patient. Histologic confirmation was available in 54 instances. Lesions ranged in diameter from 3 to 75 mm.

Leiomyomas are the most commonly encountered focal intramural masses in the upper gastrointestinal tract. They are differentiated ultrasonographically by their presence within the fourth ultrasound layer, corresponding to the muscularis propria. They are hypoechoic and usually expand the hypoechoic fourth layer but do not disrupt the boundaries between the third and fourth or fourth and fifth layers (Fig. 122-5). Occasionally, leiomyomas are seen as well-marginated hypoechoic masses between the second and third layers. In these instances, the tumor has probably arisen from the muscularis mucosae.[57] Most small leiomyomas are round; lesions over 5 cm in diameter may be lobulated.[55] Duct-like structures within hypoechoic leiomyomas may be small blood vessels.[22] Other hypoechoic areas within a leiomyoma may be produced by tumor necrosis.[55,59] Hyperechoic areas within the leiomyoma may indicate hyaline degeneration.[59] Although most leiomyomas occur in the esophagus and stomach, they have also been imaged in the duodenum and colon.[30]

Using EUS, leiomyomas may be indistinguishable from leiomyosarcomas.[55,59,60] Ultrasonographic features that sug-

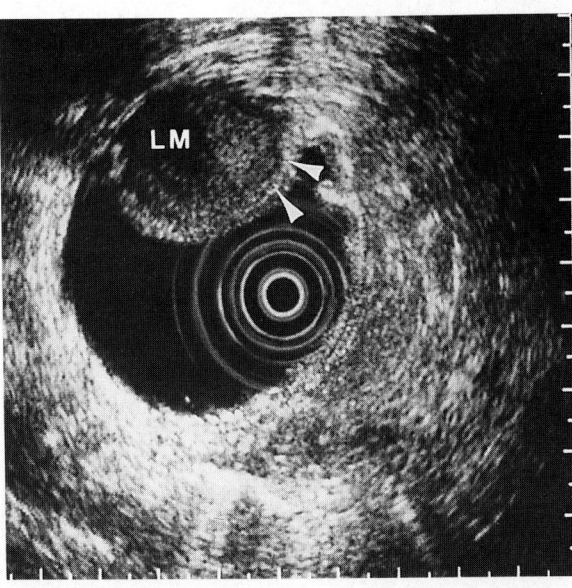

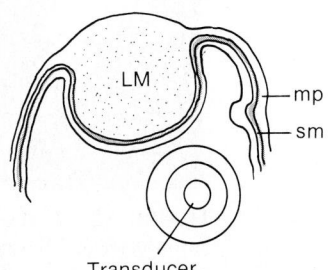

FIGURE 122-5. A gastric leiomyoma (LM) is imaged through water in the lumen of the stomach by using a 7.5-MHz ultrasound endoscope. The echogenic submucosa (sm) is pushed superficially by the tumor (*arrows*). The leiomyoma can be seen to arise from the deep hypoechoic ultrasound layer that corresponds to the muscularis propria (mp).

Transducer

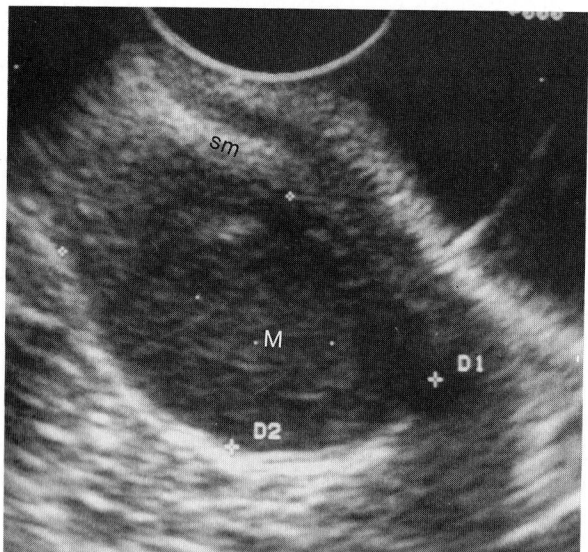

FIGURE 122-6. This hypoechoic mass (M) within the submucosa (sm) of the rectum was caused by an endometrioma. The image was made with an electronic curved array ultrasound endoscope. (Courtesy of Frank Lyons, M.D., and Amy Tsuchida, M.D., Tacoma, WA.)

gest the presence of leiomyosarcoma include irregular margins, invasion of adjacent layers, and visualization of enlarged extraintestinal lymph nodes.[22,57,60] Central ulceration or irregular hypoechoic areas corresponding to necrotic tissue may be seen in large leiomyomas (>5 cm in diameter) and leiomyosarcomas but are more common in leiomyosarcomas.[55,59]

Other causes of focal intramural lesions can be imaged with EUS. Esophageal and gastric carcinoid tumors cause well-defined hypoechoic nodules in the second, third, or fourth ultrasound layers.[22] Lipomas are differentiated by being echogenic and clearly marginated, and they are usually located in

the third (submucosal) layer.[30,56,60] Ectopic pancreas, submucosal cysts, gastric duplications, granular cell myoblastoma, and eosinophilic granuloma have also been imaged with EUS.[30,55,58,60] Endometriomas may be imaged within or adjacent to the rectal or colonic walls (Fig. 122-6).

The origins of extramural mass lesions can often be deduced by identification of contiguous structures. The aorta, liver, gallbladder, spleen, and splenic artery or vein may compress the gastrointestinal tract when enlarged or when of normal size.[55,60,62] Hepatic cysts and pancreatic pseudocysts are also identified by their surrounding organs (Fig. 122-7).

Malignant extramural lesions may compress or invade the outer layers of the gastrointestinal wall. Bronchogenic carcinoma, hepatic and pancreatic malignancies, and malignant lymph nodes have been imaged with EUS.[55,60] The location of these malignancies often suggests their origin.

The inferior resolution of transcorporeal ultrasound and CT compared with EUS predicts that EUS will be superior to these other modalities for defining and localizing focal gastrointestinal masses. Unfortunately, few studies have directly compared EUS with other imaging modalities for this purpose. In most comparisons, it is not clear that the different modalities were prospectively and independently assessed. In a large case series, transcorporeal ultrasound correctly identified only 10 intramural masses, compared with 50 intramural masses correctly identified with EUS.[60] CT may visualize a hypodense mass in the esophageal or gastric wall but cannot differentiate intramural from extramural location or the precise anatomic location of an intramural mass within the gastrointestinal wall.[22]

Esophageal Carcinoma

The diagnosis of esophageal carcinoma is usually not difficult with the use of barium radiography or routine esophagoscopy and biopsy. Staging this tumor to plan appropriate therapy

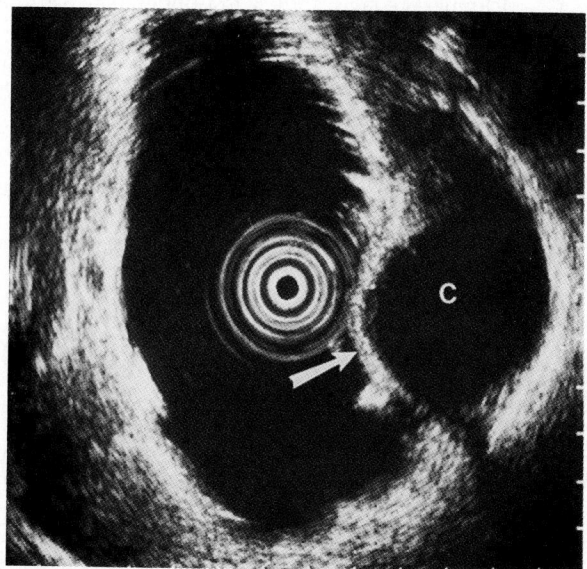

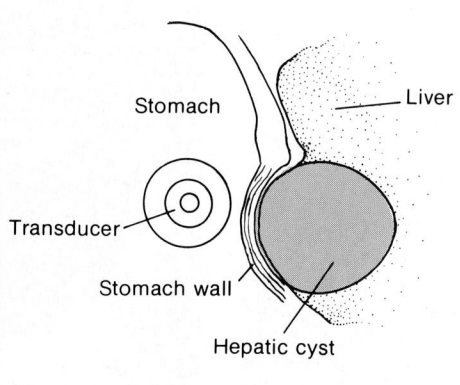

FIGURE 122-7. Extramural compression of the gastric wall (*arrow*) is caused by a hepatic cyst (C) 5 cm in diameter. The distance between adjacent lines on the scale at the right and bottom of the image represents 1 cm.

TABLE 122-2
Endoscopic Ultrasound Staging of Esophageal Carcinoma

	CORRECT ENDOSCOPIC ULTRASOUND FINDING COMPARED WITH SURGICAL PATHOLOGY*					
	Depth of Invasion				Lymph Node Involvement	
INVESTIGATOR	T1	T2	T3	T4	N0	N1
Tio[64]	7/8	7/9	25/27	20/22	13/24	46/50
Ziegler[32]	4/5	3/4	7/8	19/20		16/25
Botet[65]	2/3	2/4	19/20	23/23	9/14	35/36
Rosch[68]	4/8	7/9	20/22	4/5	8/19	17/19
Grimm[69]	9/10	12/14	28/33	5/6	17/22	37/40

* Refers to TNM staging system, in which T represents the depth of invasion (T1, submucosa; T2, muscularis propria; T3, adventitia; T4, adjacent structures) and N represents regional lymph node involvement (N0, no nodal involvement; N1, nodes involved).

is more difficult. Endoscopy or radiography defines the longitudinal extent of tumor growth but does not define depth of invasion. CT and EUS have been used to evaluate depth of invasion into the esophageal wall, detect spread to mediastinal and celiac lymph nodes, and detect invasion of other mediastinal and thoracic structures.

Information is available on the use of EUS to stage esophageal carcinoma limited to the esophageal wall. EUS is the only imaging modality that can differentiate mucosal, submucosal, and muscular involvement with esophageal carcinoma, and it can accurately determine the depth of invasion in more than 80% of early cases (Table 122-2).[32,41,63-68] EUS may also detect small areas of adenocarcinoma within Barrett's epithelium. CT cannot differentiate mucosal, submucosal, and muscular involvement by tumor.

Most patients have spread of esophageal carcinoma outside the muscularis propria at the time of presentation. EUS and CT accurately detect approximately 90% of cases with me-

diastinal invasion (Fig. 122-8).[32,63-69] EUS is more sensitive than CT in detecting aortic, pericardial, and diaphragmatic involvement with carcinoma.[63-69] The dynamic nature of EUS, with the ability to detect moving structures in real time, may contribute to the accuracy of this technique in detecting invasion of these viscera.

EUS is more accurate than CT in detecting lymph node involvement in patients with esophageal cancer.[64-69] The limitations of CT in detecting enlarged mediastinal lymph nodes in patients with esophageal cancer are well known; approximately 50% of cases of esophageal cancer are understaged by CT.[70,71] Lymph nodes as small as 5 mm in diameter can be visualized with EUS.[72] The accuracy of EUS in the detection of mediastinal lymph node involvement is approximately 70% to 80% (see Table 122-2).[64-69] Limitations of EUS in detecting lymph node involvement include false-positive results caused by enlarged inflammatory nodes and, to a lesser degree, false-negative results caused by microscopic metastases in normal-

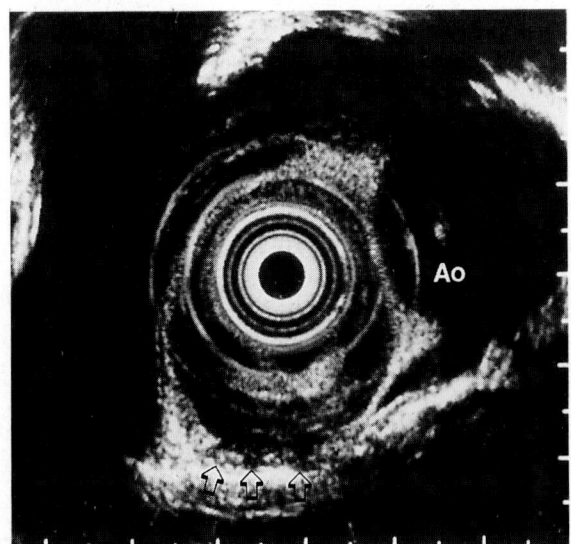
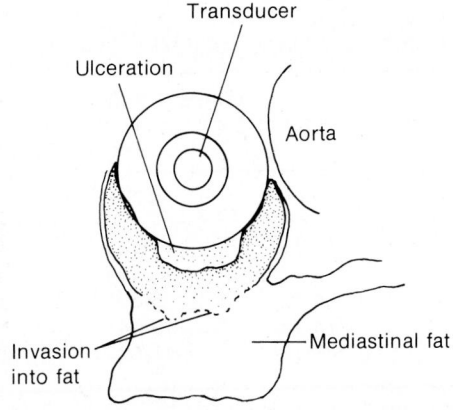

FIGURE 122-8. An ulcerated esophageal carcinoma with invasion of the mediastinal fat (*open arrows*) is imaged with a 10-MHz ultrasound endoscope.

sized nodes. CT correctly identifies the presence or absence of mediastinal lymph node involvement in only 20% to 50% of cases, with good specificity but limited sensitivity.[64-69]

EUS and CT are complementary in the detection of distant metastases from esophageal carcinoma. EUS has a sensitivity of over 90% in detecting celiac lymph node metastases when it is possible to pass the endoscope through the malignant stricture.[64] However, in comparing the overall accuracy of EUS and CT, the accuracy of both modalities is approximately 70% to 80%, because the ultrasound endoscope cannot pass through 20% to 50% of malignant strictures.[32,64-69] CT is also more sensitive than EUS in detecting hepatic metastases, especially in the right lobe.

Gastric Carcinoma

The greatest experience with EUS in the staging of gastric cancer comes from Japan, where there is a high incidence of this tumor. EUS has the potential for detecting the depth of invasion of gastric neoplasms because of the clear layers seen on ultrasound images of the gastric wall (see Fig. 122-3). Because gastric cancer confined to the mucosa and submucosa has a better outcome with surgical resection than more advanced disease, EUS can contribute significantly to the management of patients with early gastric cancer. The depth of invasion is seen as a disruption in the normal layer structure or diffuse thickening of the normal layers by infiltrating scirrhous carcinomas.[73-78]

EUS accurately predicts the depth of malignant invasion into the gastric wall in approximately 80% of patients (Table 122-3).[41,69,73,74] Accuracy rates of approximately 90% are achieved in differentiating early (i.e., confined to the mucosa or submucosa) from advanced (i.e., invasion of the muscularis propria or deeper) gastric cancer (Figs. 122-9 and 122-10). Cell type and the degree of differentiation do not appear to significantly affect staging accuracy with EUS. The depth of invasion may be overestimated if there is an ulcer scar or inflammatory reaction below the cancer.[41,74] Underestimation of the depth of invasion occurs if microscopic invasion of deeper layers occurs or the serosal ultrasound layer cannot be seen well.

The accuracy of EUS in detecting gastric cancer in extraintestinal lymph nodes is less well established. Approximately 80% of malignant regional lymph nodes are detected by EUS, but false-positive results are seen in as many as 50% of benign nodes.[20,41,75,76,78] False-negative results occur most commonly in cases of microscopic metastases in normal-sized nodes.

EUS can stage the depth of invasion and detect lymph node metastases more accurately than high-quality CT scanning.[75] When compared with pathologic evaluation of the resected specimen, EUS correctly predicted depth of invasion and lymph node involvement in 91% and 78% of cases, respectively.[75] CT scanning correctly predicted depth of invasion and lymph node involvement in 42% and 48% of cases, respectively.[75] Overall staging was significantly more accurate with EUS (73% correct) than with CT (45% correct).[75]

The invasion of gastric cancer into surrounding structures may be detected with EUS, and malignant involvement of the pancreas and liver has been described.[74] However, because of the limited penetration of EUS, CT scans are necessary for the detection of most hepatic metastases.[74,75]

An expanding role for EUS is in the guidance of endoscopic treatment of early gastric cancer.[79,80] Gastric cancer that is confined to the first two EUS layers can be ablated with a laser or resected with snare electrocautery after injection of saline into the submucosa under the lesion. When submucosal involvement is demonstrated by EUS, there is a substantial risk of regional lymph node metastases and of local recurrence after endoscopic therapy.

Recurrent carcinoma of the upper gastrointestinal tract after surgical resection may also be detected by EUS.[69,81] Recurrent tumor is suggested by nodular thickening at the anastomosis. The anastomosis in patients without recurrence is smooth and less than 6 mm thick. In 40 patients with symptoms suggesting recurrence, EUS correctly detected anastomotic recurrence in 23 of 24 and correctly predicted no recurrence in 13 of 16.[81]

Gastric Lymphoma

Lymphomas involving the stomach can present as an infiltrating or polypoid mass lesion or as a gastric ulcer.[82-84] Endoscopic biopsy may reveal the diagnosis, but biopsies may

---

TABLE 122-3
Endoscopic Ultrasound Staging of Gastric Carcinoma

	CORRECT ENDOSCOPIC ULTRASOUND FINDING COMPARED WITH SURGICAL PATHOLOGY*						
	Depth of Invasion				Lymph Node Involvement		
INVESTIGATOR	T1	T2	T3	T4	N0	N1	N2
Tio[41]	10/13	16/18	30/36	7/9	14/30	9/15	30/35
Rosch[68]	5/7	7/11	10/12	7/11	9/12	18/21	5/8
Botet[75]	4/4	6/8	30/31	6/7	10/11	15/22	14/16
Saito[77]	18/23	9/14	40/45	4/5			
Grimm[69]	28/31	41/52	28/45	17/19	40/58	11/22	41/51

* Refers to TNM staging system in which T represents the depth of invasion (T1, submucosa; T2, mucularis propria; T3, adventitia; T4, adjacent structures) and N represents regional lymph node involvement (N0, no nodal involvement; N1, nodes within 3 cm from gastric wall are involved; N2, nodes greater than 3 cm from gastric wall are involved).

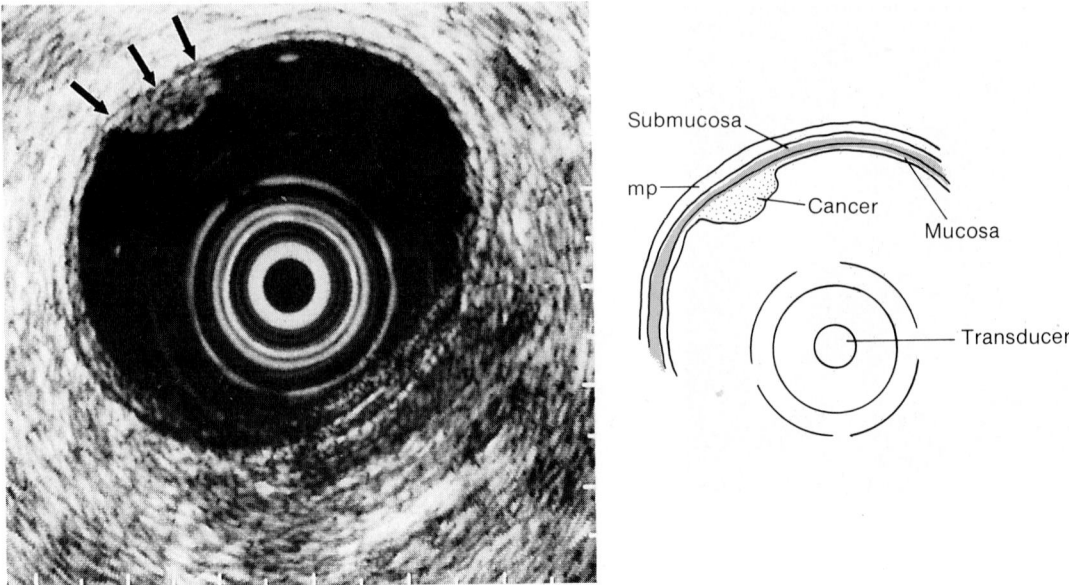

FIGURE 122-9. An early cancer of the gastric antrum is confined to the mucosa. There is no disruption of the boundary between the ultrasound layers corresponding to mucosa and submucosa (*arrows*).

be nondiagnostic when the bulk of the tumor is below the mucosa. EUS can detect the extent of lymphomatous involvement of the gastric wall in infiltrating and ulcerative gastric lymphomas (Fig. 122-11).[82-84] The depth of wall invasion, involvement of surrounding organs such as the pancreas or liver, and the presence of enlarged lymph nodes can be assessed with EUS. Reduction of tumor size after chemotherapy has also been documented by EUS imaging.[82-84]

EUS appears to be more sensitive than CT scanning in detecting the presence of intramural invasion, extragastric spread, and the presence of lymph node involvement.[82] However, these studies have involved small numbers of patients, and the use of appropriate blinds by those interpreting the images is not stated. It is also not clear that optimal CT imaging techniques, such as the use of thin sections or current-

generation instruments, have been used in these comparisons. CT may also detect lymphomatous involvement when EUS has not if the abnormality is more than 6 cm from the ultrasound transducer or if the endoscope cannot be maneuvered so that the abnormality is within the optimal focal zone of the ultrasound transducer. The two imaging techniques may be complementary; larger blinded studies using the most current equipment are needed to address this issue.

Ampullary Carcinoma

Carcinoma of the ampulla of Vater occurs infrequently compared with pancreatic cancer, but it is important to recognize the tumor because patients often present with jaundice when

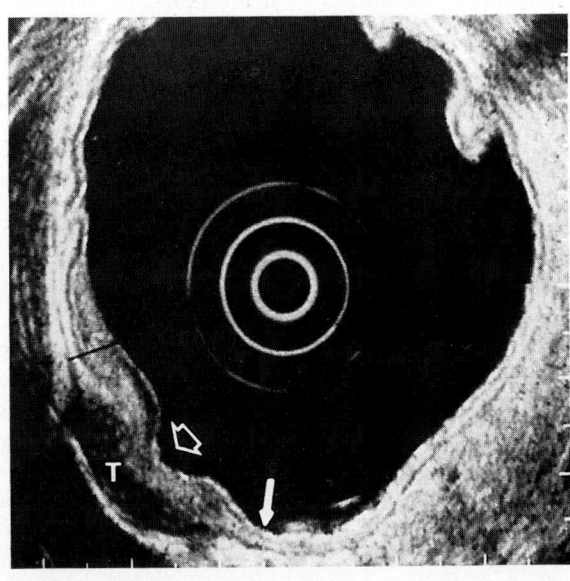

FIGURE 122-10. This advanced gastric cancer has raised borders and a central ulceration (*open arrow*). The tumor mass (T) arises from the normal wall (*arrow*), where layers corresponding to mucosa (m), submucosa (sm), and muscularis propria (mp) can be seen. The cancer can be seen to invade the fat and other tissue around the gastric wall.

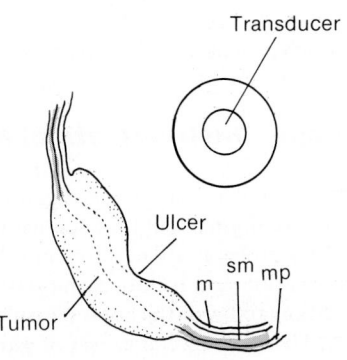

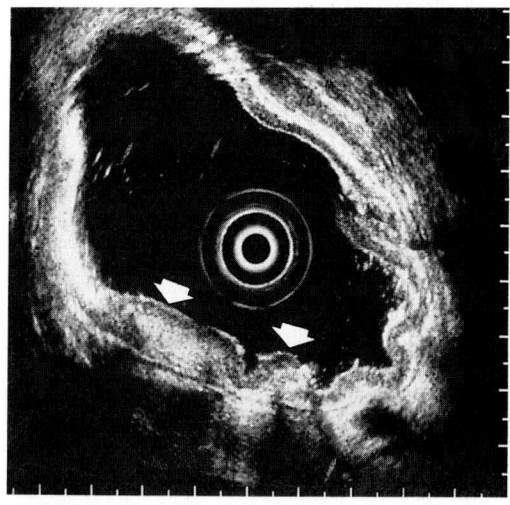

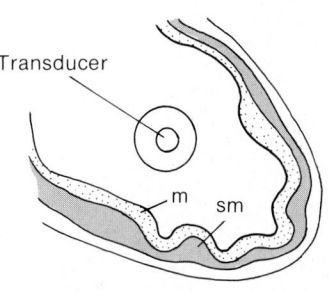

FIGURE 122-11. A gastric lymphoma has caused thickening of the ultrasound layers corresponding to mucosa (m) and submucosa (sm) in the region under the arrows.

the tumor is resectable. Five-year survival after surgical resection of ampullary cancer can be expected for approximately 40% of patients.[85] Surgery is radical and carries a mortality rate of up to 10%. It would be useful to have a preoperative assessment of those patients most likely to benefit from the surgery. Preliminary studies suggest that EUS offers more benefit than other imaging studies in the preoperative staging of these tumors.[86–89]

EUS detects the normal five layers of the duodenal wall adjacent to the papilla when imaged from the duodenum.[86] The common bile duct and pancreatic duct are seen to converge at the papilla with the portal vein lying immediately adjacent to the bile duct (see Fig. 122-4C). EUS can detect tumor masses within the papilla as small as 8 mm in diameter.[86] EUS also correctly predicts the depth of invasion of the tumor with respect to involvement of the muscularis propria or subserosa in as many as 80% of patients.[86–89] Invasion of the pancreatic parenchyma and the existence of lymph node metastases can also be detected with EUS. The limitations of EUS in the staging of ampullary carcinoma include failure to detect very small tumors, failure to visualize some liver metastases, and false-positive interpretation of some inflammatory lymph nodes.[86–89]

Most ampullary neoplasms can be accurately diagnosed by a combination of endoscopy with biopsy and ERCP. The role of EUS appears to be in demonstrating the size and depth of invasion of the tumor, the presence of involved regional lymph nodes, and the presence of portal or superior mesenteric vein invasion.[86–89] Larger studies with long-term follow-up are needed to show that the results of EUS imaging predict which patients have long-term survival after surgical resection.

Upper Gastrointestinal Wall Thickening

EUS can detect a thickened gastrointestinal wall. The upper limit of normal wall thickness has not been rigorously defined but is probably about 3 to 4 mm.[57,90] The degree of lumenal distention and balloon compression can affect layer visualization and wall thickness measurements.[8]

There are several causes of gut wall thickening, some of

which can be differentiated with EUS imaging. The first two ultrasound layers, corresponding to the mucosa, are thickened in foveolar hyperplasia, Ménétrier's disease, and gastrinoma.[57] The fourth layer, corresponding to the muscularis propria, may be thickened in response to distal obstruction.[10] All four layers may be thickened in the stomach adjacent to an ulcer or with gastric lymphoma or linitis plastica.[57,82,83]

Vascular Abnormalities

The course and mural location of esophageal and gastric varices can be determined with EUS. Varices are imaged within the submucosa and in the periesophageal or perigastric soft tissue.[37,56,91] Small submucosal varices are easily compressed and may be missed when imaging with the water-filled balloon method. After sclerotherapy, submucosal varices are obliterated, but periesophageal collaterals may not be affected.[91] The sequence of acute variceal thrombosis and organization of the thrombus after sclerotherapy has been shown with EUS.[92] All 17 patients followed with EUS in this series showed recanalization of the varices after 6 months. EUS detects gastric varices and may prove to be useful in differentiating gastric varices from large rugal folds.[56,91] Large extragastric venous collaterals in patients with portal hypertension can also be detected by EUS.

EUS has been proposed for imaging vessels within polyps to guide endoscopic resection. Tio reported a case of a 5-cm gastric polyp with 1- to 2-mm vessels in the stalk of the polyp imaged by EUS.[93] The patient required surgery to control bleeding after snare resection of the polyp.

Peptic Ulcer Disease

The depth of mucosal lesions may be difficult to gauge with routine endoscopic examination. Erosions and acute ulcers may be indistinguishable; the depth of chronic ulcers is more easily detected because the histologic layers fuse together. The depth of mucosal lesions should be determined by EUS. The second ultrasound layer is thickened around erosions, but the third layer is not penetrated.[94] Ulcers may extend into the third or fourth layer or completely through into the subserosal region.[94] The gastric wall may be diffusely thickened in the region around an ulcer; inflammatory changes may obscure the normal layered appearance of the surrounding wall.[57] EUS may also aid in differentiating benign from malignant gastric ulcers.[95]

EUS may prove to be useful in predicting the response of benign ulcers to therapy.[94] Gastric ulcers that took longer than 8 weeks to heal with H_2-receptor antagonist therapy were differentiated by their depth into the muscularis propria or subserosal region, by persistent edema in the ulcer base during healing, and by disruption of the submucosal layer in the gastric wall away from the ulcer. The finding of a disrupted submucosa away from the ulcer has been interpreted as signaling the presence of scarring from a previous ulcer.[94]

ENDOSCOPIC ULTRASONOGRAPHY OF ORGANS ADJACENT TO THE UPPER GASTROINTESTINAL TRACT

Thoracic Extraesophageal Structures

EUS may detect mediastinal or pulmonary abnormalities as incidental findings or because they compress the esophagus. Bronchogenic carcinoma may cause dysphagia by compressing or invading the esophagus. EUS may show the origin of the mass to be in the bronchus, excluding a primary esophageal lesion.[54] Other causes of esophageal compression that have been detected by EUS include mediastinal cyst, aberrant right subclavian artery, and thoracic aortic aneurysm. There are no prospective comparisons of EUS and other imaging modalities such as CT and MRI in the detection and characterization of mediastinal abnormalities.

Transesophageal echocardiography using linear and phased-array ultrasound transducers is gaining increasing acceptance for cardiac imaging. These ultrasound devices do not have visual optics and are passed and used without the benefit of endoscopy. The interested reader is referred to other sources for a discussion of this modality.[40]

Chronic Pancreatitis

The diagnosis of chronic pancreatitis is not difficult in the patient with steatorrhea, glucose intolerance, and pancreatic calcification on plain abdominal x-ray films. However, early cases may be more subtle, defying diagnosis with the use of conventional diagnostic tests. EUS has been proposed as a sensitive and specific imaging tool for the diagnosis of chronic pancreatitis. High-resolution ultrasound images of the pancreas can be made through the posterior gastric wall and through the medial wall of the duodenum.[96] Because there is no intervening intestinal gas, EUS is able to image the entire pancreas in most cases; the head and tail of the pancreas are seen more often with EUS than with transcutaneous ultrasound.[97]

The normal pancreas has a homogeneous, fine granular appearance when imaged with EUS.[97] The pancreatic duct has clearly defined walls with an overall diameter of 2 to 3 mm. Endosonographic features of chronic pancreatitis include a heterogeneous appearance of the pancreatic parenchyma with focal hypoechoic areas and other echogenic areas.[98,99] There may be enlargement of the entire gland. Ductal dilatation is readily detected with EUS; duct caliber may be irregular, with increased amplitude echoes arising from an apparently thickened duct wall (Fig. 122-12). It has been suggested that duct wall thickening may be an early sign of chronic pancreatitis.[98] Ductal strictures and intralumenal protein plugs or stones may also be imaged with EUS. Pseudocysts as small as 1 cm in diameter have been detected with EUS.[100] EUS-guided endoscopic drainage of pancreatic pseudocysts has also been described.[28]

EUS may be superior to transcorporeal ultrasound, CT, and endoscopic retrograde pancreatography (ERP) for detecting some features of chronic pancreatitis. In a series of 48 cases of chronic pancreatitis, EUS was superior to transcutaneous ultrasound and CT in detecting ductal dilatation (particularly of side branches), cysts less than 2 cm in diameter, and heterogeneous pancreatic parenchyma.[96] Pancreatic stones were visualized by EUS and CT; stones were easier to detect with EUS than with transcorporeal ultrasound because of the acoustic shadowing more apparent with the higher frequency

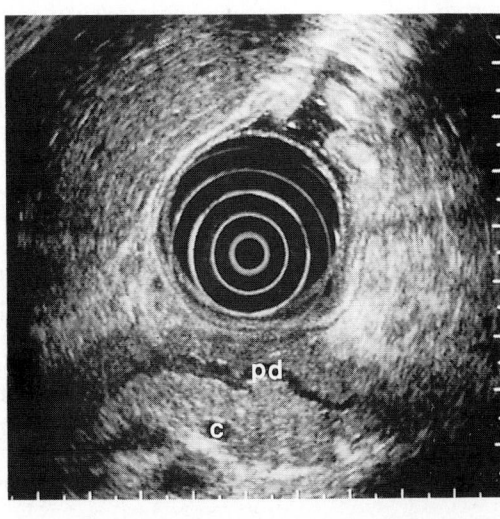 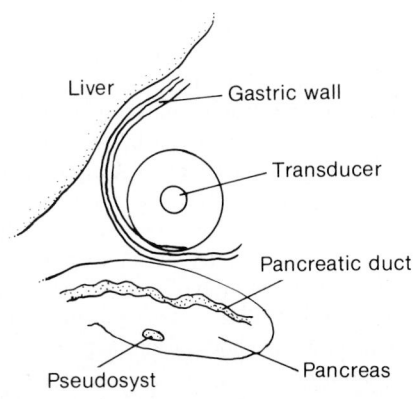

FIGURE 122-12. The pancreas of a patient with chronic pancreatitis is imaged through the posterior gastric wall with a 7.5-MHz ultrasound endoscope. A dilated pancreatic duct (pd) and a small pancreatic pseudocyst (c) are seen, as well as a heterogeneous echo texture within the pancreatic parenchyma.

Liver

Gastric wall

Transducer

Pancreatic duct

Pseudosyst

Pancreas

EUS. In most cases, ductal dilatation was better defined by ERP; however, EUS detected dilated ducts in several cases where the obstructed pancreatic duct could not be filled at ERP.

Mass lesions within a chronically inflamed pancreas may be inflammatory or malignant. It may be impossible to differentiate these possibilities with transcutaneous ultrasound, CT, and ERP. Although evaluation of EUS with rigorous, blinded, histologically confirmed studies is not available, there are endosonographic features that may help to differentiate these causes of a pancreatic mass.[101,102] Inflammatory lesions are favored by the presence of a homogenous hypoechoic mass with smooth boundaries. Malignant lesions are suggested when a heterogenous mass with irregular contours, often in a lobulated pattern, is imaged.[103] The cause of some pancreatic masses, especially those less than 3 cm in diameter, cannot be determined with any imaging modality, including EUS.[104]

Pancreatic Carcinoma

One of the first targets for EUS imaging was pancreatic cancer.[101-103] The early detection of this usually lethal neoplasm has eluded other diagnostic modalities. The increased spatial resolution of EUS may allow detection of smaller, resectable neoplasms in isolated patients with vague symptoms.[102,105] However, the expense and difficulty in using this technology are likely to impair its widespread application as a screening test for the early detection of pancreatic carcinoma.

EUS has been used to image malignant pancreatic masses, to investigate whether malignant lymph nodes are present, and to detect the presence of vascular invasion that would preclude surgical resection.[87,89,102] EUS is more sensitive than transcutaneous ultrasound, CT, and angiography in detecting masses less than 3 cm in diameter and is more accurate than the other imaging modalities in assessing tumor size.[89,102] Masses as small as 10 mm in diameter have been imaged with EUS.[102] Most pancreatic neoplasms are hypoechoic, but a few may be hyperechoic on EUS imaging. EUS may also detect cystic pancreatic neoplasms and metastases to the pancreas (Fig. 122-13).

Enlargement of lymph nodes around the porta hepatis, aorta, celiac trunk, and splenic artery can be detected with EUS. Unfortunately, there are no large studies comparing EUS detection of malignant lymph nodes with findings at laparotomy or autopsy. Accurate prediction of lymph node status in 70% to 80% of patients undergoing surgery has been reported.[87,89] EUS is more sensitive than CT in detecting regional lymph node involvement.[89,106]

Major vessel invasion by a pancreatic neoplasm precludes curative resection. The morbidity and mortality of pancreaticoduodenectomy could be prevented in a significant number of patients if a reliable method of detecting vascular invasion were available. EUS can detect portal vein and splenic vein involvement by pancreatic neoplasms (Fig. 122-14).[87,89,102] EUS is more sensitive than angiography and CT for detecting neoplastic involvement of the portal vein, including the region of its confluence with the superior mesenteric vein.[89] EUS is not as reliable for detecting major arterial (e.g., celiac, hepatic, splenic, superior mesenteric) encasement by tumor.[89]

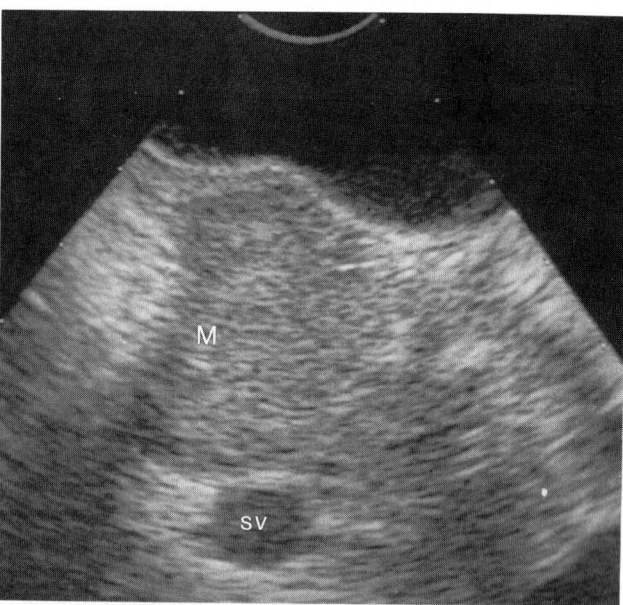

FIGURE 122-13. This hypoechoic mass (M) within the pancreas was imaged through the posterior gastric wall with an electronic curved array ultrasound endoscope. The splenic vein (sv) is seen in cross section posterior to the pancreas. The mass was later found to be caused by a metastasis from a small cell carcinoma of the lung. (Courtesy of Frank Lyons, M.D., and Amy Tsuchida, M.D., Tacoma, WA.)

Islet Cell Neoplasms

The anatomic localization of hormone-producing pancreatic tumors is important for guiding their surgical resection. Most of these neoplasms arise from islet cells within the pancreas, although a significant number are found elsewhere in the abdomen. Conventional transcorporeal imaging with ultrasound and CT detects less than one third of cases, probably because of the small size of the tumors. MRI and selective arteriography may also fail to localize the neoplasm. Careful examination of the pancreas with EUS by experienced endosonographers detects approximately 75% of islet cell neoplasms within the pancreas not found on CT scanning.[107,108] Islet cell neoplasms are usually round, homogeneous, and hypoechoic compared with surrounding pancreas. Masses as small as 5 mm in diameter have been imaged with EUS.[107,108] All patients with a clinical diagnosis of an occult islet cell neoplasm should undergo preoperative EUS to localize the neoplasm and facilitate surgical planning.

Gallbladder and Bile Ducts

The close approximation of the common bile duct and gallbladder to the duodenum and distal stomach allows EUS imaging of these organs. The detection of choledocholithiasis and the characterization and staging of bile duct and gallbladder neoplasms have been studied with EUS.

Transcutaneous ultrasound detects over 95% of gallbladder stones but may miss common duct stones in 15% to 20% of cases. EUS may detect stones in the distal bile duct by imaging

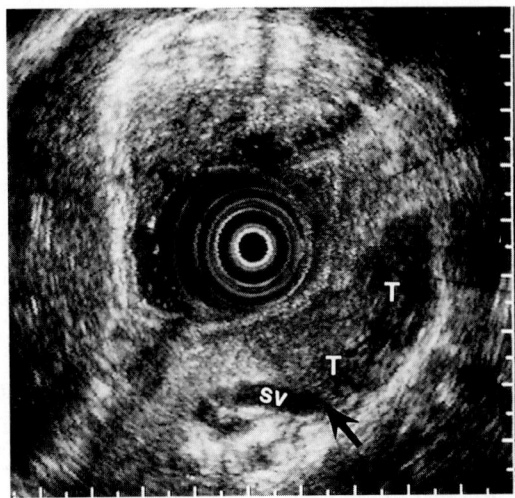
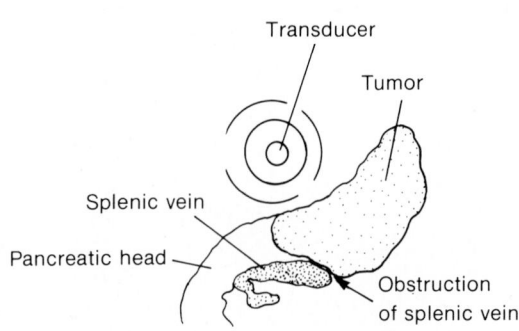

FIGURE 122-14. A carcinoma of the body of the pancreas (T) is shown (*arrow*) to obstruct the splenic vein (sv) by the use of transgastric endoscopic ultrasonographic imaging.

from the descending duodenum.[100,109,110] Common bile duct stones are most likely to be identified when EUS is being used to diagnose the cause of a dilated bile duct or jaundice when choledocholithiasis is unsuspected. If a common duct stone is suspected from transcutaneous imaging procedures or on clinical grounds, endoscopic retrograde cholangiography should be undertaken rather than EUS. Endoscopic retrograde cholangiography is more sensitive than EUS in detecting bile duct stones and allows removal of the stone after endoscopic sphincterotomy.

EUS has been used to stage carcinoma of the bile duct and gallbladder. As with pancreatic carcinoma, the detection of major portal venous invasion by the neoplasm is probably the most clinically relevant role for EUS.[111] Small-diameter catheter probes placed into the bile duct at percutaneous transhepatic cholangiography or ERCP may also prove to be useful for this indication.[112] Prospective studies are needed to define the roles of EUS, CT and angiography in staging bile duct and gallbladder neoplasms.

Liver

EUS has not been used extensively in imaging the liver. Although portions of the left lobe are imaged from the stomach and part of the right lobe from the stomach and duodenum, inadequate penetration prevents imaging of the entire liver. Transcutaneous ultrasound and CT provide a more complete examination of the liver than EUS, although no prospective comparisons of these modalities in the detection of focal liver abnormalities are available.

The application of ultrasound through a laparoscope may provide more information about the nature of hepatic mass lesions than transcorporeal imaging techniques, although rigorous comparative studies are not available. Regenerative cirrhotic nodules, hemangiomas, focal nodular hyperplasia, hepatic adenomas, and hepatomas have all been imaged with laparoscopic sonography.[45] Some ultrasonographic features may be relatively specific. For example, images of focal nodular hyperplasia may reveal a central echoic scar surrounded by a

mass with a ground glass appearance.[45] Other lesions may have multiple ultrasound appearances, making their ultrasound characterization difficult. Hepatomas may be hypoechoic, hyperechoic, or isoechoic with the surrounding liver parenchyma.[45]

TRANSRECTAL ULTRASONOGRAPHY

Ultrasound imaging from within the rectal lumen has been applied to the diagnosis of benign and malignant diseases of the rectum. The diagnosis of inflammatory bowel disease and its complications has been investigated in a small number of studies, but most experience has been accumulated in the staging of colorectal neoplasms. Most of these imaging studies are performed without the use of endoscopic viewing, but the same examination can be done with an ultrasound endoscope, and the technique and findings are similar whether or not endoscopic viewing is used.

Inflammatory Bowel Disease

Transcutaneous ultrasonography has been useful in managing patients with Crohn's disease. The detection of intraabdominal abscesses and ureteral obstruction is a common use of ultrasound in these patients, and the method has been used to detect wall thickening in patients with Crohn's disease or ulcerative colitis. Transcutaneous ultrasound can define the location and extent of intestinal involvement.[113] Changes in the ultrasound layers of the intestinal wall do not reliably differentiate ulcerative colitis from Crohn's disease.[114]

Transrectal ultrasound may also be useful in detecting perirectal complications of inflammatory bowel disease. The detailed images obtained of pararectal tissues allow detection of abscesses or fistulas. Abscesses appear as hypoechoic or anechoic areas adjacent to the rectal lumen. Fistulous tracts, with connections to skin, anus, and vagina, can also be identified with EUS.[115]

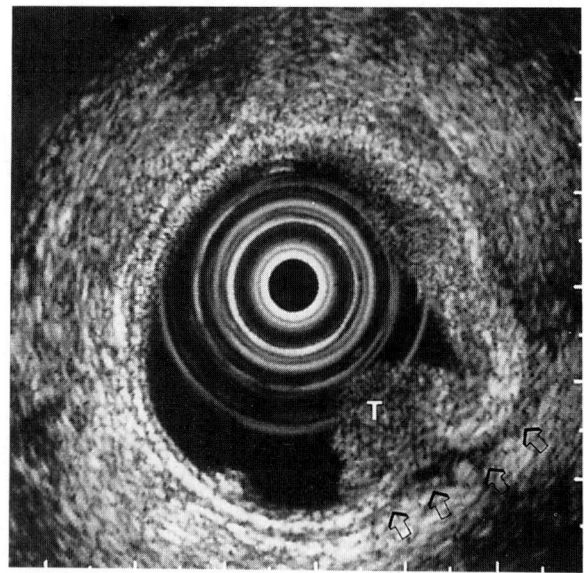

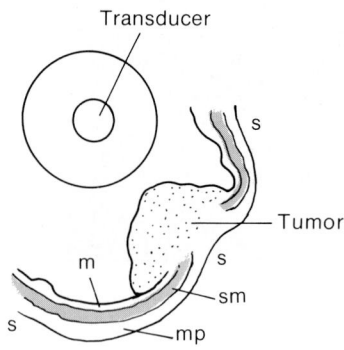

FIGURE 122-15. A polypoid rectal cancer (T) invades the submucosa (sm) but not through the muscularis propria (mp) into the subserosal fat (s). The boundary between the muscularis propria and the subserosal fat is not disrupted under the tumor (*arrows*).

Rectal Carcinoma

Transrectal ultrasonography has been studied for the preoperative staging and the detection of postoperative recurrence of rectal cancer. The depth of cancer invasion into the rectal wall and surrounding tissue and the presence of malignant perirectal lymph nodes have been evaluated with transrectal ultrasound imaging. The accuracy of this modality has been compared with CT imaging, but there are no rigorous studies showing that use of transrectal ultrasound changes patient management or influences survival from rectal cancer.

Most studies of transrectal ultrasound have used a blind ultrasound probe with no optics for visual control. The main limitation in imaging rectal cancers is lumenal obstruction by the neoplasm, which prevents passage of the ultrasound probe in about 10% of cases.[116] The use of endoscopic guidance with ultrasound endoscopes may allow the ultrasound

endoscope to be maneuvered past lesions that do not permit passage of a blind probe.[117]

Comparison of ultrasound images of resected specimens of colorectal cancer to the corresponding histologic sections has demonstrated the accuracy of ultrasound in detecting the malignant invasion.[118] Disruption of the continuity of the echogenic submucosal layer and of the echo-poor layer corresponding to the muscularis propria is a good marker for depth of invasion of the cancer.[118] Rectal cancers are usually imaged as hypoechoic masses, sometimes containing a few scattered internal echoes (Fig. 122-15).[116,118]

Most clinical studies of transrectal ultrasound staging of rectal cancer have a predominance of extensive lesions, especially those with involvement beyond the muscularis propria (Table 122-4).[43,116,117,119] Transrectal ultrasound correctly predicts invasion beyond the muscularis propria in about 85% of cases. The accuracy of detecting the extent of invasion

TABLE 122-4
Accuracy of Transrectal Ultrasound Findings Compared to Surgical Pathology Findings

INVESTIGATOR	DEPTH OF INVASION*				LYMPH NODE INVOLVEMENT			
	T1	T2	T3	T4	True Positive	True Negative	False Positive	False Negative
Hildebrandt[43]	1/3	9/9	11/11	2/2				
Hildebrandt[122]	2/3	22/24	39/45	4/4	6	14	6	1
Konishi (3 MHz)[119]	0/1	0/4	13/18					
Konishi (5 MHz)[119]	4/4	4/8	24/26					
Saitoh[116]	†	13/18	57/62	9/9	52	14	19	3
Beynon[120]	4/4	6/8	21/22	2/2	22	24	7	4
Romano[121]	1/1	6/9	9/9	4/4				
Rifkin[123]			32/49		13	70	6	13
Boyce[128]	3/3	6/8	29/32	2/2	←34/45→			
Herzog[129]	19/22	17/26	67/68	2/2			7/111	5/111

* Based on histologic examination of resected specimen.

† Combined with numbers from the next histologic level.

within the rectal wall is only about 70%. Overstaging of the extent of invasion within the wall may be caused by distortion of the ultrasound image by inflammation in the tissue layer under the cancer.[116]

Lymph node involvement by rectal cancer has also been studied with transrectal ultrasound. Ultrasound is accurate in detecting lymph node involvement in approximately 75% of cases (see Table 122-4).[119-129] As with esophageal and gastric cancer, the ultrasound appearance of malignant lymph nodes is nonspecific.[130,131] False-positive diagnoses due to enlarged inflammatory nodes and false-negative diagnoses due to microscopic invasion are common. Lymph nodes less than 5 mm in diameter are usually missed on transrectal ultrasonography.[131]

Transrectal ultrasound has been used in an effort to detect early recurrences after resection of rectal cancer. Postoperative recurrences are usually detected as mass lesions but may also have an infiltrating appearance.[121,132-135] Anastomotic and extrarectal recurrences may be detected with transrectal ultrasound at a time when CT scans are negative or equivocal.[122,132,133] Transvaginal ultrasound may also detect recurrence after abdominoperineal resection.[116] A false-positive ultrasound diagnosis of recurrence may be the result of inflammatory or fibrotic tissue.[121] EUS-guided biopsy of extraluminal masses should allow differentiation of recurrent cancer from fibrosis.[135]

Transrectal ultrasound staging of rectal cancers has been compared with clinical staging schemes that are largely based on the result of a digital rectal examination.[136-138] Ultrasound staging is more accurate than clinical staging, especially in detecting invasion beyond the muscular wall and in staging tumors proximal to the reach of the examining finger.

Rectal cancer staging with transrectal ultrasound has also been compared with staging with CT and MRI. Transrectal ultrasound and CT are both accurate in determining whether the cancer is confined within or has spread beyond the muscularis propria in 65% to 90% of cases.[121,123,137] However, CT cannot detect lesser degrees of wall invasion.[137] CT is also less accurate in detecting enlarged perirectal lymph nodes.[123] These differences in the accuracy of staging with transrectal ultrasound and CT are not clinically significant if only major surgical resection is contemplated. However, if less invasive therapies, including transanal excision and endoscopic laser therapy, are used, the additional information provided by ultrasound could aid significantly in management planning. MRI may prove to be as accurate as rectal ultrasound for staging rectal cancer.[139] The ability of MRI in differentiating fibrosis from neoplasm is a particular advantage. The availability of rectal surface coils for MRI may allow even further improvements in resolution.

Other Pelvic Organs

Gastrointestinal specialists should be aware that transrectal ultrasonography has received widespread use by urologists and radiologists for the early detection and staging of prostatic cancer. It may also have application in selected instances of bladder, uterine, and vaginal disorders, although its use in imaging these organs is less well studied. These applications are beyond the scope of this review.

TRENDS

Although EUS is a relatively new imaging modality that is still evolving, studies suggest that it is more accurate than other imaging methods in staging esophageal, gastric, and rectal cancer and in defining the cause of intramural and extramural masses of the gastrointestinal tract. EUS is also gaining acceptance as a sensitive way to detect major vascular involvement by pancreatic carcinoma. New instruments that allow EUS-directed tissue sampling are expected to further expand the indications for this procedure. Additional well-designed studies are needed to evaluate the impact of EUS on patient management and outcome.

> The reader is directed to Chapter 120, Cross-Sectional Anatomy, and Chapter 121, Ultrasonography.

REFERENCES

1. Wild JJ. The use of ultrasonic pulses for the measurement of biologic tissues and the detection of tissue density changes. Surgery 1950;27:183.
2. Wild JJ, Reid JM. Diagnostic use of ultrasound. Br J Phys Med 1956;19:248.
3. DiMagno EP, Regan PT, Wilson DA, et al. Ultrasonic endoscope. Lancet 1980;1:629.
4. Strohm WD, Phillip J, Hagenmüller F, Classen M. Ultrasonic tomography by means of an ultrasonic fiberendoscope. Endoscopy 1980;12:241.
5. Tio TL, Tytgat GNJ. Atlas of transintestinal ultrasonography. Aalsmeer, Netherlands: Mur-Kostverloren, 1986.
6. Martin RW, Silverstein FE, Kimmey MB. A 20-MHz ultrasound system for imaging the intestinal wall. Ultrasound Med Biol 1989;15:273.
7. Sasai T. Development of ultrasonic endoscope. In: Kawai K, ed. Endoscopic ultrasonography in gastroenterology. Tokyo: Igaku-Shoin, 1988:18.
8. Ødegaard S, Kimmey MB, Martin RW, et al. The effects of applied pressure on the thickness, layers and echogenicity of gastrointestinal wall ultrasound images. Gastrointest Endosc 1992;38:351.
9. Kimmey MB, Martin RW. Fundamentals of endosonography. Gastrointest Endosc Clin North Am 1992;2:557.
10. Kimmey MB, Martin RW, Haggitt RC, et al. Histologic correlates of gastrointestinal ultrasound images. Gastroenterology 1989;96:433.
11. Grech P. Mirror-image artifact with endoscopic ultrasonography and reappraisal of the fluid-air interface. Gastrointest Endosc 1993;39:700.
12. Beynon J, Foy DMA, Temple LN, et al. The endosonic appearances of normal colon and rectum. Dis Colon Rectum 1986;29:810.
13. Aibe T, Fuji T, Okita K, Takemoto T. A fundamental study of normal layer structure of the gastrointestinal wall visualized by endoscopic ultrasonography. Scand J Gastroenterol 1986;21(Suppl 123):6.
14. Wiersema MJ, Wiersema LM. High-resolution 25-megahertz ultrasonography of the gastrointestinal wall: histologic correlates. Gastrointest Endosc 1993;39:499.
15. Ødegaard S, Kimmey MB. Location of the muscularis mucosae on high frequency gastrointestinal ultrasound images. Eur J Ultrasound 1994;1:39.
16. Derch LE, Biggi E, Neumaier CE, Cicio GR. Ultrasonographic appearances of gastric cancer. Br J Radiol 1983;56:365.
17. Caletti G, Bolondi L, Labo G. Anatomical aspects in ultrasonic endoscopy for the stomach. Scand J Gastroenterol 1984;19(Suppl 94):34.

18. Konishi F, Tetsuichiro M, Takahashi H, et al. Transrectal ul-trasonography for the assessment of invasion of rectal carci-noma. Dis Colon Rectum 1985;28:889.

19. Tio TL, Tytgat GNJ. Endoscopic ultrasonography in analysing peri-intestinal lymph node abnormality. Preliminary results of studies in vitro and in vivo. Scand J Gastroenterol 1986;21(Suppl 123):158.

20. Grimm H, Hamper K, Binmoeller KF, Soehendra N. Enlarged lymph nodes: malignant or not? Endoscopy 1992;24:320.

21. Wiersema MJ, Chak A, Kopecky KK. Clinical applications of duplex and color Doppler endosonography. Gastrointest En-dosc 1993;39:259.

22. Tio TL. Endosonography in gastroenterology. Berlin: Springer-Verlag, 1988.

23. Luz G, Heyder N, Lutz H, Demling L. Endoscopic ultraso-nography—technique, orientation and diagnostic possibilities. Endoscopy 1982;14:220.

24. Rösch T, Lorenz R, Suchy R, Dancygier H, Classen M. Colonic endoscopic ultrasonography: first results of a new technique. Gastrointest Endosc 1990;36:382.

25. Vilmann P, Khattar S, Hancke S. Endoscopic ultrasound ex-amination of the upper gastrointestinal tract using a curved-array transducer. A preliminary report. Surg Endosc 1991;5: 79.

26. Vilmann P, Jacobsen GK, Henriksen FW, Hancke S. Endoscopic ultrasonography with guided fine needle aspiration biopsy in pancreatic disease. Gastrointest Endosc 1992;38:172.

27. Wiersema MJ, Chak A. Prospective comparative evaluation of a linear electronic array ultrasound endoscope and a radial me-chanical scanning ultrasound endoscope. Gastrointest Endosc 1993;39:260.

28. Grimm H, Binmoeller KF, Soehendra N. Endosonography-guided drainage of a pancreatic pseudocyst. Gastrointest Endosc 1992;38:170.

29. DiMagno EP, Regan PT, Clain JE, et al. Human endoscopic ultrasonography. Gastroenterology 1982;83:824.

30. Gordon SJ, Rifkin MD, Goldberg BB. Endosonographic eval-uation of mural abnormalities of the upper gastrointestinal tract. Gastrointest Endosc 1986;32:193.

31. Takemoto T, Aibe T, Fuji T, Okita K. Endoscopic ultrasonog-raphy. Clin Gastroenterol 1986;15:305.

32. Ziegler K, Sanft C, Zeitz M, et al. Evaluation of endosonography in TN staging of oesophageal cancer. Gut 1991;32:16.

33. Wild JJ, Foderick JW. The feasibility of echometric detection of cancer in the lower gastrointestinal tract. Am J Proctol Gas-troenterol Colon Rectal Surg 1978;16:16.

34. Rasmussen SN, Riis P. Rectal wall thickness measured by ul-trasound in chronic inflammatory diseases of the colon. Scand J Gastroenterol 1985;20:109.

35. Lutz H, Tosch W. Transgastroscopic ultrasonography. Endos-copy 1976;8:203.

36. Rosch T, Classen M. A new ultrasonic probe for endosono-graphic imaging of the upper GI tract. Preliminary observations. Endoscopy 1990;22:41.

37. Liu JB, Miller LS, Feld RI, et al. Gastric and esophageal varices: 20-MHz transnasal endoluminal US. Radiology 1993;187: 363.

38. Miller LS, Liu JB, Klenn PJ, et al. Endoluminal ultrasonography of the distal esophagus in systemic sclerosis. Gastroenterology 1993;105:31.

39. Kimmey MB, Martin RW, Silverstein FE. Clinical application of linear ultrasound probes. Endoscopy 1992;24:364.

40. Seward JB, Khandheria BK, Oh JD, et al. Transesophageal echocardiography: technique, anatomic correlations, imple-mentation, and clinical applications. Mayo Clin Proc 1988;63: 649.

41. Tio TL, Coene PPLO, Schouwink MH, Tytgat GNJ. Esophagogastric carcinoma: preoperative TNM classification with endosonography. Radiology 1989;173:411.

42. Grimm H, Binmoeller KF, Soehendra N. Ultrasonic esopha-goprobe (prototype 1). Gastrointest Endosc 1992;38:490.

43. Hildebrandt U, Feifel G. Preoperative staging of rectal cancer by intrarectal ultrasound. Dis Colon Rectum 1985;28:42.

44. Okita K, Kodama T, Oda M, Takemoto T. Laparoscopic ultra-sonography. Diagnosis of liver and pancreatic cancer. Scand J Gastroenterol 1984;19(Suppl 94):91.

45. Fukuda M, Mima S. Laparoscopic sonography in differential diagnosis of liver diseases. In: Kawai K, ed. Endoscopic ultra-sonography in gastroenterology. Tokyo: Igaku-Shoin, 1988: 119.

46. Strohm WD, Classen M. Anatomical aspects in ultrasonic en-doscopy. Scand J Gastroenterol 1984;19(Suppl 94):21.

47. Lux G, Heyder N, Lutz H. Ultrasound tomography of the upper gastrointestinal tract. Orientation and diagnostic possibilities. Scand J Gastroenterol 1984;19(Suppl 94):13.

48. Caletti G, Bolondi L, Barbara L. Instrumentation and scanning techniques. In: Kawai K, ed. Endoscopic ultrasonography in gastroenterology. Tokyo: Igaku-Shoin, 1988:1.

49. Yiengpruksawan A, Lightdale CJ, Gerdes H, Botet JF. Mucol-ytic-antifoam solution for reduction of artifacts during endo-scopic ultrasonography: a randomized controlled trial. Gas-trointest Endosc 1991;37:543.

50. Gilbert DA, DiMarino AJ, Jensen DM, et al. ASGE technology assessment status evaluation: endoscopic ultrasonography. Gastrointest Endosc 1992;38:747.

51. Han M-C, Kim C-W. Sectional human anatomy. 2nd ed. New York: Igaku-Shoin, 1989.

52. Kawai K. Endoscopic ultrasonography in gastroenterology. New York: Igaku-Shoin, 1988.

53. Rosch T, Classen M. Gastroenterologic endosonography text-book and atlas. New York: Thieme Medical Publishers, 1992.

54. Rex DK, Tarver RD, Wiersema M, et al. Endoscopic trans-esophageal fine needle aspiration of mediastinal masses. Gas-trointest Endosc 1991;37:465.

55. Yasuda K, Nakajima M, Yoshida S, et al. The diagnosis of sub-mucosal tumors of the stomach by endoscopic ultrasonography. Gastrointest Endosc 1989;35:10.

56. Caletti G, Zani L, Bolondi L, et al. Endoscopic ultrasonography in the diagnosis of gastric submucosal tumor. Gastrointest En-dosc 1989;35:413.

57. Strohm WD, Classen M. Benign lesions of the upper GI tract by means of endoscopic ultrasonography. Scand J Gastroenterol 1986;21(Suppl 123):41.

58. Boyce GA, Sivak MV Jr, Rosch T, et al. Evaluation of sub-mucosal upper gastrointestinal tract lesions by endoscopic ul-trasound. Gastrointest Endosc 1991;37:449.

59. Nakazawa S, Yoshino J, Nakamura T, et al. Endoscopic ultra-sonography of gastric myogenic tumor. A comparative study between histology and ultrasonography. J Ultrasound Med 1989;8:353.

60. Yasuda K, Nakajima M, Kawai K. Endoscopic ultrasonography in the diagnosis of submucosal tumor of the upper digestive tract. Scand J Gastroenterol 1986;21(Suppl 123):59.

61. Tio TL, Tytgat GNJ, den Hartog Jager FCA. Endoscopic ul-trasonography for the evaluation of smooth muscle tumors in the upper gastrointestinal tract: an experience with 42 cases. Gastrointest Endosc 1990;36:342.

62. Rosch T, Lorenz R, von Wichert A, Classen M. Gastric fundus impression caused by splenic vessels: detection by endoscopic ultrasound. Endoscopy 1991;23:85.

63. Tio TL, Coene PPLO, den Hartog Jager FCA, Tytgat GNJ. Preoperative TNM classification of esophageal carcinoma by endosonography. Hepatogastroenterology 1990;37:376.

64. Tio TL, Cohen P, Coene PP, et al. Endosonography and com-puted tomography of esophageal carcinoma. Preoperative clas-sification compared to the new (1987) TNM system. Gastro-enterology 1989;96:1478.

65. Botet JF, Lightdale CJ, Zauber AG, et al. Preoperative staging of esophageal cancer: comparison of endoscopic US and dy-namic CT. Radiology 1991;181:419.

66. Vilgrain V, Mompoint D, Palazzo L, et al. Staging of esophageal carcinoma: comparison of results with endoscopic sonography and CT. AJR Am J Roentgenol 1990;155:277.

67. Rice TW, Boyce GA, Sivak MV, Loop FD. Esophageal ultra-sound and the preoperative staging of carcinoma of the esoph-agus. J Thorac Cardiovasc Surg 1991;101:536.

68. Rosch T, Zenker K, von Wichert A, et al. Local staging and assessment of resectability in carcinoma of the esophagus,

stomach, and duodenum by endoscopic ultrasonography. Gastrointest Endosc 1992;38:460.

69. Grimm H, Binmoeller KF, Hamper K, et al. Endosonography for preoperative locoregional staging of esophageal and gastric cancer. Endoscopy 1993;25:224.

70. Quint LE, Glazer GM, Orringer MB, Gross BH. Esophageal carcinoma: CT findings. Radiology 1985;155:171.

71. Quint LE, Glazer GM, Orringer MB. Esophageal imaging by MR and CT: study of normal anatomy and neoplasms. Radiology 1985;156:727.

72. Murata Y, Ide H, Suzuki S, et al. The accuracy of estimation of depth of esophageal cancer invasion by endoscopic ultrasonography (EUS). Endoscopy 1988;20:22.

73. Yamanaka T, Yoshida Y, Ueno N, et al. Endoscopic ultrasonography in the diagnosis of the degree of vertical invasion of gastric cancer. Nippon Shokakibyo Gakkai Zasshi 1985;82:1865.

74. Tio TL, Schouwink MH, Cikot RJLM, Tytgat GNJ. Preoperative TNM classification of gastric carcinoma by endosonography in comparison with the pathological TNM system: a prospective study of 72 cases. Hepatogastroenterology 1989;36:51.

75. Botet JF, Lightdale CJ, Zauber AG, et al. Preoperative staging of gastric cancer: comparison of endoscopic US and dynamic CT. Radiology 1991;181:426.

76. Grimm H, Binmoeller KF, Hamper K, et al. Endosonography for preoperative locoregional staging of esophageal and gastric cancer. Endoscopy 1993;25:224.

77. Saito N, Takeshita K, Habu H, Endo M. The use of endoscopic ultrasound in determining the depth of cancer invasion in patients with gastric cancer. Surg Endosc 1991;5:14.

78. Akahoshi K, Misawa T, Fujishima H, et al. Regional lymph node metastasis in gastric cancer: evaluation with endoscopic US. Radiology 1992;182:559.

79. Takemoto T. Laser therapy of early gastric carcinoma. Endoscopy 1986;18:32.

80. Okazaki Y, Tada M. Endoscopic treatment of early gastric cancer. Semin Surg Oncol 1991;7:351.

81. Lightdale CJ, Botet JF, Kelsen DP, et al. Diagnosis of recurrent upper gastrointestinal cancer at the surgical anastomosis by endoscopic ultrasound. Gastrointest Endosc 1989;35:407.

82. Tio TL, Den Hartog Jager FCA, Tytgat GNJ. Endoscopic ultrasonography in detection and staging of non-Hodgkin lymphoma. Scand J Gastroenterol 1986;21(Suppl 123):52.

83. Tio TL, Den Hartog Jager FCA, Tytgat GNJ. Endoscopic ultrasonography of non-Hodgkin lymphoma of the stomach. Gastroenterology 1986;91:401.

84. Fujishima H, Misawa T, Maruoka A, et al. Staging and follow-up of primary gastric lymphoma by endoscopic ultrasonography. Am J Gastroenterol 1991;86:719.

85. Neoptolemos JP, Talbot IC, Carr-Locke DL, et al. Treatment and outcome in 52 consecutive cases of ampullary carcinoma. Br J Surg 1987;74:975.

86. Yasuda K, Mukai H, Dho E, et al. The use of endoscopic ultrasonography in the diagnosis and staging of carcinoma of the papilla of Vater. Endoscopy 1988;20:218.

87. Tio TL, Tytgat GNJ, Cikot RJLM, et al. Ampullopancreatic carcinoma: preoperative TNM classification with endosonography.

88. Tio TL, Mulder CJ, Eggink WF. Endosonography in staging early carcinoma of the ampulla of Vater. Gastroenterology 1992;102:1392.

89. Rosch T, Braig C, Gain T, et al. Staging of pancreatic and ampullary carcinoma by endoscopic ultrasonography. Gastroenterology 1992;102:188.

90. Bolondi L, Caletti G, Casanova P, et al. Problems and variations in the interpretation of the ultrasound feature of the normal upper and lower GI tract wall. Scand J Gastroenterol 1986;21(Suppl 123):16.

91. Caletti GC, Bolondi L, Zani L, et al. Detection of portal hypertension and esophageal varices by means of endoscopic ultrasonography. Scand J Gastroenterol 1986;21(Suppl 123):74.

92. Yasuda K, Mukai H, Nakajima M, Kawai K. Endoscopic ultrasonography in evaluating the effects of endoscopic injection sclerotherapy for esophageal varices. Gastrointest Endosc 1986;32:183.

93. Tio TL, Tytgat GNJ. Endoscopic ultrasonography of an arteriovenous malformation in a gastric polyp. Endoscopy 1986;18:156.

94. Aibe T, Takemoto T. Benign lesions of the gastrointestinal tract. In: Kawai K, ed. Endoscopic ultrasonography in gastroenterology. Tokyo: Igaku-Shoin, 1988:44.

95. Polensky A, Ziegler K, Sanft C, et al. Endosonographische Befunde benigner und maligner läsionen der Magenwand. Dtsch Med Wochenschr 1988;113:1263.

96. Lux G, Heyder N. Endoscopic ultrasonography of the pancreas. Technical aspects. Scand J Gastroenterol 1986;21(Suppl 123):112.

97. Nakazawa S, Hayashi Y, Naitoh Y, et al. Chronic pancreatitis. In: Kawai K, ed. Endoscopic ultrasonography in gastroenterology. Tokyo: Igaku-Shoin, 1988:79.

98. Wiersema MJ, Schwartz SM, Hawes RH, Rex DK. Abnormalities of pancreas parenchymal and ductular features detected by endosonography in asymptomatic subjects with a history of moderate to heavy alcohol use. Gastrointest Endosc 1993;39:336.

99. Lees WR. Endoscopic ultrasonography of chronic pancreatitis and pancreatic pseudocysts. Scand J Gastroenterol 1986;21(Suppl 123):123.

100. Dancygier H, Classen M. Endosonographic diagnosis of benign pancreatic and biliary lesions. Scand J Gastroenterol 1986;21(Suppl 123):119.

101. Sivak MV Jr, Kaufman A. Endoscopic ultrasonography in the differential diagnosis of pancreatic disease. A preliminary report. Scand J Gastroenterol 1986;21(Suppl 123):130.

102. Yasuda K, Mukai H, Fujimoto S, et al. The diagnosis of pancreatic cancer by endoscopic ultrasonography. Gastrointest Endosc 1988;34:1.

103. Dancygier H, Classen M. Pancreatic cancer. In: Kawai K, ed. Endoscopic ultrasonography in gastroenterology. Tokyo: Igaku-Shoin, 1988:72.

104. Kauffman AR, Sivak MV. Endoscopic ultrasonography in the differential diagnosis of pancreatic disease. Gastrointest Endosc 1989;35:214.

105. Yasuda K, Tanaka Y, Fujimoto S, et al. Use of endoscopic ultrasonography in small pancreatic cancer. Scand J Gastroenterol 1984;19:9.

106. Amouyal P, Amouyal G, Mompoint D, et al. Endosonography: promising method for diagnosis of extrahepatic cholestasis. Lancet 1989;2:1195.

107. Lightdale CJ, Botet JF, Woodruff JM, Brennan MF. Localization of endocrine tumors of the pancreas with endoscopic ultrasonography. Cancer 1991;68:1815.

108. Rosch TR, Lightdale CJ, Botet JF, et al. Localization of pancreatic endocrine tumors by endoscopic ultrasonography. N Engl J Med 1992;326:1721.

109. Yasuda K, Nakajima M, Kawai K. Diseases of the biliary tract and the papilla of Vater. In: Kawai K, ed. Endoscopic ultrasonography in gastroenterology. Tokyo: Igaku-Shoin, 1988:96.

110. Amougal P, Amougal G, Levy P, et al. Diagnosis of choledocholithiasis by endoscopic ultrasonography. Gastroenterology 1994;106:1062.

111. Tio TL, Tytgat GNJ. Endoscopic ultrasonography of bile duct malignancy and the preoperative assessment of local resectability. Scand J Gastroenterol 1986;21(Suppl 123):151.

112. Yasuda K, Mukai H, Nakajima M, Kawai K. Clinical application of ultrasonic probes in the biliary and pancreatic duct. Endoscopy 1992;24 (Suppl 1):370.

113. Limberg B. Diagnosis of acute ulcerative colitis and colonic Crohn's disease by colonic sonography. J Clin Ultrasound 1989;17:25.

114. Kimmey MB, Wang KY, Haggitt RC, et al. Diagnosis of inflammatory bowel disease with ultrasound: an in vitro study. Invest Radiol 1990;25:1085.

115. Tio TL, Mulder CJJ, Wijers OB, et al. Endosonography of perianal and peri-colorectal fistula and/or abscess in Crohn's disease. Gastrointest Endosc 1990;36:331.

116. Saitoh N, Okui K, Sarashina H, et al. Evaluation of echographic

diagnosis of rectal cancer using intrarectal ultrasonic examination. Dis Colon Rectum 1986;29:234.

117. Tio TL, Tytgat GNJ. Comparison of blind transrectal ultrasonography with endoscopic transrectal ultrasonography in assessing rectal and perirectal diseases. Scand J Gastroenterol 1986;21(Suppl 123):104.

118. Wang KY, Kimmey MB, Nyberg DA, et al. Colorectal neoplasms: accuracy of US in demonstrating the depth of invasion. Radiology 1987;165:827.

119. Konishi F, Tetsuichiro M, Takahashi H, et al. Transrectal ultrasonography for the assessment of invasion of rectal carcinoma. Dis Colon Rectum 1985;28:899.

120. Beynon J, Foy DMA, Roe AM, et al. Endoluminal ultrasound in the assessment of local invasion in rectal cancer. Br J Surg 1986;73:474.

121. Romano G, de Rosa P, Vallone G, et al. Intrarectal ultrasound and computed tomography in the pre- and postoperative assessment of patients with rectal cancer. Br J Surg 1985;72(Sept Suppl):S117.

122. Hildebrandt U, Feifel G, Schwarz HP, Scherr O. Endorectal ultrasound: instrumentation and clinical aspects. Int J Colorectal Dis 1986;1:203.

123. Rifkin MD, Ehrlich SM, Marks G. Staging of rectal carcinoma: prospective comparison of endorectal US and CT. Radiology 1989;170:319.

124. Holdsworth PJ, Johnston D, Chalmers AG, et al. Endoluminal ultrasound and computed tomography in the staging of rectal cancer. Br J Surg 1988;75:1019.

125. Waizer A, Zitron S, Ben-Baruch D, et al. Comparative study for preoperative staging of rectal cancer. Dis Colon Rectum 1989;32:53.

126. Roubein LD, David C, DuBrow R, et al. Endoscopic ultrasonography in staging rectal cancer. Am J Gastroenterol 1990;85:1391.

127. Goldman S, Arvidsson H, Norming U, et al. Transrectal ultrasound and computed tomography in preoperative staging of lower rectal adenocarcinoma. Gastrointest Radiol 1991;16:259.

128. Boyce GA, Sivak MV, Lavery IC, et al. Endoscopic ultrasound in the pre-operative staging of rectal carcinoma. Gastrointest Endosc 1992;38:468.

129. Herzog U, von Flue M, Tondelli P, Schuppisser JP. How accurate is endorectal ultrasound in the preoperative staging of rectal cancer? Dis Colon Rectum 1993;36:127.

130. Hulsmans FH, Bosma A, Mulder PJ, et al. Perirectal lymph nodes in rectal cancer: in vitro correlation of sonographic parameters and histopathologic findings. Radiology 1992;184:553.

131. Nielsen MB, Qvitzau S, Pedersen JF. Detection of pericolonic lymph nodes in patients with colorectal cancer: an in vitro and in vivo study of the efficacy of endosonography. AJR Am J Roentgenol 1993;161:57.

132. Mascagni D, Corbellini L, Urciuoli P, DiMatteo G. Endoluminal ultrasound for early detection of local recurrence of rectal cancer. Br J Surg 1989;76:1176.

133. Tschmelitsch J, Glaser K, Schwarz C, et al. Endosonography in the diagnosis of recurrent cancer of the rectum. J Ultrasound Med 1992;11:149.

134. Romano G, Esercizio L, Santangelo M, et al. Impact of computed tomography vs intrarectal ultrasound on the diagnosis, resectability, and prognosis of locally recurrent rectal cancer. Dis Colon Rectum 1993;36:261.

135. Nielsen MB, Pedersen JF, Hald J, Christiansen J. Recurrent extraluminal rectal carcinoma: transrectal biopsy under sonographic guidance. AJR Am J Roentgenol 1992;158:1025.

136. Nicholls RJ, Mason AY, Morson BC, et al. The clinical staging of rectal cancer. Br J Surg 1982;69:404.

137. Beynon J, Mortensen McC NJ, Foy DMA, et al. Pre-operative assessment of local invasion in rectal cancer: digital examination, endoluminal sonography or computed tomography? Br J Surg 1986;73:1015.

138. Milsom JW, Graffner H. Intrarectal ultrasonography in rectal cancer staging and in the evaluation of pelvic disease. Clinical uses of intrarectal ultrasound. Ann Surg 1990;212:602.

139. Waizer A, Powsner E, Russo I, et al. Prospective comparative study of magnetic resonance imaging versus transrectal ultrasound for preoperative staging and follow-up of rectal cancer. Preliminary report. Dis Colon Rectum 1991;34:1068.

Textbook of Gastroenterology, second edition, edited by Tadataka Yamada. JB Lippincott Company, Philadelphia © 1995.

CHAPTER 123

Applications of Computed Tomography to the Gastrointestinal Tract

Richard L. Baron

The first in vivo application of computed tomography (CT) was achieved in London in 1971. Long scan times initially limited this technique to neurologic applications, but by 1975, with a reduction in scan times to 18 seconds, significant applications were possible. Progressive improvements in CT technology have resulted in routine scan times of 1 second, with electron beam technology capable of scan times of 20 milliseconds. The basic principle of CT is to reconstruct a cross-sectional slice of the body from a set of multiple x-ray profiles with computer-aided reconstruction.[1] The resultant density or attenuation of structures is displayed on a gray-scale continuum, measurable and described in Hounsfield units (H).

Faster CT scan times have overcome the problems of respiratory motion and bowel peristalsis, and CT has become the dominant method of evaluating abdominal abnormalities. Initially used for assessing solid abdominal organs, its use in evaluating the intestinal tract is expanding. Although barium radiography and endoscopy optimally evaluate intestinal mu-

cosal abnormalities, CT is capable of evaluating intramural and extrinsic abnormalities and evaluating the extent of extralumenal neoplastic and inflammatory disease. Although barium examinations and endoscopy remain the standards for diagnosis, CT is playing an increasing role in staging the extent of disease and clarifying confusing findings. As an example, CT is used as the initial examination of choice for patients suspected of diverticulitis, replacing rather than assisting the time-honored contrast radiographic techniques.[2]

TECHNIQUES

CT scan techniques vary with the region of the body being examined. Most examinations of the abdomen require administration of oral dilute contrast (e.g., barium, water-soluble agents) 1 to 2 hours before the examination to opacify the small bowel and differentiate bowel from abnormal masses. The colon usually can be identified without contrast, but in certain instances, it may need to be opacified by retrograde filling with contrast material or air. Intravenous contrast is used to opacify vascular structures, organ parenchyma, and neoplastic masses. The combination of these contrast techniques, along with patient positioning and tailoring the CT examination, results in different protocols for investigating the many different disease processes that affect the body.

Scan techniques can be altered in several ways. Voltage, amperage, image acquisition time, field of view, reconstruction software, collimation (i.e., slice thickness), and scan intervals all affect the image results. Selecting appropriate variables depends on what clinical information is needed and the individual patient. Scan times are shortened, for example, for patients unable to maintain body positions or withhold respirations, but this is done at the expense of increased image noise and poorer contrast perception. Collimation can vary from 1 to 10 mm, depending on the spatial resolution needed. CT scanners have a spatial resolution of 0.5 to 1.5 mm, but whether an object is identifiable on CT generally depends more on its density than its size.

The introduction of slip ring technology has allowed faster acquisition of images. This technology uses a continuously rotating x-ray tube with sustained exposures up to 60 seconds while the patient is moved through the CT gantry. This improves CT capabilities by allowing faster acquisition of images and optimal use of contrast agents; obtaining continuous data acquisition because large organs can be imaged during a single breathhold; and enhancing image reconstruction capabilities.[3,4]

High-density compounds, such as metal and barium, can cause large scan artifacts, and if these materials are in the region of imaging interest, the scans should be delayed until they can be cleared. Imaging examinations should be scheduled with this in mind, particularly if tests using barium are also being considered. Such tests should be performed after the CT examination, because it may take several days for the barium to clear sufficiently to allow adequate CT examination.

COMPLICATIONS

The radiation dose from a CT examination varies with the CT scanner type and the technique used for the examination. The average skin surface dose to the patient is 1.5 to 3 cGy during a typical abdominal examination.[5] Because the x-ray beam used is tightly collimated, there is little scattered radiation and little radiation to sites distant from the area being scanned.

The most worrisome complication of a CT examination is the risk of minor reactions, such as rashes, urticaria, nausea, and vomiting, and serious reactions, such as anaphylaxis and cardiorespiratory compromise, to the intravenous contrast agents. There also is a risk of contrast-induced renal failure, and the patient's renal function should be documented before examinations requiring intravenous contrast. On the day of the examination, if intravenous contrast is to be used, patients should have nothing by mouth or only clear liquids before the examination to decrease the likelihood of vomiting and aspiration.

ESOPHAGUS

The entire length of the esophagus is usually easily identified. Although small amounts of intralumenal air can be seen in as many as 65% of patients, air-fluid levels or a fluid-filled esophagus usually indicates esophageal obstruction or dysfunction.[6] Detecting esophageal pathology often depends on identifying wall thickening and differentiating this from a collapsed, normal esophagus. This process often requires the use of air (i.e., administering an effervescent agent) or a contrast agent for distention to avoid mistaking a normal, collapsed esophagus for a pathologic condition. The normal wall thickness of the distended esophagus should not exceed 3 to 5 mm.[7,8] In cachectic patients with a paucity of mediastinal fat, it may be difficult to delineate the limits of the esophagus and to detect milder abnormalities.

Neoplasms

All esophageal neoplasms appear on CT as focal, asymmetric, soft tissue–density masses in the wall or as concentric wall thickenings. These findings are nonspecific and can be seen in benign and malignant tumors and in inflammatory conditions. Although CT is not a screening tool for esophageal diseases, some patients undergoing CT for other reasons have esophageal abnormalities detected. CT can help to delineate the abnormal masses detected on chest radiographs and prove masses to be of esophageal origin.

Benign Neoplasms

Leiomyomas appear as well-marginated soft tissue–density masses, often asymmetrically thickening the esophageal wall. This is a nonspecific appearance and is similar to that of metastatic disease and some primary malignant lesions. Intramural abscesses and duplication cysts can be differentiated by their lower attenuation, which is usually closer to water density.

Malignant Neoplasms

Carcinoma of the esophagus typically appears on CT as a focal eccentric mass or as concentric thickening of the esophageal wall (Fig. 123-1), neither of which is a specific finding. The role of CT in esophageal carcinoma includes staging the extent of disease, evaluating patients after treatment for therapy responses, and evaluating the complications of surgical therapies.

Early studies were enthusiastic about the ability of CT to stage esophageal carcinoma, but later studies showed CT to be less accurate, particularly for gastroesophageal junction tumors.[6,9] Although CT is reliable in detecting liver metastases and direct invasion into the tracheobronchial tree, it is less accurate in predicting lymph node involvement because of an inability to detect metastases in normal-sized lymph nodes.[10] The overall accuracy in detecting mediastinal invasion is 92% to 96%; the accuracy in detecting periesophageal lymph node metastases averages 65% and 87% for intraabdominal lymph nodes.[10–12] Because the esophagus normally can abut

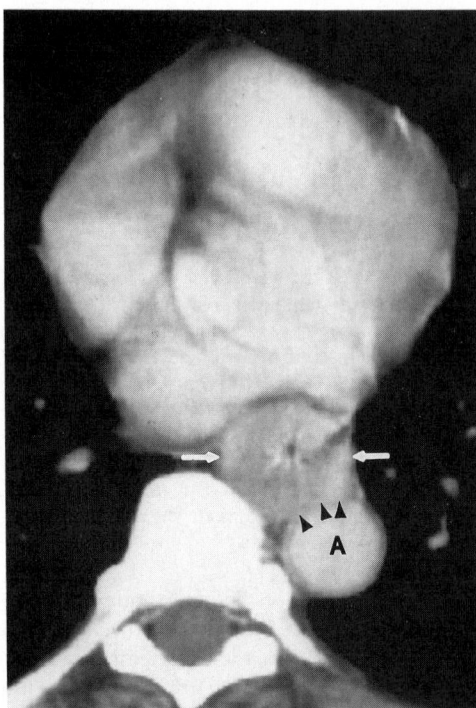

FIGURE 123-1. Esophageal carcinoma. The CT scan shows marked concentric thickening of the esophageal wall (*arrows*) and lumenal narrowing. The fat plane between the aorta (A) and the tumor is obscured over approximately 60 degrees of the aortic circumference (*arrowheads*). At surgery, there was no tumor invasion of the aorta.

the aorta without an intervening, discrete fat plane, aortic invasion by esophageal carcinoma can be a difficult CT diagnosis, although criteria for differentiating normal from abnormal scans have been suggested.[11] Despite limitations, CT is the only noninvasive screening modality able to demonstrate the extent of extralumenal disease in these patients.

CT can be used to evaluate esophageal carcinoma after therapy, particularly with a baseline CT for reference. Therapy success or failure can be based on documentation of the development of enlarged mediastinal lymph nodes or masses, lung nodules, or liver and adrenal metastases. Postsurgical complications can be detected on CT by demonstrating anastomotic leaks, which occasionally are seen only on CT scans and are not detected by standard contrast esophagography.

Lymphoma and disease metastatic to the esophagus have a similar CT appearance and cannot be differentiated from adenocarcinoma and other benign lesions based on the esophageal appearance alone. If extensive changes of mediastinal invasion or metastatic disease are present, benign lesions can be excluded.

Varices

The use of intravenous contrast with CT can aid in differentiating esophageal varices from other causes of esophageal disease.[13,14] Varices appear within the esophageal wall or in

a paraesophageal location as rounded, lobulated structures that demonstrate greater contrast enhancement than tumors or lymph nodes. The CT detection of extensive venous collaterals in other locations can aid in making the diagnosis. A characteristic CT appearance is seen in patients after sclerotherapy for esophageal varices, demonstrating a thickened esophageal wall with a low-attenuation ring.[15,16]

Esophagitis

Diffuse esophageal wall thickening can be seen in reflux, inflammatory, and infectious esophagitis.[17] Diffuse thickening has also been reported in patients with intramural pseudodiverticulosis.[18]

STOMACH

The stomach is easily identified as a fluid- and air-filled structure in the left upper abdomen. A contrast agent or air is used to distend the stomach and ensure that the wall can be evaluated without mistaking collapsed gastric folds for pathologic wall thickening. The normal gastric wall thickness varies from 3 to 10 mm, depending on the degree of gastric distention.[19] The gastroesophageal junction region can be thicker and appear as a pseudomass, usually differentiated by using lateral decubitus or prone positioning to provide maximal distention.[20]

Neoplasms

Benign Neoplasms

Small benign masses or polyps cannot be detected as separate from the normal appearance of the gastric wall. Larger adenomas are seen protruding into the contrast- or air-filled lumen. Intramural lesions, such as leiomyomas, if larger than 1.5 to 2 cm, can be seen as focal thickening of the stomach wall.[21] Generally, these soft tissue–density masses are indistinguishable, with the exception of lipomas, which are characterized by the low CT attenuation of fat.

Malignant Neoplasms

The CT appearance of adenocarcinoma of the stomach (Fig. 123-2) is varied and depends on tumor size, location, and morphologic characteristics. These lesions can appear with focal wall thickening, diffuse gastric wall thickening, small intralumenal plaques or masses, or as an ulcerating mass.

Although early studies suggested CT could accurately stage the extent of gastric carcinoma, later studies reported less than satisfactory accuracy.[10,19,22-26] In a series of 75 patients, Sussman and colleagues found CT staged 47% of patients incorrectly (i.e., 31% understaged and 16% overstaged).[26] The understaging resulted from an inability to detect metastatic lymph nodes that were too small or confluent with the primary lesion. Small metastatic nodules in the peritoneum can be difficult to detect on CT.

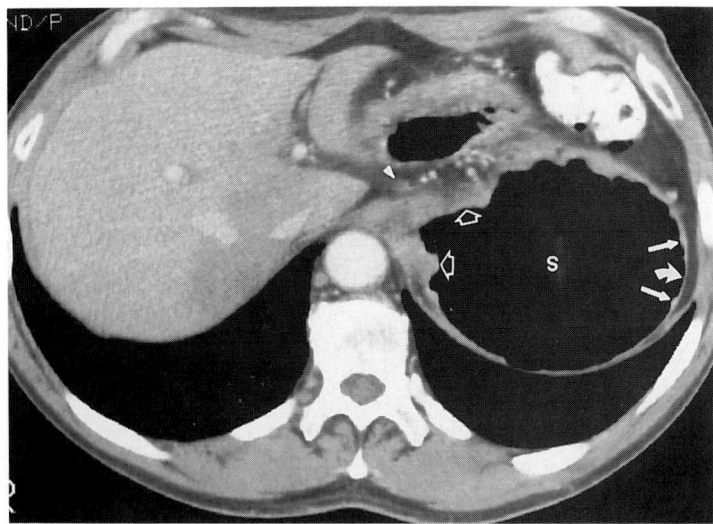

FIGURE 123-2. Adenocarcinoma of the gastric fundus. The scan was obtained with the patient in the prone position, maximizing gaseous distention of the stomach (S). The normal gastric wall (*curved arrow*) is thin, measuring 2 to 3 mm, with scattered rugal folds (*straight arrows*) seen, in contrast to the region of the gastric cardia, where the tumor is easily demarcated by the wall thickening (*open arrows*). An 8-mm-diameter lymph node (*arrowhead*) in the periserosal fat was found at surgery to contain metastatic tumor.

The preoperative role of CT in these patients is to answer questions that may affect surgery, such as detecting distant metastases or large nodal metastases, which would obviate an extensive surgical resection for cure. Postoperatively, CT can be an accurate method of patient follow-up for recurrent disease or for responses to other therapies.[27]

The large extragastric mass extension characterizing gastric leiomyosarcoma is typically seen on CT. Central necrosis often results in lower attenuation seen centrally, which is uncommon in adenocarcinoma or lymphoma.[28]

Lymphoma has an appearance similar to gastric carcinoma on CT, with focal or diffuse thickening of the gastric wall, which may contain polypoid intralumenal elements or ulceration.[29,30] Many of these patients have diffuse lymphadenopathy that suggests the diagnosis, particularly if present in the retroperitoneum.

Metastases have the nonspecific CT appearance of focal soft tissue–density masses, similar to benign and primary malignant disease.

Inflammatory Diseases

All inflammatory diseases of the stomach can produce focal or diffuse thickening of the stomach, which can simulate neoplastic disease. Peptic ulcer disease can demonstrate marked wall thickening, and occasionally the ulcer itself can be seen as an air-filled defect within the thickened wall.

Varices

Varices can cause gastric wall thickening. If patent, the vascular nature of varices usually can be ascertained with contrast-enhanced CT scans.[31]

SMALL INTESTINE

The key to evaluation of the small intestine lies in adequate opacification with orally administered contrast material. Usually, 500 to 600 mL of dilute contrast material should be administered 1 to 2 hours before examining the abdomen to provide opacification of the small bowel and avoid mistaking fluid-filled or nondistended loops for abnormal masses. CT demonstrates the plicae circulares of the jejunum with a feathery appearance, as seen on conventional small bowel radiography, but the ileum appears featureless. In both instances, the wall or fold thickness should not exceed 3 to 5 mm.

Congenital Anomalies

Although not the examination of choice to confirm rotational abnormalities of the small bowel, CT can detect positional anomalies of the intestines. With a malrotation, the duodenum fails to pass to the left aspect of the abdomen. The positions of the superior mesenteric artery and vein are often reversed.[32] The complication of intestinal volvulus may be seen with dilated, thick-walled loops of small bowel converging on a single point of mesentery.[33]

Duplication cysts can be identified on CT scans as low attenuation masses within the bowel wall.

Neoplasms

Benign tumors in the small intestine do not have a characteristic CT appearance and, in most instances, cannot be differentiated from malignant lesions. Leiomyomas, the most common such lesion, appear as rounded, soft tissue–density masses in the intestinal wall. If definitely identified within the wall, they can be differentiated from adenomas and adenocarcinomas, but this can be difficult. Lipomas are one of the few intestinal lesions that can be categorized by CT because of their low attenuation.[34]

Adenocarcinoma of the small intestine produces changes similar to adenocarcinoma elsewhere in the intestinal tract, with wall thickening and narrowing of the lumen. Obstructive changes often are seen proximally with dilated proximal bowel loops. CT can help in determining the causes of small bowel obstruction by documenting masses at the site of obstruction

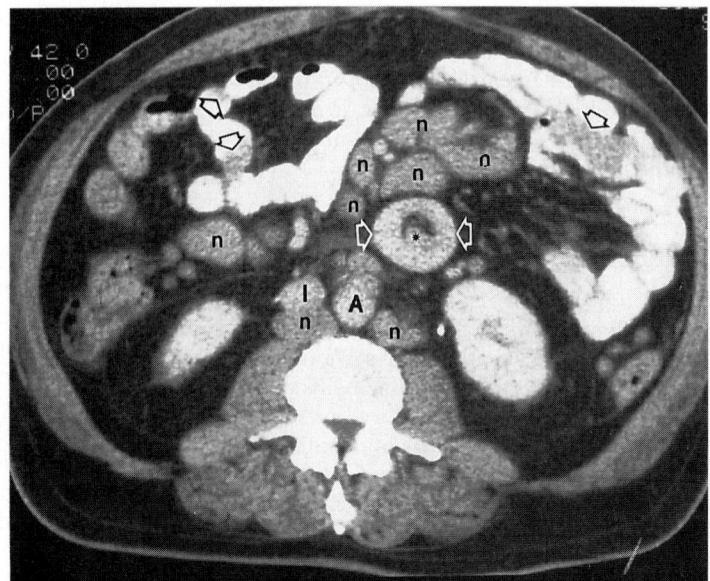

FIGURE 123-3. Lymphoma involving the small intestine and colon. Intestinal involvement is evident by multiple foci of soft tissue attenuation masses in the wall of the small intestine (*black arrows*). Bulky lymphadenopathy throughout the mesentery and retroperitoneum (n) may suggest the diagnosis of lymphoma. In this case, an enteroenteric intussusception is present with characteristic CT findings. The bowel wall is thickened (*white arrows*) and contains an intralumenal fat-density signal surrounding an intralumenal mass (*), representing the intussuscepted mesentery and intussusceptum, respectively. (A, aorta; I, inferior vena cava.)

and enabling differentiation from adhesions. Adjacent lymph node enlargement may also be a clue to the diagnosis.

Small bowel lymphoma may have similar changes of focal bowel wall thickening or nodularity (Fig. 123-3), but may be diffuse in its presentation. Bulky mesenteric adenopathy, which is not usually seen with adenocarcinoma, may be present. Despite circumferential wall thickening, the lumen may appear dilated, analogous to the aneurysmal dilatation often found on barium radiographic examinations.[29]

Although carcinoid tumors often go undetected on CT because of their small size, larger lesions are seen as soft tissue–density masses in the area of the ileum. They often are associated with lymphadenopathy and with characteristic thickening and retraction of the adjacent mesenteric fat as a result of invasion.[35]

Metastatic disease to the small bowel wall can simulate any of the lesions previously described. These may occur as blood-borne metastases within the wall or be secondary to peritoneal seeding.

Inflammatory Diseases

The inflammatory processes affecting the small bowel produce similar appearances on CT scans. For the mildest forms, CT demonstrates normal-appearing bowel. The edema and hypervascularity associated with more severe inflammatory processes produce nonspecific findings in the bowel wall.

In Crohn's disease, the early phases of mucosal limited disease do not demonstrate abnormalities on CT, but edema, wall thickening, mesenteric inflammation, and enlarged adjacent lymph nodes are detected by CT (Fig. 123-4).[36,37] The mesenteric inflammation is evidenced by fat proliferation with streaky soft tissue densities.[38] If these densities become more confluent, they are indicative of a focal phlegmon. This can be difficult to differentiate from a frank abscess, although the latter may contain air or low-attenuation areas of necrosis. Fistulas may extend from the bowel into the mesentery.[39,40]

In these complex cases, CT serves as a problem-solving tool. It can be helpful in diagnosing patients with displaced bowel loops seen on a small bowel radiographic examination by differentiating a mesenteric abscess from focal fibrofatty proliferation.

The infectious diseases that demonstrate CT findings are usually caused by *Giardia lamblia*, *Strongyloides stercoralis*, *Yersinia*, or *Mycobacterium avium* complex (formerly *Mycobacterium avium-intracellulare*). These infections usually produce nonspecific findings of bowel wall thickening, mild adenopathy, or evidence of hypersecretion. Other chronic inflammatory conditions, such as eosinophilic enteritis and nonspecific jejunitis, demonstrate similar findings, as can graft-versus-host disease.[41] Noninflammatory edema of the bowel wall, as seen in patients with congestive heart failure or hypoalbuminemia, can produce similar findings. *Mycoplasma*

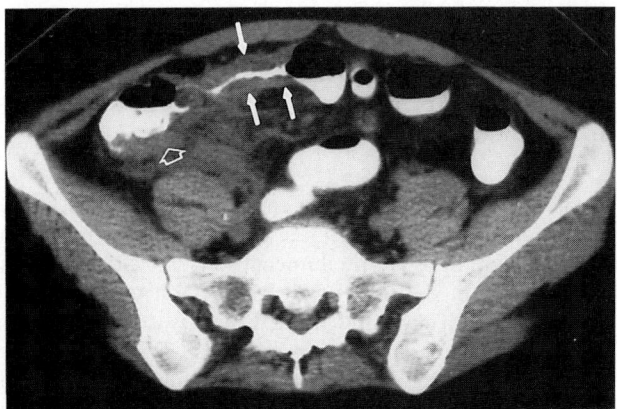

FIGURE 123-4. Crohn's disease of the terminal ileum and cecum. The CT scan shows circumferential thickening of the distal ileum (*arrows*) and focal thickening of the cecal (*open arrow*) wall. Chronic phlegmonous changes are seen on CT as infiltrating, streaky densities in the adjacent mesenteric fat.

infection occurring in patients with acquired immunodeficiency syndrome (AIDS) often produces characteristic low-attenuation enlargement of retroperitoneal and mesenteric lymph nodes.[42] Whipple's disease, in addition to nonspecific bowel wall thickening, may also demonstrate low-attenuation lymph nodes on CT scans.

Vascular Diseases

CT findings are diagnostic for only 26% of patients with ischemic disease.[43] Early changes are nonspecific, with mild bowel wall thickening and lumen dilatation. Collections of air may be seen in the bowel wall or portal venous system with infarction, although gas in the intestinal wall is nondiagnostic, because benign causes of pneumatosis have a similar CT appearance.[44] However, in a sick patient, the early diagnosis of bowel infarction may be made by detecting these changes by CT.[45]

Polyarteritis nodosa and other vasculitides can produce focal or diffuse wall thickening. Radiation-induced changes represent a focal vasculitis with wall thickening evident on CT in the area of the radiation port.[46] Focal wall thickening can be accentuated by hemorrhage into the small bowel wall in these cases or in other conditions that can cause small bowel hemorrhage, such as hemophilia, Henoch-Schönlein purpura, or uncontrolled anticoagulation medication.

CT can be helpful in evaluating complications of aortic graft surgery.[47] Experience with aortoduodenal fistulas after surgery has largely been anecdotal, but one study of 6 patients found abnormal CT findings in all of them.[48] The fistula itself was not demonstrated, but findings of aortic graft infection (e.g., perigraft fluid collections, gas) contiguous with the duodenum were present, and in the clinical setting of intestinal bleeding, this suggests the diagnosis. Gas has been reported in the aortic bed for as long as 2 weeks after surgery without evidence of infection, but beyond this period, it should raise the suspicion of graft infection.[49] The capability of CT to suggest this diagnosis may be critical, because the bleeding is usually intermittent and may not be demonstrated at angiography. However, the lack of CT findings does not exclude the possibility of a fistula, particularly if the duodenum abuts the postoperative aorta, as it does often.

Intussusception

Typical findings of ileocolic or enteroenteric intussusception can be demonstrated by CT (see Fig. 123-3). The most common CT finding is an intralumenal soft tissue–density mass separated from the bowel wall by a region of low density compatible with fat, representing the intussusceptum and the intussuscepted mesentery, respectively.[50] CT is unable to detect the underlying cause of intussusception and cannot differentiate benign from malignant causes unless the lead mass is a large lipoma.[51] Merine and colleagues reported CT to be more accurate in making the diagnosis than a barium small bowel study, reporting a 100% sensitivity in a retrospective series of 9 patients.[50]

Obstruction

CT findings of obstruction are similar to traditional radiographic findings: disparate dilatation of proximal bowel loops compared with more distal ones. Comparative studies have shown that CT is superior to plain film radiography in detecting intestinal obstruction and in determining the cause of obstruction. Studies have shown a sensitivity of 90% to 95% in detecting obstruction, with no false-positive examinations.[52,53] In the study by Fukuya and associates, 6 of 30 patients with obstruction were diagnosed by CT and not by plain film studies.[53] CT offers more information on the cause of obstruction by visualizing extralumenal abnormalities. CT findings of small bowel volvulus and strangulating obstruction with ischemic bowel have been characterized by the lack of a surrounding mass at the site of obstruction, with edematous mesenteric folds from dilated intestinal loops converging radially toward the site of torsion.[54]

COLON

The normal colon and rectum with typical haustral markings are usually well-delineated by surrounding fat. Although the normal wall thickness in a well-distended colon is 3 mm or less, a collapsed or fecal-filled colon, particularly the cecum, can be difficult to differentiate from neoplastic changes. A colon preparation and air insufflation should be used for investigating the colon.[55] In routine abdominal scanning without a bowel preparation, retrograde administration of contrast through the rectum may avoid confusion from lack of distention and adherent feces.

Neoplasms

Benign Neoplasms

Lipomas can be diagnosed by their characteristic low-attenuation appearance.[56] All other benign lesions large enough to be detected appear as nonspecific soft tissue–density masses in the colonic wall.

Malignant Neoplasms

The CT appearance of colorectal carcinomas depends on the lesion size and the technique used. The colon must be well distended to avoid mistaking collapsed bowel wall for abnormal thickening or possible neoplasm. Generally, carcinomas appear as soft tissue–density wall thickenings focally or circumferentially (Fig. 123-5). Larger lesions with necrosis may show heterogeneity with low-attenuation areas centrally. These appearances are nonspecific and can be simulated by other malignant lesions (e.g., lymphoma, metastases) and benign lesions. For more accurate detection of smaller lesions, air insufflation after a colon preparation is necessary, increasing carcinoma detection from 68% to 95% in one series.[55,57,58] The detection rates are reported from selected, retrospectively studied populations, in which patients with more advanced disease would be expected to have undergone CT, and do not

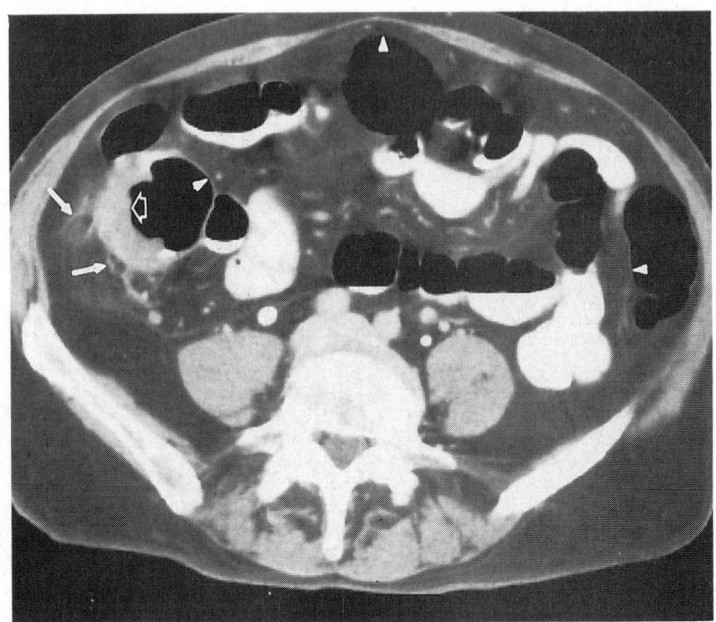

FIGURE 123-5. Colon carcinoma. The scan was obtained with concomitant rectal administration of air, resulting in colonic distention and demonstrating the normal wall thickness of 1 to 3 mm in several locations (*arrowheads*). Asymmetric wall thickening of the cecum at the site of the tumor is identified (*open arrow*). The margins of the tumor demonstrate streaky infiltration into the adjacent fat (*arrows*), proven at surgery to be local extension of tumor into the periserosal fat.

represent the detection rate that could be achieved in a screening population.

More advanced malignancies show pericolonic extension grossly as a soft tissue mass or with streaky infiltration into the adjacent fat (see Fig. 123-5).[58-60] Invasion of adjacent structures can be detected on CT, as can metastases to lymph nodes, liver, adrenal glands, mesentery, and omentum. CT is more accurate than a contrast radiographic examination in detecting perforated colorectal neoplasms and in differentiating these from benign inflammatory processes.[61]

Early CT studies suggested CT might be an accurate method for staging colorectal carcinoma.[62-64] Larger studies documented major problem areas with CT staging, proving it unreliable as a routine staging modality.[58,65-68] These problems included the inability of CT to determine the degree of bowel wall involvement (i.e., Dukes' A or B lesions), the inability to detect lymph node metastases in normal-sized lymph nodes, and poor sensitivity in detecting small foci of pericolonic fat invasion. Tumor invasion into pericolonic fat was accurately staged in only 58% to 77% of these cases, mostly because of CT understaging. The CT sensitivity for lymph node metastasis detection was 22% to 73%.

Because the main limitation of CT staging is understaging the extent of local disease, with few overstaging problems, it can be used in problem situations to plan surgical or other treatments.[58] If extensive disease is shown locally, limited resections may be planned, or radiation or chemotherapy can be used before surgery. CT can be helpful in assessing patients being considered for resection of liver metastases. Angiographically assisted CT is the most accurate method of documenting the extent of liver metastatic disease.[69,70]

Accuracies of 87% to 95% have been reported for CT detection of recurrent colorectal carcinoma.[65,66,68,71] CT plays a central role in evaluating recurrent disease after abdominoperineal resection. Because of the absence of a rectum, local recurrence cannot be evaluated by endoscopy or barium radiography. CT is capable of demonstrating locally recurrent pelvic masses, lymphadenopathy, and liver metastases. Pelvic recurrence typically presents as a globular mass in the presacral space, normally occupied by fat in the absence of the rectum. Postoperative or radiation-induced changes usually have an ill-defined infiltrating appearance.[72] Occasionally, postoperative or radiation-induced changes can result in a presacral mass that is difficult to differentiate from recurrent tumor, and CT-guided biopsy may be necessary for the diagnosis.[73,74] Serial CT scans may show a decrease in the size of the postsurgical inflammatory changes, but in 40% of patients, these remain stable.[73] A baseline postoperative CT scan helps in the follow-up evaluation of these patients by demonstrating a neoplastic change as an enlarging mass.

CT is more accurate than laboratory tests in detecting the early changes of recurrent colorectal carcinoma. In one series, carcinoembryonic antigen levels were abnormal in only 6 of 11 patients with locally recurrent disease that was detected by CT.[75]

Inflammatory Diseases

CT can help in detecting and evaluating a variety of inflammatory processes affecting the colon. Regardless of the cause, the CT findings of inflammation are similar and consist of bowel wall thickening with adjacent streaky infiltration of pericolonic fat. A frank abscess of low attenuation may be seen adjacent to the colon.

In patients with suspected diverticulitis, CT can be helpful in differentiating pericolonic phlegmon from frank abscess.[2,76] Pericolonic phlegmon is characterized by streaky densities in the pericolonic fat and is easily differentiated from an abscess with a soft tissue–density wall and low-density center (Fig. 123-6). The colon wall is usually thickened, making it difficult

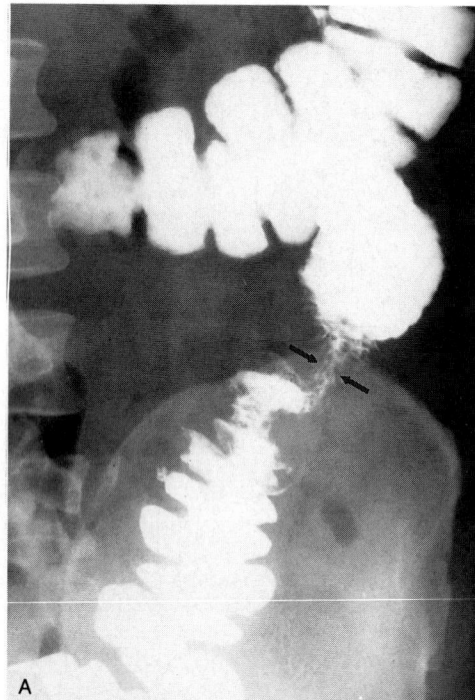
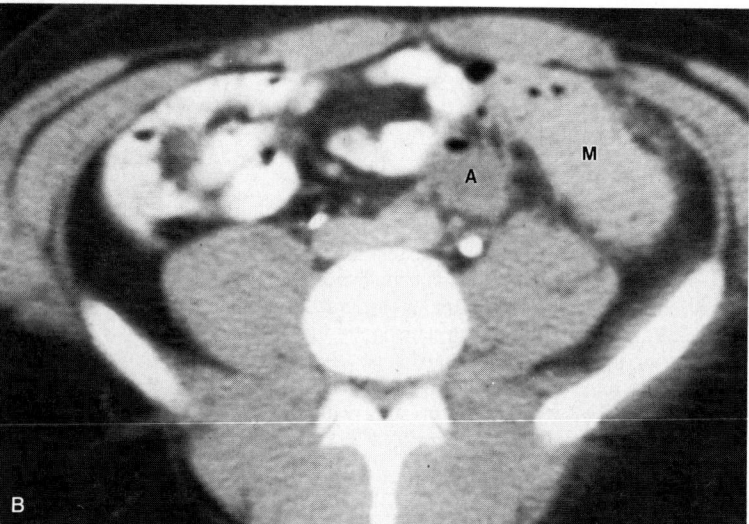

FIGURE 123-6. Diverticulitis involving the descending colon. (**A**) Barium enema examination revealed a focal area of narrowing (*arrows*), without an associated mass visualized, compatible with the clinical suspicion of diverticulitis. (**B**) CT scan performed 24 hours later confirms the focal thickening of the colon wall with effacement of the lumen, creating the effect of a soft-tissue attenuation mass (M). The scan demonstrates an adjacent abscess (A) typified by the air-fluid level centrally. The CT scan is superior in evaluating the extent of diverticulitis because it can demonstrate abnormalities remote from the bowel wall.

to differentiate from a perforated neoplasm with adjacent inflammation.[61]

The ability of CT to demonstrate the extent of disease has resulted in its increased use for patients with suspected diverticulitis. Controversy exists over whether CT or a contrast enema examination is more sensitive in diagnosing diverticulitis.[2,76] In acutely ill patients suspected of diverticulitis, Cho and associates found CT to be more sensitive than barium enema (93% versus 80%) in diagnosing diverticulitis.[2] For patients without diverticulitis, CT was able to provide a correct diagnosis in a larger number of cases than barium enema, even for some requiring emergent surgery.

The diagnosis of appendicitis is usually established by clinical presentation and physical examination, although 20% to 30% of patients present with atypical findings. For these patients, CT can be helpful in establishing the diagnosis. Barakos and colleagues reported using CT successfully to triage patients suspected of perforation for various therapies.[77] CT can differentiate a localized phlegmon from a liquefied abscess and display the extent of complicated abscesses.

The inflammatory changes of appendicitis appear similar on CT to those of diverticulitis, except they are centered on the appendix in the right lower abdomen.[78] The most frequent finding is an inflammatory mass, usually in close apposition to the cecum but occasionally remote. Appendicoliths can be identified in 25% of patients, and an abnormal appendix can be visualized in 18%.[78] Occasionally, it can demonstrate only thickening of the wall of the distal ileum, simulating Crohn's

disease. Overall, CT demonstrated intraabdominal abnormalities in 92% of patients in one series, which were specific for appendicitis in 79%.[78]

Although CT is not the screening examination of choice, inflammatory diseases of the colon may produce characteristic abnormalities.[79] Although colon wall thickening is a nonspecific finding, ulcerative colitis tends to produce inhomogeneous thickening with low-attenuation areas in the wall. Granulomatous colitis tends to result in a thicker wall, which is usually seen as a homogeneous soft tissue density. In either case, adjacent areas of phlegmon or abscess may be detected by demonstrating infiltration of the pericolonic fat or frank abscess formation.

In the appropriate clinical setting, neutropenic colitis has a characteristic location, with heterogeneous thickening of the right colon wall and often with adjacent pericolonic inflammation.[80] Pseudomembranous colitis typically shows bowel wall thickening with prominent haustral folds, similar to the barium radiography findings.[81] Radiation-induced and ischemic changes in the colon are similar to those described for the small intestines.

LIVER

A variety of CT techniques for examining the liver have been described, and the techniques chosen should optimize the evaluation of specific clinical problems.

Non–contrast-enhanced CT is used for patients allergic to iodinated contrast material. This technique is generally considered to be less accurate in detecting liver lesions than optimal contrast-enhanced techniques, particularly because the common secondary sources of tumor (e.g., colon, lung, pancreas) are hypovascular lesions.[82,83] For detecting suspected hypervascular neoplasms, such as hepatocellular carcinoma or metastases from hypervascular primary tumors such as kidney and breast sarcomas, it is imperative to obtain non–contrast-enhanced images of the liver.[84,85]

Intravenous contrast agents can be delivered in several ways for liver evaluation. Studies have shown that enhancement of normal liver parenchyma by rapid and sustained administration of contrast (40–50 g of iodine over 1 to 2 minutes) generally affords the highest lesion detection rates. This method, known as dynamic incremental bolus CT, has become the screening method of choice for most liver lesions.[82,86–88] The technique provides approximately 2.5 minutes of maximal enhancement of the normal liver parenchyma, optimizing the detection of hypovascular lesions. With slower rates of contrast infusion or slightly delayed imaging times, the equilibrium of contrast within the liver and the lesions may be reached, obscuring the liver lesions; this is the least optimal technique for liver lesion detection and should be avoided.

With helical or spiral CT, images of the entire liver can be acquired in 30 seconds. This affords the opportunity to image the liver during the arterial phase of contrast, when hypervascular tumors may be best seen. Most hypovascular tumors are best seen during the period of peak liver enhancement, and helical CT enables imaging the entire liver during this peak.

CT can detect liver metastases in 72.5% to 100% of these patients; these rates are superior to the success rates for ultrasound (82%) or scintigraphy (86%).[65,89–92] Carefully performed studies comparing CT with surgical correlation have shown that 80% to 90% of malignancies are probably detected with optimally performed screening CT.[92,93] These results are similar to those reported for magnetic resonance imaging (MRI).[93,94]

Several studies correlated pathologic examination of resected liver specimens with preoperative CT and MRI detection of liver lesions.[69,70,93] Dynamic incremental bolus CT detected only 38% of lesions in one series, failing to detect all lesions less than 1 cm in diameter and most lesions less than 2 cm.[70] In contrast, MRI (using a variety of pulse sequences) detected 52% of lesions. Other CT techniques, such as delayed high-dose CT scanning and angiography-assisted CT scanning, have higher accuracies in detecting liver lesions.

Delayed high-dose CT requires scanning the liver 4 to 6 hours after a large intravenous iodine load (60 g). The normal liver tissue secretes 1% to 2% of the iodine load into the biliary system, resulting in enhancement of normal liver parenchyma for several hours after injection. In contrast, focal hepatic lesions do not retain iodine. Although the overall normal liver enhancement in delayed liver scanning is low (20 H), it does afford an alternative method of detecting liver lesions. Controlled studies have found it to have a higher sensitivity rate than dynamic incremental CT.[70,95,96]

If documenting the number and location of liver metastases is imperative, such as before contemplated resection of isolated metastatic lesions, the highest sensitivity for detection is achieved by angiography-assisted CT. CT-angiography requires placement of a catheter in the hepatic artery, with subsequent scanning during contrast administration through the catheter. CT-portography requires placement of a catheter in the superior mesenteric artery or splenic artery, with subsequent contrast opacification of the portal venous system, bypassing the hepatic arterial system (Fig. 123-7). CT-portography has a higher sensitivity than CT-angiography, but CT-portography has less specificity. Many nonneoplastic lesions can produce defects on CT-portography. Peterson and associates found that, although some of these defects could be categorized as benign based on their appearances, many others simulated neoplasms, requiring biopsy for confirmation.[97]

Reported accuracies for angiography-assisted CT have shown a sensitivity of 81% to 91% in detecting specific liver lesions.[69,70,98] In controlled studies, this was the highest detection sensitivity, exceeding MRI and routine CT techniques.[69,70]

Extensive research into lipid-soluble contrast agents has been reported. These ethiodized oil emulsions (e.g., EOE-13) are more sensitive than dynamic contrast-enhanced liver CT scanning in detecting metastatic lesions, equalling that of CT-portography and delayed high-dose CT.[96,99–101] However, because of contrast reactions and production difficulties, this agent remains experimental.[102]

Diffuse Diseases

Fatty Infiltration

Fatty infiltration of the liver may occur in a diffuse or focal distribution. The fat accumulation lowers the CT attenuation of the liver. Normally, the liver has an attenuation level 6 to 12 H higher than the spleen, but with fatty infiltration, this relation is reversed.[103] The administration of contrast may obscure these changes, because the spleen is enhanced to a greater degree than the liver early during bolus contrast administration. If the fat deposition is focal, it can be confused with more significant lesions, such as metastases. The lack of a mass effect on vascular branches and the rapid change with time can be helpful in differentiating these lesions.[104,105]

Cirrhosis

Characteristic CT features can be seen in patients with advanced cirrhosis. The right lobe and medial segment of the left lobe are often decreased in size, but the lateral segment of the left lobe and caudate lobe are enlarged.[106] Lobar ratios that quantify these changes have been reported.[107] Normal livers demonstrate a transverse caudate lobe width to transverse right lobe width ratio of 0.37. If the ratio is greater than 0.65, cirrhosis can be diagnosed at the 96% confidence level.[107] Cirrhosis often shows additional changes, including irregular, nodular liver margins and inhomogeneous parenchymal contrast enhancement.[108] The intrahepatic fissures and the porta hepatis may appear widened because of the decreased size of the liver parenchyma.[107] Associated changes of portal hypertension, with varices and venous collaterals, commonly occur.

Screening programs have found a high incidence (up to

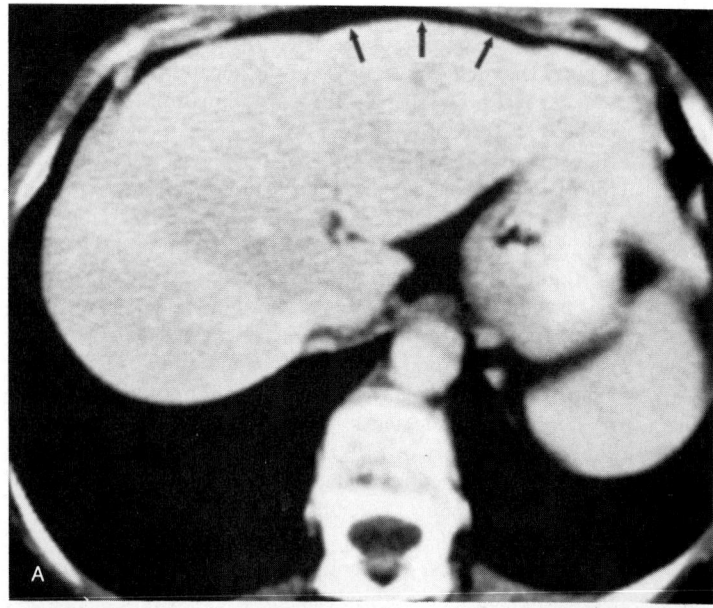

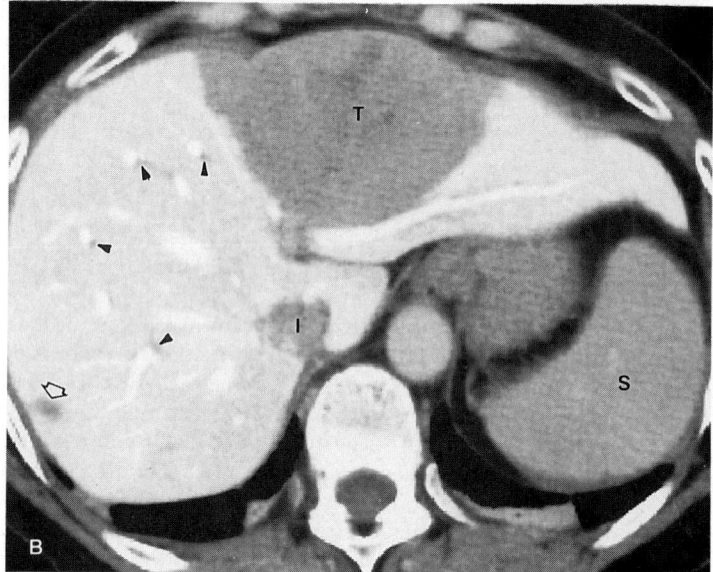

FIGURE 123-7. Hepatocellular carcinoma is demonstrated best by an angiography-assisted CT scan. **(A)** The CT scan with intravenous contrast administered using the dynamic incremental bolus technique shows a large tumor in the left lobe of the liver. The tumor is predominantly isodense with the adjacent contrast-enhanced normal hepatic parenchyma. The tumor is identifiable by the protruding margin of the mass (*arrows*). **(B)** A CT scan obtained in the same patient with contrast injected by way of an angiographic catheter in the superior mesenteric artery. The large tumor (T) is not enhanced by the contrast delivered from the portal venous system and is easily seen as a hypodense mass compared with the marked enhancement in the normal liver parenchyma. A smaller malignant nodule is identified in the right lobe of the liver (*open arrow*) that was not seen on the standard contrast CT examination. Normal intrahepatic bile ducts are seen coursing adjacent to the portal venous branches (*arrowheads*). The inferior vena cava (I) or spleen (S) has not yet enhanced to a significant degree, confirming that the contrast delivered to the liver has not come from the hepatic arterial system.

10%) of hepatocellular carcinoma in patients with advanced cirrhosis.[109,110] The distorted liver appearance caused by cirrhosis obscures many small tumors on CT scans. Miller and associates reported detecting hepatocellular carcinoma in only 68% of cirrhotic patients with tumor.[110] Confounding the difficulty in detecting small tumors is the fact that confluent, mass-like focal fibrosis in advanced cirrhosis simulates tumor on CT scans.[111] An awareness of the characteristic location (i.e., anterior and medial segments) and appearance of fibrosis (i.e., wedge shaped, radiating from the porta hepatis with associated capsular retraction) enables the diagnosis of fibrosis to be made and avoids unnecessary biopsy.[111]

Other Diffuse Diseases

Iron deposition and hemochromatosis, whether primary or secondary, increase the attenuation of the liver and spleen on CT scans.[112] The hepatic density on CT is more specific for iron overload than for serum ferritin measurement.[113]

Other processes leading to an increased attenuation of liver parenchyma include glycogen storage disease, amiodarone toxicity, and gold storage after gold treatment for rheumatoid arthritis.[114–116] Despite high serum copper levels, the CT scan of the liver does not show significant elevations over normal attenuation measurements in patients with Wilson's disease.[117]

Cysts

Cysts can be differentiated on CT scans from other significant lesions by their homogeneous low attenuation (0–10 H) and smooth margins without a perceptible wall. Their CT appearance may cause concern, particularly for smaller lesions, because of artifactually higher attenuation measurements from volume averaging. Although most necrotic metastases are not homogeneous, rare cases producing low attenuation can simulate a benign appearance.[118] The degree of resolution obtainable using 1.5- to 3-mm collimation overcomes most of these problems.

Neoplasms

Benign Neoplasms

Hemangiomas are common benign lesions, often identified on CT or ultrasound examinations as incidental findings. Strict CT criteria for the diagnosis of hemangiomas have been suggested, including a hypodense appearance on non–contrast-enhanced CT images, contrast enhancement of the lesion beginning peripherally and progressing centrally over time, and complete enhancement isodense with normal liver parenchyma on delayed scans.[119] Approximately 55% of hemangiomas fulfill these criteria, compared with 1.6% of metastatic lesions, resulting in a high specificity for these criteria.[119,120] Obtaining dynamic CT images at the same level in the liver over time appears to be the only way to document these criteria and to make an accurate CT diagnosis of a hemangioma.[119-121] This makes it difficult to diagnose a hemangioma during a screening CT survey of the entire liver.

Hepatic adenomas and focal nodular hyperplasia are vascular lesions that can present with a variety of CT appearances that are often indistinguishable. Both lesions usually demonstrate homogeneous, increased attenuation during imaging immediately after bolus contrast administration, which rapidly decreases to isodense or slightly hypodense areas.[122,123] The detection of hemorrhage can suggest the diagnosis of adenoma, although hepatomas and other malignant lesions can undergo spontaneous hemorrhage. Similarly, the identification of a central, stellate, low-density area may be helpful in the diagnosis of hyperplasia, but it is seen only in a minority of patients.[123] Patients with fibrolamellar hepatoma may demonstrate a similar, central low density.[124]

Malignant Neoplasms

Hepatocellular carcinoma (i.e., hepatoma) can appear on CT scans as a focal, solitary mass; a multifocal process; or as a diffuse, infiltrating process (Fig. 123-8). These lesions appear hypodense or isodense with normal liver on non–contrast-enhanced images; after contrast administration, they are predominantly hypodense. Because of the vascular nature of these tumors, transient regions of marked contrast enhancement can often be identified if dynamic scan techniques are used. Large lesions are almost always detected on routine CT examinations; lesions smaller than 3 cm can be difficult to detect.[125] Matsui and colleagues reported a sensitivity of 58% for CT in such cases, compared with 63% for ultrasound and 16% for radionuclide scans.[126] CT-portography was able to detect 95% of these lesions in their series, paralleling the increased sensitivity of lesion detection reported for this technique. Several Japanese centers are using angiographic instillation of iodized oil as an adjunct for CT detection of hepatoma lesions, predominantly in detecting additional liver lesions.[127-129] Vascular invasion often occurs with hepatomas and can be identified on CT, occurring in the portal vein in 11% to 37% of patients.[130,131]

Although precise guidelines for estimating surgical resectability of these lesions do not exist, CT can help in staging the disease of patients considered for resection.[131] LaBerge and associates reported CT to be superior to ultrasound in delineating the extent of hepatic involvement and extrahepatic involvement, although ultrasound was superior in detecting vascular invasion.[131] The most accurate technique appears to be intraoperative ultrasound, but this cannot be used as a screening tool.[132]

Liver metastases demonstrate a variety of CT appearances. Hypovascular lesions typically appear hypodense compared with adjacent enhanced liver parenchyma, although vascular lesions can appear hypodense, isodense, or hyperdense, depending on the timing of contrast administration and scanning. Hypervascular metastatic lesions, as are found in renal cell carcinoma, islet cell tumors, leiomyosarcoma, or thyroid carcinoma, may be better demonstrated on non–contrast-enhanced CT.[84] Metastatic lesions do not have a pathognomonic appearance and can be simulated by hepatomas, hemangiomas, abscesses, complicated cysts, and hematomas.

Abscesses

CT has become the screening procedure of choice for detecting pyogenic liver abscesses, with detection rates as high as 97%.[133-135] The typical CT features of a pyogenic abscess include a mass hypodense with normal liver parenchyma, often with a contrast-enchanced rim. Gas collections affect approximately 20% of cases, and internal septations may be seen.[135] The mass usually is of higher density than simple cysts, but overlap in these densities can make it difficult to differentiate a simple cyst from an abscess.[135] Primary and metastatic liver lesions can have similar appearances, and aspiration of all potential liver abscesses is required for accurate diagnosis.

Hepatic fungal abscesses usually present on CT as multiple, small, low-density, nonenhancing lesions spread throughout the liver.[136] Although CT is a sensitive tool for detecting these lesions, active disease can evade CT visualization.[137] Many of these lesions do not clear after successful treatment and reflect fibrotic scarring, demonstrating the lack of specificity for CT as a tool in following treatment response in patients with this disease.[137]

Amebic abscesses appear similar to pyogenic lesions as a low-density lesion, usually solitary, but with 20% of patients demonstrating multiple lesions.[138] Echinococcal infection (i.e., hydatid cysts) also appears as low-density cysts, often with internal septations and daughter or inclusion cysts, creating the appearance of a cyst within a cyst. Calcification may be seen in the cyst wall or septations.[139]

Vascular Diseases

Portal Vein Thrombosis

Portal vein thrombosis can be detected on CT scans by visualizing decreased intralumenal portal vein attenuation values, accompanied on dynamic contrast scans with ringed enhancement from opacification and thickening of the vaso vasorum.[140] Fresh thrombosis may demonstrate an increased density of the thrombus on non–contrast-enhanced scans, but in most cases, the dynamic scan techniques after intravenous contrast administration optimally show the thrombosed vein.[140,141] Chronically extensive collateral formation involving the porta hepatis is called cavernous transformation.[140] The evolution of acute portal vein thrombosis may result in focal liver parenchymal abnormalities compatible with portal

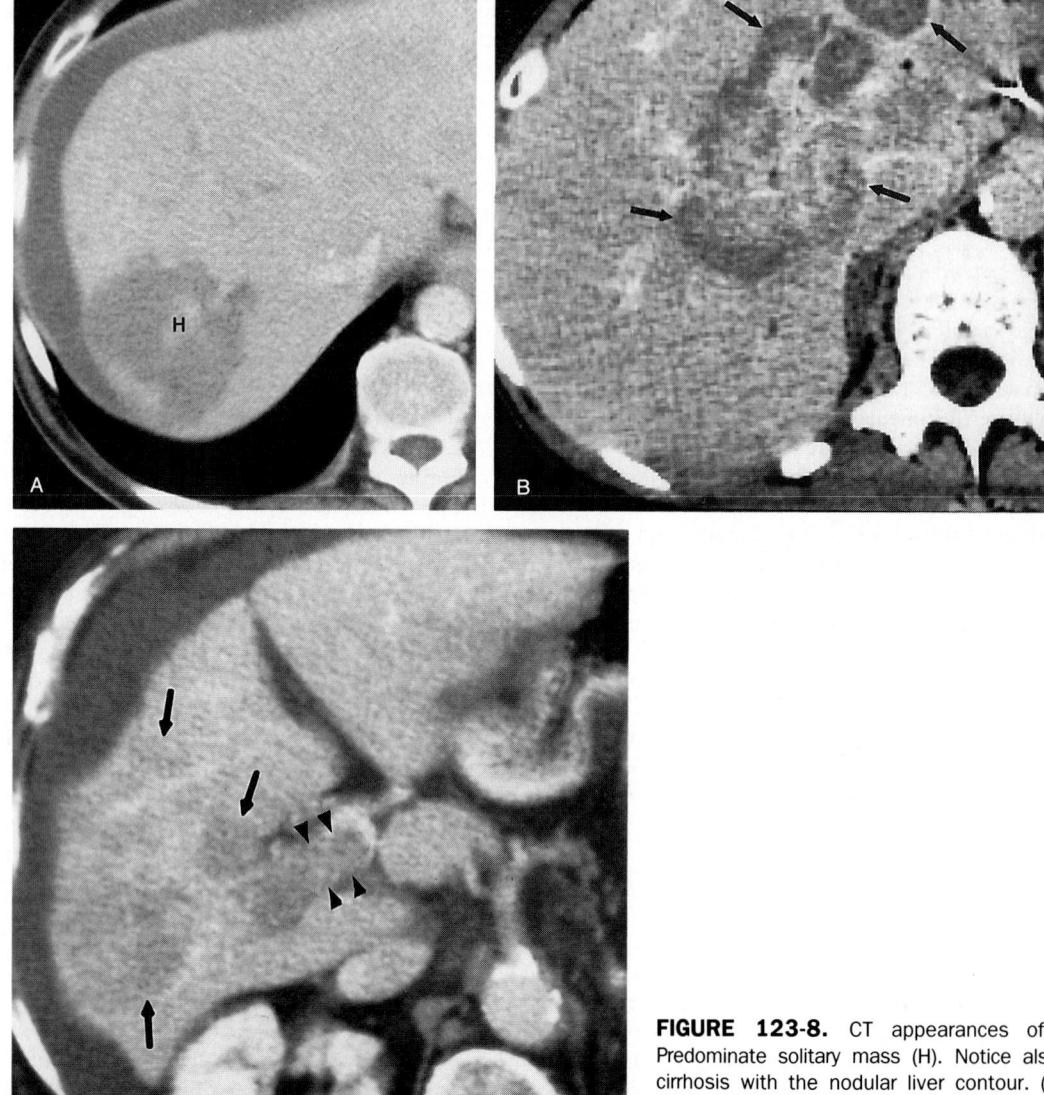

FIGURE 123-8. CT appearances of hepatomas. **(A)** Predominate solitary mass (H). Notice also the changes of cirrhosis with the nodular liver contour. **(B)** Multifocal, discrete liver masses (*arrows*). **(C)** Ill-defined, infiltrating lesion (*arrows*). Tumor invasion and thrombosis of the portal vein (*arrowheads*) are demonstrated in this intravenous contrast–enhanced scan.

infarctions.[140] The changes appear similar whether caused by a primary vascular abnormality with intrinsic thrombosis or secondary tumoral obstruction of the portal venous system, such as hepatocellular carcinoma.[142]

Although CT is capable of demonstrating these abnormalities in most cases, Doppler duplex sonography or MRI are the screening examinations of choice for documenting this abnormality.[141,143]

Hepatovenous Occlusive Disease

CT reveals a variety of findings in hepatovenous occlusive disease (i.e., Budd-Chiari syndrome). Although CT, MRI, and Doppler ultrasound can suggest the diagnosis, venogra-

phy remains the gold standard for evaluation and diagnosis.[144–150] Because of their noninvasive nature and optimal demonstration of vessel morphology and flow without the use of intravenous contrast, MRI and Doppler ultrasound are preferred for screening examinations of suspected patients. Non–contrast-enhanced CT findings include hepatomegaly with a hypodense parenchyma that spares the caudate lobe and perihilar regions of the left lobe.[144] After intravenous contrast administration, the liver parenchyma demonstrates a mottled enhancement pattern. Initially, the greatest contrast enhancement is seen in the caudate lobe and the periportal regions of the left lobe, but a reversal of this pattern is seen on later images.[144,145] Delayed images generally show a homogeneous enhancement pattern of the liver.[145] Although direct visualization of thrombus within the hepatic vein or inferior vena cava can be demonstrated, in most cases, the hepatic veins are not visualized and may be the clue to the diagnosis.[144,145]

Trauma Disorders

With its ability to display and evaluate the entire cross-sectional abdomen without hidden areas, CT has achieved a preeminence in the imaging of trauma patients. It has been shown to be the best method of detecting and evaluating the extent of liver trauma and in some centers has replaced peritoneal lavage as the preliminary investigation.[151–155] Federle and Jeffrey reported only one false-negative and two false-positive results in detecting hemoperitoneum using CT screening for 300 trauma patients.[156] From the same institution, Wing and colleagues reported a sensitivity of 100% and an accuracy of 97.6% in detecting intraabdominal injury.[155]

CT findings of liver trauma include foci of low or high attenuation indicating hemorrhage, usually in contact with some portion of the liver surface.[157] If there has not been a prior peritoneal lavage, the presence of hemoperitoneum can be seen on CT with free intraperitoneal fluid accumulations.

With the advent of CT, there has been a trend toward nonoperative therapy for isolated, blunt hepatic injuries, using constant hemodynamic monitoring and serial clinical and laboratory assessments.[152,153,158,159] Serial CT examinations play an essential role by demonstrating healing of the liver lesions and resorption of hemoperitoneum. Failure to demonstrate these changes may indicate continued bleeding.[158,160]

BILIARY TRACT

As with ultrasound, the key to the diagnosis of biliary tract pathology with CT is intrahepatic or extrahepatic bile duct dilatation. The intrahepatic ducts were not normally visualized with earlier CT scanners and, if seen, usually indicated biliary obstruction.[161,162] The resolution of modern scanners enables visualization of intrahepatic ducts in 40% of normal patients; these should not be confused with ductal dilatation.[163] The extrahepatic bile ducts are identified normally in 80% of patients and usually have diameters of 4 to 10 mm.[164] Based on prior ultrasound studies, ductal diameters larger than this probably indicate obstruction.[165,166] As with ultrasound, the phenomena of dilatation without obstruction and obstruction without dilatation can occur and require cholangiography in many cases to document obstruction unless findings other than bile duct dilatation are suggestive.[167]

Comparative studies have shown that CT is comparable to ultrasound in its ability to detect biliary obstruction and generally exceeds ultrasound in the ability to predict the level and cause of biliary obstruction, although some controversy still exists.[162,168–170] Ultrasound remains the screening examination of choice for suspected biliary obstruction because of easier availability, lower cost, and lack of intravenous contrast agents. If a high degree of suspicion for obstruction exists and if malignancy is strongly suspected, CT is the examination of choice, because it allows the staging of extent of disease in a standard, reproducible fashion.

Congenital Anomalies

Congenital anomalies of the biliary tract are diagnosed definitively with cholangiography. CT and ultrasound can suggest the possibility of a congenital abnormality in patients presenting with biliary tract signs and symptoms.

Congenital anomalies of the gallbladder are rare, mostly consisting of positional variants. The gallbladder can be seen in the left abdomen or in suprahepatic, intrahepatic, and other rare locations. CT can identify these anomalies if the gallbladder is not seen in its usual location at sonography.

Congenital cystic diseases of the biliary tree include choledochal cysts, choledochoceles, and Caroli's disease. CT can often be diagnostic by demonstrating the dilated biliary tree. In Caroli's disease, CT can reveal the branching nature of the lesions and their contiguity with dilated intrahepatic bile ducts, allowing differentiation from multiple cysts or abscesses of the liver. Choledochal cysts demonstrate focal dilatation of the extrahepatic bile ducts that may be mild and simulate a dilated duct or may be as large as 15 cm in diameter. The clue to the diagnosis may be the marked disparity between the extrahepatic and intrahepatic duct dilatation, making duct dilatation due to obstruction less likely. With all unusual cystic abnormalities of the biliary tree, administration of a biliary contrast agent before scanning may demonstrate accumulation of contrast and confirm the biliary tree as the origin of the mass.[171]

The complications of these congenital abnormalities, including abscess and carcinoma, may be detected with CT.[172]

Gallbladder Disease

CT is an excellent method of demonstrating gallbladder wall abnormalities. Thickening of the gallbladder wall, although nonspecific, can be a clue to underlying pathology. Air within the gallbladder wall or lumen, which can be mistaken for stones on ultrasound, can be well demonstrated by CT in cases of emphysematous cholecystitis.[173] Unusual right upper quadrant abdominal calcifications can be clarified with CT. CT can document the location of these as stones within the gallbladder, within the gallbladder wall (e.g., porcelain gallbladder), or extrinsic to the gallbladder.

Neoplasms

Gallbladder carcinoma is usually far advanced when patients are first seen by a physician, and the CT scans reflect these changes. The most common appearance is that of total replacement of the gallbladder lumen by a soft tissue–density mass. Less common appearances include focal gallbladder wall thickening or polypoid intralumenal masses, similar to those seen with ultrasound.[174–177] Gallbladder wall thickening is a nonspecific finding and can be seen in other conditions, such as hepatitis, pancreatitis, cholecystitis, and hypoproteinemia, and alone, it cannot be used as an indicator of malignancy. The extent of tumor can be depicted on CT in the common regions of spread, including liver, lymph node, and peritoneal metastases and invasion of adjacent organs such as liver and duodenum.[178]

Disease can metastasize to the gallbladder by direct invasion from adjacent organs, usually by means of porta hepatis metastasis, and most often occurs in gastric and pancreatic carcinoma. Blood-borne metastases are uncommon but can be seen in patients with melanoma. These appear as focal wall thickening or polypoid intralumenal lesions.

Cholecystolithiasis

Although sonography is the accepted procedure of choice for the diagnosis of gallstones, it cannot be used to determine the chemical composition of gallstones.[179,180] Therapeutic advances, such as chemical dissolution and shock wave lithotripsy, have generated interest in the ability of CT to determine the chemical composition of gallstones and to predict the efficacy of these nonsurgical gallstone therapies.[181-183] CT enables the physician to visualize 74% to 79% of gallstones; the remainder are isodense with bile and cannot be delineated.[182,184] Gallstones can be categorized by their CT density and CT pattern, which correlate with dissolution with chenodeoxycholic acid and *m*-tertbutyl ether (MTBE).[181-184] Although some investigators have found a correlation between the gallstone CT attenuation value and calcium content, others have not.[182,185] A firm correlation between gallstone CT density and cholesterol content has been confirmed by several investigators.[181,182,185]

Some investigators are using CT as a screen to predict successful dissolution with MTBE and to predict stone fragmentation with lithotripsy.[186-188] Whether CT becomes an accepted tool for these treatments awaits further investigation.

Cholecystitis

Although CT is not a screening tool for cholecystitis, patients with a confusing presentation may undergo CT scanning as the initial diagnostic examination. In one series of complicated cholecystitis, gallbladder disease was suspected clinically at presentation in only 7 of 23 patients.[189] CT can be helpful in differentiating gallbladder carcinoma from complicated cases of cholecystitis.[190]

The most common CT findings in cholecystitis are gallbladder wall thickening (>3 mm) and cholelithiasis.[191] These findings are not specific nor sensitive indicators and are also found with gallbladder carcinoma and hyperplastic cholecystosis. Other CT findings suggestive of the diagnosis include an increased density of the bile (>20 H) and loss of clear definition of the gallbladder wall.[191,192] Air within the gallbladder wall or lumen in the absence of a history of prior enteric anastomosis or sphincterotomy is virtually pathognomonic of complicated cholecystitis.[173] A low-density halo around the gallbladder may indicate edema or minimal fluid collections and is a useful clue in differentiating complicated cholecystitis from carcinoma on CT scans.[190]

Bile Duct Diseases

Neoplasms

Primary bile duct cancers (i.e., cholangiocarcinoma) usually cause obstruction of the biliary tree, which is visible on CT. Masses near the porta hepatis often achieve a sizable mass with or without invasion of the liver parenchyma and are usually identifiable. More distal lesions usually are small and may not be visualized on CT images. In these cases, acute obstruction of the bile duct is seen without associated mass or calculus, typical of a malignant process, in contrast to the normal tapered termination. Visualized on CT, cholangiocarcinoma most often is infiltrating, causing duct stenosis, and less commonly is exophytic or intralumenal.[193] In the series reported by Thorsen and colleagues, CT was able to predict the level of obstruction in 100% of cases but visualized the mass itself in only 25%.[177] Thickening of the bile duct wall may be detected just proximal to the level of obstruction and may suggest the proper diagnosis.[164]

CT and ultrasound are useful in the preoperative assessment of the extent of disease and resectability. In the series by Nesbit and colleagues, CT had a sensitivity equal to that of cholangiography in detecting abnormalities indicative of unresectability (44%); if combined with cholangiography, the sensitivity of detection increased to 64%, demonstrating the complementary information these modalities render.[193] CT was superior to ultrasound in detecting the extralumenal spread of disease (44% versus 19%). In a large series from Korea, CT was superior to ultrasound in visualizing bile duct tumors (40% versus 21%).[169]

Metastases involving the lymph nodes in the area of the porta hepatis can cause obstruction of the bile ducts and simulate cholangiocarcinoma, as can other extrinsic masses in the porta hepatis.

Inflammatory Diseases

Acute cholangitis is usually found in patients with underlying biliary tract obstruction. Most patients demonstrate dilated intrahepatic and extrahepatic bile ducts. Suppurative material within the bile ducts may be seen on CT scans as high-density areas. Bile duct wall thickening usually appears to be diffuse and concentric, often demonstrating marked contrast enhancement.[164] Gas can be seen as low-attenuation collections within the biliary tree in cases of infection with gas-forming organisms. Acute suppurative cholangitis can progress to frank liver abscesses, demonstrated on CT scans as low-density areas in the liver in contiguity with the biliary tree.

The characteristic findings seen by means of cholangiography in primary and secondary sclerosing cholangitis can also be demonstrated on CT scans. Intrahepatic duct stenoses, dilated peripheral ducts with no apparent connection to the central ducts, and irregular intrahepatic duct dilatation with a beaded appearance are characteristic CT findings of sclerosing cholangitis.[182] CT findings in the extrahepatic ducts in this condition include duct wall thickening and irregularity, as well as duct wall enhancement after intravenous contrast.[164,182] Complications in this disorder, including cirrhosis and cholangiocarcinoma, should be searched for on CT images.

Other less common causes of infection can produce characteristic CT images. Recurrent pyogenic cholangitis (i.e., Oriental cholangiohepatitis) is found in patients of lower socioeconomic status from Asia. The CT findings are marked intraheaptic and extrahepatic bile duct dilatation, large ductal calculi, and debris.

Unusual agents, such as cytomegalovirus and *Cryptosporidium*, can cause inflammation of the biliary tract in AIDS patients, resulting in changes on CT, ultrasound, and cholangiography similar to those of sclerosing cholangitis, with bile duct wall thickening; multiple, diffuse stricture formation; and duct wall contrast enhancement.[194]

Stone Disease

The noninvasive diagnosis of common bile duct stone disease is a challenging imaging task that requires meticulous ultrasound or CT techniques to achieve high detection rates. If the specific imaging question is to assess the possibility of duct stones, the examination of choice is cholangiography, which has an accuracy approaching 100%. Most patients, however, present with signs or symptoms suggesting biliary obstruction, and the task is to determine whether biliary obstruction is present and, if so, to determine the level of obstruction and its cause. In these cases, ultrasound and CT can be used as screening tools. Although most series suggest a higher detection rate for CT, ultrasound is the screening examination of choice because of availability, lower cost, and the lack of use of intravenous contrast agents. The reported CT sensitivity for common duct stone detection varies from 45% to 90%.[161,162,195–197] The higher figures reflect series with selected patient populations, often patients with known dilated ducts in whom it is easier to visualize stones.

The CT appearance of common duct stones depends on the chemical composition of each stone. Densely calcified stones can be seen as high-attenuation structures within the duct lumen, but most duct stones are isodense with soft tissue or water on CT scans.[197] Nonetheless, using thin collimation scans at close intervals in the region of the distal duct can detect as many as 76% of common duct stones (Fig. 123-9).[197]

Several processes can simulate duct stones on CT, and care must be taken to avoid misdiagnosis. Critically placed pancreatic calculi, oral contrast in an adjacent duodenal diverticulum, residual contrast material from a prior cholangiogram, and papillary ductal neoplasms can simulate choledocholithiasis.

PANCREAS

Since the earliest applications of CT to the trunk in 1975, the pancreas has been one of the organs most successfully imaged by CT, and CT has become the imaging method of choice in most cases of suspected pancreatic abnormalities.[198–201] The entire cross-sectional abdomen can be well visualized on one image to delineate the extent of inflammatory and neoplastic disease and the relation between these processes and adjacent organs, assisting in therapy planning.

In patients with abundant retroperitoneal fat, the pancreas can be delineated throughout its course in the retroperitoneum. In most patients, oral and intravenous contrast is necessary to identify and separate the duodenum and splenic vein. The pancreas can undergo fatty involution, which occurs as an aging phenomenon, with obstructive atrophy, and as a

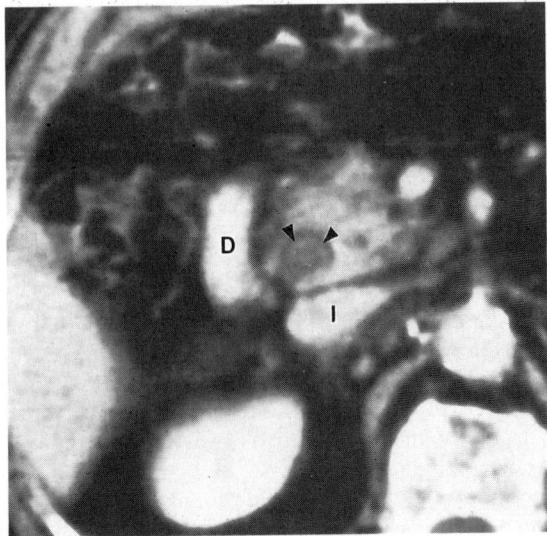

FIGURE 123-9. Common bile duct stone is seen as a predominantly low-attenuation density surrounded by a faint rim of increased density (*arrowheads*). Surrounding the stone and the key to the diagnosis is a thin rim of water-density bile, allowing visualization of the stone rim separate from the duct wall. (D, duodenum; I, inferior vena cava).

sequela of chronic pancreatitis.[202] This can make it difficult to visualize the pancreas on CT scans. Initially, CT detection of pancreatic disease relied on changes in the size and shape of the pancreas. The improvements in scanner technology and optimal use of intravenous contrast allow detection of small tumors, which do not distort the pancreatic contours, but are seen because of their different enhancement characteristics compared with normal pancreatic parenchyma. Optimal CT technique uses thin collimation (3–5 mm), rapid injection of contrast material (best performed with a power injector), and rapid scanning during the phase of greatest pancreatic parenchymal enhancement.

Anatomic Variants

Pancreas divisum is the most common congenital anomaly of the pancreas. Although this anomaly most often goes unrecognized on CT scans, the pancreatic head can appear enlarged and simulate a mass lesion. In some cases, findings suggesting the diagnosis can be seen, including visualizing separate ventral and dorsal ducts without union and visualizing the ventral and dorsal pancreatic moieties on the same craniocaudal level, occasionally separated by a fat cleft.[203]

Agenesis of the dorsal pancreatic duct is identified with CT by visualizing only the head of the pancreas without a body or tail portion, and the condition may be confused with a mass in the head of the pancreas with proximal pancreatic atrophy.[204] Annular pancreas can be suggested by a soft tissue density surrounding the duodenum at the level of and continuous with the head of the pancreas. This may appear on the CT scan as pancreatic head enlargement without a narrowed duodenum.

Neoplasms

Adenocarcinoma

CT has become the screening examination of choice for ad-enocarcinoma of the pancreas. Large series have confirmed the accuracy and sensitivity of CT in detecting these lesions and documenting the extent of disease.[200,205] CT images display the cross-sectional abdomen in its entirety with reproducible landmarks allowing easy surgical correlation and follow-up comparisons. No areas are obscured on the CT images. For smaller series, ultrasound has been highly accurate, but most centers use ultrasound, not as the screening examination, but for evaluating the subgroup of patients for whom the CT results were confusing or inconclusive; for these patients, ultrasound can be valuable in excluding, confirming, or characterizing masses.[206,207]

The most common CT finding in adenocarcinoma is a focal mass isodense with the pancreas on noncontrast images and hypodense after intravenous contrast administration (Fig. 123-10). The presence of a dilated common bile duct that terminates abruptly, rather than gradually, is the hallmark of pancreatic carcinoma and corresponds to the similar finding on cholangiography, although a soft tissue–density calculus can cause a similar CT appearance.[161,195,197] A carcinoma not distorting the head or body of the pancreas may cause proximal dilatation of the pancreatic duct or may produce atrophy and fatty replacement of the upstream portions of the pancreas, allowing CT to suggest the diagnosis. Detecting evidence of spread to the lymph nodes, around vascular structures, or to the liver may also assist in making the diagnosis.[208] A false-positive CT diagnosis of pancreatic carcinoma has been reported for 8% of patients meeting these criteria; this group included patients with focal pancreatitis, metastatic lesions, normal pancreas, lymphoma, and islet cell carcinoma.[205] This stresses the need for confirmation of the lesion, which can be

performed by percutaneous biopsy under CT or ultrasound guidance or by serial CT evaluations.

CT is highly accurate in staging the extent of pancreatic carcinoma and detecting liver metastases, lymphadenopathy, arterial and venous encasement, and direct extension into adjacent organs.[205,208,209] None of 42 tumors determined to be nonresectable by CT were found to be resectable at surgery in one large series.[205] CT has been more accurate than angiography in demonstrating tumor involvement of major peripancreatic vessels.[205,209] If vascular involvement is equivocal by CT and surgical intervention is contemplated, angiography should be performed. CT cannot detect metastases to small, normal-sized lymph nodes or small or microscopic areas of adjacent invasion. A CT scan showing no apparent disease other than within the pancreas often understages the extent of disease. Freeny and colleagues showed that all 7 of such patients in their series had nonresectable disease at surgery.[205]

In this disease, for which the prognosis is poor and life expectancy is short, CT is a cost-effective, rapid method of diagnosing, staging, and documenting the diagnosis.

Islet Cell Tumors

Islet cell tumors can be differentiated from adenocarcinoma of the pancreas because of their different CT appearance. Because of their rich vascularity, they rarely undergo central necrosis, unlike adenocarcinomas. Even the hormonally inactive lesions, which typically attain large sizes before becoming clinically apparent, do not demonstrate the central low density from necrosis so typical of adenocarcinomas. Differentiation is added by the lack of arterial encasement in islet cell tumors, although venous encasement can occur.[210,211] The calcification that occurs in many of these lesions is rare in adenocarcinoma.

Although the nonfunctioning tumors typically attain

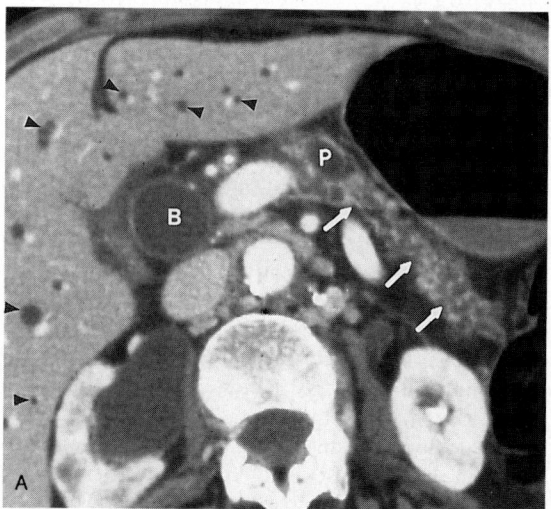
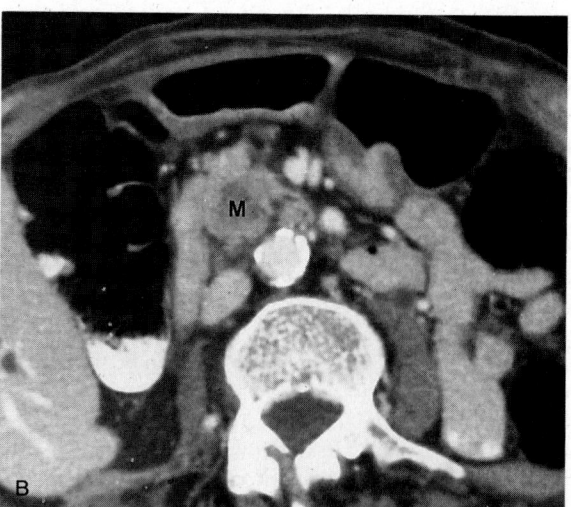

FIGURE 123-10. Pancreatic adenocarcinoma. (**A**) CT scan through the body and tail of the pancreas shows a dilated main pancreatic duct (P), with atrophy of the pancreatic parenchyma (*arrows*). Marked dilatation of the common bile duct (B) and dilated intrahepatic biliary radicles (*arrowheads*) are present, (**B**) A CT scan at the level of the pancreatic head shows a small hypodense mass (M) rounding the contours of the uncinate process.

large sizes, functioning islet cell tumors are usually less than 2 cm in diameter.[212,213] Similar to angiographic findings, these lesions can enhance dramatically and appear as high-density lesions. Approximately 80% of pancreatic lesions are seen on CT scans, although insulinomas are detected less often, with reported sensitivities of 30% to 66%.[214-219] Although CT has a relatively high sensitivity for detecting pancreatic lesions, extrapancreatic lesions are seen less often.[214,220] Wank and associates found only 35% of extrapancreatic gastrinomas on CT.[214]

Although an abnormal CT scan is helpful in locating primary tumors and staging the extent of metastatic disease, a normal CT scan does not exclude a primary extrapancreatic lesion. Successes of MRI and ultrasound in detecting gastrinomas have been reported, but one study showed CT to have a significantly higher detection rate for primary and metastatic lesions.[221]

Galiber and associates identified 61% of insulinoma cases with CT.[219] Because these lesions are small and often do not alter the contour of the pancreas, the diagnosis requires optimal CT technique with dynamic contrast injections. CT performed with an angiographic catheter in the dorsal pancreatic or superior mesenteric artery can be helpful in detecting hypovascular tumors.[222,223] Although transabdominal ultrasound has a detection rate for insulinomas as high as 61%, intraoperative ultrasound has the highest rate of imaging success, with a sensitivity of 84%. Intraoperative ultrasound combined with surgical palpation has detected 100% of lesions in one series.[219] If a patient has biochemical and clinical evidence of an insulinoma not seen on CT, ultrasound, or angiography screening, intraoperative ultrasound is the most accurate method of localizing the tumor. This raises the question whether extensive preoperative studies with low sensitivities are worthwhile.

Cystic Neoplasms

Cystic pancreatic neoplasms are classified as microcystic (glycogen-rich) or macrocystic (mucin-producing) tumors. The classification of these tumors is based on relative cyst size; cyst size can vary in these two categories.[224]

The microcystic adenomas are typified by innumerable cysts, ranging in size from less than 1 mm to 2 cm and not exhibiting malignant potential.[225] CT images reflect these changes, found most often in the older population.[226] The mass may appear as a soft tissue density or may contain small low-density regions correlating with the cystic changes seen pathologically. The central connective tissue may calcify and appear on CT in a characteristic central, often radiating pattern.[226,227] The lesions can occur throughout the pancreas but have a predilection for its head.

Macrocystic adenomas occur predominantly in the body and tail of the pancreas and are characterized on CT images by low-density masses that are usually larger than 2 cm and that correlate with the cystic changes seen pathologically. The visible septations that can separate the cystic areas can simulate multiple cysts. If the septations are thin and not visible on CT, the lesion can simulate a single cyst or pseudocyst. Because of the malignant potential of these lesions, this discrimination is important and is usually possible with modern CT

techniques. The septations and wall of these lesions can calcify, but unlike the microcystic adenomas, the calcification tends to be peripheral. These lesions can be difficult to differentiate from necrotic adenocarcinoma, cystic lesions of the pancreas from von Hippel-Lindau syndrome, lymphangioma,[228] or a complicated pseudocyst.

Mucinous cystic tumors sometimes communicate with the pancreatic duct, and the duct enlarges as a result of excessive mucin accumulation.[229] Rarely, flat, mucin-producing, benign or malignant tumors arise in the duct wall, but they are too small to be seen radiologically. The excessive mucin production results in marked pancreatic ductal dilatation, which is the only finding on CT scans. If such tumors arise in the peripheral branches of the pancreatic duct, the resulting dilatation of clustered, tortuous peripheral branches can simulate a separated, cystic tumor. This tumor has been referred to as a ductectatic tumor, referring to the visualization of the tortuous, dilated ducts seen using CT and cholangiography.[230]

Pancreatitis

CT has changed dramatically the ability to diagnose and evaluate the extent of pancreatitis. CT can visualize the morphologic changes within the pancreas and the development and extent of surrounding fluid collections.[35,231-233] Although ultrasound has also been able to evaluate the pancreas and is often helpful in evaluating patients with pancreatitis, the associated bowel ileus and overlying bowel gas hinders the ultrasound examination. CT is superior to ultrasound in diagnosing and evaluating the extent of abnormalities in these patients.[162,168,234-236]

CT can be useful in confirming the diagnosis of pancreatitis in patients with confusing clinical presentations and in delineating the extent of disease in those suspected of having complications such as retroperitoneal fluid collections, pseudocysts, or abscess. There is an association between the CT findings and the severity of disease, as judged by clinical outcome or the clinical criteria described by Ranson; however, Vernacchia and colleagues did not find a correlation between early CT appearances and subsequent abscess development.[235,237-240] Although general correlations exist, individual patients may exhibit marked differences between CT appearances and outcomes.[237,238] Necrosis of pancreatic parenchyma has been the CT finding most often associated with subsequent complications and death, particularly if combined with other CT findings (Fig. 123-11).[239] The CT findings of pancreatitis may persist after the clinical symptoms have cleared.[233]

The CT scans of approximately 30% of patients with pancreatitis are normal.[232,236] Changes may appear as diffuse or focal and may demonstrate pancreatic enlargement, edema with a lower attenuation value of the pancreas, ill-defined pancreatic margins, or fluid and inflammatory changes in the peripancreatic region or extrapancreatic locations. Focal changes can be difficult to differentiate from pancreatic carcinoma. In severe cases, the inflammatory process can extend beyond the margins of the pancreas and into the lesser sac, anterior pararenal spaces, and the mesentery. This condition is also called phlegmonous pancreatitis.[232,241,242] Although phlegmonous changes may be differentiated from fluid collections by their increased attenuation, their CT appearance

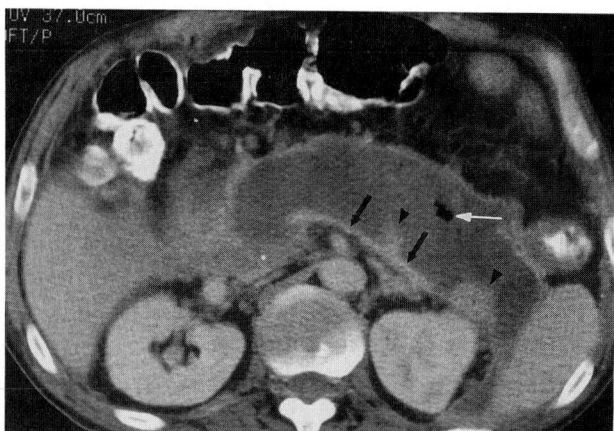

FIGURE 123-11. Acute pancreatitis with pancreatic necrosis. The CT scan at the level of the body of the pancreas reveals diffuse enlargement of the pancreas. The pancreas is seen as a fluid attenuation mass, representing necrosis replacing pancreatic parenchyma throughout the entire pancreas, sparing only small residula foci (*arrowheads*). Some infection and gas is present (*white arrow*) within the necrotic tissue. The splenic vein (*black arrows*) delineates the posterior aspect of the pancreas.

may simulate fluid caused by edema. The phlegmonous changes seen on CT can persist for months after the patient's clinical symptoms have cleared.[233]

CT is the best method of detecting and delineating the extent of peripancreatic fluid collections in complicated pancreatitis.[231] These fluid collections do not represent pseudocysts, because they lack distinct rims or margins; they are evolving, low-density collections, changing shape, size, and location. Pseudocysts, whether intrapancreatic or extrapancreatic, appear on CT as round or oval, low-density masses with a thick, well-delineated capsule. Occasionally, pseudocysts demonstrate a slightly higher density and suggest hemorrhage or infection. As with other complications of pancreatitis, CT is more sensitive than ultrasound in detecting and characterizing pseudocysts of the pancreas.[234]

Pancreatic abscess can be a complication of pancreatitis, occurring in pancreatic phlegmon or a pseudocyst. It is best detected and evaluated by CT, which is more accurate than ultrasound in detecting small foci of gas, the hallmark of the diagnosis. Unfortunately, gas is present in the minority of pancreatic abscesses and may occur without an abscess as a consequence of fistulization from adjacent bowel.[243-246] Most abscesses appear on CT images with the nonspecific findings of ill-defined, low-density areas or fluid collections, and accurate diagnosis requires needle aspiration guided by ultrasound or CT. With the aggressive use of CT imaging and guided aspiration allowing an early diagnosis of pancreatic abscess, the mortality rate for this disorder has decreased from 40% to 19%.[244]

The changes of chronic pancreatitis can be seen on CT scans in 85% of cases and include parenchymal atrophy, parenchymal and ductal calcifications, pancreatic ductal dilatation, pseudocyst formation, and findings of biliary obstruction.[247] Chronic pancreatitis can appear as a focal mass simulating neoplastic changes, and CT-guided biopsy or serial examinations can be helpful in differentiating these processes.

Other findings that suggest the diagnosis of chronic pancreatitis include irregular dilatation of the pancreatic duct, rather than the smooth dilatation seen with carcinoma, and a ratio of duct width to gland width of 0.5 or less.[248]

Pseudocysts

Unlike the fluid collections or effusions associated with acute pancreatitis, pseudocysts are surrounded by a dense fibrous capsule.[35] These lesions usually are homogeneous and isodense with water on CT scans. Infection or hemorrhage may be indicated if the the CT attenuation values of the pseudocyst contents appear to be increased. These lesions can occur within the pancreatic parenchyma or in extrapancreatic locations after the course of chronic inflammatory changes outside of the pancreas. Although ultrasound detects most intrapancreatic pseudocysts, CT is superior in visualizing extrapancreatic pseudocysts.[234]

Transplantation

The normal pancreas transplant appears on CT as a small, soft tissue–density mass in the lower abdomen or pelvis. CT is not able to detect transplant rejection but does play a role in detecting and diagnosing postoperative fluid collections or abscesses.[249] As with all intraabdominal fluid collections, the CT appearance cannot diagnose infection, which requires aspiration.

INTERVENTIONAL USES OF COMPUTED TOMOGRAPHY

Masses, fluid collections, or abscesses seen on CT can be biopsied or drained under CT guidance. CT affords a total view of the cross-sectional abdomen and can direct endoscopic or open surgical pathways away from critical structures, such as overlying bowel or lung. Unlike fluoroscopy or ultrasound, it does not give real-time guidance. For this reason, the use of CT for the biopsy of lung lesions should be reserved for cases in which the suspected lesion cannot be seen adequately except with CT.

In addition to directing catheter placement in abscesses, CT can be used for following the patient's course after abscess drainage, guiding injection of catheters with dilute contrast before follow-up scanning, and evaluating the size of lesions. CT scans can also reveal potential communications with other structures, such as bowel and biliary or pancreatic ducts.

The reader is directed to Chapter 120, Cross-Sectional Anatomy.

REFERENCES

1. Hendee WR. Cross sectional medical imaging: a history. Radiographics 1989;9:1155.
2. Cho KC, Morehouse HT, Alterman DD, Thornhill BA. Sigmoid

diverticulitis: diagnostic role of CT—comparison with barium enema studies. Radiology 1990;176:111.

3. Zeman RK, Fox SH, Silverman PM, et al. Helical (spiral) CT of the abdomen. AJR Am J Roentgenol 1993;160:719.

4. Urban BA, Fishman EK, Kuhlman JE, et al. Detection of focal hepatic lesions with spiral CT: comparison of 4- and 8-mm interscan spacing. AJR Am J Roentgenol 1993;160:783.

5. Brasch RC, Cann CE. Computed tomographic scanning in children: II. An updated comparison of radiation dose and resolving power of commercial scanners. AJR Am J Roentgenol 1982;138:127.

6. Halber MD, Daffner RH, Thompson WM. CT of the esophagus: I. Normal appearance. AJR Am J Roentgenol 1979;133:1047.

7. Moss AA, Schnyder PA, Thoeni RF, et al. Esophageal carcinoma: pretherapy staging by computed tomography. AJR Am J Roentgenol 1981;136:1051.

8. Reinig JW, Stanley JH, Schabel SI. CT evaluation of thickened esophageal walls. AJR Am J Roentgenol 1981;140:931.

9. Quint LE, Glazer GM, Orringer MB, Gross BH. Esophageal carcinoma: CT findings. Radiology 1985;155:171.

10. Thompson WM, Halvorsen RA, Foster WL, et al. Computed tomography for staging esophageal and gastroesophageal cancer: reevaluation. AJR Am J Roentgenol 1983;141:951.

11. Picus D, Balfe DM, Koehler RE, et al. Computed tomography in the staging of esophageal carcinoma. Radiology 1983;146:433.

12. Halvorsen RA, Thompson WM. Computed tomographic staging of gastrointestinal tract malignancies. Part I. Esophagus and stomach. Invest Radiol 1987;22:2.

13. Clark KE, Foley WD, Lawson TL, et al. CT evaluation of esophageal and upper abdominal varices. J Comput Assist Tomogr 1980;4:510.

14. Ishikawa T, Tsukune Y, Ohyama Y, et al. Venous abnormalities in portal hypertension demonstrated by CT. AJR Am J Roentgenol 1980;134:271.

15. Halden WJ, Harnsberger HR, Mancuso AA. Computed tomography of esophageal varices after sclerotherapy. AJR Am J Roentgenol 1983;140:1195.

16. Mauro MA, Jaques PF, Swantkowski TM, et al. CT after uncomplicated esophageal sclerotherapy. AJR Am J Roentgenol 1986;146:1.

17. Reinig JW, Stanley JH, Schabel SI. CT evaluation of thickened esophageal walls. AJR Am J Roentgenol 1983;140:931.

18. Pearlberg JL, Sandler MA, Madrazo BL. Computed tomographic features of esophageal intramural pseudodiverticulosis. Radiology 1983;147:189.

19. Lee RK, Sheedy PF. Computed tomography of the gastrointestinal tract. CRC Crit Rev Diagn Imaging 1980;18:121.

20. Thompson WM, Halvorsen RA, Williford ME, et al. Computed tomography of the gastroesophageal junction. Radiographics 1982;2:179.

21. Megibow AJ, Balthazar EJ, Hulnick DH, et al. CT evaluation of gastrointestinal leiomyomas and leiomyosarcomas. AJR Am J Roentgenol 1985;144:727.

22. Balfe DM, Koehler RE, Karstaedt N, et al. Computed tomography of gastric neoplasms. Radiology 1981;140:431.

23. Moss AA, Schnyder P, Candardjis G, Margulis AR. Computed tomography of benign and malignant gastric abnormalities. J Clin Gastroenterol 1980;2:401.

24. Freeny PC, Marks WM. Adenocarcinoma of the gastroesophageal junction: barium and CT examination. AJR Am J Roentgenol 1982;138:1077.

25. Cook AO, Levine BA, Sirinek KR, Gaskill HV. Evaluation of gastric adenocarcinoma: abdominal computed tomography does not replace celiotomy. Arch Surg 1986;121:603.

26. Sussman SK, Halvorsen RA, Illescas FF, et al. Gastric adenocarcinoma: CT versus surgical staging. Radiology 1988;167:335.

27. Mullin D, Shirkhoda A. Computed tomography after gastrectomy in primary gastric carcinoma. J Comput Assist Tomogr 1985;9:30.

28. Scatarige JC, Fishman EK, Jones B, et al. Gastric leiomyosarcoma: CT observations. J Comput Assist Tomogr 1985;9:320.

29. Megibow AJ. Gastrointestinal lymphoma: the role of CT in diagnosis and management. Semin Ultrasound CT MR 1986;7:43.

30. Buy J-N, Moss AA. Computed tomography of gastric lymphoma. AJR Am J Roentgenol 1982;138:859.

31. Balthazar EJ, Megibow AJ, Naidich D, LeFleur RS. Computed tomographic recognition of gastric varices. AJR Am J Roentgenol 1984;142:1121.

32. Nichols DM, Li DK. Superior mesenteric vein rotation: a CT sign of midgut malrotation. AJR Am J Roentgenol 1983;141:707.

33. Fisher JK. Computed tomographic diagnosis of volvulus in intestinal malrotation. Radiology 1981;140:145.

34. Ormson MJ, Stephens DH, Carlson HC. CT recognition of intestinal lipomatosis. AJR Am J Roentgenol 1985;144:313.

35. Siegelman SS, Copeland BE, Saba GP, et al. CT of fluid collections associated with pancreatitis. AJR Am J Roentgenol 1980;134:1121.

36. Goldberg HI, Gore RM, Margulis AR, et al. Computed tomography in the evaluation of Crohn's disease. AJR Am J Roentgenol 1983;140:277.

37. Gore RM, Cohen MI, Vogelzang RL, et al. Value of computed tomography in the detection of complications of Crohn's disease. Dig Dis Sci 1985;30:701.

38. Frager DH, Goldman M, Benevenatano TC. Computed tomography in Crohn's disease. J Comp Assist Tomogr 1983;7:819.

39. Goldman SM, Fishman EK, Gatewood OMB, et al. CT in the diagnosis of enterovesical fistulae. AJR Am J Roentgenol 1985;144:1229.

40. Kerber GW, Greenberg M, Rubin JM. Computed tomography evaluation of local and extraintestinal complications of Crohn's disease. Gastrointest Radiol 1984;9:143.

41. Jones B, Fishman EK, Framer SS, et al. Computed tomography of gastrointestinal inflammation after bone marrow transplantation. AJR Am J Roentgenol 1986;146:691.

42. Jeffrey RB Jr, Nyberg DA, Bottles K, et al. Abdominal CT in acquired immunodeficiency syndrome. AJR Am J Roentgenol 1986;146:7.

43. Alpern MB, Glazer GM, Francis IR. Ischemic or infarcted bowel: CT findings. Radiology 1988;166:149.

44. Connor R, Jones B, Fishman EK, Siegelman SS. Pneumatosis intestinalis: role of computed tomography in diagnosis and management. J Comput Assist Tomogr 1984;8:269.

45. Federle MP, Chun G, Jeffrey RB Jr, et al. Computed tomographic findings in bowel infarction. AJR Am J Roentgenol 1984;142:91.

46. Fishman EK, Zinreich ES, Jones B, Siegelman SS. Computed tomographic diagnosis of radiation ileitis. Gastrointest Radiol 1984;9:149.

47. Hilton S, Megibow AJ, Naidich DP, Bosniak MA. Computed tomography of the postoperative abdominal aorta. Radiology 1982;145:403.

48. Mark AS, Moss AA, McCarthy S, McCowin M. CT of aortoenteric fistulas. Invest Radiol 1985;20:272.

49. Haaga J, Baldwin GN, Reich NE, et al. CT detection of infected synthetic grafts: preliminary report of a new sign. AJR Am J Roentgenol 1978;131:317.

50. Megibow A, Balthazar E, Cho K, et al. Bowel obstruction: evaluation with CT. Radiology 1991;180:313.

51. Fukuya T, Hawes D, Lu C, et al. CT diagnosis of small-bowel obstruction: efficacy in 60 patients. AJR Am J Roentgenol 1992;158:765.

52. Merine DS, Fishman EK, Jones B, et al. Enteroenteric intussusception: CT findings in nine patients. AJR Am J Roentgenol 1987;128:1129.

53. Donovan AT, Goldman SM. Computed tomography of ileocecal intussusception: mechanism and appearance. J Comput Assist Tomogr 1981;6:630.

54. Balthazar E, Birnbaum B, Megibow A, et al. Closed-loop and strangulating intestinal obstruction: CT signs. Radiology 1992;185:769.

55. Megibow AJ, Zerhouni EA, Hulnick DH, et al. Air contrast techniques in gastrointestinal computed tomography. AJR Am J Roentgenol 1985;145:418.

56. Megibow AJ, Redmond PE, Bosniak MA, Horowitz L. Diagnosis of gastrointestinal lipomas by CT. AJR Am J Roentgenol 1979;133:743.

57. Megibow AJ, Zerhouni EA, Hulnick DH, et al. Air insufflation of the colon as an adjunct to computed tomography of the pelvis. J Comput Assist Tomogr 1984;8:797.

58. Balthazar EJ, Megibow AJ, Hulnick D, Naidich DP. Carcinoma of the colon: detection and preoperative staging by CT. AJR Am J Roentgenol 1988;150:301.

59. Kelvin FM, Maglinte DDT. Colorectal carcinoma: a radiologic and clinical review. Radiology 1987;164:1.

60. Thompson WM, Halvorsen RA. Computed tomographic staging of gastrointestinal malignancies. Part II. The small bowel, colon, and rectum. Invest Radiol 1987;22:96.

61. Hulnick DH, Megibow AJ, Balthazar EJ, et al. Perforated colorectal neoplasms: correlation of clinical, contrast enema, and CT examinations. Radiology 1987;164:611.

62. Mayes GB, Zornoza J. Computed tomography of colon carcinoma. AJR Am J Roentgenol 1980;135:43.

63. Van Waes P, Koehler PR, Feldberg M. Management of rectal carcinoma: impact of computed tomography. AJR Am J Roentgenol 1983;140:1137.

64. Thoeni RF, Moss AA, Schnyder P, Margulis AR. Detection and staging of primary rectal and rectosigmoid cancer by computed tomography. Radiology 1981;141:135.

65. Freeny PC, Marks WM, Ryan JA, Bolen JW. Colorectal carcinoma evaluation with CT: preoperative staging and detection of postoperative recurrence. Radiology 1986;158:347.

66. Thompson W, Halvorsen RA, Foster WL, et al. Preoperative and postoperative CT staging of rectosigmoid carcinoma. AJR Am J Roentgenol 1986;146:703.

67. Grabbe E, Lierse W, Winkler R. The perirectal fascia: morphology and use in staging of rectal carcinoma. Radiology 1983;149:241.

68. Adalsteinsson B, Gimelius B, Graffman S, et al. Computed tomography in staging rectal carcinoma. Acta Radiol 1985;26:45.

69. Nelson RC, Chezmar JL, Sugarbaker PH, Bernardino ME. Hepatic tumors: comparison of CT during arterial portography, delayed CT, and MR imaging for preoperative evaluation. Radiology 1989;172:27.

70. Heiken JP, Weyman PJ, Lee JKT, et al. Detection of focal hepatic masses: prospective evaluation with CT, delayed CT, CT during arterial portography, and MR imaging. Radiology 1989;171:47.

71. Moss AA, Thoeni RF, Schnyder P, Margulis AR. Value of computed tomography in the detection and staging of recurrent rectal carcinoma. J Comput Assist Tomogr 1981;5:870.

72. Lee JKT, Stanley RJ, Sagel SS, et al. CT appearance of the pelvis after abdominoperineal resection for rectal carcinoma. Radiology 1981;141:737.

73. Kelvin FM, Korobkin M, Heaston DK, et al. Pelvis after surgery for rectal carcinoma: serial CT observations with emphasis on non-neoplastic features. AJR Am J Roentgenol 1983;141:959.

74. Butch RJ, Wittenberg J, Mueller PR, et al. Presacral masses after abdominoperineal resection for colorectal carcinoma: the need for needle biopsy. AJR Am J Roentgenol 1985;144:309.

75. McCarthy SM, Barnes D, Deveney K, et al. Detection of recurrent rectosigmoid carcinoma: prospective evaluation of CT and clinical factors. AJR Am J Roentgenol 1985;144:577.

76. Johnson CD, Baker ME, Rice RP, et al. Diagnosis of acute colonic diverticulitis: comparison of barium enema and CT. AJR Am J Roentgenol 1987;148:541.

77. Barakos JA, Jeffrey RB Jr, Federle MP, et al. CT in the management of periappendiceal abscess. AJR Am J Roentgenol 1986;146:1161.

78. Balthazar EJ, Megibow AJ, Hulnick D, et al. CT of appendicitis. AJR Am J Roentgenol 1986;147:705.

79. Gore RM, Marn CS, Kirby DF, et al. CT findings in ulcerative, granulomatous and indeterminate colitis. AJR Am J Roentgenol 1984;143:279.

80. Frick MP, Maile CW, Crass JR, et al. Computed tomography of neutropenic colitis. AJR Am J Roentgenol 1984;143:763.

81. Fishman EK, Kavuru M, Jones B, et al. Pseudomembranous colitis: CT evaluation of 26 cases. Radiology 1991;180:57.

82. DuBrow RA, David CL, Libshitz HI, Lorigan JG. Detection of hepatic metastases in breast cancer: the role of nonenhanced and enhanced CT scanning. J Comput Assist Tomogr 1990;14:366.

83. Foley WD, Berland LL, Lawson TL, et al. Contrast enhancement technique for dynamic hepatic computed tomographic scanning. Radiology 1983;147:797.

84. Berland LL, Lawson TL, Foley WD, et al. Comparison of pre- and post-contrast CT in hepatic masses. AJR Am J Roentgenol 1982;138:853.

85. Bressler EL, Alpern MB, Glazer GM, et al. Hypervascular hepatic metastases: CT evaluation. Radiology 1987;162:49.

86. Paushter DM, Zeman RK, Scheibler ML, et al. CT evaluation of suspected hepatic metastases: comparison of techniques for IV contrast enhancement. AJR Am J Roentgenol 1989;152:267.

87. Foley WD. Dynamic hepatic CT. Radiology 1989;170:617.

88. Burgener FA, Hamlin DJ. Contrast enhancement of hepatic tumors in CT: comparison between bolus and infusion techniques. AJR Am J Roentgenol 1983;140:291.

89. Brendel A, Leccia F, Drouillard J, et al. Single photon emission computed tomography (SPECT), planar scintigraphy, and transmission computed tomography: a comparison of accuracy in diagnosing focal hepatic disease. Radiology 1984;153:527.

90. Knopf DR, Torres WE, Fajman WJ, et al. Liver lesions: comparative accuracy of scintigraphy and computed tomography. AJR Am J Roentgenol 1982;138:623.

91. Alderson PO, Adams DF, McNeil BJ, et al. Computed tomography, ultrasound and scintigraphy of the liver in patients with colon or breast carcinoma: a prospective comparison. Radiology 1983;149:225.

92. Ferrucci JT, Freeny PC, Stark DD, et al. Advances in hepatobiliary radiology. Radiology 1988;168:319.

93. Peterson MS, Baron RL, Dodd GD III, et al. Hepatic parenchymal perfusion defects detected with CTAP: imaging-pathologic correlation. Radiology 1992;185:149.

94. Stark DD, Wittenberg J, Butch RJ, Ferrucci JT. Hepatic metastases: randomized, controlled comparison of detection with MR imaging and CT. Radiology 1987;165:399.

95. Chezmar JL, Rumancik WM, Megibow AJ, et al. Liver and abdominal screening in patients with cancer: CT versus MR imaging. Radiology 1988;168:43.

96. Bernardino ME, Erwin BC, Steinberg HV, et al. Delayed hepatic CT scanning: increased confidence and improved detection of hepatic metastases. Radiology 1986;159:71.

97. Miller DL, Simmons JT, Chang R, et al. Hepatic metastasis detection: comparison of three CT contrast enhancement methods. Radiology 1987;165:785.

98. Soyer P, Levesque M, Elias D, et al. Detection of liver metastases from colorectal cancer: comparison of intraoperative US and CT during arterial portography. Radiology 1992;183:541.

99. Reinig JW, Dwyer AJ, Miller DL, et al. Liver metastasis detection: comparative sensitivities of MR imaging and CT scanning. Radiology 1987;162:43.

100. Sugarbaker PH, Vermess M, Doppman JL, et al. Improved detection of focal lesions with computerized tomographic examination of the liver using ethiodized oil emulsion (EOE-13) liver contrast. Cancer 1984;54:1489.

101. Miller DL, Rosenbaum RC, Sugarbaker PH, et al. Detection of hepatic metastases: comparison of EOE-13 CT and ^{99m}Tc-MAA scintigraphy. AJR Am J Roentgenol 1983;141:931.

102. Miller DL, Vermess M, Doppman JL, et al. CT of the liver and spleen with EOE-13: review of 225 examinations. AJR Am J Roentgenol 1984;143:235.

103. Piekarski J, Goldberg HI, Royal SA, et al. Difference between liver and spleen CT numbers in the normal adult: its usefulness in predicting the presence of diffuse liver disease. Radiology 1980;137:727.

104. Baker MK, Wenker JC, Cockerill EM, Ellis JH. Focal fatty infiltration of the liver: diagnostic imaging. Radiographics 1985;6:923.

105. Baker ME, Silverman PM. Nodular focal fatty infiltration of

the liver: CT appearance. AJR Am J Roentgenol 1985;145:79.

106. Torres WE, Whitmire LF, Gedgaudas-McClees K, Bernardino ME. Computed tomography of hepatic morphologic changes in cirrhosis of the liver. J Comput Assist Tomogr 1986;10:47.

107. Harbin WP, Robert NJ, Ferrucci JT. Diagnosis of cirrhosis based on regional changes in hepatic morphology. Radiology 1980;135:273.

108. Waller RM, Oliver TW, McCain AH, et al. Computed tomography and sonography of hepatic cirrhosis and portal hypertension. Radiographics 1984;4:677.

109. Oka H, Kurioka N, Kanno T, et al. Prospective study of early detection of hepatocellular carcinoma in patients with cirrhosis. Hepatology 1990;12:680.

110. Miller WJ, Dodd GD III, Baron RL, Federle MP. CT sensitivity and specificity in detecting malignancy in cirrhotic patients with pathologic correlation. Radiology 1991;181(P):95.

111. Ohtomo K, Baron RL, Dodd GD III, et al. Confluent hepatic fibrosis in advanced cirrhosis: Appearance at CT. Radiology 1993;188:31.

112. Mitnick JS, Bosniak MA, Megibow AJ, et al. CT in β-thalassemia: Iron deposition in the liver, spleen, and lymph nodes. AJR Am J Roentgenol 1981;136:1191.

113. Howard JM, Ghent CN, Carey LS, et al. Diagnostic efficacy of hepatic computed tomography in the detection of body iron overload. Gastroenterology 1983;84:209.

114. Doppman JL, Cornblath M, Dwyer A, et al. Computed tomography of the liver and kidneys in glycogen storage disease. J Comput Assist Tomogr 1982;6:67.

115. Markos J, Veronese ME, Nicholson MR, et al. Value of hepatic computerized tomographic scanning during amiodarone therapy. Am J Cardiol 1985;56:89.

116. DeMaria M, DeSimone G, Laconi A, et al. Gold storage in the liver: appearance on CT scans. Radiology 1986;159:355.

117. Dixon AK, Walsh JM. Computed tomography of the liver in Wilson disease. J Comput Assist Tomogr 1984;8:46.

118. Barnes PA, Thomas JL, Bernardino ME. Pitfalls in the diagnosis of hepatic cysts by computed tomography. Radiology 1981;141:129.

119. Freeny PC, Marks WM. Hepatic hemangioma: dynamic bolus CT. AJR Am J Roentgenol 1986;159:685.

120. Freeny PC, Marks WM. Patterns of contrast enhancement of benign and malignant hepatic neoplasms during bolus dynamic and delayed CT. Radiology 1986;160:613.

121. Itai Y, Furui S, Araki T, et al. Computed tomography of cavernous hemangioma of the liver. Radiology 1980;137:149.

122. Mathieu D, Bruneton JN, Drouillard J, et al. Hepatic adenomas and focal nodular hyperplasia: dynamic CT study. Radiology 1986;160:53.

123. Welch TJ, Sheedy PF, Johnson CM, et al. Focal nodular hyperplasia and hepatic adenoma: comparison of angiography, CT, US, and scintigraphy. Radiology 1985;156:593.

124. Brandt DJ, Johnson CD, Stephens DH, Weiland LH. Imaging of fibrolamellar hepatocellular carcinoma. AJR Am J Roentgenol 1988;151:295.

125. Takashima T, Matsui O, Suzuki M, Ida M. Diagnosis and screening of small hepatocellular carcinomas: comparison of radionuclide imaging, ultrasound, computed tomography, hepatic angiography, and α₁-fetoprotein assay. Radiology 1982;145:635.

126. Matsui O, Takashima T, Kadoya M, et al. Dynamic computed tomography during arterial portography: most sensitive examination for small hepatocellular carcinomas. J Comput Assist Tomogr 1985;9:19.

127. Yumoto Y, Jinno K, Tokuyama K, et al. Hepatocellular carcinoma detected by iodized oil. Radiology 1985;154:19.

128. Ohishi H, Uchida H, Yoshimura H, et al. Hepatocellular carcinoma detected by iodized oil: use of anticancer agents. Radiology 1985;154:25.

129. Nakakuma K, Tashiro S, Hiraoka T, et al. Hepatocellular carcinoma and metastatic cancer detected by iodized oil. Radiology 1985;154:15.

130. Teefey SA, Stephens DH, James EM, et al. Computed tomography and ultrasonography of hepatoma. Clin Radiol 1986;37:339.

131. LaBerge JM, Laing FC, Federle MP, et al. Hepatocellular carcinoma: assessment of resectability by computed tomography and ultrasound. Radiology 1984;152:485.

132. Hayashi N, Yamamoto K, Tamaki N, et al. Metastatic nodules of hepatocellular carcinoma: detection with angiography, CT and US. Radiology 1987;165:61.

133. Buchman TG, Zuidema GD. The role of computed tomographic scanning in the surgical management of pyogenic hepatic abscess. Surg Gynecol Obstet 1981;153:1.

134. Rubinson HA, Isikoff MB, Hill MC. Diagnostic imaging of hepatic abscesses: a retrospective analysis. AJR Am J Roentgenol 1980;135:735.

135. Halvorsen RA, Korobkin M, Foster WL, et al. Variable CT appearance of hepatic abscesses. AJR Am J Roentgenol 1984;142:941.

136. Callen PW, Filly RA, Marcus FS. Ultrasonography and computed tomography in the evaluation of hepatic microabscesses in the immunosuppressed patient. Radiology 1980;136:433.

137. Shirkhoda A, Lopez-Berestein G, Holbert JM, Lunga MA. Hepatosplenic fungal infection: CT and pathologic evaluation after treatment with liposomal amphotericin B. Radiology 1986;159:349.

138. Landay MJ, Setaiwan H, Hirsch G, et al. Hepatic and thoracic amebiasis. AJR Am J Roentgenol 1980;135:449.

139. Kalovidouris A, Pissiotic C, Pontifex G, et al. CT characterization of multivesicular hydatid cysts. J Comput Assist Tomogr 1986;10:428.

140. Mathieu D, Vasile N, Grenier P. Portal thrombosis: dynamic CT features and course. Radiology 1985;154:737.

141. Miller VE, Berland LL. Pulsed Doppler duplex sonography and CT of portal vein thrombosis. AJR Am J Roentgenol 1985;145:73.

142. Vigo M, De Faveri D, Biondetti PR, et al. CT demonstration of portal and superior mesenteric vein thrombosis in hepatocellular carcinoma. J Comput Assist Tomogr 1980;4:627.

143. Zirinsky K, Markisz JA, Auh YH, et al. MR imaging of portal venous thrombosis: correlation with CT and sonography. AJR Am J Roentgenol 1988;150:283.

144. Mathieu D, Vasile N, Menu Y, et al. Budd-Chiari syndrome: dynamic CT. Radiology 1987;165:409.

145. Vogelzang RL, Anschuetz SL, Gore RM. Budd-Chiari syndrome: CT observations. Radiology 1987;163:329.

146. Becker CD, Scheidegger J, Marincek B. Hepatic vein occlusion: morphologic features on computed tomography and ultrasonography. Gastrointest Radiol 1986;11:305.

147. Menu Y, Alison D, Lorphelin J-M, et al. Budd-Chiari syndrome: US evaluation. Radiology 1985;157:761.

148. Grant EG, Perrella R, Tessler FN, et al. Budd-Chiari syndrome: the results of duplex and color Doppler imaging. AJR Am J Roentgenol 1989;152:377.

149. Hricak H, Amparo EG, Fisher MR, et al. Abdominal venous system: assessment using MR. Radiology 1985;156:415.

150. Stark DD, Hahn PF, Trey C, et al. MRI of the Budd-Chiari syndrome. AJR Am J Roentgenol 1986;146:1141.

151. Federle M. CT of abdominal trauma. CRC Crit Rev Diagn Imaging 1981;19:257.

152. Meyer AA, Crass RA, Lim RC Jr, et al. Selective non-operative management of blunt liver injury using computed tomography. Arch Surg 1985;120:550.

153. Moon KL, Federle MP. Computed tomography in hepatic trauma. AJR Am J Roentgenol 1983;141:309.

154. Goldstein AS, Sclafani SJA, Kupferstein NH, et al. Diagnostic superiority of computed tomography in the evaluation of acute abdominal trauma. J Trauma 1985;25:938.

155. Wing VW, Federle MP, Morris JA, et al. Clinical impact of CT for blunt abdominal trauma. AJR Am J Roentgenol 1985;145:1191.

156. Federle MP, Jeffrey RB Jr. Hemoperitoneum studied by computed tomography. Radiology 1983;148:187.

157. Savolaine ER, Grecos GP, Howard J, White P. Evolution of CT findings in hepatic hematoma. J Comput Assist Tomogr 1985;9:1090.

158. Mirvis SE, Whitley NO, Vainwright JR, Gens DR. Blunt hepatic

trauma in adults: CT-based classification and correlation with prognosis and treatment. Radiology 1989;171:27.

159. Brick SH, Taylor GA, Potter BM, Eichelberger MR. Hepatic and splenic injury in children: role of CT in the decision for laparotomy. Radiology 1987;165:643.

160. Foley WD, Cates JD, Kellman GM, et al. Treatment of blunt hepatic injuries: role of CT. Radiology 1987;164:635.

161. Baron RL, Stanley RJ, Lee JKT, Koehler RE, Levitt RG. Computed tomographic features of biliary obstruction. AJR Am J Roentgenol 1983;140:1173.

162. Baron RL, Stanley RJ, Lee JKT, et al. A prospective comparison of the evaluation of biliary obstruction using computed tomography and ultrasonography. Radiology 1982;145:91.

163. Liddell RM, Baron RL, Ekstrom JE, et al. CT depiction of normal intrahepatic bile ducts and pancreatic ducts. Radiology 1989;173(P):146.

164. Schulte SJ, Baron RL, Teefey SA, et al. CT of the extrahepatic bile ducts: wall thickness and contrast enhancement in normal and abnormal ducts. AJR Am J Roentgenol 1990;154:79.

165. Sample WF, Sarti DA, Goldstein LI, et al. Grayscale ultrasonography of the jaundiced patient. Radiology 1978;128:719.

166. Cooperberg PL, Li DKB, Sauerbrei EE. Accuracy of common hepatic duct size in the evaluation of extrahepatic biliary obstruction. Radiology 1980;135:141.

167. Zeman RK, Dorfman GS, Burrell MI, et al. Disparate dilatation of the intrahepatic and extrahepatic bile ducts in surgical jaundice. Radiology 1981;138:129.

168. Honickman SP, Mueller PR, Wittenberg J, et al. Ultrasound in obstructive jaundice: prospective evaluation of site and cause. Radiology 1983;147:511.

169. Choi BI, Lee JH, Han MC, et al. Hilar cholangiocarcinoma: comparative study with sonography and CT. Radiology 1989;172:689.

170. Gibson RN, Yeung E, Thompson JN, et al. Bile duct obstruction: radiologic evaluation of level, cause, and tumor resectability. Radiology 1987;160:43.

171. Berger PE, Kuhn JP. Computed tomography of the hepatobiliary system in infancy and childhood. Radiol Clin North Am 1981;19:431.

172. Montana MA, Rohrmann CA Jr. Cholangiocarcinoma in a choledochal cyst: preoperative diagnosis. AJR Am J Roentgenol 1986;147:515.

173. McMillin K. Computed tomography of emphysematous cholecystitis. J Comput Assist Tomogr 1985;9:330.

174. Itai Y, Araki T, Yoshikawa K, et al. Computed tomography of gallbladder carcinoma. Radiology 1980;137:713.

175. Yeh H-C. Ultrasonography and computed tomography of carcinoma of the gallbladder. Radiology 1979;133:167.

176. Weiner SN, Koenigsberg M, Morehouse H, Hoffman J. Sonography and computed tomography in the diagnosis of carcinoma of the gallbladder. AJR Am J Roentgenol 1984;142:735.

177. Thorsen MK, Quiroz F, Lawson TL, et al. Primary biliary carcinoma: CT evaluation. Radiology 1984;152:479.

178. Engels JT, Balfe DM, Lee JKT. Biliary carcinoma: CT evaluation of extrahepatic spread. Radiology 1989;172:35.

179. Carroll BA. Gallstones: in vitro comparison of physical, radiographic, and ultrasonic characteristics. AJR Am J Roentgenol 1978;131:223.

180. Filly RA, Moss AA, Way LW. In vitro investigation of gallstone shadowing with ultrasound tomography. J Clin Ultrasound 1979;7:255.

181. Hickman MS, Schwesinger WH, Bova JD, Kurtin WE. Computed tomographic analysis of gallstones. Arch Surg 1986;121:289.

182. Baron RL, Rohrmann CA Jr, Lee SP, et al. CT evaluation of gallstones in vitro: correlation with chemical analysis. AJR Am J Roentgenol 1988;151:1123.

183. Baron RL, Kuyper SJ, Lee SP, et al. In vitro dissolution of gallstones with MTBE: correlation with characteristics at CT and MR imaging. Radiology 1989;173:117.

184. Barakos JA, Ralls PW, Lapin SA, et al. Cholelithiasis: evaluation with CT. Radiology 1987;162:415.

185. Rajagopal S, Bills P, Keightley A, et al. Predictive value of computed tomography (CT) scanning of the gall bladder in determining gall stone type. Gut 1988;29:A1487.

186. VanSonnenberg E, Casola G, Zakko SF, et al. Gallbladder and bile duct stones: percutaneous therapy with primary MTBE dissolution and mechanical methods. Radiology 1988;169:505.

187. Valette PJ, Barkun AN, Ponchon T, Cathignol D. Radiologic variables that determine the success of in vitro solitary gallstone lithotripsy. Radiology 1989;173(P):245.

188. Schulte SJ, Baron RL, Kuyper SJ. Piezoelectric biliary lithotripsy: factors affecting gallstone fragmentation. Radiology 1989;173(P):245.

189. Terrier F, Becker CD, Stoller C, Triller JK. Computed tomography in complicated cholecystitis. J Comput Assist Tomogr 1984;8:58.

190. Smathers R, Lee JKT, Heiken JP. Differentiation of complicated cholecystitis from gallbladder carcinoma by computed tomography. AJR Am J Roentgenol 1984;143:255.

191. Kane RA, Costello P, Duszlak E. Computed tomography in acute cholecystitis: new observations. AJR Am J Roentgenol 1983;141:697.

192. Jenkins PF, Golding RH, Cooperberg PL. Sonography and computed tomography of hemorrhagic cholecystitis. AJR Am J Roentgenol 1983;140:1197.

193. Nesbit GM, Johnson CD, James EM, et al. Cholangiocarcinoma: diagnosis and evaluation of resectability by CT and sonography as procedures complementary to cholangiography. AJR Am J Roentgenol 1988;151:933.

194. Dolmatch BL, Laing FC, Federle MP, et al. AIDS-related cholangitis: radiographic findings in nine patients. Radiology 1987;163:313.

195. Pedrosa CS, Casanova R, Lezana AH, Fernandez MC. Computed tomography in obstructive jaundice. Part II: the cause of obstruction. Radiology 1981;139:635.

196. Jeffrey RB Jr, Federle MP, Laing FC, et al. Computed tomography of choledocholithiasis. AJR Am J Roentgenol 1983;140:1179.

197. Baron RL. Common bile duct stones: reassessment of criteria for CT diagnosis. Radiology 1987;162:419.

198. Stephens DH, Hattery RR Jr, Sheedy PF. Computed tomography of the abdomen: early experience with the EMI body scanner. Radiology 1976;119:331.

199. Haaga RJ, Alfidi RJ, Zelch MG, et al. Computed tomography of the pancreas. Radiology 1977;120:589.

200. Hessel HJ, Siegelman SS, McNeil BJ, et al. A prospective evaluation of computed tomography and ultrasound of the pancreas. Radiology 1982;143:129.

201. Bernardino ME, Barnes PA. Imaging the pancreatic neoplasm. Cancer 1982;50:2681.

202. Heuck A, Mauback PA, Reiser M, et al. Age-related morphology of the normal pancreas on computed tomography. Gastrointest Radiol 1987;12:18.

203. Zeman RK, McVay LV, Silverman PM, et al. Pancreas divisum: thin-section CT. Radiology 1988;169:393.

204. Shah KK, DeRidder P, Schwab RE, Alexander TJ. CT diagnosis of dorsal pancreas agenesis. J Comput Assist Tomogr 1987;11:170.

205. Freeny PC, Marks WM, Ryan JA, Traverso LW. Pancreatic ductal adenocarcinoma: diagnosis and staging with dynamic CT. Radiology 1988;158:347.

206. Campbell JP, Wilson SR. Pancreatic neoplasms: how useful is evaluation with US? Radiology 1988;167:341.

207. Ormson MJ, Charboneau JW, Stephens DH. Sonography in patients with a possible pancreatic mass shown on CT. AJR Am J Roentgenol 1987;148:551.

208. Megibow AJ, Bosniak MA, Ambos MA, Beranbaum ER. Thickening of the celiac axis and/or superior mesenteric artery: a sign of pancreatic carcinoma on computed tomography. Radiology 1981;141:449.

209. Jafri SZH, Aisen AM, Glazer GM, Weiss CA. Comparison of CT and angiography in assessing resectability of pancreatic carcinoma. AJR Am J Roentgenol 1984;142:525.

210. Bok EJ, Cho KJ, Williams DM, et al. Venous involvement in islet cell tumors of the pancreas. AJR Am J Roentgenol 1984;142:319.

211. Eelkema EA, Stephens DH, Ward EM, Sheedy PF. CT features of nonfunctioning islet cell carcinoma. AJR Am J Roentgenol 1984;143:943.

212. Gunther RW, Klose KJ, Ruckert K, et al. Islet-cell tumors: detection of small lesions with computed tomography and ultrasound. Radiology 1983;1148:485.

213. Gunther RW, Klose KJ, Ruckert K, et al. Localization of small islet-cell tumors. Gastrointest Radiol 1985;10:145.

214. Wank SA, Doppman JL, Miller DL, et al. Prospective study of the ability of computed axial tomography to localize gastrinomas in patients with Zollinger-Ellison syndrome. Gastroenterology 1987;92:905.

215. Krudy AG, Doppman JL, Jensen RT, et al. Localization of islet cell tumors by dynamic CT: comparison with plain CT, arteriography, sonography, and venous sampling. AJR Am J Roentgenol 1984;143:585.

216. Rossi P, Baert A, Passariello R, et al. CT of functioning tumors of the pancreas. AJR Am J Roentgenol 1985;144:57.

217. Stark DD, Moss AA, Goldberg HI, Deveney CW. CT of pancreatic islet cell tumors. Radiology 1984;150:491.

218. Dunnick NR, Long JA Jr, Krudy AG, et al. Localizing insulinomas with combined radiographic methods. AJR Am J Roentgenol 1980;135:747.

219. Galiber AK, Reading CC, Charboneau JW, et al. Localization of pancreatic insulinoma: comparison of pre- and intraoperative US with CT and angiography. Radiology 1988;166:405.

220. Norton JA, Sugarbaker PH, Doppman JL, et al. Aggressive resection of metastatic disease in selected patients with malignant gastrinoma. Ann Surg 1986;203:352.

221. Frucht H, Doppman JL, Norton JA, et al. Gastrinomas: comparison of MR imaging with CT, angiography, and US. Radiology 1989;171:713.

222. Fink IJ, Krudy AG, Shawker TH, et al. Demonstration of an angiographically hypovascular insulinoma with intraarterial dynamic CT. AJR Am J Roentgenol 1985;144:555.

223. Merine DS, Fishman EK, Kuhlman JE, et al. CT angiographic evaluation of pancreatic islet cell tumors. Radiology 1989;173(P):318.

224. Warshaw A, Compton C, Lewandrowski K, et al. Cystic tumors of the pancreas: new clinical, radiologic, and pathologic observations in 67 patients. Ann Surg 1990;212:432.

225. Compagno J, Oertel JE. Microcystic adenomas of the pancreas (glycogen-rich cystadenomas). Am J Clin Pathol 1978;69:289.

226. Friedman AC, Lichtenstein JE, Dachman AH. Cystic neoplasms of the pancreas: radiological-pathological correlation. Radiology 1983;149:45.

227. Freeny PC, Lawson TL. Radiology of the pancreas. New York: Springer-Verlag, 1982:526.

228. Pandolfo I, Scribano E, Gaeta M, et al. Cystic lymphangioma of the pancreas: CT demonstration. J Comput Assist Tomogr 1985;9:209.

229. Itoh S, Ishiguchi T, Ishigaki T, et al. Mucin-producing pancreatic tumor: CT findings and histopathologic correlation. Radiology 1992;183:81.

230. Itai Y, Ohhashi K, Nagai H, et al. "Ductectatic" mucinous cystadenoma and cystadenocarcinoma of the pancreas. Radiology 1986;161:697.

231. Donovan PJ, Sanders RC, Siegelman SS. Collections of fluid after pancreatitis: evaluation by computed tomography and ultrasonography. Radiol Clin North Am 1982;20:653.

232. Mendez G Jr, Isikoff MB, Hill MC. CT of acute pancreatitis: interim assessment. AJR Am J Roentgenol 1980;135:463.

233. Hill MC, Barkin JS, Isikoff MB, et al. Acute pancreatitis: clinical vs. CT findings. AJR Am J Roentgenol 1982;139:263.

234. Williford ME, Foster WL, Halvorsen RA, Thompson WM. Pancreatic pseudocyst: comparative evaluation by sonography and computed tomography. AJR Am J Roentgenol 1983;140:53.

235. Nordestgaard AG, Wilson SE, Williams RA. Early computerized tomography as a predictor of outcome in acute pancreatitis. Am J Surg 1986;152:127.

236. Silverstein W, Isikoff MB, Hill MC, Barkin J. Diagnostic imaging of acute pancreatitis: prospective study using CT and sonography. AJR Am J Roentgenol 1981;137:497.

237. Balthazar EJ, Ranson JHC, Naidich DP, et al. Acute pancreatitis: prognostic value of CT. Radiology 1985;156:767.

238. Ranson JHC, Balthazar E, Caccavale R, Cooper M. Computed tomography and the prediction of pancreatic abscess in acute pancreatitis. Ann Surg 1985;201:656.

239. Balthazar EJ, Robinson DL, Megibow AJ, Ranson JHC. Acute pancreatitis: value of CT in establishing prognosis. Radiology 1990;174:331.

240. Vernacchia FS, Jeffrey RB Jr, Federle MP, et al. Pancreatic abscess: predictive value of early abdominal CT. Radiology 1987;162:435.

241. Jeffrey RB Jr, Federle MP, Laing FC. Computed tomography of mesenteric involvement in fulminant pancreatitis. Radiology 1983;147:185.

242. Dembner AG, Jaffe CC, Simeone J, Walsh J. New computed tomographic sign of pancreatitis. AJR Am J Roentgenol 1979;133:477.

243. Federle MP, Jeffrey RB Jr, Crass RA, van Dalsem V. Computed tomography of pancreatic abscesses. AJR Am J Roentgenol 1981;136:879.

244. Crass RA, Meyer AA, Jeffrey RB Jr, et al. Pancreatic abscess: impact of computerized tomography on early diagnosis and surgery. Am J Surg 1985;150:127.

245. Torres WE, Clements JL, Sones PJ, Knopf DR. Gas in the pancreatic bed without abscess. AJR Am J Roentgenol 1981;137:1131.

246. Alexander ES, Clark RA, Federle MP. Pancreatic gas: indication of pancreatic fistula. AJR Am J Roentgenol 1982;139:1089.

247. Ferrucci JT, Wittenberg J, Black EB, et al. Computed body tomography in chronic pancreatitis. Radiology 1979;130:

248. Karasawa E, Goldberg HI, Moss AA, et al. CT pancreatogram in carcinoma of the pancreas and chronic pancreatitis. Radiology 1983;148:489.

249. Maile CW, Crass JR, Frick MP, et al. CT of pancreas transplantation. Invest Radiol 1985;20:609.

Textbook of Gastroenterology, second edition, edited by Tadataka Yamada. JB Lippincott Company, Philadelphia © 1995.

CHAPTER 124

Magnetic Resonance Imaging

Edith H. Kang   Jeffrey J. Brown

Magnetic resonance (MR) imaging was developed from the theory of nuclear MR long used in the field of analytic chemistry. The first images of living humans were reported in 1977 by Damadian and associates.[1] Today MR imaging, because of its excellent soft tissue contrast and multiplanar capability, has become the next revolutionary phase in medical imaging following on the heels of ultrasonography and computed tomography (CT).

THEORETICAL CONSIDERATIONS

Image characteristics in MR imaging are described by signal intensity, which is roughly analogous to the terms *attenuation* or *density* in CT and echogenicity in ultrasonography (US). However, the factors that influence signal intensity are much more complex than those determining image contrast in conventional radiography. The following section explores some of these factors in a simplified manner. More extensive references on MR physics are available.[2-4]

The Proton

Magnetic resonance images are derived from hydrogen nuclei in the body. Any element with an odd number of protons or neutrons (unpaired nucleons) theoretically can produce a sig-

nal. Hydrogen is chosen for imaging because of its high MR sensitivity and its abundance in the body in both water and fat. The hydrogen nucleus consists of a single proton. This proton, when placed in an external magnetic field, acts like a tiny bar magnet (i.e., it possesses a magnetic dipole moment). For a group of protons placed in an external magnetic field, called B_0, slightly more than half become aligned in the direction of B_0; the remainder are aligned in the opposite direction. The net magnetization, however, is in the same direction as B_0 (Fig. 124-1). In reality the protons do not align exactly with B_0 but precess around it, much akin to a spinning top (Fig. 124-2).

Radiofrequency Pulses

When a radiofrequency (RF) pulse is applied at the appropriate frequency, called the resonant frequency, the protons absorb and release energy as a RF wave. The resonant frequency is determined by the rate of precession of the protons in the magnetic field. In turn, the rate of precession is proportional to the strength of the magnetic field. The RF signal emitted by the protons then is used to form the diagnostic image.

T1 and T2 Relaxation Times

The net equilibrium magnetization can be considered as a vector quantity with its direction aligned with B_0 in the longitudinal plane and its magnitude proportional to the strength

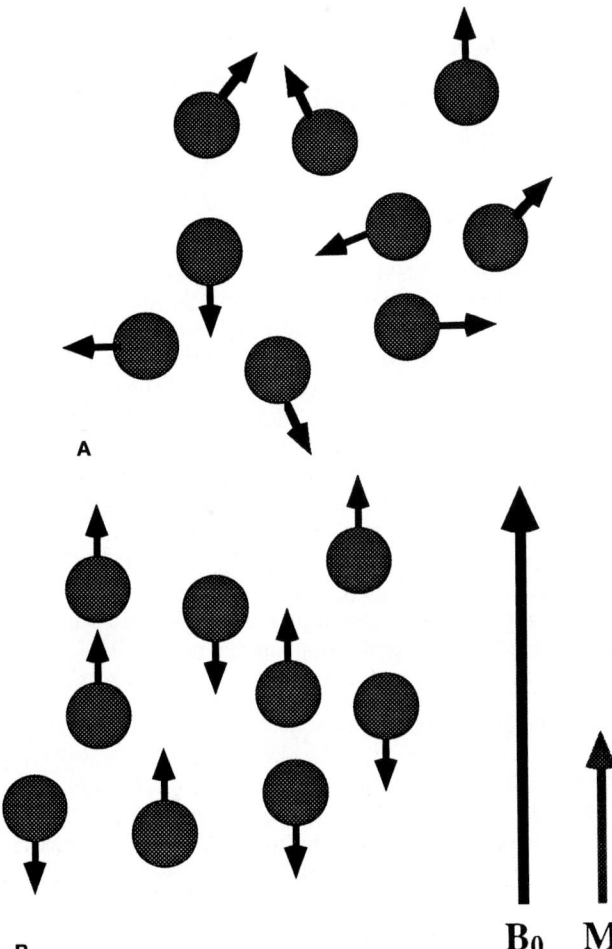

FIGURE 124-1. (**A**) Protons oriented randomly in space (**B**) act like tiny bar magnets when placed in an external magnetic field, B_0. Slightly more than one half of the protons become aligned in the direction of B_0; the remainder are aligned in the opposite direction. The net magnetization can be described by the vector quantity, M.

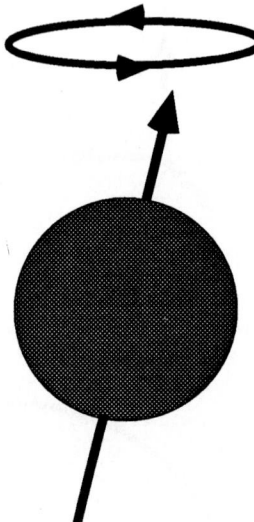

FIGURE 124-2. Protons precess around the direction of B_0 like a spinning top.

The rate of dephasing is described by the relaxation time T2 (Fig. 124-5).

Image Formation

Spatial localization is provided by the use of gradients that are additional magnetic fields superimposed on the main magnetic field B_0. There are gradients for the X, Y, and Z directions, each of which varies linearly from one end to the other. Slight differences in magnetic field strength from point to point are created by these gradients. Because the resonant frequency of a proton and its resultant RF signal are dependent on the magnetic field strength, the application of these gradients can be used to provide spatial localization to generate an image. The most common method of image reconstruction involves the two-dimensional Fourier transform.

Usually multiple acquisitions are required to produce adequate spatial resolution and adequate signal-to-noise levels

of B_0. The effect of an appropriate RF pulse is to tip the magnetization to some degree into the transverse plane. A 90-degree RF pulse tips the magnetization 90 degrees from the longitudinal or Z direction into the transverse or X-Y plane where signal can be measured (Fig. 124-3).

The net magnetization vector returns to equilibrium along the Z axis; in other words, longitudinal magnetization regrows or is recovered with time. The rate of recovery of longitudinal magnetization is exponential and is described by the longitudinal relaxation time T1 (Fig. 124-4). A second property of the magnetization vector after application of a 90-degree RF pulse is described by T2 relaxation. Once the vector has been tipped into the transverse plane, the transverse magnetization, like the individual protons that comprise it, precesses around the Z axis. The rate of precession of individual protons are influenced by slight imperfections in the homogeneity of the external magnetic field and by variations in the dipole-dipole interactions in different molecular environments experienced by different protons. The small magnetization vectors representing individual protons precess at different rates, resulting in dephasing and a loss in transverse magnetization.

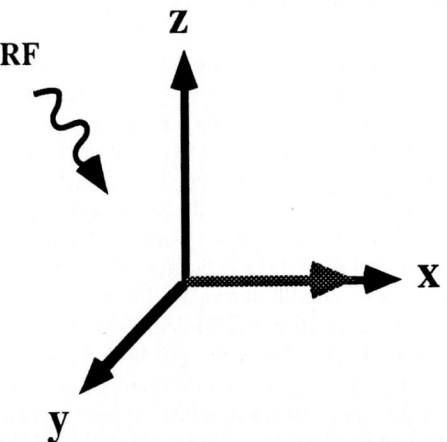

FIGURE 124-3. The application of a 90-degree radiofrequency pulse tips the magnetization vector M into the transverse plane.

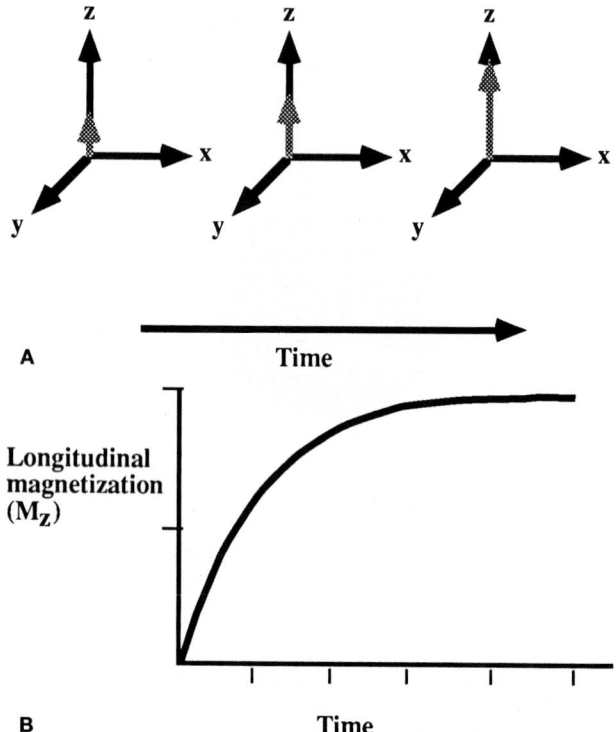

FIGURE 124-4. **(A)** With time, the net magnetization vector returns to equilibrium along the Z axis. **(B)** This rate of recovery can be described by the longitudinal relaxation time T1.

for diagnostic imaging. Imaging times for conventional MR imaging typically are longer than for CT. An sequence in MR imaging may last anywhere from a few seconds to more than 10 minutes. Consequently motion artifact from respiration, blood flow, peristalsis, and patient motion poses a significant problem and can degrade image quality. Advanced MR imaging techniques, such as echo planar imaging, acquire images in a fraction of a second, but these techniques are experimental and not yet in clinical use.

Image Contrast

T1 and T2 relaxation times, as well as the proton density of a given tissue, are the main intrinsic factors determining signal intensity. T1 and T2 can be thought of simplistically as having opposite effects: T1 relaxation is a process of recovery of longitudinal magnetization; T2 relaxation is a process of decay of transverse magnetization.[2] Tissues with a short T1 are bright whereas tissues with a short T2 are dark.

Other factors that determine the signal intensity of a given tissue can be controlled by the operator. These include the repetition time, TR, and the echo time, TE. TR is defined as the time between one 90-degree RF pulse and the next. TE is defined as the time from the 90-degree RF pulse to the time the signal is collected. The timing of both TR and TE affect the signal intensity displayed for different tissues. In standard spin echo (SE) pulse sequences, which are the most commonly used sequences in clinical imaging, a short TR (250–500 milliseconds) and a short TE (8–15 milliseconds) produce a T1-

weighted image. A long TR (>1500 milliseconds) and a long TE (>60 milliseconds) produce a T2-weighted image. A proton density or balanced image is produced by a long TR, allowing maximal T1 relaxation, and a short TE, allowing little T2 decay.

Pulse Sequences

Other commonly used pulse sequences include inversion recovery, gradient echo (GRE), and chemical shift imaging. Inversion recovery imaging provides excellent contrast between pathologic and normal tissue but is limited by a relatively long imaging time and limited number of slices available. GRE imaging can be used as a fast imaging method that can be performed during a breath hold, decreasing motion artifact. GRE sequences also are used in the evaluation of blood flow within vessels. Chemical shift imaging relies on the slight difference in the resonant frequency of protons in fat ($-CH_2-$) and protons in water (H_2O). With this technique, areas containing fat can be differentiated from surrounding tissue. New techniques allowing faster imaging times include fast SE and echoplanar imaging.

Tissue Contrast

On a standard SE T1-weighted pulse sequence, fat, which has a short T1 value, has the brightest signal. Liver is brighter (more hyperintense) than is the spleen and skeletal muscle.

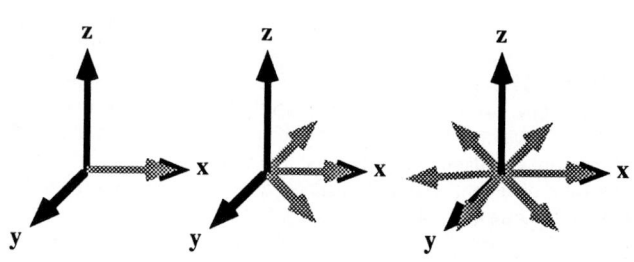

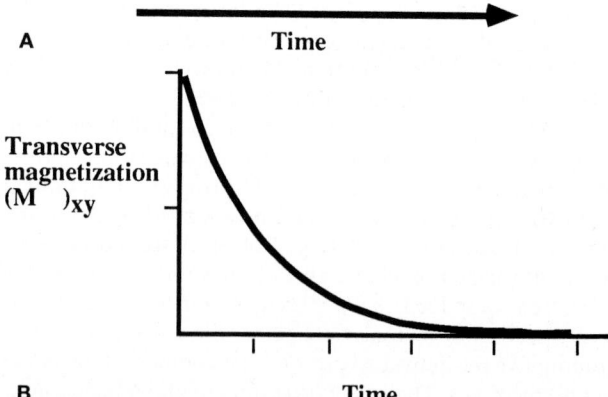

FIGURE 124-5. **(A)** Because protons precess at slightly different frequencies, with time the vector of each individual proton acquires a different phase resulting in a loss of phase coherence. **(B)** The rate of dephasing can be described by the relaxation time T2.

The pancreas is close in signal intensity to the liver or slightly darker (more hypointense). Intrahepatic bile ducts usually are not seen unless they are pathologically enlarged. Usually hepatic vessels appear darker than liver.

On a T2-weighted SE sequence, fluid, which has a long T2 value, has the brightest signal. Therefore cerebrospinal fluid, dilated bile ducts, and urine in the bladder all are bright. Fat is the next brightest tissue. On T2-weighted images, the spleen and pancreas have brighter signals than do the liver and skeletal muscle.

Many pathologic processes, both neoplastic and inflammatory, produce increased tissue water content. This results in an increase in both T1 and T2 relaxation times, and pathologic processes usually appear darker than a normal liver appears on T1-weighted images and brighter than a normal liver appears on T2-weighted images. The spleen can be used as a good internal standard for intrahepatic pathologic processes because many focal hepatic lesions follow the same signal intensity pattern as spleen on SE images.

Flowing blood can have a complex appearance but usually is dark on SE images. However, because of techniques used to reduce motion artifact from pulsating vessels, flowing blood can appear bright on T2-weighted images. Substances that can be hypointense on both T1- and T2-weighted images include air, calcium, cortical bone, and iron. Gadolinium (Gd) chelates (e.g., Gd-DTPA) are the only MR contrast agents approved for human use. These agents cause T1 shortening and, therefore, increased signal intensity of various tissues. They equilibrate rapidly with the extracellular fluid space in a manner similar to iodinated contrast materials used in CT.

Hemorrhage also has a complex appearance on SE images depending on many factors, including the age of the hematoma, the strength of the magnetic field, and the location of the hematoma. Hematomas in closed spaces such as the central nervous system evolve differently than those in spaces more accessible to macrophages such as the peritoneal cavity. Usually hyperacute hematomas appear similar to fluid, i.e., dark on T1-weighted images and bright on T2-weighted images. In subacute hematomas, the presence of methemoglobin causes T1 shortening and, hence, a bright signal. In chronic hematomas, the presence of hemosiderin causes low signal intensity on both T1- and T2-weighted images.

TECHNICAL FACTORS

Clinical MR scanners commonly range in magnetic field strength from 0.35 to 1.5 T. In contrast, the magnetic field of the earth is about 0.00006 T. Most clinical MR imaging units employ superconducting magnets requiring liquid helium to maintain temperatures adequate for superconductivity (about 4°K). The diameter of the bore of the imaging system varies but usually is in the range of 50 to 60 cm with a bore length of about 2 meters.

Surface coils can be used to increase the signal-to-noise ratio and improve image quality at the expense of field of view. A surface coil acts like a receiver antenna producing high signal intensity images from tissues close to the coil. Surface coils are commonly used for extremity and spine imaging but are rarely used in abdominal imaging because of their limited field of view.

CONTRAINDICATIONS AND RISKS

The major biologic effect of exposure to RF energy is heat deposition. The acceptable levels of RF power deposition are regulated by the Food and Drug Administration. Within these guidelines, no significant biologic effect has been demonstrated. The major risk of MR imaging is the magnet's effect on ferromagnetic objects both internal and external to the patient. Loose ferromagnetic objects can be accelerated toward the magnet, becoming dangerous projectiles. Cardiac pacemakers are an absolute contraindication to MR imaging because the strong external magnetic field interferes with the magnetic relays required for pacemaker function. In fact, pacemakers can be affected by a magnetic field as weak as 5 G (1T = 10,000 G). The presence of ferromagnetic cerebral aneurysm clips or cochlear implants also are absolute contraindications to MR imaging examination. Shrapnel located in vital positions (e.g., intraocular) is another contraindication to MR imaging. Most cardiac valves, most orthopedic devices, and noncerebral vascular clips are considered safe provided a sufficient period of time has elapsed for fixation of the device by scarring and fibrosis. More complete listings are available and should always be consulted if a question arises.[5]

During pregnancy, MR imaging can be performed if other nonirradiating diagnostic modalities such as US cannot answer the clinical question. Although no teratogenic effects from MR imaging have been shown, the full potential of possible effects of fetal exposure to strong magnetic fields and RF energy remain unexplored.

Finally, because of the small size of the imaging bore, 5% to 10% of patients will be claustrophobic. Oral or, occasionally, intravenous sedation may be necessary to allow the patient to complete the examination. Sedation or general anesthesia usually is required for infants and young children.

CLINICAL INDICATIONS

Use of MR imaging in the abdomen has lagged behind its use in the musculoskeletal and central nervous systems. This is partly because of image degradation in the abdomen from respiratory and bowel peristaltic motion artifacts. In addition, CT and US remain less expensive alternatives for abdominal imaging. However, MR is the best imaging technique for a few specific abdominal applications, and with the development of faster imaging pulse sequences and bowel- and organ-specific contrast agents, its role should continue to increase in importance in the future.

Standard SE pulse sequences have been the workhorse sequences for abdominal imaging. T1- and T2-weighted transaxial images, occasionally with coronal images, are widely used in abdominal imaging, although imaging in oblique planes can be useful in the evaluation of specific organs such as the pancreas. Fat saturation techniques can be added to increase the contrast range of tissues in the upper abdomen. Fast T1-weighted sequences are available to allow imaging during suspended respiration, which eliminates respiratory artifact. These sequences allow dynamic image acquisition during bolus injection of intravenous contrast agents similar to dynamic CT. GRE images are used for the evaluation of vascular anatomy and vessel patency. Flow direction also can be determined with this technique.

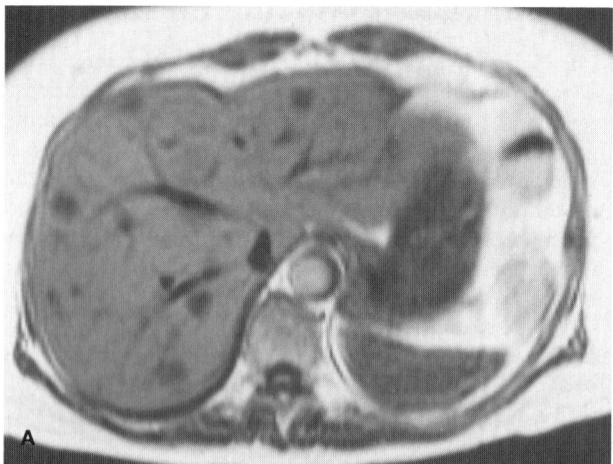
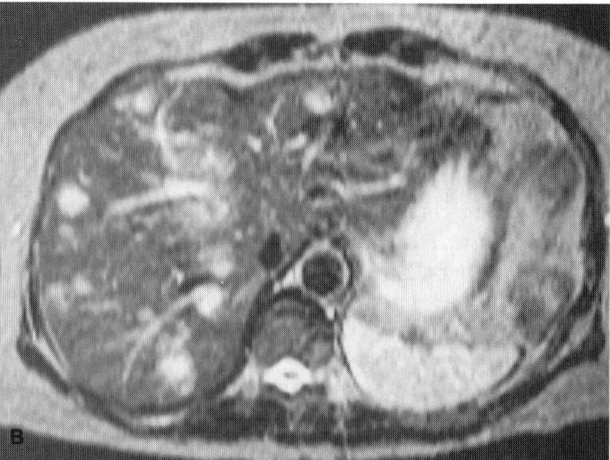

FIGURE 124-6. Multiple hepatic metastases in a patient with endometrial carcinoma are (**A**) hypointense compared with liver on the T1-weighted transaxial image and (**B**) hyperintense to liver on the T2-weighted image.

LIVER

In evaluating both focal and diffuse liver disease, MR imaging can be used. It has been used in the detection of primary and metastatic neoplasia, the characterization of focal hepatic lesions, the evaluation of hepatic vasculature, and the evaluation of preliver and postliver transplantation candidates.

Malignant Focal Hepatic Lesions

The liver is the most common site of metastatic disease in the abdomen. Because surgical resection can prolong survival in patients with certain types of malignancies such as adenocarcinoma of the colon, detecting the presence of metastatic disease and the specific size and location of focal metastases provides important information relating to treatment. MR imaging has been shown to be as or more sensitive than contrast-enhanced CT in the detection of focal hepatic lesions.[6,7] MR imaging is, however, less sensitive than CT with arterial portography, a more invasive procedure usually reserved for patients undergoing hepatic resection.

Most metastases have a higher water content than normal liver parenchyma and therefore appear darker than surrounding liver on T1-weighted images and brighter than liver on T2-weighted images (Fig. 124-6). The presence of irregular margins and lesion heterogeneity also are signs suggestive of malignancy.[8] A target appearance on T2-weighted images with a ring of brighter signal surrounding the lesion has been described as another sign of malignancy.[9] The ring of high signal is thought to represent edema in surrounding hepatic tissue.[10]

Hepatocellular carcinoma has a varied appearance on MR imaging. The lesion typically is hypointense compared with liver on T1-weighted images (Fig. 124-7); however, approx-

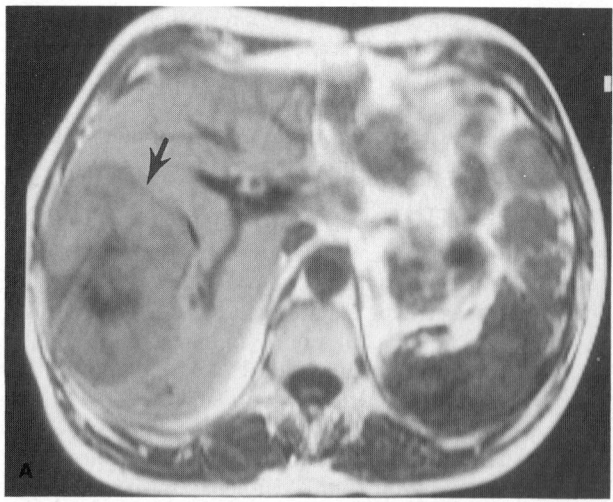
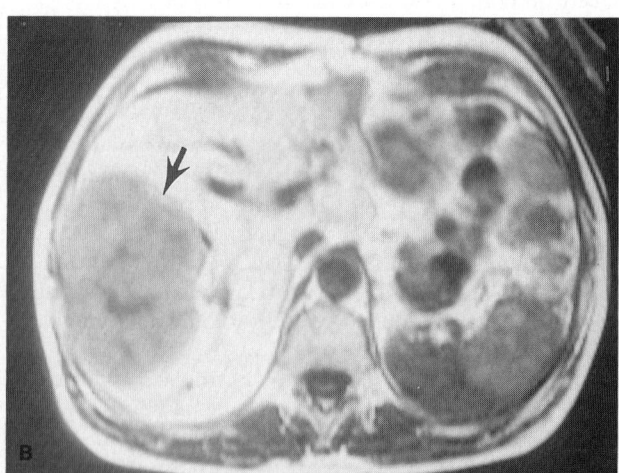

FIGURE 124-7. Transaxial T1-weighted images of the liver (**A**) before and (**B**) after the administration of manganese dipyridoxal diphosphate demonstrate a hypointense hepatocellular carcinoma in the right lobe of the liver (*arrows*).

imately one third of lesions demonstrate hyperintensity compared with liver.[11-13] The bright signal presumably is because of fatty degeneration, a feature that is commonly present in hepatocellular tumors. This may be a helpful sign to differentiate hepatocellular carcinoma from other focal hepatic lesions, which rarely are hyperintense with liver on T1-weighted images.[11,13] On T2-weighted images, hepatocellular carcinoma demonstrates increased signal intensity compared with normal liver. Other features commonly seen with hepatocellular carcinoma include a pseudocapsule that appears as a dark rim around the tumor mass on T1-weighted images, the presence of daughter nodules, and vascular invasion.

However, T1 and T2 values usually cannot be used to differentiate between different malignant cell types. Most primary and metastatic tumors have a similar appearance: hypointense on T1-weighted images and hyperintense on T2-weighted images compared with liver. In addition, the presence of necrosis or hemorrhage can alter the signal intensity of a lesion, and certain highly vascular metastases occasionally can mimic benign lesions such as cysts or hemangiomas.

The use of intravenous Gd-DTPA with fast pulse sequences allowing dynamic acquisition of images has been shown to increase both the sensitivity for detection of focal hepatic lesions, and the specificity of lesion characterization.[7,14,15] Usually metastases show irregular enhancement patterns (Fig. 124-8) compared with the more orderly centripetal enhancement pattern of benign cavernous hemangiomas, as discussed in the next section.

Benign Focal Hepatic Lesions

Simple cysts are common incidental findings in hepatic imaging. As on CT, cysts on MR imaging have a well-defined smooth border. Because cysts contain predominantly water, they are homogeneously hypointense compared with liver on T1-weighted images and markedly hyperintense on T2-weighted images, i.e., brighter than the spleen. The signal intensity of a simple cyst follows the signal of cerebrospinal fluid in the spinal canal, which is a useful marker for the behavior of water on almost any MR pulse sequence of the abdomen. Also, as on CT, cysts on MR imaging do not enhance after administration of intravenous contrast material (Fig. 124-9). Complicated cysts containing hemorrhage or having a high protein content can appear bright on T1-weighted images. US may be helpful in confirming the presence of a cyst when it does not follow these expected criteria or when the lesion is small enough that volume averaging with adjacent liver may artificially change the signal intensity of the lesion.

Hemangiomas are the most common benign hepatic neoplasms, present in 7.3% of the population in autopsy studies.[16] Therefore it is clinically important to be able to differentiate benign cavernous hemangiomas from metastases. Technetium Tc 99m–labeled red blood cell scanning with single photon emission CT traditionally has had the highest specificity for hemangiomas larger than 2 to 3 cm. However, MR imaging has been found to have an accuracy rate of about 90% for differentiating metastases from cavernous hemangiomas.[9,16]

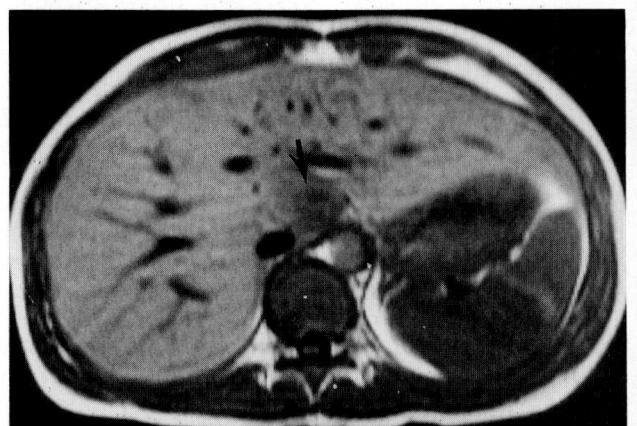

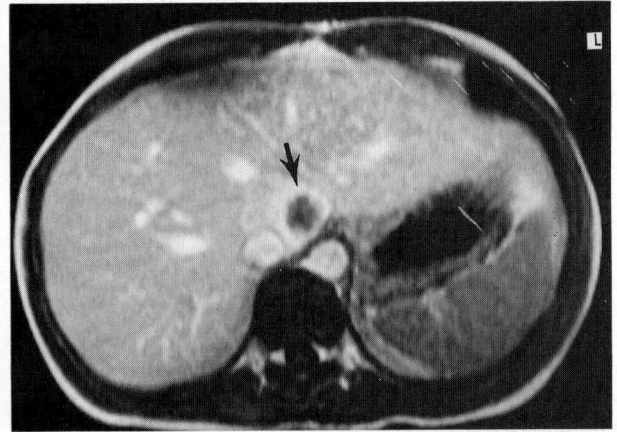

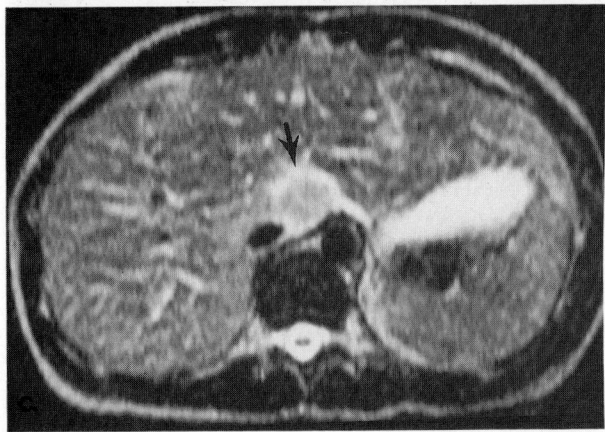

FIGURE 124-8. T1-weighted transaxial images of the liver (**A**) before and (**B**) after the administration of intravenous gadolinium-DTPA demonstrate irregular enhancement of a metastatic lesion (*arrow*) in a patient with cervical carcinoma. (**C**) The T2-weighted transaxial image demonstrates the target appearance typical of metastatic lesions (*arrow*).

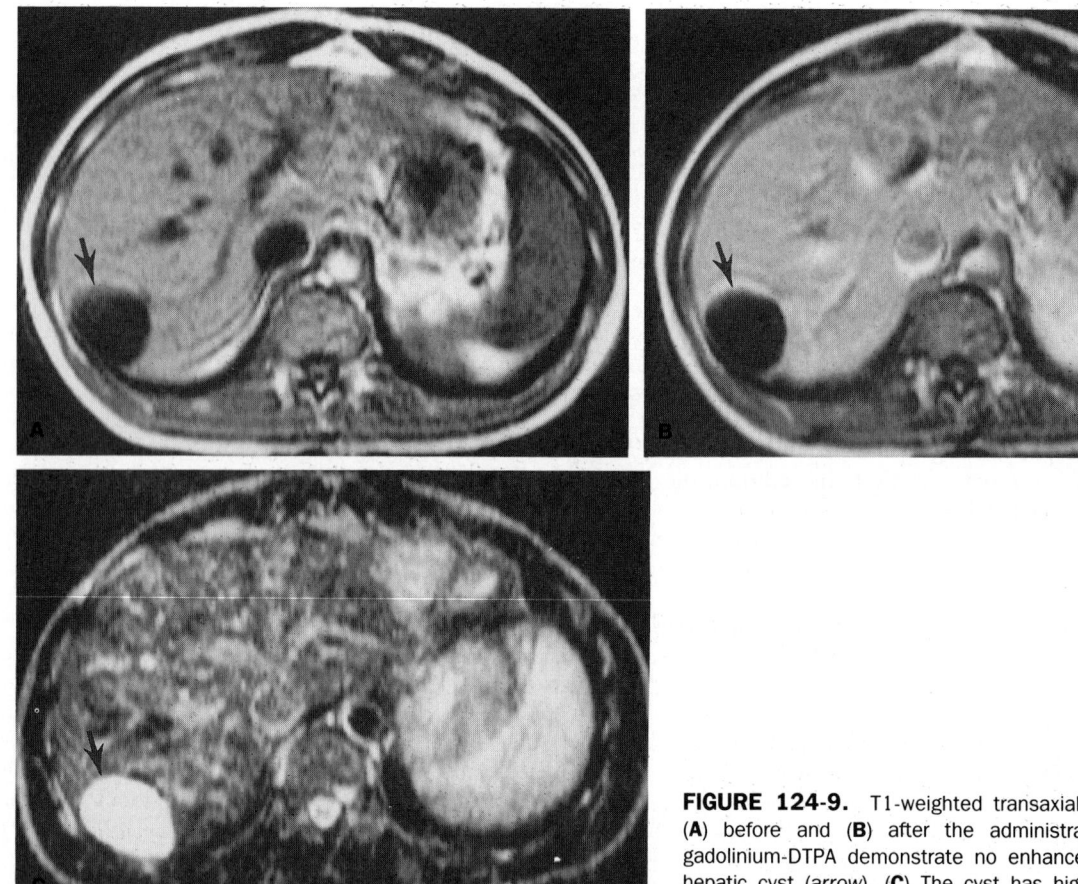

FIGURE 124-9. T1-weighted transaxial images of the liver (**A**) before and (**B**) after the administration of intravenous gadolinium-DTPA demonstrate no enhancement of the simple hepatic cyst (*arrow*). (**C**) The cyst has high signal intensity on the T2-weighted image (*arrow*), which is consistent with fluid.

The addition of intravenous Gd-DTPA with dynamic imaging should increase the specificity of MR imaging for characterization of cavernous hemangiomas.[15]

Cavernous hemangiomas appear as well-circumscribed masses, often with lobulated margins, and are homogeneous in signal intensity. The lesions are hypointense compared with liver on T1-weighted images and become brighter relative to liver parenchyma on more heavily T2-weighted images. On proton density–weighted images, cavernous hemangiomas are isointense or slightly hyperintense compared with liver in contrast to simple cysts, which mimic CSF and are, therefore, hypointense compared with liver. After the administration of intravenous Gd-DTPA, cavernous hemangiomas enhance as they do on dynamic CT with iodinated contrast. The lesions show peripheral enhancement early with concentric filling-in from periphery to center on subsequent images, reaching isointensity or hyperintensity compared with liver on later scans (Fig. 124-10). Large lesions, as on CT, may not enhance completely because of the presence of central scarring or thrombosis.

Focal nodular hyperplasia classically appears homogeneous and isointense with liver on both T1- and T2-weighted pulse sequences. The lesion commonly has a central scar that is most often hyperintense on T2-weighted images.[17-19] Focal nodular hyperplasia enhances early after intravenous gadolinium administration during the hepatic arterial phase of enhancement; the central scar typically enhances several minutes

later. However, focal nodular hyperplasia does not have the classic appearance in up to 50% of cases.[19] Atypical features include lack of a central scar, hypointensity of the scar on T2-weighted images, and increased signal intensity compared with liver on T2-weighted images. In addition, other hepatic tumors such as hepatic adenoma, hepatocellular carcinoma (especially the fibrolamellar subtype), and giant cavernous hemangioma also may have a central scar. Therefore the MR appearance of focal nodular hyperplasia is not specific enough to preclude biopsy in individual cases. Hepatic adenoma is another benign tumor that has a nonspecific appearance on MR imaging and can be indistinguishable from malignancy.[11]

Fatty Infiltration

Fatty infiltration of the liver on CT causes decreased attenuation compared with normal liver. When fatty infiltration is focal, the area of low attenuation can be difficult to distinguish from neoplasm. Although fatty infiltration on SE MR images occasionally appears as an area of relative hyperintensity, standard SE images are relatively insensitive to fatty infiltration, allowing the differentiation between fatty infiltration and neoplasm to be made more easily. One of the reasons for this relative insensitivity is believed to be that fatty infiltration often is accompanied by inflammatory changes that cause increased water content (e.g., alcoholic hepatitis).

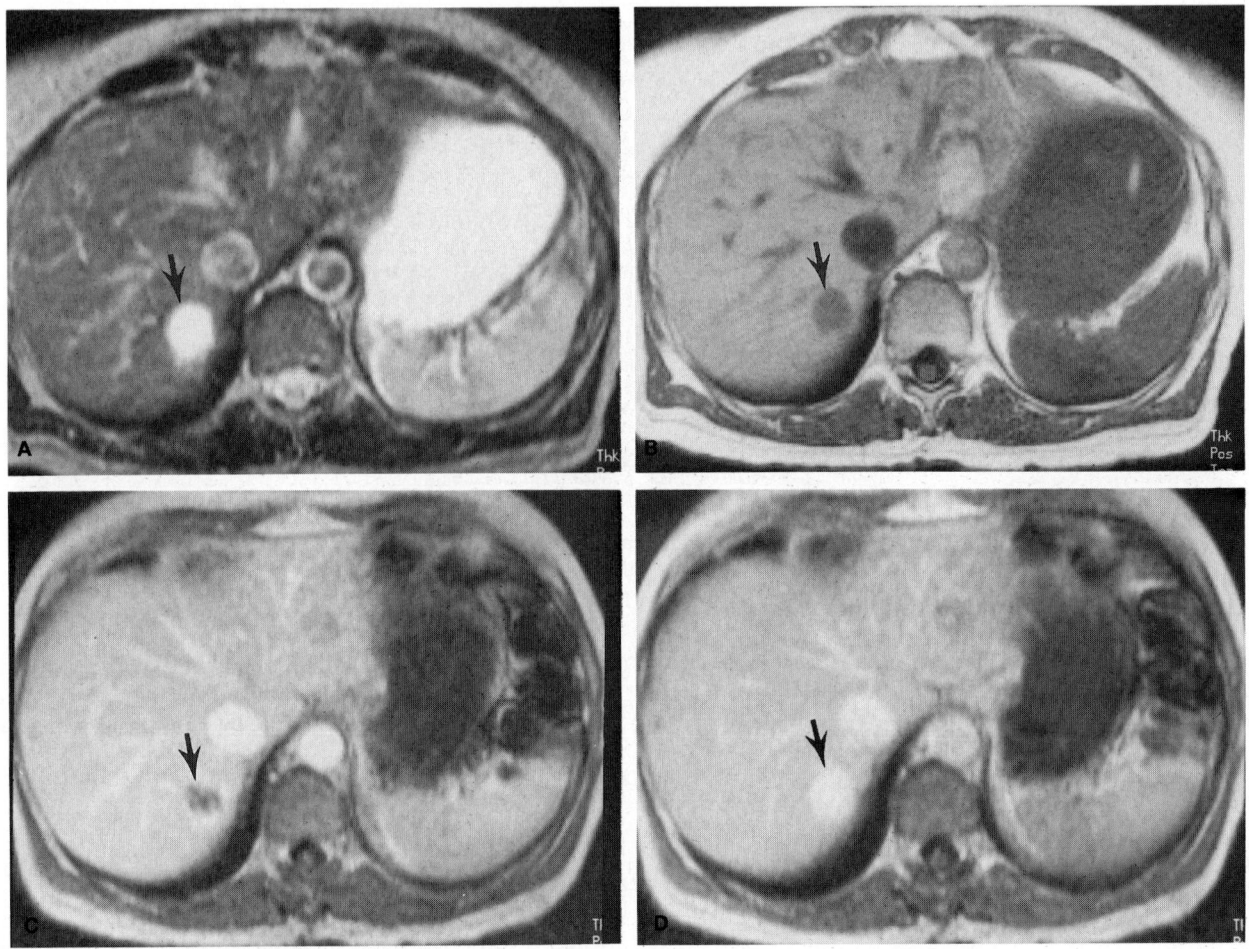

FIGURE 124-10. (**A**) Transaxial T2-weighted image of the liver shows a lesion in the right lobe of the liver with markedly hyperintense signal (*arrow*). T1-weighted transaxial images (**B**) before and sequentially (**C, D**) after the administration of intravenous gadolinium-DTPA demonstrate the classic centripetal enhancement pattern seen with cavernous hemangiomas (*arrows*). In **D** the final image shows complete, homogeneous enhancement of the hemangioma.

The T1 shortening caused by extra fat is, therefore, canceled out by the T1 lengthening of extra water, resulting in no significant change in overall signal intensity.[9,20]

The use of chemical shift imaging allows further confirmation of the presence of fatty infiltration. By using chemical shift techniques, images can be obtained when water and fat protons are 180 degrees out of phase. Therefore any volume of tissue that contains both water and fat will be dark. Fatty infiltration appears hypointense relative to normal liver on *opposed phase* chemical shift images and isointense or hyperintense to liver on conventional *in-phase* T1-weighted images (Fig. 124-11).[20,21]

Idiopathic Hemochromatosis and Hemosiderosis

The deposition of iron as hemosiderin in idiopathic hemochromatosis as well as in hemosiderosis results in marked T2 shortening. This results in decreased signal in the affected hepatic parenchyma that is more pronounced on T2-weighted images and GRE images. Detectable signal intensity changes occur with as little as 1.2 mg of iron per gram of tissue.[22,23] However, attempts to quantify iron content within the liver have not been successful clinically.[9]

In primary or idiopathic hemochromatosis, multiple organs are affected including liver, pancreas, and heart, all of which are hypointense on T2-weighted images. The spleen, however, usually is spared. In secondary hemochromatosis or hemosiderosis, excess iron is deposited in the reticuloendothelial system, and the spleen also shows the effects of T2 shortening (Fig. 124-12).

Cirrhosis

The characteristic morphologic changes of cirrhosis are demonstrated by MR imaging (Fig. 124-13). These include a nodular contour, small right hepatic lobe, and prominence of the caudate and left hepatic lobes. Ascites often is present in patients with cirrhosis and is seen as decreased signal intensity on T1-weighted images and increased signal intensity on T2-

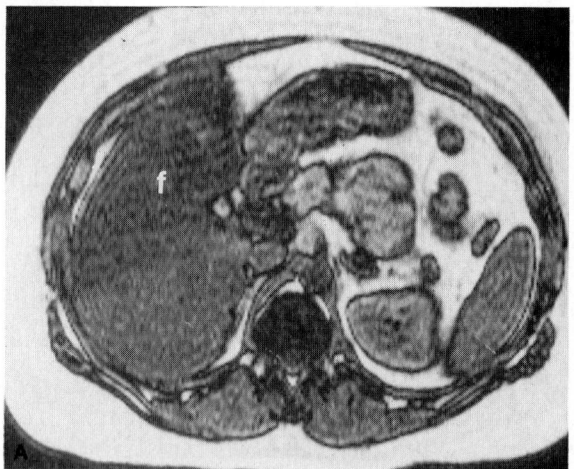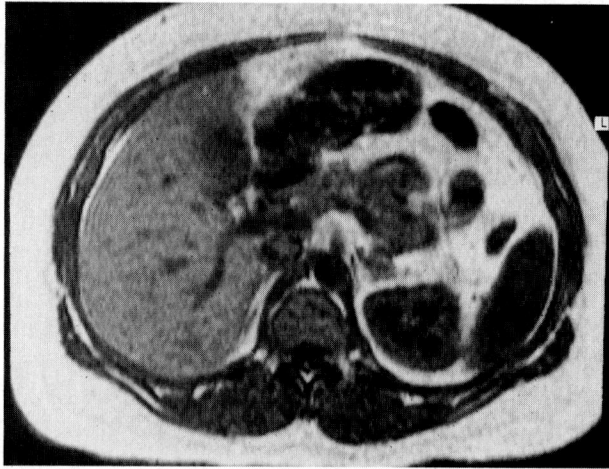

FIGURE 124-11. Transaxial (**A**) opposed-phase chemical shift image of the liver demonstrates a segmental area of decreased signal consistent with increased hepatic fat (f) when compared with (**B**) the in-phase image in a patient with fatty infiltration after chemotherapy for bronchogenic carcinoma.

weighted images surrounding the liver. Degenerating nodules can be seen as low-intensity nodules on T2-weighted images because of their iron content.[22]

Vascular Disease of the Liver

Hepatic veins can be evaluated for patency using SE and GRE images. MR imaging of patients with Budd-Chiari syndrome demonstrates small or absent hepatic veins, constriction of the intrahepatic portion of the inferior vena cava, and small comma-shaped intrahepatic collateral vessels.[23]

The portal vein also can be evaluated for patency and flow direction using GRE imaging (Fig. 124-14). MR imaging demonstrates venous collaterals[24] and portal vein occlusion, both of which can be seen in patients with portal venous hypertension. Invasion of the portal vein by tumor can be evaluated as well. Portosystemic shunts can be evaluated for patency. However, shunts with a high metal content or those associated with steel embolization coils cannot be evaluated by MR imaging. The metal creates a signal void, obscuring the region of the shunt (Fig. 124-15).[25]

Liver Transplantation

At many centers MR imaging is used to evaluate potential candidates for liver transplantation. Portal and hepatic venous anatomy and vessel patency can be determined without submitting the patient to the risks and discomfort of conventional angiography.[26] In addition, the liver can be examined for focal hepatic lesions such as hepatocellular carcinoma, and the host liver volume can be calculated. At the Mallinckrodt Institute of Radiology in St. Louis, MR imaging has replaced CT and US in the evaluation of preliver transplant candidates.

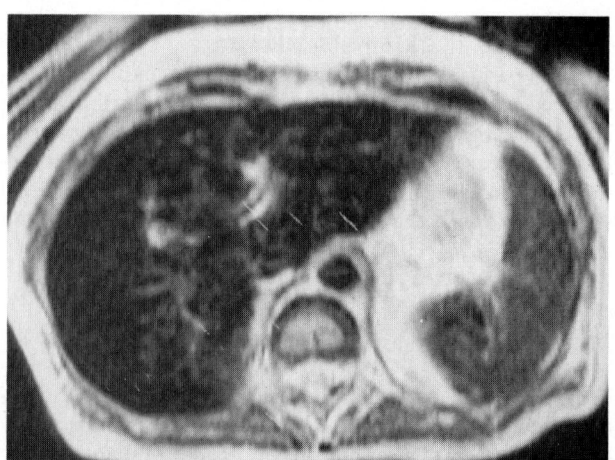

FIGURE 124-12. Transaxial T2-weighted image of the abdomen demonstrates diffusely decreased signal intensity in the liver and spleen in a patient with secondary hemochromatosis.

Hepatic Contrast Agents

Hepatic contrast agents can be classified into three major categories: extracellular agents, particulate agents, and liver-specific agents. Gd-DTPA is the prototype extracellular contrast agent and acts similarly to iodinated contrast material in CT. Particulate agents include superparamagnetic iron oxide particles that are taken up by the reticuloendothelial system and cause decreased signal intensity of normal hepatic parenchyma on T2-weighted and GRE images. This increases the conspicuousness of focal hepatic malignancies that do not contain Kupffer's cells.[27,28] Liver-specific agents include manganese dipyridoxal diphosphate (Mn-DPDP), which is taken up specifically by hepatocytes. Mn-DPDP causes T1 shortening, resulting in increased signal intensity of normal liver parenchyma on T1-weighted images and greater conspicuousness of focal liver lesions, which usually are hypointense.[27,29] Iron oxide particulate agents and Mn-DPDP are undergoing clinical trials.

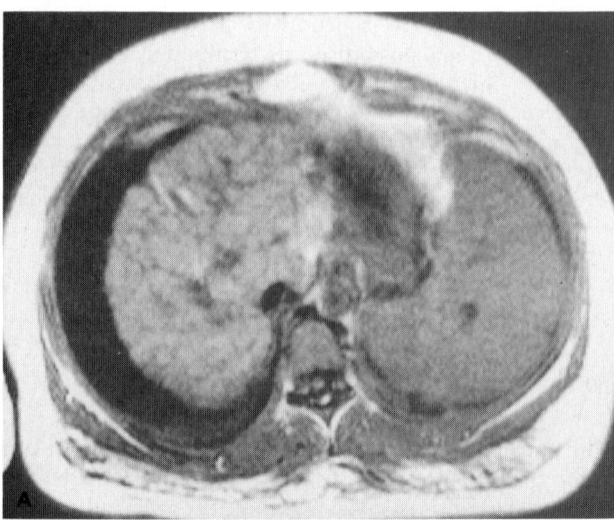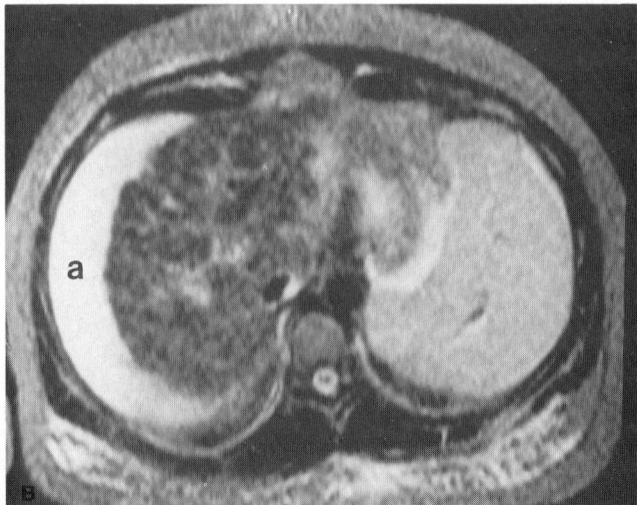

FIGURE 124-13. Transaxial (**A**) T1- and (**B**) T2-weighted images of the liver in a patient with cirrhosis demonstrating a small liver with a nodular contour and associated splenomegaly. The bright signal on the T2-weighted image surrounding the liver is ascitic fluid (a).

BILIARY SYSTEM

Dilated bile ducts demonstrate decreased signal intensity on T1-weighted images and increased signal intensity on T2-weighted images compared with the surrounding liver or pancreas. Occasionally dilated bile ducts may be difficult to distinguish from adjacent portal vessels on SE images; in these cases, GRE images demonstrating blood flow can be helpful in distinguishing the two structures.

The appearance of the gallbladder depends on the concentration of the bile. Concentrated bile found in fasting patients appears hyperintense compared with liver on T1- and T2-weighted images. Fresh bile found in nonfasting patients, however, behaves like water, i.e., hypointense on T1-weighted images and hyperintense on T2-weighted images. T1 short-

ening occurs in concentrated bile because of an increase in the proportion of water molecules bound to macromolecules.[30] Gallstones appear hypointense on all sequences because of their solid nature.

Cholangiocarcinoma appears as a soft tissue mass of decreased signal intensity compared with liver on T1-weighted images and increased signal intensity on T2-weighted images, similar to other malignant disease in the liver (Fig. 124-16). An early study demonstrated that MR imaging was equivalent to CT in defining the extent of cholangiocarcinoma, although CT better demonstrated the intrahepatic biliary ductal dilatation.[31]

The role of MR imaging in the evaluation of the biliary system still is evolving. US still is the screening examination of choice in the evaluation of patients with suspected biliary

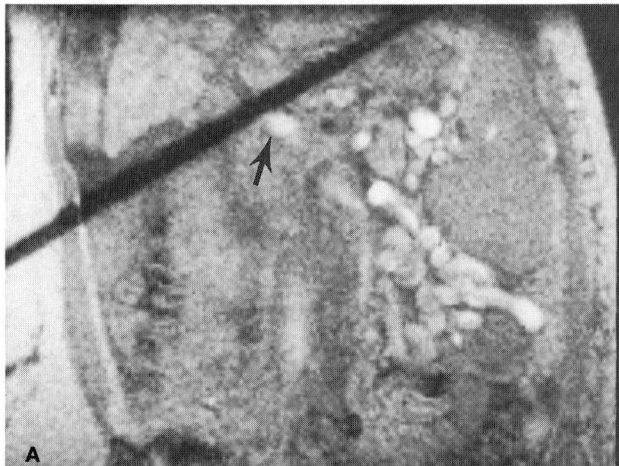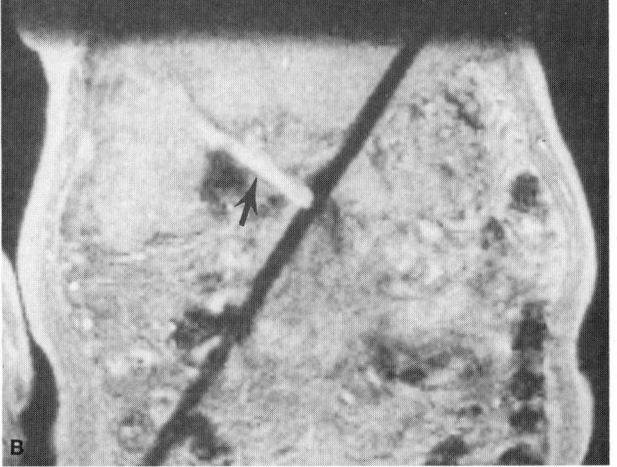

FIGURE 124-14. Coronal gradient echo images through the portal vein are obtained with a presaturation band to eliminate flow within hepatic arteries. A second presaturation band is placed perpendicular to the portal vein to determine flow direction. (**A**) Image demonstrates hepatopetal portal venous flow (*arrow*) in a patient with cirrhosis with numerous venous collaterals. (**B**) Image demonstrates hepatofugal flow (*arrow*) in a patient with alcoholic cirrhosis.

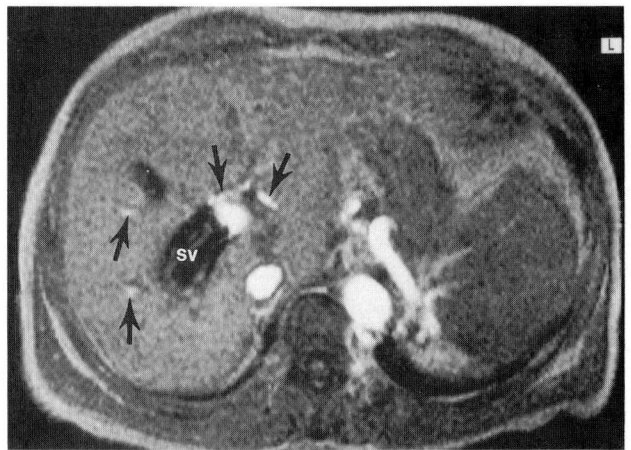

FIGURE 124-15. Transaxial gradient echo image of the liver demonstrates high signal intensity from flowing blood within hepatic vessels (*arrows*). Metal in the patient's transjugular intrahepatic portosystemic shunt causes a signal void (SV), obscuring this region of the liver.

disease. However, new sequences involving GRE imaging with three-dimensional postprocessing techniques are being evaluated for biliary imaging.[32] This method allows cholangiographic-type images to be produced in patients with obstructive jaundice without the risks of endoscopic retrograde cholangiopancreatography or percutaneous transhepatic cholangiography and may change the role of MR imaging in evaluating the biliary system in the future (Fig. 124-17).

PANCREAS

Inflammatory Disease

The morphologic changes in acute pancreatitis on MR imaging are similar to those seen on CT. These include enlargement of the pancreas, indistinctness of the pancreatic borders, edema in the peripancreatic fat, and the presence of peripancreatic fluid collections. Fluid collections and edema are hypointense on T1-weighted images and hyperintense on T2-

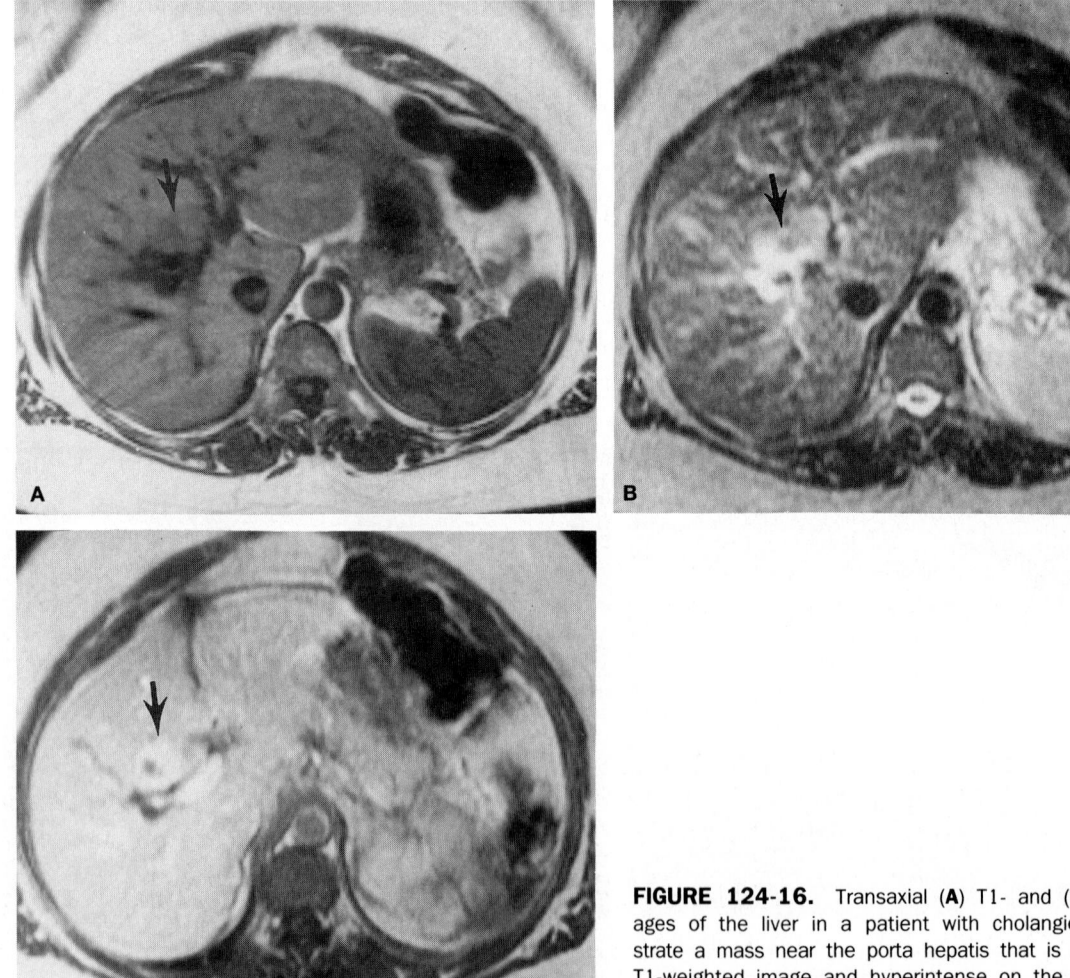

FIGURE 124-16. Transaxial (**A**) T1- and (**B**) T2-weighted images of the liver in a patient with cholangiocarcinoma demonstrate a mass near the porta hepatis that is hypointense on the T1-weighted image and hyperintense on the T2-weighted image (*arrows*). (**C**) The lesion shows irregular enhancement after administration of intravenous gadolinium-DTPA.

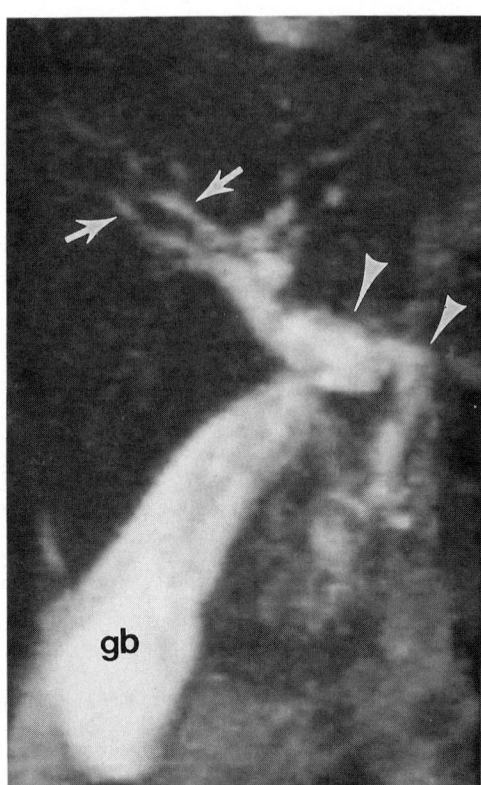

FIGURE 124-17. Coronal cholangiographic magnetic resonance image in a patient with ampullary stenosis demonstrates dilated intrahepatic (*arrows*) and extrahepatic (*arrowheads*) bile ducts and a distended gallbladder (gb).

weighted images. The pancreas itself may demonstrate hypointensity on T1-weighted images and hyperintensity on T2-weighted images when acutely inflamed.

In chronic pancreatitis, the pancreas may be hypointense on T1-weighted images. Pancreatic ductal dilatation can be seen. In addition, decreased enhancement after Gd-DTPA administration has been described.[33] Pancreatic calcification appears dark on all pulse sequences and is more difficult to identify than on CT. Focal chronic pancreatitis also can be impossible to differentiate from adenocarcinoma without biopsy.[34]

Pancreatic pseudocysts appear as well-defined areas of hypointensity on T1-weighted images and marked hyperintensity on T2-weighted images, paralleling the appearance of cerebrospinal fluid in the spinal canal. Complicated pseudocysts, however, can have variable signal intensities depending on the presence of proteinaceous material or hemorrhage. Pseudocyst images are not enhanced by administration of intravenous Gd-DTPA.

Neoplasm

Pancreatic adenocarcinoma is seen as a hypointense mass compared with normal pancreatic parenchyma on T1-weighted images (Fig. 124-18). Its appearance on T2-weighted images is variable; hypointense, isointense, and hyperintense

tumors all have been described.[34,35] Complications of carcinoma including encasing of vascular structures, local invasion, and lymphadenopathy all can be seen with MR imaging. Islet cell tumors also are hypointense on T1-weighted images compared with normal parenchyma, but can be markedly hyperintense on T2-weighted images. However, it is usually impossible to distinguish between islet cell tumors from adenocarcinoma on the basis of imaging characteristics alone.[34]

Early studies stated that MR imaging had no specific advantages over CT in the evaluation of pancreatic neoplasms.[35] However, with the development of faster imaging techniques and the use of intravenous Gd-DTPA contrast enhancement and fat suppression techniques, several authors have suggested that MR imaging is at least as accurate as CT and may be superior to CT in staging pancreatic cancer.[33,34] MR imaging certainly is helpful in cases where iodinated contrast for CT is contraindicated and in situations in which CT is unable to answer the clinical question.

SPLEEN

Standard SE imaging of splenic pathologic features is limited by the fact that most neoplasms have T1 and T2 relaxation times similar to the spleen. In addition, respiratory motion artifact can compromise image quality. Therefore focal splenic lesions have been traditionally more difficult to identify on SE MR imaging than on CT.[36] More recent experience, however, with faster imaging techniques performed during suspended respiration and the use of intravenous Gd-DTPA has increased the sensitivity of MR imaging for the detection of splenic abnormalities.[37]

BOWEL

Magnetic resonance imaging of the gastrointestinal tract is limited by peristalsis leading to motion artifact and by the lack of an inexpensive gastrointestinal contrast agent. Perflubron is the only approved gastrointestinal contrast agent.

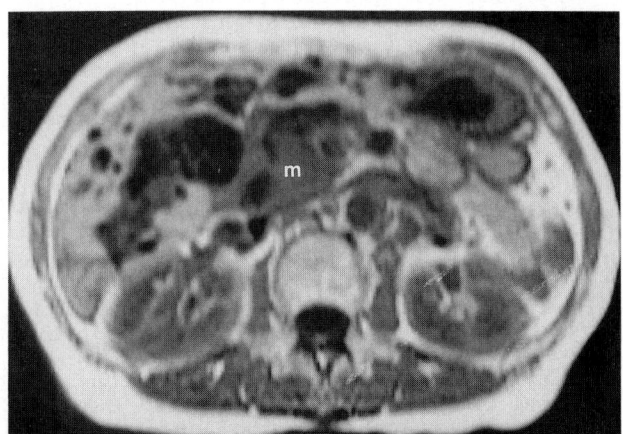

FIGURE 124-18. Transaxial T1-weighted image of the pancreas demonstrates a large hypoechoic mass (m) in the head of the pancreas in this patient with adenocarcinoma.

Several other oral MR contrast agents are under investigation. These agents help distinguish bowel from surrounding structures in the abdomen and clarify visualization of the bowel wall. Oral contrast agents may produce either *negative contrast*, showing decreased signal intensity within the bowel lumen, or *positive contrast*, causing increased intralumenal signal. Substances such as kaolin compounds,[38] Gd-DTPA,[39] solutions of magnetic particles,[40,41] barium,[42] and perfluorocarbon liquids[43] are under investigation. Glucagon can be administered to decrease bowel peristalsis.[43] Early clinical studies have suggested a role for MR imaging in the evaluation of inflammatory bowel disease and its complications,[44,45] but its precise role in gastrointestinal imaging has yet to be determined.

CLINICAL IMPLICATIONS

Although CT is still more commonly used as the first-line imaging modality for neoplastic disease in the liver, MR imaging is at least as sensitive as CT for detecting focal hepatic lesions and should replace CT in patients with contraindications to iodinated contrast material, such as contrast allergy or renal insufficiency. MR imaging is also used as a problem-solving modality when CT or US are nondiagnostic. In the remainder of the abdomen, the role of MR imaging still is evolving. Faster imaging techniques and organ-specific contrast agents should increase the applications of MR imaging in the rest of the abdomen in the future.

> The reader is directed to Chapter 114, General Considerations, and Chapter 120, Cross-Sectional Anatomy.

REFERENCES

1. Damadian R, Goldsmith M, Minkoff L. Fonar image of the live human body. Physiol Chem Phys Med NMR 1977;9:97.
2. Hendrick RE, Kanal E, Osborn AG. Basic MR physics. In: Kressel HY, Modic MT, Murphy WA, eds. Syllabus special course: MRI 1990. Oakbrook, IL: RSNA Publications, 1990:7.
3. Edelman RR, Kleefield J, Wentz KU, et al. Basic principles of magnetic resonance imaging. In: Edelman RR, Hesselink JR, eds. Clinical magnetic resonance imaging. Philadelphia: WB Saunders, 1990:3.
4. Curry TS, Dowdey JE, Murry RC, Christensen EE. Christensen's physics of diagnostic radiology. 4th ed. Philadelphia: Lea and Febiger, 1990.
5. Shellock FG, Curtis JS. MR imaging and biomedical implants, material, and devices: an updated review. Radiology 1991;180: 541.
6. Heiken JP, Weyman PJ, Lee JKT, et al. Detection of focal hepatic masses: prospective evaluation with CT, delayed CT, CT during arterial portography, and MR imaging. Radiology 1989;171:47.
7. Semelka RC, Shoenut JP, Kroeker MA, et al. Focal liver disease: comparison of dynamic contrast-enhanced CT and T2-weighted fat-suppressed, FLASH, and dynamic gadolinium-enhanced MR imaging at 1.5 T. Radiology 1992;184:687.
8. Brown JJ, Lee JM, Lee JKT, et al. Focal hepatic lesions: differentiation with MR imaging at 0.5 T. Radiology 1991;179:675.
9. Mattrey R, Trambert M, Edelman RR. MR imaging of the upper abdomen and adrenal glands. In: Edelman RR, Hesselink JR, eds. Clinical magnetic resonance imaging. Philadelphia: WB Saunders, 1990:860.
10. Lee MJ, Saini S, Compton CC, et al. MR demonstration of edema adjacent to a liver metastasis: pathologic correlation. AJR Am J Roentgenol 1991;157:499.
11. Rummeny E, Weissleder R, Stark DD, et al. Primary liver tumors: diagnosis by MR imaging. AJR Am J Roentgenol 1989;152:63.
12. Itoh K, Nishimura K, Togashi K, et al. Hepatocellular carcinoma: MR imaging. Radiology 1987;164:21.
13. Rosenthal RE, Davis PL. MR imaging of hepatocellular carcinoma at 1.5 Tesla. Gastrointest Radiol 1992;17:49.
14. Schmiedl U, Kolbel G, Hess CF, et al. Dynamic sequential MR imaging of focal liver lesions: initial experience in 22 patients at 1.5 T. J Comput Assist Tomogr 1990;14:600.
15. Hamm B, Fischer E, Taupitz M. Differentiation of hepatic hemangiomas from metastases by dynamic contrast-enhanced MR imaging. J Comput Assist Tomogr 1990;14:205.
16. Birnbaum BA, Weinreb JC, Megibow AJ, et al. Definitive diagnosis of hepatic hemangiomas: MR imaging versus Tc-99m-labeled red blood cell SPECT. Radiology 1990;176:95.
17. Mattison GR, Glazer GM, Quint LE, et al. MR imaging of hepatic focal nodular hyperplasia: characterization and distinction from primary malignant hepatic tumors. AJR Am J Roentgenol 1987;148:711.
18. Mathieu D, Rahmouni A, Anglade M, et al. Focal nodular hyperplasia of the liver: assessment with contrast-enhanced turboFLASH MR imaging. Radiology 1991;180:25.
19. Vilgrain V, Flejou J, Arrive L, et al. Focal nodular hyperplasia of the liver: MR imaging and pathologic correlation in 37 patients. Radiology 1992;184:699.
20. Kreft BP, Tanimoto A, Baba Y, et al. Diagnosis of fatty liver with MR imaging. J Magn Reson Imag 1992;2:463.
21. Heiken JP, Lee JKT, Dixon WT. Fatty infiltration of the liver: evaluation by proton spectroscopic imaging. Radiology 1985;157:707.
22. Murakami T, Kuroda C, Marukawa T, et al. Regenerating nodules in hepatic cirrhosis: MR findings with pathologic correlation. AJR Am J Roentgenol 1990;155:1227.
23. Stark DD, Hahn PF, Trey C, et al. MRI of the Budd-Chiari syndrome. AJR Am J Roentgenol 1986;146:1141.
24. Johnson CD, Ehman RL, Rakela J, et al. MR angiography in portal hypertension: detection of varices and imaging techniques. J Comput Assist Tomogr 1991;15:578.
25. Bernardino ME, Steinberg HV, Pearson TC, et al. Shunts for portal hypertension: MR and angiography for determination of patency. Radiology 1986;158:57.
26. Finn JP, Edelman RR, Jenkins RL, et al. Liver transplantation: MR angiography with surgical validation. Radiology 1991;179: 265.
27. Saini S, Modic MT, Hamm B, et al. Advances in contrast-enhanced MR imaging. AJR Am J Roentgenol 1991;156:235.
28. Reimer P, Kwong KK, Weisskoff R, et al. Dynamic signal intensity changes in liver with superparamagnetic MR contrast agents. J Magn Reson Imag 1992;2:177.
29. Hamm B, Vogl TJ, Branding G, et al. Focal liver lesions: MR imaging with Mn-DPDP: initial clinical results in 40 patients. Radiology 1992;182:167.
30. Demas BE, Hricak H, Moseley M, et al. Gallbladder bile: an experimental study in dogs using MR imaging and proton MR spectroscopy. Radiology 1985;157:453.
31. Dooms GC, Kerlan RK, Hricak H, et al. Cholangiocarcinoma: imaging by MR. Radiology 1986;159:89.
32. Wallner BK, Schumacher KA, Weidenmaier W, et al. Dilated biliary tract: evaluation with MR cholangiography with a T2-weighted contrast-enhanced fast sequence. Radiology 1991;181: 805.
33. Semelka RC, Kroeker MA, Shoenut JP, et al. Pancreatic disease: prospective comparison of CT, ERCP, and 1.5-T MR imaging with dynamic gadolinium enhancement and fat suppression. Radiology 1991;181:785.
34. Vellet AD, Romano W, Bach DB, et al. Adenocarcinoma of the pancreatic ducts: comparative evaluation with CT and MR imaging at 1.5 T. Radiology 1992;183:87.
35. Steiner E, Stark DD, Hahn PF, et al. Imaging of pancreatic neoplasms: comparison of MR and CT. AJR Am J Roentgenol 1989;152:487.

36. Hahn PF, Weissleder R, Stark DD, et al. MR imaging of focal splenic tumors. AJR Am J Roentgenol 1988;150:823.

37. Mirowitz SA, Brown JJ, Lee JKT, et al. Dynamic gadolinium-enhanced MR imaging of the spleen: normal enhancement patterns and evaluation of splenic lesions. Radiology 1991;179:681.

38. Mitchell D, Vinitski S, Mohamed FB, et al. Comparison of Kaopectate with barium for negative and positive enteric contrast at MR imaging. Radiology 1991;181:475.

39. Laniado M, Kornmesser W, Hamm B, et al. MR imaging of the gastrointestinal tract: value of Gd-DTPA. AJR Am J Roentgenol 1988;150:817.

40. Hahn PF, Stark DD, Saini S, et al. Ferrite particles for bowel contrast in MR imaging: design issues and feasibility studies. Radiology 1987;164:37.

41. Rinck PA, Smevik O, Nilsen G, et al. Oral magnetic particles in MR imaging of the abdomen and pelvis. Radiology 1991;178:755.

42. Li KCP, Tart RP, Fitzsimmons J, et al. Barium sulfate suspension as a negative oral MRI contrast agent: in vitro and human optimization studies. J Magn Reson Imag 1991;9:141.

43. Brown JJ, Duncan JR, Heiken JP, et al. Perfluoroctylbromide as a gastrointestinal contrast agent for MR imaging: use with and without glucagon. Radiology 1991;181:455.

44. Semelka RC, Shoenut JP, Silverman R, et al. Bowel disease: prospective comparison of CT and 1.5-T pre- and postcontrast MR imaging with T1-weighted fat suppressed and breath-hold FLASH sequences. J Magn Reson Imag 1991;1:625.

45. Koelbel G, Schmiedl U, Majer MC, et al. Diagnosis of fistulae and sinus tracts in patients with Crohn disease: value of MR imaging. AJR Am J Roentgenol 1989;152:999.

Textbook of Gastroenterology, second edition, edited by Tadataka Yamada. JB Lippincott Company, Philadelphia © 1995.

CHAPTER 125

Positron Emission Tomography

Markus Schwaiger   Thomas J. Colturi

Imaging Principles
  Resolution
  Radionuclide Production
  Principles of Radiochemistry
  Physiologic Imaging With Radionuclides
Technical Applications
  Image Acquisition

Data Analysis
Tracer Kinetic Modeling
Clinical Applications
  Central Nervous System and Cardiac Disease
  Gastroenterologic Disease
Risks and Cost

Positron emission tomography (PET) represents a new imaging approach that permits measurement of physiologic and biochemical processes within various human organs. PET differs from conventional scintigraphic procedures such as single photon emission tomography by its unique data acquisition, which allows quantitative measurement of regional tissue radioactivity.[1] PET uses radioisotopes of natural elements, oxygen-15, carbon-11, and nitrogen-13. These natural radioisotopes retain their normal biologic function and can be used to synthesize numerous positron-emitting radiopharmaceuticals. PET imaging provides quantitative information regarding normal physiologic features and can detect pathophysiologic alterations that occur in disease states. In most diseases, biochemical abnormalities occur before anatomic changes; PET scans may detect these early biochemical changes before other imaging modalities.

Most PET studies have been performed in research environments[2,3]; however, it has become apparent that this information also is useful in the clinical evaluation of individual patients. This chapter familiarizes the reader with the technical background of PET; reviews the clinical application of PET in neurologic, cardiac, and oncologic diseases; and finally, addresses its possible application in the physiology and pathophysiology of gastrointestinal organs.

IMAGING PRINCIPLES

Imaging of regional tracer concentration is accomplished by the unique properties of positron decay and annihilation. Positron-emitting radionuclides have a nuclear imbalance characterized by an excess of protons. To restore stability to the nuclear structure, a proton is converted to a neutron and a positron is emitted. This energetic positron traverses a few millimeters through the tissue until it becomes thermalized by electrostatic interaction between the electrons and the atomic nuclide of the media, and then combines with a free electron to form a two-particle atom-like entity called a positronium. The positronium quickly decays by annihilation, which is the complete conversion of the positron and electron mass into energy, and generates a pair of photons. Conservation of energy and momentum of the positronium before annihilation require the photons to travel in nearly opposite directions (180 degrees apart) with an energy of 511 keV each (Fig. 125-1).

This unique characteristic of positron annihilation is exploited for image formation. The opposed photons from positron decay can be detected (Fig. 125-2) by using pairs of colinearly aligned detectors. Photons interact with these aligned detectors within a predefined time window and are registered as radioactive events (coincidence counting). The detector pairs of a PET system are installed in a ring-form pattern, which allows measurement of radioactivity along lines through the organ of interest at a series of angles and radial distances. This angular information subsequently is used to reconstruct tomographic images of regional radioactivity distribution (Fig. 125-3; see Color Fig. 108).

The major objective of PET, therefore, is to label physiologically active substrates with positron-emitting radionuclides and acquire transverse sectional images of the radionuclide distribution throughout the organ of interest. State-of-the-art positron emission tomographs consist of multiple, closely packed rings of detectors that enable simultaneous imaging of several image planes. Coincident events between rings of the camera are acquired to generate cross-data, which minimizes data gaps between imaging planes. Such data acquisition allows almost complete data sampling in three dimensions.

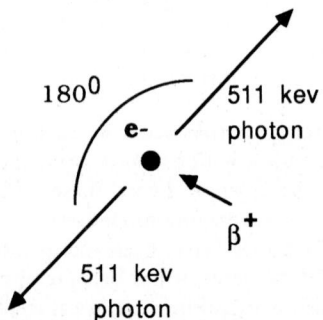

FIGURE 125-1. Annihilation reaction. During positron decay, the positively charged particle is emitted from the nucleus, which interacts with electron. During this annihilation reaction a mass of postparticles is converted into energy in the form of two 511-keV photons.

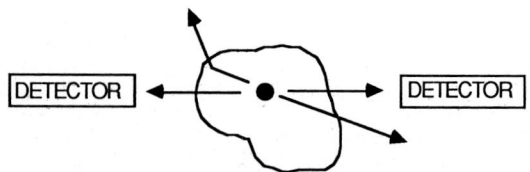

FIGURE 125-2. Coincidence detection. Positron emission tomography employs the principle of coincidence detection. Radioactive events are only registered if photons hit two opposite detector pairs within a narrow time window. Positron emission tomography cameras consist of multiple detector pairs, most commonly aligned in a circular fashion. Detection of radioactive events from multiple angles allows three-dimensional location, which is used for image reconstruction.

Resolution

Images produced by PET are spatial maps of radioactivity distribution within tissue slices, analogous to autoradiograms obtained from selected tissue in animal experiments. The PET method, unlike autoradiography, is noninvasive and thus may be used in clinical research. A second difference between PET and tissue autoradiography is in anatomic resolution. Typical film autoradiographic methods for detection of ^{3}H and ^{14}C provide 50 to 100 mm resolution, allowing clear separation of regional tissue subtypes, such as brain nuclei, from surrounding fiber tracts. The spatial resolution of current PET instrumentation is approximately 5 to 10 mm. This resolution limitation results from the number and geometry of detectors in the instrument, and from the number of counts acquired in the image and their statistical precision. These factors vary between tomographs of different design and from study to study, because of varying image acquisition times and tissue radioactivity levels. The ultimate theoretical limit of PET resolution, however, is the distance traveled by the positron in tissue before the annihilation reaction. Maximum tissue ranges vary according to the initial positron energy (Table 125-1).

As a consequence of the limited spatial resolution, small regions and thin structures such as gastric or intestinal wall cannot be fully resolved. If anatomic structures smaller than the resolution are imaged, the *true* tracer concentration in such structures will be underestimated.[4] Partial volume effect therefore limits the quantification of tracer in small structures. On the other hand, PET studies in large organs such as liver, kidney, pancreas, and spleen are not affected. Reconstructed PET data therefore reflect average isotope concentrations in the imaged tissue. However, if the dimensions of the given organ of interest are defined by an imaging technique with high spatial resolution such as computed tomography or magnetic resonance imaging, correction factors can be applied to compensate for partial volume effect.

Radionuclide Production

Carbon-11, nitrogen-13, oxygen-15, and fluorine-18 are the most common positron-emitting radionuclides, all of which have a short physical half-life ranging from 122 seconds for oxygen-15, to 110 minutes for fluorine-18 (see Table 125-1).

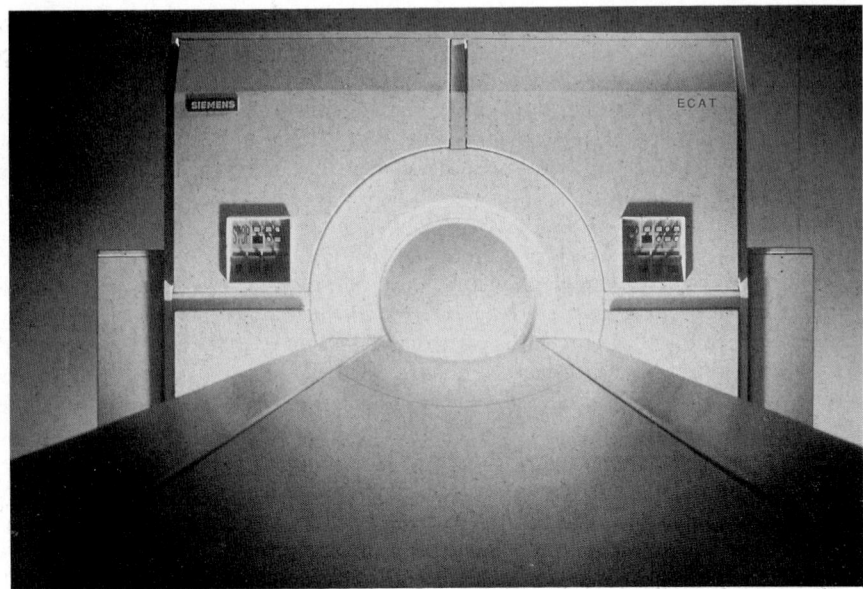

FIGURE 125-3. (See Color Fig. 108.) Positron emission tomography camera (Siemens/CTI 931, Chicago, IL) used for whole-body imaging. This instrument consists of eight detector rings of 512 detectors each, allowing simultaneous imaging of 15 planes, of which is 6.75 mm thick.

These radionuclides do not occur naturally; they must be produced using a nuclear reaction. The predominant and most efficient production method is to modify the nuclear structure of specific stable radionuclides by accelerated particle bombardment with either protons or deuterons. A cyclotron is a particle accelerator employed most often for radioisotope production in PET imaging.[5]

A cyclotron consists of a pair of pie-shaped electrostatic structures called Dees situated between two magnetic pole plates. A plasma ion source creates charged species of hydrogen or deuterium, which are injected into the center of the cyclotron. Alternating electric fields on the Dee structure accelerate the passage of the charged particles between the Dees, while a constant magnetic field constrains the particles to a circular path. With each cycle of the alternating field the particles gain energy and orbit within the cyclotron cavity at a larger radius. Therefore, each particle follows a spiral path through the cyclotron to the extractor, which electrostatically deflects the particle out of the cyclotron.

The particle beam then is directed into a target containing the stable nuclides that will be converted into radioactive positron-emitting nuclides. Target materials then are taken to the chemistry laboratory for radiopharmaceutical synthesis. Cyclotrons vary in their construction and offer different abilities in terms of particles accelerated (protons, deuterons, or

helium nuclei, and helium). Basic needs of PET radiochemistry can be met by any of the available options, but the choice of cyclotron usually is highly individual and carefully integrated with planned clinical and research objectives of a given PET program.[6]

Few positron-emitting radionuclides are generator produced. A generator consists of a parent-daughter radionuclide pair in an apparatus, which permits a separation and extraction of the daughter compound from the parent. The daughter radionuclide is replenished continuously by decay of the parent. The generator system used most often is a molybidium 99–technetium Tc 99m generator.[7] Generators are available for the following positron-emitting compounds: germanium-68–gallium-68, strontium-82–rubidium-82, and zinc-62–copper-62.[8] Germanium-68 has a half-life of 275 days and decays 100% by electron capture to gallium-68, which has a half-life of 68 minutes and decays 88% by positron emission. There is a gallium-68 radiopharmaceutical for almost all technetium radiopharmaceuticals used in nuclear medicine today, including labeled red bood cells, platelets, and albumin. Rubidium-82 has a short half-life of only 76 seconds and is used to evaluate organ blood flow. Rubidium-82 is considered a potassium analog and behaves like thallium-201, which is used extensively for the evaluation of myocardial blood flow.[9] Generators are easier to use than a cyclotron, which requires considerably more space and trained personnel.

Principles of Radiochemistry

The preparation of radiopharmaceuticals for PET requires a dedicated radiopharmaceutical facility. Because of the short half-lives of the isotopes, novel adaptations of synthetic procedures are needed to prepare useful amounts of molecules that are sometimes complex. Because there are positron-emitting radionuclides of oxygen, carbon, and nitrogen, it is theoretically possible to label any organic compound of interest, be it a natural substance or synthetic drug. The pos-

TABLE 125-1
Positron-Emitting Radionuclides

NUCLIDE	HALF-LIFE (min)	ENERGY (MeV)	RANGE (mm H_2O)
Carbon-11	20.4	0.96	4.1
Oxygen-15	2.1	1.72	8.2
Nitrogen-13	10.0	1.19	5.4
Fluorine-18	109.7	0.64	2.4
Rubidium-82	1.3	3.35	13.2

sibilities of producing PET radionuclides are tremendous. Fluorine, although not often found in naturally occurring molecules, can be readily substituted for a hydrogen or hydroxyl group and is a favorite of radiochemists designing new pharmaceuticals. With these four radionuclides, a vast number of positron-emitting tracers can be synthesized and used in clinical studies.

Time, yields, purities, and specific activities are important considerations in the synthesis of radiotracers for PET. As a rule, synthesis must be completed within three half-lives of the radionuclide, and even then the maximal radiochemical yield is only 12.5%. The problem is particularly obvious for tracers like oxygen-15, which has a 2-minute half-life. Very few complex radiochemical syntheses can be completed within the allotted 6 minutes; however, time restrictions on radio-isotopes synthesized with fluorine-18 are not as great. Fluorine has a half-life of 110 minutes and over 300 different fluoro-18 compounds have been reported.[6]

Sufficient yields parallel the problem of time. PET studies may use greater amounts of radiotracers than imaging procedures using single photon agents. Synthetic procedures therefore must be efficient enough to supply reliably large doses of radiopharmaceuticals. Radiochemical purity requirements are similar to those of any radiopharmaceutical intended for human use. Purity is particularly critical for radiotracers used in conjunction with the tracer kinetic model. A small amount of impurities with different pharmacokinetic behavior can complicate the application of such tracer kinetic models to in vivo data.

Finally, there are considerations of specific activities, defined as the ratio of radioactivity to the mass of the compound present. PET radiopharmaceuticals fall into three classes of compounds: innocuous, such as water or glucose, for which specific activities need not be considered; compounds known to be toxic, such as carbon monoxide, for which the need for high specific activities is obvious; and radiotracers for the study of processes where the biologic system is of limited capacity, such as receptor systems, for which specific activities are most important. The final specific activity needed may dictate the synthetic route chosen, because the attainable specific activity of synthetic precursors and synthetic methods may vary widely.

Physiologic Imaging With Radionuclides

Various chemical and biosynthetic procedures have been used to label several hundred biologic substrates and drugs with positron-emitting isotopes.[6,7,9,10] These labeled compounds constitute a large potential resource for development of PET bioassay methods. It is beyond the scope of this chapter to review all radioisotopes for PET imaging. The types that have been used in oncology, neurosciences, and cardiology, and which may be of importance in gastroenterology, include isotopes for the evaluation of organ blood flow, substrate and amino acid metabolism, receptor systems, and radiolabeled monoclonal antibodies.

Organ Blood Flow

Noninvasive evaluation of regional blood flow to organs is important since many diseases affect the delivery of oxygen and other nutrients necessary for energy production. In animal experiments a number of techniques such as microspheres and flow probes measure blood flow. However, although these techniques enable sophisticated measurements, they are invasive and cannot be transferred easily to the clinical situation. In comparison, noninvasive approaches to study regional organ flow in humans are crude and only provide qualitative evaluation. Ultrasound Doppler measurements and new angiographic techniques assess flow velocities in arteries. The PET scan measures regional tracer concentration and permits the quantification of tissue perfusion in milliliters per minute per gram of organ.[11-16] The recent availability of high-resolution PET instrumentation that reduces imaging artifacts and the introduction of numerous flow tracers promise a marked improvement of regional flow determinations.

Microaggregated albumin microspheres labeled with gallium-68 or carbon-11 can be used to assess accurately organ blood flow.[12] The microspheres have to be injected into the left atrium or left ventricle, limiting the clinical application of this technique to the research laboratory.

In clinical studies, two types of intravenous flow tracers are available for the assessment of regional blood flow.[17,18] Examples of the first type are rubidium-82 and ^{13}N-ammonia. These tracers are extracted from plasma and trapped in tissue in proportion to blood flow. In organs such as the myocardium and kidneys, there is a high first-pass extraction (about 80% for ^{13}N-ammonia and 65% for rubidium-82).[19-21] Tissue trapping is energy dependent and the clearance of these tracers from tissue is a function of blood flow. Rubidium-82 is a potassium analog partially sharing the sodium-potassium transport mechanism, whereas ^{13}N-ammonia is converted to ^{13}N-glutamine by glutamine synthetase reaction.[20] The tissue retention fraction of both tracers is inversely related to flow, limiting flow estimates at high flow rates. The rapid plasma extraction and slow tissue clearance are advantageous and allow clear separation of tissue activity from vascular activity. The main advantage of rubidium-82 is that it is generator produced and can be used independent of the cyclotron. The short half-life (76 seconds) permits repeat measurements at brief intervals with low radiation exposure.

The second type of flow tracers are inert diffusable substances such as ^{15}O-water and ^{11}C-butanol.[22] These tracers accumulate and clear from organs as a function of flow. ^{15}O-water is the most widely used inert flow tracer, and it is avidly extracted by tissue, with a first-pass extraction fraction close to 100%. Animal studies have shown that this high extraction is maintained as a function of flow, indicating that the distribution of ^{15}O-water is limited by flow rather than diffusion.[13,14] In addition to this favorable physiologic property, ^{15}O-water has a short physical half-life (2 minutes) and allows repetitive flow measurements in short intervals. Using dynamic PET scanning, blood and tissue activity can be differentiated, and quantification of regional blood flow can be achieved with reasonable accuracy, as demonstrated experimentally in brain, heart, and lung.

Substrate Metabolism

One of the major advantages of PET is the ability to measure quantitatively substrate metabolism. The most commonly used metabolic tracer for PET imaging is fluorine-18 deoxyglucose (FDG).[23-25] FDG is a glucose analog that is transported into tissue and phosphorylated in a manner identical to glucose. However, FDG-6-phosphate is trapped in tissue and accumulates in proportion to exogenous glucose use (Fig. 125-4). The rate of the dephosphorylation of FDG-6-phosphate is low in the brain, heart, and tumors, but varies in other organs.[10] Liver tissue, for example, has higher concentrations of phosphatase, which hydrolase FDG-6-phosphate. A three-compartmental tracer kinetic model for FDG has been developed with rate constants for transport as well as phosphorylation, which allows the quantitative assessment of regional glucose use.[26–28] These metabolic measurements using FDG have been validated in the brain and the heart, demonstrating the possibility of in vivo quantification of glucose metabolism in these organs by PET.[26,27,29]

Several other metabolic tracers have been used to characterize substrate metabolism in the heart. In contrast to the brain, which primarily depends on glucose use, the heart derives its energy from a variety of substrates. Under fasting conditions, long chain fatty acids are the primary source of energy. Therefore, ^{11}C-palmitate as a marker of fatty acid metabolism has been extensively used in the evaluation of cardiac metabolism.[30–34]

Recently ^{11}C-acetate has been introduced for the assessment of oxidative metabolism.[35,36] This tracer enters the TCA cycle directly, and the label is released in the form of carbon dioxide. ^{11}C-acetate appears to be a preferred substrate for the TCA cycle.[35] Correlation between the washout of activity from the heart after ^{11}C-acetate administrations and myocardial oxygen consumption showed a linear relationship over a wide range of myocardial oxygen consumption.[35,36] These data indicate that ^{11}C-acetate is a promising tracer for the noninvasive evaluation of tissue oxygen consumption.

Several other metabolic tracers, such as ^{11}C-labeled or ^{13}N-labeled amino acids, have been proposed for studying tissue amino acid metabolism.[37] In the brain, radiolabeled leucine has been used to measure protein synthesis using tracer kinetic modeling.[38]

In oncology, ^{11}C-methionine and ^{11}C-tyrosine have been employed for the identification of rapidly growing tumors.

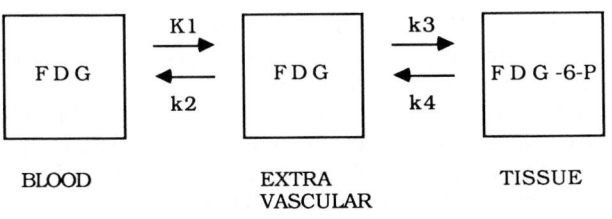

FIGURE 125-4. Compartment model for fluorine-18 deoxyglucose (FDG). This model describes the transmembraneous transport (K1, k2) as well as the phosphorylation (k3, k4) of FDG in tissue.

Current research focuses on the comparison of FDG and labeled amino acid for the diagnostic workup of patients with cancer.[39] ^{11}C-thymidine is a promising tracer for the assessment of nucleic acid metabolism, because of the biologic significance of DNA replication and cell division rates in tumor tissue. Such metabolic probes are useful in the diagnosis and in the monitoring of the response of malignant tissue to therapy.

Other metabolic pathways, such as polyamine metabolism and tissue glucose amine, have been studied with PET in small patient populations.

Tumor tissue may be rendered hypoxic during rapid growth, which may affect its reactivity to radiation. Therefore, the identification of tissue hypoxia appears interesting for the in vivo tissue characterization. Rasey and associates developed ^{18}F-misonidazole for PET imaging. This tracer accumulates in viable, hypoxic cells that contain nitroreductase enzymes.[40]

Finally, chemotherapeutic agents labeled with positron emitters provide in vivo pharmacokinetics in normal and cancer tissue. ^{18}F-fluorodeoxyuridine and ^{18}F-tamoxifen have been introduced for this purpose.[41]

Tissue Receptors

Radioactive labeled receptor agonists or antagonists are commonly used for the in vitro assay of receptor systems. The use of positron-emitting receptor ligands allows the in vivo measurement of receptor systems.[42–53] A considerable number of receptor ligands have been synthesized[44–52] (Table 125-2). It is feasible to localize cerebral dopamine, opiate, serotonin, benzodiazepine, and muscarinic cholinergic receptors using PET. Peripheral receptor systems studied by PET include the α- and β-adrenergic receptors as well as the muscarinic cholinergic receptors.[53,54] Most of these studies were performed in the heart and have not been extended to other organs.

Initially, the relative distribution of ligand binding has been explored and related to the in vitro studies employing autoradiography.[43] These more qualitative studies allow the definition of the anatomic location of receptor binding and the comparison of tracer uptake in the right and left hemispheres of the brain. However, the quantification of binding sites by PET should be possible, allowing the noninvasive assessment of receptor densities.[55]

The selection of ligands for receptor measurements is the most important step in the successful development of in vivo binding techniques and places greater restriction on the properties of an acceptable tracer than in vitro binding assays. First, the selected tracer must have high specific affinity for a single receptor type or subtype. Antagonist drugs are preferred, because antagonist binding is more closely described by a simple association and dissociation reaction simplifying tracer kinetic modeling. In addition, the nonspecific tissue binding of this ligand is important, because it affects the ability to measure specific binding sites. Minimal nonspecific binding, compared with specific binding, and rapid clearance from nonspecific binding sites are the preferred characteristics.

Applications of in vivo receptor ligand binding methods are potentially diverse, ranging from studies of disease or therapy related alterations in the number of binding sites to dynamic tests of synaptic function. The latter is based on measurements of changes in free receptor sites caused by al-

TABLE 125-2
Receptor Ligands Imaged in the Human Brain by Positron Emission Tomography

RECEPTOR TYPE	LIGAND	REFERENCE
Dopamine, D2	[^{18}F]Spiperone	Tsurumi, 1990[41]
	[^{11}C]Methylspiperone	Frost, 1986[42]
	[^{18}F]Methylspiperone	Young et al, 1986[43]
	[^{76}Br]Bromospiperone	Perlmutter et al, 1987[44]
	[^{11}C]Pimozide	Wagner et al, 1983[45]
	[^{11}C]Raclopride	Arnett et al, 1986[46]
Opiate	[^{11}C]Carfentanil	Baron et al, 1986[47]
Cholinergic, muscarinic	[^{11}C]Scopolamine	Baron et al, 1985[48]
Benzodiazepine	[^{11}C]Ro 15-1788	Farde et al, 1986[49]
	[^{11}C]Suriclone	
Serotonin, S2	[^{11}C]Methylspiperone	Frost et al, 1985[50]
	[^{11}C]-2-Br-LSD	

tered levels of endogenous neurotransmitter. Therefore either physiologic or pharmacologic challenges that alter presynaptic activity or modify binding of the endogenous transmitter may produce changes indirectly in radioligand binding to receptor sites. Because of the short half-lives of the positron-emitting radioisotopes, ligand studies can be combined with PET studies of flow or other tissue function. The combination of tracers of presynaptic function such as ^{18}F-dopamine or ^{18}F-norepinephrine analogs with postsynaptic ligand studies are promising; they allow the characterization of neurotransmission and differentiation of the effect of disease on presynaptic and postsynaptic sites.[56,57]

Antibody Labeling With Radionuclides

Radioactive labeled monoclonal antibodies are used to identify the location and extent of several tumors in experimental and clinical studies. In addition, radioactive-labeled antimyosin antibody identifies acutely necrotic tissue in the heart.[58] It is not clear if the kinetics of antibody binding and the clearance of the antibody from blood allows imaging with relatively short-lived radioisotopes employed for PET imaging. Animal studies using iodine-124 (half-life, 4.2 days) suggest a potential of ^{124}I-monoclonal antibody for tumor imaging.[59]

TECHNICAL APPLICATONS

Image Acquisition

To exploit fully the quantitative capabilities of PET, the images have to be corrected for photon attenuation.[1] Regional correction factors are derived from transmission images obtained before the injection of the radioisotopes. These transmission scans are produced by placing a ring source around the body of the patient and measuring the absorption by the tissue. The transmission scan is followed by emission scans after the intravenous injection of radiolabeled tracers. Current image instrumentation allows for variable data acquisition with high temporal resolution. Images can be either obtained in frame mode, predefined number of images of defined du-

ration, or by list mode. This acquisition method continuously acquires data, which can be retrospectively sorted, based on time or other signals such as electrocardiogram gate, to generate a temporal sequence of images. The usual acquisition time after the injection of 10 to 20 mCi of radiotracer is 10 to 15 minutes for static images and varies from seconds to minutes for dynamic data acquisition. Depending on the protocol the usual imaging time ranges from 1 hour to 2.5 hours.

Data Analysis

Multislice PET scanners generate a large number of data during one study. Archiving, storage, and data transfer are important in PET data management because of the quantity of data generated. For the qualitative management of tracer distribution, images are analyzed as in conventional nuclear medicine; hard copies or computer displays of selected images are evaluated visually. More sophisticated data analysis includes the application of regions of interest over parts of the organ of interest. These regions can be copied to a large number of dynamic images and used to generate time-activity curves, which are subsequently used for tracer kinetic modeling. New software development concentrates on the three-dimensional reconstruction of PET information and on the correlation of PET images with those of other image modalities such as magnetic resonance imaging and computed tomography. Another advantage of three-dimensional data management is the correction for interindividual changes in organ orientation, which is necessary for standardized data analysis. Finally, the three-dimensional display software allows the organ to be seen as a whole, improving our interpretation of regional alterations in tracer distribution.

Tracer Kinetic Modeling

The primary strength of PET is the ability to use tracer kinetic models to yield measurements of physiologic processes in absolute units.[60] To measure such processes after the intravenous injection or inhalation of positron-labeled compounds, appropriate mathematic tracer kinetic models based on the principals of tracer and competitive enzyme kinetics are used. Models exist for the measurement of local rates of blood flow, membrane transport, metabolism, measurement of blood volume, pH, and receptor binding.[60] The tracer kinetic models provide a framework that describes the kinetics of the process under study and the mathematic equation calculating the rates of these processes. Such models reduce complex biologic systems into a few compartments and estimate the rates of processes in those compartments in three ways: by using information about the delivery of the labeled compound into the compartment; by serially determining the activity in blood; and by determining the delivery, accumulation, and clearance of the compound in tissue by serial imaging of the organ.

An example of kinetic sampling approach is shown in Figure 125-4 for the glucose analog FDG. Carbon 14–labeled deoxyglucose initially was employed by Sokoloff and colleagues[23] in animal experiments using autoradiography to develop a tracer kinetic model method for determining cerebral glucose use. The use of deoxyglucose represents an approach with a substrate analog to isolate a segment (transport and phosphorylation) of a complex reaction sequence and to permit accurate estimates of the rate of these processes. The labeling of deoxyglucose with fluoro-18 provided a positron-emitting form of this glucose for its application in human subjects.

Once a tracer kinetic model has been validated, the operation of the model can be incorporated in the PET computer system and used to convert tomographic images into specific rates of activity for physiologic processes. PET scans with FDG and the appropriate kinetic model produce data that are converted to glucose metabolism per minute per gram of tissue.

CLINICAL APPLICATIONS

Central Nervous System and Cardiac Disease

The PET scan allows measurement of cerebral blood flow, blood volume, oxygen and glucose use, amino acid use, alteration of the blood-brain barrier, and neurotransmitter processes at presynaptic and postsynaptic sites.[2] PET scans with flow tracers or metabolic tracers have proven useful in the evaluation of patients with epilepsy.[61,62] In patients with poorly controlled seizures, the interictal PET scan can detect hypometabolic or hypoperfused brain zones that are responsible for seizure onset.[62] These zones usually appear normal on computed tomography scans; the PET scan has been used to guide surgical intervention. PET scans also have helped evaluate patients with suspected cerebrovascular disease and dementia[63-67] (Fig. 125-5).

The major area of clinical application is the metabolic characterization of brain tumors. The relative FDG uptake in tumor tissue compared with surrounding normal brain tissue has been used to grade the malignancy of the tumor, yielding important diagnostic and prognostic information in these patients. Such metabolic tissue characterization may be especially useful in patients undergoing radiation or surgical therapy to identify recurrence of tumor growth.

The clinical application of PET in cardiac patients concentrates on the evaluation of coronary artery disease.[3] PET perfusion studies with flow tracers (rubidium-82 or ^{13}N-ammonia) are more accurate than the noninvasive studies now used.[17,18,68] Combination of flow tracers with metabolic tracers has been shown to identify myocardial ischemia on a cellular level.[69,70] The PET scan can determine whether compromised myocardial tissue is ischemic or infarcted and the

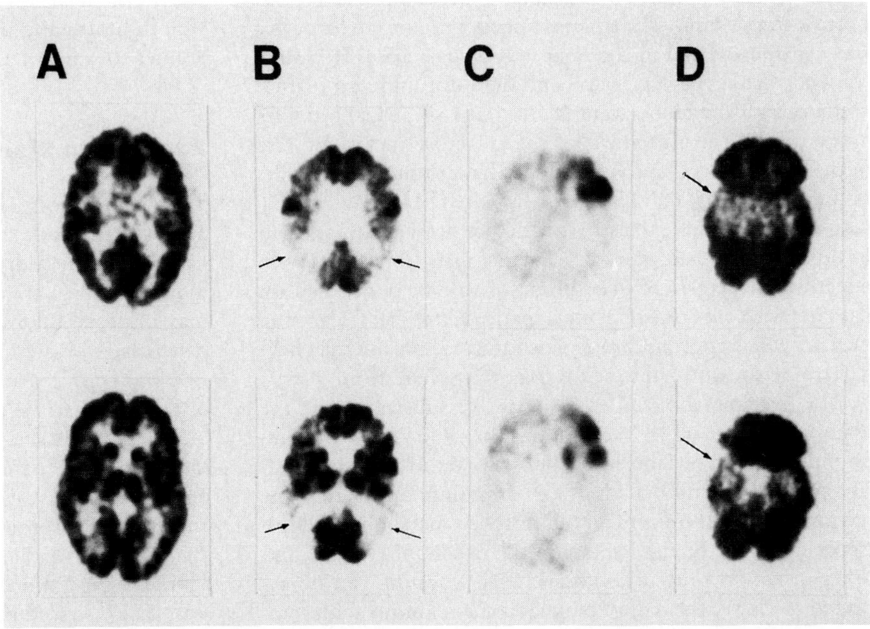

FIGURE 125-5. Cross-sectional brain images after intravenous injection of fluorine-18 deoxyglucose (FDG); four examples are shown. (**A**) Normal distribution of FDG in healthy volunteer. Notice the clear delineation of cerebral structures. (**B**) A patient with Alzheimer's disease is characterized by decreased metabolic activity (FDG uptake) in the parietal cortex (*arrows*). (**C**) Neonate with drug-resistant seizure disorder. FDG was injected during ictus. Notice the markedly increased glucose utilization in the seizure focus. (**D**) Example of a patient with epileptic seizure disorder. The seizure focus reveals hypometabolism during the interical phase (temporal lobes *arrows*).

extent of these processes. With the introduction of therapeutic strategies to revascularize ischemic myocardium, the identification of tissue viability in patients with previous myocardial infarction has gained increasing clinical importance. This test provides a high predictive value for tissue recovery after revascularization, and therefore is being used to select patients with impaired left ventricular function for bypass surgery or angioplasty.[69,71]

Gastroenterologic Disease

The basic principles of PET scanning can be applied to any discipline, and because of the unique physiologic information it provides, PET will be a useful research and clinical tool in gastroenterology.[17,61,72–80] Advances in this area require a collaborative effort between the specialists in nuclear medicine, radiochemists, and gastroenterologists. Preliminary studies suggest that PET will be useful in evaluating liver disease, pancreatic function, and gastrointestinal malignancy.

Liver Disease

Although PET scanning does not display the liver's anatomic structure as well as computed tomography or ultrasound, PET does reveal the function of biochemical-physiologic processes in the liver.[81,82] It therefore offers the promise of a true in vivo measurement of liver function. The term *liver function tests* often refers to hepatic enzymes, bilirubin, or albumin. Although severe abnormalities may indicate hepatic disease, these tests may be normal when significant hepatic dysfunction exists. Investigators have attempted to measure hepatic function better by measuring substances that are selectively metabolized by the liver. The rate of clearance of galactose is one such test. The galactose clearance test has been used in the evaluation of cirrhosis, and the results have correlated well with the prognosis of the disease.[83]

The positron-emitting tracer, 2-deoxy-2[18F]fluoro-D-galactose (18F-FDGal), can be used to measure galactose metabolism by the liver.[84] This tracer is similar to the use of FDG glucose in the brain. The tracer is transported into hepatocytes and phosphorylated in the same way as galactose. It is then trapped within the hepatocyte and does not undergo further metabolism. Therefore, accumulation of 18F-FDGal provides a quantitative measurement of the galactose metabolic rate in the liver. In liver injury, as induced by carbon tetrachloride, accumulation of 18F-FDGal is impaired. Hopefully PET scanning will be able to assess the degree of liver damage and to determine hepatic reserve.[85] Further tests in patients with hepatitis, cirrhosis, and liver tumors should be performed. In patients with cirrhosis or acute hepatic failure, PET scanning may provide important prognostic information and may help determine the optimal time for liver transplantation.

The liver metabolizes a wide range of substrates and the major advantage of PET scanning is the wide variety of compounds that can be labeled with positron-emitting isotopes.[6] The use of ^{11}C-amino acids or ^{13}N-ammonia may clarify the role of the liver in amino acid and nitrogen metabolism. These tracers also can be used to study the effects of ethanol and other drugs on protein synthesis. PET scanning can be expected to clarify the role of branched chain amino acids, am-

monia, and γ-amino butyric acid in hepatic encephalopathy.[86] The liver also plays a central role in cholesterol and fatty acid metabolism. These substrates can be labeled with positron-emitting isotopes and their role in lipid disorders can be studied. Labeled lipoproteins have been synthesized, and PET scanning allows the quantification of lipoprotein receptors.[87] PET also may be helpful in further evaluating the metabolic abnormalities in atherosclerosis. The beneficial effects of diet and drug therapy on lipid metabolism could be assessed by PET scanning. Other inborn errors of metabolism as well as the hepatic porphyrias could be studied.[88]

PET scans also may prove useful in the quantitative study of hepatobiliary function. The use of ^{99m}Tc-iminodiacetic acid derivatives has become widespread in the rapid diagnosis of acute cholecystitis and acute biliary obstruction. The hepatobiliary iminodiacetic acid scan, however, has not been helpful in the evaluation of chronic cholestatic conditions and does not accurately measure hepatic excretory rate. The positron-emitting isotope, gallium-68 has been complexed with derivatives of iminodiacetic acid.[85,89] Preliminary studies suggest that quantitative measurement of hepatic uptake and excretion are possible. Further studies may be helpful in defining the factors that regulate biliary secretion. Serial measurements of the hepatic excretory rate may be helpful in following the course of patients with chronic cholestatic syndromes. In patients with primary biliary cirrhosis, the response to medical therapy with steroids, penicillamine, or prostaglandins could be followed. In sclerosing cholangitis, the effect of dilatation of biliary strictures could be assessed by serial measurement of excretory rates.

Also, PET may be helpful in the investigation of drug metabolism and drug toxicity. The mechanism of hepatotoxic agents such as acetaminophen, isoniazide, carbon tetrachloride, and D-galactose can be elucidated. The use of radiolabeled drugs will elucidate their metabolic clearance. The kinetics and regulatory properties of hepatic drug metabolizing enzymes can be studied. In addition, information regarding the therapeutic benefit of drugs such as steroids, penicillamine, and prostaglandins can be determined.[82] One may expect that within the next few years enough information on liver function in health and disease will be accumulated through PET studies to warrant a major PET commitment to hepatology.

Pancreatic Disease

The diagnosis of pancreatic disease is difficult because of the anatomic location of the gland and the fact that function must be seriously disturbed before exocrine function tests are modified. PET with cyclotron-produced radiopharmaceuticals may improve the morphologic and functional study of the pancreas.

Noninvasive scans of the pancreas have taken advantage of the fact that the pancreas uses free amino acids from the blood to synthesize digestive enzymes. In 1961 the selenomethionine-75 pancreatic scan was introduced.[90] Selenomethionine-75 is an analog of L-methionine with the gamma-emitting ^{75}Se-isotope substituted for the sulfur atom. This alteration of the chemical structure alters the biochemical behavior of the amino acid, which limits the usefulness of this scan. The ^{75}Se-scan has been discarded at most centers because of the low fractional uptake in the pancreas and very low specificity for pancreatic disease.[91,92]

Investigators have attempted to overcome the limitations of ^{75}Se-scans by using amino acids labeled with carbon-11 and nitrogen-13.[93] These positron-emitting amino acids require a cyclotron for their production but retain their natural configuration and follow normal metabolic pathways. Amino acids used in pancreatic imaging include the following: ^{11}C-tryptophan,[93] ^{11}C-valine,[94,95] ^{11}C-methionine,[96,97] and ^{13}N-glutamate.[98] After intravenous injection, these tracers are rapidly cleared from plasma and accumulate in the pancreas.

Tracer concentration in other abdominal organs progressively declines. These changes result in a favorable target-to-nontarget ratio for pancreatic imaging. All portions of the pancreatic gland—the head, body, and tail—can be routinely identified. If an appropriate kinetic model is available that reflects the metabolic behavior of the labeled amino acid, then PET scanning can provide a detailed image of morphologic features and quantitative measurement of amino acid uptake and protein synthesis.[99,100]

Positron emission tomography scanning with ^{11}C-L-methionine was used to assess possible pancreatic disease in 100 patients.[97] In patients in whom a definitive diagnosis was achieved, PET showed a sensitivity rate of 85.0%, a specificity rate of 97.8%, and an accuracy rate of 91.8%. The PET scan was abnormal in 100% of pancreatic cancers, in 83% of chronic pancreatitis, and in 67% of acute pancreatitis. The lack of sensitivity for acute pancreatitis was due mainly to the fact that several PET scans were performed 4 to 5 weeks after the acute episode, by which time functional abnormalities had probably resolved. A problem is that PET scanning with ^{11}C-methionine is unable to differentiate pancreatic cancer from chronic pancreatitis. In both conditions there often is a marked decrease or complete absence of tracer accumulation in the pancreas. For pancreatic cancer, an ideal imaging agent would concentrate selectively in the malignancy, thus allowing accurate staging without laparotomy. Unfortunately, at this time no such tracer exists.

Animal studies have shown that PET images of the pancreas are affected by various feeding protocols.[98] The cephalic, gastric, and intestinal phases of pancreatic exocrine function are regulated by a variety of neurogenic and hormonal factors. PET scanning provides a noninvasive way of quantifying the neurohumoral factors that regulate pancreatic protein synthesis. PET can be used in experimental pancreatitis to investigate various pharmacologic or hormonal alterations. Pancreatic PET scanning with tracers other than amino acids may provide additional information regarding pancreatic function. Studies of blood flow, oxygen use, and receptor density can be quantified. These studies are helpful in research for defining normal physiologic characteristics, and are useful in studying disease states where functional alterations occur before structural changes.

Oncologic Disease

Positron emission tomography is emerging as a potentially useful imaging approach in oncology. With the further development of suitable radiotracers, it is expected that PET will enhance the detection and staging of tumors and will be useful in assessing prognosis and response to therapy.[101] Tracer approaches can be used to describe tumor biologic features uniquely. Flow, metabolism, and specific cell surface binding sites (i.e., receptors) can be targeted and quantitatively assessed by PET.

Tumors also have been characterized by measurement of blood flow.[102,103] Primary hepatocellular carcinoma (hepatoma) is the most common primary hepatic malignancy, and it has been shown that PET with ^{13}N-ammonia is useful for hepatoma imaging.[104] Early accumulation of ^{13}N-ammonia appears to correlate well with the early and rich vascular supply to the hepatoma from the hepatic artery, whereas normal liver tissue accumulates ^{13}N-ammonia primarily from the portal vein.

The most important metabolic radiotracer used in oncology is FDG. Rapidly proliferating tumor cells metabolize glucose under aerobic and anaerobic conditions. Malignant transformation of cells is associated with a high glycolytic rate. This tumor-specific change in substrate metabolism was described more than 60 years ago in the biochemical observations of Warburg and Meyerhoff.[105] The proposed explanations for this phenomenon include increased concentration of glycolytic enzymes such as hexokinase in tumors compared with normal tissue or increased glucose transport into tumors. Increased expression of the glucose transporters in malignant cells in the presence of elevated levels of transporter mRNA has been proposed as metabolic correlates of malignant cells. Indeed, Flier and associates[106] described high levels of glucose transport and transporter mRNA in red fibroplast transfected with activated ras or sarc oncogenes.

Metabolic imaging of tumors with FDG was first applied in patients with brain tumors, demonstrating a relationship of tumor growth rate and metabolic activity as defined by regional FDG uptake. Although a similar correlation between tumor growth rate and FDG uptake has not been found in peripheral tumor tissue, most investigations support the notion that the extent of FDG uptake in tumor tissue is closely correlated to the distribution of viable malignant cells. Based on the high contrast of tumor FDG uptake to surrounding tissue, FDG imaging has been employed in many human tumors. Such an approach is useful in the diagnosis of primary tumors and may be more important in the noninvasive staging of tumor extent. Several studies suggest high sensitivity of the FDG method in the detection of metastases.[107,108] A quantification of regional glucose use in tumors using the previous tracer kinetic model has been shown to differentiate benign from malignant lesion in the liver.[109]

Studies using PET of patients with breast cancer suggest that metabolic information may be useful in the assessment of response to therapy.[110] PET therefore may provide the diagnostic workup of patients and also act as a noninvasive tool to monitor the response of therapy and to detect early recurrence of tumors. Because of these promising first results, several large clinical trials are underway to assess the efficacy of FDG PET imaging in staging various tumor diseases. Although preliminary results indicate the diagnostic superiority of PET imaging over computed tomography and magnetic resonance imaging, the future clinical role of PET imaging with FDG in the workup of patients with cancer has to be defined by these studies.[111] Figures 125-6 and 125-7 show whole-body imaging of FDG distribution in a normal volunteer and in a patient with a metastatic colorectal cancer.

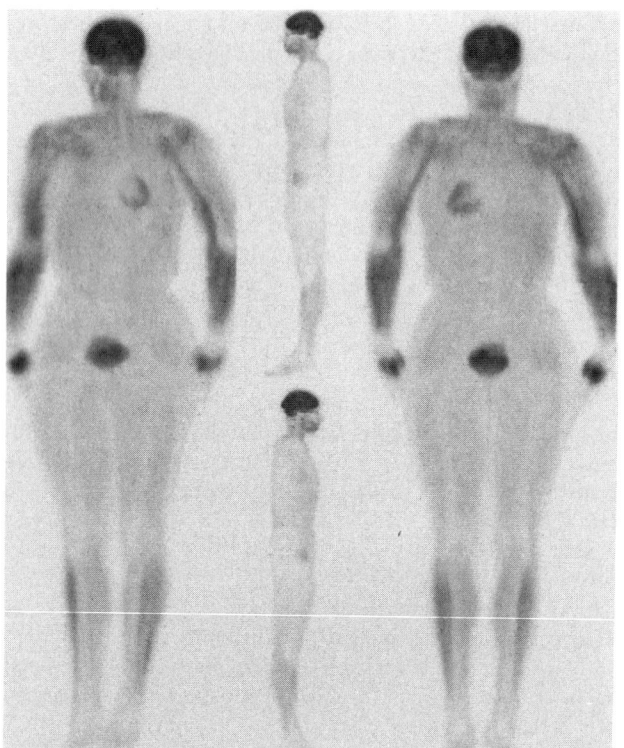

FIGURE 125-6. Images of whole-body positron emission tomography after fluorine-18 deoxyglucose (FDG) administration in a normal volunteer. The intense FDG uptake in the brain is consistent with metabolic pattern of high glucose uptake in the brain. No tracer retention is seen in the liver in this normal volunteer.

Neuroendocrine tumors are characterized by the production of peptides or amines. Radiolabeled precursors can be used to assess the capacity of primary tumor or metastasis for synthesizing specific substances. ^{11}C-labeled 5-hydroxtryptophan as precursor of serotonin has been shown to visualize carcinoid tumors and liver metastases. Tracer accumulation in tumor tissue correlated with response to therapy.[112] The use of ^{11}C-hydroxyephedrine, a norepinephrine analog, has provided clear demarcation of pheochromacytoma very early after tracer injection extending the experience previously acquired with the single photon agent ^{123}I-metaiodobenzylguadine.[113]

In detecting tumors, PET can take advantage of the fact that distinctive tumor antigens are expressed by malignancies during the course of their growth and development. Carcinoembryonic antigen is a glycoprotein that is expressed normally in the fetal gut, and has been identified in colon, lung, breast, and pancreatic cancers. Other tumor-associated antigens have been discovered that subserve important functions in the growth and development of the tumor cell. Examples include the transferin receptor that is ubiquitous on growing tumor cells, the interleukin-2 receptor on malignant T cells, and the bombesin receptor produced by small cell carcinoma of the lung. These membrane-fixed glycoproteins serve as a specific focus for the binding of essential growth factors for the tumor cell. Although no extensive studies have used PET,

these distinctive glycoproteins obviously could be imaged using positron-emitting labeled monoclonal antibodies.[114]

In breast cancer, the measurement of estrogen and progesterone receptors has important therapeutic implications, and recently the positron-emitting tracer, F-Fluro-17B-estradiol, has been synthesized. This labeled ligand allows detection of tumor cells that possess this receptor.[115] PET scanning with such tracers allows for the detection of primary and metastatic lesions and may provide noninvasive means of predicting response to therapy targeting such tumor surface binding sites (tamoxifen).

RISKS AND COST

Truly PET is a noninvasive procedure. The only significant risk involved is the radiation exposure. However, the short physical half-life of most positron-emitting radionuclides minimizes absorbed radiation to the patient.

Most PET facilities are located in academic centers and have been installed with support of extramural funding. The costs to acquire a whole-body PET unit averages $2 million. These hardware costs are exceeded by the need of room modifications and on-site installation of a cyclotron. The cost can be reduced by relying on generator-produced radioisotopes. However, a rubidium generator lasts only about 6 weeks and the cost to replace one is about $20,000. The average cost of a cyclotron installation averages about $1.5 million but may vary significantly depending on the specification for a given

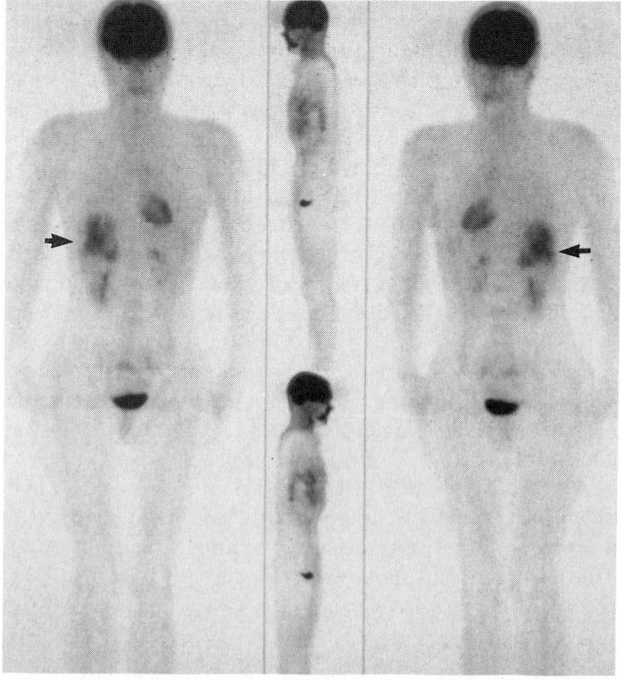

FIGURE 125-7. Anterior (left) and posterior (right) images of whole-body positron emission tomography after fluorine-18 deoxyglucose administration of patient with metastatic colorectal cancer. Focal tracer uptake in the liver provides metabolic evidence of metastases (*arrows*).

institution. In addition, a cyclotron radiopharmacy facility increases the cost of PET significantly. Published economic studies on the operation of PET centers reveals that a volume of about six to eight patients a day with an average charge of about $1500 per patient are necessary to maintain a PET facility without extramural funding. The viability of a PET facility clearly depends on the demonstration of the unique clinical utility of PET to address specific clinical problems. Several PET centers are being installed that will concentrate on the clinical application of PET, and future economic data will show the cost effectiveness of these centers.

The reader is directed to Chapter 114, General Considerations; and Chapter 120, Cross-Sectional Anatomy.

REFERENCES

1. Hoffman EJ, Phelps ME. Positron emission tomography: principles and quantification. In: Phelps ME, Mazziotta J, Schelbert H, eds. Positron emission tomography and autoradiography: principles and applications for the brain and heart. New York: Raven Press, 1986:237.

2. Mazziotta JC, Phelps ME. Positron emission tomography studies of the brain. In: Phelps ME, Mazziotta J, Schelbert H, eds. Positron emission tomography and autoradiography: principles and applications for the brain and heart. New York: Raven Press, 1986:493.

3. Schelbert HR, Schwaiger M. PET studies of the heart. In: Phelps ME, Mazziotta J, Schelbert H, eds. Positron emission tomography and autoradiography: principles and applications for the brain and heart. New York: Raven Press, 1986:581.

4. Hoffman EJ, Huang SC, Phelps ME. Quantitation in positron emission computed tomography: effect of object size. Part I. J Comput Assist Tomogr 1979;3:299.

5. Hoop B Jr, Laughlin JS, Tilbury RS. Cyclotrons in nuclear medicine. In: Hine GJ, Sorenson JA, eds. Instrumentation in nuclear medicine. Vol 2. New York: Academic Press, 1974: 407.

6. Fowler JS, Wolf AP. Positron emitter-labeled compounds: priorities and problems. In: Phelps ME, Mazziotta JC, Schelbert HR, eds. Positron emission tomography and autoradiography: principles and applications for the brain and heart. New York: Raven Press, 1986:391.

7. Sorenson JA, Phelps ME, eds. Production of radionuclides. In: Physics in nuclear medicine. 2nd ed. New York: Grune & Stratton, 1987:143.

8. Green MA, Mathias CJ, Welch MJ, et al. Copper-62-labeled pyruvaldehyde bis(N⁴-methylthiosemicarbazonato) copper (II): synthesis and evaluation as a positron emission tomography tracer for cerebral and myocardial perfusion. J Nucl Med 1990;31:1989.

9. Gennaro GP, Neirinckx RD, Bergner B, et al. A radionuclide generator and infusion system for pharmaceutical quality Rb-82. Am Chem Symp Ser 1984;241:135.

10. Barrio JR. Biochemical principles in radiopharmaceutical design and utilization. In: Phelps ME, Mazziotta JC, Schelbert HR, eds. Positron emission tomography and autoradiography: principles and applications for the brain and heart. New York: Raven Press, 1986:451.

11. Martin WR, Raichle ME. Cerebellar blood flow and metabolism in cerebral hemisphere infarction. Ann Neurol 1983;14:168.

12. Beller GA, Alten WJ, Cochavi S, et al. Assessment of regional myocardial perfusion by positron emission tomography after intracoronary administration of Ga-68 labeled albumin microspheres. J Comput Assist Tomogr 1979;3:447.

13. Bergman SR, Fox KAA, Rand AL, et al. Quantification of re-gional myocardial blood flow in vivo with H₂O-15. Circulation 1984;70:724.

14. Raichle ME, Markham J, Larson K, et al. Measurement of local cerebral blood flow in man with positron emission tomography. J Cereb Blood Flow Metab 1981;1(Suppl 1):S19.

15. Huang SC, Schwaiger M, Carson RE, et al. Quantitative measurement of myocardial blood flow with oxygen-15 water and positron computed tomography: an assessment of potential and problems. J Nucl Med 1985;25:616.

16. Shah A, Schelbert HR, Schwaiger M, et al. Measurement of regional myocardial blood flow with N-13 ammonia and positron emission tomography in intact dogs. J Am Coll Cardiol 1985;5:92.

17. Gould KL, Goldstein RA, Mullani NA, et al. Non-invasive assessment of coronary stenosis by myocardial perfusion imaging during pharmacologic coronary vasodilation: clinical feasibility of positron cardiac imaging without a cyclotron using generator-produced rubidium-82. Part VIII. J Am Coll Cardiol 1986;7: 775.

18. Schelbert HR, Phelps ME, Hoffman EJ, et al. Regional myocardial perfusion assessed with N-13 labeled ammonia and positron emission computerized axial tomography. Am J Cardiol 1979;43:209.

19. Budinger TF, Yano Y, Derenzo SE, et al. Rb-82 myocardial positron emission tomography (abstract). J Nucl Med 1979;20: 602.

20. Bergman SR, Hack S, Tewson T, Welch MJ, Sobel RE. The dependence of accumulation of N-13 NH3 by myocardium on metabolic factors and its implications for the quantitative assessment or perfusion. Circulation 1980;61:34.

21. Mullani NA, Goldstein RA, Gould KL, et al. Perfusion imaging with rubidium-82: measurement of extraction and flow with external detectors. Part I. J Nucl Med 1983;24:898.

22. Raichle ME, Eichling JO, Straatmann MG, et al. Blood brain barrier permeability of ¹¹C labeled alcohols and ¹⁵O labeled water. Am J Physiol 1976;230:543.

23. Sokoloff L, Reivich M, Kennedy C, et al. The (14C)-deoxyglu-cose method for the measurement of local cerebral glucose utilization: theory, procedure and normal values in the conscious and anesthetized albino rat. J Neurochem 1977;28:897.

24. Ido T, Wan CN, Casella V, et al. Labeled 2-deoxy-D-glucose analogs: 18F-labeled 2-deoxy-2-fluoro-D-glucose, 2-deoxy-2-fluoro-D-mannose and 14C-2-deoxy-2-fluoro-D-glucose. J Label Compds Radiopharmacol 1978;24:174.

25. Huang S-C, Phelps ME, Hoffman EJ, et al. Non-invasive determination of local cerebral metabolic rate of glucose in man. Am J Physiol 1980;238:E69.

26. Siiteri PK. Receptor binding studies. Science 1984;223:191.

27. Krivokapich J, Huang SC, Phelps ME, et al. Estimation of rabbit myocardial metabolic rate for glucose using fluorodeoxyglucose. Am J Physiol 1982;243:H884.

28. Marshall RC, Huang SC, Nash WW, Phelps ME. Investigation of th 18-fluorodeoxyglucose tracer kinetic model to accurately measure the myocardial metabolic rate for glucose during ischemia: preliminary notes. J Nucl Med 1983;24:1060.

29. Ratib O, Phelps ME, Huang SC, et al. Positron tomography with deoxyglucose for estimating local myocardial glucose metabolism. J Nucl Med 1982;23:577.

30. Hoffman EJ, Phelps ME, Weiss ES, et al. Transaxial tomographic imaging of canine myocardium with ¹¹C-palmitic acid. J Nucl Med 1977;18:57.

31. Schon HR, Schelbert HR, Najafi A, et al. C-11 labelled palmitic acid for the non-invasive evaluation of regional myocardial fatty acid metabolism with positron computed tomography: kinetics of C-11 palmitic acid in acutely ischemic myocardium. Part II. Am Heart J 1982;103:548.

32. Schelbert HR, Henze E, Schon HR, et al. C-11 palmitic acid for the noninvasive evaluation of regional myocardial fatty acid metabolism with positron computed tomography: in vivo demonstration of impaired fatty acid oxidation in acute myocardial ischemia. Part IV. Am Heart J 1983;106:736.

33. Klein MS, Goldstein RA, Welch MJ, Sobel BE. External assessment of myocardial metabolism with C-11 palmitate in rabbit hearts. Am J Physiol (Heart Circ Physiol) 1979;237:H51.

34. Goldstein RA, Klein MS, Welch MJ, Sobel BE. External assessment of myocardial metabolism with C-11 palmitate in vivo. J Nucl Med 1980;21:342.

35. Brown M, Marshall DR, Sobel BE, Bergmann SR. Delineation of myocardial oxygen utilization with carbon-11-labeled acetate. Circulation 1987;76:687.

36. Buxton DB, Schwaiger M, Nguyen A, et al. Radiolabeled acetate as a tracer of myocardial tricarboxylic acid cycle flux. Circ Res 1988;63:628.

37. Henze E, Schelbert HR, Barrio JR. Evaluation of myocardial metabolism with N-13 and C-11 labeled amino acids and positron computed tomography. J Nucl Med 1982;23:671.

38. Phelps ME, Barrio JR, Huang SC, et al. Criteria for the tracer kinetic measurement of cerebral protein synthesis in humans with positron CT. Ann Neurol 1984;15(Suppl):S192.

39. Daemen BJG, Elsinga PH, Paans AMJ, et al. Radiation-induced inhibition of tumor growth as monitored by PET using L-[1-C11]tyrosine and fluorine-18-fluorodeoxyglucose. J Nucl Med 1992;33:373.

40. Rasey JS, Koh W, Grierson JR, et al. Radiolabeled fluoromisonidazole as an imaging agent for tumor hypoxia. Int J Radiat Oncol Biol Phys 1989;17:985.

41. Tsurumi Y, Kameyama M, Ishiwata K, et al. F-18 fluoro-2' deoxyuridine (FUdR) as a tracer of nucleic acid metabolism in brain tumors. J Neurosurg 1990;72:110.

42. Frost JJ. Studies of neurotransmitters and neuroreceptors by emission-computed tomography: focus on neuroreceptors. Trends Pharmacol Sci 1986;(Dec):490.

43. Young AB, Frey KA, Agranoff BW. Receptor assays: in vitro and in vivo. In: Phelps ME, Mazziotta JC, Schelbert HR, eds. Positron emission tomography and autoradiography: principles and applications for the brain and heart. New York: Raven Press, 1986:73.

44. Perlmutter JS, Kilbourn MR, Raichle MR, Welch MJ. MPTP-induced up-regulation of in vivo dopaminergic radioligand-receptor binding in humans. Neurology 1987;37:1575.

45. Wagner HN, Burns HD, Dannals RF, et al. Imaging dopamine receptors in the human brain by positron tomography. Science 1983;221:1264.

46. Arnett CD, Wolf AP, Shiue C-Y, et al. Improved delineation of human dopamine receptors using [18F]-N-methylspiroperidol and PET. J Nucl Med 1986;27:1878.

47. Baron JC, Maziere B, Loch C, et al. Loss of striatal·[76Br]bromospiperone binding sites demonstrated by positron tomography in progressive supranuclear palsy. J Cereb Blood Flow Metab 1986;6:131.

48. Baron JC, Comar D, Zarifian E, et al. Dopaminergic receptor sites in human brain: positron emission tomography. Neurology 1985;35:16.

49. Farde L, Hall H, Ehrin E, Sedvall G. Quantitative analysis of D2 dopamine receptor binding in the living human brain by PET. Science 1986;231:258.

50. Frost JJ, Wagner HN, Dannals RF, et al. Imaging opiate receptors in the human brain by positron tomography. J Comput Assist Tomogr 1985;9:231.

51. Frey KA, Koeppe RA, Jewett DM, et al. The in vivo distribution of [11C]scopolamine in human brain determined by positron emission tomography (abstract). Soc Neurosci 1987;13:1658.

52. Persson A, Ehrin E, Eriksson L, et al. Imaging of [C-11]-labeled RO 15-1788 binding to benzodiazepine receptors in the human brain by positron emission tomography. J Psychiatr Res 1985;19:609.

53. Robinson RG, Mayberg HS, Wong DF, et al. Relationship of post-stroke depression to PET scan asymmetry in cortical serotonin receptors. Soc Neurosci 1987;13:851.

54. Syrota A, Dormont D, Berger J, et al. C-11 ligand binding to adrenergic and muscarinic receptors of the human heart studied in vivo by PET (abstract). J Nucl Med 1983;24:201.

55. Frey KA, Hichwa RD, Ehrenkaufer RLE, Agranoff BW. Quantitative in vivo receptor binding: III. tracer kinetic modeling of muscarinic cholinergic receptor binding. Proc Natl Acad Sci USA 1985;82(19):6711.

56. Wieland DM, Rosenspire KC, Hutchins GD, et al. Neuronal mapping of the heart with 6-[18F]fluorometaraminol. J Med Chem 1990;33:956.

57. Wieland DM, Hutchins GD, Rosenspire KC, et al. [C-11]Hydroxyephedrine (HED): a high specific activity alternative to 6-[F-18]fluorometaraminal (FMR) for heart neuronal imaging. J Nucl Med 1989;30(5):767.

58. Mintun MA, Welch MJ, Siegel BA, et al. Breast cancer: PET imaging of estrogen receptors. Radiology 1988;169:45.

59. Bakir MA, Eccles SA, Babich JW, et al. c-erbB2 protein over-expression in breast cancer as a target for PET using iodine-124-labeled monoclonal antibodies. J Nucl Med 1992;33:2154.

60. Huang S-C, Phelps ME. Principles of tracer kinetic modeling in positron emission tomography and autoradiography. In: Phelps ME, Mazziotta JC, Schelbert HR, eds. Positron emission tomography and autoradiography: principles and applications for the brain and heart. New York: Raven Press, 1986:287.

61. Kuhl DE, Engel J Jr, Phelps ME, Selin C. Epileptic patterns of local cerebral metabolism and perfusion in humans determined by emission computed tomography of 18FDG and 13NH3. Ann Neurol 1980;8:348.

62. Engel J Jr, Kuhl DE, Phelps ME, Crandall PH. Comparative localization of epileptic foci in partial epilepsy by PCT and EEG. Ann Neurol 1982;12:529.

63. Benson DF, Kuhl DE, Phelps ME, et al. Positron emission tomography in the diagnosis of dementia. Trans Am Neurol Assoc 1981;106:1.

64. Cutler NR, Durara R, Creasey H, et al. Brain imaging: aging and dementia. Ann Intern Med 1984;202:355.

65. Ackerman RH, Alpert NM, Davis SM, et al. Positron emission tomography of stroke patients. In: Heiss WD, Phelps MD, eds. Positron emission tomography of the brain. New York: Springer-Verlag, 1983:113.

66. Baron JC, Bousser MG, Comar D, et al. Noninvasive tomographic study of cerebral blood flow and oxygen metabolism in vivo: potentials, limitations and clinical applications in cerebral ischemic disorders. Eur Neurol 1981;20:273.

67. Lenzi GL, Frackowiak RS, Jones T. Cerebral oxygen metabolism and blood flow in human cerebral ischemic infarction. J Cereb Blood Flow Metab 1982;2:321.

68. Stewart RE, Schwaiger M, Molina E, et al. Comparison of rubidium-82 PET and thallium-201 SPECT imaging for the detection of coronary artery disease. Am J Cardiol 1991;67:1303.

69. Schwaiger M, Brunken R, Grover-McKay M, et al. Regional myocardial metabolism in patients with acute myocardial infarction assessed by positron emission tomography. J Am Coll Cardiol 1986;8:800.

70. Marshall RC, Tillisch JH, Phelps ME, Huang S-C. Identification and differentiation of resting myocardial ischemia and infarction in man with positron computed tomography 18F-labeled fluorodeoxyglucose and N-13 ammonia. Circulation 1981;64:766.

71. Eitzman D, Al-Aouar ZR, Kanter HL, et al. Clinical outcome of patients with advanced coronary artery disease following positron emission tomography viability studies. J Am Coll Cardiol 1990;20:559.

72. Council on Scientific Affairs. Jacobson HG, ed. Positron emission tomography: a new approach to brain chemistry. JAMA 1988;260:2704.

73. Baron JC. Positron tomography in cerebral ischemia: a review. Neuroradiology 1985;27:509.

74. Kuhl DE, Metter EJ, Riege WH, et al. Local cerebral glucose utilization in elderly patients with depression, multiple infarct dementia and Alzheimer's disease. J Cereb Blood Flow Metab 1983;3(Suppl 1):S494.

75. Ackerman RH, Alpert NM, Correia JA, et al. Importance of monitoring metabolic function in assessing the severity of a stroke insult (CBF: An epiphenomenon?). J Cereb Blood Flow Metab 1981;1(Suppl 1):S502.

76. Council on Scientific Affairs. Jacobson, HG, ed. Report of scientific affairs: application of positron emission tomography in the heart. JAMA 1988;259:2438.

77. Schelbert HR, Wisenberg G, Phelps ME, et al. Noninvasive assessment of coronary stenoses by myocardial imaging during pharmacologic coronary vasodilation: detection of coronary

artery disease in man with intravenous N-13 ammonia and positron computed tomography. Part VI. Am J Cardiol 1988;49:1197.

78. Brunken R, Tillisch J, Schwaiger M, et al. Regional perfusion, glucose metabolism, and wall motion in patients with chronic electrocardiographic Q wave infarctions: evidence for persistence of viable tissue in some infarct regions by positron emission tomography. Circulation 1986;73:951.

79. Brunken R, Schwaiger M, Grover-McKay M, et al. Positron emission tomography detects tissue metabolic activity in myocardial segments with persistent thallium perfusion defects. J Am Coll Cardiol 1987;10:557.

80. Tillisch J, Brunken R, Marshall R, et al. Reversibility of cardiac wall motion abnormalities predicted by positron tomography. N Engl J Med 1986;314:884.

81. Aisen AM, Martel W, Glazer GM, Carson PL. Hepatic imaging: positron emission tomography, digital angiography, and nuclear magnetic resonance imaging. Hepatology 1986;3:1024.

82. Smith JJ. Role of positron emission tomographic scanning in the diagnosis of liver disease. Semin Liver Dis 1989;9:86.

83. Myren J, Kievulf P. The intravenous galactose tolerance test as indicator of the extent of fibrosis in patients with cirrhosis of the liver. Scand J Gastroenterol 1969;4:453.

84. Ishiwata K, Ido T, Imahori Y, et al. Accumulation of 2-deoxy-2-18fluoro-D-galactose in the liver by phosphate and uridylate trapping. Nucl Med Biol 1988;15:271.

85. Fukuda H, Matsuzawa T, Tada M, et al. 2-deoxy-2-18fluoro-D-galactose: a new tracer for the measurement of galactose metabolism in the liver by positron emission tomography. Eur J Nucl Med 1986;11:444.

86. Thomas HC, Jones EA, ed. Recent advantages in hepatology, 2. Edinburgh: Churchill Livingstone, 1986.

87. McMillin-Wood JB. Biochemical approaches to metabolism: application to positron emission tomography. Circulation 1985;72(5 Pt. 2):IV145.

88. Budinger TF. PET without a local cyclotron. PET/SPECT '87. Department of Energy. Washington, DC: Office of Health and Environmental Research, 1987:184.

89. Schuhmacher J, Matys R, Hauser H, et al. A Ga-68-labeled tetrabromophthalein (Ga-68 BP-IDA) for positron imaging of hepatobiliary function: concise communication. J Nucl Med 1983;24:593.

90. Blau M, Bender MA. 75-Se-Selenomethionine for visualization of the pancreas by isotope scanning. Radiology 1962;78:974.

91. Partain CL, Staab EV, McCartney WH. Multiple imaging modalities for the study of pancreatic disease. Semin Nucl Med 1979;9:36.

92. Agnew JE, Maze M, Mitchell CJ. Pancreatic scanning. Br J Radiol 1976;49:979.

93. Kirchner PT, Ryan J, Zalutsky M, Harper PV. Positron emission tomography for the evaluation of pancreatic disease. Semin Nucl Med 1980;10:374.

94. Hubner KF, Andrews GA, Buonocore E, et al. Carbon-11-labeled amino acids for rectilinear and positron tomographic imaging of the human pancreas. J Nucl Med 1979;20:507.

95. Buonocore E, Hubner KF. Positron-emission computed tomography of the pancreas: a preliminary study. Radiology 1979;133:195.

96. Syrota A, Comar D, Cerf M, et al. [11C]Methionine pancreatic scanning with positron emission computed tomography. J Nucl Med 1979;20:778.

97. Syrota A, Duquesnoy N, Paraf A, Kellershohn C. The role of positron emission tomography in the detection of pancreatic disease. Radiology 1982;143:249.

98. Kubota K, Fukuda H, Yamada K, et al. Experimental pancreas imaging study with 13N-glutamate using positron computer tomography. Eur J Nucl Med 1983;8:528.

99. Ishiwata K, Vaalburg W, Elsinga PH, et al. Comparison of L-[11C]-methionine and L-methyl-[11C]-methionine for measuring in vivo protein synthesis rates with PET. J Nucl Med 1988;29:1419.

100. Ishiwata K, Vaalburg W, Elsinga PH, et al. Metabolic studies with L-[14C]tyrosine for the investigation of a kinetic model to measure protein synthesis rates with PET. J Nucl Med 1988;29:524.

101. Jacobson HG, ed. Positron emission tomography in oncology. JAMA 1988;259:2126.

102. Beaney RP. Positron emission tomography in the study of human tumors. Semin Nucl Med 1984;14:324.

103. Beaney RP, Lammertsma AA, Jones T, et al. Positron emission tomography for in vivo measurement of regional blood flow, oxygen utilization and blood volume in patients with breast carcinoma. Lancet 1984;1:131.

104. Hayashi N, Tamaki N, Yonekura Y, et al. Imaging of the hepatocellular carcinoma using dynamic positron emission tomography with nitrogen-13 ammonia. J Nucl Med 1985;26:254.

105. Warburg O. The metabolism of tumors. New York: Richard R. Smith, 1931:129.

106. Flier JS, Mueckler MM, Usher P, Lodish HF. Elevated levels of glucose transport and transporter messenger RNA are induced by *ras* and *sarc* ongocgenes. Science 1987;235:1492.

107. Haberkorn U, Strauss LG, Dimitrakopoulou A, et al. Fluorodeoxyglucose imaging of advanced head and neck cancer after chemotherapy. J Nucl Med 1993;34:12.

108. Adler LP, Crowe JP, Al-Kaisi NK, Sunshine JL. Evaluation of breast masses and axillary lymph nodes with [F-18] 2-deoxy-2-fluoro-D-glucose PET. Radiology 1993;187:743.

109. Okazumi S, Isono K, Enomoto K, et al. Evaluation of liver tumors using fluorine-18-fluorodeoxyglucose PET: characterization of tumor assessment of effect of treatment. J Nucl Med 1992;33:333.

110. Wahl RL, Henry CA, Ethier SP. Serum glucose effects on tumor and normal tissue accumulation of 18F-fluoro-2-deoxy-D-glucose (FDG) in rodents with mammary carcinoma. Radiology 1992;183:643.

111. Jabour BA, Choi Y, Hoh CK, et al. Extracranial head and neck: PET imaging with 2-[F-18] fluoro-2-deoxy-D-glucose and MR imaging correlation. Radiology 1993;186:27.

112. Eriksson B, Bergstrom M, Lilja A, et al. Positron emission tomography (PET) in neuroendocrine gastrointestinal tumors. Acta Oncol 1993;32(2):189.

113. Shulkin BL, Wieland DM, Schwaiger M, et al. PET scanning with hydroxyephedrine: a new approach to the localization of pheochromocytoma. J Nucl Med 1992;33:1125.

114. Larson SM, Carrasquillo JA, Reynolds JC. Radioimmunodetection and radioimmunotherapy. Cancer Invest 1984;2:363.

115. Mathias CJ, Broadack JW, Kilbourn MR, et al. Biodistribution and metabolism of 16-alpha-[18F]fluoro-17-beta-estradiol. J Nucl Med 1985;26:127.

Textbook of Gastroenterology, second edition, edited by Tadataka Yamada. JB Lippincott Company, Philadelphia © 1995.

CHAPTER 126

Applications of Radionuclide Imaging in Gastroenterology

Arnold F. Jacobson

Theoretical Considerations
  Radionuclides
  Radiopharmaceuticals
  Radiation Dose
Technical Applications
  Imaging Systems
  Computers
Imaging Applications
  Liver

Hepatobiliary System
Gastric Mucosa
Gastrointestinal Bleeding
Gastrointestinal Tract Motility Studies
Salivary Glands
Inflammatory and Infectious Diseases
Oncologic Applications
Nonimaging Uses of Radiotracers

Nuclear Medicine is a distinct imaging specialty that encompasses a wide variety of diagnostic and therapeutic applications of radioactive isotopes (radionuclides) and provides important and often unique anatomic and physiologic information. Major clinical applications of radionuclide imaging in gastroenterology include studies for diagnosis of the following disorders: cavernous hemangiomas of the liver; acute cholecystitis and diseases of the hepatobiliary system; gastrointestinal (GI) bleeding; gastric and esophageal motility disorders; and inflammatory, infectious, and malignant processes involving the liver, bowel, and abdominal cavity. Clinical and research applications of radionuclide imaging are many and varied, and this chapter provides an overview of established current and promising new methods in nuclear medicine.

THEORETICAL CONSIDERATIONS

Radionuclide imaging is performed after administration of a radiolabeled compound that localizes to a specific organ system or the location of an ongoing physiologic process. Only structures in which the radiolabeled compound accumulates can be seen externally and thereby evaluated. Fundamentally, the normal biodistribution of the administered material results in a standardized structural image, with alterations in this normal distribution, seen as decreased or increased accumu-

lation of the labeled compound, providing information concerning abnormal anatomic or physiologic processes.

Radionuclides

The basis for choosing the radionuclides used in nuclear medicine are the characteristics of the emitted radiation, and either the biologic properties of the element itself, which allow its use in vivo, such as iodine for thyroid imaging, or the physical and chemical properties of the element, which allow it to be linked to appropriate compounds or pharmaceuticals, typically as a chelate in a complex. To be usable for imaging, an internally administered radioisotope must produce either γ-photons (from the atomic nucleus) or characteristic x-rays (from electron transitions between the atomic orbital shells) of sufficient energy that the majority will travel through and escape from the body unattenuated. Isotopes with primarily lower energy photons (< 50–60 keV) or particulate radiation such as beta particles (electrons) usually are avoided, because these emissions increase the radiation dose to the patient without contributing to the diagnostic images. There is also a higher energy limit for photons that can be imaged, primarily because the greater penetrating power of high-energy photons renders effective detection difficult. Although radionuclides with photons of 60 to 400 keV are used in nuclear medicine[1] (Table 126-1), noticeable deterioration is apparent in image quality for those with energies more than 200 keV.

TABLE 126-1
Radionuclides in Common Use in Nuclear Medicine

RADIONUCLIDE	PRINCIPAL PHOTON ENERGIES (keV)*	HALF-LIFE (h)	PARTICULATE EMISSIONS†	ENERGY COLLIMATION
Gallium-67	93, 185, 300	78	Minimal	Medium
Technetium-99m	140	6	Minimal	Low
Indium-111	172, 247	67	Minimal	Medium
Iodine-123	31, 159	13	Minimal	Low
Iodine-131	364	193	Significant	High
Xenon-133	31, 81	127	Minimal	Low
Thallium-201	69, 71, 80, 167	73	None	Low

* Energy > 30 keV and ≥ 10% photon yield (mean number/distintegration).

† β-Particles or internal conversion electrons with mean energies > 100 keV.

Adapted from Sorenson JA, Phelps ME. Physics in nuclear medicine. 2nd ed. Orlando: Grune & Stratton, 1987:298.

Radiopharmaceuticals

The success of a nuclear medicine imaging procedure is dependent on how well the radiopharmaceutical used targets the organs or the physiologic processes of interest. Whereas a radiopharmaceutical rarely has the ideal properties for any specific imaging application, individual compounds, and sometimes classes of compounds, have been developed to meet a variety of needs in nuclear medicine imaging. Structural modifications to a prototype compound, such as adding different organic side groups or altering the stereochemistry of a chelation, are used to improve imaging characteristics by means of increases in radiochemical binding efficiency or targeted biologic extraction, a good example of which is the evolution of the iminodiacetic acid (IDA) hepatobiliary agents, which has occurred during the last two decades (see Hepatobiliary System).

Technetium (^{99m}Tc) has proven particularly suitable for incorporation into stable complexes and chelates, and techniques have been developed that allow all necessary chemical reactions to take place in a single vial. The vial typically contains the compound to be labeled and various reducing agents and stabilizers, to which ^{99m}Tc in the form of pertechnetate (TcO_4-)—the chemical form in which this isotope is supplied from a device called a generator—is added. After thorough mixing, more than 95% of the radionuclide typically is attached to the desired compound.

Side effects resulting from administration of nuclear medicine radiopharmaceuticals are extremely rare, with a reported incidence of minor nonspecific or possible allergic reactions of 2 per 100,000 doses.[2] Strict adherence to proper techniques for handling blood products also has minimized incidents associated with reinjection of radiolabeled blood components. Whereas use of radiolabeled proteins of both human and mouse origin in newer investigational radiopharmaceuticals raises the possibility of allergic or anaphylactic reactions, results from clinical trials have shown an excellent safety profile consistent with that of conventional nuclear medicine compounds.

Radiation Dose

The primary determinants of the internal dosimetry of a radiopharmaceutical are its biodistribution and biologic half-life, and the physical half-life and the characteristics of the radiation emissions of the radionuclide. Shorter-lived photon-emitting radionuclides attached to compounds that are rapidly cleared from the target organ and the body usually result in the lowest radiation doses. The dominant role of ^{99m}Tc in nuclear medicine, although attributable in part to the element's favorable chemical properties, also is due to its emission of a single γ-photon with good energy for imaging, minimal coemissions of low-energy electrons, and short half-life (see Table 126-1), all of which contribute to minimizing the patient radiation dose. Target organ doses from most routine nuclear medicine procedures are comparable with those received from radiologic procedures such as barium radiographic studies or contrast computed tomography (CT).

TECHNICAL APPLICATIONS

Imaging Systems

Virtually all clinical nuclear medicine imaging is performed using the gamma camera. The principal components of this device are as follow: a large, flat crystal of sodium iodide in which incoming γ- and x-ray photons are absorbed and converted into flashes of light; a matrix of photomultiplier tubes that detect and amplify these scintillations; and electronic circuitry that determines the location at which the scintillation occurred (X-Y coordinates) and its intensity, reflecting the energy deposited by the absorption event.[1] Crystals in modern cameras are typically 0.63 or 0.95 cm (0.25 or 0.38 inches) thick and circular, rectangular, or square, with maximum dimensions ranging from 30 to 61 cm.

To obtain an exact image of the radiotracer distribution in a region, it is necessary to limit the detected photons as much as possible to those emitted perpendicular to the desired imaging plane. Because γ-photons are emitted isotropically (in all directions with essentially equal probability), a collimator—essentially a sheet of lead containing a number of small holes through which photons traveling toward the camera at a 90-degree angle can pass relatively unattenuated while photons approaching at other angles are absorbed—is placed in front of the camera face. Collimators vary in design, both in the thickness of the lead sheet and the size of the holes, allowing the imager to select between high counts–lower resolution (high-sensitivity collimation) versus reduced counts–higher resolution (high-resolution collimation) images, depending on the specific needs of the study. In addition, because a greater thickness of lead is required to obtain adequate absorption of higher energy scatter and off-angle photons, low-, medium-, and high-energy collimators are used for different isotopes, depending on the highest energy photon (see Table 126-1).

The final scintigraphic image reflects the distribution of scintillation events (counts) detected across the face of the γ-camera crystal during the course of an acquisition. Images may be acquired with the camera stationary, producing separate spot images of regions of the body, or with either the camera or imaging table moving, resulting in a single image of the total-body distribution of the administered radiopharmaceutical. Typical spot images contain 200,000 to 1,000,000 counts, whereas whole-body images are composed of several million. Although image quality usually improves as the number of counts increases, there are practical limits to the total time an acquisition can be continued to achieve a target count number, particularly for more seriously ill patients and those who have difficulty remaining still. Acquisition times for spot images usually are limited to a maximum of 10 minutes. Whereas as few as 10,000 counts are sometimes present in late delayed images and studies in which only a small amount of radiotracer can be used, adequate interpretation of such images usually is possible.

Although planar gamma camera imaging may be considered analogous to conventional radiography, cross-sectional imaging analogous to x-ray CT or magnetic resonance (MR) imaging also can be done using radionuclide techniques. This method is usually referred to as single photon emission computed tomography (SPECT). SPECT is typically performed using a rotating gamma camera and either a stop-and-shoot acquisition, with 32 to 128 planar views obtained while the camera traverses a 180- or 360-degree rotational arc around the patient, or an acquisition obtained during a continuous rotation. SPECT data are processed using reconstruction algorithms similar to those used in CT or MR imaging. Images are displayed as standard axial cross-sectional views, and in sagittal and coronal planes.

Although the majority of SPECT systems in use have a single camera head, multi-head SPECT systems have become increasingly popular. Both two- and three-head SPECT systems are commonly used, the former with 180-degree opposed heads, the latter with heads separated by 120 degrees. These new systems can acquire studies two to three times faster than a single-head camera, because a complete rotational arc is no longer necessary. Improved contrast and spatial resolution also can be achieved through the increased total number of counts, which can be accumulated with these multi-headed systems. Whereas in-plane spatial resolution with a single-

head SPECT system is typically on the order of 10 to 15 mm, resolution of 7 to 10 mm can be achieved using multi-head systems.

Computers

The computer is an integral part of the modern nuclear medicine imaging system, and provides quantitative capabilities that are difficult to duplicate by other radiologic methods. Each photon detected by the gamma camera is recorded in computer memory as a count in a digital picture element (pixel) matrix of selected size, each pixel encompassing a range of X-Y coordinates. Frequently used matrices for spot images are 64 by 64 and 128 by 128 pixels, whereas a whole-body image might be stored in a 256-by-1024 pixel matrix. Using the stored digital images, regions of interest can be drawn using a cursor on the computer display screen, allowing determination of the number of counts detected within those regions. These data then can be used for quantification of organ ratios, which reflect the biodistribution of the administered radiotracer. When image acquisitions are dynamic, with typical frame durations ranging from 0.25 seconds to 1 minute, each individual image is stored in sequence in the computer memory, allowing later display of the pattern of change in activity distribution over time. Regions of interest also can be drawn to allow determination of uptake, filling, and emptying rates of physiologic interest.

IMAGING APPLICATIONS

Liver

The prototypic nuclear medicine study pertaining to the GI system may be the liver-spleen scan. This was one of the first nuclear medicine procedures to gain acceptance for examining the abdomen, and was widely used for evaluation of the liver before the routine availability of abdominal ultrasound and CT. Conventional radionuclide imaging of the liver relies on the function of the hepatic Kupffer cells, and their ability for phagocytosis of appropriately sized particulate material injected intravenously. The material used is a colloidal preparation labeled with ^{99m}Tc, either sulfur or albumin colloid.[3] After intravenous injection, these agents are rapidly cleared (half-time [T$_{1/2}$], 2–3 minutes) by the liver (80%–85% extraction), the spleen (10%–15% extraction), and the bone marrow (1%–5% extraction). With significant liver disease, hepatic uptake of colloid is impaired and there are proportionate increases in uptake in the spleen and bone marrow.[4]

Whereas colloid scintigraphy was at one time an important method for identifying space-occupying lesions and infiltrative processes in the liver, such as primary and secondary tumors, abscesses, and cirrhosis, this method is infrequently used and is often limited to difficult imaging situations, such as obese patients in whom sonography may be inadequate and whose weight exceeds the limit of the CT or MR imaging tables. Occasionally patients thought to have more severe cirrhosis than is evident from liver function tests are studied, with the degree of shift of colloid uptake to the spleen and marrow used as an indication of disease severity.[4] This method also can be used to evaluate lesions that are thought to be either focal nodular hyperplasia, which normally show colloid uptake,[5] or adenomas, which usually do not.[6] Analysis of dynamic acquisitions for relative liver and spleen flow and uptake can provide estimates of the proportion of hepatic arterial and portal venous flow, which may be of value in monitoring effectiveness of therapy for portal hypertension and other liver pathologic processes.[7,8] Colloid scintigraphic delineation of the liver margins also can aid in interpretation of nuclear medicine infection imaging for suspected subdiaphragmatic or perinephric abscess, or tumor imaging to establish whether an abdominal mass lesion is intrahepatic or extrahepatic.

Although not specifically a GI imaging application, colloid scintigraphy remains a useful method for examining the spleen, particularly in patients with prior splenectomy. Colloid imaging is specific for discriminating splenic tissue from foci of infection or tumor, neither of which should show uptake, with SPECT of the abdomen being of particular use.

The high solubility of xenon in fat allows the use of inhaled xenon 133 gas for assessment of the degree of fatty infiltration in the liver. After rebreathing of 20 mCi of xenon 133 for 5 minutes, anterior imaging of the liver is performed during washout of the radioactive gas from the lungs. Presence of significant liver activity beyond 3 minutes during the washout phase indicates fatty changes, with the intensity of activity correlated with the liver fat content on biopsy.[9,10]

Alternative radiopharmaceuticals have been developed that are more specific for hepatocyte uptake and can be used to quantify functional hepatic parenchyma. One such investigational radiopharmaceutical is ^{99m}Tc-galactosyl-neoglycoalbumin, which binds to hepatic binding protein on the hepatocyte surface, and whose uptake is directly related to hepatic function.[11,12] Whether this or similar compounds will eventually have a role in routine clinical imaging remains to be determined.

Cavernous hemangiomas are the most common benign liver tumor, and are often observed as incidental findings on abdominal sonography and CT. When these lesions are either atypical in appearance on sonography, or are observed in patients with known liver disease or extrahepatic malignancy in whom metastatic involvement of the liver must be excluded, imaging of the liver with ^{99m}Tc-labeled red blood cells (RBCs) provides an excellent means for confirming their identification. This method relies on the greater blood pool within the hemangioma than in the surrounding liver parenchyma. Similar to the delayed enhancement of hemangiomas seen on contrast CT, the characteristic scintigraphic finding for hemangiomas is mildly decreased or normal-labeled RBC activity immediately after injection, followed by progressive increase in activity over the next 20 to 30 minutes.[13,14] Whereas observation of this pattern of enhancement on planar imaging is virtually pathognomonic for hemangioma, smaller lesions, or those that are located deeply within the liver parenchyma, may not always be seen. Increased sensitivity for detection of such hemangiomas is provided by liver SPECT, which is typically performed 1 to 2 hours after the labeled RBC injection to maximize lesion enhancement. Hemangiomas appear as distinct focal areas of increased activity compared with the surrounding liver parenchyma[15,16] (Fig. 126-1). Major blood vessels must be distinguished from parenchymal hepatic lesions, particularly centrally near the portal and hepatic veins, but this usually is readily done by means of examination of sequential image slices.

For lesions larger than 2 cm, sensitivity of SPECT RBC imaging for hemangioma identification exceeds 90%, equivalent to the performance of contrast CT and MR imaging.[17,18] Hemangiomas as small as 1.4 cm can be reliably identified on SPECT with a multi-head camera.[19] Although some smaller hemangiomas can be imaged with SPECT,[17,20] verification of the identity of lesions smaller than 1.5 cm probably is best accomplished with CT or MR imaging.

Hepatobiliary System

Whereas labeled colloid and RBCs allow examination of the liver reticuloendothelial and vascular components, hepatocyte function and the hepatobiliary system are best studied with a ^{99m}Tc-labeled IDA compound.[21] As one of the earliest of these compounds was the dimethyl-substituted IDA desig-

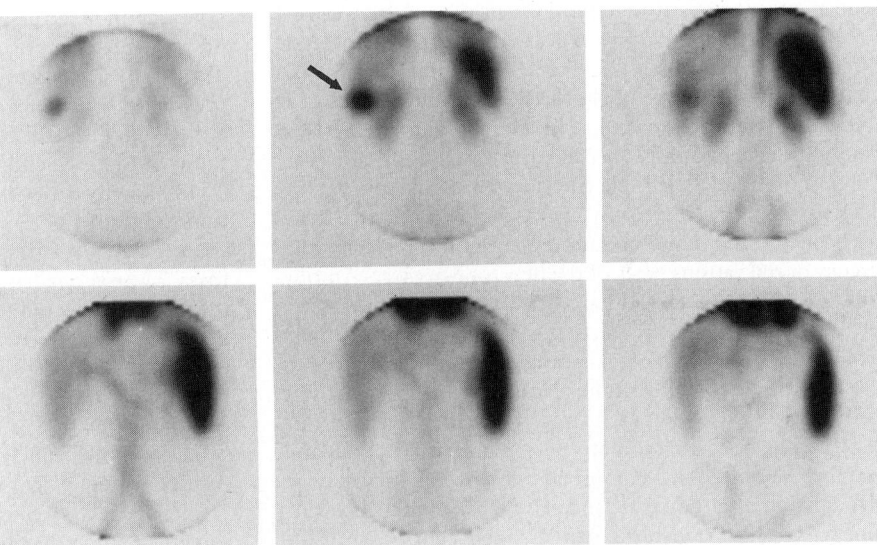

FIGURE 126-1. Sequential coronal images from single-photon emission computed tomography (posterior to anterior, *upper left* to *lower right*) from a labeled red blood cell scan of the liver show a focal region of increased activity (*arrow*) in the right lobe representing a 3-cm cavernous hemangioma initially identified on sonography.

nated as HIDA (the H standing for hepatic), the study was afterward often referred to as a HIDA scan. The HIDA agent has since been supplanted by superior substituted IDA compounds, and the imaging study is correctly designated as hepatobiliary scintigraphy or cholescintigraphy.

The IDA compounds enter the hepatocyte by means of a carrier-mediated pathway, the mechanism of which is very similar to that of bilirubin. Whereas significantly elevated serum bilirubin levels resulted in competitive inhibition of uptake of earlier IDA derivatives such as HIDA, the current compounds (disofenin, mebrofenin) have improved physiologic characteristics and can demonstrate adequate liver uptake and excretion at bilirubin levels as high as 20 to 30 mg/dL.[21]

For hepatobiliary imaging, 3 to 5 mCi of a ^{99m}Tc-labeled IDA compound is administered intravenously (up to 10 mCi may be used for patients with significantly elevated bilirubin levels), followed by anterior abdominal imaging, either as a dynamic acquisition or a series of static views, over the next 60 minutes. A normal study shows rapid uptake of the radiotracer into the liver, with virtually all cardiac blood pool activity cleared by 5 minutes after injection, followed by the liver excretory phase, with sequential visualization of intrahepatic bile ducts, the common hepatic duct, the cystic duct, gallbladder, common bile duct, and small bowel (Fig. 126-2). All of these structures typically are seen by 30 minutes after injection, although visualization of activity in the gallbladder and small bowel within 60 minutes is considered normal.

Whereas relative visualization time of the gallbladder and small bowel are not definitely correlated with most hepatobiliary pathologic disease, an association exists between patterns of bile flow and sphincter of Oddi characteristics. At low basal pressure of the sphincter of Oddi, most hepatic bile is excreted directly into the small intestine with a relatively smaller amount entering the gallbladder, typically resulting in activity being seen in the small bowel before the gallbladder. However, up to 20% of normal individuals have a relatively high resting sphincter of Oddi tone, which potentiates early filling of the gallbladder and results in absence of bowel visualization during the first 60 minutes of a hepatobiliary scan.[22] For such individuals, normalcy of the hepatobiliary system can be demonstrated through stimulation of the gallbladder, either by a fatty ingestion, which releases endogenous cholecystokinin, or an intravenously administered cholecystagogue such as sincalide (Kinevac, Squibb, Princeton, NJ), the terminal octapeptide of cholecystokinin, which produces gallbladder contraction and sphincter of Oddi relaxation (among other physiologic occurrences), with resultant visualization of radiolabeled bile entering the small bowel.

Hepatobiliary scintigraphy can be used to evaluate both parenchymal liver function and the structural integrity and patency of the various parts of the hepatobiliary tree. Among applications of this method are studies of infants with suspected biliary atresia,[23] patients with primary biliary cirrhosis[24,25] and sclerosing cholangitis,[26,27] and individuals who have undergone liver transplantation.[28,29] Time-activity curves for selected regions of interest in the liver and bile ducts can be used to estimate rates of hepatic uptake and clearance and bile flow. Abnormal bile flow kinetics may be an indication of intrahepatic and extrahepatic biliary obstruction, rejection in transplant patients, and congenital or ac-

quired ductal anomalies. Diameters of larger bile ducts can be estimated from scintigraphic images, albeit with lower precision than using ultrasound or CT, and whereas gallstones, strictures, and other intralumenal ductal lesions cannot themselves be identified, their effect usually can be observed in the form of retained activity in dilated intrahepatic or extrahepatic ducts. Common bile duct obstruction results in a typical pattern of intrahepatic cholestasis and gallbladder nonvisualization, particularly if the obstruction is more than 24 hours in duration.[30,31]

The most common use for hepatobiliary scintigraphy is to evaluate for the presence of acute cholecystitis. Acute cholecystitis and the associated obstruction of the cystic duct, whether mechanical or functional, are reflected on hepatobiliary scintigraphy by absence of gallbladder visualization. In the presence of signs and symptoms such as right upper quadrant tenderness, elevated leukocyte count, fever, and gallstones or wall thickening on gallbladder sonography, nonvisualization of the gallbladder by 60 minutes has a sensitivity greater than 95% for the diagnosis of acute cholecystitis.[32-35]

The most common reason for a false-positive hepatobiliary scan is chronic cholecystitis, where low rates of bile flow into the gallbladder may result in early nonvisualization. In the past, typical practice was to continue imaging these patients up to 2 to 4 hours after injection, because a significant percentage of patients with chronic cholecystitis eventually had sufficient bile flow into the gallbladder to demonstrate visualization. More recently, intravenous administration of a low dose of morphine (typically 0.04 mg/kg), which causes contraction of the sphincter of Oddi, increased intraductal pressure, and increased bile flow into the gallbladder, has been successfully employed to produce gallbladder visualization in the majority of patients without acute cholecystitis. If the gallbladder is not seen by 60 minutes, morphine is administered, and imaging is continued for 30 minutes. Persistent failure to see the gallbladder during this time further supports the diagnosis of acute cholecystitis.

In patients with early rapid excretion of the tracer from the liver, a second dose of the radiotracer may be given before administration of morphine to provide the activity necessary to produce gallbladder visualization if the cystic duct is patent. Conversion of a true-positive into a false-negative study does occasionally occur using morphine, most likely as a result of dislodgement of a stone because of the increased intraductal pressure. Nevertheless, sensitivity of gallbladder nonvisualization on morphine-augmented cholescintigraphy in patients thought to have acute cholecystitis is 93% to 95%.[36,37]

In patients with gallbladder nonvisualization, a secondary sign suggestive of a more severe pathologic process is a persistent region of activity in the liver adjacent to the gallbladder fossa. The *rim sign* has been attributed to edema and localized inflammation in the liver, causing impaired clearance of labeled bile, and is most often noticed in association with more complicated cholecystitis with transmural involvement, such as gangrenous or perforated gallbladder[38-40] (see Fig. 126-2). Although this sign is only moderately specific, its presence should alert the clinician to the potential need for more urgent surgical or equivalent intervention.

Hepatobiliary scintigraphy, similar to sonography, must be performed in the fasting state, because postprandially, the

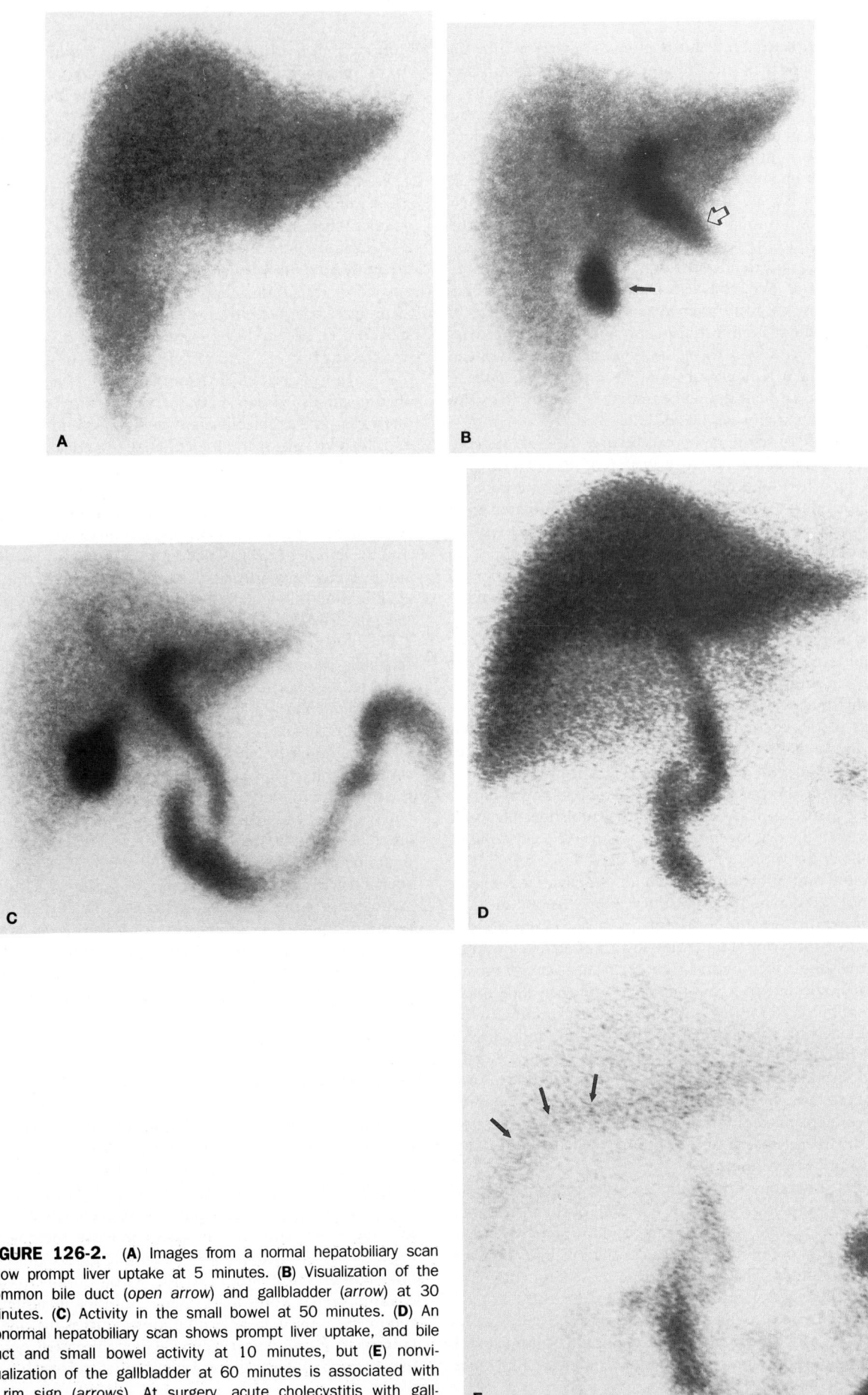

FIGURE 126-2. **(A)** Images from a normal hepatobiliary scan show prompt liver uptake at 5 minutes. **(B)** Visualization of the common bile duct (*open arrow*) and gallbladder (*arrow*) at 30 minutes. **(C)** Activity in the small bowel at 50 minutes. **(D)** An abnormal hepatobiliary scan shows prompt liver uptake, and bile duct and small bowel activity at 10 minutes, but **(E)** nonvisualization of the gallbladder at 60 minutes is associated with a rim sign (*arrows*). At surgery, acute cholecystitis with gallbladder necrosis was found.

gallbladder is contracted and bile flow is diverted into the small bowel, producing a false-positive finding of gallbladder nonvisualization.[41] A minimum fast of 4 hours usually is recommended before initiation of a study. However, false-positive study findings can occur after prolonged fasting, such as in patients in intensive care and those on total parenteral nutrition, presumably because the gallbladder becomes atonic and contains viscous, sludgy bile, which limits entry of new hepatic bile even though the cystic duct is patent.[42,43] Intravenous sincalide pretreatment of patients who have taken nothing orally for extended periods (>24–48 hours) has been advocated to produce sufficient emptying of the gallbladder to allow filling to occur after injection of the radiotracer.[44] Although regular administration of sincalide has been reported to reduce sludge formation in patients on prolonged periods of total parenteral nutrition,[45] a consensus on whether sincalide pretreatment should be routine in hepatobiliary imaging of such patients has not been reached.

Hepatobiliary scintigraphy can be used to evaluate congenital or acquired structural anomalies of the biliary tree or to examine for abnormalities resulting from operative or traumatic injury. Choledochal cysts are seen as isolated areas of increased retention of tracer corresponding to the involved region of the bile duct,[46,47] whereas sclerosing cholangitis results in multiple scattered areas of retention secondary to ductal stenoses.[26,27] Bile leakage results in visualization of the tracer outside the normal ductal pathways, and scintigraphy can be helpful in evaluating patients thought to have bile peritonitis or postoperative or posttraumatic liver or bile duct injury.[48] In addition, the pattern of bile flow can be examined in postgastrectomy patients to assess the functional characteristics of the efferent and afferent limbs, the latter often being better demonstrated scintigraphically than by radiographic studies with orally administered contrast.

The most common functional evaluation in hepatobiliary imaging involves measurement of the gallbladder response to stimulation by endogenous or exogenous cholecystokinin or its analogs. After administering the ^{99m}Tc-labeled IDA compound and allowing sufficient time thereafter for liver clearance and maximum gallbladder filling, the oral meal or the intravenous agent is given. Images in the anterior or occasionally an anterior oblique view are acquired on computer while the gallbladder gradually contracts and activity moves into the cystic and common bile ducts and then the bowel. Regions of interest for the gallbladder and background in the adjacent hepatic parenchyma are then drawn, and the net change in gallbladder activity over time is determined. A gallbladder ejection fraction, usually representing the maximum change produced by the stimulus [(maximum counts − minimum counts)/maximum counts) × 100%] then is calculated and compared against results for normal controls studied under the same test conditions.[49]

Cholescintigraphy using intravenously injected sincalide has gained widespread acceptance as a clinical and research examination method. Sincalide can be administered as either a bolus over 1 to 3 minutes or as a continuous infusion over 15 to 60 minutes. The sincalide dose most frequently employed is 0.02 μg/kg, although the higher dose of 0.04 μg/kg may be needed to elicit a response in some patients. In comparison with the bolus technique, sincalide administered as a continuous infusion produces more complete gallbladder

contraction, has better reproducibility, produces less symptoms, and is more physiologic, analogous to the sustained elevation of endogenous cholecystokinin, which occurs after a meal. In a comparison of bolus injections (0.02 μg/kg) and 30-minute infusion protocols in 23 normal volunteers, the mean gallbladder ejection fractions were 56% and 70%, respectively, with the infusion gallbladder ejection fractions higher in 21 subjects (91%), being less than 40% in 10 bolus studies but only 3 infusion studies.[50]

Sincalide-augmented hepatobiliary imaging has been used to study patients with abdominal symptoms thought to be related to acalculous biliary disease. Some investigators have demonstrated a definite correlation between low gallbladder ejection fraction and symptom relief after cholecystectomy, which suggests this method may be useful for identifying patients who might benefit from surgery.[51-53] However, conflicting published data have shown no correlation between the presurgical gallbladder ejection fraction and either severity of gallbladder histopathologic changes[54] or relief of symptoms after cholecystectomy.[55] These contradictory results highlight the complexity of the pathologic processes that affect the gallbladder, and also the multiple causes that can be responsible for nonfocal abdominal pain. Even though biliary dyskinesia and the failure of the gallbladder to respond to sincalide cannot be considered normal, patients with normal sonographic examination of the gallbladder and no symptoms still may have diminished gallbladder contraction in response to sincalide.[50] Although sincalide-augmented cholescintigraphy is reliable as a measurement technique, its results should be interpreted in conjunction with physical examination, laboratory and other radiologic data before pursuing either medical or surgical treatment.

Scintigraphy has proven useful for examining patients thought to have biliary pain on the basis of dysfunction of the sphincter of Oddi. Delayed excretion of radiolabeled bile and decreased gallbladder contraction in response to sincalide are associated with sphincter of Oddi dysfunction documented manometrically.[56,57] Sphincter dysfunction also may be associated with a paradoxic response to sincalide, i.e., increased sphincter pressure resulting in increased activity in the common bile duct after administration of the cholecystagogue. Several studies have shown significant improvement in bile flow dynamics after sphincterotomy or sphincteroplasty, with symptom relief also correlated with abnormal preoperative emptying kinetics.[57-59]

Gastric Mucosa

Radionuclide imaging of the stomach and gastric mucosa usually is limited to investigations to identify ectopic gastric mucosa associated with suspected Meckel's diverticula in children and young adults with abdominal pain and GI bleeding. ^{99m}Tc-pertechnetate is actively extracted and excreted by the mucous-secreting cells in gastric mucosa, thereby providing a means for locating sites of ectopic gastric mucosa.[60,61] For a Meckel's scan, 30 to 100 μCi/kg of ^{99m}Tc-pertechnetate is administered, followed by serial anterior imaging of the abdomen for the next 30 to 60 minutes. Just as the circulating radiotracer is progressively extracted by the gastric mucosa in the stomach, a Meckel's diverticulum that contains gastric mucosa will show enhancement of activity over time. Appearance of a focus of pertechnetate uptake outside of the stomach within 10 to 20 minutes, typically in the right lower quadrant of the abdomen, usually is indicative of a Meckel's diverticulum. Oblique views of the abdomen and views with the stomach or bladder blocked with lead sometimes are done to enhance the visualization of small focal accumulations in the lower abdomen. Intravenous administration of pentagastrin, glucagon, and cimetidine before pertechnetate injection are capable of improving visualization of Meckel's diverticula by means of increasing uptake and delaying local clearance of the radiotracer, respectively.[62,63] Summary data, mostly from studies without premedication, have shown a sensitivity of 85% and specificity of 95% for detection of Meckel's diverticula with pertechnetate scanning.[60]

Gastrointestinal Bleeding

One gastroenterologic nuclear medicine study usually performed on an urgent or emergent basis is the GI bleeding study. The underlying principle of GI bleeding scintigraphy is that an intravascular tracer in circulation at the time of active bleeding will extravasate into the bowel, thereby allowing identification of the bleeding site. Two radiopharmaceutical agents have been primarily used to investigate for sites of GI bleeding, ^{99m}Tc-labeled colloid and ^{99m}Tc-labeled RBCs. The relative utility of each of these agents is discussed in the next paragraphs.

The theoretical advantage of ^{99m}Tc-labeled colloid as an agent for GI bleeding studies is that it is rapidly cleared from circulation by the liver and spleen, such that the site of extravasated bowel activity and then subsequent movement of this intralumenal blood are readily identified because of the low tissue background.[64] Rates of bleeding as low as 0.05 mL/minute have been identified using sulfur colloid imaging in an animal model in which the radiotracer was introduced into the bowel at a controlled rate by means of a catheter.[65] The major disadvantage of labeled colloid as a bleeding tracer is that the same rapid clearance from the blood, which allows high-contrast imaging, also results in only a few minutes of opportunity for identification of the bleeding site. Since GI hemorrhage frequently is an intermittent process and patients are often referred for a scintiscan many hours after their initial presentation with bleeding complaints, it is likely that active bleeding will not be occurring during any short period of study. As such, if an initial colloid study fails to identify bleeding, additional sequential tracer injections may be needed to improve sensitivity. Because repeated injections usually are not practical, the intermittent nature of GI bleeding limits the utility of colloid as a study agent.

The most commonly used radiotracer for identification of GI bleeding sources is ^{99m}Tc-labeled RBCs. Cells are labeled by a method that does not involve intravenous administration of ^{99m}Tc-pertechnetate (either a modified in vitro or totally in vitro kit technique), because injected pertechnetate is extracted and secreted by the gastric mucosa and eventually ends up in the bowel contents in the absence of bleeding (see previous discussion concerning Meckel's scanning under the section "Gastric Mucosa"). Once reinjected, the labeled RBCs remain in circulation for as long as the cells are viable, which

allows for an imaging interval limited only by the physical half-life of ^{99m}Tc. After injection of 20 to 25 mCi of ^{99m}Tc-labeled RBCs, anterior abdominal imaging is performed for 60 to 120 minutes, depending on the initial findings and the relative stability of the patient. Imaging may be performed as a continuous dynamic acquisition, typically 1 frame per minute, or as a series of static views at 5-minute intervals. Anterior oblique and lateral views sometimes are also obtained to aid in localizing the bleeding site. In the presence of active bleeding, labeled cells enter the bowel lumen and are seen as a focal area of increased activity. The two critical features of a positive bleeding study are this identification of a focal accumulation of blood, followed by observation of the intralumenal movement of this activity to more specifically localize the bleeding site (Fig. 126-3).[66] If the patient is too unstable to remain for an extended period in the nuclear medicine department, or if angiographic or surgical procedures to stop the bleeding are pending, it may be necessary to terminate the study as soon as a positive finding is identified, but under most circumstances, further images demonstrating movement of labeled blood allow more accurate discrimination of small from large bowel sources. Dynamically acquired images viewed as a cine loop are particularly effective for demonstrating passage of intralumenal labeled RBCs through the bowel.[67]

Intralumenal accumulation of activity during the initial imaging session identifies bleeding sites in the stomach, small bowel, or colon with high accuracy, although when bleeding is occurring at a slow rate, the site identified by other means (angiography, endoscopy, surgery) may be a few centimeters proximal or distal to the location initially seen on the scan. This occurs as a result of antegrade and retrograde movement of blood in the bowel, with the initial site seen on the scan being a location near the bleeding focus where sufficient radiolabeled blood has pooled to allow it to be seen above the abdominal blood pool background.

Active bleeding sites are seen during the first 1 to 2 hours of imaging in about one third of the cases.[68–70] For patients whose studies give negative results at this point, options include proceeding with other investigations (endoscopy, angiography, surgery), or obtaining later delayed views. The results on later delayed views indicate whether active bleeding has occurred during the interval between imaging sessions, and several sequences of images frequently are obtained over the course of the 24 hours after the original labeled RBC injection, during which time imaging is feasible (see Fig. 126-3). Because *old* blood that entered the bowel before the injection of the labeled cells does not show up as a positive scan finding, any intralumenal labeled RBCs could have entered the bowel only after the start of the study. Stool or blood passed per rectum also can be examined using either the gamma camera or a well counter to detect the presence of ^{99m}Tc, and this is an extremely sensitive method for identifying very small amounts of bleeding that may not have been evident on the abdominal images.

Among patients whose early images yield negative results, later delayed images demonstrate intralumenal labeled RBCs in 20% to 46%, overall about one third of all patients studied.[66,69–71] However, the location(s) where blood is seen on delayed images often does not reflect the site of entry into the bowel. Although the bleeding site is unlikely to be significantly distal to the location where blood is seen (allowing

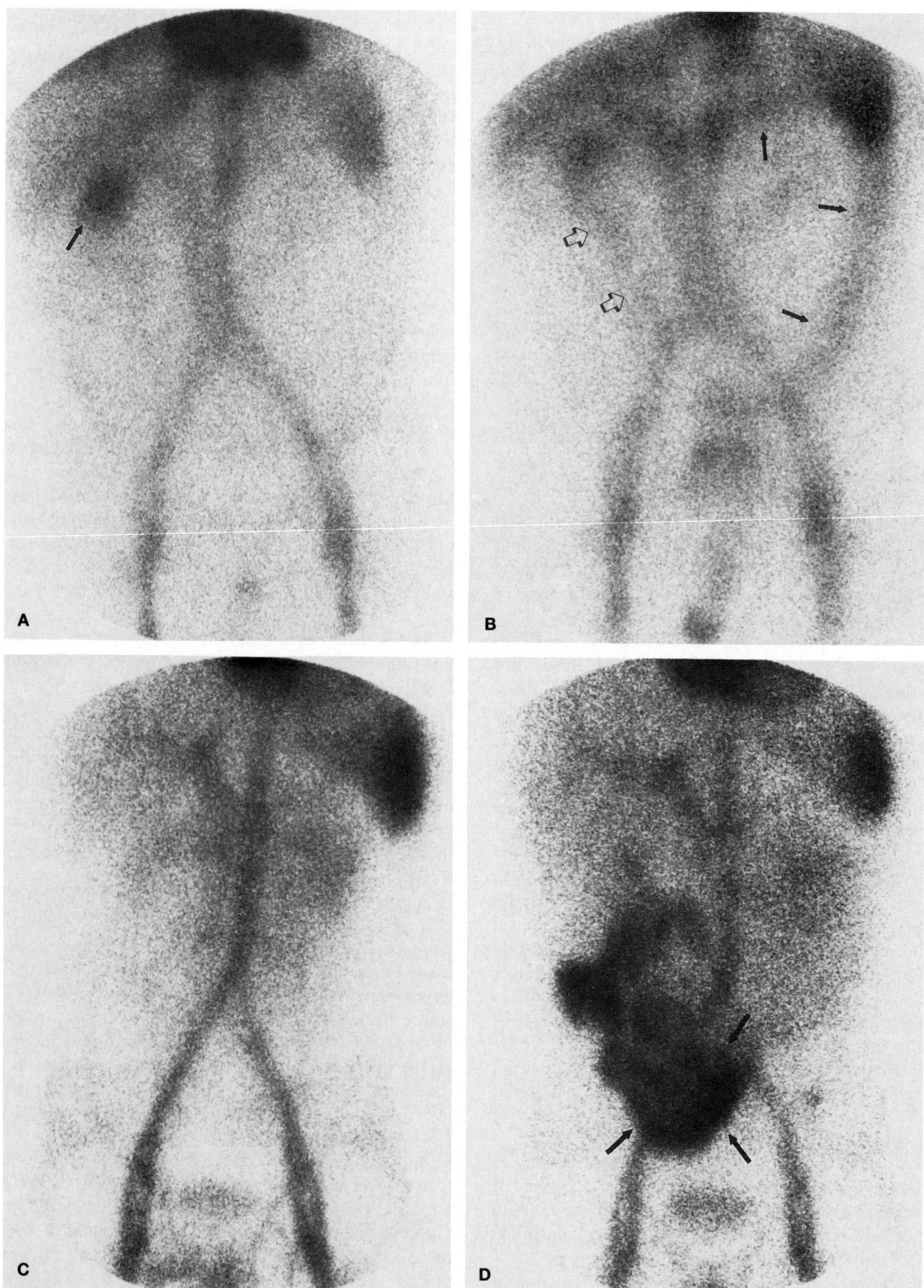

FIGURE 126-3. Anterior abdominal images from two labeled red blood cell gastrointestinal bleeding studies are shown. (**A**) Focal accumulation of activity is seen in the right upper quadrant (*arrow*) at 10 minutes after injection at the site of an anastamotic bleed in the right colon, with (**B**) labeled red blood cells seen in the ascending (*open arrows*), transverse, and descending colon (*arrows*) on a later image at 60 minutes as a result of both retro- and antegrade movement of blood. (**C**) The images on the right show no definite extravasation at 60 minutes, but (**D**) diffuse intralumenal blood is seen in the distal small bowel (*arrows*) at 4 hours and (**E**) throughout the colon (*open arrows*) at 5 hours. Angiography demonstrated active bleeding at the site of duodenal ulcers seen previously at endoscopy. All scintigraphic images show normal blood pool activity in the liver, heart, and spleen (*left* to *right* at the top of each image) and in the major abdominal blood vessels.

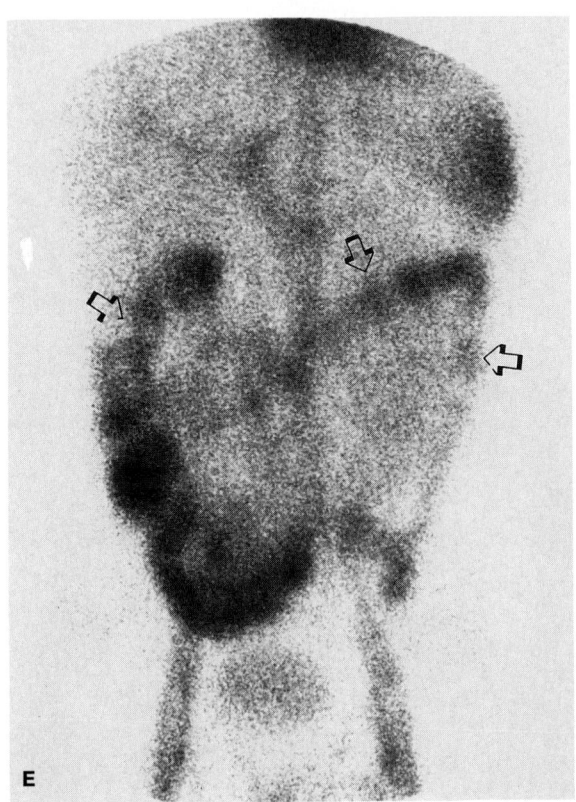

FIGURE 126-3. (Continued)

for the possibility of retrograde flow), it is not possible to exclude any source proximal to that location. Diffuse activity frequently is seen in the colon on 18- to 24-hour delayed images, but in my experience, as many as half of identified sources of bleeding in such patients will be in the upper GI tract.[70] Nevertheless, positive delayed images do provide objective evidence of the presence of bleeding during the study interval, and such patients tend to have more complicated courses, requiring greater amounts of blood transfusions and more frequent intervention by angiography or surgery than do patients whose early and late images give negative findings.[66,70] Occasionally in a patient with early negative images, later delayed, low-count rate images show a site that appears to have increasing activity suggestive of active bleeding. Such a patient can undergo reinjection with either labeled colloid or a second dose of labeled RBCs and undergo further imaging to facilitate identification of the bleeding site.[72]

Patients who have no intralumenal blood identified on scintigraphy to 24 hours tend to be the ones admitted with a single episode of bleeding, who often have no significant positive findings on their workup and no further episodes of bleeding. Negative findings from a GI bleeding study with both early and late images suggests a good prognosis for patients who present with an isolated episode of melena or hematochezia.[70]

The sensitivity for detection of bleeding using labeled RBCs is about 0.1 to 0.2 mL/minute[69] compared with 0.5 mL/minute for angiography. Even when preceded by positive results from a bleeding scan, angiograms typically show contrast extravasation in less than half of the patients studied.[66,69,73]

This reflects both the intermittent nature of most GI bleeding and the reality that even in the best organized imaging departments, bleeding may stop in the interval, regardless of how short, between the completion of the bleeding scan and the initiation of angiography.

Other approaches that have been used to identify bleeding sources have included scintigraphic studies in association with intravenous heparin to increase the likelihood of bleeding,[74] and intraarterial injections of radiolabeled material through angiographic catheters in patients with angiograms that had negative results. Identification of bleeding sites based on hemostasis rather than bleeding itself also has been investigated, with Indium-111–labeled platelets used to identify the hemostatic plug at sites that previously bled.[75]

Gastrointestinal Tract Motility Studies

Gastric Emptying

Movement of the contents of the tubular alimentary tract can be monitored using radionuclides, the best known method involving the study of gastric emptying. Both liquid and solid gastric emptying are readily examined by means of serial abdominal images in anterior or posterior projections for 60 to 120 minutes after ingestion of a suitable labeled material after an overnight fast.[76,77] Images can be acquired dynamically as a continuous sequence, or sequential static images can be obtained every 15 minutes, including both anterior and posterior views to allow calculation of the geometric mean. Regions of interest are drawn around the gastric silhouette to obtain the time-activity curve for emptying, from which a $T_{1/2}$ can be determined and compared against results for normal subjects with the same test meal (Fig. 126-4). The pattern of emptying also can be analyzed on the time-activity curve, including determination of the duration of emptying delay associated with solids (lag phase). Regions of interest can be drawn for portions of the stomach (fundus, antrum) to assess peristaltic behavior that may contribute to any observed abnormalities.

Liquid-phase gastric emptying studies are relatively simple, with approximately 100 to 300 μCi of ^{99m}Tc-labeled colloid or ^{111}In-DTPA administered in 150 to 300 mL of water, juice, or another suitable liquid. Imaging usually can be completed within 60 minutes, with normal $T_{1/2}$ in the range of 15 to 45 minutes. When liquid-phase emptying is abnormal, no further study may be necessary, but otherwise, examination of solid emptying usually is appropriate.

A variety of test meals have been used for solid emptying studies, typically labeled with 300 to 1000 μCi of ^{99m}Tc-colloid. The labeled compound should not dissociate or separate from the solid test meal in the stomach; if this occurs, the study becomes equivalent to examining liquid emptying, i.e., mainly gastric juices and whatever liquid was consumed with the meal, in the presence of solids rather than monitoring solid emptying itself. Investigators previously used methods such as injecting a chicken with ^{99m}Tc-sulfur colloid, killing the chicken several minutes later, and them removing and cooking the in vivo–labeled chicken liver to use as part of a test meal. A more practical method for routine clinical imaging involves injecting labeled colloid into an egg through

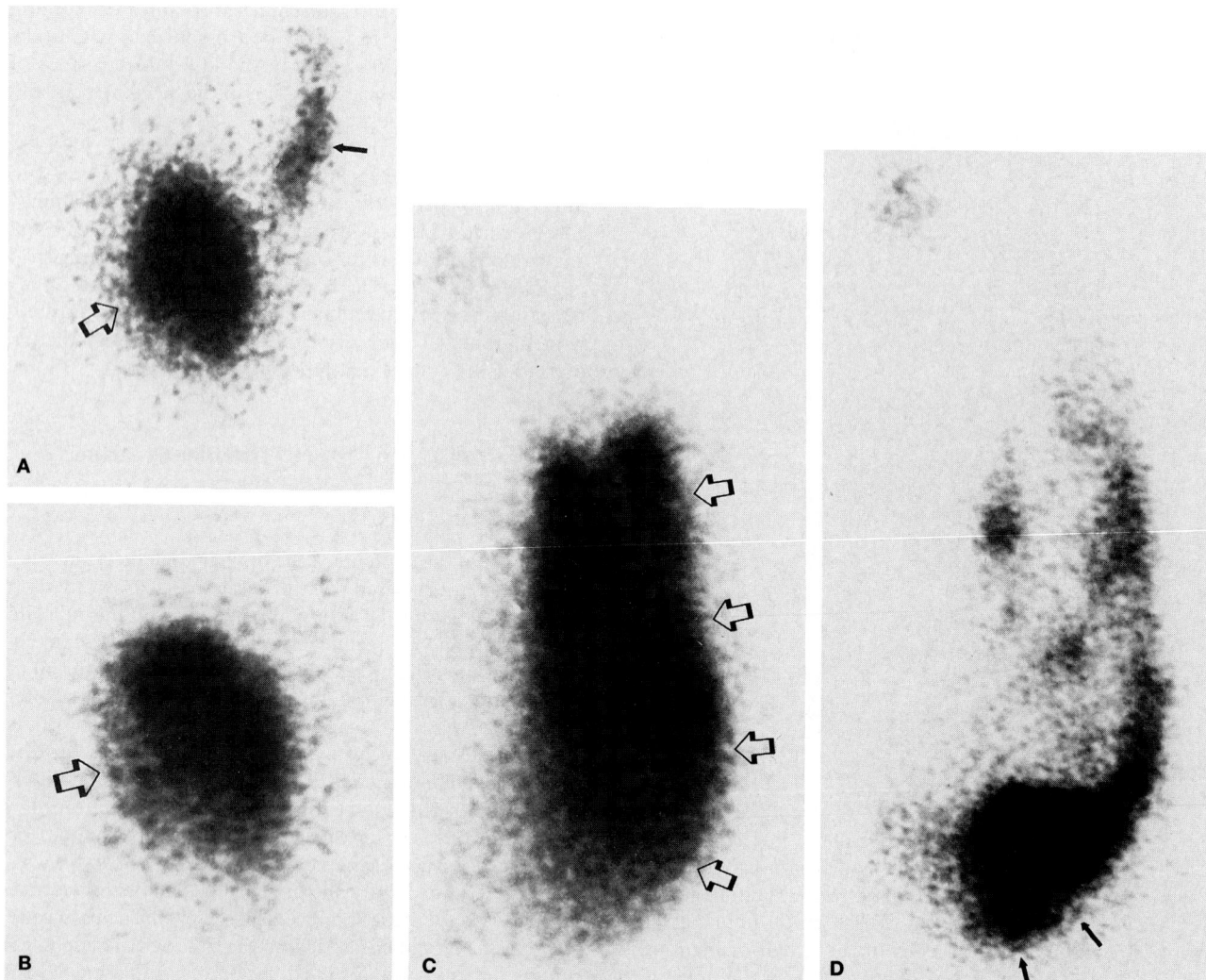

FIGURE 126-4. Posterior images of the stomach (*open arrows*) at (**A**) 5 and (**B**) 80 minutes after ingestion of radiolabeled solid meal demonstrate no significant emptying. Activity in the esophagus (*arrow*) on initial image indicates gastroesophageal reflux. (**C**) The posterior chest images on the right are from an erythromycin-augmented liquid gastric emptying study in a patient 3 weeks after esophagectomy with gastric pull-up with persistent vomiting but no obstruction on barium swallow radiographs. At 30 minutes, a large amount of activity remains in the intrathoracic stomach (*open arrows*). (**D**) After intravenous administration of 100 mg of erythromycin, significant gastric emptying is seen, with activity in the proximal small bowel (*arrows*). Faint activity in the upper left of the images represents a radioactive marker at the sternal notch.

the shell and then cooking the egg, thereby binding the radiotracer in the coagulated protein. Other solids used for test meals have included liver pâté, beef stew, and scrambled eggs.

Solid gastric emptying studies are performed in essentially the same manner as for liquids, but a longer imaging acquisition—typically 60 to 120 minutes—usually is required. Overlap between the stomach and the adjacent small bowel, or occasionally a loop of large bowel if transit is rapid, sometimes occurs, requiring a change in the camera obliquity. However, combined anterior and posterior acquisitions with calculation of geometric mean stomach activity is preferred.

Normal curves and $T_{1/2}$ for gastric emptying depend on the composition (calories, fat content) and total mass of the test meal. Although some test meals may be considered standard,

it is always best to study normal volunteers with the specific meal that will be used to evaluate patients to establish reliable normal limits. $T_{1/2}$ data for solid gastric emptying for different sized test meals range from 68 to 277 minutes,[78,79] with $T_{1/2}$ usually less than 120 minutes for the smaller meals in common clinical use.[80]

Simultaneous measurement of gastric emptying for liquids and solids is possible using a dual isotope technique, with the solid labeled with ^{99m}Tc-colloid and the liquid labeled with ^{111}In-DTPA. Anterior and posterior images are acquired after consumption of the liquid and solid together, with different energy windows used to separate data from ^{99m}Tc and ^{111}In, thereby allowing individual solid and liquid calculations. Although ingestion of liquids is minimized for measuring solid emptying alone, the dual isotope technique allows examination of the manner in which liquids affect solid emptying and vise versa. The dual isotope technique is more physiologic in that ingestion of solids in the absence of any liquids is relatively rare, and allows a more complete analysis of gastric motility in the same period of time required for a standard solid-only emptying study.[80]

The quantitative nature of gastric emptying studies makes them well-suited for examining the response to drugs given to improve motility, such as in patients with gastroparesis. A baseline study usually is performed first, followed by a second study after the achievement of a therapeutic level of a drug such as metoclopramide. This provides an elegant method to correlate clinical response to therapy with a quantitative measure of function.[81] More recently, improvement in gastric motility after the use of erythromycin, a stimulator for the motilin receptors in the stomach, has been demonstrated with radionuclide techniques.[82] Such studies may be particularly helpful in postsurgical patients, such as those who have previously undergone esophagectomy with gastric pull-up, in whom conventional barium swallow radiographs may demonstrate no evidence of mechanical obstruction (see Fig. 126-4).

Gastroesophageal Reflux

Gastroesophageal reflux can be readily identified qualitatively on the images from a conventional gastric emptying study, and can be quantified from the amount of activity in esophageal regions of interest. A more specific imaging technique for assessing gastroesophageal reflux involves use of an inflatable abdominal binder. After ingesting 300 μCi of ^{99m}Tc-colloid in 300 mL acidified orange juice in the upright position, baseline images of the chest and upper abdomen are obtained to assure initial esophageal clearance of tracer activity. The patient then is fitted with the abdominal binder and positioned supine under the gamma camera. Imaging then is performed while the binder is inflated in stepwise fashion, producing incremental increases in intraabdominal pressure. Intraabdominal pressure required to induce gastroesophageal reflux has been quantified in normal volunteers, and the control data have been used to evaluate results in symptomatic individuals.[83] Regions of interest are drawn over the esophagus to judge the timing and intensity of any reflux observed, and ratios of peak esophageal and gastric activity can be calculated to provide a further quantitative measure.

In patients thought to have pulmonary aspiration secondary to gastroesophageal reflux, a radiolabeled meal can be consumed in the evening before bedtime. After a normal night of sleep, the patient undergoes imaging to determine if radiotracer is present in the tracheobronchial tree or the lungs. The presence of any significant activity in the respiratory system is objective evidence of the occurrence of aspiration.[83] This study can be repeated after medical or surgical intervention to reduce gastroesophageal reflux and aspiration to assess the effectiveness of the measures taken.

Esophageal Motility

Tracer techniques can be used to examine esophageal motor function and esophageal transit. The patient usually is instructed to take a small quantity of ^{99m}Tc-labeled liquid into the mouth and then asked to swallow while dynamic gamma camera images of the anterior chest are obtained at a high frame rate, usually one to three images per second. Additional imaging at 15 seconds per frame for up to 10 minutes, with a dry swallow at the beginning of each frame, also may be performed. Time-activity curves then are obtained for three segments of the esophagus (proximal, middle, and distal), and the timing and coordination of the passage of the tracer is examined. Neuromuscular and collagen-vascular diseases produce characteristic patterns of delayed tracer clearance, whereas diffuse esophageal spasm results in discoordinate changes in regional activity. Data from normal volunteers frequently are used for comparison with results obtained when patients are studied.[84]

Salivary Glands

Nuclear medicine techniques can be used to examine the physiologic behavior of the salivary glands.[85] This is done using ^{99m}Tc-pertechnetate, which is taken up by the secretory cells of the salivary glands similar to chloride or iodide ions. After injection of 5 to 10 mCi, anterior and lateral images of the head and neck can document the location and relative function of the various glands. Stimulation of saliva secretion with an acidic substance such as lemon juice can be used to evaluate for possible effects of ductal anomalies, stones, or malignancy on gland clearance. Time-activity curves for regions of interest over the salivary glands also can be used to estimate rates of saliva production and excretion.

Inflammatory and Infectious Diseases

Labeled leukocytes are the scintigraphic agent of choice for investigating inflammatory processes involving the bowel.[86] Granulocytes or mixed leukocyte populations usually are separated from 30 to 60 mL of blood, and labeled in vitro with either ^{99m}Tc or ^{111}In. There is far greater experience with ^{111}In-leukocytes, which have been in wide clinical use for more than 10 years, but use of this radionuclide can be technically demanding. Its longer half-life (67 hours versus 6 hours for ^{99m}Tc) results in an increased radiation dose per millicurie administered, particularly to the spleen, and the higher energies of its two major photon emissions make it necessary to use medium energy collimation (see Table 126-1), with the resultant lower sensitivity than ^{99m}Tc. Although these limitations have led to the use of only small quantities of ^{111}In (0.3–1.0 mCi) for leukocyte imaging, with the expected significant statistical constraints on image quality, this method nevertheless has had considerable success in identifying infection and inflammation in the abdomen.[87]

After leukocyte labeling with ^{111}In-oxine, which requires approximately 2 hours, the cells are reinjected and imaging is performed 2 to 24 hours later. Delayed imaging at 18 to 24 hours allows clearance of normal intravascular activity, particularly noticeable in the lungs early after reinjection, and greater accumulation of labeled leukocytes at abnormal sites, which are typically defined more clearly on later views. Nevertheless, same-day imaging at 2 to 6 hours after injection is of acceptable quality for abdominal sites where blood pool background is not a major constraint.[86]

The characteristic abnormal finding on a labeled leukocyte scan is increased focal uptake at sites of infection or inflammation, with the degree of uptake sometimes scored relative to activity at sites of normal uptake such as the liver or bone marrow (Fig. 126-5). When increased activity is seen in the bowel, it is necessary to ascertain whether the leukocyte accumulation is in the bowel wall, such as might be seen in active inflammatory bowel disease or pseudomembranous colitis, or in the bowel lumen, either sloughed from a local inflammatory process, or transported from a more proximal site in the bowel, or from locations such as the nasopharynx or the respiratory tract. GI bleeding or swallowed blood such as from hemoptysis also can result in intralumenal-labeled leukocyte activity. When initial images demonstrate activity in a section of bowel, additional views usually are obtained a few hours or a day later, because intralumenal activity changes its location, configuration, and intensity over time, whereas inflammation or infection in the bowel itself displays a relatively fixed distribution. Bowel cleansing also can be used to aid in determining whether activity is intralumenal or intramural.

Because of the imaging and dosimetric superiority of ^{99m}Tc, considerable effort has been made to label leukocytes with this radionuclide. Recently the brain imaging agent ^{99m}Tc-HMPAO, a lipophilic substance that crosses cell membranes with relative ease, has been successfully used for in vitro labeling of leukocytes.[88] The leukocyte labeling efficiency for ^{99m}Tc-HMPAO is lower than for ^{111}In, but the higher total dose of ^{99m}Tc that can be used compensates for this. Using 10 mCi of ^{99m}Tc-HMPAO, even an average labeling efficiency of 50% to 60% results in considerable gain in photon fluence and detected count rate relative to an injected dose of 0.5 to 1.0 mCi ^{111}In-labeled cells. ^{99m}Tc-HMPAO leukocyte imaging usually is begun 1 to 4 hours after injection, with later delayed views obtained only if a diagnostic question remains. Earlier imaging is important because hepatobiliary excretion of HMPAO results in the presence of nonspecific bowel activity in most patients who undergo imaging more than 6 hours after injection. Results with early ^{99m}Tc-HMPAO-leukocyte imaging of inflammatory bowel disease may be superior to those for ^{111}In-leukocytes,[89] particularly for less severe disease, where a low sensitivity for the latter agent has been reported.[90]

Other applications of labeled leukocytes in the abdomen include the identification of abscesses, both intraabdominal and retroperitoneal, and infectious processes involving the spleen or the kidneys. SPECT of the abdomen sometimes is used to aid in discrimination of overlapping structures, particularly for correlation with CT and MR images. Labeled leukocyte imaging also can be used to confirm the diagnosis of acute cholecystitis in patients with chronic or acalculous gallbladder disease, and to identify appendicitis in patients with equivocal physical and laboratory findings.[91]

Gallium-67 has been used for infection imaging for many years. Imaging usually is performed 2 to 3 days after intravenous administration of 5 to 10 mCi of ^{67}Ga citrate. This radionuclide is avidly bound to iron-binding proteins such as transferrin, and localizes at sites of inflammation and infection primarily because of increased capillary permeability.[92] Gallium seldom is used for examination of the abdomen because of its normal physiologic excretion into the bowel, which sometimes requires that images be obtained on several consecutive days to determine whether activity seen in the abdomen is within the bowel lumen or represents a pathologic lesion.

A new agent under investigation for imaging inflammatory or infectious processes is radiolabeled nonspecific immunoglobulin IgG. This protein can be labeled with ^{99m}Tc or ^{111}In, and has the same advantage as ^{67}Ga as compared with labeled leukocytes, namely elimination of the need to draw and process blood samples. Although nonspecific localization of this material occurs at most sites of active inflammation, preliminary experience has been positive with respect to the identification of infection as well.[93] Further evaluation will determine the role of this agent as a replacement for labeled leukocytes.

Oncologic Applications

Various radionuclide methods are used to evaluate for the presence and extent of malignancies. ^{67}Ga has been used for many years in tumor imaging, and GI applications include identification of hepatocellular carcinoma and assessment of the extent of abdominal involvement by lymphoma. In as-

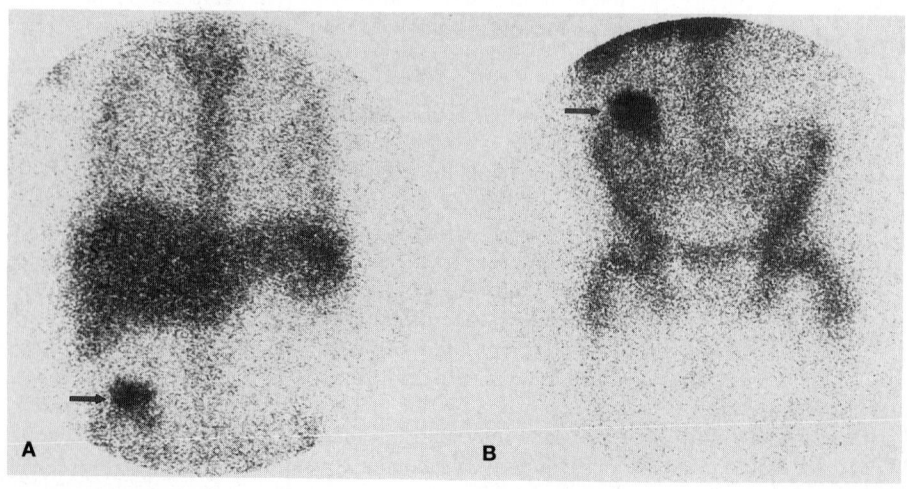

FIGURE 126-5. Anterior (**A**) chest and abdomen and (**B**) pelvis images from ^{111}Indium leukocyte scan show normal biodistribution of activity in the liver, spleen, and bone marrow, and abnormal focal increased uptake in the right lower quadrant (*arrows*). Contrast-enhanced computed tomography and subsequent surgery confirmed the presence of an abscess in this location secondary to a perforated diverticulum.

sociation with colloid liver imaging showing absence of normal parenchymal uptake or a CT or MR examination with a hepatic lesion of uncertain character, focal increased uptake of ^{67}Ga suggests the possibility of hepatocellular carcinoma.[94] In patients with gallium-avid lymphoma (avidity ranges from 50%–100%, depending on cell type),[95] active tumor can be discriminated from scar, and unsuspected sites of malignancy sometimes can be identified, especially with the use of SPECT.

A promising class of investigational radiopharmaceutical agents for imaging GI malignancy is the monoclonal antibodies. These agents are directed against specific cellular antigens, and have been portrayed as potential *magic bullets* for the diagnosis and treatment of malignancy. This characterization has proven overly optimistic, variously because of the difficulty of producing antibodies of high specificity, the heterogeneity of tumor tissues with respect to cellular antigens, and the sometimes limited access of intravenously administered substances to viable tumor tissue. Nevertheless, great interest remains in the use of radiolabeled antibodies against substances such as carcinoembryonic antigen, which is produced by many types of tumors including colon cancer. Both primary and secondary colon carcinoma have undergone successful imaging with anti-carcinoembryonic antibodies labeled with ^{131}I, ^{111}In, ^{123}I, and ^{99m}Tc, with overall sensitivity as high as 88%.[96] The technique usually is less sensitive in the liver, where tumor often is reflected as a region of decreased uptake,[97] likely as a result of inadequate delivery of antibody to hypoperfused or necrotic tissue. The primary value of antibody imaging may be to identify occult malignancy and clarify findings seen by CT and MR imaging with respect to distinguishing scar or fibrosis from recurrent tumor. A similar approach is used in PET imaging (see Chapter 125), where blood flow and metabolic activity are used to judge whether a lesion is malignant or benign.

The only monoclonal antibody imaging product currently approved by the FDA for use in the United States is an anti–tumor-associated glycoprotein–72 antibody labeled with [111]In (OncoScint, Cytogen-Knoll, Princeton, NJ), whose sensitivity and specificity for colorectal carcinoma have been reported as 69% and 77%, respectively.[98] This is a whole antibody that demonstrates slow clearance from the circulation and considerable normal hepatobiliary excretion into the bowel. These characteristics require an imaging approach similar to that used with ^{67}Ga, with several consecutive days of imaging starting on the second day after injection sometimes needed to differentiate intralumenal bowel contents from focal accumulation by tumor. OncoScint images must be reviewed with care to assure appropriate interpretation. Nevertheless, there have been impressive demonstrations of abnormalities, such as diffuse peritoneal involvement by tumor, that were not identified by CT, MR imaging, or laparoscopy (Fig. 126-6). The clinical impact of this antibody product, released in early 1993, has been small to date, but OncoScint and other new monoclonal antibody tumor imaging agents likely will become routinely used in nuclear medicine in the coming years.

Although initially intended as diagnostic agents, tumor antibody products may have a significant potential for therapy, with ^{99m}Tc and ^{111}In replaced by β-emitting isotopes such as ^{131}I and [186]Re. Clinical trials are underway to investigate the therapeutic potential of such antibody agents.

A new category of radiopharmaceuticals that has shown

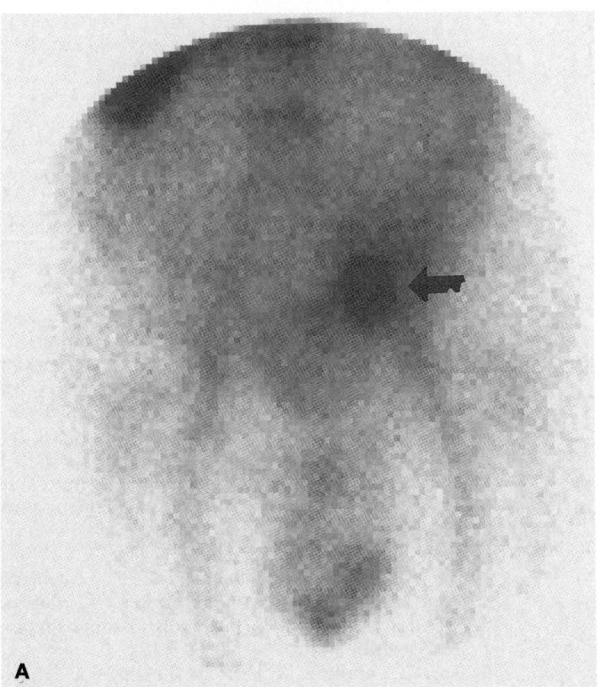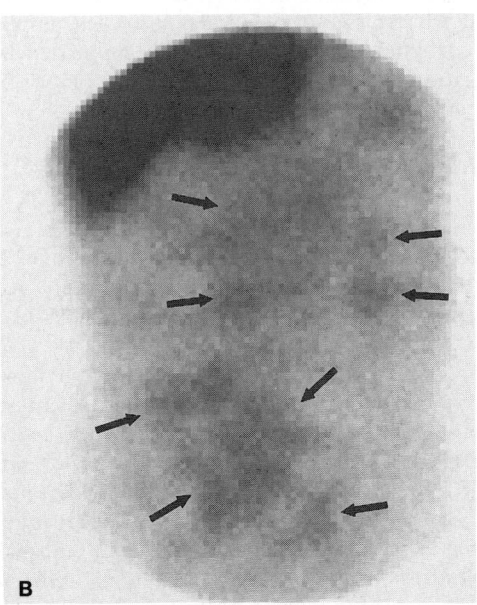

FIGURE 126-6. OncoScint images of the anterior abdomen and pelvis in two patients with colorectal carcinoma demonstrate **(A)** uptake in a sigmoid colon primary (*arrow*) and **(B)** diffuse peritoneal metastases (*arrows*). Normal liver uptake is present in the upper left of the two images. (From Maguire RT. OncoScint image atlas. In: Maguire RT, van Nostrand D, eds. Diagnosis of colorectal and ovarian carcinoma. Application of immunoscintigraphic technology. New York: Marcel Dekkel, 1992:141.)

promise for oncologic imaging applications is the radiolabeled peptides. The nonbiologic origin of these compounds provides considerable flexibility in their development for imaging of cell surface receptors and may offer an advantage over monoclonal antibodies with regard to potential immune-mediated reactions. In mid-1994, the FDA approved the first radiolabeled peptide for tumor imaging, ^{111}In-pentreotide (OctreoScan, Mallinckrodt, St. Louis, MO). The primary component of this compound is octreotide, an analog of somotastatin that binds to somatostatin receptors on cell surfaces. OctreoScan can therefore be used for imaging of neuroendocrine tumors whose cells possess somatostatin receptors. Tumors involving the gastrointestinal system that have been successfully imaged with OctreoScan include pancreatic APUDomas (i.e., gastrinoma, insulinoma, glucagonomas) and carcinoids.[98a] OctreoScan and future cell surface receptor imaging compounds may prove to be of considerable value in the staging and follow-up of many malignant tumors, and particularly for detection of functioning occult metastases, which are often difficult to localize using conventional anatomic imaging methods.

Imaging of intraperitoneally administered radiolabeled materials has several applications relevant to oncology. A small amount of liquid labeled with ^{99m}Tc-colloid can be injected, and abdominal images obtained to examine whether the tracer diffuses uniformly throughout the peritoneal cavity. The uniformity of flow provides a measure of how well intraperitoneal chemotherapy will reach sites of malignant involvement and therefore can be helpful in determining whether this will be an effective form of therapy. Likewise, imaging of labeled material instilled into the peritoneal cavity can be used to identify peritoneal leaks and communication between the peritoneal and pleural spaces, such as through an intralymphatic communication or a diaphragmatic defect. Movement of labeled ascitic fluid from the abdomen into the chest occurs relatively slowly, typically over several hours, when lymphatics are involved, and relatively rapidly, within minutes, when a diaphragmatic defect is present.[99]

NONIMAGING USES OF RADIOTRACERS

Most routine uses of radiotracers in nuclear medicine involve imaging of internal organ anatomy and physiology. Nevertheless, nonimaging uses of radiotracers occasionally provide valuable diagnostic information, and several examples of such uses relating to the GI tract are presented.

Schilling's test is used to ascertain whether vitamin B_{12} deficiency is the result of intrinsic factor deficiency or intestinal malabsorption of other causes. Vitamin B_{12} labeled with an isotope of cobalt is administered orally in a capsule, and the presence of adequate intrinsic factor in the stomach is judged based on the amount of labeled vitamin B_{12}, which is absorbed and excreted in the urine. In an individual with normal secretion of intrinsic factor by the gastric parietal cells, more than 9% of an ingested dose of labeled vitamin B_{12} will be excreted in the urine in 24 hours. If a low amount of labeled vitamin B_{12} is measured in a 24-hour urine specimen, especially if lower than 4% of the ingested dose, then part 2 of the test is performed, which involves a second 24-hour urine collection after ingestion of radiolabeled vitamin B_{12} and in-

trinsic factor together. If vitamin B_{12} malabsorption reflects pernicious anemia or intrinsic factor deficiency, then vitamin B_{12} excretion should be normal on the second part of the test. If, on the other hand, vitamin B_{12} deficiency is secondary to malabsorption, because of bacterial overgrowth or a mucosal deficiency in the terminal ileum, for instance, the amount of labeled vitamin B_{12} excreted in the 24-hour urine collection will remain low. Both parts of Schilling's test also can be done in 1 day by means of simultaneous administration of two different forms of vitamin B_{12}: one labeled with cobalt-58 and no intrinsic factor, and the other with cobalt-57 and intrinsic factor. The 24-hour urine collection is performed, and dual isotope measurements are made. Part 1 of Schilling's test is sometimes repeated after treatment of the presumed cause of vitamin B_{12} deficiency to determine if the mucosal effects of this deficiency have been reversed. This follow-up study sometimes is called a Schilling's test part 3.

Bacteria that produce high levels of urease can result in the breakdown of ingested carbon-14 urea, with production of ^{14}C-labeled CO_2, which can be detected and quantified in exhaled gases. A recent report showed good correlation between levels of exhaled labeled CO_2 and the presence and severity of *Helicobacter pylori* infection in patients with gastritis.[100] Future applications of this and similar radiotracer methods may provide opportunities for noninvasive detection and quantification of GI tract infections.

The reader is directed to Chapter 120, Cross-Sectional Anatomy.

REFERENCES

1. Sorenson JA, Phelps ME. Physics in nuclear medicine. 2nd ed. Orlando: Grune & Stratton, 1987:298.
2. Silberstein E. Incidence of adverse reactions to radiopharmaceuticals (abstract). J Nucl Med 1992;33:1025.
3. Klingensmith WC, Spitzer VM, Fritzberg AR, et al. Normal appearance and reproducibility of liver-spleen studies with Tc-99m sulfur colloid and Tc-99m microalbumin colloid. J Nucl Med 1983;24:8.
4. Drum DE, Beard JO. Liver scintigraphic features associated with alcoholism. J Nucl Med 1978;19:154.
5. Tanasescu D, Brachman M, Rigby J, et al. Scintigraphic triad in focal nodular hyperplasia. Am J Gastroenterol 1984;79:61.
6. Lubbers PR, Ros PR, Goodman ZD, et al. Accumulation of technetium-99m sulfur colloid by hepatocellular adenoma: scintigraphic-pathologic correlation. AJR 1987;148:1105.
7. Biersack HJ, Torres J, Thelen M, et al. Determination of liver and spleen perfusion by quantitative sequential scintigraphy: results in normal subjects and in patients with portal hypertension. Clin Nucl Med 1981;5:218.
8. Martin-Comin J, Mora J, Figueras J, et al. Calculation of portal contribution to hepatic blood flow with 99mTc-microcolloids: a noninvasive method to diagnose liver graft rejection. J Nucl Med 1988;29:1776.
9. Patel S, Sandler CM, Rauschkolb EN, et al. 133Xe uptake in a focal hepatic fat accumulation: CT correlation. AJR Am J Roentgenol 1982;138:541.
10. Yeh S-H, Wu L-C, Wang S-J, et al. Xenon-133 hepatic retention ratio: a useful index for fatty liver quantification. J Nucl Med 1989;30:1708.
11. Vera DR, Stadalnik RC, Trudeau WL, et al. Measurement of receptor concentration and forward-binding rate constant via

radiopharmacokinetic modeling of technetium-99m-galacto-syl- neoglycoalbumin. J Nucl Med 1991;32:1169.

12. Virgolini I, Muller C, Hobart J, et al. Liver function in acute viral hepatitis as determined by a hepatocyte-specific ligand: 99mTc-galacyosyl-neoglycoalbumin. Hepatology 1992;15: 593.

13. Front D, Royal HD, Israel O, et al. Scintigraphy of hepatic hemangiomas: the value of Tc-99m labeled red blood cells: concise communication. J Nucl Med 1981;22:684.

14. Groshar D, Ben-Haim S, Dips S, et al. Spectrum of scintigraphic appearance of liver hemangiomas. Clin Nucl Med 1992;17: 294.

15. Brodsky RI, Friedman AC, Maurer AH, et al. Hepatic cavernous hemangioma: diagnosis with 99m-Tc labeled red cells and single photon emission CT. AJR Am J Roentgenol 1987;148:125.

16. Tumeh SS, Benson C, Nagel JS, et al. Cavernous hemangioma of the liver: detection with single-photon emission computed tomography. Radiology 1987;164:353.

17. Birnbaum BA, Weinreb JC, Megibow AJ, et al. Definitive diagnosis of hepatic hemangiomas: MR imaging versus Tc-99m-labeled red blood cell SPECT. Radiology 1990;176:95.

18. Nelson RC, Chezmar JL. Diagnostic approach to hepatic hemangiomas. Radiology 1990;176:11.

19. Ziessman HA, Silverman PM, Patterson J, et al. Improved detection of small cavernous hemangiomas of the liver with high-resolution three-headed SPECT. J Nucl Med 1991;32: 2086.

20. Brown RKJ, Gomes A, King W, et al. Hepatic hemangiomas: evaluation by magnetic resonance imaging and technetium-99m red blood cell scintigraphy. J Nucl Med 1987;28:1683.

21. Krishnamurthy GT, Turner FE. Pharmacokinetics and clinical application of technetium 99m-labeled hepatobiliary agents. Semin Nucl Med 1990;20:130.

22. Williams W, Krishnamurthy GT, Brar HS, et al. Scintigraphic variations of normal biliary physiology. J Nucl Med 1984;25: 160.

23. Majd M, Reba RC, Altman RP. Hepatobiliary scintigraphy with 99m-Tc PIPIDA in the evaluation of neonatal jaundice. Pediatrics 1981;67:140.

24. Aburano T, Yokoyama K, Shuke N, et al. The role of Tc-99m IDA hepatobiliary and Tc-99m colloid hepatic imaging in primary biliary cirrhosis. Clin Nucl Med 1991;16:4.

25. Keefe EB, Lieberman DA, Krishnamurthy S, et al. Primary biliary cirrhosis: Tc-99m IDA planar and SPECT scanning. Radiology 1988;166:143.

26. Ament AE, Bick RJ, Miraldi FD, et al. Sclerosing cholangitis: cholescintigraphy with Tc-99m-labeled DISIDA. Radiology 1984;151:197.

27. Rodman CA, Keeffe EB, Lieberman DA, et al. Diagnosis of sclerosing cholangitis with technetium 99m-labeled iminodiacetic acid and single photon emission computed tomographic scintigraphy. Gastroenterology 1987;92:777.

28. Kuni CC, Engeler CM, Makhleh RE, et al. Correlation of technetium-99m-DISIDA hepatobiliary studies with biopsies in liver transplant patients. J Nucl Med 1991;32:1545.

29. Gelfand MJ, Smith HS, Ryckman FC, et al. Hepatobiliary scintigraphy in pediatric liver transplant recipients. Clin Nucl Med 1992;17:542.

30. Klingensmith WC, Kuni CC, Fritzberg AR. Cholescintigraphy in extrahepatic biliary obstruction. AJR Am J Roentgenol 1982;139:65.

31. Egbert RN, Braunstein P, Lyons KP, et al. Total bile duct obstruction: prompt diagnosis by hepatobiliary imaging. Arch Surg 1983;118:709.

32. Weissman HS, Badia J, Sugarman L, et al. Spectrum of 99m-Tc IDA cholescintigraphic patterns in acute cholecystitis. Radiology 1981;138:167.

33. Mauro MA, McCartney WH, Melmed JR. Hepatobiliary scanning with 99mTc-PIPIDA in acute cholecystitis. Radiology 1982;142:193.

34. Freitas JE, Coleman RE, Nagle CE, et al. Influence of scan and pathologic criteria on the specificity of cholescintigraphy: concise communication. J Nucl Med 1983;24:876.

35. Fink-Bennett D, Freitas JE, Ripley SD, et al. The sensitivity of hepatobiliary imaging and real-time ultrasonography in the detection of acute cholecystitis. Arch Surg 1985;120:904.

36. Kistler AM, Ziessman HA, Gooch D, et al. Morphine-augmented cholescintigraphy in acute cholecystitis: a satisfactory alternative to delayed imaging. Clin Nucl Med 1991;16: 404.

37. Fink-Bennett D, Balon H, Robbins T, et al. Morphine-augmented cholescintigraphy: its efficacy in detecting acute cholecystitis. J Nucl Med 1991;32:1231.

38. Brachman MB, Tanasescu DE, Ramanna L, et al. Acute gangrenous cholecystitis: radionuclide diagnosis. Radiology 1984; 151:209.

39. Smith R, Rosen JM, Gallo LN, et al. Pericholecystic hepatic activity in cholescintigraphy. Radiology 1985;156:797.

40. Swayne LC, Ginsberg HN. Diagnosis of acute cholecystitis by cholescintigraphy: significance of pericholecystic hepatic uptake. AJR Am J Roentgenol 1989;152:1211.

41. Klingensmith WC, Spitzer VM, Fritzberg AR, et al. The normal fasting and postprandial diisopropyl-IDA Tc 99m hepatobiliary study. Radiology 1981;141:771.

42. Larsen MJ, Klingensmith WC, Kuni CC. Radionuclide hepatobiliary imaging: nonvisualization of the gallbladder secondary to prolonged fasting. J Nucl Med 1982;23:1003.

43. Jacobson AF, Teefey SA, Lee SP, et al. Frequent occurrence of new hepatobiliary abnormalities after bone marrow transplantation: results of a prospective study using scintigraphy and sonography. Am J Gastroenterol 1993;88:1044.

44. Patterson FK, Kam JW. Practical hepatobiliary imaging using pre-treatment with sincalide in 139 hepatobiliary studies. Clin Nucl Med 1985;10:333.

45. Sitzmann JV, Pitt HA, Steinborn PA, et al. Cholecystokinin prevents parenteral nutrition induced biliary sludge in humans. Surg Gynecol Obstet 1990;170:25.

46. Huang M-J, Liaw Y-F. Intravenous cholescintigraphy using Tc-99m-labeled agents in the diagnosis of choledochal cyst. J Nucl Med 1982;23:113.

47. Camponovo E, Buck JL, Drane WE. Scintigraphic features of choledochal cyst. J Nucl Med 1989;30:622.

48. Weissmann HS, Chun KJ, Frank M, et al. Demonstration of traumatic bile leak with cholescintigraphy and ultrasonography. AJR Am J Roentgenol 1979;133:843.

49. Krishnamurthy GT, Bobba VR, Kingston E. Radionuclide ejection fraction: a technique for quantitative analysis of motor function of the human gallbladder. Gastroenterology 1981;80: 482.

50. Ziessman HA, Fahey FH, Hixson DJ. Calculation of a gallbladder ejection fraction: advantage of continuous sincalide infusion over the 3-minute infusion method. J Nucl Med 1992;33:537.

51. Zech ER, Simmons LB, Kendrick RR, et al. Cholecystokinin enhanced hepatobiliary scanning with ejection fraction calculation as an indicator of disease of the gallbladder. Surg Gynecol Obstet 1991;172:21.

52. Yap L, Wycherley AG, Morphett AD, et al. Acalculous biliary pain: cholecystectomy alleviates symptoms in patients with abnormal cholescintigraphy. Gastroenterology 1991;101: 786.

53. Kloiber R, Molnar CP, Shaffer EA. Chronic biliary-type pain in the absence of gallstones: the value of cholecystokinin cholescintigraphy. AJR Am J Roentgenol 1992;159:509.

54. DeCamp JR, Tabatowski K, Schauwecker DS, et al. Comparison of gallbladder ejection fraction with histopathologic changes in acalculous biliary disease. Clin Nucl Med 1992;17: 784.

55. Westlake PJ, Hershfield NB, Kelly JK, et al. Chronic right upper quadrant pain without gallstones: does HIDA scan predict outcome after cholecystectomy? Am J Gastroenterol 1990;85:986.

56. Zeman RK, Burrell MJ, Dobbins J, et al. Postcholecystectomy syndrome: evaluation using biliary scintigraphy and endoscopic retrograde cholangiopancreatography. Radiology 1985;156: 787.

57. Lee RGL, Gregg JA, Koroshetz AM, et al. Sphincter of Oddi

stenosis: diagnosis using hepatobiliary scintigraphy and endoscopic manometry. Radiology 1985;156:793.

58. Roberts-Thomson IC, Toouli J, Blanchett W, et al. Assessment of bile flow by radioscintigraphy in patients with biliary-type pain after cholecystectomy. Aust NZ J Med 1986;16:788.

59. Shaffer EA, Hershfield NB, Logan K, et al. Cholescintigraphic detection of functional obstruction of the sphincter of Oddi: effect of papillotomy. Gastroenterology 1986;90:728.

60. Sfakianakis GN, Conway JJ. Detection of ectopic gastric mucosa in Meckel's diverticulum and in other aberrations by scintigraphy: I. Pathophysiology and 10-year clinical experience. J Nucl Med 1981;22:647.

61. Sfakianakis GN, Conway JJ. Detection of ectopic gastric mucosa in Meckel's diverticulum and in other aberrations by scintigraphy: II. Indications and method. A 10-year experience. J Nucl Med 1981;22:732.

62. Sfakianakis GN, Anderson GF, King DR, et al. The effect of gastrointestinal hormones on the pertechnetate imaging of ectopic gastric mucosa in experimental Meckel's diverticulum. J Nucl Med 1981;22:678.

63. Yeker D, Buyukunal C, Benli M, et al. Radionuclide imaging of Meckel's diverticulum: cimetidine versus pentagastrin plus glucagon. Eur J Nucl Med 1984;9:316.

64. Alavi A. Detection of gastrointestinal bleeding with 99mTc-sulfur colloid. Semin Nucl Med 1982;12:126.

65. Alavi A, Dann RW, Baum S, et al. Scintigraphic detection of acute gastrointestinal bleeding. Radiology 1977;124:753.

66. Winzelberg GG, McKusick KA, Froelich JW, et al. Detection of gastrointestinal bleeding with 99mTc-labeled red blood cells. Semin Nucl Med 1982;12:139.

67. Maurer AH, Rodman MS, Vitti RA, et al. Gastrointestinal bleeding: improved localization with cine scintigraphy. Radiology 1992;185:187.

68. Bunker SR, Lull RJ, Tanasescu DE, et al. The superiority of 99mTc RBC over 99mTc-sulfur colloid in the detection and localization of gastrointestinal hemorrhage. AJR Am J Roentgenol 1984;143:543.

69. Smith R, Copely DJ, Bolen FH. 99mTc RBC scintigraphy: correlation of gastrointestinal bleeding rates with scintigraphic findings. AJR Am J Roentgenol 1987;148:869.

70. Jacobson AF, Cerqueira MD. Prognostic significance of late imaging results in technetium-99m-labeled red blood cell gastrointestinal bleeding studies with early negative images. J Nucl Med 1992;33:202.

71. Gupta S, Luna E, Kingsley S, et al. Detection of gastrointestinal bleeding by radionuclide scintigraphy. AJR Am J Roentgenol 1984;79:26.

72. Jacobson AF. Delayed positive gastrointestinal bleeding studies with technetium-99m-red blood cells: utility of a second injection. J Nucl Med 1991;32:330.

73. Markisz JA, Front D, Royal HD, et al. An evaluation of 99mTc-labeled red blood cell scintigraphy for the detection and localization of gastrointestinal bleeding sites. Gastroenterology 1982;83:394.

74. Chaudhuri TK, Brantly M. Heparin as a pharmacologic intervention to induce positive scintiscan in occult gastrointestinal bleeding. Clin Nucl Med 1984;9:187.

75. Schmidt KG, Rasmussen JW, Grove O, et al. The use of indium-111-labelled platelets for scintigraphic localization of gastrointestinal bleeding, with special reference to occult bleeding. Scand J Gastroenterol 1986;21:407.

76. Malmud LS, Fisher RS, Knight LC, et al. Scintigraphic evaluation of gastric emptying. Semin Nucl Med 1982;12:116.

77. Datz FL, Christian PE, Hutson WR, et al. Physiological and pharmacological interventions in radionuclide imaging of the tubular gastrointestinal tract. Semin Nucl Med 1991;21:140.

78. Christian PE, Moore JG, Sorenson JA, et al. Effects of meal size and correction technique on gastric emptying time: studies with two tracers and opposed detectors. J Nucl Med 1980;21:883.

79. Christian PE, Moore JH, Datz FL. Comparison of Tc-99m labeled liver and liver pate' as markers for solid-phase gastric emptying. J Nucl Med 1984;25:364.

80. Vitti RA, Malmud LS, Fisher RS. Gastric emptying. In: Freeman L, ed. Freeman & Johnson's clinical radionuclide imaging. 3rd ed. Orlando: Grune & Stratton, 1986:1694.

81. Choe AI, Ziessman HA, Fleischer DE. Tumor-associated gastroparesis with esophageal carcinoma: use of intravenous metoclopramide during radionuclide gastric emptying studies to predict clinical response. Dig Dis Sci 1989;34:1132.

82. Burt M, Scott AM, Yeh SDJ, et al. The effects of intravenous erythromycin on gastric emptying following esophagogastrectomy (abstract). J Nucl Med 1993;34:11.

83. Malmud LS, Vitti RA, Fisher RS. Gastroesophageal reflux. In: Freeman L, ed. Freeman and Johnson's clinical radionuclide imaging. 3rd ed. Orlando: Grune & Stratton, 1986:1669.

84. Malmud LS, Vitti RA, Fisher RS. Esophageal transit and clearance scintigraphy. In: Freeman L, ed. Freeman and Johnson's clinical radionuclide imaging. 3rd ed. Orlando: Grune & Stratton, 1986:1654.

85. Mishkin FS. Radionuclide salivary gland imaging. Semin Nucl Med 1981;11:258.

86. Froelich JW, Swanson D. Imaging of inflammatory processes with labeled cells. Semin Nucl Med 1984;14:128.

87. Knochel JP, Koehler PR, Lee THG, et al. Diagnosis of abdominal abscesses with computed tomography, ultrasound, and In-111 leukocyte scans. Radiology 1980;137:425.

88. Roddie ME, Peters AM, Danpure HJ, et al. Inflammation: imaging with Tc-99m HMPAO-labeled leukocytes. Radiology 1988;166:767.

89. Arndt J-W, van der Sluys Veer A, Blok D, et al. Prospective comparative study of technetium-99m-WBCs and Indium-111-granulocytes for the examination of patients with inflammatory bowel disease. J Nucl Med 1993;34:1052.

90. Tolia V, Kuhns LR, Chang C-H, et al. Comparison of Indium-111 scintigraphy and colonoscopy with histologic study in children for evaluation of colonic chronic inflammatory bowel disease. J Pediatr Gastroenterol Nutr 1991;12:336.

91. DeLaney AR, Raviola CA, Weber PN, et al. Improving diagnosis of appendicitis: early autologous leukocyte scanning. Arch Surg 1989;124:1146.

92. Tsan M. Mechanism of gallium-67 accumulation in inflammatory lesions. J Nucl Med 1985;26:88.

93. Rubin RH, Fischman AJ, Callahan RJ, et al. 111In-labeled nonspecific immunoglobulin scanning in the detection of focal infection. N Engl J Med 1989;321:935.

94. Serafini AN, Jeffers LJ, Reddy KR, et al. Early recognition of recurrent hepatocellular carcinoma utilizing gallium-67 citrate scintigraphy. J Nucl Med 1988;29:712.

95. Andrews GA, Hubner KF, Greenlaw RH. Ga-67 citrate imaging in malignant lymphoma: final report of cooperative group. J Nucl Med 1978;19:1013.

96. Bischof-Delaloye A, Delaloye B, Buchegger F, et al. Clinical value of immunoscintigraphy in colorectal carcinoma patients: a prospective study. J Nucl Med 1989;30:1646.

97. Abdel-Nabi HH, Schwartz AN, Higano CS, et al. Colorectal carcinoma: detection with Indium-111 anticarcinoembryonic-antigen monoclonal antibody ZCE-025. Radiology 1987;164:617.

98. Collier BD, Abdel-Nabi H, Doerr RJ, et al. Immunoscintigraphy performed with In-111-labeled CYT-103 in the management of colorectal cancer: comparison with CT. Radiology 1992;185:179.

98a. Krenning EP, Kwekkeboom DJ, Reubi JC, et al. 111In-octreotide scintigraphy in oncology. Digestion 1993;54(Suppl 1):84.

99. Jacobson AF, Cerqueira MD, Breitz HB, et al. Pleuroperitoneal communication associated with malignant ascites: a potential cause for new pleural effusion suggestive of pulmonary embolism. Clin Nucl Med 1990;15:317.

100. Debongnie JC, Pauwels S, Raat A, et al. Quantification of *Helicobacter pylori* infection in gastritis and ulcer disease using a simple and rapid carbon-14-urea breath test. J Nucl Med 1991;32:1192.

Textbook of Gastroenterology, second edition, edited by Tadataka Yamada. JB Lippincott Company, Philadelphia © 1995.

CHAPTER 127

Angiography

Kyung Cho

Since the introduction of the newer imaging modalities such as computed tomography (CT), ultrasound (US), magnetic resonance (MR) imaging, and radionuclide scintigraphy, diagnostic angiography has been used less frequently in the evaluation of gastrointestinal (GI) disease. Visceral angiography is performed to establish a specific diagnosis, to evaluate tumor resectability, and to obtain the necessary information about the normal and aberrant hepatic arterial system. Although dynamic CT scanning, MR imaging, and radionuclide angiography are capable of visualizing blood vessels, angiography remains the most accurate means of diagnosing mesenteric vascular disease, portal hypertension, and GI hemorrhage. Whereas diagnostic angiography has been performed less frequently in the last decade, its therapeutic application has expanded to a wide variety of pathologic conditions. This chapter reviews the vascular anatomy, and techniques and current role of visceral angiography in the diagnosis and treatment of GI disease.

TECHNICAL CONSIDERATIONS

Conventional film-screen and digital subtraction techniques are used in visceral angiography. Superselective catheterization, the magnification technique, and photographic subtraction are used when vascular details are necessary. Standard film-screen angiography provides better spatial resolution and fewer motion artifacts than the digital subtraction technique. Digital subtraction angiograms can be obtained with intravenous or intraarterial administration of contrast material. The intravenous digital subtraction angiography (DSA) has little role in visceral angiography because of poor spatial resolution, misregistration artifacts, and vessel superimposition. Intraarterial DSA is more useful because it requires a smaller amount of contrast medium, provides better spatial resolution, and causes less discomfort to patients (Fig. 127-1). Usually intraarterial DSA is used in patients with renal insufficiency to see blood vessels for vascular anatomy and to assess

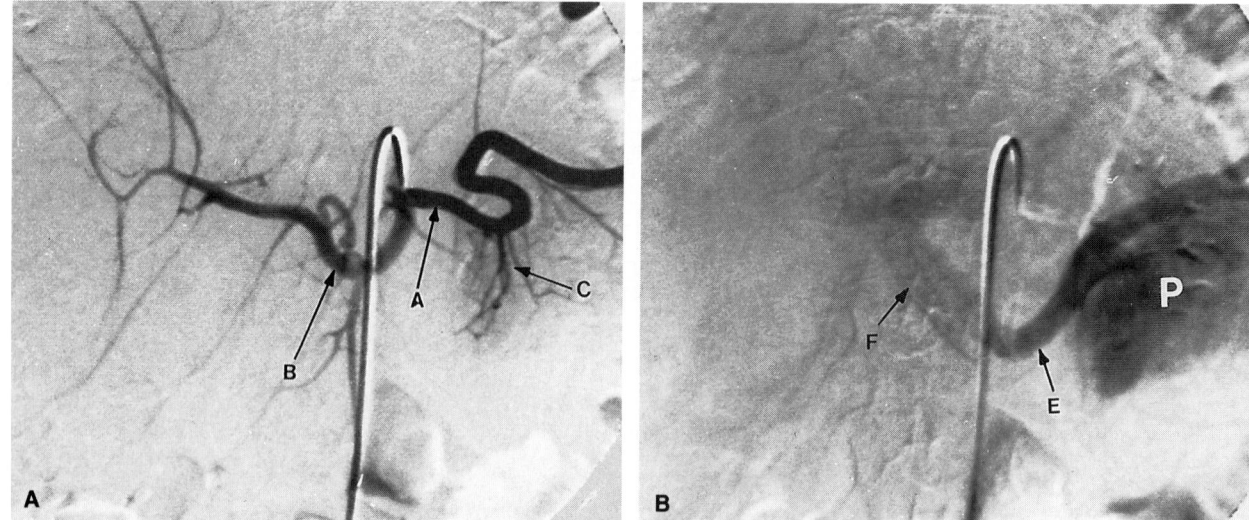

FIGURE 127-1. Intraarterial digital subtraction angiogram of the celiac artery in a patient with hepatic metastases from a colon cancer. **(A)** Arterial phase demonstrates the splenic (A), and hepatic (B), and pancreatica magna (C) arteries. A large avascular metastasis is demonstrated in the right lobe of the liver. **(B)** Venous phase demonstrates the splenic (E) and portal (F) veins, and parenchymal staining of the body of the pancreas (P). The portal vein branches in the right lobe of the liver are compressed by the tumor.

progress during intervention procedures. Intraarterial DSA images may be viewed on a video monitor during and after injection of contrast material, eliminating the delay of film processing. Selected images may be stored on a single sheet of film, reducing the film and chemical costs associated with the cut film runs of conventional angiography. Finally, the ability to cut contrast material loads by one third to one half of those used in conventional angiography reduces the risks of renal toxicity and fluid overload.

The two types of radiographic contrast agents used for angiography are the conventional high osmolar (ionic) and the newer low osmolar (nonionic) contrast agents. The nonionic contrast agents are more expensive but cause less pain and "burning" sensations. It remains controversial whether the lower osmolar contrast agents are safer and less nephrotoxic. A recent multicenter clinical study comparing adverse effects of ionic and nonionic contrast agents demonstrated that nonionic contrast materials cause fewer and less severe adverse effects.[1]

Patient Preparation

Before the procedure, the vascular radiologist explains the potential risks and benefits of the procedure and availability of alternative tests to the patient and obtains a written consent. On the day of the procedure the patient is allowed to take fluids by mouth, and an intravenous line is placed to hydrate the patient. A mild sedative and an analgesic are given 30 minutes before the procedure. During the procedure, electrocardiogram, blood pressure, oxygen saturation, and pedal pulse are monitored. General anesthesia and heavy sedation are not required for routine visceral angiography. The patient may feel slight to moderate discomfort at the puncture site

during and after the procedure and a burning sensation during the injection of contrast material. The use of more expensive nonionic contrast agents has moderately decreased such discomfort.

Angiography can be safely performed on an outpatient basis. Outpatient angiography is cost-effective because the patient returns home on the same day of procedure and may resume normal activity on the following morning. Laboratory studies required before the procedure include an electrocardiogram and renal function and coagulation studies. Patient preparation for outpatient angiography is the same as that used for inpatients. After the procedure the patient is observed in a radiology recovery room located in the vicinity of the angiography suites. Ambulation begins 4 hours after the procedure, and the patient is discharged with an attendant. The attendant is advised to stay with the patient until the following morning and instructed to take certain measures if a complication arises.

Seldinger's Percutaneous Catheter Introduction

Angiography is performed using the percutaneous technique introduced by Seldinger in 1953.[2] The technique is as follows: the common femoral artery is punctured using an 18- or 19-gauge Seldinger-type needle through a small skin incision after the skin has been anesthetized with lidocaine 2%. The needle is withdrawn slowly until blood starts to spurt, and the guidewire is inserted through the needle into the abdominal aorta. A preshaped catheter is introduced over the guidewire. Catheter tip configurations depend on the vessel of interest, such as a pigtail-like tip for aortic injections or special bends at the tip for selective arterial injections.

The technique used for catheterization of the inferior vena cava and hepatic vein is similar to that for arterial catheterization. The right femoral vein is punctured percutaneously using the Seldinger-type needle. While the cannula is slowly withdrawn, gentle aspiration is applied using a 10-mL syringe containing a few milliliters of heparinized saline. Once free blood aspiration is obtained, the guidewire is inserted into the inferior vena cava, and the catheter is advanced over the guidewire. If thrombosis has occurred in the femoral veins or inferior vena cava, the catheter is introduced by way of an antecubital, brachial, or jugular vein. After withdrawal of the venous catheter, gentle manual compression of the puncture site is required. The patient is allowed to get up after 4 hours of bed rest.

Transhepatic Portal Vein Catheterization

Percutaneous transhepatic portal vein catheterization[3] is a useful method for evaluating portal hemodynamics, localizing occult islet cell tumors, and controlling gastroesophageal variceal bleeding. Before puncture of the portal vein, portal vein patency is verified on the venous phases of celiac or superior mesenteric angiography. The puncture site usually is chosen in the midaxillary line, about halfway between the costophrenic angle and the inferolateral margin of the liver to avoid injury to the lung and intraabdominal viscera. After the procedure has been completed, the catheter track is sealed near the hepatic capsule with a gelatin sponge to arrest bleeding from the puncture site.

General Angiographic Approach

Biplane aortography is performed using a pigtail catheter for the evaluation of the origins of the celiac and superior mesenteric arteries. Otherwise, visceral angiography begins with catheterization of the celiac and superior mesenteric arteries. Oblique films are obtained as needed for better evaluation of the abnormality and vascular anatomy. Superselective catheterization of the branches of the visceral arteries is performed as needed: splenic, dorsal pancreatic, and gastroduodenal arterial catheterization for the evaluation of pancreatic cancer, and left gastric arterial catheterization for gastric bleeding. The size of the artery and the flow rate are estimated by a test injection to determine the amount and injection rate of the contrast material for the angiogram. Usually the injection rate of the celiac and superior mesenteric arteries ranges from 8 to 12 mL/second. The total volume of contrast material ranges from 32 to 48 mL. A lower injection rate is used in angiography of the branches of the visceral arteries. A serial angiogram is obtained for a duration of 24 to 30 seconds: two films per second for 3 seconds for the arterial phase, one film per second for 3 seconds for late arterial and capillary phases, and one film every 3 seconds for 18 seconds for the venous phase.

Visualization of the portal venous system is essential in angiographic study for evaluating intraabdominal masses, vascular diseases, and portal hypertension. The presence or absence of a venous abnormality plays an important role in determining whether the arteriographic abnormality is neoplastic or arteriosclerotic in nature. Visualization of the portal vein requires the injection of a large volume of contrast medium (40–60 mL of 76% contrast medium) into the superior mesenteric or splenic artery with the injection of vasodilators. This method is called *arterial portography* and has eliminated the need for injection of contrast material into the spleen for splenoportography and direct portal vein catheterization.

Balloon Occlusion Angiography

Arterial portography can be obtained using a double-lumen, end-hole balloon catheter in the superior mesenteric artery. The study is performed with the injection of contrast medium distal to balloon occlusion at a rate of 6 mL/second for 10 seconds while obtaining serial exposures.[4] This results in excellent visualization of the portal venous system. Wedged hepatic venous pressure can be obtained using a balloon occlusion catheter. The balloon occlusion catheter can be introduced into one of the major hepatic veins from the femoral vein and advanced 4 to 5 cm into the hepatic vein; the balloon then is inflated. After confirming occlusion of the vein by the balloon with the injection of a small amount of contrast medium under fluoroscopy, pressure measurement is taken. This gives wedged hepatic venous pressure, reflecting portal venous pressure in the presence of postsinusoidal block. A balloon occlusion hepatic venogram then is obtained with the injection of contrast medium at a rate of 4 to 5 mL/second for a total volume of 10 to 20 mL to see the hepatic veins and sinusoids, and to produce reflux of the contrast medium through the sinusoids into the portal vein.[5] This method is useful in the preoperative evaluation for portacaval shunt operation.

Postangiography Patient Care

Under normal conditions, manual compression to the groin after withdrawal of the catheter results in cessation of the bleeding within 10 to 15 minutes. Pressure dressings are used for patients with hypertension and the propensity to bleed. The patient may resume a normal diet after the procedure. After a transfemoral catheterization, bed rest is ordered until the following morning. Vital signs, the pedal pulse, and the puncture site are checked every 15 minutes for 1 hour and then every hour for 6 hours.

RISKS AND CONTRAINDICATIONS

The overall complication rates of transfemoral and transaxillary angiography are 1.73% and 3.29%, respectively.[6] The complications of transfemoral angiography include the following: puncture site complications (0.47%); complications related to catheter manipulation (0.64%); contrast material reactions (0.03%); contrast material toxicity (renal failure; 0.01%); and systemic complications (cardiac, 0.29%; neurologic, 0.17%). Brachial nerve injury is the most serious complication of the transaxillary artery catheterization. Nerve injury is less likely to occur with a brachial artery puncture because the brachial plexus is not as close to the brachial artery as it is to the axillary artery. The use of intraarterial nitroglycerin and calcium channel blockers during the transbrachial catheterization has reduced arterial spasm and thrombosis of the brachial artery. Mortality related to the angiographic procedures other than reactions to contrast agents is extremely rare.

The overall mortality associated with the intravenous use of the ionic contrast agents is 1 in 40,000.[7] The incidence of various forms of reaction and the death rate probably are lower with the low-osmolar contrast agents. The risk factors involved in the use of contrast material are renal failure, a history of previous reactions (major and minor), and allergic diathesis. Adequate hydration and the administration of mannitol help to reduce the incidence of the nephrotoxicity of the contrast medium. Pretreatment with a steroid for 2 consecutive days before and on the day of the procedure has been advocated to prevent reaction to contrast agents in patients with a history of this complication.

There are no absolute contraindications to visceral angiography. Relative contraindications include severe coagulopathy, recent myocardial infarction, congestive heart failure, renal failure, and pregnancy. Patients undergoing brachial or axillary artery puncture, translumbar aortic puncture, or percutaneous transhepatic procedures are at increased risk of hemorrhagic complications in the presence of coagulopathy or hypertension. Depending on the urgency and nature of the procedure, coagulopathies should be reversed with appropriate treatment by discontinuing anticoagulant therapy or administering platelets, protamine, or fresh frozen plasma. In patients with congestive heart failure and renal failure, intraarterial DSA is used to decrease the amount of contrast material necessary for the procedure.

VASCULAR ANATOMY OF THE ABDOMINAL VISCERA

Visualization of the visceral arterial anatomy and its variations is especially useful in planning surgery for intraabdominal masses, portal hypertension, aneurysms, and the intraoperative placement of hepatic artery infusion catheters. Angiography is the most accurate means of depicting the origins and branching pattern of the visceral arteries.

Arterial Vasculature

The arterial supply of the abdominal viscera is derived from the celiac and superior and inferior mesenteric arteries. They originate in the ventral surface of the aorta below the aortic hiatus of the diaphragm. The superior mesenteric artery arises from the aorta 1 to 2 cm below the celiac and above the renal arteries, and courses anterior to the third portion of the duodenum and the left renal vein. The inferior mesenteric artery arises from the aorta near the level of the L3-4 interspace of the spine.

The celiac artery gives its first branch to the stomach (left gastric artery) and divides into the splenic and common hepatic arteries. Occasionally the inferior phrenic or dorsal pan-

creatic artery originates from the celiac axis. One or more branches of the celiac artery may originate from sources other than the celiac axis. Rarely the left gastric artery originates from the aorta and the splenic from the superior mesenteric artery.

The common hepatic artery divides into the proper hepatic and gastroduodenal arteries, and the former bifurcates into the right and left hepatic arteries. The right hepatic artery divides into the anterior and posterior segmental arteries when it enters the liver; each of the segmental arteries gives off arterial branches to the superior and inferior subsegments of the liver. The left hepatic artery divides into the superior and inferior subsegmental branches. The middle hepatic artery arises from the left hepatic, right hepatic, or proper hepatic artery.

In about half of the cases, one or more branches of the hepatic artery arise from sources other than the celiac-hepatic artery (Fig. 127-2). An aberrant hepatic artery may be replaced (substituting for the celiac-hepatic) or it may be an accessory (additive to a celiac-hepatic artery). The replaced hepatic artery usually is a lobar artery, whereas the accessory hepatic artery is a segmental or subsegmental artery. From a functional standpoint, the term *accessory hepatic artery* is incorrect because it supplies a specific area of the liver. According to Michels' dissection of 200 cadavers,[8] aberrant right hepatic arteries occur in 26% of patients (replaced, 18%; accessory, 8%), most frequently originating from the superior mesenteric artery (17%); aberrant left hepatic arteries occur in 27% of patients (replaced, 15.5%; accessory, 11.5%), most frequently from the left gastric artery (13%).

The gastroduodenal artery usually originates from the common hepatic artery. In 25% of the population it may have an aberrant origin. The three main branches originating from the gastroduodenal artery are the posterior superior pancreaticoduodenal (posterior arcade), anterior superior pancreaticoduodenal (anterior arcade), and right gastroepiploic arteries. The posterior and anterior arcade arteries join inferomedially before forming an anastomosis with the inferior pancreaticoduodenal (IPD) artery, which usually originates in common with a jejunal branch from the superior mesenteric artery. The branches of the gastroduodenal artery supply arterial blood to the stomach, duodenum, pancreas, and bile duct. In the presence of a celiac artery occlusion, the pancreaticoduodenal arcade arteries function as the major collateral pathway to the liver from the superior mesenteric artery. Normally gastroduodenal blood flows away from the liver (hepatofugal), but with stenosis or occlusion in the celiac or common hepatic artery, the blood flow is reversed (hepatopetal). Preoperative recognition of flow reversal in the gastroduodenal artery is important in planning resection of pancreatic head tumors and for placement of hepatic artery catheters. DSA with a low injection rate is useful in the evaluation of arterial hemodynamics because high-pressure injection used during conventional angiography may alter arterial hemodynamics, resulting in transient reversal of the flow.

The superior mesenteric artery supplies the pancreas, duodenum, small intestine, cecum, ascending colon, and the proximal half of the transverse colon. The inferior pancreaticoduodenal and occasionally the dorsal pancreatic arteries originate from the proximal portion of the superior mesenteric artery. The other branches of the superior mesenteric artery

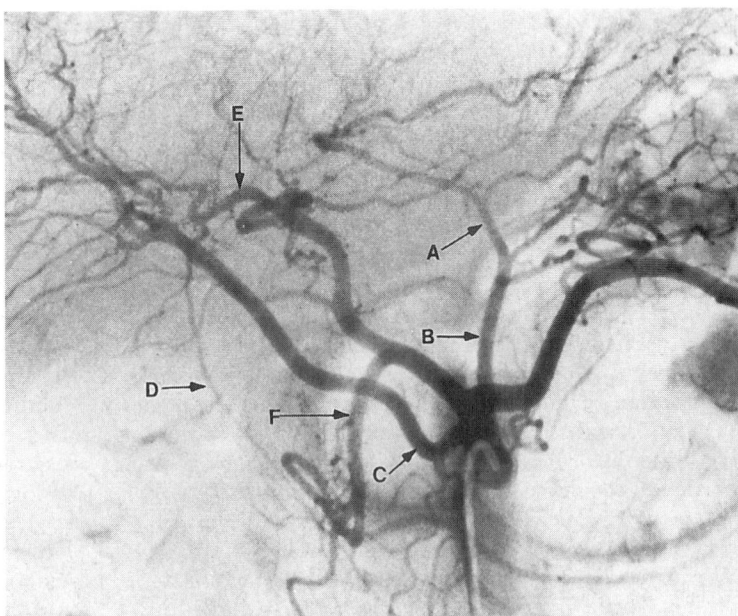

FIGURE 127-2. Hepatic artery variations. Arterial phase of a celiac arteriogram (subtraction technique) shows an accessory left hepatic artery (A) from the left gastric (B) and the right hepatic artery (C) from the celiac trunk. The middle hepatic artery (E) originates from the left hepatic artery, which is the sole branch of the common hepatic artery. (D, falciform artery; F, gastroduodenal artery.)

are the middle colic, jejunal, ileal, right colic, and ileocolic arteries.

The inferior mesenteric artery courses caudally and to the left for up to 5 cm before giving off its first major branch, the left colic artery. The ascending branch of the left colic artery supplies the descending colon and a variable amount of the splenic flexure. The inferior mesenteric artery gives off several additional branches to the descending and sigmoid colon before terminating in the superior hemorrhoidal artery. Anastomoses between the inferior mesenteric artery and middle colic branches of the superior mesenteric artery and inferior hemorrhoidal branches of the internal iliac artery are important in the setting of mesenteric ischemia or atherosclerotic disease of the distal aorta or proximal iliac arteries.

Portal Venous System

The portal vein begins behind the head of the pancreas in the confluence of the superior mesenteric and splenic veins. While it ascends along the hepatoduodenal ligament, the portal vein lies dorsal and to the left of the bile duct, and to the right of the hepatic artery. It is joined by the left gastric, right gastric, posterior superior pancreaticoduodenal, and cystic veins. The right branch of the portal vein is shorter than the left and divides into the anterior and posterior segmental branches. The left portal branch divides into the superior and inferior subsegmental branches after giving off branches to the caudate and quadrate lobes. The umbilical vein joins the left portal vein at its bifurcation into the subsegmental branches. The inferior mesenteric vein joins the splenic or, less frequently, the superior mesenteric vein just before they join in the mesenteric confluence.

The portal venous system receives venous blood from the GI tract, the pancreas, the spleen, the gallbladder, and the omentum. Normally the portal vein blood flows toward the liver (hepatopetal), and reversal in flow (hepatofugal) in any tributaries of the portal venous system indicates the presence

of portal hypertension. Reversal of portal vein flow may be partial or complete. The partial reversal of portal flow may occur in the extrahepatic or intrahepatic branches of the portal venous system. In complete reversal, usually associated with severe hepatic vein obstruction or after nonselective portosystemic shunts, the portal vein is the principal outflow conduit of the liver, and hepatic artery blood leaves the liver through the portal vein. Angiographic demonstration of the flow direction in the main portal vein is essential for planning portosystemic shunt surgery.

Hepatic Veins

The hepatic veins begin in the center of the hepatic lobules as intralobular veins. These veins join together to form sublobular veins. The hepatic veins are intersegmental or interlobar in course: the right hepatic vein lies in the intersegmental fissure of the right hepatic lobe, dividing it into the anterior and posterior segments; the middle hepatic vein lies in the interlobar fissure and the left hepatic vein lies between the medial and lateral segments of the left hepatic lobe. The hepatic veins converge posteriorly and run near the hepatic capsule before emptying into the inferior vena cava.

The accessory hepatic veins, which originate from the right and caudate lobes, are small and empty into the inferior vena cava between the main hepatic and renal veins. They function as collaterals in hepatic vein occlusion.

ARTERIAL DISEASE

Noninvasive imaging studies are performed more frequently to evaluate intraabdominal vascular diseases. MR angiography can adequately demonstrate the abdominal aorta and its branches, and portal venous system. However, arteriography remains the gold standard in the diagnosis of visceral arterial disease. It can provide the necessary vascular information regarding the exact origin of the lesion, its hemodynamics, and association with adjacent vascular structures.

Acute Mesenteric Ischemia

Acute mesenteric ischemia is a medical emergency. Delay of diagnosis and proper treatment of this condition results in bowel necrosis with high mortality.[9] Awareness of mesenteric ischemia leads to an early diagnosis and treatment of the condition. Plain abdominal radiographic findings in early mesenteric ischemia are nonspecific, but in the late stage, a thickened bowel wall, ileus, and portal vein gas may be demonstrated.[10] Noninvasive diagnostic imaging techniques such as CT and scintigraphy are not sufficiently sensitive in the diagnosis of mesenteric ischemia. Angiography is diagnostic and should be performed urgently.[11,12]

The two major types of acute mesenteric ischemia are occlusive and nonocclusive ischemia. The etiology of occlusive mesenteric ischemia includes embolism, atherosclerotic plaques, aortic dissection, neoplasms, and vasculitis. In superior mesenteric artery embolism, the occlusion may be proximal or distal to the middle colic artery. Arteriosclerosis usually involves the origin of the superior mesenteric artery, allowing collateral development through the marginal artery from the inferior mesenteric artery. Involvement of the superior mesenteric artery by aortic dissection is rare and should be evaluated with intraarterial DSA.

Nonocclusive mesenteric ischemia has been recognized with increasing frequency in the last decade and is caused by a significant reduction in mesenteric blood flow secondary to cardiac failure or hypovolemic shock. The typical angiographic findings include diffuse mesenteric arterial constriction, slowing of mesenteric arterial flow, and decreased parenchymal staining. Intravenous glucagon or intraarterial infusion of papaverine into the superior mesenteric artery through an indwelling transfemoral catheter is used to relieve the mesenteric vasoconstriction.

Colonic Ischemia

Colonic ischemia may be caused by decreased perfusion to the bowel in a low flow state or surgical ligation of the inferior mesenteric artery during abdominal aortic reconstruction or abdominoperineal resection surgery.[13] In some cases, gentle endoscopy and barium enema may be useful in this diagnosis. The angiographic findings may be nonspecific: in the early stage the mesenteric arteries are constricted and blood flow is slowed with decreased parenchymal vascularity; in the late stage the colon may appear hypervascular with prominent intramural arteries and increased accumulation of contrast material in the wall of the bowel (Fig. 127-3). Preoperative angiography is necessary to see the mesenteric circulation because ligation of the inferior mesenteric artery in the patient with a stenosis in the superior mesenteric distribution may result in mesenteric ischemia.

Intestinal Angina

At least two of the three splanchnic arteries usually have significant occlusive disease before the syndrome of intestinal angina occurs.[14] Duplex US with spectral analysis of the pulsed-wave Doppler scan frequently is used for screening patients thought to have chronic mesenteric artery occlusive

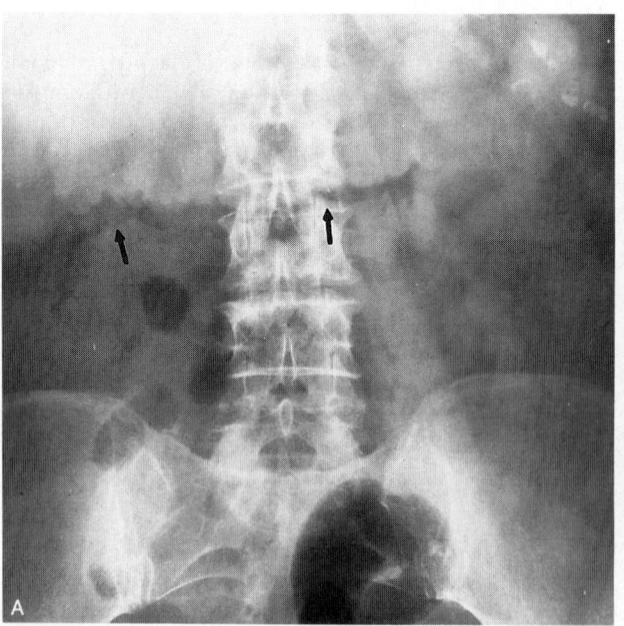
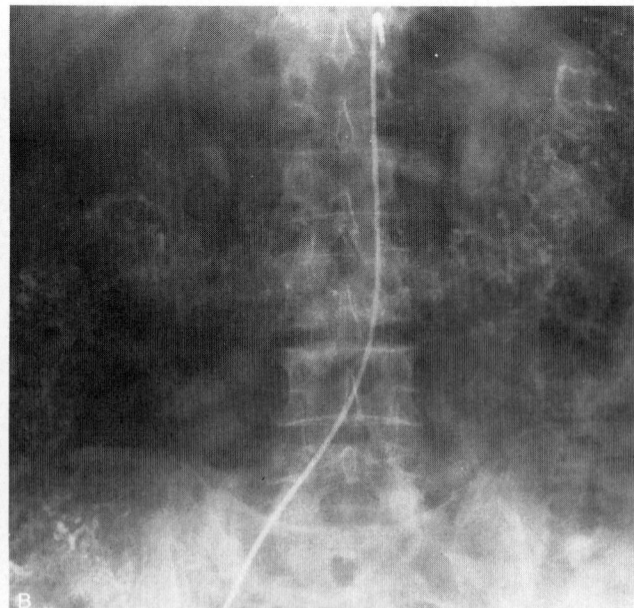

FIGURE 127-3. Ischemic colitis. **(A)** Plain film shows concave indentations along both walls of the transverse colon and ''thumbprinting,'' secondary to intramural bleeding (*arrows*). **(B)** Parenchymal phase of a superior mesenteric angiogram obtained 3 days after the radiograph shows hypervascularity throughout the colon. There was no arterial occlusive disease.

disease. Demonstration of a patent superior mesenteric artery or an insignificant stenosis of the superior mesenteric artery with patent celiac artery should exclude the diagnosis of chronic mesenteric ischemia.[15] Visceral angiograms are necessary to confirm the stenosis or occlusion of the mesenteric arteries, but it may not be possible to establish the cause-effect relation of the mesenteric arterial stenosis and ischemia. In mesenteric arterial occlusion, the collaterals may produce flow defects in the superior mesenteric artery, giving the misleading diagnosis of embolism.

Pancreatic carcinoma, mesenteric metastases, and carcinoid tumors may clinically mimic the syndrome of intestinal angina. They may cause or coexist with the narrowing of the celiac and superior mesenteric arteries.

Celiac Axis Compression

Celiac axis compression syndrome is controversial as a cause of abdominal pain. The celiac axis may be narrowed or, in severe cases, occluded by the median arcuate ligament of the diaphragm. Surgical correction of the lesion by decompression or reconstruction of the vessel usually ameliorates the pain. Celiac axis stenosis frequently is an incidental finding, with a reported incidence rate of 12% to 49%.[16,17] A lateral aortogram is necessary to confirm the diagnosis and demonstrates a concave impression on the craniad aspect of the celiac axis. The compression usually is accentuated during deep expiration. A celiac angiogram demonstrates flow defects in the branches of the celiac artery. A superior mesenteric angiogram demonstrates marked collateral circulation to the celiac artery through the pancreaticoduodenal arcades and transverse pancreatic and dorsal pancreatic arteries.

Vasculitis

Mesenteric vasculitis rarely causes intestinal angina, infarction, and GI bleeding. The angiographic findings vary with the type of vasculitis. In polyarteritis nodosa, celiac and superior mesenteric angiograms demonstrate occluded small- and medium-sized arteries and microaneurysms (Fig. 127-4). In ergot or digitalis toxicity the mesenteric artery branches are narrowed or occluded with collaterals. Crohn's disease, carcinoid tumor, and Takayasu's disease rarely are causes of mesenteric vasculitis.[18] The newer imaging modalities are insensitive when diagnosing vasculitis. Angiography is necessary to demonstrate small- and medium-sized arteries and aneurysms and should include bilateral renal, celiac, and superior mesenteric angiograms.

Splanchnic Artery Aneurysms

Splanchnic artery aneurysms and pseudoaneurysms are rare and often are found incidentally during angiographic studies for other indications. Although CT and MR imaging are capable of demonstrating splanchnic aneurysms, angiography is used to identify the exact site of the aneurysm and its relation to adjacent vascular structures. Treatment of splanchnic aneurysms with surgical resection or embolization is necessary

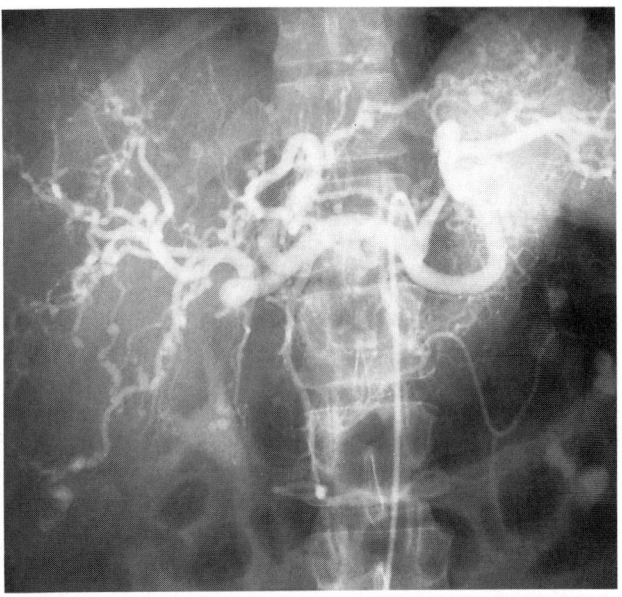

FIGURE 127-4. Multiple microaneurysms in polyarteritis nodosa. Arterial phase of a celiac angiogram shows numerous aneurysms involving the hepatic and pancreatic arteries.

to prevent catastrophic hemorrhage.[19] Aneurysms occur virtually in all splanchnic arteries.

Splenic artery aneurysms are common, accounting for 60% of all visceral artery aneurysms.[20] They occur four times more frequently in women than men and are multiple in 20% of patients. Causes include atherosclerosis, medial fibrodysplasia, multiple pregnancy, pancreatitis, portal hypertension, polyarteritis nodosa, and trauma. In portal hypertension, aneurysms tend to occur at the bifurcation of the intrasplenic branches of splenic artery. Most atherosclerotic splenic artery aneurysms are asymptomatic. Asymptomatic calcified aneurysms require no treatment. On the other hand, aneurysms occurring in pregnant women or that are associated with pancreatitis require treatment because of their propensity to bleed.

The hepatic artery is the second most common site for splanchnic aneurysm, accounting for 20% of all splanchnic aneurysms.[20] Most hepatic pseudoaneurysms are traumatic in origin and are secondary to blunt or penetrating abdominal trauma, liver biopsy, or the placement of a transhepatic biliary drainage catheter or hepatic arterial infusion catheter.[21] Most spontaneous aneurysms occur in the common hepatic or right hepatic artery. The main complications of the hepatic artery aneurysms are bleeding into the bile duct or peritoneal cavity, or rupture into the portal vein.

Mesenteric aneurysms are arteriosclerotic and may cause GI bleeding or mesenteric ischemia. Celiac axis aneurysms account for 4% of all visceral aneurysms and should be differentiated from pseudocysts when encountered during ultrasonography or nonenhanced CT scanning. A lateral aortogram using intraarterial DSA is necessary to confirm the diagnosis of aneurysms arising from the origins of the celiac and superior mesenteric arteries.

Gastroduodenal and pancreatic arterial aneurysms occur in patients with pancreatitis and pseudocysts and may cause GI and intraperitoneal hemorrhage. Aneurysms rarely rupture into the pancreatic duct or a pseudocyst. Contrast-enhanced

CT usually differentiates pseudocysts and aneurysms. Angiography is required to delineate the vascular anatomy and the exact origin of the aneurysm before surgical treatment or percutaneous embolotherapy.

Abdominal Trauma

Trauma to the abdomen may be penetrating or blunt. Patients who are unstable hemodynamically after a penetrating abdominal trauma should undergo exploratory laparotomy immediately. Otherwise most traumatized patients require radiologic studies to assess the extent of the injury. CT is the initial study used for the evaluation of abdominal trauma. Angiography is indicated to determine the exact site and extent of vascular injury after CT has demonstrated evidence for vascular injury or when a penetrating injury has occurred in the vicinity of major vessels.

VENOUS DISEASE

Occlusion of the portal, mesenteric, splenic, and hepatic veins may be asymptomatic or associated with ascites, hepatic failure, or GI hemorrhage. The newer imaging modalities can diagnose occlusion of the portal and splenic vein by demonstrating intraabdominal varices and aneurysms in the portal venous system.[22] Duplex scanning is useful in the assessment of patency and direction of blood flow of the portal vein and portosystemic shunts. The portal venous phases of the celiac and superior mesenteric angiograms are used to evaluate portal vein occlusion and aneurysm. In addition, an inferior vena cavogram and hepatic venogram are obtained if Budd-Chiari syndrome is suspected.

Portal Vein Occlusion

Portal vein occlusion may be nonneoplastic or neoplastic. Causes of nonneoplastic portal vein obstruction are cirrhosis, intraabdominal inflammatory disease, and omphalitis.[23] Neoplasms invading the portal venous system are hepatocellular carcinoma, cholangiocarcinoma, pancreatic carcinoma, and rarely, metastatic tumors.

The characteristic angiographic findings of portal vein occlusion are large collateral veins in the hepatoduodenal ligament during the portal venous phase of the superior mesenteric angiogram (Fig. 127-5). If the intrahepatic portal venous branches are occluded, the collaterals continue to run along the intrahepatic bile ducts, giving the appearance of railroad tracks.[24] Neither CT nor US are helpful in diagnosing intrahepatic portal vein occlusion. In mesenteric vein thrombosis, numerous tiny collateral veins are demonstrated throughout the mesentery without visualization of the superior mesenteric vein during the venous phase of the superior mesenteric angiogram.

The angiographic abnormality of portal vein occlusion due to neoplasms varies with the type of neoplasm. Pancreatic and biliary cancers cause localized narrowing or occlusion of the portal vein without associated tumor vessels. In contrast,

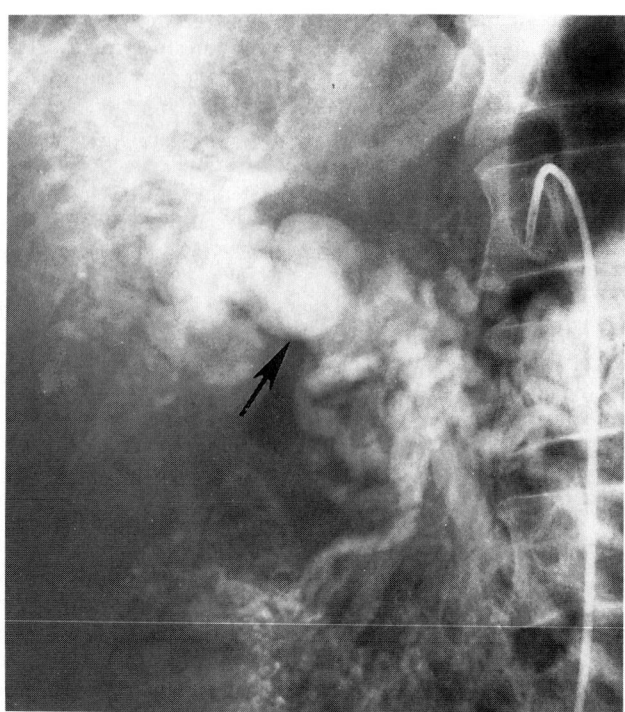

FIGURE 127-5. Portal vein occlusion. Portal venous phase of a superior mesenteric angiogram (oblique view) demonstrates tortuous venous collaterals (*arrow*) running along the hepatoduodenal ligament adjacent to the occluded portal vein. The collateral veins reconstitute intrahepatic portal venous branches. (From Reuter SR, Redman HC, Cho KJ. Gastrointestinal angiography. 3rd ed. Philadelphia: WB Saunders, 1986:121.)

portal invasion by hepatocellular carcinoma has a characteristic appearance, with abnormal vascular channels coursing within the portal vein branches in the vicinity of the tumors. Arteriovenous shunting may occur with portal vein invasion by tumors.[25]

Splenic Vein Occlusion

Splenic vein occlusion frequently is caused by pancreatitis, pancreatic tumors, and peripancreatic or retroperitoneal tumors. This entity usually is silent clinically but may cause hypersplenism or gastric bleeding. The incidence rate of gastric variceal bleeding in splenic vein occlusion varies, ranging from 11% to 65%.[26,27] The presence of gastric varices without esophageal varices suggests the diagnosis of splenic vein occlusion. Biopsy of the stomach in patients with splenic vein occlusion may result in catastrophic hemorrhage. The diagnosis can be made by dynamic CT and duplex scanning. Angiography should be performed when the noninvasive studies are inconclusive or when additional vascular information is needed. The typical angiographic findings are venous collaterals by means of the short gastric-coronary and gastroepiploic veins, and nonopacification of the splenic vein during the venous phase. Splenectomy is performed to treat variceal hemorrhage. In asymptomatic patients no specific therapy is required.

Budd-Chiari Syndrome

In Budd-Chiari syndrome, a significant portion of the hepatic venous system is obstructed by thrombosis, neoplasms, or sclerosis. Rarely the congenital membrane in the inferior vena cava causes obstruction of the hepatic vein.[28] Factors associated with hepatic vein thrombosis are polycythemia, paroxysmal nocturnal hemoglobinuria, and oral contraceptives. Diffuse hepatic vein thrombosis causes abdominal pain, hepatosplenomegaly, ascites, and portal hypertension. In contrast, localized occlusion of the hepatic vein may be difficult to recognize because the symptoms may be nonspecific and mild. In the chronic stage of the disease, even liver biopsy may not reveal the characteristic centrilobular sinusoidal dilatation and congestion.

Various imaging studies have been used for the diagnosis of hepatic venous outflow obstruction. Radionuclide scintigraphy may reveal nonspecific nonhomogeneous isotopic uptake by the liver and increased uptake by the enlarged caudate lobe. US with color-flow Doppler scan may reveal thrombi in the hepatic veins and inferior vena cava and intrahepatic venous collaterals.[29] CT usually is used as the initial test and may reveal nonuniform contrast enhancement of the liver parenchyma and enlarged caudate lobe (Fig. 127-6).[30] Increased central venous pressure from right-sided heart failure may produce a contrast enhancement pattern similar to that of Budd-Chiari syndrome. MR imaging is useful in identifying the underlying lesions such as hepatic and vena caval thrombi and congenital membrane.

Angiography is the most important procedure for the diagnosis of the Budd-Chiari syndrome. Superior mesenteric and celiac angiograms are obtained to see the portal vein and exclude hepatic neoplasms. An inferior vena cavogram is obtained using digital subtraction technique. A hepatic venogram is obtained with the injection of contrast material into the obstructed hepatic vein. This usually demonstrates the typical collateral channels, which have the appearance of a spiderweb. If catheterization of the right hepatic vein is unsuccessful, catheterization of the accessory hepatic vein should be performed to see collateral veins. Portal vein occlusion occurs in 10% to 20% of patients with hepatic vein occlusion.[31] The arteriographic abnormality of the hepatic vein occlusion usually is nonspecific and may mimic hepatic metastases, hepatitis, orthotopic transplant rejection, cirrhosis, or hemangiomas.

Percutaneous translumenal angioplasty and stent placement have been used to treat Budd-Chiari syndrome resulting from obstruction of the hepatic segment of the inferior vena cava.[32,33] Restenosis or reocclusion occurs frequently at the angioplasty site. The use of metallic stents improves patency after angioplasty. The transhepatic approach may be used for angioplasty and stent placement for right hepatic vein occlusion causing Budd-Chiari syndrome.[34] The transjugular intrahepatic portosystemic shunt (TIPS) procedure has been used to treat intractable ascites and bleeding varices from hepatic venous occlusive disease.[35]

GASTROINTESTINAL DISEASE

Barium examination and endoscopy are the most common diagnostic tests for GI disease. CT is useful in evaluating inflammatory and neoplastic diseases of the GI tract and mesentery. Angiography has little value in evaluating GI neoplasms but remains useful in the diagnosis and staging of small intestinal tumors. Other indications for angiography

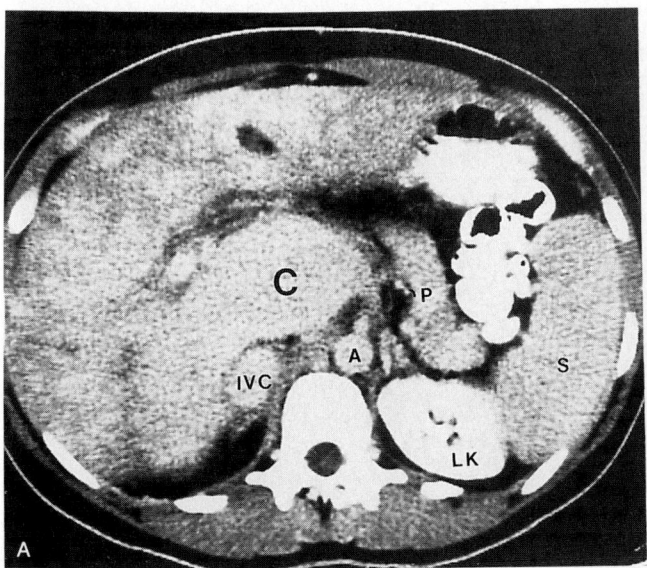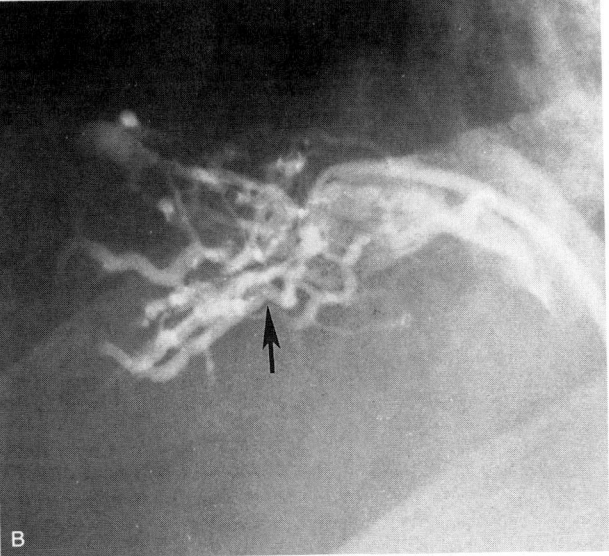

FIGURE 127-6. Budd-Chiari syndrome. **(A)** Computed tomographic scan of the liver with contrast enhancement shows nonuniform enhancement of the liver parenchyma and enlarged caudate lobe (C). (A, aorta; IVC, inferior vena cava, LK, left kidney; S, spleen.) **(B)** Wedged hepatic venogram. Contrast medium was injected into the occluded hepatic vein demonstrating numerous collateral veins (*arrow*) pathognomonic of hepatic vein occlusion.

are to diagnose vascular disease, to demonstrate a vascular road map before surgery or transcatheter therapy, and to locate the site of GI hemorrhage.

During the last decade, angiography has assumed an important role in the diagnosis and treatment of acute GI hemorrhage. Endoscopy plays an important role in the diagnosis of upper GI hemorrhage; radionuclide scintigraphy with tagged red blood cells is more useful in the detection of lower GI bleeding. Angiography is performed for the diagnosis and treatment of the bleeding when endoscopy or radionuclide scintigraphy demonstrates active bleeding (Fig. 127-7). Angiography must be performed as soon as possible after endoscopy or scintigraphy produce positive results because GI bleeding usually is intermittent. According to animal studies, selective angiography can detect the site of arterial bleeding at a rate as low as 0.5 mL/minute. Angiography is not useful in diagnosing capillary or venous hemorrhage because of the dilution of the contrast material injected intraarterially.

Barium studies and endoscopy are the most frequently used procedures for the diagnosis of chronic GI bleeding. Angiography is especially useful in identifying vascular malformation and vascular neoplasms occurring in the small intestine. Intraoperative localization of vascular lesions of the small bowel may be difficult. To facilitate the intraoperative localization, a catheter is placed subselectively in the mesenteric branch artery for the injection of methylene blue.

Upper Gastrointestinal Bleeding

In upper GI bleeding, celiac and superior mesenteric angiograms are obtained. If a bleeding site is identified the bleeding artery is catheterized for embolization. If a bleeding site is not identified, left gastric and gastroduodenal arteriograms are obtained. If the source of bleeding still has not been identified and nasogastric aspiration reveals dark blood, a catheter is placed in the left gastric artery for the next 6 to 12 hours. In patients with intermittent bleeding, the bleeding may be precipitated by intraarterial administration of heparin, vasodilators, and thrombolytic agents for localization and treatment.[36,37] In selected patients with massive upper GI bleeding with normal arteriographic studies, prophylactic embolization of the left gastric artery may be effective in preventing rebleeding.[38]

The common causes of upper GI bleeding are peptic ulceration of the esophagus, stomach, and duodenum, Mallory-Weiss tears, gastritis, and gastroesophageal varices. Angiography usually is not helpful in determining the cause of upper GI hemorrhage. Hemorrhagic gastritis is the most common cause of capillary bleeding and may demonstrate hypervascular stomach with dilated gastric arteries and increased parenchymal staining. Peptic ulceration is the most common cause of arterial bleeding and usually produces no angiographic abnormality. The bleeding into the stomach usually arises from the left gastric artery and occasionally from the short gastric, right gastric, and gastroepiploic arteries. The bleeding into the duodenum may originate from the celiac or superior mesenteric artery or from both arteries. Angiographically the arterial bleeding appears as a localized accumulation of contrast material extravasation during the arterial phase of the angiogram. The escaped contrast material persists throughout the venous phase and may outline the mucosa. Selective arterial embolization is an effective means of controlling the bleeding from peptic ulceration; embolization of the left gastric artery is performed to control bleeding into the stomach, and embolization of the gastroduodenal artery is done to control

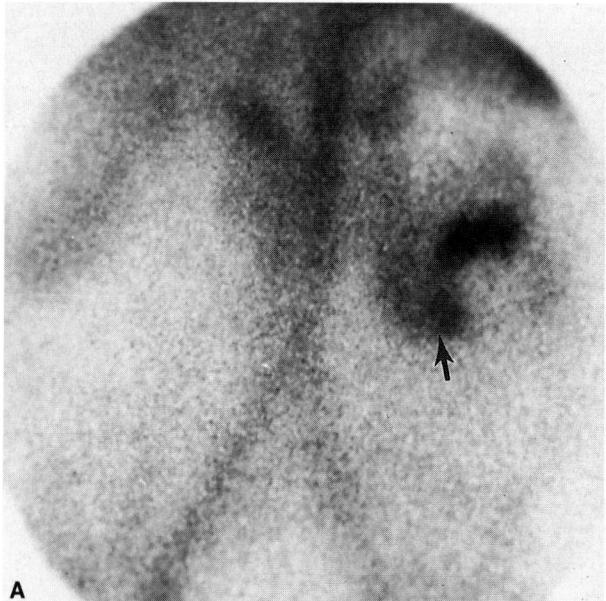
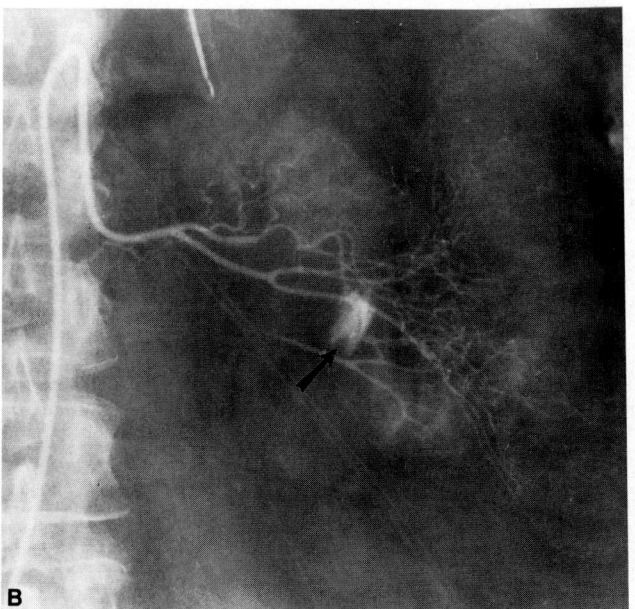

FIGURE 127-7. Massive bleeding into the jejunum. **(A)** Radionuclide scan with technetium 99m–labeled red cell shows extravasation of radionuclide (*arrow*) in the left upper abdomen. **(B)** Selective arteriogram of the jejunal artery before embolization shows extravasation (*arrow*) of the contrast medium. Angiography was essential in identifying the exact site of bleeding. (From Reuter SR, Redman HC, Cho KJ. Gastrointestinal angiography. 3rd ed. Philadelphia: WB Saunders, 1986:284.)

duodenal bleeding. Gelfoam, Ivalon, and microcoils are the most frequently used embolic agents.

Endoscopy is useful in detecting the bleeding into the biliary tract (hemobilia) and pancreatic duct (hemosuccus pancreaticus), and angiography is used to diagnose the cause of the bleeding. Liver biopsy, trauma, percutaneous transhepatic biliary drainage, tumor, and ruptured intrahepatic aneurysms are the causes of hemobilia. Hepatic artery embolization is the most effective means of treating hemobilia. Splenic artery aneurysm may rupture into the pancreatic duct and cause GI bleeding. Aortoenteric fistula rarely causes GI bleeding, and the duodenum is the most common site of the fistula. Biplane aortogram should be obtained, and it may show a false aneurysm at the aortic anastomotic site.

In patients with bleeding from esophageal varices, angiography is indicated to exclude an arterial source for the bleeding and to see the portal venous system. Angiography cannot detect bleeding varices because of the dilution of contrast material. Intravenous infusion of vasopressin and endoscopic sclerotherapy can effectively control the bleeding. Percutaneous transhepatic coronary vein embolization may be used if other forms of therapy fail to arrest the bleeding.

The technique of percutaneous creation of intrahepatic portosystemic shunt recently has been developed. The TIPS has been shown to be effective in controlling variceal bleeding in patients with cirrhosis and portal hypertension.[39,40] The procedure is a modification of that used for transjugular liver biopsy and portography. After puncture of the portal vein, the liver parenchyma is dilated and metallic stents are placed between the right hepatic vein and portal vein. Creation of an 8- to 10-mm shunt usually lowers the portosystemic pressure gradient to below 12 mm Hg. The TIPS has a 90% immediate success rate in patients with patent hepatic and portal veins, and a 30-day mortality rate is about 30%. Recurrent bleeding usually is secondary to development of shunt stenoses or occlusion. Procedural complications include bacteremia, renal failure, and inadvertent punctures of hepatic arteries, capsules, or bile ducts. The TIPS plays a role as a bridge to liver transplantation. Further experience and follow-up studies are necessary to determine long-term effectiveness.

Lower Gastrointestinal Bleeding

The causes of lower GI hemorrhage are diverticula, angiodysplasia, tumors, aneurysms, trauma, and varices. In lower GI hemorrhage, a superior mesenteric angiogram is performed to detect bleeding from the small intestine and from the right side of the colon. A celiac arteriogram is performed to evaluate the stomach and duodenum because the duodenum can be the source for lower GI bleeding. An inferior mesenteric arteriogram is obtained to evaluate the left side of the colon and rectum.

Endoscopy and barium examination are necessary to establish the diagnosis of chronic, intermittent lower GI bleeding but are less useful during acute bleeding. Retained barium in the GI tract may interfere with radionuclide scintigraphy and angiography. Angiography plays an important role in the diagnosis and management of acute and chronic bleeding. The angiographic diagnosis of acute bleeding is established by demonstrating a localized accumulation of escaped contrast material during the arterial phase of the mesenteric angiogram.

Selective intraarterial infusion of vasopressin is an effective means of controlling the bleeding.[41] Once the bleeding site has been demonstrated, vasopressin is infused into the bleeding artery at 0.2 U/minute. After 20 to 30 minutes of vasopressin infusion, repeat angiography is obtained to assess the result of the infusion. If bleeding has ceased, vasopressin infusion is continued at the same rate for 24 hours, and the rate is decreased to 0.1 U/minute for an additional 4 to 6 hours. If the bleeding persists after a 20-minute infusion of vasopressin, the infusion rate is increased to 0.4 U/minute. If bleeding has ceased and the mesenteric vessels show moderate vasoconstriction, the infusion is continued at the same rate for 24 hours before reducing to 0.2 U/minute and subsequently to 0.1 U/minute. The side effects of vasopressin include myocardial infarction, oliguria, and intestinal infarction. Because of a potential risk of infarction, mesenteric branch embolization has been limited to the bleeding vessels too large to be controlled by vasopressin. However, superselective embolization of the bleeding artery using a 0.99-mm (3-Fr) coaxial catheter such as Tracker-18 is effective in controlling bowel bleeding with minimal risk of infarction.[42]

Angiodysplasia

Three types of angiodysplasia occur in the GI tract: vascular ectasia, arteriovenous malformations, and capillary telangiectasia.[43] The clinical presentation and angiography allow identification of each type of angiodysplasia.

The vascular ectasia usually occurs along the antimesenteric border of the cecum and the ascending colon in elderly patients (older than 60 years of age). Endoscopy and angiography are useful in identifying the lesions. The angiographic findings of colonic vascular ectasia are small vascular clusters and blush in the wall of the colon, and early, dense opacification of the draining vein (Fig. 127-8).[44] Angiography is highly specific for vascular ectasia, but its sensitivity is unknown. Normal mesenteric angiography usually is accepted for exclusion of vascular ectasia, although the data for this assumption are not available. The vascular ectasia without arteriovenous shunting may not be identified by angiography. More than one vascular ectasia is frequently found at microscopic examination of the injected specimen in patients in whom one vascular ectasia has been identified by the preoperative angiogram. This suggests that angiography is less sensitive than endoscopy in detecting colonic vascular ectasia. Colonic resection is the definitive method of treatment. Injection of a silicone rubber solution (Microfil, Canton Bio-Medical, Boulder, CO) into the artery of the resected specimen facilitates localization of the lesion during pathologic examination.

Arteriovenous malformations are of developmental origin and usually affect people younger than 50 years of age. The angiographic findings are diagnostic, including tortuous, dilated arteries with early, prominent veins. The lesions frequently are found in the small intestine and vary in size. An angiogram of high quality and magnification technique is necessary to differentiate vascular malformations from vascular tumors.

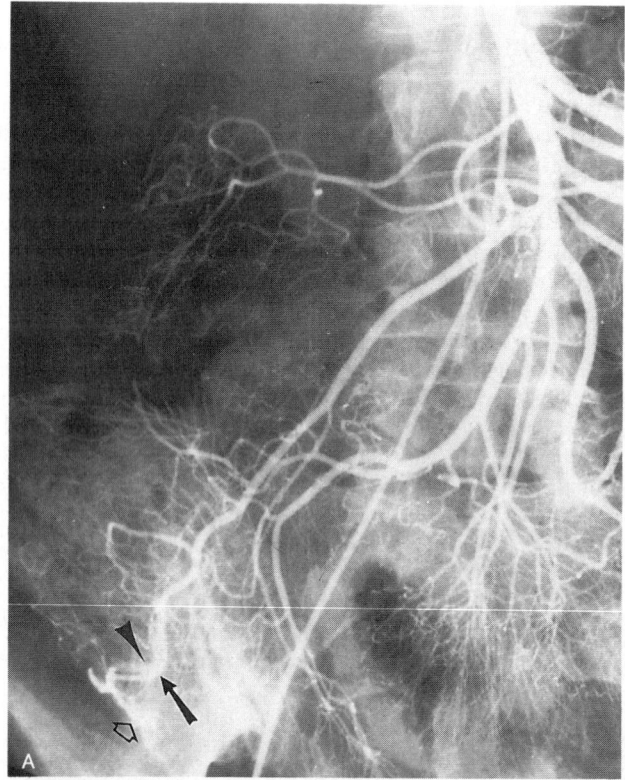

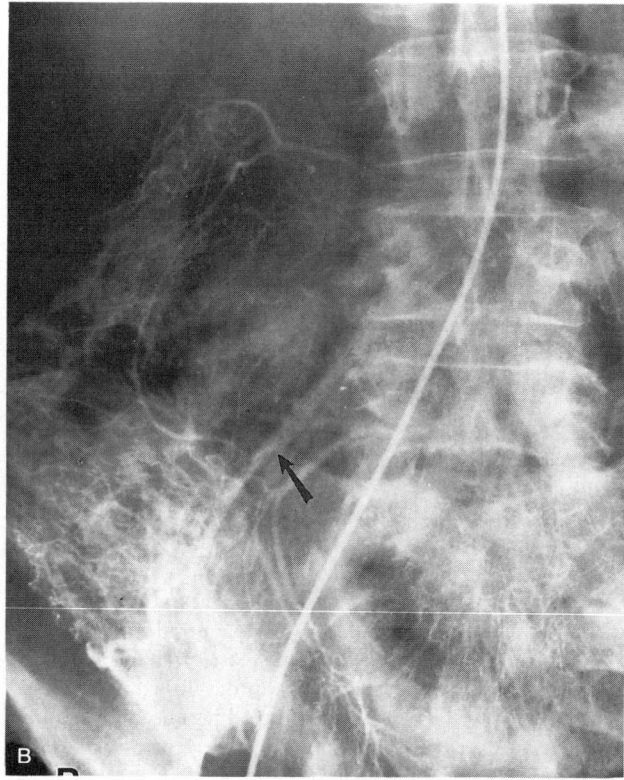

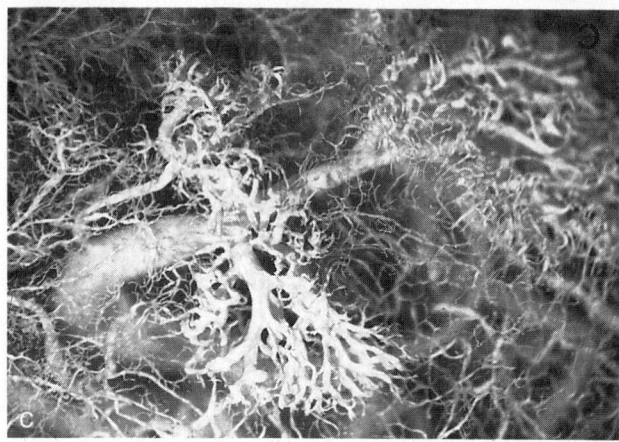

FIGURE 127-8. Vascular ectasia of the cecum. **(A)** Arterial phase of superior mesenteric angiogram in a 70-year-old woman with recurrent lower gastrointestinal bleeding. A small vascular lesion (*open arrow*) is demonstrated in the antimesenteric border of the cecum with simultaneous opacification of an entering artery (*arrow*) and a draining vein (*arrowhead*). **(B)** Capillary phase of same angiogram. Notice the early, densely opacified draining vein (*arrow*). The veins from other parts of the bowel have not been opacified. **(C)** Microfil cast of the resected specimen shows the vascular ectasia and multiple dilated submucosal veins.

Capillary telangiectasia of the GI tract may be a part of the systemic presentation of Osler-Weber-Rendu disease. The angiographic findings usually are subtle, including tiny areas of blush without arteriovenous shunting. Magnification angiography is essential. Hepatic angiogram may demonstrate dilated hepatic arteries and increased hepatic parenchymal staining.

Meckel's Diverticula

Meckel's diverticula rarely cause lower GI hemorrhage, and the main complication is bleeding. Barium examination and nuclear scintigraphy with technetium Tc 99m are used for diagnosis. Angiographically, Meckel's diverticula may appear as a short segment of bowel with increased contrast material accumulation supplied by an abnormal branch from the superior mesenteric artery.

Rectal Trauma

Bleeding may complicate fecal disimpaction, rectal tube placement, and endoscopic polypectomy. Inferior mesenteric angiography is performed for localization and treatment of the bleeding.

Intestinal Varices

Intestinal varices rarely cause lower GI hemorrhage and usually occur in patients with portal hypertension. Radionuclide scintigraphy and dynamic CT are useful in detecting large varices. Angiography provides the necessary information regarding the location and extent of the varices. The venous phase of superior mesenteric angiogram should be carefully evaluated for the diagnosis of intestinal varices. Transhepatic portal vein catheterization is the most useful method for evaluating the entire portal venous system and may be necessary in selected cases. Resection of the varices and portal decompression surgery are the most common forms of treatment for intestinal varices associated with portal hypertension. Transhepatic variceal embolization is a palliative, temporarily effective treatment for variceal hemorrhage. Recurrent hemorrhage usually is caused by recanalization of the varices after embolization or development of collaterals. The TIPS can be used in patients who have failed to conventional treatment and who are not candidates for surgical therapy.

Neoplasms of the Small Intestine

Leiomyomatous Tumors

Leiomyomatous tumors of the small bowel may present with acute or chronic GI bleeding (Fig. 127-9). Barium examination often is unrewarding, and CT may demonstrate larger tumors. Angiography, however, is useful in diagnosing the small bowel leiomyomas. These tumors usually are hypervascular with abundant tumor vessels and dense blush. The

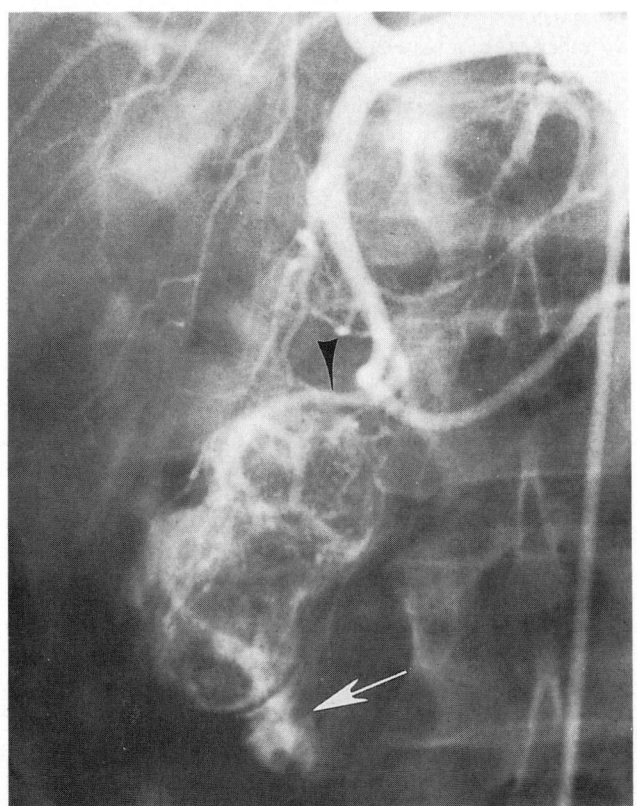

FIGURE 127-9. Bleeding leiomyoma of the duodenum. Gastroduodenal arteriogram in a 27-year-old woman with upper gastrointestinal hemorrhage. The leiomyoma in the second portion of the duodenum receives blood supply from the dilated anterior pancreatic arcade artery (*arrowhead*). Notice extravasation of the contrast medium into the duodenum (*arrow*). Gelfoam embolization successfully controlled the bleeding from the tumor and the tumor was excised 4 weeks later. (From Cho KJ, Reuter SR, Angiography of duodenal leiomyomas and leiomyosarcomas. AJR Am J Roentgenol 1980;135:31.)

draining veins usually are densely opacified. Differentiation between benign and malignant tumors cannot be made angiographically unless venous invasion or metastasis is demonstrated.[45]

Carcinoid Tumors

Most carcinoid tumors occur in the GI tract. They are rarely found in the pancreas, ovary, bile duct, liver, and thymus. Once the diagnosis is established by clinical presentation and biochemical studies, determining the site and staging the tumor are important for surgical resection. Primary carcinoid tumors usually are small and rarely detected before surgery. CT is the initial diagnostic procedure and has the ability to assess the mesenteric invasion and metastasis to the regional lymph nodes and liver.[46] Iodine-131 meta-iodo-benzylguanidine (MIBG) scanning, which is used for localizing pheochromocytomas, also can localize intestinal and bronchial carcinoid tumors.[47] MR imaging is a sensitive test for detecting hepatic metastases, but it is less helpful in detecting extrahepatic involvement.[48]

Angiography is used for diagnosis and staging of the carcinoid tumors. The angiographic findings include retraction, kinking, and occlusion of the mesenteric arteries. Carcinoid tumors metastatic to the liver usually are hypervascular with abundant neovascularity. Venous sampling with hormone assay is useful for localizing occult carcinoid tumors, especially those occurring in the ovary and lungs. Selective hepatic artery embolization is relatively safe and effective for palliating hepatic metastases from carcinoid tumors.[49]

PANCREATIC DISEASE

The role of angiography in evaluating pancreatic disease has considerably decreased with the availability of the newer diagnostic imaging modalities. CT, endoscopic retrograde cholangiopancreatography, and percutaneous aspiration biopsy usually are used for diagnosing and managing pancreatic carcinoma. CT is the initial radiologic method used for diagnosing pancreatic lesions, but it has limitations in visualizing small tumors and vascular invasion.[50] MR imaging usually is not used in evaluating pancreatic disease because of poor resolution and imaging artifacts caused by respiratory motion, bowel peristalsis, and aortic pulsations.[51]

When evaluating pancreatic lesions, angiography is performed for obtaining a specific diagnosis, determining tumor resectability, localizing islet cell adenomas, and delineating vascular anatomy in the preoperative evaluation of pancreatitis and pseudocysts.

Technical Considerations

Adequate visualization of the peripancreatic and intrapancreatic arteries and the portal venous system is important in evaluating pancreatic lesions. Selective and subselective angiograms of the celiac and superior mesenteric arteries are obtained; the splenic artery is injected to see the body and tail of the pancreas, the gastroduodenal artery for the head of the pancreas, and the dorsal pancreatic artery for the entire pancreas. High-dose splenic and superior mesenteric angiograms with the intraarterial injection of a vasodilator are obtained to see the splenic, superior mesenteric, and portal veins. When a pancreatic angiogram is performed for evaluating resectability of pancreatic cancers, only celiac and superior mesenteric angiograms are necessary.

Angiographic Diagnosis

Adenocarcinoma

Early detection of cancer arising in the pancreas remains difficult because of the nonspecificity of the presenting symptoms. Most cancers of the pancreas are nonresectable because of local spread to the adjacent structures and lymph nodes. CT or US are the initial diagnostic procedure for patients thought to have cancer of the pancreas. Patients with a suspicious pancreatic mass on this initial test should undergo endoscopic retrograde cholangiopancreatography with cytologic examination, or percutaneous aspiration biopsy under US or CT guidance. If necessary, angiography is performed to establish the definitive diagnosis and determine resectability of the lesion before palliative procedures or exploratory celiotomy. Patients with severe jaundice and dilated bile ducts demonstrated by US should be considered to undergo a biliary drainage procedure through endoscopic retrograde cholangiopancreatography or percutaneous transhepatic approach before angiography or surgical treatment. The angiographic criteria for nonresectability include involvement of any one of the major peripancreatic arteries (the splenic, hepatic, and superior mesenteric arteries) or veins (superior mesenteric, splenic, and portal veins; Fig. 127-10).

An appropriate algorithmic approach with a logical sequence of testing and the use of outpatient procedures when possible results in rapid diagnosis of pancreatic cancer with an accuracy rate greater than 90% at a relatively low cost.[52] Dynamic CT is useful in staging pancreatic cancer; it is nearly 100% accurate in predicting tumor unresectability but is slightly less accurate in predicting tumor resectability.[53]

Cystic Tumors

Cystic tumors of the pancreas are uncommon lesions, accounting for 10% to 15% of all pancreatic cystic lesions[54]; the remaining cysts are retention cysts or pseudocysts. Cystic tumors are rarely associated with von Hippel-Lindau disease. The lesions are classified as microcystic adenomas and mucinous macrocystic tumors. The latter tumors are malignant or potentially malignant. US or CT can provide the definitive diagnosis; therefore, angiography is reserved for determination of resectability and delineation of vascular anatomy for planning surgical resection. Angiographically, microcystic adenomas usually are hypervascular with abundant tumor vessels and blush, whereas mucinous cystic tumors are hypovascular with sparse tumor vessels. Angiography aids in differentiating cystic tumors from pseudocysts. Celiac and superior mesenteric angiography enables the physician to see most pancreatic cystic tumors, but occasionally subselective angiography with

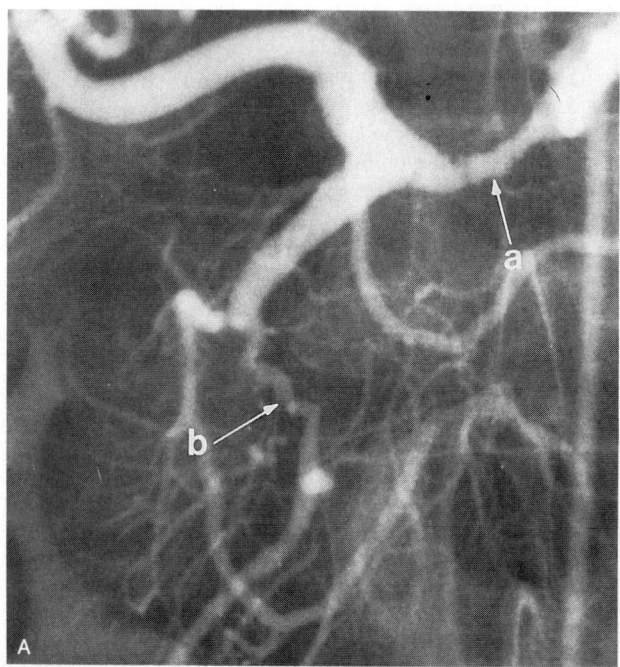
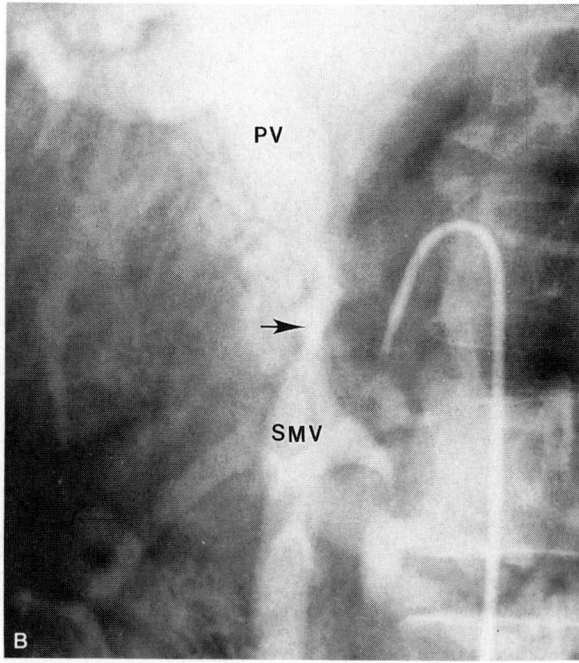

FIGURE 127-10. Unresectable pancreatic cancer. (**A**) Hepatic arteriogram (magnification technique). The common hepatic (a) and proximal gastroepiploic (b) arteries are encased by a tumor in head of the pancreas. (**B**) Portal venous phase of a superior mesenteric angiogram (oblique view). The junction of the superior mesenteric and portal veins is invaded by the tumor (*arrow*). (PV, portal vein; SMV, superior mesenteric vein; from Shields JJ, Porter DJ, Brady TM, Cho KJ. Angiography of pancreatic disease. In: Dent TL, ed. Pancreatic disease. New York: Grune & Stratton, 1981:93.)

direct magnification and photographic subtraction may be required to detect subtle neovascularity.

Pancreatic Endocrine Tumors

Preoperative localization of pancreatic endocrine tumors is essential in successful surgical treatment of islet cell adenomas, because small adenomas within the pancreas are not readily palpable at surgery. If adenomas are not visible or palpable at surgery, surgical search for such occult tumors causes extensive manipulation and dissection of the pancreas, and a "blind" distal pancreatectomy may have to be performed with the risk of missing adenomas in the remaining part of the pancreas and extrapancreatic sites.

Several radiologic methods have been used for localizing the tumors including US, CT, MR imaging, arteriography, and venous sampling with hormone assay. The sensitivity of each method depends primarily on the size, location, and cell type of the tumors. Localizing gastrin-producing adenomas is difficult because they are usually avascular angiographically and frequently occur extrapancreatically.

Usually US imaging is insensitive in localizing small adenomas. Intraoperative US, on the other hand, is 84% more sensitive in localizing small adenomas. However, this technique has not been widely used clinically.[55] CT is capable of detecting large islet tumors, but it is relatively insensitive in localizing small adenomas.[55-57] MR imaging is not useful in localizing small islet tumors.[58]

Angiography remains the most accurate means of localizing islet cell adenomas of the pancreas. The angiographic study includes celiac and superior mesenteric angiograms; subselective magnification angiograms of the splenic, dorsal pancreatic, and gastroduodenal arteries; and photographic subtraction. Intraarterial DSA may be used (Fig. 127-11). Angiographically, islet cell tumors appear as a localized area of contrast material accumulation (tumor blush) with or without tumor vessels. Malignant islet cell tumors may grow into the portal vein. Most hepatic metastases from islet cell carcinomas are hypervascular and are readily detected by hepatic angiography. Angiography is sensitive in localizing insulinomas (accuracy, 60%–90%), but it is less sensitive in detecting gastrin-producing tumors.[56,59] Other endocrine tumors, such as VIPoma, polypeptide-producing tumors, glucagonoma, and somatostatinoma are usually larger and hypervascular with abundant tumor vessels.

Percutaneous transhepatic venous sampling with hormone assay is a useful method for localizing occult islet cell tumors.[60] This usually pinpoints the source of abnormal hormone secretion to the head, body, or tail of the pancreas, or to the liver, and helps the surgeon to avoid unnecessary blind resection of the pancreas.[61] Simultaneous arterial and venous sampling from the splenic, superior mesenteric, and portal veins can detect localized elevation of hormone value near the tumor site; adenomas of the body and tail of the pancreas cause a step-up of hormone concentration in the splenic vein, and those of the pancreatic head cause step-ups in the superior mesenteric and portal veins. Simultaneous blood sampling from the hepatic and portal veins helps to determine the presence of hepatic metastases from gastrinomas and primary endocrine tumor of the liver.

In the review of 30 cases of transhepatic sampling for or-

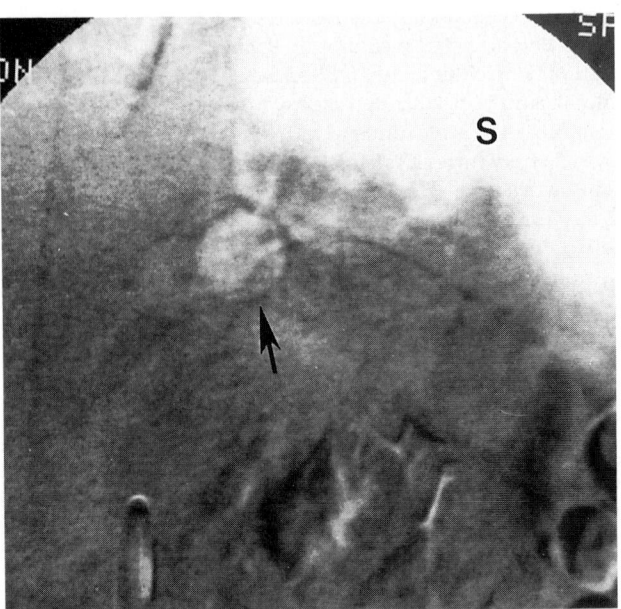

FIGURE 127-11. Islet cell adenoma in a patient with hyperinsulinism. Parenchymal phase of a splenic angiogram (digital subtraction technique) demonstrating a 1-cm diameter tumor blush in the distal body of the pancreas. (S, splenic parenchymal staining.)

ganic hyperinsulinism at the University of Michigan Medical Center, venous sampling correctly localized all insulinomas in 28 patients with a single adenoma and in 2 patients with multiple adenomas and islet cell hyperplasia. When the pancreas is involved by islet cell adenomatosis, islet cell hyperplasia, or nesidioblastosis, multiple sites of step-ups are found in the portal venous system. Transhepatic sampling is less rewarding when localizing gastrin-producing tumors. When gastrinomas are associated with multiple endocrine neoplasia type I, the pancreas often is involved diffusely with multiple tumors, microadenomatosis, and islet cell hyperplasia.[62] Sampling cannot differentiate the gastrinomas in the pancreatic head from those in the duodenal wall, peripancreatic tissue, or lymph nodes. Simultaneous sampling from the portal and hepatic veins, and selective sampling from the different parts of the hepatic veins are necessary to localize hepatic metastases or primary hepatic tumors.

Transhepatic catheterization is an invasive procedure requiring the introduction of a catheter into the portal vein transhepatically, and into the aorta and hepatic vein transfemorally. The experience and technical skills of the angiographer and the availability of radioimmunoassay of various gastroenteropancreatic hormones are essential for the success of the sampling method. The potential complications of the procedure are subcapsular hepatic hematoma, intraperitoneal bleeding, pneumothorax, and puncture of the gallbladder with bile leakage. Before withdrawing the catheter from the hepatic capsule, a gelatin sponge is injected to control the bleeding from the liver.

Recently Imamura and associates[63] introduced the selective arterial secretin injection test for localizing occult gastrinomas. It involves injection of 30 U of secretin into the splenic, gastroduodenal, proper hepatic, and superior mesenteric arteries, and blood sampling from the hepatic vein and from a peripheral artery to measure the changes of gastrin concentration. A rise (higher than 50%) in gastrin concentration in the hepatic vein after the selective intraarterial injection of secretin localizes the tumor to the part of the pancreas supplied by the artery injected: the gastroduodenal and superior mesenteric artery for the head of the pancreas, and the splenic artery for the body or tail. The selective arterial secretin injection test is more sensitive than transhepatic portal venous sampling for localizing occult gastrinomas. It is particularly useful in localizing small duodenal wall gastrinomas but is less sensitive in detecting occult hepatic metastases.[64] Transhepatic portal venous sampling still is useful in detecting occult hepatic metastases.

Surgery is the treatment of choice for endocrine tumors. Distal subtotal pancreatectomy is necessary for treating islet cell hyperplasia, nesidioblastosis, or multiple benign adenomas. Selective arterial embolization can be used as an alternative to surgery when angiography shows vascular insulinoma with a supplying artery. It involves the injection of small embolic particles into the tumor vascular bed through a catheter placed superselectively in the artery supplying the tumor.[65] This procedure is not possible if the tumor is avascular or if the supplying artery cannot be catheterized. The potential risks are incomplete removal of a potentially malignant tumor, pancreatitis, and GI ischemia.

Pancreatic Arteriovenous Malformations

Arteriovenous malformations are rare vascular lesions. They may occur as an isolated lesion or in association with Osler-Weber-Rendu disease. The malformation is a rare cause of GI bleeding. It may bleed directly into the intestine or into the pancreatic duct. Portal hypertension and varices associated with the malformation may be the causes of the bleeding. Angiography is important in the preoperative diagnosis and localization of the lesion. The lesion should be differentiated from chronic pancreatitis and vascular neoplasms.

Inflammatory Disease

Ultrasound should be the primary diagnostic mode for the diagnosis of pancreatitis and pancreatic pseudocysts. CT complements the US and is especially useful in delineating the association of pancreatic pseudocyst with adjacent organs. Angiography has little diagnostic use in patients with pancreatitis because the diagnosis is well established clinically, but plays an important role in evaluating patients with complications of pancreatitis, such as pseudocyst or hemorrhage.[66]

Angiography is not accurate in detecting pancreatic pseudocysts (24% false-negative rate) because small or primarily extrapancreatic pseudocysts often produce no significant arteriographic abnormalities. The angiographic abnormalities are arcuate stretching of intrapancreatic and peripancreatic arteries combined with a parenchymal defect in the capillary phase of the angiogram. In about half the cases of pseudocyst, peripancreatic venous narrowing or occlusion is found. Hemorrhages associated with pancreatitis may be of venous or arterial origin. Venous hemorrhage usually results from gastric varices associated with splenic or portal vein occlusion. Arterial hemorrhage is a rare but life-threatening complication

of pancreatitis, usually secondary to rupture of intrapancreatic and peripancreatic aneurysms. CT and US should be used to detect pseudocyst formation, arterial bleeding, or pseudoaneurysm formation. Color-flow Doppler US can detect turbulent arterial blood flow within the pseudoaneurysm, and MR imaging can confirm the presence of flow within the aneurysm. Arteriography is indicated for the diagnosis of arterial bleeding and pseudoaneurysm, and selective embolization should be used as a definitive or preoperative temporizing procedure.[67]

HEPATIC DISEASE

Nonimaging and imaging methods are used to detect hepatic masses. Liver function tests and carcinoembryonic antigen measurements are insensitive in detecting small liver lesions and lack the ability to provide the definitive diagnosis. ^{99m}Tc sulfur colloid scanning is less sensitive than CT in detecting smaller lesions. Sonography is sensitive in detecting cystic or echogenic lesions. CT is the most useful screening method for hepatic lesions and has the ability to distinguish a cystic from solid hepatic lesion. Bolus dynamic CT with CT-arterial portography is the most sensitive imaging modality for detecting intrahepatic metastases.[68] Doppler US and color-flow Doppler imaging are complementary procedures and provide useful information on the vascularity and hemodynamics of liver tumors. Color-flow Doppler is used to document blood flow and flow direction in the hepatic artery, hepatic veins, portal veins, and collateral venous pathways. Angiography still is important in evaluating liver tumors for the diagnosis and resectability of the tumor. MR imaging is sensitive in detecting certain liver lesions, but it is not used as a screening tool.

The role of hepatic angiography in the evaluation of hepatic mass lesions has decreased significantly with the advent of the newer imaging modalities. Angiography is performed to establish the definitive diagnosis and to determine the vascularity and resectability of tumors.

Technical Considerations

Hepatic angiography includes celiac, superior mesenteric, and hepatic angiography, inferior vena cavography, and hepatic venography. The venous phase of superior mesenteric angiogram is used to evaluate portal venous invasion by hepatic tumors. In selective hepatic angiography, a vasoconstrictor may be used to enhance tumor vascularity by altering intrahepatic arterial blood flow. Infusion hepatic angiography with a slow, long injection of the contrast medium may be used to detect hypovascular hepatic metastases. Delayed CT with the intraarterial injection of iodized oil (Lipiodol Andre Guerbet, France) into the hepatic artery is useful in detecting small hepatocellular carcinomas.[69]

Hepatic Circulation

Knowledge of hepatic circulation is important in the performance and interpretation of hepatic angiograms and in planning for hepatic arterial catheter placement in patients with hepatic malignancy. The liver receives a dual blood supply: about 75% of the total hepatic blood flow comes from the portal vein, and the remaining 25% comes from the hepatic artery. The relation between the portal vein and hepatic artery is reciprocal: a decrease in portal blood flow results in immediate compensatory increase in the hepatic arterial flow.[70] Hepatic arterial embolization in patients with diminished portal flow in cirrhosis and obstructive jaundice must be undertaken cautiously because the liver in these conditions depends primarily on the arterial blood.

ANGIOGRAPHIC DIAGNOSIS

Hepatic Neoplasms

Cavernous Hemangioma

Cavernous hemangiomas, the most common benign hepatic tumors, are composed of large sinusoidal spaces with fibrosis and thrombosis. They are often found incidentally but may be responsible for intrahepatic or intraperitoneal bleeding. Most lesions are clinically innocuous and require no therapy. The definitive diagnosis of these lesions is important to eliminate the need for biopsy or surgery. CT, US, and MR imaging are useful for obtaining a diagnosis.[71] Delayed labeled red blood cell–single photon emission computed tomography scanning has been shown to provide the correct diagnosis in 85% of cases, and it is also useful in differentiating hemangiomas from hepatocellular carcinomas.[72]

Angiography is the gold standard for the diagnosis of cavernous hemangiomas. The characteristic findings are areas of dense pooling of contrast material that persist into the venous phase (Fig. 127-12). When angiography fails to demonstrate an abnormality in patients thought to have cavernous hemangioma from previous CT, dynamic CT should be performed with the intraarterial injection of contrast material.

Adenoma

Adenomas are uncommon tumors, occurring mostly in young women with a history of taking oral contraceptives. Because of their tendency to bleed, adenomas should be excised.[73] The findings of hepatic adenomas on CT, US, and MR imaging are nonspecific. Angiographically, hepatic adenomas usually are vascular with abnormal vessels entering the tumors from the periphery and tumor blush. The definitive diagnosis cannot be established on the basis of the angiographic abnormality. Bleeding adenomas may be avascular, and radionuclide scan can be useful for localizing the tumor.

Focal Nodular Hyperplasia

Focal nodular hyperplasia is a benign, nonneoplastic lesion that usually is innocuous clinically. Angiographically, lesions are hypervascular with abundant abnormal vessels with granular contrast agent accumulation, and multiple septa radiating from the central area of scar.[74] Magnification technique and vasoconstrictive pharmacoangiography are used to enhance visualization of the nodular pattern of focal nodular hyperplasia. Sulfur colloid scan should be used in all patients

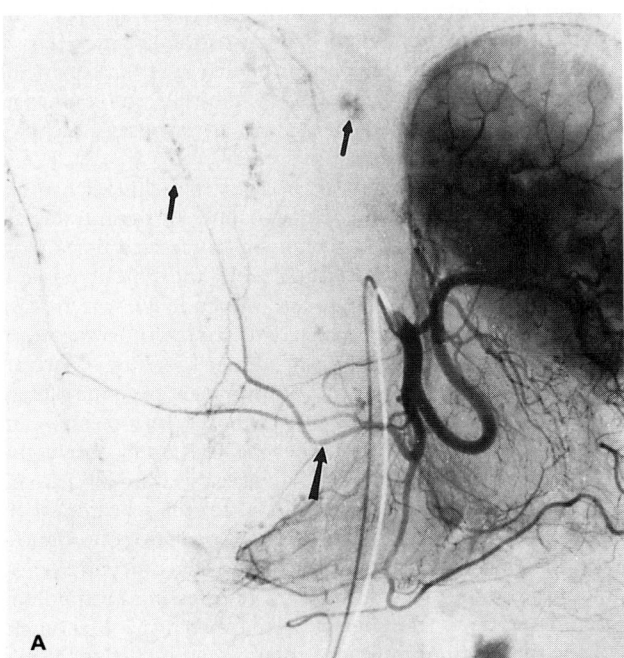 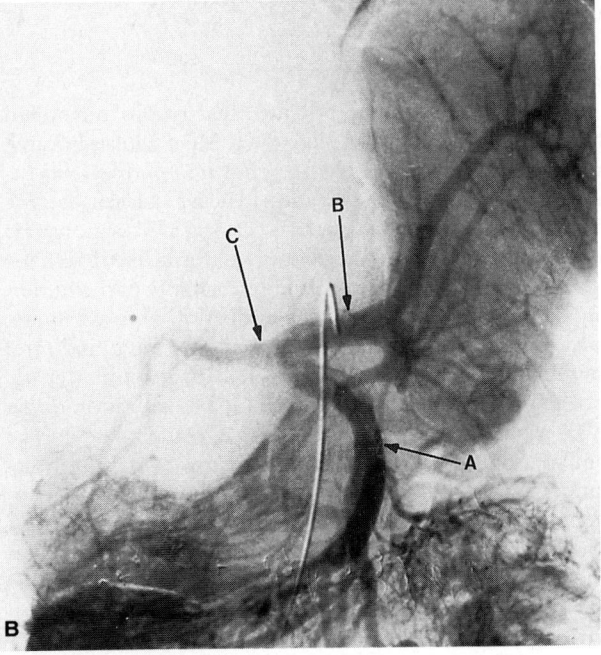

FIGURE 127-12.   Cavernous hemangioma of the liver. (**A**) Arterial phase of a celiac angiogram (subtraction technique) demonstrates a large mass with scattered pools of contrast medium (*arrows*). The hepatic artery branches are stretched and attenuated (*larger arrow*). (**B**) Portal venous phase of a superior mesenteric angiogram (subtraction technique) demonstrates occlusion of portal venous branches in the right lobe of the liver (C). The main portal vein (A) and its left portal radicle (B) are well opacified.

thought to have focal nodular hyperplasia because positive scan results are diagnostic. CT and MR imaging are capable of visualizing the central scar and radiating septa of focal nodular hyperplasia.

Biliary Cystadenoma

Biliary cystadenomas usually occur in middle-aged women and are often multiloculated. Ultrasonography can demonstrate smaller cysts and solid structures within biliary cystadeomas.[75] Angiography is performed to define hepatic arterial anatomy and determine surgical resectability. The angiographic findings usually are nonspecific and may demonstrate subtle neovascularity and rim-like staining in the wall of the tumor.

Malignant Neoplasms

Hepatocellular Carcinoma

Hepatocellular carcinoma, the most common primary malignancy of the liver, has a poor prognosis. Surgical resection offers the only possibility for cure. ^{99m}Tc sulfur colloid scans can detect the tumor but are nonspecific. CT is more useful in evaluating patients with hepatic tumors because it can demonstrate the tumor and its relation to intersegmental fissures. CT with the intraarterial injection of iodized oil into the hepatic artery is useful in detecting small, multiple hepatomas. Angiography confirms the diagnosis of the mass detected by CT and demonstrates its blood supply. Most hepatomas are hypervascular angiographically with coarse tumor vessels. Hepatomas frequently invade the portal vein, and portal vein involvement indicates unresectability of the tumor.

Cholangiocarcinoma

Cholangiocarcinoma is most frequently scirrhous in type and obliterates the lumen of the bile duct. Most cholangiocarcinomas are diagnosed in late stages and are nonresectable because of the invasion of the hepatic parenchyma, hepatic artery, and portal vein. Ultrasonography is performed to demonstrate dilated bile ducts. Cholangiography is performed to determine the level of biliary obstruction and resectability of the tumor. Angiography also is used for the evaluation of resectability, and invasion of the portal vein and hepatic artery indicates nonresectability of the tumor. Percutaneous transhepatic portogram may be necessary for detailed visualization of the portal vein when surgical resection is contemplated. The combination of radiation, chemotherapy, and biliary decompression is used for the treatment of nonresectable cholangiocarcinoma. The diagnosis of hilar cholangiocarcinoma (Klatskin's tumors) usually is presumed from the cholangiographic findings. Because benign fibrosing disease can mimic Klatskin's tumors, pathologic diagnosis of the tumor is required when surgical resection or liver transplantation is contemplated.[76] A negative result of bile cytologic study is unreliable in excluding malignancy. An atherectomy catheter such as ATHEROTRACK (ACS, Mountain View, CA) may be used to obtain tissue from the bile duct.

Metastatic Hepatic Neoplasms

Metastatic neoplasms of the liver are the most common hepatic malignancies and are rarely suitable for surgical resection. Hepatic metastases from renal cell carcinomas, islet cell carcinomas, carcinoid tumors, and medullary thyroid carcinomas are hypervascular, and other metastases are less vascular. CT frequently is used to detect hepatic metastases, but it is insensitive in detecting small lesions. Angiography is more sensitive in detecting hypervascular metastases than CT or radionuclide scanning. Angiography is performed to determine resectability of hepatic metastases and anomalies in the hepatic arterial system before the surgical placement of hepatic arterial catheters for infusion chemotherapy.

PANHEPATIC ANGIOGRAPHY

Increased resistance to the flow of portal vein blood is the principal cause of portal hypertension. The location of the blockage in portal blood flow may be intrahepatic or extrahepatic. Cirrhosis is the most common cause of the intrahepatic sinusoidal block. Hepatic vein (postsinusoidal) and portal vein (presinusoidal) occlusion produce the extrahepatic block to portal vein flow. An increase in portal vein blood flow secondary to splenomegaly and arterioportal fistula rarely causes portal hypertension (hyperkinetic).

The term *panhepatic angiography* is used for the angiographic study performed for the evaluation of portal hypertension. It includes celiac, superior mesenteric, hepatic, and splenic angiograms; wedged hepatic and left renal venograms; and manometry. Panhepatic angiography determines hepatic arterial variations, assesses portal hemodynamics, and excludes hepatoma. Visualization of aberrant hepatic arteries is important because accidental ligation of the hepatic artery in the presence of portal hypertension may result in hepatic necrosis. Furthermore, the presence of the replaced right hepatic artery from the superior mesenteric artery poses a technical difficulty for portacaval shunt surgery.

The hepatic angiogram is necessary to exclude hepatomas and helps determine the hemodynamics of the intrahepatic portal flow. In advanced cirrhosis with reversed portal flow, the portal veins may be visualized in the venous phase of hepatic arteriogram. High-dose superior mesenteric and splenic angiograms are necessary to see the superior mesenteric, splenic, and portal veins, and portosystemic collaterals. In alcoholic cirrhosis, pressure measurement from the catheter wedged in the hepatic vein reflects portal vein pressure and is useful in determining whether the location of obstruction is intrahepatic or extrahepatic. However, wedged hepatic vein pressure is not a useful determinant for the selection of the type of shunt surgery. It is also a poor predictor of prognosis and survival after a shunt surgery.[77] Wedged hepatic venography is the most accurate means of assessing morphologic features of the hepatic sinusoids and parenchyma. Manometry of the right atrium, inferior vena cava, and left renal vein is important because the presence of significant elevation of infrahepatic inferior vena caval pressure may result in incomplete decompression of portal hypertension after portacaval shunt surgery. Likewise, if the left renal vein pressure is elevated, the surgeon may decide to perform another type of shunt rather than a Warren's distal splenorenal shunt. In the presence of a hepatoma, portosystemic shunt surgery of any type is not warranted.

TRANSCATHETER THERAPY

The three commonly used vascular interventions for treatment of mesenteric arterial disease are percutaneous translumenal angioplasty, transcatheter embolotherapy, and thrombolytic therapy.

Surgical therapy (endarterectomy and bypass surgery) for superior mesenteric artery obstruction has significant mortality and recurrence rates.[18] Translumenal angioplasty is a safe and effective alternative to surgery in treating intestinal angina resulting from arteriosclerotic stenosis of the superior mesenteric artery.[19] Repeat angioplasty should be performed for recurrent stenoses. The authors have successfully dilated mesenteric artery stenoses in seven patients without complications. The total number of patients with the narrowing of the celiac and superior mesenteric arteries treated with percutaneous translumenal angioplasty is small, and no long-term follow-up study is available. The basic technique of mesenteric angioplasty is the same as for peripheral angioplasty. After catheterization of the superior mesenteric artery using a diagnostic catheter, a soft-tipped guidewire is used to cross the stenosis, and a stiffer wire (Rosen's wire) is advanced into the superior mesenteric artery. Over the guidewire, a high-pressure balloon catheter (usually 6-mm balloon) is advanced and inflated to 74 to 118 psi. The patient may feel slight abdominal discomfort during the inflation of the balloon. Heparin sodium, 3000 to 5000 U intraarterially, is given immediately after the stenosis is crossed and does not need to be converted. Calcium channel blockers and nitroglycerin are used to prevent arterial spasm. Celiac axis stenosis caused by median arcuate ligament compression is not amenable to angioplasty and thus requires surgery.

Percutaneous translumenal angioplasty is indicated in the Budd-Chiari syndrome caused by the membrane in the inferior vena cava and stenosis of the hepatic vein.[31] The method is not useful in patients with diffuse hepatic vein thrombosis and sclerosis. The potential complications of angioplasty are venous perforation and pulmonary embolism. Percutaneous transhepatic angioplasty and stent placement have been used to treat portal vein stenosis and postoperative stricture of the portal vein in patients with liver transplantation.[78,79]

Transcatheter embolization is an alternative to surgery in treating aneurisms of the hepatic and splenic arteries.[21] Occlusion of the hepatic artery by embolization is safe and well tolerated because the hepatic sinusoidal perfusion can be maintained by collateral circulation and the portal venous blood. The spleen receives adequate collateral blood flow through the pancreatic arteries after occlusion of the extrasplenic part of the splenic artery. Steel coil is the most frequently used occluding agent and produces arterial occlusion equivalent to surgical ligation. Injection of thrombin into an aneurysm promotes clot formation. A coaxial catheter system, such as Tracker-18 catheter, is extremely useful in embolization of the peripheral visceral arteries.

Intraarterial infusion of fibrinolytic agents is an effective means of recanalizing acute thrombotic occlusion of the coronary, peripheral, and pulmonary arteries. The method also has been used to lyse visceral artery thrombosis.[20] Urokinase is preferred to streptokinase. Thrombolytic therapy should not be used in acute mesenteric ischemia because delay of surgical treatment may result in bowel necrosis.

THERAPEUTIC ANGIOGRAPHY FOR HEPATIC LESIONS

Hepatic angiography is used for treatment of a variety of hepatic lesions including hepatic cancers, traumatic hemorrhage, hemobilia, arteriovenous fistula, aneurysms, and hepatic artery anastomotic stenosis of liver transplants.

Hepatic Arterial Infusion Chemotherapy

Hepatic malignancies account for 20% to 25% of cancer deaths in the United States, and metastases are the most common malignancy of the liver. Liver involvement by metastatic disease is a major cause of patient morbidity and mortality, and the prognosis of the untreated patients is dismal.[80] Surgical resection is the treatment of choice for localized cancer in the liver and can offer long-term survival. Unfortunately most patients with metastatic hepatic cancers are unsuitable for surgical resection. Only 5% to 20% of patients with primary hepatic cancers and 5% of patients with secondary hepatic cancers are candidates for surgery.[81] Therefore, other therapeutic methods have been introduced including systemic and intraarterial chemotherapy, irradiation, embolization, and chemoembolization.

Systemic chemotherapy in patients with metastatic colorectal carcinoma usually is ineffective, with a response rate of 24%.[82] Regional delivery of antineoplastic agents through the selectively placed arterial catheter produces higher tumor response than systemic infusion. Despite the controversy of its role in treating hepatic cancers, hepatic arterial chemotherapy is used with increasing frequency. The rationale for hepatic arterial infusion chemotherapy is based on the knowledge of cell kinetics, the pharmacokinetics of drugs, and the difference in the blood supply between the normal livers and tumors. Cancer cells proliferate through a series of phases, known as the cell cycle. Chemotherapeutic agents may be nonphase specific, phase specific, and cycle specific, and scheduling of drugs is important in hepatic arterial chemotherapy.[83] Floxuridine, a drug frequently used for colorectal cancer metastatic to the liver, is a phase-specific agent and, therefore, is administered using the infusion method. About 90% of floxuridine, when administered into the artery, is extracted from the blood by the liver. Intraarterial drug infusion results in a higher drug concentration in the tumor than the in surrounding normal liver.[84]

The important factors that should be considered in hepatic arterial chemotherapy are hepatic arterial anatomy, hepatic arterial hemodynamics, correct catheter placement, and a proper drug delivery system. To ensure total liver perfusion and drug delivery to the tumor site, the hepatic arterial anatomy and hemodynamic status are meticulously evaluated using intraarterial DSA and conventional angiography. Multiple hepatic arteries can be converted to a single hepatic artery using the transcatheter embolization technique to facilitate catheter placement. The gastroduodenal artery may be occluded by embolization to decrease extrahepatic perfusion of drugs.

Hepatic arterial catheters can be placed through a percutaneous approach from the femoral or brachial artery, or surgically. The introduction of the totally implantable pump has improved regional chemotherapy with surgical catheter placement.[85] Radionuclide flow study using ^{99m}Tc macroaggregated serum albumin is the most accurate means of assessing hepatic perfusion pattern after catheter placement.

The use of smaller catheters and the advances in catheterization technique have decreased the complication rates of hepatic arterial chemotherapy. The complications of percutaneous catheter placement are brachial artery thrombosis, hepatic artery thrombosis, catheter displacement, and puncture site bleeding. The complications of surgical catheter placement are hepatic artery thrombosis, incorrect catheter placement, catheter occlusion, and pump malfunction. Complications related to the toxicity of chemotherapeutic agents are chemical hepatitis, biliary sclerosis, chemical cholecystitis, and gastroduodenal inflammation and ulceration.

Embolotherapy of Hepatic Tumors

Hepatic artery embolization is used to palliate hepatic tumors when the tumors are unresponsive to hepatic arterial chemotherapy.[86] Hepatic arterial embolization results in selective destruction of the tumors exclusively dependent on arterial supply while maintaining the vitality of the normal liver with portal vein blood. Small particles such as polyvinyl alcohol (Ivalon, 150–250 μm) are used to occlude peripheral arteries to decrease the development of collateral blood flow. Hepatic artery embolization can effectively control symptoms related to abnormal hormone production in patients with carcinoid and islet cell tumors metastatic to the liver. This method also may be used to control variceal bleeding secondary to portal vein occlusion and arteriovenous shunting by hepatocellular carcinoma.

Hepatic artery embolization may be associated with the *postembolization syndrome:* abdominal pain, nausea, vomiting, and fever lasting for 2 to 7 days. Mild abnormal liver function values are common. Other complications include hepatic necrosis and gallbladder infarction.

Chemoembolization and Radiation Therapy

Chemoembolization is the combination of intraarterial infusion of chemotherapeutic agents and arterial embolization of tumor vascular bed. The rationale for this method is that concurrent embolization increases the effect of the drug by prolonging exposure of the tumor to the drug and tumor anoxia produced by occlusion while minimizing systemic drug effects. A variety of occluding materials have been used including ethylcellulose microcapsules, microspheres, gelatin

sponge, Ivalon, and iodized oil. Mitomycin C, doxorubicin (Adriamycin), cisplatin, and floxuridine are among drugs used for chemoembolization. Hepatic arterial chemoembolization, with Ivalon particles of 150 to 250 μm before and after selective injection of cisplatin, has been shown to be effective in treating hepatic metastases.[87]

Injection of iodized oil (Lipiodol) into the hepatic artery results in selective accumulation of the oil within most vascular hepatic tumors. This phenomenon has been exploited to selectively deliver antineoplastic agents and radioactive isotopes to hepatic cancers with intraarterial injection of a mixture of iodized oil and antineoplastic agents or radioactive iodized oil solution.[88,89] Chemoembolization is effective in patients with hepatic metastases of neuroendocrine tumors. Intraarterial injection of iodized oil and doxorubicin into tumor vessels is effective in palliating patients with hepatic islet cell or carcinoid tumor metastases. This method causes less morbidity than embolization of particulate material and permits repeat embolization because the supplying arteries remain patent after embolization.[90,91] A chemoembolic mixture is composed of 40 to 60 mg of doxorubicin dissolved in 10 mL of contrast medium and 20 mL of Ethiodol. The mixture is injected into the hepatic artery after an injection of the appropriate dosage of epinephrine. Epinephrine constricts normal hepatic arterioles and produces preferential shunting of the chemoembolic agent to the tumor bed.

Embolotherapy for Nonneoplastic Hepatic Lesions

Embolization is used to treat a variety of nonneoplastic hepatic lesions including traumatic bleeding, hemobilia, arterioportal fistulas, and hepatic artery aneurysms. The recent availability of coaxial catheter systems, such as Tracker's catheters, has made it possible to place the catheter in the peripheral hepatic artery and deliver occluding agents to the abnormal vessels. Various materials have been used including gelatin sponge (Gelfoam), Ivalon (size 250–590 μm), and steel coils. The important factors to be considered in selecting material for embolization are the desired level and duration of occlusion and potential complications. There are no absolute contraindications to hepatic transcatheter therapy. Portal hypertension, portal vein occlusion, and hepatic failure because of diffuse hepatic metastases are the relative contraindications to hepatic arterial occlusive therapy.

FORTHCOMING ADVANCES

With advances in noninvasive imaging techniques, particularly spiral CT, angiography will be used less in evaluating GI disease. Angiography will continue to be used in the preoperative evaluation of vascular disease, portal hypertension, neoplasms of the pancreas and liver, and GI hemorrhage. Therapeutic applications of angiography will expand in the treatment of GI bleeding, vascular abnormalities, hepatic neoplasms, and mesenteric vascular obstruction. The use of special coaxial catheter systems in subselective catheterization and vascular interventions will be further explored.

The reader is directed to Chapter 22, Gastrointestinal Blood
Flow; Chapter 30, Approach to the Patient With Gross Gas-
trointestinal Bleeding; Chapter 31, Approach to the Patient With
Occult Gastrointestinal Bleeding; Chapter 98, Tumors of the
Biliary Tree; and Chapter 128, Interventional Radiology.

REFERENCES

1. Wolf GL, Arenson RL, Cross AP. A prospective trial of ionic vs nonionic contrast agents in routine clincial practice: comparison of adverse effects. AJR Am J Roentgenol 1989;152:939.
2. Seldinger SI. Catheter replacement of the needle in percutaneous arteriography: a new technique. Acta Radiol 1953;39:368.
3. Lunderquist A, Vang J. Transhepatic catheterization and obliteration of the coronary vein in patients with portal hypertension and esophageal varices. N Engl J Med 1974;291:646.
4. Phillips DA, Adams DF, Beckmann CF, Abrams HL. Balloon occlusion superior mesenteric arteriography for improved venous opacification: a clinical trial. AJR Am J Roentgenol 1982;138:445.
5. Novak D, Bützow GH, Becker K. Hepatic occlusion venography with a balloon catheter in portal hypertension. Radiology 1977;122:623.
6. Hessel SJ, Adams DF, Abrams HL. Complications of angiography. Radiology 1981;138:273.
7. Witten DM, Hirsch FD, Hartman GW. Acute reactions to urographic contrast medium: incidence, clinical characteristics and relationship to history of hypersensitivity states. AJR Am J Roentgenol 1973;119:832.
8. Michels NA. Blood supply and anatomy of the upper abdominal organs. Philadelphia: JB Lippincott, 1955:139.
9. Kaufman SL, Harrington DP, Siegelman S. Superior mesenteric artery embolization: an angiographic emergency. Radiology 1977;124:625.
10. Tomchik FS, Wittenberg J, Ottinger LW. The roentgenographic spectrum of bowel infarction. Radiology 1970;96:249.
11. Odurny A, Sniderman KW, Colapinto RF. Intestinal angina: percutaneous transluminal angioplasty of the celiac and superior mesenteric arteries. Radiology 1988;167:59.
12. Flickinger EG, Johnsrude IS, Ogburn NL, et al. Local streptokinase infusion for superior mesenteric artery thromboembolism. AJR Am J Roentgenol 1983;140:771.
13. Ernst CB, Hagihara PF, Daugherty ME, et al. Ischemic colitis incidence following abdominal aortic reconstruction: a prospective study. Surgery 1976;80:417.
14. Hollier LH, Bernatz PE, Pairolero PC, et al. Surgical management of chronic intestinal ischemia: a reappraisal. Surgery 1981;90:940.
15. Flinn WR, Rizzo RJ, Park JS, Sandager GP. Duplex scanning for assessment of mesenteric ischemia. Surg Clin North Am 1990;70:99.
16. Bron KM, Redman HC. Splanchnic artery stenosis and occlusion. Radiology 1969;92:323.
17. Colapinto RF, McLoughlin MJ, Weisbrod GL. The routine lateral aortogram and the celiac axis compression syndrome. Radiology 1972;103:557.
18. Kirschbaum JD. Abdominal aortitis with stenosis (Takayasu's disease) and occlusive superior mesenteric arteritis associated with renal artery stenosis and hypertension: case report and review of the literature. Am Heart J 1970;80:811.
19. Baker KS, Tisnado J, Cho SR, et al. Splanchnic artery aneurysms and pseudoaneurysms: transcatheter embolization. Radiology 1987;163:135.
20. Stanley JC, Whitehouse WM Jr. Splanchnic artery aneurysms. In: Rutherford RB, ed. Vascular surgery. Philadelphia: WB Saunders, 1984:798.
21. Kadir S, Athanasoulis CA, Ring EJ, et al. Transcatheter embolization of intrahepatic arterial aneurysms. Radiology 1980;134:335.
22. Schwerk WB. Portal vein thrombosis: real-time sonographic demonstration and follow-up. Gastrointest Radiol 1986;11:312.
23. Belli L, Sansalone CV, Asemi P, et al. Portal thrombosis in cirrhotics: a retrospective analysis. Ann Surg 1986;203:286.
24. Cho KJ, Lunderquist A. The peribiliary vascular plexus: the microvascular architecture of the bile duct in the rabbit and in clinical cases. Radiology 1983;147:357.
25. Okuda K, Musha H, Yoshida T, et al. Demonstration of growing casts of hepatocellular carcinoma in the portal vein by celiac angiography: the thread and streaks sign. Radiology 1975;117:303.
26. Sutton JP, Yarborough DY, Richards JT. Isolated splenic vein occlusion. Arch Surg 1970;100:623.
27. Cho KJ, Martel W. Recognition of splenic vein occlusion. AJR Am J Roentgenol 1978;131:439.
28. Furui S, Yamauchi T, Ohtomo K, et al. Hepatic inferior vena cava obstructions: clinic results of treatment with percutaneous transluminal laser-assisted angioplasty. Radiology 1988;166:673.
29. Ralls PW, Johnson MB, Radin DR, et al. Budd-Chiari syndrome: detection with color doppler sonography. AJR Am J Roentgenol 1992;159:113.
30. Becker CD, Scheidegger J, Marincek B. Hepatic vein occlusion: morphologic features on computed tomography and ultrasonography. Gastrointest Radiol 1986;11:305.
31. Cho KJ, Geisinger KR, Shields JJ, et al. Collateral channels and histopathology in hepatic vein occlusion. AJR Am J Roentgenol 1982;139:703.
32. Walker HS, Rholl KS, Register TE, Arina van Breda. Percutaneous placement of a hepatic vein stent in the treatment of Budd-Chiari syndrome. J Virol 1990;1:23.
33. Sato M, Yamada R, Tsuji K, et al. Percutaneous transluminal angioplasty in segmental obstruction of the hepatic inferior vena cava: long-term results. Cardiovasc Intervent Radiol 1990;13:189.
34. Fujimoto M, Moriyasu F, Someda H, et al. Budd-Chiari syndrome: recanalization of an occluded hepatic vein with percutaneous transluminal angioplasty and a metallic stent. J Virol 1993;4:257.
35. Peltzer MY, Ring EJ, LaBerge JM, et al. Treatment of Budd-Chiari syndrome with a transjugular intrahepatic portosystemic shunt. J Virol 1993;4:263.
36. Glickerman DJ, Kowdley KV, Rosch J. Urokinase in gastrointestinal tract bleeding. Radiology 1988;168:375.
37. Reeves TQ, Osborne TM, List AR, Civil ID. Dieulafoy disease: localization with thrombolysis-assisted angiography. J Virol 1993;4:119.
38. Lang EV, Picus D, Marx MV, et al. Massive upper gastrointestinal hemorrhage with normal findings on arteriography: value of prophylactic embolization of the left gastric artery. AJR Am J Roentgenol 1992;158:547.
39. Zemel G, Katzen BT, Becker GJ, et al. Percutaneous transjugular portosystemic shunt. JAMA 1991;266:390.
40. LaBerge JM, Ring EJ, Gordon RL, et al. Creation of transjugular intrahepatic portosystemic shunts with the Wallstent endoprosthesis: results in 100 patients. Radiology 1993;187:413.
41. Baum S, Rösch J, Dotter CT, et al. Selective mesenteric arterial infusion in the management of massive diverticular hemorrhage. N Engl J Med 1973;288:1269.
42. Guy GE, Shetty PC, Sharma RP, et al. Acute lower gastrointestinal hemorrhage: treatment by superselective embolization with polyvinyl alcohol particles. AJR Am J Roentgenol 1992;159:521.
43. Moore JD, Thompson NW, Appelman HD, et al. Arteriovenous malformations of the gastrointestinal tract. Arch Surg 1976;111:381.
44. Baum S, Athanasoulis CA, Waltman AC, et al. Angiodysplasia of the right colon: a cause of gastrointestinal bleeding. Am J Roentgenol 1977;129:789.
45. Cho KJ, Reuter SR. Angiography of duodenal leiomyomas and leiomyosarcomas. AJR Am J Roentgenol 1980;135:31.
46. Gould M, Johnson RJ. Computed tomography of abdominal carcinoid tumor. Br J Radiol 1986;59:881.
47. Adolph JMK, Kimmig BN, Georgi P, et al. Carcinoid tumors:

CT and I-131 meta-iodo-benzylguanidine scintigraphy. Radiology 1987;164:199.

48. Kressel HY. Strategies for magnetic resonance imaging of focal liver disease. Radiol Clin North Am 1988;26:607.

49. Carrasco CH, Charnsangavej C, Ajani J, et al. The carcinoid syndrome: palliation by hepatic artery embolization. AJR Am J Roentgenol 1986;147:149.

50. Freeny PC, Ball TJ, Ryan J. Impact of new diagnostic imaging methods on pancreatic angiography. AJR Am J Roentgenol 1979;133:619.

51. Steiner E, Stark DD, Hahn PF, et al. Imaging of pancreatic neoplasms: comparison of MR and CT. AJR Am J Roentgenol 1989;152:487.

52. Freeny PC, Ball TJ. Rapid diagnosis of pancreatic carcinoma: an algorithmic approach. Radiology 1978;127:627.

53. Freeny PC, Marks WM, Ryan JA, Traverse LW. Pancreatic ductal adenocarcinoma: diagnosis and staging with dynamic CT. Radiology 1988;166:125.

54. Friedman AC, Lichtenstein JE, Dachman AH. Cystic neoplasms of the pancreas: radiological-pathological correlation. Radiology 1983;149:45.

55. Galiber AK, Reading CC, Charboneau JW, et al. Localization of pancreatic insulinoma: comparison of pre- and intraoperative US with CT and angiography. Radiology 1988;66:405.

56. Rossi P, Baert A, Passariello R, et al. CT of functioning tumors of the pancreas. AJR Am J Roentgenol 1985;144:57.

57. Wank SA, Doppman JL, Miller DL, et al. Prospective study of the ability of computed axial tomography to localize gastrinomas in patients with Zollinger-Ellison syndrome. Gastroenterology 1987;92:905.

58. Tscholakoff D, Hricak H, Thoeni R, et al. MR imaging in the diagnosis of pancreatic disease. AJR Am J Roentgenol 1987;148:703.

59. Maton PN, Miller DL, Doppman JL, et al. Role of selective angiography in the management of patients with Zollinger-Ellison syndrome. Gastroenterology 1987;92:913.

60. Ingemansson S, Lunderquist A, Lunderquist I, et al. Portal and pancreatic vein catheterization with radioimmunologic determination of insulin. Surg Gynecol Obstet 1975;141:705.

61. Cho KJ, Vinik AI, Thompson NW, et al. Localization of the source of hyperinsulinism: percutaneous transhepatic portal and pancreatic vein catheterization with hormone assay. AJR Am J Roentgenol 1982;139:237.

62. Growniak JV, Shapiro B, Vinik AI, et al. Percutaneous transhepatic venous sampling of gastrin: value in sporadic and familial islet-cell tumors and G-cell hyperfunction. N Engl J Med 1982;307:293.

63. Imamura M, Takahashi K, Adachi H, et al. Usefulness of selective arterial secretin injection test for localization of gastrinoma in the Zollinger-Ellison syndrome. Ann Surg 1987;205:230.

64. Thom AK, Norton JA, Doppman JL, et al. Prospective study of the use of intraarterial secretin injection and portal venous sampling to localize duodenal gastrinomas. Surgery 1992;112:1002.

65. Uflacker R. Arterial embolization as definitive treatment for benign insulinoma of the pancreas. J Virol 1992;3:639.

66. Walter J, Chuang VP, Bookstein JJ, et al. Angiography of massive hemorrhage secondary to pancreatic disease. Radiology 1977;124:337.

67. Boudghene F, L'Herminé, Bigot JM. Arterial complications of pancreatitis: diagnostic and therapeutic aspects in 104 cases. J Virol 1993;4:551.

68. Karl RC, Morse SS, Halpert RD, Clark RA. Preoperative evaluation of patients for liver resection: appropriate CT imaging. Ann Surg 1993;217:226.

69. Yumoto Y, Jinno K, Tokuyama K, et al. Hepatocellular carcinoma detected by iodized oil. Radiology 1985;154:19.

70. Reuter SR, Redman HC, Cho KJ. Gastrointestinal angiography. 2nd ed. Philadelphia: WB Saunders, 1986:385.

71. Freeny PC, Marks WM. Hepatic hemangioma: dynamic bolus CT. AJR Am J Roentgenol 1986;147:711.

72. Kudo M, Hirasa M, Takakuwa H, et al. Small hepatocellular carcinomas in chronic liver disease: detection with SPECT. Radiology 1986;159:697.

73. Baum JK, Holtz F, Bookstein JJ, et al. Possible association between benign hepatomas and oral contraceptives. Lancet 1973;2:926.

74. Casarella WJ, Knowles DM, Wolff M, et al. Focal nodular hyperplasia and liver cell adenoma: radiologic and pathologic differentiation. AJR Am J Roentgenol 1978;131:393.

75. Forrest ME, Cho KJ, Shields JJ, et al. Biliary cystadenomas: sonographic-angiographic-pathologic correlations. AJR Am J Roentgenol 1980;135:723.

76. Verbeek PCM, van Leeuwen DJ, de Wit LT, et al. Benign fibrosing disease at the hepatic confluence mimicking Klatskin tumors. Surgery 1992;112:866.

77. Reynolds TB. The role of hemodynamic measurements in portosystemic shunt surgery. Arch Surg 1974;108:276.

78. Mathias K, Bolder U, Löhlein D, Jäger H. Percutaneous transhepatic angioplasty and stent implantation for prehepatic portal vein obstruction. Cardiovasc Intervent Radiol 1993;16:313.

79. Olcott EW, Ring EJ, Roberts JP, et al. Percutaneous transhepatic portal vein angioplasty and stent placement after liver transplantation: early experience. J Virol 1990;1:17.

80. Bengmark S, Hafstrom L. The natural history of primary and secondary malignant tumors of the liver: prognosis for patients with hepatic metastases from colonic and rectal carcinoma by laparotomy. Part I. Cancer 1969;23:198.

81. Niederhuber JE, Ensminger WD. Surgical considerations in the management of hepatic neoplasia. Semin Oncol 1983;10:135.

82. Kemeny N. The systemic chemotherapy of hepatic metastases. Semin Oncol 1983;10:148.

83. Stagg RJ, Lewis BJ, Friedman MA, et al. Hepatic arterial chemotherapy for colorectal cancer metastatic to the liver. Ann Intern Med 1984;100:736.

84. Ramming KP. The effectiveness of hepatic artery infusion in treatment of primary hepatobiliary tumors. Semin Oncol 1983;10:199.

85. Balch CM, Urist MM, McGregor ML. Continuous regional chemotherapy for metastatic colorectal cancer using a totally implantable infusion pump: a feasibility study in 50 patients. Am J Surg 1983;145:285.

86. Chuang VP, Wallace S. Hepatic artery embolization in the treatment of hepatic neoplasms. Radiology 1981;140:51.

87. Wallace S, Carrasco CH, Charnsangavej C, et al. Hepatic artery infusion and chemoembolization in the management of liver metastases. Cardiovasc Intervent Radiol 1990;13:153.

88. Kobayashi H, Hidaka H, Kajiya P, et al. Treatment of hepatocellular carcinoma by transarterial injection of anticancer agents in iodized oil suspension or of radioactive iodized oil solution. Acta Radiol Diagnosis 1986;27:139.

89. Matsuo N, Uchida H, Nishimine K, et al. Segmental transcatheter hepatic artery chemoembolization with iodized oil for hepatocellular carcinoma: antitumor effect and influence on normal tissue. J Virol 1993;4:543.

90. Ruszniewski P, Rougier P, Roche A, et al. Hepatic arterial chemoembolization in patients with liver metastases of endocrine tumors: a prospective phase II study in 24 patients. Cancer 1993;71:2624.

91. Stokes KR, Stuart K, Clouse ME. Hepatic arterial chemoembolization for metastatic endocrine tumors. J Virol 1993;4:341.

Textbook of Gastroenterology, second edition, edited by Tadataka Yamada. JB Lippincott Company, Philadelphia © 1995.

CHAPTER 128

Interventional Radiology

David J. Glickerman

Biliary Intervention
   Percutaneous Transhepatic Cholangiography
   Percutaneous Transhepatic Biliary Drainage
   Dilatation of Benign Biliary Strictures
   Metallic Biliary Stents
   Percutaneous Cholecystostomy
Percutaneous Biopsy
   Technique
   Indications
   Contraindications and Risks
   Results
   Alternative Techniques to Biopsy
Percutaneous Abscess and Fluid Collection Drainage
   Technique

Hepatic Abscess
Pancreatic Abscess and Fluid Collections
Diverticular Abscess
Abscesses With Fistulas
Abscesses and Crohn's Disease
Transjugular Intrahepatic Portosystemic Shunt
   Patient Preparation and Technique
   Indications
   Contraindications and Risks
   Clinical Implications
Percutaneous Enterostomy
   Percutaneous Radiologic Gastrostomy
      and Gastrojejunostomy
   Percutaneous Cecostomy

The field of interventional radiology has flourished over the last 30 years, and a number of procedures have evolved that are complementary to those performed by gastroenterologists and general surgeons. In caring for patients with complex problems, close consultation between the gastroenterologist, surgeon, and the interventional radiologist will frequently result in the fashioning of a better treatment plan than could be devised by any one specialist working in isolation. This chapter discusses the application of percutaneous biliary interventions, needle biopsy, percutaneous drainage of abscesses and other fluid collections, percutaneous enterostomy, and one of the newer procedures in interventional radiology, the transjugular intrahepatic portosystemic shunt.

BILIARY INTERVENTION

Percutaneous Transhepatic Cholangiography

The role of diagnostic percutaneous transhepatic cholangiography (PTC) has diminished over the last two decades because of advances in computed tomography (CT), ultrasound (US), magnetic resonance imaging (MR), and endoscopic retrograde cholangiopancreatography (ERCP).

The cross-sectional imaging modalities noninvasively evaluate the biliary tree and discern the presence or absence of biliary ductal dilatation, and frequently pinpoint a site of obstruction. CT, US, and MR also produce information about the extraductal soft tissues that is not provided by a contrast cholangiogram. This information about the patency of visceral arteries and veins, and the presence or absence of a periductal mass and hepatic or nodal metastases usually is essential in planning percutaneous, endoscopic, or operative therapies. When the noninvasive modalities do not provide sufficient detail about ductal pathologic conditions, introduction of contrast into the biliary tree is indicated.

The morbidity and mortality of fine-needle PTC are similar to those of ERCP,[1-3] and the cost of PTC at most institutions is significantly lower. Therefore, PTC is the procedure of choice in the setting of biliary obstruction when surgical decompression is planned. When percutaneous or endoscopic decompression is being considered using information gleaned from noninvasive modalities (CT, US, MR), the choice of diagnostic procedure should be based on which is most likely to be safe and successful. If the appropriate diagnostic technique is chosen, the therapeutic procedure can be performed at the same sitting. When the intrahepatic ducts are not dilated the success rate of PTC is lower[1] and ERCP is the procedure of choice, unless postsurgical anatomy (e.g., Billroth II gastrojejunostomy or choledochojejunostomy) is present, which reduces the success rate of ERCP.

Indications

The following are indications for PTC:

- distinction of obstructive from nonobstructive jaundice when noninvasive modalities are inconclusive
- identification of the cause of ductal obstruction when non-invasive modalities are inconclusive
- delineation of congenital anomalies
- pressure flow studies[4]
- documentation of communication of hepatic abscess with the biliary tree[5]
- visualization of ductal anatomy before percutaneous transhepatic biliary drainage (PTBD).

Contraindications and Risks

Uncorrectable coagulopathy, history of severe reaction to iodinated contrast medium, and the presence of a vascular tumor or arteriovenous malformation are relative contraindications. Risks include bleeding, sepsis, bile leakage, and death with a 3% morbidity rate and a 0.1% mortality rate.[1]

Technique

Coagulation studies are obtained on all patients and significant abnormalities are corrected by the administration of fresh frozen plasma, platelets, or both. Because of the high incidence of bacterial colonization of the biliary tree in patients with biliary obstruction,[6] broad-spectrum intravenous antibiotics are administered before the procedure and for 48 hours afterward.[7-9] Possible regimens include cefazolin for afebrile patients and an antipseudomonal penicillin[10] (e.g., mezlocillin) or imipenem cilastatin for febrile patients.

For visualization of the right hepatic ducts and the extrahepatic ducts, a puncture site is chosen in the right midaxillary line. The patient is placed in the supine position, and the location of the lateral costophrenic angle is observed with the patient holding a maximal inspiration. If only a diagnostic PTC is to be performed, a puncture site is chosen one intercostal space below the costophrenic angle. If placement of a drainage catheter is anticipated, a puncture site caudal to the tenth rib is chosen, if possible, to avoid the pleural reflection and obviate the possible development of a biliary-pleural fistula.[11] The puncture site is also placed in the middle or caudal portion of an intercostal space to avoid the intercostal vessels.

A 21- or 22-gauge needle is directed, in a plane parallel to the table top, to a position 3 cm cephalad to the hilum of the liver. The position of the hilum is estimated fluoroscopically by observing the position of the dome of the liver and the air in the first and second portions of the duodenum. The stylet is removed and the needle is connected through a connecting tube to a contrast-filled syringe. The needle is slowly withdrawn while small 0.5-mL boluses of contrast medium are injected.

When the needle tip is in the hepatic parenchyma, the contrast agent remains adjacent to the needle tip. When the tip is in a hepatic artery or portal vein, the contrast agent washes out promptly to the liver periphery. When the tip is in a hepatic vein, the contrast agent washes out promptly toward the vena cava. When the tip is in a biliary duct, contrast material flows away slowly to reveal branching ducts.

If no bile ducts have been encountered by the time the needle has been withdrawn to within 2 to 3 cm of the liver edge, the stylet is reinserted and the needle readvanced to a slightly different position. With dilated ducts, the biliary tree can be accessed almost always within several needle passes.[12] When the intrahepatic ducts are not dilated, additional needle passes frequently are required.

For optimal visualization of the left hepatic ducts, or if a left-sided drainage is anticipated, a skin puncture site is chosen below the xyphoid process with the help of real time US. A peripheral location in a duct of the lateral segment of the left lobe is chosen to be the puncture site so that if drainage is desired, the catheter will have a long segment with multiple side holes within the hepatic duct above the obstruction. The needle is angled parallel to the duct in the axial plane toward the hilum of the liver and at a 30- to 50-degree angle to the table top. The needle is advanced under real time US guidance and its position is confirmed with injection of contrast medium.

If the site of obstruction has previously been determined by cross-sectional imaging and PTBD is to be performed, only a small amount of contrast agent is injected to assist guidewire placement. If a diagnostic study is to be performed, first an attempt is made to aspirate as much bile as possible, although typically little or no bile can be aspirated through the fine needle because of the viscosity of bile. Any bile obtained is sent for a Gram's stain and culture and sensitivity tests. Iodinated contrast medium such as Conray 60 (Mallinkrodt, St. Louis, MO) is slowly injected and the contrast medium can be seen to flow into the most dependent ducts. Distention of the biliary tree is minimized to avoid causing bacteremia. By tilting the table, the radiologist takes advantage of the higher specific gravity of the contrast medium, allowing it to flow to opacify ducts not seen with the patient in the supine position. Radiographs are obtained in multiple obliquities and the needle is removed. The patient is placed on bed rest for 6 hours and vital signs are monitored.

Results

Fine-needle PTC is successful in 98% of patients with dilated ducts and 70% of patients with nondilated ducts.[1]

Percutaneous Transhepatic Biliary Drainage

Leger and associates[13] first described the concept of percutaneous biliary drainage in 1952; numerous techniques have since been developed to deal with benign and malignant stenoses. Percutaneous therapy must be compared with the surgical and endoscopic alternatives, taking into account effectiveness, morbidity, mortality, and cost. In choosing the appropriate treatment, factors to consider include life expectancy, medical conditions that may limit the ability to tolerate a surgical procedure, and the patient's willingness to have an external catheter or to undergo regular catheter or stent changes.

Theoretical Considerations

The primary indication for PTBD is palliation of obstruction of the biliary tree by tumor, most commonly pancreatic adenocarcinoma, causing sepsis, worsening hepatic dysfunction, or intolerable pruritus. Resection for cure is not possible for most of these patients. If resection is not possible because of the extent of the tumor demonstrated by imaging studies or because of concomitant medical conditions precluding an extensive operation, a method of palliation must be chosen.

Patients with pancreatic cancer obstructing the common bile duct who undergo surgical biliary bypass, such as choledochojejunostomy or cholecystojejunostomy, have a 20% to 33% perioperative mortality rate[14–16] and a mean survival of 6 months. Given the limited life expectancy of most of these patients, nonoperative palliation should be considered. Although several retrospective studies have suggested that operative palliation of malignant biliary obstruction is more effective than endoscopic or radiologic palliation, these retrospective studies had selection bias with healthier patients undergoing operation. Several randomized controlled trials have shown that endoscopically and radiologically placed biliary endoprostheses are as efficacious as operative bypass for the treatment of malignant biliary obstruction.[14,17,18] Patients undergoing nonoperative palliation trade off readmission for endoprosthesis exchange (and cholangitis) with a shorter initial hospitalization compared with patients undergoing operative decompression.

Once nonoperative palliation is selected as the appropriate treatment for a given patient, the choice between a percutaneous internal-external drainage catheter and an endoscopically or percutaneously placed plastic or metal endoprosthesis must be made. In many cases an internal-external drainage catheter is preferable because once the tube is capped, most patients find it to be a minimal hindrance, and the presence of the tube allows simple, outpatient catheter replacement at regular intervals (4–6 months).

The internal-external catheter also is preferred in the situation of hilar lesions because injection of contrast agent or catheter exchange and manipulation can be useful for diagnosis and treatment of obstruction of the contralateral lobe. Endoprostheses can be placed after internal-external drainage in patients unhappy with a protruding catheter or who are uncooperative and likely to dislodge their catheter. In patients who have a percutaneously placed catheter, a plastic endoprosthesis can be placed percutaneously or perorally by means of a combined radiologic-endoscopic approach.

If a decision is made to initially place an endoprosthesis, percutaneous and endoscopic placement must be weighed. In patients with a Billroth II gastrojejunostomy or a choledochojejunostomy, percutaneous placement should be undertaken because of the difficulty of endoscopic manipulation. Percutaneous placement is more likely to be successful in patients with hilar lesions as well. The only randomized trial comparing endoscopic and percutaneous plastic endoprostheses[19] concluded that endoscopic stent placement was safer and more likely to succeed. This study has been criticized, however, because the 61% rate of early complications for percutaneous placement was considerably higher than the rate for other published studies reviewed in the same report (6%–58%), and the 76% rate of successful percutaneous stent insertion was lower than that reported for the other reviewed studies (82%–100%). Further randomized, controlled trials would be useful to further clarify the best approach to placing biliary endoprostheses.

Technique

The patient is prepared and the needle puncture is performed as for PTC. After a small injection of contrast agent confirms the placement of the 21- or 22-gauge needle tip into a suitable intrahepatic duct, a platinum-tip 0.046-cm mandril wire is advanced into the biliary tree. Over this wire, a three-part coaxial introducer set with a 1.98-mm (6-Fr) outer diameter (Meditech, Boston, MA) is advanced into the biliary tree. The stiffener and inner dilator are removed and while the 0.046-cm wire remains in place, bile is allowed to drain or is aspirated through the large-end hole of the introducer.

Bile aspiration may be performed with the guidewire in place by attaching a flexible 41.02-cm connecting tube to a 20-mL syringe, placing the end of the guidewire into the connecting tube and attaching the tube to the introducer. This method also may be used to inject contrast medium while maintaining guidewire position. Care is taken not to distend the biliary tree to reduce the risk of sepsis. A 0.097-cm guidewire then is placed alongside the 0.046-cm wire and the introducer is removed, keeping both wires in position. The 0.046-cm wire is secured out of the way as a safety wire, in case access with the larger wire is lost.

A 1.82-mm (5.5-Fr) torque control catheter with an angle at its tip is introduced over the 0.097-cm wire. This catheter then is manipulated to within 2 or 3 cm of the point of obstruction. An angled hydrophilic 0.097-cm guidewire is inserted through the 1.82-mm catheter, and by taking advantage of the steering ability of the catheter and wire, the point of obstruction is gently probed.

In most cases, the guidewire and catheter can be advanced into the duodenum, and after exchange for an extra stiff guidewire, a dilator is passed through the obstruction. The dilator is removed, and an 2.64- to 3.96-mm (8–12 Fr) internal-external drainage catheter is advanced so that its pigtail coils in the duodenum. The internal-external drainage catheter is chosen or modified so that numerous side holes are present within the biliary tree, above the point of obstruction, but none are in the extraductal hepatic parenchyma. To reduce risk of hemobilia, no side holes should be present in the hepatic parenchyma.

Most biliary drainage catheters have a suture within them that prevents the pigtail tip of the catheter from uncoiling when the suture is tied or locked at the catheter hub. This Cope loop[20] functions as a retaining device to prevent catheter displacement. The catheter is secured to the skin and irrigated with normal saline every 6 hours for the first day, and once daily thereafter. For the first day the catheter is connected to a drainage bag to allow maximal drainage, which reduces the risk of sepsis. On the second day the catheter is capped to allow internal drainage only. Once internal drainage has been established, placement of a biliary endoprosthesis, if desired, is straightforward.

If the 1.82-mm catheter and guidewire do not easily traverse the occlusion, an external drainage catheter is placed above the obstruction and the catheter is allowed to drain externally for 2 to 3 days. After a period of decompression, the obstruction can almost always be crossed and an internal-external drain can be placed.

If the drainage is being performed for the treatment of biliary sepsis, no attempt is made to traverse the obstruction. Rather, an external drainage catheter is placed above the obstruction for drainage, and a more definitive procedure will be performed in several days. Catheter and guidewire manipulation in purulent bile should be minimized because of the profound bacteremia that can ensue.

Indications

Indications for PTBD are as follow:

- palliation of neoplasms causing biliary obstruction
- treatment of cholangitis
- nonoperative removal of common bile duct or intrahepatic stones when ERCP is unsuccessful
- access for dilatation of benign strictures.

Contraindications

An uncorrectable coagulopathy is a contraindication to PTBD. Prominent ascites is a relative contraindication because the liver is displaced from the abdominal wall. This displacement can cause buckling of guidewires and catheters between the abdominal wall and liver, making the procedure difficult. Also, in patients with ascites, a risk exists of creating a peritoneal-cutaneous fistula with chronic leakage of ascitic fluid. Paracentesis can be performed before PTBD to minimize these problems.

Other serious complications of PTBD include sepsis, cholangitis, bile leakage, hemorrhage, pancreatitis, peritonitis, and death. Immediate significant complications are seen in 5% to 10% of patients.[21]

Results

With modern guidewire and catheter technology, nearly all malignant biliary obstructions can be traversed, although some may require an initial period of external drainage before the obstructions can be crossed. In patients with malignant biliary obstruction, bilirubin levels fall quickly (2–3 mg/day) after decompression and patients drained for sepsis defervesce within 24 hours.[12]

Dilatation of Benign Biliary Strictures

The group of patients with benign biliary strictures is heterogeneous. The more common benign strictures include the following:

- iatrogenic bile duct injuries, most frequently after cholecystectomy or cholecystectomy and common bile duct exploration
- anastomotic stenoses
- stenoses from primary sclerosing cholangitis
- stenoses from other inflammatory processes, including

chronic pancreatitis, cholelithiasis, and oriental cholangiohepatitis.

Percutaneous balloon dilatation of benign strictures can be performed from a percutaneous transhepatic route, through a mature T-tube tract, or by means of a percutaneous transjejunal route if a Roux-en-Y choledochojejunostomy has been created with a subcutaneously placed limb.[22] Dilatation through an existing T-tube tract or by means of a transjejunal approach avoids the potential complications of transhepatic puncture. The usefulness of temporary stent placement after percutaneous cholangioplasty is debated, and even among those who favor using stents, the stent size and appropriate duration of having the stents in place is controversial.

Long-term patency rates of percutaneous cholangioplasty are 67% to 93% for anastomotic strictures,[23–25] 76% to 88% for iatrogenic strictures,[23,24] and 42% to 54% for strictures of primary sclerosing cholangitis.[23,26]

Metallic Biliary Stents

Expandable metallic biliary stents (EMBS) offer promise for treatment of selected patients with obstruction of the intrahepatic and extrahepatic biliary ducts. Their small constrained diameter and their large expanded diameter allows placement through a small transhepatic tract of a stent of much larger caliber than any polyethylene stent. EMBS have less surface area than plastic stents and become incorporated into the duct wall in most patients after 2 months[27]; these two properties should result in less stent occlusion from bile encrustation. A major disincentive to the use of EMBS has been their purchase price: approximately $900 for a 6.8-cm Wallstent (Schneider, Inc., Plymouth, MN), $665 for a 3-cm Palmaz stent (Johnson and Johnson, Warren, NJ), and $450 for a 6-cm Gianturco-Rösch stent (Cook, Inc., Bloomington, IN). For long stenoses and for hilar lesions, multiple stents frequently are required.

Three types of metallic stents are commercially available in the United States for transhepatic use in the biliary tree. The Gianturco-Rösch Z stent is made of 0.026-cm stainless steel wire bent in a zigzag configuration and soldered end to end. Each stent body has its maximal expansion diameter limited by a monofilament nylon suture, which passes through the bends in the wire. The suture also serves to connect one stent body to the next to create multiple-bodied stents of greater length (Fig. 128-1).

These stents are available in diameters from 6 to 12 mm and in total lengths from 1.5 to 9 cm. These stents are self-expandable and provide continuous expansile force until they reach their maximal diameter. They are introduced through sheaths with diameters of 2.80 to 3.3 mm (8.5–10 Fr).

The Wallstent is a self-expandable stent made of woven stainless steel mesh that forms a cylinder (Fig. 128-2). This stent is available in lengths of 4.2, 6.8, and 9.6 cm in diameters of 8 and 10 mm. The Wallstent is delivered through a 2.31-mm (7-Fr) catheter inside a 2.31-mm sheath.

Although the Wallstent is self-expandable, its expansile force is relatively weak and frequently requires expansion with a balloon catheter to achieve its full diameter. Once it is fully expanded, the wire ends of the stent tend to catch in the wall of the duct and prevent further collapse of the stent.

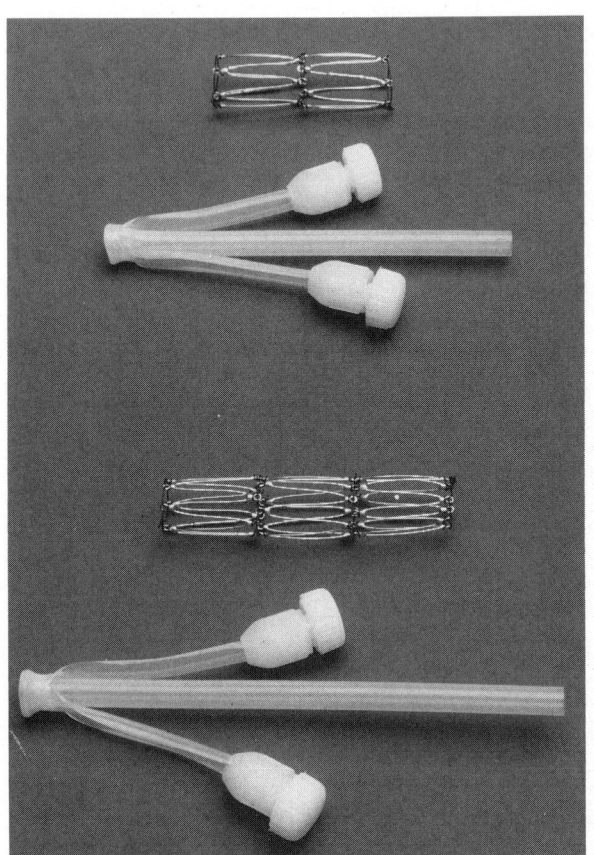

FIGURE 128-1. Two and three-body Gianturco-Rösch stents and their loading devices.

The Palmaz stent is a balloon expandable stent made of a stainless steel tube with etched slits in it (Fig. 128-3). The Palmaz stent is available in a variety of lengths and two diameter ranges with expanded diameters from 4 to 12 mm. The stent is mounted on a deflated balloon catheter that is advanced into the obstruction through a sheath. The sheath is withdrawn and the balloon is inflated, dilating the stent to the diameter of the balloon. Balloon stent systems require a 2.31- to 3.3-mm (7–10 Fr) sheath for insertion.

The standard nonoperative treatment for palliation of malignant biliary obstruction has been placement of a transhepatic internal-external drainage catheter or an endoscopically or radiologically placed plastic stent. The problems associated with a drainage catheter and the main problems of plastic stents—migration and occlusion with sludge—have prompted the investigation of EMBS. Several authors have reported favorable results using EMBS in terms of low complication rates and ease of placement.[28–30] In these studies, however, patient survival was not long enough to document an advantage in the patency rate of EMBS compared with historic controls of plastic stents.

One randomized trial of 4.62-mm (14-Fr) plastic stents versus radiologically placed Wallstents for malignant hilar obstructions demonstrated significantly fewer reinterventions in patients treated with EMBS.[31] As an additional advantage, in hilar lesions, EMBS allow placing stents in both lobes from a single transhepatic puncture. No other randomized trial of plastic stents versus radiologically placed EMBS has yet been reported. Two studies comparing endoscopically placed EMBS and plastic stents for malignant obstruction of the distal common bile duct concluded that EMBS have a significantly greater patency rate and are cost effective because of the decreased need for reintervention.[32,33]

Evaluation of EMBS for benign biliary strictures has been undertaken more conservatively than for malignant disease. This is appropriate because most EMBS cannot be removed after several weeks, even with operation, unless the entire stent segment of duct is completely resected. EMBS do not allow surgical anastomosis to the stented portion of duct. The two authors with the largest published series of benign biliary strictures treated with EMBS suggest their use with benign disease only after balloon dilatation has failed and after operation has failed or is not feasible.[34,35]

Balloon dilatation works well, is less expensive than placing stents, and will not interfere with a future operation, as might a metallic stent. Maccioni and associates[35] report a 69% 3-year patency rate in a series of patients composed of anastomotic stenoses and iatrogenic bile duct injuries. No data are available on the long-term patency rate of EMBS.

Percutaneous Cholecystostomy

Percutaneous cholecystostomy (PC) is a procedure whose niche in treating patients with gallbladder disease seems well established. Over the last decade, the high prevalence of cholelithiasis and cholecystitis drove the search for minimally invasive procedures that might be safer, less costly, and would have a shorter recuperative period than cholecystectomy. Nonsurgical procedures including extracorporeal shock wave lithotripsy, ingestion of bile acids, and percutaneous cholecystolithotomy have been investigated.

Gallstones often are larger than safely created percutaneous tracts, so methods have evolved to shrink or fragment the stones so that they can be extracted percutaneously. These methods include contact dissolution using methyl-tert-butyl ether or mono-octanoin, mechanical lithotripsy, electrohydraulic lithotripsy, and laser lithotripsy. Aside from the cost and multiple sittings required for many of these procedures, their main failing was that the gallbladder remained in situ to reform stones in 20% to 50% of patients,[36] and with an increased risk of gallbladder carcinoma.[37] The rapid evolution of laparoscopic cholecystectomy has supplanted these percutaneous techniques in most circumstances, because laparoscopic cholecystectomy does not leave the gallbladder in place. PC has been most useful in severely ill patients who may not tolerate open or laparoscopic cholecystectomy.

Technique

Intravenous antibiotics are given and coagulopathies are corrected before the procedure. Ideally the procedure is performed in the angiography suite with a combination of ultrasonic guidance for gallbladder puncture and fluoroscopy for guidewire and catheter placement. Alternatively the procedure can be performed with CT guidance, but this is slower and more awkward than US guidance because the patient must be moved repetitively in and out of the CT gantry. CT

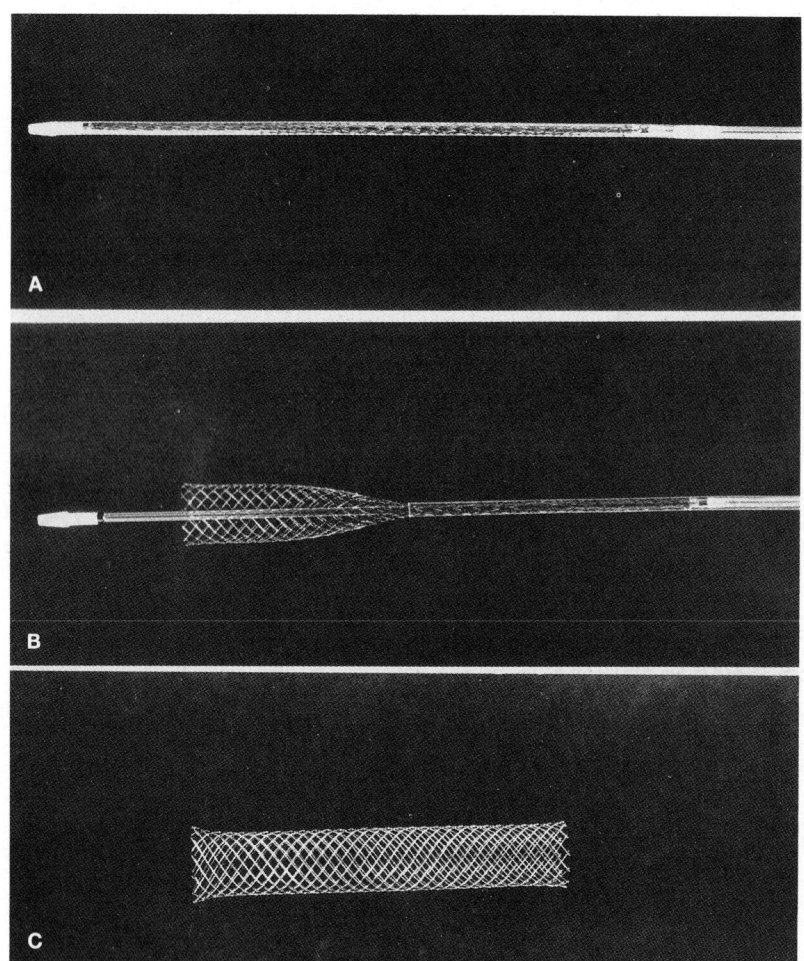

FIGURE 128-2. The Wallstent (**A**) in its constrained, elongated form, between two coaxial catheters and (**B**) partially deployed with the outer catheter partially pulled back over the inner catheter. (**C**) The fully deployed stent.

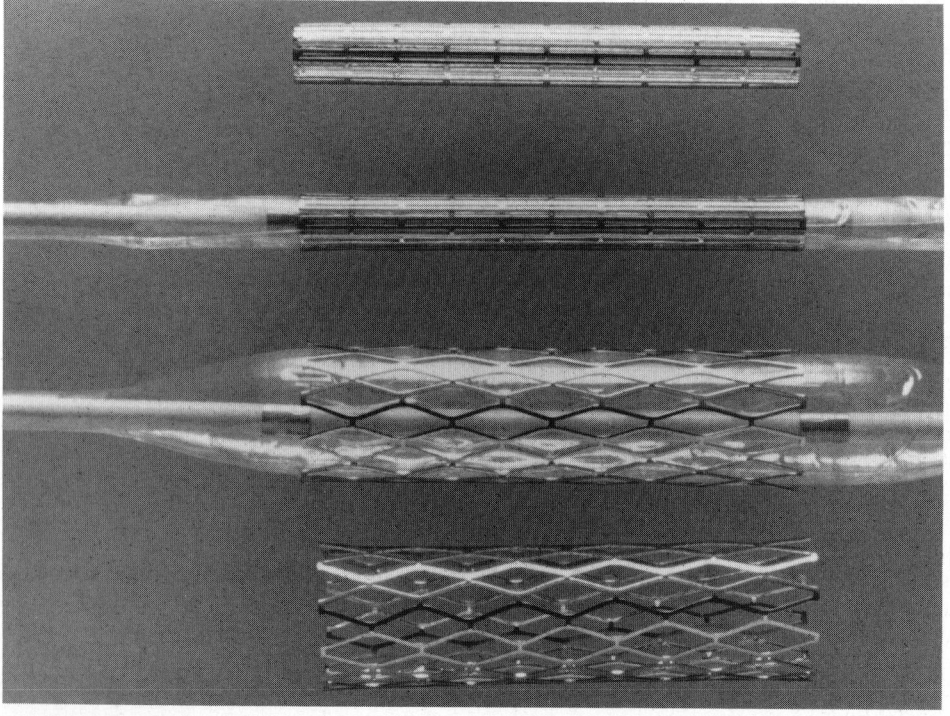

FIGURE 128-3. The Palmaz stent. From *top* to *bottom:* the stent, the stent mounted on an angioplasty balloon, the stent expanded to the size of the balloon on balloon inflation, the stent after removal of the balloon.

is useful for puncture of a contracted, stone-filled gallbladder. Extremely ill patients may be treated at their bedside with the entire procedure guided by US. The procedure is performed under local anesthesia through a 5-mm skin incision.

Percutaneous cholecystostomy initially was performed by means of a transhepatic approach in an attempt to puncture the gallbladder through the bare area of the liver and avoid the possible complication of bile peritonitis.[38] Transhepatic puncture does not, however, assure puncture through the bare area, and transhepatic transperitoneal punctures are common.[39] Subhepatic puncture has been shown to be safe[40,41] and avoids the risk of bleeding from hepatic injury.

A variety of techniques are used for PC including the standard Seldinger technique with needle puncture, guidewire placement, removal of the needle, tract dilatation, and advancement of a drainage catheter over the guidewire into the gallbladder. Another technique more suitable for use at the bedside involves the use of a trocar. A tapered catheter with an inner stiffener and a central mandril with a sharp point is advanced in one step into the gallbladder under US guidance.

Another technique appropriate for bedside use involves a long, 22-gauge needle with a Teflon 1.98-mm (6-Fr) catheter loaded on the back of the needle[42] (Hawkins Accordion catheter, Cook, Inc.; Fig. 128-4). The needle is placed into the gallbladder under US guidance and its mandril is removed. Injection of a small volume of saline and observation with US can be used to confirm the intralumenal position of the needle tip if the bile is too viscous to be aspirated through the long 22-gauge needle. A 0.046-cm guidewire is advanced through the needle and the needle tip is positioned in the center of the gallbladder. The catheter is advanced over the needle-wire unit into the gallbladder. The needle and guidewire are removed and the monofilament suture present within the catheter is tightened to accordion the catheter into a Z-shaped self-retaining configuration. In most patients, the time from application of local anesthetic to completion of the procedure is less than 10 minutes.

Bile is obtained for aerobic and anaerobic bacterial cultures and the catheter is secured to the skin. The cultures are not taken to confirm or exclude cholecystitis, but to determine antibiotic therapy if the cultures are positive. Although a small amount of contrast medium may be injected to confirm catheter position, if the PC is being performed for cholecystitis, a cholecystogram should not be performed at this time to reduce the risk of gallbladder distention and bacteremia. The catheter then is connected to gravity drainage. The use of a self-retaining catheter (Cope loop or accordion type) is essential to reduce the risk of catheter dislodgement and bile leakage.

A diagnostic cholecystocholangiogram can be performed to evaluate cystic duct patency and cholelithiasis after 48 hours and after the patient's condition stabilizes. Options for defin-

itive therapy include cholecystectomy, percutaneous stone removal or, if the patient had acalculous cholecystitis and cystic duct patency is confirmed, eventual removal of the catheter with no further treatment. The catheter cannot be removed until its tract is mature or bile leakage can occur. Patients with transhepatic PC catheters have mature tracts at 20 days.[43] If a question exists about the maturity of the tract, it can be evaluated under fluoroscopy with injection of contrast medium. For patients with severe nonbiliary problems the catheter frequently is left in place until other medical problems resolve.

Indications

The following are indications for PC:

- suspected cholecystitis in severely ill patients unlikely to tolerate cholecystectomy
- sepsis of unknown cause and a distended gallbladder in critically ill patients[44]
- acalculous cholecystitis[45]
- obstructive jaundice because of distal common bile duct obstruction when PTBD and endoscopic drainage are unsuccessful[46]
- diagnostic cholecystocholangiography in patients without dilated intrahepatic ducts or in whom PTC and ERCP are not successful
- gallstones requiring percutaneous removal or dissolution, in selected patients.

Contraindications and Risks

Relative contraindications include the visualization of a necrotic or perforated gallbladder wall on US examination, and depending on the severity, an uncorrectable bleeding diathesis.

Percutaneous cholecystostomy is a safe procedure despite its frequent application in extremely ill patients. An 8% complication rate includes bile leakage, vasovagal reaction, catheter dislodgement, hemorrhage, and a 0.5% procedure-related mortality rate.[47] In comparison, emergency surgical cholecystostomy has a mortality rate of 8%.[48]

Results

Percutaneous cholecystostomy for presumed cholecystitis in critically ill patients is useful for diagnosis and treatment. Although initially it was thought that Gram's stain and culture of aspirated gallbladder contents would be useful to diagnose cholecystitis, many of these patients are already on broad-spectrum antibiotics. The 48% sensitivity rate of Gram's stain and 38% sensitivity rate of bile culture are sufficiently low to

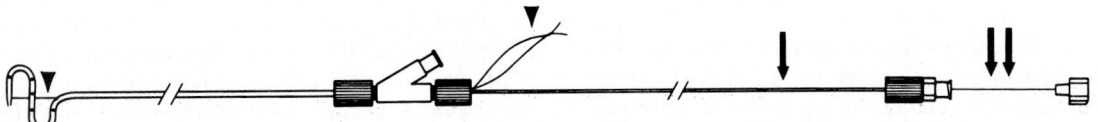

FIGURE 128-4. The Hawkins Accordion catheter. Retention suture (*arrowheads*), cannula of the 22-gauge needle (*single arrow*), and the needle stylet (*double arrows*).

make gallbladder aspiration a procedure of limited value.[49] However, PC is useful as a clinical diagnostic test. Essentially all patients who have cholecystitis without a necrotic gallbladder wall will defervesce and normalize their leukocyte count after drainage.[45,50]

Severely ill patients who have ultrasonographic evidence of a necrotic gallbladder wall (intralumenal membranes, Type II or III pericholecystic fluid)[51] are less likely to respond to PC and should undergo immediate operation or a trial of PC with operation to follow if no clinical improvement is seen in 24 hours, depending on the patient's risk of surgery. In patients without a necrotic gallbladder wall and no response to PC, cholecystitis is excluded and the search for a nongallbladder source of sepsis should continue.

Clinical Implications

The diagnosis of cholecystitis in severely ill patients continues to be a challenge. Physical examination and assessment of tenderness is unreliable in patients unresponsive to pain because of neurologic conditions and in patients who are intubated and sedated. Radionuclide hepatobiliary scans have a high false-positive rate for cholecystitis in this patient population. US findings, including gallbladder wall thickening and a striated gallbladder wall, are nonspecific for cholecystitis and are seen with other conditions common in this patient population including congestive heart failure, renal failure, liver disease, and hypoalbuminemia.[52] When cholecystitis is suspected in severely ill patients, the threshold for performing PC should be low because it is a low-risk, potentially lifesaving procedure.

Future Considerations in Percutaneous Gallbladder Intervention

The search for less invasive, safer, and more cost effective methods to treat cholelithiasis and cholecystitis continues. Patients recover faster from laparoscopic cholecystectomy than from *open* cholecystectomy. Laparoscopic cholecystectomy requires a general anesthetic, which precludes its use in extremely fragile patients. Also, it is not feasible in some patients who have had abdominal operations and adhesions. In these two groups of patients in particular, the concept of percutaneously ablating the gallbladder so that it is reduced to a fibrous scar is appealing.

Sclerosing agents have been ineffective in humans, perhaps because of the inability of sclerosing agents to eliminate all mucosal cells, particularly those deep in Aschoff-Rokitansky sinuses.[53] Yedlicka and associates[54] have demonstrated that ablation of the gallbladder with boiling radiographic contrast medium is possible in humans. The thermal injury created is transmural and may be more effective than using sclerosing agents.

Because of the multiple sessions required for cholecystostomy, percutaneous cholelithotomy and gallbladder ablation, these percutaneous procedures will not supplant cholecystectomy. Further work may demonstrate that gallbladder ablation is efficacious in patients unable to undergo cholecystectomy.

PERCUTANEOUS BIOPSY

Percutaneous image-guided sampling of abdominal lesions is a safe and effective method of obtaining material for cytologic or histologic analysis, and for microbiologic and chemical analysis of fluid collections. Advances in CT and US have allowed accurate localization of smaller and more subtle lesions, and experience has demonstrated the safety of percutaneous biopsy through windows previously thought to be unsafe. Sites in the abdomen and pelvis that are commonly biopsied percutaneously include liver, pancreas, kidney, adrenal gland, lymph node, gallbladder, extravisceral soft tissues masses, and bone. Less common sites for biopsy include spleen[55,56] and bowel.[57,58]

A variety of transcatheter biopsy techniques have been developed for use when percutaneous needle biopsy is contraindicated.

Technique

The optimal imaging modality for guiding a needle biopsy depends on the position and conspicuity of the lesion, the patient's body habitus, the ability to introduce radiopaque contrast medium adjacent to the lesion, and the experience of the radiologist.

Patients are prepared according to the type of imaging that will be used to guide their biopsies, and whether they will receive intravenous contrast medium. Patients undergoing US-guided biopsies usually fast for 8 hours before their procedure because gas in the small bowel limits visualization of structures deep to the bowel.

Patients undergoing biopsy have their prothrombin time, activated partial thromboplastin time, and platelet count checked and corrected if necessary. Patients who are to receive intravenous contrast medium are hydrated and have their blood urea nitrogen and creatinine levels checked. Most patients do not require a sedative, but those who are unusually anxious or find it painful to lie in the required position are given midazolam, fentanyl, or both.

Fluoroscopy in multiple planes, most frequently with a C-arm, provides easy and efficient guidance for biopsy of large, superficially located lesions. Fluoroscopic landmarks such as distance from a particular bony structure or position adjacent to a radiopaque stent can be used to position the needle. If an indwelling biliary catheter is present, contrast medium can be introduced to allow fluoroscopically guided biopsy of biliary duct lesions. Fluoroscopy also is useful for biopsy of abnormal lymph nodes identified at lymphangiography that still contain lymphangiographic contrast medium.

Real time ultrasonography has many advantages for intraabdominal biopsy. Perhaps its greatest advantage is that, unlike CT, it allows continuous monitoring of the course of the needle while it is being advanced, allowing instant readjustment of the needle path as necessary. US guidance may be applied when the lesion is ultrasonographically visible and a needle path that avoids gas-filled bowel exists, because the soft tissue–gas interfaces reflect most of the sound waves and preclude visualization of the needle tip and the lesion. US also is advantageous when the ideal needle path is at a steep

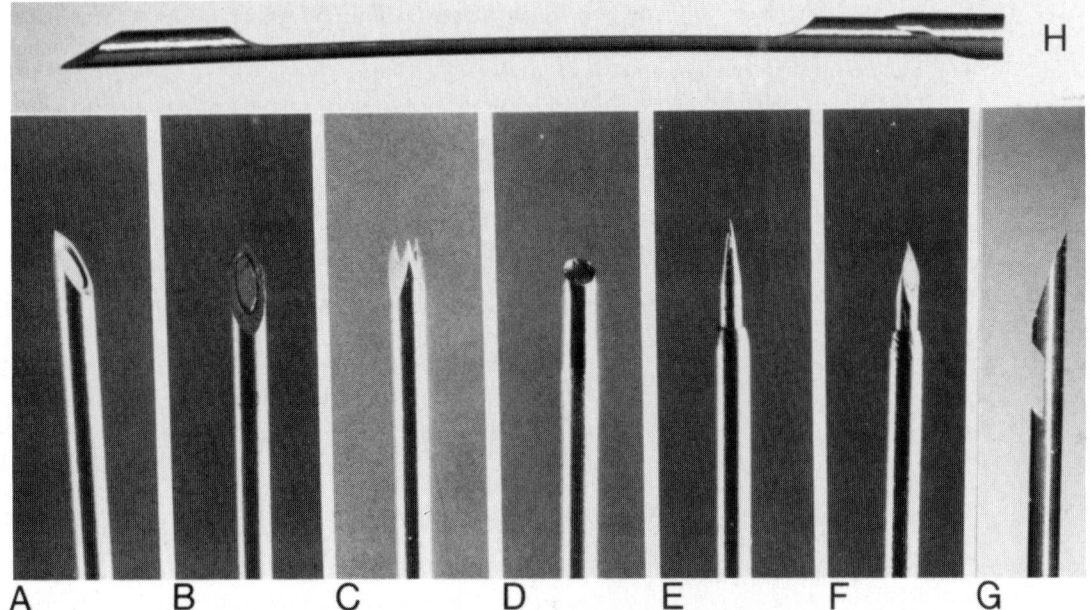

FIGURE 128-5. Needles available for percutaneous aspiration and biopsy include (**A**) Chiba needle; (**B**) spinal needle; (**C**) Franseen needle; (**D**) Turner needle; (**E**) Madayag needle; (**F**) Green needle; (**G**) Westcott needle with the stylet removed for clarity; and (**H**) TruCut needle. (Adapted from Moss AA, Gamsu G, Genant HK, eds. Computed tomography of the body. Philadelphia: WB Saunders, 1983:1089.)

angle to the axial plane because such an angle makes CT guidance more difficult. However, US guidance is difficult in obese patients because fat degrades the US image.

Computed tomography is most frequently used to guide biopsies that cannot be performed reliably with fluoroscopy or US. CT usually is the imaging modality of choice for small, deep-seated lesions. Oral, intravenous, and rectal contrast medium is administered as needed for lesion visualization. To perform CT-guided biopsies, a localizing radiopaque grid is placed on the skin covering the region of the skin entry site as estimated from prior scans, and a scan at the level of the lesion is repeated. A needle path is chosen, preferably in the axial plane, and the skin puncture site is marked on the skin. The depth of the lesion and the angle between the needle path and a vertical line through the lesion is measured.

The needle is advanced to the appropriate depth with visual approximation of the appropriate angle or using one of several devices available for this purpose. The patient then is replaced in the CT gantry and scans are obtained to show the position of the needle tip. If the needle tip is not in the correct location, it is repositioned and additional scans are obtained. These steps are repeated until the needle is in the desired position.

Computed tomography requires the most patient cooperation of the three modalities described because patients must not only be capable of holding their breath, but must hold it reproducibly in the same phase of respiration for the initial imaging and for needle placement. CT also has the disadvantage of frequently requiring the administration of intravenous iodinated contrast medium to allow lesion discrimination from normal tissue. Administration of iodinated contrast medium has its own small but real risks.

MR has limited application for guiding abdominal biopsies. Its use in the abdomen is limited to lesions that are visualized only with MR and perhaps when CT guidance would be most appropriate, but there is a need to limit exposure to ionizing radiation.[59]

The types of needles available for percutaneous biopsy are nearly as numerous as the types of diseases for which biopsy is performed (Fig. 128-5). Needles can be classified into those that obtain material for cytologic analysis and those that obtain tissue for histologic analysis. Needles from 25-gauge to 14-gauge are used: the smaller sizes predominantly for aspiration cytologic study and the larger ones for obtaining a core of tissue.

Aspiration cytologic study with a skinny needle (20–25 gauge) is the most frequently performed percutaneous biopsy. When a tissue core is desirable, the spring-loaded mechanically triggered biopsy needles (guns) are used. These needles have a TruCut-type design, and once in position, the inner and/or outer parts (depending on the manufacturer) of the needle are advanced rapidly forward by a preloaded spring-mechanism. These guns offer the benefit of producing less pain than the TruCut needle, and some 18-gauge guns produce a specimen as good as that obtained with a 14-gauge TruCut needle.[60]

A needle path is chosen that avoids lung, gallbladder, and spleen and, if possible, bowel and vascular structures. Passing 21-gauge needles through the stomach and small and large bowel is safe.[61] Some institutions are routinely placing 18-gauge needles through bowel without complication.* It appears judicious to avoid transgressing bowel in immunocompromised patients and those with ascites.

Local anesthetic and a small dermatatotomy precede needle

---

* Dawson SL, personal communication, March 1993.

placement. The needle may then be advanced directly into position. If a larger needle is being used, a skinny needle may be first positioned within the lesion, then the larger needle may be placed parallel to the smaller needle. This allows the needle repositionings common with CT guidance to take place with the smaller needle, and allows the larger needle to be properly positioned on the first pass. A coaxial needle technique also is useful for small or difficult lesions. The technique involves placement of a larger needle up to the lesion with the biopsy performed through a smaller inner needle. This allows simple repetitive sampling by removing only the smaller inner needle, assessing its yield and, if necessary, replacing the inner needle and repeating the biopsy.

Indications

The indications for needle biopsy of abdominal and pelvic lesions are legion but can be reduced to one guiding principal: if the material obtained will alter therapy, needle biopsy should be undertaken. The risk of needle biopsy is low but real; therefore, biopsy should not be performed if therapy will not be altered by the biopsy results.

The choice of obtaining a specimen by aspiration biopsy or a by larger core biopsy depends on the radiologist's experience, the availability of a skilled cytopathologist, the lesion targeted for biopsy, and the clinical situation. In most cases an aspiration biopsy is adequate to make the diagnosis of malignancy, although specific tumor characterization may require a core of tissue. Aspiration biopsy is useful in diagnosing acute liver transplant rejection, but core biopsy is more useful in diagnosing chronic rejection.[62] Cores of tissue should be obtained routinely whenever the cellular architecture is important for microscopic diagnosis (e.g., diffuse liver disease, likely benign focal liver lesions, lymphoma).

Contraindications and Risks

A patient who will not lie still is an absolute contraindication to image-guided needle biopsy. It is impossible to target a moving lesion, and there is the risk of visceral injury. For biopsy of abdominal lesions, patients must be capable of holding their breath for a minimum of 10 seconds so that respiratory excursion of the lesion is suspended during needle placement.

A bleeding diathesis is a relative contraindication depending on the severity of the diathesis, the location of the lesion, lesion vascularity, and the size of the needle required. Frequently, administration of plasma, platelets, or vitamin K may be used to correct the coagulopathy. If a coagulopathy would otherwise contraindicate biopsy and the lesion is intrahepatic, transvenous biopsy or biopsy with embolization of the needle tract (plugged biopsy) can be performed.

Suspected echinococcal cyst and hemangiomas have been listed as contraindications to needle biopsy; however, after unintended aspirations of such lesions were reported, several authors reported series of safe biopsy of these two entities.[63–66]

Echinococcal cysts clearly have a risk of anaphylaxis with spontaneous and operative rupture, but only one report exists

of anaphylaxis during percutaneous aspiration.[67] Pruritus as a minor allergic reaction has been observed.[66] When serologic tests are equivocal, a fluid collection is present after surgical drainage of hydatid disease, or percutaneous drainage of known hydatid disease is contemplated, percutaneous aspiration is not contraindicated. The needle path should first transverse a segment of normal liver to reduce the risk of intraperitoneal spillage of cyst contents.

Cavernous hemangiomas are the most common benign liver tumors. Their appearance at CT frequently is typical; however, a small hemangioma may be difficult to differentiate from a metastasis. This distinction is important in patients with known primary malignancy. A skinny needle (20-gauge) core biopsy is effective for histologic diagnosis of hemangioma and is safely performed.[65] A needle path traversing normal liver before reaching the lesion is recommended to reduce the possibility of hemorrhage.

Percutaneous needle biopsy is a relatively safe invasive procedure with a reported mortality rate between 0.03% and 0.1%.[68] The most common causes of death are hemorrhage sepsis and in the case of pancreatic biopsy, pancreatitis as well. Severe pancreatitis after pancreatic biopsy occurs in less than 3% of patients[69] and is more common when biopsy is performed on a normal pancreas. Needle tract tumor seeding after intraabdominal biopsy is a rare occurrence that happens on the order of 0.006% of the time according to four large retrospective studies.[68] Traversing normal parenchyma before entering a lesion may reduce the risk of seeding.

Hemorrhage is the most common complication of liver biopsy. Hemorrhage may occur as intraabdominal bleeding or hemobilia after creation of an arteriobiliary fistula. Hemobilia after needle biopsy frequently can be treated with superselective hepatic arterial embolization. Severe intraabdominal bleeding may be more common if the needle does not initially traverse normal parenchyma.

Results

Image-guided hepatic biopsy using skinny needles is accurate in the diagnosis of malignancy in over 90% of patients.[70] Accurate diagnosis of hemangioma can be made 100% of the time using a 20-gauge coring needle.[65]

Skinny needle biopsy of the pancreas has been reported to be accurate 60% to 90% of the time. The coexistence of pancreatic carcinoma and pancreatitis may result in biopsy of the inflammatory area, which frequently cannot be distinguished by CT or US from the neoplastic area. The possibility of sampling error suggests that an initial negative result from percutaneous pancreatic biopsy should not be accepted, and either a repeat percutaneous biopsy or an operative biopsy should be performed as warranted by clinical circumstances.

Percutaneous image-guided aspiration biopsy of lymph nodes has been performed more often than large core biopsy for evaluation of lymphadenopathy. Fine-needle (skinny needle) aspiration of lymph nodes using cytologic examination for detection of metastatic carcinoma is highly accurate.[71] The accuracy of detecting lymphoma is approximately 80%.[71] Accurate typing of lymphoma by fine-needle aspiration remains problematic but advances in immunocytochemistry[72] and flow cytometry[73] may prove helpful. The accuracy of percutaneous core biopsies for classifying lymphomas remains to be determined.

Alternative Techniques to Biopsy

A number of catheter-based techniques have evolved that are useful in specific situations when percutaneous needle biopsy is difficult or contraindicated.

Transvenous Liver Biopsy

If coagulopathy or marked ascites are present, transvenous biopsy is the procedure of choice for evaluating diffuse liver disease (e.g., cirrhosis, hepatitis, hemochromatosis) because the needle does not transverse the liver capsule, avoiding hemorrhage.[74] A 2.97-mm (9-Fr) catheter is advanced into a hepatic vein from the transjugular approach. Through this catheter, a long, 16-gauge modified Ross needle is advanced into a right hepatic vein over a guidewire. The wire is removed and the position of the needle tip is confirmed. The needle is advanced 3 cm into the liver parenchyma while suction is applied. The needle is removed and the specimen is examined visually. If the size of the specimen is inadequate the needle can be reinserted and another biopsy specimen obtained.[75] This technique is successful in 64% to 97% of patients.[76]

Major complications occur in 2% of patients and include cardiac arrhythmias and intraperitoneal hemorrhage from inadvertent capsular puncture.[76] A conceptually similar technique uses flexible biopsy forceps from a transjugular or transfemoral venous route.

An improved transvenous biopsy needle combining a TruCut-type needle on the end of a flexible coaxial cable has been described.[77] This needle yields better specimens than the modifications of the Ross needle[78] and should be commercially available shortly.†

Plugged Liver Biopsy

When a histologic core of liver tissue is needed and coagulopathy or marked ascites preclude standard percutaneous liver biopsy, embolization of the needle tract within the liver is useful for preventing bleeding from the liver capsule puncture site. Embolization of the tract is performed with a Gianturco coil[79] or with gelatin sponge plugs[80] (Fig. 128-6). Plugging the tract with clotting factors has been performed[81] and use of a hemostatic protein polymer sheath has been tested in swine.[82] The use of electrocautery of the needle tract has undergone preliminary evaluation.[83]

The two techniques in most common clinical use use coils or gelatin sponge. These materials may be introduced through the outer part of a TruCut-type needle after the inner obturator and specimen have been removed, or through a vascular sheath fitted over the needle before biopsy. Introducing the embolus through a vascular sheath is useful because the sheath is much more flexible than the needle cannula and is less likely to cause injury while the patient breathes and the liver moves. The potential disadvantage of using the sheath is that a larger

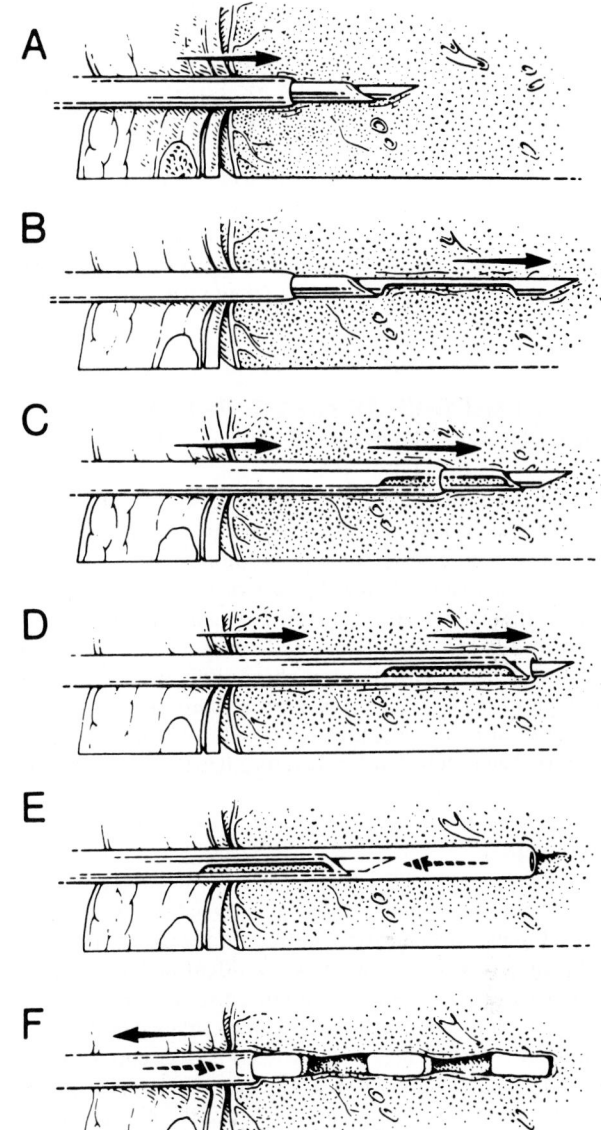

FIGURE 128-6. The technique of plugged liver biopsy using gelatin foam. (**A**) The sheathed needle is inserted. (**B, C**) The biopsy specimen is obtained. (**D**) The sheath is advanced over the needle tip to allow plugging of the deepest part of the needle path. (**E**) The needle and specimen are removed and the specimen is examined. If the specimen is inadequate the needle can be reinserted into the sheath and another specimen can be obtained. (**F**) The needle tract is embolized with gelatin foam pieces. The contrast injected with the pieces allows visualization of the otherwise radiolucent Gelfoam. The first and second pieces occlude the biopsy site, and the third piece, placed just a few millimeters from the liver edge, prevents bleeding from the liver capsule. (From Chuang VP, Alspaugh JP. Sheath needle for liver biopsy in high-risk patients. Radiology 1988;166:261.)

hole is made in the liver capsule than would be made by the needle alone. Fluoroscopic or ultrasonographic monitoring allows embolization of the entire intrahepatic tract rather than of the the biopsy site alone.

Plugged liver biopsy has several advantages and disadvantages compared with transvenous liver biopsy. Plugged biopsy

---

† Rösch J, personal communication, July 1993.

is faster, usually less costly, and does not require the same level of technical skill and experience required for transvenous biopsy. Plugged biopsy can be performed with imaging guidance to obtain a core sample of a focal lesion. Transvenous biopsy is not useful for most focal hepatic lesions because of the inability to precisely steer the transvenous needle. The published experience with plugged liver biopsy is too small to allow an accurate comparison of the risks of plugged liver biopsy with transvenous biopsy.[84] However, the authors of the two largest published series of plugged biopsies[85,86] recommend transvenous biopsy for patients with severe coagulation disorders.

PERCUTANEOUS ABSCESS AND FLUID COLLECTION DRAINAGE

Since first introduced by Gronvall and associates in 1977,[87] percutaneous abscess drainage (PAD) has gained widespread acceptance by internists, surgeons, radiologists, and patients despite the lack of randomized prospective studies comparing surgical and percutaneous drainage.[88] This acceptance is based on the readily apparent efficacy and safety of PAD compared with the alternative of surgical therapy in most situations. The indications for PAD have continued to expand and the contraindications have continued to shrink while the technique has been refined and experience has been gained.

Technique

Computed tomography is widely acknowledged as being the best technique for identifying intraperitoneal and retroperitoneal abscesses. Once an abscess is identified and the radiologists and referring gastroenterologist or surgeon decide that PAD is indicated, the abscess can be drained with CT or US guidance. Occasionally, if an abscess is large and relatively superficial, a drainage catheter can be placed with fluoroscopy if a puncture site is marked on the patient's skin during diagnostic CT.

The diagnostic CT is useful for planning the ideal catheter route. It should be as short as possible and should avoid vascular and neural structures, lung, pleura, intestines, bladder, ureters, and unless the abscess is intraparenchymal, solid organs. CT is most frequently the guidance procedure of choice because it facilitates the discrimination of bowel loops from abscess, it enables the radiologist to perform diagnostic and therapeutic procedures at the same sitting, and it allows fast and accurate confirmation of effective drainage of complex collections.

Ultrasound is most useful for retroperitoneal, hepatic, and splenic drainage, and in situations where the ideal path is at a steep angle to the axial plane. If the abscess and adjacent important structures can be distinguished, drain placement can be performed with real time guidance.

All patients undergoing abscess drainage receive intravenous broad-spectrum antibiotics before catheter placement to reduce the risk of sepsis after the bacteremia that may occur with catheter placement. A prothrombin time, activated partial thromboplastin time, and a platelet count are obtained before the diagnostic CT in anticipation of possible drain placement.

Bleeding diatheses are corrected with plasma, platelets, or coagulation factors as needed. After the diagnostic CT, the procedure is discussed with the patient, including the possibility of placing multiple catheters and the expected range of duration of catheter drainage.

Depending on the patient's personality, condition, and planned catheter course, analgesic or anxiolytic drugs may be given intravenously. Local anesthetic is administered, a needle is directed into the fluid collection, and a sample is obtained. If the sample is grossly purulent or foul smelling, a drainage catheter is placed. If it is not, an immediate Gram's stain is performed. If the presence of leukocytes or bacteria confirm an abscess, the drain is placed. If the fluid shows no evidence of infection, fluid may be obtained for other diagnostic studies and the needle removed. If no fluid can be aspirated despite an appropriately placed needle of adequate caliber, either aspiration biopsy or core biopsy is performed.

There are two principal methods for abscess catheter placement: The Seldinger and trocar techniques. Seldinger technique involves placing a guidewire through the initial needle, removing the needle over the wire, and sequential advancement of dilators and a drainage catheter. The trocar technique uses a drainage catheter with an inner stiffener and central pointed trocar. The trocar catheter is advanced in a single pass, parallel to the initial needle, and to the same depth. The trocar technique obviates guidewire exchange and tract dilatation, and also theoretically reduces the risk of leakage of pus into a noncontaminated space during guidewire exchange. When the acceptable window of access is narrow, the Seldinger technique may be preferred to avoid unintentional passage of the trocar catheter into a vital structure.

Frequently used PAD catheters range in size from 2.64 to 5.28 mm (8–16 Fr). The size of the catheter depends on the viscosity of the fluid to be drained and whether significant debris is likely to be present. Single- or double-lumen (sump) catheters may be used, based predominantly on the preference of the radiologist. Single-lumen catheters are connected to gravity drainage. Sump catheters may be left to gravity or low suction. Some radiologists use self-retaining catheters[89] similar to those used for nephrostomy tube placement, whereas others do not recommend using self-retaining catheters.[90]

After the drainage catheter is placed, the abscess cavity is drained using a syringe connected to the catheter. The cavity is irrigated until clear using volumes of saline much smaller than the volume of fluid initially obtained. Small volumes are mandatory to prevent bacteremia that may ensue if the abscess wall is distended. A repeat scan is obtained to confirm adequate drainage. If an undrained collection remains, an additional catheter is placed. Postprocedure orders include monitoring vital signs, recording the catheter output daily, and flushing the catheter with 10 mL of saline every 4 to 6 hours for the first day and once daily after the first day.

Hepatic Abscess

Pyogenic Abscess

Bacteria can be introduced into the liver by means of the biliary tree, the bloodstream (arterial or portal venous), contiguous spread from adjacent structures, and directly by penetrating trauma or operation. The most common cause of hepatic abscess has been hepatic and biliary surgery. In fairness to surgeons, this shift reflects a decreased frequency of hepatic abscess from diverticulitis and appendicitis because the surgical and medical treatment of the latter diseases has improved. When a pyogenic liver abscess forms, PAD in conjunction with antibiotic treatment is safe and succeeds in approximately 90% of patients.[88] Apparent loculation of a hepatic abscess is not a contraindication to drainage because nearly always, the loculi communicate, and effective drainage can be achieved.

Echinococcal Cyst

Aspiration of hepatic hydatid cysts was once considered contraindicated because of the perceived risk of peritoneal seeding and anaphylaxis. The traditional treatment of hydatid cysts has been surgical; however, a number of authors have demonstrated the safety and efficacy of therapeutic cyst aspiration.[66,91-93] The diagnosis of hydatid cyst is made by imaging studies, serologic study, or aspiration of the cyst. Patients with infected hydatid cysts, Type IV cysts, and cysts in communication with the biliary tree are treated surgically.[91]

The percutaneous procedure is performed under CT or US guidance with the needle traversing normal liver first en route to the cyst to reduce the risk of peritoneal spillage of cyst contents. Fluid from the cyst is aspirated and a scolecidal agent, such as alcohol or hypertonic saline, is injected through the needle to partially refill the cyst. After 5 to 20 minutes the scolecidal agent is withdrawn and the needle is removed. Ethanol and hypertonic saline do not cause a sclerosing cholangitis if a biliary communication exists.[94] This procedure is of greatest value in patients for whom operation would present a great risk and in patients in whom pericystectomy is precluded by the adherence of the cyst to major vascular or biliary structures.[93,95]

Amebic Abscess

The role of percutaneous aspiration or catheter drainage for the treatment of hepatic amebic abscess remains controversial. One group in the United States has shown that nearly all hepatic amebic abscesses can be cured by antimicrobial drugs alone, reserving percutaneous drainage for patients with bacterial superinfection and juxtacardiac lesions, which have the risk of intrapericardial rupture.[96] The same group has shown in a randomized trial that there is not a significant difference in clinical benefit between patients treated solely with amebicidal drugs and patients treated with amebicidal drugs and a single percutaneous aspiration.[97] A retrospective study in Italy compared medical therapy alone; combined surgery and medical therapy; and abscess aspirations or catheter drainage and intralesional and oral amebicidal drugs.[98] This study showed a marked reduction in time to defervescence and in hospital stay in the percutaneously treated group. In areas of the world where amebiasis is endemic, the benefits of percutaneous aspiration or catheter drainage has been shown for selected patients.[99,100] These patients include those with abscesses of more than 6 cm and those who have failed one course of medical therapy.

Pancreatic Abscess and Fluid Collections

Management of patients with pancreatic fluid collections, which complicate acute pancreatitis, chronic pancreatitis, or pancreatic trauma, requires close communication and interaction between the gastroenterologist, surgeon, and radiologist to achieve optimal patient care. Whatever initial combination of medical, surgical, or percutaneous treatment is chosen, a suboptimal response may require prompt institution of alternative therapy, often in the domain of one of the other specialists.

Classification of the different types of pancreatic fluid collection is essential in evaluating outcomes of percutaneous and operative interventions.

Usually, physicians are in accord regarding the definitions of sterile pseudocyst and infected pseudocyst. Pseudocysts, whether infected or not, are cured by percutaneous drainage in 70% to 90% of patients.[101,102] The response rate may be higher in infected than in noninfected pseudocysts.[103] Indications for percutaneous drainage include pseudocyst infection, pain associated with a pseudocyst greater than 4 to 5 cm, and a pseudocyst causing bile duct or gastric outlet obstruction. An asymptomatic pseudocyst larger than 10 cm also warrants percutaneous drainage to avoid serious complications.[103] Somatostatin analogs reduce output from pseudocyst drainage catheters and may prove useful in reducing the duration of catheter drainage.[101]

Although the definition of an infected pseudocyst is fairly clear, various authors use different and overlapping definitions of other secondary pancreatic infections.[104] Pancreatic abscess and infected pancreatic necrosis should be distinguished because of their differing outcomes and treatment.[104] CT with bolus administration of contrast medium is the most useful for identifying pancreatic necrosis, and a needle biopsy is useful for confirming or refuting the presence of infected necrosis. If the definition of pancreatic abscess applies to pancreatic infections that are predominantly liquid with a minimal amount of necrotic material, and infected pancreatic necrosis applies to pancreatic infections composed predominantly of solid necrotic debris and lesser amounts of fluid, then pancreatic abscess is best treated percutaneously and infected pancreatic necrosis is best treated surgically.[104,105] In many of these ill patients, surgical resection and drainage, and percutaneous drainage play an important and complimentary role at different times in the courses of their illnesses.

Diverticular Abscess

Percutaneous abscess drainage plays an important role in treating certain patients with complications of diverticulitis.[106,107] Patients with phlegmonous changes around the colon can be managed medically. Patients with small pericolic abscesses can be treated with en bloc resection at the time of their colectomy, and patients with peritonitis require a two-stage operation. Patients who have larger pericolic, pelvic, or retroperitoneal abscesses may benefit from PAD. This subset of patients would require staged operations if PAD were not available. PAD provides for resolution of septic complications and healing of the abscess such that a delayed single-stage operation can be performed. As with all cases of PAD, if signs of sepsis do not improve within 24 to 48 hours of PAD and intravenous antibiotics, immediate operation should be undertaken unless catheter repositioning or replacement has a high likelihood of effecting improvement.

Abscesses With Fistulas

The identification of fistulas associated with an abdominal or pelvic abscess frequently is not made on imaging studies before drainage or even at the time of drainage.[108] After several days, if the quantity of drainage remains over 50 mL/day or if the character of the drainage changes and visually or chemically resembles stool, small bowel secretions, pancreatic juice, bile, or urine, then identification of the fistula can be attempted by injecting contrast medium into the abscess cavity under fluoroscopic observation. If this is unsuccessful, an attempt can be made to identify the fistula from its other end by filling the suspected organ of origin with contrast medium, e.g., a barium enema is performed if a colonic origin is suspected, or a PTC or ERCP if a biliary communication is present.

The presence of a fistula does not preclude definitive PAD in most circumstances. If a downstream stenosis is present in the hollow viscus or if a foreign body or neoplasm is present at the site of perforation, then closure of the fistula will not occur without surgical intervention.[109] Low-output fistulas of less than 200 mL/day appear to be more likely to heal than high-output fistulas. Because most high-output fistulas tend to arise from the biliary tree, pancreatic duct, or small bowel, this is reasonable considering the digestive effects of gastric juice, pancreatic juice, and bile on tissue and their interference with healing.[110] High-output fistulas may be treated more effectively by converting them to low-output fistula with nasoenteric intubation and suction, total parenteral nutrition, and H_2 blocker therapy. Catheterization of the fistula itself and advancement of a drainage catheter into the viscus is extremely useful in diverting drainage from the fistulous tract and allowing resolution.[110]

When a fistula is present in association with a percutaneously drained abscess, the duration of catheter drainage usually is longer than if no fistula is present. Drainage for several months may be necessary; however, most of these patients can be managed as outpatients. If a patient's social situation precludes outpatient treatment, operative treatment should be considered to avoid the costs and risks associated with prolonged hospitalization.

Abscesses and Crohn's Disease

The role of PAD in Crohn's disease is debated,[88,111] but several points are clear. Postoperative abscesses with or without fistulas and hepatic abscesses in patients with Crohn's disease respond well to PAD.[112,113] Abscesses in association with transmural disease of the bowel but without visible fistulas also appear to respond.[114] It is unclear what the response rate is for abscesses with fistulas from transmural disease. Nevertheless, these patients may benefit from palliation with PAD before definitive operation. PAD may control septic complications and allow improvement of nutritional status with a course of parenteral nutrition before operation.[88,111] As in

treatment of diverticular disease, PAD may allow conversion of a two-stage operation into a single-stage operation.

TRANSJUGULAR INTRAHEPATIC PORTOSYSTEMIC SHUNT

Esophageal variceal bleeding has long posed a therapeutic challenge to surgeons, interventional radiologists, and gastroenterologists. If these patients only had bleeding varices, the task of the medical profession would be much simpler. However, these patients frequently have mild to severe liver failure with coagulopathy, hypoalbuminemia, and ascites; frequently are malnourished; and have multisystem failure. Conservative medical management, endoscopic variceal sclerotherapy and banding, esophageal balloon tamponade, and surgical portosystemic shunting all have an important role in caring for these patients. The clinical application of the transjugular intrahepatic portocaval shunt (TIPS) is relatively recent and its role in caring for this diverse and challenging patient population remains to be determined.

The first attempt at creating a percutaneous portosystemic communication was described by Rösch and associates in 1969.[115] Later work by this group[116] confirmed the feasibility of the shunt in 34 dogs and in three human cadavers. In the dogs, shunts occluded quickly and at that time the authors accurately predicted, "The internal shunt requires more research and study particularly in regards to material development." Colapinto and associates[117] were the first to apply the technique to patients but because no suitable stent was available, their patients received only balloon dilatation of the tract and the shunts rapidly occluded.[118] Palmaz and associates[119,120] and Rösch and associates[121] placed expandable metallic stents in the intrahepatic tract in animal models to increase shunt patency. Richter and associates[122] in 1989 was the first to create a portosystemic shunt in a human using a metallic stent. Since that report, interest in TIPS has burgeoned and at least seven centers have experience with over 100 patients each.

Patient Preparation and Technique

Endoscopy is performed to identify the bleeding site. If variceal bleeding or evidence of recent variceal bleeding is seen, the involved gastroenterologist, interventional radiologist, and surgeon confer and decide whether a TIPS is indicated.

If the patient is actively bleeding, every attempt (including medical management, endoscopic sclerotherapy or banding, and esophageal balloon tamponade) is made to control bleeding before the TIPS procedure.

Patency of the portal vein is confirmed using US with color flow. If the US examination gives equivocal results or suggests portal vein occlusion, the status of the portal vein is assessed with contrast CT or with arterial portography. If the portal vein is occluded, TIPS can be performed successfully and safely, although the procedure is more difficult and may require transhepatic puncture of the portal vein.[123]

The TIPS procedure can be performed with intravenous sedation without endotracheal intubation in cooperative patients, although some groups prefer the use of a general anesthetic in all patients. The presence of an anesthesiologist is helpful because moderately deep intravenous sedation is required for some patients during tract dilatation and the availability of someone skilled in airway management is reassuring.

Venipuncture of a jugular vein is performed. The right internal jugular vein usually is chosen because it allows the straightest course to the hepatic veins. However, if the right internal jugular vein cannot be accessed, the right external jugular vein or the left internal or external jugular vein can be used. A 3.3-mm (10-Fr) sheath is advanced over a guidewire into the right atrium or distal inferior vena cava, and a 1.65-mm (5-Fr) catheter is introduced coaxially. Pressures are measured in the right atrium, inferior vena cava, and the chosen hepatic vein, most often the right hepatic vein. The catheter is advanced into a wedged position, and a wedged hepatic venogram performed. In many patients, reflux of the contrast medium can be seen in the portal vein; this contrast-medium reflux is useful for guiding portal vein puncture. A 16-gauge Colapinto needle (Fig. 128-7) is advanced over the guidewire through a 2.97-mm (9-Fr) catheter into the hepatic vein. The guidewire is removed and the needle is advanced with fluoroscopic guidance into the visualized or expected position of the right main portal vein. The needle is withdrawn until blood can be aspirated, and contrast medium is injected to visualize the vascular structure entered.

When the portal vein is entered a guidewire is introduced and advanced into the superior mesenteric or splenic vein. The 2.97-mm (9-Fr) catheter is advanced over the needle and guidewire into the portal vein. If advancement of this catheter is impeded by an exceedingly fibrotic liver, the catheter is advanced as far as possible, and after the needle is removed, a 1.65-mm (5-Fr) catheter is advanced into the superior mesenteric or splenic vein. Portal and central venous pressures are measured and a portal venogram is performed (Fig. 128-8) to identify anatomic structures and varices, which may require embolization later in the procedure. The 2.97-mm (9-Fr) catheter is removed, and an 8-mm balloon catheter is placed in the hepatic tract, advanced slightly into the right main portal vein, and inflated. The balloon is deflated, withdrawn, and reinflated so that the entire tract is dilated.

The length of the tract is measured with a guidewire and a 10-mm diameter Wallstent (see Fig. 128-2) of appropriate length is advanced into position, bridging the distance from the portal to the hepatic vein. Sometimes more than one stent must be used to cover the tract. The stents are then dilated with a 10-mm balloon to assure their maximal expansion. Portal and systemic venous pressures are measured and another portal venogram is obtained (see Fig. 128-8). The residual pressure gradient, the angiographically determined flow into varices, and the patient's bleeding status determine whether embolization of varices is performed with Gianturco coils using a catheter in place through the TIPS.

A short vascular sheath usually is left in place in the neck

for 24 hours. If no rebleeding occurs the sheath is removed. If bleeding does recur the sheath is used for access for reassessment of the shunt, variceal embolization, or creation of a second shunt.[124]

A follow-up US examination is obtained before discharge from the hospital. Patients return for repeat US at 3, 6, 9, and 12 months after shunt placement and at 6 and 12 months for portal venography and pressure measurements. Patients who are seen to be occluded at ultrasonography are considered for recanalization and revision of their shunts. Patients with a 50% or greater stenosis in their shunts or a portosystemic gradient greater than 15 mm Hg undergo redilitation of the shunt with placement of additional stents as necessary.

Indications

The clearest indication for TIPS is control of variceal bleeding in patients with end-stage liver disease who are candidates for liver transplantation and whose bleeding cannot be controlled with medical treatment and sclerotherapy.[125] If sclerotherapy is not successful, a TIPS can be created and because the stents are intrahepatic, the transplant procedure is not made more difficult or more risky as is the case when most surgical portosystemic shunts are present. Because planned transplantation limits the time the TIPS must remain patent, questions about long-term TIPS patency do not affect this indication.

Possible other indications include the following:

- control of esophageal, gastric, small bowel, or colonic variceal bleeding from intrinsic liver disease or portal vein thrombosis
- control of bleeding from portal gastroenteropathy
- treatment of intractable ascites.

Decisions regarding the appropriateness of these indications await further clinical trials.

Contraindications and Risks

Absolute contraindications to TIPS include the following:

- fulminant hepatic failure
- severe hepatic encephalopathy prior to the onset of bleeding despite medical management
- active hepatic infection or bacteremia.

Because of the necessity for close patient follow-up and the frequency of shunt stenosis requiring reintervention, patients who will not return for follow-up should not be considered good candidates for TIPS. The risks of TIPS vary greatly with the patient's bleeding status at the time of shunt creation. In patients who are actively bleeding and who un-

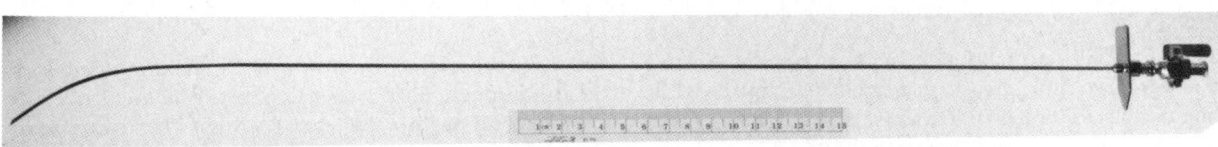

FIGURE 128-7. Colapinto needle.

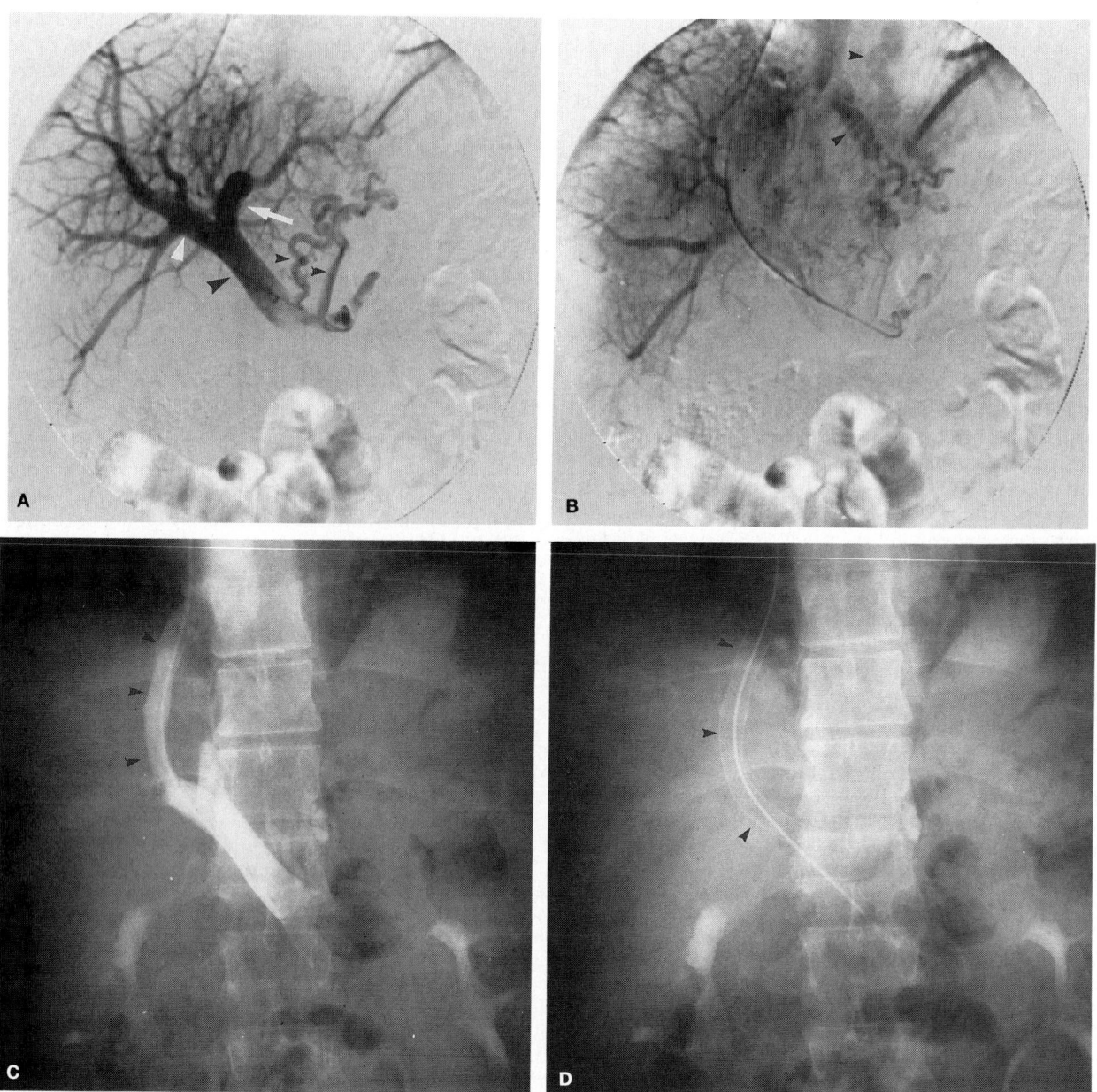

FIGURE 128-8. Transjugular intrahepatic portosystemic shunt. (**A**) Portal venogram obtained after the 1.7-mm (5-Fr) catheter has been placed at the confluence of the splenic and superior mesenteric veins. An image obtained from the middle of filming sequence shows two coronary veins (*small black arrowheads*), the main portal vein (*large black arrowhead*), the right portal vein (*white arrowhead*), and the left portal vein (*white arrow*). Observe the extensive filling of the intrahepatic portal vein branches. (**B**) An image obtained from later in the same sequence shows filling of esophageal varices (*arrowheads*). This patient's varices were graded as 4+ endoscopically. (**C**) Portal venogram after completion of the shunt with the catheter at the confluence of the splenic and superior mesenteric veins. Brisk filling of the transjugular intrahepatic portosystemic shunt is seen (*arrowheads*). Notice the loss, as expected, of hepatopedal flow in the intrahepatic portal vein branches and diminished flow in the coronary veins. (**D**) A later image from the same sequence shows the position of the two overlapping Wallstents (*arrowheads*) in place from the right main portal vein to the right hepatic vein.

dergo TIPS, a 55% mortality rate has been seen.[126] Fortunately, aggressive nonsurgical management can control bleeding in 90% to 95% of all patients, greatly reducing the numbers of patients requiring emergent TIPS.[126]

Complications include contrast agent–induced renal fail-

ure, liver capsule perforation with intraabdominal bleeding, stent migration, and encephalopathy. The incidence rate of de novo encephalopathy after TIPS is 11%.[127] In almost all cases, the encephalopathy occuring after TIPS is not severe and can be controlled medically.[127a]

Clinical Implications

The promise of a percutaneously created portosystemic shunt, which may avoid some of the morbidity and mortality associated with surgical shunts, is exciting; however, many questions remain to be answered. It is clear that patients with TIPS require intensive follow-up for at least 2 years after shunt placement, with shunt revision frequently being required. Primary shunt patency at 1 year after placement is only 30% to 50%[127b,127c]; however, with careful monitoring and treatment of shunt stenoses with balloon dilitation, additional stent placement, or both, a primary assisted patency rate of 85% can be acheived at 1 year after placement.[127b] Some patients require more than one reintervention. The long-term patency rate of TIPS remains to be determined. Unless the stenosis rate of TIPS can be reduced, either with covered stents or pharmacologic therapy, TIPS will have to be thought of as a temporary treatment of portal hypertension. Even as a temporary treatment, TIPS is useful to control variceal bleeding and stabilize patients who will undergo liver transplantation. As a method to control bleeding in Child's class C patients when other therapy has failed, TIPS is useful. In these patients, who have short life expectancies, a durable procedure is not required.

The relative role of operative versus percutaneous portal decompression remains to be determined for patients with longer life expectancies who, for medical or social reasons, are not transplant candidates. Operative shunts are clearly more durable than TIPS, so it must be determined whether TIPS with frequent follow-up and reintervention or surgical shunts result in longer survival or better quality of life.

Likewise, the role of sclerotherapy and TIPS remains to be determined, pending the results of randomized controlled studies. Both procedures require repetitive reintervention and have their own risks.

PERCUTANEOUS ENTEROSTOMY

Percutaneous Radiologic Gastrostomy and Gastrojejunostomy

Percutaneous radiologic gastrostomy and gastrojejunostomy were introduced independently by Ho,[128] Tao and Gillies,[129] and Wills and Oglesby[130] in 1983, 3 years after the introduction of percutaneous endoscopic gastrostomy. Many of the benefits of percutaneous radiologic gastrostomy are identical to those of its endoscopic predecessor. The complications and discomfort of long-term nasoenteric tubes are avoided, as are the risks of laparotomy and general anesthesia required to create a surgical gastrostomy. As with the endoscopic placement, several techniques and variations of radiologic placement exist, each with its own proponent.

Additionally, a variety of modifications of the radiologic technique allow placement of gastrostomy or gastrojejunostomy tubes when endoscopic placement is not feasible.

Technique

A prothrombin time, activated partial thromboplastin time, and a platelet count are obtained. A nasogastric tube is placed the evening before the procedure, or if a nasoenteric feeding tube is present it is left in place. Barium is administered through this tube the evening before the procedure to opacify the transverse colon at fluoroscopy the following day. If a nasogastric or orogastric tube cannot be placed because of esophageal obstruction, no barium is administered in advance of the procedure. The patient is given nothing by mouth or through the nasogastric tube except for medications beginning at midnight before the procedure.

Before the procedure, intravenous access is obtained, in case it may be needed, and the left lobe of the liver is visualized with US and its position marked on the skin with ink. The abdomen then is examined fluoroscopically. If insufficient barium or air is present in the transverse colon to allow its fluoroscopic visualization, barium is given per rectum to achieve this goal. The nasoenteric tube is adjusted as necessary so that it is within the stomach and air is introduced to inflate the stomach. Glucagon is administered to reduce the egress of air from the stomach. Distention of the stomach brings its anterior wall closer to the anterior abdominal wall, displaces the small and large bowel, and brings the stomach out from under the costal margin to facilitate puncture. Inflation also allows fluoroscopic visualization of the stomach.

If no nasoenteric tube can be passed blindly because of esophageal obstruction, in nearly all cases, a small-bore tube or catheter can be placed through the obstruction using standard angiographic techniques. If no tube will traverse an esophageal obstruction, then the entire procedure, or at least the gastric puncture and guidewire placement, can be performed under CT, which allows visualization of a fluid-filled or empty stomach that cannot be seen at fluoroscopy.[131]

The puncture site is chosen fluoroscopically so that the needle enters the body of the stomach away from the greater curve, avoiding the gastroepiploic vessels, epigastric vessels, the colon, and the left lobe of the liver. Oblique fluoroscopy is useful to confirm that the stomach abuts the anterior abdominal wall without intervening structures at the puncture site. The chosen puncture site is anesthetized with lidocaine and a skin incision large enough to admit the selected tube is made. Gastropexy sutures (Brown-Mueller T-fasteners) may be placed with a modified 18-gauge needle (Fig. 128-9),[132] although their use is not mandatory even for placement of large gastrostomy tubes.[133,134] Under fluoroscopic guidance, an 18-gauge needle attached to a 10-mL syringe half filled with water-soluble contrast medium is advanced into the stomach with a brisk motion during aspiration with the syringe. Entry into the stomach is observed by free aspiration of air and is confirmed by injection of contrast medium and visualization of rugal folds. A 0.097-cm guidewire is advanced into the stomach and the tract is dilated. A peel-away sheath is placed.

If a gastrojejunostomy tube is to be placed, an angiographic catheter and a long torqueable guidewire are used to traverse the pylorus and advance the guidewire through the duodenum into the proximal jejunum. The gastrojejunostomy catheter then is advanced over the guidewire into the jejunum and the peel-away sheath is removed.

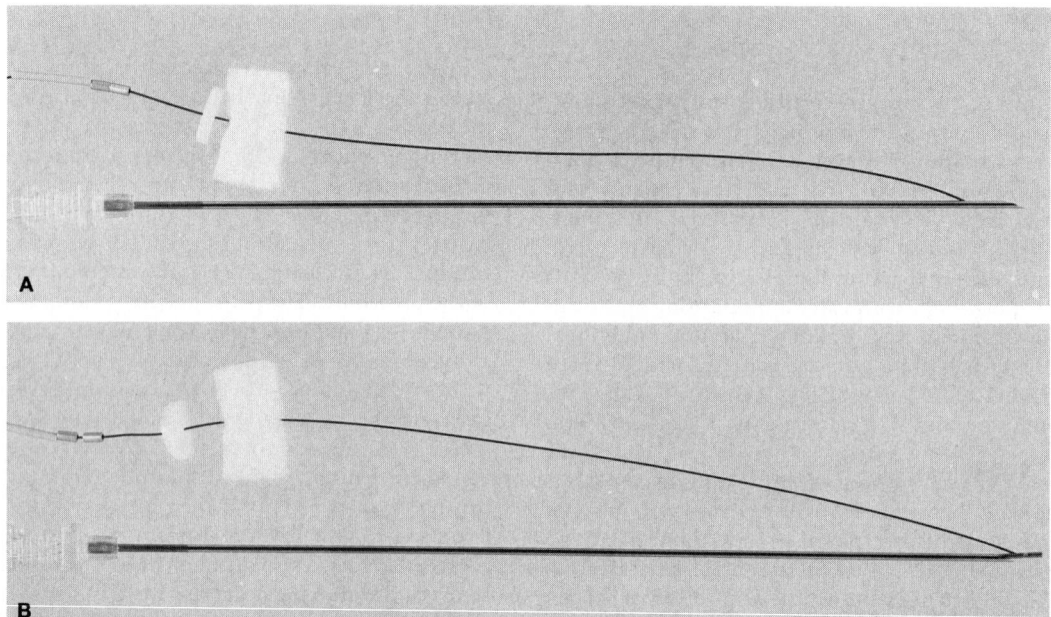

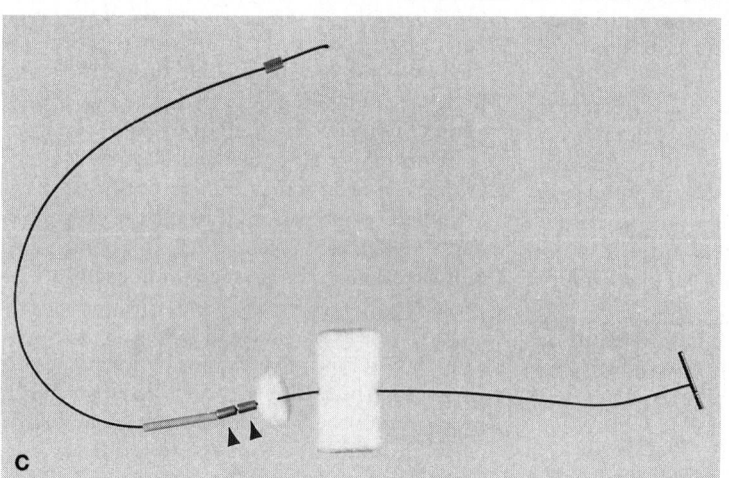

FIGURE 128-9. Brown-Mueller T-fasteners. (**A**) T-fastener loaded in introducing needle. (**B**) T-fastener being pushed out of the needle. (**C**) After placement, gentle tension is placed on the suture and the two metal bands (*arrowheads*) are firmly crimped, securing the anterior wall of the stomach to the anterior abdominal wall. When the suture is cut off at the skin, the T-fastener passes through the gastrointestinal tract.

Catheters from 2.64 to 8.58 mm (8–26 Fr) are used for gastrostomy, with the smallest catheters used in the pediatric population for feeding and the largest catheters used in adults for gastric decompression. Retention devices include balloons, Cope loops, and Malecot tips (Fig. 128-10). Injection of contrast medium confirms the final position of the gastrostomy or gastrojejunostomy tube.

The gastrostomy or gastrojejunostomy tube is secured at the skin with a Molnar disk or friction fitting to a stoma adhesive. If for any reason there is a high risk of catheter dislodgement, the tube may be sutured to the skin. The patient is observed for 6 hours for signs of bleeding or peritoneal irritation. If a gastrostomy tube has been placed, it is left open to gravity drainage overnight and tube feedings begin the following morning. If a gastrojejunostomy has been placed, tube feedings may begin immediately. The stitches (and gastropexy fasteners, if used) are removed after 10 days. The tract usually is mature enough by 7 to 10 days so that if the tube is accidentally dislodged, the tract can be recatheterized and a de novo gastrostomy avoided if replacement is performed within 24 hours.

Feeding Gastrostomy Versus Feeding Gastrojejunostomy

Because adequate data is not yet available, radiologists remain divided into two camps: those who place gastrostomy tubes in the majority of patients and gastrojejunostomy tubes only when gastroesophageal reflux is proven, and those who place gastrojejunostomy tubes in all patients. The most serious complication of tube feedings is aspiration pneumonia. Pneumonia can result from aspiration of oropharyngeal secretions, gastric juice, or gastric juice and tube feedings. Some evidence exists that surgical gastrostomies induce reflux; however, percutaneous radiologic gastrostomy does not induce reflux.[135] No study has demonstrated that endoscopic or radiologic percutaneous gastrojejunostomy results in less aspiration than percutaneous gastrostomy. Continual aspiration is a common problem after percutaneous endoscopic gastrojejunostomy,[136] and there is no reason to believe that this will be any different with the radiologic technique.

Gastrojejunostomy tubes require greater maintenance than do gastrostomy tubes. Whereas gastrostomy tubes can be

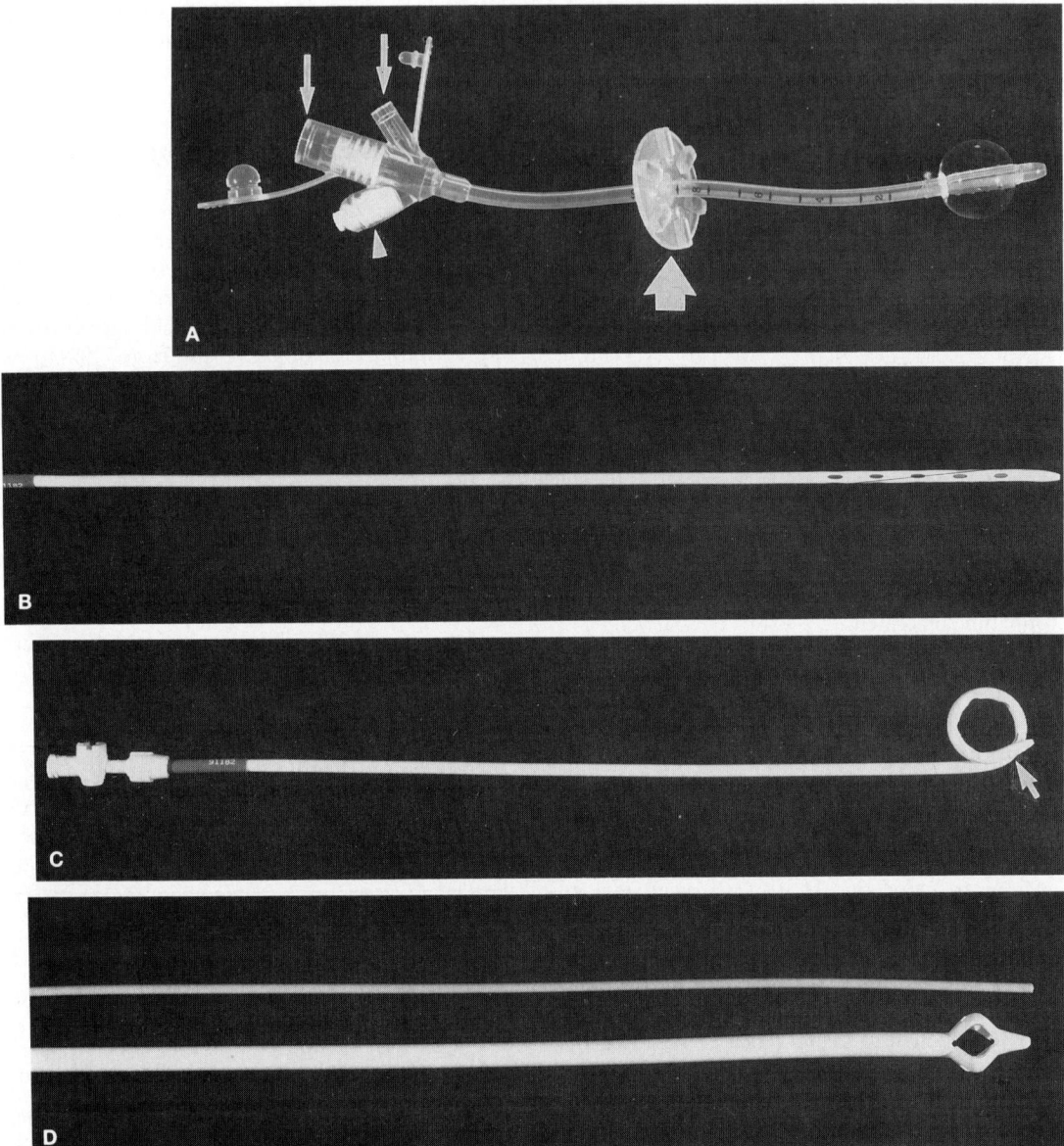

FIGURE 128-10. Three tubes used for percutaneous gastrostomy. (**A**) A 5.28-mm (16-Fr) silicone rubber gastrostomy tube. Notice the two feeding or drainage ports (*thin arrows*) connected to the same lumen to accept different connectors, balloon inflation port (*arrowhead*), and friction fitting (*broad arrow*) for securing tube to skin and for preventing migration of the balloon to the pylorus. (**B**) A 3.96-mm (12 Fr) catheter with Cope loop. The catheter is mounted on its inner stiffener, as it would be before placement. The retention suture can be seen coursing diagonally across the catheter near its tip. (**C**) A 3.96-mm (12-Fr) catheter with Cope loop after its pigtail has been reformed. The arrow marks where the retention suture leaves the catheter near its tip and reenters the catheter. When this suture is secured at the catheter hub the pigtail is prevented from uncoiling. (**D**) A 7.92-mm (24-Fr) catheter with Mallecot tip and the straightening catheter used for its insertion and removal.

changed by a nurse at the bedside, gastrojejunostomy tubes must be replaced fluoroscopically, commonly requiring the patient to be moved from nursing home to hospital. Until recently, gastrojejunostomy tubes have occluded more frequently than gastrostomy tubes because the jejunostomy portion of the tubes have been limited in size to 3.3 to 3.96 mm (10–12 Fr). Poorly crushed pill fragments or concretions of tube feedings may block the smaller tube and necessitate tube replacement. The greater length of gastrojejunostomy tubes may also contribute to this problem.

Fortunately, single-lumen, soft 4.62- to 5.94-mm (14–18 Fr) gastrojejunostomy tubes recently have become available. Dual-lumen gastrojejunostomy tubes have been available, with the claim that by feeding through the jejunal lumen and placing the gastric lumen to drainage, reflux can be reduced. However, because of the course of gastrojejunostomy tubes, the gastric side holes are in the body of the stomach, and because in the supine position fluid accumulates in the fundus, little drainage results. If gastroesophageal reflux and aspiration occur in a patient with a gastrojejunostomy tube, or in a patient with intractable gastroparesis,[137] a better result may be achieved with two tubes, one advanced into the jejunum for feeding and one into the gastric fundus for decompression. If gastrojejunostomy tube placement is desired, radiologic placement is simpler than endoscopic placement.

Indications

The indications for placement of a gastrostomy or gastrojejunostomy tube are as follows:

• long-term enteric feeding in patients unable to eat or who eat without aspirating for any reason
• decompression of chronic small bowel obstruction from abdominal carcinomatosis[134]
• palliation of vomiting and severe gastroesophageal reflux secondary to linitis plastica–type gastric carcinoma[138]
• treatment of severe intractable gastroparesis.[139]

Contraindications

The following are contraindications for gastrostomy or gastrojejunostomy tube placement:

Unacceptable bleeding risk, such as occurs from coagulopathy that cannot be corrected with vitamin K, plasma, clotting factors, or platelet transfusion, or from gastric varices.

Inaccessible stomach from prior gastric pull up, total gastrectomy, or partial gastrectomy with extremely small gastric remnant; or from interposed liver or spleen because of hepatomegaly or splenomegaly, or interposed colon or small bowel (in many of these cases where no acceptable path can be seen at fluoroscopy, a path can be found with CT guidance).

Clinically unstable patients (e.g., those with sepsis, multisystem failure). Gastrostomy tube placement should be deferred until these problems resolve. These patients should receive nasoenteric or parenteral nutrition as indicated.

Patients with limited life expectancy.

Ascites is no longer considered a contraindication.[140] Pericatheter ascitic leak can be avoided with preprocedural paracentesis and, if necessary, postprocedural paracentesis to promote skin healing. Gastropexy sutures (T-fasteners) are used in patients with marked ascites to prevent catheter dislodgement by preventing increasing amounts of ascites from displacing the stomach from the anterior abdominal wall.[140] Bacterial seeding of the ascitic fluid remains a potential problem.

Complications and Results

A compilation of four major published series of radiologic gastrostomy and gastrojejunostomy tube placement[141] in a total of 635 patients revealed a procedure-related mortality rate of 1% and a major complication rate of 5%. Major complications included peritonitis requiring laparotomy, bleeding requiring transfusion, external leakage, aspiration, and deep abdominal wall infection. Minor complications occurred in 5% of patients. No prospective study has been performed to compare radiologic with endoscopic gastrostomy.

Percutaneous radiologic gastrostomy or gastrojejunostomy can be performed in essentially all patients in whom the procedure is not contraindicated.

Percutaneous Cecostomy

Percutaneous cecostomy is an alternative to surgical and endoscopic decompression of the cecum in cases of colonic obstruction and pseudoobstruction (Ogilvie's syndrome).[142,143] Small 2.31- to 2.97-mm (7–9 Fr) catheters can be placed through the peritoneum with a Seldinger or trocar technique for decompression of gas,[143] and large 7.92- to 9.9-mm (24–30 Fr) catheters can be placed for drainage of liquid stool after placement of T-fasteners, as used for gastrostomy tube placement.[142]

This technique is applicable for patients with Ogilvie's syndrome who require decompression and in whom endoscopic decompression fails, and in patients with colonic obstruction whose medical condition precludes operation. In the latter situation, percutaneous cecostomy may be used as a temporizing measure until the patient's medical condition improves enough to allow operation, or as palliation for patients who will never tolerate an operation.[142]

The reader is directed to Chapter 22, Gastrointestinal Blood Flow; Chapter 30, Approach to the Patient With Gross Gastrointestinal Bleeding; Chapter 120, Cross-Sectional Anatomy; and Chapter 127, Angiography.

REFERENCES

1. Harbin WP, Mueller PR, Ferucci JT Jr. Transhepatic cholangiography: complications and use patterns of the fine-needle technique. Radiology 1980;135:15.
2. Reiertsen O, Skjt J, Jacobsen CD, et al. Complications of fiberoptic gastrointestinal endoscopy: five years' experience in a central hospital. Endoscopy 1987;19:1.
3. Bilbao MK, Dotter CT, Lee TG, et al. Complications of endoscopic retrograde cholangiopacreatography (ERCP). Gastroenterology 1976;70:314.
4. vanSonnenberg E, Ferrucci PR, Neff CC, et al. Biliary pressure: manometric and perfusion studies of percutaneous THC and percutaneous biliary drainage. Radiology 1983;148:41.
5. Castaneda-Zuniga WR, Irving JD, Herrera MA, et al. Biliary tract intervention. In: Castaneda-Zuniga WR, Tadavarthy SM, eds. Interventional radiology, 2nd ed. Baltimore: Williams & Wilkins, 1992:1054.
6. Lewis RT, Goodall G, Marien B, et al. Biliary bacteria, antibiotic use and wound infection in surgery of the gallbladder and common bile duct. Arch Surg 1987;122:44.
7. Pitt HA, Postier RG, Cameron JC. Biliary bacteria: significance and alterations after antibiotic therapy. Arch Surg 1982;117:445.
8. Chetlin SH, Elliott DW. Biliary bacteremia. Arch Surg 1971;102:303.
9. Spies JB, Rosen JR, Lebowitz AS. Antibiotic prophylaxis in vascular and interventional radiology: a rational approach. Radiology 1988;166;381.
10. Grecht NB, Henry NK, Hoffman WW, et al. Prospective randomized comparison of mezlocillin therapy alone with combined ampicillin and gentamicin therapy for patients with cholangitis. Arch Intern Med 1989;149:1279.

11. Neff CC, Mueller PR, Ferucci JT Jr, et al. Serious complications following transgression of the pleural space in drainage procedures. Radiology 1984;152:335.

12. Ferucci JT, Mueller PR, Harbin WP. Percutaneous transhepatic biliary drainage: technique, results and applications. Radiology 1980;135:1.

13. Leger L, Zara M, Arbay N, et al. Cholangiographie et drainage biliaire par ponction trans-hepatique. Presse Med 1952;60:936.

14. Bornman PC, Harries-Jones EP, Tobias R, et al. Prospective controlled trial of transhepatic biliary endoprosthesis vs. bypass surgery for incurable carcinoma of head of pancreas. Lancet 1986;1(8472):69.

15. Feduska NJ, Dent TL, Lindenauer SM. Results of palliative operations for carcinoma of the pancreas. Arch Surg 1971;103:330.

16. Sarr MG, Cameron JL. Surgical palliation of unresectable carcinoma of the pancreas. World J Surg 1984;8:906.

17. Andersen JR, Sorensen SM, Kruse A, et al. Radomised trial of endoscopic endoprosthesis versus operative bypass in malignant obstructive jaundice. Gut 1989;30:132.

18. Shepherd HA, Royle G, Ross APR, et al. Endoscopic biliary endoprosthesis in the palliation of malignant obstruction of the distal common bile duct: a randomized trial. Br J Surg 1988;75:1166.

19. Speer AG, Cotton PB, Russell RC, et al. Randomised trial of endoscopic versus percutaneous stent insertion in malignant obstructive jaundice. Lancet 1987;2(8550):57.

20. Cope C. Improved anchoring of nephrostomy catheters: loop technique. Am J Roentgenol 1980;135:402.

21. Wittich GR, vanSonnenberg E, Simeone JF. Results and complications of percutaneous biliary drainage. Semin Intervent Radiol 1985;2:39.

22. Russell E, Yrizarry JM, Huber JS, et al. Percutaneous transjejunal biliary dilatation: alternate management for benign strictures. Radiology 1986;159:209.

23. Mueller PR, vanSonnenberg E, Ferrucci JT Jr, et al. Biliary stricture dilatation: multicenter review of clinical management in 73 patients. Radiology 1986;160:17.

24. Williams HJ Jr, Bender CE, May GR. Benign postoperative biliary strictures: dilation with fluoroscopic guidance. Radiology 1987;163:629.

25. Millis JM, Tompkins RK, Zinner MJ, et al. Management of bile duct strictures: an evolving strategy. Arch Surg 1992;127:1077.

26. Skolkin MD, Alspaugh JP, Casarella WJ, et al. Sclerosing cholangitis: palliation with percutaneous cholangioplasty. Radiology 1989;170:199.

27. Hausegger KA, Kleinert R, Lammer J, et al. Malignant biliary obstruction: histologic findings after treatment with self-expandable stents. Radiology 1992;185:461.

28. Gordon RL, Ring EJ, LaBerge JM, et al. Malignant biliary obstruction: treatment with expandable metallic stents. Follow-up of 50 consecutive patients. Radiology 1992;182:697.

29. Lameris JS, Stoker J, Nijs HGT, et al. Malignant biliary obstruction: percutaneous use of self-expandable stents. Radiology 1991;179:703.

30. Adam A, Chetty N, Roddie M, et al. Self-expandable stainless steel endoprostheses for treatment of malignant biliary obstruction. Am J Roentgenol 1991;156:321.

31. Wagner HJ, Knyrim K, Vakil N, et al. Plastic endoprostheses versus metal stents in the palliative treatment of malignant hilar biliary obstruction: a prospective and randomized trial. Endoscopy 1993;25:213.

32. Knyrim K, Wagner HJ, Pausch J, et al. A prospective, randomized, controlled trial of metal stents for malignant obstruction of the common bile duct. Endoscopy 1993;25:207.

33. Davids PHP, Groen AK, Rauws EAJ, et al. Randomised trial of self-expanding metal stents for distal malignant biliary obstructon. Lancet 1992;340:1488.

34. Coons, H. Metallic stents for the treatment of biliary obstruction: a report of 100 cases. Cardiovasc Intervent Radiol 1992;15:367.

35. Maccioni F, Rossi M, Rossi M et al. Metallic stents in benign

biliary strictures: three-year follow-up. Cardiovasc Intervent Radiol 1992;15:360.

36. Picus D, Hicks ME, Darcy MD, et al. Percutaneous cholecystolithotomy: analysis of results and complications in 58 consecutive patients. Radiology 1992;183:779.

37. So CB, Givney RG, Scudamore CH. Carcinoma of the gallbladder: a risk associated with gallbladder-preserving treatments for cholelithiasis. Radiology 1990;174:127.

38. van Sonnenberg E, Wittich GR, Casola G, et al. Diagnostic and therapeutic percutaneous gallbladder procedures. Radiology 1986;160:23.

39. Nemcek AA Jr, Bernstein JE, Vogelzang RL. Percutaneous cholecystostomy: does transhepatic puncture preclude a transperitoneal catheter route? J Vasc Intervent Radiol 1991;2:543.

40. Cope C. Percutaneous subhepatic cholecystostomy with removable anchor. Am J Roentgenol 1988;151:1129.

41. Gillams A, Curtis SC, Donald J, et al. Technical considerations in 113 percutaneous cholecystolithotomies. Radiology 1992;183:163.

42. Caridi JG, Hawkins IF Jr, Hawkins MC. Single-step placement of a self-retaining "accordion" catheter. Am J Roentgenol 1984;143:337.

43. D'Agostino HB, van Sonnenberg E, Sanchez RB, et al. Imaging of the percutaneous cholecystostomy tract: observations and utility. Radiology 1991;181:675.

44. Lee MJ, Saini S, Brink JA, et al. Treatment of critically ill patients with sepsis of unknown cause: valve of percutaneous cholecystostomy. Am J Roentgenol 1991;156:1163.

45. Vauthey JN, Lerut J, Martini M, et al. Indications and limitations of percutaneous cholecystostomy for acute cholecystitis. Surg Gynecol Obstet 1993;176:49.

46. vanSonnenberg E, D'Agostino HB, Casola G, et al. The benefits of percutaneous cholecystostomy for decompression of selected cases of obstructive jaundice. Radiology 1990;176:15.

47. McGahan JP, Lindfors KK. Percutaneous cholecystostomy: an alternative to surgical cholecystostomy for acute cholecystitis? Radiology 1989;173:481.

48. Jurkovich GJ, Dyess DL, Ferrara JJ. Cholecystostomy: expected outcome in primary and secondary biliary diseases. Am Surg 1988;54:40.

49. McGahan JP, Lindfors KK. Acute cholecystitis: diagnostic accuracy of percutaneous aspiration of the gallbladder. Radiology 1988;167:669.

50. Vogelzang RL, Nemcek AA. Percutaneous cholecystostomy: diagnostic and therapeutic efficacy. Radiology 1988;168:29.

51. Teefey SA, Baron RL, Radke HM, et al. Gangrenous cholecystitis: new observations on sonography. J Ultrasound Med 1991;10:603.

52. Teefey SA, Baron RL, Bigler SA. Sonography of the gallbladder: significance of striated (layered) thickening of the gallbladder wall. Am J Roentgenol 1991;156:945.

53. Becker CD, Burhenne HJ. Percutaneous ablation of the cystic duct and the gallbladder: experimental and early clinical results. Semin Roentgenol 1991;26:259.

54. Yedlicka JW, Coleman CC, Peterson C. Thermal ablation of the gallbladder. J Vasc Intervent Radiol 1992;4:367.

55. Taavitsainen M, Koivuniemi A, Helminen J, et al. Aspiration biopsy of the spleen in patients with sarcoidosis. Acta Radiol 1987;28:723.

56. Kager PA, Rees PH. Splenic aspiration: review of the literature. Trop Geogr Med 1983;35(2):111.

57. Abbitt PL. Percutaneous fine-needle aspiration of bowel wall abnormalities under ultrasonic guidance. J Clin Ultrasound 1991;19:310.

58. Solbiati L, Montali G, Croce F, et al. Fine-needle aspiration biopsy of bowel lesions under ultrasound guidance: indications and results. Gastrointest Radiol 1986;11:172.

59. van Sonnenberg E, Hajek P, Gylys-Marin V, et al. A wire-sheath system for MR guided biopsy and drainage: laboratory studies and experience in 10 patients. Am J Roentgenol 1988;151:815.

60. Hopper KD, Baird DE, Reddy VV. Efficacy of automated

biopsy guns versus conventional biopsy needles in the pygmy pig. Radiology 1990;176:671.

61. Brandt KR, Charboneau JW, Stephens DH, et al. CT- and US-guided biopsy of the pancreas. Radiology 1993;187:99.

62. Lautenshlager I, Hockerstedt K, Hayry P. Fine-needle aspiration biopsy in the monitoring of liver allografts. Transplant Int 1991;4:54.

63. Livraghi T, Bosoni A, Giordano F, et al. Diagnosis of hydatid cyst by percutaneous aspiration: valve of electrolyte determinations. J Clin Ultrasound 1985;13:333.

64. Solbiati L, Livraghi T, DePra L, et al. Fine-needle biopsy of hepatic hemangioma with sonographic guidance. Am J Roentgenol 1985;144:471.

65. Cronan JJ, Esparza AR, Dorfman GS, et al. Cavernous hemangioma of the liver: role of percutaneous biopsy. Radiology 1988;166:135.

66. Bret PM, Fond A, Bretagnolle M, et al. Percutaneous aspiration and drainage of hydatid cysts in the liver. Radiology 1988;168:617.

67. Fornari F, Civardi G, Cavanna L, et al. Complications of ultrasonically guided fine-needle abdominal biopsy: results of a multicenter Italian study and review of the literature. Scand J Gastroenterol 1989;24:949.

68. Smith EH. Complications of percutaneous abdominal fine-needle biopsy. Radiology 1991;178:253.

69. Neuerburg J, Gunther R. Percutaneous biopsy of pancreatic lesions. Cardiovasc Intervent Radiol 1991;14:43.

70. Fernandez MP, Murphy FB. Hepatic biopsies and fluid drainages. Radiol Clin North Am 1991;29:1311.

71. Lawrence DD, Carrasco CH, Fornage B. Percutaneous lymph node biopsy. Cardiovasc Intervent Radiol 1991;14:55.

72. Suhrland MJ, Wieczorek R. Fine-needle aspiration biopsy in the diagnosis of lymphoma. Cancer Invest 1991;9:61.

73. Chernoff WG, Lampe HB, Cramer H, et al. The potential clinical impact of the fine-needle aspiration/flow cytometric diagnosis of malignant lymphoma. J Otolaryngol 1992; 21(Suppl 1):1.

74. Rösch J, Lakin PC, Antonovic R. Transjugular approach to liver biopsy and transhepatic cholangiography. N Engl J Med 1973;289:227.

75. Goldman ML, Gonzalez AC, Galambos JT. The transjugular technique of hepatic venography, cholangiography and obliteration of esophageal varices. Radiology 1978;128:325.

76. Gamble P, Colapinto RF, Stronell RD, et al. Transjugular liver biopsy: a review of 461 biopsies. Radiology 1985;157:589.

77. Gilmore IT, Bradley RD, Thompson RPH. Improved method of transvenous liver biopsy. Br Med J 1978;2(6132):249.

78. Bull HJM, Gilmore IT, Bradley RD, et al. Experience with transjugular liver biopsy. Gut 1983;24:1057.

79. Allison DJ, Adam A. Percutaneous liver biopsy and track embolization with steel coils. Radiology 1988;169:261.

80. Chuang VP, Alspaugh JP. Sheath needle for liver biopsy in high risk patients. Radiology 1988;166:261.

81. Rodriguez-Fuchs CA, Bruno M. Plugging liver biopsy sites with coagulation factors. Lancet 1987;2(8567):1087.

82. Gazelle GS, Haaga JR, Halpern EF. Hemostatic protein polymer sheath: improvement in hemostasis at percutaneous biopsy in the setting of platelet dysfunction. Radiology 1993;187:269.

83. Kim EH, Kopecky KK, Cummings OW, et al. Electrocautery of the tract after needle biopsy of the liver to reduce blood loss: experience in the canine model. Invest Radiol 1993;28:228.

84. Jackson JE, Adam A, Allison DJ. Transjugular and plugged liver biopsies. Bailllieres Clin Gastroenterol 1992;6:245.

85. Zins M, Vilgrain V, Gayno S, et al. US guided percutaneous liver biopsy with plugging of the needle track: a prospective study in 72 high risk patients. Radiology 1992;184:841.

85. Tobin MV, Gilmore IT. Plugged liver biopsy in patients with impaired coagulation. Dig Dis Sci 1989;34:13.

87. Gronvall J, Gronvall S, Hegedus V. Ultrasound guided drainage of fluid containing masses using angiographic catheterization techniques. Am J Roentgenol 1977;129:997.

88. Lambiase RE. Percutaneous abscess and fluid drainage: a critical review. Cardiovasc Intervent Radiol 1991;14:143.

89. van Sonnenberg E, D'Agostino HB, Casola G, et al. Percutaneous abscess drainage: current concepts. Radiology 1991;181:617.

90. Dondelinger RF, Kurdziel JC, Boverie J. Percutaneous management of intraperitoneal, hepatic and other fluid collections. Bailllieres Clin Gastroenterol 1992;6:273.

91. Khuroo MS, Zarger SA, Mahajan R. Echinococcus granulosus cysts in the liver: management with percutaneous drainage. Radiology 1991;180:141.

92. Acunas B, Rozanes I, Celik L, et al. Purely cystic hydatid disease of the liver: treatment with percutaneous aspiration and injection of hypertonic saline. Radiology 1992;182:541.

93. Giorgio A, Tarantino L, Francica G, et al. Unilocular hydatid liver cysts: treatment with US-guided, double percutaneous aspiration and alcohol injection. Radiology 1992;184:705.

94. Langer JC, Rose DD, Keystone JS, et al. Diagnosis and management of hydatid disease of the liver: a 15 year North American experience. Ann Surg 1984;199:412.

95. Leese T, Bismuth H. Surgical management of space-occupying lesions of the liver: hydatid disease. Bailllieres Clin Gastroenterol 1989;3:272.

96. Ralls PW, Barnes PF, Johnson MR, et al. Medical treatment of hepatic amebic abscess: rare need for percutaneous drainage. Radiology 1987;165:805.

97. Van Allen RJ, Katz MD, Johnson MB, et al. Uncomplicated amebic liver abscess: prospective evaluation of percutaneous therapeutic aspiration. Radiology 1992;183:827.

98. Filice C, Di Perri G, Stroselli M, et al. Outcome of hepatic amebic abscesses managed with three different therapeutic strategies. Dig Dis Sci 1992;37:240.

99. Singh JP, Kashyap A. A comparative evaluation of percutaneous catheter drainage for resistant amebic liver abscesses. Am J Surg 1989;158:58.

100. Freeman O, Akamaguna A, Jarikre LN. Amoebic liver abscess: the effect of aspiration on the resolution or healing time. Ann Trop Med Parasitol 1990;84:281.

101. D'Agostino HB, van Sonnenberg E, Sanchez RB, et al. Treatment of pancreatic pseudocysts with percutaneous drainage and octreotide: work in progress. Radiology 1993;187:685.

102. Gumaste VV, Dave PB. Pancreatic pseudocyst drainage: the needle or the scalpel (editorial). J Clin Gastroenterol 1991;13:500.

103. vanSonnenberg E, Wittich GR, Casola G, et al. Percutaneous drainage of infected and noninfected pancreatic pseudocyst: experience in 101 cases. Radiology 1989;170:757.

104. Fedorak IJ, Ko TC, Djuricin G, et al. Secondary pancreatic infections: are they distinct clinical entities? Surgery 1992;112:824.

105. Freeny PC, Lewis GP, Traverso LW, et al. Infected pancreatic fluid collections: percutaneous catheter drainage. Radiology 1988;167:435.

106. Saini S, Mueller PR, Wittenberg J, et al. Percutaneous drainage of diverticular abscess: an adjunct to surgical therapy. Arch Surg 1986;121:475.

107. Stabile BE, Puccio E, van Sonnenberg E. Preoperative percutaneous drainage of diverticular abscesses. Am J Surg 1990;159:99.

108. Papanicolaou N, Mueller PR, Ferucci JT, et al. Abscess-fistula association: radiologic recognition and percutaneous management. Am J Roentgenol 1984;143:811.

109. Schuster MR, Crummy AB, Wojtowycz MM, et al. Abdominal abscesses associated with enteric fistulas: percutaneous management. J Vasc Interv Radiol 1992;3:359.

110. McLean GK, Mackie JA, Freiman DB, et al. Enterocutaneous fistulae: interventional radiologic management. Am J Roentgenol 1982;138:615.

111. vanSonnenberg E, D'Agostino HB, Sanchez RB et al. Percutanous abscess drainage (editorial). Radiology 1992;184:27.

112. Casola G, vanSonnenberg E, Neff C, et al. Abscesses in Crohn disease: percutaneous drainage. Radiology 1987;163:19.

113. Safrit HD, Mauro MA, Jaques PF. Percutaneous abscess drainage in Crohn's disease. Am J Roentgenol 1987;148: 859.

114. Lambiase RE, Cronan JJ, Dorfman GS, et al. Percutaneous drainage of abscesses in patients with Crohn disease. Am J Roentgenol 1988;150:1043.

115. Rösch J, Hanafee WN, Snow H. Transjugular portal venography and radiologic portacaval shunt: an experimental study. Radiology 1969;92:1112-1114.

116. Rösch J, Hanafee W, Snow H, Barenfus M, et al. Transjugular intrahepatic portacaval shunt. Am J Surg 1971;121:588.

117. Colapinto RF, Stronell RD, Birsch SJ, et al. Creation of an intrahepatic portosystemic shunt with a Gruntzig balloon catheter. Can Med Assoc J 1982;126:267.

118. Abecassis M, Gordon JD, Colapinto RF, et al. The transjugular intrahepatic portosystemic shunt (TIPS): an alternative for the management of life-threatening variceal hemorrhage. Hepatology 1985;5:1032A.

119. Palmaz JC, Sibbitt RR, Reuter SR, et al. Expandable intrahepatic portacaval shunt stenosis: early experience in the dog. Am J Roentgenol 1985;145:821.

120. Palmaz JC, Garcia F, Sibbitt RR, et al. Expandable intrahepatic portacaval shunt stents in dogs with chronic portal hypertension. Am J Roentgenol 1986;147:1251.

121. Rösch J, Uchida BT, Putnam JS, et al. Experimental portacaval anastomosis: use of expandable Gianturco stents. Radiology 1987;162:481.

122. Richter GM, Palmaz JC, Noldge G, et al. The transjugular intrahepatic portosystemic stent-shunt (TIPSS). Radiologe 1989;29:406.

123. Radosevich PM, Ring EJ, LaBerge JM, et al. Transjugular intrahepatic portosystemic shunts in patients with portal vein occlusion. Radiology 1993;186:523.

124. Haskal ZJ, Ring EJ, LaBerge JM, et al. Role of parallel transjugular intrahepatic portosystemic shunts in patients with persistent portal hypertension. Radiology 1992;185:813.

125. Ring EJ, Lake JR, Roberts JP, et al. Using transjugular intrahepatic portosystemic shunts to control variceal bleeding before liver transplantation. Ann Intern Med 1992; 116:304.

126. Helton WS, Belshaw A, Althaus S. Critical appraisal of the angiographic portacaval shunt (TIPS). Am J Surg 1993;165: 566.

127. Richter G. TIPS: The Heidelberg University experience. Western Angiographic and Interventional Society Annual Meeting, Portland, Oregon, October 1993.

127a. Sanyal AJ, Freedman AM, Shiffman ML, et al. Portosystemic encephalopathy after transjugular intrahepatic portosystemic shunt: results of a prospective controlled study. Hepatology 1994;20(1 Pt 1):46.

127b. Haskal ZJ, Pentecost MJ, Soulen MC, et al. Transjugular intrahepatic portosystemic shunt stenosis and revision: early and midterm results. Am J Roentgenol 1994;163(2):439.

127c. Lind CD, Malisch TW, Chong WK, et al. Incidence of shunt occlusion or stenosis following transjugular intrahepatic portosystemic shunt placement. Gastroenterology 1994; 106(5):1277.

128. Ho CS. Percutaneous gastrostomy for jejunal feeding. Radiology 1983;149:595.

129. Tao HH, Gillies RR. Percutaneous feeding gastrostomy. Am J Roentgenol 1983;141:793.

130. Wills JS, Oglesby JT. Percutaneous gastrostomy. Radiology 1983;149:449.

131. Sanchez RB, van Sonnenberg E, D'Agostine HB, et al. CT guidance for percutaneous gastrostomy and gastroenterostomy. Radiology 1992;184:201.

132. Saini S, Mueller PR, Gaa J, et al. Percutaneous gastrostomy with gastropexy: experience in 125 patients. Am J Roentgenol 1990;154:1003.

133. Deutsch LS, Kannegieter L, Vanson DT, et al. Simplified percutaneous gastrostomy. Radiology 1992;184:181.

134. O'Keefe F, Carrasco CH, Charnsangavej C, et al. Percutaneous drainage and feeding gastrostomies in 100 patients. Radiology 1989;172:341.

135. Olson DL, Krubsack AJ, Stewart ET. Percutaneous enteral alimentation: gastrostomy versus gastrojejunostomy. Radiology 1993;187:105.

136. Kadakia SC, Sullivan HO, Staraes E. Percutaneous endoscopic gastrostomy or jejunostomy and the incidence of aspiration in 79 patients. Am J Surg 1992;164:114.

137. Yeung EY, Ho CS. Percutaneous radiologic gastrostomy. Baillieres Clin Gastroenterol 1992;6:297.

138. Wills JS. Percutaneous gastrostomy: applications in gastric carcinoma and gastroplasty dilatation. Am J Roentgenol 1986;147:826.

139. Yeung EY, Mac Phadyen N, Ho CS. Intractable gastroparesis: treatment with percutaneous fluoroscopically guided gastrostomies. Am J Gastroenterol 1992;87:651.

140. Lee MJ, Saini S, Brink JA, et al. Malignant small bowel obstruction and ascites: not a contraindication to percutaneous gastrostomy. Clin Radiol 1991;44:332.

141. Ho CS, Yeung E. Percutaneous gastrostomy and transgastric jejunostomy. Am J Roentgenol 1992;158:251.

142. Morrison MC, Lee MJ, Stafford, SA, et al. Percutaneous cecostomy: controlled transperitoneal approach. Radiology 1990;176:574.

143. vanSonnenberg E, Varney RR, Casola G, et al. Percutaneous cecostomy for Ogilvie syndrome: laboratory observations and clinical experience. Radiology 1990;175:679.

Textbook of Gastroenterology, second edition, edited by Tadataka Yamada. JB Lippincott Company, Philadelphia © 1995.

CHAPTER 129

Laparoscopy

H. Worth Boyce, Jr.   H. Juergen Nord   George Berci

DIAGNOSTIC LAPAROSCOPY

After a decade of excitement over the diagnostic potential for abdominal ultrasonography (US) and computed tomography (CT), it appears that clinicians are just beginning to recognize the limitations of these imaging methods. When results are positive, these imaging methods permit guided fine-needle aspiration or needle biopsy with high diagnostic accuracy. However, well-controlled comparison studies are proving that a significant number of patients with metastatic lesions smaller than 1 cm in diameter are not accurately evaluated or staged by imaging methods alone. Exploratory laparoscopy, after a decade of unfortunate disinterest by many clinicians, is re-entering the diagnostic arena and, once again, should become recognized as an accurate and safe method for intraabdominal diagnosis (Figs. 129-1 through 129-4; see Color Figs. 109 through 112). With the introduction of laparoscopic chole-cystectomy in 1986 and the "rediscovery" of laparoscopy by surgeons, the field of operative laparoscopy has rapidly expanded to the point where most laparoscopies are therapeutic and performed by surgeons.

History and Development

Laparoscopy is one of the oldest gastrointestinal endoscopic procedures, dating back to the turn of the century. The concept of inspection of the abdominal cavity was introduced by Kelling with his presentation of *The Inspection of the Esophagus and Stomach With Flexible Instruments* on September 21, 1901, in Hamburg.[1,2] He recognized the importance of the pneumoperitoneum, carried out experiments on dogs, and examined 2 patients. In 1910 Jacobaeus reported on the clinical usefulness of the procedure and first used the term *laparoscopy*.[3] For the first 25 years, cystoscopes that had 90-degree side-viewing optics were used. Kalk improved instrumentation and introduced the oblique, 50-degree optics, which are the preferred instruments, especially for examination of the liver.[4]

Although the initial examinations relied primarily on visual impressions and reports, Henning and Keilhack made use of the single-lens reflex camera for objective photodocumentation.[5] Black-and-white pictures were rapidly followed by color photographs. Further improvements included the design of optics and light sources. Computer-designed glass rod and conventional lenses improved image, clarity, and brightness. Today instant photodocumentation using color prints of digitized images and electronic recording of video images with lightweight chip cameras provide an immediate objective record for the patient's chart and for referring physicians, and the option for viewing later by videotape.

Accessory procedures also have undergone rapid and significant improvements. In 1929 Kalk first performed guided needle biopsies of the liver for histologic examination, and Ruddock, the father of laparoscopy in the United States, introduced forceps biopsy of the liver followed by coagulation.[6] Tissue sampling with a biopsy forceps has become irreplaceable for evaluating focal hepatic disease and for peritoneal disorders and diseases of other organs. A proliferation of other procedures followed, such as transhepatic cholangiography or cholangiograms through direct puncture of the gallbladder and splenoportography.[7-9] Even retroperitoneal organs like the pancreas can be partially inspected by laparoscopy and

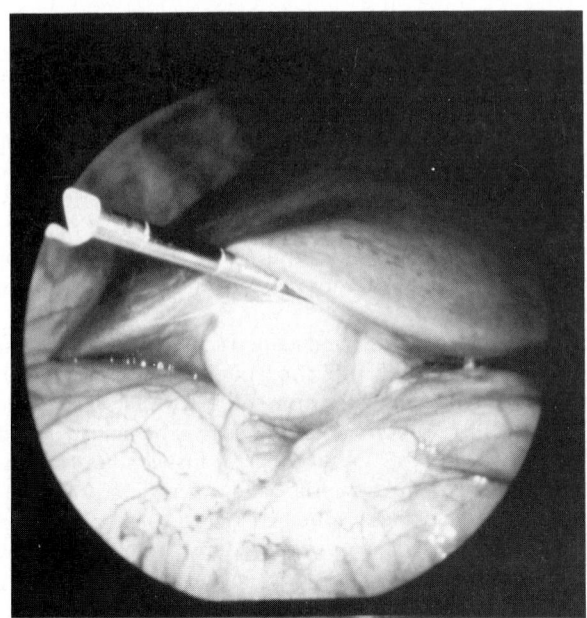

FIGURE 129-1. (See Color Fig. 109.) View of a normal right upper quadrant shows the liver margin elevated by a palpating probe passed by way of a 4-mm second-puncture trocar. Elevation of the liver margin provides a clear view of the gallbladder and permits inspection for hidden focal lesions such as metastases. The omentum (*lower left*) and the gastric antrum (lower right) are visible.

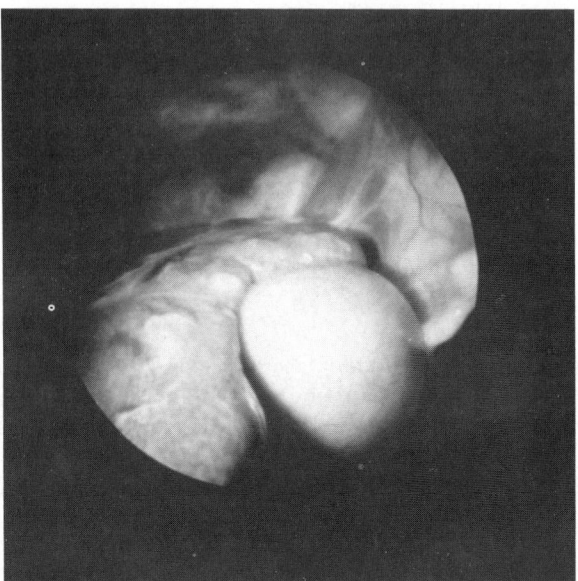

GURE 129-3. (See Color Fig. 111.) The right hepatic lobe has a dark green lobular pattern indicative of severe cholestasis. The gallbladder is distended and tense as a result of common bile duct obstruction; this is known as Cóurvoisier's sign. Along the medial margin of the right hepatic lobe are many 2- to 3-mm diameter metastases from carcinoma of the pancreas, which were not detected by imaging studies before laparoscopy. Laparotomy was avoided and an endoscopically placed biliary stent provided relief of bile duct obstruction.

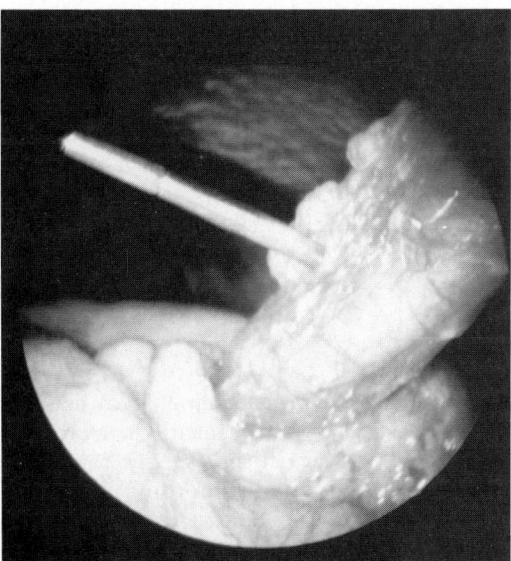

FIGURE 129-2. (See Color Fig. 110.) The round and falciform ligaments and the medial right hepatic lobe surfaces are covered with many small metastases from carcinoma of the stomach. Metastases on the anterior gastric wall are shown just below the round ligament (*bottom, center*). All staging studies before laparoscopy, including computed tomography, indicated that disease was limited to the stomach. This laparoscopic diagnosis prevented an unnecessary laparotomy.

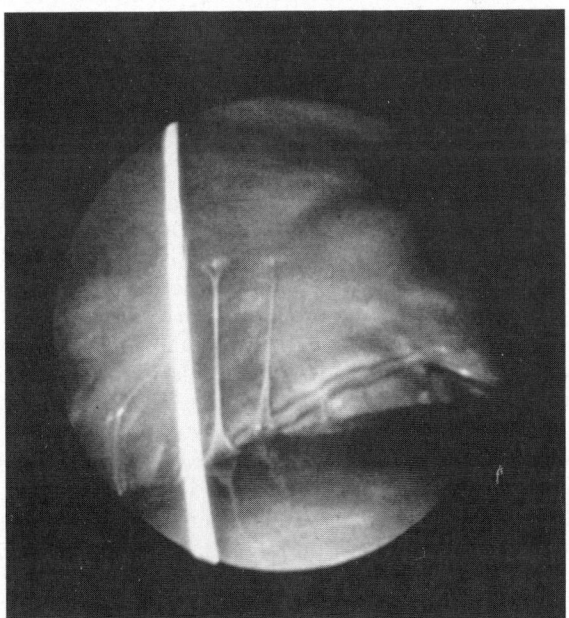

FIGURE 129-4. (See Color Fig. 112.) This view of the right hepatic lobe reveals several violin-string adhesions between the liver and peritoneum as a result of gonococcal perihepatitis. This young woman presented with recurrent, focal, perihepatic pain typical of the Curtis-Fitz-Hugh syndrome after developing gonococcal salpingitis.

safely undergo biopsy.[10,11] Today a multitude of accessories has been introduced for the various endoscopic operative procedures from appendectomy to Nissen fundoplication and bowel resection.

Laparoscopy has been developed and refined into an important procedure that plays a significant role in the evaluation and therapy of intraabdominal disorders.

Technical Applications

Instruments

Equipment for exploratory laparoscopy is less complicated than modern flexible fiberoptic endoscopes. The basic design principles have not appreciably changed in more than 50 years. A routine abdominal exploration can be performed with a minimum of equipment that costs less than a standard fiberoptic endoscope.[12-14]

Laparoscopic equipment consists of instruments for creating the pneumoperitoneum in addition to telescopes, trocar, light source, and accessory instruments. Gas is introduced into the abdominal cavity using a special needle (Veres) that allows sharp penetration of the abdominal wall. Once inside the abdominal cavity, a blunt, atraumatic obturator extends from the needle tip. Nitrous oxide is the preferred gas for gastroenterologic laparoscopy. This gas does not irritate the peritoneum and is absorbed faster than room air, which was used in the past. CO_2 causes abdominal pain from peritoneal irritation in patients who are examined under conscious sedation, which is preferred for diagnostic laparoscopy. Gynecologists and surgeons prefer CO_2 because it does not support combustion when electrocoagulation is used. However, many clinicians have used nitrous oxide during application of electrosurgical procedures with laparoscopy and believe it to be safe as well. Automatic insufflators that allow monitoring of intraabdominal pressure, gas flow rate, and volume of gas insufflated are convenient and have added to procedure safety.

Telescopes, defined as rigid metal tubes containing a series of optical lenses, come as forward-viewing 0-degree optics or oblique-viewing 50-degree optics. The latter type is preferred because it allows en face viewing of the hepatic surface, and through rotation provides a panoramic view. Telescopes are connected to high-intensity light sources by way of flexible fiberoptic light transmission cables. An array of accessory equipment is available including instruments for fluid aspiration, brush cytologic study, and needle and forceps biopsy. Electrocoagulation accessories are available, but their use for controlling bleeding is seldom necessary in diagnostic laparoscopy. An endoscopy table that allows head, foot, and lateral tilting is helpful. Laparoscopy requires sterile technique and instruments; however, performance of gastrointestinal diagnostic laparoscopy in the operating room is not necessary or desirable. Surgical and anesthesia backups are not required for diagnostic laparoscopy.[12-14]

Technique

Laparoscopy is performed after an 8-hour fast. The procedure is carried out using local anesthesia and sedation. The most important aspects of the technique are proper patient selection and preparation, and selection of the site for the insertion of the pneumoperitoneum needle and trocar. An opening is created by way of a 1-cm skin incision, and the abdominal wall is penetrated with a trocar and cannula. The usual site is above and left of the umbilicus, avoiding vascular structures, staying at least 5 cm from any mass or organ edge and 3 to 5 cm from any scar. Through insertion of the pneumoperitoneum needle and gas insufflation, a gas cupula is created that lifts the abdominal wall from the underlying structures, thereby creating an adequate space for insertion and manipulation of the telescope.

The movement of the telescope combined with patient positioning allows full inspection of the abdominal cavity. Exploration is aided by a palpating probe (see Fig. 129-1; see Color Fig. 109). Abnormal structures may be palpated, and organs may be lifted (e.g., the liver for inspection of its undersurfaces). The palpating probe and other accessory instruments, like cytology brushes and biopsy devices, may be passed through the channel of an operating endoscope or, preferably, through a smaller accessory trocar introduced at a separate site, usually in the right upper abdomen. Visual diagnosis can be enhanced by aspiration of fluid, brushing of abnormal surfaces for cytologic examination, and biopsy using various needles and forceps. After completion of the procedure and after adequate hemostasis of biopsy sites has been ensured, the pneumoperitoneum is removed. The instrument sites are closed with one or two sutures or skin clips. The small incision leaves a barely visible scar. Patients may be discharged on the same day. After liver biopsy, overnight monitoring in a short-stay observation unit is preferable.

Documentation

The laparoscopic results, including normal anatomic and pathologic findings, should be documented (see Figs. 129-1 through 129-4; see Color Figs. 109 through 112). These photographs are invaluable to referring physicians, consultants, and students. The entire procedure can be viewed on a video screen and recorded on VHS videotape using a lightweight video camera coupled to the telescope ocular. Digitized color images can be printed within 60 seconds, which can be attached to the patient chart and endoscopy report.

Indications

The use of exploratory laparoscopy should be defined relative to its role in the overall diagnostic plan. Therefore, all other diagnostic options and the patient's specific condition have to be taken into consideration. Unfortunately, medical diagnostic laparoscopy is not taught in most medical training programs and is not available in most hospitals. When available, expertise may vary. Furthermore, whereas laparoscopy usually is a low-risk procedure, this risk is directly related to the examiner's experience and the frequency with which the procedure is performed. In this era of cost containment, the procedure's accuracy, risks, and expense have to be compared with other diagnostic studies. Its high diagnostic accuracy and low risk make it a desirable alternative in many cases.

Focal Liver Disease

The patient with suspected focal liver disease is a common problem facing clinicians. This may occur in several clinical settings. The patient may have a known primary carcinoma, and liver metastases are suspected on clinical grounds or because of abnormal liver function studies. An unsuspected focal defect may have been noticed during hepatic sonography or CT scan done for other reasons. Finally, in a patient with known primary carcinoma, there may be no direct clinical evidence of hepatic metastases, and imaging studies of the liver may be normal, but the absence or presence of metastases may have a major impact on the patient's management (e.g., surgical resection for cure versus no surgery and palliative treatment). Therefore, it is of paramount importance that the true nature of a proven or suspected focal defect of the liver be determined with the most reliable test that can provide histologic confirmation. Laparoscopy appears ideally suited in these patients.[15]

Cancer Staging

The most common tumors that metastasize to the liver are colon, pancreas, breast, and lung. With the recent advances in surgical management and progress in radiation and chemotherapy, the exact tumor extent must be determined through proper staging. In cases of liver or peritoneal involvement, curative resection usually is not appropriate, and palliative treatment must be considered. In patients with carcinoma of the pancreas presenting with obstructive jaundice who at laparoscopy are found to have liver, omental, or peritoneal implants, use of endoscopic stents on the obstructed bile duct might offer the best palliation; in a patient with limited disease, an attempt of curative resection may be appropriate. The value of laparoscopy in this setting is the avoidance of unnecessary surgery through careful preoperative staging.[16,17] Whereas laparoscopy and image-guided biopsies are comparable in their diagnostic yield, if lesions have been seen on CT scan or US, laparoscopy is more sensitive in finding additional smaller lesions, omental seeding, and peritoneal spread. Laparoscopy is capable of isolating small omental lesions that might even escape detection at the time of exploratory laparotomy.[18,19]

In cancer of the pancreas and esophagus—tumors that are usually associated with alcohol abuse—laparoscopy can settle the question as to whether the hepatic abnormalities are from tumor or chronic alcoholic liver disease, such as cirrhosis. Laparoscopy has been well established as a dependable tool for tumor staging in patients with Hodgkin's disease and non-Hodgkin's lymphoma.[20] Because the lesions, especially in Hodgkin's lymphoma, frequently are small, laparoscopy can identify tumors not seen on CT scan or sonography. In cases of nonspecific surface changes, multiple biopsies from each lobe are recommended. Because the treatment schedule for various stages of Hodgkin's disease has undergone some recent changes and might vary in different institutions, the consultant gastroenterologist should confer with the oncologist. Hepatic involvement in Hodgkin's disease usually is an indication for chemotherapy, therefore laparoscopy is clearly indicated. Results of staging laparoscopy are comparable with those of exploratory surgery.[21] If splenectomy is part of the staging workup, laparotomy should be chosen rather than laparoscopy. Laparoscopy is valuable in the follow-up of patients after therapy.

Chronic Liver Disease

Laparoscopy with guided biopsy is the most reliable way to diagnose cirrhosis of the liver. However, percutaneous liver biopsy is the more frequently the first test. The sampling error with percutaneous biopsy is significant, especially if a Menghini-type aspiration needle is used.[22] The main problems with a percutaneous biopsy are a fragmented specimen and false-negative results, which often result from biopsy of a regenerating nodule. Laparoscopy, especially when combined with laparoscopic direct vision biopsy, far exceeds percutaneous blind biopsy in sensitivity and specificity.[23] Laparoscopy has additional advantages besides the high diagnostic yield. Portal hypertension, especially early changes, are easily recognized. A complicating hepatocellular carcinoma may be detected and confirmed by biopsy. Laparoscopy should be considered and hepatoma ruled out in a patient with known cirrhosis whose condition suddenly deteriorates. Serologic markers frequently are positive but not always. Although metastatic disease is less common in the cirrhotic liver, it does occur.[24]

The diagnosis of portal hypertension is easily made at laparoscopy by observation of the collateral vessels that regularly are present with this condition. In the abdomen without prior surgery or peritonitis, collateral vessels first are seen in the region of the phrenicolic and falciform ligaments. Other typical locations are the periumbilical area and about any adhesion between visceral and parietal peritoneum. Enlarged, tortuous veins in the gastroepiploic, ovarian, cecal, and gallbladder regions also are common. The spleen usually is significantly enlarged.

Even in chronic hepatitis a percutaneous biopsy is not necessarily a reliable test. Different degrees of inflammation may be present in both lobes, and in a certain number of cases even different diagnoses will be found in the right and left lobes.[25]

At a time when new therapies for hepatitis B and C are emerging, a definitive diagnosis must be established at the outset.

Ascites of Unknown Cause

In many cases the cause of ascites can be determined by simple studies of the paracentesis fluid; these must include, among others, bacterial cultures, amylase determination to exclude pancreatic ascites, and cytologic study of a cell block obtained by centrifugation of the fluid. A transudate is more common with portal hypertension, constrictive pericarditis, and congestive heart failure, whereas an exudate is more likely seen in infectious or neoplastic disorders; however, there are exceptions. If careful study of the ascitic fluid does not yield a diagnosis, exploratory laparoscopy is indicated. CT scan and US usually are unrewarding in evaluating the omentum and the peritoneum. Laparoscopy allows a definitive diagnosis in a high percentage of cases.[26–28] The most common findings are unsuspected cirrhosis, metastatic cancer, and tuberculous peritonitis. Ovarian carcinoma is one of the most common causes of peritoneal seeding, especially to the undersurfaces of the diaphragm. These sites warrant careful exploration in all cases of ascites of unknown cause.[29]

Abdominal Pain

It is unfortunate that most physicians believe that peritoneal adhesions should not be considered a cause for abdominal pain. This belief results in some patients having to endure years or a lifetime without finding a physician who understands the clinical aspects of adhesion-related abdominal pain well enough to take an adequate medical history. Adhesions are responsible for pain in a small number of patients. If the history is strongly suggestive, laparoscopy can confirm the diagnosis and in some cases allows therapy by electrosurgical lysis of adhesions. The patient may be disabled either by the severity of pain itself or the psychologic trauma caused by chronic, unexplained pain. Cancer phobia often is the patient's main problem. If the diagnosis can be established with certainty, many patients accept tolerable levels of discomfort and no invasive therapy is required.

In this situation, the usual evaluation of chronic abdominal pain frequently is nonrevealing and frustrating. The clinical history often suggests the diagnosis of a focal cause, usually adhesion related. Typically the physician fails to ask the proper questions or does not listen carefully to the patient's description. After a thorough laboratory, radiologic, and fiberendoscopic evaluation of these patients, laparoscopy can provide useful information.[12,14,30,31] Adhesions are common after surgery but also are found in patients without surgery who have had inflammatory and neoplastic processes. They are an uncommon cause of pain, but in some patients, they may cause debilitating chronic, recurrent pain. The site of focal pain is marked on the skin with gentian violet before laparoscopy.[12] At laparoscopy, the suspected area can be stimulated by traction on the adhesion to reproduce the pain. If a positive response is elicited, adhesiolysis may be appropriate. Equally important is a negative finding on exploratory laparoscopy, which excludes other significant organic causes for the patient's abdominal pain. The frequency of gynecologic causes for abdominal pain stresses the importance of careful pelvic exploration at the time of *gastroenterologic* laparoscopy.[31]

Hospital admission for observation for presumed acute appendicitis is a common occurrence. Acute appendicitis remains one of the more difficult diagnoses to make preoperatively with confidence. Diagnosis is especially difficult in women in the reproductive age group, with confirmation of suspected appendicitis proven at operation in only 50% to 60% of cases. Laparoscopy can resolve many of these cases.

Fever of Unknown Origin

The most common causes for fever of unknown origin are infection, malignancy, and collagen vascular disease. In the patient's workup, the physician usually is faced with the clinical situation where surgical exploration is considered to be the next step. Laparoscopy is a useful low-risk procedure in this setting and should be seriously considered in patients with fever of unknown origin, especially those with symptoms

or signs suggesting abdominal disease.[32] Adequate plans must be made for special tissue collection and cultures by having the proper fixatives and culture media available in the laparoscopy procedure room.

Risks and Contraindications

Laparoscopy is a remarkably safe procedure, considering its invasive nature. In six surveys and 17 series between 1954 and 1981 involving 204,591 cases, the overall complication rate was 1.86% with a mortality rate of 0.05%, which has remained remarkably stable for close to three decades. Serious complications, including the need for surgical intervention, occurred in 0.15%.[33] Complications are higher for physicians new to laparoscopy or for those who infrequently perform procedures. In training programs, residents performing laparoscopy under supervision have a good safety record.[34,35] Laparoscopic complication rates are significantly lower than morbidity and mortality rates related to exploratory surgery. Laparoscopy is a safe procedure with few contraindications. Because it is performed using local anesthesia and only conscious sedation, it is well tolerated even by debilitated patients.

Significant coagulopathy represents a contraindication. Because the liver biopsy site can be inspected for adequate clot formation and can be compressed and coagulated if necessary, laparoscopy still can be performed with a prothrombin time of 4 seconds over control and a platelet count of 50,000/mm³. However, normal coagulation studies are no safeguard against bleeding. A detailed history of any bleeding tendency in the patient or the in family is more important than laboratory studies. If any suspicion arises, additional clotting factors should be determined. Even though liver bleeding time does not appear to correlate directly with routine clotting studies, length of biopsy cylinder, or underlying liver disease, it is be wise not to ignore any abnormality in these parameters.[36] The physician who performs laparoscopy, image-guided biopsy, or "blind" needle liver biopsy must be aware that blood in the peritoneal cavity produces few diagnostic signs until large volumes accumulate. Therefore, the general status of the patient, weakness, light-headedness or tachycardia alone may be the only early indication. Abdominal wall infections are an absolute contraindication because they prevent sterile trocar insertion into the abdominal cavity. An acute abdomen or intestinal obstruction with abdominal distention precludes safe laparoscopy unless it is performed in a surgical setting.

Adhesions may limit abdominal exploration but do not represent a contraindication.[37] A veil of adhesion usually is attached to the undersurface of a surgical scar and may involve intestinal loops as well. If the trocar site is kept at least 3 to 5 cm from any scar, no problems should arise. Lower abdominal operations like an appendectomy and pelvic and sigmoid colon surgery usually do not present a problem if the main focus of interest is the liver and upper abdomen. An uncomplicated cholecystectomy may prevent examination of the right hepatic lobe, but the left lobe usually is well seen. Adhesions after transverse colectomy or gastrectomy may totally prevent examination of the upper abdomen. A long, xiphoid-to-pubis surgical scar with underlying adhesion may require two trocar passage sites to allow adequate examination on both sides of the abdomen. The second site is punctured only after the examination on one side proves the need for further exploration. These special clinical situations present more limitations of laparoscopy than contraindications. Before the procedure the patient should be informed of likely limitations caused by previous surgery and the possible need for two or more trocar sites.

A history of perforated viscus or generalized peritonitis, especially tuberculous peritonitis and, in some cases, Crohn's disease, are contraindications because of the extensive adhesions that present a significant risk for perforation of viscera and bleeding.

Morbid obesity is more of a limitation than a contraindication to laparoscopy. Obese abdominal walls make trocar insertion and manipulation difficult. Omental fat can markedly limit the intraabdominal view.

Chronic obstructive lung disease and congestive heart failure are relative contraindications. Here the procedure risk has to be balanced against the need for the laparoscopic information. If the patient can lie flat for 20 to 30 minutes, the procedure usually can be accomplished. Sedation should be kept to a minimum. Careful monitoring including pulse oximetry and cardiovascular responses are especially important in such patients.

Tense ascites prevents laparoscopy because there is usually no space for an adequate pneumoperitoneum. Exudative ascites can be safely drained before laparoscopy. A transudate from portal hypertension requires sensible mobilization therapy over time and proper patient stabilization before laparoscopy.

Results

Metastases Staging in Focal Liver Disease

Surgical and autopsy series have shown that when liver metastases are present, the liver surface is involved about 90% of the time.[16,38] By using proper techniques and a palpating probe to lift the right and left hepatic lobe for inspection of the undersurface, and by positioning the patient properly, about two thirds of the hepatic surface can be inspected and at laparoscopy[39] (see Fig. 129-2; see Color Fig. 110). The value of laparoscopy lies in the fact that lesions as small as 1 to 2 mm can be identified and can undergo biopsy.[12,14,18]

The histologic confirmation of focal defects on imaging studies is of major importance for prognosis and management. Whereas focal and contour abnormalities on hepatic scintigram in the past gave rise to a wide spectrum of differential diagnoses, hepatic sonography and CT scan have been able to resolve many of these issues. Simple or multiple hepatic cysts, a relatively common laparoscopic finding usually without clinical significance, are reliably diagnosed by these methods. The same is true for hemangiomas, which may present a significant hazard to percutaneous blind biopsy. CT scan with rapid infusion of intravenous contrast material usually gives a characteristic image. Laparoscopy rarely is needed for further clarification. Smaller hemangiomas are a common incidental finding. The laparoscopic features of multicystic appearance and bluish color are characteristic, and diagnostic biopsy is contraindicated. Other lesions for which scans are diagnostic when combined with modalities, such as serologic study, include amebic abscess and echinococcal cysts. Pyogenic liver abscess usually is diagnosed by US or CT scan with image-guided aspiration and drainage after amebiasis has been excluded.

The real value of laparoscopy lies in the fact that other benign lesions can undergo biopsy and be differentiated from malignancy, especially in cases of early small foci. Benign lesions include scars, focal fatty infiltration, tuberculosis, sarcoidosis, cholangiofibromas, peliosis, focal nodular hyperplasia, and others.[40] Excellent textbooks and atlases offer many examples.[41-44]

The most notable indication for laparoscopy is the evaluation of patients with suspected hepatic and peritoneal metastases. No other method, short of surgical laparotomy or postmortem examination, has the sensitivity and specificity of laparoscopy for hepatic and peritoneal metastases. The literature is replete with reports that support its use for this purpose. The accuracy rate of laparoscopy consistently has been reported over the last 30 years to be in the range of 88% to 95%.[26,45,46] Accuracy figures are unacceptably low only in reports of retrospective studies that presented data from chart reviews and procedures that did not use proper technique, such as failure to use a palpating wand to improve visualization of liver and other surfaces.[47]

When there is a need to know whether metastases to the liver and peritoneum are present and imaging methods with biopsy have failed to confirm their presence, direct examination of the abdominal viscera and peritoneum offers the most accurate and safe alternative.[48] Extensive abdominal metastases rarely should be diagnosed by laparotomy unless there is another reason for surgical intervention.

Recent reports have confirmed the value and safety of cytologic sampling by needle or brush during laparoscopy for the diagnosis of intraabdominal malignancy.[49-52] Cytologic study by abrasion or aspiration during laparoscopy in 927 patients was reported by Cusso and associates.[50] Cytologic study produced slightly more positive results, with an accuracy rate of 93.1%, than did biopsy at a rate of 86.4%, but the combined use of these sampling methods provided a diagnostic accuracy rate of 97.6%. An earlier report by Hajdu and associates on 1650 liver aspirates and laparoscopic brushings found an overall accuracy rate for cytologic examination of 96% with a sensitivity rate of 94% and a specificity rate of 100%.[49]

Cancer Staging

Carcinoma of the esophagus. Surgical resection for squamous cell and adenocarcinoma of the esophagus is associated with the highest mortality for any major elective operation. Proper staging for these lesions is essential because most patients have lost significant body weight and are considered among the worst of operative candidates. The finding of abdominal metastases is an absolute contraindication to resection of esophageal cancer because surgical resection for palliation only offers no advantages over other palliative measures.

Dagnini and associates reported the results of laparoscopic staging in 369 patients with cancer of the esophagus (280 cases) and cardia (89 cases).[17] They found single or multiple metastases to the liver, peritoneum, omentum, stomach, and lymph nodes in 52 patients (14%) and metastasis to the gastric wall or to the regional lymph nodes in 36 patients (9.7%). In the 250 patients who subsequently underwent laparotomy, false-negative findings by laparoscopy were documented in only 4.4%: 2.8% for liver, 1.2% for peritoneum, and 0.4% for omentum. In this series, the findings of severe portal hypertension led to rejection for surgical resection in 6.7% of esophageal cancer cases.

Carcinoma of the stomach. Gastric adenocarcinoma carries a dismal prognosis and requires complete staging evaluation before any decision is made regarding therapy. Laparoscopy has been shown to be the most sensitive method for proving the presence of liver and other abdominal metastases of this disease.[53] Any decision to operate on a patient with metastases should be based only on the strong indication for surgery to palliate severe gastric obstruction or bleeding in a patient whose general health is relatively good. Laparoscopy also may be helpful in a patient with positive findings on CT or US for which no histologic confirmation of metastasis has been obtained. A false-positive result on an imaging study without biopsy could lead to a decision not to operate on a person who may have a chance of cure.

The overall accuracy or efficiency rate of laparoscopy for metastatic gastric cancer is 96.5% (see Fig. 129-2; see Color Fig. 110).[53] This result is 5% to 20% superior to results from imaging methods used for this purpose, depending on the technique used.

As many as 40% of patients in one series with gastric cancer, who were considered resectable by the usual staging criteria, were found unresectable by laparoscopy; distant abdominal metastases were found in 12.5%.[54] The laparoscopic impression of resectability was confirmed at surgery in 87%.

Carcinoma of the gallbladder. Carcinoma of the gallbladder may present with one or a variety of clinical problems, rarely with clinical, laboratory, or radiologic findings that would make the physician strongly suspicious of this diagnosis. In the largest series of patients with gallbladder carcinoma studied by laparoscopy, gallbladder carcinoma was suspected clinically in only 10%.[55] Of 98 cases reported, the gallbladder could be completely examined in 48 patients but was partially hidden by adhesions in 21 and completely obscured by a mass of adhesions in 29. Evidence of metastasis was found in 89 of the 98 patients, so the fact that the organ was obscured totally or partially by adhesions created little problem in confirming the presence of malignancy. The diagnostic accuracy of carcinoma of the gallbladder by direct observation only is no better than 50%; however, with the high percentage of metastases usually present, a positive diagnosis by biopsy may be achieved in 90% of patients. The combined use of US and laparoscopy has a reported diagnostic accuracy rate of 100%.[56] Accurate assessment of resectability also is possible by laparoscopy.[54]

Hodgkin's disease and lymphoma. The use of laparoscopy for staging Hodgkin's disease is particularly valuable.[20,57] At initial presentation and with recurrence after therapy, this disease may present as tiny, 1- to 2-mm nodules over the liver surface.[58] Another clinical concern in this disease is the frequency of false-positive diagnosis of liver involvement in

higher than 20% of cases based on liver test and scan abnormalities.[59] The report by Coleman and researchers provides support for the opinion that laparoscopy has excellent overall accuracy and can be a valuable adjunct for staging Hodgkin's disease.[21] They reported on 34 patients evaluated by staging laparoscopy with 4 of these being confirmed by guided biopsy to have hepatic Hodgkin's disease. Multiple biopsies should be done to assist the pathologist in finding Reed-Sternberg cells to confirm the diagnosis. Laparotomy was performed on the 30 patients with negative results on laparoscopy, and only 1 was found to have Hodgkin's disease in the liver. A study from Italy on 121 patients with Hodgkin's disease also revealed an accuracy rate of about 80% for laparoscopy compared with staging laparotomy, which is the gold standard for this disease.[60]

Hepatocellular carcinoma. The prevalence of viral hepatitis and alcoholism throughout the world has led to an alarming increase in the frequency of hepatocellular carcinoma. This lesion accounts for 1% to 2% of all malignancies and has a 3 : 1 male preponderance. US- and CT-guided fine-needle aspiration have a sensitivity of only about 80%; i.e., 20% of patients have a false-negative result by this approach. This is especially a problem when this malignancy occurs in a cirrhotic liver. Needless laparotomy must be avoided in these patients because of their poor prognosis.

Jeffers and associates recently reviewed the results of laparoscopy in 27 patients with hepatocellular carcinoma evaluated over a 3-year period.[61] They used a laparoscopy-guided 22-gauge Chiba needle aspiration technique, moving this fine needle gently up and down through the lesion two or three times. They obtained 100% accuracy in establishing a cytologic diagnosis. Multiple lesions in 21 of 27 (78%), advanced cirrhosis in 23 of 27 (85%), and peritoneal metastases in 2 of 27 (7%) confirmed an unresectable status in all 27 patients.

Small focal hepatic lesions as small as 1 mm, and smaller than 1 mm with the magnifying laparoscope, are detectable by laparoscopy. So-called millimeter hepatoma is rare but can only be detected by biopsy of any atypical white or yellow spot seen during laparoscopy. Small foci of malignant neoplasms in inoperable patients may be amenable to local therapy by laparoscopically controlled microwave coagulation or alcohol injection.

The outcome of diagnostic laparoscopy for hepatocellular carcinoma is not yet established but appears to offer the most by its relative sensitivity for determining suitable candidates for hepatic resection or transplantation. No other procedure except exploratory laparotomy can answer the common questions relative to hepatic and peritoneal micrometastasis that are critical to making appropriate clinical decisions.[62,63] Although ultrasound is the most sensitive imaging technique for hepatocellular carcinoma, it is inferior to laparoscopy for the diagnosis of cirrhosis. In one report, cirrhosis was recognized in only 35 of 42 cases detected by laparoscopy. Small peritoneal metastases not found by ultrasound were confirmed by laparoscopy.[64]

Laparoscopy makes its greatest contribution to patients by avoiding needless surgery in these patients who, in most instances, have such a dismal prognosis.[65] Another advantage of laparoscopy is that the diagnosis of any primary or secondary cancer in the liver that seems potentially resectable can be confirmed without biopsy, avoiding any risk of malignant seeding.[66,67]

Adenocarcinoma of the pancreas.   Warshaw and associates clearly have shown the value and accuracy of laparoscopy for staging pancreatic cancer.[18,19] In their initial report, 40 patients were evaluated by all of the usual methods, were found to have no evidence of metastatic disease, and were considered for surgical exploration. In 14 of the 40 patients (35%), 1- to 2-mm metastases were found at laparoscopy and verified by biopsy. Because of these positive findings, therapy was altered in all 14 patients. For example, 2 of the patients had obstructive jaundice and received palliate treatment with biliary stents. The 26 patients with negative results from laparoscopy underwent laparotomy, and only 3 were found to have metastases not noticed at laparoscopy. In the the authors' opinion, two of the three cases of metastases likely were missed because a probe to allow inspection of the inferior surface of the liver was not used early in the study. In their latest report, they have further strengthened the indication for laparoscopy in staging pancreatic cancer.[19] They compared the value of CT, MR, angiography and laparoscopy and were able to identify correctly 90% of unresectable lesions. In 27 of 88 patients, small liver and peritoneal metastases were confirmed. CT missed all but two of these metastases, but laparoscopy with biopsy confirmed metastases in 22 or 23 (96%) instances.

Cuschieri reported on 73 patients undergoing laparoscopy for preoperative evaluation of pancreatic cancer.[68] Forty-two of the 73 patients were correctly staged as having incurable or inoperable disease. However, laparotomy performed in the 9 patients judged resectable by laparoscopy revealed that only 4 were resectable. Target biopsy or fine-needle cytologic study at laparoscopy confirmed the histologic diagnosis in 61 of 65 patients (92%). The goal in managing pancreatic cancer is to attempt cure for the minority shown to have disease limited to the pancreas, to provide palliation through surgery only for those who are not treatable by safer methods, and most importantly, to avoid physically stressing patients by needless surgery under the guise of palliation.

Adenocarcinoma of the colon.   When the carcinoembryonic antigen level rises above normal in patients who have undergone resection for colon cancer, a significant number are found to have liver metastases. Surgeons have considered second-look laparotomy to be the best way of evaluating for such recurrence.[69] If CT or US with guided biopsy gives negative results, laparoscopy offers a reasonable, low-risk alternative. If metastases to liver or peritoneum are confirmed, an unnecessary laparotomy can be avoided.

Adenocarcinoma of the breast.   Laparoscopy has been shown to be a useful complementary examination for staging breast cancer. Most benefit from this procedure is derived from its use in women believed to have the disease localized to the breast at the time of diagnosis. In one report, 8.5% of such patients were found to have metastases smaller than 1 cm visible in the liver after prior clinical evaluation, including imaging techniques, had not revealed evidence of liver involvement.[70] This finding converted presumed localized disease to a stage IV disease and ensured the correct decision regarding therapy.

The time saved by early detection allows proper treatment to be instituted, possibly months before the liver is found to be involved with metastases, based on symptoms or laboratory tests.

Carcinoma of the lung.   Laparoscopy has proven helpful in staging carcinoma of the lung. In 131 patients with small cell lung cancer evaluated by laparoscopy with liver biopsy and US with fine-needle aspiration, a total of 33 (25%) were found to have liver involvement.[71] In 104 patients in whom both examinations were considered *successful,* i.e., complete, laparoscopy confirmed 86% and US 79% with liver metastases. Seven percent had false-negative findings by laparoscopy and 14% had false-negative findings by hepatic US.

Carcinoma of the ovary.   The diagnosis and staging of ovarian cancer are prime indications for exploratory laparoscopy. This insidious, often occult, disease can become clinically manifest in many ways, often mimicking less severe diseases or functional disorders. Recent progress in therapy for this malignancy has made accurate staging and surveillance imperative for a successful outcome.

Ovarian cancer has a propensity for metastasizing to the peritoneum. These metastases tend to be small lesions and seem to prefer early localization to the undersurface of the right diaphragm.

Dagnini and colleagues reported the results of laparoscopy in 143 patients with ovarian cancer.[72] They used this endoscopic approach in four groups of patients: presurgical staging; postsurgical staging, which was incomplete at the time of the original operation; follow-up at the end of prescribed treatment; and restaging, carried out 8 to 36 months after apparent remission and after therapy was suspended.

The results by group were impressive: group 1, all 25 patients were found to have metastases; group 2, 45 patients had no evidence of metastases at prior surgery; in 35, laparoscopy also gave negative results, but in 10 (22%) metastases were confirmed and the staging was changed; group 3, in 50 patients with metastases confirmed before therapy, 17 had negative findings for abdominal ovarian malignancy; in 30 patients in whom results had previously been negative for metastases, the development of metastases was confirmed in 4; group 4, metastases were documented in 10 of 36 patients; metastases were suspected by clinical findings in only 5 of these patients with positive results.

Laparoscopy Versus Ultrasonography and Computed Tomography

Clinicians formerly chose between liver chemical studies, scintigrams, and biopsy—percutaneous, laparoscopic, or open—to evaluate patients with hepatic disease. Choices now include sonography, CT scan, and image-directed percutaneous biopsies. Cost considerations enter into the decision making as well. Often a patient undergoes multiple tests, including repeat examinations, before a definitive study is done, which adds to the cost and frequently delays diagnosis and treatment unnecessarily.

Most patients usually have a battery of screening liver tests followed by sonography or CT scan. A patient should not undergo laparoscopy without some prior imaging study. If a focal abnormality is detected, the clinician should decide which is the most accurate, safe, and cost-effective way to establish a correct diagnosis. The choices are percutaneous blind biopsy, image-directed biopsy, laparoscopy with guided biopsy, or open surgical biopsy. Surgical biopsy, bypassing other tests, rarely is indicated except in cases where the absence or presence of liver metastases would not alter the need for a surgical resection of the primary lesion, e.g., in a patient with obstructing colon cancer.

Postoperative adhesions and deep-seated lesions are not significant hindrances to laparoscopy.[15,71] The advantage of laparoscopy is the biopsy capability for small lesions and the detection of additional abnormalities like omental and peritoneal spread, which usually are missed by the other methods (see Fig. 129-3; see Color Fig. 111).[18,68] Another limitation of scan-directed fine-needle aspiration is the small caliber of the needle, which provides material for a cytologic smear only, rather than a core for true histologic examination.

Ultrasonography-guided fine-needle aspiration of a localized lesion appears comparable with laparoscopy and guided biopsy in sensitivity and specificity.[50,71] The same comparability is true for CT-directed and laparoscopy-directed biopsies.[15]

Brady and colleagues reported a well-designed prospective study comparing CT- and laparoscopy-guided percutaneous liver biopsy.[15] In patients with focal lesions on CT, the sensitivity rate for laparoscopy was 86% and for CT, 75%. This difference was not statistically significant. Both were 100% specific. Accuracy rate of laparoscopy was 93% and for CT it was 80%. Most important was the finding that the predictive value of a CT that gave negative results for focal hepatic lesions was only 50% compared with 89% for laparoscopy. Laparoscopy performed in 19 patients with a negative or normal result on CT scan revealed a normal liver in 8, benign disease in 5, and malignancy in 4. From this study it was concluded that blind-needle biopsy is 100% sensitive for metastases when there is 75% or higher involvement of the right lobe, and that CT-directed biopsy of focal lesions is a reasonably sensitive and less invasive procedure than laparoscopy for obtaining histologic confirmation. However, laparoscopy is at least equally sensitive and overall more accurate and has a far superior predictive value when results are negative than does the CT scan.

Brady and associates later expanded their study to patients with suspected liver or peritoneal metastases who had a negative finding on CT scan.[73] Malignancy was documented in 12 of 25 (48%) patients. Among 8 patients with exudative ascites and negative findings on abdominal CT plus at least one fluid cytologic study with negative results, 6 had peritoneal metastases at laparoscopy. The remaining 7 patients had benign liver disease documented by laparoscopy-guided biopsy. This study further emphasizes the fact that laparoscopy clearly is the preferred diagnostic procedure in patients with suspected abdominal malignancy when imaging studies with guided biopsy do not provide a positive diagnosis.[74]

Chronic Hepatitis and Cirrhosis

The availability of treatment for chronic hepatitis B and C has created more demand for diagnostic precision. Assessment of therapeutic response is impossible without accurate data on baseline liver histologic examination after therapy with interferon. The degree of hepatic inflammation and the presence or absence of cirrhosis are pertinent unknowns in any treatment protocol. This problem is readily resolved in most cases by direct vision-guided biopsies. Blind liver biopsies have been shown to be unreliable for the diagnosis of chronic hepatitis, which can be a patchy disease, and for cirrhosis, which has long been recognized by laparoscopists as difficult to exclude with blind-needle biopsy.[25,75–77]

Guided liver biopsies from both lobes during laparoscopy have shown different degrees of inflammation in 11 of 64 patients reported by Jeffers and colleagues.[25] In 5 of 64 patients the guided biopsy revealed a different diagnosis in the different lobes. High false-negative rates for biopsy diagnosis of cirrhosis associated with chronic hepatitis compared with laparoscopic diagnosis—23 of 41 versus 41 of 41—should clearly indicate the unreliability of biopsy alone for pretherapy and posttherapy examinations in therapeutic trials.[75]

It has been accepted that an average blind percutaneous liver biopsy, measuring 1.2 mm × 2.0 cm, representing between 1 of 50,000 and 1 of 100,000 of the total normal liver mass, is highly reliable for confirming a diagnosis of acute hepatitis or steatosis. Unfortunately this excellent reliability does not extend to less diffuse or focal diseases such as chronic hepatitis, granulomatous hepatitis, cirrhosis, and neoplasms, both primary and metastatic. Reports of the false-negative rates for cirrhosis vary from 10% to 67%.[78,79]

In another study, posthepatitic, macronodular cirrhosis could not be confirmed by blind percutaneous biopsy in 67% of patients known to have the condition by prior biopsy.[80]

Inspection of the liver surface with biopsy under direct visual control provides a diagnostic accuracy of 100% for cirrhosis and over 85% to 95% for other focal lesions including metastatic carcinoma. Laparoscopy usually resolves the differential diagnostic dilemma between focal neoplasm and cirrhosis that is relatively common in the alcoholic patient. A focal defect on CT scan may be caused by chronic alcoholic liver disease, such as cirrhosis, or by a malignancy metastatic to the liver, such as pancreatic or esophageal cancer, which are commonly associated with alcohol abuse.

Laparoscopy may provide additional helpful clinical information in patients with obscure illness suggestive of hepatic origin. Diseases such as schistosomiasis, echinococcosis, tuberculosis, and amebiasis usually are evaluated initially by CT or US, and in some, significant clinical confusion remains that could be resolved by direct inspection and liver biopsy.

Hepatic infections can present severe illness with difficulty in diagnosis, especially in immunocompromised hosts in whom hepatomegaly, ascites, fever, and abdominal pain may originate from many causes.[81] Focal hepatic candidiasis is being recognized as an increasingly significant problem in some patients.[82]

Retroperitoneal Disease

Although laparoscopy has not been considered a primary and reliable method for diagnosis of retroperitoneal disease, a report by Salky and colleagues has provoked reconsideration of this belief.[83] They reported on the results of laparoscopy in 19 of 316 (6%) patients in whom the indication was for diagnosis of retroperitoneal disease. The prerequisites used for laparoscopy were palpable lesions on abdominal examination or a CT or US finding positive for retroperitoneal disease. Barium contrast studies revealing displacement or compression of hollow viscera also were a reliable criterion for selection of patients for laparoscopy. Laparotomy was avoided in 16 of 19 patients because tissue sufficient for accurate histologic diagnosis was obtained by laparoscopy. In spite of this study, retroperitoneal disease usually is not considered a prime indication for laparoscopy.

Peritoneal Metastases

Laparoscopy is the best procedure for diagnosis of malignancy metastatic to the peritoneum. The only competing method is surgical exploration, which is associated with high morbidity, mortality, and high cost. Some evidence exists that exploratory laparotomy is less accurate than laparoscopy for diagnosis of small foci of multiple lesions or tiny, widely scattered peritoneal metastases. Even the most current CT and US methods have been proven ineffective for determining presence or extent of peritoneal metastases.[15,18]

Ascites of Unknown Cause

Diagnosis of the cause of ascites, especially the exudative type, is a major indication for laparoscopy. The results of its use have been clearly documented in many reports. Trujillo reported the results of laparoscopy in the evaluation of 48 patients with exudative ascites.[26] Results of prior blind peritoneal biopsy were normal in 5 patients, and cytology by paracentesis gave normal results in 25. The diagnoses in 43 (89%) patients at laparoscopy established a cause for the ascites: tuberculous peritonitis, 8; metastatic carcinoma to peritoneum, 11; hepatic cirrhosis, 14; ovarian cancer, 9; and chronic adhesive peritonitis secondary to prolonged peritoneal dialysis, 1. No pathologic disease in the peritoneum was found in 5 patients, but subsequently a diagnosis of polyserositis was made in 4 and constrictive pericarditis in 1 patient.[26]

A report by Coupland and associates indicates a success rate of 80.5% in establishing the cause of ascites, 90.9% for hepatomegaly, and 82.5% for abdominal masses.[27]

Suspected tuberculous infection of the peritoneum long has been recognized as a prime indication for diagnostic laparoscopy. Ascitic fluid often is nondiagnostic, and when positive results are found by culture of the acid-fast bacillus, there is a 3- to 4-week delay. Laparoscopy provides a diagnosis by direct vision laparoscopy within a few minutes and also serves to rule out other abdominal and peritoneal disorders. A report on 145 patients has clearly emphasized the clinical features and accuracy of laparoscopic diagnoses.[84] Only 18% of patients were found to have active pulmonary tuberculosis. Peritoneal tuberculosis will likely be seen more frequently with the recent increase in pulmonary tuberculosis in immunocompromised and immune competent persons.

Abdominal Pain

Acute and chronic perihepatitis. Acute right upper quadrant pain secondary to acute peritonitis, or perihepatitis, or more subacute or chronic pain secondary to perihepatic adhesions is called the Curtis-Fitz-Hugh syndrome. Classically, both types of the disorder are related to pelvic infection, that is, bacterial salpingitis, usually gonococcal. The syndrome may simulate acute appendicitis, acute cholecystitis, or pyelonephritis and has been reported in one homosexual man with gonorrheal infection and an immunodeficiency syndrome compatible with acquired immunodeficiency syndrome. The diagnosis was confirmed by the finding of typical perihepatic adhesions at laparoscopy.[85]

Laparoscopy has proven to be the only nonsurgical method to confirm the diagnosis of the Curtis-Fitz-Hugh syndrome (see Fig. 129-4; see Color Fig. 112). In addition to confirming perihepatitis with or without adhesions, the pelvic organs can be inspected for evidence of inflammation.[86] A recent study from the United Kingdom reports six cases presenting as acute surgical emergencies mimicking other acute disorders. Five of the six cases dated back to a difficult or complicated termination of pregnancy. All six cases were diagnosed by laparoscopy.[87]

Chronic adhesive peritonitis. One of the most common concerns relative to laparoscopic technique is placement of the trocar insertion site in patients with scars, and likely adhesions, secondary to previous abdominal surgery. Adhesions rarely cause difficulty with laparoscopy when proper patient selection is used.[88] Experience has shown that complications related to adhesions from surgery are rare if the pneumoperitoneum and trocar placement sites are kept 3 to 5 cm from the closest margin of a surgical incision.[12–14] The major risks here would be puncture of adherent bowel or laceration of a collateral vessel in a patient with portal hypertension. Postoperative adhesions rarely are clinically significant causes of pain, but when they are, the patient may go for years untreated because many physicians believe adhesions never cause symptoms.

Orlando and associates reported their observations on laparoscopy in 250 patients who had undergone previous abdominal surgery.[37] This number represented 12.5% of their series of 2000 laparoscopies performed to evaluate liver disease. The whole surface of the liver was visible in 45.3% but only partially visible in 46.2% in patients who had upper abdominal surgery. After cholecystectomy the right liver lobe is only partly visible in 50% of patients, but the left lobe is nearly always visible. This fact must be taken into consideration during planning and performance of the procedure. Lower abdominal surgery was associated with complete visibility of the liver in 97.5% of patients. Interestingly, patients with prior exploratory laparotomy had the highest incidence of nonvisibility of the liver: 28.5%. This finding likely resulted from the fact that abdominal pain from some form of peritonitis prompted the surgery and produced the adhesions. In their 1750 patients without abdominal surgery, only 4.1% were found to have adhesions.[37]

Marin and colleagues reported the use of prelaparoscopic US to detect abdominal adhesions and thereby assist in proper site selection for instrument insertion.[89] The ultrasound examination was performed after pneumoperitoneum. The site and extent of adhesions were determined and later confirmed during laparoscopy in almost all instances.

Adhesion-related abdominal and pelvic pain. The gynecologist sees many more adhesion-related pain syndromes earlier than other physicians and usually accepts this possibility more readily. Persistent pelvic or abdominal pain of at least 6 months' duration, in the same location, of a sharp or stabbing nonradiating nature, that is increased by activity that may produce jarring or stretching between abdominal or pelvic organs and the parietal peritoneum, often is related to adhesions. The clinician must use specific criteria and an observation period of several months before proceeding to laparoscopy. If this is done, the diagnostic yield can be good. Kresch and colleagues reported results of laparoscopy in 100 women with pelvic pain that persisted in the same location for at least 6 months and compared these findings in 50 asymptomatic women who had laparoscopy for tubal ligation.[90] Overall, 83% of the group with pelvic pain had abnormal pelvic organs compared with 29% of the asymptomatic group. Adhesions were the most common pathologic finding in the symptomatic group, accounting for pain in 38%, and pelvic endometriosis was the cause for pain in 32%. The majority of patients with chronic pelvic pain from adhesions had prior abdominal-pelvic surgery or had a history of pelvic inflammatory disease.

One report on 27 patients, 19 with suspected acute appendicitis, resulted in avoidance of laparotomy in 15 patients.[91] The appendix was seen in 24 of 27 with help from a palpating probe passed through a separate site in the right lower quadrant. Five of the 12 patients who underwent surgery had the type of incision changed because of the laparoscopic diagnosis. Twenty-two of the 27 laparoscopies provided a diagnosis. Hospital stay for the 15 patients in whom surgery was avoided was only 1.7 days compared with 5.6 days for those with acute appendicitis. Safety of laparoscopy in such patients also was demonstrated because a single small wound hematoma was the only complication.

Sugarbaker and colleagues reported a reduction in diagnostic errors in patients with acute abdominal pain from 22% in the laparotomy-only group to 4% in the laparoscopy group.[92] The performance of unnecessary laparotomy was reduced, obviously because of laparoscopic accuracy. When the appendix is not seen or a diagnosis is not established by laparoscopy, a laparotomy is indicated. Obviously, a false-negative finding from laparoscopy and avoidance of laparotomy could be disastrous.

In another report, 36 women in the fertile age group with nondiagnostic pelvic examinations and with a diagnosis of acute appendicitis were subjected to laparoscopy before surgery.[93] As a result of the laparoscopy, one third of the patients were found to have acute gynecologic disease not requiring operation, and surgery was cancelled.

Pelvic Pain in Children and Adolescents

The use of laparoscopy in children and adolescents has provided a high diagnostic yield, especially in those with acute and chronic pelvic pain.[94] In this study by Wolfman and Kreutner,[94] one group of patients had pelvic pain, 36 (43%) had acute, and 48 (57%) had chronic pain. Eighty-nine percent of those with acute pain had pelvic pathologic findings, whereas 73% of those with chronic pain had pathologic findings. The most common finding in patients with acute pain was functional ruptured or unruptured cysts of the ovary in 31%. Pelvic inflammatory disease at 25% and problems with intrauterine pregnancy at 19% were next in frequency. Only

14% of patients had ectopic pregnancy. The most common diagnosis in all patients with chronic pain was pelvic inflammatory disease in 33%, followed by normal results from examination in 27% and endometriosis in 19%. The combination of pelvic pain and a palpable mass usually indicated pelvic inflammatory disease in 39% or a cyst in 39%, whereas patients with dysmenorrhea usually had endometriosis. Another indication for laparoscopy during adolescence was to investigate primary and secondary amenorrhea. Based on laparoscopic findings in this report, 11.6% of the total 112 patients were found need a laparotomy.

Vercellini and associates have confirmed the value of laparoscopy for evaluating chronic pelvic pain that is defined as constant or intermittent, cyclic or acyclic pain that persists for 6 months or more and includes dysmenorrhea, deep dyspareunia, and intermenstrual pain.[95] Nearly 60% of 47 patients between 11 and 19 years of age had treatable pelvic disease.

In the adolescent with pelvic pain, the documentation of disease or normalcy has significant practical and psychologic implications. Laparoscopic examination is an important component of the orderly evaluation of these patients.[96,97]

Fever of Undetermined Origin

Laparotomy is indicated in patients with a fever of undetermined origin who have symptoms or signs of abdominal disease.[98] The results of laparoscopy as a substitute for laparotomy in such patients are related to the selection criteria. In one report, 60 of 70 patients with unexplained fever had signs of abdominal disease or abnormal liver tests.[32] Laparoscopy was helpful in 76.6% of these 60 patients but was helpful in only 2 of 10 (20%) of patients with normal findings from abdominal examination and liver tests. Laparoscopy proved of special value when fever was caused by neoplasm, necrotizing angiitis, chronic active hepatitis, and granulomatous liver lesions. It also helped establish the diagnosis in 15 of 21 patients (71.4%) whose fever was caused by infection. Surgery was avoided in 82.8% of these 70 patients. Surgery was performed in 12 patients, in 6 of these to treat disorders found at laparoscopy.

Most authors agree that an exploratory laparoscopy should be done before surgical exploration in patients with abdominal signs and symptoms who have had negative results from complete evaluation, including appropriate imaging and serologic studies.[99]

Cost Analysis

Although many laparoscopies are performed as part of a more extensive in-hospital evaluation, the largest cost saving has resulted from the recognition that the technique can be performed safely in an outpatient setting. When liver biopsy is performed, patients are observed in a short-stay observation unit, usually overnight. Table 129-1 shows costs in dollars as of October 1988 in a large urban teaching hospital in southeastern United States, including all institution charges and physician fees, such as for the gastroenterologist, pathologist, radiologist, anesthesiologist, and surgeon. Indirect costs like travel expenses, loss of time from work, and recuperation are

TABLE 129-1
Cost Analysis for Liver Biopsy

	LENGTH OF STAY	PHYSICIAN CHARGES*	INSTITUTION CHARGES*	TOTAL CHARGES*
Percutaneous liver biopsy	23 h	310	247	557
Laparoscopy without liver biopsy	8 h	850	456	1306
Laparoscopy with liver biopsy	23 h	985	631	1616
Computed tomography–directed biopsy	23 h	455	823	1278
Exploratory surgery with biopsy	3 d	2,135	2,481	4616

* US $ (Oct. 1988).

Data from a major urban teaching hospital, southeastern United States.

not included. Whereas absolute costs may vary from region to region and from one institution to another, the relative differences should remain fairly constant.[100]

Percutaneous liver biopsy is the least expensive procedure, whereas laparoscopy with guided biopsy is approximately three times more costly. This is appropriate considering the low yield of percutaneous biopsy in focal liver disease coupled with the additional benefits of laparoscopy provided by the capability for multiple biopsies, control of bleeding, and total abdominal exploration including examination of peritoneum and omentum with a low false-negative rate.

These additional benefits of laparoscopy justify the additional cost over CT scan–directed biopsy in special clinical situations. The real value of laparoscopy becomes apparent when costs, morbidity, and mortality are compared with those of exploratory surgery, which unfortunately is the only alternative to proper diagnostic laparoscopy in many hospitals in this country. The increasing use of laparoscopy by surgeons may solve this problem.

Recommendations

Many patients are subjected to major abdominal surgery to resolve relatively simple problems that could have been managed by laparoscopy. Unfortunately, many communities have no physician or surgeon adequately trained in diagnostic laparoscopy.

Gynecologists, and more recently, general surgeons, often are the only persons available to perform the procedure, and they are hindered by their relative unfamiliarity with nonsurgical abdominal diseases. Gastroenterologists, gynecologists, and general surgeons should be trained to perform diagnostic laparoscopy.

THERAPEUTIC LAPAROSCOPY

Laparoscopy has seen an explosion since the introduction of laparoscopic cholecystectomy into the United States by Muehe in 1986.[101] Diagnostic laparoscopy is an important procedure in clinical medicine, and therapeutic laparoscopy is the newest development in this field. The first and best-understood application of laparoscopic therapy is laparoscopic cholecystectomy. However, a variety of other techniques are being evaluated or used. These include laparoscopic antireflux procedures, appendectomy, hernia repair, colectomy, vagotomy, and hysterectomy. Because technology is developing so rapidly, the information available on these techniques is not yet complete.

Issues include morbidity, mortality, cost, disability, discomfort, and time away from work compared with gold standard approaches. It is hoped that as each new application is considered, these issues will be studied in well-designed and controlled studies. Other issues include the following: who should do the procedure; what training and certification are required; what are the indications for each procedure; and how the laparoscopic procedure compares with the standard approach. In the following sections the status of laparoscopic cholecystectomy is presented. This is an exciting new approach to the therapy of gallstones. It demonstrates some of the important issues that must be considered with the introduction of each new laparoscopic approach to medical problems.

History and Development

More than 60 years ago, Ruddock, an American internist,[102] and Zoeckler, a gastroenterologist,[103] introduced laparoscopy. Internists and gastroenterologists were more interested in flexible endoscopy and new imaging techniques. Surgeons also were not interested in laparoscopy at that time, and training was minimal. Of the surgical specialists, gynecologists were the first group to recognize and use laparoscopic therapy.[104] In some hospitals, one third of gynecologic procedures in operating rooms are laparoscopic. Hysterectomy and other procedures that were previously performed as open procedures increasingly are assisted by laparoscopy. Oncologists reported the use of laparoscopy as early as 1962,[105,106] but surgeons still were reluctant to accept it.

Muhe reported laparoscopic cholecystectomy in 1986,[101] followed by the surgeons Dubois and associates,[107] Perissat and colleagues,[108] and Reddick and Olsen.[109] During the last 3 years the technique has expanded, and now hospitals have performed thousands of laparoscopic cholecystectomies and many laparoscopic common bile duct explorations.[110]

Patients began to demand laparoscopic cholecystectomy, and surgeons had to learn the techniques of this procedure as quickly as possible.[111,112] A National Institutes of Health Consensus Statement on the topic of gallstones and laparoscopic cholecystectomy stated that "in comparison with open cholecystectomy, laparoscopic cholecystectomy provides a safe and effective treatment for most patients with symptomatic gallstones and has become the treatment of choice for many patients."[113] This is influenced by a 1- to 2-day hospital stay compared with 3 to 7 days for open cholecystectomy; less discomfort and pain postoperatively; smaller scars; slightly lower cost; and 7 to 14 days away from work and usual activities compared with 20 to 40 days for the open cholecystectomy approach.

Technical Applications

Training in Laparoscopic Cholecystectomy

The techniques for laparoscopic cholecystectomy are different than for open exploration, and therefore retraining is necessary. Working while watching a television monitor is required, as well as using new tactile sensations. Training and experience are critical for this technique, as is judgment regarding when to convert the procedure to an open cholecystectomy. There was concern about whether the courses offered to teach laparoscopic cholecystectomy were adequate for training. Consequently the Society of American Gastrointestinal Endoscopic Surgeons organized guidelines for training, standards of practice, and obtaining privileges.[112] The National Institutes of Health organized a Consensus Conference in 1992 to discuss laparoscopic cholecystectomy.[113] It was also necessary to incorporate laparoscopic techniques into the training of surgical residents. Some of the initial difficulties involved a shortage of trained and experienced teachers. This problem is less acute now because more people are experienced in laparoscopic techniques. The National Institutes of Health estimates that as of 1992, more than 15,000 surgeons have been trained in laparoscopic cholecystectomy.

Because a small but unavoidable number of laparoscopic cholecystectomies must be urgently converted to open procedures, the operator must be experienced and have hospital privileges to perform open biliary tract surgery. This conversion is not from a complication of laparoscopic cholecystectomy but must be considered when severe bleeding occurs, or if the anatomy of the biliary tree is aberrant or cannot be clearly identified at the time of laparoscopic cholecystectomy. The laparoscopist must be prepared and capable of performing open biliary surgery with cholecystectomy and common bile duct exploration.

Experienced laparoscopists suggest that surgeons with limited experience probably should not perform laparoscopic cholecystectomy on patients with acute cholecystitis, jaundice, common duct stones, cirrhosis, obesity, and previous abdominal surgery. After performing 25 to 50 laparoscopic procedures, the physician can begin to approach these more complex cases.

Instruments

Laparoscopic surgical procedures have required development of a new set of instruments. These include graspers, insufflators, and new imaging systems.[114,115] The cost of these instruments must be factored into analyses when laparoscopic

cholecystectomy is compared with open surgical cholecystectomy. Operating room time may be longer with the laparoscopic technique than with open surgery. However, hospitalization and disability times are reduced with the laparoscopic approach, which balances the cost equation.

Technique

The operator should be trained and familiarized with the equipment. All equipment should be reviewed and checked for proper functioning. Informed consent is essential, including discussing the possibility of conversion to an open procedure. The conversion rate from a laparoscopic to an open procedure is estimated to be 3% to 6% for elective cases.[116] In acutely ill patients, conversion may be required more often. The procedure is imaged on a television monitor, which magnifies the image and allows the entire team to watch and assist. It is recommended that the procedure be videotaped so that it can be reviewed routinely. Fluoroscopy must be available for routine cholangiography during laparoscopy.

General anesthesia is used with endotracheal intubation. A nasogastric tube is placed, as is a Foley catheter. During the procedure, physiologic parameters are monitored. If hypercapnia develops and cannot be corrected with increased ventilation, the procedure must be stopped and the pneumoperitoneum desufflated. If the situation stabilizes, the procedure can be resumed with a lower pressure pneumoperitoneum.

First it is necessary to create an optimal pneumoperitoneum with CO_2 gas. A trocar with a spring tip is used. The spring prevents injury to intraabdominal organs after the trocar is inserted blindly into the peritoneal cavity. Once the pneumoperitoneum is established, the remainder of the instruments are inserted under visual control.

The abdominal organs are inspected and the gallbladder is located. Adhesions present are dissected free. It is recommended that no structure be grasped or transected before it is identified. If unusual anatomy is encountered and cannot be clarified, it is suggested that the procedure be converted to an open operation. Rather than a failure, this decision is considered sound judgment.

Intraoperative cholangiography should be available. Modern digitized fluoroscopy and cholangiography avoid some of the problems found in older operating room units. Older units were mobile but difficult to position, with long exposure times, no fluoroscopy, the problem of inadvertent overfilling, and the risk of missing small stones. The films often were not informative, and the procedure was unnecessarily slow. The new units provide fluoroscopy with filming capability as well. Just a few minutes are needed to obtain a cholangiogram.

Fluoroscopy allows clarification of the 10% of patients with anomalous anatomy and can reduce the likelihood of unnecessary ductal injuries, such as the short cystic duct. This duct is present and drains into the right hepatic duct in 2% of patients and into the common hepatic duct in 1% of patients. Sometimes confusion exists between the cystic duct and the common bile duct. Contrast cholangiography with fluoroscopy can resolve this problem and also can identify stones in the common duct, determine the size and number of stones, and direct therapy during the laparoscopy or afterward when an endoscopic approach is used to remove the stones, such as endoscopic retrograde cholangiopancreatography (ERCP) or endoscopic retrograde sphincterotomy.[117]

Unsuspected common bile duct stones occur in 5% to 10% of patients despite normal liver function tests.[118] These stones should be removed either during laparoscopy with the application of laparoscopic choledocholithotomy or after the procedure, with ERCP. If the laparoscopic removal technique is to be applied, fluoroscopy is essential to determine the size and number of stones, the location of the stones, the anatomy and size of the ducts, and to assist with stone removal. Laparoscopic choledocholithotomy probably will become an important skill for surgical laparoscopists to enable them to solve the patient's gallstone problem at one session.

Indications

The indications for laparoscopic cholecystectomy are the same as for open cholecystectomy. Approximately 80% of cholecystectomies are accomplished with the laparoscope.[113] Usually it is not recommended that asymptomatic gallstones be removed in any patients. Once symptoms occur, it is anticipated that symptoms will recur in most patients; therefore gallbladder removal is recommended. In these symptomatic patients it is estimated that 25% will develop complications over 10 to 20 years. This can be compared with patients with asymptomatic gallstones in whom it is estimated that only 10% will develop symptoms in the 5 years after diagnosis and only 20% will develop symptoms in the 20 years after diagnosis. Overall, the laparoscopic approach is thought to be useful in 85% to 90% of patients with symptoms from gallstones who would otherwise be candidates for open surgical cholecystectomy.

Laparoscopic cholecystectomy is thought to be useful in some clinical circumstances with gallstone-related complications such as acute cholecystitis and resolved gallstone pancreatitis. In some complicated clinical presentations, however, laparoscopic cholecystectomy is contraindicated. These include cholangitis with septic shock, gallbladder cancer, advanced cirrhosis with portal hypertension, severe coagulopathy, peritonitis, and acute pancreatitis.[113] Obesity is only a contraindication if the abdominal wall is so thick that the instruments are too short to reach the gallbladder and perform the necessary surgery. Obesity may also make the procedure more difficult because of a heavy omentum that must be manipulated to image the gallbladder.

Use of laparoscopic cholecystectomy in pregnancy is not yet fully understood. The exact risk of laparoscopic cholecystectomy in the first trimester is unknown. In the second trimester, laparoscopic cholecystectomy may be useful, but the surgeon must be prepared to handle complications if they occur. In the third trimester, laparoscopic cholecystectomy is not recommended because of potential risk to the uterus.

Overall, the indications for removal of the gallbladder are not changed by the availability of laparoscopic cholecystectomy.

Difficult Clinical Circumstances

Usually the indications for laparoscopic cholecystectomy are the same as for traditional open cholecystectomy. However, the following difficult clinical presentations deserve comment.

Acute Cholecystitis

The diagnosis of acute cholecystitis usually is made from the clinical presentation and the ultrasound, which often shows a thick gallbladder wall, edema, and inflammation with a "halo" effect. The likelihood of technical problems during laparoscopy is increased if acute inflammation is present. Adhesions must be carefully dissected, and adjacent organs, such as the colonic hepatic flexure and duodenum, must be carefully examined. The infundibulum of the gallbladder may be adherent to the common duct. The possibility of perforation or damage to adherent organs is increased during dissection. If the dissection is not progressing well, it is often best to convert to an open cholecystectomy. A laparoscopic cholecystocholangiogram may be helpful to identify the anatomy.

Empyema of the Gallbladder

Empyema of the gallbladder requires decompression of the gallbladder with a direct puncture into the distended organ. A plastic bag placed around the gallbladder is essential because an infected gallbladder can spill and contaminate the peritoneal cavity before it is removed from the abdominal wall. If the gallbladder is necrotic, conversion to an open procedure is recommended. If bile does leak, copious irrigation of the right gutter is recommended. Clinically, even acutely ill patients often experience rapidly defervescence after removal of the inflamed gallbladder.

Cirrhosis or Severe Fatty Infiltration

Because of the weight and position of the liver, cirrhosis or severe fatty infiltration may interfere with visualization of Calot triangle, an essential maneuver in laparoscopic cholecystectomy. Conversion to an open procedure must be considered.

Risks and Contraindications

Bleeding

Oozing may necessitate placing a drain in the subhepatic space at the end of the procedure. If sudden arterial bleeding occurs, hemostatic maneuvers must be done quickly. Care must be taken during application of a clip or suture to the bleeding artery to be certain that no adjacent organs or structures, such as the bile duct, are injured. If several attempts to control bleeding fail, conversion to an open procedure is essential.

Bile Leakage

An accessory duct can enter the gallbladder through the liver bed. During dissection, a small opening can be seen through which bile appears. It is recommended that the liver bed be inspected several times before the already dissected gallbladder is removed. If bile leakage is seen at a small duct, it often can be coagulated or a suture can be placed to close the leak. If bile pooling is seen in the area of the common bile duct or cystic duct stump, and if the source cannot be found, the patient should have open exploration. Fluoroscopy and cholangiography also may show extravasation of contrast and indicate a leak. Furthermore, if during cholangiography contrast does not appear in the proximal ductal system, obstruction by a misplaced clip may be responsible. If these injuries or obstructions are noticed, immediate open exploration can be used to repair the problem. Bile spillage occurring during the procedure usually can be managed with irrigation and fluid removal from the right pericolic gutter. If necessary, a drain tube can be placed in the subhepatic area.

Common Duct Stones

Common duct stones can be removed during laparoscopic cholecystectomy by way of the cystic duct. This is successful if the stones are small and if the cystic duct can be safely dilated. Cholangiography can identify the stones, and if necessary the cystic duct can be dilated with a balloon catheter under fluoroscopic control. Small flexible choledochoscopes, with an operating diameter of 2.8 to 3.3 mm, also can assist with management of retained stones. Wire baskets can grasp and remove stones through the cystic duct. In the case of a large stone, a pulse dye laser or electrohydrolytic lithotriptor can fracture the stone, allowing the fragments to be removed under endoscopic control.[119]

After stone removal, a cholangiogram is obtained to confirm that there are no more stones. The cystic stump then can be closed. This can be accomplished quickly with an excellent success rate.[120] If problems occur the procedure can be converted to an open procedure. It is also possible to leave a small catheter in the common duct by way of the cystic duct. This allows a cholangiogram on the eighth postoperative day. If the radiograph gives negative results, the tube is pulled the following week. If a stone is discovered on the follow-up tube cholangiogram, ERCP with sphincterotomy with possible assistance from wires passed through the drainage tube in the common duct can be performed to remove the stone. If small stones are located in the cystic duct or common duct, it may be possible to irrigate with warm saline after intravenous administration of glucagon to flush out the stones. This is followed by a cholangiogram to confirm the disappearance of the stone.[121]

An alternative approach for stone removal is laparoscopic choledocholithotomy. The common duct can be opened during laparoscopy after a cholangiogram confirms large calculi. This technique is difficult but can remove large or multiple stones even from the proximal ducts. After removal, a T-tube is placed and secured with sutures or the duct can be closed primarily with a small catheter placed through the cystic duct for drainage of the common duct. Overall, laparoscopic stone removal will eventually approach the success of choledocholithotomy during open surgery.[121]

If a stone is left and cannot be removed, a drainage tube is placed into the cystic duct to make it easier to perform ERCP and endoscopic retrograde sphincterotomy postoperatively.

Complications

The mortality rate for laparoscopic cholecystectomy is less than 1%, as is the mortality for open cholecystectomy.[113] The morbidity rate for laparoscopic cholecystectomy is 2% to 5%

compared with 4% to 8% for the open procedure. These statistics are influenced by the indications for the procedures and the overall risk category of the patient. Ductal injury is reported to occur more frequently with laparoscopic cholecystectomy than with open surgery. Open surgery is associated with injuries in 0.1% to 0.2% of patients.[122] In laparoscopic cholecystectomy, the rate of ductal injury is higher at 0.2% to 0.6%.

Interestingly, only 10% of ductal injuries such as bile leak are recognized in the first week. They usually present as acute biliary peritonitis. Two thirds of patients with ductal injury present with strictures, as long as 1 year after the laparoscopic cholecystectomy. Most of these injuries are associated with technical problems, judgment errors, or failure to recognize ductal anatomic anomalies. Fluorocholangiography can reduce these injuries because it can detect anatomic variations, such as aberrant cystic duct drainage, before an injury occurs. If an injury does occur, intraoperative cholangiography can discover the leak or detect the obstructed duct by nonfilling of the proximal ductal system, so that these problems can be fixed immediately by conversion to an open laparotomy.

If a ductal injury is recognized, it should be repaired immediately with open exploration. The outcome is better with immediate repair than with delayed repair several days later when an anastomosis must be attempted in an infected environment. Thermal injuries from lasers or electrocautery may interfere with the blood supply and result in development of a leak or stricture formation.[123] ERCP proves essential in the diagnosis and assessment of bile leak.

Because most patients have no symptoms after laparoscopic cholecystectomy, any symptom on the first postoperative day, such as nausea or pain, even if vague, is justification for an emergency hepatic iminodiacetic acid scan. If the scan gives negative results, the patient is observed carefully for 1 more day to rule out an accidental enterotomy. If the hepatic iminodiacetic acid scan is positive, an emergency ERCP is recommended. If a leak is found, use of stents by means of ERCP is recommended.[124] This is followed by an immediate CT scan. If an accumulation of bile is seen, percutaneous drainage is recommended. If this is not successful, open drainage or laparoscopic drainage is indicated. If these complications are missed in a patient with vague symptoms for several days, the patient may present with peritonitis, cholangitis, or sepsis with high rate of associated morbidity and mortality. Late sequelae also may occur.[125,126] Strictures, cholangitis, and secondary biliary cirrhosis with portal hypertension are serious long-term consequences of complications of biliary surgery.[127]

During dissection of the gallbladder, especially if it is acutely inflamed, a perforation can occur with spillage of stones, especially small stones. These stones should be located and removed to prevent an intraabdominal abscess from forming around the calculus several months later.[127a,*]

Clips can migrate; therefore chromic catgut sutures are recommended to close the cystic duct. A migrated clip can be the nidus for a common bile duct stone.[128]

Injury can occur to the intestine with the use of a 2-mm pneumoperitoneum needle. If such an injury is recognized during laparoscopy, the area is irrigated and aspiration is performed repeatedly. The area is examined carefully. It is rec-

---

* Scott-Conner CEH, personal communication, June 1992.

ommended that a nasogastric tube remain in place and the patient remain in the hospital with nothing taken orally for 24 to 48 hours with close observation. Usually these small holes close spontaneously. Trocar injury to other abdominal organs have been described, including injury to the aorta. If recognized by sudden hypotension or shock, immediate exploration can repair the injury. Trocar or enterotomy injuries may not be recognized immediately, especially in the elderly patient. Development of an ileus on the second postoperative day is an indication of a problem that must be treated. After a laparoscopic cholecystectomy, the abdominal cavity is carefully inspected for blood or leakage of bile or intestinal contents. However, occasionally an injury will occur and not be detected at the end of the procedure; therefore close postoperative observation is essential.[129]

Bleeding is suspected if tachycardia, hypotension, or other signs of hemorrhage occur, or if hematocrit values change significantly. Bleeding from the cystic artery or liver bed must be considered and treated as an emergency.

Minor complications include infection of the umbilical trocar site and rare umbilical hernias. If large trocar sites are closed subcutaneously, hernias can be prevented.

Overall, excellent training and willingness to convert to an open procedure can reduce the risks of laparoscopic cholecystectomy to a minimum.

Laparoscopy and Biliary Endoscopy

Sphincterotomy and ERCP are important techniques associated with laparoscopic cholecystectomy.[130] These techniques are especially important if the surgeon is unable to perform laparoscopic choledocholithotomy or unwilling to convert to an open procedure. Intraoperative cholangiography is important to detect stones and to confirm removal of stones in the event that endoscopic retrograde sphincterotomy and stone removal were performed before the laparoscopic cholecystectomy.[131]

In high-risk patients, ERCP can be useful, especially in those who have severe underlying disease such as cholangitis or jaundice. Ideally stones in the gallbladder and common duct should be resolved in one session at laparoscopy. This will be more easily accomplished when laparoscopic choledocholithotomy is more widely used. Careful removal of all common duct stones also will reduce the likelihood of later stricture formation.

For diagnosis and therapy, ERCP is essential postoperatively if a retained stone is found, if leakage of bile occurs, or if a stricture is found. ERCP is one of the most important tools in the physician's armamentarium in the postoperative period of a patient with biliary complications.

Other Applications of Laparoscopic Therapy

Laparoscopic therapy has other applications in addition to cholecystectomy, but it is too early in the development of these procedures to draw conclusions about how they compare with surgical procedures. The reports are few and follow-up periods are short. Safety, efficacy, and cost-benefit ratios are not yet assessed.

Inguinal Hernia Repair

Inguinal hernias can be treated on an outpatient basis in most instances, under local anesthesia with intravenous sedation. Patients are discharged the same day. Using laparoscopy, the extraperitoneal approach is changed to an intraperitoneal approach requiring general anesthesia. This is associated with significantly increased operating room costs for the laparoscopic approach because of the added instruments and increased time in the operating room. The issue is whether the risk of general anesthesia and the increased operating room time will be balanced by lower recurrence rates and less postoperative disability. It is possible that bilateral or recurrent hernias will be better indications for laparoscopic surgery than a simple unilateral inguinal hernia.

Anti–Gastroesophageal Reflux Procedures

Repair of hiatal hernia and antireflux procedures are promising areas for patients with severe reflux esophagitis who might otherwise need to remain on medications for their lifetimes. Laparoscopic Nissen's repair or other procedures can be accomplished and improve reflux symptoms. Preoperative assessment is critical so that the procedure can be tailored to the patient's anatomy and physiologic needs. The initial data are promising, but more time is needed to obtain an objective picture.

Colectomy or Partial Colectomy

Laparoscopic colectomy is technically difficult, time consuming, and requires a team approach. More data are needed to assess this procedure and to compare it with open surgery over longer periods of follow-up than are available. Efficiency, safety, and cost must be studied in comparison with open approaches.

Future Applications

This is an exciting time in the evolution of laparoscopic surgical techniques. As each new application is presented, outcome data must be examined regarding the overall safety, effectiveness, cost-benefit ratio, patient discomfort, and required physician training compared with conventional open surgical techniques. Many physicians believe that the majority of intraabdominal procedures will eventually be accomplished laparoscopically. More work in comparative studies and instrument design will be required to reach this objective.

The reader is directed to Chapter 43, Approach to the Patient With Ascites; Chapter 100, Abdominal Cavity: Anatomy, Structural Anomalies, and Hernias; Chapter 102, Diseases of the Mesentery and Omentum; and Chapter 103, Diseases of the Peritoneum.

REFERENCES

1. Kelling G. Über die Besichtigung der Speiseröhre und des Magens mit biegsamen Instrumenten. Presentation at the 73. Versammlung Dtsch Naturf Ärzte, Hamburg, 1901.

2. Kelling G. Über die Besichtigung der Speiseröhre und des Magens mit biegsamen Instrumenten. Verh Dtsch Ges Naturf Ärzte 1902;73:117.

3. Jacobaeus HC. Über die Möglichkeit die Zystoskopie bei Untersuchungen seröser Höhlungen anzuwenden. Münch Med Wochenschr 1910;57:2090.

4. Kalk H. Erfahrungen mit der Laparoskopie (Zugleich mit Beschreibung eines neuen Instrumentes). Z Klin Med 1927;111:303.

5. Henning N, Keilhack H. Farbenphotographie der Magenhöhle. Dtsch Med Wochenschr 1938;54:1328.

6. Ruddock JC. Peritoneoscopy. West J Surg 1934;42:392.

7. Royer M, Colombato LO, Nazure PA. Peritoneoscopic cholangiography with manometric control. Gastroenterology 1954;26:626.

8. Wannagat L. Indikationen der direkten Cholezysto-Cholangiographie und Cholangiographie. Dtsch Med Wochenschr 1969;41:2111.

9. Wannagat L. Die Splenoportographie. Leber Magen Darm 1973;3:3.

10. Meyer-Burg J. The inspection, palpation and biopsy of the pancreas by peritoneoscopy. Endoscopy 1972;4:99.

11. Ishida H. Peritoneoscopy and pancreas biopsy in the diagnosis of pancreatic disease. Gastrointest Endosc 1983;29:211.

12. Boyce HW Jr. Laparoscopy In: Schiff L, ed. Diseases of the liver. Vol. 1. 7th ed. Philadelphia: JB Lippincott, 1993:226.

13. Boyce HW Jr, Palmer ED. Techniques of clinical gastroenterology. Springfield, IL: Charles C Thomas, 1975.

14. Nord HJ. Technique of laparoscopy. In: Sivak M, ed. Gastroenterologic endoscopy. Philadelphia: WB Saunders, 1987:994.

15. Brady PG, Goldschmid S, Chappel G, et al. A comparison of biopsy techniques in suspected focal liver disease. Gastrointest Endosc 1987;33:289.

16. Hogg L, Pack GT. Diagnostic accuracy of hepatic metastases at laparotomy. Arch Surg 1956;72:251.

17. Dagnini G, Caldironi MW, Marin G, et al. Laparoscopy in abdominal staging of esophageal carcinoma: a report of 369 cases. Gastrointest Endosc 1986;32:400.

18. Warshaw AL, Tepper JE, Shipley WU. Laparoscopy in the staging and planning of therapy for pancreatic cancer. Am J Surg 1986;151:76.

19. Warshaw AL, Gu Z, Wittenberg J, et al. Preoperative staging and assessment of resectability of pancreatic cancer. Arch Surg 1990;125:230.

20. DeVita VT, Bagley CM, Goodell B, et al. Peritoneoscopy in the staging of Hodgkin's disease. Cancer Res 1971;31:1746.

21. Coleman M, Lightdale CJ, Vinciguerra VP, et al. Peritoneoscopy in Hodgkin's disease: confirmation of results by laparotomy. JAMA 1976;236:2634.

22. Pagliaro L, Rinaldi F, Craxi A, et al. Percutaneous blind biopsy versus laparoscopy with guided biopsy in the diagnosis of cirrhosis: a prospective randomized trial. Dig Dis Sci 1983;28:39.

23. Nord HJ. Biopsy diagnosis of cirrhosis: blind percutaneous versus guided direct vision techniques. A review. Gastrointest Endosc 1982;28:102.

24. Zotti S, Piccigallo E, Rampinelli L, et al. Primary and metastatic tumors of the liver associated with cirrhosis: a study based on laparoscopy and autopsy. Gastrointest Endosc 1986;32:91.

25. Jeffers LJ, Findor A, Thung SN, et al. Minimizing sampling error with laparoscopic guided liver biopsy of the right and left lobes. Gastrointest Endosc 1991;37:A266.

26. Trujillo NP. Peritoneoscopy and guided biopsy in the diagnosis of intraabdominal disease. Gastroenterology 1976;71:1083.

27. Coupland GAE, Townend DM, Martin CJ. Peritoneoscopy: use in assessment of intraabdominal malignancy. Surgery 1981;89:645.

28. Villa F, de Guzman S, Steigman F. Peritoneoscopic findings in ascites. Gastrointest Endosc 1968;14:48.

29. Bagley CM, Young RC, Schein PS, et al. Ovarian cancer metastatic to the diaphragm: frequently undiagnosed at laparotomy. Am J Obstet Gynecol 1973;116:397.

30. Gaisford W. Laparoscopy in management of chronic abdominal pain. Second International Symposium, Laparoscopy: Diagnostic and Therapeutic Techniques, Lake Buena Vista, Florida, Dec 3–5, 1985.

31. Yuzpe A. Gynecologic laparoscopy for the gastroenterologist. In: Sivak M, ed. Gastroenterologic endoscopy. Philadelphia: WB Saunders, 1987:1125.

32. Solis-Herruzo JA, Benita V, Morillas JD. Laparoscopy in fever of unknown origin: study of seventy cases. Endoscopy 1981;13:207.

33. Nord HJ. Complications of laparoscopy. Endoscopy 1992;24:693.

34. O'Kieffe DA, Boyce HW Jr. Peritoneoscopy: has this procedure come of age? Med Ann DC 1972;41:437.

35. Phillips RS, Reddy KR, Jeffers LJ, Schiff ER. Experience with diagnostic laparoscopy in a hepatology training program. Gastrointest Endosc 1987;33:417.

36. Ewe K. Bleeding after liver biopsy does not correlate with indices of peripheral coagulation. Dig Dis Sci 1981;26:388.

37. Orlando R, Lirussi F, Okoliczanyi L. Validity of laparoscopy after abdominal surgery. Endoscopy 1987;19:150.

38. Foster JH, Berman MM. Solid liver tumors. Philadelphia: WB Saunders, 1977.

39. Whitcomb FF, Gibb SP, Boyce HW. Peritoneoscopy for the diagnosis of left lobe lesions of the liver. Arch Intern Med 1978;138:126.

40. Vogel HM, Fredrich K, Koch H. Ultrasound in cholangiofibromas of the liver detected by laparoscopy. Endoscopy 1988;18:185.

41. Beck K. Color atlas of laparoscopy. 2nd ed. Philadelphia: WB Saunders, 1984.

42. Henning H, Look D. Laparoskopie. Atlas and Lehrbuch. Stuttgart: Thieme, 1985.

43. Dagnini G. Clinical laparoscopy. Padua: Picin, 1980:307.

44. Bruguera M, Bordas JM, Rodes J. Atlas of laparoscopy and liver biopsy. Philadelphia: WB Saunders, 1979:215.

45. Ruddock JC. Peritoneoscopy. South Surg 1939;8:113.

46. Kuster G, Biel F. Accuracy of laparoscopic diagnosis. Am J Med 1966;42:388.

47. Danielson KS. Tomography and peritoneoscopy for detection of liver metastases: review of Mayo Clinic experience. J Comput Assist Tomogr 1983;7:230.

48. Leuschner M, Leuschner U. Diagnostic laparoscopy in focal parenchymal disease of the liver. Endoscopy 1992;24:689.

49. Hajdu SI, D'Ambrosio FG, Fields V, Lightdale CJ. Aspiration and brush cytology of the liver. Semin Diagn Pathol 1986;3:227.

50. Cusso X, Marti-Vicente A, Mon'es-Xiol J, Vilardell F. Laparoscopic cytology: an evaluation. Endoscopy 1988;20:102.

51. Vilardell F. The value of laparoscopy in the diagnosis of primary cancer of the liver. Endoscopy 1977;9:20.

52. Grossman E, Goldstein MJ, Koss LG, et al. Cytologic examination as an adjunct to liver biopsy in the diagnosis of hepatic metastases. Gastroenterology 1972;62:56.

53. Possik RA, Franco EL, Pires DR, et al. Sensitivity, specificity, and predictive value of laparoscopy for the staging of gastric cancer and for the detection of liver metastases. Cancer 1986;58:1.

54. Kriplani AK, Kapur BML. Laparoscopy for pre-operative staging and assessment of operability in gastric carcinoma. Gastrointest Endosc 1991;37:441.

55. Dagnini G, Marin G, Patella M, et al. Laparoscopy in the diagnosis of primary carcinoma of the gallbladder. Gastrointest Endosc 1984;30:289.

56. Kriplani A, Jayant S, Kapur B. Laparoscopy in primary carcinoma of the gallbladder. Gastrointest Endosc 1992;38:326.

57. Beck K, Dischler W. Die diagnostische Bedeutung der Laparoskopie beim Morbus Hodgkin. In: Stacher A, ed. Leukämien und maligne Lymphome. München: Urban & Schwarzenberg, 1972.

58. Bagley CM, Thomas LB, Johnson RE, Chretien PB, DeVita VT. Diagnosis of liver involvement by lymphoma: results of 96 consecutive peritoneoscopies. Cancer 1973;3:840.

59. Givler RL, Brunk SF, Hass CA, Gulesserian HP. Problems of interpretation of liver biopsy in Hodgkin's disease. Cancer 1971;28:1335.

60. Beretta G, Spinelli P, Ritke F, et al. Sequential laparoscopy and laparotomy combined with bone marrow biopsy in staging Hodgkin's disease. Cancer Treat Rep 1976;60:1231.

61. Jeffers L, Spieglman G, Reddy R, et al. Laparoscopically directed fine needle aspiration for the diagnosis of hepatocellular carcinoma: a safe and accurate technique. Gastrointest Endosc 1988;34:235.

62. Kameda Y, Shinji Y, Nishiuchi M, et al. Detection of minute hepatocellular carcinoma with fatty metamorphosis by laparoscopy. Endoscopy 1988;20(suppl):A29.

63. Brady PG. Laparoscopy and ultrasonography in the diagnosis of hepatocellular carcinoma (editorial). Gastrointest Endosc 1989;35:577.

64. Gandolfi L, Muratori R, Salmi L, et al. Laparoscopy compared with ultra-sonography in the diagnosis of hepatocellular carcinoma. Gastrointest Endosc 1989;35:507.

65. Nord HJ, Brady PG. Endoscopic diagnosis and therapy of hepatocellular carcinoma. Endoscopy 1993;25:126.

66. Lightdale CJ. Laparoscopy for cancer staging. Endoscopy 1992;24:682.

67. Watanabe M, Shimada Y, Nagooka S, et al. A case of laparoscopically detected cholangiocarcinoma of a few millimeters in size, with portal fibrosis. Endoscopy 1987;19:39.

68. Cuschieri A. Laparoscopy for pancreatic cancer: does it benefit the patient? Eur J Surg Oncol 1988;14:41.

69. Attiyeh RR, Stearns MW Jr. Second look laparotomy based on CEA elevations in colorectal cancer. Cancer 1981;47:2117.

70. DeSouza LJ, Shinde SR. The value of laparoscopic liver examination in the management of breast cancer. J Surg Oncol 1980;14:97.

71. Hansen SW, Jensen F, Pedersen NT, et al. Detection of liver metastases in small cell lung cancer: a comparison of peritoneoscopy with liver biopsy and ultrasonography with fine-needle aspiration. J Clin Oncol 1987;5:255.

72. Dagnini G, Marin G, Caldironi MW, et al. Laparoscopy in staging, follow-up and restaging ovarian carcinoma. Gastrointest Endosc 1987;33:80.

73. Brady PG, Peebles M, Goldschmid S. Role of laparoscopy in the evaluation of patients with suspected hepatic or peritoneal malignancy. Gastrointest Endosc 1991;37:27.

74. Nord HJ, Boyd WP. Diagnostic laparoscopy. Endoscopy 1992:133.

75. Jeffers LJ, Findor A, Thung SN, et al. Minimizing sampling error with laparoscopic guided biopsy of right and left lobes. Gastrointest Endosc 1991;37:A266.

76. Vajro P, Hadchouel P, Hadchouel M, et al. Incidence of cirrhosis in children with chronic hepatitis. J Pediatr 1990;117:392.

77. Orlando R, Lirussi F, Okoliksanyi L. Laparoscopy and liver biopsy: further evidence that two procedures improve the diagnosis of liver cirrhosis. J Clinical Gastroenterol 1990;12:47.

78. Lindner H. Grenzen und Gefahren der perkutanen Leberbiopsie mit der Menghini-Nadel. Dtsch Med Wochenschr 1967;92:1751.

79. Vido I, Wildhirt E. Korrelation des laparoskopischen und histologischen Befundes bei chronischer Hepatitis und Leberzirrhose. Dtsch Med Wochenschr 1969;94:1633.

80. Soloway RD. Observer error and sampling variability tested in evaluation of hepatitis and cirrhosis by liver biopsy. Am J Dig Dis 1971;16:1082.

81. Jeffers LJ, Algate I, Reddy KR, et al. Laparoscopic findings in AIDS and ARC patients. Gastrointest Endosc 1991;37:A267.

82. Gordon SC, Watts JC, Veneri RJ, et al. Focal hepatic candidiasis with perihepatic adhesions: laparoscopic and immunohistologic diagnosis. Gastroenterology 1990;98:214.

83. Salky BA, Bauer JJ, Gelernt IM, et al. The use of laparoscopy in retroperitoneal pathology. Gastrointest Endosc 1988;34:227.

84. Manohar A, Simjee AE, Haffejee AA, et al. Symptoms and investigative findings in 145 patients with tuberculous peritonitis diagnosed by peritoneoscopy and biopsy over a five year period. Gut 1990;31:1130.

85. Winkler WP, Kotler DP, Saleh J. Fitz-Hugh and Curtis syndrome in a homosexual man with impaired cell-mediated immunity. Gastrointest Endosc 1985;31:28.

86. Cano A, Fernandez C, Scapa M, Boixeda D, Plaza G. Gonococcal perihepatitis: diagnostic and therapeutic value of laparoscopy. Am J Gastroenterol 1984;79:280.

87. Foster HM. Curtis-Fitz-Hugh syndrome: the new mimicking disease? Ann R Coll Surg Engl 1986;68:271.

88. Pleissner T, Berndt H, Gutz H-J. Laparoscopy following abdominal operations. Endoscopy 1978;10:187.

89. Marin G, Bergano S, Miola E, Caldironi MW, Dagnini G. Prelaparoscopic echography used to detect abdominal adhesions. Endoscopy 1987;19:147.

90. Kresch AJ, Seifer DB, Sachs LB, Barrese I. Laparoscopy in 100 women with chronic pelvic pain. Obstet Gynecol 1984;64:672.

91. Anderson JL, Bridgewater FHG. Laparoscopy in the diagnosis of acute lower abdominal pain. Aust NZ J Surg 1981;51:462.

92. Sugarbaker PH, Sanders JH, Bloom BS, Wilson RE. Preoperative laparoscopy in diagnosis of acute abdominal pain. Lancet 1975;1:442.

93. Deutsch AA, Zelikovsky A, Reiss R. Laparoscopy in the prevention of unnecessary appendicectomies: a prospective study. Br J Surg 1982;69:336.

94. Wolfman WL, Kreutner K. Laparoscopy in children and adolescents. J Adolesc Health Care 1984;5:261.

95. Vercellini P, Fedele L, Arcaini L, et al. Laparoscopy in the diagnosis of chronic pelvic pain in adolescent women. Reprod Med 1989;34:827.

96. Anteby A, Schenker J, Poleshuk Z. The value of laparoscopy in acute pelvic pain. Ann Surg 1974;181:484.

97. Goldstein DP. Acute and chronic pelvic pain. Adolesc Gynecol 1989;36:573.

98. Keller JW, Williams RD. Laparotomy for unexplained fever. Arch Surg 1965;90:494.

99. Henning H. Value of laparoscopy in investigating fever of unexplained origin. Endoscopy 1992;24:687.

100. Nord HJ. Laparoscopy. In: Fleischer D. Diagnostic and therapeutic endoscopy: a resource manual. Manchester, MA: American Society of Gastrointestinal Endoscopy, 1989.

101. Muhe E. Die Erste Cholezystektomie durch das Laparoskope. Langenbecks Arch Klin Chir 1986;369:804.

102. Ruddock JD. Peritoneoscopy. Surg Gynecol Obstet 1937;65:523.

103. Zoeckler SJ. Peritoneoscopy: a reevaluation. Gastroenterology 1958;34:969.

104. Frangenheim H. Laparoscopy in diagnostic gynecology. Endoscopy. New York: Appleton-Century-Crofts, 1976.

105. Berci G. Peritoneoscopy. Br Med J 1962;1:562.

106. Berci G. Laparoscopy for oncology. In: Moossa Ar, Robson MD, Schimpff SC, eds. Comprehensive textbook of oncology. Baltimore: Williams & Wilkins, 1989:210.

107. Dubois F, Berthelot G, Levard H. Cholecystectomies par coelioscopie. Presse Med 1989;18:980.

108. Perissat J, Collet D, Belliard R. Gallstones: laparscopic treatment—cholecystectomy, cholecystectomy and lithotripsy. Surg Endosc 1990;4:1.

109. Reddick EJ, Olsen DO. Laparoscopic laser cholecystectomy: a comparison with mini-laparoscopic cholecystectomy. Surg Endosc 1989;3:131.

110. Phillips E, Berci G, Carroll B, et al. The importance of intraoperative cholangiography during LC. Am J Surg 1990;56:792.

111. Berci G, Sackier JM, Paz-Partlow M. Laparoscopic cholecystectomy mini access surgery: reality or utopia? Postgrad Gen Surg 1990;2:50.

112. Society of American Gastrointestinal Endoscopic Surgeons (SAGES) Standards of Practice in Gastrointestinal Endoscopy for Surgeons. SAGES publication, 1990.

113. NIH Consensus Statement. Gallstones and laparoscopic cholesystectomy. Vol 10. No 3. Washington, DC: National Institutes of Health Office of Medical Applications Research, 1992.

114. Berci G. Laparoscopic surgery. In: Problems in general surgery. Philadelphia: JB Lippincott 1991:284.

115. Cuschieri A, Berci G. Laparoscopic biliary surgery. 2nd ed. Boston: Blackwell Scientific Publications, 1992.

116. Sackier JM. The complicated laparoscopic cholecystectomy case. Gastrointest Endosc Clin North Am 1993;3(2):283.

117. Berci G. Biliary ductal anatomy and anomalies: the role of intraoperative cholangiography (IOC) during laparoscopic cholecystectomy. Surg Clin North Am 1991;72(5):1069.
118. Berci G, Hamlin JA. Operative biliary radiology. Baltimore: Williams & Wilkins, 1981.
119. Berci G. Intraoperative biliary endoscopy. In: Haubrich W, Schaffner F, et al, eds. Bockus gastroenterology, 5th ed. Philadelphia: WB Saunders, 1994.
120. Berci G, Phillips E. Laparoscopic cholecystectomy and choledocholithiasis. In: Braasch J, Tompkins R, eds. Surgical disease of the biliary tract and pancreas. Chicago: Mosby, Yearbook, 1994.
121. Shimi S, Banting S, Cushieri A. Transcystic drainage after laparoscopic exploration of common bile duct. Mini Invasive Ther 1992;1:273.
122. Lillimore KD, Pitt HA, Cameron JL. Current management of benign bile duct strictures. In: Advances in surgery. Chicago: Mosby, 1992;25:119.
123. Moossa AR, Easter DW, Van Sonnenberg E, et al. Laparoscopic injuries to the bile duct. Ann Surg 1992;215:203.
124. Kozarek R. Endoscopic management of bile duct injury. Gastrointest Endosc Clin North Am 1993;3:261.
125. Moossa AR, Easter DW, Van Sonnenberg E, et al. Laparos-
copic injuries to the bile duct: a cause for concern. Ann Surg 1992;215:203.
126. Davidoff AM, Pappas TN, Murray EA, et al. Mechanisms of major biliary injury during laparoscopic cholecystectomy. Ann Surg 1992;215:196.
127. Morgenstern L, Berci G, Pasternak E. Bile leakage after biliary tract surgery: a laparoscopic perspective. Surg Endosc 1993;7:432.
127a. Wilton PB, Andy OJ Jr, Peters JJ, et al. Laparoscopic cholecystectomy. Surg Endosc 1993;7:537.
128. Janson JA, Cotton PB. Endoscopic treatment of a bile duct stone containing a surgical staple. HPB Surg 1990;3:67.
129. Airan M, Appel M, Berci G, et al. Retrospective a prospective multi-institutional laparoscopic cholecystectomy study organized by the Society of American Gastrointestinal Endoscopic Surgeons (SAGES). Surg Endosc 1992;6:169.
130. Cotton PB, Lehman G, Vennes J. Endoscopic sphincterotomy complications and their management: an attempt at consensus. Gastrointest Endosc 1991;37:383.
131. Fletcher DR. Laparoscopic cholecystectomy: role of preoperative and postoperative endoscopic retrograde cholangiopancreatography and endoscopic sphincterotomy. Gastrointest Endosc Clin North Am 1993;3:249.

Textbook of Gastroenterology, second edition, edited by Tadataka Yamada. JB Lippincott Company, Philadelphia © 1995.

CHAPTER 130

Endoscopic Mucosal Biopsy

Rodger C. Haggitt   Cyrus E. Rubin

Technical Considerations
Indications for and Interpretations
of Endoscopic Biopsy
  Premalignant and Malignant Gastrointestinal Lesions
  Benign Esophageal Disease
  Diffuse Benign Gastric Mucosal Abnormalities

  Discrete Gastric Lesions
  Disease of the Proximal Small Bowel and Ileum
  Disease of the Colon
Contraindications and Risks
Cost Effectiveness

Endoscopy is an excellent tool for visualizing gross mucosal lesions, but only histologic evaluation of a biopsy provides a definitive diagnosis. Furthermore, endoscopically normal-appearing esophageal, gastric, small intestinal, or colonic mucosa may on biopsy reveal a variety of clinically significant histologic abnormalities. These include various inflammatory lesions, dysplasia, carcinoma, and many other conditions.

Before the introduction of flexible fiberendoscopy, much

of the stomach, duodenum, and colon were inaccessible to biopsy under direct visual control. The histologic diagnosis of mucosal disease was limited to blind suction biopsy techniques, biopsy by way of rigid tubular endoscopes, and laparotomy. The practice of gastroenterology and of gastrointestinal pathology has been revolutionized by the development of long, flexible, coherent, fiberoptic bundles in the mid-1950s by Lawrence Curtis, an undergraduate physics student at the University of Michigan working with Dr. Basil Hirschowitz, a young gastroenterologist with prophetic vision and missionary zeal. As a result of their pioneering efforts,[1] samples can be obtained of whatever is seen through the fiberendoscope; moreover, an increasing number of diseases can be treated without recourse to surgery.[2,3]

TECHNICAL CONSIDERATIONS

Endoscopic biopsy diagnoses are often suboptimal because many gastroenterologists do not realize how much diagnostic accuracy could be enhanced if the samples taken were large enough, sufficient in number, correctly oriented, separately labeled, properly fixed, step-serial sectioned, and appropriately stained.

Biopsy specimens taken with the large 3.4-mm diameter forceps through a large-channel upper endoscope or most colonoscopes are twice the size of those taken with smaller forceps through a standard-diameter endoscope. As a result, these biopsy specimens are easier to orient, have proportionately less crush artifact, permit more precise evaluation of architecture, and are more likely to sample small focal lesions. Yet these larger biopsies cause no more complications than those using a standard-sized forceps.

The specific number of samples that should be obtained depends on whether the disease being evaluated is patchy or diffuse in distribution, and whether it is endoscopically visible, like a polyp, or invisible, as may be dysplasia or early carcinoma.

The biopsy specimens should be unfolded and oriented with the cut side down onto a suitable substrate (monofilament plastic mesh, gelfoam, or a cucumber slice) before fixation. Such careful orientation is best performed by a trained assistant because the endoscopist and endoscopy assistant are too busy with the ongoing procedure. Orienting the biopsy so that it can be sectioned perpendicular to the mucosal surface facilitates architectural evaluation of esophageal stratified squamous epithelium, of small intestinal villi, and of colonic crypts; architectural distortion in a well-oriented biopsy specimen is of considerable diagnostic importance. Pedunculated polyps and larger pieces of tissue removed with electrocautery snares should be marked for future orientation with a needle inserted perpendicular to the cut side of a sessile polyp or through the core of a pedunculated polyp's stalk. After preliminary fixation, larger polyps should be divided perpendicular to the mucosal surface through the long axis of the stalk to ensure complete fixation and to maintain orientation.

To provide accurate clinicopathologic correlation and to facilitate rebiopsy of suspicious areas, the locations of biopsy sites should be clearly indicated by placement of the samples in separately labeled bottles of fixative.

Formalin fixation provides suboptimal nuclear detail because it does not preserve nucleoproteins adequately. Furthermore, it is such a delicate fixative that it does not protect the tissue from the disruptive effects of tissue processing. Pierre Masson's statement in 1928 about formalin is still true today, "Formol itself fixes the (endocrine) granules well but fixes the tissues very badly. (I am perhaps alone in this opinion but the greater my experience the more I am convinced of its truth)."[4]

For this reason some pathologists have shifted to Bouin or B-5 solution or other formalin-based fixatives containing metallic cations such as mercury, copper, and zinc, or acids such as picric and acetic acid. By precipitating and denaturing the tissue proteins more extensively, artifacts of uneven shrinkage are minimized and the tissue is hardened to withstand the harsh treatment during embedding and sectioning. Better nucleoprotein preservation enhances the nuclear detail so essential for the diagnosis of dysplasia and cancer. We use a modified Bouin solution called Hollande solution, which preserves red cell membranes and the granules of eosinophils better than does Bouin solution.

During paraffin embedding, up to four different biopsy specimens can be oriented on edge together to permit step-serial sectioning perpendicular to the mucosal surface. By trimming the block close to the tissue, ribbons of at least 20 to 30 serial sections of each specimen may be obtained from multiple levels in the more central, oriented core of the biopsy (Fig. 130-1).[5] We examine three stained slides containing two

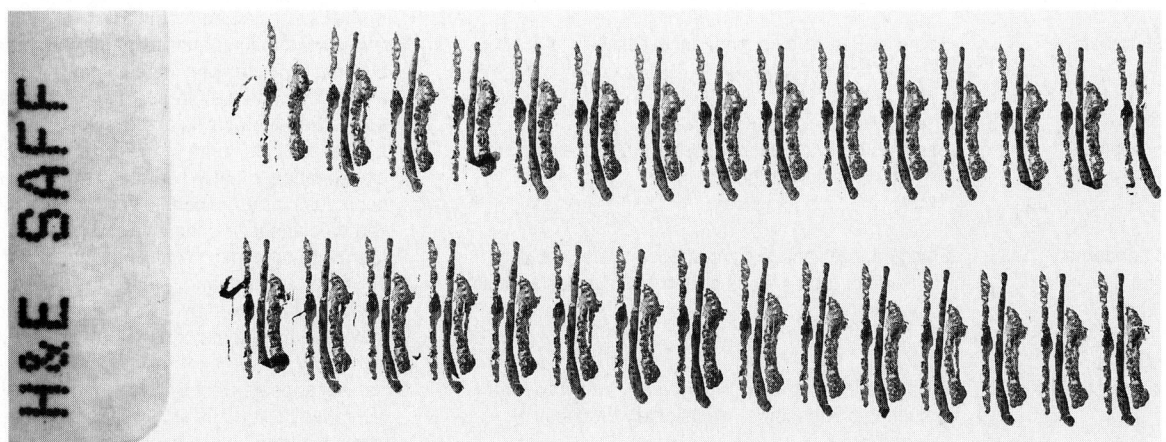

FIGURE 130-1. A single microscopic slide containing two ribbons of serial sections of three biopsy specimens with a total of 87 sections. Such serial sections make it easier to detect focal lesions including small granulomas, cryptitis, and early carcinomatous invasion of the lamina propria.

such ribbons each, for a total of more than 180 biopsy sections, and save two unstained slides for possible additional stains or ancillary techniques such as immunohistochemical study. Personal experience has shown that this approach is feasible as a routine procedure in university and community hospitals if their staffs are sufficiently trained and motivated. This extra effort makes it easier to detect focal lesions such as small epithelioid granulomas, early crypt abscesses, early malignant invasion, and abnormalities of glandular architecture.

Properly performed, the hematoxylin-eosin stain is highly informative. We routinely supplement the hematoxylin-eosin stain with Alcian blue at pH 2.5 to reveal acid intestinal mucus and with saffron to reveal collagen. The addition of Alcian blue is helpful for detecting the occasional invading signet-ring cell containing stainable acid mucus and for staining the goblet cells required for recognizing the specialized metaplastic epithelium of Barrett's esophagus. Adding saffron helps identify the collagen deposition characteristic of diseases such as collagenous sprue, collagenous colitis, and solitary rectal ulcer syndrome.

Confusing artifacts affecting mucosal histologic study may be induced by laxative use in patients when preparing for endoscopy,[6] by irritating fluids introduced from inadequately cleaned endoscopes,[7] by traumatic handling of biopsy specimens, and by improper tissue processing. Most errors in biopsy diagnosis are related to unappreciated artifacts or overinterpretation of normal variations. These will be described in the following section.

INDICATIONS FOR AND INTERPRETATIONS OF ENDOSCOPIC BIOPSY

Premalignant and Malignant Gastrointestinal Lesions

Esophageal squamous carcinoma, esophageal adenocarcinoma, cardia carcinoma, gastric adenocarcinoma, sporadic colon cancer, and cancer in ulcerative colitis (UC) occur more frequently in certain patient populations; endoscopic screening for early cancer is therefore warranted in these patients. Detecting precancerous dysplasia before invasive malignancy has developed is even more desirable (Table 130-1).

Dysplasia is defined as an unequivocal neoplastic morphologic alteration of gastrointestinal epithelium so that it exhibits cytologic abnormalities similar or identical to those seen in cancer; such altered epithelium is confined within the basement membranes of the epithelium of the esophagus (Figs. 130-2 and 130-3) or of the glands of the stomach (Fig. 130-4) or colon (Fig. 130-5). Dysplasia may be seen within grossly normal-appearing flat mucosa or within mucosa with varying degrees of abnormality, the most obvious of which is the discrete, grossly visible mass of a sessile or pedunculated adenoma (Fig. 130-6).

To be certain of the diagnosis of dysplasia, the neoplastic-appearing cells with abnormal nuclei should involve the deeper part of the crypt or gland, and should also extend to involve

---

TABLE 130-1
Premalignant Lesions

TYPE OF DYSPLASIA	HISTOLOGIC FEATURES	CLINICAL FEATURES
Esophageal squamous dysplasia	Noninvasive neoplastic basal cells that do not mature as they move superficially	Early diagnosis of squamous cancer requires biopsy of grossly invisible dysplasia in prediposed patients
Barrett's esophageal dysplasia	Loss of mucus secretion, neoplastic nuclear changes, nuclear stratification, distorted architecture, no invasion	Esophageal adenocarcinoma is rapidly increasing in frequency in American Caucasian men; early diagnosis requires extensive biopsy of all Barrett's specialized metaplasia
Cardia dysplasia	Same as Barrett's esophageal dysplasia	Cardia carcinoma in Caucasian American men is also rapidly increasing in frequency and is often associated with a short segment of Barrett's specialized metaplasia and dysplasia
Gastric dysplasia	Same as Barrett's esophageal dysplasia; associated with multifocal atrophic gastritis	Intestinalized carcinoma of the distal stomach is disappearing in the West, but is still common in nonindustrialized nations; early gastric cancer can be diagnosed endoscopically
Colonic adenoma	Enlarged, pallisading, cigar-shaped nuclei; tubular, villous, or tubulovillous patterns of dysplasia within an adenoma	Precursor to sporadic colon cancer and to familial polyposis coli; patients with distal colonic adenomas revealed by flexible sigmoidoscopy may have carcinoma or premalignant polyps proximally
Chronic ulcerative colitis	Dysplasia in a flat nonpolypoid area; similar to that seen in an adenoma, occasionally produces a gross lesion	Dysplasia appears after 8 to 10 y of extensive ulcerative coliits; it is an indication for colectomy when confirmed by an experienced gastrointestinal pathologist

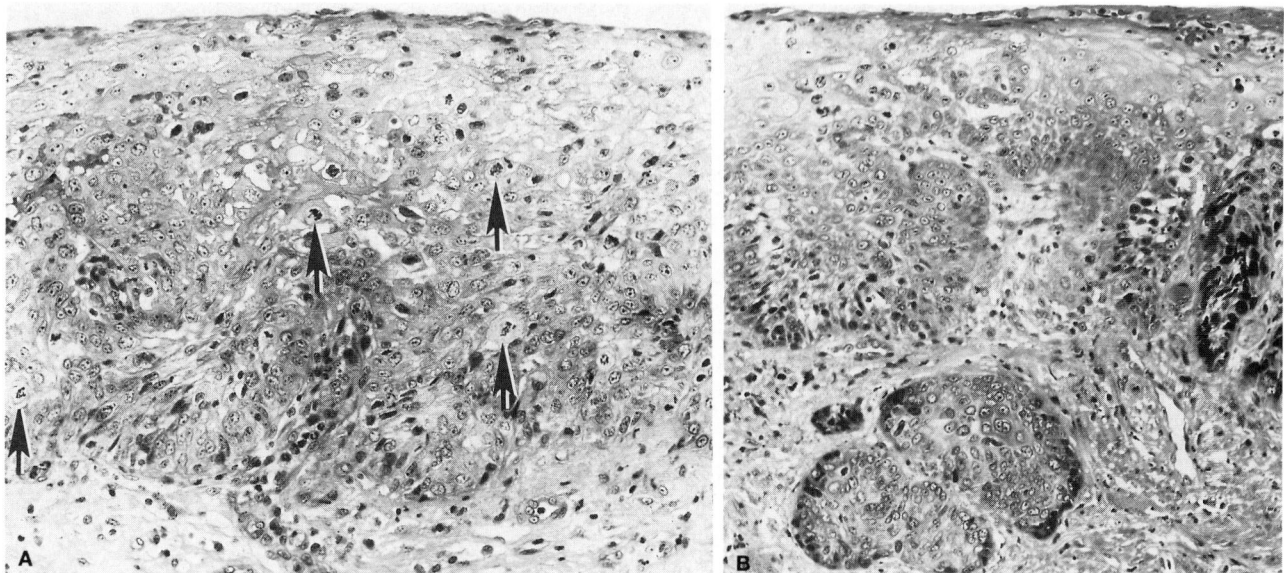

FIGURE 130-2. Esophageal squamous dysplasia and early carcinoma. (**A**) Squamous dysplasia. The papillae of the lamina propria are irregular and the mucosa has increased numbers of cells per unit area. The nuclei of the epithelial cells are crowded and hyperchromatic and overlap each other. The cells fail to mature while they move toward the luminal surface, and numerous mitotic figures are present at all levels of the mucosa (*arrows*). (**B**) An esophageal biopsy specimen from another mucosal area of the same patient shows both esophageal squamous dysplasia and early invasion of the lamina propria. This section shows tongues of dysplastic squamous epithelium extending into the lamina propria, some of which have become detached to form discrete nests of early invasive carcinoma.

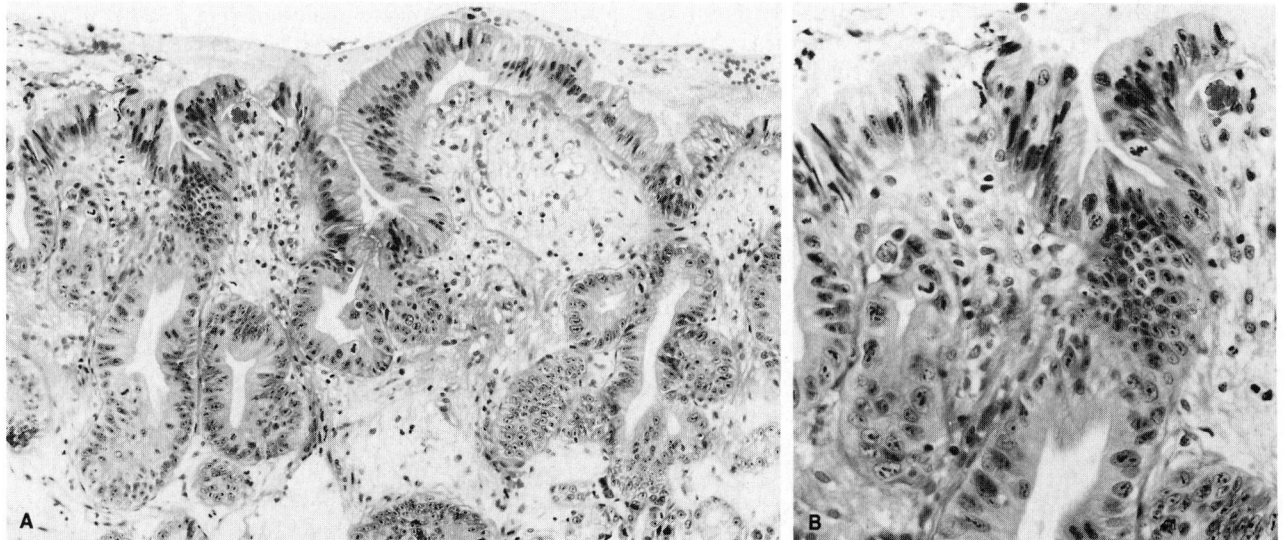

FIGURE 130-3. (**A**) Barrett's esophagus with high-grade dysplasia. The glandular architecture is distorted, as evidenced by the irregular contour of the glands and their lumens and by epithelial buds projecting from glands. The cells lining the glands have abnormal nuclei that are enlarged and hyperchromatic and have a focal loss of polarity. Epithelium with these nuclear abnormalities extends onto the mucosal surface. (**B**) The cytologic abnormalities are better seen at higher power. Notice the irregular-shaped nuclei with prominent nucleoli and the crowding of abnormal cells on the mucosal surface.

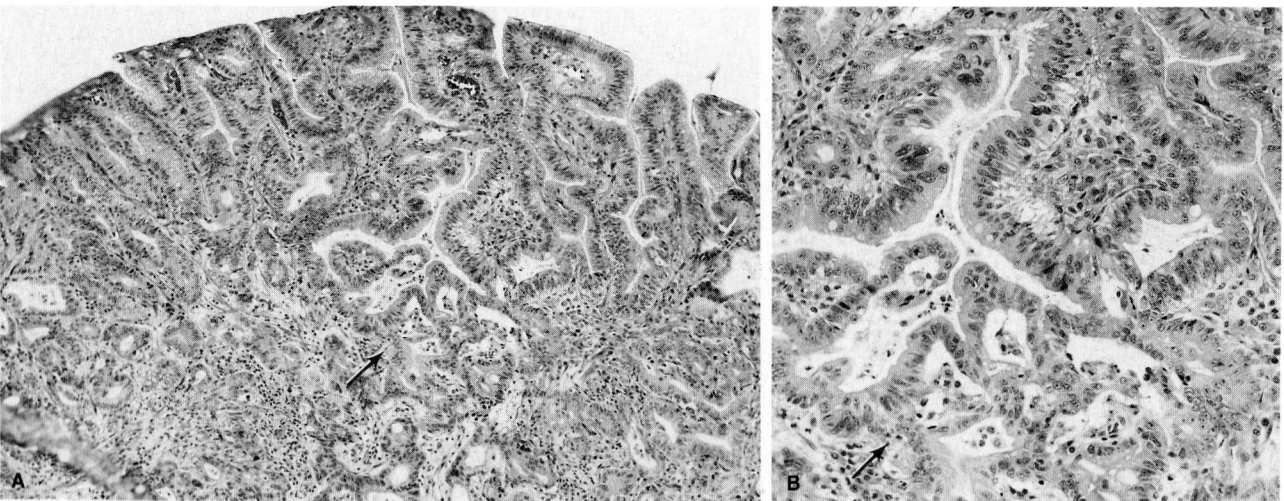

FIGURE 130-4. (A) Gastric biopsy specimen shows high-grade dysplasia without invasion in its upper portion, but with gross distortion of glandular architecture forming a complex network of gland-like spaces deeper in the biopsy specimen (*arrow*). (B) The architectural distortion is better seen at higher magnification, and the cytologic abnormalities of the nuclei lining the distorted glands can be better recognized. This gross distortion of the architectural pattern suggests invasion of the lamina propria.

the surface epithelium. Architectural features that are also helpful in diagnosing dysplasia include distorted glands, intralumenal budding, and the formation of back-to-back glands.[8]

Surveillance practices are based on several assumptions regarding dysplasia: dysplasia is a histologically recognizable precursor of cancer; cancer may eventually develop from dysplasia although its natural history is variable; and more frequent surveillance of patients with dysplasia is justified because carcinoma can be detected while it is still curable by surgical excision. In selected cases, particularly in UC, dysplasia itself may be an indication for surgical resection.

Biopsy surveillance does present problems. Even for experts the histologic diagnosis of dysplasia is regularly reproducible only when it is of a high grade.[9,10] The diagnosis of low-grade dysplasia (Fig. 130-7; see Fig. 130-17) and of changes that are indefinite for dysplasia is associated with a higher degree of observer variation.[9] Furthermore, it may be difficult in a superficial biopsy specimen to differentiate high-grade dysplasia from early invasive carcinoma (Fig. 130-8). Single epithelial cells that have extended beyond the basement membranes of their glands of origin to invade the mucosal lamina propria indicate that high-grade dysplasia has progressed to intramucosal carcinoma (Fig. 130-9). For these reasons, major

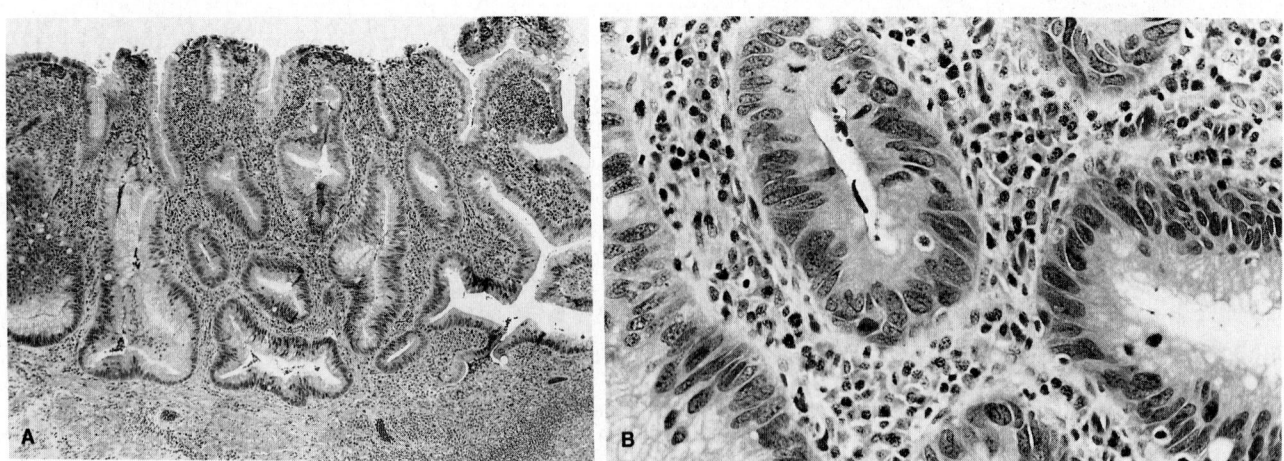

FIGURE 130-5. (A) High-grade dysplasia complicating chronic ulcerative colitis. Notice the distorted glandular architecture, almost complete absence of goblet cell mucus, and marked crowding and stratification of nuclei. (B) At higher power the cytologic abnormalities can be readily identified. The nuclei are markedly enlarged compared with the size of the nuclei in the lamina propria and they vary markedly in size and shape. A beginning loss of nuclear polarity also is seen.

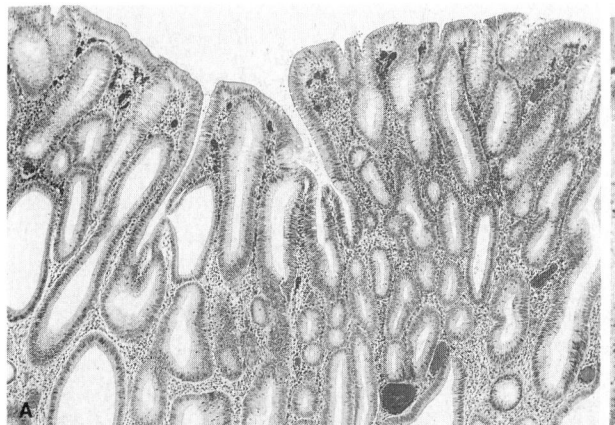
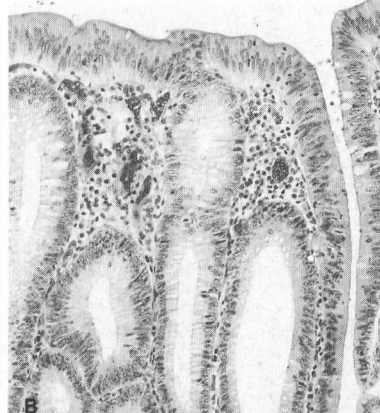
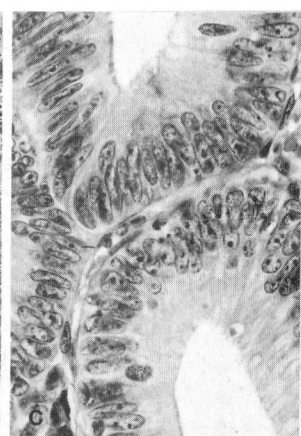

FIGURE 130-6. Colonic tubular adenoma. **(A)** Notice the characteristic tubular architecture. **(B, C)** Cytologic features of the neoplastic cells lining the tubules. Nuclear enlargement, crowding, and stratification and the focal diminution in mucus production are seen. These changes indicate low-grade dysplasia within a tubular adenoma.

clinical decisions based on biopsy interpretations should be made only after seeking a second opinion from a pathologist with wide experience in the diagnosis of gastrointestinal dysplasia and cancer. More objective techniques such as flow cytometric quantification of DNA may complement the histologic diagnosis of dysplasia.[11,12]

After the diagnosis of dysplasia has been made, the next problem is to decide when to excise the organ harboring it to preclude the development of incurable carcinoma. Most clinicians now agree that colectomy is indicated as soon as definite high-grade dysplasia develops in chronic UC. Three reasons support this attitude:

Colectomy is effective treatment for UC.
Colectomy is associated with low mortality.
Symptomatic carcinoma in UC is often incurable by the time it is diagnosed.

High-grade dysplasia or intramucosal carcinoma in Barrett's esophagus provides an opportunity to prevent or cure an almost uniformly fatal adenocarcinoma,[13,14] yet the proper course of action is unclear when only high-grade dysplasia is found after extensive biopsy. There are three reasons for this perplexity:

Barrett's esophagus with dysplasia is more common in older patients who are often poor surgical risks.
Partial esophagectomy, except when performed by exceptionally experienced and skillful physicians, has a sizable morbidity and mortality.
The length of time it takes dysplasia to become carcinoma in Barrett's esophagus is not yet established prospectively.

If only high-grade dysplasia is found after the extremely thorough sampling of the Barrett's mucosa recommended in our

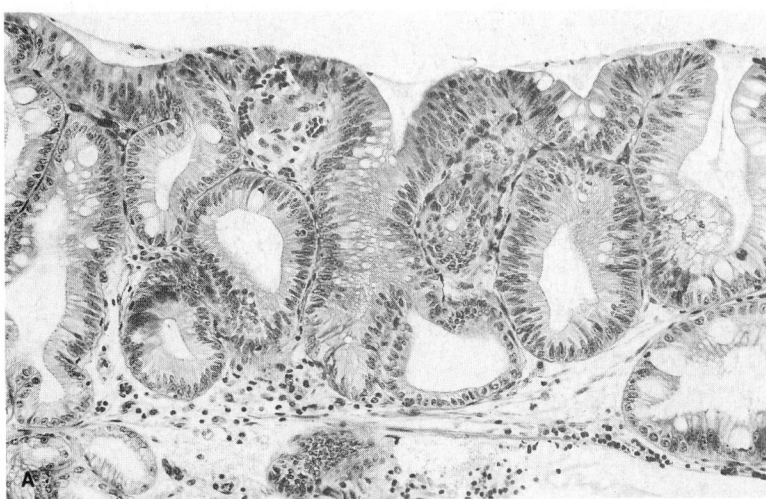
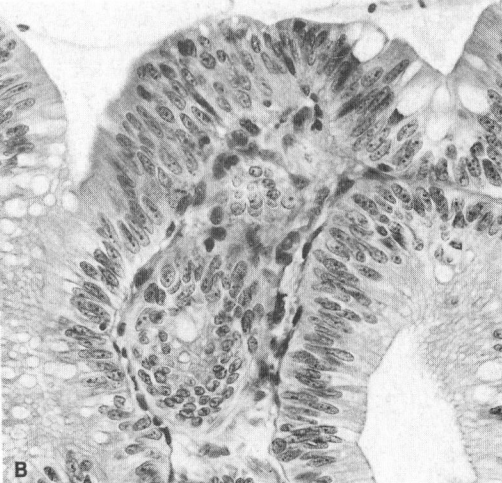

FIGURE 130-7. Barrett's esophagus with low-grade dysplasia. **(A)** The glands are irregular in size and shape and there is decreased mucus production. Some goblet cells of the nonneoplastic, Barrett's specialized metaplastic epithelial precursor to dysplasia still can be identified. **(B)** Observe the crowding, stratification, and enlargement of the dysplastic nuclei that extend to the luminal surface. The changes are less severe than those seen in high-grade dysplasia.

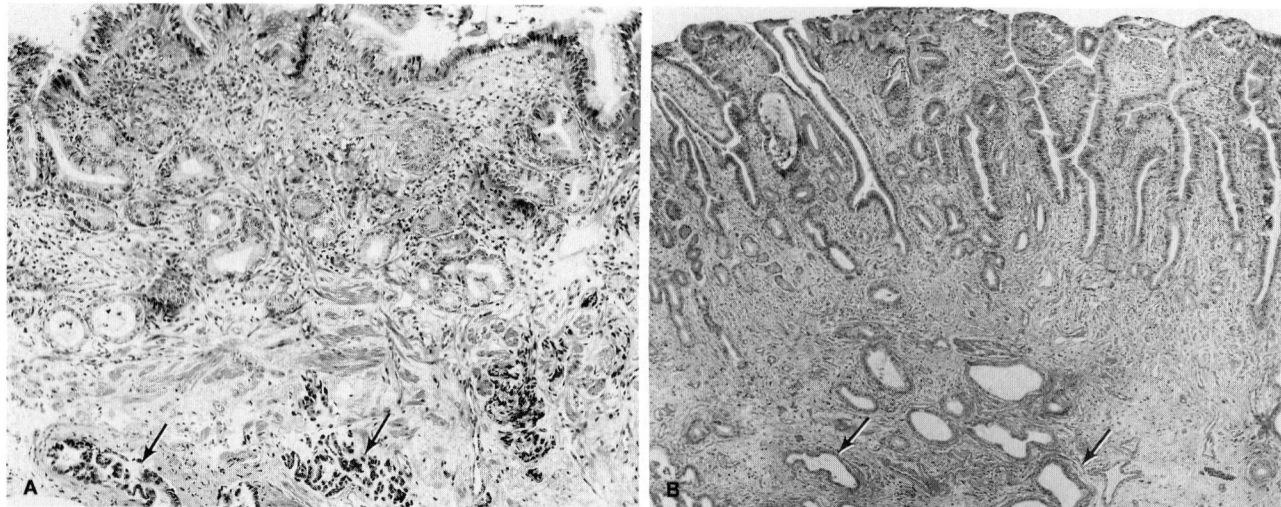

FIGURE 130-8. Possible invasive cancer in a biopsy specimen from a patient with Barrett's esophagus. The corresponding area in the surgical specimen shows definite submucosal invasion. (**A**) The upper portion of the biopsy specimen above the muscularis mucosae shows only high-grade dysplasia, whereas in the lower portion of the specimen, slightly dilated, darkly stained glands (*arrows*) extend into a widened and splayed muscularis mucosae. Because of the limited depth of the specimen, invasion through the muscularis mucosae into the submucosa cannot be confirmed, but it was suspected. (**B**) The surgical specimen from the same area clearly shows the dilated glands invading into the submucosa (*arrows*).

research protocol, esophagectomy may not have to be carried out to exclude a clinically undetected carcinoma.[14]

Perhaps the greatest problem in surveillance is to decide when a time-consuming and expensive program to detect dysplasia and early carcinoma is justified. Curable gastrointestinal cancer undoubtedly can be detected by extensive endoscopic biopsy of suitable populations undergoing surveil-

lance. But such examinations of large populations are so costly and time-consuming as to be impractical. Therefore the goal is to select the highest risk patients within a susceptible population to increase the relatively low yield of surveillance. In endemic regions with a high incidence of squamous esophageal carcinoma (parts of China, Iran, South Africa) or gastric cancer (Columbia, Japan), surveillance is justified and may

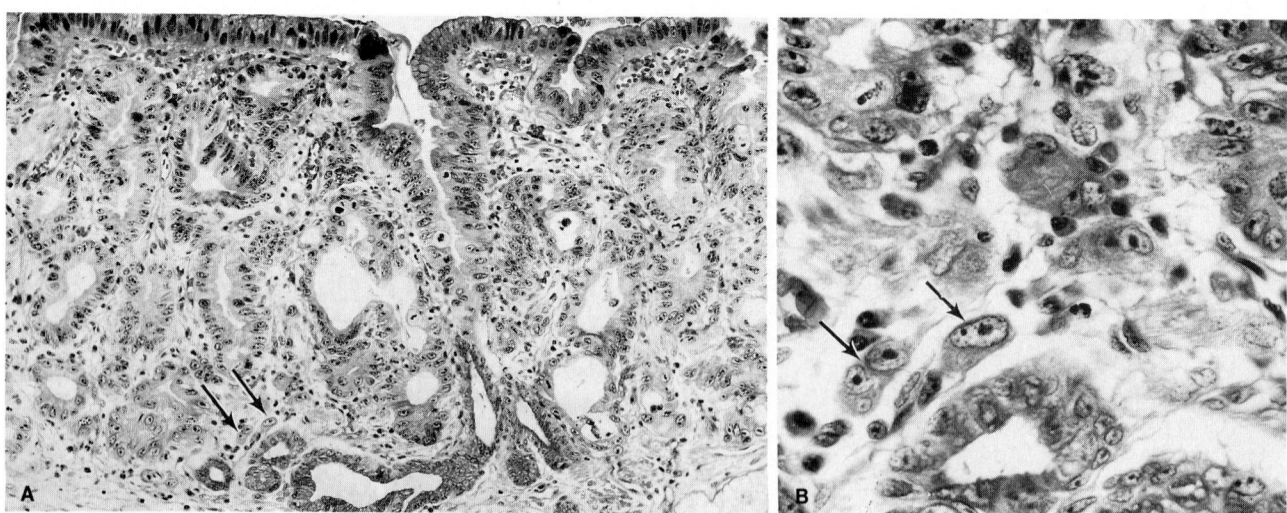

FIGURE 130-9. (**A**) Low-power and (**B**) high-power views of Barrett's esophagus with high-grade dysplasia and intramucosal carcinoma. Marked distortion of the glandular architecture and prominent nuclear abnormalities are seen. Invasion of the lamina propria by individual glandular epithelial cells represents intramucosal carcinoma (*arrows*).

be rewarding.[15,16] In the Western countries there are three conditions with potential for early detection of gastrointestinal cancer:

- Barrett's esophagus
- colonic adenomas
- chronic UC.

Even in these three conditions, the yield of dysplasia or early carcinoma is low enough that better techniques are needed to select subsets of patients whose high cancer risk warrants the time, effort, expense, and discomfort of close surveillance.

Aside from the previously mentioned conditions, far fewer early esophageal and gastric carcinomas are diagnosed in the Western countries than in high-risk populations. Does this reflect the different biologic character of these malignancies in different environments or the unfamiliarity of gastroenterologists from Western countries with early, subtle lesions? Both factors probably contribute. For example, because gastric cancer associated with atrophic gastritis and intestinal metaplasia is a major problem in Japan, their endoscopists are sensitive to minimal mucosal changes warranting biopsy, and they regularly diagnose early, curable disease.[16] The incidence of gastric adenocarcinoma associated with chronic atrophic gastritis with intestinal metaplasia is decreasing in the socioeconomically secure population of the Western countries so that surveillance programs in this group are not cost effective. The disease is diagnosed mostly when it is symptomatic and incurable. That there is an early curable phase of gastric cancer with atrophic gastritis and intestinal metaplasia in the Western countries is attested to by reports of early endoscopic biopsy diagnoses of potentially curable lesions in the United States.[17] Unquestionably, biopsy specimens of minimal gastric lesions should be taken more often. The yield will be low, but the cancers found will more often be curable.

A history of squamous carcinomas of the mouth, pharynx, or nose merits surveillance for esophageal squamous carcinoma. Smoking and alcohol consumption, although risk factors for squamous esophageal carcinoma, are so common in the Western countries that they cannot be used as a basis for surveillance. Although other predisposing conditions for esophageal squamous carcinoma exist, they are too rare to be of major importance in detecting treatable disease. They include long-standing achalasia or lye stricture, Plummer-Vinson syndrome, and tylosis. Squamous dysplasia in any of these conditions is worth detecting (see Fig. 130-2A). It resembles cancer cytologically but there is no evidence of invasion. Characteristically the neoplastic cells in the basal layer in squamous dysplasia do not mature as they migrate toward the lumenal surface.

Adenocarcinoma of the esophagus is almost always a complication of Barrett's esophagus. The definition of Barrett's esophagus may depend on an arbitrary minimal length of columnar lining within the distal tubular esophagus—3 cm or more—or on histologic evidence that the columnar lining contains Barrett's specialized metaplasia (Fig. 130-10).[8] We prefer the latter histologic definition because we believe that esophageal adenocarcinoma develops only in patients who have antecedent Barrett's specialized metaplasia. Barrett's specialized metaplasia comprises a spectrum of epithelial changes,[18] with the sine qua non for diagnosis being the presence of goblet cells containing acid mucus that stains intensely with Alcian blue at pH 2.5. The columnar cells in this type of metaplasia vary in appearance from normal gastric surface cells containing neutral mucus, to abnormal cells containing some acid mucus staining lightly with Alcian blue, to the invariably present goblet cells that stain intensely with Alcian blue. Also seen are cells resembling intestinal absorptive cells, except that their brush borders are poorly developed and their cytoplasm often contains secretory mucus granules.

Dysplasia and carcinoma in the columnar-lined tubular esophagus probably develop only in esophagi with Barrett's specialized metaplasia, which is their presumed precursor.[19]

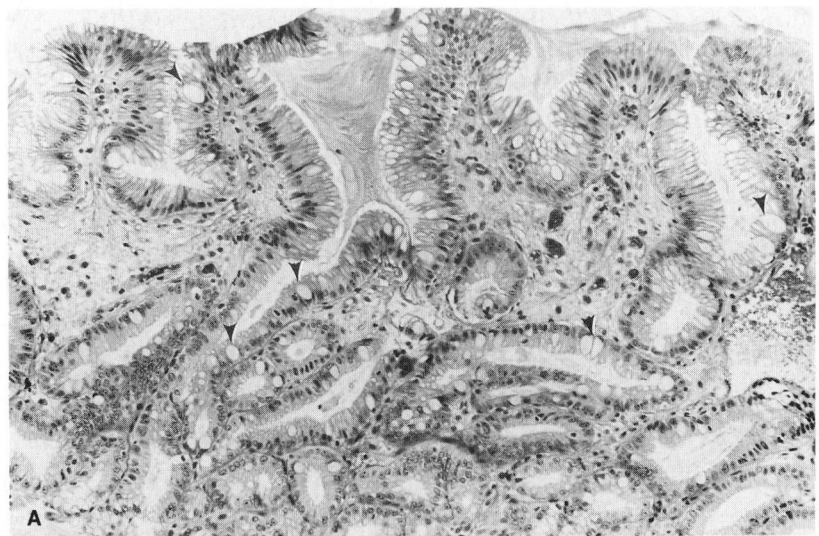
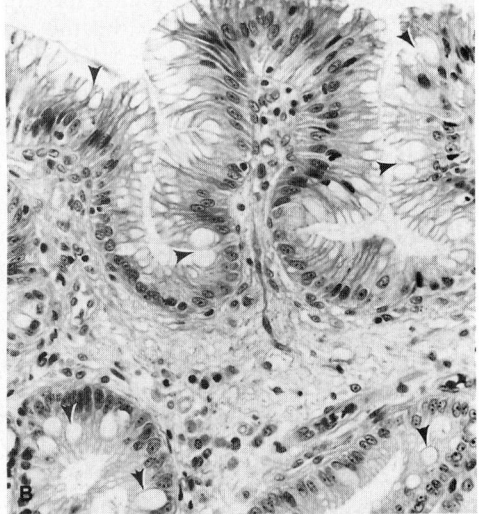

FIGURE 130-10. (A) Low-power and (B) high-power views of Barrett's esophagus show specialized metaplastic epithelium with diagnostic goblet cells (*arrowheads*). The cells between the goblet cells resemble gastric surface cells by light microscopic examination. No evidence of dysplasia is seen.

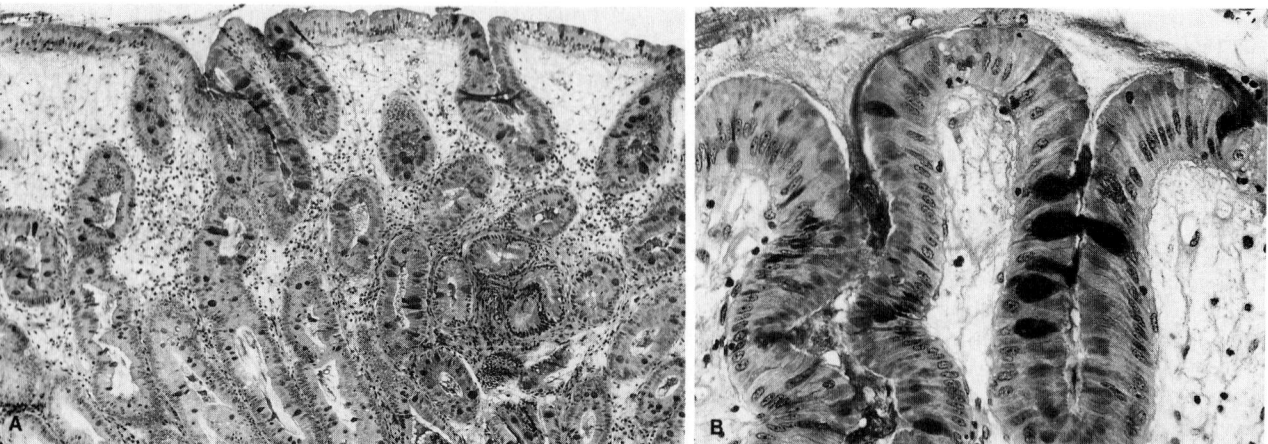

FIGURE 130-11. **(A)** Low-power and **(B)** high-power views of multifocal atrophic gastritis that has progressed to diffuse intestinal metaplasia. No residual normal gastric glands are present; they have been replaced by glands in which the acid mucin–containing Alcian blue–positive goblet cells appear black. The cells between the goblet cells have a spectrum of appearances ranging from a strong resemblance to intestinal absorptive cells to an appearance similar to gastric surface mucous cells except that the mucus stains with Alcian blue at pH 2.5. This indicates that the mucus is acidic rather than neutral, as in normal gastric surface cells.

The distal 2 or 3 cm of the tubular esophagus in healthy persons and in patients with regurgitant esophagitis without Barrett's metaplasia may normally have a columnar lining of cardiac or some fundic glands. Patients with Barrett's esophagus or severe regurgitant esophagitis almost invariably have a hiatal hernia. When biopsy is performed on the hernia above the diaphragm because it is presumed to be esophagus, columnar epithelium is obtained but it is fundic gland mucosa lining the herniated stomach. Such columnar epithelium must not be confused with Barrett's specialized metaplasia.

How can potentially curable adenocarcinoma be detected in Barrett's esophagus? The first rule is to recognize that dysplasia and early intramucosal carcinoma (see Fig. 130-9) are often grossly invisible.[13] The second rule is to repeatedly biopsy the whole length of Barrett's specialized metaplasia within the tubular esophagus from the lower esophageal sphincter to the upwardly displaced squamocolumnar junction at the ora serrata. Large, properly processed and expertly interpreted biopsy specimens increase diagnostic sensitivity and specificity. The finding of dysplasia is worrisome and warrants repeated, extensive biopsy surveillance to detect early, potentially curable intramucosal adenocarcinoma. If early carcinoma is found, the entire columnar-lined portion of the esophagus must be removed.

There are four main types of gastric cancer: The first is the gastric adenocarcinoma that usually occupies the more distal end of the stomach and often is accompanied by atrophic gastritis with intestinal metaplasia (Figs. 130-11 and 130-12) and hypochlorhydria or achlorhydria. Because this type of cancer forms glands that resemble those of a colonic cancer, it is called the intestinal type of gastric cancer. The second type of gastric cancer is called the diffuse type because it does

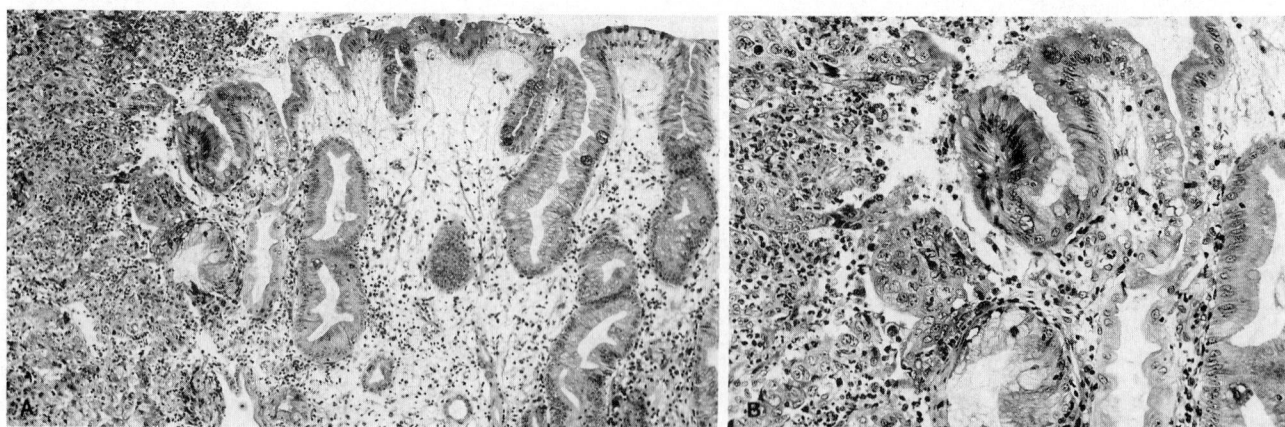

FIGURE 130-12. **(A)** Low-power and **(B)** high-power views of advanced multifocal atrophic gastritis with intestinal metaplasia and an associated adenocarcinoma. The absence of recognizable gastric pyloric or fundic glands indicates atrophy whereas the goblet and absorptive cells identify intestinal metaplasia. To the left of **A** and **B**, sheets of cells with malignant-appearing nuclei infiltrate the lamina propria.

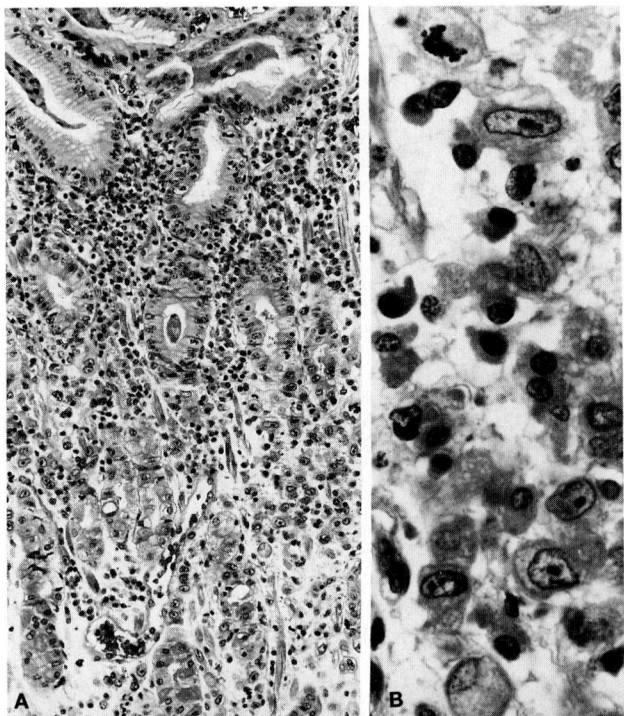

FIGURE 130-13. Gastric biopsy specimen of a minute lesion that was barely visible endoscopically. (**A**) Low-power magnification illustrates how subtle adenocarcinoma of the stomach can be. The inflamed lamina propria contains infiltrating malignant cells that are difficult to recognize because they are interspersed with inflammatory cells. (**B**) The high-power view makes these infiltrating, malignant cells readily apparent.

not form glands. It may be curable when detected early by a biopsy targeted at a minuscule lesion (Fig. 130-13). The intestinal type of gastric adenocarcinoma, which previously was the most common, is now occurring less frequently in the Western world. In contrast, the third type of proximally located cardia carcinoma is increasing in frequency. It is associated with normal fundic glands and normal or excessive secretion of acid. The fourth type, gastric lymphoma, is a much less common cancer than is gastric adenocarcinoma. Nevertheless, it is well worth diagnosing when confined to the stomach because it is often curable by surgical excision or chemotherapy or both, even when the tumor is large. Gastric Kaposi's sarcoma is being seen more often because of acquired immunodeficiency syndrome (AIDS).

Cardia carcinoma warrants more diagnostic effort because of its increasing incidence.[20-22] It has clinical and epidemiologic features in common with Barrett's esophagus[23] and often originates from a short distal segment of Barrett's specialized metaplasia. These short segments of Barrett's esophagus can be missed easily during endoscopy for regurgitant esophagitis. This emphasizes the desirability of thorough biopsy sampling of obvious longer segments of Barrett's esophagus and also of possible shorter segments at the esophagogastric junction. A jaggedly serrated irregular ora serrata is more likely to harbor a short segment of Barrett's specialized metaplasia. The finding of definite dysplasia in such a short segment is a red flag indicating the need for extensive sampling to be certain that

early carcinoma is not present. We have diagnosed several patients with early cardia carcinomas in this manner who were probably cured by surgical excision (Fig. 130-14).

Gastric Kaposi's sarcoma often is missed by shallow biopsies, although experienced endoscopists often suspect the diagnosis grossly in patients with human immunodeficiency virus infection. The diagnostic histologic picture is one of spindle cells containing clusters or individual hyaline inclusions and erythrocytes within slit-like openings between the spindle cells (Fig. 130-15).

Surveillance endoscopy can detect grossly invisible dysplasia or early carcinoma in flat colonic mucosa in chronic UC. There is a risk of dysplasia or cancer when the disease is of more than 8 years' duration and when it extends proximal to the sigmoid colon. Because dysplasia and cancer may be invisible endoscopically and localized to small areas of the mucosa, an extensive biopsy protocol to sample the whole length of the colon should be used. A total of 33 biopsies of the colonic mucosa is needed to achieve 90% confidence that dysplasia will be detected if present.[24] We therefore recommend four biopsies in each 10-cm segment of colon from the cecum to the sigmoid and four in each 5-cm segment of the sigmoid and rectum. The reason for intensifying the sampling in the sigmoid colon and rectum is that dysplasia and cancer are more frequently located there.[25,26] Additional biopsy specimens of any visible lesions are taken.

After 8 years of disease the only safe alternative to surveillance is colectomy, an approach that is unacceptable to patients who feel relatively or completely well. If and when dysplasia is found and confirmed by a second opinion from a specialist in gastrointestinal pathology, most clinicians recommend colectomy to prevent development of cancer or to cure an early endoscopically inapparent cancer. If two successive, thorough, annual colonoscopies are considered to give negative results for dysplasia by a pathologist with wide experience with dysplasia in UC, then it is probably justified to delay the next surveillance for 2 years.

Unfortunately there are special problems in the diagnosis of dysplasia in UC. Marked inflammatory or regenerative epithelial atypia in an actively inflamed mucosa may be difficult or even impossible to differentiate from precancerous dysplasia (Fig. 130-16). In this situation the patient's colitis should be treated vigorously and the biopsies repeated when the inflammation has subsided. In some patients, active inflammation continues in spite of appropriate therapy and the biopsy specimens remain difficult to interpret; such patients are possible candidates for surgery. Experienced gastrointestinal pathologists usually can agree on the diagnosis of high-grade dysplasia in UC, but significant interobserver variation occurs in the diagnoses of *low-grade dysplasia* and *indefinite for dysplasia*.[10] (Fig. 130-17) This means that it may be difficult or impossible to select patients with incipient or early dysplasia for more intensive surveillance. Preliminary prospective data suggest that flow cytometric detection of aneuploidy in biopsy specimens detects neoplastic transformation earlier than histologic methods and may serve as a useful earlier marker of patients with the greatest risk of cancer.[24]

Colonic adenomas are precursors of sporadic colon cancer or may already contain carcinoma (Fig. 130-18). When an adenomatous polyp is found on sigmoidoscopy, an increased risk exists of more adenomas or of cancer elsewhere in the

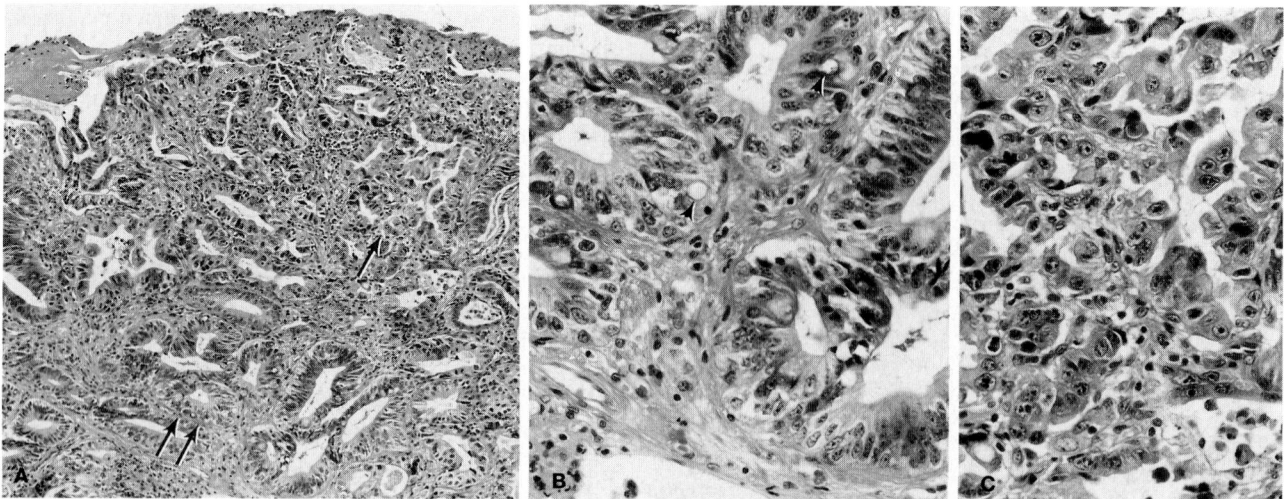

FIGURE 130-14. Early, potentially curable adenocarcinoma of the gastric cardia. **(A)** At low-power magnification both high-grade dysplasia and a focus of intramucosal carcinoma (*single arrow*) are present. Residual goblet cells suggest the presence of Barrett's specialized metaplastic epithelium (*double arrows*). **(B)** The area previously marked with double arrows shows the enlarged goblet cells that define this dysplastic epithelium as originating from Barrett's specialized metaplasia (*arrowheads*). **(C)** In the area marked in **A** with a single arrow, malignant cells infiltrating the lamina propria are evident.

colon; this usually prompts colonoscopic examination of the whole length of the colon. On the other hand, as many as 50% of patients older than 50 years of age may have a small adenoma,[27] and this may be discovered on screening sigmoidoscopy. Is it cost effective to perform a complete colonoscopy in all such patients when relatively few have a synchronous colonic cancer? It would be useful to have criteria for selecting older patients at higher risk for sporadic colon cancer who need a screening colonoscopy; however, there is no way to select such older patients.

The following sections describe the status of biopsy di-

agnosis for the organs accessible to the endoscope: the esophagus, stomach, duodenum, terminal ileum, and colon.

Benign Esophageal Disease

Heartburn is one of the most common symptoms occurring in humans. Mostly it is caused by gastroesophageal reflux disease (GERD), an entity that may be difficult to diagnose, even by endoscopic biopsy. Esophageal infections with inflammation and erosions may cause painful swallowing and

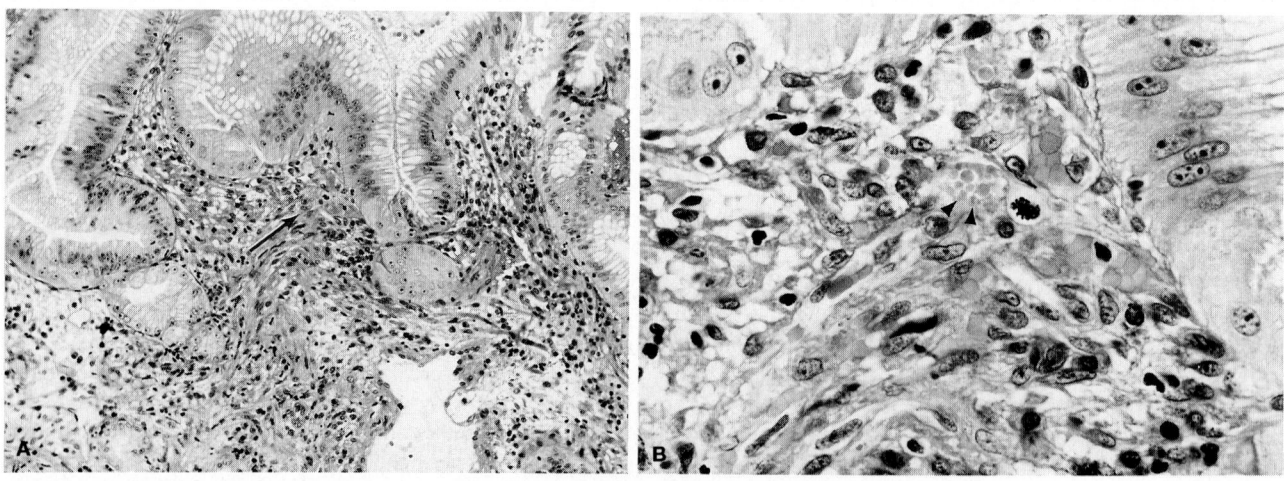

FIGURE 130-15. Gastric biopsy specimen from a patient with Kaposi's sarcoma. **(A)** The lamina propria contains infiltrating spindle cells of the sarcoma and a dilated vessel at the bottom. The arrow marks the area shown **(B)** at higher power. Observe the spindle cells that compose the lesion and the red blood cells in the slit-like spaces between individual spindle cells. The arrowheads denote intracytoplasmic hyaline inclusions that are highly characteristic of Kaposi's sarcoma. Note the mitotic figure immediately to the right of the arrowheads.

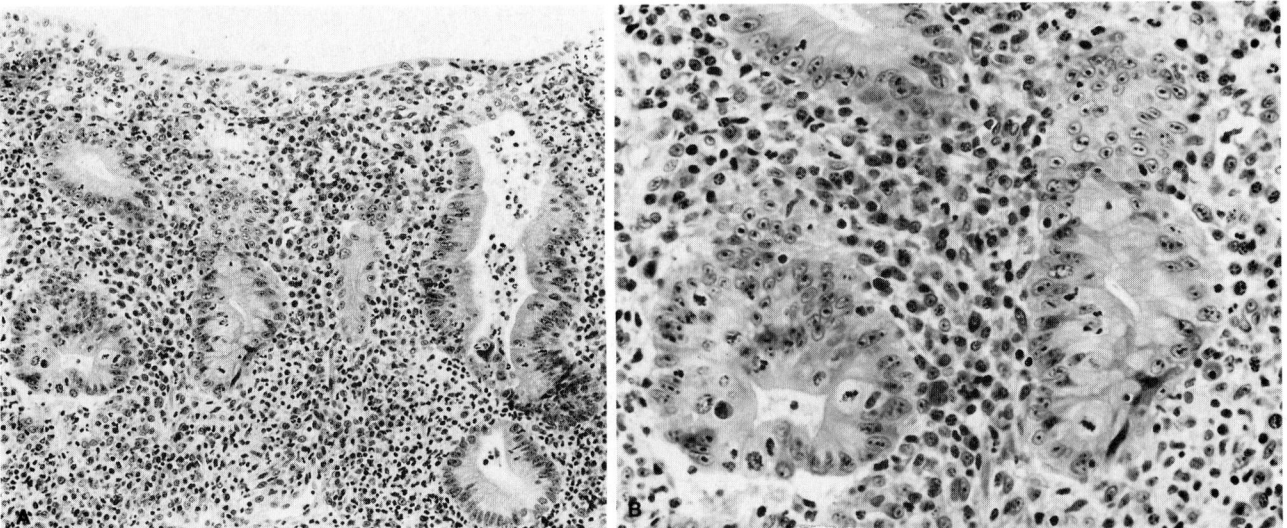

FIGURE 130-16. Colonic biopsy specimen in active ulcerative colitis. (**A**) Notice the polymorphonuclear leukocytes within the crypt epithelium, the crypt abscess, the distortion of the crypt architecture, and the marked chronic inflammatory infiltrate within the lamina propria. (**B**) Reactive epithelial changes that resemble dysplasia can be seen. Notice the occasional polymorphonuclear leukocytes within the crypt epithelium and the nuclear enlargement, crowding, stratification, and numerous mitotic figures in the crypt epithelium.

bleeding; these occur principally in persons with immunosuppression. Less common causes of painful inflammation are localized injuries from pills that impacted in the esophagus during swallowing and from acid or alkaline corrosives that were ingested accidentally or in a suicide attempt. Such acute injuries are best diagnosed by history and by acute endoscopic examination without biopsy.

When friability, bleeding, and erosions are endoscopically evident in suspected GERD, the histologic diagnosis usually is obvious because the biopsy specimen shows erosions and active inflammation with polymorphonuclear leukocytes (Fig.

130-19). Such patients require biopsy only to rule out infections or malignant lesions masquerading as regurgitant esophagitis. The main problem in GERD is reflux symptoms in patients who have some positive test results for reflux disease, but whose esophagus appears normal endoscopically or at the most, reddened, which is an undependable subjective finding. Many think that histologic evidence of hyperplasia of the squamous epithelium is an early indicator of reaction to injury that is useful in the diagnosis of reflux esophagitis[28-31]; in comparison with normal mucosa (Fig. 130-20A), there is lengthening of the papillae of the lamina propria (Fig.

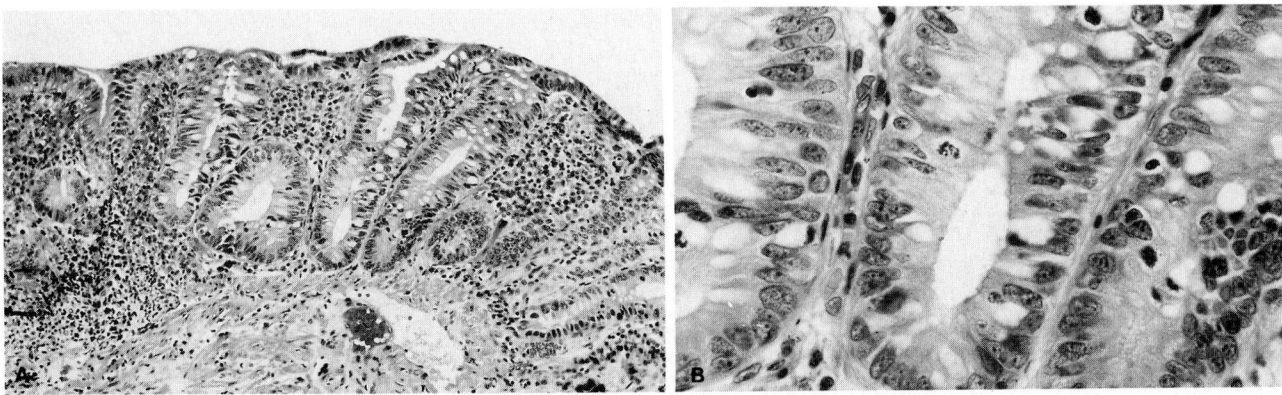

FIGURE 130-17. Ulcerative colitis with low-grade dysplasia. (**A**) Notice the relatively well-preserved crypt architecture and the mild chronic inflammatory infiltrate within the lamina propria. There is no evidence of active inflammation. Notice the decreased number of goblet cells and nuclear crowding and stratification. (**B**) At high-power magnification, the nuclear hyperchromasia, crowding, and stratification can be readily seen. Notice the *dystrophic* goblet cells that fail to communicate with the lumenal surface. Such goblet cells are characteristic but not diagnostic of dysplasia.

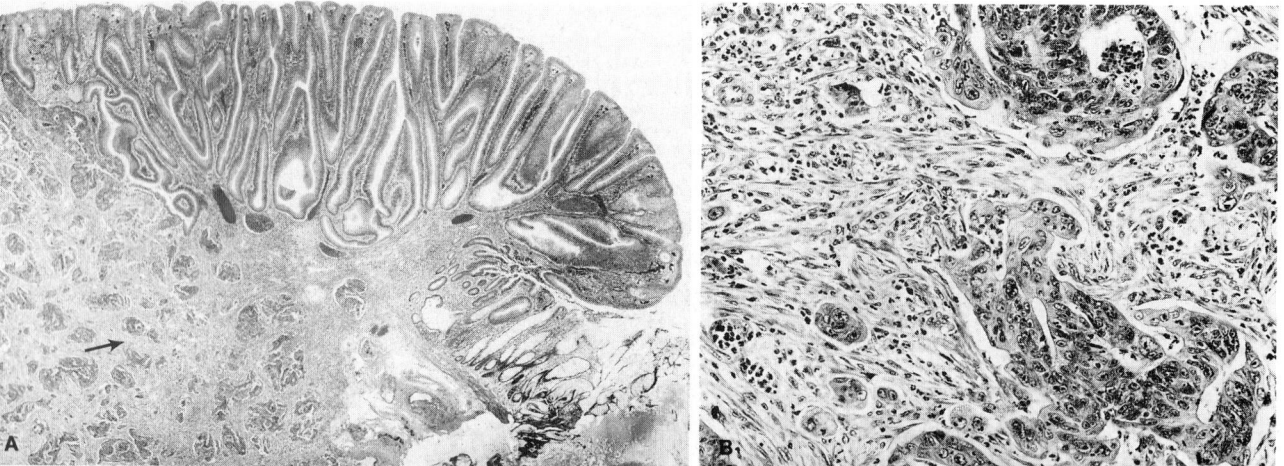

FIGURE 130-18. Electrocautery snare biopsy specimen of a sessile colonic adenoma with invasive carcinoma. (**A**) Normal mucosa distorted by electrocautery artifact is shown (*lower right*). The upper portion of the tissue is composed of villous adenoma, and (*lower left*) an invasive adenocarcinoma infiltrates below the muscularis mucosae into the submucosa. (**B**) The prominent desmoplastic stromal reaction elicited by the invading carcinoma can be readily seen.

130-20*B*) and thickening of the basal layer (Fig. 130-20*C*) in hyperplasia. For several reasons the accuracy of this histologic indicator of esophagitis remains controversial:

Most biopsy specimens taken with the standard-sized forceps are difficult to orient or are too small for accurate diagnosis of hyperplasia.

More than half of normal persons without GERD have hyperplasia in the distal 2.5 cm of their tubular esophagus and one fifth have it proximal to 2.5 cm.[32]

Fifteen percent of patients with obvious symptoms of reflux and positive tests for reflux show neither histologic evidence of active inflammation nor hyperplasia.[29]

A biopsy showing hyperplasia, like all other tests for GERD, is far from 100% accurate.

The presence of several eosinophils per individual section of squamous epithelium[33] is thought by some to be an indicator of reflux because in many patients it correlates with symptoms of GERD and positive tests for reflux.

Active esophagitis can progress to stricture or ulceration, or heal with reepithelialization. The squamous epithelium may regrow, or the eroded area may be replaced by specialized metaplastic columnar epithelium, known as Barrett's esophagus.

Endoscopy in severe GERD almost always reveals a hiatal hernia if the endoscopist knows how to look for it.[34,35] It is recognizable as an inflatable bag-like segment of stomach above the diaphragm that is demarcated distally by the diaphragmatic pinchcock, which contracts with sniffing, and proximally by the terminal portion of the tubular esophagus.

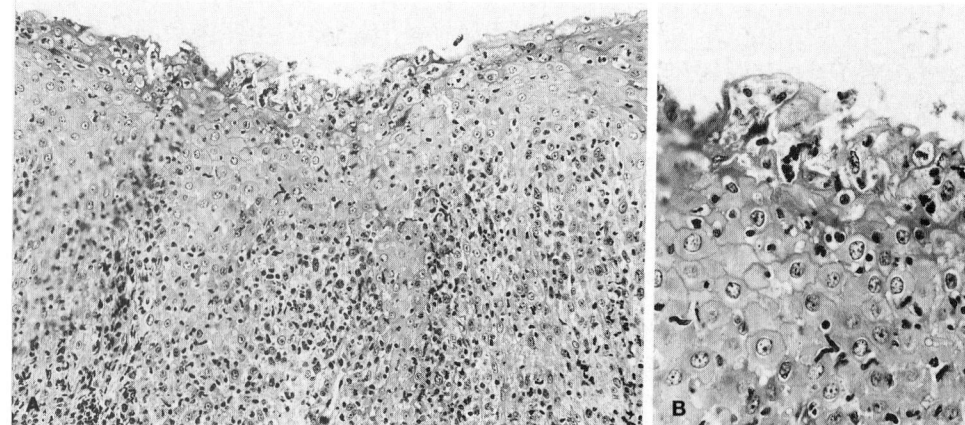
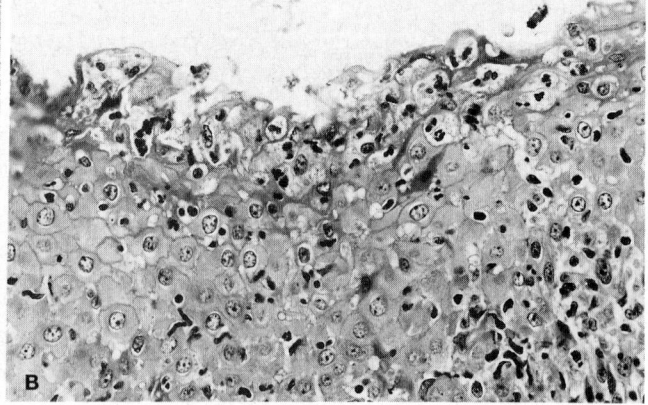

FIGURE 130-19. (**A**) Active esophagitis in gastroesophageal reflux disease in which polymorphonuclear neutrophils and lymphocytes infiltrate the surface of the squamous mucosa and the lamina propria, obscuring the interface between the mucosa and the underlying lamina propria. (**B**) Prominent epithelial hyperplasia is evidenced by the enlarged, hyperchromatic, and more numerous nuclei seen best at higher magnification.

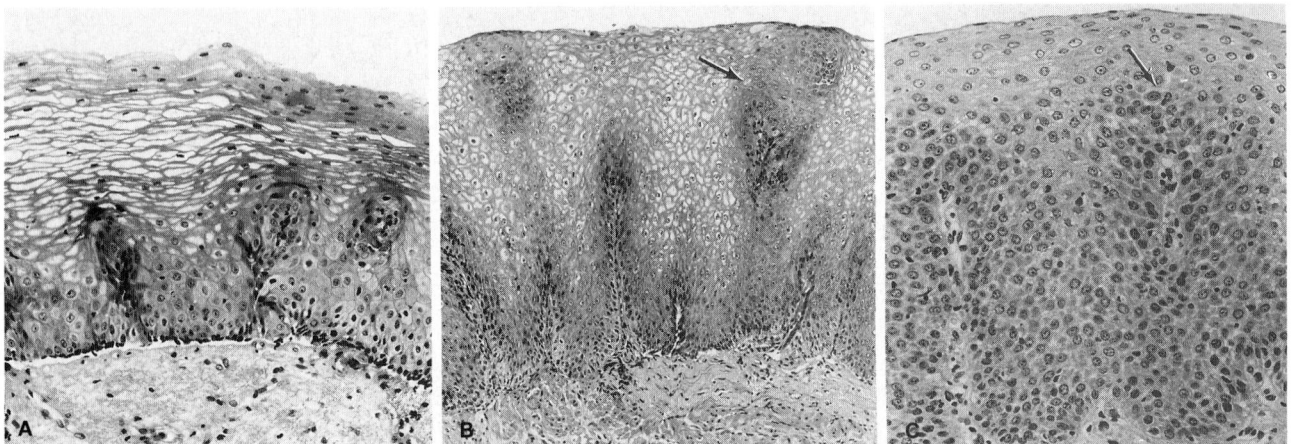

FIGURE 130-20. Biopsy specimens of normal and hyperplastic esophageal mucosa. (**A**) Normal squamous mucosa of the esophagus. The papillae of the lamina propria extend through approximately 50% of the thickness of the mucosa and the basal zone occupies a small portion of the mucosa. (**B**) Hyperplasia of the mucosa is indicated by lengthening of the papillae of the lamina propria, some of which extend close to the lumenal surface (*arrow*). In addition, the basal zone is markedly hyperplastic and occupies more than 25% of the thickness of the mucosa. (**C**) A profound degree of hyperplasia can be seen with the basal zone occupying two thirds of the thickness of the mucosa and with papillae of the lamina propria extending a similar distance through the mucosa (*arrow*).

The hernia can be shown to be stomach by biopsy revealing normal fundic glands (Fig. 130-21), with cardiac glands seen near the junction with the tubular esophagus (Fig. 130-22). Endoscopic recognition that biopsy specimens were taken from a hernia prevents an erroneous diagnosis of Barrett's esophagus based on a biopsy showing columnar epithelium from a hiatus hernia presumed to be tubular esophagus.

Endoscopic biopsies of the tubular esophagus also allow diagnosis of the various possible complications of GERD such as benign stricture, peptic esophageal ulcer, and Barrett's esophagus, which in turn may have its own complications of

Barrett's precancerous dysplasia and esophageal adenocarcinoma (see Fig. 130-8*A*).

Esophageal infections are rare in immunocompetent persons, but immunocompromised patients are susceptible to infections by cytomegalovirus (CMV), herpes simplex virus (HSV), and *Candida* organisms (Fig. 130-23), and more rarely by varicella zoster virus.[36,37] A spectrum of endoscopic appearances is possible with these infections, some of which are indistinguishable from reflux esophagitis. Biopsies, brushings, and viral cultures are indicated to make these specific diagnoses. Such infections are increasing in frequency because

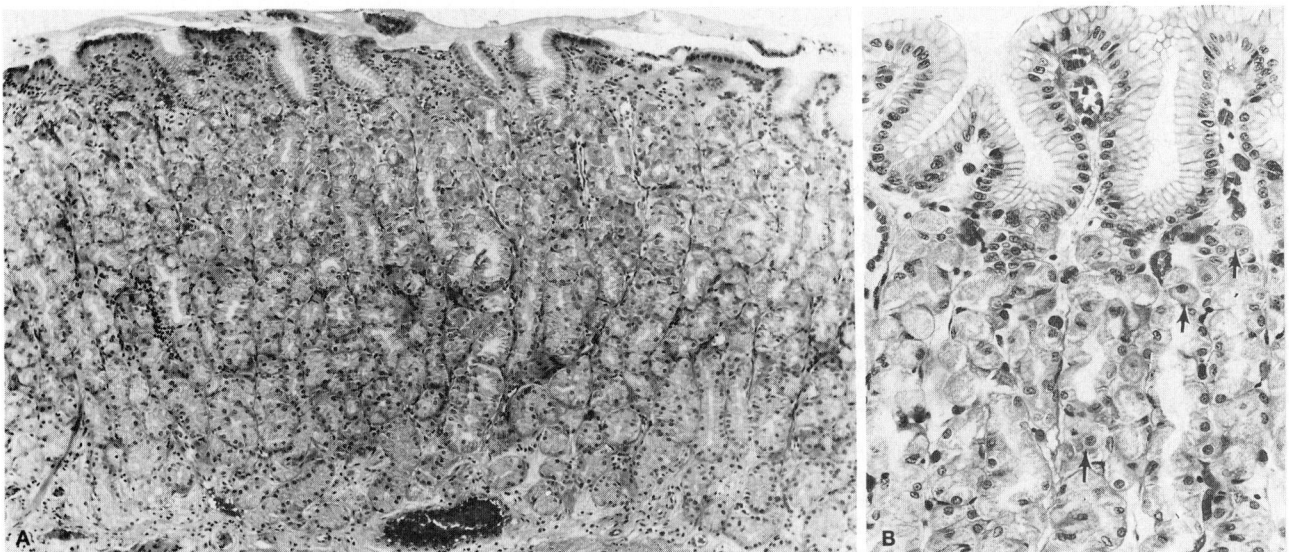

FIGURE 130-21. Biopsy specimen of a typical hiatal hernia pouch. (**A**) The gastric fundic mucosa is normal. The surface is covered by normal gastric surface mucus cells that dip into normal shallow foveolae. (**B**) The lamina propria contains no recognizable inflammatory infiltrate and numerous parietal cells are visible in the normal fundic glands (*arrows*).

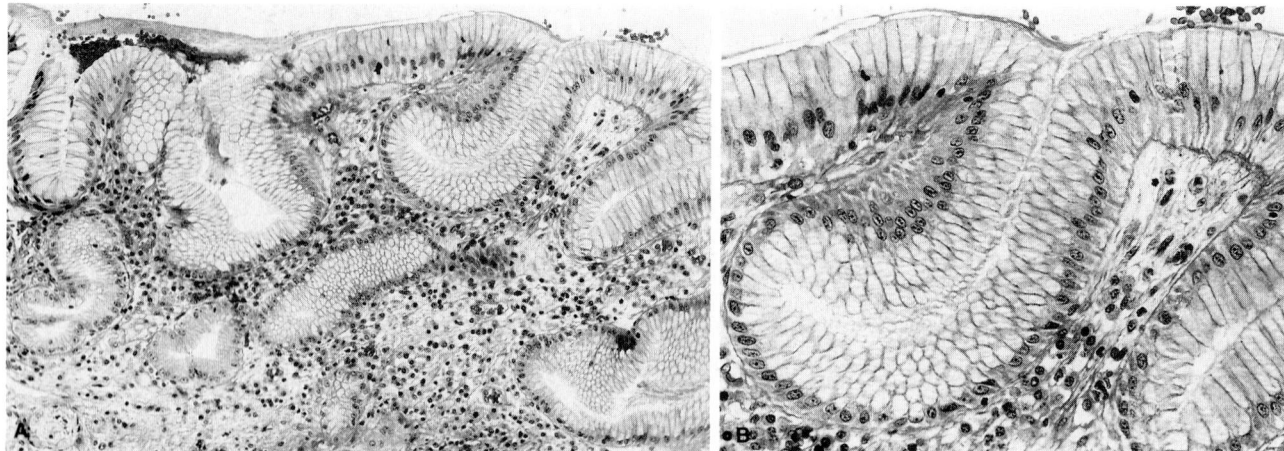

FIGURE 130-22. Normal gastric cardia. (**A**) The surface epithelium, foveolae, and glands are lined by cells producing mucus. The lamina propria contains a mild increase in lymphocytes and plasma cells, a feature found in the majority of normal biopsy specimens from this portion of the stomach. (**B**) The appearance of the epithelial mucus cells covering the surface and lining the foveolae is well illustrated at higher magnification.

of AIDS and several iatrogenic types of immunosuppression: chemotherapy, organ transplant, and others. The budding yeasts and pseudohyphae (see Fig. 130-23A) of *Candida* organisms may be recognized, especially in biopsy specimens stained with periodic acid-Schiff (see Fig. 130-23B). The presence of such pseudohyphae within the tissue indicates invasive infection but its absence does not exclude it, especially if clinical evidence shows dissemination. CMV can best be found in the mesenchymal cells of the granulation tissue in the base of ulcers, whereas HSV is located in the epithelium at the ulcer's edge.

Isolated enlarged cells containing CMV may be difficult to find histologically. The characteristic features of CMV are cytomegaly with a large viral inclusion with a surrounding

halo occupying most of the nucleus, and granular inclusions in the cytoplasm (see Fig. 130-23C). Cells infected by HSV are smaller than those infected with CMV, and the inclusions are only nuclear and not cytoplasmic. The histologic manifestations of HSV in the squamous epithelium include multinucleated epithelial giant cells (see Fig. 130-23D) and multiple small eosinophilic particles of HSV in hollow-appearing *ground glass* nuclei (see Fig. 130-23D). Varicella zoster virus closely resembles the histologic features of HSV. Greater sensitivity and specificity in diagnosing CMV, HSV, and varicella zoster virus in biopsy specimens can be achieved by using a panel of specific monoclonal antibodies to viral antigens, by performing in situ hybridization with specific nucleotide probes, or by shell vial centrifugation culture. Amplification

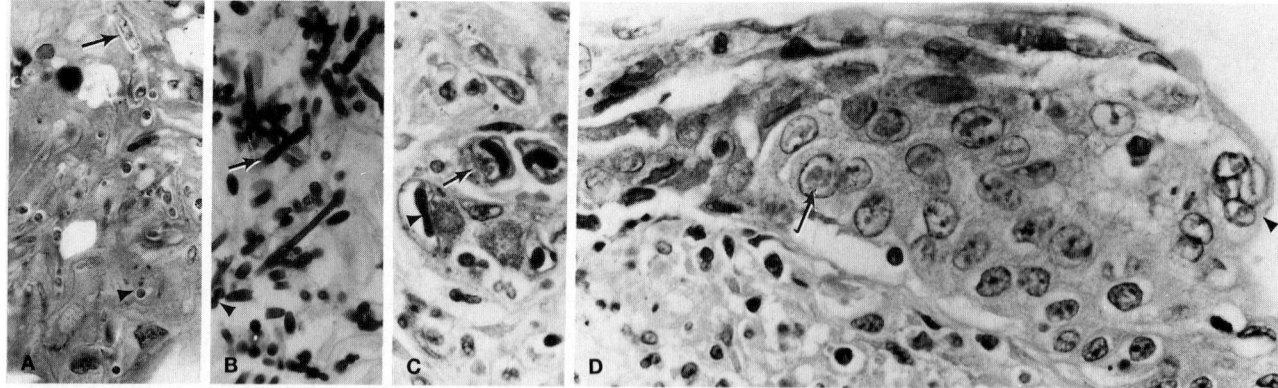

FIGURE 130-23. Esophageal biopsy specimens from various opportunistic infections. (**A**) High-power magnification illustrates esophageal squamous mucosa in which there are budding yeasts (*arrowhead*) and infiltrating pseudohyphae of *Candida* organisms (*arrow*). (**B**) Periodic acid-Schiff stain for carbohydrates highlights the budding yeasts (*arrowhead*) and pseudohyphae of *Candida* organisms (*arrow*). (**C**) A high-power photomicrograph of esophageal mucosa in which cytomegalovirus is present. The arrowhead indicates a diagnostic inclusion body with a surrounding halo within the nucleus of an enlarged mesenchymal cell. This cell and the one marked by the arrow also contain granular cytoplasmic inclusions. (**D**) The characteristic findings of herpes simplex virus infection: ground glass nuclei, a Cowdry type A inclusion body (*arrow*) and multinucleated giant cells (*arrowhead*).

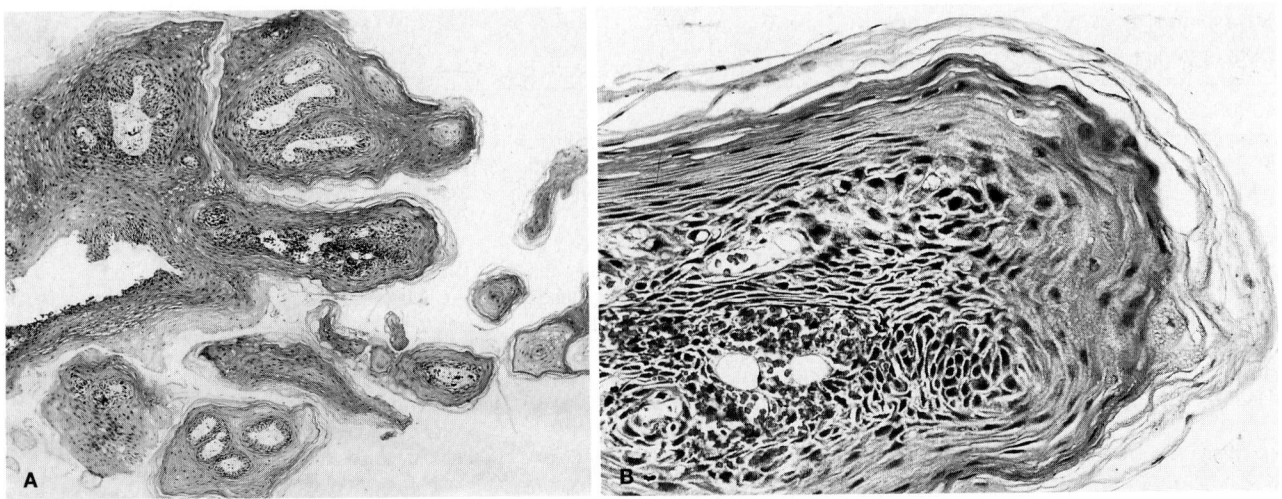

FIGURE 130-24. Esophageal biopsy specimen of a squamous papilloma. (**A**) Papillary (finger-like) projections are characteristic. (**B**) The central fibrovascular cores of the papillae are covered by lamellated, benign, squamous epithelium.

of fragments of the viral genome by the polymerase-catalyzed chain reaction recently has markedly increased the sensitivity and specificity of detection of these pathogens.

A variety of other benign conditions are diagnosable by endoscopic biopsy. The most common is the clinically unimportant entity of glycogenic acanthosis.[38] This condition is diagnosed by biopsy of small white nodules or plaques that can be shown to contain excess cytoplasmic glycogen within squamous cells, as revealed by periodic acid-Schiff–stained granules that disappear after glycogenolysis with diastase. Other rare esophageal diseases are difficult to diagnose by endoscopic biopsy alone: sarcoidosis, Crohn's disease, Behcet's disease, graft-versus-host disease, and the esophageal lesions seen in patients with bullous skin disease.

Clinically significant benign esophageal tumors are uncommon. The most frequent tumor is submucosal leiomyoma, which requires a deeper biopsy for diagnosis than is usually obtainable. A squamous papilloma is a warty growth composed of finger-like projections of benign squamous epithelium (Fig. 130-24). Inflammatory fibroid polyps contain active inflammation and eosinophils in a prominent fibrovascular stroma. A submucosal tumor of polygonal cells filled with fine granules suggests a granular cell tumor (Fig. 130-25). Lipomas are difficult to diagnose by biopsy because they are submucosal and covered by normal mucosa.

Diffuse Benign Gastric Mucosal Abnormalities

Gastritis

This section reviews the state of biopsy diagnosis of gastritis and of the other benign diffuse gastric mucosal abnormalities that often are inappropriately called *gastritis* even though they do not contain inflammatory cells such as polymorphonuclear leukocytes, seen in active inflammation, or excess numbers of plasma cells, seen in chronic inflammation (Table 130-2).

Why has gastritis always been a problem for physicians? One reason is that a large segment of the population has gas-

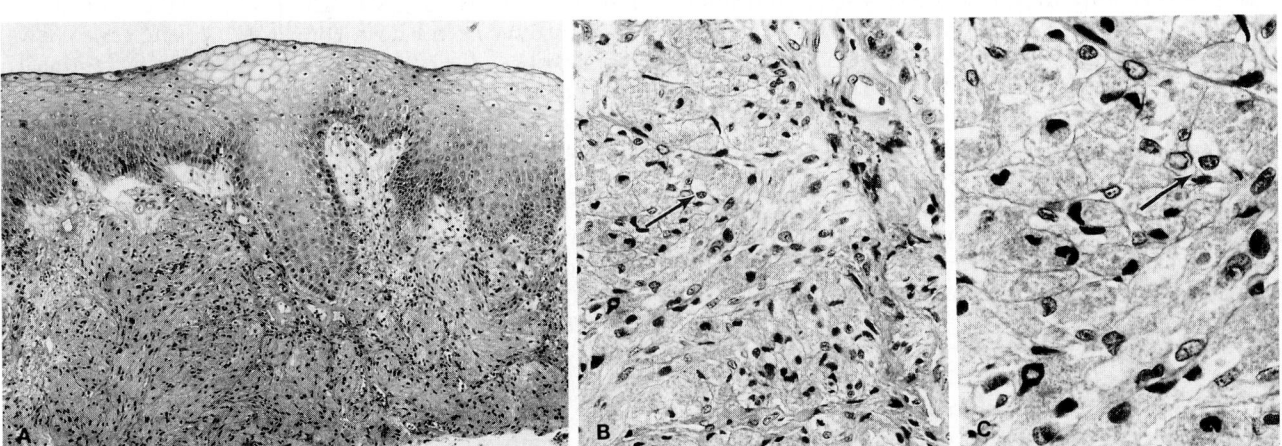

FIGURE 130-25. Granular cell tumor of the esophagus. (**A**) The lamina propria contains sheets of polygonal cells with granular cytoplasm. The area marked by arrows is progressively enlarged in **B** and **C**.

TABLE 130-2
Diffuse Benign Gastric Mucosal Abnormalities

DIAGNOSIS	HISTOLOGIC FEATURES	CLINICAL FEATURES
Diffuse antral gastritis	Almost 100% HP+, diffuse interfoveolar inflammation, deeper pyloric glands intact, milder inflammation in fundus	Asymptomatic or associated with prepyloric or DU; predominates in Caucasian middle-class persons in the United States where DU is common; reversible with HP eradication
Multifocal atrophic gastritis	Starts in multiple foci at antrofundic junction, spreads and progresses to glandular atrophy with intestinal metaplasia, only inflammation reversible with HP treatment; atrophy and intestinalization irreversible	Common in socioeconomically depressed populations, associated with GU and gastric cancer, but DU uncommon
Chronic fundal atrophic gastritis or atrophy	Chronic inflammation progresses to partial or complete loss of parietal and chief cells, and diffuse intestinal or pyloric gland metaplasia	May be autoimmune with parietal cell destruction leading to loss of secretion of HCl and intrinsic factor with resultant pernicious anemia
Hemorrhage and erosions (erosive gastropathy)	Erosions, superficial hemorrhage; edema and little or no inflammation; foveolar hyperplasia	Multiple causes: NSAIDs, alcohol, stress, hypoperfusion, iatrogenic
Vascular ectasia	Red spots or stripes, containing dilated mucosal capillaries, AV anastomoses in submucosa	Can be idiopathic but is seen more often in cirrhosis and renal failure; can bleed substantially
Infections (opportunistic)	CMV, HSV, Candida, TB, and syphilis	Most common in AIDS and other immunosuppressed states
Hypertrophies	Ménétrier disease; few or no parietal and chief cells; foveolar hyperplasia	Protein-losing enteropathy
	Gastrinoma; many parietal and chief cells	Elevated blood gastrin and excess gastric acid secretion
	Severe DU diathesis (hypertrophic hypersecretory gastropathy)	Normal blood gastrin, excess acid secretion
Postgastrectomy	Stomach: normal fundic glands; stoma: foveolar hyperplasia, epithelial regenerative atypia and no dysplasia	Not a carcinoma precursor in the United States

AIDS, acquired immunodeficiency syndrome; AV, atreriovenous; CMV, cytomegalovirus; DU, duodenal ulcer; GU, gastric ulcer; HCl, hydrochloric acid; HP, Helicobacter pylori; HSV, herpes simplex virus; NSAIDs, nonsteroidal antiinflammatory drugs; TB, tuberculosis; +, positive.

tritis histologically, but many have neither symptoms nor definable disease. Furthermore, without biopsy proof, many physicians misuse the term gastritis as a diagnostic wastebasket for any obscure digestive upset. Even with a positive biopsy, considerable doubt may exist that the mucosal abnormality found is related to the patient's illness, because the histologic picture of gastritis may be present before symptoms develop or may persist after recovery. It is generally accepted that no reliable endoscopic appearance corresponds to the histologic diagnosis of gastritis except for the visible erosions in so-called erosive gastritis. But why call these hemorrhagic erosions gastritis when the biopsy specimens show mucosa that often is uninflamed or at the most, mildly inflamed? Many investigators now believe that Helicobacter may well be the primary cause of most forms of gastritis, most peptic ulcers,[39,40] and even gastric carcinoma and lymphoma.[41] The controversies regarding these possible etiologic relationships will be gradually resolved when more objective data become available from populations living in widely varying environments in the developing and developed world. The wide geographic variation in the types of gastritis, ulcer, and cancer associated with HP suggests a multifactorial etiology of these diseases. One certainty is that the discovery of HP has rejuvenated the study of gastritis by making the whole subject more relevant clinically.

The association between antral gastritis and duodenal ulcer (DU) in the developed world has been known for a long time, well before the existence of HP was recognized. It is accepted that almost 100% of patients with DUs in the United States have an HP-infected diffuse antral gastritis. Furthermore, successful pharmacologic eradication of HP causes gradual reversal of this gastritis and long term, possibly permanent healing of the associated DU. This is why HP therapy in ulcer has caused such excitement. Formerly DUs were healed only temporarily, or their recurrence was minimized by continual acid suppressive therapy. Now cure of DUs is possible. One caveat is the apparent inability to eradicate HP permanently in certain environments, such as those found in Peru,[42] where the public water supply may contain these organisms.[43]

Little doubt exists that Helicobacter is an important pathogen. What has not been determined is whether it is the main cause of duodenal and gastric ulcers, or just one of several important factors contributing to their pathogenesis. The areas of Helicobacter research that most need more objective and methodic study are the several types of HP-infected gastritis and their different kinds of associated ulcer disease and gastric cancer. Such studies require multiple biopsy specimens of the whole length of the stomach taken in a standardized way to determine the diagnostic differences in histopathologic features and distribution of gastritis.

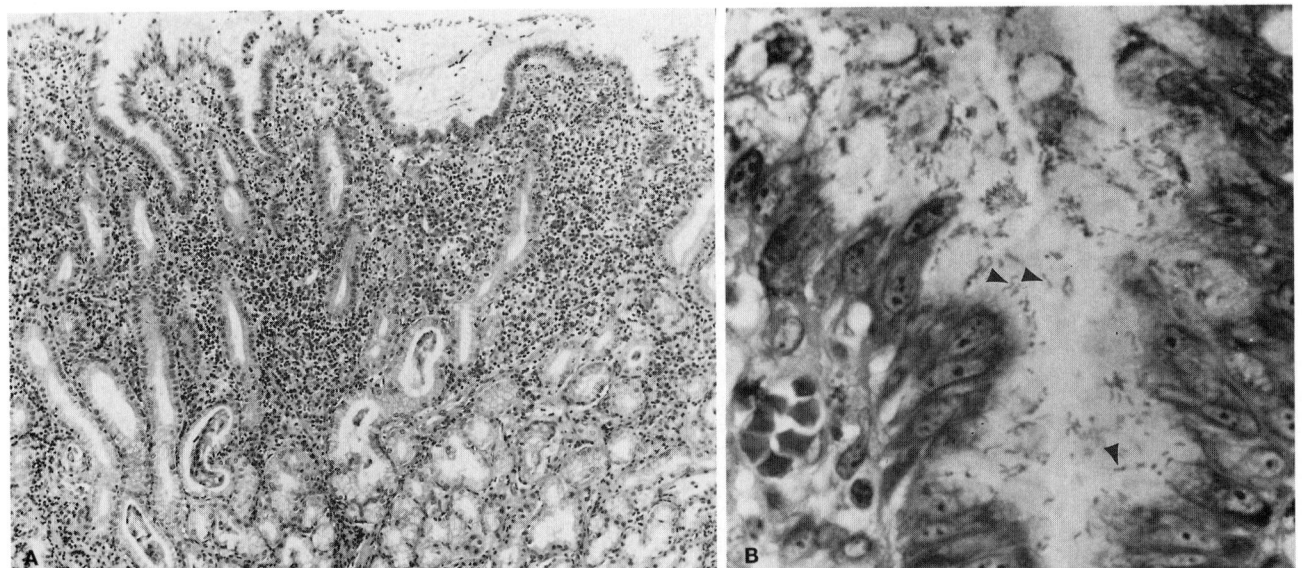

FIGURE 130-26. Diffuse antral gastritis. (**A**) A marked inflammatory infiltrate in the lamina propria of the upper portion of the mucosa is associated with an apparent reduction in the number of glands. Ample numbers of pyloric glands are present in the rest of the uninflamed mucosa. Although they cannot be recognized at this magnification, neutrophils infiltrate the glandular epithelium. (**B**) Examination of the surface and foveolar epithelium at higher power discloses numerous curved bacilli that are *Helicobacter pylori* (arrowheads). Notice the presence of the organisms in the mucous layer adjacent to the surface of the gastric surface mucus cells.

The classification of the various types of gastritis associated with HP infection is an evolving process that does not justify a final dogmatic diagnostic categorization. Even a preliminary pathogenetic description of HP-infected gastritis must take into account the wide geographic variations in its histologic appearance in populations that differ environmentally and socioeconomically. Not only are the types of gastritis different, but the prevalence and intensity of HP infection in many developing countries is greater and earlier in onset than in developed ones. Surprisingly, DU is uncommon despite the higher level of HP infection in nonindustrialized nations and, unlike the United States, the intestinal type of gastric cancer remains a frequent problem (see Fig. 130-12). The description of HP-infected gastritides proposed by Correa and associates appeals to us because it makes sense clinically. They point out that the predominant form of HP-infected gastritis in middle-class Caucasians in the United States is a diffuse antral gastritis (DAG), whereas the main type of gastritis in many parts of nonindustrialized nations is a multifocal atrophic gastritis (MAG).[44] As in most biologic phenomena, the differences between DAG and MAG are not absolute. Mixtures do occur. For example, varying degrees of MAG, at times superimposed on DAG, are typical in certain segments of the United States population, such as the elderly, Hispanics, African Americans, Asians, Polynesians, and Eastern European immigrants.[44] Much work on the environmental and socioeconomic variations in gastric pathology remains to be done. For example, it appears that DAG does not progress to MAG in middle-class Americans, whereas DAG is thought to progress to MAG in Peruvian[45] and Finnish[46] populations.

Typically DAG shows excessive infiltration with plasma cells and lymphocytes throughout the antrum. Characteristically the pyloric glands deeper within the mucosa are retained, and intestinal metaplasia is minimal or absent; HP almost always is present (Fig. 130-26). DAG also may involve the body of the stomach to varying extent, but it is milder and the fundic glands remain intact (Fig. 130-27). Although DAG in patients infected with HP is present in almost 100% of individuals with DUs in the United States, HP in the duodenal bulb adjacent to an ulcer is seen in less than half of patients with a DU, and then only when there is gastric surface cell metaplasia in the duodenal mucosa.

Multifocal atrophic gastritis is the predominant HP-associated gastritis in many nonindustrialized communities. It can best be diagnosed by multiple biopsies of the antrum, antrofundic junction, and fundic gland area. Correa finds HP-infected MAG by endoscopic biopsy, even in teenaged patients in the Colombian Andes*; whereas the Peruvians find 50% of children to have HP-infected *superficial antral gastritis,* probably DAG, that progresses to atrophic gastritis as they grow older.[45] Stemmerman and Hayashi[47] and Correa and associates[44] have observed that MAG is not a diffuse disease initially but one that begins at the antrofundic junction in multiple foci of glandular loss (atrophy), gastritis, and intestinal metaplasia. This process may spread so that the end stage shows diffuse atrophy with intestinal metaplasia (see Fig. 130-11). Thus the picture evolves with time and changes appearance and distribution. Notice that gastric ulcers have a predilection for the antrofundic junction, where MAG is most obvious. Eradication of HP with antibiotics reverses the inflammation of MAG but has little effect on the atrophy or intestinal metaplasia.

---

* Correa P, personal communication.

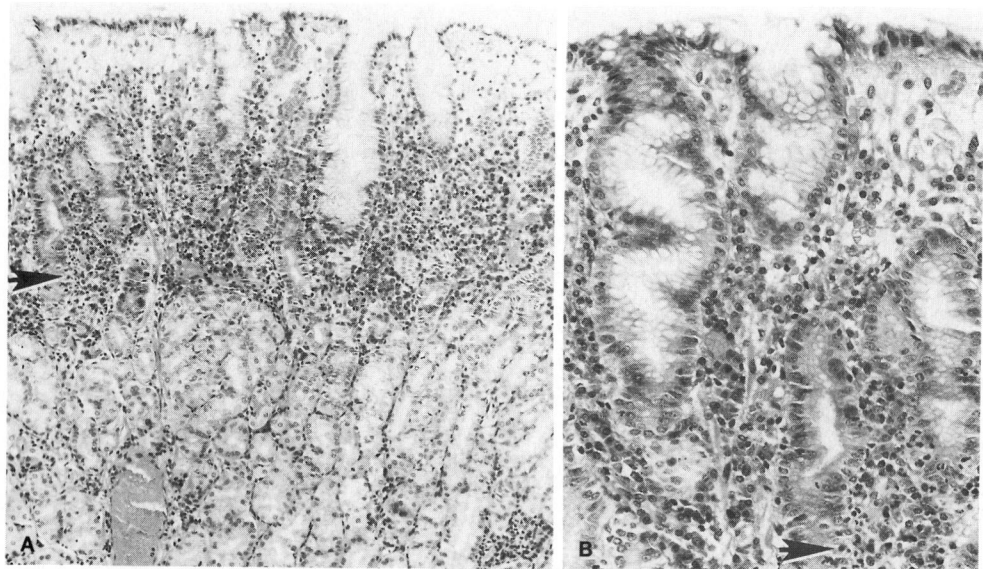

FIGURE 130-27. Spread of diffuse antral gastritis to the body of the stomach. **(A)** The inflammatory infiltrate is less severe than that seen in the antrum and is primarily limited to the most superficial mucosa. **(B)** The region indicated by the arrow is shown at higher magnification. Notice the neutrophilic infiltration of the epithelium and the decreased quantity of mucus within the surface and foveolar epithelium. The fundic glands are intact. *Helicobacter pylori* were present at the surface.

Because the diagnosis of DAG or MAG depends on the distribution and nature of the mucosal abnormalities, at least 8 to 10 biopsy specimens representative of the whole length of the stomach are needed for definitive diagnosis. This requires modification of current clinical practices. Only methodic endoscopic biopsy research in different geographic areas and populations of high and low socioeconomic status will establish the differing patterns of gastritis and associated ulcer and cancer. This information will be invaluable in planning further research on pathogenesis of these gastritis-associated diseases.

The marked differences between the types of gastritis and the incidence of DU, gastric ulcer, and the intestinal type of gastric cancer in the Western and nonindustrialized nations indicates that HP is not the only etiologic influence in ulcerogenesis. Environmental differences also exert a critical influence on the types of gastritis and associated diseases that develop. The etiology of *Helicobacter*-associated illnesses is multifactorial and possibly dependent on different factors such as the level of sanitation, dietary differences, environmental carcinogens, ingestion of nonsteroidal anti-inflammatory drugs (NSAIDs), smoking, genetic variation, and differences in HP virulence. Also remember that many more healthy individuals without ulcers or cancer are infected with HP than those who have these diseases.

It is well-known that many gastric ulcers develop within surrounding mucosa showing chronic gastritis, and about 70% of these gastric ulcers in the United States develop within HP-infected gastritis that frequently contains intestinal metaplasia. The 30% of gastric ulcers in uninflamed mucosa are caused mostly by NSAIDs; the mucosa surrounding these presumed NSAID-caused gastric ulcers often is uninflamed, free of HP, and exhibits foveolar hyperplasia (Fig. 130-28). *Helicobacter* gastritis is so widespread in patients without ulcers

that many NSAID-caused ulcers probably develop within gastric mucosa with preexisting HP-infected gastritis. Therefore a large proportion of gastric ulcers in the United States are associated with NSAIDs.

Although a clear relationship exists in the United States between most DUs and diffuse antral gastritis in patients infected with HP, the DUs that are rarely secondary to gastrinomas or short bowel syndrome do occur and are not usually associated with HP. In addition, most DUs heal in patients with HP-infected diffuse antral gastritis after acid-suppressive therapy alone; however, unless HP is eradicated the recurrence rate is high.

A number of interesting facts are known about HP infection in gastritis. Histologically the HP only grow near the surface of the gastric mucous cells, often within the layer of mucus covering them. The HP are not obviously invasive, although the underlying surface mucous cells may show injury by light and electron microscopic study.[40] Despite the almost 100% coexistence of HP, DAG, and DU in the United States, the only sites that may be infected by HP within an ulcerated duodenal bulb are areas of gastric surface cell metaplasia; HP do not grow on the surface of duodenal intestinal epithelium. Although focal gastric surface mucous cell metaplasia of the duodenum usually may be seen within the duodenal bulb, some believe that it may be more widespread in DU, providing more sites for HP to grow (Fig. 130-29). This probably does not explain how HP causes DU because less than 50% of DU patients have HP in the duodenum. A more attractive hypothesis to explain the relationship between HP and DU is the fact that patients with HP-infected DAG secrete an increased amount of gastrin, which decreases once the *Helicobacter* has been eradicated.[48] Therefore gastrin hypersecretion in response to HP infection may cause ulcers by increasing acid secretion.

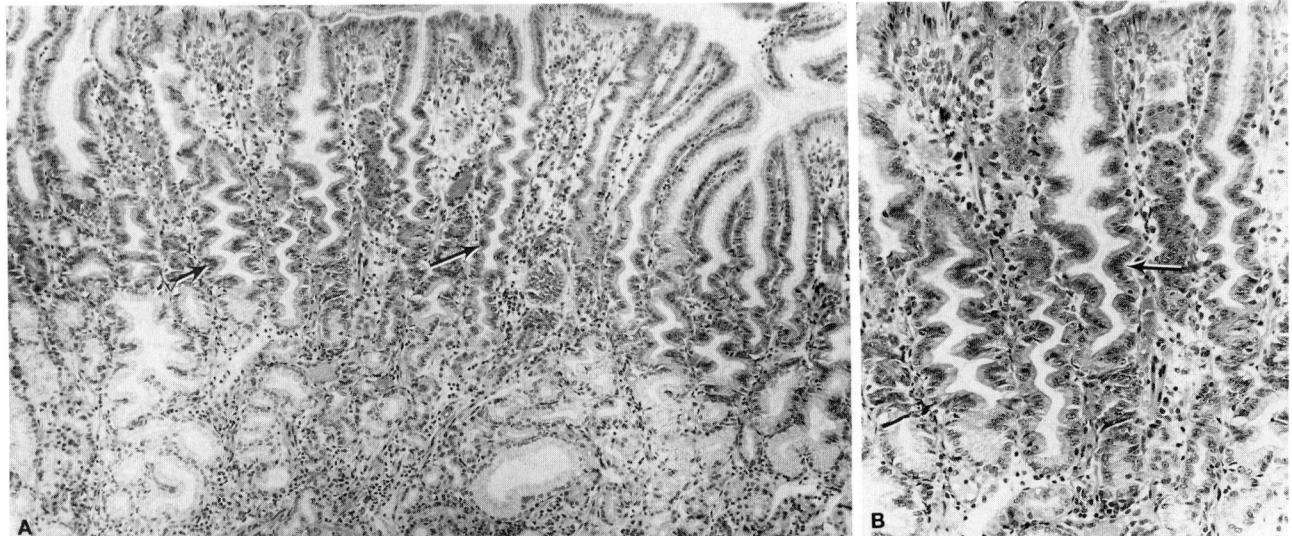

FIGURE 130-28. Gastric biopsy specimen shows foveolar hyperplasia associated with ingestion of nonsteroidal anti-inflammatory drugs. (**A**) Notice the corkscrew configuration of the elongated gastric foveolae (*arrows*) and the lack of gastritis indicated by the paucity of inflammatory cells within the lamina propria. (**B**) The foveolar hyperplasia and corkscrew configuration are seen at higher magnification (*arrow*). Notice the nuclear crowding and decreased quantity of mucus in the foveolar epithelium. No *Heliobacter pylori* were present.

Despite the increased incidence of the intestinal type of gastric cancer in nonindustrialized nations, many more individuals have no evidence of cancer despite the presence of HP-infected multifocal atrophic gastritis.[44,46,49] Other etiologic influences must be required for the development of cancer of the stomach. Does multifocal atrophic gastritis with intestinal metaplasia represent an end stage of diffuse antral gastritis with HP, or is it a manifestation of an entirely different process? Clear answers to these questions are not available, but either explanation may prove to be true in different etiologic milieus.[50,51]

Multifocal atrophic gastritis infected with HP is far more

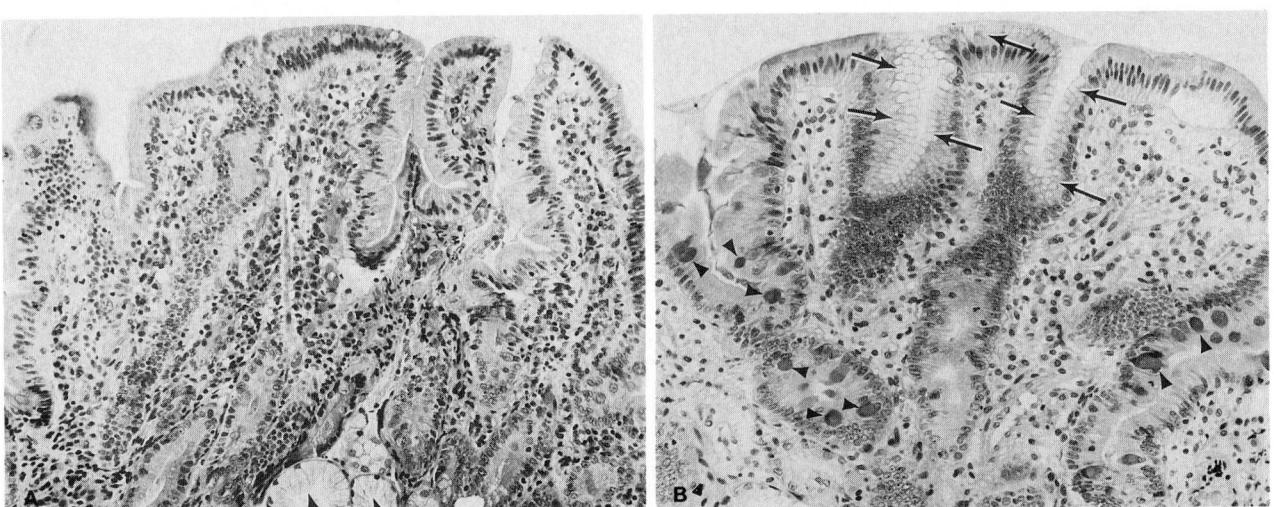

FIGURE 130-29. Normal duodenal mucosa (**A**) without and (**B**) with (*arrows*) gastric surface metaplasia. The irregular configuration and shortening of the villi are not abnormal in the duodenum. The quantity of lymphocytes and plasma cells within the lamina propria is highly variable in duodenal biopsy specimens, and the amount shown in the lamina propria is within normal limits. Notice the Brunner's glands at the bottom (*arrowheads*). (**B**) The small intestinal goblet cells appear as gray-black circular areas of acidic mucus (*arrowheads*). The arrows delineate two glands in which there is gastric surface metaplasia. Contrast the clear mucus within the gastric surface mucus cells with the darkly stained mucus within the goblet cells in the adjacent intestinal glands. (Hematoxylin and eosin plus Alcian blue stains at pH 2.5)

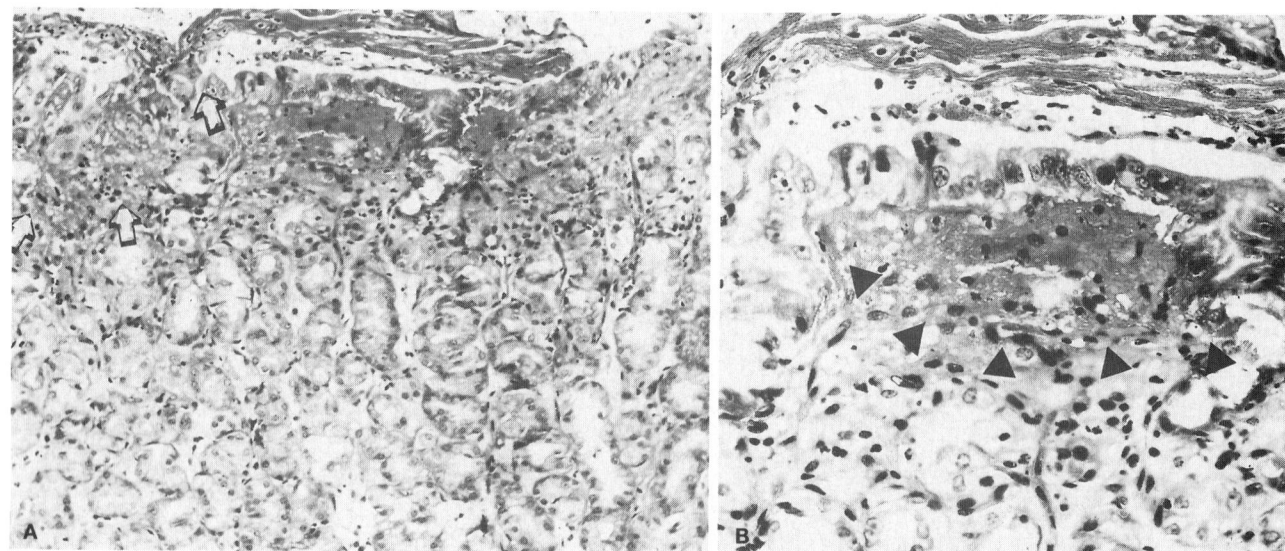

FIGURE 130-30. Gastric fundic mucosa in hemorrhagic (erosive) gastropathy. **(A)** There is a focus of erosion (*open arrows*) of the surface epithelium with fibrinopurulent exudate adherent to the mucosal surface. Notice the absence of inflammation within the gastric mucosa proper. Adjacent to the erosion, a focus of subepithelial hemorrhage (*arrowheads*) can be seen and **(B)** is marked at higher magnification (*arrowheads*).

common than fundic atrophy without HP in which evidence exists of autoimmune destruction of parietal cells with resultant achlorhydria and loss of intrinsic factor to mediate vitamin B_{12} absorption; this leads to pernicious anemia.[52]

Other Diffuse Mucosal Lesions

In some diffuse mucosal abnormalities, relatively little or no inflammation is present. Such abnormalities include hemorrhagic erosions, vascular ectasia, some opportunistic infections, mucosal hypertrophies, and postgastrectomy changes.

Erosions and hemorrhages are easily recognizable at endoscopy and usually are called *erosive gastritis*. On endoscopy, biopsy shows histologic evidence of widespread superficial hemorrhage under the surface epithelium (Fig. 130-30) in addition to erosions[53] (see Fig. 130-30). Active inflammation may or may not be seen. The erosions may have an appearance of superficial ischemic necrosis with pseudomembranes. Healing erosions may show foveolar hyperplasia. This pathologic picture of erosions and superficial hemorrhage has multiple causes: stress from burns, trauma, or severe illness; injury from drugs, especially NSAIDs and alcohol; ischemia from shock or arteriosclerotic narrowing of the celiac axis or its branches; and trauma from previous passage of tubes or endoscopes. When a patient with mucosal erosions develops severe hemorrhage requiring consideration for surgery, one or more of the erosions has probably progressed to a deeper acute ulcer that has eroded into a large submucosal blood vessel.[54]

Vascular ectasia of the gastric mucosa may bleed substantially.[55] They are seen more often in patients with cirrhosis or renal failure. Gastric vascular ectasias are made of dilated mucosal capillaries (Fig. 130-31) that extend to the surface and that owe their enlargement to increased arteriovenous anastomoses and other vascular abnormalities in the submucosa.[56] So-called *watermelon stomach* is probably a related

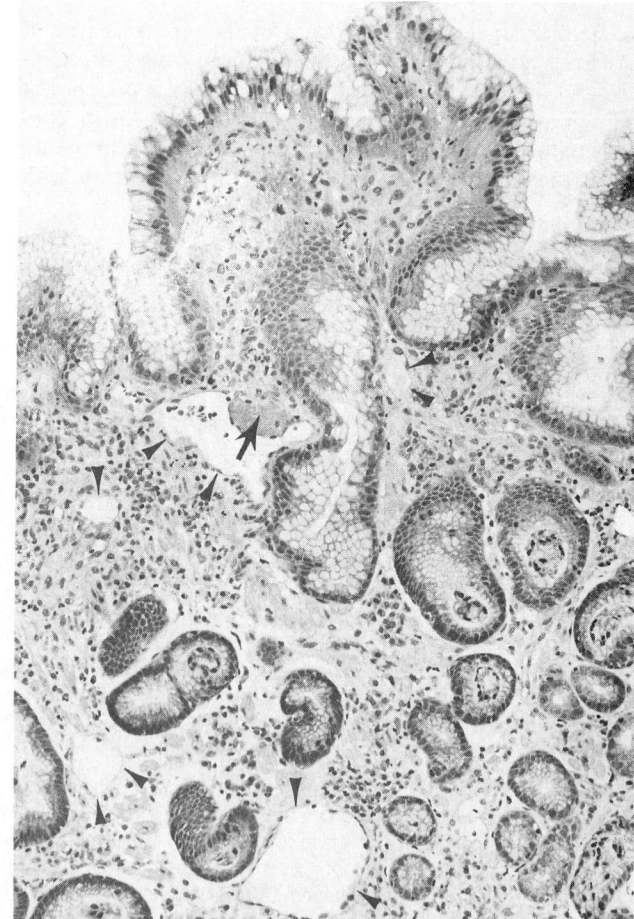

FIGURE 130-31. Gastric antral vascular ectasia. Dilated capillaries are present in the lamina propria (*arrowheads*). In one of these, a small fibrin thrombus attached to the capillary wall can be seen (*arrow*).

variant recognizable endoscopically as red linear stripes on the crests of folds in the distal stomach radiating toward the pylorus; they are made up of dilated capillaries containing fibrin thrombi (see Fig. 130-31).[57]

With the epidemic of AIDS and the many types of iatrogenic immunosuppression, opportunistic infection of the gastrointestinal tract has become more frequent, and gastric involvement is common. *Candida,* mycobacteria, CMV, and HSV all produce recognizable histologic findings whose sensitivity and specificity can be increased by special stains, immunocytochemical techniques, or shell vial centrifugation culture. Polymerase-catalyzed amplification of fragments of viral and bacterial genomes greatly increases the sensitivity of detecting these pathogens.

A variety of diffuse gastric mucosal *hypertrophies* are recognized as large folds by endoscopy. There are three causes of such folds:

- Ménétrier's disease
- gastrinoma
- hypertrophic hypersecretory gastropathy.

These lesions usually are impossible to sample deeply enough at endoscopy for definitive histologic diagnosis. In the proper clinical setting, the diagnosis of Ménétrier's disease is suggested by a convoluted cerebriform appearance of the gastric mucosa with excess secretion of thick, proteinaceous mucus endoscopically, a protein-losing gastropathy, and a biopsy specimen showing foveolar hyperplasia, little inflammation, and few or no parietal cells (Fig. 130-32). The patient may have a gastrinoma if there are heavy folds and grossly obvious acid hypersecretion during endoscopy, ample numbers of parietal and chief cells in the biopsy, and a clearly elevated serum gastrin level. A biopsy specimen with ample numbers of fundal gland parietal and chief cells and no serum gastrin elevation usually indicates a severe DU diathesis, which is probably synonymous with the nebulous entity called hypertrophic hypersecretory gastropathy.

Concern about malignancy developing near the gastroenterostomy stoma many years after partial gastrectomy is the result of European experience, where the risk is greatest 20 years or more after gastrectomy.[58] Epidemiologic study[59] and a personal unpublished endoscopic biopsy survey suggest that the situation in the United States is different: dysplasia is not present near the stoma and no increased frequency of malignant transformation exists. The mucosa near the stoma 20 or more years after gastrectomy in American patients shows only benign changes such as foveolar hyperplasia (see Fig. 130-27), regenerative atypia, and occasionally herniation of benign glands through the muscularis mucosae.

The symptomatic postgastrectomy patient who has voluminous regurgitation of bile-stained fluid into the gastric remnant presents a special problem. When do such patients have alkaline or bile reflux gastritis warranting reoperation to minimize duodenogastric regurgitation? The use of biopsy to answer this question probably is not appropriate because the characteristic histologic picture of reflux gastritis is nonspecific: foveolar hyperplasia with relatively little inflammation and some depletion of mucus. This picture may be seen in asymptomatic and symptomatic postgastrectomy patients and may occur in other unrelated conditions such as NSAID injury.

Two other diseases with unusual gastric mucosal inflammatory responses are seen. The first is granulomatous gastritis.[60] The most common cause is Crohn's disease; even giant cells without a clear granuloma suggest Crohn's disease in the stomach and duodenum (Fig. 130-33). These patients seem to have isolated gastric Crohn's disease but eventually multiple endoscopic biopsies reveal duodenal, terminal ileal, or colonic Crohn's disease in most of them. If the patient is older than 40 years of age and if the granulomas are confined to the stomach, the entity of isolated granulomatous gastritis must be considered. Another unusual reason for gastric granulomas is sarcoidosis, but diagnosis of this disease requires evidence of a multisystem disease. Multiple large granulomas

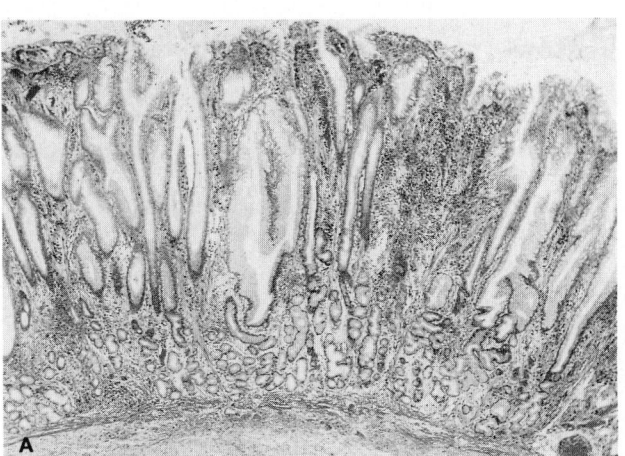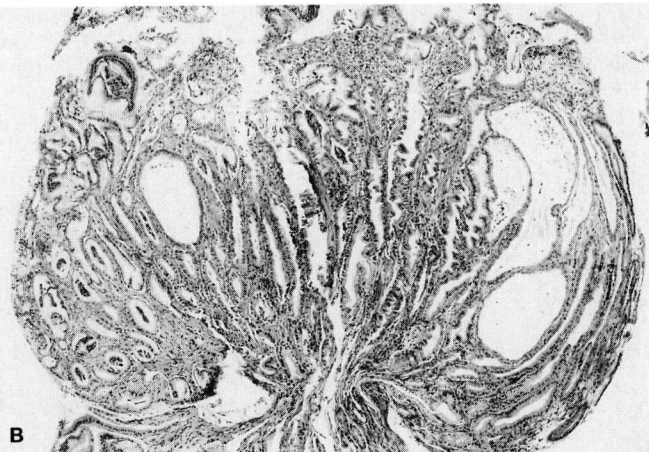

FIGURE 130-32. Ménétrier's disease. **(A)** A section of the gastric body taken from a resected stomach. The gastric pits or foveolae are strikingly elongated and irregular in configuration. This appearance is produced by a profound hyperplasia of the foveolar cells that extend into the glands and replace the parietal and chief cells so that the body mucosa is now composed exclusively of mucus-producing foveolar cells. **(B)** An endoscopic biopsy specimen from a patient with Ménétrier's disease; in addition to the marked foveolar hyperplasia that produces a corkscrew appearance of the pits, there are dilated glands, another feature commonly seen in Ménétrier's disease.

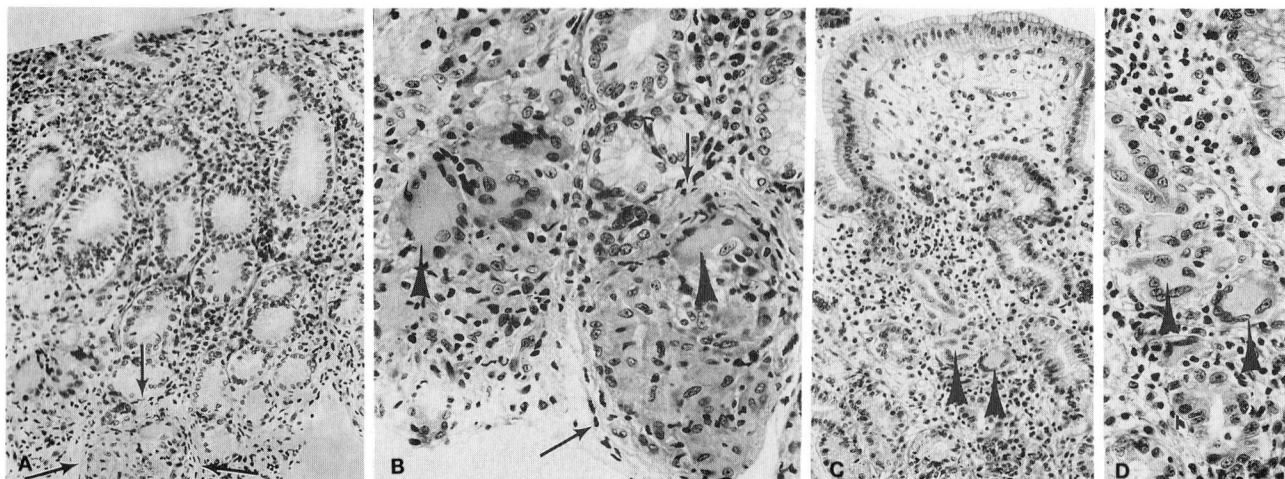

FIGURE 130-33. Granulomatous gastritis in a patient with Crohn's disease. (**A**) A discrete epithelioid granuloma is seen (*arrows*) and (**B**) at higher magnification (*arrows*). This granuloma is composed of a compact aggregate of epithelioid histiocytes with a multinucleated giant cell (*arrowhead*). In the stomach such granulomas usually prove to be associated with Crohn's disease. Isolated multinucleated giant cells are present just to the left of the discrete granuloma (*arrowhead*). (**C, D**) Multinucleated giant cells (*arrowheads*) can be seen in association with a few epithelioid histiocytes but no discrete granuloma. In the stomach and duodenum, giant cells like these are strongly suggestive of Crohn's disease.

containing necrotic centers suggest the possibility of tuberculosis and warrant a Ziehl-Neelsen stain with careful search for acid-fast bacilli.

The second unusual type of inflammatory response is seen with gastric involvement in eosinophilic gastroenteritis. This may be confined to the gastroduodenal mucosa, or it may be a component of a more diffuse submucosal or peritoneal eosinophilic gastroenteritis. Scattered eosinophils in the lamina propria are normal, but clumps of eosinophils, particularly when they infiltrate the epithelium, suggest eosinophilic gastritis, provided there is also marked elevation of the eosinophil count in the peripheral blood.

Despite the excitement regarding HP and the evolving understanding of the nongastric mucosal lesions, the precise clinical significance of some of these histopathologic entities remains uncertain.

Discrete Gastric Lesions

The most common gastric polyp, accounting for perhaps 80% of all gastric polyps, is the benign hyperplastic polyp (Table 130-3).[61,62] These polyps usually are recognized endoscopically because of their characteristic features: they are small,

TABLE 130-3
Discrete Gastric Lesions

TYPE OF POLYP	HISTOLOGIC FEATURES	CLINICAL FEATURES
Hyperplastic	Foveolar hyperplasia, irregular cystic glands, and inflamed edematous stroma	Endoscopically multiple mesa-like sessile lesions; superficial erosions on the crests of folds; may contain adenomatous areas or cancer
Fundic gland	Sessile, small, multiple, fundal glands with cysts	Seen sporadically and in familial polyposis coli; not premalignant
Adenomatous	Usually solitary, > 2 cm, antral	Rare; premalignant or already malignant; often associated with dysplasia and cancer elsewhere in stomach
Juvenile polyposis	Cystic glands	In generalized juvenile polyposis, cancer is rare and only seen in associated adenomatous tissue
Peutz-Jeghers	Excess arborized smooth muscle, disorganized glands	Pigmented buccal and lip spots, small bowel polyps, increased frequency of cancer in the stomach, colon, and especially in nongastrointestinal sites
Cronkhite-Canada	Cystic glands, edematous lamina propria	Older than 60 yr, diarrhea, protein loss, skin changes; not premalignant
Inflammatory fibroid	Benign spindle cell tumor with inflammation and infiltration with eosinophils	May obstruct gastric outlet (prior misnomer: eosinophilic granuloma)
Other rare tumors	See text	

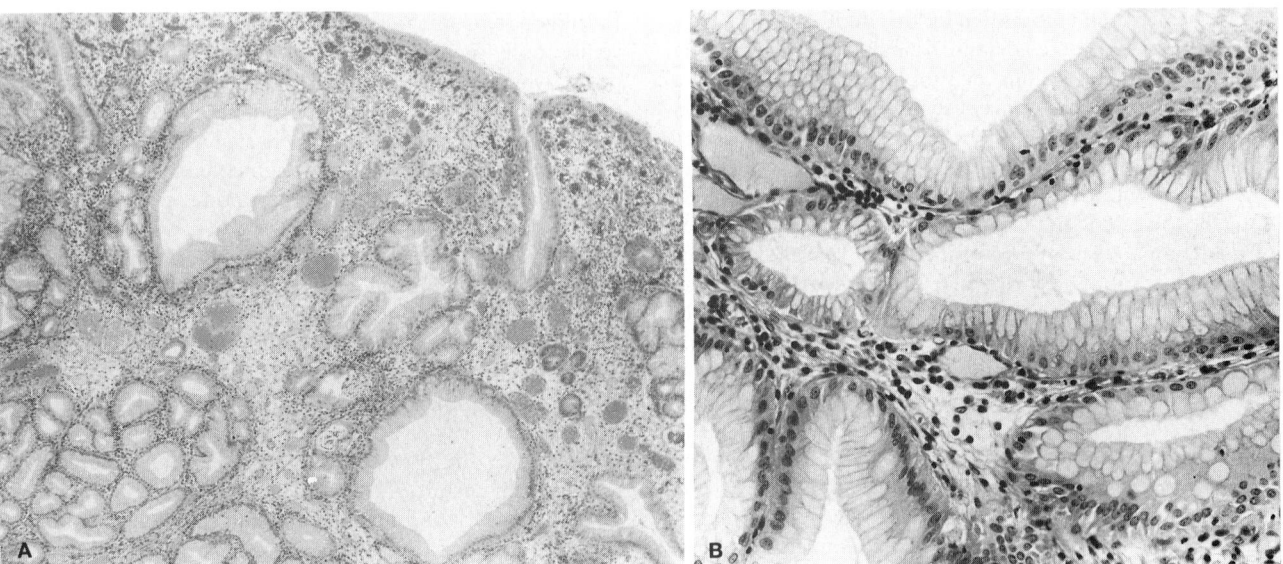

FIGURE 130-34. Hyperplastic gastric polyp. (**A**) The low-power view shows the dilated, irregular-shaped gastric glands lined with hyperplastic foveolar cells. Notice the inflamed, edematous stroma in which there are numerous dilated capillaries. (**B**) Higher magnification shows the hyperplastic foveolar cells lining the glands composing the polyp.

usually less than 2 cm in diameter; frequently multiple; and distributed on the crests of folds throughout the whole stomach. They have a sessile, mesa-like shape with an erosion or healed dimple on their top. So-called varioliform gastritis may be a variant of the same lesion. Less frequently a solitary or larger pedunculated hyperplastic polyp develops. Rather than being biopsied, they should be excised in toto because such hyperplastic polyps occasionally may contain foci of adenoma or carcinoma,[63] and they are occasionally associated with carcinoma elsewhere in the stomach; this is probably a chance relationship because of the fact that hyperplastic polyps and gastric cancer tend to arise in a background of multifocal atrophic gastritis. Foveolar hyperplasia, irregular-shaped cystic glands, and edema of the lamina propria are the typical but nonspecific histologic findings (Fig. 130-34). In spite of the synonymous name, hyperplastic polyps in the stomach are histologically different from those in the colon and are probably completely unrelated. When hyperplastic polyps have superficial erosions, there may be inflammatory atypia that may be misdiagnosed as dysplasia in a small biopsy specimen. It is rarely necessary to remove a whole sessile hyperplastic polyp with a snare for diagnosis because its typical endoscopic appearance is almost diagnostic. The less common, larger, pedunculated hyperplastic polyp can be snared with a low risk of complications and should be removed completely for diagnosis, as should all pedunculated polyps.

In the United States, adenomatous polyps of the stomach (Fig. 130-35) are uncommon, usually solitary, greater than

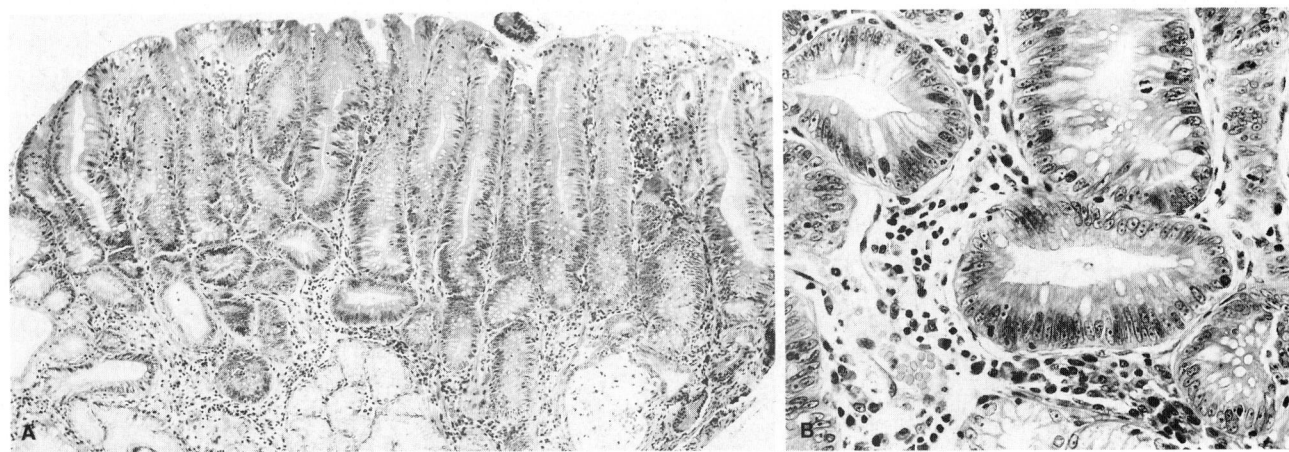

FIGURE 130-35. Gastric adenoma. (**A**) This biopsy sample of a polyp shows crowded tubular structures lined with dysplastic epithelial cells. Notice the uninvolved gastric glands at the bottom of the photograph. (**B**) Neoplastic epithelium at higher power. Observe the diminished mucus secretion and the crowded, hyperchromatic, slightly stratified nuclei.

1 cm in diameter, and most often located in the antrum. They closely resemble colonic adenomatous polyps histologically and may be tubular, villous, or tubulovillous. The mucosa surrounding gastric adenomas usually demonstrates multifocal atrophic gastritis and intestinal metaplasia. Gastric adenomas frequently contain a focus of carcinoma and also may be associated with carcinoma elsewhere in the stomach.[62,63] Strangely, the gastric adenomatous polyps associated with familial adenomatous polyposis of the colon have a lower than 3% prevalence of carcinoma, unlike the associated adenomas of the duodenum near the papilla of Vater that are frequently malignant, with a prevalence higher than 12%.[64–66] Pedunculated adenomatous polyps must be excised to exclude the diagnosis of focal carcinoma. Because precancerous dysplasia or early carcinoma may be present in the flat mucosa adjacent to the solitary adenoma, as well as within it, multiple biopsies of the apparently uninvolved surrounding mucosa are indicated. If the polyp contains carcinoma, and especially if dysplasia is present in the surrounding mucosa, simple endoscopic polypectomy may not be adequate therapy, and distal gastric resection with careful frozen section evaluation of the resection margins may be required.

Fundic gland polyps may carpet the fundus and body of the stomach. They consist of small sessile mucosal elevations made up of fundic glands that contain normal parietal and chief cells. Some of these glands are cystically dilated (Fig. 130-36).[67,68] Fundic gland polyps were first identified in association with familial adenomatous polyposis of the colon,[66] but are recognized to be more common in otherwise healthy, asymptomatic persons in whom they are discovered incidentally on an upper gastrointestinal radiograph or endoscopy.[67,69] These small polyps frequently can be excised in toto for diagnosis with a large biopsy forceps. They have no malignant potential and do not require continued endoscopic biopsy surveillance.

Polyps with histologic similarities to hyperplastic polyps are seen in three intestinal polyposis syndromes[70]:

- juvenile polyposis
- Peutz-Jeghers syndrome
- Cronkhite-Canada syndrome.

Juvenile polyps of the stomach are part of a generalized juvenile polyposis syndrome, in contrast to the solitary juvenile polyp, which is confined to the colon. Gastric cancer is rare in juvenile polyposis and has been described only within an associated adenoma. Peutz-Jeghers syndrome has characteristic clinical features including pigmented spots on the lips and buccal mucosa, multiple small bowel polyps, and less commonly, gastric or colonic polyps. These polyps may cause an obstruction or bleed. Gastrointestinal cancers occur with some increased frequency in Peutz-Jeghers syndrome in the stomach and colon; however, cancers of nongastrointestinal origin are even more common in these patients.[71] Cronkhite-Canada syndrome is a rare, acquired, generalized, nonneoplastic gastrointestinal polyposis syndrome.[72] The stomach is almost always involved; the patients are usually in their 60s and have diarrhea, protein loss, alopecia, and characteristic skin and nail changes.

Inflammatory fibroid polyps of the stomach may be pedunculated or sessile and may cause obstruction.[73] They are benign proliferations of spindle cells with local infiltration by eosinophils without an elevated eosinophil count in the peripheral blood. Formerly they were misnamed eosinophilic granulomas. Inflammatory fibroid polyps usually are asymptomatic until they reach a size large enough to obstruct the gastric outlet.

Kaposi's sarcoma in AIDS presents endoscopically as multiple violaceous, flat, macular lesions or as nodules that may have a surface that resembles a *strawberry* or *elephant hide*, or infrequently as *volcano* lesions with a superficial erosion at their peaks. Their histologic features and gross appearance are described in Premalignant and Malignant Gastrointestinal Lesions (see Fig. 130-15).

Other rare lesions include intramural, extramucosal tumors derived from muscle, fibrous tissue, nerve, or fat. Endoscopically all may show bridging mucosal folds extending from the tumor to the surrounding mucosa, like the flying buttresses of an ancient cathedral. It is often difficult to sample deeply enough during biopsy of these extramucosal lesions to provide a diagnosis. Many ulcerate and bleed; obstruction occurs in some. A variety of blood vessel tumors may be seen. Pancreatic rests occasionally are evident on gross inspection.

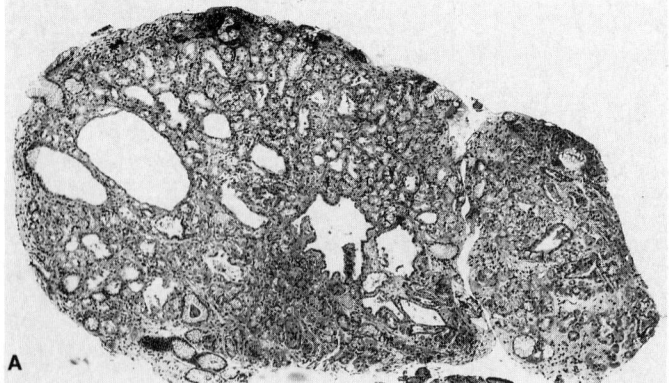 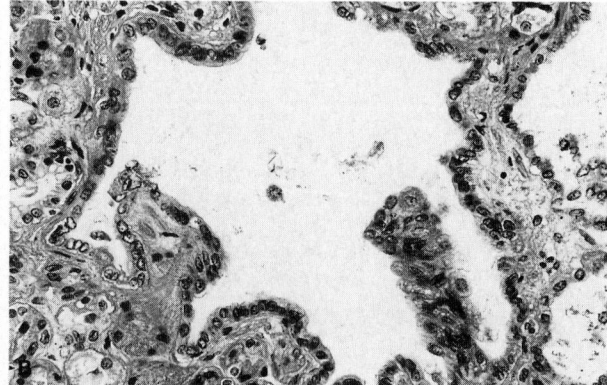

FIGURE 130-36. Fundic gland polyp of the stomach. **(A)** This endoscopic biopsy specimen from a small polyp shows dilated, irregular shaped fundic glands. **(B)** The nature of the cells lining the gland can be recognized; they include parietal cells and chief cells. Although not seen in this particular field, foveolar cells also may be present.

Short of total excision, gastric polyps may be difficult to diagnose histologically. Fortunately, gastric polyps often are pedunculated, and therefore can be easily excised for diagnosis with an electrocautery snare. Sessile lesions that cannot be excised as easily and safely with the endoscope may be diagnosable by multiple large biopsy specimens taken with a snare.

Gastric leiomyosarcoma, lymphoproliferative disorders with or without an ulcer, and adult hypertrophic pyloric stenosis usually are impossible to diagnose with certainty using superficial endoscopic biopsy; surgical resection or ancillary techniques such as immunocytochemical study or gene rearrangement studies for lymphoma to demonstrate monoclonality may be required for definitive diagnosis.

Carcinoids are diagnosable by their monotonously similar small round cells growing in cords, glands, or nests and invading the lamina propria and submucosa (Fig. 130-37). They are more common in pernicious anemia where they are indolent, rarely metastasize, and may regress after antrectomy.[74] The biologic behavior of other gastric carcinoids is difficult to predict, but metastasis usually does not occur until they exceed 2 cm in diameter.

Endocrine cells normally are present in the gastric mucosa and can be recognized by their granules and by their reversed polarity to the epithelial cells. Endocrine cell hyperplasia may be a carcinoid precursor and can be seen in pernicious anemia and atrophic gastritis when there is a chronically elevated serum gastrin.[75] Presumably it is caused by a trophic drive from the excess gastrin.

Disease of the Proximal Small Bowel and Ileum

The bulb, second, and third portions of the duodenum are accessible to endoscopic biopsy with a standard-length upper gastrointestinal endoscope.[76] Biopsy specimens of the terminal ileum often can be sampled using the colonoscope. The duodenojejunal junction can be sampled by blind suction biopsy

to provide larger sized, more easily interpretable specimens than those provided by proximal duodenal endoscopic biopsy, but at a cost of increased time and special skill. Even more time and skill are required to sample the whole length of the small bowel safely with the hydraulic suction biopsy tube. Because of the relative ease of taking endoscopic biopsy specimens, these two suction biopsy methods have fallen into disuse except for research or for special clinical problems. Biopsy specimens taken by endoscopy can be satisfactory for diagnosis provided they are large enough, taken in the distal second portion of the duodenum or in the proximal third portion, carefully unfolded and oriented, and step-serial sectioned.

The normal proximal duodenum may differ histologically from the rest of the small bowel (see Fig. 130-29).[77] Even in a normal duodenum, villi may be distorted or absent, especially in the bulb and over areas of the mucosa that contain Brunner's glands (see Fig. 130-29, *arrowheads*) penetrating through the muscularis mucosae. The number of lymphocytes and plasma cells in the lamina propria is greater in the normal duodenal bulb than in the rest of the small bowel. Foci of gastric surface cell metaplasia (see Fig. 130-29, *arrows*) normally may cover portions of the villi of the duodenal bulb. There are three major benign causes of nodular lesions within the bulb and proximal second portion of the duodenum:

- Brunner's gland hyperplasia
- Pyloric gland heterotopia
- Fundal gland heterotopia.

Because duodenitis cannot be diagnosed reliably by the endoscopic appearance of the duodenal bulb, biopsies are required to document this condition. Because the content of lymphocytes and plasma cells in the lamina propria of the bulb varies so much among normal persons, the histologic diagnosis of duodenitis requires evidence of active injury to the epithelium, usually in the form of neutrophilic infiltration of the crypt or surface epithelium (Fig. 130-38, *arrows*). Many of the same diffuse reactions seen in the stomach also may occur in the bulb, including hemorrhagic-erosive lesions, op-

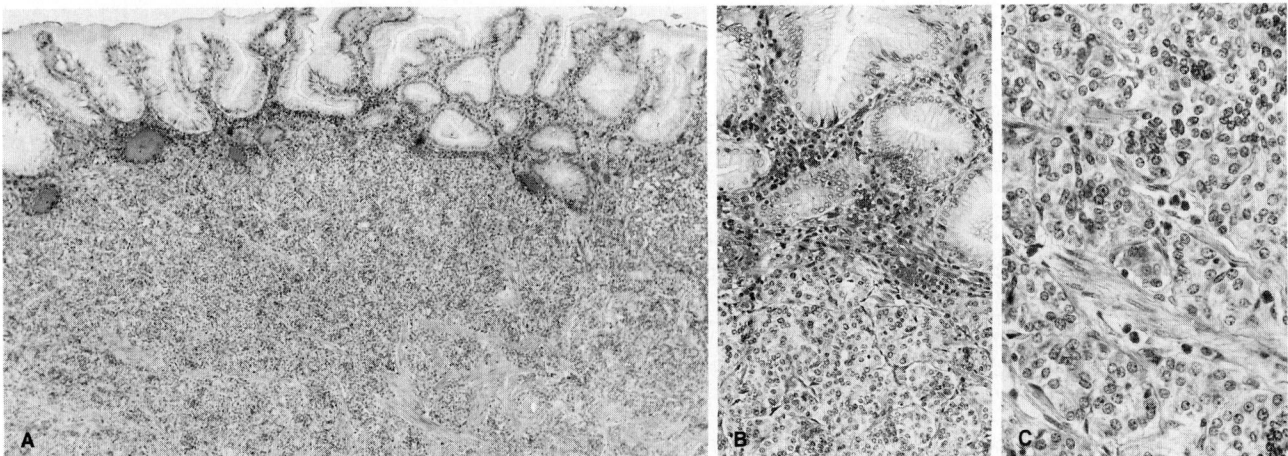

FIGURE 130-37. Gastric carcinoid. **(A)** Small nests, glands, and sheets of neoplastic cells have replaced most of the mucosa and invade into the muscularis mucosae and submucosa. **(B)** A higher magnification reveals nests of carcinoid cells in the lamina propria beneath the gastric pits. **(C)** At the highest magnification the small, round, uniform nuclei with the finely stippled chromatin pattern characteristic of carcinoid can be seen.

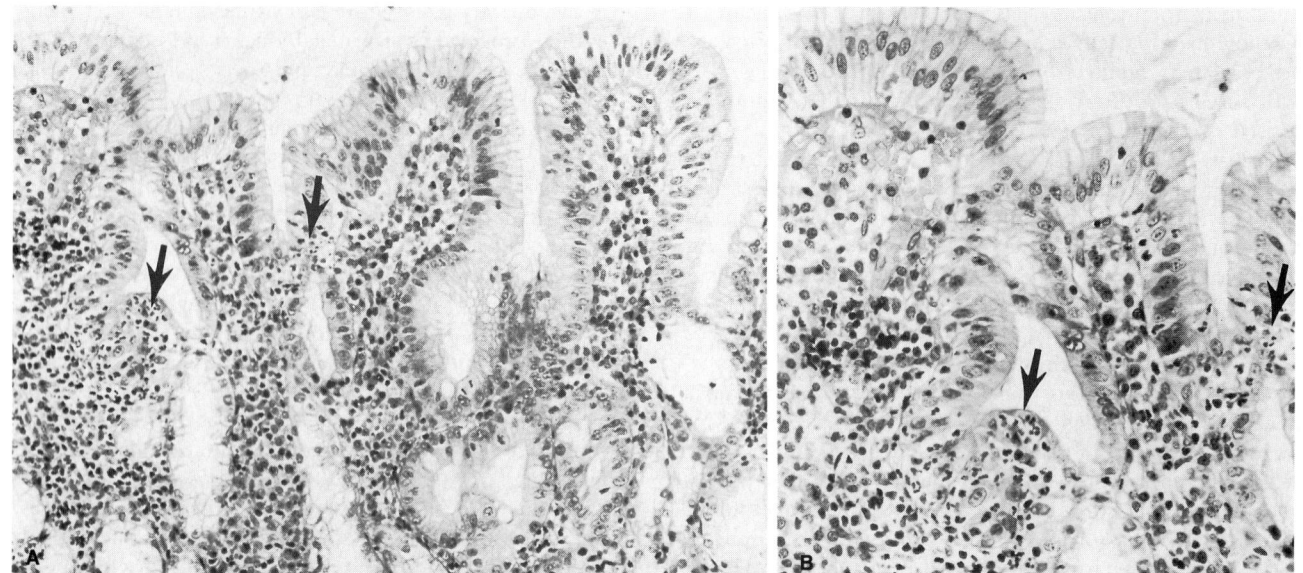

FIGURE 130-38. This duodenal biopsy sample shows active duodenitis. (**A**) There is a focus of neutrophilic infiltration of a gland (*arrows*). Notice the gastric surface cell metaplasia involving most of the surface cell of this biopsy specimen. Two glands to the right of center contain goblet cells and are normal intestinal glands, whereas the remainder of the glands are lined completely by cells that contain clear mucus and that represent gastric surface cells. Brunner's glands that have extended into the lamina propria are seen below; such findings also are seen in normal biopsy specimens of the duodenal bulb. (**B**) Higher magnification of the gland infiltrated by neutrophils, indicating active inflammation.

portunistic and other infections, and eosinophilic or granulomatous inflammation. For these reasons, we recommend that biopsy specimens taken to diagnose various kinds of more diffuse small intestinal mucosal disease also be taken as far distal to the bulb as possible, that is, in the distal second portion or proximal third portion of the duodenum. Biopsies of the crests of the valvulae conniventes should be done with the largest biopsy forceps passed through the operating endoscope. At least three or four large specimens should be taken and properly oriented before step-serial sectioning. This

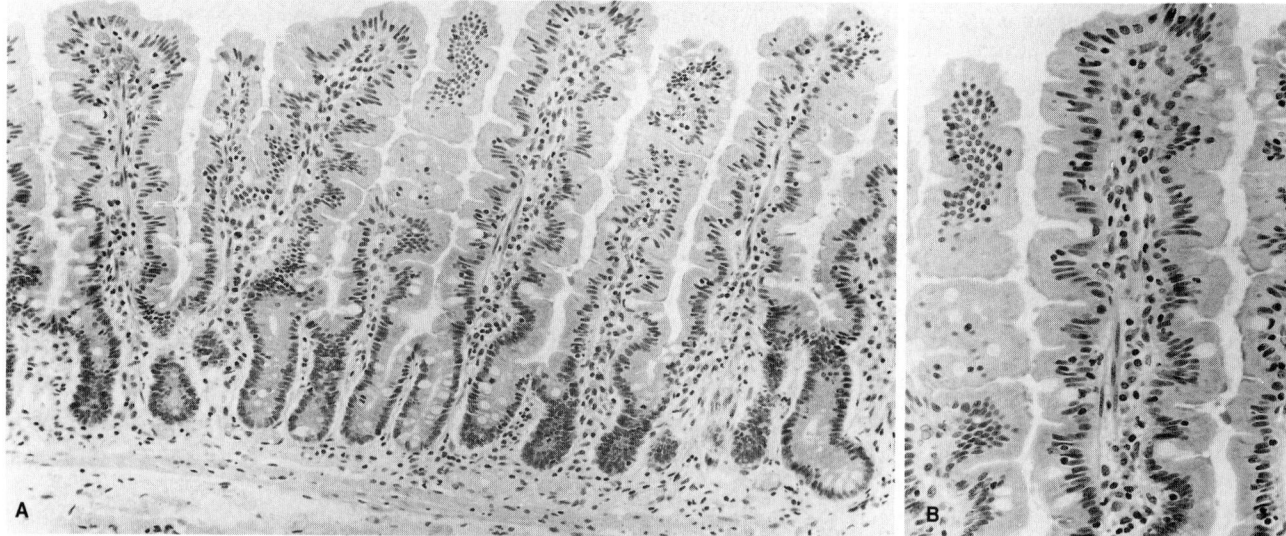

FIGURE 130-39. Biopsy specimen of normal distal duodenum. (**A**) The tall, slender villi are about three times as tall as the crypts are deep. Epithelial cells covering the villi consist predominantly of absorptive cells with scattered goblet cells. The nuclei of the surface epithelial cells are lined up in a uniform, picket fence–like arrangement. The lamina propria contains small numbers of lymphocytes and plasma cells. (**B**) The surface epithelium and lamina propria at higher magnification. The slender, fusiform cells in the lamina propria represent smooth muscle cells normally found in the cores of small bowel villi.

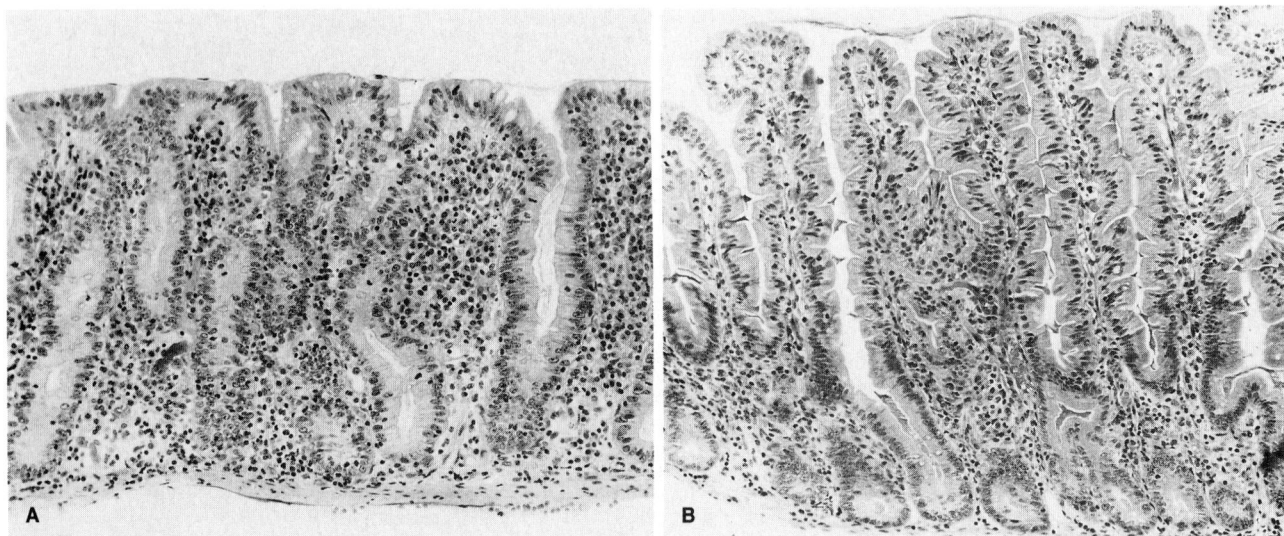

FIGURE 130-40. Celiac sprue. (**A**) Observe the flat mucosal surface in this biopsy specimen. The villi are effaced, and the crypts have become elongated. The lamina propria contains a prominent infiltrate of chronic inflammatory cells, and lymphocytes infiltrate the surface epithelium. (**B**) The appearance of this same patient's mucosa after an absolutely gluten-free period of 3 weeks, during which time total parenteral nutrition was administered. The villi have returned to a normal appearance and the inflammatory infiltrate within the lamina propria and surface epithelium has receded. Compare the abnormal appearance of the surface epithelial cells in **A** with those seen in **B**.

extra effort is essential to maximize the diagnostic sensitivity because so much depends on changes in the villous architecture, which is best judged in well-oriented sections.[77]

Distal duodenal or proximal jejunal biopsy specimens may show normal villi (Fig. 130-39), a flat appearance with complete absence of villi (Fig. 130-40A), or variably abnormal villi. In addition, the biopsy specimen may exhibit a diagnostic histologic picture or a nonspecific one (Table 130-4). The nonspecific flat biopsy specimen seen in untreated celiac sprue and in refractory or unclassified sprue (see Fig. 130-40A) typically shows virtual absence of villi, injured surface epithelium, and lengthened, parallel, closely packed crypts with increased numbers of mitotic figures. The lamina propria in most flat biopsy specimens has a marked excess of round cells that are mostly plasma cells. Polymorphonuclear leukocytes may or may not be present in small numbers. Celiac and unclassified sprue have the same nonspecific flat appearance. However, celiac sprue responds to exclusion of gluten from the diet (Fig. 130-40A,B), whereas unclassified and refractory sprue do not.

Collagenous sprue resembles the nonspecific flat lesion of the two preceding diseases but has a thickened subepithelial collagen table beneath the surface epithelium (Fig. 130-41); this disease usually is unresponsive to treatment and often fatal.[78]

Superficially, hypogammaglobulinemic sprue resembles the diagnostically nonspecific flat lesion of celiac sprue (Fig. 130-42A) except that the excess numbers of round cells in the lamina propria are mostly lymphocytes with virtually no plasma cells (Fig. 130-42B), a marked contrast to the increased numbers of plasma cells seen in the flat lesions of celiac sprue. The flat biopsy specimen of hypogammaglobulinemic sprue is one end of the spectrum of small bowel lesions seen in common variable immunodeficiency, the other end being be-

nign lymphoid hyperplasia with lymphoid nodules. The most common lesion is a mixture of lymphoid hyperplasia and variable villous abnormalities (Fig. 130-43A). Loss of villi is caused by the frequent infection with *Giardia lamblia,* an organism easily missed in histologic sections (Fig. 130-43B, C) but well visualized in Giemsa-stained smears of mucus adherent to the biopsy specimens (see Fig. 130-43C). Pharmacologic eradication of the *Giardia* cures the malabsorption of these patients and restores their villi (Fig. 130-42C) but not their lamina propria plasma cells (see Fig. 130-42B).[79]

Five diseases with a nonspecific picture of a variable abnormality of villous architecture are seen. The term *variably abnormal villi* is defined as villous architecture that varies in its severity in different patients, and even in the same patient, from absent villi, to moderately or mildly distorted villi, to normal villi. The diagnosis in these nonspecific histologic pictures depends on the clinical history and the response to specific treatments. Stasis syndrome with bacterial overgrowth responds to intermittent antibiotic treatment. The small bowel in inhabitants of nonindustrialized countries shows nonspecific abnormalities of varying severity when compared with the standard normal in an industrialized country (Fig. 130-44). The severity of the abnormality correlates with the socioeconomic level of the nonindustrialized country. The abnormality disappears after prolonged residence in an industrialized country.

Patients with tropical sprue in a nonindustrialized country tend to have an exaggeration of the nonspecific small intestinal abnormalities seen in their fellow inhabitants without overt malabsorption; the malabsorption and intestinal lesion respond to folate and antibiotics. The histologic severity of the lesion in tropical sprue also tends to mirror the developmental level of the country in which it occurs. The abnormalities in

TABLE 130-4
Proximal Small Bowel Lesions

DIAGNOSTIC CLASSIFICATION*	DISEASES	CLINICAL FEATURES
Nondiagnostic flat lesion	Celiac sprue	Responds to gluten-free diet
	Refractory sprue	Untreatable
Histologically diagnostic flat lesion	Collagenous sprue	Untreatable, often fatal
	Hypogammaglobulinemic sprue	Treat giardiasis: villi return
Nondiagnostic, variably abnormal villi	Stasis syndrome	Antibiotics help
	Zollinger-Ellison syndrome	H_2 and proton pump inhibitors effective
	Tropical sprue	Folate and antibiotics curative
	Graft-versus-host	May respond to cyclosporin and steroids
	Geographic variation	Histologic improvement after prolonged residence in a developed country
Histologically diagnostic, variably abnormal villi	Whipple's disease	Responds to antibiotics
	Crohn's disease with epithelioid granulomas or giant cells	Usually occurs in conjunction with gastric Crohn's disease
	Eosinophilic gastroenteritis	Blood eosinophils increased; intermittent digestive symptoms
	Lymphangiectasia	Congenital or acquired
	Common variable immunodeficiency	Treat giardiasis: villi return, malabsorption improves
	Primary intestinal lymphoma with malabsorption	Confined to intestine and its lymph nodes, disease in nonindustrialized nations
	Mycobacterium avium intracellulare infection	Opportunistic infection seen in acquired immunodeficiency syndrome
Rare conditions	See text	

* Histologic description in text.

Zollinger-Ellison syndrome are caused by acid peptic injury; they respond to H_2 blockers or proton pump inhibitors. Acute graft-versus-host disease, unless severe, responds to large doses of steroids or cyclosporin.

The final group of diseases has variably abnormal villi with specific, diagnostic, histologic features; in the mixed lesion of common variable immunodeficiency there are virtually no plasma cells. In Whipple's disease (Fig. 130-45), the mucosa is stuffed with macrophages that are periodic acid-Schiff positive but negative for acid-fast bacilli, unlike the other infection with many macrophages with which it may be confused: *Mycobacterium avium* complex. Infection with *M avium* complex is opportunistic, with an acid-fast bacillus seen in patients with AIDS (Fig. 130-46).

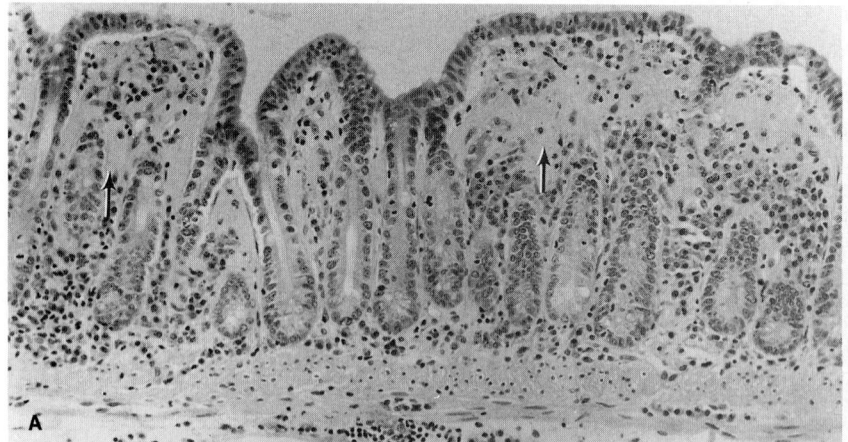
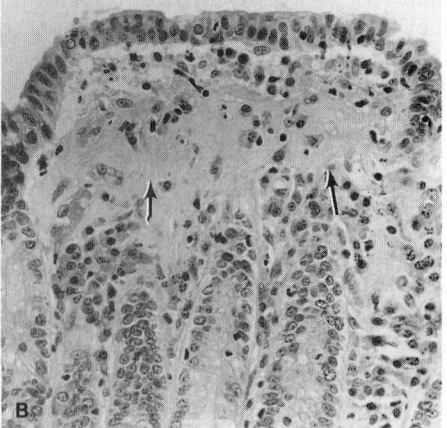

FIGURE 130-41. Collagenous sprue. **(A)** The mucosal surface is flat; the villi are absent; and the crypts are elongated. An abnormally thick layer of collagen lies beneath the surface epithelium (*arrows*). Lymphocytes and plasma cells infiltrate the lamina propria, the collagen, and the surface epithelium. **(B)** The markedly thickened subepithelial collagen table can be better seen at higher power. Observe the abnormal surface epithelium.

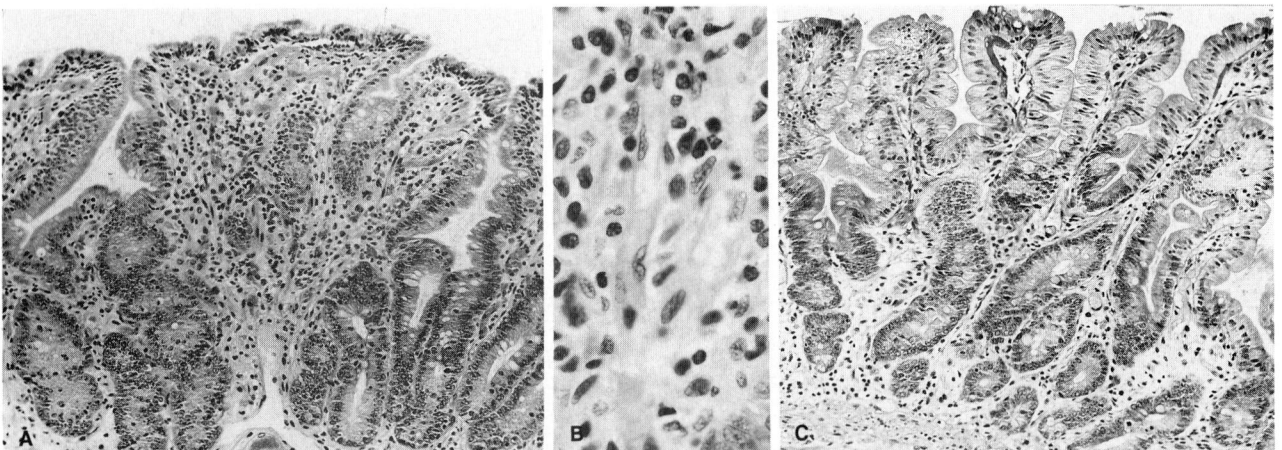

FIGURE 130-42. Hypogammaglobulinemic sprue is a variant of common variable immunodeficiency. (A) This biopsy sample of the small intestine has a flat mucosal surface with marked elongation of the crypts and a moderate inflammatory infiltrate within the lamina propria. At this magnification, it is identical with the biopsy specimens shown in Figure 130-40 from a patient with celiac sprue. (B) At higher magnification inspection of the inflammatory infiltrate in the lamina propria reveals absence of plasma cells, a finding indicative of hypogammaglobulinemic sprue. Although none was seen in this biopsy specimen, *Giardia* organisms were identified in a Giemsa-stained smear made form the mucus adherent to the biopsy specimen. (C) After treatment for giardiasis, the mucosal villi returned to a normal appearance. Virtual absence of plasma cells from the lamina propria was not reversed by eradication of the *Giardia* organisms.

An unusual manifestation of Crohn's disease may be flat duodenal mucosa (Fig. 130-47). When giant cells or granulomas are not found and when the lesion is diffusely flat, it is often confused with celiac sprue. Some hint of the diagnosis in duodenal Crohn's in a flat biopsy specimen is the intensity of the acute inflammatory response histologically with polymorphonuclear leukocytes, crypt abscesses, and destruction of glands. The clinical story and the lack of response to a gluten-free diet also may be helpful. Other rarer diseases with granulomas are sarcoidosis and tuberculosis. In sarcoidosis, other organs also are involved with noncaseating granulomas. The granulomas of tuberculosis are more numerous and larger and have necrosis and acid-fast bacilli demonstrable by Ziehl-Neelson stain.

Eosinophilic gastroenteritis of the duodenum usually is patchy and often requires multiple biopsies for detection; it has clumps of mucosal eosinophils and a markedly elevated eosinophil count in the peripheral blood. Lymphangiectasia may be congenital or acquired and has multiple dilated lymphatics distorting the villous architecture (Fig. 130-48).

Primary intestinal lymphoma associated with malabsorption (Fig. 130-49) is seen mostly in patients from underdeveloped countries and usually is confined to the intestine and its lymph nodes. When the villi are destroyed in lymphoma, the biopsy may be confused with the nondiagnostic flat lesion of celiac sprue. Two features should prevent this error: the destruction of many of the crypts suggesting an invasive malignant process, and the atypical morphologic features of the

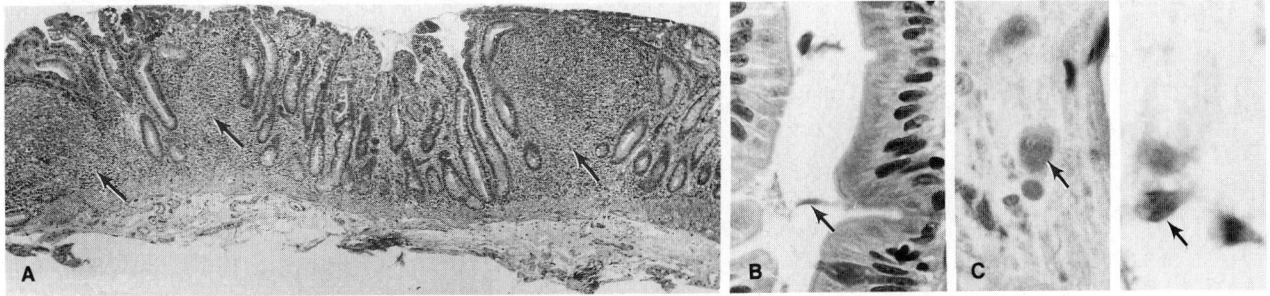

FIGURE 130-43. The typical appearance of a biopsy specimen of the small intestine in common variable immunodeficiency. (A) The biopsy shows mild lymphoid hyperplasia (*arrows*) and a mixed variable abnormality of the villous architecture. (B, C) Tissue sections show infection with *Giardia lamblia*, the usual infection in patients with common variable immunodeficiency. (B) Longitudinal sections of *Giardia lamblia* are seen. (C) Organisms that have been sectioned en face. Observe the two nuclei within the *Giardia* organism. Giardiasis is detected most easily in Giemsa-stained smears of mucus adherent to the biopsy (*right*). The *arrows* point to a characteristic pear-shaped organism in which two nuclei are visible.

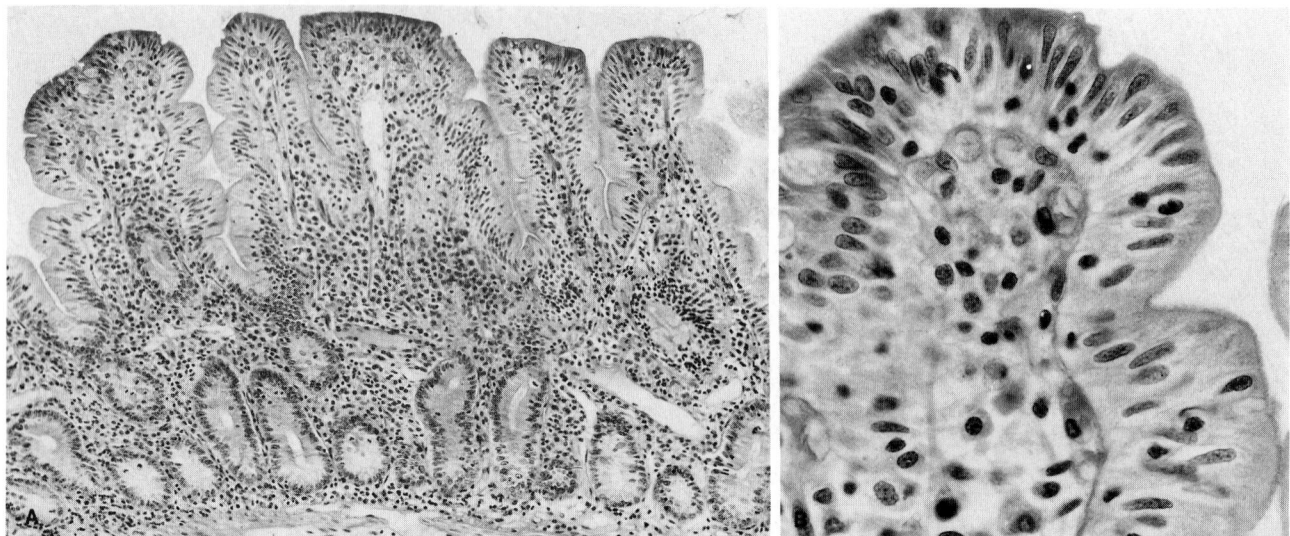

FIGURE 130-44. Geographic variation in small bowel mucosal morphologic features. (**A**) The villi are abnormal in a nonspecific manner in this biopsy specimen from an asymptomatic inhabitant of a developing country. (**B**) Observe the blunted, shortened villi and the prominent infiltrate of lymphocytes and plasma cells in the lamina propria and the surface epithelium.

lymphoid cells in the lamina propria.[80] This disease has a prelymphomatous stage in which there is diffuse infiltration of the mucosa by plasma cells without overtly malignant lymphoid cells. In this so-called immunoproliferative small intestinal disease, the infiltrating cells may synthesize abnormal α-heavy chain immunoglobulin.[81]

There are a few diseases with normal villi in which diagnostic histologic features may be seen. Amyloidosis is recognized after staining with Congo red by its dichroic bire-fringence in polarized light, producing a green and reddish orange color. The various storage diseases have a predilection for ganglion cells, macrophages, or endothelial cells; these cells usually are vacuolated and require special histochemical examination for diagnosis. If the absence of plasma cells is not recognized, the small bowel biopsy in X-linked immunodeficiency can easily be confused with normal villi, because normal villi are present and lymphoid nodules are absent.

At least six potentially fatal opportunistic infections with

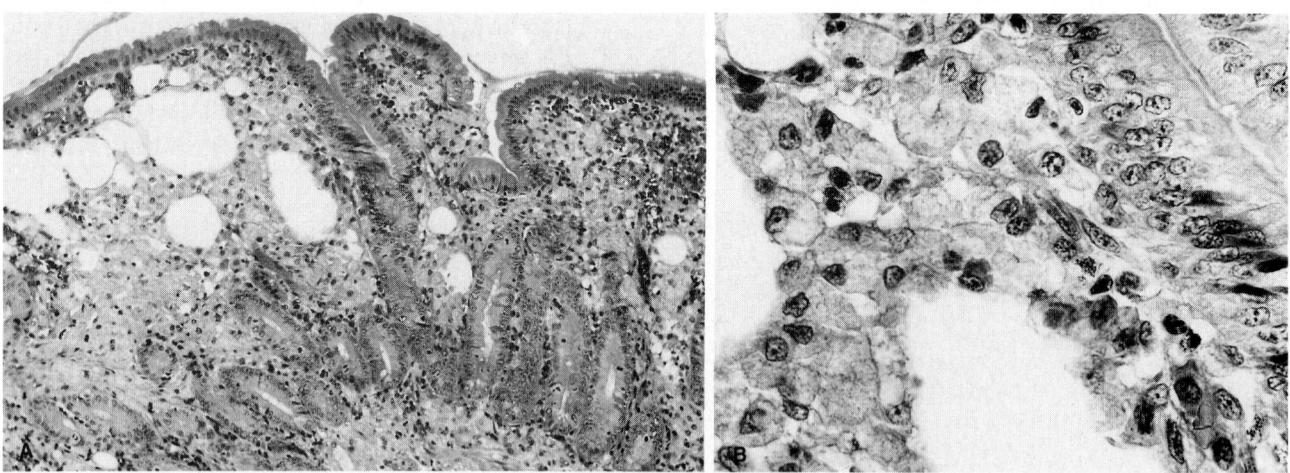

FIGURE 130-45. Whipple's disease. (**A**) Notice the marked distortion of the villous architecture with very broad villi on the left. The lamina propria is heavily infiltrated by macrophages with abundant cytoplasm. The clear spaces represent dilated blocked lacteals filled with lipid. The surface epithelium remains essentially normal. (**B**) Foamy macrophages at higher magnification are visible. By electron microscopic study, the abundant pale cytoplasm of these macrophages can be seen to contain bacilli and breakdown products of bacterial cell membranes within lysosomes. Observe the completely normal surface epithelium (*upper right*).

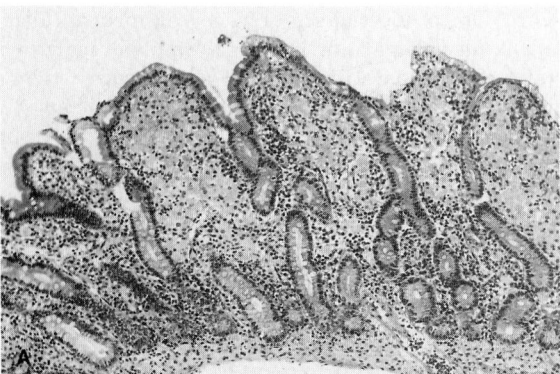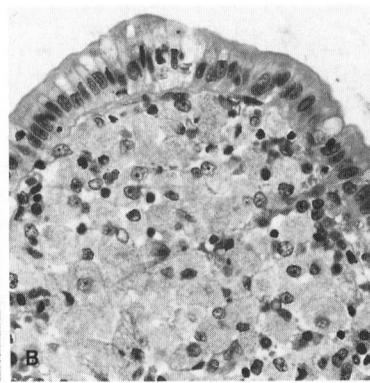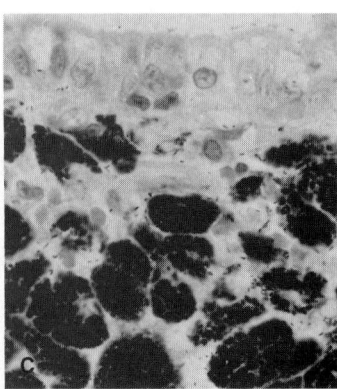

FIGURE 130-46. Small bowel biopsy specimen from a patient with acquired immunodeficiency syndrome who was infected with *Myobacterium avium* complex. (**A**) Notice the shortened, broad villi and the lamina propria packed full of macrophages. (**B**) Macrophages within the lamina propria are seen at higher magnification. With a hematoxylin-and-eosin stain, this appearance is indistinguishable from that of Whipple's disease. (**C**) Ziehl-Neelsen stain identifies the acid-fast nature of the bacilli within the macrophages and in the lamina propria.

specific histologic features are seen in the small bowel of immunosuppressed patients: strongyloidiasis, cryptosporidiosis (Fig. 130-50), candidiasis, cytomegalovirus, and infections with *Isospora belli* and *M avium* complex (see Fig. 130-46). Other infections that may be seen in the duodenum of immunologically competent and immunosuppressed patients include giardiasis and histoplasmosis.

Rare, flat lesions with nonspecific histologic features that are not listed in Table 130-4 include the idiosyncratic small bowel injuries by different food proteins, which are extremely rare in adults; childhood kwashiorkor as documented in Chile[82]; and familial enteropathy, a fatal flat lesion that is present at birth and that leads to the rapid death of the infant.[83]

Other rare lesions with specific histologic features not mentioned in Table 130-4 include A-β-lipoproteinemia with normal villi and fat-filled, vacuolated, fasting absorptive cells; chronic granulomatous disease with normal villi and typical clumps of vacuolated pigmented macrophages in the lamina propria; Waldenström macroglobulinemia with variably abnormal villi containing clumps of specific macroglobulin in the lamina propria; and severe vitamin B_{12} or folate deficiency with its reversible epithelial macrocytosis and mild abnormalities of villous architecture.

Peutz-Jeghers hamartomas, although rare, are most often seen in the small bowel, with their characteristic branching smooth muscle interspersed with benign glands (Fig.

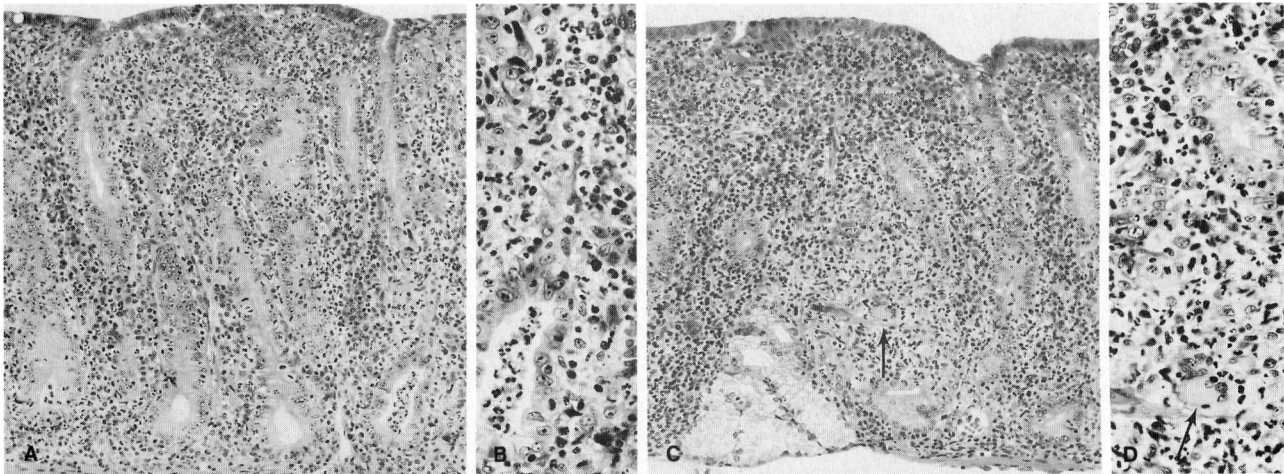

FIGURE 130-47. Duodenal biopsy specimen from a patient with Crohn's disease. (**A**) Notice the flat mucosal surface and markedly elongated crypts. (**B**) The intense inflammatory infiltrate includes numerous neutrophils that have produced a crypt abscess, shown here at higher magnification. (**C**) In another biopsy specimen from the same patient, a focus of granulomatous inflammation is present. A multinucleated giant cell is surrounded by macrophages and neutrophils (*arrow*). (**D**) Higher-power magnification of the giant cell shown in **C**.

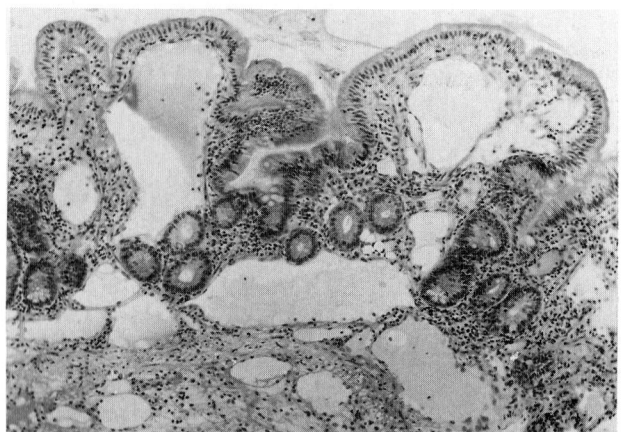

FIGURE 130-48. Congenital lymphangiectasia. The villous architecture in this small bowel biopsy specimen is distorted by dilated lymphatic channels that extend through the muscularis mucosae into the submucosa at the bottom of the photograph. Apart from the distorted architecture, the mucosa is normal.

130-51). Adenomas and adenocarcinomas of the small bowel are rare except in familial polyposis where they have a predilection for the area surrounding the papilla of Vater. The diagnosis of carcinoma in an endoscopically visible periampullary lesion may be impossible because of the superficial nature of endoscopic biopsies. Kaposi's sarcoma may be seen in AIDS; its gross appearance and histologic features are described in Premalignant and Malignant Gastrointestinal Lesions.

Experience with biopsy of the terminal ileum is accumulating, but our knowledge of the diagnostic possibilities does not yet have the underpinning of large numbers and long experience, as is the case in the proximal jejunum and duodenum. Undoubtedly, rare ileal diseases and new, more common ones will become firmly established as a result of future

experience. One of the major problems is an incorrect diagnosis of chronic inflammation in normal lymphoid aggregates and nodules associated with normal Peyer patches. Crohn's disease often is initially confined to the terminal ileum. Because UC involving the entire colon may be accompanied by *backwash* ileitis that can have a similar histologic appearance to Crohn's disease, granulomas are required for the endoscopic biopsy diagnosis of Crohn's disease when ileal disease is associated with colitis. Unfortunately, epithelioid granulomas diagnostic of Crohn's disease are not seen as frequently in the ileum as in the rectum. Tuberculosis may be diagnosable by histologic demonstration of the organisms. *Yersinia* infection may be suspected because of its characteristic necrotizing lesions of the gut lymphoid tissue (Fig. 130-52). Partially obstructive diaphragms of the terminal ileum have been described secondary to NSAID injury; characteristically they are covered with normal ileal mucosa except at the eroded, narrowed edge of the diaphragm.[84] Seronegative arthritis may have an acute or chronic inflammatory terminal ileal lesion and may resemble or be associated with Crohn's disease.[85]

Disease of the Colon

The most common clinical indication for performing a biopsy of the colon at endoscopy is to help differentiate the various types of colitis. Other reasons for colonic endoscopic biopsy include the diagnosis of dysplasia in chronic UC, the diagnosis of various types of nonneoplastic and neoplastic polyps, and the confirmation of a gross endoscopic diagnosis of carcinoma before undertaking surgical excision. Colonic endoscopic biopsy also may be helpful in a patient who has colonic symptoms possibly of organic origin such as severe diarrhea that awakens the patient from sleep, but in whom there is a normal appearance by colonoscopy. The detection in biopsy specimens of nonspecific but definite histologic abnormalities such as early crypt abscesses confirms the organic nature of the

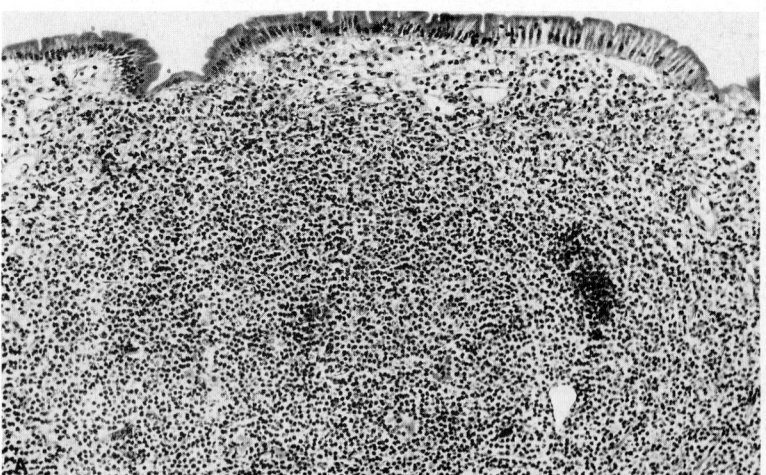
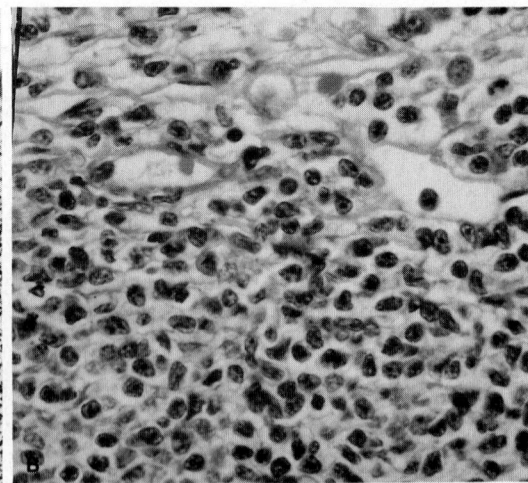

FIGURE 130-49. Small intestinal lymphoma. **(A)** The absence of crypts is noteworthy and probably reflects the destruction of the glandular architecture by the diffuse infiltrate of small lymphocytes. **(B)** At higher magnification, the monotonous, atypical appearance of the lymphoid infiltrate can be readily seen.

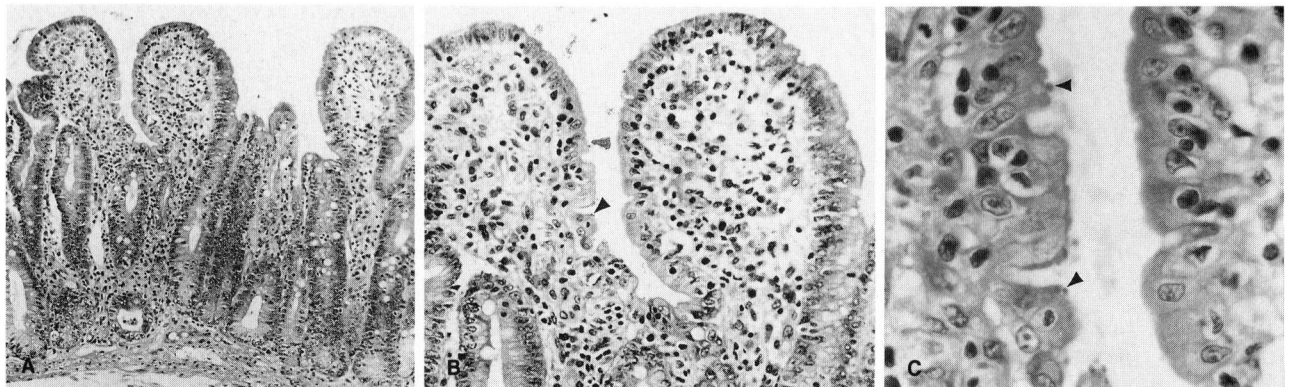

FIGURE 130-50. Cryptosporidiosis in an immunosuppressed individual. (**A**) The low-power view illustrates the shortened, blunted villi, and the elongated crypts reflect an inflammatory process in the mucosa. (**B**) Infiltration of the lamina propria and surface epithelium by lymphocytes is evident. Cryptosporidia are barely visible at this magnification (*arrowheads*). (**C**) The organisms are best seen in the high-power magnification. They appear as small, round, gray dots adherent to the apical surface of the absorptive cells. Cryptosporidia also may produce disease in normal persons, but the process is acute and self-limited rather than chronic.

symptoms. We consider such patients to have *early nonspecific colitis* whose specific diagnosis becomes apparent only in future biopsy specimens after the passage of time.

Types of Colitis

A variety of histologic findings such as crypt abscesses, isolated giant cells, active inflammation of the lamina propria with polymorphonuclear leukocytes, and regenerative epithelial atypia are all nonspecific abnormalities that may be seen in many colitides, including idiopathic UC, Crohn's colitis, acute self-limited colitis (ASLC), and other, less common types of colitis (Table 130-5).

Ileocolitis is the most common form of intestinal Crohn's disease; colitis confined to the colon is the least common. Crohn's colitis usually is segmental in distribution and infrequently is diffuse. The most dependable histologic feature supporting the diagnosis of Crohn's colitis is an epithelioid

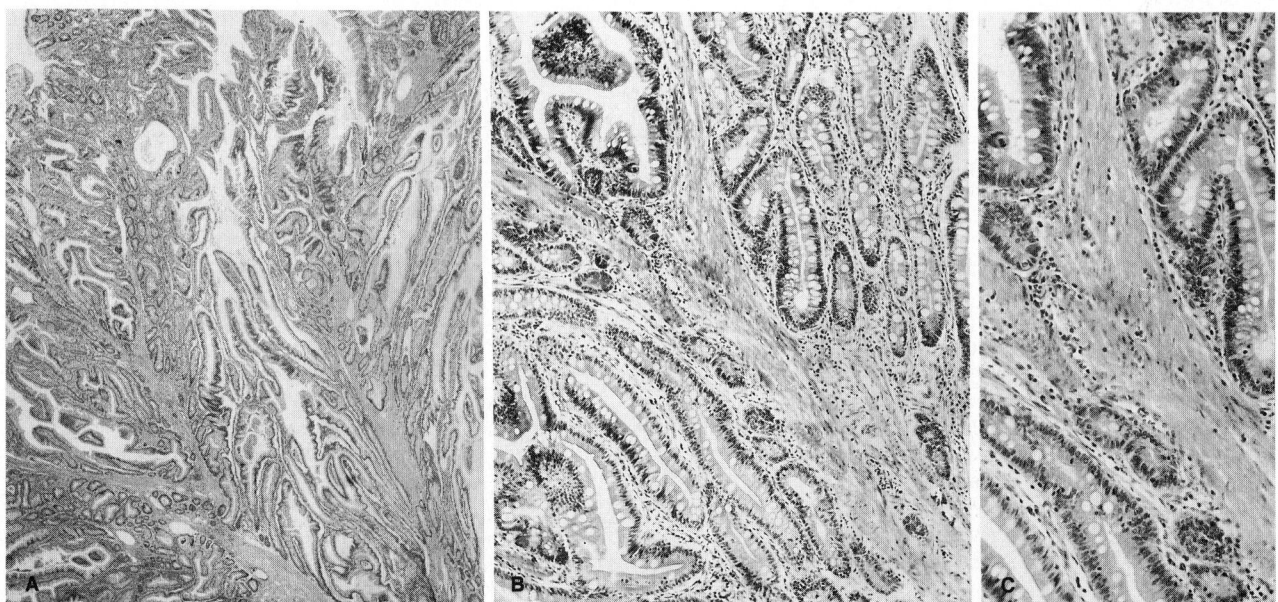

FIGURE 130-51. Small bowel hamartomatous polyp from a patient with Peutz-Jeghers syndrome. (**A**) The low-power view shows the complex, branched configuration of the hamartoma. (**B, C**) The abnormal arrangement of normal tissue elements is seen. Normal-appearing epithelium lines tubules and covers villi. A thick band of smooth muscle divides the field diagonally. (**C**) This smooth muscle band and the normal-appearing epithelium are shown at higher magnification.

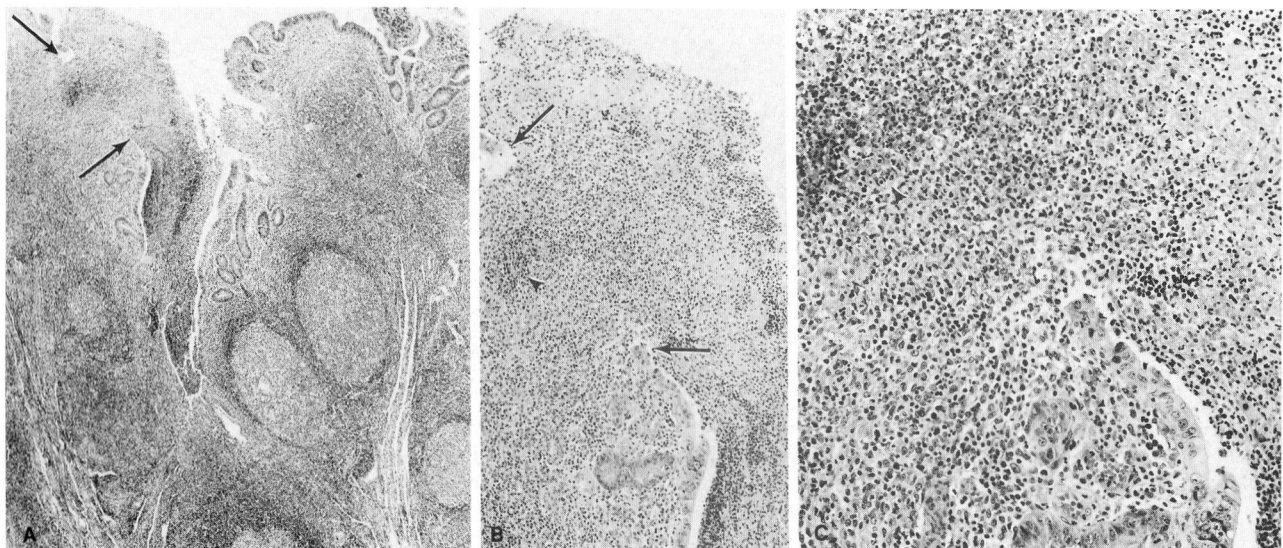

FIGURE 130-52. Yersiniosis of terminal ileum. (**A**) The low-power view shows a Peyer's patch in which there is erosion of the surface epithelium with adherent exudate (*arrows*). (**B**) This erosion is shown at higher power. The margins of the eroded surface epithelium are indicated by the arrows. The inflammatory exudate extends into the underlying lymphoid tissue, in which there is a focus of necrosis (*arrowhead*). (**C**) The focal necrosis (*arrowhead*) is better seen at higher power.

granuloma (Fig. 130-53).[86] Such granulomas in biopsy specimens are uncommon and often small and may require at least two biopsies, step-serial sectioning, and a careful search for detection.[87] Even then, only about one third of patients with Crohn's colitis have granulomas detected on biopsy. Without epithelioid granulomas the diagnosis must depend on the segmental nature of the disease, histologically documented rectal sparing, if present, and the focal nature of the active inflammation histologically. Small foci of a few distorted, actively inflamed crypts may alternate with normal mucosa in the same biopsy. Because of the segmental or even focal nature of Crohn's colitis, a few normal biopsy specimens do not rule out the disease. Crohn's disease has a lower risk of carcinoma than UC.

TABLE 130-5
Types of Colitis

DIAGNOSIS	HISTOLOGIC FEATURES	CLINICAL FEATURES
Early nonspecific colitis	Mild, nonspecific, active inflammation with preserved architecture	Differentiates organic from functional diarrhea
Ulcerative colitis	Diffuse inflammation and crypt distortion	Rectum involved along with a variable length of contiguous colon
Crohn's colitis	Epithelioid granuloma or focal active inflammation	Disease usually segmental; rectal sparing frequent
ASLC	Crypt architecture intact	Mostly infectious
Opportunistic infections	CMV, MAC, cryptosporidia, HSV, TB, histoplasma	Defects in humoral or cell-based immunity
Other infections	Amebae, schistosomes	Migrants, travelers
Antibiotic-related	Pseudomembranes or only ASLC-like lesions	*Clotridium difficile* toxin to positive
Solitary rectal ulcer	Diffuse collagen, erosions, excess muscle bands, pleated crypts	Confused with Crohn's colitis or cancer
Ischemic colitis	Superficial, hemorrhagic necrosis; can progress or reverse	Any cause of colonic hypoperfusion
Collagenous colitis	Subepithelial collagen band >10–15 μm thick	Idiopathic watery diarrhea
Other colitides		
Diversion	Mild colitis	Reversed by restoring bowel continuity
Radiation	Ischemia and vascular wall thickening	Unpredictable time of clinical onset after irradiation
Iatrogenic	Acute colitis, variable severity	Enema or laxative preparation for colonoscopy, contaminated wash fluids, chemotherapy

ASLC, acute self-limited colitis; CMV, cytomegalovirus; HSV, herpes simplex virus; MAC, *Mycobacterium avium* complex, TB, tuberculosis.

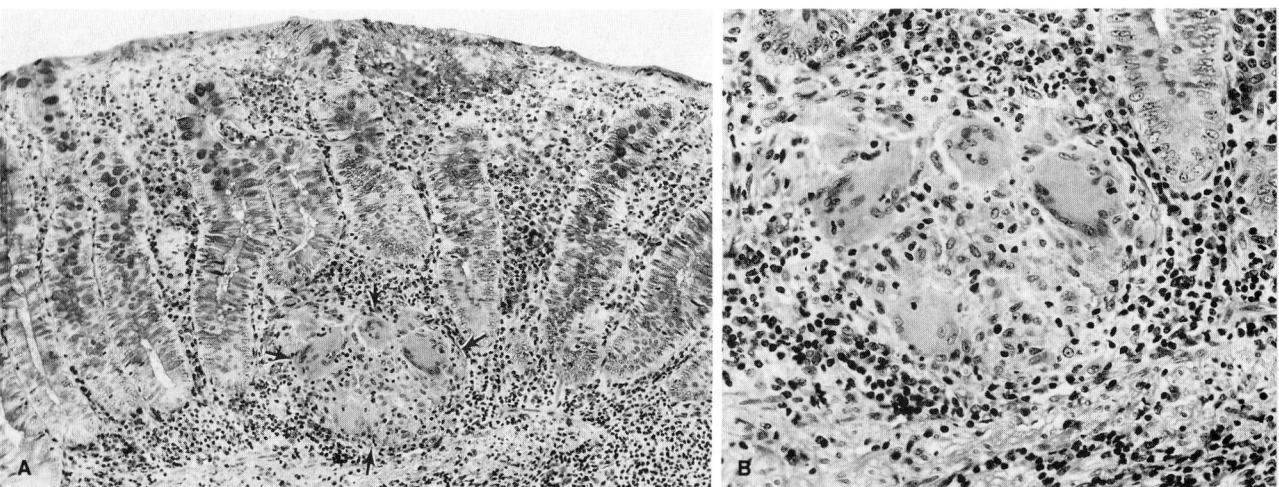

FIGURE 130-53. Crohn's disease of the colon. (**A**) This biopsy specimen contains a discrete epithelioid granuloma (*arrows*) composed of multinucleated giant cells and epithelioid histiocytes, (**B**) seen at higher power. Although inflammation surrounds the granuloma and involves some of the lamina propria, the mucosa at the left side of panel (**B**) is essentially normal, indicating that Crohn's colitis is commonly focal in distribution.

Biopsies from patients with idiopathic UC usually show distorted crypt architecture and diffuse nonspecific inflammation, but apparent focal inflammation may be seen when the disease begins to remit or when a patient with inactive disease develops focal activation of the colitis. UC can involve variable lengths of colon but almost always involves the rectum and spreads proximally to a varying extent. Distortion of cryptal architecture is the hallmark of idiopathic inflammatory bowel disease in general and of UC in particular. In active disease, increased numbers of lymphocytes, plasma cells, and some polymorphonuclear leukocytes are almost always seen in the lamina propria; crypt abscesses involving crypt epithelium and lumina are common (Fig. 130-54*A, B*). Unless the patient has been successfully treated with steroid enemas

or the disease is fulminant, the rectum is almost always involved and usually is the last area to heal. In patients who have clinically well-documented UC, the rectum may appear relatively or completely normal endoscopically, especially if corticosteroid enemas have been administered. However, such patients almost always have histologic evidence of active disease or the residual distortion of crypt architecture of prior active disease.[88] Therefore a rectal biopsy is important in evaluating patients' colitis.

Histologically the inflammation in UC is diffuse and nonspecific. Histologic features diagnostic of Crohn's disease are absent.[77] Isolated giant cells without granulomas may be seen, but these are nonspecific. Foreign body giant cell granulomas associated with crypt abscesses are relatively common in UC

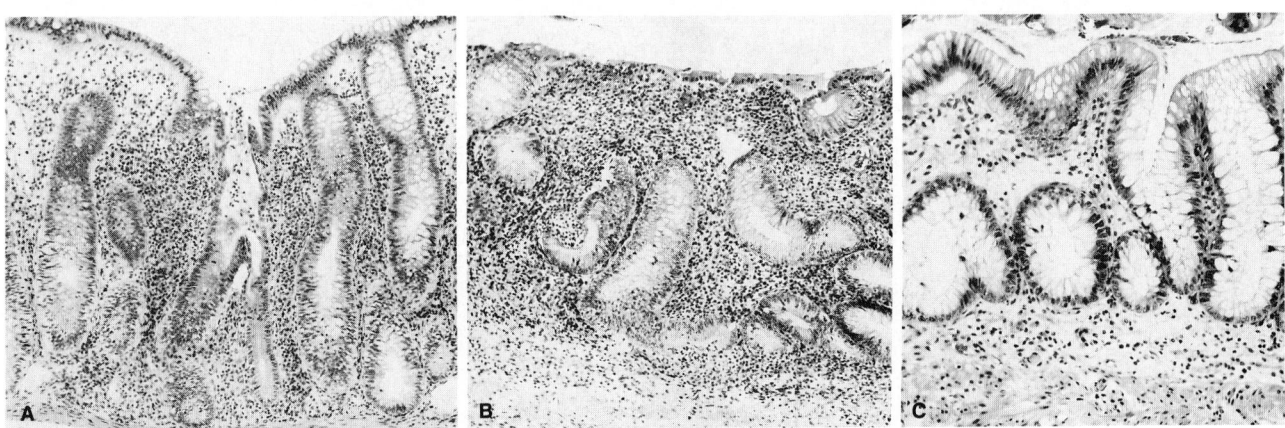

FIGURE 130-54. Ulcerative colitis. (**A**) The biopsy specimen shows early disease in which the inflammatory infiltrate varies in intensity and the distortion of the crypt architecture has not yet become diffuse; the crypt seen in the center of the biopsy sample is branched and contains neutrophils infiltrating its epithelium and lumen. (**B**) A biopsy specimen from a patient with fully developed disease with diffuse inflammation and distortion of the crypt architecture. (**C**) Atrophic mucosa in a patient with inactive ulcerative colitis; there is distortion of the crypt architecture but no inflammation.

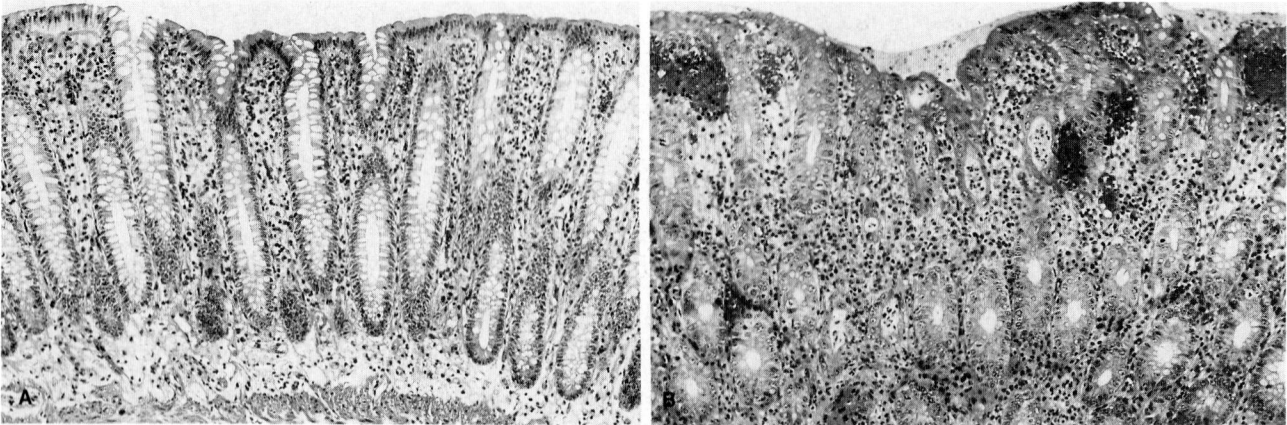

FIGURE 130-55. Acute self-limited colitis in a patient with salmonellosis. (**A**) Normal mucosa for comparison with (**B**) the histologic appearance of the mucosa in acute self-limited colitis. In acute self-limited colitis the crypts remain as straight, evenly spaced tubules, but there is a mixed inflammatory infiltrate of neutrophils and round cells in the lamina propria as well as accumulation of neutrophils within the crypt lumina to form crypt abscesses. Another feature of acute self-limited colitis well illustrated by the biopsy specimen in **B** is the absence of mucus secretion in the actively inflamed mucosa.

and represent a reaction to mucus released from destroyed epithelial cells. The true epithelioid granulomas of Crohn's colitis should be sought in areas not associated with crypt destruction. When UC has healed, all that may remain is glandular architectural distortion with or without partial glandular atrophy (Fig. 130-54C); furthermore, occasionally patients with UC have residual active inflammation in a focal distribution that can only be differentiated from the focal inflammation of Crohn's colitis by noticing the diffuse nature of the surrounding crypt distortion and atrophy. Many patients with continuing, clinically active disease will have had a colectomy before 8 years have elapsed. At this point in patients with healed or relatively inactive disease, continued regular colonoscopic biopsy surveillance for dysplasia and early cancer should be started.

The gross endoscopic appearance of the mucosa in the acute self-limited colitides usually is indistinguishable from that of idiopathic UC. The salient differential histologic finding separating ASLC from UC is the retention of normal crypt architecture in ASLC (Fig. 130-55) and the distortion of crypt architecture in UC.[89] In addition, in ASLC polymorphonuclear leukocytes are the predominant inflammatory cells in the lamina propria, crypts, and surface epithelium. In the general United States population, the most common enteric pathogens cultured in the acute self-limited colitides are *Campylobacter jejuni, Salmonella, Escherichia coli* O157:H7, and *Shigella*.[90] Cultures are essential for planning appropriate treatment. When none of these pathogens is identified, the causative organism may be an invasive *E coli* that cannot be distinguished from nonpathogenic *E coli* without tissue cul-

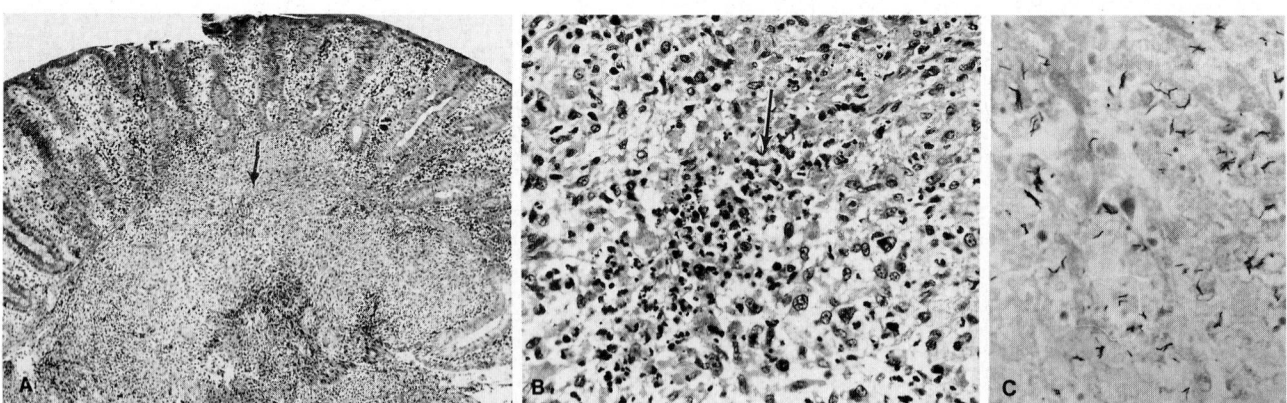

FIGURE 130-56. Colonic tuberculosis in a patient with acquired immunodeficiency syndrome. (**A**) The biopsy specimen shows inflammation of the colonic mucosa with multiple, large, confluent granulomas. The arrow points to a focus of necrosis within a granuloma. (**B**) This is seen at higher power in panel **B**. Necrosis within granulomas should always suggest an infectious agent. (**C**) Ziehl-Neelsen stain in which acid-fast bacilli of *Myobacterium tubuculosis* are evident. The tissue response to *Myobacterium avium* complex differs in that granulomas and diffuse granulomatous inflammation with discrete aggregates of epithelioid histiocytes are not seen; rather, there is diffuse infiltration of macrophages with foamy cytoplasm filled with acid-fast bacilli (see Fig. 130-46).

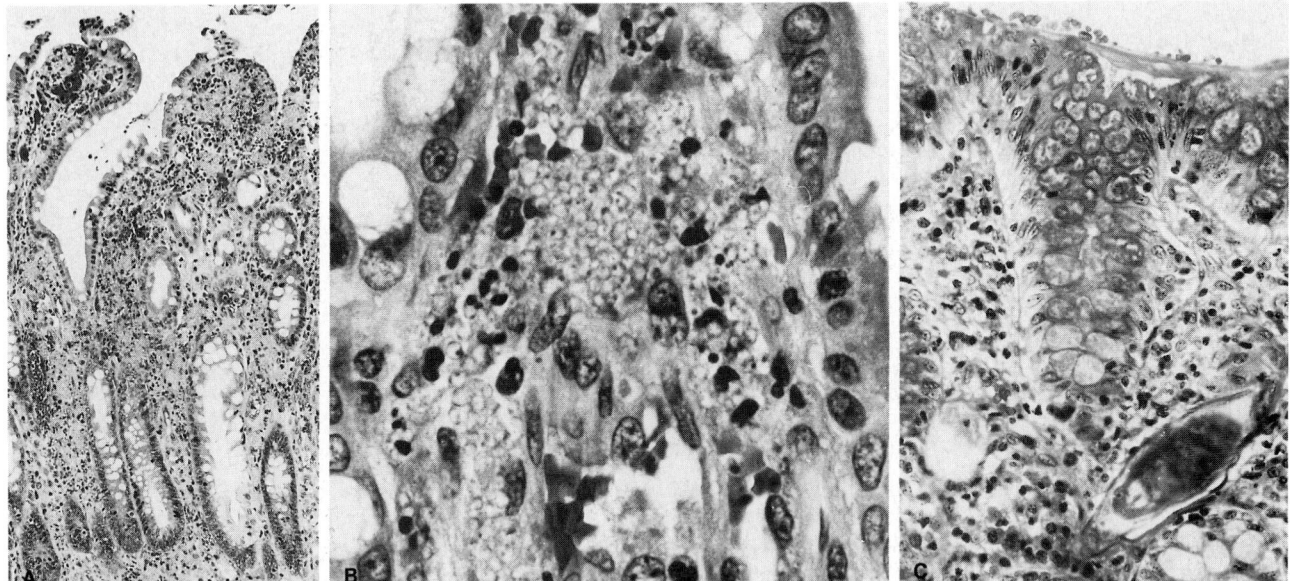

FIGURE 130-57. Colonic histoplasmosis in a patient with disseminated histoplasmosis in acquired immunodeficiency syndrome. (**A**) Distorted glandular architecture and an inflammatory infiltrate in the lamina propria are shown. (**B**) Inspection of the inflamed lamina propria at higher power reveals a foamy or bubbly appearance caused by numerous *Histoplasma* organisms within the cytoplasm of macrophages. The organisms are seen as clear vacuoles, many of which contain a dark central dot representing the nucleus. (**C**) Biopsy specimen from a patient with schistosomiasis. The ovum is clearly identified in the lamina propria and can be diagnosed as a schistosome, but speciation is not possible except in the rare circumstance in which the plane of section passes through a lateral spine of *Schistosoma mansoni.*

ture assays or DNA probing. The histologic picture seen in various bacterial causes of ASLC is essentially the same, but *E coli* 0157:H7 may have histologic features suggesting ischemia.[91]

Sexually transmitted rectal infections include gonorrhea, herpes simplex, chlamydia, syphilis, amebiasis, and the various other enteric pathogenic bacteria.[92] The *persisting* opportu-

nistic infections in AIDS each have characteristic organisms: cryptosporidia, *M avium* complex, and rotavirus in children. Cytomegalovirus, herpes simplex virus, tubercle bacilli (Fig. 130-56), and *Histoplasma* (Fig. 130-57) also are seen. Schistosomal colitis (see Fig. 130-57) is an important and extremely common problem in the rest of the world but is only occasionally seen in foreigners or international travelers in the

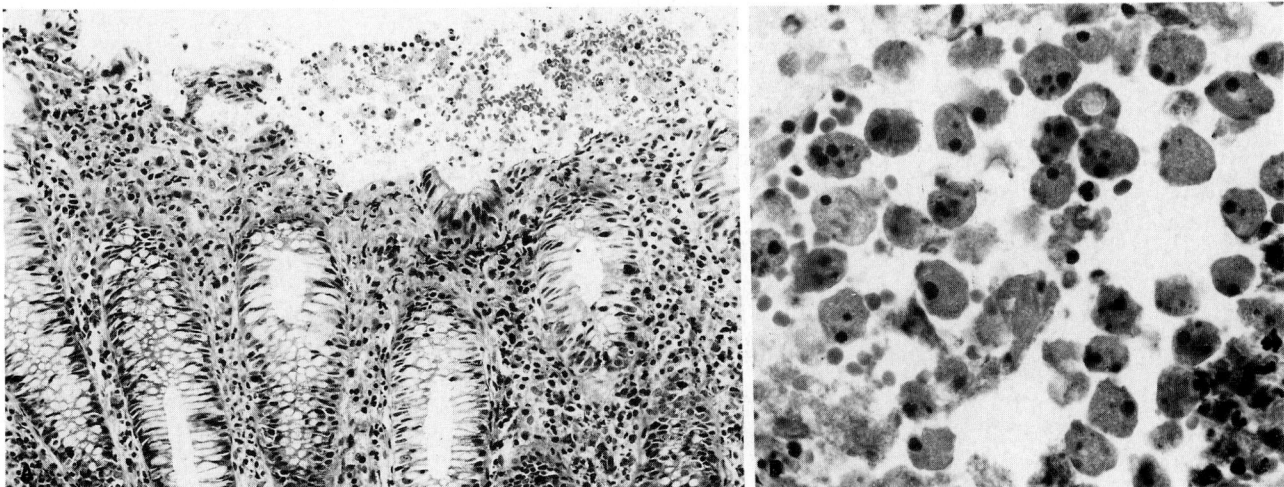

FIGURE 130-58. Amebic colitis. (**A**) The mucosa shows diffuse inflammation of the lamina propria and an eroded surface. The material adherent to the surface includes erythrocytes and numerous amebic organisms. (**B**) These are seen at high power. The organisms are large cells, measuring approximately 30 μm in diameter, which have a relatively small nucleus compared with the cytoplasmic volume. Phagocytized red blood cells are visible as black round structures within several of the amebae.

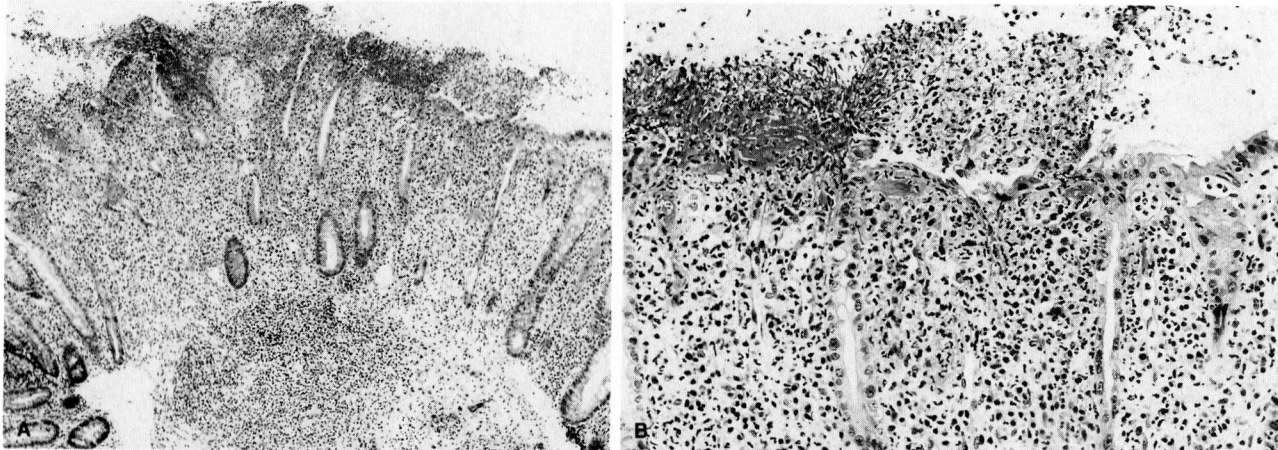

FIGURE 130-59. Pseudomembranous colitis due to *Clostridium difficile*. (**A**) This biopsy specimen shows features of an acute self-limited colitis with inflammation of the lamina propria, erosion of the surface epithelium, and adherent fibrinopurulent exudate (pseudomembrane), but preservation of the crypt architecture. Most of the inflammatory cells are neutrophils. (**B**) The erosion of the surface epithelium, the pseudomembrane, and the predominantly neutrophilic infiltration are well illustrated at high-power magnification.

United States. It is diagnosed by finding the characteristic eggs, often within epithelioid granulomas. A section through the edge of a granuloma may miss the egg and be confused with Crohn's colitis, but inspection of serial sections can overcome this problem. Amebic colitis (Fig. 130-58) in non-endemic areas of the United States is seen mostly in travelers returning from tropical countries, in migratory workers, and in homosexual men. When this infection is suspected special care must be taken while taking and handling the biopsy specimen to avoid removing adherent mucus containing amebae. Do not orient such specimens; just drop them into fixative and let the technician attempt orientation after fixation.

The most common antibiotic-related colitis is caused by overgrowth of *Clostridium difficile*, which secretes a specific toxin. Although colitis caused by *C difficile* usually is called pseudomembranous colitis (Fig. 130-59), only 50% of patients have pseudomembranes and pseudomembranes are also seen in other colitides. With or without pseudomembranes, the histologic picture may be indistinguishable from ASLC. A hemorrhagic right-sided colitis that is usually self-limited may rarely result from treatment with certain antibiotics.[93]

Solitary rectal ulcer syndrome may be confused with the ulcers of Crohn's disease or with an ulcerated carcinoma because of the hard, lumpy tissue palpable around the ulcer.[94] The thickened, eroded mucosa on the edge of the ulcers is filled with diffuse collagenous granulation tissue,[95] excess

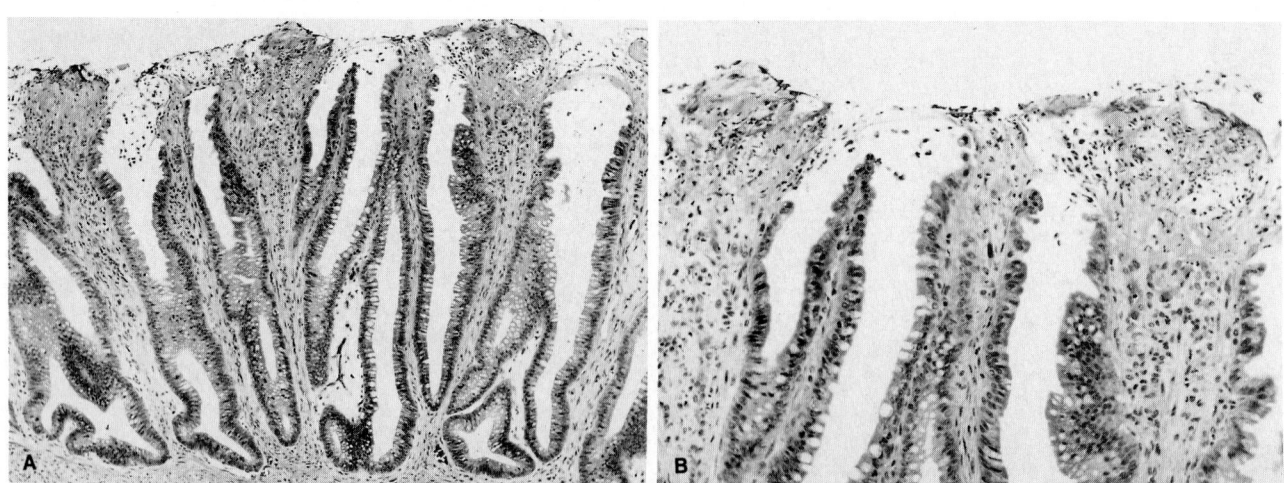

FIGURE 130-60. Solitary rectal ulcer syndrome. (**A**) The biopsy specimen shows erosion of the surface epithelium, obliteration of the lamina propria by fibrosis, granulation tissue and smooth muscle, and gross distortion of the glandular architecture. Hyperplasia of the glandular epithelium also is seen. (**B**) At higher power the eroded surface epithelium and obliteration of the lamina propria by collagenous granulation tissue and fibroblasts is better seen. Observe the epithelial hyperplasia that occasionally results in the misinterpretation of these lesions as adenomas or even cancer.

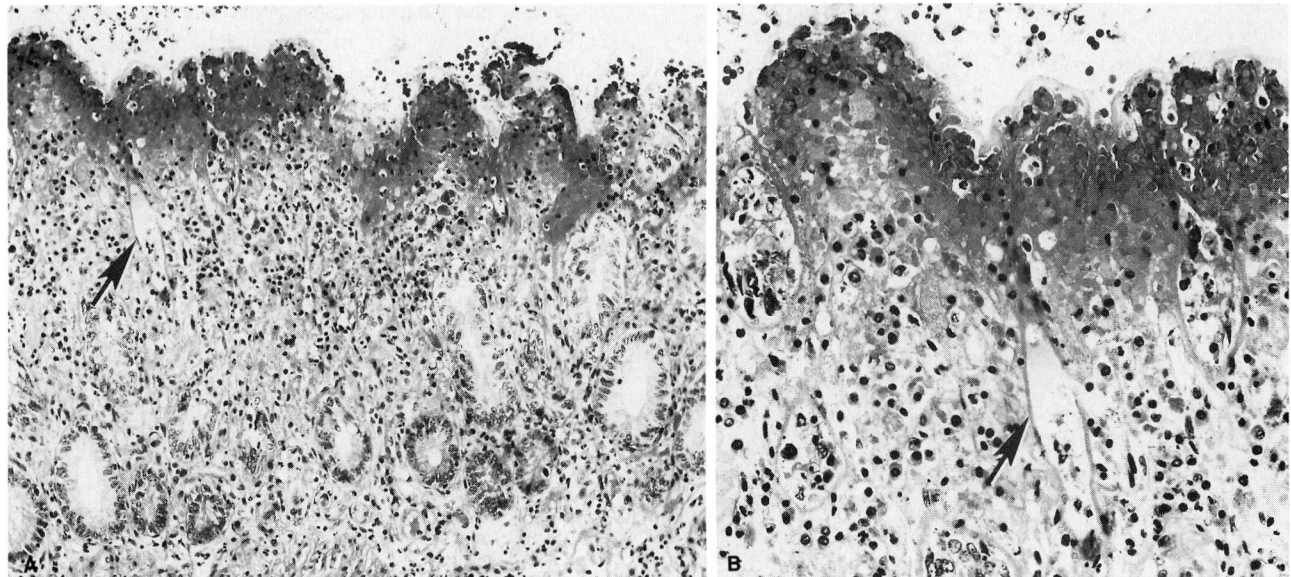

FIGURE 130-61. Ischemic colitis. (**A**) The upper part of the mucosa is necrotic whereas the deeper portion remains viable. The dark band along the surface of the mucosa represents hemorrhage. The arrow points to a crypt basement membrane devoid of epithelial cells because they have become necrotic and sloughed off (crypt ghost). Notice the relatively mild inflammatory infiltrate. (**B**) The eroded surface epithelium, superficial hemorrhage, and crypt ghosts (*arrow*) are seen at higher power.

muscle bundles, and lengthened crypts with epithelial hyperplasia (Fig. 130-60). Ten to fifteen percent of patients with solitary rectal ulcer syndrome may have cystic glands penetrating into the submucosa to form so-called colitis cystica profunda; these ectopic glands are benign and have no desmoplastic stromal reaction surrounding them to suggest invasive malignancy.

Ischemic colitis from vascular hypoperfusion can have a wide variety of causes.[96,97] Clinically its diagnosis can be difficult and biopsy often is required. In patients with acute ischemic injury, the bowel wall may be friable and biopsy specimens therefore should be taken using minimal pressure to avoid perforation. If the rectum is involved, the biopsy spec-

imen should be taken distal to the peritoneal reflection. A purplish black appearance to the mucosa suggests gangrene, and the endoscopy should be immediately terminated without biopsy. The histologic appearance in ischemia depends on whether the process is acute, healing, or healed. In acute disease, there is superficial, hemorrhagic necrosis and erosions with relative sparing of the cells at the crypt bases (Fig. 130-61). The process may progress to destroy the full thickness of the mucosa; ghosts of glands may remain (see Fig. 130-61) and regrow with subsequent complete mucosal restitution. In others the infarction may progress deeper into the bowel wall and a stricture may form during healing. If infarctive necrosis extends all the way through the wall, an

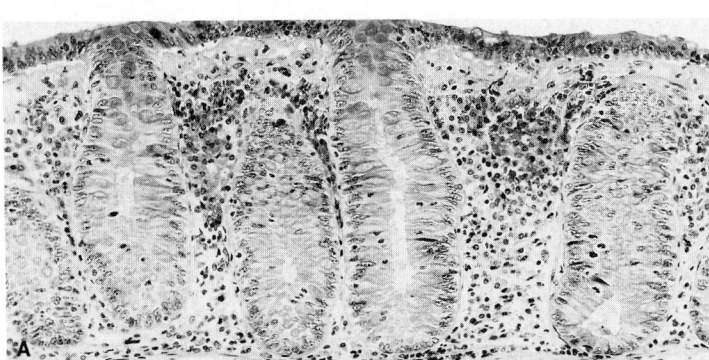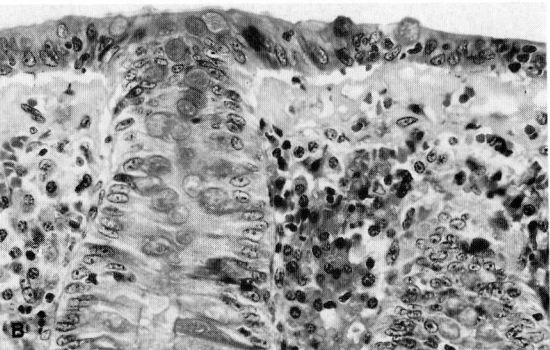

FIGURE 130-62. Collagenous colitis. (**A**) This biopsy specimen shows normal glandular architecture, a possible increase in the number of plasma cells in the upper portion of the lamina propria, and a markedly thickened subepithelial collagen band. The surface epithelium is infiltrated by lymphocytes. (**B**) These changes are seen better at higher power. Observe the lacey or reticulated appearance of the thickened subepithelial collagen table and the abnormal surface epithelium that is infiltrated by lymphocytes.

acute perforation may occur. The healed and healing mucosa may show atrophy, glandular distortion, and patchy distribution of collagenous scar. Various stages of this process may be seen simultaneously. An ischemic picture may also be seen in obstructed colons and in the presence of uremia.[96] The *non–antibiotic-related* pseudomembranous enterocolitis that occasionally follows a catastrophic illness also may be of ischemic origin.

The hallmark of collagenous colitis is a thickened subepithelial collagen band under the surface epithelium (Fig. 130-62). Clinically this condition is characterized by watery diarrhea whose cause and treatment are not established. In addition, there is often little or no colitis histologically or endoscopically. However, a few cases have been observed prospectively to progress from an earlier colitis to a later uninflamed collagenous colitis.[98] Some believe a condition called microscopic or lymphocytic colitis is a precursor or a variant of collagenous colitis, in which there is a reported excess of lymphocytes in the lamina propria and within the surface epithelium,[99] a finding that is most difficult to assess because of the wide normal variation in round cell number within the lamina propria and surface epithelium.[100] Disagreement exists regarding the thickness of the subepithelial collagen band required for a diagnosis of collagenous colitis.[101] Some think that a thickness of more than 5 μm makes the diagnosis, but the more conservative opinion is that a 10- to 15-μm thickness warrants a tentative diagnosis and more than 15 μm indicates a definite diagnosis of collagenous colitis.[102] The rectum may be spared and the lesion may be patchy.[101] Therefore colonoscopic sampling of the more proximal colon may be necessary for diagnosis of patchy collagenous changes.

There are a variety of other colitides. Diversion colitis usually is a mild colitis that occurs when the colon is excluded from the fecal stream.[103] Restoration of the fecal stream to the diverted colon reverses the process. Radiation colitis has an acute mucosal phase resembling acute ischemia and a more chronic mesenchymal phase with atypical fibroblasts, scarring,

and telangiectatic capillaries that may have hyalinized walls (Fig. 130-63).[104,105] It is an unpredictable process that may become clinically manifest at any time from months to years after irradiation.

Finally, a number of colitides are iatrogenic. Endoscopes may be inadequately rinsed after use of sterilizing solutions or wash water may be contaminated. For example, a pseudolipomatous lesion caused by the accumulation of gas bubbles is evident after inadvertent exposure to hydrogen peroxide (Fig. 130-64).[106] Residual glutaraldehyde sterilizing solution can cause colitis.[107] Less dramatic are the changes produced by various methods of cleansing the colon in preparation for colonoscopy. Many cleansing enemas can cause active surface inflammation and edema.[6] A bisacodyl enema may produce a confusing picture that can easily be considered colitic (see Fig. 130-64).[108] Gastrografin used as an enema instead of barium is hypertonic and highly irritating. A variety of chemotherapeutic agents can cause extensive mucosal injury. This is especially well documented with 5-fluorouracil.[109] Colitis associated with bone marrow transplantation is complex; the early lesion is caused by the preparatory irradiation and chemotherapy and the later lesions represent graft-versus-host reaction or opportunistic infections.[110]

Benign and Malignant Tumors

The diagnosis of benign and malignant tumors of the colon and the recognition of precancerous dysplastic lesions depend largely on endoscopic biopsy (Table 130-6). The grossly invisible dysplasia in the flat mucosa of UC has been mentioned above. A benign adenomatous polyp is an example of discrete, visible dysplasia. Total excision of polyps for histologic evaluation is the only reliable diagnostic method.

There are four common kinds of colonic mucosal polyps[70]:

1. Benign hyperplastic polyps
2. Adenomas with or without a focus of adenocarcinoma

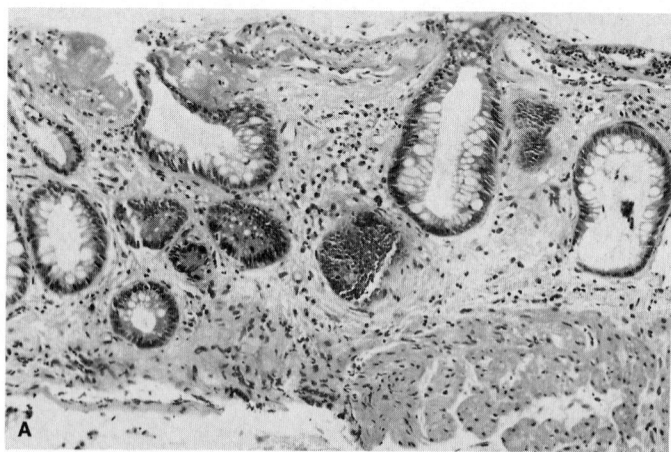
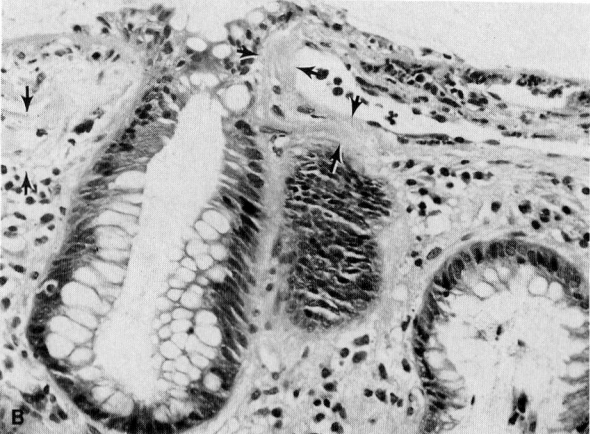

FIGURE 130-63. Colitis after therapeutic radiation. (**A**) After radiation the chronic changes in the mucosa are atrophic and may resemble inactive ulcerative colitis. (**B**) Fibrosis of the lamina propria and hyalinization of vascular walls are shown by the arrows. These ectatic vessels with hyalinized walls serve to distinguish radiation colitis from inactive ulcerative colitis. The surface epithelium in this biopsy sample is eroded; this may be an artifact because it is not a consistent finding in radiation colitis. Acute radiation changes, not shown here, may be indistinguishable from ischemia.

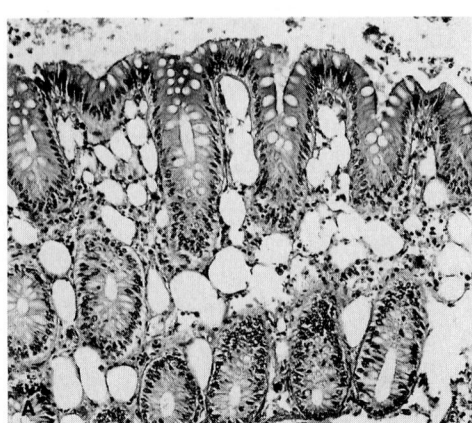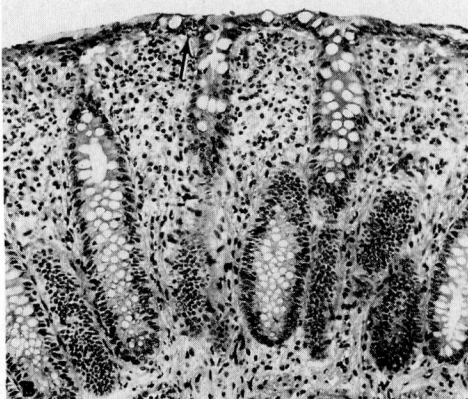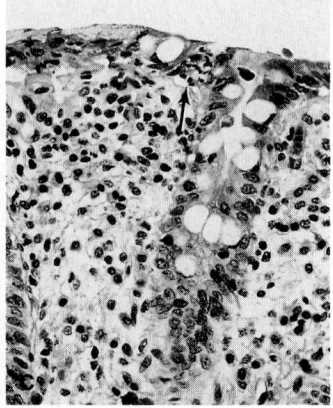

FIGURE 130-64. Pseudolipomatosis and other artifacts. (**A**) Pseudolipomatosis of the lamina propria after inadvertent exposure to hydrogen peroxide left after cleaning the wash channel of the colonoscope. The bubbles in the lamina propria represent gas bubbles caused by the release of nascent oxygen when hydrogen peroxide contacted the mucosa. These bubbles can be differentiated from fat cells because they lack a cell membrane and vary markedly in size. (**B**) The mucosa in a patient who has received a bisacodyl enema. The surface epithelium is flattened and contains focal infiltrates of neutrophils (*arrow*). (**C**) Focal neutrophilic infiltration of the abnormal surface epithelium at higher power (*arrow*).

3. Hamartomatous polyps
4. Inflammatory polyps.

Only adenomas are neoplastic. Benign hyperplastic polyps usually are less than 0.5 cm in diameter and often are multiple. They are not premalignant. Only polypectomy can differentiate them with certainty from adenomas.[111] Their frond-like, serrated, nondysplastic epithelial surface is diagnostic (Fig. 130-65). They are hyperplastic because they have an increased number of epithelial cells per unit length, and the excess cells, squeezed into a shorter distance, buckle and cause a serrated surface.[112] Deeper in their crypts the epithelium may be crowded and depleted of mucus; when cut tangentially, such crypts may be confused with an adenoma. The histologic appearance of a colonic hyperplastic polyp is different from that of a gastric hyperplastic polyp. Occasionally an adenoma may grow in a hyperplastic polyp-like pattern; however, the significance of such lesions is the same as that for any other adenoma.[113]

Adenomas are benign neoplasms that are dysplastic, that is, made up of neoplastic cells confined within the basement membranes of glands. Grossly they are pedunculated or sessile.

TABLE 130-6
Colonic Polyps

TYPE OF POLYP	HISTOLOGIC FEATURES	CLINICAL FEATURES
Hyperplastic	Benign, hyperplastic epithelial layer with serrated lumens	No malignant potential
Adenoma		
Tubular	Branching neoplastic glands	Least likely to contain cancer
Villous	Villi, often sessile	Rare, most likely to contain cancer
Tubulovillous	Mixed tubular and villous	Most common, intermediate chance of cancer
Hamartoma		
Single juvenile	Peduculated, cystic	Can self-amputate, can bleed
Multiple juvenile	May have associated adenomas	Stomach and small bowel also involved; rare cancer in adenomas
Peutz-Jeghers	Ramified smooth muscle bundles	Labial and buccal melanotic spots; small bowel most involved; rare cancer in associated adenomas
Pseudopolyp	Residual inflamed island of mucosa	No malignant potential

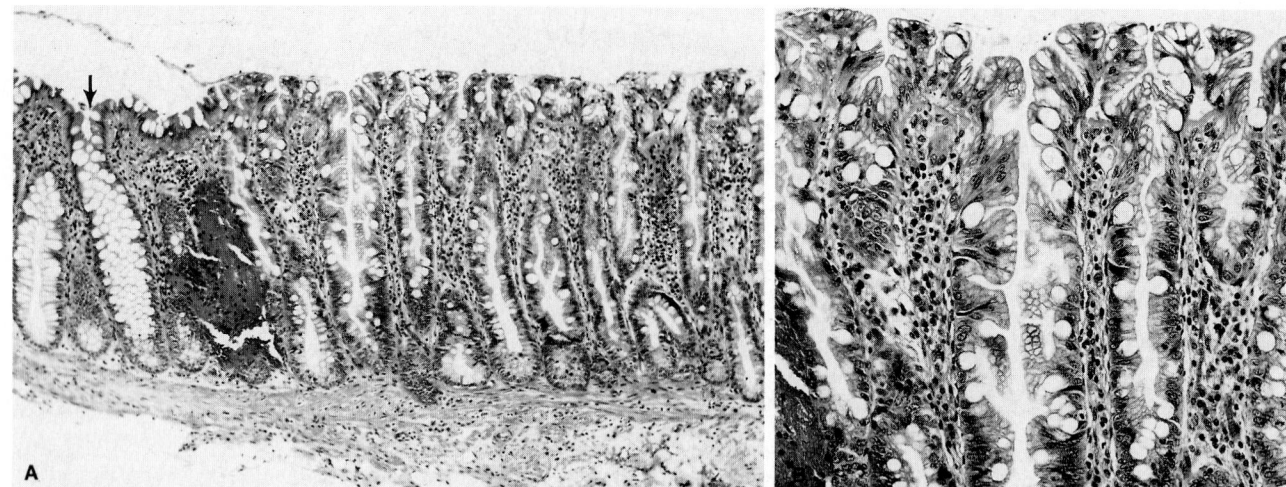

FIGURE 130-65. Hyperplastic colonic polyp. **(A)** This section passes through the junction of normal mucosa and the hyperplastic polyp (*arrow*). The lumen of the normal crypts has a straight appearance whereas the crypt lumena within a hyperplastic polyp have a serrated or stellate profile. **(B)** Inspection of the higher power shows that this serrated appearance is due to crowding of excess numbers of normal, nonneoplastic epithelial cells, causing them to form tufts that project into the lumen and from the lumenal surface.

The pedicle usually is covered by normal mucosa. The cytoplasm of the adenomatous epithelium is more basophilic and contains decreased or no goblet cell mucus; the nuclei may be hyperchromatic, enlarged, cigar-shaped, and crowded together in palisade formation. There are three types of adenomas. First, tubular adenomas contain branched tubules visible as circular acinar structures (see Fig. 130-6). Tubular adenomas tend to be small and are less likely to contain a focus of carcinoma. The second and far less common villous adenomas are typically larger and sessile, made up mostly of finger-like villi, and more likely to contain a focus of carcinoma (see Fig. 130-18). The third type of adenomas contains a mixture of tubular and villous components. Adenomas more than 2 cm in diameter are more likely to be malignant regardless of their histologic type.[114] The adenomas of familial adenomatous polyposis of the colon look the same as those of sporadic adenoma initially but there are at least 100 of them, and in virtually all patients, progression to cancer eventually occurs if the colon is not removed prophylactically.[70]

Adenomas may be confused with hyperplastic polyps if they have a serrated glandular pattern.[111] The neoplastic appearance of the adenomatous epithelium should prevent this confusion. True mixtures of hyperplasia and adenoma in the same polyp are rare.

The only way to detect a small focus of carcinoma within an adenoma is to remove it completely for histologic examination. If a carcinoma within a polyp extends deep to a line joining the layers of muscularis mucosae of the adjacent normal mucosa, there is some risk of lymph node involvement.[115] Whether a segmental resection to remove potentially positive lymph nodes should be performed requires careful consideration of the patient's clinical condition and the potential risks, benefits, and costs. Pedunculated adenomatous polyps lend themselves to complete curative removal with an electrocautery snare even if they contain an invasive carcinoma, provided it does not extend to the attachment of the pedicle

to the underlying flat mucosa.[115] Such lesions have at most a 1% to 2% likelihood of lymph node metastasis. Sessile adenomas containing invasive carcinoma are less likely to be cured by endoscopic excision because they often extend into the submucosa of the underlying bowel and the likelihood of lymph node metastasis is higher (see Fig. 130-18). The pitfall of incorrectly diagnosing invasive cancer must be avoided when normal glands have been mechanically displaced into the submucosa of a pedunculated polyp, so-called *pseudoinvasion*.[116,117] Truly invasive glands are often surrounded by desmoplastic stroma rather than the normal lamina propria of entrapped benign glands.

The hamartomas are an abnormal mixture of benign cells that only rarely contain cancer, and then only in associated adenomatous tissue. The most common hamartoma is the single pedunculated juvenile polyp in a child younger than 10 years of age (Fig. 130-66). It is less common in older children and adults. Familial juvenile polyposis is seen in patients older than 10 years of age, may involve the whole gastrointestinal tract, and is associated with a small risk of carcinoma.[70] The juvenile polyposis of infancy may be fatal but fortunately is rare. Peutz-Jeghers polyps of the colon are less common and the polyps of Cowden's disease are rare.[70] Histologically, juvenile and Cowden's polyps are more cystic, and Peutz-Jeghers polyps contain highly ramified branching smooth muscle with a large benign epithelial component.

Postinflammatory polyps, also known as *pseudopolyps,* are common in areas of healed or partially healed UC or Crohn's colitis and may be found after ischemic or infectious colitis. These polyps often represent islands of variably inflamed residual mucosa in a "sea" of surrounding, previously sloughed, healed mucosa. Pseudopolyps may have a filiform, sessile, or pedunculated configuration. Polyps composed of collagenous granulation tissue may be seen adjacent to a solitary rectal ulcer.

Colonic cancer showing invasion with surrounding des-

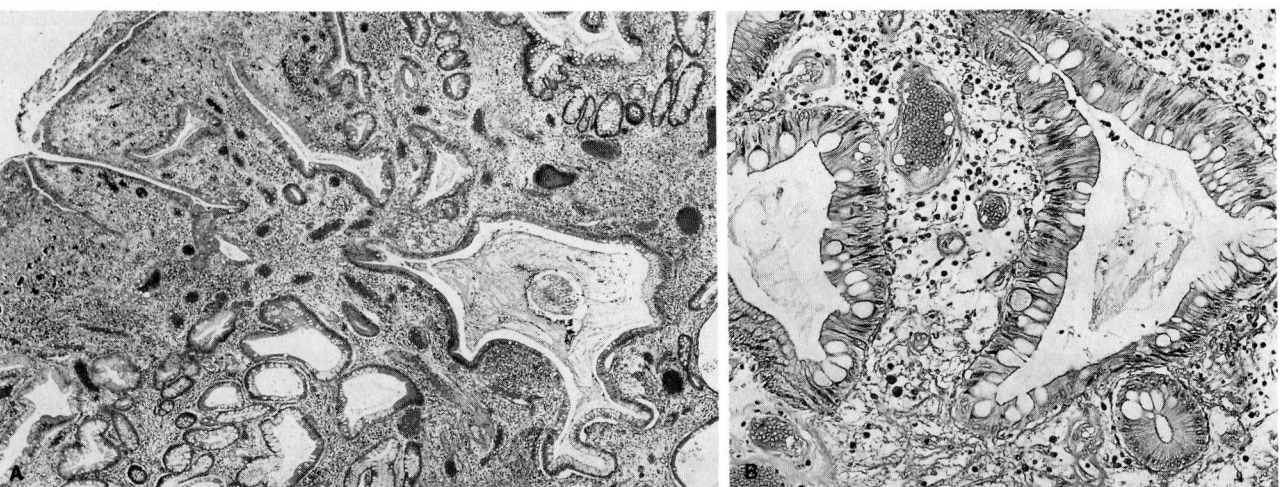

FIGURE 130-66. Juvenile polyp. **(A)** The lesion is composed of dilated, irregular-shaped glands **(B)** lined by epithelium of an essentially normal appearance. The lamina propria is inflamed and edematous and contains numerous congested vessels.

moplasia (see Fig. 130-18) is best diagnosed by colonoscopy. Colonoscopy is indicated in patients with any of the following: gross or occult rectal bleeding, previous resection for cancer or an adenoma, a history of colon cancer in first-degree relatives, UC of over 8 years' duration, relatives of patients with the colon cancer family syndrome, and all family members of patients with familial adenomatous polyposis coli.

Adenocarcinoma of the colon is common and has a 50% survival rate after surgical resection. It is curable when diagnosed early, before distant metastasis develops. Grossly, the lesser the depth of invasion, the better the prognosis (Dukes' classification). Unlike the esophagus and the stomach, neoplastic cells that invade only the lamina propria and do not penetrate the muscularis mucosae are not considered to be biologically malignant because lymph node metastasis in such lesions has never been convincingly reported.[114] Poor histologic differentiation of a carcinoma and the presence of tumor in lymphatics also are of adverse prognostic import.

Lipomas, fibromas, leiomyomas, and Kaposi's sarcoma in AIDS are usually submucosal in location and are less frequently diagnosable by biopsy. Angiomas can be sampled by hot biopsy but there is some risk of bleeding. Benign, enlarged lymphoid nodules can be mistaken for neoplasms or polyposis. These nodules may be idiopathic or a reaction to infection, or they may be the benign lymphoid hyperplasia of common variable immunodeficiency. The latter is diagnosed by the virtual absence of plasma cells from the lamina propria of the adjacent colonic mucosa.

Occasionally tumors metastatic to the colon may be recognizable as such if they retain the characteristic morphologic features of their primary site.

Carcinoids almost always are histologically invasive and have the characteristic appearance of monotonously similar, small round nuclei growing in cords, glands, or nests. Many carcinoids smaller than 2 cm are indolent and do not require segmental resection, especially if they can be completely resected locally. If they recur or enlarge, segmental resection may be required.

Other diagnoses by biopsy include melanosis coli, a benign

collection of lipofuscin-containing macrophages caused by laxatives, and pneumatosis cystoides intestinalis, marked by gross lumps on colonoscopy that contain gas-filled spaces in the submucosa lined by giant and epithelioid cells.[60]

CONTRAINDICATIONS AND RISKS

Major risks of biopsy are those associated with endoscopy rather than biopsy per se, that is, excessive sedation, inadvertent aspiration, myocardial infarction, and instrumental perforation. With appropriate measures and experience, most of these complications are avoidable. Complications of biopsy such as significant bleeding and perforation are rare and are no more frequent with the large than with the smaller standard-sized forceps. The biopsy forceps should always be extended to the biopsy site under direct visual control. Rather than pushing the forceps into the mucosa, the biopsy spike should be gently impaled on the mucosa and air aspirated from the lumen to draw mucosa into the cups of the biopsy forceps, which are then closed; this is called *turn and suck* technique.[118] Unlike the stiff cutting instruments that obtain deeper biopsy specimens through a sigmoidoscope, the double-cup forceps pinches the mucosa and removes it by avulsion, including at the most a sliver of submucosa. Therefore the deeper submucosa containing the larger blood vessels is almost always avoided.

Situations exist in which endoscopy is permissible or desirable but in which biopsy is contraindicated. For example, esophagoscopy may be indicated despite a coagulopathy in an immunosuppressed patient when the patient develops a fever, hematemesis, odynophagia, or unexplained nausea and vomiting. Although biopsy is contraindicated, gentle brushing should be used to detect treatable opportunistic infections such as with *Candida* organisms, HSV, or CMV. If a vascular lesion such as a possible angioma or a vascular variant of Kaposi's sarcoma must undergo biopsy for diagnosis, endoscopic control of bleeding can be accomplished with electrocautery, thermal probe, or sclerosant injection. To reduce the risk of bleeding, aspirin and NSAIDs should be discontinued for an appropriate interval before biopsy.

Inadvertent biopsy of a varix is rare because portal hypertension usually is suspected. In this situation biopsy specimens of the distal esophagus should be taken only when they are absolutely essential for patient management and when the site of biopsy is carefully chosen to avoid a possible varix.

Many clinicians prefer to defer biopsy of the edge of a bleeding gastric ulcer until bleeding has stopped and healing has started. When looking for cancer, it is best to biopsy four quadrants of the edge of a gastric ulcer at the junction between the mucosa and the ulcerated area. It is not particularly risky if it is certain that the ulcer is chronic and scarred. Biopsy of the thin base of a possible acute ulcer is hazardous.

Colonic biopsy of flat mucosa is safe but remember that the colonic wall is thinner than that of the rest of the gastrointestinal tract. Biopsy specimens taken proximal to the peritoneal reflection should have their depth limited by using the *turn-and-suck* aspiration technique. Biopsy specimens of adequate diameter and depth can be obtained with this technique.

Occasionally larger or deeper biopsies are required for diagnosis. Removal of portions of a lesion that protrude into the lumen with an electrocautery snare usually is safe except for lipomas. However, excising a fold that has to be pulled into the snare with a second forceps can produce complications.

COST EFFECTIVENESS

Taking a sufficient number of adequate-sized biopsy specimens and orienting and processing them in the manner suggested is more costly than routine biopsy. A large-caliber operating endoscope must be used, causing more discomfort and requiring more time for adequate premedication. An extra assistant is needed to orient the specimens correctly while they are taken. The endoscopy may take longer if the number of specimens is to be optimal for diagnosis. Step-serial sectioning and special staining also require extra effort and expense.

Is this compulsive approach cost effective? This question has not been studied systematically. Those who have been exposed to both approaches firmly believe that the more compulsive technique detects more focal lesions, may be more accurate in the diagnosis of dysplasia and early carcinoma, and permits better evaluation of abnormalities of villous, crypt, and squamous mucosal architecture. Such architectural changes are significant diagnostically.

An incorrect diagnosis of cancer followed by an operation is costly, especially if complications occur, or death. Similarly, it is difficult to estimate the cost and distress of the patients and their families that could be avoided if an early, curable cancer had been diagnosed in time. The same considerations apply to more accurate biopsy diagnosis of certain other diseases. The problem is that there may be no way to know which patients need this extra effort at the time of endoscopic biopsy. Ideally all biopsy specimens should be taken and processed as suggested to increase diagnostic accuracy and improve patient care.

The reader is directed to Chapter 141, Applications of New Technologies in Tissue Examination.

REFERENCES

1. Hirshowitz BL. Historical profiles: a personal history of the fiberscope. Gastroenterology 1979;76:864.
2. Morrissey JF. Gastrointestinal endoscopy: 20 years of progress. The 1982 A/S/G/E distinguished lecture. Gastrointest Endosc 1983;29:53.
3. Gibbs DD. The history of gastrointestinal endoscopy. In: Schiller KFR, Salmon PR, eds. Modern topics in gastrointestinal endoscopy. London: Heinemann, 1976:1.
4. Masson P. Carcinoids and nerve hyperplasia of the appendicular mucosa. Am J Pathol 1928;4:181.
5. Haggitt RC, Rubin CE. Endoscopy and endoscopic biopsy. In: Ming S-C, Goldman H, eds. Gastrointestinal pathology. Philadelphia: WB Saunders, 1992:37.
6. Meisel JL, Bergman D, Graney D, et al. Human rectal mucosa: proctoscopic and morphologic changes caused by laxatives. Gastroenterology 1977;72:1274.
7. Jonas G, Mahoney A, Johnson M, et al. Chemical colitis due to endoscope cleaning solutions: a mimic of pseudomembranous colitis. Gastroenterology 1988;95:1403.
8. Spechler SJ, Goyal RK. Medical progress: Barrett's esophagus. N Engl J Med 1986;315:362.
9. Reid BJ, Haggitt RC, Rubin CE, et al. Observer variation in the diagnosis of high grade dysplasia in Barrett's esophagus. Hum Pathol 1988;19:166.
10. Riddell RH, Goldman H, Ransohoff DF, et al. Dysplasia in inflammatory bowel disease: standardized classification with provisional clinical applications. Hum Pathol 1983;14:931.
11. Reid BJ, Haggitt RC, Rubin CE, et al. Barrett's esophagus: correlation between flow cytometry and histology in detection of patients at risk for adenocarcinoma. Gastroenterology 1987;93:1.
12. Reid BJ, Blount PL, Rubin CE, Levine DS, Haggitt RC, Rabinovitch PS. Flow-cytometric and histological progression to malignancy in Barrett's esophagus: prospective endoscopic surveillance of a cohort. Gatroenterology 1992;102:1212.
13. Reid BJ, Weinstein WM, Lewin KJ, et al. Endoscopic biopsy can detect high-grade dysplasia or early adenocarcinoma in Barrett's esophagus without grossly recognizable neoplastic lesions. Gastroenterology 1988;94:81.
14. Levine DS, Haggitt RC, Blount PL, et al. An endoscopic biopsy protocol can differentiate high-grade dysplasia from early adenocarcinoma in Barrett's esophagus. Gastroenterology 1993;105:40.
15. Huang G, Shao L, Zhang D, et al. Diagnosis and treatment of early esophageal carcinoma. Chin Med J (Engl) 1981;94:229.
16. Nagayo T. Histogenesis and precursors of human gastric cancer: research and practice. Berlin: Springer-Verlag, 1986:153.
17. Green PHR, O'Toole KM, et al. Increasing incidence and excellent survival of patients with early gastric cancer: experience in a United States medical center. Am J Med 1988;85:658.
18. Levine DS, Rubin CE, Reid BJ, et al. Specialized metaplastic columnar epithelium in Barrett's esophagus: a comparative transmission electron microscopic study. Lab Invest 1989;60:418.
19. Haggitt RC, Dean PJ. Adenocarcinoma in Barrett's epithelium. In: Spechler SJ, Goyal R, eds. Barrett's esophagus: pathophysiology, diagnosis, and management. New York: Elsevier, 1985:153.
20. Antonioli DA, Goldman H. Changes in location and type of gastric adenocarcinoma. Cancer 1982;50:775.
21. Blot WJ, Devesa SS, Kneller RW, Fraumeni JF. Rising incidence of adenocarcinoma of the esophagus and gastric cardia. JAMA 1991;265:1287.
22. Pera M, Cameron AJ, Trastek VF, et al. Increasing incidence

of adenocarcinoma of the esophagus and esophagogastric junction. Gastroenterology 1993;104:510.

23. MacDonald WC, MacDonald JB. Adenocarcinoma of the esophagus and/or gastric cardia. Cancer 1987;60:1094.

24. Rubin CE, Haggitt RC, Burmer GC, et al. DNA aneuploidy in colonic biopsies predicts future development of dysplasia in ulcerative colitis. Gastroenterology 1992;103:1611.

25. Woolrich AJ, DaSilva MD, Korelitz BI. Surveillance in the routine management of ulcerative colitis: the predictive value of low-grade dysplasia. Gastroenterology 1992;103:431.

26. Choi PM. Predominance of rectosigmoid neoplasia in ulcerative colitis and its implication on cancer surveillance (letter). Gastroenterology 1993;104:666.

27. Rickert RR, Auerback O, Garfinkel L, et al. Adenomatous lesions of the large bowel: an autopsy survey. Cancer 1979;43:1847.

28. Ismail-Beigi F, Horton PF, Pope CE II. Histological consequences of gastroesophageal reflux in man. Gastroenterology 1970;58:163.

29. Ismail-Beigi F, Pope CE II. Distribution of the histological changes of gastroesophageal reflux in the distal esophagus of man. Gastroenterology 1974;66:1109.

30. Behar J, Sheahan D. Histologic abnormalities in reflux esophagitis. Arch Pathol 1975;99:387.

31. Johnson LF, Demeester TR, Haggitt RC. Esophageal epithelial response to gastroesophageal reflux. Am J Digest Dis 1978;23:498.

32. Weinstein WM, Bogoch ER, Bowes KL. The normal human esophageal mucosa: a histological reappraisal. Gastroenterology 1975;68:40.

33. Tummala V, Barwick KW, Sontag SJ, et al. The significance of intraepithelial eosinophils in the histologic diagnosis of gastroesophageal reflux. Am J Clin Pathol 1987;87:43.

34. Boyce WH. The esophagogastric junction: 25 years looking and learning. A/S/G/E distinguished lecture, New Orleans, May 1984.

35. Dodds WJ, Hogan WJ, Helm JF, et al. Pathogenesis of reflux esophagitis. Gastroenterology 1981;81:376.

36. McDonald GB, Sharma P, Hackman RC, et al. Esophageal infections in immunosuppressed patients after marrow transplantation. Gastroenterology 1985;88:1111.

37. Spencer GD, Hackman RC, McDonald GB, et al. A prospective study of unexplained nausea and vomiting after marrow transplantation. Transplantation 1986;42:602.

38. Bender MD, Allison J, Cuartas F, et al. Glycogenic acanthosis of the esophagus: a form of benign epithelial hyperplasia. Gastroenterology 1973;65:373.

39. Dixon MF. *Campylobacter pylori* and chronic gastritis. In: Rathbone BJ, Heatley RV, eds. *Campylobacter pylori* and gastroduodenal disease. Oxford: Blackwell Scientific Publications, 1989.

40. Rauws EAJ, Tytgat GNJ. *Campylobacter pylori*. Amsterdam: WC Ouden, 1989.

41. Graham DY. *Campylobacter pylori* and peptic ulcer disease. Gastroenterology 1989;96(Suppl 2):615.

42. Leon BR, Recavarren AS, Ramirez R. El aporte peruano a la investigacion sobre *Helicobacter pylori*. Rev Medica Herediana 1991;2(4):173.

43. Klein PD, Gastrointestinal Physiology Working Group, Grahm DY, et al. Water source as risk factor for *Helicobacter pylori* infection in Peruvian Children. Lancet 1991;337:1503.

44. Correa P, Muñoz N, Cuello C, et al. The role of *Campylobacter pylori* in gastro-duodenal disease. In: Finoglio-Preiser C, ed. Progress in surgical pathology. Vol 10. Philadelphia: Field and Wood, 1989.

45. Recavarren-Arce S, Leon-Barua R, Cok J, et al. *Helicobacter pylori* and progressive gastric pathology that predisposes to gastric cancer. Scand J Gastroenterol 1991;26:51.

46. Siurala M, Varis K, Wiljasalo M. Studies of patients with atrophic gastritis: a 10–15 year followup. Scand J Gastroenterol 1966;1:40.

47. Stemmermann GN, Hayashi T. Intestinal metaplasia of the gastric mucosa: a gross and microscopic study of its distribution in various disease states. J Natl Cancer Inst 1968;40:627.

48. Levi S, Beardshall K, Swift I, et al. *Helicobacter pylori*, hypergastrinaemia, and duodenal ulcers: effect of eradicating the organism. Br Med J 1989;299:1504.

49. Cheli R, Santi L, Giancamerla G, et al. A clinical and statistical follow-up study of atrophic gastritis. Dig Dis 1933;18:1061.

50. Ihamaki T, Saukkonen M, Siurala M. Long term observations of subjects with normal mucosa and with superficial gastritis: results of 23–27 years follow-up examination. Scand J Gastroenterol 1979;13:771.

51. Whitehead R, Truelove SC, Gear MWL. The histological diagnosis of chronic gastritis in fiberoptic gastroscope biopsy specimens. J Clin Pathol 1972;25:1.

52. Strickland RG, Mackay IR. A reappraisal of the significance of chronic gastritis. Dig Dis 1973;18:426.

53. Laine L, Weinstein WM. Subepithelial hemorrhages and erosions of human stomach. Dig Dis Sci 1988;33:490.

54. Czaja AJ, McAlhany JC, Pruitt BA. Acute gastrointestinal disease after thermal injury: an endoscopic evaluation of incidence and natural history. N Engl J Med 1974;291:925.

55. Quintero E, Pique JM, Bombi JA, et al. Upper gastrointestinal bleeding caused by gastrointestinal vascular malformation: incidence, diagnosis and treatment. Dig Dis Sci 1986;31:897.

56. Hashizumi M, Tanaka K, Inokuchi K. Morphology of gastric microcirculation in cirrhosis. Hepatology 1983;3:1008.

57. Suit PF, Petras RE, Bauer TW, et al. Gastric antral vascular ectasia: a histologic and morphometric study of "the watermelon stomach." Am J Surg Pathol 1987;11:750.

58. Lindegardh G, Hans-Olav A, Helmick C, et al. Stomach cancer after partial gastrectomy for benign ulcer disease. N Engl J Med 1988;319:195.

59. Schafer LW, Larson DE, Melton J III, et al. The risk of gastric carcinoma after surgical treatment for benign ulcer disease. N Engl J Med 1983;309:1210.

60. Haggitt RC. Granulomatous disease of the gastrointestinal tract. In: Ioachim H, ed.: Pathology of granulomas. New York: Raven Press, 1983:257.

61. ReMine SG, Hughes RW, Weiland LH. Endoscopic gastric polypectomies. Mayo Clin Proc 1981;56:371.

62. Nagayo T. Histogenesis and precursors of human gastric cancer: research and practice. Berlin: Springer-Verlag, 1986:109.

63. Ming SC. The classification and significance of gastric polyps. In: Yardley JH, Morson BC, Abell MR, eds. The gastrointestinal tract (International Academy of Pathology Monograph). Baltimore: Williams & Wilkins, 1977.

64. Bussey HJR. Familial polyposis coli. Baltimore: Johns Hopkins University Press, 1975:66.

65. Sarre RG, Frost AG, Jagelman DG, et al. Gastric and duodenal polyps in familial adenomatous polyposis: a prospective study of the nature and prevalence of upper gastrointestinal polyps. Gut 1987;28:308.

66. Watanabe H, Enjoji M, Yao T, et al. Gastric lesions in familial adenomatosis coli: their incidence and histologic analysis. Hum Pathol 1978;9:269.

67. Iida M, Yao T, Watanabe H, et al. Spontaneous disappearance of fundic gland polyposis: report of three cases. Gastroenterology 1980;79:725.

68. Lee RG, Burt RW. The histopathology of fundic gland polyps of the stomach. Am J Clin Pathol 1986;86:498.

69. Tatsuta M, Okuda S, Tamura H, et al. Gastric hamartomatous polyps in the absence of familial polyposis coli. Cancer 1980;45:818.

70. Haggitt RC, Reid BJ. Hereditary gastrointestinal polyposis syndromes. Am J Surg Pathol 1986;10:871.

71. Giardiello FM, Welsh SB, Hamilton SR, et al. Increased risk of cancer in the Peutz-Jeghers syndrome. N Engl J Med 1987;316:1511.

72. Daniel ES, Leidwig SL, Lewin KJ, et al. The Cronkhite-Canada syndrome: an analysis of clinical and pathologic features and therapy in 55 patients. Medicine 1982;61:293.

73. Kim YI, Woo HK. Inflammatory fibroid polyps of gastrointestinal tract: evolution of histologic patterns. Am J Clin Pathol 1988;89:721.

74. Hirschowitz BI, Griffith J, Pellegrin D, Cummings OW. Rapid regression of enterochromaffinlike cell gastric carcinoids

in pernicious anemia after antrectomy. Gastroenterology 1992;102:1409.

75. Roucayrol A-M, Cattan D. Evolution of fundic argyrophil cell hyperplasia in nonantral atrophic gastritis. Gastroenterology 1990;99:1307.

76. Dandalides SM, Carey WD, Petras R, et al. Endoscopic small bowel mucosal biopsy: a controlled trial evaluating forceps size and biopsy location in the diagnosis of normal and abnormal mucosal architecture. Gastrointest Endosc 1989;35:197.

77. Perera DR, Weinstein WM, Rubin CE. Small intestinal biopsy. Hum Pathol 1975;6:157.

78. Weinstein WM, Saunders DR, Tytgat GN, et al. Collagenous sprue: an unrecognized type of malabsorption. N Engl J Med 1970;283:1297.

79. Ament ME, Rubin CE. The relation of giardiasis to abnormal intestinal structure and function in gastrointestinal immuno-deficiency syndromes. Gastroenterology 1972;62:216.

80. Eidelman S, Parkins RA, Rubin CE. Abdominal lymphoma presenting as malabsorption: a clinico-pathologic study of nine cases in Israel and a review of the literature. Medicine 1966;15:111.

81. Khojasteh A, Haghshenass M, Haghighi P. Immunoproliferative small intestinal disease: a "third world lesion." N Engl J Med 1983;308:1401.

82. Brunser O, Reid A, Monkeberg F, et al. Jejunal biopsies in infant malnutrition: with special reference to mitotic index. Pediatrics 1966;38:605.

83. Davidson GP, Cutz E, Hamilton JR, et al. Familial enteropathy: a syndrome of protracted diarrhea from birth, failure to thrive and hypoplastic villous atrophy. Gastroenterology 1978;75:783.

84. Bjarnason I, Price AB, Zanelli G, et al. Clinicopathological features of nonsteroidal anti-inflammatory drug-induced small intestinal strictures. Gastroenterology 1988;94:1070.

85. De Vos M, Cirvelier C, Mielants H, et al. Ileocolonoscopy in seronegative spondyloarthropathy. Gastroenterology 1989;96:339.

86. Surawicz CM, Meisel JL, Ylvisaker T, et al. Rectal biopsy in the diagnosis of Crohn's disease: value of multiple biopsies and serial sectioning. Gastroenterology 1981;81:66.

87. Surawicz CM. Serial sectioning of a portion of a rectal biopsy detects more focal abnormalities: a prospective study of patients with inflammatory bowel disease. Dig Dis Sci 1982;27:434.

88. Spiliadis CA, Spiliadis CA, Lennard-Jones JE. Ulcerative colitis with relative sparing of the rectum: clinical features, histology and prognosis. Dis Colon Rectum 1987;30:334.

89. Surawicz CM, Belic L. Rectal biopsy helps to distinguish acute self-limiting colitis from idiopathic inflammatory bowel disease. Gastroenterology 1984;86:104.

90. MacDonald KL, O'Leary MJ, Cohen ML. *Escheridia coli* 0157:H7, an emerging gastrointestinal pathogen: results of a one-year prospective, population-based study. JAMA 1988;259:3567.

91. Griffin PM, Olmstead LC, Petras RE. *Escherichia coli* 0157:H7-associated colitis: a clinical and histological study of 11 cases. Gastroenterology 1990;99:142.

92. Quinn TC, Stamm WE, Goodell SE, et al. The polymicrobial origin of intestinal infections in homosexual men. N Engl J Med 1983;309:576.

93. Silverstein FE, Tytgat GNJ. Atlas of gastrointestinal endoscopy. Philadelphia: WB Saunders, 1988;1123.

94. Rutter KRP, Riddell RH. The solitary ulcer syndrome of the rectum. Gastroenterology 1975;4:505.

95. Levine DS, Surawicz CM, Ajer TN, et al. Diffuse excess mucosal collagen in rectal biopsies facilitates the differential diagnosis of solitary rectal ulcer syndrome from other inflammatory bowel diseases. Dig Dis Sci 1988;33:1345.

96. Boley SJ, Brandt LJ, Veith FJ. Ischemic disorders of the intestine. Curr Probl Surg 1978;15:1.

97. Bynum TE, Jacobson ED. Vascular disorders of the large bowel. In: Kirsner JB, Shorter RG, eds. Diseases of the colon, rectum and anal canal. Baltimore: Williams & Wilkins, 1987:539.

98. Teglbjaerg PS, Thaysen EH, Jensen HH. Development of collagenous colitis in sequential biopsy specimens. Gastroenterology 1984;87:703.

99. Lazenby AJ, Yardley JH, Giardiello FM, et al. Lymphocytic ("microscopic") colitis: a comparative histopathologic study with particular reference to collagenous colitis. Hum Pathol 1989;20:18.

100. Levine DS, Haggitt RC. Normal histology of the colon. Am J Surg Pathol 1989 13;966:1989.

101. Jessurun J, Yardley JH, Giardiello FM, et al. Chronic colitis with thickening of the subepithelial collagen layer (collagenous colitis): histopathologic findings in 15 patients. Hum Pathol 1987;18:839.

102. Gledhill A, Cole FM. Significance of basement membrane thickening in the human colon. Gut 1984;25:1085.

103. Glotzer DJ, Glick ME, Goldman H. Proctitis and colitis following diversion of the fecal stream. Gastroenterology 1981;80:438.

104. Berthrong M, Fajardo LF. Radiation injury in surgical pathology: alimentary tract. Part II. Am J Surg Pathol 1981;5:153.

105. Weisbrot IM, Liber AF, Gordon BS. The effects of therapeutic radiation on colonic mucosa. Cancer 1975;36:931.

106. Snover DC, Sandstad J, Hutton S. Mucosal pseudolipomatosis of the colon. Am J Clin Pathol 1985;84:575.

107. Jonas G, Mahoney A, Murray J, et al. Chemical colitis due to endoscope cleaning solutions: a mimic of pseudomembranous colitis. Gastroenterology 1988;95:1403.

108. Saunders DR, Haggitt RC, Kimmey MB, et al. Morphological consequences of bisacodyl on normal human rectal mucosa: effects of a prostaglandin E1 analog on mucosal injury. Gastrointest Endosc 1990;36:101.

109. Floch MH, Hellman L. The effect of five-fluorouracil on rectal mucosa. Gastroenterology 1965;48:430.

110. McDonald GB, Sale GE. The human gastrointestinal tract after allogenic marrow transplantation. In: Sale GE, Shulman HM, eds. The pathology of bone marrow transplantation. New York: Masson, 1984:77.

111. Norfleet RG, Ryan ME, Wyman JB. Adenomatous and hyperplastic polyps cannot be reliably distinguished by their appearance through the fiberoptic sigmoidoscope. Dig Dis Sci 1988;33:1175.

112. Hayashi T, Yatani R, Apostol J, et al. Pathogenesis of hyperplastic polyps of the colon: a hypothesis based on ultrastructure and in vivo cell kinetics. Gastroenterology 1974;66:347.

113. Longacre TA, Fenoglio-Preiser CM. Mixed hyperplastic adenomatous polyps/serrated adenomas. Am J Surg Pathol 1990;14:524.

114. Muto T, Bussey HJR, Morson BC. The evolution of cancer of the colon and rectum. Cancer 1975;36:2251.

115. Haggitt RC, Glotzbach RE, Soffer EE, et al. Prognostic factors in colorectal carcinomas arising in adenomas: implications for lesions removed by endoscopic polypectomy. Gastroenterology 1985;89:328.

116. Allen DC, Biggart JD. Misplaced epithelium in ulcerative colitis and Crohn's disease of the colon and its relationship to malignant mucosal changes. Histopathology 1986;10:37.

117. Muto T, Bussey HJR, Morson BC. Pseudo-carcinomatous invasion in adenomatous polyps of the colon and rectum. J Clin Pathol 1973;26:25.

118. Levine DS, Reid BJ. Endoscopic biopsy technique for acquiring larger mucosal samples. Gastrointest Endosc 1991;37:332.

Textbook of Gastroenterology, second edition, edited
by Tadataka Yamada. JB Lippincott Company,
Philadelphia © 1995.

CHAPTER 131

Microbiologic Studies

Phillip I. Tarr   Christina M. Surawicz

Infections of the gastrointestinal tract, the hepatobiliary system, and the pancreas are encountered frequently in gastroenterologic practice. The diagnostic approach to a patient with possible or confirmed infection of the gastrointestinal tract depends on the patient's age, medical and travel history, epidemiologic associations, and sexual practices. After a careful history and examination, the physician must turn to one or more of a variety of microbiologic tests to identify the pathogens responsible for the patient's illness. Familiarity with the range of bacteriologic, serologic, virologic, histologic, and nucleic acid technologies involved in microbiologic diagnosis is, therefore, useful to the gastroenterologist.

Unfortunately the yield of microbiologic investigations is often low, resulting in high aggregate costs for many tests. However, since these tests chiefly involve stool analyses or determining serologic status, their costs in individual cases are small, and the risks are negligible. Positive findings may lead to specific therapy and avert the risk and expense of other diagnostic procedures or therapeutic interventions. For this reason, consideration should be given to microbiologic diagnosis in a wide variety of intestinal, hepatobiliary, and pancreatic disorders, even though many investigations will yield negative results.

This chapter reviews the major microbiologic tests available to clinicians practicing in North America in 1993, provides guidelines for their use and interpretation, and indicates their limitations. Specific diagnostic considerations for individual pathogens are covered in greater detail in chapters on gastrointestinal infections.

MICROBIOLOGIC TECHNIQUES FOR DIAGNOSING CLASSES OF PATHOGENS

Bacteria

General Considerations

Bacterial infections can be diagnosed by microscopic study, culture, identification of bacterial products, such as antigens or toxins, or by characteristic histologic findings. Bacteria are, of course, too small to visualize with the naked eye. However, several macroscopic observations increase the likelihood of a bacterial pathogen being present in a body fluid. For example, the observation of gross blood in diarrheal stools, especially if accompanied by abdominal pain or fever, increases the likelihood that a patient has a bacterial enteric infection.[1] The presence of occult blood frequently is associated with inflammatory cells.[2]

Microscopic examination of the stool to detect specific bacterial pathogens is of limited value because of its polymicrobial composition. However, carbol-fuchsin Gram stain[3] or methylene blue stain[4] can identify vibrio-like organisms, suggesting that subsequent stool culture will yield *Campylo-*

bacter jejuni. Furthermore, darkfield examination of the stool has been proposed to predict subsequently positive findings for cholera in cultures.[5] These practices are rarely used in North America.

Microscopic examination of the stool to detect fecal leukocytes uses methylene blue stain or Gram stain. Several studies have demonstrated that when fecal leukocytes are present, a culture positive for bacteria is more likely.[6,7] If possible, it is preferable to stain mucous in the submitted specimen. However, the presence or absence of fecal leukocytes or occult blood in acute diarrheal stools should not be used to determine which specimens should be sent for bacteriologic culture.

In body fluids that normally are sterile, microscopic examination often is critical in determining a diagnosis, especially if patients have received antibiotics that might interfere with culture, or if a fastidious organism such as a *Mycobacterium* is a likely etiologic agent. In practice, this most frequently occurs when aspiration is performed on intraabdominal abscesses, at which time the microscopic examination of the fluid should include Gram stain, and in many cases, mycobacterial stains.

Detecting Bacteria by Culture

Bacterial culture usually involves placing an aliquot of the specimen on solid media for stool or tissue, or in liquid media for blood and ascites; and incubation under conditions that favor or distinguish various pathogens. Biochemical tests are subsequently performed to identify the genus and species, and if necessary, serotyping is performed.

Cultures should be placed on the appropriate growth or selective media as soon as possible after being obtained. Ascitic fluid should be placed into broth culture at the bedside after paracentesis.[8] If an interval of 2 or more hours will elapse between sampling and plating, specimens should be stored at 4°C and placed in appropriate transport media: thioglycolate broth for Campylobacter and Cary-Blair medium for other enteric pathogens. Even though stains can be performed and interpreted rapidly, bacterial culture necessitates a minimum of overnight incubation. For many organisms that infect the gastrointestinal tract, identification might require an additional 2 or 3 days. Sensitivities of organisms to antibiotics are determined, if indicated, obligating an additional 24 hours of effort in the microbiology laboratory.

It is rarely necessary for the gastroenterologist to specify the culture techniques to the microbiologist, but a familiarity with the media used is sometimes helpful in understanding the yield and limitations of the test requested. Therefore a brief review of microbiologic techniques is helpful to the clinician who frequently orders tests. The most frequent bacterial test requested in gastroenterologic practice is a stool culture, which in North America should include techniques to detect *C jejuni, Escherichia coli* O157:H7, *Salmonella, Shigella,* and *Yersinia. Aeromonas* species (*Aeromonas hydrophila, Aeromonas caviae,* and *Aeromonas sobria*), and, to a lesser extent, *Plesiomonas shigelloides,* are also frequently sought. If epidemiologically indicated, attempts are made to isolate *Vibrio cholera* and *Vibrio parahaemolyticus* from the stool.

Usually laboratories detect *Salmonella* and *Shigella* using *Salmonella-Shigella* agar plates and an enrichment broth for *Salmonella.* These media favor the growth of gram-negative

flora and are incubated aerobically so that obligate anaerobes do not grow. *Salmonella* and *Shigella* ferment lactose slowly, and the indicator dye in the agar fails to turn pink after 24 hours, thereby identifying these nonlactose-fermenting organisms. Additional biochemical, functional, and serotyping studies confirm these genera and assign species, usually within an additional 24 hours. Enteroinvasive *E coli* also frequently fail to ferment lactose, appearing as colorless colonies on lactose-MacConkey agar.[9]

To detect *C jejuni,* a microaerophilic environment of 5% oxygen or a candle jar and elevated temperatures of 42°C are used with media containing antibiotics to suppress other flora. To detect *Yersinia enterocolitica* and *Yersinia pseudotuberculosis,* stool specimens are streaked on selective agar containing cefsulodin, irgasan, and novobiocin, and the plates are incubated between 25°C and 35°C. *Yersinia* are also nonlactose fermenters. If vibrios are suspected on epidemiologic or clinical grounds, stools should be plated on thiosulfate-citrate-bile salt-sucrose (TCBS) agar in addition to blood agar. TCBS agar also can be used to distinguish *V cholera* from noncholera vibrios, such as *V parahaemolyticus.* Serologic and biochemical tests are needed to confirm the species and serotype after initial identification on TCBS agar.

E coli O157:H7, the most frequently isolated member of the enterohemorrhagic *E coli* group, can be distinguished from most other *E coli* because organisms belonging to this serotype fail to ferment sorbitol. *E coli* O157:H7 are identified on sorbitol-MacConkey agar plates, analogous to lactose-MacConkey agar used to detect nonlactose-fermenting enteric organisms.[10] The authors recommend that all stools submitted for bacterial culture be screened for this pathogen, and that this be a reportable infection. At a minimum, stools from all patients with acute bloody diarrhea should be plated on sorbitol-MacConkey agar. Many hospitals in the area of Seattle, Washington, include sorbitol-MacConkey agar in the routine screen for bacterial enteric pathogens, and this practice, in combination with a statewide reporting requirement, led to the early detection of a massive multisource outbreak of infection with *E coli* O157:H7 in early 1993.[11] Institutions that have adopted this approach in North America have observed that the yield of *E coli* O157:H7 equals or exceeds the yield for other classic bacterial enteric pathogens.[12–15]

Methods to detect *Aeromonas* species and *P shigelloides* remains unsatisfactory. One method to determine their presence in stool cultures is to flood the colonies on a blood agar plate with oxidase reagent. These organisms, as well as vibrios, are oxidase positive, unlike *Enterobacteriaceae.*

Staphylococcus aureus, once thought to be the cause of antibiotic-associated colitis, is occasionally isolated as the predominant fecal organism, especially in patients on antibiotics.[16] Considerable variation exists in whether this organism is even reported by microbiology laboratories to the clinician. The precise role of *S aureus* in diarrhea in this setting is unknown. Less debatable is the role of *S aureus* in food poisoning. This organism can produce one or more heat-stable toxins, which can induce diarrhea, vomiting, and abdominal pain. Because the ingestion of preformed toxin is sufficient to cause the disease, cultures of food, rather than stool, should be performed. *Clostridium perfringens* and *Bacillus cereus* cause diarrhea with or without vomiting, and these pathogens are present in stool. Quantification of the number of spores for

C perfringens, or colony-forming units for *Bacillus cereus*, per gram of stool or vomitus is necessary to incriminate these agents as the cause of a patient's disease, because these organisms can be present in low numbers in the stool of asymptomatic people.[17] Public health authorities usually are involved in these investigations.

Clostridium difficile, the predominant cause of antibiotic-associated pseudomembranous colitis, is recoverable from the stools of patients using selective media (cycloserine and cefoxitin) and anaerobic incubation.[18] The yield is higher than for tests that rely on toxin detection. To complicate the matter, some people, particularly infants, can have *C difficile* organisms and their toxin in their stool in the absence of symptoms.[19]

Detecting Bacterial Products

Bacterial products, such as antigens or toxins, can be used to make a surrogate diagnosis of infection with the appropriate pathogen. The detection of bacterial toxins using a tissue culture approach is a tedious way to determine if toxigenic bacteria are present in a patient's stool or other body substances. This approach seeks the toxin phenotype from culture supernatants or from fecal filtrates. Depending on the toxin suspected, various target systems are used. In clinical practice, only tests for detecting cytotoxin B of *C difficile* are used frequently. This test involves the application of stool filtrates to one of a variety of cell lines. If antiserum to the cytotoxin of *Clostridium sordellii* or *C difficile* neutralizes the cytotoxicity, a specific effect is detected, thus implicating *C difficile*. Shiga-like cytotoxins, or verocytotoxins, occasionally are detected using cultured Vero's cells, but the most efficient way to diagnose infection with cytotoxin-producing *E coli* other than *E coli* O157:H7 has not been established. *E coli* capable of producing heat-labile and heat-stable toxins can be detected using a wide variety of in vivo and in vitro toxin assays.[20]

Antibody-based techniques to detect bacterial toxins, and in particular, *C difficile* toxin, are proliferating, especially in laboratories that cannot maintain a tissue culture facility.[21] Detection of bacteria with specific antibody to serotype occasionally is used to identify specific pathogens in stool.[22] However, serotyping is most frequently used on bacterial colonies that grow on agar.

Histopathologic Techniques for Detecting Bacterial Infection

Most bacterial infections of the gastrointestinal tract involve the colon; histologic examination usually will not give a specific diagnosis, but it may be helpful in distinguishing an acute self-limited colitis, likely of infectious origin, from early inflammatory bowel disease, which often is the most frequent question in differential diagnosis. Colorectal biopsy is helpful because in acute self-limited colitis crypt architecture usually is normal, and lamina propria inflammation is predominantly superficial and acute, although mild increases in chronic cells also may be seen (Fig. 131-1).[23-25]

In contrast, inflammatory bowel disease, especially ulcerative colitis, is characterized by distorted architecture, even early in the course of disease; lamina propria inflammation is acute and chronic. Other histologic features that are much more frequent in inflammatory bowel disease and uncommon in acute self-limited colitis are basilar plasmacytosis, basilar lymphoid aggregates, and basilar lymphoid hyperplasia (Fig. 131-2). Epithelioid granulomas usually indicate Crohn's disease but can also be seen in *Chlamydia trachomatis* and syphilitic proctitis. These usually are seen in the setting of sexually transmitted proctitis.

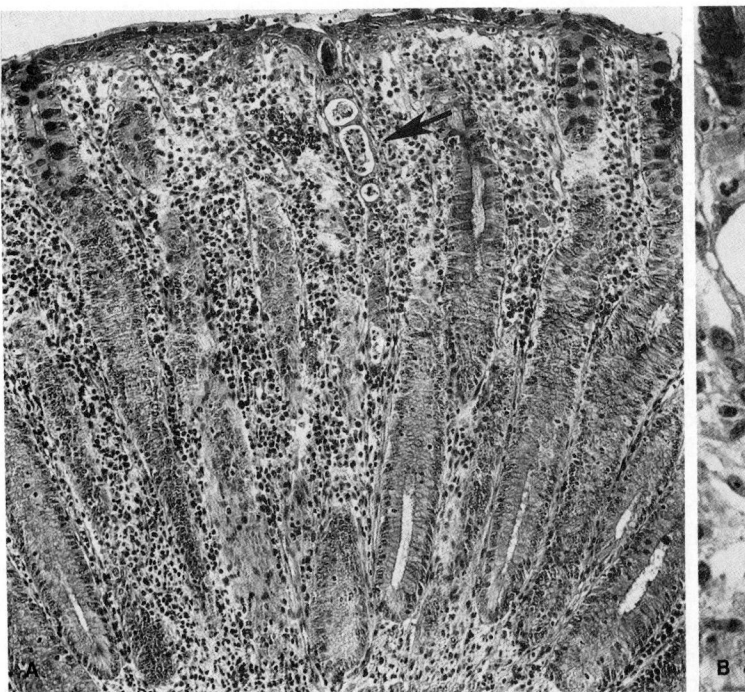
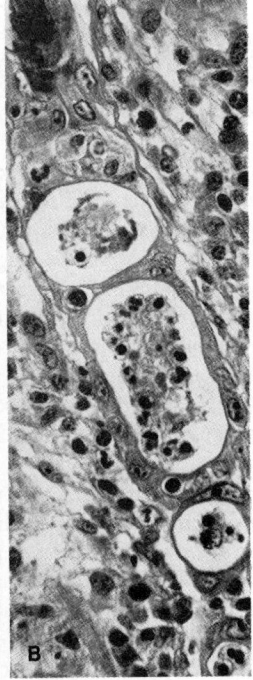

FIGURE 131-1. Biopsy specimen of colorectal mucosa from a patient with acute, self-limited, infectious-type colitis caused by *Campylobacter jejuni*. (**A**) Notice the normal architecture, acute lamina propria inflammation, and cryptitis (*arrow*). (**B**) Higher magnification.

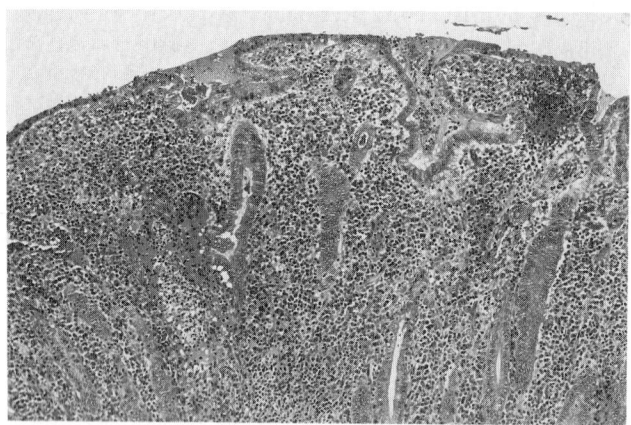

FIGURE 131-2. Colorectal biopsy specimen from a patient with ulcerative colitis shows distorted crypt architecture, chronic lamina propria inflammation, and basilar plasmacytosis, all of which are typical of inflammatory bowel disease and rare in acute self-limited colitis.

Specific histologic features may suggest infection with *C difficile* and *E coli* O157:H7. In the former, pseudomembranes are diagnostic, with superficial edema. These pseudomembranes, composed of fibrin, polymorphonuclear cells, and debris, seem to emanate or "erupt" from the mucosa, which may be relatively uninflamed unless colitis is severe.

Colitis from *E coli* O157:H7, which is often right sided, may mimic ischemia, both clinically and histologically when superficial necrosis is present.

Viruses

General Considerations

The diagnosis of viral infections of the gastrointestinal and hepatobiliary systems depends on demonstration of characteristic histologic features or specific antigens in biopsy tissues, detection of viral antigens in serum or stool, growth of the virus in cell cultures, observation of diagnostic antibodies to viral antigens, electron microscopic imaging of the virus particle, or nucleic acid hybridization technology.

The direct cultivation of viruses from stool is difficult and rarely is performed to diagnose enteric infections, although stool cultures for enteroviruses are performed in the context of systemic illness. In contrast, viral cultures of the biopsy or brushing specimens of lesions from upper and lower gastrointestinal tract sites, usually from immunocompromised hosts, frequently are used to diagnose viral mucosal infection, particularly infections caused by herpes simplex virus and cytomegalovirus.

Viral antigens can be detected in stool and mucosal biopsy specimens and in tissue culture cells soon after infection with herpes simplex virus, cytomegalovirus, and adenovirus. The use of monoclonal antibodies to detect these antigens in centrifuge cultures can provide presumptively positive results 1 or more days before microscopic evidence of viral infection of the cells is present.[26] Electron microscopic study can detect viral particles with distinctive morphologic features in stool, and the sensitivity of this technique can be increased using immune sera, called immune electron microscopic study.[27]

Recovery of Viruses by Culture

Viral cultures of body substances are variably helpful in diagnosing infection. Viral cultures of the stool are not useful in diagnosing acute enteric infection, except for enteroviruses. Enterovirus recovery is possible from stool, and illnesses with systemic findings suggestive of infection with these viruses, such as rash, headache, or photophobia, are best diagnosed by viral rectal and throat cultures. Despite their name and intestinal venue, enteroviruses usually cause extraintestinal illnesses more often than diarrhea or vomiting, except in bone marrow transplant recipients where gastroenteritis is frequent in enteroviral infection.[28]

The isolation of viruses from body substances that are normally sterile is frequently helpful to the clinician. In particular, the recovery of cytomegalovirus from blood or urine suggests systemic cytomegalovirus infection, which can have gastrointestinal and hepatic consequences. It is often helpful, however, to correlate a viral culture with appropriate histologic findings. Viral culture consists of placing the specimen in transport media if a mucosal biopsy is obtained, followed by inoculation of tissue culture cells. Viruses do not propagate extracellularly, so tissue culture is necessary for accurate diagnosis. Viral antigens may be detected in tissue culture cells after infection with herpes simplex virus, cytomegalovirus, and adenovirus using monoclonal antibodies, providing presumptively positive results 1 or more days before microscopic evidence of viral infection of the cells is present.[26] Viral cultures usually are incubated for several weeks after inoculation before issuing a final negative result. However, most viral cultures give positive results within 7 to 10 days of inoculation. The laboratories to which cultures are sent can advise the physician of the likelihood of a culture giving a positive result after a given duration of incubation.

Viral cultures are available to most physicians in the developed world. Viral cultures should be obtained on biopsy and brushing specimens of mucosal ulcers in immunocompromised patients, and patients with acute, severe esophagitis. The specimen should be placed in sterile viral transport medium containing appropriate antibacterial and antifungal agents to inhibit growth of contaminants. The medium should be frozen until immediately before use and sent to the virology laboratory as soon as possible after inoculation. Biopsy specimens from several sites can be grouped in batches for viral cultures to save expense to the patient.

The use of surveillance virus cultures to assess colonization as a marker for distal gastrointestinal infection might be useful, especially in immunocompromised patients. For example, a throat culture positive for herpes simplex virus in bone marrow transplant recipients accurately predicts herpes esophagitis.[29] Conversely, patients without antibodies to cytomegalovirus and whose throats remain free from colonization with this virus are unlikely to have cytomegalovirus esophagitis. However, the slow growth of cytomegalovirus from colonized sites such as the oropharynx, rather than from urine or infected tissue, make a negative throat culture difficult to interpret.

Imaging of Viruses

Electron microscopic study is an adjunct or alternative to culture in detecting viruses, and is used most frequently in examining fecal specimens. In addition, some noncultivatible viruses such as Norwalk agent have sufficiently distinctive morphologic features to be discerned in the stool. Institutions that can maintain an electron microscope can probably support a virology culture service, leaving electron microscopic study for diagnosing noncultivatible viruses. Immune electron microscopic study, which uses antibodies present in convalescent sera to enhance the morphologic features of viral agents in stool obtained during the acute illness, is chiefly a research tool.[27]

Detecting Viral Antigens

Rotavirus is the most common agent detected in stools by antigen assay. For many diagnostic laboratories, this virus is the only enteric viral pathogen sought by antigen detection. A role for adenovirus in diarrhea also is evolving. *Enteric* adenoviruses, types 40 and 41, and astroviruses might be important causes of gastrointestinal illness in young children,[30,31] and these viruses also can be detected by seeking characteristic antigens in stool. Viral antigens also can be detected by using appropriate antibodies in tissue culture cells inoculated with specimens containing viruses, providing a presumptive diagnosis before cytopathic effects are seen.[26,32] Finally, viral antigen diagnosis can be used to identify viruses in biopsy specimens. Immunofluorescent detection of viral antigens such as adenovirus, cytomegalovirus, and herpes simplex virus can be useful, especially if the tissue is from a region of the body that is normally sterile. False-positive reactions tend to occur in body substances that are not normally sterile, because of cross-reacting antigens on other microbes or because of nonspecific antibody binding to proteins on bacteria, such as staphylococcal protein A, or to Fc receptors of inflammatory cells. In such situations, viral culture is preferable for the diagnosis of viral infection. The value of antigen detection is of greatest clinical use in diagnosing infection with herpes simplex virus and cytomegalovirus because of the availability of antiviral agents for these pathogens.

Serologic Studies to Detect Viruses

Serologic studies may be used to diagnose selected infections. Paired antibody studies may demonstrate a rise in titer to viral pathogens. Often serologic studies must be combined with antigen detection in diagnosing hepatitis. For some agents, such as hepatitis A and hepatitis C, antibody studies are the only widely available diagnostic tests at this time, although excellent data can be obtained from rigorously conducted studies using the polymerase chain reaction.[33] For hepatitis B, serologic study is adjunctive to antigen detection, helping to distinguish various stages of infection and providing prognostic information.

Serologic study is also useful in diagnosing and treating viral mucosal infections by determining the presence and the class of antibodies directed against specific pathogens. The level of antibodies may be quantified by serial dilution or by enzyme-linked immunosorbent assay. Paired evaluation of acute and convalescent specimens seeks a significant rise in antibody levels against a specific pathogen as quantified by serial dilutions or by enzyme-linked immunosorbent assay. Because of day-to-day variation in these tests, paired specimens should be assayed simultaneously, if possible, to discern interpretable differences. As an alternative to paired sera, immunoglobulin class–specific titers can be drawn to determine acute versus chronic, persistent, or resolved infection. Absent titers to viral antigens such as herpes simplex virus and cytomegalovirus have a high negative predictive value in diagnosing mucosal disease, especially when combined with negative results from surveillance throat cultures. Negative titers assume that the infection has been present long enough to elicit an antibody response and that the patient can mount an antibody response. The appearance of antibodies to cytomegalovirus or herpes simplex virus antigens in a previously seronegative person should be interpreted in the context of the transfusion history of the recipient and the serologic status of the donors. Serial antibody quantification may be needed to determine if the antibodies are passively or actively acquired.

To interpret the presence or absence of antibodies to specific agents, several qualifying circumstances must be considered:

Prepositive: specific antibodies have yet to be formed.
False negative: specific antibodies have not been formed.
False positive: the detected infection has resolved, is not germane to the patient's problem, represents a cross-reactive antibody to a different pathogen, or reflects the polyclonal activation of the patient's B cells.

Histopathologic Techniques for Detecting Viral Infections

Biopsy diagnosis of viral infection is used most frequently in evaluating esophagitis and colitis. In the esophagus, herpes simplex virus can cause a self-limited esophagitis in immunocompetent individuals, and herpes simplex virus and cytomegalovirus can cause esophagitis in immunosuppressed patients. Herpes simplex virus can cause a self-limited distal proctitis, which usually is a sexually transmitted disease, and a chronic proctitis and perianal ulceration in the setting of human immunodeficiency virus infection. Self-limited colitis from cytomegalovirus infection has been described in immunocompetent individuals,[34,35] but cytomegalovirus is more frequently found in the immunosuppressed.

Histologic diagnosis relies on detection of viral inclusions, which can be diagnostic. The typical cytomegalovirus cell is a large cell with intranuclear inclusion surrounded by a clear halo; the cytoplasm may be clumped, indicating the cytoplasmic component of the virus (Fig. 131-3). The endothelial cells are most frequently affected, but glandular epithelial cells also can be infected, especially in the stomach. In contrast, the herpes simplex virus cell has an intranuclear inclusion, but no cytoplasmic inclusions (Fig. 131-4). The intranuclear, or *Cowdry Type A,* inclusion is smaller than that seen with cytomegalovirus infection, and thus may be more difficult to detect. Other histologic features that may be more helpful are multinucleated giant cells and cells with ground glass nuclei.

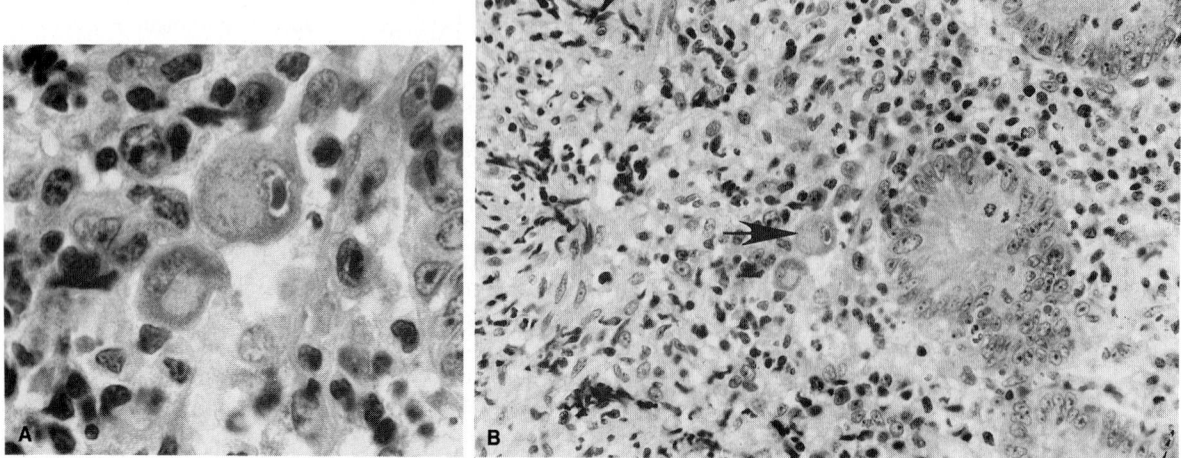

FIGURE 131-3. Colorectal biopsy specimen from a patient with cytomegalovirus colitis. (**A**) High-power view. A dense intranuclear inclusion with a clear surrounding halo and enlarged granular cytoplasmic component is present. (**B**) Typical cytomegalovirus inclusions are harder to see under low-power magnification (*arrow*). (From Surawicz CM. Infectious colitis. Can J Gastroenterol 1989;3:165.)

In addition to viral inclusions, other histologic findings are nonspecific. Cytomegalovirus can cause focal or diffuse colitis or ulceration; cytomegalovirus inclusions can be seen in otherwise normal mucosa. Other histologic features of herpes simplex virus proctitis can include intense lamina propria inflammation.

The pathologist may have difficulty making a diagnosis of viral involvement when no diagnostic cells are seen. Other diagnostic methods include in situ hybridization[36] and rapid viral culture, i.e., shell vial.[26] In situ hybridization can detect cytomegalovirus-infected cells without diagnostic inclusions.[37] Immunocytochemical study has been suggested to improve diagnosis.[38,39] The role of these adjunct tests is not clear, but many pathologists believe that careful review of serial sections for diagnostic viral inclusions remains the gold standard for diagnosis.

Parasites

General Considerations

The diagnosis of parasitic infections presents a dilemma for physicians. Symptoms caused by parasites often are nonspecific, and infestations may be asymptomatic. Laboratory diagnosis depends on observer competence and experience, which may be variable. Positive results may or may not explain the patient's symptoms. Finally, modern air travel enables patients with exotic infections to present to the most staid of practices. Parasitic infections should be considered if patients are epidemiologically at risk, or if unexplained signs, symptoms, or laboratory findings consistent with such infections are present. Parasites of relevance to gastrointestinal practice are legion, but the range of diagnostic tests is limited and

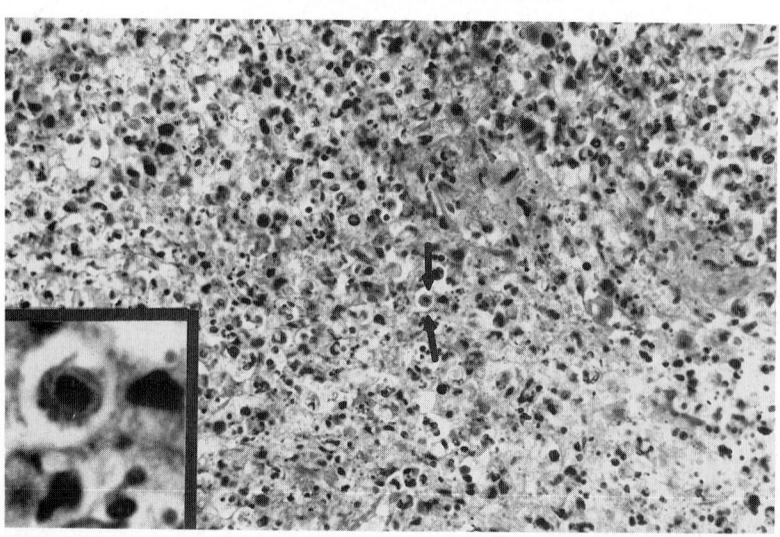

FIGURE 131-4. Typical viral inclusion of herpes simplex virus type 2 shows a Cowdry type A intranuclear inclusion (*arrows, inset*) without the cytoplasmic enlargement characteristic of cytomegalovirus. (From Surawicz CM, Graham DY. Viral colitis. In: Phillips SF, Pemberton JH, Shorter RG, eds. The large intestine: physiology, pathophysiology, and disease. New York: Raven Press 1991:429.)

consists of examination of body fluids and tissues for ova, parasites, parasite antigens, and serologic tests.

Examining Body Fluids for Parasites

Direct examination of the stool can detect various protozoal nematodal pathogens, such as round worm, and platyhelminthic pathogens, such as trematodes and cestodes. Various stages of the life cycles of these eukaryotic parasites are seen when staining or by directly examining wet mounts of fresh stool. For some parasites, only the eggs are present in the feces.

A complete evaluation of stool for ova and parasites involves the examination of fresh and fixed specimens. Semisolid or diarrheal stools generally are more productive of trophozoites, whereas solid stools may be adequate for detecting protozoal cysts. If stool cannot be examined soon after collection, appropriate fixatives such as merthiolate-iodine-formaldehyde,[40] 10% formalin, or polyvinyl alcohol should be used. Barium or bismuth should not be administered to the patient for at least 1 week before examination for parasites because of interference with visualization. Special stains usually are unnecessary, but may improve the detection of *Cryptosporidium*. Although it is traditional to obtain three stools on three separate days before declaring a patient to be free of intestinal parasites, we frequently observe the near-simultaneous submission of three stools before the report of the first stool is available. This wasteful practice should be discouraged. If the first stool has treatable pathogens in it, the test should not be repeated to find additional parasites.[41]

Lumenal contents of the small bowel, obtained by string test,[42] duodenal aspiration, or mucosal biopsy, are occasionally necessary to diagnose infection with *Giardia lamblia* or *Strongyloides* when stool examination gives negative results.

The cellophane tape test occasionally is used to detect ova of pinworms.[43] This test consists of the application of the adhesive side of transparent (not translucent) tape to the perianal skin and subsequent microscopic examination for ova of *Enterobius vermicularis*. It is otherwise difficult to detect the presence of this pathogen because examination of the stool frequently fails to detect the worm or its eggs.

Entamoeba histolytica can cause liver abscesses. Such abscesses usually do not have demonstrable parasites under direct examination, although the yield is reportedly higher if material obtained toward the end of aspiration is sent for microscopic examination.[44]

Parasite Antigen Detection

Because some intestinal parasitic infections elude multiple attempts at stool diagnosis, antigen detection tests have been proposed to detect parasite-specific molecules in the stool, thus obviating small bowel biopsy or aspiration.[45] The positive predictive value of this test in a general symptomatic population, rather than in a population with proven giardiasis, has not been determined. Therefore we do not believe that clinical decisions should be made on the basis of parasite antigen detection in stools. Patients who are suspected of having a parasite, even if one is not diagnosed on direct examination of the stool for parasites, should receive appropriate empiric therapy. The additional expense of antigen detection is not justified, especially because the number of types of such tests for multiple parasites is proliferating.

Serologic Diagnosis of Parasitic Infections

Serologic diagnosis of parasitic infections can be useful in selected settings. As with all serologic tests, the clinician must determine the likelihood that a positive result pertains to the situation at hand. For example, the finding of antibodies to *E histolytica* in a patient with acute bloody diarrhea who has lived for many years in Mexico is not helpful in diagnosing the diarrhea, because the antibodies may represent prior infection, and their presence should not stop the search for other pathogens. For several parasitic infections, a positive serologic finding is reliable and useful. Such pathogens include *Toxoplasma gondii* in infants with conjugated hyperbilirubinemia where treatment should begin as soon as the diagnosis is made; *Trypanosoma cruzi* infection in patients with megaesophagus and a travel history to Central or South America; and the echinococcus of hydatid disease presenting as liver abscess, where needle aspiration may be contraindicated. In infections caused by each of these organisms, a positive serologic test result would direct appropriate therapy—chemotherapy or surgical extirpation—when tissue is difficult or dangerous to obtain, or when histopathologic study might not be diagnostic.

Negative results for parasite serologic study can be helpful in excluding *E histolytica* or echinococcus in the differential diagnosis of liver abscesses, or in excluding *Strongyloides stercoralis* infection in eosinophilia. The availability of parasite serologic study varies in different centers and for different parasites. However, most tests can be performed at the Centers for Disease Control in Atlanta, or in an increasing number of private reference parasitology laboratories. However, the physician may not be able to wait for negative serologic study results to be reported back in many situations before starting empiric therapy or referring a patient for surgery.

Histopathologic Techniques for Detecting Parasitic Infections

Mucosal biopsy aids diagnosis of parasitic infection when a specific organism is detected. Small intestinal parasites detected by biopsy include *G lamblia*, *Cryptosporidium*, *Isospora belli*, and *Microsporidia*. Colonic parasites include *Schistosoma* species and *E histolytica*. Parasitic infection of the esophagus and stomach are extremely uncommon. *G lamblia* is present on the lumenal surface, but does not invade the mucosa. *Giardia* does not usually cause abnormalities in the small intestinal mucosa. However, in individuals with immunodeficiency syndromes, in whom this infection is common, small bowel mucosa may show some flattening of villi and chronic lamina propria inflammation; these changes often revert to normal after the *Giardia* organisms are eradicated.

Giardia and *Cryptosporidia* may be difficult to detect in biopsy specimens of the small bowel; biopsy usually is performed if the infection is suspected but stool examination gives negative results. In the small intestine, *Cryptosporidia* may be associated with blunting of the villi and increased eosinophils in the lamina propria; diagnosis is made by finding organisms on the mucosal surface.[46]

I belli also causes a self-limited diarrhea. The organism usually is detected in acid-fast bacillus stains of the stool. The diagnosis also can be made when organisms are detected in epithelial cells of the small intestine. Giemsa stains aid identification of the characteristic flask-shaped oocysts. Mild alteration of villous architecture and chronic inflammation also may be present. The parasite *Enterocytozoon bieunsi* (microsporidia) has been detected in biopsy specimens of the small bowel of individuals infected with human immunodeficiency virus[47]; many have chronic diarrhea. The organisms are best detected by electron microscopic study, but they have been detected in stool specimens and even by light microscopic study of small intestinal mucosa.[48] However, electron microscopic examination remains the gold standard. Whether this parasite always causes diarrhea or altered mucosa has not yet been determined. Cryptosporidia and microsporidia have been associated with acquired immunodeficiency syndrome–related cholangiopathy.

Most other intestinal parasites, such as hookworm, ascaris, or tapeworm, are detected in stool. Of those which can be detected in intestinal biopsy specimens, *Schistosoma* species is the most common. Schistosome ova produce foreign body granulomas. Strongyloides causes chronic inflammation from adult worms and eggs in the mucosa.

Amebiasis frequently involves the colon. *E histolytica* may be detected in smears of mucus obtained at rigid sigmoidoscopy, or in colorectal biopsy specimens. The gross appearance of shallow ulcers correlates with microulceration over lymphoid follicles, but otherwise minimal inflammation is present. The organisms usually are in the superficial areas of ulcerated mucosa, but can be found in mucosa, submucosa, and surface exudate (Fig. 131-5). The trophozoites are usually 10 to 30 μm, making them several times larger than lymphocytes, which can be useful as a point of reference. The cytoplasm often is foamy; the nucleus is small and round. Usually little reaction occurs around these superficial ulcers, although the ulcers may become deep, with submucosal involvement, perforation, and fibrosis. The areas of colon most frequently involved are cecum, appendix, and rectosigmoid.

Schistosoma organisms may involve the colon, with the eggs of the worm inciting a granulomatous reaction in biopsy material (Fig. 131-6). Aside from foreign body granulomas, little histologic alteration is present.

Fungi

General Considerations

Fungal infection should be considered in the differential diagnosis of hepatic masses and esophageal inflammation, especially in immunosuppressed individuals. These infections frequently are treatable, but treatment may require prolonged therapy with toxic agents. Therefore effort should be made to establish the specific diagnosis and the exact fungal cause.

Fungal Smear and Culture

Mucosal specimens for fungal analysis of organs that are not normally sterile usually are performed from biopsy tissue or from brushings. A smear of the characteristic exudates of mucosal fungal infections often provides a presumptive diagnosis. Fungal and viral infection, especially from herpes simplex virus and cytomegalovirus, can coexist, and the presence of mucosal fungal infection should not stop the search for additional pathogens, which often are better diagnosed by biopsy.

Fungal cultures are obtained by placing the appropriate specimen on growth media. Usually the inoculum size and the fungus being sought determine the rapidity with which positive culture results are reported. The identification of a commensal fungus from a body fluid or tissue that is not normally sterile, without histologic or gross evidence of abnormality, should be interpreted cautiously. Conversely, the isolation of a fungus from a body substance or fluid that is normally sterile, in particular, blood cultures, should always be taken seriously.

Fungal speciation often takes several additional days to perform after a positive culture result. Fungal speciation may

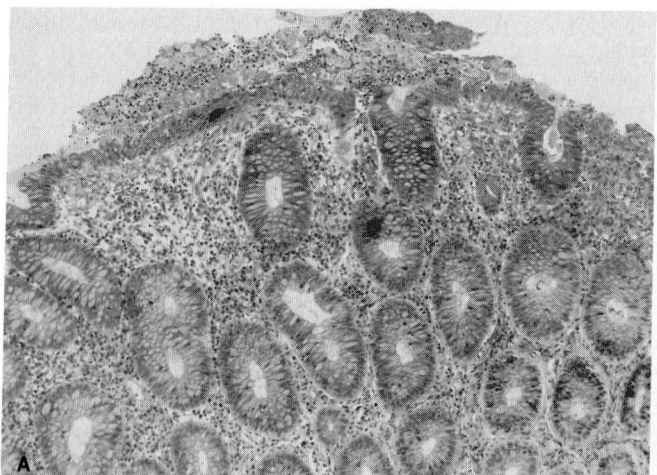
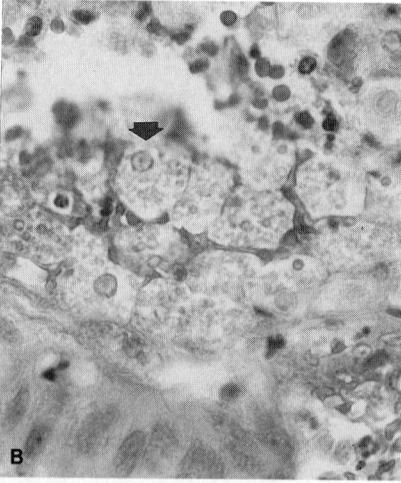

FIGURE 131-5. (**A**) Rectal biopsy specimen from a patient with amebiasis shows exudate adherent to the specimen's surface. (**B**) Higher magnification reveals *Entamoeba histolytica* trophozoites (*arrow*) in the surface mucus. (From Surawicz CM. Infectious colitis. Can J Gastroenterol 1989;3:165.)

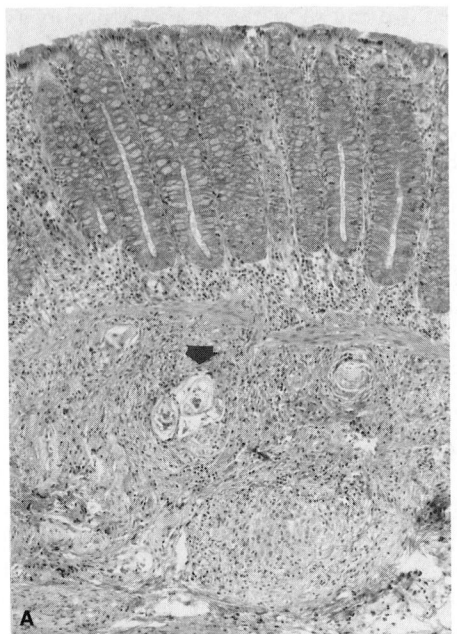
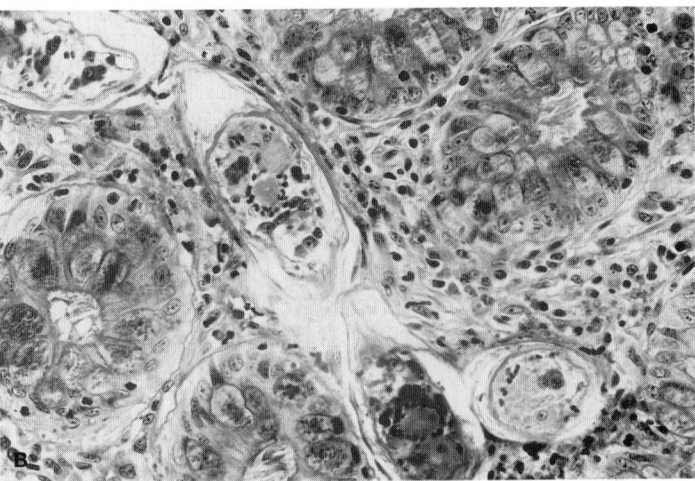

FIGURE 131-6. Rectal biopsy specimen from a man with schistosomiasis. **(A)** Normal mucosa with foreign-body granulomas in the submucosa (*arrow*). **(B)** Higher magnification reveals granuloma formation around schistosome ova. (From Surawicz CM. Infectious colitis. Can J Gastroenterol 1989;3:165.)

be important prognostically and therapeutically because different fungi may have different susceptibilities to antifungal agents.

Fungal Diagnosis by Direct Visualization

The classic cotton ball exudate of candidiasis of the esophagus often is sufficient for making a diagnosis. It is our practice, however, to brush or biopsy these specimens for confirmation. Aspergillomas can present as discreet ulcerations that can cause massive gastrointestinal bleeding, and biopsies often are necessary for diagnosis.

Detection of Fungal Products for Diagnosis

Fungi can be difficult to isolate because of the inherent growth characteristics of the organism or because of antifungal treatment administered before obtaining the specimen for culture. Unfortunately, despite much interest in identifying fungal products in body fluids as a rapid diagnostic technique,[49] such methods have not been widely adopted in clinical practice.

Histopathologic Techniques for Detecting Fungal Infections

Most fungal infections of the gastrointestinal tract occur in the immunocompromised person and involve the esophagus, where *Candida* organisms most frequently cause esophagitis. In biopsy specimens, pseudohyphae can be seen on routine sectioning; periodic acid-Schiff or silver stains can improve detection.

Other histologic features suggesting fungal infection are granulomas seen in blastomycosis and histoplasmosis. In his-

toplasmosis, the lamina propria may be infiltrated by macrophages filled with the organism. Actinomycosis causes ulcers that may cause fistulas; sulfur granules are characteristic.

Adjunctive Diagnostic Tests

The gastroenterologist should consider extraintestinal and extrahepatic processes when certain infections are considered or diagnosed. Blood cultures are indicated if patients with enteric illnesses are febrile or might be incapable of developing a febrile response to infection, such as infants or immunocompromised patients. Many bacterial enteric pathogens can invade the bloodstream, and such invasion may mandate antibiotic therapy. In addition, damage to the bowel during infectious enteritis can precipitate bacteremia with resident flora.[50] Also, metastatic infection should be considered in bacteremic patients with enteric infections, particularly in the case of infants or immunocompromised patients with *Salmonella* enteritis who are at risk of developing meningitis or osteomyelitis with this organism. Patients infected with *E coli* O157:H7 or *Shigella dysenteriae* should be watched closely in the week after the onset of diarrhea for hematologic evidence of the hemolytic uremic syndrome.

A pelvic examination should be performed on young women with right upper quadrant pain. Findings suggestive of salpingitis should raise the possibility of perihepatitis, and cervical cultures should be performed to recover *C trachomatis* and *Neisseria gonorrhoeae*. Some authorities believe that laparoscopy is desirable to confirm the impression of perihepatitis in this setting because of the difficulty in excluding a surgically remediable disease.[51] Serologic tests for syphilis should be performed if patients have a sexually transmitted disease such as proctocolitis or salpingitis. Unless adequate follow-up is assured, empiric therapy should always cover *Treponema pallidum.*

Tuberculosis skin tests should be obtained on all patients whose presentations are consistent with mycobacterial disease, and appropriate controls should be applied at the same time to exclude anergy. Occasionally a systemic infection suggests serious undiagnosed intraabdominal pathologic processes. The recovery of multiple organisms of bowel origin in blood cultures should raise the possibility of an intraabdominal abscess or other gastrointestinal or hepatobiliary sites as the source of a patient's bacteremia. The recovery of *Streptococcus bovis* or *Clostridium septicum* from a blood culture raises the possibility of colonic adenocarcinoma.

TECHNIQUES FOR MICROBIOLOGIC EVALUATION OF GASTROINTESTINAL AND HEPATOBILIARY SYSTEMS

The office and procedure suites of gastroenterologists should be prepared for the processing of specimens for microbiologic analysis. The most important element in specimen collection and processing is rapid transport to the laboratory. Although mucosal biopsy specimens may be fixed and allowed to wait at room temperature before being sent to the laboratory, it is not advisable to delay transport of culture specimens. Tissues submitted for bacterial culture should be placed in a cup and moistened with a small amount of nonbacteriostatic saline. Stool specimens are preferably submitted in a cup rather than on a swab. If a delay is not avoidable, a swab of the stool should be placed in thioglycolate medium, which is preferable for isolation of *Campylobacter* organisms, and Cary-Blair medium for other enteric pathogens. Peritoneal fluid should be inoculated into a blood culture bottle at the bedside. Bacterial toxins, with the exception of *C difficile* toxin, are rarely sought in clinical laboratories. A sterile specimen cup should be rapidly transported to the laboratory if a bacterial toxin needs to be sought.

Viruses usually are transported to the laboratory in viral transport media. This medium contains temperature-sensitive antibiotics and should be kept frozen until used. Calcium alginate swabs, which are frequently used for urethral cultures, should not be used for rectal cultures seeking viruses, because they may inhibit herpes simplex virus growth. Biopsy specimens also should be inoculated into viral transport medium. If viruses are to be cultured directly from the blood, a tube containing ethylene diamine tetraacetic acid (EDTA) should be used and rapidly transported to the laboratory.

Usually special transport medium is not used for fungal cultures. Sterile specimen cups are adequate for transport of body substances or tissues to the laboratory for fungal culture.

Parasites should be sought from fresh specimens. Stool should not be refrigerated for more than 2 hours before analysis. If a prolonged interval cannot be avoided between the collection of the stool specimen and analysis, a fixative should be considered. However, these fixatives are toxic if ingested, and adults should be cautioned about their toxicity to avoid accidental poisoning of children in the household.

If a duodenal aspirate or string test is employed to detect small bowel pathogens, the retrieved string should be placed in a specimen cup and submitted to the laboratory as soon as possible. Similarly, a mucosal biopsy specimen to detect pathogens also should be placed in a sterile urine cup and moistened with nonbacteriostatic saline. Histopathologic study of such specimens also is helpful, so a duplicate biopsy specimen should be placed in formalin or other fixative.

Patients frequently do not have sterile specimen cups at home to submit stool to the laboratory. If patients cannot obtain a sterile specimen cup before coming to the office, a clean vessel usually is adequate. Once again, rapid transport is the most important component of adequate specimen collection.

Table 131-1 summarizes the above procedures.

INDICATIONS

In performing any test, the physician must consider the risk, yield, expense, and the likelihood that the test will lead to a change in patient management. The indications for each test vary from patient to patient. For example, massive lower gastrointestinal bleeding would almost never be from a viral infection in an immunocompetent patient, but cytomegalovirus would be a prime causal candidate in a patient who has recently had an organ or a bone marrow transplant.

The risk, yield, and expense of microbiologic diagnosis in various clinical situations are discussed later in this chapter. This section considers clinical syndromes where the finding of a positive result would benefit the patient. Indications are provided for microbiologic examination in industrialized countries. Diagnosis in individual patients is much less frequently performed in developing countries where therapy is administered on an empiric or algorithmic basis, derived from epidemiologic studies of the etiology of enteric infections.

Diarrhea

For almost all cases of diarrhea, a precise cause is unnecessary because most illness is self-limited. The principles of good hydration and hygiene should be applied to any patient with diarrhea. However, stool cultures are obtained frequently, although their yield is notoriously low. Several attempts to identify the factors that increase the yield of stool cultures have been reported. DeWitt and associates[1] determined that in urban North American children, abrupt onset of diarrhea, greater than four stools per day, absence of vomiting before the onset of diarrhea, and the presence of leukocytes in the stool increase the chances of recovering a bacterial pathogen. Thorson and colleagues[4] have reported that in Virginia, patients whose history included fever, bloody diarrhea, tenesmus, abdominal pain, or raw seafood ingestion and whose stools contained leukocytes had an increased likelihood of having a bacterial pathogen in their stool. This study also emphasized the importance of seeking *C jejuni* in all bacterial enteric cultures.

The presence of fecal leukocytes has been proposed as a simple test in acute diarrhea to determine which stools are likely to yield bacterial pathogens on the more expensive subsequent stool culture.[1,6,7] However, on the basis of our experience in Seattle, we do not exclude a stool from culture if

TABLE 131-1
Procedures for Microbiologic Evaluations Performed by Gastroenterologists

AGENT SOUGHT	SPECIMEN	MATERIAL NEEDED
Bacteria	Stool	Sterile specimen cup, rapid transport time to laboratory
	Rectal swab	Moistened transport system for regular bacterial pathogens
		Gonococcal transport medium (if indicated)
		Dacron or cotton swab in plastic sheath cut into chlamydial transport medium (if indicated)*
	Liver	Nonbacteriostatic saline to transport specimen to laboratory in sterile urine cup; coordinate distribution with pathologic study and microbiologic study before biopsy
	Bile	Rapid transport to laboratory; culture for aerobic and anaerobic pathogens.
	Mucosal biopsy (stomach)	Nonbacteriostatic saline and rapid transport to laboratory
	Mucosal biopsy (proctocolitis)	Nonbacteriostatic saline and rapid transport to laboratory, chlamydial transport medium, gonococcal transport medium
	Peritoneal fluid	Blood culture bottle inoculated at bedside
	Abscess	Rapid transport to the laboratory; culture for aerobic and anaerobic pathogens
Bacterial toxins	Stool	Sterile specimen cup and rapid transport to laboratory
Viruses	Stool	Swab of stool or rectum placed into viral transport medium† (calcium alginate swabs may inhibit herpes simplex virus growth)
	Mucosal biopsy	Viral transport medium; smear or brushings on glass slides for cytologic study
	Throat culture	Viral transport medium
	Liver	Viral transport medium
	Blood	EDTA tube, rapid transport to laboratory
Viral antigens	Stool	Sterile specimen cup
Fungus	Stool	Sterile specimen cup
	Mucosal biopsy	Sterile specimen cup with nonbacteriostic saline
	Liver biopsy	Sterile specimen cup with nonbacteriostatic saline
Parasites	Stool	Submit as fresh as possible; may be refrigerated for up to 2 h before analysis; consider supplying fixative if a prolonged interval will occur between collection and analysis
	Duodenal aspirate or string test	Sterile urine cup, submit as soon as possible
	Mucosal biopsy	Sterile urine cup, nonbacteriostatic saline; histopathologic study is also helpful

* Wood and calcium-alginate swabs inhibit the growth of *Chlamydia* and are not recommended for obtaining specimens for this pathogen. Swabs grossly contaminated with fecal material should not be submitted.

† Viral transport medium contains temperature-sensitive antibiotics and should be kept frozen until immediately before use.

EDTA, ethylenediamine tetraacetic acid.

fecal leukocytes are not observed.[15] Table 131-2 shows the association between detectable fecal leukocytes and bacterial enteric pathogens in all stool submitted to the Microbiology Laboratory of Children's Hospital and Medical Center, Seattle, Washington, between 1985 and 1990. Each bacterial enteric pathogen was accompanied by fecal leukocytes in some, but not all cases; fecal leukocytes were absent in 46.7% of stools containing bacterial pathogens. Fecal leukocytes were absent from 10 (27.8%) of the 36 specimens containing *Shigella,* the classically invasive bacterial enteric pathogen. Fecal occult blood, a surrogate test for fecal leukocytes,[2] also is often absent in children with proven bacterial enteric pathogens.[52] Stool specimens without fecal leukocytes should be sent for bacterial cultures if the clinical situation is appropriate. Perhaps a lactoferrin detection test will more sensitively indicate stools that may have bacterial pathogens.[53] Of course, fecal leukocytes in patients with chronic diarrhea suggest underlying inflammatory bowel disease.

A bacterial stool culture is of little value in evaluating chronic diarrhea in an immunocompetent patient unless en-

TABLE 131-2
Stool Cultures Containing Fecal Leukocytes Among Cultures Testing Positive for Selected Pathogens

ORGANISM	PATIENTS WITH POSITIVE CULTURES RESULTS	PATIENTS WITH FECAL LEUKOCYTES (%)
Campylobacter jejuni	114	56 (49.1)
Salmonella sp	95	40 (42.1)
Escherichia coli O157:H7	81	53 (65.4)
Shigella sp	36	26 (72.2)
Yersinia enterocolitica	27	13 (48.1)

All stools submitted to the microbiology laboratory for bacterial enteric cultures at the Children's Hospital and Medical Center (Seattle, WA) between 1985 and 1990 were stained for fecal leukocytes. Patients with fecal leukocytes are listed as a function of the pathogen isolated.

From Tarr PI, Clausen CR, Christie DL. Bacterial and protozoal gastroenteritis (letter). N Engl J Med 1992;326:489.

teropathogenic (enteroadherent) *E coli* can be detected. Homosexual men with human immunodeficiency virus infection may be chronically infected with pathogens that are more typically associated with acute diarrhea, such as *Shigella, Salmonella,* and *C jejuni, Campylobacter*-like organisms (i.e. *Helicobacter* [formerly *Campylobacter*] *cinaedi* and *Helicobacter fennelliae*).[54] These organisms should be sought in the stool culture of homosexual men with chronic diarrhea, although their presence may represent carriage rather than persistent infection. Food handlers and health care workers should be screened for asymptomatic colonization of bacterial enteric pathogens if any questions arise about their carrier status because of the risk of dissemination to susceptible populations.

Quantitative aerobic and anaerobic cultures of jejunal aspirates are probably the most reliable method to detect bacterial overgrowth syndrome. Analysis of the jejunal aspirate for short-chain fatty acids are specific indicators of bacterial overgrowth of the small bowel and might obviate the more expensive quantitative cultures. However, this technique lacks sensitivity. Other less invasive investigations to detect bacterial overgrowth, such as hydrogen breath tests, lack sensitivity and specificity[55] and are not widely available. In practice, bacterial overgrowth usually is diagnosed indirectly with a trial of empiric antibiotics.

Even though a positive bacterial stool culture might not lead to specific therapy, there is sometimes considerable value to establishing the cause of a severe diarrheal illness. For example, a patient with severe, acute colitis could be spared colonoscopy by finding *E coli* O157:H7 in the stool. Detection of parasites in stools is of greater benefit to many patients than bacterial cultures because treatment is frequently more efficacious. Chronic diarrhea and malabsorption are more likely to be diagnosed and treated by examining the stool for parasites than for pathogenic bacteria. Patients with human immunodeficiency virus or other immunodeficient conditions and diarrhea represent a group where a broad polymicrobial approach to diagnosis encompassing bacterial, viral, parasitic, and fungal pathogens is necessary.

In the authors' opinions, the detection of rotavirus is of little value in clinical medicine and should be reserved for epidemiologic and etiologic studies of diarrhea and for identifying infected inpatients so that the use of cohorts can be implemented to reduce nosocomial transmission. Finding rotavirus antigen in the stool would not alter the physician's approach to the patient and does not preclude the presence of other pathogens.

Candida has been proposed as a cause of diarrhea in patients with acquired immunodeficiency syndrome[56] and in the elderly.[57] However, stool cultures for fungi are more often used to determine whether colonization has occurred in an immunocompromised patient. Fungal colonization of the gastrointestinal tract signifies risk for systemic fungal infection. Surveillance fungal cultures of susceptible patients might be useful in monitoring selective bowel decontamination. Budding yeast or hyphae on stains of stool suggest replicating fungi in the gastrointestinal tract and sometimes are used as presumptive evidence of mucosal infection.

The sampling of duodenal contents occasionally is warranted for the diagnosis of parasitic infections manifest as diarrhea. This can be performed using the string test[42] or by aspiration of duodenal contents or mucosal biopsy. Stron-

TABLE 131-3
Indications for Microbiologic Investigation of the Stool

SYNDROME	TEST INDICATED
Diarrhea, acute (nonbloody, no fever, no abdominal pain)	None
Diarrhea, acute (with fever)	Bacterial stool culture*
Diarrhea, acute (with gross blood, with or without fever)	Bacterial stool culture*
Diarrhea, acute (if antibiotic exposure or toxic appearance without antibiotic exposure)	Bacterial stool culture,* plus *Clostridium difficile* toxin
Diarrhea, chronic (over 2 wk)	Bacterial stool culture, if enteropathogenic *Escherichia coli* can be detected by tissue culture assay or gene probing
	Ova and parasites
	Clostridium difficile toxin (whether or not antibiotic exposure has occurred)
Steatorrhea, malabsorption	Ova and parasites
Diarrhea in a returned traveler or newly arrived refugee	Bacterial stool culture*
	Ova and parasites
Diarrhea, homosexual man	Bacterial stool culture*
	Ova and parasites

* Bacterial stool culture should seek at a minimum *Escherichia coli* O157:H7 and *Salmonella, Shigella,* and *Campylobacter* species. We also encourage attempts to isolate *Yersinia* species and, if indicated epidemiologically, *Vibrio* species.

gyloidiasis and giardiasis are the most common small bowel infections diagnosed using the string test.

Table 131-3 lists diarrheal conditions and subgroups where microbiologic evaluation is warranted. This table is meant to be only a guide, because hard data concerning the yield and efficacy of these tests are lacking. In some situations, empiric therapy without a causative agent is safe, inexpensive, and diagnostic, especially when an accurate diagnosis is difficult or impossible to establish. Examples of the use of empiric therapy include the use of an oral, nonabsorbable antibiotic to treat enteropathogenic *E coli* or metronidazole to treat bacterial overgrowth syndrome.

Nosocomial Diarrhea

Diarrhea that develops in hospitalized patients rarely is from enteric pathogens; evaluation with standard stool culture and ova and parasite examinations is unnecessary.[58] *C difficile* is the most common nosocomial pathogen of the gastrointestinal tract. Diagnosis is made by stool culture or cell culture assay for cytotoxin B (Fig. 131-7). Other frequent causes of diarrhea in hospitalized patients include medications, such as liquid elixirs containing sorbitol, and tube feedings. Antibiotics can alter fecal flora and cause diarrhea in the absence of *C difficile*. A reasonable approach to nosocomial diarrhea includes exclusion of *C difficile* and evaluation of medications.[58]

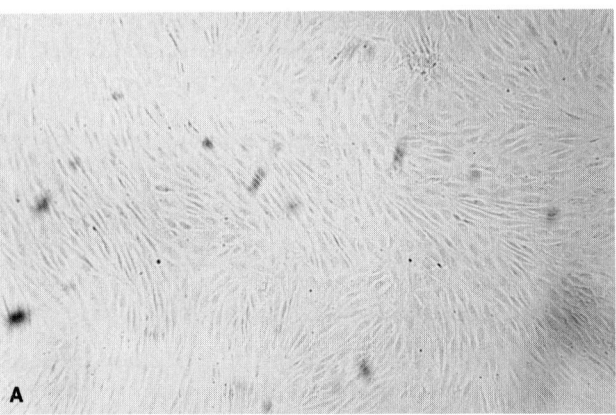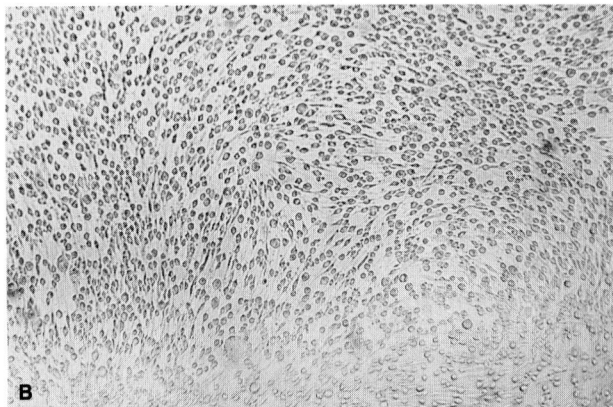

FIGURE 131-7. Toxic effect of *Clostridium difficile* in human diploid fibroblasts. **(A)** Control. **(B)** After inoculation with *Clostridium difficile* toxin. (Original magnification ×780; courtesy of Anne Cent).

Inflammatory Bowel Disease

Routine stool culture should be performed in patients experiencing an exacerbation of inflammatory bowel disease to exclude infection with a common enteric pathogen such as *Salmonella, Shigella* or *Campylobacter*. Stool examinations and serologic study for amebae should be done at lease once in all patients with inflammatory bowel disease to exclude amebiasis, which can mimic ulcerative colitis.[59,60] *C difficile* and sometimes the toxin may be present in stools from patients with inflammatory bowel disease. This probably reflects alteration in fecal flora from drugs used to treat such patients, and in most cases it does not appear to be a pathogen. However, in an individual with severe or refractory disease and cytotoxin in stools, it may be prudent to consider therapy to eradicate *C difficile*.[61,62]

Esophagitis

Esophageal symptoms in immunocompromised patients, which may be manifest only as nausea and vomiting, should be investigated thoroughly for an infectious cause.[63] Infectious esophagitis in such patients is most frequently caused by herpes simplex virus, cytomegalovirus, or *Candida albicans,* and usually occurs in the setting of immunosuppression. Mixed infections can occur. Esophagitis is easily treatable when caused by herpes simplex virus and *Candida,* and possibly treatable when caused by cytomegalovirus. Therefore efforts should be made to establish the presence of these agents. Biopsy specimens of ulcers, which are obtained only if the patient does not have a bleeding diathesis, are usually diagnostic of viral infections. Brushings of lesions have a low yield for cytomegalovirus and a higher yield for fungi, herpes simplex, and varicella-zoster virus, but may be the only option in a thrombocytopenic patient. These brushings should be smeared on a glass slide for stains and cytologic study. We do not routinely send esophageal biopsy specimens or brushings for bacterial culture because of the difficulty interpreting these specimens in the absence of well-defined criteria for the diagnosis of bacterial esophagitis, although in immunocompromised patients bacterial esophagitis might be an overlooked disorder.[64]

Parenchymal and Cholestatic Liver Disease

The microbiologic evaluation of liver diseases in adults consists chiefly of hepatitis A, B, C, D, and E serologic study, hepatitis B antigen detection, and cytomegalovirus serologic study and culture. In selected patients, bacterial, mycobacterial, fungal, parasitic, and viral studies are also performed. For example, infants with conjugated hyperbilirubinemia should always be evaluated for toxoplasmosis, syphilis, and extrahepatic *E coli* infections, although these infections are rarely considered in adult cholestasis. Occasionally patients with systemic viral (cytomegalovirus, Epstein-Barr virus, and yellow fever virus) and bacterial (syphilis, leptospirosis, and Q fever) infections can have prominent hepatitis. Furthermore, hepatic dysfunction can be present in multiple organ system failure caused by severe systemic infections. Finally, nonhepatic infections might result in mild, self-limited hepatic injury through unknown mechanisms.[65,66]

Hepatitis associated with herpes viruses and adenoviruses occurs more frequently in immunosuppressed patients. Rarely is the liver the only site from which viruses can be grown, and the growth of a virus from the biopsy specimen may add little to the growth of these viruses from other sites, especially blood. If sufficient biopsy material is obtained, a viral culture to diagnose hepatic inflammation is appropriate, but the viral culture should not be obtained at the expense of adequate histopathologic and immunohistologic study. This is particularly important in liver transplant patients, in whom immunopathologic study frequently distinguishes hepatitis because of cytomegalovirus from rejection.

Cholecystitis

Blood cultures should be obtained on febrile patients with suspected cholecystitis. Conversely, cholecystitis or indolent ascending cholangitis should be suspected as a source of bacteremia in patients whose physical examinations may not reveal the signs of biliary infection, such as the elderly.

Systemic Infection

A variety of systemic infections can be diagnosed by microbiologic studies of the liver. Liver biopsy has been described as one of the most useful invasive procedures in the evaluation of fevers of undetermined origin after less invasive procedures have failed to establish the cause.[67] Diffuse hepatic involvement can occur in a wide variety of systemic infections that are manifest as fevers of undetermined origin. Most prominent among the causes of such fever is miliary tuberculosis, which underscores the need to perform mycobacterial cultures on liver biopsy specimens obtained in the evaluation of fever. In hepatic tuberculosis, granulomas are frequent but caseating granulomas are rare and acid-fast stains often give negative results. Also, many other diseases cause hepatic granulomas.

Notice that physical findings may be minimal even in cholangitis, especially in elderly patients. Also, biochemical values in patients with diffusely infected livers may be normal or near normal. A mildly elevated alkaline phosphatase may be the only clue to hepatic involvement in fevers of undetermined origin, and sometimes even this value is normal.

Bacterial cultures should be performed on liver biopsy specimens in evaluating all fevers of undetermined origin, because cholangitis can present in this manner, particularly in the elderly. A variety of granulomatous disorders that are best diagnosed histologically can also cause fevers of undetermined origin, necessitating an adequate histopathologic study of the biopsy material. An organized, preplanned approach to handling and allocating the biopsy material is mandatory in evaluating the liver as the site of the infection.

Peritonitis

Infections of the peritoneum are almost always caused by bacteria or fungi. Primary, or spontaneous, bacterial peritonitis usually occurs in cirrhotic or nephrotic patients with preexisting ascites and is rarely caused by anaerobes. Polymicrobial peritoneal infections usually result from a perforated hollow abdominal organ, with aerobic and anaerobic bacterial spillage. Ascitic fluid obtained by paracentesis should be placed in a blood culture bottle if rapid transport to the microbiology laboratory is not possible.[8] Pneumococcal antigens should be sought in the ascitic fluid or in the patient's urine to diagnose systemic infection with this common cause of primary peritonitis, especially if the patient has received antibiotics that might interfere with culture efficiency. Fungal cultures of the peritoneum should be obtained in patients with peritonitis who have recently had abdominal operations, have indwelling peritoneal dialysis catheters, or are suspected of having a perforated hollow abdominal viscus.

Pancreatitis

Viruses, parasites, and bacteria can precipitate acute pancreatitis, particularly in the developing world and in children. Usually bacteria cause pancreatitis in sepsis syndromes and in toxigenic colitis.[68] If common precipitants of pancreatitis such as alcohol, drugs, or biliary lithiasis are excluded, it is reasonable to obtain stool for ova and parasites if the patient is epidemiologically at risk of having a parasite that could obstruct the common bile duct. Fluid aspirate from pseudocysts should be sent for bacterial culture.

Gastrointestinal Bleeding

Gastric and Duodenal Ulcers

Persistent infection of the stomach with *Helicobacter pylori* is associated with failure to heal duodenal ulcers. Histologic evaluation of the gastric mucosa to detect gastritis and associated organisms remains the most reliable method of diagnosis. Biopsy of the gastric mucosa after observing a duodenal ulcer during endoscopy might be helpful if the patient's history does not clearly implicate nonsteroidal antiinflammatory drugs as the risk factor for the ulcer. Serologic study has been disappointing in identifying infected patients.[69,70]

Gastrointestinal Bleeding in Immunocompromised Patients

Infections are a particularly important cause of gastrointestinal bleeding in immunocompromised patients. Bleeding can be because of discrete viral lesions, particularly cytomegalovirus, herpes simplex virus, or adenovirus ulcers, or fungal ulcerations, especially aspergillomas. If the site is localized, surgical resection is sometimes possible.

Occult Chronic Gastrointestinal Blood Loss

Chronic gastrointestinal blood loss may be because of parasites, particularly hookworm. Ova and parasites should be sought in patients with unexplained anemia, especially if they are epidemiologically at risk by virtue of age or location.

Constipation and Motility Disorders

Gastroenterologists rarely consider infections as a cause of constipation. However, infection with *T cruzi* can result in hypomotility, manifest as megacolon and megaesophagus. If patients are epidemiologically at risk by virtue of travel history or if they have received blood transfusions, infection with *T cruzi* should be considered. Serologic study and biopsy are appropriate tests for this infection.

Patients with typhoid fever more frequently complain of constipation than of diarrhea,[71] but this is rarely the sole presenting complaint. If a patient has other signs or symptoms suggestive of infection with *Salmonella typhi,* the absence of diarrhea should not prevent the physician from ordering a stool culture.

Epstein-Barr virus infection is occasionally incriminated as a cause of profound hypomotility syndromes.[72] There is no diagnostic histopathologic correlate of this infection in the gastrointestinal tract. However, Epstein-Barr virus serologic results can indicate if a patient has been infected with this agent, and whether or not the infection is recent.

CONTRAINDICATIONS AND RISKS

There is negligible risk to sampling stool or serum for diagnostic tests outlined above. A slightly greater risk for mucosal biopsy reflects the minimal morbidity of the endoscopy and biopsy. This risk is increased in patients with bleeding diatheses. The gastroenterologist should bear in mind that thrombocytopenia is a dynamic side effect of cancer chemotherapy, and the gastroenterologist and oncologist should be aware of the need to keep the platelet count above 50,000/mm^3 for the 2-week period after the biopsy. Anticoagulants, aspirin, and nonsteroidal antiinflammatory drugs should be discontinued in this interval. Brushings of ulcers have a lower microbiologic yield than endoscopic biopsy specimens but are considerably safer to perform if patients are thrombocytopenic, do not have a platelet count supportable above 50,000/mm^3 for the 2 weeks after the biopsy, or have prolonged bleeding or coagulation times. Needle liver biopsies to diagnose infection should be performed only after diagnostic alternatives have been exhausted such as serologic study, blood cultures, stool examination, and rectal biopsy.

INTERPRETING POSITIVE AND NEGATIVE TEST RESULTS

The sensitivity of microbiologic testing is a function of a variety of factors, including freshness and quantity of specimen, timing of the specimen collection, site of the collection, the skill of the microbiology laboratory, and the awareness of the physician and the microbiologist of the spectrum of organisms that might be responsible for a given presentation. Antecedent diagnostic procedures, such as barium studies, and therapeutic attempts, as with antiinfectives, also decrease sensitivity. In considering a test, the physician should remember that negative test results can also be helpful. For example, if *C difficile* or *Salmonella* are excluded as causes of a patient's diarrhea, the risk to the patient of taking empiric antibiotics is lessened.

The sampling of stool for bacterial enteric pathogens can be an insensitive test. For example, the analysis of a stool culture for *Salmonella, Shigella,* or *E coli* O157:H7 might involve the inspection of 100 or 200 isolated colonies on an agar plate. Assuming a patient's stool has 10^8 colony-forming units of coliform bacilli per gram, a pathogen that is present at a concentration of a million colony-forming units per gram of stool could be overlooked. This would be most important in patients who are suspected of being carriers of bacterial enteric pathogens. For this reason, we do not believe that a negative result from a stool culture should be accepted as definitive proof that infection has not occurred, or that a patient is not a carrier of a bacterial enteric pathogen.

The specificity and sensitivity of gastrointestinal and hepatobiliary microbiologic tests evolve while "new" pathogens are proposed and as "old" pathogens are shown to have variable pathogenic potential. Furthermore, as these new pathogens are treated, serologic findings become difficult to interpret. As an example of a new pathogen, *Blastocystis hominis* has been incriminated as a cause of diarrhea. The findings of this agent in the stool of a patient with diarrhea should be considered in the clinical context. If a patient with *B hominis* has nonbloody diarrhea and no other bacterial enteric patho-

gens are present, treatment with metronidazole is appropriate. If the same patient were to be febrile, have painful bloody diarrhea, and to appear toxic, further evaluation is necessary before treatment. Similarly, the finding of this protozoan in an asymptomatic patient whose stool is being examined as a screening test on return from the tropics does not require treatment. Other organisms appear to have variable pathogenicity. *G lamblia* is an undisputed cause of diarrhea, yet its presence may not always be associated with symptoms, and its eradication may not always be accompanied by resolution of symptoms.[73]

The case of *H pylori* illustrates some of the problems of serologic diagnosis.[74] Antibodies to this pathogen were initially reported as being sensitive and specific, with good correlation to gastric biopsy results. However, after the formulation of test kits to determine antibodies to *H pylori*, widespread practice has not validated this test when correlated with gastric biopsies.[69,70] If antibodies to *H pylori* in future tests can be validated as sensitive and specific in the diagnosis of current gastric infection with this agent, and if past versus present infection can be distinguished by analysis of antibody class or of epitope-specific antibody, serologic study would be preferable to esophagogastroduodenoscopy and gastric biopsy. However, the use of serologic study to monitor the adequacy of therapy and to detect recurrent infection will become more difficult as increasing numbers of patients with *H pylori* are diagnosed and treated but retain their immunologic marker of infection.

COSTS

It is difficult to determine the relative cost, specificity, sensitivity, and risk-benefit ratios for microbiologic investigations used to detect the many pathogens infecting the gastrointestinal and hepatobiliary systems. These tests are sought in conjunction with a wide variety of clinical circumstances, and their low yield is forgiven because they are usually safe and, if results are positive, can lead to specific therapy or forestall more expensive and hazardous intervention. The example of bacterial stool cultures illustrates the difficulty of cost assessment of a commonly used diagnostic test. In 1989, 3722 stool cultures were performed at three University of Washington teaching hospitals (Children's Hospital and Medical Center, University of Washington Medical Center, and Harborview Medical Center) at a weighted average cost of $63.89 per specimen. Table 131-4 lists the 165 pathogens isolated, for a yield of 4.4%. It cost $1441 to diagnose a bacterial enteric infection in Seattle in 1989, similar to the figure quoted by Koplan and associates[75] in 1980, taking into account inflation. However, many sigmoidoscopies, endoscopies, small bowel biopsies, and laparotomies might have been averted by the finding of a pathogen to explain severe diarrhea, fecal leukocytes, or peritoneal inflammation. The savings produced by a positive stool culture finding are difficult to factor into such calculations of cost effectiveness.

The yield of an examination of the stool for ova and parasites was higher. In 1989, 3196 stool samples were submitted to the microbiology laboratories at these three institutions, at a weighted average cost of $30.96 per specimen. Two hundred ninety-seven (9.3%) of the specimens contained a

TABLE 131-4
Number of Bacterial Pathogens Isolated From Stools*

No. of stools submitted for bacterial enteric pathogens	3722
No. of stools with pathogens	165
Yield of stool culture	4.4%
Pathogens isolated	
Campylobacter jejuni	77
Salmonella species	51
Escherichia coli O157:H7	15
Shigella species	11
Yersinia enterocolitica	5
Aeromonas species	5
Vibrio cholerae (non 01)	1
Total	165

* Children's Hospital and Medical Center, University of Washington Medical Center, and Harborview Medical Center, Seattle, Washington, 1989.

Data courtesy of Carla Clausen, M.D., Gertrude Schmidt, and Marie Coyle, M.D., Seattle, WA.

pathogen, which corresponds to a cost of $333.19 per examination with a positive result. The pathogens detected are listed in Table 131-5. The value of an ova and parasite examination is amplified by the greater efficacy of antiparasitic chemotherapy compared with antibacterial chemotherapy for many enteric pathogens.

FUTURE APPLICATIONS

Unlike clinical chemistry and hematology, microbiologic examination of the gastrointestinal and hepatobiliary systems uses technology that has been available for most of the century. The principles of staining, serologic study, and culture, although applied to an expanding number of pathogens, is little changed from the time of Pasteur and Koch. Microbiologic diagnosis is labor intensive, expensive relative to the yield, and necessarily slow because of the growth and staining characteristics inherent to each organism. Recombinant DNA technology might improve the sensitivity and speed of diagnostic microbiologic study.[76]

The amplification of targeted sequences specific to enteric pathogens using polymerase chain reaction enables the rapid identification of a wide variety of enteric and hepatic pathogens. Such a rapid approach might adapt what is an epidemiologic research tool to clinical diagnostic practice. The speed with which polymerase chain reaction can be performed, the greatly increased sensitivity of detection of specific amplified sequences, and the use of a single technology, such as nucleic acid detection by hybridization or visualization, to identify diverse pathogenic species in a variety of tissues or body substances will significantly alter the practice of diagnostic microbiology. However, 10 years after the initial report of the polymerase chain reaction,[77] there are disappointingly few applications of this technique in clinical practice. The problems appear to be rooted in the extreme sensitivity of this technique, leading to false-positive results, obligating strict negative controls. It is possible that selected reference laboratories will provide polymerase chain reaction–based di-

agnosis of pathogens because of the rigorous quality control needed for appropriate interpretation of results.

The next decade will likely bring the expansion of recently introduced technology to a wider range of pathogens. Antigen detection, which is successful in detecting rotavirus in stool and hepatitis B and D viremia, will be applied to an increasing number of pathogens infecting the alimentary tract and the liver. Specific and avid antibodies are the necessary reagents needed for each pathogen, and monoclonal antibody technology reduces the lot-to-lot variability of diagnostic immunoglobulins. Additionally, genetic evidence of replicating pathogens will become more central to diagnosis. There is already extensive use of hepatitis B viral DNA quantitative assays as an index of viral replication.

Serologic tests will improve with the use of increasingly purified and characterized antigens, thus reducing false-positive results. Cloned antigens should ensure an adequate supply of target molecules for serologic assays, which is a particularly difficult problem for parasites and viruses that cannot be easily grown in vitro.

As in many areas of infectious diseases, new agents of human disease will continue to be discovered. For example, of the pathogens listed in this chapter, *Aeromonas, B hominis, C jejuni, Campylobacter*-like organisms, *C trachomatis, C difficile, Cryptosporidia, E coli* 0157:H7, *G lamblia, H pylori*, hepatitis C, D, and E, human immunodeficiency virus, *I belli, Microsporidia*, Norwalk agent, *Plesiomonas*, rotavirus, and *Y enterocolitica*, were unknown or considered to be unimportant human pathogens before 1970. Each pathogen presents its own diagnostic problems and opportunities and therapeutic imperatives. While pathogens and tests proliferate, so will costs, thereby increasing the pressure for the rapid, reproducible

TABLE 131-5
Probable or Definite Pathogenic Parasites Identifed in Stools*

Number of stools submitted for ova and parasite examination	3196
Number with pathogenic parasites	297
Yield	9.3%
Pathogens identified	
Blastocystis hominis	81
Giardia lamblia	79
Hookworm species	66
Clonorchis sinensis	31
Strongyloides stercoralis	28
Entamoeba histolytica	13
Hymenolepsis nana	13
Trichuris trichiura	13
Ascaris lumbricoides	11
Isospora belli	9
Cryptosporidium species	6
Taenia species	3
Total	353†

* Children's Hospital and Medical Center, University of Washington Medical Center, and Harborview Medical Center, Seattle, Washington, 1989.

† More than one parasite was identified in some patients.

Data courtesy of Carla Clausen, M.D., Gertrude Schmidt, and Marie Coyle, M.D., Seattle, WA.

diagnostic methods that do not require as much labor as microbiologic investigations.

The reader is directed to Chapter 26, The Gastrointestinal Microflora; Chapter 38, Approach to the Patient With Diarrhea; Chapter 46, Approach to Gastrointestinal Problems in the Immunocompromised Patient; Chapter 74, Bacterial Overgrowth; Chapter 84, Bacterial Infections of the Colon; and Chapter 141, Applications of New Technologies in Tissue Examination.

REFERENCES

1. DeWitt TG, Humphrey KF, McCarthy P. Clinical predictors of acute bacterial diarrhea in young children. Pediatrics 1985;75:551.
2. Vogtlin J, Stalder H, Hurzeler L, et al. Modified guaiac test may replace search for faecal leukocytes in acute infectious diarrhoea. Lancet 1983;2:1204.
3. Radetsky M. Laboratory evaluation of acute diarrhea. Pediatr Infect Dis J 1986;6:230.
4. Thorson SM, Lohr JA, Dudley S, Guerrant RL. Value of methyleneblue examination, dark-field microscopy, and carbol-fuchsin Gram stain in the detection of *Campylobacter* enteritis. J Pediatr 1985;106:941.
5. Benenson AS, Islam MR, Greenough WB. Rapid identification of *Vibrio cholerae* by darkfield microscopy. Bull WHO 1964;30:827.
6. Harris JC, Dupont HL, Hornick RB. Leukocytes in diarrheal illness. Ann Intern Med 1972;76:697.
7. Guerrant RL, Shields DS, Thorson SM, et al. Evaluation and diagnosis of acute infectious diarrhea. Am J Med 1985;78(Suppl 6B):91.
8. Runyon BA, Antillon MR, Akriviadis EA, McHutchison JG. Bedside inoculation of blood culture bottles with ascitic fluid is superior to delayed inoculation in the detection of spontaneous bacterial peritonitis. J Clin Microbiol 1990;28:2811.
9. Toledo MRF, Trabulsi LR. Correlation between biochemical and serological characteristics of *Escherichia coli* and results of the Sereny test. J Clin Microbiol 1983;17:419.
10. March SB, Ratnam S. Sorbitol-MacConkey medium for the detection of *Escherichia coli* 0157:H7 associated with hemorrhagic colitis. J Clin Microbiol 1986;23:869.
11. Centers for Disease Control. Emerging infectious diseases. MMWR CDC Surveillance Summary 1993;42:257.
12. Gransden WR, Damm S, Anderson JD. Verocytotoxin-producing *Escherichia coli* 0157:H7 and diarrhea. Ann Intern Med 1985;103:160.
13. MacDonald KL, O'Leary MJ, Cohen ML, et al. *Escherichia coli* 0157:H7, an emerging gastrointestinal pathogen. Results of a one-year, prospective, population-based study. JAMA 1988;259:3567.
14. Marshall WF, McLimans CA, Yu PKW, et al. Results of a 6-month survey of stool cultures for *Escherichia coli* 0157:H7. Mayo Clin Proc 1990;65:787.
15. Tarr PI, Clausen CR, Christie DL. Bacterial and protozoal gastroenteritis (letter). N Engl J Med 1992;326:489.
16. Batts DH, Silva J, Fekety R. Staphylococcal enterocolitis. Curr Chemother Infect Dis 1980;2:944.
17. Thorne GM. Diagnosis of infectious diarrheal diseases. Infect Dis Clin North Am 1988;2:747.
18. George WL, Sutter VL, Citron D, Finegold SM. Selective and differential medium for isolation of *Clostridium difficile*. J Clin Microbiol 1979;9:214.
19. Larson HE, Barclay FE, Honour P, Hill ID. Epidemiology of *Clostridium difficile* in infants. J Infect Dis 1982;145:727.
20. Echeverria P, Taylor DN. New approaches to diagnosis of enteric infections. In: Farthing MJG, Keusch GT, eds. Enteric infection. New York: Raven Press, 1989:417.
21. Peterson LR, Holter JJ, Shanholtzer CJ, et al. Detection of *Clostridium difficile* toxins A (enterotoxin) and B (cytotoxin) in clinical specimens. Am J Clin Pathol 1986;86:208.
22. Tison DL. Culture confirmation of *Escherichia coli* serotype 0157:H7 by direct immunofluorescence. J Clin Microbiol 1990;28:612.
23. Surawicz CM, Belic L. Rectal biopsy helps to distinguish acute self limited colitis from idiopathic inflammatory bowel disease. Gastroenterology 1984;86:104.
24. Nostrant TT, Kumar NB, Appelman HD. Histopathology differentiates acute self-limited colitis from ulcerative colitis. Gastroenterology 1987;92:318.
25. Surawicz CM, Haggitt RC, Husseman M. Rectal biopsy differentiates acute self limited colitis from acute inflammatory bowel disease. Gastroenterology 1993;104:A786.
26. Gleaves CA, Reed EG, Hackman RC, Meyers JD. Rapid diagnosis of invasive cytomegalovirus by examination of tissue specimens in centrifuge cultures. Am J Clin Pathol 1987;88:354.
27. Kapikian AZ, Dreustay JL, Purcell RH. Immune electron microscopy as a method for the detection, identification and characterization of agents not cultivatable in an in vitro system. In: Rose NR, Friedman H, eds. Manual of clinical immunology. 2nd ed. Washington, DC: American Society of Microbiology, 1980:70.
28. Yolken RH, Bishop CA, Townsend TR, et al. Infectious gastroenteritis in bone-marrow-transplant recipients. N Engl J Med 1982;306:1009.
29. Spencer GD, Hackman RC, McDonald GB, et al. A prospective study of unexplained nausea and vomiting after marrow transplantation. Transplantation 1986;42:602.
30. Yolken RH, Lawrence F, Leister F, et al. Gastroenteritis associated with enteric type adenovirus in hospitalized infants. J Pediatr 1982;101:21.
31. Herrmann JE, Taylor DN, Echeverria P, Blacklow NR. Astroviruses as a cause of gastroenteritis in children. N Engl J Med 1991;324:1756.
32. Lautenschlager I, Suni J, Ahonen J, et al. Detection of cytomegalovirus by the early-antigen immunofluorescence test versus conventional tissue culture. Eur J Clin Microbiol Infect Dis 1989;8:610.
33. Gretch D, Lee W, Corey L. Use of aminotransferase, hepatitis C antibody, and hepatitis C polymerase chain reaction RNA assays to establish the diagnosis of hepatitis C virus infection in a diagnostic virology laboratory. J Clin Microbiol 1992;30:2145.
34. Surawicz CM, Myerson D. Self-limited cytomegalovirus colitis in immunocompetent individuals. Gastroenterology 1988;94:194.
35. Rabinowitz M, Bassan I, Robinson MJ. Sexually transmitted cytomegalovirus proctitis in a woman. Am J Gastroenterol 1988;83:885.
36. Roberts WH, Hammond S, Sneddon JM, et al. In situ DNA hybridization for cytomegalovirus in colonoscopic biopsies. Arch Pathol Lab Med 1988;11:1106.
37. Myerson D, Hackman RC, Nelson JA, et al. Widespread presence of histologically occult cytomegalovirus. Human Pathol 1984;15:430.
38. Wu GD, Shintaku IP, Chien K, et al. A comparison of routine light microscopy, immunohistochemistry, and in situ hybridization for the detection of cytomegalovirus in gastrointestinal biopsies. Am J Gastroenterol 1989;84:1517.
39. Goodgame RW, Genta RM, Estrada R, et al: Frequency of positive tests for cytomegalovirus in AIDS patients: endoscopic lesions compared with normal mucosa. Am J Gastroenterol 1993;88:338.
40. Brown HW, Neva FA. Technical diagnostic methods. In: Brown HW, Neva FA, eds. Basic clinical parasitology. Norwalk, CT: Appleton-Century-Crofts, 1983:315.
41. Morris AJ, Wilson ML, Reller LB. Application of rejection criteria for stool ovum and parasite examinations. J Clin Microbiol 1992;30:3213.
42. Beal CB, Viens P, Grant RGL, Hughes JM. A new technique for sampling duodenal contents. Am J Trop Med Hyg 1970;19:349.
43. Brown HW, Neva FA. Intestinal nematodes of human beings.

In: Brown HW, Neva FA, eds. Basic clinical parasitology. Norwalk, CT: Appleton-Century-Crofts, 1983:105.

44. Bruckner DA. Amebiasis. Clin Microbiol Rev 1992;5:356.

45. Rosoff JD, Stibbs HH. Physical and chemical characterization of a *Giardia lamblia*–specific antigen useful in the coprodiagnosis of giardiasis. J Clin Microbiol 1986;24:1079.

46. Current WL, Reese NC, Ernst JV, et al. Human cryptosporidiosis in immunocompetent and immunodeficient persons: studies of an outbreak and experimental transmission. N Engl J Med 1983;308:1252.

47. Cali A, Owen RL. Intracellular development of *Enterocytozoon,* a unique microsporidian found in the intestine of AIDS patients. J Protozool 1990;37:145.

48. Simon D, Weiss LM, Tanowitz HB, et al. Light microscopic diagnosis of human microsporidiosis and variable response to octreotide. Gastroenterology 1991;100:271.

49. De Repentigny L. Serodiagnosis of candidiasis, aspergillosis, and cryptococcosis. Clin Infect Dis 1992;14:S11.

50. Haltalin KC, Nelson JD. Coliform sepsis complicating shigellosis in children. JAMA 1965;192:441.

51. Eschenbach DA, Wolner-Hanssen P. Fitz-Hugh Curtis syndrome. In: Holmes KK, Mardh PA, Sparling PF, et al., eds. Sexually transmitted diseases. New York: McGraw-Hill, 1990:621.

52. Huicho L, Sanchez D, Contreras M, et al. Occult blood and fecal leukocytes as screening tests in childhood infectious diarrhea: an old problem revisited. Pediatr Infect Dis J 1993;12:474.

53. Guerrant RL, Araujo V, Soares E, et al. Measurement of fecal lactoferrin as a marker of fecal leukocytes. J Clin Microbiol 1992;30:1238.

54. Quinn TC, Stamm WE. Proctitis, proctocolitis, enteritis, and esophagitis in homosexual men. In: Holmes KK, Mardh PA, Sparling PF, et al., eds. Sexually transmitted diseases. New York: McGraw-Hill, 1990:663.

55. Corazza GR, Menozzi MG, Strocchi A, et al. The diagnosis of small bowel bacterial overgrowth. Gastroenterology 1990;98:302.

56. Quinn TC, Stamm WE, Goodell SE, et al. The polymicrobial origin of intestinal infections in homosexual men. N Engl J Med 1983;309:576.

57. Danna PL, Urban C, Bellin E, Rahal JJ. Role of candida in pathogenesis of antibiotic-associated diarrhoea in elderly inpatients. Lancet 1991;337:511.

58. Siegel DL, Edelstein PH, Nachamkin I. Inappropriate testing for diarrheal diseases in the hospital. JAMA 1990;263:979.

59. Patel AS, DeRidder PH. Amebic colitis masquerading as acute inflammatory bowel disease: the role of serology in its diagnosis. J Clin Gastroenterol 1989;11:407.

60. Korelitz BI. When should we look for amebae in patients with inflammatory bowel disease? (editorial). J Clin Gastroenterol 1989;11:373.

61. Meyers S, Mayer L, BoHune E, et al. Occurrence of *Clostridium difficile* toxin during the course of inflammatory bowel disease. Gastroenterology 1981;80:697.

62. Seaver RL. Screening for *Clostridium difficile* in chronic inflammatory bowel disease. J Clin Gastroenterol 1986;8:397.

63. McDonald GB, Sharma P, Hackman RC, et al. Esophageal infections in immunosuppressed patients after marrow transplantation. Gastroenterology 1985;88:1111.

64. Walsh TJ, Belitsos NJ, Hamilton SR. Bacterial esophagitis in immunocompromised patients. Arch Intern Med 1986;146:1345.

65. Zimmerman HJ, Fang M, Utili R, et al. Clinical conference: jaundice due to bacterial infection. Gastroenterology 1979;77:362.

66. Miller DJ, Keeton GR, Webber BL, Saunders SJ. Jaundice in severe bacterial infection. Gastroenterology 1976;71:94.

67. Petersdorf RG, Beeson PB. Fever of unexplained origin: report on 100 cases. Medicine 1961;40:1.

68. Grodinsky S, Telmesani A, Robson WLM, et al. Gastrointestinal manifestations of hemolytic uremic syndrome: recognition of pancreatitis. J Pediatr Gastroenterol Nutr 1990;11:518.

69. Westblom TU, Madan E, Gudipati S, et al. Diagnosis of *Helicobacter pylori* infection in adult and pediatric patients by using pyloriset: a rapid latex agglutination test. J Clin Microbiol 1992;30:96.

70. Hoek FJ, Noach LA, Rauws EAJ, Tytgat GNJ. Evaluation of the performance of commercial test kits for detection of *Helicobacter pylori* antibodies in serum. J Clin Microbiol 1992;30:1525.

71. Stuart BM, Pullen RL. Typhoid. Clinical analysis of three hundred and sixty cases. Arch Intern Med 1946;78:629.

72. Vassallo M, Camilleri M, Caron BL, Low PA. Gastrointestinal motor dysfunction in acquired selective cholinergic dysautonomia associated with infectious mononucleosis. Gastroenterology 1991;100:252.

73. Pickering LK, Woodward WE, DuPont HL, Sullivan P. Occurrence of *Giardia lamblia* in children in day care centers. J Pediatr 1984;104:522.

74. Perez-Perez GI, Dworkin B, Chodos J, Blaser MJ. *Campylobacter pylori* antibodies in humans. Ann Intern Med 1988;109:11.

75. Koplan JP, Fineberg HV, Ferraro MJB, Rosenberg ML. Value of stool cultures. Lancet 1980;2:413.

76. Wolcott MJ. Advances in nucleic acid-based detection methods. Clin Microbiol Rev 1992;5:370.

77. Mullis K. The unusual origin of the polymerase chain reaction. Sci Am 1990;240:56.

Textbook of Gastroenterology, second edition, edited
by Tadataka Yamada. JB Lippincott Company,
Philadelphia © 1995.

CHAPTER 132

Evaluation of Gastrointestinal Motility: Methodologic Considerations

John W. Wiley   Timothy T. Nostrant   Chung Owyang

Esophageal Manometry and 24-Hour pH Monitoring
Technical Aspects of Esophageal Manometry
Technical Aspects of pH Studies
Indications, Contraindications, and Clinical Applications
Gastroduodenal Manometry
Gastroduodenal Motility in the Fasting and Fed States
Technical Aspects
Indications and Contraindications
Data Interpretation
Clinical Situations That Affect Gastroduodenal Motility
Electrogastrography
Electrophysiologic Basis of Gastric Motility
Technical Aspects
Indications and Contraindications

Interpreting the Electrogastrogram
Clinical Situations That Affect the Electrogastrogram
Colonic Scintigraphy
Technical Aspects
Indications and Contraindications
Data Interpretation
Clinical Application
Anorectal Manometry
Technical Aspects
Indications and Contraindications
Data Interpretation
Clinical Applications
Future Applications

Interest in evaluating gastrointestinal motility has continued to grow in recent years because of the recognition that abnormalities of gastrointestinal motor function may contribute directly or indirectly to a number of common clinical problems, and because advances in monitoring techniques have allowed relatively noninvasive recording of gastrointestinal motility under physiologic conditions. This chapter emphasizes the developments in the application of esophageal manometry, electrogastrography, gastroduodenal manometry, colonic scintigraphy, and anorectal manometry to evaluate gastrointestinal motility. The evaluation of esophageal motility and gastric emptying using nuclear scintigraphy is discussed elsewhere (see Chaps. 54 and 60).

This chapter discusses how best to use these monitoring techniques. Aspects of each technique include the following:

What kind of information can be obtained from each technique?

What are the physiologic events that each technique records?

How is each procedure performed?

What are the indications and contraindications for performing each test?

How are data interpreted that are obtained with each test, that is, what are the criteria for normal and abnormal results?

How is each test used in the clinical setting?

What might the future have in store for gastrointestinal motility testing?

ESOPHAGEAL MANOMETRY AND 24-HOUR pH MONITORING

Esophageal manometry and 24-hour pH testing are accepted clinical and investigative tools for the study of esophageal dysfunction.[1,2] These procedures are most frequently performed in evaluating patients with dysphagia who have no evidence of mechanical obstruction and in persons with suspected noncardiac chest pain or gastroesophageal reflux. Generalized motor disorders of the gastrointestinal tract, such as scleroderma and chronic intestinal pseudoobstruction, can affect the esophagus. Confirmation of the diagnosis frequently can be made by esophageal manometry.

Technical Aspects of Esophageal Manometry

Equipment

Esophageal motility testing requires intubation of the esophagus with a recording catheter, which is connected to a physiograph. The clinician must choose between two major systems of recording catheters available: water perfused or solid state.

The standard system in most esophageal motility laboratories uses a water-perfused catheter system connected indirectly to a physiograph through a series of transducers.[3,4] Pressure is recorded at predetermined recording orifices; the signal from each orifice is changed into electrical current at external transducers and retransformed into a pen deflection at the physiograph. The major advantages of this system are the initial comparatively low cost, rapid repair of malfunctioning external transducers, and the extensive experience with the system. The major disadvantage of the water-perfused system is variability in recording accuracy when measuring transient high-pressure events such as upper esophageal sphincter pressure and pharyngeal upper esophageal sphincter coordination. This disadvantage can be overcome by using low-compliance microcapillary tubing and perfusing with a low-friction pneumohydraulic pump, which allows recording of all intraesophageal events at acceptable perfusion rates.[5] Other disadvantages are the constant need for recalibration and the possible need for a separate pH recording system.

The second system is a solid-state recording catheter with multiple, small-diameter intralumenal transducers that directly interface with the physiograph. The major advantages of the solid-state system are ease of use, minimal need for calibration, accuracy of recording, and the capability of performing simultaneous motility-pH recordings. Major disadvantages of the intralumenal transducer system are the high initial cost and the potential downtime for the system if one or more transducers are damaged. However, newer systems have been used for more than 4 years and 2000 examinations, without significant repair. Another disadvantage is the fixed nature of the transducer position, although solid-state recorders can be made to order, albeit at greater expense. Both systems can measure intraesophageal events with acceptable precision and have been used extensively by many motility centers.

Recent technical advances permit continuous monitoring of lower esophageal sphincter pressure (LESP). This led to examination of the relation between acid reflux and transient spontaneous relaxation of the lower esophageal sphincter (LES). The systems described previously cannot adequately measure LESP or relaxation continuously because of movement of this sphincter during respiration. To circumvent this problem, Dent developed a 6-cm sleeve catheter to straddle the LES throughout its entire range of motion.[6] This device monitors the maximal pressure sensed at any point on the sleeve. Although manometric sleeve catheters are available commercially, their use is predominantly in the research laboratory.

The choice of the physiograph to record pressure events is also important because this represents the major cost in any manometric system. The physiograph should satisfy the following requirements: at least four separate pressure-recording channels, including an extra channel for swallow sensor or event marker; variable paper speeds from 1 to 10 mm/second; full-scale recording for pressures between 0 and 400 mm Hg; and a recording channel for pH testing.[1]

Recording Procedure

Before attempting intubation, all of the necessary accessories must be on hand. Nasal topical anesthesia should be used: topical cocaine or viscous lidocaine are the most common agents employed. Tissue paper, an emesis container, and a 30-mL water cup should be available. Reassuring the patient and a step-by-step explanation of the procedure are prerequisites for obtaining consistently good recordings. Short-term oral intubation studies using a manometric catheter passed through a mouthpiece can be used in place of nasal studies and may be more comfortable for patients.[7]

Lower esophageal sphincter measurements. After gastrointestinal intubation is accomplished, all recording sites should be positioned in the stomach. This can be confirmed by seeing a positive deflection during abdominal breathing or compression. LESP usually is measured first. Two techniques are used. The first is the rapid pull-through technique.[8] The catheter is withdrawn at a rate of 1 cm/second while the patient suspends respiration until the distal three recording sites give LESP readings. The three distal sites are again placed in the stomach, and the cycle is repeated two more times. Mean and peak pressures are recorded from these nine measurements as that pressure above intragastric pressure. The second approach is the station pull-through technique. This method involves withdrawing the catheter in 0.5- to 1.0-cm increments and leaving it in each position for a few seconds. LESP and relaxation can be measured by this technique. Values from rapid pull-through LESP are usually 2 to 3 cm higher than those obtained with station pull-through technique.[9]

Relaxation of the LES requires that a distal recorder be stationed in the LES and a more proximal recording orifice be stationed in the lower esophagus to measure completeness of relaxation and coordination of relaxation with esophageal peristalsis. Relaxation should be complete, with a drop to intragastric pressure, and coordinated for more than 90% of wet swallows.

Esophageal body measurements. After LES manometry is completed, all recording sites are withdrawn into the esophagus. The most distal recording site is placed 2 cm above the upper border of the LES. Because recording sites are separated by 5 cm and three sites are usually used, the distal 15 cm of the esophagus can be recorded. This segment represents the smooth muscle portion of the esophagus. Water is given with each swallow because esophageal body pressure is most reliably recorded after a bolus.[1] A total of 10 wet swallows is used to measure distal esophageal, or smooth muscle, body pressure. The striated muscle portion and the junction of the striated and the smooth muscles can be measured by sequentially withdrawing the catheter in 3-cm intervals and recording five wet swallows and again withdrawing the catheter 3 cm and repeating five wet swallows.

Measurements of the esophageal body contractions include amplitude of contraction, duration of contraction, and percentage of abnormal contractions. Esophageal peristalsis is observed. Simultaneous contractions (contractions in multiple segments at the same time), spontaneous activity (pressure waves in the esophagus without swallowing), or repetitive contractions (three peaks) are considered abnormal. Failure of peristalsis increases somewhat with age but usually occurs in less than 15% of all wet swallows.[10]

Upper esophageal sphincter measurements.   Upper esophageal sphincter pressure and ability to relax are measured. Techniques used for the upper esophageal sphincter are the same as used for the LES. Recording speed may have to be increased from the usual 2.5 mm/second to 5 to 10 mm/second to record upper esophageal sphincter relaxation adequately. Coordination and completeness of relaxation are almost 100%. If a question of incomplete relaxation is present, different recording sites placed in the upper esophageal sphincter may demonstrate more complete relaxation. Because measurement of the upper esophageal sphincter may require withdrawing the catheter almost completely, only two recording orifices should be used to measure upper esophageal sphincter pressure, and more swallows should be performed to give a reliable pressure measurement. Continuous monitoring of the upper esophageal sphincter has been reported.[11] Upper esophageal sphincter pressure values recorded with this technique tend to be lower than the values obtained with the method described previously.

This completes the technique of basic esophageal manometry. Special circumstances, such as a suspicion of striated muscle disorders of the upper esophagus, for example, dermatomyositis, may require more attention to the proximal esophagus, but the most of the clinician's time is spent recording from the distal esophageal segment. At the completion of the standard manometric examination, provocative tests, such as bethanechol, edrophonium, or balloon distention, can be performed to induce chest pain in patients sent for the evaluation of noncardiac chest pain. The mechanism by which provocative agents induce chest pain is unknown, and the use of provocative agents is experimental.[12]

Technical Aspects of pH Studies

Standard Tests

After standard manometry is completed, pH studies are obtained. The first test is acid clearance. A 15-mL bolus of 0.1 normal hydrochloric acid is injected into the esophagus 5 cm above the LES. The patient is asked to dry swallow every 30 seconds until the pH is restored to the baseline level. This requires at least 15 dry swallows. Poor acid clearance is seen predominantly in conditions that disrupt peristalsis (i.e., achalasia, diffuse esophageal spasm, and scleroderma) or in disorders affecting salivation (i.e., scleroderma and the sicca syndrome) because these conditions can disturb bolus movement or esophageal acid neutralization.

The Bernstein examination allows the clinician to determine if acid in the esophagus induces chest pain or discomfort. Infusions of 0.1 normal hydrochloric acid or saline should

be done in a blinded manner by using a three-way stopcock connected to both reservoirs that are located behind the patient. Saline infused at a rate of 120 drops/minute for 5 minutes should be the initial perfusate. Acid infusions at the same rate should then be started and saline should be stopped. Acid infusion should continue until symptoms begin or until 30 minutes have elapsed. If acid, but not saline, produces chest pain or heartburn, gastroesophageal reflux is likely. If both acid and saline or saline alone induces pain, the patient may have a hypersensitive esophagus. If neither produces pain, acid reflux is not the source of chest pain. Saline washout, to evaluate pain relief after acid-induced pain, is no longer considered essential to the diagnosis of acid-induced chest pain. Simultaneous recording of esophageal body pressures may show dysmotility as a mechanism for acid-induced chest pain.

To determine if gastroesophageal reflux is present, standard acid reflux testing is performed. The pH probe is placed 5 cm above the LES, and the patient is placed in the supine, right side, left side, and prone positions. In each of these positions, the patient is asked to perform Valsalva's maneuver and to move into the knee-chest position. Both maneuvers increase intraabdominal pressure and increase the possibility of overcoming a weak sphincter. These maneuvers are repeated in the basal state and after loading the stomach with 300 mL of 0.1 normal hydrochloric acid. Reflux of acid, seen as a drop in pH to less than 4, in any position in the basal state, or in two positions after acid loading, is considered pathologic reflux.[13] Sensitivity of this examination in patients with chronic reflux symptoms approaches 90%.

After esophageal manometry and pH testing are completed, the patient should be observed for 30 minutes. Heartburn usually responds to antacids. More serious complications such as bleeding or perforation are rare: we have not seen any in over 3000 examinations to date at the University of Michigan Medical Center.

Ambulatory 24-Hour pH and Pressure Recording

The development of microcomputer-based data collection has revolutionized pH monitoring of the distal esophagus.[14] Ambulatory outpatient evaluation under true-life conditions gives a better determination of whether acid in the esophagus is associated with symptoms.[15] Johnson and DeMeester have established normal values with upper ranges of normal in young healthy subjects.[16] Use of receiver operating characteristic curves has increased the upper ranges of normal without sacrificing sensitivity and specificity.[17]

Six monitoring systems are available in this country.[18] All systems have demonstrated reasonable durability, and the life expectancy of each recording catheter is five to eight examinations.[18] Glass or antimony electrodes are frequently used. Reference electrodes must be attached to the patient with a conducting jelly for proper measurements. Newer recording catheters contain the reference electrode, eliminating the errors often seen with dislodgement of the reference electrode.

The pH electrode is placed 5 cm above the upper border of the LES. Until recently, localization of the LES required manometric testing before pH recording. Using a standard electrode to measure the step-up in esophageal pH while the recording catheter crosses the LES allows placement accuracy of within 1 to 2 cm, when compared with positioning guided by manometry.[19] This pH recording technique may be an acceptable alternative to standard manometric placement for 24-hour pH recording in patients who cannot tolerate esophageal manometrics or in an office practice where manometric equipment is too costly for routine use. The ideal duration of recording has not been established. To differentiate patients with reflux from normal subjects, recording times of 12 and 24 hours have been more successful than shorter recording periods of only 3 hours postprandially.[20,21]

When interpreting an ambulatory pH profile, total time that the pH is less than 4 and the number of episodes lasting longer than 5 minutes have the best positive-negative predictive value.[20,21] Symptom correlation with pH drops is also crucial in defining acid reflux as a cause for chest pain.[22] Correlation is rarely 100%, and multiple indexes have been used. Association of chest pain with pH less than 4 in 75% or more of painful episodes is considered strong evidence for acid-induced chest pain.[22]

In the last 10 years, ambulatory monitoring of esophageal body pressure has become available. This is done in conjunction with ambulatory esophageal pH monitoring. Current equipment and software does not allow continuous monitoring of LESP or upper esophageal sphincter pressure. The primary indication for ambulatory pressure monitoring has been noncardiac chest pain. Massive data acquisition requiring intensive scrutiny, lack of standardized definitions for peristaltic and nonperistaltic waves, and inability to define what is normal hampers use of research information for clinical patient care. An increased diagnostic yield of only 5% is anticipated in unselected patients when compared with more standard diagnostic examinations. Patients with daily but noncontinuous pain, and patients admitted to the coronary care unit with acute pain may form select groups with improved diagnostic yields from ambulatory pressure monitoring. Unfortunately, even in these groups, only 55% of patients will have their pain during monitoring.[23] The high cost of this equipment and the time-intensive nature of pressure monitoring is likely to limit use to specialized centers for chest pain.

Indications, Contraindications, and Clinical Applications

The primary indication for esophageal manometry and 24-hour pH testing is to evaluate esophageal dysfunction when anatomic causes such as esophagitis, tumors, or strictures, or congenital abnormalities such as rings, webs, or diverticula are not present. Most persons present with dysphagia or chest pain. Indications for esophageal manometry and pH monitoring are presented in Table 132-1.

Esophageal manometry is mandatory in patients with suspected achalasia. This is particularly true in patients before pneumatic dilatation or cardiomyotomy because patients with nonspecific esophageal dysmotility can present with dysphagia, which mimics achalasia.[24] Response to standard achalasia treatment in patients with nonspecific esophageal dysmotility has been less than in patients with classic achalasia findings. Manometry has had less use in patients with presumed diffuse esophageal spasm. Classic findings of esopha-

---

TABLE 132-1
Indications for Esophageal Manometry and 24-Hour pH Monitoring

Indications for Esophageal Manometry
Patients with oropharyngeal dysphagia and normal anatomic studies
   Cricopharyngeal achalasia (poor UES relaxation)
   Pharyngeo–upper esophageal sphincter dyscoordination
      Low-amplitude pharyngeal contractions
      Early or later pharyngeal contraction
      Early upper esophageal body contraction
Patients with esophageal dysphagia but normal anatomic studies
   Primary esophageal body dysmotility
      Achalasia
      Diffuse esophageal spasm
      Nutcracker esophagus
      Hypertensive lower esophageal sphincter
      Nonspecific esophageal dysmotility
      Secondary esophageal body of dysmotility
      Collagen vascular diseases
      Amyloidosis
      Secondary achalasia
      Chronic intestinal pseudoobstruction
      Laser treatment for esophageal cancer
      Sclerotherapy
      Hypothyroidism
Patients with noncardiac chest pain
   Primary esophageal body dysmotility

Indications for 24-hour pH monitoring
Patients with noncardiac chest pain
Refractory acid reflux symptoms: evaluate treatment efficacy
Preoperative and postoperative evaluation for antireflux surgery
Patient with atypical presentations of acid reflux (ENT, pulmonary)

ENT, ear-nose-throat; UES, upper esophageal sphincter.

---

geal spasm such as simultaneous contractions, multiphasic waves, and spontaneous activity but preserved peristalsis are not frequently seen in patients with esophageal chest pain.[10,25,26] Usually esophageal manometry is performed to help exclude an esophageal source for chest pain. Motility disorders, other than diffuse esophageal spasm, that can cause chest pain and dysphagia include nutcracker esophagus and hypertensive LES. Although specific manometric criteria exist for each of these diagnoses, the physiologic basis for the symptoms in patients having these manometric findings remains to be elucidated. Achalasia and diffuse esophageal spasm are contrasted with a normal esophageal motility study in Figure 132-1. Examples of nutcracker esophagus and hypertensive LES are shown in Figure 132-2.

Twenty-four–hour pH monitoring of the distal esophagus has helped to establish that excessive acid exposure in this region is associated with chest pain. Young patients with no history of dysphagia or weight loss do not need pH testing to evaluate typical pyrosis or regurgitation. Twenty-four–hour pH testing is indicated in patients presenting with typical reflux symptoms who do not respond to treatment. Patients presenting with cervical dysphagia, cough, recurrent sore throat, or aspiration with a normal result from pulmonary and otorhinolaryngology evaluation also constitute a patient group in whom pH monitoring may define the cause for the

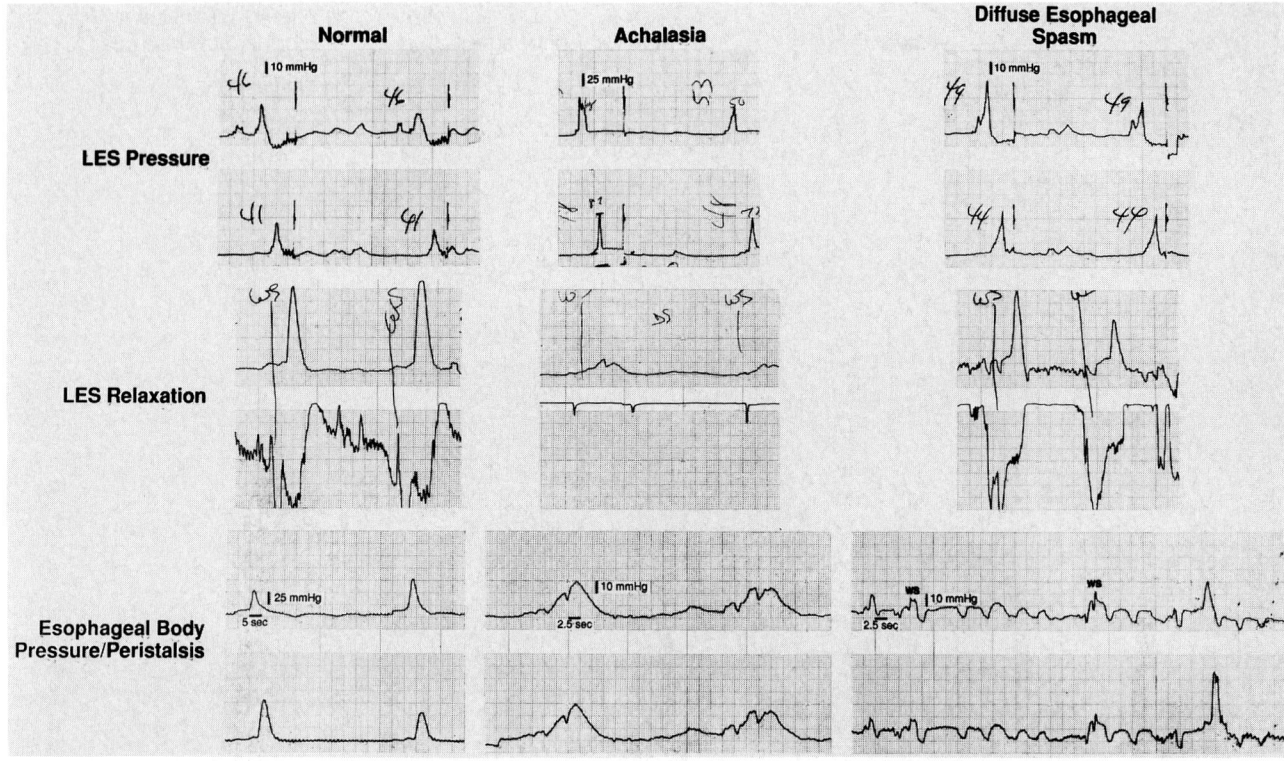

FIGURE 132-1. Comparison of esophageal manometrics of normal subjects and of patients with achalasia and diffuse esophageal spasm (DES). Lower esophageal sphincter pressure (LESP) is normal in patients with DES (range, 15–35 mm Hg). Usually, LESP is elevated to higher than 40 mm Hg in patients with achalasia. Relaxation of LES is normal in patients with DES but absent or incomplete in those with achalasia. Esophageal body motility is peristaltic in normal subjects, totally nonperistaltic in patients with achalasia, and incompletely peristaltic (some maintained peristalsis) in patients with DES. Esophageal body pressure is decreased in patients with achalasia and variable in those with DES.

symptoms.[26] Before antireflux surgery, all patients should undergo pH monitoring of the distal esophagus. This establishes the occurrence of acid reflux and whether the presence of acid in the distal esophagus is the source for symptoms, because up to 10% of patients presenting for antireflux surgery do not have acid reflux.[27] In addition, this permits objective evaluation of the surgeon's ability to prevent acid reflux in the early and the late postoperative period. Examples of upright, supine, and combined acid reflux are compared with a normal pH study in Figure 132-3.

The use of esophageal function testing in patients with generalized gastrointestinal motility disorders such as scleroderma and chronic intestinal pseudoobstruction is in its infancy. Testing should be confined to three groups of patients. The first are those in whom confirmation of esophageal disease supports the diagnosis. Although manometric findings are not highly specific for scleroderma, they are reasonably sensitive and occasionally can be helpful in supporting the diagnosis. The most common clinical patterns seen in scleroderma are shown in Figure 132-4. Esophageal manometry and 24-hour pH monitoring also can be useful in evaluating patients in whom a therapeutic change will be forthcoming, depending on the findings. Examples include 24-hour pH monitoring in patients with scleroderma and recalcitrant esophagitis or patients with chronic idiopathic intestinal

pseudoobstruction and dysphagia in whom pneumatic dilatation is a treatment option. The last group includes patients in whom documentation of how the disease affects esophageal function may improve the physician's understanding of the mechanisms underlying symptoms and general knowledge of the disease process. This group is the least likely to be candidates for monitoring, and should be monitored only at established research motility laboratories.

Major contraindications for esophageal manometry are few and involve esophageal obstruction or large diverticula because of the risk of perforation. Barium studies or endoscopy are prerequisites of manometric studies. The major reason for not doing esophageal manometry is if the information will not affect management. Esophageal manometry and pH testing are not required in all patients with typical reflux symptoms or noncardiac chest pain. A treatment course, coupled with careful exclusion of chest wall pain or panic attacks, should be attempted before manometry is performed. Approximately 20% to 40% of patients referred with dysphagia or chest pain require manometric evaluations.[12]

The role of provocative tests in patients with suspected esophageal chest pain is controversial. The initial approach is to use agents that provoke chest pain. The most commonly employed provocative agent is edrophonium, based on its safety, but the yield of positive results is typically low.[12] Other

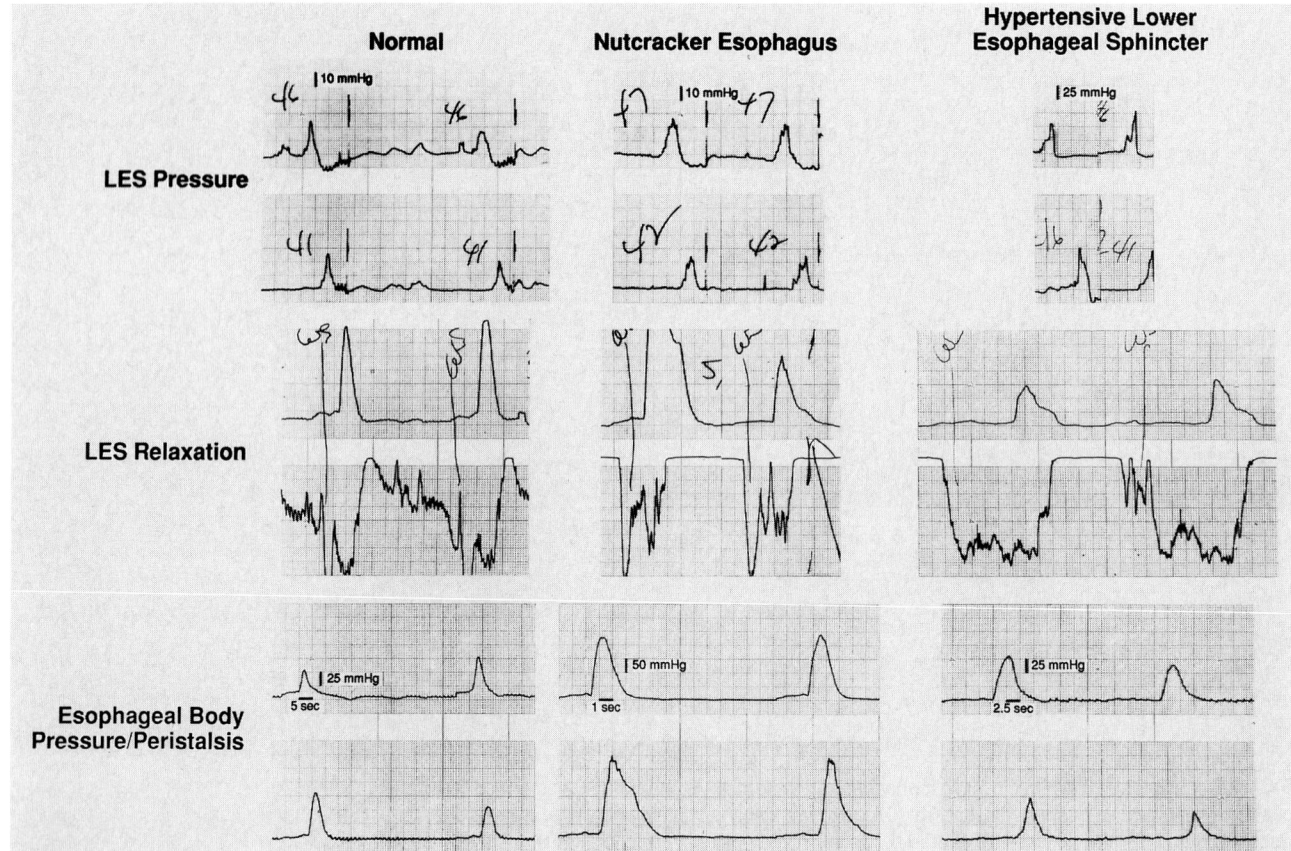

FIGURE 132-2. Comparison of esophageal manometrics of normal subjects and of patients with nutcracker esophagus and hypertensive lower esophageal sphincter (LES). The LES pressure is normal in patients with nutcracker esophagus but elevated by more than 40 mm Hg in those with hypertensive lower esophageal sphincter. Usually, LES relaxation is normal in patients with nutcracker esophagus and hypertensive LES. Esophageal body pressure is elevated to more than 180 mm Hg in patients with nutcracker esophagus and normal in those with hypertensive LES.

provocative agents such as high-dose bethanechol have been used in patients with suspected noncardiac chest pain, that is, normal epicardial vessels at cardiac catheterization, because of a higher yield of positive studies and an excellent safety record in this subset of patients.[24] Examples of esophageal recordings before and after provocation with bethanechol are shown in Figure 132-5. The indications for esophageal manometry and 24-hour pH monitoring are summarized in Table 132-1.

GASTRODUODENAL MANOMETRY

Gastroduodenal manometry is established in the research arena and has provided clinically useful information regarding normal and abnormal contraction *patterns* in this region. The technique is proving to be helpful in diagnosing motility disturbances by localizing and characterizing abnormal motor patterns. This information can be useful in identifying the cause of the motility problem.

Gastroduodenal Motility in the Fasting and Fed States

Gastroduodenal manometry is used to assess the presence of *interdigestive migratory motor complex* (IMMC) activity in the fasting state and the occurrence of a typical fed pattern, postprandially. In the fasting state, the stomach and small intestine of many species, including humans, demonstrate a cyclic, periodic contractile pattern termed the IMMC.[28] This peristaltic motor activity slowly sweeps the gastrointestinal tract, from its origin at the gastric *pacemaker* down to the ileum. The IMMC is typically divided into four phases:

Phase 1—a period of quiescence.
Phase 2—irregular motor activity.
Phase 3—a brief period of regular contractions often termed *activity fronts* or simply *phase 3 activity*, representing the migratory complex that sweeps the upper gastrointestinal tract in a peristaltic manner.
Phase 4—a brief period of irregular activity, which is occasionally noticed before the quiescence of phase 1.

Normal PH Study

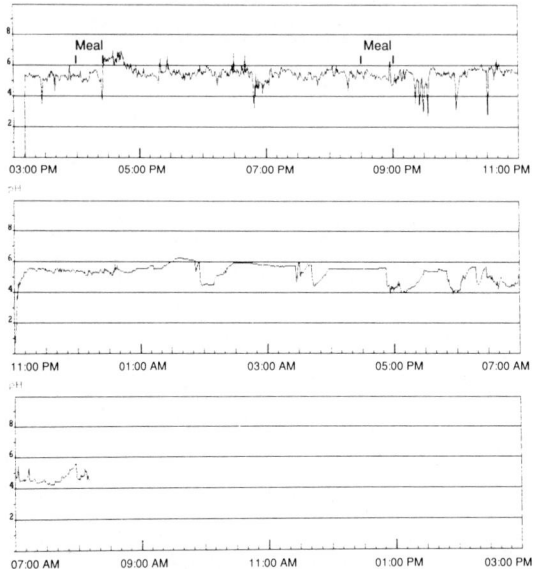

Upright and Supine Reflux

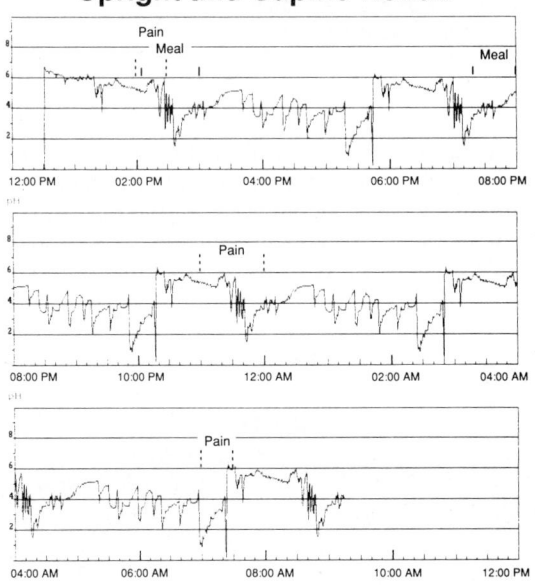

Upright Reflux

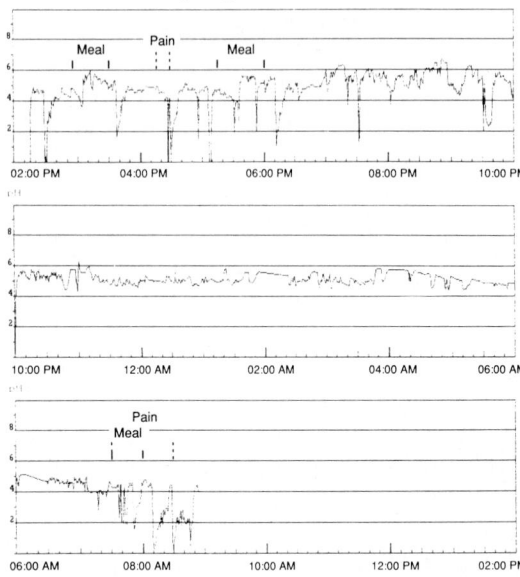

FIGURE 132-3. Comparison of 24-hour pH profiles in normal subjects, in patients with upright reflux, and in patients with combined upright and supine reflux. A normal pH study shows reflux (pH < 4) after meals and none when the patient is asleep. Patients with upright reflux have exaggerated reflux after meals and when upright but none when the patient is supine. Patients with combined reflux have acid in the esophagus after meals and when supine.

After ingestion of nutrients, IMMC activity is inhibited and replaced by a *fed pattern,* the characteristics of which vary with the type, composition, and amount of nutrients consumed.[29] For example, liquid nutrients decrease the amplitude of contractions in the antrum and generate irregular motor activity in the small intestine, whereas ingestion of solid food produces high-amplitude contractions in the distal antrum and motor pattern similar to that generated by liquid nutrients in the small intestine. Figure 132-6 depicts examples of normal fasting and fed intralumenal pressure patterns. Normal phase 2 activity is demonstrated, culminating in a phase 3 complex in the antrum and duodenum. Phase 3 contractions occur at a rate of 3 per minute in the antrum and more rapidly, 11 to 12 per minute, in the duodenum. Occasionally a normal phase 3 activity front begins in the proximal duodenum and not in

the stomach, although this usually is preceded by strong antral phase 2 activity. Figure 132-6 also shows irregular but persistent phase 2 activity. This phasic motor activity is characteristically observed postprandially in the distal antrum and proximal small intestine. Repetitive pressure activity with an amplitude more than 50 mm Hg is usually noticed in the antrum at a rate of three per minute, and persistent, irregular activity is noticed in the duodenum.

Technical Aspects

Gastroduodenal manometry requires upper gastrointestinal intubation with a specially adapted polyvinyl catheter on which miniature pressure transducers are mounted, or, alter-

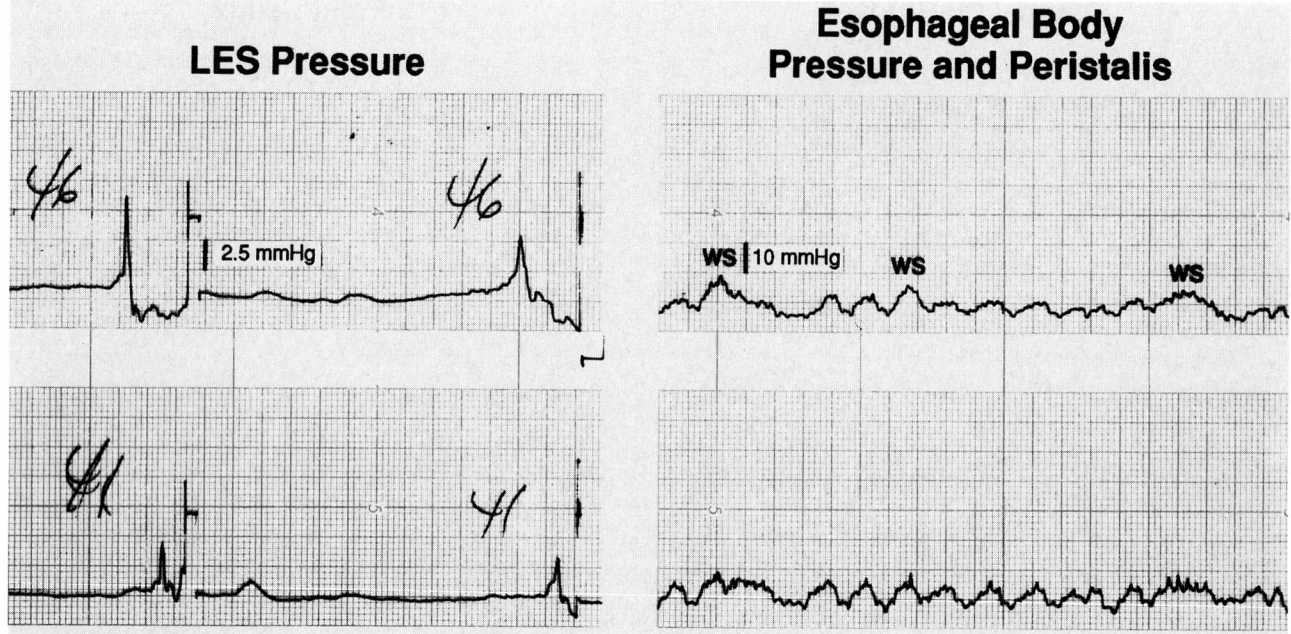

FIGURE 132-4. Esophageal manometrics in patients with scleroderma. Low pressures of the lower esophageal sphincter and nonperistaltic low-amplitude waves are the most common abnormalities in patients with scleroderma.

natively, manometric perfusion catheters are assembled together as a multilumen tube. The monitoring probe is guided into the proximal jejunum under fluoroscopic guidance. Manometric devices using miniature transducers or the pneumohydraulic perfusion system provide similar information on gastrointestinal motor activity. The miniature *strain-gauge* transducers are prone to puncture of the thin, exposed, pressure-sensitive diaphragm located at the end of the transducer, whereas the pneumohydraulic perfusion systems are susceptible to compliance problems resulting from cracks or

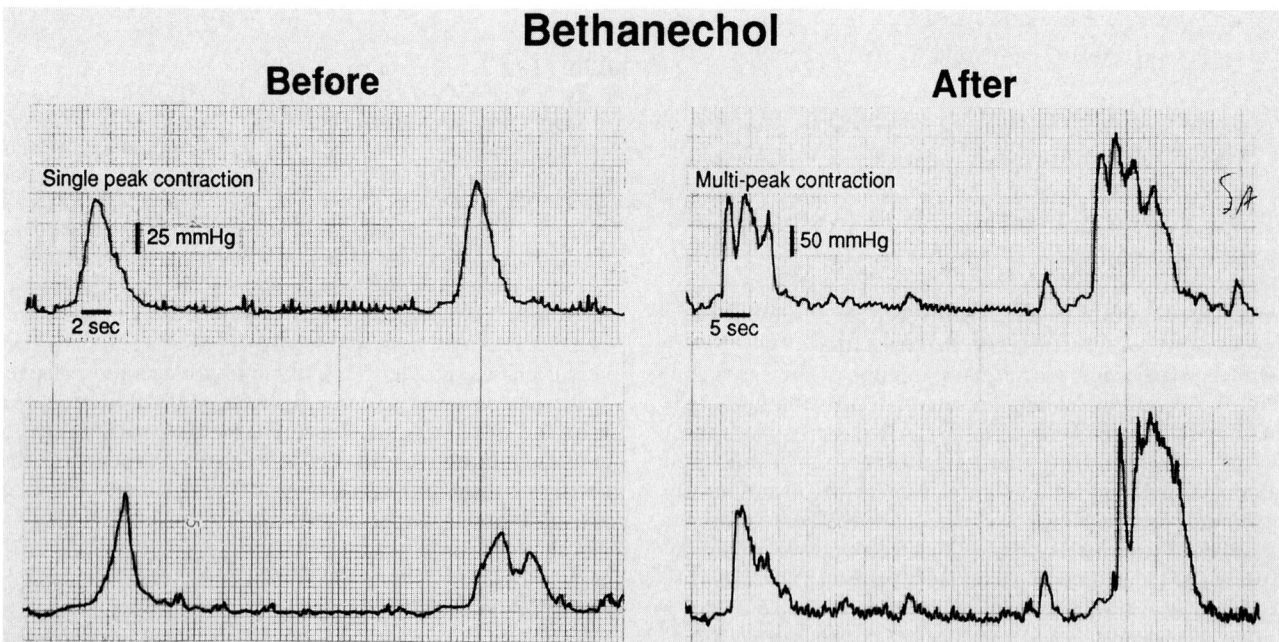

FIGURE 132-5. Esophageal manometrics before and after bethanechol provocation. Amplitude and duration of contraction are increased. Abnormal types of contraction (multiphasic, ≤ three peaks) also are increased.

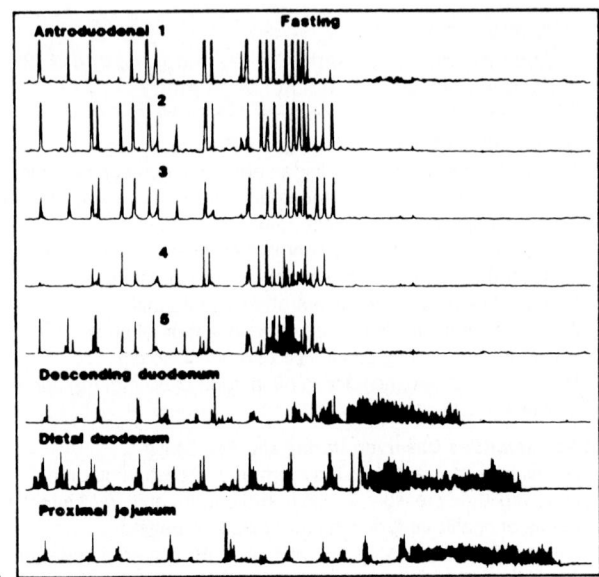
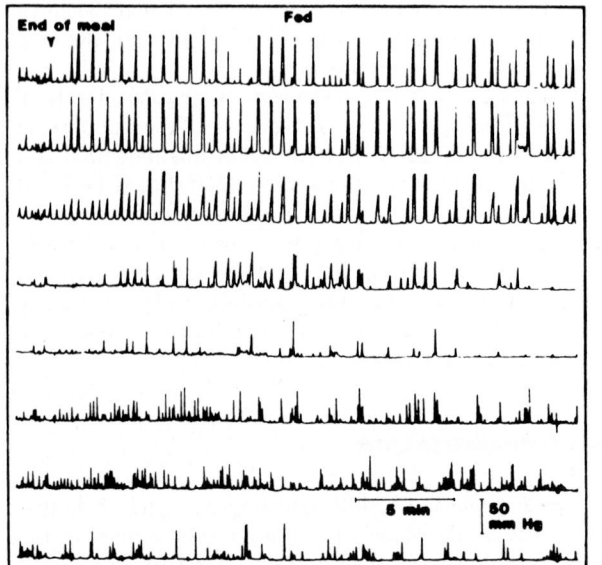

FIGURE 132-6. Normal gastrointestinal motility. **(A)** Normal fasting interdigestive migrating motor complex. Notice phase 3 activity in the antrum, pressure activity gradually moving into the duodenum, and gradual change in configuration of the waves while they move through the antroduodenal junction. **(B)** Normal fed activity. Notice irregular but persistent phasic pressure activity in the distal antrum and proximal small bowel. (From Malagelada J-R, Camilleri M, Stanghellini V. Manometric diagnosis of gastrointestinal motility disorders. New York: Thieme, 1986:45.)

leaks in the system or plugging of the tubing. Both techniques measure changes in intralumenal pressure, which is an indirect assessment of smooth muscle contractions. In patients in whom a gastroduodenal motility disorder is strongly suspected, it is occasionally necessary to position the recording probe in the duodenum with an endoscope and manually advance the catheter into the proximal jejunum.

Assessing gastroduodenal motility requires the capability to monitor pressure changes from 6 to 12 recording sites including the antrum, pylorus, duodenum, and proximal jejunum. The spacing of the recording sites along the manometric tube depends on the objectives of the study. For example, if the goal of the examination is to monitor the contractile patterns of the pylorus, several recording sites should be positioned close together to ensure satisfactory recordings from the pyloric channel. Pressure-sensitive transducer sleeves have been built into manometric tubes to record from the pyloric sphincter region.[30] These devices decrease the problem of recording from sphincter regions because of movement of the manometric tube. Manometric sites should be spaced 1 cm apart across the gastroduodenal junction and at 10-cm intervals in the small intestine. A commonly used arrangement involves positioning five closely spaced recording sites to monitor antral, pyloric, and proximal duodenal motility while three sites are spaced more widely for assessment of distal duodenal and proximal jejunal motility. The manometric recording system includes a polygraph with sufficient channels to monitor each recording site. The pressure transducers must be calibrated at the beginning and end of each study to ensure the accuracy and uniformity of data within and between studies.

Indications and Contraindications

Patients who have an upper gastrointestinal motility disturbance often experience unexplained nausea, vomiting, and abdominal pain in the fasting state or postprandially. Unfortunately, mild to moderate gastrointestinal symptoms are of limited value for predicting the outcome of manometric studies because patients with normal manometry results may report similar symptoms to those whose studies give abnormal results.[31] The presence of gastrointestinal symptoms and evidence of collagen-vascular, metabolic, urologic, neurologic, and psychiatric disorders increase the likelihood of abnormal manometric findings.[31] Gastroduodenal manometry is indicated in a patient with suggestive symptoms after mechanical obstruction has been ruled out with endoscopy or radiologic studies; appropriate consultations and work-ups have been performed to evaluate possible endocrine-metabolic, neurologic, and psychiatric disorders; and documentation of delayed gastric emptying or impaired small intestine transit is available. Gastroduodenal manometry can be helpful in making the diagnosis of a motility disorder by demonstrating an abnormality in motor activity and localizing the involved region. For example, characteristic features of an abnormal motility pattern may help distinguish whether the cause of the disturbance is an intestinal myopathy versus an enteric or extrinsic neuropathy (see Clinical Situations That Affect Gastroduodenal Motility). In addition, the technique can be useful in monitoring the patient's course and response to therapy, such as with the use of prokinetic medications. These results rarely indicate the need for additional procedures such as laparotomy, to rule out previously undetected anatomic abnormalities, or biopsy, to obtain a full-thickness intestinal specimen to rule out an infiltrative or degenerative process affecting the integrity of the neuromuscular elements.

The major contraindication to performing gastroduodenal manometry is related to the peroral passage of the manometric tube into the jejunum. If anatomic abnormalities such as a diverticulum or fistula are suspected, they should be ruled out before performing this procedure. Persons with respiratory diseases or a hypersensitive gag reflex may tolerate the procedure poorly. Patients who have undergone certain gastrointestinal surgical procedures such as a Billroth II antrostomy can be difficult to evaluate because of problems in passing the manometric tube into the jejunum.

Data Interpretation

The typical recording session lasts approximately 5 hours. Three hours are devoted to recording motor activity in the fasted state followed by ingestion of a standard meal and 2 hours of postprandial recording. It is useful to develop a systematic approach for evaluating the motor activities observed in the fasting and postprandial states. The motility pattern normally observed during the fasting state, the IMMC, is often examined for the following features: the mean cycle duration or period of time between phase 3 complexes; the duration of each phase, the amplitude and propagation velocity of phase 3 complexes in different regions of the stomach and small intestine; and the rate of contractions during phase 3 activity.[32,33] Useful qualitative information is derived from visual inspection of the tracing to determine if phase 3 activity is present; if phase 3 activity initiates from the gastric pacemaker or an ectopic site; if the time intervals for the various phases of the IMMC are appropriate; and if the complex propagates in a normal (aboral) or abnormal (retrograde) manner.

The pressure activity pattern observed in the fed state is determined by the solid-versus-liquid composition of the meal and the nutrient content. Therefore composition of the meal must be standardized to exclude meal composition as a variable between studies. Usually inhibition of IMMC activity occurs postprandially, replaced by phasic pressure waves in the antrum and irregular, phasic contractions in the small intestine. Pressure activity is often quantified in the form of a motility index, which reflects the amplitude and frequency of contractions for a defined period of time.

Interpretation of gastroduodenal manometric tracings is complicated by the intrinsic variability of the fasting and fed motor patterns. A number of IMMC parameters including the duration of its constituent phases, the velocity of propagation of the phase 3 activity front, and the duration of inhibition by food demonstrate considerable variability between persons as well as within the same individual when evaluated serially.[34,35] A number of motor patterns, such as the presence of jejunal-clustered contractions, which have been proposed to be a characteristic feature of the irritable bowel syndrome, apparently can be influenced by emotional and physical stress, including the anxiety associated with having the examination.[34,36,37] Abnormalities that have been reported in the fasting and fed motility patterns are summarized in Table 132-2.

TABLE 132-2

Abnormalities Reported in the Fasting and Fed Motility Patterns on Gastroduodenal Manometry

Abnormalities Observed During the Fasting State
Bursts of phasic activity having an abnormal duration (>2 min), amplitude (>20 mm Hg) and frequency (10–12/min), which are nonpropagation and distinct from phase 3 activity
Sustained (>30 min) poorly coordinated phasic activity, which is isolated to one or more segments of the intestine
Low-amplitude contractions but otherwise normal
Absent, incomplete, or retrograde propagation of phase 3 complexes covering a distance of at least 30 cm
Prolonged (>3 min) increase in basal tone (>30 mm Hg) during phase 3 activity

Abnormalities Observed During the Fed State
Persistence of a fasting-like pattern after ingestion of a meal
Low-amplitude pressure waves in the antrum and small intestine
Bursts of phasic contractions that fail to propagate
Premature return of IMMC activity within 90 min after ingestion
Broad-based contractions occurring in the presence of increased tone, sometimes termed, *minute clusters*

IMMC, interdigestive migratory motor complex.

Adapted from Malagelada J-R, Camilleri M, Stanghellini V. Manometric diagnosis of gastrointestinal motility disorders. New York: Thieme-Stratton, 1986:54.

Clinical Situations That Affect Gastroduodenal Motility

Disturbances of intestinal motility can result in several distinct abnormalities on manometry. Gastrointestinal manometry can be useful to distinguish motility patterns that are typically observed with intestinal myopathy versus enteric or extrinsic neuropathy. Diseases associated with an intestinal myopathy often demonstrate normal motor patterns but with abnormally low pressures. In contrast, diseases that affect the enteric or extrinsic neural pathways can demonstrate abnormalities in the configuration and propagation of the IMMC or failure to convert from the fasting to fed motor pattern postprandially. For example, diseases such as myotonic dystrophia[38,39] and late progressive systemic sclerosis[40–42] that affect intestinal smooth muscle can present with symptoms and signs consistent with chronic intestinal pseudoobstruction, such as abdominal distention, pain, and weight loss in the absence of mechanical obstruction. Manometry often reveals a localized region of infrequent, weak contractions, particularly in the postprandial state in the presence of a relatively normal fasting motility pattern (Fig. 132-7). This pattern can be contrasted with the patient who may also present with a pseudoobstruction-like picture but whose disease affects the intrinsic or extrinsic neural pathways that regulate gastrointestinal motility.[43] In this situation, abnormalities of fasting and postcibal motility are observed. In the fasting state, abnormalities in the configuration and propagation of phase 3 complexes are observed (Fig. 132-8).

Gastroduodenal manometry is typically performed on patients who present with evidence of gastroparesis. Manometrically, these patients often demonstrate antral hypomotility.

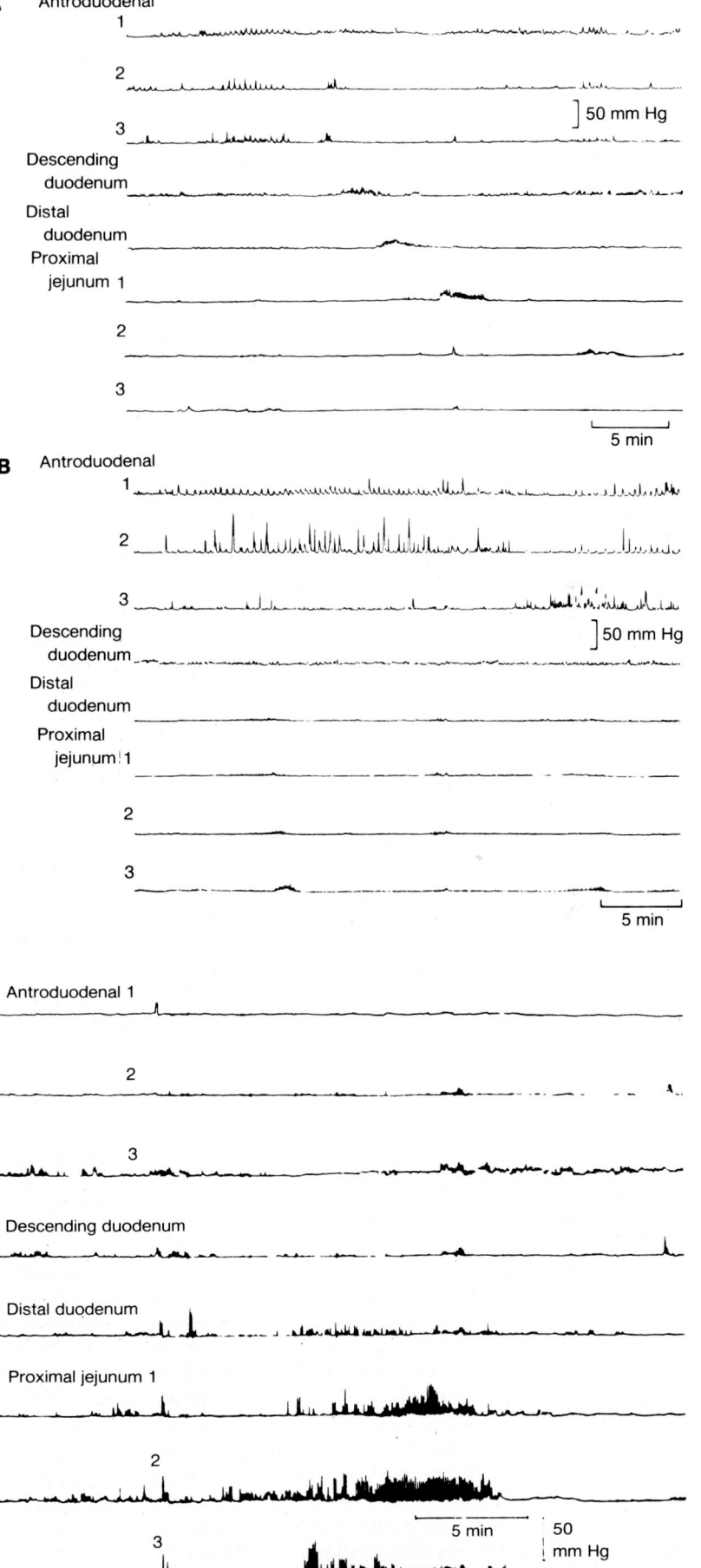

FIGURE 132-7. Myogenic chronic intestinal pseudoobstruction in a 71-year-old man with recurrent episodes of vomiting, abdominal pain, and constipation for 1 year. Radiologic examination revealed markedly dilated intestinal loops without mechanical obstruction. Full-thickness specimens taken from terminal ileum and sigmoid colon at exploratory laparotomy showed smooth muscle degeneration with replacement of muscle fibers by fibrous tissue. (**A**) Fasting tracing shows low amplitude but normal propagation of migrating motor complex and virtual absence of activity in the most distal jejunal port. (**B**) In the fed phase, antropyloric activity is mostly preserved, with waves of normal amplitude and frequency. In contrast, there is virtual absence of phasic pressure activity in the intestine. (From Malagelada J-R, Camilleri M, Stanghellini V. Manometric diagnosis of gastrointestinal motility disorders. New York: Thieme, 1986:98.)

FIGURE 132-8. Chronic sensory and autonomic neuropathy with gut dysmotility in a 34-year-old woman with weakness in the extremities, speech impairment, and dysphasia for 10 years. At the time of study, she had episodes of diarrhea, abdominal pain, and labile blood pressure with hypertensive crises followed by hypotension. There was evidence of autonomic dysfunction with sympathetic and parasympathetic involvement, and a peripheral sensory neuropathy involved upper and lower extremities. Fasting tracing reveals simultaneous bursts of phase 3–like activity in the proximal small bowel. (From Malagelada J-R, Camilleri M, Stanghellini V. Manometric diagnosis of gastrointestinal motility disorders. New York: Thieme, 1986:126.)

During the fasting state, phase 3 activity may be absent in the antrum, but the most common abnormality is postcibal antral hypomotility. Characteristically, the antral phasic pressure waves occur less frequently and with less force, that is, decreased amplitude. Nuclear scintigraphy studies indicate that this motility disorder often is associated with delayed gastric emptying of solid food.[44,45] Antral hypomotility is observed in a wide range of clinical situations including the following: persons with diabetes mellitus, generally type 1 with evidence of autonomic neuropathy[46–51]; patients receiving adrenergic agonists,[52–54] cholinergic antagonists,[55,56] and opiate agonists[57]; occasionally after certain surgical procedures including fundoplication,[58] vagotomy alone or with pyloroplasty,[59,60] and cardiomyotomy for achalasia[61]; and idiopathic gastroparesis.[62,63]

Localized, uncoordinated bursts of tonic and phasic activities can occur in the small intestine that blur the distinction between fasting and fed motility patterns. Examples of diseases that can present in this manner include early scleroderma[40–42]; diabetes mellitus[46–51]; amyloidosis[64–67]; visceral autonomic neuropathies and degenerative conditions involving the autonomic system such as idiopathic orthostatic hypotension, Shy-Drager syndrome, and pandysautonomias[68–71]; and lesions involving the central nervous system, especially the brain stem.[72–75] Notice that patients with intestinal dysmotility may have normal gastric manometric patterns but demonstrate delayed gastric emptying, supporting the view that these two tests can be complementary.

After partial gastrectomy and gastroenteric anastomosis, most persons do not experience long-term problems with intestinal dysmotility. However, some patients experience a profound motility disturbance involving fasting and fed activities.[76] Although no pathognomonic findings are seen on manometry, typically localized areas of intense activity alternate with regions of quiescence. The subset of patients who have been treated for postoperative gastric stasis with the Roux-en-Y procedure bears mentioning. Evidence suggest that the Roux limb itself may contribute to delayed emptying from the gastric remnant in some of those who had the procedure, perhaps because of loss of electrical synchrony in the implanted jejunal efferent limb.[77]

Patients who have received radiation therapy for abdominal malignancies and who develop radiation enteritis can exhibit abnormal gastroduodenal manometric findings, especially localized, poorly coordinated, either high- or low-amplitude pressure activity. Antral hypomotility can be observed and, in the presence of uncoordinated small intestinal activity, may be associated with intractable vomiting.[78–81]

A number of infectious processes can present with pseudoobstruction-like symptoms and signs and, therefore, are thought to be attributable in part to disturbances of gastrointestinal motility. These disorders may affect the intrinsic or autonomic neural pathways that regulate gastrointestinal motility and include infectious mononucleosis,[82] herpes varicella-zoster,[83] botulism B,[84] secondary bacterial overgrowth in the small intestine,[85] and the Guillain-Barré syndrome.[86]

Malignancies involving the posterior abdominal wall may interfere with the autonomic neural pathways to the gastrointestinal tract, producing a chronic ileus. Extraabdominal ma-

lignancies such as oat cell carcinoma of the lung can be associated with a paraneoplastic syndrome, which produces a clinical and manometric picture consistent with intestinal pseudoobstruction.[87,88]

Metabolic abnormalities associated with disturbances of gastrointestinal motility include hyperthyroidism and hypothyroidism and hyper- and hypoparathyroidism. Some reports suggest that rapid gastric emptying and rapid intestinal transit occur in hyperthyroidism.[89–91] Patients with hypothyroidism are at risk of developing pseudoobstruction, paralytic ileus, and megacolon.[92,93] Persons afflicted with hyperparathyroidism frequently report having symptoms of abdominal pain, nausea, vomiting, gastroesophageal reflux, and constipation possibly related to defective neurotransmission.[94,95] Hypoparathyroidism can be associated with intestinal pseudoobstruction and regional areas of tetany.[96] Patients with malnutrition and anorexia nervosa frequently have delayed gastric emptying, especially of solid meals.[97] The etiology of the disorder is not known, but disturbances of autonomic function have been reported.[98] Clinical situations associated with abnormalities of gastrointestinal manometry are summarized in Table 132-3.

In summary, gastroduodenal manometry is typically performed on patients with a suspected motility problem after metabolic, mucosal, and obstructive disturbances have been ruled out. Many patients will present with unexplained nausea, vomiting, and abdominal pain. Documentation of abnormal gastric emptying should be attempted before performing gas-

---

TABLE 132-3
Clinical Situations Associated With Abnormalities on Gastroduodenal Manometry

Patients Who Present With Symptoms and Signs of Gastroparesis and Demonstrate Absent Phase 3 Activity or Postcibal Antral Hypomotility on Manometry

Diabetes mellitus, type I with autonomic neuropathy

Drugs: adrenergic agonists, cholinergic antagonists, and opiate agonists

Postoperatively: fundoplication, vagotomy ± pyloroplasty, and cardiomyotomy for achalasia

Idiopathic

Disturbances of Intestinal Motility Presenting Clinically as Chronic Intestinal Pseudoobstruction

Manometry reveals localized region of infrequent, weak contractions, particularly in the postcibal state in the presence of relatively normal fasting motility pattern

Myotonic dystrophia

Late progressive systemic sclerosis

Manometry reveals abnormalities in both fasting and poscibal motility; in the fasting state, abnormalities in the configuration and propagation of phase 3 complexes are observed, whereas in the small intestine, localized, poorly coordinated bursts of tonic and phasic activities are seen

Early scleroderma

Diabetes mellitus

Amyloidosis

Visceral autonomica neuropathies, degenerative conditions involving the autonomic nervous system and lesions involving the central nervous system

troduodenal manometry. Gastrointestinal manometry can be useful in characterizing a motility disturbance as a neuropathic or myopathic process. This information can be helpful in making decisions regarding therapeutic measures.

ELECTROGASTROGRAPHY

Electrogastrography (EGG) measures gastric electrical activity. Interest in this technique has increased recently with the demonstration that gastric electrical patterns can be monitored noninvasively and that several clinical syndromes are associated with abnormal electrical patterns that may not be diagnosed using other available techniques for assessing upper gastrointestinal motility.

Electrophysiologic Basis of Gastric Motility

The development of a gastric contraction requires that electrical events occur at the membrane of smooth muscle cells. The electrophysiologic properties of gastric smooth muscle cells vary, depending on the region of stomach. Myoelectrical activity in the proximal one third of the stomach is characterized by a steady, nonfluctuating, transmembrane potential associated with slow contractions occurring every 1 to 3 minutes. The electrical changes observed in this region are small in magnitude and usually not seen during EGG. The distal two thirds of the stomach and small intestine demonstrate slow, phasic changes in membrane potential. This cyclic change in electrical potential has been called various names including basal electrical rhythm (BER), slow waves, pacesetter potential, and control potential.

The term BER is gaining acceptance and is used in this discussion. The BER appears to originate from the longitudinal muscle layer or nonneural boundary cells between the longitudinal and circular layers.[99–101] An important feature of the BER is that it represents cyclic depolarization of the

smooth muscle cells in the absence of associated peristaltic contractions (Fig. 132-9). Rapid depolarization of the smooth muscle membrane is necessary for a contraction to occur. This event is referred to as an action potential or electrical response activity (see Fig. 132-9). Peristaltic contractions in the gastric body and proximal antrum are associated with an increase in the amplitude and duration of the depolarization plateau above the threshold for smooth muscle contraction. In the distal antrum and small intestine, contractions are associated with electrical spikes or action potentials superimposed on the depolarization plateau.

The maximal frequency that gastrointestinal smooth muscle can contract is established by the frequency of the BER in that region. In the stomach the frequency of the BER is established by a *pacemaker* site located in the proximal body along the greater curvature.[102] In humans the BER propagates longitudinally and circumferentially from this site at a frequency of approximately three cycles per minute. In the duodenum the frequency increases to 11 to 12 cycles per minute, which is established by a different pacemaker. Passage of the BER between the stomach and duodenum is prevented by the pylorus, which acts as a functional barrier. Propagation of the BER occurs myogenically by way of gap junctions between adjacent smooth muscle cells. Occurrence of peristaltic contractions is influenced by several factors including the presence of a fed or fasted state, the neurotransmitter and hormonal milieu, and, most likely, the presence of local regulatory, or paracrine, substances. The presence of these regulatory substances appears to influence the sensitivity of smooth muscle cells to contract by decreasing or increasing the occurrence of plateau potentials. The force of contraction is determined by the amplitude and duration of the plateau potential.

The cause of gastric dysrhythmias at the cellular level is not known. However, in vitro studies on antral tissue removed from a patient with marked gastric retention revealed a tachygastria-like electrical pattern that normalized after treatment with the prostaglandin inhibitor indomethacin.[103] Application of prostaglandin E_2 resulted in return of the

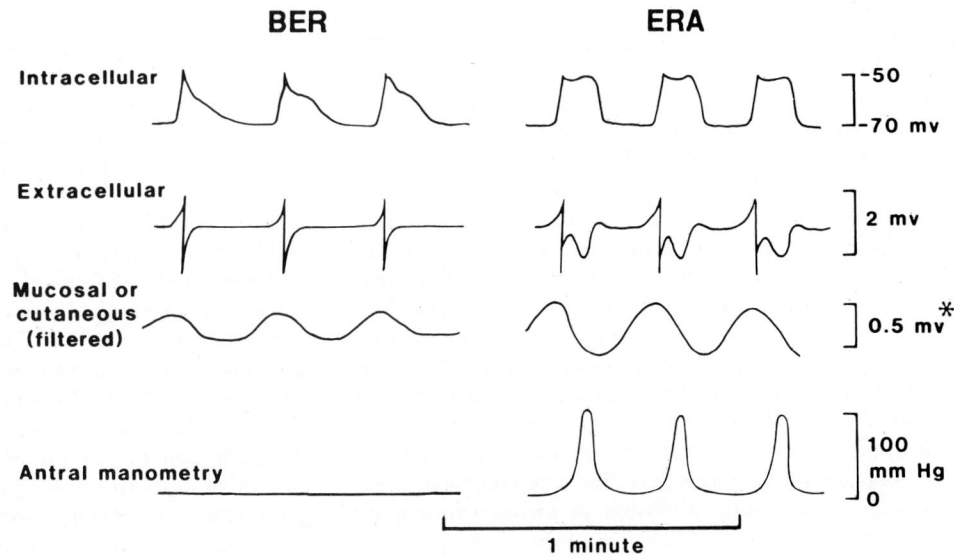

FIGURE 132-9. Stylized representation of intracellular, extracellular, and mucosal or cutaneous (filtered) electrogastrographic signals, with accompanying manometric activity. Basal electrical activity (BER) and electrical response activity (ERA) are represented. Basal electrical activity may cause some contractile activity but does not result in gastric peristalsis and usually is not detected by manometry. Voltage shown is for cutaneous recording; mucosal recordings approach 2 mV. (From Abell TL, Malagelada J-R. Electrogastrography: current assessment and future perspective. Dig Dis Sci 1988;33:983.)

tachygastria-like electrical pattern. This suggests that some gastric dysrhythmias may result from disorders associated with enhanced prostaglandin activity.

Technical Aspects

Three techniques have been used to record electrical activity of the stomach. These include serosal, mucosal, and cutaneous EEG. This chapter emphasizes cutaneous EGG because this technique is noninvasive and, therefore, more suitable for evaluation of humans. Serosal recordings require a laparotomy for surgical placement of the recording electrodes. Mucosal recordings require intubation and attachment of the recording electrode to the gastric lining by suction or by using magnetic force to hold the electrode in position.[104,105] Mucosal recordings reflect the *true* extracellular gastric electrical activity better than cutaneous recordings and appear to be less susceptible to interference from extragastric electrical signals from duodenal, colonic, cardiac, and respiratory sources.[106] However, the suction electrodes are prone to detachment from the mucosa, especially during postprandial monitoring, which limits application of this approach. This problem led to the development of a technique in which the internal electrodes are maintained in apposition with the anterior gastric wall using magnetic force.[105] Proper positioning of the recording electrodes is confirmed fluoroscopically. Optimally, at least three internal electrodes should be used, which permits assessment of the direction of electrical propagation: antegrade versus retrograde conduction. Respiratory movements are recorded concurrently with a pneumobelt transducer. Using this recording technique, EGG signals have been recorded for 6 hours in the fasting and fed state, which represents a significant improvement in the duration of recordings compared with those obtained with suction electrodes. Problems with this technique are encountered when the stomach is located underneath the rib cage while in the supine position and with morbidly obese person. In both situations, the likelihood of internal electrode detachment increases.

Cutaneous recording requires the placement of electrodes across the anterior abdominal wall, along the *antral axis,* which represents the imaginary line along the proximal to distal portion of the stomach. Usually four electrodes are positioned in the left upper quadrant along the antral axis line equidistant from the xiphoid and the umbilicus. Fluoroscopy is helpful for electrode positioning because of individual variability in stomach size and shape. *Monopolar* recording devices, those with one active and one ground electrode, and *bipolar* recording devices, those with two active and one ground electrode, have been used for cutaneous EGG. However, the quality of recordings obtained with the bipolar configuration appears to be better because of the advantageous signal-to-noise ratio it provides.[104] The electrodes are coated with electrode jelly before positioning on the patient's skin. The electrical activity detected by cutaneous electrodes reflects potential differences over large areas of the stomach and, therefore, the summation of electric potentials generated by many gastric smooth muscle cells. The signal monitored represents the basal electrical rhythm in the noncontracting stomach and electrical response activity in the contracting stomach. The cutaneous EGG signal correlates well with the frequency but not the amplitude of serosal recordings.

The electrical signals monitored during cutaneous EGG usually require some form of filtering to decrease undesired signals from other sites, such as the duodenum, colon, heart, and lungs.[107,108] However, this involves a trade-off because filtering can result in the loss of useful data. In addition, cutaneous monitoring may increase the likelihood of missing focal gastric electrical disturbances because they are hidden by the signal from the normally depolarizing gastric smooth muscle cells.

The normal gastric electrical signal in the human occurs at frequency of approximately three to four cycles per minute. This is equivalent to 0.05 Hz. The typical EGG filter partially eliminates signals having frequencies more than 0.2 Hz (12 cycles per minute) and less than 0.03 Hz (1.8 cycles per minute). In addition to filtering, the EGG signal is amplified and recorded along with other signals, such as manometric data, on a polygraph.[109,110] Contemporary recording systems include an analog-to-digital converter, which allows storage of data on a computer disk or magnetic tape for subsequent analysis.

Mucosal and cutaneous recordings can be analyzed visually for information regarding frequency, amplitude, and configuration of waveforms. However, computer-based analytic techniques have become the norm because they expedite analysis of large amounts of data and generate useful information from recordings unsuitable for visual interpretation because of obscure signals. Most methods used to analyze EGG signals employ some form of spectral analysis incorporating one of several available mathematical models such as the Fast Fourier Transformation, which transforms the signal from the time domain to a frequency spectrum.[111-113]

A *power spectrum* of the recorded signals is obtained (Fig. 132-10). The fundamental frequency, three cycles per minute or 0.05 Hz in humans, is represented with greater power because this frequency contributes a greater portion of the recorded signal frequencies. Other electrical frequencies originating from the duodenal, colonic, respiratory, or cardiac sources may be represented, but at a lower power. One drawback of this approach is loss of the ability to determine when specific events occurred during the recording period. For example, it is typically necessary to record data for several minutes to compute the *transform,* which generates the frequencies present during the recording interval and, therefore, hinders correlation of the EGG data with manometric data and the patient's symptoms. This limitation has been partially alleviated by the development of running spectral analysis.[114] In this approach, the power spectra of brief overlapping stretches of the EGG signal are computed and presented as a function of time. Although easy to perform, this approach is susceptible to problems associated with inaccurate or erratic spectral estimates because of the recording time required to generate an accurate Fast Fourier Transformation. Dysrhythmias of brief duration will not be detected reliably using this approach. This issue is addressed in part by *adaptive spectral analysis* that improves the detection of short-duration dysrhythmias using adaptive autoregressive moving-average modeling.[115]

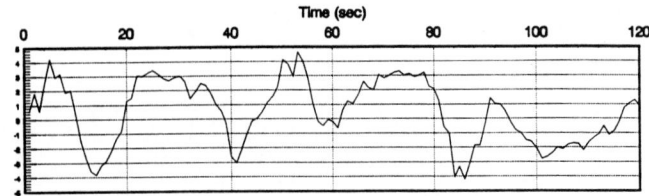

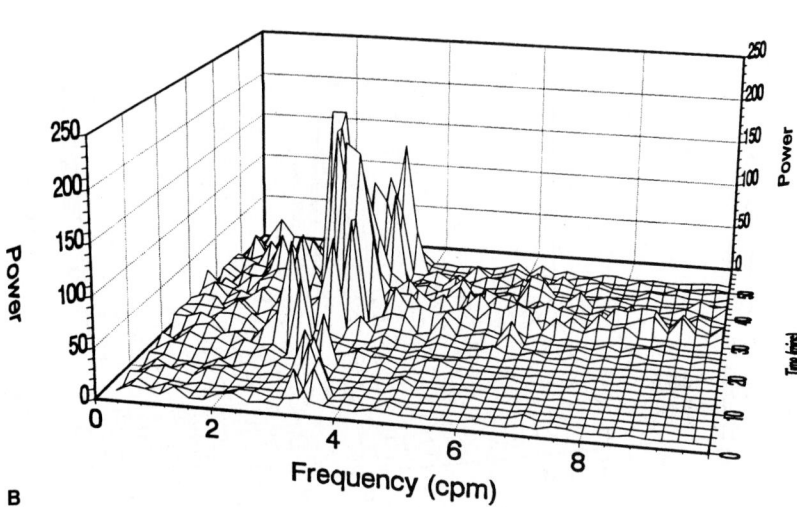

FIGURE 132-10. The results of an electro-gastrographic study of a healthy volunteer. **(A)** The raw slow-wave signal after ingestion of a 500-kcal mixed solid-liquid meal. The signal appears as a regular sinusoidal wave with a period of approximately 20 seconds. The raw signal can be analyzed by power spectral analysis to determine the dominant slow wave frequency at any given time during the record-ing. **(B)** The pseudo–three-dimensional plot from the power spectral analysis. With fasting the slow wave was regular at 3 cpm, but of low intensity. With meal ingestion, at 15 min-utes there was a transient decrease in slow-wave frequency and a prolonged increase in signal amplitude at 3 cpm. (Courtesy of William Hasler, M.D., Ann Arbor, MI.)

Indications and Contraindications

Because of its level of refinement, EGG should be limited to medical centers with the technical expertise to conduct and interpret these studies. The indication for performing EGG is similar to that for gastroduodenal manometry, namely, a patient who presents with a history of unexplained nausea, vomiting, and evidence of impaired gastric emptying. EGG is usually performed in conjunction with gastroduodenal ma-nometry. EGG complements gastroduodenal manometry and gastric emptying studies by providing additional information that may reveal the basis for disturbed gastric motility.

Interpreting the Electrogastrogram

The normal gastric electrical signal in the human is established by the gastric pacemaker at a frequency of three to four cycles per minute. The characteristic shape of the electrical waveform detected during EGG varies, depending on the location of the recording electrode: internal (mucosal or serosal) versus external (cutaneous) electrogastrogram. Abnormalities have been described involving both increased rates, or tachygastria, and decreased rates, or bradygastria, of electrical pacemaker activity. Tachygastria, defined as more than three cycles per minute, and bradygastria, defined as less than two cycles per minute, should be present for at least 1 minute.[116] Other elec-trical abnormalities include the presence of a dysrhythmia associated with an irregular resting membrane potential and abnormal wave configuration and a *mixed* or so-called tachy-bradyarrhythmia.[116] Tachygastria frequently develops at an

ectopic site in the distal antrum and propagates in a retrograde manner.[117] Gastric contractions are often absent in the pres-ence of tachygastria because of deformed BER, resulting in the failure of the plateau potential to reach threshold poten-tial.[110,118] In contrast, bradygastria arises in the corpus and antrum and propagates aborally.[119]

Clinical Situations That Affect the Electrogastrogram

The amplitude of slow wave activity detected by cutaneous EGG increases during gastric contractions in the fasting and fed states. The relation between postprandial gastric emptying and the cutaneous electrogastrogram in primates has been examined; the EGG amplitude but not the frequency corre-lated significantly with gastric emptying.[120]

Tachygastria and other dysrhythmias have been reported in patients with unexplained nausea, bloating, and vomiting (Fig. 132-11)[117]; symptomatic ulcer patients[121]; children with nonulcer dyspepsia and delayed gastric emptying[122]; pregnant women who were experiencing nausea (Fig. 132-12)[123]; dia-betics with chronic nausea, vomiting, and delayed gastric emptying in the fasting state[113]; and in normal subjects in whom motion sickness is induced experimentally.[124,125]

Preliminary studies suggest that treatment of idiopathic gastroparesis with metoclopramide was associated with res-olution of the patient's gastrointestinal discomfort and tach-ygastria.[126] Administration of domperidone to a person with diabetic gastroparesis resulted in normalization of the patient's bradygastria and improvement in symptoms.[126]

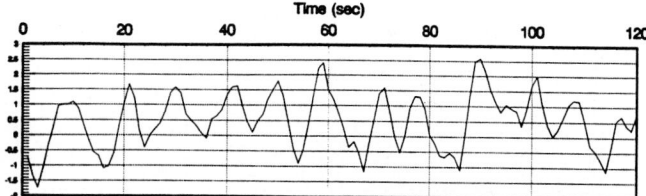

A

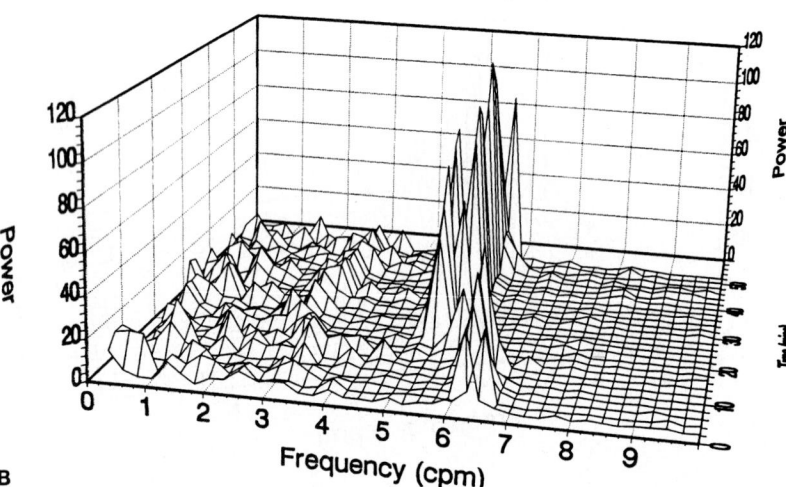

B

FIGURE 132-11. Electrogastrography (EGG) was used to evaluate a 28-year-old woman with persistent nausea, bloating, and fullness who had previously undergone a solid phase gastric emptying scan, which gave normal results. (**A**) A low-amplitude raw EGG signal after ingestion of a 250-kcal liquid meal with a period of approximately 10 seconds. The raw EGG signal was evaluated with power spectral analysis. (**B**) The pseudo–three-dimensional plot demonstrates the presence of a dominant slow-wave frequency that is higher (5 to 6 cpm) than in the healthy volunteer (see Fig. 132-10). This patient showed evidence of tachygastria, which was associated with antral hypomotility on a simultaneously performed manometric study. (Courtesy of William Hasler, M.D., Ann Arbor, MI.)

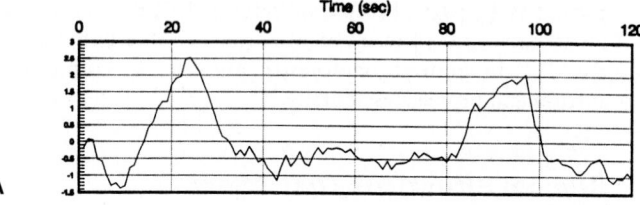

A

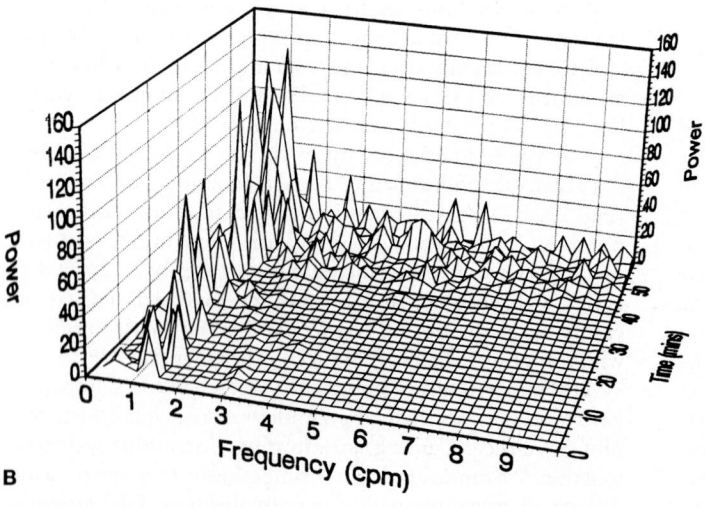

B

FIGURE 132-12. Women with nausea in the first trimester of pregnancy can exhibit marked slow-wave disturbances. Electrogastrography was performed on a 22-year-old woman in the eleventh week of pregnancy. (**A**) Large but infrequent slow waves are seen on the raw tracing. Pseudo–three-dimensional plotting of the power spectral analysis demonstrates that the bulk of the slow wave signal is in the frequency range from 0.75 to 2 cpm. This pregnant patient exhibited bradygastria in association with her first trimester nausea. (Courtesy of William Hasler, M.D., Ann Arbor, MI.)

In summary, the electrogastrogram can be a useful diagnostic tool in the evaluation of patients with unexplained nausea, vomiting, and delayed gastric emptying. The EGG should be considered in individuals with delayed gastric emptying after metabolic and structural abnormalities have been ruled out. EGG can provide information regarding whether a gastric dysrhythmia presenting in the form of tachygastria, bradygastria, or a combined tachybradyarrhythmia is the cause of the motility disturbance. This information is not readily derived from manometry. The technique also may prove to be useful for following a patient's course and response to therapy.

COLONIC SCINTIGRAPHY

During the last decade, the techniques of nuclear scintigraphy have been applied to monitor motility patterns and transit in the small intestine and colon. This section focuses on colonic scintigraphy, a relatively new technique to quantify fecal movements. Dysfunction of colonic motility is believed to be important factor in a number of common abnormalities, including the irritable bowel syndrome and idiopathic constipation. Understanding of the normal motility patterns of the colon has lagged behind other regions of the gastrointestinal tract, largely because of technical problems in monitoring the colon under physiologic conditions. Some of these technical issues have been addressed with colonic scintigraphy. Other methods to assess colonic motor function are associated with a number of methodologic problems including a lack of a quantifiable measurement, high radiation exposure, introduction of foreign body artifact by the measuring system, and the fact that recording methods do not allow monitoring under physiologic conditions.

Historically, colonic transit has been measured radiographically after ingestion of radiopaque markers. A predetermined number of markers are administered orally and abdominal roentgenograms are obtained to follow the transit of the markers.[127,128] These studies indicate that the mean colon transit in healthy individuals ranges between 35 and 40 hours. However, considerable intersubject variation exists. Roentgenograms are obtained beginning 1 to 4 days after the subject ingests the markers. Therefore this method is limited to the evaluation of suspected, prolonged colonic transit. Assessment of accelerated colonic transit with this technique would require serial abdominal radiograms soon after ingestion of the markers. This would probably represent an unacceptable level of radiation exposure.

Technical Aspects

Usually γ-emitting radionuclide markers have been used to assess colonic transit because they are associated with low radiation exposure, can be imaged noninvasively, and are comfortable to the patient. Several markers have been studied including iodine-131–cellulose,[129] indium-111–diethylene triamine pentaacetic acid (DTPA),[130] and technetium Tc 99m pellets or semisolids.[131] ^{131}I-fiber has the disadvantages of a long half-life, difficult preparation, and relatively high radiation exposure. ^{111}In-DTPA is not absorbed from the gastrointestinal tract and possesses a half-life of 68 hours that allows adequate imaging of patients with colonic inertia. [99m]Tc, with a half-life of 6 hours, is well suited to evaluate patients in whom rapid colonic transit is suspected, but the tracer may not be present for a sufficient period of time to image some patients with colonic inertia.

An advantage of using a γ-emitting radionuclide marker compared with traditional roentgenography is that serial scans can be obtained without increasing the radiation exposure to the patient. Historically, nuclear scintigraphic studies of colonic transit required orocecal intubation to place the radioisotope directly into the colon to avoid dispersion of the radiolabel during passage through the proximal gut. The recent development of placing ^{111}In-labeled ion-exchange polystyrene pellets in a medication capsule coated with a layer of the pH-sensitive polymer, methacrylate, has facilitated performing these studies in a noninvasive manner.[132] This approach takes advantage of the pH gradient in the small intestine (mean duodenal pH, 6.5; mean ileal pH, 7.4).[133] In vitro studies indicate that the capsule will dissolve in approximately 1 hour at a pH between 7.2 and 7.4.[132] In about 95% of cases the capsule dissolves as predicted and deposits the radiolabeled pellets directly into the ascending colon.[132] A comparison of ^{131}I-cellulose and ^{111}In-DTPA revealed that ^{111}In-DTPA resulted in images of higher resolution, improved counting characteristics, a decrease in absorbed dose to the patient, and minimal urinary excretion.[134] Furthermore, ^{111}In-DTPA and radiolabeled physiologic cellulose fibers had indistinguishable colonic transit patterns.

Indications and Contraindications

Clinically, colonic scintigraphy has most often been employed in the assessment of constipation and to quantify the severity of colonic inertia. However, because it allows serial imaging without increased radiation exposure, the technique is well suited to assess the possibility of rapid colonic transit, for example, in patients with diarrhea-prone irritable bowel syndrome or hyperthyroid conditions. It is also likely to find a role in assessing therapeutic response, such as in the use of prokinetic agents for treating colonic inertia.

Colonic scintigraphy is a safe technique under most circumstances. However, if concern exists about the presence of an obstructive process, this should be ruled out because it would severely limit the usefulness of the study. Orocecal intubation is a relatively invasive procedure that is not well tolerated by some patients. If ^{131}I-cellulose is employed as the tracer, Lugol's iodine, or a similar agent, should be administered two drops three times a day for 7 days beginning 2 days before tracer ingestion to block thyroidal uptake of radioiodine.

Data Interpretation

The colon is divided into several regions of interest, for example, ascending, transverse, descending, and rectosigmoid. The raw gamma counts are routinely corrected for depth, using geometric mean of anterior and posterior counts; isotope decay; and Compton scattering.[135] Colonic transit is assessed by identifying the geometric center, which represents the weighted mean of the proportions of counts in each of the regions of interest, as well as feces at predetermined time points, for example at 4, 12, and 24 hours. Each of the regions of interest and the feces at predetermined points are assigned a number that serves as a weighting factor. The proportion of counts in each region is multiplied by the weighting factor and the sum calculated.[130] Using this approach, a low geometric center indicates that most of the radiolabel resides near the cecum whereas a high geometric center suggests that most of the label is located in the distal colon. The rate of emptying from each region of interest also can be calculated. An alternative approach has been described that relies on merging multiple images of the colon recorded on multiple days to generate a composite image of the colon.[134] The composite image is used to identify up to 11 regions of interest, which are joined together with straight-line segments when necessary to form a continuous *colon line* from cecum to rectum. The counts at a particular point along the colon are obtained by summing the counts in the pixels of a line perpendicular to the colon line. A graphic representation of the distribution of activity is obtained that allows the *mean position of activity* in the colon to be calculated. Advocates of this approach suggest that this method avoids some inherent difficulties associated with the geometric center approach, namely, that geometric center analysis does not take into account interpatient differences in colon shape, total length, length of each segment, and interoperator variability in drawing the regions of interest. Difficulties can arise in the approach using the mean position of the activity when the rectum overlaps the cecum on the composite image, which makes drawing the colon line problematic. Figure 132-13 (see Color Fig. 113) depicts a colonic scintigraphy study in a healthy volunteer using the tracer ^{111}In-DTPA delivered to the cecum by means of orocecal intubation. The passage of the tracer through the colon is demonstrated along with representative regions of interest and the mean position of activity versus time.

Clinical Application

Colonic scintigraphy should be performed only at referral centers with experience in nuclear medicine and should be viewed as a potentially promising clinical technique. However, until safe orally deliverable tracers, such as the methacrylate-coated capsules containing ^{111}In-DTPA microspheres, become more readily available and imaging studies become more competitively priced, this methodology will remain primarily a research technique. Colonic scintigraphy has been particularly useful in improving understanding of normal colon transit patterns which, in turn, has provided the foundation for appreciating abnormal motor patterns associated with various gastrointestinal disorders. For example, scintigraphic techniques have revealed the following: chyme is delivered from the ileum into the cecum in boluses, which is impaired in patients with myopathic pseudoobstruction[136]; and emptying of the proximal colon is delayed in idiopathic constipation[137] and rapid in patients with diarrhea-prone irritable bowel syndrome.[138] Colonic scintigraphy has been most frequently employed in research studies to compare colonic

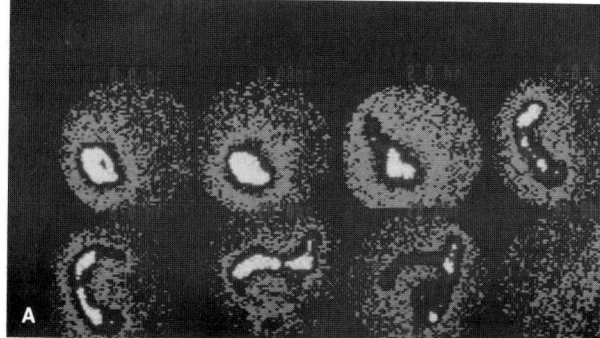

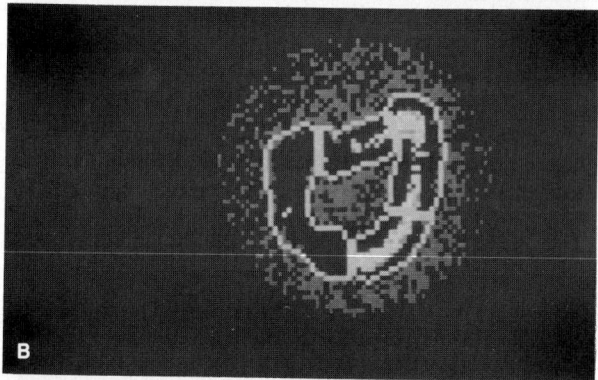

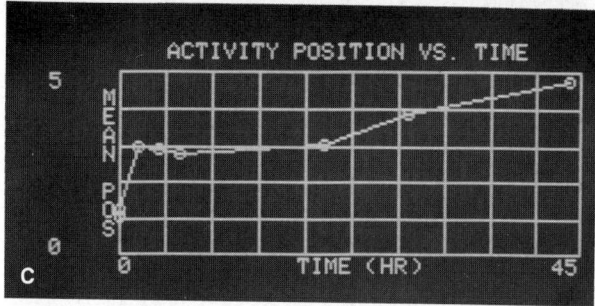

FIGURE 132-13. (See Color Fig. 113.) Colonic scintigraphy study using [111]Indium-DPTA. The tracer was delivered to the cecum by means of orocecal intubation in a healthy man. **(A)** Passage of the tracer through the colon. Beginning at the time of installation of the tracer (0 hour), scans were performed at the times indicated above the images. **(B)** Typical regions of interest (ROIs) in a representative cumulative scan of the colon. In this study, the colon was partitioned into four ROIs that correspond to the ascending, transverse, descending, and rectosigmoid regions of the colon. Assessment of the amount of tracer in the feces after defecation represents a fifth ROI. **(C)** The mean position of tracer activity versus time in a representative colonic scintigraphy study. The colon was partitioned into ROIs as described previously. In this study, the mean activity of the tracer passed from the ascending to descending colon in 0.8 to 2 hours and accumulated in the rectosigmoid colon over the ensuing 28 hours. (Courtesy of Mark Sims, M.D., Ann Arbor, MI.)

transit in healthy volunteers and individuals with unexplained constipation. Colonic transit in healthy volunteers and constipated individuals has been studied using orally administered ^{111}In-DTPA, and clear differences were observed between the groups with normal and constipated persons based on total and segmental percent retention over 4 days. The half-clearance times for normal and constipated patients were 28.6 ± 11.1 and 68.0 ± 24.9, respectively (mean hour ± SD, $P < 0.001$).[134] Whole bowel transit in normal subjects and patients with irritable bowel syndrome was examined using a nondisintegrating capsule and radiolabeled resin particles.[131] Colonic transit of the capsule was faster than the particles and, on average, patients with the diarrhea-prone irritable bowel syndrome demonstrated faster transit than normal subjects.

In summary, the optimal approach to assess colonic transit should be quantifiable, reproducible, physiologic, easy to perform, and should generate clinically relevant results. In addition, the method should be safe and demonstrate a favorable cost-benefit profile. At its level of development, colonic scintigraphy satisfies several of these criteria. Whereas the approach typically requires access to a γ-camera, it is easy to perform, well tolerated, physiologic, and generates clinically useful information. This is particularly true when the newer orally administered tracers such as ^{111}In-DTPA are employed. Critical examination of cost-benefit ratios will remain an issue until scintigraphic imaging becomes more competitively priced. Colonic scintigraphy is obtained in evaluating patients with idiopathic constipation, but it can also provide useful information in patients with suspected rapid colonic transit.

Although it lacks the accuracy and physiologic attributes of the radionuclide approach, the traditional radiographic technique employing multiple radiopaque markers and a single abdominal radiograph remains a cost-effective method to evaluate patients with suspected colonic inertia.[139] Finally, when evaluating a patient in whom a problem with colonic motility is suspected, the clinician should always consider the possibility that a more generalized disorder of gastrointestinal motor function is present.

ANORECTAL MANOMETRY

Anorectal manometry is used in the clinical assessment of patients in whom a problem with defecation is suspected. The technique is helpful in evaluating the most distal components of the anorectal sphincter mechanism: the internal and external sphincter muscles.[140]

No single methodologic approach for the study of anorectal function has gained uniform acceptance. Various techniques, including rectal compliance, electromyography, radiographic defecography, and anorectal manometry, have been used alone and in combination to examine anorectal function. This section focuses on the methods and interpretation of studies evaluating the anal sphincter mechanism.

Technical Aspects

Direct pressure-sensitive microtransducers and perfused probes have been used to record anal sphincter pressure. The former eliminates the need for a fluid perfusion system by positioning the sensor device at the point at which pressure is to be monitored. Potential drawbacks include the relatively high cost and susceptibility of the solid-state microtransducer system to malfunction. The latter approach relies on the per-fusion of a noncompressible fluid, such as water, at a constant rate through low-compliance catheters. Change in pressure is monitored as change in the resistance to flow that the sphincter offers to the constant flow.

Several technical issues must be kept in mind when performing anorectal manometry, particularly with the perfused catheter system. These include the potential for inducing recording artifacts because of probe rigidity, probe diameter, and the infusion rate. For example, a rigid probe is easier to position but can deform the anal canal and thereby produce an artifact. The diameter of the probe introduces some distortion of the anal canal by its very placement; therefore it is advisable to use the smallest probe diameter, which is 4 to 8 mm, that allows adequate contact with the opposing surfaces of the canal. From a practical standpoint, this is not an important issue unless dealing with a patient who has a markedly patulous sphincter. In this situation, it may be necessary to use a larger diameter probe of 10 to 20 mm. Infusion rates usually are 0.3 to 1.0 mL/minute/channel. During a routine study taking 15 to 45 minutes to complete, considerable fluid accumulation can occur with the rectum when using a mutilumen probe with 3 to 12 channels per probe. This can alter the reproducibility of the results during the recording period.

The pressure profile of the anal sphincter is obtained using a station pull-out or continuous pull-out technique. The state pull-out approach involves positioning the probe several centimeters above the anal verge and measuring the pressure at various intervals, usually 1 cm, while removing the probe. Because moving the probe itself induces changes in sphincter pressure, a stabilization period of 30 seconds is observed before recording the pressure at each interval. The advantage of this approach is the accuracy of the pressure recordings at each interval. This is potentially offset by the absence of the entire pressure profile and failure to identify accurately the point of maximal squeeze pressure. With the continuous pull-out technique, the probe is positioned above the canal and subsequently pulled through the sphincter at a constant rate, producing a continuous pressure profile along the longitudinal axis of the anal canal. To help avoid recording artifacts with this approach, a mechanical pulling device must be used to ensure consistency and reproducibility. The probe should be rendered as frictionless as possible with the liberal use of lubricant.

An important modification of these recording techniques involves positioning and distention of a balloon within the rectum to examine the rectal-anal inhibitory reflex.[141] This is often referred to as balloon reflex manometry. Distention of the rectum by stool, or artificially with a balloon, should evoke relaxation of the internal anal sphincter. The balloon catheter assembly is positioned 10 to 15 cm above the anal verge and distended to a volume greater than 60 mL to initiate the inhibitory reflex. Either two small balloons or the perfused catheter system are positioned in the anal canal to monitor the internal and external sphincter response to distention of the rectal balloon. Relaxation should be observed only at the level of the internal sphincter. A typical persuasion apparatus used to perform balloon reflex manometry is shown in Figure 132-14. Normal proximal sphincter response to increased rectal pressure during balloon distention is depicted in Figure 132-15.

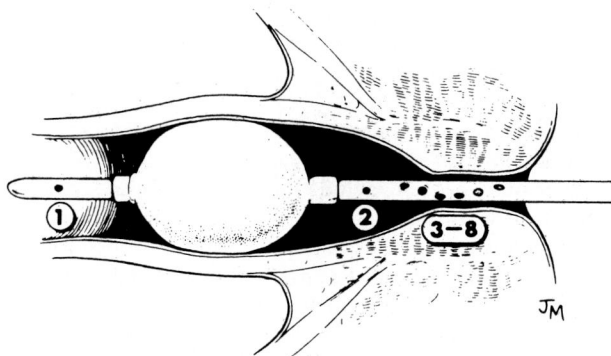

FIGURE 132-14. Perfused multilumen probe for balloon reflex manometric study. The balloon, positioned 10 to 15 cm above the anal verge, is capable of distending through at least 60 mL. Orifices 1 and 2 record intraluminal rectal pressure. Orifices 3 through 8 are located within the sphincter at 0.5-cm intervals. (From Coller JA. Clinical application of anorectal manometry. Gastroenterol Clin North Am 1987;16:27.)

Indications and Contraindications

The decision to perform anorectal manometry should be based on the patient's clinical history and the likelihood that an evaluation of the sphincter mechanism will yield information useful in management of the patient's problem. The decision to proceed with anorectal manometry is based on the patient's history and the physical examination of the anorectal area. Notice that use of the examiner's finger as a pressure probe is highly inaccurate compared with objective measurements of sphincter function.[142]

Most patients complain of constipation or incontinence. A number of problems can be assessed adequately on the basis of clinical history, physical examination, and routine laboratory tests. Examples include irritable bowel syndrome, maldigestion, and thyroid dysfunction. A specific example involving the anal sphincter mechanism in which anorectal manometry would not indicated is the presence of an acute anal fissure. This condition is associated with a deviation from the normal mean resting anal sphincter pressure,[143] but performance of manometry would not contribute any useful information beyond that obtained from the physical examination.

When constipation is associated with the perception of increased pelvic or rectal pressure, incomplete evacuation, or difficulty initiating defecation, there is an increased likelihood that anorectal manometry may be a useful diagnostic aid. On the other hand, if resting sphincter tone appears normal or elevated in the presence of incontinence, balloon reflex manometry is indicated to evaluate the possibility of decreased threshold or increased sensitivity to rectal distention.

Data Interpretation

Manometric studies of the anal canal are typically plotted on an X-Y recorder, which presents a visual comparison of the various channels relative to one another. Unfortunately, subsequent quantitative analysis is often manually performed, which is laborious and time consuming. However, micro-

computer software packages have been developed that use an analog-to-digital converter to process and store data, and to facilitate subsequent analysis of the pressure recordings (MMS-200, Narco Biosystems, Houston, TX). A typical microcomputer-generated tracing of the resting longitudinal anorectal sphincter pressure profile is depicted in Figure 132-16. The proximal end of the sphincter is that point at which the pressure is clearly above the intralumenal rectal pressure. This occurs when the perfusion orifices are withdrawn from the intralumenal rectum into the anal sphincter musculature. The normal sphincter length varies from 2.5 to 5.0 cm. A high-pressure zone is observed while the perfusion apparatus passes the distal portion of the internal sphincter muscle. The high-pressure zone is defined as that portion of the sphincter that demonstrates pressures greater than one half the maximal pressure. The point of maximal pressure is located in the distal proton of the high-pressure zone, approximately 1 to 1.5 cm from the distal end of the sphincter musculature. The normal average maximal resting pressure in the adult ranges from 65 to 85 mm Hg above rectal intralumenal pressure when measured with a perfused multichannel probe using the continuous pull-out technique. Usually a modest lowering of the resting pressure occurs with aging.[144]

Recent studies evaluating the longitudinal pressure profile of the anal canal with multichannel, radically positioned probes reveal evidence for radial pressure asymmetry. In the proximal sphincter, the posterior quadrant exhibits pressure predominance, whereas in the distal sphincter, the anterior quadrant demonstrates predominance.[145] Therefore the longitudinal pressure profile reveals that the resting sphincter is a somewhat distorted cylinder with a gentle gradient of pressure, which shifts from posterior to anterior with movement from the rostral to the caudal end of the sphincter.

In addition to the resting sphincter pressure profile, patients undergoing anorectal manometry often have the maximal voluntary squeeze pressure evaluated. This test is thought to reflect the contribution of the striated external sphincter. A voluntary squeeze should produce an increase of 50% to 100% over the average maximal resting pressure. Absolute normal values or ranges for voluntary squeeze pressure have not been agreed on in the literature, although women tend to have lower values than men.[144] The point of maximal pressure is located in the distal portion of the sphincter, similar to the situation at rest. When evaluating external sphincter function with the voluntary squeeze maneuver, several technical issues should be kept in mind. The examiner must clearly state to the patient what is required to perform a voluntary

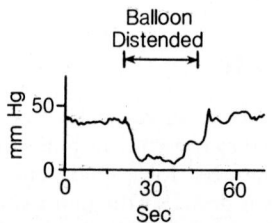

FIGURE 132-15. Normal internal anal sphincter relaxation response to balloon distention in the rectum. The balloon was located 15 cm above the anal verge and distended to 60 mL for the time shown. (Courtesy of Jeff Barnett, M.D., Ann Arbor, MI.)

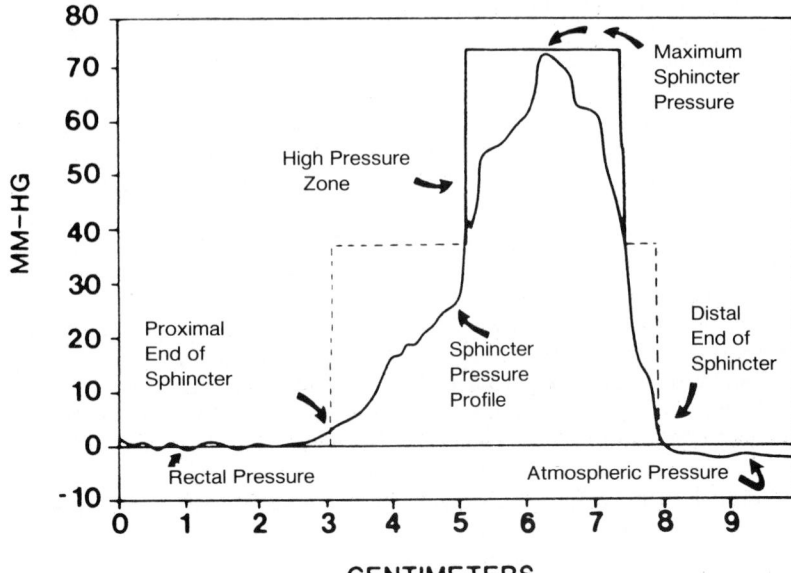

FIGURE 132-16. Typical longitudinal pressure profile of the resting anorectal sphincter. Pressures have been equated to a zero rectal pressure. The pressures from an eight-channel multilumen probe during continuous resting pullout have been averaged at each point along the sphincter by microcomputer. (From Coller JA. Clinical application of anorectal manometry. Gastroenterol Clin North Am 1987;16:20.)

squeeze. This is best achieved by placing a finger into the anal canal and instructing the patient regarding the appropriate voluntary squeeze effort. The squeezing effort results in movement of the anal canal due because of the involvement of pelvic musculature; therefore the probe should move freely with the sphincter to maintain the same position within the canal, which allows accurate comparison of resting and voluntary squeeze pressure at the same point. The external sphincter can sustain a voluntary squeeze for about 1 minute, after which fatigue occurs; therefore the probe should be withdrawn within 30 to 40 seconds to obtain an accurate indication of the longitudinal pressure profile during voluntary squeeze.

Clinical Applications

Anorectal manometry is useful in the initial evaluation of patients with constipation and in the person with incontinence. The technique also may be useful to monitor progression of a disorder that affects anal sphincter function or the response to therapeutic interventions such as biofeedback in the appropriate patient with incontinence.

Constipation

When anorectal manometry reveals a normal or high average maximal resting pressure, the examiner should proceed with balloon reflex manometry to evaluate whether the internal sphincter relaxes in response to rectal distention. If rectal distention fails to initiate relaxation of the internal sphincter, the diagnosis of Hirschsprung's disease should be considered (Fig. 132-17).[146] If the inhibitory reflex is present but demonstrates a high threshold for initiation, a problem with rectal compliance or afferent (sensory) pathways may be present. This pattern is observed in some patients with acquired megacolon or spinal cord injuries.[147] If the patient shows a deficient increase in voluntary squeeze pressure, abnormalities of sacral

root innervation to the external sphincter should be considered.[148,149]

Some patients with constipation demonstrate a low average maximal resting pressure and normal rectal distention-mediated inhibition of the internal sphincter. In this scenario, the examiner should consider other anatomic abnormalities in the anorectal mechanism, such as accentuated puborectalis angulation or internal rectal prolapse to explain the defecation problem. In addition, the constipated patient with low resting sphincter pressure deserves special mention because of the problems these persons face if an inappropriate sphincterotomy is performed. This procedure could potentially leave the patient with persistent constipation and iatrogenic loss of anal sphincter control.

Incontinence

Assessment of resting and sphincter pressures, voluntary squeeze response, and balloon reflex manometry can be used to identify the location of abnormalities in anorectal function associated with incontinence. These findings can be helpful in directing therapy. For example, when the incontinent patient exhibits normal or elevated resting sphincter pressures,

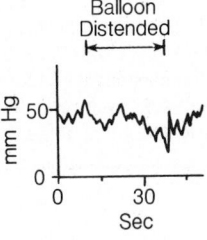

FIGURE 132-17. Patient with Hirschsprung's disease. Tracing depicts failure of normal internal and sphincter relaxation in response to rectal balloon distention. The balloon is positioned 15 cm above the anal verge and distended to 60 mL for the time shown. (Courtesy of Jeff Barnett, M.D., Ann Arbor, MI.)

balloon reflex testing should be performed to rule out decreased threshold or increased sensitivity to rectal distention. Demonstration of these abnormalities suggests that a problem in rectal compliance underlies the incontinence.

The typical patient with incontinence related to anorectal dysfunction and no history of trauma has low resting anal sphincter pressures. The voluntary squeeze response can help localize a problem in anal sphincter control to the internal or external sphincter. If a normal increase in tone is noticed with voluntary squeeze, this suggests that the problem resides in the internal sphincter, which can occur after hemorrhoid surgery or with diseases that affect the autonomic nervous system or smooth muscle cell function such as diabetes mellitus and progressive systemic sclerosis.[150,151] If a diminished or absent response to voluntary squeeze is observed, dysfunction of the external sphincter should be considered. This can be seen in patients with a neuropathy secondary to long-standing defecatory straining, sacral nerve impairment, and disorders affecting striated muscle.[150–154]

FUTURE APPLICATIONS

In the future, esophagogastrointestinal manometric testing will see increased use as a diagnostic tool and to monitor response to therapy while refinements in recording technology allow greater application to the ambulatory setting. For example, newly developed techniques allow continuous ambulatory monitoring of esophageal pH and motility. This may lead to a more precise determination of the cause of unexplained chest pain. Recent studies suggest that 60% of chest pain events may not be esophageal in origin and that the remaining 40% are more often acid-induced rather than related to primary dysmotility. These studies have substantially diminished the role of dysmotility in chest pain.[25]

It is likely that these techniques will be helpful in evaluating patients in whom so-called functional disorders of gastrointestinal motility are suspected, such as irritable bowel syndrome. These patients may be hypersensitive to stressful situations that occur in their day-to-day routines; therefore, the capability of monitoring motility patterns in the ambulatory setting may prove to be useful.

The reader is directed to Chapter 4, Smooth Muscle of the Gut; Chapter 7, Esophageal Motor Function; Chapter 9, Motility of the Small Intestine; Chapter 10, Motility of the Large Intestine; Chapter 28, Approach to the Patient With Dysphagia; Chapter 29, Approach to the Patient With Noncardiac Chest Pain; Chapter 39, Approach to the Patient With Constipation; Chapter 54, Motility Disorders of the Esophagus; Chapter 60, Disorders of Gastric Emptying; Chapter 69, Dysmotility of the Small Intestine; and Chapter 82, Motility Disorders of the Colon.

REFERENCES

1. Castell DO. Historical perspectives and current use of esophageal manometry. In: Castell DO, Richie JE, Dalton CB, eds. Esophageal motility testing. Amsterdam: Elsevier, 1987:3.
2. Castell DO, Wu WC, Ott DJ. Gastroesophageal reflux disease, pathogenesis, diagnosis therapy. New York: Futura, 1985:1.
3. Steff JJ, Dodds WJ, Hogan WJ, et al. Intraluminal esophageal manometry: an analysis of variables affecting recording fidelity of peristaltic pressures. Gastroenterology 1974;67:221.
4. Dodds WJ. Instrumentation and methods for intraluminal esophageal manometry. Arch Intern Med 1976l 126:515.
5. Arndorfer RC, Steff JJ, Dodds WJ, et al. Improved infusion system for intraluminal esophageal manometry. Gastroenterology 1977;73:23.
6. Dent J. A new technique for continuous sphincter pressure measurement. Gastroenterology 1976;71:263.
7. Castell DO, Richter JE, Dalton CB. Esophageal motility testing. Amsterdam: Elsevier, 1987:35.
8. Dodds WJ, Hogan WJ, Steff JJ, et al. A rapid pull through technique for measuring lower esophageal sphincter pressure. Gastroenterology 1975;68:437.
9. Welch RW, Drake ST. Normal lower esophageal sphincter: a comparison of rapid versus slow pull through techniques. Gastroenterology 1980;78:144.
10. Richter JE, Wu WC, Johns DN, et al. Esophageal manometry in 95 healthy adult volunteers: variability of pressure with age and frequency of "abnormal" contraction. Dig Dis Sci 1987;32:583.
11. Kahrilas PJ, Dent J, Dodds WJ, et al. A method for continuous monitoring of upper esophageal sphincter pressure. Dig Dis Sci 1987;32:121
12. Richter JE, Bradley LA, Castell DO. Esophageal chest pain: current controversies in pathogenesis, diagnosis and therapy. Ann Intern Med 1989;110:66.
13. Behar J, Biancani P, Sheahan DG. Evaluation of esophageal tests in the diagnosis of reflux esophagitis. Gastroenterology 1976;71:9.
14. Emde C, Garner A, Blum AL. Technical aspects of intraluminal pH-metry in man: current status and recommendations. Gut 1987;28:1177.
15. Allen ML, Orr WC, Woodruff DM, et al. Validation of an ambulatory esophageal pH monitoring system. Am J Gastroenterol 1988;83:287.
16. Johnson LF, DeMeester TR. Twenty-four hour pH monitoring of the distal esophagus. A quantitative measure of gastroesophageal reflux. Am J Gastroenterol 1974;62:325.
17. Schindlebeck NE, Heinrich C, Konig A, et al. Optimal thresholds, sensitivity and specificity of long term pH-metry for the detection of gastroesophageal reflux disease. Gastroenterology 1987;93:85.
18. McLauchlan G, Rawling JM, Lucan ML, et al. Electrodes for 24 hr pH monitoring: a comparative study. Gut 1987;28:935.
19. Klauser AC, Henrich CA, Schindlebeck NE, et al. Long term esophageal pH-metry: prior manometry is not necessary for positioning the electrode. Gastroenterology 1989;96:259A.
20. Pooro Bianchi G, Pace F. Comparison of three methods of intra-esophageal pH recordings in the diagnosis of gastroesophageal reflux. Scand J Gastroentrol 1988;23:743.
21. Rosen SN, Pope CE. Extended esophageal pH monitoring: an analysis of the literature and assessment of its role in the diagnosis and management of gastroesophageal reflux. J Clin Gastroenterol 1989;11:260.
22. Weiner GS, Richter JE, Cooper JB, et al. The symptom index: a clinically important parameter of ambulatory 24-hour esophageal pH monitoring. Am J Gastroenterol 1988;83:350.
23. Smout AJPM. Ambulatory monitoring of esophageal pH and pressure. In: Castell DO, ed. The esophagus. Boston: Little Brown & Co, 1992:161.
24. Vantrappen G, Janssens J, Hellemans J, et al. Achalasia, diffuse esophageal spasm and related motility disorders. Gastroenterology 1979;76:450.
25. Nostrant TT, Sans J, Huber T. Bethanechol increases the diagnosis yield in patients with esophageal chest pain. Gastroenterology 1986;91:1141.
26. Katz PO, Dalton CB, Richter JE, et al. Esophageal testing of patients with non-cardiac chest pain or dysphagia. Ann Intern Med 1987;106:593.
27. Ossakow SJ, Elta G, Bogdassarian R, et al. Esophageal reflux

and dysmotility at the basis for persistent cervical symptoms. Ann Otol Rhinol Laryngol 1987;96:287.

28. Szurszewski JH. A migrating electrical complex of the canine small intestine. Am J Physiol 1963;217:1757.

29. Reinke DA, Rosenbaum AA, Bennett DR. Patterns of dog gastrointestinal contractile activity monitored in vivo with extraluminal force transduces. Am J Dig Dis 1967;12:1757.

30. Houghton LA, Read NW, Heedle R, et al. Motor activity of gastric antrum, pylorus and duodenum under fasted condition and after a liquid meal. Gastroenterology 1988;94:1276.

31. Malagelada J-R, Stanghellini V. Manometric evaluation of functional upper gastrointestinal symptoms. Gastroenterology 1985;88:1223.

32. Rees WDW, Malagelada J-R, Miller LJ, Go VLW. Human interdigestive and postprandial gastrointestinal motor and gastrointestinal hormone patters. Dig Dis Sci 1982;27:321.

33. Kerlin P, Phillips S. Variability of motility of the ileum and jejunum in healthy humans. Gastroenterology 1982;82:694.

34. Quigley EMM, Donovan JP, Lane MJ, Gallagher TF. Antroduodenal manometry: usefullness and limitations as an outpatient study. Dig Dis Sci 1992;37:20.

35. Dooley CP, DiLorenzo C, Valenzuela JF. Variability of the migrating motor complex in the human. Dig Dis Sci 1992;37:23.

36. Kumar D, Wingate DL. The irritable bowel syndrome: a paroxysmal motor disorder. Lancet 1985;2:973.

37. Kellow JE, Gill RC, Wingate DL. Prolonged ambulant recordings of small bowel motility demonstrate abnormalities in the irritable bowel syndrome. Gastroenterology 1990;98:1208.

38. Lewis TD, Daniel EE. Gastroduodenal motility in a case of dystrophia myotonica. Gastroenterology 1981;81:145.

39. Nowak TV, Anuras S, Brown BP, et al. Small intestinal motility in myotonic dystrophy patients. Gastroenterology 1984;86:808.

40. Cohen S (moderator). The gastrointestinal manifestations of scleroderma: pathogenesis and management. Gastroenterology 1980;79:155.

41. Peachey RD, Creamer B, Pierce JW. Sclerodermatous involvement of the stomach and the small and large bowel. Gut 1969;10:285.

42. Rees WDW, Leigh RJ, Christofides ND, et al. Interdigestive motor activity in patients with systemic sclerosis. Gastroentoelogy 1982;83:575.

43. French JM, Hall G, Parish DJ, et al. Peripheral and autonomic nerve involvement in primary amyloidosis associated with uncontrollable diarrhoea and steatorrhoea. Am J Med 1965;39:277.

44. Malagelada J-R, Camilleri M, Stanghellini V. Manometric diagnosis of gastrointestinal motility disorders. New York: Thieme-Stratton, 1986:54.

45. Malagelada J-R. Quantification of gastric solid-liquid discrimination during digestion of ordinary meals. Gastroenterology 1977;72:1264.

46. Loo FD, Palmer DW, Soergel KH, et al. Gastric emptying in patients with diabetes mellitus. Gastroenterology 1984;86:485.

47. Campbell IW, Heading RC, Tothill P, et al. Gastric emptying in diabetic autonomic neuropathy. Gut 1977;88:462.

48. Camilleri M, Malagelada J-R. Abnormal intestinal motility in diabetics with gastroparesis syndrome. Eur J Clin Invest 1984;14:420.

49. Kristensson K, Nordborg C, Olsson Y, et al. Changes in the vagus nerve in diabetes mellitus. Acta Pathol Microbiol Scand [A] 1971;79:684.

50. Dotevall G, Fagerberg S-E, Langer L, et al. Vagal function in patients with diabetic neuropathy. Acta Med Scand 1972;191:21.

51. Feldman M, Schiller LR. Disorders of gastrointestinal motility associated with diabetes mellitus. Ann Intern Med 1983;98:378.

52. Rees MR, Clark RA, Holdsworth CD, et al. The effect of β-adrenoreceptor agonists and antagonists on gastric emptying in man. Br J Clin Pharmacol 1980;10:551.

53. Bear R, Steer K. Pseudo-obstruction due to clonidine. Br Med J 1976;1:197.

54. Valenzuela JE. Dopamine as a possible neuro-transmitter in gastric relaxation. Gastroenterology 1976;71:1019.

55. Hay AM, Man WK. Effect of metoclopramide on guinea pig stomach: critical dependence on intrinsic stores of acetylcholine. Gastroenterology 1979;76:492.

56. Vasconez LO, Adams JT, Woodward ER. Treatment of reluctant postvagotomy stomach with bethanechol. Arch Surg 1970;100:693.

57. Sandgren JE, McPhee MS, Greenberger NJ. Narcotic bowel syndrome treated with clonidine: resolution of abdominal pain and intestinal pseudo-obstruction. Ann Intern Med 1984;101:331.

58. Stanghellini V, Malagelada J-R. Gastric manometric abnormalities in patients with dyspeptic symptoms after fundoplication. Gut 1983;24:790.

59. Kalbasi H, Hudson FR, Herring A, et al. Gastric emptying following vagotomy and antrectomy and proximal gastric vagotomy. Gut 1975;16:509.

60. Kraft RO, Fry WJ, DeWeese MD. Postvagotomy gastric atony. Arch Surg 1964;88:865.

61. Vantrappen G, Janssens J. To dilate or to operate? This is the question. Gut 1983;24:1013.

62. You CH, Chey WY, Lee KY, Menguy R, Bortoff A. Gastric and small intestinal myoelectric dysrhythmia associated with chronic intractable nausea and vomiting. Ann Intern Med 1981;95:449.

63. Malagelada J-R, Camilleri M. Unexplained vomiting: a diagnostic challenge. Ann Intern Med 1984;101:211.

64. Gilat T, Spiro HM. Amyloidosis and the gut. Am J Dig Dis 1968;13:619.

65. Carrizosa J, Lin KY, Myerson RM. Gastrointestinal neuropathy in familial amyloidosis: report of a case with severe diarrhea without steatorrhea or malabsorption. Am J Gastroenterol 1973;59:541.

66. Monteiro JG. The digestive system in familial amyloidotic polyneuropathy. Am J Gastroenterol 1973;60:47.

67. Ikeda S-I, Makishita H, Oguchi K, et al. Gastrointestinal amyloid deposition in familial amyloid polyneuropathy. Neurology (NY) 1982;32:1364.

68. Camilleri M, Malagelada J-R, Stangehellini V, et al. Gastrointestinal motility disturbances in patients with orthostatic hypotension. Gastroenterology 1985;88:1852.

69. Khurana RK, Nelson E, Azzarelli B, et al. Shy-Drager syndrome: diagnosis and treatment of cholinergic dysfunction. Neurology (NY) 1980;30:805.

70. Low PA, Dyck PJ, Lambert EH, et al. Acute panautonomic neuropathy. Ann Neurol 1983;13:412.

71. Drachman DA, Diamond ER, Hart CW. Posturally-evoked vomiting: association with posterior fossa lesions. Ann Otol Rhinol Laryngol 1977;86:97.

72. Wood JR, Camilleri M, Low PA, et al. Brainstem tumor presenting as an upper gut motility. Gastroenterology 1985;89:1411.

73. Reynolds BJ, Eliasson SG. Colonic pseudo-obstruction in patients with stroke. Ann Neurol 1977;1:305.

74. Schomer DL. Current concepts in neurology: partial epilepsy. N Engl J Med 1983;309:536.

75. Mitchell WG, Greenwood RS, Messenheimer JA. Abdominal epilepsy: cyclic vomiting as the major symptom of simple partial seizures. Arch Neurol 1983;40:251.

76. Malagelada J-R, Rees WDW, Mazzotta LJ, et al. Gastric motor abnormalities in diabetic and postvagotomy gastroparesis: effect of metoclopramide and bethanechol. Gastroenterology 1980;78:286.

77. Mathias JR, Fernandez A, Sninksy CA, et al. Nausea, vomiting, and abdominal pain after Roux-en-Y anastomosis: motility of the jejunal limb. Gastroenterology 1985;88:101.

78. Conklin JL, Anuras S. Radiation-induced recurrent intestinal pseudo-obstruction. Am J Gastroenterol 1981;75:440.

79. Colwell HA, Gladstone RJ. A note on the action of gamma rays on the nerve-cells of the Auerbach's and Meissner's plexus. Br J Radiol 1936;9:620.

80. Conrad RA. Effects of x-irradiation on intestinal motility of the rat. Am J Physiol 1951;165:375.

81. Novak JM, Collins JT, Donowitz M, et al. Effects of radiation on the human gastrointestinal tract. J Clin Gastroenterol 1979;1:9.

82. Yahr MD, Frontera AT. Acute autonomic neuropathy: its occurrence in infectious mononucleosis. Arch Neurol 1975;32:132.

83. Wyburn-Mason M. Visceral lesions in herpes zoster. Br Med J 1959;1:678.

84. Jenzer G, Mumenthaler M, Ludin HP, et al. Autonomic dysfunction in botulism B: a clinical report. Neurology (Minneapolis) 1975;25:150.

85. Vantrappen G, Janssens J, Hellemans J, et al. The interdigestive motor complex of normal subjects and patients with bacterial overgrowth of the small intestine. J Clin Invest 1977;59:1158.

86. Lichetenfeld P. Autonomic dysfunction in the Guillain-Barré syndrome. Am J Med 1971;50:772.

87. Ahmed MN, Carpenter S. Autonomic neuropathy and carcinoma of the lung. Can Med Assoc J 1975;113:410.

88. Schuffler MD, Baird HW, Fleming CR, et al. Intestinal pseudo-obstruction as the presenting manifestation of small-cell carcinoma of the lung: a paraneoplastic neuropathy of the gastrointestinal tract. Ann Intern Med 1983;98:129.

89. Shirer JW. Hypermotility of the gastrointestinal tract in hyperthyroidism: a study of 42 cases. Am J Med Sci 1933;186:73.

90. Neporent MI, Spesivtseva VG. Motor function of gastrointestinal tract before and after I^{131} therapy in patients with thyrotoxicosis (translation suppl). Fed Proc 1963;22:T1177.

91. Wiley ZD, Lavigne ME, Liu KM, et al. The effect of hyperthyroidism on gastric emptying rates and pancreatic exocrine and biliary secretion in man. Am J Dig Dis 1987;23:1003.

92. Brown TR. The effect of hypothyroidism on gastric and intestinal function. JAMA 1931;97:511.

93. Kowalewski K, Kolodej A. Myoelectrical and mechanical activity of stomach and intestine in hypothyroid dogs. Am J Dig Dis 1977;22:235.

94. Eversman JJ, Farmer RG, Brown CH. Gastrointestinal manifestations of hyperparathyroidism. Arch Intern Med 1967;119:605.

95. Gardner EC Jr, Hersh T. Primary hyperparathyroidism and the gastrointestinal tract. South Med J 1981;74:197.

96. Clarkson BO, Kowlessar OD, Horwith M, Sleisenger MH. Clinical and metabolic study of a patient with malabsorption and hypoparathyroidism. Metabolism 1960;9:1093.

97. Dubois A, Gross HA, Ebert MH, et al. Altered gastric emptying and secretion in primary anorexia nervosa. Gastroenterology 1979;77:319.

98. Abell TL, Lucas AR, Brown ML, et al. Gastric electrical dysrhythmias, in anorexia nervosa (AN) (abstract). Gastroenterology 1985;88:1300.

99. Daniel EE, Honour AJ, Bogoch A. Electrical activity of the longitudinal muscle of dog small intestine studied in vivo using microelectrodes. Am J Physiol 1960;198:113.

100. Suzuki N, Prosser CL, Dahms V. Boundary cells between longitudinal and circular layer: essential for electrical slow waves in cat intestine. Am J Physiol 1986;250:G287.

101. Hara Y, Kubota M, Szurszewski JH. Electrophysiology of the smooth muscle of the small intestine of some mammals. J Physiol (Lond) 1986;372:501.

102. Hinder RA, Kelly KA. Human gastric pacesetter potential: site of origin, spread, and response to gastric transsection and proximal gastric vagotomy. Am J Surg 1977;133:29.

103. Sanders KM, Menguy R, Chey WY et al. One explanation for human antral tachygastria (abstract). Gastroenterology 1979;76;1234.

104. Stern RM, Koch KL, eds. Electrogastrography: methodology, validation and applications. New York: Praeger, 1985.

105. Abell TL, Malagelada JR. Glucagon-evoked gastric dysrhythmias in humans shown by an in humans shown by an improved electrogastrographic technique. Gastroenterology 1985;88:1932.

106. Hamilton JW, Bellahsene BE, Reichelderfer M, et al. Human electrogastrograms: comparison of surface and mucosal recordings. Dig Dis Sci 1986;31:33.

107. Kentie MA, Van der Schee EJ, Grashuis JL, Smout AJPM. Adaptive filtering of canine electrogastrographic signals: system design. Part I. Med Biol Eng Comput 1981;19:759.

108. Van der Schee EJ, Kentie MA, Grashuis JL, Smout AJPM. Adaptive filtering of canine electrogastrographic signals: filter performance. Part 2. Med Biol Eng Comput 1981;19:765.

109. Abell TL, Tucker R, Malagelada J-R. Simultaneous electromanometry in man. In: Stern RM, Koch KL, eds. The electrogastrogram: research studies and applications. New York: Praeger, 1985:78.

110. You CH, Chey WY. Studies of electromechanical activity of the stomach in humans and in dogs with particular attention to tachygastria. Gastroenterology 1985;86:1460.

111. Linkens DA. Methods of analyzing rhythmic electrical potentials in the gastrointestinal tract. In: Duthie HL, ed. Gastrointestinal motility in health and disease. Baltimore: University Park Press, 1978:235.

112. Van der Schee EJ, Grashuis JL. Application of running spectrum analysis as analysis to electrogastrographic signals recorded from dog and man. In: Weinbeck M, ed. Motility of the digestive tract. New York: Raven Press, 1982:241.

113. Pfista CJ, Hamilton JW, Nagel N, et al. Use of spectral analysis in the detection of frequency differences in the electrogastrograms of normal and diabetic subjects. IEEE Trans Biomed Eng 1988;35:935.

114. Van der Schee EJ, Grashuis JL. Running spectrum analysis as an aid in the representation and interpretation of electrogastrographic signals. Med Biol Eng Comput 1987;25:57.

115. Chen J, McCallum RW. Electrogastrography: measurement analysis and prospective applications. Med Biol Eng Comput 1991;29:339.

116. Abell TL, Malagelada JR. Electrogastrographic study of patients with unexplained nausea, bloating and vomiting. Gastroenterology 1980;79:311.

117. You CH, Lee KY, Chey WY, et al. Electrogastrographic study of patients with unexplained nausea, bloating and vomiting. Gastroenterology 1980;79:311.

118. Telander RL, Morgan KG, Kreulen DL, et al. Human gastric atony with tachygastria and gastric retention. Gastroenterology 1978;75:497.

119. Kim CH, Azpiroz F, Malagelada J-R. Characteristics of spontaneous and drug induced gastric dysrhythmias in chronic canine model. Gastroenterology 1986;90:421.

120. Bruley Des Varannes S, Mizrahi M, Dubois A. Relation between postprandial gastric emptying and cutaneous electrogastrogram in primates. Am J Physiol 1991;261:G248.

121. Walker BB, Sandman CA. Physiological response patterns in ulcer patients: phasic and tonic components of the electrogastrogram. Psychophysiology 1977;14:393.

122. Cucchiara S, Riezzo G, Minella R, et al. Electrogastrography in non-ulcer dyspepsia. Arch Dis Child 1992; 67:613.

123. Riezzo G, Pezzolla F, Darconza G, Giorgio I. Gastric myoelectrical activity in the first trimester of pregnancy: a cutaneous electrogastrographic study. Am J Gastroenterol 1992; 87:702.

124. Stern RM, Koch KL, Stewart WE, et al. Spectral analysis of tachygastria recorded during motionsickness. Gastroenterology 1980;92:92.

125. Stern RM, Koch KL, Leibowitz HW, et al. Tachygastria and motion sickness. Aviat Space Environ Med 1985;56:1074.

126. Koch KL. Gastric dysrhythmias and the current status of electrogastrography. Practical Gastroenterol 1989;13:37.

127. Arhan P, Devroede G, Jehannin B, et al. Segmental colonic transit time. Dis Colon Rectum 1981;24:625.

128. Chaussade S, Roche H, Khyari A, et al. Mesure du temps de transit colique (TTC): description of validation d'une nouvelle technique. Gastroenterol Clin Biol 1986;10:385.

129. McLean RC, Smart RC, Gaston-Parry D, et al. Colon transit scintigraphy in health and constipation using oral Iodine-131-cellulose. J Nucl Med 1990;31:985.

130. Krevsky B, Malmud LS, D'evcole F, et al. Colonic transit scintigraphy: a physiologic approach to quantitative measurement of colonic transit in humans. Gastroenterology 1986;91:1102.

131. Hardy JG, Wood E, Clark AG, Reynolds JR. Whole-bowel

transit in patients with the irritable bowel syndrome. Eur J Nucl Med 1986;11:393.

132. Proano M, Camilleri M, Phillips SF, et al. Transit of solids through the human colon: regional quantification of the unprepared bowel. Am J Physiol 1990;258:G856.

133. Evans DR, Pye G, Bramley R, et al. Measurement of gastrointestinal pH profiles in normal ambulant human subjects. Gut 1988;29:1035.

134. Smart RC, McLean RG, Gaston-Parry D, et al. Comparison of oral iodine-131-cellulose and indium-111-DTPA as tracers for colon transit scintigraphy: analysis by colon activity profiles. J Nucl Med 1991;32:1668.

135. Malagelada JR, Robertson JS, Brown ML, et al. Intestinal transit of solid and liquid components of a meal in health. Gastroenterology 1984;87:1255.

136. Camilleri M, Brown ML, Malagelada J-R. Impaired transit of chyme in chronic intestinal pseudoobstruction: correction by cisapride. Gastroenterology 1986;91:619.

137. Stivland T, Camilleri M, Vassull M, et al. Scintigraphic measurement of regional gut transit in idopathic constipation. Gastroenterology 1991;101:107.

138. Vassall M, Camilleri M, Phillips SF, et al. Transit through the proximal colon influences stool weight in the irritable bowel syndrome. Gastroenterology 1992;102:102.

139. Metcalf AM, Phillips SF, Zinsmeister AR, et al. Simplified assessment of segmental colonic transit. Gastroenterology 1987;92:40.

140. Hancock AF. Measurement of anal pressure and motility. Gut 1976;17:645.

141. Schuster MM, Hookman P, Hendrix TR. Simultaneous manometric recording of the internal and external and sphincter reflexes. Bull Johns Hopkins Hosp 1965;116:79.

142. Read N, Harford WV, Schmulen AC, et al. A clinical study of patients with fecal incontinence and diarrhea. Gastroenterology 1979;76:747.

143. Gibbons CP, Read NW. Anal hypertonia in fissures: cause or effect? Br J Surg 1986;73:443.

144. McHugh SM, Diamant NE. Effect of age, gender, and pacity on anal canal pressures: contribution of impaired anal sphincter function to fecal incontinence. Dig Dis Sci 1987;32:726.

145. Taylor BM, Bert RW, Phillips SF. Longitudinal and radial variations of pressure in the human and anal sphincter. Gastroenterology 1984;86:693.

146. Hurst AF. Anal achalasia and megacolon (Hirschsprung's disease; idiopathic dilation of colon). Guys Hosp Rev 1934;84:317.

147. Verdiron A, Devroede G, Boucroucha M, et al. Megarectum. Dig Dis Sci 1988;33:1164.

148. Gunterberg B, Kewenter J, Peterson I, Steiner B. Anorectal function after major resections of the sacrum with the bilateral or unilateral sacrifice of sacral nerves. Br J Surg 1976;63:546.

149. Devroede G, Lamarche J. Functional importance of extrinsic para-sympathetic innervation to the distal colon and rectum in man. Gastroenterology 1974;66:273.

150. Henry MM. Pathogenesis and management of fecal incontinence in the adult. Gastroenterol Clin North Am 1987;16:35.

151. Miller R, Bartolo DC, Row A, et al. Anal sensation and the continence mechanism. Dis Colon Rectum 1988;31:433.

152. Wald A, Tanuguntla K. Anorectal sensorimotor dysfunction in fecal incontinence and diabetes mellitus. N Engl J Med 1984;310:1322.

153. Kiff ES, Barnes RPH, Swash M. Evidence of pudenal nerve neuropathy in patients with perineal descent and chronic straining at stool. Gut 1984;25:1279.

154. Rogers J, Henry MM, Misiewicz JJ. Combined sensory and motor deficit in primary neuropathic fecal incontinence. Gut 1988;29:5.

Textbook of Gastroenterology, second edition, edited by Tadataka Yamada. JB Lippincott Company, Philadelphia © 1995.

CHAPTER 133

Tests of Gastric and Exocrine Pancreatic Function and Absorption

Eugene P. DiMagno

Tests of Gastric Acid Secretion
Historical Perspectives
Role in Clinical Practice
Measurement of Basal and Maximal Acid Output

Tests of Pancreatic Function
Invasive Tests
Noninvasive Tests

This chapter provides the clinician with a perspective of gastric and exocrine pancreatic secretory tests used in the diagnosis and management of patients with gastrointestinal disorders. Discussion includes development of these tests, how their use has changed over time, their advantages in a large clinical practice, and pitfalls to avoid, together with a brief description of how each test is performed.

Tests of gastric secretion have decreased in importance. In specific instances, however, they are helpful and may even be necessary to make an appropriate clinical decision. Examples of these instances include the need to determine the status of vagal innervation, of parietal cells after vagotomy, and of acid secretion in patients who have hypergastrinemia or who are being treated for a gastrinoma. Tests of gastric secretion should be available in tertiary centers, but even in these locations, they are usually not required more than 25 to 50 times a year. Performing fewer tests than this may be associated with inaccuracy and increased expense. For these reasons, expanding the availability of these tests appears inappropriate.

Clearly, invasive pancreatic function tests are of superior diagnostic accuracy than any of the noninvasive tests; their sensitivity and specificity of 90% or greater cannot be matched by any of the noninvasive tests. The only impediment to the widespread use of invasive tests is the necessity of gastrointestinal intubation. However, well-trained gastrointestinal assistants can perform the entire test (i.e., intubation, intestinal perfusion, intravenous hormone administration, collection of timed duodenal samples, analysis of enzyme, and infusion of marker concentration and calculation of output). The complexity of the test can therefore be overcome and handled well by paramedical personnel and should not prevent invasive tests from being performed when they are needed. However, because they are required no more frequently than gastric and secretory tests, and for the reasons mentioned previously, their use should probably be restricted to medical centers that have a large referral of patients with difficult gastrointestinal problems.

To circumvent the complexities of the invasive tests, investigators have been attempting to develop sensitive, specific, noninvasive tests that are easy to perform. Several problems have arisen, however, as part of this effort. The sensitivity and specificity of each of the noninvasive tests are suspect, and investigators do not know whether a superior test exists or how most of the tests compare with invasive tests. Unfortunately, these problems will likely go unsolved, because only a large trial in which patients would undergo invasive and multiple noninvasive pancreatic function tests would yield valid results.

Other overlooked characteristics of some noninvasive tests include technical difficulties and the length of time required of both medical personnel and the patient. Accurate, timed collections of urine, blood, or breath carried over many hours are not easy to obtain, and the necessity of a prolonged collection period (6 hours in many patients, and up to several days in some) is a severe constraint as the medical profession continues to be appropriately concerned about cost–benefit issues.

Because of these considerations, my colleagues and I have opted to continue using the cholecystokinin octapeptide–(CCK-OP-) stimulated pancreatic function test. This test can be completed in 2 to 3 hours, with the results made available by midafternoon, allowing the patient to undergo other diagnostic tests on the same day. This test yields the highest sensitivity and specificity of any pancreatic function test.

TESTS OF GASTRIC ACID SECRETION

Historical Perspectives

Tests of gastric acid secretion have been used diagnostically by gastroenterologists for many decades. They have been used to aid in the diagnosis of many upper gastrointestinal lesions, to help select the type of surgical procedure for gastric and duodenal ulcers, and to determine postoperatively the completeness of a vagotomy. The most commonly used tests are the basal and pentagastrin-stimulated gastric secretion tests. In the past, the most commonly performed test was the induction of hypoglycemia by insulin to stimulate vagally mediated gastric acid secretion. Previously, other secretagogues, such as histamine and betazole, were used, but because of their association with side effects (i.e., hypertension, pain at site of injection, flushing, nausea, abdominal cramps, dizziness, and palpitations), they have been supplanted by pentagastrin. The insulin test of vagal function (Hollander's test) is rarely used; for example, at the Mayo Clinic, it was performed only once between 1987 and 1988. Similarly, other tests of gastric secretion are no longer used clinically (e.g., meal stimulation, tubeless tests of gastric secretion) or are only used for research purposes (e.g., modified sham feeding, intragastric titration).

Historically,[1] tests of gastric secretion were performed to provide answers to three questions: How many parietal (or chief) cells are there in the stomach? Are some or all of these cells innervated by branches of the vagus nerve? How much acid is secreted? The answers to these questions aided the clinician in diagnosing pernicious anemia, distinguishing between benign and malignant gastric ulcers, evaluating patients with ulcer dyspepsia but normal x-ray films, selecting appropriate operations in patients with duodenal ulcers, and evaluating and assessing the type of reoperation needed for patients who developed recurrent ulceration after surgery for duodenal ulcer. Today, most of these clinical problems can be satisfactorily addressed without performing gastric secretory tests.

Previously, the diagnosis of pernicious anemia was made when macrocytic anemia was accompanied by absolute gastric anacidity in response to a maximal stimulus of gastric acid secretions. Gastric secretory tests have become obsolete, however, and measurement of serum vitamin B_{12} is the preferred screening test for pernicious anemia. Tests of gastric acid secretion were also performed to help distinguish between benign gastric ulcer and gastric carcinoma (20% of gastric carcinomas are accompanied by gastric anacidity, but these are bulky infiltrating tumors); this differentiation is now made with confidence by performing endoscopy with biopsy and cytology. Similarly, before the availability of fiberoptic endoscopy, gastric secretory tests were used in patients who had nonulcer dyspepsia and normal upper gastrointestinal x-ray films, because gastric acid hypersecretion in this situation could indicate a duodenal ulcer. Today, endoscopy, not gastric analysis, is used to exclude peptic ulceration in patients who have nonulcer dyspepsia and normal x-ray films. In fact, in many institutions, endoscopy is replacing radiologic exami-

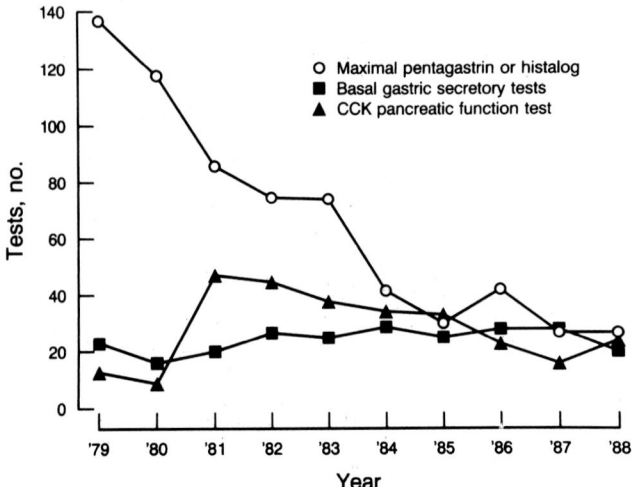

FIGURE 133-1. Patients who underwent gastric and pancreatic secretory tests from 1979 to 1988 at the Mayo Clinic. All patients undergoing maximal pentagastrin or Histalog testing (Histalog was replaced by pentagastrin in 1982) also had a basal secretory test. (CCK, cholecystokinin.)

nation of the upper gastrointestinal tract as a first-line test for the evaluation of patients with dyspepsia.

Role in Clinical Practice

At the Mayo Clinic, where tests of acid secretion are readily available, the use of gastric secretory tests has decreased dramatically over the past decade (Fig. 133-1), mostly because

of a decrease in the number of maximal output tests. Gastric secretory tests continue to be performed to determine whether patients who have undergone surgery for ulcer disease and who have complications are secreting acid (22 [28%] of 80 patients; Table 133-1). Most of these patients have both basal and maximal output tests of acid secretion. Even in patients with recurrent ulceration after gastric surgery, however, the frequency and importance of gastric analysis have declined, because the ulcers can often be healed with H_2-blocking drugs,[2] and surgical treatment may not be necessary.[3]

If an operation is necessary in a patient with recurrent ulceration, measurements of basal, maximal, and perhaps insulin-stimulated acid output, as well as serum gastrin, should be obtained. The results of these tests should allow the surgeon to determine whether reoperation will require an antrectomy, partial gastrectomy, revagotomy, or both antrectomy and revagotomy (Table 133-2). Some surgeons perform an antrectomy without revagotomy for patients who develop a recurrent ulcer after vagotomy. These surgeons do not use the results of gastric secretory tests to plan the reoperation. Others use the guidelines outlined in Table 133-2 to plan the reoperation.

I am not enthusiastic about using these tests before the first operation for peptic ulcer disease to exclude the possibility of a gastrinoma or G-cell hyperplasia in a patient with a duodenal ulcer, or about using the results of gastric analysis to select the type of operation. We measure serum gastrin in all patients undergoing an ulcer operation. After this test, if there still remains a question of whether a gastrinoma is present, we perform a secretin stimulation test to measure gastrin; only in unusual circumstances is gastric analysis necessary.

Previously, surgeons would perform gastric analysis before the first operation for peptic ulcer disease to select the type

TABLE 133-1
Indications for Basal and Maximal Gastric Acid Output Tests Done in 1987 and 1988 at the Mayo Clinic*

		BASAL OUTPUT	MAXIMAL ACID OUTPUT
Is Zollinger-Ellison (ZE) syndrome present?			
Hypergastrinemia only		10	9
Hypergastrinemia with duodenitis or ulcer		3	1
Normal gastrin but ? Ze		14	7
Monitor treatment of Ze		17	3
Postoperative gastric surgery			
Recurrent ulcer		14	11
Gastritis, esophagitis, ? acid secretion		8	7
Miscellaneous		14	5
? HCl for ketoconazole absorption	3		
? Hypersecretion esophagitis	3		
Gastric polyps	1		
Menetrier's disease	1		
Preoperative ulcer surgery	3		
NTS unresponsive to treatment, ? acid hypersecretion	1		
Evaluation of Rx in non ZE DU	1		
Gastric atony with cholecystectomy	1		
Total		80	43

* Ninety-three gastric analyses were performed in the 80 patients. Thirteen patients, particularly the patients with ZE (gastrinoma; n = 9) had more than one test, usually to assess the repsonse to treatment. All patients who had a maximal acid output had a basal test of acid secretion.

DU, duodenal ulcer; NTS, nontropical sprue; Rx, treatment.

TABLE 133-2
Results of Tests of Gastric Secretions and Planning Reoperation in Patients With Recurrent Ulcers After Vagotomy

CAUSE	ACID SECRETION AFTER VAGOTOMY			REOPERATION
	Basal	*Maximal*	*Insulin*	
High parietal cell mass	↓	↑	↓	Partial gastrectomy
Remaining vagal innervation	↑	↑ →	↑	Repeat vagotomy with or without antrectomy
Excess antral gastrin	↑	↑ →	↓	Antrectomy

↓, low; →, normal; and ↑ high levels of acid output.

of operation, but gastric analysis is now done rarely for this purpose (4% of all gastric analyses; see Table 133-1). For example, a surgeon might have elected to perform partial gastric resection and vagotomy in patients with hypersecretion and highly selective proximal gastric vagotomy in patients with normal secretion. Evidence shows, however, that the recurrence rate after highly selective proximal gastric vagotomy is not higher in hypersecretory patients compared with patients who have normal secretion.[4] The following results were obtained from studies of patients who underwent highly selective proximal gastric vagotomy: 1 of 25 patients had recurrent ulceration when the acid output was lower than 25 mmol/hour, compared with 3 of 10 patients who had an output of 25 mmol/hour or higher;[5] 19% of patients had recurrent ulceration after vagotomy and pyloroplasty when preoperative maximal acid output was higher than 45 mmol/hour;[6] and 8.6% of patients who underwent vagotomy and antrectomy, or vagotomy and drainage, had recurrent ulceration when the maximal output was 25 mmol/hour or higher.[7]

The trend is to avoid preoperative tests of gastric secretion. Although controversy may persist regarding the use of preoperative gastric analysis to select the type of operation, the issue is not likely to be settled without large prospective studies. Also, the controversy may never be settled satisfactorily, because the question has become less important; the advent of effective medical treatment has been associated with a decrease in the frequency of gastric surgery. All of the previously mentioned studies were performed before the use of H$_2$-blocking drugs or omeprazole became widespread.

The second most common reason to perform gastric analysis, in our experience, is to judge the response of H$_2$-blocker or omeprazole therapy in patients with gastrinomas (17 [25%] of 80 patients; see Table 133-1). Consensus is that basal acid output of 10 mmol/hour or lower obtained before the next dosing indicates adequate control of Zollinger-Ellison syndrome.[8] Another important reason for obtaining a basal acid secretory test is to determine whether achlorhydria is present in patients who are referred for hypergastrinemia and have no evidence or history of peptic ulcer disease. The majority of these patients also received pentagastrin to ensure that no acid was secreted even after stimulation.

The remaining reasons for obtaining basal tests are varied. Fourteen patients in the miscellaneous group had the test performed to evaluate the possibility of hypersecretion of acid despite usual medical treatment for various disorders, including esophagitis (3 patients), nontropical sprue (1 patient), and a duodenal ulcer (1 patient). An unusual reason to obtain basal acid was to determine whether an intragastric acidic pH was present, which is necessary for the antibiotic ketoconazole to be absorbed (3 patients).

In summary, a few indications remain for tests of gastric secretion in the modern practice of gastroenterology (Table 133-3). Although the tests are no longer used routinely in

TABLE 133-3
Indications for Gastric Secretory Studies

Duodenal ulcer patients who
　Fail appropriate medical therapy
　Have recurrent postoperative ulceration
　Have enlarged gastric folds
　Have diarrhea
　Have hyperparathyroidism
Zollinger-Ellison syndrome patients who continue to have ulceration even with treatment (adjust treatment to maintain low basal acid)
Hypergastrinemia (see Table 133-4)

TABLE 133-4
Appropriateness of Gastric Acid Secretory Test to Differentiate Among Classes of Hypergastrinemia

Inappropriate: Associated With Hypersecretion of Acid
Gastrinoma (Zollinger-Ellison syndrome)
Antral G-cell hyperfunction
Isolated retained antrum
Massive small-bowel resection (rare)
Pheochromocytoma (rare)

Appropriate: Associated With Normal or Low Gastric Secretion
Pernicious anemia
Atrophic gastritis
Gastric ulcer
Gastric cancer
Postvagotomy
Renal failure

Appropriate: Associated With Hypersecretion of Acid
Gastric outlet obstruction

patients with duodenal or gastric ulcers, they may be used in special circumstances in which determination of the status of acid secretion is clinically important, such as in determining whether vagal innervation of parietal cells is intact after a presumed vagotomy, assessing the status of secretion in patients with hypergastrinemia (Table 133-4), and evaluating the effects of treatment in patients with gastrinoma.

Measurement of Basal and Maximal Acid Output

In preparing patients for measurements of basal acid output and maximal acid output, treatment with pharmaceutical agents that may affect the results of the test should be discontinued, unless the indication for the test is to determine the acid secretory response to the treatment. A clear liquid supper should be eaten the evening before the test, and no food or liquid should be ingested for 12 hours before the test. H_2 antagonists or anticholinergics and antacids should be

discontinued 72 and 12 hours before the test, respectively. If, however, the objective of the test is to determine the effectiveness of an H_2 antagonist on acid secretion, the drug should be continued and the basal output of gastric acid should be performed 1 hour after administration of the morning dose.

The test is performed in the morning after an overnight fast. A double-lumen 5.94-mm (18-Fr) gastric sump tube with a perfusion tube cemented to the side is placed into the antrum of the stomach under fluoroscopic control. After intubation, the patient is placed supine with the head slightly elevated, and the gastric tube is connected to continuous suction at 80 mm Hg. Radioactive chromic chloride ($^{51}CrCl_3$) in normal saline is perfused into the stomach at a rate of 0.33 mL/minute so that the adequacy of recovery of gastric contents can be measured accurately. During the basal (i.e., nonstimulated) period, four 15-minute collections are obtained. Volume and pH are recorded for each 15-minute collection while the pooled 15-minute collections are used to measure the total acid output by titrating to pH 7, which is referred to as

---

TABLE 133-5
Invasive Tests of Exocrine Pancreatic Function Requiring Gastrointestinal Intubation

TEST	WHAT IS MEASURED	SPECIAL TECHNIQUES AND REQUIREMENTS	APPROXIMATE RANGES FOR DIAGNOSIS OF CHRONIC PANCREATIC DISEASE	
			Sensitivity (%)*	Specificity (%)†
Indirect Tests				
Pancreatic secretion in response to intraluminal stimuli Lundh's test meal EAA	Activity of pancreatic enzymes in duodenal samples	Gastroduodenal intubation for collection of duodenal samples. Lundh's test meal is swallowed or EAA are perfused into duodenum. A nonabsorbable marker is also perfused into the duodenum to quantify outputs, and samples are collected for 90–120 min. Gastric contents are aspirated only during the EAA test.	75–85	75–85
Direct Tests‡				
Pancreatic secretion in response to exogenous hormones Secretin CCK, CCK-OP	HCO$_3$, amylase activity and volume of duodenal samples Trypsin, lipase, activity in duodenal samples (outputs quantified by infusing nonabsorbable marker into duodenum)	Gastroduodenal intubation followed by collection of duodenal samples, continuous aspiration of gastric contents and administration of hormone by intravenous injection of constant infusion. Markers with duodenal perfusion, if used, allow quantification of output.	85–90	80–90
Secretin and CCK	Same as for secretin, CCK, and CCK-OP			

CCK, cholecystokinin; CCK-OP, cholecystokinin octapeptide; EAA, essential amino acids.

* Tests do not separate chronic pancreatitis from cancer of the pancreas. In patients with pancreatic cancer in the head of the pancreas, there is 90% sensitivity; with cancer in the body or tail, sensitivity is 75%.

† False-positive tests in patients with small bowel disease duodenal acidification.

‡ False-negative tests occur in patients with calcific pancreatitis (10%) carcinomas that do not obstruct the proximal pancreatic duct; false-positive tests occur in severely malnourished patients, and in patients with nontropical sprue, and malignancies arising from gastrointestinal organs other than the pancreas.

the *titratable acidity*. The concentration of hydrogen ions or hydrogen ion activity (pH) is not the same as the titratable acidity.

If a maximal pentagastrin stimulation test is to be performed after the basal collection, pentagastrin is administered intravenously (6 μg/kg). Sequential 15-minute samples of gastric secretion are collected. Each sample is immediately analyzed for volume and pH and is retitrated to a pH of 7. Total amount of hydrochloric acid is calculated in millimoles per 15 minutes. At least four 15-minute specimens must be collected after pentagastrin is administered. If the acid output continues to rise, collections are continued for an additional 30 minutes (total time, 90 minutes). Once the peak acid secretion is achieved and at least four specimens have been collected, the test is terminated, and the tube is removed.

TESTS OF PANCREATIC FUNCTION

Pancreatic function tests fall into two general categories: invasive tests (Table 133-5) and noninvasive tests (Table 133-6). Invasive tests are the classic gold standard tests of

TABLE 133-6
Noninvasive Tests of Pancreatic Function*

TEST	WHAT IS MEASURED	SPECIAL TECHNIQUES AND REQUIREMENTS	SENSITIVITY IN PANCREATIC INSUFFICIENCY (%) Mild	Severe	SPECIFICITY (%)
^{13}C-labeled corn starch breath test	Breath $^{13}CO_2$	Give ^{13}C-labeled starch or glucose orally in 250 mL H_2O on separate days (2 days apart). Measure breath $^{13}CO_2$ q 30 min × 6 h (isotope ratio, mass spectrophotometer). Calculate ratio of cumulative 6 h $^{13}CO_2$ glucose: $^{13}CO_2$ starch.	†	†	†
Cholesteryl octanoate breath test	Breath $^{14}CO_2$	Give ^{14}C cholesteryl octanoate orally, Measure breath $^{14}CO_2$ for 6 h.	†	†	†
Mixed triglyceride test	Breath $^{13}CO_2$	Give 1,3-distearyl, 2 [carboxyl-^{13}C] octanoyl glycerol orally. Measure breath $^{13}CO_2$ q 30 min × 6 h (isotope ratio, mass spectrophotometer). Express as cumulative $^{13}CO_2$ per 6 h.	†	†	†
H_2 breath test	Breath H_2	Measure basal fasting H_2. Give 100 g rice starch in 250 mL. Measure breath H_2 every 20–30 min for 2 h. Rise ≥20 ppm indicates abnormal positive test result.	0?	100	50–100
NBT-PABA test	Urine PABA	Administration of *N*-benzoyl-L-tyrosyl *p*-aminobenzoic acid with timed meal and urine collection	46	71	39–100‡
Pancreolauryl test	Urinary fluorescein	2-day test: 1st day fluorescein dilaurate given, 2nd day free fluorescein given—both days with test mean urine collected 10 h.	40	79	39–97‡
Dual-labeled Schilling's test	24-h urine collection ^{57}CO and ^{58}CO measured with gamma counter	Orally administer a) intrinsic factor [^{57}CO] cobalamin; b) hog R protein [^{58}CO] cobalamin and c) cobinamide (prevents endogenous R protein from removing [^{57}CO] cobalamin from intrinsic factor). 1 mg cobalamin given IM after oral test solution given	†	†	†
Plasma PP	PP during fasting or intravenous CCK	Measure plasma concentrations of PP by radio immunoassay	†	†	†
Plasma amino acids during CCK	Plasma amino acids	Administer CCK by constant intravenous infusion for 1 h. Measure plasma amino acids before and after 30 and 60 min of IV CCK.	†	†	†

CCK, cholecyplokinin; PP, pancreatic polypeptide.

* Synthetic compounds are administered that are hydrolyzed by pancreatic enzymes, absorbed by the small intestine and measured in blood or urine or plasma hormones or amino acids measured during administration of CCK intravenously.

† Incompletely tested.

‡ Depends on the character of the control groups. See text for reasons for false-positive tests. The 100% specificity rates are from studies in which control groups were normal subjects. Lower rates are from studies where control groups included patients with other gastrointestinal diseases (e.g., inclusion of patients with malabsorption secondary to conditions other than pancreatic insufficiency would greatly reduce specificity of the starch H_2 breath test) or diabetes and chronic obstructive lung disease (in the case of breath tests) or an assumption by the author of this chapter of what specificity would be if the control gorup included these patients.

TABLE 133-7
Indication for Performing Cholecystokinin Pancreatic Function Tests Done in 1987 and 1988 at the Mayo Clinic*

		NUMBER OF PATIENTS (%)	GROUP
Do patients with abdominal pain and normal imaging tests have chronic pancreatitis?		10 (24)	1
Is malabsorption due to pancreatic insufficiency?		17 (42)	2
Is severe pancreatic insufficiency contributing to malabsorption in presence of nonpancreatic conditions associated with malabsorption?		7 (17)	
Diabetes mellitus	3		3
Nontropical sprue	2		4
Postoperative gastric resection	2		5
Is severe pancreatic insufficiency present in pantients with diarrhea, but no steatorrhea?		7 (17)	
Chronic pancreatitis	4		6
Other diarrhea without steatorrhea	3		7
Total		41 (100)	

* The number and percentage of patients undergoing cholecystokinin CCK tests are listed for each group (last column). The values of the CCK test for each group are given in Fig. 133-7.

pancreatic function, but they are difficult to perform because they require gastrointestinal intubation to collect duodenal samples for analysis of enzymes, bicarbonate, and volume. Therefore, a number of simple noninvasive tests have been devised. Noninvasive tests are simpler and cheaper than invasive tests but, unfortunately, are not as reproducible, sensitive, or specific. Noninvasive tests are of three types:

1. Measurement of unabsorbed food or pancreatic enzymes in stool.
2. Measurement of products of food digestion or synthetic compounds that are hydrolyzed by intralumenal pancreatic enzymes, absorbed by the gut, and appear in blood, urine, or breath.
3. Measurement of plasma concentrations of hormones or amino acids that are significantly different in patients with a chronic pancreatic disease.

Selection of a particular pancreatic function test depends on the clinical question and on the characteristics of the test. At the Mayo Clinic, CCK-OP–stimulated pancreatic function tests are performed to answer four questions (Table 133-7):

1. Do patients with abdominal pain and normal results of imaging tests have chronic pancreatitis?

2. Is malabsorption due to pancreatic insufficiency?
3. Is severe pancreatic insufficiency also present (<10% normal enzyme outputs) and contributing to malabsorption or diarrhea in patients with nonpancreatic diseases or conditions associated with malabsorption?
4. In patients with an uncertain cause of diarrhea but no steatorrhea, is pancreatic insufficiency present?

In patients whose malabsorption is secondary to pancreatic exocrine insufficiency and whose response to treatment has been suboptimal, pancreatic function tests are sometimes also used to assess the adequacy of pancreatic enzyme replacement treatment, and to determine the extent of exocrine pancreatic insufficiency before pancreatic resection.

At my institution, pancreatic function tests represent the fourth line of testing in the diagnosis of pancreatic diseases (Fig. 133-2). Pancreatic function tests should be performed if the diagnosis of pancreatic disease remains a possibility, even after noninvasive imaging tests (i.e., ultrasonography, computed tomography scan) and invasive imaging tests (i.e., endoscopic retrograde cholangiopancreatography) have yielded normal or inconclusive results. Invasive tests of pancreatic function are ordinarily performed for this purpose, because only invasive tests can measure the entire range of

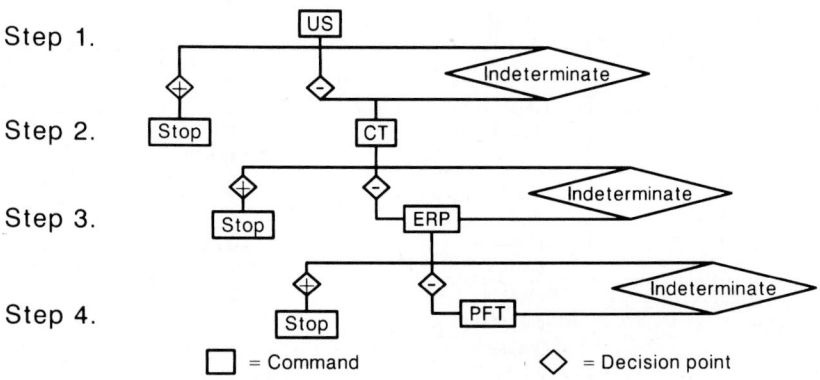

FIGURE 133-2. Algorithm for diagnosis of pancreatic cancer if ultrasonography (US), computed tomography (CT), endoscopic retrograde pancreatogram (ERP), and pancreatic function test (PFT) are available. When the combination of US and ERP is used, sensitivity is 87% (either test positive) and specificity is 77% (both tests negative) when the tests are used in parallel. (Data from Gowland M, Kalantzis N, Warwick F, Braganza J. Relative efficiency and predictive value of ultrasonography and endoscopic retrograde pancreatography in diagnosis of pancreatic disease. Lancet 1981;2:190.)

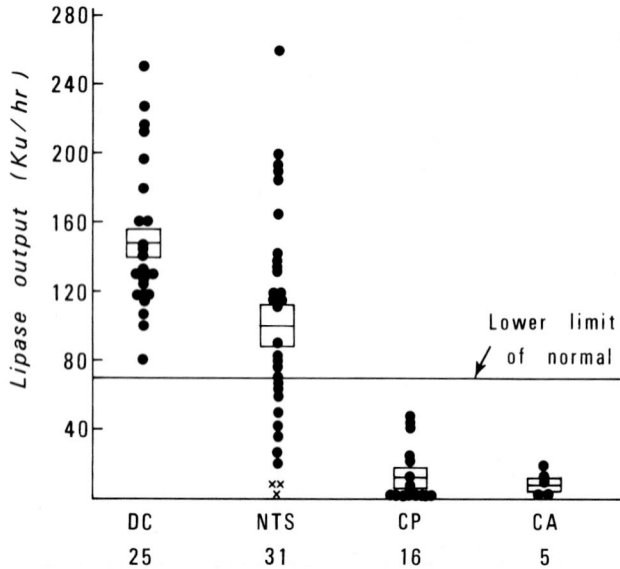

FIGURE 133-3. Cholecystokinin-stimulated outputs of lipase in four groups of subjects: disease control (DC), nontropical sprue (NTS), chronic pancreatitis with pancreatic insufficiency (CP), and pancreatic cancer with pancreatic insufficiency (CA). Mean ± SE values for each group are depicted by rectangles. Lower limit of normal for lipase outputs in our laboratory is shown. (x, patients with pancreatic enzyme outputs less than 10% of normal and in whom severe pancreatic insufficiency contributes to malabsorption; from Regan PT, DiMagno EP. Exocrine pancreatic insufficiency in celiac sprue: a cause of treatment failure. Gastroenterology 1980;78:484.)

pancreatic function and ensure adequate sensitivity and specificity for detection of disease. They are 90% sensitive and specific,[9] but they may yield false-negative results in patients with calcific pancreatitis, and false-positive results in patients with nontropical sprue[10] (Fig. 133-3) and malignancies arising from the gastrointestinal organs other than the pancreas (Fig. 133-4).

Pancreatic enzyme output is abnormal in 90% of patients with cancer of the pancreatic head and in 75% of patients with cancer of the pancreatic body and tail.[11] My colleagues and I[11] have found that in the detection of pancreatic cancer, measurement of enzyme output and bicarbonate in response to CCK are more accurate than measurement of bicarbonate in response to secretin. (Lipase may be more sensitive than trypsin, particularly for detection of pancreatitis; see Fig. 133-4.)

Invasive tests that depend on meals of specified composition or infusion of nutrients into the small bowel to stimulate exocrine pancreatic secretion may be less specific than intravenously administered hormones because they depend on hormonal secretion from the intestinal tract to stimulate pancreatic secretion. For example, postprandial pancreatic enzyme secretion is low in patients who have diseases that affect the mucosa of small bowel[12] (Fig. 133-5), because the gastrointestinal hormones that stimulate pancreatic secretion (i.e., CCK, secretin) are synthesized in and secreted from the mucosa.

Noninvasive tests that yield abnormal results only when enzyme secretion into the duodenum is markedly decreased (<10% normal) may be used to determine whether malab-

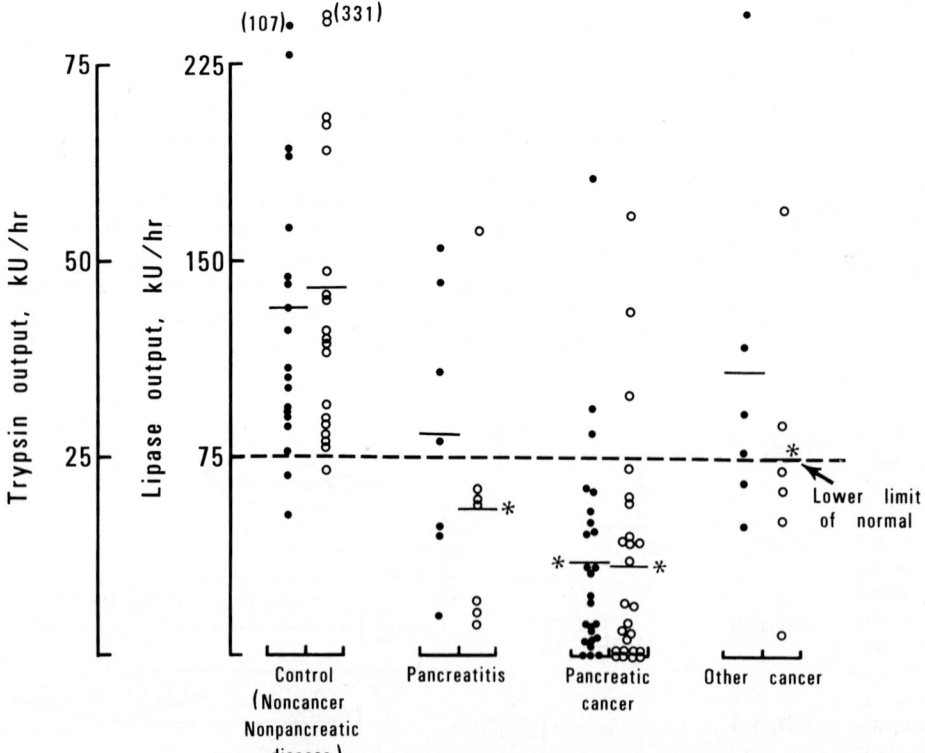

FIGURE 133-4. Trypsin (●) and lipase (○) outputs in 10^3 units per hour (kU/hr) in response to intravenous cholecystokinin (15 Crick-Harper-Raper units/kg/hour) in patients with nonmalignant nonpancreatic disease, pancreatitis, pancreatic cancer, and other cancers. Horizontal line in each column indicates the mean. (*, $P < 0.01$ compared with control patients; from DiMagno EP, Malagelada J-R, Moertel CG, Go VLW. Prospective evaluation of the pancreatic secretion of immunoreactive carcinoembryonic antigen, enzyme, and bicarbonate in patients suspected of having pancreatic cancer. Gastroenterology 1977;73:457.)

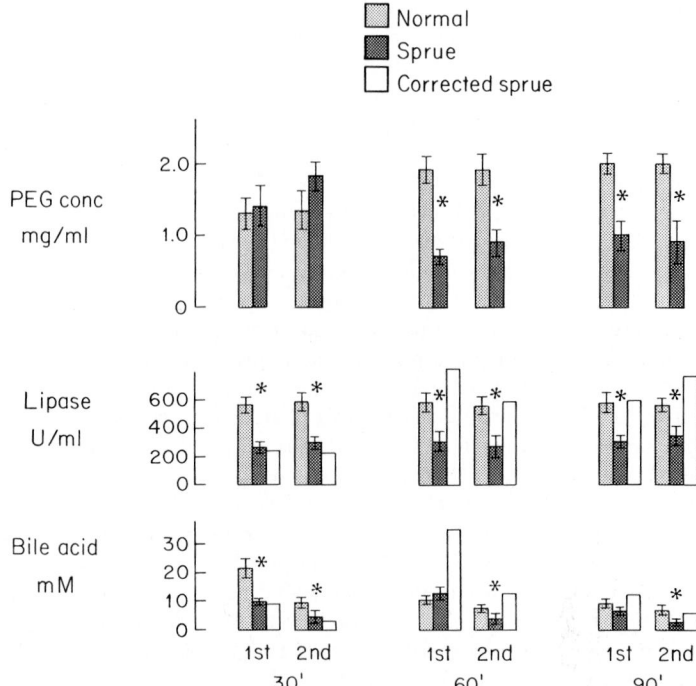

FIGURE 133-5. Concentrations of polyethylene glycol (PEG), lipase, and bile acids ±SE after first and second meals in health and sprue, together with values for lipase and bile acids corrected for dilution. (*, $P < 0.05$; from DiMagno EP, Go VLW, Summerskill WHJ. Impaired CCK-P2 secretion, intraluminal dilution and maldigestion of fat in sprue. Gastroenterology 1972;63:25.)

sorption is due to severe exocrine pancreatic insufficiency and whether patients with known chronic pancreatitis have severe exocrine insufficiency. Abnormal results indicate pancreatic insufficiency when extrapancreatic diseases associated with abnormal test results can be excluded. However, a normal result does not exclude pancreatic disease, and we prefer to determine whether steatorrhea is due to pancreatic insufficiency by performing an invasive test of pancreatic function in which enzyme outputs are quantified. Because CCK-stimulated enzyme outputs can be related accurately to malabsorption[13] (Fig 133-6), we prefer them to bicarbonate output in the assessment of pancreatic function.

Noninvasive tests can also be used to determine whether treatment with pancreatic enzyme is adequate. Such tests include two-stage measurement of fecal fat, measurement of breath triolein and hydrogen, and N-benzoyl-L-tyrosyl-p-aminobenzoic acid (NBT-PABA) and pancreolauryl tests with and without pancreatic enzyme replacement. However, noninvasive tests cannot detect early chronic pancreatic disease (i.e., before malabsorption appears) and, therefore, can only be considered preliminary tests in diagnosing chronic pancreatic diseases.

Occasionally, symptomatic steatorrhea persists despite optimum treatment with pancreatic enzymes. In such instances, the clinician can perform the simple diagnostic maneuver of testing various adjuvant regimens (e.g., addition of H_2 blockers, antacids, or microencapsulated enteric-coated preparations) by performing a noninvasive test such as fecal fat or triolein breath tests with and without the adjuvant treatment (two-stage tests). If enough lipase is being given (>10% of normal amounts), the usual reason for failing to abolish steatorrhea is persistent postprandial intralumenal acidic conditions[14] despite the addition of H_2 blockers or antacids. Thus, if symptoms of steatorrhea persist, intragastric and intraduodenal pH measurements during adjuvant treatments

may be necessary so that dose adjustments of the H_2 blockers or antacids can be made to alkalinize the upper gastrointestinal tract.

Over the past decade, the number of pancreatic function tests performed for clinical purposes has remained relatively stable, ranging from 9 to 48 per year (see Fig. 133-1). The clinical reasons for performing pancreatic function tests during 1987 and 1988 are given in Table 133-7. During 1987

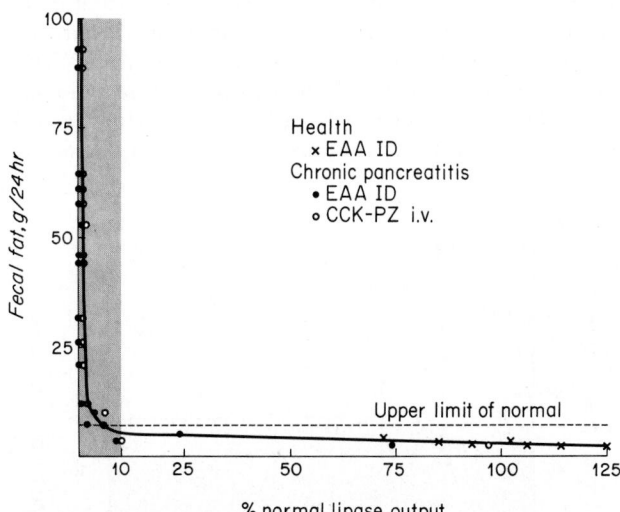

FIGURE 133-6. Relation between steatorrhea and lipase output. Steatorrhea (24-hour fecal fat more than 7 g/day when 100 g of fat is ingested daily) does not occur until lipase output is reduced below 10% of normal. (CCK-P2 i.v., intravenous cholecystokinin-pancreotymin; EAA ID, essential amino acids, 78mM; from DiMagno EP, Go VLW, Summerskill WHJ. Relations between pancreatic enzyme outputs and malabsorption in severe pancreatic insufficiency. N Engl J Med 1973;288:813.)

and 1988, 24%, 42%, 17%, and 17% of the tests were performed to answer the first through the fourth diagnostic questions, respectively (see Table 133-7).

The CCK test is extremely helpful in answering these diagnostic questions (Fig 133-7). For example, in group 1 patients, the diagnosis of pancreatic disease was made in 3 of 10 patients only after performing the CCK test (all imaging test results were normal), whereas in group 2, 4 (24%) of the 17 patients with steatorrhea were found to have malabsorption secondary to pancreatic insufficiency; failure to find pancreatic insufficiency as a cause for malabsorption led to diagnosis of bacterial overgrowth in 5 patients and nontropical sprue in 1 patient. The remaining patients had connective tissue or vascular lesions (3 patients), bone marrow transplant (1 patient), agnogenic myeloid metaplasia (1 patient), hypoparathyroidism (1 patient), and Crohn's disease (1 patient). In groups 3 to 7, 5 (36%) of 14 patients were found to have pancreatic insufficiency. None of the 4 patients with chronic pancreatitis who complained of diarrhea (group 6) but who did not have steatorrhea had enzyme outputs lower than 10% of normal. Overall, of all the patients who had a pancreatic function test, the test clarified whether chronic pancreatitis was present or whether malabsorption was due to severe pancreatic insufficiency in 11 (27%) of the 41 patients.

Invasive Tests

Invasive tests require gastroduodenal intubation to collect samples for measuring pancreatic enzyme or bicarbonate secretion into the duodenum. The gastric tube is necessary to aspirate gastric secretions constantly, because acid in the duodenum stimulates exocrine pancreatic secretion but may also inactivate pancreatic enzyme activity. After tubes are in place, the pancreas is stimulated by intravenous administration of a hormone, by ingestion of a meal, or by infusion of a nutrient, or nutrients, into the small intestine. Invasive tests (see Table 133-5) are used to quantify exocrine pancreatic secretion directly. The normal ranges of pancreatic secretion for the commonly used invasive secretory tests are given in Table 133-8.

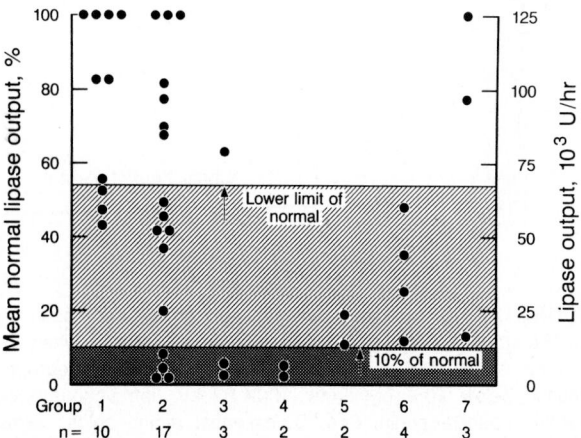

FIGURE 133-7. Lipase output of the various groups of patients (see Table 133-7) undergoing cholecystokinin pancreatic function test.

TABLE 133-8	
Reported Normal Ranges of Pancreatic Responses to Secretory Tests	

1. Secretin test*
   Volume: 117–392 (mL/80 min)
   Bicarbonate concentrations: 88–137 (mEq/L)
   Bicarbonate output: 16–33 (mEq/80 min)
   Amylase output: 439–1921 (U/80 min)
2. Secretin + CCK (lower limts of normal; mean − 2 SD)†
   Volume: 151 (mL/60 min)
   Bicarbonate concentratioin: 70 (mmol/h)
   Bicarbonate output: 11.3 (mmol/60 min)
   Amylase output: 131 (Units during 30 min of CCK)
3. CCK test†
   Trypsin output: 25–54 (Ku/h)
   Lipase output: 77–322 (Ku/h)
4. Lundh's test‡
   Mean tryptic activity: 61 (IU/L)

CCK; cholecystokinin.

* Dreiling DA, Hollander F. Studies in pancreatic function. II. A statistical study of pancreatic secretion following secretin in patients without pancreatic disease. Gastroenterology 1950;15:620.

† Howat HT, Braganza JM. Assessment of pancratic dysfunction in man. In: Howat HT, Sarles H, eds. The exocrine pancreas. Philadelphia: WB Saunders, 1979:129.

‡ DiMagno EP, Go VLW, Summerskill WHJ. Relations between pancreatic enzyme outputs and malabsorption in severe pancreatic insufficiency. N Engl J Med 1973;288:813–815.

Adapted from Mottaleb A, Kapp F, Noguera ECA, et al. The Lundh test in the diagnosis of pancreatic disease: A review of five years' experience. Gut 1973;14: 835.

My colleagues and I routinely infuse a nonabsorbable marker into the duodenum to quantitate enzyme output according to recovery of the marker. Unless we are conducting rigorous protocol studies, we do not infuse a second marker into the stomach to quantify gastric acid output and duodenogastric reflux. During clinical tests, the gastric marker is not required, because duodenogastric reflux is negligible in most cases, and nearly complete gastric aspiration can be accomplished with the gastric tube positioned in the antrum.

By perfusing a marker into the duodenum, the clinician can calculate accurate outputs of pancreatic secretions without requiring complete or almost complete aspiration of duodenal content. Without the use of a duodenal marker, accurate measurement of pancreatic enzyme outputs can be obtained only if the duodenal tubes are constructed so that they can carry large volumes and if they are positioned in the duodenum so that they remove 85% or more of duodenal content. Almost complete aspiration of duodenal contents, however, might alter pancreatic responses, particularly when meals are given or nutrients are perfused into the duodenum either as clinical tests of pancreatic function or during physiologic studies. In our experience, continuous aspiration of the duodenum and removal of most of the duodenal content during nutrient stimulation of pancreatic enzyme secretion lead to a steady decline in pancreatic enzyme secretion. The most physiologic and accurate way to measure pancreatic secretion is to use a duodenal marker to calculate outputs and to sample, but not attempt complete aspiration of, the duodenal contents.

Noninvasive Tests

Fecal Fat Measurement

Quantitative fecal fat collection is the gold standard test for malabsorption. The test requires a 48- to 72-hour stool collection. During this period, and preferably for several days before the stool collection, a constant known quantity of dietary fat is eaten. Normally, 7% or less of the ingested fat appears in stool (coefficient of absorption $\geq$ 93%). For example, when a diet that includes 100 g of fat is ingested, fecal fat excretion greater than 7 g/24 hours is considered abnormal.

In contrast to its use in detection of malabsorption, the quantitative collection of fecal fat is an insensitive and nonspecific test of pancreatic function. Only end-stage pancreatic insufficiency (< 10% secretory capacity remaining) can be detected.[13] In addition, many patients with nonpancreatic causes of malabsorption have excessive fecal fat, which accounts for the nonspecificity of the test for the detection of pancreatic diseases. The result of a two-stage test (i.e., quantitative fecal fat collection with and without exogenous pancreatic enzyme replacement), however, can be used to differentiate steatorrhea secondary to pancreatic insufficiency from other causes of malabsorption and can also be used to judge whether pancreatic enzyme treatment is effective.

The simple qualitative test for fat in the stool, microscopic examination of a single stool sample for oil, is almost as sensitive as a quantitative stool collection for fat (94%).[15] Quantitative evaluation of fecal nitrogen is less sensitive than quantitative evaluation of fecal fat for detection of pancreatic malabsorption, because secretion of trypsin decreases more slowly than secretion of lipase, and in chronic pancreatitis, increased fecal nitrogen (azotorrhea) occurs later than steatorrhea.[16]

Fecal Chymotrypsin Measurement

Chymotrypsin is stable in stools for days, even when the stools are stored at room temperature; chymotrypsin is also easy to measure. New, simple colorimetric methods are as sensitive as automatic titration assay, the previously favored test, and they are much easier to perform. The sensitivity of fecal chymotrypsin measurement is between 41% and 64% in patients with mild to moderate insufficiency.[17,18] Specificity ranges from 50% to 90% and is related to the population studied. False-positive results occur in various diseases associated with malabsorption, including nontropical sprue, Crohn's disease, and cirrhosis, and in patients who have had a Billroth II gastrectomy.

Advocates of this test admit that it is sensitive only for advanced pancreatic disease, but point out that because it is simple, it is also useful in monitoring progression or remission of established disease.

Triolein Breath Test

The measurement of breath $^{14}CO_2$ after ingestion of ^{14}C triolein can be used to detect malabsorption of fat. Therefore, as with fecal fat, the measurement of breath $^{14}CO_2$ is abnormal in patients with chronic pancreatic disease when pancreatic insufficiency is advanced. However, multiple steps are involved in the pathway from ingestion of ^{14}C triolein to exhalation of $^{14}CO_2$, including lipolysis, mucosal absorption, hepatic metabolism, and pulmonary function. Therefore, mucosal, hepatic, and pulmonary abnormalities, as well as metabolic abnormalities (e.g., diabetes mellitus, obesity) are associated with low excretion of $^{14}CO_2$ after ingestion of ^{14}C triolein.[15] Thus, diseases other than chronic pancreatitis or pancreatic cancer that are associated with malabsorption can cause an abnormal test result.

A two-stage test described previously (see Fecal Fat Measurement) may improve sensitivity for detection of steatorrhea secondary to pancreatic disease.[19]

Cholesteryl Octanoate Breath Tests and Mixed Triglyceride Breath Tests

Two novel breath tests[20,21] have been developed to assess exocrine pancreatic function. They are based on the hypothesis that sensitivity and specificity in diagnosing pancreatic disease may be improved by the use of substrates engineered so that they are hydrolyzed by a specific pancreatic lipase. For both tests, a ^{13}C- or ^{14}C-labeled substrate is hydrolyzed by its specific lipase, is absorbed, and is metabolized by the liver, and $^{13}CO_2$ or $^{14}CO_2$ is measured in breath, respectively.

Cholesteryl-[1-^{14}C] octanoate, the substrate for the cholesteryl octanoate breath test, is hydrolyzed by pancreatic carboxylester lipase.[20] In the single report of the cholesteryl octanoate breath test, 2 of 3 patients with mild steatorrhea (7–11 g fat/24 hours) had normal test results, whereas all 7 patients with severe steatorrhea (> 11 g fat/24 hours) had abnormal test results.

1,3-Distearyl, 2 [carboxyl-^{13}C] octanoyl glycerol is the substrate for the mixed triglyceride breath test. In this test, the long-chained fatty acids in the 1 and 3 positions are hydrolyzed by pancreatic lipase, which is the rate-limiting step in the digestion of this triglyceride. Vantrappen and colleagues,[21] who developed this test, have reported an excellent correlation between lipase output in the duodenum and the 6-hour cumulative $^{13}CO_2$ excretion in breath, with a sensitivity of 0.89 and a specificity of 0.81 when patients with pancreatic disease were compared with normal controls. However, many false-positive test results were reported for patients with nonpancreatic steatorrhea (7 [32%] of 22 patients), liver disease (5 [42%] of 12 patients) and diabetes (2 [22%] of 9 patients).

The sensitivity and specificity of these tests cannot be assessed. In many patients with bile acid deficiency, however, false-positive results of both tests probably occur because activity of carboxylester lipase requires bile acids, which are necessary for efficient fat absorption. In addition, any breath test based on measurement of breath $^{13}CO_2$ or $^{14}CO_2$ after intestinal hydrolysis of a substrate, absorption of a product, and metabolism by the liver may be associated with false-positive results in patients with diabetes mellitus or obesity, or in patients with diseases (or resection) of the small intestine, liver, or lungs.

Hydrogen Breath Test

With the advent of commercially available, inexpensive, and dedicated breath hydrogen detectors, analysis of breath hydrogen is simple, requires less than 1 minute, and is inexpensive. If 50 g of cooked rice starch is given to patients with severe pancreatic insufficiency, abnormal levels of breath hydrogen are exhaled within 1 to 2 hours (> 20 ppm), whereas normal subjects have no significant increase in breath hydrogen. Although breath hydrogen analysis is a sensitive noninvasive test for carbohydrate malabsorption, it is an insensitive test for detecting pancreatic insufficiency because the test result is abnormal only when pancreatic insufficiency is severe. False-positive results arise in patients who have small bowel bacterial overgrowth or primary maltose deficiency, but this condition is rare. A two-stage test, as described for the triolein breath test and fecal fat tests, has also been described.

In a comparison between the rice flour hydrogen breath test and the NBT-PABA test (see NBT-PABA Test), Patel and associates[22] found that specificity of both tests was 100% in normal subjects and that sensitivity of the hydrogen breath test was 50% and 67% in patients with chronic pancreatitis due to alcohol (n = 14) and tropical pancreatitis (n = 6), respectively, whereas the NBT-PABA test was abnormal in only 29% and 17% of these groups, respectively. In this study, 100 g of uncooked rice flour in 360 mL of water was given, and an increase in breath hydrogen levels of 10 ppm or greater that persisted for at least 45 minutes was considered a positive test result.

Similar results with the hydrogen breath test after administration of 100 g of rice starch have been reported by Kerlin and associates,[23] who found an increase in breath hydrogen in 12 (71%) of 17 patients with pancreatic diseases. However, Hiele and colleagues[24] detected a significant increase of breath H_2 in only 6 (37.5%) of 16 patients with pancreatic disease. These investigators gave patients only 50 g of rice starch; perhaps the decreased sensitivity was due to reduced starch load, but no studies have been performed to test whether different amounts of starch ingested affect sensitivity of the test. Overall, the sensitivity of the hydrogen breath test appears to be between 35% and 70%, but the sensitivity in a group of patients depends on the number of patients with severe pancreatic insufficiency. The hydrogen breath test, nevertheless, may be at least as sensitive and specific as the NBT-PABA test.

The hydrogen breath test has been used with different substrates (glucose or lactulose) to diagnose bacterial overgrowth. The glucose and lactulose tests had sensitivities of 62% and 68% and specificities of 83 and 44%, respectively, when compared with cultures of jejunal aspirates as the gold standard.[25] Because a false-positive result with the glucose hydrogen breath test may occur in up to 44% of patients with celiac disease, use of this test is limited to etiologic investigation of malabsorption.

^{13}C-Labeled Starch Breath Test

A variant of the starch hydrogen breath test[25] takes advantage of naturally occurring ^{13}C in corn starch, and ^{13}C glucose and ^{13}C corn starch were used to measure rates of glucose metabolism and starch digestion and absorption in 13 normal subjects and in 16 patients who had chronic pancreatitis (n = 15) or who had undergone pancreatectomy for pancreatic cancer (n = 1). Because endocrine insufficiency in patients with pancreatic disease alters the rate of glucose metabolism, the measurement of breath $^{13}CO_2$ after corn starch ingestion must be corrected by measurement of breath $^{13}CO_2$ after glu-

cose administration. Thus, a 2-day test was required. In the test, 50 g of ^{13}C glucose and 50 g of ^{13}C corn starch, each in 250 mL of water, were administered on separate days (the order of administration does not affect the test results). During each test, breath $^{13}CO_2$ was measured at basal levels and then every 30 minutes for 6 hours. The ratio of the cumulative 6-hour breath $^{13}CO_2$ measurement with glucose to the same measurement with starch was used as an indicator of starch digestion and absorption. The ratio was abnormal only when amylase secretion was less than or equal to 10% of normal (7 [44%] of 16 of their patients with pancreatic disease).

Similarly, my colleagues and I showed that in normal humans, reduction of amylase activity to 10% or less of normal was associated with starch malabsorption. In these studies, an amylase inhibitor partially purified from white beans[26] was administered orally.[27] Thus, tests of carbohydrate malabsorption detect only end-stage pancreatic disease. Appropriately, the developers of the ^{13}C-labeled starch breath test concluded, "Clearly the $^{13}CO_2$ breath test is not a diagnostic test for pancreatic disease, but evaluates starch absorption in a new way."

Among the human pancreatic enzymes, amylase secretion may be more variable in normal subjects. It is the most resistant to intralumenal inactivation and may be preserved during the development of pancreatic insufficiency and during aboral small intestinal transit.[28] Early in our experience, we found that measurement of amylase outputs after CCK administration was not as sensitive as trypsin and lipase outputs in the detection of pancreatic disease. We therefore do not measure amylase secretion routinely when performing pancreatic function tests. We have found that measurement of amylase secretion (and presumably synthesis) is much more responsive than measurement of trypsin and lipase secretion to dietary manipulations in normal humans,[29] and to induced carbohydrate malabsorption in humans[30] and dogs.[31] In response to amylase inhibition or infusion of carbohydrate into the distal small intestine, amylase secretion increases, but the secretion of trypsin and lipase decreases or remains unchanged. By a variety of mechanisms, humans maintain amylase activity within the gut lumen in preference to other pancreatic enzymes. Thus, noninvasive carbohydrate tests of pancreatic function are not sufficiently sensitive to be practical in diagnosing pancreatic disease.

NBT-PABA Test

The most commonly used tubeless (i.e., noninvasive) test of pancreatic function is based on the hydrolysis of NBT-PABA, a synthetic tripeptide, by chymotrypsin (see Table 133-6). p-Aminobenzoic acid (PABA) is formed by chymotrypsin hydrolysis of NBT-PABA within the small intestine and is absorbed by the intestine, conjugated by the liver, and excreted in urine. Urinary excretion and plasma concentrations of PABA indirectly indicate the amount of intralumenal chymotrypsin. Concentrations of arylamine (i.e., PABA and its metabolites) are measured in urine and serum (see Table 133-6). Certain drugs (acetaminophen, benzocaine, chloramphenicol, lidocaine, phenacetin, procaine, sulfonamide, sulfonylurea, and thiazides) and foods (prunes and cranberries) interfere with the measurement of arylamines; these drugs and foods and exogenous pancreatic enzymes that contain chymotrypsin should not be ingested the day of, and 3 days before, the test is performed. Measuring serum concentrations of PABA provides the same specificity and sensitivity as the urine test.[32] Because obtaining a single blood sample 150 minutes after ingestion of NBT-PABA is easier than obtaining a timed urine collection, the former may become the preferred method.

The appropriate dose of NBT-PABA, the proper duration of the urine collection, and whether NBT-PABA should be given in conjunction with stimulation of pancreatic secretion are partially resolved questions. In the United States, the consensus is that 500 mg of NBT-PABA and a 6-hour collection of urine best discriminate normal humans from those with chronic pancreatitis. In Europe, however, administration of 1 g of NBT-PABA is more common. Administration of NBT-PABA with a meal is recommended, although this practice has not become standard. The normal appearance of PABA in blood and its subsequent excretion into urine represent a physiologic process that involves a number of steps. Therefore, diseases in other organs, or the removal of those organs, may cause abnormal test results. Absorption of PABA may be decreased in patients with mucosal small-bowel disease or Crohn's disease, or in patients who have undergone gastrointestinal surgery. Impaired hepatic function may lead to decreased conjugation of PABA, thereby lowering plasma concentrations and decreasing urinary secretion. Patients with renal insufficiency also have lower excretion of PABA into urine. In addition, 50% of patients with primary diabetes mellitus have an abnormal test result.

Several modifications of the test have been employed to overcome its nonspecificity. Administration of free PABA on a separate day (NBT-PABA–PABA test), or of a labeled ^{14}C-PABA tracer dose simultaneously with NBT-PABA (NBT-PABA–[14]C PABA test), may segregate patients with malabsorption secondary to disorders of the small intestine from those with pancreatic insufficiency. In patients with disorders of the small intestine, PABA excretion is abnormal on both days of the NBT-PABA–PABA test; excretion of both PABA and ^{14}C PABA are abnormal when the NBT-PABA–[14]C PABA is used. By contrast, patients with pancreatic insufficiency have reduced PABA excretion only when NBT-PABA is administered (NBT-PABA–PABA test); when the NBT-PABA–[14]C-PABA test is used, unlabeled PABA excretion is decreased. Simultaneous measurement of creatinine clearance also has been used to correct for renal function. All these modifications probably increase specificity of the test but make it more complex, lengthy, and expensive and do not increase sensitivity (Table 133-9).

The NBT-PABA test has been reported to be 37% to 100% sensitive[33-36] for the detection of chronic pancreatitis. This wide range occurs because the sensitivity of the test depends on the patient's degree of pancreatic insufficiency. In patients with severe insufficiency and malabsorption, the test produces abnormal results 80% to 90% of the time. Unfortunately, in patients who have early pancreatic disease, no malabsorption, and mild to moderate decreases in chymotrypsin secretion, the sensitivity is too low (40%) to be helpful. However, in selected referral populations, the sensitivity may be higher. For example, Lankisch and associates[32] found that the serum and urine tests of NBT-PABA were 86% sensitive in patients with moderate pancreatic insufficiency (i.e., reduced bicar-

TABLE 133-9
Sensitivity and Specificity of Pancreatic Function Tests

TEST	SENSITIVITY (%)	SPECIFICITY (%)
Invasive Tests		
Direct	85–90	85–90
Secretin		
CCK-OP		
Secretin CCK		
Indirect	75–85	75–85
Lundh's test		
Essential amino acids		
Noninvasive Tests		
NBT-PABA	46–86	39–100
Pancreolauryl test	40–93	39–97
Dual-labeled Schilling's test	67–83	?100
Cholesteryl octanoate breath test	100	?100

CCK, cholecystokinin, CCK-OP, N-benzoyl-L-tyrosyl-P-aminobenzoic acid; NBT-PABA, cholecystokinin octapeptide.

bonate concentration and enzyme output without steatorrhea), and 88% sensitive in patients with severe pancreatic insufficiency (i.e., with steatorrhea present). The specificity was 71% in patients with nonpancreatic disease. This study did not include patients with mild pancreatic insufficiency (i.e., moderate reduction of enzyme output without steatorrhea), and this test and other noninvasive tests are least sensitive in this group of patients.

Pancreolauryl Test

The pancreolauryl test is based on the same principle as the NBT-PABA test. Fluorescein dilaurate is a poorly soluble synthetic ester that is hydrolyzed by pancreatic arylesterases to water-soluble fluorescein, which is absorbed by the small intestine, conjugated by the liver, and excreted into urine.

The test is conducted by administering fluorescein dilaurate midway through a breakfast consisting of 50 g of white bread, 20 g of butter, and one cup of tea. To increase the flow of urine, 0.5 L of tea should be consumed before breakfast, and 1 L should be consumed 3 to 5 hours after. Urine is collected for 10 hours after breakfast, and the free fluorescein that has been secreted into urine is measured. Two days later, the same sequence is followed except that free fluorescein, rather than the fluorescein dilaurate, is given with breakfast. The ratio of fluorescein recovered during the first day to the amount recovered when free fluorescein alone is administered, expressed as a percentage, is an index of pancreatic function. Normal test values are greater than 30%; test values between 20% and 30% are inconclusive.

The specificity of the pancreolauryl test is between 46% and 97%,[17,37-41] because false-positive results occur in patients with mucosal small-bowel disease, Crohn's disease, or gastrointestinal surgery. In addition, liver diseases are associated with false-positive results, because bile acids may be necessary for efficient digestion and absorption of the fluorescein dilaurate. Furthermore, some patients with pancreatic insufficiency, particularly in the presence of bacterial overgrowth, may have false-negative test results, because the ester may be hydrolyzed by the intestinal mucosa and by bacteria.

In patients with severe pancreatic insufficiency, the sensitivity of the pancreolauryl tests may be as high as 79%. With mild to moderate degrees of insufficiency, the sensitivity drops precipitously to 40%. However, Lankisch and colleagues[32] reported a 100% and 93% sensitivity in patients with moderate and severe pancreatic insufficiency for the serum and urinary pancreolauryl tests. The pancreolauryl test may offer a slightly higher sensitivity and specificity than the NBT-PABA test (Table 133-10).

Dual-Labeled Schilling's Test

R protein and intrinsic factors are cobalamin-binding proteins in gastric juice. Cobalamin is first bound by R protein. Later, cobalamin is transferred to intrinsic factor after R protein is partially digested by pancreatic enzymes. Normally, equal amounts of intrinsic factor–cobalamin and R protein–cobalamin are absorbed. By contrast, patients with pancreatic insufficiency have normal absorption of intrinsic factor–cobalamin but malabsorption of R protein–cobalamin.

The dual-labeled Schilling's test is performed by administering 0.2 nmol of human intrinsic factor [^{57}CO] cobalamin, 0.2 nmol of hog R protein [^{58}CO], 0.4 nmol of free human intrinsic factor, and 200 nmol of cobinamide together as an oral cocktail. Cobinamide binds only to R protein and prevents endogenous R protein from removing [^{57}CO] cobalamin from intrinsic factor. After the oral solutions are given, 1 mg of cobalamin is given intramuscularly, and urine is collected for 24 hours.

The ratio of [^{58}CO] cobalamin to [^{57}CO] cobalamin in urine indicates pancreatic function (see Table 133-6). Low ratios are found in patients with pancreatic insufficiency, and they correlate with decreased secretion of pancreatic trypsin[42] and bicarbonate.[43] The sensitivity and specificity of this test are uncertain, because the test has been evaluated in only a few studies.[42,43] However, in Brugge's original study,[42] the sensitivity in 18 patients with moderate pancreatic insufficiency (no symptoms and presumably no steatorrhea) and in 19 patients with severe (symptomatic) pancreatic insufficiency was

26% and 100%, respectively, and the specificity was 82% in 11 patients with nonpancreatic gastrointestinal diseases. The false-positive test results occurred in a patient with Crohn's disease and ileal resection and in a patient with bacterial overgrowth. Chen and associates[43] reported similar results. In 9 patients with mild pancreatitis and in 8 patients with severe pancreatitis, as judged by endoscopic retrograde pancreatography, the sensitivity was 44% and 87%, respectively. All 8 patients who had normal results of endoscopic retrograde cholangiopancreatography had a normal dual-labeled Schilling's test result (specificity of 100%).

The dual-labeled Schilling's test may be more sensitive and specific than the NBT-PABA test (see Table 133-10). Chen and associates[43] found that the results of the dual-labeled Schilling's test correlated with the results of endoscopic retrograde pancreatography and of pancreatic function tests, whereas the NBT-PABA test results did not. Similarly, in patients with normal results of endoscopic retrograde pancreatography or of direct pancreatic function tests, the dual-labeled Schilling's test was negative in 100% and 83% of patients, respectively. By comparison, the NBT-PABA test was normal in 67% and 58% of patients, respectively. The increased specificity of the dual-labeled Schilling's test may occur because it is not affected by liver or renal dysfunction.

Plasma Concentrations of Pancreatic Polypeptide During Fasting and Cholecystokinin Administration

Koch and colleagues[44] and others[45] have shown that plasma concentrations of pancreatic polypeptide during fasting and CCK administration are diminished in patients with chronic pancreatitis and pancreatic cancer.

A fasting level of less than 125 pg/mL is sensitive but relatively nonspecific for detection of chronic pancreatitis or pancreatic cancer and has a high negative but a low positive predictive value. Although a low fasting concentration is present in 88% of patients with chronic pancreatitis or pancreatic cancer, it also occurs in 35% of normal subjects. In contrast, a fasting concentration of 125 pg/mL or greater excludes pancreatic cancer or chronic pancreatitis with 85 to 90% confidence.[44]

TABLE 133-10
Sensitivity and Specificity of Pancreatic Function Tests

	NBT-PABA* (%)	PLT† (%)	SCHILLING'S* (%)	SECRETIN-CCK* (%)
Sensitivity				
Chronic pancreatitis				
Moderate	33	93	67	100
Severe	67	100	83	100
Specificity	71	100	100	100

CCK, cholecystokinin; NBT-PABA, N-benzoyl-L-tyrosyl-P-aminobenzoic acid; PLT, pancreolauryl test.

* Data from Chen W-L, Morishita R, Eguchi T, et al. Clinical usefulness of dual-labeled Schilling test for pancreatic exocrine function. Gastroenterology 1989;96:1337.

† Data from Lankisch PG, Brauneis J, Otto J, Göke B. Pancreolauryl and NBT-PABA tests. Are serum tests more practicable alternatives to urine tests with diagnosis of exocrine pancreatic insufficiency? Gastroenterology 1986;90:350.

Koch and colleagues believe, however, that pancreatic polypeptide levels are not specific enough to use routinely in assessing pancreatic function.

Plasma Amino Acid With Cholecystokinin

Domschke and colleagues[46] and Heptner and colleagues[47] have reported that plasma amino acids fall in normal subjects during constant intravenous CCK administration, but that the decrease is smaller in patients with pancreatic disease. Domschke and colleagues[46] reported a significant correlation between the amino acid tests and chymotrypsin output: 67% of patients with 20% to 40% of normal chymotrypsin output had an abnormal test result, whereas all patients with greater loss of chymotrypsin secretion had an abnormal amino acid test result. Gullo and associates[48] reported that measurement of plasma amino nitrogen, which is a simpler method of measuring total plasma amino acid concentration than measurement of individual amino acids during intravenous administration of CCK, is a sensitive indicator of pancreatic function in patients with pancreatic diseases. This test, called the amino acid consumption test (AACT), is simple (two blood samples—fasting and after 60 minutes of intravenous administration of CCK) but lacks sufficient sensitivity and specificity. My colleagues and I have found that during infusion of CCK-OP, the AACT is not an accurate measure of exocrine pancreatic function as assessed by direct measurement of pancreatic secretion.[49] Similarly, Kemmer and associates recently reported that the AACT did not reliably discriminate between patients with normal and abnormal pancreatic function as classified by the pancreolauryl test.[50]

All the noninvasive tests of pancreatic function are satisfactory for diagnosing severe pancreatic insufficiency when steatorrhea is present. In the presence of mild pancreatic insufficiency (only slight reduction of pancreatic secretion), the sensitivity of noninvasive tests likely ranges from 0 (measurement of fecal fat, triolein breath test) to 40% (remaining tests), but the pancreolauryl, NBT-PABA, and dual-labeled Schilling's tests may be up to 85% sensitive in patients with moderate pancreatic insufficiency (50%–90% reduction of pancreatic secretion). Of these tests, the pancreolauryl and dual-labeled Schilling's tests may be more sensitive and specific for the diagnosis of chronic pancreatitis, but there are not enough data to make this claim with certainty. Of all the noninvasive tests, the most attractive may be the serum pancreolauryl and the cholesteryl octanoate breath tests because they are simple and convenient to perform and may be more sensitive and specific than the other noninvasive tests.

> The reader is directed to Chapter 13, Gastric Secretion; Chapter 15, Pancreatic Secretion; Chapter 32, Approach to the Patient with Unexplained Weight Loss; Chapter 61, Acid-Peptic Disorders; and Chapter 91, Chronic Pancreatitis.

REFERENCES

1. Baron JH. When should a clinician perform gastric analysis? J Clin Gastroenterol 1981;3:87.
2. Gugler R, Lindstaedt H, Miederer S, et al. Cimetidine for anastomotic ulcers after partial gastrectomy. N Engl J Med 1979;301:1077.
3. Festen HPM, Lamers CBH, Driessen WMM, Van Tongeren JHM. Cimetidine in anastomotic ulceration after partial gastrectomy. Gastroenterology 1979;76:83.
4. Johnston D, Pickford IR, Walker BE, Goligher JC. Highly selective vagotomy for duodenal ulcer: do hypersecretors need antrectomy? Br Med J 1975;1:716.
5. Joffe SN. Is there a role for gastric secretory testing before ulcer surgery? Surg Gynecol Obstet 1981;152:421.
6. Kronborg O. Influence of the number of parietal cells on risk of recurrence after truncal vagotomy and drainage for duodenal ulcer. Scand J Gastroenterol 1972;7:423.
7. Robbs VJ, Bank S, Marks IN, Louw JH. Selection of operation for duodenal ulcer based on acid secretory studies—a reappraisal. Br J Surg 1973;60:601.
8. Bonfils S, Jensen RT, Malagelada J, Sandil F. Zollinger-Ellison syndrome management: a protocol for strategy. Gastroenterology International 1989;2:9.
9. DiMagno EP, Malagelada J-R, Taylor WP, Go VLW. A prospective comparison of current diagnostic tests in pancreatic cancer. N Engl J Med 1977;297:737.
10. Regan PT, DiMagno EP. Exocrine pancreatic insufficiency in celiac sprue: a cause of treatment failure. Gastroenterology 1980;78:484.
11. DiMagno EP, Malagelada J-R, Moertel CG, Go VLW. Prospective evaluation of the pancreatic secretion of immunoreactive carcinoembryonic antigen, enzyme, and bicarbonate in patients suspected of having pancreatic cancer. Gastroenterology 1977;73:457.
12. DiMagno EP, Go VLW, Summerskill WHJ. Impaired CCK-PZ secretion, intraluminal dilution and maldigestion of fat in sprue. Gastroenterology 1972;63:25.
13. DiMagno EP, Go VLW, Summerskill WHJ. Relations between pancreatic enzyme outputs and malabsorption in severe pancreatic insufficiency. N Engl J Med 1973;288:813.
14. Regan PT, Malagelada J-R, DiMagno EP, et al. Comparative effects of antacids, cimetidine, and enteric coating on the therapeutic response to oral enzymes in severe pancreatic insufficiency. N Engl J Med 1977;297:854.
15. Newcomer AD, Hofmann AF, DiMagno EP, et al. Triolein breath test: a sensitive and specific test for fat malabsorption. Gastroenterology 1979;76:6.
16. DiMagno EP, Malagelada J-R, Go VLW. Relationship between alcoholism and pancreatic insufficiency. Ann NY Acad Sci 1975;252:200.
17. Lankisch PG, Schreiber A, Otto J. Pancreolauryl test: evaluation of a tubeless pancreatic function test in comparison with other indirect and direct tests for exocrine pancreatic function. Dig Dis Sci 1983;28:490.
18. Ammann RW, Akovbiantz A, Haecki W, et al. Diagnostic value of the fecal chymotrypsin test in pancreatic insufficiency, particularly chronic pancreatitis: correlation with the pancreozymin-secretion test, fecal fat excretion and final clinical diagnosis. Digestion 1981;21:281.
19. Perez MM, Newcomer AD, Moertel CG, Go VLW, DiMagno EP. Assessment of weight loss, food intake, fat metabolism, malabsorption, and treatment of pancreatic insufficiency in pancreatic cancer. Cancer 1983;52:346.
20. Cole SG, Rossi S, Stern A, Hofmann AF. Cholesteryl octanoate breath test. Gastroenterology 1987;93:1372.
21. Vantrappen GR, Rutgeerts PJ, Ghoos YF, Hiele MI. Mixed triglyceride breath test: a noninvasive test of pancreatic lipase activity in the duodenum. Gastroenterology 1989;96:1126.
22. Patel VP, Jain NK, Agarwal N, et al. Comparison of bentiromide test and rice flour breath hydrogen test in the detection of exocrine pancreatic insufficiency. Pancreas 1986;1:172.
23. Kerlin P, Wong L, Harris B, Capra S. Rice flour, breath hydrogen, and malabsorption. Gastroenterology 1984;87:578.
24. Hiele M, Ghoos Y, Rutgeerts P, Vantrappen G. Starch digestion in normal subjects and patients with pancreatic disease, using a $^{13}CO_2$ breath test. Gastroenterology 1989;96:503.
25. Corazza GR, Menozzi MG, Strocchi A, et al. The diagnosis of

small bowel bacterial overgrowth. Gastroenterology 1990;93: 302.

26. Layer P, Carlson GL, DiMagno EP. Partially purified white bean amylase inhibitor reduces starch digestion in vitro and inactivates intraduodenal amylase in humans. Gastroenterology 1985; 88;1895.

27. Layer P, Zinsmeister AR, DiMagno EP. Effects of decreasing intraluminal amylase activity on starch digestion and postprandial gastrointestinal function in humans. Gastroenterology 1986;91: 41.

28. Layer P, Go VLW, DiMagno EP. Fate of pancreatic enzymes during small intestinal aboral transit in humans. Am J Physiol 1986;251(Gastrointest Liver Physiol 14):G475.

29. Boivin M, Lanspa SJ, Zinsmeister AR, et al. Are diets associated with different rates of human interdigestive and postprandial pancreatic enzyme secretion? Gastroenterology 1990;99: 1763.

30. Jain NK, Boivin M, Zinsmeister AR, DiMagno EP. The ileum and carbohydrate mediated feedback regulation of postprandial pancreaticobiliary secretion in normal humans. Pancreas 1991;6: 495.

31. Tohno H, Bentley KJ, Sandberg RJ, et al. Is postprandial regulation of amylase secretion (A) by carbohydrate (CHO) in the ileum a response to gastric emptying (GE) of solids or liquids? Pancreas 1988;3:620.

32. Lankisch PG, Brauneis J, Otto J, Göke B. Pancreolauryl and NBT-PABA tests. Are serum tests more practicable alternatives to urine tests in the diagnosis of exocrine pancreatic insufficiency? Gastroenterology 1986;90:350.

33. Arvanitakis C, Greenberger NJ. Diagnosis of pancreatic disease by a synthetic peptide: a new test of exocrine pancreatic function. Lancet 1976;1:663.

34. Gyr K, Stalder GA, Schiffman I, et al. Oral administration of a chymotrypsin-labile peptide—a new test of exocrine pancreatic function in man (PFT). Gut 1976;17:27.

35. Mitchell CJ, Hemphrey CS, Bullen AW, et al. Improved diagnostic accuracy of a modified oral pancreatic function test. Scand J Gastroenterol 1979;14:737.

36. Tetlow VA, Lobley RW, Herman K, Braganza JM. A one-day oral pancreatic function test using a chymotrypsin-labile peptide and a radioactive marker. Clin Trials J 1980;17:121.

37. Boyd EJS, Cumming JGR, Cuschieri A, et al. Prospective comparison of the fluorescein-dilaurate test with the secretin-cholecystokinin test for pancreatic exocrine function. J Clin Pathol 1982;35:1240.

38. Kay G, Hine P, Braganza J. The pancreolauryl test: a method of assessing the combined functional efficacy of pancreatic esterase and bile salts in vivo. Digestion 1982;24:241.

39. Malfertheiner P, Peter M, Junge Un, Ditschuneit H. Der orale Pankreasfunktionstest mit FDL in der Diagnose der chronischen Pankreatitis. Klin Wochenschr 1983;61:193.

40. Ventrucci M, Gullo L, Daniele C, et al. Pancreolauryl test for pancreatic exocrine insufficiency. Am J Gastroenterol 1983;73: 806.

41. Cavallini G, Piubello W, Brocco G, et al. Reliability of the Bz-Ty-PABA and the pancreolauryl test in the assessment of exocrine pancreatic function. Digestion 1983;27:129.

42. Brugge WR, Goff JS, Allen NC, et al. Development of a dual label Schilling test for pancreatic exocrine function based on the differential absorption of cobalamin bound to intrinsic factor and R protein. Gastroenterology 1980;78:937.

43. Chen W-L, Morishita R, Eguchi T, et al. Clinical usefulness of dual-label Schilling test for pancreatic exocrine function. Gastroenterology 1989;96:1337.

44. Koch MB, Go VLW, DiMagno EP. Can pancreatic polypeptide detect diseases of the exocrine pancreas? Mayo Clin Proc 1985;60: 259.

45. Owyang C, Scarpello JH, Vinick AI. Correlations between pancreatic enzyme secretion and plasma concentrations of human pancreatic polypeptide in health and in chronic pancreatitis. Gastroenterology 1982;83:55.

46. Domschke S, Heptner G, Kolb S, et al. Decrease in plasma amino acid level after secretin and pancreozymin as an indicator of exocrine pancreatic function. Gastroenterology 1986;90:1031.

47. Heptner G, Domschke S, Domschke W. Exocrine pancreatic function after gastrectomy. Gastroenterology 1989;97:147.

48. Gullo L, Pezzili R, Ventrucci M. Cerulein-induced plasma amino acid decrease: a simple, sensitive, and specific test of pancreatic function. Pancreas 1989;4:619.

49. Maringhini A, Nelson DK, Jones JD, DiMagno EP. Is the plasma amino acid consumption test an accurate test of exocrine pancreatic insufficiency. Gastroenterology 1994;106:488.

50. Kemmer TP, Malfertheiner P, Häberle H, et al. Die diagnostische Wertigkeit des Aminosäuren-absorptionstests beim Nachweis einer exokrinen Pankreasfunktionsstörung. Z Gastroenterol 1992;30:391.

Textbook of Gastroenterology, second edition, edited by Tadataka Yamada. JB Lippincott Company, Philadelphia © 1995.

CHAPTER 134

Psychiatric Evaluation and Management in Gastrointestinal Illness

Carol S. North

Evaluation of Psychiatric Disorders in Patients With Gastrointestinal Complaints
Mood Disorders
Anxiety Disorders
Personality Disorders
Somatization Disorder
Other Somatoform Disorders
Factitious Disorders
Malingering
Psychologic Factors Affecting Physical Condition

Gastrointestinal Conditions and Psychiatric Associations
Peptic Ulcer
Ulcerative Colitis
Crohn's Disease
Irritable Bowel Syndrome
Esophageal Spasm Syndrome
Colostomy and Ileostomy
Miscellaneous Gastrointestinal Disorders

Gastrointestinal disorders having documented associations with psychiatric disorders include irritable bowel syndrome, esophageal spasm, functional dyspepsia, psychogenic nausea and vomiting, and Crohn's disease. Such psychiatric association, however, does not prove that these conditions are psychosomatic but should serve as a reminder to screen for psychiatric disorders in patients with these conditions. The major psychiatric disorders most commonly associated with functional GI disorders include major depression, anxiety disorders, and somatization disorder. These psychiatric conditions are frequently missed in patients with medical illnesses, and their treatment cannot only reduce morbidity significantly but can also be expected to contribute to better outcome of the physical condition. With basic knowledge of psychiatric diagnosis and appropriate use of psychotropic medication, many psychiatric conditions can be managed without referral to a psychiatric specialist.

It is important for clinicians to avoid the pitfall of treating individual psychiatric symptoms such as anxiety or insomnia; instead, appropriate focus on treatment of diagnosable psychiatric disorders yields greater success. Appropriate psychiatric diagnosis can only be made by careful history-taking to determine whether the patient's symptoms qualify him for a particular psychiatric diagnosis by currently accepted criteria. When treating diagnosed psychiatric disorders, the appropriate psychotropic agent must be selected, and it should be pre-

scribed in sufficiently vigorous doses for therapeutic efficacy. Specifically, this requires daily doses of up to 300 mg for most tricyclic antidepressants (nortriptyline requires about one half this dose) and a trial of at least 2 to 3 weeks once a therapeutic dose is achieved. Appreciation that the pharmacotherapeutic profile for the use of antidepressant medication is unique from that of the benzodiazepines helps the physician avoid errors such as treating with antidepressant doses too small to be effective. Medication should be prescribed that is appropriate to the particular psychiatric disorder and not aimed at individual symptoms. For example, anxiety symptoms and complaints of insomnia that are secondary to major depression are more appropriately treated with an antidepressant than with a benzodiazepine as the primary agent. Familiarity with specific side effects such as the prominent sedation characteristic of amitriptyline can aid in the selection of an appropriate agent for the individual situation.

The near future cannot be expected to produce technology that will allow psychiatric diagnosis through any particular laboratory or psychometric procedure. Physicians have to continue to rely on clinical information achieved through personal examination of the patient to arrive at a psychiatric diagnosis by the established criteria. New pharmacotherapeutic agents with greater efficacy and different side effect profiles continue to be introduced into the market, allowing more choices for the unique characteristics of each case.

Literature on psychiatric aspects of gastrointestinal (GI) medicine is voluminous and complicated by the fact that historically there have been many different ways of examining the interplay of psychiatric factors and GI conditions. This chapter describes evaluation and management of specific psychiatric disorders encountered in the practice of gastroenterology, using the medically oriented model of psychiatry as a source of information and focus. This information should help clinicians to recognize the most frequent psychiatric conditions encountered in GI practice and to manage most of these conditions or know when to refer cases to psychiatric specialists.

In the past 15 to 20 years, the field of psychiatry has experienced a shift in focus to reidentify with the rest of medicine. Associated with this shift, psychiatric illness has been reconceptualized to constitute a set of ideas often referred to as the medical model.[1] This model is based on an appreciation of distinct psychiatric disorders and their differences, paralleling the concept of distinct and identifiable diseases basic to the study of medicine. Psychiatric illness cannot be adequately investigated without its delineation into distinct syndromes. The current standard nosology of psychiatric illness is the *Diagnostic and Statistical Manual of Mental Disorders, 4th edition, revised (DSM-IV)*.[2]

The availability of reliable diagnostic criteria provided in *DSM-IV* has enabled subsequent development of structured diagnostic interviews, such as the Diagnostic Interview Schedule.[3] With these techniques, diagnostic reproducibility in psychiatry has been shown to be comparable to routine tests in other areas of medicine such as the electrocardiogram.[4] Increasing acceptance and use of such techniques have enabled recent advances in diverse areas of psychiatric research. Standardized criteria and structured interviews are necessary methodologic tools for the exploration of the relation of psychiatric illness to GI disease.[5]

An important caveat in the recognition of psychologic symptoms in GI illness is to avoid jumping to the conclusion of causation in the mere presence of data only indicating an association. Today it is recognized that physical illness may directly induce psychologic symptoms, in contrast to the reverse idea that certain illnesses are a product of psychosomatic origins.[6] For example, the occurrence of anxiety in an ulcerative colitis patient anticipating surgery may represent a common human response to stress generated by the illness, rather than a cause of the exacerbation of illness. It cannot be disputed that stress may exacerbate any physical illness, further complicating efforts to untangle the variables involved in the relation of psychiatric symptoms to GI illness. Common psychologic accompaniments to physical illness include symptoms of depression or anxiety, as well as a range of other emotions such as anger, sadness, or fear. In most persons, these reactions are transitory, do not indicate the presence of serious psychiatric disorder, and can often be resolved by a physician who takes the time to share genuine concern and interest in the patient. Knowing the basics of psychiatric diagnosis, the average gastroenterologist, general internist, or family physician should be able to recognize and manage the majority of psychiatric conditions that present with gastroenterologic complaints.[7] Knowledge of psychiatric diagnosis can also aid in determining when referral to a psychiatrist is warranted.

EVALUATION OF PSYCHIATRIC DISORDERS IN PATIENTS WITH GASTROINTESTINAL COMPLAINTS

About one third of the general population develop a psychiatric disorder in their lives.[8,9] Rates are even higher for persons with chronic medical illness, with a 42% lifetime prevalence of psychiatric disorders documented in this population.[9] Hence, in conducting research on the rates of psychopathology in patients with chronic GI illness, it is crucial to have a population of medically ill controls to avoid contamination by measurement of the nonspecific psychiatric effects of chronic medical illness.

Establishing a psychiatric diagnosis is a critical first step for clinical and research investigations.[1] Accurate diagnosis is also essential for determining prognosis and designing treatment. A clinician can be easily misled by symptoms such as anxiety or diarrhea from determining the greater meaning of these symptoms within the context of psychiatric diagnosis. Identification of psychiatric disorders greatly enhances the primary physician's repertoire in managing patients with gastroenterologic complaints, considering that the majority of these complaints are functional, and the majority of functional GI disorders occur in the context of a psychiatric disorder.[10]

Although it is easier to order psychologic testing or to have patients fill out self-report inventories, there is no substitute for time spent with the patient to determine the presence of criterion symptoms of specific psychiatric disorders. Psychologic tests such as the Minnesota Multiphasic Personality Inventory (MMPI), the Rorschach inkblot test, the Thematic Apperception Test (TAT), and the Beck Depression Inventory (BDI) have their place. However, failure to recognize their limitations and proper applications has led to invalid conclusions in numerous studies, and reliance on them can lead to inadequate clinical management.

Psychologic tests with established reliability are appropriate for the assessment of IQ, cognition, and personality factors, but not in determining psychiatric diagnosis. Patients with somatization disorder, for example, often report high rates of depressive symptoms and would score very high on the BDI. Clinicians using this instrument for diagnostic purposes could mistakenly classify these patients as having a primary depressive disorder and miss the important diagnosis of somatization disorder. If a psychiatric diagnosis is so puzzling that psychologic testing is being considered, the patient should probably be referred to a psychiatrist.

Just as a clinical interview is necessary for making a psychiatric diagnosis, direct patient contact regarding symptoms and medication effects is necessary to provide sufficient feedback for directing the treatment regimen. Depressed patients, for example, should be monitored for any changes in the criterion symptoms of depression, such as fluctuations in mood, sleep, appetite, and energy. Evidence of medication side effects and certain crucial symptoms, such as suicidality, should also be elicited.

Just as there are no psychologic tests that make psychiatric diagnoses, there are no laboratory tests available to do this either. Although a positive dexamethasone suppression test for depression and enlarged cerebral ventricular size by computed tomography for schizophrenia correlate positively with the presence of these psychiatric diagnoses, these tests are neither sufficiently sensitive nor specific enough to permit diagnosis on the basis of their results.

This chapter describes several psychiatric disorders that commonly accompany GI complaints and focuses on techniques for diagnosis and treatment of each. Substance abuse disorders and eating disorders are not included in this discussion because these disorders are discussed elsewhere in this text (see Chaps. 32 and 50).

Mood Disorders

Mood disorders represent the most common of the major psychiatric conditions.[11] In *DSM-IV*, these disorders are divided into bipolar mood disorders and unipolar depressive disorders.[2] Occurrence of a manic episode, whether or not history of a depressive episode is present, automatically qualifies the mood disorder as bipolar. Unipolar depression, also called major depression, is characterized by depressive episodes only.

Approximately 5% of men and 9% of women suffer from mood disorder during their lives.[11] Unipolar depression is far more common than the bipolar type, with only one in ten mood disorder patients ever experiencing a manic episode. Peak age of onset for mood disorders is early in the third decade,[2] although the age of risk extends throughout life. The illness tends to be episodic, typically with full recovery and good function between episodes. The length of episodes can vary, usually briefer in mania (days to months) than in depression (usually 6 months or longer).

Manic episodes usually begin suddenly in an otherwise well-adjusted person, with rapid escalation over a few days, and they must last at least 1 week to qualify for a definite diagnosis. Typically, the patient has poor insight that he or she is ill. Poor judgment and hyperactivity associated with a manic episode can rapidly progress to serious consequences such as financial losses and embarrassing or illegal behaviors; hence, mania should be managed without delay by a psychiatrist, often with hospitalization. A manic episode is characterized by a distinct change in mood that is classically euphoric or irritable, often associated with decreased need for sleep, hyperactivity, grandiosity, and loud, rapid speech. Delusions and hallucinations commonly occur in mania, and the physician should avoid the mistake of diagnosing schizophrenia just because of the presence of these psychotic symptoms. Hypomania is similar to mania but with a lesser degree of impairment, usually not severe enough to warrant hospitalization. Treatment consists of lithium, antipsychotic medication, or both; nonresponders sometimes improve with carbamazepine (Tegretol), valproic acid (Depakote), or electroconvulsive therapy.

Mania may follow childbirth or psychosocial stresses, and an episode can be precipitated by antidepressant medication. Organic syndromes resembling mania can result from certain psychoactive substances such as amphetamines or steroids. The clinician should always consider this possibility when a patient on steroids develops acute mania, depression, or psychotic symptoms. An acutely psychotic patient may be suffering from mania, intoxication, a postictal state, or a variety of medical and psychiatric conditions.

A major depressive episode represents a change from the person's usual state or level of functioning, and it must last at least 2 weeks to qualify for a definite diagnosis. The hallmark of major depression is depressed mood, often with irritability; otherwise, loss of interest or pleasure (i.e., anhedonia) in almost all activities must be present for the diagnosis. Change in mood is neither necessary nor sufficient for a diagnosis of depression, and mood is not the only disordered function in major depression.

According to one study, 97% of patients with depression complained of fatigue or low energy[12]; other common symptoms include change in appetite and weight, which is usually decreased but sometimes increased; insomnia or, less frequently, excessive need for sleep; physical agitation or retardation; feelings of worthlessness, low self-esteem, or guilt; impaired concentration; and thoughts of death or suicide. Occasionally, patients may experience psychotic symptoms such as hearing voices or having delusions usually related to depressive ideas. Table 134-1 lists the *DSM-IV* criteria for major depression. Because depression is common in gastroenterologic practice, the clinician may want to keep a list of these symptoms handy for inquiry when major depression is suspected.

The etiology of mood disorder is unknown, but it runs in families. Genetic factors have been documented in family

---

TABLE 134-1
Diagnostic Criteria for Major Depressive Episode

A. At least five of the following symptoms have been present nearly every day during the same 2-week period and represent a change from previous functioning; at least one of the symptoms is either (1) depressed mood, or (2) loss of interest or pleasure. Do not include symptoms that are clearly due to a physical condition, mood, incongruent delusions or hallucinations, incoherence, or marked loosening of associations.
  1. Depressed mood most of the day
  2. Markedly diminished interest or pleasure in all, or almost all, activities most of the day
  3. Significant weight loss or weight gain when not dieting (e.g., more than 5% of body weight in a month), or decrease or increase in appetite
  4. Insomnia or hypersomnia
  5. Psychomotor agitation or retardation (observable by others, not merely subjective feelings of restlessness or being slowed down)
  6. Fatigue or loss of energy
  7. Feelings of worthlessness or excessive or inappropriate guilt (which may be delusional; not merely self-reproach or guilt about being sick)
  8. Diminished ability to think or concentrate, or indecisiveness
  9. Recurrent thoughts of death (not just fear of dying), recurrent suicidal ideation without a specific plan, or a suicide attempt or a specific plan for committing suicide
B. Symptoms cause clinically significant distress or impairment in social, occupational, or other important areas of function.
C. Symptoms are not due to direct physiological effects of a substance or a general medical condition.
D. Symptoms are not due to bereavement.

Adapted from American Psychiatric Association Diagnostic and statistical manual of mental disorders. 4th ed. Washington, DC: American Psychiatric Association, 1994.

studies, twin studies, and adoption studies.[12] Chronic physical illness may predispose to major depression, and, in the practice of gastroenterologic medicine, conditions such as Crohn's disease and irritable bowel syndrome have been specifically associated with increased rates of depression beyond those seen in association with other chronic medical illnesses (see Gastrointestinal Conditions and Psychiatric Associations). Other medical conditions associated with elevated rates of depressive symptoms are pneumonia and other infections, pernicious anemia, diabetes, thyroid and parathyroid disorders, Cushing's disease, Addison's disease, systemic lupus erythematosus, and neurologic disorders including intracranial tumors and dementias.[2,6,13]

Substance abuse, particularly alcohol and cocaine dependence, may predispose to depression. Depression may also follow childbirth, ranging from ordinary baby blues to psychotic postpartum depression, and depression may also follow stressful events such as death of a loved one or divorce. An organic depressive syndrome may be precipitated by psychoactive substances such as reserpine, propranolol, cimetidine, or occasionally, steroids.[2]

The most serious complication of depression is suicide, which is completed in about 15% of persons experiencing major depression during their lifetime.[14] Thus, it is crucial that the physician performs a diagnostic inquiry in any patient with symptoms related to depression such as discouragement, insomnia, and fatigue, and includes with this inquiry an exploration of the possibility of suicide. Over two thirds of suicide completers warn others of their intent,[15] and patients with suicidal thoughts usually admit these to a physician if asked.[16]

Once the patient admits to suicidal ideas, further inquiry is needed to determine if these ideas are currently present. Seriousness of these ideas is assessed by asking about whether the patient has intent to harm himself and whether he has a lethal plan. Because the majority of persons who commit suicide contact a physician within weeks or even hours before their death,[15] the physician may be the greatest source of intervention. However, due to lack of awareness, physicians often fail to inquire further when signs of depression are present.

Greatest risk of suicide occurs in males over age 40, currently unmarried, with concurrent substance abuse, a history of recent personal loss, history of prior suicide attempts, especially if recent, and communication of suicidal intent.[11,17] The two psychiatric disorders most frequently associated with completed suicide are alcoholism and mood disorder.[18]

Treatment of depression in uncomplicated cases can be managed without referral to a psychiatrist. The most common errors in pharmacologic treatment are the use of inappropriate psychotropic agents, inadequate doses of the appropriate agent, and inadequate length of trial.[19]

The following agents should not be used for the primary treatment of depression: anxiolytic agents, such as benzodiazepines (e.g., diazepam [Valium], chlordiazepoxide [Librium], alprazolam [Xanax]), and sedative hypnotics. The agents of choice in treating depression are any of the tricyclic antidepressant medications and some of the newer tetracyclic or nontricyclic drugs. Widely used tricyclic antidepressants include amitriptyline (Elavil) and imipramine (Tofanil). The usual starting dose is 25 to 50 mg/day, generally at bedtime,

particularly for amitriptyline, which is more sedating. Usually the dose is rapidly advanced over a period of days (as tolerated) to 150 mg/day, and the patient is reassessed.

A therapeutic response does not occur for 2 or 3 weeks after therapeutic dosage is achieved; lack of clinical response in the first few days of treatment does not indicate therapeutic failure. If there is no response after 2 weeks at 150 mg, the dosage is increased as tolerated in increments of 50 mg, waiting 2 weeks at each dosage level for a response. This process is continued until a clinical response occurs or until a dosage of 300 mg is reached. For the patient who is nonresponsive after an adequate trial, a serum tricyclic level may aid in determining whether the lack of response is due to insufficient blood level or to treatment failure.

Unlike the benzodiazepines, antidepressants have a dosage threshold below which there is no beneficial effect. Hence, failing to advance the dosage beyond 50 or 100 mg automatically dooms the treatment plan to failure. Once a therapeutic response has been achieved, duration of therapy should be 4 to 6 months. At that time, the drug dosage may be tapered over 2 to 3 weeks, and the patient should be observed carefully for a reemergence of depressive symptoms.

The most common side effects are anticholinergic and include dry mouth, constipation, blurred vision, urinary hesitancy, and sexual dysfunction. Weight gain is another side effect, which may understandably reduce compliance in some patients. Amitriptyline is the most anticholinergic tricyclic, making it less desirable as a first-choice antidepressant. Doxepin (Sinequan) is less anticholinergic but almost as sedating, making it a reasonable alternative if sedation is desired. Desipramine (Norpramin) is the least anticholinergic of the tricyclics.

The most dangerous side effects include cardiac arrhythmias, orthostatic hypotension, and diminished sweating. Compared to other tricyclic antidepressant agents, nortriptyline (Pamelor) is associated with fewer problems with orthostasis.[20] Therefore it is an especially attractive agent for geriatric patients and patients with chronic medical illness, specifically cardiovascular disease. Nortriptyline differs from the other tricyclics in that the doses used are about half the others.

The arrhythmogenic properties of tricyclic antidepressants make these medications potentially dangerous for certain cardiac patients. These drugs affect cardiac conduction in much the same way as the group I antiarrhythmic agents, such as quinidine and procainamide. Their effect is greatest on the distal portion of the His-Purkinje system, with electrocardiographic manifestations of increased PR interval, increased QRS duration, and sinus tachycardia. The general rule with tricyclic antidepressants is that these agents might be expected to improve the condition of premature ventricular contraction, but would worsen bundle branch block, anterior hemiblock, and other conduction defects. Overdose of tricyclic antidepressants in amounts of only a 10- to 15-day supply of daily dosage can be lethal, which should be considered when prescribing these medications to patients who may be at risk for suicide attempts.

The nontricyclic agent fluoxetine (Prozac) is far safer in such situations because it is not associated with anticholinergic, orthostatic, or cardiotoxic side effects and is virtually never fatal in overdoses. It is therefore a relatively safe choice for patients with cardiac problems and for patients who may be at increased risk for suicide. Its main side effects are upper GI symptoms such as nausea and dyspepsia, and headache. GI side effects can be reduced by administering it with food. Fluoxetine can be very activating, and therefore is given as a 20 mg dose in the morning or twice early in the day. Patients who find it too activating with this dosage schedule may find it tolerable if concomitantly administered a benzodiazepine to cover the initial period of jitteriness before tolerance to this side effect is achieved. In some cases, patients who have difficulty tolerating fluoxetine's side effects can be managed with lower doses; given the long half life of this agent, patients can be managed with a 20 mg dose of fluoxetine every other day or every third day.

Another nontricyclic agent, trazodone (Desyrel), is sedating and is therefore useful as a bedtime agent in doses similar to those of most tricyclic antidepressants, but some patients may require and can tolerate up to 600 mg a day. A potential advantage is sedation, a side effect that may benefit patients with insomnia. Unwelcome cases of priapism, sometimes irreversible without surgery, have made this drug unpopular as a first-choice agent of therapy for male patients. Initial reports indicated relatively few problems with cardiotoxicity, but subsequent indications of occasional ventricular arrhythmias and orthostatic hypotension further limit this drug's usefulness.

Other new agents include bupropion (Wellbutrin) and sertraline (Zoloft). Both can be somewhat activating. Bupropion is associated with seizures and therefore must be given in carefully spaced, divided doses, up to four times a day, with a maximum recommended dosage of 450 mg per 24-hour period. The most frequent side effect of sertraline is diarrhea, and it is prescribed in doses of 50 to 200 mg a day, usually early in the day.

In patients who are poorly tolerant or unresponsive to adequate antidepressant therapy, psychiatric consultation is recommended. Psychiatric referral is also necessary for patients expressing intent to harm themselves or others and for those with psychotic symptoms such as hallucinations and delusions. The latter patients will require neuroleptic medication along with the antidepressant, or electroconvulsive therapy. Lithium is sometimes used as an adjunct to antidepressant treatment, although the initiation of treatment and monitoring is much more complicated with this agent. Electroconvulsive therapy is considered the most effective form of treatment for depression, and it is often used when pharmacotherapy is unsatisfactory or in the presence of psychotic symptoms. Contrary to its reputation, electroconvulsive therapy is a safe and not particularly unpleasant mode of treatment, and in many cases (e.g., cardiac disease, pregnancy) it is much safer than antidepressant medications.

Psychotherapy is important in treatment of depression. Supportive psychotherapy, consisting of compassionate listening to the patient discuss symptoms and problems, is often enough to ameliorate stress to a more tolerable level while the antidepressant regimen is proceeding. A large part of psychotherapy also consists of educating the patient about the psychiatric disorder, the prognosis, and medication and its expected side effects, which greatly enhances compliance and speeds recovery. It is common for patients to want to take a pill when they are feeling most upset and seeking immediate symptom relief, while neglecting regular doses. Unnecessary delays in the treatment may be avoided by explaining to patients how antidepressant medication works (i.e., about the therapeutic threshold). Providing information about common side effects and how to cope with them may prevent patient abandonment of the medication as a result of disillusionment.

Anxiety Disorders

Symptoms of anxiety commonly accompany serious medical illness, and anxiety disorders are also common in the general population.[8] In gastroenterologic practice, anxiety symptoms commonly occur in association with irritable bowel syndrome and esophageal spasm syndrome. In DSM-IV, anxiety disorders include panic disorders and generalized anxiety disorder.

Panic Disorder

This disorder affects 2% of women and around 1% of men in the general population.[21] Average age of onset is in the mid 20s, although this may vary. Panic attacks typically begin with sudden feelings of fear and apprehension, which frequently build to terror and a sense of impending doom. During these circumscribed attacks, patients experience, by definition, at least four of the following thirteen symptoms: difficulty breathing, dizziness, palpitations, shaking, sweating, choking, nausea, feelings of unreality, paresthesias, hot flashes or chills, chest pain, fear of dying, and fear of going crazy.[2]

The majority of patients with this disorder will also have a lifetime history of major depression,[22] and panic disorder occurs in about one of five patients with major depression. In addition, more than one third of patients with panic disorder develop agoraphobia.[21]

Differential diagnosis of panic disorder includes effects of pharmacologic agents such as amphetamines, theophylline, and caffeine. Medical disorders known to cause anxiety and panic symptoms include pheochromocytoma, thyroid and parathyroid disorders, Cushing's disease, hypoglycemia, neurologic disorders, porphyria, pneumonia, hyperventilation, angina pectoris, cardiac arrhythmias, and mitral valve prolapse.[6,13] Other conditions must be ruled out by careful medical evaluation of patients with anxiety complaints, always keeping in mind that conditions such as mitral valve prolapse may coexist with an anxiety disorder in the same patient.

Anxiety and panic symptoms also commonly occur in somatization disorder, alcoholism, and withdrawal from drugs. A well-known complication of anxiety disorders is abuse of alcohol and other substances; barbiturate and benzodiazepine abuse occur frequently, often iatrogenically induced through overzealous prescription by well-meaning physicians.

Treatment of panic disorder is accomplished with specific pharmacologic agents that have been shown effective in double-blind trials. The first group is tricyclic antidepressants, with imipramine having been best documented, although there is evidence that other agents including desipramine, nortriptyline, amitriptyline, and doxepin may also be useful[22] in doses in the range as those considered effective for major depression.

Monoamine oxidase inhibitors are also useful but are less attractive than tricyclic antidepressants in the treatment of panic disorder, due to the potential for hypertensive crisis induced by ingestion of tyramine, requiring a special low-tyramine diet and avoidance of sympathomimetic agents. This same problem complicates the otherwise very effective treatment of major depression with monoamine oxidase inhibitors.

Nontricyclic antidepressant agents such as fluoxetine have also been recommended for the management of panic disorder in patients with functional bowel disease.[23,24] Trazodone and bupropion have not been shown to be effective, however.[23]

High-potency benzodiazepines such as alprazolam (Xanax), lorazepam (Ativan), and clonazepam (Klonopin) have been found to be as effective as tricyclic antidepressants and monoamine oxidase inhibitors in the treatment of panic disorder, and diazepam (Valium) has also been demonstrated to be useful. Although abuse potential is considered low, drawbacks to the use of benzodiazepines include difficulty tapering these agents and tolerance.[23,25,26] Benzodiazepines are not recommended for patients with a history of substance abuse, personality disorders, and chronic benign pain syndromes (e.g., back pain, headaches) and in patients with a family history of substance abuse. Controversy continues over the potential of benzodiazepines for tolerance, abuse, and general utility for prolonged therapy.[27]

Although major tranquilizers such as chlorpromazine (Thorazine) and thioridazine (Mellaril) lack the abuse potential of benzodiazepines, they may not be as effective, and chronic use is limited by their potential for serious side effects such as tardive dyskinesia, a movement disorder that is not always reversible on termination of the drug. Antipsychotic medications might be a reasonable second choice agent for short-term (i.e. <4 weeks) treatment of anxiety disorders in patients who have contraindications for benzodiazepines. The low-potency agents mentioned previously may have less potential compared with high-potency agents such as haloperidol (Haldol) for movement disorders.[28]

In addition to pharmacotherapy, behavioral treatment including systematic desensitization, flooding techniques, and progressive relaxation are thought to be useful adjuncts as well as primary procedures in the treatment of panic disorder.[26] Psychotherapy, especially utilizing cognitive-behavioral techniques, may also be very helpful.[26,29–31] Consensus remains, however, that pharmacotherapy is central to the management of panic disorder.[32]

Generalized Anxiety Disorder

This is a relatively newly defined disorder which first appeared in the *DSM-IV* in 1980. It occurs in about 5% of the population, with a slight male preponderance.[33] It tends to start in the early 20s, but it can start at any age. It is characterized by generalized, persistent anxiety without circumscribed panic attacks. According to *DSM-IV*, generalized anxiety disorder is defined as excessive worry and anxiety that are difficult to control about a number of events or activities and are associated with at least three of the following six symptoms: restlessness or feeling keyed up or on edge; being easily fatigued; difficulty concentrating or mind going blank; irritability; muscle tension; and sleep disturbance. The symptoms must last for at least 6 months, cause significant distress or impairment in social, occupational, or other important areas of functioning, and be independent of effects of substance abuse or medical conditions.[2]

These patients are less likely to receive psychiatric treatment than are patients with panic disorder. They more often present to cardiologists, pulmonary specialists, and gastroenterologists, infrequently seeking out psychiatric treatment. One fourth of patients with generalized anxiety disorder will also develop panic disorder.[34] The majority will also develop major depression.[34] The differential diagnosis of generalized anxiety disorder is the same as for panic disorder.

Imipramine and benzodiazepines such as alprazolam and diazepam have been shown to have similar efficacy for the treatment of generalized anxiety disorder, although the benzodiazepines may have a faster onset of action.[35] In addition, a newer agent of the azapirone category, buspirone (Buspar), appears useful for the management of generalized anxiety disorder, without the risks of tolerance and withdrawal associated with benzodiazepines.

Beta blockers such as propranolol may also be useful in anxiety disorders, especially for predominant autonomic symptoms such as tremor, but in general they are not found to be as useful as antidepressants or alprazolam.[34] Anxiety disordered patients may be helped by eliminating caffeine from their diets, as its anxiogenic effects may contribute to anxiety and panic symptoms.

Personality Disorders

Personality disorders are a collection of behaviors or traits that are longstanding, typically beginning in childhood, and that impair social or occupational function or cause subjective distress. Some consider this a pejorative term, because the most extreme and easily recognized patients with this diagnosis have undesirable traits and can be difficult and unpleasant to manage.[34] Personality disorders, however, are quite varied, and can range from the most unpleasant overdramatic, obnoxious, criminal, and dangerous types to ones that are merely chronically anxious, dependent, and unmotivated. Patients particularly with the latter types of personality disorders can often be pleasant and yield satisfying results in the treatment setting. *Neurosis* is an outdated term for a class of patients now largely described as having personality disorders.

Personality disorders are common, with 10% to 20% of the population meeting criteria for one of the 11 specific personality disorders.[34,36] As currently defined in *DSM-IV,* these disorders overlap extensively within individuals, and many patients who meet criteria for one diagnosis also qualify for others.[36–40] Personality disorders frequently accompany other psychiatric disorders, especially substance abuse[41] and eating disorders,[42] but also commonly accompany major depression and anxiety disorders.[43]

Unfortunately, the nosological classification of personality disorders is not yet sufficiently established.[39,44,45] This problem makes the study of these disorders very difficult, and as a result there has been little systematic research on personality disorder in gastrointestinal illness.

Personality disorders are prevalent in patients with functional gastrointestinal disorders. In particular, irritable bowel syndrome, chronic abdominal pain disorders, and psychogenic vomiting are commonly associated with personality problems or with neurosis,[10,46,47] and with a variety of interpersonal and psychosocial problems and multiple other psychiatric disorders,[48–51] a pattern associated with personality disorders. Laxative abusers would be expected to have excess rates of personality disorders, and laxative abuse is a well known behavior of patients with eating disorders.

Personality disorder greatly complicates the treatment of medical and psychiatric conditions. The prognosis is compromised by problems of noncompliance and often difficult doctor-patient relationships. Patterns of missing appointments and calling with a crisis at inconvenient times characterize the health care–seeking behavior of many of these patients; others regularly use emergency departments for treatment during crises in lieu of regular follow-up, which might have prevented the crisis. Physicians may find these patients unpleasant and demanding, and may have to expend extra effort to maintain quality care.

These patients also have increased risk for iatrogenic substance abuse due to the chronic nature of their complaints, and their use of abusable substances should be limited and closely monitored. Excessive demands for narcotics and benzodiazepines should automatically alert the physician to the possibility of a personality disorder.

Because these patients characteristically evoke strong reactions in others, feelings of anger or other emotion toward a patient can provide a valuable indicator of the possibility of personality disorder for further exploration. The role of the practitioner in these cases is first to recognize the disorder, and to manage the behavioral problems by setting limits on demands for attention, favors, and abusable drugs. Maintenance of firm rules regarding fees, roles, and schedules may be necessary. Personality disorders are generally lifelong conditions; the efficacy of psychotherapy on long-term outcome is not documented.

Somatization Disorder

Somatization disorder is characterized by a long, dramatic, and complex medical history of multiple somatic symptoms without medical explanation. The older label of hysteria is no longer applied to this disorder. The importance of this disorder is the havoc it can play in medical management if it is not recognized. The diagnosis requires onset prior to 30 years of age, with social or occupational or other signs of impairment due to the presence of symptoms in four symptom groups (Table 134-2). To qualify as a positive symptom on this list, it has to be medically unexplainable, have had a significant effect on the patient's life or required medical attention, and have occurred at times other than during a panic attack. There are seven screening symptoms on the list, and, if two are positive, there is a high likelihood that the disorder is present.

Although somatization disorder is relatively uncommon in the general population (<2%),[8] it is seen more frequently in large medical centers because patients search for an explanation of their multiple unexplainable symptoms in many medical specialties.[50] Somatization disorder is also more prevalent in less educated, lower socioeconomic populations.[51] This is a stable diagnosis, and, after years of follow-up, 90% of patients with this diagnosis continue to have the same syndrome without discovery of medical disorders to explain their symptoms.[52]

Somatization disorder is almost exclusively a disorder of

TABLE 134-2
Criteria for Diagnosis of Somatization Disorder

A. Multiple physical complaints or feeling sickly, beginning before age 30 years and lasting several years that result in treatment being sought or significant impairment in social, occupational or other important areas of function.

B. Each of the following criteria must have been met with symptoms* occurring at any time during the illness:
   1. Four pain symptoms (of at least four different sites or functions)
   2. Two gastrointestinal symptoms (other than pain)
   3. One sexual or reproductive symptom (other than pain)
   4. One pseudoneurological symptom (other than pain)

* Not fully explained by effects of known general medical condition or a substance; or complaint or impairment are in excess of what would be expected from history, physical examination, or laboratory findings.

Adapted from American Psychiatric Association. Diagnostic and statistical manual of mental disorders. 4th ed. Washington, DC: American Psychiatric Association, 1994.

---

women. When somatoform symptoms appear in men, caution in making this diagnosis is advised because men often develop serious medical or psychiatric conditions over time accounting for the symptoms.[53,54]

The somatoform symptoms typically begin before age 20 and almost always by age 30.[55] Thus, caution is warranted in considering this diagnosis in a woman who first develops somatoform symptoms later in life. The condition remains chronic, with only rare remissions, and a year seldom passes without medical attention. Somatization disorder runs in families, occurring in 10% to 20% of first-degree female relatives; male relatives show increased rates of antisocial personality disorder and substance abuse.[2] Through the process of assortative mating (i.e., finding partners who complement or provide counterpoint to their characteristics), women with somatization disorder tend to attach themselves to men who are sociopathic, alcoholic, or both.[56,57] Their marriages also have high rates of discord and dissolution.[53,58] Patients with somatization disorder very often have a personality disorder,[2] and some experts think the disorder should be reclassified as a personality disorder.[58]

Patients with somatization disorder can find ample opportunity to consult internists about GI symptoms, because the criteria include seven symptoms referable to the GI system, including: vomiting, abdominal pain, nausea, bloating/flatulence, diarrhea, food intolerances, and burning rectal pain. Somatization disorder was discovered in 17% of irritable bowel subjects in one study[59] and 28% in another.[60] Somatization disorder has also been found to be present in 20% of patients with esophageal contraction abnormalities.[61] Organic and pseudoorganic conditions most easily confused with somatization disorder include psychomotor epilepsy, symptoms of migraine, chronic fatigue syndrome, and complaints of hypoglycemia or multiple allergies.[13] In fact, many patients with documented somatization disorder also report these problems, and many patients with these other syndromes meet full criteria for somatization disorder.[62–65]

Many patients with somatization disorder report chronic

abdominal or pelvic pain, and as a result undergo multiple gastroenterologic and gynecologic surgeries. A history of sexual abuse in childhood is present in nearly two thirds of women with chronic pelvic pain, and almost half have experienced sexual abuse as adults.[66] A study of women with functional GI disorders found that more than half had been sexually or physically abused.[48] Sexual and physical abuse are highly associated with a variety of major psychiatric disorders and especially with somatization and personality disorders.[67-69] Therefore sensitive questioning about history of abuse may help identify such patients.

The significance of somatization disorder in primary care is that the diagnosis is frequently missed[70] or misdiagnosed as depression, anxiety, or another psychiatric disorder. In one study, only 9% of patients with somatization disorder were detected by their treating physicians at a tertiary care hospital.[71]

Whenever a woman presents with a dramatic or complicated medical history of unexplainable polysymptomatic complaints, a high index of suspicion for the diagnosis of somatization disorder is indicated. The physician may find it useful to keep a copy of the *DSM-IV* symptom criteria for such occasions. Because many patients with somatization disorder either fail to volunteer symptoms or may even deny having had them,[57] it may be necessary to collect symptoms over time or to add data from additional sources.[72] Information from family members and independent medical records is often required before the diagnosis can be established. Patients with somatization disorder are frequently but not always dramatic and histrionic in their symptom descriptions. Obtaining an accurate history may be particularly difficult and time-consuming due to the vague and circumstantial speech that is typical of these patients.

Failure to recognize this disorder results in multiple and often unnecessary surgeries, hospitalizations, and treatment procedures,[55] usually without lasting improvement in symptoms or with subsequent appearance of new symptoms. Chronic failure of these patients to improve, coupled with demands for further medical action and suggestions of physician incompetence as the reason for the medical failures, can make these patients among the most frustrating and confusing encountered by physicians.[72]

Patients with somatization disorder are also prone to develop problems with abuse of and dependence on the pain medication and benzodiazepines they receive for their complaints of pain and psychologic symptoms. Well-meaning physicians may unknowingly contribute to their morbidity in their efforts to help by failing to identify the diagnosis of somatization disorder.[70] Related to their frequent depressive complaints and chronic incapacity, these patients may often threaten or attempt suicide, although completed attempts are uncommon unless substance abuse is also present.[2,57]

One study found that almost all patients with somatization disorder also met criteria for an additional lifetime psychiatric diagnosis, most frequently depression, which occurred in 87%.[73] In fact, patients with somatization disorder have been found to report higher rates of depressive symptoms than do patients diagnosed with major depression.[74]

Patients with somatization disorder tend to have little insight into their condition,[57] and they often resist the imposition of a psychiatric approach to their complaints.[55] They may, however, appreciate the opportunity to consult with a psychiatrist under the guise of helping them with their frequent psychologic complaints such as symptoms of depression and anxiety, or in helping them cope with the stress of their multiple medical symptoms.

A study demonstrated more than a 50% drop in health care costs of patients with somatization disorder after psychiatric consultation.[75] In treating patients with this disorder, conservative management of medical complaints is recommended with the basic rule that no surgical or otherwise invasive action should be taken until physical signs can be verified.[57] This is not to say that these patients' complaints do not ever represent serious illness. Patients with somatization disorder are not immune to medical conditions, and it is important not to overlook this possibility.[70]

Therapy for patients with somatization disorder is best focused on symptomatic relief, being careful to avoid potential iatrogenic complications. A systematic effort must be made to keep the patient from doctor-shopping, while at the same time avoiding demands to perform additional surgical procedures or add medications unless medical indication is documented. It is helpful to keep in mind that patients with somatization disorder have elevated rates of complications from medications and surgical procedures.

These patients frequently request anxiolytic medications such as diazepam. Because many of them may have received benzodiazepines from other physicians who were unaware of the psychiatric diagnosis, they may insist that they need Valium and that it is the only drug that ever helped them. For such patients, hydroxyzine (Atarax, Vistaril) may alleviate symptoms of anxiety and emotional upset while avoiding problems of tolerance. At the same time, the act of prescribing medication may relay the message to the patient that the physician has taken the symptoms seriously enough to prescribe something for symptom relief. Doses of 25 to 100 mg of hydroxyzine up to three times a day provide sensations of relaxation or sedation. Patients with somatization disorder are often suggestible and thus may benefit from placebo enhancement. Patients who are bothered by side effects such as sedation may require lower doses. Small doses (25–50 mg) of trazodone (Desyrel) can be similarly helpful in its nonspecific sedative effects, and, in patients who also meet criteria for depression, antidepressant medication in adequate doses can improve the depression.

Somatization disorder patients also benefit from regularly scheduled physician appointments for the chance to talk about their symptoms and frustrations without having to produce physical complaints to earn the physician's attention.[57] It is often very reassuring to have a regular physician who acknowledges their suffering with all of their physical symptoms.

The physician must recognize that patients with somatization disorder are not consciously malingering or faking. They lack insight into their symptoms and fully believe that they are experiencing the things they report. Somatization disorder is an established psychiatric disorder that results in considerable disability and suffering. Thus, it would be a mistake for the physician to confront the patient with an accusation of malingering, because the patient will conclude that the physician is wrong and does not understand, leading to more doctor-shopping. Their symptoms are very real to them, and any allegation of the contrary is countertherapeutic.

Just as it is important not to miss the diagnosis of somatization disorder, it is equally important to avoid overdiagnosis. Not all patients with histrionic or dramatic complaints have somatization disorder, nor do all patients with conversion symptoms. To label such patients as hysterical without the supporting evidence of chronic unexplainable polysymptomatic complaints risks missing serious medical illness.

Katon and colleagues[76] have identified a group of patients with less severe forms of somatization who report 4 to 12 medically unexplained symptoms and who are high utilizers of medical care. These patients have frequent associated depressive and anxiety syndromes that when successfully treated may result in decreased physical complaints and reduced hypochondriacal concern.

Other Somatoform Disorders

Like somatization disorder, other somatoform disorders constitute an unconscious process, which is not the same as voluntary malingering or faking. Somatoform pain disorder, formerly termed psychogenic pain disorder, is a syndrome of chronic pain unexplained by medical evaluation or inconsistent with known principles of pathophysiology or neuroanatomy. Hypochondriasis is characterized by preoccupation with having a serious disease, but there is no physical evidence. Conversion symptoms are physical symptoms that lack evidence of any physical disorder or known pathophysiologic mechanism; classically, these symptoms are called pseudoneurologic, and suggest neurologic disease, such as blindness, paralysis, aphonia, or deafness. Although somatoform pain disorder, hypochondriasis, and conversion symptoms appear similar to somatization disorder, they lack its polysymptomatic picture.

Conversion symptoms are common in somatization disorder, comprising 12 of the 35 criterion symptoms and representing a complete category of symptoms listed for making this diagnosis. However, conversion symptoms are not unique to somatization disorder; they occur in every psychiatric disorder and occasionally in persons without a psychiatric diagnosis.[77] Conversion symptoms also occur in patients with antisocial personality, alcoholism, and drug abuse and frequently in major depression.[51,78]

Factitious Disorders

Gastrointestinal symptoms can be a manifestation of factitious disorders in which symptoms are intentionally faked to assume the sick role. Although these behaviors are deliberate and intentional, the person seems unable to refrain from compulsive repetition of the behavior. This disorder is more common in males and typically begins in early adulthood. Common gastroenterologic presentations are hematemesis and severe right lower quadrant pain with nausea and vomiting. Symptom presentation is often dramatic and embellished, but, when pushed for details, these patients are typically vague, inconsistent, and evasive.

Predisposing factors are a history of true medical disorders that have required extensive medical treatment, employment in a health-related capacity such as a laboratory technician or nurse, and maladaptive personality traits. Often substance abuse and sometimes iatrogenic analgesic abuse are present.

In its chronic form, called Munchausen's syndrome, a lifelong pattern of repeated hospitalizations results when the patient becomes adept at presenting factitious physical symptoms that are credible enough to gain medical intervention. Unnecessary operations and treatments may result in iatrogenic medical complications. The presence of multiple surgical scars, sometimes presenting as a gridiron abdomen, should arouse suspicion of a factitious disorder.

Once medical investigation reveals no pathology behind the physical complaints, the patient may proceed to develop other symptoms for further evaluation. In the hospital, they are characteristically noncompliant, demanding, attention-seeking, and disruptive. They often display evidence of considerable knowledge of medical and hospital procedures. If confronted with proof that the symptoms are factitious, patients deny it and typically make no delay in getting discharged against medical advice. Admission to another hospital may be accomplished later the same day. Occasional patients may travel widely, gaining admission to various medical centers, and hence they may be difficult to detect.

Malingering

Like factitious disorders, malingering involves faking symptoms, but the difference is that in malingering there is an external motivator, such as obtaining a warm hospital bed for the night, avoiding work, obtaining financial compensation for disability, or obtaining drugs. A high index of suspicion is indicated when symptoms occur in a medicolegal context such as in referrals for forensic evaluation or for disability compensation. Antisocial personality disorder is commonly present in malingerers.

Psychologic Factors Affecting Physical Condition

The *DSM-IV*[2] has a category for physical disorders that can be demonstrated by standard medical evaluation, yet are affected by psychologic factors. In the past, these conditions were classified as psychosomatic or psychophysiologic. A syndrome must have a documented temporal relation between the disorder and the psychologic factor involved to be placed in this category. These disorders may include medical diagnoses such as migraine headache, arthritis, and neurodermatitis, or they may represent isolated physical findings or symptoms such as nausea and vomiting or tachycardia.

GASTROINTESTINAL CONDITIONS AND PSYCHIATRIC ASSOCIATIONS

Abdominal pain, poor appetite and weight loss, diarrhea, and constipation can be symptoms of psychiatric disorders, and careful investigation of both GI and psychiatric possibilities are needed to determine the source of symptoms in any given case. In the following pages, psychiatric associations of specific GI conditions are discussed.

Peptic Ulcer

Only indirect evidence has been collected to suggest an association between emotional factors and peptic ulcer disease. Animal model studies of stress-induced ulceration have been used to support claims of emotional origins,[79,80] but these claims are based on loosely postulated connections. In humans with peptic ulcer disease, hypersecretion of gastric acid has been shown to parallel sustained anxiety and to resolve with alleviation of the stressful stimulus and the anxiety[81]; however, formal psychiatric evaluation was not obtained on these subjects. No clinical association between peptic ulcer disease and any psychiatric illness has been adequately demonstrated in a controlled data-oriented study. One systematic study failed to show that life stress, as measured by life-events scales, is a significant risk factor for the exacerbation of chronic peptic ulcer disease.[82] One controlled study showed that peptic ulcer patients have an increase in depressive symptoms, but this study did not examine actual psychiatric diagnoses.[83]

Ulcerative Colitis

In the last 60 years since the association between psychologic factors and ulcerative colitis was first suggested, a voluminous literature has accumulated. Most of this literature, particularly the earlier work, is based on theoretical and anecdotal findings, each accepting the assertions of a psychosomatic relation described in prior papers and proceeding to delineate a specific psychologic mechanism for the unchallenged ideas of etiology. Recent data-oriented studies challenge the long-accepted view of ulcerative colitis as a psychosomatic condition.

Three recent studies using structured interviews to make psychiatric diagnoses by well-defined criteria have documented no excess of psychiatric disorders in ulcerative colitis patients compared to medically ill controls,[84] healthy controls,[85] or the general population.[86] In some patients, psychologic stressors may appear to provoke relapses of ulcerative colitis.

To document an association between stressful life events and GI exacerbations in inflammatory bowel disease patients, however, a prospective research design is necessary. A 2-year prospective study of life events and inflammatory bowel disease has failed to identify association of life events and GI exacerbations[87]; similar negative findings have been reported in another study.[88] A prospective study of ulcerative colitis and Crohn's disease patients by Duffy and colleagues[89] found that health-related stress was associated with disease activity, but other kinds of stress were not found to be contributory. A prospective study by von Wietersheim and colleagues[90] found no association of life event stress with disease activity in ulcerative colitis and Crohn's disease patients.

Crohn's Disease

Crohn's disease has also collected a voluminous literature addressing its psychosomatic aspects. This literature is likewise composed largely of theoretical and anecdotal reports. However, a study by Helzer and colleagues[91] using structured interviews to make psychiatric diagnoses by accepted criteria demonstrated significantly higher lifetime prevalence rates of psychiatric disorders in Crohn's disease patients than in controls (52% versus 30%). The only diagnosis that was significantly more prevalent in Crohn's patients was major depressive disorder (36% versus 18%). The authors cautioned against inferring psychosomatic causation from their findings, especially because psychiatric diagnoses did not correlate with duration or severity of the bowel disease, and no temporal relation in either direction was present. Moreover, use of the Eysenck Personality Questionnaire in this same study failed to find an association between personality traits and Crohn's disease.

Tarter and colleagues,[85] using the Diagnostic Interview Schedule, reported significantly higher lifetime prevalence rates of three psychiatric disorders in Crohn's disease patients compared to healthy controls. These diagnoses were generalized anxiety disorder (42% versus 14%), panic disorder (27% versus 0%), and major depression (19% versus 0%). Due to this apparent association of psychiatric disorders and Crohn's disease, physicians should be alert to the possibility of psychiatric disorders, particularly depression and anxiety disorders, in Crohn's disease patients. Regardless of impact on the course of the GI disease, recognition and treatment of these psychiatric disorders are important in their own right.

A prospective study of Crohn's disease by Garrett and colleagues found a significant relation between daily stress and self-rated disease activity, but this relation was present in only 3 of the 10 subjects in that study.[92] Incidentally, all 10 subjects in the study were selected from a support group for individuals with inflammatory bowel disease, who may be poorly representative of Crohn's disease patients in general. Temporal directionality was not addressed in this study and therefore it cannot be determined whether disease activity was a product or a source of the reported stress.

Irritable Bowel Syndrome

Although up to 15% of the population suffers from symptoms of irritable bowel syndrome, most persons do not consult a physician.[93,94] In spite of this, symptoms of irritable bowel syndrome are the most common GI complaints brought to the attention of physicians[10] and the most common problem referred to gastroenterologists.[95] Irritable bowel syndrome is also the second leading cause of industrial absenteeism due to illness.[96,97] As was the case with inflammatory bowel disease, the pathogenesis of irritable bowel syndrome is unknown, and, again, a large collection of literature debates the issue of psychosomatic factors in this condition.

Three studies using well-defined criteria for psychiatric diagnosis, two of which used structured interviews, found that the overwhelming majority of irritable bowel patients (70%, 72%, and 93%, respectively) had a lifetime history of psychiatric disorder.[59,60,98] The most common psychiatric conditions in these patients were somatization disorder, anxiety disorders, major depression, and undiagnosed psychiatric disorder. The psychiatric symptoms presented simultaneously with or had preceded irritable bowel symptoms in 86% of subjects.[59,60] Because of the high rates of psychopathology reported with irritable bowel syndrome, the clinician should routinely screen for psychiatric disorder and institute appropriate treatment or referral according to the diagnosis.[46] Drossman and Thompson[46] concluded that individuals with irritable bowel syndrome who consult physicians have increased depression, anxiety, and somatization; those who do not consult physicians are no different from the normal population.

Antidepressant medications have been reported as useful in the treatment of irritable bowel syndrome, potentially due to both antidepressant and antimuscarinic properties as well as to placebo effects.[99] Effective doses are reportedly lower (25–50 mg) than for treatment of depressive disorders,[10] and in these subtherapeutic doses for antidepressant effect, their benefit would presumably be unrelated to their antidepressant properties. It is important to differentiate irritable bowel patients who have psychiatric illness from those who do not, because these patients will require the full therapeutic doses of antidepressant medication typically used for the treatment of major depression and anxiety disorders.

Although patients with diarrhea-predominant irritable bowel syndrome may do best with traditional tricyclic antidepressant agents such as imipramine and desipramine, patients with sensitivity to anticholinergic effects or with constipation-predominant irritable bowel symptoms may do better with agents such as fluoxetine at 5 to 20 mg/day, or with sertraline at 50 to 100 mg/day, which can be associated with diarrhea symptoms.[24]

Esophageal Spasm Syndrome

Parallels have been drawn between this disorder and irritable bowel syndrome, both in regard to physiologic factors and to psychiatric aspects.[100,101] A controlled study[61] using accepted criteria for psychiatric diagnosis demonstrated significantly higher lifetime prevalence rates of psychiatric diagnoses in patients with esophageal contraction abnormalities compared to controls (84% versus 32%). Generalized anxiety disorder and panic disorder were responsible for the majority of psychiatric disorders in the patient group; 20% met criteria for somatization disorder, and most of these had an anxiety disorder or depression as well. In most cases, psychiatric symptoms were thought to have preceded the onset of symptoms related to esophageal spasm. Clouse[100] has suggested that esophageal spasm and irritable bowel syndrome may represent aspects of a related peripheral dysfunction, possibly in direct relation to a psychiatric disorder, in some patients, considering the high rates of psychiatric illness in both GI diseases.

A study by Katon and colleagues[102] found that patients with chest pain who had normal coronary angiographic studies had high rates of panic disorder (43%) and current major depression (36%), significantly higher rates than patients with documented coronary artery disease. The bulk of these patients with negative coronary angiographic studies are thought to have esophageal disease.[102,103]

Trazodone has been found to be useful in the treatment of contraction abnormalities of the esophagus, regardless of the presence or absence of an identifiable psychiatric disorder.[104]

Colostomy and Ileostomy

Although a survey of patients undergoing colostomy for rectal cancer revealed higher rates of depression, sexual problems, and social isolation than in cancer patients undergoing surgery without colostomy,[105] documentation of the relation between colostomy and these problems has not been duplicated in patients with inflammatory bowel disease. Ulcerative colitis patients have been shown to adjust quite well to a colostomy,[106] although psychologic distress, sexual difficulties, and embarrassment have been reported.[107] Advice from patients who have made a good adjustment to an ostomy by way of a local ostomy club can be helpful to patients undergoing this kind of surgery.[108]

Miscellaneous Gastrointestinal Disorders

Functional nonulcer dyspepsia has been shown to be associated with psychiatric disorders in 87% of functional dyspepsia patients in one study, and 67% of the patients with functional dyspepsia met criteria for an anxiety disorder.[109] Symptoms of functional dyspepsia may overlap with those of psychogenic nausea and vomiting, and it has been hypothesized that the latter syndrome may represent a motor disorder in response to acute stress.[100] Alpers[10] has observed frequent depressive symptoms in patients with psychogenic nausea and vomiting, although there are no controlled studies. Little is known about psychopathology in proctalgia fugax.

Any of the functional GI disorders may occur as part of somatization disorder. Swallowing difficulty, for example, is one of the criterion symptoms of somatization disorder. In the past, this symptom, termed globus hystericus, was considered the essence of hysteria. In a patient with inability to swallow, a label of somatization should never be applied before adequate physical investigation and psychiatric evaluation have documented other criteria for somatization disorder.

The reader is directed to Chapter 27, Psychosocial Factors in the Care of Patients With Gastrointestinal Disorders; Chapter 32, Approach to the Patient with Unexplained Weight Loss; Chapter 50, Approach to the Patient with Drug or Alcohol Dependency; and Chapter 81, Irritable Bowel Syndrome.

REFERENCES

1. Guze SB, Helzer JE. The medical model and psychiatric disorders. In: Cavenar JO, ed. Psychiatry. vol. 1. Philadelphia: JB Lippincott, 1985:1.
2. American Psychiatric Association. Diagnostic and statistical manual of mental disorders. 4th ed. Washington DC: American Psychiatric Association, 1994.
3. Robins LN, Helzer JE, Croughan J, Ratcliff KS. National Institutes of Mental Health diagnostic interview schedule: its history, characteristics, and validity. Arch Gen Psychiatry 1981;38:381.
4. Helzer JE, Clayton PJ, Pambakian R, Reich TM, Woodruff RA, Reveley MA. Reliability of psychiatric diagnosis. II. The test-retest reliability of diagnostic classification. Arch Gen Psychiatry 1977;34:136.
5. Clouse RE, Alpers DH. The relationship of psychiatric disorder to gastrointestinal illness. Annu Rev Med 1986;37:283.
6. Gelder M, Gath D, Mayou R. Oxford textbook of psychiatry. New York: Oxford University Press, 1983.
7. Guze SB. Mental disease classification: significance for primary physicians. Hosp Pract 1980;8:77.

8. Robins LN, Helzer JE, Weissman MM, et al. Lifetime prevalence of specific psychiatric disorders in three sites. Arch Gen Psychiatry 1984;41:949.

9. Wells KG, Golding JM, Burnam MA. Psychiatric disorder in a sample of the general population with and without chronic medical conditions. Am J Psychiatry 1988;145:976.

10. Alpers DH. Functional gastrointestinal disorders. Hosp Pract 1983;18:139.

11. Goodwin DW, Guze SB. Psychiatric diagnosis. 4th ed. New York: Oxford University Press, 1989.

12. Winokur G. Depression: The facts. New York: Oxford University Press, 1981.

13. Tomb DA. Psychiatry for the house officer. 3rd ed. Baltimore: Williams & Wilkins, 1988.

14. Guze SB, Robins E. Suicide and primary affective disorders. Br J Psychiatry 1970;117:437.

15. deLong W, Robins E. The communication of suicidal intent prior to psychiatric hospitalization: a study of 87 patients. Am J Psychiatry 1961;117:695.

16. Murphy GE. The physician's responsibility for suicide. II. Errors of omission. Ann Intern Med 1975;82:305.

17. Murphy GE, Robins E. Social factors in suicide. J Am Med Assoc 1967;199:303.

18. Robins E, Murphy GE, Wilkerson RG, Gassner S, Kayes J. Some clinical considerations in the prevention of suicide based on a study of 134 successful suicides. Am J Public Health 1959;49:888.

19. Helzer JE. Psychiatric aspects of inflammatory bowel disease. In: Kodner IJ, Fry RD, Roe JP, eds. Colon, rectal, and anal surgery: current techniques and controversies. St Louis: CV Mosby, 1985:329.

20. Roose SP, Glassman AH, Giardina EV, et al. Nortriptylene in depressed patients with left ventricular impairment. J Am Med Assoc 1986;256:3253.

21. Eaton WW, Dryman A, Weissman MW. Panic and phobia. In: Robins LN, Regier DA, eds. Psychiatric disorders in America: the Epidemiologic Catchment Area Study. New York: The Free Press, 1991:155.

22. Katon W. Panic disorder in the medical setting. Washington DC: American Psychiatric Press, 1991.

23. Lydiard B. Pharamcological treatment. Psychiatr Ann 1988;18:468.

24. Lydiard B. Anxiety and the irritable bowel syndrome. Psychiatr Ann 1992;22:612.

25. King D, Nicolini H, de la Fuente JR. Abuse and withdrawal of panic treatment drugs. Psychiatr Ann 1990;20:525.

26. Lesser IM. The treatment of panic disorders: pharmacologic aspects. Psychiatr Ann 1991;21:341.

27. Woods JH, Katz JL, Winger G. Use and abuse of benzodiazepines: issues relevant to prescribing. J Am Med Assoc 1988;260:3476.

28. Chou JCY, Sussman N. Neuroleptics in anxiety. Psychiatr Ann 1988;18:172.

29. Andrews G, Crino R. Behavioral psychotherapy of anxiety disorders. Psychiatr Ann 1991;21:358.

30. Gelder MG. Psychological treatment of panic anxiety. Psychiatr Ann 1990;20:529.

31. Rapee RM, Barlow DH. Cognitive-behavioral treatment. Psychiatr Ann 1988;18:473.

32. Brown JT, Mulrow CD, Stoudemire GA. The anxiety disorders. Ann Intern Med 1984;100:558.

33. Blazer DG, Hughes D, George LK, Swartz M, Boyer R. Generalized anxiety disorder. In: Robins LN, Regier DA, eds. Psychiatric disorders in America: the Epidemiologic Catchment Area Study. New York: The Free Press, 1991:180.

34. Andreasen NC, Black DW. Introductory textbook of psychiatry. Washington DC: American Psychiatric Press, 1991.

35. Rickels K, Schweizer E. The treatment of generalized anxiety disorder in patients with depressive symptomatology. J Clin Psychiatry 1993;54(Suppl):20.

36. Zimmerman M, Coryell W. DSM-III personality disorder diagnoses in a nonpatient sample. Arch Gen Psychiatry 1989;46:682.

37. Widiger TA, Rogers JH. Prevalence and comorbidity of personality disorders. Psychiatr Ann 1989;19:132.

38. Widiger TA, Frances AJ, Harris M, Jacobsberg LB, Fyer M, Manning D. Comorbidity among axis II disorders. In: Oldham JM, ed. Personality disorders: new perspectives on diagnostic validity. Washington DC: American Psychiatric Press, 1991:147.

39. Skodol AE, Rosnick L, Kellman D, Oldham JM, Hyler SE. Validating structured DSM-III-R personality disorder assessments with longitudinal data. Am J Psychiatry 1988;145:1297.

40. Pfohl B, Coryell W, Zimmerman M, Stangl D. DSM-III personality disorders: diagnostic overlap and internal consistency of individual DSM-III criteria. Compr Psychiatry 1986;27:21.

41. Nace EP, Davis CW, Gaspari JP. Axis II comorbidity in substance abusers. Am J Psychiatry 1991;148:118.

42. Gartner AF, Marcus RN, Halmi K, Loranger AW. DSM-III-R personality disorders in patients with eating disorders. Am J Psychiatry 1989;146:1585.

43. Pfohl B, Black DW, Noyes RN, Coryell WH, Barrash J. Axis I and axis II comorbidity findings: implications for validity. In: Oldham JM, ed. Personality disorders: new perspectives on diagnostic validity. Washington DC: American Psychiatric Press, 1991:165.

44. Livesley WJ. The classification of personality disorder. I: the choice of category concept. Can J Psychiatry 1985;30:353.

45. Livesley WJ. Trait and behavioral prototypes of personality disorder. Am J Psychiatry 1986;143:728.

46. Drossman DA, Thompson WG. The irritable bowel syndrome: review and a graduated multicomponent treatment approach. Am Coll Physicians 1992;116:1009.

47. Leibovich MA. Psychogenic vomiting: psychotherapeutic considerations. Psychother Psychosom 1973;22:263.

48. Drossman DA, Leserman J, Nachman G, et al. Sexual and physical abuse in women with functional or organic gastrointestinal disorders. Ann Intern Med 1990;113:828.

49. Creed F, Craig T, Farmer R. Functional abdominal pain, psychiatric illness, and life events. Gut 1988;29:235.

50. Barker A, Mayou R. Psychological factors in patients with nonspecific abdominal pain acutely admitted to a general surgical ward. J Psychosom Res 1992;36:715.

51. Colgan S, Creed F, Klass H. Symptom complaints, psychiatric disorder, and abnormal illness behavior in patients with upper abdominal pain. Psychol Med 1988;18:887.

52. Woodruff RA, Clayton PJ, Guze SB. Hysteria: studies of diagnosis, outcome, and prevalence. J Am Med Assoc 1971;215:425.

53. Perley M, Guze SB. Hysteria—the stability and usefulness of clinical criteria. N Engl J Med 1962;266:421.

54. Cloninger CR, Martin RL, Guze SB, Clayton PJ. A prospective follow-up and family study of somatization in men and women. Am J Psychiatry 1986;143:873.

55. Guze SB, Perley MJ. Observations on the natural history of hysteria. Am J Psychiatry 1963;19:960.

56. Woerner P, Guze SB. A family and marital study of hysteria. Br J Psychiatry 1968;114:161.

57. Murphy GE. The clinical management of hysteria. J Am Med Assoc 1982;247:2559.

58. Pennebaker JW, Watson D. The psychology of somatic symptoms. In: Kirmayer LJ, Robbins JM, eds. Current concepts of somatization: research and clinical perspectives. Washington DC: American Psychiatric Press, 1991:21.

59. Young SJ, Alpers DH, Norland CC, Woodruff RA. Psychiatric illness and the irritable bowel syndrome: practical implications for the primary physician. Gastroenterology 1976;70:162.

60. Liss JL, Alpers D, Woodruff RA. The irritable colon syndrome and psychiatric illness. Dis Nerv Sys 1973;34:151.

61. Clouse RE, Lustman PJ. Psychiatric illness and contraction abnormalities of the esophagus. N Engl J Med 1983;309:1337.

62. Kruesi MJ, Dale J, Strauss SE. Psychiatric diagnoses in patients who have chronic fatigue syndrome. J Clin Psychiatry 1989;50:53.

63. Taerk GS, Toner BB, Salit IE, Garfinkel PE, Ozersky S. Depression in patients with neuromyasthenia (benign myalgic encephalitis). Int J Psychiatr Med 1987;17:49.

64. Black DW, Rathe A, Goldstein RB. Environmental illness: a controlled study of 26 subjects with "20th century disease". J Am Med Assoc 1990;264:3166.

65. Goldenberg DL. Psychiatric and psychologic aspects of fibromyalgia syndrome. Rheum Dis Clin North Am 1989;15:105.

66. Walker E, Katon W, Harrop-Griffiths J, Holm L, Russo J, Hickok LR. Relationship of chronic pelvic pain to psychiatric diagnoses and childhood sexual abuse. Am J Psychiatry 1988;145:75.

67. Ogata SN, Silk KR, Goodrich S, Lohr NE, Western D, Hill EM. Childhood sexual and physical abuse in adult patients with borderline personality disorder. Am J Psychiatry 1990;147:1008.

68. Brown GR, Anderson B. Psychiatric morbidity in adult inpatients with childhood histories of sexual and physical abuse. Am J Psychiatry 1991;148:55.

69. Jacobson A, Richardson B. Assault experiences of 100 psychiatric inpatients: evidence of the need for routine injury. Am J Psychiatry 1987;144:908.

70. Quill TE. Somatization disorder: one of medicine's blind spots. J Am Med Assoc 1985;254:3075.

71. deGruy F, Crider J, Hashini DK, Dickinson P, Mullins HC, Troncale J. Somatization disorder in a university hospital. J Fam Pract 1987;25:579.

72. Guze SB, Cloninger CR, Martin RL, Clayton PJ. A follow-up and family study of Briquet's syndrome. Br J Psychiatry 1986;149:17.

73. Liskow B, Othmer E, Penick E, de Souza C, Gabrielli W. Is Briquet's syndrome a heterogenous disorder? Am J Psychiatry 1986;143:626.

74. deSouza C, Othmer E, Gabrielli W, Othmer S. Major depression and somatization disorder: the overlooked differential diagnosis. Psychiatr Ann 1988;18:340.

75. Smith GR, Monson RA, Rey DC. Psychiatric consultation in somatization disorder. N Engl J Med 1986;314:1407.

76. Katon WK, Lin E, Von Korff M, Russo J, Lipscomb P, Bush T. Somatization: a spectrum of severity. Am J Psychiatry 1991;148:34.

77. Guze SB. The role of follow-up studies: their contribution to diagnostic classification as applied to hysteria. Semin Psychiatry 1970;2:392.

78. Guze SB, Woodruff RA, Clayton PJ. A study of conversion symptoms in psychiatric outpatients. Am J Psychiatry 1971;128:643.

79. French MD, Porter RW, Cavanaugh EB, Langmire RL. Experimental gastroduodenal lesion induced by stimulation of the brain. Psychosom Med 1957;3:209.

80. Adler R. Psychosomatic research in animals. In: Hill OW, ed. Modern trends in psychosomatic medicine. London: Butterworth, 1976.

81. Peters MN, Richardson CT. Stressful life events, acid hypersecretion, and ulcer disease. Gastroenterology 1983;84:114.

82. Piper DW, MacIntosh JH, Ariotti DE, Fenton BH, MacLennan R. Life events and chronic duodenal ulcer: A case control study. Gut 1981;22:1011.

83. Walker P, Luther J, Samloff IM, Feldman M. Life events stress and psychosocial factors in men with peptic ulcer disease. Gastroenterology 1988;94:323.

84. Helzer JE, Stillings WA, Chammas S, Norland CC, Alpers DH. A controlled study of the association between ulcerative colitis and psychiatric diagnoses. Dig Dis Sci 1982;27:513.

85. Tarter RE, Switala J, Carra J, Edwards KL, van Thiel DH. Inflammatory bowel disease: psychiatric status of patients before and after disease onset. Int J Psychiatry Med 1987;17:173.

86. Andrews H, Barczak P, Allan RN. Psychiatric illness in patients with inflammatory bowel disease. Gut 1987;28:1600.

87. North CS, Alpers DH, Helzer JE, Spitznagel EL, Clouse RE. Do life events or depression exacerbate inflammatory bowel disease? A prospective study. Ann Intern Med 1991;114:381.

88. Campbell D, Shannon S, Collins SM. The relationship between personality, stress, and disease activity in ulcerative colitis (abstract). Gastroenterology 1986;90:1364.

89. Duffy LC, Zielezny MA, Marshall JR, et al. Relevance of major stress events as an indicator of disease activity prevalence in inflammatory bowel disease. Behav Med 1991;Fall:101.

90. von Wietersheim J, Kohler T, Feiereis H. Relapse-precipitating life events and feelings in patients with inflammatory bowel disease. Psychother Psychosom 1992;58:103.

91. Helzer JE, Chammas S, Norland CC, Stillings WA, Alpers DH. A study of the association between Crohn's disease and psychiatric illness. Gastroenterology 1984;86:324.

92. Garrett VD, Brantley PJ, Jones GN, McKnight GT. The relation between daily stress and Crohn's disease. J Behav Med 1991;14:87.

93. Thompson WG, Heaton KW. Functional bowel disorder in apparently healthy people. Gastroenterology 1980;79:283.

94. Sandler RS, Drossman DA, Nathan HP, McKee DC. Symptom complaints and health seeking behavior in subjects with bowel dysfunction. Gastroenterology 1984;87:314.

95. Kirsner JB, Palmer WL. The irritable colon. Gastroenterology 1958;34:491.

96. Almy TP. What is "irritable colon?" Am J Dig Dis 1957;2:93.

97. Ruoff M. The irritable colon syndrome. In: Lindner AE, ed. Emotional factors in gastrointestinal illness. Amsterdam: Excerpta Medica, 1973:156.

98. Fava GA, Pavan L. Large bowel disorders: II. Psychopathology and alexithymia. Psychother Psychosom 1976;27:100.

99. Clouse RE, Alpers DH. Abdominal pain: could it be irritable bowel syndrome? Female Patient 1987;12:13.

100. Clouse RE. Anxiety and gastrointestinal illness. Psychiatr Clin North Am 1988;11:399.

101. Clouse RE, Eckert TC. Gastrointestinal symptoms of patients with esophageal contraction abnormalities. Dig Dis Sci 1986;31:236.

102. Katon W, Hall ML, Russo J, et al. Chest pain: relationship of psychiatric illness to coronary arteriographic results. Am J Med 1988;84:1.

103. Clouse RE. Psychiatric interactions with the esophagus. Psychiatr Ann 1992;22:598.

104. Clouse RE, Lustman PJ, Eckert TC, Ferney DM, Griffith LS. Low-dose trazodone for symptomatic patients with esophageal contraction abnormalities: a double-blind, placebo-controlled trial. Gastroenterology 1987;92:1027.

105. Devlin HB, Plant JA, Griffin M. Aftermath of surgery for anorectal cancer. Br Med J 1971;3:413.

106. Wirsching M, Druner HU, Herrmann G. Results of psychosocial adjustment to long-term colostomy. Psychother Psychosom 1975;26:245.

107. Burnham WR, Leonard-Jones JE, Brooke BN. Sexual problems among married ileostomists. Gut 1977;18:673.

108. Druss RG, O'Connor JF, Prudden JF, Stern LD. Psychologic response to colectomy. Arch Gen Psychiatry 1968;18:53.

109. Magni G, Mario F, Bernasconi G, Mastropaelo G. DSM-III diagnoses associated with dyspepsia of unknown cause. Am J Psychiatry 1987;144:1222.

Textbook of Gastroenterology, second edition, edited by Tadataka Yamada. JB Lippincott Company, Philadelphia © 1995.

CHAPTER 135

Gastrointestinal Dilation

Richard A. Kozarek

Historically, treatment of gastrointestinal stenoses with dilation has been limited to accessible anatomic areas, primarily the esophagus or anorectum. With the advent of endoscopically or radiographically placed polyethylene balloons, a variety of gastric, colonic, biliary, and anastomotic strictures have become amenable to such therapy. Moreover, additional dilating modalities, particularly the development of hollow-core polyvinyl dilators, have radically changed the approach to esophageal bougienage. The primary goal associated with dilation of any stenosis is lumenal enlargement and amelioration of obstructive symptoms. Such symptoms are obviously contingent on the stricture site and may include dysphagia, jaundice, or cholangitis, as well as varied types of abdominal pain.

Whereas all of the current dilating systems achieve efficacy by either stricture stretch or fracture, there are very few data regarding mechanisms of action with individual dilating systems. Nor are there good prospective data comparing endoscopically facilitated dilation with alternative treatment modalities, particularly surgery. Finally, despite widespread application of this technology, there are few studies comparing efficacy and side effects of various dilating systems. This chapter compares the various technologies with regard to ease and site of application, patient tolerance, cost-benefit ratio, and available safety and efficacy data. It also defines potential future scenarios for dilation.

THEORETICAL CONSIDERATIONS

The basic goals of stricture dilation include safe and efficacious lumenal enlargement and prevention of restenosis.[1] The latter may include pharmacologic maneuvers such as the use of H_2 receptor antagonists, substituted benzimidazoles, or prokinetic agents after esophageal bougienage for a reflux-induced stricture.[2] It may include mechanical means such as placement of an esophageal prosthesis after dilation of an esophageal malignancy or an endoscopically placed biliary stent after dilation of a postoperative biliary stricture.[3,4] It may also include subsequent surgical resection, plasty, or bypass of the dilated area. On occasion one can, for example, convert an obstructing rectosigmoid malignancy, which has a high operative risk in an unprepped situation, into a nonemergent condition after dilation (or laser photoablation) and subsequent colon preparation.

The exact mechanisms of lumenal enlargement remain uncertain with many of the available dilating systems. Two basic theories have been espoused for stricture dilation: circumferential stretch and stricture split. The former presupposes considerable elasticity in circumferential fibrous tissue; the latter presupposes an inherent stenosis rigidity in which dilation is effected by one or several longitudinal tears. It seems unlikely that a 3-mm diameter pylorus can be dilated to 10 or 15 mm without a significant laceration of scirrhous tissue and potentially of muscle, but there are few good postdilation studies of gross anatomy or histology available. The exceptions include two papers that have defined gross longitudinal tears and histologic disruption of collagen and circular muscle after esophageal bougienage for fibrous stenoses and achalasia.[5,6]

Available dilating modalities can be divided into mercury bougies, guidewire-directed dilators, polyethylene balloons, and miscellaneous types (Table 135-1, Figs. 135-1 through 135-4).[2,7] Mercury-filled dilators, ranging in size from 3 to 20 mm (10–60 Fr), can be subdivided into the original, blunt-

TABLE 135-1
Dilators for Gastrointestinal Stenoses

Mercury Bougies
Blunt-tip (Hurst)
Tapered-tip (Maloney)

Guidewire-Directed
Metal olives (Jackson-Plummer; Eder-Puestow, including triple olive
  adaptation)
Hollow-core polyvinyl (Savary-Gillard, American)
Neoplex stepped-diameter (Celestin)
Spindle-shaped (Keymed advanced dilator)

Polyethylene Balloons
TTS
Guidewire facilitated
Hybrid TTS-guidewire

Latex Balloons
Brown-McCardy
Mosher

Miscellaneous
Woven silk (Jackson, Phillips)
Graded, plastic oversheath
Tapered-tip endoscope
Balloon or tape affixed to endoscope shaft
Electronic-mechanical (Starck variant)

TTS, through the scope.

tipped Hurst bougies and a tapered-tip variant called Maloney bougies. As initially described, these dilators were passed blindly.

Historically, guidewire-directed dilators have included Jackson-Plummer bougies and Eder-Puestow dilators, the latter originally described in 1955. Variants of the latter system include triple olives, in which multiple metal olives of increasing diameter are placed on the same dilating shaft.[8] Four additional wire-guided dilating systems have been marketed: the Keymed advanced dilator, consisting of three spindle-shaped silicone bougies on stainless steel shafts; the stepped neoplex (Celestin) dilator; and two types of hollow-core polyvinyl systems, the Savary-Gillard and the American. The Celestin dilating system consists of two tapered dilators that reach a maximum diameter of 12 and 18 mm, respectively. The Savary-Gillard system consists of bougies ranging in size from 5 to 18 mm (15–54 Fr). The American dilating system (Bard Inc., Mentor, Ohio) ranges in size from 7 to 20 mm (21–60 Fr). In contrast to the barium-impregnated American dilators, Savary-Gillard dilators are longer and have a more gradually tapered tip. As a result, they require a full loop of guidewire within the stomach to prevent dilator impaction on the tip of the guidewire. They are also considerably less radiopaque and more difficult to visualize fluoroscopically.

In addition to the above, a number of less often used technologies have been advocated for stenosis dilation, limited only by the ingenuity of the individual endoscopist or equipment manufacturer. These include tapered-tip endoscopes, mechanical dilators with the ability to monitor the width and force of dilation, and variably tapered plastic sheaths that fit over conventional pediatric or adult endoscopes.[3] Attaching a polyethylene balloon to a bronchoscope or pediatric endoscope or placing a bolus of tape onto an endoscope shaft[9,10]

have also been advocated. Historically, cork and woven silk dilators have also been used, the latter since at least the 16th century, when Thomas Willis used a cork-tipped whalebone to treat a probable achalasia patient.[11]

A major advance in addition to guidewires has been the development of polyethylene balloons for use in the gastrointestinal tract.[12] Such balloons allow dilation of previously inaccessible strictures. Graded and fixed-diameter polyethylene balloons range between 4 and 40 mm, the smaller restricted for use in the pancreaticobiliary tree and the latter limited to treatment of achalasia. Such balloons are fixed on 2.5-mm (7-Fr) catheter shafts that range between 100 and 200 cm in length. They can be passed over an endoscopically or radiographically placed guidewire or directly through the scope (TTS). Biliary balloons, ranging in size from 4 mm to 10 mm in diameter, are a hybrid and as such are used TTS but also over a guidewire. A full dilation set includes balloons of variable length and diameter, 5- to 30-mL syringes, guidewires, and a manometer to delineate balloon pressure during inflation; optional are a dilating gun to maintain pressure and stopcocks to ensure a constant pressure during inflation.

TECHNICAL APPLICATION

In general, directed bougienage, using either radiography or endoscopy or a combination of the two, should prove both safer and more effective than blind dilation.[13] This is particularly true for sharply angulated, extremely tight, or proximal esophageal stenoses, and it should be an invariable rule with more distal stenoses, including those in the stomach, bile duct, and colon. For dilation, these general principles must be balanced against the availability of fluoroscopy, the added cost of endoscopic or fluoroscopic control of bougienage, and the physician's previous experience with a particular dilating modality. Endoscopically facilitated guidewire placement and subsequent bougienage need not always require fluoroscopic control if copious guidewire has been placed into the stomach and attention is given to ensure that guidewire displacement does not occur on endoscope withdrawal.[14]

Of obvious importance technically is the degree of lumenal enlargement that can be undertaken safely in a single dilating session. There remains a maxim in esophageal bougienage

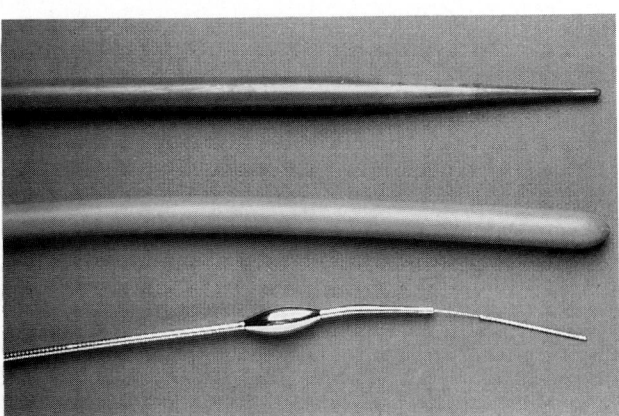

FIGURE 135-1. Standard dilating systems for esophageal bougienage: Maloney (*top*), Hurst (*middle*), Eder-Puestow (*bottom*). The latter two are obsolete but are still widely used.

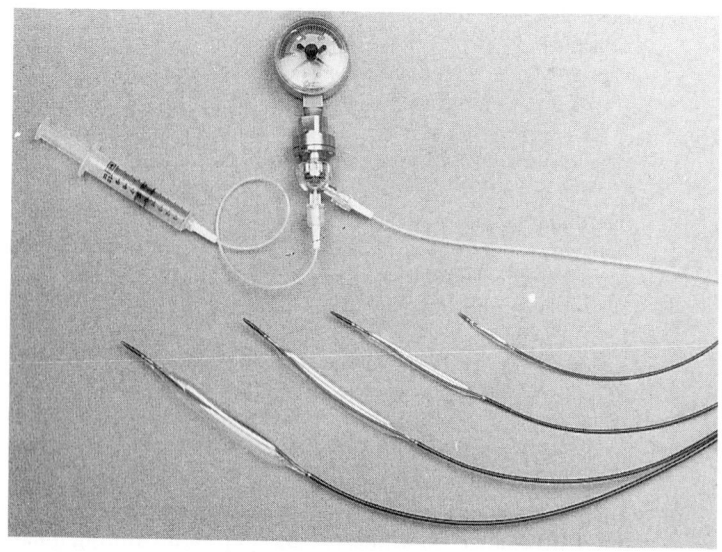

FIGURE 135-2. Polyethylene balloon dilating kit includes mercury manometer and injection syringe. Balloons are passed over an endoscopically or radiographically placed guidewire.

that one should increase a lumenal stenosis by no more than 2 mm (6 Fr) in a single dilation session.[1] Although it is based on common sense and an attempt to avoid such complications as bleeding and perforation, this adage does not necessarily hold true for most rings or webs and some pliable, reflux-induced strictures. The degree of lumenal enlargement should be contingent not only on the stricture itself (i.e., membranous or fibrotic) but on the degree of associated lumenal ulceration and the risks and benefits of alternative treatment modalities. These decisions cannot be made by a review of the scanty literature discussing side effects of bougienage but require a great deal of common sense on the part of the physician.

Esophageal Strictures

Taking esophageal stenosis as the prototype, there are three basic dilation systems in widespread use: mercury bougies, guidewire-directed dilators, and polyethylene balloons. Most patients who present with dysphagia have had previous esophagoscopy, although a few with lower esophageal rings may have had barium studies alone. With rings, webs, and mild reflux stenosis, mercury bougienage after a 6-hour fast

and pharyngeal anesthesia can often be done using a single 16 to 18 mm (48–54 Fr) Maloney dilator.[15] Such dilators can be passed in the upright or lateral decubitus position. Although ideally done under fluoroscopic control to avoid kinking or retroflexion, many such esophageal dilations can be performed safely without these capabilities.

Long, angulated, or eccentric esophageal strictures, as well as severe (<7 mm) stenoses, are best handled with a guidewire dilating system. Patients require an initial endoscopy to define the stricture's cause and characteristics. These include length, diameter, pliability, eccentricity, and the presence of associated pseudodiverticula. Because a small increase in bleeding and perforation rates has been observed when biopsies were performed before bougienage, and because a biopsy of the entire length of the stricture can be performed after dilation, my colleagues and I delay tissue sampling until immediately after the dilation proper. This ensures that the entire length of the stricture is sampled. Whereas most of the historic experience has been obtained using 5 to 15 mm (16–45 Fr) Puestow olives, this particular dilating system has been supplanted by hollow-core polyvinyl dilators in most centers.

Use of polyvinyl dilators always requires guidewire placement.[13] This is usually done in conjunction with initial endoscopy, at which time a piano-style wire with a spring tip

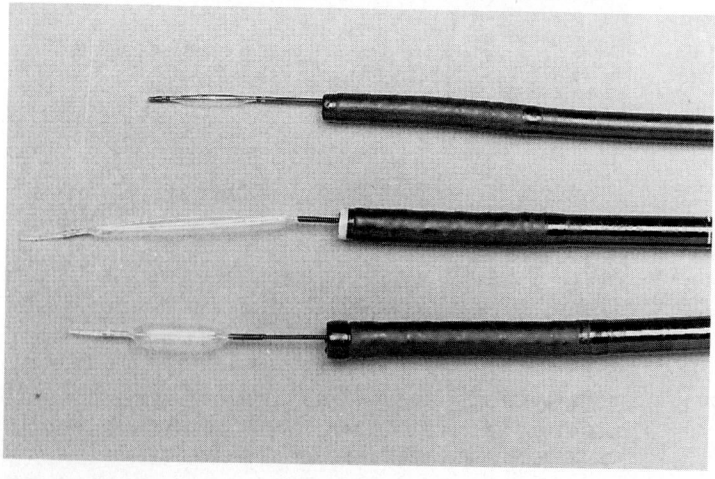

FIGURE 135-3. Through-the-scope polyethylene dilating balloons are available in various lengths and diameters. The biliary balloon (*top*) is a hybrid that passes through the scope but over the guidewire.

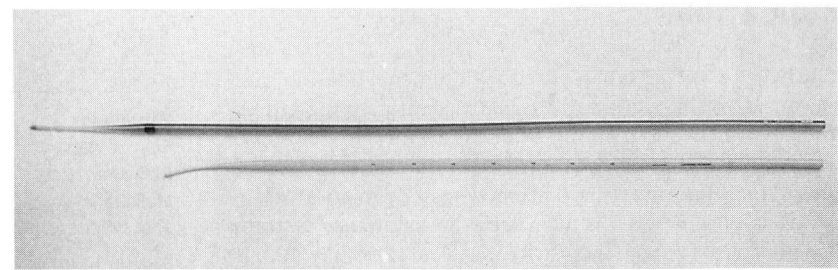

FIGURE 135-4. Hollow-core polyvinyl dilators. The Savary-Gillard dilator (*top*) is longer, more tapered, and less radiopaque than the American dilator (*bottom*).

can be passed through the stricture and fed freely into the stomach as ascertained fluoroscopically. Alternatively, the wire can sometimes be passed radiographically without the use of an endoscope. After baseline endoscopy and stricture sizing, a dilator approximately the size of the stricture is passed, making sure the guidewire is fixed and the head is bent forward. This is followed by one or two additional dilators, for an increment of up to 3 or 4 mm (10–12 Fr) contingent on stricture, before repeat endoscopy and stricture biopsy. Because of their gradual taper, polyvinyl dilators can pass through most stenoses with relative ease. The hesitation that is felt with these systems is related more to dilator friction over the guidewire than to the stricture itself. The characteristic "pop" associated with the use of metal olives is absent.

Moderate stenoses (7–13 mm) can be dilated using either mercury bougies under fluoroscopic control or polyvinyl dilators. The latter systems can be used without radiographic monitoring in some of these patients. This requires a certain level of expertise to ensure that the guidewire has advanced far enough into the stomach and is not inadvertently withdrawn at the time of endoscope removal. This is best done by feeding the guidewire forward simultaneously with endoscope or bougie withdrawal and having an assistant fix the wire at the level of the patient's mouth. In addition to the above modalities, polyethylene balloons have also been used to dilate moderate esophageal strictures. The technique is described in the section on nonesophageal strictures; the major points of contention in using balloon technology within the esophagus are the need for fluoroscopic control to ensure full balloon inflation and the rapidity with which a stricture may be dilated.[7,13]

Nonesophageal Strictures

Most nonesophageal strictures require balloon dilation, although stenotic gastric stapling orifices and anastomotic strictures of the rectosigmoid can be enlarged with polyvinyl dilators. Using pyloric stenosis as a representative stricture, I recommend using TTS balloons whenever possible. Advantages include direct stricture visualization, improved placement control, and immediate evaluation of the dilated stenosis.[12] Moreover, the attempt to pass balloons over an endoscopically placed guidewire in tight pyloric or proximal colonic stenoses is often unsuccessful because such balloon dilators lose their mechanical advantage for placement in a dilated stomach or redundant colon.

The use of a TTS dilator requires endoscopic approximation of the stricture size and selection of a balloon that is 1 to 2 mm (3–6 Fr) larger. Both balloon and dilator shaft should be coated with silicone, and negative pressure should be ap-

plied to the balloon using a 10- to 20-mL syringe. These measures, as well as avoiding excessive angulation of the endoscopic tip, allow dilator passage until all or part of the balloon is visualized. The balloon is centered in the stenotic pylorus under a combination of endoscopic and fluoroscopic control. The latter also helps prevent damage of the bulb apex or C loop wall related to excessive pressure of the balloon tip or extreme balloon angulation.

Although air can be used for inflation, a 10% to 25% contrast solution allows better visualization fluoroscopically and a more uniform balloon dilation. Technical efficacy in dilation requires obliteration of the balloon waist with pressures ranging from 30 psi (2 atm) for a 15-mm balloon to 45 psi (3 atm) for a 10-mm balloon. More recently, low-profile balloons with bursting pressures between 4 and 8 atm have been marketed. Although they are theoretically more efficacious, data concerning their use have been sparse. There is no evidence that 2 minutes of continued inflation is more advantageous than 15 seconds after the balloon waist has been effaced. I usually use 30 seconds of dilation and redilate a second or third time after repositioning of the balloon. After dilation has been effected, complete evacuation of the balloon and straightening of the endoscope tip are required to allow retrieval. Additional larger dilating balloons can then be used, but the degree of lumenal enlargement in a single session remains a matter of common sense and is contingent on size of the initial stenosis, presence and degree of active ulceration, and patient discomfort with initial dilation. The ultimate goal is to dilate with a 15-mm balloon and follow up with complete endoscopic inspection of the pylorus and duodenum. This goal sometimes requires two or three dilating sessions separated by an interval of several days if the obstruction is acute or several weeks if it is chronic.

In contrast to pyloric dilation, dilation of biliary stenoses uses a combination of TTS and guidewire technology with balloon placement over a guidewire and directly through the duodenoscope. Four- and 6-mm balloons are readily passed through a 2.8-mm endoscope channel; 8- to 10-mm balloons require an instrument with at least a 3.2-mm biopsy channel. After baseline cholangiogram and stricture localization, a 0.035-in guidewire is passed through the stenosis and into the intrahepatic biliary tree. Sequential balloons can be passed, and dilation can be effected as already described. In contrast to larger balloons, which can fracture at 30 to 45 psi, biliary balloons, because of their smaller diameter, usually can withstand pressures two to three times these values. An additional difference in dilating biliary stenoses as opposed to pyloric stenoses is the frequent requirement for subsequent stent placement. This is particularly true in postoperative strictures, in malignancies, and with the nonmembranous stenoses that can be seen in sclerosing cholangitis.

INDICATIONS

The benefits and risks associated with lumenal dilation must be considered in relation to alternative treatment modalities. Such treatment modalities may include antireflux surgery or gastric resection for a reflux stricture and vagotomy-pyloroplasty for pyloric stenosis. They may include dilation by nonendoscopic methods, as typified by the percutaneous, transhepatic approach to biliary strictures. And they may include other endoscopic approaches to various types of stenoses, such as laser photoablation, electrocautery, and prosthesis placement. Finally, the pharmacologic implications of dilation of certain strictures must be kept in mind. For instance, reflux-related esophageal strictures and many pyloric stenoses require long-term H_2 blockade and possible use of a prokinetic agent as well.[2] Dilation of a stenosis associated with Crohn's disease usually requires adjustment of corticosteroid dosage to minimize the inflammatory response and stricture reformation.

Indications for dilation are contingent on the anatomic area involved. In the esophagus, symptoms are most often dysphagia and food impaction, although atypical chest pain, aspiration, and odynophagia may also be seen. Indications for pyloric dilation are usually recurrent nausea and vomiting, weight loss, abdominal pain, and severe reflux. Most biliary stenoses present with jaundice or, more commonly, recurrent episodes of cholangitis. Progressive cholestasis without jaundice may also be seen, particularly in sclerosing cholangitis. Small bowel and distal colonic stenoses may require dilation for intractable obstipation, progressive diminution in stool size, pain, and recurrent bowel obstruction. The causes of the above and of a variety of miscellaneous stenoses are listed in Table 135-2.

CONTRAINDICATIONS AND RISKS

Contraindications to gastrointestinal dilation include such concerns as lack of informed consent, acute abdomen, and the presence of a deeply ulcerated stenosis for which the risks of dilation significantly outweigh the benefits. There may also be patient- and lesion-specific contraindications, as, for example, in the case of acute myocardial ischemia or acute pancreatitis in a patient undergoing dilation of a dominant pancreatic stenosis. Both the physician and the patient must be aware of alternative treatment modalities and the possible need for subsequent long-term ancillary measures. The latter may include H_2 blockade and prokinetic agents for esophageal and pyloric stenoses or periodic stent exchange for pancreaticobiliary stenoses. Data on alternative treatment modalities include, for example, a retrospective series on pyloric stenosis patients treated with resective surgery, highly selective vagotomy, or vagotomy with pyloroplasty.[16] This series by Gleysteen and Droege had a combined morbidity of 32% and mortality of 6% for all surgical modalities. A reoperative rate of approximately 10% was found, and a long-term symptom relief rate was not defined. Delayed postoperative gastric emptying, which did not require reoperation, was recorded in 25% of patients.

Risks of gastrointestinal dilation include problems associated with endoscopic procedures, such as medication reaction, vasovagal reaction, oxygen desaturation, and arrhythmia, as well as the risk of aspiration for upper gastrointestinal en-

TABLE 135-2
Indications for Gastrointestinal Dilation

Esophagus
Ring or web
Reflux stricture
Malignancy
Miscellaneous (e.g., caustic ingestion, motility disorders)

Stomach
Pyloric stenosis
Anastomotic stricture
Gastric stapling stenosis
Miscellaneous (e.g., acid ingestion, proximal malignancy)

Small Bowel
Duodenum (web, acid-peptic stricture)
Ileum (Crohn's, NSAID-induced stenosis)

Biliary Tree
Anastomotic stricture
Inflammatory stricture (sclerosing cholangitis, stone-induced)
Malignancy
Sphincter dysfunction or spasm

Colon
Anastomotic stenosis
Inflammatory stricture (IBD, diverticular, radiation-induced)

Miscellaneous
Isolated stenosis pancreatic duct
Stenotic gastrostomy, enterostomy, or colostomy stoma

NSAID, nonsteroidal anti-inflammatory drugs; IBD, inflammatory bowel disease.

doscopy.[17] There are additional small risks of bleeding and perforation with diagnostic endoscopy or colonoscopy alone. The site- and lesion-specific risks associated with dilation itself have usually been defined as an increased incidence of bleeding and lumenal perforation, particularly in the esophagus, stomach, small bowel, and colon. The procedure may also be associated with significant cholangitis or pancreatitis if dilation is applied to the pancreaticobiliary tree.[18] The more rigid polyvinyl dilators are very effective at dilating but have a slightly increased risk of perforation. These dilators must be used with a guidewire. With the exception of the esophageal dilation, the incidence of these complications in various settings is poorly defined.

ASSESSMENT OF RESULTS

Esophagus

Because of the frequency as well as the accessibility of benign and malignant esophageal strictures, most of the data on gastrointestinal dilation have derived from esophageal bougienage, especially with a combination of the Puestow and mercury dilating systems. This combination, using sequential bougies over a period of days to months, has been associated with a 70% to 100% improvement in dysphagia in more than 850 patients with benign esophageal strictures compiled from various series.[3,13,15,19]

Reported complications in these 850 patients included 16 (0.2%) perforations, 5 major bleeding episodes, 2 aspirations, and 1 death. This compares with the perforation rates of 0.4% for mercury dilators and 0.6% for metal olives reported in the 1976 American Society for Gastrointestinal Endoscopy (ASGE) survey by Silvis and colleagues.[17] Such perforations are usually in the cervical esophagus and related to improper dilator introduction or in the thoracoabdominal esophagus just proximal to the stenosis and related to dilator or guidewire kinking.[1] Less frequently, the stricture itself splits, as may be seen with achalasia (1%–5% perforation rate).[1]

In addition, a number of series have assessed the use of balloon dilators for esophageal stenoses. Graham and Smith were successful in increasing lumenal size from 7.8 to 15.1 mm in 10 patients with benign strictures, and from 8.7 to 15.2 mm in 12 patients with malignant esophageal strictures.[20] The procedure was undertaken in a single session and without fluoroscopy, and no complications were reported. Lindor and colleagues treated benign and malignant esophageal strictures in 88 patients and were technically successful in 93% of the dilations.[21] These authors reported a 3% minor complication rate and 91% symptomatic improvement over a mean of 10 months. Additional series have been reported in adults and children,[22–25] as have trials comparing balloon technology to Eder-Puestow[26] or Savary[27] dilators. Comparable system efficacy has generally been reported, although the Eder-Puestow dilators have been associated with an increased risk of complications.[26]

In an attempt to place hydrostatic balloon dilators into clinical perspective with respect to efficacy and side effects, I undertook a questionnaire of 3000 ASGE members in 1985.[18] Of 1093 replies, 240 endoscopists were using this recently introduced technique, which did not yet include TTS balloons. A total of 617 esophageal dilations were reported, with an 85% technical success rate and 85% acute symptomatic relief rate. The complication rate was 2.1%, comprising 11 hemorrhages requiring transfusion and 2 perforations. These data suggested that either balloons were not as safe as previously available dilating systems or that their use was limited to extremely complex or angulated stenoses. More likely, there was a learning curve associated with their introduction and application.

Data using the newer, guidewire-directed dilating systems is limited. In a randomized, prospective trial comparing Eder-Puestow and Celestin dilators in 72 patients, there was no significant difference with regard to long-term symptom relief, although the Celestin system was thought to be quicker and cause less pharyngeal trauma. A single perforation occurred with the Celestin system.[28] A second paper reviewed 302 dilations in 100 patients with benign esophageal strictures using this system.[29] The two reported perforations were medically managed and were thought to be related to esophageal laceration with the endoscope and not the dilator proper. An additional series reported a 10% perforation rate with the Celestin system.[3]

Finally, although hollow-core polyvinyl dilating systems have supplanted metal olives in most U.S. centers, data are even more sparse with these systems.[7,13,19,27,30] Dumon and colleagues have reported their experience in 300 patients with benign and malignant esophageal stenosis, claiming efficacy in all and only one perforation.[31] Their claim regarding increased ease and safety of use compared with the Puestow olive system has been widely accepted but never subjected to a controlled trial.

Stomach

The only large series reported for gastric dilation have been limited to polyethylene balloon dilation, and series defining long-term follow-up remain sparse. Since the initial description by Benjamin and associates reporting a successful hydrostatic dilation in a single patient with pyloric stenosis and gastric outlet obstruction,[32] several series have been published using this technique.[33–36] McLean and colleagues radiographically dilated 94 gastrointestinal strictures in 92 patients over a period of 6 years, with a mean follow-up of 389 days in 80 patients.[37] Thirty-three of these patients had various forms of gastric stenosis. Technically, 25 of the 33 were successfully dilated, and 70% were symptom-free at 1 year. Hogan and colleagues were technically successful in dilating 13 of 15 patients with pyloric and anastomotic gastric stenoses, had no complications, and reported that most patients were symptom-free 2 years after dilation.[38]

In the 1985 ASGE survey, 545 patients were reported to have had balloon dilation for a variety of reasons, including pyloric stenosis, gastroenterostomy strictures, and small gastric stapling orifices.[18] Technical success rates were purported to be 81%, with an acute symptomatic relief rate of 76% (66% in pyloric stenosis, 72% in stenotic gastroenterostomy orifices, and 85% in patients with strictures of gastric stapling anastomoses). There was a 0.9% complication rate, with four perforations and one major hemorrhage. Despite such data, the long-term symptomatic relief rate in patients undergoing balloon dilation for gastric obstruction remains poorly defined.[39,40] In 23 patients treated for pyloric or anastomotic gastric stenoses in our institution followed for a mean of 31 months, 13 (60%) continue to be asymptomatic, 5 have had subsequent resective or bypass surgery, 3 have died of unrelated causes, and 2 continue to have chronic obstructive symptoms.[36] Additional case reports or small series have reported successful balloon dilation of postoperative,[39] tubercular,[40] or Crohn's-associated[41] gastric outlet obstructions.

Bile Duct

Although surgical therapy has been the traditional approach to the treatment of benign biliary tract strictures, numerous series suggest that stricture recurrence approximates 20% to 30%.[42] Because of this, transhepatic balloon dilation was initially used in high-risk surgical patients and, more recently, in good operative candidates. May and associates used this technique in 74 patients with inflammatory, postoperative, or anastomotic stenoses and in 14 patients with sclerosing cholangitis with a dominant stricture.[43,44] Mueller and colleagues described 73 patients with biliary-enteric and postcholecystectomy strictures.[45] Although relief of pruritus, cholangitis, and jaundice was impressive in these series, significant complications occurred in one third and restenoses in 5% to 30%. Moreover, questions regarding the utility of and need for prolonged internal or external stenting after such dilations were not answered.

Based on these data, endoscopically facilitated balloon dilation of the biliary tree has been used increasingly in hope of providing good efficacy with a lower complication rate.[4] Geenen and associates treated 25 patients with postoperative

strictures, 23 with balloon dilation and 18 with stent placement, for up to 2 years.[46] Using clinical symptoms, liver enzymes, degree of ductal dilation, and stricture diameter as
indices, 18 of 23 patients were reported to have a good result
at 4 years. Other series by Ponchon and associates[47] and by
Berkelhammer and colleagues[48] reported roughly comparable
results, as did the largest series to date, reported by Davids
and his Amsterdam colleagues.[49] These authors used balloon
dilation and placement of endoprostheses of 2 to 3.5 mm
(10 Fr) for repair of bile duct injury. The procedure was successful in 66 (94%) of 70 patients; 83% of patients followed
long term (mean 42 months) retained a good or excellent
result. Johnson and colleagues described 10 patients with
sclerosing cholangitis who underwent endoscopic sphincterotomy (10 patients), balloon dilation of a dominant stricture
(8 patients), and endoprosthesis placement (3 patients).[50]
There was a significant improvement in liver function tests
and in rate of hospitalization for recurrent episodes of cholangitis. There are a plethora of additional small series and
individual case reports using this technology.[51-53] An additional 46 cases of postcholecystectomy strictures and 15 cases
of sclerosing cholangitis strictures were recorded in the ASGE
survey. A technical success rate of approximately 75% was
followed by radiographic and symptomatic improvement in
two thirds to three quarters of patients, and a 7% complication
rate was seen.[18]

Anastomotic and malignant stenoses have also been successfully dilated endoscopically, usually in association with
subsequent endoprosthesis placement. There is considerable
debate, however, regarding use of these balloons within the
sphincter of Oddi proper. Because it has been postulated as
useful for the ampullary spasm–papillary stenosis symptom
complex, Siegel and Guelrud reported on 24 patients in whom
they dilated the sphincter of Oddi using a 6-mm balloon at
6 atm.[54] Only two of their patients subsequently underwent
endoscopic sphincterotomy, and improvement in biochemical
tests and symptoms was implied. Numerous additional case
reports have also suggested that this is a useful tool.[55] In contrast, the ASGE survey, although recording a significant percentage of symptomatically improved patients, reported a 35%
complication rate. This included 40 cases of cholangitis and
22 cases of pancreatitis in 200 instances of sphincter dilation.[18]
A single prospective controlled trial using balloon or sham
dilation for biliary dyskinesia showed no difference between
the two groups with respect to clinical improvement or follow-
up sphincter pressures at 3 and 12 months.[56] There was, however, a 25% incidence of pancreatitis in patients undergoing
balloon dilation.

Pancreas

There have been no large series using hydrostatic balloons in
the pancreas, although postoperative, posttraumatic, and
chronic pancreatitis stenoses have been dilated on an individual basis.[57] Two thirds of the 36 patients described in the
ASGE survey experienced symptomatic relief, and a 19% incidence of pancreatitis as a complication was reported.[18] In
limited personal experience, pancreatic duct stenoses have invariably restenosed after balloon dilation, and I currently restrict its application as a temporizing modality only.

Small Bowel

Because of the problems of access to the small intestine, there
are few data regarding dilation of proximal small bowel strictures.[58] There are, however, multiple series using balloon
technology to dilate ileal or anastomotic ileocolonic strictures
in Crohn's disease.[59,60] For instance, Blomberg and colleagues
dilated 27 anastomotic strictures in patients with Crohn's
disease[61]; no complications were noted, and at a follow-up
ranging from 7 to 38 months, 18 patients remained free from
obstructive symptoms. Breysem and associates were successful
in effecting balloon dilation in 16 of 18 Crohn's stenoses.[62]
Fourteen patients experienced immediate symptomatic relief,
and long-term success was reported in 9 patients. No complications were seen. In contrast, among the ureteroenteric
anastomotic strictures which have been dilated, 70% of 37
benign stenoses recurred within 6 months in one report, and
84% within a year.[63]

Colon

Most reported colonic dilations have been used for rectal or
anastomotic stenoses.[63-69] Linares and associates dilated 33
anorectal strictures in Crohn's disease patients using a variety
of techniques; half of these patients experienced short- or long-
term symptomatic relief.[66] Pietropaolo and colleagues dilated
42 patients with postoperative strictures with either balloons
or bougies.[67] There was no morbidity or mortality in the series,
and a 2.4% failure rate was cited. Finally, Venkatesh and colleagues successfully dilated 25 patients with anastomotic
strictures, although 71 (84%) required multiple dilations.[68]
Several additional authors have reported successful colon dilation for a variety of stenoses such as anastomotic, Crohn's,
and diverticular strictures. In the ASGE survey, 64 patients
underwent balloon dilation for colon strictures: 44 anastomotic strictures, 5 malignant, 5 diverticular, 3 inflammatory
bowel disease, and 7 miscellaneous.[18] There was a 79% technical success rate, and 56% of patients had acute symptomatic
relief. There were three perforations and two bleeding episodes, for a 7.8% complication rate.

CLINICAL IMPLICATIONS

The ability to dilate a stenosis does not imply that dilation is
the procedure of choice in every instance. Although there are
adequate data available to support H_2 receptor blockade and
periodic esophageal bougienage as adequate therapy for many
patients with a reflux-induced stenosis,[2] such data cannot be
generalized to a 30-year-old patient with a midesophageal
stricture in a Barrett's epithelium, in whom an antireflux procedure may be preferable. Nor does the ability to dilate the
pylorus dictate that this is the procedure of choice in the young
patient with a hypersecretory state in whom lifelong pharmacologic suppression of acid would be required. Likewise,
patients with a gastric outlet obstruction caused by a deep
and active ulcer crater who do not respond to conventional
management (e.g., nasogastric suction, acid suppression) may
be better handled with a surgical drainage or resective
procedure.

Esophageal Stenoses

There are several considerations involved in choosing an appropriate dilating method for the esophagus. If the various types of dilators had equal efficacy and safety profiles for bougienage of routine esophageal stenoses (an unproven assumption), the physician would tend to use the most cost-effective system. On the other hand, if inherent advantages are assumed for a particular system, there is a tendency to increase its use. The claimed advantages of balloon dilators over other systems have included ease of passage, dilation of the stricture alone, and radial as opposed to vector force applied to a stenotic wall.[13] Ideally, such balloons should be safer and more effective, claims that cannot be substantiated with available data. If fluoroscopy is used to ensure waist dilation, total costs using this technology in our institution are threefold higher than dilation with polyvinyl dilators and eightfold higher than mercury bougienage.[3] Given this and the fact that such balloons, particularly the TTS variety, have a limited life span of one to ten uses, balloon technology is better limited to areas of the gut not accessible to other types of dilators. The exception to this statement is achalasia, in which polyethylene balloons have proven both effective and much easier to pass than conventional dilating systems.[70]

Webb has tried to place the multitude of dilating systems into perspective.[71] He used Maloney dilators in 78% and Eder-Puestow dilators in 21% of his patients in 1985; he currently uses mercury dilators in 56%, hydrostatic balloons in 24%, and Savary dilators in 20% of patients with benign esophageal stenoses. In our institution, on the other hand, Savary-type dilators are used in two thirds of all esophageal stenoses.[72]

Nonesophageal Stenoses

The major question for nonesophageal stenoses is the appropriateness of stenosis dilation compared with alternative treatment modalities. Using pyloric stenosis as an example, available series are small, data are limited, and follow-up of dilated patients has been suboptimal. Nevertheless, a 60% to 65% good-to-excellent symptomatic response at 1 to 2 years can be expected,[23,34,36] and this should be compared with the results of drainage or resective therapy for benign gastric outlet obstruction.[16] A recent cost analysis comparing pyloric balloon dilation with vagotomy and pyloroplasty at our institution has been published and updated.[36] Although these data show balloon dilation to be extremely cost-effective in the short term at one tenth of the total costs for vagotomy and pyloroplasty, they do not take into consideration the long-term H_2 blockade usually required after endoscopic therapy.[73]

Additional unanswered questions include the need for subsequent stent placement after dilation of pancreaticobiliary stenoses, the relative efficacy of balloons as opposed to polyvinyl dilators for amenable rectal or sigmoid stenoses, and the rapidity with which stenoses at various sites can be safely dilated.

FUTURE APPLICATIONS

The future of gastrointestinal dilation is contingent on further experience with the newer dilating systems such as balloons and polyvinyl dilators. Both expanded clinical experience and controlled clinical trials should allow improved definition of the indications, benefits, and risks for individual dilating systems and for specific stenotic lesions.

There are also likely to be additional technologic combinations using dilators and various thermal modalities. Just as bipolar tumor probes have conjoined Eder-Puestow dilators with multipolar electrocautery to treat concentric esophageal or rectal neoplasms, similar electrodes can be implanted on balloons or polyvinyl dilators. A new approach is to take a quartz laser fiber and surround the tip with a balloon. The balloon keeps the fiber tip in the center of the lumen. These catheters may ultimately allow treatment of nonresectable biliary, gastroesophageal, or rectal neoplasms by transmission of laser energy.

The future of gastrointestinal dilation may also include the development of dilators that can detect a fall in wall tension or resistance within a tissue during dilation. This fall in tension may predict that the dilation is adequate and that further lumenal enlargement may be unnecessary and hazardous. Devices such as these should improve technical safety.

Finally, dilation will be increasingly used in conjunction with expandable stent technology, potentially even in the setting of benign stenoses. These expandable stents, currently undergoing refinement both in the endoprostheses themselves and in their delivery systems, hold at least the potential of prolonged stricture patency, which would preclude the need for repeated dilation sessions.[74]

The reader is directed to Chapter 28, Approach to the Patient With Dysphagia; Chapter 35, Approach to the Patient With Gas and Bloating; and Chapter 115, Upper Gastrointestinal Endoscopy.

REFERENCES

1. Talman AB, Boyce HW. Complications of esophageal dilation and guidelines for their prevention. Gastrointest Endosc 1981;27:320.
2. Starlinger M, Appel WH, Schemper M, Schiessel R. Long-term treatment of peptic esophageal stenosis with dilatation and cimetidine, factors influencing clinical result. Eur Surg Res 1985;17:207.
3. Kozarek RA. Esophageal dilation and prostheses. Endosc Rev 1987;4:9.
4. Kozarek RA. Endoscopic management of bile duct injury. Gastrointestinal Endoscopy Clinics of North America 1993;3:261.
5. Aste H, Munizzi F, Saccomanno S, Pugliese V. "Splitting" and stretching dilation of esophageal strictures. Endoscopy 1983;15:41.
6. Wong RK, Johnson LF. Achalasia. In: Castell DO, Johnson LF, eds. Esophageal function in health and disease. New York: Elsevier Biomed, 1983:99.
7. Cox JGC, Dakkak M, Bucton GK, Bennett JR. Dilators for esophageal stricture—a description of a new bougie and a comparison of current instruments. Gastrointest Endosc 1989;35:551.
8. Goldberg RI, Manten HO, Barkin JS. Esophageal bougienage with triple metal olive dilators. Gastrointest Endosc 1986;32:226.
9. Frimberger E. Endoscopic treatment of benign esophageal stricture. Endoscopy 1983;15:199.
10. Lehman GA, O'Connor KW. Endoscopic tape dilator—a simple and inexpensive method to dilate upper gastrointestinal strictures. J Clin Gastroenterol 185;7:208.
11. Luna LL. Endoscopic therapy of benign esophageal stricture. Endoscopy 1983;15:203.

12. Kozarek RA. Endoscopic Grüntzig balloon dilation of gastrointestinal stenoses. J Clin Gastroenterol 1985;6:401.
13. American Society for Gastrointestinal Endoscopy. Esophageal dilation. Guidelines for clinical application. (ASGE publication no. 1023). Gastrointest Endosc 1991;32:122.
14. Kadakia SC, Cohan CF, Starnes EC. Esophageal dilation with polyvinyl bougies using a guidewire with markings without the aid of fluoroscopy. Gastrointest Endosc 1991;37:183.
15. Harrison ME, Sanowski RA. Mercury dilation of benign strictures. Hepatogastroenterology 1992;39:497-501.
16. Gleysteen JJ, Droege EA. Expedient surgical treatment of chronic ulcer stenosis. A case for proximal gastric vagotomy. J Clin Gastroenterol 1988;10:619.
17. Silvis SE, Nebel O, Rogers G, et al. Endoscopic complications: results of the 1974 American Society for Gastrointestinal Endoscopy survey. JAMA 1976:235:928.
18. Kozarek RA. Hydrostatic balloon dilation of gastrointestinal stenoses: a national survey. Gastrointest Endosc 1986;32:15.
19. Anand BS. Eder-Puestow and Savary dilators. Hepatogastroenterology 1992;39:494.
20. Graham DY, Smith JL. Balloon dilatation of benign and malignant strictures. Gastrointest Endosc 1985;31:171.
21. Lindor KD, Ott BJ, Hughes RW Jr. Balloon dilatation of upper digestive tract strictures. Gastroenterology 1985;89:345.
22. London RL, Trotman BW, DiMarino AJ Jr, et al. Dilation of severe esophageal strictures by an inflatable balloon catheter. Gastroenterology 1985;89:545.
23. McLean GK, Cooper GS, Hartz WH, et al. Radiologically guided balloon dilation of gastrointestinal strictures. Part I. Technique and factors influencing procedural success. Radiology 1987;165:35.
24. Myer CM III, Ball WS Jr, Bisset GS III. Balloon dilation of esophageal strictures in children. Arch Otolaryngol Head Neck Surg 1991;117:529.
25. Goenka AS, Dasilva MS, Cleghorn GJ, et al. Therapeutic upper gastrointestinal endoscopy in children: an audit of 443 procedures and literature review. J Gastroenterol Hepatol 1993;8:44.
26. Yamamoto H, Hughes RW Jr, Schroeder KW, et al. Treatment of benign esophageal stricture by Eder-Puestow or balloon dilators: a comparison between randomized and prospective non-randomized trials. Mayo Clin Proc 1992;67:228.
27. Shemesh E, Czerniak A. Comparison between Savary-Gillard and balloon dilation of benign esophageal strictures. World J Surg 1990;14:518.
28. Fellows IW, Raina S, Holmes GKT. Celestin dilation of benign esophageal strictures: a review of 100 patients. Am J Gastroenterol 1986;81:1052.
29. Hine KR, Hawkey CJ, Atkinson M, Holmes GKT. Comparison of the Eder-Puestow and Celestin techniques in dilating benign oesophageal strictures. Gut 1984;25:1100.
30. Desai DC, Swaroop VS, Mohandas KM, et al. Out-patient esophageal dilation: an experience in 130 patients using Savary-Gillard dilators. Indian J Gastroenterol 1992;11:65.
31. Dumon JR, Meric B, Sivak MV, et al. A new method of esophageal dilation using Savary-Gillard bougies. Gastrointest Endosc 1985;31:379.
32. Benjamin SB, Cattau EL, Glass RL. Balloon dilation of the pylorus: therapy for gastric outlet obstruction. Gastrointest Endosc 1982;28:253.
33. Heymans HSA, Bartelsman JWFM, Herweijer TJ. Endoscopic balloon dilatation as treatment of gastric outlet obstruction in infancy and childhood. J Pediatr Surg 1988;23:139.
34. Griffin SM, Chung SCS, Leung JWG, Li AKC. Peptic pyloric stenosis treated by endoscopic balloon dilatation. Br J Surg 1989;76:1147.
35. Hegedüs V, Poulson PE. Balloon dilatation of alimentary tract strictures. Acta Radiol Diagn 1986;27:681.
36. Kozarek RA, Botoman VA, Patterson DJ. Endoscopic management of gastric outlet obstruction. Gastrointest Endosc 1990;36:558.
37. McLean GK, Cooper GS, Hartz WH, et al. Radiologically guided balloon dilation of gastrointestinal strictures. Part II. Results of long-term follow-up. Radiology 1987;165:41.
38. Hogan RB, Hamilton JK, Potter DE. Preliminary experience with hydrostatic balloon dilation of gastric outlet obstruction. Gastrointest Endosc 1986;32:71.
39. Desai DC, Swaroop VS, Mohandas KM, et al. Outpatient dilation of anastomotic strictures of the upper gastrointestinal tract. Indian J Gastroenterol 1992;11:16.
40. Vij JC, Ramesh GN, Choudhary V, Malhotra V. Endoscopic balloon dilation of tuberculous duodenal strictures. Gastrointest Endosc 1992;38:511.
41. Murthy UK. Repeated hydrostatic balloon dilation in obstructive gastroduodenal Crohn's disease. Gastrointest Endosc 1992;37:484.
42. Lillemoe KD, Pitt HA, Cameron JL. Current management of benign bile duct strictures. Adv Surg 1992;25:119.
43. May GR, Bender CE, LaRusso NF, Wiesner RH. Nonoperative dilation of dominant strictures in primary sclerosing cholangitis. Am J Radiol 1985;145:1061.
44. Williams HV, Bender CE, May GR. Benign postoperative biliary strictures: Dilation with fluoroscopic guidance. Radiology 1987;163:629.
45. Mueller PR, van Sonnenberg E, Ferrucci JT Jr, et al. Biliary stricture dilation: Multicenter review of clinical management in 73 patients. Radiology 1986;160:17.
46. Geenen DJ, Geenen JE, Hogan WJ, et al. Endoscopic therapy for benign bile duct strictures. Gastrointest Endosc 1989;35:367.
47. Ponchon T, Gallez J-F, Valette PJ, et al. Endoscopic treatment of biliary tract fistulas. Gastrointest Endosc 1989;35:490.
48. Berkelhammer C, Kortan P, Haber GB. Endoscopic biliary prostheses as treatment for benign postoperative strictures. Gastrointest Endosc 1989;35:95.
49. Davids PHP, Rauws EAJ, Coene PPLO, et al. Endoscopic stenting for postoperative biliary strictures. Gastrointest Endosc 1992;38:12.
50. Johnson GK, Geenen JE, Venu RP, Hogan WJ. Endoscopic treatment of biliary duct strictures in sclerosing cholangitis; follow-up assessment of a new therapeutic approach. Gastrointest Endosc 1987;33:9.
51. Foutch PG, Harlan JR, Hoefer M. Endoscopic therapy for patients with postoperative biliary leak. Gastrointest Endosc 1993;39:416.
52. Kozarek R, Gannan R, Baerg R, et al. Endoscopic approach to biliary leak following laparoscopic cholecystectomy. Arch Intern Med 1992;152:1040.
53. Traverso LW, Kozarek RA, Ball TJ, et al. Endoscopic retrograde cholangiopancreatography after laparoscopic cholecystectomy. Am J Surg 1993;165:581.
54. Siegel JH, Guelrud M. Endoscopic cholangiopancreatoplasty: hydrostatic balloon dilation in the bile duct and pancreas. Gastrointest Endosc 1983;29:99.
55. Kozarek RA. Biliary dyskinesia. Are we any closer to defining the entity? Gastrointestinal Endoscopy Clinics of North America 1993;3:167.
56. Bader M, Geenen JE, Hogan WJ, et al. Endoscopic balloon dilatation of the sphincter of Oddi in patients with suspected biliary dyskinesia: results of a prospective randomized trial. Gastrointest Endosc 1986;32:158.
57. Kozarek RA. Endoscopic therapy in chronic pancreatitis. In: Beger HG, Büchler M, Malfertheiner P, eds. Standards in pancreatic surgery. New York: Springer-Verlag, 1993:332.
58. Johnstone AJ, Hendry GMA, Orr JD. Case report: duodenal and jejunal strictures treated with balloon dilatation through a duodenostomy. Clinical Radiology 1992;45:208.
59. Williams AJK, Palmer KR. Endoscopic balloon dilatation as a therapeutic option in the management of intestinal strictures resulting from Crohn's disease. Br J Surg 1991;78:453.
60. Fregonese D, DiFalco G, DiToma F. Balloon dilatation of anastomotic intestinal stenoses: long-term results. Endoscopy 1990;22:249.
61. Blomberg B, Rolny P, Järnerot G. Endoscopic treatment of anastomotic strictures in Crohn's disease. Endoscopy 1991;23:195.
62. Breysem J, Janssens JF, Coremans G, et al. Endoscopic balloon dilation of colonic and ileocolonic Crohn's strictures: long-term results. Gastrointest Endosc 1992;38:142.
63. Shapiro MJ, Banner MP, Amendola MA, et al. Balloon catheter dilation of ureteroenteric strictures: long-term results. Radiology 1988;168:385.
64. Dinneen MD, Motson RW. Treatment of colonic anastomotic

strictions with "through the scope" balloon dilators. J R Soc Med 1991;84:264.

65. Oz MC, Forde KA. Endoscopic alternatives in the management of colonic strictures. Surgery 1990;108:513.

66. Linares L, Moreira LF, Andrews H, et al. Natural history and treatment of anorectal strictures complicating Crohn's disease. Br J Surg 1988;75:653.

67. Pietropaolo V, Masoni L. Ferrara M, Montori A. Endoscopic dilation of colonic postoperative strictures. Surg Endosc 1990;4:26.

68. Venkatesh K, Ramanujam PS, McGee S. Hydrostatic balloon dilatation of benign colonic anastomotic strictures. Dis Colon Rectum 1992;35:789.

69. Gamliel Z, Wesson D. Prograde dilatation with Tucker bougies: a technique for managing postoperative rectal strictures. J Pediatr Surg 1991;26:1285.

70. Gelfand MD, Kozarek RA. An experience with polyethylene balloons for pneumatic dilation in achalasia. Am J Gastroenterol 1989;84:924.

71. Webb WA. Esophageal dilation: personal experience with current instruments and techniques. Am J Gastroenterol 1988;83:471.

72. Kozarek RA. Esophageal dilation (editorial). Mayo Clin Proc 1992;677:299.

73. Kozarek RA. Endoscopic therapy for gastric outlet obstruction. Are balloons a bust? (editorial). J Clin Gastroenterol 1993;17:2.

74. Kozarek RA. Expandable endoprostheses for gastrointestinal stenoses. Gastrointestinal Endoscopy Clinics of North America 1994;4:279.

Textbook of Gastroenterology, second edition, edited by Tadataka Yamada. JB Lippincott Company, Philadelphia © 1995.

CHAPTER 136

Percutaneous Endoscopic Gastrostomy

Jeffrey L. Ponsky

Methods
  The Pull Technique
  The Push Technique
  The Introducer Technique
  Comparison of Methods
  Percutaneous Endoscopic Jejunostomy

Removal and Replacement of PEGs
Complications
Considerations in Choosing Percutaneous Gastrostomy
  Indications
  Contraindications

Percutaneous endoscopic gastrostomy (PEG) was developed as an alternative to operative gastrostomy and first introduced in 1980. The method has become widely practiced and shown to be a safe and effective means of providing long-term enteral nutrition. Other applications, such as gastric decompression and as a biliary conduit, have also been used. Modifications of the original technique have been introduced and may offer unique advantages in particular clinical situations.

Complications have been acceptably low and mostly of an infectious nature; careful attention to the details of technique and to patient follow-up can avert most of these. Endoscopic gastrostomy also compares favorably with surgical gastrostomy in effectiveness, safety, and cost.

As our experience with this procedure increases, and as new materials and techniques become available, the indications for PEG may expand in the future. The importance of this technique is that it establishes a route for the adminis-

tration of enteral nutrition in patients with a variety of disease states for whom nutritional support is often a critical problem.

The importance of nutritional support for the ill has been repeatedly emphasized in the past two decades. Advancements in the area of parenteral nutrition have been lifesaving. More recently, interest has been renewed in providing nutrition by the enteral route, where feasible, because this method is safe and less costly. Advances in the development of enteral formulas have provided numerous specialized mixtures of nutrients tailored to a patient's needs and absorptive capacity.

The concept of a surgically created fistula between the stomach and abdominal wall was first conceived by Egeberg in 1837 and attempted by Sellidot in 1849. A variety of surgical approaches to the creation of the gastrostomy were developed, culminating in the more popular Janeway and Stamm methods.[1] The Janeway gastrostomy involved the formation of a tube of gastric wall brought out through the abdomen to create a permanent gastric stoma. The Stamm gastrostomy employed concentric pursestring sutures placed in the anterior gastric wall through which was placed a rubber catheter. The sutures were tied around the catheter, and it was brought out through the abdominal wall. Both of these methods were effective in creating a gastrocutaneous fistula to be used for feeding or decompression. Use of these techniques was somewhat limited, however, because patients requiring gastrostomy were often poor surgical candidates. These procedures required laparotomy, often with general anesthesia.

Thus, delivery of enteral nutrition was most often by means of nasoenteric tubes. These tubes, frequently of large caliber, were constructed of stiff rubber or plastic. More recent designs have provided smaller caliber and softer materials. Nutrition by way of nasoenteric tubes may be quite effective but is associated with numerous frustrations and complications. Frequent plugging of the tubes may require replacement, and it is not unusual for the tubes to become dislodged. Esophagitis may develop as a result of irritation of the esophagus by the tube, and because the tube may render the esophagogastric junction incompetent, gastroesophageal reflux often results. Aspiration pneumonia is a frequent complication of tube feeding. Long-term use of nasoenteric tubes may also lead to parotitis and erosion of nasal cartilage.

In 1980, the technique of PEG was introduced.[2] This method allowed the formation of a tube gastrostomy without the need for laparotomy or general anesthesia. Safety of the procedure was ensured by endoscopic visualization of the tube insertion. The original method described for PEG has been called the pull technique.[3] Two modifications of the original method have been introduced and have gained some popularity. These are referred to as the push technique and the introducer technique.[4,5] All these methods have been shown to be safe and effective.

Complications of percutaneous gastrostomy, although not frequent, are known to occur and are well documented. Careful attention to patient selection and the details of the method may help to reduce the incidence of undesirable outcomes.

The increasing ease by which enteral access is established with percutaneous gastrostomy has led to tremendous growth in the application and use of this procedure. Moral and ethical dilemmas arise as the technique is applied to an increasingly debilitated population of patients. Further study of the technique and its long-term outcome may provide answers to some of these problems.

METHODS

The Pull Technique

The patient is not fed for 8 hours before the procedure, and a single preoperative dose of an intravenous antibiotic, usually a cephalosporin, is given. The supine position is used; therefore, it is imperative that someone be assigned to suction the posterior pharynx when secretions accumulate. The patient is given intravenous sedation, and the mouth and pharynx are swabbed with an antiseptic solution in an attempt to remove accumulated debris and decrease the bacterial population. The abdomen is washed and draped in a sterile fashion. The room lights are turned down as the gastroscope is passed into the stomach. Transillumination of the abdominal wall

by the light of the scope is an indication that intervening structures have been displaced and that the stomach lies in contact with the abdominal wall. The site selected for placement of the gastrostomy should be one at which transillumination is well seen.

Finger pressure by the assistant at this point produces a clear indentation of the gastric wall as seen by the endoscopist (Fig. 136-1). This indentation should be covered by an open polypectomy snare, passed through the endoscope. Local anesthetic is injected into the abdominal wall at the proposed area of puncture, and a 1-cm incision is made in the skin of the abdomen. An intravenous cannula is thrust through the incision and into the gastric lumen. If the polypectomy snare was correctly positioned, the thrusting needle will enter the center of its loop. If not, the snare is quickly looped around the cannula and tightened near the point where the cannula exits the gastric mucosa. A long, stout suture or wire is passed through the needle into the gastric lumen, and the snare is moved from around the cannula to tighten around the suture itself (Fig. 136-2). The suture is pulled with the endoscope from the patient's stomach out of the mouth. The drainage end of the gastrostomy tube is affixed to the suture at the patient's mouth. The tube is well lubricated, and pull is begun on the abdominal end of the long suture so that the gastrostomy tube moves down the esophagus and exits the abdominal wall (Fig. 136-3). The gastroscope is reinserted to check the position of the head of the tube, and care is taken to avoid excessive tension on the head of the catheter. The endoscope

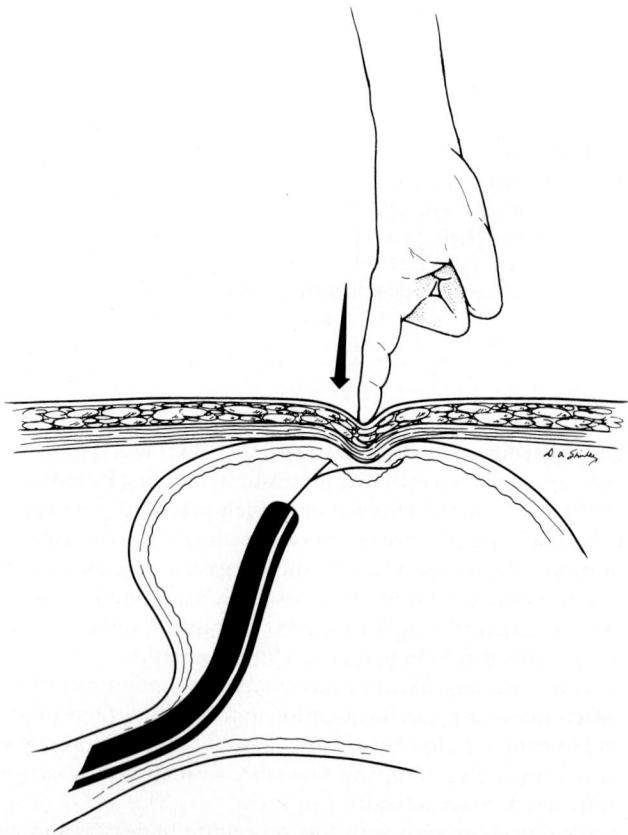

FIGURE 136-1. The endoscopist observes a distinct indentation of the gastric wall as the assistant applies finger pressure to the abdominal wall at the proposed site of puncture.

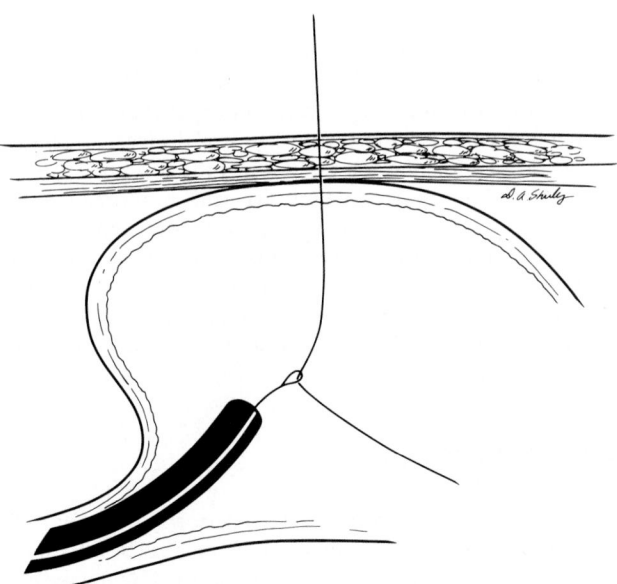

FIGURE 136-2. The snare is tightened around the suture and pulled out of the patient's mouth with the gastroscope.

is removed, and an outer bolster is applied, which holds the gastric and abdominal walls in close contact. Feedings are begun the next day.

The Push Technique

This method differs little from the pull technique. The patient is prepared, and the puncture is performed in the same manner. In this procedure, a long guidewire is grasped with the snare and pulled from the patient's mouth. A special gastrostomy tube with a long tapered dilator end is pushed over the guidewire. Both ends of the wire must be held under tension as the tube is pushed down the esophagus and exits the abdominal wall. Once the tube emerges from the abdominal wall, it may be grasped and pulled the rest of the way into its final position. The gastroscope is reinserted to ensure that the head of the catheter lies in contact with the gastric mucosa. An outer crossbar or faceplate is added to fix the abdominal and gastric walls together.

The Introducer Technique

Percutaneous methods for the insertion of central venous catheters and cardiac pacemakers have been adapted to the performance of gastrostomy in the introducer method. Developed by Russell and colleagues,[5] this method allows percutaneous placement of a gastrostomy tube without passing the tube through the oropharynx and with only a single insertion of the endoscope. The gastroscope is passed into the stomach, and the room lights are dimmed. Transillumination of the abdominal wall and finger pressure at the point of best transillumination are used to identify the proper site for puncture. Once the site for insertion has been agreed on, the skin is anesthetized and a small incision is made. A needle is introduced into the gastric lumen, and a guidewire is passed through the needle. The needle is removed, and an introducer with an outer, peel-away sheath is passed over the guidewire

into the stomach (Fig. 136-4). The wire and introducer are removed, leaving only the sheath in the stomach. A urinary catheter is introduced through the sheath, and its balloon is inflated (Fig. 136-5). The sheath is removed, and the balloon of the catheter is pulled up to the gastric mucosa. The catheter is either sutured to the skin, or an outer faceplate is applied to hold the gastric and abdominal walls in approximation.

Comparison of Methods

All of the above techniques for the performance of percutaneous gastrostomy have been widely used and found effective. Each provides benefits that should be considered in choosing a method for a particular patient.[6]

The pull technique provides a great deal of control for the physician. The puncturing needle is stabilized with the surrounding snare, ensuring that loss of air from the gastric lumen does not result in loss of the puncturing needle. The gastrostomy tube is pulled down the esophagus and out of the abdominal wall in a direction that apposes the gastric and abdominal walls. This should minimize leakage around the puncture site. The push method adds the stability of a guidewire to act as a trolley on which the tube can ride as it passes through the alimentary tract. Both of these methods have the potential of introducing oral bacteria into the tissues of the abdominal wall. Thus, infection is a potential threat with these techniques. Both require a second passage of the endoscope to ensure correct positioning of the catheter head against the gastric wall.

The introducer method enjoys the advantage of a direct puncture insertion of the tube. This avoids the potential risk of infection from oral flora. This method also permits insertion of a gastrostomy in patients with narrow lesions of the esophagus without the fear of disrupting such lesions while the catheter is positioned. However, in this method, the forces of insertion push the stomach away from the abdominal wall and may lead to the creation of a submucosal tunnel in the stomach without puncture of the mucosa. Loss of control of the punctured stomach and leakage of gastric contents are also more likely to occur. The tubes used for this procedure are of small diameter and suffer from premature extrusion secondary to deflation of the balloon catheter.

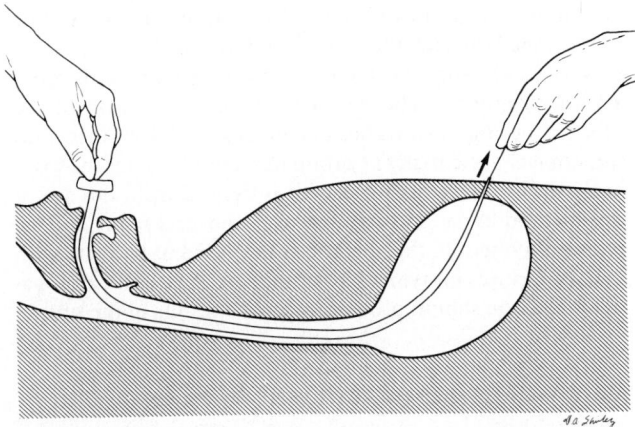

FIGURE 136-3. The assistant pulls on the abdominal end of the suture, and the gastrostomy tube proceeds down through the esophagus and stomach to exit the abdominal wall.

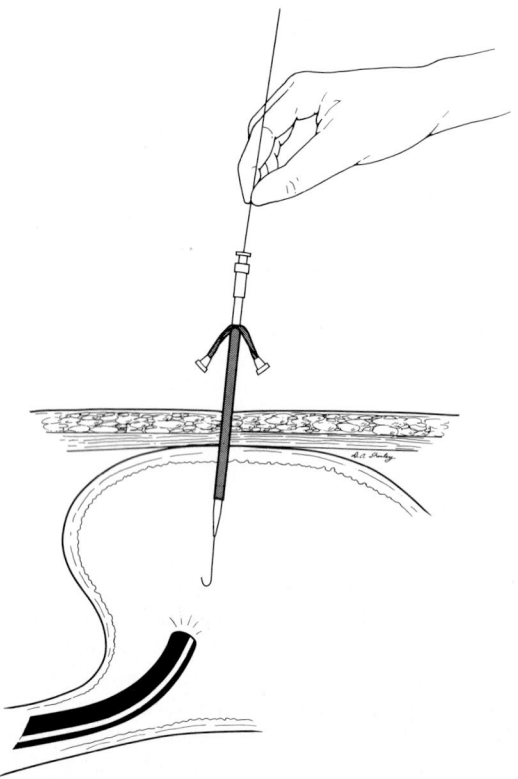

FIGURE 136-4. The introducer and its outer sheath are passed over the guidewire into the gastric lumen.

In practice, each of these methods has been demonstrated effective with a low rate of complications. Experienced endoscopists are familiar with all of these techniques and select the one with which they are most comfortable and which best suits the needs of the patient.

Percutaneous Endoscopic Jejunostomy

Percutaneous endoscopic jejunostomy is a modification of PEG, intended to accomplish concomitant jejunal feeding and gastric decompression. The method is similar to that of PEG, the gastric tube, acting to anchor the apparatus and decompress the stomach while a parallel longer enteric tube is positioned through the pylorus and used to deliver feeding solutions.[7] Present tube designs are imperfect, and tube problems are common. The thin jejunal feeding portion of the tube has been known to occlude or migrate backwards, into the stomach, essentially negating its value. Also, recent work has demonstrated that no benefit is derived from the use of this method in patients with gastroesophageal reflux and aspiration. Presently, this method is best used in patients with delayed gastric emptying. Newer tube designs, and better patient selection should provide improved results in the future.

Removal and Replacement of PEGs

Some PEG tube designs require endoscopic extraction of the intragastric portion at the time of tube replacement or removal. Designs are presently available which permit extraction

by means of external traction without the need for endoscopy.[8] Although PEG tubes may be replaced with balloon tip catheters, these tubes generally last only a short time, and have been known to migrate and obstruct the pyloric channel. Use of a mushroom-tip catheter or a skin-level device is preferable.

Gauderer and colleagues developed the concept of a skin-level gastrostomy device.[9] This device, with an antireflux valve, permits a cosmetic solution to gastrostomy feedings (Fig. 136-6). It may be placed after removal of a previous gastrostomy tube or at the time of the creation of the initial PEG. A standard tube is often preferable to the skin-level device in patients that require custodial care as it is more easily accessed by nursing personnel.

COMPLICATIONS

Complications occur with a frequency of approximately 6% to 10%.[10] Although most are minor, some may be life-threatening. The most common problems after percutaneous gastrostomy are infections caused by the escape of oral and gastric flora into the tissues of the abdominal wall. Infection usually becomes evident as erythema around the gastrostomy tube site several days after the procedure. There is usually local tenderness, slight edema of the skin, and the patient often demonstrates a low-grade fever and leukocytosis. Early recognition and incision and drainage of the area by means of a small skin incision under local anesthesia most often resolve

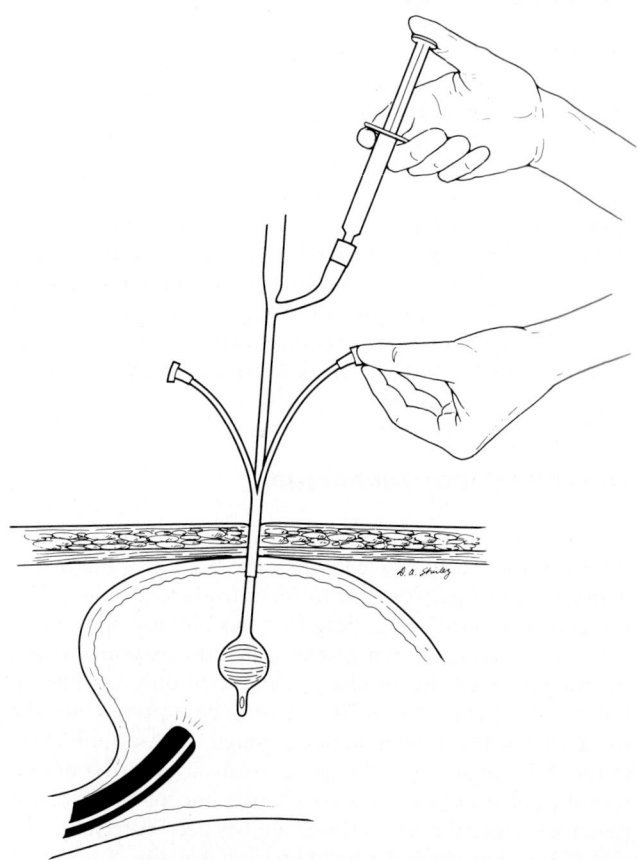

FIGURE 136-5. The introducer and guidewire are removed, and a balloon catheter is inserted through the sheath. The balloon is inflated, and the sheath is peeled away.

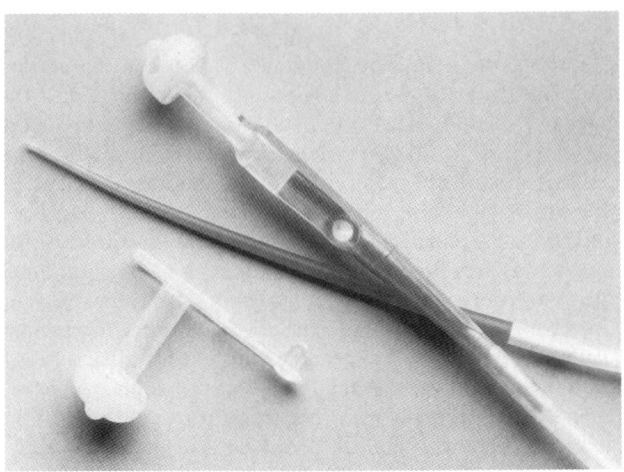

FIGURE 136-6. Skin-level gastrostomy devices provide important cosmetic benefits in selected patients. These devices may be placed after the initial tract has matured, or they may be placed at the time the gastrostomy is performed. A skin-level device (*bottom*). A modification of a skin-level device for one-step placement (*top*).

the problem. Failure to identify and treat this problem at an early stage may result in necrotizing infections of the abdominal wall and death.

Necrosis of the tissue of the abdominal wall which is interposed between the head of the tube and the outer bolster may play a major role in the occurrence of infection at a PEG site. Excessive tension applied to the bolster acts as a tourniquet producing ischemia of the underlying tissue. Loose contact is all that is required between the outer bolster and skin.

It is a good idea to begin systemic antibiotics for all infections around the tube and to continue them until the infection is resolved. Infectious complications can be minimized by the prophylactic administration of a single preoperative and a single postoperative dose of an intravenous cephalosporin.[11] Also, an adequate skin incision in the abdominal wall allows room around the gastrostomy tube for the egress of bacteria. Swabbing of the oropharynx with an antiseptic solution before the procedure to remove debris would also seem judicious, although its value has not been tested.

Extrusion of the head of the tube from the gastric lumen into the subcutaneous tissue has been frequently encountered. This is almost certainly due to excessive tension that has been applied to the tube. To prevent leakage of gastric contents and ensure adhesion of the stomach to the abdominal wall, the physician may pull up on the gastronomy tube and push downward on the outer bolster. Although this fixes the stomach to the abdominal wall, it also produces ischemia of the intervening abdominal wall tissue with subsequent necrosis. This can be avoided by ensuring that no tension is present when the head of the catheter is placed in contact with the gastric mucosa and that the outer bolster only loosely approximates the skin. Such approximation of the gastric and abdominal walls results in satisfactory adhesion without tissue necrosis.

Leakage of feedings into the peritoneal cavity may occur after percutaneous gastrostomy. This is usually the result of separation of the gastric and abdominal walls and often is

due to necrosis of the abdominal wall tissue due to excessive tension on the catheter. Patients who develop abdominal tenderness, fever, or leukocytosis should be evaluated for leakage and the resultant peritonitis. This may be done by instilling water-soluble contrast material into the gastrostomy tube under fluoroscopic guidance. Intraperitoneal extravasation indicates something has gone awry. If the contrast study indicates that the head of the tube remains in the stomach and that the extravasation is around the tube, the tube may be pulled up on a bit more tension to seal the leak, placed to drainage, and intravenous fluids and antibiotics can be administered. If the contrast study reveals complete separation of the gastric and abdominal walls with dislodgement of the tube from the stomach, the tube should be pulled from the abdominal wall, a nasogastric tube should be inserted to effect gastric drainage, and intravenous fluids and antibiotics should be begun. If at any time the patient's condition begins to deteriorate or signs of peritonitis worsen, exploratory laparotomy with operative repair should be performed.

Gastrocolic fistula has rarely been known to occur after percutaneous gastrostomy. This may be due to puncture of the colon at the time of gastrostomy or pinching of the colon between the gastric and abdominal walls with subsequent necrosis of the colonic wall and fistula formation. This complication usually becomes apparent after several weeks with the development of severe diarrhea after feeding. It may be documented with an upper gastrointestinal series or barium enema. In nearly all cases, the condition may be treated by removing the gastrostomy tube. The fistula closes rapidly once the tube is removed.

Progressive enlargement of the gastrostomy stoma around the gastrostomy tube may occur in some patients. Although this, too, may be the result of excessive tension on the tube, it is also occasionally seen in patients in whom the gastrostomy tract is well established. Poor nutritional status may play a part in the development of this problem. The temptation in dealing with this problem is to remove the gastrostomy tube and replace it with a larger one that fills the hole. This solves the problem for a short time, but the tract soon enlarges again. A better solution is to remove the tube entirely and allow the tract to close. After it has closed a bit, a new, smaller tube may be inserted.

Pneumoperitoneum is a frequent occurrence after percutaneous gastrostomy. This may be the result of air escaping around the puncturing needle. Routine x-ray films of the abdomen after gastrostomy are unwarranted. Air in the abdominal cavity has been shown to last for up to 5 weeks after gastrostomy. Patients found to have pneumoperitoneum after gastrostomy must be clinically evaluated. In the absence of abdominal tenderness, leukocytosis, or fever, there is no need for further evaluation of the gastrostomy. However, the patient who demonstrates any of these should be evaluated by a water-soluble contrast study through the gastrostomy tube for signs of separation or intraperitoneal extravasation.

Good skin care is important after gastrostomy. It is common to see a foreign body reaction around the tube with some exudate or granulation tissue. This is usually easy to handle. The exudate is merely swabbed away with hydrogen peroxide. The site should be left open to the air. Granulation tissue may be cauterized with silver nitrate. Occlusive dressings should be avoided because they lead to maceration of the underlying skin.

Percutaneous gastrostomy is a simple procedure with few severe complications. Close attention to detail and rapid assessment of potential problems minimize unsatisfactory outcomes.

CONSIDERATIONS IN CHOOSING PERCUTANEOUS GASTROSTOMY

Indications

PEG may be indicated as a means of delivering alimentation in patients who are unable to take oral nutrition but who possess a functional gastrointestinal tract. Such patients include those with neurologic disorders and tumors of the oropharynx.

In children, neurologic impairment may be the result of birth trauma, subsequent injury, or progressive nervous system disease. Percutaneous gastrostomy has been advantageous in allowing parents and nursing personnel to care for these children without the need for repeated nasogastric intubation or laparotomy for surgical gastrostomy. A number of these patients improve sufficiently to resume oral feedings and allow removal of the gastrostomy.

Adults with neurologic impairment due to injury or disease are also candidates for percutaneous gastrostomy. These conditions may be progressive or reversible and include maladies such as head trauma, stroke, multiple sclerosis, amyotrophic lateral sclerosis, and pseudobulbar palsy.

Tumors of the oropharynx restrict the intake of food and impair the swallowing mechanism. Patients with these tumors often benefit from placement of a percutaneous gastrostomy. The gastrostomy may be placed before radical surgery and radiation therapy, or at a time when supplemental feedings become necessary.

Other indications for percutaneous gastrostomy have been identified. The method has been used to return external biliary drainage to the gastrointestinal tract.[12] In patients with malignant biliary obstruction in whom transhepatic biliary drainage has been established, the drainage catheter may be connected to a percutaneous gastrostomy. In this way, the biliary secretions are channeled back into the intestinal tract, allowing for normal digestion and averting fluid losses. The gastrostomy has been used to provide supplemental nighttime feedings in children with malabsorption and inflammatory bowel disease. It has also been used as a route for chronic delivery of unpalatable medications to young children.

Patients with chronic bowel obstruction secondary to carcinomatosis or radiation enteritis have benefited by the placement of a percutaneous gastrostomy for gastric decompression. Although the gastrostomy does not completely empty the stomach, it usually serves as a vent sufficient to prevent nausea and vomiting.

The percutaneous gastrostomy catheter may also be modified with a jejunal feeding tube placed through its lumen or alongside it. The jejunal tube may be used to feed the patient, and the gastrostomy port is used for gastric decompression. This modification, known as percutaneous endoscopic jejunostomy, is useful in patients with severe gastroesophageal reflux or gastric atony.

Contraindications

From a purely technical standpoint, PEG is contraindicated if an endoscope cannot be passed into the stomach or if the light of the endoscope cannot be seen to transilluminate the abdominal wall. Massive ascites is also a contraindication, because adhesion of the stomach to the abdominal wall is less likely to occur. Correctable obstruction of the intestinal tract and intraabdominal sepsis are also contraindications to the procedure. Previous abdominal surgery is not a contraindication to percutaneous gastrostomy but adds to its risk. The operator must make certain that adequate transillumination of the abdominal wall is present, thus ensuring the absence of intervening organs. Percutaneous gastrostomy may be accomplished in patients with ventriculoperitoneal shunts if the area of the shunt is carefully avoided.

PEG should not be performed in rapidly deteriorating patients with multiple system organ failure, or in cases where systemic sepsis is present. In such cases, an unsatisfactory outcome is likely. These patients can usually be managed with nasoenteric feedings until they have improved. Gastrostomy may be placed if it is still indicated. It is most unfortunate that the technique has been applied to patients who have short life expectancies or who are critically ill. Such use is unfair to the patients and serves to discredit the method.[13]

> The reader is directed to Chapter 48, Approach to the Patient Requiring Nutritional Supplementation.

REFERENCES

1. Gauderer MWL, Stellato TA. Gastrostomies: evolution, techniques, indications and complications. Curr Probl Surg 1986; 23(9):657.
2. Gauderer MWL, Ponsky JL, Izant RJ Jr. Gastrostomy without laparotomy. A percutaneous endoscopic technique. J Pediatr Surg 1980;15:872.
3. Ponsky JL, Gauderer MWL. Percutaneous endoscopic gastrostomy: a non-operative technique for feeding gastrostomy. Gastrointest Endosc 1981;27:9.
4. Sacks BA, Vine HS, Palestrant AM, et al. A non-operative technique for establishment of a gastrostomy in the dog. Invest Radiol 1983;18:485.
5. Russell TR, Brotman M, Forbes N. Percutaneous gastrostomy: a new simplified and cost-effective technique. Am J Surg 1984;148:132.
6. Ponsky JL. Techniques of percutaneous gastrostomy: a comparison. In: Ponsky JL, ed. Techniques of percutaneous gastrostomy. New York: Igaku-Shoin, 1988:111.
7. Ponsky JL, Aszodi A. Percutaneous endoscopic jejunostomy. Am J Gastroenterol 1984;79:113.
8. Ponsky JL. Percutaneous endoscopic gastrostomy: techniques of removal and replacement. Gastrointest Endosc Clin North Am 1992;2(2):215.
9. Gauderer MWL, Picha GJ, Izant RJ Jr. The gastrostomy "button"—a simple, skin-level, nonrefluxing device for long-term enteral feedings. J Pediatr Surg 1984;19:803.
10. Strodel WE, Ponsky JL. Complications of percutaneous gastrostomy. In: Ponsky JL, ed. Techniques of percutaneous gastrostomy, New York: Igaku-Shoin, 1988:63.
11. Jonas SK, Neimark S, Panwalker AP. Effect of antibiotic prophylaxis in percutaneous endoscopic gastrostomy. Am J Gastroenterol 1985;80:438.
12. Ponsky JL, Aszodi A. External biliary-gastric fistula: a simple method for recycling bile. Am J Gastroenterol 1982;77:939.
13. Taylor CM, Larson DJ, Ballard LR, et al. Who should receive placement of percutaneous endoscopic gastrostomy (PEG) feeding tubes? Gastroenterology 1991;100:A12.

Textbook of Gastroenterology, second edition, edited by Tadataka Yamada. JB Lippincott Company, Philadelphia © 1995.

CHAPTER 137

Endoscopic Control of Upper Gastrointestinal Variceal Bleeding

Harvey S. Young   Suzanne M. Matsui   Peter B. Gregory

Historical Perspectives
Anatomic Considerations
Natural History of Variceal Bleeding
  Esophageal Varices
  Extraesophageal Varices
Sclerotherapy Techniques
  Endoscope
  Sclerosants
  Sclerotherapy Schedule
  Accessories and Balloon Compression
  Evaluation

  Mechanism of Action
  Efficacy
  Esophageal Varices
  Ectopic Varices
  Contraindication and Risks
Elastic Band Ligation
  Technique
  Mechanism of Action
  Efficacy
  Contraindications and Risks

Variceal hemorrhage has been a challenging clinical problem for many years. The resurgence and refinement of endoscopic therapies have provided further insight into the natural history of esophageal varices and has improved the overall management of this problem. For patients with acutely bleeding esophageal varices, emergency sclerotherapy or variceal ligation are good adjunctive therapies to the usual supportive treatment. With the extensive practice and training that have occurred in the last decade, most gastroenterologists are now capable of performing these procedures. However, these two techniques are not very effective in stopping bleeding from gastric varices. Endoscopic injection of Histoacryl is the only promising endoscopic technique available for bleeding gastric varices at present. The overall efficacy and safety of this technique are yet to be confirmed. A new treatment modality, transjugular intrahepatic portosystemic shunt (TIPS), has the potential to stop bleeding from esophageal and gastric varices, as well as portal hypertensive gastropathy, and may emerge as the treatment of choice for patients with patent portal veins. The long-term safety and efficacy of TIPS, and comparisons of TIPS to sclerotherapy or ligation, are still pending.

Both long-term sclerotherapy and band ligation are able to lower recurrent bleeding rates in patients with variceal bleeding. Their efficacies in this respect are better than medical observation, but are inferior to shunt surgery. Band ligation, combined with low volume sclerotherapy may be more effec-

tive than either endoscopic technique alone. Repeated sclerotherapy improves long-term survival in these patients, but the effect is probably modest. Whether band ligation is superior to sclerotherapy in this regard is yet to be confirmed. However, band ligation is associated with a lower risk of esophageal stricture formation compared to sclerotherapy. At present, it is reasonable to recommend either long-term sclerotherapy or band ligation for most patients who have bled from esophageal varices. This is especially applicable to patients with noncirrhotic portal hypertension and those with good liver function. For patients who rebleed and cannot be stopped by sclerotherapy or band ligation, TIPS or shunt surgery are alternative treatment options. Shunt surgery poses additional technical difficulties during liver transplantation. Therefore, for transplant candidates, endoscopic therapies still play an important role in controlling variceal bleeding until transplantation is performed. However, the deep esophageal ulcerations induced by sclerotherapy may increase the risk of sepsis in posttransplant patients, and endoscopic band ligation or TIPS may be better suited for these patients.

Prophylactic therapy for patients with esophageal varices to prevent the first variceal bleed is still undergoing evolution. Endoscopic sclerotherapy is clearly not beneficial. The role of band ligation in prophylactic therapy is not yet defined. Treatment with beta blockers appears to be the only safe alternative. However, the fundamental problem in this field is our inability to reliably identify patients at high risk of bleeding from esophageal varices.

HISTORICAL PERSPECTIVES

Endoscopic control of variceal bleeding has gone through significant evolution over the last fifty years. In 1939, Crafoord and Frenckner[1] first reported the use of sclerotherapy for bleeding esophageal varices. Using a rigid esophagoscope and a specially designed needle, they successfully introduced a sclerosant, quinine-uretan, into the varices of a young woman with portal hypertension. After a month-long course of sclerotherapy, they were able to obliterate her varices. Several other physicians of that era[2-5] adopted this procedure and found encouraging results in subsets of patients who had esophageal varices without concomitant gastric varices and in those with better baseline hepatic function.

In the mid 1940s, however, the portacaval shunting procedure introduced by Whipple[6,7] and Blakemore[8] diverted attention away from endoscopic sclerotherapy. Over the next two to three decades, shunt surgery was performed frequently. It was shown to be capable of lowering the risk of recurrent hemorrhage from varices, but it failed to prolong patient survival. In addition, it was associated with undesirable rates of hepatic encephalopathy or hepatic failure, particularly in those patients who already had reduced hepatic reserve.[9-13]

As the shortcomings of shunt surgery became widely known, endoscopic sclerotherapy again emerged as an attractive alternative in the treatment of bleeding esophageal varices.

Over the past fifteen years, endoscopic sclerotherapy once again has been established as the first-line therapy for variceal bleeding.

In 1986, Van Stiegmann and colleagues[14] introduced a new endoscopic ligation technique for control of variceal bleeding. This technique is now emerging as a good alternative to endoscopic sclerotherapy.

ANATOMIC CONSIDERATIONS

The portal circulation in normal individuals is a high-flow (1000–1200 mL/minute), low-pressure system ($\approx$7 mm Hg) and provides the liver with 60% to 70% of its total oxygen supply.[15] Both intrahepatic and extrahepatic abnormalities that increase the resistance to blood flow in this system result in portal hypertension. Once portal hypertension develops, extrahepatic collateral venous channels between the portal and systemic circulations dilate and form varices (Fig. 137-1).

Varices can be found along the entire gastrointestinal tract in patients with portal hypertension. Those most likely to bleed are found in the distal esophagus and proximal stomach. The varices in the distal 5 cm of the esophagus are easily identified by endoscopy because of their superficial location in the lamina propria.[16] Gastric varices, on the other hand, are located in the submucosa and are not as easily visualized.[17] Anatomical studies of the lower esophagus have provided insight into why varices in the distal 5 cm of the esophagus are most apt to bleed and why the current practice of endoscopic

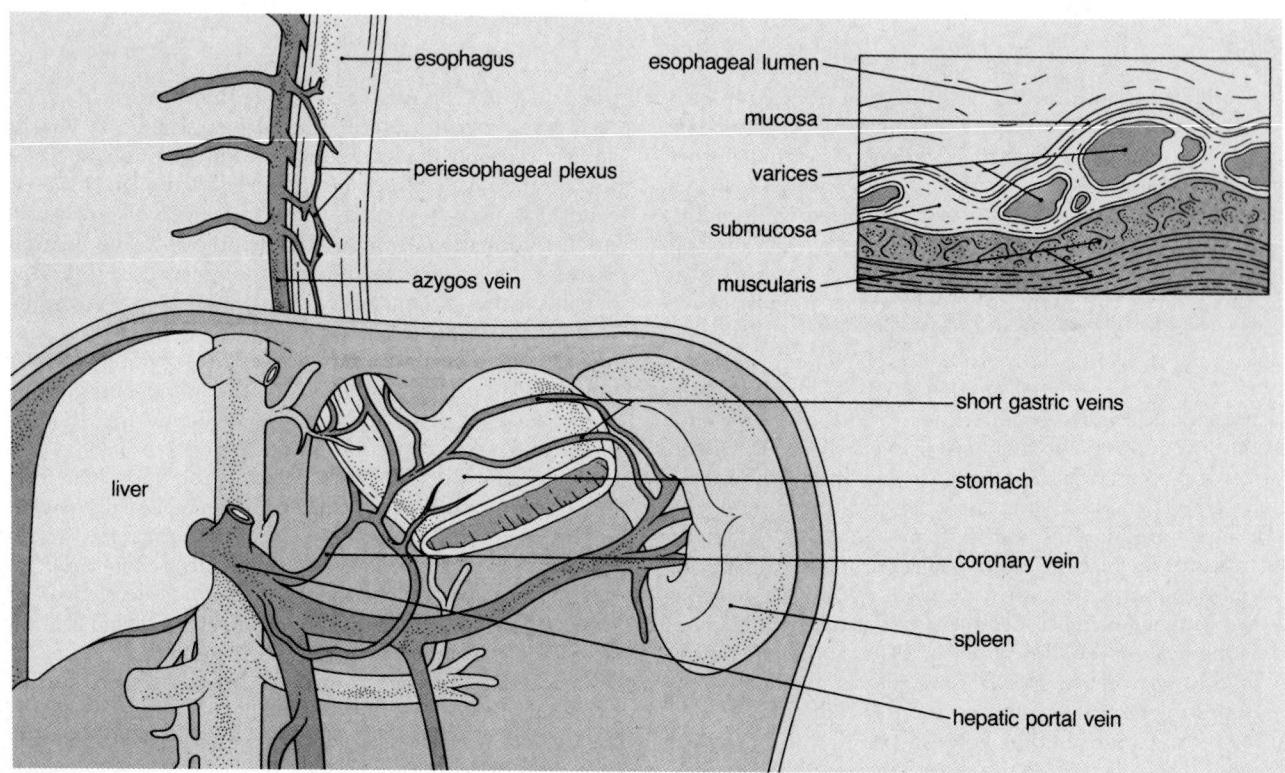

FIGURE 137-1. The portal venous system and esophageal varices. (From Silverstein FE, Tytgat GNJ. Atlas of gastrointestinal endoscopy. 2nd ed. New York: Gower Medical, 1991.)

therapy is likely to be successful in obliterating these varices. Our current understanding of the venous anatomy of this region derives from the pioneering work of Butler in 1951[18] and from recent studies which have used more sophisticated, high-resolution techniques.[19-24]

In normal patients, four distinct venous zones have been identified in the distal esophagus and proximal stomach (Fig. 137-2). Of these, the palisade zone and the perforating zone are considered the most important in the development and rupture of esophageal varices. The palisade zone begins at the gastroesophageal junction and extends 2–3 cm cephalad. The veins within this zone are longitudinally arranged in the lamina propria. Blood flow within the palisade zone is bidirectional and accommodates the variable pressures at the gastroesophageal junction associated with the respiratory cycle, coughing, and Valsalva maneuvers. Thus, blood from the

palisade zone alternately drains into the gastric zone (i.e., into the portal system) and into the perforating zone, which extends 3–5 cm proximal to the gastroesophageal junction. In the perforating zone, four distinct layers of veins[19] have been identified (Fig. 137-3). Fine, superficial, arborizing intraepithelial veins drain capillary beds in the epithelium into a superficial venous plexus. Blood subsequently flows into three to five, larger caliber, deep intrinsic veins. Blood from these intraesophageal veins is directed into periesophageal veins through perforating veins which have valves to encourage directional flow.

These normal vascular relations are altered significantly in the patient with portal hypertension. Dilatation and high pressures in the periesophageal veins cause the valves in the perforating veins to become incompetent, allowing retrograde flow into the deep intrinsic veins and its tributaries. This re-

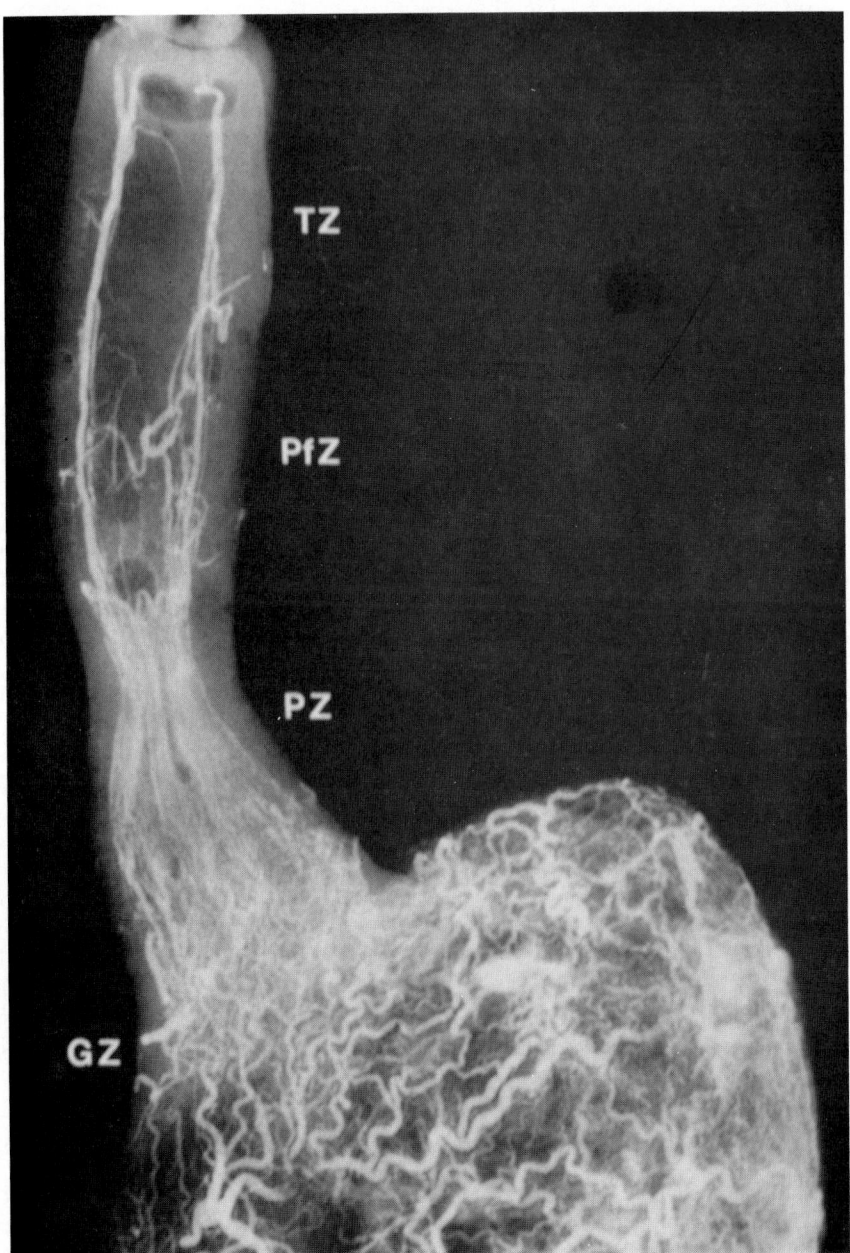

FIGURE 137-2. Radiograph of the venous zones in the human gastroesophageal junction. (GZ, gastric zone; PfZ, perforating zone; PZ, palisade zone; TZ, truncal zone; from Vianna A, Hayes PC, Moscoso G, et al. Normal venous circulation of the gastroesophageal junction. Gastroenterology 1987;93:876.)

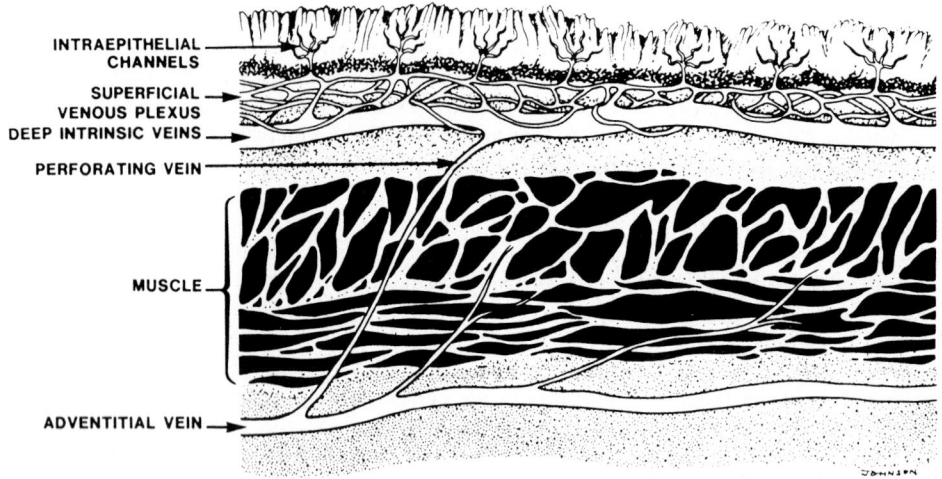

INTRAEPITHELIAL
CHANNELS

SUPERFICIAL
VENOUS PLEXUS

DEEP INTRINSIC VEINS

PERFORATING VEIN

MUSCLE

ADVENTITIAL VEIN

FIGURE 137-3. The layers of veins at the human distal esophagus. (From Kitano S, Terblanche J, Kahn J, et al. Venous anatomy of the lower oesophagus in portal hypertension: practical implications. Br J Surg 1986;73:525.)

sults in increased blood flow and turbulence in the intrinsic venous trunks. The dilated deep intrinsic veins displace the superficial venous plexus and assume a subepithelial position. These are the tortuous, large variceal trunks seen at endoscopy.[19] Dilatation of the intraepithelial veins result in the endoscopically recognizable cherry red spots, red wales, or varices upon varices.[25] The dilatation and increased pressure in the perforating zone influences blood to flow caudally into the palisade zone. The palisade zone, however, must also accommodate the increased gastrosplenic blood flow associated with portal hypertension. Consequently, blood flow in the palisade zone is more turbulent in patients with portal hypertension. High pressures and turbulent flow in superficially located dilated vessels in the distal 5 cm of the esophagus (i.e., the palisade and perforating zones) contribute to the likelihood of rupture of these varices.

The current practice of endoscopic therapy for variceal bleeding is directed at obliterating the varices of the distal esophagus and gastroesophageal junction which are most likely to bleed. This is accomplished by injecting the sclerosant in or around the varices to cause thrombosis of these channels and mucosal fibrosis around them, or by ligation of these variceal channels with endoscopically applied rubber bands. However, the incompetent perforating veins which connect the intrinsic venous trunks to the periesophageal veins are not effectively obliterated and new collateral channels may form in the distal esophagus.

NATURAL HISTORY OF VARICEAL BLEEDING

Esophageal Varices

The finding of esophageal varices in cirrhotic patients carries a grim prognosis.[26] It is estimated that 50% of these patients will bleed from their varices at some time in their lives.[27,28] Factors that can predict which patient will bleed and when this event will occur have not been fully elucidated. The magnitude of the elevation of portal pressure appears predictive in that patients whose portal pressure is above 10 to 12 mm Hg have an increased risk of bleeding compared to those whose portal pressures are below this level.[29,30] However, an

elevation in portal pressure does not necessarily mean that the pressure in esophageal varices is also high, because individual patients may differ in the type and degree of collateral circulation.[31] Red color signs (i.e., cherry red spots, red wale markings, or hematocystic spots) and blue varices, which may indicate thin overlying mucosa, have been associated with a history of variceal bleeding.[25] This relation in still debatable. In a prospective trial, only 19% of patients with these variceal stigmata bled from esophageal varices over a 2-year period.[32] Large varices are associated with an increased likelihood of variceal hemorrhage. An average of 30%, and as many as 83%, of patients who have large varices bleed from them in the 25 months following their discovery.[29,30,33–37]

When bleeding from esophageal varices occurs, it usually stops spontaneously, at least temporarily, in up to two thirds of patients.[38] Still, 30% to 40% of these patients are at risk for rebleeding within 2 to 3 days[26] and 60% rebleed within 1 week.[26,39,40] Mortality in the first week following the index bleed hovers around 25%, with rebleeding and liver failure accounting for most of the deaths.[41]

Most studies have found a correlation between the extent of liver failure in patients with bleeding esophageal varices, as expressed by the Child's classification, and mortality.[42] Survival statistics are best for patients with minimal liver dysfunction (Child's group A) and worst for the sickest patients (Child's group C). For the Child's group C patients, the one month mortality is greater than 45%, 1-year survival is 35%, and 2-year survival is 23%. Early rebleeding may be an overt reflection of the degree of liver failure and has been correlated with death within 30 days.

Graham and Smith have shown that the bleeding-associated mortality rate is highest in the first days to weeks after the variceal bleed and returns to baseline by 3 to 4 months.[26] Therefore, therapeutic interventions are likely to have the most influence on survival if introduced in the early period following the bleed.

Extraesophageal Varices

Extraesophageal or ectopic varices have been found at almost any level of the gastrointestinal tract and in the peritoneum, biliary tree, and genitourinary tract. Ectopic varices are found in the range of 1% to 3% in cirrhotic patients and 20% to 30% in patients with extrahepatic portal hypertension. Patients with portal hypertension who have also had abdominal surgery are more likely to develop these varices in adhesions or enterostomal sites.[43] All of these varices have the potential to cause significant hemorrhage. We will confine our discussion to ectopic varices of the upper gastrointestinal tract.

Gastric Varices

In patients with portal hypertension, gastric varices are predominantly supplied by dilated short gastric veins and are frequently found with esophageal varices.[15] Gastric varices may form as a result of increased resistance to cephalad flow through the palisade zone at the gastroesophageal junction in these patients.[20] Isolated gastric varices are found in patients with splenic vein thrombosis.[15]

Gastric varices may be more difficult to identify at endoscopy because they are generally situated deeper than esophageal varices and may resemble rugal folds. In acutely bleeding patients, the fundus is frequently obscured by a pool of blood and small gastric varices may not be easily detected.

In much of the literature, gastric varices are reported together with esophageal varices rather than as a separate entity. Therefore, the incidence, frequency of bleeding, and natural history of gastric varices have not been defined precisely. Incidence rates of 16% to 70% have been reported in patients with portal hypertension and cirrhosis.[17] Whether the mere presence of gastric varices influences survival is unknown. However, patients who bleed from gastric varices appear to have a higher mortality. Bleeding gastric varices present a therapeutic challenge because they are part of an extensive collateral network, making hemostasis and ultimate obliteration difficult.[44]

Duodenal Varices

Aside from esophagogastric varices, duodenal varices are one of the more commonly reported digestive tract varices in portal hypertension. The incidence of these varices is not known, but duodenal varices represented one third of the bleeding ectopic varices reported by Lebrec and Benhamou.[43] These varices may be less likely to rupture because they are found deeper in the gut wall than esophageal varices. Duodenal varices are found more often in individuals with extrahepatic portal hypertension where the varices serve to bypass the obstructed segment. In patients with intrahepatic portal hypertension, duodenal varices form between the afferent branches of the portal vein, such as the superior mesenteric vein, and the inferior vena cava.[45]

Patients with bleeding duodenal varices commonly present with hematemesis or melena. During emergency endoscopy, these varices may be difficult to identify and concomitant esophagogastric varices that are more readily visualized may be assumed to be the source of bleeding. Angiography or dynamic CT scan may be needed to confirm the diagnosis.[43]

SCLEROTHERAPY TECHNIQUES

Sclerotherapy techniques have been modified significantly since Crafoord and Frenckner's initial report.[1] The development of fiberoptic endoscopy has done much to advance the practice of sclerotherapy. Although sclerotherapy has gained wide acceptance around the world over the last 15 years, no uniform technique is practiced by all endoscopists. There is considerable variation in the choice of endoscopes, needles, sclerosants, injection sites, treatment schedules and accessories used by individual endoscopists.

Endoscope

During the initial resurgence of sclerotherapy, the patient was given general anesthesia and the rigid endoscope was used to perform the procedure. Enthusiasts of the rigid endoscope have reported excellent results with this instrument.[46-49] They cite as advantages the capacity of the rigid instrument to suction large amounts of blood, compress bleeding varices, and facilitate injection by allowing the protrusion of a varix into the slotted tip. However, the ease with which the flexible endoscope can be used more than offsets the theoretical advantages of the rigid instrument. Moreover, the importance of variceal compression and a slotted tip have not been confirmed. Acute and chronic maintenance sclerotherapy may be carried out equally well with the rigid or the flexible endoscope, but the complication rate is higher with the rigid instrument regardless of the endoscopist's level of experience.[50,51]

The flexible endoscope is currently the instrument of choice in both emergency and elective sclerotherapy. The intravenous sedation used for endoscopy with flexible instruments is safer for patients with poor liver function than the general anesthesia that is required for endoscopy with rigid esophagoscopes. The judicious use of endotracheal intubation is recommended during emergency sclerotherapy to prevent aspiration in patients with active variceal bleeding. The procedure can be performed on an outpatient basis during chronic maintenance sessions.

Sclerosants

Dosage

Over the past 50 years, many sclerosants or combinations of these agents have been used for variceal sclerotherapy. Selection of these agents has largely been extrapolated from experiences with the sclerosis of varicosities in the lower extremities or hemorrhoids. Many investigators believe that the ideal sclerosant should first induce rapid thrombosis to provide acute hemostasis, followed by fibrosis of the variceal channel with minimal damage to the surrounding esophageal tissue and with minimal systemic side effects. Some argue that necrosis of tissue surrounding the variceal channel is necessary to achieve a permanent obliteration of these vessels.[52] Agents that have been tested fall into 2 major categories: the physical irritants such as the fatty acids (e.g., sodium morrhuate, ethanolamine oleate, polidocanol) and the dehydrating compounds such as the alkyl salt sodium tetradecyl sulfate, ethanol, hypertonic glucose, and 3% phenol.[53] Cefazolin, quinine, or topical bovine thrombin have also been tried empirically.

In clinical practice, the choice of sclerosant has largely

remained a matter of personal preference and has been dependent on the availability of the particular sclerosants in various countries. In the United States, sodium morrhuate and sodium tetradecyl have been the agents of choice. Ethanolamine, which has just been approved by the Food and Drug Administration for sclerotherapy in the United States, has been used exclusively in Britain and South Africa. Polidocanol (Aethoxyskerol) is the sclerosant of choice in Austria and Germany.

Only very few direct comparisons of these agents have been made. Using a canine model, Jensen and colleagues[55,154] compared the acute hemostatic efficacy of 5% sodium morrhuate, 5% ethanolamine oleate, 1.5% sodium tetradecyl sulfate, cefazolin, 95% and 47% ethanol, and a mixture of 0.5% sodium tetradecyl sulfate and 50 U/mL thrombin in 50% dextrose (TTD). All of these agents produced acute hemostasis in 98 to 100% of cases after a single 2 ml intravariceal injection of these sclerosants into a bleeding varix. Using a similar model, different sclerosants were compared with respect to their efficacy in achieving variceal obliteration and frequency of complications following a single variceal injection.[56] Cefazolin, 47% ethanol, and TTD were found to be no more effective than the saline control in obliterating varices. 95% ethanol and a mixture of 0.75% tetradecyl plus 47% ethanol were of borderline efficacy, but alcohol had an 80% ulceration rate. Sclerosants that were significantly better than saline injection were 1.5% sodium tetradecyl sulfate, 5% sodium morrhuate, and a combination of 1% tetradecyl plus 32% ethanol and saline (TES). They recommended the TES solution because its ulceration rate was only 10%, whereas the other two agents had ulceration rates of 30 to 40%.

Prospective randomized clinical comparisons of some of these agents have been reported recently. Kitano and colleagues[57] compared 5% ethanolamine to 1% polidocanol. They suggested that 5% ethanolamine required fewer sclerotherapy sessions and therefore less time to achieve eradication of the varices. The overall variceal obliteration rates were the same. However, early rebleeding and ulcerations induced by sclerotherapy were significantly greater with polidocanol. This finding cannot be directly compared to previous results of polidocanol from Germany because different sclerotherapy techniques were used.

In a separate study, Kitano and colleagues[58] compared 5% ethanolamine to 2% sodium tetradecyl sulfate and again found that ethanolamine appeared to induce less ulceration and bleeding, and was able to obliterate varices faster than tetradecyl. Chung and colleagues[59] recently compared 3% sodium tetradecyl with 5% ethanolamine. These agents were equally effective in stopping variceal hemorrhage, but sodium tetradecyl sulfate obliterated the varices in significantly fewer sessions. The ulceration rates were the same.

Bhargava and colleagues[60] compared 1.5% sodium tetradecyl sulfate to polidocanol. Both sclerosants achieved the same rate of variceal obliteration. However, sodium tetradecyl sulfate was associated with a significantly higher rates of deep esophageal ulceration, dysphagia and stricture formation. Paoluzi and colleagues[61] conducted a prospective comparison of absolute alcohol to polidocanol. This study was stopped after enrolling eleven patients because unacceptably large ulcers were induced by the alcohol injection.

The interpretation of the results in these studies is made more difficult because of differences in injection technique, populations studied and end points. At this point in time, there are no data to dictate which agent is the best sclerosant. It is likely that any one of a large number of sclerosants are equally effective.

Sodium morrhuate, sodium tetradecyl sulfate, ethanolamine or ethanol are usually injected directly into the varix. Depending on the size of the varix, 0.5 to 2 ml of the selected sclerosant is used in each injection. The total volume used per sclerotherapy session is usually around 10 to 20 ml. Polidocanol, on the other hand, is injected into the submucosa around the varix. Each time 0.5 to 1.5 ml is injected and 40 to 60 ml of polidocanol is used per sclerotherapy session.

Soehendra and colleagues have pioneered the use of a liquid tissue adhesive, isobutyl 2-cyano-acrylate (Histoacryl), for intravariceal injections into bleeding esophageal and gastric varices.[54] This liquid polymer solidifies instantly in blood and lead to immediate obliteration of the varix. This adhesive plug sloughs off in a few weeks, leaving a fibrotic scar at the injection site. Histoacryl is diluted with Lipiodol (0.5 : 0.8 mL) prior to injection in order to prevent the adhesive from hardening too fast and to allow fluroscopic monitoring. The biopsy channel and tip of the endoscope should be treated with silicon oil to prevent sticking of Histoacryl to the instrument. A single, 0.5 ml dose of this solution is injected intravascularly into each esophageal variceal channel through a regular sclerotherapy needle. Two to three injections of 0.5 mL each are often required for large varices in the gastric fundus. After each injection of 0.5 mL of the Histoacryl solution, the sclerotherapy needle must be thoroughly rinsed with distilled water. Initial hemostasis using Histoacryl has been achieved for both esophageal and gastric variceal bleeding.[62] The early postsclerotherapy variceal rebleeding rate observed was 12%, significant improvement over the 30% rebleeding rate found in a historic control group using 1% Polidocanol as the sclerosant. In addition, esophageal perforation and stricture formation rates were lower in the Histoacryl treated patients. However, controlled trials that compare the efficacy and complication rates of Histoacryl with other sclerosants are not yet available.

Injection Site

As alluded to in the previous section, there are also differences in opinion regarding the correct injection site. Intravariceal injection was the first method described[1] and is still used by most endoscopists around the world, especially in the United States and England. Injection is carried out initially at the bleeding site. All the variceal channels are then injected at the gastroesophageal junction. Finally, the variceal channels are injected again 3 to 5 cm proximally.[63]

Other endoscopists inject the sclerosant alongside the varix or paravariceally. This technique is based on the work of Wodak[64] who advocated the preservation of esophageal varices which he considered to be essential collaterals for decompressing portal hypertension. The aim of paravariceal injection is to create a layer of fibrosis covering the variceal channels. Injections are carried out starting at the cardia and repeated 30 to 50 times, producing a helical arrangement of weals as the endoscope is withdrawn. The injections are limited to the distal esophagus unless there is a more proximal bleeding site.

This technique is currently the method of choice in Germany, Austria and other European countries. Direct comparison of these two methods, however, has been limited. Sarin and his colleagues recently reported a prospective comparison of these two injection techniques in 54 patients using 50% ethanol as the sclerosant.[65] They concluded that intravariceal injection is superior to paravariceal injection in controlling active variceal bleeding and achieving more rapid obliteration of all variceal channels. Despite a higher variceal recurrence rate in the intravariceal group, the rebleeding rates were similar between the two groups. Paravariceal injection was associated with a higher incidence of retrosternal pain after sclerotherapy. Future studies, especially ones that use more commonly injected sclerosants, are needed to confirm these findings. Although the issue of intravariceal versus paravariceal injection is far from resolved, most experienced endoscopists are aware that they are not always able to inject the intended target site. A mixture of intravariceal and paravariceal injections is the usual end result in each sclerotherapy session, especially during treatment for acute bleeding.

On the basis of a recently completed study of the variceal anatomy, Kitano and colleagues have proposed yet another injection method.[66] Varices are initially obliterated by intravariceal injection of ethanolamine. This is followed by intentional submucosal injection to create superficial ulcerations and to denude the mucosa at the distal esophagus. Subsequent reepithelialization of these ulcerations obliterate the submucosal space in which new varices may develop. Using this technique, they reported a recurrent bleeding rate of 4.9%, and no variceal recurrence in a median follow-up period of 14.6 months in 155 patients. These rates are outstanding when compared to the 40% recurrent bleeding rate[67] and 60% variceal recurrence rate[67,68] that are associated with the previously described methods. Despite the obvious differences in patient population, instrument and sclerosant, Kitano and colleagues' results remain impressive and await confirmation.[66]

Sclerotherapy Schedule

Sclerotherapy, as a long-term treatment, requires repeated injection sessions to achieve obliteration of varices. Despite the popularity of the procedure in the past 15 years, no uniform follow up sclerotherapy schedule has emerged. After the initial treatment, subsequent sclerotherapy sessions have been scheduled at various intervals, ranging from a few days to a few weeks.[67–72] Westaby and colleagues[73] compared a weekly sclerotherapy schedule to sclerotherapy every three weeks. They did not observe any difference in rates of variceal obliteration and recurrent bleeding between the two schedules. Ulcerations at the injection sites were seen more frequently on the weekly schedule, but the incidence of other complications was similar on both schedules. However, using ethanol as the sclerosant, Sarin and colleagues[74] reported faster obliteration of varices and a subsequent lower rebleeding rate with a weekly sclerotherapy schedule compared to a three week schedule. They also noted a higher ulceration rate with the weekly schedule which led to postponement of sclerotherapy sessions in 25% of these patients.

As ulcerations appear to be inevitable with current sclero-therapy techniques, it is reasonable to recommend that follow-up sessions be done no more frequently than once a week. The ideal schedule, however, has yet to be defined. After the varices are obliterated, most endoscopists do follow-up endoscopies every 3 to 6 months. If varices recur, sclerotherapy should be reinstituted according to the initial treatment schedule until they are obliterated once again.

Accessories and Balloon Compression

Many accessories have been developed for use with the flexible endoscope in the hope of incorporating some of the potential advantages of the rigid endoscope. Devices such as flexible overtubes and balloon catheters have been designed to provide either proximal or distal variceal compression during sclerotherapy.[75–77] Initial uncontrolled studies endorsed the additional merit of these devices, but prospective randomized evaluations of these devices have been limited and their usefulness remains controversial.[78] In current practice, most endoscopists use the freehand technique, because these accessories are somewhat cumbersome to use.

Some investigators have proposed the use of radiopaque contrast material or fluorescein in the sclerosant to improve the accuracy of injection into the varix.[79] However, it is not clear that accurate intravascular injection is crucial to the efficacy of sclerotherapy. Most endoscopists, therefore, seldom use sclerosant markers in their routine practice.

When a patient is being treated with long-term sclerotherapy, visual inspection by the endoscopist is the usual method in deciding whether all variceal channels have been obliterated. Hosking[80] recently reported that this visual inspection had a 25% error rate in determining the patency of the variceal channel when compared to an intravariceal manometric measurement. This interesting result awaits confirmation.

Many commercial needle injectors are now available. The needle size varies from 23 to 25 gauge, and its length ranges from 2 to 5 mm. Needles longer than 5 mm have been associated with an increased in incidence of bacteremia after sclerotherapy.[81] Most of these needles are retractable into a flexible plastic sheath. The type of needle used appears to rely upon the endoscopist's personal preference. There is little prospective comparison of the various models.

Evaluation

Although the concept of endoscopic sclerotherapy for varices appears to be straightforward, the clinical practice of the technique has yet to be standardized. The importance of the many technical variables outlined above in determining the efficacy of sclerotherapy is not well understood. Many investigators believe that these factors are of secondary importance compared to the overall clinical status of the patient when sclerotherapy is performed.[82,83]

The sclerotherapy patient should usually anticipate a long-term treatment program. In the U.S., the patient will probably undergo two to three sclerotherapy sessions during the index hospitalization after an acute episode of variceal hemorrhage. Two to three subsequent sessions will be performed in the following 4 to 8 weeks before the variceal channels are obliterated. The patient will return for follow up endoscopies every 3 to 6 months, presumably for the rest of his or her life as esophageal varices recur in up to 60% of these patients.[67,68] It is obvious that this treatment program requires a tremendous amount of commitment from both the patient and physician.

Mechanism of Action

Despite the rapid proliferation of reports describing the efficacy of sclerotherapy on varices, precise information on sclerotherapy's mechanism of action is scanty. Most of this information is derived from studies on sclerotherapy of esophageal varices in animal models, autopsy specimens or patients undergoing radiologic examinations.[72,84-87] The effect of sclerotherapy on gastric varices or other ectopic varices has not been well studied.

The ability of sclerotherapy to stop active hemorrhage was initially thought to be due to acute venous thrombosis induced by the sclerosant, as is the case when varicose veins are injected. However, Chung and colleagues[63] pointed out that, unlike peripheral varicosities, esophageal varices have a much higher blood-flow rate and no functioning valves. Sclerosant injected into esophageal varices may dissipate rapidly. Several studies in which contrast material was mixed with the sclerosant showed that most of the sclerosant injected into the varices was cleared cephalad.[88-90] This occurred despite compression with a balloon placed cephalad to the injection site.[88] Sclerosant-induced venous thrombosis is therefore not a likely explanation for the acute hemostatic effect of intravascular sclerotherapy. In addition, when sclerosants are intentionally injected around the varices, the rate of acute hemostasis is the same as that seen with intravascular injection.[91] This observation further supports the view that acute venous thrombosis is probably not the principal hemostatic mechanism. Another hypothesis suggests that esophageal and vascular smooth muscle spasm induced by the sclerosant may be the key factor in initial hemostasis.[65] The mechanical compression effect of submucosal edema created by sclerotherapy may also be responsible for acute hemostasis.

Autopsy studies indicate that venous thrombosis, mucosal ulceration and acute inflammatory reactions can be found in the injection site as soon as two days after sclerotherapy.[86,92-94] Thrombosis is not limited to the superficial varices but may involve varices in all layers. The ulceration usually involves the submucosa or the inner layer of the muscularis propria, but may extend transmurally. As the acute inflammatory reactions subside, fibrosis develops and leads to obliteration of the variceal channels. The timing of this change is variable, ranges from two weeks to several months after sclerotherapy.[86,93,94]

Efficacy

Sclerotherapy has been used as emergency treatment for initial hemostasis, as short-term and chronic treatment to prevent recurrent bleeding, and finally as prophylaxis to prevent the first episode of bleeding esophageal varices. Although there are a large number of uncontrolled series in the published literature, this discussion will focus on the available prospective randomized controlled trials in order to estimate the efficacy of endoscopic sclerotherapy in these clinical situations.

The efficacy of sclerotherapy on ectopic varices is primarily reported in uncontrolled studies. It is difficult to analyze the results of these reports as the natural history of these ectopic varices is not well known, and their frequency of bleeding is not well established.

Endoscopic sclerotherapy is one of the few endoscopic hemostatic techniques that has become available in the past 15 years. In a canine esophageal varices model, sclerotherapy was shown to be superior to the argon laser, heater probe, multipolar and monopolar electrodes in controlling bleeding. Its efficacy was equivalent to the Nd:YAG laser.[55] However, experience with the endoscopic Nd:YAG laser for variceal hemorrhage in humans has been limited, and comparison of Nd:YAG laser to sclerotherapy in this setting has not been reported.[95]

Esophageal Varices

Emergency Sclerotherapy

As many as one third of patients presenting with variceal hemorrhage may have active bleeding during the initial diagnostic endoscopy.[83] This group of patients has a high mortality rate and large blood transfusion requirement. Vasoconstrictive agents and balloon tamponade have been the standard treatment in this situation in many centers. The efficacy of these modalities is still controversial. Uncontrolled studies have indicated that sclerotherapy performed as a first-line therapy is highly successful.[46,96,97]

Data from six controlled trials comparing emergency sclerotherapy to either tamponade alone,[98-100] vasopressin with or without tamponade,[101] vasopressin plus nitroglycerin,[102] or somatostatin[103] are listed in Table 137-1. In all of these studies, sclerotherapy was used as the sole experimental emergency hemostatic therapy when actively bleeding esophageal varices were found during the initial diagnostic endoscopy. These procedures were performed within 24 hours after the patients were admitted to the hospital. Sclerotherapy was more effective in controlling bleeding than all the alternate therapies, with the exception of somatostatin. This difference was statistically significant in two[98,99] of these studies, and a positive trend was noted in the other three.[100-102] Sustained hemostasis during the acute hospitalization also appeared to be better in the sclerotherapy groups. However, this was not the case when sclerotherapy was compared to vasopressin plus nitroglycerin in Westaby's study.[102] This could be due to the fact that all the patients who received vasopressin initially in this study were treated with sclerotherapy 12 hours later. When early rebleeding occurred, sclerotherapy was also able to arrest the bleeding more frequently. In Shields and colleagues' study,[103] somatostatin appeared to be as efficacious and safe as sclerotherapy in terms of initial hemostasis, prevention of early rebleeding and hospital mortality.

Emergency sclerotherapy did not improve the patients' acute mortality rate either during the index hospitalization or within 30 days after admission in all of these studies. How-

TABLE 137-1
Emergency Sclerotherapy for Actively Bleeding Esophageal Varices

STUDY	NUMBER OF PATIENTS	TYPE OF TREATMENT	INITIAL HEMOSTASIS (%)	P	REBLEEDING (%)	P	HOSPITAL OR 1-MO MORTALITY (%)	P	DEATHS SECONDARY TO VARICEAL BLEEDING (%)	P
Barsoum, 1982	50	Sclerotherapy*	74		26		26		†	
				<0.01		<0.01				<0.05
	50	Tamponade	42		58		42		†	
Soderlund, 1985	28	Sclerotherapy and vasopressin	89		57		28		11	
				NS		NS		NS		<0.05
	31	Vasopressin with or without tamponade	74		52		36		30	
Paquet and Feussner, 1985	21	Sclerotherapy	95		20		10			
				NS		NS		NS		
	22	Tamponade	73		44		37			
Moretó et al, 1988	23	Sclerotherapy	100		17		30		9	
				NS		<0.05		NS		<0.05
	20	Tamponade	80		55‡		30‡		30	
Westaby et al, 1989	33	Sclerotherapy	88		31		27		9	
				<0.05		NS		NS		<0.05
	31	Vasopressin and nitroglycerin	65		31§		39§		26	
Shields et al, 1992	41	Sclerotherapy	98		17		20			
				NS		NS		NS		
	39	Somatostatin	97		23		31			

NS, not significant.

* Rigid endoscopy under general anesthesia.

† Actual number not listed in paper.

‡ Sclerotherapy used upon rebleeding.

§ All received sclerotherapy 12 hours after randomization.

From Soderlund C, Ihre T. Endoscopic sclerotherapy versus conservative management of bleeding oesophageal varices. Acta Chir Scand 1985;151:449.

ever, the frequency of persistent variceal hemorrhage as the principal cause of death was less in the sclerotherapy groups in four studies.[98,99,101,102]

The overall long-term survival was better in the sclerotherapy group in Paquet and Feussner's study.[100] In this study, the control group did not receive any further long-term therapy, whereas the treatment group continued to receive sclerotherapy. This improvement in overall survival was not observed in the other four studies where the control group received sclerotherapy for rebleeding episodes.

These studies indicate that emergency sclerotherapy can be performed safely during the initial diagnostic endoscopy. Emergency sclerotherapy is similar to, if not better than, somatostatin, tamponade and vasopressin in the initial control of bleeding. This hemostatic effect also appears to last longer. However, one must realize that sclerotherapy is more difficult to perform as an emergency procedure than as an elective procedure. Overall survival does not appear to be impaired if the initial hemorrhage is controlled by other means as long as sclerotherapy or other forms of long-term treatment are available in follow-up. It is premature to conclude that sclero-

therapy must be the first choice for emergency treatment. If an experienced endoscopist is not readily available, alternative approaches are acceptable during the first 24 hours of variceal hemorrhage.

Acute Short-Term Sclerotherapy

Once the patient with variceal bleeding is resuscitated and the bleeding has stopped either spontaneously or following somatostatin, vasopressin, or tamponade, sclerotherapy is the most commonly used treatment. Two or three sclerotherapy sessions are often performed during the initial hospitalization. Prospective controlled comparison of this treatment strategy to more traditional medical or surgical therapies are summarized in Table 137-2.[70,104–106] Larson and colleagues[104] conducted the first U.S. randomized study on 82 patients comparing the effect of short-term sclerotherapy to medical supportive measures. In a 2-week follow up, only 23% of the sclerotherapy patients rebled, whereas 53% of the control group had recurrent bleeding. However, the mortality of the two groups was similar during this period. This lack of effect

TABLE 137-2
Short-Term Sclerotherapy for Esophageal Variceal Bleeding

STUDY	NUMBER OF PATIENTS	TYPE OF TREATMENT	REBLEEDING (%)	REBLEEDING P	ACUTE MORTALITY (%)	ACUTE MORTALITY P	DEATHS SECONDARY TO VARICEAL BLEEDING (%)	DEATHS SECONDARY TO VARICEAL BLEEDING P
Larson et al, 1986	44	Sclerotherapy	23		5		2.5	
	38	Vasopressin with or without tamponade	53	<0.001	13	NS	10	NS
Copenhagen Project, 1984	93	Sclerotherapy	37		50			
	94	Tamponade with or without vasopressin	30	NS	50	NS		
Cello et al, 1987	32	Sclerotherapy	25		50		NA	
	32	Portacaval shunt	19	<0.009	56	NS	0	NA
Burroughs et al, 1989	50	Sclerotherapy	25		44			
	51	Esophageal stapling	7	<0.05	35	NS		

NA, not available; NS, not significant.

on acute mortality was similar to observations in a much larger study from Copenhagen.[70]

This short-term sclerotherapy strategy had been compared to emergency portal caval shunt in 52 Child's class C patients by Cello and colleagues.[105] Both groups had a grim mortality rate of over 50% during the index hospitalization. Although the acute rebleeding rate was higher in the sclerotherapy group, the total transfusion requirement and health care cost per patient were significantly higher in the shunt group.

Burroughs and colleagues[106] compared sclerotherapy to staple esophageal transection in 101 patients who had not responded to vasopressin in the first 24 to 35 hours after hospital admission. Twelve percent of the transection group developed recurrent bleeding during the first 5 days after the procedure, whereas 38% of patients who received a single sclerotherapy session rebled. Further control of rebleeding was achieved in 82% of the sclerotherapy patients after three treatment sessions. The complication rates were the same in the two groups, with a 10% procedure-related death rate. The 6-week mortality rates were also similar, 35% and 44%, respectively. These findings are comparable to an earlier report by Huizinga and colleagues in which staple transection surgery was performed in a more elective manner.[106a]

In summary, short-term sclerotherapy appears to be better than medical supportive treatment for short term hemostasis. It does not improve the short-term survival of patients bleeding from esophageal varices. Shunt surgery, staple esophageal transection, and sclerotherapy are comparably effective in high-risk patients.

Long-Term Sclerotherapy

Table 137-3 summarizes the data from controlled trials comparing chronic sclerotherapy to various medical, radiological, and surgical therapies.[67,68,70,98,101,107-120]

Sclerotherapy Versus Conservative Medical Therapy

The results of seven controlled trials comparing long-term sclerotherapy to supportive medical treatment are now available in the English literature.[67,68,70,98,101,107,108] These seven studies differ from each other with respect to the instrument used and the diagnosis and severity of the patients' underlying liver disease. Despite these differences, all of these studies showed a significantly lower risk of recurrent bleeding, especially bleeding from esophageal varices, in patients treated with sclerotherapy. The recurrent bleeding rate was 30% to 50% in the sclerotherapy groups, which was significantly lower than the 70% to 80% rate in the control groups. This effect, however, was usually not evident until variceal obliteration had been achieved, usually in 1 to 3 months.

The effect of repeated sclerotherapy on the long-term overall survival of these patients is more controversial. Only three of these trials demonstrated an improvement in survival in treated patients.[67,70,98] Skeptics of these three positive studies are quick to point out that Barsoum[98] primarily studied patients with schistosomiasis, and Westaby and colleagues' study[67] only included patients who had survived the first 2 to 5 days, and excluded 23% of patients who were determined to be too ill to enroll in the study. In the Copenhagen study,[70] improved survival in the sclerotherapy group was only evident for those patients who survived the first 40 days after the initial bleed. The four negative studies[68,101,107,108] also have features in their trial that may have influenced their outcome. In Terblanche and colleagues' study,[68] the control group was treated with acute sclerotherapy in addition to tamponade and medical support. Korula and colleagues' study was marred by a high drop out rate.[107] The VA Cooperative Sclerotherapy Trial[108] studied only alcoholic men. The natural history of diseases associated with alcoholism may have offset the ben-

TABLE 137-3
Long-Term Sclerotherapy for Esophageal Variceal Bleeding

STUDY	TREATMENT	NUMBER OF PATIENTS	FOLLOW-UP (months)	REBLEEDING (%)	P	LONG-TERM MORTALITY (%)	P
Sclerotherapy Versus Medical Therapy							
Barsoum, 1982	Sclerotherapy	50	12–48	26	<0.001	30	<0.05
	Medical	50		58		52	
Terblanche et al, 1983	Sclerotherapy	37	12–60	58	NS	62	NS
	Medical	38		77		68	
Copenhagen et al, 1984	Sclerotherapy	93	9–52	48	NS*	65	0.03
	Medical	94		54		79	
Westaby et al, 1985	Sclerotherapy	56	19–68	55	<0.01	32	<0.01
	Medical	60		80		53	
Soderlund and Ihre, 1985	Sclerotherapy	57	12–54	56	NS†	56	NS
	Medical	50		66		70	
Korula et al, 1985	Sclerotherapy	53	12–24		†	33	NS
	Medical	57				33	
Gregory et al, 1990	Sclerotherapy	122	60	55	NS‡	63	NS
	Medical	131		63		56	
Sclerotherapy Versus Surgical Therapy							
Teres, Bordas et al, 1987	Sclerotherapy	55	27	37	<0.02	27	NS
	Distal splenorenal shunt	57		14		23	
Henderson et al, 1990	Sclerotherapy and distal splenorenal shunt§	37	30–84	59	<0.001	35	<0.02
	Distal splenorenal shunt	35		3		57	
Spina et al, 1990	Sclerotherapy	20	24	35	<0.04	10	NS
	Distal splenorenal shunt	20		5		5	
Rikkers et al, 1993	Sclerotherapy	30	87	60	<0.001	74	<0.05
	Distal splenorenal shunt	30		17		47	
Cello et al, 1987	Sclerotherapy	32	18	87	<0.001	50	NS
	Distal splenorenal shunt	32		19		56	
Planas et al, 1991	Sclerotherapy	41	21	40	<0.002	21	NS
	Distal splenorenal shunt	41		3		17	
Kitano et al, 1992	Sclerotherapy	32	40	3	NS	13	NS
	Distal splenorenal shunt	32		16		22	
	Transection	32		16		16	
Triger et al, 1992	Sclerotherapy	51	53	69	NS	36	NS
	Transection‖	46		64		33	
Sclerotherapy Versus Radiologic Therapy							
Terabayashi et al, 1987	Sclerotherapy	33	15	18	<0.005	15	<0.05
	Transhepatic embolization	33		64		57	
Sclerotherapy Versus Pharmacologic Therapy							
Fleig et al, 1987	Sclerotherapy	36	12–24	28	NS	8	NS
	Propranolol	34		29		15	
Teres, Bosch et al, 1987	Sclerotherapy	46	11	21	0.02	31	NS
	Propranolol	45		45		21	
Westaby et al, 1987	Sclerotherapy	52	6–48	42	NS	27	NS
	Propranolol	48		52		27	
Alexandrino et al, 1988	Sclerotherapy	31	15–57	63	NS‡	29	NS
	Propranolol	34		84		32	
Dollet et al, 1988	Sclerotherapy	28	14–58	64	NS	54	NS
	Propranolol	27		44		44	
Rossi et al, 1991	Sclerotherapy	26	19	50	NS	23	NS
	Propranolol	27		48		26	
Dasarathy et al, 1992	Sclerotherapy	45	30–36	42	<0.05	22	NS
	Propranolol	46		67		41	
Westaby et al, 1986	Sclerotherapy	27	6	30	NS	26	NS
	Sclerotherapy and propranolol	26		27		35	

(continued)

TABLE 137-3. *(Continued)*

STUDY	TREATMENT	NUMBER OF PATIENTS	FOLLOW-UP (months)	REBLEEDING		LONG-TERM MORTALITY	
				(%)	P	(%)	P
Vickers et al, 1987	Sclerotherapy	34	10–58	29	NS	26	NS
	Sclerotherapy and propranolol	35		45		37	
Jensen and Krarup, 1989	Sclerotherapy	16	6	75	<0.05		
	Sclerotherapy and propranolol	15		20			
Lundell et al, 1990	Sclerotherapy	22		11	NS		
	Sclerotherapy and propranolol	19		12			
Bertoni et al, 1990	Sclerotherapy	14		28	NS	21	NS
	Sclerotherapy and nadolol	14		7		7	
Gerunda et al, 1990	Sclerotherapy	30	6	23	NS	10	NS
	Sclerotherapy and nadolol	30		20		3	
Vinel et al, 1992	Sclerotherapy	36	3	39	<0.005	14	NS
	Sclerotherapy and propranolol	39		18		13	
O'Connor et al, 1989	Sclerotherapy and propranolol	31	24–65	68	NS	55	NS
	Propranolol	31		87		81	

NS, not significant.

* Bleeding episode per patient was significantly less in sclerotherapy patients after 40 days of therapy.

† Bleeding episode per patient was significantly less in sclerotherapy patients.

‡ Rebleeding from esophageal varices was significantly less in sclerotherapy patients.

§ Shunt surgery was performed after sclerotherapy failed in 59% of patients.

‖ Emergency sclerotherapy was the initial treatment for all patients.

eficial effect of sclerotherapy. Indeed, these four negative trials all had a higher proportion of patients with alcoholic liver disease than the three positive trials. In a recent meta-analysis of these long-term studies, Infante-Rivard and colleagues suggest that sclerotherapy may indeed reduce mortality by 25%.[120a]

Sclerotherapy Versus Surgical Therapy

Long-term sclerotherapy has been compared to the distal splenorenal shunt surgery in four studies.[115–118] The rebleeding rate of 3% to 20% in the surgery groups was significantly better than the 40% to 50% rate in the sclerotherapy groups in all of these studies. The long-term mortality was not significantly different between the sclerotherapy and the surgery groups in the initial analysis of three of these studies.[115,117,118] The late result of Rikkers and colleagues, however, suggested that mortality was reduced in the surgery group.[111] In contrast, the Atlanta study[109] reported a decrease in long-term mortality in the sclerotherapy group. In this study, 59% of the sclerotherapy patients subsequently had the distal splenorenal shunt for recurrent bleeding. Meta-analysis of these four studies[119] confirms that distal splenorenal shunt reduces the rebleeding rate when compared to sclerotherapy. The overall long-term mortality, however, was only marginally decreased in the distal splenorenal shunt group. This trend of survival improvement

was more apparent in patients with nonalcoholic liver disease. The incidence of encephalopathy was slightly, but not significantly increased in the surgery group.

Sclerotherapy has been compared to portacaval shunt in two studies.[105,112] Rebleeding rates were significantly less in the surgery groups. However, the long-term mortality rates were similar between the sclerotherapy and surgery groups. The incidence of encephalopathy was increased in the surgery group.

When compared to esophageal transection with gastric devascularization, sclerotherapy resulted in similar rebleeding and long-term mortality rates.[113,114]

Sclerotherapy Versus Radiographic Therapy

Percutaneous transhepatic embolization of esophageal varices is not commonly practiced in the United States, but it is quite popular in Japan. A randomized controlled trial comparing sclerotherapy to percutaneous transhepatic embolization in patients with nonalcoholic cirrhosis showed that sclerotherapy was superior in preventing recurrent variceal bleeding and was associated with a lower mortality rate.[120] In a recent study in which the patients were predominantly alcoholics with Child's C status, those treated with sclerotherapy plus propranolol also appeared to have less recurrent bleeding and a slightly better survival rate than those treated with transhepatic embolization plus propranolol.[117] TIPS is a promising technique for stopping variceal bleeding.[121] Studies comparing sclerotherapy to TIPS are in progress.

Sclerotherapy Versus Pharmacologic Therapy

Long-term sclerotherapy was compared to propranolol in eight studies.[116,118,122–127] Most of the patients in these studies were in the Child's class A or B categories. Meta-analysis of these trials suggested that the recurrent bleeding rates and long-term survival were similar between the sclerotherapy and the propranolol groups.

As sclerotherapy's ability to reduce the rebleeding rate is only evident after varices are obliterated, addition of beta blockers prior to variceal obliteration is thought to be potentially beneficial. Two[128,129] of the seven studies[129–134] comparing sclerotherapy alone to sclerotherapy plus beta blockers suggested that the rebleeding rates in the combined therapy groups indeed were lower. However, meta-analysis of all these studies failed to show an improvement in rebleeding rates and survival in the groups treated with sclerotherapy plus beta blockers.

Prophylactic Sclerotherapy

The concept of prophylactic therapy to prevent the first episode of variceal hemorrhage in patients with esophageal varices is attractive because of the high mortality associated with each bleeding episode. Prophylactic shunt surgery failed to improve survival in these patients.[135] The revival of sclerotherapy has renewed an interest in prophylactic therapy because sclerotherapy has been considered a less invasive procedure associated with a lower morbidity. Thirteen trials comparing prophylactic sclerotherapy to placebo have now been published in the English literature. Three studies show that sclerotherapy reduces the risk of variceal bleeding and improves survival,[36,37,136] whereas the other ten studies fail to demonstrate these beneficial effects of prophylactic sclerotherapy (Table 137-4).[137–146]

The bleeding rates of the control groups in the three positive trials were uniformly higher (42%–66%) than in the negative trials (15%–40%). In these three studies, Paquet[36] used his previously reported endoscopic criteria to select patients with higher bleeding risks and Piai and colleagues used the more complex Japanese system. Witzel and colleagues[37] did not use any selection criteria but reported a direct correlation of bleeding risk to variceal size. Among the negative trials, Santangelo and colleagues[138] also used Paquet's criteria[36] to select patients at high risk but the observed rate of bleeding was not as high. In this study, higher bleeding-associated mortality was observed in the patients treated with prophylactic sclerotherapy. Although the VA Cooperative trial[143] and Sauerbruch and colleagues[139] enrolled predominantly patients with large varices, bleeding rates in the control groups were significantly lower than in Witzel and colleagues' study[37]; these two studies failed to demonstrate a beneficial effect of prophylactic sclerotherapy and there was excess mortality in the treated patients in the VA study.

In a recent meta-analysis of data from these studies, as well as data from six other studies that were published in non-

English literature (2) or in abstracts (4), the effectiveness of prophylactic sclerotherapy remains undetermined.[147] Efficacy of prophylactic sclerotherapy can only be demonstrated in patients with a potential bleeding rate of over 50%. However, no reliable selection criteria for patients with this high bleeding risk can be derived from the studies that demonstrated efficacy with sclerotherapy. If the patient's potential bleeding rate is only around 30%, which is the average rate in most trials studying prophylactic treatment, the complications of sclerotherapy are likely to mask any of its beneficial effects. At present, sclerotherapy is not recommended for prevention of the first episode of variceal bleeding. For prophylactic therapy, the effectiveness of β blockers is more well-established.[147] However, addition of β blocker to sclerotherapy does not improve the efficacy.[146]

Ectopic Varices

In the early 1970s, many enthusiasts of sclerotherapy directly applied this technique to bleeding gastric varices. They quickly realized that the same technique that seemed to be so effective in treating esophageal varices was disappointingly ineffective in treating gastric varices.[44] It was difficult to arrest acute hemorrhage from gastric varices. In addition, the large number of collaterals associated with gastric varices made it more difficult to completely obliterate the variceal channels. Consequently, sclerotherapy was ineffective in preventing recurrent hemorrhage. And finally, ulcerations at the injection site seemed to be more severe compared to those seen with esophageal variceal sclerotherapy. Recently, interest in sclerotherapy for gastric varices has been rekindled; encouraging results using large volumes of the common sclerosants for esophageal varices[44] and the use of isobutyl-2-cyano-acrylate[54,62] have been reported. However, further studies are needed before sclerotherapy in gastric varices can be endorsed.

Sclerotherapy has been used in the treatment of various bleeding ectopic varices such as duodenal, rectal and colonic varices.[45,148–151] Experience in these settings has been limited and general guidelines cannot be established. Based upon the success reported in the various case studies, sclerotherapy may be a reasonable alternative treatment for these ectopic varices. Techniques such as ligation of peristomal varices, colectomy for colonic varices and portacaval shunt have been used.[43]

Contraindication and Risks

There are very few contraindications to sclerotherapy. As with upper endoscopy, perforation of the GI tract is an absolute contraindication. The presence of deep ulcerations at previous injection sites indicates that further sessions of sclerotherapy should be postponed until the ulcers have healed adequately. Coagulopathy is not considered a contraindication, because most patients with portal hypertension have some degree of coagulopathy.

Successful sclerotherapy depends to a large extent on patient cooperation. In the setting of acute variceal hemorrhage, an agitated patient should be sedated and endotracheal intubation should be used to protect the airway as necessary. The presence of gastric varices does not preclude sclerotherapy

TABLE 137-4
Prophylactic Sclerotherapy for Esophageal Varices

STUDY	TREATMENT	NUMBER OF PATIENTS	FOLLOW-UP (mo)	BLEEDING (%)	BLEEDING P	MORTALITY (%)	MORTALITY P	DEATHS DUE TO VARICEAL BLEEDING (%)	DEATHS DUE TO VARICEAL BLEEDING P	DEATHS DUE TO OTHER CAUSES (%)	DEATHS DUE TO OTHER CAUSES P
Paquet, 1982	Sclerotherapy	32	24	6	<0.01	6	<0.01				
	Control	33		66		42					
Witzel et al, 1985	Sclerotherapy	56	25	9	<0.01	21	<0.01	4	<0.01	17	NS
	Control	53		57		55		36		19	
Koch et al, 1986	Sclerotherapy	30	36	30	NS	37	NS	0	<0.05	31	NS
	Control	30		33		33		20		13	
Piai et al, 1988	Sclerotherapy	71	24	14	<0.001	22	<0.01	7	<0.01	15	NS
	Control	69		42		38		28		10	
Santangelo et al, 1988	Sclerotherapy	49	13	35	<0.05	24	NS	18*	NS	6	NS
	Control	46		15		24		4*		20	
Sauerbruch et al, 1988	Sclerotherapy	68	22	28	NS	35	NS	15	NS	21	NS
	Control	65		37		47		17		30	
Potzi et al, 1989	Sclerotherapy	41	40	29	NS	24	NS	12	NS	12	NS
	Control	41		34		46		22		24	
Russo et al, 1989	Sclerotherapy	21	17	0	NS	0	NS	0	NS	0	NS
	Control	20		15		15		10		5	
Andreani et al, 1990	Sclerotherapy	42	24	21	NS	43	NS	5	NS	38	NS
	Control	41		32		44		10		34	
VA Cooperative Variceal Sclerotherapy Group, 1991	Sclerotherapy	143	22	22	NS	32	<0.006	7*	NS	25	<0.01
	Control	138		17		17		4*		13	
Triger et al, 1991	Sclerotherapy	33	14–107	39	NS	61	NS	18	NS	43	NS
	Control	35		40		60		11		49	
De Franchis et al, 1991	Sclerotherapy	55	24	36	NS	34	NS	13*	NS	21	NS
	Control	51		37		47		21*		26	
PROVA, 1991	Sclerotherapy	73	15	25	NS	25	NS	7	NS	18	NS
	Control	72		25		22		11		11	

NS, not significant.

* Deaths due to all types of upper gastrointestinal bleeding.

for bleeding esophageal varices. Although obliteration of esophageal varices could theoretically increase the risk of bleeding from gastric varices, the true incidence of this sequela is probably low.

Sclerotherapy is a safe procedure but complications are not infrequent. The actual incidence of sclerotherapy-induced morbidity and mortality is difficult to determine due to the large variation in technique used in different studies.[152] The most common complications associated with sclerotherapy are transient and self limiting. Over half of the patients undergoing sclerotherapy may experience sore throat, low-grade fever, dysphagia and retrosternal pain after sclerotherapy, but these symptoms usually subside after a few days. More serious complications may develop in 10% to 15% of these patients,[152,153] immediately after sclerotherapy or in the weeks or months following treatment. The complications seen in sclerotherapy patients may be categorized as those limited to the esophagus, those involving the lungs and the thoracic cavity, and those affecting distant organs or the entire body (i.e., systemic or distant). Table 137-5 lists these complica-

TABLE 137-5
Complications of Endoscopic Variceal Sclerotherapy

TIME OF COMPLICATION	LOCATION OF COMPLICATION (RATE IN %)		
	Esophagus	Pulmonary or Thoracic	Systemic or Distant
Early (1–2 d)	Substernal pain (40–50) Traumatic perforation (2–4)	Aspiration pneumonia 5 Pleural effusion 50 ARDS* Chylothorax* Subcutaneous emphysema* Pneumothorax* Mediastinitis*	Fever (10–50) Bacteremia (4–50) Pneumatosis intestinalis* Pneumoperitoneum* Spinal cord paralysis* Coronary spasm* Bradyarrhythmia* Ventricular arrythmia* Pericarditis*
Intermediate (1–4 wk)	Ulceration (25–75) Bleeding (2–13) Perforated (2–4) Intramural hematoma* Monilial esophagitis*	Bronchoesophageal fistula*	Bowel pseudoobstruction*
Late (>1 mo)	Stricture (2–30) Dysmotility 4		Spontaneous splenorenal shunt* Brain abscess* Perinephric abscess* Duodenal varices* Rectal varices* Colonic varices* Cardiac tamponade*

ARDS, adult respiratory distress syndrome.

* Case reports.

tions, their temporal relation to the procedure and their estimated incidence.

Esophageal Complications

All the currently used sclerosants are ulcerogenic at the injection site.[136,155] Mucosal erosions develop at the injection sites 2 to 4 days after each sclerotherapy session in almost every patient.[156] These lesions occur with both intravariceal and paravariceal injections.[65,136,155,156] Deep ulcerations develop at these sites at reported rates of 5% to 78%.[65,107,136,155,156] These ulcers appear 4 to 7 days after the injection and commonly cause follow-up treatments to be postponed.[73,74] Significant bleeding from these ulcers may develop in 2% to 13% of these patients.[152] Ulcer formation does not appear to correlate with the choice of sclerosant or injection technique. However ulcerations may occur more frequently if sclerotherapy sessions are carried out in close succession.[73,74] Preliminary data from a recent randomized study suggest that sucralfate suspension may promote healing of these ulcers.[157]

Acute esophageal perforation may occur in 2% to 5% of patients and usually presents shortly after a sclerotherapy session.[70,158] This complication occurs more often when the rigid endoscope is used.[50] These patients usually respond to antibiotics although some may require chest tube drainage. Delayed esophageal perforation resulting from necrosis of transmural ulcerations may prove fatal.[159–161] This complication usually develops 1 to 4 weeks after sclerotherapy, but its true incidence is unknown.

Esophageal strictures develop months after sclerotherapy in 2% to 20% of treated patients.[101,116,137–139,158] An incidence as high as 53% has been reported.[162] Stricture formation appears to correlate with the number of sclerotherapy sessions and the amount of sclerosant used.[162] Most of these patients are successfully treated with mercury-filled or balloon dilators. Bleeding seldom develops with these dilatations.[163] Another 4% of patients may have persistent dysphagia without stricture after sclerotherapy.[162] This may be due to esophageal dysmotility induced by sclerotherapy.[152,164–166]

Other esophageal complications that have been described include intramural hematoma, pseudotumor, granuloma, mucosal bridges and monilial esophagitis.[153] These probably represent the spectrum of esophageal responses to the necrotizing sclerosant.

Pulmonary and Thoracic Complications

Aspiration pneumonia develops in about 5% of patients.[70,99,100,102,107] Most episodes of aspiration occur during emergency sclerotherapy. The judicious use of endotracheal intubation is essential during sclerotherapy for massive variceal hemorrhage.

Pleural effusions may be detected in close to 50% of patients shortly after sclerotherapy.[167] They may occur in either pleural cavity or bilaterally. Most of these effusions are small and resolve spontaneously. Only about 2% of these patients require therapeutic thoracentesis.[153] The development of pleural effusions appears to increase in proportion to the amount of sclerosant injected.[167] Bacon and colleagues[167] have demonstrated that these effusions are exudates and suggest that the inflammation of the mediastinal parietal pleura induced by injection of sclerosant in the esophagus may cause this effect. The true pathogenic mechanism of these effusions is still not fully understood.

Adult respiratory distress syndrome has been described in a few patients after sclerotherapy with sodium morrhuate or sodium tetradecyl sulfate.[152,168] The etiology of this pulmonary complication is unclear. Monroe's[169] initial hypothesis that sodium morrhuate may affect pulmonary hemodynamics has not been validated by subsequent animal and clinical studies.[71,170]

A variety of other pulmonary complications such as chylothorax, pneumothorax, acute respiratory failure due to gastric distention, subcutaneous emphysema, and bronchoesophageal fistula have been described in a small number of patients.[152]

Systemic and Distant Complications

After sclerotherapy, 20% to 50% of patients may develop a low grade fever that lasts for 24 to 48 hours.[63,171] The etiology of fever in these patients is not known but has been attributed to an acute inflammatory response to the sclerosants.[172] The development of fever does not appear to correlate with the presence of bacteremia and antibiotic therapy is not necessary.[173] However, if the fever persists for more than 2 days or high spiking temperatures develop, a search for an infectious focus should be carried out, and antibiotic treatment is indicated.

One might imagine that a procedure in which a substance is injected through an instrument that is contaminated by oral flora into varices that have systemic connections would result in a high incidence of septic complications. Transient bacteremia has been documented by blood culture studies in 4% to 50% of patients,[173–175] and peaks at 5 minutes after sclerotherapy.[173] The bacteria recovered have been oral flora or bacteria that have contaminated the endoscopic equipment during storage. It is not clear whether the transient bacteremia rate is higher in sclerotherapy than in uncomplicated upper endoscopy.[176] Clinically significant sepsis, as a result of this transient bacteremia, is presumably infrequent, but rates as high as 16% to 30% have been reported.[177,178] Distant dissemination of oral flora causing brain or perinephric abscesses have been described.[179,180] Surprisingly, there is no solid evidence to associate sclerotherapy with an increased incidence of bacterial peritonitis. Due to the conflicting data on the septic complication rate of sclerotherapy, there are no strict guidelines for prophylactic antibiotics for patients undergoing sclerotherapy. However, it is prudent to administer prophylactic antibiotics in patients with prosthetic heart valves.[176]

Cardiac complications associated with sclerotherapy are uncommon. Acute development of ventricular arrhythmia, coronary spasm, and persistent bradyarrhythmia requiring pacemaker placement have been described in patients undergoing sclerotherapy.[181,182] Pericarditis has been reported in three patients a few days after sclerotherapy,[183] and cardiac tamponade developed in another patient 6 months after sclerotherapy as a consequence of chronic pericarditis.[184]

Acute dissemination of the injected sclerosant has been incriminated in the development of spinal cord paralysis and mesenteric venous thrombosis.[185,186] Pneumatosis intestinalis has also been described as an acute complication of sclerotherapy.[187]

Bleeding from gastric, duodenal, colonic, rectal varices, and portal vein thrombosis has been attributed to altered hemodynamics of the portal system after months of sclerotherapy for esophageal varices.[188–191] The actual frequency of these complications is unknown. A recent study suggests that a spontaneous splenorenal shunt may develop after sclerotherapy in 40% of patients with extrahepatic portal hypertension.[192] This shunt appears to effectively prevent recurrent variceal bleeding.

Mortality

Deaths attributable to acute complications of sclerotherapy is probably about 1% to 2%.[104,153,158,171,192] However, procedure related deaths as high as 10% were reported in the Copenhagen study.[70] Most of the patients undergoing sclerotherapy are seriously ill and the cause of death is often multifactorial. Recurrent bleeding, perforation and pulmonary complications are frequently associated with acute mortality after sclerotherapy.

ELASTIC BAND LIGATION

The concept of endoscopic variceal ligation is an extension of the widely used band ligation technique for hemorrhoids. This technique is designed with the intention of reducing the complications associated with endoscopic sclerotherapy.

Technique

The current, commercially available, variceal ligator was designed by Van Stiegmann and colleagues.[14] It consists of a housing cylinder which can be mounted onto the tip of most flexible endoscopes. Inside this housing cylinder is a banding cylinder with one preloaded rubber O ring on its distal end. The banding cylinder can slide inside the housing cylinder to release the rubber ring. This sliding mechanism is operated by pulling a trip wire that is attached to the banding cylinder by a special notch and inserted through the biopsy channel of the endoscope. During the ligation process, the target variceal channel is drawn into the ligator's chamber by suction applied through the endoscope. The rubber ring, once released, ensnares the variceal pedicle (Figs. 137-4 and 137-5). For variceal channels that are actively bleeding, ligations are started at or near the bleeding sites. For nonbleeding channels, the process should be started at the gastroesophageal junction and proceed cephalad. For most small varices, one ligation at the distal esophagus is adequate. For larger varices, a second ligation is needed within a few centimeters above the first ligation site.

In general, it is easier to ligate the larger varices and more difficult to treat varices that are less than 3 mm in diameter. An average of 5 to 10 ligations are usually performed in the initial session, with progressively decreasing numbers in sub-

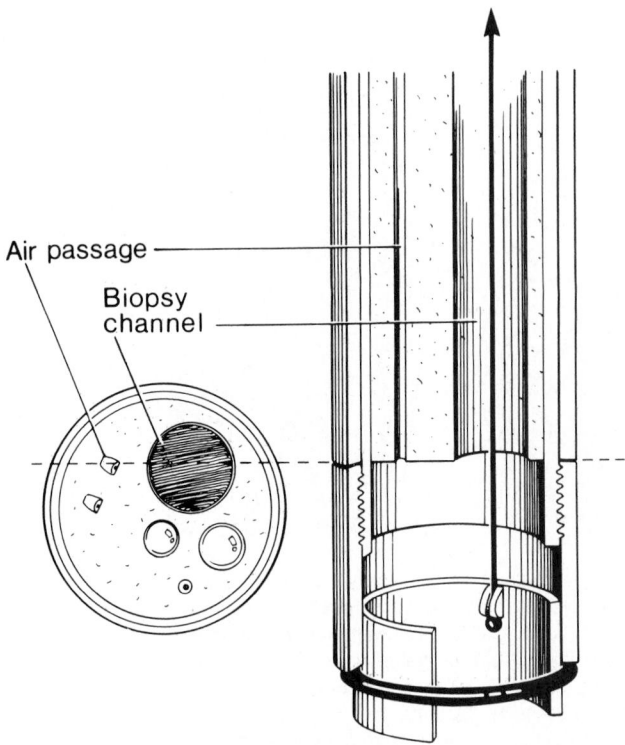

FIGURE 137-4. The endoscopic ligating device and distal tip of endoscope. The device has threaded ends so it may be attached directly to the endoscope. The trip wire (*arrow*) runs retrograde through the biopsy channel and exits the biopsy channel port. The elastic O ring is at the far end of the banding cylinder. (From Stiegmann GV, Goff JS. Endoscopic esophageal varix ligation: preliminary clinical experience. Gastrointest Endosc 1988;34: 113.)

sequent sessions. As only one rubber ring can be loaded onto the ligator each time, the endoscope must be removed for reloading and then reinserted into the patients as many times as needed for effective ligation in a given session. This process is facilitated by use of a 25 cm overtube to splint the cricopharyngeus. Twenty to thirty minutes are usually required to complete all the ligations in each session. Follow-up ligation sessions are repeated in seven to fourteen days and then every two to four weeks until the varices are obliterated. Four to six treatment sessions are usually required.[193]

Mechanism of Action

Hemostasis by band ligation is achieved initially by strangulation of the variceal channel. In a canine model,[194] the ligated varix initially blanched and then became cyanotic within 3 to 7 minutes. Ischemic necrosis of the mucosa and submucosa developed within 24 hours. The banded tissue sloughed off in 3 to 7 days, leaving a shallow ulcer measuring 10 to 12 mm in diameter and 1 to 2 mm in depth. These ulcers healed in 21 days, leaving only minimal residual varices, and without full thickness esophageal injury. Complete healing occurred in 60 days. These early endoscopic and pathological findings have been observed in human studies as well.[195,196]

Efficacy

The efficacy of variceal band ligation in controlling active esophageal variceal bleeding and preventing recurrent bleeding was initially demonstrated in an uncontrolled study by the Denver group.[193] The initial hemostasis rate by ligation was 86%, and a rebleeding rate of 46% in a 15 month follow-up period. The complication rate was only 3%. These findings were confirmed by a recent U.S. multicenter trial comparing variceal ligation to sclerotherapy.[197] In this study, ligation and sclerotherapy achieved similar initial hemostasis rates for active variceal bleeding (86% and 77%, respectively). In a 10-month follow-up period, 36% of the ligation group and 48% of the sclerotherapy group rebled. This difference, however, did not reach statistical significance. A similar London trial also suggested a trend in the reduction of rebleeding rate by ligation compared to sclerotherapy.[198] About 70% of these patients rebled from esophageal varices that were not yet obliterated.

The overall mortality rate in the ligation group was significantly lower than the sclerotherapy group (28% versus 45%). This difference was predominantly seen in patients of the Child's A and B status, whereas no mortality difference was seen in the Child's C patients. More than one half of the deaths occurred within 30 days after the index bleed. The lower mortality rate in the ligation group was thought to be due to the fewer cases of rebleeding and pulmonary infections in this group. The use of an overtube during the ligation was thought to have lowered the pulmonary complications rates. Indeed, analysis of a similar trial from Los Angeles suggested that when an overtube was also used for sclerotherapy, the pulmonary complication rates were similar between the ligation and sclerotherapy groups.[199]

On average, fewer treatment sessions are needed to obliterate the varices in the ligation group (4 ± 2 versus 5 ± 2). This trend was also reported in the London and Los Angeles trials.

As most of the rebleeding developed in patients whose varices had not yet been obliterated, and this may account for the early mortalities, addition of low dose sclerotherapy to ligation was proposed to accelerate variceal obliteration. Preliminary results of this approach from an uncontrolled study from Denver[200] and a randomized controlled trial from France[201] suggested that complete variceal obliteration could be achieved in 1 to 3 sessions. Long-term follow up on these patients is pending.

In summary, variceal ligation appears to be as efficacious as sclerotherapy in controlling active esophageal variceal bleeding. This technique is also at least as good as, if not superior to, sclerotherapy in the prevention of recurrent bleeding and improvement in survival. However, confirmation of these results by other ongoing studies are needed. In view of the low procedure-related complication rate, variceal ligation may have a role in the prophylaxis of the first variceal bleed. However, this is yet to be proven.

Contraindications and Risks

The general contraindication in performing variceal ligation are the same as those described for upper endoscopy and sclerotherapy. In addition, because the ligation process de-

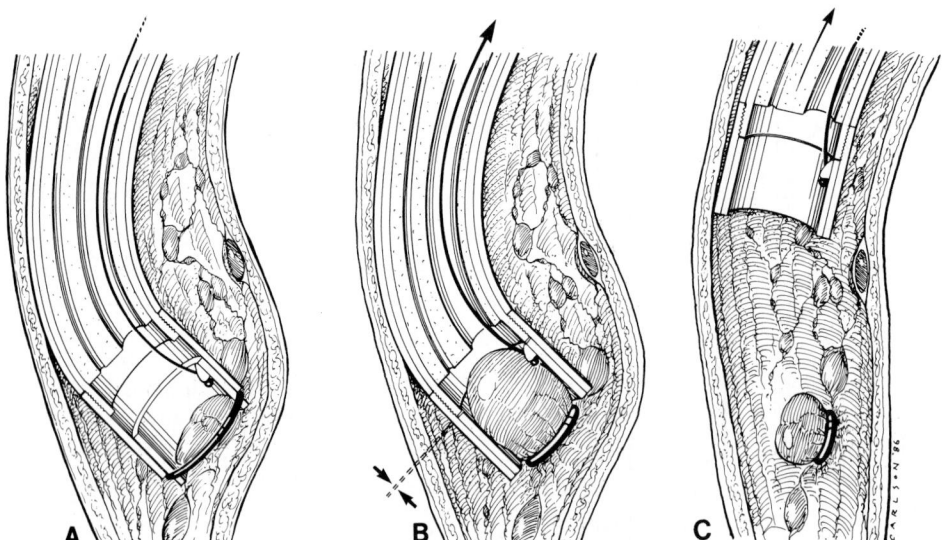

FIGURE 137-5. Endoscopic band ligation of esophageal varices. (**A**) The target varix is drawn into the banding cylinder by suction through the endoscope. (**B**) After the varix is fully drawn into the banding cylinder, the trip wire is pulled, moving the banding cylinder toward the endoscope and releasing the elastic O ring around the neck of the varix. (**C**) The ligated varix is discharged from the cylinder by withdrawing the endoscope and air insufflation. The endoscope and ligation device are withdrawn and reloaded, and any additional necessary ligations are performed. Reinsertion of the endoscope is facilitated by use of an endoscopic overtube. (From Stiegmann GV, Goff JS. Endoscopic esophageal varix ligation: preliminary clinical experience. Gastrointest Endosc 1988;34:113.)

pends on aspirating the esophageal mucosa in to the banding cylinder, the esophageal wall must be pliable. Previous scarring or stricture of the distal esophagus may decrease the success rate of the procedure.

The clinically significant complications associated with variceal ligation, as anticipated by the original designers, occur only at the rate of 2% to 3%.[193,197] This is significantly lower than the 22% associated with sclerotherapy.

A number of local esophageal complications associated with ligation have been described. Transient substernal discomfort that may last 24 to 48 hours has been reported by most patients. Large but shallow ulcerations at the ligation sites is a natural process of the therapy.[202] However, as the injury to the esophageal wall at the ligation site spares the muscularis, transmural ulceration and stricture formation are rare after variceal ligation. Only 2% of the patients developed esophageal stricture in the first 100 patients studied in Denver, and none was seen in the U.S. multicenter trial.[193,197] At present, only one case of bleeding from a deep ulcer induced by ligation has been reported.[203] Transient esophageal obstruction due to the banded variceal pedicle or spasm has been reported.[204,205] Esophageal laceration and perforation during passage of the overtube, which was not seen in the U.S. multicenter trial, have now been reported.[203,205-207] This complication is thought to be related to pinching of the esophageal wall in the gap between the overtube and the endoscope when the overtube slides over the endoscope. This problem may be avoided if a 45Fr tapered dilator is used as the introducer for the overtube.[207] A better overtube is now being designed by the manufacturer of the ligator.

Infectious complications related to variceal ligation include

bacteremia, pneumonia and peritonitis. In a small study of 17 patients, only one blood culture was positive for Staphylococcus epidermis 5 minutes after the ligation.[208] The patient was asymptomatic. Pneumonia after ligation have been reported in the rate of 2% to 10%.[197,199] This lower rate is probably the result of using the overtube during the procedure. Peritonitis has been reported in up to 15% of patients after ligation.[199]

Mortality directly due to ligation has been reported in two patients, one was due to pneumonia and the other due to esophageal perforation.[197,203]

The reader is directed to Chapter 30, Approach to the Patient With Gross Gastrointestinal Bleeding; Chapter 115, Upper Gastrointestinal Endoscopy; and Chapter 138, Endoscopic Control of Nonvariceal Upper Gastrointestinal Hemorrhage.

REFERENCES

1. Crafoord C, Frenckner P. New surgical treatment of varicous veins of the oesophagus. Acta Otolaryngol (Stockh) 1939;27:422.
2. Macbeth R. Treatment of oesophageal varices in portal hypertension by means of sclerosing injections. Br Med J 1955∞:877.
3. Moersch HJ. Treatment of esophageal varices by injection of a sclerosing solution. J Am Med Assoc 1947;135:754.
4. Patterson CO, Rouse MO. The sclerosing therapy of esophageal varices. Gastroenterology 1947;9:391.
5. Fearon B, Sass-Kortsak A. The management of esophageal var-

ices in children by injection of sclerosing agents. Ann Otol Rhinol Laryngol 1959;68:906.

6. Whipple AO. The problem of portal hypertension in relation to the hepatosplenopathies. Ann Surg 1945;22:449.
7. Whipple AO. The rationale of portacaval anastomosis. Bull NY Acad Med 1946;22:251.
8. Blakemore AH, Lord JWJ. The technique of using vitallium tubes in establishing portacaval shunts for portal hypertension. Ann Surg 1975;122:477.
9. Conn HO. Therapeutic portacaval anastomosis: to shunt or not to shunt. Gastroenterology 1974;67:1065.
10. Orloff MJ, Bell RHJ, Hyde PV, et al. Longq term results of emergency portacaval shunt for bleeding esophageal varices in unselected patients with alcoholic cirrhosis. Ann Surg 1980;192:325.
11. Reuff B, Degos F, Degos JD, et al. A controlled study of therapeutic portacaval shunt in alcoholic cirrhosis. Lancet 1976;1:655.
12. Reynolds TB, Donovan AJ, Mikkelsen WP, et al. Results of a 12-year randomized trial of portacaval shunt in patients with alcoholic liver disease and bleeding varices. Gastroenterology 1981;80:1005.
13. Resnick RH, Iber FL, Ishihara AM, et al. A controlled study of the therapeutic portacaval shunt. Gastroenterology 1974;67:843.
14. Van Stiegmann G, Cambre T, Sun JH. A new endoscopic elastic band ligation device. Gastrointest Endosc 1986;32:230.
15. Sherlock S. Disease of the liver and biliary system. 8th ed. Oxford: Blackwell Scientific, 1989:151.
16. Butler H. Gastro-oesophageal haemorrhage in hepatic cirrhosis. Thorax 1952;7:159.
17. Sarin SK, Sachdev G, Nanda R, et al. Endoscopic sclerotherapy in the treatment of gastric varices. Br J Surg 1988;75:747.
18. Butler H. Veins of oesophagus. Thorax 1951;6:276.
19. Kitano S, Terblanche J, Kahn J, et al. Venous anatomy of the lower oesophagus in portal hypertension: practical implications. Br J Surg 1986;73:525.
20. Vianna A, Hayes PC, Moscoso G, et al. Normal venous circulation of the gastroesophageal junction. Gastroenterology 1987;93:876.
21. Spence RAJ, Terblanche J. Venous anatomy of the lower oesophagus: a new perspective on varices. Br J Surg 1987;74:659.
22. Hashizume M, Kitano S, Sugimachi K, et al. Three-dimensional view of the vascular structure of the lower esophagus in clinical portal hypertension. Hepatology 1988;8:1482.
23. Mc Cormack TT, Rose JD, Smith PM, et al. Perforating veins and blood flow in oesophageal varices. Lancet 1983;24:1442.
24. Noda T. Angioarchitectural study of esophageal varices—with special reference to variceal rupture. Virchows Arch 1984;404:381.
25. Beppu K, Inokuchi K, Koyanagi N, et al. Prediction of variceal hemorrhage by esophageal endoscopy. Gastrointest Endosc 1981;27:213.
26. Graham DY, Smith JL. The course of patients after variceal hemorrhage. Gastroenterology 1981;80:800.
27. Koff RS. Benefit of endoscopy in upper gastrointestinal bleeding in patients with liver disease. Dig Dis Sci 1981;26:12.
28. Galambos JT. Esophageal variceal hemorrhage: diagnosis and an overview of treatment. Semin Liver Dis 1982;2:211.
29. Garcia-Tsao G, Groszmann RJ, Fisher RL, et al. Portal pressure, presence of gastroesophageal varices and variceal bleeding. Hepatology 1985;5:419.
30. Lebrec D, De Fleury P, Rueff B, et al. Portal hypertension, size of esophageal varices, and risk of gastrointestinal bleeding in alcholic cirrhosis. Gastroenterology 1980;79:1139.
31. Rector WG, Reynolds TB. Risk factors for haemorrhage from oesophageal varices and acute gastric erosions. Clin Gastroenterol 1985;14:139.
32. Inokuchi K. Prophylactic portal non-decompressive surgery in patients with oesophageal varices. Ann Surg 1984;200:61.
33. Baker LA, Smith C, Lieberman G. The natural history of esophageal varices—a study of 115 cirrhotic patients in whom varices were diagnosed prior to bleeding. Am J Med 1959;26:228.
34. Dagradi A. The natural history of esophageal varices in patients with alcoholic liver cirrhosis. Am J Gastroenterol 1972;57:520.
35. Palmer ED, Brick BI. Correlation between the severity of esophageal varices in portal cirrhosis and their propensity towards hemorrhage. Gastroenterology 1956;30:85.
36. Paquet K. Prophylactic endoscopic sclerosing treatment of the esophageal wall in varices—a prospective controlled randomized trial. Endoscopy 1982;14:4.
37. Witzel L, Wolbergs E, Merki H. Prophylactic endoscopic sclerotherapy of oesophageal varices. Lancet 1985;1:773.
38. Fleischer D. Etiology and prevalence of severe persistent upper gastrointestinal bleeding. Gastroenterology 1983;84:538.
39. Olsson R. The natural history of esophageal varices: a retrospective study of 224 cases with liver cirrhosis. Digestion 1972;6:65.
40. Peterson WL, Barnett CC, Smith HJ, et al. Routine early endoscopy in upper gastrointestinal-tract bleeding. A randomized, controlled trial. N Engl J Med 1981;304:925.
41. Bernuau J, Rueff B. Treatment of acute variceal bleeding. Clin Gastroenterol 1985;14:185.
42. Schalm SW, van Buuren HR. Prevention of recurrent variceal bleeding: non-surgical procedures. Clin Gastroenterol 1985;14:209.
43. Lebrec D, Benhamou J-P. Ectopic varices in portal hypertension. Clin Gastroenterol 1985;14:105.
44. Trudeau W, Prindiville T. Endoscopic injection sclerosis in bleeding gastric varices. Gastrointest Endosc 1986;32:264.
45. Sauerbruch T, Weinzierl M, Dietrich HP, et al. Sclerotherapy of a bleeding duodenal varix. Endoscopy 1982;14:187.
46. Paquet KJ. Sclerotherapy of bleeding oesophageal varices by means of endoscopy. Endoscopy 1978;10:7.
47. Johnston GW, Rodgers HW. A review of 15 years' experience in the use of sclerotherapy in the control of acute haemorrhage from oesophageal varices. Br J Surg 1973;60:797.
48. Hennessy TPJ, Stephens RB, Keane FB. Acute and chronic management of esophageal varices by injection sclerotherapy. Surg Gynecol Obstet 1982;155:375.
49. Terblanche J, Yakoob HI, Bornman PC, et al. Acute bleeding varices: a five-year prospective evaluation of tamponade and sclerotherapy. Ann Surg 1981;1:521.
50. Bornman P, Kahn D, Terblanche J, et al. Rigid versus fiberoptic endoscopic injection sclerotherapy. Ann Surg 1988;208:175.
51. Reilly JJJ, Schade RR, Roh MS, et al. Esophageal variceal sclerosis. Surg Gynecol Obstet 1982;155:497.
52. Schuman B. Alcohol for variceal injection—pure but not so simple. Gastrointest Endosc 1988;34:434.
53. Mathur SK, Naik SR, Supe AN, et al. Endoscopic esophageal variceal sclerotherapy using 3% aqueous phenol. Gastrointest Endosc 1992;38:152.
54. Soehendra N, Nam V, Grimm H, et al. Endoscopic obliteration of large esophagogastric varices with bucrylate. Endoscopy 1986;18:25.
55. Jensen D, Silpa M, Tapia J, et al. Comparison of different methods for endoscopic hemostasis of bleeding canine esophageal varices. Gastroenterology 1983;1983:1455.
56. Jensen L, Dybdahl H, Juhl C, et al. Endoscopic sclerotherapy of esophageal varices in an experimental animal mode—a histomorphologic study. Scand J Gastroenterol 1986;21:725.
57. Kitano S, Iso Y, Koyanagi N, et al. Ethanolamine oleate is superior to polidocanol (aethoxysklerol) for endoscopic injection sclerotherapy of esophageal varices: a prospective randomized trial. Hepatogastroenterology 1987;34:19.
58. Kitano S, Yamaga H, Hashizume M, et al. Trial of sclerosing agents in patients with oesophageal varices. Br J Surg 1988;75:751.
59. Chung SCS, Lo KK, Sung JY, et al. Which sclerosant for variceal injection: a prospective randomised double blind trial of STD vs ethanolamine. Gastroenterology 1988;94:A530.
60. Bhargava DK, Singh B, Dogra R, et al. Prospective randomized comparison of sodium tetradecyl sulfate and polidocanol as variceal sclerosing agents. Gastrointest Endosc 1992;87:182.

61. Paoluzi P, Pietroiusti A, Ferrari S, et al. Absolute alcohol in esophageal vein sclerosis. Gastrointest Endosc 1988;34:400.
62. Soehendra N, Grimm H, Maydeo A, et al. Endoscopic sclerotherapy—personal experience. Hepatol Gastroenterol 1991;38:220.
63. Chung R, Lewis J, Camara D. A technique of sclerotherapy. Surg Gastroenterol 1983;2:303.
64. Wodak E. Osophagus varigen bei portaler Hypertension: Ihre Therapie und Prophylaxe. Wein Med Wochenschr 1960;110:581.
65. Sarin S, Nanda R, Scahdev G, et al. Intravariceal versus paravariceal sclerotherapy: a prospective, controlled, randomized trial. Gut 1986;28:657.
66. Kitano S, Koyanagi N, Iso Y, et al. Prevention of recurrence of esophageal varices after endoscopic injection sclerotherapy with ethanolamine oleate. Hepatology 1987;7:81.
67. Westaby D, Macdougall R, Williams R. Improved survival following injection sclerotherapy for esophageal varices: final analysis of a controlled trial. Hepatology 1985;5:827.
68. Terblanche J, Kahn D, Campbell J, et al. Failure of repeated injection sclerotherapy to improve long-term survival after oesophageal variceal bleeding. Lancet 1983;1328.
69. Cello JP, Grendell JH, Crass RA, et al. Endoscopic sclerotherapy versus portacaval shunt in patients with severe cirrhosis and variceal hemorrhage. N Engl J Med 1984;311:1589.
70. Copenhagen Esophageal Varices Sclerotherapy Project. Sclerotherapy after first variceal hemorrhage in cirrhosis. N Engl J Med 1984;311:1594.
71. Korula J, Baydur A, Sassoon C, et al. Effect of esophageal variceal sclerotherapy (EVS) on lung function. Arch Intern Med 1986;146:1517.
72. Soderlund C, Backman L, Erwald R, et al. Sclerotherapy of esophageal varices: an endoscopic and portographic study. Hepatology 1984;4:877.
73. Westaby D, Melia W, Macdougall B, et al. Injection sclerotherapy for oesophageal varices: a prospective randomised trial of different treatment schedules. Gut 1984;25:129.
74. Sarin S, Sachdev G, Nanda R, et al. Comparison of the two time schedules for endoscopic sclerotherapy: a prospective randomised controlled study. Gut 1986;27:710.
75. Clark A, Westaby D, Silk D, et al. Prospective controlled trial of injection sclerotherapy in patients with cirrhosis and recent variceal hemorrhage. Lancet 1980;2:552.
76. Wang K, Yang P, Hutcheon D, et al. A new method of injection sclerotherapy of esophageal varices. Gastrointest Endosc 1983;29:38.
77. Sciaretta G, Verri A, Maiguti P. A new endoscopic balloon for sclerotherapy in active bleeding from esophageal varices. Endoscopy 1985;17:113.
78. Westaby D, Macdougall BRD, Melia W, et al. A prospective randomized study of two sclerotherapy techniques for esophageal varices. Hepatology 1983;3:681.
79. Hine K, Toghill P, Morris D, et al. Fluorescein mixed with sclerosant improves the accuracy of endoscopic injection of oesophageal varices. Lancet 1984_:322.
80. Hosking S, Robinson P, Johnson A. Usefulness of manometric assessment of varices in maintenance sclerotherapy. Gastroenterology 1987;93:846.
81. Snady H, Korsten MA, Waye JD. The relationship of bacteremia to the length of the injection needle in endoscopic variceal sclerotherapy. Gastrointest Endosc 1985;31:243.
82. Lieberman DA. Sclerotherapy for bleeding esophageal varices after randomized trials. West J Med 1986;145:481.
83. Terblanche J, Burroughs AK, Hobbs KEF. Controversies (first of two parts) in the management of bleeding esophageal varices. N Engl J Med 1989;320:1393.
84. Ayres S, Goff J, Warren G. Endoscopic sclerotherapy for bleeding esophageal varices: effects and complications. Ann Intern Med 1983;98:900.
85. Jensen L, Laurberg S, Juhl C, et al. Esophageal collagen content and mechanical strength after endoscopic sclerotherapy of esophageal varices. Scand J Gastroenterol 1987;22:743.
86. Soehendra N, De Hee K, Kempeneers I, et al. Morphological

alterations of the esophagus after endoscopic sclerotherapy of varices. Endoscopy 1983;15:291.
87. Tihansky D, Reilly J, Schade R, et al. The esophagus after injection sclerotherapy of varices. Radiology 1984;1984:43.
88. Grobe J, Kozarek R, Sanowski R, et al. Venography during endoscopic injection sclerotherapy of esophageal varices. Gastrointest Endosc 1984;30:6.
89. Rose J, Crane M, Smith P. Factors affecting successful endoscopic sclerotherapy for oesophageal varices. Gut 1983;24:946.
90. Barsoum MS, Khattar NY, Risk-Allah MA. Technical aspects of injection sclerotherapy of acute oesophageal variceal haemorrhage as seen by radiography. Br J Surg 1978;65:588.
91. Paquet K. Endoscopic paravariceal injection sclerotherapy of the esophagus—Indications, technique, complications: results of a period of 14 years. Gastrointest Endosc 1983;29:310.
92. Ayres S, Goff J, Warren G, et al. Esophageal ulceration and bleeding after flexible fiberoptic esophageal vein sclerosis. Gastroenterology 1982;83:131.
93. Helpap B, Bollweg L. Morhologic changes in the terminal oesophagus with varices, following sclerosis of the wall. Endoscopy 1981;13:229.
94. Evans DMD, Jones DB, Cleary BK, et al. Oesophageal varices treated by sclerotherapy: a histopathological study. Gut 1982;23:615.
95. Fleischer D. Endoscopic Nd:YAG laser therapy for active esophageal variceal bleeding. Gastrointest Endosc 1985;31:4.
96. Fleig WE, Stange EF, Ruettenauer K, et al. Emergency endoscopic sclerotherapy for bleeding esophageal varices: a prospective study in patients not responding to balloon tamponade. Gastrointest Endosc 1983;29:8.
97. Lewis JW, Chung RS, Allison JG. Injection sclerotherapy for control of acute variceal hemorrhage. Am J Surg 1981;142:592.
98. Barsoum M. Tamponade and injection sclerotherapy in the management of bleeding oesophageal varices. Br J Surg 1982;69:76.
99. Moretó M, Zaballa M, Bernal A, et al. A randomized trial of tamponade or sclerotherapy as immediate treatment for bleeding esophageal varices. Surg Gynecol Obstet 1988;167:331.
100. Paquet K-J, Feussner H. Endoscopic sclerosis and esophageal balloon tamponade in acute hemorrhage from esophagogastric varices: a prospective controlled randomized trial. Hepatology 1985;5:580.
101. Soderlund C, Ihre T. Endoscopic sclerotherapy v conservative management of bleeding oesophageal varices. Acta Chir Scand 1985;151:449.
102. Westaby D, Hayes PC, Gimson AES, et al. Controlled clinical trial of injection sclerotherapy for active variceal bleeding. Hepatology 1989;9:274.
103. Shields R, Jenkins SA, Baxter JN, et al. A prospective randomized controlled trial comparing the efficacy of somatostatin with injection sclerotherapy in the control of bleeding oesophageal varices. J Hepatol 1992;16:128.
104. Larson AW, Cohen H, Zweban B, et al. Acute esophageal variceal sclerotherapy: results of a prospective randomized controlled trial. J Am Med Assoc 1986;255:497.
105. Cello JP, Greendell JH, Crass Ra, et al. Endoscopic sclerotherapy versus portacaval shunt in patients with severe cirrhosis and acute variceal hemorrhage. N Engl J Med 1987;316:11.
106. Burroughs AK, Hamilton G, Phillips A, et al. A comparison of sclerotherapy with staple transection of the esophagus for the emergency control of bleeding from esophageal varices. N Engl J Med 1989;321:857.
106a. Huizinga WK, Angorn IB, Baker LW. Esophageal transection versus injection sclerotherapy in the management of bleeding esophageal varices in patients at high risk. Surg Gyn Obstet 1985;160:539.
107. Korula J, Balart L, Radvan G, et al. A prospective, randomized controlled trial of chronic esophageal variceal sclerotherapy. Hepatology 1985;5:584.
108. Gregory PB, VA Cooperative Variceal Sclerotherapy Group. Sclerotherapy for male alcoholics with cirrhosis who have bled

from esophageal varices: results of a randomized multicenter clinical trial. Sydney: World Congress of Gastroenterology Proceedings, 1990.

109. Henderson JM, Kutner MH, Millikan WJ, et al. Endoscopic variceal sclerosis compared with distal splenorenal shunt to prevent recurrent variceal bleeding in cirrhosis. A prospective, randomized trial. Ann Intern Med 1990;112:262.

110. Spina GP, Santambrogio R, Opocher E, et al. Distal splenorenal shunt versus endoscopic sclerotherapy in the prevention of variceal rebleeding. Ann Surg 1990;211:178.

111. Rikkers LF, Jin G, Burnett DA, et al. Shunt surgery versus endoscopic sclerotherapy for variceal hemorrhage: late results of a randomized trial. Am J Surg 1993;165:27.

112. Planas R, Boix J, Broggi M, et al. Portacaval shunt versus endoscopic sclerotherapy in the elective treatment of variceal hemorrhage. Gastroenterology 1991;100:1078.

113. Kitano S, Iso Y, Hashizume M, et al. Sclerotherapy vs esophageal transection vs distal splenorenal shunt for the clinical management of esophageal varices in patients with Child class A and B liver function: a prospective randomized trial. Hepatology 1992;15:63.

114. Triger DR, Johnson AG, Brazier JE, et al. A prospective trial of endoscopic sclerotherapy vs oesophageal transection and gastric devascularisation in the long term management of bleeding oesophageal varices. Gut 1992;33:1553.

115. Teres J, Bordas J, Bravo D, et al. Sclerotherapy vs distal splenorenal shunt in the elective treatment of variceal hemorrhage: a randomized controlled trial. Hepatology 1987;7:430.

116. Fleig W, Stange E, Hunecke R, et al. Prevention of recurrent bleeding in cirrhotics with recent variceal hemorrhage: prospective randomized comparison of propanolol and sclerotherapy. Hepatology 1987;7:355.

117. O'Connor K, Lehman G, Yune H, et al. Comparison of three nonsurgical treatments for bleeding esophageal varices. Gastroenterology 1989;96:900.

118. Alexandrino PT, Alves MM, Pinto-Correia J. Propranolol or endoscopic sclerotherapy in the prevention of recurrence of variceal bleeding: a prospective, randomized controlled trial. J Hepatol 1988;7:175.

119. Spina GP, Henderson JM, Rikkers LF, et al. Distal splenorenal shunt versus endoscopic sclerotherapy in the prevention of variceal rebleeding. J Hepatol 1992;16:338.

120. Terabayashi H, Ohnishi K, Tsunoda T, et al. Prospective controlled trial of elective endoscopic sclerotherapy in comparison with percutaneous transhepatic obliteration of esophageal varices in patients with nonalcoholic cirrhosis. Gastroenterology 1987;93:1205.

120a. Infante-Rivard C, Asnaola S, Villeneuve J. Role of endoscopic variceal sclerotherapy in the long-term management of variceal bleeding: a meta-analysis. Gastroenterology 1989;96:1087.

121. LaBerge JM, Ring EJ, Gordon RL, et al. Creation of transjugular intrahepatic portosystemic shunts with the Wallstent endoprosthesis: results in 100 patients. Radiology 1993;187:413.

122. Dollet JM, Champigneulle B, Patris A, et al. Sclerotherapie endoscopique contre propranolol apres hemorrage par rupture de varices oesophagennes chez le cirrhotique. Gastroenterol Clin Biol 1988;12:234.

123. Liu JD, Jeng YS, Chen PH, et al. Endoscopic injection sclerotherapy and propranolol in the prevention of recurrent variceal bleeding. Sydney: Proceedings of the World Congress of Gastroenterology, 1990;1181.

124. Rossi V, Cales P, Burtin P, et al. Prevention of recurrent variceal bleeding in alcoholic cirrhotic patients: prospective controlled trial of propranolol and sclerotherapy. J Hepatol 1991;12:283.

125. Teres J, Bosch J, Bordas JM, et al. Endoscopic sclerotherapy versus propranolol in the elective treatment of variceal bleeding: preliminary results of a randomized controlled trial (abstract). J Hepatol 1987;5:S210.

126. Westaby D, Polson RJ, Gimson AES, et al. Propranolol—a primary role for the prevention of recurrent variceal bleeding in compensated cirrhotic. Hepatology 1987;7:1030.

127. Dasarathy S, Dwivedi M, Bhargava DK. A prospective randomized trial comparing repeated endoscopic sclerotherapy and propranolol in decompensated (Child class B and C) cirrhotic patients. Hepatology 1992;16:89.

128. Lundell L, Leth R, Lind T, et al. Evaluation of propranolol for prevention of recurrent bleeding from esophageal varices between sclerotherapy sessions. Acta Chir Scand 1990;156:711.

129. Westaby D, Melia W, Hegarty J, et al. Use of propranolol to reduce the rebleeding rate during injection sclerotherapy prior to variceal obliteration. Hepatology 1986;6:673.

130. Bertoni G, Fornaciari G, Beltrami M, et al. Nadolol for prevention of variceal rebleeding during the course of endoscopic injection sclerotherapy: A randomized pilot study (letter). J Clin Gastroenterol 1990;12:364.

131. Gerunda GE, Neri D, Cangrandi F, et al. Nadolol does not reduce early rebleeding in cirrhotic undergoing endoscopic variceal sclerotherapy: a multicenter randomized controlled trial (abstract). Hepatology 1990;12:988.

132. Jensen LS, Krarup N. Propranolol in prevention of rebleeding from esophageal varices during the course of endoscopic sclerotherapy. Scand J Gastroenterol 1989;24:339.

133. Vickers C, Rhodes J, Hillenbrand P, et al. Prospective controlled trial of propranolol and sclerotherapy for prevention of rebleeding from esophageal varices (abstract). Gut 1987;28:A1359.

134. Vinel JP, Lamoulilette H, Cales P, et al. Propranolol reduces the rebleeding rate during injection sclerotherapy: results of a randomized study. Gastroenterology 1992;102:1760.

135. Conn HO, Lindenmuth WW, May CJ, et al. Prophylactic portacaval anastomosis: a tale of two studies. Medicine 1972;51:27.

136. Piai G, Cipolletta L, Claar M, et al. Prophylactic sclerotherapy of high-risk esophageal varices: results of a multicentric prospective controlled trial. Hepatology 1988;8:1495.

137. Koch H, Henning H, Grimm H, et al. Prophylactic sclerosing of esophageal varices—results of a prospective controlled study. Endoscopy 1986;18:40.

138. Santangelo W, Dueno M, Estes B, et al. Prophylactic sclerotherapy of large esophageal varices. N Engl J Med 1988;318:814.

139. Sauerbruch T, Wotzka R, Kopcke W, et al. Prophylactic sclerotherapy before the first episode of variceal hemorrhage in patients with cirrhosis. N Engl J Med 1988;319:8.

140. Potzi R, Bauer P, Reichel W, et al. Prophylactic endoscopic sclerotherapy of oesophageal varices in liver cirrhosis. A multicenter prospective controlled randomized trial in Vienna. Gut 1989;30:873.

141. Russo A, Giannone G, Magnano A, et al. Prophylactic sclerotherapy in nonalcoholic liver cirrhosis: preliminary results of a prospective controlled randomized trial. World J Surg 1989;13:149.

142. Andreani T, Poupon RE, Balkau BJ et al. Preventive therapy of first gastrointestinal bleeding in patients with cirrhosis: results of a controlled trial comparing propranolol, endoscopic sclerotherapy and placebo. Hepatology 1990;12:1413.

143. The VA Cooperative Variceal Sclerotherapy Group. Prophylactic sclerotherapy for esophageal varices in men with alcoholic liver disease—a randomized, single-blind, multicenter clinical trial. N Engl J Med 1991;324:1779.

144. Triger DR, Smart HL, Hosking SW, et al. Prophylactic sclerotherapy for esophageal varices: Long-term results of a single-center trial. Hepatology 1991;13:117.

145. De Franchis R, Primignani M, Arcidiacono PG, et al. Prophylactic sclerotherapy in high-risk cirrhotic selected by endoscopic criteria. A multicenter randomized controlled trial. Gastroenterology 1991;101:1087.

146. The PROVA Study Group. Prophylaxis of first hemorrhage from esophageal varices by sclerotherapy, propranolol or both in cirrhotic patients: a randomized multicenter trial. Hepatology 1991;14:1016.

147. Pagliaro L, D'Amico G, Sorensen TIA, et al. Prevention of first bleeding in cirrhosis. A meta-analysis of randomized trials of nonsurgical treatment. Ann Intern Med 1992;117:59.

148. Wang M, Desigan G, Dunn D. Endoscopic sclerotherapy for

bleeding rectal varices: a case report. Am J Gastroenterol 1985;80:779.

149. Weiserbs DB, Zfass AM, Messmer J. Control of massive hemorrhage from rectal varices with sclerotherapy. Gastrointest Endosc 1986;32:419.

150. Kirkpatrick JR, Shoenut JP, McFlikier AB. Successful injection sclerotherapy for bleeding duodenal varix in intrahepatic portal obstruction. Gastrointest Endosc 1985;31:259.

151. Gertsch P, Blumgart LH. Cure of a bleeding duodenal varix by sclerotherapy. Br J Surg 1988;75:717.

152. Schuman BM, Beckman JW, Tedesco FJ, et al. Complication of endoscopic injection sclerotherapy: a review. Am J Gastroenterol 1987;82:823.

153. Marzuk P, Schwartz J. Endoscopic sclerotherapy for esophageal varices. Ann Intern Med 1984;100:608.

154. Jensen D, Machicado G, Silpa M. Esophageal varix hemorrhage and sclerotherapy—animal studies. Endoscopy 1986;18:18.

155. Sarles HE, Sanowski RA, Talbert G. Course and complications of endoscopic variceal sclerotherapy: a prospective study of 50 patients. Am J Gastroenterol 1985;80:595.

156. Kahn D, Bornmann P, Terblanche J. Incidence and management of complications after injection sclerotherapy: a ten-year prospective evaluation. Surgery 1989;105:160.

157. Tabibian N, Smith J, Graham D. Sclerotherapy-associated esophageal ulcers: Lessons from a double-blind, randomized comparison of sucralfate suspension versus placebo. Gastrointest Endosc 1989;35:312.

158. MacDougall B, Theodossi A, Westaby D, et al. Increased long-term survivial in variceal haemorrhage using injection sclerotherapy. Lancet 1982;1:124.

159. Bacon B, Camara D, Duffy M. Severe ulceration and delayed perforation of the esophagus after endoscopic variceal sclerotherapy. Gastrointest Endosc 1987;33:311.

160. McGrew W, Goodin J, Stuck W. Fatal complication of endoscopic sclerotherapy: *Serratia marcescens* bacteremia with delayed esophageal perforation. Gastrointest Endosc 1985;31:329.

161. Vickers CR, O'Connor HJ, Quintero GA, et al. Delayed perforation of the esophagus after variceal sclerotherapy and hepatic transformation. Gastrointest Endosc 1989;35:459.

162. Sorensen T, Burcharth F, Pedersen ML, et al. Esophageal stricture and dysphagia after endoscopic sclerotherapy for bleeding varices. Gut 1984;25:473.

163. Haynes WC, Sanowski RA, Foutch PG, et al. Esophageal strictures following endoscopic variceal sclerotherapy: clinical course and response to dilation therapy. Gastrointest Endosc 1986;32:202.

164. Soderlund C, Thor K, Wiechel K. Oesophageal motility after sclerotherapy for bleeding varices. Acta Chir Scand 1985;151:249.

165. Sauerbruch T, Wirsching B, Leisner B, et al. Esophageal function after sclerotherapy of bleeding varices. Scand J Gastroenterol 1982;17:745.

166. Ogle S, Kirk C, Bailey R, et al. Oesophageal function in cirrhotic patients undergoing injection sclerotherapy for oesophageal varices. Digestion 1978;18:178.

167. Bacon B, Bailey-Newton R, Connors A. Pleural effusions after endoscopic variceal sclerotherapy. Gastroenterology 1985;88:910.

168. Crawford D, Ryan D. Acute respiratory insufficiency after endoscopy for bleeding oesophageal varices. Br Med J 1984;288:1639.

169. Monroe P. Acute respiratory failure after sodium morrhuate esophageal sclerotherapy. Gastroenterology 1983;85:693.

170. Bailey-Newton R, Connors A, Bacon B. Effect of endoscopic variceal sclerotherapy on gas exchange and hemodynamics in humans. Gastroenterology 1985;89:368.

171. Hughes RW, Larson DE, Viggiano TR, et al. Endoscopic variceal sclerosis: a one year experience. Gastrointest Endosc 1982;28:62.

172. Barsoum M, Mooro H, Bolous F, et al. The complications of injection sclerotherapy of bleeding oesophageal varices. Br J Surg 1982;69:79.

173. Sauerbruch T, Holl J, Ruckdeschel G, et al. Bacteremia associated with endoscopic sclerotherapy of oesophageal varices. Endoscopy 1985;17:170.

174. Camara D, Gruber M, Barde C, et al. Transient bacteremia following endoscopic injection sclerotherapy of esophageal varices. Arch Intern Med 1983;143:1350.

175. Low D, Shoenut J, Kennedy J, et al. Infectious complications of endoscopic injection sclerotherapy. Arch Intern Med 1986;146:569.

176. Camara D. Bacteremia and injection sclerotherapy. Arch Intern Med 1986;146:458.

177. Lange S, Laughlin B, Hughes RW, et al. Septic complications of variceal hemorrhage and ethanolamine sclerotherapy of varices. Gastrointest Endosc 1983;29:191.

178. Gerhartz H, Sauerbruch T, Weinzierl M, et al. Nosocomial septicemia in patients undergoing sclerotherapy for variceal hemorrhage. Endoscopy 1984;16:129.

179. Cohen FL, Koerner RS, Taub SJ. Solitary brain abscess following endoscopic injection sclerosis of esophageal varices. Gastrointest Endosc 1985;31:331.

180. Ritchie M, Lightdale C, Botet J. Bilateral perinephric abscesses: a complication of endoscopic injection sclerotherapy. Am J Gastroenterol 1987;82:670.

181. Charng M, Wang A, Chang M, et al. Coronary spasm complicating sclerotherapy of esophageal varices. Chest 1988;93:204.

182. Perakos P, Cirbus J, Camara D. Persistent Brady arrhythmia after sclerotherapy for esophageal varices. South Med J 1984;77:531.

183. Knauer C, Fogel M. Pericarditis: complication of esophageal sclerotherapy. Gastroenterology 1987;93:287.

184. Tabibian N, Schwartz J, Smith J, et al. Cardiac tamponade as a result of endoscopic sclerotherapy: report of a case. Surgery 1987;102:546.

185. Seidman E, Weber A, Morin C, et al. Spinal cord paralysis following sclerotherapy for esophageal varices. Hepatology 1984;4:950.

186. Thatcher B, Sivak M, Ferguson D, et al. Mesenteric venous thrombosis as a possible complication of endoscopic sclerotherapy: a report of two cases. Am J Gastroenterol 1986;81:126.

187. DeMarino G, Sumkin J, Leventhal R, et al. Pneumatosis intestinalis and pneumoperitoneum after sclerotherapy. Am J Roentgenol 1988;151:953.

188. Foutch PG, Sivak MV. Colonic variceal hemorrhage after endoscopic injection sclerosis of esophageal varices: a report of three cases. Am J Gastroenterol 1984;79:756.

189. Keane R, Britton D. Massive bleeding from rectal varices following repeated injection sclerotherapy of oesophageal varices. Br J Surg 1986;73:120.

190. Eleftheriadis E. Duodenal varices after sclerotherapy for esophageal varices. Am J Gastroenterol 1988;83:439.

191. Goodale RL, Silvis SE, O'Leary JF, et al. Early survival after sclerotherapy for bleeding esophageal varices. Surgery 1982;155:523.

192. Dilawari J, Raju G, Chawla Y. Development of large spleno-adrenorenal shunt after endoscopic sclerotherapy. Gastroenterology 1989;97:421.

193. Stiegmann GV, Goff JS, Sun JH, et al. Endoscopic ligation of esophageal varices. Am J Surg 1990;159:21.

194. Stiegmann GV, Sun JH, Hammond WS. Results of experimental endoscopic esophageal varix ligation. Am Surgeon 1988;54:105.

195. Stiegmann GV, Goff JS. Endoscopic esophageal varix ligation: preliminary clinical experience. Gastrointest Endosc 1988;34:113.

196. Marks RD, Arnold MD, Baron TH. Gross and microscopic findings in the human esophagus after esophageal variceal band ligation: a postmortem analysis. Am J Gastroenterol 1993;88:272.

197. Stiegmann GV, Goff JS, Michaletz-Onody PA, et al. Endoscopic sclerotherapy as compared with endoscopic ligation for bleeding esophageal varices. N Engl J Med 1993;326:1527.

198. Gimson AES, Ramage JK, Panos MZ, et al. Randomized trial

of variceal banding ligation versus injection sclerotherapy for bleeding oesophageal varices. Lancet 1993;342:391.

199. Laine L, El-Newihi HM, Migikovsky B, et al. Endoscopic ligation compared with sclerotherapy for the treatment of bleeding esophageal varices. Ann Intern Med 1993;119:1.

200. Reveille RM, Goff JS, Stiegmann GV, et al. Combination endoscopic variceal ligation (EVL) and low volume endoscopic sclerotherapy (ES) for bleeding esophageal varices: a faster route to variceal eradication? Gastrointes Endosc 1991;37:243.

201. Koutsomanis D. Endoscopic variceal ligation combined with low-volume sclerotherapy: a controlled study. Gastroenterology 1992;102:A835.

202. Young MF, Sanowski RA, Rasche R. Comparison and characterization of ulcerations induced by endoscopic ligation of esophageal varices versus endoscopic sclerotherapy. Gastrointes Endsoc 1993;39:119.

203. Johnson PA, Campbell DR, Antonson CW, et al. Complications associated with endoscopic band ligation of esophageal varices. Gastrointest Endosc 1993;39:181.

204. Stiegmann GV. Endoscopic ligation: now and the future. Gastrointest Endosc 1993;39:203.

205. Saltzman JR, Arora S. Complications of esophageal variceal band ligation. Gastrointest Endosc 1993;39:185.

206. Goldschmiedt M, Haber G, Kandel G, et al. A safety maneuver for placing overtubes during endoscopic variceal ligation. Gastrointest Endosc 1992;38:399.

207. Berkelhammer C, Madhav G, Lyon S, et al. "Pinch" injury during overtube placement in upper endoscopy. Gastrointest Endosc 1993;39:186.

208. Tseng CC, Green RM, Burke SK, et al. Bacteremia after endoscopic band ligation of esophageal varices. Gastrointest Endosc 1992;38:336.

Textbook of Gastroenterology, second edition, edited by Tadataka Yamada. JB Lippincott Company, Philadelphia © 1995.

CHAPTER 138

Endoscopic Control of Nonvariceal Upper Gastrointestinal Hemorrhage

Dennis M. Jensen

Severe upper gastrointestinal (UGI) bleeding is a common, and serious medical-surgical problem.[1,2] Most patients with severe UGI bleeding are admitted to hospitals for observation and care. Early endoscopy has been performed for accurate diagnosis of severe UGI bleeding for more than twenty years. Nevertheless, the reported mortality for this condition has not changed in over 30 years in spite of accurate diagnostic

endoscopy and major improvements in intensive care unit (ICU), medical, and surgical management. Mortality remains about 10% for UGI bleeding in the United States.[3–5]

Over the last 5 to 10 years, major advances have occurred in the endoscopic treatment of patients with severe UGI hemorrhage. Combined endoscopic diagnosis and treatment of ulcer and esophageal varix bleeding has improved outcomes of patients with severe UGI bleeding in some centers. Primarily, progress has been made because of innovative ideas for therapy, advances in technology, new laboratory research results, and carefully performed randomized controlled studies (RCS). Endoscopic applications have most often been to bleeding ulcers which are the most frequent cause of severe UGI bleeding in the United States.[1,6,7] With these advances and results, there is a better understanding about which patients with nonvariceal UGI bleeding will benefit most and least from these therapies; what are the best techniques and limitations of each new therapy; and what are the safety, efficacy, and cost of these therapies relative to routine medical-surgical treatment.[7] The purpose of this chapter is to discuss the clinically applicable techniques and results of endoscopic hemostasis for nonvariceal UGI hemorrhage.

PATIENT SELECTION

Endoscopic hemostasis will not benefit all patients hospitalized for nonvariceal UGI hemorrhage. Patients who are not at risk for continued bleeding or rebleeding are unlikely to benefit from the treatments and yet are at risk of complications and increased medical cost resulting from an unnecessary therapeutic procedure. For endoscopic hemostasis, one must select the patients at risk for continued bleeding or rebleeding and assess the possible benefit to them. Data about UGI bleeders with ulcers, Mallory-Weiss tears and UGI angiomata will be reviewed to help select patients likely to benefit from endoscopic treatment. Patients with UGI hemorrhage from Dieulafoy's lesion or UGI tumors will also be discussed briefly.

Severe UGI bleeding is a serious medical-surgical emergency. At the UCLA Center for the Health Sciences in Los Angeles, serious UGI bleeding represents the most common diagnosis for admission to the medical ICU.* Nevertheless, most UGI bleeders are admitted to the ward for care. The latter group appears to have stopped bleeding by the time of hospital admission and often do not rebleed.

Whereas other investigators have evaluated or treated all UGI bleeders admitted to the hospital for observation, the CURE Hemostasis Research Group has focused its attention on defining the relations between clinically severe bleeding, endoscopic stigmata and short-term (i.e., first 30 days) outcomes. Patients admitted to an ICU for severe bleeding have been our primary concern. The most common diagnoses for patients admitted to an ICU for UGI bleeding are listed on Table 138-1.

These patients were assessed as part of RCSs of sclerotherapy for control of variceal hemorrhage or thermal devices for ulcer hemostasis. In each case, the endoscopic appearance of the lesions was described in accordance with stigmata of recent hemorrhage for: ulcers,[8,9] varices,[7,10] and Mallory-Weiss tears. All patients were managed with modern ICU care and had transfusions of red cells, platelets and fresh frozen plasma as necessary. These results are similar to the rates of continued bleeding and rebleeding reported in male veterans by Fleischer.[11]

---

* Bellamy P, personal communication, March 1994.

TABLE 138-1
CURE Hemostasis Research Group Results—Diagnosis and Rates of More Bleeding for ICU Patients

FINAL DIAGNOSIS*	FREQUENCY OF DIAGNOSIS (%)	MORE BLEEDING† (%)
Peptic ulcers	50.5	28
Esophagogastric varices	22	46
UGI angiomata	7.5	7
Mallory-Weiss tears	6	17
UGI cancers	5	10
Gastric or duodenal erosions	4.5	0
Other	4.5	11

UGI, upper gastrointestinal.

* Final diagnosis as a rate in 200 consecutive patients with severe UGI bleeding admitted to UCLA or West Los Angeles VA intensive care units was made by emergency endoscopy, surgery, or autopsy.

† More bleeding indicates clinically significant bleeding requiring continued intensive care unit management, transfusions, emergency intervention (surgery or therapeutic endoscopy) during initial hospitalization.

Ulcer Patient Selection—London Data

Swain and coworkers performed three different RCSs with argon laser,[8] Nd:YAG laser,[9] and heater probe.[12] The risks of further bleeding were carefully defined by their controls (i.e., medically managed patients) based upon initial endoscopic appearance or stigmata. Endoscopy was performed early upon hospital admission in all patients with UGI bleeding. Endoscopy and treatment were performed in an endoscopy unit equipped with lasers and later with heater probe, rather than in an ICU. Gentle washing of the ulcer base was used to wash off nonadherent clots and localize the precise bleeding point.[8,9,12] They carefully determined stigmata of recent hemorrhage at the initial, diagnostic endoscopy, stratified by these different endoscopic stigmata, and treated approximately half the patients with different endoscopic thermal methods (i.e., laser or heater probe) and the other half were treated medically (i.e., controls). Inpatients who developed UGI bleeding were not included in their studies. The control groups (i.e., no endoscopic treatment) for each stigma of recent hemorrhage defined the prognosis for further bleeding (Table 138-2).

The prevalence of the different stigma varied from 6.8% for nonbleeding, flat, red or black spots to 54.7% for nonbleeding visible vessels. Swain and coworkers defined a nonbleeding visible vessel as a raised area in the ulcer crater, resistant to washing, usually unique and often in the center of the ulcer crater (Fig. 138-1; see Color Fig. 114). Swain and coworkers considered visible vessels, either bleeding or nonbleeding, to be major stigmata of recent hemorrhage because of the high rebleeding rates of 70.6% and 50.6%, respectively. All other stigmata (i.e., clots or flat spots with or without bleeding) or oozing bleeding without a visible vessel had significantly lower rates of rebleeding varying from 0 (i.e., flat nonbleeding spot) to 36% (i.e., nonbleeding clot). Based upon the high rebleeding rates on medical management, patients who might benefit most from endoscopic hemostasis are those with major stigmata of hemorrhage (i.e., active bleeding or

TABLE 138-2
London Studies Rebleeding Rates for Ulcer Patients With Stigmata of Recent Hemorrhage

ENDOSCOPIC STIGMATA	PREVALENCE (%)	REBLEEDING RATE (%)
Major Stigmata		
Bleeding visible vessel	11.5	70.6
Nonbleeding visible vessel	54.7	50.6
Minor Stigmata		
Bleeding overlying clot	7.4	9.0
Nonbleeding overlying clot	7.4	36.0
Bleeding flat spots	6.8	10.0
Nonbleeding flat spots	12.2	0.0
Total	100	39.9

Rebleeding rates from peptic ulcers according to stigmata of recent hemorrhage for 148 patients admitted to a London hospital with recent upper gastrointestinal bleeding, endoscoped early, and managed medically. Patients with each stigma of recent hemorrhage were combined from three randomized controlled trials of ulcer hemostasis with argon laser,[8] Nd:YAG laser,[9] and heater probe.[12]

TABLE 138-3
Outcomes of Intensive Care Unit Patients With Severe Ulcer Bleeding

ENDOSCOPIC APPEARANCE	PERCENT OF TOTAL	MORE BLEEDING* (%)
Active bleeding†	16	88
Nonbleeding visible vessel	22	50
Nonbleeding clot	15	33
Gray slough, flat red or black spot	14	7
Clean ulcer base	33	3

This CURE study included 100 patients admitted to an intensive care unit with severe bleeding whose ulcer could be identified on emergency endoscopy.[1,7] All patients received an H_2-receptor antagonist and sucralfate or antiacids but did not have therapeutic endoscopy.

* Refers to more bleeding requiring transfusion of red blood cells.

† Includes patients with arterial-type bleeding, from a visible vessel, from the base of the ulcer crater, or from under an adherent clot; does not include oozing from granulation tissue on the side of the ulcer.

nonbleeding visible vessels). Other investigators have relied upon these data to select patients for randomization or treatment on prospective studies.

Selection of Peptic Ulcer Patients for Hemostasis—CURE Data

The rates of continued bleeding or rebleeding from the peptic ulcers of patients evaluated in CURE Hemostasis studies and treated medically with H_2 antagonists, sucralfate or antacids in an ICU depended upon appearance of the ulcer base on initial endoscopy (Table 138-3). Further, clinically significant bleeding occurred 3% to 7% of the time for clean ulcers or those with gray slough or flat red or black spots. By contrast,

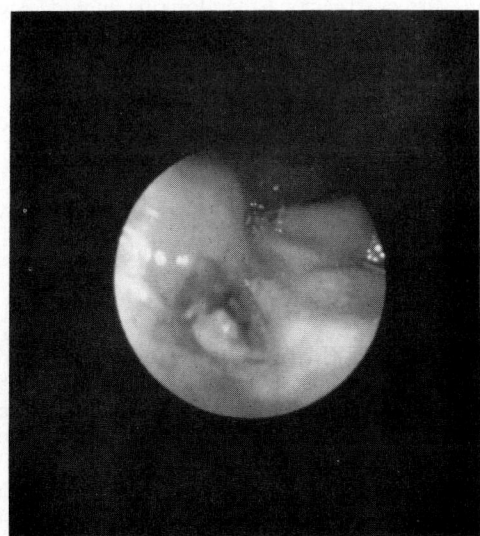

FIGURE 138-1. (See Color Fig. 114.) Nonbleeding visible vessel in a benign ulcer crater.

ulcers with overlying nonbleeding clots rebled one third of the time. For patients with nonarterial oozing bleeding in the absence of a visible vessel or adherent clot, further bleeding on medical therapy occurred 10% of the time. Patients with major stigmata of ulcer hemorrhage had much higher rates of continued bleeding or rebleeding. Patients with active arterial bleeding from a visible vessel, the base of an ulcer or under an adherent clot rebled 88% of the time. Clinically significant rebleeding rates were 50% for nonbleeding visible vessel patients on medical management. The higher rates of continued bleeding for the active bleeders in the CURE study when compared to the London study probably related to the clinical severity and the later endoscopies in the former group after transfusion or ICU care.

Patients at the highest risk of more bleeding from ulcers (i.e., those with major stigmata of hemorrhage) were selected for treatment in CURE studies—those with active arterial bleeding at initial endoscopy or with nonbleeding visible vessels. Patients with nonbleeding clots, oozing bleeding without a visible vessel or adherent clot and other lesser stigmata of hemorrhage (i.e., gray slough or flat spots) were not randomized on initial endoscopy but were later considered for treatment if rebleeding occurred. In our opinion, a similar approach to selection for endoscopic hemostasis of patients with severe ulcer bleeding can be recommended at the present time to others treating patients in clinical practice or on therapeutic trials.

PRINCIPLES OF ARTERIAL HEMOSTASIS

The histopathology of bleeding gastric ulcers has been reported by Swain and Johnston from resected benign ulcers.[13,14] Careful histopathology and injection of barium into the penetrating arteries were the methods used by the investigators to define the location, size, and histopathology of the arteries which had bled.[13] The visible vessels correlated with a pseudoaneurysm of the penetrating artery or with an organizing clot in the side hole of the underlying artery. The location of

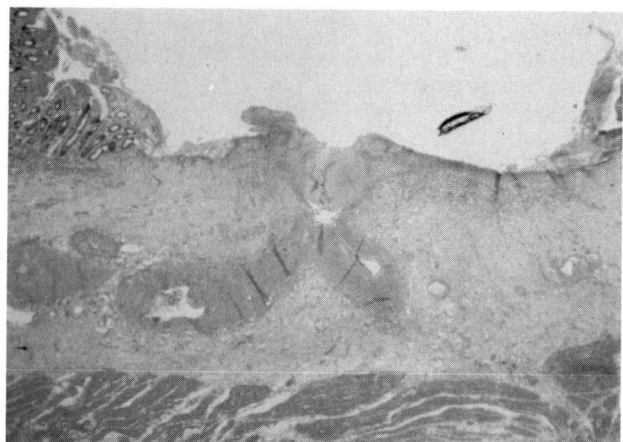

FIGURE 138-2. (See Color Fig. 115.) Histopathology of a nonbleeding visible vessel in a resected chronic gastric ulcer. There is a side hole in the artery, and an organizing clot protrudes into the ulcer crater from this hole. The artery is nearest to the ulcer base at the visible vessel site. (Courtesy of C. Paul Swain, M.D., London, UK.)

the penetrating artery was nearest to the ulcer base at the site of the visible vessel and coursed below the base at variable angles from that bleeding point (Fig. 138-2; see Color Fig. 115). The actual artery under gastric ulcers was most often a secondary or tertiary branch rather than the main artery such as the left gastric artery. The mean internal diameter of the arteries was only 0.7 mm with a range of 0.3 to 1.8 mm.

Recently Swain has reported upon the histopathology of duodenal ulcers from patients with fatal UGI hemorrhages.[15] The relation of the vessel to the ulcer base and the histopathology of the visible vessel were similar to resected gastric ulcer visible vessels. However, the mean diameter of the arteries was 1.0 mm with a range of 0.1 to 3.54 mm.

About one third of the vessels were larger than 2.0 mm. About 25% penetrated into the pancreas and 20% were giant ulcers, greater than 20 mm in diameter. No similar data are available for nonfatal DU bleeds because the duodenum is

not resected during DU surgery and artery sizes are difficult to accurately measure at surgery.

The goal of endoscopic hemostasis is to effectively coagulate this underlying artery.[7,16] The general principles are to apply firm pressure with a contact probe (i.e., heater probe or bipolar electrocoagulation) directly upon the visible vessel by way of endoscopy in an attempt to interrupt blood flow in the artery then apply enough heat to weld the walls of the artery together.[16] Intrinsic arterial hemostasis will then occur in patients with normal platelet coagulation. In the laboratory, this method enables the investigator to weld gut arteries together which are as large as 2.5 mm in diameter (Fig. 138-3; see Color Fig. 116). Conversely, one can fire a laser from a distance or fulgurate with a monopolar electrode. Arterial hemostasis with these devices depends upon tissue heating, tissue edema, artery compression and contraction of the artery[16-19] rather than coaptation (Fig. 138-4; see Color Fig. 117).

Based upon experimental observations, four different mechanisms of action of injection agents for arterial hemostasis are proposed.[20] These include arterial compression, muscle spasm, arteriolar constriction and in situ fixation (Table 138-4). Any of the mechanisms may result in arterial thrombosis if the effects are sustained, if intrinsic coagulation is activated, and if clot lysis does not occur. These mechanisms are also supported by the histopathologic observations of Rutgeerts[21] and Asaki[22] and the microcirculation data in animals reported by Guth and Smith.[23]

INDICATIONS, CONTRAINDICATIONS, AND TIMING OF ENDOSCOPY

In patients with clinical evidence of severe UGI bleeding, emergency panendoscopy for diagnosis and endoscopic treatment is indicated, if the results of the examination would change the management of the patient. When the risks to the patient outweigh the most favorable benefits of the procedure, either emergency or elective panendoscopy of the patient with severe UGI bleeding is contraindicated.[1-2,4-6] Other contraindications for emergency panendoscopy include suspected

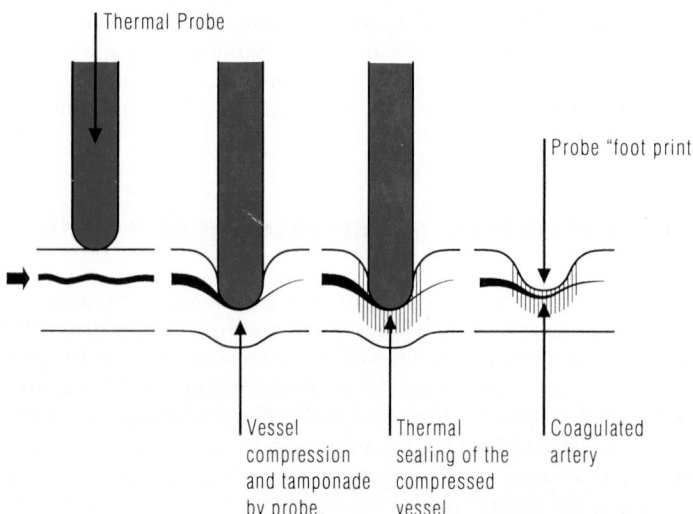

FIGURE 138-3. (See Color Figure 116.) Tamponade of coaptation and effective coagulation of a submucosal artery by a contact probe. Patent artery (*left*). Vessel compression by tamponade (*center*). Coagulated vessel and probe imprint (*right*). (From Johnston JH, Jensen DM, Auth D. Experimental comparison of endoscopic yttrium-aluminum-garnet laser, electrosurgery, and heater probe for canine gut arterial coagulation: The importance of vessel compression and avoidance of tissue erosion. Gastroenterology 1987;92:1101.)

ZONAL HEATING

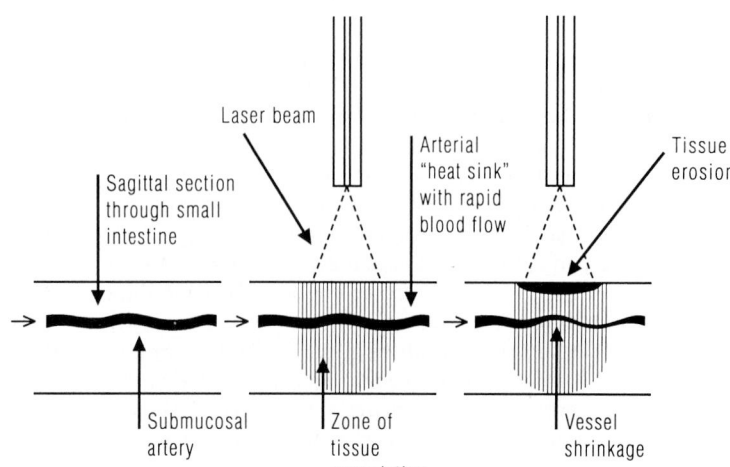

FIGURE 138-4. (See Color Fig. 117.) Zonal heating and coagulation with laser. Patent artery (*left*). En face coagulation of tissue transmurally without artery coagulation (*center*). Vessel shrinkage, tissue coagulation, and tissue erosion (*right*). (From Johnston JH, Jensen DM, Auth D. Experimental comparison of endoscopic yttrium-aluminum-garnet laser, electrosurgery, and heater probe for canine gut arterial coagulation: the importance of vessel compression and avoidance of tissue erosion. Gastroenterology 1987;92:1101.)

perforation, lack of informed consent, and an uncooperative patient for whom the examination may be impossible or dangerous. A relative contraindication for endoscopic hemostasis of nonvariceal lesions is irreversible, serve coagulopathy, especially with platelet function abnormalities.

The timing of panendoscopy for diagnosis and possible treatment varies considerably among investigators and health care systems; two extremes are exemplified by investigators in London and Los Angeles. For patients with suspected bleeding peptic ulcer disease, Swain and coworkers perform panendoscopy early, while patients are in transit from the admission area to the hospital ward.[8,9,12] We prefer to perform emergency endoscopy after resuscitation in an ICU and only for patients with evidence of continued bleeding or rebleeding because we believe that these patients are the most likely to benefit from emergency endoscopy and treatment.[1,7,10] All

other patients who stop bleeding except those with portal hypertension and suspected esophagogastric varices are examined electively in an endoscopy unit within 12 to 24 hours of admission.[10] The reported risk of emergency panendoscopy for diagnosis of UGI hemorrhage is approximately 10 times the risk of elective examination for similar patients in a large ASGE study.[3,4,6]

Specific indications for endoscopic treatment of nonvariceal lesions in the patient with clinically significant UGI hemorrhage are: control of active bleeding from ulcers, Mallory-Weiss tears, UGI angiomata, Dieulafoy's lesion,[24] and UGI tumors[25]; and prevention of rebleeding from ulcers or Dieulafoy's lesion with nonbleeding visible vessels or UGI angiomata. The rationale is that these are the patients most likely to benefit from the therapy when the outcomes, risks and costs are evaluated.

TABLE 138-4
Proposed Mechanisms of Action of Sclerosing Agents for Arterial Hemostasis*

MECHANISM	EFFECT	AGENTS
Physical		
Arterial compression	Compression of artery by adjacent solution with temporary reduction of arterial flow and resultant mucosal injury; volume dependent	All solutions
Pharmacologic		
Muscle spasm	Smooth muscle (bowel wall) spasm with temporary arterial flow reduction and mucosal injury; volume dependent	Polidocanol
Arteriolar constriction	Temporary reduction in submucosal arteriolar flow with resultant mucosal injury	Polidocanol, epinephrine
Chemical		
In situ fixation	Artery and tissue coagulation and injury; volume dependent	ETOH, TES

* Different mechanisms of action and effects of sclerosing agents for arterial hemostasis are listed, based on experimental observations.[20]

ETOH is 98% ethyl alcohol. TES is a mixture with final concentration of 1% tetradecyl sulfate, 32% ethanol, and 0.3% normal saline.

METHODS AND TECHNIQUES

Surgery

The principles of ulcer surgery for bleeding are to first control the active bleeding and then to perform an acid reducing or standard ulcer operation.[26,27] Control of bleeding is accomplished by ligation or oversewing the bleeding artery in the ulcer base. For duodenal ulcer, oversewing the bleeding site is often accompanied by pyloroplasty and truncal vagotomy. Alternatively, antrectomy and vagotomy are combined with oversewing of the duodenal ulcer bleeding site. The rebleeding rate is 5% to 10%. For a bleeding gastric ulcer partial gastric resection including removal of the ulcer without vagotomy is associated with an early rebleeding rate of less than 10%. The operative mortality of emergency ulcer surgery for bleeding depends upon the age and concomitant medical problems of the patients.[2,5,26,27] Laparoscopic surgery is a new type of therapy for the elective treatment of selected patients with recurrent duodenal ulcer hemorrhage.[28] CURE affiliated surgeons are performing posterior truncal vagotomy and highly selective arterior vagotomy after endoscopic control of duodenal ulcer bleeding. Young patients with a recurrent DU hemorrhage who have failed medical management are being considered for such therapy. Although the long-term recurrence rates of bleeding and symptomatic DU are not known, patients prefer to be considered for laparoscopic surgery because of its low morbidity and mortality.[29] Also, patients lose less time from work or usual activities with laparoscopic than open surgery.

General Endoscopic Techniques for Hemostasis

A therapeutic endoscope with two suction channels greatly facilitates diagnostic and therapeutic endoscopy for patients with severe UGI bleeding. Several commercially available video endoscopes are available with a 3.7- and 2.8-mm suction channel (Olympus) or a smaller channel (Pentax). Also, Olympus has a prototype 13-mm-diameter fiberoptic endoscope with two 3.7-mm suction channels. While a probe or catheter is in one channel, the other channel is available to suction fluid or blood. Although single channel video or fiberoptic instruments are adequate for diagnosis of active bleeders, they are often inadequate for treatment of actively bleeding nonvariceal lesions. The suction channel is blocked by the large probe and will not suction adequately during the endoscopic treatment. Therefore, the actively bleeding lesion and precise bleeding point, or both, are obscured by blood or clots.

Visualization is facilitated by suctioning excess fluid or blood from the area, positioning of the patients so that the blood flows away from the ulcer base, Dieulafoy lesion, or Mallory-Weiss tear and placing a tamponade probe at the bleeding point while suctioning the ulcer base or Mallory-Weiss tear. When clots obscure the active bleeding point, irrigating the area, changing the position of the patient, suctioning the clots, pushing them off with the probe, or, on occasion, pulling them off with a polyp grasper is necessary just before tamponade and coagulation. Blind treatment around the ulcer or nonvariceal lesion without tamponade of the bleeding point is often not effective for coagulation of active arterial bleeding.

The equipment and techniques of application are one of the most important determinants of outcome for patients with arterial bleeding who are treated with endoscopic thermal devices or injection sclerosis. These should be standardized before any prospective studies, particularly RCSs, are initiated. Lack of standardization of techniques among different investigators or endoscopists will result in variable outcomes. We have been able to train skilled endoscopists to use similar techniques for randomized hemostasis studies. This standardization has been possible through the application of different techniques under similar experimental laboratory conditions and in comparative clinical studies that have been preparatory to controlled or randomized studies.[16,30–33]

Nd:YAG Laser Coagulation

For hemostasis of bleeding ulcers, high power YAG lasers are required.[9,12,16,17,33–36] The power output from the quartz lightguides is adjustable from 0 to 120 watts. Several different commercially available instruments now feature disposable or reusable lightguides with metal tips; these can be used with standard fiberoptic or video endoscopes. Coaxial CO_2 gas under footswitch control blows away blood during treatment of actively bleeding lesions. Removal of CO_2 gas and fluid is greatly facilitated by a two channel, therapeutic endoscope. Most continuous wave, high-power (i.e., >100-watt output from the lightguide) Nd:YAG lasers are water-cooled units that require three-phase electrical outlets and high-voltage lines with high amperage. Special electrical outlets and water connections, and physically heavy Nd:YAG units combine to create a hemostasis unit that is not portable.[1]

Based upon laboratory and nonrandomized clinical results,[16,31,33] our choice of parameters for endoscopic hemostasis of active peptic ulcer, Dieulafoy's lesion, tumor, or Mallory-Weiss bleeding with Nd:YAG laser would be: high power, 75 to 85 watts; treatment distance, 1 to 2 cm; as en face as possible; short-duration coagulation pulses, 0.3 to 0.5 seconds; and removal of clots and blood via a therapeutic dual channel endoscope, irrigation, positioning, suctioning or accessories before coagulation.

The preferred pattern of coagulation with Nd:YAG laser would be to rim the actively bleeding point circumferentially in four or five areas 2 to 3 mm from the actual bleeding point, within the ulcer base, tumor, or Mallory-Weiss tear or next to be the Dieulafoy's lesion. The shots are directed by the aiming light and are fired until bleeding is controlled. The purpose of this method is to coagulate the feeding artery under the bleeding ulcer, tumor, Dieulafoy's lesion, or Mallory-Weiss tear by shrinkage, tissue edema, and activation of intrinsic arterial coagulation.[16–19,31]

After control of the active bleeding, the point is washed clean and the area of active bleeding is relocated. Withdrawal of the laser catheter to a treatment distance of 3 to 4 cm and firing several shots at the previously bleeding point is recommended by some investigators.[9,12,16,34–36] The same recommendations are followed for nonbleeding visible vessels in chronic ulcers or Dieulafoy's lesion with recent, severe UGI bleeding.[9,12,34–36]

For GI angiomata there is often thinning of the bowel wall transmurally with age or atrophy. Under controlled experimental conditions, the depth of coagulation with YAG laser is greater than other thermal methods such as argon laser, heater probe or bipolar electrocoagulation, unless the latter two are applied with very firm pressure.[16,32,33] The frequency of transmural injury is also increased with bowel distention, which reduces wall thickness.[32,33] Therefore, there is a greater risk of transmural coagulation, prolonged ulceration, or perforation with Nd:YAG laser treatment of GI angiomata.[37–41] Because of these risks, some gastroenterologists prefer to coagulate GI angiomata with thermal devices other than Nd:YAG laser. However, most endoscopists who treat gut angiomata with YAG laser recommend: lower power than treatment of bleeding ulcers (40–50 watts); short pulses (0.5–1 seconds), treatment distance of 1 to 4 cm; coagulation (whitening) of the entire angioma from the periphery to center; avoidance of vaporization or continued treatment or retreatment to the same spot; and avoidance of bowel distention during treatment.[16,31,33,37–41]

Argon Laser

For emergency hemostasis of bleeding ulcers, high power argon lasers are necessary with power outputs in the range of 8–12 watts from the lightguide.[8,16,30,33,42–44] Such units are not mobile because of their electrical requirements (i.e., three-phase, 440-V, high-amperage), their size, and the fragility of alignment. Similar to YAG lasers, flexible quartz lightguides of 200 to 400 μm are disposable or recleavable. Coaxial CO_2 gas is necessary to blow away blood from the actively bleeding ulcer prior to firing the argon laser because the blue-green wave length is absorbed by hemoglobin (Fig. 138-5; see Color Fig. 118). Treatment of overlying blood with argon laser will preclude coagulation of the underlying artery.[8,42–44] Because the argon laser units are not portable, similar to Nd:YAG lasers, patients with severe UGI bleeding who require emergency endoscopy and UGI hemostasis must be transported to the laser unit for treatment.

The specific limitations and guidelines for endoscopic treatment of bleeding ulcers by argon laser are: treatment distance of 1 to 3 cm (lightguide tip to target); coagulation (whitening) of bleeding lesions rather than vaporization (producing holes); adequate CO_2 gas backpressure at the target to visualize the bleeding point and clear away blood that oth-

erwise absorbs the argon laser energy; as en face orientation as possible; 8 to 10 watts of output from the lightguide with 10-degree full-angle of divergence; clearance of blood and clots from the bleeding target prior to treatment; and treatment directly on bleeding points and, if that is unsuccessful, coagulation immediately around the bleeding point to facilitate hemostasis.[30,33,44]

A two-channel therapeutic endoscope with standard 2.8-mm and large 3.7-mm suction channels greatly facilitates treatment by allowing simultaneous suctioning of blood, fluid, or CO_2 gas and coagulation of bleeding lesions with argon laser. Localization of the bleeding point and preparation of it for treatment (i.e., clearing it of blood and fluid and getting it in an en face position) are much more difficult than the actual endoscopic treatment. Position changes of the patient and target water irrigation of bleeding lesions are often necessary to accomplish the preparation of lesions prior to endoscopic treatment. All of these guidelines were used clinically in two controlled trials of argon laser for bleeding peptic ulcers and yielded excellent clinical results.[8,44] Similar guidelines are used for treatment of bleeding Mallory-Weiss tears.[42,44]

For any thermal method, including argon laser, a significantly lower amount of thermal energy is required for coagulation of gut angiomata than bleeding ulcers. General guidelines for argon laser treatment of UGI angiomata are power setting of 5 to 7 watts, treatment distance of 1 to 4 cm, and avoidance of gut distention.[33,37,38,45,46] Coagulation of the entire angioma rather than erosion or vaporization is the immediate goal of endoscopic treatment. Because the blue-green wavelength is absorbed by hemoglobin[8,30,33] or red color, the endoscopist must wash away overlying blood or clots before treatment in order to coagulate the mucosal or submucosal angiomata. Coagulation from the periphery of the angioma toward the center is recommended.[37,45,46] When angiomata are tangential with a forward viewing endoscope, a side-viewing or oblique-viewing endoscope will facilitate coagulation of bleeding or nonbleeding UGI angioma.[37,45,46]

Monopolar Electrocoagulation

For successful endoscopic hemostasis of bleeding ulcers, monopolar electrocoagulation (MPEC) standard probes, modified probes, or the hydrothermal probe all require more skill than any other thermal modality. Also, efficacy and tissue damage are much less predictable and controllable. An analog computer does not alter patterns of tissue injury nor increase ease of endoscopic use.[47] Monopolar probes often stick to the tissue during coagulation. Pulling the probe away from the lesion after coagulation can cause rebleeding at the site.[1,7,16,32,33] Although constant water or saline irrigation facilitates visualization of the bleeding points, tissue coagulation and hemostasis may be more difficult.[33,48,49]

Nevertheless, experienced endoscopists have reported good to excellent results of MPEC for emergency hemostasis of nonvariceal UGI lesions.[49–55] Specific guidelines for endoscopic MPEC are: as en face as possible, although some tangential treatment is possible with newer probes; 50 to 100 watts/pulse; short, 0.5-second pulses; target washing to identify the exact bleeding points, tamponade of these, and target coagulation; simultaneous suctioning of blood and ir-

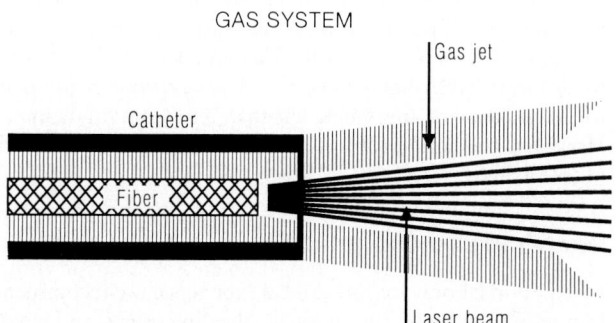

GAS SYSTEM

FIGURE 138-5. (See Color Fig. 118.) Laser catheter with coaxial CO_2 gas around a central quartz light guide. (Courtesy of Charles Enderby, Ph.D., Mountainview, CA.)

rigation solution; and a two-channel endoscope rather than a single-channel therapeutic endoscope, especially if the liquid probe is used.[48,49]

When specific guidelines are used with MPEC, efficacy for ulcer treatment is good to excellent.[49-55] Although some tamponade is possible at endoscopy with monopolar coagulation, ulcers with high bleeding rates and those tangentially oriented are difficult to control and tissue damage may be extensive.[32,33,48] MPEC is also more difficult to use than the newer commercially available thermal probes such as BICAP and heater probe.

MPEC is not extensively used for coagulation of UGI angiomata. The real or perceived increased risk of transmural injury and the availability of newer and safer devices such as bipolar electrocoagulation or heater probe have limited the use of MPEC for UGI angioma hemostasis.

Bipolar or Multipolar Electrocoagulation

For chronic ulcers with major stigmata, we recommend firm tamponade directly on the visible vessel with a 3.2 mm probe, suctioning of excess blood and fluid, and coagulation with 5- to 10-second pulses with a power setting of 4 to 5 watts on a 50-watt generator. Repositioning and recoagulation is performed until hemostasis occurs and the visible vessel is flattened (Figs. 138-6 and 138-7; see Color Figs. 119 and 120).[1,7,16,32,33,56-59] These guidelines are similar to the techniques of Laine in his clinical trials.[60,61] For bleeding Mallory-Weiss tears, the active bleeder is moderately tamponaded and three, 1-second pulses are delivered before changing probe position. Coagulation with the side of the probe (i.e., tangentially) is at least as effective as en face coagulation.[62] Tamponade with the newer Gold probe is more effective than the BICAP probe because the Gold probe is more rigid.[59] This

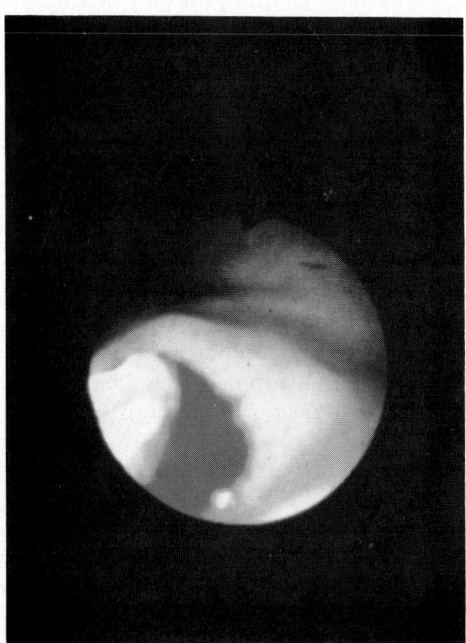

FIGURE 138-6. (See Color Fig. 119.) BICAP treatment of a bleeding ulcer. Tamponade of the ulcer is performed with the large probe in a tangential approach.

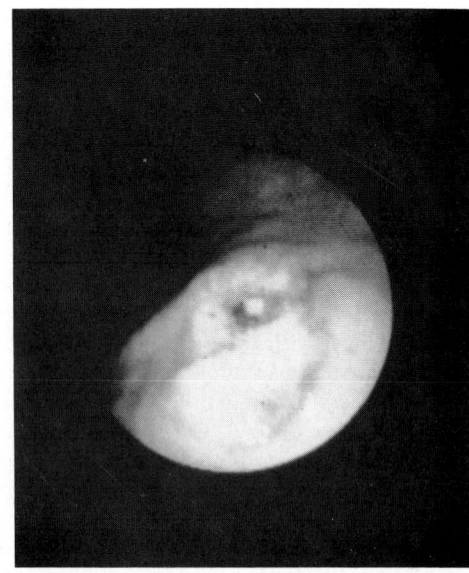

FIGURE 138-7. (See Color Fig. 120.) A coagulated vessel in an ulcer crater is seen after BICAP (Circon ACMI, Stamford, CT) coagulation of an actively bleeding ulcer (see Fig. 138-6).

difference is significant for tangential treatment of bleeding ulcers via endoscopy.[63]

For bleeding ulcers, the large probes with 3.2-mm diameters have several advantages over small probes with 2.4-mm diameters: tamponade is more effective because of the stiffness of the BICAP probe, washing is more efficient, and the coagulation volume zone is greater.[33] The disadvantage is that large-channel endoscopes with suction channels 3.5 to 3.7 mm in diameter are required for treatment, but these may not be available in all hospitals.

Whereas firm tamponade may be necessary for endoscopic artery coaptation and successful coagulation of bleeding peptic ulcers, this technique should not be applied to angiomata which are associated with reduced bowel wall thickness. Power settings of multipolar probes for treatment of UGI angiomata should be lower than for ulcers because of the risk of transmural coagulation.[33] In experimental studies, the transmural thickness of the normal canine stomach uninflated is 4 to 5 mm, whereas the duodenum and jejunum are 3 to 4 mm.[33] In comparison, elderly patients with chronic diseases insufflated during endoscopy may have transmural thickness of 2 to 3 mm or less in the UGI tract. For treatment of UGI angiomata with bipolar electrocoagulation, we recommend a power setting of 2 to 3 on the dial and 1-second pulses for the 50 watt BICAP generator.[33,37] A small probe is adequate for coagulation of angiomata less than 3 to 4 mm in diameter. However, the large probe is recommended for larger lesions (Table 138-5).[33,37,39]

Heater Probe Coagulation

Based upon laboratory and clinical experience, we recommend firm tamponade of the actively bleeding ulcer and coagulation with four, 30-J pulses before repositioning the probe.[16,33,57,62,64,65] Firm tamponade and coagulation are feasible with both the tip (en face) and the side (tangential) of

TABLE 138-5
Endoscopic Technical Parameters for Heater Probe and Bipolar Electrocoagulation Endoscopic Lesions and Stigmata*

	PEPTIC ULCER		MALLORY-WEISS TEAR	DIEULAFOY'S LESION		UPPER GASTROINTESTINAL ANGIOMA	
	Active Bleeding	Nonbleeding Visible Vessel	Active Bleeding	Active Bleeding	Nonbleeding Visible Vessel	Active Bleeding	Nonbleeding Visible Vessel
Heater Probe							
Probe size†‡	Large	Large	Large or small	Large	Large	Large versus small	Large versus small
Pressure§	Very firm	Very firm	Moderate	Firm	Firm	Moderate	Light
Power setting (J)	30	30	20	30	30	15	15
Number of pulses per tamponade station‖	4	4	3	4	4	2–3	2
End point	Bleeding stops	Visible vessel flattened and white	Bleeding stops	Bleeding stops	Visible vessel flattened and white	Bleeding stops	Lesion white
Bipolar Coagulation (Bicap or Gold Probe)							
Probe size†‡	Large	Large	Large or small	Large	Large	Large versus small	Large versus small
Pressure§	Very firm	Very firm	Moderate	Firm	Firm	Moderate	Light
Power setting							
BICAP I	3	3	3	3	3	2	2
BICAP II (watts)	20	20	20	20	20	15	15
Pulse duration per tamponade station (sec)‖	10	10	4	10	10	2	2
End point	Bleeding stops	Visible vessel flat	Bleeding stops	Bleeding stops	Visible vessel flat	Bleeding stops	Visible vessel flat

* These are general guidelines that have been standardized from CURE laboratory and randomized endoscopic studies.[1,7,20,24,25,32,33,37,39,46,56–59,62–65,75,78,93,98] Power, pressure, and power duration settings must be reduced for small, acute, or very deep upper gastrointestinal bleeding lesions. The CURE Hemostasis Research Group recommends checking probes prior to endoscopic application and resuscitation of the patient before and during endoscopy. Surgical consultation on all patients with severe upper gastrointestinal hemorrhage is recommended before endoscopic coagulation. If endoscopic therapy fails to control active bleeding or prevent rebleeding, continued resuscitation of the patient and gastrointestinal surgery are recommended.

† Single or double large-channel endoscopes are recommended for all emergency panendoscopies for severe upper gastrointestinal hemorrhage. Large-diameter thermal probes (~3.2 mm in diameter) are recommended for all nonvariceal bleeding lesions or nonbleeding visible vessels except for small arteries (spurts) in Mallory-Weiss tears (<0.5 mm in diameter) or small upper gastrointestinal angiomata (<3 mm in diameter).

‡ Small endoscopic thermal probes (~2.4 mm in diameter) have less tamponade capability, washing capacity, and volume of coagulation than large probes and are only recommended with coagulation through large-channel endoscopes for small Mallory-Weiss tear spurts (<0.5 mm, stream) or small upper gastrointestinal angiomata (<3 mm diameter).

§ Pressure refers to the tamponade pressure exerted en face or tangentially by way of the contract probe, directly on the bleeding lesion or nonbleeding visible vessel. Sufficient pressure to stop the bleeding before coagulation is recommended for those with active bleeding.

‖ Pulses per tamponade station are the number of coagulation pulses applied to the bleeding point after tamponade before changing the probe position. The pulse duration is set on the power unit for bipolar electrocoagulation, but pulse duration depends on the power setting and probe size for the heater probe.

the heater probe catheter. Large, 3.2-mm-diameter probes are recommended. Suctioning of pooled water and blood from the area of treatment facilitates effective hemostasis. For severe actively bleeding ulcers a two channel therapeutic endoscope will be necessary for simultaneous coagulation and suctioning. Similar guidelines are recommended for treatment of patients with actively bleeding UGI tumors[25] or Dieulafoy's lesion[24] and patient with recent, severe, UGI hemorrhage and a non-bleeding visible vessel in a chronic ulcer or Dieulafoy's lesion on endoscopy.

For Mallory-Weiss tears, the arteries are often small, less than 1 mm, and the thickness of the esophageal wall is reduced.[65] We recommend moderate tamponade with application of 20-J pulses before repositioning the probe.[33,62,65] For telangiectasia or angioma, a lower setting (5–10 J) and light contact pressure rather than firm tamponade are recommended.[33,37,45] This relates to the thinness of the bowel wall with angioma in contrast to the thickened wall with most chronic ulcers (see Table 138-5).

Injection Coagulation

Most investigators inject ulcers with commercially available disposable sclerotherapy catheters with retractable needles through single channel, small endoscopes. For injection sclerosis of bleeding ulcers, we prefer a disposable, small-diameter (1.8–2.0 mm) sclerotherapy catheter with 25- or 26-gauge needle that protrudes 4 to 5 mm from the tip and a therapeutic endoscope with either one or two large channels. Even with a single channel therapeutic endoscopic (3.7-mm-diameter biopsy channel), suctioning of fluid is possible during treatment because the catheter has such a small diameter.

The purpose of sclerotherapy of bleeding ulcers, Dieulafoy's lesion, UGI tumors, or Mallory-Weiss tears is to control active bleeding or prevent rebleeding. Most investigators inject 1 to 3 mm circumferentially around the bleeding point in four to six areas to raise an edema cuff and compress the bleeding vessel (see Fig. 138-2; see Color Fig. 115). Lesions that are inaccessible or tangential to an end viewing therapeutic endoscope may be difficult or impossible to inject. However, injections that are given submucosally immediately behind the bleeding site with a large volume of solution may bring the lesion into view for en face treatment.[66] For ulcers, tumors, Dieulafoy's lesion or Mallory-Weiss tears which are too tangential for injection, two other options are possible: use of heater probe or bipolar electrocoagulation, because these coagulate well tangentially; or select a different endoscope (i.e., side-viewing or smaller caliber) which may afford en face treatment. For example, Lin and coworkers reported that bleeding ulcers high on the lesser curvature of the stomach or in the superior duodenal bulb were tangential and significantly more difficult to treat and control with injection than heater probe coagulation.[67]

As with sclerosing agents for esophageal varices, the choice of agents for bleeding ulcers or nonbleeding visible vessels by most investigators remains empirical.[20,21] Agents which have been reported to be effective are dilute epinephrine (1:10,000–1:20,000) in saline,[20,21,66–69] ethyl alcohol,[22,67,70,71] polidocanol,[69] other variceal sclerosing agents,[20] hypertonic saline,[72] thrombin,[73] or various combinations of these.[69,74,75] Very few randomized clinical studies have compared efficacy

and safety of agents. Whereas many agents appear effective clinically, the injury patterns for peptic ulcer injection are unknown. Randall and colleagues of CURE reported a controlled study of different sclerosing agents for coagulation of canine gut arteries.[20]

Based upon those experimental data and the proposed mechanism of action of sclerosing agents for arterial hemostasis (see Table 138-4), we have chosen sequential injection treatment. Dilute epinephrine (1:20,000) in normal saline is injected in and around the active bleeding point as described above. As a single treatment, the total volume has not been limited for bleeding ulcers, Dieulafoy's lesion, UGI tumors, or Mallory-Weiss tears yet more than 90% can be controlled with 20 cc or less injected. The mechanism of action appears to be compression of the artery by the solution. The epinephrine reduces the back bleeding commonly seen with multiple injections in and around the bleeding site. After controlling the active bleeding, or for prevention of rebleeding in the ulcer with the nonbleeding visible vessel after one major UGI hemorrhage, 0.1 to 0.2 mL aliquots of ethanol are injected to cause chemical in situ fixation (see Table 138-4) and coagulation of the underlying artery.[20,21] Volumes of ethanol greater than 1 to 2 mL increase the risk of extensive tissue damage.[20,67,71,72] In our experience, initial efficacy of injection of ulcers with active bleeding has been good and with nonbleeding visible vessels has been excellent. We had one perforation from alcohol injection of a patient with an adherent clot on an ulcer and an underlying visible vessel, as part of a randomized, controlled multicenter study.[75]

Retreatment is recommended by some endoscopists. Chung and colleagues endoscoped all patients 24 hours after initial sclerosis and empirically retreated all ulcers which had endoscopic evidence of further bleeding with epinephrine.[68] Others have retreated with repeat injection after patients had clinical evidence of significant rebleeding.[66,69,70] There are no clinical prospective studies which describe the comparative healing rates of injected versus noninjected ulcers, nor histopathologic effects of different sclerosing agents on the artery or associated tissues, although these effects have been studied in dogs.[21]

Microwave Coagulation

Endoscopic microwave coagulation has been evaluated in laboratory[76] and randomized comparative studies for hemostasis of bleeding ulcers.[77] A 1-magnetron generator for endoscopic use produces microwaves of 2450 MHz in frequency and 12 cm in wave length.[76,77] Although a coaxial cable was used to transmit microwave energy through the biopsy channel of an endoscope in Japan, microwave coagulation has not been as extensively studied or applied endoscopically in other countries as other thermal devices. However, the safety and efficacy have been reported to be similar to injection, heater probe, or bipolar electrocoagulation in comparative studies.[76,77]

The guidelines for endoscopic use in patients with bleeding ulcers, nonbleeding visible vessels, oozing ulcers, or ulcers with adherent clots were: use of a 2.4-mm-diameter Teflon-coated coaxial cable with a 3- × 1-mm needle; 40 watts of output for 10 seconds using an automatic timer; use of six 10-second pulses of microwaves; after coagulation, use of a dissociation device producing 16 to 20 mA of direct current for 5 seconds, which reduces sticking.[77] In one randomized study of 127 ulcer patients with different stigmata of hemorrhage, there were no significant differences in effectiveness or safety between endoscopic injection and microwave coagulation.[77]

Combination Injection and Thermal Coagulation

In a recent survey of endoscopists by the author, 65% used combination epinephrine injection and then thermal coagulation with either heater probe or bipolar electrocoagulation for hemostasis of actively bleeding ulcers.[78] However, there are very few data about combination endoscopic therapy for bleeding, nonvariceal lesions. Also, utilization of separate injectors and thermal coagulation probes adds to the cost and perhaps the endoscopy time. Rutgeerts suggested that preinjection with epinephrine improved the primary hemostasis rates of actively bleeding ulcers with Nd:YAG laser and BICAP in one small study.[79] But this was relative to historical controls. There are no data on combination treatments such as epinephrine injection and thermal coagulation for nonbleeding visible vessels or adherent clots on ulcers. Nevertheless, there are some theoretical advantages for combining treatments such as injection and thermal coagulation which have different mechanisms of action. An injector-Gold probe was recently developed which combines a retractable needle with a bipolar probe. In laboratory studies of bleeding ulcers, the injector-Gold probe was more convenient and faster for ulcer hemostasis than separate injectors and thermal probes.[78] The efficacy was excellent. Further prospective, comparative clinical studies are warranted to evaluate whether combination therapy is superior to injection or thermal treatment alone for control of active bleeding or prevention of rebleeding for bleeding nonvariceal lesions.

CLINICAL RESULTS AND COSTS

This chapter provides a review of and discusses RCSs and prospective randomized studies. These types of studies eliminate bias and allow the reader to interpret the trials in light of a control group, which characteristically has routine medical or surgical management. There are remarkable regional differences in outcomes independent of treatment. An example is the continued bleeding rates for ulcers found on initial endoscopy to be actively bleeding. For CURE studies 88% to 93% of patients with active arterial ulcer bleeding on initial endoscopy had continued bleeding,[1,44,57,62,64] whereas with medical treatment for the Swain studies[8,9,12] the rate was 70.6% (see Table 138-2) and in a Hong Kong study of sclerotherapy 41% of patients continued bleeding with medical treatment.[68]

An enormous number of variables make interpretation or extrapolation of hemostasis results for ulcer bleeding extremely difficult. One is the definition of active ulcer bleeding. In the CURE study, this was active arterial bleeding, which accounted for less than 10% rate of permanent hemostasis on medical management.[1,44,57,62,64] The Hong Kong study included nearly 80% of patients with oozing bleeding without

visible vessels or clots whose rate of hemostasis on medical therapy was 73%.[68] Another reason for difference among studies is the variability of the control group. Some other common problems are the small size of many studies, the lack of blinding for further medical-surgical management after randomization, the failure to standardize the endoscopic technique of hemostasis before initiation of the study, the failure to stratify or balance important baseline variables (e.g., age of the patients, surgical risk, endoscopic stigmata) that influence outcomes independent of treatment, and patients' selection relative to the clinical severity of the UGI bleeding.

Hemostasis of Bleeding Ulcers

Nd:YAG Laser Coagulation

Several randomized, controlled studies with YAG laser have been reported from different countries.[9,12,79–86] Four of the eight randomized, prospective studies have reported statistically significant reductions in rebleeding,[9,12,83,84,86] need for emergency ulcer surgery,[9,84,86] transfusion requirement[9,12,86] or mortality.[9] The other four did not report such significant differences between medical and YAG laser treated patients.[80–82,85]

The different entry criteria, techniques, and type of stigmata included may reconcile some of these different results. Reports by Ihre,[80] Escourrou[81] and Rohde[82] were negative studies; they randomized patients with severe UGI bleeding without first determining accessibility of the bleeding ulcer to Nd:YAG laser treatment. This may have significantly influenced subsequent outcome. For example, in the Ihre trial,[80] 23 patients were randomized to Nd:YAG laser treatment but in 8 the laser treatment was not possible because of poor access or other technical reasons.

Patients who were severely ill were excluded from entry in the Krejs study because they could not be transported to the laser unit.[85] The majority of patients randomized had nonbleeding visible vessels or minor stigmata of recent hemorrhage such as clots or flat spots (total, 140 patients), rather than active arterial bleeding (36 patients). For all patients randomized or for the subgroups of active bleeding or nonbleeding visible vessels, there were no significant differences in outcomes (i.e., rebleeding, emergency surgery, or mortality). These patients had a low risk for rebleeding with medical treatment. The rate of continued bleeding in the active bleeding subgroup was 31% and the rebleeding with other stigmata was 18%. Krejs and coworkers reported four major complications of Nd:YAG laser treatment. Precipitation of uncontrollable major hemorrhage requiring surgery was the most dramatically related to Nd:YAG laser photocoagulation. It is not known if standardization of laser techniques or more experience would have altered the results of the Dallas Nd:YAG laser study by Kriejs.

Rutgeerts and coworkers randomized patients with oozing bleeding from ulcers or other nonbleeding stigmata (i.e., visible vessels or adherent clot) into a YAG laser versus medical therapy.[83] Patients with spurting bleeding were excluded from randomization. There was a significant difference in the control of oozing bleeding of Nd:YAG laser (100% of 38 patients) versus medical treatment (78% hemostasis in 32 patients) for the subgroup of oozing ulcers. However, there were no significant differences in bleeding recurrence, emergency operation, or mortality for either oozing bleeding or the clot–visible vessel ulcer subgroups. One might argue that the patients most likely to benefit from Nd:YAG laser treatment, the active arterial bleeders, were excluded from randomization and this may have influenced results.

Rutgeerts also randomized Mallory-Weiss tears or erosions with oozing bleeding or clot–visible vessels. For the 12 controls, the rebleeding rate (20%) did not significantly differ from the Nd:YAG laser group (9%) of 11 patients. The rates of operation and mortality also did not differ significantly. Similar to the ulcer control groups of Rutgeerts, the risk of rebleeding was much too low to expect a significant benefit of Nd:YAG laser treatment. No major complications were reported of Nd:YAG laser treatment.

The largest randomized, controlled Nd:YAG laser study for severe ulcer bleeding was reported by Swain and coworkers.[9] Sixty-one gastric and 62 duodenal ulcers with stigmata of recent hemorrhage accessible to endoscopic treatment were randomized (Table 138-6). They reported significant reductions in rebleeding rate, need for emergency surgery, and mortality in ulcer patients with stigmata of recent hemorrhage accessible to laser treatment. Four nonbleeding visible vessel patients (16%) bled during Nd:YAG laser treatment but all could be controlled with further laser treatment. No perforations occurred in laser treated patients.

In this Swain study, the patients with major stigmata benefitted significantly. For the spurting subgroup, rebleeding was significantly reduced (2 of 10 treated versus 7 of 9 medical). The nonbleeding visible vessels represented the largest subgroup with significant rebleeding reduction (4 of 35 treated versus 21 of 38 medical). In the subgroup with overlying clot, there were few rebleeds (1 of 11 laser versus 2 of 11 medical) and no benefit of treatment. For other stigmata (e.g., spots, slough), few medical patients rebled and there was no benefit of treatment (rebleeding in 0 of 16 laser versus 1 of 12 medical). This study is as important from the prognostic point of view (i.e., significance of various stigmata of recent hemorrhage on initial diagnostic endoscopy) as it is from the therapeutic standpoint. The Nd:YAG laser significantly benefitted only patients with major stigmata of hemorrhage.

Argon Laser Coagulation

Three RCSs of argon laser for hemostasis of severe ulcer bleeding have been reported.[8,42-44] The first study was performed in Barcelona where patients with major and minor

TABLE 138-6
Laser Versus Medical Treatment in Ulcer Patients With Stigmata of Recent Hemorrhage

	MEDICAL	LASER
Total number of patients	61	62
Rebleeding (%)	39	8*
Emergencey surgery (%)	31	8*
Mortality (%)	13	1.6*

* P < 0.05.

Data from Swain CP, Kirkham JS, Salmon PR, Brown SG, Northfield TC. Controlled trial of Nd-YAG laser photocoagulation in bleeding peptic ulcers. Lancet 1 1986;8490:1113.

stigmata of recent hemorrhage were randomized to argon laser or medical management.[43] There were no significant differences between treatments in any outcomes—rebleeding rates, emergency surgery or mortality—for subgroups or all laser versus all medical patients. For the 15 spurters treated with laser the continued bleeding rate was 33% which did not significantly differ from the 13 medical patients whose rate was 69%. Rebleeding rates were 20% laser and 50% medical. Urgent surgery rates for the spurters were 53% laser and 69% medical. The rebleeding rates for the 19 nonbleeding visible vessel patients was 42% and the 16 medical patients was 50%. The 73 medical patients with nonbleeding spots had a low risk of rebleeding (12%) and no differences were evident after argon laser treatment.

There are three major criticisms of this study which may have influenced outcomes: inaccessibility to laser treatment, which was assessed before randomization, was not an exclusion; the primary hemostasis rates for active bleeders were low and rebleeding rates for all ulcers treated were high relative to other argon laser studies,[8,42-44] suggesting lack of standardization of treatment or inexperience with argon laser treatment of the therapeutic endoscopists; and inclusion of a large group with minor stigmata (73 patients) at low risk for rebleeding and fewer patients with major stigmata (63 patients).

In Swain's RCS using the argon laser,[8] 76 patients were stratified by major and minor stigmata of recent hemorrhage similar to their Nd:YAG laser study previously discussed.[9] All the problems of the Barcelona argon laser were obviated in this study: accessibility, standardization of treatment, experience with lasers, and adequate numbers of high risk patients. Thirty-nine gastric, 33 duodenal, and 4 stomal ulcers accessible to laser treatment were randomized. The study included 11 patients with arterial bleeding, 41 with nonbleeding visible vessel, 7 with overlying clot, and 17 with flat spots or slough.

There was a significant difference in mortality for all laser versus medical groups treated. However, all the deaths and 89% of the rebleeds (25 of 28) occurred in patients with major stigmata. Rebleeding rates in the argon laser treated ulcers were significantly less than medical patients with nonbleeding visible vessels (4 of 17 laser versus 13 of 24 medical) and the combined bleeding and nonbleeding visible vessel subgroups (8 of 24 laser versus 17 of 28 medical). As a major complication, precipitation of uncontrollable bleeding during argon laser treatment occurred in 12% of patients (2 of 17) with nonbleeding visible vessels. Both patients required emergency surgery.

Argon laser significantly reduced mortality from bleeding peptic ulcers accessible to laser treatment.[8] However, it is difficult to explain why 7 of 19 medical patients who rebled died whereas there were no deaths among the 8 laser-treated patients who rebled. Attempts to identify bias between the two groups suggested that they were well matched for other factors known to affect mortality rate such as age, hypotension on admission, initial hemoglobin level, and number of gastric versus duodenal ulcers.[2,8]

In a smaller controlled trial of spurting ulcer bleeding and nonbleeding visible vessels with one prior rebleed, the CURE group reported significant differences in outcomes for argon laser treated patients.[42,44] For argon laser treated patients vs. medical patients, the results were: further significant hemorrhage in 29% (2 of 7) [versus 78% (7 of 9)], mean units of

RBC transfused after randomization, 1.3 (versus 6.8); emergency surgery for hemostasis, 0% (versus 56%); major complications, 0% (versus 22%); and mortality, 0% (versus 11%). The mean direct cost of care was $6850 for the argon laser patients and $12,342 for the medical-surgical patients. Using a graded score of outcome criteria, there was a significant difference between argon laser and medical groups.[42,44]

Despite the significant differences in some studies of argon or Nd:YAG lasers, Brunetaud and Jensen predicted that the limitations of high-powered lasers for emergency hemostasis (e.g., lack of portability, expense of equipment, requirement of technical support, inability to treat lesions tangentially, inability to tamponade effectively even with special tips) would limit their use to a small fraction of all patients with ulcer hemorrhage.[42]

Monopolar Electrocoagulation

Three controlled trials of liquid or dry MPEC were reported from different countries.[49,51,55] In Michigan, Papp randomized 32 patients with severe UGI hemorrhage and nonbleeding visible vessels in ulcers to dry MPEC or medical treatment.[51] Both gastric (17 total) and duodenal ulcers (15 total) were included. Eighty-one percent of the medical patients rebled and of these, 56% had emergency surgery and 25% were coagulated with MPEC. This is a very high rate of rebleeding for nonbleeding visible vessel patients. Papp reported significant differences in rebleeding rates for dry MPEC versus medical groups (6% versus 81%), the need for emergency surgery (6% versus 65%), as well as the direct cost ($3157 versus $4732) and length of hospitalization (8.3 versus 15.3 days). There was one death in the medical group (6%) and non in the dry MPEC group. No complications occurred.

Freitas and coworkers of Portugal randomized 78 patients with active bleeding (21 patients) or stigmata of recent hemorrhage (57 patients) to liquid MPEC versus medical therapy.[49] Patients with either spurting bleeding (6 patients) or oozing bleeding (15 patients) were randomized. There were no significant differences in outcomes in this subgroup of patients with a high risk for rebleeding. Nor was there any benefit for patients with central flat spots who had a low risk of rebleeding (0 of 11 MPEC versus 2 of 15 medical). Only in the subgroup of nonbleeding visible vessels was there a significant benefit of MPEC in rebleeding rates (21% versus 53%) and need for emergency surgery (14% versus 47%). No complications occurred from therapy. This RCT confirms the results of Papp for nonbleeding visible vessel treatment with MPEC.

Moreto and coworkers of Spain randomized patients with bleeding gastric ulcers to treatment with liquid monopolar coagulation or medical management.[55] Thirty-seven patients with visible vessels either spurting bleeding (12 patients) or nonspurting bleeding (25 patients) in either gastric (81%) or stomal ulcers (19%) were included. For the small subgroup of spurting visible vessel patients (12 total), there was a significant reduction in rebleeding (0 of 6 MPEC versus 6 of 6 medical therapy) but no difference in mortality (1 of 6 MPEC versus 2 of 6 medical). For the nonspurting visible vessel group, there were no significant differences in rebleeding (1 of 10 MPEC versus 5 of 15 medical) or mortality (0 of 10 MPEC versus 1 of 15 medical).

When the authors analyzed all the MPEC-treated versus medical patients together, they reported significant differences in rebleeding (1 of 16 MPEC versus 11 of 21 medical), emergency surgery (0 of 16 MPEC versus 8 of 21 medical), and postendoscopy transfusion requirements (1.6 units MPEC versus 3.4 units medical). Most of the statistical benefit seemed to result from the small, spurting subgroup treated with MPEC rather than the larger nonspurting subgroup. There were no complications of the MPEC. Limitations of this study are exclusion of all duodenal ulcers, exclusion of deep gastric ulcers or those with large visible vessels, exclusion of two patients randomized in the study, inability to coagulate tangentially with the MPEC probe and frequent utilization of side-viewing endoscope to get en face, and failure to clarify the subgroup of nonspurting visible vessels. For the patients analyzed, only the spurting bleeders appeared to benefit significantly from MPEC. This result contrasted to the other two RCT of MPEC, which reported an improvement only for the nonbleeding visible vessel subgroup.[49,51]

Bipolar Electrocoagulation

Several RCSs from different countries have been reported with differing results with BICAP. Three showed a significant benefit[57,60,61] of BICAP compared to medical treatment, and four others did not.[87–90] In two recent studies from Los Angeles, Laine reported that BICAP was safe and effective for control of active ulcer bleeding[60] and prevention of rebleeding for nonbleeding visible vessels in ulcers.[61] The large probe was used in these studies which included hospitalized patients with severe UGI bleeding. Similar techniques were applied via endoscopy. A mean of at least 40 seconds of electrocoagulation per ulcer was used in both studies at a dial setting of 5 or 6 on a 50-watt generator. Patients with actively bleeding lesions (ulcer 24, Mallory-Weiss tear 17, angiomas 3) were randomized to treatment with BICAP or medical treatment without endoscopic treatment. The patients with significant rebleeding had urgent surgery. BICAP significantly reduced postrandomization RBC transfusions (6.4 versus 2.4 units), emergency surgery rates (57% versus 14%), hospital days (7.2 versus 4.4 days), and direct costs ($7,550 versus $3,420) but did not significantly change mortality (13% versus 0%).

Patients with nonbleeding visible vessels in ulcers were randomized by Laine in another USC study (Table 138-7).[61] There were significant improvements with BICAP treatment in rebleeding rates, RBC transfused after randomization, need for emergency surgery, hospital days, and direct costs.[61] No major complications occurred.

O'Brien, using a small BICAP probe, improved rebleeding rates in some patients in a RCS.[87] Patients were stratified based upon initial stigmata as active bleeding from a visible vessel, nonbleeding visible vessel or adherent clot. In comparison to medical therapy, significantly fewer BICAP patients rebled (17% BICAP versus 33% medical). However, BICAP treatment did not reduce emergency surgery or mortality rates and did not benefit patients with adherent clot.

Three other RCSs from the United Kingdom did not demonstrate a positive effect of BICAP coagulation compared to medical treatment.[88–90] Major problems with these studies included inclusion of many patients with minor stigmata in all three of the studies, lack of standardization of entry criteria and endoscopic hemostasis techniques, use of the small (2.4-mm-diameter) probe rather than the large (3.2-mm) probe in

TABLE 138-7
Medical Versus Bicap Treatment for Nonbleeding Visible Vessels

	MEDICAL	BICAP
Number of patients	37	38
Rate of rebleeding (%)	41	18*
Number of patients receiving red blood cell transfusions	3.0	1.6*
Emergency surgery (%)	30	8*
Number of hopsital days	6.2	4.3*
Direct cost (U.S. $)	5630	3790
Mortality (%)	0	3

Post-randomization outcomes are for patients with nonbleeding visible vessels. Means or rates are shown.

* P < 0.05.

Data from Laire L. Multipolar electrocoagulation in the treatment of peptic ulcers with nonbleeding visible vessels: a prospective controlled trial. Ann Int Med 1989;110:510.

two studies, and application of less total BICAP energy than the USC studies and often at higher dial settings. It is likely that the study design and technical issues related to the different outcome with BICAP than in the USC studies. Laine standardized his protocol and endoscopic hemostasis techniques. Furthermore, he singlehandedly performed all the randomizations and treatments in his studies.

Heater Probe Coagulation

Three RCSs of heater probe from different countries were reported.[12,57,64,91] Two reported significant benefits of heater probe[64,91] and one did not.[12] Matthewson and coworkers reported a study of heater probe versus Nd:YAG laser versus standard medical-surgical management of patients with severe ulcer bleeding.[12] In this study, 143 consecutive patients with stigmata of recent hemorrhage accessible to endoscopic diagnosis and treatment were randomized. At the time of initial endoscopy, patients were stratified for active bleeding, nonbleeding visible vessel, overlying clot, and red or black spots and randomized to Nd:YAG laser treatment (44 patients), heater probe coagulation (57 patients), and control–no endoscopic treatment (42 patients). In their initial report, the authors analyzed all patients together with major or minor stigmata by different treatments.[12] For all treatments of minor and major stigmata, they reported that YAG laser was associated with a lower frequency of rebleeding than control (20% versus 42%) whereas heater probe was not (28% heater probe versus 42% control).

For the subgroups of patients with major or minor stigmata, there were no significant differences in outcomes with the different treatments. The rebleeding rates for the 31 Nd:YAG patients with major stigmata was 26% compared to 33% for the 42 heater probe patients or 47% for the 32 medical patients.[12] Nor were there significant differences for the 38 patients with minor stigmata of recent hemorrhage in rebleeding rates: heater probe 13%, Nd:YAG laser 8% and medical 30%.

There was one ulcer perforation among the heater probe treated patients. For Nd:YAG laser, bleeding was precipitated

during treatment of about 20% of the nonbleeding stigmata such as nonbleeding visible vessels or flat spots. In every case the authors were able to control the active bleeding by further Nd:YAG laser treatment with no perforations. They did not investigate ulcer healing rates for any of the treatment groups.

Heater probe significantly lowered rebleeding rates in a study of 43 patients in Scotland with either active ulcer bleeding or nonbleeding visible vessels.[91] Twenty patients were treated with heater probe and 23 with medical therapy. No mortality occurred in either medical or heater probe patients.

In a large study in Los Angeles, patients with active spurting bleeding (47 total) or nonbleeding visible vessels (78 total) were randomized to either heater probe, BICAP, or medical-surgical therapy.[57,62,64] Initial hemostasis rates with heater probe and BICAP for spurting bleeding were 93% to 95%, compared with 14% for the medical group. Yet, only the heater probe subgroup benefitted with significant reductions in postrandomization bleeding, units of RBC transfused, mean ICU days, and emergency surgery rates compared to medical patients.[57,64] For the subgroup with nonbleeding visible vessels, heater probe treatment significantly decreased postrandomization rates of rebleeding, red cell transfusion and emergency surgery. No major complications of heater probe or BICAP occurred. CURE investigators observed that both heater probe and BICAP were a significant advance over lasers for emergency hemostasis because of portability, tamponade capability permitting coaptation coagulation, ability to coagulate tangentially, washing capacity, efficacy and expense.[1,7,44,62,64]

Standardization of the endoscopic treatment parameters such as probe size, tamponade pressure, site of application, and total energy applied may have influenced results of these heater probe studies as much as inclusion of high risk patients, experience and skill of the endoscopists, and size of the study.[57,62,64] For example, Matthewson and coworkers effected coagulation around the bleeding site or stigmata first with firm pressure whereas CURE investigators treated directly on the visible vessel or active bleeding site after very firm tamponade. The small probe was used in 26% of Matthewson's cases and less than 5% of CURE patients. The joules per tamponade station varied from 60 to 90 J in London to 120 to 150 J in Los Angeles. These technical differences may account for some of the treatment results, especially with contact probes such as heater probe or BICAP.[1,7,16,32,33,62,64]

Injection Sclerosis

Several randomized, prospective trials of injection compared with other treatments have been reported. Chung and colleagues of Hong Kong recently reported a RCS of sclerotherapy for patients admitted with actively bleeding ulcers.[68] Sixty-eight patients with actively bleeding ulcers were randomized to receive either endoscopic injection of epinephrine or no endoscopic treatment. Both oozing ulcers (72%) and spurting ones (28% of total) were injected with 0.5-mL aliquots of 1:10,000 epinephrine in multiple sites (maximum, 20 mL) in and around the bleeding point until all bleeding was controlled.

All patients were reendoscoped in 24 hours and those in the treatment group with bleeding were reinjected (Table 138-8). The spontaneous hemostasis rate was 59% for the control patients treated with standard medical therapy, which is sig-

TABLE 138-8
Efficacy of Sclerotherapy for the Treatment of Active Ulcer Bleeding

	CONTROL	SCLEROTHERAPY
Number of patients	34	34
Initial hemostasis (%)	0	100*
Repeat injection (%)	0	18
Definitive hemostasis (%)	59	85
Emergency surgery (%)	41	15*
Number of patients receiving red blood cell transfusion	5.9	3.8*
Number of hospital days	12.8	7.3
Mortality (%)	6	9

Results are post-randomization rates or means for different outcomes during hospitalization.

* $P < 0.05$.

Data from Chung SCS, Leng JWC, Steele RJC, Gofts TJ, Li AKC. Endoscopic injection of adrenaline for actively bleeding ulcers: a randomized trial. Br Med J 1988;296:163.

nificantly higher than the 14% spontaneous hemostasis rate for severe ulcer bleeders in the large CURE RCSs.[44,57,62,64] The overall difference is because of the large number of oozers who did not rebleed on medical therapy and did not require emergency surgery (71%). However, 70% (7 of 10) of control patients with spurting bleeding in the Hong Kong study required emergency surgery compared to 33% (3 of 9) of the injected group. This was the first RCS published for injection of bleeding ulcers, and it demonstrated a significant benefit of epinephrine injection in active ulcer bleeders.

A randomized comparison of injection with epinephrine alone, epinephrine followed by polidocanol, or epinephrine followed by Nd:YAG laser therapy in ulcer patients with active bleeding or nonbleeding visible vessels was reported.[69] An improved hemostasis rate with the sequential epinephrine followed by polidocanol injections was demonstrated. In view of these good to excellent results, the simplicity, portability, inexpense, and low incidence of reported complications, injection therapy seems very promising.

Comparisons of Injection Versus Thermal Hemostasis of Ulcers

Several large randomized studies prospectively comparing injection with thermal devises have been reported. Lin and coworkers of Taiwan reported a prospective randomized study of injection sclerosis versus heater probe for treatment of ulcer patients with severe UGI bleeding and major stigmata of recent hemorrhage.[67] Seventy-five patients with either active bleeding or nonbleeding visible vessel were treated with injection (34 patients) or heater probe (41 patients). All patients also had routine medical management.

Overall, 71% of injection patients (24 of 34) had permanent hemostasis compared to 95% of heater probe patients (39 of 41). The difference was reported to be significant. The authors reported that patients with ulcers on the lesser curvature of the stomach or superior aspect of the duodenal bulb had higher permanent hemostasis rates with heater probe

(100%, or 15 of 15 patients) than injection (45%, or 5 of 11 patients). This related to the ease of tangential coagulation with heater probe compared to the difficulty of approaching such lesions for injected tangentially. No major complications were reported for either heater probe or injection.

Chung and coworkers randomized 122 patients with active ulcer bleeding, 58 patients to heater probe coagulation and 64 patients to injection.[92] Duodenal ulcers were found in 64% of heater probe and 74% injection patients. Spurting arterial bleeding was described in 31% of both injection and heater probe patients, whereas 42% of heater probe and 50% of injection patients had hypotension on presentation. Twenty-four hours after randomization, all patients were reendoscoped. Those with any bleeding were retreated with the same modality as previously. Patients who had severe rebleeding clinically, required more than eight units total transfusions, or who had four more units of blood transfusion for continued bleeding after randomization were sent for emergency ulcer surgery.

The initial hemostasis rate of 95% with injection was significantly higher than heater probe (85% initial hemostasis rate). Overall, permanent hemostasis with injection occurred in 78% of patients and for 81% of heater probe patients. Other outcomes for heater probe versus injection did not differ significantly: emergency surgery rates (19% versus 22%), mean RBC transfused (3.7 versus 4.7), median hospital days (6 versus 5), and mortality (6.9% versus 3.1%). The authors concluded that heater probe and epinephrine injection were equally effective for hemostasis of actively bleeding ulcers. There were no major complications of injection for bleeding ulcers. Two perforations resulted from heater probe treatments. Both occurred in patients who were treated twice, once at randomization and again 24 hours later upon surveillance endoscopy. In their opinion, epinephrine injection was technically easier to perform than heater probe and may be safer if early retreatment is necessary. Their opinion contrasted with that of Lin and colleageus who reported better results for tangential coagulation with heater probe than injection.[67]

Results with any hemostasis modality will depend upon technique, experience and practice. The safety of retreatment with heater probe depends upon the thickness of the ulcer base and the strength of the previously coagulated area. Recoagulation of acute, thin ulcers within 24 hours of initial treatment may be hazardous compared to recoagulation of chronic ulcers with thick fibrotic bases.[1,7,33,38,86]

Hemostasis of Mallory-Weiss Tears

For bleeding Mallory-Weiss tears, there are few data from prospective or randomized trials about stigmata of recent hemorrhage and the benefits and risks of endoscopic hemostasis.[62,65] Laine reported on a small subgroup of patients with active arterial bleeding from Mallory-Weiss tear treated with bipolar electrocoagulation or medical therapy.[60] There was a significant benefit to the patients treated with the BICAP probe in terms of lower rates of continued bleeding, fewer transfusions, and a lower rate of emergency surgery for hemostasis. In a recent CURE study which prospectively compared the rates of continued bleeding by stigmata of recent hemorrhage and treatments,[93] Mallory-Weiss tear patients who had severe UGI hemorrhage and active arterial bleeding but did not have portal hypertension had an endoscopic hemostasis rate of 100% compared to 40% for medically managed Mallory-Weiss tear patients. In Mallory-Weiss tear patients without portal hypertension, nonbleeding visible vessel or adherent clots had rebleeding less than 20% of the time on medical management. Therefore, we and others recommend treatment of actively bleeding Mallory-Weiss tear but not other patients with nonbleeding visible vessel or adherent clot unless the patient has already rebled from the same lesion.[60,65,93]

Hemostasis of Dieulafoy's Lesion

Dieulafoy's lesion was characterized more than a hundred years ago pathologically as a large artery protruding through the mucosa, unassociated with a peptic ulcer but causing severe UGI hemorrhage.[24,94] Skilled endoscopists now diagnose Dieulafoy's lesion when an actively bleeding visible vessel without an ulceration is seen at emergency panendoscopy in a patient with severe UGI bleeding.[24,94] Less often a non-bleeding visible vessel or adherent clot with a nonbleeding visible vessel underneath is found and diagnosed as Dieulafoy's lesion when no other bleeding site can be recognized.[24,94] Endoscopic treatment is feasible for Dieulafoy's lesions and small series report good primary hemostasis with injection or various thermal techniques.[24,94,95] There have been no large studies and no prospective, randomized studies of different endoscopic therapies for either control of active arterial bleeding or prevention of rebleeding (nonbleeding visible vessel). In some CURE patients with severe arterial bleeding from Dieulafoy's lesions, primary hemostasis could not be achieved by single therapy alone (i.e., injection or thermal). Combination therapy with epinephrine injection and bipolar electrocoagulation was successful in these cases.[3] In our CURE study of Dieulafoy's lesions, rebleeding rates were about 50% after single modality therapy.[24]

Hemostasis of Bleeding UGI Tumors

A CURE prospective, case-control study was performed to assess clinical outcomes of endoscopic hemostasis in 42 patients with severe UGI bleeding due to malignancy compared to 524 patients with severe UGI bleeding due to peptic ulcers.[25] Initial hemostasis of bleeding tumors was 100% and for peptic ulcers was 99% with injection, bipolar, or heater probe coagulation. No patients required emergency surgery. 57% of tumor patients who received endoscopic hemostasis underwent elective surgery within 30 days of the initial bleeding, compared to 6% of peptic ulcer patients who received endoscopic hemostasis. The 30-day mortality rate was 29% for treated tumors compared to 17% for peptic ulcers, and the 1-year mortality rates were 100% and 32% respectively. Emergency endoscopic treatment was equally successful for hemostasis of bleeding malignant ulcers and benign peptic ulcers. Endoscopic hemostasis allowed patients with UGI malignanices to be medically stabilized before elective surgery. Severe bleeding from UGI tumors was a poor prognostic sign with high short-term and long-term mortality rates.

A recent report of endoscopic treatment of bleeding gas-troduodenal malignancies in 15 patients from the Mayo Clinic concluded that endoscopic hemostasis was often ineffective and had a high risk of complications.[96] However, that study differed from the CURE study in that only 45% of patients received treatment for active bleeding compared to 100% of our patients and Nd:YAG laser was used to treat 36% of patients compared to no laser use in our study. The indication for treatment is important as it is unknown whether the endoscopic stigmata of early rebleeding applied to peptic ulcers are applicable to tumors. The Mayo study also reported 2 perforations. Nd:YAG lasers have been associated with higher rates of transmural injury in the canine stomach than bipolar electrocoagulation.[32] Perforation rates of 5% to 10% have been reported with Nd:YAG laser treatment of esophageal cancer.[97]

Hemostasis of UGI Angiomata

There are no reported RCSs of endoscopic hemostasis for bleeding UGI angiomata or telangiectasia of Osler-Weber-Rendu Syndrome (OWR). However, several prospective studies were reported.[37,39-41,45,46,98] The CURE Hemostasis Group reported the largest prospective study (104 patients) of endoscopic treatment for bleeding UGI angiomata.[37,39,45,98] Both UGI angiomata and OWR telangiectasia were included. Criteria for a definitive diagnosis of AVM as the bleeding site were endoscopic active bleeding or stigmata of recent UGI bleeding on the AVM (e.g., clot, erosion, spot) or hematemesis with clean angioma on endoscopy and no other UGI bleeding source.[37,98] Incidental angioma were the subgroup for patients with chronic GI bleeding and angioma on panendoscopy when the criteria for angioma as the definite bleeding source were not met. Treatment was with argon laser (22 patients), BICAP (50 patients) or heater probe (37 patients). Patient outcomes were compared for a mean of 2.5 years before (on medical management) versus 2.5 years after (on endoscopic treatment) coagulation (Table 138-9). There were no major complications.

Patients with documented UGI bleeding from OWR telangiectasia or UGI angioma had good palliation with endoscopic hemostasis. There were significant increases in hematocrits whereas transfusion requirements and hospitalizations for bleeding decreased significantly. Treatment of incidental angioma did not reduce GI bleeding or benefit those patients. Endoscopic treatment with heater probe or BICAP was technically easier than argon laser but all were safe and equally effective. The CURE group also reported that the estimated cost of hospitalization and blood transfusions was reduced at least twofold by endoscopic hemostasis compared to medical management.[98]

Rutgeerts and coworkers reported the long-term treatment results of GI angioma with Nd:YAG laser.[40] Twenty-five patients with OWR or UGI angiomas were treated and prospectively evaluated. During a mean of 11.5 months of follow-up, there were significant reductions in bleeding episodes and RBC transfused. Two patients (8%) had complications of treatment, one a chronic duodenal ulcer and one perforation treated conservatively.[40]

Brunetaud and coworkers reported 53 patients with UGI angioma and chronic GI bleeding treated with argon laser.[99]

TABLE 138-9
Palliative Results of Endoscopic Hemostasis by Argon Laser, Bicap, or Heater Probe

	UPPER GASTROINTESTINAL ANGIOMA	OSTER-WEBER-RENDU TELANGIECTASIA	INCIDENTAL
Total patients	68	23	13
Mean URBC/y			
Before hemostasis	4.8	9.5	5.8
After hemostasis	1.1*	2.0*	7.6
Mean Number of Gastrointestinal Bleeds/y			
Before hemostasis	1.6	2.6	1.9
After hemostasis	0.4*	0.6*	3.4
Mean Hematocrit (mL/dL)			
Before hemostasis	25	27	23
After hemostasis	37*	35*	24

URBC/y, units of red cells transfused per year.

* $P < 0.05$.

Data from references 37, 39, and 98.

All 43 UGI-AVM patients had bleeding controlled after a mean of two laser sessions. All the 10 OWR patients stopped bleeding after an average of 4.3 laser treatment sessions. Overall the treatment benefitted these patients, as judged by a major decrease in blood transfusions. No major complications occurred.

Using argon, Nd:YAG lasers, or both, Bown and coworkers treated 18 patients who had severe UGI bleeding from angiomata.[41] Seventy-eight percent of patients (5 OWR, 9 UGI-angioma) had their transfusion requirements reduced after one or more laser treatments. Four patients (22%) had surgery, two for failure of laser hemostasis and two because on rebleeding a laser was not available. Seven patients (39%) had an exacerbation of GI bleeding as a complication that might be attributable to laser treatment. The investigators concluded that both lasers were effective. In their opinion, Nd:YAG laser may be more effective for long-term results than argon laser because of its ability to obliterate the vascular component in the submucosa. However, there is a higher risk of deeper ulceration and delayed hemorrhage with the Nd:YAG laser than with the argon laser.

FUTURE DEVELOPMENTS

Despite the incredible progress in the last 10 years, there are several problems related to nonvariceal UGI bleeding which warrant further investigation and solutions. These will require new instruments, new studies of healing and histopathology of bleeding lesions, cost assessments, additional RCSs and further training of therapeutic endoscopists.

One problem of endoscopic diagnosis and treatment is clots. Better endoscopic accessories are needed for removal of large or small clots that obscure bleeding lesions. One solution for large clots might be a high speed rotary device which can spin the fibrin onto a catheter and leave liquid blood to suction.

Better technology is needed to endoscopically image the gut wall and the vessels which underlie nonvariceal lesions.

The commercially available 7.5- to 12-MHz ultrasound endoscopes do not appear to be sensitive enough to visualize the small submucosal arteries or arterioles associated with most peptic ulcers, Mallory-Weiss tears, or UGI angiomata. It is not known if improvement in ultrasound endoscopes or development of higher frequency ultrasound endoscopy probes will increase vessel resolution or distinguish coagulated from uncoagulated vessels. A careful correlation with the histopathology of bleeding ulcers, Mallory-Weiss tears and angiomata is warranted as has been reported for normal gut wall or other UGI pathology.[100,101]

Endoscopic instrumentation to accurately quantitate blood flow of vessels underlying lesions before and after coagulation might help guide endoscopic hemostasis. Endoscopic Doppler probes have been developed and used in a few case reports to facilitate ulcer or Dieulafoy lesion hemostasis.[102,103] Whereas most bleeding ulcers, Dieulafoy's lesions, Mallory-Weiss tears and angiomata can be controlled initially by new thermal or injection techniques, rebleeding rates particularly of ulcers remain high. Adequate coagulation on initial treatment of the vessels underlying these nonvariceal lesions undoubtedly would result in reduced rebleeding rates.

Another area for study is the morphology of bleeding UGI lesions. More clinical prospective studies of the healing patterns after endoscopic hemostasis with different techniques versus medical therapy alone are warranted. Also, the transmural histopathology of bleeding Dieulafoy's lesion, UGI tumors, UGI angiomata, and Mallory-Weiss tears should be studied as a guide to endoscopic treatment, similar to studies of bleeding gastric or duodenal ulcers.[13–15]

Another area for future investigation is to determine the recurrence rates of ulcer rebleeding during long-term medical management, after endoscopic hemostasis. Long-term recurrence rates of patients managed medically have been infrequently studied since the introduction of endoscopic coagulation and H_2-receptor antagonists.[104–106] CURE prospective and RCSs indicate high recurrence rates of peptic ulcer bleeding. Patients who heal their ulcers after a severe ulcer bleed and are not treated with maintenance H_2-receptor antagonists or ulcer surgery had a cumulative recurrence rate of recurrent ulcer bleeding at 30 months of 30% compared to 0% for surgery and 6% for full doses of H_2-receptor antagonist.[105,106]

The role of open ulcer surgery, either emergency or elective, and laparoscopic surgery require redefinition since the introduction of endoscopic treatment for emergency hemostasis and H_2-receptor antagonists for healing and maintenance.[26–29,105,106]

The direct and indirect costs of medical, endoscopic, and surgical treatment can and should be quantitated and compared.[107,108] These cost assessment of short- and long-term treatments will be important for improving the care of high risk patients.

More widespread training in emergency hemostasis of skilled endoscopists and gastroenterology fellows will be required to change current clinical practices and mortality from UGI hemorrhage. Teaching standarized endoscopic techniques for safe and effective diagnosis and treatment will be necessary.[32,62]

CONCLUSIONS

Teaching endoscopists to recognize and treat patients with major stigmata of hemorrhage (i.e., active bleeding or nonbleeding visible vessel) rather than minor stigmata is necessary to improve patient outcomes. The former patients have a high risk of rebleeding and need for emergency surgery and may benefit from safe and effective endoscopic hemostasis. Treatment of minor stigmata does not benefit patients but increases the cost of health care.[62]

Over the last decade, the endoscopic treatment of nonvariceal bleeding has progressed significantly. We now have a much better idea of which patients will benefit from endoscopic therapy: those with clinically severe ulcer bleeding and major stigmata of recent hemorrhage (i.e., active bleeding or nonbleeding visible vessels). These are the patients at high risk for continued bleeding or rebleeding and, in the past, had high rates of emergency surgery for hemostasis.

Actively bleeding Mallory-Weiss tears, Dieulafoy's lesions, UGI tumors, and UGI angiomata might also be considered in this group. Patients who are unlikely to benefit from endoscopic hemostasis are ulcer patients with no stigmata or minor stigmata of recent hemorrhage (i.e., nonbleeding flat spots, clots, or slough). Unnecessary therapy increases their risk of an unnecessary therapeutic procedure and the likelihood receiving a larger medical bill. Patients with documented GI bleeding from UGI angiomata have good palliation of their chronic, recurrent bleeding from endoscopic hemostasis and should be considered for endoscopic hemostasis and long-term follow-up.

Argon and Nd:YAG lasers, MPEC, bipolar electrocoagulation, heater probe, and injection sclerotherapy are effective techniques for hemostasis of nonvariceal bleeding. Based upon experimental, histologic, and clinical studies, the guidelines and limitations for application of each endoscopic technique have been determined. Tamponade, coaptation, and tangential treatment appear to be advantages of newer (e.g., bipolar, heater probe) over older techniques (e.g., lasers, MPEC).

An NIH consensus conference on ulcer hemorrhage was held and reported.[109,110] Positive results from randomized,

controlled studies were reported with YAG laser, heater probe, bipolar electrocoagulation and injection for patients with actively bleeding ulcers or nonbleeding visible vessels.[110] In the hands of individual experts or experienced groups of investigators who have standardized endoscopic treatment and performed RCT in high risk patients, all previously studied endoscopic devices have been shown to be effective and safe in at least one RCS. More recently metanalyses of RCSs of ulcer hemorrhage have noted significant improvements with endoscopic hemostasis. However, this improvement was only with bleeding ulcers and ulcers with nonbleeding visible vessels only.[111,112] Significant reductions in rebleeding rates, transfusion requirements, need for emergency surgery, or direct costs have been reported. Rarely have significant reductions in mortality been reported in RCSs. The frequency of severe complications from endoscopic hemostasis has been low, although precipitation of severe bleeding is a problem with endoscopic lasers.

The newer endoscopic hemostasis devices (e.g., bipolar electrocoagulation, heater probe) appear to have several major advantages over older devices (e.g., argon or Nd:YAG laser, MPEC) for emergency hemostasis of nonvariceal UGI lesions. These include tamponade and coaptation capabilities, ability to coagulate tangentially as well as en face, portability, relative inexpense, and absence of an erosive effect on tissue or arteries.

Standardization and teaching of these techniques to skilled endoscopists are feasible. Injection sclerotherapy shares many of these advantages over lasers or MPEC. Whether the recent advances in technology and positive results of some investigators will ultimately translate into better widespread care for the nonvariceal bleeder is unknown. A significant reduction in mortality from nonvariceal hemorrhage will depend upon more widespread training and application of standardized endoscopic techniques and current knowledge to more patients at high risk for continued bleeding or rebleeding.

Acknowledgment

The CURE laboratory research included was in part funded by Veteran's Administration Funds (Merit Review). The CURE Clinical research was in part funded by NIH-NIDDK Grants R01-33273 and CORE Grant 41301. The author wishes to thank Assumpta Oturu for the word processing.

The reader is directed to Chapter 30, Approach to the Patient With Gross Gastrointestinal Bleeding; Chapter 31, Approach to the Patient With Occult Gastrointestinal Bleeding; Chapter 116, Colonoscopy and Flexible Sigmoidoscopy; and Chapter 117, Endoscopic Retrograde Cholangiopancreatography, Endoscopic Sphincterotomy and Stone Removal, and Endoscopic Biliary and Pancreatic Drainage.

REFERENCES

1. Kovacs TOG, Jensen M. Endoscopic control of gastroduodenal hemorrhage. Ann Rev Med 1987;38:267.
2. Schiller KFR, Truelove SC, Williams DG. Haematemesis and melena with special reference to factors influencing the outcome. Br Med J 1970;27:7.

3. Silverstein FE, Gilbert DA, Tedesco FJ, Buenger NK, Persing J. The national ASGE survey on upper gastrointestinal bleeding. I. Study design and baseline data. Gastrointest Endosc 1981;27(2):73.

4. Silverstein FE, Gilbert DA, Tedesco FJ, Buenger NK, Persing J. The national ASGE surgery on upper gastrointestinal bleeding. II. Clinical prognostic factors. Gastrointest Endosc 1981;27(2):80.

5. Allan R, Dykes P. A study on the factors influencing mortality rates from gastrointestinal hemorrhage. Q J Med 1976;180:533.

6. Gilbert DA, Silverstein FE, Tedesco FJ, Buenger NK, Persing J. The national ASGE survey on upper gastrointestinal bleeding. III. Endoscopy in upper gastrointestinal bleeding. Gastrointest Endosc 1981;27(2):94.

7. Kovacs TOG, Jensen DM. Endoscopy of upper gastrointestinal bleeding. In: Cotton PB, Tytgat GNJ, Williams CB, eds. Annual of gastrointestinal endoscopy. London: Gower Academic, 1988:37.

8. Swain CP, Bown SG, Storey DW, Kirkham JS, Northfield TC, Salmon PR. Controlled trial of argon laser photocoagulation in bleeding peptic ulcers. Lancet 1981;2(8259):1313.

9. Swain CP, Kirkham JS, Salmon PR, Bown SG, Northfield TC. Controlled trial of Nd-YAG laser photocoagulation in bleeding peptic ulcers. Lancet 1986;1(8490):1113.

10. Kovacs TOG, Jensen DM. Current management of patients with bleeding esophageal varices. Gastroenterol Forum 1989;2(2):2.

11. Fleischer D. Etiology and prevalence of severe persistent upper gastrointestinal bleeding. Gastroenterology 1989;84:538.

12. Matthewson D, Swain CP, Bland M, Kirkham JS, Bown SG, Northfield TC. Randomized comparison of Nd-YAG laser, heater probe, and no endoscopic therapy for bleeding peptic ulcer. Gastroenterology 1990;98:1239.

13. Swain CP, Storey DW, Bown SG, et al. Nature of the bleeding vessel in recurrently bleeding gastric ulcers. Gastroenterology 1986;90:595.

14. Johnston JH. The sentinel clot and invisible vessel: pathologic anatomy of bleeding peptic ulcer. Gastrointest Endosc 1984;30:313.

15. Swain CP, Kalabakas A, Grandison A, et al. Size and pathology of vessel and ulcer in patients with fatal bleeding from duodenal ulcer (abstract). Gastroenterology 1990;98:A133.

16. Johnston JH, Jensen DM, Auth D. Experimental comparison of endoscopic yttrium-aluminum-garnet laser, electrosurgery, and heater probe for canine gut arterial coagulation: the importance of vessel compression and avoidance of tissue erosion. Gastroenterology 1987;92:1101.

17. Gorisch W, Boergen KP. Heat-induced contraction of blood vessels. Lasers Surg Med 1982;2:1.

18. Sigel B, Dunn MR. The mechanism of blood vessel closure by high frequency electrocoagulation. Surg Gynec Obstet 1965;121:823.

19. Sigel B, Hatke FL. Physical factors in electrocoaptation of blood vessels. Arch Surg 1967;95:54.

20. Randall GM, Jensen DM, Hirabayashi K, Machicado GA. Controlled study of different sclerosing agents for coagulation of canine gut arteries. Gastroenterology 1989;96:1274.

21. Rutgeerts P, Geboes K, Vantrappen G. Experimental studies of injection therapy for severe non-variceal bleeding in dogs. Gastroenterology 1989;97:610.

22. Asaki S, Nishimura T, Satoh A, Goto Y. Endoscopic control of gastrointestinal hemorrhage by local injection of absolute ethanol: a basic assessment of the procedure. Tohoku J Exp Med 1982;140:339.

23. Guth PH, Smith SE. Vasoactive agents and the gastric microcirculation. Microvasc Res 1974;8:125.

24. Narayan S, Jensen DM, Kovacs, TOG, et al. Upper Gastrointestinal bleeding from Dieulafoy's lesion compare to peptic ulcer (abstract). Gastrointest Endosc 1992;38:239.

25. Savides TJ, Jensen DM, Randall GM, et al. The role of endoscopy in the treatment of severe upper gastrointestinal bleeding from tumors compared to peptic ulcers (abstract). Gastrointest Endosc 1993;39:288.

26. Dronfield MW, Atkinson M, Langman MJ. Effect of different operation policies on mortality from bleeding peptic ulcer. Lancet 1979;1(8126):1126.

27. Schrock TR. Does endoscopy affect the surgical approach to the patient with upper gastrointestinal bleeding? Dig Dis Sci 1981;26(Supp 7):27.

28. Shapiro S. Gardon LA. Laparoscopic vagotomy. Gastrointest Endoss Clin North Am 1993;3(2)319.

29. Kathouda N, Movie J. A new technique of surgical treatment of chronic duodenal ulcer without laparotomy by video-coelioscopy. Am J Surg 1991;161:361.

30. Johnston JH, Jensen DM, Mautner W, Elashoff J. Argon laser treatment of bleeding canine gastric ulcers: limitations and guidelines for endoscopic use. Gastroenterology 1981;80:708.

31. Johnston JH, Jensen DM, Mautner W, Elashoff J. YAG laser treatment of experimental bleeding canine gastric ulcers. Gastroenterology 1980;79:1252.

32. Johnston JH, Jensen DM, Mautner W. Comparison of endoscopic electrocoagulation and laser photocoagulation of bleeding canine gastric ulcers. Gastroenterology 1982;82:904.

33. Jensen DM. GI endoscopic hemostasis and tumor palliation—experimental results and techniques. In: Jensen DM, Brunetaud JM, ed. Medical laser endoscopy. Dordecht, The Netherlands: Kluwer Academic Publishers, 1990:45.

34. Rutgeerts P, Vantrappen G, Broeckaert L, et al. Controlled trial of YAG laser treatment of upper digestive hemorrhage. Gastroenterology 1982;83:410.

35. Kiefhaber P, Kiefhaber K, Haber F, Nath G. Endoscopic neodymium YAG laser coagulation in gastrointestinal hemorrhage. Endoscopy 1986;18(Suppl 2):46.

36. Johnston JH, Sones JQ, Long BW, Posey EL. Comparison of heater probe and YAG laser in endoscopic treatment of major bleeding from peptic ulcers. Gastrointest Endosc 1985;31:175.

37. Machicado GA, Jensen DM. Upper gastrointestinal angiomata: diagnosis and treatment. Gastrointest Endosc Clin North Am 1991;1:241.

38. Johnston JH. Complications of endoscopic laser therapy. In: Fleischer D, Jensen DM, Bright-Asare P, eds. Therapeutic laser endoscopy in gastrointestinal disease. Boston: Martinus Nijhoff, 1983:173.

39. Jensen DM, Machicado GA. Upper gastrointestinal angiomata: diagnosis and treatment. In: Jensen DM, Brunetaud JM, eds. Medical laser endoscopy. Dordrecht, The Netherlands: Kluwer Academic Publishers, 1990:71.

40. Rutgeerts P, Van Gompel F, Geboes K, Vantrappen G, Broekaert L, Coremans G. Long-term results of vascular malformations of the gastrointestinal tract by Neodymium-YAG laser photocoagulation. Gut 1985;26:586.

41. Bown SG, Swain CP, Storey DW, et al. Endoscopic laser treatment of vascular abnormalities of the upper gastrointestinal tract. Gut 1985;26:1338.

42. Brunetaud JM, Jensen DM. Current status of argon laser hemostasis of bleeding ulcers. Endoscopy 1986;18(Suppl 2):40.

43. Vallon AG, Cotton PB, Laurence BH, Armengol-Miro JR, Salord-Oses JC. Randomized trial of endoscopic argon laser photocoagulation in bleeding peptic ulcers. Gut 1981;22(3):228.

44. Jensen DM, Machicado GA. Argon laser for severe ulcer hemorrhage: health and economic considerations. In: Jensen DM, Brunetaud JM, eds. Medical laser endoscopy. Dordrecht, The Netherlands: Kluwer Academic Publishers, 1990:119.

45. Smith JW, Jensen DM. Gastrointestinal angiomas: source of recurrent bleeding. Postgrad Med 1987;82(8):171.

46. Jensen D, Bown S. Gastrointestinal angiomata: diagnosis and treatment with laser therapy and other endoscopic modalities. In: Fleischer D, Jensen DM, Bright-Asare P, ed. Therapeutic laser endoscopy in gastrointestinal disease. Boston: Martinus-Nijhoff, 1983:151.

47. Piercey JRS, Auth DC, Silverstein FE, et al. Electrosurgical treatment of experimental bleeding gastric ulcer: development of a computer control and better electrode. Gastroenterology 1978;74:527.

48. Swain CP, Mills TN, Shemesh E, et al. Which electrode? A comparison of four endoscopic methods of electrocoagulation in experimental bleeding ulcers. Gut 1984;25(12):1424.

49. Frietas D, Donato A, Monteiro JG. Controlled trial of liquid monopolar electrocoagulation in bleeding peptic ulcers. Am J Gastroenterol 1985;80:853.

50. Papp JP. Endoscopic treatment of gastrointestinal bleeding: electrocoagulation. In: Sivak MV, ed. Gastrointestinal endoscopy. Philadelphia: WB Saunders, 1987:143.

51. Papp JP. Endoscopic electrocoagulation in the management of upper gastrointestinal tract bleeding. Surg Clin North Am 1982;62:797.

52. Sugawa C, Shier M, Lucas CE, Walt AJ. Electrocoagulation of bleeding in the upper part of the gastrointestinal tract: a preliminary experimental clinical report. Arch Surg 1975;110(8):975.

53. Gaisford WD. Endoscopic electrohemostasis of active upper gastrointestinal bleeding. Am J Surg 1979;137:47.

54. Wara P. Endoscopic electrocoagulation of major bleeding from peptic ulcer. Acta Chir Scand 1985;151:29.

55. Moreto M, Zaballa M, Ibanez S, Setien F, Figa M. Efficacy of monopolar electrocoagulation in the treatment of bleeding gastric ulcer: a controlled trial. Endoscopy 1987;19(2):54.

56. Jensen DM, Machicado GA, Silpa M, Van Deventer G, Sue M, Kovacs TOG, English S, Reedy T, Elashoff J. BICAPR vs. heater probe for hemostasis of severe ulcer bleeding (abstract). Gastrointest Endosc 1986;32:143.

57. Jensen DM. Heater probe for endoscopic hemostasis of non-variceal UGI bleeding. In: Schuman B, Sugawa C, Lucas C, eds. Gastrointestinal bleeding. New York: Igaku-Shoin, 1992:298.

58. Jensen D, Hirabayashi K, CURE Hemostasis Research Group. A study of coagulation depths with BICAPR and heater probe to improve endoscopic hemostasis of bleeding peptic ulcers (abstract). Gastrointest Endosc 1989;35(2):181.

59. Jensen DM, Hirabayashi K. A comparative study of coagulation depths and efficacy of arterial coagulation for Gold probe (abstract). Am J Gastroenterol 1989;84:1161.

60. Laine L. Multipolar electrocoagulation in the treatment of active upper gastrointestinal hemorrhage. N Engl J Med 1987;316:1613.

61. Laine L. Multipolar electrocoagulation in the treatment of peptic ulcers with non-bleeding visible vessels: a prospective controlled trial. Ann Intern Med 1989;110:510.

62. Jensen DM. New developments in the diagnosis and treatment of severe upper gastrointestinal bleeding. In: Tytgat GNJ, Van Blankenstein M, eds. Current topics in gastroenterology and hepatology. Georg Thieme, 1990;4.

63. Jensen DM, Hirabayashi K. A randomized controlled endoscopic study of Gold probe for hemostasis of bleeding canine ulcers (abstract). Am J Gastroenterol 1989;84:1162.

64. Jensen DM. Heat probe for hemostasis of bleeding peptic ulcers: techniques and results of randomized controlled trials. Gastrointest Endosc 1990;36:S42.

65. Kovacs TOG, Jensen DM. Endoscopic diagnosis and treatment of bleeding Mallory-Weiss tears. Gastrointest Endosc Clin North Am 1991;1:387.

66. Soehendra N, Grimm H, Stenzel M. Injection of nonvariceal bleeding lesions of the upper gastrointestinal tract. Endoscopy 1985;17:129.

67. Lin HJ, Tsai VT, Lee DS, et al. A prospectively randomized trial of heat probe thermocoagulation versus pure alcohol injection in non-variceal peptic ulcer hemorrhage. Am J Gastroenterol 1988;83:283.

68. Chung SCS, Leung JWC, Steele RJC, Crofts TJ, Li AKC. Endoscopic injection of adrenalin for actively bleeding ulcers: a randomized trial. Br Med J 1988;296:1631.

69. Rutgeerts P, Broekaert L, Coremans G, et al. Randomized comparison of three hemostasis modalities for severely bleeding peptic ulcers: epinephrine 0.01% injection alone (1), epinephrine + polidocanol 1% injection (2), epinephrine injection followed by YAG laser (3) (abstract). Gastrointest Endosc 1987;33:148.

70. Sugawa C, Ikeda T, Fujita Y, Walt AJ. Endoscopic hemostasis of upper gastrointestinal bleeding by local injection of ninety-eight percent dehydrated ethanol. Surg Gynecol Obstet 1986;162:159.

71. Otani T, Tatska T, Kanamura K, et al. Intramural injection of ethanol under direct vision for the treatment of protuberant lesions of the stomach. Gastroenterology 1975;69:123.

72. Hirao M, Kobayashi T, Masuda K, et al. Endoscopic local injection of hypertonic saline-epinephrine solution to arrest hemorrhage from the upper gastrointestinal tract. Gastrointest Endosc 1985;31:313.

73. Fuchs KH, Wirtz HJ, Schaube H, Elfeldt R. Initial experience with thrombin as injection agent for bleeding gastroduodenal lesions. Endoscopy 1986;18:146.

74. Chen PC, Wu CS, Liaw YF. Hemostatic effect of endoscopic local injection with hypertonic saline-epinephrine solution and pure ethanol for digestive tract bleeding. Gastrointest Endosc 1986;32:319.

75. Jensen DM, Kovacs TOG, Randall GM, et al. Initial results of randomized controlled study of non-bleeding adherent clots in patients with severe ulcer hemorrhage (abstract). Gastrointest Endosc 1993;39:279.

76. Michaletz P, Judge D. Microwave energy compared with heater probe and BICAP in canine models of peptic ulcer hemorrhage. Gastroenterology 1989;97:676.

77. Panes J, Viver J, Forne M. Randomized comparision of endoscopic microwave coagulation and endoscopic sclerosis in treatment of bleeding peptic ulcers. Gastrointest Endosc 1991;37:611.

78. Jutabha R, Jensen DM, Hirabayashi K. Randomized controlled study of injector-Gold probe for hemostasis of bleeding gastric ulcers in a canine model (abstract). Gastrointest Endosc 1993;39(2):252(A17).

79. Rutgeerts P, Vantrappen G, Van Hootegem P, et al. Neodymium-YAG laser photocoagulation versus multipolar electrocoagulation for treatment of bleeding ulcers. A randomized comparison. Gastrointest Endosc 1987;33:199.

80. Ihre T, Johansson C, Seligson U, et al. Endoscopic YAG laser treatment in massive upper gastrointestinal bleeding. Scand J Gastroenterol 1981;16:633.

81. Escourrou J, Frexinos J, Bommelaer G, et al. Prospective randomized study of YAG photocoagulation in gastrointestinal bleeding. In: Atsumi K, Nimsakul N, eds. Proceedings of Laser Tokyo '81. Tokyo: The Japan Society for Laser Medicine, 1981:5.

82. Rohde M, Thon K, Fischer M, et al. Results of a defined therapeutic concept of endoscopic neodymium-YAG laser therapy in patients with upper gastrointestinal bleeding. Br J Surg 1980;67:360.

83. Rutgeerts P, Vantrappen G, Broeckhaert L, et al. Controlled trial of YAG laser treatment of upper digestive hemorrhage. Gastroenterology 1982;83:410.

84. MacLeod I, Mills PR, Mackenzie JF, et al. Neodymium YAG laser photocoagulation for major haemorrhage from peptic ulcers and single vessels. Br Med J 1983;286:345.

85. Krejs GJ, Little KH, Westergaard H, Hamilton JK, Polter DE. Laser photocoagulation for the treatment of acute peptic ulcer bleeding: a randomized controlled clinical trial. N Engl J Med 1987;316:1618.

86. Swain CP. Results, complications, and techniques of laser treatment for bleeding peptic ulcers: conclusions and recommendations after two controlled trials. In: Jensen DM, Brunetaud JM, eds. Medical laser endoscopy. Dordrecht, The Netherlands: Kluwer Academic Publishers, 1990:135.

87. O'Brien JD, Day SJ, Burnham WR. Controlled trial of small bipolar probe in bleeding peptic ulcers. Lancet 1986;1(8479):464.

88. Kernohan RM, Anderson JR, McKelvey ST, Kennedy T. A controlled trial of bipolar electrocoagulation in patients with upper gastrointestinal bleeding. Br J Surg 1984;71(11)889.

89. Goudie BM, Mitchell KG, Birnie GG, Mackay C. Controlled trial of endoscopic bipolar electrocoagulation in the treatment of bleeding peptic ulcers (abstract). Gut 1984;25:A1185.

90. Brearley S, Hawker PC, Dykes PW, Keighley MR. Per-endoscopic bipolar diathermy coagulation of visible vessels using a 3.2 mm probe—a randomised clinical trial. Endoscopy 1987;19(4):160.

91. Fullerton GM, Birnie GG, MacDonald A, Murray WR. Con-

trolled study of heater probe in bleeding peptic ulcers. Br J Surg 1989;76:541.

92. Chung S, Leung JW, Sung JY, Lo KK, Li AK. Injection or heat probe for bleeding ulcers. Gastroenterology 1991;100:33.

93. Jensen DM, Kovacs TOG, Machicado GA, Randall GM, Sue M, CURE Hemostasis Unit. Prospective study of the stigmata of hemorrhage and endoscopic and medical treatment of bleeding Mallory Weiss tears (abstract). Gastrointest Endosc 1992;38:235.

94. Veldhuyzen Van Zanten SJO, Bartelsman JFWM, Schipper MEI, Tytgat GNJ. Recurrent massive haematemesis from Dieulafoy vascular malformations—a review of 101 cases. Gut 1986;27:213.

95. Miko TL, Thomazy VA. The caliber-persistent artery of the stomach: a unifying approach to gastric aneurysm, Dieulafoy's lesion and submucosal arterial malformation. Hum Pathol 1988;19:914.

96. Loftus EV, Alexander GL, Balm RK. Endoscopic treatment of bleeding gastroduodenal malignancies (abstract). Gastrointest Endosc 1993;39:269.

97. Johnston JH. Complications of gastrointestinal laser endoscopy. In: Jensen DM, Brunetaud JM, eds. Medical laser endoscopy. Dordrecht, The Netherlands: Kluwer Academic Publishers, 1990:207.

98. Jensen DM. Gastrointestinal angiomata. In: Gastrointestinal endoscopy. Diagnostic and therapeutic procedures. An information resource manual. Manchester, MA: American Society for Gastrointestinal Endoscopy, 1989:36.

99. Brunetaud JM, Maunoury V, Cochelard D, Cortot A, Paris JD. Laser treatment for vascular malformations of the digestive tract. In: Jensen DM, Brunetaud JM, eds. Medical laser endoscopy. Dordrecht, The Netherlands: Kluwer Academic Publishers, 1990:93.

100. Tio TL, Tytgat GNJ. Endoscopic ultrasonography of normal and pathologic upper gastrointestinal wall structure. Compar-

ison of studies in vivo and in vitro with histology. Scand J Gastroenterol Suppl 1986;21(123):27.

101. Silverstein F, Kimmey M, Martin R, et al. Ultrasound and the intestinal wall: experimental methods. Scand J Gastroenterol Suppl 1989;21(123):34.

102. Kohler B, Riemann JF. The endoscopic Doppler: its value in evaluating gastroduodenal ulcers after hemorrhage and as an instrument of control of endoscopic injection therapy. Scand J Gastroenterol 1991;26:471.

103. Jaspersen D. Dieulafoy's disease controlled by Doppler ultrasound endoscopic treatment. Gut 1993;34:857.

104. Jensen DM, Machicado GA, Kovacs TOG, Randall GM, Reedy T. Long-term recurrence rates of peptic ulceration and rebleeding with H2 maintenance, surgery, and no maintenance therapy (abstract). Gastroenterology 1989;96:A239.

105. Egan JV, Jensen DM. Long-term management of patients with bleeding ulcers: rationale, results, and economic impact. Gastrointest Endosc Clin North Am 1991;1(2):367.

106. Jensen DM, You S, Jensen ME, et al. Randomized controlled study of ranitidine maintenance for patients with a recent duodenal ulcer hemorrhage. N Engl J Med 1994;330:382.

107. Jensen DM. Economic and health aspects of peptic ulcer disease and H2 receptor antagonists. Am J Med 1986;8(Suppl 4B):42.

108. Jensen DM. Economic assessment of peptic ulcer disease. Scand J Gastroenterol Suppl 1988;23(146):214.

109. NIH consensus development conference: therapeutic endoscopy and bleeding ulcers. J Am Med Assoc 1989;262:1369.

110. Proceedings of the consensus conference on therapeutic endoscopy in bleeding ulcers. Gastrointest Endosc 1990;36(Suppl):51.

111. Cook, DJ, Guyatt GH, Salena BJ, Laine L. Endoscopic therapy for acute non-variceal upper gastrointestinal hemorrhage: a meta-analysis. Gastroenterology 1992:102.

112. Sacks HS, Chalmers TC, Blum AL, Berrier J, Pegano D. Endoscopic hemostasis. An effective therapy for bleeding peptic ulcers. J Am Med Assoc 1990;264:494.

Textbook of Gastroenterology, second edition, edited by Tadataka Yamada. JB Lippincott Company, Philadelphia © 1995.

CHAPTER 139

Endoscopic Therapy for Sessile Lesions

Gregory G. Ginsberg   David Elliot Fleischer

Therapeutic Principles
Thermal Modalities
Nonthermal Modalities
Other Therapeutic Techniques
Clinical Principles
Precursor Lesions
Objectives of Treatment
Considerations in Patient Selection for Endoscopic Therapy

Esophageal Lesions
Patient Evaluation
Dilation of Esophageal Cancer
Endoscopic Laser Therapy for Esophageal Cancer
Bipolar Electrocoagulation
Endoscopic Intubation
Comparative Studies

(continued)

Gastric Lesions
  Gastric Polyps
  Early Gastric Cancer
  Advanced Gastric Cancer
  Metastatic Tumors to the Stomach
Duodenal Lesions

Colorectal Lesions
  Diminutive Adenomatous Polyps
  Flat Adenoma
  Sessile Colorectal Polyps
  Large Sessile Adenomas
  Endoscopic Treatment of Colorectal Cancers

A natural extension of the improved diagnostic capabilities afforded by flexible endoscopy has been the development of therapeutic innovations applied, usually under direct vision, through the endoscope's working channel. A wide range of endoscopic interventions has evolved to meet the challenges of managing tumors of the lumenal gastrointestinal tract.

In its simplest terms, endoscopic therapies do one of the following: resect, destroy, or displace tissue. Endoscopic tumor resection is generally performed via diathermic snare resection, although multiple forceps biopsies may suffice for diminutive lesions. Tumor destruction or ablation is facilitated by thermal (i.e., electrocautery or laser), chemical, afterloading (i.e., intralumenal radiotherapy), or photodynamic means. Although performed with a curative intent in some instances, more often, ablative therapies are employed for palliation, usually of bleeding or lumenal obstruction. Tumor displacement is always palliative and brought about by mechanical dilation or more permanently by the insertion of a plastic or metallic endoprosthesis. Multiple modalities may be used in combinations or at different intervals in the face of disease progression.

This chapter provides a review of the modalities available for endoscopic treatment of sessile neoplastic lesions of the digestive tract. Means of accurate diagnosis, staging and patient selection will be addressed. The role of endoscopic therapy for the prevention, cure, and palliation of esophageal, gastric, proximal small bowel, and colorectal cancer is discussed. Data from prospective controlled trials, is provided, where available, and the personal experience of the authors is given emphasis. Limitations, cost considerations and specific guidelines are offered for several options.

Endoscopic therapy of sessile lesions may be curative when the neoplasm is benign or contains early carcinoma with favorable histologic characteristics. Endoscopic therapy for palliation of advanced gastrointestinal malignancies has several appealing aspects: it averts the need for surgery and general anesthesia; side effects are minimal; it is performed under direct vision; it has no maximum dose, so that repeated treatments can be performed if necessary; and quality of life is generally improved. Disadvantages are that typically, only the intralumenal portion of the tumor is treated; technical success does not always assure functional success; and survival is not prolonged. With the growing tendency to explore minimally invasive treatments, the role of endoscopic therapies for sessile lesions is sure to increase.

THERAPEUTIC PRINCIPLES

Thermal Modalities

Tissue response to thermal energy is dependent on temperature and absorption (Table 139-1). Low level tissue heating up to 45°C is defined as *hyperthermia*. When applied over several minutes, tissue injury may occur. Long treatment times and the absence of immediately visible tissue effects are disadvantages. Currently endoscopic applications for hyperthermic therapy remain investigational.

Tissue heating to temperatures between 45°C and 99°C results in *coagulation*. Coagulation necrosis can be achieved within a matter of seconds and the tissue effect, at least on the surface, can be observed immediately. Tissue coagulation is caused by protein denaturization and the destruction of cellular components, resulting in structural alterations and cell death. Tissue desiccation and shrinkage is produced and a whitening is observed. Shrinkage of the tissue leads to constriction of the involved blood vessels with resultant thrombosis. This feature enables primary hemostasis as well as prevention of rebleeding. Sloughing of the coagulated tissue occurs in several days leaving an ulceration with fibrosis and lymphocytic infiltration. At the periphery of a coagulation necrosis injury, a rim of hyperemic tissue may be seen acutely. This is the result of radiant thermal injury to the surrounding

TABLE 139-1
Temperature and Tissue Effects

TEMPERATURE (°C)	HISTOLOGIC EVENT	ENDOSCOPIC APPEARANCE
45	Cell death, edema	Erythema
60	Protein coagulates	Whitening
80	Collagen shrinkage	Puckering
100	Tissue water boils	Vaporization causes divot
210	Desiccated tissue burns	Charring, glowing embers

tissue. Histologically, edema, hemorrhage and vasodilatation are present; subsequently necrosis occurs.[1]

When tissue is rapidly heated to above 100°C, *vaporization* results. At these temperatures, tissue fluids and water vaporize, proteins denature, smoke is created, and carbonization may occur. Obliteration of tissue, as evidenced by a divot, may be produced. Radiant heat transmitted to the surrounding tissue causes coagulation necrosis and hemostasis at the edges of the vaporized defect.

At temperatures greater than 210°C, *incandescence* occurs as dehydrated tissue burns. There is no role for the use of temperatures in this range for therapeutic endoscopy.

Electrosurgery

Electrosurgical current, at frequencies greater than 100,000 cycles per second, causes excitation of molecular particles imparting a kinetic energy which raises the cellular temperature. The heat directed to the tissue is dependent on the *resistance* offered by the tissue to current flow, the *current density* itself, and the *duration* of current application.[2] Generally, a longer duration of energy application results in more heat generated and a greater depth of tissue effect.

Total heat attained in a tissue will increase directly with the resistance. Water is a good conductor, offering low resistance, and therefore decreases heating effect. Once tissue water has been evaporated, dry desiccated tissue has a high resistance and is subject to increased heating effect, which may result in undesirable injury to surrounding tissue.

The current density is the effect on heating of the cross-sectional area of the tissue through which the current is flowing. Current density varies indirectly with the cross-sectional area. A thin diameter snare wire allows a high current density and thus greater temperature in the adjacent tissue. The broad grounding pad used in monopolar electrosurgery provides a large cross-sectional area and thus a low current density with no significant tissue heating at the exit site.

Monopolar electrodes. Monopolar devices used in endoscopic therapy include the diathermic snare and the hot biopsy forceps. The monopolar device in contact with the tissue surface forms one pole from which current flows. A grounding plate affixed to the patient's skin completes the circuit. Because of the differential in current density at the site of contact with the device versus the grounding plate, tissue heating is concentrated near the monopolar electrode. Both coagulation and cutting can be accomplished with monopolar therapy. These effects may be roughly selected for by the application of a continuous (CUT) or intermittently pulsed (COAG) current. A blended current is produced when these two types of current are mixed in varying ratios. When a monopolar device is held near, but not in contact with, the tissue surface, a spark may be generated. Use of this technique, called *fulguration,* results in surface desiccation and coagulation necrosis. Depth of tissue injury, however, is difficult to predict or control. A tissue specimen is not retrieved for histologic assessment, and the technique is not generally used with flexible endoscopy.

Diathermic snare. Electroresection using a diathermic snare is commonly utilized. The procedure can be performed to completely resect a polypoid lesion, perform piecemeal polypectomy, reduce a large tumor mass, or provide tissue for histologic confirmation. A wire loop which acts as a monopolar electrode is used to ensnare the tissue for resection. Techniques for standard polypectomy are described elsewhere in this book. One method utilizing alternate application of COAG and CUT currents allows initial desiccation followed by cutting to secure hemostasis. Alternatively, use of a blended current may allow cutting and coagulation in one maneuver. A comparison of blended versus CUT current failed to demonstrate a statistically significant difference in the incidence of complications between the two with respect to major and minor bleeding, transmural burn, and perforation.[3] The timing of major bleeding, however, was significantly different: all of the major hemorrhages were immediate when blended current was used; all were delayed 2 to 8 days when pure COAG current was used.

When performing snare resection of sessile lesions or when performing a mucosal strip biopsy, adjunctive techniques may be used to improve results. Injection of physiologic saline into the submucosa at the base of the lesion creates a pillow effect, lifting the lesion away from the muscularis mucosae and allowing a purchase for ensnarement. Others have utilized double channeled endoscopes, with which a lesion may be ensnared via instrumentation through one working channel while a forceps is placed through the second channel to grasp and elevate the lesion. The authors have not found the latter technique easy to perform or very beneficial.

Hot-biopsy forceps. Small polyps, generally 5 mm or less in diameter, can be removed with a hot biopsy forceps. The jaws of the forceps have a blunted rather than sharp, surface to allow grasping rather than cutting of the tissue. The polyp is grasped and tented away from the mucosa. Generation of the electrosurgical current produces coagulation necrosis at the pseudostalk. A specimen suitable for histologic assessment is retrieved, hemostasis is achieved, and residual abnormal tissue may be destroyed within the extent of the tissue injury. Small (2.3 mm) and large (3.2 mm) diameter forceps are available. However, prospective studies evaluating the efficacy of the hot biopsy forceps for eradicating residual polypoid tissue have not yielded favorable results.[4,5]

Multipolar electrocoagulation. In bipolar and multipolar electrocautery both active electrodes are contained on the device tip. With this technique a circuit is completed when current passes through the tissue between two adjacent electrodes. Low powers are used and a grounding plate is unnecessary. When desiccation occurs in the contact tissue, resistance increases, effectively limiting the extent and depth of tissue injury. The depth of tissue injury is typically equal to the center-to-center distance between the electrodes.

Multipolar hemostatic probes, used effectively for endoscopic treatment of bleeding lesions, have been used to treat bleeding from neoplastic tissue. Multipolar electrode cautery devices, other than the BICAP tumor probe (Circon-ACMI, Stamford, CT), have been used to ablate tumor by producing coagulation necrosis. However, its use in this capacity has been limited because the depth of effect is shallow and tissue tends to stick to the tip requiring frequent cleaning. Conversely, heated contact probes also used for endoscopic hemostasis, do not allow adequate dissipation of heat for effective tumor ablation.

BICAP tumor probe. The BICAP tumor probe is similar in appearance to an Eder-Puestow dilator. In place of the metal olive, however, is a multipolar electrocoagulation unit. The standard kit consists of five probes. Four probes have electrical contact plates arranged circumferentially allowing a 360-degree radius of coagulation. The contact portion of the probes are 6, 9, 12, and 15 mm in diameter. The fifth probe is 15 mm in diameter, and has a 180-degree hemicircumferential configuration of the electrical plates. Tumor probes are used primarily in the palliation of circumferential esophageal malignancies and are discussed in detail in that section. They have also been used to treat rectal cancers.

Laser

The term *laser* is an acronym for light amplification by stimulated emission of radiation. Laser energy is created and harnessed when electrons in an active medium are bombarded by photons from an energy source. Electrons in the active medium are raised to a higher energy state. When they are struck again while at an elevated energy level, a pair of photons is released. This reaction takes place in a nearly closed space cylinder with mirrors on either side which reflect the photons. Repeated stimulation results in an amplified production of photons, which is then harnessed as photoelectric energy. A defect in one of the reflecting mirrors allows the release of a column of light energy which can be intensely focused and precisely aimed. The light energy emitted is monochromatic and unique to the active medium from which it is produced. Tissue effects vary based on the distinct characteristics of the tissue-wavelength interaction of the laser in use. Neodymium: yttrium aluminum garnet (Nd:YAG) and argon lasers have been used for endoscopic therapy of GI malignancies. With the Nd:YAG laser the active medium is a solid; with the argon laser it is a gas. Initial investigation of the use of lasers in endoscopic therapy included both the Nd:YAG and the argon lasers, however, the Nd:YAG has become the favored technology.

When laser light strikes tissue it can be absorbed, scattered, reflected or transmitted. Usually some combination of these effects is observed. The tissue response depends on the wavelength-specific interaction of the laser with the specific absorption characteristics of the tissue components, most significantly water and hemoglobin. Reflected and transmitted energy cause no tissue effects. Direct absorption results in excitation at the molecular level and the generation of heat. A variable portion of laser energy, not directly absorbed by the target tissue, may be scattered and absorbed by the immediately surrounding tissue—this, too, is dependent on the specific laser wavelength-tissue interaction. Although some scatter is necessary for hemostasis, peripheral tissue injury increases relative to the total amount of scatter.

The thermal effect is dependent on the power in watts, the duration, and the distance, or spot size, of the laser beam. Although contact laser probes have been used in endoscopic laser therapy (ELT), the noncontact mode predominates. A focal distance of approximately 10 mm. typically yields the optimal spot size and tissue effect. With the Nd:YAG laser at a 1-cm distance, lower-power settings (30–50 watts) produce photocoagulation. High-power settings (80–100 watts) will produce photoablation of tissue. A rim of coagulation necrosis typically surrounds the zone of photoablation. The power setting is adjusted to obtain the desired effect. The application may be continuous or interrupted. Interrupted, pulsed, application may yield greater directed tissue effect with decreased conduction of heat energy to the surrounding tissue.

Lasers have been used for both curative and palliative therapy for esophageal, gastric, duodenal and colorectal lesions. Advantages are the capacity to vaporize tissue in addition to producing coagulation necrosis; large areas of tumor can be treated in a single session; the noncontact mode avoids the problem of tissue sticking to the device; extensive worldwide experience has demonstrated it to be a safe and effective tool for endoscopic therapy of GI tumors. Disadvantages are the production of smoke; concern over the possibility of carcinogens or viral particles in the smoke plume; damage to endoscopic equipment; and cost. Smoke can be minimized with avoidance of charring the tissue. A dual channel endoscope is efficient in suctioning smoke through the second working channel. Damage to the endoscope can be avoided by attention to the location of the laser fiber tip outside the working channel when firing. Risk of ocular injury and the need for special eye safety wear is no longer an issue with the use of videoendoscopes. All modern videoendoscopes are laser coated; however, when using Nd:YAG at high power or other lasers in the visible light spectrum, the videoprocessor may be overpowered, resulting in an image white-out during firing of the laser. The involved industries need to develop improved filters to overcome this problem. Initial equipment costs are high, and repair costs can also be considerable, however, once a laser is in place and operational, its use is not significantly more costly than other treatment modalities.

Contact tips may also be utilized.[6,7] These are synthesized with coated ceramic materials that allow concentration of the laser energy at the contact surface. Synthetic coatings minimize, or eliminate, the problem of debris sticking to the tip surface. Contact laser tips, depending on their design, can be used to cut, coagulate or vaporize tissue. Potential advantages are that: lower energy levels are required (12–20 watts); less smoke is produced; and the depth of tissue effect may be more reliably controlled. Generally, however, it takes longer to treat the same volume of tissue than with a noncontact mode.

Naveau and colleagues[8] evaluated the use of a naked, or bare-tipped, fiber imbedded 2 to 3 mm into tumor to obtain cavitation and vaporization. When compared with the non contact coaxial fiber technique, the method using the naked fiber achieved maximal endoscopic benefit in fewer treatment sessions and at a lower financial cost. This technique has not been advanced by others.

Nonthermal Modalities

Chemical Injection

Chemical injection therapy is attractive because it is cheap, simple and readily available. A variety of chemical agents have been used for palliation of GI malignancies, to both debulk the tumor as well as for the treatment of bleeding from tumor. These have included chemotherapeutic agents (e.g., 5-fluorouracil) and chemical sclerosants such as polidocanol, ethanol, and sodium morrhuate. Tissue destruction is brought about by chemical necrolysis. Hemostasis is achieved by the combination of edema, vasoconstriction, and thrombosis.

Disadvantages are the inability to control the depth of tissue injury and the lack of immediately visible tissue effect to guide therapy. Only small series have been reported.

Photodynamic Therapy

The biological effects of photodynamic therapy (PDT) are photochemical and different from those induced by heat. Photosensitizing drugs are administered which have some selectivity to localize preferentially in severely dysplastic cells. The photsensitizing agent is then activated by laser induced fluorescence applied in close proximity to the lesion. Activation by light produces a local cytotoxic effect mediated by singlet oxygen. Dye lasers are typically used because they can deliver a selective wavelength of light energy specific to the absorptive peak of the photosensitizer. The extent of necrosis is dependent on tissue concentration of the photosensitizing agent and the dose of laser light given. Necrotic tissue sloughs and is replaced by normal regenerative tissue. A potential advantage of PDT is that due to a lack of effect on tissue collagen, even in full thickness necrosis, there is no risk of perforation because the mechanical strength of the lumenal wall is not reduced. Another advantage is that large areas may be treated at a single setting.

Hematoporphyrin derivatives have been the most widely investigated sensitizing agents, but are far from ideal. Unfortunately the difference in the concentration of sensitizing agent between the tumorous tissue and the tissue from which it arose is small, and that difference is in the vascular stromal cells and not the tumor cells themselves. Thus selective eradication of individual tumor cells, with preservation of normal cells, at the advancing edge of the lesion is not feasible. Severe hemorrhage has been reported following PDT to advanced tumors. Another disadvantage of PDT is that of photosensitivity of skin to ambient light such that direct sunlight must be avoided. The cost of PDT is high and the lasers are finicky.

Currently the use of PDT has been restricted. It has been applied for the treatment of esophageal, gastric and colon cancers. When used as palliative therapy, recanalization of advanced esophageal tumors has been reported. PDT is more suited for the eradication of early tumors rather than advanced ones.

Intracavitary Irradiation

Endoscopy has been used to place intralumenal isotopes directly in contact with or adjacent to a lesion. The advantage in enabling close approximation of the dose is that surrounding tissue can be spared the effects of radiation. The initial encouraging results of laser therapy in patients with carcinomas of the esophagus and cardia and of brachytherapy have not been reproduced.

Other Therapeutic Techniques

Resection

Resection employs the use of instruments to separate and remove the abnormal tissue from the surrounding normal tissue. Its distinct advantage over ablative therapy is that tissue resection provides a specimen for pathologic review, allowing a confirmatory histologic diagnosis and assessment of the margins. For benign neoplasms and malignant lesions that have not metastasized, total endoscopic resection with demonstrable clean margins is curative in most instances. Generally electrcoagulation is required to provide hemostasis at the site of resection. Electrocoagulation may also serve to destroy residual abnormal tissue at the base of the lesion not removed with the resected specimen.

The best example of endoscopic resection therapy is the diathermic snare polypectomy of a pedunculated or small sessile colonic adenoma with contained carcinoma in situ (CIS). The lesion is readily accessible with a colonoscope. The abnormal tissue can be visually distinguished from the surrounding normal mucosa. The entire lesion can be removed by a minimally invasive technique which is safe, relatively inexpensive, and can be performed on an outpatient basis, with conscious sedation. The resected specimen is submitted to the pathologist for histologic diagnosis of its malignant nature and confirmation of clean margins. In the presence of favorable histologic features, this approach to management results in curative therapy.[9,10] Favorable histologic features are defined as: the absence of CIS; or well- or moderately well-differentiated CIS, with no invasion of lymphatics, and a clean margin of 2 to 3 mm. When unfavorable histologic features such as moderately or poorly differentiated CIS, invasion into vasculature or lymphatics, invasion into the stalk or to the resected margin are present, a cancer operation should be performed if the patient is a candidate.

Piecemeal polypectomy is used to resect large lesions which are unsuitable for standard snare polypectomy. In contrast to complete polypectomy the snare is used to selectively remove portions of the intralumenal lesion. In this way, broad sessile lesions may be resected, the base coagulated, and tissue submitted for histologic interpretation, including an assessment of the margins.[11] Piecemeal snare resection may also be used as a debulking procedure, decreasing tumor volume, thereby facilitating further treatment.[12,13]

Endoscopic strip biopsy was first described by Tada and colleagues[14] and developed for resection of flat or depressed lesions (Fig. 139-1). The technique has subsequently been applied to sessile and broad-based polypoid lesions. A small volume (2–4 mL) of physiologic saline is injected into the submucosa beneath the lesion with an endoscopic needle (see Fig. 139-1); use of hypertonic saline-epinephrine and 50% dextrose solutions have been described as well. This elevates the lesion so that it can then be resected by snare cautery in the usual method for endoscopic polypectomy. The horizontal separation of the lesion from the underlying tissue minimizes the extent of excision needed to resect the specimen. This technique increases the resistance to high frequency alternating current, so that the effects of electrocoagulation are more closely limited to the submucosa. The lesion may be resected in its entirety or in a piecemeal fashion. Specimens are retrieved and the margins of resection can be assessed histologically. This technique allows removal of a large portion of the mucosa, while preventing serious complications such as bleeding or perforation.

Any mucosal lesion that can be safely removed en toto endoscopically, should be managed as such. Reliance on forceps biopsy sampling alone, without complete resection of the lesion, may result in false-negative results, as focal areas of neoplasia or even carcinoma may be missed. Lesions in the

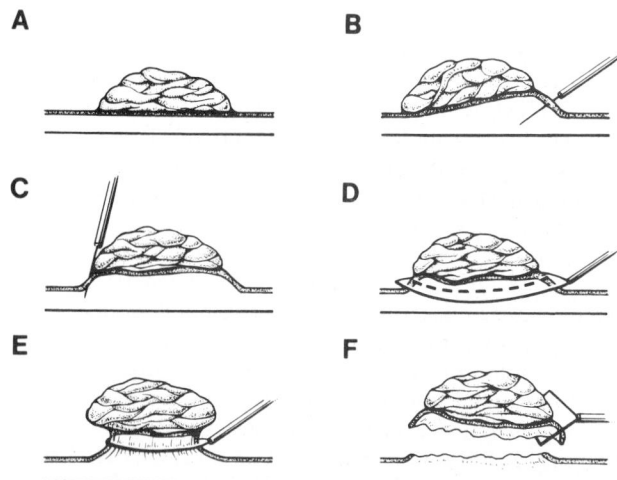

FIGURE 139-1. Strip biopsy technique. **(A)** Sessile lesion is limited to mucosa. **(B, C)** Physiologic saline is injected into the submucosa around the periphery of the lesion, creating a pillow effect. **(D, E)** The lesion is resected using a loop snare. **(F)** The entire specimen is retrieved.

colon, stomach and duodenum are generally amenable to this approach. Neoplastic lesions in the esophagus, on the other hand, do not generally lend themselves to endoscopic resection.

Endoscopic ultrasound (EUS) has improved diagnostic and staging capabilities for gastrointestinal neoplasms. Although not a substitute for histologic determination, EUS can dis-

tinguish depth of invasion allowing an assessment of whether a lesion may be amenable to endoscopic resection (Fig. 139-2). EUS allows accurate staging and assessment of resectability in carcinoma of the esophagus, stomach, duodenum, and rectosigmoid.[15,16] CT scanning should be obtained to complement local tumor and lymph node staging obtained by EUS and for the assessment of distant metastasis.

Ablation

Total destruction and eradication of neoplastic tissue can be accomplished by inducing necrosis or vaporization. Laser phototherapy can yield photocoagulation, with subsequent necrosis and sloughing, or primary photoablation. Nd:YAG laser (1062 nm) therapy is the most frequently utilized means for tumor ablation. Indications for Nd:YAG laser photoablation include palliative irradiation to reduce tumor mass and to recanalize obstructing lesions in the upper and lower GI tract; and for curative eradication of sessile villous adenomas in the stomach, duodenum and colorectum.

PDT is another means of tumor destruction. This method exploits the ability of a photoactive drug to be retained in tumors relative to adjacent normal tissue. Laser light activation (630 nm) of the photosensitizer results in a chemical reaction causing cell death and subsequent tumor destruction.

Displacement

Tumor displacement is accomplished by the use of lateral shearing forces to stretch and tear the abnormal tissue. It is hoped that the displacement will convey some memory to

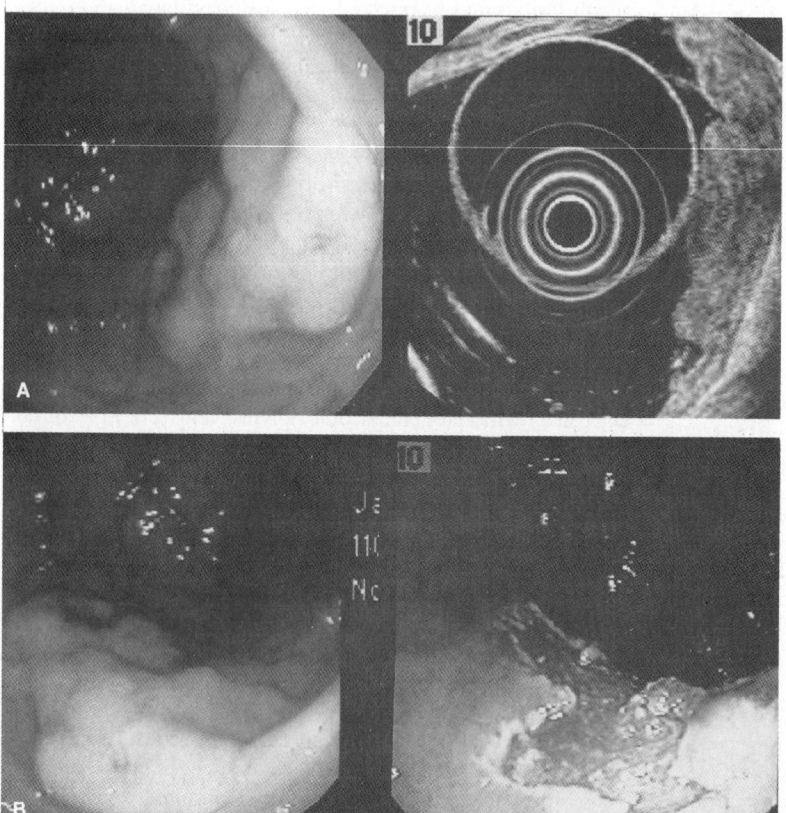

FIGURE 139-2. Large sessile rectal lesion. **(A)** Endoscopic ultrasonography demonstrates a T1 lesion without invasion into the muscularis propria. **(B)** Piecemeal snare resection was curative.

the tissue to provide a prolonged duration of effect. Temporary displacement can usually be accomplished with dilation using a number of mechanical devices. Dilation may be performed adjunctively to facilitate more definitive thermal or stent therapy. More permanent displacement is accomplished with the insertion of a rigid or expandable endoprosthesis into the stenotic region. This is done almost exclusively for palliation of cancers of the esophagus and gastroesophageal junction. In addition to maintaining lumenal patency, intubation may be used to seal enterorespiratory fistulas in the setting of esophageal or bronchogenic carcinoma. Case reports of expandable metal stents being placed in the colon and nonesophageal upper gastrointestinal tract are appearing in the literature.[17,18]

A variety of dilating systems have been utilized and are widely available. Mercury filled rubber bougies have been used for nonobstructing esophageal and rectal lesions. Tapered polyvinyl dilators that can be passed over a guidewire are the most popular means of dilating tight strictures of the esophagus and esophagogastric junction. A flexible spring-tip guidewire is passed through the stricture under fluoroscopic guidance. Progressively larger diameter dilators are then passed over the guidewire to dilate the stricture. This technique is described in detail in the section on endoscopic therapy for esophageal cancers.

Eder-Puestow and, similarly, KeyMed Advanced dilators consist of smooth metal olives of various diameters fixed to a flexible shaft which can be passed over a guidewire. Some experts prefer this system for the initial dilation of long, tight, and tortuous malignant esophageal strictures.[19]

Through-the-scope (TTS) pneumatic or hydrostatic balloon dilators direct their shearing forces in a radial, rather than longitudinal, axis and are a safe and effective alternative means of dilating complex malignant strictures.[20] They may be used for dilating tight, angulated esophageal stenosis, and for gastric and colorectal neoplasms. TTS balloon dilators pass through the channel of the endoscope and can be inserted into the stenotic segment under endoscopic guidance. The actual dilation can be monitored both endoscopically and fluoroscopically. In the authors' experience, balloon dilators have not been as effective as tapered polyvinyl dilators for treatment of malignant strictures.

CLINICAL PRINCIPLES

Precursor Lesions

All neoplasms originate from a focus of abnormal cells. In some cases, premalignant or early malignant lesions may be distinguished by their macroscopic appearance at endoscopy as distinct from the surrounding normal mucosa. Barrett's mucosa and the colonic adenomatous polyp-to-cancer sequence are two prominent examples.

Barrett's esophagus has been identified as a precursor lesion for adenocarcinoma of the esophagus and the esophagogastric junction.[21] The aim of endoscopic surveillance is to identify CIS or premalignant changes (i.e., high-grade dysplasia). When carcinoma, and in some cases high grade dysplasia, is identified in Barrett's epithelia, surgical resection is recommended. The use of the Nd:YAG and argon lasers to ablate

Barrett's mucosa with subsequent replacement by normal squamous mucosa, has been recently reported.[22-24] Proponents believe this may be a means by which this potentially premalignant condition may be eradicated.

Squamous cell carcinoma of the esophagus does not present with a macroscopically appreciable premalignant lesion. The best chance for long term survival in patients with squamous cell carcinoma of the esophagus is when the lesion is identified early and curative resection can be performed. Aggressive screening programs in Asian populations where esophageal squamous cell carcinoma is endemic have been successful in increasing the percentage of early stage cancers at the time of diagnosis.[25] The endoscopic application of vital stains, such as Lugol's solution, to identify malignant or dysplastic epithelia, and to clearly demarcate the extent of surface spread, is partly responsible for their good results. Experience with endoscopic mucosal resection techniques as primary therapy for dysplastic mucosal lesions in the esophagus, and other portions of the upper GI tract, is gaining in Japan.[26] No such high risk populations for squamous cell carcinoma have been identified in Western societies to warrant widespread endoscopic screening. There are several conditions that have been associated with a higher incidence of squamous cell carcinoma of the esophagus: Plummer-Vincent syndrome, tylosis, achalasia, and prior caustic ingestion. The greatest association is with laryngeal and oropharyngeal cancers. There may be a synergistic association seen with combined cigarette and alcohol use.

Adenomatous gastric polyps are true neoplasms and are considered premalignant with a reported incidence of malignant transformation ranging from 6% to 75%.[27] Pedunculated polyps greater than 2 cm in diameter and sessile lesions are more often associated with carcinomatous conversion. Hyperplastic gastric polyps are associated with a much lower risk malignant potential. However, all gastric polyps amenable to snare resection should be removed in this fashion as it renders the entire specimen for histologic exam, thus avoiding the potential for sampling error incurred with forceps biopsy.[28] Furthermore, in most instances snare resection of a gastric polyp is effectively curative.

The endoscopic management of pedunculated and small sessile colorectal polyps is well established. Snare resection for invasive adenocarcinoma contained in an adenomatous polyp is curative if favorable histologic features are present (i.e., low-grade carcinoma with free margins of resection and no evidence of lymphatic invasion). When the pathology of the resected specimen reveals unfavorable criteria (i.e., high-grade carcinoma at or near the resected margin or lymphatic invasion), a cancer operation is generally recommended. For large sessile villous adenomas of the colon and rectum that cannot be easily removed by snare resection, surgery remains the first option. However, patients who are poor surgical candidates or who are unwilling to undergo partial colectomy, may be considered for endoscopic snare resection or laser ablation therapy with intent to cure.

Objectives of Treatment

When complete resection or destruction of a precancerous neoplasms or early stage malignancy (i.e., T1 or T2, N0 stage) is achieved, endoscopic therapy may be curative. Lesions amenable to endoscopic therapy with a curative intent may be identified: in patients who present early on with symptoms related to the lesion; as an incidental finding during evaluation for symptoms unrelated to the presence of the lesion; or during surveillance endoscopy for a premalignant condition. Endoscopic resection with retieval of the entire specimen for pathologic interpretation is preferred. Endoscopic ablation techniques are often easier to perform, however, no histologic specimen is provided.

In nearly all instances, for patients who present with locally contained gastrointestinal tract malignancies surgical resection is generally preferred. Alternatively, patients with T1 or T2, N0 lesions who are poor operative candidates or who refuse surgery may be candidates for endoscopic therapy with an intent to cure. In patients with more advanced lesions, palliatiative surgical resection gennerally provides the best results. However, surgical resection with a palliative intent is accompanied by increased morbidity and mortality when compared to endoscopic therapy and is not typically associated with a prolongation or improved quality of life.

The following are the desired goals of palliative therapy:

- reestablish or maintain lumenal patency and enteral nutrition
- rapid effect
- long-lasting effect
- well tolerated by patient
- keep costs low
- low rate of complications
- outpatient procedure (minimize hospitalizations).

Endoscopic palliative therapy meets many of these goals. It is generally performed on an outpatient basis, using conscious sedation. Mortality rates are exceedingly low and the morbidity is quite acceptable. Patient discomfort is generally minimal. Results are achieved quickly, usually in one or two sessions, and in many instances are long-lasting. Costs are typically lower than other modalities.

Palliation of symptoms, without influencing survival, can usually be obtained by partial destruction of the tumor by endoscopic therapy. Because destruction is only partial, repeated sessions are likely to be required depending on the rate of tumor growth and the patient's overall condition. Treatment aimed at both palliation of symptoms and prolongation of life require more extensive destruction of the primary tumor and may be performed as a component of multimodality therapy including radiation or chemotherapy.

Factors influencing the decision between endoscopic therapy and surgical resection include: the stage of the tumor, its location and morphology, the overall prognosis of the disease, the patient's age, the presence of comorbid disease, assessment of resectability versus operability, and the morbidity and mortality associated with the operative procedure.

Considerations in Patient Selection for Endoscopic Therapy

Following staging, patients are typically divided in two groups: those with nonmalignant or local-regional disease in whom the lesion is potentially curable, and those with extensive or metastatic disease in whom palliation is the goal. As expected, patients with poor performance status at the initiation of endoscopic therapy are less likely to achieve a good functional outcome.[29] Specifically, premorbid patients, in whom life-1expectancy is less than 1 month, are unlikely to receive meaningful benefit from endoscopic therapy.

EUS staging of local tumor extent and regional lymph node involvement is a considerable improvement over conventional staging tools. It allows more accurate identification of patients with unresectable disease who might be best served with endoscopic palliation. Furthermore, EUS may allow accurate identification of those lesions amenable to primary curative endoscopic therapy.[30]

When early lesions are identified, surgical resection offers the best chance for curative therapy. Unfortunately, the majority of patients with upper GI malignancies have extensive disease at the time of presentation. The 5-year survival rate for upper GI cancers ranges from 9% to 16%.[31] Many patients presenting with upper gastrointestinal tract malignancies are elderly, have comorbid diseases, and are malnourished—each an independent variable for poor outcome. Resectability may be hampered because these tumors frequently invade or encase surrounding vital structures. Therefore, palliative endoscopic therapy plays a major role in the management of patients with symptoms due to upper GI malignancies. Dysphagia, obstruction and bleeding are the most common symptoms. Endoscopic therapy with an intent to cure should be reserved for nonmalignant lesions and for early lesions in patients unwilling or unable to withstand surgery.

Colorectal cancer is more often identified at an earlier stage and has a better outlook.[31] Colorectal cancers also have a more favorable result following palliative surgical resection. Again, however, many patients are elderly and frail and wish to avoid major surgery, particularly the abdominoperineal resection for rectosigmoid lesions. Others will find the consideration of a colostomy unacceptable. Recurrence following surgery is not uncommon and frequently is not amenable to repeat resection. Noncancerous neoplasms (e.g., villous adenomas) may be adequately managed endoscopically. Therefore, endoscopic therapy with an intent to cure may be applicable for benign colorectal neoplasms and focal carcinomas in patients unwilling or unable to withstand surgery. Palliative endoscopic therapy is appropriate for patients with symptoms related to advanced or recurrent disease. Obstruction, bleeding, mucus discharge, and tenesmus are the most common symptoms.

ESOPHAGEAL LESIONS

In the United States and Europe, the majority of patients who present with symptoms related to esophageal cancer already have advanced disease. For this reason, survival seldom exceeds one year. Reasons for this include the absence of a serosal layer, the presence of a rich lymphatic drainage system, and the proximity to a number of vital structures that prohibits a wide excision. Many patients delay seeking medical attention in spite of the onset of symptoms and thus are in poor condition at the time of initial presentation.

In parts of the world where squamous cell carcinoma is endemic, aggressive screening programs have increased the incidence of early stage cancers at the time of detection. In the West, early cancers (e.g., CIS or invasive cancer limited to the mucosa without lymphatic spread) may be detected in patients with Barrett's esophagus undergoing surveillance endoscopy with biopsies. EUS has allowed more accurate staging of local invasion in esophageal cancers.[32] Improved long-term survival is likely to be achieved when the cancer is diagnosed at an early stage, T1 or T2, N0.[31]

Surgery remains the best option for patients in whom the possibility of a curative resection exists. Two types of operative approachs are performed, transthoracic and transhiatal. Success rates are best at centers where a high volume of esophageal surgery is performed. Endoscopic mucosal resection,[33] ELT[34] and PDT[35] for early esophageal cancers have been described, but should be reserved for patients who are otherwise ill-suited for surgical resection.

The majority of patients present with advanced disease. In these patients palliation is the main goal. Patients typically present with dysphagia, initially to solids, and subsequently to liquids as well. They may also present with esophageal obstruction, bleeding, or complications related to esophagorespiratory fistula formation. Malnutrition and sialorrhea may accompany late stages of disease.

There are a number of modalities available for the palliative management of esophageal cancer. These include surgical resection, radiotherapy, chemotherapy and endoscopic therapy. Less than 50% of patients can be resected and palliative resection is associated with mortality rates of 7% to 29%, and perioperative morbidity is considerable.[36-40] External beam radiation achieves temporary response in 25% of patients, with more than 50% of responders developing local recurrence.[37,41] Several weeks are required before the beneficial effects of radiation therapy are seen. Patients in whom recurrent symptoms develop cannot receive additional radiation therapy. Chemotherapy achieves a partial response rate of 50% but not without considerable side effects.[42] Combination radiotherapy and chemotherapy have not significantly improved these results. Furthermore, in one recent study,[43] severe side effects were experienced in 44% of patients, and life-threatening side effects were seen in 20%. Because of poor results and considerable morbidity associated with the aforementioned therapies, endoscopic palliation is attractive.

Several endoscopic modalities have been demonstrated as effective for the palliation of esophageal cancers. These include laser ablation, BICAP tumor probe therapy, and endoprosthesis placement. Endoscopic therapy is generally effective, of relative low cost, typically performed on an outpatient basis, and offers rapid and often prolonged relief of symptoms. The principal goal of endoscopic palliative therapy is to maintain a patent esophageal lumen. Other aims may be the management of esophagorespiratory fistulas, regurgitation and pulmonary aspiration, hemorrhage, pain, and malnutrition. As there is no intent to cure, patients eligible for endoscopic therapies should include those with unresectable or inoperable tumors and those with recurrent disease.

Patient Evaluation

Patient should undergo radiographic imaging studies including a barium swallow and a CT scan or MRI in addition to upper endoscopy. Blood work should include a CBC and bio-chemical tests with particular attention to liver-associated enzymes. EUS should be performed for thorough staging, allowing stratification of patients into classification based on the TNM system. The barium swallow defines the location and the length of the lesion. It is also the best method to map out angulations and distortions of the lumen. A barium swallow may also demonstrate the presence of a tracheoesophageal fistula. Endoscopy serves to establish or confirm the diagnosis of cancer allowing tissue biopsy. It allows direct evaluation of the lesion to determine whether it is exophytic or submucosal, polypoid or sessile, asymetric or circumferential. It also determines the lesion's position in relation to the upper esophageal sphincter and the gastroesophageal junction. CT scanning is most useful for the evaluation of metastatic disease to the liver, lungs and lymph nodes. A CT scan can also identify airway compression and the presence of pleural effusions. MRI of the chest does not appear to offer any additional information. EUS has been demonstrated to be more accurate for local tumor staging by depth of invasion and direct extension, as well as for local and celiac lymph node staging. It is unknown whether improved tumor staging afforded by EUS will contribute to a better patient outcome.

Dilation of Esophageal Cancer

Dilation is generally an effective means of providing temporary relief of dysphagia in patients with esophageal cancer. Dilating equipment currently used include polyvinyl dilators (e.g., Savary-Guilliard, American type), metal olives (e.g., Eder-Puestow), hydrostatic TTS balloons, Key-Med advanced dilators, and mercury filled rubber bougies (e.g., Maloney, Hurst). Advantages of dilation include simplicity, low cost, wide availability, short procedure time and relative safety. Most patients get initial benefit from dilation therapy. Successful palliation may be highly dependent on the anatomic location and physical characteristics of the tumor.[44,45] Dilation is a useful adjunct to other treatments including endoscopic interventions as well as external beam radiation or chemotherapy. Esophageal dilation is typically performed on an outpatient basis. Initial dilation of a tight stenosis may require sequential sessions before dysphagia is relieved. Typically patients remain at home between sessions. The main disadvantage of dilation therapy is that its relief is often short-lived and as the disease progresses, symptom-free intervals decrease in length requiring more frequent sessions.[46] The majority of patients find dilation therapy, alone, inadequate for satisfactory palliation.

In most instances, dilation should be performed over a guidewire with scored markings. If the pediatric or standard endoscope can be passed through the tumor, the guidewire can be advanced under direct visualization into the distal stomach and the endoscope removed. This is done by advancing the guidewire 10 cm and then withdrawing the endoscope by 10 cm until the endoscope is completely withdrawn. With the guidewire tip placed in the antrum, typically three markings, indicating 60 cm, are seen at the level of the incisors. When the endoscope cannot be passed through the lesion, the guidewire should be advanced under fluoroscopic control into the antrum. The guidewire should pass easily and its position confirmed fluoroscopically within the gastric air bubble. Subsequent dilation should also observed under fluoroscopic control. If placement of the guidewire into the stomach cannot be assured, dilation should not be performed as adverse results could be disastrous. With a well-positioned guidewire, progressively larger, tapered polyvinyl dilators can be passed over the guidewire. This technique is effective for passage through tight strictures and long or tortuous strictures. An assistant holds the exposed end of the guidewire, maintaining back traction while the lubricated dilator is passed through this strictured area. The guidewire position should be maintained and can be checked by fluoroscopic control and by the scored markers on the guidewire.

Initial diameter of the dilator should be estimated, based on endoscopic visualization. Effective and safe dilation is more art than science. Determining the ideal extent of dilation during a given session is subjective. Dilation should be gradual and not abrupt. Underdilation, with incomplete symptom relief requiring a repeat session, is preferable to overaggressive dilation that may result in a perforation. We recommend the start-low-and-go-slow philosophy. It is generally recommended that when using a taper-tip system, after the first degree of resistance is felt with an increased diameter dilator, two sequentially increased size dilators may be used. A small amount of bleeding may be expected.

There was some initial enthusiasm for hydrostatic balloon dilators, however, most clinicians have found the technique to be less effective and less predictable. They are generally not useful for longer tumors. Mercury filled rubber bougies can be used once the lumen has been rendered patent and known to be straight. The occasional patient can be trained to perform self dilation to maintain lumenal patency at home.

Endoscopic Laser Therapy for Esophageal Cancer

When ELT is being considered, the goals of therapy need to be identified. Relief of dysphagia, maintenance of lumenal patency and resumption of oral nutrition are the most reasonable goals. Favorable and unfavorable characteristics for ELT have been identified.[47] Characteristics that favor successful ELT include its endoscopic appearance as mucosal, exophytic or polypoid. These characteristics: allow better distinction between normal and abnormal tissue; allow more precise aiming of the laser beam; and allow alignment of the laser beam in the axis of the lumen, reducing the risk of perforation. Examples include: asymetric, noncircumferential tumors; polypoid masses; soft fleshy lesions; recurrences at surgical resection sites; and tumor overgrowth of endoprostheses (Fig. 139-3). Lesions causing complete lumenal obstruction may also be treated with ELT.

Submucosal or extrinsic lesions are less amenable to ELT because the extent of tumor is difficult to appreciate endoscopically, and overlying normal mucosa must be treated, which results in pain and increases the risk of perforation. Straight segments are more easily treated and have better outcomes than angulated segments (Fig. 139-4). Short tumor segments, less than 6 cm, are more effectively treated than longer segments. Lesions that occur in close proximity to the upper esophageal sphincter are difficult to treat because aiming the laser beam is more difficult in this location. Likewise, lesions at the gastroesophageal junction, which are horizontal in orientation, are more difficult to treat because of difficulty in aiming.

Technique

A surveillance endoscopy should precede ELT using a small diameter endoscope. Where possible, the entire tumor should be viewed endoscopically to assess its actual length, its exophytic versus submucosal character, its relation to the upper esophageal sphincter and the gastroesophageal junction. When the endoscope cannot be passed through the lumen due to narrowing, a guidewire should be placed and dilation be performed to allow passage of the endoscope. This enables treatment in a retrograde fashion. The advantage being that the entire tumor may be treated in a single session.[48] When feasible, the retrograde method is preferred.[49] The endoscope is passed beyond the malignant stricture. Laser treatment is begun at the distal tumor margin proceeding cephalad until the most proximal margin is treated. For annular lesions, circumfirential treatment should be applied at each level. ELT, in addition to tumor ablation and coagulation necrosis, often produces some tissue edema and swelling which may result in transient lumenal narrowing. This disadvantage may be encountered when treatment is directed in an antegrade manner. When complete lumenal obstruction is present, ELT in a antegrade fashion is necessary. The retrograde technique may be difficult because the endoscope needs to be maneuvered in a narrowed channel. Smoke is produced and carbon debris may accumulate on the endoscope optics where compromise visibility requiring removal of the endoscope for cleaning of the lens. When using coaxial gas, distention of the stomach may occur. Patient discomfort becomes greater when the presence of the endoscope in the esophageal lumen or narrowing of the lumen due to treatment effect prevents the patient from expelling this gas. We overcome this by using a large channel or double channel therapeutic endoscope with allows adequate suction while the laser fiber is in place.

In the antegrade method,[50] the laser beam is focused at the proximal margin of the tumor from above. Again, annular lesions are treated in a circumferential pattern, beginning at the center of the lumen and working outward. The laser is used to drill a lumen through the obstruction. Advantages are that smoke and air can be easily evacuated; the beam may be more easily directed parallel to the lumen; and largediameter, two channel endoscopes can be used to facilitate evacuation of smoke and air. The disadvantage, as noted above, is that edema at the proximal margin caused by thermal injury, may impede passage of the endoscope distally so that the entire lesion may not be treated in a single session.

ELT may be performed, using the Nd:YAG laser, at highpower settings (80–100 watts) using 1-second pulsed or continuous duration. With the laser fiber distanced approximately one cm from the tissue, a combination of vaporization and coagulation necrosis occurs. At lower powers (40–50 watts) using similar technique, coagulation necrosis occurs with little tissue ablation. Although the latter has been considered safer by some, it takes longer to destroy an equivalent amount of tumor and in our experience does not offer an advantage.

Contact laser tips have also been used. Sapphire and ceramic tips of varying shapes are used to concentrate laser energy into a thermal delivery device.[51] Lower powers from 10 to 40 watts may be used. The advantages of contact technique

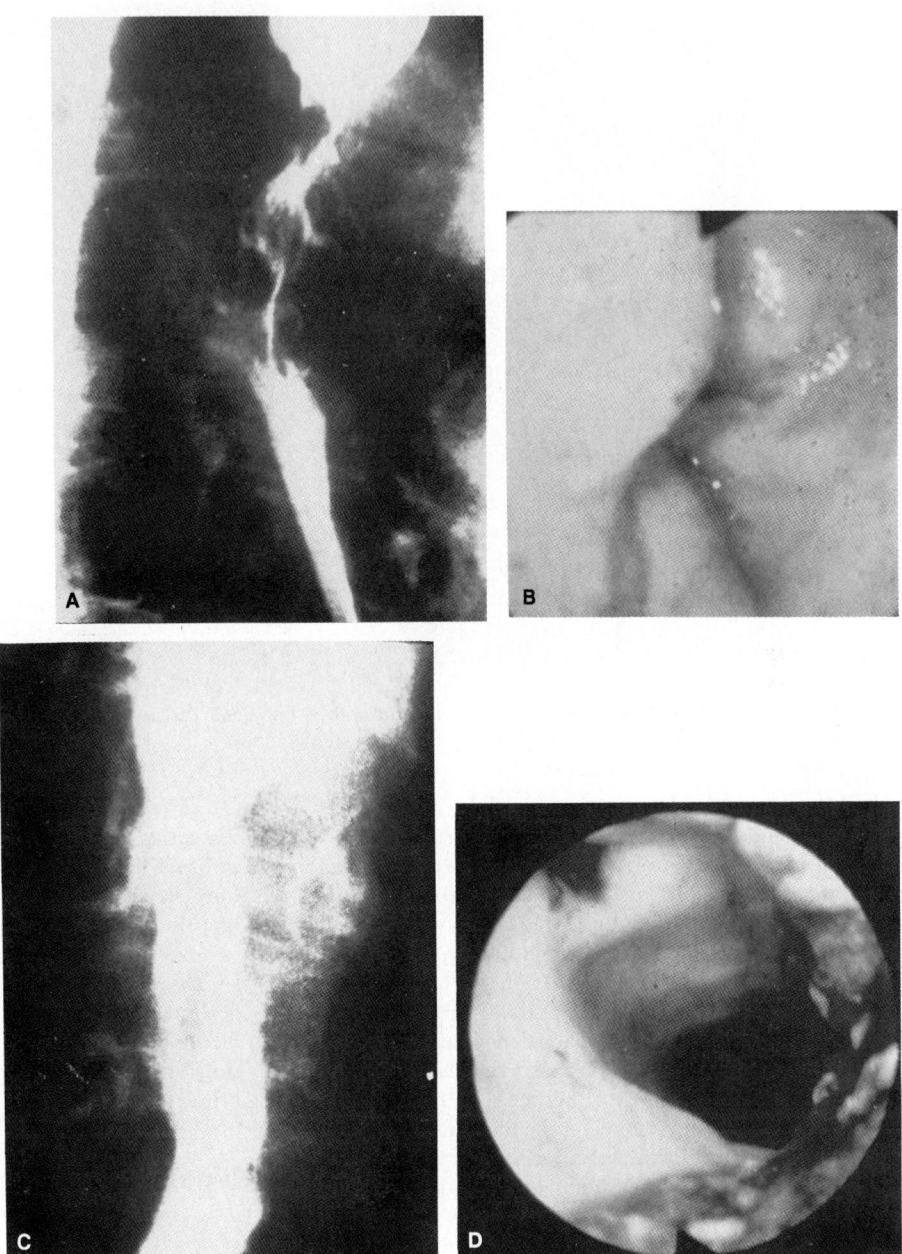

FIGURE 139-3. (**A**) Radiographic and (**B**) endoscopic views of narrowed lumen due to esophageal cancer. (**C**) Radiographic and (**D**) endoscopic views after laser therapy.

is that it allows more precise, selective tissue injury and decreased smoke production. The disadvantage is that the treatment spot size is considerably smaller so that treatment sessions take longer. The tip may become coated with adherent debris which diminishes effectiveness and requires treatment interruption for cleaning. The noncontact method allows painting broader areas so that treatment times are typically shorter.

Postendoscopic Procedure

After treatment the patient is kept NPO overnight. Dysphagia is often initially made worse after ELT due to narrowing of the lumen by tissue edema. A trial of clear liquids may be resumed the following day and the diet advanced as tolerated. If further treatment sessions are required to maintain lumenal

patency, the patient is kept NPO and on intravenous hydration. It is uncommon to require more than three sessions to obtain lumenal patency. Patient's are routinely treated 48 hours after the prior session until maximal lumenal patency is achieved. The occasional patient may experience chest pain and odynophagia briefly post procedure. A low-grade fever and mild elevation of the leukocyte count may be expected. Should adverse signs or symptoms persist, or increase in severity, a chest x-ray film should be obtained to rule out perforation as evidenced by pneumomediastinum or pneumothorax.

On the subsequent endoscopic procedure performed 48 hours after the prior, surveillance endoscopy should be, again undertaken. The effects of the previous session appear as coagulated, necrotic tissue. This must be debrided and numerous modalities can facilitate this. Equipment used for debridement

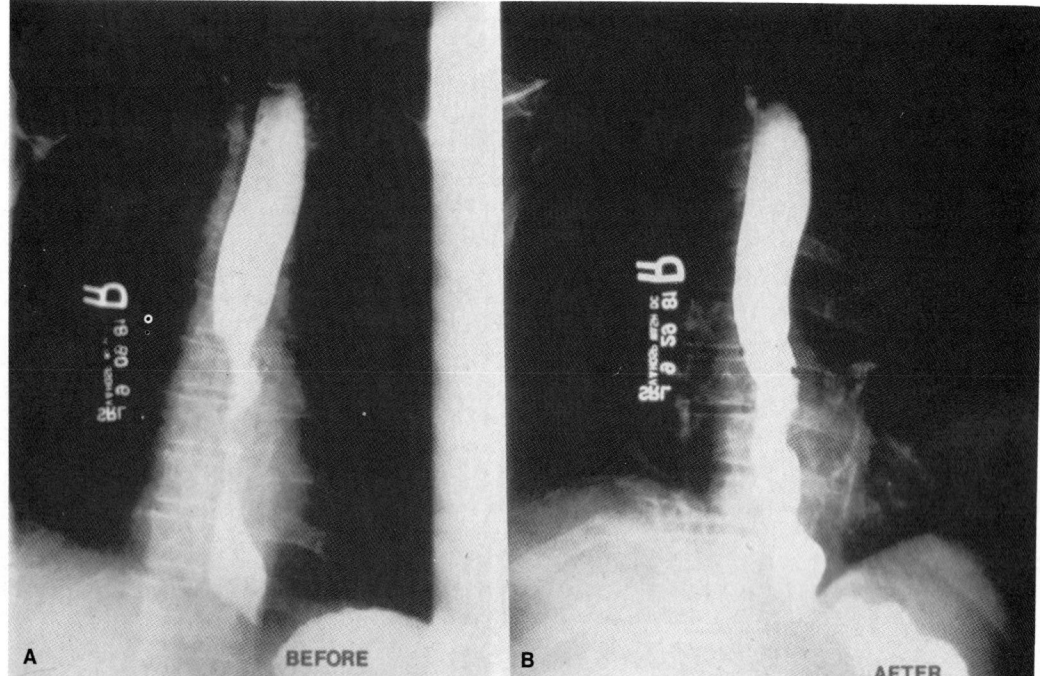

FIGURE 139-4. Esophagram of patient with esophageal cancer (**A**) before and (**B**) after laser treatment. Note the increased lumenal diameter after therapy.

include: the endoscope, biopsy forceps, Dormia baskets, polyp graspers, endoscopic brushes, water jets, large caliber suction tubes, and polyvinyl dilators. Dilators allow concomitant debridement along with dilation. Bougienage with the endoscope or with a tapered dilator is fast, easy, and effective. Repeat sessions should be continued until the lumen diameter has been increased to 11 to 13 mm allowing passage of a standard endoscope. Once lumenal patency has been achieved to the desired extent, a follow-up endoscopy should be carried out in 3 to 4 weeks to assess the need for repeat ELT. A contrast barium swallow is recommended after completion of a laser therapy to document the effects of therapy and to rule out perforation. The diet should include liquid nutritional supplements. Patients are instructed to chew foods well, to avoid stringy foods and to drink large amounts of liquids after eating solid foods.

Results

The success of ELT for palliation of esophageal malignancy is well documented.[29,34,47,52-59] ELT results in technical success with lumenal patency in 97% of cases, however, functional success defined by relief of dysphagia occurs in only 70% to 85%.[29] This difference is attributable to neuromotor damage from tumor invasion and treatment induced fibrosis of the esophageal musculature. Sixty to seventy percent of patients remain free of dysphagia for 3 to 6 weeks. Only 20% to 25% remain symptom free for three months or beyond. Follow up monthly endoscopy was performed by Maunoury and colleagues[60] after initial successful therapy, and repeat ELT was performed based on the endoscopic findings. With this approach symptomatic relief persisted for a mean of 4.2 months and 76% of patients remained palliated until death.

Rutgeerts and colleagues[34] demonstrated that laser therapy improved patients quality of life by allowing them to eat and improve their performance status. Effects on survival remain questionable.[61]

Overall complications occurred in 4.1% of cases from a survey which included 1359 cases.[62] Perforation occurred in 2%; the procedure-related mortality was 1%; the incidence of fistula or hemorrhage, 1%; and sepsis, 0.5% to 1%. Perforations are more likely to occur in patients who have undergone prior radiation therapy.

Bipolar Electrocoagulation

The BICAP tumor probe is a multipolar electrocautery device similar in appearance to an Eder-Puestow dilator (Fig. 139-5). Electrical plates are arranged circumferentially around an olive-shaped metal cylinder attached to flexible shaft with scored 1 cm distance markers on it. A flexible spring-tip, which acts as a guide, screws into the electrically active multipolar probe. The thermal probes range in size from 6 mm to 15 mm. The assembled apparatus has a central lumen which enables the system to be passed over a guidewire. The shaft is connected to an electrical power source which allows the generation of an electrosurgical current, which is then delivered circumferentially from the probe. Although the depth of coagulation effect varies with the power settings and the duration of application, the tumor probe produces a predictable depth of injury. This is because contact with nondesiccated tissue is required to complete the circuit. As tissue is heated and water evaporates, tissue resistance increases, and current flow diminishes.

Fluoroscopic guidance is required in most cases. A sur-

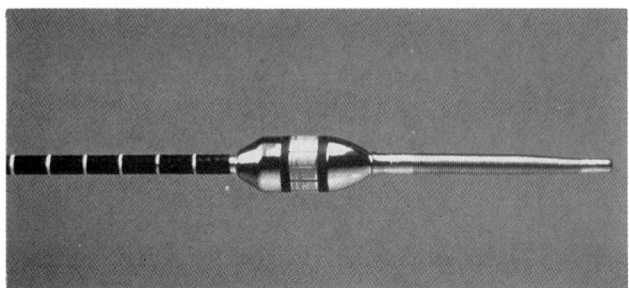

FIGURE 139-5. The BICAP tumor probe (Circon-ACMI, Stamford, CT) has a distal flexible tip, metal olive with active electrode, and proximal bendable shaft.

veillance endoscopy is performed and the locations of the proximal and distal tumor margins are measured with the endoscope with respect to their distance from the incisors. Fluoroscopic markings are placed using external radiopaque markers. If the large, 15 mm probe cannot be inserted into the strictured lumen, an attempt at dilation to allow passage of this probe should be performed. If the lumen cannot be dilated to 15 mm., the smaller probes can be used. In all cases, the tumor probe of maximal diameter that can be readily passed into the stenotic lesion should be employed (Fig. 139-6). As in ELT, a retrograde approach is recommended. A guidewire is placed endoscopically or under fluoroscopic guidance into the stomach. The tumor probe is then passed over top of the guidewire and through the area of lumenal narrowing. The tumor probe is then withdrawn until resistance is initially met. This should coincide with the radiographic markings and the endoscopic measurements of the distal tumor margin. Under fluoroscopy, the probe is then pulled back in retrograde fashion so that the electrosurgical component of the tumor probe is in contact with the malignant tissue. The active electrode is 1.5 cm in length and so

by withdrawing the tumor probe at 1 cm intervals, a small amount of overlap is achieved and a uniform tissue injury is delivered to the zone, extending 1 to 2 mm circumferentially. Powers of 50 watts are generally used and the probe is left at each station for 15 seconds. The probe should be withdrawn and activated until the entire tumor has been treated. Short segments have been treated in the antegrade fashion under endoscopic vision with a small diameter endoscope placed alongside the flexible shaft.

The treated tissue demonstrates a circumferential white coagulum (Fig. 139-7). A chest x-ray film should be obtained following the procedure to rule out pneumomediastinum or pneumothorax. The patient is kept NPO overnight and observed in the hospital. The following day a contrast esophagram is performed to exclude a perforation. At follow-up endoscopy 48 hours postprocedure, necrotic debris is removed by means similar to those described following laser therapy. Further therapy is based on clinical results.

The BICAP tumor probe is best suited for symmetrical, circumferential tumors. It is ill-suited for asymmetric tumors, tortuous segments and tight strictured tumors. The esophageal wall should be at least 5 mm thick in all directions to allow a margin of safety. Advantages are its relative low cost, and its ability to treat a large extent of tumor in a single setting. Inadvertent treatment of opposing or marginal nonmalignant tissue may result in pain and stricture. Another disadvantage is that it is essentially a blind procedure.

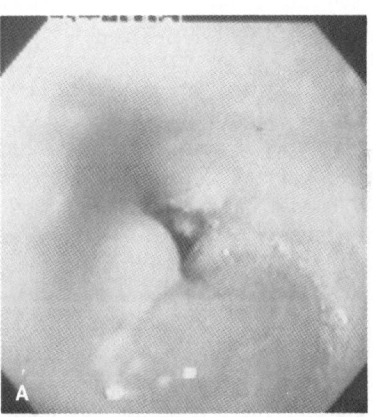
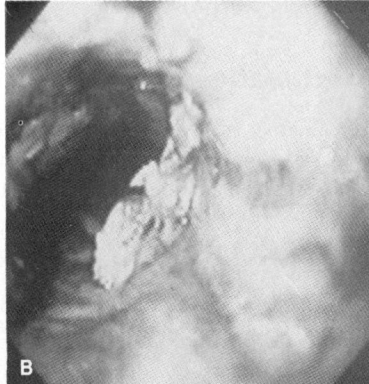

FIGURE 139-7. Squamous cell carcinoma of the esophagus. (**A**) In the endoscopic view, the lumen is narrowed, and there is a proximal mass lesion. (**B**) After tumor probe treatment, the lumen is patent.

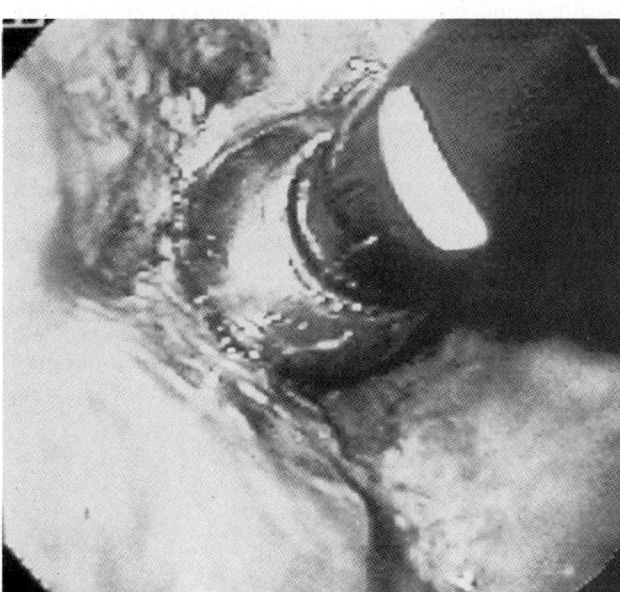

FIGURE 139-6. Tumor probe inserted into lumenal stricture due to esophageal cancer.

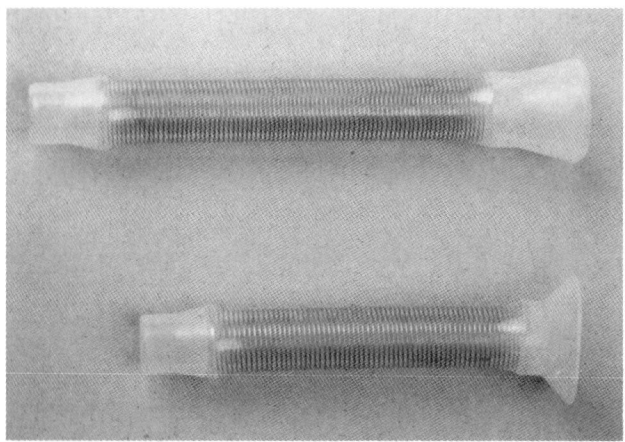

FIGURE 139-8. Esophageal prostheses may have a normal upper flange (*top*) or a low profile flange (*bottom*).

The BICAP tumor probe has not had as extensive use as a laser and stent therapy for esophageal cancers. Johnston and colleagues[63] in a multicenter trial demonstrated technical success with increased lumenal diameter and significant improvement in dysphagia grade in posttreatment assessment. The mean number of treatment sessions was 1.7, with a mean duration of palliation of 7.6 weeks. Major complications, tracheoesophageal fistula and delayed hemorrhage, occurred in 20%. Fleischer and colleagues[64] reported stricture formation in 12.5%. Jensen and colleagues,[65] in a comparison with Nd: YAG laser therapy, reported a functional success rate of 86%. They found the technique effective for cervical lesions. Fistula formation occurred in one patient (7%). They emphasized not using of the BICAP tumor probe for treatment of noncircumferential tumors. Maunoury and colleagues[60] prospectively selected 38 patients with roughly uniform circumferential stenosis, both exophytic and submucosal lesions, for treatment with the BICAP tumor probe and reported successful therapy in 87% after the initial session. All failures were in distal esophageal lesions. No complications occurred during the initial treatment session, one patient developed a tracheoesophageal fistula during follow-up treatment. They concluded that the BICAP tumor probe offers a palliative solution for the minority of patients with submucosal, circumferential, and tight strictures.

Endoscopic Intubation

Because thermal ablative therapies required repeat sessions, alternative modalities to palliate dysphagia and maintain lumenal patency have been sought. Peroral stenting provides rapid and maintained lumenal patency, allowing the pleasures of food intake, and reducing sialorrhea and the risks of aspiration. Esophageal endoprostheses have enjoyed varying levels of patient and physician enthusiasm over the years. Esophageal endoprostheses or stents are available in a variety of materials including: latex or silicone rubber, polyvinyl chloride, and other plastic materials. Expandable metallic stents are currently being evaluated for application in the esophagus. The presence of an obstructing lesion or an esophagorespiratory fistula is an indication for stent placement.

The original stents were custom, homemade endoprostheses fabricated from polyvinyl tubing such as tygon with an outside diameter of 14.7 mm, an inside diameter of 12.5 mm, and a wall thickness of 1.6 mm. The length of the segment could be determined by the specific length of the tumor with additional 2 to 3 cm added to each end to form the cuff. Today, a variety of commercially available stents in varying sizes, diameters and flange shapes are available. Metallic rings or spirals have been added to many devices to improve their rigidity, thus resisting kinking or compression (Fig. 139-8). A dedicated, cuffed, fistula prosthesis has been developed with an expandable foam sponge in its mid portion to seal tracheoesophageal fistulas. Two primary methods for placing esophageal stents have evolved. One mechanism deploys the stent on a polyvinyl dilator with a pusher tube (Fig. 139-9). The other, pioneered by Atkinson,[66] employs the Nottingham introducer system. This consists of a hollow-lumen, semirigid shaft, onto which is mounted an expandable metal olive which keeps the prosthesis in place. The former technique, described in below, is the method the authors find safest and most effective. Several large studies are reported and conclude that intubation is a highly efficient means of restoring lumenal patency and relieving dysphagia.[67-70]

Stent Placement

A surveillance endoscopy using a small caliber endoscope is performed and precise measurements of the proximal and distal margins of the tumor are obtained from the incisors. Fluoroscopic correlation should be obtained with radiographic markers placed on the skin. It is important to measure the location of the upper and lower esophageal sphincters and the specific location of an esophagorespiratory fistula, if present. The diameter of most prostheses is 14 to 16 mm. The esophageal lumen, therefore, must be dilated to at least 15 mm. For rigid, fixed tumors, a dilator, at least one size larger than the stent's outside diameter should be used. For soft, fleshy tumors, one size below that diameter may be preferable. This helps prevent stent migration which might occur if the lumen is over dilated. For rigid tumors, serial dilations may

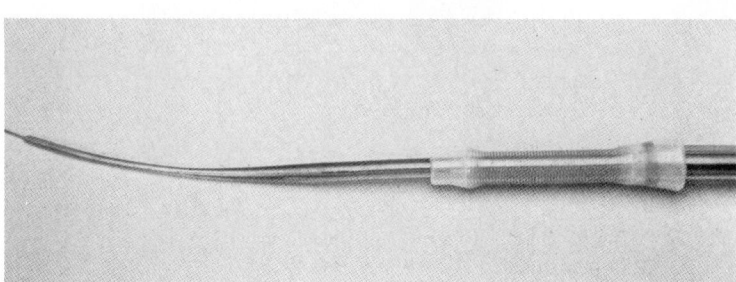

FIGURE 139-9. Stent over a stabilizing dilator.

be required over several days prior to insertion of the stent. Equipment necessary for endoprosthesis placement, besides the stent itself, include: a modified, 100-cm long, 33-Fr polyvinyl dilator, or one just smaller than the internal diameter of the stent; a springtip guidewire; a pusher tube; two strands of 3.0 silk suture at least 60 cm in length; silicone lubricant; an indelible marker; and accessories for stent removal, if necessary.

The procedure is performed under fluoroscopic guidance. A guidewire is passed into the antrum and the lumen is dilated to the appropriate diameter. Typically, conscious sedation using meperidine and midazolam is used. The patient is placed in the left lateral decubitus position, although some endoscopists prefer to have the patient supine. The elongated dilator is passed through the pusher tube and the stent is passed over top of the dilator and engaged with pusher tube. Two needle holes are made through the proximal cuff of the stent through which the 3.0 silk suture is fed. This is held tethered to the side of the pusher tube and allows rapid removal of the stent should airway compression result after placement. The interface between the pusher tube and the proximal stent cuff is lubricated with silicone to allow easy disengagement. The pusher tube has been marked with the indelible marker to identify key points of the stent at tumor engagement. After dilation to the appropriate diameter, the guidewire is left in place and the entire apparatus is then inserted over the guidewire and advanced until initial resistance is met. This represents the distal cuff engaging with the proximal margin of the tumor and should correlate with the endoscopic measurements and the radiographic markers. Gentle and persistent pressure is then applied to advance the stent into position. A subtle give is appreciated when the central shaft of the stent is engaged in the tumor and the distal cuff is passed beyond the distal margin of the tumor. The endoscope should then be passed through the pusher tube and the stent location confirmed endoscopically, as well as fluoroscopically. If the endoscopy reveals that the stent has been placed too proximally, the pusher tube can be reengaged and the stent advanced to the appropriate position. If the stent had been placed too far distally, it can be withdrawn by placing traction on the attached silk sutures. The endoscope itself can be used for repositioning the stent by placing the tip of the scope in the stent lumen and angling the tip with left right control to engage the stent. The stent can then be pushed or pulled to reposition it into the appropriate location. A pneumatic balloon device has also been developed to engage the stent for repositioning. Other mechanisms used to withdraw the stent have included loops snares and alligator forceps.

When proper stent placement has been confirmed, and there is no airway compression, the deployment apparatus can be removed. First, the silk suture is removed, then, with a gentle twisting motion, the pusher tube disengaged from the stent and withdrawn. This should be done under fluoroscopic guidance to confirm that the stent does not moved while the pusher tube is being withdrawn. A chest x-ray film should be obtained postprocedure to document the stent location and be used as a reference if the question of stent migration arises. Evidence of pneumomediastinum or pneumothorax should be sought on this film. The patient should be kept NPO and be maintained with the head of the bed in a 45 degree elevated position. Antitussive pharmaceuticals may be required to inhibit coughing or hiccuping which may cause dislodgment or stent migration. On the following day, a repeat chest x-ray film is obtained, and if unremarkable, a dilute contrast study obtained to demonstrate stent patency and rule out fistula formation. The diet may then be initiated with liquids and advanced. The patients are advised to chew foods well, to avoid stringy foods, and to take copious liquids to help wash through the stent.

An alternative mechanism for stent insertion uses the Nottingham Introducer System. The delivery device has a flanged tip that can be expanded to engage the stent or be contracted to release it. The patient is prepared and the stent is delivered in a similar manner as detailed above. This device can also be useful in repositioning stents that have migrated or were ill-positioned at primary insertion.

Complications

Tracheal compression by the endoprosthesis is the most acute complication of stent placement and the physician must be in a position to quickly remove the stent or advance it into the stomach to relieve airway compression. Migration is the most common complication encountered after a stent has been successfully placed. Stent migration occurs in approximately 10% to 40% of patients, with proximal migration occurring most frequently. Repositioning by the techniques described above is often successful. However, if the stent is the wrong size, stent removal or advancement into the stomach should be considered with a subsequent insertion of a more appropriate sized stent.

Free reflux may occur when the stent protrudes beyond the lower esophageal sphincter. Tumor overgrowth may occur at both the distal and proximal ends. This may be treated effectivly with laser therapy.[71] In rare instances, stents have eroded into the aorta which is a terminal event. Perforation has been reported to occur in up to 12% following stent insertion. When diagnosed early, the majority of instrumental perforations can be successfully managed with conservative therapy consisting of institution of NPO orders, broad-spectrum antibiotics, and adequate aspiration above and below the perforation site.[72]

Fistula Prosthesis

A specialized, cuffed, fistula prosthesis has been developed and is commercially available. The prosthesis is a standard Wilson-Cook silicone rubber tube with a metal coil to retain its shape. The cuff is formed by a circumferential foam-rubber sponge contained in a silicone sheath. The stent is deployed with the cuff in a compressed state created by a vacuum syringe. Once the stent is in place, the vacuum is released and the cuff self-inflates, expanding to a diameter of 4 cm, and effectively sealing the fistula track.[73] Modified endoprosthesis with a floppy[74] or large upper funnel[75] have also been reported to successfully manages esophagorespiratory fistulas. The latter may offer an advantage over the cuffed tube in the management of cervical esophageal lesions. All of these systems may afford symptomatic relief for an otherwise desperate situation.

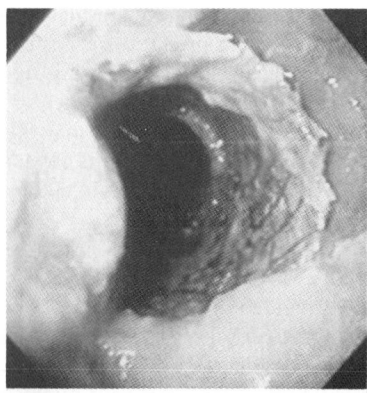

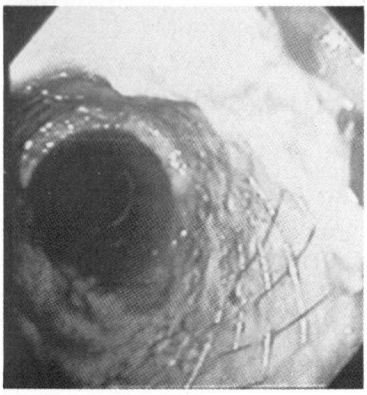

FIGURE 139-10. Endoscopic views of an expandable metal prosthesis in a patient with esophageal cancer.

Expandable Metal Esophageal Stents

The concept of a self-expanding metallic stent is appealing for several reasons. The stent can be inserted, atraumatically, into a narrow-diameter lumen, thus reducing the risk of perforation associated with actual insertion or preinsertion dilation. The stent is thin-walled and expands to a diameter greater than that achieved with conventional plastic stents, offering a greater internal lumen diameter (Figs. 139-10 and

139-11). Lastly, the expansile nature and imbedding feature of the mesh latticework should reduce the incidence of stent migration. Several types of metallic endoprostheses have been developed and are in various stages of clinical trial. The main drawback of metal mesh stents is the occurrence of tumor ingrowth through the latticework. This is being addressed by developing stents with a more tightly woven mesh or with internal or external coatings.[76] The Wallstent, described below, has been studied most extensively. Other designs under investigation are a modified Gianturco stent,[77] and two stents made of the memory metal Nitinol—the Ultraflex, based on the Strecker stent design, is a mesh tube of knitted metal filaments encased in a surrounding gelatine membrane which dissolves when placed in contact with esophageal secretions; and the Instent which is a spiral tube of coiled metal ribbon that may be removable.

The Wallstent is a woven tubular mesh of stainless alloy filaments. It is flexible and self-expanding. The predeployment diameter is 6 mm, and expands to 20 mm when deployed. It will be available in lengths of 6 and 10 cm. Knyrim and colleagues[78] reported a randomized trial comparing the results of palliation of malignant dysphagia with a Wallstent (post-deployment diameter, 16 mm) versus a 16-mm-diameter plastic prosthesis. Palliation was equal in both groups, however, there were fewer complications, and no fatal complications, in the Wallstent group. The reduction in complications resulted in decreased hospital stay and translated into lower costs. Tumor ingrowth or overgrowth was the most common cause of recurrent dysphagia in the Wallstent group (24%) and was managed effectively with ELT. Self-expanding metal prostheses, by solving the problem of procedure related complications, would greatly enhance the role of intubation for palliation of esophageal cancers.

Comparative Studies

The mainstays of endoscopic palliation of esophageal cancer have been the Nd:YAG laser and the plastic stent. Both modalities have their advantages and disadvantages. Ideally, stents

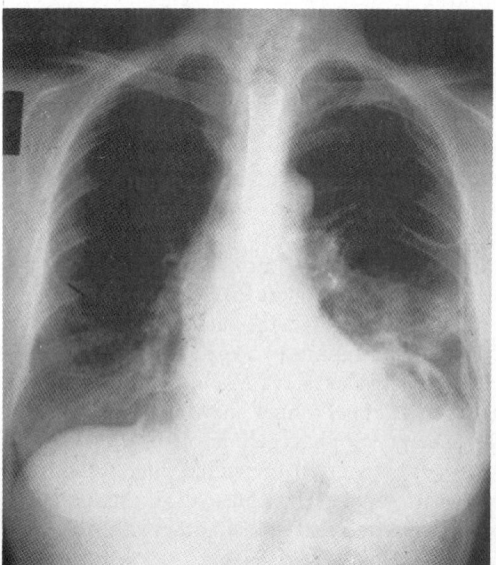

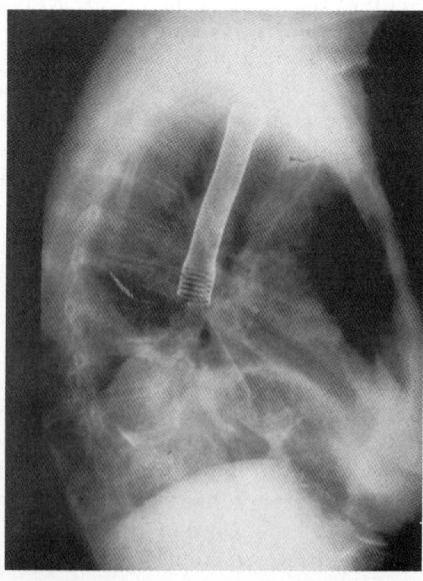

FIGURE 139-11. Radiographs show the expandable metal stent used for the treatment of esophageal cancer.

provide rapid and long lasting palliation. They are preferred for longer, infiltrating, submucosal, or extrinsic tumors, and are used for sealing esophagorespiratory fistulas.[79] Repeat procedures are less frequently required.[70] Disadvantages include a high complication rate and procedure related mortality. ELT is best suited for bulky intralumenal tumors. After laser therapy patients are more likely to resume a normal diet. However, repeat laser therapy sessions are usually required to manage recurrent dysphagia, and these sessions become increasingly difficult and uncomfortable for the patient.[80] The approach to palliation of esophageal cancers is best decided on an individual basis. The choice, and ultimate success, of therapy are based on the treatment objectives, the anatomy and characteristics of the tumor, and the local expertise. For these reasons, the results from trials comparing these two accepted techniques are difficult to evaluate; several of these series are described below.

Hahl and colleagues[81] reported a retrospective evaluation of 96 patients; 69 treated with laser and 27 with an endo-prosthesis. Laser therapy effectively reduced tumor bulk in 87%, but a functional success (i.e., patient is able to resume a normal or near-normal diet) was achieved in only 55%. Stent insertion was successful in 89%, and all achieved functional success. In the laser treated group the overall complication rate was 8.7%. There were no fatal complications, and the 1-year survival was 12%. The stented group had a complication rate of 48%; there were 3 (11%) procedure-related deaths; and the 1-year survival was 0%. The authors conclude that both techniques are effective, but that mortality and complications were lower with laser therapy. It should be noted, however, that the patients receiving stents in this non-randomized study had considerably more advanced stage disease (100% endoscopically impassable lesions in the stent group versus 50% in the laser group) which certainly affected outcome.

Barr and colleagues,[82] in a randomized trial, compared laser therapy alone versus laser therapy followed by stent insertion. They concluded that both methods were equally effective in relieving dysphagia; however, dysphagia scores fluctuated more in the laser only group. Overall, there was no significant difference in quality of life assessment. Significantly fewer complications occurred in the laser group (10%) versus the laser plus stent group (40%), but most complications responded to conservative management.

Carter and colleagues[83] randomized 40 patients with inoperable esophageal cancer to laser therapy versus intubation. Their results were analysed on an intention-to-treat basis and patients were followed to death. All patients treated by laser achieved patency; there was one failed stent insertion. The laser treated group had a significantly better functional success, as assessed by swallowing grade, both after treatment and before death. There was no significant difference in survival or inpatient hospitalization time. There were three perforations and one tracheoesophageal fistula formation in the laser treated group, including one procedure-related death. There were no perforations or deaths due to intubation.

Loizou and colleagues,[84] in a prospective, nonrandomized two-center trial compared 43 patients treated with laser with 30 patients treated with stent insertion. The two groups were comparable for age and tumor length, location, and histology. Improvement in dysphagia grade for thoracic esophageal tu-

mors was similar in the two groups both initially and over the long term. For tumors at the esophagogastric junction, stent insertion was superior. Improved quality-of-life scores correlated with improvement in dysphagia grade. Patients treated with laser were more likely to eat a normal diet over the long term. Laser treated patients required, on average, more procedures and days in the hospital. The perforation rate was lower in the laser group (2% versus 13%; $P < 0.02$); no treatment-related deaths occurred in either group. The authors suggest for patients who are anorex, or in poor general condition, that a stent be used because it provides rapid and lasting relief of symptoms and obviates the need for further sessions. For reasonably fit patients, they suggest initial laser therapy because it may result in a better quality of life, by allowing near-normal swallowing function. If the patient achieves only a mediocre results from attempted laser palliation, stent insertion should be considered early during follow-up.

Laser recanalization and esophageal intubation are both effective and acceptable means of palliating inoperable esophageal and esophagogastric carcinomas. Best results are achieved when the two methods are used in complementary fashion by experienced endoscopists.

GASTRIC LESIONS

Gastric cancer is the second most common malignancy worldwide. Although its incidence in the United States has markedly diminished over the past several decades, it remains the second most common gastrointestinal malignancy in the United States. Ninety-five percent of gastric cancers are adenocarcinomas and Lauren has classified them into two distinct types: diffuse and intestinal.[85] The diffuse, or infiltrative, form is derived from stratified goblet cells that undergo histologic transformation into signet ring cell carcinoma. This variety of gastric cancer does not have a well recognized precursor lesion and does not typically lend itself to endoscopic therapies. The intestinal, or epidemic, variety occurs on the background of chronic gastritis leading to gastric atrophy with intestinal metaplasia. In some patients the intestinal metaplasia will evolve further through dysplasia to cancer. Vital staining may become a means by which intestinal metaplasia may be distinguished from normal mucosa.[86,87] The dysplastic epithelium may be differentiated macroscopically during endoscopy when it protrudes into the lumen, as a polyp. The intestinal variety of gastric cancer may be more amenable to endoscopic therapy and is discussed below.

Endoscopic therapy for gastric lesions may be employed for resection of benign polyps. In patients with early cancers who are poor surgical candidates, and patients with advanced disease who are unwilling or unable to undergo surgical resection. Endoscopic therapy may also be performed for palliation of bleeding or obstruction in advanced disease.

Gastric Polyps

Gastric polyps may precede the development of gastric cancer, although less commonly than their colon counterparts. Gastric polyps may present with bleeding, obstruction, or abdominal pain. However, up to 50% are asymptomatic and are unexpected findings when endoscopy is performed to evaluate symptoms unrelated to the presence of a polyp.[88] The majority of gastric polyps are hyperplastic, comprising 70% to 90% in most published series.[89,90] The risk of malignant transformation in a hyperplastic polyp is low. Of 477 hyperplastic gastric polyps removed by endoscopic polypectomy by Daibo and colleagues,[91] 10 (2.1%) contained focal carcinoma. An additional 19 (4.0%) contained dysplasia without a foci of carcinoma. Adenomatous polyps, are true neoplasms and are considered premalignant with a reported incidence of malignant transformation ranging from 6 to 75%.[92] The risk of malignancy is greatest in adenomatous polyps ≥ 2 cm in diameter. Most gastric polyps less than 5 mm in diameter can be completely removed with forceps biopsy resection, whereas those greater than 5 mm can generally be safely and effectively removed by endoscopic snare excision. When feasible, gastric polyps should be removed completely as specimens obtained by forceps biopsy alone may fail to correctly characterize polyp histology or may fail to identify a focus of early carcinoma.[93,94] When CIS is present and limited to the resected specimen without invasion into the base, endoscopic polypectomy is curative. When the resected specimen reveals invasion into the stalk or is poorly differentiated, a cancer operation should be recommended with local lymph node resection.

Gastric polypectomy technique is similar to that for colonic polypectomy and is typically performed as an outpatient procedure. Glucagon may be administered to reduce peristalsis and facilitate polyp retrieval. Because of increased vasculature, bleeding occurs more commonly after gastric polypectomy than it does in the colon. Pedunculated polyps with a thick stalk should be considered for injection of dilute epinephrine solution into the stalk to reduce the likelihood of bleeding. Bleeding from a polypectomy site, in most cases can be managed endoscopically. Grasping the resected pedicle with the snare and tightening with or without further electrocautery is one effective means. Other therapies include injection of vasoconstrictors, alcohol, or other sclerosants; electrocautery with hemostatic probes, and Nd:YAG laser photocoagulation. In rare instances surgery may be required.

Care must be taken to prevent the resected specimen from being dropped into the airway upon retrieval. Polyps 5 mm or less can generally be withdrawn through the working channel. For larger lesions, the resected polyp should be resnared or captured in a polyp grasper to allow safe retrieval. Another technique utilizes an overtube to protect the airway. This mechanism is preferred when multiple or piecemeal polypectomy is to be performed.

Ulceration at the polypectomy site can be expected and patients are placed on acid-suppressive therapy, although the value of this measure is unknown. Perforation after excision of true epithelial gastric polyps is rare due to the thickness of the gastric wall. The risk of perforation is higher for submucosal lesions.

Ghazi and colleagues,[95] reported endoscopic resection of 443 gastroduodenal polyps, 63% sessile and 37% pedunculated. Pedunculated and sessile polyps less than 1.5 cm were excised in one piece. Larger sessile polyps were excised in a piecemeal fashion. Bleeding from the polypectomy site occurred in one patient and stopped spontaneously. The Mayo Clinic reported results of 48 consecutive endoscopic gastric polypectomies.[93] Uncontrolled bleeding occurred in two patients who required surgical ligation. We reported results from snare resection of 26 gastric polyps greater than 5 mm in diameter. In two resected polyps, forceps biopsy sampling had either mischaracterized the polyp or failed to demonstrate the presence of focal carcinoma.[28] Bleeding requiring endoscopic therapy occurred in four patients, all treated successfully.

Early Gastric Cancer

In Western countries, the diagnosis of early stage gastric cancer is unusual. However, in Japan, where the incidence of gastric cancer is high, aggressive endoscopic screening programs have resulted in a 30% incidence of early gastric cancer detection compared to only 3% to 6% in the United States.[96,97] The distinction of early gastric cancer, as defined in Japan, implies a curable stage of the disease.[98] These are carcinomas limited to the gastric mucosa and submucosa, irrespective of the presence or absence of lymph node metastases.[99]

The five year survival for early gastric cancers after surgical resection is 90%. Therefore, in the United States surgical resection should be the procedure of choice. In Japan, small protruding early cancers in which EUS confirms intramucosal invasion only, endoscopic techniques of ablation and resection are being evaluated. Strip-biopsy using a diathermic snare with or without submucosal saline injection is one option. Laser ablation of the tumor is also being used as a single modality, or in combination with snare resection. Snare resection allows tissue submission for assessment of resected margins. Biopsies of the treated area are performed following laser ablation to assess persistence of carcinomatous tissue. Other modalities have included PDT and injection of local inflammatory mediators.

The distinction of early gastric cancers previously was made on the basis of the macroscopic appearance at endoscopy. EUS has improved accuracy of staging for gastric cancer. This improved accuracy of staging allows more meaningful assessment of patient response to specific therapies and allows identification of patients who may be candidates for endoscopic therapy with intent to cure. Yasuda and colleagues found the overall accuracy of EUS for gastric cancer to be 78%.[100] Most importantly, the accuracy for staging early gastric cancers was 91%. Furthermore, they identified a correlation between the depth of gastric invasion and the presence of lymph node metastasis. Only 1% of patients with T1 lesions had positive lymph nodes at resection. Endoscopic laser treatment, with intent to cure, was performed in 28 patients staged as early cancers (i.e., limited to the mucosa by EUS). They report a curative success rate of 96%. In 8 patients, in whom EUS demonstrated submucosal extent of the lesion, the cure rate was 63%. Others have applied lasers, primarily the Nd: YAG, for curative treatment for early gastric cancers with intent to cure in patients with early cancers who are inoperable due to concurrent medical conditions.[6,101] The staging in these series did not include EUS and their results are less favorable.

Hirao and colleagues[102] used the strip biopsy technique for resection of 83 early gastric cancers. Of these, cancer was limited to the mucosa in 74, whereas in the remaining 9, cancer invaded the submucosa as well. In all patients with

T1 lesions, in whom the resected margins were free of infiltration, there was no evidence of recurrence during follow-up of 3 to 54 months. The mean follow-up time was not reported. Karita and colleagues describe single and successive strip biopsy resection for gastric cancers up to 20 mm and 50 mm in diameter respectively.[103]

Haruma and colleagues[104] used a combination of endoscopic methods in 42 patients with 44 early gastric cancers who were not surgical candidates. Snare resection or strip biopsy alone was performed on 17, Nd:YAG laser photoablation alone on 12, and combined therapy in 15. Endoscopic therapy alone was successful in 35 of the 44 lesions. Of those judged completely cured by initial endoscopic therapy there was no evidence of local recurrence or lymph node metastasis during the mean follow-up time of 37 months. Some of these patients also received local injection of OK-432, a biological response modifier derived from streptococci. Injection of OK-432 results in marked infiltration of inflammatory cells into the submucosal layer thought to be effective in eliminating tumor cells.[105]

Teixeira and colleagues[106] evaluated the efficacy of endoscopic therapy in patients with gastric cancer who were more than 80 years old. The authors used a variety of modalities to suit the characteristics of the lesion. Nd:YAG laser irradiation was used on 12 lesions, snare polypectomy on 8, OK-432 injection in 8, and strip biopsy on 2. In 13 patients in whom curative treatment was attempted, a curative response was achieved in 11 (85%). Furthermore, adequate palliation was successful in those patients who failed curative endoscopic therapy.

Hayata and colleagues[107] used PDT to treat 17 patients with early gastric cancers by endoscopic classification. Thirteen patients subsequently underwent operative resection. Of 10 patients deemed to have demonstrated a complete response, only 6 specimens proved histologically tumor free.

In summary, endoscopic therapy for early gastric cancers, with intent to cure, is feasible in patients who are poor operative candidates due to comorbid disease or advanced age. The addition of EUS as an accurate staging tool may permit the use endoscopic therapy as a first line treatment for early gastric cancer.

Advanced Gastric Cancer

Most gastric cancers are advanced at the time of presentation. Although surgical resection remains the treatment of choice for all gastric cancers if there is a potential for cure, it also offers the best palliative therapy for advanced gastric cancers. It is the best means for maintaining lumenal patency and enteral nutrition, and for the control of bleeding. However, resectability rates for gastric cancer vary from 31 to 66%, and palliative resection is associated with an operative mortality rate of 8 to 29%. In nonsurgical candidates (i.e., those with significant comorbid disease or unresectable tumors) palliative endoscopic therapies may be applied.

Gastric cancers may cause acute gastrointestinal bleeding or may result in anemia secondary to chronic GI blood loss. Fleischer first described use of the Nd:YAG laser for hemostasis of GI bleeding from gastric cancer[108] using low to intermediate powers, 50 to 70 watts, in the noncontact mode, for photo-

coagulation of the tumor surface. Endoscopic therapy for bleeding gastric cancers has not been demonstrated to affect survival. However, it is useful for stabilizing the patient and providing hemostasis while more definitive therapy is being planned. Suzuki and colleagues[109] reported successful hemostasis using Nd:YAG laser therapy in 17 of 18 cases of massive bleeding from upper gastrointestinal cancers.

Endoscopic management of bleeding from tumors is effective for lesions less than 5 cm in diameter. It is less likely to be effective in large tumors (>8 cm). We have also used injection therapy with dilute epinephrine or ethyl alcohol for temporary control of bleeding from gastric cancers. The BICAP cautery probe and heater probe have also been used. All these modalities are likely to increase surface ulceration on the lesion and rebleeding is not uncommon. Therefore, these modalities should be reserved for patients who are unacceptable surgical risks or who otherwise choose not to undergo surgical resection for palliation.

When bulky gastric cancers cause lumenal obstruction, at the gastroesophageal junction or the gastric outlet, Nd:YAG laser therapy can be used to ablate tissue and regain lumenal patency. A mean of three treatment sessions may be required, with functional success achieved in 73% of patients with gastric cancer of the cardia, with a low complication rate.[108] Palliation of lumenal obstruction in antral cancers with endoscopic therapy is less successful (50%).[109] In antral cancers, even when a large sized lumen is achieved, gastric motility disturbance due to tumor invasion compromises gastric emptying. Surgical resection and bypass are preferred in this occurrence as it offers more effective and longer lasting palliation.

Metastatic Tumors to the Stomach

Metastatic tumors to the stomach are unusual but pose clinical problems when symptomatic. Significant GI bleeding occurs in approximately 20% of the patients with gastric metastases. The most common cancer metastatic to the stomach is melanoma, followed by breast, colon, and lung. Lesions typically have a volcano-like appearance with heaped-up margins and an umbilicated central ulceration. Bull's-eye or target lesion is another descriptive term. Histologic diagnoses require deep biopsies from the edge of the ulcer crater. Endoscopic treatment is generally for palliation of bleeding. This can be effectively accomplished when the lesion is small, less than 3 cm in diameter. For larger lesions endoscopic therapy may be effective in stabilizing the patient while arranging more definitive therapy. Endoscopic therapy has included injection with epinephrine or alcohol, laser photocoagulation, and heater probe or BICAP electrocoagulation. Bleeding frequently recurs and therefore more definitive therapy should be considered after stabilization with endoscopic means. Bleeding not amenable to endoscopic therapy may be managed by arteriographic embolization.

DUODENAL LESIONS

Villous adenomas and adenocarcinoma of the duodenum and major papilla are uncommon in the general population. Their incidence is considerably higher in patients with familial polyposis syndromes—25% to 100% of patients with familial adenomatous polyposis. Histopathology based on tissue sampling from forceps biopsies is notoriously inaccurate and therefore, snare resection or surgery should be performed to exclude cancer or as primary therapy.

Ryan and colleagues[110] reviewed 19 cases of villous lesions of the duodenum. Sixteen involved the ampulla of Vater; 3 were nonampullary duodenal adenomas. Malignant elements were contained in 63%. Endoscopic biopsy had a false negative rate for malignancy of 56%. Similar false negative rates for forceps biopsy alone are reported by Yamaguchi and colleagues.[111] Seifert and colleagues[112] retrospectively reviewed the clinical course of 12 adenomas and 35 carcinomas of the papilla of Vater, and 21 nonampullary duodenal adenomas. Among the 12 ampullary adenomas, 30% were found to contain carcinoma at surgery or in follow-up. Among ampullary carcinomas, the diagnostic yield of forceps biopsy was increased by 30% when sphincterotomy was performed and deep biopsies were obtained. Only 9.5% of nonampullary duodenal adenomas developed carcinoma.

Ampullary adenomas have a high rate of malignant conversion, 5.5% to 35%.[113,114] Surgical resection of these lesions carries considerable morbidity due to their proximity to the pancreas and biliary tree. EUS, although evaluated in small numbers, appears useful in distinguishing early lesions and the absence of local lymph node metastasis.[115] Patients with benign adenomas or early adenocarcinomas may be amenable to local excision rather than broad excision for. It may also identify those lesions that are unresectable for cure which may be managed with endoscopic palliation. In the majority of cases, endoscopic therapy for ampullary adenomas and adenocarcinoma is palliative.

The optimal therapy for patients with ampullary carcinoma who can tolerate surgery, is a Whipple procedure. This procedure provides biliary drainage and avoids late gastric outlet obstruction due to duodenal stenosis. However the procedure has a mortality rate of 4% to 13% and considerable morbidity. In patients who are poor operative risks or who are unwilling to undergo operative resection, endoscopic sphincterotomy with or without endoprosthesis placement is effective in maintaining biliary patency. Lambert and colleagues[116] did not find Nd:YAG laser photodestruction as a complement to sphincterotomy and stent placement to be very effective in 8 patients with ampullary carcinoma.

For patients with nonampullary duodenal carcinoma, surgical resection is the procedure of first choice. However, Obata and colleagues[117] report curative endoscopic resection of an early duodenal cancer using the strip biopsy technique, in a patient unsuitable for surgery due to comorbid disease, with 10-month follow-up.

For patients with ampullary and nonampullary duodenal adenomas, without evidence of carcinoma, local surgical resection is generally preferred, however, endoscopic removal is an option. Nonampullary adenomas less than 2.5 cm may be removed by standard snare polypectomy or with the strip biopsy technique.[118] However, the duodenal wall is relatively thin and the risk of perforation is greater than in the rectum or stomach. A side viewing duodenoscope should be used to distinguish the major and minor papilla before attempting resection. In patients deemed unfit for surgery, larger lesions may be treated with piecemeal snare resection,[119] or laser

ablation.[120] Recurrence rate is high; therefore, repeat therapy is often required.

Endoscopic therapy for true ampullary adenomas, aside from sphincterotomy and stent insertion, has included endoscopic snare papillectomy[121] and laser ablation.[116] Binmoeller and colleagues[121] reported results of endoscopic papillectomy performed on 25 patients with ampullary lesions deemed benign by endoscopic criteria. Procedure-related complications (bleeding, 2; pancreatitis, 3) occurred in 20%. During a follow up period of 2 to 7 years, only 4 patients required an operation. Of six recurrences, half responded to further endoscopic therapy. Lambert and colleagues[116] achieved complete tumor destruction in 7 of 8 patients with ampullary adenomas followed from 14 to 53 months. A recurrence was observed at 2 years in one patient. At this time, these modalities should be reserved for patients who either refuse surgery or in whom considerable comorbid disease makes them unsuitable for an extensive surgical procedure.

COLORECTAL LESIONS

Any discussion of endoscopic therapy for colorectal neoplasms needs to distinguish therapy directed towards nonmalignant, sessile adenomas and true colorectal cancers. Curative endoscopic treatment of small, flat adenomas and villous adenomas of less than 2.5 cm in diameter is generally accepted. Adenomas greater than 3 cm may be appropriately managed by endoscopic piecemeal resection or surgical segmental resection. Large villous adenomas unamenable to snare resection, due to their size or location in the thin walled right colon, in patients unfit for or unwilling to undergo operative resection, can be effectively managed by laser photoablation.

The standard treatment of colorectal cancer is surgical. However, many patients with colorectal cancer are elderly, or have associated medical conditions that increase the risk of operative resection.

Patients who present with widely metastatic disease may opt for endoscopic palliation over surgical palliation. Lastly, in some individuals, the consideration of a colostomy is unacceptable. Endoscopic electrosurgical and laser therapies provide effective alternatives to surgery in the majority of these patients.

Diminutive Adenomatous Polyps

Cold forceps biopsies are typically adequate for complete resection of diminutive (<5 mm) adenomatous polypoid lesions. Under direct vision, the entire polyp, or a portion of it, is positioned between the open jaws of the forceps. The lesion is then grasped by closing the jaws. Gentle traction pulls the lesion away from the bowel wall resecting the tissue within the biopsy cups. Lesions larger than the lateral diameter of the biopsy forceps cups may require several biopsies to resect the entire specimen. The risk of perforation is considered negligible. Some oozing of blood can be expected, however, this is usually self limited. With this technique, orientation for the pathologist may be difficult and there may be considerable crush artifact. However, the presence of high grade dysplasia or CIS in diminutive adenomatous polyps is rare.

The use of hot biopsy forceps has been recommended for simultaneous biopsy and coagulation of diminutive polypoid lesions. It is proposed that this would more likely eradicate residual adenomatous tissue left from the resected specimen. A status evaluation of this technique by the American Society for Gastrointestinal Endoscopy Technology Assessment Committee[122] concluded that evidence was lacking to demonstrate that the incidence of colorectal cancer was diminished, that complete obliteration of residual neoplastic tissue at the base of a resected diminutive polyp was accomplished with the use of the hot biopsy forceps.

Tappero and colleagues[123] describe the use of cold snare excision of small, colorectal polyps. In their series of 210 consecutive patients, a total of 288 small polyps of 5 mm or less in diameter were transected with a polypectomy snare but without applying electrical energy. They reported no bleeding or perforation complications with this technique. Fifty-six percent of the polyps were adenomas, and severe dysplasia was seen in 4.3% adenomas. There were no polyps with invasive cancer. However, follow up of patient's with severe dysplasia is not available nor was an effort made by the authors to assess the presence of residual polypoid tissue after resection.

Woods and colleagues[124] evaluated BICAP coagulation and compared it to cold forceps biopsy for eradication of diminutive colorectal polyps. They detected residual polypoid tissue at repeat endoscopy in 21% and 29% respectively, despite apparent eradication of the polyp at the time of initial therapy. Based on these findings, bipolar eradication is not recommended for primary management of diminutive colorectal polyps.

Flat Adenoma

The improvement in colonoscopic images and video endoscopy have improved the diagnostic yield of colonoscopy. This has led to the description of flat adenomas, which are defined histologically as showing slightly elevated plaques of adenomatous mucosa never more than twice the thickness of the adjacent mucosa. The periphery of these lesions show radial extension of the dysplastic epithelium in the superficial lumenal portion of the mucosa without vertical extension to the base of crypts. Flat adenomas are relatively common lesions in patients presenting for colonoscopy (12%).[125] The flat adenoma is a benign colorectal neoplasm, however, it has drawn great interest because of its reported, higher malignant potential.

Muto and colleagues[126] reported that 42% of flat adenomas, most less than 1 cm in size, contained high grade dysplasia. A similar prevalence of high grade dysplasia was seen among 29 flat adenomas reported by Wolber and Owen[127] in which 41% of lesions contained high grade dysplasia compared to only 4% of polypoid tubular adenomas. Others[128,129] have reported a much lower incidence of severe atypia.

Kuramota[130] recommends multiple hot biopsies to resect and coagulate the tissue base. Alternatively, the strip biopsy technique is recommended by Karita and colleagues.[131] This is facilitated by the injection of 2 to 4 mL of saline solution into the submucosa beneath and surrounding the lesion. This creates an artificial elevation of the lesion on a pillow of saline

and yields a margin for resection between the lesion and the muscularis mucosa. This method has been safe in our experience and yields a resected specimen suitable for histologic evaluation including the ascertainment of tumor free margins. There is, however, no data to support the notion that this technique is superior to other means of retrieving flat adenomas.

Sessile Colorectal Polyps

For sessile polyps greater than 5 mm and less than 20 mm, snare resection of the lesion is the procedure of choice. The wire loop is placed around the rim of the lesion and closed to draw the entire lesion within the snare. The ensnared lesion is then tented away from the bowel wall, creating a pseudostalk. Using a pure coagulating or blended current the lesion is resected (Fig. 139-12).

All adenomatous polyps are dysplastic by definition. Approximately 5% to 7% of adenomatous polyps contain CIS. Polyps containing CIS are thought to be uniformly cured by electrosurgical snare polypectomy.[132] Polyps containing invasive carcinoma, that is carcinoma penetrating the muscularis propria, have a mean occurrence of 4.7% of adenomatous polyps (2.6%–9.4%).[133] The incidence of lymph node metastasis from a polyp containing invasive carcinoma varies from 8.5% to 17%.[133] The likelihood of the lesion being cured by electrosurgical snare polypectomy is high when the following favorable criteria are met: the polyp is completely excised; the

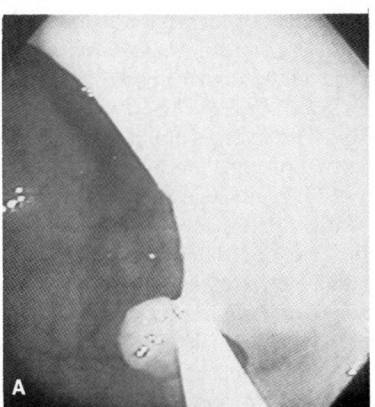

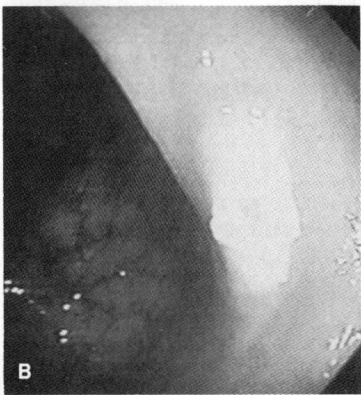

FIGURE 139-12. (A) A small sessile colon polyp is removed by snare. (B) Coagulum is present after removal of the polyp.

cancer is not poorly differentiated; and the cancer does not show vascular and lymphatic invasion. Favorable distance for the carcinoma free margin varies in the literature from 1 mm to 3 mm from the diathermy burn.[134] Follow-up endoscopy should be performed at three months to insure that no adenomatous tissue remains at the polypectomy site.

When favorable criteria are not met, the risk of developing local recurrence or distant metastasis from the polypectomy site must be weighed against the potential risks of elective colon resection. The risk of death from elective colon cancer resection ranges from 0.2% to 10% depending on the patient's age and comorbid disease. Coverlizza and colleagues,[133] in a review of 17 series, determined that in patients with unfavorable histologic characteristics, the average metastatic rate was reported at 8.5%. Ten to seventeen percent of malignant polyps have histologic evidence of vascular or lymphatic invasion, and metastasis is noted in 25%. If the polyp histology is poorly differentiated carcinoma, the incidence of metastasis is 50%.

Sessile adenomatous polyps that contain invasive carcinoma pose a difficult dilemma for the clinician. Little data is available on efficacy of endoscopic therapy for malignant, sessile polyps. They may be missed often at endoscopy and may present with advanced disease. These sessile lesions are not as easily removed endoscopically and, therefore, more patients undergo surgical resection. Cranley[134] reviewed 9 endoscopic studies to evaluate the frequency of cancer at surgery or follow-up of sessile malignant polyps removed endoscopically. Sessile malignant polyps with favorable histologic features had a 4.1% incidence of cancer at surgery or follow-up compared to 20.6% in those with unfavorable histology. Russell and colleagues[135] reported an incidence of metastasis from sessile malignant polyps at 15%. A decision analysis by Wilcox and Beck concluded that all sessile, malignant polyps should be resected if the patient is a good surgical risk.[136]

In summary, sessile and pedunculated polyps containing CIS are cured by polypectomy providing that the polyp is completely excised. Pedunculated polyps containing invasive cancer are usually cured if favorable histologic features are present. In this case, the risk of metastatic disease is approximately 1%. Sessile polyps containing invasive carcinoma may have a higher risk of early metastasis. Thus, endoscopic resection alone, even when favorable histologic features are present, may not be adequate, therefore, segmental resection should be considered in these patients. Recommendations for surgical resection vary depending on the patient's age and comorbid conditions. In younger patients, less than 49 years of age, mortality approaches 0%, mortality is 1.6% for patients age 50 to 69 years, but elderly patients over the age of 75 have a mortality rate of 4% to 10%.[137]

Large Sessile Adenomas

Large sessile benign colonic adenomas, are those greater than 2 to 3 cm. in diameter without overt evidence of malignancy. Endoscopic snare resection, and in some cases laser ablation, have evolved as alternatives to conventional surgery for the treatment of these lesions. The term large is based only on technical criteria of endoscopic removal and not on clinical

or pathologic grounds. Endoscopic appearance cannot reliably distinguish those lesions that may contain focal or infiltrative carcinoma. There are, however, overt endoscopic features that favor malignancy including ulceration, hard texture, and fixation. Snare biopsy of large chunks provides more tissue for histologic interpretation than is provided by forceps biopsy alone. Adequate tissue should be submitted to the pathologist to evaluate the presence of carcinoma prior to considering endoscopic therapy. EUS can identify tumor invasion and disruption of the normal colonic wall architecture. These features, when present, may help distinguish the lesion as malignant versus benign.

The majority of villous and tubulovillous adenomas are located in the rectum and rectosigmoid. These lesions are best suited for endoscopic therapy because they are easily accessible with a minimum of patient preparation. Conscious sedation may not be required and the retroperitoneal reflection minimizes the risk of perforation. Finally, these lessions are more often referred for endoscopic therapy because the conventional surgical alternative, abdominal peritoneal resection, is less appealing than the simpler segmental resection required for more proximal lesions. Operative mortality after abdominoperineal resection is approximately 5% and approximately 7% after rectal resection. Morbidity is reported as high as 53%. Other surgical options include transanal and transsacral resection but both of these modalities incur the risk of general anesthesia. Rectal fistulas occur in up to 21% of patients following a transsacral approach. The rate of recurrence following transanal resection is 6% to 42% and complications occur in approximately 13%.[138-140]

Large villous adenomas in the more proximal colon are traditionally managed with segmental resection. Endoscopic piecemeal resection is an alternative to surgery. This is more technically challenging as the endoscope may need to be repeatedly advanced to, and withdrawn from, the lesion when retrieving multiple resected specimens. Care must be taken to avoid overinsufflation which may result in thinning of the colonic wall, theoretically increasing the risk of perforation. Endoscopic piecemeal resection may be offered to patients with advanced age, comorbid disease, or those simply wishing to avoid the morbidity and mortality associated with surgical resection and the associated risks of general anesthesia. The risks of perforation and bleeding, and perhaps the need for emergent surgery, must be weighed against the potential benefits of endoscopic therapy.

Endoscopic therapy for colorectal neoplasms is typically performed on an outpatient basis using flexible video endoscopes. In patients with rectosigmoid lesions, many centers feel that per rectal enemas provide adequate preparation. For all other lesions, a peroral bowel lavage and conscious sedation are used. The two techniques of piecemeal snare excision and laser photoablation have been described with the greatest enthusiasm in the literature.

Nivatvongs and colleagues[141] reported the results of piecemeal snare polypectomy of 28 large sessile polyps. Polyps ranged from 2 to 6 cm. Five polyps were in the right colon, two in the transverse, six in the proximal sigmoid, and 15 in the rectum and rectosigmoid area. Eight specimens contained carcinoma. Five of these eight patients underwent surgical resection and no residual tumor was found. Of the remaining 20 patients without carcinoma, five had residual adenomatous tissue or recurrence, with a follow-up from 6 months to 6 years (mean, 18 months). All were managed with additional electrocoagulation therapy and no further malignancies developed. They had one complication, bleeding soon after the procedure, which stopped spontaneously.

Bedogni and colleagues[142] reported 66 colonoscopic piecemeal excisions of large pedunculated and sessile polyps greater than or equal to 3 cm. in size, deemed to be benign on the basis of their endoscopic features. Forty-five of these were sessile; 34 were in the rectum and sigmoid area, the remainder in the more proximal colon. Of 36 patients with sessile adenomas who had colonoscopic follow-up, residual or recurrent disease was observed in 16.5%. Only three complications (4.5%) were recorded; bleeding in two patients, and serosal burn in one patient, all managed medically. Karita and colleagues[131] used the strip biopsy technique described earlier to resect 21 adenocarcinomas (including cancer in adenoma), 46 sessile adenomas, 3 metaplastic polyps, and 1 juvenile polyp. Of the 71 lesions, 68 were completely resected in a single strip biopsy procedure. However, no long-term follow-up data is available. Mild postpolypectomy bleeding occurred in one patient. Walsh and colleagues[143] performed colonoscopic piecemeal resection of 132 sessile polyps with a mean size of 3 cm. Of these, adenomas recurred or persisted in 28%, most of which were successfully reresected. Nearly one half of all recurrent polyps occurred after at least one negative intervening exam. Mean follow-up of 3.7 years was achieved in 77% of patients. Complications, bleeding and probable microperforation, occurred in 3% and were managed medically. When surgical resection was performed for invasive carcinoma in the colonoscopically resected specimen, no tumor was found in 41% of the surgical specimens. These data demonstrate that endoscopic piecemeal snare excision of sessile colorectal adenomas can be safe and effective. Surgical resection does not appear to offer advantages over endoscopic resection when the entire lesion can be completely resected by endoscopic means. Surveillance colonoscopy is required following endoscopic piecemeal excision of sessile adenomas to detect and manage residual disease and local recurrences.

Several centers, primarily European, have reported their substantial experience with endoscopic laser photocoagulation as primary treatment for villous adenomas of the colorectum. Techniques for ELT of colorectal neoplasms are detailed in the following section. Brunetaud and colleagues[144] treated 56 patients with rectal villous adenomas using argon and Nd: YAG lasers. Complete tumor ablation was documented in 42 of the 56 treated patients. Treatment was well tolerated with no major complications. Treatment duration, that is number of sessions, as well as recurrences varied directly with the annular size of the tumor. Lesions that encompassed less than one third of the lumenal circumference (C1) were most easily treated, and had the fewest recurrences. Those lesions greater than two thirds of lumenal circumference (C3) had the highest incidence of recurrence and required the greatest number of sessions. Among 47 patients in whom thorough follow-up was available, 89% had successful treatment. In five patients who did not achieve good results, the failure was due to the development of histologic changes suggestive of carcinoma. Adenomas recurred in 19% of patients who underwent additional laser therapy. Of these, the majority occurred in C3 lesions.

Brunetaud and colleagues[145] later reported their 9-year retrospective experience with endoscopic laser treatment in 264 patients with benign rectosigmoid villous adenomas. Indications for laser therapy were medical contraindications to surgery, recurrences after nonlaser therapy, and individuals in whom surgical resection was thought to be too drastic for a small lesion found benign on biopsy. Prior nonlaser treatment included: surgery, radiation therapy and electrocoagulation. Some lesions were debulked by diathermic snare prior to laser therapy. Treatment was completed in 226 patients with total tumor destruction attained in 92% with an average of six laser sessions over four months. Carcinoma was detected in 7% on biopsy specimens obtained during laser treatment and benign villous tissue persisted in one percent. During a mean follow-up of 26 months, adenomas recurred in 13% after ablation and epithelialization. This treatment was well tolerated with no major complications. Similarly, the circumferential extension of the tumor base was the only factor predicting the duration of treatment, the rate of cancer detected during treatment and the rate of complications. Complications included: bleeding, asymptomatic stenosis, and post-treatment fever. There were no major bleeding episodes or perforations. A cost analysis determined that the direct cost of laser treatments was 28% to 40%, that of surgery treatment for lesions of identical size.

Mathus-Vliegen and Tytgat reported 241 patients with colorectal adenomas who were unsuitable for, or refused surgery who presented with incompletely removed polyps, or lesions unsuitable for endoscopic polypectomy.[146] Full evaluation was possible in 196 patients. Greatest success was achieved in small (C1) and intermediate (C2) sized lesions with ultimate ablation in 93% and 85% respectively. In large (C3) lesions, greater than two thirds of the circumference of the lumen, only 56% of patients ultimately had successful ablation. However, symptoms of excessive mucous discharge, bleeding, incontinence and diarrhea were successfully eradicated when 75% or more of the tumor was ablated. There were no treatment-associated deaths. Bleeding and stenosis occurred in 7% of patients. Their follow-up lasted a mean of greater than three years and in some patients, up to 10.5 years (Fig. 139-13).

Low and Kozarek described the technique of snare cautery debridement prior to Nd:YAG total ablation of broad based adenomas of the colorectum.[147] They reported 46 patients who underwent piecemeal resection of large, sessile villous adenomas followed by immediate laser photoablative therapy. This technique provides copious tissue for histologic analysis, decreases the amount of residual neoplasm requiring laser treatment, and has a potential to improve laser efficacy. In their series, eradication required mean of 2.1 treatment sessions. They found that this technique improved treatment efficacy without concomitant increase in complication rate.

Because laser tissue destruction precludes complete histologic evaluation of polyp tissue, it should be reserved for lesions that cannot be removed completely by endoscopic polypectomy in patients with serious contraindications to surgery or who refuse surgery. Laser ablation may also be applicable in patients with residual or recurrent villous adenoma after previous, nonlaser therapy, and for ablation of rectal stump polyps in patients with familial polyposis coli after subtotal colectomy and ileoanal anastomosis.

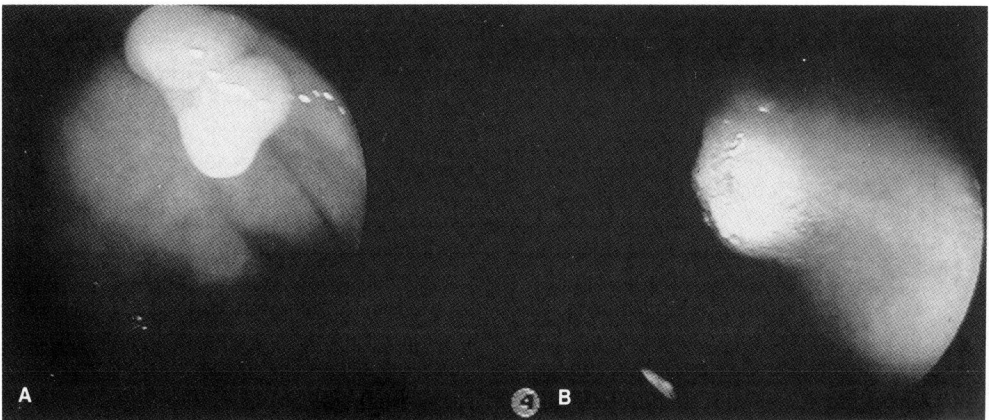

FIGURE 139-13. Familial polyposis in patient with an iliorectal anastomosis. (**A**) Polyp is seen prior to laser treatment. (**B**) After the first laser pulses, coagulative changes are seen.

Endoscopic Treatment of Colorectal Cancers

Surgical resection is the treatment of choice in colorectal carcinoma for both cure and palliation. When patients present with lumenal obstruction, widspread or recurrent disease, or are otherwise unfit or unwilling to undergo an operation, ELT provides effective palliation.

Small C1 lesions of less than 2 to 3 cm may be completely treated in a single session. Larger lesions typically require several sessions, generally treated every 48 hours until the initial treatment goal is realized. For T1 and some T2 lesions curative therapy may be achieved and, therefore, the treatment goal is complete eradication of all neoplastic tissue. For most patients, however, referred for endoscopic management of malignant colorectal lesions, palliation is the goal. Treatment endpoints for palliation of colorectal neoplasms include cessation of bleeding, maintaining lumenal patency and diminishing mucous discharge.

Those patients most likely to benefit from laser treatment would be those with unresectable metastasis and those in whom coexisting medical conditions make surgery an unduly high risk. And, finally, those patients, whom after consultation with the surgeon, find the risks of surgical resection or the prospect of a colostomy unacceptable. As for benign lesions, adenocarcinomas of the rectosigmoid are the most amenable to endoscopic therapy for the same reasons: they are easily accessible, a minimum of preparation is required to apply therapy, and the retroperitoneal anatomy reduces the risk of free perforation. Treatment is generally performed on an outpatient basis and enema preparation is typically adequate, at least for distal colonic lesions which are the majority. Lesion characteristics that pose technical difficulties for laser therapy include: circumfirential lesions at the rectosigmoid angle, long lesions and lesions near the anal verge. Obstructing lesions may be initially dilated to allow passage of a small, caliber endoscope.

Most laser endoscopists use noncontact Nd:YAG lasers at high power (70–90 watts). We generally use a double channel, or large channel, endoscope so that smoke and coaxial gas can be suctioned from the field around the laser fiber improving visibility and avoiding over distention. Mellow describes the placement of a thin suction catheter intermittently into the rectum to help remove smoke and debris from the field.[148]

The Nd:YAG laser is applied until blanching of the tumor surface occurs. In this way, coagulation necrosis is induced with a minimization of smoke and charring which hamper further therapy (Fig. 139-14). Brunetaud uses an argon laser for flat, sessile lesions and lesions close to the anus at 10 watts for the treatment of residual, flat lesions to the point of tissue vaporization.[144] Conversely, the Nd:YAG laser was used to treat bulky tumors. Delayed necrosis can be expected after using Nd:YAG laser with considerable loss of tumor volume in follow-up compared to that observed at the time of coagulation therapy. Once the initial treatment goal has been achieved, the patient returns in 4 to 8 weeks for reevaluation. Repeat treatments depend on the tumor's regrowth characteristics and the recurrence or absence of symptoms.

Mathus-Vliegen and Tytgat treated 63 patients with advanced colorectal cancer because of obstruction (16 patients), bleeding (32 patients), and combined bleeding and obstruction (15 patients).[146] Lumenal patency was restored in 94%, hemostasis achieved in 88%, and effective treatment in 87% of patients with combined obstruction and bleeding. Palliation was evident after 2 to 3 sessions. Minor complications (i.e., transient stenosis and laser-induced bleeding) occurred in 19%. There was one treatment-associated death, resulting from a pararectal abcess.

Eckhauser reported the results of 55 patients with colorectal cancers treated with ELT, 48 presenting with obstruction and 7 with bleeding.[149] Successful photocoagulation obviated the need for further blood transfusions in those patients treated for bleeding. Among those with obstruction, 31 patients underwent preresectional recanalization, allowing peroral bowel lavage and avoiding initial operative diversion. The majority of these lesions were above the peritoneal reflection. Although survival did not appear to be affected, length of hospital stay and cost were significantly reduced. Another 17 patients with imminent obstruction were nonresectable due to regional or metastatic disease and underwent palliative laser therapy. Ten were above, and 7 below the peritoneal reflection. A mean of 3 treatment sessions was required for successful recannulation in all cases and performance status was improved. Perforation occurred in one patient in the preresection group.

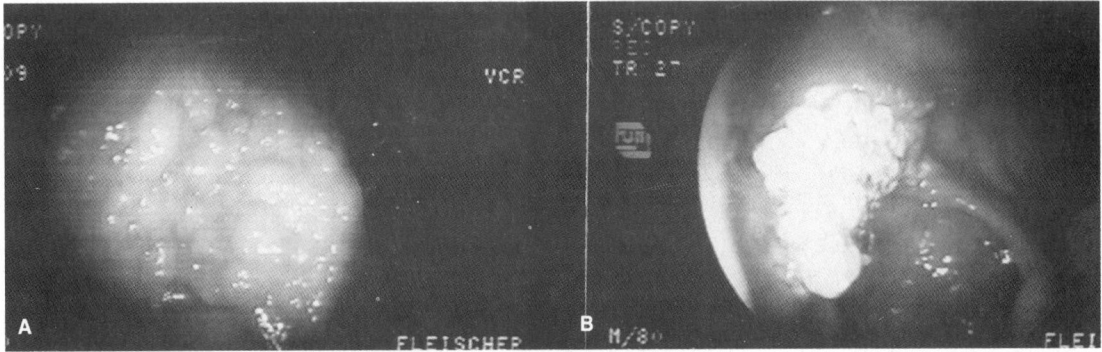

FIGURE 139-14. (**A**) Nd:YAG laser ablation of cecal villous adenoma in a patient who was not a candidate for surgery. (**B**) The desired effect of coagulation necrosis is achieved.

Finally, in a survey of 7 European laser centers, 181 patients underwent laser palliation, 60 for obstruction, 81 for bleeding, and 40 referred for both obstruction and bleeding.[150] The success rate for palliation of obstruction was 89%. There were 4 complications in this group, with 2 deaths (1 perforation, 1 uncontrolled bleeding). These results compare favorably to the morbidity and mortality of a surgical colostomy. Bleeding responded to laser coagulation in 90% with a complication rate of 11% and no deaths. Similar results for palliation of obstruction and cessation of bleeding from advanced colorectal cancer have been reported by others.[151,152]

Nd:YAG laser therapy has been highly successful for the palliative management of bleeding or obstructing colorectal cancer. It has converted this otherwise hopeless situation into a manageable and responsive condition. In a comparison to surgery for palliation of adenocarcinoma of the rectum, the cost of ELT was significantly less; and hospital stay, intensive care time and complications were significantly lower in the laser group compared to the surgical group.[153] Preresection laser recanalization for obstructing lesions allows a formal bowel prep, and definitive one-stage operation, requiring a shorter hospital stay and lower total cost.[154]

Primary laser therapy for small, rectal carcinomas with an intent to cure may be achieved with ELT. Among 19 patients that Brunetaud treated who had small cancers, defined as less than 3 cm in length with lumenal circumference less than one third, 17 had no known local or metastatic disease on a mean follow-up of 37 months.[155] Escourrou[156] reported 18 patients with successful endoscopic destruction without recurrence of the mean follow-up of 13 months. Dittrich and colleagues[152] treated 9 patients with early (T1,Nx,MO) carcinoma who were unfit for, or refused, abdominoperineal resection. Two patients died of other causes, the remaining 7 were alive at a mean survival time of 25.5 months. Autopsies of the two patients who died revealed no evidence of colon cancer. All these authors agree that laser therapy for curative intent should be reserved for special cases in which surgery is not an option.

The reader is directed to Chapter 57, Esophageal Neoplasms; Chapter 65, Tumors of the Stomach; Chapter 85, Colonic Polyps: Benign and Premalignant Neoplasms of the Colon; Chapter 115, Upper Gastrointestinal Endoscopy; and Chapter 116, Colonoscopy and Flexible Sigmoidoscopy.

REFERENCES

1. Ginsberg G, Gupta P, Newsome J, Brennecke L, Fleischer D. A new laser for therapeutic gastrointestinal endoscopy: initial investigation of the KTP/532 laser in a canine model (abstract). Am J Gastroenterol 1992;87:1339.
2. Odell R. Principles of electrosurgery. In: Sivak M, ed. Gastroenterologic endoscopy. Philadelphia: WB Saunders 1987.
3. Van Gossum A, Cozzoli A, Adler M, Taton G, Crenier M. Colonoscopic snare polypectomy: analysis of 1485 resections comparing two types of current. Gastrointest Endosc 1992;38:472.
4. Vanagunas A, Pothen J, Nimesh V. Adequacy of "hot biopsy" for the treatment of diminutive polyps: a randomized trial. Am J Gastroenterol 1989;84:383.
5. Peluso F, Golodner F. Follow-up of hot biopsy forceps treatment of diminutive colonic polyps. Gastrointest Endosc 1991;37:604.
6. Suzuki S, Aoki J, Shiina Y, et al. New ceramic endoprobes for endoscopic contact irradiation with Nd:YAG laser: experimental and clinical applications. Gastrointest Endosc 1986;32:282.
7. Radford C, Ahlquist D, Gostout C, et al. Prospective comparison of contact with noncontact Nd:YAG laser therapy for palliation of esophageal carcinoma. Gastrointest Endosc 1989;35:394.
8. Naveau S, Poynyard T, Zourabichvili O, Poitrine A, Chaput J. A randomized study of a coaxial fiber versus a naked fiber for endoscopic Nd:YAG laser therapy of esophageal and rectal tumors. Gastrointest Endosc 1989;35:201.
9. Cranley J, Petras R, Carey W, Paradis K, Sivak M. When is endoscopic polypectomy adequate therapy for colonic polyps containing invasive carcinoma? Gastroenterol 1986;91:419.
10. Williams C, Whiteway J, Jass J. Practical aspects of endoscopic management of malignant polyps. Endoscopy 1987;19:31.
11. Walsh R, Ackroyd F, Shellito P. Endoscopic resection of large sessile polyps. Gastrointest Endosc 1992;38:303.
12. Brunetaud J, Mosquet L, Houcke M, et al. Villous adenoma of the rectum: results of endoscopic treatment with argon and Nd:YAG lasers. Gastrointest Endosc 1985;89:832.
13. Low P, Kozarek R. Snare cautery debridement prior to Nd:YAG photoablation improves treatment efficiency of broad-based adenomas of the colorectum. Gastrointest Endosc 1989;35:288.
14. Tada M, Shimada T, Yanai H, et al. New technique of gastric biopsy (in Japanese with English abstract). Stom Intest 1984;19:1107.
15. Rosch T, Lorenz R, Zecker K, et al. Local staging and assessment of resectability in carcinoma of the esophagus, stomach and duodenum by endoscopic ultrasonography. Gastrointest Endosc 1992;38:460.
16. Cho E, Nakajima M, Yasuda K, Ashihara T, Kawai K. Endoscopic ultrasonography of colorectal cancer invasion. Gastrointest Endosc 1993;39:521.
17. Kozarek R, Ball T, Patterson D. Metallic self-expanding stent application in the upper gastrointestinal tract: caveats and concerns. Gastrointest Endosc 1992;38:1.

18. Itabashi M, Hamano S, Asahina K. Self-expanding stainless steel stent application in the rectosigmoid stricture. Dis Colon Rectum 1993;36:508.
19. Tytgat G, Bartelsman J, Verdmeyden J. Dilation and prosthesis for obstructing esophagogastric carcinoma. Gastrointest Endosc Clin North Am 1992;2:415.
20. Graham D, Tabibian N, Schwartz J, Lacey Smith J. Evaluation of the effectiveness of through-the-endoscope balloons as dilators of benign and malignant gastrointestinal strictures. Gastrointest Endosc 1987;33:432.
21. Spechler S, Robbins A, Bloomfield Rubins H, et al. Adenocarcinoma and Barrett's esophagus. An overrated risk? Gastroenterol 1984;87:927.
22. Brandt L, Kauvar D. Laser-induced transient regression of Barrett's epithelium. Gastrointest Endosc 1992;38:619.
23. Sampliner R, Hixson L, Fennerty M, Garewal H. Regression of Barrett's esophagus by laser ablation in an anacid environment. Dig Dis Sci 1993;38:365.
24. Berenson M, Johnson T, Markowitz N, Buchi K, Samowitz W. Restoration of squamous mucosa after ablation of Barrett's esophageal epithelium. Gastroenterology 1993;104:1686.
25. Sugimachi K, Kitamura K, Baba K, Ikebe M, Kuwano H. Endoscopic diagnosis of early carcinoma of the esophagus using Lugol's solution. Gastrointest Endosc 1992;38:657.
26. Inoue H, Takeshita K, Hori H, et al. Endoscopic mucosal resection with a cap-fitted panendoscope for esophagus, stomach, and colon mucosal lesions. Gastrointest Endosc 1993;39:58.
27. Harju E. Gastric polyposis and malignancy. Br J Surg 1986;73:632.
28. Ginsberg G, Al-Kawas F, Reilly H, Fleischer D, Benjamin S. Should all gastric polyps be removed (abstract)? Am J Gastroenterol 1992;87:1268.
29. Mellow M, Pinkus H. Endoscopic laser therapy for malignancies affecting the esophagus and gastroesophageal junction: analysis of technical and functional efficacy. Arch Intern Med 1985;145:1443.
30. Yasuda K, Kiyota K, Nakajima M, et al. Fundamentals of endoscopic laser therapy for GI tumors—new aspects with endoscopic ultrasonography. Endoscopy 1987;19:1.
31. Boring C, Squires T, Tong T. Cancer statistics, 1993. CA Cancer J Clin 1993;43:7.
32. Tio T, Coene P, Luiken G, et al. Endosonography in the clinical staging of esophagogastric carcinoma. Gastrointest Endosc 1990;36:S2.
33. Kawano T, Miyake S, Yasun M, et al. A new technique for endoscopic esophageal mucosectomy using a transparent overtube with intralumenal negative pressure. Dig Endosc 1991;3:159.
34. Rutgeerts P, Van Trappen G, Broeckaert L, et al. Palliative Nd:YAG laser therapy for cancer of the esophagus and gastroesophageal junction: impact on quality of remaining life. Gastrointest Endosc 1988;34:87.
35. Patrice T, Foultier M, Yactayo S, et al. Endoscopic photodynamic therapy with hematoporphyrin derivative for primary treatment of gastrointestinal neoplasms in inoperable patients. Dig Dis Sci 1990;35:545.
36. Kasai M, Mori S, Watanabe T, Follow-up results after resection of thoracic oesophageal carcinoma. World J Surg 1978;2:543.
37. Koch N, Lewin E, Petterson S. Carcinoma of the thoracic oesophagus: a review of 146 cases. Acta Chir Scand 1967;133:375.
38. Fein R, Kelson D, Geler N, et al. Adenocarcinoma of the esophagus and gastroesophageal junction: prognostic factors and results of therapy. Cancer 1985;56:2512.
39. Belsey R. Palliative management of esophageal carcinoma. Am J Surg 1980;139:789.
40. Conlan A, Nicolaou N, Hammond C, et al. Retrosternal gastric bypass for inoperable esophageal cancer: a report of 71 patients. Ann Thorac Surg 1983;36:396.
41. Parker E, Gregorie H. Carcinoma of the esophagus: longterm results. J Am Med Assoc 1976;235:1018.
42. Kelson D. Chemotherapy for local, regional and advanced esophageal cancer. Cancer: principles and practices of oncology updates 1988;2:1.
43. Herskovic A, Martz K, Al-Sarraf M, et al. Combined chemotherapy and radiotherapy compared to radiotherapy alone in patients with cancer of the esophagus. N Engl J Med 1992;326:1598.
44. Boyce H Jr. Nonsurgical measures to relieve distress of late esophageal carcinoma. Geriatrics 1973;28:97.
45. Heit H, Johnson L, Siegel S, et al. Palliative dilation for dysphagia in esophageal carcinoma. Ann Intern Med 1978;89:629.
46. Tytgat G, den Hartog Jager F. To dilate or intubate? Gastrointest Endosc 1983;29:58.
47. Fleischer D, Sivak M. Endoscopic Nd:YAG laser therapy as palliation for esophagogastric cancer: parameters affecting initial outcome. Gastroenterol 1985;89:827.
48. Pietraffitta J, Dwyer R. New laser technique for the treatment of malignant esophageal obstruction. J Surg Oncol 1987;35:157.
49. Pietraffitta J, Bowers G, Dwyer R. Prograde versus retrograde endoscopic laser therapy for the treatment of malignant esophageal obstruction: a comparison of techniques. Lasers Surg Med 1988;8:288.
50. Fleischer D, Kessler F, Haye O. Endoscopic Nd:YAG laser therapy for carcinoma of the esophagus: a new palliative technique. Am J Surg 1982;143:280.
51. Suzuki S, Aoki J, Shiina Y, Nomiyama T, Miwa T. New ceramic endoprobes for endoscopic contact irradiation with Nd:YAG laser: experimental studies and clinical applications. Gastrointest Endosc 1986;32:282.
52. Fleischer D, Kessler F. Endoscopic Nd:YAG laser therapy for carcinoma of the esophagus: a new form of palliative treatment. Gastroenterol 1983;85:600.
53. Mellow M, Pinkas H. Endoscopic therapy for esophageal carcinoma with Nd:YAG laser: prospective evaluation of efficacy, complications and survival. Gastrointest Endosc 1984;30:334.
54. Cello J, Gerstenberger P, Wright T, et al. Endoscopic neodymium-YAG laser palliation of nonresectable esophagel malignancy. Ann Intern Med 1985;102:610.
55. Pietrafitta J, Dwyer R. Endoscopic laser therapy of malignant esophageal obstruction. Arch Surg 1986;121:395.
56. Bown S, Hawes R, Mattewson K, et al. Endoscopic laser palliation for advanced malignant dysphagia. Gut 1987;28:799.
57. Buset M, des Marez B, Baize M, et al. Palliative endoscopic management of obstructive esophagogastric cancer: laser for prosthesis? Gastrointest Endosc 1987;33:357.
58. Krasner N, Barr H, Skidmore C, et al. Palliative laser therapy for malignant dysphagia Gut 1987;28:792.
59. Richter J, Hilgenberg A, Chistensen M, et al. Endoscopic palliation of obstructive esophagogastric malignancy. Gastrointest Endosc 1988;34:454.
60. Maunoury V, Brunetaud J, Cochelard, et al, Endoscopic palliation for inoperable malignant dysphagia: long term follow up. Gut 1992;33:1602.
61. Stange E, Dyalla J, Fleig W. Laser treatment of upper gastrointestinal tract carcinoma: determinants of survival. Endoscopy 1989;21:254.
62. Ell C, Demling L. Laser therapy of tumor stenosis in the upper gastrointestinal tract: an international inquiry. Lasers Surg Med 1987;7:491.
63. Johnston J, Fleischer D, Petrini J, et al. Palliative bipolar electrocoagulation therapy of obstructing esophageal cancer. Gastrointest Endosc 1987;33:349.
64. Fleischer D, Ranard R, Kanath R, et al. Stricture formation following BICAP tumor probe therapy for esophageal cancer. Gastrointest Endosc 1987;33:183(A).
65. Jensen D, Macchicado G, Randall G, et al. Comparison of low-power YAG laser and BICAP tumor probe for palliation for esophageal cancer stricture. Gastroenterology 1988;94:1263.
66. Atkinson M, Ferguson R, Ogilvie A. Management of malignant dysphagia by intubation at endoscopy. J Soc Med 1979;72:894.
67. Tytgat G, Bartelsman J, Den Hartog Jager F, Huibregtse K, Mathus-Vliegen E. Upper intestinal and biliary tract endoprosthesis. Dig Dis Sci 1986;31(Suppl):S57.
68. Gasparri G, Casalegno P, Camandona M, et al. Endoscopic insertion of 248 prosthesis in inoperable carcinoma of the

esophagus and cardia: short-term and long-term results. Gastrointest Endosc 1987;33:354.

69. Buset M, des Marez B, Baize M, et al. Palliative endoscopic management of obstructive esophagogastric cancer: laser or prosthesis? Gastrointest Endosc 1987;33:357.

70. Richter J, Hilgenberg A, Christensen M, et al. Endoscopic palliation of obstructive esophagogastric malignancy. Gastrointest Endosc 1988;34:454.

71. Sargeant I, Loizou L, Tulloch M, Thorpe S, Bown S. Recanalization of tube overgrowth: a useful new indication for laser palliation of malignant dysphagia. Gastrointest Endosc 1992;38:165.

72. Hine K, Atkinson M. The diagnosis and management of perforations of esophagus and pharynx sustained during intubation of neoplastic esophageal strictures. Dig Dis Sci 1986;31:571.

73. Sargeant I, Thorpe S, Bown S. Cuffed esophageal prosthesis: a useful device in desperate situations in esophageal malignancy. Gastrointest Endosc 1992;38:669.

74. Loizou L, Rampton D, Bown S. Treatment of malignant strictures of the cervical esophagus by endoscopic intubation using modified endoprostheses. Gastrointest Endosc 1992;38:158.

75. Buess G, Schellong H, Kometz B, et al. A modified prosthesis for the treatment of malignant esophagotracheal fistula. Cancer 1986;61:1679.

76. Fleischer D, Bull-Henry K. A new coated self-expanding metal stent for malignant esophageal strictures. Gastrointest Endosc 1992;38:494.

77. Schaer J, Katon R, Ivancev K, Uchida B, Rosch J, Binmoller K. Treatment of malignant esophageal obstruction with silicone-coated metallic self-expanding stents. Gastrointest Endosc 1992;38:7.

78. Knyrim K, Wagner H, Bethge N, Keymling M, Vakil N. A controlled trial of an expansile meta stent for palliation of esophageal obstruction due to inoperable cancer. N Engl J Med 1993;329:1302.

79. Anderson D, Wright P. Laser recanalization versus endoscopic intubation in the palliation of malignant dysphagia. Br J Surg 1990;77:1151.

80. Lightdale C, Zimbalist E, Winawer S. Outpatient management of esophageal cancer with Nd:YAG laser. Am J Gastroenterol 1987;82:46.

81. Hahl J, Salo J, Ovaska J, Haapiainen R, Kalima T, Schroder T. Comparison of endoscopic Nd:YAG laser therapy and oesphageal tube in palliation of oesophagogastric malignancy. Scand J Gastroenterol 1991;26:103.

82. Barr H, Krasner N, Raouf A. Prospective randomized trial of laser therapy only and laser therapy followed by endoscopic intubation for the palliation of malignant dysphagia. Gut 1990;31:252.

83. Carter R, Smith J, Anderson J. Laser recanalization versus endoscopic intubation in the palliation of malignant dysphagia: a randomized prospective study. Br J Surg 1992;79:1167.

84. Loizou L, Grigg D, Atkinson M, Robertson C, Bown S. A prospective comparison of laser thrapy and intubation in endoscopic palliation for malignant dysphagia. Gastroenterol 1991;100:1303.

85. Lauren P, The two histological main types of gastric carcinoma: diffuse and so-called intestinal type carcinoma. Acta Pathol Microbial Scand 1965;64:31.

86. Weinstein W. Vital staining of esophageal and gastric mucosa: not vital but may be helpful. Gastrointest Endosc 1992;38:723.

87. Fennerty M, Sampliner R, McGee D, et al. Intestinal metaplasia of the stomach: identification by a selective mucosal staining technique. Gastrointest Endosc 1992;38:696.

88. Neimark S, Rogers A. Gastric polyps: a review. Am J Gastroenterol 1982;77:585.

89. Seifert E, Gail K, Weismuller J. Gastric polypectomy. Endoscopy 1985;15:8.

90. Deppish L, Rona V. Gastric epithelial polyps: a 10-year study. J Clin Gastroenterol 1989;11:110.

91. Diabo M, Itabashi M, Hirota T. Malignant transformation of gastric hyperplastic polyps. Am J Gastroenterol 1987;82:1016.

92. Harju E. Gastric polyposis and malignancy. Br J Surg 1986;73:632.

93. Remine S, Hughes R, Weiland L. Endoscopic gastric polypectomies. Mayo Clin Proc 1981;56:371.

94. Fabry T, Frankel A, Way J. Gastric polyps. J Clin Gastroenterol 1982;4:23.

95. Ghazi A, Ferstenberg H, Shinya H. Endoscopic gastroduodenal polypectomy. Ann Surg 1984;200:175.

96. Tsukuma H, Mishima T, Oshima A. Prospective study of "early" gastric cancer. Int J Cancer 1983;31:421.

97. Lawrence M, Shiu M. Early gastric cancer: twenty eight years of experience. Ann Surg 1991;213:.

98. Yoshimori M. The natural history of early gastric cancer. Jpn J Clin Oncol 1989;19:89.

99. Sakita T, Iizuka T, Kato H, et al. The development of endoscopic diagnosis of early carcinoma of the stomach. Jpn J Clin Oncol 1971;1:113.

100. Yasuda K, Nakajima M, Kawai K. Endoscopic diagnosis and treatment of early gastric cancer. Gastrointest Endosc Clin North Am 1992;2(3):495.

101. Imaoka W, Ida K, Katoh T, et al. Is curative endoscopic treatment of early gastric cancer possible? Endoscopy 1987;19(Suppl 1):7.

102. Hirao M, Masuda K, Asanuma T, et al. Endoscopic resection of early gastric cancer and other tumors with local injection of hypertonic saline-epinephrine. Gastrointest Endosc 1988;34:264.

103. Karita M, Tada M, Okita K. The successive strip biopsy partial resection technique for large early gastric and colon cancers. Gastrointest Endosc 1992;38:174.

104. Haruma K, Sumii K, Inoue K, Teshima H, Kajiyama G. Endoscopic therapy in patients with inoperable early gastric cancer. Am J Gastroenterol 1990;85:522.

105. Nakazawa S, Yoshino J, Kijima Y, et al. The endoscopic intratumor administration of OK-432 in gastric cancer unsuitable for surgery. Endoscopy 1989;21:168.

106. Teixeira C, Haruma K, Teshima, et al. Endoscopic therapy for gastric cancer in patients more than 80 years old. Am J Gastroenterol 1991;86:725.

107. Hayata Y, Kato H, Ojitsu, et al. Photodynamic therapy with hematoporphyrin derivative in cancer of the upper gastrointestinal tract. Semmin Surg Oncol 1985;1:1.

108. Fleischer D, Sivak M. Endoscopic Nd:YAG laser therapy as palliative treatment for advanced adenocarcinoma of the gastric cardia. Gastroenterol 1984;87:815.

109. Suzuki H, Miho O, Watanabe Y, et al. Endoscopic laser therapy in the curative and palliative treatment of upper gastrointestinal cancer. World J Surg 1989;13:158.

110. Ryan D, Schapiro R, Warshaw A. Villus tumors of the duodenum Ann Surg 1986;203:301.

111. Yamaguchi K, Enjoji M, Kitamura K. Endoscopic biopsy has limited accuracy in diagnosis of ampullary tumors. Gastrointest Endosc 1990;36:588.

112. Seifert E, Schulte F, Stolte M. Adenoma and carcinoma of the duodenum and papilla of Vater: a clinicopathological study. Am J Gastroenterol 1992;87:37.

113. Yamaguchi K, Enjonji M. Carcinoma of the ampulla of Vater: a clinicopathologic study and pathologic staging of 104 cases of carcinoma and 5 cases of adenoma. Cancer 1987;59:506.

114. Hayes D, Bolton J, Willis G, et al. Carcinoma of the ampulla of Vater. Ann Surg 1987;206:572.

115. Tio L, Tytgat G, Cicot R, Houthoff H, Sars P. Ampullopancreatic carcinoma: preoperative TNM classification with endosonography. Radiology 1990;175:455.

116. Lambert R, Ponchon T, Chavaillon A, Berger F. Laser treatment of tumors of the papilla of Vater. Endoscopy 1988;20:227.

117. Obata S, Suenaga M, Araki K, et al. Use of strip biopsy in a case of early duodenal cancer. Endoscopy 1992;24:232.

118. Delpy J, Bruneton J, Drouillard J, Lecompte P. Nonvaterian duodenal adenomas: report of 24 cases and review of the literature. Gastrointest Radiol 1983;8:135.

119. Braga M, Stella M, Zerbi A, et al. Giant villous adenoma of the duodenum. Br J Surg 1986;73:924.

120. Paraf F, Naveau S, Zourabichvili O, et al. Endoscopic laser

therapy for duodenal villous adenoma. Dig Dis Sci 1989;34:1466.

121. Binmoeller K, Boaventura S, Ramsperger K, Soehendra N. Endoscopic snare excision of benign adenomas of the papilla of Vater. Gastrointest Endosc 1993;39:127.

122. Gilbert D, DiMarino A, Jensen D, et al. Status evaluation: hot biopsy forceps. Gastrointest Endosc 1992;38:753.

123. Tappero G, Gaia E, DeGiuli P, et al. Cold snare excision of small colorectal polyps. Gastrointest Endosc 1992;38:310.

124. Woods A, Sanowski R, Wadas D, Manne R, Friess S. Eradication of diminutive polyps: a prospective evaluation of bipolar coagulation versus conventional biopsy removal. Gastrointest Endosc 1989;35:536.

125. Lanspa S, Smyrk T, Lynch H, Jenkins J. The flat adenoma: significance and management. Gastrointest Endosc Clin North Am 1993;3(4):649.

126. Muto T, Kamaiya J, Zawada T, et al. Small "flat adenomas" of the large bowel with special reference to its clinicopathologic features. Dis Colon Rectum 1985;28:847.

127. Wolber R, Owen D. Flat adenomas of the colon. Hum Pathol 1991;22:70.

128. Lanspa S, Rouse J, Smyrk T, et al. Epidemiologic characteristics of the flat adenomas of Muto: a prospective study. Dis Colon Rectum. 1992;35:543.

129. Matsumoto T, Iida M, Kuano Y, et al. Minute non-polypoid adenoma of the colon detected by colonoscopy: correlation between endoscopic and histologic findings. Gastrointest Endosc 1992;38:645.

130. Kuramota S, Ihara O, Sakai S, et al. Depressed adenoma in the large intestine: endoscopic features. Dis Colon Rectum 1990;33:108.

131. Karita M, Tada M, Okita K, Kodama T. Endoscopic therapy for early colon cancer: the strip biopsy resection technique. Gastrointest Endosc 1991;37:128.

132. Haggitt R, Glotzbach R, Soffer E, Wruble L. Prognostic factors in colorectal carcinomas arising in adenomas: implications for lesions removed by endoscopic polypectomy. Gastroenterology 1985;89:328.

133. Coverlizza S, Rise M, Ferrari, A, et al. Colorectal cancers containing invasive carcinoma: pathologic assessment of lymph node metastatic potential. Cancer 1989;64:1937.

134. Cranley J. Proper management of the patient with a malignant colorectal polyp. Gastrointest Endosc Clin North Am 1993;3(4):661.

135. Russell J, Chu D, Russell M, et al. When is polypectomy sufficient treatment for colorectal cancer in a polyp? Am J Surg 1990;160:665.

136. Wilcox G, Beck J. Early invasive cancer in adenomatous colonic polyps ("malignant polyps"): evaluation of the therapeutic options by decision analysis. Gastroenterology 1987;92:1159.

137. Greenburg A, Saik R, Coyle J, et al. Mortality and gastrointestinal surgery in the elderly. Arch Surg 1981;116:788.

138. Said S, Huber P, Pichlmaier. Technique and clinical results of endorectal surgery. Surgery 1993;113:65.

139. Grahm R, Garnsey L, Jessup J. Local excision of rectal carcinoma. Am J Surg 1990;160:306.

140. Delile P, Marche C, Edelman G. Les tumors villeuses du colon et du rectum: problemes diagnostiques et therapeutiques. Ann Chir 1977;31:829.

141. Nivatvongs S, Snover D, Fang D. Piecemeal snare excision of large sessile colon and rectal polyps: is it adequate? Gastrointest Endosc 1984;30:18.

142. Bedogni G, Bertoni G, Ricci E, et al. Colonic excision of large and giant colorectal polyps. Dis Colon Rectum 1986;29:831.

143. Walsh R, Ackroyd F, Shellito P. Endoscopic resection of large sessile colorectal polyps. Gastrointest Endosc 1992;38:303.

144. Brunetaud J, Mosquet L, Houcke M, et al. Villus adenoma of the rectum: results of endoscopic treatment with argon and Nd:YAG lasers. Gastroenterology 1985;89:832.

145. Brunetaud J, Maunoury V, Cochelard D, et al. Endoscopic laser treatment for rectosigmoid villous adenoma: factors affecting the results. Gastroenterology 1989;97:272.

146. Mathus Vliegen E, Tytgat G. The potential and limitations of laser photoablation of colorectal adenomas. Gastrointest Endosc 1991;37:9.

147. Low D, Kozarek R. Snare cautery debridement prior to Nd:YAG photoablation improves treatment efficacy of broad-based adenomas of the colorectum. Gastrointest Endosc 1989;35:288.

148. Mellow M. Endoscopic therapy of colorectal neoplasms. Gastrointest Endosc Clinics North Am 1993;3(4):737.

149. Eckhauser M. Laser therapy of gastrointestinal tumors. World J Surg 1992;16:1054.

150. Mathus-Vliegen E, Tytgat G. Laser ablation and palliation in colorectal malignancy: results of a multicenter inquiry. Gastrointest Endosc 1986;32:393.

151. Chia Y, Ngoi S, Goh P. Endoscopic Nd:YAG laser in the palliative treatment of advanced low rectal carcinoma in Singapore. Dis Colon Rectum 1991;34:1093.

152. Dittrich K, Armbruster Hoffer F, Tuchmann A, Dinsti K. Nd:YAG laser treatment of colorectal malignancies: an experience of 4 ½ years. Lasers Surg Med 1992;12:199.

153. Mellow M. Endoscopic laser therapy as an alternative to palliative surgery for adenocarcinoma of the rectum—comparison of costs and complications. Gastrointest Endosc 1989;35:283.

154. Eckhauser M, Imbembo A, Mansour E. The role of pre-resectional laser recanalization for obstructing carcinomas of the colon and rectum. Surgery 1989;106:710.

155. Brunetaud J, Maunoury V, Cochelard D, et al. Laser palliation for rectosigmoid cancers. Int J Colorect Dis 1989;4:6.

156. Escourrou J, Delvaux M, deBellison, et al. Laser for curative treatment of rectal cancer: indications and follow-up (abstract). Gastrointest Endosc 1988;34:195.

Textbook of Gastroenterology, second edition, edited by Tadataka Yamada. JB Lippincott Company, Philadelphia © 1995.

CHAPTER 140

Exploratory Laparotomy

Mika Sinanan

Exploratory laparotomy is defined as a surgical procedure carried out through an abdominal incision for the diagnosis of intraabdominal pathology. Exploration of the abdomen also forms a part of most *therapeutic* abdominal surgical procedures where the primary objective is surgical correction of a previously defined problem. Although an accurate estimate of the number of exploratory laparotomies performed is difficult to achieve, the National Hospital Discharge Survey of 1987 listed 103,000 laparotomies and more than 1.3 million other common abdominal procedures where laparotomy was carried out in the course of a specific therapeutic intervention.[1] The clear benefits of abdominal surgery include accurately identifying and removing malignant or complicated benign neoplasms, repairing obstructed or perforated viscera, draining infection, stopping bleeding, and beneficially altering physiological function. What is less evident are the acute and long-term adverse consequences of the surgical wound, stress response, and coincident anesthetic. This chapter provides a basis for comparing the risks and benefits of exploratory laparotomy with other diagnostic procedures, a comparison that is essential in formulating strategy for the management of patients with complex abdominal pathology.

Laparotomy is often considered among the most costly, invasive, and morbid of diagnostic techniques available. However, although serious adverse consequences can occur, they are relatively rare and can often be anticipated and avoided. Cholecystectomy is an example of a laparotomy procedure performed across a wide range of patient risk categories. The negligible mortality and low, less than 5% surgical mor-

bidity of cholecystectomy in several recent reviews indicate the relative safety with which laparotomy can be performed.[2-4] In weighing the value of exploratory laparotomy as a diagnostic procedure, the accuracy and cost-efficiency of diagnosis, corollary therapeutic benefit, and an accurate estimate of risk in the individual patient must all be assessed.

THEORETICAL CONSIDERATIONS

Surgical Stress Response

Surgical trauma during laparotomy is *always* associated with an acute injury response. Elective procedures of short duration may have minimal consequences. However, laparotomy for acute, severe disease such as resection of a complex abdominal cancer or a perforated viscus often requires prolonged anesthesia with significant tissue injury and profound metabolic derangement. Visceral exposure during surgery disrupts fluid, electrolyte, and thermal homeostasis. Evaporative, urinary, and respiratory fluid losses as well as tissue edema and blood loss contribute to an ongoing fluid requirement.[5,6] Electrolyte losses from the circulation must also be replaced. The anesthesiologist anticipates and corrects these deficiencies as completely as possible in addition to providing analgesia, amnesia, and somatic muscle relaxation essential to the conduct of the operation. Recognition of the magnitude of the surgical injury and improvements in both intraoperative and postoperative resuscitation of patients is largely responsible for the improving results of surgical therapy over the past 20 years.

Stages of Recovery

Recovery after laparotomy occurs in stages similar to recovery from other types of traumatic injury.[7] As might be expected, the duration and magnitude of each stage is determined by the general health of the patient, the severity of the illness, and the conduct of the operation. Progression through all stages may be accelerated in a healthy patient with a minimal procedure. Alternatively, progression to recovery can be halted by a complication, for example infection, that requires further treatment. Manifestations of the process also differ by age and gender,[8] but the sequence of hormonal and metabolic changes is remarkably consistent even in the elderly.[9,10] The perioperative energy metabolism that fuels this process is quite distinct from the ketosis and hypometabolism that develop from starvation alone.[11]

The first stage is one of relative hypovolemia that develops immediately after surgery. It is associated with pain from the surgical site together with tissue hypoxia and acidosis which persist until the circulating volume is reestablished, generally within 24 hours of the procedure. An abrupt increase in ACTH, growth hormone, and antidiuretic hormone levels is followed by increases in catecholamines, cortisol, and glucagon[12] due to sympathetic and adrenal activation. Both neural[13] and cytokine factors[14] including IL-1β and IL-6[15] have been implicated in this process. Oxygen consumption is increased along with circulating levels of glucose, free fatty acids, and glycerol but alanine, glutamine, and both the insulin level and peripheral tissue insulin sensitivity are depressed.[8,11,16]

The next stage, one of tissue catabolism, is associated with an increase in the metabolic rate and both oxygen and glucose consumption, together with a negative nitrogen balance.[6] Structural protein and fat stores are consumed in proportion to the severity of the injury, to patient nutritional condition, and to the requirements of the healing wound. Significant lean body mass may be lost during this stage which ends with an increase in physical activity and resumption of eating. The catabolic phase usually lasts from 1 to 5 days. Early supplemental nutrition may be required in patients with severe preoperative malnutrition after a difficult procedure or when complications have occurred, but most patients can tolerate up to a week without food.[17]

The third, anabolic stage is marked by replenishment of protein and fat stores due to improved nutrition, continued elevation of growth hormone, and a rise in insulin levels.[12] Weight, physical activity, strength, and endurance rise toward normal, preoperative levels. Wound strength increases and postoperative fatigue resolves.[18,19] Although all other metabolic factors may be back to normal within several months, wound healing and maximal tensile strength in the incision are generally not achieved for 6 to 9 months.[20]

The risk of complications or death after laparotomy depends on more than just intraoperative, technical factors in the conduct of the operation. Surgical complications often occur when basic physiological systems, perhaps already chronically impaired, become further compromised by the disease or the surgical procedure required for treatment. This cumulative injury may prevent spontaneous recovery. Thus a patient being considered for surgery must have sufficient physiological reserve to withstand and recover from the procedure and heal. Factors that impact on an individual's physiological reserve include extremes of age, weight, or nutrition, compromise of one or more major organ systems: cardiac, pulmonary, renal, hepatic, immune, and endocrine (Table 140-1). Careful assessment of these factors as well as a knowledge of the physiological consequences of laparotomy thus become important in anticipating the effects of surgery and estimating risk in the individual patient.[21]

Organ System Effects of Laparotomy

Anesthesia and the surgical procedure both have physiological effects that are, of necessity, difficult to separate. However, the minimal cardiopulmonary effects of a general anesthetic during minor soft-tissue surgery procedures and surgery on an extremity suggest that surgical trauma during thoracic or abdominal procedures is a major cause of dysfunction in these systems.[22]

Heart

Laparotomy increases myocardial oxygen demand but also induces physiological changes that potentially decrease oxygen supply to the heart. The elevated catecholamines associated with surgical stress cause a relative tachycardia and an increase in the systemic vascular resistance.[23] Associated hypertension, anemia, sympathomimetic drugs, and possible cessation of beta blocking drugs contribute to an increase in oxygen demand.[24] In contrast, hypoxia, episodic hypotension, anemia, and shifts in cardiac filling pressure all tend to decrease cardiac output and myocardial oxygen supply. The sum of these events, together with surgically-induced hypercoagulability and coronary artery spasm, increases the risk of myocardial injury and arrhythmias for a period of up to 1 week after surgery.[25] Although preexisting cardiac disease is a major determinant of postoperative complications,[26] laparotomy alone, particularly in the upper abdomen, remains an independent risk factor associated with a 15 to 25 fold increase in cardiac morbidity.[27]

TABLE 140-1
Factors Influencing Physiologic Reserve

Extremes of age
Severe malnutrition or obesity
Major organ failure
    Pulmonary
    Cardiac
    Hepatic
    Renal
    Multisystem (i.e., posttrauma, thermal injury)
    Hematologic (i.e., postchemotherapy)
Alcohol or drug dependency
Endocrinopathy
    Corticosteroid therapy
    Adrenal insufficiency
    Diabetes mellitus
    Hyperthyroidism or hypothyroidism

Lung and Airway

General inhalational anesthesia and laparotomy together are associated with profound effects on lung function. Increased venous admixture and the combined effects of gas trapping, small airway closure, and alveolar collapse are *intraoperative* events that lead to relative hypoxemia, a 15 to 25% decrease in functional residual capacity (FRC), and a decline in lung compliance that may reach 50%.[28] Adequate oxygenation is usually maintained by increasing the inspired oxygen concentration. In the postoperative period, hypoxemia persists, but for different reasons. Early postoperative hypoxemia has been attributed to a combination of residual anesthetic drug effects, surfactant damage, suppressed ventilatory drive from intraoperative hyperventilation, and both residual shunt and ventilation-perfusion mismatch that continue for several hours after recovery from an anesthetic.[22,28] Tissue oxygen demands increase after abdominal surgery but incisional pain, the increased work of breathing, and other, previously mentioned factors may prevent adequate compensation, thus potentiating the relative hypoxemia.[29] Although many of these effects are transient, lung function after laparotomy may be disrupted long into the postoperative period especially in those with chronic lung disease or an upper abdominal incision.[30]

The patient recovering from laparotomy has a pattern of shallow, monotonous breathing that is only partially related to pain from the procedure. Postoperative spirometry shows that FRC is the most profoundly affected lung volume. FRC is decreased by up to 30% on postoperative day 1 and takes up to 5 days to return to normal.[22,31] Acute neuromuscular compromise of the abdominal wall and diaphragm, together with surfactant losses from endotracheal intubation and an abnormal breathing pattern, reduce pulmonary compliance.[32–34] Regionally, small airway closing capacity exceeds FRC so that alveolar collapse and atelectasis develop, causing shunt and arterial hypoxemia.[22,29] In addition, thickened secretions from hypovolemia, a poor cough, and compromised mucociliary clearance, contribute to bacterial stasis that may serve as a nidus for infection in the airway.[35]

Kidney

Both inhalational and narcotic anesthetics increase the filtration fraction of the kidney by decreasing glomerular filtration and renal plasma flow.[36] Increased intraabdominal pressure from a tight abdominal closure and hypovolemia have both been shown to reduce postoperative renal perfusion.[37] Creatinine clearance in the perioperative period is therefore reduced and, even in patients with previously normal kidney function, may progress to overt renal failure in up to 0.1% of laparotomy patients.[38]

Liver

The combination of anesthetic drug effects,[39] increased sympathetic tone, and splanchnic vasoconstriction from hypovolemia during laparotomy also reduces hepatic blood flow.[40] Although the normal liver is quite tolerant of ischemia, a subsequent reperfusion injury may profoundly affect hepatic metabolism.[41–45] For example, impaired hepatic mixed func-

tion oxidases can generate toxic drug metabolites that may worsen the liver injury or cause an exaggerated or unexpected response to other medications.[40,46] Hepatic injury after laparotomy rarely achieves clinical significance in the healthy patient. However, in patients with acute hepatitis, cirrhosis, or extensive cancer replacement of the hepatic parenchyma, hepatic injury after laparotomy may be lethal.

Coagulation

Abdominal surgery activates the coagulation system regionally in operated tissues and pathologically in the deep venous system of some patients. Immobility and peripheral vasodilation from the anesthetic create static venous pools of blood that, together with endothelial damage from circulating vasoactive amines, may result in clot formation. Long duration of anesthesia, patient age over 40, and the presence of cancer increase the risk of peripheral deep venous thrombosis (DVT) and pulmonary embolism (PE) after laparotomy.[47,48] Rarely, a diffuse coagulopathy develops in the perioperative period due to a drug or transfusion reaction. Coagulopathy can also develop after massive blood loss, hypothermia, and dilution of clotting factors during surgery.[49,50]

Immune System

After laparotomy, white blood cells and elements of the immune system are responsible for clearance of particulate matter and bacteria from both wound and peritoneum. This process is essential for healing and occurs by neutrophil phagocytosis, drainage through diaphragmatic lymphatics, fibrin sequestration, and inactivation of pathogens by the immune system.[51] In the postoperative period, impairment of cellular[52–54] and humoral[55,56] immunity as well as decreased complement, fibronectin, and white cell phagocytosis[57] have all been shown to occur and last for up to 4 weeks, depending on the severity of the surgical trauma. Some authors have suggested that postoperative attenuation of neutrophil and immune function may be a modulated, physiological response,[58] influenced in part by growth factors from the healing wound[59] or other circulating factors.[57] A modulated response might protect the host against an excessive inflammatory response. Other authors have shown that perioperative immunosuppression, especially after blood product transfusions,[60] is associated with an increase in septic complications,[61,62] cancer recurrence after curative resection,[63–65] and death.[66,67]

Endocrine System

With the rare exception of patients who have glandular tissue ablated at surgery (i.e., total pancreatectomy resulting in diabetes mellitus), postoperative endocrinopathy is usually a result of preexisting defects in pancreatic endocrine, thyroid, or adrenal function. Safe recovery from laparotomy requires intact thyroid and adrenal function. Both acute, severe hyperthyroidism (i.e., thyroid storm) or a deficiency of thyroid or adrenal cortical hormones can cause profound metabolic abnormalities and cardiovascular collapse. These effects emphasize the critical role that endocrine organs play in the normal surgical stress response.[68,69]

Intestinal Motility

Postoperative ileus is another physiological consequence of laparotomy. Anesthesia and the surgical incision both decrease spontaneous intestinal electrical activity and motility. Activation of CNS reflex pathways and the sympathetic system are considered responsible for ileus rather than the length of anesthesia or handling of the bowel during surgery.[70] The entire intestinal system must function for a patient to tolerate nutrition other than an elemental, totally absorbed diet. In most patients, motility returns quickly in the small bowel, after 1 to 2 days in the stomach, and 1 or 2 days later in the colon[71] but the usual clinical parameters of flatus and passage of stool correlate poorly with this resumption of motility.[72] Rarely, ileus persists as a pathological condition for weeks or months after laparotomy. This is a type of intestinal pseudo-obstruction which usually improves but may take weeks or months to resolve.

TECHNICAL APPLICATION

Based on the preceding discussion, preoperative clinical assessment should suggest those complications for which a given patient is at increased risk.[21] The patient, family, and referring physician can then be fully informed regarding the risks of surgery. Preoperative measures can also be taken to improve the safety of the procedure, if patient status and the surgical condition permit. At a minimum, every patient considered for laparotomy should be evaluated for anesthetic, intubation, and cardiopulmonary risk. Identification of specific risks also encourages closer postoperative monitoring for expected problems.

Preoperative Assessment and Preparation

Age, prior general anesthetics, drug reactions or allergies, the nature and acuity of the surgical illness, and the general health of the patient are all considered in the anesthetic assessment. Neck extension, ease of intubation, status of the teeth, and

positioning for surgery are assessed in planning airway management. Clearly, cardiac and pulmonary disorders, which are considered in separate sections later in this chapter, are also of major importance in assigning anesthetic risk.[73] With this information, each patient is graded according to the Dripps ASA Physical Status Scale (Table 140-2),[74] which indicates prospectively the perioperative mortality risk of anesthesia and guides both anesthetic management and postoperative monitoring. Recently, other clinical assessments such as the APACHE II score[75] combining age, chronic health parameters, and a number of acute physiological variables have provided a better correlation with morbidity and mortality. Unfortunately, application of such scoring systems to the individual patient is still imprecise.[76-78]

For patients suspected of significant cardiac disease, Goldman has described and prospectively validated a *cardiac risk index* that is widely employed.[23] The cardiac risk index is calculated by adding points from several categories:

- age older than 70 years
- myocardial infarction (MI) within 6 months
- clinical evidence for congestive failure (e.g., S_3 or jugular distention)
- aortic stenosis
- significant arrhythmias as detected by electrocardiogram
- poor general medical condition
- major vascular, thoracic, or abdominal procedure
- emergency procedures.

These factors generate a score that correlates with cardiac morbidity and overall mortality after surgery.[79] Patients who achieve a high score (class III or IV) on the cardiac risk index should wait at least 6 months after their last MI before having elective surgery. Prior to surgery, congestive failure, angina, arrhythmias, hypertension, and significant aortic stenosis should be evaluated and treated, because each of of these conditions is an independent predictor for adverse outcome by multivariate analysis.[26]

Chronic obstructive, restrictive, and vascular diseases (i.e., pulmonary hypertension) of the lung are associated with the complications of atelectasis, lung infections, and hypoxemia after surgery.[27,32,34,80] A long history of smoking or prior breathing problems are the most common indications for

---

TABLE 140-2
Anesthesia Physical Status Scale

CLASS	DESCRIPTION	PERIOPERATIVE MORTALITY (%)*
I	Normal, healthy person	0.08
II	Mild systemic disease	0.27
III	Severe systemic disease, not incapacitating	1.8
IV	Incapacitating disease that is life-threatening	7.8
V	Moribund patient, not expected to live 24 h regardless of treatment	9.4
E	Emergency surgery	

* Perioperative (30-day) mortality due to complications of anesthesia in patients with chronic disease. This scale does not include mortality due to complications of surgical treatment.

Adapted from Derrington, M.C. and Smith, G. A review of studies of anaesthetic risk, morbidity and mortality. Br J Anaesth 1987; 59:817.

preoperative pulmonary evaluation. Patients with an abnormal breathing pattern during simple bedside maneuvers[35] or after mild exertion such as walking one flight of stairs also deserve evaluation.

Pulmonary function tests include spirometry and arterial blood gas (ABG) measurements that supplement but do not replace clinical evaluation of the patient. A forced expiratory volume at 1 second approaching the low, critical value of 1 L, a maximal breathing capacity under 50% of the normal, predicted value, and ABG showing significant arterial hypoxia ($PaO_2 \leq 50$ mm Hg) or hypercapnia ($PaCO_2 \geq 45$ mm Hg) are all predictive of postoperative pulmonary complications.[35,81] In the patient with chronic lung disease, measures to reduce perioperative morbidity include cessation of smoking, preferably for 3 weeks, inhaled bronchodilators, theophylline, antibiotics for chronic bronchitis, expectorants, and physiotherapy. Most interventions are continued into the postoperative period. After surgery, good pain control is essential to pulmonary recovery. Inspiratory breathing exercises, early ambulation, and careful fluid management also reduce the incidence of postoperative pulmonary failure.[33,34]

Preparation for surgery also includes consideration of special risks from bleeding, abnormal coagulation, malnutrition, or infection. Coagulation is tested and corrected.[82] Patients are asked to refrain from aspirin ingestion for 1 to 3 weeks and extra measures are taken for the patient on therapeutic anticoagulation. Immobile or elderly patients, those with cancer, a prior history of DVT, or PE constitute a high-risk group[47,83,84] that benefit from special measures such as perioperative low-dose heparin therapy and pneumatic leg compression.[48,85] In the nonemergent setting, a period of nutritional repletion in severely malnourished patients reduces complications and improves wound healing.[86-88] Any active infection that is incidental to the surgical disease (e.g., pneumonia, soft tissue, or urinary tract infections) should be appropriately treated to avoid secondary, surgical wound sepsis.[89] In elective patients for whom surgery may include entry into the intestine or biliary tract, infectious complications are also reduced by preoperative intravenous antibiotics[90-93] and a complete mechanical and antibiotic bowel preparation before colonic procedures.[94,95]

Acutely ill patients are approached somewhat differently. Surgery usually cannot be delayed for bowel preparation or treatment of chronic health conditions. Thus, every attempt should be made to correct intravascular volume, electrolyte, and clotting abnormalities prior to surgery. Adequate preparation for intraoperative monitoring and resuscitation includes, where necessary, available blood for transfusion. Antibiotics with appropriate enteric and anaerobic coverage are started before the incision in septic patients and in those cases where contamination of the surgical wound is anticipated.[96] Anesthetic preparation should be appropriate to the severity of the anticipated surgical injury.

Once the patient is in the operating room, great care is taken with surgical positioning, padding to avoid pressure injury, measures for keeping the patient warm, and skin preparation. Relevant preoperative x-ray films and other studies are reviewed and a set of specific goals developed for the operation. This helps ensure that all appropriate diagnostic steps, tissue samples, and procedures are completed to return the patient to health. It should be evident that even in the patient

who is otherwise healthy, thorough preoperative preparation is critical to achieving a good outcome.

Procedure

Although details of anesthetic management are beyond the scope of this chapter, anticipating the severity of postoperative pain may guide the selection of anesthetic. The type of incision is dictated by patient factors such as prior incisions, stomas, or wounds, as well as the indication for surgery. Transverse or oblique incisions often work well for regional access to discrete mass lesions or specific organ disease (e.g., cholecystolithiasis) while minimizing postoperative pain and pulmonary problems.[97] However, in the patient with unclear pathology or diffuse symptoms, a midline incision has the greatest versatility for complete abdominal exploration.

During exploratory laparotomy, all peritoneal and retroperitoneal organs are investigated. The surface of the liver, spleen, and gut from esophageal hiatus to proximal rectum are inspected. The caliber of the intestine along its length is noted and and palpated for evidence of lumenal masses in patients suspected of obstruction or tumor. Both kidneys are palpated as are the pancreas, gallbladder, retroperitoneal portions of the colon, aorta, pelvic viscera in the female, and urinary bladder. In a laparotomy for cancer, lymphadenopathy is sought in the gut mesentery and in the retroperitoneum. The common sites of peritoneal carcinomatosis along the diaphragm and in the pelvic cul-de-sac are scrutinized. Evidence of infection, inflammation, injection, ischemia, firm or abnormally hard tissues, unusual nodules or plaques, and pathological tissue adherence are all noted. Normal peritoneal fluid is straw-colored and clear, with just enough volume to lubricate peritoneal surfaces. When the peritoneal fluid is excessive or has an odor or unusual character, an exudative process, liver disease, chyle leak, or a pancreatic juice leak should be sought. Biopsies of abnormal tissues and aspirates of peritoneal fluid are sent for histology and, where necessary, cytology, bacterial culture, or chemical analysis, taking care to preserve the samples appropriately. A systematic approach to exploration of the peritoneum is important to attain the full value of the procedure.

Following the diagnostic phase, therapeutic maneuvers should be carried out to achieve the goals set out preoperatively, as modified by the exploratory findings. Treatment may include control of bleeding, repair or bypass of obstruction, resection of cancer, ischemic or inflammatory tissues, repair of dysmotility or other dysfunctional tissue or organs, and drainage of pus. In all patients, care must be taken to maintain normal temperature and hemostasis, and to protect the tissues from drying or contamination. Foreign body material and excessive tension or pressure on tissues are avoided by following the surgical principles of Halsted.[98] Preserving tissue integrity and blood supply are among the most important technical factors in reducing the incidence of anastomotic dehiscence, wound breakdown, fistulas, and hernia formation.

Recovery

Following recovery from anesthesia, breathing exercises and mobilization to sitting and walking are instituted as soon as possible. This minimizes the pulmonary problems, skin pressure sores, and the DVT risk of prolonged bed rest. Good pain control is essential for the patient to move about and cough. Pain regimens in the past have relied on intermittent dosing of narcotics by the nursing staff but more recent innovations in analgesia with the epidural catheter,[99] transcutaneous narcotic patches,[100] and patient-controlled anesthesia (PCA)[101,102] have markedly improved the *potential* efficacy of pain management. Prospective studies show that optimal pain control reduces postoperative stress and improves outcome.[103] Unfortunately, insufficient treatment due to ignorance, an unreasonable fear of respiratory depression, or fear of dependency, still occurs in up to 30 to 60% of patients.[104]

During the recovery period, the patient is followed by serial examinations for resumption of normal gut function and wound healing, as well as anticipated postoperative complications. In particular, lung function and signs of leg swelling or calf tenderness are assessed daily until the patient is ambulating and breathing normally. Intravenous fluids are continued until an oral diet is resumed. Diuresis of excess fluid usually occurs about the second or third day unless complications intervene. A number of clinical findings including failure to diurese, unexplained tachycardia, prolonged ileus, glucose intolerance, fever, wound erythemia or discharge, and excessive abdominal pain or tenderness, may signal development of a septic complication and must be investigated. Complications presenting during the first 2 to 3 days include those due to anesthesia, cardiopulmonary dysfunction, and surgical bleeding. Anastomotic breakdown, wound complications, and sepsis usually become evident later.

INDICATIONS

The advantages of laparotomy are definitive diagnosis by direct inspection, biopsy, and exclusion of alternative diagnoses suggested by prior diagnostic studies and the potential for immediate surgical treatment.

In the *living* patient, careful and thorough operative exploration of the abdomen combined with histopathologic study of tissue biopsies is the gold standard to which all other, less direct diagnostic techniques for abdominal pathology, including laparoscopy, must be compared. Laparotomy is indicated for diagnosis when a calculation has been made that the benefits of surgical intervention in a given patient outweigh the potential risks, complications, and costs of the procedure, when no other technique provides equal safety and accuracy of diagnosis, and when there is a reasonable likelihood that effective surgical treatment for the condition is possible. The experienced surgeon may detect subtle changes in tissue texture or appearance at laparotomy, prompting further directed investigation that may reveal obscure neoplastic, ischemic, or inflammatory processes long before other diagnostic techniques and at a time when curative treatment is still potentially feasible. In other situations, marked or widespread pathologic tissue changes might be easily detectable by other means but laparotomy often offers the best opportunity for definitive treatment if the process is surgically correctable. The only exception may be in those patients with endoscopically treatable, mucosal lesions of the gastrointestinal tract. Several studies emphasize the diagnostic value of laparotomy where there is a significant risk of missed or in-

correct diagnoses of abdominal pathology which can result in increased mortality.[105,106] In contrast, blind abdominal exploration in the septic, gravely ill ICU patient without some evidence for an abdominal process has not been shown to influence survival.[107]

Patients presenting with an acute abdomen are among those who benefit most from concomitant surgical treatment of their condition. Laparotomy is often the first and only diagnostic procedure for these patients other than physical examination. In some cases, determining the cause of the illness and carrying out immediate treatment may provide the only chance for survival.[108] Medical advances including improvements in diagnostic laparoscopy,[109–111] radiologic imaging,[112,113] and interventional treatment techniques[114,115] have reduced the necessity for laparotomy, however an appropriately directed abdominal exploration remains the most reliable method for diagnosing and treating obscure or acute, catastrophic intraabdominal illness.

The range of specific diagnoses and procedures carried out in or through the peritoneal space numbers in the hundreds. However surgical pathology of the abdomen can be organized into several common categories (Table 140-3).

CONTRAINDICATIONS AND RISKS

The contraindications to laparotomy are, for the most part, relative rather than absolute. They primarily reflect the inherent risks of anesthesia, the surgical stress response, and the surgical wound. It is rare that the underlying health of a patient is so severely compromised or the risks of the procedure so prohibitive that he or she is absolutely not a candidate for laparotomy. Severe pulmonary compromise may lead to postoperative ventilator dependency and a high cardiac risk index predicts a potentially difficult postoperative course. Good operative technique minimizes surgical bleeding, but if transfusion of blood products is necessary, the risks of immune suppression[116] and viral infection (1 in 3300 per unit for hepatitis C and about 1 in 200,000 or less per unit for hepatitis B and human immunodeficiency virus)[117] should not preclude surgical therapy. Drug reaction, anesthetic, infection, wound, and bowel obstructive complications occur but again, anticipation and early aggressive treatment of these problems should minimize their impact.

If the indication for laparotomy is compelling and no good alternative treatment exists, the combination of preoperative resuscitation, modern anesthesia, expedient surgery, and postoperative intensive care can bring most patients through surgery. On the other hand, improvements in medical, endoscopic, laparoscopic, and interventional radiologic treatment now offer many alternatives that can achieve the same goals and may obviate the necessity for laparotomy, at least until the patient status has improved.

One important contraindication to laparotomy is chronic abdominal pain. Patients presenting with chronic pain should be clinically evaluated and cautiously investigated by noninvasive techniques, as directed by the clinical findings. Early psychosocial evaluation is critical. In appropriate patients, pathological processes such as those detailed in Table 140-3 should be sought and, if present, may become an indication for laparotomy. However, specific diagnoses leading to

TABLE 140-3
Indications for Laparotomy

INDICATION	OBJECTIVES OF SURGICAL MANAGEMENT
Acute abdomen	Diagnosis and treatment
Visceral abdominal trauma	Diagnosis and treatment
Acute hemorrhage	Control intraabdominal hemorrhage
	Define and control gastrointestinal source
Infection	Diagnosis
	Drainage or debridement
Inflammation	Diagnosis
	Ulcer disease: vagotomy and gastric drainage, repair perforation
	Cholecystitis/biliary colic: cholecystectomy
	Inflammatory bowel disease: resection or bypass
	Intestinal ischemia: revascularization, resection
Intestinal obstruction	Mechanical: repair
	Dysmotility syndrome: diagnosis, intestinal resection
Neoplasm	Diagnosis, staging
	Palliative bypass
	Resection

chronic pain are usually suggested by the initial clinical evaluation rather than exploratory radiographic studies.[118] Laparotomy or laparoscopy performed for the *sole indication* of chronic abdominal pain without preoperative identification of any specific, treatable lesion, defines unexpected pathology in less than 50% of cases and changes management in less than 40%.[119,120] In particular, the evidence is equivocal that peritoneal adhesions, one of the most common diagnoses postulated in these patients, cause abdominal pain.[121] Even when adhesions are present, symptoms rarely improve in the long term after adhesiolysis.[122,123]

Cardiopulmonary Complications

The cardiac complications of laparotomy including MI, ventricular arrhythmias, congestive failure, and death occur in 5.2% of unselected patients after noncardiac surgery.[124] Patients with a low or moderate cardiac risk index (Goldman class I and II, discussed previously) have a cardiac event risk of less than 5%. Those with no prior history of MI have an infarction rate of 0.1% to 0.65% and a mortality with infarction of 30% to 60%. In patients with a higher cardiac risk index (Goldman class III and IV), up to 50% will suffer postoperative cardiac complications. Perioperative reinfarction occurs in 4.3% of patients with a prior history of MI, with a mortality of 30% to 50%.[125] Once the decision has been made to take a high-risk cardiac patient to surgery, intensive monitoring and steps to minimize surgical stress, acute volume or blood pressure shifts, anemia, tachycardia, hypoxemia, and pain are critical in sustaining cardiac function through to recovery.

Atelectasis, hypoxemia, or pneumonia occur in over 20% of all patients undergoing abdominal surgery[34] and in up to 76% of those undergoing upper abdominal surgery.[33] Although respiratory dysfunction is common and often prolongs recovery, it is rarely lethal. The pulmonary consequences of abdominal surgery (see Theoretical Considerations) and the

preoperative assessment of patients with pulmonary disease (see Technical Application) have previously been discussed. Vigorous breathing exercises,[34] correction of preoperative protein depletion,[80] and avoidance of the upper midline incision[30,126] are the principal means of circumventing these complications in patients with otherwise normal lung function.

Complications of Anesthesia and Analgesia

Minor morbidity after anesthesia includes nausea, sore throat, chipped teeth, muscle pains, urinary retention, disorientation, and headache. One or more of these problems occurs in 10% of patients and for the most part, resolve rapidly. Major anesthetic morbidity including MI, aspiration, loss of airway, and pulmonary failure occurs in less than 0.5% of patients.[74] Nerve palsy, malignant hyperthermia, or idiosyncratic drug reactions such as an acute drug allergy or postanesthesia hepatitis are exceedingly rare but among the more troublesome sequelae of anesthesia. Many of the major complications attributed to general anesthesia are cardiopulmonary in nature or due to progression of preexisting, advanced systemic disease. In some patients, regional techniques of spinal[127] or epidural anesthesia[103] are effective alternatives. Unfortunately, these techniques also cause systemic effects, especially hypotension. Intraoperative deaths *directly* related to anesthesia occurred in only 0.01% of patients undergoing all types of surgery in a recent study, but abdominal surgery was an independent risk factor for higher mortality.[73]

Narcotic analgesics that are commonly administered for postoperative pain have a variety of side effects that may overlap the effects of anesthesia. One or more symptoms of nausea, vomiting, pruritus, urinary retention, respiratory depression, and a depressed state of consciousness occur in over 50% of patients during the recovery period.[128] Adequate medication for pain relief is essential. Measures to titrate the dose and interval, the route and type of narcotic, and to aggressively treat side effects with antiemetics are all important in improving patient comfort. New, effective nonnarcotic analgesics such as ketorolac are tolerated better and should find increased application in the future.

Complications of Wound Healing

Normal wound healing represents a complex sequence of cellular and biochemical events that have been the subject of several recent reviews.[129-132] Normal healing includes hemostasis and local release of multiple growth factors by platelets and macrophages. These factors stimulate processes of angiogenesis, epithelial cell growth, fibroblast procollagen deposition, and wound contraction in sequence. Disruption of the healing wound is the most common *technical* complication of laparotomy. Infection, dehiscence, hernia formation, and anastomotic breakdown are all forms of wound disruption. Although mechanical factors, contamination, desiccation, or ischemic injury to tissues account for most wound problems, it is important to recognize that other factors such as malnutrition,[88] hypoxia, diabetes, corticosteroid treatment, radiation or chemotherapy, and other causes of abnormal immune function[133-135] may also contribute to failure in the surgical wound.

Surgical wound infections occur in proportion to the degree of bacterial wound contamination from skin, hollow viscera, and breaks in sterile technique.[136] A long preoperative hospitalization, skin shaving, a prolonged procedure (>2 hours), use of open drains through the wound, abdominal surgery and variations in surgical technique, as well as other patient factors (≥3 surgical or medical diagnoses recorded on discharge) also increase the risk of wound infection.[135,137,138] Overall, a 4.1% incidence of surgical wound infection has been reported. This ranges from 1.5% to 3% in clean operations (e.g., hernia or breast surgery with no contamination or visceral penetration) to 13% to 40% in dirty or infected procedures (e.g., drainage of infection, entry into unprepared bowel).[137,138] The increased length of stay and associated morbidity from wound infections is striking. Improvements in patient preparation,[92] technical conduct of procedures,[89] and appropriate antibiotic prophylaxis for patients undergoing emergency abdominal,[139] elective biliary,[93,140] colonic,[91] or other abdominal procedures[90,141] have all been shown to minimize the long-term risk of wound infection, even as surgical intervention is extended to increasingly high-risk populations.

Wound dehiscence (i.e., disruption of fascia in the immediately postoperative period) occurs in 1% to 3% of patients after major abdominal surgery with an associated mortality that may reach 35%.[96,142] Incisional hernias develop in up to 8% of patients and most require repair with a second operation. Many of the factors predisposing to wound infection are also risk factors for dehiscence or incisional hernia but mechanical and technical factors predominate. These include wound infection, abdominal distention, pulmonary disease, type of wound closure, and closure under tension. Any wound closure where suture tension exceeds the capillary perfusion pressure (25–30 mm Hg) of the tissue is prone to disruption from ischemia. Surgical practices that minimize contamina-

tion and tension in the closure, as well as use of monofilament suture, a mass closure technique incorporating all fascial elements of the abdominal wall, or a paramedian incision[143] have effectively reduced acute wound disruption.[142] Similar pathophysiological considerations apply to bowel anastomoses where disruption or stricture of the healing wound may be an even more catastrophic event.[144]

Deep Venous Thrombosis and Pulmonary Embolism

DVT occurs more after abdominal surgery than is commonly recognized. Postoperative ^{125}I-fibrinogen leg scanning detects DVT in up to 40% of unselected laparotomy patients over age 40 when no prophylaxis is used. Many, if not most, of these patients are virtually asymptomatic.[47] Both patient factors and the type of procedure influence the risk of thrombotic and thromboembolic disease. Defining a low-risk category, less than 10% of healthy patients under age 40 having short (<30 minutes), elective procedures will develop calf vein thrombosis. When no DVT precautions are taken, the proximal deep veins become involved in less than 1% of this group. Up to 80% of older patients with cancer, a prior history of DVT or PE, and a long anesthesic period will suffer calf vein thrombosis and 10% to 20% of this group will develop proximal deep vein involvement if no prophylactic measures are employed.[48,83] Other independent risk factors for DVT include female sex, cigarette smoking, and varicose veins.[47,84] Although the risk of fatal PE is less than 0.01% in the low-risk group, the incidence of this feared complication rises to 1% to 5% in the latter, high-risk group.

All surgical patients but particularly those considered at increased risk should routinely be monitored for calf or leg pain and tenderness, asymmetric leg swelling, unexplained fever, and dyspnea. Duplex scanning of the venous system, ventilation-perfusion lung scan, or pulmonary angiography should be considered in patients with worrisome findings.[145,146] Fortunately, early ambulation and other prophylactic measures in high-risk patients can substantially reduce the risk of DVT and PE. Mechanical calf compression, IV low-molecular-weight dextran, and various other types of anticoagulation have all been proven effective at reducing the risk of DVT when started before surgery and continued until the patient is again ambulatory.[48] In one of the most commonly employed regimens, subcutaneous heparin (5000 U) is administered two or three times daily throughout the perioperative period. This reduces the incidence of DVT by a factor of four with minimal risk of wound hematoma or bleeding during surgery.[47,85] Often mechanical and anticoagulant regimens are combined for supplementary benefit in high-risk patients.

Bowel Obstruction

Abdominal surgery results in an inevitable injury to the peritoneal membrane. Overhealing of injured, ischemic peritoneum after surgery is the most common (80%) cause of abdominal adhesions in man.[147] Adhesive small bowel obstruction occurs after 3% of all laparotomies, 20% of these within 1 month of operation, and a further 10% within the first year. Unfortunately, the risk of obstruction is lifelong.[148,149] Procedures below the transverse mesocolon, for example, colonic, small bowel, or appendiceal resection, have a higher risk of small bowel obstruction.[150] Delicate handling of the tissues and avoidance of ischemic injury are important surgical techniques in avoiding subsequent obstruction. There is the possibility of specific pharmacotherapy for adhesions in the future.[149] Early postoperative small bowel obstruction resolves in over 60% of patients with nonoperative management.[151,152] However, patients with prolonged obstruction or obstruction complicated by gangrenous bowel require urgent correction of fluid and electrolyte abnormalities followed by immediate laparotomy to limit complications and mortality that otherwise approach 26% and 5% respectively.[153,154]

ASSESSMENT OF RESULTS

Measures of efficacy for any procedure include cost, morbidity, and the impact of the procedure on patient health. Although laparotomy is costly and has many physiological consequences and risks, skillful surgical exploration and treatment often provide a decisive advantage in comparison with other diagnostic modalities. Acute, severe abdominal processes; those where the differential diagnosis includes urgent, life-threatening abdominal disorders; and those where the diagnosis is incomplete and the patient's health is inexorably declining despite treatment, are all conditions where a clear resolution of diagnostic uncertainty by laparotomy or laparoscopy should strongly be considered. Advances in laparoscopic instrumentation and technique will increase the diagnostic accuracy and options for treatment by this technique in coming years.[109,155,156] Despite the economic pressures of the current era, safe and efficient return of the patient to health should always be the final objective.

Costs

Laparotomy is the most expensive diagnostic procedure for abdominal pathology. Time in the operating room (OR) costs $12 to $15/minute in U.S. currency, not including professional fees, anesthesia or items such as prostheses or disposable instruments. Hospital costs and fees for several types of procedures have been reviewed and are summarized in Table 140-4.[2,157–159] Extrapolating from these figures, a relatively straightforward laparotomy that takes 1.5 hours of operating

room time and requires 5 days of inpatient treatment should cost approximately $8700, estimating hospitalization, radiology, and laboratory costs of $5500, operating room costs of $1200, and anesthesia and surgeon professional fees of $2000. However, these figures must be considered in context. If an accurate diagnosis can be achieved and definitive therapy instituted, if duplicate studies and ineffective treatment can be avoided, and if earlier recovery to health and work[159] can be achieved, laparotomy becomes among the most cost effective of interventions.

Technical Skill

Surgery is a technical art and the results of surgical therapy depend on skillful technique. This is infrequently emphasized. Operator-dependent factors such as excessive tension on tissues, inadequate hemostasis, technically poor anastomosis, excessive manipulation or inadequate margins in cancer surgery, and prolonged operative time, increase the risks of cancer recurrence,[160] complications, and death.[161] Institutional and individual surgeon experience with a given procedure or complex diagnosis have an important influence on mortality.[162] Both the physician and patient seeking to know whether laparotomy is the best diagnostic and therapeutic intervention for a given problem must include the skill and experience of the surgeon as well as the ancillary resources of the institution as crucial factors in patient outcome.

CLINICAL IMPLICATIONS

In addition to a diagnostic role in acute abdominal disease, laparotomy has an established role in evaluating a number of neoplastic, infectious, and inflammatory conditions that affect the abdominal organs.

Cancer Staging

Staging laparotomy is an important diagnostic technique in a number of abdominal cancers, both before and after initiation of treatment. Despite improvements in radiographic imaging, subtle involvement of abdominal organs and retroperitoneal lymph nodes in patients with Hodgkin's lymphoma can often be determined only by direct inspection and resectional biopsy at laparotomy.[163] Similarly, a recent report suggests that laparotomy provides a more accurate measure

---

TABLE 140-4
Cost of Laparotomy

PROCEDURE	OPERATING ROOM COSTS ($)	HOSPITAL COST U.S. ($)*	LENGTH OF STAY (d)	PROFESSIONAL FEE U.S. ($)	REFERENCE
Adhesiolysis		10,960	11.4	904	157
Colectomy	3100	12,000	8		158
Cholecystectomy		4000–6000	4.9–6		2, 159

* Includes OR costs.

of resectability than preoperative radiographic studies in patients with nonductal pancreatic tumors.[164] In contrast, second-look laparotomy for recurrent colorectal carcinoma is useful only in radiographically selected patients.[165] Resection of recurrent colorectal cancer at laparotomy improves survival but only when preoperative radiographic studies indicate that the disease is both localized and resectable.[166,167] Laparotomy also appears useful in the staging of patients with bulky rectal cancer prior to radiation treatment,[168] for early diagnosis of primary small bowel tumors,[169] and in the follow-up of women after chemotherapy or radiotherapy for ovarian carcinoma.[170,171] These studies support continued application of diagnostic laparotomy in selected patients with abdominal malignancy.

Intraabdominal Sepsis

Sepsis from intraabdominal sources may be due to infectious or inflammatory disorders. Untreated intraabdominal infection is usually lethal[115] and uncontrolled inflammatory disease of the intestine usually leads to severe complications. The purpose of laparotomy in intraabdominal sepsis is accurate definition of the cause of sepsis and drainage or removal of the septic focus.[96] In the current era, radiologic diagnosis and percutaneous or endoscopic alternatives for treatment have been widely advocated and are often successful,[155] but in fragile patients who have no margin for error, in those with progressive sepsis despite nonoperative treatment, and most importantly, in those who present with massive, overwhelming sepsis from an abdominal source, the only reasonable intervention is laparotomy. Not all patients in this group will have surgically correctable disease, but failure to operate early in these patients will more often lead to mortality from untreated infection than from complications from unnecessary laparotomy.[172]

An extensive literature supports aggressive, early exploration of the abdomen when definitive drainage of intraabdominal infection cannot otherwise be achieved. Laparotomy, often repeated over several days, has been advocated in sick, ICU patients for control of massive intraabdominal infection or traumatic injury, and for surveillance of ischemic bowel and fragile anastomoses.[173–175] Early postoperative complications of intraabdominal infection, bleeding, or wound dehiscence are also best treated by immediate relaparotomy.[176] Exploration and debridement in septic patients with necrotizing pancreatitis usually offers the only chance for survival.[177] Laparotomy also improves survival in AIDS patients with selected abdominal diseases. Cytomegalovirus enterocolitis and perforation, complicated lymphoma of the small bowel, gastrointestinal Kaposi's sarcoma, and mycobacterial or other opportunistic infections of the peritoneum and retroperitoneum in these patients can all be effectively treated with laparotomy.[178–181] Perforated peptic ulcer disease seems to occur increasingly in older, sicker patients and urgent laparotomy is the only intervention that may reduce the 24% mortality associated with this disease.[182] Similarly, localizing peritonitis or deterioration while under medical therapy in patients with neutropenic enterocolitis,[183,184] pseudomembranous enterocolitis,[185,186] or toxic colitis from idiopathic inflammatory disease,[187] should lead to urgent laparotomy. The crucial,

lifesaving benefits of early diagnosis and immediate, definitive therapy in each of these septic conditions emphasize the role of exploratory laparotomy for advanced abdominal disease.

The reader is directed to Chapter 34, Approach to the Patient With Abdominal Pain; Chapter 36, Approach to the Patient With Acute Abdomen; and Chapter 100, Abdominal Cavity: Anatomy, Structural Anomalies, and Hernias.

REFERENCES

1. Graves EJ. Detailed diagnosis and procedures, National Hospital Discharge Survey, 1989. National Center for Health Statistics. Vital Health Stat 1991;13:108.
2. Gilliland TM, Traverso LW. Modern standards for comparison of cholecystectomy with alternative treatments for symptomatic cholelithiasis with emphasis on long term relief of symptoms. Surg Gynecol Obstet 1990;170:39.
3. Herzog U, Messmer P, Tondelli P. Surgical treatment for cholelithiasis. Surg Gynecol Obstet 1992;175:238.
4. Clavien PA, Sanabria JR, Mentha G, et al. Recent results of elective open cholecystectomy in North American and European centers. Ann Surg 1992;216:618.
5. Roberts JP, Roberts JD, Skinner C, et al. Extracellular fluid deficit following operation and its correction with Ringer's Lactate. Ann Surg 1985;202:1.
6. Hill GL, Douglas RG, Schroeder D. Metabolic basis for the management of patients undergoing major surgery. World J Surg 1993;17:146.
7. Cuthbertson D, Tilstone WJ. Metabolism during the post-injury period. Adv Clin Chem 1969;12:1.
8. Hakanson E, Rutberg H, Jorfeldt L, Wiklund L. Endocrine and metabolic responses after standardized moderate surgical trauma: influence of age and sex. Clin Physiol 1984;4:461.
9. Watters JM, Redmond ML, Desai D, March RJ. Effects of age and body composition on the metabolic responses to elective colon resection. Ann Surg 1990;212:89.
10. Blichert-Toft M, Christensen V, Engquist A, et al. Influence of age on the endocrine-metabolic response to surgery. Ann Surg 1979;190:761.
11. Nordenstrom J, Sonnenfeld T, Arner P. Characterization of insulin resistance after surgery. Surgery 1989;105:28.
12. Alberti KGMM, Batstone GF, Foster KJ, Johnston DG. Relative role of various hormones in mediating the metabolic response to injury. JPEN J Parenter Enteral Nutr 1980;4:141.
13. Brandt MR, Fernandes A, Mordhorst R, et. al. Epidural analgesia improves postoperative nitrogen balance. Br Med J 1978;1:1106.
14. Naito Y, Tamai S, Shingu K, et al. Responses of plasma adrenocorticotropic hormone, cortisol, and cytokines during and after upper abdominal surgery. Anesthesiology 1992;77:426.
15. Baigrie RJ, Lamont PM, Kwiatkowski D, Dallman MJ, Morris PJ. Systemic cytokine response after major surgery. Br J Surg 1992;79:757.
16. Parry-Billings M, Baigrie RJ, Lamont PM, Morris PJ, Newsholme EA. Effects of major and minor surgery on plasma glutamine and cytokine levels. Arch Surg 1992;127:1237.
17. Dempsey DT, Mullen JL, Buzby GP. The link between nutritional status and clinical outcome: can nutritional intervention modify it? Am J Clin Nutr 1988;47:352.
18. Christensen T, Stage JG, Galbo H, Christensen NJ, Kehlet H. Fatigue and cardiac and endocrine metabolic response to exercise after abdominal surgery. Surgery 1989;105:46.
19. Christensen T, Kehlet H. Postoperative fatigue. World J Surg 1993;17:220.
20. Hunt TK. The physiology of wound healing. Ann Emerg Med 1988;17:1265.
21. Pettigrew RA, Hill GL. Indicators of surgical risk and clinical judgement. Br J Surg 1986;73:47.

22. Craig DB. Postoperative recovery of pulmonary function. Anesth Analg 1981;60:46.
23. Weitz HH, Goldman L. Noncardiac surgery in the patient with heart disease. Med Clin North Am 1987;71:413.
24. Mangano DT. Perioperative cardiac morbidity. Anesthesiology 1990;72:153.
25. Goldman L. Supraventricular tachyarrhythmias in hospitalized adults after surgery. Chest 1978;73:450.
26. McIntyre RW, Hart A. Perioperative ischemia and infarction: Noncardiac surgery. Anesth Clin North Am 1988;6:527.
27. Pedersen T, Eliasen K, Henriksen E. A prospective study of risk factors and cardiopulmonary complications associated with anaesthesia and surgery: risk indicators of cardiopulmonary morbidity. Acta Anesthesiol Scand 1990;34:144.
28. Marshall BE, Wyche MQJ. Hypoxemia during and after anesthesia. Anesthesiology 1972;37:178.
29. Siler JN, Rosenberg H, Mull TD, Kaplan JA, Bardin H, Marshall BE. Hypoxemia after upper abdominal surgery: comparison of venous admixture and ventilation/perfusion inequality components, using a digital computer. Ann Surg 1974;179:149.
30. Ali J, Khan TA. The comparative effects of muscle transection and median upper abdominal incisions on postoperative pulmonary function. Surg Gynecol Obstet 1979;148:863.
31. Meyers JR, Lembeck L, O'Kane H, Baue AE. Changes in functional residual capacity of the lung after operation. Arch Surg 1975;110:576.
32. Ali J, Weisel RD, Layug AB, Kripke BJ, Hechtman HB. Consequences of post-operative alterations in respiratory mechanics. Am J Surg 1974;128:376.
33. Roukema JA, Carol EJ, Prins JG. The prevention of pulmonary complications after upper abdominal surgery in patients with noncompromised pulmonary status. Arch Surg 1988;123:30.
34. Bartlett RH, Bazzaniga AB, Geraghty TR. Respiratory maneuvers to prevent postoperative pulmonary complications. JAMA 1973;224:1017.
35. Tisi GM. Preoperative identification and evaluation of the patient with lung disease. Med Clin North Am 1987;71:399.
36. Charlson ME, MacKenzie CR, Gold JP, Ales KL, Shires GT. Postoperative renal dysfunction can be predicted. Surg Gynecol Obstet 1989;169:303.
37. Patell C, Hall J, Dobb G. Impaired renal functioon due to raised intraabdominal pressure. Intensive Care Med 1990;16:328.
38. Wait RB, Kahng KU. Renal failure complicating obstructive jaundice. Am J Surg 1989;157:256.
39. Sear JW. Adverse effects of analgesics and intravenous anesthetic agents. Acta Anaesthesiol Belg 1988;39(Suppl 2):97.
40. Gholson CF, Provenza, Bacon BR. Hepatologic considerations in patients with parenchymal liver disease undergoing surgery. Am J Gastroenterol 1990;85:487.
41. Komatsu H, Koo A, Ghadishah E, et al. Neutrophil accumulation in ischemic reperfused rat liver: evidence for a role for superoxide free radicals. Am J Physiol 1992;262:G669.
42. Rodriguez AA, LaMorte WW, Hanrahan LM, et al. Liver viability after ischemia-reperfusion. Arch Surg 1991;126:767.
43. Poggetti RS, Moore FA, Moore EE, Bensard DD, Anderson BO, Banerjee A. Liver injury is a reversible neutrophil-mediated event following gut ischemia. Arch Surg 1992;127:175.
44. Kobayashi H, Nonami T, Kurokawa T, Sugiyama S, Ozawa T, Takagi H. Effects of preceding ischemic time on the recovery course of energy metabolism in rat liver. Biochem Int 1990;22:227.
45. Hampton WA, Townsend MC, Haybron DM, Shirmer WJ, Fry DE. Effective hepatic blood flow and hepatic bioenergy status in murine peritonitis. J Surg Res 1987;42:33.
46. Schirmer WJ, Schirmer JM, Townsend MC, Fry DE. Femur fracture with associated soft-tissue injury produces hepatic ischemia. Arch Surg 1988;123:412.
47. Lowe GDO, McArdle BM, Carter DC, et al. Prediction and selective prophylaxis of venous thrombosis in elective gastrointestinal surgery. Lancet 1982;1:409.
48. Merli GJ, Martinez J. Prophylaxis for deep vein thrombosis and pulmonary embolism in the surgical patient. Med Clin North Am 1987;71:377.
49. Shen GK, Rappaport W. Control of nonhepatic intra-abdominal hemorrhage with temporary packing. Surgery 1992;174:411.
50. Sharp KW, Locicero RJ. Abdominal packing for surgically uncontrolled hemorrhage. Ann Surg 1992;215:467.
51. Mavroudis C, Malangoni MA, Katzmark SL, Montgomery R, Schrodt CR, Polk HC Jr. The comparative clearance rates of the pleural and peritoneal cavities. Arch Surg 1988;123:157.
52. Tarpley JL, Twomey PL, Catalona WJ, Cretien PB. Suppression of cellular immunity by anesthesia and operation. J Surg Res 1977;22:195.
53. Park SK, Brody JI, Wallace HA, Blakemore WS. Immunosuppressive effect of surgery. Lancet 1971;1:53.
54. Roth JA, Golub SH, Grimm EA, Eiber FR, Morton DL. Effects of operation on immune response in cancer patients: sequential evaluation of in vitro lymphocyte function. Surgery 1976;79:46.
55. Lennard TW, Shenton BK, Borzotta A, et al. The influence of surgical operations on components of the human immune system. Br J Surg 1985;72:771.
56. Post-operative immunosuppression (editorial). Lancet 1974;2:817.
57. Feliciano DV, O'Gorman RB, Bitondo CG, Cruse PA, Matthews RH, Matthews KS. Lymphocyte function and abdominal operations. Trauma vs elective surgery. Arch Surg 1987;122:697.
58. Wakefield CH, Carey PD, Foulds S, Monson JRT, Guillou PJ. Polymorphonuclear leukocyte activation. Arch Surg 1993;128:390.
59. Eggermont AMM, Steller EP, Marquet RL, Jeekel J, Sugarbaker PH. Local regional promotion of tumor growth after abdominal surgery is dominant over immunotherapy with interleukin-2 and lymphokine activated killer cells. Cancer Detect Prev 1988;12:421.
60. Salo M. Immunosuppressive effects of blood transfusion in anaesthesia and surgery. Acta Anaesthesiol Scand Suppl 1988;89:26.
61. Ford CD, VanMoorleghem G, Menlove RL. Blood transfusions and postoperative wound infection. Surgery 1993;113:603.
62. Agarwal N, Murphy JG, Cayten CG, Stahl WM. Blood transfusion increases the risk of infection after trauma. Arch Surg 1993;128:171.
63. Wu H, Little AG. Perioperative blood transfusions and cancer recurrence. J Clin Oncol 1988;6:1348.
64. Biebuyck JF. The possible immunosuppressive effects of perioperative blood transfusions in cancer patients. Anesthesiology 1988;68:422.
65. Tartter PI. The association of perioperative blood transfusion with colorectal cancer recurrence. Ann Surg 1992;216:633.
66. Christou NV. Host-defense mechanisms in surgical patients: a correlative study of the delayed hypersensitivity skin-test response, granulocyte function and sepsis. Can J Surg 1985;28:39.
67. Christou NV, Rode H, Larsen D, Loose L, Broadhead M, Meakins JL. The walk-in anergic patient. How best to assess the risk of sepsis following elective surgery. Ann Surg 1984;199:438.
68. Roizen MF, Hensel P, Lichtor JL, Schreider BD. Patients with disorders of thyroid function. Anesth Clin North Am 1987;5:277.
69. Lampe GH, Roizen MF. Anesthesia for patients with abnormal function at the adrenal cortex. Anesth Clin North Am 1987;5:245.
70. Waldhausen JHT, Shaffrey ME, Skenderis BSI, Jones RS, Schirmer BD. Gastrointestinal myoelectric and clinical patterns of recovery after laparotomy. Ann Surg 1990;211:777.
71. Livingston EH, Passaro EP. Postoperative ileus. Dig Dis Sci 1990;35:121.
72. Schippers E, Holscher AH, Bollschweiler E, Siewert JR. Return of interdigestive motor complex after abdominal surgery. Dig Dis Sci 1991;36:621.
73. Pedersen T, Eliasen K, Henriksen E. A prospective study of mortality associated with anesthesia and surgery: risk indicators of mortality in hospital. Acta Anesthesiol Scand 1990;34:176.
74. Derrington MC, Smith G. A review of studies of anesthetic risk, morbidity and mortality. Br J Anaesth 1987;59:815.

75. Gagner M. Value of preoperative physiologic assessment in outcome of patients undergoing major surgical procedures. Surg Clin North Am 1991;71:1141.

76. Monson JR, Darzi A, Carey PD, Guillou PJ. Prospective evaluation of laparoscopic-assisted colectomy in an unselected group of patients. Lancet 1992;340:831.

77. Nespoli A, Ravizzini C, Trivella M, Segala M. The choice of surgical procedure for peritonitis due to colonic perforation. Arch Surg 1993;128:814.

78. Rutledge R, Fakhry SM, Rutherford EJ, et al. Acute physiology and chronic health evaluation (APACHE II) score and outcome in the surgical intensive care unit: An analysis of multiple intervention and outcome variables in 1,238 patients. Crit Care Med 1991;19:1048.

79. Goldman L. Multifactorial index of cardiac risk in noncardiac surgery: ten-year status report. J Cardiothorac Anesth 1987;1:237.

80. Windsor JA, Hill GL. Risk factors for postoperative pneumonia: the importance of protein depletion. Ann Surg 1988;208:209.

81. Dunn WF, Scanlon PD. Preoperative pulmonary function testing for patients with lung cancer. Mayo Clin Proc 1993;68:371.

82. Weaver DW. Differential diagnosis and management of unexplained bleeding. Surg Clin North Am 1993;73:353.

83. Kakkar VV, Howe CT, Nicolaides AN, Renney JTG, Clarke MB. Deep vein thrombosis of the leg. Is there a "high risk" group? Am J Surg 1970;120:527.

84. Sue-Ling HM, McMahon MJ, Johnston D, Philips PR, Davies JA. Pre-operative identification of patients at high risk of deep venous thrombosis after elective major abdominal surgery. Lancet 1986;1:1173.

85. Koppenhagen K, Adolf J, Matthes M, et al. Low molecular weight heparin and prevention of postoperative thrombosis in abdominal surgery. Thromb Haemost 1992;67:627.

86. The Veterans Affairs Total Parenteral Nutrition Cooperative Study Group. Perioperative total parenteral nutrition in surgical patients. N Engl J Med 1991;325:525.

87. Windsor JA, Hill GL. Weight loss with physiologic impairment. A basic indicator of surgical risk. Ann Surg 1988;207:290.

88. Windsor JA, Knight GS, Hill GL. Wound healing response in surgical patients: recent food intake is more important than nutritional status. Br J Surg 1988;75:135.

89. Nichols RL. Prevention of infection in high risk gastrointestinal surgery. Am J Med 1984;76(5A):111.

90. Kaiser AB. Antimicrobial prophylaxis in surgery. N Engl J Med 1986;315:1129.

91. Stone HH, Hooper CA, Kolb LD, Gehener CE, Dawkins EJ. Antibiotic prophylaxis in gastric, biliary and colonic surgery. Ann Surg 1976;184:443.

92. Clarke JS, Condon RE, Bartlett JG, Gorbach SL, Nichols RL, Ochi S. Preoperative oral antibiotics reduce septic coomplications of colon operations. Ann Surg 1977;186:251.

93. Kaufman Z, Engelberg M, Eliashiv A, Reiss R. Systemic prophylactic antibiotics in elective biliary surgery. Arch Surg 1984;119:1002.

94. Beck DE, Harford FJ, DiPalma JA, Brady CEI. Bowel cleaning with polyethylene glycol electrolyte lavage solution. South Med J 1985;78:1414.

95. Washington JAI, Dearing WH, Judd ES, Elveback LR. Effect of preoperative antibiotic aregimen on development of infection after intestinal surgery: prospective, randomized double-blind study. Ann Surg 1974;180:567.

96. Gallinaro RN, Polk HCJ. Intra-abdominal sepsis: the role of surgery. Clin Gastroenterol 1991;5:611.

97. Armstrong PJ, Burgess RW. Choice of incision and pain following gallbladder surgery. Br J Surg 1990;77:746.

98. Halsted WS. The training of the surgeon. Bull Johns Hopkins Hosp 1904;15:267.

99. Badner NH. Epidural agents for postoperative analgesia. Anesth Clin North Am 1992;10:321.

100. Sandler AN. New techniques of opioid administration for the control of acute pain. Anesth Clin North Am 1992;10:271.

101. Lehmann KA. Methods of postoperative acute pain management. Acta Anaesthesiol Belg 1988;39(Suppl 2):53.

102. White FP. Use of patient-controlled anesthesia for management of acute pain. JAMA 1988;259:243.

103. Yeager MP, Glass DD, Neff RK, Brinck-Johnsen T. Epidural anesthesia and analgesia in high-risk surgical patients. Anesthesiology 1987;66:729.

104. Oden RV. Acute postoperative pain: Incidence, severity, and the etiology of inadequate treatment. Anesth Clin North Am 1989;7:1.

105. Barendregt WB, de Boer HH, Kubat K. The results of autopsy of patients with surgical diseases of the digestive tract. Surg Gynecol Obstet 1992;175:227.

106. Persson AV, Davis RJ, Villavicenncio JL. Deep venous thrombosis and pulmonary embolism. Surg Clin North Am 1991;71:1195.

107. Sinanan MN, Maier RV, Carrico CJ. Laparotomy for intraabdominal sepsis in patients in an intensive care unit. Arch Surg 1984;119:652.

108. Sinanan MN. Acute abdomen and appendix. In: Greenfield LJ, Mulholland MW, Oldham KT, Zelenock GB, eds. Surgery. Scientific principles and practice. Philadelphia: JB Lippincott, 1993:1120.

109. Lightdale CJ. Laparoscopy for cancer staging. Endoscopy 1992;24:682.

110. Sackier J. Diagnositc laparoscopy in nonmalignant disease. Surg Clin North Am 1992;72:1033.

111. Jeng KS, Chiang HJ. Delayed formation of gallstone after transcatheter arterial embolization for hepatocellular carcinoma. Is elective cholecystectomy advisable during hepatectomy? Arch Surg 1989;124:1319.

112. Hoogewoud HM, Rubli E, Terrier F, Hassler H. The role of computerized tomography in fever, septicemia and multiple system organ failure after laparotomy. Surg Gynecol Obstet 1986;162:539.

113. Black WC, Welch HG. Advances in diagnostic imaging and overestimations of disease prevalence and the benefits of therapy. N Engl J Med 1993;328:1237.

114. Jaques P, Mauro M, Safrit H, Yankaskas B, Piggott B. CT features of intraabdoominal abscesses: prediction of successful percutaneous drainage. AJR Am J Roentgenol 1986;146:1041.

115. Levinson M. Percutaneous versus opern operative drainge of intra-abdominal abscesses. Infect Dis Clin North Am 1992;6:525.

116. Salo M. Immunosuppressive effects of blood transfusion in anaesthesia and surgery. Acta Anesthesiol Scand Suppl 1988;89:26.

117. Dodd R. The risk of transfusion-transmitted infection. N Engl J Med 1992;327:419.

118. Kreitner KF, Mildenberger P, Maurer M, Heintz A. The value of imaging techniques in the diagnosis of non-specific abdominal pain in young patients. Aktuelle Radiol 1992;2:234.

119. Nagy AG, James D. Diagnostic laparoscopy. Am J Surg 1989;157:490.

120. Easter DW, Cuschieri A, Nathanson LK, Lavelle-Jones M. The utility of diagnostic laparoscopy for abdominal disorders. Arch Surg 1992;127:379.

121. Trimbos JB, Trimbos Kemper GC, Peters AA, van der Does CD, van Hall EV. Findings in 200 consecutive asymptomatic women, having a laparoscopic sterilization. Arch Gynecol Obstet 1990;247:121.

122. Ikard RW. There is no current indication for laparoscopic adhesiolysis to treat abdominal pain. South Med J 1992;85:939.

123. Mecke H. Pelviscopic adhesiolysis in chronic pelvic pain—laser versus conventional techniques. Geburtshilfe Frauenheilkd 1992;52:47.

124. Goldman L. Assessment of the patient with known or suspected ischaemic heart disease for non-cardiac surgery. Br J Anaesth 1988;61:38.

125. Haagensen R, Steen PA. Perioperative myocardial infarction. Br J Anaesth 1988;61:24.

126. Garc'ia Valdecasas JC, Almenara R, Cabrer C, et al. Subcostal

incision versus midline laparotomy in gallstone surgery: a prospective and randomized trial. Br J Surg 1988;75:473.

127. Carpenter RL, Caplan RA, Brown DL, Stephensen C, Wu R. Incidence and risk factors for side effects of spinal anesthesia. Anesthesiology 1992;76:906.

128. Etches RC. Complications of acute pain management. Anesth Clin North Am 1992;10:417.

129. Howell JM. Current and future trends in wound healing. Emerg Med Clin North Am 1992;10:655.

130. Kingsnorth AN, Slavin J. Peptide growth factors and wound healing. Br J Surg 1991;78:1286.

131. Orgill D, Demling RH. Current concepts and approaches to wound healing. Crit Care Med 1988;16:899.

132. Herndon DN, Hayward PG, Rutan RL, Barrow RE. Growth hormones and factors in surgical patients. Adv Surg 1992;25:65.

133. Ehrlichman RJ, Seckel BR, Bryan DJ, Moschella CJ. Common complications of wound healing. Prevention and management. Surg Clin North Am 1991;71:1323.

134. Peterson PK. Host defense abnormalities predisposing the patient to infection. Am J Med 1984;76(5A):2.

135. Christou NV. Predicting infectious morbidity in elective operations. Am J Surg 1993;165(Suppl 2A):52S.

136. Pollock AV, Evans M. Microbiologic prediction of abdominal surgical wound infection. Arch Surg 1987;122:33.

137. Haley RW, Culver DH, Morgan WM, White JW, Emori TG, Hooton TM. Identifying patients at high risk of surgical wound infection. Am J Epidemiol 1985;121:206.

138. Cruse PJE, Foord R. The epidemiology of wound infection. Surg Clin North Am 1980;60:27.

139. Richards DG, Clark RG, Rowlands BJ, Moore PJ, Eyre-Brook I, Kay PH. Antibiotic prophylasix against wound infection in emergency abdominal surgery. J Roy Coll Surg Edinb 1981;26:232.

140. Lykkegaard Nielsen M, Moesgaard F, Justesen T, Scheibel JH, Lindenberg S. Wound sepsis after elective cholecystectomy. Scand J Gastroenterol 1981;16:937.

141. Ulualp K, Condon RE. Antibiotic prophylaxis for scheduled operative procedures. Infect Dis Clin North Am 1992;6:613.

142. Gibney EJ. Asymptomatic gallstones. Br J Surg 1990;77:368.

143. Cahalane MJ, Shapiro ME, Silen W. Abdominal incision: decision or indecision? Lancet 1989;1:146.

144. Ravo B. Colorectal anastomotic healing and intracolonic bypass procedure. Surg Clin North Am 1988;68:1267.

145. Nicolaides A, Kalodiki E. Duplex scanning in post-operative surgical patients. Haemostasis 1993;23(Suppl 1):72.

146. Mattos MA, Londrey GL, Leutz DW, et al. Color-flow duplex scanning for the surveillance and diagnosis of acute deep venous thrombosis. J Vasc Surg 1992;15:366.

147. Ellis H. Internal overhealing: the problem of intraperitoneal adhesions. World J Surg 1980;4:303.

148. Weigelt JA, Kingman RG. Complications of negative laparotomy for trauma. Am J Surg 1988;156:544.

149. Menzies D. Peritoneal adhesions. Incidence, cause, and prevention. Surg Annu 1992;24(Pt 1):27.

150. Stewart RM, Page CP, Brender J, Schwesinger W, Eisenhut D. The incidence and risk of early postoperative small bowel obstruction. A cohort study. Am J Surg 1987;154:643.

151. Pickleman J, Lee RM. The management of patients with suspected early postoperative small bowel obstruction. Ann Surg 1989;210:216.

152. Quatromoni JC, Rosoff L, Halls JM, Yellin AE. Early postoperative small bowel obstruction. Ann Surg 1980;191:72.

153. Stewardson RH, Bombeck CT, Nyhus LM. Critical operative management of small bowel obstruction. Ann Surg 1978;187:189.

154. Landercasper J, Cogbill TH, Merry WH, Stolee RT, Strutt PJ. Long-term outcome after hospitalization for small-bowel obstruction. Arch Surg 1993;128:765.

155. Paterson Brown S. Strategies for reducing inappropriate laparotomy rate in the acute abdomen. Br Med J 1991;303:1115.

156. Berci G. Elective and emergent laparoscopy. World J Surg 1993;17:8.

157. Ray NF, Larsen JWJ, Stillman RJ, Jacobs RJ. Economic impact of hospitalizations for lower abdominal adhesiolysis in the United States in 1988. Surg Gynecol Obstet 1993;176:271.

158. Falk PM, Beart RWJ, Wexner SD, et al. Laparoscopic colectomy: a critical appraisal. Dis Colon Rectum 1993;36:28.

159. Stoker ME, Vose J, O'Mara P, Maini BS. Laparoscopic cholecystectomy. A clinical and financial analysis of 280 operations. Arch Surg 1992;127:589.

160. Phillips RKS, Hittinger R, Blesovsky L, Fry JS, Fielding LP. Local recurrence following "curative" surgery for large bowel cancer: I. The overall picture. Br J Surg 1984;71:12.

161. Pettigrew RA, Burns HJG, Carter DC. Evaluating surgical risk: the importance of technical factors in determining outcome. Br J Surg 1987;74:791.

162. Hannan EL, O'Donnell JF, Kilburn H, Bernard HR, Yazici A. Investigation of the relationship between volume and mortality for surgical procedures performed in New York State hospitals. JAMA 1989;262:503.

163. Huang PP, Urist M. Evaluation of abdominal Hodgkin's disease. Surg Oncol Clin North Am 1993;2:207.

164. De Jong SA, Pickleman J, Rainsford K. Nonductal tumors of the pancreas. The importance of laparotomy. Arch Surg 1993;128:730.

165. Bleday R, Steele GJ. Second-look surgery for recurrent colorectal carcinoma: is it worthwhile?. Semin Surg Oncol 1991;7:171.

166. Wanebo HJ, Vezeridis MP, Llaneras MR. Evaluation of a patient prior to second-look surgery. Semin Surg Oncol 1991;7:133.

167. Sardi A, Minton JP, Nieroda C, Sickle-Santanello B, Young D, Martin EWJ. Multiple reoperations in recurrent colorectal carcinoma. An analysis of morbidity, mortality, and survival. Cancer 1988;61:1913.

168. Buhre LM, Verschueren RC, Mehta DM, Oldhoff J. Staging laparotomy for inoperable or borderline operable cancer of the rectum. Dis Colon Rectum 1987;30:352.

169. Brophy C, Cahow CE. Primary small bowel malignant tumors. Unrecognized until emergent laparotomy. Am Surg 1989;55:408.

170. Rome RM, Fortune DW. The role of second-look laparotomy in the management of patients with ovarian carcinoma. Aust NZ J Obstet Gynaecol 1988;28:318.

171. Hand R, Fremgen A, Chmiel JS, et al. Staging procedures, clinical management, and survival outcome for ovarian cancer. JAMA 1993;269:1119.

172. Sutherland FR, Temple WJ, Snodgrass T, Huchcroft SA. Predicting the outcome of exploratory laparotomy in ICU patients with sepsis or organ failure. J Trauma 1989;29:152.

173. Garcia Sabrido JL, Tallado JM, Christou NV, Polo JR, Valdecantos E. Treatment of severe intra-abdominal sepsis and/or necrotic foci by an 'open-abdomen' approach. Zipper and zipper-mesh techniques. Arch Surg 1988;123:152.

174. Bohnen JM, Mustard RA. A critical look at scheduled relaparotomy for secondary bacterial peritonitis. Surg Gynecol Obstet 1991;172Suppl:25.

175. Burch JM, Ortiz VB, Richardson RJ, Martin RR, Mattox KL, Jordan GLJ. Abbreviated laparotomy and planned reoperation for critically injured patients. Ann Surg 1992;215:476.

176. Pusajo JF, Bumaschany E, Doglio GR, et al. Postoperative intra-abdominal sepsis requiring reoperation. Arch Surg 1993;128:218.

177. Ranson JHC. The role of surgery in the management of acute pancreatitis. Ann Surg 1990;211:382.

178. Williams RA, Wilson SE. Gastrointestinal disorders requiring surgical treatment in patients with AIDS. Compr Ther 1992;18:9.

179. Macho JR. Gastrointestinal surgery in the AIDS patient. Gastroenterol Clin N A 1988;17:563.

180. Davidson T, Allen Mersh TG, Miles AJ, et al. Emergency laparotomy in patients with AIDS. Br J Surg 1991;78:924.

181. Wilson SE, Robinson G, Williams RA, et al. Acquired immune deficiency syndrome (AIDS). Indications for abdominal surgery, pathology, and outcome. Ann Surg 1989;210:428.

182. Gunshefski L, Flancbaum L, Brolin RE, Frankel A. Changing

patterns in perforated peptic ulcer disease. Am Surg 1990;56:270.

183. Koea JB, Shaw JHF. Surgical management of neutropenic enterocolitis. Br J Surg 1989;76:821.

184. Glenn J, Funkhouser WK, Schneider PS. Acute illnesses necessitating urgent abdominal surgery in neutropenic cancer patients: description of 14 cases and review of the literature. Surgery 1989;105:778.

185. Medich DS, Lee KK, Simmons RL, Grubbs PE, Yang HC, Showalter DP. Laparotomy for fulminant pseudomembranous colitis. Arch Surg 1992;127:847.

186. Morris JB, Zollinger RM, Stellato TA. Role of surgery in antibiotic-induced pseudomembraneoous enterocolitis. Am J Surg 1990;160:535.

187. Hawley PR. Emergency surgery for ulcerative colitis. World J Surg 1988;12:169.

Textbook of Gastroenterology, second edition, edited by Tadataka Yamada. JB Lippincott Company, Philadelphia © 1995.

CHAPTER 141

Applications of New Technologies in Tissue Examination

David M. Hockenbery

Identification of Infectious Agents
Immunoblotting
Solid-Phase Immunoassays
Immunocytochemistry
Polymerase Chain Reaction
In situ Hybridization
Evaluation of Cancer and Cancer Risk
Detection of Aneuploidy
Cell Cycle Analysis
Specific Genetic Alterations in Cancer
Southern Blot and RFLP
Loss of Heterozygosity
DNA Sequencing

Oligonucleotide Hybridization
Mutation-Specific PCR
Sample Processing
Polymerase Chain Reaction
In situ Hybridization
Immunocytochemistry
Molecular Approaches to Therapy
Gene Therapy
Adoptive Immunotherapy
Intracellular Immunization
Models of Disease
Transgenic Mice
Homologous Recombination

New techniques to identify, quantitate, and discriminate important genetic and cellular hallmarks in human disease are rapidly being developed. The sensitivity and specificity inherent in immunologic recognition is utilized in the antibody-based methodologies of solid-phase immunoassays, immunoblots, and immunohistochemistry to detect novel protein antigens or conformational epitopes. The polymerase chain reaction (PCR) uses flanking oligonucleotides to anneal to unique DNA or RNA sequences and prime repetitive DNA synthesis and amplification of target sequences to easily detectable levels. In situ hybridization using nucleic acid probes enables specific detection of cellular or viral sequences in tissue sections.

Measurement of cellular DNA content by flow cytometry is of prognostic and predictive value for certain human neoplasias. Identification of mutations in DNA sequences is fundamentally important for linkage mapping of inherited disease syndromes. Southern blot hybridization of genomic DNA is used to detect restriction fragment length polymorphisms (RFLPs) as well as loss of heterozygosity (LOH) indicating deletions at specific loci which may represent tumor suppressor genes. Mutations encoding alterations in the protein sequences of disease-associated genes are defined by DNA sequencing and can be detected using several strategies adaptable to multiple tissue samples, including oligonucleotide hybridization, and various PCR-based approaches.

Identification of new infectious agents and disease-associated gene products translates into new targets for therapeutic intervention. Newer approaches attempt to directly modify pathophysiologic processes in tissues of interest, through gene therapy, adoptive immunotherapy, and intracellular immunization. Finally, transgenic manipulations can create animal models of human disease by overproduction, mutation, or ablation by homologous recombination of disease-associated genes.

Advances in molecular and cellular biology research have made possible many new diagnostic and therapeutic tools for human disease. Central to the success of these techniques is a new and better understanding of the molecular and genetic basis of individual diseases, achieved by advances in gene mapping and cloning technology. This has enabled the design of tests and treatments with greater specificity and sensitivity directed at the underlying causative agent or cellular defect. Medical science has responded to the identification of disease-specific gene products or mutations by devising both simpler and more sensitive detection methods. Of great potential importance, research tools are now available for the creation of animal and cellular models of human disease incorporating specific genetic alterations and susceptibilities to infectious agents which should speed the discovery of more effective therapies.

The ability to detect and follow disease-specific genes or gene products is useful in several ways. Molecular tests can be used to diagnose disease, or subclassify diseases based on the molecular lesion in a highly specific and sensitive way. Specific markers of disease activity and host response can yield prognostic information. Inherited or acquired predisposition to disease can be assessed to infer risk of disease and design screening or interventional strategies. Treatment response can be followed with sensitive assays for residual disease.

In this chapter, specific goals in tissue examination will serve to introduce individual techniques. Although considerable overlap in the utility of these methods exists, strategies for detection of viral genes and gene products, for example, differ from those for detection of single nucleotide mutations in cellular genes.

IDENTIFICATION OF INFECTIOUS AGENTS

Strategies for the detection of microbial genes and gene products depend upon specific reagents that bind to unique sequence or structural determinants. These may supplement or serve in lieu of culture methods or routine histologic examination. Modifications allow tissue localization of infection, determination of latent versus active infection, and detection of mutations of microbial genomes of prognostic or therapeutic significance. The ability to amplify conserved microbial sequences such as ribosomal RNA by PCR has proven useful to identify novel infectious agents which cannot be grown in culture.

Immunoblotting

This method to identify proteins or antibodies by immunoreactivity typically employs sodium dodecyl sulfate (SDS)-polyacrylamide gel electrophoresis as an initial step. Protein samples are denatured by heating in the presence of the anionic detergent SDS to allow complex formation between SDS and protein. SDS binds to proteins in proportion to their molecular weight. The SDS molecules contribute a negative charge and uniform charge-mass ratio for all sample proteins. Migration of protein-SDS complexes toward the anode during electrophoresis is therefore inversely related to protein molecular weights, rather than isoelectric properties of individual proteins. Proteins are then transferred to nitrocellulose paper electrophoretically, preserving their pattern of migration. The nitrocellulose blot is successively incubated with primary antibody and secondary reagents which are radioactively labeled with ^{125}I or covalently coupled to enzymes such as alkaline phosphatase and horseradish peroxidase. Antibody-containing complexes which have bound to specific proteins on the blot can be visualized by development with enzyme substrates yielding a color reaction product (Fig. 141-1). Recent modifications to the technique have included chemiluminescent substrates for alkaline phosphatase and horseradish peroxidase, enabling rapid detection on photographic film.[1]

Most uses of immunoblots in clinical practice test for specific antibodies in patient sera against protein samples of the infectious agent in question. These tests are widely used in secondary tests for anti-HIV antibodies and in second-generation tests for hepatitis C antibodies.[2,3]

Solid-Phase Immunoassays

Solid-phase immunoassays use antibodies or antigens immobilized in plastic wells in a microtiter plate or on nitrocellulose paper to capture cognate antigens or antibodies. Binding is recognized with an enzyme-conjugated secondary

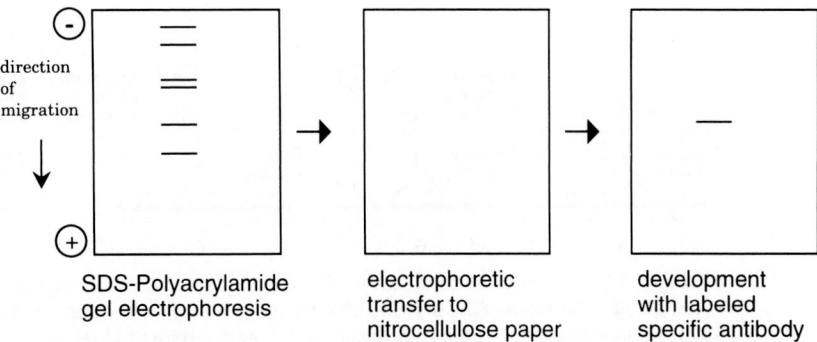

direction of migration

SDS-Polyacrylamide gel electrophoresis

electrophoretic transfer to nitrocellulose paper

development with labeled specific antibody

FIGURE 141-1. Immunoblotting procedure.

antibody, whose color reaction product can be scanned and quantitated in an automated plate reader, or ^{125}I-conjugated antibody. Basic variations in binding and detection strategies are antibody capture, antigen capture, and two antibody sandwich techniques.[4] Modifying the assay to include known amounts of labeled competing antigen and titrations of unknown samples can provide quantitative results. This rapid assay is used for primary testing for anti-HIV antibodies and first- and second-generation tests for hepatitis C antibodies.[5,6]

Immunocytochemistry

As opposed to indirect measures of immunologic exposure to an etiologic agent, the ability to detect exogenous proteins, particularly viral, in tissue sections is helpful in demonstrating an active process in sites and cells of interest, and of general interest as a research tool. The ability of antibodies to recognize specific epitopes is dependent on the survival of the epitopes during the fixation process, and balanced against the desire for optimal morphology using strong fixatives. Antigen retrieval methods may allow recovery of hidden epitopes in aldehyde-fixed samples, including archival material.[7]

Amplification of the signal resulting from primary antibody can be achieved with multivalent secondary reagents. Two methods are in common use (Fig. 141-2).

1. The peroxidase-antiperoxidase method uses a bridging secondary antibody which can bivalently bind to Fc portions of the primary antibody and an antiperoxidase antibody, which itself binds two peroxidase molecules as a complex.
2. The avidin-biotin complex method uses the avidin protein, which possesses tetravalent high-affinity binding sites for a biotin molecule to amplify the signal. The primary or secondary antibody is multiply biotinylated through covalent coupling to free amino groups. The avidin is com-

plexed to horseradish peroxidase or alkaline phosphatase in a preformed complex of avidin and biotinylated enzyme.

Antibodies against many infectious agents producing gastrointestinal or hepatic disease are available for immunohistochemistry, including herpes simplex types I and II, cytomegalovirus, varicella-zoster, hepatitis B, and *Chlamydia*.

Polymerase Chain Reaction

PCR uses the ability of sequence-specific oligodeoxynucleotides to bind to a single-target DNA and prime repetitive cycles of overlapping DNA synthesis between the primers to detect unique DNA sequences.[8] The exponential amplification allowed by the semiconservative replication of each DNA strand between the primers, providing two DNA double-stranded fragments from each template at the beginning of a cycle of DNA synthesis, yields a 10^6-fold or greater increase in copy number of the amplified segment. This is sufficient for cloning of the DNA fragment or direct dideoxy sequencing. A single copy of a DNA sequence from a single haploid cell (e.g., spermatozoa) can be detected.[9] For comparison, detection of unique sequences by Southern blotting has a lower limit of sensitivity of 10^5 copies.

Oligonucleotide primers, complementary to sequences on opposite DNA strands which flank the region to be amplified, are chosen. The sensitivity of the assay is often dependent on the choice of primers, reflecting sequence conservation and competition due to nonspecific binding. Comparison of primers from hepatitis C 5' untranslated, core, NS3, NS3/4 and NS5 regions showed variation of sensitivity for cDNA amplification in chronic hepatitis C patients from 20% to 90% with the 5' untranslated region primers most sensitive.[10] The 5' to 3' direction of the primers bound to the DNA sequence should be towards the opposite primer, such that primer extension from the 3' ends traverses the sequence of

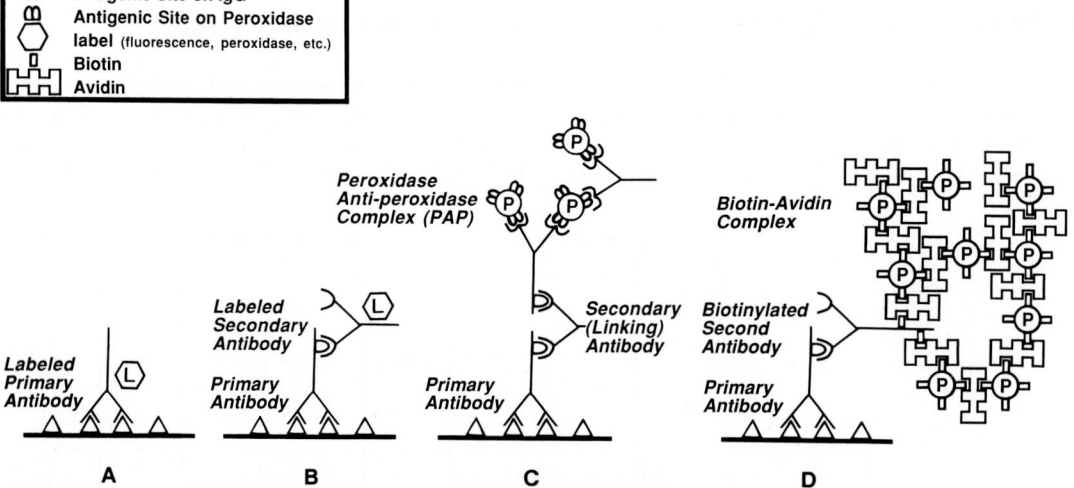

FIGURE 141-2. Various techniques of immunocytochemistry. (Adapted from Gosselin EJ, Cate C, Pettengill OS, Sorenson GD. Immunocytochemistry: its evolution and criteria for its application in the study of epon-embedded cells and tissue. Am J Anat 1986;175:135.)

interest. The polymerase reaction involves successive cycles of DNA denaturation, annealing of primers to DNA, and primer extension, typically at 3 separate temperatures. One cycle results in new DNA synthesis extending from the 3′ end of each primer beyond the second primer sequence on the opposite strand (Fig. 141-3). A second cycle denatures the nascent and template strands to allow new primers to anneal. The availability of cloned DNA polymerases from thermophilic bacteria which survive at denaturing temperatures permits a single addition of polymerase enzyme for multiple cycles. A second round of PCR with a second set of nested primers is often used to increase sensitivity and specificity, as nonspecific amplification products for the first set will not have complementary sequences for the second set.[11]

The initial template for PCR may be an RNA sequence when information on mRNA expression or detection of RNA viral genomes is desired.[12] The first step involves first strand cDNA synthesis with reverse transcriptase. Subsequent amplification steps can proceed with thermostable DNA polymerase as in standard PCR.

The amplified product may be detected by ethidium bromide staining of an agarose or polyacrylamide gel at a sensitivity of 5 to 10 μg. The size of the amplified band can be determined by comparison to DNA molecular weight standards run in an adjacent lane and used as a check against the predicted size of the product. Alternatively, an internal DNA sequence fragment can be used as a probe in a Southern blot to verify the amplified sequence and boost the sensitivity for detection. Finally, DNA sequence can be obtained directly from the PCR product to confirm its identity. DNA sequencing of PCR products from the pre-core region of hepatitis B has identified mutations which prevent e antigen production and correlate with severe hepatitis.[13,14] The ability to amplify ribosomal DNA sequences using generic primers to conserved sequences among all bacterial species has led to the identification of new bacterial agents responsible for the clinical syndromes of bacillary angiomatosis and peliosis hepatis (i.e., *Rochalimaea henselae*) and Whipple's disease.[15,16] The unique

sequence of ribosomal DNA determined in this manner allows classification of new pathogens which are unable to be cultured.

PCR assays have been clinically useful for hepatitis C RNA detection, and have proven more sensitive than standard assays for detection of CMV and hepatitis B.[17-20] A decided advantage is the ability to amplify gene sequences from tissue, including paraffin-embedded specimens and from cell samples on microscope slides, providing great versatility to this technique.[21,22] This allows the use of archived material for analysis, and the potential benefit of direct assay of the target tissue or purified cell populations rather than blood samples. A caveat to PCR detection of microbial genes is the extreme sensitivity of this method. The predictive value for disease of an amplifiable product, which may represent a limited quantity of organisms or virions in the sample and without further information on viability or infectivity of the microbe in question, remains to be determined for many applications. Quantitative PCR tests can be designed with an internal control PCR template of known quantity and should yield information on the clinical importance of positive tests at the lower limits of detection.[23]

In situ Hybridization

A complementary approach to immunohistochemical methods to detect microbial gene expression in tissues uses RNA or DNA probes complementary to gene sequences of interest to hybridize to nucleic acid sequences in tissue sections.[24] Bound probe is visualized by detection of radionuclide incorporated in the probe or enzymatic detection coupled to the hybridizing sequences via modified nucleotides incorporated in the RNA probe. This methodology makes it possible to proceed directly from a new gene sequence to tissue localization without the time and effort of deriving antibodies against protein products encoded by the gene. It also allows parallel screening of sequences from several regions of a mi-

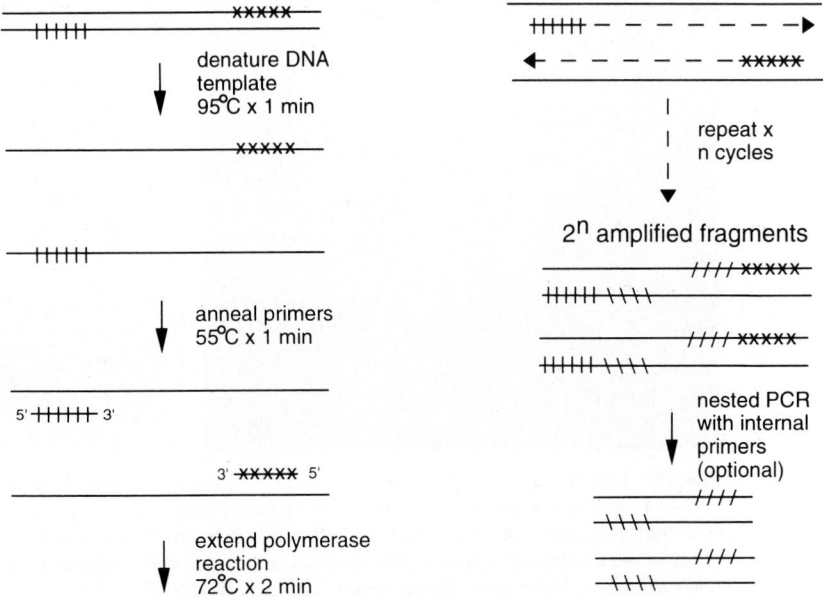

FIGURE 141-3.   Polymerase chain reaction.

crobial genome for optimal sensitivity and background. The sensitivity enables detection of 10 to 100 mRNA molecules/cell.

The basic method uses paraformaldehyde-fixed or frozen tissue sections cut as frozen or wax-embedded sections 8 to 10 μ thick and mounted on slides. The sections are treated with a protease to increase the accessibility of RNA bound to protein, and subsequently with acetic anhydride to modify protein groups which may bind nonspecifically to nucleic acid probes. In the case of riboprobes, a single-stranded antisense RNA probe complementary to the RNA of interest is synthesized from a plasmid template containing the sequence of interest and an adjacent bacteriophage RNA polymerase initiation site (e.g., T3, T7, SP6). DNA double-stranded probes can be made by nick translation or random primed synthesis of a DNA fragment (see Southern Blot). A radioactive nucleotide (35S-UTP) or biotinylated nucleotide is included in the polymerase reaction to uniformly label the probe throughout its length. 35S is most often used as the radioactive isotope because of its lower-energy beta emission, which produces a better-localized autoradiography signal. Nonradioactive probes can also be prepared with biotinylated or digoxigenin-labeled nucleotides. Digoxigenin is a steroid hapten which can be covalently attached to nucleotides and recognized by specific monoclonal antibodies.[25] In some cases, it

may be preferable to partially hydrolyze the probe to smaller lengths (approximately 100–300 base pairs) for the hybridization. Oligonucleotide DNA probes may also be used.

The probe is heat denatured in hybridization buffer containing formamide to reduce secondary structure of probe and incubated with the tissue section at 37°C to 55°C for several hours. The sections are washed according to the desired stringency of hybridization, with buffers of variable salt concentration and temperature to remove nonspecific binding. Treatment with RNase is usually included for riboprobes to degrade single-stranded (i.e., nonhybridized) probe. For radioactive probes, the slides are processed for autoradiography by dipping each slide in molten emulsion solution, allowing it to dry, and incubating at 4°C for the required exposure time (2 days–6 weeks). The slides are processed in photographic developer and fixer and counterstained. The activated silver grains in the emulsion are visualized by dark field microscopy which can be compared to the histologic appearance under light field.

Tissue sections can be examined for viral genomes and have proven useful for herpesviruses (e.g., herpes simplex, cytomegalovirus), adenoviruses, papillomavirus, and hepatitis B virus (Fig. 141-4). Single-stranded riboprobes are able to distinguish hepatitis B viral RNA from single-stranded replicative DNA.[26]

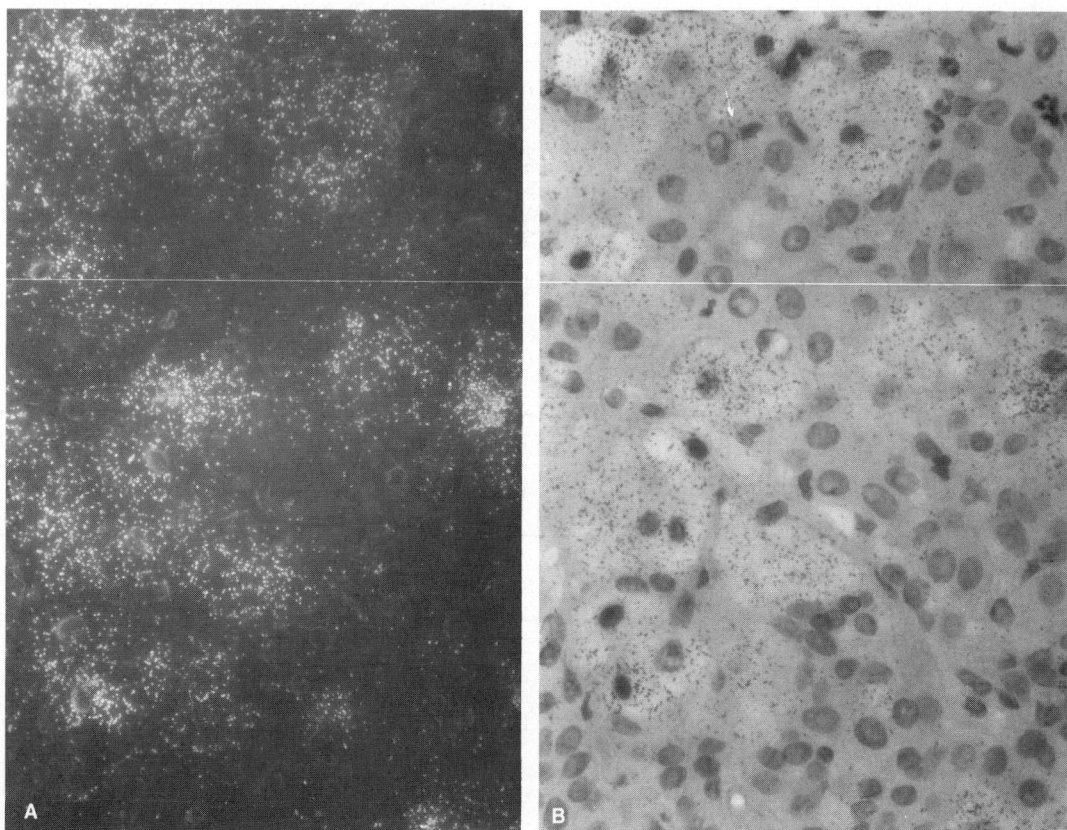

FIGURE 141-4. In situ hybridization signal of ^{35}S-labeled antisense riboprobe to hepatitis B virus RNA in liver biopsy specimen from a patient with fibrosing cholestatic hepatitis syndrome following orthotopic liver transplantation. **(A)** Dark field and **(B)** light field microscopy show signal localized to ballooning hepatocytes undergoing cytolysis. (Hematoxylin and eosin stain; original magnifications ×400; courtesy of Andrew Mason, M.D.; and Robert Perrillo, M.D., St. Louis, MO.)

EVALUATION OF CANCER AND CANCER RISK

Detection of Aneuploidy

Alterations in the chromosomal content and structure of cancer cells are believed to contribute to the unregulated growth behavior through effects on gene expression. Genomic instability is also a fundamental attribute of transformed cells. The chromosomal composition of cancer cells can be determined in two ways, karyotypic analysis and flow cytometry using DNA-binding fluorescent probes.

The number and identity of chromosomes is evaluated by examination of metaphase chromosome preparations stained with dyes such as Giemsa to reveal banding patterns characteristic of each of 22 autosomes and the sex chromosomes.[27] The banding pattern may also reveal chromosomal rearrangements such as deletions, insertions, translocations, and inversions. In additions to being markers of genetic instability characteristic of cancer cells, these rearrangements may mark specific genes at sites of chromosome breakage which are deregulated and act as cellular oncogenes. The requirement for metaphase nuclei restricts this application to cell lines derived from cancers or some rapidly growing tumors.

Flow cytometry measures cell-bound fluorescence and light scatter as dispersed cells or nuclei are passed singly past a focused excitation light source. Fluorophores can be coupled to antibodies to visualize cell surface or intracellular antigens, or designed to target intracellular compartments or yield information on metabolic pathways or intracellular milieu. Several DNA-binding fluorescent reagents are available which are useful for flow cytometric analysis of DNA ploidy. These intercalate between DNA bases or otherwise bind to DNA and provide a fluorescent signal proportional to the total cellular DNA or number of chromosomes. Cells with aneuploid DNA contents can be recognized by fluorescent signals different than a diploid population or multiples thereof, which may represent G2 cells or multinucleate cells (Fig. 141-5A).[28] Cal-

ibration can be performed with a normal cell population such as chicken erythrocytes or human peripheral lymphocytes. Near-diploid populations within 5% to 10% of the diploid peak may not be reliably detected.

Cell Cycle Analysis

Another parameter frequently measured by flow cytometry is the fraction of cells in S phase as a measure of cells undergoing DNA synthesis, equivalent to a thymidine labeling index. Cycling cell populations show a G1 diploid peak, a G2 tetraploid peak and a trough of cells between G1 and G2 representing cells undergoing DNA synthesis with continuously increasing DNA content (Fig. 141-5B). Various curve-fitting algorithms are used to arrive at cell cycle phase fractions within the population.[28] Increased S-phase or S + G2–phase fraction correlates poorly with prognosis for many tumor types.

The identification of intracellular antigens expressed in cycling cells has provided complementary assays to flow cytometry analysis of DNA content. The antigens in most common use are Ki-67 and proliferating cell nuclear antigen (PCNA). Ki-67 is a nuclear matrix antigen expressed predominantly during S and G2 phase.[29] PCNA is an auxiliary protein of DNA polymerase delta, expressed during S phase.[30] In addition to immunohistochemistry on tissue sections, these antigens can be assessed by flow cytometry using appropriate cell fixation and permeabilization methods.

Specific Genetic Alterations in Cancer

A central tenet of modern cancer biology is that the underlying defect responsible for the cancer cell phenotype lies in the introduction of new genes or mutations in cellular genes. A large body of current research concerns refinements in techniques to detect these genetic changes, for their potential usefulness in diagnosis, treatment and prevention of cancer.

FIGURE 141-5. DNA content histograms. (**A**) Abnormal DNA content histogram shows a large aneuploid population with a DNA content of 3.3 N. (**B**) Normal DNA content histogram from a patient who had Barrett's metaplasia without dysplasia. Cells in the G0/G2 phase of the cell cycle are represented by the large peak with a DNA content of 2 N. Cells in the G2 interval are represented by the 4 N peak, which typically contains 6% or less of the cells in the biopsy specimen when processed with a single-step detergent technique and adequately syringed to eliminate aggregations of G0/G1 cells. The S phase is represented by the plateau between 2 N and 4 N. (Courtesy of Brian Reid, M.D., and Peter Rabinovitch, M.D., Seattle, WA.)

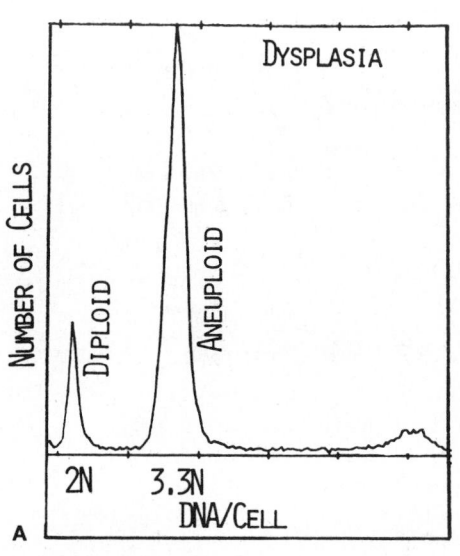

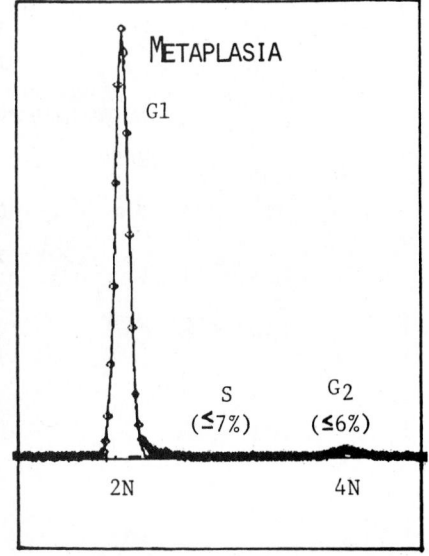

Southern Blot and RFLP

The majority of human cancers appear to be associated with mutation, deletion, or rearrangement of human cellular genes. Most of the known cancer-associated genes (i.e., oncogenes or tumor-suppressor genes) have been identified by positional cloning, on the basis of chromosomal translocations or deletions which serve as physical markers, or by their transforming ability when introduced into cell lines. Additional genes are being sought in cancer-prone families, including familial clustering with low penetrances and nonclassic Mendelian inheritance.

Extremely important to this effort are efforts to construct linkage maps of the human genome, with loci defined by RFLPs. Restriction enzymes are bacterial endonucleases which cleave DNA at specific short (4–10 bp) sequences. Genomic DNA digested with a restriction enzyme yields many different sized fragments which can be aligned according to size by electrophoresis in an agarose gel and transferred to a DNA binding paper by capillary or vacuum-mediated fluid transfer, in a procedure called a Southern blot.[24] Double-stranded DNA bound to the blotting paper can be denatured to enable hybridization with a unique sequence probe in hybridization buffer. The DNA fragment used as a probe can be radioactively labeled by nick translation, using DNAse to create single-stranded gaps which are filled in by DNA polymerase utilizing ^{32}P-labeled deoxynucleotides, or by random priming, using a mixture of random hexamer oligonucleotides to anneal to the denatured fragment and prime new DNA synthesis. Nonradioactive probes can be prepared with digoxigenin or biotin-labeled dUTP. The pattern of bands visualized with the probe represent the fragments of restriction enzyme-digested genomic DNA identical or homologous to the probe sequence.

RFLPs represent insertions, deletions, or mutations at restriction enzyme sites on different alleles of a gene which produce different patterns and sizes of bands on a Southern blot with a genomic DNA probe. The pattern of bands on a Southern blot for an individual represents the superposition of hybridizing fragments for each of two alleles of the gene sequence probed. By testing family members, especially offspring, one sees allelic segregation of the pattern of bands from each chromosome, enabling their recognition (Fig. 141-6). A comparison of two probed sequences or loci with RFLPs shows that all combinations of polymorphic patterns will show up in the offspring if the loci are on different chromosomes (i.e., independent assortment). If both loci are on the same chromosome, one allelic pattern for the first locus will segregate in the offspring linked to one of the allelic patterns for the second locus. Opportunities to disrupt this pattern occur, however, during each meiotic division during spermatogenesis and oogenesis. Meiotic recombinations can occur between pairs of chromosomes, such that alleles no longer remain linked on the same chromosome. The frequency at which this occurs is roughly proportional to the chromosomal distance separating the loci.

Genetic distance between loci can be estimated by calculating the likelihood ratio or odds ratio, at each meiotic opportunity for recombination that can be scored, for the hypotheses of linkage at a certain recombination frequency or no linkage. The logarithm of the odds ratio (LOD) multiplied by the observed frequency of the linkage result observed is tallied for each family. LOD scores are added for each indi-

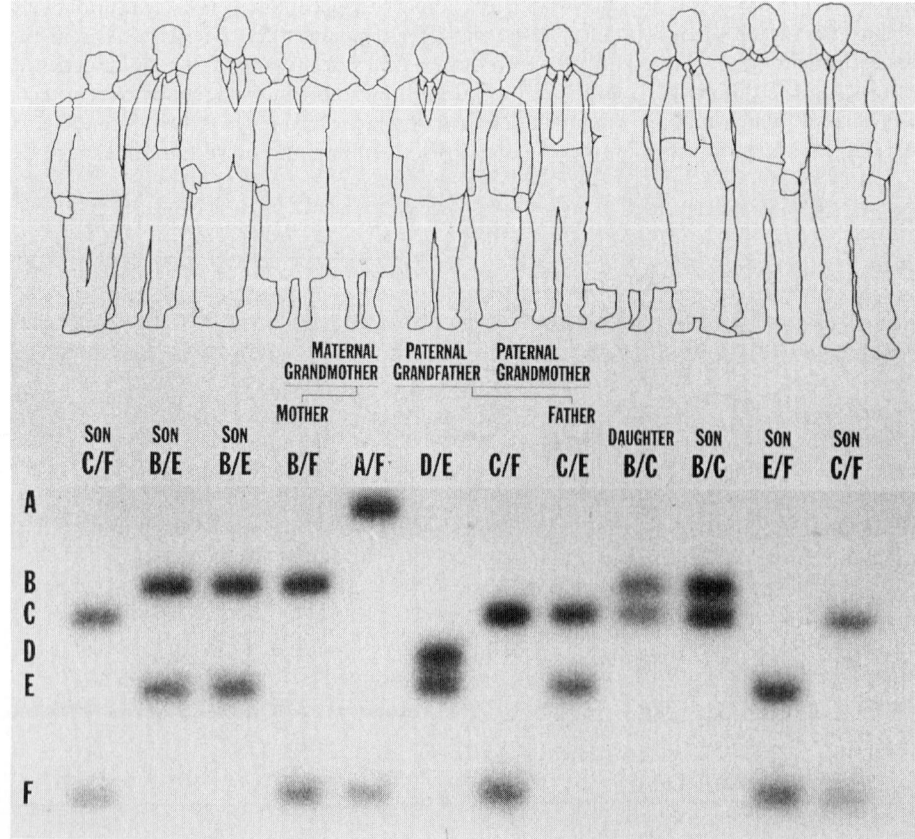

FIGURE 141-6. Restriction fragment length polymorphism analysis by Southern blot of DNA samples from three generations shows segregation of alleles A through F. (Courtesy of DNA Diagnostic Lab, Eccles Institute of Human Genetics, University of Utah, Salt Lake City, UT.)

vidual whose meiotic recombination in offspring can be scored (Fig. 141-7). A LOD score >3 is considered significant for the linkage hypothesis tested. Genetic loci with RFLPs in the population studied can be linked in this manner to create an RFLP genomic linkage map. Linkage between any heritable trait, such as disease susceptibility, can be tested to RFLP positions on such a map and used to establish the chromosomal location of the disease gene in question and narrow its position to the vicinity of a closely linked RFLP locus in preparation for cloning strategies.[31]

Loss of Heterozygosity

A well recognized genetic change leading to cancer involves deletion or mutational inactivation of tumor-suppressor genes, such as p53, Rb, DCC, and APC. Additionally, cancer cells have been demonstrated to undergo allelic deletions at many loci. The recognition of deletion events at candidate genes usually requires RFLPs within the gene or closely linked loci. Southern blot analysis of tumor cell DNA compared to nonmalignant tissue from the same patient reveals loss of one polymorphic band if sequence homologous to the probe is deleted. Deletion of nonpolymorphic loci can be suspected from loss of band intensity in the tumor sample compared to a second locus preserved in both samples.

DNA Sequencing

The genetic alteration which predisposes to cancer for some common cancer genes is a point mutation in the coding sequence which alters a single amino acid. This change may activate protein function, as in ras oncogenes, or cause a loss of function, as in tumor suppressor genes such as p53. These mutations have necessitated development of assays specific for single nucleotide changes in a DNA sequence.

The determination of DNA sequence is the most direct and sensitive method for detecting mutations in a cloned DNA fragment, although additional strategies are required for screening for mutations in genomic DNA samples representing the sequence contributions of two alleles. DNA sequence is obtained from a purified DNA sequence by either of two methods, dideoxy sequencing or chemical sequencing.[24] Both methods involve the generation of a ladder of DNA oligonucleotide single-strand fragments, each terminating at successive nucleotide positions from a common origin. Using different strategies, fragments with the same terminal deoxynucleotides can be pooled and run in a single lane of a high-resolution denaturing sequencing polyacrylamide gel, able to resolve single-nucleotide differences over 300 to 500 nucleotides. With four adjacent lanes representing different terminal deoxynucleotides, a continuous sequence ladder can be read from the gel.

Dideoxy sequencing uses a DNA polymerase (e.g., T7 DNA polymerase) to extend a labeled single strand from a primer annealed to template DNA. Random chain termination is caused by addition of a low abundance dideoxynucleotide to the reaction, which prevents further extension after its incorporation. Four separate reactions with a different dideoxynucleotide serve to label the fragments. Radionucleotides are commonly incorporated during the polymerase reaction for autoradiography. Protocols using thermostable polymerases allow for better product extension by destabilizing secondary structure in the template, and allow direct sequencing with smaller amounts of template DNA. Nonradioactive alternatives include chemiluminescent substrates for alkaline phosphatase using avidin-biotin interactions to bind biotinylated

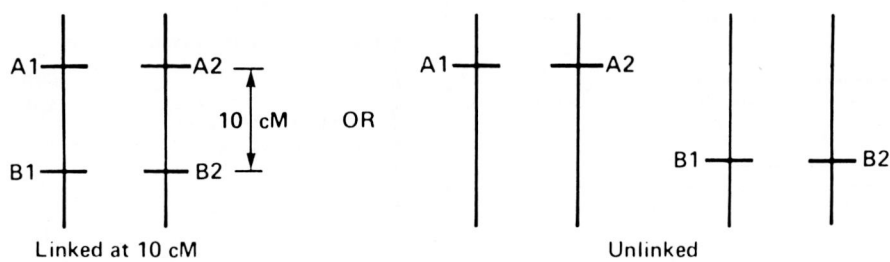

Possible Genotypes	Frequency of Genotype		Ratio of Odds	Expected Contribution to LOD Score	
	If Linked	If Unlinked	Ratio of Odds (linked/unlinked)	If Linked	If Unlinked
A2B2	0.90	0.50	9/5	0.9 log 9/5	0.5 log 9/5
A2B1	0.10	0.50	1/5	0.1 log 1/5	0.5 log 1/5
			Expected LOD Score =	+0.16 or	−0.22

FIGURE 141-7. Logarithm of the odds (LOD) score from a single meiosis. The contribution of one meiosis to the LOD score calculation is shown. One centimorgan is a genetic map unit denoting a recombination frequency of 1% during a single meiosis. (From Donis-Keller H, Botstein D. Recombinant DNA methods: applications to human genetics. In: Childs B, Holtzman NA, Kazazian HH Jr, Valle, DC, eds. Molecular genetics in medicine. New York: Elsevier, 1988.)

deoxynucleotides incorporated in the synthesized DNA strand, and various fluorescent labels, which can tag each dideoxy terminator distinctly and enable discrimination of different fluorescent signals in a single gel lane. This approach has been successfully applied to automated sequencing protocols, with a detector reading fluorescent peaks as the oligonucleotide fragments migrate past the detector on the gel (Fig. 141-8).

Chemical sequencing by the Maxim-Gilbert technique uses nucleotide-specific chemical modifications of an end-labeled DNA strand and subsequent piperidine treatment to cleave at modified sites. The initial modifications occur at low frequency and yield a similar ladder of oligodeoxynucleotide lengths detected by their common radiolabeled end. Chemical sequencing can be applied to small oligonucleotides with no requirement for a primer and is not limited by secondary structure or primary sequence difficulties which can interfere with primer extension in the dideoxy method.

Oligonucleotide Hybridization

Southern blots can be performed with radiolabeled oligonucleotides 20 to 30 nucleotides in length conforming to the wild-type sequence or a mutated sequence differing at one nucleotide. Stringent hybridization and wash conditions can be carefully chosen to limit each probe's binding to its specific genomic sequence. Ras mutations at specific codons have been detected in colon adenoma and carcinoma specimens using this method.[32]

Mutation-Specific PCR

Several variations on the standard PCR technique are available to detect single nucleotide mutations in a target sequence. These include use of internal restriction enzyme sites spanning the mutation, design of mutation-specific primers, oligonucleotide ligation assay, single-strand conformational polymorphism (SSCP) analysis, denaturant gradient gel electrophoresis (DGGE), and mismatch analysis. These methods differ in their overall applicability, requirement for prior knowledge of the mutation, sensitivity, and complexity.

Certain mutations in ras and p53 have fallen within restriction enzyme sites enabling a restriction enzyme digest of the PCR fragment to determine the presence of the mutation (Fig. 141-9). The obvious disadvantage of this method is the limited number of mutations which fit this criteria.

Primers incorporating a mutation, usually at the 3'-most position can be used to differentially amplify a mutated target sequence under stringent conditions, compared to the nonmutated primer. This method requires prior knowledge of the mutation and empiric determination of hybridization conditions.

The oligonucleotide ligation assay tests the ability of two adjacent oligonucleotides which hybridize to one strand of amplified DNA to be ligated to each other.[33] The oligonucleotides are designed so that the single nucleotide mutation to be tested is incorporated at the 5' or 3' end of one of the oligonucleotides at the joining site. By controlling the temperature and salt concentration of the ligation reaction, the success of the reaction will be dependent on the matching of

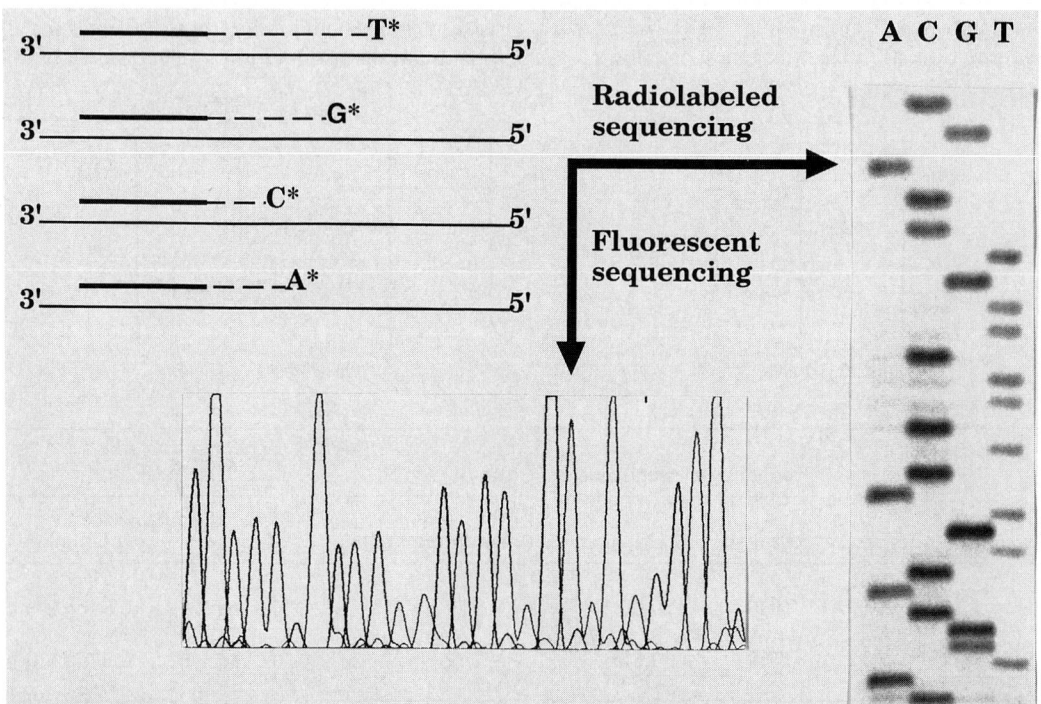

FIGURE 141-8. Dideoxy DNA sequencing using radiolabeled nucleotides or fluorescent tagged dideoxynucleotide chain terminators. Radiolabeled reactions are separated in four lanes of sequencing gel corresponding to the dideoxynucleotide terminator. Fluorescent sequencing reaction is read by an automated sequencer after electrophoresis in a single lane, using a different fluorescent tag for each dideoxynucleotide. (Courtesy of Jerry Radich, M.D., Seattle, WA.)

A. p53 exon 7

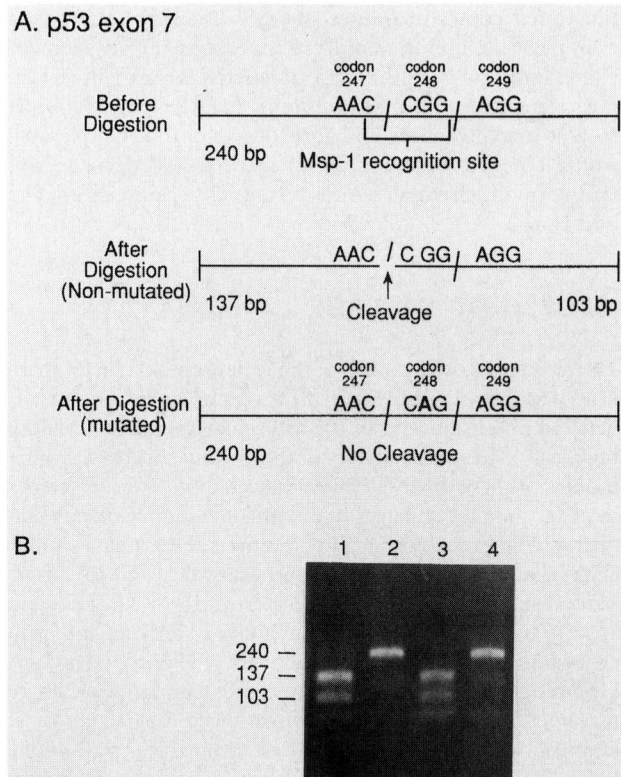

electrophoresed on a polyacrylamide gel with an increasing concentration gradient of denaturants (e.g., urea, formamide), there is an abrupt slowing of migration when the first strand melting occurs. Mutations affect the position in the gradient at which this dissociation begins, thereby changing the final distance that the fragment migrates on the gel. Modifications to this technique include the addition of a G+C clamp sequence, a PCR-directed addition of a high-melting-temperature GC-rich sequence to the end of the PCR-amplified fragment, to allow detection of mutations which affect the final complete strand dissociation into single-stranded DNA.[36] Additionally, gels with constant denaturant concentration can be used with predicted and experimentally determined optimal concentrations for maximal separation between mutated and wild type sequences.[37]

Mismatch analysis uses chemical modification and cleavage of mismatched base pairs to identify single-nucleotide changes in PCR amplified fragments.[38] A wild type fragment is 5′ end labeled with ^{32}P-ATP and T4 polynucleotide kinase, denatured and reannealed with an unlabeled mutated fragment to form heteroduplexes. Nonannealing cytosines and thymines can be modified with hydroxylamine and osmium tetraoxide, respectively. Subsequent treatment with piperidine cleaves at modified bases. The presence and position of single-nucleotide mutations can be recognized by electrophoresis on sequencing denaturing polyacrylamide gels.

SAMPLE PROCESSING

Polymerase Chain Reaction

The sensitivity of PCR permits amplification of DNA and RNA from extremely small amounts of tissue and after partial degradation of DNA in stored and fixed samples. Routine PCR of single-copy genes in genomic DNA requires only 50 ng of DNA or 10^4 cells.[39] Protocols for PCR analysis of human DNA in cotton-swabbed samples, endoscopic biopsies, whole blood (10 μL), and stool samples are available.[40-42] Crude lysates from detergent and protease-solubilized cells are sufficient for most applications. DNA amplification is possible from air-dried blood smears, ethanol-fixed tissue, and 5- to 10-μ, formalin-fixed, paraffin-embedded sections.[21]

In situ Hybridization

Previous requirements for frozen tissue sections are no longer necessary for most applications and many investigators have used paraformaldehyde-fixed specimens with resultant improvements in morphology. Combinations of PCR and in situ methodologies have been tried successfully, possibly extending the usefulness of this technique to rare DNA and RNA sequences and less than optimally prepared tissues.[43]

Immunocytochemistry

The availability of antigen retrieval methods for enhancement of low signal intensities and detection in archival materials increases the range of this method.[7]

FIGURE 141-9. Polymerase chain reaction detection of mutation by restriction analysis. Digestion of p53 exon 7 amplification product with Msp1. **(A)** Amplification of exon 7 yields 240 bp product. Recognition of the Msp1 site (CCGG) permits digestion at codon 248 in nonmutated specimens, yielding 137 and 103 bp fragments. When codon 248 is mutated (in this case a G → A mutation), the enzyme site is not recognized, and the 240 bp product remains intact. **(B)** Agarose gel shows the results. Lanes 1 and 3 represent sites without evidence of mutation, lanes 2 and 4 represent sites with mutation. (Courtesy of Teri Brentnall, M.D., and Cyrus Rubin, M.D., Seattle, WA.)

the terminal nucleotides. The reaction products can be visualized by gel electrophoresis by radioactively labeling one oligonucleotide , or if the other oligonucleotide can be coupled to a solid phase support, the bound radioactivity can be measured. This method is applicable to any known single-base mutation, requires three oligonucleotides, including mutated and wild-type sequences, and optimization of the reaction for individual sequence variants.

SSCP analysis relies on the ability of single-base changes in a single-stranded DNA fragment to alter migration during electrophoresis in nondenaturing gels.[34] PCR products which are radioactively labeled during synthesis are denatured and electrophoresed on nondenaturing polyacrylamide gels. This is a very sensitive screening method for detecting unknown point mutations in amplified sequences.

DGGE uses the property of strand dissociation or melting of a double-stranded DNA fragment at increasing concentrations of denaturing agents to separate fragments by electrophoresis with a single nucleotide change.[35] A mutation within a melting domain affects the required denaturant concentration to cause strand dissociation. When a DNA fragment is

MOLECULAR APPROACHES TO THERAPY

Knowledge of the molecular pathogenesis of disease states and essential steps in host antipathogen and antitumor responses has led to attempts to manipulate target tissues by molecular approaches to repair cellular defects or improve disease outcome. Three approaches using evolving molecular and cellular biology techniques will be highlighted.

Gene Therapy

Theoretically, the identification of hereditary or acquired diseases due to the loss of a functioning gene product afford the opportunity to transfer a normal gene product into the affected cell or tissue lineage and permanently cure the disease.[44] Examples of defective genes and their target tissues are adenosine deaminase, a rare cause of immunodeficiency syndrome, and T lymphocytes; LDL receptor, which causes familial hypercholesterolemia, and hepatocytes; and cystic fibrosis transmembrane regulator (CFTR) and bronchial epithelial cells. Additional goals of gene therapy include introduction of cytokine genes into tumor-infiltrating lymphocytes to enhance immune response and tumor lysis, and cell marking with new gene products to aid in evaluation of experimental protocols. Most commonly, retroviral vectors are being used in animal and human gene therapy protocols. Retroviral vectors replace all viral gene sequences with the gene to be expressed and a selectable gene to enrich for cells which have incorporated the retroviral vector sequences. Flanking the replacement genes are the long-terminal repeat sequences (LTR) of the retrovirus which mediate chromosomal integration of the retroviral DNA intermediate within target cells. The retroviral construct is introduced by DNA transfection into a packaging cell line that has the missing retroviral genes necessary for viral assembly, retroviral RNA packaging, and infection of a target cell with subsequent LTR-mediated integration of the desired gene sequences. The helper virus produced by the packaging cell line which carries the genes to be expressed does not lead to productive infection in the target cells because the essential viral gene sequences are not included in the assembled virions.

Adoptive Immunotherapy

The ability to propagate and expand T lymphocytes in vitro and enhance their function by administration of cytokines has led to antitumor effects following patient infusion. The natural extension of this technique is to expand and activate CD8+ T cell clones reactive to defined viral or tumor antigens. Initial trials of this approach have proven effective against CMV infections in bone marrow transplant patients.[45]

Intracellular Immunization

Identification of specific viral DNA sequences necessary for viral replication or accumulation of viral gene products provides the possibility of inhibiting essential viral processes by diluting out the viral target sequences with additional non

functional copies introduced by gene transfer. A potential example is the HIV transactivation response (TAR) element, which interacts with the viral transactivator protein (tat) to greatly increase viral transcription.[46] A TAR element coupled to a strong promoter and introduced into T lymphocytes would compete for tat-TAR interactions and decrease viral transcription, essentially immunizing cells against future viral infection.

MODELS OF DISEASE

The rapid pace of discovery of the genes responsible for many inherited diseases and familial cancers holds the promise of detailed understanding of the molecular and cellular defects involved. Already available is the means to create animal models of these diseases, for easy availability of experimental material and first attempts to modify or eliminate disease with pharmacologic or biologic interventions. Transgenic animals enable overexpression of gene products targeted to specific tissues or cell lineages. Mice with overexpressed oncogenes as transgenes have been instrumental in studying the properties and interactions of these genes in whole animal models. Homologous recombination refers to the site-specific replacement of a modified gene introduced into a cell for its endogenous counterpart. This strategy enables the homozygous deletion or knock-out of a single gene, creating models of human diseases which are due to loss of function of a single gene. Evolving techniques should allow introduction of single-nucleotide mutations resulting in subtler alterations in gene function.

Transgenic Mice

DNA fragments including the protein coding sequence for the gene to be expressed, tissue-specific promoter and enhancer, and RNA splice and termination sequences are ligated to form the transgene construct. Fertilized eggs are harvested from a recently impregnated female mouse. A single oocyte is held by suction against a fine polished glass pipet tip, while a second glass needle is used to impale the eggs and inject the transgene construct in solution into the pronucleus (Fig. 141-10). Injected eggs are transferred to the uterus of a pseudopregnant female mouse. Approximately 10% of offspring will carry the transgene. One or multiple copies of the transgene integrate in a head to tail orientation usually at a single site located randomly in the mouse genome. The transfer of transgene DNA to the fertilized egg before cell division occurs usually results in all cells of the transgenic offspring carrying the transgene, including the germline, which enables establishment of a transgenic line. Transgene status is usually ascertained by Southern blot or PCR analysis of tail DNA.

Homologous Recombination

Mammalian cells integrate extrachromosomal DNA into homologous sites by a process called homologous recombination at a low frequency of 10^{-2} to 10^{-3} compared to nonhomologous sites of integration.[47] This necessitates a selection strat-

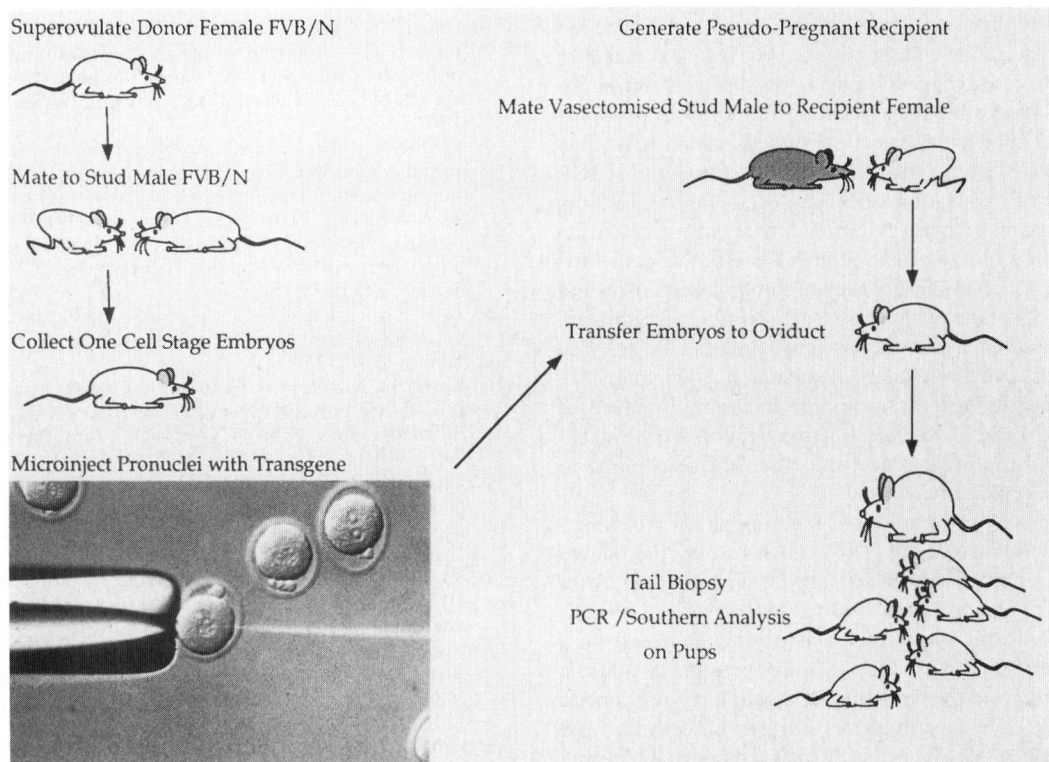

FIGURE 141-10. Methodology for producing transgenic mice by pronuclear microinjection of DNA. (Courtesy of Grant MacGregor, M.D., Atlanta, GA.)

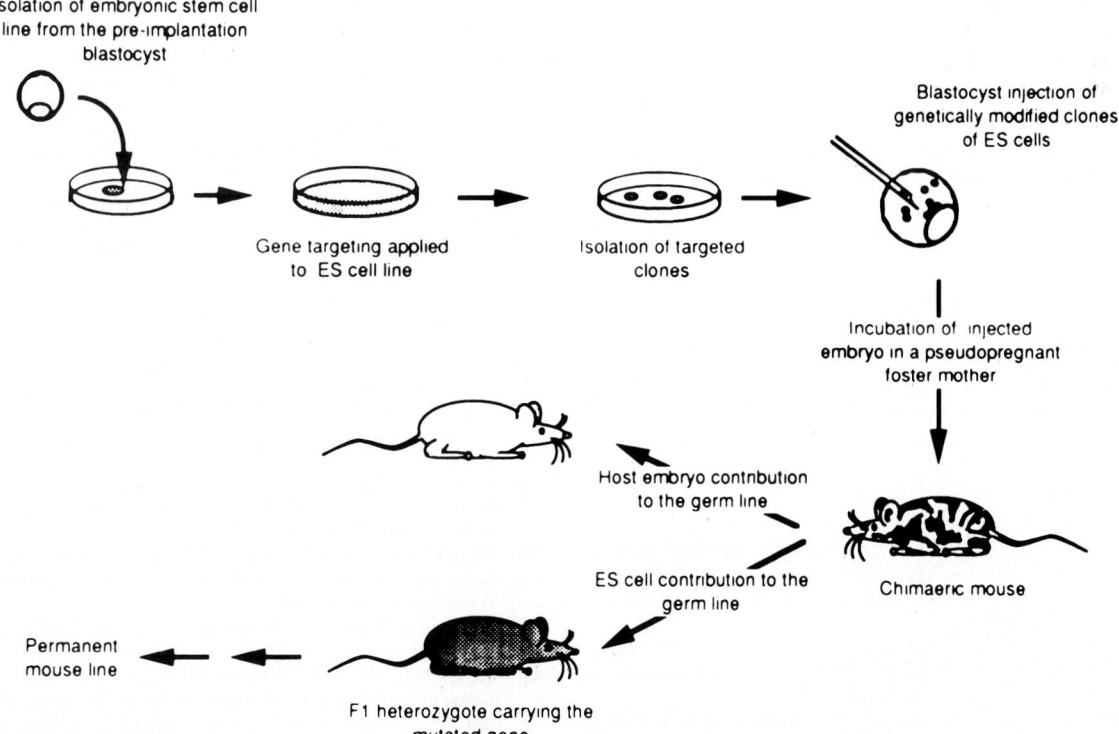

FIGURE 141-11. Homologous recombination is used to create gene-ablated mouse models. (From Bradley A, Hasty P, Davis A, Ramirez-Solis R. Modifying the mouse: design and desire. Biotechnology (NY) 1992;10:534.)

egy to identify those cells in which the introduced gene has correctly replaced one endogenous copy. The usual means of disabling the inserted gene copy is to replace internal sequences with a selectable marker such as neomycin phosphotransferase. This enables selection of cells which have integrated the transfected gene. Negative selection against cells with nonhomologous integration can be achieved by adding a selectable gene, such as thymidine kinase, to the construct outside the homologous gene sequences. Homologous integrations will preferentially use the homologous sequences and delete the tk portion of the construct. Nonhomologous integrants will often retain the tk genes and can be selected against with the thymidine kinase substrate, ganciclovir. Additional screening will be required, including pooling of transfected clones, PCR analysis using primers from the endogenous and modified gene copy, and Southern blots, to confirm gene replacement.

The cells used for homologous recombination are embryonic, totipotential stem cells (ES) which can be maintained in an undifferentiated state in cell culture (Fig. 141-11). After identication of an appropriate clone, the transfected ES cells are injected into the cavity of a blastocyst obtained from a day 3.5 gestation. The blastocysts can be reimplanted into a pregnant uterus and the resulting litters will include chimeric mice, with cellular contribution from the ES cells and the normal blastocyst cells. This can be easily recognized by using ES cells from a different genetic background than the blastocyst recipients, such that two coat colors will be present in chimeric mice. If the ES cells contribute to the germline, offspring can be generated with all cells derived from the ES cell line and possessing one inactivated allele. Matings between two of these offspring will generate 25% homozygotes with both copies inactivated.

This strategy has been successfully applied to the cystic fibrosis gene, CFTR, which is mutated in human patients resulting in a nonfunctional truncated protein. Mice homozygous for insertional disruptions in the endogenous CFTR gene develop cellular, electrophysical and pathologic changes of cystic fibrosis, including meconium ileus and intestinal obstruction.[48]

The reader is directed to Chapter 26, The Gastrointestinal Microflora; Chapter 46, Approach to Gastrointestinal Problems in the Immunocompromised Patient; and Chapter 131, Microbiologic Studies.

REFERENCES

1. Beck S, Koster H. Applications of dioxetane chemiluminescence probes to molecular biology. Anal Chem 1990;62:2258.
2. Sloand EM, Pitt E, Chiarello RJ. HIV testing: state of the art. JAMA 1991;266:2861.
3. van der Poel CL, Cuypers HTM, Reesink HW, et al. Confirmation of hepatitis C virus infection by new four-antigen recombinant immunoblot assay. Lancet 1991;337:317.
4. Harlow E, Lane D. Antibodies: a laboratory manual. Cold Spring Harbor: Cold Spring Harbor Laboratory, 1988.
5. van der Poel CL, Reesink HW, Schaasberg W, et al. Infectivity of blood seropositive for hepatitis C virus antibodies. Lancet 1990;335:558.
6. Chien DY, Choo Q-L, Tabrizi A, et al. Diagnosis of hepatitis C virus (HCV) infection using an immunodominant chimeric polyprotein to capture circulating antibodies: reevaluation of the role of HCV in liver disease. Proc Natl Acad Sci USA 1992;89:10011.
7. Shi SR, Key ME, Kalra KL. Antigen retrieval in formalin-fixed, paraffin-embedded tissues: an enhancement method for immunohistochemical staining based on microwave oven heating of tissues sections. J Histochem Cytochem 1991;39:741.
8. Saiki RK, Gelfand DH, Stoffel S, et al. Primer-directed enzymatic amplification of DNA with a thermostable DNA polymerase. Science 1988;239:487.
9. Li H, Gyllensten UB, Cui X, et al. Amplification and analysis of DNA sequences in single human sperm and diploid cells. Nature 1988;335:414.
10. Castillo I, Bartolome J, Quiroga JA, Carreno V. Comparison of several PCR procedures for detection of serum HCV-RNA using different regions of the HCV genome. J Virol Methods 1992;38:71.
11. Okamoto H, Okada S, Sugiyama Y, et al. Detection of hepatitis C virus RNA by a two-stage polymerase chain reaction with two pairs of primers deduced from the 5' noncoding region. Jpn J Exp Med 1990;60:215.
12. Kawasaki ES. Amplification of RNA. In: Ennis MA, Gelfand DH, Sninsky JJ, White TJ, eds. PCR protocols: a guide to methods and applications. San Diego: Academic Press, 1990:21.
13. Brunetto MR, Stemler M, Schodel F. Identification of HBV variants which cannot produce precore derived HBeAg and may be responsible for severe hepatitis. Ital J Gastroenterol 1989;21:151.
14. Omata M, Ehata T, Yokosuka O, Hosoda K, Ohto M. Mutations in the precore region of hepatitis B virus DNA in patients with fulminant and severe hepatitis. N Engl J Med 1991;324:1699.
15. Relman DA, Loutit JS, Schmidt TM, Falkow S, Tompkins LS. The agent of bacillary angiomatosis: an approach to the identification of uncultured pathogens. N Engl J Med 1990;323:1573.
16. Wilson KH, Blitchington R, Frothingham R, Wilson JAP. Phylogeny of the Whipple's-disease-associated bacterium. Lancet 1991;338:474.
17. Lazizi Y, Elfassi E, Pillot J. Detection of hepatitis C virus sequences in sera with controversial serology by nested polymerase chain reaction. J Clin Microbiol 1992;30:931.
18. Shibata D, Martin WJ, Appleman MD, et al. Detection of cytomegalovirus DNA in peripheral blood of patients infected with human immunodeficiency virus. J Infect Dis 1988;158:1185.
19. Kaneko S, Miller RH, Feinstone SM, et al. Detection of hepatitis B virus DNA in patients with chronic hepatitis using the polymerase chain reaction assay. Proc Natl Acad Sci USA 1989;86:312.
20. Wright TL, Mamish D, Combs C, et al. Hepatitis B virus and apparent non-A, non-B hepatitis. Lancet 1992;339:952.
21. Impraim CC, Saiki RK, Ehrlich HA, Teplitz RL. Analysis of DNA extracted from formalin-fixed, paraffin-embedded tissues by enzymatic amplification and hybridization with sequence-specific oligonucleotides. Biochem Biophys Res Commun 1987;142:710.
22. Yap EPH, McGee JO. Slide PCR: DNA amplification from cell samples on microscopic glass slides. Nucl Acids Res 1991;19:4294.
23. Kaneko S, Murakami S, Unoura M, Kobayashi K. Quantitation of hepatitis C virus RNA by competitive polymerase chain reaction. J Med Virol 1992;37:278.
24. Ausubel FM, Brent R, Moore DA, et al. Current protocols in molecular biology. New York: Greene Publishing Associates and Wiley-Interscience, 1987.
25. Boehringer Mannheim Biochemicals. Biochemical applications manual. Indianapolis: Boehringer Mannheim, 1989.
26. Mason AL, Wick M, White HM, et al. Increased hepatocyte expression of hepatitis B virus transcription in patients with features of fibrosing cholestatic hepatitis. Gastroenterology 1993;105:237.
27. Yunis JJ. Mid-prophase chromosomes: the attainment of 2000 bands. Hum Genet 1981;56:293.
28. Rabinovitch PS. Practical considerations for DNA content and

cell cycle analysis. In: Bauer KD, Duque RE, Sharkey TV, eds. Clinical flow cytometry: principles and application. Baltimore: Williams & Wilkins, 1993:117.

29. Lopez F, Belloc F, Lacombe F, et al. Modalities of synthesis of Ki67 antigen during the stimulation of lymphocytes. Cytometry 1991;12:42.

30. Bravo R, Frank R, Blandell PA, Macdonald-Bravo H. Cyclin/ PCNA is the auxiliary protein of DNA polymerase d. Nature 1987;326:515.

31. Bodmer WF, Bailey C, Bodmer J, et al. Localization of the gene for familial adenomatous polyposis on chromosome 5. Nature 1987;328:614.

32. Bos JL, Fearon ER, Hamilton SR, et al. Prevalence of ras gene mutations in human colorectal cancers. Nature 987;327:293.

33. Landegren U, Kaiser R, Sanders J, Hood L. A ligase-mediated gene detection technique. Science 1988;241:1077.

34. Orita M, Suzuki Y, Sekiya T, Hayashi K. Rapid and sensitive detection of point mutations and DNA polymorphisms using the polymerase chain reaction. Genomics 1989;5:874.

35. Myers RM, Lumelsky N, Lerman L, Maniatis T. Detection of single base substitutions in total genomic DNA. Nature 1985;313:495.

36. Sheffield VC, Cox DR, Lerman LS, Myers RM. Attachment of a 40-base-pair G+C-rich sequence (GC-clamp) to genomic DNA fragments by the polymerase chain reaction results in improved detection of single-base changes. Proc Natl Acad Sci USA 1989;86:232.

37. Borresen AL, Hovig E, Smith-Sorensen B, et al. Constant denaturant gel electrophoresis as a rapid screening technique for p53 mutations. Proc Natl Acad Sci USA 1991;88:8405.

38. Montandon AJ, Green PM, Giannelli F, Bentley DR. Direct detection of point mutations by mismatch analysis: applications to haemophilia B. Nucl Acid Res 1989;17:3347.

39. Saiki RK. Amplification of genomic DNA. In: Innis MA, Gelfand DH, Sninsky JJ, White TJ, eds. PCR protocols: a guide to methods and applications. San Diego: Academic Press, 1990:13.

40. Kawasaki ES. Sample preparation from blood, cells, and other fluids. In: Innis MA, Gelfand DH, Sninsky JJ, White TJ, eds. PCR protocols: a guide to methods and applications. San Diego: Academic Press, 1990:146.

41. Lohr M, Brenner DA, Rooney JF, Nelson JA. Application of the polymerase chain reaction in gastroenterological endoscopy. Endoscopy 1992;24:779.

42. Sidransky D, Tokino T, Hamilton SR, et al. Identification of ras oncogene mutations in the stool of patients with curable colorectal tumors. Science 1992;256:102.

43. Nuovo GJ, Gorgone GA, MacConnell P, Margiotta M, Gorevic PD. In situ localization of PCR-amplified human and viral cDNAs. PCR Methods Appl 1992;2:117.

44. Miller AD. Human gene therapy comes of age. Nature 1992;357: 455.

45. Greenberg PD, Goodrich JM, Riddell SR. Adoptive immunotherapy of human cytomegalovirus infection: potential role in protection from disease progression. Transplant Proc 1991;23: 97.

46. Sullenger BA, Gallardo HF, Ungers GE, Gilboa E. Overexpression of TAR sequences renders cells resistant to human immunodeficiency virus replication. Cell 1990;63:601.

47. Bradley A, Ramirez-Solis R, Zheng H, Hasty P, Davis A. Genetic manipulation of the mouse via gene targeting in embryonic stem cells. In: Postimplantation development in the mouse. Ciba Foundation symposium 165. Chichester: Wiley, 1992: 256.

48. Dorin JR, Dickenson P, Alton EW, et al. Cystic fibrosis in the mouse by targeted insertional mutagenesis. Nature 1992;359: 211.

Index

Page numbers followed by *f* indicate figures; those followed by *t* indicate tabular material. Page numbers in boldface indicate major discussions.

A

AA. *See* Amyloidosis, secondary
AAPC. *See* Attenuated adenomatous polyposis coli
Abdomen. *See also* Acute abdomen
  anatomy. *See* Abdominal cavity; *specific organ*
  auscultation, 786, 802. *See also* Bowel sounds
  imaging, 2654*f*, 2654–2655. *See also specific modality*
  inspection, 739, 801, 801*t*
  palpation, 739. *See also* Abdominal tenderness; Murphy's sign; Rebound tenderness
  radiographic examination (x-rays), 761, 806–807, 807*f*, 870. *See also* Radiologic examination
    with intra-abdominal abscess, 2291
  trauma. *See* Abdominal trauma
Abdominal abscess. *See* Abscess(es), intra-abdominal
Abdominal aorta, 2495*f*
Abdominal aortic aneurysm, 795
  pain with, 786
  ruptured
    clinical features, 795, 2316
    diagnostic studies, 2316
    differential diagnosis, 2316
    epidemiology, 2316
    etiology, 2316
    retroperitoneal bleeding with, 2316–2317
    treatment, 795, 2316–2317
Abdominal aortography, in Zollinger-Ellison syndrome, 1437
Abdominal bloating. *See* Bloating
Abdominal bruit. *See* Bruit(s)
Abdominal cavity, **2278–2288**
  anatomy, 2280–2282
    cross-sectional, **2646–2649**
  congenital anomalies, 2280–2281
  embryology, **2278–2280**, 2279*f*
  ultrasound evaluation, **2684–2686**
    correlative imaging, 2685–2686
    technical applications, 2684
Abdominal compartments, 2280
Abdominal cramping
  in celiac disease, 1648–1649
  in inflammatory bowel disease, 1774
  with VIPoma syndrome, 2135
Abdominal distention, 801. *See also* Lactose, intolerance; Malabsorption; Pseudoobstruction
  with acute abdominal pain, 786
  in celiac disease, 1648–1649
  in immunocompromised patient, 1001
  with intestinal ischemia, 2500
  with intestinal obstruction, 786, 798
  in irritable bowel syndrome, 82, 1835

  nausea and, 734
  pathogenic mechanisms, 1863
Abdominal epilepsy, 2439
Abdominal fluid collections. *See* Fluid collection(s)
Abdominal ligaments. *See specific ligament*
Abdominal mass(es). *See also* Tumor(s)
  with colonic ulcers, 1821
  contrast radiology, indications for, 2643
  with omental and mesenteric tumors, 2303
  with omental torsion, 2304
  with pancreatic cancer, 2120
  with pancreatic cyst, 2062
  with pneumatosis intestinalis, 1826
  with small bowel tumor, 1699*t*
  in Whipple's disease, 1636
Abdominal migraine, 761, 2439
Abdominal nerves. *See also specific organ(s), innervation;* Vagus nerve(s)
  nociceptive, 752
  nonnociceptive, 752
Abdominal pain, **750–771**, 904, 1861. *See also* Dyspepsia; Pelvic pain; Visceral pain
  and abnormal liver chemistries, 911
  acute, **757–760**. *See also* Acute abdomen
    abdominal distention with, 786
    abdominal examination with, 759
    atypical, 758–760
    facial expression and, 759
    gynecologic causes, 787
    history-taking with, 757–758
    laboratory findings in, 760
    physical findings with, 758–760
    in pregnancy, 1028–1030
      nonobstetric causes, 1029–1030
      obstetric causes, 1030
    relieving and aggravating factors, 758
    subjective characterization, 757–758
    temporal considerations, 758, 786
  with acute diabetic acidosis, 2428
  with acute mesenteric ischemia, 2500, 2501*t*
  adhesion-related, 2822
    laparoscopy for, 2827–2828
  associated symptoms, 785–786
  of bacterial colitis, 1891
  with bacterial overgrowth, 1677
  in celiac disease, 1648–1649
  character, 750
  of choledocholithiasis, 2196
  chronic, **760–768**. *See also* Pain, chronic
    characteristics, 765
    idiopathic, 762
    intermittent, 760–761
      causes, 760, 760*t*
      diagnosis, 760–761
      patient evaluation with, 760–761
      treatment, 761

  intractable, 760, 762–768
    biofeedback for, 767
    clinical features, 762–764, 763*t*
    diagnosis, 765–766
    epidemiology, 764
    hypnosis for, 767
    management, 766*t*, 766–768
    pathogenesis, 764–765, 765*f*
    patient evaluation, 765–766
    prognosis for, 764
    psychotherapy with, 767–768
    relaxation training for, 767
  management, 761–762, 766*t*, 766–768, 3044–3045
  neurophysiology, 757
  psychologic responses to, 760
  syndromes, **2403–2407**, 2406*t*
  undiagnosed, 762
  unrelenting, 761–762
    diagnosis, 761
    drug therapy for, 761–762
    nerve destruction therapy for, 762
    patient evaluation with, 761
    transcutaneous electrical nerve stimulation for, 762
    treatment, 761–762
  with chronic pancreatitis, 2095, 2167
  with constipation, 869
  in Crohn's disease, 1757, 1757*t*
    in children, 1798
  in Cronkhite-Canada syndrome, 1960
  with cystic duct remnant, 2267
  with defecation, 760
  in diabetes mellitus, 2428
  diagnostic laparoscopy for, 2822, 2827–2828
  with diarrhea, 826, 826*t*
  with diverticulitis, 1881
  with duodenal ulcer perforation, 1530
  duration, 758, 786
  economic impact, 750
  in elderly, 970
  epigastric, 755
  gas and, 773–774
  with groin hernia, 2283
  gynecologic causes, 2822
  health impact, 750
  in HIV-infected (AIDS) patient, 2310–2311, 2338
  in ileus, 798
  in immunocompromised patient, 1001–1002
  intensity, 750
  with intra-abdominal abscess, 2291
  in irritable bowel syndrome, 1833–1834
    treatment, 1850
  laparoscopy with, 2822, 2827–2828
  lateralized, 755
  in liver transplant recipient, 1002

1

Brown-Mueller T-fasteners, 2811, 2812f, 2814
Brown pigment stones
  bacteria and, 2214
  chemical composition, 2192t, 2192–2193
  clinical associations, 2192t, 2192–2193
  pathogenesis, 2192–2193, 2214, 2215f
BRS-3 receptor, 55
Bruber's syndrome, with pancreatic cysts, 2062
Brucellosis (Brucella infection)
  granulomas in, 2431t–2432t
  pancreatitis caused by, 2072
Bruit(s), 911
  abdominal, 739
  with pancreatic cancer, 2120
Brunner's gland(s), 1310, 1310f, 1557, 2862f
  formation, 549
  hamartomas, 1696
  hyperplasia, 1484, 1484f, 2861
  hypertrophy, in renal failure, 2444
  submucosal, color fig 28
Brush border, 143
  cytoskeleton, 1561
  damage, 824t
    mechanisms, 821
  membrane, electrochemical gradient across, 473f
Brush-border carbohydrase(s), 410–422, 411t.
    See also Brush-border hydrolase(s);
    specific enzyme
  integrated function, 417
Brush-border hydrolase(s). See also Brush-border
    carbohydrase(s); Brush-border
    peptidase(s); specific enzyme
  oligopeptide hydrolysis by, 458f, 460f, 460–
    461
Brush-border peptidase(s), 461t
  oligopeptide hydrolysis by, 458f, 460f, 460–
    461
Bruton's X-linked agammaglobulinemia,
    gastrointestinal involvement in, 995
BSP. See Sulfobromophthalein
BSS. See Bismuth subsalicylate
Buboes, in Chlamydia trachomatis infection, 1906
Buccopharyngeal aponeurosis, 160
Budd-Chiari syndrome, 2433, 2437–2438, 2780
  angiography in, 2781, 2781f
  ascites in, 930
  computed tomography in, 2718
  etiology, 2664
  magnetic resonance imaging in, 2738
  percutaneous transluminal angioplasty in, 2791
  ultrasound examination in, 2664
Budesonide enemas, in ulcerative colitis, 1780
Bulimia nervosa, 727–729, 741, 1547, 2442
  clinical manifestations, 728
  complications, 1120, 1120t
  delayed gastric emptying in, 1323
  diagnosis, 728
  diagnostic criteria, 728t
  epidemiology, 723, 727
  etiology, 727
  pathogenesis, 727–728
  physical manifestations, 2442t
  signs and symptoms, 1120, 1120t
  small bowel dysmotility with, 1594
  and substance abuse, 1120
  treatment, 728–729
Bulk-forming agents
  mechanism of action, 851t
  side effects, 851t
Bullae, 801t
Bullous pemphigoid
  esophageal involvement, differential diagnosis,
    1293
  esophageal involvement in, 1292t, 1292–1293
  gastrointestinal involvement in, 963
  pathophysiology, 1292–1293
Bullous skin disease, gastrointestinal involvement
    in, 962–963. See also specific disease

Buprenorphine (Temgesic SL), dosage and
    administration, for pancreatic cancer,
    2125t
Bupropion (Wellbutrin), 2945
Burkitt's lymphoma, 582
Burn(s)
  esophageal, 2564
  gastric, 2564
  oropharyngeal, 1285–1286
  outcome, effects of enteral dietary regimens on,
    498
Buspar. See Buspirone
Buspirone (Buspar), 633
  for chronic abdominal pain, 762
  for generalized anxiety disorder, 2946
Busulfan, gastrointestinal side effects, 990
Butterfly dermatitis, 801t
Button batteries. See Batteries
Butylated hydroxyanisole, anticancer effects,
    1984, 1984t
Butylated hydroxytoluene, anticancer effects,
    1984
N-Butyl-2-cyanoacrylate (histoacryl), for variceal
    bleeding, 2552–2553
Butyrophenone(s), 633
  for nausea and vomiting, 744t, 746
Butyrovibrio, in colonic flora, 609
B vitamins. See Vitamin B
Byler's disease, 900
Bypass enteritis syndrome, after jejunoileal
    bypass, 1687

C

Ca²⁺. See Calcium
CA 19-9, 1931, 2121
  in pancreatic cancer, 2102, 2121
  in pseudocysts, 2085
Ca²⁺-ATPase pump. See ATPase(s), Ca²⁺-
Cachectin. See also Tumor necrosis factor
  in sepsis, 503
Cachexia, cancer, 1985
Cadmium, 1058
Café-au-lait spots, in Cowden's disease, 1959
Caffeine
  effects on resting energy expenditure, 509
  metabolism, 600t
  as stimulus of acid secretion and serum gastrin,
    303
CAGA gene, 1357
CAGE test, 1115
Cajal's cells, 1162
Calbindin
  D, 477
  neurons reactive for, 12
Calcification
  in hereditary pancreatitis, 2167, 2167f
  metastatic, 2445
  pancreatic, 2120
  tumors that demonstrate, 2666
Calcitonin, 225
  effects, on gastric emptying, 199
  gene expression, 33, 33f
  intracerebroventricular injection, inhibition of
    pentagastrin and meal-stimulated gastric
    acid secretion, 304
  secretory effects, 341t
  tumors secreting, 837
Calcitonin gene-related peptide, 8t, 225, 622
  in appetite regulation, 485
  in biliary tract, 263
  effects
    on gastric emptying, 198–199
    on lower esophageal sphincter, 174, 175t
    on pancreatic secretion, 368, 373t, 458–459
  in esophageal and lower esophageal sphincter
    neurons, 162
  gene expression, 33, 33f

as inhibitory neurotransmitter, 76, 174, 373t
  and intestinal maturation, 559
  intracerebroventricular injection, inhibition of
    pentagastrin and meal-stimulated gastric
    acid secretion, 304
  as neurotransmitter, 76
  release, 27
Calcitriol. See also 1,25-Dihidroxyvitamin D₃
  synthesis, 473
Calcium. See also Smooth muscle, activator
    calcium
  absorption, 2381
    in elderly, 976
    maturation, 556
  in acetylcholine-induced inward current, 244
  biliary, and gallstone formation, 2191
  bioavailability, 476
  and colon cancer, 1976
  cytoplasmic, in colonic contraction, 244–245
  cytosolic, 89, 91, 149
    concentrations, 95
    during contraction of isolated cells, 93–94,
      94f
    effects on bile formation, 391
    measurement, 95
    regulation, 92–93, 93f, 95f, 95–96
  deficiency, 841t, 1048t, 1051–1052
    in short bowel syndrome, 1685–1686
  dietary, 476
    absorption, 476–477, 477t
      decreased, 477–478
      disorders, 477–478, 478t
      increased, 477
    sources, 476
  effects on pancreatic secretion, 377
  in esophageal smooth muscle contraction, 171,
    172f
  extrusion mechanisms, in plasma membrane,
    95
  in gallbladder muscle function, 265
  and gastrin release, 1433
  intake, in nutritional support (TPN), 1073
  intracellular
    in intracellular signal transduction, 307–310
    regulation, 335
  losses, 1045
  malabsorption
    in celiac disease, 1649
    with short bowel syndrome, 1690
    with tropical sprue, 1632–1633
  mobilization, 92–93
    in cells of longitudinal muscle layer, 94–95
  in pancreatic juice, 362
  and pancreatic secretion, 369–372
  protective effect, against colon adenomas and
    cancers, 1917
  requirements, 1051
    for acetylcholine induced contraction of
      esophageal circular muscle, 171
  as second messenger, in intracellular signaling,
    341t, 342
  sequestration, 103
  serum. See also Hypercalcemia; Hypocalcemia
    in pancreatitis, 2080
  in spike potential activity, 210
  supplementation, 1051–1052
    indications for, 477
    with short bowel syndrome, 1690
  supplements, 1051, 1051t
  transport, 87–88
    transcellular, 477
  uptake and release, in smooth muscle cells, 88
Calcium acetate, 1051t
Calcium bilirubinate, formation, 2214, 2215f
Calcium carbonate
  pharmacology, 1390
  as stimulus of acid secretion and serum gastrin,
    303
  stones, and chronic pancreatitis, 2676

Clostridium difficile (infection), 1630, 1891. *See also* Pseudomembranous (entero)colitis, *Clostridium difficile*
in bone marrow recipient, 993–994
carriage, 1899
(entero)colitis, 688, **1897–1903**, 2874
in bone marrow recipient, 994
in cancer patient, 990
clinical features, 1899–1901
diagnosis, 1901
epidemiology, 1899
etiology, 1897–1898
fulminant, 1900
immunity, 1898–1899
in immunocompromised patient, treatment, 1009
pathogenesis, 1898
relapse, 1902–1903
therapy, 1901–1902
treatment, 1902–1903
in colonic flora, 610
colonization
of antibiotic-treated patient, 615
in infants, 1899
colonoscopy in, 1901
in Crohn's disease, 1901
cytotoxin, 1898
detection, 2885
titer, 1901
diagnosis, 2885, 2894
diarrhea, 826t, 827, 1899, 1900t
chronic, 830
in elderly, 979
in immunocompromised patient, 1000
nosocomial, 831
differential diagnosis, 2355
in elderly, 975
endotoxin, 2499
enterotoxin, 1898
secretory effects, 341t
and exacerbations of inflammatory bowel disease, 1756
exotoxins, 1898
histopathology, 2886
in HIV-infected (AIDS) patient, treatment, 2324t
in immunocompromised patient, 1001–1002
anorexia with, 999–1000
bleeding caused by, 1003
fever with, 1006
in inflammatory bowel disease, 1901, 2895
interaction with colonic flora, 613
latex bead agglutination assay, 1901
manifestations, 1899, 1900t
in marrow transplant recipient, 2441
nontoxicogenic, 1898
nosocomial, 1899, 1899f
hospital control measures, 1903
transmission, 1149–1150
pathogenicity, 1898
properties, 1897–1898
and protein-losing gastroenteropathy, 1728
sigmoidoscopy in, 1901
stool culture for, 1901
stool cytotoxin assay, 1901
strains, 1898
toxin, 2330
antibodies to, 1898, 1898f
detection, 1149
toxin A, 1898, 1901
toxin B, 1898, 1901
transmission, 1899
in ulcerative colitis, 1901
weakly toxicogenic, 1898
Clostridium perfringens (infection)
acute jejunitis caused by, 1726
alpha-toxin, 1615
antibiotic-associated diarrhea, 1615

beta-toxin, 1615
diagnosis, 2884–2885
diarrhea, 826t, 1606, 1615
enterotoxin, 1614–1615
food poisoning, 1609t–1610t, 1614–1615
clinical features, 1615
diagnosis, 1615
differential diagnosis, 1615
pathogenesis, 1614
in immunocompromised patient, 1001–1002
in intra-abdominal abscesses, 2290, 2290t
Clostridium septicum (infection)
in blood culture, 2892
in bone marrow recipient, 993–994
iliopsoas abscess, treatment, 1009
in immunocompromised patient, 989, 993–994, 1001
bleeding caused by, 1003
diarrhea caused by, 1000
treatment, 1009
typhlitis caused by, 1001–1002, 1009
CLOtest, for *Helicobacter pylori, color fig 30,* 1352, 1353f, 1462
Clotrimazole
adverse effects, 1246
for esophageal candidiasis, 1246
for immunocompromised patient
for *Candida* infections, 1010
for mucosal fungal infections, 1010
prophylaxis, 1008
Clotting factors
assessment in liver disease, 913
deficits, 2433
CNNA. *See* Culture-negative neutrocytic ascites
Coagulation, 3012–3013. *See also* Prothrombin time
effects of exploratory laparotomy on, 3041
Coagulation necrosis, 3012–3013
Coagulopathy
in abetalipoproteinemia, 2390
and paracentesis, 933
Cobalamin. *See* Vitamin B$_{12}$
Cobalt, 1058
Cobblestone appearance, 1767
in eosinophilic gastroenteritis, 2465
Cocaine, 1113
abuse/dependence, 1117–1118
clinical features, 1118
diagnosis, 1118
treatment, 1118
abuse potential, 1118
adverse effects, in small bowel, 1722
body packers, gastrointestinal problems in, 1722
detection, in screening tests, 1122
freebasing, 1117
gastrointestinal effects, 2445
hepatotoxicity, 1117
intoxication, signs and symptoms, 1121t
ischemic colonic injury due to, 1818
metabolism, 1117
neuronal effects, 1117
pharmacology, 1115t, 1117
tolerance, 1118
withdrawal syndrome, 1118
COCA1 locus, 1987
Coccidioides
ascites formation with, 929
hepatic, in immunocompromised patient, 1005
Coccidioidomycosis
diagnosis, 2337
granulomas caused by, 2431t
retroperitoneal, 2318
Coccidiosis, small bowel biopsy in, 845t
Coccygeus muscle, 2656
Coccygodynia (pain in coccyx), 2046
functional, 2046
organic, 2046

Codeine
abuse, 1117
constipating effects, 1117
dosage and administration, for pancreatic cancer, 2125t
mechanism of action, 851t, 1847
metabolism, 600t, 1117
for short bowel syndrome, 1687
side effects, 851t
Coffee, and pancreatic cancer, 2115–2116
Coincidence detection, in positron emission tomography, 2744f
Colapinto needle, 2809, 2809f
Colchicine
effects
on acid secretion, 310
on nutrient absorption, 342t, 832, 1045, 1725
for familial Mediterranean fever, 2403
malabsorption caused by, 1045
steatorrhea caused by, 832
Cold-induced thermogenesis. *See* Thermogenesis, cold-induced
Cold lavage, for treating upper GI bleeding, 674
Colectomy
for colonic inertia, 876
cost, 3047t
in elderly, 981
emergency, for toxic megacolon, 1786
for familial adenomatous polyposis, 1951
with ileorectal anastomosis
in attenuated adenomatous polyposis coli, 1954
in familial adenomatous polyposis, 1951
in familial juvenile polyposis coli, 1958
ileostomy after, malignancy with, 1703t
indications for, 2841
laparoscopy in, 2833
with malignant polyps, 1934–1936
metabolic effects, 1682
with mucosal proctectomy and ileoanal pouch, for familial adenomatous polyposis, 1951
operative morality, 1935
partial, laparoscopy in, 2833
prophylactic, 1109
with juvenile polyposis, 1958
subtotal, with ileoproctostomy, in Crohn's disease, 1789
for toxic megacolon, 1790
in ulcerative colitis, 1786, 1799, 2841, 2845
Colestipol, for antibiotic-associated colitis and diarrhea, 1902
Colic
biliary. *See* Biliary colic
definition, 758
intestinal, 790
lead, 2432
with obstruction, 758, 798–799
renal, 758
Colic artery
left, 1739, 1741f, 2495f
middle, 1739, 1741f, 2494f–2495f
right, 1739, 1741f, 2494f–2495f
Colic vein(s)
middle, 2056, 2056f
superior right, 2056f
Coliforms, in small intestine flora, 609
Colipase
deficiency, 2385t
in fat malabsorption, 2097
pancreatic, 363, 430
deficiency, **2169**
properties, 431t
Colitic arthritis, with Crohn's disease, 1758–1759

of diffuse benign gastric mucosal abnormalities, 2851–2858
of discrete gastric lesions, 2858*t*, 2858–2861
in erosive gastropathy, 2852*t*, 2856, 2856*f*
esophageal, in opportunistic infections, 2849–2850, 2850*f*
of gastric cancer, 2846*f*
with gastric hypertrophy, 2852*t*
with gastric infection, 2852*t*
with gastric vascular ectasia, 2852*t*, 2856, 2856*f*
in gastritis, 2851–2856, 2852*t*, 2853*f*–2855*f*
in gastroesophageal reflux disease, 2847–2849, 2848*f*
in hiatal hernia, 2848–2849, 2849*f*
of ileum, 2861–2868
indications for, **2838–2879**
interpretation, **2838–2879**
orientation, 2837
in parasitic infections, 2889–2890
postgastrectomy, 2852*t*
of premalignant or malignant lesions, 2838–2846
of proximal small bowel, 2861–2868
risks, **2879–2880**, 2897
specimen
    fixation, 2837
    paraffin embedding, 2837
technical considerations, 2837*f*, **2837–2838**
Endoscopic pancreatography, in acute pancreatitis, 2078
Endoscopic papillotomy, 2218–2219
for sphincter of Oddi dysfunction or stenosis, 2070
Endoscopic resection therapy, 3015–3016
Endoscopic retrograde cholangiography, 2198, 2198*f*. *See also* Endoscopic retrograde cholangiopancreatography
in choledocholithiasis, 2216–2217, 2701
Endoscopic retrograde cholangiopancreatography, 843, 2198, 2199*f*, **2590–2598**
of annular pancreas, 2060
antibiotic prophylaxis and, 2591
applications, 2598
of benign bile duct strictures, 2594–2595
of biliary cysts, 2229
with Caroli's disease, 2595–2596
of cholangiocarcinoma, 2595
with choledochal cysts, 2595–2596
for choledocholithiasis, 2081
    after cholecystectomy, 2267, 2267*f*
with cholelithiasis, 2594
in chronic pancreatitis, 2101*f*, 2101–2102, 2102*f*, 2596–2597, 2597*f*
clinical implications, 2597–2598
complications, 2593, 2593*t*
    incidence, 2618, 2618*t*
consent for, 2591
cost, 2597
of cystic duct remnant, 2267
to diagnose papillary stenosis, 2241–2242
diagnostic
    complications, 2593, 2593*t*
    contraindications to, 2593
as diagnostic adjunct, 2598
endoscopic findings, 2593–2594
indications for, 921, 1760, 2260, 2592*t*, 2592–2593, 2676, 2795, 2833
infection risk with, 2623
instruments, 2591
of intrahepatic metastases, 2595
in jaundice, 905
of malignant bile duct strictures, 2595
manometry with, 2592
normal findings in, 2594, 2596
of pancreas divisum, 2061
in pancreatic cancer, 2121–2122, 2122*f*, 2123, 2123*f*, 2594, 2597, 2598*f*
with pancreatic pseudocyst, 2103

in pancreatitis, emergency treatment, 2081
pancreatitis caused by, 2073
patient positioning for, 2591
patient preparation, 2590–2591
versus percutaneous transhepatic cholangiography, 2795
of periampullary tumor, 2594
with postcholecystectomy syndrome, 2266
premedication for, 2591
preoperative, 2201
with primary sclerosing cholangitis, 2235–2236, 2236*f*
procedure, 2591
radiography with, 2591–2592
with recurrent pancreatitis and progressive jaundice, 2240*f*
results, 2593
of sclerosing cholangitis, 2595
sedation for, 2591
with sphincter of Oddi dysfunction, 2270, 2271*f*
technical considerations, 2590–2592
Endoscopic sclerotherapy. *See* Sclerotherapy
Endoscopic sphincterotomy (and gallstone removal), 2275, 2590, **2598–2604**
and acute pancreatitis, 2073
bleeding with, 2622
in chronic pancreatitis, 2105
clinical implications, 2603–2604
complications, 2602–2603
contraindications to, 2602
in elderly, 982, 2599, 2602*f*
indications for, 2601–2602
instruments, 2598–2599
with pancreas divisum, 2105
patient preparation, 2598
procedure, 2599–2601, 2600*f*–2601*f*
results, 2603
risks, 2602–2603
technical considerations, 2598–2601
Endoscopic strip biopsy, 3015, 3016*f*
Endoscopic surveillance, 1705, 2565–2566
of Barrett's esophagus, 1235, 1265, 1270, 1367, 3017, 3019
for esophageal adenocarcinoma, 1270
Endoscopic treatment. *See also* Bleeding, upper GI, endoscopic control; Sphincter of Oddi, manometry; Upper gastrointestinal endoscopy
in acute pancreatitis, 2081–2082
for chronic pancreatitis, 2105
of colonic adenomas, 3032–3033, 3034*f*
for gastric cancer, 1514
for lower GI bleeding, 690
for prevention of recurrent hemorrhage, 675–676
for sessile lesions, **3011–3038**
for upper GI variceal bleeding, **2969–2991**
Endoscopic ultrasound. *See* Ultrasound, endoscopic
Endoscopy. *See also* Endoscopic treatment
anatomical considerations, 2542
in anisakiasis, 2371
antibiotic prophylaxis in, recommendations for, 2620, 2620*t*
of anus. *See* Anoscopy
of bezoar, 1545
with caustic ingestion, 1286
of colon. *See* Colon, endoscopic examination; Colonoscopy
for diagnosis of small bowel tumors, 1701*t*, 1702–1703
in diverticulitis, 1883
duodenal bulb, 2547–2548
of duplication cysts, 1164
equipment. *See also* Endoscope(s)
    disinfection, 2548
    preventive maintenance, 2625–2626
with esophageal diverticula, 1168
fiberoptic, advantages, 2567

in gastric cancer, 1507–1508, 1511
with gastrointestinal bleeding, 2782
in graft-versus-host disease, 1291, 2467
in herpetic esophagitis, 1248
of heterotopic gastric mucosa, 1165
in immunoproliferative small-intestinal disease, 1703
infection risk with, 2623
in inflammatory bowel disease, *color fig 34*, 1761*f*, 1764–1768, 1769*f*, **1769–1770**
of lower esophageal rings, 1166–1167
with Mallory-Weiss tears, 1295–1296
medication-related complications, 2618–2621
    respiratory depression, 2619
    response to topical agents, 2619
of mesenteric ischemia, 2500
monitoring during, **2577**, 2624, 2625*t*
in obstruction and ileus, 808
pathological considerations, 2542
patient preparation, 2556–2557
in peptic ulcer disease, 1376*t*, 1376–1377
with pharyngoesophageal diverticula, 1168
postprocedure evaluation, 2624–2625
procedure-related complications, **2621–2624**
    bleeding, 2622–2623
    cardiopulmonary, 2621
    incidence, 2618, 2618*t*
    infection, 2623–2624
    instrument injury, 2618*t*, 2622, 2622*f*–2623*f*
    prevention or reduction, **2624–2626**
    recognition, 2624–2625
    types, 2618–2624
rectal, retroversion maneuver, *color fig 102*
of sigmoid colon. *See* Flexible sigmoidoscopy
in syphilitic esophagitis, 1252
upper GI. *See* Upper gastrointestinal endoscopy
in upper GI bleeding, 684, 2567
Endothelial cell(s), intestinal vasoregulation and, 529–530
Endothelin, secretory effects, 341*t*
Endotoxemia, hyperbilirubinemia associated with, 902
Endotoxin(s)
    Clostridium difficile, 2499
    of gram-negative bacteria, 2498–2499
    Shigella, 1893
Endotracheal intubation
    with caustic ingestion, 1286
    with sclerotherapy, 2973, 2981
Enema(s). *See also* Barium enema
    5-ASA, for diversion colitis, 1812
    for bowel preparation, 2576
    cleansing, colitis associated with, 2876
    colitis associated with, 1814–1815
    ethanol, 1815
    hydrofluoric acid, 1815
    hydrogen peroxide
        colitis caused by, 1815
        complications, 1815
    SCFA, with diversion colitis, 1811–1812
    small bowel, 1700, 2637, 2637*f*
        applications, 2637–2638
    vinegar, 1815
Energy, 486
    body stores, total, **499**
    expenditure. *See also* Basal energy expenditure; Resting energy expenditure
        of activity, 488, 1069
        calculated, 487
        components, 487–488
        measurement, 486–487
            by double-labeled water method, 487
        with severe pancreatitis, 2080
        for weight gain, 1069
    from food, 486
    intake, in nutritional support (TPN), 1068–1070, 1072
    losses, in urine, stool, and drainage from fistulas and wounds, 1069

Fitz-Hugh-Curtis syndrome, 930
FK506
　gastrointestinal complications with, 995
　metabolism, 600t
Flag sign, 965, 1048t
Flagyl. *See* Metronidazole
Flank tenderness, 739
Flatulence, 774–775, 2193
　increased, foodstuffs associated with, 1844,
　　1845t
Flatus. *See also* Gas
　in celiac disease, 1648–1649
　composition, 774–775
　poor control of, 2039
　selective passage of, 2039
　volume, 774–775
Flatus tube, 809
Flavin adenine dinucleotide, 1061
Flavin mononucleotide. *See* Riboflavin
Fleets Phospho Soda, 1052t
Fleroxacin, for infectious diarrhea, 829
Flexible fiberendoscopy, 2836–2837
Flexible sigmoidoscope(s), with integral
　　disposable sheath, 2572
Flexible sigmoidoscopy, **2571–2589.** *See also*
　　Colonoscopy
　applications, 870
　in chronic diarrhea, 844
　with collagenous colitis, 1809
　in diverticulitis, 1883
　indications for, 2582
　　high-yield, 2582–2584
　instrumentation, 2572
　patient positioning for, 2578
　technical considerations, 2572
　technique, 2578–2579
Flow cytometry, 1995, 2841
　in Barrett's esophagus, 1268–1269
　of cancer cells, 3057
　for cell cycle analysis, 3057
　in gastric cancer, 1510
Floxuridine, hepatic arterial infusion
　for colorectal cancer metastases, 2014
　and sclerosing cholangitis, 2234
Flu, vaccination/vaccine, 1128
Flubendazole, indications for, 2367
Fluconazole (Diflucan)
　adverse effects, 1246
　for esophageal candidiasis, 1246
　in immunocompromised patient
　　for *Candida* infections, 1010
　　for invasive fungal infections, 1010
　　for mucosal fungal infections, 1010
　　prophylactic, 1008
Flucytosine (Ancobon)
　adverse effects, 1247
　antifungal activity, 1247
　colitis caused by, 1820
　for esophageal candidiasis, 1247
　for invasive fungal infections, in
　　immunocompromised patient, 1010
Flufenamic acid, colitis caused by, 1819
Fluid(s)
　intake, in nutritional support (TPN), 1071–
　　1072
　overload, with total parenteral nutrition,
　　1077
　replacement, with obstruction, 809
　restriction, in portal hypertension–related
　　ascites, 947
　secretion, 327
　transport, in gallbladder, 394
Fluid and electrolytes
　absorption, abnormal, 814–815
　imbalance, with obstruction or ileus, 800
　secretion
　　abnormal, 815
　　salivary, **283–286**
Fluid collection(s)
　abdominal, ultrasound evaluation, 2684–2685

pancreatic
　drainage, percutaneous technique, **2807**
　magnetic resonance imaging, 2740
　in pancreatitis, 2651
peripancreatic
　computed tomography, 2724
　with pancreatitis, 2082
　in retroperitoneum, **2315–2316**
Flukes. *See also* Trematodes
　drug therapy for, 2364t
　liver. *See* Liver flukes
Flumazenil (Mazicon), 1114, 1116, 2577, 2619
　sedative effects, 2547
Fluorescein dye injection, study of small intestine
　　viability, 809–810
Fluorescent technique, evaluation of ischemic
　　bowel variability, 2502–2503
Fluoride, recommended dietary allowance, 1058
Fluorine-18, 2744–2745, 2745t
Fluorine-18 deoxyglucose
　compartment model for, 2747, 2747f
　metabolic imaging of tumors with, 2751–
　　2752, 2752f
　as metabolic tracer
　　in oncology, 2751
　　for positron emission tomography imaging,
　　　2746–2747
　tracer kinetic model, 2749
Fluorine-18 misonidazole, for positron emission
　　tomography imaging, 2747
Fluorodeoxyuridine, as radiation sensitizer, 2525
Fluoroscopy, guidance for biopsy, 2802
5-Fluorouracil
　colitis caused by, 1819–1820, 2876
　for colon cancer, 2010, 2011f, 2014
　erosive enteritis with, 1726
　for esophageal cancer
　　concomitant radiation and, 1264
　　infusional, 1263
　　neoadjuvant, 1264
　for gastric cancer, 1513
　gastrointestinal side effects, 989–990
　for metastatic pancreatic endocrine tumors,
　　2150t
　for pancreatic cancer, 2124
　as radiosensitizer, 1264, 2525
5-Fluorouracil, doxorubicin, and cisplatin (FAP)
　for gastric cancer, 1514
　for metastatic pancreatic endocrine tumors,
　　2150t
5-Fluorouracil, doxorubicin, and methyl-CCNU
　　(FAMe protocol), for gastric cancer,
　　1513
5-Fluorouracil, doxorubicin, and mitomycin C
　　(FAM protocol)
　for gastric cancer, 1513
　for pancreatic cancer, 2124
5-Fluorouracil, doxorubicin, and triazinate, for
　　gastric cancer, 1514
5-Fluorouracil and methyl-CCNU, for gastric
　　cancer, with radiation therapy, 1514
Fluoxetine (Prozac), 632–633, 2944–2945
　for alcoholism, 1116
　dosage and administration, 2945
　for panic disorder, 2946
　side effects, 2945
Flushing
　in carcinoid syndrome, 962
　with multiple endocrine neoplasia, 962
　with small bowel tumor, 1699t
　with VIPoma syndrome, 2136
f-met-leu-phe, 344
FMF. *See* Familial Mediterranean fever
FMLP, 344
Focal nodular hyperplasia
　hepatic, 2759
　　angiographic diagnosis, 2789–2790
　　computed tomography, 2717
　of liver, magnetic resonance imaging, 2736
Folacin. *See* Folic acid

Folate. *See* Folic acid
Folate conjugase, 461, 467
　endogenous substrates, 461t
　products, 461t
Folic acid (folate)
　absorption, 467–468, 468f, 473f
　　in elderly, 975
　　in neonate, 556
　anticancer effects, 1976
　brush-border carrier, 468
　deficiency, 468–469, 1048t, **1062**
　　in abetalipoproteinemia, 2390
　　in etiology of tropical sprue, 1632
　　in malnutrition, 997
　　in short bowel syndrome, 1686, 1690
　　small bowel biopsy in, 845t
　　small bowel involvement in, 2867
　homeostasis, disorders, 468–469
　malabsorption, with tropical sprue, 1632–1633
　recommended dietary allowances, 1062
　salvage pathway, 468
　sources, 467, 1062
　supplementation
　　in celiac disease, 1656
　　and cobalamin status, 469–470
　　indications for, 1725–1726
　　with inflammatory bowel disease, 468
　　in pregnancy, 469
　supplements, 1062
　toxicity, 1062
　in TPN solutions, 1073
　transport defect, 2386t
　for tropical sprue, 1634
Food(s)
　abdominal pain provocation and, 758
　adverse reactions to, 2461, 2461t
　　differential diagnosis, 2461t
　and bezoars, 1544
　characteristics, and gastric emptying, 195
　commonly implicated in food-borne illness,
　　1610t–1613t
　esophageal impaction, 1289–1290
　and flatus production, 1844, 1845t
　and gastric cancer, 1496
　Giardia in, 2350
　glycemic index, 423, 423t, 506–507
　high-oxalate, 1690
　ingestion, disorders, in elderly, **971–973**
　intake, 80
　　decreased, causes, 720t
　　regulation, 718
　intolerance, 2461
　　in irritable bowel syndrome, 1842
　palatability
　　and eating behavior, 486
　　in feeding behavior, 486
　pruritus ani caused by, 2042
　specific dynamic action, 488
　as stimulus of gastric acid secretion, 303
　thermic effect, 488
　and traveler's diarrhea, 1607–1608
Food allergens, 2462
Food allergy, 844, **2461–2464**
　classification, 2461
　clinical manifestations, 2462–2463
　diagnosis
　　skin tests, 2464
　　in vitro assays, 2464
　diagnostic criteria, 2463
　diarrhea with, 836
　immunologic reactions mediating, 2461–2462
　pancreatitis associated with, 2074
　pathogenesis, 2462
　prevalence, 2461
　prevention, 2464
　suspected
　　evaluation of patient with, 2463–2464
　　investigation, 2463t, 2463–2464
　terminology, 2461
　treatment, 2464